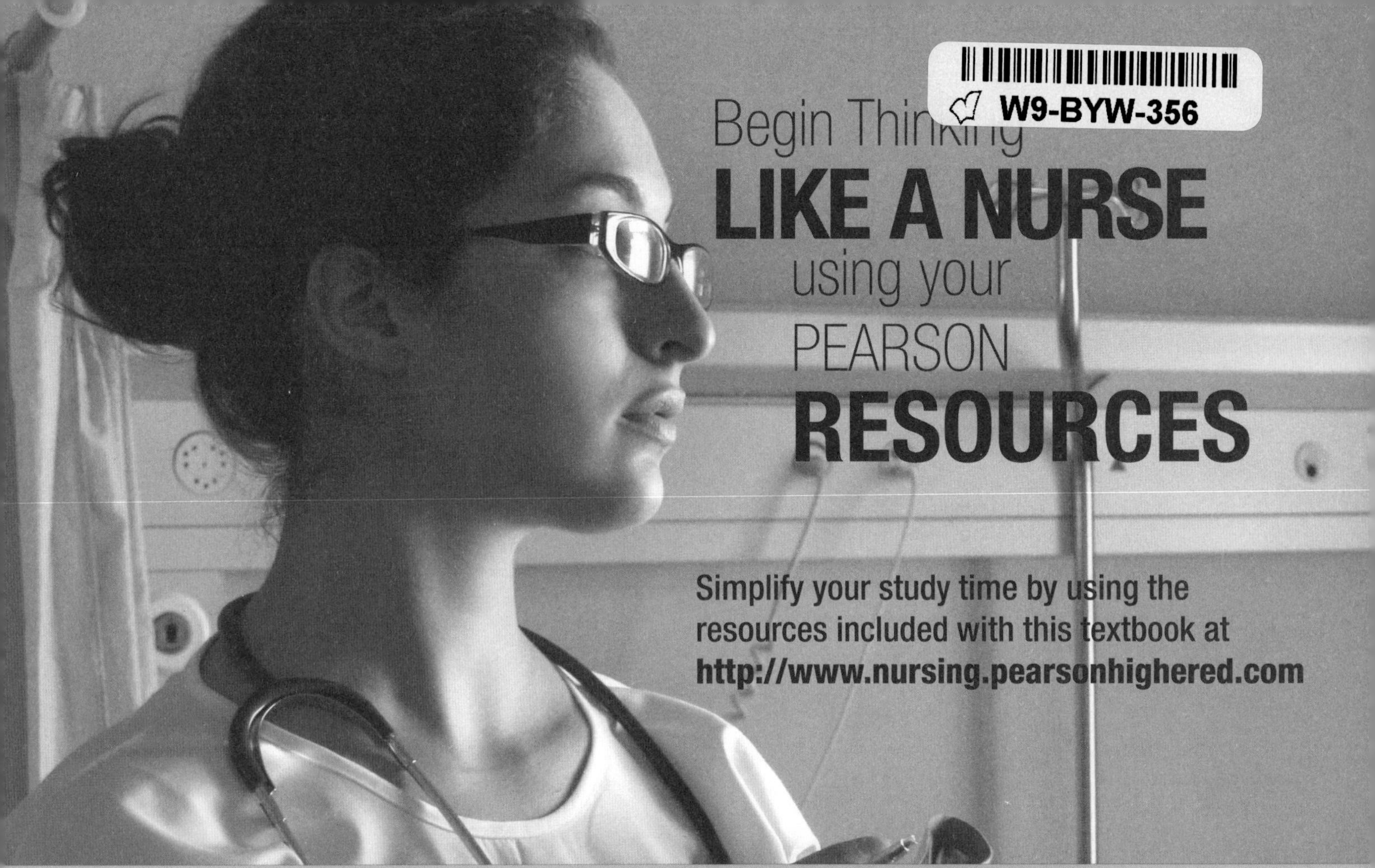

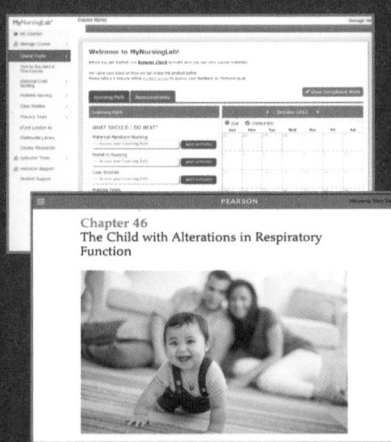
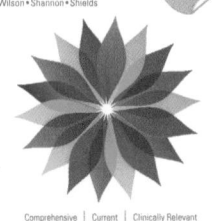

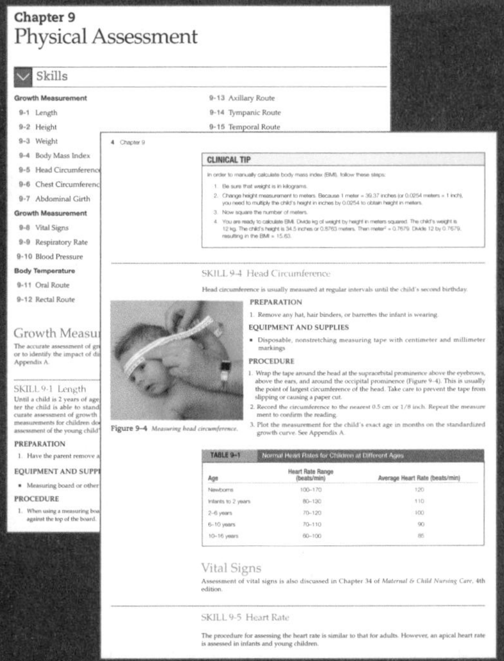

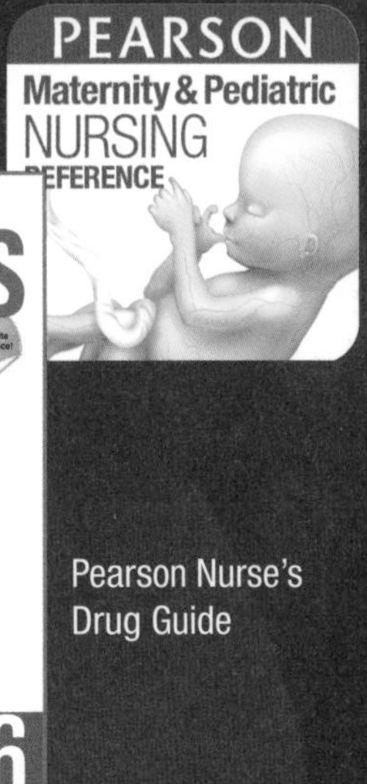

MyNursingLab®

www.mynursinglab.com
Learn more about and purchase
access to MyNursingLab.

myPEARSONstore

www.mypearsonstore.com
Find your textbook and everything
that goes with it.

MATERNAL & CHILD
NURSING CARE
Fifth Edition

Marcia L. London, RN, MSN, APRN, CNS, NNP-BC
Senior Clinical Instructor and Director of Neonatal Nurse Practitioner Program (Ret.)
Beth-El College of Nursing and Health Sciences
University of Colorado
Colorado Springs, Colorado

Patricia A. Wieland Ladewig, RN, PhD
Provost
Regis University
Denver, Colorado

Michele R. Davidson, RN, PhD, CNM, CFN
Associate Professor of Nursing and Women's Studies
Coordinator of the School of Nursing PhD Program
George Mason University
Fairfax, Virginia

Jane W. Ball, RN, CPNP, DrPH
Consultant
American College of Surgeons
Gaithersburg, Maryland

Ruth C. McGillis Bindler, RNC, PhD
Professor Emeritus
Washington State University, College of Nursing
Spokane, Washington

Kay J. Cowen, RN-BC, MSN, CNE
Clinical Professor
University of North Carolina at Greensboro School of Nursing
Greensboro, North Carolina

PEARSON

Boston   Columbus   Indianapolis   New York   San Francisco
Amsterdam   Cape Town   Dubai   London   Madrid   Milan   Munich   Paris   Montréal   Toronto
Delhi   Mexico City   São Paulo   Sydney   Hong Kong   Seoul   Singapore   Taipei   Tokyo

Publisher: Julie Levin Alexander
Publisher's Assistant: Sarah Henrich
Executive Editor: Katrin Beacom
Editorial Assistant: Erin Sullivan
Director, Publishing Operations: Etain O'Dea
Program Management Team Lead: Melissa Bashe
Program Manager: Erin Rafferty
Project Management Team Lead: Cynthia Zonneveld
Project Manager: Maria Reyes
Development Editors: Lynda Hatch and Mary Cook
Interior and Cover Designer: Mary Siener
Vice President of Sales and Marketing: David Gesell
Vice President, Director of Marketing: Margaret Waples
Senior Product Marketing Manager: Phoenix Harvey
Field Marketing Manager: Debi Doyle
Marketing Specialist: Michael Sirinides

Marketing Assistant: Amy Pfund
Media Project Manager: Karen Bretz
Manufacturing Manager: Maura Zaldivar-Garcia
Composition: Cenveo® Publisher Services
Full-Service Project Management: Bonnie Boehme, Cenveo® Publisher Services
Printer/Binder: RR Donnelley/Kendallville
Cover Printer: Lehigh-Phoenix Color/Hagerstown
Cover Image: Getty/Blend Images, Mike Kemp
Part Openers: Marcy Maloy/Getty Images, Paul Bradbury/Getty Images, ERproductions Ltd./Getty Images, Blend Images-ERproductions Ltd./Getty Images, Blend Images-Mike Kemp/Getty Images, Shannon Banal/Getty Images, Tetra Images/Getty Images, Abel Mitja Varela/Getty Images

Credits and acknowledgments borrowed from other sources and reproduced, with permission, in this textbook appear on the appropriate page within text

Notice: Care has been taken to confirm the accuracy of information presented in this book. The authors, editors, and the publisher, however, cannot accept any responsibility for errors or omissions or for consequences from application of the information in this book and make no warranty, express or implied, with respect to its contents.

The authors and publisher have exerted every effort to ensure that drug selections and dosages set forth in this text are in accord with current recommendations and practice at time of publication. However, in view of ongoing research, changes in government regulations, and the constant flow of information relating to drug therapy and drug reactions, the reader is responsible for consulting current resources for drug information to verify use, dosage, contraindications, and precautions. This is particularly important when the recommended agent is a new and/or infrequently employed drug.

A note about nursing diagnoses: Nursing diagnoses in this text are taken from Herdman, T.H. & Kamitsuru, S. (Eds.) *Nursing Diagnoses—Definitions and Classification 2015–2017.* Copyright © 2014, 1992–2014 NANDA International. Used by arrangement with John Wiley & Sons Limited. Companion website: www.wiley.com/go/nursingdiagnoses. In order to make safe and effective judgments using NANDA-I nursing diagnoses, it is essential that nurses refer to the definitions and defining characteristics of the diagnoses listed in this work.

Library of Congress Cataloging-in-Publication Data

Names: London, Marcia L., author.
Title: Maternal & child nursing care / Marcia L. London, Patricia A. Wieland Ladewig, Michele R. Davidson, Jane W. Ball, Ruth C. McGillis Bindler, Kay J. Cowen.
Other titles: Maternal and child nursing care
Description: Fifth edition. | Hoboken, NJ : Pearson Education, Inc., [2017] | Includes bibliographical references and index.
Identifiers: LCCN 2015039065| ISBN 9780134167220 (alk. paper) | ISBN 0134167228 (alk. paper)
Subjects: | MESH: Maternal-Child Nursing—methods. | Pediatric Nursing—methods.
Classification: LCC RG951 | NLM WY 157.3 | DDC 618.2/0231—dc23
LC record available at http://lccn.loc.gov/2015039065

2013032544

10 9 8 7 6 5 4 3 2 1

PEARSON

ISBN-13: 978-0-13-416722-0
ISBN-10:   0-13-416722-8

About the Authors

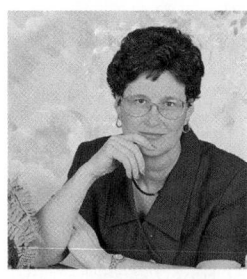

MARCIA L. LONDON received her BSN and School Nurse Certificate from Plattsburgh State University in Plattsburgh, New York, and her MSN in pediatrics as a clinical nurse specialist from the University of Pittsburgh in Pennsylvania. She worked as a pediatric nurse, and began her teaching career at Pittsburgh Children's Hospital Affiliate Program. Mrs. London began teaching at Beth-El School of Nursing and Health Science in 1974 (now part of the University of Colorado, Colorado Springs) after opening the first intensive care nursery at Memorial Hospital of Colorado Springs. She has served in many faculty positions at Beth-El, including assistant director of the School of Nursing. Mrs. London obtained her postmaster's Neonatal Nurse Practitioner certificate in 1983, and subsequently developed the Neonatal Nurse Practitioner (NNP) certificate and the master's NNP program at Beth-El. She is active nationally in neonatal nursing and was involved in the development of National Neonatal Nurse Practitioner educational program guidelines. Mrs. London pursued her interest in college student learning by taking doctoral classes in higher education administration and adult learning at the University of Denver in Colorado. She feels fortunate to be involved in the education of her future colleagues and teaches undergraduate education. Mrs. London and her husband, David, enjoy reading, travel, and hockey games. They have two sons: Craig, who lives in Florida with his wife, Jennifer, and daughter, Hannah, works with Internet companies; and Matthew, who works in computer teleresearch. Both are more than willing to give Mom helpful hints about computers.

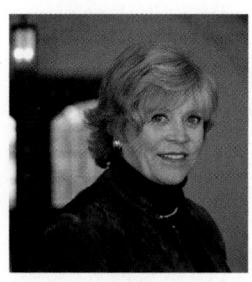

PATRICIA A. WIELAND LADEWIG received her BS from the College of Saint Teresa in Winona, Minnesota; her MSN from Catholic University of America in Washington, DC; and her PhD in higher education administration from the University of Denver in Colorado. She served as an Air Force nurse and discovered her passion for teaching as a faculty member at Florida State University in Tallahassee. Over the years, she has taught at several schools of nursing. In addition, she became a women's health nurse practitioner and maintained a part-time clinical practice for many years. In 1988, Dr. Ladewig became the first director of the nursing program at Regis College in Denver. In 1991, when the college became Regis University, she became academic dean of the Rueckert-Hartman College for Health Professions. Under her guidance, the School of Nursing added a graduate program. In addition, the college added a School of Physical Therapy and a School of Pharmacy. In 2009, Dr. Ladewig became Vice President for Academic Affairs, and in 2012, she became Provost at Regis University. She and her husband, Tim, enjoy skiing, baseball games, and traveling. However, their greatest pleasure comes from their family: son Ryan, his wife Amanda, and grandchildren Reed and Addison Grace; and son Erik, his wife Kedri, and grandchildren Emma and Camden.

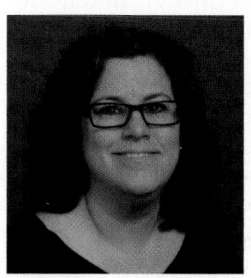

MICHELE R. DAVIDSON completed her ADN degree from Marymount University in Arlington, Virginia. She has worked in multiple women's health specialty areas including postpartum, newborn nursery, high-risk nursery, labor and delivery, reproductive endocrinology, gynecology medical-surgical, and oncology units as a registered nurse while obtaining a BSN from George Mason University in Fairfax, Virginia. Dr. Davidson earned her MSN and a nurse-midwifery certificate at Case Western Reserve University in Cleveland, Ohio, and continued to work as a full-scope nurse-midwife for 16 years. She has delivered over 1000 babies during her career as a nurse-midwife. She completed her PhD in nursing administration and healthcare policy at George Mason University (GMU) and began teaching at GMU in 1999 while continuing in her role as a nurse-midwife. Dr. Davidson serves as the Coordinator for the PhD program in the School of Nursing. She has an interest in women's mental health and focuses her research on perinatal and postpartum mood and anxiety disorders. Dr. Davidson also has an interest in the care of individuals with disabilities; she serves as a member of the Loudoun County Disability Advisory Committee and is a disability advocate in her community. She was a member of the American College of Nurse-Midwives Certification Council, the body that writes the national certification examination for certified nurse-midwives. She is a member of numerous editorial and advisory boards and has a passion for writing. In 2000, Dr. Davidson developed an immersion clinical experience for GMU students on a remote island in the Chesapeake Bay. In 2003, she founded the Smith Island Foundation, a nonprofit organization in which she served as executive director for 8 years. Dr. Davidson has also completed certifications in lactation consulting, forensic nursing, and surgical first assistant. In 2012, her book, *A Nurse's Guide to Women's Mental Health*, won an American Journal of Nursing Book Award. In her free time, she enjoys spending time with her mother, writing, gardening, Internet surfing, and spending time on Smith Island with her nurse-practitioner husband, Nathan, and their four active children, Hayden, Chloe, Caroline, and Grant. Dr. Davidson and her family love the Eastern Shore of Maryland and continue to be part-time residents of Smith Island.

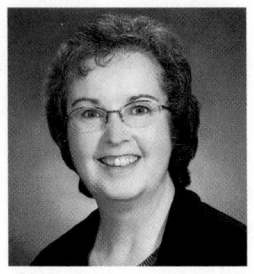

JANE W. BALL graduated from The Johns Hopkins Hospital School of Nursing in Baltimore, Maryland, and subsequently received a BS from The Johns Hopkins University in Baltimore. She worked in the surgical, emergency, and outpatient units of the Johns Hopkins Children's Medical and Surgical Center, first as a staff nurse and then as a pediatric nurse practitioner. Thus began her career as a pediatric nurse and advocate for children's health needs. She obtained both a master of public health and doctor of public health degree from the Johns Hopkins University Bloomberg School of Public Health with a focus on maternal and child health. After graduation, she became the chief of child health services for the Commonwealth of Pennsylvania Department of Health. In this capacity, she oversaw the state-funded well-child clinics and explored ways to improve education for the state's community health nurses. After relocating to Texas, she joined the faculty at the University of Texas at Arlington School of Nursing to teach community pediatrics to registered nurses returning to school for a BSN. During this time she became involved in writing her first textbook, *Mosby's Guide to Physical Examination*, which is currently in its eighth edition. After relocating to the Washington, DC, area, she joined the Children's National Medical Center to manage a federal project to teach instructors of emergency medical technicians from all states about the special care children need during an emergency. Exposure to the shortcomings of the emergency medical services system in the late 1980s with regard to pediatric care was a career-changing event. With federal funding, she developed educational curricula for emergency medical technicians and emergency nurses to help them provide improved care for children. A textbook entitled *Pediatric Emergencies, A Manual for Prehospital Providers* was developed from these educational ventures. She served as the executive director of the federally funded Emergency Medical Services for Children National Resource Center for 15 years, providing consultation and resource development for state health agencies, health professionals, families, and advocates to improve the emergency healthcare system for children. Dr. Ball is a consultant for the American College of Surgeons, assisting states to develop and enhance their trauma systems. She is also collaborating on a pediatric explosion injury electronic curriculum and virtual pediatric trauma center conceptual design as a consultant to the Uniformed Services University of the Health Sciences.

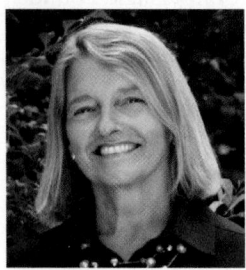

RUTH C. MCGILLIS BINDLER received her BSN from Cornell University–New York Hospital School of Nursing in New York, New York. She worked in oncology nursing at Memorial–Sloan Kettering Cancer Center in New York, and then moved to Wisconsin and became a public health nurse in Dane County. Thus began her commitment to work with children as she visited children and their families at home, and served as a school nurse for several elementary, middle, and high schools. As a result of this interest in child healthcare needs, she earned her MS in child development from the University of Wisconsin in Madison. A move to Washington State was accompanied by a new job as a faculty member at the Intercollegiate Center for Nursing Education in Spokane, now the Washington State University College of Nursing. Dr. Bindler feels fortunate to have been involved for 38 years in the growth of this nursing education consortium, which is a combination of public and private universities and offers undergraduate and graduate nursing degrees. She taught theory and clinical courses in child health nursing, cultural diversity, graduate research, pharmacology, and assessment; served as lead faculty for child health nursing; was the first director of the PhD program; and served as Associate Dean for Graduate Programs, which include Master of Nursing, Post-Masters certificates, and PhD and Doctor of Nursing Practice (DNP) programs. She recently retired from this position and serves the college and profession as a professor emeritus, continuing work with graduate students and research. Her first professional book, *Pediatric Medications*, was published in 1981, and she has continued to publish articles and books in the areas of pediatric medications and pediatric health. Her research was focused in the area of childhood obesity, type 2 diabetes, and cardiovascular risk factors in children. Ethnic diversity and interprofessional collaboration have been other themes in her work. Dr. Bindler believes that her role as a faculty member and administrator enabled her to learn continually, to foster the development of students in nursing, and to participate fully in the profession of nursing. In addition to teaching, research, publication, and leadership, she enhances her life by service in several professional and community activities, and by outdoor activities with her family.

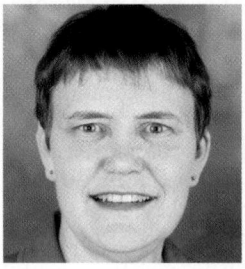

KAY J. COWEN received her BSN degree from East Carolina University in Greenville, North Carolina, and began her career as a staff nurse on the pediatric unit of North Carolina Baptist Hospital in Winston-Salem. She developed a special interest in the psychosocial needs of hospitalized children and preparing them for hospitalization. This led to the focus of her master's thesis at the University of North Carolina at Greensboro (UNCG), where she received a MS in Nursing Education degree with a focus in maternal–child nursing. Mrs. Cowen began her teaching career in 1984 at UNCG, where she continues today as clinical professor. Her primary responsibilities include coordination of the pediatric nursing course, teaching classroom content, and supervising a clinical group of students. Mrs. Cowen shared her passion for the psychosocial care of children and the needs of their families through her first experience as an author of the chapter "Hospital Care for Children" in *Child Health Nursing: A Comprehensive Approach to the Care of Children and Their Families*, published in 1993. In the classroom, Mrs. Cowen realized that students learn through a variety of teaching strategies, and she became especially interested in the strategy of gaming. She led a research study to evaluate the effectiveness of gaming in the classroom, and subsequently continues to incorporate gaming in her teaching. In the clinical setting, Mrs. Cowen teaches her students the skills needed to care for patients and the importance of family-centered care, focusing on not only the physical needs of the child but also the psychosocial needs of the child and family. During her teaching career, Mrs. Cowen has continued to work part time as a staff nurse, first on the pediatric unit of Moses Cone Hospital in Greensboro and then at Brenner Children's Hospital in Winston-Salem. In 2006, she became the part-time pediatric nurse educator in Brenner's Family Resource Center. Through this role she is able to extend her love of teaching to children and families. Through her role as an author, Mrs. Cowen is able to extend her dedication to pediatric nursing and nursing education.

Thank You!

We are forever grateful to nurse geneticist Linda Ward, PhD, APRN, the author of this book's new genetics chapter, Chapter 3, *Genetic and Genomic Influences in Maternal, Newborn, and Child Health*. We appreciate her expertise in genetic and genomic science, her superb writing skills, and her willingness to contribute such an essential chapter to our text. We also are thankful to Brenda Senger for contributing the content on mitochondrial diseases in Chapter 53 and to Janet Houser for her contribution of the *Evidence-Based Practice* features in the maternal-newborn section of this book.

We are grateful to all of the nurses, both clinicians and educators, who reviewed the manuscript of this text. Their insights, suggestions, and focus on detail helped us prepare a more relevant and useful book, one that focuses on the essential components of learning in the fields of maternal, newborn, and child health nursing.

Catherine A. Alvarez, MSN, RN-LRN
Holy Name Medical Center School of Nursing
Teaneck, New Jersey

Mary Armstrong, MSN, RN, CCRN, CPN
Carson Newman University
Jefferson City, Tennessee

Elizabeth Bettini, APRN, MSN, PCNS-BC, CHPPN
Children's National Medical Center
Washington, DC

Melissa Black, PhDc, MSN, FNP, RN
Nurse Consultant/Educator
Kaplan College

Ann M. Bowling, PhD, RN, CPNP-PC, CNE
Wright State University
Dayton, Ohio

Michele I. Bracken, PhD, WHNP-BC
Salisbury University
Salisbury, Maryland

Barbara L. Cannella, PhD, RNC-OB, APN
Rutgers University
Newark, New Jersey

Tonya Chapin, RN, MSN
Colorado Mesa University
Grand Junction, Colorado

Teresa Chase, MSN, RN
University of Kentucky
Children's Hospital
Lexington, Kentucky

Laura Clemens, BSN, RN, C-EFM
New York–Presbyterian Hospital
New York, New York

Kelley Connor, RN, MSN, CNE, CHSE
Boise State University
Boise, Idaho

Elizabeth Cordero, RN, BSN, MBA
Western Nevada College
Carson City, Nevada

Margot DeSevo, PhD, LCCE, IBCLC, RNC
Adelphi University
Garden City, New York

Holly J. Diesel, PhD, RN
Goldfarb School of Nursing at Barnes–Jewish College
St. Louis, Missouri

Karan Dublin, MEd, RN
Tyler Junior College
Tyler, Texas

Barbara S. Edwards, RN, CPN
Wake Forest Baptist Health, Brenner Children's Hospital
Winston-Salem, North Carolina

Linda B. Esposito, MSN, RN, CCRN
Wake Forest Baptist Health, Brenner Children's Hospital
Winston-Salem, North Carolina

Julie Fitzgerald, PhD, RN, CNE
Ramapo College of New Jersey
Mahwah, New Jersey

Vivienne Friday, EdD, RN
Bridgeport Hospital School of Nursing
Bridgeport, Connecticut

Julie C. Garcia, MSN, APRN, CCRP
University of Texas Health Science Center
San Antonio, Texas

Jolynn Greenhalgh, DNP, ARNP
Florida State University
Tallahassee, Florida

Deborah Henry, MSN, RN
Blue Ridge Community College
Flat Rock, North Carolina

Indra Hershorin, PhD, RN, CNE
Barry University
Miami Shores, Florida

Karen Hessler, PhD, FNP-C
University of Northern Colorado
Greeley, Colorado

Brenda K. Hoolapa, RNC-OB, MS, BSN
University of Texas
Arlington, Texas

Catherine Hrycyk, MScN, RN
De Anza College
Cupertino, California

Gina M. Idol, RN, BSN
Wake Forest Baptist Health, Brenner Children's Hospital
Winston-Salem, North Carolina

Amy Mitchell Kennedy, MSN, RN
Nurse Educator – Consultant
Newport News, Virginia

Kathleen Krov, PhD, CNM, RN, CNE
Raritan Valley Community College
North Branch, New Jersey

Meredith Krutar, MSN, FNP-BC
Carroll College
Helena, Montana

Meredith Lahl, MSN, PCNS-BC, PPCNP-BC, CPON
Cleveland Clinic
Cleveland, Ohio

Robyn Leo, MS, RN
Worcester State University
Worcester, Massachusetts

Carolyn Levi, MSN, RN
Grand Rapids Community College
Grand Rapids, Michigan

Angela P. Lukomski, RN, DNP, CPNP
Eastern Michigan University
Ypsilanti, Michigan

Diane E. Mosqueda, DNP, APRN, FNP-C, CNE
University of Texas Medical Branch
Galveston, Texas

Patricia Novak, RN, BSN, MSN
Gateway Community College
Phoenix, Arizona

Valerie O'Dell, DNP, RN, CNE
Youngstown State University
Youngstown, Ohio

Gloanna J. Peek, PhD, RN, CPNP
The University of Arizona
Tucson, Arizona

Susan Perkins, MSN, RN
Washington State University
Spokane, Washington

Linda Sue Pippin, MSN, RN-BC
Newberry College
Newberry, South Carolina

Theresa Puckett, RN, CNE
Stark State College
North Canton, Ohio

Wendi Strauss Pulse, DNP, MS, RNC-OB, C-EFM
St. Mary's Hospital and
Regional Medical Center
Grand Junction, Colorado

Colleen Quinn, RN, MSN, EdD
Broward College
Davie, Florida

Amy Roberts, MSN, RN
Minot State University
Minot, North Dakota

JoAnne Silbert-Flagg, DNP, PNP, IBCLC
Johns Hopkins University
Baltimore, Maryland

Jennifer S. Simmons, MSN, RN, CPNP-AC/PC, CPON
Wake Forest Baptist Health,
Brenner Children's Hospital
Winston-Salem, North Carolina

Anita Smith, CPNP
Wake Forest University
Winston-Salem, North
Carolina

Charla Smith, MSN, RN, CPN, CNE
Jackson State Community
College
Jackson, Tennessee

Nancy M. Smith, DNP, CRNP, FNP-BC
Salisbury University
Salisbury, Maryland

Eleanor Lowndes Stevenson, PhD, RN
Duke University
Durham, North Carolina

Linda Stone, MS, RN, CPNP, CLC
Roxbury Community College
Boston, Massachusetts

Patricia D. Suplee, PhD, RNC-OB
Rutgers University
Camden, New Jersey

Brenda Tanner, MSN, RNC-OB
Greenville Technical College
Greenville, South Carolina

Maureen P. Tippen, RN, C, MS
University of Michigan
Flint, Michigan

Teresa Tyson, RN, PhD
Winston-Salem State
University
Winston-Salem, North
Carolina

Diane K. Van Os, MS, RN
Westminster College
Salt Lake City, Utah

Amber Welborn, RN, MSN
The University of North
Carolina
Greensboro, North Carolina

Wanda Williams, PhD, RN, WHNP-BC
Rutgers University
Camden, New Jersey

Donna Wilsker, MSN, RN
Lamar University
Beaumont, Texas

Dedication

Throughout the ages, nurses have cared for families, fathers, mothers, and their children—treating, healing, soothing, educating, and advocating.

And so we dedicate this book to nurses—

> For their wisdom, expertise, and compassion
> For their willingness to challenge the system when necessary
> For their ability to remain strong during times of difficulty and stress
> And for their unfailing commitment to the families they assist.

And to nursing students everywhere—

> For seeking to serve others when so many have become self-serving
> For committing their minds and talents to a proud profession
> For accepting the challenges posed by the changes in health care
> And for daring to envision a brighter tomorrow.

Then, too, as always, we honor our beloved families—

> David London; Craig, Jennifer, and Hannah; Matthew
> Tim Ladewig; Ryan, Amanda, Reed, and Addison Grace; Erik, Kedri, Emma, and Camden
> Nathan Davidson; Hayden, Chloe, Caroline, and Grant
> Ronald Ball
> Julian Bindler; Dana, Brady, and Ivy; Ross and Cami
> Fred Cowen III, Benjamin and Marcia, Michael and Caroline

Preface

Faculty and students in today's maternal–newborn and pediatric nursing courses face a wide variety of issues and challenges. Courses are increasingly shortened, clinical experiences are more limited, and patients in hospitals are often more seriously ill. Time is precious for both students and faculty, and competence in nursing practice is essential. Changes in healthcare delivery stem from the Affordable Care Act, and new regulations offer challenges to the student and faculty member. The primary goal in this edition is to present key content in an accurate, readable format that helps students and faculty focus on what is important. This textbook helps students develop the skills and abilities they need now and in the future in an ever-changing healthcare environment. This is done through the **Learning Outcomes** listed at the beginning of each chapter and the **Focus Your Study** review feature at the end of each chapter, through the illustrations and photographs that clarify concepts more efficiently than words can do, and through the downloadable practice content at www.pearsonhighered.com/nursingresources, which depicts clinical situations and requires students to engage in critical thinking. In its structure, format, and delivery, this text provides a concise look at maternal–newborn, women's health, and pediatric nursing.

Organization

The organization of the text reflects a time-saving approach. As educators and nurses, we know how difficult it is to teach everything that students need to learn in so little time. Consequently, we sought to reduce duplication in the text by carefully integrating relevant nursing topics and cross-referencing to other chapters. For example, three introductory chapters address concepts important for maternal, newborn, and child nursing. Chapter 1 discusses introductory concepts of family-centered care, health promotion, community and home care, evidence-based practice, and legal issues, as well as the complex ethical considerations related to reproductive decisions, stem cell research, terminating life-sustaining treatment, and organ transplantation issues. Chapter 2 addresses concepts that are important for culturally appropriate care for the entire family, such as cultural norms related to childbearing and childrearing, cultural assessment, and complementary and alternative therapies. Chapter 3, written by genetics nurse specialist Linda Ward, PhD, APRN, focuses on the field of genetics and genomics. Students will learn basic concepts and apply them in the critical specialties of maternal–newborn and child nursing. These concepts will be built upon in the students' future careers as genetic causes of disease and treatments that influence the genome are increasingly developed and applied.

Subsequent chapters focus on reproductive issues and women's health, pregnancy, birth processes, postpartum care, and newborn management. The maternal–newborn chapters begin with basic theory followed by nursing assessment and nursing care for essentially healthy women or newborns. Complications of a specific period appear in the last chapter or chapters of each section. The second half of the text transitions into the pediatric care chapters. The pediatric chapters begin with introductory concepts, such as growth and development, nutrition, assessment, health promotion for children ranging from newborn to adolescents, and care of the child in the community and hospital settings. Chapters 44 through 57 cover the nursing care of children with various disorders, organized by body system.

Important Themes in This Edition

Central to this edition are several key themes that are increasingly important in nursing care of childbearing and childrearing families.

Family-Centered Nursing Care

Nursing care for pregnant women and children is a family-centered process, and family focus is essential to providing culturally competent care. The underlying philosophy of *Maternal & Child Nursing Care* is simple: We believe that family members are coparticipants in care during pregnancy, childbirth, and childrearing. Parents must be integrated into the care of an infant or child at any stage of development, as they are the central influence on the child's life. Families experience the excitement and exhilaration of welcoming a healthy infant into their home, but they also experience sorrow and concern when a health problem occurs. Nurses play a pivotal role in helping families celebrate the normal life processes associated with birth, in promoting the health of the family and child, in fostering the child's growth and development from infancy through adolescence, and in caring for the child with any health condition. We are committed to providing a text that integrates the needs of families across the continuum from conception through adolescence.

Health Promotion

As nurses and educators, we are supportive of the goals and objectives of *Healthy People 2020*. This science-based effort provides a 10-year agenda for improving the health and well-being of the nation. Throughout the text, we have incorporated content reflecting the objectives of the project as they relate to childbearing families, newborns, infants, children, and adolescents.

We also subscribe to the paradigm that all childbearing and childrearing families and children need health promotion and health maintenance interventions, no matter where they seek health care or what health conditions they may be experiencing. Families may visit offices or other community settings specifically to obtain health supervision care. Nurses may also integrate health promotion and health maintenance into the care for childbearing and childrearing families and for children with acute and chronic illness in a variety of inpatient and outpatient settings. The inclusion of *Healthy People 2020* initiatives throughout the text integrates the national public health efforts to improve healthcare outcomes and assists nursing students and nurses with integrating healthcare policy into practice. This textbook provides health promotion and health maintenance content throughout, most visibly in four chapters: Chapter 5, *Health Promotion for Women*; Chapter 34, *Health Promotion and Maintenance: General Concepts, the Newborn, and the Infant*; Chapter 35, *Health Promotion and Maintenance: The Toddler and the Preschooler*; and Chapter 36, *Health Promotion and Maintenance: The School-Age Child and the Adolescent*.

In addition, a feature entitled **Health Promotion** summarizes the needs of women from preconception to postpartum, newborns, and children with specific chronic conditions, such as asthma or diabetes. These overviews teach the student to look at the child with a chronic illness like any other child, with health maintenance needs for prevention, education, and basic care.

Nursing Care in the Community

Most maternity and pediatric nursing care occurs in the community setting, especially since most children and pregnant women are healthy and have only episodic acute health conditions. Even women with high-risk pregnancies and children with serious chronic health conditions are receiving more care in their homes and in the community. This textbook integrates community and home care throughout, including information on long-term management of complex health conditions, which are especially challenging to manage in community settings.

Five chapters provide a theoretical perspective and important tools in caring for childbearing and childrearing families in the community setting: Chapter 9, *Antepartum Nursing Assessment*; Chapter 10, *The Expectant Family: Needs and Care*; Chapter 29, *The Postpartum Family: Early Care Needs and Home Care*; Chapter 37, *Family Assessment and Concepts of Nursing Care in the Community*; and Chapter 38, *Nursing Considerations for the Child and Family with a Chronic Condition*. In addition, **Community-Based Nursing Care** is a special heading used throughout this text.

Patient and Family Education

Patient and family education remains a critical element of effective nursing care, one that we emphasize in this text. Nurses teach their patients during all stages of pregnancy and the childbearing process, during the child's health visits, and while providing care for specific conditions. Throughout the book, we include **Teaching Highlights** that present a special healthcare issue or problem and the related key teaching points for the family.

Clinical Reasoning

Nurses are faced with the responsibility to manage care for multiple families with diverse healthcare needs, and to work collaboratively with other health professionals to enhance care. Thus, nurses must be able to think critically, communicate well, and problem solve effectively.

To promote the development of clinical reasoning skills that will support nurses in challenging situations, **Clinical Reasoning** boxes provide brief scenarios that ask students to determine the appropriate response. Students can test their own decision-making skills by checking their answers to these questions against the suggested answers posted at www.pearsonhighered.com/nursingresources. Students can also access a variety of critical thinking exercises and case studies on this space.

Another feature that emphasizes these skills is the **Clinical Reasoning in Action** feature. This case study at the end of each chapter introduces a patient situation along with questions to enable the student to decide which nursing actions are appropriate. The *Instructor's Resource Manual* has more suggestions for clinical reasoning exercises for both the classroom and the clinical setting.

Evidence-Based Practice

Healthcare providers are increasingly aware of the importance of using evidence-based practice approaches as the foundation for planning and providing skilled, effective care. The approach of evidence-based practice draws on information from a variety of sources, including nursing research. To help nurses become more comfortable integrating new knowledge into their nursing practice, a discussion of evidence-based practice is included in Chapter 1.

A feature entitled **Evidence-Based Practice** further enhances the approach of using research to determine nursing actions. It describes a particular problem or clinical question and investigates the current evidence that suggests solutions to the problem. In these features, we provide an interpretation explaining the implications of the studies and then invite the student to apply clinical reasoning skills to further identify nursing care approaches.

Developing Cultural Competence

The influence of a family's culture on health beliefs and healthcare practices cannot be underestimated. Chapter 1 briefly introduces cultural issues relevant to maternity and pediatric nursing care. Additionally, we include Chapter 2, *Culture and the Family*, to directly and specifically address cultural issues.

We also emphasize cultural competence throughout the text. We highlight specific cultural issues and their application to nursing care in the **Developing Cultural Competence** features.

Other New or Expanded Concepts in This Edition

Many other important concepts are emphasized throughout this text:

- *Assessment* is an essential and core role in nursing management. Several chapters are dedicated to helping the student perform an assessment during the pregnancy continuum, including the fetus and newborn, and later through the stages of childhood. In addition, body system assessment guidelines are provided in many of the pediatric chapters.

- *Communication* is one of the most important skills that students need to learn. Effective communication is the very fiber of nursing practice. This book integrates communication skills in an applied manner where students can most benefit. It is an essential part of the **Clinical Tip** and **Teaching Highlights** boxes. The importance of communication with families and other health professionals underscores the Collaborative Care sections of this text.

- *Ensuring appropriate nutrition* during pregnancy, the newborn period, infancy, and childhood is important to promote growth, development, and health. A growing national focus on healthy nutrition patterns underscores the importance of this information. Chapters 11, 25, 28, and 32 address nutrition for pregnant women, newborns, and children.

- *Healthy People 2020* goals are included as a new feature in this edition. Many of these national goals, which are arranged by categories, have direct relevance for maternal–newborn and pediatric nurses. Relevant goals are cited throughout the text to acquaint students with national public health efforts and to assist them to make connections between care of individual families and broad-based community health care and public policy.

- **Professionalism in Practice**, another new feature, focuses on topics such as legal and ethical considerations, contemporary nursing practice issues, professional accountability, practice guidelines, patient advocacy, and home and community care considerations. This feature reflects our belief that professionalism requires astute nurses to demonstrate professional standards of moral, ethical, and legal conduct and to model the values of the nursing profession as they care for childbearing and childrearing families.

- *Patient safety* is an essential element of effective patient care. It is the focus of the Joint Commission and one of the key elements of the Quality and Safety Education for Nurses (QSEN) project, both of which are discussed in Chapter 1. To help keep safety in the forefront, the feature called *SAFETY ALERT!* calls attention to issues that could place a patient (or a nurse) at risk. Another feature, **Clinical Tip**, relates to patient safety and many other nursing concepts by providing readers with concrete suggestions for safe, effective practice.

- *Pain* is considered a vital sign, and pain management is a priority in healthcare settings. All of the chapters in Part 4, *Birth and the Family*, address pain assessment and management, and it is the primary focus in Chapter 19, *Pharmacologic Pain Management*. Pain assessment and management is also a focus in five chapters (Chapters 23, 25, 26, 29, and 30) of Part 5, *The Newborn*, and Part 6, *The Postpartum Family*. In Part 7, Chapter 40, *Pain Assessment and Management in Children*, provides tools and guidance for pain assessment in children of all ages, as well as pharmacologic and complementary therapies for pain management. We discuss applicable pain management when appropriate in other chapters in Part 7 (Chapters 41 and 43) and in each of the chapters in Part 8, *Caring for Children With Alterations in Health Status*. Current research is used as the basis for discussions and nursing management of pain throughout the text.

- A new 2-page, 16-photograph *Birth Sequence* in Chapter 18 provides a moment-by-moment visual presentation of the birth of a baby.

- Chapter 12, *Pregnancy in Selected Populations*, is a new chapter that provides expanded content on nursing care for pregnant women from potentially vulnerable populations, such as adolescents, women over 35 years of age, and those with physical or intellectual disabilities.

- Another new chapter—Chapter 3, *Genetic and Genomic Influences in Maternal, Newborn, and Child Health,* written by Linda Ward, PhD, APRN—was added to this edition to reflect an emerging understanding of genome science, its impact on health and illness in children and childbearing families, and the expanding role that nurses play in applying genetics in clinical practice.

- *End-of-life care* has rightfully gained prominence as a critical component of nursing care. Expanded focus on the care of the family and the child who is dying has been added to Chapter 41, *The Child With a Life-Threatening Condition and End-of-Life Care*. Grief and loss associated with miscarriage are addressed in Chapter 15, *Pregnancy at Risk: Gestational Onset*. Care of the family experiencing perinatal loss is presented in Chapter 21, *Childbirth at Risk: Labor-Related Complications*.

Tools That Focus Student Review to Maximize Time

Both instructors and students value learning aids that unify the objectives and concepts of a chapter as well as reinforce the overall themes in a text. In keeping with our theme of family-centered care, each chapter begins with a **Family Quote** that helps personalize and set the stage for content that follows from the family's perspective. This is followed by a list of **Learning Outcomes**. Throughout the text important terms—**Key Terms**—are bolded when they first appear to emphasize their importance to the content. All of the key terms are compiled in a **Glossary** at the end of the book.

Focus Your Study

This feature is a direct response to instructors' and students' requests that the text provide more opportunities for review. Each chapter ends with **Focus Your Study**, a feature designed to help students retain the most important concepts from a chapter in a short period of time. Students save time by having the important concepts identified for them, allowing them to use more of their study time for reviewing the concepts themselves.

Application of the Nursing Process

Nursing Management

The nursing process is emphasized throughout the nursing care chapters. The heading, **Nursing Management**, highlights nursing assessment, actions, and evaluation. In chapters with frequently seen or high-risk health issues or conditions, the expanded section on nursing management helps students understand and apply care principles more completely. The expanded section includes the subheadings Nursing Assessment and Diagnosis, Planning and Implementation, and Evaluation.

In keeping with changing approaches to nursing care management, we feature **Nursing Care Plans** throughout the text. The Nursing Care Plans address nursing care for patients who have complications, such as a woman with preeclampsia, or health conditions, such as a child with otitis media. We designed this feature to help students approach care from the nursing management perspective.

Visuals That Teach

The conviction that art can teach is evident throughout the book. There are hundreds of contemporary photographs of childbearing and childrearing families and children in healthcare and related settings throughout the textbook, as well as illustrations, all of which serve to display conditions, compare developmental stages, and depict concepts.

In particular, **Pathophysiology Illustrated** figures allow the student to see into the body and to visualize the causes and effects of conditions on childbearing women, newborns, and children. **As Children Grow** illustrations help the student visualize the important anatomic and physiologic differences between a child and an adult. These features illustrate how the child progresses through developmental stages and the important ways in which a child's development influences healthcare needs and how the child progresses through developmental stages.

Resources for Student Success

- **Online Resources** are available for download at www.pearsonhighered.com/nursingresources, which aim to further enhance the student's learning experience, build on knowledge gained from this textbook, prepare students for the NCLEX-RN® examination, and foster clinical reasoning. These resources include:
  - NCLEX-RN® Review Questions
  - Case Studies
  - Care Plans
  - Thinking Critically Questions, and more!
- The *Clinical Skills Manual for Maternity and Pediatric Nursing* is a useful resource to assist students in successful planning and performance of essential nursing skills. This manual helps to translate theoretic concepts into performance while caring for patients in a variety of health settings.
- **NEW!** Pearson's *Maternity and Pediatric Nursing Reference App*, now available for both iPhone and Android devices, provides a collection of handy tools and additional content for students and professionals looking for a quick reference in maternity or pediatrics nursing. The maternity content includes a section on **Patient/Family Teaching**, which sup-

plies useful information, tips, and strategies for educating parents and families in a variety of situations and settings. The colorful **Maternal–Fetal Growth and Development Timeline** depicts maternal/fetal development month by month and provides specific teaching guidelines for each stage of pregnancy. For pediatrics, the information provided in the **Guidance for Children and Families** section provides insight into the issues related to health maintenance, development, and family that may present from birth to adolescence.

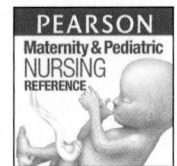

Resources for Faculty Success

Pearson Education is pleased to offer a complete suite of resources to support teaching and learning, including:

- TestGen Test Bank
- Lecture Note PowerPoints
- Classroom Response System PowerPoints
- Instructor's Resource Manual

Nursing is facing many new challenges: an ongoing nursing shortage, dramatic advances in healthcare knowledge, implementation of the Affordable Care Act, reenvisioning of nursing education needs and approaches, and natural and human-made disasters that create a critical need for skilled nurses. We believe that nursing is facing these issues and challenges with enthusiasm and commitment. Many people feel a strong desire to choose professions that make a difference—professions such as nursing. We, like you, know that expert nurses can have a tremendous impact on the lives of childbearing and childrearing families. Our goal in writing this textbook is to help prepare nurses with the skills and knowledge to make a difference—one family at a time.

Marcia L. London

Patricia W. Ladewig

Michele R. Davidson

Jane W. Ball

Ruth C. Bindler

Kay J. Cowen

Features That Help You Use This Textbook Successfully

Instructors and students alike value the in-text learning aids that we include in our textbooks. The following guide will help you use the features and resources from *Maternal & Child Nursing Care*, Fifth Edition, to be successful in the classroom, in the clinical setting, on the NCLEX-RN® examination, and in nursing practice.

Each chapter begins with **Learning Outcomes** and a chapter opening **Quote**. These personal stories illustrate the diversity of cultures, parental concerns, and family situations that nurses will encounter throughout the course of their careers.

As Children Grow boxes illustrate the anatomic and physiologic differences between children and adults. These features illustrate how the child progresses through developmental stages and the important ways in which a child's development influences healthcare needs.

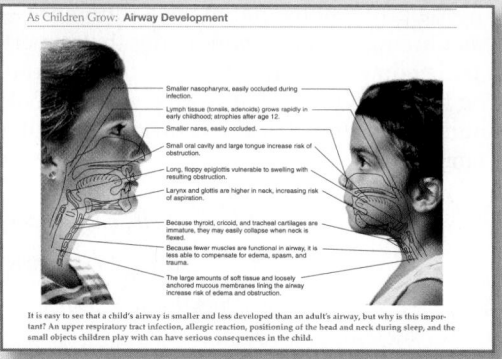

As Children Grow: Airway Development

Smaller nasopharynx, easily occluded during infection.

Lymph tissue (tonsils, adenoids) grows rapidly in early childhood; atrophies after age 12.

Smaller nares, easily occluded.

Small oral cavity and large tongue increase risk of obstruction.

Long, floppy epiglottis vulnerable to swelling with resulting obstruction.

Larynx and glottis are higher in neck, increasing risk of aspiration.

Because thyroid, cricoid, and tracheal cartilages are immature, they may easily collapse when neck is flexed.

Because fewer muscles are functional in airway, it is less able to compensate for edema, spasm, and trauma.

The large amounts of soft tissue and loosely anchored mucous membranes lining the airway increase risk of edema and obstruction.

It is easy to see that a child's airway is smaller and less developed than an adult's airway, but why is this important? An upper respiratory tract infection, allergic reaction, positioning of the head and neck during sleep, and the small objects children play with can have serious consequences in the child.

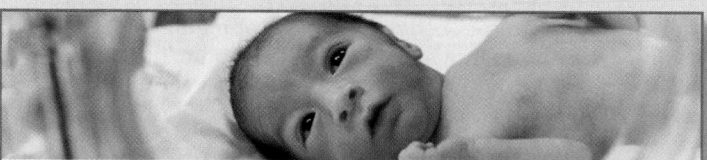

Chapter 18
The Family in Childbirth: Needs and Care

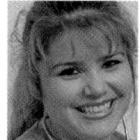

Jonathan Nourok/PhotoEdit

For as long as I can remember, I have been fascinated with birth. Currently, I am a labor and delivery nurse at our town's only hospital. I'm still fascinated with birth but a little nervous, too. You see, I was just admitted in early labor with my first child. Before I got here I worried that I would be a "bad" patient or that I would lose my cool. How silly I was. All that matters is that my baby is healthy and that I am able to take care of him effectively. (Yes. We know it is a boy!)
—Amanda, 31

⌄ Learning Outcomes

18.1 Identify admission data that should be noted when a woman is admitted to the birthing area.

18.2 Describe the nursing care of a woman and her partner/family upon admission to the birthing area.

18.3 Use assessment data to determine the nursing interventions to meet the psychologic, social, physiologic, and spiritual needs of the woman and her partner/family during each stage of labor.

18.4 Compare methods of promoting comfort during the first and second stages of labor.

18.5 Explain the immediate needs and physical assessment of the newborn following birth in the provision of nursing care.

18.6 Examine the unique needs of the adolescent during birth in the provision of nursing care.

18.7 Describe the role and responsibilities of the nurse in the management of a precipitous labor and birth.

Assessment Guides, found in the maternal–newborn chapters, assist you with diagnoses by incorporating physical assessment and normal findings, alterations and possible causes, and guidelines for nursing interventions. Assessment guides within several chapters of Part 8, *Caring for Children With Alterations in Health Status*, provide a system-oriented approach to assessing the child's health condition.

ASSESSMENT GUIDE	The Child in Respiratory Distress*
Assessment Focus	**Assessment Guideline**
Position of comfort	• Is the child comfortable lying down?
	• Does the child prefer to sit up or in the **tripod position** (sitting forward with arms on knees for support and extending the neck)?
Vital signs	• Assess the rate and depth of respirations. See Table 33–9 for age-related respiratory rates. Is **tachypnea** (abnormally rapid respiratory rate) present?
	• Assess the pulse for rate and rhythm. See Table 33–11 for age-related heart rates.
Lung auscultation	• Are breath sounds bilateral, diminished, or absent?
	• Are **adventitious sounds** (wheezes, crackles, or rhonchi) present?
Respiratory effort (work of breathing)	• Is **stridor** (audible crow-like inspiratory and expiratory breath sounds) or wheezing present? Is grunting heard on expiration?
	• Is breathing easy or labored?
	• Are retractions present or are accessory muscles used to breathe?
	• Is nasal flaring present?
	• Can the child say a full sentence or is a breath needed every few words? Is the cry strong or weak?
	• Do the chest and abdomen rise simultaneously with inspiration or is **paradoxical breathing** present in which the chest and abdomen do not rise simultaneously?
Color	• What is the color of the mucous membranes, nail beds, or skin (pink, pale, cyanotic, or mottled)?
	• Does crying improve or worsen the color?
Cough	• Is the cough dry (nonproductive), wet (productive, mucousy), brassy (noisy, musical), or croupy (barking, seal-like)?
	• Is the coughing effort forceful or weak?
Behavior change	• Is irritability, restlessness, or change in level of responsiveness present?
*Refer to Chapter 33 for the assessment techniques mentioned in this table.	

Clinical Reasoning Pregnancy Complication
Jillian Rundus is a 31-year-old G1P0 who is 35 weeks pregnant. She presents for a routine office visit with complaints of nausea and abdominal pain rating 7/10. She has had a headache and general malaise for 2 days. She denies visual changes. Upon examination, you find her to be alert and oriented and her physical examination is unremarkable with the exception of abdominal tenderness and a blood pressure of 170/110 mmHg. She has had no previous history of hypertension. Fetal heart rate ranges from 140 to 150 beats per minute.
   What should the nurse do at this time?

Clinical Reasoning boxes provide brief case scenarios that ask students to determine the appropriate response.

Clinical Reasoning in Action features at the end of each chapter propose a real-life scenario and a series of clinical reasoning questions so that you can apply to the clinical setting what you learned in class.

Clinical Reasoning in Action

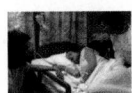

Cindy Bell, a 20-year-old gravida 2, para 1, at 40 weeks' gestation, presents to you in the birthing unit with contractions every 5 to 7 minutes. She is accompanied by her husband. Spontaneous rupture of membranes occurred 2 hours prior to admission. Cindy tells you that the fluid was colorless and clear. You orient Cindy and her family to the birthing room and perform a physical assessment, documenting that vital signs are normal. A vaginal examination demonstrates the cervix is 75% effaced, 4 cm dilated with a vertex at -1 station in the LOP position. You place Cindy on an external fetal monitor. The fetal heart rate baseline is 140 to 147 with accelerations to 156; no decelerations are noted. Contractions are 5 to 6 minutes apart, moderate intensity, and lasting 40 to 50 seconds. Cindy states she would like to stay out of bed as long as possible because lying down seems to make the contractions more painful, especially in her back.

1. Discuss the benefits of ambulation in labor.
2. Cindy would like her 5-year-old daughter to be present for the baby's birth. What would you discuss with her about the impact of having a young sibling present during labor and birth?
3. What fetal heart rate assessment will best ensure fetal well-being during the period Cindy is ambulating?
4. When a nonreassuring fetal heart pattern is detected, what remedial nursing intervention is carried out?
5. What are indications for continuous fetal monitoring in labor?

Clinical Tip
If a woman is experiencing severe fear or anxiety about a vaginal examination, advise her to slowly count to 10 during the examination while continually wiggling her toes. This source of distraction may lessen her fear and anxiety. It also enables the woman to have a sense of control.

Clinical Tip features offer hands-on suggestions and clinical tips. These are placed at locations in the text that will help you apply them. They include topics such as legal and ethical considerations, nursing alerts, and home and community care considerations.

Developing Cultural Competence boxes highlight specific cultural issues and their application to nursing care.

Developing Cultural Competence Using Cultural Information Effectively
Although it is important to avoid stereotyping, race and ethnicity may provide valuable starting information about cultural, behavioral, environmental, and medical factors that might affect a pregnant woman's health. With this general knowledge as a framework, it is essential to ask the woman about specific practices in her culture to determine their meaning for her.

EVIDENCE-BASED PRACTICE | Risk Factors for Adolescent Pregnancy

Clinical Question
What are risk factors for adolescent pregnancy in vulnerable populations?

The Evidence
Unplanned pregnancy for an adolescent can result in a host of adverse outcomes for both mother and baby. These risks are even higher among vulnerable populations. Two research studies focused on identifiable risk factors in specific vulnerable populations in an effort to target preventive efforts effectively. Researchers conducted an integrated literature review of 18 research studies that identified risk factors for teen pregnancy among African American adolescents. A second study used a predictive model to study risk factors among nearly 300 adolescents in the child welfare system/foster homes. Taken together, these studies form a strong basis of evidence. Lee, Cintron, & Kocher (2014) found that five major factors contributed to adolescent pregnancy among African American youth: substance use, gender roles, peer influences, parental involvement, and level of knowledge about sexual health. Of these, substance use was also a predictive factor for teens in the welfare system, but in this population, delinquency was also a risk factor (Helfrich & McWey, 2014). In the latter study, the timing of pregnancy was also identified; pregnancy occurred, on average, within 3 years of a predictive event.

Best Practice
Knowing specific predictive factors for a population enables the development of risk-specific educational programs for the prevention of adolescent pregnancy. These data suggest that supports need to be wide reaching and include reducing substance abuse, encouraging parental involvement, and integration of peer support into interventions.

Clinical Reasoning
How can the nurse determine risk factors of teen pregnancy for a specific population? How can parents and peers be involved in adolescent pregnancy prevention programs?

Evidence-Based Practice boxes present recent nursing research, discuss implications, and challenge you to incorporate this information into your nursing practice through nursing actions.

Growth and Development

Strategies for communicating with school-age children include the following:

- Provide concrete examples of pictures or materials to accompany verbal descriptions.
- Assess knowledge before planning teaching.
- Allow child to select rewards following procedures.
- Teach techniques such as counting or visualization to manage difficult situations.
- Include child in discussions and history with parent.
- Be honest in explanations and all communications.

Growth and Development boxes, found exclusively in the pediatric chapters, provide information about the different responses of children at various ages to health conditions.

Healthy People 2020

(BDBS-18.4) Reduce the proportions of persons who develop adverse events due to alloimmunization among persons with hemoglobinopathies

Healthy People 2020 goals are cited throughout the text to acquaint students with national public health efforts and to assist them to make connections between care of individual families and broad-based community health care and public policy. The coding in front of each objective identifies the specific chapter—for example, "Maternal, Infant, and Child Health" (MICH); "Adolescent Health" (AH); and "Injury and Violence Prevention" (IVP)—and number of the objective for the *Healthy People 2020* initiative. See the *Healthy People 2020* website to find chapter abbreviations for all *Healthy People 2020* objectives listed in our text.

A feature entitled **Health Promotion** summarizes the needs of children with specific chronic conditions, such as asthma or diabetes. These overviews teach you to look at the child with a chronic illness like all children, with health maintenance needs for prevention, education, and basic care.

Health Promotion The Child With Bronchopulmonary Dysplasia

Health Supervision

- Assess blood pressure to detect abnormal findings associated with pulmonary hypertension.
- Coordinate vision screening by an ophthalmologist every 2 to 3 months during the first year of life. Myopia and strabismus are common in premature infants.
- Coordinate pulmonary function tests annually or as needed for clinical condition.
- Perform hearing and other screening tests as recommended for age.

Growth and Developmental Surveillance

- Assess growth and plot measurements on a growth chart corrected for gestational age. Even if length and weight are lower than normal, monitor for continued growth following the growth curves.
- Perform a developmental assessment, correcting for gestational age.

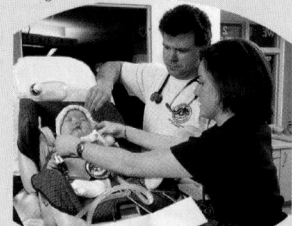

Nutrition

- Review caloric intake. Ensure that increased calories are provided to support growth. Assess feeding difficulties related to oral motor function associated with long-term enteral feeding. Refer to a nutritionist as necessary.

Physical Activity

- Organize care to provide rest periods during the day.
- Give parents ideas for promoting the infant's motor development, such as reaching for and moving toward toys and objects of interest.

Family Interactions

- Identify ways to coordinate nighttime care to reduce child and family sleep disturbances.
- Provide discipline appropriate for developmental age.

Disease Prevention Strategies

- Reduce exposure to infections. Encourage selection of a childcare provider who cares for a small number of children, if one is used. If possible, avoid the use of childcare centers during RSV season.
- Immunize the child with the routine vaccine schedule based on chronologic age.
- Administer the 23-valent pneumococcal vaccine at 2 years of age.
- Provide monthly injections of palivizumab throughout the RSV season.

Condition-Specific Guidance

- Develop an emergency care plan for times when the infant's condition rapidly worsens.

A **Medications Used to Treat** feature in tabular format provides an overview of the types of medications that can be used for a specific condition and nursing considerations associated with their use.

Medications Used to Treat: Asthma

QUICK RELIEF MEDICATIONS, ROUTE, AND ACTION	NURSING MANAGEMENT
Short-acting beta$_2$-agonists (SABA) Albuterol, levalbuterol, pirbuterol *Metered-dose inhaler or nebulizer* Relaxes smooth muscle in airway leading to rapid bronchodilation (within 5–10 min) and mucus clearing. Drug of choice for acute therapy and prevention of exercise-induced bronchospasm.	• Use before inhaled steroid, wait 1–2 min between puffs, wait 15 min to give inhaled steroid. Child should hold breath 10 sec after inspiring. Then rinse mouth and avoid swallowing medication. Use a spacer. • Differences in potency exist, but all products are comparable on a per puff basis. • Dose-related side effects include tachycardia, nervousness, nausea and vomiting, headaches. • Regular use more than 2 days a week for symptom control indicates a loss of control and need for additional therapy.

Nursing Care Plan: The Woman With Preeclampsia

1. Nursing Diagnosis: *Fluid Volume: Deficient*, related to fluid shift from intravascular to extravascular space secondary to vasospasm (NANDA-I © 2014)

GOAL: Client is restored to normal fluid volume levels.

INTERVENTION	RATIONALE
• Encourage woman to lie in the left lateral recumbent position.	• The left lateral recumbent position decreases pressure on the vena cava, thereby increasing venous return, circulatory volume, and placental and renal perfusion. Angiotensin II levels are decreased when there is improved renal blood flow, which helps to promote diuresis and lower blood pressure.
• Assess blood pressure every 1 to 4 hours as necessary.	• Frequent monitoring will assess for progression of the disorder and allow for early intervention to ensure maternal and fetal health and well-being.
• Monitor urine for volume and proteinuria every shift or every hour per agency protocol.	• Monitoring provides information to assess renal perfusion. Proteinuria is the last cardinal sign of preeclampsia to appear. As the disorder worsens, the capillary walls of the glomerular endothelial cells stretch, allowing protein molecules to pass into the urine. Normally, urine does not contain protein. Readings of 3+ and 4+ indicate loss of 5 g or more protein in 24 hours. Urinary output decreases when there is a reduction of the glomerular filtration rate. Urinary output that falls below 30 mL per hour or less than 700 mL in a 24-hour period should be reported.
• Assess deep tendon reflexes and clonus.	• Hyperreflexia may occur as preeclampsia worsens. Eliciting deep tendon reflexes provides information about CNS status and is also used to assess for magnesium sulfate toxicity. Reflexes are graded on a scale of 0 to 4+ using the Deep Tendon Reflex Rating Scale. A rating of 4+ is abnormal and indicates hyperreflexia. A rating of 0 or no response is also abnormal and is seen with high maternal serum magnesium levels. Clonus, an abnormal finding, is present if the foot "jerks" or taps the examiner's hand, at which time the examiner counts the number of taps or beats. The presence of clonus indicates a more pronounced hyperreflexia and is indicative of CNS irritability.
• Assess for edema.	• Edema develops as fluid shifts from the intravascular to the extravascular spaces. Edema is assessed either by weight gain (more than 3.3 lb (1.5 kg)/month in the second trimester or more than 1.1 lb (0.5 kg)/week in the third trimester) or by assessing for pitting edema (assessed by using finger pressure to a swollen area, usually the lower extremities, and grading on a scale of 1+ to 4+).
• Administer magnesium sulfate per infusion pump as ordered.	• As preeclampsia worsens, the risk of an eclamptic seizure increases. Magnesium sulfate is the treatment of choice for seizures because of its CNS depressant action. As a secondary effect, magnesium sulfate relaxes smooth muscles and may therefore decrease the blood pressure. Magnesium sulfate is contraindicated in women with myasthenia gravis.
• Assess for magnesium sulfate toxicity.	• Side effects of magnesium sulfate are dose related. Therapeutic levels are in the range of 4.8–8.4 mg/dL. As maternal serum magnesium levels increase, toxicity may occur. Signs of toxicity include decreased or absent deep tendon reflexes (DTRs), urine output below 30 mL/hr, respirations below 12, and confusion.
• Provide a balanced diet that includes 80–100 g/day or 1.5 g/kg/day of protein.	• A diet rich in protein is necessary to replace protein that is excreted in the urine.

EXPECTED OUTCOME: The signs and symptoms of preeclampsia will diminish as evidenced by decreased blood pressure, urine protein levels of zero, and a return of the DTRs to normal.

Nursing Care Plans are also provided. They address nursing care for women who have complications such as preeclampsia or diabetes mellitus, as well as for high-risk newborns and children. We designed this information to enhance your preparation for the clinical setting.

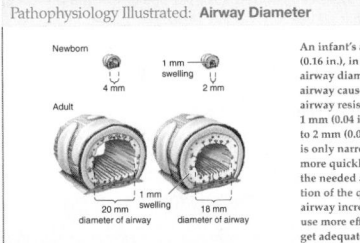

Pathophysiology Illustrated: **Airway Diameter**

Pathophysiology Illustrated boxes feature unique drawings that illustrate conditions on a cellular or organ level, and may also portray the step-by-step process of a disease. These images visually explain the pathophysiology of certain conditions to increase your understanding of the condition and its treatment.

Professionalism in Practice **Asthma Management by School Nurses**

The National School Nurses Association joined eight organizations in a position statement to improve asthma management in school settings. School nurses are encouraged to implement a comprehensive asthma plan for the management of students with asthma in the school setting that includes identifying and monitoring all students with asthma and obtaining their asthma action plans. School nurses are additionally encouraged to collaborate with school officials to adopt and implement an environmental assessment and management plan that addresses environmental asthma triggers (American Lung Association, 2013). See Chapter 37 for more information on nursing care in the school setting.

Professionalism in Practice focuses on important topics related to contemporary nursing practice issues, including legal and ethical considerations. This feature reflects a commitment to quality improvement in all aspects of care.

SAFETY ALERT!
If there is no fetal reaction to the scalp stimulation test and a Category II or Category III fetal heart rate tracing persists, the nurse should contact the physician/CNM to come to the woman's bedside and perform further evaluation.

The *SAFETY ALERT!* features present essential information that calls attention to issues that could place a patient or a nurse at risk and provide guidance on maintaining a safe environment for all patients and healthcare providers.

TEACHING HIGHLIGHTS	Home Care Instructions for the Infant Requiring a Cardiorespiratory Monitor

Apnea Equipment
- Review how the monitor operates, the lead wires, placement of skin electrodes and pulse oximetry sensor, and how to set the event recorder. Keep the battery fully charged, and keep the manual for troubleshooting handy.

Emergency Preparation
- Have an emergency plan and complete an emergency information form about the infant's health problem. Notify the telephone company, electric company, local ambulance service, and the local emergency department (to get priority service status).
- Post the emergency response phone numbers by all phones and save in cell phones, along with the phone numbers for the healthcare provider, medical equipment company, power company, neighbor, and key family members.
- Take a cardiopulmonary resuscitation (CPR) course.

Safety Precautions
- Place monitor on firm surface; keep away from other appliances (television, microwave oven) and water.
- Ensure that alarms are audible from all locations.
- Double-check that the monitor and event recorder are on before putting the infant down for a nap or at bedtime.
- Thread cable and wires through lower end of infant's clothes.
- Ensure integrity of leads, monitor cable, and power cord (replace if frayed).

Routine Care
- Explain the reasons for the apnea monitor and frequency of use. Use it whenever the infant sleeps. Review the manual for troubleshooting.
- Show how to attach and detach infant chest leads and belt. Evaluate the skin for irritation or sores under the electrodes, and move the electrode if skin is irritated. Use no oils or lotions on the chest.

Responding to an Alarm
- Observe the infant for breathing first to determine if this is a real event or a loose lead.
- Stimulate the infant if respirations are absent or infant is lethargic. Start by calling the infant's name and gently touching, proceeding to vigorous touch if needed.
- If no response, proceed with CPR and call 9-1-1.
- If a loose lead is suspected, determine if electrode patches are loose. Check the wires from the electrode or monitor cable. Check the power supply. Is the monitor malfunctioning?

Teaching Highlights present special healthcare issues or problems and the related key teaching points to address with the family.

Women With Special Needs Contraceptive Counseling

Many healthcare providers assume that women with developmental disabilities are not sexually active and, therefore, do not need contraceptive counseling. Women with developmental disabilities need education on sexual issues, including conception and pregnancy prevention. A level of functioning assessment should be performed to determine if the woman is capable of using different types of contraceptives effectively. Contraceptive choices should be discussed and provided as needed.

Women With Special Needs features serve as alerts that women with individualized needs may require modified plans of care.

Each chapter ends with **Focus Your Study**, which outlines the main points of the chapter and a list of **References**.

Where relevant, SKILLS found in the companion book, *Clinical Skills Manual for Maternity and Pediatric Nursing*, are cited.

Focus Your Study

- Major treatment modes for children with mental health disorders include individual therapy, family therapy, and group therapy.

- Therapeutic strategies for treatment of children and adolescents with mental health disorders include play therapy, art therapy, cognitive behavioral therapy (CBT), visualization, and hypnosis.

- Nurses conduct mental health assessments, prevent disorders when possible, participate in intervention to treat disorders, and evaluate outcomes of treatment.

- Autism spectrum disorder is the major type of pervasive developmental disorder and is manifested by abnormal behavior, social interaction, and communication.

- Attention deficit hyperactivity disorder is characterized by developmentally altered behaviors involving inattention and hyperactivity.

- Mood disorders in childhood and adolescence are commonly manifested as depression or bipolar disorder.

- Several anxiety disorders occur in children and adolescents, most notably generalized anxiety, separation anxiety, panic, obsessive-compulsive disorder, social phobia, conversion reaction, and posttraumatic stress disorder (PTSD).

- Behavioral therapy and selective serotonin reuptake inhibitors (SSRIs) are used in treatment of anxiety; prescription drug use in children must be closely monitored.

- Suicide is a significant cause of death among youth; nurses play a key role in identifying youth at risk, instituting prevention programs, and counseling families and friends of suicide victims.

- Nurses play a role in identifying children with potential learning disabilities, referring for diagnosis, and partnering with the family to provide a positive learning experience for the child.

- Intellectual disability is subaverage intellectual and adaptive functioning, and may be caused by chromosomal, genetic, or environmental factors.

- A multidisciplinary team plans the care for children with intellectual disability and periodically evaluates the child's progress and the family's needs.

Acknowledgments

Nursing is a dynamic, exciting healthcare profession. As curricula develop, many nursing programs have begun to teach nursing of childbearing families and nursing of children together in a single course. This combined format requires that faculty approach these two fields with a similar framework and philosophy, and with similar teaching methods, so that students can maximize learning. With this fifth edition, we have created a tool that will enable students to master these two critical areas of nursing—the care of childbearing families and the care of children. Creating a dynamic and integrated text would not be possible without the skill and dedication of a host of people.

We are grateful to the nurses who contributed to this text. Linda Ward, PhD, APRN, is an assistant professor at Washington State University College of Nursing and the author of Chapter 3, *Genetic and Genomic Influences in Maternal, Newborn, and Child Health*. Linda is a graduate of the National Institutes of Health Summer Genetics Institute and has been proactive in integrating genetic and genomic content into nursing curricula. Brenda Senger, PhD, RN, undergraduate program director and assistant professor at the School of Nursing and Human Physiology at Gonzaga University, engages in research about mitochondrial disease and contributed the material on this subject matter in Chapter 53, *The Child With Alterations in Endocrine Function*.

We are also grateful to Janet Houser, PhD, RN, Academic Dean of the Rueckert-Hartman College for Health Professions at Regis University, Denver, Colorado, for developing the **Evidence-Based Practice** boxes that are presented in the women's health and maternal–newborn sections of this textbook.

We would personally like to thank several people. Our thanks go to Julie Levin Alexander, our publisher. Julie is committed to excellence and creativity. She is the driving force behind the exciting changes occurring at Pearson Health Science and is truly a creative futurist in publishing.

For this edition, we have been blessed to have two developmental editors who worked together astonishingly well: Lynda Hatch for the maternal–newborn chapters and Mary Cook for the pediatric chapters. Lynda and Mary challenged us creatively, ensured consistency, and kept us on track. They have been supportive, innovative, and unflappable during the long months of hard work. Thank you both for all you have done!

Special thanks to the people of Cenveo® Publisher Services for coordinating production and moving things forward so effectively.

Finally, we all wish to thank our other coauthors. As six individuals, but two teams, we came together with our own ideas, writing styles, and vision for this book. Over five editions we have grown closer in our collaboration, with productive discussions of important issues that have ultimately resulted in a new and different text for maternal, newborn, and child health nursing. We hope that this book and associated learning aids will be a useful tool for legions of nursing students to come.

Marcia L. London

Patricia W. Ladewig

Michele R. Davidson

Jane W. Ball

Ruth C. Bindler

Kay J. Cowen

Detailed Contents

32 Infant, Child, and Adolescent Nutrition 777

33 Pediatric Assessment 806

Chapter 1
Contemporary Maternal, Newborn, and Child Health Nursing

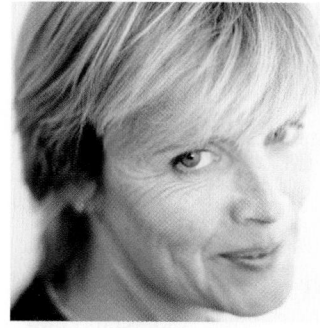

Justin Pumfrey/Getty Images

My younger son turned 21 today—officially a man now. I remember so well the night he was born in a birthing room at our local hospital. I watched my husband rock our baby and talk to him just minutes after his birth. Over the years we sought emergency health care for our son several times—when he was diagnosed with asthma as a high school freshman, when he fell skateboarding and needed surgery to put three pins in his wrist, when he fell snowboarding and dislocated his shoulder. Active kids do get their share of bumps! It is easy to take good health care for granted, but we shouldn't. It can make all the difference.
—Marjorie, 47

∨ Learning Outcomes

1.1 Identify the nursing roles available to maternal-newborn and pediatric nurses.

1.2 Summarize the use of community-based nursing care in meeting the needs of childbearing and childrearing families.

1.3 Summarize the current status of factors related to health insurance and access to health care.

1.4 Relate the availability of statistical data to the formulation of further research questions.

1.5 Delineate significant legal and ethical issues that influence the practice of maternal-child nursing.

1.6 Discuss the role of evidence-based practice in improving the quality of nursing care for childbearing families.

Skilled nurses care for people, care about people, and use their expertise to help people care for themselves. This is the essence of nursing. Most nurses experience special moments professionally; that is, times in which they know that they have practiced the essence of nursing and, in doing so, have touched the lives of others. For nurses who work with childbearing families or with children and their families, the rewards that come from skilled nursing practice can be especially rich.

This chapter focuses on introductory concepts related to the nurse and childbearing families, newborns, infants, children, and adolescents.

Nursing Roles in Maternal-Child Nursing

Traditionally, **maternal-child nursing** refers to the care of women during pregnancy, birth, and postpartum, as well as the care of newborns, infants, children, and adolescents. However, this designation is somewhat misleading because it fails to acknowledge clearly the consideration due to fathers, partners, and family members. As nurses who work with families quickly learn, a holistic, inclusive approach is crucial to effective nursing care.

The nursing process provides the framework for delivery of direct nursing care. The nurse assesses the client—whether childbearing woman, newborn, infant, child, or adolescent—and identifies the nursing diagnoses that describe the responses of the individual and family to the condition or area of needed knowledge. The nurse then implements and evaluates nursing care. This care is designed to meet specific physical and psychosocial needs. For children, the care is tailored to the individual developmental stage, giving the child additional responsibility for self-care with increasing age.

Nurses play a major role in minimizing the psychologic and physical stress experienced by childbearing families and by children and their families. This often involves listening to concerns, being present during stressful or emotional experiences, and implementing strategies to help the individual and family members cope. Nurses help families by suggesting ways to support their loved ones in the hospital, in community settings, and in the home. Nurses also suggest ways to support families with informational resources, family support groups, referral for healthcare services, and, in some cases, respite care.

Client education is a major component of maternal-child nursing. During pregnancy, nurses provide anticipatory guidance to prepare the woman and her partner, if he or she is involved, for the changes that each month brings. For example, the woman is taught self-care measures to relieve personal discomforts and learns to identify the warning signs that she should report. Both partners receive information on the psychologic changes of pregnancy that they may experience. Education for the laboring woman focuses on activities that help her deal successfully with a challenging experience—childbirth—whereas postpartum teaching addresses the needs of the woman and her newborn to prepare them for discharge.

In pediatric nursing, education is especially challenging because nurses must be prepared to work with children at various levels of understanding and to include family members in all aspects of care. As client educators, nurses help children adapt to the hospital setting and prepare them for various nursing and medical procedures.

When a child is ill, most hospitals encourage a parent to stay with the child and to provide much of the direct and the supportive care under the guidance of a nurse. Nurses teach parents to watch for important signs and responses to therapies, to increase the child's comfort, and even to provide advanced care. Taking an active role during hospitalization helps prepare the parent to assume total responsibility for care after the child leaves the hospital.

Nurses also serve as advocates, acting to safeguard and advance the interests of families. To be an effective advocate, the nurse must be aware of the individual's needs, the family's needs and resources, and the healthcare services available in the hospital and the community. The nurse can then assist the family to make informed choices about these services and to act in their best interests. Nurses must also ensure that the policies and resources of healthcare agencies meet the psychosocial needs of childbearing women and of children and their families.

Collaborative practice is a comprehensive model of health care that uses a multidisciplinary team of health professionals to provide high-quality, cost-effective care. In maternal-newborn settings the team generally includes certified nurse-midwives (see later discussion), physicians, nurse practitioners, nurses, and other health specialists such as pharmacists, lactation consultants, or childbirth educators. Similarly, the multidisciplinary team assembled when a child has a significant health problem or handicapping condition may include physicians, nurses, pediatric nurse practitioners, social workers, physical and occupational therapists, and other specialists. The team's goal is to create an

Developing Cultural Competence Adapting the Reading Level of Client Education Materials

Among U.S. adults, 20% read at a fifth-grade level or below; however, this rate varies by cultural group with higher rates of poor literacy being seen among Latinos, Blacks, and Asians (Pontius, 2013). This means that many childbearing women and parents have difficulty using and understanding health information. Healthcare materials need to be provided in the appropriate language and at the appropriate reading level; for example, a sixth-grade reading level for individuals with a low literacy level (Pontius, 2014). Printed materials to educate children and families about a health condition might be readily available, but they often are written at too high a reading level. Even though printed material may be available in the primary language of the client and family, do not assume that the family has reading skills in that language.

When developing client education materials with a lower reading level:

- Use short, familiar words with one or two syllables and short sentences.

- Substitute simple language for a medical term.

- Use pictures or graphics to give directions when possible.

- Use lists and tables to simplify content.

- Use "must" to express a requirement.

- Divide the content into small sections and use headers.

- Color code information to help readers understand its importance.

- Use a computer program to evaluate the reading level of materials you develop.

interprofessional plan designed to meet the child's medical, nursing, developmental, educational, and psychosocial needs. Because nurses spend large amounts of time providing nursing care for the client and family, they often are better informed than other healthcare professionals about the family's wishes and resources. As a member of the team, the nurse serves as an advocate to ensure that the plan of care considers the family's wishes and contains appropriate services.

Case management is a process of coordinating the delivery of health-care services in a manner that focuses on both quality and cost outcomes. This is often a collaborative practice with other healthcare providers designed to promote continuity of care. The nurse case manager has control over the use of healthcare resources that are considered appropriate for the client's condition and links the client and family to these services. The goal is to help the individual and family have the best healthcare outcome and decrease fragmentation of care, while controlling the cost of healthcare services. In maternal-child nursing, case management is often used for a complicated high-risk pregnancy and for long-term care of children with chronic conditions.

Discharge planning is a form of case management. Effective discharge planning promotes a smooth, rapid, and safe transition into the community and improves the results of treatment begun in the hospital. To be a discharge planner, the nurse needs to know about community medical resources, appropriate

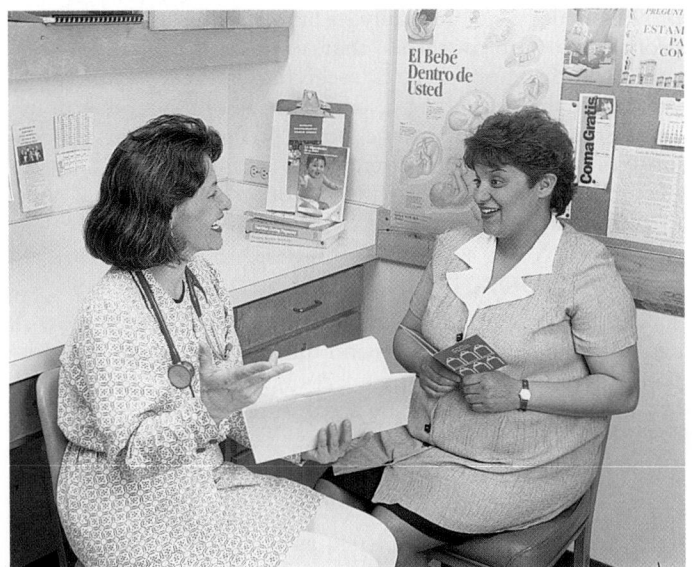

Figure 1–1 A certified nurse-midwife confers with her client.

home care agencies and community resources, reliable Internet sites, educational interventions, and services reimbursed by the individual's health plan or other financial resources.

In addition, several advanced-practice roles are available to maternal-child nurses with additional education. A **nurse practitioner (NP)**, who has specialized education in a **Doctor of Nursing Practice (DNP)** program or a master's degree program, often provides ambulatory care services to pregnant women, newborns, children, adolescents, and families. The area of specialization determines the NP's title, so there are family nurse practitioners, neonatal nurse practitioners, pediatric nurse practitioners, women's health nurse practitioners, and so forth. NPs focus on physical and psychosocial assessments, including history, physical examination, and certain diagnostic tests and procedures. They make clinical judgments and begin appropriate treatments, seeking physician consultation when necessary. A **clinical nurse specialist (CNS)** has a master's degree and specialized knowledge and competence in a specific clinical area. They often are found on mother-baby units, on pediatric units, and in intensive care units assisting staff to provide excellent, evidence-based care. The **certified nurse-midwife (CNM)** is educated in the two disciplines of nursing and midwifery and is certified by the American College of Nurse-Midwives. The CNM is prepared to manage independently the care of women at low risk for complications during pregnancy, birth, and the postpartum period, as well as the care of healthy newborns (Figure 1–1).

The **nurse researcher** has an advanced doctoral degree, typically a PhD, and assumes a leadership role in generating new research. Nurse researchers are typically found in university settings, although more and more hospitals are employing them to conduct research relevant to client care, administrative issues, and the like.

Family-Centered Maternal-Child Care

Family-centered care—that is, nursing care characterized by an emphasis on the family and the family's choices about their birth experience—is a hallmark of contemporary childbirth.

Fathers and partners are active participants, not simply bystanders; siblings are encouraged to visit and meet the newest family member, and they may even attend the birth.

New definitions of family are evolving. For example, the family of a single mother may include her mother, her sister, another relative, a close friend, a same-sex partner, or the father of the child. Many cultures also recognize the importance of extended families, and several family members may provide care and support. See Chapter 2 for an in-depth discussion of family and culture.

In pediatric settings, family-centered care is a dynamic, deliberate approach to building collaborative relationships between health professionals and families that is respectful of their diversity and beliefs about the nature of children's health conditions and ways to manage them. It is designed to meet the emotional, social, and developmental needs of children and families seeking health care. The family is the principal caregiver and center of strength and support for the child (Figure 1–2). As partners in the child's care, the family needs to learn about the child's condition and participate in decisions regarding his or her care. The Society of Pediatric Nurses and the American Nurses Association have established practice guidelines for family-centered care (Table 1–1).

Contemporary Childbirth

Contemporary childbirth is characterized by an increasing number of choices about the birth experience. The family can make choices about the primary caregiver (physician, CNM, or certified midwife); the use of a *doula* to provide labor support (see Chapter 10 for more information about doulas); and birth-related experiences such as the method of childbirth preparation, position for birth, and use of analgesia and anesthesia, as well as breastfeeding and child care choices.

Many women elect to have their pregnancy and birth managed by a CNM. Midwives who are not registered nurses but who complete a direct-entry midwifery education program

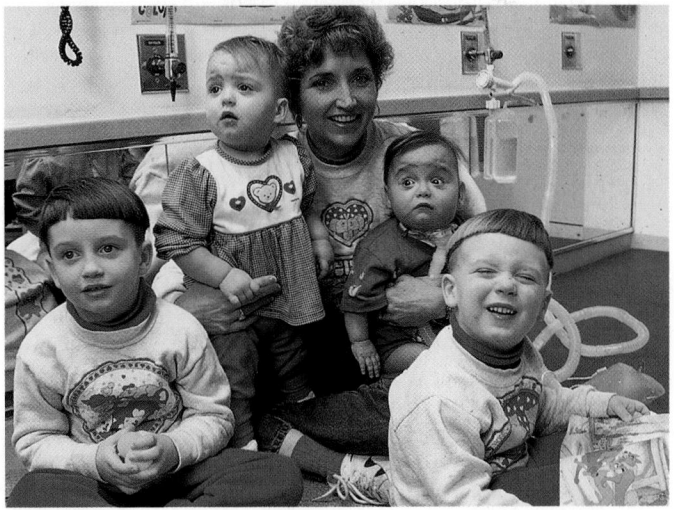

Figure 1–2 Many facilities now encourage family visitation for children with health problems who require long-term hospitalization. Extended family visits enable parents to learn about the child's care and provide siblings with opportunities to interact with the hospitalized child.

TABLE 1–1 Concepts of Family-Centered Care

- The family is acknowledged as the constant in the child's life and a partner in the child's health care.

- The family, child, and health professionals work together in the best interest of the child and the family. Over time, the child assumes a partnership role in his or her health care.

- Health professionals listen to and respect the skills and expertise that the family brings to the relationship.

- Trust is a fundamental element of the relationship between the family, child, and health professionals.

- Communication occurs in an open, unbiased manner and is ongoing.

- Families, children, and health professionals make decisions regarding the child's care in a collaborative manner in all healthcare settings and for all types of health care needed (e.g., health promotion, health maintenance, acute care, chronic condition care, and end-of-life care). Negotiation may be involved in collaborative decision making.

- The child is supported to learn about and participate in his or her health care and decision making. The adolescent is supported to assume a partnership role in his or her health care and in the transition to adult health care.

- The racial, ethnic, cultural, and socioeconomic background of the family and child, as well as family traditions, are honored. Health professionals work to integrate these values and the preferences of the family and child when planning and providing health care.

- Family-to-family and peer support are encouraged.

- Healthcare settings develop policies, procedures, practices, and systems that are family friendly and family centered; they support the choices the family and child will make regarding care.

- Health information for children and families is available and provided to match the range of cultural and linguistic diversity in the community as well as the health literacy levels.

Source: Data from Lewandowski, L. A., & Tesler, M. D. (Eds.). (2008). Family-centered care: Putting it into action. *The SPN/ANA Guide to Family-Centered Care.* Washington, DC: American Nurses Publishing; Committee on Hospital Care, & Institute for Patient and Family-Centered Care. (2012). Patient and family-centered care and the pediatrician's role. *Pediatrics, 129*(2), 394–404; Hughs, D. (2014). *A review of the literature pertaining to family-centered care for children with special health care needs.* Retrieved from http://lpfch-cshcn.org/publications/research-reports/a-review-of-the-literature-pertaining-to-family-centered-care-for-children-with-special-health-care-needs/

that meets the standards established by the American College of Nurse-Midwives (ACNM) may take a certification exam to become a *certified midwife (CM)*. In 2012, CNMs and CMs attended 7.9% of all births in the United States and 11.8% of all vaginal births (ACNM, 2014). Education and certification standards are the same for CNMs and CMs. As of 2010, a graduate degree is required (ACNM, 2014).

The North American Registry of Midwives (NARM) is also a certification agency. Midwives certified through NARM may have been prepared through a formal educational program at a college, university, or midwifery school. NARM also has a path to certification for experienced midwives who have nonconventional or extensive training and experience. These midwives are eligible to use the credential *certified professional midwife (CPM)* (NARM, 2014).

The place of birth is an important decision. Birthing centers and special homelike labor-delivery-recovery-postpartum (LDRP) rooms in hospitals have become increasingly popular. Some women choose to give birth at home, although healthcare

professionals do not generally recommend this approach. Most professionals are concerned that, in the event of an unanticipated complication, delay in receiving emergency care might jeopardize the well-being or even the life of the mother or her baby. Some CNMs do attend home births; however, the majority of home births are attended by CMs, CPMs, or lay midwives. In 2012, less than 1% (0.89%) of births occurred at home (MacDorman, Mathews, & Declerq, 2014).

Contemporary Care of Children

As of 2012, more than 83.7 million children under 20 years of age live in the United States, and they account for 26.7% of the population (U.S. Census Bureau, 2013). (See Figure 1–3 for a distribution of the population by age group.)

Pediatric nursing is a specialized area of nursing that focuses on caring for children in many different settings within the hospital and the community. These settings include the following:

- Various hospital units, such as pediatric units, intensive care units, emergency departments, radiology, rehabilitation units, and specialty care clinics

- Physician offices, healthcare centers, and clinics

- Schools, child care centers, detention centers, and camps

- The child's home

Pediatric health care occurs along a continuum that reflects not only the various settings of care, but also the complexity and range of care needed by individual children and their families. For example, all children need health promotion and health maintenance care, but some children need care for chronic conditions, acute illnesses and injuries, and even end-of-life care. See Figure 1–4 for the model of pediatric health care used in this textbook.

Managing the child's transition from the hospital to another setting involves planning the discharge, implementing interdisciplinary plans, ensuring that the family understands the aspects of care they need to provide, helping the family to develop an emergency care plan in the event their child has an unexpected healthcare crisis, and collaborating with a broad range of healthcare professionals.

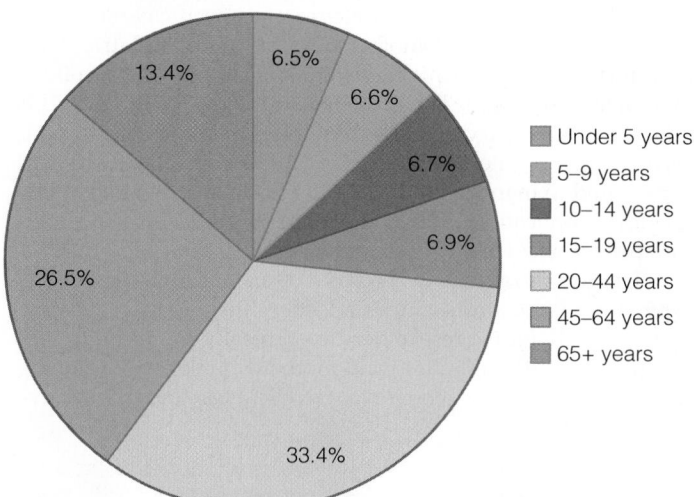

Legend:
- Under 5 years
- 5–9 years
- 10–14 years
- 15–19 years
- 20–44 years
- 45–64 years
- 65+ years

Values shown: 6.5%, 6.6%, 6.7%, 6.9%, 13.4%, 26.5%, 33.4%

Figure 1–3 In 2012, children from birth to 19 years of age accounted for almost 27% of the total population of the United States.

SOURCE: Data from U.S. Census Bureau. (2013). *Current Population Survey, Annual Social and Economic Supplement, 2012.* Retrieved from http://www.census.gov/population/age/data/2012comp.html

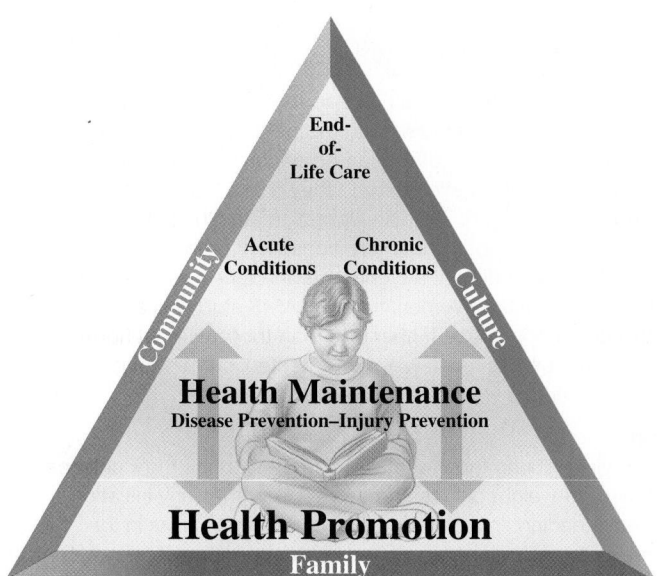

Figure 1–4 The Bindler-Ball Continuum of Pediatric Health Care for Children and Their Families. The outer bars represent the family, cultural, and community influences on the care that the child receives, either through the services sought by the family or the services provided in the community. Cultural influences include the family's values and beliefs and the cultural competence of the nurse in caring for a child and family.

The inner categories represent the range of health care needed by children. All children need health promotion and health maintenance services, represented by the base of the triangle. Notice the arrows representing the upward and downward movement between the levels of care as the child's condition changes.

Children may be healthy with episodic acute illnesses and injuries. Some children develop a chronic condition for which specialized health care is needed. A child's chronic condition may be well controlled, but acute episodes (such as with asthma) or other illnesses and injuries may occur, and the child also needs health promotion and health maintenance services. Some children develop a life-threatening illness and ultimately need end-of-life care. A healthy child may also experience a catastrophic injury leading to death and the family needs supportive end-of-life care.

SOURCE: Bindler & Ball, 2007.

Maternal-Child Care in the Community

Primary care is the focus of much attention as caregivers search for a new, more effective direction for health care. Primary care includes a focus on health promotion, illness prevention, and individual responsibility for one's own health. These services are best provided in community-based settings. Healthcare payers are beginning to recognize the importance of primary care in containing costs and maintaining health. Community-based healthcare systems that provide primary care and some secondary care are becoming available in schools, workplaces, homes, churches, clinics, transitional care programs, and other ambulatory settings.

The growth and diversity of health payer plans offer both opportunities and challenges for women's and children's health care. Opportunities for improved delivery of screening and preventive services exist in community-based models of coordinated and comprehensive well-woman and well-child care. A challenge that health payer plans face is how to relate to essential community providers of care, such as family-planning clinics, women's health centers, and child health centers, that offer a unique service or serve groups of women and children with special needs (adolescents, women and children with disabilities, and ethnic or racial minorities).

Community-based care remains an essential element of health care for uninsured or underinsured individuals, as well as for individuals who benefit from programs such as Medicare, Medicaid, or the Children's Health Insurance Program (CHIP). Some of these programs are broad based, such as those offered through public health departments, while others, such as parenting classes for adolescents, are geared to the needs of a specific population.

Maternal-child nurses are especially sensitive to these changes in healthcare delivery because the vast majority of health care provided to childbearing and childrearing families takes place outside of hospitals in clinics, offices, and community-based organizations. In addition, maternal-child nurses offer specialized services such as childbirth preparation classes, sibling classes, and parenting classes.

Healthcare reform has increased the emphasis on the need for individuals to have a *medical home* or *healthcare home*—a continuous, comprehensive, family-centered, and compassionate source of health care. This is especially important for children throughout their developmental years. Criteria for a medical or healthcare home for children include being well known by a physician or nurse who provides the usual source of sick care and having access to specialty care and other services or therapies. In addition, the healthcare provider spends adequate time communicating clearly with the family, provides help with care coordination when needed, respects the family's values and partners with the family in the child's care, and provides interpreters when necessary. An estimated 54.4% of U.S. children have a healthcare home that meets these criteria (Health Resources and Services Administration, 2014).

The current trend toward shorter hospital stays can end in the discharge of individuals who still require support, assistance, and teaching. Health care provided in a client's home helps fill this gap. Home care also enables newborns, infants, children, and women to remain at home with conditions that formerly would have required hospitalization.

Nurses are major providers of home care services. Home care nurses perform direct nursing care and also supervise unlicensed assistive personnel who provide less skilled levels of service. In a home setting, nurses use their skills in assessment, intervention, communication, teaching, problem solving, and organization to meet the needs of childbearing and childrearing families. They also play a major role in coordinating services from other providers, such as physical therapists or lactation consultants.

Postpartum and newborn home visits help ensure a satisfactory transition from the birthing center to the home. This positive trend meets the needs of childbearing families and should become standard practice. See Chapter 29 for discussion of home care and guidance about making a home visit. Information on home care is also provided as appropriate throughout this text.

Many children with serious chronic conditions and disabilities assisted by technology are now cared for at home by families rather than by long-term hospitalization. After studies

EVIDENCE-BASED PRACTICE | Home Visiting Services and Birth Outcomes

Clinical Question
Can prenatal home visiting services improve birth outcomes, even in high-risk populations?

The Evidence
Poor birth outcomes have negative consequences on families and communities. Home nursing visits during the prenatal period have been proposed as one way to achieve better birth outcomes.

Two studies focused on the effects of prenatal home visits on adequacy of prenatal care, low birth weight, preterm labor, initiation of breastfeeding, breastfeeding duration, and preventable risk factors for newborn morbidity, such as smoking. One study was a cross-sectional analysis of data from the state Pregnancy Risk Assessment and Monitoring System (PRAMS) that included 1 year of data and 407 women. The second study focused on high-risk pregnancies in a population of African American women; in this study, monthly home visits were part of a maternal health program emphasizing racial equity and case management. State data representing more than 9300 women were used in the latter study and used a matched-comparison design. These studies, taken together, comprise a strong level of evidence.

Women in both studies had a reduced incidence of low birth weight when compared with mothers who had no home visits. In the population of African American women, better birth weight was achieved even though they had a higher prenatal smoking rate (Kothari, Zielinski, James, et al., 2014). Women with home visits sought out more consistent prenatal care and initiated breastfeeding at a higher rate than their counterparts without home visits. Women in the PRAMS study initiated postnatal contraception at a higher rate than those without home visits, although this result was not detected in the population of African American women (Shah & Austin, 2014).

Best Practice
Home visits during the prenatal period can reduce the incidence of low-birth-weight babies and can support the early initiation of breastfeeding. In high-risk populations, home visits in the context of case management and culturally appropriate care can improve birth outcomes even in the presence of risk factors.

Clinical Reasoning
What might be the elements of a prenatal program that are modified to be culturally appropriate? How can prenatal home visits demonstrate cost effectiveness when designing overall maternal-child care?

---

in the 1980s found that home health care was substantially less expensive than hospital care, Congress amended laws to permit payment of home care services with federal funds, such as through Medicaid. Children with conditions considered fatal 15 years ago are thriving with home care and are participating in family, community, and school life. See Chapter 38.

Complementary Care

Interest in complementary care, previously termed complementary and alternative therapies (CAM), continues to grow nationwide and affects the care of childbearing and childrearing families. Complementary care includes a wide array of therapies, such as acupuncture, acupressure, therapeutic touch, biofeedback, massage therapy, meditation, herbal therapies, and homeopathic remedies. Concepts related to the use of complementary care by families are presented in more detail in Chapter 2.

Access to Health Care

Healthcare issues are at the top of policy and legislative agendas. Cost, access, and quality of health care have become the "bywords" of the times. In 2011, healthcare expenditures in the United States were $2.3 trillion, a 4.1% increase over the previous year (National Center for Health Statistics [NCHS], 2014).

Almost all adults over age 65 are covered by Medicare; so the vast majority of the uninsured are under age 65. In 2012, the percentage of people ages 18 to 44 covered by private insurance declined from 68.7% in 2002 to 61.4% in 2012. This decrease has been offset, however, by increases in the percentage of people with Medicaid, which increased from 7.1% to 11.6% during this same 10-year period (NCHS, 2014).

The Affordable Care Act bridges a portion of the gap. It ends pre-existing condition exclusions for children, eliminates annual limits on insurance coverage, and keeps young adults covered for a longer period. It also provides more affordable health insurance options including tax credits for middle- and low-income families. These credits cover a major portion of the cost (U.S. Department of Health and Human Services, 2015).

Congress created the Children's Health Insurance Program (CHIP) in 1997 and reauthorized it in 2009 to provide health insurance for children when their family's income is too high to qualify for Medicaid but inadequate to pay for private insurance coverage. An estimated 43 million children have health insurance coverage through Medicaid and CHIP (Centers for Medicare and Medicaid Services, 2014a). The average income eligibility criteria among the states is 241% of the federal poverty level for families to obtain free or low-cost health coverage for their children (Centers for Medicare and Medicaid Services, 2014b).

For women who become pregnant, early prenatal care is one of the most important approaches available to reduce adverse pregnancy outcomes. In 2008, 70.7% of pregnant women in the United States who had live births began prenatal care in the first trimester. However, these percentages vary significantly among groups, with Black or African American, Hispanic or Latina, and Native American women less likely to receive early and adequate prenatal care than White and Asian women (NCHS, 2013).

Healthy People 2020 Goals

For 30 years the federal government's *Healthy People* program has been providing science-based, national agendas for improving the health of all Americans. "The Healthy People initiative is grounded in the principle that setting national objectives and monitoring progress can motivate action, and indeed, in just the last decade, preliminary analyses indicate that the country has either progressed toward or met 71% of its *Healthy People* targets" (U.S. Department of Health and Human Services, 2011, p. 1). In December 2010, the next 10-year effort, *Healthy People 2020*, was launched. *Healthy People 2020* is grouped by topic area and objectives.

Maternal-newborn, pediatric, and women's health nurses focus directly on many of the topics, including the following:

- Maternal, newborn, infant, and child health
- Adolescent health (new)
- Family planning
- Injury and violence prevention
- Lesbian, gay, bisexual, and transgender health (new)
- Sexually transmitted infections

Because of the role women play in maintaining their family's health, many other topics may also be of importance to them, such as immunization and infectious diseases, diabetes, and nutrition and weight status, to name but a few. Nurses of all disciplines will find it helpful to become familiar with the 2020 topics and objectives, which may be found at the *Healthy People* website. To increase your familiarity with the objectives, look for the *Healthy People 2020* feature that identifies relevant objectives for topics presented throughout the text.

Culturally Competent Care

The population of the United States daily becomes more diverse. Approximately 47% of all children younger than 18 years of age are from families of minority populations (Federal Interagency Forum on Child and Family Statistics, 2013). Thus, it is vitally important for a nurse who cares for women and children to recognize the importance of a family's cultural values and beliefs, which may be quite different from those of the nurse.

Specific elements that contribute to a family's value system include the following:

- Religion and social beliefs
- Presence and influence of the extended family, as well as socialization within the ethnic group
- Communication patterns
- Beliefs and understanding about the concepts of health and illness
- Permissible physical contact with strangers
- Education

When the family's cultural values are incorporated into the care plan, the family is more likely to accept and comply with the needed care, especially in the home care setting. It is important for nurses to avoid imposing personal cultural values on the families and children in their care. By learning about the values of the different ethnic groups in the community, nurses can develop an individualized nursing care plan for each child and family.

Because of the importance of culturally competent care, this topic is discussed in more depth in Chapter 2 and throughout the book in special boxed features.

Developing Cultural Competence Values Conflicts

Conflicts can occur within a family when the traditional rituals and practices of the family do not conform to current healthcare practices. Nurses need to be sensitive to these potential conflicts when managing a child's health care, especially after the child has been discharged from the hospital. When cultural values are not part of the nursing care plan, parents may be forced to decide whether the family's beliefs should take priority over the healthcare professional's guidance.

Statistical Data and Maternal-Child Care

Health-related statistics provide an objective basis for projecting client needs, planning the use of resources, and determining the effectiveness of specific treatments. Statistics are used to help identify certain healthcare trends and high-risk target groups. The following sections discuss descriptive statistics that are particularly important to maternal-child health care.

Birth Rate

Birth rate refers to the number of live births per 1000 people in a given population. Worldwide, birth rates vary dramatically as Table 1–2 indicates. In the United States in 2013, the birth rate was 12.6. Birth rates decreased for women in all age groups between 15 and 29 years of age. The rate for women ages 30 to 39 increased, the rate for women for women ages 40 to 44 was unchanged, while the rate for women ages 45 to 49 increased (Martin, Hamilton, & Osterman, 2014).

The statistics do raise questions. For example: What is the impact of cultural differences and changing societal values on birth rates? Do birth rates change when access to information on contraception increases? What role does government policy, such as China's legislation limiting births to one child per family, play?

Maternal Mortality

The **maternal mortality rate** is the number of deaths from causes related to or aggravated by pregnancy or the management of pregnancy during the pregnancy cycle (including the 42-day postpartum period) per 100,000 live births. It does not include deaths of pregnant women due to external causes such as accidents, homicides, and suicides. Since 1986, the Centers for Disease Control and Prevention (CDC) has tracked pregnancy-related deaths. **Pregnancy-related deaths** are defined

TABLE 1–2 Live Birth Rates and Infant Mortality Rates for Selected Countries*

COUNTRY	BIRTH RATE	INFANT MORTALITY RATE
Afghanistan	38.8	117.2
Argentina	16.9	10.0
Australia	12.2	4.4
Cambodia	24.4	51.4
Canada	10.3	4.7
China	12.2	14.8
Egypt	23.4	22.4
Germany	8.4	3.5
Ghana	31.4	38.5
India	19.9	43.2
Iraq	26.9	37.5
Japan	8.1	2.1
Mexico	19.0	12.6
Russia	11.9	7.1
United Kingdom	12.2	4.4
United States	12.6*	6.0*

*Based on 2013 final data.

Source: Data from *The World Fact Book 2014*. Washington, DC: The Central Intelligence Agency. Retrieved from https://www.cia.gov/library/publications/the-world-factbook/geos/uk.html

as the death of a woman while pregnant or within 1 year of the termination of pregnancy (regardless of the length of the pregnancy or the site of implantation) from any cause aggravated by pregnancy or related to it (NCHS, 2013). The pregnancy-related mortality rate in the United States in 2009 was 17.8 deaths per 100,000 live births, which was the highest level reported since surveillance began. Black women have a significantly higher risk of maternal death than White women: 35.6 deaths per 100,000 live births as compared to 11.7 deaths for White women and 17.6 deaths for women of other races (NCHS, 2013).

Factors influencing the long-term decrease in maternal mortality include the increased use of hospitals and specialized healthcare personnel by maternity clients, the establishment of care centers for high-risk mothers and infants, the prevention and control of infection with antibiotics and improved techniques, the availability of blood products for transfusions, and the lowered rates of anesthesia-related deaths. Additional factors may be identified by asking the following research questions: Is there a correlation between maternal mortality and age? Is there a correlation between maternal mortality and availability of health care? Is economic status a factor in maternal mortality?

Healthy People 2020

(MICH-5) Reduce the rate of maternal mortality

Infant Mortality

The **infant mortality rate** is the number of deaths of infants under 1 year of age per 1000 live births in a given population. *Neonatal mortality* is the number of deaths of infants less than 28 days of age per 1000 live births, *perinatal mortality* includes both neonatal deaths and fetal deaths per 1000 live births, and *fetal death* is death in utero at 20 weeks or more gestation.

In 2013, the infant mortality rate in the United States was 5.96 per 1000 live births (Figure 1–5) (Kochanek, Murphy, Xu, et al., 2014). Infant mortality rates are higher among infants born in multiple births, infants born prematurely, and those

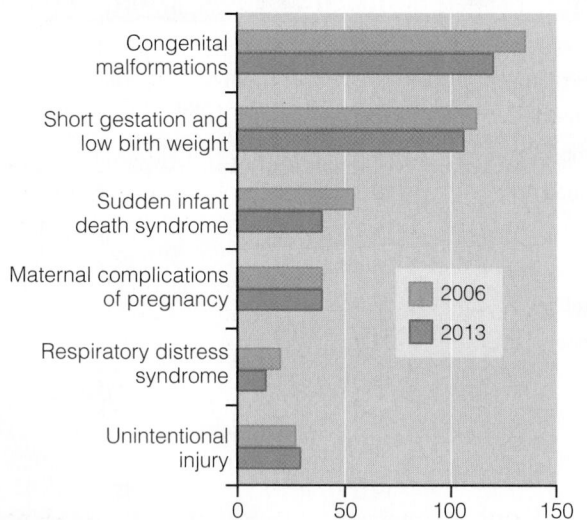

Figure 1–5 Infant mortality rates for the six leading causes of infant death in the United States, 2006 and 2013.

SOURCE: Heron, M., Hoyert, D. L., Murphy, S. L., Xu, J., Kochanek, K. D., & Tejada, B. (2009). Deaths: Final data for 2006. *National Vital Statistics Reports, 57*(14), 1–136; Kochanek, K. D., Murphy, S. L., Xu, J., & Arias, E. (2014). Mortality in the United States, 2013. *NCHS Data Brief*, No. 178. Retrieved from http://www.cdc .gov/nchs/data/databriefs/db178.pdf

born to unmarried mothers; rates are also higher for infants of teen mothers and mothers 40 years of age and older (Mathews & MacDorman, 2012).

The U.S. infant mortality rate continues to be of concern because the United States' rate is higher than that of most European countries as well as Australia, New Zealand, Japan, Korea, and Israel. Much of the infant mortality rate can be attributed to the high percentage of preterm births in the United States (MacDorman, Mathews, Mohangoo, et al., 2014). Healthcare professionals, policy makers, and the public continue to stress the need for better prenatal care, coordination of health services, and provision of comprehensive maternal-child services in the United States.

Table 1–2 identifies infant mortality rates for selected countries. As the data indicate, the range is dramatic among the countries listed. Information about birth rates and mortality rates is limited for some countries because of a lack of organized reporting mechanisms.

The information raises questions about access to health care during pregnancy and after birth and about standards of living, nutrition, and sociocultural factors. Additional factors affecting the infant mortality rate may be identified by considering the following research questions: What are the leading causes of infant mortality in each country? Why do mortality rates differ among racial groups?

Pediatric Mortality

The most common cause of death for U.S. children between 1 and 19 years of age is injury. Congenital malformations, cancer, and diseases of the heart are the most common medical causes of death.

Although unintentional injury is the leading cause of death, it is disturbing that intentional injury (homicide and suicide) is a major cause of death for the nation's children. The major causes of unintentional injury mortality in childhood include motor vehicle accidents (passengers and pedestrians), drowning, fires and burns, suffocation, and poisoning. Table 1–3 illustrates the leading causes of injury deaths by age group. Many injury prevention programs have been implemented by state health departments, healthcare facilities, and national organizations to reduce the number of children who die unnecessarily.

Healthy People 2020

(MICH-3) Reduce the rate of child deaths

Pediatric Morbidity

Morbidity—an illness or injury that limits activity, requires medical attention or hospitalization, or results in a chronic condition—also varies according to the age of the child. In 2011, children under 18 years of age accounted for more than 5.6 million hospitalizations, and the number of hospitalizations in this age group decreased 26% since 1997. Infants less than 1 year of age accounted for 4.2 million of these hospitalizations. Most of these hospitalizations were related to birth, but other leading causes of hospitalization included acute bronchitis, hemolytic jaundice, pneumonia, and short gestation/low birth weight (Pfuntner, Wier, & Stocks, 2013). Figure 1–6 illustrates the five leading causes of hospitalization of children 1 through 17 years of age in 2011. Diseases of the respiratory system account for the greatest number of hospitalizations when pneumonia and asthma hospitalizations are combined. Mood disorders hospitalizations have increased 68% since 1997.

TABLE 1–3 Five Leading Causes of Injury Death by Age Group, 2013*

AGE GROUP	RANKING				
	FIRST	SECOND	THIRD	FOURTH	FIFTH
Under 1 year	Suffocation	Homicide, unspecified cause	Homicide, specified cause	Motor vehicle	Undetermined suffocation
1 to 4 years	Drowning	Motor vehicle	Suffocation	Homicide	Fire, burns
5 to 9 years	Motor vehicle	Drowning	Fire, burns	Homicide, firearm	Suffocation
10 to 14 years	Motor vehicle	Suicide, suffocation	Suicide, firearms	Homicide, firearms	Drowning
15 to 19 years	Motor vehicle	Homicide, firearm	Suicide, suffocation	Suicide, firearms	Poisoning

Source: Data from National Center for Health Statistics. (2015). *10 leading causes of injury deaths, United States 2013.* Retrieved from http://www.cdc.gov/injury/wisqars/fatal.html

*Darker shading indicates unintentional injuries.

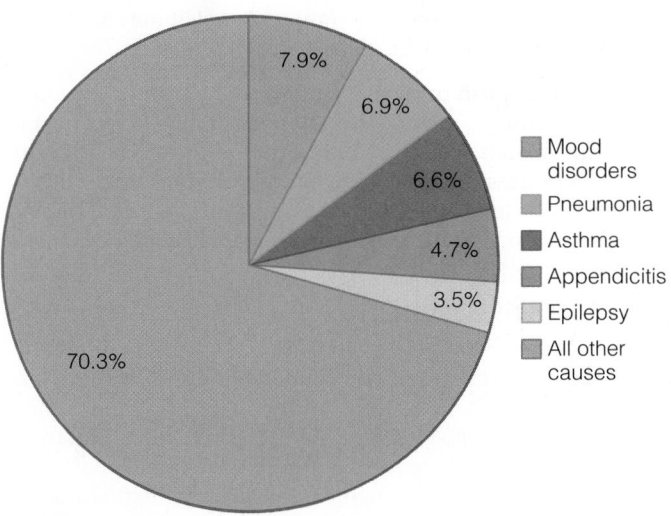

Figure 1–6 The leading causes of hospitalization for children 1 to 17 years of age in the United States in 2011 presented as a percentage of all causes of hospitalization in this age group.

SOURCE: Data from Pfuntner, A., Wier, L. M., & Stocks, C. (2013). Most frequent conditions in U.S. hospitals, 2011. *H-CUP Statistical Brief # 162.* Retrieved from http://www.hcup-us.ahrq.gov/reports/statbriefs/sb162.pdf

Implications for Nursing Practice

Nurses can use statistics in a number of ways. For example, they can use statistical data to:

- Determine populations at risk.
- Assess the relationship between specific factors.
- Help establish databases for specific client populations.
- Determine the levels of care needed by particular client populations.
- Evaluate the success of specific nursing interventions.
- Determine priorities in caseloads.
- Estimate staffing and equipment needs of hospital units and clinics.
- Apply for funding to support health needs.

Nurses who use statistical information are better prepared to promote the health needs of maternal, newborn, and pediatric clients and their families.

Legal Considerations in Maternal-Child Nursing

Scope of Practice

Scope of practice is defined as the limits of nursing practice set forth in state statutes. Although some state practice acts continue to limit nursing practice to the traditional responsibilities of providing client care related to health maintenance and disease prevention, most state practice acts cover expanded practice roles that include collaboration with other health professionals in planning and providing care, physician-delegated diagnosis and prescriptive privileges, and the delegation of direct care tasks to other specified licensed and unlicensed personnel. A nurse must function within the scope of practice or risk being accused of practicing medicine without a license.

Standards of Nursing Care

Standards of care establish minimum criteria for competent, proficient delivery of nursing care. Such standards are designed to protect the public and are used to judge the quality of care provided. Legal interpretation of actions within standards of care is based on what a reasonably prudent nurse with similar education and experience would do in similar circumstances.

The American Nurses Association (ANA) has published standards of practice for maternal-child health. ANA, the National Association of Pediatric Nurse Practitioners, and the Society of Pediatric Nurses (2008) collaborated on the development of standards for pediatric clinical nursing practice. The ANA and the National Association of Neonatal Nurses also published the scope and standards of practice for neonatal nursing (2008). Specialty organizations such as the Association of Women's Health, Obstetric and Neonatal Nurses (AWHONN) continue to set the standards of professional nursing practice in the care of women and newborns. Agency policies, procedures, and protocols also provide appropriate guidelines for care standards. For example, **clinical practice guidelines** are comprehensive interdisciplinary care plans for a specific condition that describe the sequence and timing of interventions that should result in expected client outcomes. Clinical practice guidelines are adopted within a healthcare setting to reduce variation in care management, to limit costs of care, and to evaluate the effectiveness of care.

While standards of care do not carry the force of law, they have important legal significance. Any nurse who fails to meet appropriate standards of care invites allegations of negligence or malpractice. Practicing within the guidelines established by an agency or following local or national standards decreases the potential for litigation.

Patient Safety

The Joint Commission, a nongovernmental agency that audits the operation of hospitals and healthcare facilities, has identified patient safety as an important responsibility of healthcare providers and provides an annual list of specific patient safety goals. Specific criteria that healthcare facilities must meet for accreditation can be found on the Joint Commission website.

Safety is a major focus of nursing education programs. The Quality and Safety Education for Nurses (QSEN) project, established in 2005, is designed "to meet the challenge of preparing future nurses who will have the knowledge, skills, and attitudes (KSAs) necessary to improve continuously the quality and safety of the healthcare systems within which they work" (QSEN, 2011, p. 1). The project focuses on competencies in six areas:

1. Client-centered care
2. Teamwork and collaboration
3. Evidence-based practice
4. Quality improvement
5. Safety
6. Informatics

To support the efforts of the Joint Commission and to draw special attention to the importance of the QSEN project's emphasis on safety, key issues related to safety are noted throughout this text with the words **SAFETY ALERT!** in red.

Infants and children are at a higher risk for medical error than adults and also may be more vulnerable to harm from errors made. Most errors in medical care within hospitals are "systems" errors related to equipment, complex procedures, fragmented care, and lack of standardized procedures (see Figure 1–7). Incorrect dosing

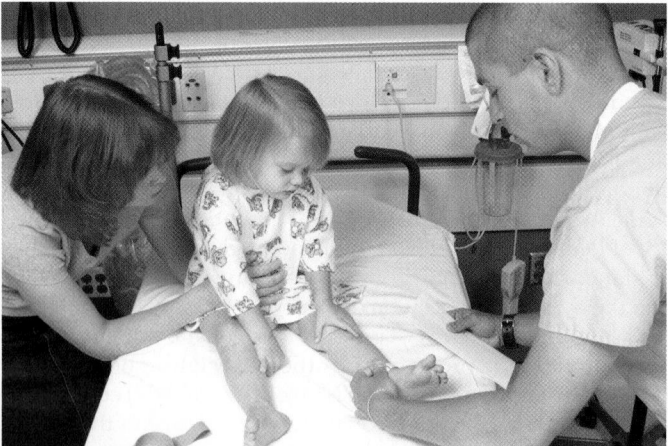

Figure 1–7 **An important client safety action is to verify the identity of the child prior to performing any procedure or administering medication. The nurse needs two forms of identification. In this case, the child's identification bracelet is compared to the name and birth date on the laboratory test form, and the parent also confirms the child's identity.**

is a commonly reported medication error and reasons for this increased risk among children include the following:

- Medication dosage is based on weight or body surface area, often making dosage calculations more complex. The misplacement of a decimal point in the medication dosage calculation can result in an overdose that can cause harm to a child or even death.

- Children often need suspensions or liquid preparations, adding to the dosage calculation complexity. Not only must the correct dose be calculated, but also the amount of liquid preparation with that dose. Some medications are in concentrations that require dilution, further complicating the accurate medication dosage calculation.

- Off-label medications (those not yet approved for use in children by the U.S. Food and Drug Administration [FDA]) are sometimes prescribed, thus the appropriate pediatric dose and adverse effects are unknown.

- Young children cannot communicate well if they are having a reaction to the medication.

Limited English proficiency may also be a potential source of medical error for childbearing women and children. In such cases, a risk exists for errors in interpretation—either of what the health professional says or what the family member understands. Healthcare facilities are actively working to implement strategies that will reduce medical errors in all child clients.

Informed Consent

Informed consent is a legal concept that protects a person's right to autonomy and self-determination by specifying that no action may be taken without that individual's prior understanding and freely given consent. Although this policy is actively enforced for major procedures, surgery, or regional anesthesia, it pertains to any nursing, medical, or surgical intervention. To touch a person without consent (except in an emergency) constitutes *battery*. Consent is not informed unless the client, or parent (or guardian) in the case of a child, understands the recommended procedures or treatments, their rationales, the benefits of each, alternative treatments, and any associated risks. When possible, it is important to have translators available for non–English-speaking women and families.

The person who is ultimately responsible for the treatment or procedure, usually the physician, should provide the information necessary to obtain informed consent. In such cases, the nurse's role is to witness the client's signature (or the parent's signature for a child) giving consent. The nurse may also serve as a witness if clients or parents give verbal consent by telephone. If the nurse determines that the individual does not understand the procedure or risks, the nurse must notify the physician, who must then provide additional information to ensure that the consent is informed. The nurse also responds to questions asked by adult clients or by parents and children. Anxiety, fear, pain, and medications that alter consciousness may influence an individual's ability to give informed consent. An oral consent is legal, but written consent is easier to defend in a court of law. Adolescents under 18 or 21 years of age, depending on state law, can legally give informed consent in the following circumstances (American Academy of Pediatrics, 2011):

- The minor is a parent or is pregnant.
- The adolescent is a legally **emancipated minor** (self-supporting adolescent under 18 years of age not subject

to parental control; for example, not living at home, married, on active duty in the military, or incarcerated). In most states, a pregnant teen is considered emancipated.

- In some states, **mature minors** (14- to 18-year-old adolescents who are able to understand treatment risks) can give independent consent for treatment or refuse treatment for some limited conditions such as testing and treatment for sexually transmitted infections, family planning, drug and alcohol abuse, blood donation, and mental health care (Coleman & Rosoff, 2013).

Refusal of a treatment, medication, or procedure after appropriate information is provided also requires that the individual sign a form releasing the physician and clinical facility from liability resulting from the effects of such a refusal. Refusal of blood transfusions by Jehovah's Witnesses is an example of such refusal.

Nurses are responsible for educating clients about any nursing care. Before each nursing intervention, the maternal-child nurse lets the individual and/or family know what to expect, thus ensuring cooperation and obtaining consent. Afterward the nurse documents the teaching and the learning outcomes in the person's record. The importance of clear, concise, and complete nursing records cannot be overemphasized. These records are evidence that the nurse obtained consent, performed prescribed treatments, reported important observations to the appropriate staff, and adhered to acceptable standards of care.

Because children are not considered competent to make healthcare decisions, parents, as the legal custodians of minor children, are customarily requested to give informed consent on behalf of a child. Both children and parents must understand that they have the right to refuse treatment at any time. In an emergency, consent for treatment to preserve life or limb is not required. When parents are divorced, some states limit the parental rights to give informed consent to the parent with custody. When parents have joint custody, in most cases, either parent may give consent. The nurse should obtain legal advice from the facility's designated legal experts for complex family issues related to guardianship, divorced parents disagreeing over care, or a caregiver who is not the legal guardian.

Parents or guardians have absolute authority to make choices about their child's health care except in certain cases. Specifically:

- When the parents' choice of treatment does not permit life-saving treatment for the child
- When there is a potential conflict of interest between the child and parents, such as with suspected child abuse or neglect

In some cases, the court may be requested to appoint a proxy decision maker for the child or to determine that the child is capable of making a major treatment decision.

Children should become more actively involved in decision making about treatment procedures as their reasoning skills develop. Children too young to give informed consent can be given age-appropriate information about their condition and asked about their care preferences. Their parents, however, make ultimate decisions about their care.

With regard to children's participation in research, federal guidelines state that children 7 years of age and older must receive information about a research project and give *assent* (the voluntary agreement to participate in a research project or to accept treatment) before they are enrolled. Children should be given adequate time to ask questions and be told that they have the right to refuse to participate in the study. The child is then asked if he or she wishes to participate. If the child assents, parents then provide signed permission for the child to participate in the research project.

Growth and Development

By 7 or 8 years of age, a child is able to understand concrete explanations about informed consent for research participation. By age 11, a child's abstract reasoning and logic abilities are advanced. By age 14, an adolescent can weigh options and make decisions regarding consent as capably as an adult.

Right to Privacy

The *right to privacy* is the right of a person to keep his or her person and property free from public scrutiny. To protect this right for clients and families, only those responsible for their care should conduct an examination or discuss their case.

The right to privacy is protected by state constitutions, statutes, and common law. The ANA, the National League for Nursing (NLN), and the Joint Commission have adopted professional standards protecting the privacy of clients. Healthcare agencies should also have written policies dealing with client privacy. The Health Insurance Portability and Accountability Act of 1996 (HIPAA), which was fully implemented in 2002, also has a provision to guarantee the security and privacy of health information.

Laws, standards, and policies about privacy specify that information about an individual's treatment, condition, and prognosis can be shared only by health professionals responsible for his or her care. Information considered vital statistics (name, age, occupation, and so on) may be revealed legally, but is often withheld because of ethical considerations. The client should be consulted as to what information may be released and to whom.

Professionalism in Practice   Adolescents and Confidentiality

Breaching confidentiality is a potential problem for adolescents, who are just learning whom they can trust in the healthcare system. Current electronic health records that provide access to parents and adolescents regarding personal health care have no current criteria for limiting access by parents to data regarding care adolescents have sought privately as a mature minor (American Academy of Pediatrics, 2012). Make sure you openly discuss the limits of confidentiality in electronic health records as well as mandatory reporting requirements with the client and family. Inadvertent disclosure of personal information may lead to psychologic, social, or physical harm in some clients.

Patient Self-Determination Act

The federal Patient Self-Determination Act directs healthcare institutions to inform hospitalized clients about their rights, which include expressing a preference for treatment options and making **advance directives** (writing a living will or authorizing a durable power of attorney for healthcare decisions on the individual's behalf). Nurses often discuss these issues with clients and their families. Minor children and their parents should also be informed of their rights. Adolescents with serious acute or chronic conditions with a higher risk of death should be encouraged to talk with their parents about their healthcare wishes and to prepare advance directives jointly.

Do-not-resuscitate (DNR) (or *allow natural death [AND]*) orders have become more common for children with terminal illnesses in which no further aggressive treatments are available or desired. In many cases, these children are cared for at home or in a hospice program. Implementation of DNR orders for such children then becomes a community issue—to ensure that resuscitation measures are not initiated by any emergency care provider when the child has a life-threatening event. State health policies must be developed so children with these signed orders are easily identified and appropriate documentation of the orders is on file.

Ethical Issues in Maternal-Child Nursing

Although ethical dilemmas confront nurses in all areas of practice, those related to pregnancy, birth, newborns, and children seem especially difficult to resolve.

Maternal-Fetal Conflict

Until fairly recently the fetus was viewed legally as a nonperson. Mother and fetus were viewed as one complex client—the pregnant woman—of which the fetus was an essential part. However, advances in technology have permitted the physician to treat the fetus and monitor fetal development. The fetus is increasingly viewed as a client separate from the mother. This focus on the fetus intensified in 2002 when President George W. Bush announced that "unborn children" would qualify for government healthcare benefits. This move was designed to promote prenatal care, but it represented the first time that any U.S. federal policy had defined childhood as starting at conception.

Most women are strongly motivated to protect the health and well-being of their fetus. In some instances, however, women have refused interventions on behalf of the fetus, and forced interventions have occurred. These include forced cesarean birth, coercion of mothers who practice high-risk behaviors, such as substance abuse, to enter treatment; and, perhaps most controversial, mandated experimental in utero therapy or surgery in an attempt to correct a specific birth defect. These interventions infringe on the autonomy of the mother. They may also be detrimental to the baby if, as a result, maternal bonding is hindered, the mother is afraid to seek prenatal care, or the mother is herself harmed by the actions taken.

Attempts have also been made to criminalize the behavior of women who fail to follow a physician's advice or who engage in behaviors (such as substance abuse) that are considered harmful to the fetus. This raises two thorny questions:

1. What practices should be monitored?
2. Who will determine when the behaviors pose such a risk to the fetus that the courts should intervene?

The American College of Obstetricians and Gynecologists (ACOG) Committee on Ethics has affirmed the fundamental right of pregnant women to make informed, uncoerced decisions about medical interventions and has taken a direct stand against coercive and punitive approaches to the maternal-fetal relationship (ACOG, 2005).

Both ACOG and the American Academy of Pediatrics recognize that cases of maternal-fetal conflict involve two clients, both of whom deserve respect and treatment. Such cases are best resolved by using internal hospital mechanisms, including counseling, the intervention of specialists, and consultation with an institutional ethics committee. Court intervention should be considered a last resort, being appropriate only in extraordinary circumstances.

Abortion

Since the 1973 *Roe v. Wade* Supreme Court decision, elective abortion has been legal in the United States. Abortion can be performed until the period of viability; that is, the point at which the fetus can survive independently of the mother. After that time, abortion is permissible only when the life or health of the mother is threatened. Before viability, the rights of the mother are paramount; after viability, the rights of the fetus take precedence.

Personal beliefs, cultural norms, life experiences, and religious convictions shape people's attitudes about abortion. Ethicists have thoughtfully and thoroughly argued positions supporting both sides of the question. Nevertheless, few issues spark the intensity of response seen when the issue of abortion is raised.

At present, the decision about abortion is to be made by the woman and her physician. Nurses (and other caregivers) have the right to refuse to assist with the procedure if abortion is contrary to their moral and ethical beliefs. However, if a nurse works in an institution where abortions may be performed, the nurse can be dismissed for refusing to assist. To avoid being placed in a situation contrary to personal ethical values and beliefs, it is important to identify the practices of an institution before going to work there. A nurse who refuses to participate in an abortion because of moral or ethical beliefs has a responsibility to ensure that someone with similar qualifications is available to provide appropriate care for the client. Clients must never be abandoned, regardless of a nurse's beliefs.

Intrauterine Fetal Surgery

Intrauterine fetal surgery, an example of therapeutic research, is a therapy for anatomic lesions that can be corrected surgically and are incompatible with life if not treated. Examples include surgery for myelomeningocele and some congenital cardiac defects. The procedure involves opening the uterus during the second trimester (before viability), performing the planned surgery, and replacing the fetus in the uterus. The risks to the fetus are substantial, and the mother is committed to cesarean births for this and subsequent pregnancies (because the upper, active segment of the uterus is entered). The parents must be informed of the experimental nature of the treatment, the risks of the surgery, the commitment to cesarean birth, and alternatives to the treatment.

As in other aspects of maternity care, caregivers must respect the pregnant woman's autonomy. The procedure involves health risks to the woman, and she retains the right to refuse any surgical procedure. Healthcare providers must be careful that their zeal for new technology does not lead them to focus unilaterally on the fetus at the expense of the mother.

Reproductive Assistance

Assisted reproductive technology (ART) is the term used to describe highly technologic approaches used to produce pregnancy. *In vitro fertilization* and *embryo transfer (IVF-ET)*, a therapy offered to selected infertile couples, is perhaps the best known ART technique.

Multifetal pregnancy may occur with ART because the use of ovulation-inducing medications typically triggers the release of multiple eggs that, when fertilized, produce multiple embryos, which are then implanted. Multifetal pregnancy increases the risk of miscarriage, preterm birth, and neonatal morbidity and mortality. It also increases the mother's risk of complications, including cesarean birth. To help prevent a high-order multifetal pregnancy (presence of three or more fetuses), the American Society for Reproductive Medicine (ASRM) has issued guidelines to limit the number of embryos transferred. These guidelines are designed to decrease risk while allowing for individualized care (ASRM & Society for Assisted Reproductive Technology, 2013).

This practice raises ethical considerations about the handling of the unused embryos. However, when a multifetal pregnancy does occur, the physician may suggest that the woman consider fetal reduction, in which some of the embryos are aborted to give the remaining ones a better chance for survival. Clearly this procedure raises ethical concerns about the sacrifice of some so that the remainder can survive.

Prevention should be the first approach to the problem of multifetal pregnancy. It begins with careful counseling about the risks of multiple gestation and the ethical issues that relate to fetal reduction. No physician who is morally opposed to fetal reduction should be expected to perform the procedure; however, physicians should be aware of the ethical and medical issues involved and be prepared to respond to families in a professional and ethical manner (ACOG, 2013).

Surrogate childbearing is another approach to infertility. Surrogate childbearing occurs when a woman agrees to become pregnant for a childless couple. She may be artificially inseminated with the male partner's sperm or a donor's sperm or may receive a gamete transfer, depending on the infertile couple's needs. If fertilization occurs, the woman carries the fetus to term and releases the newborn to the couple after birth.

These methods of resolving infertility raise ethical issues about candidate selection, responsibility for a child born with a congenital defect, and religious objections to artificial conception. Other ethical questions include the following:

- What should be done with surplus fertilized oocytes?
- To whom do frozen embryos belong?
- Who is liable if a woman or her offspring contracts HIV from donated sperm?
- Should children be told about their conception?

Embryonic Stem Cell Research

Human stem cells can be found in embryonic tissue and in the primordial germ cells of a fetus. Research has demonstrated that in tissue cultures these cells can be made to differentiate into other types of cells such as blood, nerve, or heart cells, which might then be used to treat problems such as diabetes, Parkinson and Alzheimer diseases, spinal cord injury, or metabolic disorders. The availability of specialized tissue or even organs grown from stem cells might also decrease society's dependence on donated organs for organ transplants.

Positions about embryonic stem cell research vary dramatically, from the view that any use of human embryos for research is wrong to the view that any form of embryonic stem cell research is acceptable, with a variety of other positions that fall somewhere in between these extremes. Other questions also arise: What sources of embryonic tissue are acceptable for research? Is it ever ethical to clone embryos solely for stem cell research? Is there justification for using embryos remaining after fertility treatments?

The question of how an embryo should be viewed—with the status in some way of a person or in some sense of property (and, if property, whose?)—is a key question in the debate. Ethicists recognize that it is not necessary to advocate full moral status or personhood for an embryo in order to have significant moral qualms about the instrumental use of a human embryo in the "interests" of society. The issue of consent, which links directly to an embryo's status, also merits consideration. In truth, the ethical questions and dilemmas associated with embryonic stem cell research are staggeringly complex and require careful analysis and thoughtful dialogue.

Making Treatment Decisions for Children

Technology makes it possible to sustain the lives of children who previously would have died, thus creating many ethical issues. Conflict often arises between health professionals and parents when parents choose to withhold therapy or to request aggressive therapy on behalf of their child and the health professionals have a different opinion about treatment. Nurses often face ethical dilemmas when providing care to such a child, especially as they witness parents struggling to decide among treatment options.

When making treatment decisions in pediatrics, healthcare professionals need to determine whether their responsibility is limited to the child or includes the interests of the parents. The healthcare institution's ethics committee often plays a role in resolving conflicts about treatment decisions. Courts should make ethical decisions only when healthcare professionals and parents are unable to agree about providing or withholding treatment.

Terminating Life-Sustaining Treatment

The Child Abuse and Treatment Act of 1984, also known as the Baby Doe Regulations, defines withholding of medically indicated treatment for an infant with a life-threatening condition as medical neglect, except when care is futile (Douglas & Dahnke, 2013). Parents of such infants are usually the ultimate decision makers about the infant's care. Factors important to parents in making their decision include the infant's quality of life, degree of pain and suffering, likelihood for improvement, and physician recommendations. Physicians may believe treatment will help the infant and improve the quality of life (sometimes defined as a meaningful existence or an ability to develop human relationships). Conflict may arise when parents choose to withdraw therapy or request aggressive therapy when the healthcare providers' recommendations differ. An ethical consultation may be needed to resolve conflicts.

Organ Transplantation Issues

The death of a child can benefit several other children through organ transplantation, and organ transplantation has become an accepted therapeutic option for some life-threatening conditions. Children between 11 and 17 years of age account for nearly 45% of all children waiting for a transplant (Health Resources and Services Administration & Organ Procurement and Transplant Network, 2011). The National Organ Transplant Act (PL 98-507) generated laws, regulations, and guidelines for organ collection and transplantation. The limited supply of organs has created numerous ethical issues: Which individuals on a waiting list should receive the organs available? Should a child with multiple congenital anomalies or abnormal chromosomes be eligible for a transplant? Should families be permitted to pay donor families for organs? Should the family's ability to pay for an organ transplant give a child higher priority for an organ? Should parents conceive another child hoping that the new baby is a potential stem cell donor for a child with an illness? If so, what pressures does this knowledge place on each child as he or she grows older?

Genetic Testing of Children

Genetic testing and screening of children are now possible for detection of carrier status or for presymptomatic detection of a specific condition, such as Duchenne muscular dystrophy. When genetic testing is considered, both the risks and benefits of receiving the results of the genetic test should be discussed when seeking informed consent. Genetic screening of newborns, such as for inborn errors of metabolism, cystic fibrosis, sickle cell disease, and other conditions, routinely occurs. In this case, the early identification of the genetic condition will have a clear benefit to the child, a system is in place to confirm the diagnosis, and treatment and follow-up are available for affected newborns. See Chapter 3 for more information on genetic testing.

Evidence-Based Practice in Maternal-Child Nursing

Evidence-based practice—that is, nursing care in which all interventions are supported by current, valid research evidence—is emerging as a force in health care. It provides a useful approach to problem solving and decision making and to self-directed, client-centered, lifelong learning. Evidence-based practice builds on the actions necessary to transform research findings into clinical practice by also considering other forms of evidence that can be useful in making clinical practice

decisions. These other forms of evidence may include statistical data, quality measurements, risk management measures, and information from support services such as infection control.

As practicing clinicians, nurses need to meet three basic competencies related to evidence-based practice:

1. Recognize which clinical practices are supported by sound evidence, which practices have conflicting findings as to their effect on client outcomes, and which practices have no evidence to support their use.
2. Use data in their clinical work to evaluate outcomes of care.
3. Appraise and integrate scientific bases into practice.

Nurses need to know what data are being tracked in their workplaces and how care practices and outcomes are improved as a result of quality improvement initiatives. However, there is more to evidence-based practice—competent, effective nurses learn to question the very basis of their clinical work.

Throughout this text we have provided *snapshots* of evidence-based practice related to childbearing women and families. We believe that these *Evidence-Based Practice* features will help you understand the concept more clearly and may challenge you to question the usefulness of some of the routine care you observe in clinical practice. That is the impact of evidence-based practice—it moves clinicians beyond practices of habit and opinion to practices based on high-quality, current science.

Clinical Reasoning

It can be challenging to use evidence, analyze information, and make sound decisions that result in safe, effective client care.

Scenarios provide a realistic way of enabling students to apply concepts. The *Clinical Reasoning* feature found throughout the chapters and the *Clinical Reasoning in Action* feature at the end of every chapter in this text presents a client scenario and asks clinical reasoning questions to help students formulate how they would handle the issues raised and how they would apply concepts they have learned in the chapter.

Focus Your Study

- Many nurses working with childbearing and childrearing families are expert practitioners who are able to serve as role models for nurses who have not yet attained the same level of competence.

- Case management is a process of coordinating the delivery of healthcare services in a manner that focuses on both quality and cost outcomes.

- Contemporary childbirth is family centered, offers choices about birth, and recognizes the needs of siblings and other family members.

- In pediatric settings, *family-centered care* is a dynamic, deliberate approach to building collaborative relationships between health professionals and families that is respectful of their diversity and beliefs about the nature of children's health conditions and ways to manage them.

- The U.S. healthcare system is facing a variety of challenges including the high cost of health care and the need for cost containment while retaining quality, the large numbers of uninsured and underinsured people, high infant mortality rates as compared with other industrialized nations, and a high incidence of poverty, especially among children and households headed by women.

- The nurse who provides culturally competent care recognizes the importance of the family's value system, acknowledges that differences occur among people, and seeks to respect and respond to ethnic diversity in a way that leads to mutually desirable outcomes.

- Statistical data can also reveal trends that require research to determine cause, to analyze the implications of specific findings for given populations, to explore relationships between specific factors, and to evaluate the success of specific nursing interventions.

- A nurse must practice within the scope of practice or be open to the accusation of practicing medicine without a license. The standard of care against which individual nursing practice is compared is that of a reasonably prudent nurse.

- Nursing standards provide information and guidelines for nurses in their own practice, in developing policies and protocols in healthcare settings, and in directing the development of quality nursing care.

- Informed consent—based on knowledge of a procedure and its benefits, risks, and alternatives—must be secured before providing treatment. Parents have authority to provide informed consent for all their children, except in cases when an adolescent is an emancipated minor or can be treated for specific conditions as a mature minor.

- Maternal-fetal conflict may arise when the fetus is viewed as a person of equal rights to those of the mother and external agents attempt to force the mother to accept a therapy she wishes to refuse or similarly attempt to restrict a mother's actions to support the well-being of the fetus.

- Abortion can be performed until the age of viability. Caregivers have the right to refuse to perform an abortion or assist with the procedure.

- Assisted reproductive technology (ART) is a term that describes the highly technologic approaches used to produce pregnancy. A variety of procedures are available to help infertile couples achieve a pregnancy. However, some of these procedures provoke serious ethical dilemmas.

- Embryonic stem cell research using human stem cells obtained from a human embryo is marked by controversy. On the one hand, it raises the possibility of treatment for a variety of major diseases such as diabetes, Parkinson disease, and Alzheimer disease. On the other hand, ethicists question the ethical implications of using embryonic tissue—especially tissue obtained specifically for stem cell research.

- Federal "Baby Doe" regulations were developed to protect the rights of infants with severe defects.

- Evidence-based practice—that is, nursing care in which all interventions are supported by current, valid research evidence—is emerging as a positive force in health care.

Clinical Reasoning in Action

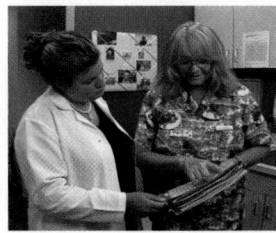

You are working as a prenatal nurse in a local clinic. Before entering a client's room, you review the medical record for pertinent information such as cultural background, significant family members, weeks of gestation, test results, birth plan, and education for health promotion. You greet each client and family member by name and ask how they are coping with the pregnancy. Depending on the trimester of the pregnancy, you review the discomforts or concerns of the mother and family and what they may expect. You examine the mother, including fundal height, fetal heart rate and fetal position if appropriate, maternal blood pressure, weight gain, and urine analysis.

With each client, you discuss the community resources available, such as prenatal classes, lactation consultants, and prenatal exercise or yoga classes. Based on the information you obtain, you might refer the mother to social services or the Special Supplementary Food Program for Women, Infants, and Children (WIC program) as appropriate. At the end of the clinic session, you review the status of the clients you saw with the collaborating physician.

1. How would you define the terms *family* and *family-centered care*?
2. Describe how the nursing process provides the framework for the delivery of direct nursing care.
3. How would you describe the concept of community-based care?
4. How would you describe culturally competent care?

References

American Academy of Pediatrics (AAP). (2011). Policy statement: Consent for emergency medical services for children and adolescents. *Pediatrics, 128*(2), 427–433.

American Academy of Pediatrics. (2012). Policy statement: Standards for health information technology to ensure adolescent privacy. *Pediatrics, 130*(5), 987–990.

American College of Nurse-Midwives (ACNM). (2014). *Essential facts about midwives*. Retrieved from http://www.midwife.org/Essential-Facts-about-Midwives

American College of Obstetricians and Gynecologists (ACOG). (2005). *Maternal decision making, ethics, and the law* (Committee Opinion No. 321). Washington, DC: Author.

American College of Obstetricians and Gynecologists (ACOG). (2013). *Multifetal pregnancy reduction* (Committee Opinion No. 553). Washington, DC: Author.

American Nurses Association, National Association of Pediatric Nurse Practitioners, & Society of Pediatric Nurses. (2008). *Pediatric nursing: Scope and standards of practice*. Silver Spring, MD: Nurses books. org.

American Society for Reproductive Medicine (ASRM) and the Society for Assisted Reproductive Technology. (2013). Criteria for number of embryos to transfer: A committee opinion. *Fertility and Sterility, 99*, 44–46.

Bindler, R. C., & Ball, J. W. (2007). The Bindler-Ball healthcare model: A new paradigm for health promotion. *Pediatric Nursing, 33*(2), 121–126.

Centers for Medicare and Medicaid Services. (2014a). *Medicaid: Children*. Retrieved from http://www.medicaid.gov/Medicaid-CHIP-Program-Information/By-Population/Children/Children.html

Centers for Medicare and Medicaid Services. (2014b). *2013 poverty level guidelines*. Retrieved from http://www.medicaid.gov/Medicaid-CHIP-Program-Information/By-Topics/Eligibility/Downloads/2013-Federal-Poverty-level-charts.pdf

Coleman, D. L., & Rosoff, P. M. (2013). The legal authority of mature minors to consent to general medical treatment. *Pediatrics, 131*(4), 786–793.

Committee on Hospital Care, & Institute for Patient and Family-Centered Care. (2012). Patient- and family-centered care and the pediatrician's role. *Pediatrics, 129*(2), 394–404.

Douglas, S. M., & Dahnke, M. D. (2013). Creating an ethical environment for parents and health providers dealing with the treatment dilemmas of neonates at the edge of viability. *Journal of Neonatal Nursing, 19*, 33–37.

Federal Interagency Forum on Child and Family Statistics. (2013). *America's children: Key national indicators of well-being, 2013*. Retrieved from http://childstats .gov/americaschildren/index.asp

Health Resources and Services Administration, Maternal and Child Health Bureau. (2014). *The health and wellbeing of children: A portrait of the states and nation 2011–2012*. Retrieved from http://mchb.hrsa .gov/nsch/2011-12/health/index.html

Health Resources and Services Administration & Organ Procurement and Transplant Network. (2011). *Transplants in the U.S. by recipient age, and current U.S. waiting list by age*. Retrieved from http://optn .transplant.hrsa.gov/

Heron, M., Hoyert, D. L., Murphy, S. L., Xu, J., Kochanek, K. D., & Tejada, B. (2009). Deaths: Final data for 2006. *National Vital Statistics Reports, 57*(14), 1–136.

Hughs, D. (2014). *A review of the literature pertaining to family-centered care for children with special health care needs*. Retrieved from http://lpfch-cshcn.org /publications/research-reports/a-review-of-the -literature-pertaining-to-family-centered-care-for -children-with-special-health-care-needs/

Kochanek, K. D., Murphy, S. L., Xu, J., & Arias, E. (2014). Mortality in the United States, 2013. *NCHS Data Brief*, No. 178. Retrieved from http://www.cdc.gov /nchs/data/databriefs/db178.pdf.

Kothari, C., Zielinski, R., James, A., Charoth, R., & Sweezy, L. (2014). Improved birth weight for black infants: Outcomes of a Healthy Start Program. *American Journal of Public Health, 104*(S1), S96–S104.

Lewandowski, L. A., & Tesler, M. D. (Eds.). (2008). Family-centered care: Putting it into action. *The SPN/ANA Guide to Family-Centered Care*. Washington, DC: American Nurses Publishing.

MacDorman, M. F., Mathews, T. J., & Declerq. (2014). Trends in out-of-hospital births in the United States, 1990–2012. *NCHS Data Brief, No. 144*. Hyattsville, MD: National Center for Health Statistics.

MacDorman, M. F., Mathews, T. J., Mohangoo, A. D., & Zeitlin, J. (2014). International comparisons of infant mortality and related factors: United States and Europe, 2010. *National Vital Statistics Reports, 63*(5), 1–7.

Martin, J. A., Hamilton, B. E., & Osterman, M. J. K. (2014). Births in the United States, 2013. *NCHS Data Brief*, No. 175. 1–8.

Mathews, T. J., & MacDorman, M. F. (2012). Infant mortality statistics from the 2008 period linked birth/infant death data set. *National Vital Statistics Report, 60*(5), 128.

National Center for Health Statistics (NCHS). (2013). *Pregnancy Mortality Surveillance System*. Retrieved from http://www.cdc.gov/reproductivehealth /maternalinfanthealth/pmss.html#5

National Center for Health Statistics (NCHS). (2014). *Health, United States, 2013. With Special Feature on Prescription Drugs*. Hyattsville, MD: Author.

National Center for Health Statistics (NCHS). (2015). *10 leading causes of injury deaths, United States 2010*. Retrieved from http://www.cdc.gov/injury/wisqars /fatal.html

North American Registry of Midwives (NARM). (2014). *Equivalency applicants: Important: Updates to CPM eligibility requirements*. Retrieved from http://narm .org/equivalency-applicants/

Pfuntner, A., Wier, L. M., & Stocks, C. (2013). Most frequent conditions in U.S. hospitals, 2011. *H-CUP Statistical Brief #162*. Retrieved from http://www .hcup-us.ahrq.gov/reports/statbriefs/sb162.pdf

Pontius, D. J. (2013). Health literacy part 1: Practical techniques for getting your message home. *NASN School Nurse, 28*(5), 246–252.

Pontius, D. J. (2014). Health literacy part 2: Practical techniques for getting your message home. *NASN School Nurse, 29*(1), 30–42.

Quality and Safety Education for Nurses (QSEN). (2011). *About QSEN*. Retrieved from www.qsen.org/ about _qsen.php

Shah, M., & Austin, K. (2014). Do home visiting services received during pregnancy improve birth outcomes? Findings from Virginia PRAMS 2007–2008. *Public Health Nursing, 31*(5), 405–413.

U.S. Census Bureau. (2013). *Current Population Survey, Annual Social and Economic Supplement, 2012*. Retrieved from http://www.census.gov/population /age/data/2012comp.html

U.S. Department of Health and Human Services. (2011). *Healthy People 2020*. Retrieved from http://www .healthypeople.gov/2020/about/default.aspx

U.S. Department of Health and Human Services. (2015). *Key features of the Affordable Care Act by year*. Retrieved from http://www.hhs.gov/healthcare/facts /timeline/timeline-text.html

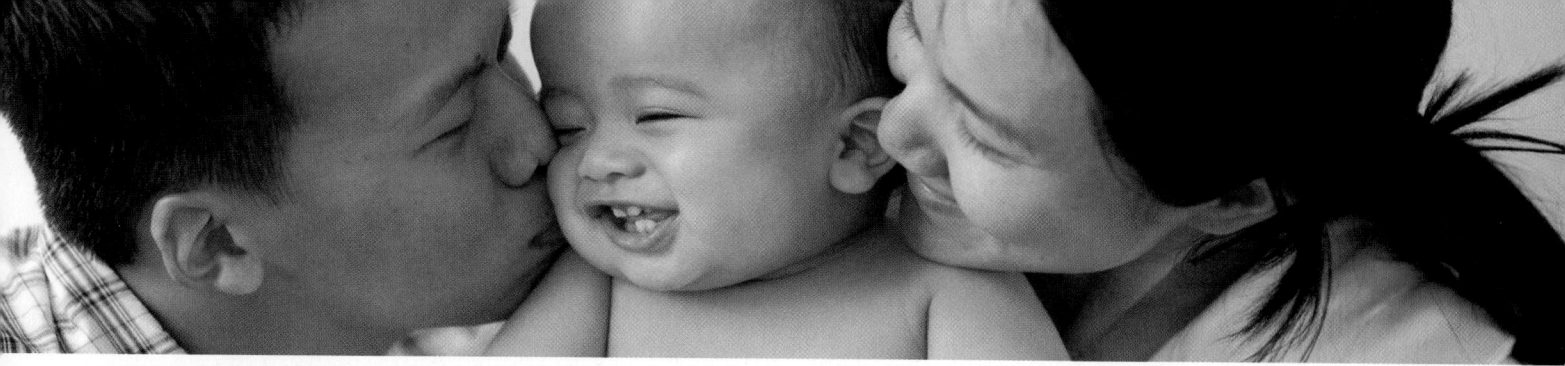

Chapter 2
Culture and the Family

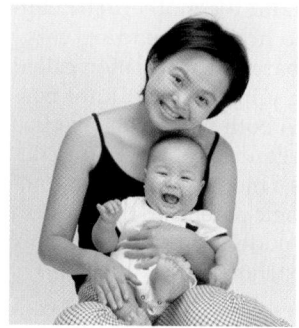

Ken Usami/Getty Images

My parents came here from China when I was 3. They wanted the chance to make a better life, and they wanted another child. Needless to say, although I have always felt loved and cherished, I know how thrilled they were when my brother was born. Sometimes I feel as though I am walking a line between their ways and the ways I have learned growing up in this country. My husband is Chinese but he, too, grew up here. We are expecting our second baby in a few months. We talk often about which Chinese ways we want to retain and which new ways make more sense. I am not sure that my parents will understand, however. To them, the old ways are always best.

—Li Wei, age 29

⌄ Learning Outcomes

2.1 Compare the characteristics of different types of families.

2.2 Identify the stages of a family life cycle.

2.3 Identify prevalent cultural norms related to childbearing and childrearing.

2.4 Summarize the importance of cultural competency in providing nursing care.

2.5 Discuss the use of a cultural assessment tool as a means of providing culturally sensitive care.

2.6 Identify key considerations in providing spiritually sensitive care.

2.7 Differentiate between complementary and alternative therapies.

2.8 Determine the benefits and risks of complementary and alternative therapies.

2.9 Summarize complementary therapies appropriate for the nurse to use with childbearing and childrearing families.

Individuals do not live in isolation. Their values, beliefs, behaviors, decisions, attitudes, and biases are shaped by many factors, including their families, their culture, and their religious beliefs.

This chapter begins with a brief discussion of family types, functioning, and assessment. It then addresses the impact of culture on the family and concludes with a brief examination of some of the complementary and alternative therapies a family might use.

The Family

The U.S. Census Bureau defines a **family** as two or more individuals who are joined together by marriage, birth, or adoption and live together in the same household (U.S. Census Bureau, 2013). More broadly, however, families are generally characterized by bonds of emotional closeness, sharing, and support.

Families are guided by a common set of values or beliefs about the worth and importance of certain ideas and traditions. These values often bind family members together, and these values are greatly influenced by external factors, including cultural background, social norms, education, environmental influences, socioeconomic status, and beliefs held by peers, coworkers, political and community leaders, and other individuals outside the family unit. Because of the influence of these external factors, a family's values may change considerably over the years.

Types of Families

Families are diverse in structure, roles, and relationships. Various types of families—both those considered traditional and nontraditional—exist in contemporary American society. This section identifies common types of family structures.

- In the *nuclear family,* children live in a household with both biologic parents and no other relatives or persons. One parent may stay home to rear the children while one parent works, but more commonly, both parents are employed by choice or necessity. Two-income families must address important issues such as child care arrangements, household chores, and how to ensure quality family time. *Dual-career/dual-earner families* are now considered the norm in modern society.

- The *child-free family* is a growing trend. In some cases, a family is child free by choice; in other cases, a family is child free because of issues related to infertility.

- In an *extended family,* a couple shares household and childrearing responsibilities with parents, siblings, or other relatives. Families may reside together to share housing expenses and child care. However, in many cases, the child may be residing with the grandparent and one parent because of issues associated with unemployment, parental separation, parental death, or parental substance abuse. Grandparents may raise children owing to the inability of parents to care for their own children.

- An *extended kin network family* is a specific form of an extended family in which two nuclear families of primary or unmarried kin live in proximity to each other. The family shares a social support network, chores, goods, and services.

- The *single-parent family* is becoming increasingly common. In some cases, the head of the household is widowed, divorced, abandoned, or separated. In other cases, the head of the household, most often the mother, remains unmarried. Single-parent families often face difficulties because the sole parent may lack social and emotional support, need assistance with childrearing issues, and face financial strain (Figure 2–1).

- The *single mother by choice family* represents a family composed of an unmarried woman who chooses to conceive or adopt without a life partner (Maggio, 2013). Although these families are statistically included in the single-parent family

statistics, they differ significantly in that these women typically are older, college educated, and financially stable and have contemplated pregnancy significantly prior to conceiving (Single Mothers by Choice, 2013).

- The *blended,* or *reconstituted nuclear, family* includes two parents with biologic children from a previous marriage or relationship who marry or cohabitate. This family structure has become increasingly common because of high rates of divorce and remarriage. Potential advantages to the children may include better financial support and a new supportive role model. Stresses can include lack of a clear role for the stepparent, lack of acceptance of the stepparent, financial stresses when two families must be supported by stepparents, and communication problems.

- A *binuclear family* is a post-divorce family in which the biologic children are members of two nuclear households, with coparenting by the father and the mother. The children alternate between the two homes, spending varying amounts of time with each parent in a situation called coparenting, usually involving joint custody. Joint custody is a legal situation in which both parents have equal responsibility and legal rights, regardless of where the children live. The binuclear family is a model for effective communication. It enables both biologic parents to be involved in a child's upbringing and provides additional support and role models in the form of extended family members.

- A *heterosexual cohabitating family* describes a heterosexual couple who may or may not have children and who live together outside of marriage. This may include never-married individuals as well as divorced or widowed persons. While some individuals choose this model for personal reasons, others do so for financial reasons or to seek companionship.

- *Gay* and *lesbian families* include those in which two adults of the same sex live together as domestic partners with or without children, and those in which a gay or lesbian single parent rears a child. Children in these families may be from a previous heterosexual union, or be born to or adopted by one or both member(s) of the same-sex couple. A biologic child may be born to one of the partners through artificial insemination or through a surrogate mother. Children who are adopted or born into lesbian and gay families are highly valued, as with heterosexual families. Evidence suggests that children reared by same-sex couples are as well adjusted as those born into heterosexual families and have positive peer relationships (Haney-Caron & Heilbrun, 2014).

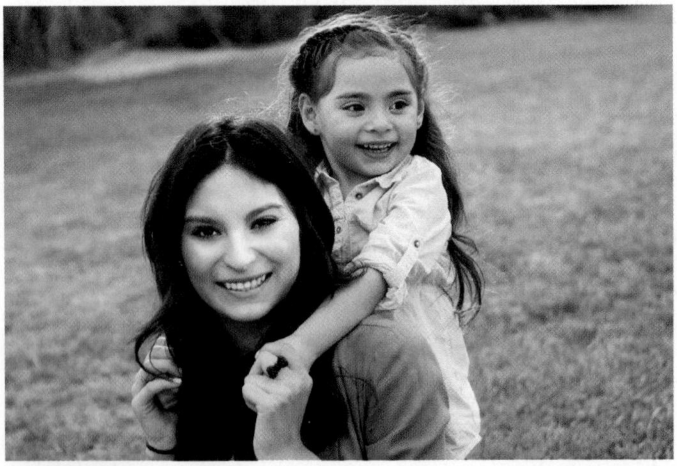

Figure 2–1 **Single-parent families account for nearly one third of all U.S. families. What types of challenges do single-parent families face?**

SOURCE: © Phase4Photography/Fotolia.

Clinical Tip

It is important to establish which parent has legal custody, current visitation policies, and other variables (e.g., restraining orders and supervised visitation) when communicating information to parents about their children. Certain legal issues may prohibit the nurse from sharing some information with the noncustodial parent.

Family Development Frameworks

Family development theories use a framework to categorize a family's progression over time according to specific, typical stages in family life. These are predictable stages in the life cycle of every family, but they follow no rigid pattern. Duvall's (1977) eight stages in the family life cycle of a traditional nuclear family have been used as the foundation for contemporary models of

TABLE 2–1 Eight-Stage Family Life Cycle

STAGES	CHARACTERISTICS
Stage I	Beginning family, newly married couples*
Stage II	Childbearing family (oldest child is an infant through 30 months of age)
Stage III	Families with preschool children (oldest child is between 2.5 and 6 years of age)
Stage IV	Families with schoolchildren (oldest child is between 6 and 13 years of age)
Stage V	Families with teenagers (oldest child is between 13 and 20 years of age)
Stage VI	Families launching young adults (all children leave home)
Stage VII	Middle-aged parents (empty nest through retirement)
Stage VIII	Family in retirement and old age (retirement to death of both spouses)

*Keep in mind that this was the norm at the time the model was developed, but today families form through many different types of relationships.

Source: Adapted from Duvall, E. M. (1977). *Marriage and family development* (5th ed.). Philadelphia, PA: Lippincott; Duvall, E. M., & Miller, B. C. (1985). *Marriage and family development* (6th ed.). New York, NY: Harper Row; Coehlo, D. P. (2015). Family child health nursing. In J. R. Kaakinen, D. P. Coehlo, R. Steele, A. Tabacco, & S. M. H. Hanson, *Family health care nursing: Theory, practice, and research* (5th ed., pp. 387–432). Philadelphia, PA: F. A. Davis.

the family life cycle that describe the developmental processes and role expectations for different family types. Table 2–1 lists Duvall's eight stages to illustrate important developmental transitions that occur at some point in most families.

Other family development models have been developed to address the stages and developmental tasks facing the unattached young adult, the gay and lesbian family, those who divorce, and those who remarry. Textbooks on families and developmental psychology provide further information on this topic.

Family Assessment

The nurse's understanding of a family's structure helps provide insight into the family's support system and needs. A *family assessment* is a collection of data about the family's type and structure, current level of functioning, support system, sociocultural background, environment, and needs.

To obtain an accurate and concise family assessment, the nurse needs to establish a trusting relationship with the woman or child and the family. Data are best collected in a comfortable, private environment, free from interruptions.

Basic information should include the following:

- Name, age, sex, and family relationship of all people residing in the household
- Family type, structure, roles, and values
- Cultural associations, including cultural norms and customs related to childbearing, childrearing, and infant feeding
- Religious affiliations, including specific religious beliefs and practices related to childbearing
- Support network, including extended family, friends, and religious and community associations
- Communication patterns, including language barriers

The nurse also gathers information about the health of individual family members because health status can have a major impact on family functioning. When possible, it is helpful to have information about the family's home environment as well. In many cases, this information is gathered during client interviews. However, a home visit provides far more data about family relationships, roles, needs, and preparation for a new baby. See Chapter 37 for more information about family assessment.

Cultural Influences Affecting the Family

When caring for families, it is critical to consider the influence of culture, which may affect how a family responds to health-related issues. **Culture** has many definitions and is currently described as:

the combination of a body of knowledge, a body of belief and a body of behavior. It involves a number of elements, including personal identification, language, thoughts, communications, actions, customs, beliefs, values, and institutions that are often specific to ethnic, racial, religious, geographic, or social groups. (National Institutes of Health [NIH], 2013)

Culture is characterized by certain key elements, including the following:

- *Culture is based on shared values and beliefs.* Each culture identifies and articulates its shared values and beliefs. Expected behaviors and roles emerge that are consistent with those values and beliefs. A belief system suggests what preventive health measures and treatment for diseases are sought and accepted. It may also state the importance of children, of the family, of other individuals, and of the collective group, all of which can influence the choices people in the culture make regarding health.

- *Culture is learned and dynamic.* A child is born into a culture and starts learning the beliefs and practices of the group from birth. Children who are members of two cultural groups, such as African and immigrant, learn about both groups as they grow and develop. Immigrants have moved from one country to another to live and may face challenges when integrating the rules of the dominant culture. Children who have family members from two or more cultural groups integrate parts of the worldview from each group. Therefore, although culture is connected with groups, each individual's manifestation of his or her own cultural background will be unique. Culture evolves and adapts as new members are born into or join the group, and as the surrounding social and physical environments change. For example, as first-generation immigrants enter a new country, they generally closely follow the cultural patterns of their native lands. As their children grow, the youth maintain some of the family cultural patterns but begin to incorporate some of the new culture (Figure 2–2).

- *Culture is integrated into life and uses symbols.* Culture is integrated through social institutions such as schools, houses of worship, friendships, families, and occupations. This provides a variety of opportunities for learning about one's culture. The sense of integration may be disrupted or harder to maintain if individuals move frequently and as cultures intertwine with each other. Symbols are an important way that many cultures communicate with each other and with the outside world. Language, dress, music, tools, and nonverbal gestures are symbols a culture uses to display and transmit the culture.

Race refers to a group of people who share biologic similarities such as skin color, bone structure, and genetic traits. Examples of races include White (sometimes called Caucasian

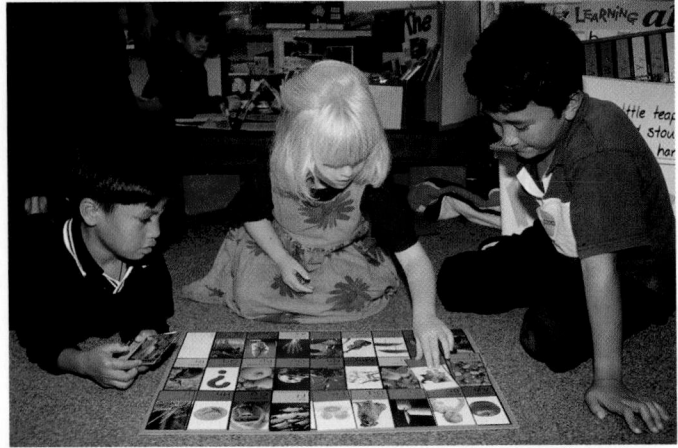

Figure 2–2 **Preschoolers from various cultural backgrounds play together. How can nurses partner with families to assist children to understand and respect cultural differences?**

or European American), Black (sometimes called African American in the United States), Hispanic, natives (such as Native Americans, Alaskan Native, Hawaiian Native, and First Nation people of Canada), and Asian.

Ethnicity describes a "cultural group's sense of identification associated with the group's common social and cultural heritage" (Spector, 2013, p. 357). Examples of ethnic groups include Hmong, Jews, and Irish Americans. Even the mainstream or majority of groups usually identify with an ethnic group. Some beliefs and practices are common among certain ethnic groups, but it is important to avoid **stereotyping** individuals; that is, assuming that all members of a group have the same characteristics. The nurse should assess the woman or child and family to see which characteristics common to a group are possessed by the client rather than assume that because individuals identify themselves as a specific ethnicity they must practice certain customs.

Acculturation refers to the process of modifying one's culture to fit within the new or dominant culture. **Assimilation** is related to acculturation and is described as adopting and incorporating traits of the new culture within one's practice (Spector, 2013). Acculturation frequently occurs when people leave their country of origin and immigrate to a new country. Often acculturation is associated with improved health status and health behaviors, especially if the immigration is associated with improved socioeconomic status, which leads to better nutrition and access to health care. This is frequently true for people who immigrate to the United States from a developing country. On the other hand, health sometimes declines with acculturation. For example, obesity is a problem that is growing rapidly within the United States and particularly among immigrant populations.

Family Roles and Structure

A family's organization and the roles played by individual family members are largely dependent on cultural influence. The family structure defines acceptable roles and behavior of family members. For example, culture may determine who has authority (head of household) and is the primary decision maker for other members of the family. Additionally, the role of decision maker may change according to specific decisions. In some cultures, decisions regarding the family's health care are primarily

the responsibility of the female family member, while other decisions are male dominated. Family dominance patterns may be *patriarchal*, as may be seen in Appalachian cultures; *matriarchal*, as may be seen in African American cultures; or more *egalitarian* (equal), as may be seen in European American cultures. Nurses need to be alert to the roles and functions in families since teaching may need to be directed to those responsible for decision making in order to promote health for all family members.

Culture also defines gender roles, the role of the elderly, and the role of the extended family. For example, Native Americans may consult tribal elders (considered part of the extended family) before agreeing to medical care for a pregnant woman or for a child. In some cultures, major decisions for the family, including a child's health care, include input from grandparents and other extended family members (Figure 2–3). Grandparents may even assume responsibility for care of the children in the family. In these cases, nurses must direct teaching for health promotion and demonstration for treatment procedures to the grandparent.

Family goals are also determined by cultural values and practices, as are family member roles and childbearing and childrearing practices and beliefs.

Health Beliefs, Approaches, and Practices

Three views of health described by Andrews and Boyle (2012) are magico-religious, scientific, and holistic. In reality, many people ascribe to a view that combines more than one of these belief systems, but it is helpful to examine them separately.

In the *magico-religious belief paradigm*, health and illness are determined by supernatural forces such as God, gods, magic, spirits, or fate. A miscarriage, for example, or the illness of a pregnant woman or of a child may be perceived as a punishment for actions. Children of preschool age and early school age usually have this view of illness; some adults also believe that higher or supernatural powers determine health and illness. It is wise to ask both children and their families what they think caused an illness or how they believe they can stay well. People who believe in this paradigm may gain comfort from prayer, healing rituals,

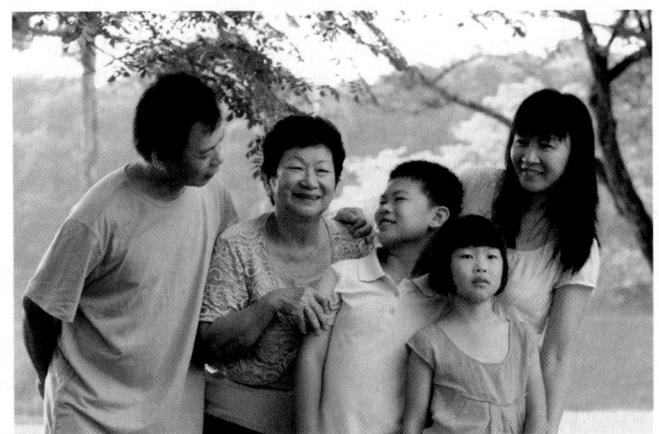

Figure 2–3 **Many cultures value the input of grandparents and other elders in the family or group. In this multigenerational family, the grandmother's guidance is highly valued and significantly influences the family's childrearing practices.**

SOURCE: Wong yu liang/Fotolia.

and faith healing. Young children who, because of their developmental level, believe that they have caused their own illness can be expressly told that it was not something they did that caused the illness. This may help decrease their feelings of guilt.

The *scientific* or *biomedical health paradigm* assumes that physiology explains all illness and life itself (Andrews & Boyle, 2012). Biochemical reactions and the genomic code are used to explain all health states. Illness is always caused by viruses, bacteria, or damage to the body in this framework. This approach is often called "Western medicine." Families who hold this view expect a traditional Western medical intervention, such as medication, treatment, or surgery, to treat the specific health problem. Within this belief system, it is very difficult to understand certain health conditions. Families may struggle to "explain" an illness by wondering if the child was exposed to something harmful during fetal life or exposed to something in the environment. A reason for the condition is needed to understand it.

Most physicians, nurses, and other healthcare professionals adhere primarily to the biomedical or scientific theories to explain and treat illnesses. However, certain therapies such as therapeutic touch, biofeedback, and other nontraditional methods that are more common in a holistic health paradigm are gaining popularity within these professions. For the family with this belief system, health professionals sometimes need to emphasize that certain conditions have no known cause, and should suggest treatments other than traditional Western medicine if other approaches may be helpful.

Balance and harmony of the body and nature are important concepts in the *holistic health belief*. It is believed that illness results when the natural balance or harmony is disturbed. Infections and other illnesses gain entry into the body when it is not in balance. This health belief is most common in North American Indian and Asian cultures (Andrews & Boyle, 2012). Increasingly the ideas of holism are being integrated into Western health care and combined with other approaches. An example of integration of approaches is use of a medication or radiation for illness in combination with adequate rest and a diet that is designed to increase immune function.

An associated holistic health belief is the hot and cold theory of disease, which subscribes to the thought that illnesses and diseases are a result of disruption in the hot and cold balance of the body. Therefore, consuming foods of the opposite variety can cure or prevent specific hot and cold illnesses. Hot and cold therapies related to healing are practiced in some African American, Asian, Latino, Arab, Muslim, and Caribbean cultures (Andrews & Boyle, 2012) (see Table 2–2).

Healthcare Practitioners

The family seeking care for the child may choose one or a combination of magico-religious, holistic, or biomedical healthcare providers. The use of *folk healers* varies according to the culture. Although the healer's role and position in the community differ among cultures, healers do share commonalities. Healers speak the language of the cultural group, use common methods of communication for the culture, and live in the same community.

Mexican Americans may seek healing by a *curandero* (male healer) or *curandera* (female healer), who is a holistic

TABLE 2–2 Hot and Cold Conditions and Foods

HOT CONDITIONS	COLD FOODS USED TO TREAT HOT CONDITIONS	COLD CONDITIONS	HOT FOODS USED TO TREAT COLD CONDITIONS
Diarrhea	Barley water	Cancer	Beef
Fever	Chicken	Earaches	Cheese
Constipation	Dairy products	Headaches	Eggs
Infection	Raisins	Musculoskeletal conditions	Grains (other than barley)
Kidney problems	Fish	Pneumonia	Liquor
Liver conditions	Cucumber	Menstrual cramps	Pork
Sore throats	Fresh fruits	Malaria	Onions
Stomach ulcers	Fresh vegetables	Arthritis	Spicy foods
	Goat meat	Rhinitis	Chocolate
		Colic	Warm water with honey

Source: Data from Purnell, L. D. (2014). *Guide to culturally competent health care* (3rd ed.). Philadelphia, PA: F. A. Davis; Purnell, L. D. (2013). *Transcultural health care: A culturally competent approach* (4th ed.). Philadelphia, PA: F. A. Davis; Spector, R. E. (2013). *Cultural diversity in health and illness* (8th ed.). Upper Saddle River, NJ: Pearson.

healer who deals with physical, psychologic, and social problems (Spector, 2013). The curandero/a's holistic treatment may include use of herbs, laying on of hands, massaging the afflicted area, cleansing the body with herbs, preparing an amulet to be worn, burning a candle with a specific prayer printed on the candle jar, or calling the spirit of a saint to bless the individual. Essential to the curandero/a and the family is the faith the family has in his or her abilities. Families may combine *curanderismo* (Hispanic medical system) with a Western approach for some conditions. For example, a child with seizures may be given medications for the disorder obtained from Western care and may be fed a tea that the healer believes will treat the condition.

Puerto Ricans may use an *espiritistas*, a healer who communicates with spirits for the physical and emotional development of the client. Mexican Americans may use this type of healer when the ailment is thought to be caused by witchcraft. However, use of an *espiritistas* is frowned on in some Hispanic cultures (Purnell, 2014). A *sobador* is an individual who uses massage and manipulation to treat clients with joint and muscle problems, and is another type of healer who might be used by Mexican Americans (Zoucha & Zamarripa, 2013).

African Americans often combine Western and traditional beliefs about illness. Some believe in spirits as causes of illness and may use powders, oils, and ceremonies to maintain health.

Native Americans may seek healing from a **shaman**, "a woman or man who enters an altered state of consciousness, at will, to contact and utilize another type of reality to acquire knowledge and power and to help other people" (Fontaine, 2015, p. 341). Because Native Americans generally believe in the balance of nature and a state of harmony, they seek advice to identify what they have done to disrupt their body harmony. The healer will then prescribe the required treatment for restoration of balance and harmony. Teas, other herbal products, sweats, smudges, meditation, and other approaches are common. Returning to one's family, home, and roots may produce a sense of balance.

Impact of Religion and Spirituality

The terms *religion* and *spirituality* mean different things to different people. Many people view religion, which is sometimes termed *faith-based belief*, as an organized system that shares a common set of beliefs and practices about the significance, cause, and purpose of life and the universe. Religion is usually centered on the belief in or worshipping of a supernatural being or Supreme Being (such as God or Allah). **Spirituality** refers to the individual's experience and own interpretation of his or her relationship with a Supreme Being. Children are spiritual beings and generally express their spirituality through behavior such as imaginative play, art, dance, and song (Lascar, 2013). Prayer, one of the most common expressions of religious faith, is a frequently used therapy in which many children and families engage (Lambert, Fincham, & Graham, 2011; Wachholtz & Sambamoorthi, 2011).

A family's religious beliefs, affiliation, and practices can deeply influence their experiences and attitudes toward health care, childbearing, and childrearing. Members of certain religious groups such as Christian Scientists may attempt to avoid all medical interventions, whereas others such as Jehovah's Witnesses may refuse specific interventions, such as blood transfusions. Roman Catholics may refuse contraception. In most cases, families gain comfort from acknowledgment of and respect for their religious beliefs and practices in the healthcare setting. However, the agnostic (one who has doubts about the existence of a transcendent being) or the atheist (one who believes that there is no higher power) may be offended if care providers assume that references to God or to a higher power will be comforting.

A religious or spiritual history is often completed when a woman is admitted to a clinic or labor setting or when a child is admitted to the hospital. The assessment can include questions about current spiritual beliefs and practices and preferences for religious rituals. Whenever possible the nurse should attempt to accommodate religious rituals and practices requested by the family.

Considering the diversity of religious beliefs, it is not unusual for nurses to encounter childbearing families whose beliefs conflict with their own. This is not problematic as long as the nurse avoids attempts to influence the family's decision making. For example, a nurse who does not believe in baptism should avoid revealing this to a Catholic seeking baptism for her stillborn newborn. Nurses should also examine their religious beliefs related to genetic screening procedures, use of assisted reproductive technology to achieve pregnancy, abortion, use of technology to support life in a severely compromised newborn or a terminally ill child, and even less dramatic issues such as methods of contraception, circumcision, infant feeding, and disciplinary practices for children.

Although spirituality and faith-based belief are generally positive in supporting families to maintain and restore health, at times they can have potentially negative effects for children. Certain groups may blame individuals for their own illnesses, and children may develop guilt as a result. Abuse may result from parental religious beliefs about corporal punishment and discipline. If a religious group denies lifesaving treatments, courts may intervene to ensure care for the child.

Although adherence to a religious tradition is predominant in the United States, it should not be assumed that all individuals believe in or practice organized religion. Approximately 20% of Americans do not identify with any religious group or consider themselves followers of any specific religion (Pew Research Center, 2012). The nurse should always ask the family if they follow a faith tradition and if they would like a leader from that faith to visit when in the hospital (Figure 2–4).

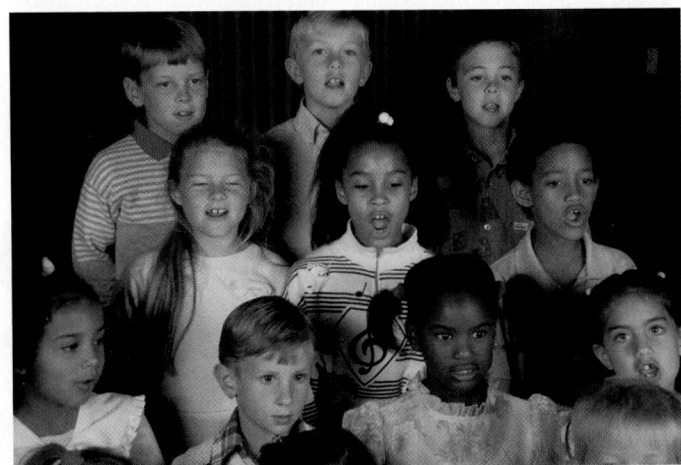

Figure 2–4 Today, very few communities are limited to one culture. The children in this multicultural choir are representative of the changes in demographics of many Western countries. Even though they may differ in cultural background, a common thread is found in their religious preference.

SOURCE: Myrleen Ferguson/PhotoEdit.

Adolescents may follow different faith traditions than their parents and should be asked the question individually.

Collaboration between the healthcare team and family is essential to providing care congruent with the child's and family's expectations. Although spirituality is important for many families, it is often overlooked as a healing strategy. Illness and injury may cause the family to turn to spiritual guidance as a method of understanding and coping. Assessment of the family's and child's spiritual needs is an important aspect of nursing care. The nurse must respect the family's view and avoid being judgmental about their beliefs. Partnering with the child and family to incorporate their traditional practices and beliefs with prescribed therapies will help to ensure the delivery of safe and effective care for the child.

In many institutions, nurses can ask to be reassigned to a different client if their religious beliefs are in conflict because of health care being provided or refused by the client and family. However, if other personnel are not available, it is the nurse's responsibility to provide sensitive, appropriate, and nonjudgmental care to that client.

Childbearing Practices

Children are generally valued all over the world, not only for the joy they bring, but also because they ensure continuation of the family and cultural values. This valuing of children may manifest itself in different ways. Families in the United States and many Western countries commonly have only one or two children out of a desire to provide the children with the best home and education they can afford and to spend as much free time with them as possible. In contrast, in many cultures throughout the world, it is common to have as many children as possible.

In some cultures a woman who gives birth achieves a higher status, especially if the child is male. This is especially true in the traditional Chinese culture and in some Middle Eastern cultures (Bulte, Heerink, & Zhang, 2011). Similarly, in the western United States, people of the Mormon faith view motherhood as the primary responsibility of a woman's life, comparable with the male role of priesthood (Chen, 2014). In Mexican American society and among many other Latino groups, having children is evidence of the male's virility and is a sign of manliness or *machismo*, a desired trait.

Culture may also influence attitudes and beliefs about contraception. For example, a study in India revealed that while some Muslims may use birth control, they do not believe in sterilization because it is a permanent method (Algur, Kazi, & Yadavannavar, 2013). Other Muslims might not practice contraception because children are highly valued, and it is believed that the traditional role of women is to bear children. In Chinese society, on the other hand, where government policy limits the number of children a couple can have, contraception is common.

Health values and beliefs are also important in understanding reactions and behavior. Certain behaviors can be expected if a culture views pregnancy as a sickness, whereas other behaviors can be expected if the culture views pregnancy as a natural occurrence. For example, because Native Americans, African Americans, and Mexican Americans generally view pregnancy as a natural and desirable condition, prenatal care may not be a priority. In other cultures, pregnancy may be seen as a time of increased vulnerability. In Orthodox Judaism, for example, it is a man's responsibility to procreate, but it is a woman's right, not her obligation, to do so. This is because, according to Orthodox Jewish law, the health of the mother, both physically and mentally, is of primary concern, and she should never be obliged to do something that threatens her life.

Individuals of many cultures take certain protective precautions based on their beliefs. For example, many Southeast Asian women fear that they will have a complicated labor and birth if they sit in a doorway or on a step. Thus, they tend to avoid areas near doors in waiting rooms and examining rooms. In the Mexican American culture, the belief is common that *mal aire,* or bad air, may enter the body and cause harm. Preventive measures, such as keeping the windows closed or covering the head, are used. Some Latinos may place a raisin on the cord stump of a newborn to prevent drafts from entering their bodies.

A **taboo** is a behavior or thing that is to be avoided. Many cultures, including those found in the United States, have taboos centered on the unborn baby or newborn that are meant to ensure that the baby will survive. For example, it is common among Muslims to avoid naming the baby until after birth; similarly, many Orthodox Jewish women wait to set up the nursery until after the baby is born.

In developing countries, mortality rates among infants and young children are extremely high; thus certain traditions focus on protecting the baby from evil spirits. For example, many Muslim parents will pin an amulet such as a blue stone or a verse from the Qur'an to the newborn's clothing as protection. Following birth, it is common for a male family member to whisper prayers in the newborn baby's ear to declare faith and protect the baby (Algur et al., 2013).

Childrearing Practices

In some families, children are expected to take on responsibilities early and may be expected to take on tasks such as management of their own chronic disease and nutritional intake. In other families, children are given long periods to grow up and are not expected to manage healthcare needs. Directing teaching to a child with diabetes in the latter family type may not be appropriate. Nurses often provide information and ask about developmental milestones for children; however, there may be variations in family goals and it is not unusual for children to accomplish various tasks at younger or older ages. For example, it is commonly expected that children are weaned by 1 year of age and toilet trained at about 2 years of age, but this is not always the case. The nurse should ask about the norms in the family and whether the child is developing according to the parents' expectations. As long as the child is progressing in motor, language, and social tasks, some variation is expected due to cultural norms.

Views about alternative lifestyles such as sexual orientation and single parenting are also established by the family's values and beliefs. Understanding such values assists the nurse in providing sensitive care. Examples of childrearing practices common to particular cultures are listed in Table 2–3. Realize that the practices listed are common in these cultures, but not necessarily practiced by all members of that culture.

Culture and Nursing Care

Healthcare providers are often unaware of the cultural characteristics they themselves demonstrate. Without cultural awareness, caregivers tend to project their own cultural responses onto foreign-born clients; clients from different socioeconomic, religious, or educational groups; or clients from different regions of the country. This projection leads care providers to assume that the clients are demonstrating a specific behavior for the same reason that they themselves would. Moreover, healthcare providers often fail to realize that medicine has its own culture, which has been dominated historically by traditional middle-class values and beliefs.

TABLE 2-3 Childrearing Practices of Selected Cultures

CULTURE	CHILDREARING PRACTICES
African American	Grandmothers play an important role in the care of children.
	Children are expected to demonstrate respectfulness, conformity to rules, obedience, and good behavior.
	Extended family is very important.
Amish	The family contains, on average, seven children.
	Childrearing is regarded as the highest priority for parents.
	Grandparents often provide care to children.
	Children are expected to continue with the Amish tradition.
	Children are expected to follow the rules as prescribed by the church district.
Appalachian	Large families are common.
	Strict parenting practices and physical punishment are common.
	Grandparents frequently provide care to children.
Arab American	The father is typically the disciplinarian.
	The child's character is considered a reflection of the family's influence.
	Children are expected to respect their elders and to have good behavior.
	Adolescents are expected to do well in their studies.
	Discipline may include physical punishment and shaming.
Chinese American	The family may lavish resources on child.
	Children typically depend on family for all needs and may not be expected to earn their own money as adolescents.
	Male children are often more valued than female children.
	Children may be taught to avoid displaying their emotions/feelings.
	Children are expected to assist parents in the home (chores).
	High educational achievement is expected.
Mexican American	Children are closely protected and are not encouraged to leave the home.
	Extended family members frequently live close by.
	Children are expected to demonstrate respect for parents and elderly family members.
	Discipline may include physical punishment.
	Education is a priority.
Navajo Indian	Grandmothers are important decision makers in the family.
	Infants may be kept in a cradleboard to protect them.
	Children are allowed to make decisions about their care.

Source: Data from Purnell, L. D. (2013). *Transcultural health care: A culturally competent approach* (4th ed.). Philadelphia, PA: F. A. Davis; Purnell, L. D. (2014). *Guide to culturally competent health care* (3rd ed.). Philadelphia, PA: F. A. Davis.

Ethnocentrism is the conviction that the values and beliefs of one's own cultural group are the best or only acceptable ones. It is characterized by an inability to understand the beliefs and worldview of another culture. To a certain extent, everyone is guilty of ethnocentrism, at least some of the time. Thus, the nurse who values stoicism during labor may be uncomfortable with the more vocal response of some Latin American women. Another nurse may be disconcerted by a Southeast Asian woman who believes that pain is something to be endured rather than alleviated and who is intent on maintaining self-control in labor.

Healthcare providers sometimes believe that if members of other cultures do not share Western values and beliefs, they should adopt them. For example, a nurse who believes strongly in equality of the sexes may find it difficult to remain silent if a woman from a Middle Eastern culture defers to her husband in decision making. It is important to remember that pressure to defy cultural values and beliefs can be stressful and anxiety provoking for these women.

Developing Cultural Competence Culture Shock

The experience that people have in attempting to understand or adapt to a culture that is fundamentally different from their own culture is known as *culture shock*. The person may experience feelings of discomfort, powerlessness, anxiety, and disorientation. Immigrants to the United States may experience culture shock when differences or conflicts arise between their own values, beliefs, and customs and the ways of their new surroundings. The nurse should assess childbearing women, children, and their families who have recently immigrated for indications of culture shock. Referring the family to counseling or support from representatives of the family's culture, such as a translator or community group, may be helpful.

To address issues of cultural diversity in the provision of health care, emphasis is being placed on developing **cultural competence**—that is, the ability to understand and effectively respond to the needs of individuals and families from different cultural backgrounds. "Cultural competence is a complex combination of knowledge, attitudes, and skills" (Spector, 2013, p. 356). It involves identifying and integrating the family's health beliefs, practices, and cultural and linguistic needs into client care (National Institutes of Health, 2013).

Culturally Influenced Responses

The nurse can begin developing cultural competence by becoming knowledgeable about the cultural differences and practices of various groups. Nurses who are knowledgeable about differences and who take them into account in planning and providing nursing care will be far more effective caregivers than those who do not.

BIOLOGIC DIFFERENCES

Genetic and physical differences occur among cultural groups and can lead to disparity in needs and care. Differences include blood type, body build, skin color, drug metabolism, and susceptibility to certain diseases. Other disparities occur because of fundamental differences between genders, ages, and races. For example, male children are more likely to manifest pyloric stenosis and attention deficit disorder, whereas female children more often have congenital hip dysplasia and systemic lupus erythematosus. Age provides another biologic variation, as infants are more likely to manifest the cancer neuroblastoma, whereas adolescents have a higher incidence of Hodgkin disease. Race is also connected with certain disease processes. Sickle cell disease occurs predominantly in African Americans. African Americans also have a higher incidence of hypertension. American Indians have the highest incidence of diabetes by percentage of population in the United States. However, type 1 diabetes is more common in Whites, whereas type 2 diabetes has a higher incidence in Hispanics and American Indians. Thalassemia, another type of anemia, is most common in Mediterranean people. Lactose intolerance is common in Mexican Americans, African Americans, American Indians, and Asians (Giger, 2013).

Nurses need to understand other genetic characteristics in order to perform culturally competent nursing assessments and interventions. Differences in skin color and tone may make cyanosis, pallor, and jaundice difficult to recognize and describe. Mongolian spots are darkened skin on the lower back and buttocks of some babies with dark skin tones. Variations in texture of hair require different approaches to hygiene among various racial groups.

COMMUNICATION PATTERNS

Communication is the method by which members of cultural groups share information and preserve their beliefs, values, norms, and practices. To ensure effective care, it is essential for families to be able to communicate with nurses and other healthcare providers. This becomes an issue when the family does not speak the language of the health professionals. In such cases, it is best if the healthcare facility provides translators. Children are most likely to speak both the language of the parents and the healthcare providers and may appear to be likely interpreters. However, it is recommended that children never be used to interpret in healthcare situations due to the confidentiality needs of both parent and child. Additionally, if children are used as interpreters, it can create an imbalance in power that could adversely affect parental authority. Signs, posted literature, and brochures should also be available in the languages of the children and families served. Even when children speak the language of the healthcare providers, written material must be provided at a level that the family can read and understand.

Language can also affect health literacy skills because a large number of instructions are given in writing, including prescriptions and directions on medication bottles, signs hanging in health facilities, consent forms for procedures and surgery, insurance forms, directions for techniques or procedures, future appointment dates, and health promotion materials. Nurses need to verify what the client and family can read and whether alternative ways of providing the information are needed. For example, nurses could verbally give the information and provide paper and pencil so that the family can take notes in their own language. Translation services should be available in all healthcare settings.

Variations in communication among cultures are reflected in their word meaning, voice inflection and quality, and verbal styles. Culture not only influences the manner in which feelings are expressed, but also which verbal and nonverbal expressions of communication are considered appropriate. An individual's willingness to discuss certain topics or to express or conceal certain thoughts and feelings is also influenced by cultural norms. Some groups may be expected to remain quiet when experiencing pain, while other cultures may loudly and dramatically express pain.

Clinical Tip

Speaking and reading may not occur in the same language. For example, an immigrant may read and speak fluently in his or her primary language and speak but not read the language of the new country. The immigrant's child may read and speak the language of the present country and speak but not read the native language of the family. Always ask about both reading and speaking preferences.

Use of first names and surnames varies among cultural groups, so nurses should not make assumptions, because the use of a person's first name may be considered disrespectful. Address family members respectfully, usually using terms such as Mr., Mrs., and Ms. If the person has a title such as doctor, judge, or senator, it should be used. The nurse should ask what the person prefers to be called and record this in the health record for future reference. In some cultures such as Korean, Cambodian, and Filipino, the first name used is actually the family name. Asking for the "family name" rather than the "last name" may clarify this practice.

Nonverbal Communication. Nonverbal communication refers to body language such as posture, gestures, facial expressions, eye contact, and touch, as well as the use of silence. The nurse's use of nonverbal communication may hinder or help communication. Gestures and body language may be misunderstood or misinterpreted. Eye contact has different meanings among cultures. European Americans, for example, value eye contact with communication and interpret this as a sign of sincerity and interest. In other cultures, such as Asian and Native American, sustained eye contact may be considered rude or disrespectful. Some African Americans may misinterpret direct eye contact as aggressive behavior (Purnell, 2013, 2014).

Silence is considered a sign of respect in some cultures. Among those groups, offering an immediate response to a question may be viewed as being disrespectful since an instant reply could indicate that no thought was given to the matter. Nurses should watch for patterns in various cultures and alter their approach to be more congruent. For example, many nurses commonly nod and say "yes" or "oh, I see" when a client is speaking. This may seem disruptive to some cultures. If the listener is silent and does not use such patterns of agreement, the nurse should alter his or her response to match more closely the acceptable method of communication for the family.

Touch. The appropriateness of touch varies with each culture. For example, an Asian may consider touching an unfamiliar person of the opposite gender to be inappropriate, whereas touch between men and women may be viewed as appropriate by another culture. Adults commonly feel that it is acceptable to touch children of all ages, but this may not be accurate. It is best to look for responses from the family to touch and progress accordingly.

Space. An individual's sense of personal space also differs by culture. Space refers to the physical distance and relationships between the individual and other persons and objects in the environment. Cultures may have specific spatial preferences, such as personal distance and social distance. Some cultures tend to prefer close contact with less space since they use touch as a form of communication. The nurse should be alert for how close a child-bearing woman or a child comes to other individuals and try to maintain this space during interactions. Nursing procedures often cause the space barrier to be broken. Nurses need to touch clients to take vital signs, administer injections, change dressings, and the like. This does not mean that close touch is appropriate at all times. It is essential to tell all clients before touching them for procedures so they understand what is happening.

TIME ORIENTATION

Cultures have specific values and meanings regarding time orientation. Cultural groups may place emphasis on the events of the past, those events that occur in the present, or those events that will occur in the future. Children reflect the time orientation of their families and the cultures in which they live. Time is also influenced by development, so that young children sometimes do not understand the use of clocks, the importance ascribed to being "on time," or other time orientations.

Cultures that are oriented predominantly to the past may want to begin healthcare encounters with lengthy descriptions of past healthcare treatments, family history of diseases, or individual past experiences with health. There may be little interest in learning methods of adapting to or maintaining a new plan of care.

For cultures that are oriented predominantly to the present, little consideration may be given to either the past or the future. For example, adolescents commonly focus on the present, and may not engage in preventive health practices for long-term health. Therefore, short-term goals often provide more incentive to adolescents.

Cultures that are oriented predominantly to the future may not focus on what is important at the present time. For example, the family may focus on the dreams they had for a child's education or sports performance and have trouble setting present goals for treatment of a disease such as juvenile arthritis. One commonly hears that it was a big adjustment to learn to "take one day at a time." Not living up to the family's expectation for their future success may be difficult for a child who has developed an illness that has a chronic course.

Time also refers to punctuality about schedules and appointments. In the United States, the predominant culture respects being on time and considers time valuable and not to be wasted. Other cultures may not emphasize a concern for time. This may be manifested by a family's inability to follow timed medication schedules or treatments or to show up as scheduled for an appointment. In these cases, it is not intended as a sign of disrespect.

NUTRITION

Nutritional practices begin even before birth, as many cultural groups have beliefs that determine foods that are healthy to eat or should be avoided during pregnancy. Nutritional habits and patterns vary among cultures and are related to both religious practices and health beliefs. Certain cultures and religions have restrictions related to specific foods and preparation methods.

Ritualistic behaviors involving eating and drinking, for example, on special occasions and holidays, are observed by most cultures. Many religions recommend fasts during specific holy seasons, such as Lent for Roman Catholics, Yom Kippur for Jews, and Ramadan for Muslims; however, in most cases, small children, pregnant women, older adults, and sick individuals are not required to fast.

Additionally, some cultures value large size or may associate a healthy child with being "large." Other cultures value slimness and look down on individuals who are obese. Both of these views influence family eating patterns and expectations for the child; the child's self-esteem can therefore be influenced. The U.S. culture honors being slim in the media but reinforces eating and large size by the availability of fast food and positive image of large sports stars such as some football players, which can result in confusion about health and body image.

Nutrition may also be essential to the culture's practices for health promotion and care during illness. Health problems associated with specific cultures that may require dietary changes are also identified. Nutrition can be closely related to environmental situations, and families with few resources may not be able to obtain or eat cultural foods because of lack of access or financial issues. Nutrition plays a powerful role in maintaining health, so resources for nutritious and desired foods may be needed.

Nursing Management

The focus of nursing care is assessment of cultural influences on the client's health. The nurse providing culturally competent care to the woman or child and family considers all facets of their culture. Identification of cultural influences as well as cultural barriers will enable the nurse to provide culturally competent nursing care and management. See *Evidence-Based Practice: Investigating Culture and Healthcare Barriers*.

Nursing Assessment

Assessment of the woman or child and family includes determining the family's cultural healthcare beliefs and practices. Questions may include the following:

- Who in the family must be consulted before decisions are made about a person's care?
- Does the client, or do the parents of a child, see primarily in the present or do they have a futuristic time orientation?
- What type of health provider is most appropriate for (or preferred by) the woman, the child, or the family?
- Does the family have beliefs or traditions that may affect the plan of care?

Several cultural assessment tools (including self-assessment tools) are available to assist nurses in gathering this information as well as information about their own cultural competencies. These tools are becoming increasingly common at healthcare

---

Professionalism in Practice **Standards of Practice for Culturally Competent Nursing**

Standards of Practice for Culturally Competent Nursing were developed to guide nursing practice. These standards focus on clinical practice, education, administration, and research. Emphasis is placed on the importance of providing culturally competent care to all clients and families (Douglas et al., 2011). Identify and learn more about the cultures in the community where you practice nursing care so that you can provide culturally competent care to your clients.

EVIDENCE-BASED PRACTICE | Investigating Culture and Healthcare Barriers

Clinical Question
What barriers to providing accessible health care exist among ethnically diverse families with children?

The Evidence
Ferayorni, Sinha, and McDonald (2011) examined demographic characteristics, socioeconomic status, access to care, perceived barriers to care, compliance with follow-up care, and unmet health needs in foreign-born children who visited a pediatric emergency department. Parents of 385 children were interviewed during a visit to the emergency department and by telephone 1 week after the visit. Twenty-three percent of these children did not have health insurance. Compared to children with health insurance, those who did not have coverage were less likely to have a regular healthcare provider and a regular place for health and dental care. Parents of 31% of uninsured children cited a perceived barrier to care. Barriers reported most often were language, lack of insurance and inability to pay, and transportation. Parents of 26 children reported unmet healthcare needs, with a slightly higher prevalence among uninsured children as opposed to insured children. Dental care was the most commonly reported unmet healthcare need. Uninsured children who were foreign born were primarily Spanish speaking, poorer, and had poor access to health care. This population was also more likely to use the emergency department for its healthcare needs.

Adorador, McNulty, Hart, et al. (2011) examined perceived barriers to immunizations in 108 Latino mothers of children in a low-income clinic. Results of the immunization survey revealed that 92% of mothers thought their children were up-to-date on their immunizations, when health records indicated that only 42% were up-to-date. Barriers to immunizations identified by these mothers included the child being sick, transportation issues, no health insurance, affordability, language concerns, and child care issues.

Taylor, Nicolle, and Maguire (2013) conducted interviews with 38 healthcare professionals to determine their perceptions of the barriers that ethnic minorities who spoke poor or no English encountered when seeking health care. Five key themes emerged from the interviews: language; low literacy; retention of information; lack of understanding; and attitudes, gender attitudes, and health beliefs.

Best Practice
Socioeconomic status is a theme in two of these studies. These families may not have health insurance, a regular healthcare provider, or adequate transportation. Nurses need to refer families to sources for healthcare services and then follow up to be sure the families were able to access care. Referrals to community health centers and instructions for transportation to the health setting are important for many families. A need for understandable information is another theme among most groups. Explaining why an immunization is needed as well as providing information about the child's condition are important nursing roles. Interpreters may be needed to provide this information. Referring the family to others from the same ethnic or racial group and assisting them in navigating complex systems such as school and social services may also be necessary. Cultural differences and practices were also cited as a barrier to health care. It is essential that healthcare providers become familiar with other cultures and be accepting of practices that are safe for the child. By being open to practices of other cultures, healthcare providers will find families more willing to share openly about how they treat their children. This may lead to an opportunity for education related to unsafe practices.

Clinical Reasoning
What is the process that immigrant families in your state or province must follow to secure health care for their children? How would you help to guide someone through this process? What cultural groups are common in your community? Do you speak their language? If not, what measures should you take to ensure that they understand the teaching offered in clinical settings? What type of support groups will be helpful for families when they have a child with special healthcare needs?

---

agencies as providers act in response to the expectation of culturally competent care. The nurse who respects cultural diversity is an asset to the childbearing and childrearing family as they adjust to their new role. Establishing a trusting relationship enables the nurse to assist the family in meeting educational needs.

The use of North American Nursing Diagnosis Association (NANDA) nursing diagnoses to describe situations specifically related to culture may in itself be culturally biased because the foci of these diagnoses are based on Western cultural beliefs. Diagnoses such as *Communication: Verbal, Impaired* or *Knowledge, Deficient* should not be used solely because a person does not speak English. Is someone who speaks a different language "impaired" in communication?

Specific nursing diagnoses are dependent on the reason the family seeks contact with healthcare professionals, ranging from a pregnancy to a child's health promotion and health maintenance (e.g., immunizations) to the care of a child with a chronic or terminal illness. Examples include the following (NANDA-I © 2014):

- *Health Management, Family, Ineffective,* related to mistrust of healthcare personnel

- *Fear* related to separation from support system in stressful situation such as hospitalization

- *Spiritual Distress* related to discrepancy between spiritual beliefs and prescribed treatment

- *Family Processes, Interrupted,* related to a shift in family roles due to illness

The planning and implementation of nursing care for the culturally diverse family depend specifically on the findings of the previous assessments. Nurses need to partner with the family to establish a safe, effective, and desirable plan of care. Nurses can ensure access to an interpreter if needed and evaluate whether the match with a particular interpreter is appropriate for the child and family.

Recognizing the influence of culture on one's beliefs, values, and healthcare practices is essential for the nurse to deliver culturally competent care. Nurses demonstrate appropriate strategies for delivering culturally sensitive care when they develop techniques in assessing the influence of culture on the pregnant woman or the child and family and incorporate that information into an individualized plan of care.

Culturally competent nurses find effective ways to partner with the family to assist them in determining how they can incorporate prescribed therapies with their healthcare practices. Ensure that the woman herself or the child and family understand the problem or illness, treatment, and health-promotion activities. Apply culturally sensitive techniques when dispelling any cultural myths.

Nurses can also collaborate with a multidisciplinary team, including social workers and language specialists, to assist the family in receiving assistance with barriers to care such as transportation, financial issues, remote access, and others.

Complementary and Alternative Therapies and the Family

Through most of the 20th century in the United States, it was rare for European American childbearing families to consult anyone except their obstetrician for advice about their pregnancy, birth, and postpartum period. Similarly, most childrearing families closely followed the advice of their pediatrician about all aspects of child care. Although such clients are still encountered today, nurses are more likely to care for families who integrate other types of practitioners and therapies with traditional Western medicine.

Although the terms *complementary* and *alternative* are often used interchangeably, they have different meanings and applications. A **complementary therapy** may be defined as any procedure or product that is used as an adjunct to conventional medical treatment (Mitchell, 2013; National Center for Complementary and Alternative Medicine [NCCAM], 2013). Although complementary therapies were not available in clinics and hospitals until the past few decades, therapies such as acupuncture, acupressure, and massage therapy are now often used with conventional medical care, and many health insurance plans cover at least a portion of the cost of such therapies.

In contrast, an **alternative therapy** is usually considered a substance or procedure that is used in place of conventional medicine (NCCAM, 2013). It usually has not undergone rigorous scientific testing in this country, although it might have been thoroughly tested in other countries. Alternative therapies are not usually available in conventional clinics and hospitals, and their costs are not typically covered under most health insurance policies. An example of an alternative therapy is the use of herbal medicines instead of biomedicines for the treatment of a child's health condition. In other words, the child would not receive traditional Western medical care for the condition, such as surgery, radiation, prescribed medications, or other medical interventions.

The dramatic increase in complementary and alternative therapies that began in the final decade of the 20th century was probably the result of a combination of several factors:

- Increased consumer awareness of the limitations of conventional Western medicine
- Increased international travel
- Increased media attention
- Advent of the Internet

In this century, it seems clear that Western health care will see an ever-increasing integration between conventional medicine and complementary therapies. Some obvious examples of this new integration in perinatal settings include the acceptance of certain herbal teas for antepartum discomforts; the use of massage, Reiki, or therapeutic touch during the first stage of labor; music during childbirth; and the increased emphasis on skin-to-skin mother-to-baby bonding in the immediate postpartum period.

Further evidence of this increased integration is the establishment in 1992 of the Office of Alternative Medicine (OAM) at the National Institutes of Health. The OAM was mandated by Congress to promote research into complementary and alternative therapies and dissemination of information to consumers. In 1998, the OAM was incorporated into a new National Center for Complementary and Alternative Medicine (NCCAM) with an expanded mission and increased funding. Many studies of complementary and alternative therapies are currently under way at NCCAM.

Benefits and Risks

Complementary and alternative therapies have many benefits for women and children. Many complementary and alternative therapies emphasize prevention and wellness, and place a higher value on holistic healing than on physical cure.

SAFETY ALERT!
Complementary and alternative therapies must be assessed for safety, including positive and negative benefits, cost, efficacy, and clinical usefulness. The use of herbs and natural products raises many issues, of which these are just a few: standards of products, misleading claims, and safety related to megadoses of some products.

Determine the family's use of complementary and/or alternative therapies such as the type of remedies and healthcare practices used. Also determine the side effects, risks, and other implications to the child receiving this type of therapy. Work with the family to ensure safe practices with the use of complementary and/or alternative therapies.

Types of Complementary and Alternative Therapies

Numerous forms of complementary and alternative therapies are available. Only a few of the most commonly used approaches are presented here.

HOMEOPATHY
Homeopathy is a healing approach in which a sick person is treated with small doses of medicines that would cause illness when given to someone who is healthy. Traditional Western (or allopathic) medicine generally gives medicine or treatments that suppress symptoms. Analgesics for pain or antibiotics for infection are examples of such treatments. In homeopathy, the symptoms are viewed as the body's method of healing, and small doses of medications are given to enhance the symptoms (Fontaine, 2015; Spector, 2013).

NATUROPATHY
Naturopathy is a form of medicine that utilizes the healing forces of nature and is commonly referred to as *natural medicine*. It is more precisely defined as a healing system that combines safe and effective traditional means of preventing and treating human disease with the most current advances in modern medicine (American Association of Naturopathic Physicians [AANP], 2014). Many naturopathic physicians are eclectic, employing a variety of therapies in their practice. These might include clinical nutrition, botanical medicine, homeopathy, natural childbirth, hydrotherapy, naturopathic manipulative therapy, pharmacology, minor surgery, and public health measures (AANP, 2014).

TRADITIONAL CHINESE MEDICINE

Traditional Chinese medicine (TCM) developed more than 3000 years ago in the Chinese culture and then gradually spread with modifications to other Asian countries. The underlying focus of TCM is prevention, although diagnosis and treatment of disease also play an important role.

TCM seeks to ensure the balance of energy, which is called *chi* or *qi* (pronounced "chee"). Chi is the invisible flow of energy in the body that maintains health and energy and enables the body to carry out its physiologic functions. Chi flows along certain pathways or meridians.

Another important concept in TCM is that of *yin* and *yang*, opposing internal and external forces that, together, represent the whole.

TCM includes the following therapeutic techniques:

- *Acupuncture* uses very fine (hairlike) stainless steel needles to stimulate specific acupuncture points, depending on the client's medical assessment and condition.
- *Acupressure* (Chinese massage) uses pressure from the fingers and thumbs to stimulate pressure points.
- *Herbal therapy* is an important part of TCM, but it is sometimes difficult to locate a skilled herbalist because there are relatively few in the United States and other English-speaking countries.
- *Qigong* (pronounced "chee-goong") is a self-discipline that involves the use of breathing, meditation, self-massage, and movement. Typically practiced daily, the movements are nontiring and are designed to stimulate the flow of chi.
- *T'ai chi* (pronounced "ty-chee") is a form of martial art. It originally focused on physical fitness and self-defense, but it is currently used primarily to improve health (Fontaine, 2015).
- *Moxibustion* involves the application of heat from a small piece of burning herb called *moxa (Artemisia vulgaris)*. The moxa stick is typically burned at the lateral side of the mother's little toe. In TCM moxibustion has many uses. For example, studies from China demonstrate good success when moxibustion is used to help turn a fetus who is breech to a vertex presentation (Vas et al., 2013).

MIND-BASED THERAPIES

Biofeedback is a method used to help individuals learn to control their physiologic responses based on the concept that the mind controls the body. An individual is attached to a system of highly sensitive instruments that relay information about the body back to that person. Currently, biofeedback has more than 150 applications for disease prevention and the restoration of health. The effectiveness of biofeedback has been proven in countless studies, and it is now considered a conventional therapy more than a complementary one.

Hypnosis, whether guided by a trained hypnotherapist or induced through self-hypnosis, is a state of great mental and physical relaxation during which a person is very open to suggestions. In this state, the individual is able to modify body responses. Pregnant women who receive hypnosis before childbirth have reported shorter, less painful labors and births.

Visualization is a complementary therapy in which a person goes into a relaxed state and focuses on, or "visualizes," soothing or positive scenes such as a beach or a mountain glade. Visualization helps reduce stress and encourage relaxation.

Guided imagery is a state of intense, focused concentration used to create compelling mental images. It is sometimes considered a form of hypnosis. Guided imagery is useful in imagining a desired effect such as weight loss or in mentally rehearsing a new procedure or activity.

CHIROPRACTIC

Chiropractic, the third largest independent health profession in the United States (behind medicine and dentistry), is based on concepts of manipulation to address health problems that are thought to be the result of abnormal nerve transmissions (subluxation) caused by misalignment of the spine. Spinal manipulation is the most common procedure performed by chiropractors (American Chiropractic Association, 2014). Chiropractors also stress the importance of proper nutrition and regular exercise to good health. Chiropractic is widely available, and popular demand has earned it a higher level of insurance coverage than most other alternative therapies.

MASSAGE THERAPY

Massage has been used for centuries as a form of therapy. *Massage therapy* involves manipulation of the soft tissues of the body to reduce stress and tension, increase circulation, diminish pain, and promote a sense of well-being. Different techniques have been developed, including Swedish massage, shiatsu massage, Rolfing, and trigger point massage. Most forms use techniques such as pressing, kneading, gliding, circular motion, tapping, and vibrational strokes.

Certain massage therapists specialize in massage for women during pregnancy. Massage is often helpful as women adapt to the discomforts of their changing bodies. Certified nurse-midwives often use perineal massage prior to labor to stretch the muscles of the perineum around the vaginal opening and thereby prevent tearing of the tissues during childbirth. During labor, massage of the back and buttocks by the nurse, labor coach, or doula can help the woman relax and may help decrease her discomfort.

Infant massage is also growing in popularity in the United States, and many parents have learned to massage their infants and young children (Figure 2–5). Massage also plays a role in therapy for children with a variety of conditions, including eczema.

HERBAL THERAPIES

Herbal therapy, or herbal medicine, has been used since ancient times to treat illnesses and ailments. Well-known herbal remedies include ginger, rosemary, ginseng, ginkgo, chamomile, oil of evening primrose, echinacea, garlic, lemon balm, and black cohosh.

Herbs are categorized as dietary supplements and are controlled by the Dietary Supplement Health and Education Act of 1994. They do not require approval by the Food and Drug Administration (FDA) as do prescription and over-the-counter

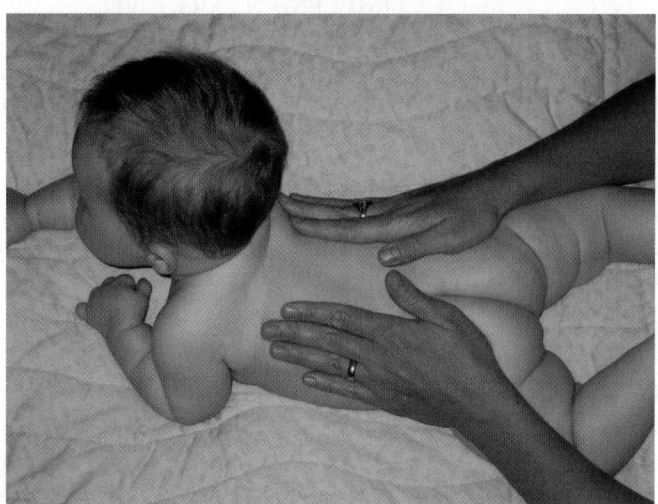

Figure 2–5 **Infant massage.**

medications; however, the FDA does have the authority to pull a product off the market if it is proven to be unsafe (FDA, 2014).

SAFETY ALERT!

The use of herbs during pregnancy is an especially important consideration for nurses working with childbearing families. Pregnant and lactating women interested in using herbs are best advised to consult with their healthcare provider before taking any herbs, even as teas. Lists identifying common herbs that women are advised to avoid or use with caution during pregnancy and lactation are available. Certain herbs may be harmful to children with some conditions (e.g., renal disorders), or they may interact with prescribed medication, and should not be used.

In cases when the family's cultural practice is placing the child in a hazardous situation, civil courts may intervene to provide care for the child; for example, by mandating a life-preserving chemotherapy procedure for a child even when the family is opposed to treatment. Support families in their beliefs and healthcare practices, but remain alert for any care that could be harmful for the child and report it promptly.

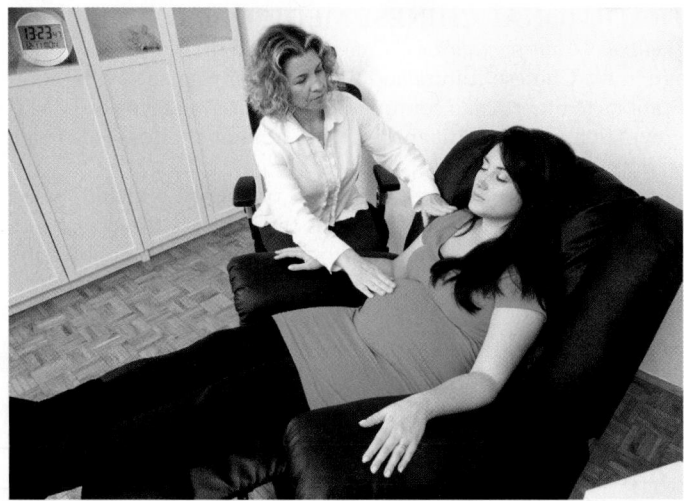

Figure 2–6 During pregnancy, therapeutic touch is often helpful in easing pain and reducing anxiety.

SOURCE: Dean Bertoncelj/Shutterstock.

Developing Cultural Competence Herbalism

The World Health Organization estimates that 80% of the earth's population depends on plants to treat common ailments. Herbalism is an essential part of traditional Indian, Asian, Native American, and naturopathic medicines. Many homeopathic remedies are also developed from herbs (University of Maryland Medical Center, 2012).

THERAPEUTIC TOUCH

Therapeutic touch is based on the belief that people are a system of energy with a self-healing potential. The therapeutic touch practitioner, often a nurse, can unite his or her energy field with that of the client's, directing it in a specific way to promote well-being and healing. Healing is promoted when the body's energies are in balance. By passing their hands over the client, without touching the client, healers can identify energy imbalances (Fontaine, 2015).

Like many other conventional and complementary therapies, therapeutic touch should be applied cautiously to pregnant women, newborns, and children by trained providers (Figure 2–6).

OTHER TYPES OF COMPLEMENTARY AND ALTERNATIVE THERAPIES

This discussion only touched on some of the most common forms of complementary and alternative therapies. Other examples include Ayurveda (the traditional medicine of India), meditation, craniosacral therapy, reflexology, hydrotherapy, hatha yoga, regular physical exercise, aromatherapy, color and light therapy, music and sound therapies, magnetic therapy, and Reiki, to name a few. Readers interested in these therapies are referred to specialty texts.

Nursing Care of the Family Using Complementary Therapies

Some form of complementary and alternative medicine (CAM) is currently being used by two thirds of adults in the United States. Women use CAM more often than men do, as do people with higher educational levels (Fontaine, 2015).

The reality that families may use CAM and not reveal it raises some concern. Certain CAM modalities such as biofeedback, acupuncture, aromatherapy, and massage are not likely to cause adverse effects. However, the possibility exists that there might be interactions between herbal therapies and other medications prescribed by the healthcare provider (Fontaine, 2015). Complications may also develop from the use of vitamin supplements.

The use of CAM in the care of children must be addressed because of the limited research with this age group and developmental variations that may influence efficacy and safety. While many CAM therapies may have been proven effective in adults, they may have little effect on children, or even be harmful.

Nurses who create a climate of respect and openness tend to be more effective in gathering information about a family's use of complementary or alternative therapies. The nurse should use a nonjudgmental approach in assessing pregnant women and families for the use of CAM. Identify the expected outcome of the herbal or dietary supplement. Ask specifically about the use of herbs and other supplements, as the pregnant woman, parent, or child may not think to include them in their list of medications.

Nurses should use complementary modalities that are in the scope of their nursing practice and the nursing practice act in their state. Their use should also be supported by evidence-based research (Fontaine, 2015). Nurses working with a pregnant woman might use acupressure wristbands for the treatment of nausea. Other therapies nurses often employ include progressive relaxation, exercise and movement, therapeutic touch, visualization and guided imagery, prayer, meditation, music therapy, massage, storytelling, aromatherapy, and journaling.

Nurses who use complementary modalities should document their use within the context of nursing practice. This is most effective when the modality is identified as an intervention to address a specific nursing diagnosis or identified client need. Thus, music therapy might be used for a laboring woman or a child to help address the identified nursing diagnosis of *Pain, Acute* (NANDA-I © 2014). Nurses have a role in conducting and supporting research on CAM. Because of the variety of CAM therapies in use, research is needed in a host of areas. The results of research on CAM can be found in professional journals and at the National Institutes of Health website. As the evidence supporting the use of certain interventions grows, nurses and other healthcare providers are incorporating the results as part of their evidence-based practice.

Focus Your Study

- The family is defined as two or more individuals who are joined together by marriage, birth, or adoption and live together in the same household.

- Nuclear families consist of a mother, father, and children.

- Dual-career/dual-earner families comprise the majority of contemporary families in the United States.

- Child-free families are a growing trend in American culture.

- Extended family members can play an active role in family life, decision making, and family roles.

- Extended kin network families share a social support network, chores, goods, and services.

- Single-parent families account for almost one third of all U.S. families.

- The single mother by choice family represents a family composed of an unmarried woman who chooses to conceive or adopt without a life partner.

- The blended, or reconstituted nuclear, family includes two parents with biologic children from a previous marriage or relationship who marry or cohabitate.

- A binuclear family is a post-divorce family in which the biologic children are members of two nuclear households, with coparenting by the father and the mother.

- A heterosexual cohabiting family describes a heterosexual couple who may or may not have children and who live together outside of marriage.

- Gay and lesbian families include those in which two adults of the same sex live together as domestic partners with or without children and those in which a gay or lesbian single parent rears a child.

- Family development theories use a framework to categorize a family's progression over time according to specific, typical stages in family life.

- A family assessment provides an in-depth tool to collect pertinent family life information that can assist the nurse in planning care.

- Culture plays a significant part in a family's development, assignment of roles, and observance of traditions, customs, and taboos.

- Cultural norms influence a family's beliefs about the importance of children, pregnancy, health practices, and infant feeding.

- Providing culturally competent care involves recognizing the importance of the childbearing family's value system, acknowledging that differences occur among people, and respecting and responding to ethnic diversity in a way that leads to mutually desirable outcomes.

- A cultural assessment can assist the nurse in identifying cultural norms and in providing culturally appropriate nursing care. It should focus on factors that will influence the practices of the childbearing and childrearing family with regard to health needs and may include a religious history.

- Providing spiritually sensitive care involves determining the current spiritual and religious beliefs and practices that will affect the mother and baby, accommodating these practices where possible, and examining one's own spiritual or religious beliefs to be more aware and able to provide nonjudgmental care.

- A complementary therapy is an adjunct to conventional medical treatment, whereas an alternative therapy is used in place of prescribed medical therapy.

- CAM therapies have several benefits. Many of them emphasize prevention and wellness, place a higher value on holistic healing than on physical cure, are noninvasive, and have few side effects. In addition, many are more affordable and available than conventional therapies.

- Risks of using CAM therapies include lack of standardization, lack of regulation and research substantiating safety and effectiveness, inadequate training and certification of some healers, and financial and health risks of unproven methods.

- Homeopathy is a healing system that uses like to cure like; that is, homeopathic remedies are minute dilutions of substances that, if ingested in larger amounts, would produce effects *similar* to the symptoms of the disorder being treated.

- Traditional Chinese medicine (TCM) seeks to ensure the balance of energy, called *chi* or *qi*. TCM techniques include acupuncture, acupressure, herbal therapy, qigong, t'ai chi, and moxibustion.

- Biofeedback is a method used to help individuals learn to control their physiologic responses based on the concept that the mind controls the body.

- Hypnosis, whether guided by a trained hypnotherapist or induced through self-hypnosis, is a state of great mental and physical relaxation during which a person is very open to suggestions.

- Guided imagery is a state of intense, focused concentration used to create compelling mental images.

- Chiropractic, a profession practiced by licensed chiropractors, is based on concepts of manipulation, especially spinal manipulation.

- Massage therapy involves manipulation of the soft tissues of the body to reduce stress and tension, increase circulation, diminish pain, and promote a sense of well-being.

- Herbal therapy has been used since ancient times; well-known herbal remedies include ginger, rosemary, ginseng, ginkgo, chamomile, oil of evening primrose, echinacea, garlic, lemon balm, and black cohosh.

- Therapeutic touch is based on the belief that people are a system of energy with a self-healing potential. The therapeutic touch practitioner, often a nurse, can unite his or her energy field with that of the client's, directing it in a specific way to promote well-being and healing.

- Many nurses are open to and supportive of complementary and alternative therapies. Nurses who incorporate such therapies into their practice must be certain that they are practicing within the framework of their nursing practice and act with the informed consent of their clients.

Clinical Reasoning in Action

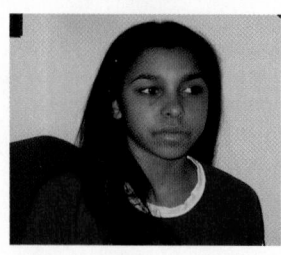

While working in an inner-city clinic for adolescents, you meet a new client, a 14-year-old Latina girl named Juanita. Her parents accompany her to the clinic. None of them speak English. Through an interpreter, Juanita tells you that she recently moved here with her parents. They have brought her here today because she has a sore throat. The curandero they took her to see prescribed the herbal remedy echinacea, but her throat is still sore. The rapid test you perform for strep throat is positive and the healthcare provider prescribes an antibiotic.

1. According to the national standards for culturally and linguistically appropriate services in health care set by the government, what are examples of important standards of care you as the nurse can provide in the care of this adolescent?

2. How can you, as the nurse, take steps to achieve cultural competence?

3. How would you, as the nurse, be able to address some of the disparities that can exist when this client comes to the clinic?

4. What are some examples of common food preferences in the Latino-American culture?

References

Adorador, A., McNulty, R., Hart, D., & Fitzpatrick, J. J. (2011). Perceived barriers to immunizations as identified by Latino mothers. *Journal of the Academy of Nurse Practitioners, 23,* 501–508.

Algur, V. S., Kazi, S., & Yadavannavar, M. (2013). Family planning practices among rural health training centers beneficiaries. *International Journal of Current Research and Review, 5*(1), 64–68.

American Association of Naturopathic Physicians (AANP). (2014). *What is naturopathic medicine?* Retrieved from http://www.naturopathic.org/content.asp?contentid=59

American Chiropractic Association. (2014). *Spinal manipulation.* Retrieved from http://www.acatoday.org/content_css.cfm?CID=1083

Andrews, M. M., & Boyle, J. S. (2012). *Transcultural concepts in nursing care* (6th ed.). Philadelphia, PA: Lippincott Williams & Wilkins.

Bulte, E., Heerink, N., & Zhang, X. (2011). China's one-child policy and "the mystery of missing women": Ethnic minorities and male-biased sex ratios. *Oxford Bulletin of Economics and Statistics, 73*(1), 21–39.

Chen, C. H. (2014). Diverse yet hegemonic: Expressions of motherhood in "I'm a Mormon" ads. *Journal of Media and Religion, 13* (1), 31–47.

Coehlo, D. P. (2015). Family child health nursing. In J. R. Kaakinen, D. P. Coehlo, R. Steele, A. Tabacco, & S. M. H. Hanson, *Family health care nursing: Theory, practice, and research* (5th ed., pp. 387–432). Philadelphia, PA: F. A. Davis.

Douglas, M. K., Pierce, J. U., Rosenkoetter, M., Pacquiao, D., Callister, L. C., Hattar-Pollara, M., . . . Purnell, L. (2011). Standards of practice for culturally competent nursing care: 2011 Update. *Journal of Transcultural Nursing, 22*(4), 317–333.

Duvall, E. M. (1977). *Marriage and family development* (5th ed.). New York, NY: Harper & Row.

Duvall, E. M., & Miller, B. L. (1985). *Marriage and family development* (6th ed.). New York, NY: Harper & Row.

Ferayorni, A., Sinha, M., & McDonald, F. W. (2011). Health issues among foreign born uninsured children visiting an inner city pediatric emergency department. *Journal of Immigrant and Minority Health, 13*(3), 434–444.

Food & Drug Administration (FDA). (2014). *Dietary supplements: What you need to know.* Retrieved from http://www.fda.gov/Food/ResourcesForYou/Consumers/ucm109760.htm

Fontaine, K. L. (2015). *Complementary and alternative therapies for nursing practice* (4th ed.). Upper Saddle River, NJ: Pearson.

Giger, J. N. (2013). *Transcultural nursing: Assessment & intervention* (6th ed.). St. Louis, MO: Elsevier Mosby.

Haney-Caron, E., & Heilbrun, K. (2014). Lesbian and gay parents and determination of child custody: The changing legal landscape and implications for policy and practice. *Psychology of Sexual Orientation and Gender Diversity, 1*(1), 19–29.

Lambert, N. M., Fincham, F. D., & Graham, S. M. (2011). Understanding the layperson's perception of prayer: A prototype analysis of prayer. *Psychology of Religion and Spirituality, 3*(1), 55–65.

Lascar, E. (2013). *The role of spiritual care in CPC programmes.* Retrieved from http://www.ehospice.com/internationalchildrens/ArticleView/tabid/10670/ArticleId/3929/language/en-GB/Default.aspx

Maggio, J. (2013). *Peace and the single mom.* New York, NY: Choose NOW Publishing.

Mitchell, M. (2013). Women's use of complementary and alternative medicine in pregnancy: A journey to normal birth. *British Journal of Midwifery, 21*(2), 100–106.

National Center for Complementary and Alternative Medicine (NCCAM). (2013). *Complementary, alternative, or integrative health: What's in a name?* Retrieved from http://nccam.nih.gov/health/whatiscam#cvsa

National Institutes of Health. (2013). *Cultural competency.* Retrieved from http://www.nih.gov/clearcommunication/culturalcompetency.htm

Pew Research Center. (2012). *"Nones" on the rise: One-in-five adults have no religious affiliation.* Retrieved from http://www.pewforum.org/2012/10/09/nones-on-the-rise/

Purnell, L. D. (2013). *Transcultural health care: A culturally competent approach* (4th ed.). Philadelphia, PA: F. A. Davis.

Purnell, L. D. (2014). *Guide to culturally competent health care* (3rd ed.). Philadelphia, PA: F. A. Davis.

Single Mothers by Choice. (2013). *About single mothers by choice.* Retrieved from http://www.singlemothersbychoice.org/

Spector, R. E. (2013). *Cultural diversity in health and illness* (8th ed.). Upper Saddle River, NJ: Pearson.

Taylor, S. P., Nicolle, C., & Maguire, M. (2013). Cross-cultural communication barriers in health care. *Nursing Standard, 27*(31), 35–43.

University of Maryland Medical Center. (2012). *Herbal medicine.* Retrieved from http://www.umm.edu/altmed/articles/herbal-medicine-000351.htm

U.S. Census Bureau. (2013). *Definition: Household and family.* Retrieved from http://www.census.gov/cps/about/cpsdef.html

Vas, J., Aranda-Regules, J. M., Modesto, M., Ramos-Monserrat, M., Barón, M., Aguilar, I., . . . Rivas-Ruiz, F. (2013). Using moxibustion in primary health care to correct non-vertex presentation: A multicentre randomised controlled trial. *Acupuncture Medicine, 31*(1), 31–38. doi:10.1136/acupmed-2012-010261

Wachholtz, A., & Sambamoorthi, U. (2011). National trends in prayer use as a coping mechanism for health concerns: Changes from 2002 to 2007. *Psychology of Religion and Spirituality, 3*(2), 67–77.

Zoucha, R., & Zamarripa, C. A. (2013). People of Mexican heritage. In L. D. Purnell, *Transcultural health care: A culturally competent approach* (4th ed., pp. 374–390). Philadelphia, PA: F. A. Davis.

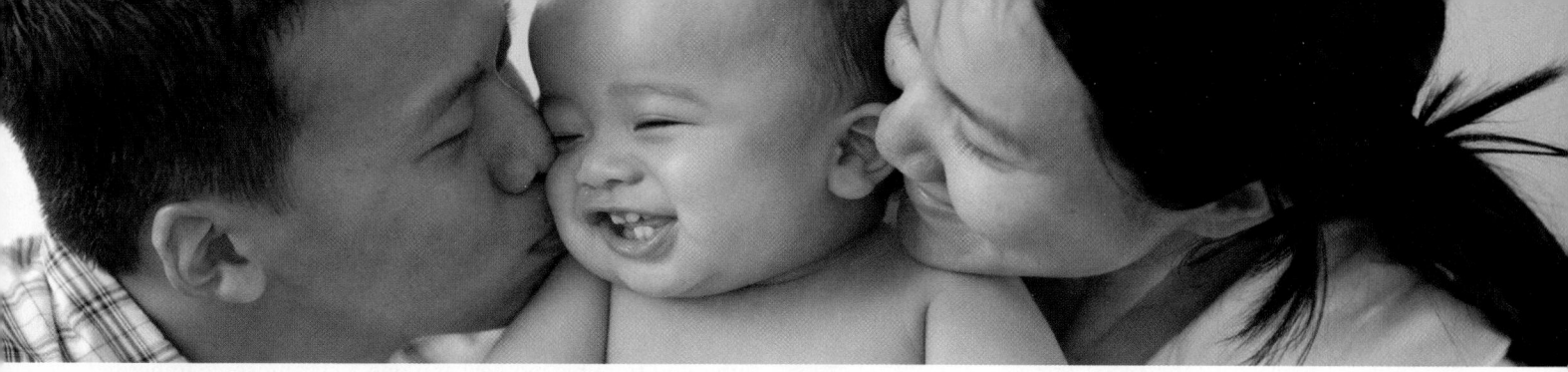

Chapter 3
Genetic and Genomic Influences in Maternal, Newborn, and Child Health

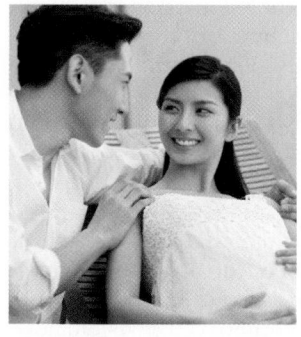

Lane Oatey/Blue Jean Images/
Getty Images

We are now 12 weeks' pregnant and have been on cloud nine until today, when we learned our baby might have Down syndrome. We really never considered that possibility—what do we do now? Our physician suggested we could have chorionic villus sampling (CVS) or amniocentesis to find out for sure, but there is a small chance of miscarrying our baby. She also mentioned a newer blood test that is extremely accurate but still not perfect. Our world is upside down. Do we want to know? What would be the benefit, unless we were going to end our pregnancy? We don't know anyone with Down syndrome, or anyone who has raised a child with Down syndrome, or what that would be like. Our happiness has really turned into turmoil.

—Jessica, age 30

⌄ Learning Outcomes

3.1 Understand foundational concepts of genetics and genomics, including how DNA influences health and illness.

3.2 Explain mechanisms by which alterations in DNA cause disease.

3.3 Distinguish between single-gene (Mendelian) and multifactorial diseases and health conditions.

3.4 Identify characteristics of common inheritance patterns of single-gene conditions.

3.5 Describe the uses, implications, and limitations of various prenatal and postnatal types of genetic tests that are offered to childbearing families and children, distinguishing between screening and diagnostic tests.

3.6 Explain ways that nurses can advocate for and support clients and families undergoing genetic testing.

3.7 Describe the role of the nurses in assessing and communicating genetic risk, including eliciting a family history, creating a genetic pedigree, and incorporating genetics into physical assessment.

3.8 Identify children or families who might benefit from genetic information and services or referral to a genetic professional, and explain the nurse's role in supporting the family undergoing genetic counseling.

3.9 Discuss ethical, legal, and social implications of genomic health care.

Pregnancy and childbirth usually take their normal course and a healthy baby is born without problems. Three to five percent of pregnancies, however, result in the birth of a child with some sort of birth defect or genetic disorder. Genetic problems may become evident during pregnancy, at birth, or during the newborn period, or may not appear for some time. The Human Genome Project, which was completed in 2003, brought rapid progress in genome science and an understanding that essentially all diseases and health conditions have a genetic component. It is predicted that health care will increasingly be personalized, based on each individual's genetic information. **Genomics**, the study of all human genes including their interactions with each other and with environmental factors, is now considered to be a central science for nursing practice. All registered nurses should be able to identify, refer, support, and care for children and families affected by conditions or diseases with a genetic component. This chapter presents information nurses must understand to provide competent care in the genome era of health care.

Genetic Basics

A basic knowledge of the cell, cell division, DNA, chromosomes, and genes is essential to deliver the genetic standard of care to children, adolescents, and their families.

Cells and DNA

The **cell** is the basic unit of life and the working unit of all living systems. Life starts when a sperm and ovum combine to form a single cell, which develops to form a human body made up of trillions of cells. These cells share common features such as a nucleus that contains the DNA and **organelles** such as mitochondria. Cells are specialized in appearance and function, according to their location. For example, pancreatic cells function much differently than nerve cells.

All human cells, except red blood cells, contain a complete set of DNA molecules, which are long sequences of nucleotides. A nucleotide is a base with an attached sugar and phosphate group. Four different bases, designated A, C, T, and G, make up DNA. The order, or sequence, of these bases provides exact instructions for protein building. The entire DNA in a human cell is referred to as the **human genome**. Most of the DNA is organized into **chromosomes**, which are contained in the cell nucleus. A small amount of DNA is found in the mitochondria and will be discussed later in this section. Each person's genome is unique, with the exception of monozygotic twins, who are derived from the same fertilized ovum and therefore share identical DNA.

The nucleus of each cell (except gametes) contains about 6 feet of DNA that is tightly wound and packaged into 23 pairs of chromosomes, making a complete set of 46 chromosomes. The set includes 22 pairs of **autosomes**, which are by tradition numbered according to size, with chromosome 1 being the largest. There are two copies of each autosome, one inherited from the mother and the other from the father. Copies of a chromosome pair are called **homologous chromosomes**. The 23rd chromosome pair, the **sex chromosomes**, determines an individual's sex. A female has two copies of the X chromosome (one copy inherited from each parent), and a male has one X chromosome (inherited from his mother) and one Y chromosome (inherited from his father). The structure and number of chromosomes can be shown by preparing a **karyotype**, or picture of an individual's chromosomes. Figure 3–1 depicts a normal male and female karyotype. A karyotype is usually obtained from specially treated and stained peripheral blood lymphocytes, but a fetal karyotype can be obtained by sampling amniotic fluid or placental tissue.

Cell Division

Mitosis and meiosis are the two types of cell division in humans. **Mitosis** takes place in somatic or tissue cells of the body, allowing the formation of new cells. Cell division by mitosis results in two cells called *daughter cells* that are genetically identical to the original cell and to each other. Mitosis is responsible for rapid human growth in early life and also replaces cells lost daily from skin surfaces and the lining of gastrointestinal and respiratory tracts.

Meiosis is also known as *reduction cell division*. Meiosis occurs only in the reproductive cells of the testes and ovaries and results in the formation of sperm and ova, **(gametes)**. Meiosis is similar to mitosis in that it is a form of cell division; however, through a series of complex mechanisms, the amount of genetic material is reduced to half. Each gamete contains a single copy of each of the 22 autosomes, plus a single sex chromosome. This is critical to ensure that when two gametes combine during fertilization, the correct total number of chromosomes (46) is present in the offspring's cells. The other purpose of meiosis is to make new combinations of genetic material through processes of crossing over and independent assortment. New combinations are necessary to promote diversity in the human population. **Crossing over** results in an exchange or shuffling of

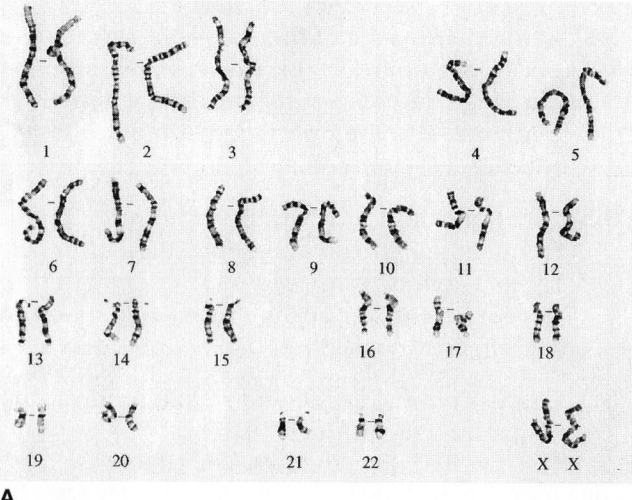

A

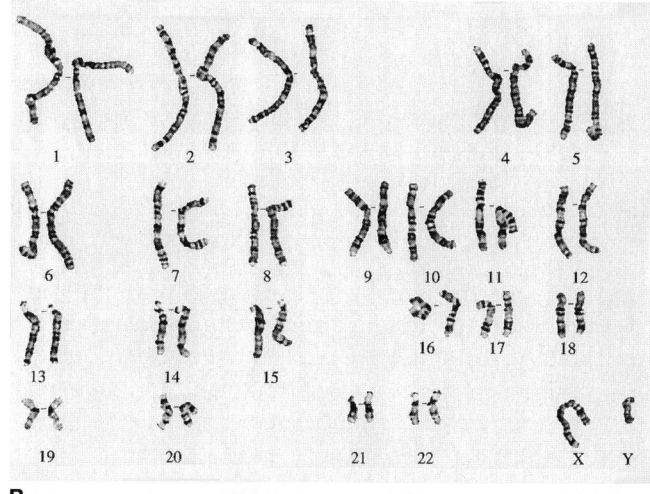

B

Figure 3–1 A karyotype is a picture of an individual's chromosomes. It depicts the number and structure of the 22 pairs of autosomes and the sex chromosomes. *A*, Female. *B*, Male.

SOURCE: Courtesy of the Greenwood Genetic Center, Greenwood, SC.

material between homologous chromosomes, so that sperm and ova contain a patchwork of genetic material from an individual's maternal and paternal chromosomes. **Independent assortment** means that chromosome pairs segregate randomly into one or another gamete, further enhancing the genetic diversity that is possible at fertilization.

Chromosomal Alterations

Alterations in chromosomes sometimes occur during cell division (meiosis or mitosis) and are classified as alterations in either chromosome number or chromosome structure. The clinical consequences of both types of alterations vary according to the amount of DNA involved.

ALTERATIONS IN CHROMOSOME NUMBER

An increase or decrease in chromosome number is called **aneuploidy**. Aneuploidy is the result of an error during cell division, most often when **nondisjunction** occurs during meiosis. With nondisjunction, pairs of homologous chromosomes do not separate before migrating into egg or sperm cells. This creates a gamete with either two copies or no copies of a particular chromosome. When such a gamete is fertilized by a normal gamete with all 23 chromosomes, a **zygote** that is **monosomic** (missing one member of a chromosome pair) or **trisomic** (having three homologous chromosomes instead of the usual two) results.

Humans do not tolerate either extra or missing DNA very well, and most monosomic or trisomic conceptions result in early pregnancy loss. For example, Turner syndrome (45,X) is the only monosomic condition that is compatible with life. Trisomies involving chromosomes with small numbers of genes may result in live births. Down syndrome is the most common trisomy abnormality seen in children. The presence of the extra chromosome 21 produces distinctive clinical features and a variety of cognitive and physical impairments. Early intervention and clinical practice guidelines developed specifically for children with Down syndrome have improved their health and quality of life and extended their life expectancy (see Chapter 55). Babies are occasionally born with trisomy 13 (Patau syndrome) or trisomy 18 (Edwards syndrome). The prognosis for these conditions is extremely poor; most children die within the first 3 months of life because of cardiac and respiratory complications. However, about 8% to 10% of these children survive the first year; therefore, the family needs to plan for the possibility of long-term care of a severely affected infant (Wu, Springett, & Morris, 2013). It is not a coincidence that the three trisomy conditions that are not universally lethal involve duplication of chromosomes containing the smallest number of genes; other trisomies are lethal. (Pierce, 2014).

Mosaicism. Monosomy and/or trisomy can also occur during cell division (mitosis) after fertilization, resulting in an individual with two, or occasionally more, separate cell lines with different chromosomal makeup. This is known as **mosaicism**. The earlier in development the error occurs, the more cells that will be abnormal. The converse is also true. The degree to which a person is affected by this chromosomal error varies. For example, an individual with mosaic Down syndrome may have a higher intelligence level than children whose every cell has three copies of chromosome 21, and children who are mosaic for trisomy 13 or trisomy 18 tend to survive longer than children with the full trisomy.

Aneuploidies of the Sex Chromosome. In order to understand aneuploidies of the X and Y chromosome, the nurse should know that Y has few genes, none of which is critical to life. In contrast, the X chromosome has many critical genes that would be duplicated in females (compared to males) if it were not for a

phenomenon called *X-inactivation.* Early in female embryonic development, within a week of fertilization, one of her X chromosomes is inactivated. This results in equalizing the expression of genes on the X chromosome between the two sexes. Because of X-inactivation and the lack of critical genes on the Y chromosome, aneuploidies involving sex chromosomes are much better tolerated than autosomal aneuploidies. The most common sex chromosome aneuploidies are Turner syndrome in females (45,X) and Klinefelter syndrome in males (47,XXY). Girls with Turner syndrome have short stature, may not develop secondary sex characteristics, and are usually infertile, while men with Klinefelter syndrome tend to be tall with reduced testosterone production, resulting in delayed puberty, breast enlargement, and infertility.

ALTERATIONS IN CHROMOSOME STRUCTURE

Abnormalities of chromosome structure involve only parts of the chromosome and generally occur in the form of an inversion, translocation, deletion, or duplication.

Inversion. A chromosomal **inversion** occurs when a chromosome breaks in two places and the piece between the breaks turns end-for-end and reattaches within the same chromosome. An inversion changes the DNA sequence for that portion of the chromosome. Inversion often results in *balanced* rearrangements because the amount of DNA in the chromosome remains normal. The clinical consequences of an inversion depend on how much chromosomal material is involved and where the inversion occurs. For example, an inversion that occurs between genes may have no effect on health, while an inversion within the gene that codes for factor VIII, a clotting factor, is an important cause of hemophilia A.

Translocation. Translocation occurs when two, usually nonhomologous, chromosomes exchange segments of DNA. A translocation that results in a correct amount of chromosomal material but a new arrangement is a *balanced translocation*. The individual who has a balanced rearrangement has all the chromosomal material present and therefore does not usually have any physical or mental disabilities. However, individuals with a balanced translocation are at high risk to produce gametes with unbalanced rearrangements. This leads to increased risk of pregnancy loss or having children with mental and/or physical disabilities owing to missing or extra genetic material. A common *unbalanced translocation* is responsible for about 4% of children diagnosed with Down syndrome (Schaaf, Zschocke, & Potocki, 2012). When a child with Down syndrome is born, it is important to determine if the cause is nondisjunction or translocation. Translocation, while unrelated to maternal age, carries a significantly greater recurrence risk with subsequent pregnancies. Clinically, the two types of Down syndrome are indistinguishable, and chromosome analysis is required to determine the cause.

Deletion and Duplication. Chromosomal alterations sometimes occur when unequal crossing over or abnormal segregation causes a chromosome to have a missing segment (deletion) or an additional segment (duplication) of genetic material. These are called *unbalanced* rearrangements. Conditions associated with unbalanced rearrangements may be incompatible with life or cause altered physical and/or mental development. An example is cri du chat syndrome, which is caused by a large deletion on chromosome 5. Children with cri du chat syndrome have microcephaly (a small head), significant intellectual disability, and an underdeveloped larynx, which causes a peculiar cry that sounds like a cat mewing (Schaaf et al., 2012).

Some deletions or duplications are too small to detect with a standard karyotype. These chromosome abnormalities, known as *microdeletions* and *microduplications,* can be detected by the use of a technology called *microarray comparative genomic hybridization* (aCGH). An aCGH analysis compares a client's DNA to that of a normal control individual and detects not only aneuploidies and large structural changes, but also submicroscopic duplications, deletions, and unbalanced rearrangements in genes (ACOG, 2013). The higher resolution of aCGH makes it useful to detect disorders typically missed by conventional cytogenetic studies.

Genes

In addition to understanding chromosomal alterations, nurses must have knowledge of genes—what they are, their function, and the consequences of gene alterations. Nurses must also understand how gene alterations are inherited in order to design appropriate nursing interventions and teach the child, adolescent, and family at risk for or with a known genetic condition. Also, as genetic influences on common diseases are better understood, knowledge of gene function and inheritance has become increasingly relevant in health promotion and health maintenance.

GENE DISTRIBUTION

A **gene** is a small segment of a chromosome that can be identified with a particular function, most commonly protein production. In humans, protein-coding DNA is organized into about 21,000 genes (Lander, 2011), which are arranged along chromosomes in a linear order. The vast majority of human DNA lies between genes; it is believed that only about 1% of the human genome is actually represented by protein-encoding genes (McCarthy, McLeod, & Ginsburg, 2013).

Genes have a specific location on a designated chromosome; this is called the *genetic locus*. Gene mapping has documented the locus for most human genes. For example, it is known that the Huntington gene is located at the tip of chromosome 4, whereas the gene associated with cystic fibrosis is on chromosome 7.

Genes that reside on autosomes (i.e., chromosomes 1 through 22) come in pairs, with one copy on each homologous chromosome. Each gene copy, or **allele**, is inherited from a different parent; therefore, pairs of alleles likely have differences in their nucleotide sequence. These differences may be so minor that they do not affect gene function at all, or they may disrupt or totally disable the gene. An individual who has two functionally identical alleles of a gene is said to be **homozygous** (*homo* = same) for that gene. An individual whose alleles for a particular gene function differently is said to be **heterozygous** (*hetero* = different) for that gene.

GENES AND PROTEINS

The 21,000 genes in the human genome are responsible for encoding hundreds of thousands of proteins that carry out all physiologic functions. Proteins form structures, transmit messages between cells, fight infection, direct genes to turn on or off, metabolize nutrients and drugs, and sense light, taste, and smell. When proteins do not function normally, health may be impaired.

The order of amino acids in a particular protein is determine by the order of nucleotides in its encoding gene. Therefore, an alteration in the DNA sequence within a gene may disrupt the amino acid sequence in the protein product of that gene. Genes are described as being *altered* or *mutated* when a change has taken place in their nucleotide sequence. Such a change may or may not result in an altered protein product. A gene alteration that disrupts the order of amino acids in that gene's protein product is called a **mutation**. A protein with an incorrect amino acid may assume the wrong three-dimensional shape and, because protein function is dependent on protein shape (or configuration), the protein may not function as expected.

GENE EXPRESSION

A gene is said to be expressed when it is actively making protein. **Gene expression** can change moment to moment in response to thousands of intracellular and extracellular signals. An example is the mechanism that stimulates cells to produce insulin after eating a candy bar. After the candy bar is eaten, a gene on chromosome 11 directs pancreatic cells to produce and secrete insulin. Although the gene for producing insulin is present in all nucleated cells of the body, it is only functional in insulin-secreting pancreatic cells. The control of gene expression is complex and poorly understood. Changes in nucleotide sequence some distance from a gene may affect its activity in making protein. Smaller, non-DNA molecules are also involved in gene expression: These **epigenetic** effects can cause genes to be overexpressed (making more than expected protein product), underexpressed (making less than expected), or expressed at a time in development when the gene is normally inactive.

Each individual's particular set of genes represents his or her **genotype**. The observable, outward expression of an individual's entire physical, biochemical, and physiologic makeup, as determined by the person's genotype and environmental factors, is referred to as **phenotype**. Phenotype may be expressed as physical appearance such as curly or straight hair or physiologic function; for example, signs or symptoms of a disease.

MITOCHONDRIAL GENES

The vast majority of human genes reside on nuclear DNA that make up chromosomes in the cell nucleus, but mitochondria (organelles involved in energy metabolism, known as the "powerhouse" of the cell) also contain a small amount of DNA. Mitochondrial DNA (mtDNA) contains 37 genes (Turnpenny & Ellard, 2012). Because mitochondria are the sites for energy production, cells requiring large amounts of energy contain more mitochondria than other cells. mtDNA is inherited from the mother in a unique *matrilineal* pattern. This occurs because sperm's mitochondria are located in the tail, which detaches at fertilization. A woman with a mitochondrial gene mutation will consequently pass that mutation to all her children, whereas an affected man will not pass the mtDNA mutation to any of his children (Turnpenny & Ellard, 2012). Clinical manifestations occurring as a result of mitochondrial gene alterations primarily affect high-energy tissues such as brain and cardiac and skeletal muscle.

HUMAN GENETIC VARIATION

The Human Genome Project and other genetic studies have shown that humans are remarkably similar to each other at the DNA level. On average, any two humans vary in less than 1% of their nucleotide sequence. Much of human variation can be attributed to single nucleotide (or "single-letter") changes in DNA sequence. DNA sequencing of hundreds of individuals around the globe has shown that these single-nucleotide changes occur at several million sites (or loci) across the genome; the rest of the genome is identical in 99% of individuals. These single-letter variations are called **single nucleotide polymorphisms**, or SNPs (pronounced "snips"). Most SNPs are benign, although collectively they are thought to account for much phenotypic variation in appearance and risk for common diseases. SNPs have been mapped to the human genome, and the resulting SNP maps are of enormous value to researchers. For example, scientists studying the genetics of type 2 diabetes mellitus have compared SNP patterns in large numbers of individuals with and without the disease to identify genetic variations associated with this common multifactorial disease. Such **genome-wide association studies** (GWAS) are uncovering the genetic contribution to common chronic conditions that cause most of the disease burden in developed countries.

In recent years, DNA research has identified **copy number variation** as an additional source of human genetic variation. In some individuals, stretches of DNA of variable size (up to 3 million bases and sometimes containing entire genes) are replicated one or more times. Copy number variants (CNVs) appear to be fairly common; on average, each person is believed to have about 100 CNVs of various sizes (Lander, 2011). A CNV that contains an entire gene may result in more than expected gene product. In some cases, copy number variation has been associated with disease or birth defects (Pierce, 2014).

Mutations and Disease

Mutations are gene alterations, and typically the term *mutation* is used to describe an alteration that threatens health. Mutations may cause the formation of an altered or defective protein or cause too much or too little protein to be made. Sometimes a mutation will cause protein to be formed at a time in development when that protein is not normally made.

Mutations can be inherited or acquired. Hereditary mutations are passed to offspring from one or both parents and are also known as *germline mutations* because the mutation exists in the reproductive cells or gametes. Consequently, the DNA in every cell of that offspring will have the mutation, which can then be transmitted to following generations.

Acquired, or somatic, mutations are DNA alterations that occur in an individual at any time throughout a lifetime after fertilization. They result from errors during cell division (mitosis) or from environmental influences such as radiation, toxins, or viral infections. Acquired mutations are also called *sporadic* or *de novo* mutations. Most cases of cancer, for example, are due to somatic mutations. Somatic mutations are not passed from one generation to another.

SINGLE-GENE (MENDELIAN) MUTATIONS

Single-gene alterations are responsible for more than 5000 hereditary diseases such as cystic fibrosis, Duchenne muscular dystrophy, and phenylketonuria (PKU) (Online Mendelian Inheritance in Man [OMIM], 2014). Each of these disorders is relatively rare, although collectively they affect 1 of every 200 newborns (Schaaf et al., 2012). Although they are of enormous consequence to affected families, they constitute a relatively small portion of the total public health burden.

Genes vary enormously in size, but all are very long, containing tens of thousands or even hundreds of thousands of base pairs. Consequently, mutations can occur at various different loci within a gene and result in a wide variety of signs and symptoms. For example, the cystic fibrosis transmembrane conductance regulator (*CFTR*) gene on chromosome 7 contains about 250,000 base pairs and encodes a protein that forms a chloride channel. More than 1000 different *CFTR* mutations that disrupt the chloride channel have been identified (Turnpenny & Ellard, 2012). Some of these mutations cause cystic fibrosis, while others are associated with milder disorders such as absence of the vas deferens, pancreatitis, and rhinosinusitis. Most genetic tests for cystic fibrosis will detect only the most common *CFTR* mutations.

Alterations as small as a single-nucleotide change are known to cause disease. Sickle cell disease is such a disorder:

A single A-for-T substitution in the *HBB* gene causes an incorrect amino acid (valine) to be inserted at a site in the protein product (β-globin) normally occupied by a different amino acid (glutamic acid). The altered β-globin protein is then incorporated into hemoglobin molecules. Under conditions of low oxygen tension, the altered β-globin causes red blood cells to assume an abnormal, sickle-like shape. This leads to vascular occlusion and hemolytic anemia (Turnpenny & Ellard, 2012).

TRINUCLEOTIDE REPEAT DISORDERS

Some genetic disorders are caused by a phenomenon known as *trinucleotide repeat expansion*. This occurs at sites within a gene where the DNA sequence consists of adjacent three-nucleotide repeats such as CAGCAGCAG. These repeat sequences tend to expand during meiosis, a feature known as **anticipation**, resulting in a larger number of repeats in subsequent generations. A larger number of repeats may be associated with disease; typically, the larger the number of repeats, the more severe the condition. More than a dozen diseases result from trinucleotide repeat expansion, including Huntington disease, myotonic dystrophy, and Friedreich ataxia. Fragile X syndrome, the most common form of inherited cognitive disability, is a trinucleotide repeat disorder caused by an increased number of CGG trinucleotide repeats in the *FMR1* gene, located at a "fragile site" on the long arm of the X chromosome. The normal number of CGG repeats is up to 60. Individuals with a repeat number ranging between 60 and 200 have a *premutation* allele, meaning that the copy number can increase during meiosis. If the CGG repeat number increases to over 200, the individual (particularly males, who have only one X chromosome) can have the syndrome.

MULTIFACTORIAL DISORDERS

Most inherited traits, such as eye and skin color, are polygenic. That is, they occur as a result of variations on several genes. Most diseases and health conditions are polygenic as well, and the expression of those altered genes is often modified by environmental influences. Such conditions are said to be **multifactorial** and include many birth defects such as cleft lip and palate, pediatric conditions such as autism and asthma, and adult-onset conditions such as cancer and heart disease. Because the term *polygenic* does not imply the influence of the environment, the term *multifactorial* is preferred terminology. The relative contribution of genetic and environmental influences varies across disorders.

GENE ALTERATIONS THAT DECREASE RISK OF DISEASE

Although gene alterations are commonly associated with disease, they can also be helpful and decrease the risk of disease. For example, having a single copy of some genes known to cause autosomal recessive disorders can provide protection against disease. Individuals with a single altered copy of the gene associated with sickle cell disease are less likely to develop malaria. Another protective gene alteration involves a deletion in the *CCR5* gene, which encodes a cell receptor to which the HIV virus binds. Persons who have two copies of the altered *CCR5* gene are almost completely resistant to infection with HIV type 1, and those who are heterozygous for the deletion (have one copy of the altered gene) experience markedly delayed progression from the point of HIV infection to the development of AIDS (Barmania, Potgieter, & Pepper, 2013). As genome research continues, more beneficial gene alterations are being identified.

Principles of Inheritance

Knowledge of inheritance prepares the nurse to offer and reinforce genetic information to children, adolescents, and their families. Genetic knowledge may be important for nurses who assist clients with care management and reproductive decision making. Basic underlying principles of inheritance that nurses can apply to risk assessment and teaching include (a) nearly all genes are paired, (b) only one gene of each pair is transmitted (passed on) from each parent to an offspring, and (c) one copy of each gene in the offspring comes from the mother and the other copy comes from the father. Understanding of Mendelian patterns of inheritance is based on these principles.

Classic Mendelian Patterns of Inheritance

Single-gene, or monogenic, disorders are known as *Mendelian disorders* because they are predictably passed on from generation to generation following Mendel's laws of inheritance. More than 5000 monogenic disorders, most relatively rare, have been catalogued. Monogenic disorders that occur as a result of a mutation on an autosome (chromosome numbers 1 through 22) are commonly inherited in an autosomal dominant or autosomal recessive pattern. Disorders due to a mutation on one of the sex chromosomes are inherited in an X-linked, or rarely Y-linked, pattern. See Table 3–1 for a description of selected Mendelian disorders.

DOMINANT VERSUS RECESSIVE DISORDERS

For some disorders, the presence of a single altered gene allele is enough to cause disease; these disorders are said to be **dominant**. An individual who is heterozygous for a dominant disorder will therefore have (or express) the disorder despite the presence of one normally functioning allele. Other disorders occur only when both alleles of a gene pair are altered. In these **recessive** disorders, the gene product produced from a single unaltered gene is sufficient to perform the expected function and maintain homeostasis. Because most human genes reside on autosomes, the most common inheritance patterns are therefore called *autosomal dominant* or *autosomal recessive*. The nurse should realize, however, that the concept of dominant and recessive genes is most useful when considering the relatively rare, single-gene conditions inherited in classic Mendelian fashion.

AUTOSOMAL DOMINANT

More than half of the known Mendelian conditions are autosomal dominant (AD). Examples include neurofibromatosis, achondroplasia (dwarfism), Marfan syndrome, Huntington disease, and familial hypercholesterolemia. By definition, AD disorders involve altered genes on autosomes rather than the sex chromosomes X and Y. Disease occurs in AD disorders despite the presence of one unaltered gene, and most individuals with AD disorders are heterozygous for the disease-producing gene. Homozygous dominant conditions can occur, but they are generally much more severe or lethal and frequently result in early pregnancy loss. For example, the child who is born homozygous for achondroplasia (dwarfism with short stature and short limbs) is much more severely affected than a heterozygous child and usually will not survive early infancy.

Inheritance Risk in Autosomal Dominant Conditions. Because the mutation that causes an AD condition occurs on an autosome rather than a sex chromosome, males and females have an equal chance of being affected. There is a 50% chance that an affected parent will pass the altered disease-producing

TABLE 3–1 Selected Genetic Conditions Inherited in a Mendelian Pattern

GENETIC CONDITION	DESCRIPTION	INHERITANCE PATTERN
Achondroplasia	Abnormal bone growth resulting in short stature	Autosomal dominant More than 80% of cases represent a new mutation
Beta-thalassemia	Reduced synthesis of hemoglobin A resulting in anemia	Autosomal recessive
Cystic fibrosis	Complex multisystem disease leading to end-stage lung disease	Autosomal recessive
Duchenne muscular dystrophy	Progressive disease leading to atrophy of skeletal and/or cardiac muscle	X-linked recessive
Fragile X syndrome	Minimal-to-moderate intellectual disability due to trinucleotide repeat expansion	X-linked recessive Anticipation is demonstrated
Gaucher disease	Several subtypes, but all are lipid storage diseases due to enzyme deficiency	Autosomal recessive
Hemophilia A	Bleeding disorder due to deficient factor VIII clotting activity	X-linked recessive About 30% of cases represent a new mutation
Marfan syndrome	Connective tissue disorder with cardiovascular, ocular, and skeletal involvement	Autosomal dominant 25% of cases represent a new mutation
Neurofibromatosis (NF-1)	Variable expression with café au lait spots and benign cutaneous and subcutaneous neurofibromas	Autosomal dominant 50% of cases represent a new mutation
Phenylketonuria (PKU)	Enzyme deficiency results in accumulation of phenylalanine, inhibiting brain and cognitive development	Autosomal recessive
Sickle cell disease	Abnormal hemoglobin causes vaso-occlusive events and chronic anemia	Autosomal recessive
Tay-Sachs disease	Fatal neurodegenerative disorder of lipid accumulation due to enzyme deficiency	Autosomal recessive

Note: Information adapted from Online Mendelian Inheritance in Man. Retrieved March 14, 2014, from http://omim.org/

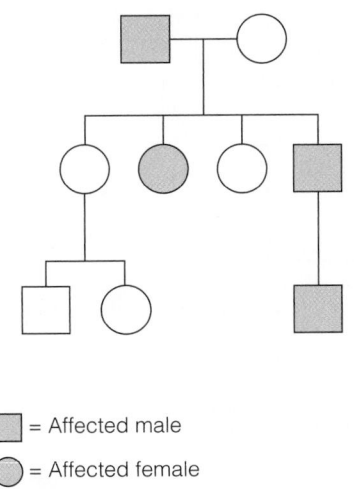

= Affected male

= Affected female

Figure 3–2 **Autosomal dominant pedigree. One parent is affected. Statistically, 50% of offspring will be affected, regardless of sex.**

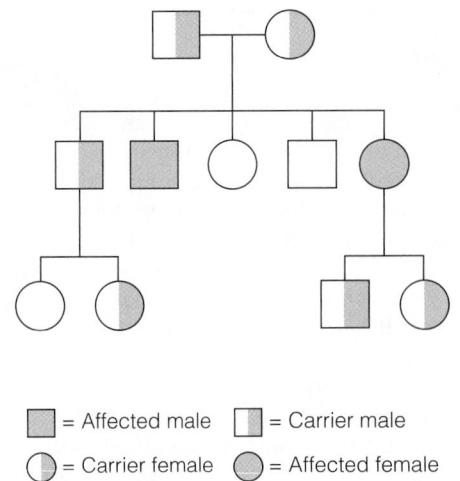

= Affected male ⬜ = Carrier male

= Carrier female ⬤ = Affected female

Figure 3–3 **Autosomal recessive pedigree. Both parents are carriers. Statistically, 25% of offspring will be affected, regardless of sex.**

gene on to a child. Nurses must remember and teach families that no matter how many of a couple's previous children inherited the altered gene, each pregnancy is an independent event with a 50% chance of having an affected child. Family histories will often reflect this 50% inheritance rate as well as both males and females being affected. An affected child always has an affected parent, who in turn also has an affected parent (Figure 3–2). See *Clinical Tip*. Exceptions to this inheritance pattern occur when the condition is due to a spontaneous new mutation, as discussed later in this chapter.

Clinical Tip

When examining a genetic pedigree, the nurse should recognize the following characteristics of autosomal dominant inheritance:

1. Both males and females are affected.
2. Males and females are usually affected in equal numbers.
3. An affected child will have an affected parent, and/or all generations will have an affected individual (appearing as a vertical pattern of affected individuals on the family pedigree).
4. Unaffected children of an affected parent will have unaffected offspring.
5. A significant proportion of isolated cases are due to a new mutation.

AUTOSOMAL RECESSIVE

Autosomal recessive (AR) conditions occur when both copies of the same gene in an individual are altered. Generally, AR conditions are more severe and have an earlier onset than conditions with other patterns of inheritance. Examples of AR conditions include cystic fibrosis, sickle cell disease, Tay-Sachs disease, and most inborn errors of metabolism. Like AD disorders, AR conditions involve genes on one of the 22 autosomes. A condition is called "recessive" when two altered gene copies gene are needed to express the condition. A child born with a recessive condition has therefore inherited one altered gene from each parent. Both parents are **carriers** of the condition (Figure 3–3). Usually carriers do not exhibit signs or symptoms; however, exceptions to this general rule are increasingly being discovered.

Sickle cell disease (SCD) provides an example: Although individuals with a single copy of the altered gene are usually asymptomatic, they can develop symptoms in situations of extreme physical exertion, dehydration, or high altitude (Bender & Hobbs, 2012). The heterozygous, or carrier, state for SCD (known as sickle cell trait) actually affords some evolutionary benefit because a single copy of the altered gene provides some resistance to malaria. Individuals whose ancestors are from malaria-endemic areas are therefore more likely to carry an altered sickle cell gene. Because carrier status usually confers no symptoms, parents are often unaware of their carrier status until they have an affected child.

Because individuals who are related are more likely to be carriers for the same rare AR conditions, children born to parents who are genetically related have an increased risk to inherit a recessive condition. Therefore, **consanguinity** should be identified when taking a family history. See *Clinical Tip*. See *Developing Cultural Competence: Consanguineous Marriages* below.

Clinical Tip

When examining a genetic pedigree, the nurse should recognize the following characteristics of autosomal recessive inheritance:

1. Both males and females are affected.
2. Males and females are usually affected in equal numbers.
3. An affected child will have an unaffected parent but may have affected siblings (appearing as a horizontal pattern of affected individuals on the family pedigree).
4. The condition may appear to skip a generation.
5. The parents of the affected child may be consanguineous (close blood relatives).
6. The family may be descendants of an ethnic group that is known to have a more frequent occurrence of a certain genetic condition.

Inheritance Risk in Autosomal Recessive Conditions.

Because AR conditions do not involve genetic material on the sex chromosomes, males and females have an equal chance

Developing Cultural Competence Consanguineous Marriages

In the United States, marriage between related individuals is generally taboo. In Western medicine, there is a well-recognized concern that a child conceived by people who are related by blood may have an increased risk for birth defects. In many other cultures, however, marriage of first cousins and others who are related by blood is customary or even preferred. Historically, consanguineous marriage has offered a number of social benefits, including stronger family ties, relative ease in finding a suitable partner, support for the woman's status, better relationships with in-laws, and better care for people in old age. In times of high overall infant mortality, the increased risk for passing on serious or life-threatening recessive disorders was likely to be overshadowed by the social security that came with a consanguineous marriage. Today, genetic counseling involves identifying consanguinity and offering risk information, carrier testing, and nondirective counseling.

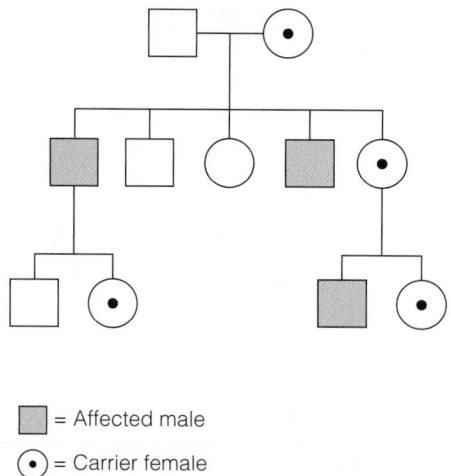

= Affected male

= Carrier female

Figure 3–4 X-linked recessive pedigree. The mother is the carrier. Statistically, 50% of male offspring will be affected, and 50% of female offspring will be carriers.

of inheriting the altered genes and exhibiting the condition. When both parents are carriers of an autosomal recessive gene alteration, each pregnancy presents the same inheritance risks. Each child born to carrier parents has a 25% chance of inheriting two copies of the altered gene and having the condition, a 50% chance of inheriting only one altered gene copy and being a carrier, and a 25% chance of inheriting both unaltered genes and thus neither being affected nor being a carrier. Remembering that each pregnancy is an independent event, these probability percentages remain constant with each pregnancy, no matter how many affected or unaffected children a family already has. This is often a difficult concept for parents to grasp, and the nurse should carefully evaluate the parent's level of understanding of this important detail about inheritance.

The transmission percentages stated previously apply when both parents are carriers of an autosomal recessive condition. Percentages will change if only one parent is a carrier or if a parent is homozygous for the condition. The nurse must be able to teach a parent about these simple inheritance percentages.

X-LINKED

X-linked conditions are the result of an altered gene on the X chromosome. Examples include hemophilia A and Duchenne muscular dystrophy. Most X-linked conditions are recessive; that is, the presence of a normal allele is sufficient to maintain health. Recall, however, that the sex chromosomes are unevenly represented in males and females. Males, with their single X chromosome, have just one copy of each gene that resides on the X chromosome. Any altered X gene will consequently be expressed in males because an unaltered allele is not present for "backup." Females have two copies of each X gene, and the unaltered gene usually compensates for an altered allele, making the female a carrier. This is not the case, however, in X-linked dominant disorders. Such disorders are rare, the most common being vitamin D–resistant rickets. In X-linked dominant conditions, heterozygous females can be affected. Otherwise, the inheritance pattern is the same as X-linked recessive inheritance (Figure 3–4). See *Clinical Tip*.

Clinical Tip

When examining a genetic pedigree, the nurse should recognize the following characteristics of X-linked inheritance:

1. More males will be affected than females.
2. An affected male will have all carrier daughters.
3. There is no male-to-male inheritance.
4. Affected males are related by carrier females.
5. Females may report varying milder symptoms of the condition.
6. A new sporadic case could occur owing to a new mutation.

Recall also that one of the X chromosomes in females is inactivated early in development. Although the inactivation of either the maternal or paternal X chromosome is random in a given cell, every daughter cell (through mitosis) will have the same X chromosome inactivated. Females therefore have a mosaic pattern of X chromosome expression; some of their cells will express genes on the paternal X, and other cells will express genes on the maternal X. Females who inherit altered genes on an X chromosome show variable expression because the gene alteration will be present in only some cells. Expression of symptoms can vary from extremely mild to a full manifestation of the condition. For example, female carriers of X-linked ocular albinism may have pigment deficiencies of their irises and ocular fundi (Turnpenny & Ellard, 2012).

Inheritance Risk in X-Linked Conditions. In families with X-linked disorders, a pattern of maternal transmission is seen. Females who are carriers of X-linked conditions have a 50% chance of passing the altered gene to their offspring. Any daughter who receives the altered gene is likely to receive an unaltered X chromosome from her father and therefore be a carrier like her mother. Sons of carrier mothers, however, have no backup X chromosome. Therefore, a son who inherits the altered X will display the condition and go on to pass that altered X to each of his daughters, who will then be carriers of the altered gene. A male can never transmit an altered gene on the X chromosome to his sons because only Y chromosomes are transmitted from fathers to sons.

Y-LINKED DISORDERS

Because the Y chromosome has very few genes, alterations on the Y chromosome are not often associated with health problems. The Y chromosome does contain genes associated with spermatogenesis, and alterations in those genes can cause male infertility (Turnpenny & Ellard, 2012).

Variability in Classic Mendelian Patterns of Inheritance

In addition to classic Mendelian inheritance patterns, nurses must be prepared to help families understand several other concepts that affect the risk for inheriting a genetic disorder. These concepts include the following common variations in traditional Mendelian patterns of inheritance.

PENETRANCE

Penetrance is the probability that a gene will be expressed phenotypically. It is an "all-or-none" concept; a gene is considered to be penetrant if it is expressed to any degree. Penetrance can be measured in the following way. In a certain group of individuals with the same genotype, what percentage of them will exhibit any signs or symptoms of the condition? If the number is less than 100%, then that condition is said to show *reduced* or *incomplete penetrance*. For example, both achondroplasia and Huntington disease exhibit 100% penetrance because every individual with one copy of the altered gene will exhibit signs and symptoms of the disease.

VARIABLE EXPRESSION

The term *expressivity* is used to describe the degree to which a phenotype is expressed. When people with the same genetic makeup (genotype) exhibit signs or symptoms with varying degrees of severity, the phenotype is described as showing *variable expression*. Variable expression is common in the autosomal dominant condition neurofibromatosis type 1 (NF-1). Although neurofibromatosis has 100% penetrance, members of the same affected family often exhibit marked variation in degree of signs or symptoms (Friedman, 2012).

NEW MUTATIONS

When there is no previous family history of a condition, the disease may be caused by a spontaneous new mutation. A new mutation is said to be sporadic or de novo. Mutation rates have been estimated for a number of inherited disorders and vary widely due to a number of factors, only some of which are understood. Diseases with high new mutation rates include NF-1, achondroplasia, Duchenne muscular dystrophy, and hemophilia A and B. Determining whether a genetic condition is due to an inherited or a de novo mutation has important implications in calculating a family's recurrence risk.

IMPRINTING

The expression of a few genetic conditions varies depending on whether the altered gene is inherited from the mother or the father. This differential gene expression is due to genomic **imprinting**. Imprinting takes place before gametes are formed, when certain genes are chemically marked as having maternal or paternal origin. After conception, the imprint controls gene expression so that only one allele, either maternal or paternal, is expressed. If the unsilenced (active) allele carries a mutation, disease may result. A well-studied example of imprinting involves a deletion in a gene on chromosome 15 that causes two very different disorders depending on whether the altered gene comes from the mother or the father. Prader-Willi syndrome, characterized by hypotonia in infancy, excessive eating habits leading to obesity, and mild-to-moderate intellectual disability, is due to a deletion on chromosome 15 that is inherited from the father. Angelman syndrome is due to a similar deletion in the same gene on chromosome 15, but it is inherited from the mother. The clinical presentation is very different. Individuals with Angelman syndrome have severe intellectual disability, absent speech, an uncoordinated gait, seizures, and a happy, sociable disposition (Schaaf et al., 2012).

Multifactorial Inheritance

Multifactorial conditions aggregate in families but do not follow the characteristic Mendelian patterns of inheritance seen with single-gene conditions. Multifactorial conditions often present with highly variable severity. Neural tube disorder, for example, ranges from spina bifida occulta to myelomeningocele to anencephaly. Often, more severe defects reflect a greater number of altered genes. Some multifactorial conditions show a sex bias. Pyloric stenosis, for example, is more common in males, whereas cleft palate is more common among females. When a member of the less commonly affected sex shows the condition, a greater number of altered genes are thought to be present. This situation confers a higher risk for recurrence of the disorder for clients and their relatives. Recurrence risk varies among multifactorial conditions but is usually less than that of Mendelian conditions. Recurrence risk is calculated from population studies and expressed as a percentage; for some disorders, recurrence risk is not easily predicted. Recurrence risk varies according to the number of affected family members, the degree of relationship, and sometimes the severity of the defect. As examples, the recurrence risk for cleft lip or cleft palate in a family with one affected child is 4%, while recurrence risk for pyloric stenosis is as high as 10% (Turnpenny & Ellard, 2012).

Although most congenital malformations are multifactorial (Table 3–2), a careful family history should always be taken because occasionally cleft lip and palate, certain congenital heart defects, and other malformations are inherited as autosomal dominant or recessive traits. Adult-onset disorders such as type 2 diabetes, hypertension, some heart diseases, and some mental illness, are also included in the multifactorial inheritance group.

Genetic Testing

Many health professionals work together in the screening, diagnosis, identification, and treatment of genetic disorders. The goals of collaborative care are early diagnosis through assessment and testing, development of an effective treatment plan combined with psychosocial support to enhance coping, and referral to a genetic specialist when needed.

Genetic tests are useful to diagnose disease, predict risk of future disease, inform reproductive decision making, and manage client care. The landscape of genetic testing is changing rapidly. New methodologies have expanded the number of conditions for which genetic testing is available and reduced the cost. Genetic nurses express concern that genetic tests are becoming available very quickly with little regulation of the companies offering them. For example, some genetic testing is offered directly to consumers

TABLE 3–2 Common Birth Defects and Conditions With a Multifactorial Cause

Neural tube defects	A neural tube defect (NTD) is a condition that occurs early during fetal development with incomplete closure of the neural tube. Severity of the disorder varies, depending on which part of the tube does not close. Anencephaly, meningomyelocele, and spina bifida are examples of NTD. Recurrence risk is increased in families with an affected child, but that risk can be modified by maternal dietary folic acid supplementation (Turnpenny & Ellard, 2012).
Congenital heart defects	Most congenital heart defects are thought to be of multifactorial cause. A number of genes have been associated with patent ductus arteriosus, atrial or ventricular septal defects, and other heart defects. In some states, newborn screening for critical congenital heart disease is performed routinely using pulse oximetry (Bradshaw & Martin, 2012).
Cleft lip and palate	Cleft lip and/or palate (CL/P) occur as a result of failure of bony fusion early in gestation. While rare gene mutations can cause CL/P, most cases are thought to be multifactorial. The more severe the malformation, the higher the family's recurrence risk is for future pregnancies (Tobias, Connor, & Ferguson-Smith, 2011).
Autism spectrum disorder	Although the etiology of autism spectrum disorder remains poorly understood, most experts believe it to be multifactorial. Twin studies suggest a strong genetic component, with 60%–90% concordance between identical twins. A number of environmental influences have been suspected to influence the development of autism as well, including environmental exposures, viral infections, and maternal stress (Johnson, Giarelli, Lewis, et al., 2013).

without benefit of oversight by a healthcare provider, nor is counseling or follow-up uniformly provided. Individuals may make hard and irrevocable life-altering decisions after receiving test results, so accuracy and reliability, along with professional counseling, are essential (Beery & Workman, 2012). Guidelines regarding who should be tested and when to test are available for some genetic conditions. However, new knowledge accumulates rapidly, and recommendations for practice often lag behind research findings by several years.

Nurses must have knowledge of available genetic tests and their implications to assist clients and their families as they weigh choices regarding genetic testing. Genetic testing can be done for screening or diagnostic purposes, can detect both chromosomal and gene-based alterations, and can be done across development, from early in the prenatal period to any time after birth. Some genetic testing is done on specimens obtained noninvasively, such as a cheek swab or peripheral blood sample; other tests require invasive procedures such as amniocentesis or biopsy. See Box 3–1.

> **Box 3–1 What Is a Genetic Test?**
>
> A genetic test involves the analysis of chromosomes, DNA, RNA, genes, or gene products (e.g., enzymes and other proteins) to detect variations related to disease or health. Whether a laboratory method is considered a genetic test also depends on the intended use, claim, or purpose of a test. For example, amino acid analysis to detect metabolic disorders such as phenylketonuria (PKU) is considered a genetic test, but the use of this same analysis to monitor general nutritional status is not (U.S. Department of Health and Human Services, 2008).

Categories of Genetic Tests

Genetic tests have been used for some time to detect heritable conditions that are passed from generation to generation. There are several categories of genetic testing, each with a unique purpose. See Table 3–3.

TABLE 3–3 Categories of Genetic Tests

TYPE OF TEST	DESCRIPTION
Diagnostic testing	Used to establish a diagnosis of a genetic disorder in an individual who is symptomatic or has had a positive screening test.
Prenatal testing	Testing to identify a fetus with a genetic disease or condition. Some prenatal testing is offered routinely; other testing may be initiated on account of family history or maternal factors.
Newborn screening	Testing of a newborn to identify the presence of a condition that requires immediate initiation of treatment to prevent death or disability.
Preimplantation testing	Following in vitro fertilization (IVF), testing to identify embryos with a particular genetic condition.
Carrier testing	Testing in an asymptomatic individual to identify carrier status for a genetic condition.
Presymptomatic and predictive testing	Offered usually to asymptomatic individuals to detect genetic conditions that occur later in life. • *Presymptomatic testing* detects mutations that, if present, are likely or certain to eventually cause symptoms (an example is Huntington disease). • *Predictive*, or *predispositional, testing* detects mutations that increase the likelihood that symptoms will develop (such as *BRCA1* and *BRCA2*).

It is especially important for nurses to understand the difference between a screening test and a diagnostic test, which lies in the purpose of the test. Screening tests are population-based tests designed to find individuals at risk for a disorder. They are designed to be very sensitive; that is, to find every case. Sensitive tests, however, will sometimes be positive in individuals who do not have the disorder; that is, false-positive tests do occur. For that reason, a positive screening test must be followed by a diagnostic test. Newborn screening provides an excellent example. Most newborns in developed countries are screened for a variety of genetic diseases, most rare. Recent advances in laboratory technology have allowed greatly expanded newborn screening with little increase in cost, and newborns in some states are tested for more than 40 rare conditions. Each positive screening test must be followed by a diagnostic test. Fortunately, most positive screening tests are falsely positive, but the cost of follow-up testing is significant both in terms of parental anxiety and financial burden (DeLuca, Zanni, Bonhomme, et al., 2013).

Diagnostic tests are performed to confirm a diagnosis when a child is suspected of having a specific disorder based on clinical presentation or screening test results.

Diagnosing Chromosomal Alterations

Cytogenetics describes the microscopic examination of chromosomes to reveal large alterations such as additions, deletions, breaks, and rearrangements or rejoinings (translocations). Prenatally, amniocentesis and chorionic villi sampling (CVS) can be undertaken to provide specimens for cytogenetic examination. After a child is born, chromosomal diagnostic examination can be accomplished with a blood, skin, or buccal cell sample. Cytogenetic testing includes karyotyping, as described earlier in this chapter, and molecular cytogenetic techniques, which are capable of detecting submicroscopic DNA variations too small to be seen on a karyotype.

Diagnosing Gene Alterations

Recent advances in molecular genetic technology along with the mapping of the human genome have resulted in tremendous expansion of available genetic testing. Genetic testing is currently available for nearly 3000 diseases, with new tests constantly being added (Lander, 2011). DNA-based tests involve sophisticated new technology that permits the detection of DNA sequence changes as small as a single nucleotide. These tests can be performed on blood, bone marrow, amniotic fluid, fibroblast cells of the skin, or buccal cells from the mouth. Genetic testing can examine DNA (to determine specific nucleotide sequence), RNA (to measure gene expression), or proteins (to analyze gene products). Some tests can be performed quickly; others require several days to weeks, or occasionally several months, before results are reported.

Genes are very long DNA sequences made up of hundreds of thousands of nucleotides (or base pairs). Alterations at various sites along a gene may alter its function and cause disease. As an example, the *CFTR* gene (which in an altered form causes cystic fibrosis) is 230,000 base pairs long, and nearly 2000 different *CFTR* mutations have been identified (Cystic Fibrosis Mutation Database, 2014). Most of these mutations are exceedingly rare; the most common (named delta F508) is found in about two thirds of affected individuals (De Boeck, Zolin, Cuppens, et al., 2014). Although DNA testing is capable of detecting any of these alterations in DNA sequence, it is not feasible to test for all of them. Currently available *CFTR* tests detect from about 23 to 98 different mutations. The chance of missing an uncommon mutation therefore varies depending on which test is selected. Also, mutation detection rates are higher in people of

European ancestry than other populations. Therefore, a "negative" CF test must be interpreted with caution and an eye on how many mutations were included in the test. This is just one of the limitations of genetic testing that nurses must understand in order to provide genetically competent care. See *The Role of the Nurse in Genetic Testing* section below.

Other Genetic Tests

Tests are available to measure gene expression, For example, **microarray analysis** can detect levels of messenger RNA in cells, which indicates which genes are "turned on" or being expressed. Microarray analysis is especially useful to examine tumor cells.

Often, genetic tests do not examine DNA directly, but are biochemical tests for gene products or metabolites of gene products. Most newborn screening tests are biochemical. For example, PKU is caused by an alteration in the gene encoding the enzyme phenylalanine hydroxylase (PAH), which breaks down dietary phenylalanine. The PKU test actually measures phenylalanine levels, which are markedly elevated in individuals with PKU. Many of these biochemical tests have been in use for years.

Prenatal Testing

Nurses who care for childbearing families may be responsible for counseling about prenatal testing for congenital or inherited conditions. Screening and invasive diagnostic testing for chromosome abnormalities should be available to all women who present for prenatal care before 20 weeks of pregnancy regardless of maternal age. Nurses therefore require current information and sufficient expertise to explain testing to families. Women should be counseled regarding the differences between screening and diagnostic testing. For example, noninvasive screening tests, such as nuchal translucency ultrasound and maternal serum screening, are designed to assess a pregnancy's risk of chromosomal abnormalities or a neural tube defect. If the risk is increased above a specific cutoff, the woman is offered invasive prenatal diagnosis. These diagnostic techniques, such as amniocentesis and CVS, obtain cells from the pregnancy to rule out or diagnose a chromosomal abnormality or certain genetic disorders. They are associated with a small risk of pregnancy complications, including miscarriage.

Several methods of prenatal testing are currently available. The tests are used for different purposes and involve varying degrees of risk.

GENETIC ULTRASOUND

Ultrasound may be used to assess the fetus for genetic or congenital problems. With ultrasound, one can visualize the fetal head for abnormalities in size, shape, and structure. Craniospinal defects (anencephalus, microcephaly, hydrocephalus), thoracic malformations (diaphragmatic hernia), gastrointestinal malformations (omphalocele, gastroschisis), renal malformations (dysplasia or obstruction), and skeletal malformations (caudal regression, conjoined twins) are just some of the disorders that have been diagnosed in utero by ultrasound.

Screening by ultrasound for congenital anomalies is best done at 16 to 20 weeks, when fetal structures have developed completely. With the addition of a fetal nuchal translucency measurement at 10 to 14 weeks, there is high correlation with fetal chromosomal abnormalities (Gilbert, 2011). The nuchal translucency is a fluid-filled space at the back of the fetal neck. An increased amount of fluid is associated with an increased risk for chromosomal abnormalities, birth defects, genetic syndromes, and poor pregnancy outcome—the larger the nuchal translucency, the higher the risk for abnormalities. There is no information documenting harm to the fetus or long-term effects with exposure to ultrasound. However, there is no guarantee of complete safety; therefore, the practitioner and the parents must evaluate the risks against the benefits on an individual basis.

MATERNAL SERUM SCREENING

Measuring specific hormones and proteins in the maternal serum during the first and/or second trimester can determine the risk for Down syndrome, trisomy 18, or open spina bifida. In the first trimester, the nuchal translucency measurement is often added to improve the detection rate for Down syndrome and trisomy 18. Detection and false-positive rates vary depending on the type of screening test that is performed and sometimes the laboratory that performs the screening.

NONINVASIVE PRENATAL TESTING

Noninvasive prenatal testing (NIPT) for chromosomal abnormalities, which examines fetal DNA circulating in maternal serum, is now available. Approximately 3% to 13% of the circulating DNA in a woman's plasma is derived from the placenta (ACOG/SMFM, 2012). Several laboratories have developed techniques to quantify fetal DNA fragments as early as 9 to 10 weeks of gestation in order to detect some of the common trisomies (including Down syndrome, trisomy 18, and trisomy 13). NIPT shows greater sensitivity and specificity than traditional maternal serum screening but is not yet meant to replace diagnostic testing such

as amniocentesis or CVS. NIPT has limitations, including limited data on low-risk pregnancies, twin gestations, and pregnancies with a vanishing twin as well as concerns about false-positive results due to maternal or placental mosaicism (ACOG/SMFM, 2012). At this time, NIPT is used as a screening test and is recommended primarily for women of advanced maternal age or other indications of a high-risk pregnancy such as fetal ultrasound findings suggestive of aneuploidy; history of prior pregnancy with trisomy 21, trisomy 18, or trisomy 13; or positive maternal serum screening. Clients with abnormal NIPT results, or those with other factors suggestive of a chromosomal abnormality, should receive genetic counseling and be given the option of standard confirmatory diagnostic testing (Devers et al., 2013).

GENETIC AMNIOCENTESIS AND CVS

Methods of prenatal diagnosis include genetic amniocentesis and CVS. Figure 3–5 illustrates these two procedures. Both tests collect cells derived from fetal origin and are therefore invasive. With amniocentesis, a needle is inserted into the amniotic fluid under continuous ultrasound guidance and a small amount of amniotic fluid is collected. Fetal cells can then be cultured and tested. With CVS, a tiny amount of placental tissue of fetal origin is obtained by inserting a needle through either the abdomen or cervix. While amniocentesis is offered after 15 weeks of gestation, CVS can be performed after 9 weeks. A variety of tests can be performed on the fetal cells collected from either procedure.

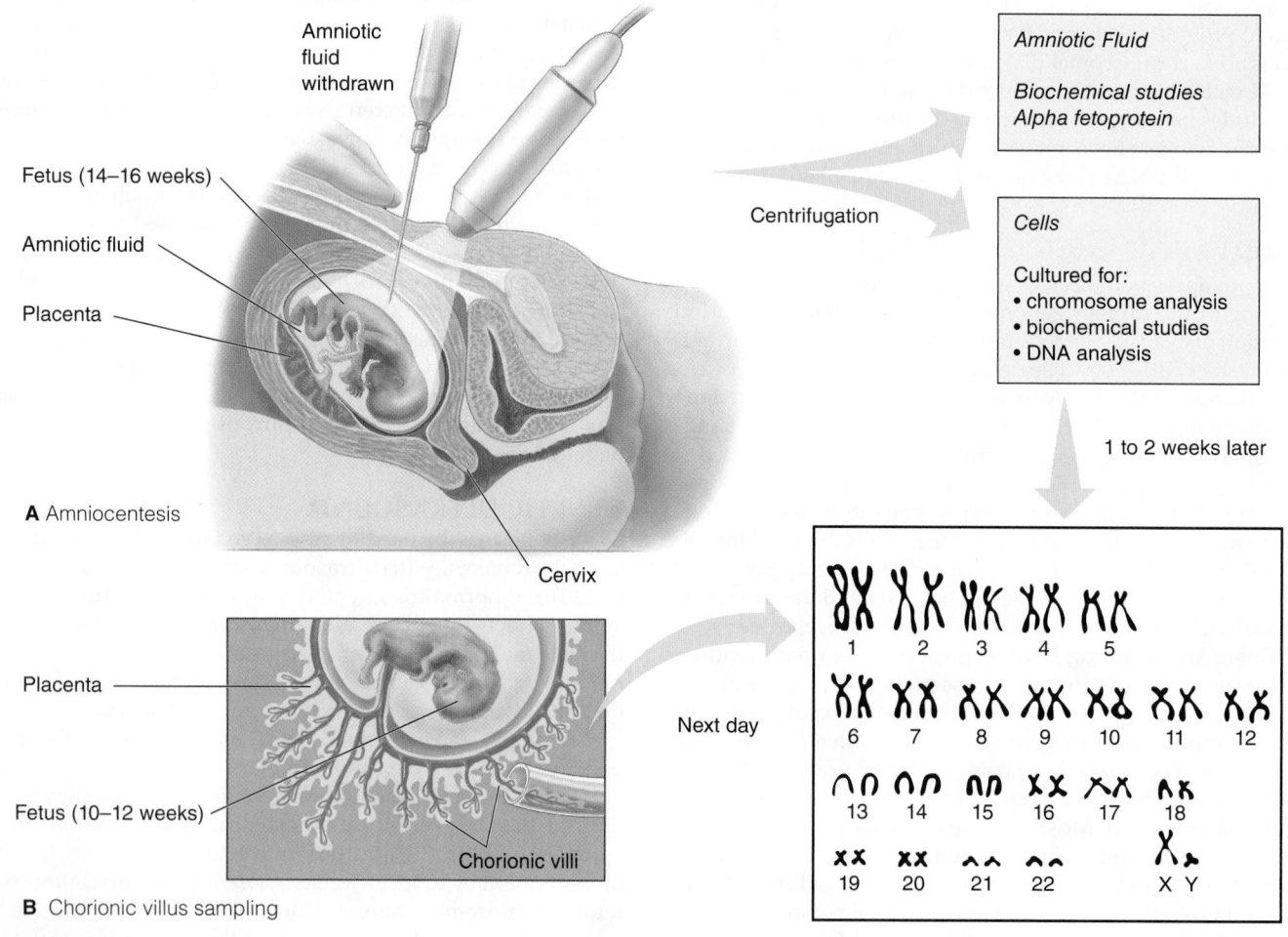

Figure 3–5 *A,* **Genetic amniocentesis for prenatal diagnosis can be done after 15 weeks' gestation. Fetal cells are cultured and tested; results take 7 to 14 days.** *B,* **Chorionic villus sampling is done after 9 weeks' gestation; results take 1 to 3 days.**

Both procedures carry a small risk for pregnancy complications, including infection and miscarriage. Although invasive diagnostic testing should be available to all women (ACOG, 2007), testing is frequently targeted to women who meet one or more of the following criteria:

1. *Maternal age 35 or older.* Women ages 35 or older are at greater risk for having children with chromosomal abnormalities. Chromosomal abnormalities because of maternal age include trisomy 21, trisomy 13, trisomy 18, XXX, or XXY. A woman's risk for having an infant with a chromosomal abnormality increases from less than 1 in 1000 at age 21 years to about 1 in 350 at age 35 and 1 in 30 at age 46 (Schaaf et al., 2012).

2. *Previous child born with a chromosomal abnormality.* Young couples who have had a child with a trisomy 21, 18, or 13 have an approximately 1% to 2% risk of a future child having a chromosomal abnormality.

3. *Parent carrying a chromosomal abnormality (balanced translocation).* A woman who carries a balanced 14/21 translocation has a risk of approximately 10% to 15% that her children will be affected with the unbalanced translocation of Down syndrome; if the father is the carrier, there is a 2% to 5% risk.

4. *Mother carrying an X-linked disease.* In families in which the woman is a known or possible carrier of an X-linked disorder such as hemophilia A or B or Duchenne muscular dystrophy, the risk of an affected male fetus is 50%. Now DNA testing may make it possible to identify affected males from nonaffected males in some disorders.

5. *Parents carrying an inborn error of metabolism that can be diagnosed in utero.* Inborn errors of metabolism disorders are detectable in utero by DNA analysis or biochemical testing; these include Fabry disease, galactosemia, Gaucher disease, homocystinuria, Hunter syndrome, Hurler syndrome, Krabbe disease, Lesch-Nyhan disease, maple syrup urine disease, metachromatic leukodystrophy, methylmalonic aciduria, Niemann-Pick disease, Pompe disease, and Tay-Sachs disease.

6. *Both parents carrying an autosomal recessive disease.* When both parents are carriers of an autosomal recessive disease, there is a 25% risk for each pregnancy that the fetus will be affected. Autosomal recessive diseases identified by amniocentesis are hemoglobinopathies such as sickle cell disease, thalassemia, and cystic fibrosis.

7. *Family history of neural tube defects.* Genetic amniocentesis is available to couples who have had a child with neural tube defects or who have a family history of these conditions, which include anencephaly, spina bifida, and myelomeningocele. Neural tube defects are usually multifactorial traits.

8. *Positive screening test.* When the first- or second-semester maternal screening test and/or ultrasound exam indicates the fetus may be affected with an aneuploidy or neural tube defect, further testing may be offered. This may be in the form of a more accurate noninvasive test (NIPT) or an invasive diagnostic test such as CVS or amniocentesis. For further discussion see Chapter 13.

PERCUTANEOUS UMBILICAL BLOOD SAMPLING

Percutaneous umbilical blood sampling (PUBS), also called *cordocentesis,* involves drawing blood from the umbilical vein under direct ultrasound guidance. It can be performed after 18 weeks' gestation and allows rapid chromosomal diagnosis and other genetics studies, but its use has diminished as other technologies have become more readily available.

Nursing Management

Nurses are on the front line of client care and need to be competent in genetic- and genomic-related health care. Specific competencies are expected of all professional nurses. These competencies include eliciting a genetic family history and depicting it in a pedigree; identifying current, credible genetic information; identifying clients and families who might benefit from referral to a genetic expert; and managing genetic information (Consensus Panel on Genetic/Genomic Nursing Competencies, 2009). This section focuses on the roles of nurses in the care of clients and families with genetic health issues.

Assessing Genetic Risk

All professional nurses should incorporate awareness of genetic risk into the assessments they perform. "Thinking genetic" is important throughout health assessment, in collecting the health history, performing the physical assessment, and interpreting assessment findings.

ASSESSING REPRODUCTIVE RISK

Nursing care for the childbearing family includes identifying women who may be at increased risk to have a child with a genetic disorder. Nurses should be aware of risk factors that indicate a couple may benefit from a genetic referral or consideration for prenatal testing. Annual examinations and other clinic appointments provide opportunities to identify women whose family history or other factors indicate risk. If couples with genetic risk factors are planning to conceive, the nurse may encourage them to consider genetic counseling before discontinuing contraception. See *Health Promotion: Couples Who May Benefit From Prenatal Diagnostic Testing* below.

Health Promotion **Couples Who May Benefit From Prenatal Diagnostic Testing**

- Women ages 35 or older at time of birth

- Couples with a balanced translocation (chromosomal abnormality)

- Family history of known or suspected Mendelian genetic disorder (e.g., cystic fibrosis, hemophilia A and B, Duchenne muscular dystrophy)

- Couples with a previous child with chromosomal abnormality

- Couples in which either partner or a previous child is affected with, or in which both partners are carriers for, a diagnosable metabolic disorder

- Family history of birth defects and/or intellectual disability (e.g., neural tube defects, congenital heart disease, cleft lip and/or palate)

- Ethnic groups at increased risk for specific disorders (see *Developing Cultural Competence: Genetic Screening Recommendations for Various Ethnic and Age Groups* below)

- Couples with history of two or more first-trimester spontaneous abortions

- Women with an abnormal maternal serum alpha-fetoprotein (MSAFP or AFP) test

- Women with a teratogenic risk secondary to an exposure or maternal health condition (e.g., diabetes)

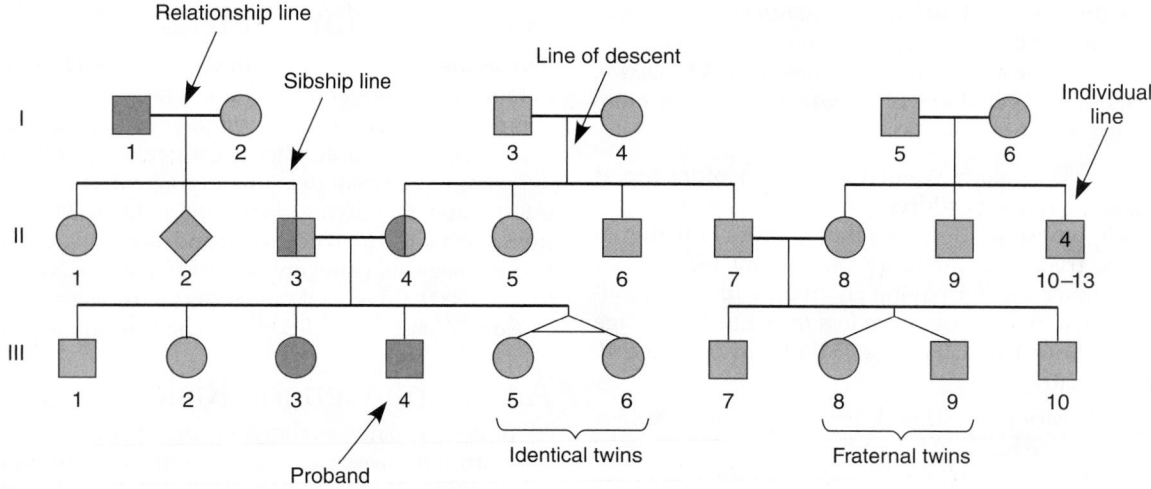

Figure 3–6   Sample three-generation pedigree.

FAMILY HISTORY AND THE GENETIC PEDIGREE

An expectation of all professional nurses is that they know how to collect a three-generation family history and record the history in a pedigree using standard symbols and terminology. Information to document in a family history includes:

- First name of all family members with age or year of birth
- Any medical conditions or diseases including age at diagnosis
- Age and cause of death
- Infertility or no children by choice
- Pregnancy complications with gestational age indicated
- Adoption status
- Ancestry
- Consanguinity

A **pedigree** is a graphic representation or diagram of a family's medical history and genetic relationships. Figure 3–6 shows a sample pedigree. Standard format and nomenclature for pedigrees, which includes multiple symbols (Figure 3–7), have been adopted (Bennett, 2010). A pedigree is constructed around a designated "index" patient, called the **proband** (if he or she is affected with the genetic disorder of interest) or **consultand** (if he or she seeks genetic counseling without being known to have the disorder). A finished pedigree provides a clear, visual representation of a family's medical data and biologic relationships at a glance. A pedigree identifies affected individuals in the immediate and extended family and can identify family members who might benefit from a genetic consultation. A pedigree can also illustrate patterns of inheritance and clusters of multifactorial conditions. On the basis of the pedigree, genetic referral and/or reproductive risk teaching for the individual and family can occur. The visual nature of a pedigree enhances a family's learning and can be used to clarify misunderstandings or misconceptions about inheritance. If completed correctly and comprehensively, a pedigree allows all healthcare professionals working with the child or family to see quickly what history and background information has been collected.

Throughout the process of gathering family history information, the nurse must protect family confidentiality. A pedigree is different from a personal health history in that it reflects information about multiple individuals, which greatly increases the risk for harm if confidentiality is broken. A pedigree may reveal sensitive details that include infertility problems, reproductive decisions, or misassigned paternity that may not be known by a current partner or other family members. Other sensitive issues include pregnancies conceived by technology, a history of suicides, drug or alcohol abuse, and same-sex relationships.

Challenges inherent in recalling the family history include failure to report conditions thought not to be genetic or attributed to other causes, or to recall conditions that have been surgically repaired and forgotten. Also, clients may be reluctant to

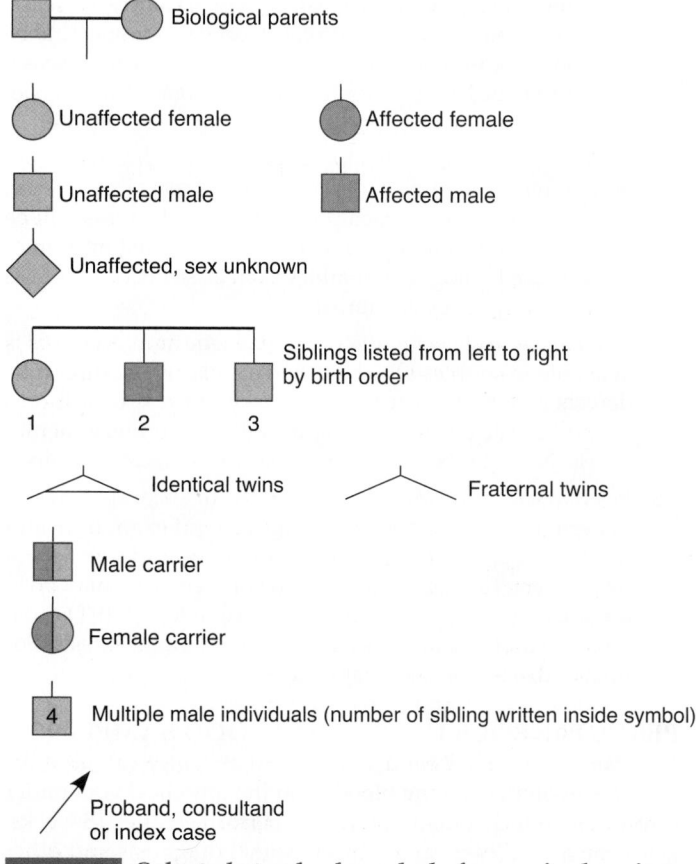

Figure 3–7   Selected standard symbols for use in drawing a pedigree.

reveal sensitive information, particularly information unknown to other family members.

Families are encouraged to collect and record their own family history in a form that can be shared within the family as well as with healthcare providers. The U.S. Surgeon General's Family History Initiative is a national campaign to promote the collection of family histories. The Initiative provides a web-based program entitled "My Family Health Portrait" that allows individuals to easily record and save their information, as well as print their family pedigree.

Clinical Tip

Follow these steps when drawing a pedigree:

I. Organization

1. Begin recording data in the middle of the sheet of paper (to allow enough room for both the maternal and paternal sides of the family).

2. Use only standard pedigree symbols (see Figure 3–7).

3. Place the male individual in a couple on the left of the relationship line; the paternal side of the family will also be on the left side of the paper.

II. Determining Family Relationships

1. Determine relationships within the family by asking questions such as:
   - Do you have a partner or are you married?
   - How many biologic brothers and sisters do you have?
   - How many children do you have? Are they with the same partner?
   - Do all the children have the same biologic father?
   - Do your siblings share the same mother and father as you?

2. Referring to "the baby's father or mother" can be helpful until the relationship between parents is established.

3. Referring to a "union" if marriage does not exist can also help communication.

III. Who Should or Should Not Be Included

1. To ensure accuracy, the pedigree should include the parents, offspring, siblings, aunts, uncles, grandparents, and first cousins of the individual seeking counseling.

2. Detailed information about the spouses of the proband's family can be omitted unless there is a history of some kind of disorder or condition.

3. Eliminating persons or information that does not contribute any valuable information can help keep the pedigree small and more manageable.

IV. Recording the Family History

1. It may be useful to determine the approximate size of the family, to plan spacing on paper.

2. Begin the drawing with the proband (the person who is seeking counseling or is affected with the genetic condition). Mark the proband with an arrow.

3. Then add the symbols for the brothers and sisters of the proband and an individual line for each. Connect the individual lines with a sibship line and add a line of descent, the relationship line for the parents, and symbols for parents of the proband.

4. Repeat this step for children of the proband and children of the proband's siblings.

5. Continue with symbols for all immediate relatives of the proband's parents and grandparents. Record ancestry or country of origin of the first generation at the top of the page.

6. Mark each symbol to designate relevant information (see Figure 3–7).

7. Create a key to contain all information relevant to interpretation of the pedigree.

8. The pedigree should include at least three generations.
   - Mark each generation with a Roman numeral along the left side of the paper with the first generation marker (I) at the top.
   - Each person in a generation should fall along the same imaginary horizontal line.

9. The pedigree should include:
   - Half-siblings, pregnancy losses, stillbirths, previous marriages, and adopted children
   - The reason for taking the pedigree (e.g., developmental disability, dysmorphology)
   - The name of the family historian (person relaying the information)

V. Other

1. **Consanguinity** may be suspected if the historian repeatedly gives the same last name on both sides of the family. Ask if any relatives in the family have ever had a child together.

VI. Completing the Pedigree

1. When completed, the pedigree should be dated and signed with the name, credentials, and position of the person drawing it.

Source: Data from Bennett, R. L. (2010). *The practical guide to the genetic family history* (2nd ed.). Copyright © 2010 John Wiley & Sons. Reproduced with permission of John Wiley & Sons, Inc.

GENETIC PHYSICAL ASSESSMENT

Nurses caring for newborns and children in any setting should also "think genetic" when performing physical assessment. An early finding by the nurse will provide the child and family with an opportunity for a genetic referral and more specialized health care. **Dysmorphology** refers to the study of human congenital defects or abnormalities of body structure that begin before birth. Traditionally, congenital anomalies have been included under the umbrella of genetic disorders whether they occur due to a gene alteration or another cause of abnormal embryonic or fetal development. Dysmorphic anomalies can occur anywhere in the body, but are perhaps most often associated with facial features. As a routine part of client assessment, the nurse should screen for both minor and major anomalies. A **minor anomaly** or malformation is an unusual morphologic feature that in itself is of no serious medical or cosmetic concern to the individual or family. The presence of a single minor anomaly is relatively common, occurring in approximately 10% of newborns, and is usually of no consequence (Turnpenny & Ellard, 2012). Some minor anomalies are merely family traits or are present in certain ethnic groups. Minor anomalies include such traits as wide-set eyes, single palmar creases, café au lait patches, low anterior hairline, preauricular (in front of the ears) pits and tags, broad face, or mild proportionate short stature. Examples of variations associated with ethnic origin include upward-slanting eyes or prominent epicanthal folds among individuals of Asian descent.

The appearance of multiple minor anomalies in an infant is of greater concern. Fewer than 1% of newborns have two minor anomalies, and fewer still have three or more. But of those newborns who do have multiple minor anomalies, many will also have a major anomaly or an underlying genetic condition. Therefore, the nurse who notes multiple minor anomalies in a newborn or child should consider the possibility of a major anomaly or an underlying genetic condition and advocate for a genetic referral. For example, a newborn who is hypotonic and has a single palmar crease with up-slanting eyes that do not resemble his parent's eyes should be evaluated for Down syndrome.

About 2% to 3% of all children have a **major anomaly**, defined as a serious structural defect present at birth that may have severe medical or cosmetic consequences, interfere with normal functioning of body systems, lead to a lifelong disability, or even cause an early death. Congenital heart defects, cleft lip and/or palate, myelomeningocele, duodenal atresia, and craniosynostosis are considered major anomalies, as is developmental disability. Some major anomalies are present at birth but are not apparent, such as deafness, various skeletal dysplasias, and some types of congenital heart defects (Turnpenny & Ellard, 2012).

A **syndrome** is a collection of multiple anomalies, major or minor, that occur in a consistent pattern and have a common cause. For example, Down syndrome causes a variety of anomalies in multiple body systems, including the eyes, ears, hair, mouth and tongue, heart, and brain. A **sequence** is a collection of anomalies that occur as a chain of events initiated by a single problem. As an example, Potter sequence begins with prenatal failure of renal development, which leads to small amounts of amniotic fluid, which in turn causes growth restriction. An **association** is a group of abnormalities of unknown cause that occur together more often than is expected by chance (Schaaf et al., 2012).

The nurse can identify clues to genetic problems by examining the child and considering the physical characteristics of the parents and other family members (see *Assessment Guide: The Child With Selected Dysmorphic Physical Features* below). Nurses may even ask to look at family photographs and examine them for common dysmorphic features and family traits. Several standardized craniofacial measurements have been defined, and tables are available displaying normal values according to age, so that dysmorphic facial features can be more easily identified. Figure 3–8 depicts some standard measurements used in describing facial features. By advocating for a genetic referral, the nurse can make a difference in the child's state of health.

The Role of the Nurse in Genetic Testing

For childbearing families, genetic screening is routinely offered in the prenatal and newborn periods and is commonly performed in the diagnostic workup for children with a variety of health problems or concerns. Many people have misconceptions about genetic testing. Nurses play an important role in teaching parents and children about the implications and limitations of genetic tests to ensure that they make informed decisions. The nurse should promote communication, autonomy, and privacy when helping families. Recognizing that genetic testing affects families, and not just individuals, the nurse should use a family perspective when assisting parents and children who are making decisions about genetic testing. Not all family members will want to know their genetic risks. All voices should be heard, and each family member's decision should be respected, whether it is to participate in genetic testing or to decline. To ensure autonomy, a nondirective approach is critical; nurses must take care to avoid imposing their own values or personal opinions onto clients and families. Finally, as with all aspects of delivering genetic nursing care, privacy and confidentiality are paramount.

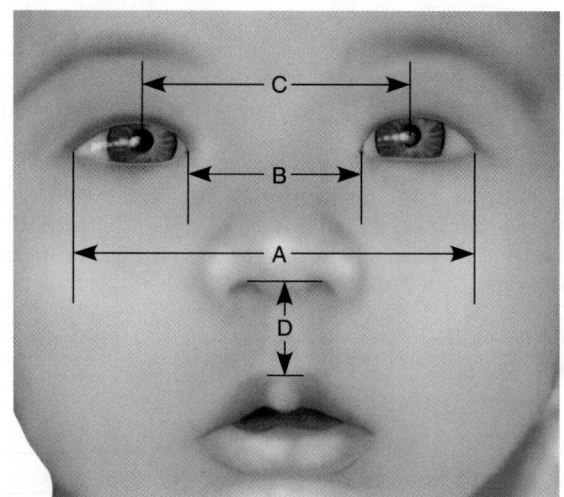

Figure 3–8 Classic facial measurements for genetic assessment with a focus on facial features. *A,* Outer intercanthal distance. *B,* Intercanthal distance. *C,* Interpupillary distance. *D,* Philtrum length.

PRENATAL GENETIC TESTING

It is essential that couples be informed before any prenatal testing is done, whether that testing is routine screening or diagnostic testing. Counseling should address the reason for the test, the potential outcomes and follow-up tests that may be indicated based on those outcomes, potential risks and benefits of testing, and limitations and implications. The nurse must recognize the emotional impact on the family of a decision to undergo or not to undergo genetic testing and ensure that any decision to undergo prenatal testing is based on autonomous decision making and informed consent.

Every pregnancy has a 3% to 4% risk of resulting in an infant with a birth defect. When an abnormality is detected or suspected before birth, an attempt is made to determine the diagnosis by assessing the family health history (via the pedigree) and the pregnancy history and by evaluating the fetal anomaly or anomalies via ultrasound. After experts on a specific disorder have been consulted, healthcare professionals can then present the parents with options. Treatment of prenatally diagnosed disorders may begin during the pregnancy, thus possibly preventing irreversible damage. In light of the philosophy of preventive health care, information that can be obtained prenatally should be made available to all couples who are expecting a baby or who are contemplating pregnancy.

With the advent of diagnostic techniques such as amniocentesis, at-risk couples who would not otherwise have a first child or additional children can decide to conceive. Following prenatal diagnosis, a couple can decide not to have a child with a genetic disease. For many couples, prenatal diagnosis is not a solution because they choose not to prevent the genetic disease by aborting the fetus. The decision about whether to use prenatal diagnosis can only be made by the family. Even when termination is not an option, prenatal diagnosis can give parents an opportunity to prepare for the birth of a child with special needs, contact the families of children with similar problems, or access support services before the birth.

Client Advocacy (or Considerations) in Prenatal Testing. The aim of prenatal screening is to provide prospective parents with information about the health of their fetus. Maternal serum screening is a noninvasive procedure that has become a

ASSESSMENT GUIDE | The Child With Selected Dysmorphic Physical Features*

Skull	Asymmetric head/face	Fontanels too large or small
	Brachycephaly (short, broad head shape) (See Figure 54–11.)	Frontal bossing (prominent central forehead)
		Microcephaly or macrocephaly
	Craniosynostosis (premature closing of skull sutures)	Micrognathia (small jaw)
	Flattened or prominent occiput	Prognathism (projection of jaw beyond that of the forehead)
Extremities	Abnormally positioned feet	Hypoplastic (very small) or absent nails
	Arachnodactyly (long fingers or toes)	Hypotonia (diminished muscle tone)
	Brachydactyly (short fingers or toes)	Loose joints
	Camptodactyly (permanent flexion of fingers or toes)	Polydactyly (extra fingers and/or toes)
	Clinodactyly (curved fingers or toes, most often the fifth finger)	Rocker bottom feet
		Single transverse palmar crease (See Figure 33–33.)
	Edema of the hands or feet	Syndactyly (webbing between fingers and toes)
	Extremely long/thin or short extremities	
Ears	Ear tags or pits	Hearing loss
	Ears that are posteriorly rotated	Low-set or malformed ears
Hair	Excessive body hair	Large section of white hair in otherwise pigmented hair
	Unusual hairline or hair distribution	Sparse or brittle hair
Eyes	Blue sclera	Extreme myopia (nearsightedness)
	Different colored eyes	Hypertelorism (widely spaced eyes)
	Down-slanting eyes	Hypotelorism (closely spaced eyes)
	Epicanthal folds inconsistent with ethnicity (See Figure 33–7.)	Short palpebral fissures (distance between inner and outer canthus of eyes)
	Extreme hyperopia (farsightedness)	Up-slanting eyes (See Figure 33–8.)
Skin	Axillary freckling	Hirsutism (excessive hair)
	Café au lait spots	Hyperelastic skin
	Excessive skin	Leaf-shaped white markings
	Extremely loose or thin skin	Syndactyly (webbing between fingers and toes)
Mouth	Cleft lip with or without cleft palate (See Figure 51–1.)	Early loss of teeth
	Large or small tongue	Late eruption of teeth
	Misshapen, missing, or extra teeth	Smooth or abnormal philtrum
		Thin upper lip
Other	Abdominal wall defect	Seizures
	Ambiguous genitalia	Short, webbed neck
	Cryptorchidism (undescended testicle)	Single umbilical artery
	Hernia (inguinal or umbilical)	Small or widely spaced nipples
	Hypospadias	Multiple fractures
	Hypogonadism	Unusual cry (catlike/mewing, hoarse, weak)
	Obesity	Unusually tall or short stature
	Scoliosis	Webbed neck

This list is not all-inclusive, but is meant to increase the nurse's awareness of assessment findings that may be significant and require a referral to a genetic specialist.

routine aspect of prenatal care. Usually, screening provides reassurance, but when screening tests are abnormal, parents must make decisions about issues that they never may have considered. Within a short time of a receiving a positive screening result, for example, parents must decide whether to have invasive diagnostic testing. Informed decision making requires acquiring significant knowledge about various testing procedures and their respective risks, limitations, and benefits, and about the disorders for which testing is being performed. As parents learn this new information, they consider the potential impact of a genetic diagnosis on their child and their family, often in the context of their perceived moral

duty regarding responsible parenthood and safeguarding the health and well-being of their family. Nurses have a critical role in encouraging clients to make informed decisions and in providing sufficient information to support informed consent. Distinct challenges are associated with this role.

- Most clients have limited health literacy related to prenatal screening, particularly in the face of evolving technology.
- Most clients also have limited understanding of the conditions for which testing is done. For example, life with Down syndrome has changed in many ways in recent

years, and up-to-date information is required for families to make informed decisions about continuing the pregnancy and either keeping the child, placing the child for adoption, or terminating the pregnancy (Van Riper, 2012).

- First-trimester screening is carried out early in pregnancy, limiting opportunities for informed consent. Still adjusting to a new pregnancy, women and their partners may be unprepared to face the emotional impact should a test result be abnormal.

- Although prenatal testing may establish a diagnosis, for example, of Down syndrome, results cannot provide specific information about the level of intellectual ability or health status of the fetus.

- Attitudes about the purpose of prenatal screening vary widely. Research indicates some women accept prenatal screening with little thought, expecting a reassuring outcome. Others have the test to gain information about the pregnancy, with no thought of intervening should the outcome be abnormal. Still others consider the purpose of a screening test to inform decisions around pregnancy termination (Fisher, 2012).

- Multiple considerations—ethical, legal, social, cultural, and religious—affect decision making related to reproductive health and must be balanced to achieve the most appropriate decision about prenatal screening.

To provide competent care, nurses must assess each client's knowledge, attitudes, and values about prenatal diagnosis and tailor the information they share in order to provide individualized care.

POSTNATAL GENETIC TESTING

Newborn screening is the most common postnatal genetic test being performed routinely to identify newborns at high risk of a variety of disorders which require immediate intervention. The panel of tests included in newborn screening has expanded greatly in recent years and varies from state to state. Although informed consent should be a part of any genetic testing, in most states newborn screening is mandated and written consent is not required. Parents are likely, therefore, to have little information about the tests that are performed or the meaning of a positive test. Nurses therefore have a key role in teaching parents about newborn screening and that a positive test does not mean that their newborn has a genetic condition. Diagnostic testing is always required to confirm a positive screening test. Most often, a positive screening test represents a false-positive result and the diagnostic test is normal.

When a child is born with anomalies, has a stormy newborn period, or does not progress as expected, a genetic evaluation may be warranted, and testing may confirm a genetic diagnosis. Questions concerning genetic disorders (cause, treatment, and prognosis) are most often first discussed in the newborn nursery or during the infant's first few months of life. To make an accurate diagnosis, the geneticist consults with other specialists, reviews the current literature, and evaluates all the available information before arriving at a diagnosis and plan of action.

One cannot expect a couple who has just learned that their child has a birth defect or genetic condition to take in any information concerning risks with future pregnancies. However, the couple should never be "put off" from genetic counseling for so long that they conceive another affected child because of lack of information. The nurse can inform parents that genetic counseling is available before they attempt to have another child.

GENETIC TESTING FOR MINORS

In order to support, advocate for, and educate children, adolescents, and their families, the pediatric nurse must have knowledge of issues related to genetic testing of minor children. Parents may request genetic testing for their minor children without foreseeing the consequences associated with a positive finding. Nurses have a critical role in providing information and anticipatory guidance for families considering genetic testing.

The primary focus of genetic testing in children is to promote the child's well-being, and guidelines generally recommend that genetic testing in children only be conducted if the results would affect medical management soon after testing. With this in mind, nurses should help families to understand clearly why a genetic test is being done.

Newborn screening is an example of testing designed to offer an immediate medical benefit for the child in terms of disease prevention or early treatment. Consensus statements by several professional groups support the mandatory offering of newborn screening to parents of all children (Ross, Saal, David, et al., 2013). Diagnostic genetic testing for children with symptoms of a genetic condition is also broadly supported because establishing a diagnosis informs health management for the child as well as reproductive decision making by the family. Predictive testing in asymptomatic children for conditions that cause morbidity at a young age or for specific health promotion, screening, or treatment is also recommended. An example is familial adenomatous polyposis (FAP). Children with a family history of FAP should be tested for the altered gene because screening by colonoscopy is recommended for affected individuals during adolescence (Munck et al., 2011). Genetic counseling and informed consent are essential prior to predictive genetic testing in minors (Ross et al., 2013).

In contrast to the above scenarios, a parent or child may request predictive genetic testing for future planning in the absence of any immediate benefit. This situation may arise with inherited adult-onset disorders such as Huntington disease, certain cancers, or familial (early-onset) Alzheimer disease. An older child who has a relative with such a disorder may wish to know whether he or she carries the altered gene to plan for a life career or to make relationship decisions such as marriage. Parents sometimes request predictive or carrier testing for their children who are well below reproductive age. Among genetics professionals, there is widespread consensus that predictive genetic testing for minors in the absence of targeted preventive, surveillance, or treatment interventions should be deferred until a child reaches the age of majority (Ross et al., 2013). In most states that age is 18 years.

Occasionally, a family member may request genetic testing for a child when the test results are entirely for the benefit of another family member, with no direct benefit to the child. This may occur during DNA linkage studies, in which multiple blood samples from both affected and unaffected individuals within a family are analyzed and compared to identify a specific DNA alteration for diagnosing a genetic condition in that particular family. Another example is genetic testing for the purpose of human leukocyte antigen (HLA) matching prior to stem cell donation. Because HLA-matched siblings are often preferred as stem cell donors, parents may request this testing, which offers no clinical benefit for the child but may benefit immediate family members. Such testing is supported by consensus in pediatric and genetic communities (Ross et al., 2013).

In recent years, advances in genetic knowledge and increasing availability of genetic testing have blurred the issues around testing in minors. Consider, for example, carrier screening. While routine carrier testing of minors is not recommended, carrier screening may be appropriate for adolescents under certain circumstances. Examples are sickle cell trait screening for some athletes and carrier screening for adolescents who are pregnant or considering reproduction. Sometimes, carrier status is identified on newborn screening, creating an issue regarding testing in minors. Although carrier status in a newborn is rarely clinically significant, it is generally agreed that carrier status should be communicated to the family (Ross et al., 2013). Predispositional testing is also complex. Consider a child who is tested and found to have a genetic predisposition to type 2 diabetes. Typically, the disease risk is moderately elevated— perhaps 2 to 3 times the population risk. Does knowledge of that genetic test have immediate medical benefit for the child? Does the potential benefit outweigh any harm that may accompany the knowledge? Issues such as these are of great interest in genomic medicine, but clear guidelines have yet to be established.

ENSURING INFORMED CONSENT AND CONFIDENTIALITY FOR GENETIC TESTING

Nurses are responsible for alerting clients and families of their right to make an informed decision prior to *any* genetic testing, with consideration of the special circumstances arising from the family's social, cultural, and community life. All genetic testing should be voluntary, and it is the nurse's responsibility to ensure that the consent process includes discussion of the risks and benefits of the test, including any physical or psychologic harm, as well as potential societal injury due to stigmatization or discrimination. Ross et al. (2013) suggest using a consent process similar to that conducted before an elective medical procedure. Providing informed consent involves more than just presenting a form and asking clients to sign; rather, nurses must ensure clients fully understand both the process of the testing and potential implications (Badzek, Henaghan, Turner, et al., 2012). For example, tests may reveal unexpected genetic alterations unrelated to the indication for which the test was ordered, and the management of such **incidental findings** should be explained during the consent process. The nurse should be aware that health insurance policies may not cover genetic testing, which is often very expensive. Even if the insurance benefit will cover the test, and despite protections afforded by law, many individuals are fearful of discrimination based on genetic test results that are included in their medical record. The pediatric nurse should inform the child and the family of their right to know who will have access to the genetic test results and of legal protections against genetic discrimination. See *Professionalism in Practice: ELSI.*

PSYCHOSOCIAL ISSUES IN GENETIC TESTING

Nurses must be prepared to assist clients and families to manage anxiety associated with genetic testing. Uncertainty and stress associated with making a decision to undertake genetic

Professionalism in Practice ELSI

Since its inception, the National Human Genome Research Institute has designated a percentage of its budget to examining the ethical, legal, and social implications (ELSI) of genetic and genomic information. Genetic testing raises many questions that have been addressed by ELSI. Genetic exceptionalism, the idea that genetic information should be treated differently than other health information, continues to be a subject of great interest and little consensus. Proponents of genetic exceptionalism point out that genetic information is unique and deserving of special consideration and protection because it is predictive, is potentially stigmatizing, and may reveal information about family members other than the client undergoing testing. The contrasting view points out that other information is also predictive (consider blood cholesterol and risk for cardiovascular disease) and stigmatizing (e.g., information about sexually transmitted infections).

Federal health privacy protection, as mandated under the federal Health Insurance Portability and Accountability Act (HIPAA) privacy rule, does not afford special protection to genetic information, treating it as being no more sensitive than other health-related information. However, by 2008, the majority of states had enacted legislation to protect people from discrimination based on genetic information and penalties for violating genetic privacy. These laws were implemented in response to concerns that individuals might be reluctant to seek potentially beneficial genetic testing without some guarantee about the confidentiality, privacy, and security of that information. For example, an individual may have health coverage for a genetic test but be unwilling to submit the claim because of concerns about the insurance company "owning" the information in the test result. Federal legislation to prohibit discrimination based on genetic information in health insurance and employment (the Genetic Information Nondiscrimination Act [GINA]) was implemented in November 2009. As a federal law, GINA offers protection to Americans in all states.

testing may extend into weeks or even months before results are available. That stress may be increased or relieved once test results are known. Although receiving favorable test results may decrease anxiety for the family or the individual, potential problems do occur and the nurse must be prepared to address them. Concerns about carrier status may interfere with development of intimacy and interpersonal relationships. A positive test result may lead to feelings of unworthiness and disturb self-image. Survivor guilt may affect children with negative results if their siblings are positive. Younger children may blame themselves, thinking they did or said something to cause the gene alteration. The adolescent carrying a gene alteration for a late-onset disease may have an increased tendency for risky behaviors. The adolescent who has inherited an altered disease-producing gene may foster resentment toward the parent who carries the altered gene. Parental guilt may exist for passing the altered gene to the child. Finally, parent–child bonds may be altered if parents become either overprotective or overly permissive. The parent and other

TEACHING HIGHLIGHTS	Nursing Responsibilities in Genetic Counseling

The nurse in genetic counseling is responsible for the following:
- Identify families at risk for genetic problems.
- Determine how the family perceives the genetic problem and what information they wish before proceeding.
- Assist families in acquiring accurate information about the specific problem.
- Act as a liaison between the family and genetic counselor.
- Assist the family in understanding and dealing with information received.
- Provide information on support groups.
- Aid families in coping with this crisis.
- Provide current, credible genetic information.
- Assure continuity of nursing care to the family.

family members may unconsciously form lowered expectations for the child or adolescent. Nurses must use counseling interventions to assist clients to process, adjust to, and use genetic information.

The Role of the Nurse in Genetic Referral

When the nursing assessment reveals a client may benefit from referral to a genetic specialist, the nurse is expected to partner with the client and facilitate the referral. This is a nursing responsibility in the same way as a referral to a dietitian or social worker. *Genetic counseling* is a communication process in which a genetic counselor, physician, or specially trained and certified nurse helps a family or individuals understand and adapt to the medical, psychologic, and familial implications of genetic contributions to disease (National Society of Genetic Counselors, 2005, reaffirmed 2011). Genetic specialists are able to answer questions regarding genetic conditions, inheritance, availability of treatment, and economic, insurance, and future implications of genetic conditions.

Genetic counseling referral is advised for any of the following categories:

- *Congenital abnormalities.* These include *developmental, cognitive, and intellectual disabilities.* Any couple who has had a child or a relative with a congenital malformation may be at increased risk and should be so informed. If a developmental, cognitive, or intellectual disability of unidentified cause has occurred in a family, there may be an increased risk of recurrence. In some cases, the genetic counselor will identify the cause of a malformation as a teratogen. The family should be aware of teratogenic substances so they can avoid exposure during any subsequent pregnancy.

- *Familial disorders.* Families should be told that certain diseases may have a genetic component and that the risk of their occurrence in a particular family may be higher than that in the general population. Such disorders as diabetes, heart disease, cancer, and mental illness fall into this category.

- *Known inherited diseases.* Families may know that a disease is inherited but not know the mechanism or the specific risk for them. An important point to remember is that family members who are not at risk for passing on a disorder should be as well informed as family members who are at risk.

- *Metabolic disorders.* Any families at risk for having a child with a metabolic disorder or biochemical defect should be referred for genetic counseling. Because most inborn errors of metabolism are autosomal recessively inherited, a family may not be identified as being at risk until the birth of an affected child.

- *Chromosomal abnormalities.* As discussed previously, any couple who has had a child with a chromosomal abnormality may be at increased risk of having another child similarly affected. This group includes families in which there is concern about a possible translocation.

When facilitating referral to a genetic specialist, the nurse should educate the client or family so they know what to expect during and after a genetic evaluation. Before the first visit, the client will usually be contacted to provide a detailed medical and family history. The client should be prepared to give as exact a family history as possible so that a detailed three-generation pedigree can be constructed. Information concerning ancestry will also be collected because some genetic disorders are more common among certain groups or individuals from a particular geographic area. (See *Developing Cultural Competence: Genetic Screening Recommendations for Various Ethnic and Age Groups* below.)

Clients should be informed that a genetic consultation visit can last several hours. During the appointment, a genetic clinical nurse, genetic counselor, and/or physician will perform an initial interview with the parents and their child. A geneticist will examine the child and possibly the parent(s) in order to establish an accurate diagnosis. Photos may be taken and tests may be ordered. The specialist will often provide preliminary information based on the data at hand, although a definitive diagnosis may not be possible at the initial visit.

After the completion of testing and careful analysis of all data, the geneticist or genetic counselor will discuss the findings with the parents and/or child and make recommendations. This may occur at a subsequent visit. The discussion will include the diagnosis (if known), the probable course of the disorder, and available management options. The inheritance pattern for the disorder and risk of recurrence with future pregnancies will also be discussed. The remainder of the counseling session is spent discussing the course of action that seems appropriate to the family in view of the risk and family goals. For couples who desire to become parents or who want a subsequent child, options include prenatal diagnosis, early detection and treatment, preimplantation genetic diagnosis or other assisted reproductive therapies, delayed childbearing until prenatal diagnosis is available or a disease can be detected and treated early to prevent irreversible damage, or, in some cases, adoption. When the parents have

Developing Cultural Competence Genetic Screening Recommendations for Various Ethnic and Age Groups

Background of Population at Risk	Disorder	Screening Test	Definitive Test
Ashkenazi Jewish, French-Canadian, Cajun	Tay-Sachs disease	Decreased serum hexosaminidase-A or DNA mutation analysis	Chorionic villus sampling (CVS) or amniocentesis for hexosaminidase-A assay or DNA mutation analysis
Ashkenazi Jewish	Cystic fibrosis, Canavan disease, familial dysautonomia, several other disorders	DNA mutation analysis	CVS or amniocentesis for DNA mutation analysis
African; Hispanic from Caribbean, Central America, or South America; Arab, Egyptian; Asian Indian	Sickle cell disease	Presence of sickle cell hemoglobin; confirmatory hemoglobin electrophoresis	CVS or amniocentesis for DNA mutation analysis
Greek, Italian	Beta-thalassemia	Mean corpuscular volume less than 80%; confirmatory hemoglobin electrophoresis	CVS or amniocentesis for DNA mutation analysis
Southeast Asian (Vietnamese, Laotian, Cambodian), Filipino	Alpha-thalassemia	Mean corpuscular volume less than 80%; confirmatory hemoglobin electrophoresis	CVS or amniocentesis for DNA mutation analysis or gene deletion studies
Women over age 35 (all ethnic groups)	Chromosomal trisomies	Prenatal serum and/or ultrasound screening	CVS or amniocentesis for cytogenetic analysis
Women of any age (all ethnic groups; particularly suggested for women from British Isles, Ireland)	Neural tube defects and selected other anomalies	Maternal serum alpha-fetoprotein (MSAFP)	Amniocentesis for amniotic fluid alpha-fetoprotein (AFP) and acetylcholinesterase assays
Caucasian (northern European, Celtic population), Ashkenazi Jewish	Cystic fibrosis	DNA mutation analysis of the cystic fibrosis transmembrane regulation (CFTR) gene	CVS or amniocentesis for DNA mutation analysis

completed the counseling sessions, the counselor sends them and the referring provider a letter detailing the contents of the sessions. The parents should keep this document for reference.

Genetic healthcare providers present the individual and the family with information to promote informed decisions. They are also sensitive to the importance of protecting the individual's autonomy. A challenge during any visit to a genetic specialist is in providing nondirective counseling. Families should be permitted to make decisions that are not influenced by any biases or values from the nurse, counselor, or geneticist. Many families are accustomed to practitioners and nurses providing direction and guidance in their decision making, and families may be uncomfortable with a nondirective approach. They may believe that the nurse or healthcare provider is withholding very bad news. Health professionals should present all indicated options and discuss the positive and negative aspects of each option, employing therapeutic listening and communication skills.

After genetic counseling, the nurse with the appropriate knowledge of genetics is in an ideal position to help couples review what has been discussed during the counseling sessions and to answer any additional questions they might have. As families return to daily living, the nurse can provide helpful information on the day-to-day aspects of caring for a child, answer questions as they arise, support parents in their decisions, and refer families to other health and community agencies.

Clinical Tip

The following are indications for pediatric referral to a genetic specialist:

- If the child or family reports a known or "believed" genetic condition in the family
- Single major or multiple minor congenital anomalies
- Dysmorphic features that are not familial
- Developmental delay or regression
- A known or suspected metabolic disorder
- Speech problems
- Learning disability
- Failure to thrive
- Delays in physical growth, unusual body proportions, or low muscle tone
- Abnormal or delayed development of secondary sex characteristics or sex organs
- Short or extremely tall stature
- Blindness or cataracts in infants or children
- Deafness
- Hypotonia in an infant or child
- Seizures in newborns or infants
- Skin lesions such as café au lait spots

The Role of the Nurse in Genetic Teaching, Psychosocial Care, and Advocacy

Nurses must be prepared to educate clients and families about genetic disorders. Consideration of a client's cultural and religious beliefs and values is important to teaching. Gene alterations may be viewed as uncontrollable, as occurring secondary to cultural beliefs such as a stranger looking at the infant, or as a "punishment." A family's readiness to learn can be influenced by cultural or religious beliefs and values. Obtaining educational materials in the primary language of the child or family will help facilitate the teaching–learning experience.

The nurse must be aware of common inheritance misconceptions such as a parent's belief that with a 25% recurrence risk, after one child is affected the next three children will be unaffected, or with a 50% recurrence risk every other child will be affected. The recurrence risk *for each pregnancy* should be continually stressed by the nurse. Families often believe that certain family members have inherited a genetic condition because they look like or "take after" a relative with a genetic condition. When new gene alterations or mutations are found or even discussed, families will often express surprise. Because no one else in the family has the condition, they perceive the trait or condition cannot be inherited. Helping families to understand genetic concepts about inheritance is fundamental to delivering competent genetic nursing care.

In order to provide holistic care, the nurse should identify the psychosocial needs and expectations of the child and family, as well as their cultural, spiritual, value, and belief systems. Denial of a genetic diagnosis is common, and nurses must be aware of the family's state of acceptance. Nurses must often help alleviate anxiety or guilt in the child or family. Anxiety related to uncertainty is common when awaiting diagnosis or test results, but individuals also experience anxiety from not understanding the future implications of a confirmed genetic disease. Guilt may be associated with knowledge of a genetic condition being "in the family." It is important for the nurse to reassure parents that the genetic condition is not the result of something they did or did not do during pregnancy. The nurse should encourage open discussion and free expression of fears and concerns. Guilt and shame are common as a family deals with the loss of the expectation and dream of a healthy child, grandchild, niece, or nephew. Reinforce to parents that genetic alterations are caused by changes within a gene and not by superstitions related to sin or other cultural beliefs. As mothers, fathers, and extended family members provide continuous care for the individual with a genetic condition, depression can result. Depression can also occur in the individual with the condition. The nurse must maintain awareness of the possibility of depression and be proactive in obtaining support for the individual or family.

The nurse also is responsible for assessing the family's coping mechanisms and available family, spiritual, cultural, and community support systems. The nurse can refer the individual or family to a support group; however, it is important to have permission from the child or family before providing a support group with their names and contact information. Electronic sources of genetic information abound and are unregulated; many of them are proprietary, offering expensive genetic testing that may have little scientific basis. Nurses should help families to select and evaluate credible websites and online discussion groups.

Another key role for the nurse is to help families with the often difficult task of communicating genetic information such as inheritance patterns to extended family members. Cultural values of autonomy and privacy come into play when a person considers whether to communicate genetic information to extended family members who may also carry the altered gene. Family members often have difficulty understanding that some genetic conditions have variable expressivity. Members of the extended family often feel shock and profound guilt upon learning that they carry the gene alteration that has caused their loved one to have a genetic condition.

The nurse must continually advocate for the child and family and support their decisions even if the decisions contradict the nurse's own ideals and morals. Therefore, careful self-assessment of feelings is essential for the nurse to recognize when one's own attitudes and values may affect care (Consensus Panel on Genetic/Genomic Nursing Competencies, 2009). Coping with genetic revelations and making genetic-related treatment decisions are difficult activities for everyone. The nurse must remember that families will need resources and support and also help in gathering information about reproductive options.

Evaluation

Expected outcomes of delivering nursing care with a genetic focus include:

- The child and family will make informed and voluntary decisions related to genetic health issues.
- The child and family will accurately identify:
  - Basic genetic concepts and simple inheritance risk probabilities
  - What to expect from a genetic referral
  - The influence of genetic factors in health promotion and health maintenance
  - Social, legal, and ethical issues related to genetic testing

Vision for the Future

Nurses are often the primary caregivers to whom children and their families turn for information, guidance, and clarification of ideas. Genetic and genomic competency among nurses is essential, not only to provide direct care but also to function as informed members of the community and greater society. As more information about the genome science becomes available to consumers—in areas such as **pharmacogenomics**, gene therapy, ethics, genetic engineering, and stem cell research—the role of nurses not only remains vital but also increases in breadth. For example, research in pharmacogenetics is leading to prescribing medications based on an individual's genomic profile. As that testing becomes the standard of care for more medications, the nurse's role expands to ensure the testing is completed and to explain results and implications to families. Nurses must acquire foundational understanding of genetic and genomic concepts, maintain currency as genomic discovery is translated to practice, and be ready to discuss trends and changes with children, adolescents, and their families.

Focus Your Study

- Nurses must understand basic concepts of genetics and genomics to deliver the expected standard of nursing care.

- When cell division does not occur as expected, chromosomal alterations in autosomes or sex chromosomes can result.

- Large chromosomal alterations can be seen in a karyotype.

- Mosaicism may cause varied clinical manifestations of chromosomal alterations.

- Gene structure or sequence is critical to the formation of proteins, which are necessary to carry out all physiologic functions.

- Alterations in gene sequence can cause the production of proteins that do not function as expected, which may threaten health.

- Different forms of a gene that occupy the same place on a pair of chromosomes are alleles.

- An individual may be identified as heterozygous or homozygous for a single gene.

- Some gene alterations cause disease, and some protect individuals from disease.

- Mitochondrial gene alterations are inherited from the mother and are primarily involved in high-energy organs such as skeletal muscles, brain, and heart muscle.

- Knowledge of the principles of inheritance allows the nurse not only to offer and reinforce genetic information to children, adolescents, and their families but also to assist them in managing their care and in making reproductive decisions.

- Multifactorial conditions do not follow Mendelian inheritance patterns.

- Several types of genetic tests are available and vary in intended use, implications, and limitations.

- Nurses have an important role in educating clients about genetic testing, promoting informed decision making, and obtaining informed consent.

- Genetic testing of minors has particular implications that require careful consideration.

- The nurse must be aware of the ethical, social, legal, cultural, and spiritual issues related to the delivery of genetic care.

- Basic genetic nursing involves initiating a referral to genetic specialists.

Clinical Reasoning in Action

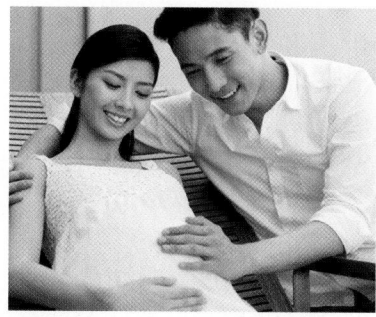

SOURCE: Lane Oatey/Blue Jean Images/ Getty Images.

Jessica Chan, age 30, is 12 weeks pregnant with her first child. She presents to the clinic with her spouse, Brian, for follow-up after a maternal serum screening test and ultrasound, which indicate an increased risk for Down syndrome. She appears anxious and is intermittently tearful. She describes their pregnancy as being planned, a source of great joy and little concern until hearing about her positive screening test. "To tell you the truth, I thought that blood test was just routine and never gave it any thought. And when we had our ultrasound, we were both just so happy to see our baby!" she says.

Although Jessica and Brian have both heard of Down syndrome, neither has personally known a person or even a family in which there is a member with Down syndrome. "We don't know what to do," says Jessica. "What are our options?"

1. How will you explain the implications and limitations of positive screening tests?

2. Jessica asks about additional tests that might provide more specific information without threatening her pregnancy. What would you tell her?

3. Jessica asks you about amniocentesis and CVS, which she was told could determine for sure whether their baby has Down syndrome. What would you tell her about those two procedures?

4. If Jessica chooses to have further testing, what particular challenges are associated with obtaining informed consent?

5. How can you tailor Jessica's and Brian's care based on their knowledge, attitudes, and values?

References

American College of Obstetricians and Gynecologists Committee on Genetics and the Society for Maternal-Fetal Medicine Committee Opinion. (2013). The use of chromosomal microarray analysis in prenatal diagnosis. Committee Opinion No. 581. *Obstetrics and Gynecology, 122,* 1374–1377.

American College of Obstetricians and Gynecologists Committee on Genetics and the Society for Maternal-Fetal Medicine Publications Committee. (2012). Noninvasive prenatal testing for fetal aneuploidy. Committee Opinion No. 545. *Obstetrics and Gynecology, 120,* 1532–1534.

American College of Obstetricians and Gynecologists Committee on Practice Bulletins. (2007). Invasive prenatal testing for aneuploidy. ACOG Practice Bulletin No. 88. *Obstetrics and Gynecology, 110,* 1459–1467.

Badzek, L., Henaghan, M., Turner, M., & Monsen, R. (2012). Ethical, legal, and social issues in the translation of genomics into health care. *Journal of Nursing Scholarship, 4*(1), 15–24.

Barmania, F., Potgieter, M., & Pepper, M. S. (2013). Mutations in C-C chemokine receptor type 5 (CCR5) in South African individuals. *International Journal of Infectious Disease, 17*(12), e1148–e1153. doi: 10.1016/j. ijid.2013.06.009

Beery, T. A., & Workman, M. L. (2012). *Genetics and genomics in nursing and health care.* Philadelphia, PA: F.A. Davis.

Bender, M. A., & Hobbs, W. (2012). *Sickle cell disease.* Retrieved March 14, 2014, from http://www.ncbi .nlm.nih.gov/books/NBK1377/

Bennett, R. L. (2010). *The practical guide to the genetic family history* (2nd ed.). Hoboken, NJ: Wiley-Blackwell.

Bradshaw, E. A., & Martin, G. R. (2012). Screening for critical congenital heart disease: Advancing detection in the newborn. *Current Opinion in Pediatrics, 24*(5), 603–608.

Consensus Panel on Genetic/Genomic Nursing Competencies. (2009). *Essentials of genetic and genomic nursing: Competencies, curricula guidelines, and outcome indicators* (2nd ed.). Silver Spring, MD: American Nurses Association.

Cystic Fibrosis Mutation Database. (2011). Retrieved March 15, 2014, from http://www.genet.sickkids.on.ca/cftr/StatisticsPage.html

De Boeck, K., Zolin, A., Cuppens, H., Olesen, H. V., & Viviani, L. (2004). The relative frequency of CFTR mutation classes in European patients with cystic fibrosis. *Journal of Cystic Fibrosis, 13*(4), 403–409. doi:10.1016/j.jcf.2013.12.003

DeLuca, J., Zanni, K. L., Bonhomme, N., & Kemper, A. R. (2013). Implications of newborn screening for nurses. *Journal of Nursing Scholarship, 45*(1), 25–33.

Devers, P. L., Cronister, A., Ormond, K. E., Facio, F., Brasington, C. K., & Flodman, P. (2013). Noninvasive prenatal testing/noninvasive prenatal diagnosis: The position of the National Society of Genetic Counselors. *Journal of Genetic Counseling, 22*(3), 291–295. doi:10.1007/s10897-012-9564-0

Fisher, J. (2012). Supporting patients after disclosure of abnormal first trimester screening results. *Current Opinions in Obstetrics and Gynecology, 24,* 109–113.

Friedman, J. M. (2012). *Neurofibromatosis 1.* Retrieved March 14, 2014, from http://www.ncbi.nlm.nih.gov/books/NBK1109/

Gilbert, E. S. (2011). *Manual of high risk pregnancy & delivery* (5th ed.). St. Louis, MO: Mosby Elsevier.

Johnson, N. L., Giarelli, E., Lewis, C., & Rice, C. E. (2013). Genomics and autism spectrum disorder. *Journal of Nursing Scholarship, 45*(1), 1–10.

Lander, E. S. (2011). Initial impact of the sequencing of the human genome. *Nature, 470,* 187–197. doi:10.1038/nature09792

McCarthy, J. J., McLeod, H. L., & Ginsburg, G. S. (2013). Genomic medicine: A decade of successes, challenges, and opportunities. *Science Translational Medicine, 5*(189), 1–17. doi: 10.1126/scitranslmed.3005785

Munck, A., Gargouri, L., Alberti, C., Viala, J., Peuchmaur, M., Lenaerts, C., . . . Meyer, M. (2011). Evaluation of guidelines for management of familial adenomatous polyposis in a multicenter pediatric cohort. *Journal of Pediatric Gastroenterology and Nutrition, 53,* 296–302.

National Society of Genetic Counselors (NSGC). (2014). *Students and prospective genetic counselors: What is genetic counseling?* Retrieved from http://www.nsgc.org/p/cm/ld/fid=43

Online Mendelian Inheritance in Man (OMIM). (2014). Baltimore, MD: McKusick-Nathans Institute for Genetics Medicine, Johns Hopkins University; Bethesda, MD: National Center for Biotechnology Information Library of Medicine. Retrieved from http://www.ncbi.nlm.nih.gov/sites/entrez?db=OMIM

Pierce, B. A. (2014). *Genetics: A conceptual approach* (5th ed.). New York, NY: W. H. Freeman and Company.

Ross, L. F., Saal, H. M., David, K. L., Anderson, R. R., American Academy of Pediatrics, & American College of Medical Genetics and Genomics. (2013). Technical report: ethical and policy issues in genetic testing and screening of children. *Genetics in Medicine, 15*(3), 234–245.

Schaaf, C. P., Zschocke, J., & Potocki, L. (2012). *Human genetics: From molecules to medicine.* Baltimore, MD: Lippincott Williams & Wilkins.

Tobias, E. S., Connor, M., & Ferguson-Smith, M. (2011). *Essential medical genetics* (6th ed.). West Sussex, UK: Wiley-Blackwell.

Turnpenny, P., & Ellard, S. (2012). *Emery's elements of medical genetics.* Philadelphia, PA: Elsevier Churchill Livingstone.

U.S. Department of Health and Human Services. (2008). *United States system of oversight of genetic testing: A response to the charge of the Secretary of Health and Human Services. Report of the Secretary's Advisory Committee on Genetics, Health, and Society (SACGHS).* Retrieved March 15, 2014, from http://osp.od.nih.gov/sites/default/files/SACGHS_oversight_report.pdf

Van Riper, M. (2012). Changing landscape of prenatal testing: Ethical and social implications for families. *American Journal of Maternal Child Nursing, 37*(3), 143.

Wu, J., Springett, A., & Morris, J. K. (2013) Survival of trisomy 18 (Edwards syndrome) and trisomy 13 (Patau syndrome) in England and Wales: 2004–2011. *American Journal of Medical Genetics, Part A 161A,* 2512–2518.

Chapter 4
Reproductive Anatomy and Physiology

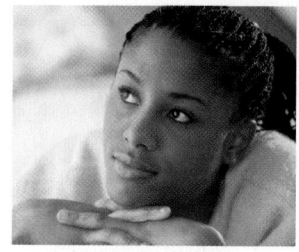

I am amazed by how little many of our students know about anatomy, physiology, and reproduction. As nurses, we must use every opportunity we have to teach young people about their bodies and those of their partners. Information is the key to helping keep them safe and well!

—**University Health Clinic Nurse**

SW Productions/Getty Images

∨ Learning Outcomes

4.1 Identify the structures and functions of the female reproductive system.

4.2 Explain the significance of specific female reproductive structures during pregnancy and childbirth.

4.3 Summarize the actions of the hormones estrogen, progesterone, and the prostaglandins that affect reproductive functioning.

4.4 Identify the two phases of the ovarian cycle and the changes that occur in each phase.

4.5 Describe the phases of the uterine (menstrual) cycle, their dominant hormones, and the changes that occur in each phase.

4.6 Identify the structures and functions of the male reproductive system.

Understanding childbearing requires more than understanding sexual intercourse, or the process by which the female and male sex cells unite. The nurse must also become familiar with the structures and functions that make childbearing possible and the phenomena that initiate it. This chapter presents the anatomic and physiologic aspects of the female and male reproductive systems.

The female and male reproductive organs are *homologous*; that is, they are fundamentally similar in structure and function. The primary functions of both female and male reproductive systems are to produce sex cells and transport them to locations where their union can occur. The sex cells, called *gametes*, are produced by specialized organs called *gonads*. A series of ducts and glands within both male and female reproductive systems contributes to the production and transport of the gametes.

Physiology of Onset of Puberty

The term *puberty* refers to the developmental period between childhood and attainment of adult sexual characteristics and functioning. The age at onset and progress of puberty vary widely, physical changes overlap, and the sequence of events can vary from person to person. (For a detailed discussion of physical changes associated with puberty, see Chapter 33.) Puberty is initiated by the maturation of the hypothalamic-pituitary-gonad complex (the *gonadostat*) and input from the central nervous system. The process, which begins during fetal life, is sequential and complex.

The central nervous system releases a neurotransmitter that stimulates the hypothalamus to synthesize and release **gonadotropin-releasing hormone (GnRH)**. GnRH is transmitted to the anterior pituitary, where it causes the synthesis and secretion of the gonadotropins **follicle-stimulating hormone (FSH)** and **luteinizing hormone (LH)** (Figure 4–1).

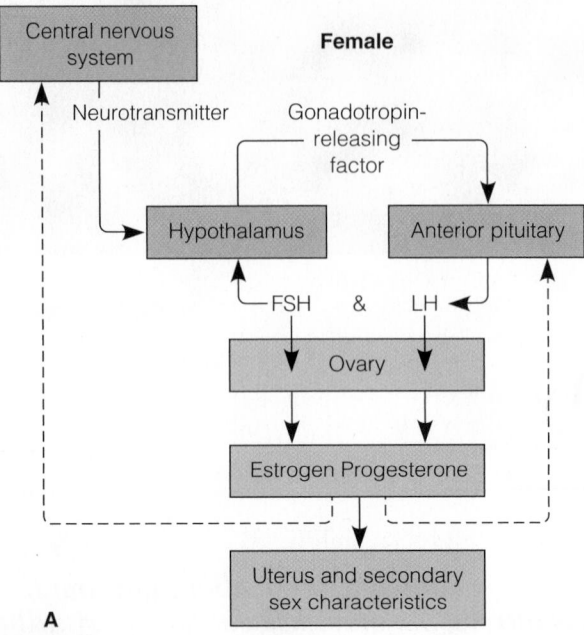

Female

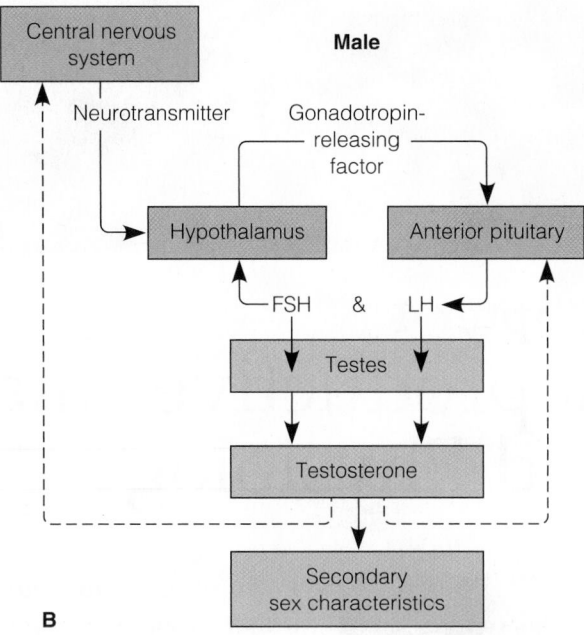

Male

A

B

Figure 4–1 Physiologic changes leading to onset of puberty. *A*, In females, and *B*, in males. Solid lines illustrate stimulation of hormone production, and broken lines illustrate inhibition. Through a neurotransmitter the central nervous system stimulates the hypothalamus, which in turn produces a gonadotropin-releasing factor that causes the anterior pituitary to produce gonadotropins (follicle-stimulating hormone, FSH; or luteinizing hormone, LH). These hormones stimulate specific structures in the gonads to secrete steroid hormones (estrogen, progesterone, or testosterone). The rise in pituitary hormone production increases hypothalamus activity. Elevated steroid hormone levels stimulate the central nervous system and pituitary gland to inhibit hormone production.

Although the gonads do produce small amounts of *androgens* (male sex hormones) and *estrogens* (female sex hormones) before the onset of puberty, FSH and LH stimulate increased secretion of these hormones. Androgens and estrogens influence the development of secondary sex characteristics. FSH and LH stimulate the processes of spermatogenesis and maturation of ova.

The external and internal female reproductive organs develop and mature in response to estrogen and progesterone. Other hormones are involved in the onset of puberty. Abnormally high or low levels of adrenocorticotropic hormone (ACTH), thyroid hormone, or growth hormone (GH) can disrupt the onset of normal puberty and the childbearing years (see Chapter 53 for a detailed discussion).

Female Reproductive System

The female reproductive system consists of the external and internal genitals and the accessory organs of the breasts. Because of its importance to childbearing, the bony pelvis is also discussed in this chapter.

External Genitals

The appearance of the external genitalia varies greatly among women. Heredity, age, race, and the number of children a woman has borne influence the size, color, and shape of her external organs. The female external genitals, also referred to as the *vulva*, include the following structures (Figure 4–2):

- Mons pubis
- Labia majora

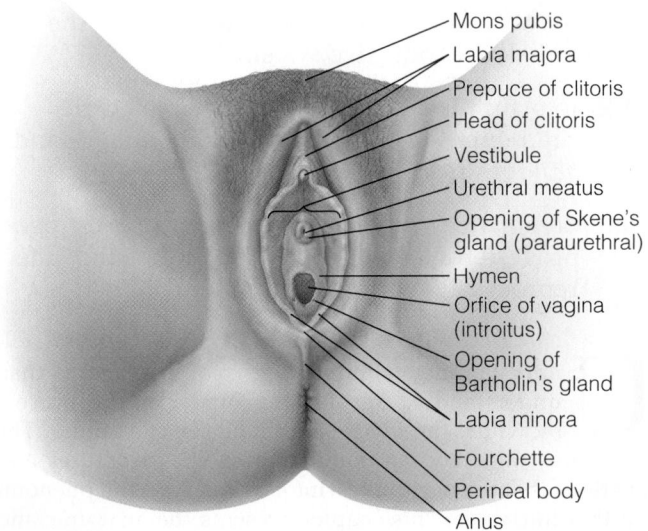

Figure 4–2 Female external genitals, longitudinal view.

- Labia minora
- Clitoris
- Urethral meatus and opening of the paraurethral (Skene) glands
- Vaginal vestibule (vaginal orifice, vulvovaginal [Bartholin] glands, hymen, and fossa navicularis)
- Perineal body

Although they are not true parts of the female reproductive system, the urethral meatus and perineal body are considered here because of their proximity and relationship to the vulva. The vulva has a generous supply of blood and nerves. As a woman ages, estrogen secretions decrease, causing the vulvar organs to atrophy.

MONS PUBIS

The *mons pubis* is a softly rounded mound of subcutaneous fatty tissue beginning at the lowest portion of the anterior abdominal wall (see Figure 4–2). The mons pubis is covered with pubic hair, typically with the hairline forming a transverse line across the lower abdomen. The mons pubis protects the symphysis pubis, especially during coitus.

Developing Cultural Competence Female Pubic Hair

Natural female pubic hair varies considerably around the world, ranging from short to long, from sparse to dense, and from straight and soft to wiry and curly. Pubic hair is short and varies from sparse and fine in Asian women to heavy, coarse, and curly in women of African descent. In color, pubic hair does not always match head hair. Many dark-haired women have lighter pubic hair often with a red tinge. Most women have wavy and curly pubic hair, even when their head hair is straight. In Asians, however, straight black head hair is matched by pubic hair that has been described as "black, short, straight and not thick but rather sparse . . . ." (Morris, 2007, pp. 192–202).

LABIA MAJORA

The *labia majora* are longitudinal, raised folds of pigmented skin, one on either side of the vulvar cleft. Their chief function is to protect the structures lying between them. The labia majora are covered by hair follicles and sebaceous glands, with underlying adipose and muscle tissue. The inner surface of the labia majora in women who have not had children is moist and looks like mucous membrane, whereas after many births, it is more skin-like. With each pregnancy, the labia majora may become less prominent.

Because of the extensive venous network in the labia majora, varicosities may occur during pregnancy, and obstetric or sexual trauma may cause hematomas (Cunningham et al., 2014). The labia majora share an extensive lymphatic supply with the other structures of the vulva, which can facilitate the spread of cancer in the female reproductive organs. Because of the nerves supplying the labia majora (from the first lumbar and third sacral segment of the spinal cord), certain regional anesthesia blocks will affect them and cause numbness.

LABIA MINORA

The *labia minora* are soft folds of skin within the labia majora that converge near the anus, forming the *fourchette*. Each labium minus has the appearance of shiny mucous membrane, being moist and devoid of hair follicles. The labia minora are rich in sebaceous glands, which lubricate and waterproof the vulvar skin and provide bactericidal secretions. Because the sebaceous glands do not open into hair follicles but open directly onto the surface of the skin, sebaceous cysts commonly occur in this area. The labia minora are composed of erectile tissue and involuntary muscle tissue. Vulvovaginitis in this area is irritating

because the labia minora have many tactile nerve endings. The labia minora increase in size at puberty and decrease after menopause because of changes in estrogen levels.

CLITORIS

The *clitoris*, located between the labia minora, is about 5 to 6 mm long and 6 to 8 mm across. Its tissue is essentially erectile. The glans of the clitoris is partly covered by a fold of skin called the *prepuce*, or clitoral hood. This area resembles an opening to an orifice and may be confused with the urethral meatus. Accidental attempts to insert a catheter in this area produce extreme discomfort. The clitoris has rich blood and nerve supplies and is the primary erogenous organ of women. It secretes *smegma*, which along with other vulval secretions has a unique odor that may be sexually stimulating to the male.

URETHRAL MEATUS AND PARAURETHRAL GLANDS

The *urethral meatus* is located 1.0 to 2.5 cm beneath the clitoris in the midline of the vestibule; it often appears as a puckered, slitlike opening. At times, the meatus is difficult to visualize because of the presence of blind dimples, small mucosal folds, or wide variations in location.

The paraurethral glands, or *Skene glands*, open into the posterior wall of the urethra close to its opening (see Figure 4–2). Their secretions lubricate the vaginal opening, facilitating sexual intercourse.

VAGINAL VESTIBULE

The vaginal vestibule is a boat-shaped depression enclosed by the labia majora and minora, which is visible when they are separated (see Figure 4–2). The vestibule contains the vaginal opening, or *introitus*, which is the border between the external and internal genitals.

The *hymen* is a thin, elastic collar or semicollar of tissue that surrounds the vaginal opening. The appearance changes during the woman's lifetime. At birth, the hymen is essentially avascular. For thousands of years, some societies have perpetuated the belief that the hymen covers the vaginal opening and thus an intact hymen is a sign of virginity. However, modern studies of female genital anatomy have revealed that the hymen surrounds rather than entirely covers the vaginal opening, and can be torn not only through sexual intercourse but also through strenuous physical activity, masturbation, menstruation, or the use of tampons, thus dispelling old beliefs. For discussion of the nurse's role in discussing these topics, see Chapter 5.

The *vulvovaginal (Bartholin) glands'* duct openings lie under the constrictor muscle of the vagina. These glands secrete a clear, thick, alkaline mucus that enhances the viability and motility of the sperm deposited in the vaginal vestibule. These gland ducts can harbor *Neisseria gonorrhoeae* and other bacteria, which can cause pus formation and abscesses in the Bartholin glands.

The vestibular area is innervated predominantly by the perineal nerve from the sacral plexus. The area is not sensitive to touch generally; however, the hymen contains numerous free nerve endings as receptors to pain.

PERINEAL BODY

The *perineal body* is a wedge-shaped mass of fibromuscular tissue found between the lower part of the vagina and the anus (see Figure 4–2). The superficial area between the anus and the vagina is referred to as the *perineum*.

The muscles that meet at the perineal body are the external sphincter ani, both levator ani (the superficial and deep transverse perineal), and the bulbocavernosus. These muscles mingle

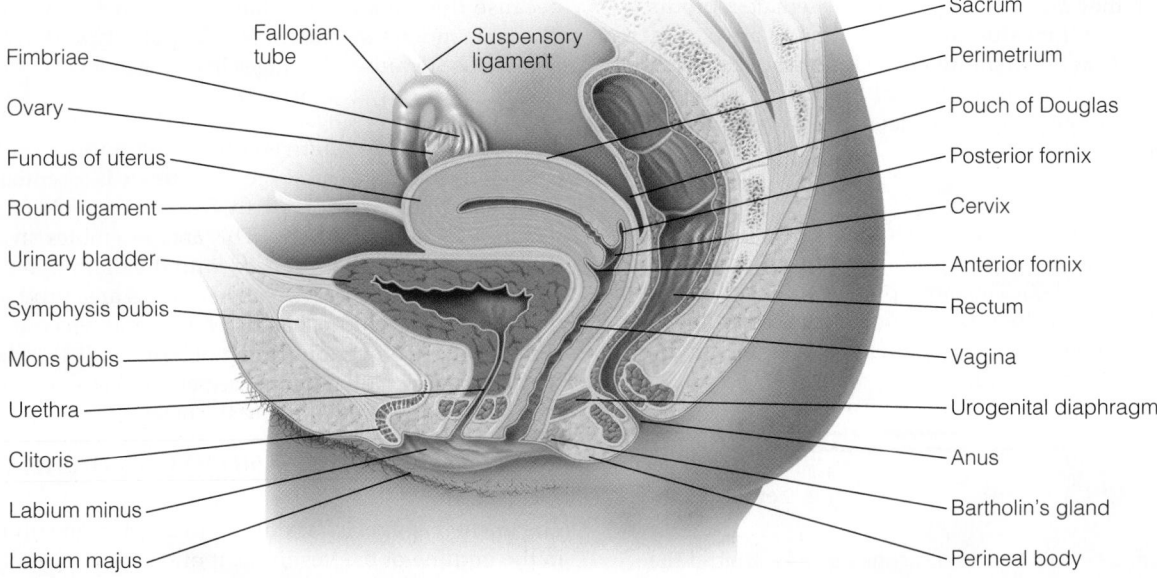

Fimbriae
Fallopian tube
Suspensory ligament
Ovary
Fundus of uterus
Round ligament
Urinary bladder
Symphysis pubis
Mons pubis
Urethra
Clitoris
Labium minus
Labium majus

Sacrum
Perimetrium
Pouch of Douglas
Posterior fornix
Cervix
Anterior fornix
Rectum
Vagina
Urogenital diaphragm
Anus
Bartholin's gland
Perineal body

Figure 4–3 Female internal reproductive organs.

with elastic fibers and connective tissue in an arrangement that allows a remarkable amount of stretching. During the last part of labor, the perineal body thins out until it is just a few centimeters thick. This tissue is often the site of lacerations or episiotomy during childbirth (see Chapter 21).

Female Internal Reproductive Organs

The female internal reproductive organs—the vagina, uterus, fallopian tubes, and ovaries—are target organs for estrogenic hormones and they play a unique part in the reproductive cycle (Figure 4–3). Certain internal reproductive organs can be palpated during vaginal examination and assessed with various instruments.

VAGINA

The **vagina** is a muscular and membranous tube that connects the external genitals with the uterus. It extends from the vulva to the uterus in a position nearly parallel to the plane of the pelvic brim. The vagina is often called the *birth canal* because it forms the lower part of the pelvic axis through which the fetus must pass during birth.

Because the cervix of the uterus projects into the upper part of the anterior wall of the vagina, the anterior wall is approximately 2.5 cm shorter than the posterior wall. Measurements range from 6 to 8 cm for the anterior wall and from 7 to 10 cm for the posterior wall (Cunningham et al., 2014).

In the upper part of the vagina, which is called the *vaginal vault*, there is a recess, or hollow, around the cervix. This area is called the *vaginal fornix*. Since the walls of the vaginal vault are very thin, various structures can be palpated through them, including the uterus, a distended bladder, the ovaries, the appendix, the cecum, the colon, and the ureters. The upper fourth of the vagina is separated from the rectum by the pouch of Douglas (sometimes referred to as the cul-de-sac of Douglas). This deep pouch, or recess, is posterior to the cervix.

When a woman lies on her back after intercourse, the space in the fornix permits the pooling of semen. The collection of a large number of sperm near the cervix at or near the time of ovulation increases the chances of pregnancy.

The walls of the vagina are covered with ridges, or rugae, crisscrossing each other. These rugae allow the vaginal tissues to stretch enough for the fetus to pass through during childbirth as well as stretch during coitus.

During a woman's reproductive life, an acidic vaginal environment is normal (pH 4–5). Secretion from the vaginal epithelium provides a moist environment. The acidic environment is maintained by a symbiotic relationship between lactic acid–producing bacilli (Döderlein bacillus, or *Lactobacillus*) and the vaginal epithelial cells. These cells contain glycogen, which is broken down by the bacilli into lactic acid. The amount of glycogen is regulated by the ovarian hormones. Any interruption of this process can destroy the normal self-cleaning action of the vagina. Such interruption may be caused by antibiotic therapy, douching, frequent intercourse, or use of vaginal sprays or deodorants. (For further discussion, see Chapter 5.) During pregnancy and increased vascularity, the vaginal secretions are markedly increased and may be mistaken for amniotic fluid (Cunningham et al., 2014). The acidic vaginal environment is normal only during the mature reproductive years and in the first days of life, when maternal hormones are operating in the newborn. A relatively neutral pH of 7.5 is normal from infancy until puberty and after menopause.

Each third of the vagina is supplied by a distinct vascular pattern (Figure 4–4). Although one would expect venous drainage going to the heart and lungs, anastomoses of the veins are present and make it possible for a pelvic embolism or carcinoma to bypass the heart and lungs and lodge in the brain, spine, or other remote part of the body.

Vaginal lymphatic fluids drain into the external and internal iliac nodes, the hypogastric nodes, and the inguinal glands. The posterior wall drains into nodes lying in the rectovaginal septum. Any vaginal infection follows these routes.

The pudendal nerve supplies what relatively little somatic innervation there is to the lower third of the vagina. Thus sensation during sexual excitement and coitus is reduced in this area, as is vaginal pain during the second stage of labor.

The vagina has three functions:

• To serve as the passage for sperm during coitus and for the fetus during birth

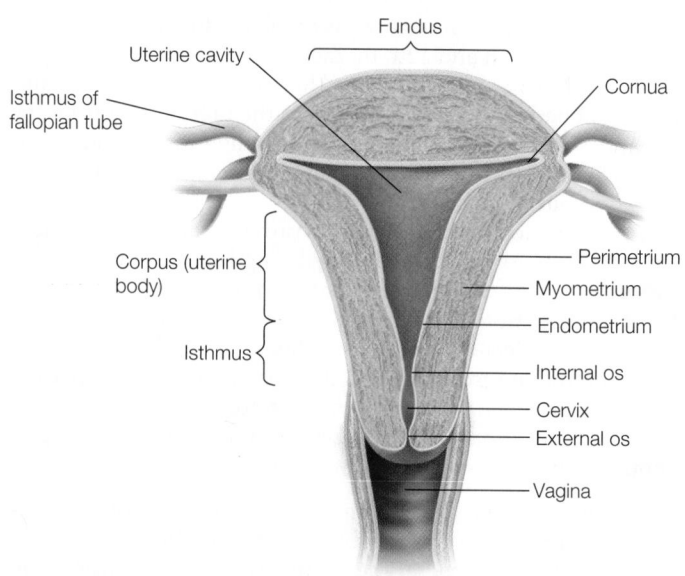

Figure 4–5 Structures of the uterus.

- To provide passage for the menstrual products from the uterine cavity to the outside of the body
- To protect against trauma from sexual intercourse and infection of the uterus, ovaries, and pelvis from pathogenic organisms

UTERUS

The **uterus** is a hollow, muscular, thick-walled organ shaped like an upside-down pear (Figure 4–5). It lies in the center of the pelvic cavity between the base of the bladder and the rectum and above the vagina. It is level with or slightly below the brim of the pelvis, with the external opening of the cervix (external os) at about the level of the ischial spines. The uterus of the never pregnant (nulligravid) mature woman weighs about 60 g and weighs more in a woman who has been pregnant. The nulligravid uterus measures 6 to 8 cm in length and 9 to 10 cm in multiparious women (Cunningham et al., 2014).

The uterus is divided into two major parts: the upper triangular portion called the **corpus**, or uterine body; and the lower cylindrical portion called the **cervix**. The corpus comprises the upper two thirds of the uterus and is composed mainly of a smooth muscle layer (myometrium). The lower third is the cervix, or neck. The rounded uppermost portion of the corpus that extends above the points of attachment of the fallopian tubes is called the **fundus**. The elongated portion of the uterus where the fallopian tubes enter is called the **cornua**.

The *isthmus* is that portion of the uterus between the internal cervical os and the endometrial cavity. The isthmus is about 6 mm above the uterine opening of the cervix (the internal os), and it is in this area that the uterine lining changes into the mucous membrane of the cervix; it joins the corpus to the cervix. The isthmus takes on importance in pregnancy because it becomes the lower uterine segment. At birth, this thin lower segment, situated behind the bladder, is the site for lower-segment cesarean births (see Chapter 22).

The blood and lymphatic supplies to the uterus are extensive. Innervation of the uterus is entirely by the autonomic nervous system. Even without an intact nerve supply, the uterus can contract adequately for birth; for example, hemiplegic women have adequate uterine contractions.

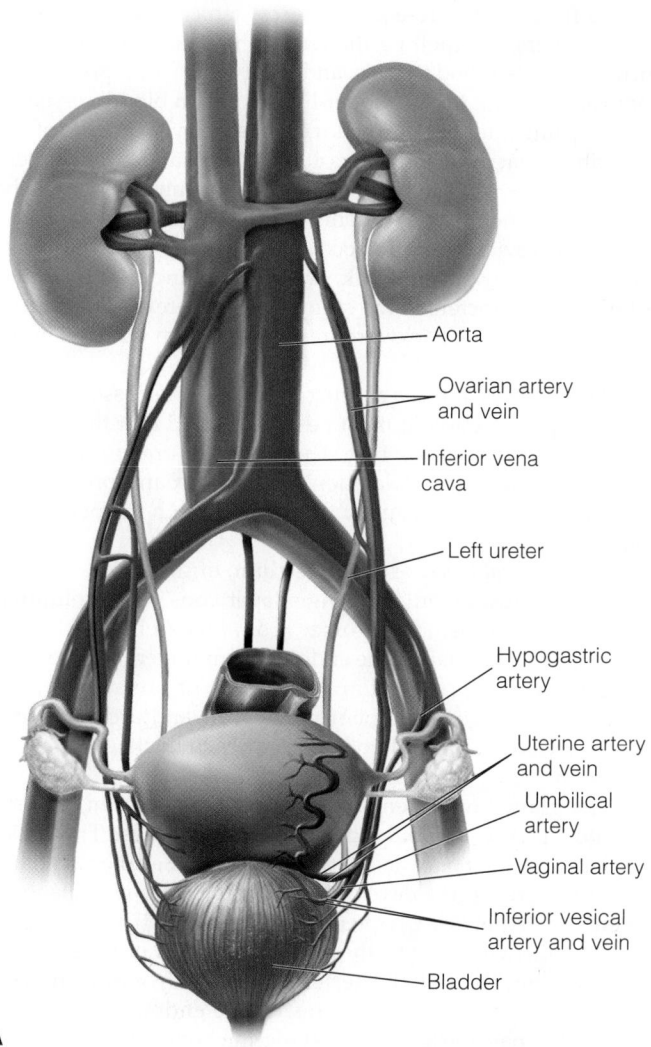

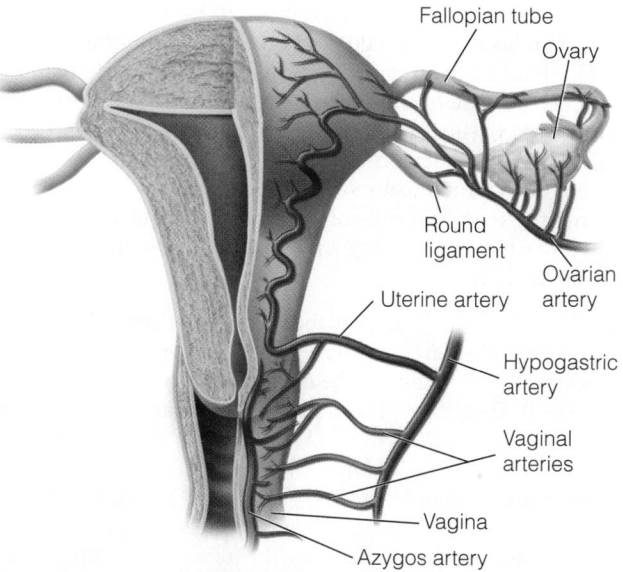

Figure 4–4 Blood supply to internal reproductive organs. *A*, Pelvic blood supply. *B*, Blood supply to vagina, ovaries, uterus, and fallopian tube.

Pain of uterine contractions is carried to the central nervous system by the 11th and 12th thoracic nerve roots. Pain from the cervix and upper vagina passes through the ilioinguinal and pudendal nerves. The motor fibers to the uterus arise from the 7th and 8th thoracic vertebrae. Because the sensory and motor levels are separate, epidural anesthesia can be used during labor and birth.

The function of the uterus is to provide a safe environment for fetal development. The uterine lining is cyclically prepared by steroid hormones for implantation of the embryo, a process known as **nidation**. Once the embryo is implanted, the developing fetus is protected until it is expelled.

Both the uterine body and the cervix are changed permanently by pregnancy. The body never returns to its prepregnant size, and the external os changes from a circular opening of about 3 mm to a transverse slit with irregular edges.

Uterine Corpus. The uterine corpus is made up of three layers. The outermost layer is the *serosal layer*, or **perimetrium**, which is composed of peritoneum. The middle layer is the *muscular uterine layer*, or **myometrium**. This muscular uterine layer is continuous with the muscle layers of the fallopian tubes and the vagina. This characteristic helps these organs present a unified reaction to various stimuli—ovulation, orgasm, or the deposit of sperm in the vagina. These muscle fibers also extend into the ovarian, round, and cardinal ligaments and minimally into the uterosacral ligaments, which helps explain the vague but disturbing pelvic "aches and pains" reported by many pregnant women.

The myometrium has three distinct layers of uterine (smooth) involuntary muscles (Figure 4–6). The outer layer, found mainly over the fundus, is made up of longitudinal muscles that cause the descent of the fetus, which places pressure on the cervical fibers leading to cervical effacement and delivery of the fetus. The thick middle layer is made up of interlacing

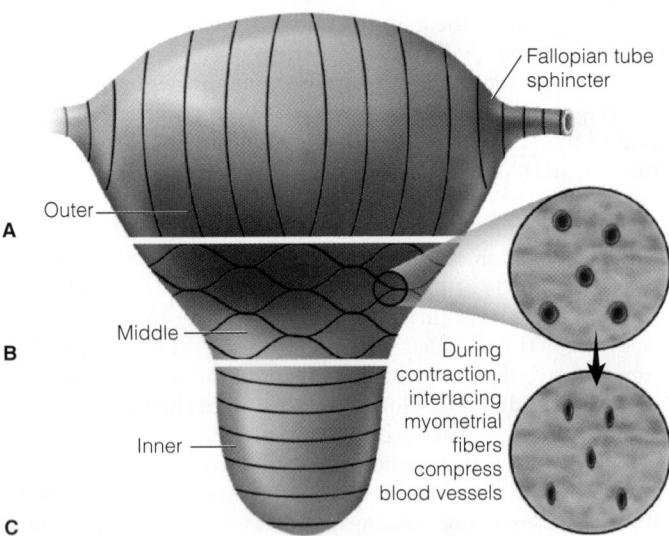

Figure 4–6 Myometrium uterine muscle layer placement and function. *A,* Outer layer (longitudinal muscles) is suited to expelling fetus. *B,* Middle layer (interlacing muscle fibers in figure-eight pattern) surrounds and constricts blood vessels to stop bleeding. *C,* Inner layer (circular muscle fibers form sphincters at fallopian tubes and internal os) prevents backflow of menstrual blood into fallopian tubes and stretches during labor as cervical dilatation occurs.

muscle fibers in figure-eight patterns, which assist the longitudinal fibers in expelling the fetus. These muscle fibers also surround large blood vessels, and their contraction produces a hemostatic action (a tourniquet-like action on blood vessels to stop bleeding after birth). The inner muscle layer consists of circular fibers that form sphincters at the fallopian tube attachment sites and at the internal os. The internal os sphincter inhibits the expulsion of the uterine contents during pregnancy but relaxes in labor as cervical dilatation occurs. An incompetent cervical os can be caused by a torn, weak, or absent sphincter at the internal os. The sphincters at the fallopian tubes prevent menstrual blood from flowing backward into the fallopian tubes from the uterus.

Although each layer of muscle has been discussed as having a unique function, it must be remembered that the uterine musculature works as a whole. The uterine contractions of labor are responsible for the dilatation of the cervix and provide the major force for the passage of the fetus through the pelvis and vaginal canal at birth.

The *mucosal layer*, or **endometrium**, of the uterine corpus is the innermost layer. This single layer consists of columnar epithelium, glands, and stroma. From menarche (first menstruation) to menopause, the endometrium undergoes monthly degeneration and renewal in the absence of pregnancy. As it responds to the governing hormonal cycle and prostaglandin influence as well, the endometrium varies in thickness from 0.5 to 5.0 mm.

The glands of the endometrium produce a thin, watery, alkaline secretion that keeps the uterine cavity moist. This endometrial "milk" not only helps sperm travel to the fallopian tubes but also nourishes the developing embryo before it implants in the endometrium (see Chapter 7).

The blood supply to the endometrium is unique. In the myometrium, the radial arteries branch off from the arcuate arteries at right angles. Once inside the endometrium, they become the basal arteries supplying the zona basalis (a layer of the endometrium) and ultimately become the coiled arteries supplying the zona functionalis (also part of the endometrium). The basal arteries are not sensitive to cyclic hormonal control; hence, the zona basalis portion remains intact and is the site of new endometrial tissue generation. The coiled arteries are extremely sensitive to hormonal control. Their response is alternate relaxation and constriction during the ischemic, or terminal, phase of the menstrual cycle. These differing responses allow part of the endometrium to remain intact while other endometrial tissue is shed during menstruation.

When pregnancy occurs and the endometrium is not shed, the reticular stromal cells surrounding the endometrial glands become the decidual cells of pregnancy. The stromal cells are highly vascular, channeling a rich blood supply to the endometrial surface.

Cervix. The narrow neck of the uterus is the **cervix**. It meets the body of the uterus at the internal os and descends about 2.5 cm to connect with the vagina at the external os (Heitmann, 2013) (see Figure 4–3). Thus it provides a protective entrance for the body of the uterus. The cervix is divided by its line of attachment into the vaginal and supravaginal areas. The *vaginal cervix* projects into the vagina at an angle of from 45 to 90 degrees. The *supravaginal cervix* is surrounded by the attachments that give the uterus its main support: the uterosacral ligaments, the transverse ligaments of the cervix (Mackenrodt ligaments), and the pubocervical ligaments.

The vaginal cervix has a pink appearance and ends at the external os. The cervical canal has a rosy red appearance and is lined with columnar ciliated epithelium, which contains

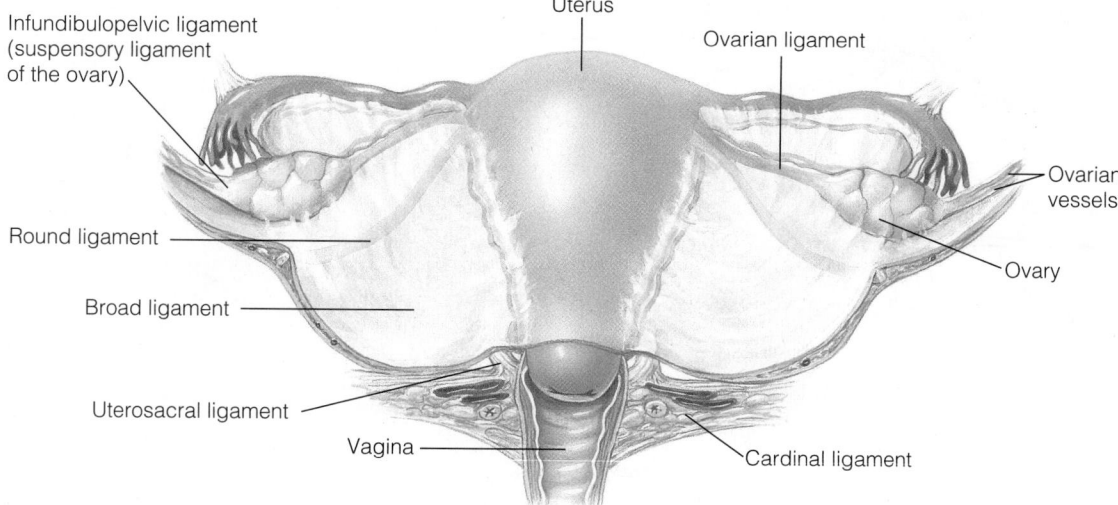

Infundibulopelvic ligament
(suspensory ligament
of the ovary)

Uterus

Ovarian ligament

Ovarian vessels

Round ligament

Ovary

Broad ligament

Uterosacral ligament

Vagina

Cardinal ligament

Figure 4–7 Uterine ligaments.

mucus-secreting glands. Most cervical cancer begins at this *squamocolumnar* junction. The specific location of the junction varies with age and number of pregnancies. Elasticity is the chief characteristic of the cervix. Its ability to stretch results from both the high fibrous and collagenous content of the supportive tissues and the vast number of folds in the cervical lining.

The cervical mucus has three functions:

- To lubricate the vaginal canal
- To act as a bacteriostatic agent
- To provide an alkaline environment to shelter deposited sperm from the acidic vaginal secretions

At ovulation, cervical mucus is clearer, thinner, more profuse, and more alkaline than at other times.

UTERINE LIGAMENTS

The *uterine ligaments* support and stabilize the various reproductive organs. The ligaments shown in Figure 4–7 are described as follows:

1. The **broad ligament** keeps the uterus centrally placed and provides stability within the pelvic cavity. It is a double layer that is continuous with the abdominal peritoneum. The broad ligament covers the uterus anteriorly and posteriorly and extends outward from the uterus to enfold the fallopian tubes. The round and ovarian ligaments are at the upper border of the broad ligament (Cunningham et al., 2014). At its lower border, it forms the cardinal ligaments. Between the folds of the broad ligament are connective tissue, involuntary muscle, blood and lymph vessels, and nerves.

2. The **round ligaments** help the broad ligament keep the uterus in place. The round ligaments arise from the sides of the uterus near the fallopian tube insertions. They extend outward between the folds of the broad ligament, passing through the inguinal ring and canals and eventually fusing with the connective tissue of the labia majora. The round ligaments are made up of longitudinal muscle and undergo hypertrophy and increase in both length and diameter during pregnancy (Cunningham et al., 2014). During labor the round ligaments steady the uterus, pulling downward and forward so that the presenting part of the fetus is moved into the cervix.

3. The **ovarian ligaments** anchor the lower pole of the ovary to the cornua of the uterus. They are surrounded by muscle fibers that allow the ligaments to contract. This contractile ability influences the position of the ovary to some extent, thus helping the fimbriae of the fallopian tubes to "catch" the ovum as it is released each month.

4. The **cardinal ligaments** are the chief uterine supports and suspend the uterus from the side walls of the true pelvis. These ligaments, also known as Mackenrodt or transverse cervical ligaments, arise from the sides of the pelvic walls and attach to the cervix in the upper vagina. These ligaments prevent uterine prolapse and also support the upper vagina.

5. The **infundibulopelvic ligament** suspends and supports the ovaries. Arising from the outer third of the broad ligament, the infundibulopelvic ligament contains the ovarian vessels and nerves.

6. The **uterosacral ligaments** provide support for the uterus and cervix at the level of the ischial spines. Arising on each side of the pelvis from the posterior wall of the uterus, the uterosacral ligaments sweep back around the rectum and insert on the sides of the first and second sacral vertebrae. The uterosacral ligaments contain smooth muscle fibers, connective tissue, blood and lymph vessels, and nerves. They also contain sensory nerve fibers that contribute to dysmenorrhea (painful menstruation) (see Chapter 5).

FALLOPIAN TUBES

The two **fallopian tubes**, also known as the *oviducts* or *uterine tubes*, arise from each side of the uterus and reach almost to the sides of the pelvis, where they turn toward the ovaries (Figure 4–8). Each tube is approximately 8.0 to 13.5 cm long. A short section of each fallopian tube is inside the uterus; its opening into the uterus is only 1 mm in diameter. The fallopian tubes link the peritoneal cavity with the uterus and vagina. This linkage increases a woman's biologic vulnerability to disease processes in the pelvis.

Each fallopian tube may be divided into three parts: the *isthmus*, the *ampulla*, and the *fimbria (ends of the infundibulum)*. The fallopian tube **isthmus** is straight and narrow, with a thick

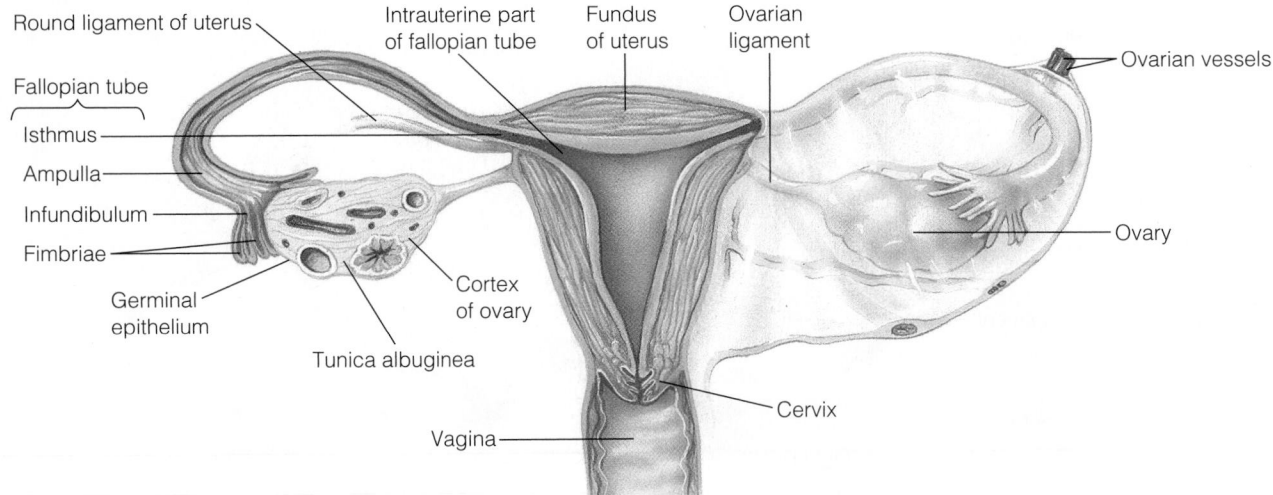

Figure 4–8 Fallopian tubes and ovaries.

muscular wall and an opening (lumen) 2 to 3 mm in diameter. It is the site of tubal ligation, a surgical procedure to prevent pregnancy (see Chapter 5).

Next to the isthmus is the curved **ampulla**, which comprises the outer two thirds of the tube. Fertilization of the secondary oocyte by a spermatozoon usually occurs here. The ampulla ends at the **fimbria**, which is a funnel-like enlargement with many finger-like projections (fimbriae) reaching out to the ovary. The longest of these, the fimbria ovarica, is attached to the ovary to increase the chances of intercepting the ovum as it is released.

The wall of the fallopian tube consists of four layers: peritoneal (serous), subserous (adventitial), muscular, and mucous tissues. The peritoneum covers the tubes. The subserous layer contains the blood and nerve supply, and the muscular layer is responsible for the peristaltic movement of the tube. The mucosal layer, immediately next to the muscular layer, is composed of ciliated and nonciliated cells, with the number of ciliated cells being more abundant at the fimbria. Nonciliated cells secrete a protein-rich, serous fluid that nourishes the ovum. The constantly moving tubal cilia propel the ovum toward the uterus. Because the ovum is a large cell, this ciliary action is needed to assist the tube's muscular layer peristalsis. Any malformation or malfunction of the tubes or cilia can result in infertility, ectopic pregnancy, or even sterility.

A well-functioning tubal transport system involves active fimbriae close to the ovary, peristalsis of the tube created by the muscular layer, ciliated currents beating toward the uterus, and the proximal contraction and distal relaxation of the tube caused by different types of prostaglandins.

A rich blood and lymphatic supply serves each fallopian tube (see Figure 4–4). Thus the tubes have an unusual ability to recover from an inflammatory process. The fallopian tubes have three functions:

- To provide transport for the ovum from the ovary to the uterus (transport time through the fallopian tubes varies from 3 to 4 days)
- To provide a site for fertilization
- To serve as a warm, moist, nourishing environment for the ovum or zygote (fertilized egg) (See Chapter 7 for further discussion.)

OVARIES

The **ovaries** are two almond-shaped structures just below the pelvic brim. One ovary is located on each side of the pelvic cavity. Their size varies among women and with the stage of the menstrual cycle. Each ovary weighs approximately 6 to 10 g and is 1.5 to 3.0 cm wide, 2 to 5 cm long, and 1.0 to 1.5 cm thick. The ovaries of girls are small, but they become larger after puberty and then decrease in size following menopause. They also change in appearance from a dull white, smooth-surfaced organ to a pitted gray organ as the woman ages. The pitting appearance on their surface is the result of scarring after ovulation. The ovaries are maintained in their position by the broad, ovarian, and infundibulopelvic ligaments. It is rare for both ovaries to be at the same level in the pelvic cavity.

There is no peritoneal covering for the ovaries. Although this lack of covering assists the mature ovum to erupt, it also allows easier spread of malignant cells from cancer of the ovaries. The ovaries are composed of three layers: the tunica albuginea, the cortex, and the medulla. The *tunica albuginea* is dense and dull white and serves as a protective layer. The *cortex* is the main functional part because it contains ova, graafian follicles, corpora lutea, the degenerated corpora lutea (corpora albicantia), and degenerated follicles. The *medulla* is completely surrounded by the cortex and contains the nerves and the blood and lymphatic vessels.

The ovaries are the primary source of two important hormones: estrogen and progesterone. *Estrogens* are associated with those characteristics contributing to femaleness, including breast alveolar lobule growth and duct development. The ovaries secrete large amounts of estrogen, while the adrenal cortex (extraglandular sites) produces minute amounts of estrogen in nonpregnant women, and the fat cells produce a secondary estrogen.

Progesterone is often called the *hormone of pregnancy* because it inhibits uterine contractions and relaxes smooth muscle to cause vasodilation, allowing pregnancy to be maintained. The interplay between the ovarian hormones and other hormones such as follicle-stimulating hormone (FSH) and luteinizing hormone (LH) is responsible for the cyclic changes that allow pregnancy to occur. The hormonal and physical changes that occur during the female reproductive cycle are discussed in depth later in this chapter.

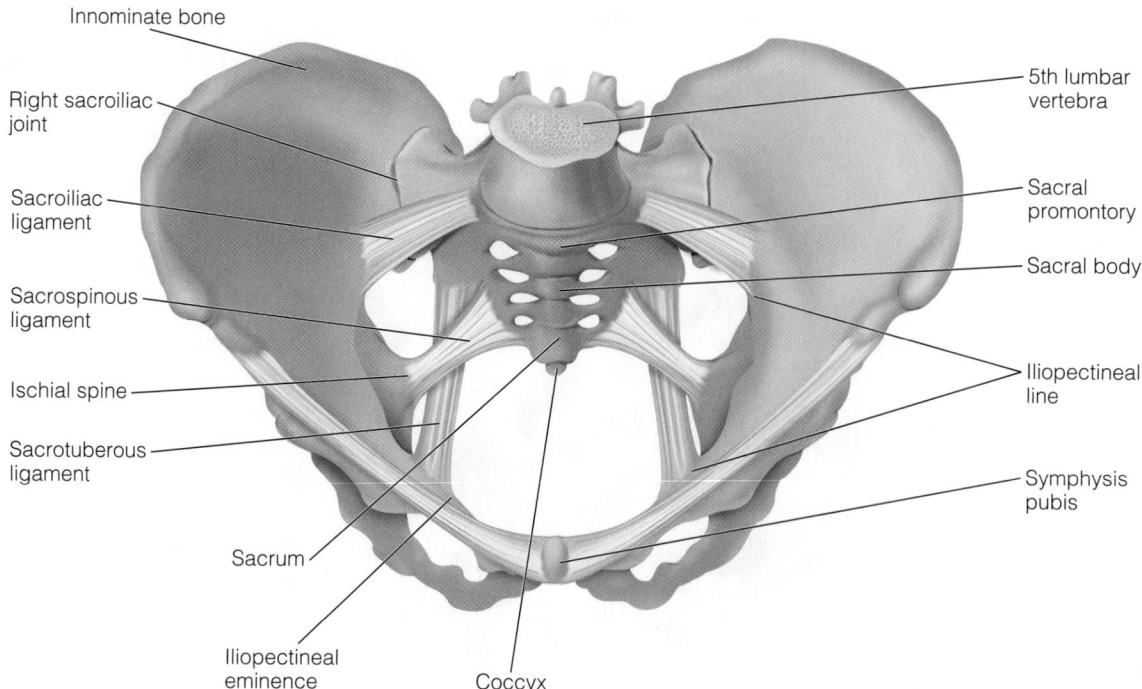

Innominate bone

Right sacroiliac joint

Sacroiliac ligament

Sacrospinous ligament

Ischial spine

Sacrotuberous ligament

Sacrum

Iliopectineal eminence

Coccyx

5th lumbar vertebra

Sacral promontory

Sacral body

Iliopectineal line

Symphysis pubis

Figure 4–9 **Pelvic bones with supporting pelvic ligaments.**

Between the ages of 45 and 55, a woman's ovaries secrete decreasing amounts of estrogen. Eventually, ovulatory activity ceases and menopause occurs.

Bony Pelvis

The female bony pelvis has two unique functions:

- To support and protect the pelvic contents
- To form the relatively fixed axis of the birth passage

Because the pelvis is so important to childbearing, its structure must be understood clearly.

BONY STRUCTURE

The pelvis is made up of four bones: two innominate bones, the sacrum, and the coccyx (or tail bone). The pelvis resembles a bowl or basin; its sides are the innominate bones, and its back is the sacrum and coccyx. Lined with fibrocartilage and held tightly together by pelvic ligaments (Figure 4–9), the four bones join at the symphysis pubis, the two sacroiliac joints, and the sacrococcygeal joints.

The *innominate bones*, also known as the *hip bones*, are made up of three separate bones: the ilium, ischium, and pubis. These bones fuse to form a circular cavity, the *acetabulum*, which articulates with the femur.

The *ilium* is the broad, upper prominence of the hip. The iliac crest is the margin of the ilium. The ischial spines, the foremost projections nearest the groin, are the site of attachment for ligaments and muscles.

The *ischium*, the strongest bone, is under the ilium and below the acetabulum. The L-shaped ischium ends in a marked protuberance, the ischial tuberosity, on which the weight of a seated body rests. The **ischial spines** arise near the junction of the ilium and ischium and jut into the pelvic cavity. The shortest diameter of the pelvic cavity is between the ischial spines. The ischial spines serve as reference points during labor to evaluate

the descent of the fetal head into the birth canal (see Chapter 16 and Figure 16–8).

The **pubis** forms the slightly bowed front portion of the innominate bone. Extending medially from the acetabulum to the midpoint of the bony pelvis, each pubis meets the other to form a joint called the **symphysis pubis**. The triangular space below this junction is known as the pubic arch. The fetal head passes under this arch during birth. The symphysis pubis is formed by heavy fibrocartilage and the superior and inferior pubic ligaments. The mobility of the inferior ligament increases during a first pregnancy and to a greater extent in subsequent pregnancies.

The sacroiliac joints also have a degree of mobility that increases near the end of pregnancy as the result of an upward gliding movement. The pelvic outlet may be increased by 1.5 to 2.0 cm in the squatting, sitting, and dorsal lithotomy positions. Relaxation of the pelvic joints is induced by the hormones of pregnancy.

The *sacrum* is a wedge-shaped bone formed by the fusion of five vertebrae. The anterior upper portion of the sacrum has a projection into the pelvic cavity known as the **sacral promontory**. This projection is another obstetric guide in determining pelvic measurements. (For a discussion of pelvic measurements, see Chapter 9.)

The small triangular bone last on the vertebral column is the coccyx. It articulates with the sacrum at the sacrococcygeal joint. The coccyx usually moves backward during labor to provide more room for the fetus.

PELVIC FLOOR

The muscular floor of the bony pelvis is designed to overcome the force of gravity exerted on the pelvic organs. It acts as a supportive structure to the irregularly shaped pelvic outlet, thereby providing stability for surrounding structures.

Deep fascia, the levator ani, and coccygeal muscles form the part of the pelvic floor known as the **pelvic diaphragm**. The

Anterior

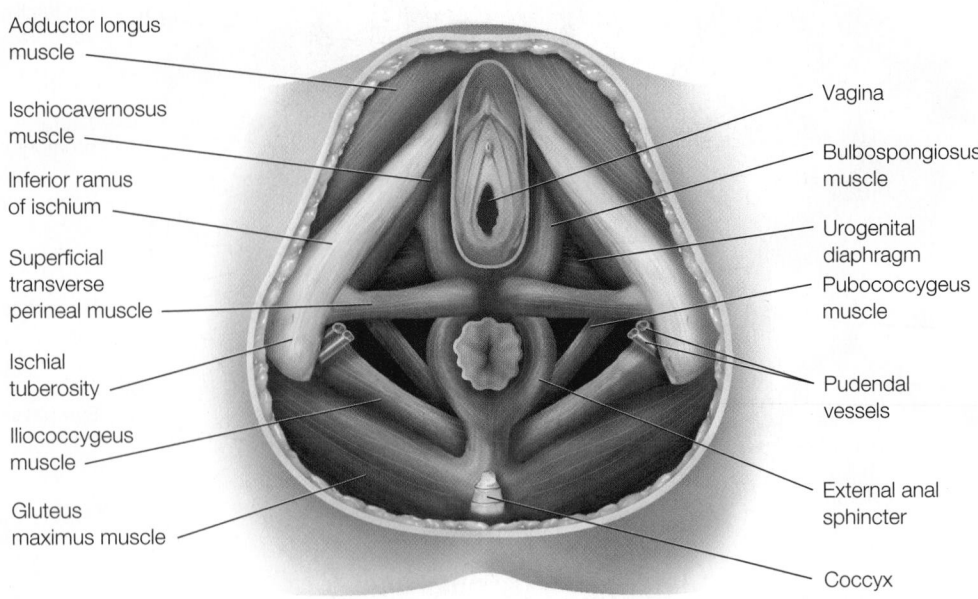

Figure 4–10 Muscles of the pelvic floor. (The puborectalis, pubovaginalis, and coccygeal muscles cannot be seen from this view.)

components of the pelvic diaphragm function as a whole, yet they are able to move over one another. This feature provides an exceptional capacity for relaxation during birth and return to prepregnancy condition following birth. Above the pelvic diaphragm is the **pelvic cavity**; below and behind it is the perineum. The sacrum is located posteriorly.

The levator ani muscle makes up the major portion of the pelvic diaphragm and consists of four muscles: the iliococcygeus, pubococcygeus, puborectalis, and pubovaginalis. The iliococcygeal muscle, a thin muscular sheet underlying the

sacrospinous ligament, helps the levator ani support the pelvic organs. Muscles of the pelvic floor are shown in Figure 4–10 and discussed in Table 4–1.

PELVIC DIVISION

The pelvic cavity is divided into the false pelvis and the true pelvis (Figure 4–11A). The **false pelvis**, the portion above the pelvic brim, or linea terminalis, serves to support the weight of the enlarged pregnant uterus and direct the presenting fetal part into the true pelvis below.

TABLE 4–1 Muscles of the Pelvic Floor

MUSCLE	ORIGIN	INSERTION	INNERVATION	ACTION
Levator ani	Pubis, lateral pelvic wall, and ischial spine	Blends with organs in pelvic cavity	Inferior rectal, second, and third sacral nerves, plus anterior rami of third and fourth sacral nerves	Supports pelvic viscera; helps form pelvic diaphragm
Iliococcygeus	Pelvic surface of ischial spine and pelvic fascia	Central point of perineum, coccygeal raphe, and coccyx		Assists in supporting abdominal and pelvic viscera
Pubococcygeus	Pubis and pelvic fascia	Coccyx		
Puborectalis	Pubis	Blends with rectum; meets similar fibers from opposite side		Forms sling for rectum, just posterior to it; raises anus
Pubovaginalis	Pubis	Blends into vagina		Supports vagina
Coccygeus	Ischial spine and sacrospinous ligament	Lateral border of lower sacrum and upper coccyx	Third and fourth sacral nerves	Supports pelvic viscera; helps form pelvic diaphragm; flexes and abducts coccyx

Posterior

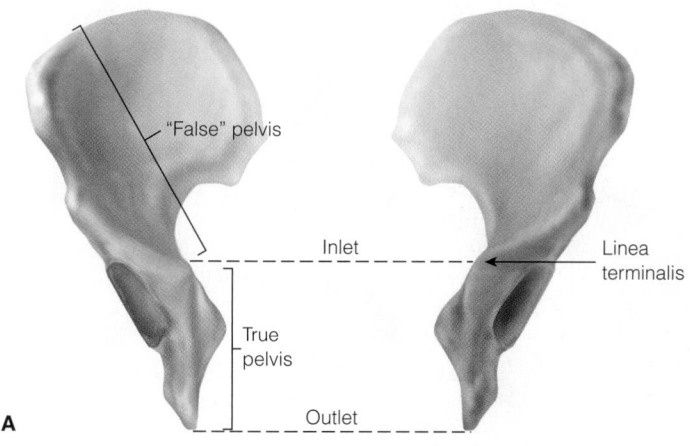

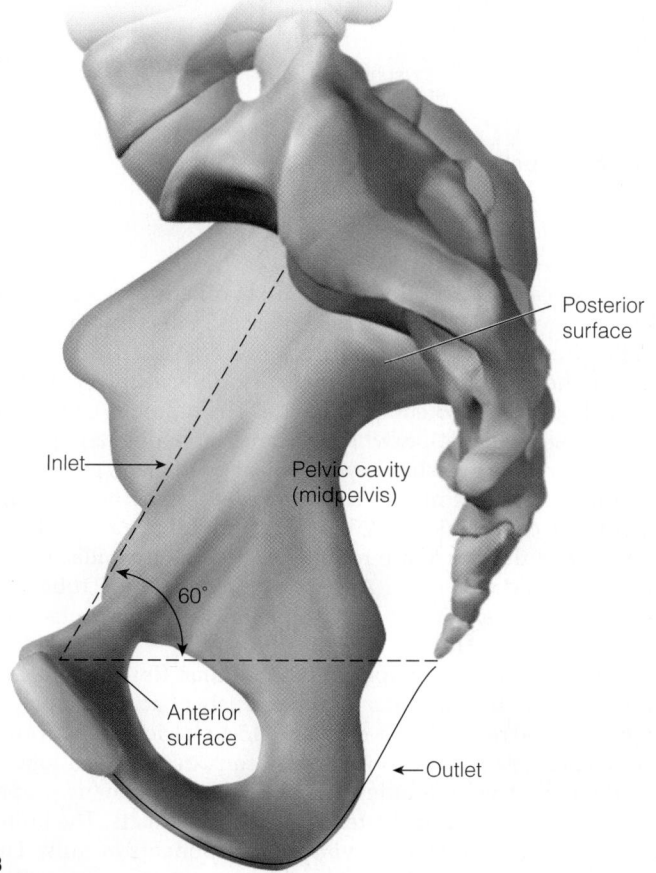

Figure 4–11 Female pelvis. *A,* False pelvis is a shallow cavity above the inlet; true pelvis is the deeper portion of the cavity below the inlet. *B,* True pelvis consists of inlet, cavity (midpelvis), and outlet.

The **true pelvis** is the portion that lies below the pelvic brim. The bony circumference of the true pelvis is made up of the sacrum, coccyx, and innominate bones and represents the bony limits of the birth canal. The relationship between the true pelvis and the fetal head is of paramount importance: The size and shape of the true pelvis must be adequate for normal fetal passage during labor and at birth. The true pelvis consists of three parts: the inlet, the pelvic cavity, and the outlet (Figure 4–11*B*). Each part has distinct measurements that aid in evaluating the adequacy of the pelvis for childbirth. Measurement

techniques are discussed in Chapter 9. The effects of inadequate or abnormal pelvic diameters on labor and birth are discussed in Chapter 16.

The **pelvic inlet** is the upper border of the true pelvis and is typically rounded in the female. The size and shape of the pelvic inlet are determined by assessing three anteroposterior diameters. The **diagonal conjugate** extends from the subpubic angle to the middle of the sacral promontory and is typically 12.5 cm. The diagonal conjugate can be measured manually during a pelvic examination. The **obstetric conjugate** extends from the middle of the sacral promontory to an area approximately 1 cm below the pubic crest. Its length is estimated by subtracting 1.5 cm from the length of the diagonal conjugate (Figure 4–12). The fetus passes through the obstetric conjugate, and the size of this diameter determines whether the fetus can move down into the birth canal in order for engagement to occur. The true (anatomic) conjugate, or **conjugate vera**, extends from the middle of the sacral promontory to the middle of the pubic crest (superior surface of the symphysis). One additional measurement, the transverse diameter, helps determine the shape of the inlet. The **transverse diameter** is the largest diameter of the inlet and is measured by using the linea terminalis as the point of reference.

The midpelvis, or *pelvic cavity (canal),* is a curved canal with a longer posterior than anterior wall. During labor, the descent of the fetal head into the true pelvis can be described by station and the midpelvis and ischial spines serve to mark zero station (Cunningham et al., 2014). A change in the lumbar curve can increase or decrease the tilt of the pelvis and can influence the progress of labor because the fetus has to adjust itself to this curved path as well as to the different diameters of the true pelvis.

The **pelvic outlet** is at the lower border of the true pelvis. The size of the pelvic outlet can be determined by assessing the outlet *transverse diameter.* The anteroposterior diameter of the pelvic outlet increases during birth as the presenting part pushes the coccyx posteriorly at the mobile sacrococcygeal joint. Decreased mobility, a large head, and/or a forceful birth can cause the coccyx to break. As the baby's head emerges, the long diameter of the head (occipital frontal) parallels the long diameter of the outlet (anteroposterior).

The transverse diameter *(bi-ischial or intertuberous)* extends from the inner surface of one ischial tuberosity to the other. In the pelvic outlet, the transverse diameter is the shortest diameter and becomes even shorter if the woman has a narrowed pubic arch. The pubic arch is of great importance because the fetus must pass under it during birth. If it is narrow, the baby's head may be pushed backward toward the coccyx, making extension of the head difficult. This situation, known as *outlet dystocia,* may require the use of forceps or a cesarean birth. The shoulders of a large baby may also become wedged under the pubic arch, making birth more difficult (see Chapter 22). The clinical assessment of each of these obstetric diameters is discussed further in Chapter 9.

PELVIC TYPES

The Caldwell-Moloy classification of pelvises is widely used to differentiate bony pelvic types (Caldwell & Moloy, 1933). The four basic types are *gynecoid, android, anthropoid,* and *platypelloid* (see Figure 16–1). However, variations in the female pelvis are so great that classic types are not usual. Each type has a characteristic shape, and each shape has implications for labor and birth, which are discussed in detail in Chapter 21.

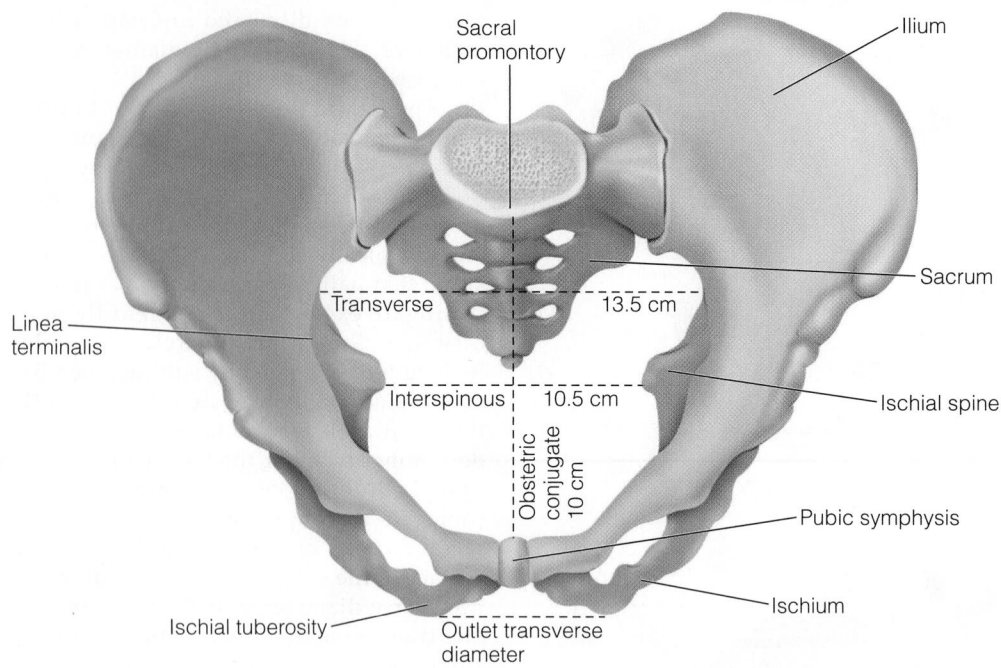

Figure 4–12 Pelvic planes: coronal section and diameters of the bony pelvis.

Breasts

The *breasts*, or *mammary glands*, considered accessories of the reproductive system, are specialized sebaceous glands (Figure 4–13). They are conical and symmetrically placed on the sides of the chest. The pectoral and anterior serratus muscles underlie each breast. Suspending the breasts are fibrous tissues, called *Cooper ligaments*, which extend from the deep fascia in the chest outward to just under the skin covering the breast. Frequently,

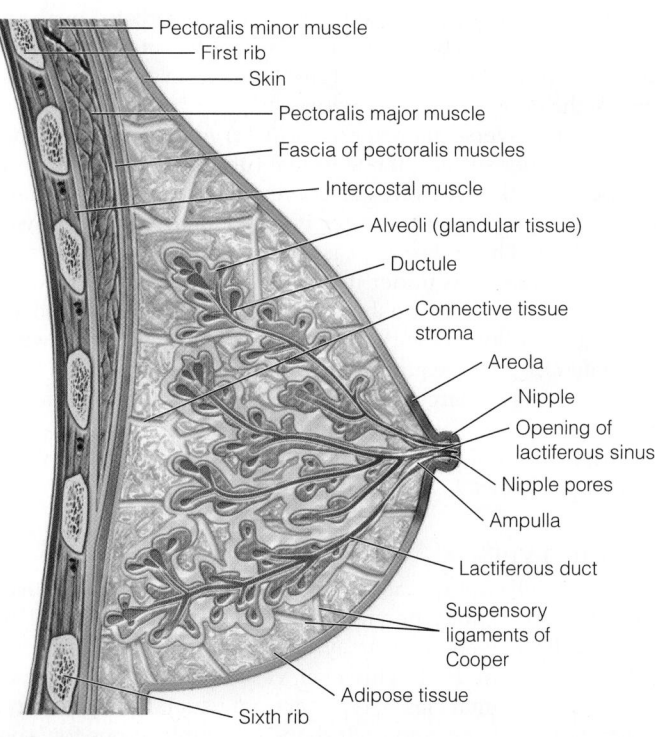

Figure 4–13 Anatomy of the breast.

the left breast is larger than the right. In different racial groups, breasts develop at slightly different levels in the pectoral region of the chest.

In the center of each mature breast is the **nipple**, a protrusion about 0.5 to 1.3 cm in diameter. The nipple is composed mainly of erectile tissue, which becomes more rigid and prominent during the menstrual cycle, sexual excitement, pregnancy, and lactation. The nipple is surrounded by the heavily pigmented **areola**, which is 2.5 to 10.0 cm in diameter. Both the nipple and the areola are roughened by small papillae called *tubercles of Montgomery*. As a baby suckles, these tubercles secrete a fatty substance that helps lubricate and protect the nipple (Karam, 2013).

The breasts are composed of glandular, fibrous, and adipose tissue. The glandular tissue consists of acini, or alveoli, which are arranged in a series of 15 to 24 lobes separated from each other by adipose and fibrous tissue. Each lobe is made up of several lobules that are made up of many grape-like clusters of alveoli clustered around tiny ducts. The lining of these ducts secretes the various components of milk. The ducts from several lobules share common openings, called *nipple pores*, and open on the surface of the nipple. The smooth muscle of the nipple causes erection of the nipple on contraction (Karam, 2013).

The biologic function of the breasts is to:

- Provide nourishment and protective maternal antibodies to newborns and infants through the lactation process.

- Be a source of pleasurable sexual sensation.

The Female Reproductive Cycle

The **female reproductive cycle (FRC)** is composed of the ovarian cycle, during which ovulation occurs, and the uterine (menstrual) cycle, during which menstruation occurs. These two cycles take place simultaneously (Figure 4–14).

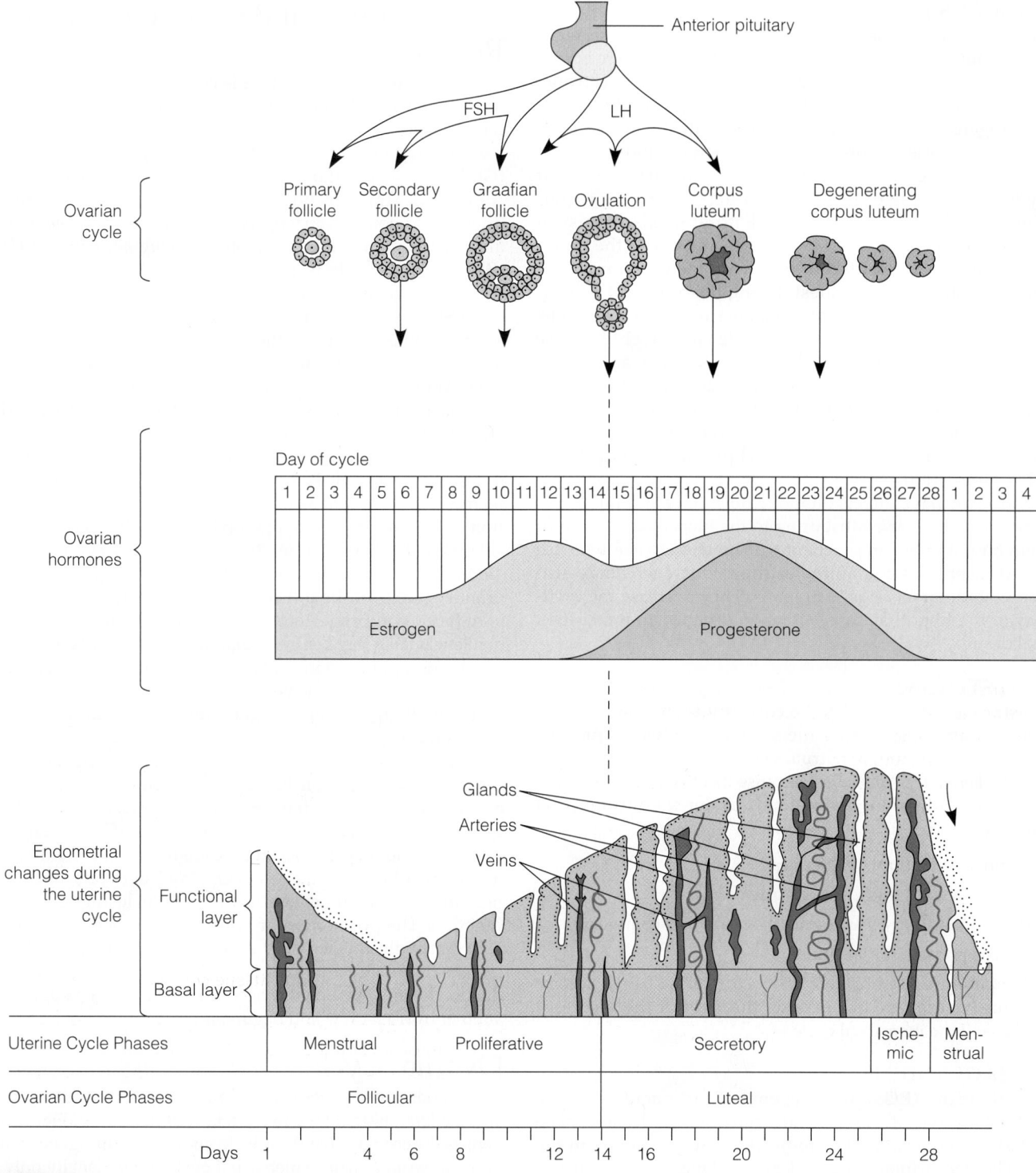

Figure 4-14 Female reproductive cycle: interrelationships of hormones with the four phases of the uterine cycle and the two phases of the ovarian cycle in an ideal 28-day cycle.

Effects of Female Hormones

After menarche, a woman undergoes a cyclic pattern of ovulation and menstruation for a period of 30 to 40 years. Menstruation is an orderly process under neurohormonal control. Each month multiple oocytes mature, with one rupturing from the ovary, and entering the fallopian tube. The ovary, vagina, uterus, and fallopian tubes are major target organs for female hormones.

The ovaries produce mature gametes and secrete hormones (see discussion in Chapter 7). Ovarian hormones include estrogen, progesterone, and testosterone. The ovary is sensitive to follicle-stimulating hormone (FSH) and luteinizing hormone (LH). The uterus is sensitive to estrogen and progesterone. The relative proportion of these hormones to each other controls the events of both ovarian and menstrual cycles.

ESTROGENS

Estrogens are hormones that are associated with characteristics contributing to "femaleness." The major estrogenic effects are primarily the result of three classic estrogens: estrone, β-estradiol, and estriol. The major estrogen is β-estradiol.

Estrogens control the development of the female secondary sex characteristics: breast development (including breast alveolar lobule growth and duct development), growth of body hair, widening of the hips, and deposits of tissue (fat) in the buttocks and mons pubis. Estrogens also assist in the maturation of the ovarian follicles and cause the endometrial mucosa to proliferate following menstruation. The amount of estrogens is greatest during the proliferative (follicular or estrogenic) phase of the menstrual cycle. Estrogens also cause the uterus to increase in size and weight because of increased glycogen, amino acids, electrolytes, and water. Blood supply is expanded as well. Under the influence of estrogens, myometrial contractility increases in both the uterus and the fallopian tubes, and uterine sensitivity to oxytocin increases. Estrogens inhibit FSH production and stimulate LH production.

Estrogens have effects on many hormones and other carrier proteins, such as contributing to the increased amount of protein-bound iodine in pregnant women and women who use oral contraceptives containing estrogen. Estrogens may also increase libidinal feelings in humans. They decrease the excitability of the hypothalamus, which may cause an increase in sexual desire.

PROGESTERONE

Progesterone is secreted by the corpus luteum and is found in greatest amounts during the secretory (luteal or progestational) phase of the menstrual cycle. Progesterone is often called the *hormone of pregnancy* because its effects on the uterus allow pregnancy to be maintained. Under the influence of progesterone:

- Vaginal epithelium proliferates.
- Cervix secretes thick, viscous mucus.
- Breast glandular tissue increases in size and complexity.
- Breasts prepare for lactation.
- Temperature rise of about 0.5 to 1.0°F (0.3 to 0.6°C) accompanies ovulation and persists throughout the secretory phase of the menstrual cycle.

PROSTAGLANDINS

Prostaglandins (PGs) are oxygenated fatty acids that are produced by the cells of the endometrium and are also classified as hormones. Prostaglandins have varied action in the body. The two primary types of prostaglandins are groups E and F. Generally PGE relaxes smooth muscles and is a potent vasodilator; PGF is a potent vasoconstrictor and increases the contractility of muscles and arteries. Although the primary actions of PGE and PGF seem antagonistic, their basic regulatory functions in cells are achieved through an intricate pattern of reciprocal events.

Prostaglandin production increases during follicular maturation, is dependent on gonadotropins, and seems to be critical to follicular rupture. Extrusion of the ovum, resulting from follicular swelling and increased contractility of the smooth muscle in the theca externa layer of the mature follicle, is thought to be caused in part by $PGF_{2\alpha}$. Significant amounts of PGs are found in and around the follicle at the time of ovulation.

Neurohormonal Basis of the Female Reproductive Cycle

The female reproductive cycle is controlled by complex interactions between the nervous and endocrine systems and their target tissues.

The hypothalamus secretes *gonadotropin-releasing hormone* (GnRH) to the pituitary gland in response to signals received from the central nervous system. This releasing hormone is often called both *luteinizing hormone-releasing hormone* (LHRH) and *follicle-stimulating hormone-releasing hormone* (FSHRH) (Blackburn, 2013). In response to GnRH, the anterior pituitary secretes the gonadotropic hormones *FSH* and *LH*.

FSH is primarily responsible for the maturation of the ovarian follicle. As the follicle matures, it secretes increasing amounts of estrogen, which enhance the development of the follicle (Alford & Nurudeen, 2013). (This estrogen is also responsible for the rebuilding/proliferation phase of the endometrium after it is shed during menstruation.)

Final maturation of the follicle cannot come about without the action of LH. The anterior pituitary's production of LH increases 6- to 10-fold as the follicle matures. The peak production of LH can precede ovulation by as much as 12 to 24 hours (Blackburn, 2013; Caudle, 2014). LH is also responsible for "luteinizing" the increase in production of progesterone by the granulosa cells of the follicle. As a result, estrogen production is reduced and progesterone secretion continues. Thus estrogen levels fall a day before ovulation; tiny amounts of inhibitin and progesterone are in evidence (Blackburn, 2013). **Ovulation** takes place following the very rapid growth of the follicle, as the sustained high level of estrogen diminishes and progesterone secretion begins.

The ruptured follicle undergoes rapid change, complete luteinization is accomplished, and the mass of cells becomes the **corpus luteum**. The lutein cells secrete large amounts of progesterone with smaller amounts of estradiol. (Concurrently, the excessive amounts of progesterone are responsible for the secretory phase of the uterine cycle.) On day 7 or 8 following ovulation, the corpus luteum begins to involute, losing its secretory function. The production of both progesterone and estrogen is severely diminished. The anterior pituitary responds with increasingly large amounts of FSH; a few days later LH production begins. As a result, new follicles become responsive to another ovarian cycle and begin maturing.

Ovarian Cycle

The ovarian cycle has two phases: the *follicular phase* (days 1 to 14) and the *luteal phase* (days 15 to 28 in a 28-day cycle). Figure 4–15 depicts the changes that the follicle undergoes during the ovarian cycle. In women whose menstrual cycles vary, usually only the length of the follicular phase varies because the luteal phase is of fixed length (Caudle, 2014; Cunningham et al., 2014). During the follicular phase, the immature follicle matures as a result of FSH. Within the follicle, the oocyte grows.

A mature **graafian follicle** appears on about the 14th day under dual control of FSH and LH. It is a large structure, measuring about 5 to 10 mm. The mature follicle produces increasing amounts of estrogen. In the mature graafian follicle, the cells surrounding the fluid-filled antral cavity are granulosa cells. The mass of granulosa cells surrounding the oocyte and follicular fluid is called the *cumulus oophorus*. In the fully mature graafian follicle, the *zona pellucida*, a thick elastic capsule, develops around the oocyte. Just before ovulation, the mature oocyte completes its first meiotic division (see Chapter 7 for a

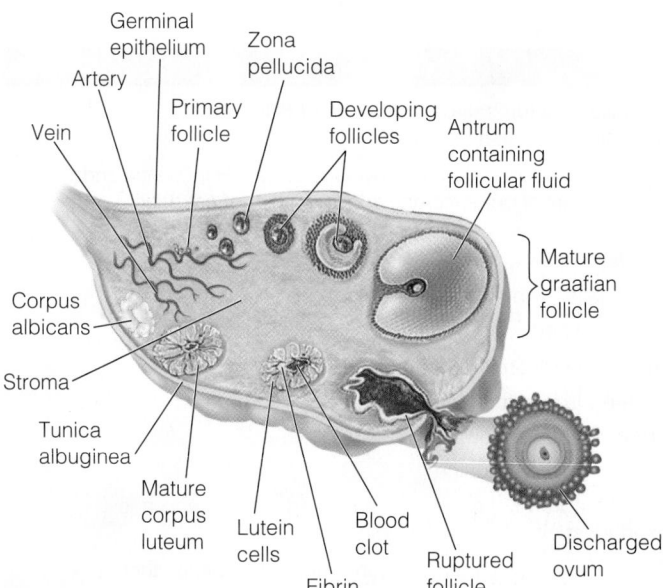

Germinal epithelium
Zona pellucida
Artery
Primary follicle
Developing follicles
Vein
Antrum containing follicular fluid
Mature graafian follicle
Corpus albicans
Stroma
Tunica albuginea
Mature corpus luteum
Lutein cells
Blood clot
Fibrin
Ruptured follicle
Discharged ovum

Figure 4–15 Various stages of development of the ovarian follicles.

description of meiosis). As a result of this division, two cells are formed: a small cell, called a *polar body*, and a larger cell, called the *secondary oocyte*. The secondary oocyte matures into the ovum (see Figure 7–1).

As the graafian follicle matures and enlarges, it comes close to the surface of the ovary. The ovary surface forms a blister-like protrusion 10 to 15 mm in diameter, and the follicle walls become thin. The secondary oocyte, polar body, and follicular fluid are pushed out. The ovum is discharged near the fimbria of the fallopian tube and is pulled into the tube to begin its journey toward the uterus (see Figure 7–3).

In some women, ovulation is accompanied by midcycle pain known as *mittelschmerz*. This pain may be caused by a local peritoneal reaction to the expelling of the follicular contents. Vaginal discharge may increase during ovulation, and a small amount of blood (midcycle spotting) may be discharged as well.

The body temperature increases about 0.5 to 1.0°F (0.3 to 0.6°C) 24 to 48 hours after the time of ovulation. It remains elevated until the day before menstruation begins. There may be an accompanying sharp basal body temperature drop before the increase. These temperature changes are useful clinically to determine the approximate time ovulation occurs (Blackburn, 2013).

Generally, the ovum takes several minutes to travel through the ruptured follicle to the fallopian tube opening. The contractions of the tube's smooth muscle and its ciliary action propel the ovum through the tube. The ovum remains in the ampulla, where, if it is fertilized, cleavage can begin. The ovum is thought to be fertile for only 6 to 24 hours. It reaches the uterus 72 to 96 hours after its release from the ovary.

The luteal phase begins when the ovum leaves its follicle. Under the influence of LH, the corpus luteum develops from the ruptured follicle. Within 2 or 3 days, the corpus luteum becomes yellowish and spherical and increases in vascularity. If the ovum is fertilized and implants in the endometrium, the fertilized egg begins to secrete **human chorionic gonadotropin** (hCG), which is needed to maintain the corpus luteum. If fertilization does not occur, within about a week after ovulation the corpus luteum begins to degenerate, eventually becoming a connective tissue scar called the *corpus albicans*. With degeneration

comes a decrease in estrogen and progesterone. This allows for an increase in LH and FSH, which triggers the hypothalamus to secrete gonadotropin-releasing hormone (GnRH) to restart the follicular phase.

Uterine (Menstrual) Cycle

Menstruation is cyclic uterine bleeding in response to cyclic hormonal changes. Menstruation occurs when the ovum is not fertilized and begins about 14 days after ovulation (in an ideal 28-day cycle) in the absence of pregnancy. The menstrual discharge, also referred to as the *menses*, or *menstrual flow*, is composed of blood mixed with fluid, cervical and vaginal secretions, bacteria, mucus, leukocytes, and other cellular debris. The menstrual discharge is dark red and has a distinctive odor.

Menstrual parameters vary greatly among individuals. Generally, menstruation occurs every 29 days, but varies from 21 to 35 days. Some women normally have longer cycles, which can skew standard calculations of the estimated date of birth (EDB) when they become pregnant. Emotional and physical factors such as illness, excessive fatigue, stress or anxiety, and vigorous exercise programs can alter the cycle interval. Certain environmental factors such as temperature and altitude may also affect the cycle. The duration of menses is from 2 to 8 days, with the blood loss averaging 25 to 60 mL, and the loss of iron averaging 0.5 to 1.0 mg daily.

The uterine (menstrual) cycle has four phases: menstrual, proliferative, secretory, and ischemic (see Figure 4–14). Menstruation occurs during the *menstrual phase*. Some endometrial areas are shed, although others remain. Some of the remaining tips of the endometrial glands begin to regenerate. The endometrium is in a resting state following menstruation. Estrogen levels are low, and the endometrium is 1 to 2 mm deep. During this part of the cycle, the cervical mucosa is scanty, viscous, and opaque.

The *proliferative phase* begins when the endometrial glands enlarge, becoming twisted and longer in response to increasing amounts of estrogen. The blood vessels become prominent and dilated, and the endometrium increases in thickness six- to eightfold. This gradual process reaches its peak just before ovulation. The cervical mucosa becomes thin, clear, watery, and more alkaline, making the mucosa more receptive to spermatozoa. As ovulation nears, the cervical mucosa shows increased elasticity. The cervical mucosa pH increases from below 7.0 to 7.5 at the time of ovulation. On microscopic examination, the mucosa shows a characteristic ferning pattern (Caudle, 2014) (see *Teaching Highlights: Methods of Determining Ovulation* in Chapter 6 and Figure 6–7).

The *secretory phase* follows ovulation. The endometrium, under estrogenic influence, undergoes slight cellular growth. Progesterone, however, causes such marked swelling and growth that the epithelium is warped into folds. The glandular epithelial cells begin to fill with cellular debris, become twisted, and dilate. The glands secrete small quantities of endometrial fluid in preparation for a fertilized ovum. The vascularity of the entire uterus increases greatly, providing a nourishing bed for implantation. If implantation occurs, the endometrium, under the influence of progesterone, continues to develop and become even thicker (see Chapter 7 for a discussion of implantation).

If fertilization does not occur, the *ischemic phase* begins. The corpus luteum begins to degenerate, and as a result both estrogen and progesterone levels fall. Areas of necrosis appear under the epithelial lining. Extensive vascular changes also occur. Small blood vessels rupture, and the spiral arteries constrict

TABLE 4–2 Summary of Female Reproductive Cycle

CYCLE	PHASE	DAYS	EVENTS
Ovarian Cycle	Follicular phase	Days 1–14	Primordial follicle matures under influence of FSH and LH up to the time of ovulation.
	Luteal phase	Days 15–28	Ovum leaves follicle; corpus luteum develops under LH influence and produces high levels of progesterone and low levels of estrogen.
Uterine (Menstrual) Cycle	Menstrual phase	Days 1–6	Estrogen levels are low. Cervical mucus is scant, viscous, and opaque. Endometrium is shed.
	Proliferative phase	Days 7–14	Endometrium and myometrium thickness increases. Estrogen peaks just before ovulation. Cervical mucus at ovulation: Is clear, thin, watery, alkaline; Is more favorable to sperm; shows ferning pattern and has increased elasticity on microscopic exam. Just before ovulation, body temperature may drop slightly, then at ovulation basal body temperature increases 0.5–1.0°F (0.3–0.6°C). Mittelschmerz and/or midcycle spotting may occur.
	Secretory phase	Days 15–26	Estrogen drops sharply, and progesterone dominates. Vascularity of entire uterus increases. Tissue glycogen increases, and the uterus is made ready for implantation.
	Ischemic phase	Days 27–28	Both estrogen and progesterone levels drop. Spiral arteries undergo vasoconstriction. Endometrium becomes pale; blood vessels rupture. Blood escapes into uterine stromal cells, gets ready to be shed.

and retract, causing a deficiency of blood in the endometrium, which becomes pale. This ischemic phase is characterized by the escape of blood into the stromal cells of the uterus. The menstrual flow begins, thus beginning the menstrual cycle again. After menstruation the basal layer remains, so that the tips of the glands can regenerate the new functional endometrial layer. For further discussion, see Table 4–2.

Male Reproductive System

The primary reproductive functions of the male genitals are to produce and transport sex cells (sperm) through and eventually out of the male genital tract and into the female genital tract. The external and internal genitals of the male reproductive system are shown in Figure 4–16.

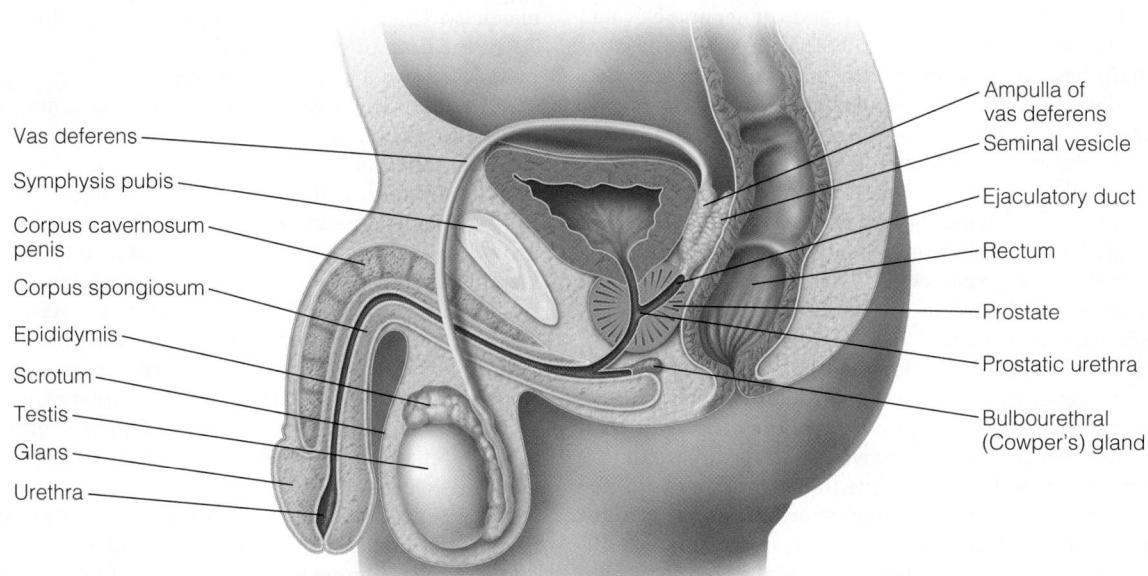

Figure 4–16 **Male reproductive system, sagittal view.**

External Genitals

The two external reproductive organs are the penis and scrotum.

PENIS

The *penis* is an elongated, cylindrical structure consisting of a body, called the *shaft*, and a cone-shaped end, called the *glans*. The penis lies in front of the scrotum. The shaft of the penis is made up of three longitudinal columns of erectile tissue: the paired *corpora cavernosa* and the *corpus spongiosum*. These columns are covered by dense fibrous connective tissue and then enclosed by elastic tissue. The penis is covered by a thin outer layer of skin.

The corpus spongiosum contains the urethra and becomes the glans at the distal end of the penis. The urethra widens within the glans and ends in a slitlike opening, located in the tip of the glans, called the *urethral meatus*. A circular fold of skin arises just behind the glans and covers it. Known as the *prepuce*, or *foreskin*, it may be removed by the surgical procedure of circumcision (see Chapter 25 for a discussion of circumcision). If the corpus spongiosum does not surround the urethra completely, the urethral meatus may occur on the ventral aspect of the penile shaft (hypospadias) or on the dorsal aspect (epispadias).

The penis is innervated by the pudendal nerve. Sexual stimulation causes the penis to elongate, thicken, and stiffen, a process called *erection*. The penis becomes erect when its blood vessels become engorged, a consequence of parasympathetic nerve stimulation. If sexual stimulation is intense enough, the forceful and sudden expulsion of semen occurs through the rhythmic contractions of the penile muscles. This phenomenon is called *ejaculation*.

The penis serves both the urinary and the reproductive systems. Urine is expelled through the urethral meatus. The reproductive function of the penis is to deposit sperm in the vagina so that fertilization of the ovum can occur.

SCROTUM

The *scrotum* is a pouchlike structure that hangs in front of the anus and behind the penis. Composed of skin and the *dartos* muscle, the scrotum shows increased pigmentation and scattered hairs. The sebaceous glands open directly onto the scrotal surface; their secretion has a distinctive odor. Contraction of the dartos and cremasteric muscles shortens the scrotum and draws it closer to the body, thus wrinkling its outer surface. The degree of wrinkling is greatest in young men and at cold temperatures and is least in older men and at warm temperatures.

Inside the scrotum are two lateral compartments. Each compartment contains a testis with its related structures. Because the left spermatic cord grows longer, the left testis and its scrotal sac hang lower than the right. A ridge (raphe) on the external scrotal surface marks the position of the medial septum and continues anteriorly on the urethral surface of the penis, disappearing in the perineal area.

The function of the scrotum is to protect the testes and the sperm by maintaining a temperature lower than that of the body. Spermatogenesis cannot occur if the testes fail to descend and thus remain at body temperature. Because it is sensitive to touch, pressure, temperature, and pain, the scrotum defends against potential harm to the testes.

Male Internal Reproductive Organs

The male internal reproductive organs include the gonads (testes or testicles), a system of ducts (epididymides, vas deferens,

ejaculatory duct, and urethra), and accessory glands (seminal vesicles, prostate gland, bulbourethral glands, and urethral glands).

TESTES

The *testes* are a pair of oval, compound glandular organs contained in the scrotum. In the sexually mature male, they are the site of spermatozoa (male gamete) production and the secretion of several male sex hormones.

Each testis is 4 to 6 cm long, 2 to 3 cm wide, and 3 to 4 cm thick and weighs about 10 to 15 g. Each is covered by an outer serous membrane and an inner capsule that is tough, white, and fibrous. The connective tissue sends projections inward to form septa, dividing the testis into 250 to 400 lobules. Each lobule contains one to three tightly packed, convoluted *seminiferous tubules* containing sperm cells in all stages of development.

The seminiferous tubules are surrounded by loose connective tissue that houses abundant blood and lymph vessels and *interstitial (Leydig) cells*. The interstitial cells produce testosterone, the primary male sex hormone. The tubules also contain Sertoli cells, which nourish and protect the spermatocytes (phase between spermatids and spermatozoa). The seminiferous tubules come together to form 20 to 30 straight tubules, which in turn form an anastomotic network of thin-walled spaces, the rete testis. The rete testis forms 10 to 15 efferent ducts that empty into the duct of the epididymis.

Most of the cells lining the seminiferous tubules undergo *spermatogenesis*, a process of maturation in which spermatocytes become spermatozoa. (Chapter 7 further discusses the process of spermatogenesis.) Sperm production varies among and within the tubules, with cells in different areas of the same tubule undergoing different stages of spermatogenesis. The sperm are eventually released from the tubules into the epididymis, where they mature further.

Like the female reproductive cycle, the process of spermatogenesis and other functions of the testes are the result of complex neural and hormonal controls. The hypothalamus secretes releasing factors that stimulate the anterior pituitary to release the gonadotropins—FSH and LH. These hormones cause the testes to produce testosterone, which maintains spermatogenesis, increases sperm production by the seminiferous tubules, and stimulates production of seminal fluid.

Testosterone is the most prevalent and potent of the testicular hormones. It is also responsible for the development of secondary male characteristics and certain behavioral patterns. The effects of testosterone include structural and functional development of the male genital tract, emission and ejaculation of seminal fluid, distribution of body hair, promotion of growth and strength of long bones, increased muscle mass, and enlargement of the vocal cords. The action of testosterone on the central nervous system is thought to produce aggressiveness and sexual drive. The action of testosterone is constant, not cyclic like that of the female hormones. Its production is not limited to a certain number of years, but it is thought to decrease with age.

The testes have two primary functions:

- To serve as the site of spermatogenesis
- To produce testosterone

EPIDIDYMIS

The *epididymis* (plural, *epididymides*) is a duct about 5.6 m long, although it is convoluted into a compact structure about 3.75 cm long. An epididymis lies behind each testis. It arises from the top of the testis, courses downward, and then passes upward, where it becomes the vas deferens.

The epididymis provides a reservoir for maturing spermatozoa. When discharged from the seminiferous tubules into the epididymis, the sperm are immotile and incapable of fertilizing an ovum. The spermatozoa usually remain in the epididymis for 2 to 10 days but can be stored in the body for up to 42 days. As the sperm move along the tortuous course of the epididymis they become both motile and fertile.

VAS DEFERENS AND EJACULATORY DUCTS

The *vas deferens*, also known as the *ductus deferens*, is about 40 cm long and connects the epididymis with the prostate. One vas deferens arises from the posterior border of each testis. It joins the spermatic cord and weaves over and between several pelvic structures until it meets the vas deferens from the opposite side. Each vas deferens terminus expands to form the *terminal ampulla*. It then unites with the seminal vesicle duct (a gland) to form the ejaculatory duct, which enters the prostate gland and ends in the prostatic urethra. The ejaculatory ducts serve as passageways for semen and fluid secreted by the seminal vesicles. The main function of the vas deferens is to squeeze the sperm rapidly from their storage sites (the epididymis and distal part of the vas deferens) into the urethra.

Men who choose to take total responsibility for birth control may elect to have a vasectomy. In this procedure, the scrotal portion of the vas deferens is surgically incised or cauterized. Although sperm continues to be produced for the next several years, they can no longer reach the outside of the body. Eventually, the sperm deteriorate and are reabsorbed.

URETHRA

The *male urethra* is the passageway for both urine and semen. The urethra begins in the bladder and passes through the prostate gland, where it is called the *prostatic urethra*. The urethra emerges from the prostate gland to become the *membranous urethra*. It terminates in the penis, where it is called the *penile urethra*. In the penile urethra, goblet secretory cells are present, and smooth muscle is replaced by erectile tissue.

ACCESSORY GLANDS

The male accessory glands secrete a unique and essential component of the total seminal fluid in an ordered sequence.

The *seminal vesicles* are two glands composed of many lobes. Each vesicle is about 7.5 cm long. They are situated between the bladder and the rectum, immediately above the base of the prostate. The epithelium lining the seminal vesicles secretes an alkaline, viscous, clear fluid rich in high-energy fructose, prostaglandins, fibrinogen, and amino acids. During ejaculation, this fluid mixes with the sperm in the ejaculatory ducts. This fluid helps provide an environment favorable to sperm motility and metabolism.

The *prostate gland* encircles the upper part of the urethra and lies below the neck of the bladder. Made up of several lobes, it measures about 4 cm in diameter and weighs 20 to 30 g. The prostate is made up of both glandular and muscular tissue. It secretes a thin, milky, alkaline fluid containing high levels of zinc, calcium, citric acid, and acid phosphatase. This fluid protects the sperm from the acidic environment of the vagina and the male urethra, which would otherwise be spermicidal.

The *bulbourethral (Cowper) glands* are a pair of small, round structures on either side of the membranous urethra. The glands secrete a clear, thick, alkaline fluid rich in mucoproteins that becomes part of the semen. This secretion also lubricates the penile urethra during sexual excitement and neutralizes the acid in the male urethra and the vagina, thereby enhancing sperm motility.

The *urethral (Littré) glands* are tiny mucus-secreting glands found throughout the membranous lining of the penile urethra. Their secretions add to those of the bulbourethral glands. See Table 4–3.

TABLE 4–3 Summary of Male Reproductive Organ Functions

ORGAN	STRUCTURE	FUNCTION
Testes	Seminiferous tubules	Contain sperm cells in various stages of development and undergoing meiosis.
	Sertoli cells	Nourish and protect spermatocytes (phase between spermatids and spermatozoa).
	Interstitial (Leydig) cells	Provide the main source of testosterone.
Ducts	Epididymides	Provide an area for maturation of sperm and a reservoir for mature spermatozoa.
	Vas deferens	Connects the epididymis with the prostate gland, then connects with ducts from the seminal vesicle to become an ejaculatory duct.
	Ejaculatory ducts	Provide a passageway for semen and seminal fluid into the urethra.
Accessory glands	Seminal vesicles	Secrete yellowish fluid rich in fructose, prostaglandins, and fibrinogen. This provides nutrition that increases motility and fertilizing ability of sperm. Prostaglandins also aid fertilization by making the cervical mucus more receptive to sperm.
	Prostate gland	Secretes thin, alkaline fluid containing calcium, citric acid, and other substances. Alkalinity counteracts acidity of ductus and seminal vesicle secretions.
	Bulbourethral (Cowper) glands	Secrete alkaline, viscous fluid into semen, aiding in neutralization of acidic vaginal secretions.
	Urethral (Littré) glands	Add secretions to those of the bulbourethral glands.

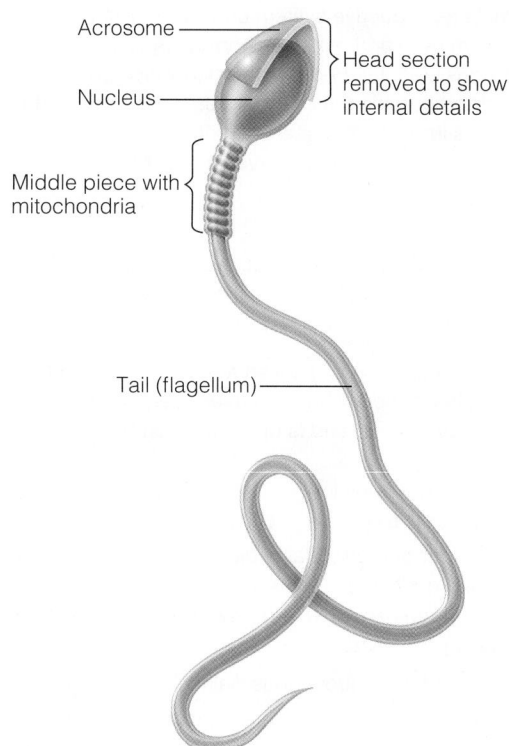

Acrosome

Nucleus

Head section removed to show internal details

Middle piece with mitochondria

Tail (flagellum)

Figure 4–17 Schematic representation of a mature spermatozoon.

SEMEN

The male ejaculate, *semen* or *seminal fluid*, is made up of spermatozoa and the secretions of all the accessory glands. The seminal fluid transports viable and motile sperm to the female reproductive tract. Effective transportation of sperm requires adequate nutrients, an adequate pH (about 7.5), a specific concentration of sperm to fluid, and an optimal osmolarity.

A spermatozoon is made up of a head and a tail (Figure 4–17). The head's main components are the acrosome and nucleus. The head carries the male's haploid number of chromosomes (23), and it is the part that enters the ovum at fertilization (see Chapter 7). The tail, or *flagellum*, is specialized for motility. The tail is divided into the middle and end piece.

Sperm may be stored in the epididymis and distal vas deferens for up to 42 days, depending primarily on the frequency of ejaculations. The average volume of ejaculate following abstinence for several days is 2 to 5 mL but may vary from 1 to 10 mL. Repeated ejaculation results in decreased volume. Once ejaculated, sperm can live for 2 or 3 days in the female genital tract.

Focus Your Study

- Reproductive activities require a complex interaction between the reproductive structures, the central nervous system, and such endocrine glands as the pituitary, hypothalamus, testes, and ovaries.

- The female reproductive system consists of the ovaries, where female germ cells and female sex hormones are formed; the fallopian tubes, which capture the ovum and allow transport to the uterus; the uterus, which is the implantation site for the fertilized ovum; the cervix, which is a protective portal for the body of the uterus and the connection between the vagina and the uterus; and the vagina, which is the passageway from the external genitals to the uterus and provides for discharge of menstrual products out of the body.

- The pelvic structure of the true pelvis consists of an inlet, cavity (midpelvis), and outlet and must be adequate for normal fetal passage during labor and birth. The midpelvis (cavity) structure includes the ischial spines which are used to mark the descent of the fetal head into the true pelvis.

- Estrogen causes endometrial mucosa to proliferate following menstruation and increases the size and weight of the uterus. It increases uterine sensitivity to oxytocin and therefore increases myometrial contractility in both the uterus and fallopian tubes. Estrogen inhibits FSH production while stimulating LH production. Progesterone decreases uterine motility

and contractility. It causes uterine endometrium to increase its nutrient store and arterial blood supply. The vaginal epithelium proliferates and the cervix secretes thick, viscous mucus. Progesterone increases breast glandular tissue and prepares the breasts for lactation. Prostaglandins are necessary for follicular rupture.

- The female reproductive cycle may be described in terms of the ovarian cycle, during which ovulation occurs, and the menstrual cycle, during which menstruation occurs. These two cycles take place simultaneously and are under neurohumoral control.

- The ovarian cycle has two phases: the follicular phase and the luteal phase. During the follicular phase, the primordial follicle matures under the influence of FSH and LH until ovulation occurs. The luteal phase begins when the ovum leaves the follicle and the corpus luteum develops under the influence of LH and prostaglandin. The corpus luteum produces high levels of progesterone and low levels of estrogen.

- The menstrual cycle has four phases: menstrual, proliferative, secretory, and ischemic. Menstruation is the actual shedding of the endometrial lining, when estrogen levels are low. The proliferative phase begins when the endometrial glands begin to enlarge under the influence of estrogen and cervical mucosal changes occur; the changes peak at ovulation. The secretory phase follows ovulation, and, influenced primarily by progesterone, the uterus increases its vascularity to make ready for possible implantation. The ischemic phase is characterized by degeneration of the corpus luteum, decreases in both estrogen and progesterone levels, constriction of the spiral arteries, and escape of blood into the stromal cells of the endometrium.

- The male reproductive system consists of the testes, where male germ cells and male sex hormones are formed; a series of continuous ejaculatory ducts through which spermatozoa are transported outside the body; accessory glands that produce secretions important to sperm nutrition, survival, and transport; and the penis, which serves as the reproductive organ of intercourse.

Clinical Reasoning in Action

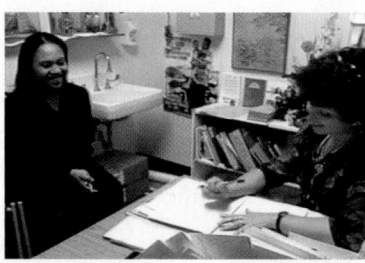

You are working in the OB/GYN clinic when Sally Smith, a 17-year-old teenager, comes in complaining of irregular menses. She believes her periods are really "messed up" and interfering with her active schedule. She wants them to be more regular and asks you for birth control. She tells you that she is a member of the swimming team and is a senior in high school. She says she is planning to start community college next year to obtain an associate degree in computer technology. You assess Sally's history as follows: menarche began at age 12; periods occur every 28 to 32 days. She usually experiences cramping in the first 2 days and the flow lasts 4 to 5 days. She uses an average of four to five tampons a day during her period. She has never been hospitalized, has no prior medical problems, and is up-to-date on her immunizations except for meningitis.

1. Based on your knowledge of menstruation, how would you describe Sally's menstrual cycle?
2. What is your primary goal in discussing Sally's menstrual cycle with her?
3. What information would you give Sally relating to her menstrual cycle?
4. What important request does Sally have?
5. Sally expresses problems dealing with the cramping she experiences with the first 2 days of her menses. What would you suggest to Sally to cope with the discomfort?

References

Alford, C., & Nurudeen, S. (2013). Physiology of reproduction in women. In A. H. DeCherney, L. Nathan, N. Lauffer, & A. S. Roman (Eds.), *Current diagnosis and treatment: Obstetrics & gynecology* (10th ed.). Boston, MA: McGraw-Hill.

Blackburn, S. T. (2013). *Maternal, fetal, & neonatal physiology: A clinical perspective* (4th ed.). St. Louis, MO: Saunders.

Caldwell, W. E., & Moloy, H. C. (1933). Anatomical variations in the female pelvis and their effect on labor with a suggested classification [Historical article]. *American Journal of Obstetrics and Gynecology, 26,* 479–505.

Caudle, P. W. (2014). Reproductive tract structure and function. In R. G. Jordan, J. L. Engstrom, J. A. Marfell, & C. L. Farley (Eds.), *Prenatal and postnatal care: A women-centered approach.* Ames, IA: Wiley Blackwell.

Cunningham, F. G., Leveno, K. J., Bloom, S. L., Spong, C. Y., Dashe, J. S., Hoffman, B. L., … Sheffield, J. S. (2014). *Williams obstetrics* (24th ed.). New York, NY: McGraw-Hill.

Heitmann, R. J. (2013). Anatomy of the female reproductive system. In A. H. DeCherney, L. Nathan, N. Lauffer, & A. S. Roman (Eds.), *Current diagnosis and treatment: Obstetrics & gynecology* (10th ed.). Boston, MA: McGraw-Hill.

Karam, A. (2013). The breast. In A. H. DeCherney, L. Nathan, N. Lauffer, & A. S. Roman (Eds.), *Current diagnosis and treatment: Obstetrics & gynecology* (10th ed.). Boston, MA: McGraw-Hill

Morris, D. (2007). The pubic hair. In D. Morris, *The Naked Woman: A study of the female body.* New York, NY: Thomas Dunne Books.

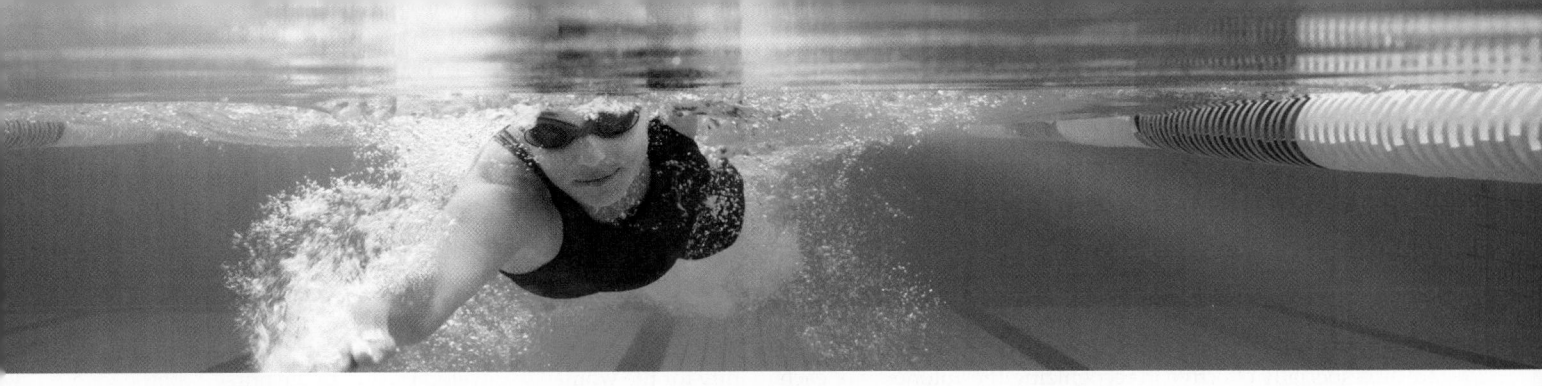

Chapter 5
Health Promotion for Women

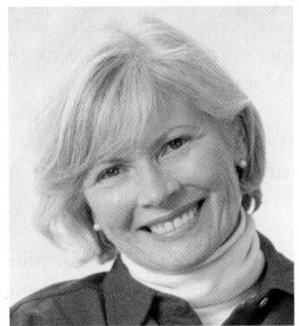

Steve Smith/Getty Images

I am 64 now, an early baby boomer. I am astonished at the changes that have occurred in women's health care in my lifetime. I remember that my mom was shocked when our family doctor taught me to do a breast exam when I turned 18. What a farsighted man. Information on sexually transmitted infections was not as generally available. AIDS was beyond our imagination. Contraceptive options were more limited, although the pill was gaining in popularity. Menopause seemed like the end of life—menopausal women were old. Today more and more of us women are becoming savvy healthcare consumers. We have more information, we have treatment options, we decide our own care. I think this is the most exciting change of all!

—Alice

∨ Learning Outcomes

5.1 Describe accurate information to be provided to girls and women so that they can implement effective self-care measures for dealing with menstruation.

5.2 Contrast the signs, symptoms, and nursing management of women with dysmenorrhea and those with premenstrual syndrome.

5.3 Compare the advantages, disadvantages, and effectiveness of the various methods of contraception available today.

5.4 Summarize major health measures to address in providing preconception counseling.

5.5 Identify basic gynecologic screening procedures indicated for well women.

5.6 Examine the physical and psychologic aspects and clinical treatment options of menopause when caring for menopausal women.

5.7 Describe the phases of the cycle of violence.

5.8 Identify the phases of the rape trauma syndrome.

5.9 Discuss the nurse's role in screening and caring for women who have experienced domestic violence or rape.

A woman's healthcare needs change throughout her lifetime. As a young girl, she needs health teaching about menstruation, sexuality, and personal responsibility. As a teen she needs information about reproductive choices and safe sexual activity. During this time she should also be introduced to the importance of healthcare practices such as regular Papanicolaou (Pap) smears. The mature woman may need to be reminded of these self-care issues and prepared for the physical changes that accompany childbirth and aging. By educating women about their bodies, their healthcare choices, and their right to be knowledgeable consumers, nurses can help

women assume responsibility for the health care they receive. This chapter provides information about selected aspects of women's health care with an emphasis on conditions typically addressed in a community-based setting.

Nursing Care in the Community

The term *women's health* refers to a holistic view of women and their health-related needs within the context of their everyday lives. It is based on the awareness that a woman's physical, mental, and spiritual status are interdependent and affect her state of health or illness. The woman's view of her situation, her assessment of her needs, her values, and her beliefs are valid and important factors to be incorporated into any healthcare intervention.

Nurses can work with women to provide health teaching and information about self-care practices in schools, during routine examinations in a clinic or office, at senior centers, at meetings of volunteer organizations, through classes offered by local agencies or schools, or in the home. Nurses oriented to community-based care are especially effective in recognizing the autonomy of each individual and in dealing with clients holistically. This holistic approach is important in addressing not only physical problems but also major health issues such as violence against women, which may go undetected unless care providers are alert for signs of it.

The Nurse's Role in Addressing Issues of Sexuality

Because sexuality and its reproductive implications are such intrinsic and emotion-laden parts of life, people have many concerns, problems, and questions about sex roles, behaviors, education, inhibitions, morality, and related areas such as family planning. The reproductive implications of sexual intercourse must also be considered. Some people desire pregnancy; others wish to avoid it. Health factors are another consideration. The increase in the incidence of sexually transmitted infections (STIs), especially HIV/AIDS and herpes, has caused many people to modify their sexual practices and activities. Women frequently ask questions or voice concerns about these issues to the nurse in a clinic or ambulatory setting. Thus the nurse may need to assume the role of counselor or educator on sexual and reproductive matters.

Nurses who assume this role must recognize their own feelings, values, and attitudes about sexuality so they can be more sensitive when they encounter the values and beliefs of others. Nurses need to have accurate, up-to-date information about anatomy and physiology and about topics related to sexuality, sexual practices, and common gynecologic problems. In addition, when a woman is accompanied by her partner, it is important that the nurse be sensitive to the dynamics of the relationship and communication patterns between the two.

Taking a Sexual History

Nurses are often responsible for taking a woman's initial history, including her gynecologic and sexual history. To be effective in this role, the nurse must have effective communication skills and should ideally conduct the interview in a quiet, private place free of distractions.

Clinical Tip

When taking a history, start your interview with less intimate areas, such as medical and surgical history, and then proceed to the sexual history toward the end of the history-taking session. This approach helps the woman develop a comfort level with you before disclosing personal information.

Opening the discussion with a brief explanation of the purpose of such questions is often helpful. For example, the nurse might say,

> As your nurse, I'm interested in all aspects of your well-being. Often women have concerns or questions about sexual matters, especially as their life situations change. I will be asking you some questions about your sexual history as part of your general health history.

This explanation helps women understand the nature of this part of their history and encourages more open, honest answers.

It may be helpful to use direct eye contact as much as possible unless the nurse knows it is culturally unacceptable to the woman. The nurse should do little, if any, writing or typing into a computer during the interview, especially if the woman seems ill at ease or is discussing very personal issues. Beginning with general questions such as "What brings you here today?" before progressing to more sensitive topics will provide an opportunity for the woman to develop trust with the nurse. Open-ended questions are often useful in eliciting information. For example, "What, if anything, would you change about your sex life?" will elicit more information than "Are you happy with your sex life now?" The nurse needs to clarify terminology and proceed from easier topics to those that are more difficult to discuss.

Throughout the interview the nurse should be alert to body language and nonverbal cues. It is important that the nurse not assume that the woman is heterosexual. Some women are open about lesbian relationships or transgender surgery; others are more reserved until they develop a sense of trust in their caregivers.

After completing the sexual history, the nurse assesses the information obtained. If there is a problem that requires further medical tests and assessments, the nurse refers the woman to a nurse practitioner, certified nurse-midwife, physician, or counselor as necessary. In many instances, the nurse alone will be able to develop a nursing diagnosis and then plan and implement therapy. The nurse must be realistic in making assessments and planning interventions. It requires insight and skill to recognize when a woman's problem requires interventions that are beyond a nurse's preparation and ability. In such situations, it is essential that the nurse make appropriate referrals.

Menstruation

Girls today begin to learn about puberty and menstruation at a young age. Unfortunately, the source of their "education" is sometimes their peers or the media; thus the information is often incomplete, inaccurate, and sensationalized. Nurses who work with young girls and adolescents recognize this and have been working hard to provide accurate health teaching and to correct misinformation they have been given about *menarche* (the onset of menses) and the menstrual cycle.

Cultural, religious, and personal attitudes about menstruation are part of the menstrual experience. Currently in the Western world, there are few customs associated with menstruation. Sexual intercourse during menses is a common practice, and is not generally contraindicated. For most couples, the decision is one of personal preference. (The physiology of menstruation is discussed in Chapter 4.)

Counseling the Premenstrual Girl About Menarche

Many young women find it embarrassing to discuss menstruation. However, the most critical factor in successful adaptation to menarche is the adolescent's level of preparedness. Information should be given to premenstrual girls over time rather than all at once. This allows them to absorb information and develop questions.

The following basic information is helpful for girls and young women:

- *Cycle length.* Cycle length is determined from the first day of one menses to the first day of the next menses. Initially, a female's cycle length may be irregular. Once established, it is about 29 days, although it may vary from 21 to 35 days. Cycle length frequently varies by a day or two from one cycle to the next, although greater normal variations may also occur.

- *Amount of flow.* The average flow is approximately 25 to 60 mL per period. Usually women characterize the amount of flow in terms of the number of pads or tampons used. Flow is often heavier at first and lighter toward the end of the period.

- *Length of menses.* Menses usually lasts from 3 to 5 days, although the length may vary, and may last up to 7 or 8 days (American College of Obstetricians and Gynecologists [ACOG], 2011b).

The nurse should make it clear that variations in age at menarche, length of cycle, and duration of menses are normal because girls may worry if their experiences vary from those of their peers. It also is helpful to acknowledge the negative aspects of menstruation (messiness, cramping, embarrassment) while stressing its positive role as a symbol of maturity and womanhood.

Cultural factors may play an important role in menstruation for girls and women of some cultures. See *Developing Cultural Competence: Islamic Women and Menstruation.*

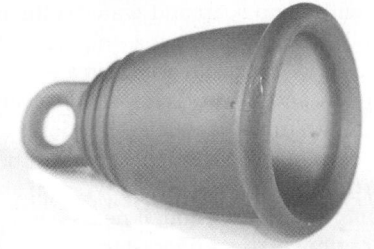

Figure 5–1 **A menstrual cup is an ecofriendly way to manage menstrual flow.**

SOURCE: Aguadeluna/Fotolia.

bleeding. Because *Staphylococcus aureus*, the causative organism of TSS, is frequently found on the hands, a woman should wash her hands before inserting a fresh tampon and should avoid touching the tip of the tampon when unwrapping it or before insertion.

Clinical Tip

If you work with teens and preteens, keep a variety of pads and tampons on hand so that you can help these young girls become familiar with the options available for dealing with menstruation. You can also put colored water in a small glass and insert a tampon to show a girl how much fluid a tampon absorbs. Girls often think that they lose far more blood with a period than they actually do.

In the absence of a heavy menstrual flow, tampons absorb moisture, leaving the vaginal walls dry and subject to injury. The absorbency of regular tampons varies. If the tampon is hard to pull out or shreds when removed, or if the vagina becomes dry, the tampon is probably too absorbent.

A woman may want to use tampons only during the day and switch to pads at night to avoid vaginal irritation. If a woman experiences vaginal irritation, itching, or soreness or notices an unusual odor while using tampons, she should stop using them and be evaluated for infection. The choice of sanitary protection—whether pads or tampons—must meet the individual's needs and feel comfortable. Cultural factors may play a role in this decision and should be considered.

VAGINAL SPRAY, DOUCHING, AND CLEANSING

Vaginal sprays are unnecessary and can cause infections, itching (pruritus), burning, vaginal discharge, rashes, and other problems. If a woman chooses to use a spray, she needs to know that these sprays are for external use only, should be used infrequently, and should never be applied to irritated or itching skin.

Douching as a hygienic practice is unnecessary because the vagina cleanses itself. Douching washes away the natural mucus and upsets the vaginal flora, which can make the vagina more susceptible to infection. Perfumed douches can cause allergic reactions. Propelling water up the vagina may force bacteria and germs from the vagina into the uterus. Women should avoid douching during menstruation because the cervix is dilated to permit the downward flow of menstrual fluids from the uterine lining. Douching is also contraindicated during pregnancy.

The secretions that bathe the vagina are odor-free while they are in the vagina; odor develops only when they mingle with perspiration and are exposed to the air. Keeping one's skin clean and

---

Developing Cultural Competence **Islamic Women and Menstruation**

Islamic women who are menstruating are not required to fast during the month of Ramadan but if they elect not to fast, they are expected to make up the missed fasting days before the next Ramadan. Because it may be harder to fast alone, many Muslim women use oral contraceptives to delay their menses until Ramadan ends (Kridli, 2011). Others choose to fast even when menstruating.

Educational Topics

PADS AND TAMPONS

Since early times women have made pads and tampons from cloth or rags, which required washing but were reusable. Commercial tampons were introduced in the 1930s.

Today, adhesive-stripped, disposable minipads and maxipads and tampons are readily available. However, the deodorants and increased absorbency that manufacturers have added to both pads and tampons may prove to be harmful. The chemical used to deodorize can create irritation of the vulva and inner aspects of the vagina. This irritation may cause an external rash or internal sores from trauma to the tender mucosal lining of the vagina.

Interest is also growing in the use of ecofriendly menstrual products, including reusable menstrual pads made of washable cotton, menstrual cups, and menstrual sponges. These products are becoming more readily available at pharmacies and major discount stores (see Figure 5–1).

The use of superabsorbent tampons has been linked to the development of toxic shock syndrome (TSS). (For more information about TSS, see Chapter 6.) Women can prevent problems by using tampons with the minimum absorbency necessary to control menstrual flow, changing them every 3 to 6 hours, and avoiding using them for vaginal discharge or light

free of bacteria with plain soap and water is the most effective method of controlling odor. Bathing is as important during menses as at any other time. A long, leisurely soak in a warm tub promotes menstrual blood flow and relieves cramps by relaxing the muscles.

A woman can ensure adequate ventilation by wearing cotton panties and clothes loose enough to permit the vaginal area to "breathe." After using the toilet, a woman should always wipe herself from front to back and, if necessary, follow up with a moistened paper towel or a premoistened wipe. If an unusual odor persists despite these efforts, a visit to one's healthcare provider is indicated. Certain conditions such as vaginitis produce a foul-smelling discharge that women often describe as having a "fishy" odor.

Associated Menstrual Conditions

New self-explanatory terminology has been developed to define a variety of menstrual irregularities. These include the following:

- Abnormal uterine bleeding (AUB)
- Heavy menstrual bleeding (HMB)
- Heavy and prolonged menstrual bleeding (HPMB)
- Intermenstrual bleeding (IMB)
- Postmenopausal bleeding (PMB)

The following terms are still used among some caregivers to define various menstrual irregularities but an International Review Panel has recommended that they be phased out (Garza-Cavazos & Loret de Mola, 2012):

- Hypomenorrhea: abnormally short duration of menses
- Hypermenorrhea: abnormally long duration of menses

- Oligomenorrhea: infrequent menses
- Polymenorrhea: too frequent menses
- Menorrhagia: excessive menstrual flow
- Metrorrhagia: bleeding between periods
- Menometrorrhagia: bleeding that is excessive in amount and duration, which occurs at either regular or irregular intervals

AMENORRHEA

Amenorrhea, the absence of menses, is classified as primary or secondary. Primary amenorrhea (menstruation has not been established by 16 years of age or within 4 years of breast development) necessitates a thorough assessment to determine its cause. Possible causes include congenital obstructions; Turner syndrome; congenital absence of the uterus, ovaries, or vagina; testicular feminization (external genitals appear female but uterus and ovaries are absent and testes are present); chronic anovulation related to polycystic ovarian syndrome, thyroid, or adrenal disorders; or absence or imbalance of hormones. Treatment depends on the causative factors. Some causes are not correctable.

Secondary amenorrhea, or the cessation of regular menses, is caused most frequently by pregnancy. Additional causes include lactation, hormonal imbalances, poor nutrition (anorexia nervosa, obesity, and fad dieting), ovarian lesions, strenuous exercise (associated with long-distance runners, dancers, and other athletes with low body fat ratios), debilitating systemic diseases, stress of high intensity or long duration, stressful life events, a change in season or climate, use of oral contraceptives, use of the phenothiazine and chlorpromazine

---

EVIDENCE-BASED PRACTICE | Amenorrhea in Female Athletes

Clinical Question

What is the incidence of amenorrhea in female athletes? What is the attitude of athletes toward amenorrhea, particularly elite athletes?

The Evidence

Hormonal changes brought about by extreme exercise and related low energy may result in menstrual dysfunction in female athletes, even those with normal eating patterns. Two studies focused on amenorrhea in female athletes. One study included 245 female athletes in National Collegiate Athletics Association (NCAA) Division 1 sports and focused both on the prevalence of menstrual irregularities and the attitudes of athletes toward amenorrhea. A second, year-long study conducted in Sweden focused on 149 elite athletes—those ranked in the top 10 nationally for their sport. These are descriptive studies, but taken together form a strong level of evidence.

In the general population, the prevalence of amenorrhea is approximately 1%. In contrast, 18% of the NCAA Division I athletes reported amenorrhea and 36% reported fewer than 10 cycles in a year (oligomenorrhea.) Twenty-five percent of the elite athletes reported a history of amenorrhea (Rost, Jacobsson, Dahlstrom, et al., 2014). Runners with lower body mass index (BMI) had a higher prevalence of amenorrhea, as did women who participated in sports with high demands on aerobic performance; for example, long distance running.

Missed or irregular menses are often the first sign of a health disturbance, yet some athletes interpret missed menses as a sign of fitness. Fifty-seven percent of the NCAA athletes believed missing menses was normal, 58% believed it was not harmful, and 67% believed it is common among all women (Myrisk, Reinn, & Harkins, 2014). This normalization of amenorrhea is problematic from a clinical standpoint in that amenorrhea is one element of the "female athlete triad" that includes menstrual dysfunction, eating disorders, and osteoporosis. The long-term consequences of menstrual irregularities can include loss of bone mineral density and a three-fold greater risk of musculoskeletal injury.

Best Practice

Coaches, athletic trainers, and athletes need education regarding the serious consequences of menstrual dysfunction and the female athlete triad in general. The most common reported cause of amenorrhea among athletes is energy deficiency brought on by consuming too few calories relative to energy expenditure. Adequate nutrition for female athletes is essential to avoid the long-term consequences of menstrual dysfunction.

Clinical Reasoning

How can the nurse affect the attitudes of athletes about normal menstrual function and the importance of adequate nutrition? How can coaches and athletic trainers be motivated to attend to menstrual dysfunction as a signal of a health disturbance?

group of tranquilizers, and syndromes such as Cushing and Sheehan syndromes.

The causative factors of amenorrhea dictate treatment. The nurse can explain that once the underlying condition has been corrected—for example, when sufficient body weight is gained—menses will resume. Athletes and women who participate in strenuous exercise routines may be advised to increase their caloric intake or reduce their exercise levels for a month or two to see whether a normal cycle ensues. If it does not, medical referral is indicated.

DYSMENORRHEA

Dysmenorrhea, or painful menstruation, occurs at, or a day before, the onset of menstruation and disappears by the end of menses. Dysmenorrhea is classified as primary or secondary.

Primary dysmenorrhea is defined as cramps without underlying disease. Prostaglandins F_2 and $F_{2\alpha}$, which are produced by the uterus in higher concentrations during menses, are the primary cause. They increase uterine contractility and decrease uterine artery blood flow, causing ischemia. The end result is the painful sensation of cramps. Dysmenorrhea typically disappears after a first pregnancy and does not occur if cycles are anovulatory.

Treatment of primary dysmenorrhea includes combined oral contraceptives, which inhibit ovulation and nonsteroidal anti-inflammatory drugs (NSAIDs) (such as ibuprofen, aspirin, and naproxen), which act as prostaglandin inhibitors. Biofeedback has also been used with some success as has acupuncture. See *Health Promotion: Self-Care Measures for Dysmenorrhea*.

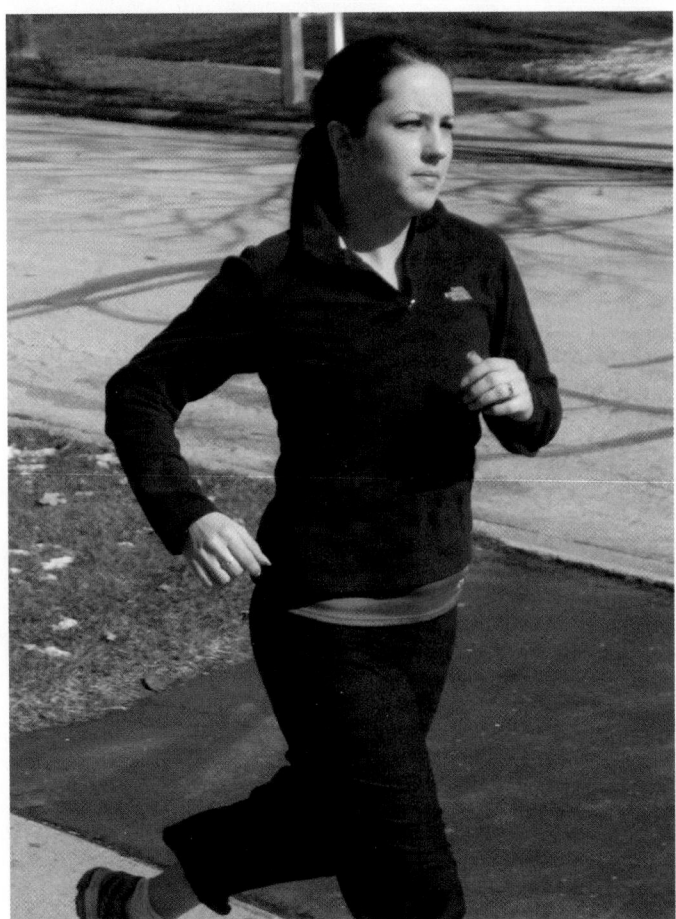

Figure 5–2 Regular exercise is an important part of therapy for dysmenorrhea.

Health Promotion Self-Care Measures for Dysmenorrhea

- Regular exercise, rest, application of heat, and good nutrition (Figure 5–2).

- Avoidance of salt to decrease discomfort from fluid retention.

- Vitamin B_6, which may help relieve the premenstrual bloating and irritability some women experience.

- Vitamin E, a mild prostaglandin inhibitor, may ease cramping.

Secondary dysmenorrhea is associated with pathology of the reproductive tract and usually appears after menstruation has been established. Conditions that most frequently cause secondary dysmenorrhea include endometriosis; residual pelvic inflammatory disease; cervical stenosis, uterine fibroids, ovarian cysts, benign or malignant tumors of the pelvis or abdomen; and the presence of an intrauterine device. Because primary and secondary dysmenorrhea may coexist, accurate differential diagnosis is essential for appropriate treatment.

For women with severe dysmenorrhea, use of continuous oral contraceptive therapy, which does not allow ovulation or menstruation to occur, may be of benefit. Hysterectomy may be the treatment of choice if there are anatomic disorders and childbearing is not desired.

PREMENSTRUAL SYNDROME

Premenstrual syndrome (PMS) refers to a symptom complex associated with the luteal phase of the menstrual cycle (2 weeks prior to the onset of menses). The symptoms must, by definition, occur between ovulation and the onset of menses. They repeat at the same stage of each menstrual cycle and include some or all of the following:

- *Psychologic:* irritability, lethargy, depression, low morale, anxiety, sleep disorders, crying spells

- *Neurologic:* classic migraine, vertigo, syncope

- *Respiratory:* rhinitis, hoarseness, and occasionally asthma

- *Gastrointestinal:* nausea, vomiting, constipation, abdominal bloating, craving for sweets

- *Urinary:* retention, oliguria

- *Dermatologic:* acne

- *Mammary:* swelling and tenderness

- *Musculoskeletal:* joint or muscle pain

Most women experience only some of these symptoms of PMS. The symptoms usually are most pronounced 2 or 3 days before the onset of menstruation and subside as menstrual flow begins, with or without treatment.

The exact cause of PMS is unknown, although evidence suggests that progesterone and estradiol levels are involved in PMS in some way. Central nervous system–mediated interactions between neurohormones and sex steroids may also account for the occurrence of PMS. Certain risk factors such as stress, traumatic life events, genetics, obesity, or a history of depression or other psychiatric disorders may predispose women to these disorders (Freeman, Halberstadt, Rickels, et al., 2011; Matsumoto, Asakura, & Hayashi, 2013).

Premenstrual dysphoric disorder (PMDD), a more serious form of PMS, is a diagnosis that may be applied to a small subgroup of women with PMS whose symptoms are primarily mood related and severe. Women with PMDD may benefit from selective serotonin reuptake inhibitors (SSRIs) such as fluoxetine hydrochloride (Prozac), sertraline hydrochloride (Zoloft), and paroxetine CR (Paxil CR).

Nursing Management

Counseling for PMS may include advising the woman to restrict her intake of foods containing methylxanthines such as chocolate, cola, and coffee; restrict her intake of alcohol, nicotine, red meat, and foods containing salt and sugar; increase her intake of complex carbohydrates and protein; and increase the frequency of meals. For women whose primary symptoms are psychologic, supplementation with B-complex vitamins, especially B_6, may decrease anxiety and depression. These women may also gain relief from complementary therapies such as vitex agnus castus (fruit of the chaste tree) and acupuncture (Kelderhouse & Taylor, 2013). Vitamin E supplements may help reduce breast tenderness. Supplementation with 1200 mg calcium daily may help relieve certain physical and psychologic symptoms. Magnesium supplements may help reduce fluid retention and bloating.

Herbal remedies may include black cohosh, ginger, red raspberry leaf, and evening primrose oil. Natural progesterone creams derived from wild yams or soybeans may provide relief to some women; however, no scientific studies have shown this to be true (Schuiling & Likis, 2013). However, underlying health conditions may contraindicate the use of herbal or vitamin supplements and must be considered when recommending them.

A program of aerobic exercise such as fast walking, jogging, and aerobic dancing is generally beneficial. In addition to vitamin supplements, pharmacologic treatments for PMS include diuretics and prostaglandin inhibitors.

Women with PMS may find it helpful to have an empathetic relationship with a healthcare professional to whom she feels free to voice concerns. Encourage the woman to keep a diary to help identify life events associated with PMS. Self-care groups and self-help literature both help women feel they have control over their bodies.

Contraception

The decision to use a method of contraception may be made individually by a woman (or, in the case of vasectomy, by a man) or jointly by a couple. The decision may be motivated by a desire to avoid pregnancy, to gain control over the number of children conceived, or to determine the spacing of future children. In choosing a specific method, consistency of use outweighs the absolute reliability of the given method.

> **Professionalism in Practice** **Family Planning**
> Globally, the question has been raised: Is family planning a basic human right? (United Nations Population Fund [UNFPA], 2012).

Decisions about contraception should be made voluntarily, with full knowledge of available choices, advantages, disadvantages, effectiveness, side effects, contraindications, and long-term effects. Many outside factors influence this choice, including cultural practices, religious beliefs, attitudes and personal preferences, cost, effectiveness, misinformation, practicality of method, and self-esteem. Different methods of contraception may be appropriate at different times for individuals or couples.

> *Healthy People 2020*
> (FP-1) Increase the proportion of pregnancies that are intended
> (FP-2) Reduce the proportion of females experiencing pregnancy despite use of a reversible contraceptive method

Fertility Awareness–Based Methods

Fertility awareness–based (FAB) methods include methods that require a woman to monitor her *fertile window* (generally between days 8 and 19 of 26- to 32-day cycles) and use a barrier method during that time. A woman is most fertile 5 days before ovulation until 1 day post-ovulation. If a woman abstains from coitus until after her fertile window has closed, she is using *natural family planning* (NFP) (Zieman, Hatcher, & Allen, 2015).

NFP is free, safe, and acceptable to many whose religious beliefs prohibit other methods. It provides an increased awareness of the body, involves no artificial substances or devices, encourages a couple to communicate about sexual activity and family planning, and, conversely, is useful in helping a couple plan a pregnancy. To be used effectively, all FAB methods require extensive initial counseling and are best suited for women with regular menstrual cycles. FAB/NFP methods may interfere with sexual spontaneity, require the couple to maintain records for several menstrual cycles (months) before beginning use, may be difficult or impossible for certain groups of women to use, and may not be as reliable in preventing pregnancy as other methods. Women for whom a FAB/NFP method might not be ideal include those with irregular menstrual cycles, those who are breastfeeding, or those in the perimenopause.

The *standard days method* is good for women with regular menstrual cycles between 26 and 32 days. Intercourse is avoided, or a barrier method used, between cycle days 8 through 19 (Zieman et al., 2015). CycleBeads or its software program is useful when using this method.

The *calendar rhythm method* (CRM) is based on the assumption that ovulation tends to occur 14 days (plus or minus 2 days) before the start of the next menstrual period. To use this method, the woman must record her menstrual cycle for 6 months to identify the shortest and longest cycles. The first day of menstruation is the first day of the cycle. The fertile phase is calculated from 18 days before the end of the shortest recorded cycle through 11 days from the end of the longest recorded cycle. The woman must abstain from intercourse during the fertile phase or use a barrier method during that time (Zieman et al., 2015).

The *Billings ovulation method* involves the assessment of cervical mucus changes that occur during the menstrual cycle. The amount and character of cervical mucus change because of the influence of estrogen and progesterone. At the time of ovulation, the mucus (estrogen-dominant mucus) is clearer, more stretchable (a quality called *spinnbarkeit*), and more permeable to sperm (Figure 5–3A). It also shows a characteristic fern pattern when placed on a glass slide and allowed to dry (Figure 5–3B). During the luteal phase, the cervical mucus is thick and sticky (progesterone-dominant mucus) and forms a network that traps sperm, making their passage more difficult.

To use the cervical mucus method, the woman abstains from intercourse for the first menstrual cycle. Each day she

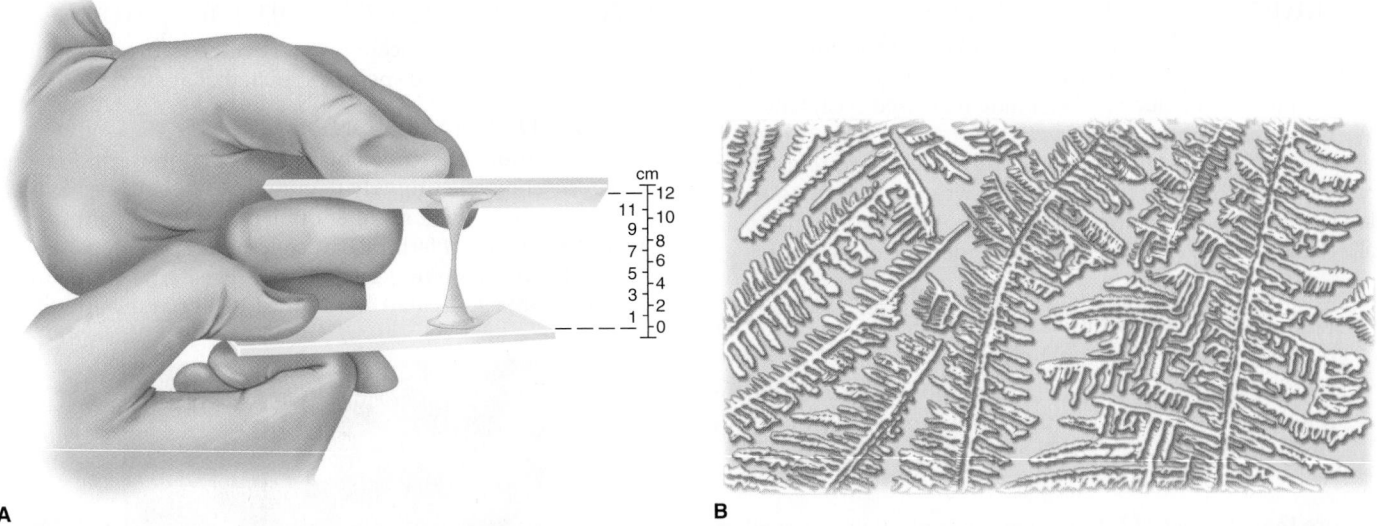

Figure 5–3 *A,* Cervical mucus showing spinnbarkeit. *B,* Characteristic fern pattern of cervical mucus at ovulation.

assesses her cervical mucus for amount, feeling of slipperiness or wetness, color, clearness, and spinnbarkeit, as she becomes familiar with varying characteristics.

The peak day of wetness and clear, stretchable mucus is assumed to be the time of ovulation. To use this method correctly, the woman should abstain from intercourse from the time she first notices that the mucus is becoming clear, more elastic, and slippery until 4 days after the last wet mucus (ovulation) day. Because this method evaluates the effects of hormonal changes, it can be used by women with irregular cycles.

The *TwoDay Method* is based on a woman's ability to distinguish the difference between progesterone-mediated and estrogen-mediated cervical mucus that is present at her introitus before she urinates, preferably in the afternoon and evening. If she notices cervical secretions of any type either yesterday or today, she is fertile *today*. If no secretions were noted today or yesterday, she is not fertile *today*—hence the name (Zieman et al., 2015).

The *symptothermal method* consists of various assessments made and recorded by the couple. These include information regarding cycle days, coitus, cervical mucus changes, and secondary signs such as increased libido, abdominal bloating,

mittelschmerz (midcycle abdominal pain), and basal body temperature. Through the various assessments, the couple learns to recognize signs that indicate ovulation.

The *basal body temperature* (BBT) method is incorporated into the symptothermal method and provides an objective record of fertile days. It requires that a woman take her BBT every morning upon awakening (before any activity) and record the readings on a temperature graph. To do this she uses a BBT thermometer. After 3 to 4 months of recording temperatures, a woman with regular cycles should be able to predict when ovulation will occur. The method is based on the fact that the temperature sometimes drops just before ovulation and almost always rises and remains elevated for several days after. The temperature rise occurs in response to the increased progesterone levels that occur in the second half of the cycle. Figure 5–4 shows a sample BBT chart of an ovulating woman. To avoid conception, the couple abstains from intercourse on the day of the temperature rise and for 3 days after. Because the temperature rise does not occur until after ovulation, a woman who had intercourse just before the rise is at risk of pregnancy.

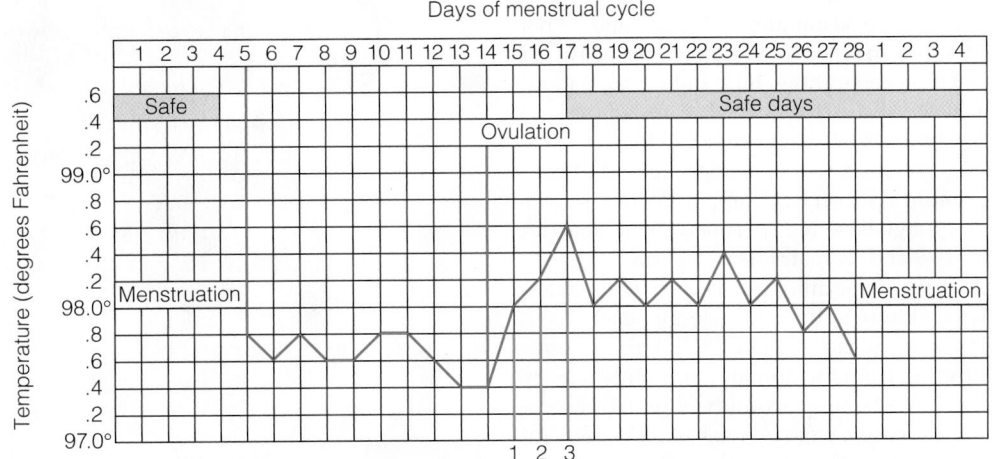

Figure 5–4 Sample basal body temperature chart.

Situational Contraceptives

Abstinence can be considered a method of contraception, and, partly because of changing values and the increased risk of infection with intercourse, it is gaining increased acceptance.

Coitus interruptus, or *withdrawal,* is one of the oldest and least reliable methods of contraception. This method requires that the male withdraw from the female's vagina when he feels that ejaculation is impending. He then ejaculates away from the external genitalia of the woman. Failure tends to occur because of the following:

- This method requires great control on the part of the man, who must withdraw just as he feels the urge for deeper penetration with impending orgasm.

- In some men, the pre-ejaculatory fluid, which a man may release as soon as his penis becomes erect, may contain small numbers of sperm. The man may not be aware that he has released pre-ejaculatory fluid.

If more than one act of intercourse takes place within a short time, the man should urinate first and wipe the tip of his penis to remove any remaining sperm.

Douching after intercourse is an ineffective method of contraception and is *not* recommended. It may actually facilitate conception by pushing sperm farther up the birth canal.

Women With Special Needs **Contraceptive Counseling**

Many healthcare providers assume that women with developmental disabilities are not sexually active and, therefore, do not need contraceptive counseling. Women with developmental disabilities need education on sexual issues, including conception and pregnancy prevention. A level of functioning assessment should be performed to determine if the woman is capable of using different types of contraceptives effectively. Contraceptive choices should be discussed and provided as needed.

Spermicides

The **spermicide** approved for use in the United States, nonoxynol-9 (N-9), is available as a cream, jelly, foam, vaginal film, and suppository. Spermicide is inserted into the vagina before intercourse. It destroys sperm by disrupting the cell membrane. Spermicides that effervesce in a moist environment offer more rapid protection, and coitus may take place immediately after they are inserted. Suppositories may require up to 30 minutes to dissolve and do not offer protection until they do so. The woman should be instructed to insert these spermicide preparations high in the vagina and maintain a supine position.

N-9 is minimally effective when used alone, but its effectiveness increases in conjunction with a barrier method of contraception such as a diaphragm, cervical cap, or male or female condom. The cervical sponge is both a spermicide and a barrier method, as it contains N-9 and its matrix traps sperm.

The major advantages of spermicides are their wide availability and low toxicity. Skin irritation and allergic reactions to spermicides are the primary disadvantages. N-9 does not offer protection against infection from the human immunodeficiency virus, which causes HIV/AIDS, or against any other STI. Moreover, N-9 may actually increase a woman's risk of HIV infection because it irritates vaginal tissue, making the tissue more susceptible to invasion by organisms (Zieman et al., 2015).

Barrier Methods of Contraception

Barrier methods of contraception prevent the transport of sperm to the ovum, immobilize sperm, or are lethal against sperm.

MALE AND FEMALE CONDOMS

The male **condom** offers a viable means of contraception when used consistently and properly (Figure 5–5). Acceptance has been increasing as a growing number of men are assuming responsibility for regulation of fertility. The condom is applied to the erect penis, rolled from the tip to the base of the shaft, before vulvar or vaginal contact. A small space must be left at the end of the

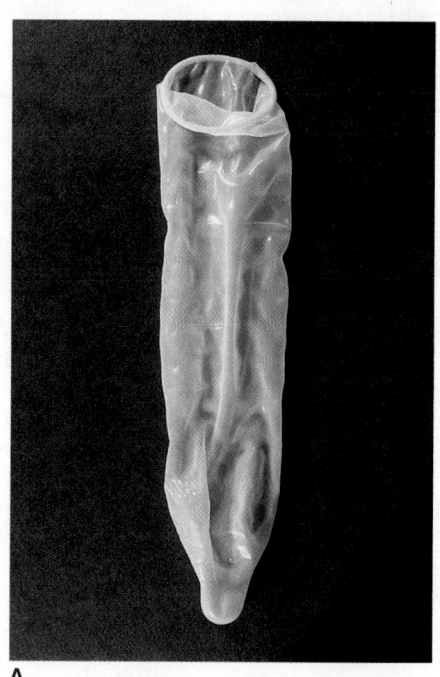

A

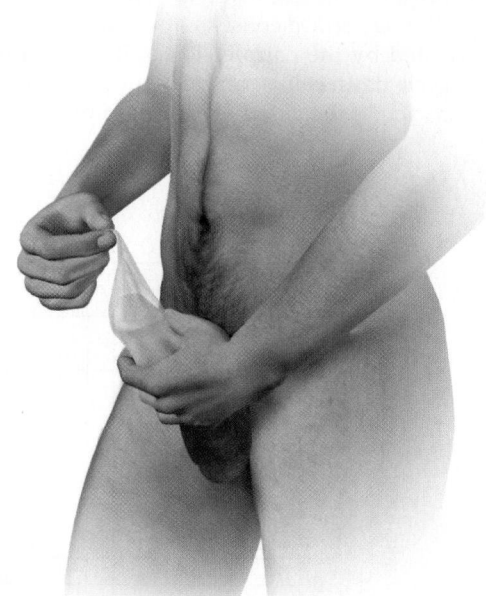

B

Figure 5–5 The male condom. *A,* Unrolled condom with reservoir tip. *B,* Correct use of a condom.

condom to allow for collection of the ejaculate, so that the condom will not break at the time of ejaculation. If the condom or vagina is dry, a water-soluble lubricant such as K-Y jelly or Astroglide should be used to prevent irritation and possible condom breakage. Oil-based lubricants such as petroleum jelly, baby oil, or hand lotion may weaken the condom and facilitate breakage.

Couples should be careful when removing the condom after intercourse. For optimal effectiveness the man should withdraw his penis from the woman's vagina while it is still erect and hold the condom rim to prevent spillage. If after ejaculation the penis becomes flaccid while still in the vagina, the man should hold onto the edge of the condom while withdrawing to avoid spilling semen and to prevent the condom from slipping off.

The effectiveness of male condoms is determined by their use. The condom is small, disposable, and inexpensive; it has no side effects, requires no medical examination, and offers visual evidence of effectiveness. Most condoms are made of latex, although polyurethane and silicone rubber condoms are available for individuals allergic to latex. All condoms, except natural "skin" condoms made from lamb's intestines, offer protection against both pregnancy and STIs. Breakage, displacement, perineal or vaginal irritation, and dulled sensation are possible disadvantages. Condoms deteriorate in hot conditions, making them susceptible to breaking. Thus, men should avoid placing them in their car glove box or in their wallets in a rear pants pocket.

The male condom is becoming increasingly popular because of the protection it offers from infections. For women, an STI increases the risk of pelvic inflammatory disease (PID) and resultant infertility. Many women are beginning to insist that sexual partners use condoms, and many women carry condoms with them.

The *Reality Female Condom* (Figure 5–6) is a thin sheath with a flexible ring at each end. The inner ring, at the closed end of

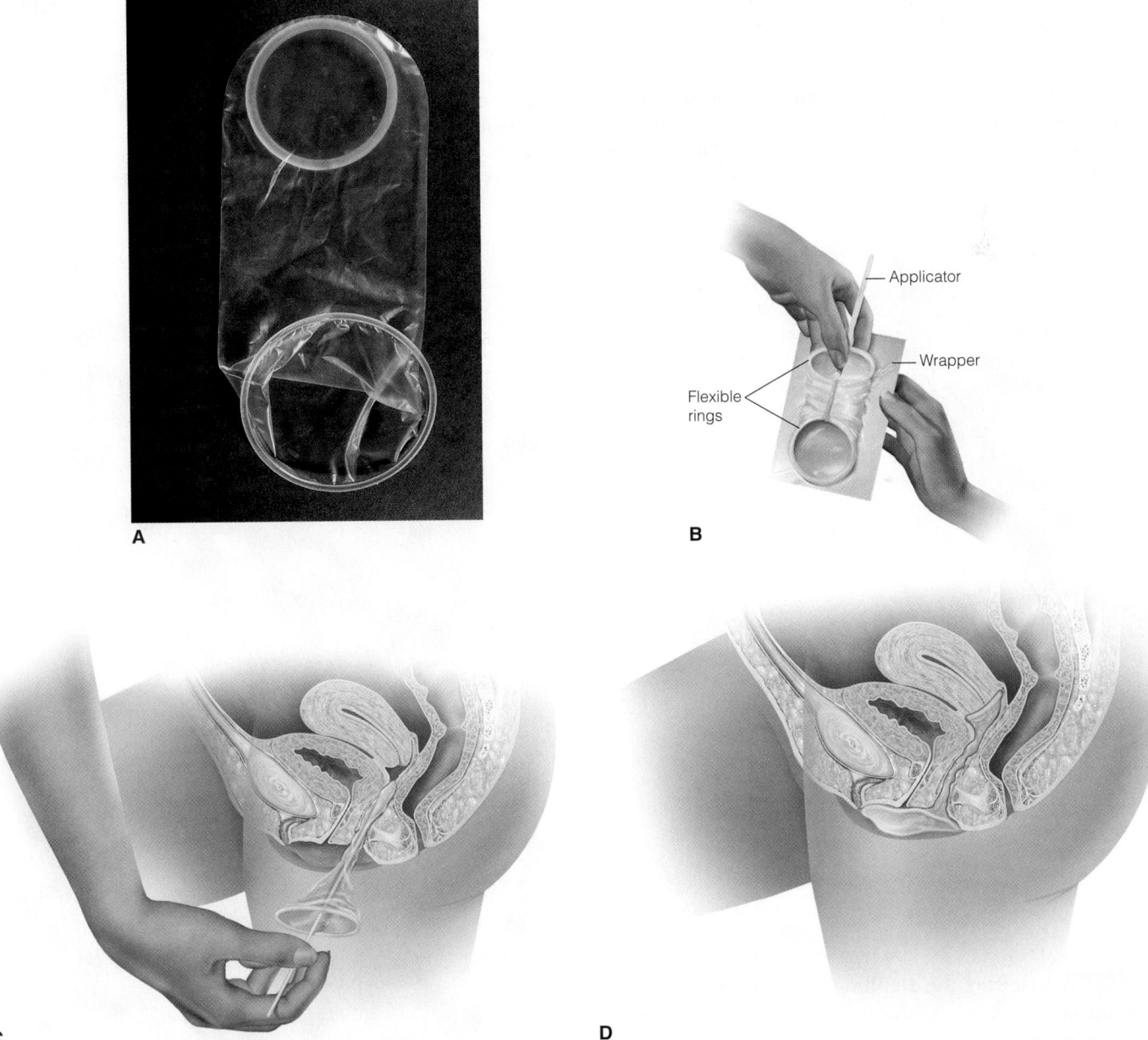

Figure 5–6 Application of the female condom. *A,* The condom. To insert: *B,* Remove condom and applicator from wrapper by pulling up on the ring. *C,* Insert condom slowly by gently pushing the applicator toward the small of the back. *D,* When properly inserted, the outer ring should rest on the folds of skin around the vaginal opening, and the inner ring (closed end) should fit loosely against the cervix.

the condom, serves as the means of insertion and fits over the cervix like a diaphragm. The second ring remains outside the vagina and covers a portion of the woman's perineum. It also covers the base of the man's penis during intercourse. Available over-the-counter and designed for one-time use, the condom may be inserted up to 8 hours before intercourse. The inner sheath is prelubricated but does not contain spermicide and is not designed to be used with a male condom. Because it also covers a portion of the vulva, it probably provides better protection than other methods against some pathogens. High cost, noisiness during intercourse, and the cumbersome feel of the device make acceptability a problem for some couples.

DIAPHRAGM AND CERVICAL CAP

The **diaphragm** (Figure 5–7) is used with spermicidal cream or jelly and offers a good level of protection from conception. The woman must be fitted with a diaphragm and instructed in its use by trained personnel. The diaphragm should be rechecked for correct size after each childbirth and whenever a woman has gained or lost 10 to 15 lb or more.

The diaphragm must be inserted before intercourse, with approximately 1 tsp (or 1.5 in. from the tube) of spermicidal jelly placed around its rim and in the cup. This chemical barrier supplements the mechanical barrier of the diaphragm. The diaphragm is inserted through the vagina and covers the cervix. The

last step in insertion is to push the edge of the diaphragm under the symphysis pubis, which may result in a "popping" sensation. When fitted properly and correctly in place, the diaphragm should not cause discomfort to the woman or her partner. Correct placement of the diaphragm can be checked by touching the cervix with a fingertip through the cup. The cervix feels like a small, firm, rounded structure and has a consistency similar to that of the tip of the nose. The center of the diaphragm should be over the cervix. If more than 6 hours elapse between insertion of the diaphragm and intercourse, additional spermicidal cream or jelly should be used. It is necessary to leave the diaphragm in place for at least 6 hours after coitus. The diaphragm should then be removed, cleaned with mild soap and water, and allowed to air dry before it is stored in its case. If intercourse is desired again within the 6 hours, another type of contraception must be used or additional spermicidal jelly placed in the vagina with an applicator, taking care not to disturb the placement of the diaphragm. Periodically, the diaphragm should be held up to the light and inspected for tears or holes.

Some couples feel that the use of a diaphragm interferes with the spontaneity of intercourse. However, this perception can be decreased if the woman inserts the diaphragm herself before intercourse.

Diaphragms are an excellent contraceptive method for women who are lactating, who cannot or do not wish to use the

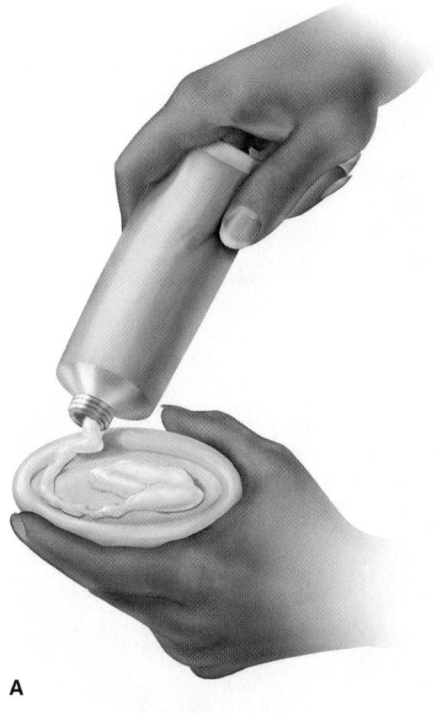

A

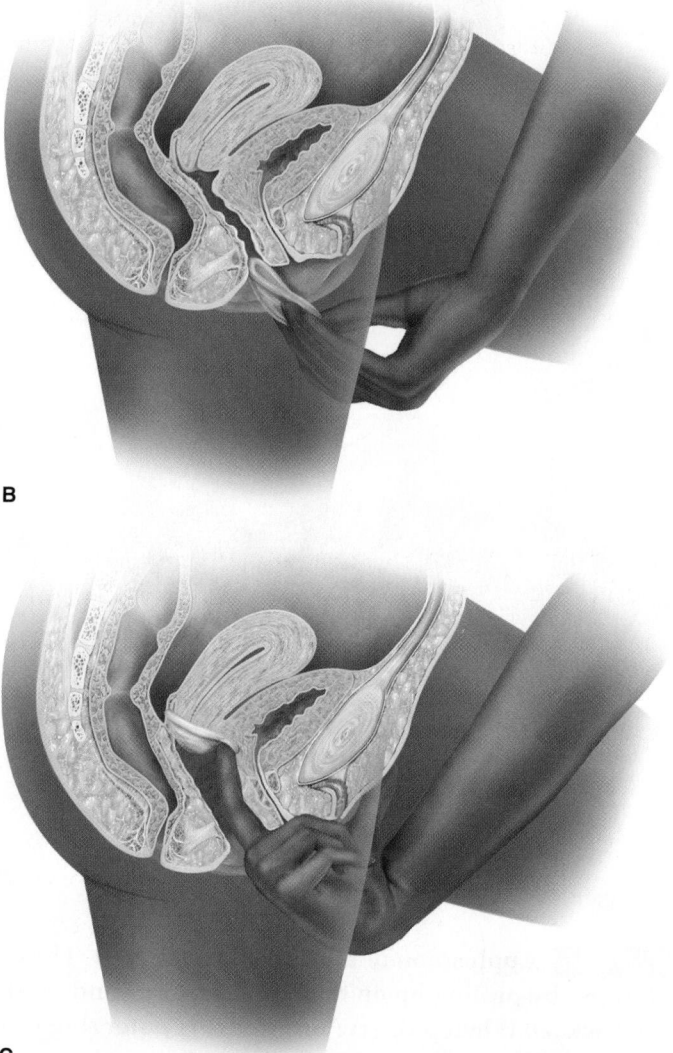

B

C

Figure 5–7 Inserting the diaphragm. *A*, Apply jelly to the rim and center of the diaphragm. *B*, Insert the diaphragm. *C*, Push the rim of the diaphragm under the symphysis pubis. Then check placement of the diaphragm. Cervix should be felt through the diaphragm.

NOTE: The diaphragm shown here is no longer manufactured, but many women who use a diaphragm will still have this model.

pill (oral contraceptives), who are smokers over age 35, or who wish to avoid the increased risk of pelvic inflammatory disease (PID) associated with intrauterine devices. A silicone diaphragm is available for women with latex allergies.

Women who object to manipulating their genitals to insert the diaphragm, check its placement, and remove it may find this method unsatisfactory. It is not recommended for women with a history of urinary tract infection because pressure from the diaphragm on the urethra may interfere with complete bladder emptying and lead to recurrent urinary tract infections.

SAFETY ALERT!

Women with a history of toxic shock syndrome should not use the diaphragm, cervical sponge, or cervical cap because they are left in place for prolonged periods. For the same reason, the diaphragm should not be used during a menstrual period or if a woman has abnormal vaginal discharge.

The *FemCap* cervical cap is reusable, looks like a small sailor's cap, and is made of soft silicone. Used with spermicidal cream or jelly, it fits snugly over the cervix and is held in place by suction. Advantages, disadvantages, and contraindications are similar to those associated with the diaphragm.

VAGINAL SPONGE

The *Today vaginal sponge*, available without a prescription, is a pillow-shaped, soft, absorbent synthetic sponge containing spermicide. It is made with a concave or cupped area on one side that fits over the cervix and has a loop for easy removal. The sponge is moistened thoroughly with water before insertion to activate the spermicide and then inserted into the vagina with the cupped side against the cervix (Figure 5–8). It should be left in place for 6 hours following intercourse and may be worn for up to 24 hours, then removed and discarded.

The sponge has the following advantages: professional fitting is not required, it may be used for multiple acts of coitus for up to 24 hours, one size fits all, and it acts as both a barrier and a spermicide. Problems associated with the sponge include difficulty removing it and irritation or allergic reactions. Some women report that the sponge absorbs vaginal secretions, contributing to vaginal dryness. For women without children, the failure rate is comparable to that of the diaphragm. The failure rate is higher for women who have borne children, possibly because of changes in the shape of the cervix (Zieman et al., 2015).

Long-Acting Reversible Contraception (LARC)

Long-acting reversible contraceptive methods include those that are used for an extended period of time, do not require user compliance, and are reversible upon discontinuation. These cost-effective methods are especially well suited for adolescents and include intrauterine contraception and the subdermal implant.

INTRAUTERINE CONTRACEPTION

Intrauterine contraception (IUC) refers to the use of a device that is designed to be inserted into the uterus by a qualified healthcare provider and left in place for an extended period, providing continuous contraceptive protection for 3 to 10 years (Figure 5–9). The following three devices used for IUC are available in the United States:

- The *copper IUC (ParaGard T 380A)* is a small, T-shaped device that has copper covering parts of its stem and arms. It provides effective contraception for 10 years,
- The *Mirena levonorgestrel intrauterine system (LNg-IUC)* is a small, T-shaped frame with a reservoir that releases levonorgestrel gradually. The Mirena provides 5 years of protection.
- The *Skyla LNg-IUC* device gradually releases levonorgestrel and has a 3-year indication. It is smaller than the Mirena and may fit into the uterus of nulliparous women more easily. The Skyla device also has a radiopaque silver ring at the top of the "T" (if the woman needs an MRI, she must notify the technician).

Both Mirena and Sklya devices are progestin-only; thus the primary cause of discontinuation is unscheduled bleeding. Women need anticipatory guidance to understand how the LNg-IUCs work and how they can affect menstrual bleeding patterns. The LNg-IUCs are excellent choices for women who are allergic to copper or who have heavy menses and desire decreased bleeding or amenorrhea.

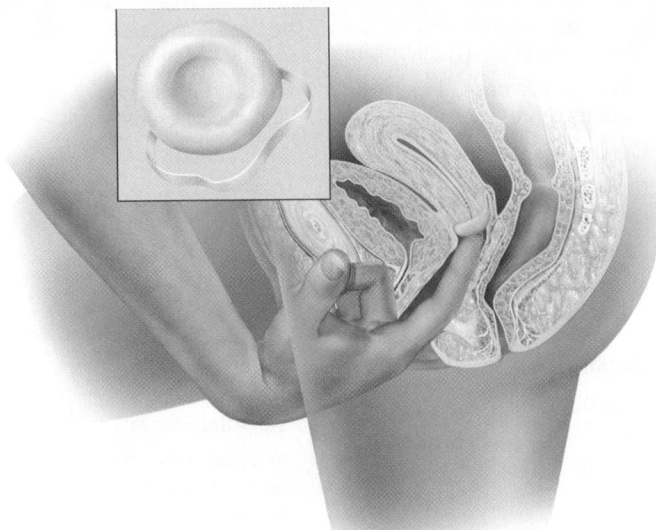

Figure 5–8 **Application of the contraceptive sponge. The contraceptive sponge is moistened well with water and inserted into the vagina with the concave portion positioned over the cervix.**

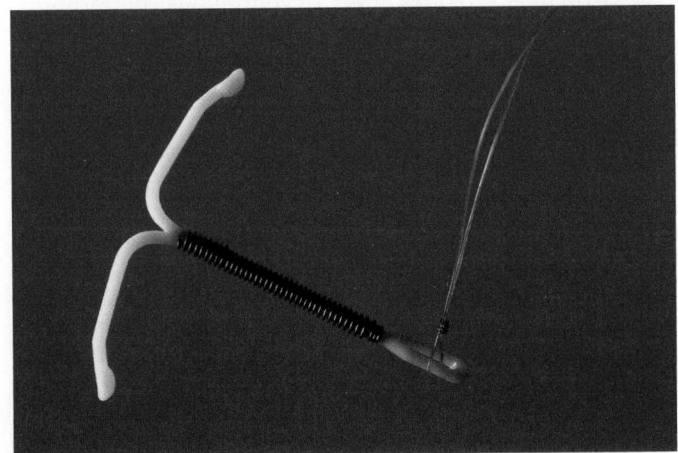

Figure 5–9 **An example of an IUC.**

SOURCE: Boucharlat/AGE Fotostock America Inc.

Traditionally, IUC was believed to act by preventing the implantation of a fertilized ovum. Thus it was considered an abortifacient (abortion-causing) method. This belief is not accurate; all IUCs are truly contraceptive. The copper IUC is known to have local inflammatory effects on the endometrium and to impair sperm from functioning properly. The Mirena and Skyla LNg-IUCs cause the lining of the uterus (endometrium) to become atrophic. Also, IUC produces a spermicidal intrauterine environment.

Advantages of IUC include high rate of effectiveness, continuous contraceptive protection, no coitus-related activity, and relative inexpensiveness over time. Possible adverse reactions to IUC include discomfort to the wearer, increased bleeding during menses, PID, perforation of the uterus, intermenstrual bleeding, dysmenorrhea, and expulsion of the device.

IUC is an excellent method of contraception for most women including adolescents. IUCs are contraindicated in women who are pregnant and in women who have an active pelvic infection (PID, endometritis, cervicitis, or pelvic tuberculosis). IUCs should not be inserted in women with cervical or endometrial cancer or gestational choriocarcinoma. The risk for IUC expulsion is greater in women with anatomic abnormalities of the uterus.

An IUC device is inserted into the uterus with its strings or tail protruding through the cervix into the vagina. It may be inserted at any time during a woman's cycle providing she is not pregnant or during the 4- to 6-week postpartum check. After insertion, the clinician instructs the woman to check for the presence of the strings once a week for the first month and then after each menses. She is told that she may have some cramping or bleeding intermittently for 2 to 6 weeks and that her first few menses may be irregular. Follow-up examination is suggested 4 to 8 weeks after insertion.

Women with IUCs should contact their healthcare providers if they are exposed to an STI or if they develop the following warning signs: late period, abnormal spotting or bleeding, pain with intercourse, abdominal pain, abnormal discharge, signs of infection (fever, chills, and malaise), or missing strings. If the woman becomes pregnant with an IUD in place, the device should be removed as soon as possible to prevent infection and miscarriage (Cunningham et al., 2014).

NEXPLANON

Nexplanon, manufactured by Merck & Co., replaces Implanon. It is a single-capsule implant inserted subdermally in the woman's nondominant upper underarm. It is impregnated with etonogestrel, a progestin, and is effective for 3 years. It acts by preventing ovulation. Nexplanon also stimulates the production of thick cervical mucus, which inhibits sperm penetration past the cervix.

Nexplanon provides effective continuous contraception removed from the act of coitus. Possible side effects include spotting, irregular bleeding or amenorrhea, an increased incidence of ovarian cysts, weight gain, headaches, fluid retention, acne, hair loss, mood changes, and depression. A minor surgical procedure is required to insert and remove the implant (Merck & Co., 2012).

Hormonal Contraception

Hormonal contraceptives are available in a variety of forms. They may be progestin-only hormones, most often using a synthetic form of progesterone called *progestin*, or a combination of estrogen and a progestin.

COMBINED ESTROGEN-PROGESTIN APPROACHES

Combined hormonal approaches work by inhibiting the release of an ovum, by creating an atrophic endometrium, and by maintaining thick cervical mucus that slows sperm transport and inhibits the process that allows sperm to penetrate the ovum.

Combined Oral Contraceptives. Combined oral contraceptives (COCs), also called *birth control pills*, are typically a combination of the hormones estrogen and progesterone. COCs are safe, highly effective, and rapidly reversible. Many COCs are available. The oral contraceptive pill ("the pill") is taken daily for 21 days, typically beginning on the Sunday after the first day of the menstrual cycle, although the woman can also start on day 1 of her menstrual cycle. In most cases, menses occurs 1 to 4 days after the last pill is taken. Seven days after taking her last pill, the woman restarts the pill. Thus the woman always begins the pill on the same day. Some companies offer a 28-day pack with seven "blank" pills so that the woman never stops taking a pill. The pill should be taken at approximately the same time each day—usually upon arising or before retiring in the evening.

Three COC formulations for extended use are available in the United States. Women taking extended use COCs have four withdrawal bleeds per year (rather than 12), or no withdrawal bleeding at all. Extended-use COCs reduce the side effects of COCs such as bloating, headache, breast tenderness, cramping, and swelling (Lentz, Lobo, Gersenson, et al., 2012). Many of these formulations are now generic, but were previously marketed as Seasonale, Seasonique, and Lybrel. Irregular pill taking is one of the major causes of unscheduled bleeding, a side effect that leads many women to discontinue COCs.

Although they are highly effective when taken correctly, COCs may produce a variety of side effects, which may be either progesterone or estrogen related (Table 5–1). The use of low-dose (35 mcg or less estrogen) preparations has reduced many of the side effects. The newer 20-mcg pills have even fewer side effects, but they may result in less contraceptive effectiveness.

Contraindications to the use of COCs include pregnancy, previous history of thrombophlebitis or thromboembolic

TABLE 5–1 Side Effects Associated With Oral Contraceptives

ESTROGEN EFFECTS	PROGESTIN EFFECTS
Alterations in lipid metabolism	Acne, oily skin
Breast tenderness, engorgement; increased breast size	Breast tenderness; increased breast size
Cerebrovascular accident	Decreased libido
Changes in carbohydrate metabolism	Decreased high-density lipoprotein (HDL) cholesterol levels
Chloasma (melasma)	
Fluid retention; cyclic weight gain	Depression
Headache	Fatigue
Hepatic adenomas	Hirsutism
Hypertension	Increased appetite; weight gain
Leukorrhea, cervical erosion, ectopia	Increased low-density lipoprotein (LDL) cholesterol levels
Nausea	
Nervousness, irritability	Oligomenorrhea, amenorrhea
Telangiectasia	Pruritus
Thromboembolic complications— thrombophlebitis, pulmonary embolism	Sebaceous cysts

disease, acute or chronic liver disease of cholestatic type with abnormal function, presence of estrogen-dependent carcinomas, undiagnosed uterine bleeding, heavy smoking, gallbladder disease, hypertension, diabetes, and hyperlipidemia. In addition, women with the following relative contraindications who use COCs need to be monitored frequently: migraine headaches, epilepsy, depression, oligomenorrhea, and amenorrhea. Women who choose this method of contraception should be fully advised of its potential side effects.

COCs also have some important noncontraceptive benefits. Many women experience relief of uncomfortable menstrual symptoms. Cramps are lessened, flow is decreased, and cycle regularity is increased. Mittelschmerz is eliminated. More important, there is a reduction in the incidence of ovarian cancer, endometrial cancer, colorectal cancer, menstrual migraines, and iron deficiency anemia. In addition, hormonal contraceptives can be effective in improving bone mineral density and in treating acne or hirsutism, pelvic pain due to endometriosis, and bleeding due to leiomyomas (ACOG, 2012a). In addition, COCs are considered a good solution to the physiologic problems some women experience during the perimenopause (such as hot flashes).

Because of the increased risk of myocardial infarction (heart attack), women over age 35 who smoke should not take COCs.

SAFETY ALERT!

The woman using COCs should contact her healthcare provider if she becomes depressed, becomes jaundiced, develops a breast lump, or experiences any of the following warning signs: severe abdominal pain, severe chest pain or shortness of breath, severe headaches, dizziness, changes in vision (vision loss or blurring), speech problems, or severe leg pain.

Other Combined Hormonal Methods. Hormones can now be administered transdermally using a *contraceptive skin patch* called Ortho Evra. Roughly the size of a silver dollar, but square, the patch is applied weekly for 3 weeks to one of four sites: her abdomen, buttocks, upper outer arm, or trunk (excluding the breasts). During the fourth week, no patch is worn and menses occurs. Users apply the first patch on the first day of their menses or on the Sunday following; if the latter is chosen a backup method for 7 days is necessary.

The patch is highly effective in women who weigh less than 198 lb. It is as safe and reliable as a COC and has a better rate of compliance. Product labeling specifies that there is a greater risk of venous thromboembolism (VTE) for women using the patch versus those taking COCs. The Food and Drug Administration (FDA) (2012) considers the patch a safe method of contraception for women not at risk of a VTE.

NuvaRing vaginal contraceptive ring (manufactured by Merck & Co.), another form of low-dose, sustained-release hormonal contraceptive, is a flexible soft ring that the woman inserts into her vagina (Figure 5–10). The ring is left in place for 3 weeks and then removed for 1 week to allow for withdrawal bleeding. One size fits virtually all women. Women who use the NuvaRing should begin its use in the same way as described for the patch. Replacement rings should be kept in the refrigerator to maintain integrity. The ring is highly effective and has minimal side effects. It can be worn during intercourse and is comfortable for both the woman and her partner.

PROGESTIN CONTRACEPTIVES

The progestin-only pill, also called the *minipill,* is another oral contraceptive. It is used primarily by nursing mothers because

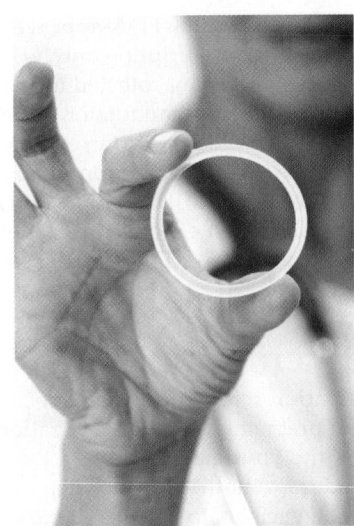

Figure 5–10 **The NuvaRing vaginal contraceptive ring.**

SOURCE: © N. Aubrier/Getty Images.

it does not interfere with breast milk production. It is also used by women who have a contraindication to the estrogen component of the combination preparation, such as history of thrombophlebitis or hypertension, but are strongly motivated to use this form of contraception. The major problems with progesterone-only pills are amenorrhea or irregular bleeding patterns.

Long-acting progestin-only contraceptives include Depo-Provera and Nexplanon, the latter of which is also considered a LARC method and was discussed previously.

Depot-medroxyprogesterone acetate (DMPA) (**Depo-Provera**) is administered by injection, provides highly effective contraception for 3 months after administration, with subsequent injections every 10 to 14 weeks. It is available in two dosings: DMPA-IM 150 mg for intramuscular use or DMPA-SC 104 mg for subcutaneous use.

DMPA, which acts primarily by suppressing ovulation, is safe, convenient, private, and relatively inexpensive. It also separates birth control from the act of coitus. It can be given to nursing mothers because it contains no estrogen. Side effects include menstrual irregularities, headache, weight gain, breast tenderness, and depression. Return of fertility may be delayed for an average of 10 months.

DMPA is associated with bone demineralization, especially during the first 2 years of use. The rate of calcium loss slows after this time, and bone loss is reversible after discontinuation of DMPA. All women should exercise daily and take 1200 mg of calcium with vitamin D.

Postcoital Emergency Contraception

Postcoital **emergency contraception (EC)**, once known as the *morning after pill*, is indicated when a woman is worried about pregnancy because of unprotected intercourse or possible contraceptive failure (e.g., broken condom, slipped diaphragm, missed COCs, or too long a time between DMPA injections).

Plan B, a progestin-only approach (levonorgestrel), is the most commonly used EC. Originally it was given in two 0.75-mg doses—the first as soon after intercourse as possible (but not longer than 72 hours) and a second dose 12 hours later. Studies suggest that a single 1.5-mg dose (Plan B One-Step) may be as effective. Next Choice is a two-pill generic form of Plan B. Both are available over-the-counter, without prescription, to any woman 15 years or older. A new FDA-approved EC, ulipristal acetate (Ella), available by prescription only, is highly effective, especially if taken soon after unprotected intercourse. Ella is a selective progesterone receptor modulator, which can be taken up to 5 days after unprotected intercourse, thus providing two additional days for use (Levy, Jager, Kapp, et al., 2014).

Placement of the copper T IUD within 5 days after unprotected intercourse is the most effective postcoital contraceptive available (Zieman et al., 2015). However, the cost is high if the IUC is used only for EC.

Operative Sterilization

Operative **sterilization** refers to surgical procedures that permanently prevent pregnancy. Before sterilization is performed on either partner, the physician provides a thorough explanation of the procedure to both. Each needs to understand that sterilization is not a decision to be taken lightly or entered into when psychologic stresses, such as separation or divorce, exist. Even though both male and female procedures are theoretically reversible, the permanency of the procedure should be stressed and understood.

Male sterilization is achieved through a relatively minor procedure called a **vasectomy**. This procedure involves surgically severing the vas deferens in both sides of the scrotum. Following vasectomy it takes about 4 to 6 weeks and 6 to 36 ejaculations to clear the remaining sperm from the vas deferens. During that period the couple is advised to use another method of birth control and to bring in two or three semen samples for a sperm count. The man is rechecked at 6 and 12 months to ensure that fertility has not been restored by recanalization. Side effects of a vasectomy include pain, infection, hematoma, sperm granulomas, and spontaneous reanastomosis (reconnecting).

Female sterilization is most frequently accomplished by **tubal ligation**. The tubes are located through a small subumbilical incision or by minilaparotomy techniques and are clipped, ligated, electrocoagulated, banded, or plugged. Tubal ligation may be done at any time. However, the postpartum period is an ideal time to perform a tubal ligation because the tubes are somewhat enlarged and easily located.

Complications of female sterilization procedures include coagulation burns on the bowel, bowel perforation, pain, infection, hemorrhage, and adverse anesthesia effects. Reversal of a tubal ligation depends on the type of procedure performed.

The *Essure* method of permanent sterilization requires no surgical incision and yields no scar. Under hysteroscopy, a stainless steel microinsert is placed into the proximal section of each fallopian tube. Within 3 months, these microinserts create a benign tissue response that occludes the fallopian tubes. Three months after placement, tubal occlusion is confirmed by hysterosalpingogram.

Male Contraception

The vasectomy and the condom, discussed previously, are currently the only forms of male contraception available in the United States. Hormonal contraception for men has yet to be developed, although studies are under way.

Nursing Management

In most cases, the nurse who provides information and guidance about contraceptive methods works with the female partner because most contraceptive methods are female oriented.

TABLE 5–2 Factors to Consider When Choosing a Method of Contraception

Effectiveness of method in preventing pregnancy	Lifestyle: How frequently does client have intercourse?

Safety of the method:
  Are there inherent risks?
  Does it offer protection against STIs or other conditions?
	Does she have multiple partners?
	Does she have ready access to medical care in the event of complications?
	Is cost a factor?

Client's age and future childbearing plans	Partner's support and willingness to cooperate
Any contraindications in client's health history	Personal motivation to use method Personal preferences, biases
Religious or moral factors influencing choice	

Because men can purchase condoms without seeing a healthcare provider, counseling and interaction with a nurse are required only with vasectomy. As a nurse, you can play an important role in helping a woman choose a method of contraception acceptable to her and to her partner.

In addition to completing a history and assessing for any contraindications to specific methods, spend time with a woman learning about her lifestyle, personal attitudes about particular contraceptive methods, religious beliefs, personal biases, and plans for future childbearing before helping the woman select a particular contraceptive method. Once the method is chosen, help the woman learn to use it effectively. Table 5–2 summarizes factors to consider when choosing an appropriate method of contraception.

Also review any possible side effects and warning signs related to the method chosen and counsel the woman about what

Clinical Reasoning Choosing a Method of Contraception

Monique Hermann, age 37, was divorced 3 years ago. Her only son, now 19, is away at college. Recently, with some trepidation, Monique began dating, and she is now enjoying an active social life. She is being seen today for advice about contraception, which had not been an issue during her marriage because her husband had had a vasectomy. She reports that she is a little nervous about becoming sexually active because until this point her husband had been her only sexual partner. Monique is very attracted to two different men but does not prefer one over the other at this point. She states that she wants a reliable method that would permit her to have intercourse at any time without having to take action beforehand because she thinks that would be embarrassing for her. Similarly, she is not interested in the patch, which is visible. She is not willing to consider a tubal ligation. She is a nonsmoker who drinks occasionally. She has no known contraindications to any available methods. Which methods of contraception might be appropriate for Monique?

TEACHING HIGHLIGHTS | Using a Method of Contraception

- Discuss factors a woman should consider when choosing a method of contraception (see Table 5–2). Note that different methods may be appropriate at different times in a woman's life.
- Review the woman's reasons for choosing a particular method and confirm the absence of any contraindications to specific methods.
- Give a step-by-step description of the correct procedure for using the method chosen. Provide opportunities for questions.
- If a technique is to be learned, such as charting BBT or inserting a diaphragm, demonstrate and then have the woman do a return demonstration as appropriate. (*Note:* If certain aspects are beyond your level of expertise, such as fitting a diaphragm, review the content about its use and confirm that the woman understands what she is to do.)
- Provide information on what the woman should do if unusual circumstances arise (e.g., she misses a pill or forgets to take a morning temperature). These can be presented in a written handout as well.
- Stress warning signs that may require immediate action by the woman and explain why these signs indicate a risk. (These should also be covered in the handout.)
- Arrange to talk with the woman again soon, either by phone or at a return visit, to see if she has any questions or has encountered any problems.

---

action to take if she suspects she is pregnant. In many cases, the nurse is involved in telephone counseling of women who call with questions and concerns about contraception. Thus it is vital to be knowledgeable about this topic and have resources available to find answers to less common questions. *Teaching Highlights: Using a Method of Contraception* provides guidelines for helping women use a method of contraception effectively.

Clinical Interruption of Pregnancy

Although abortion was legalized in the United States in 1973, controversy over moral and legal issues continues. Many people are opposed to abortion for religious, ethical, or personal reasons. Others feel that access to a safe, legal abortion is every woman's right. A number of physical and psychosocial factors influence a woman's decision to seek an abortion. Some situations may involve lack of knowledge about contraceptive options, contraceptive failure, rape, or incest.

Medical abortion provides an effective alternative to surgical abortion for many women with an unintended pregnancy. The combination of *mifepristone* (Mifeprex or RU 486), an anti-progesterone, and *misoprostol*, a prostaglandin analog that causes smooth muscle to contract, leads to complete abortion in approximately 92% of women (ACOG, 2011a). The regimen of mifepristone 600 mg orally followed in 48 hours by misoprostol 400 mcg orally is the FDA-approved regimen for use up to 49 days after the last menstrual period. About 14 days after taking the misoprostol, the woman is seen to confirm that the abortion was successful. Other regimens are used in an attempt to decrease cost, decrease time to expulsion of the products of conception, and decrease side effects, but ACOG (2011a) affirms that mifepristone-misoprostol regimens are preferable to those using methotrexate-misoprostol or misoprostol alone for medical abortion.

Surgical abortion in the first trimester is technically easier and safer than abortion in the second trimester. It may be performed by dilation and curettage (D&C), minisuction, or vacuum curettage. Second-trimester abortion may be done using dilation and evacuation (D&E), hypertonic saline, systemic prostaglandins, and intrauterine prostaglandins.

Prior to an elective abortion, women often experience clinically significant anxiety and/or depression. Research suggests that following first-trimester elective abortion, whether medical or surgical, women tend to experience significant improvements in psychologic outcomes. Depression and anxiety are reduced and quality of life improves significantly (Crandell, 2012).

Nursing Management

The nurse needs to recognize that the decision to have an abortion is a major one with psychologic implications for the woman and her partner, if he is involved. In caring for a woman who decides to have an abortion, it is important to do the following:

- Provide information about the methods of abortion and associated risks.
- Counsel the woman about available alternatives to abortion and their implications.
- Encourage the woman to talk about feelings related to her decision to end her pregnancy.
- Provide support before, during, and after the procedure.
- Monitor vital signs, intake, and output.
- Provide for physical comfort and privacy throughout the procedure.
- Teach about self-care, the importance of the postabortion checkup, and contraception review.

Preconception Counseling

One of the first questions a couple should ask before conception is whether they wish to have children. This involves consideration of each person's goals, expectations of their relationship, and desire to be a parent. At times, one individual wishes to have a child, whereas the other does not. In such situations, an open discussion is essential to reach a mutually acceptable decision. In some cases, professional counseling for the couple may be necessary.

Couples who wish to have children face a decision about the timing of pregnancy. At what point in their lives do they believe it would be best to become parents? For couples who have religious beliefs that do not support contraception or who feel that family planning is unnatural and wrong, planning the timing of pregnancy is unacceptable and irrelevant. These couples can still take steps to ensure that they are in the best possible physical and mental health when pregnancy occurs.

Preconception Health Measures

Preconception planning typically begins with a careful health assessment, including a consideration of known or suspected risks.

MODIFIABLE RISK FACTORS

The nurse encourages the woman to address modifiable health risks including the following:

- *Smoking.* Pregnancy often provides a strong incentive for women to quit smoking.
- *Alcohol.* Alcohol consumed during pregnancy can result in fetal alcohol syndrome, birth defects, and low birth weight.
- *Social drugs and street drugs.* These substances pose a real threat to the fetus and are associated with a variety of complications.
- *Caffeine.* The effects of caffeine are less clearly understood; however, as a precaution the woman is advised to avoid caffeine or limit her daily intake.
- *Medications.* A woman who uses any prescription or over-the-counter medications needs to discuss the implications of their use with her healthcare provider. It is best to avoid using any medication if possible.
- *Environmental hazards.* Because of the possible teratogenic effects of environmental hazards in the workplace, the couple contemplating pregnancy needs to determine whether they are exposed to any environmental hazards at work or in their community.

PHYSICAL EXAMINATION

It is advisable for both partners to have a physical examination to identify any health problems that might affect pregnancy so that they can be corrected if possible. These might include medical conditions, such as high blood pressure or obesity; problems that pose a threat to fertility, such as certain STIs; or conditions that keep the individual from achieving optimal health, such as anemia or colitis. If the family history indicates previous genetic disorders, or if the couple is planning pregnancy when the woman is over age 35, the healthcare provider may suggest that the couple consider genetic counseling. Some ethnic groups have higher incidences of certain genetic conditions; therefore, testing should be offered when risks are indentified.

In addition to the history and physical examination, the woman may have the following laboratory tests: urinalysis, complete blood count, blood type and Rh factor, venereal disease research laboratory (VDRL) test, Pap smear, gonorrhea culture, chlamydia screen, and rubella and hepatitis screens. Women who are not immune to rubella should be counseled about the possible effects on the fetus should infection occur during the first trimester of pregnancy. If a woman decides to receive the rubella vaccine, the nurse needs to advise her to wait 3 months before conceiving to eliminate the risk of prenatal infection. These women should be counseled to use contraception during the 3-month period to prevent pregnancy. Before conception, the woman is also advised to have a dental examination and any necessary dental work completed to avoid exposure to x-rays and the risk of infection.

Women should also be asked questions regarding their psychologic history and assessed for mental illness. Certain classes of medications may be contraindicated during pregnancy, and drug changes may be needed prior to conception to prevent adverse maternal or fetal effects.

NUTRITION

Before conception, it is advisable for the woman to be at an average weight for her body build and height. The nurse can discuss nutrition and recommend that the woman follow a nutritious diet that contains ample quantities of all the essential nutrients. Some nutritionists advocate emphasizing the following nutrients: calcium, protein, iron, B complex vitamins, vitamin C, magnesium, and folic acid. Folic acid supplementation should be initiated before conception because it decreases the incidence of neural tube defects in infants. The Centers for Disease Control and Prevention (CDC) estimates that most of these birth defects could be prevented if all women of childbearing age consume 400 mcg of folic acid daily (CDC, 2012). Consumption of a balanced diet with the appropriate distribution of the basic food groups is especially important during pregnancy. Excessive intake of certain vitamins can cause severe fetal problems and should be avoided. Nutritional counseling is warranted for women with a history of eating disorders.

EXERCISE

A woman is advised to establish a regular exercise plan beginning at least 3 months before she plans to attempt to become pregnant. The exercise should be one she enjoys and will continue. It needs to provide some aerobic conditioning and some general toning. Exercise improves the woman's circulation and general health and tones her muscles. Once an exercise program is well established, the woman is generally encouraged to continue it during pregnancy. Prepregnancy obesity, defined as a body mass index (BMI) of 30 or above, puts the woman at risk for a variety of complications; therefore, it is advisable to advocate weight reduction for obese women who want to become pregnant.

Contraception

A woman who takes birth control pills is advised to stop the pill and have two or three normal menses before attempting to conceive. This allows the natural hormonal cycle to return and facilitates dating the subsequent pregnancy. A woman using an intrauterine device is advised to have it removed and wait 1 month before attempting to conceive. This allows the endometrium to be resterilized. Other methods of contraception that women can use during the waiting period include a variety of barrier methods of contraception (condoms, diaphragm, or cervical cap with a spermicide).

Conception

Most preconception recommendations focus on helping the couple attain their best possible health state so that they do not enter pregnancy with unnecessary risks. Conception is a personal and emotional experience, and, even if a couple is prepared, the individuals may feel some ambivalence. This is a normal response, but they may require reassurance that the ambivalence will pass. The prospective parents may get so caught up in preparation and in their efforts to "do things right" that they lose sight of the pleasure they derive from each other and their lives together and cease to value the joy of spontaneity in their relationship. It is often helpful for the healthcare provider to remind an overly zealous couple that moderation is always appropriate and that there is value in "taking time to smell the roses."

Health Promotion for Women

Healthcare providers and consumers alike are becoming increasingly aware of the importance of activities that promote health and prevent illness, including lifestyle choices. In addition, the value of regular screenings to detect any health problems early cannot be overemphasized. Health screening recommendations vary by age. General screening and immunization guidelines for women can be found on the website of the CDC's Office of Women's Health.

This section focuses on some of the most commonly used screening procedures: breast self-examination and breast examination by a trained healthcare provider, mammography, Pap smear, and pelvic examination.

Breast Examination

Like the uterus, the breast undergoes regular cyclic changes in response to hormonal stimulation. Each month, in rhythm with the cycle of ovulation, the breasts become engorged with fluid in anticipation of pregnancy, and the woman may experience sensations of tenderness, lumpiness, or pain. If conception does not occur, the accumulated fluid drains away via the lymphatic network. *Mastodynia* or *mastalgia* (premenstrual swelling and tenderness of the breasts) is common. It usually lasts for 3 to 4 days before the onset of menses, but the symptoms may persist throughout the month.

After menopause, adipose breast tissue atrophies and is replaced by connective tissue. Elasticity is lost, and the breasts may droop and become pendulous. The recurring breast engorgement associated with ovulation ceases. If estrogen replacement therapy is used to counteract other symptoms of menopause, breast engorgement may resume.

Monthly **breast self-examination (BSE)** is a good method for detecting breast masses early. Women at high risk for breast cancer are especially encouraged to be attentive to the importance of early detection through routine BSE.

The value of BSE, however, has been under continual scrutiny. The U.S. Preventive Services Task Force made a recommendation in November 2009 against teaching women breast self-examination based on studies they reviewed that suggested that BSE did not reduce breast cancer mortality but resulted in additional imaging procedures and biopsies. The American College of Obstetricians and Gynecologists stresses *breast self-awareness*—the need for a woman to be aware of how her breasts normally look and feel. ACOG (2012c) identifies breast self-examination as one way for a woman to develop self-awareness. Women who choose to do BSE should have their technique reviewed during the annual examination.

Therefore, in light of the conflicting recommendations, in the course of a routine physical examination, or during an initial visit to the caregiver, women are generally taught the BSE technique. The effectiveness of BSE is determined by the woman's ability to perform the procedure correctly. See *Teaching Highlights: Breast Self-Examination.*

Clinical breast examination (CBE) by a trained healthcare provider, such as a physician, nurse practitioner, or nurse-midwife, is an essential element of a routine gynecologic examination. The ACS no longer recommends CBE for women at average risk of breast cancer (Oeffinger, Fontham, Etzioni, et al., 2015). In clinical practice, however, many caregivers advocate annual CBE for all women over 20 years of age.

Mammography

A **mammogram** is a soft-tissue x-ray of the breast without the injection of a contrast medium (Figure 5–11). It can detect lesions in the breast before they can be felt and has gained wide acceptance as a screening tool. Currently, the

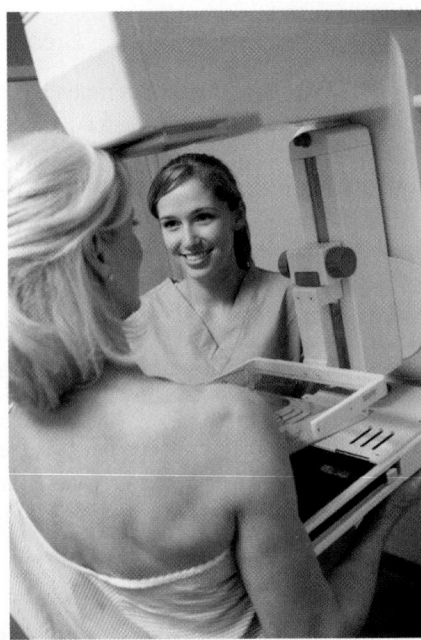

Figure 5–11 Recommended position for mammogram.

SOURCE: Monkey Business/Fotolia.

ACS recommends that all women at average risk of breast cancer begin mammograms at age 45 and continue having them once a year until age 54, then every other year (Oeffinger et al., 2015). The ACS (2013) continues to recommend both mammogram and magnetic resonance imaging (MRI) beginning at age 30 in women who are at a high risk for breast cancer due to gene mutations and/or a strong family history of breast cancer and in women who had radiation to the chest between the ages of 10 and 30 years because they often develop breast cancer at a younger age. On the other hand, the U.S. Preventive Services Task Force on Breast Cancer Screening (USPSTF, 2015; 2009) recommends biennial screening for women ages 50 to 74 years. The Task Force also states that prior to age 50 the decision to start mammography should be an individual one.

Pap Smear and Pelvic Examination

The *Pap smear* is a form of cervical cytology testing used to detect cellular abnormalities by examining a sample containing cells from the cervix and the endocervical canal. Traditionally, the test has been done by preparing a Pap smear slide. Currently, another test—the liquid-based medium Pap smear—is being used more often. In this test, no slide is prepared; instead, the Pap smear is obtained using a speculum to reveal the cervix. The cervix is visualized and a smear is obtained using a plastic spatula on the surface of the cervix and a cytobrush, which is inserted into the cervical os, or opening, to obtain cells in the cervical canal. The brush and spatula are swished in the solution to release cells. The specimen is sent to a laboratory where a special processor prepares a slide. This test has become the method of choice for cervical cancer screening. Liquid-based Pap smear preparations allow for removal of debris from the sample, such as blood and mucus, thereby increasing accuracy. Additionally, these preparations allow for human papillomavirus (HPV) screening and for some STI infection screening. Pap smear findings are reported using the Bethesda system (see Table 6–2).

In 2012, new guidelines for cervical cancer screening were issued by the U.S. Preventive Services Task Force, the ACS,

TEACHING HIGHLIGHTS | Breast Self-Examination

Describe and demonstrate the correct procedure for BSE.

Inspection

The woman should inspect her breasts by standing or sitting in front of a mirror. She should inspect them in three positions: both arms relaxed at her sides, both arms raised straight over her head, and both hands placed on her hips while she leans forward. Instruct her to note the following:

- *Size and symmetry of the breasts, and their shape, contours, and direction.* Have her check for redness or inflammation, rashes, ulceration, or nipple discharge. A blue hue with a marked venous pattern that is focal or unilateral may indicate an area of increased blood supply due to tumor. Symmetric venous patterns are normal.

- *Thickening or edema.* Skin edema is seen as thickened skin with enlarged pores ("orange peel"). It may indicate blocked lymph drainage due to tumor.

- *Surface of the skin.* Skin dimpling, puckering, or retraction when the hands are pressed together in front of the chest or against the hips suggests malignancy.

- *The nipples.* Note any deviation, flattening, broadening, or recent inversion.

Palpation

The woman should be instructed to palpate her breasts as follows:

- Lie down. Put one hand behind your head. With the other hand, fingers flattened, gently feel your breast. Press lightly (Figure 5–12A).

- Still lying down, check each breast as shown in Figure 5–12B. Follow the arrows shown in the image, moving in an up and down pattern, feeling gently for a lump or thickening. Remember to feel all parts of each breast, including the "tail" of tissue near the armpit. Repeat the process on the second breast.

- Now repeat the same process on each breast while sitting up, with your hand still behind your head (Figure 5–12C).

- Squeeze the nipple between your thumb and forefinger. Look for any discharge—clear, bloody, or milky.

Determine whether the client has any questions about her findings during this examination. If she has questions, palpate the area and attempt to identify whether it is normal.

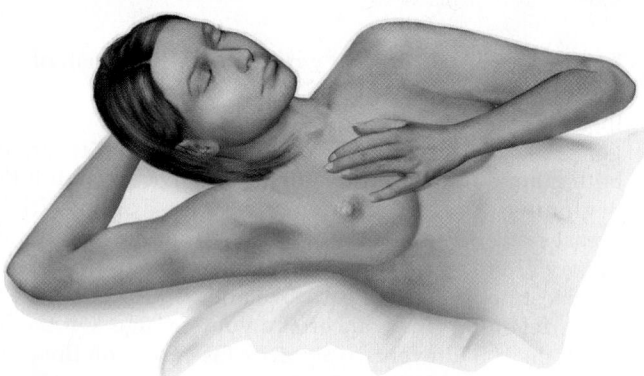

With one hand behind your head, flatten your fingers and press lightly on your breast, feeling gently for a lump or thickening.

A

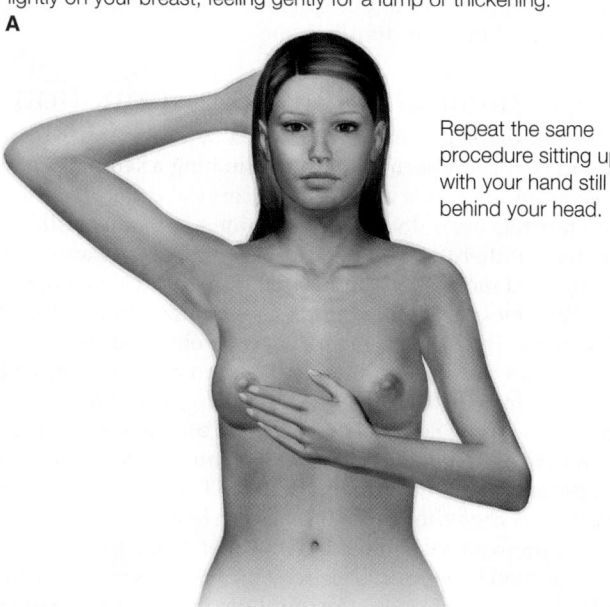

Repeat the same procedure sitting up with your hand still behind your head.

B

C

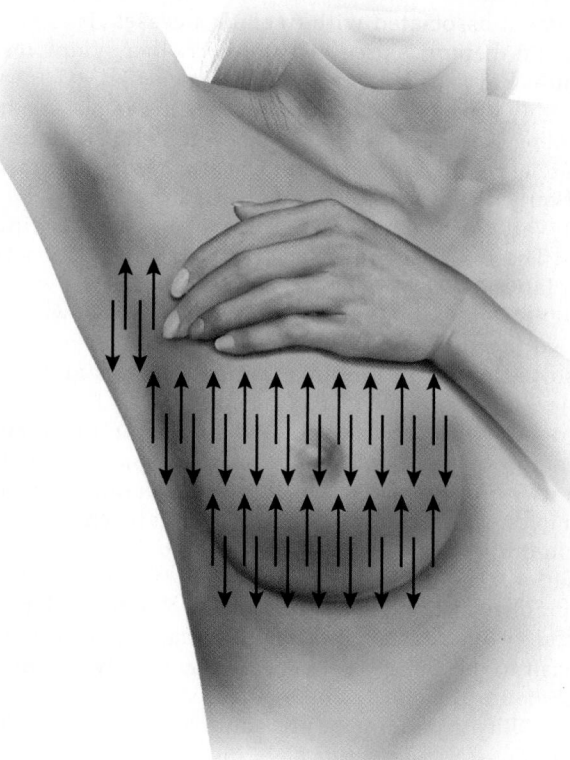

Check each breast in an up-and-down pattern, feeling all parts of the breast.

Figure 5–12 **Procedure for breast self-examination.**

TABLE 5–3 Screening for Cervical Cancer

POPULATION	TEST AND FREQUENCY
Women under age 21	No screening
Women ages 21 to 29	Screening with cytology alone every 3 years (*Note:* Co-testing for HPV is not recommended for this group because of the high prevalence of HPV.)
Women ages 30 to 65	Preferred approach: screen with cytology and HPV testing every 5 years Acceptable approach: test with cytology alone every 3 years
Women over age 65 who have had adequate prior screening and are not at high risk	Do not screen
Women who have undergone hysterectomy and have no history of high-grade precancer or cervical cancer	Do not screen

Source: U.S. Preventive Services Task Force. (2013). Cervical cancer screening guidelines for average-risk women. Retrieved from http://www.cdc.gov/cancer/cervical/pdf/guidelines.pdf

and other groups. These guidelines are found in Table 5–3. It is important to recognize that these recommendations are population-based guidelines reflecting statistical analysis. As such, they are not appropriate for all women. Each woman needs to consult her healthcare provider about the best approach to screening based on her risk factors, history, preexisting conditions, and signs and symptoms.

Clinical Tip

Whenever you teach about pelvic examination and cervical cytology testing, be sure the woman understands that she should not douche for at least 24 hours beforehand. Douching is the use of a medicated solution or water to clean the vagina. Douching can interfere with the accuracy of the Pap smear. Occasionally, a healthcare provider will specifically request that a woman use a douche before a Pap smear; douching should be done only in this circumstance.

Healthy People 2020

(C-15) Increase the proportion of women who receive a cervical cancer screening based on the most recent guidelines

(C-18.2) Increase the proportion of women who were counseled by their healthcare providers about Pap tests

---

The *pelvic examination* lets the healthcare provider assess a woman's vagina, uterus, ovaries, and lower abdominal area. It is often performed after the Pap smear but may also be performed without a Pap for diagnostic purposes. Women sometimes perceive the pelvic examination as uncomfortable and embarrassing and may delay having yearly gynecologic examinations. This avoidance may pose a threat to life and health.

To make the pelvic examination less threatening and thus improve health-seeking behavior, healthcare providers can offer the woman a mirror to watch the procedure, point out anatomic parts to her, and position and drape her to allow eye-to-eye contact with the examiner. Healthcare providers can encourage the woman to participate by asking questions and giving feedback.

Nurse practitioners, CNMs, and physicians all perform pelvic examinations. Nurses assist the healthcare provider and the woman during the examination. See Assisting with a Pelvic Examination in the *Clinical Skills Manual* `SKILLS`.

Menopause

Menopause, defined as the absence of menses for a full year, is a time of transition for a woman, marking the end of her reproductive abilities. *Climacteric,* or *change of life* (often used synonymously with menopause), refers to the psychologic and physical alterations that occur around the time of menopause. Today, the median age at menopause is 50 to 51 years, and the average life span of a woman in the United States is over 80 years. Thus the average woman will live one third of her life after menopause.

A woman's psychologic adaptation to menopause and the climacteric is multifactorial. She is influenced by her own expectations and knowledge, physical well-being, family views, marital stability, and sociocultural expectations. While some women still accept the negative emotional connotations society once attached to menopause, that view has changed dramatically. Today, women in this age group are generally active, engaged, and fit. They simply regard menopause as a new stage of life and a time of personal growth and fulfillment.

Perimenopause is the term applied to the time before menopause when ovarian function wanes and hormonal deficiencies begin to produce symptoms. Symptoms of perimenopause may be nonexistent or bothersome. They may include PMS, hot flashes, irregular periods, insomnia, decreased libido, vaginal dryness, and mood changes.

Contraception remains a concern during perimenopause. Combined hormonal methods (the pill, patches, and vaginal rings) are popular among healthy nonsmokers because many women also benefit from the noncontraceptive effects, including regulation of menses, relief of symptoms of estrogen deficiency, and a decreased risk of endometrial and ovarian cancers. Other contraceptive options for perimenopausal women include sterilization, IUCs, progestin-only methods, and barrier methods such as male and female condoms, diaphragm, cervical cap, and spermicides.

The physical characteristics of menopause are linked to the shift from a cyclic to a noncyclic hormonal pattern. The age at onset may be influenced by nutritional, cultural, or genetic factors. The onset of menopause occurs when estrogen levels become so low that menstruation stops.

Generally, ovulation ceases 1 to 2 years before menopause, but individual variations exist. Atrophy of the ovaries occurs gradually. FSH levels rise, and less estrogen is produced. Menopausal symptoms include atrophic changes in the vagina, vulva, and urethra and in the trigonal area of the bladder.

Many menopausal women experience a vasomotor disturbance commonly known as *hot flashes,* a feeling of heat arising from the chest and spreading to the neck and face. The hot flashes are often accompanied by profuse sweating (*night sweats*) and sleep disturbances. These episodes may occur as often as 20 to 30 times a day and generally last 3 to 5 minutes. Some women also experience dizzy spells, palpitations, and weakness. Many women find their own most effective ways to deal with the hot flashes. Some report that using a fan or drinking a cool liquid helps relieve distress; others seek relief through hormone therapy. In addition, many women use complementary therapies (see later discussion).

The uterine lining (endometrium) and uterine muscle layer (myometrium) atrophy, as do the cervical glands. The uterine cavity constricts. The fallopian tubes and ovaries atrophy. The vaginal mucosa loses its elasticity and becomes thinner and smoother. As a result, intercourse can be painful, but this problem may be overcome by using lubricating gel. Dryness of the mucous membrane can lead to burning and itching. The vaginal pH level increases as the number of Döderlein bacilli decreases.

Vulvar atrophy occurs late, and the pubic hair thins, turns gray or white, and may ultimately disappear. The labia shrink and lose their heightened pigmentation. Pelvic fascia and muscles atrophy, resulting in decreased pelvic support. The breasts become pendulous and decrease in size and firmness.

Sexual functioning generally declines with age, although more than 75% of the middle-aged women in the Study of Women's Health Across the Nation (SWAN) (Santoro & Sutton-Tyrrell, 2011) cited sex as being moderately to extremely important. Contributing factors to the decline in both interest and occurrence of sexual activity are widespread. Pain during intercourse due to lack of lubrication and thinning vaginal walls is a common cause. Other factors may include a lack of partners, stress in current relationships, psychosocial factors, and a decline in general health. Completing a good sexual history will help the nurse to assess the woman's sexual health and allow the woman to ask questions and express concerns or frustrations.

Long-range physical changes may include **osteoporosis**, a decrease in the bony skeletal mass. This change is associated with lowered estrogen levels, lack of physical exercise, inadequate vitamin D, and a chronic low intake of calcium. However, the greatest influencing factor is a family history of osteoporosis. Moreover, the estrogen deprivation that occurs in menopausal women may significantly increase their risk of *coronary heart disease,* which is the number one killer of women in the United States. Loss of protein from the skin and supportive tissues causes wrinkling. Postmenopausal women frequently gain weight, which may be due to excessive caloric intake or to lower caloric need with the same level of intake.

Women With Special Needs Assisting the Older Woman With a Physical Disability

More than 50% of women over the age of 65 have a physical disability. The most common disabilities in this age group are related to arthritis or rheumatism. Older women with physical disabilities may need assistance getting onto the examination table for a gynecologic examination. The nurse should assist the woman into a semi-Fowler position and move both legs simultaneously to stirrups to prevent muscle strain or injury.

Memory and cognitive function change with advancing age. It may be that declining estrogen levels might contribute to loss of this function as well as to the development of dementia. This change is also influenced by lifestyle, genetics, and socioeconomic status. In the United States, Alzheimer disease (AD) is the most common form of dementia. AD is estimated to affect 5.2 million Americans. Projections indicate that by the year 2025, 7.1 million Americans over the age of 65 will have AD

(Alzheimer's Association, 2013). This projected increase represents a major health concern for the country.

Healthy People 2020

(DIA-1) (Developmental) Increase the proportion of persons with diagnosed Alzheimer disease and other dementias, or their caregivers, who are aware of the diagnosis

(DIA-2) (Developmental) Reduce the proportion of preventable hospitalizations in persons with diagnosed Alzheimer disease and other dementias

---

Clinical Therapy

Menopausal hormone therapy (MHT), formerly called *hormone replacement therapy (HRT)*, refers to the administration of specific hormones, usually estrogen therapy (ET) alone or a combination estrogen-progestogen therapy (EPT), to alleviate menopausal symptoms. ET is used for women who have had a hysterectomy, whereas EPT is used for women with an intact uterus. When estrogen is given alone, it can produce endometrial hyperplasia and increase the risk of endometrial cancer. Thus, in women who still have a uterus, estrogen is opposed by giving a progestin, often Provera, continuously or sequentially.

For over a decade, the use of MHT had decreased significantly because of a large study that suggested that the risks of MHT outweighed the benefits, particularly the increased risk of breast cancer, thromboembolic disease, and stroke. In light of findings from more recent clinical trials, that study has been called into question. In late 2012, the International Menopause Society convened a global panel to develop recommendations about the clinical management of menopausal hormone therapy. Among their recommendations were the following (de Villiers et al., 2013):

- MHT remains the most effective therapy for moderate-to-severe menopausal vasomotor symptoms (hot flashes and night sweats). For symptomatic women younger than age 60 or within 10 years after menopause, the benefits are likely to outweigh the risks.

- The decision to use MHT is an individual one based on quality of life, health priorities, and personal risk factors (age, time since onset of menopause, risk of venous ischemic heart disease, thromboembolism, and breast cancer).

MHT is effective for the prevention of fractures related to osteoporosis in women who are at risk before age 60 or within 10 years of menopause. MHT can be prescribed in a number of ways, including orally; transdermally (patch); intramuscularly; topically as a gel, lotion, or vaginal cream; or through a vaginal ring. It is given in a continuous manner as a daily administration of both estrogen and progestogen, or as a cyclic or sequential therapy, with estrogen use daily and a progestogen added on a set sequence. Combination estrogen-progestogen preparations are also available.

Postmenopausal women experiencing decreased libido may experience improved sexual desire, responsiveness, and frequency when testosterone is added to their MHT. Options for providing testosterone in doses low enough for women are still limited. Estratest, a combined estrogen-androgen pill, is used by some women. Custom-compounded testosterone preparations are available by prescription, and work is underway on low-dose testosterone patches.

Before starting MHT, a woman should undergo a thorough history; a physical examination, including Pap smear;

measurement of cholesterol, lipid, and liver enzyme levels; and a baseline mammogram. An initial endometrial biopsy is indicated for women with an increased risk of endometrial cancer; biopsy is also indicated if excessive, unexpected, or prolonged vaginal bleeding occurs. Women taking estrogen should be advised to stop immediately if they develop headaches, visual changes, signs of thrombophlebitis, or chest pain.

COMPLEMENTARY AND ALTERNATIVE THERAPIES

For women who do not wish to take MHT or who have medical contraindications to it, a variety of approaches have been proposed as alternative or complementary treatment or preventive measures for the discomforts of the perimenopausal and postmenopausal years. Research suggests that mind-body practices such as yoga, t'ai chi, and meditation are helpful in reducing many of the common symptoms of menopause for some women; acupuncture may also help reduce the severity of symptoms (National Center for Complementary and Alternative Medicine [NCCAM], 2012). Women may also seek relief through diet and nutrition, specifically a high-fiber, low-fat diet with supplements of calcium and vitamins D, E, and B complex.

Phytoestrogens, plant substances with estrogen-like properties, have been studied extensively to determine their effectiveness in relieving menopausal symptoms. The two main classes of phytoestrogens are isoflavones such as soy, and lignans, found in flaxseed, legumes, whole grains, fruits, and vegetables. Of these, soy has been the focus of the most study, primarily because Asian women, who typically have a diet rich in soy, have a far lower incidence of vasomotor symptoms at menopause than American or European women. A meta-analysis and systematic review found that the use of phytoestrogens is associated with a decrease in hot flash frequency but not in other symptoms of menopause when compared to a placebo (Chen, Lin, & Liu, 2014). Research into the use of phytoestrogens continues.

A great deal of attention has been given to "bioidentical" hormones because of current views, which are not supported by medical literature, that these "more natural" hormones are safer and more effective. A bioidentical hormone refers to a hormone that is structurally identical to those found in the body; more specifically, those produced by the ovaries. These hormones are compounded by a specialty pharmacy and are not approved by the FDA, nor have they been proven to have a better safety profile, and their use is not recommended (de Villiers et al., 2013).

Dihydroepiandrosterone (DHEA) is a dietary supplement that is changed in the body to the hormones estrogen and testosterone. It has been suggested that DHEA might have antiaging effects and might help in improving decreased sexual arousal, mood, cognition, and bone density, although the results of randomized controlled trials and observational studies are mixed and further study is needed (Rutkowski, Sowa, Rutkowski-Talipska, et al., 2014).

Weight-bearing exercises such as walking, jogging, tennis, and low-impact aerobics help increase bone mass and decrease the risk of osteoporosis. Exercise also improves cholesterol profiles and contributes to overall health. Pelvic floor, or Kegel, exercises can help maintain vaginal muscle tone and increase blood circulation to the perineal area. Vaginal lubricants and adequate foreplay can be helpful in maintaining a satisfactory sexual experience. Stress management and relaxation techniques such as biofeedback, meditation, yoga, visualization, and massage may provide a sense of well-being.

The following botanicals are often mentioned for treating menopausal symptoms but results are mixed (NCCAM, 2012):

- Black cohosh has received attention for its possible effectiveness but preliminary research suggests that it is no more effective than a placebo in relieving symptoms. In rare cases, it has been associated with liver inflammation.
- Red clover is sometimes used to reduce hot flashes but research has failed to demonstrate its effectiveness.
- Ginseng may help relieve mood symptoms and sleep disturbances but has not been effective in treating hot flashes.
- Kava has not been shown to relieve hot flashes, but it may decrease anxiety. Like black cohosh, it has been associated with liver disease.

PREVENTION AND TREATMENT OF OSTEOPOROSIS

One of every two White women over age 50 and one in five men will have an osteoporosis-related fracture. Osteoporosis is less common in African Americans, but those with the diagnosis have the same fracture risk (National Osteoporosis Foundation [NOF], 2013). Osteoporosis is a largely preventable disease, however, and a source of significant risk for fracture and subsequent health decline. *Healthy People 2020* addresses the issue of osteoporosis in general and hip fracture in particular. Table 5–4 identifies risk factors associated with osteoporosis.

Healthy People 2020

(AOCBC-10) Reduce the proportion of adults with osteoporosis

(AOCBC-11) Reduce hip fractures among older adults

Bone mineral density (BMD) testing is useful in identifying individuals who are at risk for osteoporosis. The NOF (2013) recommends BMD testing of all women ages 65 and older and all men ages 70 and older. BMD testing may also be indicated for premenopausal or postmenopausal women with risk factors; certain medical conditions such as eating disorders, thyroid disorders, leukemia, rheumatoid arthritis, and multiple sclerosis; and for those women on certain medications such as corticosteroids or anticonvulsants.

Prevention of osteoporosis is a primary goal of care. Perimenopausal and postmenopausal women are advised to have a daily calcium intake of 1200 mg (NAMS, 2012). Most women require supplements to achieve this level. Vitamin D

TABLE 5–4 Risk Factors for Osteoporosis

- Advanced age
- Being female
- European American or Asian ethnic origin
- Being thin (weight less than 127 lb and/or having a small frame)
- Family history of osteoporosis, especially a maternal hip fracture
- Inactive lifestyle
- Nulliparity
- Early onset of menopause
- Consistently low intake of calcium; vitamin D deficiency
- Cigarette smoking, moderate to heavy alcohol intake
- Use of certain medications such as anticonvulsants, corticosteroids, chemotherapy, barbiturates

supplements (800 to 1000 International Units per day) may also be indicated for those at risk of deficiency. Women are also advised to participate regularly in exercise, to consume only modest quantities of alcohol and caffeine, and to stop smoking. Alcohol and smoking have a negative effect on the rate of bone resorption.

Women's height should be measured at each visit because a loss of height is often an early sign that vertebrae are being compressed because of reduced bone mass. The effectiveness of estrogen in preventing osteoporosis is well documented. However, because of the increased risks associated with long-term use of MHT, other pharmacologic agents are being used more frequently to prevent and treat osteoporosis. These include the following:

- *Bisphosphonates* are calcium regulators that act by inhibiting bone resorption and increasing bone mass. Alendronate (Fosamax) and risedronate (Actonel) are commonly prescribed. Zoledronic acid (Zometa) is administered IV once a year and seems to achieve the same results in treating osteoporosis as other bisphosphonates taken daily or weekly without the troublesome gastrointestinal side effects.

- *Selective estrogen receptor modulators* (SERMs) such as raloxifene (Evista) preserve the beneficial effects of estrogen, including its protection against osteoporosis, but do not stimulate uterine or breast tissue.

- Salmon *calcitonin* is a calcium regulator that may inhibit bone loss. Administered as a nasal spray, its value is less clear than that of the other medications listed.

- *Parathyroid hormone,* taken daily as a subcutaneous injection, activates bone formation, which results in substantial increases in bone density.

- *Receptor activator of nuclear factor kappa-B ligand* (RANKL) *inhibitor* (denosumab, brand name Prolia) decreases bone resorption and increases bone mass and strength. It is administered subcutaneously every 6 months.

Nursing Management

Most menopausal women deal well with this developmental phase of life, although some women may need counseling to adjust successfully. Nurses and other health professionals can help menopausal women achieve high-level functioning at this time in life. Of major importance is the nurse's ability to understand and provide support for the woman's views and feelings. Use an empathetic approach in counseling, health teaching, and when providing physical care.

Explore the question of the woman's comfort during sexual intercourse. In counseling, it may be appropriate to say, "After menopause many women notice that their vagina seems drier and intercourse can be uncomfortable. Have you noticed any changes?" This gives the woman information and may open discussion. Then go on to explain that dryness and shrinking of the vagina can be addressed by use of a water-soluble jelly. Use of estrogen, orally or in vaginal creams, may also be indicated. Increased frequency of intercourse will maintain some elasticity in the vagina. When assessing the menopausal woman, address the question of sexual activity openly but tactfully because the woman may have been socialized to be reticent about discussing sex.

The crucial need of women in the menopausal period of life is for adequate information about the changes taking place in their bodies and in their lives. Supplying that information provides both a challenge and an opportunity for nurses.

Violence Against Women

Violence against women is a major health concern in society today. Violence affects women of all ages, races, ethnic backgrounds, socioeconomic levels, educational levels, and walks of life. Two of the most common forms of violence are domestic violence, also called *intimate partner violence* or *relationship violence,* and sexual assault. Worldwide, 35% of women have experienced intimate partner violence or nonpartner sexual violence at some time in their lives; estimates suggest that 38% of all female murders are committed by an intimate partner (World Health Organization [WHO], 2013).

Violence against women is a major health concern. In addition to causing injuries, associated physical and mental health outcomes, and fatalities, violence costs the healthcare system millions of dollars annually. In response to this epidemic, healthcare providers are becoming more knowledgeable about actions they should take to identify women at risk, implement preventive measures, and provide effective care.

Healthy People 2020

(IVP-39) (Developmental) Reduce violence by current or former partners

(IVP-40) (Developmental) Reduce sexual violence

Domestic Violence

Domestic violence or **intimate partner violence (IPV)** is defined as a pattern of coercive behavior and methods used to exert power and control by one individual over another in an adult domestic or intimate relationship. This section focuses on domestic violence experienced by women in heterosexual relationships, although gay and lesbian individuals do experience domestic violence in their relationships as well.

Although the incidence has decreased significantly in the past decade, IPV is still staggeringly common in the United States, where almost one in four women (22.3%) will experience at least one act of severe physical violence during her lifetime. Psychologic aggression by an intimate partner is even more common—47.1% of women will experience at least one act of psychologic aggression during their lifetimes (Breiding et al., 2014). The incidence of domestic violence is highest in women ages 18 to 34, but it does occur in all age groups (Catalano, 2012). The woman may be married to her abuser, or she may be living with, dating, or divorced from him. Domestic violence takes many forms, including verbal attacks, insults, intimidation, threats, sexual violence, emotional abuse, social isolation, economic deprivation, intellectual derision, ridicule, stalking, and physical attacks and injury. Physical battering includes slapping, kicking, shoving, punching, forms of torture, attacks with objects or weapons, and sexual assault. Women who are physically abused can also suffer psychologic and emotional abuse.

CYCLE OF VIOLENCE

In an effort to explain the experience of battered women, Walker (1984) developed the theory of the *cycle of violence.* Battering takes place in a cyclic fashion through three phases:

1. *Tension-building phase.* The batterer demonstrates power and control in this phase, which is characterized by anger, arguing, blaming the woman for external problems, and possibly minor battering incidents. The woman may blame herself and believe she can prevent the escalation of the batterer's anger by her own actions.

2. *Acute battering incident.* Typically triggered by some external event or internal state of the batterer, it is an episode of acute violence distinguished by lack of control, lack of predictability, and major destructiveness. The cycle of violence can be interrupted before the acute battering incident if proper interventions take place.

3. *Tranquil, loving phase.* Sometimes termed the *honeymoon period*, this phase may be characterized by extremely kind and loving behavior on the part of the batterer as he tries to make up with the woman, or it may simply be manifested as an absence of tension and violence. Without intervention this phase will end and the cycle of violence will continue. Over time the violence increases in severity and frequency.

CHARACTERISTICS OF BATTERED WOMEN

Battered women often hold traditional views of gender roles. Many were raised to be submissive, passive, and dependent and to seek approval from male figures. Some battered women were exposed to violence between their parents, whereas others first experienced it from their partners. Many battered women do not work outside the home. As part of the manipulation of batterers, they are isolated from family and friends and totally dependent on their partners for their financial and emotional needs.

Women with physically abusive partners nearly always experience psychologic abuse as well, and have been told repeatedly by their batterers that the family's problems are all their fault. Many believe their batterers' insults and accusations. As these women become more isolated, they find it harder to judge who is right. Eventually they fully believe in their inadequacy, and their low self-esteem reinforces their belief that they deserve to be beaten. Battered women often feel a pervasive sense of guilt, fear, and depression. Their sense of hopelessness and helplessness reduces their problem-solving ability. Battered women may also experience a lack of support from family, friends, and their religious community.

CHARACTERISTICS OF BATTERERS

Batterers come from all backgrounds. They often have feelings of insecurity, socioeconomic inferiority, powerlessness, and helplessness that conflict with their assumptions of male supremacy. Emotionally immature and aggressive men have a tendency to express these overwhelming feelings of inadequacy through violence. Many batterers feel undeserving of their partners, yet they blame and punish the very women they value.

Battered women often describe their husbands or partners as lacking respect toward women in general, having come from homes where they witnessed abuse of their mothers or were themselves abused as children, and having a hidden rage that erupts occasionally. Batterers accept traditional macho values, yet when they are not angry or aggressive, they appear childlike, dependent, seductive, manipulative, and in need of nurturing. They may be well respected in the community. This dual personality of batterers reflects the conflict between their belief that they must live up to their macho image and their feelings of inadequacy in the role of husband or provider. Combined with low frustration tolerance and poor impulse control, their pervasive sense of powerlessness leads them to strike out at life's inequities by abusing women.

Nursing Management

Nurses often come in contact with abused women but fail to recognize them, especially if their bruises are not visible. Women at high risk for battering often have a history of alcohol or drug abuse, child abuse, or abuse in the previous or present relationship.

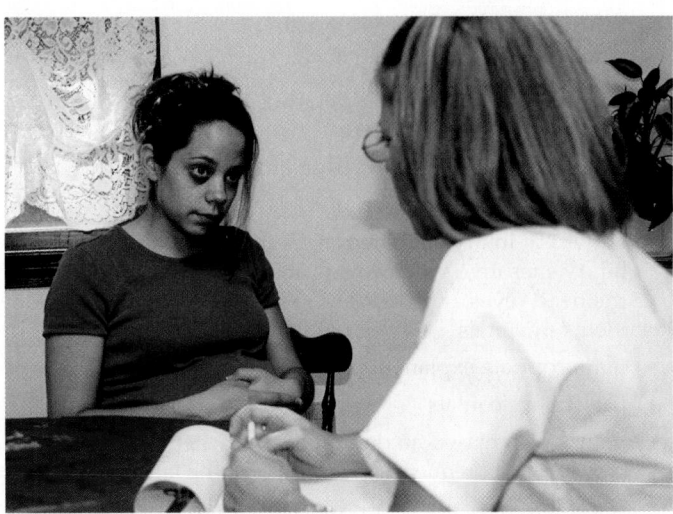

Figure 5–13 Screening for domestic violence should be done privately.

Other possible signs of abuse include expressions of helplessness and powerlessness; low self-esteem revealed by the woman's dress, appearance, and the way she relates to healthcare providers; signs of depression evidenced by fatigue, hopelessness, and somatic problems such as headache, insomnia, chest pain, back pain, or pelvic pain; and possible suicide attempts. In addition, the abused woman may have a history of missed or frequently changed appointments, perhaps because she had signs of abuse that kept her from coming in or because her partner prevented it.

Because female partner abuse is so prevalent, many caregivers now advocate *universal screening of all female clients at every health encounter.* Screening should be done privately, with only the caregiver and client present, and in a safe and quiet place. Specific language leads to higher disclosure rates. Possible screening questions include the following:

1. During the past year, have you been slapped, kicked, hit, choked, or hurt physically by someone?

2. Has your partner or anyone else ever forced you to have sex?

3. Are you afraid of an ex-partner or anyone at home?

During the screening, assure the woman that her privacy will be respected (Figure 5–13). It is essential to remain nonjudgmental. Create a warm, caring climate conducive to sharing, and demonstrate a willingness to talk about violence. A battered woman may interpret your willingness to discuss violence as permission for her to discuss it as well.

It is important to consider cultural and religious factors that may impact a woman's willingness to disclose abuse. See *Developing Cultural Competence: Supporting Immigrant Women Who Suffer Abuse.*

Developing Cultural Competence Supporting Immigrant Women Who Suffer Abuse

Immigrant women who experience IPV may be reluctant to report it for fear of deportation. Nurses need to be aware that the "U" nonimmigrant visa permits immigrants who have been victims of IPV or other crimes to remain in the United States legally if it is justified on humanitarian grounds, is in the public interest, or ensures family unity (ACOG, 2012b).

When a woman seeks care for an injury, be alert to the following cues of abuse:

- Hesitation in providing detailed information about the injury and how it occurred
- Inappropriate affect for the situation
- Delayed reporting of symptoms
- Pattern of injury consistent with abuse, including multiple injury sites involving bruises, abrasions, and contusions to the head (eyes and back of the neck), throat, chest, abdomen, or genitals
- Inappropriate explanation for the injuries
- Lack of eye contact
- Signs of increased anxiety in the presence of the possible batterer, who frequently does much of the talking

When a battered woman comes in for treatment, she needs to feel safe physically and secure in talking about her injuries and problems. If a man is with her, ask or tell him to remain in the waiting room while the woman is examined. A battered woman also needs to regain a sense of predictability by knowing what to expect and how she can interact. Provide sufficient information about what to expect in terms the woman can understand.

In providing care, let the woman work through her story, problems, and situation at her own pace. Reassure the woman that she is believed and that her feelings are reasonable and normal. Anticipate the woman's ambivalence (due to her fear and possible love–hate relationship with her batterer), but also respect the woman's capacity to change and grow when she is ready. Thus any assessment should include information about a woman's strengths and support systems. The woman may need help identifying specific problems and developing realistic ideas for reducing or eliminating those problems. In all interactions, stress that no one should be abused and that the abuse is not the woman's fault.

Community-Based Nursing Care

Inform any woman suspected of being in an abusive situation of the services available in the community. A battered woman may need the following:

- Medical treatment for injuries
- Temporary shelter to provide a safe environment for her and her children
- Counseling to raise her self-esteem and help her understand the dynamics of violence
- Legal assistance for protection from or prosecution of the batterer
- Financial assistance to obtain shelter, food, and clothing
- Job training or employment counseling

If the woman returns to an abusive situation, encourage her to develop an exit plan for herself and her children, if any. As part of the plan, she should:

- Pack a change of clothes for herself and the children, including toilet articles and an extra set of car and house keys stored away from her house with a friend or neighbor.
- Ask a neighbor to call the police if violence begins.
- Have money, identification papers (driver's license, social security cards), checkbook, bank account information, other financial records (such as mortgage papers, rent and utility receipts, automobile title, insurance policies and numbers), and information about the children to help her enroll them in school.
- Have a plan for where she will go, regardless of the day or time.
- Identify friends and family who know about the situation and will help her. Ask that she establish a code word for danger with those family and friends.
- Have a planned escape route and emergency telephone numbers she can call, including personal numbers, the local police, a phone hotline, and a women's shelter if one is available in the community.

Working with battered women is challenging, and many healthcare providers feel frustrated and impotent when the women repeatedly return to their abusive situations. Nurses must realize that they cannot rescue battered women; battered women must decide on their own how to handle their situations. Effective nurses provide battered women with information that empowers them in decision making and supports their decisions, knowing that incremental assistance over the years may be the only alternative until the battered women are ready to explore other options.

> **Professionalism in Practice** Client Advocacy
>
> Client advocacy is a nursing responsibility that extends beyond individual nurse-client relationships. Nurses can follow and become involved in legislative advocacy for issues related to domestic violence and other issues related to women's health through participation in their local and state chapters of the American Nurses Association, by being aware of current issues, by following the progress of specific bills online, by writing to their legislators, and by exercising their right to vote.

Sexual Assault

Broadly, **sexual assault** is involuntary sexual contact with another person. **Rape** is forced sexual intercourse as a result of physical force or psychologic coercion. *Forced sexual intercourse* refers to vaginal, oral, or anal penetration by a body part or by an object.

Sexual assault remains one of the most underreported violent crimes in the United States. In 2012, only an estimated 28% of rapes or sexual assaults were reported to the police, making the actual number of victims significantly higher (Truman, Langton, & Planty, 2013). Over 78% of victims know their offender; about 40% of assailants had been drinking or using drugs prior to the assault. Although both men and women can be sexually assaulted, research indicates that 91% or approximately 9 of every 10 rape or sexual assault victims are female (Planty, Langton, Krebs, et al., 2013).

No woman of any age, cultural or ethnic background, or socioeconomic status is immune, but statistics indicate that young, unmarried women; women who are unemployed or have low family income; and students have the highest incidence of sexual assault or attempted assault.

Why do men rape? Of the many theories put forth, none provides a completely satisfactory explanation. So few assailants are actually caught and convicted that a clear characteristic of the assailant has not been developed. However, rapists tend to be emotionally weak and insecure and may have difficulty maintaining interpersonal relationships. Many assailants also have trouble dealing with the stresses of daily life. Such men may become angry and overcome by feelings of powerlessness. They then commit a sexual assault as an expression of power or anger.

Acquaintance rape, which occurs when the assailant is someone with whom the victim has had previous nonviolent interaction, is the most common form of rape. One type of acquaintance rape, **date rape**, which occurs between a dating couple, is an increasing problem on high school and college campuses. In some cases, an assailant uses alcohol or other drugs to sedate his intended victim. One drug, flunitrazepam (Rohypnol), has gained notoriety as a date rape drug. Gamma hydroxybutyrate (GHB), ketamine, methylenedioxymethamphetamine (MDMA, Ecstasy), clonazepam, and scopolamine have also been identified as date rape drugs that are used to incapacitate a woman. More recently, prescription drugs have been used in combination with alcohol to facilitate many sexual assaults. Because these drugs frequently produce amnesia, the woman may be unable to remember details of her assault, thereby making prosecution more difficult.

Awareness of the prevalence of date rape and violence against women on college campuses has increased significantly in the wake of several high-profile rape cases at American universities. Title IX legislation, best known for its requirement that all colleges and universities that receive federal funds provide equal opportunities for women in athletic programs, facilities, educational programs, and the like, also addresses the issue of sexual harassment and violence against women. In April 2011, the Department of Education's Office of Civil Rights issued a "Dear colleague" letter that specifically states that higher education institutions are required to "take immediate and effective steps to end sexual harassment and sexual violence" (Office of the Assistant Secretary, DOE, 2011). Today, campuses have a Title IX compliance officer and are actively working to provide education to students, faculty, and staff about these issues.

RESPONSES TO SEXUAL ASSAULT

Sexual assault is a *situational crisis.* It is a traumatic event that the survivor cannot be prepared to handle because it is unforeseen. Following an assault the victim generally experiences a cluster of symptoms, described by Burgess and Holmstrom (1979) as the *rape trauma syndrome,* that last far beyond the rape itself. These phases are described in Table 5–5. Although the phases of response are listed individually, they often overlap, and individual responses and their duration may vary. A fourth phase—integration and recovery—has also been suggested (Holmes, 1998).

Research suggests that survivors of sexual assault may exhibit high levels of posttraumatic stress disorder, the same disorder that developed in many of the veterans of the Vietnam War. Posttraumatic stress disorder is marked by varying degrees of intensity. Assault victims with this disorder often require lengthy, intensive therapy to regain a sense of trust and feeling of personal control.

Nursing Management

Survivors of sexual assault often enter the healthcare system by way of the emergency department. Thus the emergency department nurse is often the first person to counsel them. Because the values, attitudes, and beliefs of the healthcare provider necessarily affect the competence and focus of the health care, it is essential that you clearly understand your feelings about sexual assault and assault survivors and resolve any conflicts that may

TABLE 5–5 Phases of Recovery Following Sexual Assault

PHASE	RESPONSE
Acute phase (disorganization)	Fear, shock, disbelief, desire for revenge, anger, anxiety, guilt, denial, embarrassment, humiliation, helplessness, dependence, self-blame, wide variety of physical reactions, lost or distorted coping mechanisms
Outward adjustment phase (denial)	Survivor appears outwardly composed, denying and repressing feelings (e.g., she returns to work, buys a weapon); refuses to discuss the assault; denies need for counseling
Reorganization	Survivor makes many life adjustments, such as moving to a new residence or changing her phone number; uses emotional distancing; may engage in risky sexual behaviors; may experience sexual dysfunction, phobias, flashbacks, sleep disorders, nightmares, anxiety; has a strong urge to talk about or resolve feelings; may seek counseling or remain silent
Integration and recovery	Time of resolution; survivor begins to feel safe and be comfortable trusting others; places blame on assailant; may become an advocate for others

exist. In many communities, a specially trained sexual assault nurse examiner (SANE) coordinates the care of survivors of sexual assault, gathers necessary forensic evidence, and is then available as an expert witness when assailants are tried for the crime.

The first priority in caring for a survivor of a sexual assault is to create a safe, secure environment. Gather admission information in a quiet, private room. Reassure the woman that she is safe and not alone. Assess the survivor's appearance, demeanor, and ways of communicating for the purpose of planning care. Initially the woman is evaluated to determine the need for emergency care. Obtaining a careful, detailed history is essential. After the woman has received any necessary emergency care, complete a forensic chart and kit.

Give the woman a thorough explanation of the procedures to be carried out and have her sign a consent form for the forensic examination and collection of materials. Sexual assault kits contain all the necessary supplies for collecting and labeling evidence. The woman's clothing should be collected and bagged, swabs of stains and secretions taken, hair samples and any fingernail scrapings collected, blood samples drawn, tissue swabs obtained, and photographs taken of any injuries. Vaginal and rectal examinations are performed, along with a complete physical examination for trauma. The woman is offered prophylactic treatment for STIs. If the assailant's HIV status is not known, the woman may be offered postexposure prophylaxis with HIV antiviral medications. In such cases, consultation with an HIV specialist is advised. Question the woman about her menstrual cycle and contraceptive practices. If she could become pregnant as a result of the rape, she should be offered postcoital contraceptive therapy.

Throughout the experience you should act as the sexual assault survivor's advocate, providing support without usurping decision making. You need not agree with all the survivor's decisions but should respect and defend her right to make them.

The family members and friends on whom the survivor calls also need nursing care. The reactions of the family will depend on the values to which they ascribe. Many families or partners blame the survivor for the assault and feel angry with her for not having been more careful. They may also incorrectly view the assault as a sexual act rather than an act of violence. They may feel personally wronged and see the survivor as devalued or unclean. Their

reactions may compound the survivor's crisis. By spending some time with family members before their first interaction with the survivor, you can perhaps reduce their anxiety and absorb some of their frustrations, sparing the woman further trauma.

PROSECUTION OF THE ASSAILANT

Legally, sexual assault is considered a crime against the state, and prosecution of the assailant is a community responsibility. The survivor, however, must begin the process by reporting the assault and pressing charges against her assailant. In the past, the police and the judicial system were notoriously insensitive in dealing with survivors. However, many communities now have classes designed to help police officers work effectively with sexual assault survivors or have special teams to carry out this important task.

Many women who have sought to use the judicial process have had such a traumatic experience that they refer to it as a second assault. The woman may be asked repeatedly to describe the experience in intimate detail, and her reputation and testimony may be attacked by the defense attorney. In addition, publicity may intensify her feelings of humiliation, and, if her assailant is released on bail or found not guilty, she may fear retaliation.

The nurse acting as a counselor needs to be aware of the judicial sequence to anticipate rising tension and frustration in the survivor and her support system. The woman needs consistent, effective support at this crucial time.

Health Promotion **Counseling After Sexual Assault**

Sexual assault counseling, provided by qualified nurses or other counselors, is a valuable tool in helping the survivor come to terms with her assault and its impact on her life. In counseling, the woman is encouraged to explore and identify her feelings and determine appropriate actions to resolve her problems and concerns. The counselor must avoid reinforcing the prevalent myth that the assault was somehow the woman's fault. The fault lies with the assailant. The counselor also plays an important role in emphasizing that the loss of control the woman experienced during the rape was temporary and that the woman can regain a feeling of control over life.

Focus Your Study

- Nurses should provide girls and women with clear information about menstrual issues, such as the use of pads and tampons (including warnings regarding deodorant and absorbency); vaginal spray and douching practices; and self-care comfort measures during menstruation, such as maintaining good nutrition, exercising, and applying heat and massage.

- Dysmenorrhea usually begins at, or a day before, the onset of menses and disappears by the end. Hormone therapy (e.g., combined oral contraceptives), nonsteroidal anti-inflammatory drugs, or prostaglandin inhibitors can alleviate dysmenorrhea. Self-care measures include improving nutrition, exercising, applying heat, and getting extra rest.

- Premenstrual syndrome occurs most often in women over age 30. The most pronounced symptoms occur 2 to 3 days before onset of menstruation and subside as menstruation starts, with or without treatment. Medical management usually includes prostaglandin inhibitors and calcium supplementation. Self-care measures include improving nutrition (taking vitamin B complex and E supplements and avoiding methylxanthines, which are found, for example, in chocolate and caffeine; undertaking a program of aerobic exercise; and participating in self-care support groups. In some cases, pharmacologic agents such as SSRIs may be indicated.

- The FAB method of NFP is a "natural," noninvasive method of contraception often used by people whose religious beliefs prevent them from using artificial methods.

- Barrier contraceptives such as the contraceptive sponge, diaphragm, FemCap, and condom act by blocking the transport of sperm. These methods are often used in conjunction with a spermicide.

- N-9, the spermicide available in the United States, is far less effective in preventing pregnancy when it is not used with a barrier method.

- The Mirena and Skyla levonorgestrel-releasing IUCs (LNg-IUCs) are both hormonal and mechanical contraceptives. Their action is similar to that of the copper IUC, but they also secrete a progestin, levonorgestrel, that helps the endometrium to become atrophic, the cervical secretions to become thick, and the menstrual flow to be decreased.

- COCs are combinations of estrogen and a progestin. When taken correctly, they are one of the most effective and reversible methods of contraception. They also provide noncontraceptive benefits such as less acne and decreased scheduled bleeding.

- The progestin-only subdermal implant, Nexplanon, is an excellent choice for women desiring long-term contraception who cannot take estrogen.

- Other combined hormonal options (estrogen and progestin) such as the patch (Ortho Evra) and the vaginal ring (NuvaRing) have broadened the range of contraceptive options available.

- The long-acting progestin-only injections, Depo-Provera IM 150 mg and Depo-Provera SC 104 mg, are available for lactating women or those who cannot take estrogen.

- Permanent sterilization is accomplished by tubal ligation for women and vasectomy for men. Although theoretically reversible, clients are advised that the method should be considered irreversible. Essure offers a nonoperative approach to permanent blockage of the fallopian tubes.

- The termination of pregnancy through abortion may now be achieved by either medical or surgical means.

- A mammogram is a soft tissue x-ray examination of the breast taken without the injection of a contrast medium. Currently both ACS and ACOG recommend that all women over age 40 have an annual mammogram.

- Preconception counseling can be used to identify risk factors and unhealthy behaviors before a pregnancy occurs. Healthful lifestyle changes can be employed.

- Pap smear screening is recommended for all women 21 years of age and older. Several factors put a woman at high risk for an abnormal Pap smear: intercourse at a young age, multiple partners, history of immunotherapy, long-term COC use, smoking, and previous history of dysplasia. HPV is highly associated with abnormal Pap smears.

- Menopause is a physiologic, maturational change in a woman's life. Physiologic changes include the cessation of menses and a decrease in circulating hormones. Hormonal changes sometimes bring unsettling emotional responses. The more common physiologic symptoms are hot flashes, palpitations, dizziness, and increased perspiration at night. The woman's anatomy also undergoes changes, such as atrophy of the vagina, reduction in size and pigmentation of the labia, and myometrial atrophy. Osteoporosis becomes an increasing concern.

- Osteoporosis is becoming a significant health problem in the United States. Prevention is the preferred approach to addressing the issue. This includes adequate calcium intake and regular weight-bearing exercise. For women who have already developed osteoporosis, medications are available as a treatment option.

- MHT is recommended for the treatment of vasomotor symptoms in women under age 60 or within 10 years of menopause. The decision to begin MHT should be made jointly by the woman and her caregiver based on a careful analysis of the risks and benefits.

- Domestic violence is very common. One in three to one in four women will experience violence at the hands of an intimate partner during their lifetime.

- Batterers use psychologic, physical, and sexual abuse to maintain power and control in abusive relationships.

- Battering occurs in a cyclic pattern called the *cycle of violence*, which increases in frequency and severity over time.

- Women in abusive relationships who belong to cultural and linguistic minority communities and immigrant women face additional barriers when attempting to access services. The nurse must work to provide culturally aware and competent care.

- Estimates suggest that the majority of sexual assaults are not reported to the police. Rapes and sexual assaults committed by strangers are more likely to be reported to the police than rapes or sexual assaults committed by nonstrangers, including intimate partners, other relatives, and friends or acquaintances.

- Rape is an act of violence acted out sexually. Most sexual assaults are expressions of a need for power and control.

- Following sexual assault, the victim will usually experience an assortment of symptoms known as *rape trauma syndrome*. Recent research also links the effects of rape to posttraumatic stress disorder. Nursing actions to assist rape victims are encompassed in the roles of healthcare provider, advocate, and educator.

Clinical Reasoning in Action

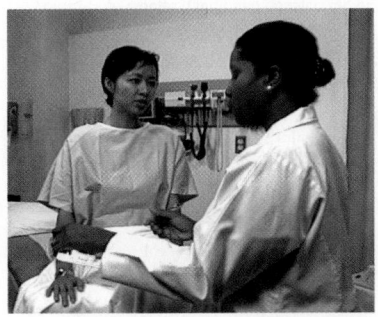

You are working at a local clinic when Joy Lang, age 20, presents for her first pelvic examination. You obtain the following GYN history: menarche age 12, menstrual cycle 28–30 days lasting 4–5 days, heavy 1 day, then lighter. She tells you that she needs to use superabsorbent tampons on the first day of her period, and then she switches to a regular absorbency tampon for the remaining days. She confirms that she changes the tampon every 6 to 8 hours, never leaving it in overnight. She denies premenstrual syndrome, dysmenorrhea, or medical problems and says that she is not taking any medication on a regular schedule. She tells you that she recently got married, but would like to wait before getting pregnant. She would like to discuss birth control methods. Joy tells you that doctors make her nervous and she admits to being anxious about her first pelvic examination.

1. What position is best to relax Joy's abdominal muscles for the pelvic examination?

2. What precaution should be taken when obtaining a Pap smear?

3. Explain the purpose of the Pap smear.

4. What factors do you include in a discussion of the type of birth control that Joy could practice?

References

Alzheimer's Association. (2013). *2013 Alzheimer's disease facts and figures.* Retrieved from http://www.alz.org/downloads/facts_figures_2013.pdf

American Cancer Society (ACS). (2013). American Cancer Society recommendations for early breast cancer detection in women without breast symptoms. Retrieved from http://www.cancer.org/cancer/breastcancer/moreinformation/breastcancerearlydetection/breast-cancer-early-detection-acs-recs

American College of Obstetricians and Gynecologists (ACOG). (2009, reaffirmed 2011a). *Medical management of abortion* (ACOG Practice Bulletin No. 67). Washington, DC: Author.

American College of Obstetricians and Gynecologists (ACOG). (2010, reaffirmed 2012a). *Noncontraceptive uses of hormonal contraceptives* (ACOG Practice Bulletin No. 110). Washington, DC: Author.

American College of Obstetricians and Gynecologists (ACOG). (2011b). *Menstruation* (ACOG Patient Education Pamphlet No. AP049). Washington, DC: Author.

American College of Obstetricians and Gynecologists (ACOG). (2012b). Intimate partner violence. (ACOG Committee Opinion No. 518). Washington, DC: Author.

American College of Obstetricians and Gynecologists (ACOG). (2012c). *Screening for breast problems.* Retrieved from http://www.acog.org/~/media/For%20Patients/FAQ178.pdf?dmc=1&ts=20120526T1508258847

Breiding, M. J., Smith, S. G., Basile, K. C., Walters, M. L., Chen, J., & Merrick, M. T. (2014). Prevalence and characteristics of sexual violence, stalking, and intimate partner violence victimization—National Intimate Partner and Sexual Violence Survey, United States, 2011. *Morbidity and Mortality Weekly Report (MMWR), 63*(SS08), 1–18.

Burgess, A. W., & Holmstrom, L. L. (1979). *Rape: Crisis and recovery.* Englewood Cliffs, NJ: Prentice-Hall.

Catalano, S. (2012). *Intimate partner violence, 1993–2010.* Retrieved from http://www.bjs.gov/content/pub/pdf/ipv9310.pdf

Centers for Disease Control and Prevention (CDC). (2012). *Folic acid: Recommendations.* Retrieved from http://www.cdc.gov/ncbddd/folicacid/recommendations.html

Chen, M-N., Lin, C-C., & Liu, C-F. (2014). Efficacy of phytoestrogens for menopausal symptoms: A meta-analysis and systematic review. *Climacteric, 17,* 1–10.

Crandell, L. (2012). Psychological outcomes of medical versus surgical elective first trimester abortion. *Nursing for Women's Health, 16*(4), 296–307.

Cunningham, F. G., Leveno, K. J., Bloom, S. L., Spong, C. Y., Dashe, J. S., Hoffman, B. L., . . .& Sheffield, J. S.(2014). *Williams obstetrics* (24th.). New York, NY: McGraw-Hill.

de Villiers, T. J., Gass, M. L. S., Haines, C. J., Hall, J. E., Lobo, R. A., Pierroz, D. D., & Rees, M. (2013). Global consensus statement on menopausal hormone therapy. *Climacteric, 16,* 203–204.

Freeman, E., Halberstadt, S., Rickels, K., Legler, J., Lin, H., & Sammel, M. (2011). Core symptoms that discriminate premenstrual syndrome. *Journal of Women's Health, 20*(1), 29–35.

Garza-Cavazos, A., & Loret de Mola, J. R. (2012). Abnormal uterine bleeding: New definitions and contemporary terminology. *The Female Patient, 37*(7), 27–36.

Holmes, M. M. (1998). The clinical management of rape in adolescents. *Contemporary OB/GYN, 43*(5), 62–78.

Kelderhouse, K., & Taylor, J. S. (2013). A review of treatment and management modalities for premenstrual dysphoric disorder. *Nursing for Women's Health, 17*(4), 294–305.

Kridli, S. (2011). Health beliefs and practices of Muslim women during Ramadan. *MCN, The American Journal of Maternal/Child Nursing, 36*(4), 216–221.

Lentz, G. M., Lobo, R. A., Gersenson, D. M., & Katz, V. L. (2012). *Comprehensive gynecology* (6th ed.). Philadelphia, PA: Elsevier.

Levy, D. P., Jager, M., Kapp, N., & Abitbol, J. (2014). Ulipristal acetate for emergency contraception: Postmarketing experience after use by more than 1 million women. *Contraception, 89*(5), 431–433.

Matsumoto, T., Asakura, H., & Hayashi, T. (2013). Biopsychosocial aspects of premenstrual syndrome and premenstrual dysphoric disorder. *Gynecological Endocrinology, 29*(1), 67–73.

Merck & Co., Inc. (2012). Nexplanon prescribing information. Retrieved from http://www.nexplanon-usa.com/en/consumer/main/prescribing-information.asp

Myrisk, K., Reinn, R., & Harkins, M. (2014). The prevalence of and attitudes toward oligomenorrhea and amenorrhea in Division I female athletes. *International Journal of Athletic Therapy & Training, 19*(6), 41–17.

National Center for Complementary and Alternative Medicine (NCCAM). (2012). *Get the facts: Menopausal symptoms and complementary health practices.* Retrieved from http://nccam.nih.gov/health/menopause/menopausesymptoms#hed2

National Osteoporosis Foundation (NOF). (2013). *Clinician's guide to prevention and treatment of osteoporosis.* Washington, DC: Author.

North American Menopause Society (NAMS). (2012). *FRAX®: A tool for estimating your fracture risk.* Retrieved from http://www.menopause.org/ for-women/menopauseflashes/frax-sup-sup-a- tool-for-estimating-your-fracture-risk

Oeffinger, K.C., Fontham, E.T.H., Etzioni, R., Herzig, A., Michaelson, J.S., Shih, Y.T.,...& Walter, L. (2015). Breast cancer screening for women at average risk: 2015 guideline update from the American cancer society. *Journal of the American Medical Society (JAMA), 314*(15), 1599–1614.

Office of the Assistant Secretary, Department of Education. (2011). Dear colleague letter. Retrieved from http://www2.ed.gov/about/offices/list/ocr/letters/colleague-201104.html

Planty, M., Langton, L., Krebs, C., Berzofsky, M., & Smiley-McDonald, H. (2013). *Female victims of sexual violence, 1994–2010.* Retrieved from http://www.bjs.gov/content/ pub/pdf/fvsv9410.pdf

Rost, M., Jacobsson, J., Dahlstrom, O., Hammar, M., & Timpka, T. (2014). Amenorrhea in elite athletics athletes: Prevalence and associations to athletics injury. *British Journal of Sports Medicine, 48*(7), 560–674.

Rutkowski, K., Sowa, P., Rutkowski-Talipska, J., Kuryliszyn-Moskal, A., & Rutkowski, R. (2014). Dehydroepiandrosterone (DHEA): Hypes and hopes. *Drugs, 74*(11), 1195–1207.

Santoro, N., & Sutton-Tyrrell, K. (2011). The SWAN song: Study of women's health across the nation. *Obstetric & Gynecologic Clinics of North America, 38*(3), 417–423.

Schuiling, K. D., & Likis, F. E., (2013) *Women's gynecologic health.* (2nd ed.). Burlington, MA: Jones and Bartlett Learning.

Truman, J., Langton, L., & Planty, M. (2013). *Criminal victimization, 2012.* Retrieved from http://www.bjs.gov/content/pub/pdf/cv12.pdf

U.S. Food and Drug Administration (FDA). (2012). Ortho Evra (norelgestromin/ethinyl estradiol information). Retrieved from http://www.fda.gov/Drugs/DrugSafety/PostmarketDrugSafetyInformationforPatientsandProviders/ucm110402.htm

U.S. Preventive Services Task Force. (2009). Final recommendation statement: Breast cancer: Screening. Retrieved from http://www.uspreventiveservicestaskforce.org Page/Document/RecommendationStatementFinal/breast-cancer-screening

U.S. Preventive Services Task Force. (2015). Breast cancer screening draft recommendations. Retrieved from http://screeningforbreastcancer.org

Walker, L. (1984). *The battered woman syndrome.* New York, NY: Springer.

World Health Organization. (WHO). (2013). Global and regional estimates of violence against women: Prevalence and health effects of intimate partner violence and non-partner sexual violence. Retrieved from http://apps.who.int/iris/bitstream/10665/85239/1/9789241564625_eng.pdf

Zieman, M., Hatcher, R. A., & Allen, A. Z. (2015). *Managing contraception 2015–2016.* Tiger, GA: Bridging the Gap Foundation.

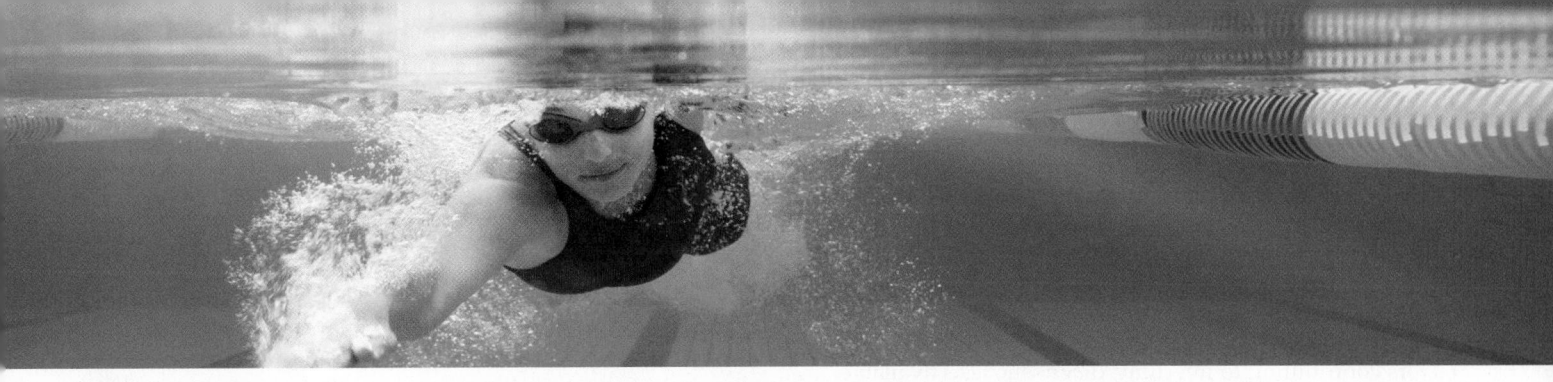

Chapter 6
Common Gynecologic Problems

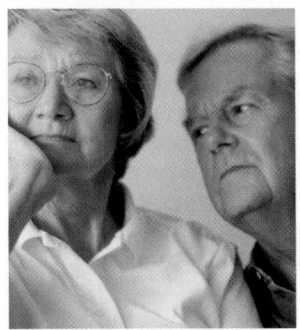

Don Klumpp/Getty Images

I was 58 when I learned that I had human papillomavirus infection. My first reaction was denial. I had been a virgin when I married and always thought I had the world's best marriage. When I confronted my husband of 30 years, I learned that he had been unfaithful to me with three different women over the course of our marriage. At first, I was ready to walk away. But my husband begged for a second chance, we saw a counselor for almost 6 months, and eventually rebuilt our life together. Many women would call me a fool but I know that, for me, it was important to save something I had committed to—for better or for worse—and to practice the forgiveness so many preach but fail to follow.

—Leonora

∨ Learning Outcomes

6.1 Contrast the contributing factors, signs and symptoms, treatment options, and nursing care management of women with common benign breast disorders.

6.2 Explain the signs and symptoms, medical therapy, and implications for fertility of endometriosis.

6.3 Discuss the signs and symptoms, treatment options, and health implications of polycystic ovarian syndrome (PCOS).

6.4 Summarize the risk factors, treatment options, and nursing interventions for women with toxic shock syndrome.

6.5 Compare the causes, signs and symptoms, treatment options, and nursing care for women with vulvovaginal candidiasis versus bacterial vaginosis.

6.6 Compare the common sexually transmitted infections with regard to their etiology, treatment options, nursing care, and methods of prevention.

6.7 Summarize the pathology, signs and symptoms, treatment, nursing care, and implications for future fertility of pelvic inflammatory disease (PID).

6.8 Identify the implications of an abnormal finding during a pelvic examination in the provision of nursing care.

6.9 Contrast the causes, signs and symptoms, treatment options, and nursing care for women with cystitis versus pyelonephritis.

6.10 Compare the signs and symptoms and treatment options of the three forms of pelvic relaxation—cystocele, rectocele, and uterine relaxation.

6.11 Contrast laparoscope-assisted vaginal hysterectomy and abdominal hysterectomy with regard to indications for use and the advantages and disadvantages of each procedure.

6.12 Compare the essential components of fertility with the possible causes of infertility.

6.13 Summarize the indications for the tests and associated treatments, including assisted reproductive technologies, that are performed in an infertility workup.

6.14 Relate the physiologic and psychologic effects of infertility on a couple to the nursing care management indicated for them.

The contemporary woman is likely to encounter various major or minor gynecologic or urinary problems during her lifetime. Some of these problems may be minor and easily treated, whereas others may be more serious. This chapter provides information about a variety of gynecologic conditions, with an emphasis on problems commonly addressed in community-based settings. It also addresses the issue of infertility and its impact on couples who dream of having a baby but have been unable to conceive or carry a pregnancy to term. It considers factors contributing to infertility, diagnostic tests available, and therapies to address the problem.

Care of the Woman With a Benign Disorder of the Breast

This section deals with the most common breast disorders women encounter. For information on breast cancer, consult a medical-surgical nursing textbook.

Fibrocystic Breast Changes

Fibrocystic breast changes, also known as *benign breast disease (BBD)*, is the most common of the benign breast disorders. It is most prevalent in women 20 to 50 years of age. *Fibrosis* is a thickening of the normal breast tissue. *Cyst* formation that may accompany fibrosis is considered a later change in the condition. The exact etiology of fibrocystic breast changes is unclear. Generally, fibrocystic changes are not a risk factor for breast cancer. In some rare cases, if the change is proliferative and results in hyperplasia or buildup of the cells of the breast ducts, atypia may occur.

The woman with fibrocystic breast changes often reports pain, tenderness, and swelling that occur cyclically and are most pronounced just before menses. Physical examination may reveal only mild signs of irregularity, or the breasts may feel dense, with areas of irregularity and nodularity. Women often refer to this irregularity as "lumpiness." Some women may also have expressible nipple discharge. Although unilateral discharge and serosanguineous discharge are the most worrisome findings, all breast discharge should be investigated further.

If the woman has a large, fluid-filled cyst, she may experience a localized painful area as the capsule containing the accumulated fluid distends coincident with her cycle. However, if small cysts form, the woman may experience not a solitary tender lump but a diffuse tenderness. A cyst may often be differentiated from a malignancy because a cyst is more mobile (easily moved with palpation) and tender and is not associated with skin retraction (pulling) in the surrounding tissue.

Mammography, sonography, magnetic resonance imaging (MRI), palpation, and fine-needle aspiration are used to confirm fibrocystic breast changes and rule out malignancy. Often, fine-needle aspiration is the treatment as well, affording relief from the tenderness or pain. Treatment of palpable cysts is conservative; invasive procedures such as biopsy are used only if the diagnosis is questionable.

Women with mild symptoms may benefit from restricting sodium intake and taking a mild diuretic during the week before the onset of menses. This counteracts fluid retention, relieves pressure in the breast, and helps decrease the pain. In other cases, a mild analgesic is necessary. In severe cases, the hormone inhibitor danazol is often helpful because it suppresses follicle-stimulating hormone (FSH) and luteinizing hormone (LH), resulting in anovulation. However, it can cause undesirable side effects including masculinization. Women who do not respond to other treatment approaches may be given a trial of bromocriptine, a prolactin inhibitor.

Some researchers suggest that methylxanthines (found in caffeine-containing products, such as coffee, tea, colas, and chocolate, and in some medications) may contribute to the development of fibrocystic breast changes and that limiting intake of these substances will help decrease fibrocystic changes.

Other Benign Breast Disorders

Fibroadenoma is a common benign tumor seen in women in their teens and early 20s. It has not been significantly associated with breast cancer. Fibroadenomas are freely movable, solid tumors that are well defined, sharply delineated, and rounded, with a rubbery texture.

Ultrasound is the best method for imaging women under age 35 with a palpable mass because of the density of their breast tissue. Most women can be observed and followed every 6 months with ultrasound for 2 years then once yearly thereafter. Some clinicians may prefer surgical excision to prove that it is benign (Lee, 2009).

The term for nipple discharge not associated with lactation (production of milk for breastfeeding) is **galactorrhea**. Nonclinically significant nipple discharge occurs in women who have fibrocystic changes in the breast, who are using contraceptives, or who are on hormone therapy. Certain medications that are used to treat psychiatric disorders have a side effect of galactorrhea.

The most common types of nipple discharge occur in both breasts, are secreted from several ducts, and vary in color from white to brown. The likelihood of malignancy increases with the presence of a spontaneous discharge arising from a single duct in one breast that is watery or bloody in nature; all unexplained nipple discharge warrants further investigation.

Intraductal papillomas, most often occurring during the menopausal years, are tumors growing in the terminal portion of a duct or, sometimes, throughout the duct system within a section of the breast. Symptoms may include a unilateral mass or a spontaneous, and often bloody, nipple discharge.

The majority of papillomas present as solitary nodules. These small, ball-like lesions may be detected on mammography but often are nonpalpable. A papilloma is often frightening to the woman because her primary symptom is a discharge from the nipple that may be serosanguineous or brownish green due to old blood. The location of the papilloma within the duct system and its pattern of growth determine whether nipple discharge will be present. Papillomas are typically benign but they are generally excised to rule out the possibility of cancer.

Duct ectasia (comedomastitis), an inflammation of the ducts behind the nipple, commonly occurs during or near the onset of menopause and is not associated with malignancy. The condition typically occurs in women who have borne and breastfed children. It is characterized by a thick, sticky nipple discharge and by burning pain, pruritus, and inflammation. Nipple retraction may also be noted, especially in postmenopausal women. Treatment is conservative, with drug therapy aimed at symptomatic relief. The major central ducts of the breast occasionally have to be excised.

Nursing Management
For the Woman With a Breast Disorder

Nursing Assessment and Diagnosis

During the period of diagnosis of any breast disorder, the woman may be anxious about a possible change in body image or a diagnosis of cancer. Use therapeutic communication to assess the significance the woman places on her breasts, her current emotional status, coping mechanisms used during periods of stress, knowledge and beliefs about cancer, and other variables that may influence her coping and adjustment.

Nursing diagnoses that may apply to a woman with a benign disorder of the breast include the following (NANDA-I © 2014):

- *Knowledge, Readiness for Enhanced,* about diagnostic procedures for breast disorders related to an expressed desire to understand procedures
- *Anxiety* related to threat to body image

Planning and Implementation

During the prediagnosis period, clarify misconceptions and encourage the woman to express her anxiety. Once a diagnosis is made, ensure that the woman understands her condition, its association to breast malignancy, and the treatment options. Also point out that frequent professional breast examinations and regular mammograms help detect any abnormalities. Although recommendations about the importance of monthly breast self-examination (BSE) have been modified (see Chapter 5; also see Teaching Breast Self-Examination in the *Clinical Skills Manual* SKILLS), most professionals agree that women should be familiar with their own breasts so that they are able to note changes should they occur.

Evaluation

Expected outcomes of nursing care include the following:

- The woman is able to discuss her fears, concerns, and questions during the period of diagnosis.
- The diagnosis is made quickly and accurately, and treatment is initiated if indicated.

Care of the Woman With Endometriosis

Endometriosis, a condition characterized by the presence of endometrial tissue outside the endometrial cavity, occurs in about 10% of reproductive-age women (Schindler, 2011). Endometriosis has been found almost everywhere in the body, including the vagina, lungs, cervix, central nervous system, and gastrointestinal tract. The most common location, however, is the pelvic cavity. This tissue responds to the hormonal changes of the menstrual cycle and bleeds in a cyclic fashion. The bleeding results in inflammation, scarring of the peritoneum, and formation of adhesions.

Endometriosis may occur at any age after puberty, but it is most common in women between ages 20 and 45. The exact cause of endometriosis is unknown. Proposed theories include retrograde menstrual flow, hereditary tendency, gene mutations, and a possible immunologic defect (American College of Obstetricians & Gynecologists [ACOG], 2014).

The most common symptom of endometriosis is pelvic pain, which is often dull or cramping. Usually the pain is related to menstruation itself and is often thought to be dysmenorrhea by the affected woman. However, the pain of dysmenorrhea usually begins right before menses starts and lasts for a day or 2, decreasing as prostaglandin levels decrease (ACOG, 2012). **Dyspareunia** (painful intercourse) and abnormal uterine bleeding are other common signs. The condition is often diagnosed when the woman seeks evaluation for infertility. Bimanual examination may reveal a fixed, tender, retroverted uterus and palpable nodules in the cul-de-sac. Diagnosis is confirmed by laparoscopy.

Treatment may be medical, surgical, or a combination of the two. In women with minimal disease and symptoms, treatment

---

EVIDENCE-BASED PRACTICE | Interventions for Pain Relief and Subfertility Among Women With Endometriosis

Clinical Question

What interventions are effective for relief of pain among women diagnosed with endometriosis? What treatment options for subfertility are available and effective for these women?

The Evidence

Women with diagnosed endometriosis often experience pain and difficulty becoming pregnant. A team of Cochrane reviewers summarized the evidence from 17 published systematic reviews of the effectiveness of interventions for both conditions. Systematic reviews, particularly those published in the scientifically rigorous Cochrane Reviews, form the highest quality of evidence, and this meta-synthesis of these reviews is the strongest available evidence.

Suppression of menstrual cycles with gonadotrophin-releasing hormone (GnRH), a levonorgestrel-releasing intrauterine device (LNG-IUD), and danazol were all beneficial interventions. Laparoscopic treatment and excision of endometriomata were also effective in relieving pain. Nonsteroidal anti-inflammatory medications did not provide conclusive relief, and there was no evidence of benefit from long-term hormonal treatment after surgery (Brown & Farquhar, 2014). None of the alternative medical treatments (acupuncture, herbal medicines, vitamins) was effective in pain relief.

Treatment with GnRH agonists for 3 months improved pregnancy rates, but no other medical treatments were found to be effective. Excisional surgery and laparoscopic removal of excess tissue resulted in improved spontaneous pregnancy rates 9 to 12 months after surgery. Ablative surgery was not effective in improving pregnancy rates and neither were diagnostic laparoscopic procedures. None of the alternative medical treatments had any effect on pregnancy rates in these women.

Best Practice

Medical and surgical treatments can be effective in reducing the pain associated with endometriosis and can enhance fertility within 9 to 12 months. Women can be counseled that fertility after surgical removal of endometriomata is possible. Medical treatment after surgery is not helpful and is unnecessary. Over-the-counter and alternative treatments are not effective; effective medical treatment is focused on the suppression of menstrual cycles through hormonal treatments.

Clinical Reasoning

Why does menstrual suppression affect the pain of endometriosis? Why would surgical removal of endometriomata improve fertility among these women?

Medications Used to Treat: Endometriosis

- *Combined oral contraceptives* (COCs), which suppress menstruation, can be used in women who do not desire fertility.

- *Progestins* such as medroxyprogesterone acetate (MPA) exert an antiendometriotic effect and ultimate atrophy. The medication is administered intramuscularly every 3 months; the effectiveness of the treatment is evaluated every 3 to 6 months. Side effects may include nausea, weight gain, fluid retention, and breakthrough bleeding.

- *Danazol* is a testosterone derivative that suppresses ovulation and causes amenorrhea. It is intended for short-term therapy. Because of adverse effects on lipid metabolism and significant side effects such as weight gain, hirsutism, acne, oily skin, vaginal dryness, hot flashes, reduced libido, voice changes, clitoral enlargement, and decreased breast size, many clinicians have moved away from danazol to other treatment options.

- *GnRH analogs* such as *nafarelin acetate* (given as a metered nasal spray twice daily) and *leuprolide acetate* (Lupron, given once a month as an intramuscular injection), are gaining popularity because many women tolerate them better than danazol and their results in treating endometriosis are comparable. GnRH analogs suppress the menstrual cycle through estrogen antagonism. This may result in the hypoestrogen side effects of hot flashes, vaginal dryness, headache, breast reduction, and loss of bone density. Consequently, the use of GnRH agonists should be limited to 6 months (Schindler, 2011).

includes observation, analgesics, and nonsteroidal anti-inflammatory drugs (NSAIDs). See *Medications Used to Treat: Endometriosis* for a list of medications used to treat endometriosis.

In more advanced cases, surgery may be done to remove endometrial implants and break up adhesions. If severe dyspareunia or dysmenorrhea is a symptom, the surgeon may perform a presacral neurectomy to relieve the pain. In advanced cases in which childbearing is not an issue, treatment may be a hysterectomy (removal of the uterus) with bilateral salpingo-oophorectomy (removal of the fallopian tubes and ovaries).

Nursing Management

For the Woman With Endometriosis

Nursing Assessment and Diagnosis

Be aware of the symptoms of endometriosis and elicit an accurate history. If a woman is being treated for endometriosis, assess the woman's understanding of the condition, its implications, and the treatment alternatives.

Nursing diagnoses that may apply to a woman with endometriosis include the following (NANDA-I © 2014):

- *Pain, Acute*, related to peritoneal irritation secondary to endometriosis

- *Coping: Family, Compromised*, related to depression secondary to infertility

Planning and Implementation

Be available to explain the condition, its symptoms, treatment alternatives, and prognosis. Help the woman evaluate treatment options and make appropriate choices. If the woman begins taking medication, review the dosage, schedule, possible side effects, and any warning signs. A woman with endometriosis is often advised not to delay pregnancy because of the increased risk of infertility. The woman may wish to discuss the implications of this decision on her life choices, relationship with her partner, and personal preferences. Be a nonjudgmental listener and help the woman consider her options.

Evaluation

Expected outcomes of nursing care include the following:

- The woman is able to discuss her condition, its implications for fertility, and her treatment options.

- After considering the alternatives, the woman chooses appropriate treatment options.

Care of the Woman With Polycystic Ovarian Syndrome

Polycystic ovarian syndrome (PCOS) is a complex endocrine disorder of ovarian dysfunction that is evidenced by menstrual dysfunction, signs of androgen excess (typically hirsutism, acne), and infertility.

The most common clinical signs and symptoms of PCOS include:

- *Menstrual dysfunction.* Irregular menses, ranging from total absence of periods (amenorrhea) to intermittent or infrequent periods (oligomenorrhea), are the hallmarks of PCOS. Anovulation is usually a chronic problem with PCOS and may present as a history of menstrual irregularities.

- *Hyperandrogenism.* Women with PCOS consistently have elevated serum androgen levels. These elevated androgen levels often lead to clinical manifestations such as hirsutism (excessive hair growth), acne, deepening voice, and increased muscle mass.

- *Obesity.* About half of women with PCOS are clinically obese (Smith & Taylor, 2011). The obesity is generally of the android type, with an increased hip-to-waist ratio.

- *Hyperinsulinemia.* Women with PCOS may be insulin resistant. This insulin resistance, characterized by the failure of insulin to enter the cells appropriately, places these women at increased risk for impaired glucose tolerance and type 2 diabetes mellitus (ACOG, 2014).

- *Infertility.* The majority of women who have been diagnosed with PCOS struggle with some degree of infertility related to anovulation.

Clinical Therapy

If a woman presents with complaints of hirsutism, menstrual irregularities, acne, difficulty conceiving, and unexplained weight gain, several other disorders must be ruled out. Important disorders to consider include thyroid disease, congenital adrenal hyperplasia, Cushing syndrome, hyperprolactinemia, primary ovarian failure, and androgen-producing tumors (ACOG, 2014). The diagnostic process is fourfold: history, physical examination, laboratory studies, and imaging.

Once PCOS is diagnosed, the goals for treatment include:

- Decreasing the effects of hyperandrogenism (e.g., hirsutism, acne)

- Restoring reproductive functioning for women desiring pregnancy

- Protecting the endometrium (increased risk for uterine cancer)

- Reducing long-term risks, specifically type 2 diabetes and cardiovascular disease.

If pregnancy is not an immediate goal, menstrual irregularities can be treated with a COC or cyclic progesterone. COCs help to regulate menstrual cycles; provide a balance between estrogen and progesterone, thereby protecting the endometrium and decreasing the risk of uterine cancer, and may improve acne by inhibiting ovarian androgen production.

Antiandrogens such as spironolactone (Aldactone) may be used to decrease symptoms of androgen excess. Metformin (Glucophage) improves tissue sensitivity to insulin, inhibits glucose production in the liver, and improves glucose uptake by fat and muscle cells. It improves ovarian function, reduces the degree of hyperandrogenism, restores normal ovulation in women with PCOS, and is associated with an improved ability to lose weight. In addition, lifestyle changes are important. Modifications should include weight loss, regular exercise, balanced diet, and smoking cessation.

If initial approaches to helping a woman with PCOS become pregnant fail, assisted reproductive technology (ART) may be recommended using in vitro fertilization, intrauterine insemination, or intracytoplasmic sperm injection. This may be combined with gonadotropin therapy (McFarland, 2012).

Long term, PCOS may increase a woman's risk for developing type 2 diabetes, hypertension, cardiovascular disease, endometrial cancer, breast cancer, and ovarian cancer. Additionally, the woman with PCOS may struggle with significant emotional responses to this chronic disorder. She will likely face issues related to body image, infertility, problematic menses, and depression.

Nursing Management

The nurse plays a vital role in the identification of PCOS and its evaluation, management, and follow-up. The signs of PCOS, especially hirsutism, negatively impact women's feelings of femininity, and they may feel physically inferior and lack self-confidence (Weiss & Bulmer, 2011). You can help women recognize these feelings and find ways to develop a more positive body image. You also have an important role in providing accurate information, education, and counseling for a woman diagnosed with PCOS. Finally, because the woman with PCOS is at risk for developing long-term complications, you and subsequent nurses can play a key role in follow-up and continuity of care throughout the life of a woman facing this challenging disorder.

Care of the Woman With Toxic Shock Syndrome

Toxic shock syndrome (TSS) is primarily a disease of women often occurring at or near menses or during the postpartum period. The causative organism is a toxin released by a strain of *Staphylococcus aureus*. Formerly, the use of superabsorbent tampons was related to an increased incidence of TSS; however, that relationship has declined. Occluding the cervical os with a contraceptive device such as a diaphragm or cervical cap during menses may also increase the risk of TSS.

Early diagnosis and treatment are important in preventing death. For a diagnosis of TSS to be made, certain criteria must be met, including:

- Fever (often greater than 102.0°F (38.9°C)

- Hypotension (systolic BP less than 90 mmHg)

- Rash

- Multisystem involvement

The fever and a rash on the trunk present initially followed by desquamation of the skin, especially the palms and soles, which usually occurs 1 to 2 weeks after the onset of symptoms; hypotension; and dizziness. Systemic symptoms often include vomiting, diarrhea, severe myalgia, and inflamed mucous membranes (oropharyngeal, conjunctival, or vaginal). Disorders of the central nervous system, including alterations in consciousness, disorientation, and coma, may also occur. Laboratory findings reveal elevated blood urea nitrogen (BUN), creatinine, aspartate aminotransferase (AST), alanine aminotransferase (ALT), and total bilirubin levels, whereas platelets are often less than $100,000/mm^3$.

Women with TSS are gravely ill. They are hospitalized and given antibiotics and supportive therapy, including oxygen, and intravenous fluids to maintain blood pressure. Severe cases may require renal dialysis, administration of vasopressors, and intubation.

Nursing Management

Nurses play a major role in helping educate women about preventing the development of TSS. It is crucial that women understand the importance of avoiding prolonged use of tampons. Women who choose to continue using tampons may reduce their risk of TSS by alternating them with pads and avoiding overnight use of tampons.

SAFETY ALERT!

Warn women about the danger of using a diaphragm or cervical cap to trap menstrual flow for prolonged periods because of the increased risk of TSS.

Women should avoid the use of tampons for 6 to 8 weeks after childbirth. Women who use diaphragms or cervical caps should not use them during the postpartum period. Also, help make women aware of the signs and symptoms of TSS so that they will seek treatment promptly if symptoms occur.

Care of the Woman With a Vaginal Infection

Vaginitis is one of the most common reasons why women seek gynecologic care. Symptoms of vaginitis or vulvovaginitis may include increased vaginal discharge, vulvar irritation, pruritus, foul odor, dyspareunia (painful sexual intercourse), bleeding with intercourse, and pain when urine touches irritated vulvar tissue. It may be caused directly by an infection or it may result from an alteration of normal flora, as in the case of bacterial vaginosis or vulvovaginitis caused by *Candida albicans*.

Bacterial Vaginosis

Bacterial vaginosis (BV) is more prevalent among sexually active women, but it is not considered a sexually transmitted infection because it has also been detected in virginal women. BV is an alteration of normal vaginal bacterial flora that results in the loss of hydrogen peroxide–producing lactobacilli, which are normally the main vaginal flora. With the loss of this natural defense, bacteria such as *Gardnerella vaginalis*, mycoplasmas, and anaerobes overgrow in large numbers, causing vaginitis. The cause of this overgrowth is not clear, although tissue trauma from douching, frequent sexual intercourse without condom use, and an upset in normal vaginal flora are predisposing factors. BV during pregnancy may be a factor in premature rupture of the membranes and preterm birth.

The infected woman often notices an excessive amount of thin, watery, white or gray vaginal discharge with a foul odor described as "fishy." The characteristic "clue" cell is seen on a wet-mount preparation (Figure 6–1). The addition of 10% potassium hydroxide (KOH) solution to the vaginal secretions, called a "whiff" test, releases a strong, fishy odor. The vaginal pH is usually greater than 4.5.

The symptomatic woman, whether nonpregnant or pregnant, is generally treated with metronidazole (Flagyl) orally or as a vaginal cream. Alternately, tinidazole orally or clindamycin (Cleocin) orally or as vaginal cream may be used (Centers for Disease Control and Prevention [CDC], 2015). Women should avoid intercourse or use condoms during the treatment period.

Metronidazole is an antimicrobial working in an anaerobic environment. It is an antiprotozoal and antibacterial agent. See *Medications Used to Treat: Bacterial Vaginosis* for a comparison of medication regimens for treating BV. Women should avoid intercourse or use condoms during the treatment period.

Vulvovaginal Candidiasis

Vulvovaginal candidiasis (VVC), also called moniliasis or yeast infection, is one of the most common forms of vaginitis that women experience. Recurrences are frequent for some women. *Candida albicans* is the fungal species responsible for most vaginal yeast infections. Factors that contribute to VVC are the use of COCs, immunosuppressants, and antibiotics, which destroy normal bacteria that usually keep the yeast cells in check. Other factors are frequent douching, pregnancy, and diabetes mellitus.

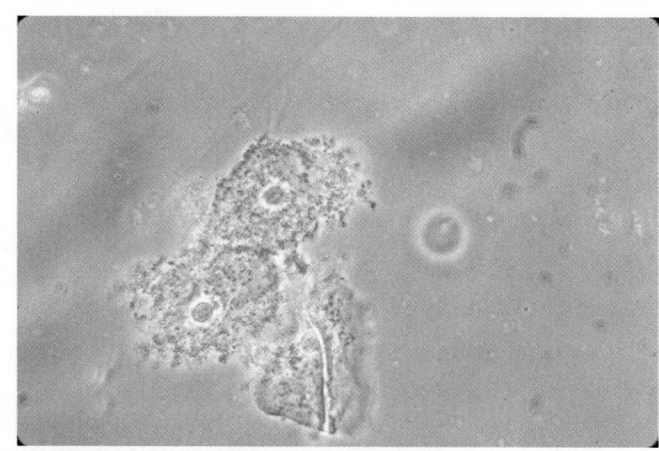

Figure 6–1 Clue cells characteristically seen in bacterial vaginosis. Unlike normal epithelial cells, which appear translucent and have a clear border, clue cells are desquamated epithelial cells with bacteria adhering to them. The presence of the bacteria makes the cell appear to be speckled with black dots. The borders are also obscured because of the bacteria.

SOURCE: Centers for Disease Control and Prevention (CDC).

The woman with VVC often complains of thick, curdy vaginal discharge, severe itching, dysuria, and dyspareunia. A male sexual partner may experience a rash or excoriation of the skin of the penis and possibly pruritus. The male may be symptomatic and the female asymptomatic.

On physical examination the woman's labia may be swollen and excoriated if pruritus has been severe. A speculum examination reveals thick, white, tenacious cheeselike patches adhering to the vaginal mucosa. Diagnosis is confirmed by microscopic examination of the vaginal discharge; hyphae and spores are usually seen on a wet-mount preparation (Figure 6–2). Other diagnostic tests include DNA probe and culture, although cultures are not used for routine diagnosis. The pH of the vagina remains 4.0 to 4.5 or less (the normal pH of the vagina is about 3.8 to 4.2). This vaginal pH level is in contrast to the pH noted with BV or *Trichomonas* infection.

Medical treatment of VVC includes intravaginal clotrimazole or miconazole cream or suppositories or tioconazole intravaginal ointment, which are available over the counter (OTC) (CDC, 2015). They are indicated for women with a history of yeast infections who are able to correctly recognize true VVC symptoms.

Prescription intravaginal agents include butoconazole, nystatin, and terconazole and orally, fluconazole. Single-dose and

---

Medications Used to Treat: Bacterial Vaginosis

NONPREGNANT AND SYMPTOMATIC PREGNANT WOMEN
- Metronidazole (Flagyl): 500 mg orally twice a day for 7 days

OR

- Metronidazole gel (0.75%): One full applicator intravaginally, once daily for 5 days.

OR

- 2% clindamycin (Cleocin) vaginal cream, one full applicator at bedtime for 7 days
- Alternative regimens: Tinidazole or clindamycin

Source: Data from Centers for Disease Control and Prevention (CDC). (2015). Sexually Transmitted Disease Treatment Guidelines, 2015. *Morbidity and Mortality Weekly Report, 64*(RR#), 1–137.

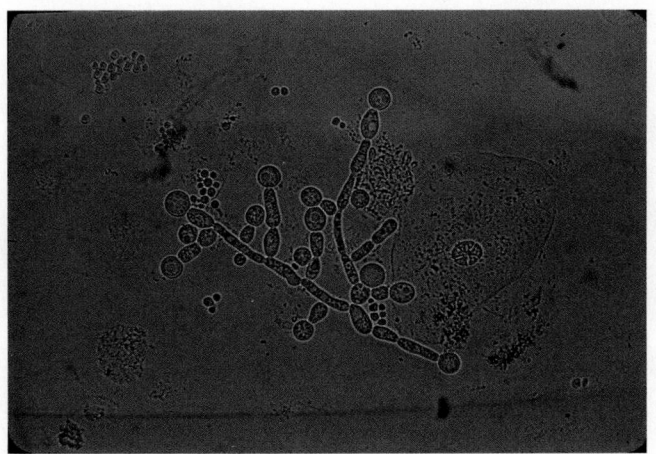

Figure 6–2 The hyphae and spores of *Candida albicans*. This is the fungus that is responsible for vulvovaginal candidiasis.

SOURCE: Centers for Disease Control and Prevention (CDC).

short-course approaches (3 days) are effective for 80% to 90% of women with uncomplicated VVC. One-day regimens include oral fluconazole or miconazole vaginal suppository. All of these treatments are effective for mild VVC (CDC, 2013d). There are also 3-day, 5-day, and 7-day treatment regimens. Women with complicated VVC may present with severe symptoms, recurrent VVC, or nonalbicans infection or be a compromised host (immunosuppression) and may require a longer course of treatment of up to 14 days with vaginal or oral azole agents (CDC, 2013d). If the vulva is also infected, the cream is applied topically. Women with recurrent infections may be advised to use oral fluconazole weekly for 6 months (CDC, 2015).

Treatment of the male partner is generally not necessary unless candidal balanitis (inflammation of the glans penis) is present. Then treatment with a topical antifungal medication is indicated (CDC, 2013d).

If a woman experiences recurrent VVC (four or more symptomatic episodes in 1 year), she should be tested for an elevated blood glucose level to determine whether a diabetic or prediabetic condition is present. Women at high risk for sexually transmitted infections should also be tested for HIV. Recurrent infection is then treated with an intensive regimen of oral and local agents for 7 to 14 days followed by maintenance antifungal therapy. Pregnant women with VVC are treated only with topical azole preparations applied for 7 days; fluconazole is contraindicated (CDC, 2013d). Infection at the time of birth may cause *thrush* (a mouth infection) in the newborn.

Nursing Management

For the Woman With VVC

Nursing Assessment and Diagnosis

Suspect VVC if a woman complains of intense vulvar itching and a curdy, white discharge. Because pregnant women with diabetes mellitus are especially susceptible to this infection, be alert for symptoms in these women. In some areas, nurses are trained to do speculum examinations and wet-mount preparations and can confirm the diagnosis themselves. In most cases, however, the nurse who suspects a vaginal infection reports it to the woman's healthcare provider.

Nursing diagnoses that might apply to the woman with VVC include the following (NANDA-I © 2014):

- *Skin Integrity, Impaired*, related to scratching secondary to discomfort of the infection
- *Knowledge, Readiness for Enhanced*, regarding information about yeast infection related to an expressed desire to learn about ways of preventing VVC

Planning and Implementation

If the woman is experiencing discomfort because of pruritus, recommend gentle bathing of the vulva with a weak sodium bicarbonate solution. If a topical treatment is being used, the woman will need to bathe the area before applying the medication. Table 6–1 provides information on ways to distinguish among the common types of vaginitis.

Also discuss with the woman the factors that contribute to the development of VVC and suggest ways to prevent recurrences, such as wearing cotton underwear and avoiding vaginal powders or sprays that may irritate the vulva. Stress the importance of completing the course of medication even during menses. Some women report that the addition of yogurt to the diet or the use of activated culture of plain yogurt as a vaginal douche helps prevent recurrence by maintaining high levels of lactobacilli. For the same reason, some clinicians recommend that women who are taking antibiotics consume yogurt or probiotics supplements (containing acidophilus and other helpful bacteria) simultaneously.

Evaluation

Expected outcomes of nursing care include the following:

- The woman's symptoms are relieved, and the infection is cured.
- The woman is able to identify self-care measures to prevent further episodes of VVC.

TABLE 6–1 Comparison of the Most Common Types of Vaginitis

TYPE OF VAGINITIS	CAUSE	APPEARANCE OF DISCHARGE	DIAGNOSTIC TEST	TREATMENT
Vulvovaginal candidiasis (moniliasis)	*Candida albicans*	Thick, curdy, like cottage cheese	Slide of vaginal discharge (treated with potassium hydroxide) shows characteristic hyphae and spores	Azole vaginal cream or suppositories
Bacterial vaginosis (*Gardnerella vaginalis* vaginitis)	*Gardnerella vaginalis*	Gray, milky	Slide of vaginal discharge shows characteristic "clue" cells	Metronidazole or clindamycin
Trichomoniasis	*Trichomonas vaginalis*	Greenish white and frothy	Saline slide of vaginal discharge shows motile flagellated organisms, OSOM Trichomoniasis Rapid Test, or Affirm VP III test	Metronidazole or tinidazole

Care of the Individual With a Sexually Transmitted Infection

The occurrence of **sexually transmitted infections (STIs)**, or *sexually transmitted diseases* (STDs), has increased during the past few decades. In fact, vaginitis and STIs are the most common reasons for outpatient, community-based treatment of women.

Children and adolescents can also become infected with sexually transmitted organisms through sexual experimentation, sexual play, molestation, and sexual abuse. Adolescents and young adults acquire half of all new STIs; one in four sexually active adolescent girls has an STI such as human papillomavirus (HPV) infection or chlamydial infection (CDC, 2014a).

Results from the CDC's *Youth Risk Behavior Surveillance—United States, 2013*, reveal that 46.8% of high school students had engaged in sexual intercourse and 40.9% of sexually active adolescents had not used a condom at last sexual intercourse (CDC, 2014c). Adolescents are considered an at-risk population because of their inexperience and lack of knowledge about STIs. They may disregard the importance of using barrier protection, may have multiple sexual partners, may have sex frequently, and often do not seek medical treatment until symptoms are well advanced.

Frequently diagnosed STIs include chlamydial infections, genital herpes (herpes simplex type 2), gonorrhea, genital warts (HPV), trichomoniasis, and syphilis. For more detailed information on the specific signs, symptoms, and treatment of males with STIs, consult a medical-surgical nursing textbook.

Trichomoniasis

Trichomoniasis is an infection caused by *Trichomonas vaginalis*, a microscopic motile protozoan that thrives in an alkaline environment. Almost all infections are acquired through sexual intimacy. Fomite transmission by shared bath facilities, wet towels, or wet swimsuits is possible, but rare. In young, sexually active women, trichomoniasis is the most common curable sexually transmitted infection, with a prevalence of approximately 3% in women (CDC, 2013d). Pregnant women with trichomoniasis may be at increased risk for premature rupture of the membranes, preterm birth, and a low-birth-weight newborn.

Approximately 70% to 85% of women with trichomoniasis are asymptomatic or have only mild symptoms (CDC, 2013d). Symptoms of trichomoniasis include a yellow-green, frothy, odorous discharge frequently accompanied by inflammation of the vagina and cervix, dysuria, and dyspareunia.

Diagnosis is made based on the following findings:

- Microscopic visualization of mobile trichomonads and increased leukocytes (Figure 6–3)
- Vaginal pH of 5.0 or higher
- Positive whiff test
- Two other tests with greater sensitivity than the wet-mount preparation are also available and are performed on vaginal secretions: the OSOM Trichomonas Rapid Test (results available in 10 minutes) and the Affirm VP III (results available in 45 minutes) (CDC, 2013d).

Recommended treatment for trichomoniasis is metronidazole (Flagyl) administered in a single 2-g dose, or tinidazole in a single 2-g oral dose, or, alternatively, metronidazole 500 mg twice daily for 7 days for both male and female sexual partners. Tinidazole has fewer gastrointestinal side effects but is more

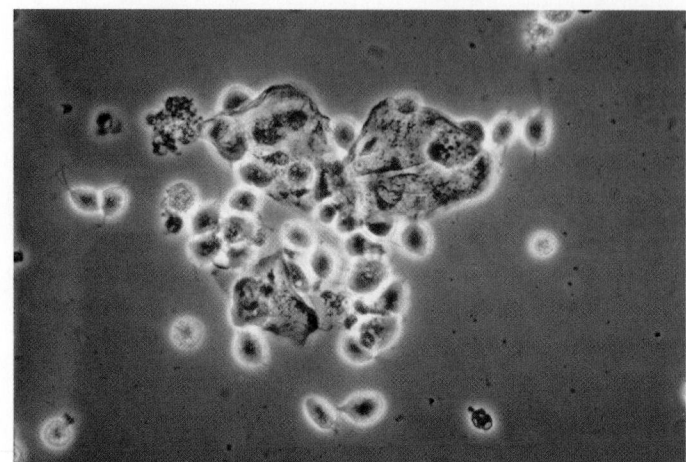

Figure 6–3 Microscopic appearance of *Trichomonas vaginalis.*

SOURCE: Centers for Disease Control and Prevention (CDC).

costly (CDC, 2015). Partners should avoid intercourse until both are cured (therapy is completed and both are symptom free).

SAFETY ALERT!

Alcohol should be avoided when taking either metronidazole or tinidazole. When combined with alcohol, both metronidazole and tinidazole can produce effects similar to those seen when alcohol is ingested while taking disulfiram (Antabuse)—abdominal pain, flushing, and tremors. The CDC (2015) recommends abstaining from alcohol for 24 hours after completing metronidazole and 72 hours after completing tinidazole.

Developing Cultural Competence Racial Disparity in STIs

Racial disparities exist in all STIs, with the highest rates being found among African Americans. In 2012, African Americans accounted for 63% of reported gonorrhea cases with known race/ethnicity and almost 40% (39.7%) of the cases of syphilis (CDC, 2014b). Although less marked, disparities also exist among Hispanics. These disparities may result, in part, because people from minority populations are more likely to seek care in public health clinics, which report STIs more accurately than private providers do. However, socioeconomic barriers to high-quality health care and to STI prevention and treatment play a role. It is essential that these barriers be addressed if such disparities are to be eliminated.

Chlamydial Infection

Chlamydial infection (or sometimes simply called *chlamydia*), caused by *Chlamydia trachomatis*, is the most commonly reported STI in the United States (CDC, 2013b). It is found most frequently in sexually active adolescents and young adults. In fact, in 2012, 70% of all reported cases of chlamydial infection occurred in people under age 25. Transmission commonly occurs through vaginal sex. A strain of *C. trachomatis* is responsible for trachoma, the world's leading cause of preventable blindness.

Healthy People 2020

(STD-2) Reduce chlamydia rates among females aged 15 to 44 years

In males, chlamydia is a major cause of nongonococcal urethritis (NGU). In females, it can cause infections similar to those that are associated with gonorrhea. Pelvic inflammatory disease, infertility, and ectopic pregnancy are associated with chlamydia. In addition, chlamydial infection is associated with an increased risk of acquiring and transmitting HIV infection. The newborn of a woman with untreated chlamydia is at risk of developing ophthalmia neonatorum, which responds to erythromycin ophthalmic ointment prophylaxis at birth. The newborn may also develop chlamydia pneumonia.

In females, signs of chlamydia include a thin or purulent discharge, burning and frequency of urination, a friable cervix (bleeds easily), and lower abdominal pain. Women, however, are often asymptomatic. Diagnosis is often made after treatment of a male partner for NGU or in a symptomatic woman with a negative gonorrhea culture. Of the laboratory tests available to diagnose chlamydia, nucleic acid amplification testing (NAAT) is the most sensitive. Other tests for diagnosis include polymerase chain reaction (PCR) assay and antigen detection (CDC, 2015). The recommended treatment is a single 1-g dose of azithromycin orally or doxycycline 100 mg orally twice daily for 7 days. Sexual partners should be treated, and couples should abstain from intercourse for 7 days. Doxycycline is contraindicated in pregnancy. The CDC (2015) recommends that pregnant women be treated with azithromycin or amoxicillin.

Because so many people with chlamydia are asymptomatic, annual screening of the following groups is recommended as a primary method of decreasing its incidence:

- Sexually active adolescent females and women ages 20 to 25, even if they are asymptomatic
- Women over age 25 who are at risk for chlamydia (history of STIs, multiple sexual partners, new sexual partner, inconsistent use of barrier contraceptives)
- High-risk pregnant women at their first prenatal visit or during the third trimester of pregnancy, or both (practitioners routinely screen all pregnant women)

Clinical Reasoning Sexually Transmitted Infections

Ella Matlosz is a 21-year-old, single woman, never pregnant, who comes to the office complaining of excessive, odorous vaginal discharge. She uses an intrauterine device (IUD) for contraception and has several sex partners. She states that she douches with a medicated douche after intercourse.

What should you tell Ella about feminine hygiene? What would you tell Ella about the relationship between contraceptives and sexually transmitted infections?

Gonorrhea

Gonorrhea is an infection caused by the bacterium *Neisseria gonorrhoeae*. If a nonpregnant female contracts the disease, she is at risk of developing pelvic inflammatory disease. If a woman becomes infected after the third month of pregnancy, the mucous plug in the cervix will prevent the infection from ascending, and it will remain localized in the urethra, cervix, and Bartholin glands until the membranes rupture. Then it can spread upward. A newborn exposed to a gonococci-infected birth canal is at risk of developing ophthalmia neonatorum. To prevent this infection, all newborns should receive eye prophylaxis at birth, generally with erythromycin ophthalmic ointment (CDC, 2013b).

Often girls and women with gonorrhea are asymptomatic. Thus it is routine to screen for this infection using a cervical culture during the initial prenatal examination. For women at high risk, the culture may be repeated during the last month of pregnancy. Cultures of the urethra, throat, and rectum may also be required for diagnosis, depending on the body orifices used for intercourse.

In females, the most common symptoms of gonorrheal infection include a purulent, greenish yellow vaginal discharge, dysuria, and urinary frequency. Some women also develop inflammation and swelling of the vulva. The cervix may appear swollen and eroded and may secrete a foul-smelling discharge in which gonococci are present. Diagnosis is confirmed by culture of swab specimens or NAAT. In males, urethritis, or inflammation of the urethra, is the cardinal symptom. This is marked by burning during urination and the presence of discharge from the urethra.

Healthy People 2020

(STD-6-1) Reduce gonorrhea rates among females aged 15 to 44 years

The preferred treatment of uncomplicated gonococcal infection is the same for nonpregnant and pregnant women, namely, a single dose of ceftriaxone 250 mg intramuscularly plus a single 1-g dose of azithromycin orally. This dual treatment is used to address the risk of coinfection with chlamydia because gonorrhea and chlamydia often occur together (CDC, 2015). All sexual partners must also be treated or the woman may become reinfected.

A test of cure is not needed if the recommended treatment is followed unless symptoms persist. However, retesting 3 months after treatment is recommended because of the risk of reinfection (CDC, 2015). Both sexual partners should be treated if either has a positive test for gonorrhea.

Herpes Genitalis

Herpes infections are caused by the herpes simplex virus (HSV). Two types of herpes infections can occur: HSV-1 (the cold sore), which can cause genital herpes through oral-genital contact, and HSV-2, which is usually associated with genital infections. The clinical symptoms and treatment of both types are the same. At least 50 million people in the United States have been diagnosed with genital HSV-2 infection—*herpes genitalis*. Even so, most people infected with genital herpes have not been diagnosed because they have mild or unrecognized infections but shed the virus intermittently (CDC, 2013a).

The primary episode of herpes genitalis is characterized by the development of single or multiple blister-like vesicles. In males, these usually occur on the penis or anal area. In females, the vesicles occur in the genital area and sometimes affect the vaginal walls, cervix, urethra, and anus. The vesicles may appear within a few hours to 20 days after exposure and rupture spontaneously to form painful, open, ulcerated lesions. Inflammation and pain secondary to the presence of herpes lesions can cause difficult urination and urinary retention. Inguinal lymph node enlargement may be present. Flulike symptoms and genital pruritus or tingling also may be noticed. Primary episodes usually last the longest and are the most severe. Lesions heal spontaneously in 2 to 4 weeks.

After the lesions heal, the virus enters a dormant phase, residing in the nerve ganglia of the affected area. Some individuals never have a recurrence, whereas others have regular recurrences. Recurrences are usually less severe than the initial episode and seem to be triggered by emotional stress, menstruation, ovulation, pregnancy, frequent or vigorous intercourse, poor health status or a generally run-down physical condition, tight clothing, or overheating. Diagnosis is most often made on the basis of the clinical appearance of the lesions, culture of the lesions, PCR identification, and HSV-specific glycoprotein G2 and glycoprotein G1 assays (CDC, 2013a).

No known cure for herpes exists. The recommended treatment of the first clinical episode of genital herpes is oral acyclovir, valacyclovir, or famciclovir. These same medications, in somewhat different dosages, are also recommended for recurrent herpes infection and for daily suppression therapy for people who have frequent recurrences. Because there is more documented information on the use of acyclovir during pregnancy, it may be administered orally to pregnant women with first-episode genital herpes or severe recurrent herpes. Its use from 36 weeks' gestation to birth may reduce the frequency of cesarean births by decreasing the incidence of recurrences at term (CDC, 2015).

Keeping the genital area clean and dry, wearing loose clothing, and wearing cotton underwear or none at all help promote healing. If herpes is present in the genital tract of a woman during childbirth, it can have a devastating effect on the newborn. Women with herpetic lesions when labor begins should give birth by cesarean to prevent neonatal herpes.

Syphilis

Syphilis, which is acquired through vaginal, oral, or anal sex, is a chronic STI caused by the spirochete *Treponema pallidum*. Syphilis is divided into early and late stages. During the early stage (primary), a chancre appears at the site where the *T. pallidum* organism entered the body. Symptoms include slight fever, loss of weight, and malaise. The chancre persists for about 4 weeks and then disappears. In 6 weeks to 6 months, secondary symptoms appear. Skin eruptions called *condylomata lata*, which resemble wartlike plaques and are highly infectious, may appear on the vulva. Other secondary symptoms are a rash on the palms of the hands and soles of the feet, acute arthritis, enlargement of the liver and spleen, nontender enlarged lymph nodes, iritis, and a chronic sore throat with hoarseness.

Syphilis may also be transmitted transplacentally. When infected in utero, the newborn exhibits secondary-stage symptoms of syphilis. Transplacentally transmitted syphilis may cause intrauterine growth restriction, preterm birth, and stillbirth. As a result of the disease's impact on the fetus in utero, serologic testing of every pregnant woman is recommended; some state laws require it. Testing is done at the initial prenatal screening and may be repeated in the third trimester. Blood studies in early pregnancy may be negative if the woman has only recently contracted the infection.

Diagnosis of syphilis is made by dark-field examination for spirochetes. Blood tests such as the Venereal Disease Research Laboratory (VDRL) test, the rapid plasma reagin (RPR) test, or the more specific fluorescent treponemal antibody absorption (FTA-ABS) test are commonly done.

For nonpregnant and pregnant women with syphilis of less than a year's duration (early latent syphilis), the CDC (2013c)

recommends 2.4 million units of benzathine penicillin G administered intramuscularly in a single dose. If syphilis is of long (more than a year) duration or of unknown duration, 2.4 million units of benzathine penicillin G is given intramuscularly once a week for 3 weeks. For nonpregnant women allergic to penicillin, doxycycline or tetracycline can be given. The pregnant woman who is allergic to penicillin should be desensitized to it in the hospital and then treated with it (CDC, 2013c).

Condylomata Acuminata (Venereal Warts)

The infection **condylomata acuminata**, also called *venereal warts*, is a common sexually transmitted condition caused by HPV. Transmission can occur through vaginal, oral, or anal sex. The infection has received considerable attention because HPV is almost always the cause of cervical cancer.

Over 100 HPV subtypes have been identified. Of these, at least 40 can infect the genital tract (CDC, 2015). HPV types 6 and 11 account for most visible genital warts, whereas high-risk HPV types such as 16 and 18 cause most of the cervical cancers (CDC, 2015).

Often an individual seeks medical care after noticing a single or multiple soft, grayish pink, cauliflower-like lesions on the penis or in the genital area (Figure 6–4). The moist, warm environment of the genital area is conducive to the growth of the warts, which may be present on the vulva, vagina, cervix, and anus. The incubation period following exposure is 3 weeks to 3 years.

Because condylomata sometimes resemble other lesions and malignant transformation is possible, all atypical, pigmented, and persistent warts should be biopsied and treatment should be instituted promptly. The CDC (2013a) does not

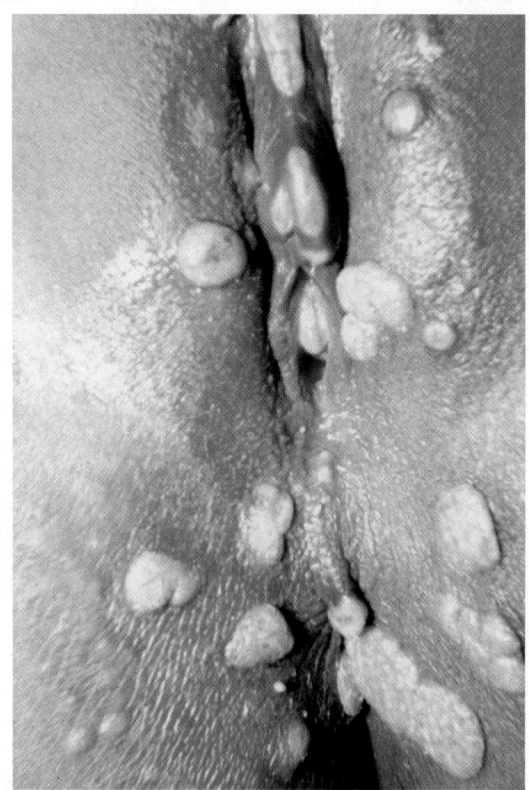

Figure 6–4 **Condylomata acuminata on the vulva.**

SOURCE: Centers for Disease Control and Prevention (CDC).

specify a treatment of choice for genital warts, but recommends that treatment be determined based on the client's preference, available resources, and experience of the healthcare provider. Client-applied therapies include podofilox solution or gel, imiquimod cream, or sinecatechin ointment.

SAFETY ALERT!

If a client-applied therapy is prescribed, the client must understand exactly how to apply the medication and must be able to identify and reach all the warts. These regimens have specific directions for application, frequency, and length of use, which the nurse should review carefully. Both imiquimod and sinecatechin ointment must be washed off after specified time periods.

Provider-administered therapies include cryotherapy with liquid nitrogen; trichloroacetic acid (TCA); bichloroacetic acid (BCA); surgical removal by tangential scissor excision, shave excision, curettage, or electrocautery; or laser surgery (CDC, 2015). Imiquimod, sinecatechins ointment, and podofilox are not used during pregnancy because they are thought to be teratogenic and in large doses have been associated with fetal death.

Two HPV vaccines are now available against HSV types 16 and 18, which cause 70% of cervical cancers. Gardasil, the first vaccine to receive Food and Drug Administration (FDA) approval, is a quadrivalent vaccine and also provides protection against types 6 and 11, which cause 90% of genital warts. The second vaccine, Cervarix, is bivalent, only offering protection against HSV types 16 and 18. Either vaccine is recommended for girls ages 11 to 12 (preferably before they are sexually active), but can be given beginning at age 9, and for 13- to 26-year-old females who did not receive or complete the three-dose vaccine series. The CDC (2015) now recommends that the three-dose HPV vaccine be routinely given to boys ages 11 to 12 to protect against HPV and also help provide indirect protection of women by reducing HPV transmission.

Women who have received the vaccine should receive regular Papanicolaou (Pap) smears as recommended. Sex partners of infected females are probably also infected but do not require treatment unless large lesions are present. The use of male or female condoms may reduce the risk of transmitting the virus to an uninfected partner.

AIDS

Acquired immunodeficiency syndrome (AIDS) is a serious, often fatal disorder caused by the *human immunodeficiency virus (HIV)*. Medical-surgical texts more fully describe care of people with HIV/AIDS. However, because HIV/AIDS has profound implications for the pregnant woman's fetus, AIDS is discussed in more detail in Chapter 14.

Nursing Management

For the Individual With a Sexually Transmitted Infection

Nursing Assessment and Diagnosis

Nurses need to become adept at taking a thorough history and identifying people at risk for STIs. Risk factors include multiple sexual partners, a partner's involvement with other partners, high-risk sexual behaviors such as intercourse without barrier contraception or anal intercourse, partners with high-risk behaviors, treatment with antibiotics while taking oral contraceptives, and young age at onset of sexual activity. Be alert for signs and symptoms of STIs and be familiar with diagnostic procedures if an STI is suspected.

When children or adolescents have a possible STI, the nurse usually encounters them and their families in the emergency department, outpatient clinic, or nursing unit. Because adolescents are often afraid of the consequences of reporting symptoms, it is important to develop good assessment skills, particularly when asking questions about sexual activity, partners, and the possibility of abuse. When a child or adolescent is diagnosed with one STI, it is important to screen for others because these diseases may coexist. Adolescents who are symptomatic may postpone care because of their discomfort with examinations and cultures. Routine screening of sexually active adolescents is recommended because many have subclinical infections or are asymptomatic.

Clinical Tip

- When a child younger than 10 years of age is found to have gonorrhea or another STI, consider the possibility of sexual abuse.
- Whenever anorectal symptoms are found in a child, suspect molestation.

Although each STI has certain distinctive characteristics, the following complaints warrant further investigation:

- Presence of a sore or lesion on the penis or vulva
- Increased vaginal discharge or malodorous vaginal discharge
- Urethral discharge (males)
- Burning with urination
- Dyspareunia
- Bleeding after intercourse
- Pelvic pain

In many instances, a woman is asymptomatic but may report symptoms in her partner, especially painful urination or urethral discharge. It is often helpful to ask the woman whether her partner is experiencing any symptoms.

Nursing diagnoses that may apply when an STI is diagnosed include the following (NANDA-I © 2014):

- *Family Processes, Interrupted*, related to the effects of a diagnosis of STI on the couple's relationship
- *Knowledge, Readiness for Enhanced*, about preventing STIs related to an expressed desire to prevent infection

---

Professionalism in Practice Attitudes About STIs

Many women deal matter-of-factly with an STI diagnosis; other women find it embarrassing and possibly even shameful. The nurse's attitude of straightforward acceptance conveys to the woman that she is still a respectable person who happens to have an infection and can help the woman deal effectively with her diagnosis and its implications.

Planning and Implementation

Some STIs such as trichomoniasis or chlamydia may cause a woman concern but, once diagnosed, are rather easily treated. Other STIs may be simple to treat medically but may carry a

TEACHING HIGHLIGHTS | Preventing STIs and Their Consequences

The risk of contracting an STI increases with the number of sexual partners. Because of the extended time between infection with HIV and evidence of infection, intercourse with an individual exposes a female or male to all the other sexual partners of that individual for the past 5 or more years. In light of this risk, it is important to take the following actions:

- Plan ahead and develop strategies to refuse sex (especially important for adolescents who may be less confident about saying "no" to casual sexual encounters). Abstinence is the best method of preventing STIs.
- Limit the number of sexual contacts and practice mutual monogamy with an uninfected partner.
- The condom is the best contraceptive method currently available (other than abstinence) for protection from STIs. Use one for every act of vaginal or anal intercourse. Other types of contraceptives such as the diaphragm, cervical cap, and spermicides also offer some protection against STIs.
- Plan strategies for negotiating condom use with a partner. Do not assume that a sexually experienced partner knows how to practice safe sex.
- Reduce high-risk behaviors. Use of recreational drugs and alcohol can increase sexual risk taking.
- Refrain from oral sex if your partner has active sores in the mouth, on the genitals, or around the anus.
- Refrain from sexual interaction when signs and symptoms of an STI are present.
- Seek care as soon as you notice symptoms and make sure your partner gets treatment if indicated. Absence of symptoms or disappearance of symptoms does not mean that treatment is unnecessary if you suspect an STI. Take the full course of all prescribed medications.
- The presence of a genital infection may lead to an abnormal Pap smear. Women with certain infections should have more frequent Pap smears according to a schedule recommended by their healthcare providers. Ask your healthcare provider if you need more frequent Pap tests.

stigma and be emotionally difficult to accept. Stress prevention with all clients and encourage them to require partners, especially new partners, to use condoms. While condoms offer protection from many STIs, they do not protect against infections like herpes and HPV, which are transmitted by direct skin-to-skin contact (Fantasia, Fontenot, Sutherland, et al., 2011). It is important to emphasize that, to be effective, condoms must remain in place during each and every act of intercourse. See *Teaching Highlights: Preventing STIs and Their Consequence.*

Refer the child with signs of an STI for evaluation of sexual assault by a facility or healthcare provider specializing in collecting evidence and providing specialized care. Similarly, refer any adolescent who has been sexually assaulted to a sexual assault nurse examiner or other healthcare provider who can collect evidence and coordinate medical treatment and mental health support.

As a nurse, you can be especially helpful in encouraging a client to explore feelings about the diagnosis. People may, for example, experience anger or feel betrayed by a partner, they may feel guilt or see their diagnosis as a form of punishment, or they may feel concern about the long-term implications for future childbearing or ongoing intimate relationships. Opportunities to discuss personal feelings in a nonjudgmental environment can be very helpful. Offer suggestions about support groups, if indicated, and assist the person in planning for future sexual activity.

Health Promotion **Information for the Woman With an STI**

In a supportive, nonjudgmental way, provide the woman who has an STI with information about the infection, methods of transmission, implications for pregnancy or future fertility, and the importance of thorough treatment. If treatment of her partner is indicated, help her understand that it is necessary to prevent a cycle of reinfection. She should also understand the need to abstain from sexual activity, if necessary, during treatment.

Evaluation

Expected outcomes of nursing care include the following:

- The infection is identified and cured, if possible; if not, supportive therapy is provided.
- The individual and partner can describe the infection, its method of transmission, its implications, and the therapy.
- The person copes successfully with the impact of the diagnosis on self-concept.

Care of the Woman With Pelvic Inflammatory Disease

Pelvic inflammatory disease (PID) is a clinical syndrome of inflammatory disorders of the upper female genital tract that includes any combination of endometritis, salpingitis (tubal infection), tubo-ovarian abscess, pelvic abscess, and pelvic peritonitis (CDC, 2015). The disease is more common in sexually active women younger than age 25. Other risk factors include multiple sexual partners, a history of PID, recent insertion of an intrauterine device, and regular douching. Perhaps the greatest problem of PID is postinfection tubal damage, which is closely associated with infertility.

The organisms most frequently identified with PID are *C. trachomatis* and *N. gonorrhoeae*, although not all cases of chlamydia or gonorrhea cause PID. Symptoms of PID include bilateral sharp, cramping pain in the lower quadrants, fever, chills, purulent vaginal discharge, irregular bleeding, malaise, nausea, and vomiting. However, it is also possible to be asymptomatic and have normal laboratory values.

Diagnosis is based on examination, cultures for gonorrhea and chlamydial infection, a complete blood count (CBC) with differential, and an RPR or VDRL test to check for syphilis. The woman may have an elevated C-reactive protein and an elevated sedimentation rate. Physical examination usually reveals direct abdominal tenderness with palpation, adnexal tenderness, and cervical and uterine tenderness with movement (chandelier sign). A palpable mass is evaluated with ultrasound. Laparoscopy may confirm the diagnosis and enable the examiner to obtain cultures from the fimbriated ends of the fallopian tubes.

Oral outpatient therapy is comparable to inpatient intravenous therapy in women with PID of mild to moderate severity (CDC, 2015). The decision to hospitalize is based on clinical judgment and severity of symptoms. Inpatient treatment includes intravenous fluids, pain medications, and intravenous antibiotics—often either cefoxitin or cefotetan plus doxycycline or clindamycin plus gentamicin. Outpatient oral therapy usually includes a single dose of ceftriaxone IM plus doxycycline orally for 14 days with or without metronidazole (CDC, 2015). Other antibiotic combinations may also be used. In addition, supportive therapy is often indicated for severe symptoms. The sexual partner should be treated. If the woman has an IUD, it is generally removed 24 to 48 hours after antibiotic therapy is started.

Nursing Management

For the Woman With Pelvic Inflammatory Disease

Nursing Assessment and Diagnosis

Be alert to factors in a woman's history that put her at risk for PID. Question the woman who has an IUD about possible symptoms, such as aching pain in the lower abdomen, foul-smelling discharge, malaise, and the like. The woman who is acutely ill will have obvious symptoms, but a low-grade infection is more difficult to detect.

Nursing diagnoses that may apply to a woman with PID include the following (NANDA-I © 2014):

- *Pain, Acute,* related to peritoneal irritation
- *Knowledge, Deficient,* related to a lack of information about the possible effects of PID on fertility

Planning and Implementation

The nurse plays a vital role in helping to prevent or detect PID. Accordingly, spend time discussing risk factors related to this infection. The woman who uses an IUD for contraception and has multiple sexual partners needs to understand clearly the risk she faces. Discuss signs and symptoms of PID and stress the importance of early detection.

Counsel the woman who develops PID on the importance of completing her antibiotic treatment and of returning for follow-up evaluation. She should also understand the possibility of decreased fertility following the infection.

Evaluation

Expected outcomes of nursing care include the following:

- The woman describes her condition, her therapy, and the possible long-term implications of PID on her fertility.
- The woman completes her course of therapy and the PID is cured.

Care of the Woman With an Abnormal Finding During Pelvic Examination

Abnormal Pap Smear Results

As discussed in Chapter 5, a Pap smear is a cervical cytology test done to screen for the presence of cellular anomalies. Although the Pap smear is useful in detecting a variety of abnormalities, it has had its greatest impact on the detection of cervical cancer. The *Bethesda system* (Table 6–2) has become the most widely used system in the United States for reporting Pap smear results. Early detection of abnormalities allows changes to be treated before cells reach the precancerous or cancerous stage. Notification of an abnormal Pap smear usually causes anxiety for a woman, so it is important that she be told in a caring way. The woman needs accurate, complete information about the meaning of the results and the next steps to be taken. She should also be given time to ask questions and express her concerns.

Colposcopy, the direct, detailed visualization and examination of the cervix, has become a common second step in many cases of abnormal Pap smears. The examination, done in an office or clinic, permits more detailed visualization of the cervix in bright light using a high-magnification microscope. The cervix can be visualized directly and again following application of acetic acid. The acetic acid causes abnormal epithelium to assume a characteristic white appearance. The colposcope can also be used to obtain a directed biopsy.

Ovarian Masses

Ovarian masses may be palpated during the pelvic examination. Between 70% and 80% of ovarian masses are benign. More than 50% are functional cysts (cysts that develop from ovarian follicles, from the corpus luteum, or from the theca luteum), occurring most commonly in women 20 to 40 years of age. Functional cysts are rare in women who take oral contraceptives. Ovarian cysts usually represent physiologic variations in the menstrual cycle. Dermoid cysts (cystic teratomas) and endometriomas, or "chocolate cysts," are common types of ovarian masses. No relationship exists between ovarian masses and ovarian cancer. However, ovarian cancer is the most fatal of all cancers in women because it is difficult to diagnose and often has spread throughout the pelvis before it is detected. Refer to medical-surgical nursing texts for an in-depth discussion of ovarian cancer.

Many women with a benign ovarian mass are asymptomatic; the mass may be noted on a routine pelvic examination. Others experience a sensation of fullness or cramping in the lower abdomen (often unilateral), dyspareunia, irregular bleeding, or delayed menstruation. Diagnosis is made on the basis of a palpable mass with or without tenderness and other related symptoms. Radiography or ultrasonography may be used to assist in the diagnosis.

The woman is often kept under observation for a month or two because most cysts resolve on their own and are harmless. Oral contraceptives may be prescribed for 1 to 2 months to suppress ovarian function. If this regimen is effective, a repeat pelvic examination should be normal. If the mass is still present after 60 days of observation and oral contraceptive therapy, a diagnostic laparoscopy or laparotomy may be considered. Tubal or ovarian lesions, ectopic pregnancy, cancer, infection, or appendicitis also must be ruled out before a diagnosis can be confirmed.

Surgery is not always necessary but is considered if the mass is larger than 6 to 7 cm in circumference; if the woman is over 40 years of age with an adnexal mass, a persistent mass, or continuous pain; or if the woman is taking oral contraceptives. Surgical exploration is also indicated when a palpable mass is found in an infant, a young girl, or a postmenopausal woman.

Women may need clear explanations about why the initial therapy is observation. A discussion of the origin and resolution of ovarian cysts may clarify this treatment plan. If a surgical treatment removes or impairs the function of one ovary,

TABLE 6–2 The Bethesda System for Classifying Pap Smears

SPECIMEN TYPE	OTHER
Indicate conventional smear (Pap smear) vs. liquid based vs. other	Endometrial cells (in a woman ≥ 40 years of age) (Specify if negative for squamous intraepithelial lesion) *Epithelial cell abnormalities*
Specimen Adequacy	SQUAMOUS CELL
Satisfactory for evaluation *(describe presence or absence of endocervical/transformation zone component and any other quality indicators [e.g., partially obscuring blood inflammation]).*	Atypical squamous cells
	—of undetermined significance (ASC-US)
Unsatisfactory for evaluation *(specify reason)*	—cannot exclude HSIL (ASC-H)
Specimen rejected/not processed *(specify reason)*	Low-grade squamous intraepithelial lesion (LSIL)
Specimen processed and examined, but unsatisfactory for evaluation of epithelial abnormality because of *(specify reason)*	—encompassing HPV/mild dysplasia/CIN-1
	High-grade squamous intraepithelial lesion (HSIL)
General Categorization (optional)	—encompassing moderate and severe dysplasia CIS/CIN-2 and CIN-3
Negative for intraepithelial lesion or malignancy.	—with features suspicious for invasion *(if invasion is suspected)*
Epithelial cell abnormality. See Interpretation/Result *(specify squamous or glandular as appropriate).*	Squamous cell carcinoma
Other: See Interpretation/Result *(e.g., endometrial cells in a woman ≥ 40 years of age).*	GLANDULAR CELL
	Atypical
Automated Review	—endocervical cells *(NOS or specify in comments)*
If case examined by automated device, specify device and result.	—endometrial cells *(NOS or specify in comments)*
	—glandular cells *(NOS or specify in comments)*
Ancillary Testing	Atypical
Provide a brief description of the test methods and report the result so that it is easily understood by the clinician.	—endocervical cells, favor neoplastic
	—glandular cells, favor neoplastic
Interpretation/Result	Endocervical adenocarcinoma in situ
Negative for intraepithelial lesion or malignancy (when there is no cellular evidence of neoplasia, state this in the General Categorization above and/or in the Interpretation/Result section of the report, whether or not there are organisms or other nonneoplastic findings)	Adenocarcinoma
	—endocervical
ORGANISMS:	—endometrial
Trichomonas vaginalis	—extrauterine
Fungal organisms morphologically consistent with *Candida* spp.	—not otherwise specified (NOS)
Shift in flora suggestive of bacterial vaginosis	*Other malignant neoplasms (specify)*
Bacteria morphologically consistent with *Actinomyces* spp.	
Cellular changes associated with herpes simplex virus	**Educational Notes and Suggestions (optional)**
OTHER NONNEOPLASTIC FINDINGS	Suggestions should be concise and consistent with clinical follow-up guidelines published by professional organizations (references to relevant publications may be included).
(Optional to report list not inclusive)	
Reactive cellular changes associated with	
—inflammation (includes typical repair)	
—radiation	
—intrauterine contraceptive device (IUD)	
Glandular cells status post-hysterectomy	
Atrophy	

Source: National Cancer Institute.

the woman needs to be assured that the remaining ovary can be expected to take over ovarian functioning and that pregnancy is still possible if desired.

Uterine Abnormalities

Endometrial polyps are pedunculated (growing on a stalk) overgrowths of the endometrium. They can occur as single or multiple growths. Polyps are common and are often accompanied by symptoms of midcycle bleeding or spotting, bleeding or spotting after intercourse, or prolonged bleeding or spotting with menstrual cycles. Polyps are generally benign, but they can occasionally coexist with carcinoma of the endometrium. Treatment is dilation and curettage (D&C) using a hysteroscope for visualization.

Fibroid tumors, or *leiomyomas*, are among the most common benign disease entities in women. By the age of 50, 70% of White women and 80% of Black women have fibroids (Rice, Secrist, Woodrow, et al., 2012).

Most uterine fibroid tumors are asymptomatic and require no treatment. The most common symptoms include pelvic pain, menstrual irregularities, and infertility. Women most often seek treatment for bleeding and pain. On pelvic examination the woman may have an irregularly shaped, enlarged uterus. Diagnosis is most often made using pelvic ultrasound and magnetic resonance imaging (MRI). Occasionally, hysterosonography is used for further evaluation (Rice et al., 2012).

Treatment for uterine fibroids varies and may include the following:

- Combined oral contraceptives to control heavy menstrual bleeding
- GnRH analogs such as Lupron to reduce the size and subsequent bleeding. GnRH analogs also may be used before surgery to reduce the size of the fibroid and decrease complications (Rice et al., 2012)
- Levonorgestrel intrauterine system (LNG-IUS) for contraception and control of excessive menstrual bleeding by suppression of endometrial growth
- MRI-guided ultrasound, which focuses high-intensity sound waves on the fibroids, resulting in clotting, necrosis, and shrinkage of the tumor
- *Myomectomy,* a surgical procedure to remove the fibroid without removing the uterus, which can preserve or improve fertility
- Uterine artery embolization (UAE), an interventional radiologic procedure in which the uterine arteries are blocked, resulting in diminished blood flow to the uterus and the necrosis of the fibroids

Hysterectomy may be indicated and can be performed laparoscopically or abdominally depending on the size of the uterus.

Endometrial cancer, most commonly a disease of postmenopausal women, has a high rate of cure if detected early. The hallmark sign is vaginal bleeding in postmenopausal women not treated with hormone replacement therapy. Endometrial biopsy, transvaginal ultrasound, and posthysterectomy pathologic examination of the uterus are used in the diagnosis. The treatment is total abdominal hysterectomy (TAH) and bilateral salpingo-oophorectomy (BSO). Radiation therapy may also be indicated depending on the stage of the cancer.

Nursing Management

Pelvic examinations and Pap smears are not done by nurses except those with special training. In most cases, nursing assessment is directed toward an evaluation of the woman's understanding of the findings and their implications and her psychosocial response.

The woman needs accurate information on etiology, symptomatology, and treatment options. Encourage her to report symptoms and keep appointments for follow-up examination and evaluation. The woman needs realistic reassurance if her condition is benign; she may require counseling and effective emotional support if a malignancy is likely. If the management plan includes surgery, she may need the nurse's support in obtaining a second opinion and making her decision about treatment.

Care of the Woman With a Urinary Tract Infection

A **urinary tract infection (UTI)**, defined as significant bacteriuria in the presence of symptoms, is one of the most common problems women experience. Estimates indicate that more than 60% of women will experience a UTI in their lifetime (Minkin, 2011). Bacteria usually enter the body by way of the urethra. The organisms are capable of migrating against the downward flow of urine. The shortness of the female urethra facilitates the passage of bacteria into the bladder. Other conditions associated with

bacterial entry are relative incompetence of the urinary sphincter, frequent enuresis (bed-wetting) before adolescence, and urinary catheterization. Wiping from back to front after urination may transfer bacteria from the anorectal area to the urethra. Voluntarily suppressing the desire to urinate is a predisposing factor. Retention overdistends the bladder and can lead to an infection. Sexual activity is a strong risk factor for UTI, especially in younger women. General poor health or lowered resistance to infection can increase a woman's susceptibility to UTI.

Asymptomatic bacteriuria (ASB) (bacteria in the urine actively multiplying without accompanying clinical symptoms) is a condition that becomes especially significant if the woman is pregnant because, if untreated, ASB can lead to pyelonephritis in the pregnant woman and low birth weight in the newborn (Cunningham et al., 2014). ASB is almost always caused by a single organism, typically *Escherichia coli*. A woman who has had a UTI is susceptible to recurrent infection. If a pregnant woman develops an acute UTI, especially with a high temperature, amniotic fluid infection may develop and retard the growth of the placenta.

Lower Urinary Tract Infection

Because UTIs are ascending, it is important to recognize and diagnose a lower UTI early to avoid the sequelae associated with an upper UTI. *Cystitis*, or inflammation of the bladder, usually occurs secondary to an ascending infection. *E. coli* is present in the majority of cases. Other common causative organisms include *Klebsiella pneumonia*, *Proteus mirabilis*, *Enterococcus* species, and *Staphylococcus saprophyticus*.

When cystitis develops, the initial symptom is often dysuria, specifically at the end of urination. Urgency and frequency also occur. Cystitis is usually accompanied by a low-grade fever (101°F [38.3°C] or lower), and hematuria is occasionally seen. Urine specimens usually contain an abnormal number of leukocytes and bacteria. Diagnosis is made with a urine culture.

Treatment depends on the causative organism. Nitrofurantoin has reemerged as an effective first-line therapy and is given twice daily for 5 days. A 3-day, twice daily course of oral trimethoprim-sulfamethoxazole (TMP-SMZ) is recommended as a viable alternative if local resistance to it is low. Fluoroquinolones (FQ) such as ciprofloxacin, levofloxacin, gatifloxacin, or norfloxacin should be reserved for treatment failures and for women with suspected upper UTI infection (Schultz & Edson, 2011).

Upper Urinary Tract Infection (Pyelonephritis)

Pyelonephritis (inflammatory disease of the kidneys) is less common but more serious than cystitis and is often preceded by lower UTI. It is more common during the latter part of pregnancy or early postpartum and poses a serious threat to maternal and fetal well-being. Women with symptoms of pyelonephritis during pregnancy have an increased risk of preterm birth and of intrauterine growth restriction.

Acute pyelonephritis has a sudden onset, with chills, high temperature of 103° to 105°F (39.6° to 40.6°C), and flank pain (either unilateral or bilateral). The right side is almost always involved if the woman is pregnant because the large bulk of intestines to the left pushes the uterus to the right, putting pressure on the right ureter and kidney. Nausea, vomiting, and general malaise may ensue. With accompanying cystitis, the woman may experience frequency, urgency, and burning with urination.

Edema of the renal parenchyma or ureteritis with blockage and swelling of the ureter may lead to temporary suppression of urinary output. This is accompanied by severe colicky (spastic, intense) pain, vomiting, dehydration, and ileus of the large bowel. Women with acute pyelonephritis generally have increased diastolic blood pressure, positive fluorescent antibody titer (FA test), low creatinine clearance, significant bacteremia in urine culture, pyuria, and presence of white blood cell casts.

Many women can be treated as outpatients or given IV fluids and one IV dose of antibiotics, then discharged on oral medications. Fluoroquinolones (FQ) are the first-line treatment in communities where FQ resistance is low, specifically ciprofloxacin, extended-release ciprofloxacin, or levofloxacin. If local FQ resistance is high, an initial dose of ceftriaxone or gentamicin is given followed by an oral FQ regimen (Colgan, Williams, & Johnson, 2011).

A woman who is severely ill or has complications may require hospitalization. She is started on IV antibiotics. Therapy also includes IV hydration, urinary analgesics such as phenazopyridine (Pyridium), pain management, and medications to manage fever. In the case of obstructive pyelonephritis, a blood culture is necessary. The woman is kept on bed rest. After the sensitivity report is received, the antibiotic is changed as necessary. If signs of urinary obstruction occur or continue, the ureter may be catheterized to establish adequate drainage.

With appropriate drug therapy, the woman's temperature should return to normal. The pain subsides and the urine shows no bacteria within 2 to 3 days. Follow-up urinary cultures are needed to determine that the infection has been eliminated completely.

Nursing Management

For the Woman With a Urinary Tract Infection

Nursing Assessment and Diagnosis

During a woman's visit, obtain a sexual and medical history to identify whether she is at risk for UTI. A clean-catch urine specimen is evaluated for evidence of asymptomatic bacteriuria (ASB).

Nursing diagnoses that may apply to a woman with an upper UTI include the following (NANDA-I © 2014):

- *Pain, Acute,* related to dysuria, systemic discomforts, or renal pain secondary to UTI
- *Fear* related to the possible long-term effects of the disease

Planning and Implementation

Give the woman information to help her recognize the signs of UTI. Also discuss hygiene practices, the advantages of wearing cotton underwear, and the need to void frequently to prevent urinary stasis. Stress the importance of maintaining a good fluid intake. UTIs usually respond quickly to treatment, but follow-up clinical evaluation and urine cultures are important. See *Teaching Highlights: Preventing Cystitis.*

Evaluation

Expected outcomes of nursing care include the following:

- The woman completes her prescribed course of antibiotic therapy.
- The woman's infection is cured.
- The woman incorporates preventive self-care measures into her daily regimen.

Pelvic Relaxation

A **cystocele** is the downward displacement of the bladder, which appears as a bulge in the anterior vaginal wall. Genetic predisposition, childbearing, obesity, and increased age are factors that may contribute to cystocele. Symptoms of stress urinary incontinence (SUI) are most common, including loss of urine with coughing, sneezing, laughing, or sudden exertion. Vaginal fullness, a bulging out of the vaginal wall, or a dragging sensation may also be noticeable.

If pelvic relaxation is mild, Kegel exercises help restore tone. The exercises involve contraction and relaxation of the pubococcygeal muscle (see the *Perineal Exercises* section in Chapter 10 for more information). Women have found these exercises helpful before and after childbirth in maintaining vaginal muscle tone. Estrogen may improve the condition of vaginal mucous membranes, especially in menopausal women.

Duloxetine, a balanced serotonin and norepinephrine reuptake inhibitor used to treat major depressive disorders and the pain of fibromyalgia or diabetic neuropathy, is the only medication shown to help decrease SUI. Although approved for the treatment of SUI in the European Union, it is not approved for that purpose in the United States. Its administration would be an off-label use (Wilson, Shannon, & Shields, 2014). Vaginal pessaries or rings may be used if surgery is undesirable or impossible or until surgery can be

---

TEACHING HIGHLIGHTS | Preventing Cystitis

Following is information for women about ways to avoid cystitis:

- If you use a diaphragm for contraception, try changing methods or using another size of diaphragm.
- Avoid bladder irritants such as alcohol, caffeine products, and carbonated beverages.
- Increase fluid intake, especially water, to a minimum of six to eight glasses per day.
- Make regular urination a habit; avoid long waits.
- Practice good genital hygiene, including wiping from front to back after urination and bowel movements.
- Be aware that vigorous or frequent sexual activity may contribute to the development of urinary tract infections.
- Urinate before and after intercourse to empty the bladder and cleanse the urethra.
- Complete medication regimens even if symptoms decrease.
- Do not use medication left over from previous infections.
- Drink cranberry juice to acidify the urine. This has been found to alleviate symptoms in some cases (Bass-Ware, Weed, Johnson, et al., 2014).

scheduled. Surgery may be considered for cystoceles considered moderate to severe.

The nurse can instruct the woman in the use of Kegel exercises. Information on causes and contributing factors and discussion of possible alternative therapies greatly help the woman.

A **rectocele** may develop when the posterior vaginal wall is weakened. The anterior wall of the rectum can then sag forward, ballooning into the vagina, pushing the weakened posterior wall of the vagina in front of it. When the woman strains to have a bowel movement, a pocket of rectum develops that traps stool, and constipation results. To defecate, a woman with a rectocele may find it necessary to press the tissue between the vagina and rectum, which elevates the rectocele.

Diagnosis is based on history and physical examination. Decisions about treatment are based on the size of the rectocele, the presence and severity of symptoms, and the woman's individual situation, including her overall health. Surgery is often indicated.

Uterine prolapse occurs when the uterus protrudes downward (drops) into the upper vagina, pulling the vagina with it. The extent of the prolapse is determined by the location of the cervix in the vagina. In severe cases, the uterus may prolapse below the vaginal introitus. The woman may report a "dragging" sensation in her groin and a backache over the sacrum, which is caused by pulling on the uterosacral ligaments. Typically, these symptoms are relieved when the woman lies down. As with cystocele, conservative treatment includes the use of topical or systemic estrogen and vaginal pessaries. Surgery for uterine prolapse often involves hysterectomy and repair of the prolapsed vaginal walls.

Care of the Woman Requiring a Hysterectomy

Hysterectomy is the surgical removal of the uterus. In the United States, it is the most common nonpregnancy-related surgical procedure that women undergo. Removal of the uterus through a surgical incision is called a *total abdominal hysterectomy* (TAH), and removal of both fallopian tubes and ovaries is called a *bilateral salpingo-oophorectomy* (BSO). When both procedures are performed at the same time, it is called a *TAH-BSO*. When the uterus is removed through the vagina, it is termed a *total vaginal hysterectomy* (TVH).

A *laparoscopic-assisted vaginal hysterectomy* (LAVH) may also be used. In this technique, the surgeon inserts the laparoscope through an incision near the umbilicus and uses it to assist with visualization and dissection to facilitate vaginal removal of the uterus. The benefit is that the surgeon can achieve results similar to those of a TAH without a large abdominal incision.

Abdominal hysterectomy is the usual treatment for several conditions, including cancer of the cervix, endometrium, or ovary; large fibroids; severe endometriosis; chronic PID; and adenomyosis. TAH is preferred when cancer is expected because it permits easier exploration of the abdomen. It is also helpful when large uterine masses are present.

Vaginal hysterectomy is generally done for pelvic relaxation, abnormal uterine bleeding, or small fibroids. Advantages of vaginal hysterectomy include earlier ambulation, less postoperative pain, less anesthesia and operative time, less blood loss, no visible scar, and a shorter hospital stay. The major disadvantage is the increased risk of trauma to the bladder.

Nursing Care Management
For the Woman Requiring a Hysterectomy

Nursing Assessment and Diagnosis

Preoperatively, the nurse needs to identify the woman's physiologic and psychologic needs as she approaches surgery. Additionally, it is important to evaluate her learning needs in relation to the surgery and its implications postoperatively. In assessing the woman, consider her age, her culture and educational level, the attitudes of her partner and family, her preoperative status, and whether the hysterectomy is being performed because of a cancer diagnosis. The significance of her reproductive health to her self-image is also a consideration.

Nursing diagnoses that may apply to a woman having a hysterectomy include the following (NANDA-I © 2014):

- *Knowledge, Deficient,* related to a lack of information about preoperative routines, postoperative activities, and expected postoperative changes

- *Fear* related to the risk of possible surgical complications

Planning and Implementation

Preoperative teaching should include information about the procedure, expected preparation, type of anesthesia to be used, possible risks and complications, postoperative care routines, and expected recovery time (Figure 6–5).

Routine postoperative care includes monitoring of physiologic and emotional responses and implementation of nursing interventions to ensure physical well-being and comfort. The woman should be aware of possible complications and when to follow up with her surgeon. Follow up with the woman regarding any psychosocial implications discussed preoperatively, such as support at home and potential for sadness or depression related to perception of changed sexuality or self-image.

Evaluation

Expected outcomes of nursing care include the following:

- The woman can discuss the reasons for her hysterectomy and the type of procedure performed, the alternatives, and aspects of self-care following surgery.

- The woman has an uneventful recovery without complications.

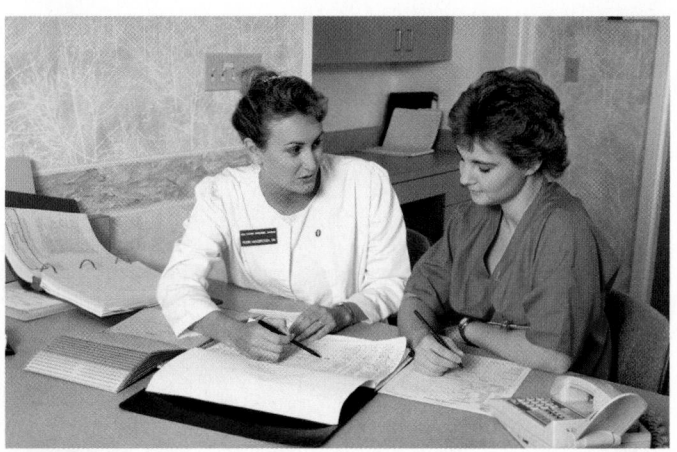

Figure 6–5 **The nurse provides information for the woman during preoperative teaching.**

- The woman participates in decision making about her care.
- The woman can identify available resources if she has physical or emotional concerns in the postoperative period.

Infertility

Infertility is defined as a failure to achieve a successful pregnancy after 12 months or more of regular, unprotected intercourse (American Society for Reproductive Medicine [ASRM], 2012a). It has a profound emotional, psychologic, and economic impact on both the affected couple and society. The term **sterility** is applied when there is an absolute factor preventing reproduction. *Subfertility* is used to describe a couple who has difficulty conceiving because both partners have reduced fertility. **Primary infertility** refers to a woman with no prior pregnancies; secondary infertility refers to couples who have been unable to conceive after one or more successful pregnancies or who cannot sustain a pregnancy.

In the United States, approximately 15% of couples in their reproductive years are infertile (ASRM, 2012e). Public perception is that the incidence of infertility is increasing, but in fact there has been no significant change in the proportion of infertile couples in the United States. What has changed is the composition of the infertile population, which has increased in the age group 25 to 44 because of delayed childbearing. The perception that infertility is on the rise may be related to the following factors (Fritz & Speroff, 2011):

- Increase in the use of assisted reproductive techniques, which has improved the prognosis for many infertile couples
- Increase in availability and use of infertility services

- Increase in insurance coverage of more socioeconomic groups for diagnosis of and treatment for infertility
- Increased number of childless women over age 35 seeking medical attention for infertility

Essential Components of Fertility

Understanding the elements essential for normal fertility can help the nurse identify the many factors that may cause infertility. The components necessary for normal fertility are correlated with possible causes of deviation in Table 6–3. Infertility can be due to a male factor (20%), a female factor (40%), or either an unknown cause (unexplained infertility) or a problem with both partners (30% to 40%) (ASRM, 2012b). Professional intervention can help approximately 65% of infertile couples achieve pregnancy.

Young couples with no history that is suggestive of reproductive disorders should be referred for infertility evaluation if they have been unable to conceive after at least 1 year of attempting to achieve pregnancy. An earlier workup is indicated in couples with positive history for fertility-lowering disease or advancing maternal age. For women over age 35, it is appropriate to refer the couple after only 6 months of unprotected intercourse without conception or earlier if clinically indicated (ASRM, 2012a).

Healthy People 2020

(MICH-17.1) Reduce the proportion of women ages 18 to 44 years who have impaired fecundity (i.e., a physical barrier preventing pregnancy or carrying a pregnancy to term)

(MICH-17.2) Reduce the proportion of men ages 18 to 44 years who have impaired fecundity

---

TABLE 6–3 Possible Causes of Infertility

NECESSARY NORMS	DEVIATIONS FROM NORMAL
Female	
Favorable cervical mucus	Cervicitis, cervical stenosis, use of coital lubricants, antisperm antibodies (immunologic response)
Clear passage between cervix and tubes	Myomas, adhesions, adenomyosis, polyps, endometritis, cervical stenosis, endometriosis, congenital anomalies (e.g., septate uterus, diethylstilbestrol [DES] exposure)
Patent tubes with normal motility	PID, peritubal adhesions, endometriosis, IUC, salpingitis (e.g., chlamydia, recurrent STIs), neoplasm, ectopic pregnancy, tubal ligation
Ovulation and release of ova	Primary ovarian failure, polycystic ovarian disease, hypothyroidism, pituitary tumor, lactation, periovarian adhesions, endometriosis, premature ovarian failure, hyperprolactinemia, Turner syndrome
No obstruction between ovary and tubes	Adhesions, endometriosis, PID
Endometrial preparation	Anovulation, luteal phase defect, malformation, uterine infection, Asherman syndrome
Male	
Normal semen analysis	Abnormalities of sperm or semen, polyspermia, congenital defect in testicular development, mumps after adolescence, cryptorchidism, infections, gonadal exposure to x-rays, chemotherapy, smoking, alcohol abuse, malnutrition, chronic or acute metabolic disease, medications (e.g., morphine, aspirin, ibuprofen), cocaine, marijuana use, constrictive underclothing, heat
Unobstructed genital tract	Infections, tumors, congenital anomalies, vasectomy, strictures, trauma, varicocele
Normal genital tract secretions	Infections, autoimmunity to semen, tumors
Ejaculate deposited at the cervix	Premature ejaculation, impotence, hypospadias, retrograde ejaculation (e.g., as can occur with diabetes), neurologic cord lesions, obesity (inhibiting adequate penetration)

Initial Investigation: Physical and Psychosocial Issues

The easiest and least intrusive infertility testing approach is used first. The nurse provides information about the most fertile times to have intercourse during the menstrual cycle. Teaching the couple the signs and timing of ovulation, the most effective times for intercourse within the cycle, and other fertility-awareness behaviors may solve the problem (see *Teaching Highlights: Suggestions for Improving Fertility*). Primary assessment, including a comprehensive history (with a discussion of genetic conditions) and physical examination for any obvious causes of infertility, is done before a costly, time-consuming, and emotionally trying investigation is initiated.

The basic infertility investigation depends on the couple's history and usually includes assessment of ovarian function, cervical mucus adequacy and receptivity to sperm, sperm adequacy, tubal patency, and the general condition of the pelvic organs. The mutual desire to have children is a cornerstone of many marriages. A fertility problem is a deeply personal, emotion-laden area in a couple's life. The self-esteem of one or both partners may be threatened if the inability to conceive is perceived as a lack of virility or femininity. It is never easy to discuss one's sexual activity, especially when potentially irreversible problems with fertility exist. The nurse can provide comfort to couples by offering a sympathetic ear, a nonjudgmental approach, and appropriate information and instructions throughout the diagnostic and therapeutic process. The first interview should involve both partners and include a comprehensive history and physical examination. Table 6–4 lists the items in a complete infertility physical workup and laboratory evaluation for both partners. A semen analysis is one of the first diagnostic tests done before moving on to more invasive diagnostic procedures involving the woman. Figure 6–6 outlines the couple's history and physical examination data, diagnostic tests usually performed, and healthcare interventions used in cases of infertility.

Assessment of the Woman's Fertility

After a thorough history and physical examination, both partners may undergo tests to identify causes of infertility. A thorough female evaluation includes assessment of the hypothalamic-pituitary axis in terms of ovulatory function, as well as structure and function of the cervix, uterus, fallopian tubes, and ovaries. See Chapter 4 for an in-depth discussion of the female reproductive cycle.

EVALUATION OF OVULATORY FACTORS

Ovulation problems are a common cause of infertility.

Testing for Ovulation. The following tests may be indicated:

- **Basal body temperature (BBT)** recording is the least expensive method for detecting ovulation, but interpretation of these charts can be complex and have wide variations depending on who is reading them.
- Several other tests have limited clinical utility, including endometrial biopsy, postcoital testing, and evaluation of cervical factors (e.g., ferning and mucus elasticity) and are not considered to be the preferred methods in the evaluation of the infertile female.
- Serum testing is generally used for assessment of ovulatory function in women with irregular menstrual cycles. A mid–luteal phase serum progesterone level should be obtained approximately 1 week before expected menstruation to document ovulation. A progesterone level greater than 3 ng/mL collected on or about day 21 for a typical 28-day cycle is evidence of recent ovulation. If the progesterone level is less than 3 ng/mL, an evaluation of anovulation is warranted. This includes measurement of serum prolactin, thyroid-stimulating hormone (TSH), FSH, and assessment for PCOS.
- Over-the-counter urinary ovulation prediction kits are also available. These kits detect LH and predict the timing of the LH surge, which reliably predict ovulation. However, they have false-positive and false-negative rates. Serum confirmation may be useful for clients unable to detect urinary LH surge.
- **Endometrial biopsy (EMB)** provides information about the effects of progesterone produced by the corpus luteum after ovulation and endometrial receptivity. EMB is reliable for determining the presence of ovulation. Histologic evidence of secretory endometrium detected by endometrial

TABLE 6–4 Initial Infertility Physical Workup and Laboratory Evaluations

FEMALE	MALE
Physical Examination	**Physical Examination**
Assessment of height, weight, blood pressure, temperature, and general health status	General health (assessment of height, weight, blood pressure)
Endocrine evaluation of thyroid for exophthalmos, lid lag, tremor, or palpable gland	Endocrine evaluation (e.g., presence of gynecomastia)
Optic fundi evaluation for presence of increased intracranial pressure, especially in oligomenorrheal or amenorrheal women (possible pituitary tumor)	Visual fields evaluation for bitemporal hemianopia (blindness in one-half of the visual field)
Reproductive features (including breast and external genital area)	Abnormal hair patterns
Physical ability to tolerate pregnancy	**Urologic Examination**
	Presence or absence of phimosis
Pelvic Examination	Location of urethral meatus
PAP smear	Size and consistency of each testis, vas deferens, and epididymis
Culture for gonorrhea if indicated and possibly chlamydia or mycoplasma culture (opinions vary)	Presence of varicocele
Signs of vaginal infections	**Rectal Examination**
Shape of escutcheon (e.g., does pubic hair distribution resemble that of a male's?)	Size and consistency of the prostate with microscopic evaluation of prostate fluid for signs of infection
Size of clitoris (enlargement caused by endocrine disorders)	Size and consistency of seminal vesicles
Evaluation of cervix: old lacerations, tears, erosion, polyps, condition and shape of os, signs of infections, cervical mucus (evaluate for estrogen effect on mucus elasticity and cervical ferning)	**Laboratory Examination**
	Complete blood count
Bimanual Examination	Sedimentation rate if indicated
Size, shape, position, and motility of uterus	Serology
Presence of congenital anomalies	Urinalysis
Presence of endometriosis	Rh factor and blood grouping
Evaluation of adnexa: ovarian size, cysts, fixations, or tumors	Semen analysis
	If indicated, testicular biopsy, buccal smear
Rectovaginal Examination	Hormonal assays, FSH, LH, prolactin
Presence of retroflexed or retroverted uterus	
Presence of rectouterine pouch masses	
Presence of possible endometriosis	
Laboratory Examination	
Complete blood count	
Sedimentation rate if indicated	
Serology	
Urinalysis	
Rh factor and blood grouping	
Rubella immunoglobulin (IgG)	
FSH level regardless of age and regularity of menstrual cycles	
If indicated, depending on age and regularity of menstrual cycles: thyroid-stimulating hormone (TSH), prolactin (PRL) levels, glucose tolerance test, hormonal assays including estradiol (E_2), LH, midluteal progesterone (MLP), dehydroepiandrosterone sulfate (DHEAS), androstenedione, testosterone, 17α-hydroxyprogesterone (17-OHP)	

biopsy shows ovulation and corpus luteum formation. However, it is not effective for diagnosing luteal phase deficiency (ASRM, 2012e).

- **Transvaginal ultrasound** is the method of choice for follicular monitoring of women undergoing induction cycles, for timing ovulation for insemination and intercourse, for

retrieving oocytes for in vitro fertilization (IVF), and for monitoring early pregnancy.

EVALUATION OF CERVICAL FACTORS

The mucous cells of the endocervix consist predominantly of water. As ovulation approaches, the ovary increases its secretion

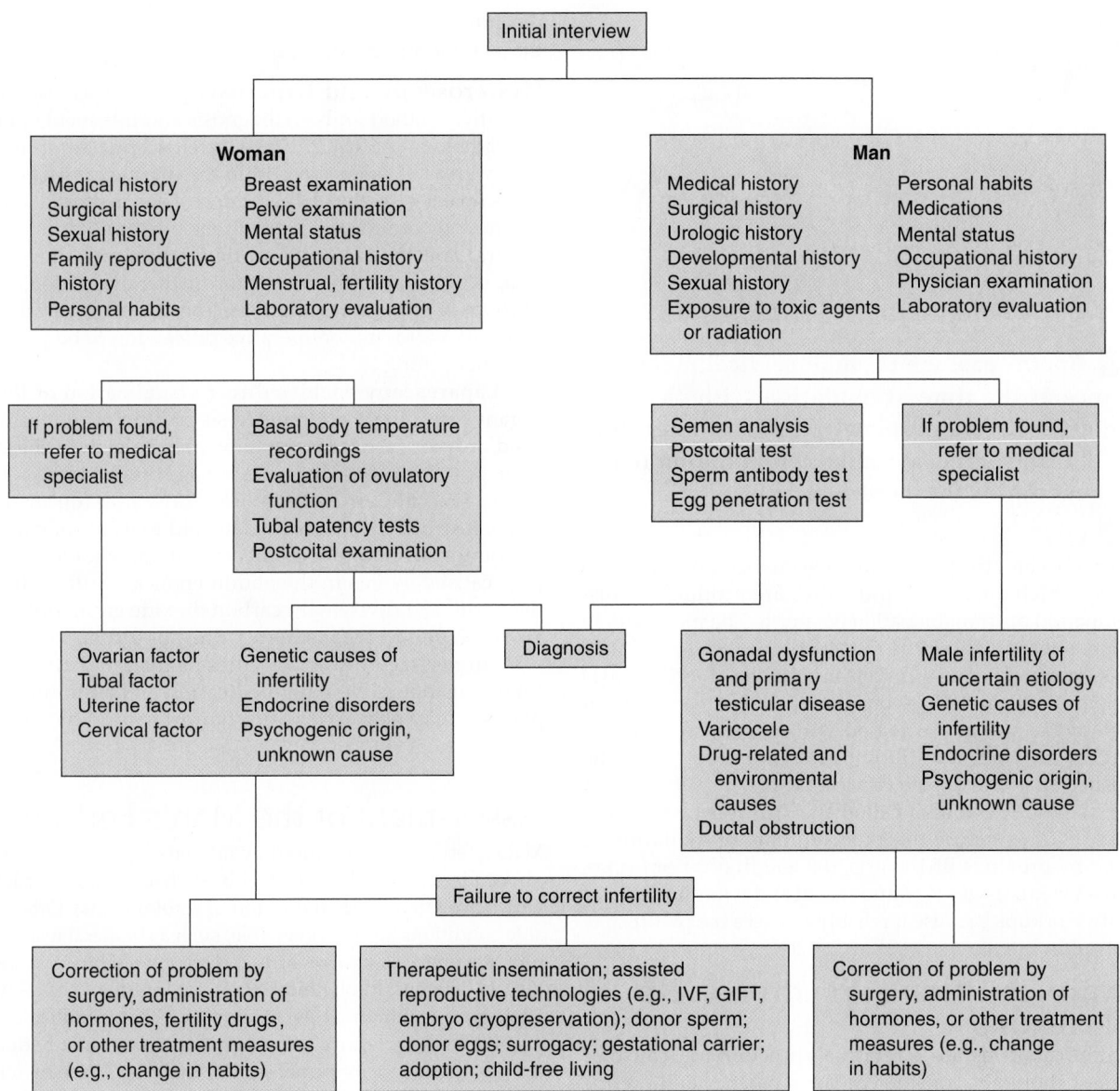

Figure 6–6   Flowchart for management of the infertile couple.

of estrogen and produces changes in the cervical mucus. The amount of mucus increases 10-fold, and the water content rises significantly. At ovulation, mucous elasticity (spinnbarkeit) increases to at least 5 cm in length and viscosity decreases. Excellent spinnbarkeit exists when the mucus can be stretched 8 to 10 cm or longer. Mucous elasticity is determined by using two glass slides (see Figure 5–3A) or by grasping some mucus at the external os.

The **ferning capacity** (crystallization) (Figure 5–3B) of the cervical mucus also increases as ovulation approaches. Ferning is caused by decreased levels of salt and water interacting with the glycoproteins in the mucus during the ovulatory period and is thus an indirect indication of estrogen production. To test for ferning, mucus is obtained from the cervical os, spread on a glass slide, allowed to air dry, and examined under the microscope. Within 24 to 48 hours postovulation, rising levels of progesterone markedly decrease the quantity of cervical mucus and increase its viscosity and cellularity. The resulting absence of spinnbarkeit and ferning capacity decreases sperm survival.

To be receptive to sperm, cervical mucus must be thin, clear, watery, profuse, alkaline, and acellular. As shown in Figure 6–7A, the mazelike microscopic mucoid strands align in a parallel manner to allow for easy sperm passage. The mucus is termed inhospitable if these changes do not occur (Figure 6–7B).

Cervical mucus inhospitable to sperm survival can have several causes, some of which are treatable. For example, estrogen secretion may be inadequate for development of receptive mucus. Cone biopsy, electrocautery, or cryosurgery of the cervix may remove large numbers of mucus-producing glands, creating a "dry cervix" that decreases sperm survival. Treatment with clomiphene citrate may have harmful effects on cervical mucus because of its antiestrogenic properties. Therapy with supplemental estrogen for approximately 6 days before expected ovulation encourages the formation of suitable spinnbarkeit. However, intrauterine insemination (IUI) is more often the most appropriate therapy to overcome these obstacles. When mucosal hostility to sperm is because of cervical infection, antimicrobial therapy may be effective.

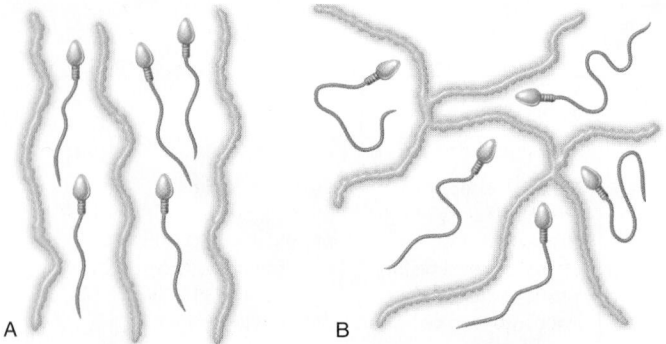

Figure 6–7 Sperm passage through cervical mucus. *A*, Appearance at the time of ovulation with channels favoring efficient sperm penetration and migration upward. *B*, Unfavorable mazelike configuration found at other times during the menstrual cycle.

The cervix can also be the site of secretory immunologic reactions in which antisperm antibodies are produced, causing agglutination or immobilization of sperm. The most widely used serum–sperm bioassay to detect specific classes of antibodies in serum and seminal fluid is immunobead testing (IBT) (Fritz & Speroff, 2011). IBT is considered clinically significant when 50% of the sperm are coated with immunobeads. The treatment for antisperm antibodies may include IUI of the man's washed sperm to bypass cervical factors.

The postcoital test, also called the **Huhner test**, is performed 1 or 2 days before the expected date of ovulation as determined by previous BBT charts, the length of prior cycles, or a urinary LH kit. Its use is controversial and it has limited use in infertility workups because it reliably assesses the presence of sperm only after intercourse (ASRM, 2012e).

EVALUATION OF UTERINE STRUCTURES AND TUBAL PATENCY

Uterine abnormalities are a relatively uncommon cause of infertility but should be considered. Tubal patency and uterine structure are usually evaluated by hysterosalpingography or laparoscopy. Other invasive tests used to evaluate only the uterine cavity are hysteroscopy and sonohysterography. Hysteroscopy may be performed earlier in the evaluation if the woman's history suggests the potential for adhesive disease or uterine abnormalities.

Hysterosalpingography. Hysterosalpingography (HSG), or *hysterography*, involves the instillation of a radiopaque substance into the uterine cavity for visualization. In addition, the dye and injection pressure used in HSG may have a therapeutic effect, causing the flushing of debris, breaking of adhesions, or induction of peristalsis by the instillation of the radiopaque substance.

HSG should be performed in the follicular phase of the cycle to avoid interrupting an early pregnancy. This timing also avoids the lush secretory changes in the endometrium that occur after ovulation, which may prevent the passage of the dye through the tubes and present a false picture of obstruction of the entry point of the fallopian tube into the uterus.

HSG causes moderate discomfort. Women can take an over-the-counter (OTC) prostaglandin synthesis inhibitor (such as ibuprofen) 30 minutes before the procedure to decrease the pain, cramping, and discomfort. HSG can also cause recurrence of pelvic inflammatory disease, so prophylactic antibiotics are recommended to prevent infection that could be triggered by the procedure (ASRM, 2012c).

Hysteroscopy and Laparoscopy. **Hysteroscopy** is the definitive method for both diagnosis and treatment of intrauterine pathology (ASRM, 2012b). Hysteroscopy permits evaluation of any areas of suspicion within the uterine cavity or fallopian tubes revealed by the HSG. It can be done in conjunction with a laparoscopy or independently in the office and does not require general anesthesia. A fiberoptic instrument called a *hysteroscope* is placed into the uterus for further evaluation of polyps, fibroids, or structural variations. The newest generation hyperscope allows for minor operative procedures to be performed in the office setting.

Laparoscopy enables direct visualization of the pelvic organs to evaluate endometriosis and pelvic adhesions. It is used only if there is strong clinical suspicion of these conditions or before considering more aggressive treatments with higher risks and/or costs (ASRM, 2012c). In routine preanesthesia instructions, the woman is told that she may have some discomfort from organ displacement and shoulder and chest pain caused by gas in the abdomen as a result of distending the peritoneal cavity with carbon dioxide gas in order to visualize the pelvic organs better. She should be informed that she can resume normal activities as tolerated after 24 hours. Using postoperative pain medication and assuming a supine position may help relieve discomfort caused by any remaining gas.

Assessment of the Man's Fertility

Male infertility can be caused by numerous factors, some of which can be identified and are reversible, such as ductal obstruction and varicocele (an abnormal dilation of scrotal veins). Other identifiable conditions are not reversible, such as bilateral testicular atrophy secondary to viral orchitis and congenital bilateral absence of the vas deferens. Idiopathic male factor infertility occurs when the etiology of an abnormal semen analysis is not identifiable.

If a male infertility factor is present, it is usually defined by the findings of an abnormal semen analysis. A semen analysis of sperm quality, quantity, and motility is the single most important diagnostic study of the male partner. The sample is usually obtained by masturbation after 3 days of abstinence. It should be done early in the couple's evaluation, before invasive testing of the woman.

Seasonal and incidental variability may be seen in count and motility in successive semen analyses from the same individual. A minimum of two separate analyses is recommended for confirmation. In cases in which a known testicular insult has occurred (infection, high fevers, or surgery), a repeat analysis may not be done for at least 2.5 months to allow for new sperm maturation.

Sperm analysis provides information about sperm motility and morphology and a determination of the absolute number of spermatozoa present (Table 6–5). Although low numbers and motility may indicate compromised fertility, other parameters, such as morphology, motion patterns, and progression, are important prognostic indicators. The quality of sperm decreases with increasing paternal age and may result in chromosomal damage. For example, fathers older than 40 years may be at an increased risk for offspring with chromosomal abnormalities or new gene mutations.

Genetic factors may affect male fertility. Men with oligospermia (semen with a low concentration of sperm) and nonobstructive azoospermia (impaired or nonexistent sperm

TABLE 6–5 Normal Semen Analysis

FACTOR	VALUE
Volume	$\geq$1.5 mL
pH	7.2–7.8
Sperm concentration	$\geq$15 × 106/mL
Total sperm count	$\geq$39 × 106
Progressive motility	$\geq$32%
Total motility	$\geq$40%
Normal morphology (strict criteria)	$\geq$4%
Vitality	$\geq$58%

Source: Cooper, T., Noonan, E., von Eckardstein, S., et al. (2010). World Health Organization reference values for human semen characteristics. *Human Reproduction Update*, 16(3), 231–245.

production) have an increased risk for chromosomal abnormalities and Y chromosome deletions (ASRM, 2012e). Spermatozoa have been shown to possess intrinsic antigens that can provoke male immunologic infertility. Any disruption in the blood–testes barrier, such as vasectomy reversals, or genital trauma, such as testicular torsion, can lead to the production of anti-sperm antibodies (ASAs) (ASRM, 2012e).

Treatment for ASAs is directed toward preventing the formation of antibodies or arresting the underlying mechanism that compromises sperm function. The treatment of choice for clinically significant ASAs is intracytoplasmic sperm injection (ICSI) in conjunction with IVF. If the man's history indicates, he may be referred to a urologist for further testing.

Methods of Infertility Management

Methods of managing infertility include pharmacologic agents, therapeutic insemination, IVF, and other assisted reproductive techniques. In addition, many couples choose adoption as their preferred response to infertility.

PHARMACOLOGIC AGENTS

The pharmacologic treatment chosen depends on the specific cause of infertility.

Clomiphene Citrate. Oral *clomiphene citrate* (Clomid, Sero-phene) is often used as first-line therapy for women with normal ovaries, a normal prolactin level, and an intact pituitary gland. It works by binding to estrogen receptors in the hypothalamus and pituitary gland. This blocks the negative feedback of circulating estrogen and stimulates a release of GnRH, LH, and FSH, thereby inducing ovulation (Wilson et al., 2014). Ovulation is restored in 70% of women treated with clomiphene, but fewer than half achieve pregnancy (Tredway, Schertz, Bock, et al., 2011).

The antiestrogenic effects of clomiphene may cause a decrease in cervical mucus production and endometrial lining development. Other side effects include vasomotor flushes, abdominal distention and ovarian enlargement secondary to follicular growth (bloating) and multiple corpus luteum formation, pain, soreness, breast discomfort, nausea and vomiting, visual symptoms (spots, flashes), headaches, dryness or loss of hair, and multiple pregnancies.

For the first course of clomiphene citrate, the woman usually takes 50 mg/day orally for 5 days from CD 3 to CD 7 or CD 5 to day CD 9. Ovulation should be confirmed to ensure that if continued doses are needed, they are at the lowest possible dose. In nonresponders, the dose may be increased to 100 mg/day to a maximum of 250 mg/day, although doses in excess of 100 mg/day are not approved by the FDA. The woman is informed

that if ovulation occurs, it is expected to occur 5 to 9 days after the last dose. The nurse determines if the couple has been advised to have sexual intercourse every other day for 1 week, beginning 5 days after the last day of medications.

The woman should be knowledgeable about side effects and call her healthcare provider if they occur. The antiestrogenic effects of this drug were discussed previously.

Although rare, visual disturbances can be permanent and should be treated immediately. When visual disturbances (flashes, blurring, spots) occur, the woman should avoid bright lighting.

Most women who conceive do so within the first 6 cycles, although the medication can be continued for 12 cycles (Propst & Wright Bates, 2012). Failure to conceive after clomiphene induction is an indication to expand the diagnostic evaluation or to change the overall treatment plan if evaluation is complete.

Gonadotropins. *Human menopausal gonadotropins (hMGs)* are indicated as a first line of therapy for anovulatory infertile women with low to normal levels of gonadotropins (FSH and LH). It is a second line of therapy in women who fail to ovulate or conceive with clomiphene citrate therapy and in women undergoing controlled ovarian stimulation with assisted reproduction.

Gonadotropin therapy requires close observation with serum estradiol levels and ultrasound. Follicle development must be monitored to minimize the risk of multiple pregnancies and to avoid ovarian hyperstimulation syndrome.

SAFETY ALERT!

Ovarian hyperstimulation syndrome (OHSS) is a potentially life-threatening complication of ovulation induction and can, in its most severe form, result in massive ovarian enlargement and multiple cysts, hemoconcentration, and third-space accumulation of fluid. This can lead to renal failure, hypovolemic shock, thromboembolism, acute respiratory distress syndrome, and death.

The daily dose of medication given is titrated based on serum estradiol and ultrasound findings, but usually starts with a dose of 50 to 100 IU daily. Human chorionic gonadotropin (hCG) is used to trigger ovulation once ovarian follicles are mature. The couple is advised to have intercourse 24 to 36 hours after hCG administration and for the next 2 days. Women who elect to undergo ovarian stimulation with gonadotropins have usually passed through all other forms of management without conceiving. Strong emotional support and thorough education are needed because of the numerous office visits and injections that are required. Often the partner is instructed, with return demonstration, to administer the daily injections. The risk of multiple gestations is higher with gonadotropin therapy than with clomiphene citrate therapy.

Letrozole. Originally developed for the treatment of advanced breast cancer in postmenopausal women, letrozole is more commonly being used off-label for ovulation induction (Pavone & Bulun, 2013). This aromatase inhibitor blocks the conversion of androgens to estrogens. When estradiol levels are low, there is less negative feedback on the hypothalamus and pituitary and increased levels of GnRH and FSH to stimulate follicular development. Letrozole can be used in women who experience side effects from or do not respond to clomiphene. Like clomiphene, it is given for 5 consecutive days starting as early as day 3 of the cycle. Data suggest that letrozole has a lower incidence of multiple gestation pregnancies compared to clomiphene and gonadotropins (Propst & Wright Bates, 2012).

Bromocriptine. High prolactin levels may impair the glandular production of FSH and LH or block their action on the ovaries. When hyperprolactinemia accompanies anovulation, the infertility may be treated with bromocriptine (Parlodel). This medication acts directly on the prolactin-secreting cells in the anterior pituitary. It inhibits the pituitary's secretion of pro-lactin, thus preventing suppression of the secretion of FSH and LH. This restores normal menstrual cycles and induces ovula-tion by allowing FSH and LH production.

GnRH. *GnRH* is a therapeutic tool for inducing ovulation, but its use is limited to women who have insufficient endogenous release of GnRH or it is used adjunctively with gonadotropin ther-apy. Pulsatile GnRH therapy is administered by continuous intra-venous infusion with a portable infusion pump. With this method, GnRH is released intravenously every 60 to 90 minutes at a dose of 2.5 to 10.0 mcg per pulse. Pulsatile GnRH is available in the United States but is used more widely in other parts of the world.

Insulin-Sensitizing Agents. Approximately 80% of anovu-latory women have PCOS, causing insulin resistance and hyper-insulinemia. Strategies to induce ovulation include weight loss followed by oral treatment with clomiphene, aromatase inhibitors including letrozole, or gonadotropin therapy. However, hyperinsu-linemia may cause these clients to be more resistant to treatment. Recently, studies have shown that oral hypoglycemia agents (e.g., metformin and rosiglitazone) can induce ovulation in women with PCOS. Clinical trials are underway to determine the appro-priateness of oral hypoglycemic agents with and without clomi-phene in the infertility setting.

THERAPEUTIC INSEMINATION

Therapeutic insemination has replaced the previously used term *artificial insemination* and involves the depositing of semen at the cervical os or in the uterus by mechanical means. *Thera-peutic husband insemination* (THI) is the current term for use of the husband's semen, and *therapeutic donor insemination* (TDI) is the current term for use of donor semen.

THI is generally indicated for the following:

- Seminal deficiencies as oligospermia (low sperm count), asthenospermia (decreased motility), and teratospermia (low percentage, abnormal morphology)
- Anatomic defects accompanied by inadequate deposition of semen such as hypospadia (a congenital abnormal male urethral opening on the underside of the penis)
- Ejaculatory dysfunction (such as retrograde ejaculation).
- Cases of unexplained infertility
- Some cases of female factor infertility, such as scant or inhospitable mucus, persistent cervicitis, or cervical stenosis

The couple undergoing genetic counseling may consider assisted reproduction techniques, such as TDI. This alternative is appropriate in several instances; for example, if the man has an autosomal dominant disease, TDI would decrease to zero the risk of having an affected child (if the sperm donor is not at risk) because the child would not inherit any genes from the affected parent. If the man is affected with a male sex-linked disorder and does not wish to continue the gene in the family (all his daughters will be carriers), TDI would be an alternative to terminating all pregnancies with a female fetus. If the man is a carrier for a balanced translocation and if termination of preg-nancy is against family ethics, TDI is an appropriate alternative. If both parents are carriers of an autosomal recessive disorder, TDI lowers the risk to a very low level or to zero if a carrier test is available. Finally, TDI may be appropriate if the family is at high risk for a multifactorial disorder or in cases of azoospermia (absence of sperm), severe oligospermia, or asthenospermia. In the past several years, indications for donor insemination have expanded to include single women or lesbians who want to become pregnant. Some states have specified the parental rights of single women and donors, but most are silent on this issue.

TDI has become more complicated and expensive in the past decade because of the need for strict screening and pro-cessing procedures to prevent transmission of a genetic defect or sexually transmitted infection to the offspring or recipient. Guidelines have been established and updated by the American Society for Reproductive Medicine (ASRM, 2013) that include mandatory medical (genetic) and infectious disease screen-ing of both donor and recipient, the need for informed consent from all parties, the need to limit the number of pregnancies per donor, and the need for accurate means of record keeping. Finally, because of the risk of transmitting infectious diseases, donated sperm must be frozen and quarantined for 6 months from the time of acquisition, and the donor must be retested before sperm can be released for use.

Numerous factors need to be evaluated before TDI is per-formed. Has every possible effort been made to diagnose and treat the cause of the male infertility? Do tests indicate nor-mal fertility and sperm–ovum transport in the woman? Has the couple had an opportunity to discuss this option with an infertility counselor to explore the issues of secrecy, disclosure, and potential feelings of loss the couple (particularly the male partner) may feel about not having a genetic child? Are there any religious constraints? After making the decision, the couple should allow themselves time to assess further their concerns and explore their feelings individually and together to ensure that this option is acceptable to both.

Developing Cultural Competence Infertility Treatments

The acceptance of infertility treatments varies widely around the world. Some belief systems do not allow various treat-ments because using a fertility treatment is considered inter-fering with God's design or because the treatment itself is seen as tainted or sinful. For example, artificial reproductive technology in predominantly Muslim countries is accepted and encouraged because adoption is not an accepted solu-tion. However, the approved methods for treating infertility are limited to use of therapeutic insemination using the husband's sperm or IVF involving the fertilization of the wife's ovum by the husband's sperm because the use of donor sperm, egg, or embryo is condemned by Islamic law (Obeisat, Gharaibeh, Owis, et al., 2012).

In Jewish cultures, infertile couples are encouraged to try all possible means to have children, including egg and sperm donation. However, owing to the *Niddah* laws of separation, Orthodox Jewish women are forbidden from engaging in sexual intercourse from the start of their menstruation until 7 days after the end of menses when they immerse themselves in a ritual bath (*mikveh*). Women with unexpected spotting or bleeding must seek the advice of a rabbi or physician, and if uterine bleeding is diagnosed, she may not participate in intercourse for 7 days thereafter (Haimov-Kochman, Adler, Ein-Mor, et al., 2012). For this reason, Jewish law has a signifi-cant impact on fertility, particularly for women with irregular and unpredictable cycles. If the infertility is because of a male factor, artificial insemination with sperm from a non-Jewish sperm donor is acceptable because "Jewishness" is conferred through the matriline. IVF and embryo transfer (ET) are also acceptable artificial insemination methods because they do not involve putting sperm into another's wife.

IN VITRO FERTILIZATION

In vitro fertilization (IVF) is selectively used in cases in which infertility has resulted from tubal factors, mucus abnormalities, male infertility, unexplained infertility, male and female immunologic infertility, and cervical factors. In IVF, a woman's ovaries are stimulated by a combination of medications, one or more oocytes are aspirated from her ovaries and fertilized in the laboratory, and then are placed into her uterus after normal embryo development has begun. These steps occur over a 2-week period of time, known as an *IVF cycle*. If the procedure is successful, the embryo continues to develop in the uterus, and pregnancy proceeds naturally.

Fertility drugs are used to induce ovulation before the process of IVF begins. Follicular growth is monitored frequently with ultrasound and hormonal assays. Monitoring usually begins around CD 5, and medications are titrated according to individual response. When the follicles have grown to an appropriate size, hCG is given to induce final egg maturation and control the induction of ovulation. Egg retrieval is performed approximately 34 to 36 hours later before ovulation occurs.

In the majority of cases, egg retrieval is performed by a transvaginal approach under ultrasound guidance (Figure 6–8A). It is an outpatient procedure performed with sedation, usually intravenous propofol but occasionally conscious sedation or a regional block is used. A needle guide that helps direct the aspirating needle through the posterior vaginal wall into the follicle is attached to the vaginal ultrasound probe (Figure 6–8B). Many follicles can be aspirated with only one puncture, and the procedure generally lasts no more than 30 minutes. Many physicians use prophylactic antibiotics to reduce the risk of infection from the procedure.

Oocytes are then mixed with spermatozoa in culture medium and fertilization is confirmed about 17 hours later by observing two pronuclei within the zygote. After fertilization, the cells will continue to divide exponentially every 12 to 14 hours so that the embryo is approximately eight cells about 72 hours after retrieval. Many programs will transfer these *cleavage stage* embryos at this time. Some programs wait until day 5 when the embryo is at the *blastocyst stage*, with the theory that better quality embryos can be transferred at a time when natural implantation would be occurring. After the procedure, the woman is advised to engage in only minimal activity for 12 to 24 hours. To optimize endometrial receptivity, progesterone supplementation is prescribed at the time of oocyte retrieval or embryo transfer to promote implantation and support the early pregnancy (Hill et al., 2013).

OTHER ASSISTED REPRODUCTIVE TECHNIQUES

Other assisted reproductive techniques include procedures for transfer of gametes, zygotes, or embryos; cryopreservation of embryos; IVF using donor oocytes; assisted embryo hatching (AH); and use of a gestational carrier.

Gamete intrafallopian transfer (GIFT) involves the retrieval of oocytes by laparoscopy; immediate placement of the oocytes in a catheter with washed, motile sperm; and placement of the gametes into the fimbriated end of the fallopian tube. Fertilization occurs in the fallopian tube as with normal conception (in vivo) rather than in the laboratory (in vitro). The fertilized egg then travels through the fallopian tube to the uterus for implantation as in normal reproduction. GIFT may be more acceptable than other procedures such as zygote intrafallopian transfer (ZIFT) to adherents of some religions (Roman Catholic Church) because fertilization does not occur outside the woman's body.

From the GIFT technology evolved procedures such as **zygote intrafallopian transfer (ZIFT)** and **tubal embryo transfer (TET)**. In these procedures, eggs are retrieved and incubated with the man's sperm. However, the eggs are transferred back to the woman's body at a much earlier stage of cell division than in IVF and, as in GIFT, are placed in the fallopian tube or tubes and not the uterus. In TET, the placement is done at the embryo stage. These procedures allow fertilization to be documented, which is not possible with GIFT, and the pregnancy rate is theoretically increased when the fertilized ovum is placed in the fallopian tube.

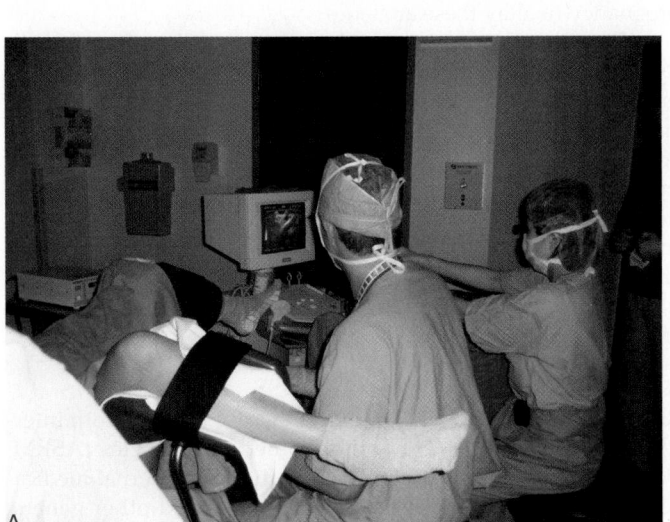

A

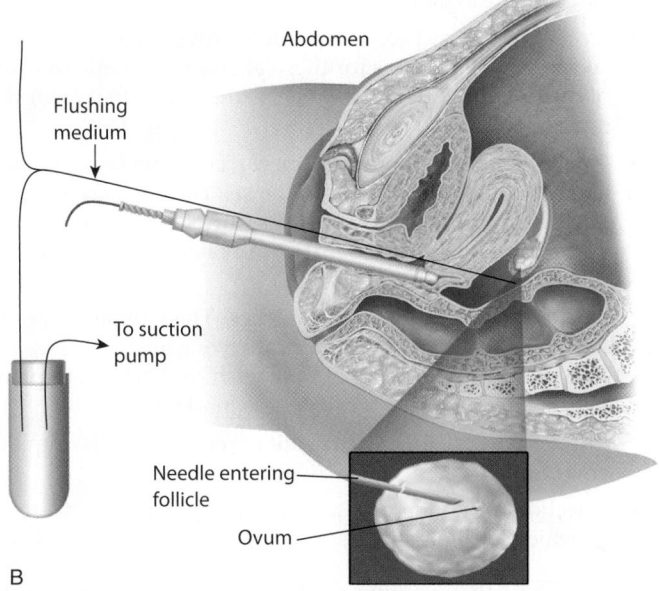

Abdomen

Flushing medium

To suction pump

Needle entering follicle

Ovum

B

Figure 6–8 *A,* **Operating room setup for ultrasound-guided oocyte retrieval.** *B,* **Transvaginal ultrasound-guided oocyte retrieval.**

AH, a micromanipulation procedure, has proved to be an effective adjunct therapy in IVF. IVF using a gestational carrier allows infertile women who are genetically sound but unable to carry a pregnancy to exercise the option of having their own biologic child. Other technologies involve oocyte donation (women donate ovum to another woman) and cryopreservation of the embryo (embryos are frozen and then thawed at a later date) (Michalakis, DeCherney, & Penzias, 2013).

PREIMPLANTATION GENETIC DIAGNOSIS

Recent advances in micromanipulation allow a single cell to be removed from the embryo for genetic study. Couples at risk for having a detectable single-gene or chromosomal anomaly may wish to undergo such *preimplantation genetic testing*, called *blastomere analysis* or, more recently, *preimplantation genetic diagnosis (PGD)*. PGD is used when one or both genetic parents carry a gene mutation or balanced chromosome rearrangement to determine whether that mutation or balanced chromosomal complement has been passed to the oocyte or embryo (Laliota, 2011).

Preimplantation genetic screening (PGS) is used when the genetic parents are known or presumed to have normal chromosomes, and their embryos are screened for aneuploidy with the purpose of increasing the likelihood of a viable pregnancy with normal chromosomes. The single cell is obtained from an eight-cell embryo by a process known as *blastomere biopsy*. The genetic content of the cell is examined using comparative genome hybridization (CGH) (Laliota, 2011). Biopsied embryos are examined so that embryos affected with a particular genetic disease or chromosomal abnormality are not placed in the mother. Both PGD and PGS can produce false-positive and false-negative results. Prenatal diagnostic testing to confirm the results is strongly encouraged (Laliota, 2011).

The diagnosis of genetic disorders before implantation provides couples with the option of foregoing the attempt to establish a pregnancy and thereby avoiding a difficult decision about terminating an affected pregnancy (Kalfoglou, Kammersell, Philpott, et al., 2013). This technology also raises several ethical issues, including the following:

- Identification of couples at risk. There is a need for criteria that identify couples at risk for diseases that constitute significant hardship and suffering so that "wrongful birth" cases can be avoided.

- Availability of and access to centers providing PGD. Should society provide access for those at risk for genetic transfer of disease but without the financial resources to pay for the services?

- Analysis of blastomeres for sex chromosome testing when a genetic disorder carried on the sex chromosomes is suspected. In X-linked diseases, the only way to prevent the disorder is to select against the blastomere with the Y chromosome.

- Identification of late-onset diseases. The Human Genome Project has aided in the identification of genetic markers for late-onset disease. Couples may wish to choose to implant blastomeres that do not carry these markers.

- Effect on the offspring as a result of removing cells from the embryo.

- Selection for nonmedical reasons and potential concern of eugenics "designer babies."

Sperm Sorting. Sperm sorting is a technology designed to separate sperm that primarily produce females or those that primarily produce males. Sorted sperm enriched with male- or female-producing sperm is then used for IUI or IVF. This technology is used to increase the likelihood of having a child of a particular gender in couples at risk for an X-linked genetic disorder or for couples interested in family balancing (gender selection when a couple has two or more children of the same gender) (Kalfoglou et al., 2013).

ADOPTION

Infertile couples consider various alternatives for resolving their infertility, and adoption is one option that may be considered at several points during the treatment process. The adoption of a healthy American infant can be difficult and frustrating, often involving long waiting periods, continual setbacks, and high costs. Thus many couples seek international adoption or consider adopting older children, children with handicaps, or children of mixed parentage because the adoption process in such cases is quicker and more children are available. Nurses in the community can assist couples considering adoption by providing information on community resources for adoption and support through the adoption process. Couples need support if they remain childless, either by choice or circumstance. Informational books, websites such as Childless by Choice, and support groups such as San Francisco RESOLVE's "living without children" are available for couples who remain childless by choice or circumstance.

PREGNANCY AFTER INFERTILITY

The feeling of being infertile does not necessarily disappear with pregnancy. Although there may be initial ecstasy, couples may face a whole new arena of fear and anxiety, and the parents-to-be often do not know where they "fit in." They may feel a great sense of isolation because those who have had no trouble conceiving cannot relate to the physical and emotional pain they endured to achieve the pregnancy. Contact with their past support system of other infertile couples may vanish when peers learn the couple has resolved their infertility. Although the desperation to become pregnant may have superseded the couple's ability to acknowledge their concerns about undergoing various treatments or procedures, questions about the repeated cycle of fertility drugs or the achievement of pregnancy through IVF technology or cryopreservation may now arise. The expectant couple may be very concerned about the potential of these treatments to adversely affect the fetus (McGrath, Samra, Zukowsky, et al., 2010). Couples may need reassurance throughout the pregnancy to allay these anxieties.

The nurse can assist couples who conceive after infertility by acknowledging their past experiences of infertility treatment; validating their fears and anxieties as they face childbirth classes, birth, and parenting issues; and providing support and education about what to anticipate physically and emotionally throughout the pregnancy. The nurse can also counsel couples that infertility because of nonstructural causes may correct itself following a successful pregnancy and birth; therefore, postchildbirth contraception counseling may be warranted. These interventions will go a long way toward normalizing the experience for the couple.

RECURRENT PREGNANCY LOSS

Recurrent pregnancy loss (RPL) is a disease distinct from infertility. It is defined by two or more failed pregnancies (ASRM, 2012d). There are several etiologies, including maternal medical complications, chromosomal abnormalities and other genetic conditions, autoimmune disorders, and thrombotic causes. However, in up to 50% of couples with RPL, an etiology will not be identified (ASRM, 2012d).

Nursing Management

Infertility therapy taxes a couple's financial, physical, and emotional resources. Treatment can be costly, and insurance coverage is limited. Years of effort and numerous evaluations and examinations may take place before conception occurs, if it occurs at all. In a society that values children and considers them to be the natural result of marriage, infertile couples face a myriad of tensions and discrimination.

Be aware of the emotional needs of the couple confronting infertility evaluation and treatment. Often an intact marriage will become stressed with intrusive infertility procedures and treatments. Constant attention to temperature charts and instructions about their sex life from a person outside the relationship naturally affects the spontaneity of a couple's interactions. Tests and treatments may heighten feelings of frustration or anger between partners. The need to share this intimate area of a relationship, especially when one or the other is identified as "the cause" of infertility, may precipitate feelings of guilt or shame. Infertility often becomes a central focus for role identity, especially for women (McGrath et al., 2010).

The couple may experience feelings of loss of control, feelings of reduced competency and defectiveness, loss of status and ambiguity as a couple, a sense of social stigma, stress on the marital and sexual relationships, and a strained relationship with healthcare providers. The couple will need to recognize and express how infertility affects their lives, and grieve the loss of potential children. They then can decide on a plan to manage their infertility (Sawatzky, 1981). Your roles can be summarized as those of counselor, educator, facilitator, and advocate.

Your ability to assess and respond to emotional and educational needs is essential to give infertile couples a sense of control and help them negotiate the treatment process. It is important to use a nursing framework that recognizes the multidimensional needs of the infertile individual or couple within physical, social, psychologic, spiritual, and environmental contexts.

Infertility may be perceived as a loss by one or both partners. Affected individuals have described this as a loss of their relationship with spouse, family, or friends; their health; their status or prestige; their self-esteem and self-confidence; their security; and the potential child. Any one of these losses may lead to depression, but in many cases the crisis of infertility evokes feelings similar to those associated with all these losses (McGrath et al., 2010). Each couple passes through several stages of feelings: surprise, denial, anger, isolation, guilt, grief, and resolution. The impact of these feelings on the couple and how fast they move into resolution, if ever, may depend on the cause and on the duration of treatment. Each partner may progress through the stages at different rates (McGrath et al., 2010).

Nonjudgmental acceptance and a professional, caring attitude on your part can go far in dissipating the negative emotions the couple may experience while going through these stages. This is also a time when you can assess the couple's relationship: Are both partners able and willing to communicate verbally and share feelings? Are the partners mutually supportive? The answers to such questions may help to identify areas of strength and weakness and to construct an appropriate plan of care.

Referral to mental health professionals is helpful when the emotional issues become too disruptive in the couple's relationship or life. The couple should be aware of infertility support and education organizations such as RESOLVE (National Infertility Association), which may help meet some of their needs and validate their feelings. Finally, individual or group counseling with other infertile couples can help the couple resolve feelings brought about by their own difficult situation.

Focus Your Study

- With fibrocystic breast changes, the cysts tend to be round, mobile, and well delineated. The woman generally experiences increased discomfort premenstrually.

- Galactorrhea (nipple discharge not associated with lactation) should be evaluated with cytologic testing.

- Endometriosis is a condition in which endometrial tissue occurs outside the endometrial cavity. This tissue bleeds in a cyclic fashion in response to the menstrual cycle. The bleeding leads to inflammation, scarring, and adhesions. The prime symptoms include dysmenorrhea, dyspareunia, and infertility.

- Treatment of endometriosis may be medical, surgical, or a combination of both. For the woman not desiring pregnancy at present, oral contraceptives are used. Women desiring pregnancy are treated with danazol or the GnRH analogs.

- Polycystic ovary syndrome (PCOS) is a disorder of unknown etiology characterized by ovulatory dysfunction, hyperandrogenism, and polycystic ovaries. Women with PCOS often experience infertility, hirsutism, and difficulty controlling their weight. They are at increased risk for type 2 diabetes and cardiovascular disease.

- Toxic shock syndrome, a rare but potentially fatal disease, is usually caused by a toxin of *Staphylococcus aureus* and is most common in women of childbearing age. There is an increased incidence in women who use superabsorbent tampons or barrier methods of contraception, such as the diaphragm and cervical cap, especially if the woman leaves them in place for extended periods of time.

- Vulvovaginal candidiasis (moniliasis), a vaginal infection most often caused by *Candida albicans*, is most common in women who use oral contraceptives, are taking antibiotics, are currently pregnant, are immunosuppressed, or have diabetes mellitus. It is generally treated with intravaginal miconazole or clotrimazole suppositories or fluconazole orally.

- Bacterial vaginosis (BV), a common vaginal infection, is diagnosed by its characteristic fishy odor and by the presence of "clue" cells on a vaginal smear. It is treated with metronidazole.

- Chlamydial infection is difficult to detect in a woman but can result in pelvic inflammatory disease (PID) and infertility. It is treated with antibiotic therapy. It often coexists with gonorrhea.

- Gonorrhea, a common sexually transmitted infection, can be asymptomatic in women initially but can cause PID if not diagnosed early. The treatment of choice is ceftriaxone intramuscularly combined with azithromycin.

- Herpes genitalis, caused by the herpes simplex virus, is a recurrent infection with no known cure. Acyclovir (Zovirax) may reduce the symptoms.

- Syphilis, caused by *Treponema pallidum*, is a sexually transmitted infection that is treatable if diagnosed. The characteristic lesion is the chancre. Syphilis can also be transmitted in utero to the fetus of an infected woman. The treatment of choice is benzathine penicillin G.

- Condylomata acuminata (genital warts) are transmitted by the human papilloma virus (HPV). Treatment is indicated because research has identified approximately 15 HPV genotypes linked with cervical cancer. The treatment chosen depends on the size and location of the warts and the woman's reproductive status. Two vaccines are now available to prevent several types of HPV.

- Pelvic inflammatory disease can be life threatening and can lead to infertility. The organisms that cause PID most frequently include *C. trachomatis* and *N. gonorrhoeae*. *Mycoplasma genitalium* and bacterial vaginosis (BV) are increasingly being noted as pathogens causing PID.

- There are three common forms of pelvic relaxation. A cystocele is a downward displacement of the bladder into the vagina. Often it is accompanied by stress incontinence. Kegel exercises may help restore tone in mild cases. A rectocele is displacement of the rectum into the vagina. Prolapse of the uterus is displacement of the uterine cervix into the vagina.

- A couple is considered infertile when they do not conceive after 1 year of unprotected coitus.

- A thorough history and physical of both partners are essential as a basis for infertility investigation.

- General fertility investigations include evaluation of ovarian function, cervical mucus adequacy and receptivity to sperm, sperm number and function, tubal patency, general condition of the pelvic organs, and certain laboratory tests.

- Among cases of infertility, 20% involve male factors, 40% involve female factors, and 30% to 40% involve either an unknown cause (unexplained infertility) or a problem with both partners.

- Medications may be prescribed to induce ovulation, facilitate cervical mucus formation, reduce antibody concentration, increase sperm count and motility, and suppress endometriosis.

- The emotional aspect of infertility may be more difficult for the couple than the testing and therapy.

Clinical Reasoning in Action

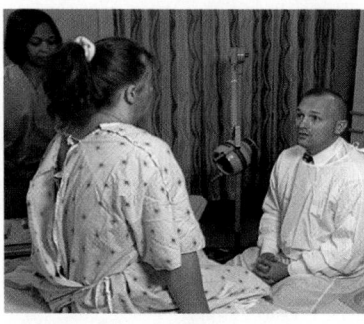

Linda Knoll, 35 years old, presents to you at the GYN clinic for her annual physical and pelvic examination. You obtain the following menstrual history: LMP 8 days ago. Periods occur every 29 days and last 5 days. She tells you that she uses superabsorbent tampons during the first 2 days of her period and then changes to regular absorbency tampons for the duration, and that she currently has an IUD in place for contraception. She tells you that her husband has been complaining for the past few months that she seems irritable, tense, and moody near "that time of the month." Linda admits that she doesn't feel well before her period and describes having low pelvic discomfort, breast tenderness, "bloating," and some constipation. She seems to cry easily 2 to 3 days before her period. She has noticed this pattern over the last 4 or 5 months. You recognize these symptoms as related to premenstrual syndrome (PMS). Linda asks you if these changes are due to female hormones.

1. How would you answer Linda's question concerning female hormones?

2. After reviewing Linda's diet with her, what would you recommend to help?

3. Linda has an IUD in place. What other type of contraceptive might help reduce the symptoms of PMS?

4. What other activities can you suggest to help Linda reduce PMS symptoms?

5. What should you tell Linda about using tampons during heavy menstrual flow?

References

American College of Obstetricians and Gynecologists (ACOG). (2012). *FAQ: Dysmenorrhea*. Retrieved from http://www.acog.org/~/media/For%20Patients/faq046.pdf?dmc=1&ts=20121227T1451215783

American College of Obstetricians and Gynecologists (ACOG). (2014). *Guidelines for women's health care.* 4th ed. Washington, DC: Author.

American Society for Reproductive Medicine (ASRM). (2012a). Diagnostic evaluation of the infertile female: A committee opinion. *Fertility and Sterility, 98*(2), 302–307.

American Society for Reproductive Medicine (ASRM). (2012b). Diagnostic evaluation of the infertile male: A committee opinion. *Fertility and Sterility, 98*(2), 294–301.

American Society for Reproductive Medicine (ASRM). (2012c). *Infertility: An overview.* Retrieved from http://www.asrm.org/patientbooklets

American Society for Reproductive Medicine (ASRM). (2012d). Multiple gestation associated with infertility therapy: An American Society for Reproductive Medicine Practice Committee opinion. *Fertility and Sterility, 97*(4), 825–834. doi:10.1016/j.fertnstert.2011.11.048

American Society for Reproductive Medicine (ASRM). (2012e). Smoking and infertility: A committee opinion. *Fertility and Sterility, 98*(6), 1400–1406. doi:10.1016/j.fertnstert.2012.07.1146

American Society for Reproductive Medicine (ASRM). (2013). Criteria for number of embryos to transfer: A committee opinion. *Fertility & Sterility, 99*(1), 44–46. doi:10.1016/j.fertnstert.2012.09.038

Bass-Ware, A., Weed, D., Johnson, T., & Spurlock, A. (2014). Evaluation of the effect of cranberry juice on symptoms associated with urinary tract infection. *Urologic Nursing, 34*(3), 121–127.

Brown, J. & Farquhar, C. (2014). Endometriosis: An overview of Cochrane Reviews. *Cochrane Database of Systematic Reviews 2014*, Issue 3. Art. No.:CD009590.

Centers for Disease Control and Prevention (CDC). (2013a). *STD curriculum for clinical educators: Genital human papilloma virus (HPV) infection module.* Atlanta, GA: Author.

Centers for Disease Control and Prevention (CDC). (2013b). *STD curriculum for clinical educators: Gonorrhea module.* Atlanta, GA: Author.

Centers for Disease Control and Prevention (CDC). (2013c). *STD curriculum for clinical educators: Syphilis module.* Atlanta, GA: Author.

Centers for Disease Control and Prevention (CDC). (2013d). *STD curriculum for clinical educators: Vaginitis module.* Atlanta, GA: Author.

Centers for Disease Control and Prevention (CDC). (2014a). *STDs in adolescents and young adults.* Retrieved from http://www.cdc.gov/std/stats12/adol.htm

Centers for Disease Control and Prevention (CDC). (2014b). *STDs in racial and ethnic minorities.* Retrieved from http://www.cdc.gov/std/stats12/minorities.htm

Centers for Disease Control and Prevention (CDC). (2014c). Youth risk behavior surveillance—United States, 2013. *MMWR, 63*(4), 1–168.

Centers for Disease Control and Prevention (CDC). (2015). Sexually transmitted diseases treatment guidelines, 2015. *Morbidity and Mortality Weekly Report, 64* (RR#), 1–137.

Colgan, R., Williams, M., & Johnson, J. R. (2011). Diagnosis and treatment of acute pyelonephritis in women. *American Family Physician, 84*(5), 519–526.

Cunningham, F. G., Leveno, K. J., Bloom, S. L., Spong, C. Y., Dashe, J. S., Hoffman, B. L., . . . Sheffield, J. S. (2014). *Williams obstetrics* (24th ed.). New York, NY: McGraw-Hill.

Fantasia, H. C., Fontenot, H. B., Sutherland, M., & Harris, A. L. (2011). Sexually transmitted infections in women: An overview. *Nursing for Women's Health, 15*(1), 46–57.

Fritz, M. A., & Speroff, L. (2011). *Clinical gynecologic endocrinology and infertility* (8th ed.). Philadelphia, PA: Lippincott Williams & Wilkins.

Haimov-Kochman, R., Adler, C., Ein-Mor, E., Rosenak, D., & Hurwitz, A. (2012). Infertility associated with precoital ovulation in observant Jewish couples: Prevalence, treatment, efficacy and side effects. *Israel Medical Association Journal (IMAJ), 14*, 100–103.

Hill, M. J., Whitcomb, W., Lewis, T. D., Wu, M., Terry, N., Decherney, A. H., . . . Propst, A. M. (2013). Progesterone luteal support after ovulation induction and intrauterine insemination: A systematic review and meta-analysis. *Fertility and Sterility, 100*(5), 1373–1380.

Kalfoglou, A., Kammersell, M., Philpott, S., & Dahl, E. (2013). Ethical arguments for and against sperm sorting for non-medical sex selection: A review. *Reproductive BioMedicine Online 26*(3), 231–239. doi:10.1016/j.rbmo.2012.11.007

Laliota, M. D. (2011). Preimplantation genetic diagnosis. In E. Seli (Ed.), *Infertility* (pp. 155–163) West Sussex, UK: Wiley-Blackwell.

Lee, E. (2009). Evidence-based management of benign breast diseases. *American Journal for Nurse Practitioners, 13*(7/8), 22–31.

McFarland, C. (2012). Treating polycystic ovary syndrome and infertility. *American Journal of Maternal/Child Nursing, 37*(2), 116–121.

McGrath, J. M., Samra, H. A., Zukowsky, K., & Baker, B. (2010). Parenting after infertility: Issues for families and infants. *American Journal of Maternal/Child Nursing, 35*(3), 156–165.

Michalakis, K. G., DeCherney, A. H., & Penzias, A. S. (2013). Assisted reproductive technologies: In vitro fertilization & related techniques. In A. H. DeCherney, L. Nathan, N. Laufer, & A. S. Roman (Eds.), *Current diagnosis & treatment: Obstetrics & gynecology* (11th ed., pp. 920–947). New York, NY: McGraw-Hill.

Minkin, M. J. (2011). Urinary tract infection 101: Diagnosis and therapy. *The Female Patient, 36*(10), 14–18.

Obeisat, S., Gharaibeh, M. K., Owis, A., & Gharaibeh, H. (2012). Adversities of being infertile: The experience of Jordanian women. *Fertility and Sterility, 98*(2), 444–449.

Pavone, M. E., & Bulun, S. E. (2013). The use of aromatase inhibitors for ovulation induction and superovulation. *Journal of Clinical Endocrinology & Metabolism, 98*(5), 1838–1844.

Propst, A., & Wright Bates, G. (2012). Evaluation and treatment of anovulatory and unexplained infertility. *Obstetrics & Gynecology Clinics of North America, 39*(4), 507–519.

Rice, K. E., Secrist, J. R., Woodrow, E. L., Hallock, L. M., & Neal, J. L. (2012). Etiology, diagnosis, and management of uterine leiomyomas. *Journal of Midwifery & Women's Health, 57*, 241–247.

Sawatzky, M. (1981). Tasks of the infertile couple. *Journal of Obstetric, Gynecologic, and Neonatal Nursing, 10*, 132.

Schindler, A. E. (2011). Dienogest in long-term treatment of endometriosis. *International Journal of Women's Health, 3*, 175–184.

Schultz, H. J., & Edson, R. S. (2011). Cystitis treatment in women, circa 2011: New role for an old drug. *Mayo Clinic Proceedings, 86*(6), 477–479.

Smith, J. W., & Taylor, J. S. (2011). Polycystic ovarian syndrome: Evidence-based strategies for managing symptoms and preventing long-term sequelae. *Nursing for Women's Health, 15*(5), 403–410.

Tredway, D., Schertz, J. C., Bock, D., Hemsey, G., & Diamond, M. (2011). Anastrozole vs. clomiphene citrate in infertile women with ovulatory dysfunction: A phase II, randomized, dose-finding study. *Fertility and Sterility, 95*(5), 1720. doi:10.1016/j.fertnstert.2010.12.064

Weiss, T. R., & Bulmer, S. M. (2011). Young women's experiences living with polycystic ovary syndrome. *Journal of Obstetric, Gynecologic & Neonatal Nursing, 40*(6), 709–718.

Wilson, B. A., Shannon, M. T., & Shields, K. M. (2014). *Prentice Hall nurse's drug guide—2015.* Upper Saddle River, NJ: Pearson Education.

Chapter 7
Conception and Fetal Development

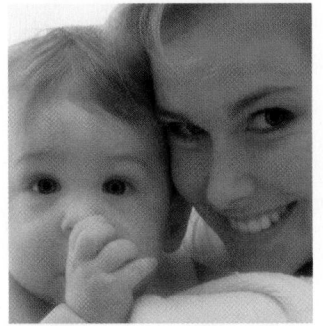

My friends tease me when I say this, but I know the moment my son was conceived. My husband and I had both been so busy at work, but finally we planned a getaway weekend. It was wonderful. We got back some of the magic as we took long walks and talked. Until that weekend, whenever we discussed having children it was always "maybe someday."

On the second night, we decided to skip the diaphragm for the first time. Our lovemaking seemed so special and magical—a true reflection of the emotional closeness we had recaptured. We are convinced that Michael is the result of that night together.

—Michelle, 29

Peter Bowater/Science Source

Learning Outcomes

7.1 Differentiate between meiotic cellular division and mitotic cellular division.

7.2 Compare the processes by which ova and sperm are produced.

7.3 Analyze the components of the process of fertilization as to how each may impact fertilization.

7.4 Summarize the processes that occur during the cellular multiplication and differentiation stages of intrauterine development and their effects on the structures that form.

7.5 Compare the factors and processes by which fraternal (dizygotic) and identical (monozygotic) twins are formed.

7.6 Describe the development, structure, and functions of the placenta and umbilical cord during intrauterine life (embryonic and fetal development).

7.7 Summarize the significant changes in growth and development of the fetus at 4, 6, 12, 16, 20, 24, 28, 36, and 40 weeks' gestation.

7.8 Identify the factors that influence congenital malformations of the various organ systems.

The human genome contains *genes*, which are units of genetic information. Genes are encoded in the DNA that makes up the chromosomes in the nucleus of each cell. These chromosomes, which determine the structure and function of organ systems and traits, are of the same biochemical substances. How then does each person become unique? The answer lies in the physiologic mechanisms of heredity, the processes of cellular division, and the environmental factors that influence our development from the moment we are conceived. This chapter explores the processes involved in conception and fetal development—the basis of human uniqueness.

Cellular Division

Each human begins life as a single cell called a *fertilized ovum*, or **zygote**. This single cell reproduces itself, and in turn each resulting cell also reproduces itself in a continuing process. The new cells are similar to the cells from which they came. Cells are reproduced by either mitosis or meiosis, two different but related processes.

Mitosis

Mitosis results in the production of diploid body (somatic) cells, which are exact copies of the original cell. During mitosis, the cell undergoes several changes, ending in cell division. As the last phase of cell division nears completion, a furrow develops in the cell cytoplasm, which divides it into two daughter cells, each with its own nucleus. Daughter cells have the same **diploid number of chromosomes** (46) and same genetic makeup as the cell from which they came. After a cell with 46 chromosomes goes through mitosis, the result is two identical cells, each with 46 chromosomes. Mitosis makes growth and development possible, and in mature individuals it is the process by which our body cells continue to divide and replace themselves.

Meiosis

Meiosis is a special type of cell division by which diploid cells in the testes and ovaries give rise to gametes (sperm and ova). These cells are different from somatic (body) cells because they contain only half of the parent cell—23 chromosomes—the **haploid number of chromosomes**.

Meiosis consists of two successive cell divisions. In the first division, the chromosomes replicate. Next, a pairing takes place between homologous chromosomes (Sadler, 2015). Instead of separating immediately, as in mitosis, the chromosomes become closely intertwined. At each point of contact, there is a physical exchange of genetic material between the chromatids (the arms of the chromosomes). New combinations are provided by the newly formed chromosomes; these combinations account for the wide variation of traits in people (e.g., hair or eye color). The chromosome pairs then separate, and the members of the pair move to opposite sides of the cell. (In contrast, during mitosis, the chromatids of each chromosome separate and move to opposite poles.) The cell divides, forming two daughter cells, each with 23 double-structured chromosomes—the same amount of DNA as a normal somatic cell. In the second division, the chromatids of each chromosome separate and move to opposite poles of each of the daughter cells. Cell division occurs, resulting in the formation of four cells, each containing 23 single chromosomes (the haploid number of chromosomes). These daughter cells contain only half the DNA of a normal somatic cell (Sadler, 2015) (Table 7–1).

Chromosomal mutations may occur during the second meiotic division; for example, if two of the chromatids do not move apart rapidly enough when the cell divides. The still-paired chromatids are carried into one of the daughter cells and eventually form an extra chromosome. Another type of chromosomal mutation can occur if chromosomes break during meiosis. The effects of the chromosomal mutations of *nondisjunction* and *translocation* are described in Chapter 3.

Gametogenesis

Meiosis occurs during **gametogenesis**, the process by which germ cells, or **gametes** *(ovum and sperm)*, are produced. These cells contain only half the genetic material of a typical body cell. Each gamete must have only the haploid number (23) of chromosomes so that when the female gamete (egg or ovum) and the male gamete (sperm or spermatozoon) unite to form the zygote (fertilized ovum), the normal human diploid number of chromosomes (46)—half from the mother and half from the father—is reestablished.

TABLE 7–1 Comparison of Mitosis and Meiosis

MITOSIS

Purpose

Produces cells for growth and tissue repair. Cell division characteristic of all somatic cells.

Cell Division

One-stage cell division

Number of Daughter Cells

Two daughter cells identical to the mother cell, each with the diploid number (46 chromosomes)

MEIOSIS

Purpose

Produces reproductive cells (gametes). Reduction of chromosome number by half (from diploid [46] to haploid [23]), so that when fertilization occurs the normal diploid number is restored. Introduces genetic variability.

Cell Division

Two-stage reduction

Number of Daughter Cells

Four daughter cells, each containing one half the number of chromosomes of the mother cell, or 23 chromosomes. Nonidentical to original cell.

Oogenesis

Oogenesis is the process that produces the female gamete, called an *ovum* (egg). As discussed in Chapter 4, the ovaries begin to develop early in the fetal life of the female. All the ova that the female will produce in her lifetime are present at birth. The ovary gives rise to oogonial cells, which develop into oocytes. Meiosis (cell replication by division) begins in all oocytes before the female fetus is born but stops before the first division is complete and remains in this arrested phase until puberty. During puberty, the mature primary oocyte proceeds (by oogenesis) through the first meiotic division in the graafian follicle of the ovary.

The first meiotic division produces two cells of unequal size with different amounts of cytoplasm but with the same number of chromosomes. These two cells are the *secondary oocyte* and a minute *polar body*. Both the secondary oocyte and the polar body contain 22 double-structured autosomal chromosomes and one double-structured sex chromosome (X).

At the time of ovulation, a second meiotic division begins immediately and proceeds as the oocyte moves down the fallopian tube. Division is again not equal, and the secondary oocyte moves into the metaphase stage of cell division, where its meiotic division is arrested until and unless the oocyte is fertilized.

When the secondary oocyte completes the second meiotic division after fertilization, the result is a mature ovum with the haploid number of chromosomes and virtually all the cytoplasm. In addition, the second polar body (also haploid) forms at this time. The first polar body has now also divided, producing two additional polar bodies. Thus, at the completion of meiosis, four haploid cells have been produced: the three polar bodies, which eventually disintegrate, and one ovum (Sadler, 2015) (Figure 7–1).

Spermatogenesis

During puberty, the germinal epithelium in the seminiferous tubules of the testes begins the process of spermatogenesis, which produces the male gamete (sperm). The diploid spermatogonium

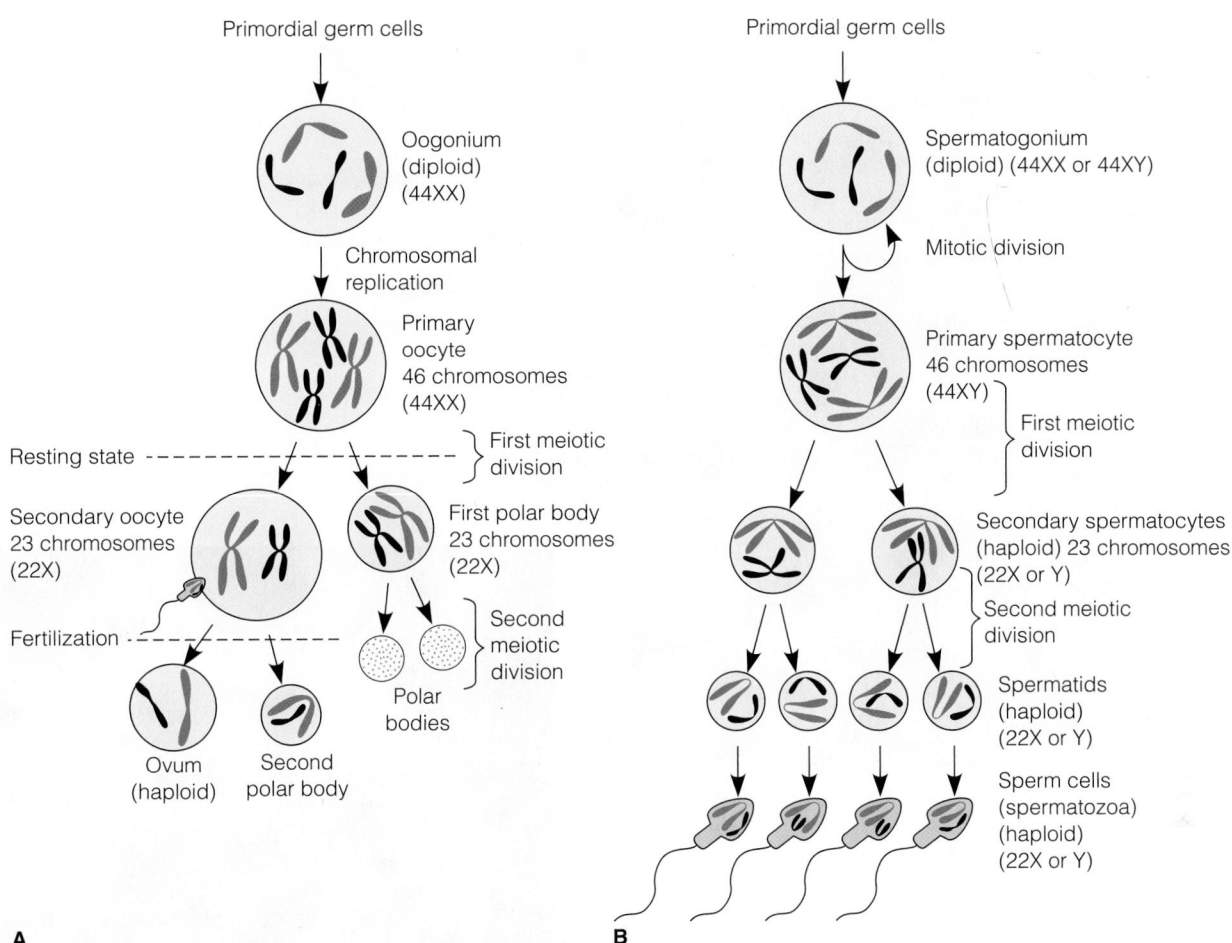

Figure 7–1 Result of gametogenesis. Gametogenesis involves meiosis within the ovary and testis. *A,* During meiosis each oogonium produces a single haploid ovum once some cytoplasm moves into the polar bodies. *B,* Each spermatogonium produces four haploid spermatozoa.

replicates before it enters the first meiotic division, during which it is called the *primary spermatocyte*. During this first meiotic division, the spermatogonium replicates and forms two cells called *secondary spermatocytes*, each of which contains 22 double-structured autosomal chromosomes and either a double-structured X sex chromosome or a double-structured Y sex chromosome. During the second meiotic division, they divide to form four spermatids, each with the haploid number of chromosomes. The spermatids undergo a series of changes during which they lose most of their cytoplasm and become sperm (spermatozoa) (see Figure 7–1*B*). The nucleus becomes compacted into the head of the sperm, which is covered by a cap called an *acrosome* that is, in turn, covered by a plasma membrane. A long tail is produced from one of the centrioles.

The Process of Fertilization

Fertilization is the process by which a sperm fuses with an ovum to form a new diploid cell, or zygote. The zygote begins life as a single cell with a complete set of genetic material, 23 chromosomes from the mother's ovum and 23 chromosomes from the father's sperm, for a total of 46 chromosomes. The following events lead to fertilization.

Preparation for Fertilization

The mature ovum and spermatozoa have only a brief time to unite. Ova are considered fertile for about 12 to 24 hours after ovulation. Sperm can survive in the female reproductive tract for 48 to 72 hours, but are believed to be healthy and highly fertile for only about 24 hours.

The ovum's cell membrane is surrounded by two layers of tissue. The layer closest to the cell membrane is called the *zona pellucida*. It is a clear, noncellular layer whose thickness influences the fertilization rate. Surrounding the zona pellucida is a ring of elongated cells, called the *corona radiata* because they radiate from the ovum like the gaseous corona around the sun. These cells are held together by hyaluronic acid. The ovum has no inherent power of movement. During ovulation, high estrogen levels increase peristalsis within the fallopian tubes, which helps move the ovum through the tube toward the uterus. The high estrogen levels also cause a thinning of the cervical mucus, facilitating movement of the sperm through the cervix, into the uterus, and up the fallopian tube.

The process of fertilization takes place in the ampulla (outer third) of the fallopian tube. In a single ejaculation, the male deposits approximately 200 to 300 million spermatozoa into the vagina, of which only 300 to 500 sperm actually reach the ampulla (Caudle, 2014; Sadler, 2015). Fructose in the semen, secreted by the seminal vesicles, is the energy source for the sperm. The spermatozoa propel themselves up the female tract by the flagellar movement of their tails. Transit time from the cervix into the fallopian tube can be as short as 30 minutes to as long as 6 days (Sadler, 2015). Prostaglandins in the semen may increase uterine smooth muscle contractions, which help

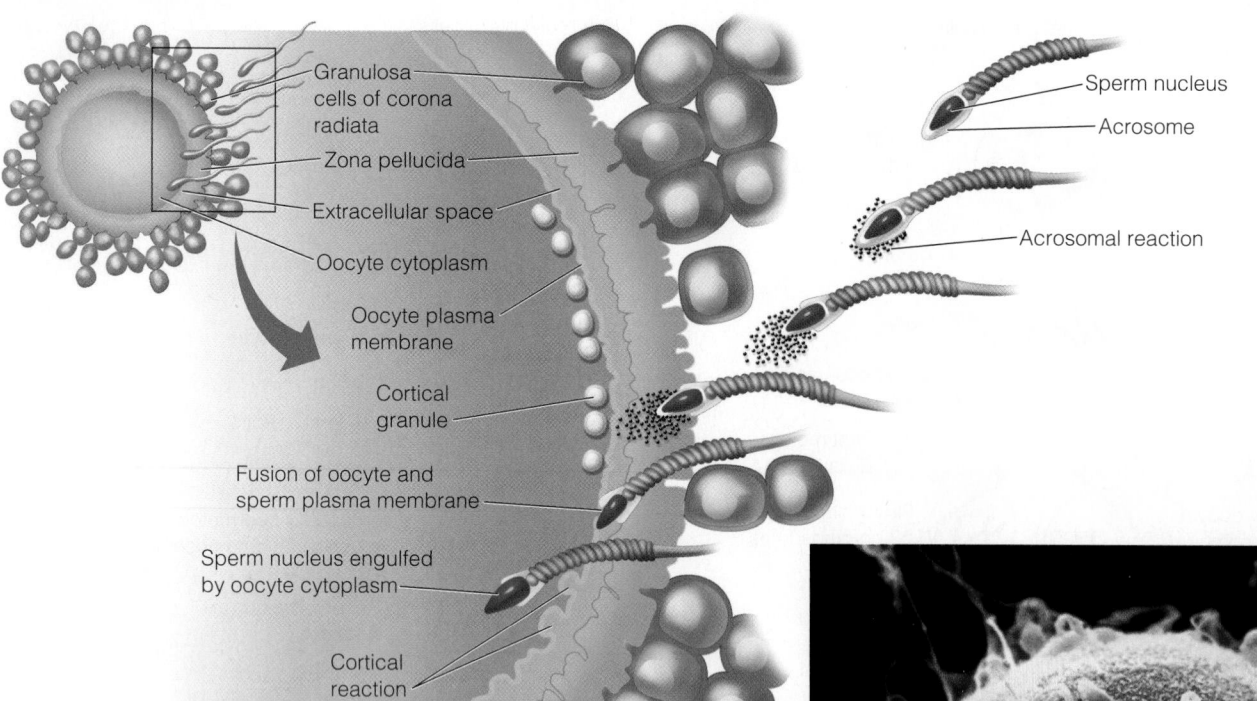

transport the sperm. The fallopian tubes have a dual ciliary action that facilitates movement of the ovum toward the uterus and movement of the sperm from the uterus toward the ovary.

The sperm must undergo two processes before fertilization can occur: capacitation and the acrosomal reaction. **Capacitation** is the removal of the plasma membrane overlying the spermatozoa's acrosomal area and the loss of seminal plasma proteins. If the glycoprotein coat is not removed, the sperm will not be able to fertilize the ovum (Sadler, 2015). Capacitation occurs in the female reproductive tract (aided by uterine enzymes) and is thought to take about 7 hours. Sperm that undergo capacitation now take on three characteristics: (1) the ability to undergo the acrosomal reaction, (2) the ability to bind to the zona pellucida, and (3) the acquisition of hypermotility.

The **acrosomal reaction** follows capacitation, whereby the acrosomes of the sperm surrounding the ovum release their enzymes (hyaluronidase, a protease called *acrosin*, and trypsin-like substances) and thus break down the hyaluronic acid in the ovum's corona radiata (Sadler, 2015). Hundreds of acrosomes must rupture before enough hyaluronic acid is cleared for a single sperm to penetrate the ovum's zona pellucida successfully.

At the moment of penetration by a fertilizing sperm, the zona pellucida undergoes cortical and zona reactions that release

lysosomal enzymes. These enzymes prevent additional sperm from entering a single ovum (Caudle, 2014) (Figure 7–2). This is known as the *block to polyspermy*. This cellular change is mediated by release of materials from the cortical granules, organelles found just below the ovum's surface, and is called the *cortical reaction*.

The Moment of Fertilization

After the sperm enters the ovum, a chemical signal prompts the secondary oocyte to complete the second meiotic division, forming the nucleus of the ovum and ejecting the second polar body. Then the nuclei of the ovum and sperm swell and approach each other. The true moment of fertilization occurs as the nuclei unite. Their individual nuclear membranes disappear, and their chromosomes pair up to produce the diploid zygote. Because each nucleus contains a haploid number of chromosomes (23), this union restores the diploid number (46). The zygote contains a new combination of genetic material that results in an individual different from either parent and from anyone else.

The sex of the zygote is determined at the moment of fertilization. The two chromosomes (the sex chromosomes) of the 23rd pair—either XX or XY—determine the sex of an individual.

The X chromosome is larger and bears more genes than the Y chromosome. Females have two X chromosomes, and males have an X and a Y chromosome. The mature ovum produced by oogenesis can have only one type of sex chromosome—an X. Spermatogenesis produces two sperm with an X chromosome and two sperm with a Y chromosome. When each gamete contributes an X chromosome, the resulting zygote is female. When the ovum contributes an X and the sperm contributes a Y chromosome, the resulting zygote is male. As discussed in more detail in Chapter 3, certain traits are termed *sex linked* because they are controlled by the genes on the X sex chromosome. Two examples of sex-linked traits are color blindness and hemophilia.

Developing Cultural Competence Iraqi
Childbirth Customs

"My sister, she did not have baby for very, very long time, you see. This is very sad where I am from [Iraq]. Her husband's family wanted him to leave her and we so feared he would. Then my sister became pregnant and it was very nice, we all so happy, you see. Then I learned my sister birthed a baby girl and I cried and cried for a week. My mother cried, too, so sad all this time no baby come and then finally to have a girl. I still feel sad for her."

Source: Excerpt from author's interview with an Iraqi woman on childbirth customs in Iraq.

Preembryonic Development

The first 14 days of development, starting the day the ovum is fertilized (conception), are called the *preembryonic stage* or the *stage of the ovum*. Development after fertilization can be divided into two phases: cellular multiplication and cellular differentiation. These phases are characterized by rapid cellular multiplication and differentiation and establishment of the primary germ layers and embryonic membranes. Synchronized development of both the endometrium and embryo is a prerequisite for implantation to succeed (Moore, Persaud, & Torchia, 2016). These phases and the process of implantation (nidation), which occurs between them, are discussed next.

Cellular Multiplication

Cellular multiplication begins as the zygote moves through the fallopian tube toward the cavity of the uterus. This transport takes 3 days or more and is accomplished mainly by a very weak fluid current in the fallopian tube resulting from the beating action of the ciliated epithelium that lines the tube.

The zygote now enters a period of rapid mitotic divisions called **cleavage**, during which it divides into two cells, four cells, eight cells, and so on. These cells, called *blastomeres*, are so small that the developing cell mass is only slightly larger than the original zygote. The blastomeres are held together by the zona pellucida, which is under the corona radiata. The blastomeres eventually form a solid ball of 12 to 32 cells called the **morula** (Moore et al., 2016).

As the morula enters the uterus, two things happen: The intracellular fluid in the morula increases, and a central cavity forms within the cell mass. Inside this cavity is an inner solid mass of cells called the **blastocyst**. The outer layer of cells that surrounds the cavity and replaces the zona pellucida is the **trophoblast**. Eventually, the trophoblast develops into one of the two embryonic membranes, called the *chorion*. The blastocyst develops into a double layer of cells called the *embryonic disc*, from which the embryo and the amnion (embryonic membrane) will develop. Figure 7–3 shows the journey of the fertilized ovum to its destination in the uterus.

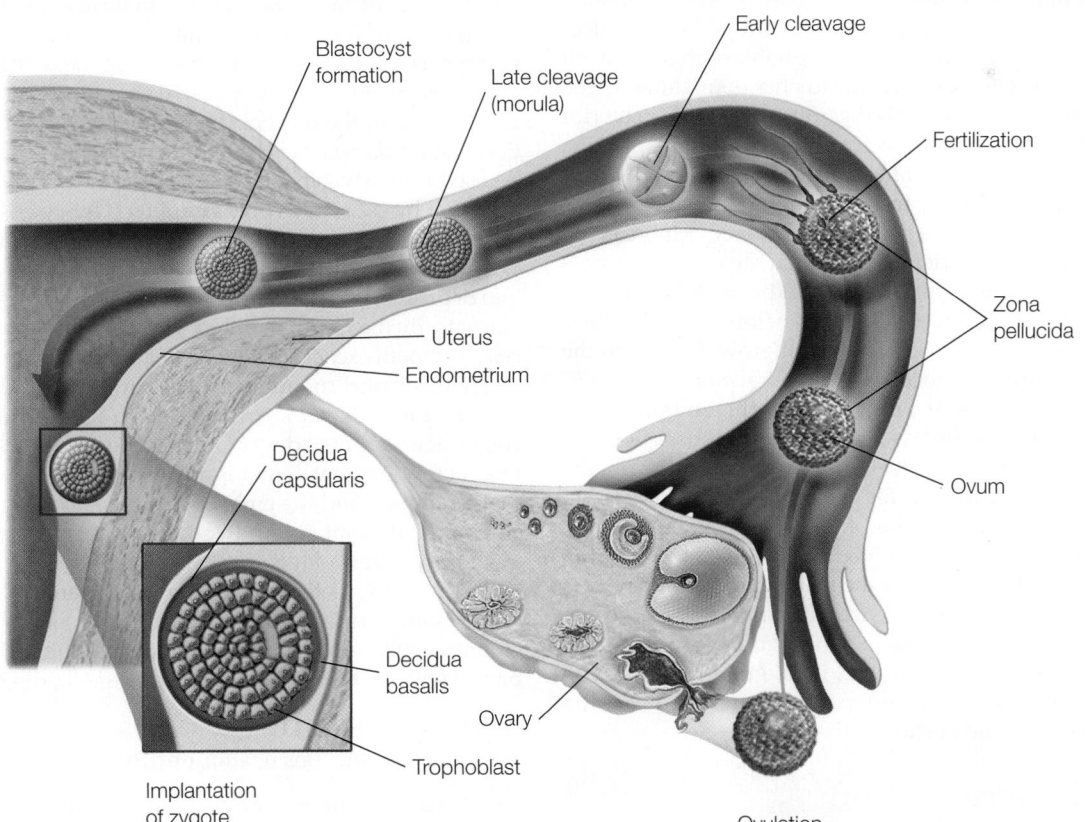

Figure 7–3 Changes in fertilized ovum from conception to implantation. During ovulation, the ovum leaves the ovary and enters the fallopian tube. Fertilization generally occurs in the outer third of the fallopian tube.

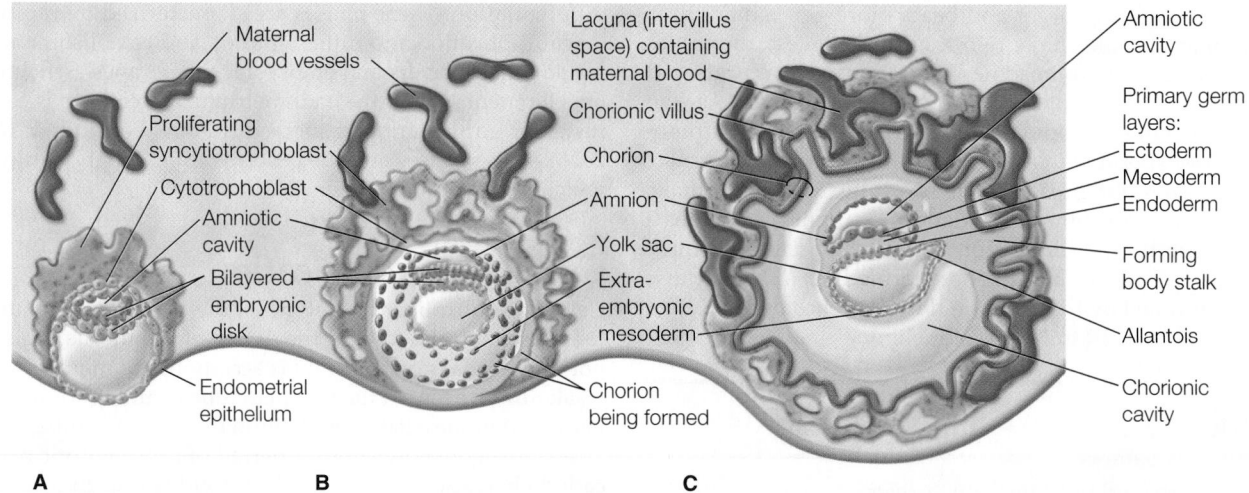

Figure 7–4 Formation of primary germ layers. *A,* Implantation of a 7½-day blastocyst in which the cells of the embryonic disc are separated from the amnion by a fluid-filled space. The erosion of the endometrium by the syncytiotrophoblast is ongoing. *B,* Implantation is completed by day 9, and extraembryonic mesoderm is beginning to form a discrete layer beneath the cytotrophoblast. *C,* By day 16, the embryo shows all three germ layers, a yolk sac, and an allantois (an outpouching of the yolk sac that forms the structural basis of the body stalk, or umbilical cord). The cytotrophoblast and associated mesoderm have become the chorion, and chorionic villi are developing.

Early pregnancy factor (EPF), an immunosuppressant protein, is secreted by the trophoblastic cells. This factor appears in the maternal serum within 24 to 48 hours after fertilization and forms the basis of a pregnancy test during the first 10 days of development (Caudle, 2014; Moore et al., 2016).

Implantation (Nidation)

While floating in the uterine cavity, the blastocyst is nourished by the uterine glands, which secrete a mixture of lipids, mucopolysaccharides, and glycogen. The trophoblast attaches itself to the surface of the endometrium for further nourishment. The most frequent site of attachment is the upper part of the posterior uterine wall. Between days 7 and 10 after fertilization, the zona pellucida disappears and the blastocyst implants itself by burrowing into the uterine lining and penetrating down toward the maternal capillaries until it is completely covered (Moore et al., 2016). The blastocyst will orient itself so that the embryonic pole is closest to the endometrial lining (Blackburn, 2013; Caudle, 2014). The lining of the uterus thickens below the implanted blastocyst, and the cells of the trophoblast grow down into the thickened lining, forming processes that are called *chorionic villi.*

Under the influence of progesterone, the endometrium increases in thickness and vascularity in preparation for implantation and nutrition of the ovum. After implantation, the endometrium is called the *decidua.* The portion of the decidua that covers the blastocyst is called the **decidua capsularis,** the portion directly under the implanted blastocyst is the **decidua basalis,** and the portion that lines the rest of the uterine cavity is the **decidua vera (parietalis).** The maternal part of the placenta develops from the decidua basalis, which contains large numbers of blood vessels (see magnified inset in Figure 7–3). The chorionic villi (discussed shortly) in contact with the decidua basalis will form the fetal portion of the placenta.

Cellular Differentiation

PRIMARY GERM LAYERS

About the 10th to 14th day after conception, the homogeneous mass of blastocyst cells differentiates into the primary germ layers (Figure 7–4). These three layers, the **ectoderm, mesoderm,** and **endoderm,** are formed at the same time as the embryonic membranes. All tissues, organs, and organ systems will develop from these primary germ cell layers (Table 7–2). For example, differentiation of the endoderm results in the formation of epithelium lining the respiratory and digestive tracts (Figure 7–5).

EMBRYONIC MEMBRANES

The **embryonic membranes** begin to form at the time of implantation (Figure 7–6). These membranes protect and support the embryo as it grows and develops inside the uterus. The first and outermost membrane to form is the **chorion.** This thick membrane develops from the trophoblast and has many finger-like projections called *chorionic villi* on its surface. These chorionic villi can be used for early genetic testing of the embryo at 8 to 11 weeks' gestation by chorionic villus sampling (CVS) (see Chapter 13). As the pregnancy progresses, the chorionic villi begin to degenerate, except for those just under the embryo, which grow and branch into depressions in the uterine wall, forming the fetal portion of the placenta. By the fourth month of pregnancy, the surface of the chorion is smooth except at the place of attachment to the uterine wall.

The second membrane to form, the **amnion,** originates from the ectoderm, a primary germ layer, during the early stages of embryonic development. The amnion is a thin protective membrane that contains amniotic fluid. The space between the membrane and the embryo is the *amniotic cavity.* This cavity surrounds the embryo and yolk sac, except where the developing embryo (germ-layer disc) attaches to the trophoblast via the umbilical cord. As the embryo grows, the amnion expands until it comes into contact with the chorion. These two slightly adherent membranes form the fluid-filled amniotic sac, also called the **bag of waters (BOW),** which protects the floating embryo.

AMNIOTIC FLUID

The primary functions of **amniotic fluid** are to:

- Act as a cushion to protect the embryo against mechanical injury
- Help control the embryo's temperature (relies on the mother to release heat)

TABLE 7–2 Derivation of Body Structures From Primary Cell Layers

ECTODERM	MESODERM	ENDODERM
Epidermis	Dermis	Respiratory tract epithelium
Sweat glands	Wall of digestive tract	Epithelium (except nasal), including pharynx, tongue, tonsils, thyroid, parathyroid, thymus, tympanic cavity
Sebaceous glands	Kidneys and ureter (suprarenal cortex)	
Nails	Reproductive organs (gonads, genital ducts)	Lining of digestive tract
Hair follicles		Primary tissue of liver and pancreas
Lens of eye	Connective tissue (cartilage, bone, joint cavities)	Urethra and associated glands
Sensory epithelium of internal and external ear, nasal cavity, sinuses, mouth, anal canal	Skeleton	Urinary bladder (except trigone)
	Muscles (all types)	Vagina (parts)
Central and peripheral nervous systems	Cardiovascular system (heart, arteries, veins, blood, bone marrow)	
Nasal cavity	Pleura	
Oral glands and tooth enamel	Lymphatic tissue and cells	
Pituitary gland	Spleen	
Mammary glands		

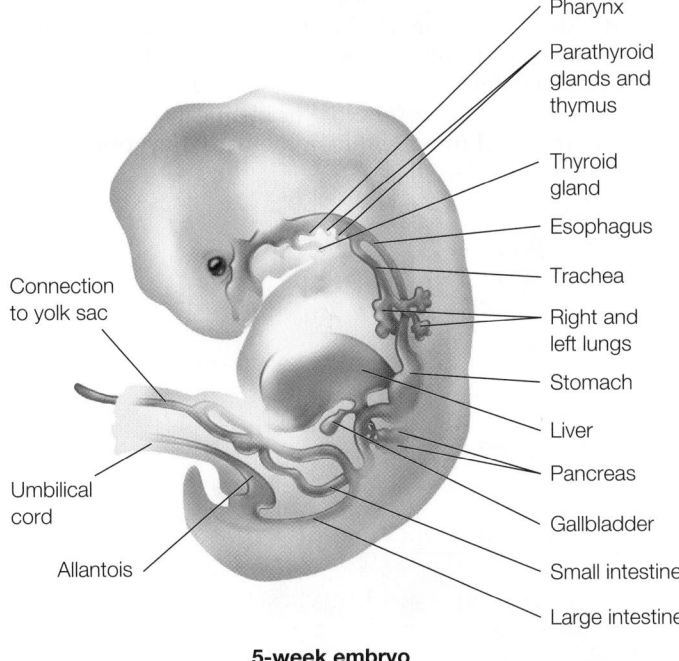

5-week embryo

Figure 7–5 **Differentiation of endoderm. Endoderm differentiates to form the epithelial lining of the digestive and respiratory tracts and associated glands.**

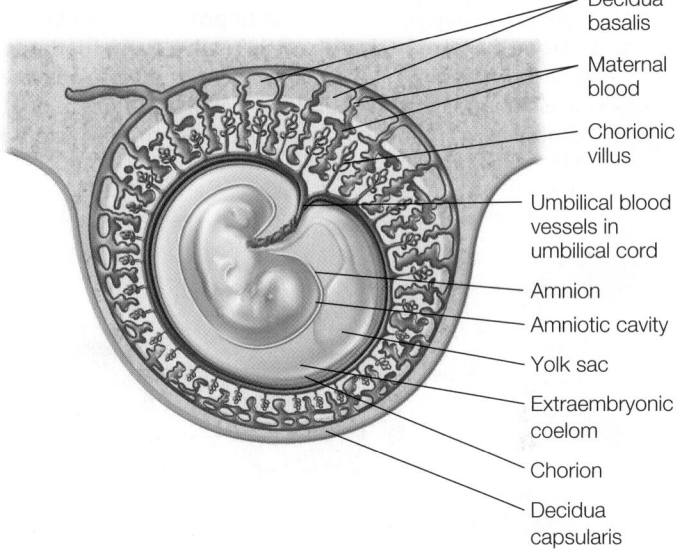

Figure 7–6 **Early development of primary embryonic membranes. At 4½ weeks, the decidua capsularis (placental portion enclosing the embryo on the uterine surface) and decidua basalis (placental portion encompassing the elaborate chorionic villi and maternal endometrium) are well formed. The chorionic villi lie in blood-filled intervillous spaces within the endometrium. The amnion and yolk sac are well developed.**

- Permit symmetric external growth and development of the embryo
- Prevent adherence of the embryo-fetus to the amnion (decreases chance of amniotic band syndrome) to allow freedom of movement so that the embryo-fetus can change position (flexion and extension), thus aiding in musculoskeletal development
- Allow the umbilical cord to be relatively free of compression
- Act as an extension of fetal extracellular space (hydropic babies have increased amniotic fluid)

- Act as a wedge during labor
- Provide fluid for analysis to determine fetal health and maturity

Amniotic fluid is slightly alkaline and contains albumin, uric acid, creatinine, lecithin, sphingomyelin, bilirubin, vernix, leukocytes, epithelial cells, enzymes, and fine hair called **lanugo**. The amount of amniotic fluid at 10 weeks is about 30 mL, and it increases to 210 mL at 16 weeks (Cunningham et al., 2014). After 28 weeks, the amniotic fluid volume ranges from 700 to 1000 mL. The amniotic fluid volume changes little until 39 weeks, after which it decreases dramatically (Black-burn, 2013). As the pregnancy continues, the fetus influences the volume of amniotic fluid by swallowing the fluid and by excreting lung fluid and urine into the amniotic fluid.

Abnormal variations in amniotic fluid volume are *oligohydramnios* (less than 400 mL of amniotic fluid) and *hydramnios* (more than 2000 mL or amniotic fluid index greater than 97.5 percentile for the corresponding gestational age). Hydramnios is also called *polyhydramnios*. See Chapter 21 for an in-depth discussion of alterations in amniotic fluid volume during childbirth.

YOLK SAC

In humans, the **yolk sac** is small and functions early in embryonic life. It develops as a second cavity in the blastocyst on about day 8 or 9 after conception. It forms primitive red blood cells during the first 6 weeks of development, until the embryo's liver takes over the process. As the embryo develops, the yolk sac is incorporated into the umbilical cord, where it can be seen as a degenerated structure after birth.

UMBILICAL CORD

As the placenta is developing, the **umbilical cord** is also being formed from the amnion (Caudle, 2014). The *body stalk*, which attaches the embryo to the yolk sac, contains blood vessels that extend into the chorionic villi. The body stalk fuses with the embryonic portion of the placenta to provide a circulatory pathway from the chorionic villi to the embryo. As the body stalk elongates to become the umbilical cord, the vessels in the cord decrease to one large vein and two smaller arteries. About 1 in 200 umbilical cords have only two vessels, an artery and a

vein; this condition may be associated with congenital malformations primarily of the renal, gastrointestinal, and cardiovascular systems (Sadler, 2015). A specialized mucoid connective tissue known as **Wharton jelly** surrounds the blood vessels in the umbilical cord (Caudle, 2014; Moore et al., 2016). This tissue, plus the high blood volume pulsating through the vessels, prevents compression of the umbilical cord in utero. The umbilical cord has no sensory or motor innervation, so cutting the cord after birth is not painful. At term (38 to 42 weeks' gestation), the average cord is 2 cm (0.8 in.) across and about 55 cm (22 in.) long. The cord can attach itself to the placenta in various sites. Central insertion into the placenta is considered normal. (See Chapter 21 for a discussion of the various attachment sites.)

Umbilical cords appear to be twisted or spiraled, which is most likely caused by fetal movement. A true knot in the umbilical cord rarely occurs; if it does, the cord will be longer than usual. More common are so-called "false knots," caused by the folding of cord vessels. A *nuchal cord* is said to exist when the umbilical cord encircles the fetal neck.

Twins

Twins normally occur in approximately 33.2 per 1000 live births in the United States (Society of Maternal-Fetal Medicine [SMFM], Moise & Argon, 2013). The current rate of twinning is attributed to delayed childbearing and the use of artificial reproductive treatments.

Twins may be either fraternal or identical (Figure 7–7). If twins are fraternal (nonidentical), they are dizygotic, which

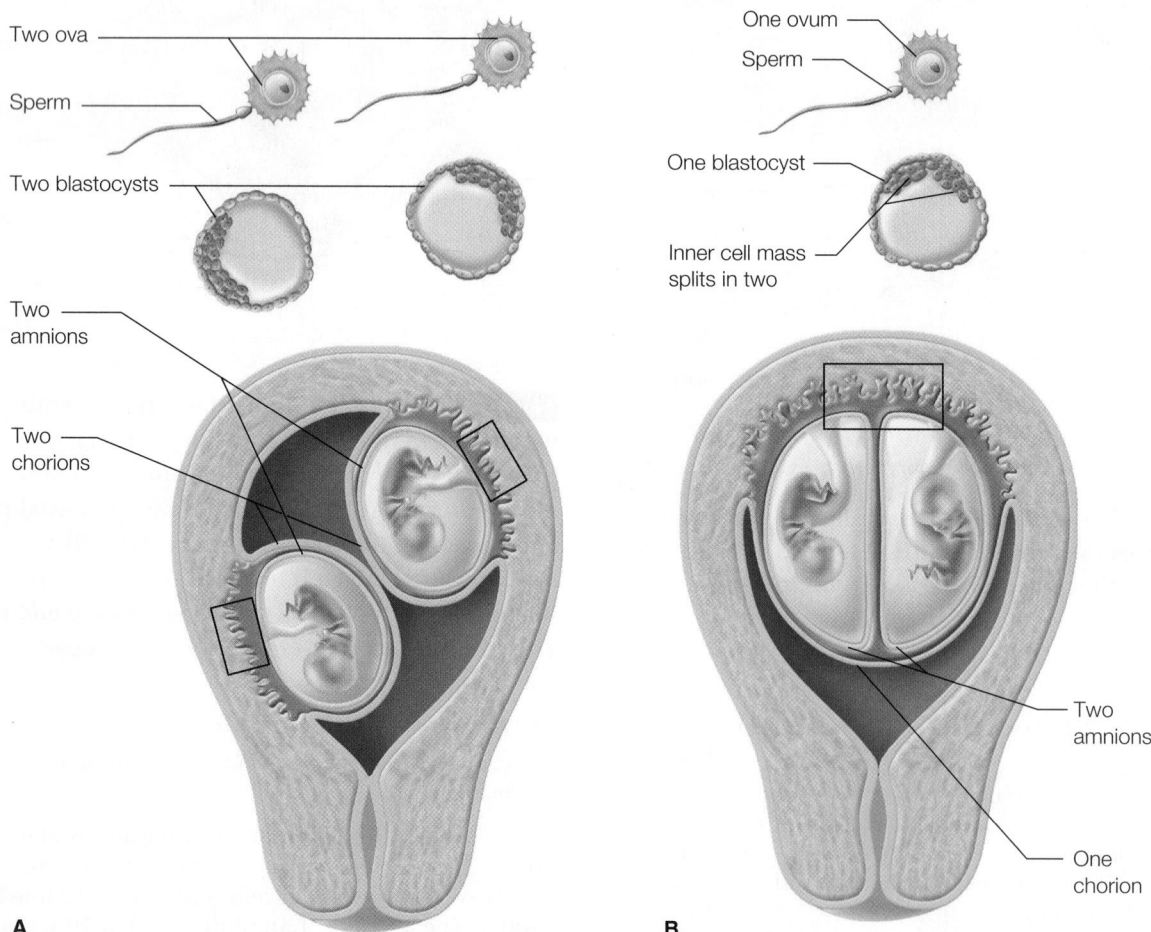

A

B

Figure 7–7 *A*, Formation of fraternal twins. (Note separate placentas.) *B*, Formation of identical twins.

means they arise from two separate ova fertilized by two separate spermatozoa. There are two placentas, two chorions, and two amnions; however, the placentas sometimes fuse and look as if they are one. Despite their birth relationship, fraternal twins are no more similar to each other than they would be to siblings born singly. They may be of the same or different sex.

Dizygotic twinning increases with maternal age up to about age 35 and then decreases abruptly. The chance of dizygotic twins increases with parity, in conceptions that occur in the first 3 months of marriage, and also with coital frequency. The chance of dizygotic twinning decreases during periods of malnutrition and during winter and spring for women living in the northern hemisphere. Studies indicate that dizygotic twins occur in certain families, perhaps because of genotype (genetic constitution) of the mother that results in elevated serum gonadotropin levels leading to double ovulation (Moore et al., 2016). Fraternal (dizygotic) twins have been reported to occur more often among African American women than among White women and more often among White women than among women of Asian origin (Moore et al., 2016). Among all groups, as parity (having given birth to a viable baby) increases, so does the chance for multiple births.

Identical, or monozygotic, twins develop from a single fertilized ovum. They are of the same sex and have the same phenotype (appearance). Identical twins usually have a common placenta. Monozygosity is not affected by environment, race, physical characteristics, or fertility.

Monozygotic twins originate from division of the fertilized ovum at different stages of early development, after the zygote consists of thousands of cells. Complete separation of the cellular mass into two parts is necessary for twin formation. The number of amnions and chorions present depends on the timing of the division:

1. If division occurs within 4 days of fertilization (before the inner cell mass and chorion have formed), two embryos, two amnions, and two chorions will develop. This dichorionic-diamniotic situation occurs about 25% of the time, and there may be two distinct placentas or a single fused placenta.

2. If division occurs about 4 to 8 days after fertilization (when the inner cell mass has formed and the chorion cells have differentiated but those of the amnion have not), two embryos develop with separate amnion sacs. These sacs will eventually be covered by a common chorion; thus there will be a monochorionic-diamniotic placenta (see Figure 7–7B).

3. If the amnion has already developed, approximately 8 to 12 days after fertilization, division results in two embryos with a common amniotic sac and a common chorion (a monochorionic-monoamniotic placenta) (Cunningham et al., 2014). This type rarely occurs (Society of Maternal-Fetal Medicine (SMFM), Moise & Argon, 2013).

Monozygotic twinning is considered a random event and occurs in approximately 3 to 4 per 1000 live births (Blackburn, 2013). The survival rate of monozygotic twins as a group is 10% lower than that of dizygotic twins, and congenital anomalies are more prevalent. Both twins may have the same malformation.

Development and Functions of the Placenta

The **placenta** is the means of metabolic and nutrient exchange between the embryonic and maternal circulations. Placental development and circulation do not begin until the third

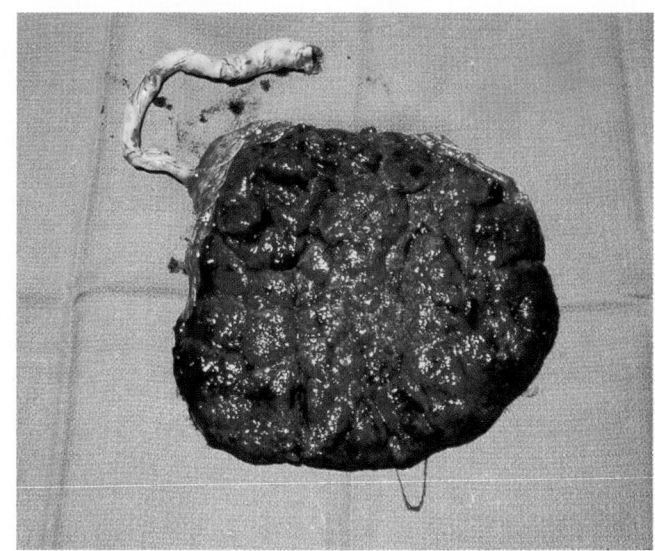

Figure 7–8 **Maternal side of placenta.**

SOURCE: M. London.

week of embryonic development. The placenta develops at the site where the embryo attaches to the uterine wall. Expansion of the placenta continues until about 20 weeks, when it covers approximately one half of the internal surface of the uterus. After 20 weeks' gestation, the placenta becomes thicker but not wider. At 40 weeks' gestation, the placenta is about 15 to 20 cm (5.9 to 7.9 in.) in diameter and 2.5 to 3.0 cm (1.0 to 1.2 in.) in thickness. At that time, it weighs about 400 to 600 g (14 to 21 oz).

The placenta has two parts: the maternal and fetal portions. The maternal portion consists of the decidua basalis and its circulation. Its surface is red and fleshlike (often called *Dirty Duncan*). The fetal portion consists of the chorionic villi and their circulation. The fetal surface of the placenta is covered by the amnion, which gives it a shiny, gray appearance (often called *Shiny Schultze*) (Figures 7–8 and 7–9).

Development of the placenta begins with the chorionic villi. The trophoblastic cells of the chorionic villi form spaces in the tissue of the decidua basalis. These spaces fill with maternal

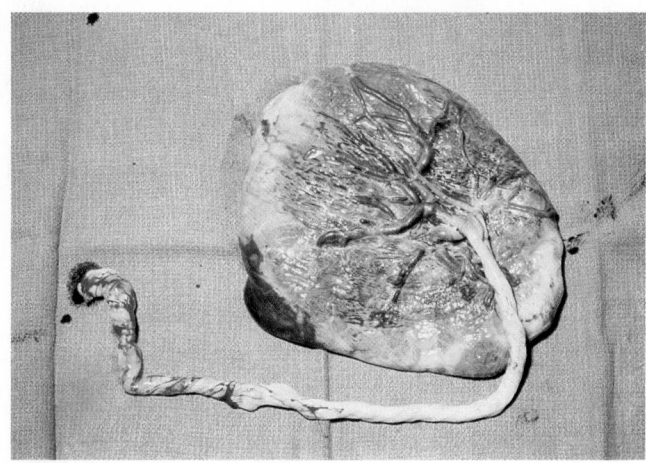

Figure 7–9 **Fetal side of placenta.**

SOURCE: M. London.

blood, and the chorionic villi grow into them. As the chorionic villi differentiate, two trophoblastic layers appear: an outer layer, called the *syncytium* (consisting of syncytiotrophoblasts), and an inner layer, known as the *cytotrophoblast* (see Figure 7–4). The cytotrophoblast thins out and disappears about the fifth month, leaving only a single layer of syncytium covering the chorionic villi. The syncytium is in direct contact with the maternal blood in the intervillous spaces. It is the functional layer of the placenta and secretes the placental hormones of pregnancy.

A third, inner layer of connective mesoderm develops in the chorionic villi, forming *anchoring villi*. These anchoring villi eventually form the *septa* (partitions) of the placenta. The septa divide the mature placenta into 15 to 20 segments called **cotyledons** (subdivisions of the placenta made up of anchoring villi and decidual tissue). In each cotyledon, the *branching villi* form a highly complex vascular system that allows compartmentalization of the uteroplacental circulation. The exchange of gases and nutrients takes place across these vascular systems.

Exchange of substances across the placenta is minimal during the first 3 to 5 months of development because the villous membrane is initially too thick, which limits its permeability. As the villous membrane thins, placental permeability increases until about the last month of pregnancy, when permeability begins to decrease as the placenta ages. In the fully developed placenta, fetal blood in the villi and maternal blood in the intervillous spaces are separated by three to four thin layers of tissue.

Placental Circulation

The completion of the maternal–placental–embryonic circulation occurs about 17 days after conception, when the embryonic heart begins functioning (Moore et al., 2016). By the end of the fourth week, embryonic blood is circulating between the embryo and the chorionic villi. The placenta has begun to function as a means of metabolic exchange between embryo and mother. By 14 weeks, the placenta is a discrete organ. It has grown in thickness as a result of growth in the length and size of the chorionic villi and accompanying expansion of the intervillous space.

In the fully developed placenta's umbilical cord, fetal blood flows through the two umbilical arteries to the capillaries of the villi, and oxygen-enriched blood flows back through the umbilical vein into the fetus (Figure 7–10). Late in pregnancy, a soft blowing sound (*funic souffle*) can be heard over the area of the umbilical cord. The sound is synchronous with the fetal heartbeat and fetal blood flow through the umbilical arteries.

Maternal blood, rich in oxygen and nutrients, spurts from the arcuate artery to the radial artery to the spiral uterine arteries and then spurts into the intervillous spaces. These spurts are produced by the maternal blood pressure. The spurt of blood is directed toward the chorionic plate, and as the blood loses pressure, it becomes lateral (spreads out). Fresh blood enters continuously and exerts pressure on the contents of the intervillous spaces, pushing blood toward the exits in the basal plate. The blood then drains through the uterine and other pelvic veins. A *uterine souffle*, timed precisely with the mother's pulse, is also heard just above the mother's symphysis pubis during the last months of pregnancy. This uterine souffle is caused by the augmented blood flow entering the dilated uterine arteries.

Braxton Hicks contractions are intermittent painless uterine contractions that may occur every 10 to 20 minutes and occur more frequently near the end of pregnancy (see Chapter 16). These contractions are believed to facilitate placental circulation by enhancing the movement of blood from the center of the cotyledon through the intervillous space. Placental blood flow is enhanced when the woman is lying on her side because

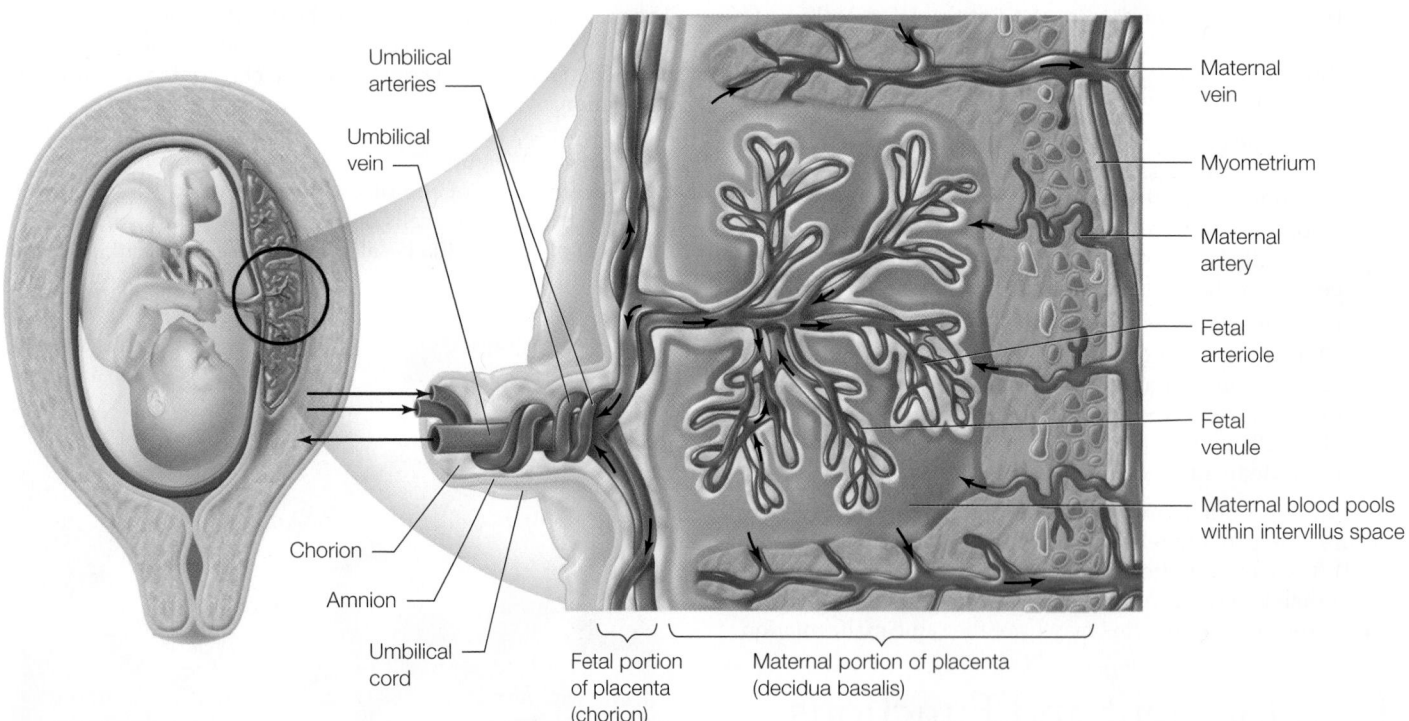

Figure 7–10 Vascular arrangement of the placenta. Arrows indicate the direction of blood flow. Maternal blood flows through the uterine arteries to the intervillous spaces of the placenta and returns through the uterine veins to maternal circulation. Fetal blood flows through the umbilical arteries into the villous capillaries of the placenta and returns through the umbilical vein to the fetal circulation.

venous return from the lower extremities is not compromised (Blackburn, 2013).

Placental Functions

Placental exchange functions occur only in those fetal vessels that are in intimate contact with the covering syncytial membrane. The syncytium villi have brush borders containing many microvilli, which greatly increase the exchange rate between maternal and fetal circulation (Blackburn, 2013; Sadler, 2015).

The placental functions, many of which begin soon after implantation, include fetal respiration, nutrition, and excretion. To carry out these functions, the placenta is involved in metabolic and transfer activities. In addition, it has endocrine functions and special immunologic properties; see discussion later in this section.

METABOLIC ACTIVITIES

The placenta performs several essential metabolic activities:

- Produces glycogen, cholesterol, and fatty acids continuously for fetal use and hormone production
- Produces numerous enzymes required for fetoplacental transfer, including sulfatase, which enhances excretion of fetal estrogen precursors, and insulinase, which increases the barrier to insulin
- Breaks down certain substances such as epinephrine and histamine (Blackburn, 2013)
- Stores glycogen and iron

TRANSPORT FUNCTION

The placental membranes actively control the transfer of a wide range of substances by a variety of transport mechanisms, such as:

- *Simple diffusion* moves substances from an area of higher concentration to an area of lower concentration. Substances that move across the placenta by simple diffusion include water, oxygen, carbon dioxide, electrolytes (sodium and chloride), anesthetic gases, and drugs. Insulin, steroid hormones originating from the adrenals, and thyroid hormones also cross the placenta but at a very slow rate. Unfortunately, many substances of abuse, such as cocaine and heroin, cross the placenta via simple diffusion. The rate of oxygen transfer across the placental membrane is greater than that allowed by simple diffusion, indicating that oxygen is also transferred by some type of facilitated diffusion transport.
- *Facilitated transport* involves a carrier system to move molecules from an area of greater concentration to an area of lower concentration. Molecules such as glucose, galactose, and some oxygen are transported by this method. The glucose level in the fetal blood ordinarily is approximately 20% to 30% lower than the glucose level in the maternal blood because the fetus is metabolizing glucose rapidly. This in turn causes rapid transport of additional glucose (facilitated by insulin) from the maternal blood into the fetal blood.
- *Active transport* can work against a concentration gradient and allows molecules to move from areas of lower concentration to areas of higher concentration. Amino acids, calcium, iron, iodine, water-soluble vitamins, and glucose are transferred across the placenta in this way. The measured amino acid content of fetal blood is greater than that of maternal blood, and calcium and inorganic phosphate occur in greater concentration in fetal blood than in maternal blood (Blackburn, 2013).

Other modes of transfer also exist. *Pinocytosis* is important for transferring large molecules such as albumin and gamma globulin. Materials are engulfed by amoeba-like cells, forming plasma droplets. *Hydrostatic* and *osmotic pressures* allow the bulk flow of water and some solutes. Fetal red blood cells pass into the maternal circulation through breaks in the capillaries and placental membrane, particularly during labor and birth. Certain cells, such as maternal leukocytes, and microorganisms, such as viruses (e.g., HIV, which causes AIDS; that causing rubella; cytomegalovirus; and poliovirus) and the bacterium *Treponema pallidum* (which causes syphilis), can also cross the placental membrane under their own power (Moore et al., 2016). Some bacteria and protozoa infect the placenta by causing lesions and then entering the fetal blood system.

Reduction of the placental surface area, as with abruptio placentae (partial or complete premature separation of an abnormally implanted placenta), decreases the area that is functional for exchange. Placental diffusion distance also affects exchange. In conditions such as diabetes and placental infection, edema of the villi increases the diffusion distance, thus increasing the distance the substance has to be transferred.

Blood flow alteration changes the transfer rate of substances. Decreased blood flow in the intervillous space is seen in labor and with certain maternal diseases such as hypertension. Mild fetal hypoxia increases the umbilical blood flow, but severe hypoxia results in decreased blood flow.

As the maternal blood picks up fetal waste products and carbon dioxide, it drains back into the maternal circulation through the veins in the basal plate. Fetal blood is hypoxic by comparison; it therefore attracts oxygen from the mother's blood. Affinity for oxygen increases as the fetal blood gives up its carbon dioxide, which also decreases its acidity.

ENDOCRINE FUNCTIONS

The placenta produces hormones that are vital to the survival of the fetus. These include human chorionic gonadotropin (hCG), human placental lactogen (hPL), also referred to as human chorionic somatomammotropin (hCS), relaxin, inhibin, and two steroid hormones, estrogen and progesterone.

The hormone hCG is similar to luteinizing hormone (LH) and prevents the normal involution of the corpus luteum at the end of the menstrual cycle. If the corpus luteum stops functioning before the 11th week of pregnancy, spontaneous abortion occurs. hCG also causes the corpus luteum to secrete increased amounts of estrogen and progesterone.

After the 11th week, the placenta produces enough progesterone and estrogen to maintain pregnancy. In the male fetus, hCG also exerts an interstitial cell–stimulating effect on the testes, resulting in the production of testosterone. This small secretion of testosterone during embryonic development is the factor that causes male sex organs to grow. hCG may play a role in the trophoblast's immunologic capabilities (its ability to keep the mother's system from rejecting the placenta and embryo). This hormone is used as a basis for pregnancy tests (see Chapter 8).

hCG is present in maternal blood serum 8 to 10 days after fertilization, just as soon as implantation has occurred, and is detectable in maternal urine at the time of missed menses. After reaching its maximum level at 50 to 70 days' gestation, hCG begins to decrease as placental hormone production increases.

Progesterone is an essential hormone for pregnancy. It increases the secretions of the fallopian tubes and uterus to provide appropriate nutritive matter for the developing morula and blastocyst. It also appears to aid in ovum transport through the fallopian tube. Progesterone causes decidual cells to develop in the uterine endometrium, and it must be present in high levels for implantation to occur. Progesterone also decreases the contractility of the uterus, thus preventing uterine contractions from causing spontaneous abortion.

Before stimulation by hCG, production of progesterone by the corpus luteum reaches a peak about 7 to 10 days after ovulation. Implantation occurs at about the same time as this peak. At 16 days after ovulation, progesterone reaches a level between 25 and 50 mg per day and continues to rise slowly in subsequent weeks. After 11 weeks, the placenta (specifically, the syncytiotrophoblast) takes over the production of progesterone and secretes it in tremendous quantities, reaching levels of more than 250 mg per day late in pregnancy.

By 7 weeks, the placenta produces more than 50% of the estrogens in the maternal circulation. *Estrogens* serve mainly a proliferative function, causing enlargement of the uterus, breasts, and breast glandular tissue. Estrogens also have a significant role in increasing vascularity and vasodilation, particularly in the villous capillaries toward the end of pregnancy. Placental estrogens increase markedly toward the end of pregnancy, to as much as 30 times the daily production in the middle of a normal monthly menstrual cycle. The primary estrogen secreted by the placenta *(estriol)* is different from the estrogen secreted by the ovaries *(estradiol)*. The placenta cannot synthesize estriol by itself. Essential precursors such as dehydroepiandrosterone sulfate (DHEAS) are provided by the fetal adrenal glands, are processed by fetal liver, and are transported to the placenta for the final conversion to estrone, estradiol, and estriol (Blackburn, 2013).

The hormone hPL is similar to human pituitary growth hormone in that hPL stimulates certain changes in the mother's metabolic processes. These changes ensure that more protein, glucose, and minerals are available for the fetus. Secretion of hPL can be detected by about 4 weeks after conception.

Relaxin acts to quiet the myometrium, facilitates the decidual reaction, remodels collagen, softens the cervix, and softens ligaments and cartilage in the skeletal system (Blackburn, 2013; Caudle, 2014). Inhibin, another glycoprotein, is produced by the trophoblast. In combination with the sex steroids, inhibin decreases the secretion of follicle-stimulating hormone from the pituitary gland, thereby stopping ovulation during the pregnancy.

IMMUNOLOGIC PROPERTIES

The placenta and embryo are transplants of living tissue within the same species and are therefore considered *homografts*. Unlike other homografts, the placenta and embryo appear exempt from immunologic reaction by the host. Most recent data suggest that the placental hormones (progesterone and hCG) suppress cellular immunity during pregnancy. One theory suggests that chorionic villi syncytiotrophoblastic tissue is immunologically inert. The chorionic villi may lack major histocompatibility (MHC) antigens and thus do not evoke rejection responses. They do, however, protect against antibody formation. Extravillous trophoblast (EVT) cells, which invade the uterine deciduas, have human leukocyte antigen (HLA-G), which is not readily recognized by sensitized T lymphocytes and natural killer cells (Blackburn, 2013).

Development of the Fetal Circulatory System

The circulatory system of the fetus has several unique features that, by maintaining the blood flow to the placenta, provide the fetus with oxygen and nutrients while removing carbon dioxide and other waste products.

Most of the blood supply bypasses the fetal lungs because they do not carry out respiratory gas exchange. The placenta assumes the function of the fetal lungs by supplying oxygen and allowing the fetus to excrete carbon dioxide into the maternal bloodstream. Figure 7–11 shows the fetal circulatory system. The blood from the placenta flows through the umbilical vein, which enters the abdominal wall of the fetus at the site that, after birth, is the umbilicus (belly button). As umbilical venous blood approaches the liver, a small portion of the blood enters the liver sinusoids, mixes with blood from the portal circulation, and then enters the inferior vena cava via hepatic veins. Most of the umbilical vein's blood flows through the **ductus venosus** directly into the fetal inferior vena cava, bypassing the liver. This blood then enters the right atrium, passes through the **foramen ovale** into the left atrium, and pours into the left ventricle, which pumps blood into the aorta. Some blood returning from the head and upper extremities by way of the superior vena cava is emptied into the right atrium and passes through the tricuspid valve into the right ventricle. This blood is pumped into the pulmonary artery, and a small amount passes to the lungs for nourishment only. The larger portion of blood passes from the pulmonary artery through the **ductus arteriosus** into the descending aorta, bypassing the lungs. Finally, blood returns to the placenta through the two umbilical arteries, and the process is repeated.

The fetus obtains oxygen via diffusion from the maternal circulation because of the gradient difference of PO_2 of 50 mmHg in maternal blood in the placenta to 30 mmHg PO_2 in the fetus. At term, the fetus receives oxygen from the mother's circulation at a rate of 20 to 30 mL per minute (Sadler, 2015). Fetal hemoglobin facilitates obtaining oxygen from the maternal circulation because it carries as much as 20% to 30% more oxygen than adult hemoglobin.

Fetal circulation delivers the highest available oxygen concentration to the head, neck, brain, and heart (coronary circulation) and a lesser amount of oxygenated blood to the abdominal organs and the lower body. This circulatory pattern leads to cephalocaudal (head-to-tail) development in the fetus.

Embryonic and Fetal Development

Pregnancy is calculated to last an *average* of 10 lunar months: 40 weeks, or 280 days. This period of 280 days is calculated from the onset of the last normal menstrual period to the time of birth. Many obstetric units in the United States and Australia use a combination of menstrual dates and ultrasonographic dates to perform this calculation. Estimated date of birth (EDB), sometimes referred to as the *estimated date of delivery* (EDD), is usually calculated by this method. Most fetuses are born within 10 to 14 days of the calculated date of birth. The postconception age (fertilization age) of the fetus is calculated to be *about* 2 weeks less, or 266 days (38 weeks) or 9.5 calendar months. The latter measurement is more accurate because it measures time from the fertilization of the ovum, or conception. See Chapter 9 for a detailed discussion of due date determination, including Nägele's rule.

The basic events of organ development in the embryo and fetus are outlined in Table 7–3. The time periods in the table are **postconception age periods**. During the period from fertilization to the end of the embryonic period (8 weeks), age is often expressed in days but can be given in weeks. During the fetal period (ninth week until birth), age is given in weeks (Moore et al., 2016). The National Institute for Health and Clinical Excellence (NICE) (2011) guidelines state that the crown-to-rump (C–R)

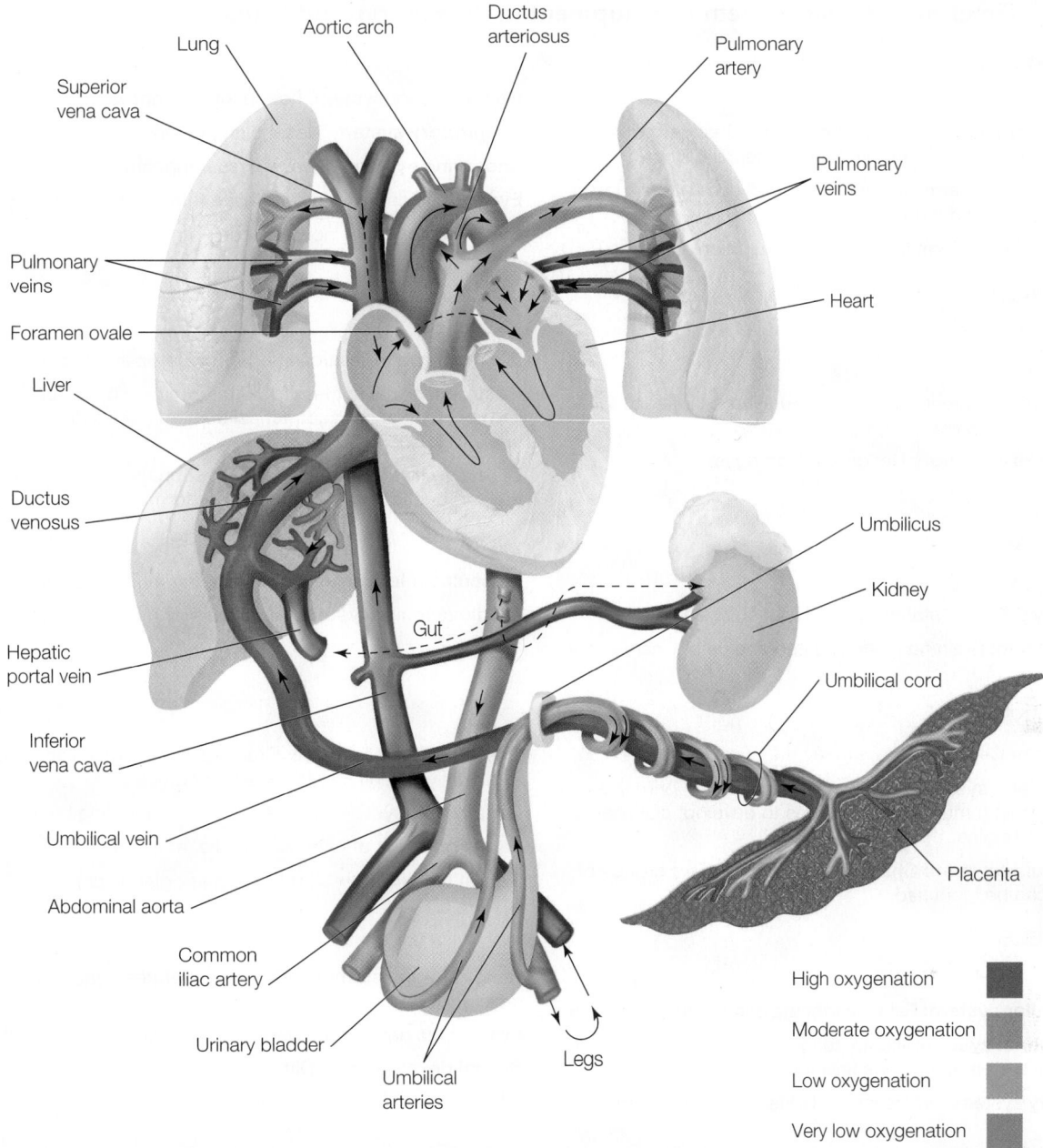

Figure 7–11 **Fetal circulation. Blood leaves the placenta and enters the fetus through the umbilical vein. After circulating through the fetus, the blood returns to the placenta through the umbilical arteries. The ductus venosus, the foramen ovale, and the ductus arteriosus allow the blood to bypass the fetal liver and lungs.**

length should be used to determine gestational age, and if the C–R length is greater than 84 mm, the head circumference (HC) should be used instead.

In review, human development follows three stages. The pre-embryonic stage, as discussed earlier in the chapter, consists of the first 14 days of development after the ovum is fertilized; then the embryonic stage covers the period from day 15 until approximately the end of the eighth week postconception, and the fetal stage extends from the end of the eighth week until birth.

Embryonic Stage

The stage of the **embryo** starts on day 15 (the beginning of the third week after conception) and continues until approximately the eighth week, or until the embryo reaches a crown-to-rump (C–R) length of 3 cm (1.2 in.). This length is usually reached

about 56 days after fertilization (the end of the eighth gestational week). During the embryonic stage, tissues differentiate into essential organs, and the main external features develop. The embryo is the most vulnerable to *teratogens* during this period. These are discussed in more depth later in the chapter.

3 WEEKS

In the third week, the embryonic disc becomes elongated and pear shaped, with a broad cephalic end and a narrow caudal end. The ectoderm has formed a long cylindrical tube for brain and spinal cord development. The gastrointestinal tract, created from the endoderm, appears as another tubelike structure communicating with the yolk sac. The most advanced organ is the heart. At 3 weeks, a single tubular heart forms just outside the body cavity of the embryo.

TABLE 7–3 Timeline of Organ System Development in the Embryo and Fetus

AGE: 2–3 WEEKS

Length: 2 mm C–R (crown-to-rump)

Nervous system: Groove forms along middle back as cells thicken; neural tube forms from closure of neural groove.

Cardiovascular system: Beginning of blood circulation; tubular heart begins to form during third week.

Gastrointestinal system: Liver begins to function.

Genitourinary system: Formation of kidneys beginning.

Respiratory system: Nasal pits forming.

Endocrine system: Thyroid tissue appears.

Eyes: Optic cup and lens pit have formed; pigment in eyes.

Ears: Auditory pit is now enclosed structure.

AGE: 4 WEEKS

Length: 4–6 mm C–R

Weight: 0.4 g

Nervous system: Anterior portion of neural tube closes to form brain; closure of posterior end forms spinal cord.

Musculoskeletal system: Noticeable limb buds.

Cardiovascular system: Tubular heartbeats at 28 days, and primitive red blood cells circulate through fetus and chorionic villi.

Gastrointestinal system: Mouth: formation of oral cavity; primitive jaws present; esophagotracheal septum begins division of esophagus and trachea.

Digestive tract: Stomach forms; esophagus and intestine become tubular; ducts of pancreas and liver forming.

AGE: 5 WEEKS

Length: 8 mm C–R

Weight: Only 0.5% of total body weight is fat (to 20 weeks).

Nervous system: Brain has differentiated and cranial nerves are present.

Musculoskeletal system: Developing muscles have innervation.

Cardiovascular system: Atrial division has occurred.

AGE: 6 WEEKS

Length: 12 mm C–R

Musculoskeletal system: Bone rudiments present; primitive skeletal shape forming; muscle mass begins to develop; ossification of skull and jaws begins.

Cardiovascular system: Chambers present in heart; groups of blood cells can be identified.

Gastrointestinal system: Oral and nasal cavities and upper lip formed; liver begins to form red blood cells.

Respiratory system: Trachea, bronchi, and lung buds present.

Ears: Formation of external, middle, and inner ear continues.

Sexual development: Embryonic sex glands appear.

AGE: 7 WEEKS

Length: 18 mm C–R

Cardiovascular system: Fetal heartbeats can be detected.

Gastrointestinal system: Mouth: tongue separates; palate folds. Digestive tract: stomach attains final form.

Genitourinary system: Separation of bladder and urethra from rectum.

Respiratory system: Diaphragm separates abdominal and thoracic cavities.

Eyes: Optic nerve formed; eyelids appear, thickening of lens.

Sexual development: Differentiation of sex glands into ovaries and testes begins.

AGE: 8 WEEKS

Length: 2.5–3.0 cm C–R

Weight: 2 g

Musculoskeletal system: Digits formed; further differentiation of cells in primitive skeleton; cartilaginous bones show first signs of ossification; development of muscles in trunk, limbs, and head; some movement of fetus now possible.

Cardiovascular system: Development of heart essentially complete; fetal circulation follows two circuits—four extraembryonic and two intraembryonic. Heartbeat can be heard with Doppler at 8–12 weeks.

Gastrointestinal system: Mouth: completion of lip fusion. Digestive tract: rotation in midgut; anal membrane has perforated.

Ears: External, middle, and inner ear assuming final forms.

Sexual development: Male and female external genitals appear similar until end of ninth week.

AGE: 10 WEEKS

Length: 5–6 cm C–R

Weight: 14 g

Nervous system: Neurons appear at caudal end of spinal cord; basic divisions of brain present.

Musculoskeletal system: Fingers and toes begin nail growth.

Gastrointestinal system: Mouth: separation of lips from jaw; fusion of palate folds.

Digestive tract: Developing intestines enclosed in abdomen.

Genitourinary system: Bladder sac formed.

Endocrine system: Islets of Langerhans differentiated.

Eyes: Eyelids fused closed; development of lacrimal duct.

Sexual development: Males: production of testosterone and physical characteristics between 8 and 12 weeks.

AGE: 12 WEEKS

Length: 8 cm C–R; 11.5 cm C–H (crown-to-heel)

Weight: 45 g

Musculoskeletal system: Clear outlining of miniature bones (12–20 weeks); process of ossification is established throughout fetal body; appearance of involuntary muscles in viscera.

Gastrointestinal system: Mouth: completion of palate.

Digestive tract: Appearance of muscles in gut; bile secretion begins; liver is major producer of red blood cells.

Respiratory system: Lungs acquire definitive shape.

Skin: Pink and delicate.

Endocrine system: Hormonal secretion from thyroid; insulin present in pancreas.

Immunologic system: Appearance of lymphoid tissue in fetal thymus gland.

AGE: 16 WEEKS

Length: 13.5 cm C–R; 15 cm C–H

Weight: 200 g

Musculoskeletal system: Teeth beginning to form hard tissue that will become central incisors.

Gastrointestinal system: Mouth: differentiation of hard and soft palate.

Digestive tract: Development of gastric and intestinal glands; intestines begin to collect meconium.

Genitourinary system: Kidneys assume typical shape and organization.

Skin: Appearance of scalp hair; lanugo present on body; transparent skin with visible blood vessels; sweat glands developing.

Eyes, ears, and nose: Formed.

Sexual development: Sex determination possible.

AGE: 18 WEEKS

Musculoskeletal system: Teeth beginning to form hard tissue (enamel and dentine) that will become lateral incisors.

Cardiovascular system: Fetal heart tones audible with fetoscope at 16–20 weeks.

AGE: 20 WEEKS

Length: 19 cm C–R; 25 cm C–H

Weight: 435 g (6% of total body weight is fat).

Nervous system: Myelination of spinal cord begins.

Musculoskeletal system: Teeth beginning to form hard tissue that will become canines and first molars. Lower limbs are of final relative proportions.

Gastrointestinal system: Fetus actively sucks and swallows amniotic fluid; peristaltic movements begin.

Skin: Lanugo covers entire body; brown fat begins to form; vernix caseosa begins to form.

Immunologic system: Detectable levels of fetal antibodies (IgG type).

Blood formation: Iron is stored and bone marrow is increasingly important.

AGE: 24 WEEKS

Length: 23 cm C–R; 28 cm C–H

Weight: 780 g

Nervous system: Brain looks like mature brain.

Musculoskeletal system: Teeth are beginning to form hard tissue that will become the second molars.

Respiratory system: Respiratory movements may occur (24–40 weeks). Nostrils reopen. Alveoli appear in lungs and begin production of surfactant; gas exchange possible.

Skin: Reddish and wrinkled, vernix caseosa present.

Immunologic system: IgG levels reach maternal levels.

AGE: 28 WEEKS

Length: 27 cm C–R; 35 cm C–H

Weight: 1200–1250 g

Nervous system: Begins regulation of some body functions.

Skin: Adipose tissue accumulates rapidly; nails appear; eyebrows and eyelashes present.

Eyes: Eyelids open (26–29 weeks).

Sexual development: Males: testes descend into inguinal canal and upper scrotum.

AGE: 32 WEEKS

Length: 31 cm C–R; 38–43 cm C–H

Weight: 2000 g

Nervous system: More reflexes present.

AGE: 36 WEEKS

Length: 35 cm C–R; 42–48 cm C–H

Weight: 2500–2750 g

Musculoskeletal system: Distal femoral ossification centers present.

Skin: Pale; body rounded, lanugo disappearing, hair fuzzy or woolly; few sole creases; sebaceous glands active and helping to produce vernix caseosa (36–40 weeks).

Ears: Earlobes soft with little cartilage.

Sexual development: Males: scrotum small and few rugae present; descent of testes into upper scrotum to stay (36–40 weeks). Females: labia majora and minora equally prominent.

(continued)

TABLE 7–3 Timeline of Organ System Development in the Embryo and Fetus (*continued*)

AGE: 38–40 WEEKS	
Length: 40 cm C–R; 48–52 cm C–H	**Skin:** Smooth and pink; vernix present in skin folds; moderate to profuse silky hair; lanugo on shoulders and upper back; nails extend over tips or digits; creases cover sole.
Weight: 3200+ g (16% of total body weight is fat).	
Respiratory system: At 38 weeks, lecithin–sphingomyelin (L/S) ratio approaches 2:1 (indicates decreased risk of respiratory distress from inadequate surfactant production if born now).	**Ears:** Earlobes firmer because of increased cartilage.
	Sexual development: Males: rugous scrotum. Females: labia majora well developed and minora small or completely covered.

Note: *Age* refers to postfertilization or postconception age. Measurements are an average.

Sources: Data from Moore, K. L., Persaud, T. V. N., & Torchia, M. G. (2016). *The developing human: Clinical oriented embryology* (10th ed.). Philadelphia, PA: Saunders/Elsevier; Sadler, T. W. (2015). *Langman's medical embryology* (13th ed.). Philadelphia, PA: Lippincott Williams & Wilkins.

4 TO 5 WEEKS

During days 21 to 32, *somites* (a series of mesodermal blocks) form on either side of the embryo's midline. The vertebrae that form the spinal column will develop from these somites. Before 28 days, arm and leg buds are not visible, but the tail bud is present. The pharyngeal arches—which will form the lower jaw, hyoid bone, and larynx—develop at this time. The pharyngeal pouches appear now; these pouches will form the eustachian tube and cavity of the middle ear, the tonsils, and the parathyroid and thymus glands. The primordia of the ear and eye are also present. By the end of 28 days, the tubular heart is beating at a regular rhythm and pushing its own primitive blood cells through the main blood vessels.

During the fifth week, the optic cups and lens vessels of the eye form and the nasal pits develop. Partitioning in the heart occurs with the dividing of the atrium. The embryo has a marked C-shaped body, accentuated by the rudimentary tail and the large head folded over a protuberant trunk (Figure 7–12). By day 35, the arm and leg buds are well developed, with paddle-shaped hand and foot plates. The heart, circulatory system, and brain show the most advanced development. The brain has differentiated into five areas, and 10 pairs of cranial nerves are recognizable.

6 WEEKS

At 6 weeks, the head structures are more highly developed and the trunk is straighter than in earlier stages. The upper and lower jaws are recognizable, and the external nares are well formed. The trachea has developed, and its caudal end is bifurcated for beginning lung formation. The upper lip has formed, and the palate is developing. The ears are developing rapidly. The arms have begun to extend ventrally across the chest, and both arms and legs have digits, although they may still be webbed. There is a slight elbow bend in the arms, which are more advanced in development than the legs. Beginning at this stage, the prominent tail will recede. The heart now has most of its definitive characteristics, and fetal circulation begins to be established. The liver starts to produce blood cells.

7 WEEKS

At 7 weeks, the head of the embryo is rounded and nearly erect (Figure 7–13). The eyes have shifted and are closer together, and the eyelids are beginning to form. The palate is near completion, and the tongue is developing in the formed mouth. The gastrointestinal and genitourinary tracts undergo significant changes during the seventh week. Before this time, the rectal and urogenital passages formed one tube that ended in a blind pouch; they now separate into two tubular structures. The intestines enter the extraembryonic coelom in the area of the umbilical cord (called *umbilical herniation*) (Moore et al., 2016). The beginnings of all essential external and internal structures are present.

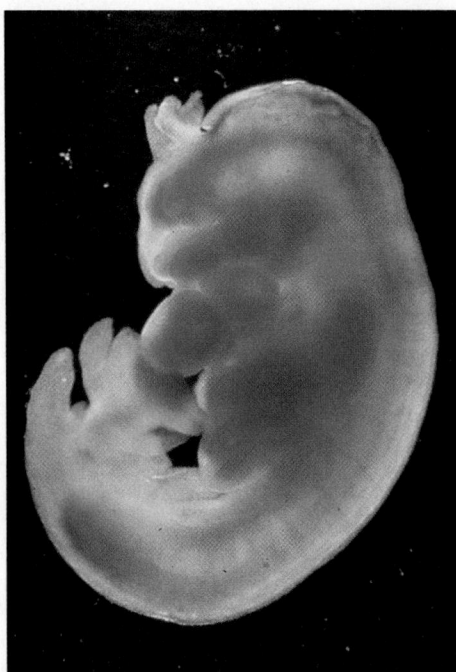

Figure 7–12 The embryo at 5 weeks. The embryo has a marked C-shaped body and a rudimentary tail.

SOURCE: Omikron/Getty Images.

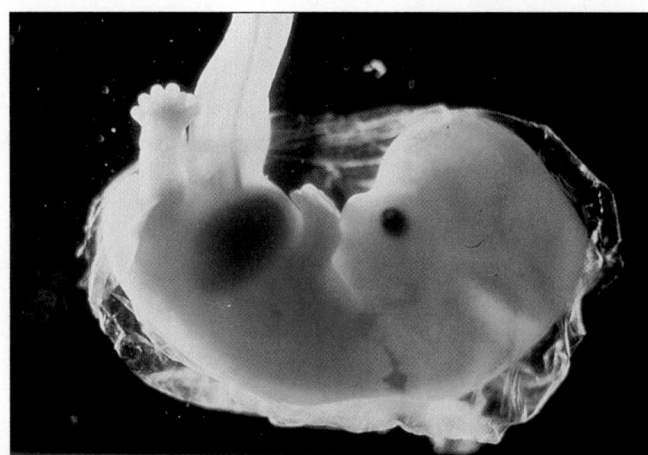

Figure 7–13 The embryo at 7 weeks. The head is rounded and nearly erect. The eyes have shifted forward and closer together, and the eyelids begin to form.

SOURCE: Petit Format/Science Source.

8 WEEKS

At 8 weeks, the embryo is approximately 3 cm (1.2 in.) C–R length and clearly resembles a human being. Facial features continue to develop. The eyelids begin to fuse. Auricles of the external ears begin to assume their final shape, but they are still set low (Moore et al., 2016). External genitals appear, but the embryo's sex is not clearly identifiable. The rectal passage opens with the perforation of the anal membrane. The circulatory system through the umbilical cord is well established. Long bones are beginning to form, and the large muscles are now capable of contracting.

Fetal Stage

By the end of the eighth week, the embryo is sufficiently developed to be called a **fetus**. Every organ system and external structure that will be found in the full-term newborn is present. The remainder of gestation is devoted to refining structures and perfecting function.

9 TO 12 WEEKS

By the end of the ninth week the fetus reaches a C–R length of 5 cm (2 in.) and weighs about 14 g (0.5 oz). The head is large and comprises almost half of the fetus's entire size (Figure 7–14). At 12 weeks, the fetus reaches 8 cm (3.2 in.) C–R length and weighs about 45 g (1.6 oz). The face is well formed, with the nose protruding, the chin small and receding, and the ear acquiring a more adult shape. The eyelids close at about the 10th week and will not reopen until about the 26- to 29-week period. Some movement of the lips suggestive of the sucking reflex has been observed at 3 months. Tooth buds now appear for all 20 of the child's first teeth (baby teeth). The limbs are long and slender, with well-formed digits. The fetus can curl its fingers toward its palm and begins to make a tiny fist. The legs are still shorter and less developed than the arms. The urogenital tract completes its development, well-differentiated genitals appear, and the kidneys begin to produce urine. Red blood cells are produced primarily by the liver. Spontaneous movements of the fetus now occur. Fetal heart rates can be ascertained by electronic devices between 8 and 12 weeks. The rate is 120 to 160 beats per minute.

13 TO 16 WEEKS

This is a period of rapid growth. At 13 weeks, the fetus weighs 55 to 60 g (1.9 to 2.1 oz) and is about 9 cm (3.6 in.) in C–R length. Lanugo, or fine hair, begins to develop, especially on the head. The skin is so transparent that blood vessels are clearly visible beneath it. More muscle tissue and body skeleton have

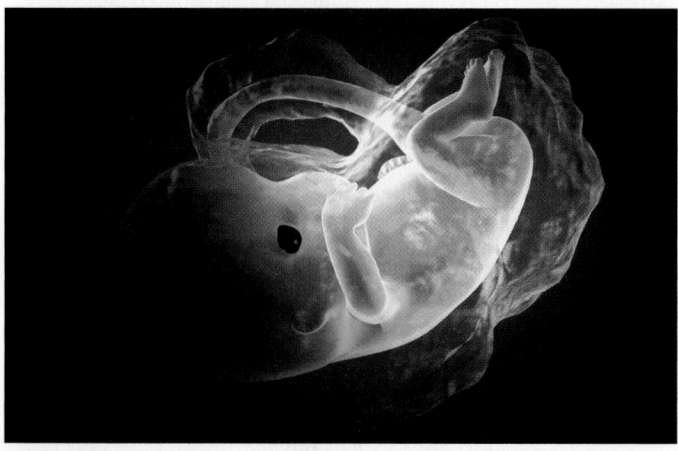

Figure 7–14 The fetus at 9 weeks. Every organ system and external structure is present.

SOURCE: MedicalRF.com/Corbis.

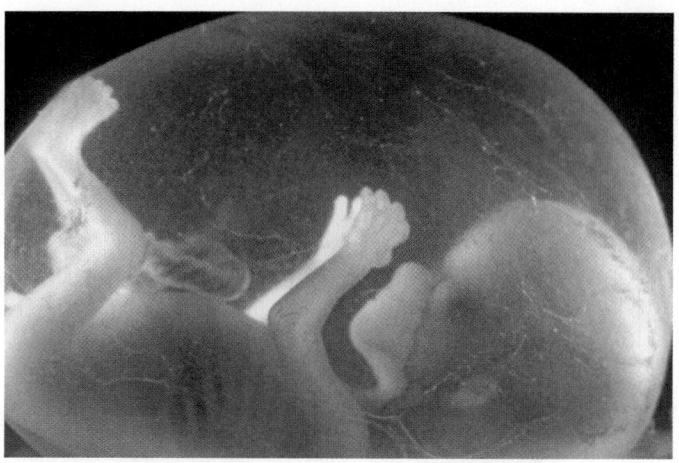

Figure 7–15 **The fetus at 14 weeks. During this period of rapid growth the skin is so transparent that blood vessels are visible beneath it. More muscle tissue and body skeleton have developed, and they hold the fetus more erect.**

SOURCE: Claude Edelmann/Science Source.

developed and hold the fetus more erect (Figure 7–15). Active movements are present; the fetus stretches and exercises its arms and legs. It makes sucking motions, swallows amniotic fluid, and produces meconium in the intestinal tract. Bronchial tubes are branching out in the primitive lungs, and sweat glands are developing. The liver and pancreas now begin producing their appropriate secretions. By the beginning of week 16, skeletal ossification is clearly identifiable.

20 WEEKS

The fetus doubles its C–R length and now measures 19 cm (7.5 in.) long. Fetal weight is between 435 and 465 g (15.2 and 16.3 oz). Lanugo covers the entire body and is especially prominent on the shoulders. Subcutaneous deposits of brown fat, which has a rich blood supply, make the skin less transparent. Brown fat is found chiefly at the root of the neck, posterior to the sternum, and in the perirenal area. Nipples now appear over the mammary glands. The head may be covered with fine, "woolly" hair, and the eyebrows and eyelashes are beginning to form. Nails are present on both fingers and toes. Muscles are well developed, and the fetus is active (Figure 7–16). The mother feels fetal movement, known as *quickening*. The fetal heartbeat is audible through a fetoscope. Quickening and fetal heartbeat can help in validating the EDB.

24 WEEKS

The fetus at 24 weeks reaches a C–R of 23 cm (9.2 in.) or crown-to-heel (C–H) length of 28 cm (11.2 in.). It weighs about 780 g (1 lb, 10 oz). The hair on the head is growing long, and eyebrows and eyelashes have formed. The eye is structurally complete and will soon open. The fetus has a reflex hand grip (grasp reflex) and, by the end of 6 months, a startle reflex. Skin covering the body is reddish and wrinkled, with little subcutaneous fat. Skin on the hands and feet have thickened, with skin ridges on the palms and soles forming distinct footprints and fingerprints. The skin over the entire body is covered with **vernix caseosa**, a protective cheeselike, fatty substance secreted by the sebaceous glands. The alveoli in the lungs are just beginning to form.

25 TO 28 WEEKS

At about 25 weeks, the fetal skin is still red, wrinkled, and covered with vernix caseosa. The brain is developing rapidly, and the

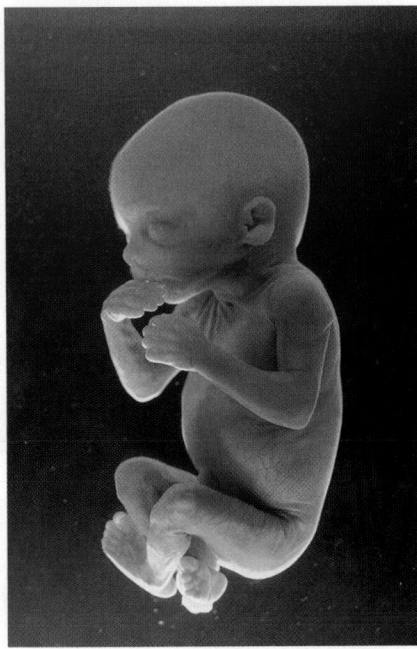

Figure 7–16 The fetus at 20 weeks. The fetus now weighs 435 to 465 g (15.2 to 16.3 oz) and measures about 19 cm (7.5 in.). Subcutaneous deposits of brown fat make the skin a little less transparent. "Woolly" hair may cover the head, and nails have developed on the fingers and toes.

SOURCE: James Stevenson/Science Source.

nervous system is complete enough to provide some degree of regulation of body functions. The eyelids, under neural control, open and close. The fetus has nails on both fingers and toes. In the male fetus, the testes begin to descend into the scrotal sac. Even though the lungs are still physiologically immature, they are sufficiently developed to provide gas exchange. A fetus born at this time will require immediate and prolonged intensive care to survive and then to decrease the risk of major handicap. The fetus at 28 weeks is about 27 cm (10.8 in.) C–R or 35 to 38 cm (14 to 15 in.) C–H and weighs 1200 to 1250 g (2 lb, 10.5 oz to 2 lb, 12 oz).

29 TO 32 WEEKS

At 30 weeks, the pupillary light reflex is present (Moore et al., 2016). The fetus is gaining weight from an increase in body muscle and fat and weighs about 2000 g (4 lb, 6.5 oz), with a C–R length of 31 cm (12.4 in.) or C–H length of about 38 to 43 cm (15 to 17 in.) by 32 weeks of age. The central nervous system (CNS) has matured enough to direct rhythmic breathing movements and partially control body temperature; however, the lungs are not yet fully mature. Bones are fully developed but soft and flexible. The fetus begins storing iron, calcium, and phosphorus. In males, the testicles may be located in the scrotal sac but are often still high in the inguinal canals.

35 TO 36 WEEKS

The fetus begins to become plump, and less wrinkled skin covers the deposits of subcutaneous fat. Lanugo begins to disappear, and the nails reach the edge of the fingertips. By 35 weeks of age, the fetus has a firm grasp and exhibits spontaneous orientation to light. By 36 weeks of age, its weight is usually 2500 to 2750 g (5 lb, 12 oz to 6 lb, 11.5 oz), and the C–H length of the fetus is about 42 to 48 cm (17 to 19 in.) or C–R 35 cm (14 in.). A baby born at this time has a good chance of surviving but may require special care, especially if there is intrauterine growth restriction.

38 TO 40 WEEKS

The fetus is considered full term at 38 weeks and up to 40 weeks after conception. The C–H length varies from 48 to 52 cm (19 to 21 in.) or C–R of 40 cm (16 in.), with males usually being longer than females. Males also usually weigh more than females. The weight at term is about 3000 to 3600 g (6 lb, 10 oz to 7 lb, 15 oz) and varies in different ethnic groups. The skin is pink and has a smooth, polished look. The only lanugo left is on the upper arms and shoulders. The hair on the head is no longer woolly but is coarse and about 1 in. long. Vernix caseosa is present, with heavier deposits remaining in the creases and folds of the skin. The body and extremities are plump, with good skin turgor, and the fingernails extend beyond the fingertips. The chest is prominent but still a little smaller than the head, and mammary glands protrude in both sexes. In males, the testes are in the scrotum or palpable in the inguinal canals.

As the fetus enlarges, amniotic fluid diminishes to about an average of 400 mL, and the fetal body mass fills the uterine cavity (Blackburn, 2013). The fetus assumes what is called its *position of comfort*, or lie. The head is generally pointed downward, following the shape of the uterus (and possibly because the head is heavier than the feet). The extremities, and often the head, are well flexed. After 5 months, patterns in feeding, sleeping, and activity become established, so at term the fetus has its own body rhythms and individual style of response. See Table 7–4 for important developmental milestones. For a detailed discussion of each body system's transition to full functioning in the newborn, see Chapter 23.

TABLE 7–4 Fetal Development: What Parents Want to Know

4 weeks:	The fetal heart begins to beat.
8 weeks:	All body organs are formed.
8–12 weeks:	Fetal heart rate can be heard by ultrasound Doppler device.
16 weeks:	Baby's sex can be seen. Although thin, the fetus looks like a baby.
20 weeks:	Heartbeat can be heard with fetoscope. Mother feels movement (quickening). Baby develops a regular schedule of sleeping, sucking, and kicking. Hands can grasp. Baby assumes a favorite position in utero. Vernix caseosa (lanolin-like covering) protects the body, and lanugo (fine hair) keeps oil on skin. Head hair, eyebrows, and eyelashes present.
24 weeks:	Weighs 780 g (1 lb, 10 oz). Activity is increasing. Fetal respiratory movements begin. Baby makes sucking movements.
28 weeks:	Eyes open and close. Baby can breathe at this time. Surfactant needed for breathing at birth is formed. Baby is two thirds its final length.
32 weeks:	Baby has fingernails and toenails. Subcutaneous fat is being laid down. Baby appears less red and wrinkled.
38+ weeks:	Baby fills total uterus. Baby gets antibodies from mother.

Factors Influencing Embryonic and Fetal Development

Factors that may affect embryonic development include the quality of the sperm or ovum from which the zygote was formed, the genetic code established at fertilization, and the adequacy of the intrauterine environment. If the environment is unsuitable before cellular differentiation occurs, all the cells of the zygote are affected. The cells may die, which causes spontaneous abortion, or growth may be slowed, depending on the severity of the situation. When differentiation is complete and the fetal membranes have formed, an injurious agent has the greatest effect on those cells undergoing the most rapid growth. Thus the time of injury is critical in the development of anomalies.

Because organs are formed primarily during embryonic development, the growing organism is considered most vulnerable to hazardous agents during the first months of pregnancy. Any agent (e.g., drug, virus, or radiation) that can cause abnormal structures to develop in an embryo is called a **teratogen**. It is important to remember that the effects of teratogens depend on the (1) fetal genotype and maternal genome, (2) stage of development when exposure occurs, and (3) dose and duration of exposure of the agent. Potential teratogens can cause malformations of the heart, limbs, eyes, and other organ systems as early as 3 weeks postconception (Moore et al., 2016). Chapter 10 discusses the effects of specific teratogenic agents on the developing fetus.

Adequacy of the maternal environment is also important during the periods of rapid embryonic and fetal development. Maternal nutrition can affect brain and neural tube development. The period of maximum brain growth and myelination begins with the fifth lunar month before birth and continues into adulthood (Blackburn, 2013). Amino acids, glucose, and fatty acids are considered to be the primary dietary factors in brain growth. A subtle type of damage that affects the associative capacity of the brain, possibly leading to learning disabilities, may be caused by nutritional deficiency at this stage. Studies in Tunisia showed that babies of mothers who were pregnant during the observance of Ramadan (the ninth month of the Islamic calendar) and practiced the required strict fasting for 29 to 30 days had reduced birth weight, head circumference, ponderal index, and placental weight (Alwasel et al., 2013). Similar results were found in studies of pregnant women fasting during Ramadan in Saudi Arabia.

Clinical Reasoning Illness During Pregnancy

Melodie Chong, in her third week of pregnancy, develops a fever of 102.4°F (39.1°C) and flulike symptoms but refuses to take any medication because she is afraid that drugs will harm her baby.

Melodie asks when her baby is most vulnerable for abnormal growth or structure. How would you answer?

Healthy People 2020

(MICH-14) Increase the proportion of women of childbearing potential with daily intake of at least 400 mcg of folic acid from fortified foods or dietary supplementation to 26.2% from the current level of 23.8%

Poor maternal nutrition may also predispose babies who were small or disproportionate at birth to the development of adult coronary heart disease, hypertension, and diabetes (Moore et al., 2016). Maternal nutrition is discussed in depth in Chapter 11.

Another prenatal influence on the intrauterine environment is maternal hyperthermia associated with sauna or hot tub use. Studies of the effects of maternal hyperthermia during the first trimester have raised concern about possible central nervous system defects and failure of neural tube closure. Cigarette smoking during pregnancy is a well-established cause of intrauterine growth restriction (IUGR) (Moore et al., 2016). Maternal substance abuse also affects the intrauterine environment and is discussed in Chapter 14.

SAFETY ALERT!

Vitamins and folic acid supplements taken before conception can reduce the incidence of neural tube defects.

Focus Your Study

- Humans have 46 chromosomes, which are divided into 23 pairs—22 pairs of autosomes and 1 pair of sex chromosomes.

- Mitosis is the process by which additional somatic (body) cells are formed. It provides growth and development of the organs and replacement of body cells.

- Meiosis produces cells called gametes (ova and sperm) that are necessary for reproduction of the species. It occurs during gametogenesis (oogenesis and spermatogenesis) and consists of two successive cell divisions (reduction division), which produce a gamete with 23 chromosomes (22 chromosomes and 1 sex chromosome)—the haploid number of chromosomes.

- Gametes must have a haploid number (23) of chromosomes so that when the female gamete (ovum) and the male gamete (spermatozoon) unite to form the zygote, the normal human diploid number of chromosomes (46) is reestablished.

- An ovum is considered to be fertile for about 12 to 24 hours after ovulation, and the sperm is believed to be capable of fertilizing the ovum for about 24 hours after it is deposited in the female reproductive tract.

- Fertilization usually takes place in the ampulla (outer third) of the fallopian tube. Both capacitation and the acrosomal reaction must occur for the sperm to fertilize the ovum. Capacitation is the removal of the plasma membrane, which exposes the acrosomal covering of the sperm head. The acrosomal reaction is the deposit of hyaluronidase in the corona radiata, which allows the sperm head to penetrate the ovum.

- Sex chromosomes are referred to as X and Y. Females have two X chromosomes, and males have an X and a Y chromosome. Y chromosomes are carried only by the sperm. To produce a female child, both the mother and the father contribute an X chromosome. To produce a male child, the mother contributes an X chromosome and the father contributes a Y chromosome.

- Intrauterine development first proceeds via cellular multiplication in which the zygote undergoes rapid mitotic division called cleavage. As a result of cleavage, the zygote divides and multiplies into cell groupings called blastomeres, which are held together by the zona pellucida. The blastomeres will eventually become a solid ball of cells called the morula. When a cavity forms in the morula cell mass, the inner solid cell mass is called the blastocyst.

- Implantation usually occurs in the upper part of the posterior uterine wall when the blastocyst burrows into the uterine lining.

- After implantation, the endometrium is called the decidua. Decidua capsularis is the portion that covers the blastocyst. Decidua basalis is the portion that is directly under the blastocyst. Decidua vera is the portion that lines the rest of the uterine cavity.

- Primary germ layers will give rise to all tissues, organs, and organ systems. The three primary germ cell layers are the ectoderm, endoderm, and mesoderm.

- Embryonic membranes are called the amnion and the chorion. The amnion is formed from the ectoderm and is a thin protective membrane that contains the amniotic fluid and the embryo. The chorion is a thick membrane that develops from the trophoblast and encloses the amnion, embryo, and yolk sac.

- Amniotic fluid cushions the fetus against mechanical injury, maintains the embryo's temperature, allows symmetric external growth, prevents adherence to the amnion, and permits freedom of movement.

- The umbilical cord contains two umbilical arteries, which carry deoxygenated blood from the fetus to the placenta, and one umbilical vein, which carries oxygenated blood from the placenta to the fetus. The umbilical cord has a central insertion into the placenta. Wharton jelly, a specialized connective tissue, prevents compression of the umbilical cord in utero.

- Twins are either dizygotic (fraternal) or monozygotic (identical). Dizygotic twins arise from two separate ova fertilized by two separate spermatozoa. Monozygotic twins develop from a single ovum fertilized by a single spermatozoon.

- The placenta, which develops from the chorionic villi and the decidua basalis, has two parts:
  - The maternal portion, consisting of the decidua basalis, is red and flesh-looking;
  - The fetal portion, consisting of chorionic villi, is covered by the amnion and appears shiny and gray.
  - The placenta is made up of 15 to 20 segments called cotyledons.

- The placenta serves metabolic functions, endocrine functions (hPL), hCG, estrogen, and progesterone), and immunologic functions. It acts as the fetus's respiratory organ, is an organ of excretion, and aids in the exchange of nutrients.

- Stages of fetal development include the preembryonic stage (the first 14 days of human development starting at fertilization), the embryonic stage (from day 15 after fertilization, or the beginning of the third week, until approximately 8 weeks after conception), and the fetal stage (from 8 weeks until birth at approximately 38 weeks postconception).

- Significant events that occur during the embryonic stage are that at 4 weeks the fetal heart begins to beat and at 6 weeks fetal circulation is established. Fetal circulation is a specially designed circulatory system that provides for oxygenation of the fetus while bypassing the fetal lungs.

- The fetal stage is devoted to refining structures and perfecting function. The following are some significant developments during the fetal stage:
  - At 8 to 12 weeks: all organ systems are formed and now require maturation.
  - At 16 weeks: the sex of the fetus can be determined visually.
  - At 20 weeks: 19 cm (7.5 in.) C–R, myelination of spinal cord begins. Suck and swallow begins, lanugo covers body, vernix caseosa begins to form; fetal heartbeat can be auscultated by a fetoscope, and the mother can feel movement (quickening).
  - At 24 weeks: 23 cm (9.2 in.) C–R, respiratory movement and surfactant production begins, brain appears mature. Vernix caseosa covers the entire body
  - At 26 to 28 weeks: the eyes reopen.
  - At 28 weeks: 27 cm (10.8 in.) C–R, nervous system begins regulation of some functions, adipose tissue accumulates rapidly. Nails, eyebrows, and eyelids are present. Eyes open and close.
  - At 32 weeks: skin appears less wrinkled and red because subcutaneous fat has been laid down.
  - At 35 to 36 weeks: 35 cm C–R, earlobes soft with little cartilage, fingernails reach the ends of fingers, few sole creases.
  - At 38 weeks: vernix caseosa is apparent only in the creases and folds of skin, and lanugo remains on upper arms and shoulders only.
  - At 38 to 40 weeks: 40 cm (16 in.) C–R, adequate surfactant, vernix caseosa in skin folds and lanugo on shoulders, earlobes firm, sex apparent.

- The embryo is particularly vulnerable to teratogenesis during the first 8 weeks of cell differentiation and organ system development. Effects of teratogens depend on the (1) maternal and fetal genotype, (2) stage of development when exposure occurs, and (3) dose and duration of exposure of the agent.

Clinical Reasoning in Action

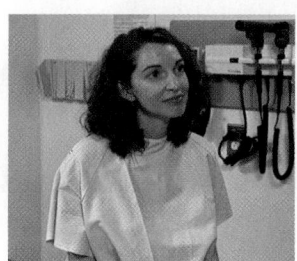

You are working at the local clinic when Frances, a 28-year-old G2 P1001 at 11 weeks' gestation, comes into the office. Frances tells you that early in the first trimester, her husband experienced a flulike syndrome and that he was later diagnosed with cytomegalovirus (CMV) pneumonia. She tells you that his physician found an enlarged supraclavicular lymph node and an ulcer on one tonsil. Laboratory testing revealed elevated liver enzymes. Further testing led to the discovery of positive CMV IgM levels. She has come today with symptoms including night sweats, persistent sore throat, joint pain, headache, vomiting, and fatigue. You obtain vital signs of temperature 99°F (37.2°C), pulse 90, respirations 14, BP 110/70. Her physical exam is normal; no lymphadenopathy is present. Her weight gain is 2 lb even though she has experienced nausea and some vomiting. She is worried that her husband's illness could be related to her current symptoms.

1. How would you respond to Frances's concern?
2. Frances asks you if her baby is formed. How would you discuss the three stages of development?
3. Frances asks when her baby is most vulnerable for developing abnormalities in growth or structure. How would you answer?
4. Frances asks what stage her baby is in. What would you tell her?

References

Alwasel, S. H., Harrath, A., Aljarallah, J. S., Abotalib, Z., Osmond, C., Al Omar, … Barker, D. J. P. (2013). Intergenerational effects of in utero exposure to Ramadan in Tunisia. *American Journal of Human Biology*. Retrieved from http://onlinelibrary.wiley.com/doi/10.1002/ajhb.22374/fulldoi:10.1002/ajhb.22374

Blackburn, S. T. (2013). *Maternal, fetal, & neonatal physiology: A clinical perspective* (4th ed.). St. Louis, MO: Saunders/Elsevier.

Caudle, P. W. (2014). Physiological foundations of prenatal and postnatal care. In R. G. Jordan, J. L. Engstrom, J. A. Marfell & C. L. Farley (Eds.) *Prenatal and postnatal care: A women-centered approach*. Ames, IA: Wiley Blackwell.

Cunningham, F. G., Leveno, K. J., Bloom, S. L., Spong, C. Y., Dashe, J. S., Hoffman, B. L., … Sheffield, J. S. (2014). *Williams obstetrics* (24th ed.). New York, NY: McGraw-Hill.

Moore, K. L., Persaud, T. V. N., & Torchia, M. G. (2016). *The developing human: Clinical oriented embryology* (10th ed.). Philadelphia, PA: Saunders/Elsevier.

National Institute for Health and Clinical Excellence (NICE) (2011). Antenatal care: Routine care for the healthy pregnant woman. Retrieved from http://www.nice.org.uk/CG62

Sadler, T. W. (2015). *Langman's medical embryology* (13th ed.). Philadelphia, PA: Lippincott Williams & Wilkins.

Society of Maternal-Fetal Medicine (SMFM); Moise, K. J., & Argon, P. S. (2013). The importance of determining choronicity in twin gestations. *Contemporary OB/GYN*, February 3, 2013, 35–43.

U.S. Department of Health and Human Services. (2011). *Healthy People 2020 topics & objectives*. Retrieved from http://www.healthypeople.gov/2020/topicsobjectives2020/default.aspx?

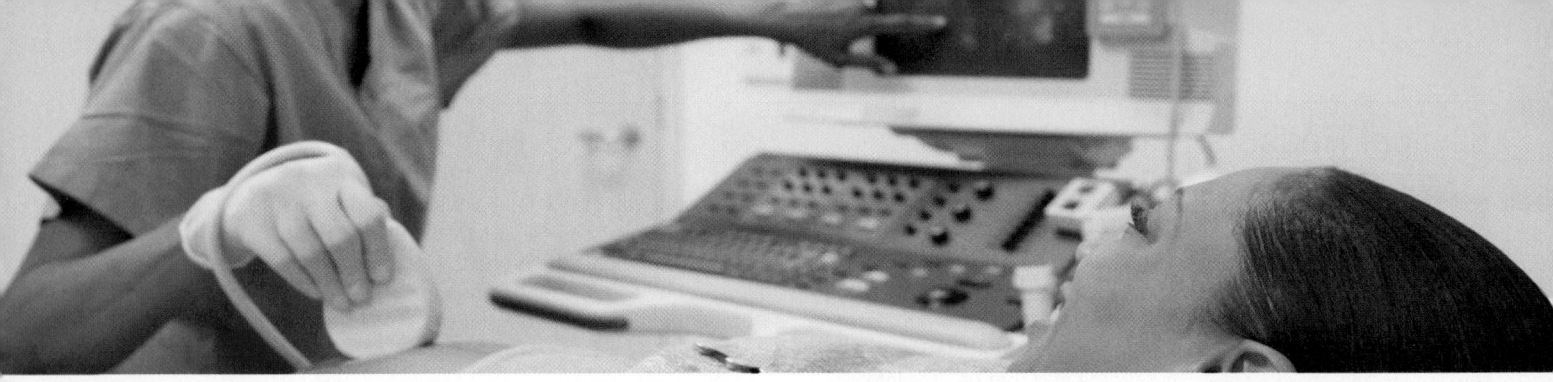

Chapter 8
Physical and Psychologic Changes of Pregnancy

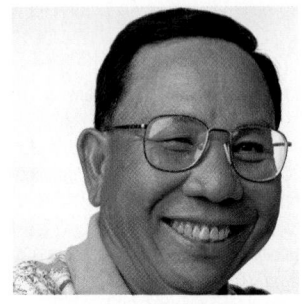

Our son and his wife just told us they are pregnant. I am going to be a grandfather! I have tried to be a good father, to give my boy love, to teach him to respect others, to show him what it means to be a real man, someone a family can count on. Guess time will tell if the lessons took—I'm betting they have.

—Patrick, 52

Kevin Peterson/Getty Images

⌄ Learning Outcomes

8.1 Describe the anatomic and physiologic changes that occur during pregnancy.

8.2 Relate the physiologic and anatomic changes that occur in the body systems during pregnancy to the signs and symptoms that develop in the woman.

8.3 Compare subjective (presumptive), objective (probable), and diagnostic (positive) changes of pregnancy.

8.4 Contrast the various types of pregnancy tests.

8.5 Examine the emotional and psychologic changes that commonly occur in a woman, her partner, and her family during pregnancy.

8.6 Summarize cultural factors that may influence a family's response to pregnancy.

Pregnancy is divided into three trimesters, each approximately a 3-month period. Each trimester brings predictable changes for both the mother and the fetus. How does pregnancy affect the woman physically and psychologically? How does it affect her family, including siblings, partner, and grandparents? This chapter describes these physical and psychologic changes and the responses of the entire family to pregnancy. It also presents the various cultural factors that can affect a pregnant woman's well-being. Subsequent chapters build on this information in describing effective approaches to planning and providing care.

Anatomy and Physiology of Pregnancy
Reproductive System

Some of the most dramatic changes of pregnancy occur in the reproductive organs.

UTERUS

Before pregnancy the uterus is a small, almost solid, pear-shaped organ measuring approximately 7.5 × 5 × 2.5 cm (3 × 2 × 1 in.) and weighing about 60 g (2 oz). At the end of pregnancy, it measures about 28 × 24 × 21 cm (11 × 9.5 × 8.25 in.) and weighs approximately 1100 g (2.75 lb); its capacity has also increased from about 10 mL to 5000 mL (5 L) or more (Cunningham et al., 2014). The change is primarily a result of the enlargement (hypertrophy) of the preexisting myometrial cells in response to the stimulating influence of estrogen and the distention caused by the growing fetus. Only a limited increase in cell number (hyperplasia) occurs. The fibrous tissue between the muscle bands increases markedly, which adds to the strength and elasticity of the muscle wall. The enlarging uterus, developing placenta, and growing fetus require additional blood flow to the uterus. By the end of pregnancy, one sixth of the total maternal blood volume is contained within the vascular system of the uterus.

Braxton Hicks contractions, which are irregular, generally painless contractions of the uterus, occur intermittently throughout pregnancy. They may be felt through the abdominal wall beginning about the fourth month of pregnancy. In later months, these contractions become uncomfortable and may be confused with true labor contractions.

CERVIX

Estrogen stimulates the glandular tissue of the cervix, which increases in cell number and becomes hyperactive. The endocervical glands secrete a thick, sticky mucus that accumulates and forms the **mucous plug**, which seals the endocervical canal and prevents the ascent of organisms into the uterus. This mucous plug is expelled at the onset of labor or before, when cervical dilatation begins. The hyperactivity of the glandular tissue also increases the normal physiologic mucorrhea, at times resulting in profuse discharge. Increased cervical vascularity also causes both the softening of the cervix (Goodell sign) and its bluish discoloration (Chadwick sign).

OVARIES

The ovaries stop producing ova during pregnancy, but the corpus luteum continues to produce hormones until about weeks 6 to 8. It secretes progesterone until about the seventh week of pregnancy, maintaining the endometrium until the placenta assumes the task. The corpus luteum then begins to disintegrate slowly.

VAGINA

Estrogen causes a thickening of the vaginal mucosa, a loosening of the connective tissue, and an increase in vaginal secretions (leukorrhea). These secretions are thick, white, and acidic (pH 3.5 to 6.0). The acid pH helps prevent bacterial infection but favors the growth of yeast organisms. Thus the pregnant woman is more susceptible to *Candida* infection than usual.

The supportive connective tissue of the vagina loosens throughout pregnancy. By the end of pregnancy, the vagina and perineal body are sufficiently relaxed to permit passage of the baby. Because blood flow to the vagina is increased, the vagina may show the same blue-purple color (Chadwick sign) as the cervix.

Clinical Tip

Beginning after the first trimester, have the woman feel her uterus periodically so that she becomes familiar with the size and the way it feels. As her pregnancy progresses, she then will be more likely to identify Braxton Hicks contractions and preterm labor, if it occurs.

BREASTS

Estrogen and progesterone cause many changes in the mammary glands. The breasts enlarge and become more nodular as the glands increase in size and number in preparation for lactation. Superficial veins become more prominent, the nipples become more erectile, and the areolae darken. Montgomery tubercles (sebaceous glands) enlarge, and striae (reddish stretch marks that slowly turn silver after childbirth) may develop.

Colostrum, an antibody-rich yellow secretion, may leak or be expressed from the breasts during the last trimester. Colostrum gradually converts to mature milk during the first few days after childbirth.

Respiratory System

Many respiratory changes occur to meet the increased oxygen requirements of a pregnant woman. The volume of air breathed each minute increases 30% to 40% (Gordon, 2012). In addition, progesterone decreases airway resistance, permitting a 15% to 20% increase in oxygen consumption, as well as increases in carbon dioxide production and in the respiratory functional reserve.

As the uterus enlarges, it presses upward and elevates the diaphragm. The subcostal angle increases, so that the rib cage flares. The anteroposterior diameter increases, and the chest circumference expands by as much as 6 cm (2.4 in.); as a result there is no significant loss of intrathoracic volume. Breathing changes from abdominal to thoracic as pregnancy progresses, and descent of the diaphragm on inspiration becomes less possible. Some hyperventilation and difficulty in breathing may occur.

Nasal stuffiness and epistaxis (nosebleeds) may also occur because of estrogen-induced edema, hypersecretion of mucus, and vascular congestion of the nasal mucosa.

Cardiovascular System

Blood volume progressively increases beginning in the first trimester, increases rapidly until about 30 to 34 weeks, and then plateaus until birth at about 40% to 50% above nonpregnant levels. This increase is a result of increases in both erythrocytes and plasma (Gordon, 2012).

During pregnancy, blood flow increases to organ systems with an increased workload. Thus blood flow increases to the uterus, placenta, and breasts, whereas hepatic and cerebral flow remain unchanged. Cardiac output begins to increase early in pregnancy and peaks at 25 to 30 weeks' gestation at 30% to 50% above prepregnant levels. It generally remains elevated in the third trimester.

The pulse may increase by as many as 10 to 15 beats per minute at term. The blood pressure decreases slightly, reaching its lowest point during the second trimester. It gradually increases to near prepregnant levels by the end of the third trimester. The enlarging uterus puts pressure on pelvic and femoral vessels, interfering with returning blood flow and causing stasis of blood in the lower extremities. This condition may lead to dependent edema and varicosity of the veins in the legs, vulva, and rectum (hemorrhoids) in late pregnancy. This increased blood volume in the lower legs may also make the pregnant woman prone to postural hypotension.

When the pregnant woman lies supine, the enlarging uterus may press on the vena cava, thus reducing blood flow to the right atrium, lowering blood pressure, and causing dizziness, pallor, and clamminess. The enlarging uterus may also press on the aorta and its collateral circulation (Cunningham et al., 2014). This condition is called **supine hypotensive syndrome**. It may also be referred to as *vena caval syndrome* or *aortocaval compression* (Figure 8–1). It can be corrected by

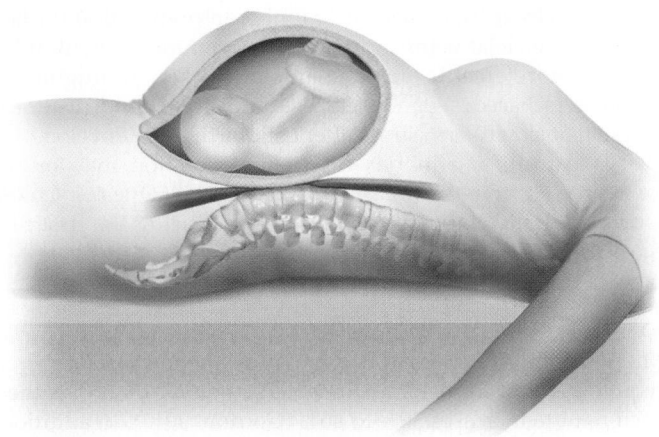

Figure 8–1 Supine hypotensive syndrome (vena caval syndrome). The gravid uterus compresses the vena cava when the woman is supine. This reduces the blood flow returning to the heart and may cause maternal hypotension.

having the woman lie on her left side or by placing a pillow or wedge under her right hip.

The total erythrocyte (red blood cell [RBC]) volume increases by about 30% in women who receive iron supplementation but only about 18% without iron supplementation. This increase in erythrocytes is necessary to transport the additional oxygen required during pregnancy. However, the increase in plasma volume during pregnancy averages about 50%. Because the plasma volume increase (50%) is greater than the erythrocyte increase (25%), the hematocrit, which measures the concentration of red blood cells in the plasma, decreases slightly (Cao & O'Brien, 2013). This decrease is referred to as the **physiologic anemia of pregnancy** (pseudoanemia).

Iron is necessary for hemoglobin formation, and hemoglobin is the oxygen-carrying component of erythrocytes. Thus the increase in erythrocyte levels results in an increased need for iron by the pregnant woman. The American College of Obstetricians and Gynecologists (ACOG, 2013a) recommendation for an iron supplement during pregnancy is 27 mg of iron daily. This can be found in most prenatal supplements. Women who were diagnosed with anemia prior to pregnancy may require more iron supplementation. Leukocyte production increases slightly to a range of 5600 to 12,200/mm^3. During labor and early postpartum, these levels may reach 25,000/mm^3 or higher (Gordon, 2012). Although the exact cause of the leukocytosis is not known, this increase is a normal finding (Cunningham et al., 2014).

Both fibrin and plasma fibrinogen levels increase during pregnancy. Although the blood-clotting time of the pregnant woman does not differ significantly from that of the nonpregnant woman, clotting factors VII, VIII, IX, and X increase; thus pregnancy is a somewhat hypercoagulable state. These changes, coupled with venous stasis in late pregnancy, increase the pregnant woman's risk of developing venous thrombosis.

Gastrointestinal System

Nausea and vomiting are common during the first trimester and may result from several factors, including elevated human chorionic gonadotropin (hCG) levels, relaxation of the smooth muscle of the stomach, and changed carbohydrate metabolism (Gordon, 2012). Gum tissue may soften and bleed easily. The secretion of saliva may increase and even become excessive (ptyalism).

Elevated progesterone levels cause smooth muscle relaxation, resulting in delayed gastric emptying and decreased peristalsis. As a result the pregnant woman may complain of bloating and constipation. These symptoms are aggravated as the enlarging uterus displaces the stomach upward and the intestines are moved laterally and posteriorly. The cardiac sphincter also relaxes, and heartburn (pyrosis) may occur because of reflux of acidic secretions into the lower esophagus. Hemorrhoids frequently develop in late pregnancy from constipation and from pressure on vessels below the level of the uterus.

The emptying time of the gallbladder is prolonged during pregnancy as a result of smooth muscle relaxation from progesterone. This, coupled with the elevated levels of cholesterol in the bile, can predispose the woman to gallstone formation. Pruritus (itching) caused by retained bile salts may also occur (Cunningham et al., 2014).

Urinary Tract

During the first trimester, the enlarging uterus is still a pelvic organ and presses against the bladder, producing urinary frequency. This symptom decreases during the second trimester, when the uterus becomes an abdominal organ and pressure against the bladder lessens. Frequency reappears during the third trimester, when the presenting part descends into the pelvis and again presses on the bladder, reducing bladder capacity, contributing to hyperemia, and irritating the bladder.

The ureters (especially the right ureter) elongate and dilate above the pelvic brim. The glomerular filtration rate rises by as much as 50% beginning in the second trimester and remains elevated until birth. To compensate for this increase, renal tubular reabsorption also increases. However, glycosuria is sometimes seen during pregnancy because of the kidneys' inability to reabsorb all the glucose filtered by the glomeruli. Glycosuria may be normal or may indicate gestational diabetes, so it always warrants further testing.

Skin and Hair

Changes in skin pigmentation commonly occur during pregnancy. They are thought to be stimulated by increased estrogen, progesterone, and α-melanocytic-stimulating hormone levels. Pigmentation of the skin increases primarily in areas that are already hyperpigmented: the areolae, the nipples, the vulva, and the perianal area. The skin in the middle of the abdomen may develop a pigmented line, the **linea nigra**, which usually extends from the pubic area to the umbilicus or higher (Figure 8–2). Facial **chloasma (melasma gravidarum)**, also known as the "mask of pregnancy," a darkening of the skin over the forehead and around the eyes, may develop. Melasma is more prominent in dark-haired women and is aggravated by exposure to the sun. Fortunately, it fades or becomes less prominent soon after childbirth when the hormonal influence of pregnancy subsides. The sweat and sebaceous glands are often hyperactive during pregnancy. **Striae (striae gravidarum** when they result from pregnancy), or stretch marks, may appear on the abdomen, thighs, buttocks, and breasts. They result from reduced connective tissue strength because of elevated adrenal steroid levels.

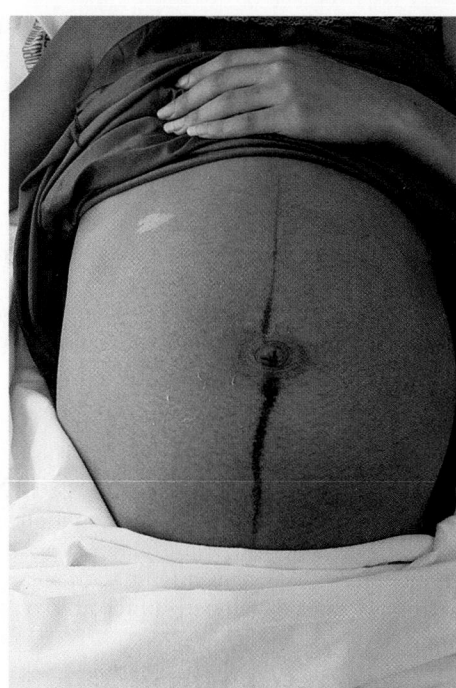

Figure 8–2 **Linea nigra.**

Vascular spider nevi, small, bright-red elevations of the skin radiating from a central body, may develop on the chest, neck, face, arms, and legs. They may be caused by increased subcutaneous blood flow in response to elevated estrogen levels.

The proportion of hair in the growing phase increases during pregnancy compared with the number of hair follicles in the resting or dormant phase. After birth the number of hair follicles in the resting phase increases sharply, and the woman may notice increased hair shedding beginning 1 to 4 months postpartum. However, practically all hair is replaced within 6 to 12 months (Cunningham et al., 2014).

Musculoskeletal System

No demonstrable changes occur in the teeth of pregnant women. The dental caries that sometimes accompany pregnancy are probably caused by inadequate oral hygiene and dental care, especially if the woman has problems with bleeding gums or nausea and vomiting.

The joints of the pelvis relax somewhat because of hormonal influences. The result is often a waddling gait. As the pregnant woman's center of gravity gradually changes, the lumbar spinal curve becomes accentuated (lordosis), and her posture changes (Figure 8–3). This posture change compensates for the increased weight of the uterus anteriorly and frequently results in low backache.

Pressure of the enlarging uterus on the abdominal muscles may cause the rectus abdominis muscle to separate, producing **diastasis recti**. If the separation is severe and muscle tone is not regained postpartum, subsequent pregnancies will not have adequate support and the woman's abdomen may appear pendulous.

Central Nervous System

Pregnant women frequently describe decreased attention, concentration, and memory during and shortly after pregnancy, but few studies have explored this phenomenon. One study did find a decline in memory that could not be attributed to depression, anxiety, sleep deprivation, or other physical changes of pregnancy. This memory loss disappeared soon after childbirth (Cunningham et al., 2014).

Metabolism

Most metabolic functions increase during pregnancy because of the increased demands of the growing fetus and its support system. For a detailed discussion of nutrient, vitamin, and mineral metabolism, see Chapter 11.

WEIGHT GAIN

The recommended total weight gain during pregnancy for a woman of normal weight before pregnancy is 11.5 to 16.0 kg (25 to 35 lb); for women who were overweight before becoming pregnant, the recommended gain is 6.8 to 11.5 kg (15 to 25 lb). Women with obesity are advised to limit weight gain to 5 to 9 kg (11 to 20 lb). Underweight women are advised to gain 12.7 to 18.1 kg (28 to 40 lb) (Institute of Medicine [IOM], 2009). A woman of normal weight should gain about 0.5 to 2.0 kg

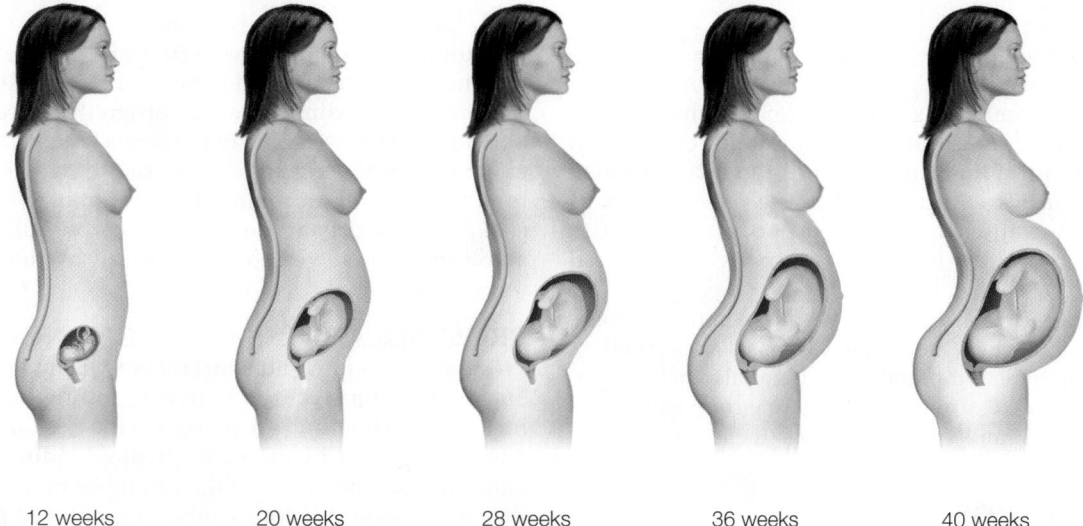

| 12 weeks | 20 weeks | 28 weeks | 36 weeks | 40 weeks |

Figure 8–3 **Postural changes during pregnancy. Note the increasing lordosis of the lumbosacral spine and the increasing curvature of the thoracic area.**

(1.1 to 4.4 lb) during the first trimester, followed by an average gain of about 0.45 kg (1 lb) per week during the last two trimesters (IOM, 2009).

ACOG (2013b) supports the IOM recommendations and recommends that healthcare providers determine a woman's body mass index (BMI) at the initial prenatal visit. Individualized care and clinical judgment should then be used to determine the appropriate weight gain.

WATER METABOLISM

Increased water retention, a basic alteration of pregnancy, is caused by several interrelated factors. The increased level of steroid sex hormones affects sodium and fluid retention. The lowered serum protein also influences fluid balance, as do increased intracapillary pressure and permeability. The extra water is needed for the fetus, the placenta, amniotic fluid, and the mother's increased blood volume, interstitial fluids, and enlarged organs.

NUTRIENT METABOLISM

The fetus makes its greatest protein and fat demands during the second half of pregnancy, doubling in weight during the last 6 to 8 weeks. Protein (contributing nitrogen) must be stored during pregnancy to maintain a constant level within the breast milk and to avoid depletion of maternal tissues. Carbohydrate needs also increase, especially during the second and third trimesters. Fats are more completely absorbed during pregnancy, and the level of free fatty acids increases in response to human placental lactogen (hPL). The levels of lipoproteins and cholesterol also increase. Because of these changes, increased levels of dietary fat or reduced carbohydrate production may lead to ketonuria in the pregnant woman.

Endocrine System

THYROID GLAND

The thyroid gland often enlarges slightly during pregnancy because of increased vascularity and hyperplasia of glandular tissue. Estrogen increases its capacity to bind thyroxine, resulting in an increase in serum protein-bound iodine. The basal metabolic rate increases by as much as 20% to 25% during pregnancy. However, within a few weeks after birth, all thyroid function returns to normal limits.

PITUITARY GLAND

Pregnancy is made possible by the hypothalamic stimulation of the anterior pituitary gland. The anterior pituitary produces follicle-stimulating hormone (FSH), which stimulates ovum growth, and luteinizing hormone (LH), which brings about ovulation. Stimulation of the pituitary also prolongs the ovary's corpus luteal phase. This maintains the endometrium in case conception occurs. Prolactin, another anterior pituitary hormone, is responsible for initial lactation.

The posterior pituitary secretes vasopressin (antidiuretic hormone) and oxytocin. Vasopressin causes vasoconstriction, which results in increased blood pressure; it also helps regulate water balance. Oxytocin promotes uterine contractility and stimulates ejection of milk from the breasts (the letdown reflex) in the postpartum period.

ADRENAL GLANDS

During pregnancy, circulating cortisol, which regulates carbohydrate and protein metabolism, increases in response to increased estrogen levels. Cortisol blood levels return to normal within 1 to 6 weeks postpartum. The adrenal glands secrete increased levels of aldosterone by the early part of the second trimester. This increase in aldosterone in a normal pregnancy may be the body's protective response to the increased sodium excretion associated with progesterone (Cunningham et al., 2014).

PANCREAS

The pregnant woman has increased insulin needs, and the pancreatic islets of Langerhans, which secrete insulin, are stressed to meet this increased demand. Any marginal pancreatic function quickly becomes apparent, and the woman may show signs of gestational diabetes mellitus (GDM). (For a discussion of GDM, see Chapter 14.)

Hormones in Pregnancy

HUMAN CHORIONIC GONADOTROPIN

The trophoblast secretes human chorionic gonadotropin (hCG) in early pregnancy. This hormone stimulates progesterone and estrogen production by the corpus luteum to maintain the pregnancy until the placenta is developed sufficiently to assume that function.

HUMAN PLACENTAL LACTOGEN

Also called *human chorionic somatomammotropin*, human placental lactogen (hPL) is produced by the syncytiotrophoblast. hPL is an antagonist of insulin; it increases the amount of circulating free fatty acids for maternal metabolic needs and decreases maternal metabolism of glucose to favor fetal growth.

ESTROGEN

Secreted originally by the corpus luteum, estrogen is produced primarily by the placenta as early as the seventh week of pregnancy. Estrogen stimulates uterine development to provide a suitable environment for the fetus. It also helps develop the ductal system of the breasts in preparation for lactation.

PROGESTERONE

Also produced initially by the corpus luteum and then by the placenta, progesterone plays the greatest role in maintaining pregnancy. It maintains the endometrium and inhibits spontaneous uterine contractility, thus preventing early spontaneous abortion. Progesterone also helps develop the acini and lobules of the breasts in preparation for lactation.

RELAXIN

Relaxin is detectable in the serum of a pregnant woman by the time of the first missed menstrual period. Relaxin inhibits uterine activity, diminishes the strength of uterine contractions, aids in the softening of the cervix, and has the long-term effect of remodeling connective tissue, which is necessary for the uterus to accommodate pregnancy (Cunningham et al., 2014). Its primary source is the corpus luteum, but small amounts are believed to be produced by the placenta and uterine decidua.

PROSTAGLANDINS IN PREGNANCY

Prostaglandins are lipid substances that can arise from most body tissues but occur in high concentrations in the female reproductive tract and are present in the decidua during pregnancy. The exact functions of prostaglandins during pregnancy are still unknown, although it has been proposed that they are responsible for maintaining reduced placental vascular resistance. Decreased prostaglandin levels may contribute to hypertension and preeclampsia. Prostaglandins may also play a role in the complex biochemistry that initiates labor.

Signs of Pregnancy

Many of the changes women experience during pregnancy are used to diagnose the pregnancy itself. They are called the subjective, or presumptive, changes; the objective, or probable, changes; and the diagnostic, or positive, changes of pregnancy.

Subjective (Presumptive) Changes

The subjective changes of pregnancy are the symptoms the woman experiences and reports. Because they can be caused by other conditions, they cannot be considered proof of pregnancy (Table 8–1). Several subjective signs can be diagnostic clues when other signs and symptoms of pregnancy are also present.

- *Amenorrhea*, or the absence of menses, is the earliest symptom of pregnancy. Missing more than one menstrual period, especially in a woman whose cycle is ordinarily regular, is an especially useful diagnostic clue.

- *Nausea and vomiting of pregnancy (NVP)* occur frequently during the first trimester. It may be mild or may cause considerable distress. Because these symptoms often occur in the early part of the day, they are commonly referred to as **morning sickness**. In reality, the symptoms may occur at any time and can range from a mere distaste for food to severe vomiting. Women who experience NVP often have a more favorable pregnancy outcome than those who do not.

- *Excessive fatigue* may be noted within a few weeks after the first missed menstrual period and may persist throughout the first trimester.

- *Urinary frequency* is experienced during the first trimester as the enlarging uterus presses on the bladder.

- *Changes in the breasts* are frequently noted in early pregnancy. These changes include tenderness and tingling sensations, increased pigmentation of the areola and nipple, and changes in the Montgomery glands. The veins also become more visible and form a bluish pattern beneath the skin.

- **Quickening**, or the mother's perception of fetal movement, occurs about 18 to 20 weeks after the last menstrual period in a woman pregnant for the first time but may occur as early as 16 weeks in a woman who has been pregnant before. Quickening is a fluttering sensation in the abdomen that gradually increases in intensity and frequency.

Clinical Tip

Some women suggest that it is easiest to imagine the fluttering associated with quickening by letting the outer tips of the eyelashes brush a finger and then imagining that same sensation deep inside the abdomen.

Objective (Probable) Changes

An examiner can perceive the objective changes that occur in pregnancy. Because these changes can have other causes, they do not confirm pregnancy (Table 8–2).

- *Changes in the pelvic organs*—the only physical changes detectable during the first 3 months of pregnancy—are caused by increased vascular congestion. These changes are noted on pelvic examination. As noted earlier, there is a softening of the cervix called the **Goodell sign**. **Chadwick sign** is a bluish, purple, or deep-red discoloration of the mucous membranes of the cervix, vagina, and vulva (some sources consider this a presumptive sign). **Hegar sign** is a softening of the isthmus of the uterus, the area between the cervix and the body of the uterus (Figure 8–4). **McDonald sign** is an ease in flexing of the body of the uterus against the cervix.

TABLE 8–1 Differential Diagnosis of Pregnancy—Subjective Changes

SUBJECTIVE CHANGES	POSSIBLE ALTERNATIVE CAUSES
Amenorrhea	*Endocrine factors:* early menopause; lactation; thyroid, pituitary, adrenal, ovarian dysfunction
	Metabolic factors: malnutrition, anemia, climatic changes, diabetes mellitus, degenerative disorders, long-distance running
	Psychologic factors: emotional shock, fear of pregnancy or sexually transmitted infection, intense desire for pregnancy (pseudocyesis), stress
	Obliteration of endometrial cavity by infection or curettage
	Systemic disease (acute or chronic), such as tuberculosis or malignancy
Nausea and vomiting	Gastrointestinal disorders
	Acute infections such as encephalitis
	Emotional disorders such as pseudocyesis or anorexia nervosa
Urinary frequency	Urinary tract infection
	Cystocele
	Pelvic tumors
	Urethral diverticula
	Emotional tension
Breast tenderness	Premenstrual tension
	Chronic cystic mastitis
	Pseudocyesis
	Hyperestrogenism
Quickening	Increased peristalsis
	Flatus ("gas")
	Abdominal muscle contractions
	Shifting of abdominal contents

TABLE 8–2 Differential Diagnosis of Pregnancy—Objective Changes

OBJECTIVE CHANGES	POSSIBLE ALTERNATIVE CAUSES
Changes in pelvic organs: • Goodell sign • Chadwick sign • Hegar sign • Uterine enlargement	Increased vascular congestion Estrogen-progestin oral contraceptives Vulvar, vaginal, cervical hyperemia Excessively soft walls of nonpregnant uterus Uterine tumors
Enlargement of abdomen	Obesity, ascites, pelvic tumors
Braxton Hicks contractions	Hematometra, pedunculated, submucous, and soft myomas
Uterine souffle	Large uterine myomas, large ovarian tumors, or any condition with greatly increased uterine blood flow
Pigmentation of skin: • Chloasma (melasma) • Linea nigra • Nipples/areolae	Estrogen-progestin oral contraceptives Melanocyte hormonal stimulation
Abdominal striae	Obesity, pelvic tumor
Ballottement	Uterine tumors/polyps, ascites
Positive pregnancy test	Increased pituitary gonadotropins at menopause, choriocarcinoma, hydatidiform mole
Palpation for fetal outline	Uterine myomas

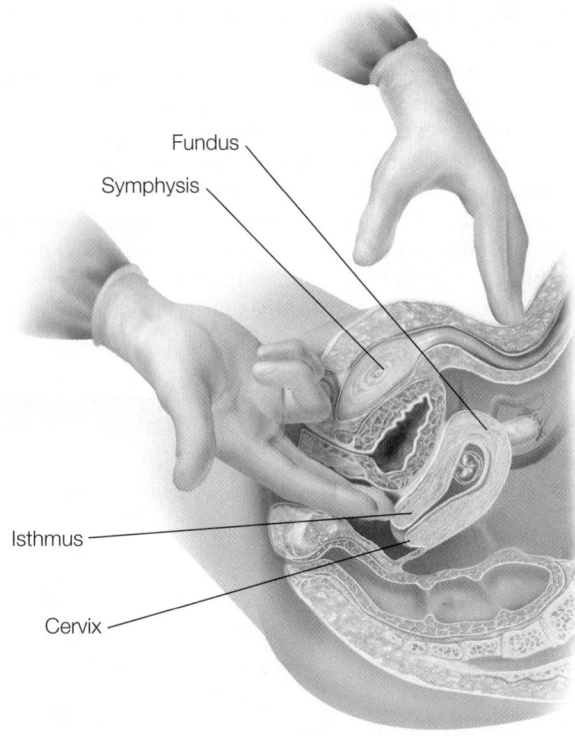

Fundus
Symphysis
Isthmus
Cervix

Figure 8–4 The presence of Hegar sign, which is a softening of the isthmus of the uterus, can be determined by the examiner during a vaginal examination.

General enlargement and softening of the body of the uterus can be noted after the eighth week of pregnancy. The fundus of the uterus is palpable just above the symphysis pubis at about 10 to 12 weeks' gestation and at the level of the umbilicus at 20 to 22 weeks' gestation (Figure 8–5).

- *Enlargement of the abdomen* during the childbearing years is usually regarded as evidence of pregnancy, especially if it is continuous and accompanied by amenorrhea.

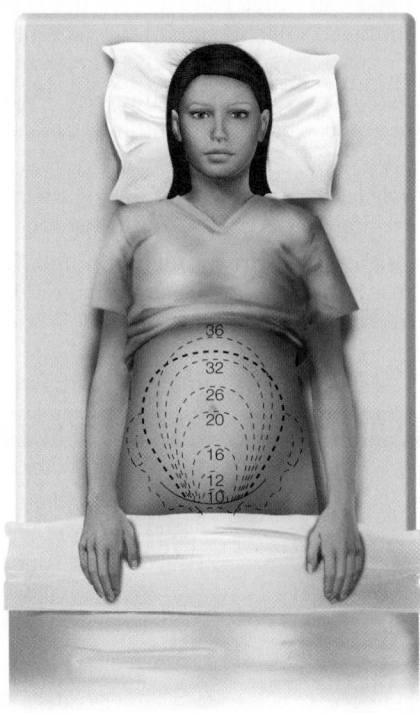

Figure 8–5 Approximate height of the fundus at various weeks of pregnancy.

- *Braxton Hicks contractions* can be palpated most commonly after the 28th week. As the woman approaches the end of pregnancy, these contractions may become uncomfortable. They are often called *false labor*.
- *Uterine souffle* may be heard when the examiner auscultates the abdomen over the uterus. It is a soft, blowing sound that occurs at the same rate as the maternal pulse and is caused by the increased uterine blood flow and blood pulsating through the placenta. It is sometimes confused with the funic souffle, a soft, blowing sound of blood pulsating through the umbilical cord. The funic souffle occurs at the same rate as the fetal heart rate.

- *Changes in pigmentation of the skin* are common in pregnancy. The nipples and areolae may darken, and the linea nigra may develop. Facial melasma (chloasma) may become noticeable, and striae may appear.
- The *fetal outline* may be identified by palpation in many pregnant women after 24 weeks' gestation. **Ballottement** is the passive fetal movement elicited when the examiner inserts two gloved fingers into the vagina and pushes against the cervix. This action pushes the fetal body up, and, as it falls back, the examiner feels a rebound.
- *Pregnancy tests* detect the presence of hCG in the maternal blood or urine. These are not considered a positive sign of pregnancy because other conditions can cause elevated hCG levels.

CLINICAL PREGNANCY TESTS

A variety of assay techniques are available to detect hCG in either blood or urine during early pregnancy. Most healthcare providers use urine screening tests because the results are immediate, the cost is minimal, the tests are reasonably accurate, and no invasive procedure (blood draw) is required.

- *β-Subunit radioimmunoassay (RIA)* uses an antiserum with specificity for the β-subunit of hCG in blood plasma. This test may not only detect pregnancy but also detect an ectopic pregnancy or trophoblastic disease.
- *Enzyme-linked immunosorbent assay (ELISA)* uses a substance that results in a color change after binding. This assay, which may be done on urine or blood, is sensitive and quick. It can detect hCG levels as early as 7 to 9 days after ovulation and conception, which is 5 days before the first missed period.
- *Fluoroimmunoassay (FIA)* uses an antibody tagged with a fluorescent label to detect serum hCG. The test, which takes about 2 to 3 hours to perform, is extremely sensitive and is used primarily to identify and follow hCG concentrations.

OVER-THE-COUNTER PREGNANCY TESTS

Home pregnancy tests are available over-the-counter at a reasonable cost. These ELISA tests, performed on urine, detect even low levels of hCG. Test instructions should be followed carefully. If the results are negative, the woman should repeat the test in 1 week if she has not started her period.

Clinical Reasoning **Evaluating Fundal Height**

At 33 weeks' gestation, Elena Martinez, G2P1, who is 5 feet 4 inches tall and weighs 144 lb (prepregnancy weight of 120 lb), is examined by her certified nurse-midwife. At that time her fundal height is measured as 33 cm. Because of a vacation trip, she is not seen again by her midwife until 36 weeks' gestation. At that time, her fundus measures 35 cm (14 in.) and she weighs 147 lb. Elena asks if there is something wrong with her baby's growth. What is your assessment?

Diagnostic (Positive) Changes

The diagnostic signs of pregnancy are completely objective, cannot be confused with a pathologic state, and offer conclusive proof of pregnancy.

- *Fetal heartbeat* can be detected with an electronic Doppler device as early as weeks 10 to 12 of pregnancy.
- *Fetal movement* is actively palpable by a trained examiner after about the 20th week of pregnancy.
- *Visualization of the fetus by ultrasound examination* confirms a pregnancy. The gestational sac can be observed by 4 to 5 weeks' gestation (2 to 3 weeks after conception). Fetal parts and fetal movement can be seen as early as 8 weeks' gestation. Transvaginal ultrasound has been used to detect a gestational sac as early as 10 days after implantation (Cunningham et al., 2014).

Psychologic Response of the Expectant Family to Pregnancy

Pregnancy is a turning point in a family's life, accompanied by stress and anxiety, whether the pregnancy is desired or not. Especially if this is their first child, the expectant couple may be unaware of the physical, emotional, and cognitive changes of pregnancy and may anticipate no problems from such a normal event. Thus they may be confused and distressed by new feelings and behaviors that are essentially normal.

For beginning families, pregnancy is the transition period from childlessness to parenthood. If the expectant woman is married or has a stable partner, she no longer is only a mate but must also assume the role of mother. Her partner, whether male or female, will become a parent, too. Career goals and mobility may be affected, and the couple's relationship takes on a different meaning to them and their families and community. If the pregnancy results in the birth of a child, the couple enters a new, irreversible stage of their life together. With each subsequent pregnancy, routines and family dynamics are again altered, requiring readjustment and realignment.

If the pregnant woman has no stable partner, she must deal alone with the role changes, fears, and adjustments of pregnancy or seek support from family or friends. She also faces the reality of planning for the future as a single parent. Even if the pregnant woman plans to relinquish her baby, she must still deal with the adjustments of pregnancy. This adjustment can be especially difficult without a good support system.

In most pregnancies, finances are an important consideration. Traditional lore relegates to the father the role of primary breadwinner, and indeed finances are often a very real concern for fathers. In today's society, however, even pregnant women with stable partners recognize the financial impact of a child and may feel concern about financial issues. For the single mother, finances may be a major source of concern.

Decisions about financial matters need to be made at this time. Will the woman work during her pregnancy and return to work after her child is born? If so, who will provide child care? Couples may also need to decide about the division of domestic tasks. Any differences of opinion must be discussed openly and resolved so that the family can meet the needs of its members.

Pregnancy can be viewed as a developmental stage with its own distinct developmental tasks. For a couple it can be a time of support or conflict, depending on the amount of adjustment each is willing to make to maintain the family's equilibrium.

During a first pregnancy, the woman and her partner plan together for the child's arrival, collecting information on how to be parents. At the same time, each continues to participate in some separate activities with friends or family members. The availability of a social support network is an important factor in psychosocial well-being during pregnancy. Most pregnant parents find that their partners are their greatest source of support followed by family and friends (Widarsson, Kerstis, Sundquist, et al., 2012). The broader social network is often a major source of advice for the pregnant woman. However, both sound and unsound information may be conveyed.

During any pregnancy, the expectant parents face significant changes and must deal with major psychosocial adjustments (Table 8–3). Other family members, especially other children of the woman or couple and the grandparents-to-be, must also adjust to the pregnancy.

For some, pregnancy is more than a developmental stage; it is a crisis. *Crisis* can be defined as a disturbance or conflict in which the individual cannot maintain a state of equilibrium. Pregnancy can be considered a *maturational crisis*, as it is a common event in the normal growth and development of the family. If the crisis is not resolved, it will result in maladaptive behaviors in one or more family members and possible disintegration of the family. Families that are able to resolve a maturational crisis will return successfully to normal functioning and can even strengthen the bonds in the family relationship.

The Mother

Pregnancy alters body image and also necessitates a reordering of social relationships and changes in roles of family members. The way each woman meets the stresses of pregnancy is influenced by her emotional makeup, her sociologic and cultural background, and her acceptance or rejection of the pregnancy. However, many women manifest similar psychologic and

TABLE 8–3 Parental Reactions to Pregnancy

FIRST-TRIMESTER	SECOND-TRIMESTER	THIRD-TRIMESTER
Mother's Reactions	*Mother's Reactions*	*Mother's Reactions*
Informs father secretively or openly.	Remains regressive and introspective, projects all preexisting problems with authority figures onto partner, may become angry if she perceives his lack of interest as a sign of weakness in him.	Experiences more anxiety and tension, with physical awkwardness.
Feels ambivalent toward pregnancy, anxious about labor and responsibility of child.		Feels much discomfort and insomnia from physical condition.
Is aware of physical changes, daydreams of possible miscarriage.	Continues to deal with feelings about motherhood; shops for nursery furniture as something concrete to do.	Prepares for birth, assembles layette, picks out names.
Develops special feelings for and renewed interest in her own mother, begins to form a personal identity as a mother.	May experience anxiety or, alternately, may be very lackadaisical and wait until ninth month to look for furniture and clothes for baby.	Dreams often about misplacing baby or not being able to give birth, fears birth of deformed baby.
	Feels movement and is aware of fetus and incorporates it into herself.	Feels ecstasy and excitement, has spurt of energy during last month.
	May dream that partner will be killed, telephones him often for reassurance.	
	Experiences more distinct physical changes; sexual desires may increase or decrease.	
Father's Reactions	*Father's Reactions*	*Father's Reactions*
Differ according to age, parity, desire for child, economic stability.	If he can cope, will give her extra attention she needs; if he cannot cope, will develop a new time-consuming interest outside of home.	Adapts to alternative methods of sexual contact.
Acceptance of pregnant woman's attitude or complete rejection and lack of communication.	May develop a creative feeling and a "closeness to nature."	Becomes concerned over financial responsibility.
Is aware of his sexual feelings, may develop more or less sexual arousal.	May become involved in pregnancy and buy or make furniture.	Daydreams about child as if older and not newborn, dreams of losing partner.
Accepts, rejects, or resents mother-in-law.	Feels for movement of baby, listens to heartbeat, or remains aloof, with no physical contact.	Renewed sexual attraction to partner.
May develop new hobby outside of family as sign of stress.	May have fears and fantasies about himself being pregnant, may become uneasy with this feminine aspect in himself.	Feels he is ultimately responsible for whatever happens.
	May react negatively if partner is too demanding, may become jealous of physician and of physician's importance to partner and her pregnancy.	

emotional responses during pregnancy, including ambivalence, acceptance, introversion, mood swings, and changes in body image.

A woman's attitude toward her pregnancy can be a significant factor in its outcome. Even if the pregnancy is planned, there is an element of surprise at first. Many women commonly experience feelings of ambivalence during early pregnancy. This ambivalence may be related to feelings that the timing is somehow wrong; worries about the need to modify existing relationships or career plans; fears about assuming a new role; unresolved emotional conflicts with the woman's own mother; and fears about pregnancy, labor, and birth. These feelings may be more pronounced if the pregnancy is unplanned or unwanted. Research indicates that women who are ambivalent about pregnancy are generally younger, less likely to have been pregnant previously, and more likely to have been a victim of sexual violence, to have experienced pregnancy coercion, to have unhealthy behaviors such as smoking, and to have psychologic risk factors. They are also more likely to experience stress and depression during pregnancy (Patel, Laz, & Berenson, 2015).

Indirect expressions of ambivalence include complaints about considerable physical discomfort, prolonged or frequent depression, significant dissatisfaction with changing body shape, excessive mood swings, and difficulty accepting the life changes resulting from the pregnancy. Many pregnancies are unintended, but not all unintended pregnancies are unwanted. A pregnancy can be unintended and wanted at the same time. For some women, an unintended pregnancy has more psychologic and social advantages than disadvantages. It provides purpose and direction to life and allows a woman to test the devotion and love of her partner and family. However, an unintended pregnancy can be a risk factor for depression. Higher levels of depression are also found in women who report more negative responses to pregnancy, who believe that the pregnancy has greater consequences, and who experience more symptoms, especially in the third trimester (Jessop, Craig, & Ayers, 2014).

Acceptance of pregnancy is influenced by many factors. Lower acceptance tends to be related to an unplanned pregnancy and greater evidence of fear and conflict. When a pregnancy is well accepted, the woman demonstrates feelings of happiness and pleasure in the pregnancy. She experiences less physical discomfort and shows a high degree of tolerance for the discomforts associated with the third trimester (Lederman & Weis, 2009).

Conflicts about adapting to pregnancy are no more pronounced for older pregnant women (age 35 and over) than for younger ones. Moreover, older pregnant women tend to be less concerned about the normal physical changes of pregnancy and are confident about handling issues that arise during pregnancy and parenting. This difference may result because mature pregnant women have more experience with problem solving.

Pregnancy produces marked changes in a woman's body within a relatively short period. Pregnant women experience changes in body image because of physical alterations and may feel a loss of control over their bodies during pregnancy and later during childbirth. These perceptions are to a certain extent related to personality factors, social network responses, and attitudes toward pregnancy. Although changes in body image are normal, they can be stressful for the woman. Explanation and discussion of the changes may help both the woman and her partner deal with the stress associated with this aspect of pregnancy.

FIRST TRIMESTER

During the first trimester, feelings of disbelief and ambivalence are paramount. The woman's baby does not seem real, and she focuses on herself and her pregnancy. She may experience one or more of the early symptoms of pregnancy, such as breast tenderness or morning sickness, which are unsettling and at times unpleasant.

At this time, the expectant mother begins to exhibit some characteristic behavioral changes. She may become increasingly introspective and passive. She may be emotionally labile, with characteristic mood swings from joy to despair. She may fantasize about a miscarriage and feel guilt because of these fantasies. She may worry that these thoughts will harm the baby in some way.

SECOND TRIMESTER

During the second trimester, quickening occurs. This perception of fetal movement helps the woman think of her baby as a separate person, and she generally becomes excited about the pregnancy even if earlier she was not. The woman becomes increasingly introspective as she evaluates her life, her plans, and her child's future. This introspection helps the woman prepare for her new mothering role. Emotional lability, which may be unsettling to her partner, persists. In some instances the partner may react by withdrawing. This withdrawal is especially distressing to the woman, because she needs increased love and affection. Once the couple understands that these behaviors are characteristic of pregnancy, they are easier to accept; however, they may be sources of stress to some extent throughout pregnancy.

As pregnancy becomes more noticeable, the woman's body image changes. She may feel great pride, embarrassment, or concern. Generally women feel best during the second trimester, which is a relatively tranquil time.

THIRD TRIMESTER

In the third trimester, the woman feels pride about her pregnancy and anxiety about labor and birth. Physical discomforts increase, and the woman is eager for the pregnancy to end. She experiences increased fatigue, her body movements are awkward, and her interest in sexual activity may decrease. The woman tends to be concerned about the health and safety of her unborn child and may worry that she will not cope well during childbirth. Toward the end of this period, there is often a surge of energy as the woman prepares a "nest" for the newborn. Many women report bursts of energy, during which they vigorously clean and organize their homes.

PSYCHOLOGIC TASKS OF THE MOTHER

Rubin (1984) identified four major tasks that the pregnant woman undertakes to maintain her intactness and that of her family and to incorporate her new child into the family system. These tasks form the foundation for a mutually gratifying relationship with her baby:

1. *Ensuring safe passage through pregnancy, labor, and birth.* The pregnant woman feels concern for both her unborn child and herself. She looks for competent maternity care to provide a sense of control. She may seek information from literature, observation of other pregnant women

and new mothers, and discussion with others. She often engages in self-care activities related to diet, exercise, alcohol consumption, and so forth. In the third trimester, she becomes more aware of external threats in the environment—a toy on the stairs, the awkwardness of an escalator—that pose a threat to her well-being. Sleep becomes more difficult and she longs for birth even though it, too, is frightening.

2. *Seeking acceptance of this child by others.* The birth of a child alters a woman's primary support group (her family) and her secondary affiliative groups. The woman slowly and subtly alters her network to meet the needs of her pregnancy. In this adjustment the woman's partner is the most important figure. The partner's support and acceptance help form a maternal identity. If there are other children in the home, the mother also works to ensure their acceptance of the coming child. The woman without a partner looks to others such as a family member or friend for this support.

3. *Seeking commitment and acceptance of herself as mother to the baby (binding-in).* During the first trimester, the child remains a rather abstract concept. With quickening, however, the child begins to become a real person, and the mother begins to develop bonds of attachment. The mother experiences movement of the child within her in an intimate, exclusive way, and bonds of love form. The mother develops a fantasy image of her ideal child. This binding-in process, characterized by its strong emotional component, motivates the pregnant woman to become competent in her role and provides satisfaction for her in the role of mother.

4. *Learning to give of oneself on behalf of one's child.* Childbirth involves many acts of giving. The man "gives" a child to the woman; she in turn "gives" a child to him. Life is given to a newborn; a sibling is given to older children of the family. The woman begins to develop a capacity for self-denial and learns to delay immediate personal gratification to meet the needs of another. Baby showers and gifts are acts of giving that increase the mother's self-esteem and help her recognize the separateness and needs of the coming baby.

Accomplishment of these tasks helps the pregnant woman develop her self-concept as mother. The expectant mother who was well nurtured by her own mother may view her as a role model and emulate her; the woman who views her mother as a "poor mother" may worry that she will make similar mistakes. A woman's self-concept as a mother expands with actual experience and continues to grow through subsequent childbearing and childrearing.

The Father

For the expectant father, pregnancy is a psychologically stressful time because he, too, must make the transition from nonparent to parent or from parent of one or more to parent of two or more. Most men handle the transition to fatherhood well, and generally any anxieties they feel resolve over time. Fathers' feelings of anxieties often stem from inadequate preparation and can be addressed by recognizing paternal needs and including fathers more in antepartum education.

Initially, expectant fathers may feel pride in their virility, which pregnancy confirms, but also have many of the same ambivalent feelings as expectant mothers. The extent of ambivalence depends on many factors, including the father's relationship with his partner, his previous experience with pregnancy, his age, his economic stability, and whether the pregnancy was planned.

In adjusting to his role, the expectant father must first deal with the reality of the pregnancy and then gain recognition as a parent from his partner, family, friends, coworkers, and society—and from his baby as well. Preliminary research suggests that fathers who perceive that they have more marital intimacy and support from their partners tend to develop stronger bonds of attachment to their babies after birth (Yu, Hung, Chan, et al., 2012). The expectant mother can help her partner adjust if she has a definite sense of the experience as their pregnancy and their baby, and not her pregnancy and her baby.

The expectant father must establish a fatherhood role, just as the woman develops a motherhood role. Fathers who are most successful at this task generally like children, are excited about the prospect of fatherhood, are eager to nurture a child, and have confidence in their ability to be a parent. Fathers may have a lack of understanding of their role if they came from dysfunctional families, if they lacked positive role models, or if there was a general lack of education available to them (Alio, Lewis, Scarborough, et al., 2013). (See Table 8–3.)

FIRST TRIMESTER
After the initial excitement attending the announcement of the pregnancy, an expectant father may begin to feel left out. He may be confused by his partner's mood changes. He might resent the attention she receives and her need to modify their relationship as she experiences fatigue and possibly a decreased interest in sex. He might also be concerned about what kind of father he will be. During this time, his child is a "potential" baby. Fathers often picture interacting with a child of 5 or 6 years, not a newborn. The pregnancy itself may seem unreal until the woman shows more physical signs.

SECOND TRIMESTER
The father's role in the pregnancy is still vague, but his involvement may increase as he watches and feels fetal movement and listens to the fetal heartbeat during a prenatal visit. For many men, seeing their baby on ultrasound is an important experience in accepting the reality of pregnancy. Like expectant mothers, expectant fathers need to confront and resolve some of their conflicts about the parenting they received. A father needs to sort out which behaviors of his own father he wants to imitate and which he wants to avoid.

The father-to-be's anxiety is lessened if both parents agree on the paternal role the man is to assume. For example, if both see his role as that of breadwinner, the man's stress is low. However, if the man views his role as that of breadwinner and the woman expects him to be actively involved in child care, his stress increases. An open, honest discussion about the expectations the parents have about their roles will help the father-to-be in his transition to fatherhood.

As the woman's appearance begins to change, her partner may have several reactions. Her appearance may decrease his sexual interest, or it may have the opposite effect. Because of the variety of emotions both partners may feel, communication and acceptance remain important.

THIRD TRIMESTER

If the couple's relationship has grown through effective communication of their concerns and feelings, the third trimester is often a rewarding time. They may attend childbirth classes and make concrete preparations for the arrival of the baby. However, if the father has developed a detached attitude about the pregnancy, it is unlikely he will become a willing participant even though his role becomes more obvious.

Concerns and fears may recur. The father may worry about hurting the unborn baby during intercourse or become concerned about labor and birth. He may also wonder what kind of parents he and his partner will be.

COUVADE

Couvade has been traditionally referred to as the observance of certain rituals and taboos by the male to signify the transition to fatherhood. This observance affirms his psychosocial and biophysical relationship to the woman and child. More recently, the term has been used to describe the unintentional development of physical symptoms such as fatigue, increased appetite, difficulty sleeping, depression, headache, or backache by the partner of a pregnant woman. Men who demonstrate couvade syndrome tend to have a higher degree of paternal role preparation and be involved in more activities related to this preparation.

Siblings

Bringing a new baby home often marks the beginning of sibling rivalry. The siblings view the baby as a threat to the security of their relationships with their parents. Parents who recognize this potential problem early in pregnancy and begin constructive actions can minimize the problem of sibling rivalry.

Preparation of the young child begins several weeks before the anticipated birth. Because they do not have a clear concept of time, young children should not be told too early about the pregnancy. From the toddler's point of view, a period of several weeks is an extremely long time. The mother may let the child feel the baby moving in her uterus, explaining that the uterus is "a special place where babies grow." The child can help the parents put the baby clothes in drawers or prepare the baby's room.

Pregnant women may find it helpful to bring their children on a prenatal visit to the certified nurse-midwife or physician to give them an opportunity to listen to the fetal heartbeat. Such a visit helps make the baby more real to the children.

Consistency is important in dealing with young children. They need reassurance that certain people, special things, and familiar places will continue to exist after the new baby arrives. The crib is an important, although transient, object in a child's life. If it is to be given to the new baby, the parents should thoughtfully help the child adjust to this change. Any move from crib to bed or from one room to another should precede the baby's birth by several weeks or more. If the new baby is to share a room with siblings, the parents must discuss this with the older child or children.

Some parents advocate *cosleeping* or *bed sharing* (one or both parents sleeping with their baby or young child), and so the crib is less of an issue. Cosleeping, which is common in many non-Western cultures, is on the increase in the United States, although it is not recommended. It is discussed further in Chapter 29.

If siblings are school-age children, pregnancy should be viewed as a family affair. Teaching should be suitable to the child's level of understanding and may be supplemented with appropriate books. Taking part in family discussions, attending sibling preparation classes, feeling fetal movement, and listening to the fetal heartbeat help the school-age child take part in the experience of pregnancy and not feel like an outsider.

Older children or adolescents may appear to have sophisticated knowledge but may have many misconceptions about pregnancy and birth. The parents should make opportunities to discuss their concerns and involve the children in preparations for the new baby.

Sibling preparation is essential, but other factors are equally important. These include the amount of parental attention the new arrival receives, the amount of attention the older child receives after the baby comes home, and parental skill in dealing with regressive or aggressive behavior. See the discussion of sibling preparation in Chapter 10.

Grandparents

The first relatives told about a pregnancy are usually the grandparents. The expectant grandparents often become increasingly supportive of the couple, even if conflicts previously existed. But it can be difficult for even sensitive grandparents to know how deeply to become involved in the childrearing process.

Because grandparenting can occur over a wide expanse of years, people's response to this role can vary considerably. Younger grandparents leading active lives may not demonstrate as much interest as the young couple would like. In other cases, expectant grandparents may give advice and gifts unsparingly. For grandparents, conflict may be related to the expectant couple's need to feel in control of their lives, or it may stem from events signaling changing roles in the grandparents' own lives (e.g., retirement, financial concerns, menopause, or death of a friend). Some parents of expectant couples may already be grandparents with a developed style of grandparenting. This influences their response to the pregnancy. Clarifying the role of the helping grandparent ensures a comfortable situation for all.

Because childbearing and childrearing practices have changed, family cohesiveness is promoted by effective communication and frank discussion between young couples and interested grandparents about the changes and the reasons for them.

Cultural Values and Pregnancy

Cultures have a universal tendency to create ceremonial rituals or rites around important life events. The rituals and customs of a group are a reflection of the group's values. In many developed countries, such as the United States, Canada, England, and Germany, populations are becoming more and more ethnically diverse as the number of immigrants continues to grow. It is not realistic or appropriate to assume that people who are new to a country or area will automatically abandon their ways and adopt the practices of the dominant culture (Dean, 2010). Consequently, the identification of cultural values is useful in planning and providing culturally sensitive care.

Generalization about cultural characteristics or values is difficult because not every individual in a culture may display these characteristics. Just as variations are seen between cultures, variations are also seen within cultures. For example, because of their exposure to the American culture, a third-generation Chinese American family might have very different values and beliefs from those of a Chinese family that has recently immigrated to the United States. For this reason, the nurse needs to supplement a general knowledge of cultural values and practices with a complete assessment of the individual's values and practices. *Developing Cultural Competence: Providing Effective Prenatal Care to Families of Different Cultures* summarizes the key actions a nurse can take to become more culturally aware.

Cultural assessment is an important aspect of prenatal care. The nurse needs to identify the prospective parents' main beliefs, values, and behaviors about pregnancy and childbearing. This includes information about ethnic background, amount of affiliation with the ethnic group, patterns of decision making, religious preference, language, communication style, and common etiquette practices. The nurse can also explore the woman's (or family's) expectations of the healthcare system. Once this information is gathered, the nurse can then plan and provide care that is appropriate and responsive to family needs. See Chapter 2 for more detail on these topics.

Developing Cultural Competence Providing Effective Prenatal Care to Families of Different Cultures

Nurses who are interacting with expectant families from a different culture or ethnic group can provide more effective, culturally sensitive nursing care by:

- Critically examining their own cultural beliefs
- Identifying personal biases, attitudes, stereotypes, and prejudices
- Making a conscious commitment to respect the values and beliefs of others
- Using sensitive, current language when describing others' cultures
- Learning the rituals, customs, and practices of the major cultural and ethnic groups with whom they have contact
- Including cultural assessment and assessment of the family's expectations of the healthcare system as a routine part of prenatal nursing care
- Incorporating the family's cultural and spiritual practices into prenatal care as much as possible
- Fostering an attitude of respect for and cooperation with alternative healers and caregivers whenever possible
- Providing for the services of an interpreter if language barriers exist
- Learning the language (or at least several key phrases) of at least one of the cultural groups with whom they interact
- Recognizing that ultimately it is the woman's right to make her own healthcare choices
- Evaluating whether the woman's healthcare beliefs have any potential negative consequences for her health

---

Focus Your Study

- Virtually all systems of a woman's body are altered in some way during pregnancy. Blood pressure decreases slightly during pregnancy. It reaches its lowest point in the second trimester and gradually increases to near normal levels in the third trimester. The enlarging uterus may exert pressure on the vena cava when the woman lies supine, causing a drop in blood pressure. This is called the vena caval syndrome or supine hypotension.

- A physiologic anemia may occur during pregnancy because the total plasma volume increases more than the total number of erythrocytes. This produces a drop in the hematocrit.

- The glomerular filtration rate increases during pregnancy. Glycosuria may be caused by the body's inability to reabsorb all the glucose filtered by the glomeruli.

- Changes in the skin include the development of chloasma; linea nigra; darkened nipples, areolae, and vulva; striae; and spider nevi.

- Insulin needs increase during pregnancy. A woman with a latent deficiency state may respond to the increased stress on the islets of Langerhans by developing gestational diabetes mellitus.

- The subjective (presumptive) signs of pregnancy are those symptoms experienced and reported by the woman, such as amenorrhea, nausea and vomiting, fatigue, urinary frequency, breast changes, and quickening.

- The objective (probable) signs of pregnancy can be perceived by the examiner but may be caused by conditions other than pregnancy.

- The diagnostic (positive) signs of pregnancy can be perceived by the examiner and can be caused only by pregnancy.

- During pregnancy the expectant woman may experience ambivalence, acceptance, introversion, emotional lability, and changes in body image.

- Rubin (1984) identified four developmental tasks for the pregnant woman: (1) ensuring safe passage through pregnancy, labor, and birth; (2) seeking acceptance of this child by others; (3) seeking commitment and acceptance of self as mother to the infant; and (4) learning to give of oneself on behalf of one's child.

- Fathers also face a series of adjustments as they accept their new role.

- Siblings of all ages require assistance in dealing with the birth of a new baby.

- Cultural values, beliefs, and behaviors influence a couple's response to childbearing and the healthcare system.

- A cultural assessment should focus on factors that will influence the practices of the childbearing family with regard to their health needs.

Clinical Reasoning in Action

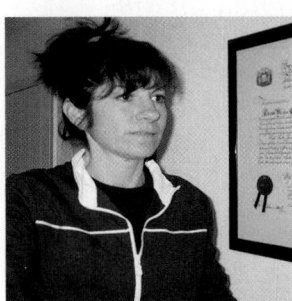

Twenty-two-year-old Jean Simmons is an aerobics instructor, G1P0 in her first trimester of pregnancy. She presents to you at the local clinic complaining of frequent nausea, urinary frequency, and fatigue. You obtain her vital signs: BP 108/60, temperature 97°F (36°C), pulse 68, respirations 12, weight 125 lb, height 64 inches. Her urine tests negative for ketones, albumin, leukocytes, and sugar. You note that Jean has lost 3 lb since her last visit. You assist the certified nurse-midwife with a physical exam, the findings of which are essentially normal. Jean says that while she knows it could become an issue, she would like to continue working as an aerobics instructor for as long as she possibly can during the pregnancy. You identify Jean's complaints as normal discomforts of pregnancy, and proceed with prenatal education.

1. What advice would you suggest to cope with the nausea of pregnancy?
2. What advice might you suggest to cope with urinary frequency?
3. What teaching would be important relating to exercise in pregnancy?
4. What symptoms related to exercise should Jean report to her physician?

References

Alio, A. P., Lewis, C. A., Scarborough, K., Harris, K., & Fiscella, K. (2013). A community perspective on the role of fathers during pregnancy: A qualitative study. *BMC Pregnancy and Childbirth, 13*(60), 1–11.

American College of Obstetricians and Gynecologists (ACOG). (2013a). *Nutrition during pregnancy [frequently asked questions faq001 pregnancy].* Retrieved from http://www.acog.org/~/media/For%20Patients /faq001.pdf?dmc=1&ts=20130711T1116342432

American College of Obstetricians and Gynecologists (ACOG). (2013b). *Weight gain during pregnancy [(ACOG Committee Opinion no. 548)].* Retrieved from http://www.acog.org/Resources_And_Publications /Committee_Opinions/Committee_on_Obstetric _Practice/Weight_Gain_During_Pregnancy

Cao, C., & O'Brien, K. O. (2013). Pregnancy and iron homeostasis: An update. *Nutrition Reviews, 71*(1), 35–51.

Cunningham, F. G., Leveno, K. J., Bloom, S. L., Spong, C. Y., Dashe, J. S., Hoffman, B. L., . . .Sheffield, J. S. (2014). *Williams obstetrics* (24th ed.). New York, NY: McGraw-Hill.

Dean, R. A., K. (2010). Cultural competence: Nursing in a multicultural society. *Nursing for women's health, 14*(1), 51–56.

Gordon, M. C. (2012). Maternal physiology. In S. G. Gabbe, J. R. Niebyl, J. L. Simpson, M. B. Landon, H. L. Galan, E. R. M. Jauniaux, & D. A. Driscoll (Eds.), *Obstetrics: Normal and problem pregnancies* (6th ed.). Philadelphia, PA: Churchill Livingstone.

Institute of Medicine (IOM). (2009). *Weight gain during pregnancy: Reexamining the guidelines.* Washington, DC: National Academies Press.

Jessop, D. C., Craig, L., & Ayers, S. (2014). Applying Leventhal's self-regulatory model to pregnancy: Evidence that pregnancy-related beliefs and emotional responses are associated with maternal health outcomes. *Journal of Health Psychology, 19*(9), 1091–1102.

Lederman, R. P., & Weis, K. (2009). *Psychosocial adaptation to pregnancy* (3rd ed.). New York, NY: Springer.

Patel, P. R., Laz, T. H., & Berenson, A. B. (2015). Patient characteristics associated with pregnancy ambivalence. *Journal of Women's Health, 24*(1), 37–41.

Rubin, R. (1984). *Maternal identity and the maternal experience.* New York, NY: Springer.

Widarsson, M., Kerstis, B., Sundquist, K., Engstrom, G., & Sarkadi, A. (2012). Support needs of expectant mothers and fathers: A qualitative study. *Journal of Perinatal Education, 21*(1), 36–44.

Yu, C. Y., Hung, C. H., Chan, T. F., Yeh, C. H., & Lai, C. Y. (2012). Prenatal predictors for father-infant attachment after childbirth. *Journal of Clinical Nursing, 21*(11/12), 1577–1583.

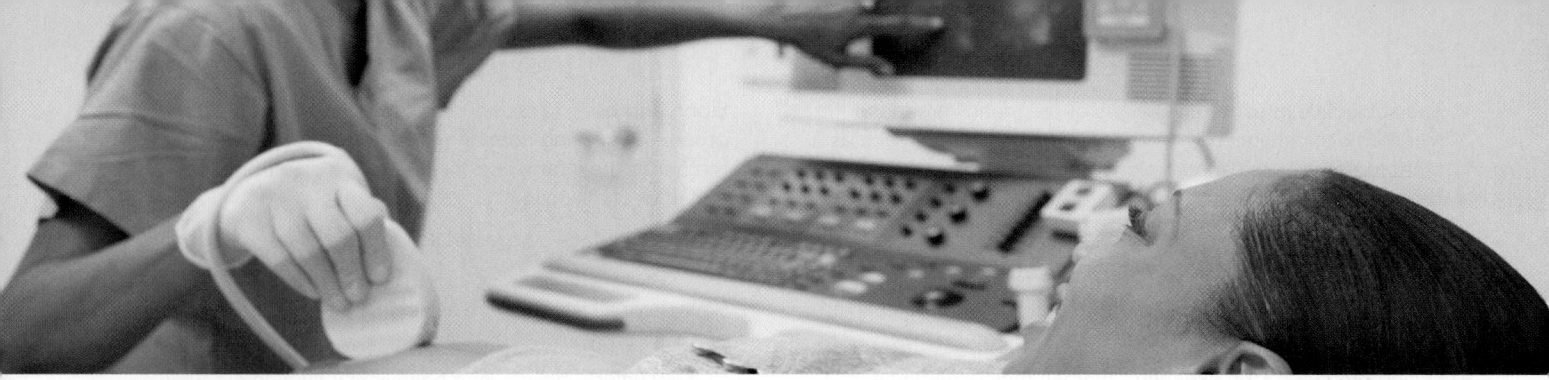

Chapter 9
Antepartum Nursing Assessment

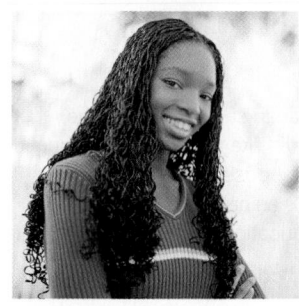

Joe McBride/Getty Images

I'm 16—just got my license—so it was weird telling my friends that my mom is pregnant. I was embarrassed (and a little jealous) at first but now I kind of like the idea of having a baby sister. Mom had an amniocentesis because she is 37, so we know it's a girl. My mom has been great about including me and telling me what is going on. I've gone to a couple of her prenatal appointments so I got to hear the heartbeat and I saw the baby moving on ultrasound. I'm surprised by how interesting I am finding everything. Don't laugh, but I think I might like to be a nurse-midwife someday.

—Krista, 16

⌄ Learning Outcomes

9.1 Summarize the essential components of a prenatal history.

9.2 Define common obstetric terminology found in the history of maternity clients.

9.3 Predict the normal physiologic changes one would expect to find when performing a physical assessment on a pregnant woman.

9.4 Calculate the estimated date of birth using the common methods.

9.5 Describe the essential measurements that can be determined by clinical pelvimetry.

9.6 Summarize the results of the major screening tests used during the prenatal period in the assessment of the prenatal client.

9.7 Relate the danger signs of pregnancy to their possible causes.

9.8 Relate the components of the subsequent prenatal history and assessment to the progress of pregnancy and the nursing care of the prenatal client.

D uring the antepartum period, the role of the nurse is determined by academic preparation, clinical expertise, and professional credentials. The RN may complete many areas of prenatal assessment. Advanced practice nurses such as certified nurse-midwives (CNMs) and nurse practitioners are able to perform complete antepartum assessments. This chapter focuses on the prenatal assessments completed initially and at subsequent visits to provide optimum care for the childbearing family.

Healthy People 2020

(MICH-1) Reduce the rate of fetal and infant deaths

(MICH-5) Reduce the rate of maternal mortality

(MICH-6) Reduce maternal illness and complications due to pregnancy (complications during hospitalized labor and delivery)

(MICH-10) Increase the proportion of pregnant women who receive early and adequate prenatal care

Initial Client History

The course of a pregnancy depends on a number of factors, including the woman's prepregnancy health, presence of disease/illness states, family history, emotional status, and past health care. A thorough history helps determine the status of a woman's prepregnancy health.

Definition of Terms

The following terms are used in recording the history of maternity clients:

- **Antepartum:** time between conception and the onset of labor; describes the period during which a woman is pregnant; used interchangeably with *prenatal*
- **Intrapartum:** time from the onset of true labor until the birth of the baby and placenta
- **Postpartum:** time from the delivery of the placenta and membranes until the woman's body returns to a nonpregnant condition; typically about 6 weeks
- **Gestation:** the number of weeks of pregnancy since the first day of the last menstrual period
- **Abortion:** birth that occurs before the end of 20 weeks' gestation or the birth of a fetus-newborn who weighs less than 500 g (Cunningham et al., 2014). Abortion is abbreviated as ab. An abortion may occur spontaneously or it may be induced by medical or surgical means. If induced, it is often termed a therapeutic abortion.
- **Stillbirth:** a baby born dead after 20 weeks' gestation
- **Term**: a word that was formerly used to identify the normal duration of pregnancy. The stand-alone use of this word is now discouraged because it represents such a wide range of time and related risk (Spong, 2013). The American College of Obstetrics and Gynecology (ACOG, 2013a) recommends that the following definitions be used:
  - **Late preterm:** births that occur between 34 0/7 through 36 6/7 weeks' gestation (ACOG, 2013c).
  - **Early term:** births occurring between 37 weeks 0 days and 38 weeks 6 days
  - **Full term:** births occurring between 39 weeks 0 days and 40 weeks 6 days
  - **Late term:** births occurring between 41 weeks 0 days through 41 weeks 6 days
  - **Postterm:** births occurring after 42 weeks
- **Preterm labor:** labor that occurs after 20 weeks' gestation but before completion of 36 weeks' gestation
- **Postterm labor:** labor that occurs after 42 weeks' gestation
- **Gravida:** any pregnancy, regardless of duration, including present pregnancy. Gravida is often abbreviated as G.
- **Nulligravida:** a woman who has never been pregnant
- **Primigravida**: a woman who is pregnant for the first time
- **Multigravida:** a woman who is in her second or any subsequent pregnancy
- **Para:** birth after 20 weeks' gestation regardless of whether the baby is born alive or dead. Para is often abbreviated as P.
- **Nullipara:** a woman who has had no births at more than 20 weeks' gestation
- **Primipara:** a woman who has had one birth at more than 20 weeks' gestation regardless of whether the baby was born alive or dead
- **Multipara:** a woman who has had two or more births at more than 20 weeks' gestation

The terms *gravida* and *para* refer to pregnancies, not to the fetus. Thus, traditionally, twins, triplets, and other multiple fetuses are counted as one pregnancy and one birth. This approach is confusing, however, because it fails to identify the number of children that a woman might have. To provide comprehensive data, a more detailed approach is used in some settings. A useful acronym for remembering the system is TPAL (King, Brucker, Kriebs, et al., 2015).

T: number of early, full, or late *term* births the woman has experienced (number of babies born at the 37 0/7 weeks' gestation or beyond)

P: number of *preterm* births (births after 20 weeks' gestation but before 37 0/7weeks' gestation, whether living or stillborn)

A: number of pregnancies ending in either spontaneous or therapeutic *abortion* (before 20 weeks' gestation)

L: number of currently *living* children to whom the woman has given birth

The following examples delineate the differences between the two systems.

1. Jean Sanchez has one child born at 39 weeks' gestation and became pregnant for a second time. The second pregnancy ended in a miscarriage at 15 weeks' gestation. Using the *traditional approach* her obstetric history would be recorded as "gravida 2 para 1 ab 1." Using the *detailed approach*, her obstetric history would be recorded as "gravida 2 para 1011."

2. Tracy Hopkins is pregnant for the fourth time. At home she has a child who was born at full term. Her second pregnancy ended at 10 weeks' gestation. She then gave birth to twins at 35 weeks. Using the *traditional approach* her obstetric history would be recorded as gravida 4 para 2 ab 1. Using the *detailed approach* her obstetric history would be recorded as "gravida 4 para 1113."

To avoid confusion, it is best for practicing nurses to clarify the recording system used at their facilities.

Clinical Tip

In general, it is best to avoid an initial discussion of a woman's gravida and para status in front of her partner. It is possible that the woman had a previous pregnancy that she has not mentioned to her partner, and revealing the information could violate her right to privacy.

Client Profile

The history is essentially a screening tool to identify factors that may place the mother or fetus at risk during the pregnancy. The following information is obtained for each pregnant woman at the first prenatal assessment:

1. Current pregnancy
   - First day of last normal menstrual period (LMP) (Is she sure of the dates or uncertain? Do her cycles normally occur every 28 days, or do her cycles tend to be longer?)

- Presence of cramping, bleeding, or spotting since LMP
- Woman's opinion about the time when conception occurred and when baby is due
- Woman's attitude toward pregnancy (Is this pregnancy planned? Wanted?)
- Results of pregnancy tests, if completed
- Any discomforts since LMP such as nausea, vomiting, urinary frequency, fatigue, or breast tenderness

2. Past pregnancies
   - Number of pregnancies
   - Number of abortions, spontaneous or induced
   - Number of living children
   - History of previous pregnancies, length of pregnancy, length of labor and birth, type of birth (vaginal, forceps-assisted, vacuum-assisted birth, or cesarean), location of birth, type of anesthesia used (if any), woman's perception of the experience, and complications (antepartum, intrapartum, and postpartum)
   - Neonatal status of previous children: Apgar scores, birth weights, general development, complications, and feeding patterns (breast milk, formula, or both). If breastfed, for how long?
   - Loss of a child (miscarriage, elective or medically indicated abortion, stillbirth, neonatal death, relinquishment, or death after the neonatal period). Cause of loss? What was the experience like for her? What coping skills helped? How did her partner, if involved, respond?
   - Blood type and Rh factor (If Rh negative, was Rh immune globulin received after birth/miscarriage/abortion? Baby's blood type)
   - Prenatal education classes and resources (books, websites); knowledge about pregnancy, childbirth, and parenting

3. Gynecologic history
   - Date of last Papanicolaou (Pap) smear; result? Any history of abnormal Pap smear; any follow-up therapy completed
   - Previous infections: vaginal, cervical, pelvic inflammatory disease (PID), or sexually transmitted infections (STIs)
   - Previous surgery (uterine, ovarian)
   - Age at menarche
   - Regularity, frequency, and duration of menstrual flow
   - History of dysmenorrhea
   - History of infertility
   - Sexual history
   - Contraceptive history (If hormonal method used, did pregnancy occur immediately following cessation of method? If not, how long after? When was contraception last used?)
   - Any issues related to infertility or fertility treatments

4. Current medical history
   - Weight (prepregnancy and current), height, body mass index (BMI) (determine recommended weight gain)

- General health, including nutrition (dietary practices such as vegetarianism; lactose intolerance; food allergies?), regular exercise program (type, frequency, and duration); monthly breast self-examination; eye examination; date of last dental examination
- Any medications presently being taken (including prescription, nonprescription, homeopathic, or herbal medications) or taken since the onset of pregnancy
- Previous or present use of alcohol, tobacco, or caffeine (Ask specifically about the amounts of alcohol, cigarettes, and caffeine [specify coffee, tea, colas, or chocolate] consumed each day.)
- Illicit drug use or abuse (Ask about specific drugs such as cocaine, crack, methamphetamines, and marijuana; planning cessation?)
- Drug allergies and other allergies (Ask about latex allergies or sensitivities.)
- Potential teratogenic insults to this pregnancy such as viral infections, medications, x-ray examinations, surgery, or cats in the home (possible source of toxoplasmosis)
- Presence of chronic disease conditions such as diabetes, hypertension, cardiovascular disease, renal problems, cancer, or thyroid disorder
- Infections or illnesses since LMP (flu, measles)
- Record of immunizations (especially rubella); up to date?
- Presence of any abnormal signs/symptoms

5. Past medical history
   - Childhood diseases
   - Past treatment for any disease condition (Any hospitalizations? Major injuries?)
   - Surgical procedures
   - Presence of bleeding disorders or tendencies (Has she received blood transfusions? Will she accept blood transfusions?)

6. Family medical history
   - Presence of diabetes, cardiovascular disease, cancer, hypertension, hematologic disorders, tuberculosis, thyroid disease
   - Occurrence of multiple births
   - History of congenital diseases or deformities
   - Occurrence of cesarean births and cause, if known

7. Genetic history (client, father of the child [FOC], and both families)
   - Birth defects
   - Recurrent pregnancy loss
   - Stillbirth
   - Down syndrome, intellectual disability, developmental delay, chromosomal abnormalities
   - Ethnic background (Mediterranean descent, Jewish, Asian)
   - Genetic disorders (cystic fibrosis, sickle cell disease/trait, muscular dystrophy).

8. Religious, spiritual, and cultural history
   - Does the woman wish to specify a religious preference on her medical record? Does she have any spiritual

beliefs or practices that might influence her health care or that of her child, such as a prohibition against receiving blood products, dietary considerations, or circumcision rites?

- What practices are important for her spiritual well-being?
- Might practices in her culture or that of her partner influence her care or that of her child?

9. Occupational history
   - Occupation
   - Physical demands (Does she stand all day, or are there opportunities to sit and elevate her legs? Any heavy lifting?)
   - Exposure to chemicals or other harmful substances
   - Opportunity for regular meals and breaks for nutritious snacks
   - Provision for maternity or family leave

10. Birth father's physical history
    - Age
    - Significant health problems
    - Blood type and Rh factor
    - Presence of genetic conditions or diseases in him or in his family history

11. Father's/partner's social history
    - Occupation
    - Educational level; methods by which he or she learns best
    - Current tobacco use, drug use, and alcohol intake
    - Thoughts/feelings about the pregnancy

12. Personal history
    - Age
    - Relationship status (Married? Birth father involved? Partner's level of involvement [if partner is not the father of the child])
    - Educational level; methods by which she learns best
    - Race or ethnic group (to identify need for prenatal genetic screening and racially or ethnically related risk factors)
    - Housing; stability of living conditions; neighborhood safety; animals in the home
    - Economic level: ability to pay bills, purchase nutritious food; use of supplemental programs such as WIC
    - Acceptance of pregnancy, whether intended or unintended
    - Any history of emotional or physical deprivation or abuse of herself or children or any abuse in her current relationship (Has she been hit, slapped, kicked, or hurt within the past year or since she has been pregnant? Is she afraid of her partner or anyone else? If yes, of whom is she afraid? [*Note:* Ask these questions when the woman is alone.])
    - History of emotional/mental health problems (depression in general, postpartum depression, anxiety, bipolar disorder)
    - Support systems
    - Personal preferences about the birth (expectations of both the woman and her partner, presence of others, and so on)

- Plans for care of newborn following birth; plans for circumcision if the baby is male.
- Feeding preference for the baby (Breast milk or formula?)

Obtaining Data

A questionnaire is often used to obtain information. Some clinics and offices send the form via e-mail or regular mail, or post the form on their website for downloading, so the woman can complete it prior to her first prenatal visit; others prefer that it be done in person. In either case, the woman should complete the questionnaire in a quiet place with a minimum of distractions. The nurse can get further information in an interview, which allows the pregnant woman to clarify her responses to questions and gives the nurse and client the opportunity to develop rapport.

SAFETY ALERT!
Because some medications may pose a risk to the fetus if taken during pregnancy, it is crucial to develop a list of all the medications the pregnant woman is currently taking as well as those she had been taking before she learned she was pregnant. This list should be given to the client's primary healthcare provider. (See discussion of classification system for medications taken during pregnancy in Chapter 10.)

The expectant father or partner can be encouraged to attend the prenatal examinations. The partner is often able to contribute to the history and may use the opportunity to ask questions or express concerns that are important to him or her.

Prenatal Risk-Factor Screening

Risk factors are any findings that suggest the pregnancy may have a negative outcome for either the woman or her unborn child. Screening for risk factors is an important part of the prenatal assessment. Many risk factors can be identified during the initial assessment; others may be detected during subsequent prenatal visits. It is important to identify high-risk pregnancies early so that appropriate interventions can be started promptly. Not all risk factors threaten a pregnancy equally; thus many agencies use a scoring sheet to determine the degree of risk. Information must be updated throughout pregnancy as necessary. Any pregnancy may begin as low risk and change to high risk because of complications.

Clinical Reasoning **Hot Tub Use in Pregnancy**
Karen Blade, a 23-year-old woman, G1P0, is 10 weeks' pregnant when she sees you for her first prenatal examination. She has been experiencing some mild nausea and fatigue but otherwise is feeling well. She asks you about continuing with her routine exercises (walking 3 miles a day and lifting light weights). She also asks about using the heated pool and a hot tub. What should you tell her?

Table 9–1 identifies the major risk factors currently recognized. The table also identifies maternal and fetal or newborn implications if the risk is present in the pregnancy.

TABLE 9–1 Prenatal High-Risk Factors

FACTOR	MATERNAL IMPLICATIONS	FETAL OR NEONATAL IMPLICATIONS
Social and Personal		
Low income level and/or low educational level	Insufficient antenatal care or late antenatal care ↑ risk preterm birth Poor nutrition ↑ risk preeclampsia	Low birth weight Prematurity Intrauterine growth restriction (IUGR)/small for gestational age (SGA)
Poor diet	Inadequate nutrition ↑ risk preterm birth ↑ risk anemia ↑ risk preeclampsia	Fetal malnutrition IUGR/SGA Prematurity
Living at high altitude	↑ hemoglobin	Prematurity IUGR ↑ hemoglobin (polycythemia)
Multiparity greater than 3	↑ risk antepartum or postpartum hemorrhage	Anemia Fetal death
Weight less than 45.5 kg (100 lb)	Poor nutrition Cephalopelvic disproportion Prolonged labor	IUGR/SGA Hypoxia associated with difficult labor and birth
Weight greater than 91 kg (200 lb)	↑ risk hypertension ↑ risk cephalopelvic disproportion ↑ risk diabetes	↓ fetal nutrition ↑ risk macrosomia
Age less than 16 years	Poor nutrition Insufficient antenatal care ↑ risk preeclampsia ↑ risk cephalopelvic disproportion	Low birth weight ↑ fetal demise
Age older than 35	↑ risk preeclampsia ↑ risk cesarean birth	↑ risk congenital anomalies ↑ chromosomal abnormalities
Smoking one pack/day or more	↑ risk hypertension ↑ risk cancer	↓ placental perfusion → ↓ O_2 and nutrients available Low birth weight IUGR/SGA Preterm birth
Use of addictive drugs	↑ risk poor nutrition ↑ risk infection with IV drugs ↑ risk HIV, hepatitis C	↑ risk congenital anomalies ↑ risk abruptio placentae ↑ risk low birth weight Neonatal withdrawal Lower serum bilirubin
Excessive alcohol consumption	↑ risk poor nutrition Possible hepatic effects with long-term consumption	↑ risk fetal alcohol syndrome
Preexisting Medical Disorders		
Diabetes mellitus	↑ risk preeclampsia, hypertension Episodes of hypoglycemia and hyperglycemia ↑ risk cesarean birth	Low birth weight Macrosomia Neonatal hypoglycemia ↑ risk congenital anomalies ↑ risk respiratory distress syndrome

Preexisting Medical Disorders (*continued*)

Cardiac disease	Cardiac decompensation	↑ risk fetal demise
	Further strain on mother's body	↑ prenatal mortality
	↑ maternal death rate	
Anemia: hemoglobin less than 11 g/dL or less than 32% hematocrit	Iron deficiency anemia	Fetal death
	Low energy level	Prematurity
	Decreased oxygen-carrying capacity	Low birth weight
Hypertension	↑ vasospasm	↓ placental perfusion
	↑ risk central nervous system irritability	→ low birth weight
	→ convulsions	Preterm birth
	↑ risk cerebrovascular accident	
	↑ risk renal damage	
Thyroid disorder	↑ infertility	↑ spontaneous abortion
Hypothyroidism	↓ basal metabolic rate, goiter, myxedema	↑ risk congenital goiter
	↑ risk miscarriage, preterm labor/birth	↑ risk IUGR/SGA
	↑ risk preeclampsia	↑ risk stillbirth
Hyperthyroidism	↓ risk postpartum hemorrhage	Mental retardation →
	↑ risk preeclampsia	cretinism
	Danger of thyroid storm	↑ incidence congenital anomalies
		↑ incidence preterm birth, IUGR/SGA
		↑ risk neonatal hyperthyroidism
		↑ tendency to thyrotoxicosis
Renal disease (moderate to severe)	↑ risk renal failure	↑ risk IUGR/SGA
		↑ risk preterm birth
Diethylstilbestrol (DES) exposure	↑ infertility, spontaneous abortion	
	↑ cervical insufficiency	↑ risk preterm birth

Obstetric Considerations

Previous Pregnancy

Stillborn	↑ emotional or psychologic distress	↑ risk IUGR/SGA
		↑ risk preterm birth
Recurrent abortion	↑ emotional or psychologic distress	↑ risk abortion
Cesarean birth	↑ possibility repeat cesarean birth	↑ risk preterm birth
		↑ risk respiratory distress
Rh or blood group sensitization		↑ risk erythroblastosis fetalis
		Hydrops fetalis
		Neonatal anemia
		Kernicterus
		Hypoglycemia
Large baby	↑ risk cesarean birth	Birth injury
	↑ risk gestational diabetes	Hypoglycemia

Current Pregnancy

Rubella (first trimester)		Congenital heart disease
		Cataracts
		Nerve deafness
		Bone lesions
		Prolonged virus shedding

(*continued*)

TABLE 9–1 Prenatal High-Risk Factors (*continued*)

FACTOR	MATERNAL IMPLICATIONS	FETAL OR NEONATAL IMPLICATIONS
Current Pregnancy (continued)		
Toxoplasmosis		Retinochoroiditis
		Convulsions, coma, microcephaly
Rubella (second trimester)		Hepatitis
		Thrombocytopenia
Cytomegalovirus		IUGR
		Encephalopathy
Herpesvirus type 2	Severe discomfort	Neonatal herpesvirus type 2
	Concern about possibility of cesarean birth, fetal infection	2% hepatitis with jaundice
		Neurologic abnormalities
Syphilis	↑ incidence abortion	↑ fetal demise
		Congenital syphilis
HIV positive	Candidal infections	Transmission of HIV
	Wasting syndrome	
	Concurrent STIs such as herpes	
	Postpartum hemorrhage, poor wound healing	
Abruptio placentae and placenta previa	↑ risk hemorrhage	Fetal or neonatal anemia
	Bed rest	Intrauterine hemorrhage
	Extended hospitalization	↑ fetal demise
Preeclampsia or eclampsia	See hypertension	↑ placental perfusion
		→ low birth weight
Multiple gestation	↑ risk postpartum hemorrhage	↑ risk preterm labor/birth
	↑ risk preterm labor	↑ risk stillbirth
	↑ risk gestational diabetes mellitus	↑ risk fetal demise, IUGR/SGA
	↑ risk placenta previa	↑ risk malpresentation
	↑ risk preeclampsia	↑ risk stillbirth
Elevated hematocrit Greater than 41% (White) Greater than 38% (Black)	Increased viscosity of blood	Fetal death rate 5 times normal rate
Spontaneous premature rupture of membranes	↑ uterine infection	Preterm birth
		Fetal demise

Note: This table is not inclusive of all potential outcomes.

Initial Prenatal Assessment

The initial prenatal assessment focuses on the woman holistically by considering physical, cultural, and psychosocial factors that influence her health. The establishment of the nurse-client relationship is a chance to develop an atmosphere conducive to interviewing, support, and education. Because many women are excited and anxious at the first antepartum visit, the initial psychosocial-cultural assessment is general.

As part of the initial psychosocial-cultural assessment, discuss with the woman any religious or spiritual, cultural, or socioeconomic factors that influence the woman's expectations of the childbearing experience. It is especially helpful to be familiar with common practices of the members of various religious and cultural groups who reside in the community.

Women With Special Needs Assessing Care Needs During Pregnancy

During the initial assessment, the woman with a disability should be questioned to determine her current level of functioning and the degree of assistance she normally requires in her everyday routine. This assists the healthcare team in planning care and interventions that may be needed. Care needs may change during pregnancy and warrant ongoing assessments of the woman's level of functioning.

After obtaining the history, prepare the woman for the physical examination. The physical examination begins with assessment of vital signs; then the woman's body is examined. The pelvic examination is performed last.

Before the examination the woman should provide a clean urine specimen for screening. When her bladder is empty, the woman is more comfortable during the pelvic examination and the examiner can palpate the pelvic organs more easily. After the woman empties her bladder, the nurse should ask her to disrobe and give her a gown and sheet or some other protective covering.

Professionalism in Practice Physical Exams and Scope of Practice

Increasing numbers of nurses, such as CNMs, nurse practitioners, and other nurses in advanced practice, are educationally prepared to perform complete physical examinations. The nurse who is not an advanced practitioner assesses the woman's vital signs, explains the procedures to allay apprehension, positions her for examination, and assists the examiner as necessary. Each nurse is responsible for operating at expected professional standards within his or her skill level, educational preparation, and knowledge base.

Thoroughness and a systematic procedure are the most important considerations when performing the physical portion of an antepartum examination. See *Assessment Guide: Initial Prenatal Assessment.* To promote completeness, the assessment guide is organized in three columns that address the areas to be assessed (and normal findings), the variations or alterations that may be observed, and nursing responses to the data. Certain organs and systems are assessed concurrently with others during the physical portion of the examination.

Clinical Tip

Gloves are worn for procedures that involve contact with body fluids such as drawing blood for laboratory work, handling urine specimens, and conducting pelvic examinations. Because of the increased incidence of latex allergies, it is becoming more common for nonlatex gloves to be used. It is important to inquire about latex allergies with any client before beginning an examination.

Nursing interventions based on assessment of the normal physical and psychosocial changes of pregnancy, evaluation of the cultural influences associated with pregnancy, and mutually defined client teaching and counseling needs are discussed further in Chapter 10.

ASSESSMENT GUIDE | Initial Prenatal Assessment

Physical Assessment/Normal Findings	Alterations and Possible Causes*	Nursing Responses to Data†
Vital Signs		
Blood pressure (BP): Less than or equal to 120/80 mmHg.	High BP (essential hypertension; renal disease; pregestational hypertension, apprehension; preeclampsia if initial assessment not done until after 20 weeks' gestation)	BP of 120–139/80–89 is considered prehypertensive. BP greater than 140/90 requires immediate consideration; establish woman's BP; refer to healthcare provider if necessary. Assess woman's knowledge about high BP; counsel on self-care and medical management.
Pulse: 60–100 beats/min; rate may increase 10 beats/min during pregnancy	Increased pulse rate (excitement or anxiety, dehydration, cardiac disorders)	Count for 1 full minute; note irregularities. Evaluate temperature, increase fluids.
Respirations: 12–20 breaths/min (or pulse rate divided by 4); pregnancy may induce a degree of hyperventilation; thoracic breathing predominant	Marked tachypnea or abnormal patterns	Assess for respiratory disease.
Temperature: 97°–99.6°F (36.2°–37.6°C)	Elevated temperature (infection)	Assess for infection process or disease state if temperature is elevated; refer to healthcare provider.
Weight		
Amount of weight gain depends on body build Underweight: 28–40 lb (12.5–18.0 kg) Normal weight: 25–35 lb (11.5–16.0 kg) Overweight: 15–25 lb (7.0–11.5 kg) Obese: 11–20 lb (5.0–9.1 kg)	Weight less than 45 kg (100 lb) or greater than 91 kg (200 lb); rapid, sudden weight gain (preeclampsia)	Evaluate need for nutritional counseling; obtain information on eating habits, cooking practices, food regularly eaten, food allergies, income limitations, need for food supplements, and pica and other abnormal food habits. Note initial weight to establish baseline for weight gain throughout pregnancy. Determine body mass index (BMI) and recommend amount of weight gain for pregnancy.

(continued)

ASSESSMENT GUIDE | Initial Prenatal Assessment (*continued*)

Physical Assessment/Normal Findings	Alterations and Possible Causes*	Nursing Responses to Data†
Skin		
Color: Consistent with racial background; pink nail beds	Pallor (anemia); bronze, yellow (hepatic disease; other causes of jaundice)	The following tests should be performed: complete blood count (CBC), bilirubin level, urinalysis, and blood urea nitrogen (BUN). If abnormal, refer to healthcare provider.
	Bluish, reddish, mottled; dusky appearance or pallor of palms and nail beds in dark-skinned women (anemia)	
Condition: Absence of edema (slight edema of lower extremities is normal during pregnancy)	Edema (preeclampsia, normal pregnancy changes); rashes, dermatitis (allergic response)	Counsel on relief measures for slight edema. Initiate preeclampsia assessment; refer to healthcare provider.
Lesions: Absence of lesions	Ulceration (varicose veins, decreased circulation)	Further assess circulatory status; refer to healthcare provider if lesion is severe.
Spider nevi common in pregnancy	Petechiae, multiple bruises, ecchymosis (hemorrhagic disorders; abuse)	Evaluate for bleeding or clotting disorder. Provide opportunities to discuss abuse if suspected.
		Refer to healthcare provider.
Moles		
Pigmentation: Pigmentation changes of pregnancy include linea nigra, striae gravidarum, melasma	Change in size or color (carcinoma)	Assure woman that these are normal manifestations of pregnancy and explain the physiologic basis for the changes.
Cafe-au-lait spots	Six or more (Albright syndrome or neurofibromatosis)	Consult with healthcare provider.
Nose		
Character of mucosa: Redder than oral mucosa; in pregnancy nasal mucosa is edematous in response to increased estrogen, resulting in nasal stuffiness (rhinitis of pregnancy) and nosebleeds	Olfactory loss (first cranial nerve deficit)	Counsel woman about possible relief measures for nasal stuffiness and nosebleeds (epistaxis); refer to healthcare provider for olfactory loss.
Mouth		
May note hypertrophy of gingival tissue because of estrogen	Edema, inflammation (infection); pale in color (anemia)	Assess hematocrit for anemia; counsel regarding dental hygiene habits. Refer to healthcare provider or dentist if necessary. Routine dental care appropriate during pregnancy.
Neck		
Nodes: Small, mobile, nontender nodes	Tender, hard, fixed, or prominent nodes (infection, carcinoma)	Examine for local infection; refer to healthcare provider.
Thyroid: Small, smooth, lateral lobes palpable on either side of trachea; slight hyperplasia by third month of pregnancy	Enlargement or nodule tenderness (hyperthyroidism)	Test to perform: thyroid-stimulating hormone (TSH). Listen over thyroid for bruits, which may indicate hyperthyroidism. Question woman about dietary habits (iodine intake). Ascertain history of thyroid problems; refer to healthcare provider.
Chest and Lungs		
Chest: Symmetric, elliptic, smaller anteroposterior (AP) than transverse diameter	Increased AP diameter, funnel chest, pigeon chest (emphysema, asthma, pulmonary disease)	Evaluate for emphysema, asthma, pulmonary disease.
Ribs: Slope downward from nipple line	More horizontal (pulmonary disease) angular bumps rachitic rosary (vitamin C deficiency)	Evaluate for pulmonary disease. Evaluate for fractures. Consult healthcare provider. Consult nutritionist.

Physical Assessment/Normal Findings	Alterations and Possible Causes*	Nursing Responses to Data†
Inspection and palpation: No retraction or bulging of intercostal spaces (ICS) during inspiration or expiration; symmetric expansion.	ICS retractions with inspirations, bulging with expiration; unequal expansion (respiratory disease)	Do thorough initial assessment. Refer to healthcare provider.
Tactile fremitus	Tachypnea, hyperpnea (respiratory disease)	Refer to healthcare provider.
Percussion: Bilateral symmetry in tone	Flatness of percussion, which may be affected by chest wall thickness	Evaluate for pleural effusions, consolidations, or tumor.
Low-pitched resonance of moderate intensity	High diaphragm (atelectasis or paralysis), pleural effusion	Refer to healthcare provider.
Auscultation: Upper lobes: bronchovesicular sounds above sternum and scapulas; equal expiratory and inspiratory phases	Abnormal if heard over any other area of chest	Refer to healthcare provider.
Remainder of chest: vesicular breath sounds heard; inspiratory phase longer (3:1)	Rales, rhonchi, wheezes; pleural friction rub; absence of breath sounds; bronchophony, egophony, whispered pectoriloquy	Refer to healthcare provider.
Breasts		
Supple: Symmetric in size and contour; darker pigmentation of nipple and areola; may have supernumerary nipples, usually 5–6 cm (2.0 to 2.4 in.) below normal nipple line	"Pigskin" or orange-peel appearance, nipple retractions, swelling, hardness (carcinoma); redness, heat, tenderness, cracked or fissured nipple (infection)	Encourage monthly self-examination; instruct woman how to examine her own breasts.
Axillary nodes nonpalpable or pellet sized	Tenderness, enlargement, hard node (carcinoma); may be visible bump (infection)	Refer to healthcare provider for evaluation of abnormal breast findings. Plan ultrasound/mammogram/MRI of breasts.
Pregnancy changes: 1. Size increase noted primarily in first 20 weeks. 2. Become nodular. 3. Tingling sensation may be felt during first and third trimester; woman may report feeling of heaviness. 4. Pigmentation of nipples and areolae darkens. 5. Superficial veins dilate and become more prominent. 6. Striae seen in multiparas. 7. Tubercles of Montgomery enlarge. 8. Colostrum may be present after 12th week. 9. Secondary areola appears at 20 weeks, characterized by series of washed-out spots surrounding primary areola. 10. Breasts less firm, old striae may be present in multiparas.		Discuss normalcy of changes and their meaning with the woman. Teach and/or institute appropriate relief measures. Encourage use of supportive, well-fitting brassiere.
Heart		
Normal rate, rhythm, and heart sounds	Enlargement, thrills, thrusts, gross irregularity or skipped beats, gallop rhythm or extra sounds (cardiac disease)	Complete an initial assessment. Explain normal pregnancy-induced changes. Refer to healthcare provider if indicated.
Pregnancy changes: 1. Palpitations may occur due to sympathetic nervous system disturbance. 2. Short systolic murmurs that increase in held expiration are normal due to increased volume.		

(continued)

ASSESSMENT GUIDE | Initial Prenatal Assessment (*continued*)

Physical Assessment/Normal Findings	Alterations and Possible Causes*	Nursing Responses to Data†
Abdomen		
Normal appearance, skin texture, and hair distribution; liver nonpalpable; abdomen nontender	Muscle guarding (anxiety, acute tenderness); tenderness, mass (ectopic pregnancy, inflammation, carcinoma)	Assure woman of normalcy of diastasis. Provide initial information about appropriate prenatal and postpartum exercises. Evaluate woman's anxiety level. Refer to healthcare provider if indicated.
Pregnancy changes:		
1. Purple striae may be present (or silver striae on a multipara) as well as linea nigra.		
2. Diastasis of the rectus muscles is seen late in pregnancy.	Size of uterus inconsistent with length of gestation (intrauterine growth restriction [IUGR], multiple pregnancy, fetal demise, incorrect estimated date of birth (EDB), abnormal amniotic fluid, hydatidiform mole)	Reassess menstrual history regarding pregnancy dating. Evaluate increase in size using McDonald method. (See Figure 9–3.) Use ultrasound to establish diagnosis.
3. Size: Flat or rotund abdomen; progressive enlargement of uterus due to pregnancy: *10–12 weeks:* Fundus slightly above symphysis pubis. *16 weeks:* Fundus halfway between symphysis and umbilicus. *20–22 weeks:* Fundus at umbilicus. *28 weeks:* Fundus three finger breadths above umbilicus. *36 weeks:* Fundus just below ensiform cartilage.		
4. Fetal heart rate: 110–160 beats/min may be heard with Doppler at 10–12 weeks' gestation; may be heard with fetoscope at 17–20 weeks.	Failure to hear fetal heartbeat with Doppler (fetal demise, hydatidiform mole)	Refer to healthcare provider. Administer pregnancy tests. Use ultrasound to establish diagnosis.
5. Fetal movement palpable by a trained examiner after the 18th week.	Failure to feel fetal movements after 20 weeks' gestation (fetal demise, hydatidiform mole)	Refer to healthcare provider.
6. Ballottement: During fourth to fifth month, fetus rises and then rebounds to original position when uterus is tapped sharply.	No ballottement (oligohydramnios)	Refer to healthcare provider.
Extremities		
Skin warm, pulses palpable, full range of motion; may be some edema of hands and ankles in late pregnancy; varicose veins may become more pronounced; palmar erythema may be present	Unpalpable or diminished pulses (arterial insufficiency); marked edema (preeclampsia)	Evaluate for other symptoms of heart disease; initiate follow-up if woman mentions that her rings feel tight. Discuss prevention and self-treatment measures for varicose veins; refer to healthcare provider if indicated.
Spine		
Normal spinal curves: Concave cervical, convex thoracic, concave lumbar	Abnormal spinal curves; flatness, kyphosis, lordosis	Refer to healthcare provider if indicated.
In pregnancy, lumbar spinal curve may be accentuated	Backache	May have implications for administration of spinal anesthetics
Shoulders and iliac crests should be even	Uneven shoulders and iliac crests (scoliosis)	Refer very young women to healthcare provider; discuss back-stretching exercise with older women.
Reflexes		
Normal and symmetric	Hyperactivity, clonus (preeclampsia)	Evaluate for other symptoms of preeclampsia.
Pelvic Area		
External female genitals: Normally formed with female hair distribution; in multiparas, labia majora loose and pigmented; urinary and vaginal orifices visible and appropriately located	Lesions, genital warts, hematomas, varicosities, inflammation of Bartholin glands; clitoral hypertrophy (masculinization)	Explain pelvic examination procedure. Encourage woman to minimize her discomfort by relaxing her hips. Provide privacy.
Vagina: Pink or dark pink, vaginal discharge odorless, nonirritating; in multiparas, vaginal folds smooth and flattened; may have episiotomy scar	Abnormal discharge associated with vaginal infections	Obtain vaginal smear. Provide understandable verbal and written instructions about treatment for woman and partner, if indicated.

Physical Assessment/Normal Findings	Alterations and Possible Causes*	Nursing Responses to Data†
Cervix: Pink color; os closed except in multiparas, in whom os admits fingertip	Eversion, reddish erosion, nabothian or retention cysts, cervical polyp; granular area that bleeds (carcinoma of cervix); lesions (herpes, human papillomavirus [HPV]); presence of string or plastic tip from cervix (intrauterine device [IUD] in uterus)	Provide woman with a hand mirror and identify genital structures for her; encourage her to view her cervix if she wishes. Refer to healthcare provider if indicated. Advise woman of potential serious risks of leaving an IUD in place during pregnancy; refer to healthcare provider for removal.
Pregnancy changes:		
1–4 weeks' gestation: enlargement in anteroposterior diameter	Absence of Goodell sign (inflammatory conditions, carcinoma)	Refer to healthcare provider.
4–6 weeks' gestation: softening of cervix (Goodell sign); softening of isthmus of uterus (Hegar sign); cervix takes on bluish coloring (Chadwick sign)		
8–12 weeks' gestation: vagina and cervix appear bluish violet in color (Chadwick sign)		
Uterus: Pear shaped, mobile; smooth surface	Fixed (pelvic inflammatory disease [PID]); nodular surface (fibromas)	Refer to healthcare provider.
Ovaries: Small, walnut shaped, nontender (ovaries and fallopian tubes are located in the adnexal areas)	Pain on movement of cervix (PID); enlarged or nodular ovaries (cyst, tumor, tubal pregnancy, corpus luteum of pregnancy)	Evaluate adnexal areas; refer to healthcare provider.
Pelvic Measurements		
Internal measurements:		
1. Diagonal conjugate at least 11.5 cm (4.5 in.) (see Figure 9–5)	Measurement below normal	Vaginal birth may not be possible if deviations are present.
2. Obstetric conjugate estimated by subtracting 1.5–2.0 cm (0.60 to 0.79 in.) from diagonal conjugate	Disproportion of pubic arch	
3. Inclination of sacrum	Abnormal curvature of sacrum	
4. Motility of coccyx; external intertuberosity diameter greater than 8 cm (3.15 in.)	Fixed or malposition of coccyx	
Anus and Rectum		
No lumps, rashes, excoriation, tenderness; cervix may be felt through rectal wall	Hemorrhoids, rectal prolapse; warts (HPV infection); nodular lesion (carcinoma)	Counsel about appropriate prevention and relief measures; refer to healthcare provider for further evaluation.
Laboratory		
Evaluation		
Hemoglobin: 12–16 g/dL; women residing in areas of high altitude may have higher levels of hemoglobin	Less than 11.0 g/dL in the first trimester, less than 10.5 g/dL in the second trimester, and less than 11.0 g/dL in the third trimester (anemia) (King et al., 2015)	Hemoglobin less than 12 g/dL requires nutritional counseling; less than 11 g/dL requires iron supplementation.
ABO and Rh typing: Normal distribution of blood types	Rh negative	If Rh negative, check for presence of anti-Rh antibodies. Check blood type of father of child; if he is Rh positive, discuss with woman the need for Rh immune globulin administration at 28 weeks, management during the intrapartum period, and possible need for Rh immune globulin after birth. (See discussion in Chapter 15.)

(continued)

ASSESSMENT GUIDE | Initial Prenatal Assessment (*continued*)

Physical Assessment/Normal Findings	Alterations and Possible Causes*	Nursing Responses to Data†
Complete Blood Count (CBC) **Hematocrit:** 38%–47% physiologic anemia (pseudoanemia) may occur	Marked anemia or blood dyscrasias	Perform CBC and Schilling differential cell count.
Red blood cells (RBC): 4.2–5.4 million/mcL		
White blood cells (WBC): 5000–12,000/mcL	Presence of infection; may be elevated in pregnancy and with labor	Evaluate for other signs of infection.
Differential Neutrophils: 40%–60%		
Bands: up to 5%		
Eosinophils: 1%–3%		
Basophils: up to 1%		
Lymphocytes: 20%–40%		
Monocytes: 4%–8%		
First-trimester aneuploidy screening (testing to detect conditions related to abnormal chromosome number): If nuchal translucency (NT) testing is available, offer first-trimester screening for Down syndrome using nuchal translucency and serum markers (PAPP-A and free β-hCG). Normal range.	Increased nuchal translucency, elevated β-hCG, and reduced pregnancy-associated plasma protein A (PAPP-A) (Down syndrome, trisomy 18, trisomy 13)	If findings are positive, genetic counseling and diagnostic testing using chorionic villus sampling (CVS) or second-trimester amniocentesis are offered.
Integrated screening: Combines first-trimester aneuploidy screening results with second-trimester quadruple (quad) screen to detect aneuploidy and neural tube defects; may be used in areas in which NT testing is not available. (See discussion in *Assessment Guide: Subsequent Prenatal Assessment.*)		
Syphilis tests: Serologic tests for syphilis (STS), complement fixation test, Venereal Disease Research Laboratory (VDRL) test—nonreactive	Positive reaction STS—tests may have 25%–45% incidence of biologic false-positive results; false results may occur in individuals who have acute viral or bacterial infections, hypersensitivity reactions, recent vaccinations, collagen disease, malaria, or tuberculosis bacterial infections	Positive results may be confirmed with the fluorescent treponemal antibody-absorption (FTA-ABS) test; all tests for syphilis give positive results in the secondary stage of the disease; antibiotic tests may cause negative test results. Refer to healthcare provider for treatment.
Gonorrhea culture: Negative	Positive	Refer for treatment.
Urinalysis (u/a): Normal color, specific gravity; pH 4.6–8	Cloudy appearance (infection; pus or tissue)	Repeat u/a; refer to healthcare provider.
	Abnormal color (porphyria, hemoglobinuria, bilirubinemia): alkaline urine (metabolic alkalemia, *Proteus* infection, old specimen)	
Negative for protein, red blood cells, white blood cells, casts	Positive findings (contaminated specimen, urinary tract infection (UTI), kidney disease)	Repeat u/a; urine culture with sensitivities if bacteria detected; refer to healthcare provider.
Negative for glucose (small degree of glycosuria may occur in pregnancy)	Glycosuria (low renal threshold for glucose, diabetes mellitus)	Assess blood glucose level; test urine for ketones.
Urine culture: Negative for bacteria	Bacteria (UTI)	If bacteria detected, refer to healthcare provider for treatment.

Physical Assessment/Normal Findings	Alterations and Possible Causes*	Nursing Responses to Data†
Rubella titer: Hemagglutination-inhibition (HAI) test–1:10 or above indicates woman is immune	HAI titer less than 1:10	Immunization will be given postpartum. Instruct woman whose titers are less than 1:10 to avoid children who have rubella.
Hepatitis B screen: For hepatitis B surface antigen (HBsAg): negative *Note:* Women with risk factors are also tested for hepatitis C (spread by direct contact with infected blood)	Positive	If positive, refer to physician. Babies born to women who test positive are given hepatitis B immune globulin soon after birth followed by first dose of hepatitis B vaccine.
HIV screen: Completed on all pregnant woman unless woman specifically opts out of screening; negative	Positive	Refer to healthcare provider.
Illicit drug screen: Offered to all women; negative	Positive	Refer to healthcare provider.
Sickle cell screen for clients of African or Latino descent: Negative	Positive; test results would include a description of cells	Refer to healthcare provider.
Pap smear: If indicated because the woman is due for the test; negative	Test results that show abnormal cells with negative or positive high-risk HPV.	Refer to healthcare provider. Discuss with the woman the meaning of the findings and the importance of follow-up. Plan colposcopy if indicated.

Cultural Assessment	Variations to Consider*	Nursing Responses to Data†
Determine the woman's fluency in written and oral English.	Woman may be fluent in language other than English.	Work with a knowledgeable translator to provide information and answer questions.
Ask the woman how she prefers to be addressed. Nickname?	Some women prefer informality; others prefer to use titles.	Address the woman according to her preference. Maintain formality in introducing oneself if that seems preferred.
Determine customs and practices regarding prenatal care:	Practices are influenced by individual preference, cultural expectations, or religious beliefs.	Honor a woman's practices and provide for specific preferences unless they are contraindicated because of safety.
• Ask the woman if there are certain practices she expects to follow when she is pregnant. • Ask the woman if there are any activities she cannot do while she is pregnant.	Some women believe that they should perform certain acts related to sleep, activity, or clothing. Some women have restrictions or taboos they follow related to work, activity, sexual, environmental, or emotional factors.	Have information printed in the language of different cultural groups that live in the area.
• Ask the woman whether there are certain foods she is expected to eat or avoid while she is pregnant. Determine whether she has lactose intolerance.	Food is an important cultural factor. Some women may have certain foods they must eat or avoid; many women have lactose intolerance and have difficulty consuming sufficient calcium.	Respect the woman's food preferences, help her plan an adequate prenatal diet within the framework of her preferences, and refer to a dietitian if necessary.
• Ask the woman whether the gender of her caregiver is of concern.	Some women are comfortable only with a female caregiver.	Arrange for a female caregiver if it is the woman's preference.
• Ask the woman about the degree of involvement in her pregnancy that she expects or wants from her support person, mother, and other significant people.	A woman may not want her partner involved in the pregnancy. For some the role falls to the woman's mother or a female relative or friend.	Respect the woman's preferences about her partner or husband's involvement; avoid imposing personal values or expectations.
• Ask the woman about her sources of support and counseling during pregnancy.	Some women seek advice from a family member, *curandera*, tribal healer, and so forth.	Respect and honor the woman's sources of support.
Psychologic Status Excitement and/or apprehension, ambivalence	Marked anxiety (fear of pregnancy diagnosis, fear of medical facility)	Establish lines of communication. Active listening is useful. Establish trusting relationship. Encourage woman to take active part in her care.

(continued)

ASSESSMENT GUIDE | Initial Prenatal Assessment (*continued*)

Cultural Assessment	Variations to Consider*	Nursing Responses to Data†
	Apathy; display of anger with pregnancy diagnosis	Establish communication and begin counseling. Use active listening techniques.
Educational Needs		
May have questions about pregnancy or may need time to adjust to reality of pregnancy		Establish educational, supporting environment that can be expanded throughout pregnancy.
Support System		
Can identify at least two or three individuals with whom woman is emotionally intimate (partner, parent, sibling, friend)	Isolated (no telephone, unlisted number); cannot name a neighbor or friend whom she can call on in an emergency; does not perceive parents as part of her support system	Institute support system through community groups. Help woman to develop trusting relationship with healthcare professionals.
Family Functioning		
Emotionally supportive	Long-term problems or specific problems related to this pregnancy, potential stressors within the family, pessimistic attitudes, unilateral decision making, unrealistic expectations of this pregnancy or child	Help identify the problems and stressors, encourage communication, and discuss role changes and adaptations. Refer to counseling if indicated.
Communications adequate		
Mutually satisfying		
Cohesiveness in times of trouble		
Economic Status		
Source of income is stable and sufficient to meet basic needs of daily living and medical needs	Limited prenatal care; poor physical health; limited use of healthcare system; unstable economic status	Discuss available resources for health maintenance and the birth. Institute appropriate referral for meeting expanding family's needs—food stamps, WIC (a federally funded nutrition program for women, infants, and children), and so forth.
Stability of Living Conditions		
Adequate, stable housing for expanding family's needs	Crowded living conditions; questionable supportive environment for newborn	Refer to appropriate community agency. Work with family on self-help ways to improve situation.

*Possible causes of alterations are identified in parentheses.

†This column provides guidelines for further assessment and initial intervention.

Determination of Due Date

Childbearing families generally want to know the "due date," or the date around which childbirth will occur. Historically, the due date has been called the *estimated date of confinement (EDC)*. However, the concept of confinement is rather negative, and many caregivers avoid it by referring to the due date as the *estimated date of delivery (EDD)*. Childbirth educators often stress that babies are not "delivered" like a package; they are born. In keeping with a view that emphasizes the normality of the process, the authors of this text refer to the due date as the **estimated date of birth (EDB)**.

To calculate the EDB, it is essential to know the first day of the last menstrual period (LMP). However, some women have episodes of irregular bleeding or fail to keep track of menstrual cycles. Thus other techniques also help to determine how far along a woman is in her pregnancy—that is, at how many weeks' gestation she is. Techniques include evaluating uterine size, determining when quickening occurs (or occurred), using early ultrasound, and auscultating fetal heart rate with a Doppler device or ultrasound. An early ultrasound should be obtained if an accurate LMP is not available to help establish an accurate EDB.

Nägele's Rule

The most common method of determining the EDB is **Nägele's rule**, which uses 280 days as the mean length of pregnancy. To use this method, begin with the first day of the LMP, subtract 3 months, and add 7 days. For example:

First day of LMP	November 21
Subtract 3 months	– 3 months
	August 21
Add 7 days	+ 7 days
EDB (of the next year)	August 28

It is simpler to change the months to numeric terms:

November 21 becomes	11–21
Subtract 3 months	–3 months
	8–21
Add 7 days	+ 7 days
EDB (of the next year)	8–28

A gestation calculator or wheel lets the caregiver calculate the EDB even more quickly (Figure 9–1).

Nägele's rule may be a fairly accurate determiner of the EDB if the woman has a history of menses every 28 days, remembers her LMP, and was not taking oral contraceptives before becoming pregnant. However, ovulation usually occurs 14 days *before* the onset of the next menses, not 14 days after the previous menses. Consequently, if a woman's cycle is irregular, or more than 28 days long, the time of ovulation may be delayed. If a woman has been using oral contraceptives, ovulation may be delayed several weeks following her last menses. Then, too, a postpartum woman who is breastfeeding may resume ovulating but be amenorrheic for a time, making calculation based on the LMP impossible. Thus Nägele's rule, although helpful, is not foolproof and, in such cases, an ultrasound is done to visualize the gestational sac and obtain measurements of the embryo-fetus to determine EDB.

Uterine Assessment

PHYSICAL EXAMINATION

When a woman is examined in the first 10 to 12 weeks of her pregnancy and her uterine size is compatible with her menstrual history, uterine size may be the single most important clinical method for dating her pregnancy. In many cases, however, women do not seek maternity care until well into their second trimester, when it becomes much more difficult to evaluate specific uterine size. In women who are obese, it is difficult to determine uterine size early in a pregnancy because the uterus is more difficult to palpate.

FUNDAL HEIGHT

Fundal height may be used as an indicator of uterine size, although this method is less accurate late in pregnancy. A tape measure is used to measure the distance in centimeters from the top of the symphysis pubis to the top of the uterine fundus (McDonald method) (Figure 9–2). Fundal height in centimeters correlates well with weeks of gestation between 22 and 34 weeks. Thus, at 26 weeks' gestation, for example, fundal height is probably about 26 cm (10.25 in.). If the woman is very tall or very short, fundal height will differ. To be most accurate, fundal height should be measured by the same examiner each time. The woman should have voided within one half hour of the examination and should lie in the same position each time. In the third trimester, variations in fetal weight decrease the accuracy of fundal height measurements.

A lag in progression of measurements of fundal height from month to month and week to week may signal intrauterine

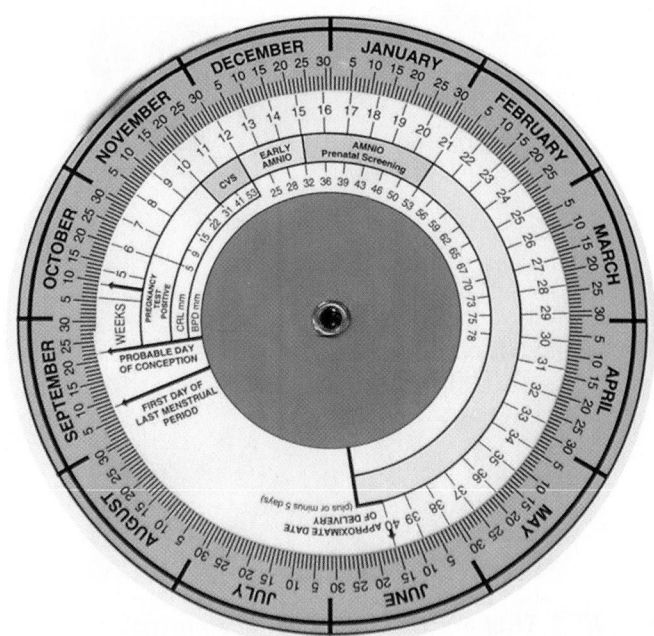

Figure 9–1 The EDB wheel can be used to calculate the due date. To use it, place the "last menses began" arrow on the date of the woman's LMP. Then read the EDB at the arrow labeled 40. In this case, the LMP is September 8, and the EDB is June 15.

growth restriction (IUGR). A sudden increase in fundal height may indicate twins or hydramnios (excessive amount of amniotic fluid).

Assessment of Fetal Development

QUICKENING

Fetal movements felt by the mother, called *quickening*, may indicate that the fetus is nearing 20 weeks' gestation. However,

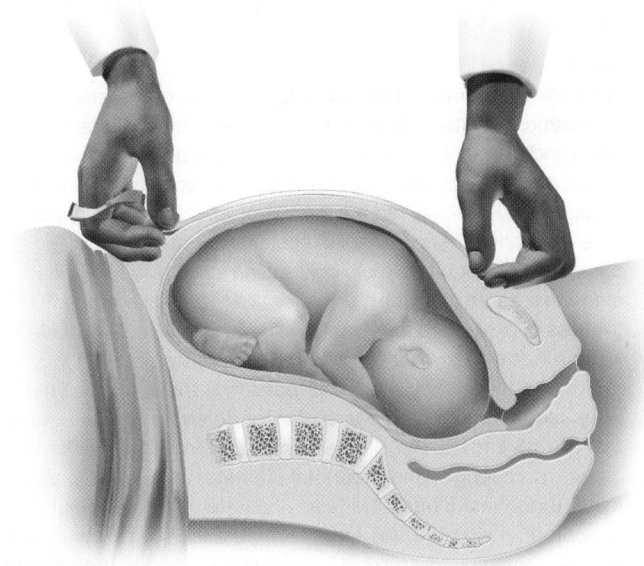

Figure 9–2 A cross-sectional view of fetal position when the McDonald method is used to assess fundal height.

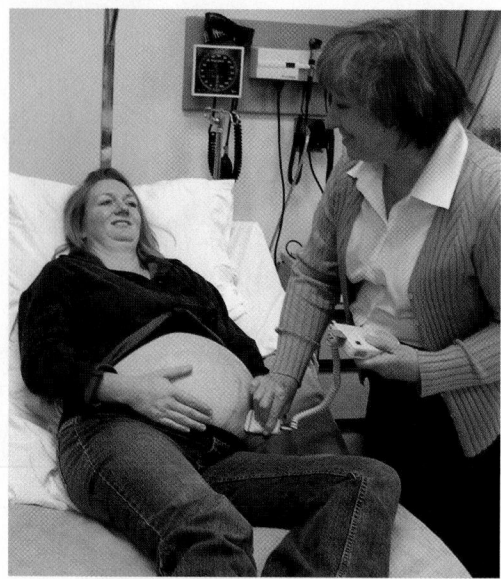

Figure 9–3 This practitioner is using an ultrasonic Doppler device to listen to the fetal heartbeat.

quickening may be experienced between 16 and 22 weeks' gestation, so this method is not completely accurate.

FETAL HEARTBEAT

The ultrasonic Doppler device (Figure 9–3) is the primary tool for assessing fetal heartbeat. It can detect fetal heartbeat, on average, at 8 to 12 weeks' gestation. The normal range for fetal heart tones (FHTs) is 110 to 160 beats/min. An ultrasound should be completed if the nurse is unable to auscultate

between 10 and 12 weeks because there may be a discrepancy in the EDB, twins, or a missed abortion. In the case of twins or a woman with obesity, it may be later before the fetal heartbeat can be detected.

ULTRASOUND

Transvaginal ultrasound is often used in early pregnancy; after about 10 weeks, transabdominal ultrasound is indicated (ACOG, 2013d). In the first trimester (up to and including 13 6/7 weeks' gestation), ultrasound can detect a gestational sac as early as 5 weeks after the LMP, fetal heart activity by 6 to 7 weeks, and fetal breathing movements by 10 to 11 weeks of pregnancy. Crown-to-rump measurements can be made to assess fetal age from 5 to 6 weeks until about 12 weeks (until the fetal head can be visualized clearly). Biparietal diameter (BPD) can then be used. BPD measurements can be made by approximately 12 to 13 weeks and are most accurate between 14 and 26 weeks, when rapid growth in the biparietal diameter occurs. (See Chapter 13 for further discussion of fetal ultrasound scanning.)

Assessment of Pelvic Adequacy (Clinical Pelvimetry)

The pelvis can be assessed vaginally to determine whether its size is adequate for a vaginal birth. This procedure, clinical pelvimetry, is performed by physicians or by advanced practice nurses such as CNMs or nurse practitioners. For a detailed description of how clinical pelvimetry is done, refer to a nurse-midwifery text. This section provides basic information about

---

EVIDENCE-BASED PRACTICE | Determination of Gestational Age Using Ultrasound

Clinical Question

Is ultrasound biometry an accurate way of determining the gestational age of a fetus?

The Evidence

Accurate gestational dating is an important part of prenatal care. Assessment of fetal growth and development, timely screening tests, and maternal preparation for birth depend on having an accurate prediction of fetal maturity. In addition, accurate assignment of gestational age may reduce the rate of labor induction for postdate pregnancy. Three Canadian obstetricians and a consulting committee of diagnostic radiologists used strict review criteria to evaluate a dozen research studies relative to the safety and effectiveness of ultrasound for gestational dating. The resulting guideline forms the strongest level of evidence for clinical practice.

The strongest evidence supports first trimester crown-rump length as the best parameter for determining gestational age (Butt & Lim, 2014). Between the 12th and 14th weeks, crown-rump length and biparietal diameter are similar in accuracy. Abdominal ultrasound is as accurate as transvaginal ultrasonography, although the latter is more accurate for visualizing early embryonic structures. If ultrasound is used in the second or third trimester, gestational age is best determined by a com-

bination of multiple biometric parameters, including biparietal diameter, head circumference, abdominal circumference, and femur length. During the second and third trimesters, no single measure best predicts gestational age. The most difficult time to determine a due date is during the third trimester. When performed accurately and precisely, ultrasound is more accurate than even a "certain" missed menstrual date for determining gestational age in spontaneous conceptions. It is the best method for estimating the birth date.

Best Practice

Ideally, every pregnant woman should be offered a first-trimester ultrasound to determine gestational age. Abdominal ultrasound is as accurate as transvaginal ultrasound and is more comfortable for the mother. Dating can still be accomplished later in the pregnancy, but ultrasound becomes a less accurate predictor as gestation progresses through the second and third trimesters.

Clinical Reasoning

What are some of the reasons that an accurate gestational age is important to prenatal care? Can a case be made for the cost-effectiveness of early ultrasound to determine an accurate birth due date?

the assessment of the inlet and outlet, which were described in detail in Chapter 4.

1. Pelvic inlet (Figure 9–4):
   - **Diagonal conjugate** (the distance from the lower posterior border of the symphysis pubis to the sacral promontory): at least 11.5 cm (4.5 in.)
   - **Obstetric conjugate** (a measurement approximately 1.5 cm (0.60 in.) smaller than the diagonal conjugate): 10.0 cm (3.9 in.) or more

2. Pelvic outlet (Figures 9–4 and 9–5):
   - Anteroposterior diameter: 9.5 to 11.5 cm (3.75 to 4.5 in.)
   - Transverse diameter (bi-ischial or intertuberous diameter): 8 to 10 cm (3.15 to 3.9 in.)

The pelvic cavity (midpelvis) cannot be accurately measured by clinical examination. Examiners estimate its adequacy.

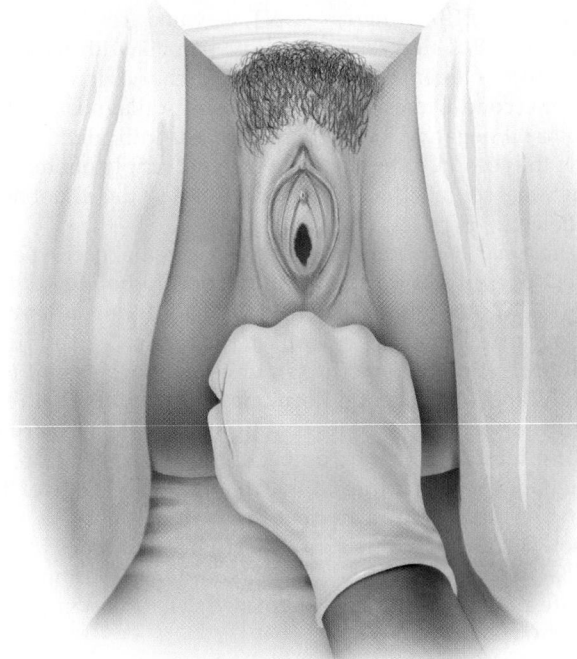

Figure 9–5 Use of a closed fist to measure the outlet. Most examiners know the distance between their first and last proximal knuckles. If they do not, they can use a measuring device.

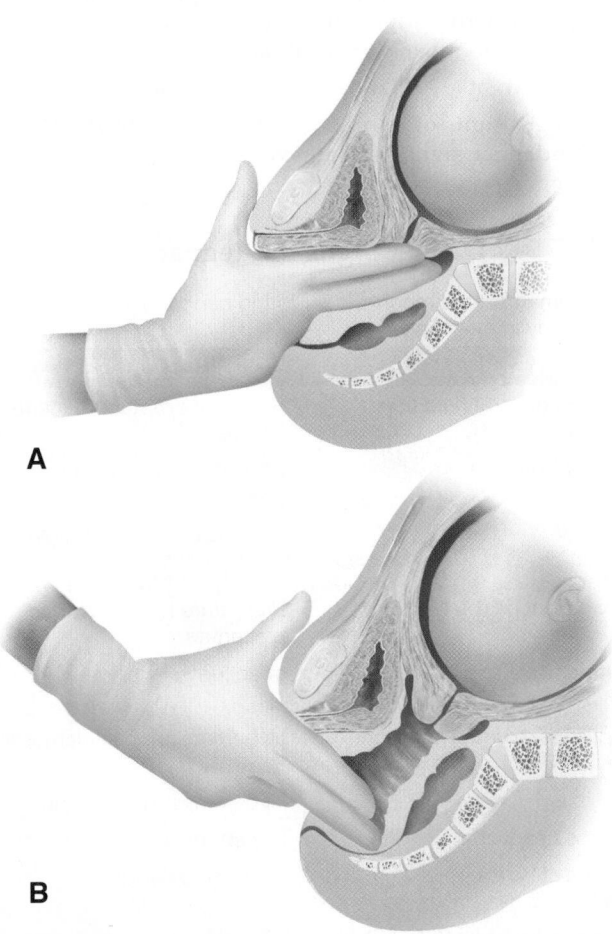

A

B

Figure 9–4 Manual measurement of inlet and outlet. *A*, Estimation of the diagonal conjugate, which extends from the lower border of the symphysis pubis to the sacral promontory. *B*, Estimation of the anteroposterior diameter of the outlet, which extends from the lower border of the symphysis pubis to the tip of the sacrum.

Screening Tests

Many screening tests are routinely performed and/or offered either at the initial prenatal visit or at a specified time during pregnancy. These tests include a Pap smear if indicated, a complete blood count, HIV screening, urine culture, rubella titer, ABO and Rh typing, and a hepatitis B screen as well as testing for sexually transmitted infections such as syphilis, chlamydial infection, and gonorrhea. The urine is screened for abnormal findings initially and at each prenatal visit.

Hemoglobin electrophoresis should be performed in women of African, Southeast Asian, and Mediterranean descent to evaluate for sickle cell disease and thalassemias. Prenatal screening for cystic fibrosis has been a routine screening test for all pregnant women for over a decade. To avoid redundant testing, caregivers should determine whether the woman was screened for cystic fibrosis during a previous pregnancy (ACOG, 2011).

A tuberculin test (either purified protein derivative [PPD] or Quantiferon Gold) should also be completed on women who are considered to be high risk. High-risk populations include women who were not born in the United States or who have a known exposure to tuberculosis and healthcare workers who care for clients with tuberculosis.

All pregnant women, regardless of age, should be offered screening for fetal chromosomal anomalies (*aneuploidy*), including Down syndrome, trisomy 18, trisomy 13, and Turner syndrome. First-trimester screening is available at many centers using ultrasound assessment of the thickness of the fetal nuchal fold (called *nuchal translucency* [NT]) combined with serum screening for free β-hCG and for pregnancy-associated plasma protein A (PAPP-A). Increased NT, elevated free β-hCG, and reduced PAPP-A suggest aneuploidy. Women with these findings are offered genetic counseling and chorionic villus sampling or second-trimester amniocentesis for diagnosis. If these tests are all negative, no further testing is indicated. Instead, during the second trimester, the woman is simply offered a test for maternal serum alpha-fetoprotein to detect the risk of neural tube defects.

The *quadruple screen* (quad screen) is a safe, useful screening test performed on the mother's serum between weeks 15 and 20 of pregnancy. The test is used to detect levels of specific serum markers—alpha-fetoprotein (AFP), human chorionic gonadotropin (hCG), unconjugated estriol (UE), and inhibin-A (a placental hormone). Test results that reveal higher than normal AFP levels might indicate an increased risk of a fetal neural tube defect, a multiple gestation, or a pregnancy that is further along than believed. Lower than normal AFP could indicate that the woman's child is at risk for Down syndrome or trisomy 18. Higher than normal levels of hCG and inhibin-A and lower than normal UE may also indicate that a woman is at increased risk of having a baby with Down syndrome.

NT evaluation requires a skilled ultrasonographer and specialized training. In areas where NT is not available, first-trimester free β-hCG screening and PAPP-A screening may be combined with second-trimester quad screening in an integrated approach to detection of aneuploidy.

Noninvasive prenatal testing for fetal aneulopoidy (trisomy), specifically trisomy 13, trisomy 18, and trisomy 21 is also available using *cell free fetal DNA (cffDNA)* from the blood of pregnant women. Cell free fetal DNA is thought to be derived from the placenta and can be collected as early as 10 weeks' gestation. Currently ACOG (2012) does not recommend this testing as routine screening for all women, but it can serve as a primary screening test for women at high risk of a trisomy.

It is important for healthcare professionals to provide parents with factual information about the results of tests that detect chromosomal defects or fetal anomalies including the false-positive and detection rates and the implications of the findings. Parents then need to decide on any course of action based on their own spiritual and cultural beliefs.

Screening for gestational diabetes mellitus (GDM) is typically completed between 24 and 28 weeks' gestation. ACOG (2013b) recommends that the testing be done using a 50 g 1-hour glucose screen. If results are abnormal, diagnostic testing using a 100-g, 3-hour oral glucose tolerance test is indicated (for a discussion of GDM, see Chapter 14). The American Diabetes Association (2011) recommends that pregnant women at average risk should have a diagnostic test 24 to 28 weeks' gestation using a 75-g 2-hour oral glucose tolerance test (OGTT). A Consensus Conference convened to evaluate the two approaches recommends the two-step approach with screening followed by diagnostic testing if screening results are abnormal, as advocated by ACOG (VanDorsten et al., 2013). A hemoglobin or hematocrit is also completed at this time to evaluate for iron deficiency anemia.

Group B streptococcus (GBS) can cause serious problems for a newborn. Consequently, rectal and vaginal swabs of the mother are taken at 35 to 37 weeks' gestation to screen for the infection. Women with GBS in the urine at any time during the pregnancy are considered to be positive and do not need a culture completed. This infection is discussed in more detail in Chapter 14.

Additional tests are completed in the event of pathologic findings or known disease states. For example, a woman with known chronic hypertension should have a 24-hour urine, metabolic panel, and uric acid completed.

Subsequent Client History

At subsequent prenatal visits the nurse continues to gather data about the course of the pregnancy to date and the woman's responses to it. The nurse also asks about:

- Adjustment of the support person and of other children, if any, in the family
- Preparations the family has made for the new baby
- Discomfort, especially the kinds of discomfort that are often seen at specific times during a pregnancy
- Physical changes that relate directly to the pregnancy, such as fetal movement
- Exposure to contagious illnesses
- Medical treatments and therapies prescribed for nonpregnancy problems since the last visit
- Consumption of prescription or over-the-counter medications or herbal supplements that were not prescribed as part of the woman's prenatal care
- Use of complementary and alternative therapies
- Danger signs of pregnancy (Table 9–2). (*Note:* Many of the danger signs indicate conditions that are potential complications.)

TABLE 9–2 Danger Signs in Pregnancy

The woman should report the following danger signs in pregnancy immediately:

DANGER SIGN	POSSIBLE CAUSE
Sudden gush of fluid from vagina	Premature rupture of membranes
Vaginal bleeding	Abruptio placentae, placenta previa
	Lesions of cervix or vagina
	"Bloody show"
Abdominal pain	Premature labor, abruptio placentae
Temperature above 101.0°F (38.3°C) and chills	Infection
Dizziness, blurring of vision, double vision, spots before eyes	Hypertension, preeclampsia
Persistent vomiting	Hyperemesis gravidarum
Severe headache	Hypertension, preeclampsia
Edema of hands, face, legs, and feet	Preeclampsia
Muscular irritability, convulsions	Preeclampsia, eclampsia
Epigastric pain	Preeclampsia, ischemia in major abdominal vessel
Oliguria	Renal impairment, decreased fluid intake
Dysuria	Urinary tract infection
Absence of fetal movement	Maternal medication, obesity, fetal death

Periodic prenatal examinations offer a chance to assess the childbearing woman's psychologic needs and emotional status. If the woman's partner attends the antepartum visits, they can also be a time to identify the partner's needs and concerns. The woman should have sufficient time to ask questions and air concerns. If a nurse provides the time and demonstrates genuine interest, the woman will be more at ease bringing up questions that she may believe are silly or has been afraid to verbalize.

Be sensitive to religious or spiritual, cultural, and socioeconomic factors that may influence a family's response to pregnancy, as well as to the woman's expectations of the healthcare system. One way to avoid stereotyping clients is simply to ask each woman about her expectations for the antepartum period. Although many women's responses may reflect what are thought to be traditional norms, other women will have decidedly different views or expectations that represent a blending of beliefs or cultures. During the antepartum period, it is also essential to begin assessing the readiness of the woman and her partner (if possible) to assume their responsibilities as parents successfully.

Subsequent Prenatal Assessment

Assessment Guide: Subsequent Prenatal Assessment provides a systematic approach to the regular physical examinations the pregnant woman should undergo for optimal antepartum care and also provides a model for evaluating both the pregnant woman and the expectant father, if he is involved in the pregnancy.

The recommended frequency of antepartum visits in an uncomplicated pregnancy is as follows:

- Every 4 weeks for the first 28 weeks' gestation
- Every 2 weeks until 36 weeks' gestation
- After week 36, every week until childbirth

During the subsequent antepartum assessments, most women demonstrate ongoing psychologic adjustment to pregnancy. However, some women may exhibit signs of possible psychologic problems such as the following:

- Increasing anxiety
- Inability to establish communication
- Inappropriate responses or actions
- Denial of pregnancy
- Inability to cope with stress
- Intense preoccupation with the gender of the baby
- Failure to acknowledge quickening
- Failure to plan and prepare for the baby (e.g., living arrangements, clothing, and feeding methods)
- Indications of substance abuse

If the woman's behavior indicates possible psychologic problems, the nurse can provide ongoing support and counseling and also refer the woman to appropriate professionals.

Clinical Tip

When assessing blood pressure, have the pregnant woman sit up with her arm resting on a table so that her arm is at the level of her heart. Expect a decrease in her blood pressure from baseline during the second trimester because of normal physiologic changes.

ASSESSMENT GUIDE | Subsequent Prenatal Assessment

Physical Assessment/Normal Findings	Alterations and Possible Causes*	Nursing Responses to Data†
Vital Signs		
Temperature: 97.0°–99.6°F (36.2°–37.6°C)	Elevated temperature (infection)	Evaluate for signs of infection. Refer to healthcare provider.
Pulse: 60–100 beats/min	Increased pulse rate (anxiety, cardiac disorders)	Note irregularities. Assess for anxiety and stress.
Rate may increase 10 beats/min during pregnancy.		
Respiration: 12–20 breaths/min	Marked tachypnea or abnormal patterns (respiratory disease)	Refer to healthcare provider.
Blood pressure: Less than or equal to 120/80 (falls in second trimester)	BP of 120–139/80–89 is considered prehypertensive. Greater than 140/90 or increase of 30 mmHg systolic and 15 mmHg diastolic (preeclampsia)	Assess for edema, proteinuria, and hyperreflexia. Refer to healthcare provider.
		Schedule appointments more frequently.
Weight Gain		
Prepregnant weight based on body mass index (BMI):		
Normal BMI: Total recommended weight gain 11.5–16 kg (25–35 lb)		
First trimester: 1.6–2.3 kg (3.5–5.0 lb)	Inadequate weight gain (poor nutrition, nausea, IUGR)	Discuss appropriate weight gain.
Second trimester: 5.5–6.8 kg (12–15 lb)	Excessive weight gain (excessive caloric intake, edema, preeclampsia)	Provide nutritional counseling. Assess for presence of edema or anemia. Refer to a dietitian as needed.
Third trimester: 5.5–6.8 kg (12–15 lb)		

(continued)

ASSESSMENT GUIDE | Subsequent Prenatal Assessment (*continued*)

Physical Assessment/Normal Findings	Alterations and Possible Causes*	Nursing Responses to Data†
Edema		
Small amount of dependent edema, especially in last weeks of pregnancy	Marked edema in hands, face, legs, and feet (preeclampsia)	Identify any correlation between edema and activities, blood pressure, or proteinuria: Refer to healthcare provider if indicated.
Uterine Size		
See *Assessment Guide: Initial Prenatal Assessment* for normal changes during pregnancy	Unusually rapid growth (multiple gestation, hydatidiform mole, hydramnios, miscalculation of EDB)	Evaluate fetal status. Determine height of fundus. Use diagnostic ultrasound.
Fetal Heartbeat		
110–160 beats/min Funic souffle	Absence of fetal heartbeat after 20 weeks' gestation (maternal obesity, fetal demise)	Evaluate fetal status.
Laboratory Evaluation		
Hemoglobin: 12–16 g/dL Pseudoanemia of pregnancy	Less than 11 g/dL (anemia)	Provide nutritional counseling. Hemoglobin is repeated at 7 months' gestation. Women of Mediterranean heritage need a close check on hemoglobin because of possibility of thalassemia.
Quad marker screen: Blood test performed at 15–21 weeks' gestation but best performed between 16 and 18 weeks' gestation. Evaluates four factors: maternal serum alpha-fetoprotein (MSAFP), unconjugated estriol (UE), hCG, and inhibin-A: normal levels	Elevated MSAFP (neural tube defect, underestimated gestational age, multiple gestation); lower than normal MSAFP (Down syndrome, trisomy 18); higher than normal hCG and inhibin-A (Down syndrome); lower than normal UE (Down syndrome)	Offered to all pregnant women. If quad screen is abnormal, further testing such as ultrasound or amniocentesis may be indicated.
Indirect Coombs test done on Rh-negative women: Negative (done at 28 weeks' gestation)	Rh antibodies present (maternal sensitization has occurred)	If Rh negative and unsensitized, Rh immune globulin given (see discussion in Chapter 15). If Rh antibodies present, Rh immune globulin not given; fetus monitored closely for isoimmune hemolytic disease.
50-g 1-hour glucose screen (done between 24 and 28 weeks' gestation)	Plasma glucose level greater than 140 mg/dL (gestational diabetes mellitus [GDM])	Refer for a diagnostic 100-g oral glucose tolerance test. Discuss implications of gestational diabetes mellitus (GDM) if diagnosis is made. Refer to healthcare provider.
Urinalysis: See *Assessment Guide: Initial Prenatal Assessment* for normal findings	See *Assessment Guide: Initial Prenatal Assessment* for deviations	Urinalysis and culture is completed at initial visit and at subsequent visits as indicated. Repeat dipstick test at each visit.
Protein: Negative	Proteinuria, albuminuria (contamination by vaginal discharge, urinary tract infection, preeclampsia)	Obtain dipstick urine sample. Refer to healthcare provider if deviations are present.
Glucose: Negative *Note:* Glycosuria may be present due to physiologic alterations in glomerular filtration rate and renal threshold	Persistent glycosuria (diabetes mellitus)	Refer to healthcare provider.
Screening for Group B streptococcus (GBS): Rectal and vaginal swabs obtained at 35–37 weeks' gestation for all pregnant women.	Positive culture (maternal infection)	Explain maternal and fetal/neonatal risks (see Chapter 15). Refer to healthcare provider for therapy.

Cultural Assessment	Variations to Consider*	Nursing Responses to Data†
Determine the mother's (and family's) attitudes about the gender of the unborn child.	Some women have no preference about the gender of the child; others do. In many cultures, boys are especially valued as firstborn children.	Provide opportunities to discuss preferences and expectations; avoid a judgmental attitude to the response.
Ask about the woman's expectations of childbirth. Will she want someone with her for the birth? Whom does she choose? What is the role of her partner?	Some women want their partner present for labor and birth; others prefer a female relative or friend.	Provide information on birth options but accept the woman's decision about who will attend.
	Some women expect to be separated from their partner once labor begins.	
Ask about preparations for the baby. Determine what is customary for the woman.	Some women may have a fully prepared nursery; others may not have a separate room for the baby.	Explore reasons for not preparing for the baby. Support the mother's preferences and provide information about possible sources of assistance if the decision is related to a lack of resources.

Expectant Mother

Psychologic status	Increased stress and anxiety	Encourage woman to take an active part in her care.
First trimester: Period of adjustment. Incorporates idea of pregnancy; may feel ambivalent or anxious, especially if she must give up desired role; usually looks for signs of verification of pregnancy, such as increase in abdominal size or fetal movement.	Inability to establish communication; inability to accept pregnancy; inappropriate response or actions; denial of pregnancy; inability to cope	Establish lines of communication. Discuss and provide anticipatory guidance regarding normalcy of feelings and actions. Establish a trusting relationship. Counsel as necessary. Refer to appropriate professional as needed.
Second trimester: Period of radiant health. Baby becomes more real to woman as abdominal size increases and she feels movement; she begins to turn inward, becoming more introspective.		
Third trimester: Period of watchful waiting. Begins to think of baby as separate being; may feel restless, uneasy, and may feel that time of labor will never come; remains self-centered and concentrates on preparing place for baby. Fears for her well-being and that of her baby.		
Educational needs:	Inadequate information	Provide information and counseling.
Self-care measures and knowledge about the following (discussed in Chapter 10): • Health promotion • Breast care • Hygiene • Rest • Exercise • Nutrition • Relief measures for common discomforts of pregnancy • Danger signs in pregnancy (see Table 9–2)		
Sexual activity: Woman knows how pregnancy affects sexual activity	Lack of information about effects of pregnancy and/or alternative positions during sexual intercourse	Provide counseling.
Preparation for parenting: Appropriate preparation	Lack of preparation (denial, failure to adjust to baby, unwanted child)	Counsel. If lack of preparation is due to inadequacy of information, provide information.

(continued)

ASSESSMENT GUIDE | Subsequent Prenatal Assessment (*continued*)

Cultural Assessment	Variations to Consider*	Nursing Responses to Data†
Preparation for childbirth: Client aware of the following: 1. Prepared childbirth techniques 2. Normal processes and changes during childbirth		If couple chooses particular technique, refer to classes Encourage prenatal class attendance. Educate woman during visits based on current physical status. Provide reading list for more specific information.
3. Problems that may occur as a result of drug and alcohol use and of smoking	Continued abuse of drugs and alcohol; denial of possible effect on self and baby	Review danger signs that were presented on initial visit.
Woman has met other physician or nurse-midwife who may be attending her birth in the absence of primary caregiver	Introduction of new individual at birth may increase stress and anxiety for woman and partner	Introduce woman to all members of group practice.
Impending labor: Client knows signs of impending labor: 1. Uterine contractions that increase in frequency, duration, and intensity 2. Bloody show 3. Expulsion of mucous plug 4. Rupture of membranes	Lack of information	Provide appropriate teaching, stressing importance of seeking appropriate medical assistance.
Expectant Father/Partner		
Psychologic status		
First trimester: May express excitement over confirmation of pregnancy and of his virility; concerns move toward providing for financial needs; energetic; may identify with some discomforts of pregnancy and may even exhibit symptoms (couvade)	Increasing stress and anxiety; inability to establish communication; inability to accept pregnancy diagnosis; withdrawal of support; abandonment of the mother	Encourage partner to come to prenatal visits. Establish line of communication. Establish trusting relationship.
Second trimester: May feel more confident and be less concerned with financial matters; may have concerns about wife's changing size and shape and her increasing introspection		Counsel. Let expectant partner know that it is normal for him to experience these feelings.
Third trimester: May have feelings of rivalry with fetus, especially during sexual activity; may make changes in his physical appearance and exhibit more interest in himself; may become more energetic; fantasizes about child but usually imagines older child; fears mutilation and death of woman and child		Include expectant partner in pregnancy activities as he desires. Provide education, information, and support. Increasing numbers of expectant partners are demonstrating desire to be involved in many or all aspects of prenatal care, education, and preparation.

*Possible causes of alterations are identified in parentheses.
†This column provides guidelines for further assessment and initial intervention.

Focus Your Study

- A complete history forms the basis of prenatal care and is reevaluated and updated as necessary throughout the pregnancy.

- The initial prenatal assessment is a careful and thorough physical examination and cultural and psychosocial assessment designed to identify variations and potential risk factors.

- Laboratory tests completed at the initial visit, such as a complete blood count, ABO and Rh typing, urinalysis/culture, Pap smear, chlamydia culture, gonorrhea culture, rubella titer, and various blood screens (such as rapid plasma reagin [RPR], HIV, and hepatitis B), provide information about the woman's health during early pregnancy and also help detect potential problems.

- The estimated date of birth (EDB) can be calculated using Nägele's rule. Using this approach, one begins with the first day of the last menstrual period, subtracts 3 months, and adds 7 days. A "wheel" may also be used to calculate the EDB.

- Accuracy of the EDB may be evaluated by physical examination to assess uterine size, measurement of fundal height, and ultrasound. Perception of quickening and auscultation of fetal heartbeat are also useful tools in confirming the gestation of a pregnancy.

- The diagonal conjugate is the distance from the lower posterior border of the symphysis pubis to the sacral promontory.

The obstetric conjugate is estimated by subtracting 1.5 to 2.0 cm (0.60 to 0.79 in.) from the length of the diagonal conjugate.

- As part of the assessment of the pelvic cavity (midpelvis), the prominence of the ischial spines is assessed, the sacrosciatic notch and the length of the sacrospinous ligament are measured, and the shape of the pelvic side walls is evaluated. Finally, the hollowness of the sacrum is determined.

- The anteroposterior diameter of the pelvic outlet is determined, the mobility of the coccyx is assessed, the suprapubic angle is estimated, and the contour of the pubic arch is evaluated to assess the adequacy of the pelvic outlet.

- The nurse begins evaluating the woman psychosocially during the initial prenatal assessment. This assessment continues and is modified throughout the pregnancy.

- Cultural and ethnic beliefs may strongly influence the woman's attitudes and apparent cooperation with care during pregnancy.

Clinical Reasoning in Action

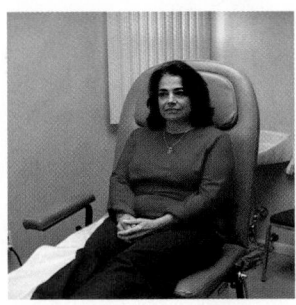

Wendy Stodard, age 40, G3P0020, comes to the obstetrician's office where you are working for a prenatal visit. Wendy has experienced two spontaneous abortions followed by a D&C at 14 and 15 weeks' gestation during the previous year. She has a history of *Chlamydia trachomatis* infection 3 years ago, which was treated with azithromycin. She is at 10 weeks' gestation. Wendy tells you that she is afraid of losing this pregnancy as she did previously. She says that she has been experiencing some mild nausea, breast tenderness, and fatigue, which did not occur with her other pregnancies. You assist the obstetrician with an ultrasound. The gestational sac is clearly seen, fetal heartbeat is observed, and crown-to-rump measurements are consistent with gestational age of 10 weeks. The pelvic examination demonstrates a closed cervix, and positive Goodell, Hegar, and Chadwick signs. You discuss with Wendy the signs of a healthy pregnancy.

1. What signs are reassuring with this pregnancy?
2. What symptoms should be reported to the obstetrician immediately?
3. What is the frequency of antepartum visits?

References

American College of Obstetricians and Gynecologists (ACOG). (2011). *Update on carrier screening for cystic fibrosis* (ACOG Committee Opinion No. 486). Washington, DC: Author.

American College of Obstetricians and Gynecologists (ACOG). 2012. *Noninvasive prenatal testing for fetal aneuploidy* (ACOG Committee Opinion No. 545). Washington, DC: Author.

American College of Obstetricians and Gynecologists (ACOG). (2013a). *Definition of term pregnancy* (ACOG Committee Opinion No. 579). Washington, DC: Author.

American College of Obstetricians and Gynecologists (ACOG). (2013b). *Gestational diabetes mellitus* (ACOG Practice Bulletin No. 137). Washington, DC: Author.

American College of Obstetricians and Gynecologists (ACOG). (2013c). *Medically indicated late-preterm and early-term deliveries* (ACOG Committee Opinion No. 560). Washington, DC: Author.

American College of Obstetricians and Gynecologists (ACOG). (2013d). *Ultrasound Exams* (ACOG Patient Education Pamphlet No. AP025). Washington, DC: Author.

American Diabetes Association (ADA). (2011). Position statement: Standards of medical care in diabetes—2011. *Diabetes Care, 34*(Suppl. 1), S11–S61.

Butt, K., & Lim, K. (2014). Determination of gestational age by ultrasound. *Journal of Obstetrics and Gynaecology Canada, 36*(2), 171–181.

Cunningham, F. G., Leveno, K. J., Bloom, S. L., Spong, C. Y., Dashe, J. S., Hoffman, B. L., ... Sheffield, J. S. (2014). *Williams obstetrics* (24th ed.). New York, NY: McGraw-Hill.

King, T. L., Brucker, M. C., Kriebs, J. M., Fahey, J. O., Gegor, C. L., & Varney, H. (2015). *Varney's midwifery* (5th ed.). Burlington, MA: Jones & Bartlett Learning.

Spong, C. Y. (2013). Defining "term" pregnancy: Recommendations from the defining "term" pregnancy workgroup. Published online May 3, 2013. doi:10.1001/jama.2013.6235

VanDorsten, J. P., Dodson, W. C., Espeland, M. A., Grobman, W. A., Guise, J. M., Mercer, B. M., ... Tita, A. T. (2013). *Diagnosing gestational diabetes mellitus: National Institutes of Health Consensus Development Conference Statement.* Retrieved from http://www.ncbi.nlm.nih.gov/pubmed/23748438

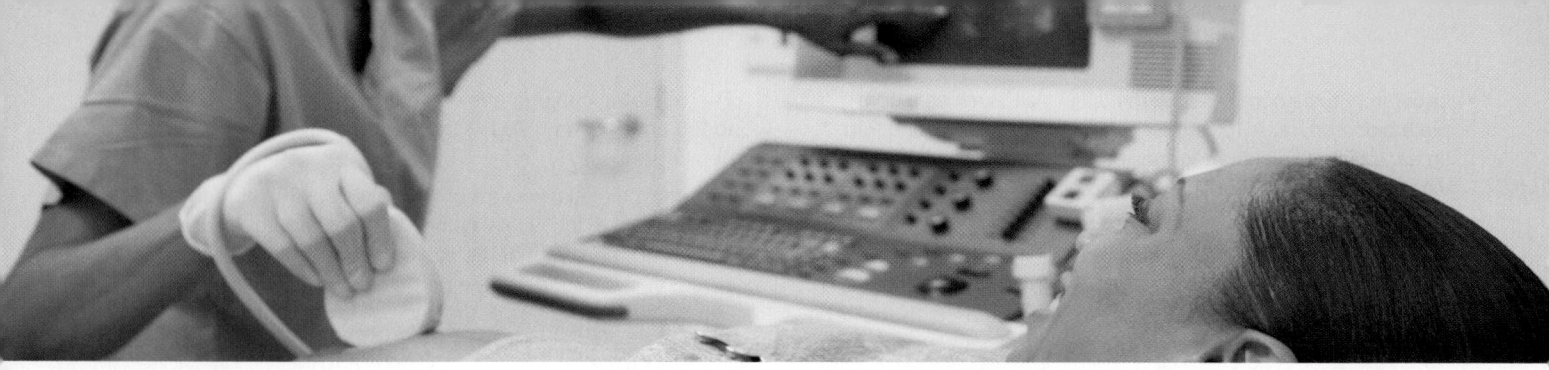

Chapter 10
The Expectant Family: Needs and Care

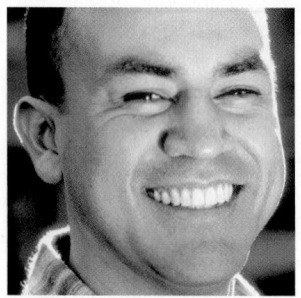

We have what I guess you would call a blended family. I have two college-age sons from my first marriage, and my wife has a 12-year-old boy. She is expecting our first child now. Because she is 38, she had an amniocentesis done and we know that this baby is a girl. How excited we all are! I don't think anything could have done more to unite us as a new family. Now if we can just agree on a name.

—Ricardo, 46

Ken Huang/Getty Images

∨ Learning Outcomes

10.1 Describe the significance of using the nursing process to promote health in the woman and her family during pregnancy.

10.2 Describe actions the nurse can take to help maintain the well-being of the expectant father and siblings during a family's pregnancy.

10.3 Discuss the significance of cultural considerations in managing nursing care during pregnancy.

10.4 Identify information that expectant parents may need to assist them in making the best decisions possible about issues related to pregnancy, labor, and birth.

10.5 Explain the basic goals of childbirth education in providing care to expectant couples and their families.

10.6 Identify the common discomforts of pregnancy and their causes.

10.7 Summarize appropriate measures to alleviate the common discomforts of pregnancy.

10.8 Delineate self-care actions a pregnant woman and her family can take to maintain and promote well-being during each trimester of pregnancy.

10.9 Identify some of the concerns that an expectant couple may have about sexual activity.

From the moment a woman finds out she is pregnant, she faces a future marked by dramatic changes—changes in her appearance, in her relationships, and in her psychologic state. In coping with these changes, she and her loved ones need to make adjustments in their daily lives.

Nurses caring for pregnant women need an up-to-date understanding of pregnancy to be effective in implementing the nursing process as they plan and provide care. With this in mind, Chapter 8 provides a database for the nurse by presenting material related to the normal physical, psychologic, social, and cultural changes of pregnancy. Chapter 9 then uses that database to begin discussing nursing care management by focusing on assessment. This chapter further addresses nursing

management as it relates to the needs of the expectant woman and her loved ones.

Nursing Care During the Prenatal Period

Nursing Diagnoses During Pregnancy

The nurse may see a pregnant woman only once every 3 to 4 weeks during the first several months of her pregnancy. Therefore, a written care plan or clinical path that incorporates the database, nursing diagnoses, and client goals is essential to ensure continuity of care.

The nurse can anticipate that, for many women with a low-risk pregnancy, certain nursing diagnoses will be made more frequently than others. The diagnoses will, of course, vary from woman to woman and according to the time in the pregnancy. After formulating an appropriate diagnosis, the nurse and woman establish related goals to guide the nursing plan and interventions.

Planning and Implementation During Pregnancy

Once nursing diagnoses have been identified, the next step is to establish priorities of nursing care. Sometimes priorities of care are based on the most immediate needs or concerns expressed by the woman. For example, during the first trimester, when she is experiencing nausea or is concerned about sexual intimacy with her partner, the woman is not likely to want to hear about labor and birth. At other times, priorities may develop from findings during a prenatal examination. For example, a woman who is showing signs of preeclampsia (a pregnancy complication discussed in Chapter 14) may feel physically well and find it hard to accept the nurse's emphasis on the need for frequent rest periods. It then becomes the responsibility of medical and nursing professionals to help the woman and her family to understand the significance of a problem and to plan interventions to deal with it.

Healthy People 2020

(MICH-10) Increase the proportion of pregnant women who receive early and adequate prenatal care

---

Health Promotion Anticipatory Guidance for the Postpartum Period

Throughout the prenatal period, the nurse shares information with the family, both verbally and through written materials. Anticipatory guidance helps the expectant couple identify and discuss issues that could be sources of postpartum stress. Issues to be addressed beforehand may include the sharing of infant and household chores, help in the first few days after childbirth, options for babysitting to allow the mother (and couple) some free time, the mother's return to work after the baby's birth, and sibling rivalry. Couples resolve these issues in different ways, but postpartum adjustment tends to be easier for couples who agree on the issues beforehand than for couples who do not confront and resolve these issues.

NURSING CARE IN THE COMMUNITY

Prenatal care, especially for women with low-risk pregnancies, is community based, typically in a clinic or a private office. The nurse in a clinic or health maintenance organization may be the only source of continuity for the woman, who may see a different physician or certified nurse-midwife at each visit. The nurse can be extremely effective in working with the expectant family by answering questions; providing complete information about pregnancy, prenatal healthcare activities, and community resources; and supporting the healthcare activities of the woman and her family. Communities often have a wealth of services and educational opportunities available for pregnant women and their families, and the knowledgeable nurse can help expectant mothers to assess and access these services.

Home Care.   Home care can be of benefit to any pregnant woman, but it is especially effective in removing barriers for women who have difficulty accessing health care. These barriers may include lack of locally available healthcare facilities, problems with transportation to the facility, or schedule conflicts with available appointment times because of employment hours or family responsibilities.

In-home nursing assessments vary according to the experience and preparation of the nurse and include current history, vital signs, weight, urine screen, physical activity, dietary intake, reflexes, tests of fetal well-being, and cervical examinations, if indicated. Once the assessments are completed, the nurse can determine the level of follow-up home care or telephone contact needed. See Chapter 29 for further discussion of home care of the childbearing family.

Currently, home care is not routinely used because of the cost, but when home care is available, it is most often used for women with prenatal complications that can be managed without hospitalization if effective nursing assessment and care are provided in the home.

Care of the Pregnant Woman's Family

The well-being of the pregnant woman is intertwined with the well-being of those to whom she is closest. Thus the nurse also addresses the needs of the woman's family. Although the expectant father is often involved in the pregnancy, his presence cannot be assumed. If he is not part of the family structure, it is important to assess the woman's support system to determine which significant people in her life will play a major role during this childbearing experience. This may be a spouse or a same sex partner. The following information still applies.

Anticipatory guidance of the expectant father, if he is involved in the pregnancy, is a necessary part of any plan of care. He may need information about the anatomic, physiologic, and emotional changes that occur for the expectant mother and father during and after pregnancy; the couple's sexuality and sexual response; and the reactions that he is experiencing. He may wish to express his feelings about the sex of the child, his ability to parent, and other topics.

If it is culturally acceptable to the couple and personally acceptable to the expectant father, refer the couple to expectant parents' classes. These classes provide valuable information about pregnancy and childbirth, using a variety of teaching strategies such as discussion, films, demonstrations with educational models, and written handouts. Some classes even give the father the opportunity to get a "feel" for pregnancy by wearing a pregnancy simulator (Figure 10–1). Such classes also offer the couple an opportunity to gain support from other couples.

The nurse assesses the father's intended degree of participation during labor and birth and his knowledge of what to expect. If the couple prefers that his participation be minimal or restricted, support their decision. Research indicates that increased focus on the father's needs during prenatal care aids his transition to fatherhood and also improves the mother's

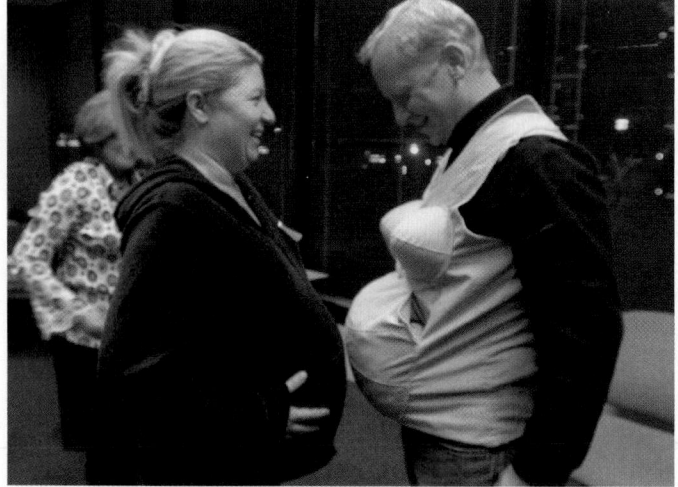

Figure 10–1 The Empathy Belly® is a pregnancy simulator that allows men and women to experience some of the symptoms of pregnancy. The "belly," which weighs 33 lb, produces symptoms such as shortness of breath, bladder pressure, shift in the center of gravity with resulting waddling gait, increased lordosis and backache, and fatigue. It also can simulate fetal kicking movements.

SOURCE: ZUMA Press/Alamy.

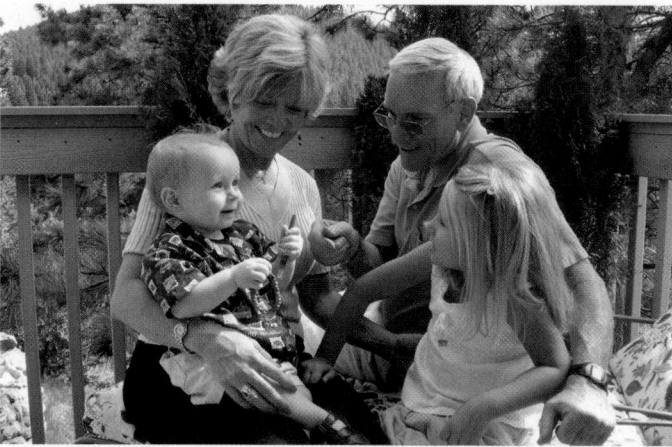

Figure 10–2 Grandparents can offer nurturing and guidance to their grandchildren, not to mention lots of fun.

stress levels and prenatal health behavior. Assessing and fostering progress in the father's journey to becoming a parent has significant long-term benefits for the man, his partner, and their child (Alio, Lewis, Scarborough, et al., 2013). In the plan for prenatal care, the nurse also incorporates a discussion about the negative feelings older children may develop. Parents may be distressed to see an older child regress to "babyish" behavior or become aggressive toward the newborn. Parents who are unprepared for an older child's feelings of anger, jealousy, and rejection may respond inappropriately in their confusion and surprise. The nurse emphasizes that open communication between parents and children (or acting out feelings with a doll if the child is too young to verbalize) helps children master their feelings. Children may feel less neglected and more secure if they know that their parents are willing to help with their anger and aggressiveness.

The nurse can encourage the couple to address relationship changes with in-laws as well as the woman's or couple's expectations of the grandparents. Although some grandparents are eager to assist with child care by babysitting, others are not (Figure 10–2). The parents should also give some thought to the best ways of dealing with possible conflicts with the grandparents over childrearing approaches. However, postpartum adjustment is easiest for couples who acknowledge potential problems and develop strategies to address them beforehand.

Cultural Considerations in Pregnancy

As discussed in Chapter 2, actions taken during pregnancy are often determined by cultural beliefs. Table 10–1 presents activities encouraged or forbidden by some specific cultures. The

table is not meant to be all-inclusive, nor is it meant to imply that all members of a given culture hold these beliefs. Rather, it offers a few examples of cultural activities that may be important to some women during the prenatal period.

In working with clients of other cultures, health professionals should be open to and respectful of others' beliefs. Effective nurses recognize that each childbearing family, shaped by culture and life experience, has expectations of both its members and the healthcare system during pregnancy and birth.

Language barriers often pose a challenge in providing effective prenatal nursing care. When possible, it is important to have an interpreter—family member, friend, or staff person—present at prenatal visits so that the nurse can provide basic information about pregnancy and prenatal care. It is essential to have printed material available in the woman's language. (See *Nursing Care Plan: Language Barriers at First Prenatal Visit*.)

Childbearing Decisions

Childbearing decisions are decisions parents face about their childbirth preferences and experiences. A method that has assisted many couples in making these choices is called a birth plan. In the birth plan, prospective parents identify aspects of the childbearing experience that are most important to them. (A sample birth plan is presented in Figure 10–3.) The birth plan helps identify available options and becomes a tool for communication among the expectant parents, the healthcare providers, and the healthcare professionals at the birth setting.

The birth plan also helps pregnant women and couples set priorities. Using the plan, they identify areas that they want to incorporate in their own birth experience. Then they can take the birth plan to a visit with their physician/certified nurse-midwife (CNM) or other healthcare provider and use it in discussing and comparing their wishes with the philosophy and beliefs of the provider. It is imperative that the couple discuss their preferences at a prenatal visit before labor. Sometimes couples may include requests that need clarification. For example, if the couple states they do not want any external monitoring, the provider needs to explain that

TABLE 10–1 Cultural Beliefs and Practices During Pregnancy

These are a few examples of cultural beliefs and practices related to pregnancy. It is important not to make assumptions about a client's beliefs because cultural norms vary greatly within a culture and from generation to generation. The nurse should observe the client carefully and take the time to ask questions. Clients will benefit greatly from the nurse's increased awareness of their cultural beliefs and practices.

BELIEF OR PRACTICE	NURSING CONSIDERATION
Home Remedies	
Pregnant women of Native American background may use herbal remedies. An example is the dandelion, which contains a milky juice in its stem believed to increase breast milk flow in mothers who choose to breastfeed (Spector, 2013). Clients of Chinese descent may drink ginseng tea for faintness after childbirth or as a sedative when mixed with bamboo leaves. Some people of African heritage may use self-medication for pregnancy discomforts—for example, laxatives to prevent or treat constipation (Purnell, 2014).	Find out what medications and home remedies your client is using, and counsel your client regarding overall effects. It is common for individuals to avoid telling healthcare workers about home remedies; the client may feel this will be judged unfavorably. Phrase your questions in a sensitive, accepting way. In some cases, you might want to suggest remedies that may be more effective—for example, eating high-fiber foods to reduce constipation. If the home remedy is not harmful, there is no reason to ask a client to discontinue this practice.
Nutrition	
Some women of Italian background may believe that it is necessary to satisfy desires for certain foods in order to prevent congenital anomalies. Also, they may believe that they must eat food that they smell, or else the fetus will move "inside," which will result in a miscarriage. Pregnant women of Vietnamese descent are considered to be in a weak, cold state and must correct this by eating and drinking hot foods during the first trimester (Purnell, 2014). So, too, people of Ethiopian descent may believe that unfulfilled cravings may cause miscarriage (Spector, 2013).	Discuss the client's beliefs and practices in regard to nutrition during pregnancy. Obtain a diet history from the client. Discuss the importance of a well-balanced diet during pregnancy with consideration of the client's cultural beliefs and practices.
Alternative Healthcare Providers	
Pregnant women of Mexican background may choose to seek out the care of a *partera* (midwife) for prenatal and intrapartum care. A partera speaks their language, shares a similar culture, and can care for pregnant women at home or in a birthing center instead of a hospital. Some people in Hispanic American communities may use the *curandero,* the holistic folk healer. The curanderos are believed to have received their gift from God and may use herbs or prescribe over-the-counter medications (Spector, 2013).	Discuss the variety of choices of healthcare providers available to the pregnant woman. Contrast the benefits and risks of different settings for prenatal care and birth. Provide reassurance that the goal of health care during pregnancy and birth is a healthy outcome for mother and baby with respect for the specific cultural beliefs and practices of the client.
Exercise	
Pregnant women of Korean descent may work hard toward the end of pregnancy to increase the chances of giving birth to a small baby (Purnell, 2014). Some people of European, African, and Mexican descent believe that reaching over the head during pregnancy can harm the baby.	Ask your client whether there are any activities she is afraid to do because of the pregnancy. Assure her that reaching over her head will not harm the baby, and evaluate other activities to their effect on the pregnancy.
Spirituality	
Navajo Indians are aware of the mind–soul connection and may try to follow certain practices to have a healthy pregnancy and birth. Practices could include focus on peace and positive thoughts as well as certain types of prayers and ceremonies. A traditional healer may assist them (Purnell, 2014). Some people of European background may tend to pay more attention to spirituality in their life to alleviate fears and ensure a safe birth.	Encourage the use of support systems and spiritual aids that provide comfort for the mother.
Birth Rituals	
In certain countries such as Algeria, Brazil, China, and Korea, the father is not present at birth. In Japan, a new mother may be confined for up to 100 days, whereas in Bangladesh, the new mother remains indoors for up to 40 days. In Iran, Iraq, and Greece, amulets may be placed on the baby or crib (Spector, 2013).	Recognize the importance of birth practices that are part of a family's tradition and honor these practices when possible.

Nursing Care Plan: Language Barriers at First Prenatal Visit

Nursing Diagnosis: *Health Maintenance, Ineffective*, related to alteration in verbal and written communication skills (NANDA-I ©2014)

GOAL: Client will demonstrate understanding of health information received during prenatal visits.

INTERVENTION	RATIONALE
• If no interpreter is available, refer to posters with pictures to explain routine care and procedures during the prenatal examination.	• Posters put words into verbal images and are helpful in communicating information.
• Provide handouts and brochures about prenatal care in the woman's native language.	• Translated handouts provide information that the client can refer to at home. This reinforces information discussed during the visit and helps the family understand what the woman will experience during the pregnancy and at each visit.
• Use teaching models to demonstrate procedures. Teaching models may include plastic pelvis, knitted uterus, fetal model, breast model, birth control devices, ultrasound equipment, and so forth.	• Visual aids help to communicate information during the examination.
• Schedule an interpreter for subsequent prenatal visits.	• If a family member cannot translate the health information to the client, an independent translator is essential to ensure that information is accurately provided. When an interpreter is used (especially a family member), the nurse should be sure that the interpreter is translating information received from the woman and not simply answering the questions for her.
• Refer the woman to prenatal classes taught in her own language, if available.	• Prenatal classes taught in the woman's language enable her to receive health information that is easily understood, which will provide a better understanding of what she should expect during pregnancy, birth, and postpartum. Prenatal classes may also provide a social outlet for clients.
• Involve other members of the healthcare team in planning and providing care.	• Cultures vary in language, nonverbal expression, dietary habits, use of time, spatial expectations, and so forth. Use of medication and blood products may also be influenced by cultural beliefs. Social workers who are familiar with the client's cultural beliefs, for example, may help the client adjust to different healthcare practices while providing suggestions to ensure prenatal care that is more in line with the woman's cultural beliefs. Dietitians may help the woman plan meals that are aligned with her cultural practices while meeting the nutritional needs of pregnancy.

EXPECTED OUTCOME: Effective communication occurs. The client will gain an understanding of basic prenatal information as evidenced by using hand gestures, by pointing to pictures on posters and translated phrases on handouts, and through an interpreter, if one is available.

intermittent monitoring could be provided but that eliminating all monitoring during labor could jeopardize both the mother and the fetus. Possible obstetric interventions that may be needed should also be part of the birth plan. They can also take the birth plan to the birth setting and use it as a basis for communicating their wishes during the childbirth experience.

Today, there are many more choices that pregnant women and couples make. Some of these are explored in Table 10–2. Although most birth experiences are close to those presented in the birth plan, at times expectations cannot be met. This may be because of the unavailability of some choices in the community or unexpected problems during pregnancy or birth. While research indicates maternal satisfaction is highest when a

planned cesarean section or vaginal birth is achieved, it is important for nurses to help expectant parents keep sight of what is realistic for their situation (Bloomquist, Quiroz, MacMillan, et al., 2011).

Healthcare Provider

One of the first decisions facing expectant parents is the selection of a healthcare provider. The nurse assists them by explaining the various options and outlining what can be expected from each. A thorough understanding of the differences of educational preparation, skill level, practice style, and general philosophy and characteristics of practice of certified nurse-midwives, obstetricians, family practice physicians, and lay

Developing Cultural Competence Pregnant Women of African American Heritage

In caring for pregnant women of African American heritage, it is helpful to consider the following general points (Purnell, 2014):

- Pregnant African American women may be guided by their extended family into common practices such as geophagia, the ingestion of dirt or clay, which is believed to reduce mineral deficiencies. This practice has implications for the focus of teaching a nurse will offer.

- Many African American families are matriarchal. Women are respected and heeded in decision making and often stress good behavior and firm parenting with their children, especially to keep them safe in dangerous situations.

- Three-generation extended families are common, and the grandmother is often highly respected for her wisdom. She may play a critical role in the care of the children.

- Certain taboos may exist, such as the belief in the need to avoid taking pictures during pregnancy to prevent stillbirths. Some women of African American descent may also believe that the purchase of infant clothing or supplies can result in a stillbirth. Thus they may appear to be unprepared for the arrival of the baby.

Professionalism in Practice Providing Culturally Sensitive Care

In providing effective, culturally sensitive care, nurses can use the following strategies (University of South Carolina, 2011):

- Take actions that help break down language barriers.
- Ask the client what she or he believes caused the illness.
- Integrate folk treatments and Western medicine as much as possible.
- Enlist the family caretaker and others as needed.
- Respect the client's beliefs.
- Provide printed materials in the client's language.

midwives is essential. The nurse can encourage expectant parents to investigate the healthcare provider's credentials, basic and special education and training, fee schedule, and availability to new clients; this is often accomplished by telephoning the provider's office.

The nurse can also help the woman/couple develop a list of interview questions for their first visit to a healthcare provider. These could include the following:

- Who is in practice with you, or who covers for you when you are unavailable?
- At what point after admission do you come to the hospital or birth setting to provide support?
- How do your partners' philosophies compare to yours?

Sample Birth Plan

Choice	Choice
Care provider:	Position during birth:
Certified nurse-midwife	On side
Obstetrician	Hands and knees
Family physician	Kneeling
Lay midwife	Squatting
Birth setting:	Birthing chair
Hospital:	Birthing bed
Birthing room	Other:
Delivery room	Family present (sibs)
Birth center	Filming of birth (videotaping)
Home	Photography of birth
Support during labor and birth:	Leboyer
Partner present	Episiotomy
Doula present	No sterile drapes
During labor:	Partner to cut umbilical cord
Ambulate as desired	Hold baby immediately after birth
Shower if desired	Breastfeed immediately after birth
Wear own clothes	No separation after birth
Use hot tub	Save the placenta
Use own rocking chair	Collect cord blood for banking
Have perineal prep	Newborn care:
Have enema	Eye treatment for the baby
Water birth	Vitamin K injection
Electronic fetal monitor	Heptovac injection
Membranes:	Breastfeeding
Rupture naturally	Formula feeding
Amniotomy if needed	Pacifier use
Labor stimulation if needed	Glucose water
Medication:	Circumcision
Identify type desired	Postpartum care:
Fluids or ice as desired	Short stay
Music during labor and birth	48-hour stay after vaginal birth
Massage	Home visits after discharge
Therapeutic touch	Home doula
Healing touch	Other:

Figure 10–3 Birth plan for childbirth choices. The columns list various choices that the couple may consider during their childbirth experience. Once the couple has considered each of the choices, they can circle the items they desire.

- How do you feel about my partner, other support person, or other children coming to the prenatal visits?
- Do you offer centering (group care) or individual prenatal care visits?
- What weight gain do you recommend and why?
- What are your feelings about (fill in special desires for the birth event, such as different positions assumed during labor, avoidance of an episiotomy, induction of labor, other people present during the birth, pain control measures, breastfeeding immediately after the birth, no separation of newborn and parents following birth, and so on)?
- If a cesarean is necessary, can my partner be present?
- What are your feelings regarding complementary treatments during labor (herbs to augment labor, use of acupressure/massage/hypnosis, use of oils for perineal massage, and so on)?

Expectant parents also need to discuss the qualities they want in a healthcare provider for the newborn. They may want to visit several pediatric healthcare providers before the birth to select someone who will meet their needs and those of their child.

TABLE 10–2 Benefits and Risks of Some Consumer and Medical Decisions During Pregnancy, Labor, and Birth

ISSUE	BENEFITS	RISKS
Breastfeeding	• No additional expense • Contains maternal antibodies • Decreases incidence of infant otitis media, vomiting, and diarrhea, hospitalizations during the first year of life, and allergies • Easier to digest than formula • Immediately after birth, promotes uterine contractions and decreases incidence of postpartum hemorrhage • Promotes maternal–infant bonding	• Transmission of maternal infections to newborn, such as HIV • Irregular ovulation and menses can cause false sense of security and nonuse of hormonal contraceptives • Increased nutritional requirement in mother

Ambulation during labor	• Comfort for laboring woman
	• May assist in labor progression by
	  • Stimulating contractions
	  • Allowing gravity to help descent of fetus
	  • Giving sense of independence and control
		• Cord prolapse with rupture of membranes unless engagement has occurred
		• Birth of baby in undesirable locations (hallways, outdoors, waiting area)
		• Inability to monitor fetal heart rate (FHR) unless telemetry unit available

Electronic fetal monitoring	• Helps evaluate fetal well-being • Helps identify fetal stress • Useful in diagnostic testing • Helps evaluate labor progress	• Supine postural hypotension • Intrauterine perforation (with internal uterine pressure device) • Infection (with internal monitoring) • Decreases personal interaction with mother because of attention paid to the machine • Mother is unable to ambulate or change her position freely
Whirlpool (jet hydrotherapy)	• Increased relaxation • Decreased anxiety • Stimulation of labor • Provides pain relief • Slight decrease in blood pressure (BP) • Increased diuresis • Decreased incidence of vacuum and forceps deliveries • Increased pain threshold • Higher satisfaction with birth • Decreased use of pain medication (Avery, 2013)	• May slow contractions if used before active labor is established • Possible risk of infection if membranes are ruptured • Slight increase in maternal temperature and pulse in tub • Hypothermia • Increases fetal heart rate (FHR) by 10–20 beats/min
Analgesia	• Maternal relaxation facilitates labor	• All drugs reach the fetus in varying degrees and with varying effects
Episiotomy	• Decreases irregular tearing of perineum • Easier to repair for practitioner	• Increased pain after birth and for 1–3 months following birth • Dyspareunia • Infection • Increased frequency of third- and fourth-degree lacerations (Cunningham et al., 2014; Groutz et al., 2011)

Prenatal Care Services

The nurse can assist expectant parents in obtaining the type of prenatal care services that are most appropriate for their personal needs. Most practitioners offer individual prenatal care services in which the woman or the woman and her family attend a clinic or office visit on a regular basis depending on her stage of pregnancy. Recently, the concept of centering, or group prenatal care, has become popular.

When empowering women to choose health-promoting behaviors, it may be helpful to consider a relatively new, innovative model for prenatal care called *CenteringPregnancy*®. CenteringPregnancy® integrates the three major components of care—health assessment, education, and support—into a unified program providing complete prenatal care to women within a group setting. It is discussed in more detail later in this chapter.

Birth Setting

The nurse can help expectant parents choose a birth setting by suggesting they tour facilities and talk with nurses there as well as talk with friends or acquaintances who are recent parents. Questions that may be asked of new parents include the following:

- What kind of support did you receive during labor? Was it what you wanted?

- Were you allowed to take an active role in decision making throughout the birth process?

- If you had a doula, was her role respected? Was she welcome in the birth setting?

- Was your birth plan respected? Did you share it with the facility before the birth? If something did not work, why do you think there were problems?

- Did the nurse offer suggestions regarding comfort measures?

- Did the healthcare team provide emotional support?

- How were medications handled during labor? Were you comfortable with this?

- Were siblings welcomed in the birth setting? At the birth? After the birth?

- Did you feel you were given ample time to spend with your baby immediately after childbirth?

- Was the nursing staff helpful after the baby was born? Did you receive self-care and infant care information? Was it in a usable form? Did you have a choice about what information you got? Did they let you decide what information you needed?

- Did you feel your choice of feeding method was supported?

The nurse helps expectant parents understand the array of choices available to them. The nurse can encourage them to consider options early in the pregnancy to allow time for talking with other parents and touring facilities.

Nurses involved in childbirth education need to include the concept of individuality when providing information to expectant parents about the process of childbirth and their own pattern of coping. The wave of the future in childbirth education is to encourage women to incorporate their natural responses into coping with the pain of labor and birth. Alternative self-care activities should be explored with the expectant couple to identify preferences.

Nurses should encourage expectant women and couples to personalize the birth setting. The woman might plan, for example, to bring items from home to enhance relaxation and comfort, such as warm socks, slippers, bath powder, lotion, or a favorite blanket. She may wish to bring photographs of children, parents, or friends who cannot be there to share the birth experience. Many expectant parents enjoy listening to tapes of favorite music or watching home videos or favorite films. Such personalization of the birth setting may give expectant parents feelings of increased serenity and empowerment.

Clinical Tip

Call the birthing facilities in your community and inquire about what choices are available in each facility so that you can answer expectant parents' questions.

Labor Support Person

Some of the first formal childbirth preparation classes were patterned after a book titled *Husband Coached Childbirth* by Dr. Robert Bradley, which was published in 1965. Since that time, husbands and other partners of expectant women have been very involved in acting as "coaches" or support persons during childbirth classes, labor, and birth. Although some men or support persons welcome the role and look forward to providing emotional and physical support, others do not. Some men may become anxious and fearful. These feelings can be related to past experiences and/or cultural factors. In these situations, the nurse provides encouragement and support to both the woman and her support person. Women who had continuous intrapartum support were less likely to have intrapartum analgesia, operative birth, or to report dissatisfaction with their childbirth experiences (Donna, 2011). A woman's satisfaction with childbirth is directly affected by the relationship with the healthcare provider, the support she received from healthcare providers,

---

EVIDENCE-BASED PRACTICE | Interventions to Reduce Childbirth Fear in Pregnant Women

Clinical Question

Can education and psychologic support reduce the fear of childbirth in healthy pregnant women?

The Evidence

Fear of the process of childbirth has been linked to adverse maternal outcomes, including high rates of surgical birth, mental health issues, and increased postpartum depression. Many women with childbirth fear may request surgical birth if they perceive their fears have not been addressed. These researchers used a randomized trial to test an antenatal intervention of psychologic support and education delivered by nurse-midwives. More than 1400 women were included in the study population. Randomized trials with large sample sizes form a strong level of evidence.

The intervention was a telephone education counseling intervention that reviewed the woman's current expectations and feelings regarding fear of childbirth. The nurse supported the expression of feelings, and provided a framework for women to identify and work through the elements of childbirth that they found frightening. The intervention focused on helping the mother develop situational supports for the birth and a plan for dealing with the childbirth experience that gave the mother control over her birth process. The women who received the intervention reported lower levels of fear and higher levels of self-efficacy and sense of control (Toohill et al., 2014). These mothers also had fewer depression symptoms and requested surgical birth with less frequency.

Best Practice

Prenatal psychologic support and education may reduce the fear of childbirth among women. Improving antenatal emotional well-being has a myriad of positive benefits and may result in an optimal childbirth experience. Providing this support leads to fewer requests for surgical births.

Clinical Reasoning

What are some of the ways that the nurse can help the mother gain a sense of control over the birth process? What might be some of the benefits of reduced childbirth fear for the mother and for the provider?

personal expectations, and her involvement with decision making. Clearly, the role of the nurse cannot be overestimated.

For centuries, women have been serving and assisting other women in childbirth. Out of this need for companionship and special support in the birthing journey, the role of the *doula* has evolved. The doula is specially trained to assist with births and to provide *labor support*, which includes emotional, physical, and informational support. The doula does not perform clinical tasks but she also acts as an advocate for the woman and her family by verbalizing their wishes to the nurses and physicians/CNMs. Continuous labor support facilitates birth; enhances the mother's memory of the experience; strengthens mother–newborn bonding; increases breastfeeding success; and significantly reduces many forms of medical intervention, including cesarean delivery and the use of analgesia, anesthesia, vacuum extraction, and forceps (Donna, 2011). A doula may also be trained to provide support and care during the postpartum period. Later postpartum benefits for the mother include increased bonding/interaction with the infant and decreased symptoms of depression. The doula may accompany the childbearing couple on a volunteer basis or may be paid a fee by the family.

Siblings at Birth

Some couples decide to have their other children present at the birth. Children who will attend a birth can be prepared through books, audiovisual materials, models, discussion, and sibling classes.

It is imperative that the child has his or her own support person or coach whose sole responsibility is tending to the needs of that child during the labor and birth experience. The support person should be familiar to the child, warm, sensitive, flexible, knowledgeable about the birth process, and comfortable with sexuality and birth. This person must be prepared to interpret to the child what is happening and to intervene when necessary. The support person should be prepared and willing to leave the birthing room at any time, should that be the child's desire. The support person for the child should assume responsibility for providing distractions such as trips to the cafeteria, visits to the nursery window, outdoor walks, and other age-appropriate activities.

Children should be given the option of relating to the birth in whatever manner they choose as long as it is not disruptive. Children should understand that it is their own choice to be there and that they may stay or leave the room as they choose. To help children recognize their needs and desires, the nurse may wish to elicit exactly what they expect from the experience. Children need to feel free to ask questions and express feelings.

Allowing children to participate in the arrival of their sibling engenders the desire to nurture "our" baby, as opposed to jealousy and rivalry directed at "Mom's" baby. The mother does not disappear mysteriously into the hospital and return with a demanding outsider. Instead, the family attending the birth together finds a new opportunity for closeness and growth by sharing in the birth of a new member.

Developing Cultural Competence Female Relatives as Caregivers

In most Middle Eastern countries, childbirth is exclusively attended to by women. A woman in labor is most commonly surrounded by female relatives and friends. It is customary for the husband to be excluded from the birthing unit. In Iran, full segregation is mandated by law. Women can only be cared for by female healthcare providers.

Classes for Family Members During Pregnancy

Childbirth classes are routinely taught by certified childbirth educators (CBEs or CCEs). These are individuals who have received specific educational preparation related to pregnancy, labor, birth, and postpartum/newborn care and issues. Many CBEs are also registered nurses; however, nursing training is not required. The majority of the certification programs do, however, require witnessing a minimum number of births.

The CBE should consider elements developed by authoritative organizations such as the Coalition for Improving Maternity Services (CIMS) when developing their own Philosophy of Childbirth for their classes. The "Mother-Friendly Childbirth Initiative" was created in 1996 by the Coalition for Improving Maternity Services (CIMS), a national alliance of more than 50 childbirth organizations and many prominent individuals. The coalition's mission is to promote a wellness model of maternity care that will improve birth outcomes and substantially reduce costs. The philosophic cornerstones of mother-friendly care are: (1) normalcy of the birthing process, (2) empowerment, (3) autonomy, (4) do no harm, and (5) responsibility (Coalition for Improving Maternity Services [CIMS], 2013).

Prenatal education programs provide important opportunities to share information about pregnancy, childbirth, coping mechanisms, and choices available for the woman and her support person. Studies have shown that prepared childbirth education programs can have a beneficial effect on performance in labor and birth. The prenatal period should be used to expose the prospective parents to up-to-date, evidence-based information about the following topics:

- Labor and birth
- Pain relief
- Obstetric complications and procedures
- Breastfeeding
- Normal newborn care
- Postpartum adjustment

The content of each class is generally directed by the overall goals of the program. For example, specific classes may address the following subjects:

- Gestational changes and fetal development
- Childbirth choices available today
- Preparation of the mother for pregnancy and birth
- Preparation for cesarean birth or for vaginal birth after cesarean
- Preparation for couples who desire an unmedicated birth
- Preparation of the grandparents or siblings for the birth
- Newborn care and safety
- Self-care during the postpartum period

The nurse who knows the types of prenatal programs available in the community can direct expectant parents to programs that meet their special needs and learning goals.

From the expectant parents' point of view, class content is best presented in chronology with the pregnancy. It is important that the classes begin by identifying the parents' needs, goals, and learning styles. Although both parents expect to learn breathing and relaxation techniques and infant care, fathers usually expect facts and mothers expect coping strategies.

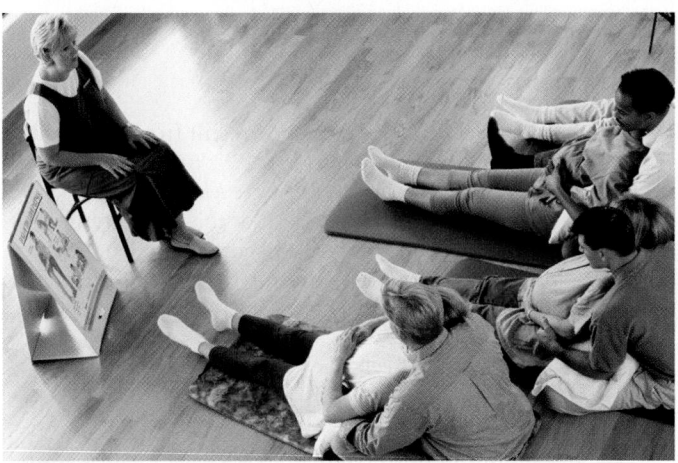

Figure 10–4 **In a group setting with a nurse-instructor, expectant parents share information about pregnancy and childbirth.**

SOURCE: Jiang Jin/Alamy.

Women's goals commonly include gaining information, reducing anxiety/increasing confidence, having their partner present and involved, and having a positive emotional experience in childbirth. Classes that provide an environment supportive of practicing newly learned techniques and the freedom to ask questions and receive explanations are beneficial in helping class participants obtain these goals (Figure 10–4). By the end of the class, parents should feel that they will be able to make appropriate and informed decisions by participating in a class where information is given in a nonjudgmental, nonthreatening environment. Classes may be divided into early and late classes so specific needs can be addressed.

Education of the Family Having Cesarean Birth

Cesarean birth is an alternative method of birth that now accounts for 32.8% of births in the United States (Martin, Hamilton, Osterman, et al., 2013). Consequently, although the need for a cesarean birth is not often known in advance, more and more childbirth preparation classes are integrating content on cesarean birth into the curriculum.

Class content should cover what the parents can expect to happen during a cesarean birth, what they might feel, and what choices are available. All pregnant women and couples should be encouraged to discuss with their physician/CNM the progression of events if a cesarean birth becomes necessary. Cesarean birth and repeat cesarean birth are discussed in detail in Chapter 22.

When expectant parents are anticipating a repeat cesarean birth, they have time to plan and prepare. Many birthing units provide preparation classes for repeat cesarean birth. Parents who have had previous negative experiences need an opportunity to describe what contributed to their feelings. They should be encouraged to identify what they would like to change and to list interventions that would make the experience more positive. Those who have had positive experiences require reassurance that their needs and desires will be met in a similar manner. All parents should be encouraged to air any fears or anxieties.

Often, a woman facing a repeat cesarean birth is concerned about postoperative pain. She needs reassurance that subsequent cesarean births are often less painful than the first. In addition, planned cesarean births involve less fatigue than unplanned procedures because they are not preceded by a long, strenuous labor. Providing this information will help the woman cope more effectively with stressful stimuli, including pain.

Preparation for Parents Desiring Trial of Labor After Cesarean Birth

Trial of labor after cesarean birth (TOLAC) was previously termed *vaginal birth after cesarean* (VBAC) and is discussed in detail in Chapter 22. Parents who have had a cesarean birth and are now anticipating a vaginal birth have unique needs. Because they may have unresolved questions and concerns about the last birth, it is helpful to begin the series of classes with an informational session. The nurse can supply information about the criteria necessary to attempt a trial of labor and identify decisions to be made regarding the birth experience. Some childbirth educators suggest that parents prepare two birth plans: one for vaginal birth and one for cesarean birth. Preparing birth plans seems to give parents some sense of control over the birth experience and tends to increase the positive aspects of the experience.

Breastfeeding Programs

Programs offering information on breastfeeding are increasing. For decades, a primary source of information has been the La Leche League. Information can also be obtained from lactation consultants, peer counselors, labor and postpartum nurses, birthing centers, hospitals, and health clinics. Online support groups can also be an important resource for breastfeeding mothers.

Healthy People 2020

(MICH-21) Increase the proportion of infants who are breastfed

---

Rates of breastfeeding in the United States are well below the *Healthy People 2020* objective of 81.9% (U.S. Department of Health and Human Services [HHS], 2013). *Healthy People 2020* has set goals not only for increasing the rate of breastfed infants, but also for increasing the availability of worksite lactation support programs to encourage mothers to continue breastfeeding following their return to work.

Classes and support groups typically include information about the following topics:

- Advantages and challenges of breastfeeding
- Techniques and positioning
- Methods of breast pumping and milk storage
- How to involve the father or partner in the feeding process, such as having him or her bring the baby to the mother for feedings, burp the baby between or after feedings, or rock the baby back to sleep
- Ways of successfully breastfeeding and returning to work

Sibling Preparation: Adjustment to a Newborn

The birth of a new sibling is a significant event in a child's life. Positive adjustment can be enhanced by attendance at formal sibling preparation classes (Figure 10–5). Typically, the classes are attended by children ages 3 to 12 years. Children younger than 3 tend to have shorter attention spans and may have difficulty participating in the class; however, many facilities will allow younger children to attend, especially if an older sibling is enrolled in the class. These classes can assist with decreasing

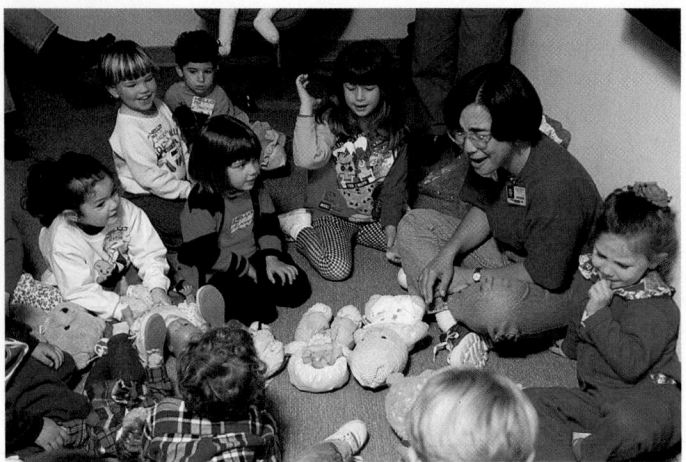

Figure 10–5 It is especially important that siblings be well prepared when they are going to be present at the birth. However, even siblings who will not be present at the birth can benefit from information about childbirth and the new baby ahead of time.

sibling rivalry and reducing children's anxiety. They help children feel that they are part of the birthing process. The classes also enable parents to identify children's concerns related to the new baby. They provide a means to facilitate communication and explore children's feelings. They also provide basic information about pregnancy, childbirth, and the characteristics and behavior of newborns. The classes usually focus on:

- Reducing anxiety in the child
- Providing opportunities for the child to express feelings and concerns
- Encouraging realistic expectations of the newborn
- Teaching the older child to be an active participant in the baby's care by showing how to safely hold the newborn, feed and burp the baby, or even change diapers

Typically, parents and their children attend the class together. Many activities are devised to help each child feel special. Time is usually allotted at the end of the class for talking with parents about coping skills and providing hints about dealing with sibling jealousy. Class content typically includes care and behavior of new babies, a practice session holding anatomically correct dolls, changing diapers, and a tour of the "bedroom" and the nursery where Mom and baby will stay. Many times, a newborn is held up at the nursery window so the children can see a "real baby." Some facilities give the children a special gift for attendance or a trip to the cafeteria for a special treat. In addition, parents may wish to take advantage of books and videos designed to help children prepare for a new sibling.

Classes for Grandparents

Grandparents are an important source of support and information for prospective and new parents. They are now being included in the birthing process more frequently. Prenatal programs for grandparents can address current roles, transitioning to a new role, beliefs regarding childbirth, and ways to support the new family unit. Grandparents can also benefit from educational information, such as the benefits of breastfeeding, and updates on infant care, such as proper sleep positions and when to introduce foods. If they plan to be integral members of the labor and birth team, they will need information about being coaches.

Common Discomforts of Pregnancy

The common discomforts of pregnancy result from physiologic and anatomic changes and are fairly specific to each of the three trimesters. See *Health Promotion: Self-Care Measures for the Common Discomforts of Pregnancy* at the end of this section for an at-a-glance summary of the common discomforts of pregnancy, their possible causes, and self-care measures that often help relieve the discomfort.

First Trimester

NAUSEA AND VOMITING

Nausea and vomiting of pregnancy (NVP) are early, common symptoms occurring in up to 80% of pregnant women (Fantasia, 2014). These symptoms appear sometime after the first missed menstrual period and usually cease by the fourth missed menstrual period. Some women develop an aversion to specific foods, many experience nausea when they get up in the morning, and others experience nausea throughout the day or in the evening.

The exact cause of NVP is unknown, but it is thought to be multifactorial. An elevated human chorionic gonadotropin (hCG) level is believed to be a major factor, but relaxation of the smooth muscle of the stomach, changes in carbohydrate metabolism, fluctuating hormone levels, fatigue, and emotional factors may also play a role.

In addition to common self-care measures for NVP, certain complementary or alternative therapies such as the use of acupressure wristbands (Figure 10–6) or the ingestion of ginger may be helpful for some women. Ginger has long been used as a traditional remedy for treating nausea and vomiting associated with early pregnancy (Tiran, 2012). Ginger is available in a variety of forms, including fresh or dried root, capsules, tea, candy, cookies, crystals, inhaled powdered ginger, and sugared ginger. It has few side effects when taken in small doses (National Center for Complementary and Alternative Medicine [NCCAM], 2012). Some women find pyridoxine (vitamin B_6) helpful. Diclegis, a combination of pyridoxine 10 mg plus doxylamine succinate 10 mg, was approved by the Food and Drug

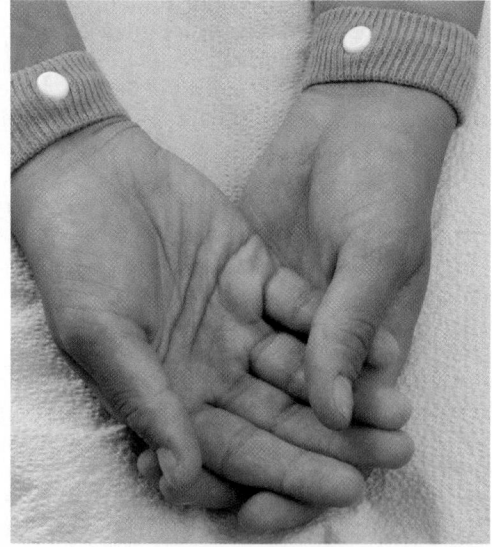

Figure 10–6 Morning sickness relief. Acupressure wristbands are sometimes used to help relieve nausea during early pregnancy.

Administration (FDA) in 2013 specifically for the treatment of NVP (Fantasia, 2014). Antihistamine H_1-receptor blockers, benzamines, and phenothiazines are considered to be safe and effective for treating refractory cases. In very severe cases, methylprednisolone, a steroid, may be used, but strictly as a last resort because it poses a potential risk to the fetus (American College of Obstetricians and Gynecologists [ACOG], 2011a).

The nurse should advise a woman to contact her healthcare provider if she vomits more than once a day or shows signs of dehydration such as dry mouth and concentrated urine. In such cases, the physician/CNM might order an antiemetic. However, antiemetics should be avoided if possible during this time because of possible harmful effects on embryo development.

Nausea and vomiting symptoms generally decrease by the 16th week of pregnancy. If they do not, hyperemesis gravidarum, which occurs in 1% to 3% of pregnancies, must be considered. Hyperemesis symptoms include weight loss, dehydration, and nutrition imbalance (ACOG, 2012).

URINARY FREQUENCY

Urinary frequency, a common discomfort of pregnancy, occurs early in pregnancy and again during the third trimester because the enlarging uterus puts pressure on the bladder. Although frequency is considered normal during the first and third trimesters, advise the woman to tell her healthcare provider about signs of bladder infection such as pain, burning with voiding, or blood in the urine. Fluid intake should never be decreased to prevent frequency. The woman needs to maintain an adequate fluid intake—at least 2000 mL (eight to ten 8-oz glasses) per day. Also, encourage her to empty her bladder frequently (about every 2 hours while awake). Frequent bladder emptying helps decrease the incidence of leakage of urine and also reduces the risk of developing a urinary tract infection.

FATIGUE

Marked fatigue is so common in early pregnancy that it is considered a presumptive sign of pregnancy. It is aggravated if the woman cannot sleep through the night because of urinary frequency. Typically, it resolves after the end of the first trimester.

BREAST TENDERNESS

Sensitivity of the breasts occurs early and continues throughout the pregnancy. Increased levels of estrogen and progesterone contribute to soreness and tingling of the breasts and increased sensitivity of the nipples.

INCREASED VAGINAL DISCHARGE

Increased whitish vaginal discharge, called **leukorrhea**, is common in pregnancy. It occurs as a result of hyperplasia of the vaginal mucosa and increased mucus production by the endocervical glands. The increased acidity of the secretions encourages the growth of *Candida albicans*, so the woman is more susceptible to monilial vaginitis.

NASAL STUFFINESS AND EPISTAXIS

Once pregnancy has progressed somewhat, elevated estrogen levels may produce edema of the nasal mucosa, which results in nasal stuffiness, nasal discharge, and obstruction. *Epistaxis* (nosebleeds) may also result. Cool air vaporizers and normal saline nasal sprays may help, but the problem is often unresponsive to treatment. Women experiencing these problems find it difficult to sleep and may resort to using medicated nasal sprays and decongestants. Such interventions may provide initial relief but can actually increase nasal stuffiness over time.

PTYALISM

Ptyalism is a rare discomfort of pregnancy in which excessive, often bitter, saliva is produced. The cause is unknown, and effective treatments are limited (King et al., 2015).

Second and Third Trimesters

The discomforts discussed in this section usually do not appear until the third trimester in primigravidas but may occur earlier with each succeeding pregnancy.

HEARTBURN (PYROSIS)

Heartburn is the regurgitation of acidic gastric contents into the esophagus. It creates a burning sensation in the esophagus and sometimes leaves a bad taste in the mouth. As many as 80% of women experience heartburn in the third trimester (King et al., 2015). Heartburn during pregnancy appears to be primarily a result of the displacement of the stomach by the enlarging uterus. The increased production of progesterone in pregnancy, decreased gastrointestinal motility, and relaxation of the cardiac (esophageal) sphincter also contribute to heartburn.

Liquid forms of low-sodium antacids are often most effective in providing relief. However, many women prefer chewable over-the-counter antacid tablets. The nurse should advise women that antacids containing aluminum may cause constipation, and antacids containing magnesium can cause diarrhea. The nurse should also let women know that they should avoid sodium bicarbonate (baking soda) and Alka-Seltzer because they may lead to electrolyte imbalance.

If maternal heartburn is severe, not relieved by antacids, and accompanied by gastrointestinal reflux, an antisecretory agent (H_2 blocker) such as ranitidine (Zantac), cimetidine (Tagamet), or omeprazole (Losec) may be helpful. To date, they have not been linked with an excessive risk of birth defects.

ANKLE EDEMA

Most women experience ankle edema in the last part of pregnancy because of the increasing difficulty of venous return from the lower extremities. Prolonged standing or sitting and warm weather increase the edema. It is also associated with varicose veins. Ankle edema becomes a concern only when accompanied by hypertension or proteinuria or when the edema is not postural in origin.

VARICOSE VEINS

Varicose veins are a result of weakening of the walls of veins or faulty functioning of the valves. Poor circulation in the lower extremities predisposes people to varicose veins in the legs and thighs, as does prolonged standing or sitting. The pregnant uterus puts pressure on the pelvic veins, preventing good venous return, so it may aggravate existing problems or contribute to obvious changes in the veins of the legs (Figure 10–7).

Surgical correction of varicose veins is not generally recommended during pregnancy. The nurse should advise the woman that treatment may be needed after she gives birth because the problem will be aggravated by a succeeding pregnancy.

Although less common, varicosities in the vulva and perineum may also develop. They produce aching and a sense of heaviness. Wearing a foam rubber commercial product that is placed across the perineum and held in place by a sanitary pad–type belt can provide support for vulvar varicosities (Cunningham et al., 2014). It is important that the pelvic area be elevated to promote venous drainage into the trunk of the body. The woman may best relieve uterine pressure on the pelvic veins by resting on her side. Blocks may also be placed under the foot of her bed to elevate it slightly.

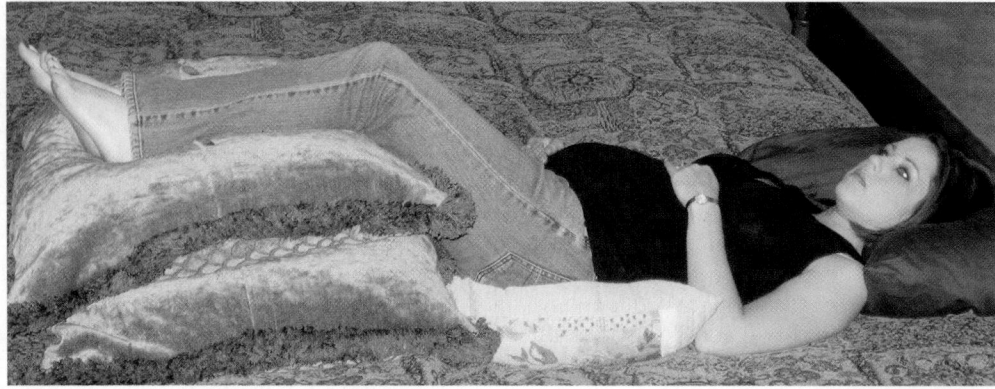

Figure 10–7 Swelling and discomfort from varicosities can be decreased by lying down with the legs and one hip elevated (to avoid compression of the vena cava).

FLATULENCE

Flatulence results from decreased gastrointestinal motility, leading to delayed emptying, and from pressure on the large intestine by the growing uterus. Air swallowing may also contribute to the problem.

HEMORRHOIDS

Hemorrhoids are varicosities of the veins in the lower rectum and the anus. During pregnancy the gravid uterus presses on the veins and interferes with venous circulation. In addition, the straining that accompanies constipation is frequently a contributing cause of hemorrhoids.

Some women may not be bothered by hemorrhoids until the second stage of labor, when the hemorrhoids appear as they push. These hemorrhoids usually become asymptomatic a few days after childbirth. Symptoms of hemorrhoids include itching, swelling, pain, and bleeding. Women who have had hemorrhoids before pregnancy will probably experience difficulties with them during pregnancy.

Some women find relief by gently reinserting the hemorrhoid. The woman lies on her side, places some lubricant on her finger, and presses against the hemorrhoid, pushing it inside the rectum. She holds the hemorrhoid in place for 1 to 2 minutes and then gently withdraws her finger. The anal sphincter should then hold it inside the rectum. The woman will find it especially helpful if she can maintain a side-lying (Sims) position for a time, so this method is best done before bed or prior to a daily rest period.

The woman should contact her healthcare provider if the hemorrhoid(s) becomes hardened and noticeably tender to touch. Rectal bleeding that is more than spotting following defecation should also be reported.

CONSTIPATION

Conditions that predispose the pregnant woman to constipation include general bowel sluggishness caused by increased progesterone and steroid metabolism; displacement of the intestines, which increases with growth of the fetus; and the oral iron supplements most pregnant women need. In severe or preexisting cases of constipation, the woman may need stool softeners, mild laxatives, or suppositories as recommended by her healthcare provider.

BACKACHE

Nearly 70% of women experience lower backache during pregnancy (King et al., 2015) primarily caused by exaggeration of the lumbosacral curve that occurs as the uterus enlarges and becomes heavier. Maintaining good posture and using proper body mechanics throughout pregnancy can help prevent backache.

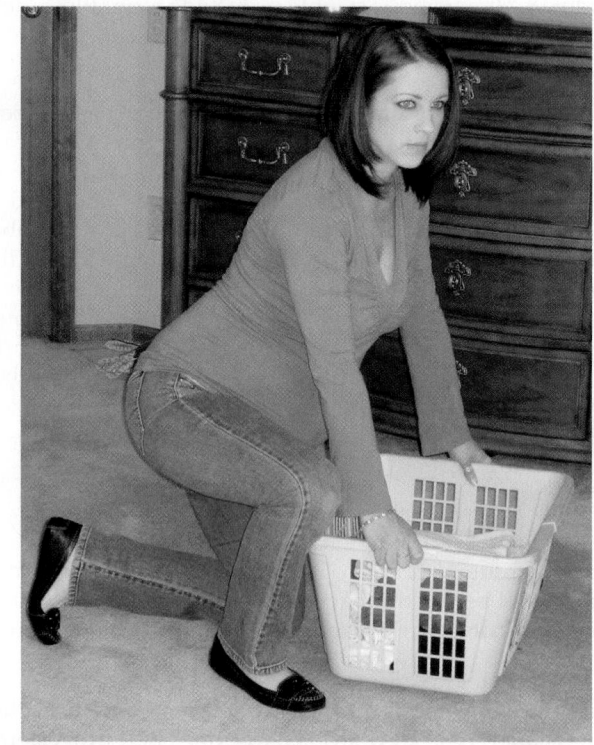

Figure 10–8 Body mechanics in pregnancy. When picking up objects from floor level or lifting objects, the pregnant woman must use proper body mechanics.

Advise the pregnant woman to avoid bending over at the waist to pick up objects and to bend from the knees instead (Figure 10–8). She should place her feet 12 to 18 inches apart to maintain body balance. If the woman uses work surfaces that require her to bend, advise her to adjust the height of the surfaces.

LEG CRAMPS

Leg cramps are painful muscle spasms in the gastrocnemius muscles. They occur most often after the woman has gone to bed at night but may occur at other times. Extension of the foot can often cause leg cramps. The nurse should warn the pregnant woman not to extend the foot during childbirth preparation exercises or during rest periods.

Stretching provides immediate relief of the muscle spasm. With the woman lying on her back, another person presses the woman's knee down to straighten her leg while pushing her foot toward her leg (Figure 10–9). The woman may also stand and put

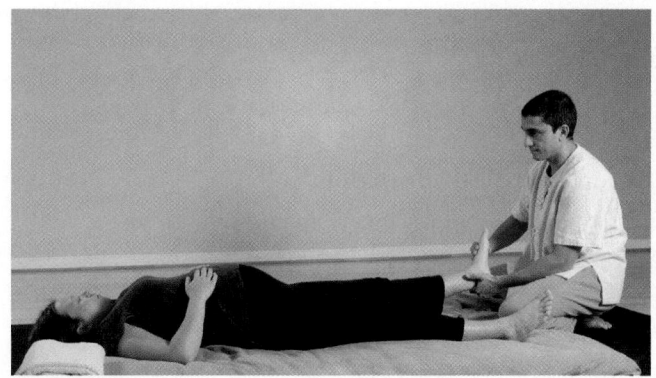

Figure 10–9 **Leg cramp relief. The expectant father can help relieve the woman's painful leg cramps by flexing her foot and straightening her leg.**

SOURCE: Yanik Chauvin/Fotolia.

her foot flat on the floor. Massage and warm packs can alleviate the discomfort of leg cramps. A diet that includes daily portions of both calcium and phosphorus may help prevent leg cramps.

FAINTNESS

Many pregnant women occasionally feel faint, especially in warm, crowded areas. Faintness is caused by a combination of changes in the blood volume and postural hypotension due to pooling of blood in the dependent veins. Sudden change of position or standing for prolonged periods can also cause this sensation, and the woman may faint.

If a woman begins to feel faint from prolonged standing or from being in a stuffy room, she should sit down and lower her head between her knees. If this procedure does not help, she should ask someone to help her to an area where she can lie down and get fresh air. The nurse should advise the woman that when getting up from a resting position, it is important to move slowly. Women whose jobs require standing in one place for long periods should march in place regularly to increase venous return from the legs.

SHORTNESS OF BREATH (DYSPNEA)

Shortness of breath occurs as the uterus rises into the abdomen and causes pressure on the diaphragm. This problem worsens in the last trimester because the enlarged uterus presses directly on the diaphragm, decreasing vital capacity. The primigravida experiences considerable relief from shortness of breath in the last few weeks of pregnancy, when **lightening** occurs, and the fetus and uterus move down in the pelvis. Because the multigravida does not usually experience lightening until labor, she tends to feel short of breath throughout the latter part of her pregnancy.

DIFFICULTY SLEEPING

Many physical factors in late pregnancy may make sleeping difficult. The enlarged uterus may make it difficult to find a comfortable position for sleep, and an active fetus may aggravate the problem. Other discomforts of pregnancy such as urinary frequency, shortness of breath, and leg cramps may also make it hard to sleep.

ROUND LIGAMENT PAIN

As the uterus enlarges during pregnancy, the round ligaments stretch and hypertrophy as the uterus rises up in the abdomen, causing pain. The woman may feel concern when she first experiences round ligament pain because it is often intense and causes a "grabbing" sensation in the lower abdomen and inguinal area. The nurse should warn the pregnant woman of this possible discomfort. Once it has been determined that the cause of the pain is not a medical complication such as appendicitis, the woman may find that applying a heating pad to the abdomen brings relief.

CARPAL TUNNEL SYNDROME

Carpal tunnel syndrome, characterized by numbness and tingling of the hand near the thumb, occurs in about 25% to 50% of pregnant women (Kimberly, Niebyl, & Johnson, 2012). It is caused by compression of the median nerve in the carpal tunnel of the wrist. The syndrome is aggravated by repetitive hand movements, such as typing, and may disappear following childbirth. Fluid retention during pregnancy and high weight gain may aggravate the condition (Gregory, Niebyl, & Johnson, 2012). Treatment usually involves splinting and avoiding aggravating movements, but surgery may be needed in severe cases if more conservative approaches are not effective.

Health Promotion During Pregnancy

Fetal Activity Monitoring

Many healthcare providers encourage pregnant women to monitor their unborn child's well-being by regularly assessing fetal activity beginning at 28 weeks' gestation. Vigorous activity generally provides reassurance of fetal well-being, but a marked decrease in activity or cessation of movement may indicate a problem that needs immediate evaluation. Fetal activity is affected by fetal sleep, sound, time of day, blood glucose levels, cigarette smoking, and some illicit drugs such as crack and cocaine. At times, a healthy fetus may be minimally active or inactive. See Chapter 13 for an in-depth discussion of maternal–fetal activity monitoring and *Teaching Highlights: What to Tell the Pregnant Woman About Assessing Fetal Activity.*

Breast Care

Whether the pregnant woman plans to formula-feed or breast-feed her baby, support of the breasts is important to promote comfort, retain breast shape, and prevent back strain, particularly if the breasts become large and pendulous. The sensitivity of the breasts in pregnancy is often relieved by good support.

A well-fitting, supportive bra has the following qualities:

- The straps are wide and do not stretch (elastic straps soon lose their tautness with the weight of the breasts and frequent washing).
- The cups hold all breast tissue comfortably.
- The bra has tucks or other devices that allow it to expand and accommodate the enlarging chest circumference.
- The bra supports the nipple line approximately midway between the elbow and shoulder but is not pulled up in the back by the weight of the breasts.

Cleanliness of the breasts is important, especially as the woman begins producing colostrum. Colostrum that crusts on the nipples can be removed with warm water. The nurse should advise the woman planning to breastfeed not to use soap on her nipples because of its drying effect.

Some women have flat or inverted nipples. True nipple inversion, which is rare, is usually diagnosed during the initial

Health Promotion **Self-Care Measures for Common Discomforts of Pregnancy**

Discomfort	Influencing Factors	Self-Care Measures
First Trimester		
Nausea and vomiting	Increased levels of human chorionic gonadotropin	Avoid odors or causative factors.
	Changes in carbohydrate metabolism	Eat dry crackers or toast before arising in morning.
	Emotional factors	Have small but frequent meals.
	Fatigue	Avoid greasy or highly seasoned foods.
		Take dry meals with fluids between meals.
		Drink carbonated beverages.
		Avoid lying supine for 2 hours after eating
Urinary frequency	Pressure of uterus on bladder in both first and third trimesters	Void when urge is felt.
		Increase fluid intake during the day.
		Decrease fluid intake only in the evening to decrease nocturia.
Fatigue	Specific causative factors unknown	Plan time for a nap or rest period daily.
	May be aggravated by nocturia due to urinary frequency	Go to bed earlier.
		Seek family support and assistance with responsibilities so that more time is available to rest.
Breast tenderness	Increased levels of estrogen and progesterone	Wear well-fitting, supportive bra.
Increased vaginal discharge	Hyperplasia of vaginal mucosa and increased production of mucus by the endocervical glands due to the increase in estrogen levels	Promote cleanliness by daily bathing.
		Avoid douching, nylon underpants, and pantyhose; cotton underpants are more absorbent; powder can be used to maintain dryness if not allowed to cake.
Nasal stuffiness and nosebleed (epistaxis)	Elevated estrogen levels	May be unresponsive, but cool air vaporizer may help; avoid use of nasal sprays and decongestants.
Ptyalism (excessive, often bitter, salivation)	Specific causative factors unknown	Use astringent mouthwashes, chew gum, or suck hard candy.
Second and Third Trimesters		
Heartburn (pyrosis)	Increased production of progesterone, decreasing gastrointestinal motility and increasing relaxation of cardiac sphincter, displacement of stomach by enlarging uterus, thus regurgitation of acidic gastric contents into the esophagus	Eat small and more frequent meals.
		Use low-sodium antacids.
		Avoid overeating, fatty and fried foods, lying down after eating, and sodium bicarbonate.
Ankle edema	Prolonged standing or sitting	Practice frequent dorsiflexion of feet when prolonged sitting or standing is necessary.
	Increased levels of sodium due to hormonal influences	Elevate legs when sitting or resting.
	Circulatory congestion of lower extremities	Avoid tight garters or restrictive bands around legs.
	Increased capillary permeability	
	Varicose veins	
Varicose veins	Venous congestion in the lower veins that increases with pregnancy	Elevate legs frequently.
	Hereditary factors (weakening of walls of veins, faulty valves)	Wear supportive hose.
	Increased age and weight gain	Avoid crossing legs at the knees, standing for long periods, garters, and hosiery with constrictive bands.

Health Promotion Self-Care Measures for Common Discomforts of Pregnancy (*continued*)

Discomfort	Influencing Factors	Self-Care Measures
Hemorrhoids	Constipation (see following discussion)	Avoid constipation.
	Increased pressure from gravid uterus on hemorrhoidal veins	Apply ice packs, topical ointments, anesthetic agents, warm soaks, or sitz baths; gently reinsert into rectum as necessary.
Constipation	Increased levels of progesterone, which cause general bowel sluggishness	Increase fluid intake, fiber in the diet, and exercise.
	Pressure of enlarging uterus on intestine	Develop regular bowel habits.
	Iron supplements	Use stool softeners as recommended by physician.
	Diet, lack of exercise, and decreased fluids	
Backache	Increased curvature of the lumbosacral vertebrae as the uterus enlarges	Use proper body mechanics.
	Increased levels of hormones, which cause softening of cartilage in body joints	Practice the pelvic tilt exercise.
	Fatigue	Avoid uncomfortable working heights, high-heeled shoes, lifting of heavy loads, and fatigue.
	Poor body mechanics	
Leg cramps	Imbalance of calcium/phosphorus ratio	Practice dorsiflexion of feet to stretch affected muscle.
	Increased pressure of uterus on nerves	Evaluate diet.
	Fatigue	Apply heat to affected muscles.
	Poor circulation to lower extremities	Rise slowly from resting position.
	Pointing the toes	
Faintness	Postural hypotension	Avoid prolonged standing in warm or stuffy environments.
	Sudden change of position causing venous pooling in dependent veins	Evaluate hematocrit and hemoglobin.
	Standing for long periods in warm area	
	Anemia	
Dyspnea	Decreased vital capacity from pressure of enlarging uterus on the diaphragm	Use proper posture when sitting and standing.
		Sleep propped up with pillows for relief if problem occurs at night.
Flatulence	Decreased gastrointestinal motility leading to delayed emptying time	Avoid gas-forming foods.
	Pressure of growing uterus on large intestine	Chew food thoroughly.
	Air swallowing	Get regular daily exercise.
		Maintain normal bowel habits.
Carpal tunnel syndrome	Compression of median nerve in carpal tunnel of wrist	Avoid aggravating hand movements.
	Aggravated by repetitive hand movements	Use splint as prescribed.
		Elevate affected arm.

prenatal assessment. Breast shields designed to correct inverted nipples are effective for some women but others gain no benefit from them. Information on breastfeeding can be found on the websites of the La Leche League, the American Academy of Pediatrics, the National Organization of Mothers of Twins Club, and other breastfeeding-focused sites.

Clothing

Traditionally, maternity clothes have been constructed with fuller lines to allow for the increase in abdominal size that occurs during pregnancy. However, in recent years, maternity clothing has changed and now also includes more clothes that are fitted with little attempt to hide the pregnant abdomen. Maternity clothing can be expensive and is worn for a relatively short time, so women can economize by sharing clothes with friends, sewing their own garments, or buying used maternity clothes.

High-heeled shoes tend to aggravate back discomfort by increasing the curvature of the lower back. Women who experience backache or have problems with balance do best to avoid them. Shoes should fit properly and feel comfortable.

Bathing

Hygiene is important because perspiration and mucoid vaginal discharge increase during pregnancy. Keep in mind, however, that cultural norms often influence bathing and cleansing practices. A pregnant woman may choose to cleanse only some portions of her body regularly or may elect to take showers or tub baths. Advise women to be careful in the tub because balance becomes a problem in late pregnancy. Rubber mats and hand grips are important safety devices. Vasodilation due to warm water may cause the woman to feel faint when she gets out of the tub, so she may need assistance, especially during the last trimester.

Employment

Pregnant women who have no complications can usually continue to work until they go into labor (American Academy of Pediatrics [AAP] & ACOG, 2012). Although pregnant women who are employed in jobs that require prolonged standing (more than 3 hours) do have a higher incidence of preterm birth, this has no effect on fetal growth. However, the workplace environment can affect maternal well-being as well as birth outcomes (Katz, 2012). Overfatigue, prolonged standing, excessive physical strain, fetotoxic hazards in the environment, and medical or obstetric complications are the major deterrents to certain types of employment during pregnancy. In the second half of pregnancy, women whose occupations involve balance should make adjustments as needed.

Fetotoxic hazards are always a concern to the expectant couple. The pregnant woman (or the woman contemplating pregnancy) who works in industry should contact her company physician or nurse about possible hazards in her work environment and should do her own reading and research on environmental hazards as well. Her partner can also find out how hazards in his workplace might affect his sperm.

Travel

Pregnant women without complications can travel as usual. Pregnant women should avoid travel if they have a history of preterm birth, bleeding, or preeclampsia or if multiple births are anticipated.

Travel by automobile can be tiring, aggravating many of the discomforts of pregnancy. The pregnant woman needs frequent opportunities to get out of the car and walk. (A good pattern is to stop every 2 hours and walk around for about 10 minutes.) She should wear both lap and shoulder belts. The lap belt should fit snugly and be positioned under the abdomen and across the upper thighs; the shoulder strap should rest comfortably between the woman's breasts. Seat belts play an important role in preventing fetal and maternal injury and death (Cunningham et al., 2014). Fetal death in car accidents is sometimes caused by placental separation (abruptio placentae) as a result of uterine distortion. Shoulder belts decrease the risk of traumatic flexion of the woman's body, making placental separation less likely.

As pregnancy progresses, long-distance trips are best taken by plane or train. Currently, occasional flying is considered safe in the absence of any obstetric or medical complications (AAP & ACOG, 2012). Before flying the woman should check with her airline to see if they have any travel restrictions because many prohibit flying after 36 weeks' gestation. To avoid the development of phlebitis or blood clots, pregnant women should drink plenty of fluid to avoid dehydration and hemoconcentration. They should also walk about the plane at regular intervals and change position frequently. Air travel is not recommended during pregnancy for women who have obstetric or medical conditions that could require emergency care or that might be exacerbated by flight (AAP & ACOG, 2012). Remind near-term women who travel to think about the availability of medical care at the destination.

Activity and Rest

Exercise during pregnancy helps maintain maternal fitness and muscle tone, leads to improved self-image, promotes regular bowel function, improves cardiovascular function, increases energy, improves sleep, relieves tension, helps control weight gain, and is associated with improved postpartum recovery. Exercise also improves symptoms of depression during pregnancy (Shivakumar, 2015). Fetal benefits include advanced neurobehavioral maturation and improved stress tolerance (Melzer, Schutz, Boulvain, et al., 2010). Normal participation in exercise can continue throughout an uncomplicated pregnancy and, in fact, is encouraged.

Exercise may play a role in the prevention of maternal and fetal complications (Ferraro, Gaudet, & Adamo, 2012). For women who are morbidly obese, exercise may assist in the prevention of gestational diabetes. Exercise is also recommended by the American Diabetes Association (2013) to assist in glycemic control for women with gestational diabetes.

The woman can check with her certified nurse-midwife or physician about taking part in strenuous sports. ACOG (2011b) recommends that women avoid activities with a high risk for falling, such as skiing, gymnastics, and horseback riding, and those activities that have a high risk of blunt trauma, such as ice hockey and basketball. Scuba diving should be avoided because of the risk of decompression sickness.

Certain conditions do contraindicate exercise. Absolute contraindications to exercise include the following (AAP & ACOG, 2012):

- Rupture of the membranes
- Preeclampsia-eclampsia
- Cervical insufficiency (cerclage)
- Persistent vaginal bleeding in the second or third trimesters

- Multiple gestation at risk for preterm labor
- Preterm labor in the current pregnancy
- Placenta previa after 26 weeks' gestation
- Chronic medical conditions that might be negatively impacted by vigorous exercise such as significant heart disease or restrictive lung disease

The following guidelines are helpful in counseling pregnant women about exercise:

- Even mild-to-moderate exercise is beneficial during pregnancy. Regular exercise—at least 30 minutes of moderate exercise daily or at least most days—is preferred (Kimberly et al., 2012).
- After the first trimester, women should avoid exercising in the supine position. In most pregnant women, the supine position is associated with decreased cardiac output. Because uterine blood flow is reduced during exercise as blood is shunted from the visceral organs to the muscles, the remaining cardiac output is further decreased. Similarly, women should also avoid standing motionless for prolonged periods (Katz, 2012).
- Light muscle strength training using lighter weights (or resistance bands) and more repetitions done once or twice per week helps improve overall fitness and does not negatively affect the fetus. Heavy weights should be avoided because they may overload joints that are looser than normal because of the effects of the hormone relaxin (Zavorsky & Longo, 2011).
- Because decreased oxygen is available for aerobic exercise during pregnancy, women should modify the intensity of their exercise based on their symptoms, should stop when they become fatigued, and should avoid exercising to the point of exhaustion.
- Non–weight-bearing exercises such as swimming and cycling are recommended and provide fitness with comfort. As pregnancy progresses and the center of gravity changes, especially in the third trimester, women should avoid exercises in which the loss of balance could pose a risk to mother or fetus. Similarly, the woman should avoid any type of exercise that has a high potential for physical contact such as basketball, soccer, and ice hockey because it could result in trauma to the woman or her fetus.
- A normal pregnancy requires an additional 300 kcal per day. Women who exercise regularly during pregnancy should be careful to ensure that their diet is adequate.
- To augment heat dissipation, especially during the first trimester, pregnant women who exercise should wear appropriate clothing that is comfortable and loose, ensure adequate hydration, and avoid prolonged overheating.
- As a result of the cardiovascular changes of pregnancy, heart rate is not an accurate indicator of the intensity of exercise for pregnant women. If a pregnant, exercising woman is unable to maintain a conversation, then the exercise effort is too high.

The woman should wear a supportive bra and appropriate shoes when exercising. She should also warm up and stretch to help prepare the joints for activity and cool down with a period of mild activity to help restore circulation and avoid pooling of blood. A moderate, rhythmic exercise routine involving large muscle groups such as swimming, cycling, or brisk walking is best. Jogging or running is acceptable for women already conditioned to these activities as long as they avoid exercising at maximum effort and overheating. Warning signs include the following (AAP & ACOG, 2012):

- Chest pain
- Vaginal bleeding
- Regular uterine contractions
- Decreased or absent fetal movement
- Leakage of amniotic fluid
- Calf pain or swelling
- Dizziness, headache, dyspnea before exertion, and muscle weakness

The woman should stop exercising if any of these symptoms occur and modify her exercise program. If the symptoms persist, the woman should contact her healthcare provider.

Clinical Reasoning Counseling About Strenuous Physical Activity

Ana Gonzalez, a 24-year-old, G1P0, is 11 weeks pregnant when she presents for her first prenatal examination. She has been a long-distance runner for 6 years. Because of her low body fat, her menses have always been irregular, and it had not occurred to Ana that she might be pregnant. Ana says she has been told that it is fine to continue any physical activity at which one is proficient, and says that she would like to continue running long distances while pregnant. What should you tell Ana about running long distances?

Adequate rest is important for both physical and emotional health. Pregnant women need more sleep, particularly in the first and last trimesters, when they tire easily. Without enough rest, pregnant women have less resilience. Finding time to rest during the day may be difficult for women who work outside the home or who have small children. The nurse can help the expectant mother examine her daily schedule to develop a realistic plan for short periods of rest and relaxation.

Sleeping becomes more difficult during the last trimester because of the enlarged abdomen, increased frequency of urination, and greater activity of the fetus. Finding a comfortable position becomes difficult. Figure 10–10 shows a position most pregnant women find comfortable. Women can also prepare for sleep with progressive relaxation techniques similar to those taught in prepared childbirth classes.

Exercises to Prepare for Childbirth

Certain exercises help strengthen muscle tone in preparation for birth and promote more rapid restoration of muscle tone after birth. A few of the more common body-conditioning exercises for pregnancy are discussed here.

The **pelvic tilt**, or pelvic rocking, helps maintain pelvic flexibility and prevent or reduce back strain as it helps strengthen abdominal muscles. To do the pelvic tilt in early pregnancy, the pregnant woman lies on her back and puts her feet flat on the floor. This flexes the knees and helps prevent strain or discomfort. She decreases the curvature in her back by pressing her spine toward the floor. With her back pressed to the floor, the woman tightens her abdominal muscles as she tightens

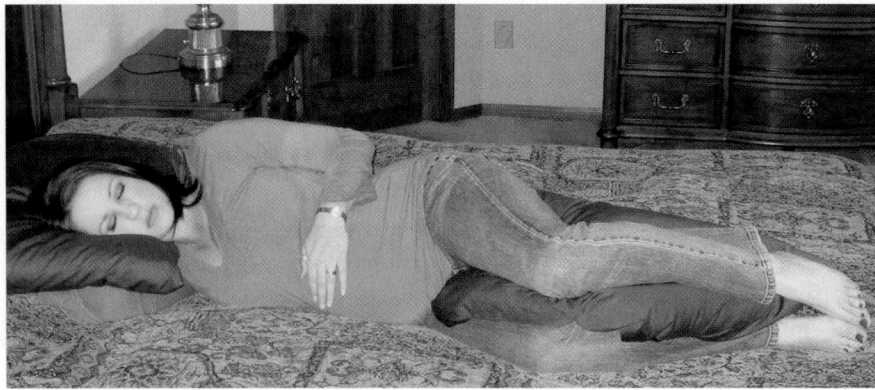

Figure 10–10 Position for relaxation and rest as pregnancy progresses.

and tucks in her buttocks. In the second and third trimesters, the woman can also do the pelvic tilt on her hands and knees (Figure 10–11), while sitting in a chair, or while standing with her back against a wall. The woman should maintain the body alignment that results when the pelvic tilt is done correctly as much as possible throughout the day.

Clinical Tip

Doing the pelvic tilt on hands and knees may aggravate back strain. Teach women with a history of minor back problems to do the pelvic tilt only in the standing position.

ABDOMINAL EXERCISES

A basic exercise to increase abdominal muscle tone is tightening abdominal muscles with each breath. It can be done in any position, but it is best learned while lying supine. With knees flexed and feet flat on the floor, the woman expands her abdomen and slowly takes a deep breath. Exhaling slowly, she gradually pulls in her abdominal muscles until they are fully contracted. She relaxes for a few seconds and then repeats the exercise. The pregnant woman should avoid the supine position after the first trimester.

Partial sit-ups strengthen abdominal muscle tone and are done according to individual comfort levels. In early pregnancy, partial sit-ups may be done with the knees flexed and the feet flat on the floor to avoid strain on the lower back. The woman stretches her arms toward her knees as she slowly pulls her head and shoulders off the floor to a comfortable level (if she has poor abdominal muscle tone, she may not be able to pull up very far). She then slowly returns to the starting position, takes a deep breath, and repeats the exercise. To strengthen the oblique abdominal muscles, she repeats the process but

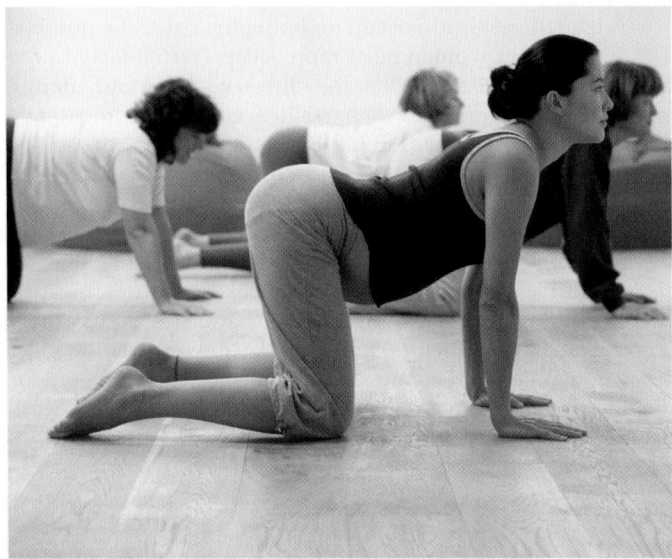

A

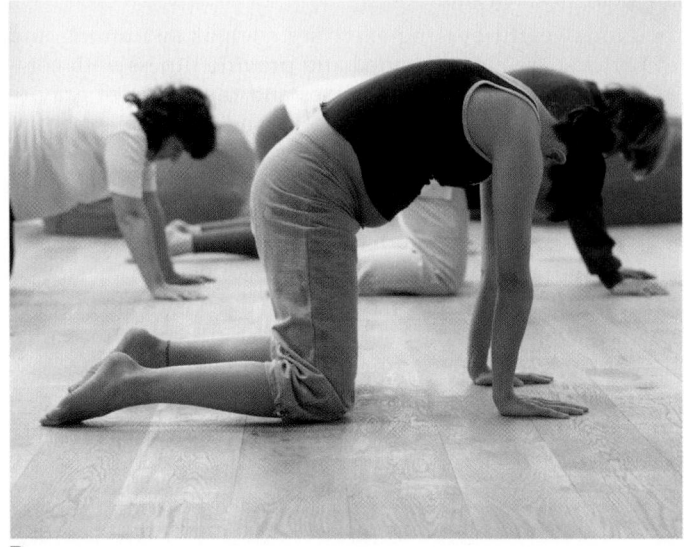

B

Figure 10–11 When the pelvic tilt is done on hands and knees, the starting position is back flat and parallel to the floor, hands below the head, and knees directly below the buttocks. *A,* For the first part of the tilt, head is up, neck is long and separated from the shoulders, buttocks are up, and pelvis is thrust back, allowing the back to drop and release on an inhaled breath. *B,* The next part of the tilt is done on a long exhalation, allowing the pregnant woman to arch her back, drop her head loosely, push away from her hands, and draw in the muscles of her abdomen to strengthen them. Note that in this position the pelvis and buttocks are tucked under, and the buttock muscles are tightened.

SOURCE: Moose Azim/Alamy.

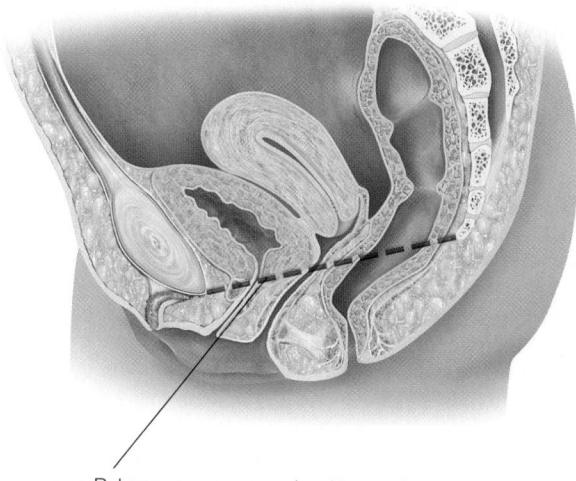

Pubococcygeus muscle with good tone

Pubococcygeus muscle with poor tone

Figure 10–12 **Kegel exercises. The woman learns to tighten the pubococcygeus muscle, which improves support to the pelvic organs.**

stretches the left arm to the side of her right knee, returns to the floor, takes a deep breath, and then reaches with the right arm to the left knee. During the second and third trimesters, these exercises can be done on a large exercise ball.

Women can do these exercises approximately 5 times in a sequence and repeat the sequence at other times during the day as desired. It is important to do the exercises slowly to prevent muscle strain and overtiring.

PERINEAL EXERCISES

Pelvic floor muscle tightening, also called **Kegel exercises**, strengthens the pubococcygeus muscle and increases its elasticity (Figure 10–12). Research indicates that Kegel exercises performed during pregnancy and postpartum increase pelvic floor muscle strength and help prevent symptoms associated with childbirth such as urinary incontinence, pelvic organ prolapse, and fecal impaction (Sut & Kaplan, 2015).

The woman can identify the specific muscle group to be exercised by stopping urination midstream. Doing Kegel exercises while urinating is discouraged, however, because this practice has been associated with urinary stasis and urinary tract infection. Childbirth educators sometimes use the following technique to teach Kegel exercises. They tell the woman to think of her perineal muscles as an elevator. When she relaxes, the elevator is on the first floor. To do the exercises, she contracts, bringing the elevator to the second, third, and fourth floors. She keeps the elevator on the fourth floor for a few seconds, and then gradually relaxes the area. If the exercise is properly done, the woman does not contract the muscles of the buttocks and thighs. Kegel exercises can be done at almost any time. Some women use ordinary events—for instance, stopping at a red light or talking on the telephone—as a cue to remember to do the exercise.

INNER THIGH EXERCISES

The nurse can advise the pregnant woman to assume a cross-legged sitting position whenever possible. This "tailor sit" stretches the muscles of the inner thighs in preparation for labor and birth. See Figure 10–13.

Sexual Activity

Because of the physiologic, anatomic, and emotional changes of pregnancy, couples usually have many questions and concerns

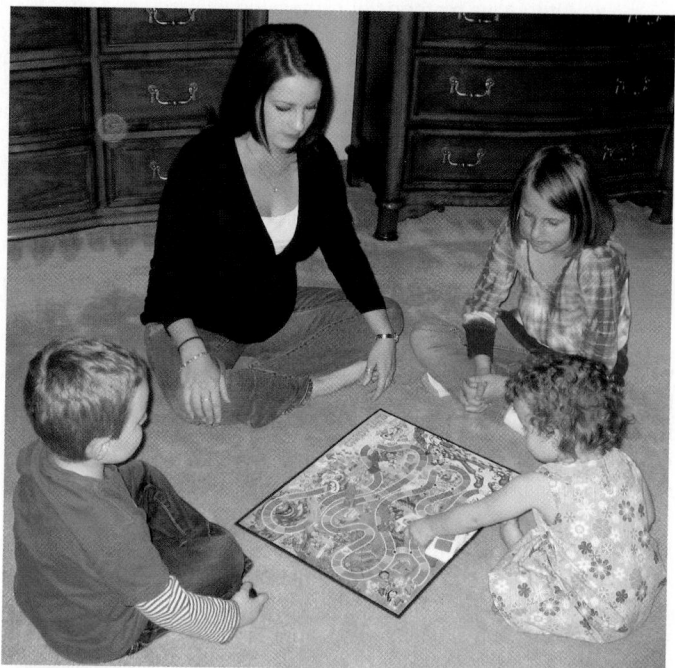

Figure 10–13 Tailor sitting. To help prepare her inner thigh muscles for labor and birth, the pregnant woman should assume a cross-legged sitting position whenever possible during the day.

about sexual activity during pregnancy. Often these questions are about possible injury to the baby or the woman during intercourse and about changes in the desire each partner feels for the other.

In the past, couples were often warned to avoid sexual intercourse during the last 6 to 8 weeks of pregnancy to prevent complications such as infection or premature rupture of the membranes. However, these fears seem to be unfounded. In a healthy pregnancy, there is no medical reason to limit sexual activity. Intercourse is contraindicated for medical reasons such as threatened miscarriage or risk of preterm labor (Cunningham et al., 2014).

The expectant mother may experience changes in sexual desire and response. Often these changes are related to the

| TEACHING HIGHLIGHTS | Sexual Activity During Pregnancy |

In starting a discussion about sexual activity during pregnancy, universal statements that give permission, such as, "Many couples experience changes in sexual desire during pregnancy. What kind of changes have you experienced?" are often effective.

In your teaching, explain the following points to the woman and her partner:

- The pregnant woman may experience changes in desire during the course of pregnancy. During the first trimester, discomforts such as nausea, fatigue, and breast tenderness may make intercourse less desirable for many women. In the second trimester, as symptoms decrease, desire may increase. In the third trimester, discomfort and fatigue may lead to decreased desire in the woman.
- Men may notice changes in their level of desire, too. This may be related to feelings about their partner's changing appearance, their belief about the acceptability of sexual activity with a pregnant woman, or concern about hurting the woman or fetus. Some men find the changes of pregnancy erotic; others must adjust to the notion of their partners as mothers.
- The woman may notice that orgasms are much more intense during the last weeks of pregnancy and may be followed by cramping.
- Because of the pressure of the enlarging uterus on the vena cava, the woman should not lie flat on her back for intercourse after about the fourth month. If the couple prefers that position, a pillow should be placed under her right hip to displace the uterus. Alternative positions such as side-by-side, female superior, or vaginal rear entry may become necessary as her uterus enlarges.
- Sexual activities that both partners enjoy are generally acceptable. It is not advisable for couples who favor anal sex to go from anal penetration to vaginal penetration because of the risk of introducing *Escherichia coli* into the vagina.
- Alternative methods of expressing intimacy and affection such as cuddling, holding and stroking each other, and kissing may help maintain the couple's feelings of warmth and closeness. If the man feels desire for further sexual release, his partner may help him masturbate to ejaculation, or he may prefer to masturbate in private.
- Sexual intercourse is contraindicated once the membranes are ruptured or if bleeding is present. Women with a history of preterm labor may be advised to avoid intercourse because the oxytocin that is released with orgasm stimulates uterine contractions and may trigger preterm labor. Because oxytocin is also released with nipple stimulation, fondling the breasts may also be contraindicated in those cases.

Stress the importance of open communication so that the couple feels comfortable expressing their feelings, preferences, and concerns. Deal with any specific questions about the physical and psychologic changes that the couple may have.

various discomforts that occur throughout pregnancy. For instance, during the first trimester, fatigue or nausea and vomiting may decrease sexual desire. During the second trimester, many of these discomforts are lessened and sexual satisfaction increases. During the third trimester, interest in sex may again decrease as the woman becomes more uncomfortable and tired. Shortness of breath, urinary frequency, leg cramps, and decreased mobility may also lessen sexual desire and activity. If they are not already doing so, the couple should consider coital positions other than male superior, such as side-by-side, female superior, and vaginal rear entry.

Sexual activity does not have to include intercourse. Many of the nurturing and sexual needs of the pregnant woman can be satisfied by cuddling, kissing, and being held. The warm, sensual feelings that accompany these activities can be an end in themselves. Her partner, however, may choose to masturbate for satisfaction.

Many factors in pregnancy also affect the sexual desires of men. The man's previous relationship with the partner, acceptance of the pregnancy, attitudes toward the partner's change of appearance, and concern about hurting the expectant mother or baby can all play a role. Some men find it difficult to view their partners as sexually appealing while they are adjusting to the concept of them as mothers. Other men find their partners' pregnancies arousing and experience feelings of increased happiness, intimacy, and closeness.

The expectant couple should be aware of their changing sexual desires, the normality of these changes, and the importance of communicating these changes to each other so that they can make nurturing adaptations. It is important that the couple feel free to express concerns about sexual activity. Use a relaxed manner when responding to questions and giving anticipatory guidance. (See *Teaching Highlights: Sexual Activity During Pregnancy*.)

Dental Care

Proper dental hygiene is important in pregnancy because ensuring a healthy oral environment is essential to overall health. In spite of such discomforts as nausea and vomiting, gum hypertrophy, and heartburn, it is important for pregnant women to maintain regular oral hygiene by brushing at least twice a day and flossing daily. Dental treatment is safe throughout pregnancy; however, the second trimester is considered the most appropriate time for dental treatment because the risk of pregnancy loss tends to be lower and the woman tends to be more comfortable. It is important to encourage the woman to have a dental checkup early in pregnancy. She should inform her dentist that she is pregnant so that she is not exposed to teratogenic substances.

Immunizations

Immunizations with attenuated live viruses, such as rubella vaccine, should not be given in pregnancy because of the teratogenic effect of the live viruses on the developing embryo. The most current recommendations on vaccines during pregnancy should be obtained from the Centers for Disease Control and Prevention website.

Women should be assessed during the preconception stage for varicella, rubella, hepatitis B, and HIV. Women anticipating global travel should pay careful attention to vaccinations that are required. There are multiple vaccinations that can be given during pregnancy; however, others are contraindicated and should not be administered (Centers for Disease Control and Prevention [CDC], 2012b).

Complementary and Alternative Therapies

As discussed in Chapter 2, many women use complementary and alternative medicine (CAM) such as homeopathy, herbal medicine, acupressure and acupuncture, biofeedback, therapeutic touch, massage, and chiropractic as part of a holistic approach to their health care. Thus the nurse should inquire about the use of CAM as part of routine antepartum assessment. Nurses working with pregnant women and childbearing families need to develop a general understanding of the more commonly used therapies to be able to answer basic questions and to provide resources as needed.

It is important for the pregnant woman to understand that herbs are considered to be dietary supplements and are not regulated as prescription or over-the-counter drugs are through the FDA. In general, it is best to advise pregnant women not to ingest any herbs, except ginger, during the first trimester of pregnancy. The website of the National Center for Complementary and Alternative Medicine is a reliable source of information about herbs, homeopathic remedies, and other alternative options.

CenteringPregnancy®

CenteringPregnancy® is a model of prenatal health care designed to empower women to choose health-promoting behaviors and, as a result, improve prenatal care outcomes. CenteringPregnancy® integrates two main components of care—*assessment* and *education*—into a unified program providing complete prenatal care to women within a group setting, thereby providing the added benefit of support (DeCesare & Jackson, 2015). This model replaces the traditional one-on-one visits. Instead, group meetings are held where moms-to-be and their partners receive care and education and form a sense of community with other group members.

Clients begin monthly meetings in small groups at 12 to 16 weeks' gestation and then meet biweekly as their due dates approach. Each group session begins with the expectant mothers taking their own blood pressure, monitoring weight gain, checking urine samples, and recording data on medical charts under the guidance of their healthcare provider or nurse. The provider then reviews each group member's information and completes any further assessments that are indicated. After all assessments have been completed, the group members convene in a circle to discuss topics such as nutrition, fetal development, common discomforts of pregnancy and possible remedies, exercise, relaxation, labor and birth procedures, parenting and relationship issues, contraception, and infant care. Both mothers and fathers report an increased investment in the pregnancy and self-care after attending group sessions.

Teratogenic Substances

Substances that adversely affect the normal growth and development of the fetus are called *teratogens*. Many substances are known or suspected teratogens, including certain medications, psychotropic drugs, and alcohol. The harmful effects of other substances, such as some pesticides or exposure to x-rays in the first trimester of pregnancy, have also been documented. It is essential to provide pregnant women with information about recognized teratogens and environmental risks.

MEDICATIONS

The use of medications during pregnancy, including prescriptions, over-the-counter drugs, and herbal remedies, is of great concern because maternal drug exposure is associated with birth defects. Many pregnant women need medication to treat infections, allergies, or other pathologic processes. In these situations, the problem can be complex. Even when a woman is highly motivated to avoid taking any medications, she may have taken potentially teratogenic medications before her pregnancy was confirmed, especially if she has an irregular menstrual cycle.

The fetus is at highest risk for gross abnormalities during the first trimester of pregnancy, when fetal organs are first developing. The classic period of teratogenesis in a woman with a 28-day cycle extends from day 31 after the last menstrual period (17 days after fertilization) to day 71 (57 days after fertilization) (Niebyl & Simpson, 2012). Many factors influence teratogenic effects, including the type of teratogen and the dose, the stage of embryo development, and the genetic sensitivity of the mother and fetus. For example, the commonly prescribed acne medication isotretinoin (Accutane) is associated with a high incidence of spontaneous abortion and congenital malformations if taken early in pregnancy.

Formerly, drugs were classified in categories A, B, C, D, and X with category X indicating that the demonstrated fetal risks clearly outweigh any possible benefit. In 2014, the FDA amended its regulations governing the labeling of prescription drugs and biologic products for women who are pregnant or lactating. These regulations became effective in June 2015. According to the new requirements, three categories have been specified (FDA, 2014):

- *Pregnancy.* If the drug is absorbed systemically, labeling must include a risk summary of adverse developmental outcomes that includes data from all relevant sources, including human, animal, and/or pharmacologic information. The labeling must also contain relevant information to help healthcare providers counsel women about the use of the drug during pregnancy. In addition, if there is a pregnancy exposure registry for the drug, the labeling should include a specific statement to that effect followed by contact information needed to obtain information about the registry or to enroll.

- *Lactation.* For drugs that are absorbed systemically, labeling must include a summary of the risks of using a drug when the woman is lactating. To the extent that information is available, the summary should include relevant information about the drug's presence in human milk, the effects of the drug on milk production, and the effects of the drug on the breastfed child.

- *Females and males of reproductive potential.* This section must include information when human or animal data suggest drug-associated effects on fertility. It should also specify when contraception or pregnancy testing is required or recommended, such as before, during, or after the drug therapy.

Although the first trimester is the critical period for teratogenesis, some medications are known to have a teratogenic effect when taken in the second and third trimesters. For example, tetracycline taken in late pregnancy is commonly associated with staining of teeth in children and has been shown to depress skeletal growth, especially in premature babies. Sulfonamides taken in the last few weeks of pregnancy are known to compete with bilirubin attachment of protein-binding sites, increasing the risk of jaundice in the newborn (Niebyl & Simpson, 2012).

Pregnant women need to avoid all medications—prescribed, homeopathic, or over-the-counter—if possible. If no alternative exists, it is wisest to select a well-known medication rather than a newer drug whose potential teratogenic effects may not be known. When possible, the oral form of a drug should be used, and it should be prescribed in the lowest possible therapeutic dose for the shortest time possible. Caution is the watchword for pregnant women who have been taking medications. The advantage of using a particular medication must outweigh the risks. Any medication with possible teratogenic effects is best avoided.

SAFETY ALERT!
It is essential that pregnant women check with their physicians/CNMs about any herbs or medications they were taking when pregnancy began and about any nonprescription drugs they are thinking of using. (See Chapter 14 for a discussion of the use of alcohol and illicit drugs during pregnancy.)

TOBACCO

In the United States, smoking during pregnancy is one of the most significant, modifiable causes of poor pregnancy outcomes. It is associated with an increased risk of spontaneous abortion, intrauterine growth restriction, low birth weight, preterm birth, premature rupture of the membranes, perinatal mortality, placenta previa, abruptio placentae, and premature rupture of membranes (Cunningham et al., 2014). Research also links maternal smoking, both during pregnancy and afterward, with an increased risk of sudden infant death syndrome (SIDS) (Niebyl & Simpson, 2012). Maternal smoking also exposes young children to other risks of secondhand smoke, including middle ear infections; acute and chronic respiratory tract illnesses such as asthma, bronchitis, and pneumonia; inflammatory bowel disease; sleep disturbances; and learning disabilities and conduct disorders (Al-Sayed & Ibrahim, 2014).

The ingredients in cigarette smoke, such as carbon monoxide, nicotine, lead, and cotinine, are toxic to the fetus and decrease the availability of oxygen to maternal and fetal tissues (Cunningham et al., 2014).

In response to public health education campaigns in the United States, smoking during pregnancy has decreased significantly. In fact, approximately 46% of women who smoke quit during pregnancy. Unfortunately, about 50% to 60% of women who quit smoking during their pregnancy resume smoking within a year after birth (ACOG, 2013a). This finding suggests that although women are aware of the potential impact of smoking on the fetus, they may be less knowledgeable about the effects of passive smoke on the baby.

Any decrease in smoking during pregnancy most likely improves fetal outcome, and researchers continue to explore approaches designed to help women quit smoking. Pregnancy may be a difficult time for a woman to stop smoking, but the nurse should encourage her to reduce the number of cigarettes she smokes daily. The perceived need to protect her unborn child may increase her motivation. Many educational resources are available for healthcare providers and consumers on smoking cessation programs through organizations such as the American Lung Association, the March of Dimes, and Healthy Mothers, Healthy Babies.

ALCOHOL

Fetuses of women who drink heavily are at increased risk of developing **fetal alcohol syndrome (FAS)**. This syndrome, which is characterized by growth restriction, facial anomalies, and central nervous system (CNS) dysfunction of varying severity, is a major cause of intellectual disability in the United States (Cunningham et al., 2014).

The effects of moderate drinking during pregnancy are unclear. Research indicates an increased incidence of lowered birth weight and some neurologic effects, such as attention deficit

disorder. Evidence suggests that the risk of teratogenic effects increases proportionally with increased average daily intake of alcohol. Although an occasional drink during pregnancy does not carry any known risk, no safe level of drinking during pregnancy has been identified; thus healthcare providers recommend that pregnant women abstain from all alcohol during pregnancy. In most cases, once a woman becomes aware of her pregnancy, she decreases her consumption of alcohol. However, the alcohol consumed after conception and before pregnancy is diagnosed remains a cause for concern. For this reason, and for their general well-being, women of childbearing age—and indeed all women—should be counseled to avoid heavy or binge drinking.

Assessment of alcohol intake is a major part of every woman's medical history. The nurse should ask questions in a direct, nonjudgmental manner. All women need to be counseled about the role of alcohol in pregnancy. If heavy consumption is involved, the nurse should refer the pregnant woman immediately to an alcohol treatment program. Counselors in these programs need to know about a woman's pregnancy before drug therapy is suggested, since certain drugs may be harmful to the developing fetus. For example, the drug disulfiram (Antabuse), often used in conjunction with alcohol treatment, is contraindicated during pregnancy because it potentiates the teratogenic effect of alcohol (Wisner et al., 2012).

CAFFEINE

While studies continue, current research reveals no evidence that moderate levels of caffeine are linked to birth defects, spontaneous abortion, or preterm birth, nor is there any clear evidence of a link between caffeine intake and intrauterine growth restriction (ACOG, 2013b). Until more definitive data are available, nurses can advise women about common sources of caffeine, including coffee, tea, colas, and chocolate, and suggest that they limit their caffeine intake to less than 200 mg/day (Cunningham et al., 2014). The average cup of brewed coffee has 100 mg, a cup of tea has 50 mg, a regular cola drink has up to 40 mg, and a normal-sized chocolate bar has up to 50 mg of caffeine.

Evaluation

Throughout the antepartum period, evaluation is an ongoing and essential part of effective nursing care. In evaluating the effectiveness of the interactions, try creative solutions that are logical and carefully thought out. Creative solutions are especially important in dealing with families from other cultures. If a practice is important to a woman and not harmful, the culturally competent nurse will not discourage it.

Be alert for situations that require referral for further evaluation. For example, a woman who has gained 4 lb in a single week does not require counseling about nutrition; she needs further assessment for preeclampsia. The nurse who has a sound knowledge of theory will recognize this need and act immediately.

Throughout the course of pregnancy, certain criteria determine the quality of care. In essence, nursing care has been effective if the following occur:

- The common discomforts of pregnancy are quickly identified and are relieved or lessened effectively.
- The woman is able to discuss the physiologic and psychologic changes of pregnancy.
- The woman uses self-care measures, if needed, during pregnancy.
- The woman avoids substances and situations that pose a risk to her or her child's well-being.
- The woman seeks regular prenatal care.

Focus Your Study

- Providing anticipatory guidance about childbirth, the postpartum period, and childrearing is a primary responsibility of the nurse caring for women in an antepartal setting.

- The nurse assesses the expectant father's knowledge level and intended degree of participation and then works with the couple to help ensure a satisfying experience.

- Culturally based practices and taboos may have a major impact on the childbearing family.

- Childbearing decisions include the healthcare provider, birth setting, support persons, and whether to include siblings in the birth experience.

- Prenatal classes may be offered early or late in the pregnancy. The class content varies depending on the type of class and the individual offering it. Expectant parents tend to want information in chronologic sequence with the pregnancy.

- Breastfeeding programs in the prenatal period offer encouragement, practical instruction, and resources for the breastfeeding family.

- Siblings are now included in the whole birthing process, and classes for them are available from many sources.

- Grandparents have unique information needs that are addressed in grandparents' classes.

- The common discomforts of pregnancy occur as a result of physiologic and anatomic changes. The nurse provides the woman with information about self-care activities aimed at reducing or relieving discomfort.

- To make appropriate self-care choices and ensure healthful habits, a pregnant woman requires accurate information about a range of subjects from exercise to sexual activity, from bathing to immunization.

- Maternal assessment of fetal activity keeps the woman "in touch" with her fetus and provides ongoing assessment of fetal status.

- Teratogenic substances are substances that adversely affect the normal growth and development of the fetus.

- A pregnant woman should avoid taking nonessential medications or using over-the-counter preparations during pregnancy.

- Evidence confirms that smoking or consuming alcohol, during pregnancy may be harmful to the fetus.

Clinical Reasoning in Action

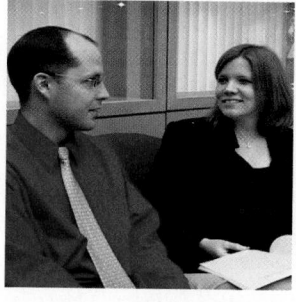

Thirty-seven-year-old Cathy Sommers, G1P0, presents to you, with her husband, at the OB physician's office at 32 weeks' gestation. Cathy tells you that she and her husband are practicing lawyers with their own firm. The couple delayed starting a family because it has been important to them to advance their careers and establish their firm. Cathy had an amniocentesis at 18 weeks' gestation because of her advanced maternal age, and the results ruled out chromosomal abnormalities. The couple knows that the baby is a boy, and they are anticipating a vaginal birth. Cathy tells you that she is experiencing more fatigue, leg cramps, and shortness of breath when climbing stairs. The physical examination, including a negative Homans sign, is within normal limits with the exception of slight ankle edema. Her weight is 150 lb, temperature 98.6°F (37.0°C), pulse 88, respirations 16, BP 126/70. You discuss pregnancy discomforts in the third trimester with Cathy and her husband.

1. What measures can you suggest to cope with fatigue?
2. Discuss measures to decrease leg cramps.
3. Discuss the physiologic changes underlying dyspnea.
4. Review Braxton Hicks contractions.

References

Alio, A. P., Lewis, C. A., Scarborough, K., Harris, K., & Fiscella, K. (2013). A community perspective on the role of fathers during pregnancy: A qualitative study. *Pregnancy and Childbirth, 13*(2), 1–11.

Al-Sayed, E. M., & Ibrahim, K. S. (2014). Second-hand tobacco smoke in children. *Toxicology and Industrial Health, 30*(7), 635–644.

American Academy of Pediatrics (AAP) and the American College of Obstetricians and Gynecologists (ACOG). (2012). *Guidelines for perinatal care* (7th ed.). Elk Grove Village, IL: Author.

American College of Obstetricians and Gynecologists (ACOG). (2011a). *Diagnosis and treatment of nausea and vomiting of pregnancy* (ACOG Practice Bulletin No. 52). Washington, DC: Author.

American College of Obstetricians and Gynecologists (ACOG). (2011b). *Exercise during pregnancy*

(Frequently Asked Questions [FAQ] 119). Washington, DC: Author.

American College of Obstetricians and Gynecologists (ACOG). (2012). *Morning sickness.* (Frequently Asked Questions [FAQ] 126). Washington, DC: Author.

American College of Obstetricians and Gynecologists (ACOG). (2013a). *Smoking cessation during pregnancy* (Committee Opinion No. 471, reaffirmed 2013). Washington, DC: Author.

American College of Obstetricians and Gynecologists (ACOG). (2013b). *Moderate caffeine consumption during pregnancy* (Committee Opinion No. 462). Washington, DC: Author.

American Diabetes Association. (2013). *How to treat gestational diabetes.* Retrieved from http://www.diabetes.org/diabetes-basics/gestational/how-to-treat-gestational.html

Avery, M. D. (2013). *Supporting a physiologic approach to pregnancy and birth: A practical guide.* Ames, IA: Wiley & Sons, Inc.

Bloomquist, J. L., Quiroz, L. H., MacMillan, D., McCullough, A., & Handa, V. L. (2011). Mothers' satisfaction with planned vaginal and planned cesarean birth. *American Journal of Perinatology, 28*(5), 383–388.

Coalition for Improving Maternity Services (CIMS). (2013). Mother-friendly childbirth initiative. Retrieved from http://www.motherfriendly.org/MFCI

Cunningham, F. G., Leveno, K. J., Bloom, S. L., Spong, C. Y., Dashe, J. S., Hoffman, B. L., ... Sheffield, J. S. (2014). *Williams obstetrics* (24th ed.). New York, NY: McGraw-Hill.

DeCesare, J. Z., & Jackson, J. R. (2015). Centering Pregnancy: Practical tips for your practice. *Archives of Gynecology and Obstetrics, 291*, 499–507.

Donna, S. (2011). *Promoting normal birth: Research, reflections and guidelines.* United Kingdom: Fresh Heart Publishing.

Fantasia, H. C. (2014). A new pharmacologic treatment for nausea and vomiting of pregnancy. *Nursing for Women's Health, 18*(1), 73–77.

Ferraro, Z. M., Gaudet, L., & Adamo, K. (2012). The potential impact of physical activity during pregnancy on maternal and neonatal outcomes. *Obstetric & Gynecologic Survey, 67*(2), 99–110.

Food and Drug Administation (FDA). (2014). *Content and format of labeling for human prescription drug and biological products: Requirements for pregnancy and lactation labeling.* Retrieved from https://s3.amazonaws.com/public-inspection.federalregister .gov/2014-28241.pdf

Gregory, K. D., Niebyl, J. R., & Johnson, T. R. B. (2012). Preconception and prenatal care: Part of the continuum. In S. G. Gabbe, J. R. Niebyl, J. L. Simpson, M. B. Landon, H. L. Galan, E. R. M. Jauniaux, & D. A. Driscoll (Eds.), *Obstetrics: Normal and problem pregnancies* (6th ed.). Philadelphia, PA: Elsevier Saunders.

Groutz, A., Hasson, J., Wengier, A., Gold, R., Skornick-Rapaport, A., Lessing, J. B., & Gordon, D. (2011). Third-and fourth-degree perineal tears: Prevalence and risk factors in the third millenium. *American Journal of Obstetrics & Gynecology, 204,* 337e.1–4.

Katz, V. (2012). Work and work-related stress in pregnancy. *Clinical Obstetrics and Gynecology, 55*(3), 765–773.

Kimberly, D. G., Niebyl, J. R., & Johnson, T. R. B. (2012). Preconception and prenatal care: Part of the continuum. In S. G. Gabbe, J. R. Niebyl, J. L. Simpson, M. B. Landon, H. L. Galan, E. R. M. Jauniaux, & D. A. Driscoll (Eds.), *Obstetrics: Normal and problem pregnancies* (6th ed.). Philadelphia, PA: Elsevier Saunders.

King, T. L., Brucker, M. C., Kriebs, J. M., Fahey, J. O., Gegor, C. L., & Varney, H. (2015). *Varney's midwifery* (5th ed.). Burlington, MA: Jones & Bartlett Learning.

Martin, J. A., Hamilton, B. E., Osterman, M. J. K., Curtin, S. C., & Mathewa, T. J. (2013). Births: Final data for 2012. *National Vital Statistics Reports, 62*(9), 1–87.

Melzer, K., Schutz, Y., Boulvain, Y., & Kayser, B. (2010). Physical activity and pregnancy: cardiovascular adaptations, recommendations and pregnancy outcome. *Sports Medicine, 40*(6), 493–507.

National Center for Complementary and Alternative Medicine (NCCAM). (2012). *Herbs at a glance: Ginger.* Retrieved from http://nccam.nih.gov/health/ginger

Niebyl, J. R., & Simpson, J. L. (2012). Drugs and environmental agents in pregnancy and lactation: Embryology, teratology, epidemiology. In S. G. Gabbe, J. R. Niebyl, J. L. Simpson, M. B. Landon, H. L. Galan, E. R. M. Jauniaux, & D. A. Driscoll (Eds.), *Obstetrics: Normal and problem pregnancies* (6th ed.). Philadelphia, PA: Elsevier Saunders.

Purnell, L. D. (2014). *Guide to culturally competent health care.* (3rd ed.). Philadelphia, PA: F. A. Davis.

Shivakumar, G. (2015). Exercise improves depressive symptoms during pregnancy. *BJOG: An International Journal of Obstetrics and Gynaecology, 122*(1), 63.

Spector, R. E. (2013). *Cultural diversity in health and illness* (8th ed.). Upper Saddle River, NJ: Prentice Hall Health.

Sut, H. K., & Kaplan, P.B. (2015). Effect of pelvic muscle floor exercise on pelvic floor muscle activity and voiding functions during pregnancy and the postpartum period. *Neurourology and Urodynamics.* doi:10.1002 /nau.22728.

Tiran, D. (2012). Ginger to reduce nausea and vomiting during pregnancy: Evidence of effectiveness is not the same as proof of safety. *Contemporary Therapies in Clinical Practice, 18,* 22–25.

Toohill, J., Fenwick, J., Gamble, J., Creedy, D., Bulst, A., Turkstra, E., & Ryding, E. (2014). A randomized controlled trial of a psycho-education intervention by midwives in reducing childbirth fear in pregnancy women. *Birth, 41*(4), 384–395.

United States Department of Health and Human Services (HHS). (2013). *Healthy People 2020.* Retrieved from http://www.healthypeople.gov/2020

University of South Carolina. (2011). *Cultural knowledge.* Retrieved from http://www.usc.edu/hsc/ebnet/Cc /knowledge/ccknow.htm

Wisner, K. L., Sit, D. K. Y., Altemus, M., Bogen, D. L., Famy, C. S., Pearlstein, T. B., … Perel, J. M. (2012). Mental health and behavioral disorders in pregnancy. In S. G. Gabbe, J. R. Niebyl, J. L. Simpson, M. B. Landon, H. L. Galan, E. R. M. Jauniaux, & D. A. Driscoll (Eds.), *Obstetrics: Normal and problem pregnancies* (6th ed.). Philadelphia, PA: Elsevier Saunders.

Zavorsky, G. S., & Longo, L. D. (2011). Adding strength training, exercise intensity, and caloric expenditure to exercise guidelines in pregnancy. *Obstetrics & Gynecology, 117*(6), 1399–1402.

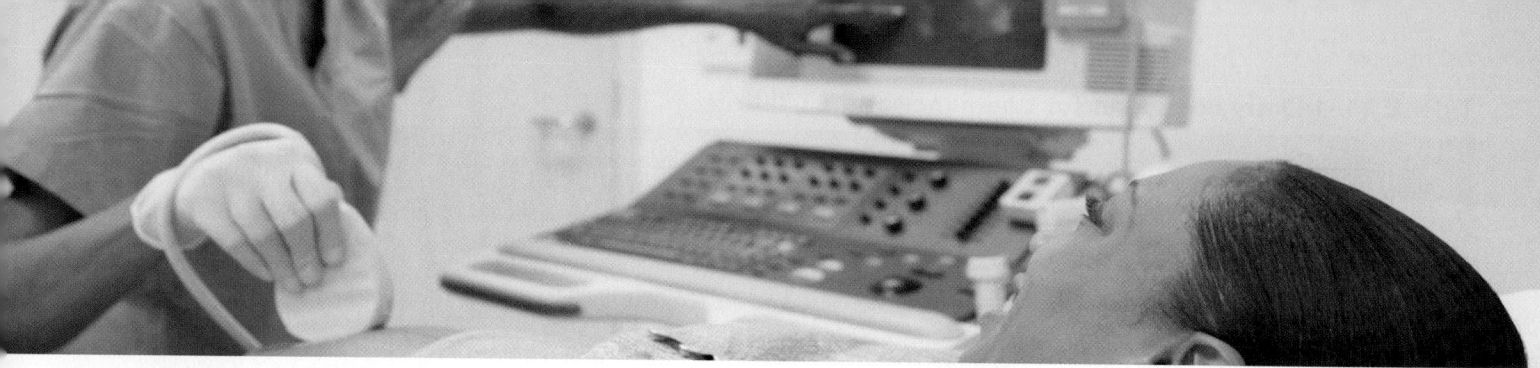

Chapter 11
Maternal Nutrition

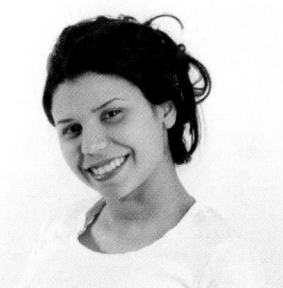

When I was young I thought nutrition was boring. Now that I am pregnant I find it endlessly fascinating. I realize how important good nutrition is for me, for my husband, and for the well-being of our child. My mother just laughs and reminds me about the times I resisted her efforts to help me develop better eating habits. Oh well, it is just another example of how smart our parents get as we get older!

—Maria, 26

Monart Designs/Fotolia

∨ Learning Outcomes

11.1 Describe the recommended levels of weight gain during pregnancy when providing nursing care for pregnant women.

11.2 Explain the significance of specific nutrients in the diet of the pregnant woman.

11.3 Compare nutritional needs during pregnancy, the postpartum period, and lactation with nonpregnant requirements.

11.4 Plan adequate prenatal vegetarian diets based on the nutritional requirements of pregnancy.

11.5 Explain the ways in which various physical, psychosocial, and cultural factors can affect

nutritional intake and status in the nursing management of pregnant women.

11.6 Compare recommendations for weight gain and nutrient intakes in the pregnant adolescent with those for the mature pregnant adult.

11.7 Describe basic factors a nurse should consider when offering nutritional counseling to a pregnant adolescent.

11.8 Compare nutritional counseling issues for breastfeeding and formula-feeding mothers.

A woman's nutritional status before and during pregnancy can significantly influence her health and the health of her fetus. In most prenatal clinics and offices, nurses offer nutritional counseling directly or work closely with the nutritionist in providing nutritional assessment and teaching. This chapter focuses on the nutritional needs of the pregnant woman. Special sections consider the nutritional needs of the pregnant adolescent and the woman after giving birth.

Fetal growth occurs in three overlapping stages:

1. Growth by increase in cell number
2. Growth by increase in cell number and cell size
3. Growth by increase in cell size alone

Nutritional problems that interfere with cell division may have permanent consequences. If the nutritional deficit occurs when cells are mainly enlarging, the changes are usually reversible when normal nutrition resumes.

Growing fetal and maternal tissues require increased quantities of nutrients. These are listed in the **Dietary Reference Intakes (DRIs)**, a broad array of dietary reference values developed jointly by the United States and Canada, as either the *Recommended Dietary Allowance (RDA)* or *Adequate Intake (AI)*. An RDA is the daily dietary intake that is considered sufficient to meet the nutritional requirements of nearly all individuals in a specific life stage and gender group. An AI is a value cited for a nutrient when there are insufficient data to calculate an estimated average requirement.

TABLE 11–1 Daily Food Plan for Pregnancy and Lactation

FOOD GROUP	NUTRIENTS PROVIDED	FOOD SOURCE	RECOMMENDED DAILY AMOUNT DURING PREGNANCY	RECOMMENDED DAILY AMOUNT DURING LACTATION
Dairy products	Protein; riboflavin; vitamins A, D, and others; calcium; phosphorus; zinc; magnesium	Milk—whole, 2%, skim, dry, buttermilk Cheeses—hard, semisoft, cottage Yogurt—plain, low-fat Soybean milk—canned, dry	Four 8-oz cups (five for teenagers) used plain or with flavoring, in shakes, soups, puddings, custards, cocoa Calcium in 1 cup milk equivalent to 1½ cups cottage cheese, 1½ oz hard or semi-soft cheese, 1 cup yogurt, 1½ cups ice cream (high in fat and sugar)	Four 8-oz cups (five for teenagers); equivalent amount of cheese, yogurt, and other dairy products
Meat and meat alternatives	Protein; iron; thiamine, niacin, and other vitamins; and minerals	Beef, pork, veal, lamb, poultry, animal organ meats, fish, eggs; legumes; nuts, seeds, peanut butter, grains in proper vegetarian combination (vitamin B_{12} supplement needed)	Three servings (one serving = 2 oz), combination in amounts necessary for same nutrient equivalent (varies greatly)	Two servings
Grain products, whole grain or enriched	B vitamins; iron; whole grain also has zinc, magnesium, and other trace elements; provides fiber	Breads and bread products such as cornbread, muffins, waffles, hotcakes, biscuits, dumplings, cereals, pastas, rice	Six to 11 servings daily: one serving = one slice bread, ¾ cup or 1 oz dry cereal, ½ cup rice or pasta	Same as for pregnancy
Fruits and fruit juices	Vitamins A and C; minerals; raw fruits for roughage	Citrus fruits and juices, melons, berries, all other fruits and juices	Two to four servings (one serving for vitamin C): one serving = one medium fruit, ½ –1 cup fruit, 4 oz orange or grapefruit juice	Same as for pregnancy
Vegetables and vegetable juices	Vitamins A and C; minerals; provides roughage	Leafy green vegetables; deep yellow or orange vegetables such as carrots, sweet potatoes, squash, tomatoes; green vegetables such as peas, green beans, broccoli; other vegetables such as beets, cabbage, potatoes, corn, lima beans	Three to five servings (one serving of dark green or deep yellow vegetable for vitamin A): one serving = ½ –1 cup vegetable, two tomatoes, one medium potato	Same as for pregnancy
Fats	Vitamins A and D; linoleic acid	Butter, cream cheese, fortified table spreads; cream, whipped cream, whipped toppings; avocado, mayonnaise, oil, nuts	As desired in moderation (high in calories): one serving = 1 tbsp butter or enriched margarine	Same as for pregnancy
Sugar and sweets		Sugar, brown sugar, honey, molasses	Occasionally, if desired	Same as for pregnancy
Desserts		Nutritious desserts such as puddings, custards, fruit whips, and crisps; other rich, sweet desserts and pastries	Occasionally, if desired	Same as for pregnancy
Beverages	Fluid	Coffee, decaffeinated beverages, tea, bouillon, carbonated drinks	As desired, in moderation	Same as for pregnancy
Miscellaneous		Iodized salt, herbs, spices, condiments	As desired	Same as for pregnancy

Note: The pregnant woman should eat regularly: three meals a day, with nutritious snacks of fruit, cheese, milk, or other foods between meals if desired. (More frequent but smaller meals are also recommended.) Four to six 8-oz glasses of water and a total of eight to ten 8-oz cups total fluid intake should be consumed daily. Water is an essential nutrient.

Women can get most of the recommended nutrients by eating a well-balanced diet each day. The basic food groups and recommended amounts during pregnancy and lactation are presented in Table 11–1.

Maternal Weight Gain

Maternal weight gain is an important factor in fetal growth and newborn birth weight. Optimal weight gain depends on the woman's body mass index (BMI) (a measure of body fat based on height and weight) and her prepregnant nutritional state. An adequate weight gain indicates an adequate caloric intake. However, it does not ensure that the woman has a good diet nutritionally. The pregnant woman must maintain the nutritional quality of her diet as her weight gain progresses.

The Institute of Medicine (IOM) (2009) has established optimum ranges of weight gain based on a woman's BMI, and the American College of Obstetricians and Gynecologists (ACOG) (2013a) supports these recommendations. The IOM's optimum ranges of weight gain are as follows:

- *Underweight woman:* BMI less than 18.5: 28 to 40 lb (12.5 to 18.0 kg)
- *Normal-weight woman:* BMI between 18.5 and 24.9: 25 to 35 lb (11.5 to 16.0 kg)
- *Overweight woman:* BMI between 25 and 29.9: 15 to 25 lb (7.0 to 11.5 kg)
- *Obese woman:* BMI equal to or greater than 30: 11 to 20 lb (5.0 to 9.1 kg)

The average maternal weight gain is distributed as follows:

11 lb (5 kg)	Fetus, placenta, amniotic fluid
2 lb (0.9 kg)	Uterus
4 lb (1.8 kg)	Increased blood volume
3 lb (1.4 kg)	Breast tissue
5 to 10 lb (2.3 to 4.5 kg)	Maternal stores

The pattern of weight gain is important. For women of normal weight, the IOM recommendations are based on a first-trimester weight gain of 1.1 to 4.4 lb (0.5 to 2.0 kg) followed by a gain of about 1 lb (0.45 kg) per week during the second and third trimesters. The rate of weight gain in the second and third trimesters needs to be slightly higher for underweight women and slightly lower for women who are overweight (0.6 lb) or obese (0.5 lb) (IOM, 2009).

The prevalence of obesity in the United States has increased dramatically over the past 25 years. The recent National Health and Nutrition Examination Survey found that in the United States more than one third of women are obese and 8% of reproductive-aged women are extremely obese (ACOG, 2013a). Pregnant women who are obese are at risk for many pregnancy complications including gestational diabetes mellitus, preeclampsia, and cesarean birth. Their fetuses are at increased risk for congenital anomalies, stillbirth, prematurity, macrosomia, and childhood obesity. Thus it is recommended that these women receive counseling on strategies to move toward and to remain at a healthful weight prior to conceiving (ACOG, 2013b).

The incidence of bariatric surgery among obese reproductive-aged women is increasing (ACOG, 2013a). Women who lose weight after weight-loss surgery are less likely to have complications during pregnancy. The need for vitamin supplementation should be evaluated as these women are at risk for deficiencies in iron, vitamin B_{12}, folate, vitamin D, and calcium. Women who have undergone gastric band surgery should be referred to their general surgeon to evaluate the need for a band adjustment.

Clinical Tip

Weight varies with time of day, amount of clothing, inaccurate scale adjustment, or weighing error. Do not overemphasize a single weight, but pay attention to the overall pattern of weight gain.

Because of the association between maternal weight gain and pregnancy outcome, most caregivers pay close attention to weight gain during pregnancy (Figure 11–1). Weight gain charts can be useful in monitoring the rate and pattern of weight gain over time.

All pregnant women should include a variety of nutrient rich foods each day to ensure they are meeting the nutritional needs of both themselves and their babies. The U.S. Department of Agriculture (USDA) offers an online tool (choosemyplate .gov) that can help expectant women customize an eating plan based on age, weight, height, physical activity, and gestation stage (Figure 11–2).

Nutritional Requirements

The RDA for almost all nutrients increases during pregnancy, although the amount of increase varies with each nutrient. These increases reflect the additional requirements of both the mother and the developing fetus.

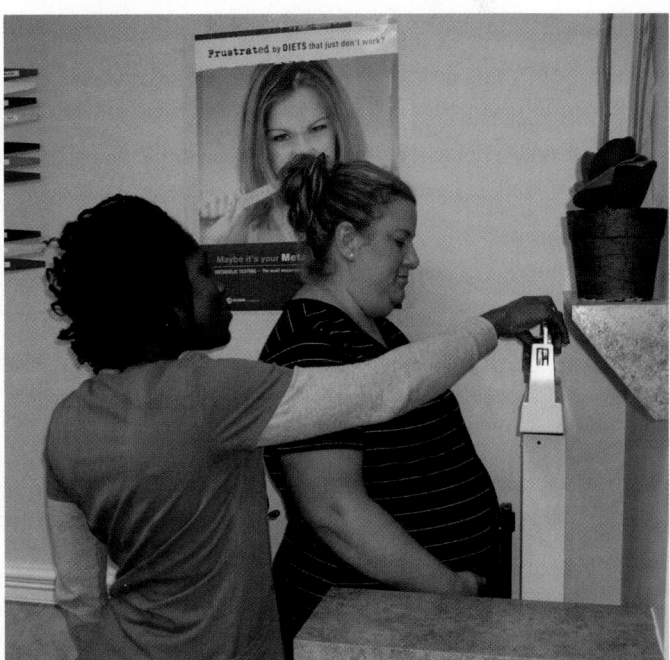

Figure 11–1 It is important to monitor a pregnant woman's weight over time.

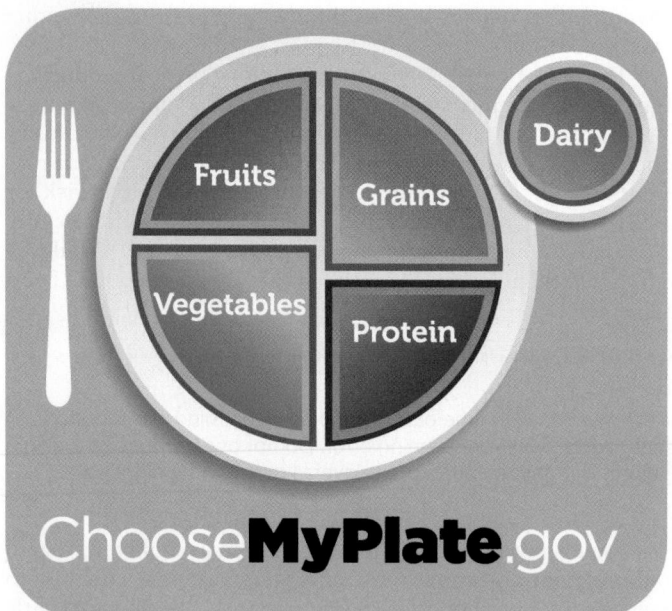

Figure 11–2 MyPlate is part of an initiative to encourage healthy eating. It illustrates the five food groups and encourages people to fill half their plates with fruits and vegetables.

SOURCE: USDA (U.S. Department of Agriculture).

Calories

The term **calorie** (cal) designates the amount of heat required to raise the temperature of 1 g of water 33.8°F (1.0°C). The **kilocalorie** (kcal) is equivalent to 1000 cal and is the unit used to express the energy value of food.

The dietary reference intakes for energy requirements during pregnancy do not change during the first trimester. During the second and third trimesters, pregnant women should consume an extra 300 kcal/day. Prepregnant weight, height, maternal age, health status, and activity level all influence caloric needs, and weight should be monitored regularly during the pregnancy. See *Teaching Highlights: Adding 300 kcal During Pregnancy.*

Carbohydrates

Carbohydrates provide the body's main source of energy as well as the fiber necessary for proper bowel functioning. If the total caloric intake is not adequate, the body uses protein for energy. Protein then becomes unavailable for growth needs. In addition, protein breakdown leads to ketosis.

The carbohydrate and caloric needs of the pregnant woman increase, especially during the last two trimesters. Carbohydrate intake promotes weight gain and growth of the fetus, placenta, and other maternal tissues. Dairy products, fruits, vegetables, and whole-grain cereals and breads all contain carbohydrates and other important nutrients.

Protein

Protein supplies the amino acids required for the growth and development of maternal tissues, such as the uterus and breasts, and to meet fetal needs. This is especially important during the last half of pregnancy, when fetal growth is greatest.

The protein requirement for a pregnant woman is 60 g/day, an increase of 14 g over nonpregnant levels. Animal products such as meat, fish, poultry, and eggs provide high-quality protein. Dairy products are also important protein sources. A quart

---

TEACHING HIGHLIGHTS | Adding 300 kcal During Pregnancy

- The notion of "eating for two" may result in overeating. Emphasize the relatively small increase in calories necessary during pregnancy.
- The additional 300 kcal/day recommended during pregnancy can be achieved by adding two milk servings and one serving of meat or alternative.
- MyPlate is designed to represent the food groups needed to make a balanced diet. Following MyPlate recommendations, women should aim to have half their plate consist of fruits and vegetables, make at least half their grains whole grains, and switch to fat-free or low-fat (1%) milk. Women are encouraged to drink water rather than sugary drinks and compare the sodium content of foods and choose foods that are lower in sodium (USDA, 2012). A balanced diet includes the following:
  - *Grains:* Six to eleven servings (one serving = 1 slice bread, ½ hamburger roll, 1 oz dry cereal, 1 tortilla, ½ cup pasta, rice, grits)
  - *Fruits:* Two to four servings; one should be a good source of vitamin C (one serving = 1 medium-sized piece of fruit, ½ cup juice)
  - *Vegetables:* Three to five servings (one serving = 1 cup raw vegetable, 1 cup green leafy vegetable, ½ cup cooked vegetable)
  - *Dairy:* Two to three servings (one serving = 1 cup milk or yogurt, 1.5 oz hard cheese, 2 cups cottage cheese, 1 cup pudding made with milk)
  - *Meats and alternatives:* Two to three servings (one serving = 2 oz cooked lean meat, poultry, or fish; 2 eggs; ½ cup cottage cheese; 1 cup cooked legumes [kidney, lima, garbanzo, or soybeans, split peas]; 6 oz tofu; 2 oz nuts or seeds; 4 tbsp peanut butter)
- Not all foods that are nutritionally equivalent have the same number of calories; it is important to consider that when making food choices.
- Consider using low-fat milk, lean cuts of meat, or fish broiled or baked instead of fried.
- Foods can be combined. For example, 1 cup spaghetti with a 2-oz meatball would count as 1 serving meat, ¾ cup spaghetti = 1 grain, and ¼ cup tomato sauce = ½ serving vegetable.
- Use a calorie-counting guide to compare the calories in a variety of foods that are equivalent, such as 2 oz beef and 2 oz fish or 1 cup low-fat milk and 1 cup whole milk.

of milk supplies 32 g of protein, more than half the average daily protein requirement. A woman can incorporate milk into her diet in a variety of dishes, including soups, puddings, custards, sauces, and yogurt. Beverages such as hot chocolate and milk-and-fruit drinks can also be included, but they are high in calories. Various kinds of hard and soft cheeses and cottage cheese are excellent protein sources, although cream cheese is considered a fat source only. Women who have allergies to milk, are lactose intolerant, or practice vegetarianism may find soy milk acceptable. It can be used in cooked dishes or as a beverage. Tofu, or soybean curd, can replace cottage cheese.

Fat

Fats are valuable sources of energy for the body and aid in the absorption of fat-soluble vitamins. Fats are more completely absorbed during pregnancy, resulting in a marked increase in serum lipids, lipoproteins, and cholesterol, and decreased elimination of fat through the bowel. Fat deposits in the fetus increase from about 2% at midpregnancy to almost 12% at term. However, fat requirements are unchanged during pregnancy and should account for about 20% to 35% of daily caloric intake, of which 10% or less should be saturated fat.

Essential fatty acids are important for the development of the central nervous system of the fetus. Of particular interest are the omega-3 fatty acids and their derivative, docosahexaenoic acid (DHA). Maternal dietary intake of DHA during pregnancy may reduce the risk of preterm birth and low birth weight, and may enhance fetal and infant brain development (Carlson, Colombo, Gajewski, et al., 2013). Oily fish provide the best source of DHA (however, see the *Mercury in Fish* section later in this chapter); other sources include fortified dairy products, and even some fortified soymilk. Plant sources of omega-3 fatty acids include soybean oil, canola oil, flaxseeds and their oil, and walnuts.

Minerals

CALCIUM AND PHOSPHORUS

Calcium and phosphorus are involved in the mineralization of fetal bones and teeth and acid–base buffering. The body absorbs and uses calcium more efficiently during pregnancy. Some calcium and phosphorus are required early in pregnancy, but most fetal bone calcification occurs during the last 2 to 3 months. Teeth begin to form at about 8 weeks' gestation and are formed by birth. The 6-year molars begin to calcify just before birth.

The identified AI for calcium for the pregnant or lactating woman, ages 19 or older, is 1000 mg/day. It is 1300 mg/day for pregnant women younger than age 19. If calcium intake is low, fetal needs will be met at the mother's expense by demineralization of bone.

A diet that includes 4 cups of milk or an equivalent dairy alternative will provide sufficient calcium. Smaller amounts of calcium are supplied by legumes, nuts, dried fruits, and dark green leafy vegetables (such as kale, cabbage, collards, and turnip greens).

The RDA for phosphorus is 700 mg/day for the pregnant or lactating woman ages 19 and older. It is 1250 mg/day for pregnant women younger than 19 years. Because phosphorus is so widely available in foods, the daily requirement is readily supplied through calcium- and protein-rich foods.

IODINE

Iodine is an essential part of the thyroid hormone thyroxine. The thyroid gland may become enlarged if iodine is not replaced by adequate dietary intake or an additional supplement. Moreover, cretinism may occur in the baby if the mother has a severe iodine deficiency. Pregnant women can meet the iodine allowance of 220 mcg/day by using iodized salt. When salt is restricted, the physician may prescribe an iodine supplement.

SODIUM

Sodium is essential for proper metabolism and the regulation of fluid balance. Sodium intake in the form of salt is never entirely restricted during pregnancy even when hypertension is present. The pregnant woman may season food to taste during cooking but should avoid using extra salt at the table. She can avoid excessive intake by eliminating salty foods such as potato chips, ham, sausages, and sodium-based seasonings.

ZINC

Zinc is needed for protein metabolism and the synthesis of DNA and RNA. It is essential for normal fetal growth and development as well as milk production during lactation. The RDA during pregnancy is 11 mg/day for women ages 19 and older. This increases to 12 mg during lactation. Sources include meats, shellfish, poultry, whole grains, and legumes.

MAGNESIUM

Magnesium is essential for cellular metabolism and structural growth. The RDA for pregnancy is 350 mg/day for women ages 19 to 30 and 360 mg for women 31 to 50 years of age. Good sources include milk, whole grains, dark green vegetables, nuts, and legumes.

IRON

Iron requirements increase during pregnancy because of the growth of the fetus and placenta and the increased maternal blood volume. Anemia in pregnancy is mainly caused by low iron stores, although it may also be caused by inadequate intake of other nutrients, such as vitamins B_6 and B_{12}, folic acid, ascorbic acid, copper, and zinc. Iron deficiency anemia is generally defined as a decrease in the oxygen-carrying capacity of the blood. Anemia leads to a significant reduction in hemoglobin in the volume of packed red cells per deciliter of blood (hematocrit) or in the number of erythrocytes. Iron deficiency anemia in pregnancy is associated with an increased incidence of preterm birth, low-birth-weight newborns, and maternal and infant mortality (Hark & Catalano, 2012).

Fetal demands for iron further contribute to symptoms of anemia in the pregnant woman. The fetal liver stores iron, especially during the third trimester. The baby needs this stored iron during the first 4 months of life to compensate for the normally inadequate levels of iron in breast milk and non–iron-fortified formulas.

To prevent anemia, the woman must balance iron requirements and intake. Adequate iron intake is a problem for nonpregnant women and a greater one for pregnant women. By carefully choosing foods high in iron, the woman can increase her daily iron intake considerably. Lean meats, dark green leafy vegetables, eggs, and whole-grain and enriched breads and cereals are the usual food sources of iron. Other iron sources include dried fruits, legumes, shellfish, and molasses.

Iron absorption is usually higher for animal products than for vegetable products. However, the woman can increase absorption of iron from nonmeat sources by combining them with meat or a food rich in vitamin C. The RDA for iron during pregnancy is 27 mg/day, but this intake is almost impossible to achieve through diet alone. Thus, in the second and third trimesters, the pregnant woman should take a daily supplement of 30 mg elemental iron (Hark & Catalano, 2012). Unfortunately, iron supplements often cause gastrointestinal discomfort, especially if taken on an empty stomach. Taking the iron supplement after a meal may help reduce this discomfort. Iron supplements may also cause constipation, so an adequate fluid intake is important in pregnancy.

Vitamins

Vitamins are organic substances needed for life and growth. They are found in small amounts in specific foods and generally cannot be synthesized by the body in adequate amounts.

Vitamins are grouped according to solubility. Vitamins A, D, E, and K dissolve in fat; vitamin C and the B-complex vitamins dissolve in water. An adequate intake of all vitamins is essential during pregnancy; however, several are required in larger amounts to fulfill specific needs.

FAT-SOLUBLE VITAMINS

The fat-soluble vitamins, A, D, E, and K, are stored in the liver and thus are available if the dietary intake becomes inadequate. The major complication related to these vitamins is not deficiency but toxicity due to overdose. Unlike water-soluble vitamins, excess amounts of vitamins A, D, E, and K are not excreted in the urine. Symptoms of vitamin toxicity include nausea, gastrointestinal upset, dryness and cracking of the skin, and loss of hair.

Vitamin A. Vitamin A is involved in the growth of epithelial cells, which line the entire gastrointestinal tract and make up the skin. It also plays a role in the metabolism of carbohydrates and fats. Without vitamin A the body cannot synthesize glycogen, and the body's ability to handle cholesterol is also affected. In addition, the protective layer of tissue surrounding nerve fibers does not form properly if vitamin A is lacking.

Probably the best known function of vitamin A is its effect on vision in dim light. A person's ability to see in the dark depends on the eye's supply of retinol, a form of vitamin A. Adequate vitamin A prevents night blindness. Vitamin A is associated with the formation and development of healthy eyes in the fetus. The RDA for vitamin A is 770 mcg/day for pregnant women ages 19 and older.

Although routine supplementation with vitamin A is not recommended, supplementation with 5000 International Units is indicated for women whose dietary intake may be inadequate, such as strict vegetarians and recent emigrants from countries where deficiency of vitamin A is endemic. Rich sources of vitamin A include deep green, deep orange, and yellow vegetables; animal sources include egg yolk, cream, butter, and fortified margarine and milk.

Vitamin D. Vitamin D is best known for its role in the absorption and use of calcium and phosphorus in skeletal development. To supply the needs of the developing fetus, the pregnant woman should have a vitamin D intake of 5 mcg/day. Main food sources of vitamin D include fortified milk, margarine, butter, and egg yolks. Drinking a quart of milk daily provides the vitamin D needed during pregnancy. Vitamin D is also obtained through the synthesis of sunlight on the skin. However, during the winter months women who live in northern latitudes are at risk for limited sun exposure, as are women who routinely wear sun protection including high sun protection factor (SPF) products and protective clothing.

Vitamin D deficiency is more common than previously recognized. While universal screening for vitamin D deficiency is not currently recommended, women at risk (vegetarians, women with limited sun exposure, ethnic and racial groups with dark skin) may be screened. If a deficiency is identified, a daily dose of 1000 to 2000 International Units is safe (ACOG, 2011).

Excessive intake of vitamin D usually comes from high-potency vitamin preparations, not from the diet. Overdoses during pregnancy can cause hypercalcemia, or high blood calcium levels, due to withdrawal of calcium from the skeletal tissue. Symptoms of toxicity include excessive thirst, loss of appetite, vomiting, weight loss, irritability, and high blood calcium levels.

Vitamin E. The major function of vitamin E, or tocopherol, is antioxidation. Antioxidants such as vitamin E protect the body's cells from the destructive effects of free radicals. Vitamin E takes on oxygen, thus preventing another substance from combining with the oxygen in a process called *oxidation*. For example, vitamin E helps spare vitamin A by preventing its oxidation in the intestinal tract and in the tissues. It decreases the oxidation of polyunsaturated fats, thus helping to retain the flexibility and health of the cell membrane. For this reason, vitamin E affects the health of all cells in the body.

Vitamin E is also involved in certain enzymatic and metabolic reactions. It is essential for the synthesis of nucleic acids required in the formation of red blood cells in the bone marrow. Vitamin E is useful in treating certain types of muscular pain and intermittent claudication, in surface healing of wounds and burns, and in protecting lung tissue from the damaging effects of smog. These functions may help explain the abundant claims and cures attributed to vitamin E, many of which have not been scientifically proved.

The recommended intake of vitamin E for pregnant women is unchanged at 15 mg/day. Vitamin E is widely distributed in foodstuffs, especially vegetable fats and oils, whole grains, greens, and eggs. Excessive intake of vitamin E has been associated with abnormal coagulation in the newborn.

Vitamin K. Vitamin K, or menadione (as used synthetically in medicine), is essential for the synthesis of prothrombin, so its function is related to normal blood clotting. It is synthesized in the intestinal tract by the *Escherichia coli* bacterium normally found in the large intestine. However, the body's need for vitamin K is not totally met by synthesis. Green leafy vegetables are excellent sources. The RDA for vitamin K, 90 mcg per day, does not increase during pregnancy.

Intake of vitamin K is usually adequate in a well-balanced prenatal diet. Problems may arise if an illness is present that results in malabsorption of fats or if antibiotics are used for an extended period, which would inhibit vitamin K synthesis by destroying intestinal *E. coli*.

WATER-SOLUBLE VITAMINS

Water-soluble vitamins are excreted in the urine. Since only small amounts are stored, adequate amounts must be consumed daily. During pregnancy the concentration of water-soluble vitamins in the maternal serum falls, whereas high concentrations are found in the fetus.

Vitamin C. The requirement for vitamin C (ascorbic acid) increases in pregnancy from 75 to 85 mg. Vitamin C's major function is to aid in the formation and development of connective tissue and the vascular system. Ascorbic acid is essential to the formation of collagen, which binds cells together. If the collagen begins to disintegrate because of a lack of ascorbic acid, cell functioning is disturbed and cell structure breaks down, resulting in muscular weakness, capillary hemorrhage, and eventual death. These are symptoms of scurvy, the disease caused by vitamin C deficiency. Surprisingly, newborns of women who have taken megadoses of vitamin C may have a rebound form of scurvy.

Maternal plasma levels of vitamin C progressively decrease during pregnancy, with values at term being about half those found at midpregnancy. It appears that ascorbic acid concentrates in the placenta; levels in the fetus are 50% or more above maternal levels.

A nutritious diet should meet the pregnant woman's needs for vitamin C without additional supplementation. Common food sources of vitamin C include citrus fruit, tomatoes, cantaloupe, strawberries, potatoes, broccoli, and other leafy greens. Ascorbic acid is readily destroyed by water and oxidation. Therefore, foods containing vitamin C must be stored and cooked properly.

The B vitamins include thiamine (B_1), riboflavin (B_2), niacin, folic acid, pantothenic acid, vitamin B_6, and vitamin B_{12}. These vitamins serve as vital coenzyme factors in many reactions such as cell respiration, glucose oxidation, and energy metabolism. The quantities needed increase as caloric intake increases to meet the metabolic and growth needs of the pregnant woman.

- **Thiamine.** Required amount increases from the prepregnant level of 1.1 mg/day to 1.4 mg/day. *Sources:* pork, liver, milk, potatoes, and enriched breads and cereals.

- **Riboflavin.** Deficiency is manifested by *cheilosis* (fissures and cracks of the lips and corners of the mouth) and other skin lesions. During pregnancy women may excrete less riboflavin and still require more because of increased energy and protein needs. An additional 0.3 to 1.4 mg/day is recommended for pregnant women ages 19 and older. *Sources:* milk, liver, eggs, enriched breads, and cereals.

- **Niacin.** Intake should increase 4 mg/day during pregnancy to 18 mg. *Sources:* meat, fish, poultry, liver, whole grains, enriched breads, cereals, and peanuts.

- **Folic acid (folate).** Required for normal growth, reproduction, and lactation, **folic acid** prevents the macrocytic, megaloblastic anemia of pregnancy, which is rarely found in the United States, but does occur. Inadequate intake of folic acid has been associated with neural tube defects (NTDs) (spina bifida, meningomyelocele) in the fetus or newborn. Although these defects are considered multifactorial, research indicates that most of these birth defects could be prevented if folic acid supplementation recommendations were followed before most women know they are pregnant (Centers for Disease Control and Prevention [CDC], 2012). Consequently, experts recommend that all women of childbearing age (15 to 45 years) consume 400 mcg of folic acid daily because half of all U.S. pregnancies are unplanned and NTDs occur very early in pregnancy (3 to 4 weeks after conception), before most women realize they are pregnant (CDC, 2012). Folic acid can be made inactive by oxidation, ultraviolet light, and heating. To prevent unnecessary loss, foods should be stored covered to protect them from light, cooked with only a small amount of water, and not overcooked. *Sources:* fresh green leafy vegetables, liver, peanuts, and whole-grain breads and cereals.

- **Pantothenic acid.** No allowance has been set during pregnancy, but 5 mg/day is considered a safe, adequate intake. *Sources:* meats, egg yolk, legumes, and whole-grain cereals and breads.

- **Vitamin B_6 (pyridoxine).** Associated with amino acid metabolism, thus a higher-than-average protein intake requires increased pyridoxine intake. The RDA during pregnancy is 1.9 mg/day, an increase of 0.6 mg over the allowance for nonpregnant women. Generally, the slightly increased need can be supplied by diet. *Sources:* wheat germ, yeast, fish, liver, pork, potatoes, and lentils.

- **Vitamin B_{12} (cobalamin).** Plays a role in the synthesis of DNA and red blood cells, and is important in maintaining the myelin sheath of nerve cells. Vitamin B_{12} is the cobalt-containing vitamin found only in animal sources. Women of reproductive age rarely have a B_{12} deficiency. However, vegetarians/vegans (see later discussion on vegetarianism) can develop a deficiency so it is essential that their dietary intake be supplemented with this vitamin. Occasionally, vitamin B_{12} levels decrease during pregnancy but increase again after childbirth. The RDA during pregnancy is 2.6 mcg/day, an increase of 0.2 mcg. A deficiency may be because of a congenital inability to absorb vitamin B_{12}, resulting in pernicious anemia. Infertility is a complication of this type of anemia. *Sources:* foods that come from animals.

Clinical Tip

More women are consuming over-the-counter (OTC) vitamin, mineral, and food supplements today than in the past. Ask about the use of any OTC supplements to help avoid potentially harmful excess intakes.

Fluid

Water is essential for life, and it is found in all body tissues. It is necessary for many biochemical reactions. It also serves as a lubricant, as a medium of transport for carrying substances in and out of the body, and as an aid in temperature control. A pregnant woman should consume at least eight to ten 8-oz glasses of fluid each day, of which four to six glasses should be water. Because of their sodium content, sodas and diet sodas should be consumed in moderation. Caffeinated beverages have a diuretic effect, which is counterproductive to increasing fluid intake.

Clinical Reasoning **Weight Gain in Pregnancy**

Jaya Singh, a 28-year-old, G1P0, is 14 weeks pregnant. The rate and total amount of her weight gain during the first trimester have been consistent with recommendations. She has gained an average of 0.5 kg (1 lb) per week during both of the past 2 weeks. Her appetite is good, and she consumes three meals per day and snacks between meals on occasion.

Jaya has altered her diet because she is concerned about excessive weight gain. She told you that she has decreased her intake from the bread and dairy groups in order to limit her caloric intake. Because she has omitted most dairy products, she has increased her consumption of salads and broccoli to provide calcium sources.

A diet history revealed the following:

Grain	3–4 servings, mainly cereal and rice
Fruit	2–4 servings, fresh fruit
Vegetables	3–5 servings, salads, peas, corn, broccoli
Meat	4–5 servings, beef, pork, chicken
Dairy	occasionally cheese, ice cream, pudding
Fats, oils,	occasionally salad dressings, margarine, desserts sweets
Beverages	8–10 servings, soda, juices, water

After assessing her diet history, what is your evaluation of Jaya's diet? How would you counsel her?

TABLE 11–2 Vegetarian Food Groups

FOOD GROUP	MIXED DIET	LACTO-OVOVEGETARIAN	LACTOVEGETARIAN	VEGAN
Grain	Bread, cereal, rice, pasta	Bread, cereal, rice, pasta	Bread, cereal, rice, pasta	Bread, cereal, rice, pasta
Fruit	Fruit, fruit juices	Fruit, fruit juices	Fruit, fruit juices	Fruit, fruit juices
Vegetable	Vegetables, vegetable juices	Vegetables, vegetable juices	Vegetables, vegetable juices	Vegetables, vegetable juices
Dairy and dairy alternatives	Milk, yogurt, cheese	Milk, yogurt, cheese	Milk, yogurt, cheese	Fortified soy milk, rice milk
Meat and meat alternatives	Meat, fish, poultry, eggs, legumes, tofu, nuts, nut butters	Eggs, legumes, tofu, nuts, nut butters	Legumes, tofu, nuts, nut butters	Legumes, tofu, nuts, nut butters

Vegetarianism

Vegetarianism is the dietary choice of many people for religious, health, or ethical reasons. There are several types of vegetarians. **Lacto-ovovegetarians** include milk, dairy products, and eggs in their diet. **Lactovegetarians** include dairy products but no eggs in their diets. **Vegans** are "pure" vegetarians who will not eat any food from animal sources.

The expectant mother who is vegetarian must eat the proper combination of foods to obtain adequate nutrients. If her diet allows, a woman can obtain ample and complete proteins from dairy products and eggs. An adequate, pure vegan diet contains protein from unrefined grains (brown rice, whole wheat), legumes (beans, split peas, lentils), nuts in large quantities, and a variety of cooked and fresh vegetables and fruits. Complete proteins can be obtained by eating different types of plant-based proteins such as beans and rice, peanut butter on whole-grain bread, and whole-grain cereal with soy milk, either in the same meal or over the day. Seeds may provide adequate protein in the vegetarian diet if the quantity is large enough. Obtaining sufficient calories to ensure adequate weight gain

may be difficult because vegan diets tend to be high in fiber and therefore filling.

Because vegans use no animal products, a daily supplement of 4 mg of vitamin B_{12} is necessary. If soy milk is used, only partial supplementation may be needed. If no soy milk is taken, daily supplements of 1200 mg of calcium and 10 mg of vitamin D are needed.

Because the best sources of iron and zinc are animal products, vegan diets may also be low in these minerals. In addition, a high-fiber intake may reduce mineral (calcium, iron, and zinc) bioavailability. Nurses need to emphasize the use of foods containing these nutrients. A vegetarian food group guide appears in Table 11–2.

Factors Influencing Nutrition

It is important to consider the many factors that affect a client's nutrition. What are the age, lifestyle, and culture of the pregnant woman? What food beliefs and habits does she have? What a person eats is determined by availability, economics, and symbolism. These factors and others influence the expectant mother's acceptance of dietary recommendations.

EVIDENCE-BASED PRACTICE | Lifestyle Interventions to Improve Dietary Behaviors of Pregnant Women

Clinical Question

Can prenatal counseling improve the nutritional intake of pregnant women? Are these interventions effective across cultures?

The Evidence

Lack of sound nutritional intake can lead to a host of problems during pregnancy. Excessive weight gain has been linked to significant morbidity for both mother and baby. Even when weight is controlled, many pregnant women do not get adequate dietary intake of fruits, vegetables, and fiber in particular. Current practice guidelines recommend aggressive management of maternal weight before, during, and after pregnancy, and it is widely supported that nutritional counseling can be effective in preventing excessive weight gain. Two studies focused on nutritional counseling as a part of prenatal care, and its effectiveness in affecting eating behavior. In one study, researchers measured whether a relationship existed between healthcare providers discussing diet with their pregnant clients and subsequent changes in dietary intake. A second study reviewed a community-based, healthcare provider–led lifestyle intervention exclusively aimed at Spanish-speaking mothers. Taken together, more than 600 mothers were included in these studies; this yields a strong level of evidence.

The researchers found that healthcare providers can influence maternal nutritional intake when they counsel mothers

about its importance during routine prenatal care (May, Suminski, Berry, et al., 2014). Mothers who were provided information in the context of healthy behaviors were more likely to engage in healthy dietary practices during pregnancy than mothers who did not receive counseling from their healthcare providers. Similar findings were yielded in the Spanish-speaking population. When mothers received culturally appropriate interventions about lifestyle modifications in the prenatal period, they were more likely to reduce daily consumption of sugar, saturated fat, and caloric intake, and to increase vegetable and fiber intake (Kieffer, Welmerink, Sinco, et al., 2014).

Best Practice

The healthcare provider can have an impact on prenatal nutrition simply by addressing healthy lifestyle issues during pregnancy. This type of prenatal counseling is effective across other cultures when provided in an appropriate language and in a culturally sensitive way.

Clinical Reasoning

What are some cultural influences on nutrition that should be considered in prenatal counseling? What are other lifestyle behaviors that should be addressed alongside nutritional counseling in prenatal support services?

Common Discomforts of Pregnancy

Gastrointestinal functioning can be altered at times during pregnancy, resulting in discomforts such as nausea, vomiting, heartburn, and constipation. Although these changes can be uncomfortable for the woman, they are seldom a major problem. These discomforts and dietary modifications that may provide relief are discussed in Chapter 10.

Complementary and Alternative Therapies

While the use of some herbal, botanical, and alternative therapies may seem like a natural and safe alternative to some individuals, the pregnant consumer should take caution. Few clinical trials exist that have examined the safety of supplements and herbs during pregnancy. Many herbs, such as black haw, chamomile, dandelion, ginger, nettle leaf, and red raspberry are considered safe for use in pregnancy. Other herbs could pose a risk (Shinde, Patil, & Bairagi, 2012). Pregnant women should be advised to consult reputable sources such as the National Center for Complementary and Alternative Medicine website about these therapies and should also speak with their healthcare providers to determine the safety of such products or therapies.

Use of Artificial Sweeteners

Foods and beverages that contain artificial sweeteners are increasingly available. Sweeteners classified as Generally Recognized as Safe (GRAS) by the U.S. Food and Drug Administration (FDA) are acceptable for use during pregnancy and include acesulfame potassium (Sweet One), aspartame (NutraSweet, Equal), saccharin (Sweet'N Low, Sugar Twin), sucralose (Splenda), and stevia (Truvia, PureVia, SunCrystals). As with other foods, moderation should be exercised in using artificial sweeteners.

Energy Drinks

Energy drinks, such as Monster Energy, Red Bull, and 5-Hour Energy, used to boost performance and delay fatigue have become increasingly popular in recent years. These beverages are soft drinks with ingredients such as caffeine, ginseng, guarana, taurine, and sugar added to provide stimulation and increase energy. Because they are classified as dietary supplements and not food, they are not subject to the same regulations and monitoring as food (Guilbeau, 2012). The caffeine content of energy drinks can be as high as 300 mg (equivalent to about three average cups of brewed coffee). Excessive intake of energy drinks can cause a variety of symptoms, including anxiety, headache, agitation, tremors, seizures, psychosis, and altered mental state (Rath, 2012).

Energy drinks have come under scrutiny for the general public because of concerns about workplace safety when drinks are used to counter the effects of inadequate sleep and reports of deaths following excessive use (Meier, 2012). Research on the effects of caffeine on pregnancy are mixed, therefore pregnant women are advised to use energy drinks cautiously and include the drink's caffeine content in calculating daily caffeine intake in order to stay within recommended levels.

Foodborne Illnesses

Because of the risk of *Salmonella* contamination in raw eggs, pregnant women are advised to avoid eating or tasting foods that may contain raw or lightly cooked eggs. Examples include cake batter, homemade eggnog, sauces made with raw eggs such as Caesar salad dressing, and homemade ice cream.

Listeria monocytogenes is another bacterium that poses a threat to an expectant mother and her fetus. *Listeria* organisms are especially challenging because they can be found in refrigerated, ready-to-eat foods such as unpasteurized milk and dairy products, meat, poultry, and seafood. To prevent listerial infection (listeriosis), pregnant women should be advised to do the following (U.S. Food and Drug Administration [FDA], 2014):

- Maintain refrigerator temperature at 40°F (4°C) or below and the freezer at 0°F (−18°C).
- Refrigerate or freeze prepared foods, leftovers, and perishables within 2 hours after eating or preparation.
- Do not eat hot dogs and luncheon meats unless they are reheated until they are steaming hot.
- Avoid soft cheeses such as feta, brie, Camembert, blue-veined cheeses, queso fresco, or queso blanco (a soft cheese often used by Hispanic women in their cooking) unless the label clearly states that they are made with pasteurized milk.
- Do not eat refrigerated patés or meat spreads, foods that contain raw (unpasteurized) milk, or drink unpasteurized milk.
- Avoid eating refrigerated smoked seafood such as salmon, trout, cod, tuna, or mackerel unless it is in a cooked dish such as a casserole. Canned or shelf-stable patés, meat spreads, and smoked seafood are considered safe to eat.

Mercury in Fish

Fish and shellfish are important parts of a healthy diet, but nearly all contain traces of mercury. Although this is not a concern for most people, some fish and shellfish contain higher levels of mercury than others, and mercury can pose a serious threat to the developing nervous system of an unborn baby or a young child.

SAFETY ALERT!
Women who are pregnant or who may become pregnant, breastfeeding mothers, and young children should not eat swordfish, shark, tilefish, or king mackerel because these fish contain high levels of methyl mercury.

Many pregnant women are aware of the mercury warning, but are far less aware of the important nutritional value of fish, especially fish high in DHA. Consequently, fish consumption has declined but a strong body of evidence supports the nutritional value of fish during pregnancy (Carlson et al., 2013). Thus pregnant women need to be encouraged to eat at least 8 oz and up to 12 oz/week (two average meals) of shellfish and fish that are lower in mercury (USDA, 2012). Commonly eaten fish that are lower in mercury include canned light tuna, shrimp, salmon, catfish, and pollack. Albacore (white) tuna has more mercury than canned light tuna; therefore only 6 oz/week of albacore tuna is recommended.

Lactase Deficiency (Lactose Intolerance)

Some individuals have difficulty digesting milk and milk products. This condition, known as **lactase deficiency (lactose intolerance)**, results from an inadequate amount of the enzyme lactase, which breaks down the milk sugar lactose into smaller digestible substances.

Lactase deficiency is found in most adults of African, Mexican, Native American, Ashkenazi Jewish, and Asian descent and, indeed, in many other adults worldwide. People of northern European heritage are usually not affected. Symptoms include abdominal distention, discomfort, nausea, vomiting, loose stools, and cramps.

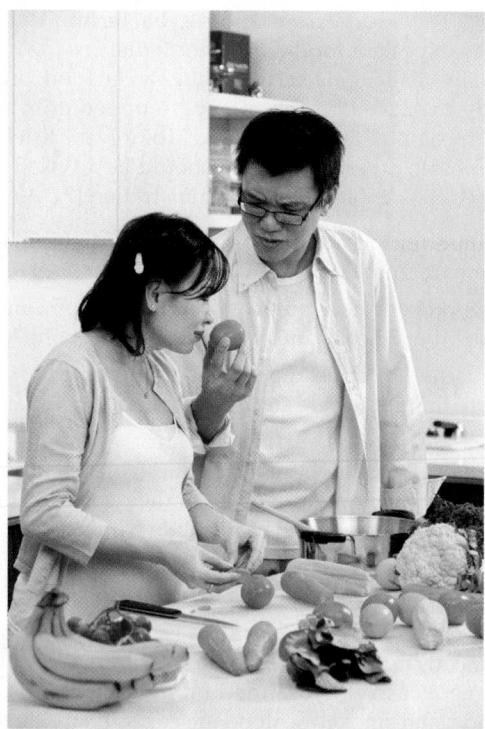

Figure 11–3 Cultural factors affect food preferences and habits.

SOURCE: © Arto/Fotolia.

In counseling pregnant women who might be intolerant of milk and milk products, be aware that even one glass of milk can produce symptoms. Milk in cooked form, such as custards, is sometimes tolerated, as are cultured or fermented dairy products such as buttermilk, some cheeses, kefir, and yogurt. Lactase deficiency need not be a problem for pregnant women because the enzyme is available over-the-counter in tablets or drops. Lactase-treated milk is also available commercially in some grocery stores.

Cultural, Ethnic, and Religious Influences

Cultural, ethnic, and religious backgrounds determine people's experiences with food and influence food preferences and habits (Figure 11–3). People of different nationalities are accustomed to eating different foods because of the kinds of foodstuffs available in their countries of origin. The way food is prepared varies, depending on the customs and traditions of the ethnic and cultural group. In addition, the laws of certain religions forbid the use of some foods and direct the preparation and serving of meals. (See *Developing Cultural Competence: The Kosher Diet.*)

Developing Cultural Competence The Kosher Diet

The kosher diet followed by many Jewish people forbids the eating of pork products and shellfish. Certain cuts of meat from sheep and cattle are allowed as are fish with fins and scales. In addition, according to kosher dietary rules, meat and dairy products should not be mixed and eaten at the same meal.

In each culture, certain foods have symbolic meaning. Generally, these symbolic foods are related to major life experiences such as birth, death, or developmental milestones. Although generalizations have been made about the food practices of ethnic and religious groups, there are many variations. The extent to which people continue to eat traditional ethnic foods and follow food-related ethnic customs is affected by their exposure to other cultures and the availability, quality, and cost of traditional foods.

When working with pregnant women from any ethnic background, it is important to understand the impact of the woman's cultural beliefs on her eating habits and to identify any beliefs she may have about food and pregnancy. Talking with the client can help determine the level of influence that traditional food customs exert. It is then possible to give dietary advice in a way that is meaningful to the woman and her family.

Psychosocial Factors

Various psychosocial factors may influence a woman's food choices. The sharing of food has long been a symbol of friendliness, warmth, and social acceptance in many cultures. Some foods and food practices are associated with status. Some foods are prepared "just for company"; others are served only on special occasions or holidays.

Socioeconomic level may be a determinant of nutritional status. Poverty-level families cannot afford the same foods that higher income families can. Thus pregnant women with low incomes are frequently at risk for poor nutrition.

Knowledge about the basic components of a balanced diet is essential. Often educational level is related to economic status, but even people on very limited incomes can prepare well-balanced meals if they know enough about nutrition.

The expectant mother's attitudes and feelings about her pregnancy influence her nutritional status. For example, foods may be used as a substitute for the expression of emotions, such as anger or frustration, or as a way of expressing feelings of joy. The woman who is depressed or does not wish to be pregnant may manifest these feelings in loss of appetite or overindulgence in certain foods.

Eating Disorders

Two serious eating disorders, anorexia nervosa and bulimia nervosa (or simply bulimia), affect millions of men and women, although they develop most commonly in adolescent girls and young women. Both conditions are psychologic disorders that can have a major impact on physiologic well-being.

Anorexia nervosa is an eating disorder characterized by an extreme fear of weight gain and fat. People with this problem have distorted body images and perceive themselves as fat even when they are extremely underweight. Their dietary intake is very restrictive in both variety and quantity. They may also engage in excessive exercise to prevent weight gain.

Bulimia is characterized by binge eating (secretly consuming large amounts of food in a short time) and purging. Self-induced vomiting is the most common method of purging; laxatives or diuretics may also be used. Individuals with bulimia nervosa often maintain normal or near-normal weight for their height, so it is difficult to know whether bingeing and purging occur.

Women with anorexia nervosa do not often become pregnant because of the physiologic changes that affect their reproductive systems. Women with bulimia can become pregnant. Their self-induced vomiting may produce many of the same complications as hyperemesis gravidarum (see Chapter 15). In both anorexia nervosa and bulimia, a multidisciplinary approach to treatment, involving medical, nursing, psychiatric, and dietetic practitioners, is indicated. Pregnant women with eating disorders need to be closely monitored and supported throughout their pregnancies.

Pica

Pica is the persistent eating of substances, such as soil or clay (geophagia), powdered laundry starch or corn starch (amylophagia), soap, baking powder, ice (pagophagia), freezer frost, burned matches, paint, or ashes that are not ordinarily considered edible or nutritionally valuable. Most women who eat such substances do so only during pregnancy.

Women who practice pica may have nutrient deficiencies because they often consume a less varied diet than they might otherwise eat. Iron deficiency anemia is the most common concern in pica. Eating laundry starch or certain types of clay may contribute to iron deficiency because they interfere with iron absorption. The ingestion of large quantities of clay could fill the intestine and cause fecal impaction; eating starch may be associated with excessive weight gain. Lead levels should be checked in women who may have eaten peeling paint.

Assessment for pica is an important part of a nutritional history. However, a woman may be embarrassed about her cravings or reluctant to discuss them for fear of criticism. Using a nonjudgmental approach, give the woman information that can help her decrease or eliminate this practice. Some women are able to switch to eating nonfat powdered milk instead of powdered laundry starch and frozen fruit juice instead of ice. Others find that sucking on hard lemon or mint candies helps decrease the craving.

Nutritional Care of the Pregnant Adolescent

Nutritional care of the pregnant adolescent is of particular concern to healthcare professionals. Many adolescents are nutritionally at risk because of a variety of complex emotional, social, and economic factors. Important nutrition-related factors to assess in pregnant adolescents include low prepregnant weight, low weight gain during pregnancy, young age at menarche, smoking, excessive prepregnant weight, anemia, unhealthy lifestyle (drugs or alcohol use), chronic disease, and history of an eating disorder.

The nutritional needs of adolescents are generally estimated by using the Dietary Reference Intakes (DRIs) for nonpregnant teenagers (ages 11 to 14 or 15 to 18) and adding nutrient amounts recommended for all women. If she is mature (more than 4 years since menarche), the pregnant adolescent's nutritional needs approach those reported for pregnant adults. However, adolescents who become pregnant less than 4 years after menarche are at risk because of their physiologic and anatomic immaturity. They are more likely than older adolescents to still be growing, which can affect the fetus's development. Thus young adolescents (ages 14 and younger) need to gain more weight than older adolescents (18 years and older) to produce babies of equal size.

In determining the optimal weight gain for the pregnant adolescent, add the recommended weight gain for an adult pregnancy to that expected during the postmenarchal year in which the pregnancy occurs. If the teenager is underweight, additional weight gain is recommended to bring her to a normal weight for her height.

Specific Nutrient Concerns

Caloric needs of pregnant adolescents vary widely. Major factors in determining caloric needs include whether growth has been completed and the physical activity level of the individual. Figures as high as 50 kcal/kg have been suggested for young, growing teens who are very active physically. A satisfactory weight gain usually confirms an adequate caloric intake.

An inadequate iron intake is a major concern with the adolescent diet. Iron needs are high for the pregnant teen due to the requirement for iron by the enlarging maternal muscle mass and blood volume. Iron supplements are definitely indicated.

Calcium is another important nutrient for pregnant adolescents. Inadequate intake of calcium is often a problem in this age group. Adequate calcium intake is necessary to support normal growth and development of the fetus as well as growth and maintenance of calcium stores in the adolescent. An extra serving of dairy products is usually suggested for teenagers. Calcium supplementation is indicated for teens who dislike milk unless they consume enough other dairy products or significant calcium sources.

Because folic acid plays a role in cell reproduction, it is also an important nutrient for pregnant teens. As previously indicated, a supplement is usually recommended for pregnant females of all ages.

Other nutrients and vitamins must be considered when evaluating the overall nutritional quality of the teenager's diet. Nutrients that have frequently been found to be deficient in this age group include zinc and vitamins A, D, and B_6. Eating a variety of foods—especially fresh and lightly processed foods—helps the teen get adequate amounts of trace minerals, fiber, and other vitamins.

Dietary Patterns

Healthy adolescents often have irregular eating patterns. Many skip breakfast, and most tend to be frequent snackers. Teens rarely follow the traditional three-meals-a-day pattern. Their day-to-day intake often varies drastically, and they eat food combinations that may seem bizarre to adults. Despite these practices, adolescents usually achieve a better nutritional balance than most adults would expect.

In assessing the diet of the pregnant adolescent, it is important to consider the eating pattern over time, not simply a single day's intake. Once the pattern is identified, counseling can be directed toward correcting deficiencies.

Counseling Issues

Counseling about nutrition and healthy eating practices is an important element of care for pregnant teenagers. Nurses can effectively provide this counseling in a community setting. It may be individualized, involve other teens, or provide a combination of both approaches. If an adolescent's family member does most of the meal preparation, it may be useful to include that person in the discussion if the adolescent agrees. Involving the expectant father in counseling may also be helpful. Clinics and schools often offer classes and focused activities designed to address this topic.

The pregnant teenager's understanding of nutrition will influence not only her well-being but also that of her child. However, teens tend to live in the present, and counseling that stresses long-term changes may be less effective than more concrete approaches. In many cases, group classes are effective, especially those with other teens.

Nursing Management

For the Pregnant Woman Desiring Optimum Nutrition

Nursing Assessment and Diagnosis

To plan an optimal diet with each woman, it is essential to assess nutritional status. The woman's medical record and a client interview provide information about the following:

- Woman's height and weight, as well as her weight gain during pregnancy

- Pertinent laboratory values, especially hemoglobin and hematocrit

- Clinical signs that have possible nutritional implications, such as constipation, anorexia, or heartburn

- Dietary history to evaluate the woman's views on nutrition as well as her specific nutrient intake

While gathering data, seek information about psychologic, cultural, and socioeconomic factors that may influence food intake. Also use the opportunity to discuss important aspects of nutrition within the context of the family's needs and lifestyle. A nutritional questionnaire is often useful in gathering and recording important facts. This information can be used to develop an intervention plan to fit the woman's individual needs. The sample questionnaire shown in Figure 11–4 has been filled in to demonstrate this process.

Once information is obtained, begin to analyze the information, formulate appropriate nursing diagnoses, and, with the woman, develop goals and desired outcomes. Nursing diagnoses might include the following (NANDA-I © 2014).

For a woman during the first trimester, the diagnosis may be *Nutrition, Imbalanced: Less than Body Requirements related to nausea and vomiting.* If a woman has excessive weight gain, the diagnosis might be *Overweight, Risk for, related to excessive caloric intake.* Be specific in addressing issues such as inadequate intake of nutrients, including iron, calcium, or folic acid; problems with nutrition because of a limited food budget; problems related to physiologic alterations, including anorexia, heartburn, or nausea; and behavioral problems related to excessive dieting, binge eating, and so on. At other times, the diagnosis *Knowledge, Readiness for Enhanced, related to nutrition* may seem most appropriate, especially if the woman asks for information about nutrition.

Planning and Implementation

After determining the nursing diagnosis, plan an approach to address any nutritional deficiencies or improve the overall quality of the diet. To be truly effective, this plan must be made in cooperation with the woman. The following example demonstrates ways to plan with the woman based on the nursing diagnosis (NANDA-I © 2014):

- *Nutrition, Imbalanced: Less than Body Requirements* related to low intake of calcium

- *Goal:* The woman will increase her daily intake of calcium to the minimum DRI level.

- *Implementation:*
  1. Plan with the woman how to add more milk or dairy products to the diet (specify amounts).
  2. Encourage the use of other calcium sources such as leafy greens and legumes.
  3. Plan for the addition of powdered milk in cooking and baking.
  4. If none of the preceding options is realistic or acceptable, consider the use of calcium supplements.

Most families can benefit from guidance about food purchasing and preparation. Advise women to plan food purchases thoughtfully by preparing general menus and a list before shopping. It is also helpful to monitor sales, compare brands, and be cautious when purchasing convenience foods, which tend to be expensive. Other techniques for keeping food costs down without jeopardizing quality include buying food in season, using bulk foods when appropriate, using whole-grain or enriched products, buying lower grade eggs (grading has no relation to the egg's nutritional value but indicates color of the shell, delicacy of flavor, and so forth), and avoiding foods from specialty shops and foods in elaborate packaging.

Health Promotion: Optimizing Maternal–Fetal Health summarizes key actions pregnant women can take to optimize maternal health and reduce the risk of birth defects.

Health Promotion **Optimizing Maternal–Fetal Health**

- Achieve appropriate weight gain based on prepregnancy weight and BMI.

- Participate in regular physical activity (at least 30 minutes of moderate, safe activity on most, if not all, days).

- Consume a variety of healthy foods that form the basic food groups, including fruits, vegetables, grains, proteins, and dairy using MyPlate as a guideline.

- Consume 8 to 12 oz of fish high in omega-3 fatty acids weekly.

- Take appropriate vitamin and mineral supplements.

- Consume caffeine in moderation.

- Avoid alcohol, tobacco, and other harmful substances.

- Follow safe food handling practices.

Source: Data from the American College of Obstetricians and Gynecologists (2013). *Nutrition during pregnancy.* Patient Education Pamphlet AP001. Washington, DC: Author.

Evaluation

Once a plan has been developed and implemented, the nurse and client may wish to identify ways of evaluating its effectiveness. Evaluation may involve keeping a food journal, writing out weekly menus, returning for weekly weigh-ins, and the like. If anemia is a special problem, periodic hematocrit assessments are indicated.

Postpartum Nutrition

Nutritional needs change following childbirth. Nutrient requirements vary depending on whether the mother decides to breastfeed. An assessment of postpartum nutritional status is necessary before nutritional guidance is given.

Postpartum Nutritional Status

Postpartum nutritional status is determined by assessing the new mother's weight, hemoglobin and hematocrit levels, clinical signs, and dietary history. As mentioned previously, an ideal weight gain during pregnancy is 25 to 35 lb (11.5 to 16.0 kg). After birth there is a weight loss of approximately 10 to 12 lb (4.5 kg to 5.4 kg). Additional weight loss is most rapid during the next few weeks as the body adjusts to the end of pregnancy. The mother's weight then begins to stabilize. This weight stabilization may take 6 months or longer.

The mother's weight should be considered in terms of ideal weight, prepregnancy weight, and weight gain during pregnancy. Refer women who want information about weight reduction to a dietitian or community-based nutritional program.

NUTRITIONAL QUESTIONNAIRE

Name Susan Longmont   **Date** 2-18-15

Age 20

Ethnic group Caucasian

Religion Protestant

Gravida 1   **Para** 0   **EDB** 9-12-15

Age of youngest child? NA

Birth weights of previous children? NA

Usual nonpregnant weight 119   **Present weight** 125

Weight gain during last pregnancy? NA

Vitamin or herbal supplements? none

Current medications? aspirin for headache

Do you smoke? yes   **How much per day?** 1-1½ packs

Have you ever had anorexia or bulimia?   **Please describe the circumstances.**

Eating patterns:

1. How many meals per day? 2   **when** 12:30 pm   6:30 pm
2. How many snacks per day? 3   **when** 10:30 am   4:00 pm   10:00 pm
3. What other foods are important to your usual diet? chocolate and candy bars
4. Amount per day 4 bars/week
5. Do you have any different food preferences now? no
6. Do you eat nonfoods such as:

		Amount
laundry starch	no	NA
ice	yes	10 cubes/day
other (name)	no	NA

7. What foods do you dislike or do not eat? spinach and dried beans
8. For added information complete a typical daily intake (24-hour recall is suggested).

Do you have special problems in food preparation such as:

1. Physical disability   yes   no ✓   Explain
2. Cooking appliances   yes   no ✓   Explain
3. Refrigeration of food   yes   no ✓   Explain

Who does the meal planning? I do.   **shopping?** We both do.

cooking? I do most of the time but my husband likes to help.

Are there transportation problems? We have only one car but we go in the evening.

Financial situation: My husband is working and going to school.

I am not working.   **Food Stamps** yes   **WIC** no

Do you have any previous nutritional problems? No. I have never paid much attention

to food before, but now I have lots of questions.

Are there any problems with this pregnancy? Nausea Yes, in the morning.

Constipation No   **Other** NA

Assessment by the nurse following the completion of the questionnaire.

Basic estimated nutrient and caloric value of typical daily intake.

Please circle one of the following:

Protein intake was	low	adequate	high
Caloric intake was	low	adequate	high
Calcium intake was	low	adequate	high
Iron intake was	low	adequate	high
Vitamin C intake was	low	adequate	high

Figure 11–4   The form shown here is a sample nutritional questionnaire used in the nursing management of a pregnant woman.

Hemoglobin and erythrocyte levels should return to normal within 2 to 6 weeks after childbirth. Iron supplements are generally continued for 2 to 3 months following childbirth to build stores depleted by pregnancy.

Constipation is a common problem following birth. To prevent it the woman should maintain a high fluid intake, which helps keep the stool soft. Dietary sources of fiber, such as whole grains, fruits, and vegetables, also help prevent constipation.

It is important to get specific information on dietary intake and eating habits directly from the woman. Visiting the mother during mealtimes provides an opportunity for unobtrusive nutritional assessment. Which foods has the woman selected? Is her diet nutritionally sound? A comment focusing on a positive aspect of her meal selection may initiate a discussion of nutrition.

Notify the dietitian about any woman whose cultural or religious beliefs require specific foods so that appropriate meals can be prepared for her. Also consider referring women with unusual eating habits or numerous questions about good nutrition to the dietitian. In addition, providing literature on nutrition ensures that the woman has a source of information at home.

During the childbearing years the risk for obesity becomes especially problematic for women. Consequently, it is critical to use the postpartum period to change behaviors and help promote effective weight management in women.

Nutritional Care of Formula-Feeding Mothers

After birth the formula-feeding mother's dietary requirements return to prepregnancy levels. If the mother has a good understanding of nutritional principles, it is sufficient to advise her to reduce her daily caloric intake by about 300 kcal and to return to prepregnancy levels for other nutrients. If the mother has a limited understanding of nutrition, now is the time to teach her the basic principles and the importance of a well-balanced diet. Her eating habits and dietary practices will eventually be reflected in the diet of her child.

If the mother has gained excessive weight during pregnancy (or perhaps was overweight before pregnancy) and wishes to lose weight, a referral to the dietitian is appropriate. The dietitian can design weight reduction diets to meet nutritional needs and food preferences. Weight loss goals of 1 to 2 lb (0.45 to 0.9 kg)/week are usually suggested.

In addition to meeting her own nutritional needs, the new mother is usually interested in learning how to provide for her infant's nutritional needs. A discussion of infant feeding that includes topics such as selecting infant formulas, formula preparation, and vitamin and mineral supplementation are appropriate and generally well received.

Nutritional Care of Breastfeeding Mothers

A breastfeeding woman needs increased nutrients. Table 11–1 provides a sample daily food guide for lactating women. It is especially important for the breastfeeding mother to consume sufficient calories because inadequate caloric intake can reduce milk volume. However, milk quality generally remains unaffected. The breastfeeding mother should increase her calories by about 200 kcal over her pregnancy requirement, or 500 kcal over her prepregnancy requirement. This results in a total of about 2500 to 2700 kcal/day for most women.

Because protein is an important ingredient in breast milk, an adequate intake while breastfeeding is essential. An intake of 65 g/day during the first 6 months of breastfeeding and 62 g/day during the second 6 months is recommended. As in pregnancy, it is important to consume adequate nonprotein calories to prevent the use of protein as an energy source.

Calcium is an important ingredient in milk production. Requirements during lactation remain the same as during pregnancy—an increase of 1000 mg/day. If the intake of calcium from food sources is not adequate, calcium supplements are recommended.

Iron is not a principal mineral component of milk; thus the needs of lactating women are not substantially different from those of nonpregnant women. However, supplementation for 2 to 3 months after childbirth is advisable to replenish maternal stores depleted by pregnancy.

Clinical Tip

Explain to breastfeeding mothers that liquids are especially important during lactation because inadequate fluid intake may decrease milk volume. Encourage them to drink at least eight to ten 8-oz glasses of fluid daily, including water, juice, milk, and soups.

In addition to counseling breastfeeding mothers on how to meet their increased nutrient needs, the nurse should discuss a few issues related to infant feeding. For example, many mothers are concerned about how specific foods they eat will affect their babies during breastfeeding. Generally, the breastfeeding mother need not avoid any foods except those to which she might be allergic. Occasionally, however, some breastfeeding mothers find that their babies are affected by certain foods. Onions, turnips, cabbage, chocolate, spices, and seasonings are commonly listed as offenders. The best advice to give the breastfeeding mother is to avoid those foods she suspects cause distress in her baby. For the most part, however, she should be able to eat any nourishing food she wants without fear that her baby will be affected. For further discussion of successful infant feeding, see Chapter 25.

Community Resources

Food is a significant portion of a family's budget, and meeting nutritional needs may be a challenge for families on limited incomes. Community-based services offered through clinics, local agencies, schools, and volunteer organizations address these needs. Increasingly, nurses play an important role in managing such community-based services, especially services focusing on client education. Most communities offer special assistance to qualifying families to meet their nutritional needs. The Supplemental Nutrition Assistance Program (SNAP), formerly referred to as the Food Stamp Program, provides an Electronic Benefit Transfer or EBT card, which is similar to a debit card, for participating households whose net monthly income is below a specified level. This card can be used to purchase food for the household each month.

The Special Supplemental Nutrition Program for Women, Infants, and Children (WIC) is designed to assist pregnant or breastfeeding women with low incomes and their children under 5 years of age. To be eligible, applicants must meet income guidelines (income at or below 185% of the U.S. poverty level), state residency requirements, and be individually determined to be nutritionally at risk by a healthcare professional (Food and Nutrition Service, 2013). The program provides food assistance, nutrition education, and referrals to healthcare providers. The food distributed, including dried beans and peas, peanut butter, eggs, cheese, milk, fortified adult and infant cereals, juice, and iron-fortified formula, is designed to provide good sources of iron, protein, and certain vitamins and minerals for people with an inadequate diet.

Focus Your Study

- Maternal weight gains averaging 25 to 35 lb (11.5 to 16.0 kg) for a normal-weight woman are associated with the best reproductive outcomes.

- If the diet is adequate, folic acid and iron are the only supplements generally recommended during pregnancy.

- Women should not restrict caloric intake to reduce weight during pregnancy.

- Pregnant women should be encouraged to eat regularly and to eat a wide variety of foods, especially fresh and lightly processed foods.

- Taking megadoses of vitamins during pregnancy is unnecessary and potentially dangerous.

- Pregnant women who eat vegetarian diets should place special emphasis on obtaining ample proteins, calories, calcium, iron, vitamin D, vitamin B_{12}, and zinc through food sources or supplementation if necessary.

- Pregnant women should avoid eating fish such as swordfish, shark, tilefish, or king mackerel, which contain high levels of mercury, and should limit their intake of fish that are lower in mercury.

- Food safety and sanitation should be a priority when preparing and storing food; foods that are known to cause foodborne illness should be avoided during pregnancy.

- Evaluation of physical, psychosocial, and cultural factors that affect food intake is essential before the nurse can determine nutritional status and plan nutritional counseling.

- Adolescents who become pregnant less than 4 years after menarche have higher nutritional needs and are considered to be at high biologic risk.

- Weight gains during adolescent pregnancy must accommodate recommended gains for a normal pregnancy plus necessary gains due to growth.

- After childbirth, the formula-feeding mother's dietary requirements return to prepregnancy levels.

- Breastfeeding mothers require an additional 200 calories above pregnancy intake and increased fluid intake to maintain ample milk volume.

Clinical Reasoning in Action

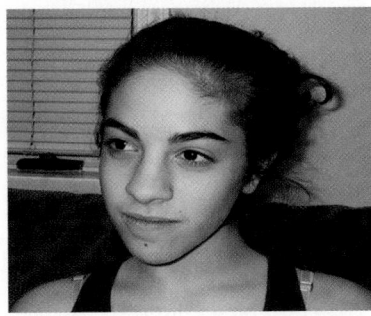

Sandra Hill is a 17-year-old at 19 weeks' gestation with her first pregnancy. She presents to you accompanied by her mother. Her mother tells you that Sandra is an active teenager who plays sports and has been taking dance lessons for 5 years. She maintains a B+ average in school.

Sandra voices concern about potential weight gain during pregnancy. She tells you that this was not a planned pregnancy and she has ambivalent feelings about it. You become concerned as she tells you that she has reduced her caloric intake over the past few months to try to keep her weight down and camouflage her pregnancy. You do a nutritional assessment and find that she is deficient in calcium, iron, and protein. Sandra seems to have irregular eating patterns and she admits to skipping breakfast often. She asks why she has to gain so much weight when you explain the nutritional needs of her baby during the pregnancy.

1. Discuss weight distribution in pregnancy.
2. Discuss foods that will increase calcium, protein, and iron in her diet.
3. Explain why folate supplementation is important.
4. What criteria will measure adequate caloric intake during pregnancy?

References

American College of Obstetricians and Gynecologists (ACOG). (2011). *Vitamin D: Screening and supplementation during pregnancy* (Committee Opinion No. 495). Washington, DC: Author.

American College of Obstetricians and Gynecologists (ACOG). (2013a). *Obesity in pregnancy* (Committee Opinion No. 549). Washington, DC: Author.

American College of Obstetricians and Gynecologists (ACOG). (2013b). *Weight gain during pregnancy* (Committee Opinion No. 548). Washington, DC: Author.

Carlson, S. E., Colombo, J., Gajewski, B. J., Gustafson, K. M., Mundy, D., Yeast, J., ... Shaddy, D. J. (2013). DHA supplementation and pregnancy outcomes. *The American Journal of Clinical Nutrition, 97*(4), 808–815.

Centers for Disease Control and Prevention (CDC). (2012). *Folic acid: Recommendations.* Retrieved from http://www.cdc.gov/ncbddd/folicacid/recommendations.html

Food and Nutrition Service. (2013). *WIC: The Special Supplemental Nutrition Program for Women, Infants, and Children.* Retrieved from http://www.fns.usda.gov/wic/default.htm

Guilbeau, J. R. (2012). Health risks of energy drinks. *Nursing for Women's Health, 16*(5), 423–428.

Hark, L., & Catalano, P. M. (2012). Nutritional management during pregnancy. In S. G. Gabbe, J. R. Niebyl, J. L. Simpson, M. B. Landon, H. L. Galan, E. R. M. Jauniaux, & D. A. Driscoll (Eds.), *Obstetrics: Normal and problem pregnancies* (6th ed.). Philadelphia, PA: Elsevier Saunders.

Institute of Medicine (IOM). (2009). *Weight gain during pregnancy: Reexamining the guidelines.* Washington, DC: National Academies Press.

Kieffer, E., Welmerink, D., Sinco, B., Welch, K., Clayton, E., Schumann, C., & Uhley, V. (2014). Dietary outcomes in a Spanish-language randomized controlled diabetes prevention trial with pregnant Latinas. *American Journal of Public Health, 104*(3), 526–533.

May, L., Suminski, R., Berry, A., Linklater, E., & Jahnke, S. (2014). Diet and pregnancy: Healthcare providers and patient behaviors. *The Journal of Perinatal Education, 23*(1), 50–56.

Meier, B. (2012). F.D.A. may tap experts on energy drinks. *New York Times.* Retrieved from http://www.nytimes.com/2012/11/28/business/fda-may-tap-experts-on-energy-drinks.html?_r=0

Rath, M. (2012). Energy drinks: What is all the hype? The dangers of energy drink consumption. *Journal of the American Academy of Nurse Practitioners, 24*(2), 70–76.

Shinde, P., Patil, P., & Bairagi, V. (2012). Herbs in pregnancy and lactation: A review appraisal. *International Journal of Pharmaceutical Sciences and Research, 3*(9), 3001–3006.

U.S. Department of Agriculture (USDA). (2012). *Maternal intake of seafood omega-3 fatty acids and infant health: A review of the evidence.* Retrieved from http://www.cnpp.usda.gov/sites/default/files/nutrition_insights_uploads/Insight46.pdf

U.S. Food and Drug Administration (FDA). (2014). *Food safety for moms-to-be: While you're pregnant—listeria.* Retrieved from http://www.fda.gov/Food/FoodborneIllnessContaminants/PeopleAtRisk/ucm083320.htm

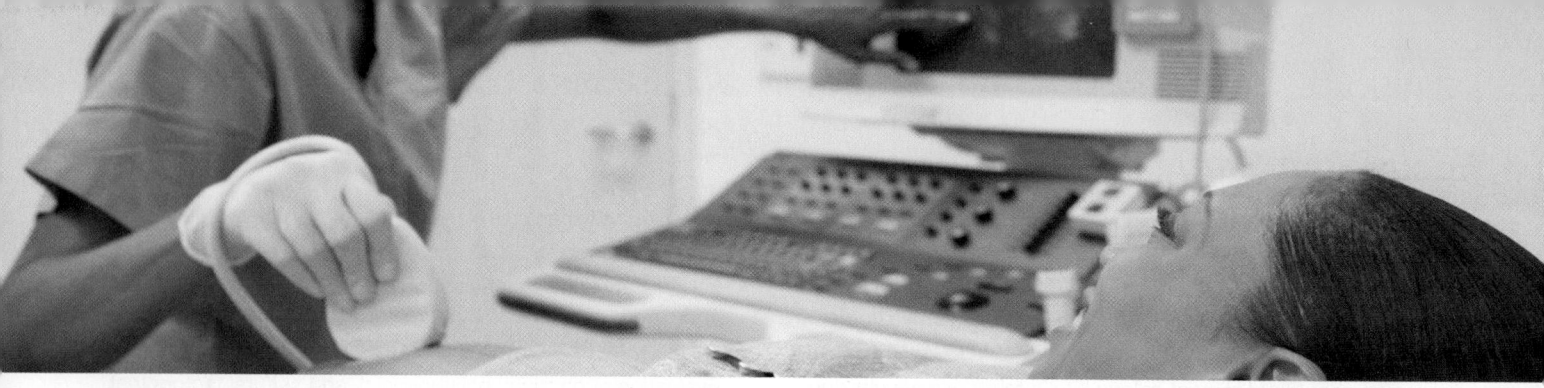

Chapter 12
Pregnancy in Selected Populations

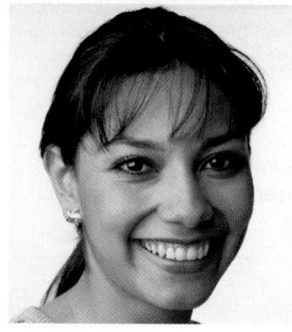

My daughter and I make quite a pair. She is 17 and pregnant with my first grandchild and I am 39 and, quite unexpectedly, pregnant with my third child. I am not sure which of us was more surprised, but we are adjusting. The important thing is that we do all we can to ensure that our babies—we are both expecting boys—stay healthy.

—Sophia, married, works as an accountant

Kevin Peterson/Getty Images

∨ Learning Outcomes

12.1 Describe the scope of the problem and the impact of adolescent pregnancy.

12.2 Identify the physical, psychologic, and sociologic risks a pregnant adolescent faces.

12.3 Delineate the characteristics of the fathers of children of adolescent mothers.

12.4 Discuss the possible reactions of the adolescent's family and social network to her pregnancy.

12.5 Describe successful community approaches to prevention of adolescent pregnancy.

12.6 Describe factors that have contributed to the increased incidence of pregnancy in women over 35 years of age.

12.7 Summarize the nursing care needs of an expectant woman over age 35.

12.8 Discuss general health care risks that a woman with a significant chronic physical disability might face during pregnancy.

12.9 Identify the key needs of a pregnant woman with an intellectual disability.

While pregnancy is a normal process, for certain women, it carries increased risk. This is especially true for adolescents, pregnant women over age 35, and women with physical and/or mental disabilities. This chapter focuses on their needs and care.

Adolescent Pregnancy

In the United States, each year about 750,000 teenage girls (ages 15 to 19) become pregnant. Of these pregnancies, about one fourth (26%) are terminated by therapeutic abortion (Alan Guttmacher Institute [AGI], 2012a). A portion of pregnancies end in miscarriage, but more than half of teens who become pregnant give birth and keep their babies.

U.S. teenage childbearing has declined steadily over the last few decades. In 2013, the birth rate (number of births per 1000 women) for adolescents ages 15 to 19 fell to 26.6, a historic low level, specifically the lowest rate reported in over half a century (Ventura, Hamilton, & Mathews, 2014). See Figure 12–1. Equally significant, these declines occurred for all race and Hispanic origin groups, although rates for Hispanic teens (46.3) and non-Hispanic Black teens (43.9) remain considerably higher than the rates for non-Hispanic White teens (20.5) (Ventura et al., 2014).

Even with this recent decline in adolescent pregnancies, the U.S. teenage birth rate remains one of the highest of any industrialized nation (exceeded only by Bulgaria [41.7] and Romania [35.2]), almost twice as high as Canada (14.1) and 6 times as high as the Netherlands (4.8) and Japan (4.5) (Ventura et al., 2014).

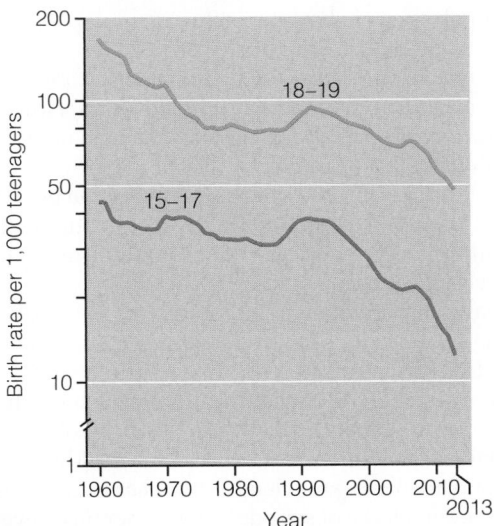

Figure 12-1 Birth rates for teenagers aged 15–17 and 18–19: United States, 1960–2013.

SOURCE: CDC/NCHS National Vital Statistics System. [Retrieved from http://www.cdc.gov/nchs/data/nvsr/nvsr63/nvsr63_04.pdf]

Healthy People 2020

(FP-8) Reduce pregnancies among adolescent females

(FP-9) Increase the proportion of adolescents aged 17 years and under who have never had sexual intercourse

(FP-12) Increase the proportion of adolescents who received formal instruction on reproductive health topics before they were 18 years old

Overview of the Adolescent Period

PHYSICAL CHANGES

Puberty—that period during which an individual becomes capable of reproduction—is a maturational process that can last from 1.5 to 6 years. The major physical changes of puberty include a growth spurt, weight change, and the appearance of secondary sexual characteristics. Menarche, or the time of the first menstrual period, usually occurs in the last half of this maturational process, with the average age between 12 and 13. The initial menstrual cycles are usually irregular and often anovulatory, although not always. Thus, contraception is important for all sexually active adolescents.

PSYCHOSOCIAL DEVELOPMENT

Many authorities have described the developmental tasks of adolescence, based on a variety of classic theories. The following are major developmental tasks of this period (Steinberg, 2014):

- Developing a sense of identity
- Gaining autonomy and independence
- Developing intimacy in a relationship
- Developing comfort with one's own sexuality
- Developing a sense of achievement

Resolution of these tasks is a developmental process that occurs over time. Although average ages for the completion of tasks have been identified, these ages are somewhat arbitrary and are affected by many factors, including culture, religion, and socioeconomic status.

In **early adolescence** (ages 14 and under), teens still see authority in their parents. However, they begin the process of gaining independence from the family by spending more time with friends. Conformity to peer group standards is important. Adolescents in this phase are very egocentric and are concrete thinkers, with only a minimal ability to see themselves in the future or to foresee the consequences of their behavior. Teens perceive their locus of control as external; that is, their destinies are controlled by others such as parents and school authorities.

Middle adolescence (ages 15 to 17 years) is the time for challenging; experimenting with drugs, alcohol, and sex are common avenues for rebellion. Middle adolescents seek independence and turn increasingly to their peer groups. They begin to move from concrete thinking to formal operational thought, but they are not yet able to anticipate the long-term implications of all their actions. These years are often a time of great turmoil for the family as the adolescent struggles for independence and challenges the family's values and expectations.

In **late adolescence** (ages 18 to 19 years) teens are more at ease with their individuality and decision-making ability. They can think abstractly and anticipate consequences. Late adolescents are capable of formal operational thought. They learn to solve problems, to conceptualize, and to make decisions. These abilities help them see themselves as having control, which leads to the ability to understand and accept the consequences of their behavior.

Factors Contributing to Adolescent Pregnancy

SOCIOECONOMIC AND CULTURAL FACTORS

Poverty is a major risk factor for adolescent pregnancy. Adolescents who do not have access to middle-class opportunities tend to maintain their pregnancies because they see pregnancy as their only option for adult status. Kearney and Levine (2012) suggest that teens who are on a low economic trajectory are more likely to become pregnant because of the lack of economic opportunity and the social marginalization that comes with poverty. Specifically, these adolescents are more likely to "drop out" of the economic mainstream and opt for early parenthood instead of investing in their own economic progress because they feel that they have little chance of advancing.

In the United States, the adolescent birth rate is higher among African American teens and Hispanic teens than among White teens. To some degree, the higher teenage pregnancy rate in these groups reflects the impact of poverty because a disproportionately high number of African American and Hispanic youths live in poverty (Yoost, Hertweck, & Barnett, 2014).

Higher levels of competence cognitively, behaviorally, and socially tend to have a protective effect on adolescent sexuality and reproductive health (House, Bates, Markham, et al., 2010). Intelligence and academic ability are positively associated with delayed sexual activity, greater use of contraception, and lower rates of pregnancy (Katz, 2011). Teens with future goals (i.e., college or job) tend to use birth control more consistently compared with other teens; if they become pregnant, they are also more likely to have abortions.

The younger the teen when she first gets pregnant, the more likely she is to have another pregnancy in her teens. Just over one third (35%) of adolescents who have had an abortion or recent birth become pregnant again within 2 years (Baldwin & Edelman, 2013). Moreover, the likelihood of repeat pregnancies increases when the teen is living with her sexual partner and has dropped out of school.

Internationally, female adolescents who are married are more likely to welcome a pregnancy in countries in which Islam is the predominant religion, where large families are desired, where social change is slow in coming, and where most childbearing occurs within marriage. Early pregnancy is less desired in countries in which the reverse is true.

Developing Cultural Competence Impact of Education on Marriage and Childbearing

Throughout the world, the higher a woman's educational level, the more likely she is to delay marriage and childbirth.

HIGH-RISK BEHAVIORS

Developmentally, adolescents, especially younger ones, are not yet able to foresee the consequences of their actions. As a result, they may have a sense of invulnerability that leads to the mistaken idea that harm will not befall them. This sense of invulnerability may also result in an overly optimistic view of the risks associated with their actions (AGI, 2012a).

Among American adolescents there is great peer pressure to become sexually active during the teen years. Premarital sexual activity is commonplace, and teenage pregnancy is more socially acceptable today than it was in the past. In fact, by age 19, 70% of all teens have had intercourse (AGI, 2012a). Sexual innuendo permeates every aspect of the popular media, but issues of sexual responsibility are commonly ignored.

Texting is a form of flirting and social behavior that has become commonplace among teens and young adults. Of particular note is the current blend of "sex and text" called "sexting" in which teens and young adults share semi-nude or nude pictures of themselves or others using cell phones, websites, and social media networks. Sexting is associated with an increased likelihood of being sexually active and of engaging in risky sexual behavior such as using drugs and alcohol before sex and having unprotected sex. Then, too, individuals in a romantic relationship are more likely to engage in sexting (Klettke, Hallford, & Mellor, 2014).

High-risk sexual behaviors, including multiple partners and lack of contraceptive use, are of concern. Research indicates that young people 15 to 24 years of age comprise 25% of the sexually experienced population in the United States. However, they account for nearly half of the new cases of sexually transmitted infections (STIs) (Centers for Disease Control and Prevention [CDC], 2011). This is particularly worrisome because many STIs, including HIV infection, are asymptomatic. Thus apparently healthy young people who are infected may not have a reason to seek health care.

Statistics have demonstrated an increased use of condoms among the adolescent population, with 68% of females aged 15 to 19 and 80% of males using condoms during their first sexual intercourse probably because of the tremendous educational efforts related to HIV infection (AGI, 2013). Adolescents, however, remain inconsistent contraceptive users. Many teens lack accurate and adequate knowledge about contraceptive options. This is a common topic of sex education programs; nevertheless, debate continues about the appropriateness of such programs in schools. Proponents advocate early sex education to provide teens with the knowledge they need to avoid unwanted pregnancy and the risk of STIs. Opponents feel that sex education is the responsibility of parents and worry that sex education in the schools will promote sexual activity. However, a review of research on sex education reveals that it does not increase initiation of sexual activity at an earlier age. In fact, it helps teens withstand the pressure to have sex too soon (AGI, 2012a). Other factors affecting the use of contraception include access or availability, cost of supplies, and concern about confidentiality.

PSYCHOSOCIAL FACTORS

Pregnancy desire tends to be higher among teens who are older, who were younger when they became sexually active, who are in a short-term relationship (which may be romanticized and intense), and who have greater perceived stress in their lives (Sipsma, Ickovics, Lewis, et al., 2011).

Family dysfunction and poor self-esteem are also major risk factors for adolescent pregnancy. Some young teenagers deliberately plan to get pregnant. A female adolescent may use pregnancy for various subconscious or conscious reasons: to punish

---

EVIDENCE-BASED PRACTICE | Risk Factors for Adolescent Pregnancy

Clinical Question
What are risk factors for adolescent pregnancy in vulnerable populations?

The Evidence
Unplanned pregnancy for an adolescent can result in a host of adverse outcomes for both mother and baby. These risks are even higher among vulnerable populations. Two research studies focused on identifiable risk factors in specific vulnerable populations in an effort to target preventive efforts effectively. Researchers conducted an integrated literature review of 18 research studies that identified risk factors for teen pregnancy among African American adolescents. A second study used a predictive model to study risk factors among nearly 300 adolescents in the child welfare system/foster homes. Taken together, these studies form a strong basis of evidence. Lee, Cintron, & Kocher (2014) found that five major factors contributed to adolescent pregnancy among African American youth: substance use, gender roles, peer influences,

parental involvement, and level of knowledge about sexual health. Of these, substance use was also a predictive factor for teens in the welfare system, but in this population, delinquency was also a risk factor (Helfrich & McWey, 2014). In the latter study, the timing of pregnancy was also identified; pregnancy occurred, on average, within 3 years of a predictive event.

Best Practice
Knowing specific predictive factors for a population enables the development of risk-specific educational programs for the prevention of adolescent pregnancy. These data suggest that supports need to be wide reaching and include reducing substance abuse, encouraging parental involvement, and integration of peer support into interventions.

Clinical Reasoning
How can the nurse determine risk factors of teen pregnancy for a specific population? How can parents and peers be involved in adolescent pregnancy prevention programs?

her parents, to escape from an undesirable home situation, to gain attention, or to feel that she has someone to love and someone that loves her. Pregnancy may also be an adolescent's form of acting out. For others, pregnancy marks an important milestone that leads to enhanced maturity, better decision making, and healthier behaviors (Herrman & Nandakumar, 2012).

Evidence suggests that teens who have a history of sexual abuse, physical abuse, or neglect are more likely to give birth as a teenager than those who have not been maltreated (Herrman, 2014). Teenage pregnancy also can result from an incestuous relationship. In the very young adolescent, incest or sexual abuse should be suspected as a possible cause of pregnancy. More teens who become pregnant, compared with teens who have not been pregnant, have been physically, emotionally, or sexually abused. In fact, maltreatment of any kind is a high-risk contributor to early teen pregnancy. Teenage pregnancy could also be caused by other nonvoluntary sexual experiences such as acquaintance rape.

Risks to the Adolescent Mother

PHYSIOLOGIC RISKS
Adolescents older than 15 years who receive early, thorough prenatal care are at no greater risk during pregnancy than women older than age 20. Unfortunately, adolescents often begin prenatal care later in pregnancy than other age groups. Thus risks for pregnant adolescents include preterm births, low-birth-weight newborns, cephalopelvic disproportion, iron deficiency anemia, and preeclampsia and its sequelae. In the adolescent age group, prenatal care is the critical factor that most influences pregnancy outcome.

Teenagers ages 15 to 19 have a high incidence of STIs, including herpesvirus, syphilis, and gonorrhea. The incidence of chlamydial infection is also increased in this age group. The presence of such infections during a pregnancy greatly increases the risk to the fetus. Other problems seen in adolescents are cigarette smoking and drug use. By the time pregnancy is confirmed, the fetus may already have been harmed by these substances.

PSYCHOLOGIC RISKS
The major psychologic risk to the pregnant adolescent is the interruption of her developmental tasks. Adding the tasks of pregnancy to her own developmental tasks creates a huge amount of psychologic work, the completion of which will affect the adolescent's and her newborn's futures. Table 12–1 suggests typical behaviors of the adolescent when she becomes aware of her pregnancy. In reviewing these behaviors, the nurse should realize that other factors may influence individual response.

TABLE 12–1 Initial Reaction to Awareness of Pregnancy

AGE	ADOLESCENT BEHAVIOR	NURSING IMPLICATIONS
Early adolescent (14 years and younger)	Fears rejection by family and peers. Enters healthcare system with an adult, most likely mother (parents still seen as locus of control). Value system closely reflects that of parents, so teen turns to parents for decisions or approval of decisions. Pregnancy probably not a result of intimate relationship. Is self-conscious about normal adolescent changes in body. Self-consciousness and low self-esteem likely to increase with rapid breast enlargement and abdominal enlargement of pregnancy.	Be nonjudgmental in approach to care. Focus on needs and concerns of adolescent, but if parent accompanies daughter, include parent in plan of care. Encourage both to express concerns and feelings regarding pregnancy and options: abortion, maintaining pregnancy, adoption. Be realistic and concrete in discussing implications of each option. During physical exam of adolescent, respect increased sense of modesty. Explain in simple and concrete terms physical changes that are produced by pregnancy versus puberty. Explain each step of physical exam in simple and concrete terms.
Middle adolescent (15–17 years)	Fears rejection by peers and parents. Unsure of whom to confide in. May seek confirmation of pregnancy on own with increased awareness of options and services, such as over-the-counter pregnancy kits and Planned Parenthood. If in an ongoing, caring relationship with partner (peer), may choose him as confidant. Economic dependence on parents may determine if and when parents are told. Future educational plans and perception of parental support or lack of support are significant factors in decision regarding termination or maintenance of the pregnancy. Possible conflict between parental and own developing value system.	Be nonjudgmental in approach to care. Reassure the adolescent that confidentiality will be maintained. Help adolescent identify significant individuals in whom she can confide to help make a decision about the pregnancy. Be aware of state laws regarding requirement of parental notification if abortion intended. Also be aware of state laws regarding requirements for marriage: usually, minimum age for both parties is 18; 16- and 17-year-olds are, in most states, allowed to marry only with consent of parents. Encourage adolescent to be realistic about parental response to pregnancy.
Late adolescent (18–19 years)	Most likely to confirm pregnancy on own and at an earlier date due to increased acceptance and awareness of consequences of behavior. Likely to use pregnancy kit for confirmation. Relationship with father of baby, future educational plans, and personal value system are among significant determinants of decision about pregnancy.	Be nonjudgmental in approach to care. Reassure the adolescent that confidentiality will be maintained. Encourage adolescent to identify significant individuals in whom she can confide. Refer to counseling as appropriate. Encourage adolescent to be realistic about parental response to pregnancy.

SOCIOLOGIC RISKS

Being forced into adult roles before completing adolescent developmental tasks causes a series of events that may result in prolonged dependence on parents, lack of stable relationships with the opposite sex, and lack of economic and social stability. Many teenage mothers drop out of school during their pregnancy, and then are less likely to complete their schooling. Similarly, they are less likely to go to college. In fact, fewer than 2% of teenagers who give birth before age 18 attain a college degree by age 30 (AGI, 2012a). In addition, teenage mothers are more likely to have big families and more likely to be single. Lack of education in turn reduces the quality of jobs available and leads to more tenuous employment and increased poverty (Herrman & Nandakumar, 2012).

Some pregnant adolescents choose to marry the father of the baby, who may also be a teenager. Unfortunately, most adolescent marriages end in divorce. This fact should not be surprising because pregnancy and marriage interrupt the adolescents' childhood and basic education. Lack of maturity in dealing with an intimate relationship also contributes to marital breakdown.

Dating violence is often an issue for teens. When surveyed, 10.3% of adolescents report some level of physical dating violence, and 10.4% experienced some form of sexual dating violence ranging from touching and kidding to forced intercourse (Kann, Kinchen, Shanklin, et al., 2014). The violence increases in pregnant teens. However, research suggests that this number is significantly lower than reality because teens are far less likely to report domestic violence than are adults.

The increased incidence of maternal complications, preterm birth, and low-birth-weight babies among teen mothers also affects society because many of these mothers are on welfare. The need for increased financial support for good prenatal care and nutritional programs remains critical.

In the United States, the results of teenage childbearing cost taxpayers $9.4 billion annually (Ventura et al., 2014). Much of this cost comes from Medicaid, state health department maternal care clinics, federal monies for Aid to Families with Dependent Children programs, the Supplemental Nutrition Assistance Program (SNAP), and direct payments to healthcare providers.

Table 12–2 identifies the early adolescent's response to the developmental tasks of pregnancy. Middle and older adolescents respond differently, reflecting their progression through developmental tasks. In addition to her maturational level, the

TABLE 12–2 The Early Adolescent's Response to the Developmental Tasks of Pregnancy

STAGE	DEVELOPMENTAL TASKS OF PREGNANCY	EARLY ADOLESCENT'S RESPONSE TO PREGNANCY	NURSING IMPLICATIONS
First trimester	Pregnancy confirmation. Seeks early prenatal care as a confirmation tool. Begins to evaluate her diet and general health habits. Initial ambivalence common. Usually supportive partner.	May delay confirmation of pregnancy until late first trimester or later. Reasons for delay may include lack of awareness that she is pregnant, fear of confiding in anyone, and/or denial. Rapid enlargement and sensitivity of breasts are embarrassing and frightening to early adolescents—may be perceived as changes of puberty. If confiding in mother, may be experiencing family turmoil in response to pregnancy.	Explain physiologic changes of pregnancy versus those associated with puberty. Explain that ambivalence is normal with any pregnancy, but recognize it as a much greater concern with adolescent pregnancy. Emphasize need for good nutrition as important for her well-being as much as baby's (prevention of preeclampsia and anemia). Use simple explanations and lots of audiovisual aids. Have adolescent listen to fetal heart rate with Doppler.
Second trimester	Changes in physical appearance begin, and fetal movement is experienced, causing pregnancy to be experienced as a reality. Begins wearing maternity clothes to accommodate the physical changes. As a result of quickening, she perceives her fetus as a real baby and begins preparing for the maternal role and new relationships with her partner and members of her family.	Some teenagers may delay validation of pregnancy until now, with family turmoil occurring at this time. Abdominal enlargement and quickening may be perceived as loss of control over body image. May try to maintain prepregnant weight and wear restrictive clothing to control and conceal changing body. Becomes dependent on her own mother for support. Egocentric; unable to develop a maternal role at this time.	Continue to discuss importance of good nutrition and adequate weight gain as noted above. Discuss ways of wearing common teenage clothing (large sweatshirts, blouses) to promote comfort but preserve adolescent image to some degree. Discuss plans being made for baby, continued educational plans, and role of teen's parents. Explain physiologic changes of pregnancy versus those associated with puberty. Explain that ambivalence is normal with any pregnancy, but recognize it as a much greater concern with adolescent pregnancy.
Third trimester	At end of second trimester, begins to view fetus as separate from self. Buys baby clothes and supplies. Prepares a place for the baby. Realistic about what baby is like. Prepares to give birth to baby. Anxiety increases as labor and birth approach and has concerns about well-being of fetus.	May focus on "wanting it to be over." May have trouble individuating fetus. May have fantasies, dreams, or nightmares about childbirth. Natural fears of labor and birth greater than with older primigravida. Probably has not been in a hospital, and may associate this with negative experiences.	Assess whether adolescent is preparing for baby by buying supplies and preparing a place in the home. Childbirth education is important. Provide hospital tour. Assess for discomforts of pregnancy, such as heartburn and constipation. Adolescent may be uncomfortable mentioning these and other problems.

amount of nurturing the pregnant adolescent receives is a critical factor in the way she handles pregnancy and motherhood.

RISKS FOR THE CHILD

Children of adolescent parents are at a disadvantage in many ways because teens are not developmentally or economically prepared to be parents. In general, children of teenage mothers are found to be at a developmental disadvantage compared with children whose mothers were older at the time of their birth. Many factors contribute to these differences, especially the adverse social and economic conditions many teenage mothers face. These factors result in high rates of family instability, disadvantaged neighborhoods, and high rates of behavior problems. In addition, these children do not do as well in school and are less likely to complete high school. Children born to adolescent mothers also have higher rates of abuse and neglect (March of Dimes [MOD], 2012).

Partners of Adolescent Mothers

Approximately half of the fathers of babies born to adolescent mothers are not teens but 20 years of age or older (Herrman, 2010). Teens in poor, recently immigrated populations are especially likely to have older partners. Adolescent males tend to become sexually active at an earlier age than females, and they have more sexual partners in their teenage years. When the father is an adolescent, he, too, has uncompleted developmental tasks for his age group and is no better prepared psychologically than his female counterpart to deal with the consequences of pregnancy. Teenage fatherhood may lead to a decrease in the years of schooling the male receives, and increases the rate of cohabitation and early marriage. It also is associated with full-time and military employment status (Fletcher & Wolfe, 2012).

In general, adolescent males tend to view an unintended pregnancy as negative because of the impact on their aspirations, life goals, and current freedoms. Attitudes toward teen pregnancy tend to be more favorable among male adolescents of lower socioeconomic status and/or lower educational level (Lohan, Cruise, O'Halloran, et al., 2010).

The adolescent who attempts to assume his responsibility as a father faces many of the same psychologic and sociologic risks as the adolescent mother. The mother and father are generally from similar socioeconomic backgrounds and have similar educational levels.

Although they may not be married, many adolescent couples have meaningful relationships. The male partners may be very involved in the pregnancy and may be present for the birth. In situations in which the adolescent father wants to assume some responsibility, healthcare providers should support him in his decision. It is also important to ensure that the pregnant adolescent has the opportunity to decide for herself whether she wants the father to participate in her health care.

Fathers are included on birth certificates far more frequently today than in the past. This inclusion helps ensure the fathers' rights and encourages them to meet their responsibilities to their children. In addition, legal paternity gives children access to military and Social Security benefits and to medical information about their fathers. In some situations, the pregnant adolescent may not want to identify or contact the father of the baby, and the male may not readily acknowledge paternity. Those situations include rape, exploitative sexual relations, incest, and casual sexual relations. If healthcare providers suspect any of the first three causes, further investigation into the situation

is important for the well-being of the pregnant adolescent, and referral to other resources should be made as appropriate.

Even if the adolescent father has been included in the health care of the adolescent mother throughout the pregnancy, it is not unusual for her to want her mother as her primary support person during labor and birth. Younger adolescents are especially likely to choose their mothers for this role. It is important to support the pregnant adolescent's wishes and to acknowledge and support the adolescent father's wishes as appropriate.

Father love is an important predictor of a child's well-being. Children whose fathers are involved and loving are more likely to have healthy self-esteem, do well in school, and avoid drug use and criminal activity than those children with fathers who are uninvolved (Kirven, 2014). Therefore, it behooves healthcare professionals to do what they can to support the efforts of adolescent fathers to be effective.

As a part of counseling, the nurse should assess the father's stressors, his support systems, his plans for involvement in the pregnancy and childbearing, and his future plans. He should be referred to social services for counseling about his educational and vocational future. When the father is involved in the pregnancy, the young mother feels less deserted, more confident in her decision making, and better able to discuss her future.

Reactions of Family and Social Network to Adolescent Pregnancy

The reactions of families and support groups to adolescent pregnancy vary widely. In families that foster children's educational and career goals, adolescent pregnancy is often a shock. Anger, shame, and sorrow are common reactions. The majority of pregnant adolescents from these families are likely to choose abortion, with the exception of teens whose cultural and religious beliefs prevent them from seeking abortions.

In populations in which adolescent pregnancy is more prevalent and more socially acceptable, family and friends may be more supportive of the adolescent parents. In many cases, the teen's friends and mother are present at the birth. The expectant parents may also have friends who are already teen parents. Some male partners of these adolescent mothers see pregnancy and the birth of a baby as signs of adult status and increased sexual prowess—a source of pride.

The mother of the pregnant adolescent is usually among the first to be told about the pregnancy. She typically becomes involved with decision making, especially with the young adolescent, about issues such as maintaining the pregnancy, abortion, and dealing with the father-to-be and his family.

Once the pregnant adolescent decides how to proceed, it is often her mother who helps her access health care, and her mother's support is essential if the teen self-image is to grow to include the notion of herself as "mother" (Turnage & Pharris, 2013). If the pregnancy is maintained, the mother may participate in prenatal care and classes and can be an excellent source of support for her daughter. She should be encouraged to participate if the mother–daughter relationship is positive. If the baby's father is involved in the pregnancy, he and the pregnant adolescent's mother may be able to work together to support the teenage mother. The nurse can update the pregnant adolescent's mother on current childbearing practices to clarify any misconceptions she might have. During labor and birth, the mother may be a key figure for her daughter, offering reassurance and instilling confidence in the teen.

The younger the adolescent when she gives birth, the more she needs her mother's support. Children of adolescent parents experience more negative outcomes, including more aggressive behavior at a younger age, when the adolescent is in constant conflict with her mother and becomes less involved in parenting.

Nursing Management

For the Adolescent Mother-to-Be

Nursing Assessment and Diagnosis

In working with adolescents, remember that oftentimes the nurse is the first contact with the healthcare system that the adolescent has. Then, too, many adolescents have never before accessed health care without a parent. Establish a knowledge base to plan interventions for the adolescent mother-to-be and family. Areas of assessment include history of family and personal physical health, developmental level and impact of pregnancy, and emotional and financial support. Also assess the family and social support network and the father's degree of involvement in the pregnancy.

As with all pregnant women, it is important to have information on the teen's general physical health. This may be the first time the adolescent has ever provided a health history. Consequently, it may be helpful to ask specific questions and give examples if she appears confused about a question. The teen's mother may be best able to answer questions about family history because the adolescent is often unaware of this information.

The following areas should be assessed:

- Family and personal health history
- Medical history
- Menstrual history
- Obstetric and gynecologic history
- Substance abuse history

It is important to assess the maturational level of each person. The adolescent's development level and the impact of pregnancy are reflected in the degree of recognition of the realities and responsibilities involved in teenage pregnancy and parenting. Also assess the mother's self-concept (including body image), her relationship with the significant adults in her life, her attitude toward her pregnancy, and her coping methods in the situation, as well as the teen's knowledge of, attitude toward, and anticipated ability to care for the coming baby. Ask specifically about dating violence. Teens are not likely to reveal dating violence unless they are asked about it.

The socioeconomic status of the pregnant adolescent often places the baby at risk throughout life, beginning with conception. It is essential to assess family and social support systems, as well as the extent of financial support available.

The nursing diagnoses applicable to pregnant women in general apply to the pregnant adolescent. Other nursing diagnoses are influenced by the adolescent's age, support systems, socioeconomic situation, health, and maturity. Examples of nursing diagnoses specific to the pregnant adolescent may include the following (NANDA-I © 2014):

- *Nutrition, Imbalanced: Less than Body Requirements,* related to poor eating habits
- *Self-Esteem, Situational Low, Risk for,* related to unanticipated pregnancy

Planning and Implementation

COMMUNITY-BASED NURSING CARE

If pregnancy occurs, early, thorough prenatal care is the strongest and most critical determinant for reducing risk for the adolescent mother and her newborn. The nurse needs to understand the special needs of the adolescent mother to meet this challenge successfully.

Many new and innovative community-based programs have evolved to provide care for high-risk clients and their partners throughout the childbearing experience and beyond. Nurses in community-based agencies can help adolescents access the healthcare system as well as social services and other support services (e.g., food banks and the Special Supplemental Nutrition Program for Women, Infants, and Children [WIC]). These nurses are also involved extensively in counseling and client teaching.

Teaching adolescents in groups according to their ages is often more effective for learning. In addition, many teens prefer teaching aids that are visual and that they can handle, such as realistic fetal models. Pregnant teens with low reading levels tend to prefer handouts and posters that have visual interest, short sentences, bulleted items, and white space (Broussard & Broussard, 2010).

Issue of Confidentiality

Most states have passed legislation that confirms the right of some minors to assume the rights of adults; they are then called **emancipated minors**. An adolescent may be considered emancipated if he or she is self-supporting and living away from home, married, pregnant, a parent, or in the military service. Even if a minor has not become formally "emancipated," all 50 states permit confidential testing and treatment for sexually transmitted infections (STIs), but only 21 states and the District of Columbia explicitly permit all minors to consent to contraception without a parent's knowledge or consent; 25 states permit minors to consent to contraception in certain circumstances (AGI, 2012e). Currently, 36 states and the District of Columbia explicitly allow some minors to consent to prenatal care; of that group, 28 states allow all minors to give consent, whereas 13 states have no relevant law or policy (AGI, 2012c). All states either explicitly allow minors to give consent for their children's medical care or have no policy about it (AGI, 2012d).

Professionalism in Practice Emancipated Minors

It is important to remember that if a pregnant minor is considered emancipated, she has the right and responsibility to consent to health care for herself and later for her child. She is entitled to respect and confidentiality in her dealings with healthcare providers. Only with her consent can other adults, including her parents, be included in communication.

Development of a Trusting Relationship
With the Pregnant Adolescent

The first visit to the clinic or caregiver's office may make the adolescent feel anxious and vulnerable. Making this first experience as positive as possible for her will encourage the adolescent to return for follow-up care and to cooperate with her healthcare providers, and will help her recognize the importance of health care for her and her baby. Developing a trusting relationship with the pregnant adolescent is essential. Honesty, respect, and a caring attitude promote self-esteem.

Clinical Tip

During the initial pelvic examination, with the consent of the examiner, offer the teen a handheld mirror. A mirror is helpful in enabling the adolescent to see her cervix, thus educating her about her anatomy. It also gives her an active role in the examination if she so desires.

Depending on the adolescent's age, this may be her first pelvic examination, an anxiety-provoking experience for any woman. Provide explanations during the procedure. A gentle and thoughtful examination technique will help the adolescent to relax.

Promotion of Self-Esteem and Problem-Solving Skills

Assist the adolescent in her decision-making and problem-solving skills so that she can proceed with her developmental tasks and begin to assume responsibility for her life and that of her newborn. Many adolescents are not aware of the legally available options for handling an unplanned pregnancy. In an open, nonjudgmental way, without imposing personal values, educate the teen about her alternatives: terminating the pregnancy, maintaining the pregnancy and parenting the baby, or relinquishing the baby for adoption. The nurse can also provide information about community resources available to help with each alternative. Once the teen has decided on a course of action, healthcare providers should respect her decision and support her efforts to achieve her goals.

Adolescents who choose to terminate a pregnancy cite reasons such as economic hardship or interference with school or a career. Teens most often involve their parents and their partners in the decision. Their involvement does not always indicate that they support the adolescent's decision. Research, however, indicates that a significant portion of pregnant teens report pressure from their mother, partner, or other family member to consider terminating the pregnancy. Teens are similar to adults in how they experience abortion. They expect to feel a range of emotions and believe they are prepared to cope with them after the abortion (Ralph, Gould, Baker, et al., 2014).

If the adolescent chooses to continue her pregnancy, describe what she can expect over the prenatal period and provide an explanation and rationale for each procedure as it occurs. This overview fosters the adolescent's understanding and gives her some control.

Early adolescents tend to be egocentric and oriented to the present. They may not think it is important that their health and habits affect the fetus. Thus it is often helpful to emphasize how these practices affect the teens themselves. Early adolescents also need help in problem solving and in visualizing the future so they can plan effectively.

Middle adolescents are developing the ability to think abstractly and can recognize that actions may have long-term consequences. They may not yet have acquired assertive communication skills, however, and may be reluctant to ask questions. Therefore, ask teens directly if they have questions. Middle adolescents can absorb more detailed health teaching and apply it.

Late adolescents can usually think abstractly, plan for the future, and function in a manner comparable to older

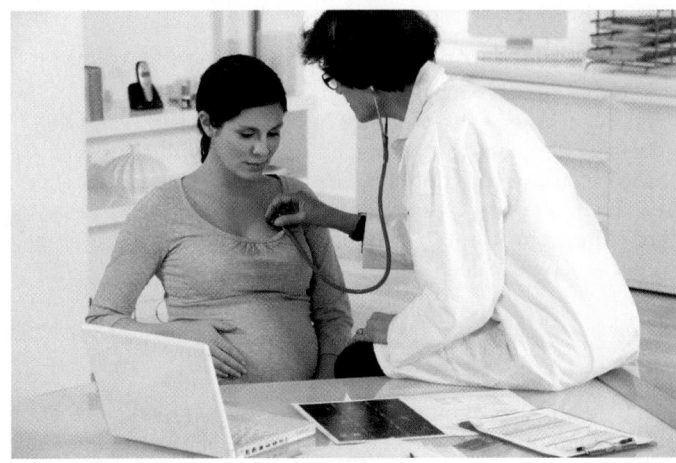

Figure 12–2 The nurse carefully assesses this pregnant teen.

SOURCE: © Auremar/Fotolia.

pregnant women. They can also handle complex information and apply it.

Promotion of Physical Well-Being

Baseline weight and blood pressure measurements are valuable in assessing weight gain and predisposition to preeclampsia (Figure 12–2). Encourage the adolescent to take part in her care by measuring and recording her own weight. Use this time as an opportunity for assisting her in problem solving. Encourage her to ask herself the following questions: "Have I gained too much or too little weight?" "What influence does my diet have on my weight?" "How can I change my eating habits?"

Introduce the subject of nutrition during measurement of baseline and subsequent hemoglobin and hematocrit values. Because the adolescent is at risk for anemia, she needs education about the importance of iron in her diet. Indeed, basic education about nutrition is a critical component of care for pregnant teens.

Preeclampsia is the most prevalent medical complication of pregnant adolescents. Blood pressure readings of 140/90 mmHg are not acceptable as the determinant of preeclampsia in adolescents. Young women ages 14 to 20 years without evidence of high blood pressure usually have diastolic readings between 50 and 66 mmHg. Gradual increases from the prepregnant diastolic readings, along with excessive weight gain, must be evaluated as precursors to preeclampsia. Establishment of baseline readings is one reason early prenatal care is vital to management of the pregnant adolescent.

Adolescents have an increased incidence of STIs. The initial prenatal examination should include gonococcal and chlamydial cultures; wet-mount prep for *Candida, Trichomonas,* and *Gardnerella;* and tests for syphilis. Although today's teens are knowledgeable about HIV/AIDS, they know much less about other STIs, especially with regard to symptoms and risk reduction, so education is important. If the adolescent's history indicates that she is at increased risk for HIV, she should be given information about it and offered HIV screening.

Discuss substance abuse with the adolescent. It is important to review the risks associated with the use of tobacco, caffeine, drugs, and alcohol. The adolescent mother should be aware of how these substances affect both her and her fetus's development.

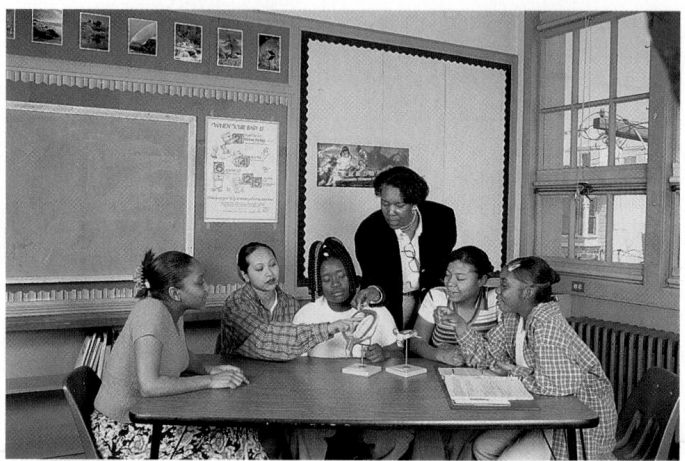

Figure 12–3 **Prenatal classes for adolescents. Young adolescents may benefit from prenatal classes designed for them.**

Ongoing care should include the same assessments that an older pregnant woman receives. Pay special attention to evaluating fetal growth by determining when quickening occurs and by measuring fundal height, fetal heart rate, and fetal movement. If there is a question of size–date discrepancy by 2 cm either way when assessing fundal height, an ultrasound is warranted to establish fetal age so that instances of intrauterine growth restriction can be detected early.

Promotion of Family Adaptation

Assess the family situation during the first prenatal visit and find out the level of involvement the adolescent wants from each of her family members and the father of the child, as well as her perception of their present support. If the mother and daughter agree, the mother should be included in the client's care. Pregnancy may change a teen's relationship with her mother from one of antagonism to one of understanding and empathy. The opportunity to renew or establish a positive relationship with their mothers is welcomed by most teens. Help the teen's mother assess and meet her daughter's needs. Some adolescents become more dependent during pregnancy, and some become more independent. The mother can ease and encourage her daughter's self-growth by understanding how best to respond to and support the adolescent.

The adolescent's relationship with her father is also affected by her pregnancy. Provide information to the adolescent's father and encourage his involvement to whatever degree is acceptable to both daughter and father.

The father of the adolescent's baby should not be forgotten in promoting the family's adaptation to the pregnancy. He should be included in prenatal visits, classes, health teaching, and the birth itself to the extent that he wishes and that is acceptable to the teenage mother. He should also have the opportunity to express his feelings and concerns and to have his questions answered.

Most childbirth educators believe that prenatal classes with other teens are best, even though they can be challenging to teach (Figure 12–3). The pregnant teen may be accompanied by her mother, her boyfriend, or her girlfriends. Those who bring girlfriends may bring a different one each time, and giggling and side conversations may occur. Such activity reflects the short attention span of the teen and is fairly typical.

Goals for prenatal classes may include some or all of the following:

- Providing anticipatory guidance about pregnancy
- Preparing participants for labor and birth
- Helping participants identify the problems and conflicts of teenage pregnancy and parenting
- Promoting increased self-esteem

- Providing information about available community resources
- Helping participants develop adaptive coping skills

To keep the attention of adolescent participants in childbirth preparation classes, it is important to use a variety of teaching strategies, including audiovisual aids, demonstrations, and games. Although parenting topics are sometimes included in prenatal classes for adolescents, teens may not retain the information because they tend to be present oriented. Parenting skills are crucial, but adolescents generally are not ready to learn about these skills until birth makes the newborn—and thus parenting—a reality.

HOSPITAL-BASED NURSING CARE

As mentioned earlier, the adolescent's mother is often present during the teen's labor and birth. The father of the baby may also be involved. Close girlfriends may arrive soon after the teen is admitted. At admission, ask the teen who will be her primary support person in labor and whom she wants involved in the labor and birth. This information may also be included on her prenatal record. The adolescent in labor has the same care needs as any pregnant woman. However, she may require more sustained care. Be readily available and answer questions simply and honestly, using lay terminology. Also help the adolescent's support people understand their roles in assisting the teen.

If the father of the baby is involved, encourage him, at his own level of comfort, to play an active role in all phases of the birth process, perhaps by supporting the teen's relaxation techniques, feeding her ice chips, timing her contractions, and coaching her with her breathing. Recommend hand-holding, back rubs, and supportive touching.

During the postpartum period, most teens do not foresee that they will become sexually active in the near future and are often adamant that they will not become pregnant again for a long time. However, the statistics demonstrate a different reality. Consequently, predischarge teaching should include information about the resumption of ovulation and the importance of contraception.

Several safe and effective contraceptive options are available for adolescents. Condoms are by far the most common method of contraception among teens and, when used consistently and correctly, they offer the added advantage of protection against STIs. Increasingly, experts are recommending a dual approach to prevent pregnancy and STIs—a condom combined with a second method of contraception. The American Academy of Pediatrics (AAP) (2014) has issued a policy statement on contraception for adolescents that advises caregivers to recommend contraceptive methods that require the least individual adherence, specifically, long-acting reversible contraception (LARC) such as progestin implants and intrauterine contraceptives (IUCs), followed by Depo-Provera (DMPA), combined oral contraceptives (COCs), and other hormone-based approaches including the vaginal ring, transdermal patch, and progestin-only pills.

Implanon and Nexplanon are both single-rod implants that may be left in place for 3 years. They are highly effective. DMPA is convenient for teens because it is easy to use. However, it does require an injection every 13 weeks.

IUC is now considered to be a safe, first-line contraceptive choice for adolescents. Research indicates that IUCs do not increase the adolescent's risk of pelvic inflammatory disease (PID) or affect her fertility (AAP, 2014), and the levonorgestrel-releasing intrauterine system (LNG-IUS) can be beneficial in teens by reducing heavy menstrual bleeding and alleviating symptoms of dysmenorrhea (Forcier & Harel, 2011).

COCs are the most popular method of contraception among teens and have few contraindications; however, they do require individual adherence. Extended or continuous-cycle pills are an option for teens who prefer amenorrhea.

SAFETY ALERT!

Nurses need to be certain that adolescents who are prescribed combined oral contraceptives (COCs) clearly understand the correct use, possible complications, warning signs, and implications of missed pills. They should also be aware that some medications, such as certain antibiotics, decrease the effectiveness of COCs.

As part of discharge planning, ensure that the teen is aware of community resources available to assist her and her family. Postpartum classes, especially with peers, can be particularly beneficial. Such classes address a variety of topics, including postpartum adaptation, infant and child development, and parenting skills.

Evaluation

Expected outcomes of nursing care include the following:

- A trusting relationship is established with the pregnant adolescent.

- The adolescent is able to use her problem-solving abilities to make appropriate choices.

- The adolescent follows the recommendations of the health-care team and receives effective health care throughout her pregnancy, the birth, and the postpartum period.

- The adolescent, her partner (if he is involved), and their families are able to cope successfully with the effects of the pregnancy.

- The adolescent is able to discuss pregnancy, prenatal care, and childbirth.

- The adolescent develops skill in child care and parenting.

Prevention of Adolescent Pregnancy

At the individual level, balanced and realistic sexual education, which includes information on both abstinence and contraception, can delay teens' onset of sexual activity, increase the use of contraception by sexually active teens, and reduce the number of their sexual partners. The AAP policy statement (2014) on contraception for adolescents addresses the role of healthcare providers in working with adolescents. The statement stresses the importance of encouraging abstinence while also providing counseling on risk-reduction approaches, including the use of condoms for every act of sexual intercourse. It points out that latex condoms also help reduce the transmission of STIs. In addition, the statement emphasizes the need to ensure ready access to contraceptive services and appropriate follow-up.

In 2012, the AAP issued a policy statement supporting the availability of emergency contraception (EC) and recommending that both male and female teens should be counseled about emergency contraception as part of routine anticipatory guidance about safe sex and family planning. In 2013, the Food and Drug Administration (FDA) approved Plan B One-Step emergency contraceptive for use by all women of childbearing potential without any age restrictions, thereby giving teens access to EC (FDA, 2013).

At the national level, the National Campaign to Prevent Teen and Unplanned Pregnancy (NCPTUP), a private, nonprofit organization made up of a broad spectrum of religious, political, social, human services, health, and academic organizations, is working to reduce teenage pregnancy by one third between 2006 and 2015 (NCPTUP, 2012b). The Association of Women's Health, Obstetric and Neonatal Nurses (AWHONN) is one of the many professional organizations that joined this group and made a commitment to focus on adolescent pregnancy prevention. Not surprisingly, the National Campaign has found that adolescent pregnancy is a multifaceted problem with no easy answers. The best approaches are local ones based on strong, community-wide involvement with a variety of programs directed at the multiple causes of the problem.

A problem in local communities continues to be conflict among different groups about how to approach adolescent pregnancy prevention. Most teens and adults believe that teens should be strongly encouraged to avoid having sex until they have completed high school, but both groups also favor providing young people with information about both abstinence and contraception (Albert, 2012). Nevertheless, some parents favor an abstinence-only approach. No evidence to date supports the effectiveness of this approach and it may have the unintended consequence of deterring teens from using contraceptives, thereby increasing the risk of sexually transmitted infections (STIs) or unintended pregnancy (AGI, 2012b). Most Americans support providing education in junior and senior high schools with information about protection against unplanned

TABLE 12–3 Recommendations for Parents to Help Their Teens Avoid Pregnancy

- Parents should be clear about their own sexual attitudes and values in order to communicate clearly with children.
- Parents need to talk with their children about sex early and often and be specific in the discussions.
- Parents should supervise and monitor their children and teens with well-established rules, expectations, curfews, and standards of behavior.
- Parents should know their children's friends and their families.
- Parents need to clearly discourage early dating as well as frequent and steady dating.
- Parents should take a strong stand against allowing a daughter to date a much older boy; similarly, they should not allow a son to develop an intense relationship with a much younger girl.
- Parents need to help children set goals for their future and have options that are more attractive than early pregnancy and childrearing.
- Parents should show their children that they value education and take school performance seriously.
- Parents need to monitor what their children are reading, listening to, and watching.
- It is especially important for parents to build a strong, loving relationship with their children from an early age by showing affection clearly and regularly, spending time with them doing age-appropriate activities, building children's self-esteem, and having meals together as a family often.

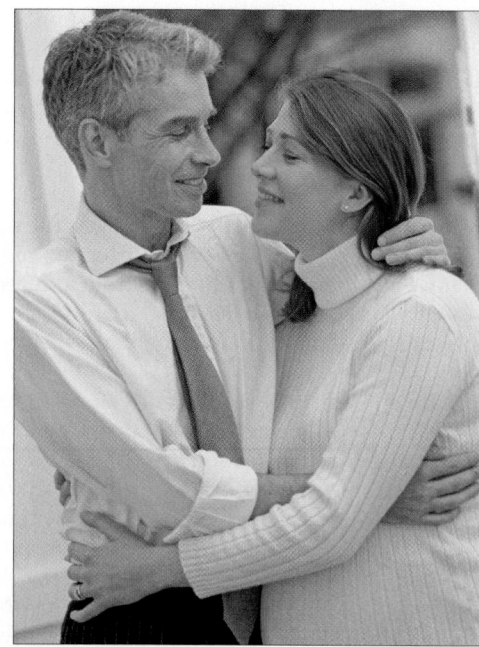

Figure 12–4 **For many older couples, the decision to have a child may be very rewarding.**
SOURCE: Ruth Jenkinson/DK Images.

pregnancy and STIs. Evidence suggests that comprehensive programs that support both abstinence and the use of contraceptives and condoms have a positive effect in delaying or reducing sexual activity or in increasing the use of condoms or other contraceptives (AGI, 2012b).

The National Campaign's task forces have identified characteristics shared by all successful programs regardless of the type of offering or community. Effective adolescent pregnancy prevention programs are long term and intensive. They also involve adolescents in program planning, include good role models from the same cultural and racial backgrounds, and focus on the adolescent male.

The National Campaign has identified a list of recommendations for parents that are designed to help teens avoid pregnancy (see Table 12–3). Nurses can use this information when working with parents (NCPTUP, 2012a).

Care of Expectant Parents Over Age 35

Today, an increasing number of women are choosing to have their first baby after age 35. In fact, in 2012, 14.9% of all births occurred to women age 35 or older (Martin, Hamilton, Osterman, et al., 2013). Many factors have contributed to this trend, including the following:

- The availability of effective birth control methods
- The expanded roles and career options available for women
- The increased number of women getting advanced education, pursuing careers, and delaying parenthood until they are established professionally
- The increased incidence of later marriage and second marriage
- The high cost of living, which causes some young couples to delay childbearing until they are more financially secure
- The increased availability of specialized reproductive technologies, which may help women previously considered infertile

There are advantages to having a first baby after age 35. Single women or couples who delay childbearing until they are older tend to be well educated and financially secure. Usually, their decision to have a baby was deliberately and thoughtfully made (Figure 12–4). Because of their greater life experiences, they also are more aware of the realities of having a child and what it means to have a baby at their age. Many of the women have experienced fulfillment in their careers and feel secure enough to take on the added responsibility of a child. Some women are ready to make a change in their lives, wanting to stay home with a new baby. Those who plan to continue working typically can afford good child care.

Medical Risks

In the United States and Canada, the risk of death has declined dramatically during the past 30 years for women of all ages. However, the risk of maternal death is higher for women over age 35 and even higher for women age 40 and older. These women are more likely to have chronic medical conditions that can complicate a pregnancy. Preexisting medical conditions such as hypertension or diabetes probably play a more significant role than age in maternal well-being and the outcome of pregnancy. In addition, the rate of miscarriage, stillbirth, preterm birth, low birth weight, and perinatal morbidity and mortality is higher in pregnant women over age 35 (Carolan, 2013). Nevertheless, while the risk of pregnancy complications is higher in women over age 35 who have a chronic condition such as hypertension or diabetes or who are in poor general health, the risks are much lower than previously believed for physically fit women without pre-existing medical problems (Cunningham et al., 2014).

Because of advances in reproductive technology, the number of women over age 45 who give birth is increasing although these women still constitute a very small percentage of overall births. While these women have a higher risk of complications than their younger counterparts, the absolute rate of stillbirth or perinatal death is still low (less than 10 per 1000) if they are healthy and free of pre-existing disease. Thus, for most, the outcome of pregnancy is positive (Carolan, 2013).

The risk of conceiving a child with Down syndrome does increase with age, especially over age 35. ACOG (2011) recommends that all pregnant women, regardless of age, be screened for Down syndrome. A quadruple screening to detect Down syndrome and trisomy 18 is often used. Noninvasive analysis of fetal nucleic acid in maternal plasma is also available for prenatal diagnosis early in the first trimester (Chiu & Lo, 2011). Alternatively, first-trimester ultrasound assessment of the thickness of fetal nuchal folds (nuchal translucency [NT]), combined with serum screens of free beta-human chorionic gonadotropin (β-hCG) and pregnancy-associated plasma protein A (PAPP-A), may be used in the detection of Down syndrome, trisomy 18, and trisomy 13. If the screening results are not in the normal range, follow-up testing using ultrasound and amniocentesis is often indicated (ACOG, 2011).

Advanced paternal age is associated with adverse fetal and neonatal outcomes (Wiener-Megnazi, Auslender, & Dirnfeld, 2012). Additionally, advanced paternal age increases the risk for autism spectrum disorders (Ben Itzchak, Lahat, & Zachor, 2011).

Special Concerns of Expectant Parents Over Age 35

No matter what their age, most expectant parents have concerns about the well-being of the fetus and their ability to parent. Expectant parents over age 35 often have additional concerns about their age, especially the closer they are to age 40. Some couples are concerned about whether they will have enough energy to care for a new baby. Of greater concern is their ability to deal with the needs of the child as they age.

The financial concerns of the older couple are usually different from those of the younger couple. The older couple is generally more financially secure, but when their "baby" is ready for college, the older couple may be close to retirement and might not have the means to provide for their child. The older couple may also be forced to face their own mortality. Certainly, the realization of one's mortality is not uncommon in midlife, but older expectant parents may confront the issue earlier as they consider what will happen as their child grows.

Older couples facing pregnancy in a late or second marriage or after therapy for infertility may find themselves somewhat isolated socially. They may feel different because they are often the only couple in their peer group expecting their first baby. In fact, many of their peers are likely to be parents of adolescents or young adults and may be grandparents as well.

Older couples who already have children may respond quite differently to learning that the woman is pregnant, depending on whether the pregnancy was planned or unexpected. Other factors influencing their response include their children's, family's, and friends' attitudes toward the pregnancy; the impact on their lifestyle; and the financial implications of having another child. Sometimes couples who had previously been married to other mates will choose to have a child together. *Blended families* are formed when "her" children, "his" children, and "their" children come together as a new family group.

Healthcare professionals may treat older expectant parents differently than they would a younger couple. They may offer older women more medical procedures, such as amniocentesis and ultrasound, than younger women. They may also discourage an older woman from using a birthing room or birthing center even if she is healthy because her age is considered to put her at risk.

The woman who has delayed pregnancy may be concerned about the limited amount of time that she has to bear children. When pregnancy does not occur as quickly as she had hoped, the older woman may become increasingly anxious as time slips away on her "biologic clock." When an older woman becomes pregnant but has a spontaneous abortion, her grief for the loss of her unborn child is exacerbated by anxiety about her ability to conceive again in the time remaining to her.

Nursing Management

For the Pregnant Woman Over Age 35

Nursing Assessment and Diagnosis

In working with a woman in her late 30s or 40s who is pregnant, make the same assessments as are indicated in caring for any woman who is pregnant. Assess physical status, the woman's understanding of pregnancy and its changes, the couple's attitudes about the pregnancy and their expectations of the impact a baby will have on their lives, their health teaching needs, the degree of support the woman has, and her knowledge of infant care.

The nursing diagnoses applicable to pregnant women in general apply to pregnant women over age 35. Examples of other nursing diagnoses that may apply include the following (NANDA-I © 2014):

- *Decisional Conflict* related to unexpected pregnancy
- *Anxiety* (moderate) related to uncertainty about fetal well-being

Planning and Implementation

Once an older couple has made the decision to have a child, respect and support the couple in this decision. As with any client, discuss risks, identify concerns, and promote strengths. Do not make the woman's age an issue. It is helpful in promoting a sense of well-being to treat the pregnancy as normal unless the woman has specific health risks.

As the pregnancy continues, identify and discuss concerns the woman may have related to her age or to specific health problems. The older woman who has made a conscious decision to become pregnant often has carefully thought through potential problems and may actually have fewer concerns than a younger woman or one with an unplanned pregnancy.

Childbirth education classes are important in promoting adaptation to the event of childbirth for expectant parents of any age. However, older expectant parents often feel uncomfortable in classes in which most of the participants are much younger. Consequently, classes for expectant parents over age 35 are now available in many communities.

Women who are over age 35 and having their first baby tend to be better educated than other healthcare consumers. These clients frequently know the kind of care and services they want and may be assertive in their interactions with the healthcare system. You should not be intimidated by these individuals, and you should not assume that anticipatory guidance and support are not needed. Instead, support the couple's strengths and be sensitive to their individual needs.

In working with older expectant couples or an older single woman, be sensitive to special needs. A particularly difficult issue these couples face is the possibility of bearing an unhealthy child or a child with a genetic disorder. As discussed previously, screening tests are available to assess for Down syndrome. Because of the risk of Down syndrome in these families, amniocentesis is often suggested or may be indicated if screening results are not in the normal range.

For couples who agree to amniocentesis, the first few months of pregnancy are a difficult time. Amniocentesis cannot be done until week 14 of pregnancy, and the chromosomal studies take roughly 2 weeks to complete. Their fear that the fetus is at risk may delay the successful completion of the psychologic tasks of early pregnancy.

You can support couples who decide to have amniocentesis by providing information and answering questions about the procedure and by providing comfort and emotional support during the amniocentesis. If the results indicate that the fetus has Down syndrome or another genetic abnormality, ensure that the couple has complete information about the condition, its range of possible manifestations, and its developmental implications.

Evaluation

Expected outcomes of nursing care include the following:

- The woman and her partner are knowledgeable about the pregnancy and express confidence in their ability to make appropriate healthcare choices.
- The expectant parents (and their children) are able to cope with the pregnancy and its implications for the future.
- The woman receives effective health care throughout her pregnancy and during birth and the postpartum period.
- The woman and her partner develop skills in child care and parenting.

Care of the Pregnant Woman With Special Needs

More than 1 million women of childbearing age report that they have a chronic physical disability (CPD) that causes them to need assistance with activities of daily living (Signore, Spong, Kroloski, et al., 2011). Of this number, approximately 163,700 women with a CPD become pregnant each year (Iezzoni, Yu, Wint, et al., 2014).

Chronic physical disabilities may include mobility difficulties that involve upper or lower extremities, arthritis, vision or hearing problems, disorders such as multiple sclerosis or cerebral palsy, heart or lung problems, and a variety of diseases. These numbers are predicted to increase because dramatic improvements in medical care are enabling women born with a CPD and those who acquire them through accident or illness to live into their childbearing years and beyond. Moreover, changes in societal attitudes have led to a decrease in stigmatization of disability, and civil rights laws such as the Americans with Disabilities Act provide increased support and acceptance for women with disabilities who seek motherhood. In addition, technologically sophisticated maternity and newborn care has made positive pregnancy outcomes more likely (Iezzoni, Yu, Wint, et al., 2013).

Women with an intellectual disability may also become pregnant and have special needs for teaching and support. Among these women there is a high incidence of unplanned pregnancy, and they often seek prenatal care late. Typically, they have lower reading and comprehension levels and are at a disadvantage when presented with complex information (Porter, Kidd, Murray, et al., 2012). Healthcare providers may perceive the pregnancy negatively, and the woman may experience social isolation and anxiety. Women with intellectual disabilities are also at increased risk of intervention by social services, which may result in the removal of the newborns from their custody.

Collectively, women with disabilities have often been discouraged from becoming mothers. Research suggests that these women often perceive themselves as "perennial outsiders" who are automatically categorized as high risk because of their disability (Walsh-Gallagher, Conkey, Sinclair, et al., 2013).

A family-centered approach is designed to optimize the childbearing experience of *all* women by providing a high-quality, individualized experience that builds on the strength of each woman rather than perceived limitations. Ideally, this begins with preconception counseling so that the woman is in optimal health before conception. The woman and her family should be advised of potential health concerns and given information about their management.

During pregnancy, professional support and a team effort are essential. The woman needs to have a sense that she is empowered to make her health care decisions and that she has a good degree of control over the experience. In many cases, care at a tertiary level facility is important to an optimal outcome.

Women With Special Needs Intimate Partner Violence

Women with disabilities are at greater risk of being victimized and of sustaining intimate partner violence. Women who rely on their partner for assistance with activities of daily living are at risk for having care withheld and of being neglected in addition to physical and mental abuse. They are also at risk for financial abuse. The nurse should provide an extensive intimate partner assessment with the woman without the partner present to determine if abuse is occurring.

Nursing Management
For the Woman With a Disability

Nursing Assessment and Diagnosis

In addition to the assessments made for all pregnant women, nursing assessment of a woman with a disability needs to be condition specific. These assessments will vary depending on the extent of the woman's disability. A discussion of every possible disability is beyond the scope of this text. Some general principles are provided here.

A woman with a mobility disorder, especially if it is extensive, as in the case of a spinal cord injury, needs careful assessment. Be alert for commonly occurring complications associated with her condition such as pressure ulcers, bladder infection, gastroesophageal reflux disease (GERD), deep vein thrombosis (DVT), stool impaction, anemia, and autonomic dysreflexia (a rapid increase in blood pressure in response to a noxious stimulus such as catheterization, or uterine contractions below the level of the spinal cord lesion) (Camune, 2013). Weight gain and changes in the woman's center of gravity may increase the risk for falls. In addition, the woman may be unaware of preterm labor and thus faces the possibility of an unattended birth.

Assess the woman with an intellectual disability for her level of understanding of instructions and printed materials. Determine her awareness of the signs of complications and of the onset of labor. Also evaluate her level of support from her partner and family members.

Nursing diagnoses that may apply include the following (NANDA I © 2014):

- *Dysreflexia, Autonomic*, related to a spinal cord injury
- *Skin Integrity, Risk for Impaired*, related to decreased or absent mobility
- *Knowledge, Deficient*, related to a documented learning disability

Nursing Plan and Implementation

Women with a disability involving a lower extremity (e.g., amputation, spinal cord injury) may need assistance in issues involving mobility such as transferring to an examination table or bed. Typically, they will have adaptive equipment. Women who use wheelchairs may find that additional weight late in pregnancy may interfere with their ability to propel their chairs (Figure 12–5). Thus it is important that the woman avoid excessive weight gain and regularly perform range of motion exercises (Signore et al., 2011).

During labor, assist the woman to change position periodically to avoid dependent edema. Be alert for signs of respiratory distress, DVT, and autonomic dysreflexia. Provide necessary adaptive equipment. Women with a loss of sensation in their lower extremities may find it difficult or impossible to push effectively and consequently have an increased incidence of cesarean birth. Women with upper extremity disorders may need assistance with, for example, position change or holding the newborn. Assist with breastfeeding as necessary.

The most important need of pregnant women with intellectual disabilities is for information that is timely, accessible, and understandable. They often find that information available for the general population is too difficult to understand. To address this need, easy-to-understand information should be available. It is also helpful for caregivers to allow extra consultation

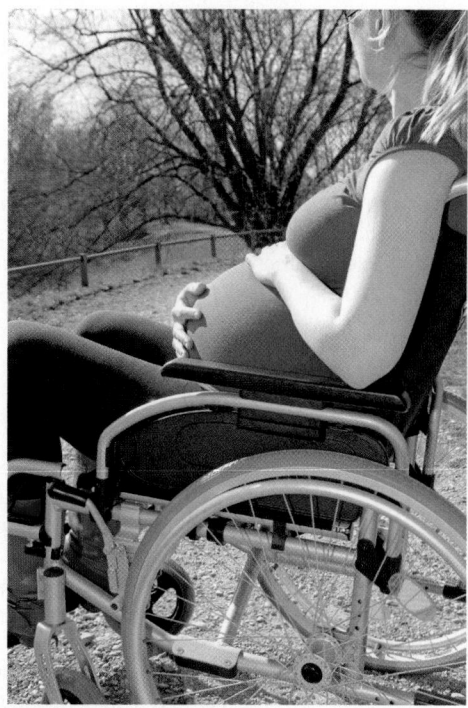

Figure 12–5 **Pregnant woman with a lower extremity disability.**

SOURCE: RioPatuca Images/Fotolia.

time and good communication aids. This might include videotaping or audio-taping information so the woman can refer to it as needed (Porter et al., 2012).

Evaluation

Expected outcomes of nursing care include the following:

- The expectant woman is able to cope with the pregnancy and its implications for the future.
- The woman receives effective health care throughout her pregnancy and during birth and the postpartum period.

Focus Your Study

- Many factors contribute to the high teenage pregnancy rate, including earlier age of first sexual intercourse, lack of knowledge about conception, lack of easy access to contraception, lessened stigma associated with adolescent pregnancy in some populations, poverty, early school failure, and early childhood sexual abuse.
- Physical risks of adolescent pregnancies include preterm births, low-birth-weight babies, cephalopelvic disproportion, iron deficiency anemia, and preeclampsia and its sequelae.
- Factors affecting an adolescent's response to pregnancy include her degree of achievement of the developmental tasks

of adolescence (which can be closely associated with age) as well as cultural, religious, and socioeconomic factors.

- Nurses working with pregnant adolescents face many challenges, including safeguarding the client's confidentiality, winning her trust, and helping to build her sense of self-esteem.
- Often the adolescent has little understanding of pregnancy, childbirth, or parenting. Consequently, education is a primary responsibility of the nurse.
- Adolescent pregnancy prevention programs should be multifaceted, target males as well as females, and involve community-wide approaches.

- Childbirth among women over 35 is becoming increasingly common. It poses fewer health risks than previously believed and offers advantages for the woman or couple who makes this choice.

- A major risk for the older expectant couple relates to the increased incidence of Down syndrome in children born to women over age 35. Screening tests and amniocentesis can provide information as to whether the fetus has Down syndrome. The couple can then decide whether they wish to continue the pregnancy.

- Common risks of a pregnant woman with a mobility disorder include pressure ulcers, bladder infection, gastroesophageal reflux disease (GERD), deep vein thrombosis (DVT), stool impaction, anemia, and autonomic dysreflexia.

- The most pressing needs of a woman with an intellectual disability who becomes pregnant are accurate information appropriate to her level of understanding and consistent emotional support.

Clinical Reasoning in Action

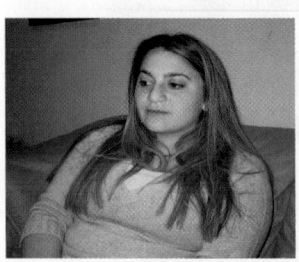

Sixteen-year-old Linda Perez and her mother present to you at the OB clinic for Linda's first prenatal visit. You determine that Linda is 20 weeks pregnant. Her weight is 135 lb, height 5 ft 4 in., T 98°F (36.6°C), P 80, R 14, BP 100/64. You assess that Linda's mother has type 2 diabetes, and that her siblings are healthy. Linda admits to having one sexual partner, and says she has never been hospitalized. Her immunizations are up-to-date, and she has never used tobacco or recreational drugs. To date, the father of the baby is not involved. Mrs. Perez is clearly upset that Linda's pregnancy is so far advanced without her knowledge. Linda is quiet and speaks only when questioned directly. You do your best to try to establish a trusting relationship with Linda and her mother by providing an atmosphere where issues can be discussed.

1. What psychologic factors contribute to teenage pregnancy?
2. Explore reasons why teenagers delay prenatal care.
3. Linda's mother asks you what factors facilitate adolescent pregnancies.
4. You assess that Linda has some anxiety concerning the birth process. She states she is not interested in prenatal classes because she is single and does not want to have natural childbirth. What would be your best response?

References

Alan Guttmacher Institute (AGI). (2012a). *Facts on American teens' sexual and reproductive health*. Retrieved from http://www.guttmacher.org/pubs/FB-ATSRH.pdf

Alan Guttmacher Institute (AGI). (2012b). *Facts on American teens' sources of information about sex.* Retrieved from http://www.guttmacher.org/pubs/FB-Teen-Sex-Ed.pdf

Alan Guttmacher Institute (AGI). (2012c). *Minors' access to prenatal care*. Retrieved from http://www.guttmacher.org/statecenter/spibs/spib_MAPC.pdf

Alan Guttmacher Institute (AGI). (2012d). *Minors' rights as parents*. Retrieved from http://www.guttmacher.org/statecenter/spibs/spib_MRP.pdf

Alan Guttmacher Institute (AGI). (2012e). *State policies in brief: Minors' access to contraceptive services*. Retrieved from http://www.guttmacher.org/statecenter/spibs/spib_MACS.pdf

Alan Guttmacher Institute (AGI). (2013). *Facts on American teens' sexual and reproductive health*. Retrieved from http://www.guttmacher.org/pubs/FB-ATSRH.pdf

Albert, B. (2012). *With one voice: America's adults and teens sound off about teen pregnancy*. Retrieved from http://thenationalcampaign.org/resource/one-voice-2012

American Academy of Pediatrics (AAP). (2012). Policy statement: Emergency contraception. *Pediatrics, 130*(6), 1174–1180.

American Academy of Pediatrics (AAP). (2014). Policy statement: Contraception for adolescents. *Pediatrics, 134,*(4), e1244–e1256.

Baldwin, M. K., & Edelman, A. B. (2013). The effect of long-acting reversible contraception on rapid repeat pregnancy in adolescents: A review. *The Journal of Adolescent Health, 52*(4 Suppl), S47–53.

Ben Itzchak, E., Lahat, E., & Zachor, D. A. (2011). Advanced parental ages and low birth weight in autism spectrum disorders—Rates and effect on functioning. *Research in Developmental Disabilities, 32*(5), 1776–1781.

Broussard, A. B., & Broussard, B. S. (2010). Teaching pregnant teens: Lessons learned. *Nursing for Women's Health, 14*(2), 104–111.

Camune, B. D. (2013). Challenges in the management of the pregnant woman with a spinal cord injury. *Journal of Perinatal and Neonatal Nursing, 27*(3), 225–231.

Carolan, M. (2013). Maternal age ≥ 45 years and maternal and perinatal outcomes: A review of the evidence. *Midwifery, 29,*479–489.

Centers for Disease Control and Prevention (CDC). (2011). *Sexually transmitted disease surveillance 2010*. Atlanta, GA: U.S. Department of Health and Human Services.

Chiu, R. W., & Lo, Y. D. (2011). Non-invasive prenatal diagnosis by fetal nucleic acid in maternal plasma: The coming of age. *Seminars in Fetal and Neonatal Medicine, 16*(2), 88–93.

Cunningham, F. G., Leveno, K. J., Bloom, S. L., Spong, C. Y., Dashe, J. S., Hoffman, B. L., ... Sheffield, J. S. (2014). *Williams Obstetrics* (24th ed.). New York, NY: McGraw-Hill.

Fletcher, J. M., & Wolfe, B. L. (2012). The effects of teenage fatherhood on young adult outcomes. *Economic Inquiry, 50*(1), 182–201.

Food and Drug Administration, (FDA). (2013). FDA approves Plan B One-Step emergency contraceptive for use without prescription for all women of child-bearing potential. Retrieved from http://www.fda.gov/NewsEvents/Newsroom/PressAnnouncements/ucm358082.htm

Forcier, M., & Harel, Z. (2011). Adolescents and the IUD: An underutilized contraception for a high-risk population. *The Female Patient, 36*(6), 22–25.

Helfrich, C., & McWey, L. (2014). Substance use and delinquency: high-risk behaviors as predictors of teen pregnancy among adolescents involved with the child welfare system. *Journal of Family Issues, 35*(10), 1322–1338.

Herrman, J. W. (2010). Assessing the teen parent family. *Nursing for Women's Health, 14*(3), 214–224.

Herrman, J. W. (2014). Adolescent girls who experience abuse or neglect are at an increased risk of teen pregnancy. *Evidence Based Nursing, 17*(3), 79.

Herrman, J. W., & Nandakumar, R. (2012). Development of a survey to assess adolescent perceptions of teen parenting. *Journal of Nursing Measurement, 20*(1), 3–20.

House, L., Bates, J., Markham, C., & Lesesne, C. (2010). Competence as a predictor of reproductive health outcomes for youth: A systematic review. *Journal of Adolescent Health, 46*(3, Suppl. 1), S7–S22.

Iezzoni, L. I., Yu, J, Wint, A. J., Smeltzer, S. C., & Eaker, J. L. (2013). Prevalence of current pregnancy among US women with and without chronic physical disabilities. *Medical Care, 51*(6), 555–562.

Iezzoni, L. I., Yu, J, Wint, A. J., Smeltzer, S. C., & Eaker, J. L. (2014). General health, health conditions, and current pregnancy among U. S. women with and without chronic physical disabilities. *Disability and Health Journal, 7,* 181–188.

Kann, L., Kinchen, S., Shanklin, S. L., Flint, K. H., Hawkins, J., Harris, W. A., ... Zaza, S. (2014). Youth Risk Behavior Surveillance—United States, 2013. *MMWR Surveillance Summaries, 63*(4), 1–172.

Katz, A. (2011). Adolescent pregnancy: The good, the bad and the promise. *Nursing for Women's Health, 14*(2), 149–152.

Kearney, M. S., & Levine, P. B. (2012). Why is the teen birth rate in the United States so high and why does it matter? *Journal of Economic Perspectives, 26*(2), 141–166.

Kirven, J. (2014). Helping teen dads obtain and sustain parental success. *International Journal of Childbirth Education, 29*(2), 85–88.

Klettke, B., Hallford, D. J., & Mellor, D. J. (2014). Sexting prevalence and correlates: A systematic literature review. *Clinical Psychology Review, 34*(1), 44–53.

Lee, Y., Cintron, A., & Kocher, S. (2014). Factors related to risky sexual behaviors and effective STI/HIV and pregnancy intervention programs for African American adolescents. *Public Health Nursing, 31*(5), 414–427.

Lohan, M., Cruise, S., O'Halloran, P., Alderdice, F., & Hyde, A. (2010). Adolescent men's attitudes in relation to pregnancy and pregnancy outcomes: A systematic review of the literature from 1980–2009. *Journal of Adolescent Health, 47*, 327–345.

March of Dimes (MOD). (2012). *Teenage pregnancy*. Retrieved from http://www.marchofdimes.com /materials/teenage-pregnancy.pdf

Martin, J. A., Hamilton, B. E., Osterman, M. J. K., Curtin, S. C., & Mathews, T. J. (2013). Births: Final data for 2012. *National Vital Statistics Reports, 62*(9), 1–87.

National Campaign to Prevent Teen and Unplanned Pregnancy (NCPTUP). (2012a). *Ten tips for parents*. Retrieved from http://www.thenationalcampaign.org /parents/ten_tips.aspx

National Campaign to Prevent Teen and Unplanned Pregnancy (NCPTUP). (2012b). *Our mission: Goal*. Retrieved from http://www.thenationalcampaign.org /about-us/our-mission.aspx

Porter, E., Kidd, G., Murray, N., Spink, A., & Anderson, B. (2012). Developing the pregnancy support pack for people who have a learning disability. *British Journal of Learning Disabilities, 40*, 310–317.

Ralph, L., Gould, H., Baker, A., & Foster, D. G. (2014). The role of parents and partners in minors' decisions to have an abortion and anticipated coping after abortion. *Journal of Adolescent Health, 54*, 428–434.

Signore, C., Spong, C. Y., Krotoski, D., Shinowara, N. L., & Blackwell, S. C. (2011). Pregnancy in women with physical disabilities. *Obstetrics & Gynecology, 117*(4), 935–947.

Sipsma, H. L., Ickovics, J. R., Lewis, J. B., Ethier, K. A., & Kershaw, T. S. (2011). Adolescent pregnancy desire and pregnancy incidence. *Women's Health Issues, 21*(2), 110–116.

Steinberg, L. (2014). *Adolescence* (10th ed.). New York, NY: McGraw-Hill.

Turnage, B. F., & Pharris, A. D. (2013). Supporting the pregnant adolescent. *International Journal of Childbirth Education, 28*(4), 72–76.

Ventura, S. J., Hamilton, B. E., & Mathews, T. J. (2014). National and state patterns of teen births in the United States, 1940–2013. *National Vital Statistics Reports, 63*(4), 1–34.

Walsh-Gallagher, D., McConkey, R., Sinclair, M., & Clarke, R. (2013). Normalising birth for women with a disability: The challenges facing practitioners. *Midwifery, 29*(4), 294–299.

Wiener-Megnazi, Z., Auslender, R., & Dirnfeld, M. (2012). Advanced paternal age and reproductive outcome. *Asian Journal of Andrology, 14*(1), 69–76.

Yoost, J. L., Hertweck, S. P., & Barnett, S. N. (2014). The effect of an educational approach to pregnancy prevention among high-risk early and late adolescents. *Journal of Adolescent Health, 55*(2), 222–227.

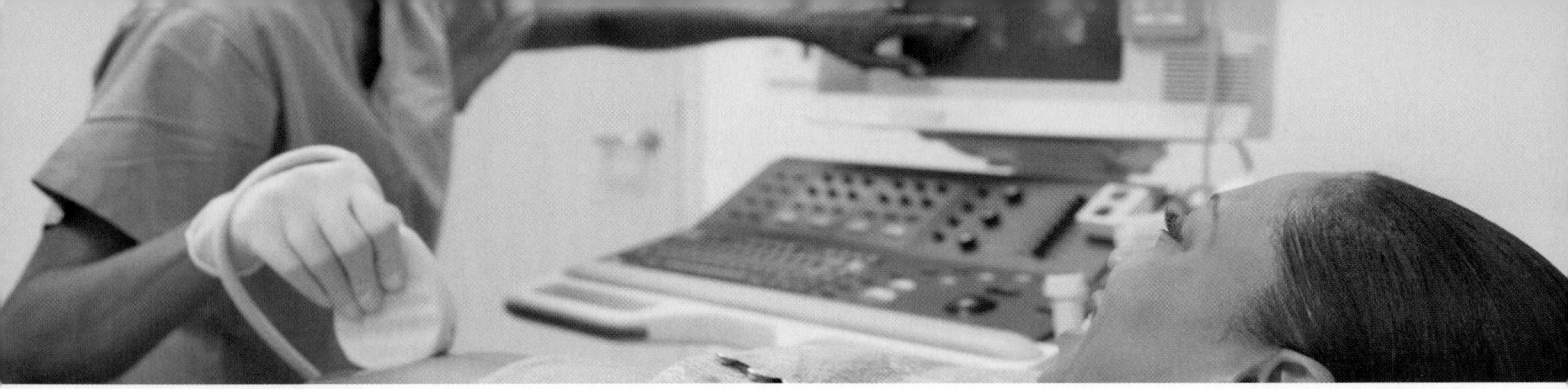

Chapter 13
Assessment of Fetal Well-Being

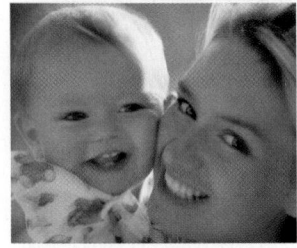

My first pregnancy was so tenuous that I didn't know from one moment to the next how it would end. I hoped for our baby's safety, but in the end the baby died. When I became pregnant the next time, I was very nervous. Being able to see the baby on ultrasound helped me so much. I knew then that our baby was alive and growing.

—Sharon, 29

Peter Bowater/Science Source

∨ Learning Outcomes

13.1 Identify pertinent information to be discussed with the woman regarding her own assessment of fetal activity and methods of recording fetal activity.

13.2 Describe the methods, clinical applications, and results of ultrasound in the nursing management of the pregnant woman.

13.3 Describe the use, procedure, information obtained, and nursing considerations for the following: first trimester combined screening, cell-free fetal DNA testing, Doppler velocimetry,

non-stress test, fetal acoustic and vibroacoustic stimulation tests, biophysical profile, and contraction stress test.

13.4 Explain the use of amniocentesis as a diagnostic tool.

13.5 Describe the tests that can be performed using amniotic fluid.

13.6 Compare the advantages and disadvantages of chorionic villus sampling (CVS).

The past few decades have produced a notable increase in the number of techniques used to assess fetal well-being. From the relatively simple maternal assessment of fetal movement to more complex diagnostic tests guided by ultrasound, each technique is used to obtain accurate and helpful data about the developing fetus. For example, specialized diagnostic tests can provide information about the normal growth of the fetus, the presence of congenital anomalies, the location of the placenta, and fetal lung maturity (Table 13–1). At times, just one test is done, and in other circumstances, a combination of testing is needed.

Some of these assessment techniques pose risks to the fetus and possibly to the pregnant woman; the risk to both should be considered before deciding to perform the test. The healthcare provider must be certain that the advantages outweigh the potential risks and added expense. In addition, the diagnostic accuracy and applicability of these tests may vary.

Although some tests are for screening purposes, meaning that they indicate the fetus *may* be at risk for a certain disorder or abnormality, others are diagnostic, meaning that they can diagnose the abnormality. Certainly not all high-risk pregnancies require the same tests. Factors that indicate a pregnancy at risk include the following:

- Maternal age less than 16 or more than 35 years
- Chronic maternal hypertension, preeclampsia, diabetes mellitus, or heart disease
- Presence of Rh alloimmunization
- A maternal history of unexplained stillbirth
- Suspected intrauterine growth restriction (IUGR)
- Pregnancy prolonged past 42 weeks' gestation
- Multiple gestation
- Maternal history of preterm labor
- Previous cervical insufficiency

TABLE 13–1 Summary of Screening and Diagnostic Tests

GOAL	TEST	TIMING
To validate the pregnancy	Ultrasound: gestational sac volume	5 and 6 weeks after last menstrual period (LMP) by transvaginal ultrasound
To determine how advanced is the pregnancy	Ultrasound: crown–rump length	6–10 weeks' gestation
	Ultrasound: biparietal diameter, femur length, abdominal circumference	13–40 weeks' gestation
To identify normal growth of the fetus	Ultrasound: biparietal diameter	Most useful from 20–30 weeks' gestation
	Ultrasound: head/abdomen ratio	13–40 weeks' gestation
	Ultrasound: estimated fetal weight	About 24–40 weeks' gestation
To detect congenital anomalies and problems	Nuchal translucency testing	11–13 weeks' gestation
	Ultrasound	18–40 weeks' gestation
	Chorionic villus sampling	10–12 weeks' gestation
	Amniocentesis	15–20 weeks' gestation
	Fetoscopy	18 weeks' gestation
	First-trimester combined screening test	11–13 weeks' gestation
	Quadruple test	Generally 15–20 weeks' gestation
	Cell-free fetal DNA testing	After 10 weeks' gestation
To localize the placenta	Ultrasound	Usually in third trimester or before amniocentesis
To assess fetal status	Biophysical profile	Approximately 28 weeks to birth
	Maternal assessment of fetal activity	Approximately 28 weeks to birth
	Non-stress test	Approximately 28 weeks to birth
	Contraction stress test	After 28 weeks
To diagnose cardiac problems	Fetal echocardiography	Second and third trimesters
To assess fetal lung maturity	Amniocentesis	33–40 weeks
	L/S ratio	33 weeks to birth
	Phosphatidylglycerol	33 weeks to birth
	Phosphatidylcholine	33 weeks to birth
	Lamellar body counts	33 weeks to birth
To obtain more information about breech presentation	Ultrasound	Just before labor is anticipated or during labor

See Chapter 8 for further discussion of prenatal at-risk factors and Chapters 14 and 15 for descriptions of various conditions that may threaten the successful completion of pregnancy.

Nursing care for the woman who is undergoing diagnostic testing focuses on outcomes to ensure that she understands the reasons for the test and its results and receives adequate support during the test (see Table 13–2). In addition, other objectives include

TABLE 13–2 Suggested Nursing Approaches to Pretest Teaching

Assess if the woman knows the reason the screening or diagnostic test is being recommended.

Examples:

"What has your doctor or nurse-midwife told you about why this test is necessary?"

"Sometimes tests are done for many different reasons. Can you tell me why you are having this test?"

"What is your understanding about what the test will show?"

Provide an opportunity for questions.
Examples:

"What questions do you have about the test?"

"Is there anything that is not clear to you?"

Explain the test procedure, paying particular attention to any preparation the woman needs before the test.
Example:

"The test that has been ordered for you is designed to _____ _____." (Add specific information about the particular test. Give the explanation using simple language.)

Validate the woman's understanding of the preparation.
Example:

"Tell me what you will have to do to get ready for this test."

Give permission for the woman to continue to ask questions if needed.
Example:

"I'll be with you during the test. If you have any questions at any time, please don't hesitate to ask."

completing the tests without complications and ensuring that the safety of the mother and her unborn child has been maintained.

Maternal Assessment of Fetal Activity

Clinicians now generally agree that vigorous fetal activity provides reassurance of fetal well-being and that marked decrease in activity or cessation of movement may indicate possible fetal compromise (or even death) requiring immediate follow-up (Blackburn, 2013). Fetal activity is typically used to monitor fetal well-being beginning at approximately 28 gestational weeks. Fetal activity monitoring has been used for some time as a low-technology, inexpensive means to evaluate fetal well-being. One study of mothers with perceived decreased fetal movement identified 80% of those fetuses with intrauterine growth restriction (King, Brucker, Kriebs, et al., 2013). A reduction of fetal movement has been associated with fetal hypoxia, fetal growth restriction, and fetal death (Malm, Lindgren, Rubertsson, et al., 2014). Although more research is needed to

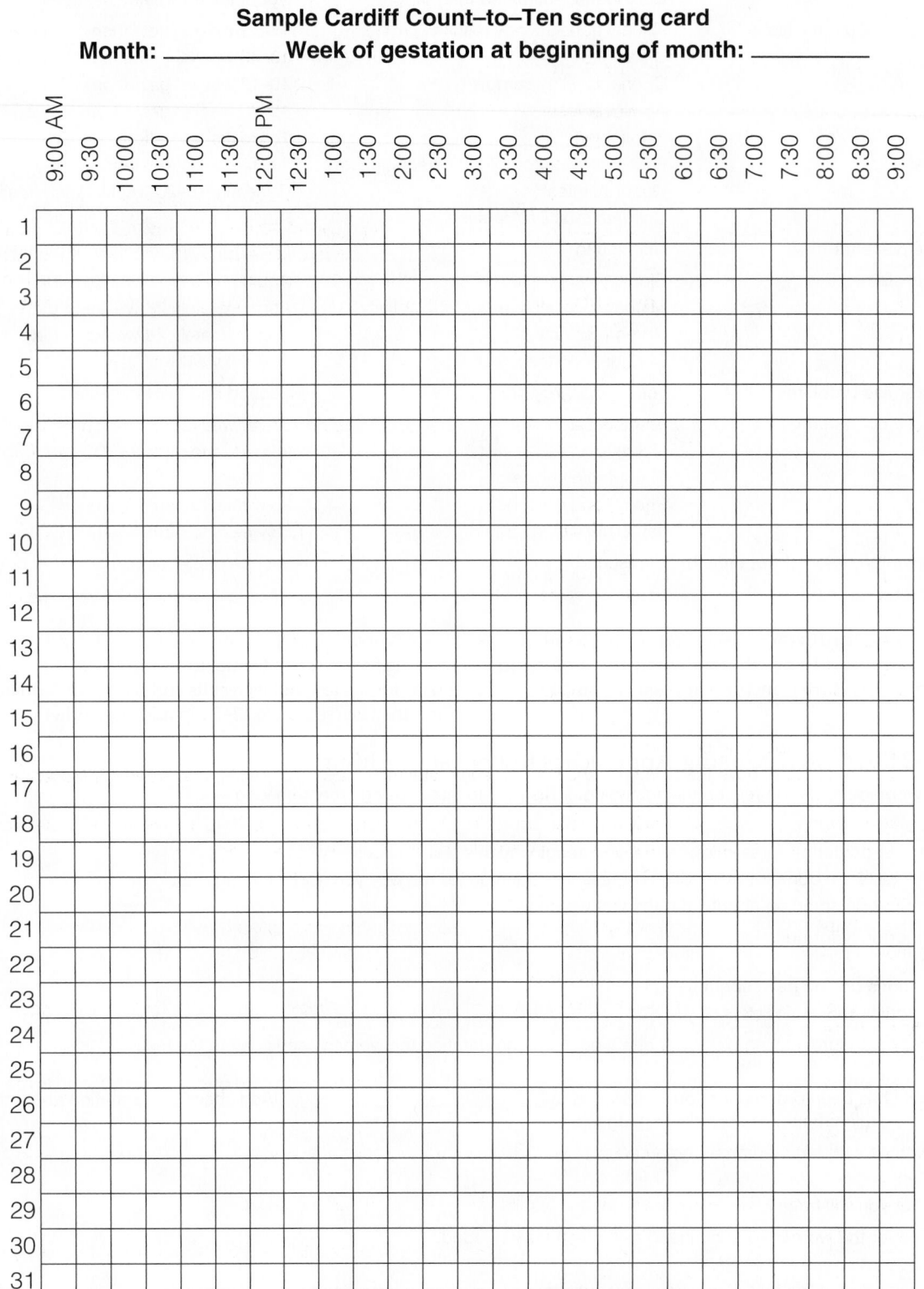

Sample Cardiff Count–to–Ten scoring card

Month: _____ Week of gestation at beginning of month: _____

Figure 13–1 An adaptation of the Cardiff Count-to-Ten scoring card for fetal movement assessment.

determine if fetal activity assessment improves neonatal outcomes, the literature does suggest that maternal monitoring does result in a decrease in perinatal mortality and decreases maternal anxiety (Malm et al., 2014).

A variety of methods for obtaining a **fetal movement count (FMC)** have been developed. They focus on having the woman keep a **fetal movement record (FMR)** using a technique such as the Cardiff Count-to-Ten method (see Figure 13–1). An FMR is noninvasive and lets the pregnant woman monitor and record movements easily and without expense. See *Teaching Highlights: What to Tell the Pregnant Woman About Assessing Fetal Activity*.

Clinical Tip

Families undergoing fetal testing experience a wide range of emotions based on personal expectations, past experiences, fears, and cultural norms. Encouraging the family to verbalize concerns, ask questions, and express any apprehensions or fears can help put the family at ease.

Women With Special Needs Women With Paralysis

Women with paralysis often warrant intermittent fetal surveillance since they are unable to feel fetal movement or premature contractions. These women are at risk for unattended birth since they cannot perceive their contractions. Their partner or healthcare provider should be trained to palpate contractions and observe for fetal movement on a regular basis.

Fetuses spend approximately 10% of their time making gross body movements. Fetal movements are directly related to the fetus's sleep–wake cycles and vary from the maternal sleep–wake cycle (Blackburn, 2013). After 38 weeks, the fetus spends 75% of its time in a quiet sleep or active sleep state. In a woman with a multiple gestation, daily fetal movements are significantly higher. The expectant mother's perception of fetal movements and her commitment to completing a fetal movement record may vary. When a woman understands the purpose of the assessment, how to complete the form, who to call with questions, and what to report—and has the opportunity for follow-up during each visit—she generally views completing the fetal movement record as an important activity. The nurse is available to answer questions and clarify areas of concern.

Ultrasound

Valuable information about the fetus may be obtained from **ultrasound** testing. Intermittent ultrasonic waves (high-frequency sound waves) are transmitted by an alternating current to a transducer, which is applied to the woman's abdomen. The ultrasonic waves deflect off tissues within the woman's abdomen, showing structures of varying densities (Figures 13–2 and 13–3).

Diagnostic ultrasound has several advantages. It is noninvasive, is painless for both the woman and the fetus, and has no known harmful effects to either. Serial studies (several ultrasound tests done over a span of time) may be done for assessment and comparison. Soft-tissue masses (such as tumors)

TEACHING HIGHLIGHTS | What to Tell the Pregnant Woman About Assessing Fetal Activity

- Explain that fetal movements are first felt around 18 weeks' gestation. From that time, the fetal movements get stronger and easier to detect. A slowing or stopping of fetal movement may be an indication that the fetus needs some attention and evaluation.

- Explain the procedure for the Cardiff Count-to-Ten method or for the daily fetal movement record. For both methods, advise the woman to:
  - Keep a daily record of fetal movement, beginning at about 27 weeks' gestation.
  - Try to begin counting at about the same time each day, about 1 hour after a meal if possible.
  - Lie quietly in a side-lying position.

- Using the Cardiff card, have the woman place an X for each fetal movement until she has recorded 10. Movement varies considerably, but most women feel fetal movement at least 10 times in 3 hours.

- Using the daily fetal movement record, have the woman count three times a day for 20 to 30 minutes each session. If there are fewer than three movements in a session, have the woman count for 1 hour or more.

- Explain when to contact the care provider:
  - If there are fewer than 10 movements in 3 hours
  - If overall the fetus's movements are slowing, and it takes much longer each day to note 10 movements
  - If there are no movements in the morning
  - If there are fewer than three movements in 8 hours

- Describe procedures and demonstrate how to assess fetal movement. Sit beside the woman and show her how to place her hand on the fundus to feel fetal movement.

- Provide a written teaching sheet for the woman's use at home.

- Demonstrate how to record fetal movements on the Cardiff Count-to-Ten scoring card or on the daily fetal movement record.
  - Watch the woman fill out the record as examples are provided. Encourage her to complete the record each day and bring it with her to each prenatal visit. Assure her that the record will be discussed at each prenatal visit, and questions may be addressed at that time if desired.
  - Provide the woman with a name and phone number in case she has further questions.
  - Evaluate learning by having the woman explain the method and by asking the woman to fill the card in using a fictitious situation. At each prenatal visit, the expectant mother's record is reviewed. This provides another opportunity for evaluation of learning and for questions and clarification.

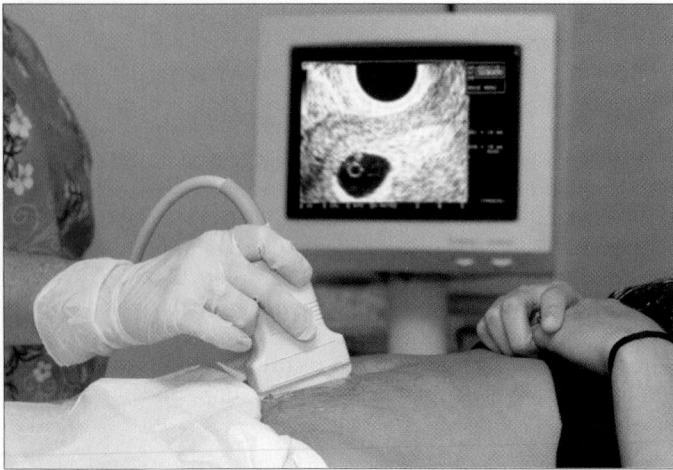

Figure 13–2 Ultrasound scanning permits visualization of the fetus in utero.

SOURCE: Steven Frame/Shutterstock.

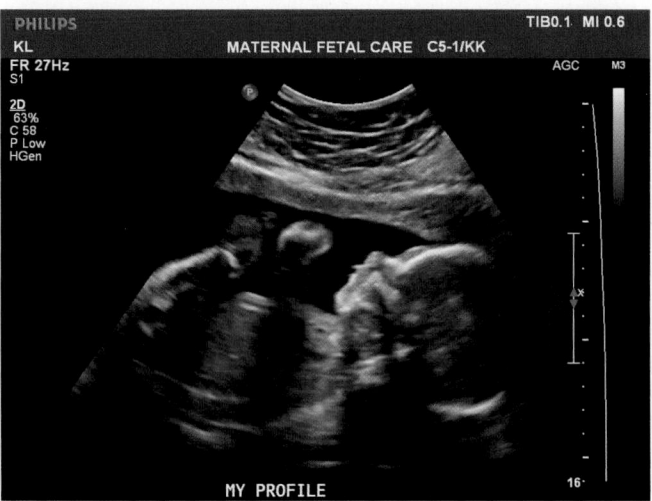

Figure 13–3 Ultrasound of the face and body of a fetus.

can be differentiated, the fetus can be visualized, fetal growth can be followed (especially in the presence of multiple gestation), cervical length and impending cervical insufficiency can be detected, and a number of other potential problems can be averted In addition, the ultrasonographer or physician immediately obtains results.

Future research in fetal well-being will be generated and enhanced by the use of *four-dimensional ultrasound*. Four-dimensional ultrasound combines the components of three-dimensional ultrasound with a fourth dimension, time, because it monitors live action. The technology produces images of photo-like quality, allowing healthcare providers to better visualize fetal structures, and providing better guidance during invasive intrauterine procedures such as amniocentesis and chorionic villus sampling (CVS) (discussed later in this chapter). However, advanced 3D/4D techniques can increase the incidence of artifacts, which could increase the need for additional scanning and increase parental anxiety (Malhotra, Shah, Kumar, et al., 2014).

Although ultrasound serves as a useful tool in monitoring the fetus throughout pregnancy, ultrasound has limitations and it cannot guarantee that a fetus does not have certain disorders or defects. Ultrasound is limited by fetal positioning and by technician or physician skill. Even though fetal problems can be diagnosed via the technology, abnormalities may, at times, go unrecognized. A "normal" ultrasound is reassuring for the parents and healthcare team, but it is important that parents realize the ultrasound or sonogram is not 100% reliable.

Procedures

The two most common methods of ultrasound scanning are transabdominal and transvaginal.

TRANSABDOMINAL ULTRASOUND

In the transabdominal approach, a transducer is moved across the woman's abdomen. The woman is often scanned with a full bladder. When the bladder is full, the examiner can assess other structures, especially the vagina and cervix, in relation to the bladder. The ability to see the lower portion of the uterus and cervix is particularly important when vaginal bleeding is noted and placenta previa is the suspected cause. The woman is advised to drink 1.0 to 1.5 quarts of water approximately 2 hours before the examination, and she is asked to refrain from emptying her bladder. If the bladder is not sufficiently filled, she is asked to drink three to four 8-oz glasses of water and is rescanned 30 to 45 minutes later.

Transmission gel is generously spread over the woman's abdomen, and the sonographer slowly moves a transducer over the abdomen to obtain a picture of the uterine contents. Ultrasound testing takes 20 to 30 minutes. The woman may feel discomfort caused by pressure applied over a full bladder. In addition, if the woman lies on her back during the test, shortness of breath can develop. This may be relieved by elevating her upper body during the test.

TRANSVAGINAL ULTRASOUND

The transvaginal approach uses a probe inserted into the vagina. Once inserted, the transvaginal probe is close to the structures being imaged and so produces a clearer, more defined image than is possible with the transabdominal approach. The improved images obtained by transvaginal ultrasound have enabled sonographers to identify structures and fetal characteristics earlier in pregnancy. Internal visualization can also be used as a predictor for preterm birth in high-risk cases. Use of the ultrasound to detect shortened cervical length or funneling (a cone-shaped indentation in the cervical os) is helpful in predicting preterm labor, especially in women who have a history of preterm birth (Cunningham et al., 2014).

After the procedure is fully explained to the woman, she is prepared in the same manner as for a pelvic examination: in the lithotomy position, with appropriate drapes to provide privacy and a female attendant in the room. It is important for her buttocks to be at the end of the table so that, once inserted, the probe can be moved in various directions. A small, lightweight vaginal transducer is covered with a specially fitted sterile sheath, a condom, or one finger of a glove. Ultrasound coupling gel is then applied to both the inside and outside of the covering, making insertion into the vagina easier and providing a medium for enhancing the ultrasound image. The transvaginal procedure can be accomplished with an empty bladder, and most women do not feel discomfort during the examination. The probe is smaller than a speculum, so insertion is usually completed with ease. The woman may feel the movement of the probe during the examination as various structures are imaged. Some women may choose to insert the probe themselves to enhance their comfort, whereas others would feel embarrassed even to be asked. The certified nurse-midwife, physician, or ultrasonographer offers the choice based on personal rapport with the woman.

Clinical Applications

Ultrasound testing can be of benefit in the following ways:

- *Early identification of pregnancy.* Pregnancy may be detected as early as the fifth or sixth week after the last menstrual period (LMP) by assessing the gestational sac and the presence of a fetal heart rate (FHR) after 6 gestational weeks.

- *Observation of fetal heartbeat and fetal breathing movements (FBMs).* FBMs have been observed as early as week 11 of gestation.

- *Identification of more than one embryo or fetus.*

- *Measurement of the biparietal diameter of the fetal head or the fetal femur length to assess growth patterns.* These measurements help determine the gestational age of the fetus and identify intrauterine growth restriction (IUGR).

- *Clinical estimations of birth weight.* This assessment helps to identify macrosomia (neonates greater than 4000 g at birth) and low-birth-weight neonates (neonates less than 2500 g at birth). Macrosomia has been identified as a predictor of birth-related trauma and is a risk factor for both maternal and fetal morbidity (Jazayeri, 2012).

- *Detection of fetal anomalies such as facial anomalies, anencephaly, and hydrocephalus (Richards, 2012).*

- *Examination of nuchal translucency in the first trimester to assess for trisomy 21 (Down syndrome) and other fetal structural anomalies (Richards, 2012).* Nuchal translucency describes an area in the back of the fetal neck that is measured via ultrasound during the first trimester of pregnancy. Fetuses with a nuchal translucency measurement of greater than 3 mm are at risk for certain birth defects, including trisomies 13, 18, and 21.

- *Examination of fetal cardiac structures (echocardiography).* The presence of fetal cardiac defects during the first-trimester nuchal translucency screening test increases the risk that the fetus has a chromosomal disorder (Miguelez, De Lourdes Brizot, Liao, et al., 2012).

- *Length of fetal nasal bone.* The length of the fetal nasal bone during the nuchal translucency test is used to indicate a risk factor for Down syndrome. Fetuses with a nonvisualized or shortened nasal bone are more likely to have trisomy 21 than those with a normal length nasal bone (Sonek, Molina, Hiett, et al., 2012).

- *Identification of amniotic fluid volume (AFV) and amniotic fluid index (AFI).* Amniotic fluid volume parameters measure the single largest pocket of amniotic fluid on ultrasonography, free of cord and fetal parts, and then measure either the greatest vertical dimension or the greatest vertical and horizontal dimensions. The vertical diameter of the largest amniotic fluid pocket in each of four quadrants is measured for AFI. The measurements are totaled to obtain the AFI in centimeters. Women with an AFI of more than 24 cm and amniotic fluid volume of equal to or greater than 8 cm are considered to have hydramnios, and women with less than 5 cm at term and the deepest vertical pocket of AFV of less than 2 cm are considered to have oligohydramnios (Magann & Ross, 2014). After 39 weeks, the amniotic fluid volume begins to decline (Magann & Ross, 2014). Both hydramnios and oligohydramnios are associated with increased risk to the fetus, including nonreassuring fetal status, intrauterine growth restriction, meconium-stained amniotic fluid, and an increase in admissions to the neonatal intensive care unit.

- *Location of the placenta.* The placenta is located before amniocentesis to avoid puncturing the placenta.

Ultrasound also is valuable in identifying and evaluating placenta previa in the following ways:

- *Placental grading.* As the fetus matures, the placenta calcifies. These changes can be detected by ultrasound and graded according to the degree of calcification. Placenta grading can be used to identify internal placenta vasculature, which can be associated with preeclampsia and chronic hypertension. It can also identify disorders such as fetal growth abnormalities, triploidy, nonimmune hydrops, and infections.

- *Detection of fetal death.* Inability to visualize the fetal heart beating and the separation of the bones in the fetal head are signs of fetal death.

- *Determination of fetal position and presentation.*

- *Accompanying procedures.* Ultrasound is used to assist with conducting amniocentesis, chorionic villus sampling, intrauterine procedures, and other procedures that will be discussed shortly.

Risks of Ultrasound

Ultrasound has been used clinically for over 40 years; to date no clinical studies verify harmful effects to the mother, the fetus, or the newborn. Many pregnant clients themselves received diagnostic ultrasound in utero with no adverse effects.

Nursing Management

It is important to inform the woman of the following:

- Ultrasound is standard of care that is performed between 18 and 20 weeks

- Ultrasound is not 100% reliable for diagnosis of some anomalies

- Other options to determine fetal well-being are often used in conjunction with ultrasound and often include combined first trimester screening, quadruple screening, chorionic villus sampling (CVS), or amniocentesis

First-Trimester Combined Screening

First-trimester combined screening is comprehensive screening testing that includes **nuchal translucency testing (NTT)** and serum screening for pregnancy-associated plasma protein-A (PAPP-A) and free beta human chorionic gonadotropin (β-hCG) to determine if a fetus is at risk for trisomies 13, 18, and 21. The combined test is more accurate than an NTT alone because it provides additional data. Using both the NTT and serum testing, the accuracy rates for diagnosis improve to 91% for assessing the risk of trisomy 21 and 98% for assessing trisomy 18 (Kagan, Wright, & Nicolaides, 2015).

Nuchal translucency testing (NTT), also known as *nuchal testing (NT)* or the *nuchal fold test*, is performed at 11 1/7 to 13 6/7 gestational weeks to screen for trisomies 13, 18, and 21 and is a component of the first-trimester combined screening (Kagan et al., 2015). Although women over the age of 35 have a higher risk of chromosomal disorders, universal screening is recommended for all women in the United States in their first and second trimesters. The test uses ultrasound to scan the translucent or clear area on the back of the fetal neck, measuring the diameter of the area. Fetuses with certain genetic disorders often have an excess accumulation of fluid that can be seen at the end of the first trimester. The results are computed using the nuchal measurement, exact gestational age, and maternal age. Fetuses that have a nuchal translucency measurement of greater than 3 mm are at risk for trisomies 13, 18, and 21, and their mothers should be offered an amniocentesis (to be discussed later).

Clinical Tip

NTT is a *screening test*, meaning it indicates that a fetus is at risk. Diagnostic testing, such as an amniocentesis, is a *diagnostic test*, which indicates that the fetus has or does not have the specific diagnosis.

NTT has several advantages over other testing options. It can be performed in the first trimester, early in a pregnancy, to determine if a fetus is *at risk* for chromosomal disorders. Unlike chorionic villus sampling (CVS) or amniocentesis, it has no risk of spontaneous abortion because it is a noninvasive test. NTT accurately detects 90% of fetuses with Down syndrome (DS) (Kagan et al., 2015). When combined with serum testing, the accuracy level increases. Many women feel anxious during pregnancy. A normal result can provide reassurance to the woman that her baby most likely does not have a chromosomal disorder.

The disadvantage is that it can provide false positives and is not diagnostic. The combined test has a 5% false-positive rate, meaning the test may indicate that the fetus is at risk for DS when in fact the fetus has normal chromosomes. Women who receive an abnormal test are then counseled to determine if they would like to have an amniocentesis for diagnostic purposes. The choice to proceed with testing is a very personal one. Some women will wish to obtain the test so they will be more prepared for the diagnosis; other women will want to discontinue the pregnancy. Some women may decide not to have additional testing.

Fetuses that have a nuchal translucency measurement above the 99th percentile are also at risk for congenital heart disease (Mogra, Alabbab, & Hyett, 2012). A fetal echocardiogram is ordered in these cases to determine if a cardiac anomaly is also present. These fetuses have been found to have various cardiac diseases including "tricuspid regurgitation and abnormal flow in the 'a' wave of the ductus venosus" (Mogra et al., 2012, p. 264). The presence of tricuspid regurgitation provides a 55% detection rate for trisomy 21, whereas the presence of ductus venous flow provides a detection rate of 65% (Shafi, 2013).

Fetuses that lack a nasal bone have a Down syndrome detection rate of 65%, and those with an abnormal facial angle as measured on ultrasound have a 45% detection rate. Clearly, combining all of these ultrasound findings and serum testing parameters dramatically increases the rate of detection. More literature is needed to move toward standardization of these testing techniques because currently the biochemical markers and nuchal translucency imaging remain the gold standard of screening testing.

Clinical Tip

When advising clients that a screening test, such as NTT, is abnormal, be sure to explain that this does not mean their baby definitely has the disorder, but rather indicates that the baby may be at risk. It is imperative for parents to understand that an abnormal NTT, or any type of screening test, is only an indication that more testing is needed to make the actual diagnosis. Advise parents that some women with abnormal test results have normal fetuses and that because the test only screens and does not actually diagnose the fetus, a fetus that screens within the normal criteria could have an unrecognized anomaly.

Cell-Free Fetal DNA Testing

In late 2011, **cell-free fetal DNA (cffDNA) testing** was introduced as a maternal screening blood test that can be obtained to test for trisomies 13, 18, and 21. The test detects circulating fetal DNA within the maternal serum, which is as high as 3% to 13% (American College of Obstetricians & Gynecologists [ACOG], 2012). The test is noninvasive and detects 98.6% of fetuses affected with Down syndrome (trisomy 21) (ACOG, 2012). The Food and Drug Administration (FDA) does not approve different types of genetic testing; however, the test is available in the United States and is being marketed by a number of distributors. ACOG (2012) recommends this as a testing option for women at an increased risk of chromosomal disorders. ACOG (2012) advises that the test should not be used for low-risk women or for women with a multiple gestation, but is appropriate for women older than 35 years of age, women with a history of a child with trisomy, and women carrying fetuses that show abnormalities on an ultrasound. In laboratory testing, false positives did occur in 0.5% of testing samples and an additional 0.6% of samples could not be definitively tested (ACOG, 2012; Palomaki et al., 2012).

Professionalism in Practice   Insurance Coverage of Testing

Cell-free fetal DNA testing may be covered by insurance carriers if the test is recommended by a healthcare provider. Nurses need to inform women of all testing options and explain the risks and benefits of each type of test. Nurses should advise the woman to call her insurance company prior to testing so the woman can make an informed decision that includes financial considerations.

Doppler Blood Flow Studies (Umbilical Velocimetry)

Umbilical velocimetry, a noninvasive ultrasound test, measures blood flow changes that occur in maternal and fetal circulation in order to assess placental function. An ultrasound beam, like that provided by the pocket Doppler (a handheld ultrasound device), is directed at the umbilical artery (in some cases a maternal vessel such as the arcuate can also be used). The signal is reflected off the red blood cells moving within the vessels and creates a "picture" (waveform) that looks like a series of waves. The highest velocity peak of the waves is the systolic measurement, and the lowest point is the diastolic velocity. To interpret the waveforms, the systolic (S) peak is divided by the end-diastolic (D) component. This calculation is called the *S/D ratio*. The normal S/D ratio is below 2.6 by 26 weeks' gestation and below 3.0 at term. A decrease in uteroplacental perfusion (because of narrowing of the vessels) causes an increase in placental bed resistance and a decrease in diastolic flow, resulting in an elevated S/D ratio (Blackburn, 2013). Elevations of 3 and above are considered abnormal. Doppler blood flow studies are helpful in assessing and managing pregnancies with suspected uteroplacental insufficiency before asphyxia occurs (Blackburn, 2013). Abnormal Doppler flow studies accompanied by a decrease in amniotic fluid have been associated with small-for-gestational-age fetuses, cesarean section for nonreassuring fetal status, 5-minute Apgar score of less than 7 (7 to 10 is the normal range), respiratory distress syndrome, NICU admission, and perinatal death (Blackburn, 2013).

Doppler blood flow studies are relatively easy to obtain. The woman lies supine with a wedge under the right hip (to promote uteroplacental perfusion). Warmed transducer gel is applied to the abdomen, and a pulsed-wave Doppler device is used to ascertain the blood flow. The Doppler flow study takes about 15 to 20 minutes. Doppler flow studies can be initiated at 16 to 18 weeks' gestation and are then scheduled at regular intervals for women at risk.

Non-Stress Test

The **non-stress test (NST)**, a widely used method of evaluating fetal status, may be used alone or as part of a more comprehensive diagnostic assessment called *a biophysical profile* (BPP) (discussed later in this chapter). The non-stress test is based on the knowledge that when the fetus has adequate oxygenation and an intact central nervous system, there are accelerations of the fetal heart rate (FHR) with fetal movement (FM). An NST requires an electronic fetal monitor to observe and record these fetal heart rate accelerations. (See discussion of accelerations in Chapter 17.) A nonreactive NST is fairly consistent in identifying at-risk fetuses (Cunningham et al., 2014). The advantages of the NST are as follows:

- It is quick to perform, permits easy interpretation, and is inexpensive.
- It can be done in an office or clinic setting.
- There are no known side effects.

The disadvantages of the NST include the following:

- It is sometimes difficult to obtain a suitable tracing.
- The woman has to remain relatively still for at least 20 minutes.
- A false positive result due to the fetal sleep cycle.

Procedure

The NST can be done with the woman in a reclining chair or in bed in a left-tilted semi-Fowler or side-lying position. Research has shown that certain maternal positions can help produce more favorable results. Women in left-tilted semi-Fowler, reclining, and left lateral positions have more fetal movement and are more likely to have a reactive tracing. Women should not be placed in a supine position because it is associated with less fetal movement, maternal back pain, and maternal shortness of breath. The nurse places the electronic fetal monitor under the woman's clothing. Privacy should be provided. The examiner places two elastic belts on the woman's abdomen. Some facilities utilize disposable mesh sashes to hold the devices in place. One belt (tocodynamometer) holds a device that detects uterine or fetal movement; the other belt holds the ultrasound transducer that detects the FHR. As the NST is done, each fetal movement is documented, so that associated or simultaneous FHR changes can be evaluated. See Assessment of Fetal Well-Being: Non-Stress Test (NST) in the *Clinical Skills Manual* SKILLS .

Interpretation of NST Results

Women with a high-risk factor will probably begin having NSTs at 30 to 32 weeks' gestation and at frequent intervals for the remainder of the pregnancy. The results of the NST are interpreted as follows:

- ***Reactive test.*** A reactive NST shows at least two accelerations of FHR with fetal movements of 15 beats per minute (beats/min), lasting 15 seconds or more, over 20 minutes (Figure 13–4). This is the desired result. (See Table 13–3.) Some practitioners may begin NSTs at 28 weeks and utilize a 10-beat increase criteria at this

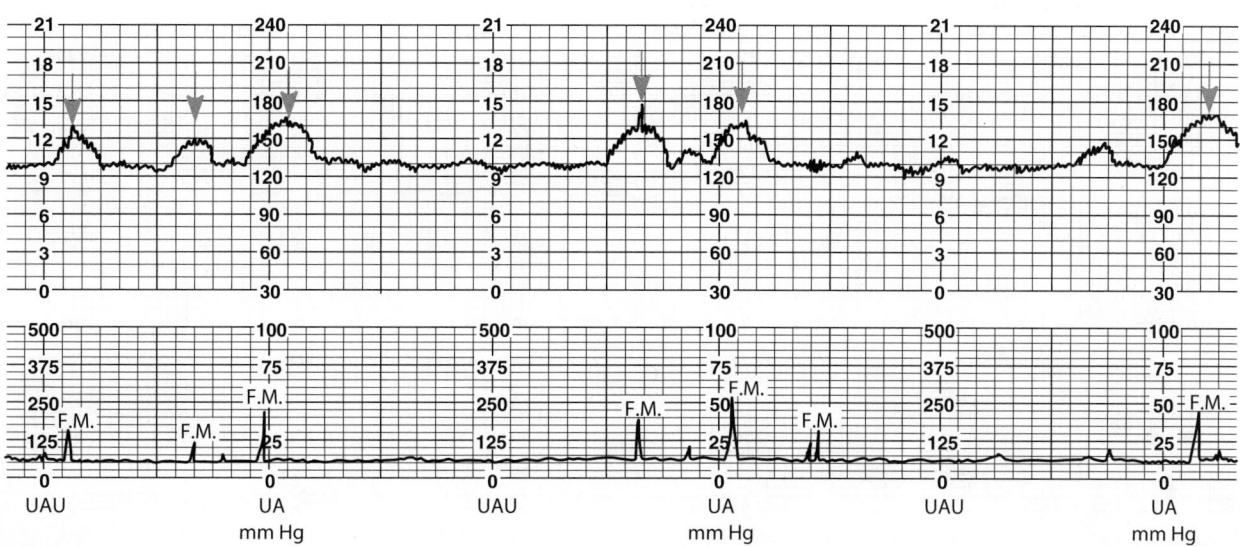

Figure 13–4 Example of a reactive non-stress test (NST). The test shows accelerations of 15 beats/min lasting 15 seconds with each fetal movement (FM). Top of strip shows fetal heart rate (FHR); bottom of strip shows uterine activity tracing. Note that FHR increases (above the baseline) at least 15 beats and remains at that rate for at least 15 seconds before returning to the former baseline.

TABLE 13–3 Non-Stress Test

Diagnostic value: Demonstrates fetus's ability to respond to its environment by acceleration of FHR with movement.

Results:

- *Reactive test:* Accelerations (at least 2) of 15 beats/min above the baseline, lasting 15 seconds or more in a 20-minute window, are present, indicating fetal well-being.
- *Nonreactive test:* Accelerations are not present or do not meet the above criteria, indicating that the fetus is at risk or asleep.

gestational age (Cunningham et al., 2014). Central nervous system maturity is required to execute a non-stress test, which is why earlier testing is not performed.

- *Nonreactive test.* In a nonreactive test, the reactive criteria are not met. For example, the accelerations do not meet the requirements of 15 beats/min or do not last 15 seconds (Figure 13–5).
- *Unsatisfactory test.* An NST is unsatisfactory if the data cannot be interpreted or there was inadequate fetal activity.

It is important that anyone who performs the NST understand the significance of any decelerations of the FHR during testing. If decelerations are noted, the physician/certified nurse-midwife (CNM) should be notified for further evaluation of fetal status. (See Chapter 17 for further discussion of FHR decelerations.)

Clinical Management

The clinical management of potential nonreassuring fetal status may vary depending on the clinical judgment of the care provider. One commonly used protocol is as follows: If the NST is reactive in less than 30 minutes, the test is concluded and rescheduled as indicated by the high-risk condition that is present. If it is nonreactive, the test time is extended for 30 minutes until the results are reactive, and then the test is rescheduled as indicated. It is estimated that 80% to 90% of nonreactive NSTs

happen because of fetal sleep states (Cunningham et al., 2014). If the FHR remains nonreactive for longer than 30 minutes, the test is typically repeated after the woman eats or the fetus is stimulated via vibroacoustic stimulation or palpation. Such measures often wake a fetus, so a reactive NST can be obtained. If a reactive test is not obtained within 30 minutes, additional testing (such as diagnostic ultrasound and biophysical profile [BPP]) or immediate birth is considered; if the NST is nonreactive and spontaneous decelerations of the FHR are present, diagnostic ultrasound and BPP are performed and birth is recommended. Many testing guidelines vary in frequency, recommending a retest either once or twice a week, depending on the at-risk condition that exists.

Nursing Management

Evaluate the woman's understanding of the NST and the possible results. Reassure the client that more frequent evaluation is used to ensure the well-being of the fetus and that reassuring fetal status means that uteroplacental circulation is providing adequate oxygenation to the fetus. Review with the woman the reasons for the NST and the procedure before beginning the test. Administer the NST, interpret the results, and report the findings to the physician/CNM and the expectant woman.

Fetal Acoustic and Vibroacoustic Stimulation Tests

Acoustic (sound) and vibroacoustic (vibration and sound) stimulation of the fetus can be used as an adjunct to the nonstress test (NST). A handheld, battery-operated device is applied to the woman's abdomen over the area of the fetal head. This device generates a low-frequency vibration and a buzzing sound. These are intended to induce movement and associated accelerations of the fetal heart rate (FHR) in fetuses with a nonreactive NST and in fetuses with decreased variability of FHR during labor. (See discussion of variability in Chapter 17.) The sound stimulus persists for 2 to 5 seconds;

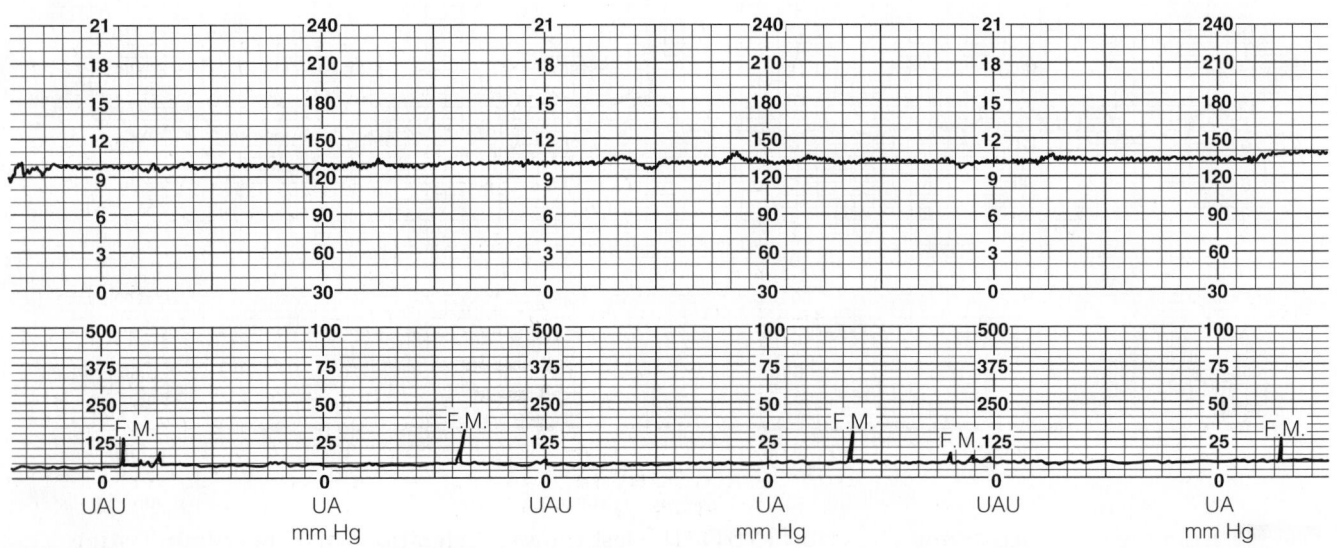

Figure 13–5 Example of a nonreactive non-stress test (NST). There are no accelerations of fetal heart rate (FHR) with fetal movement (FM). Baseline FHR is 130 beats/min. The tracing of uterine activity is on the bottom of the strip.

if no accelerations occur, it is then repeated at 1-minute intervals up to three times. Whether the fetus responds more to the vibration or to the sound is not known. Two FHR accelerations of 15 beats/min, lasting 15 seconds, in a 20-minute period indicate a reactive test (Cunningham et al., 2014). Although no evidence-based clinical trials have examined the safety and efficiency of this technique, it continues to be used, although somewhat infrequently, in clinical practice. A 2013 Cochrane Review found no adverse effects but noted that it decreased incidence of non-reactive NSTs and a reduction in testing time (Tan, Smyth, & Wei, 2013).

Advantages of the fetal acoustic stimulation test (FAST) and the vibroacoustic stimulation test (VST) are as follows:

- Both are noninvasive techniques and are easy to perform.
- Results are rapidly available.
- Time for the NST is shortened.

Biophysical Profile

The **biophysical profile (BPP)** is a comprehensive assessment of five biophysical variables and can be performed after 28 weeks (Buonocore, Bracci, & Weindling, 2012):

1. Fetal breathing movement
2. Fetal movements of body or limbs
3. Fetal tone (extension and flexion of extremities)
4. Amniotic fluid volume (visualized as pockets of fluid around the fetus)
5. Reactive fetal heart rate (FHR) with activity (reactive non-stress test [NST])

The first four variables are assessed by ultrasound scanning; FHR reactivity is assessed with the NST. By combining these five assessments, the BPP helps to either identify the compromised fetus or confirm the healthy fetus and provides an assessment of placental functioning. Specific criteria for normal and abnormal assessments are presented in Table 13–4. A score of 2 is assigned to each normal finding, and a score of 0 to each abnormal one, for a maximum score of 10. The absence of a specific activity is difficult to interpret because it may indicate central nervous system (CNS) depression or simply the resting state of a healthy fetus. Scores of 8/10 (with normal amniotic fluid) and 10/10 are considered normal. Such scores have the least chance of being associated with a compromised fetus unless a decrease in the amount of amniotic fluid is noted, in which case birth may be indicated. The use of maximum vertical pocket depth,

and not the four-quadrant AFI (amniotic fluid index), in traditional BPS is validated by current research (Jelsema, 2012). See Assessment of Fetal Well-Being: Biophysical Profile (BPP) in the *Clinical Skills Manual* SKILLS.

The BPP is indicated when there is risk of placental insufficiency or fetal compromise because of the following:

- Intrauterine growth restriction (IUGR)
- Maternal diabetes mellitus
- Maternal heart disease
- Maternal chronic hypertension
- Maternal preeclampsia or eclampsia
- Maternal sickle cell disease
- Suspected fetal postmaturity (more than 42 weeks' gestation)
- History of previous stillbirths
- Rh alloimmunization
- Abnormal estriol excretion
- Hyperthyroidism
- Renal disease
- Nonreactive NST

Contraction Stress Test

The **contraction stress test (CST)** is a means of evaluating the respiratory function (oxygen and carbon dioxide exchange) of the placenta. This provides the ability to identify risk for intrauterine asphyxia through observation of the fetal heart rate (FHR) in relation to the stress of uterine contractions (spontaneous or induced). During contractions, intrauterine pressure increases. Blood flow to the intervillous space of the placenta is reduced momentarily, thereby decreasing oxygen transport to the fetus. A healthy fetus usually tolerates this reduction well and maintains a steady heart rate. If the placental reserve is insufficient, fetal hypoxia, depression of the myocardium, and a decrease in FHR occur.

In many areas, the CST has given way to the biophysical profile. CST is still used in areas where the availability of other technology is reduced (such as during night shifts) or limited (such as at small community hospitals or birthing centers). Often, a nurse will document CST results as part of her assessment if the criteria for a CST are met; however, they are rarely ordered in standard practice owing to the wide availability of ultrasound technology.

TABLE 13–4 Criteria for Biophysical Profile Scoring

COMPONENT	NORMAL (SCORE = 2)	ABNORMAL (SCORE = 0)
Fetal breathing movements	≥1 episode of rhythmic breathing lasting ≥30 sec within 30 min	≤30 sec of breathing in 30 min
Gross body movements	≥3 discrete body or limb movements in 30 min (episodes of active continuous movement considered as single movement)	≤2 movements in 30 min
Fetal tone	≥1 episode of extension of a fetal extremity with return to flexion, or opening or closing of hand	No movements or extension/flexion
Amniotic fluid volume	Single vertical pocket >2 cm amniotic fluid index (AFI) >5 cm	Largest single vertical pocket ≤2 cm AFI ≤ 5 cm
Non-stress test	≥2 accelerations of ≥15 beats/min for ≥15 sec in 20 min	0 or 1 acceleration in 20 min

Procedure

The critical component of the CST is the presence of uterine contractions. They may occur spontaneously (which is unusual before the onset of labor), or they may be induced (stimulated) with oxytocin (Pitocin) administered intravenously (also known as an oxytocin challenge test [OCT]). A natural method of obtaining oxytocin is through the use of breast stimulation (Angelini & Lafontaine, 2013).

An electronic fetal monitor is used to provide continuous data about the FHR and uterine contractions. After a 15-minute baseline recording of uterine activity and FHR, the tracing is evaluated for evidence of spontaneous contractions. If three spontaneous contractions of good quality and lasting 40 to 60 seconds occur in a 10-minute window, the results are evaluated, and the test is concluded. If no contractions occur or they are insufficient for interpretation, oxytocin is administered or breast stimulation is performed to produce contractions of good quality. (See Chapter 22 for more information on nursing care management of oxytocin induction.) The CST should be conducted only in a setting where tocolytic medications are available if a hypersystolic pattern occurs or if labor is stimulated from the test. See Assessment of Fetal Well-Being: Contraction Stress Test (CST) in the *Clinical Skills Manual* SKILLS.

Interpretation of CST Results

The CST is classified as follows:

- *Negative.* A negative CST shows three contractions of good quality lasting 40 or more seconds in 10 minutes without evidence of late decelerations. This is the desired result. It implies that the fetus can handle the hypoxic stress of uterine contractions.

- *Positive.* A positive CST shows repetitive persistent late decelerations with more than 50% of the contractions (Figure 13–6). This is not a desired result. The hypoxic stress of the uterine contraction causes a slowing of the FHR. The pattern will not improve and will most likely get worse with additional contractions.

- *Equivocal or suspicious.* An equivocal or suspicious test has nonpersistent late decelerations or decelerations associated with hyperstimulation (contraction frequency of every 2 minutes or duration lasting longer than 90 seconds). When this test result occurs, more information is needed.

Clinical Application

A negative CST implies that the placenta is functioning normally, fetal oxygenation is adequate, and the fetus will probably be able to withstand the stress of labor. If labor does not occur in the ensuing week, further testing is done.

A positive CST with a nonreactive NST presents evidence that the fetus will not likely withstand the stress of labor. A positive CST may be able to identify compromised fetuses earlier than a nonreactive NST because of the stimulated interruption of intervillous blood flow (Blackburn, 2013). Although a negative CST is reliable in predicting fetal status, a positive result needs to be verified, such as with a biophysical profile (see Table 13–5).

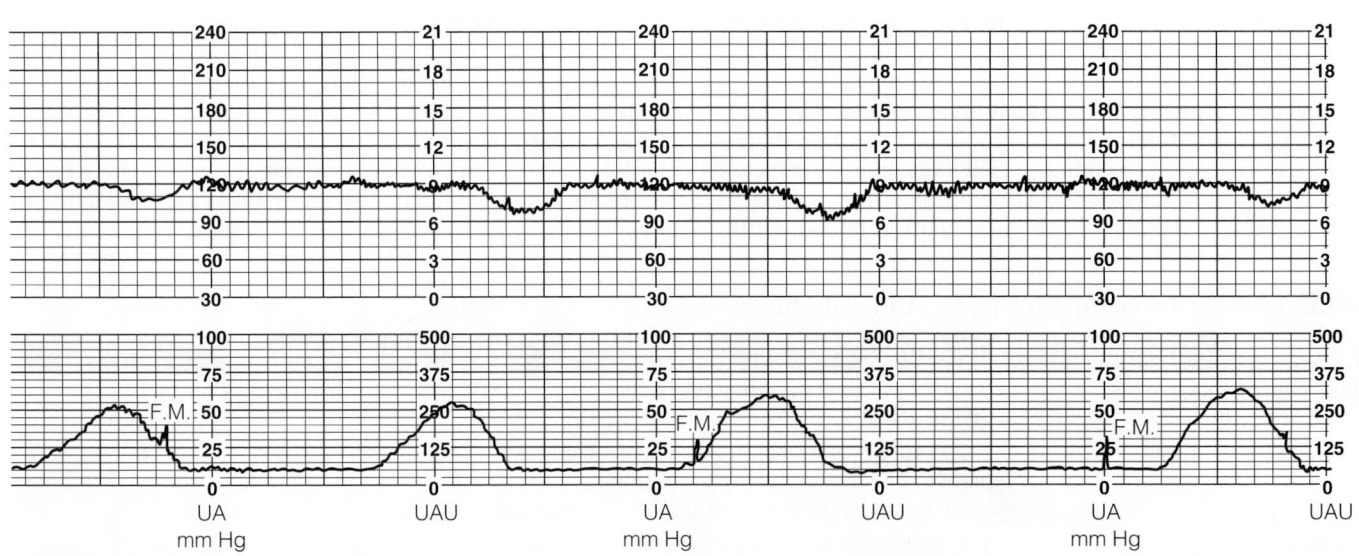

Figure 13–6 Example of a positive contraction stress test (CST). Repetitive late decelerations occur with each contraction. Note that there are no accelerations of fetal heart rate (FHR) with three fetal movements (FM). The baseline FHR is 120 beats/min. Uterine contractions (bottom half of strip) occurred four times in 12 minutes.

TABLE 13–5 Contraction Stress Test

Diagnostic value: Demonstrates reaction of FHR to stress of uterine contraction.

Results:
- *Negative test:* Stress of uterine contraction shows three contractions of good quality lasting 40 or more seconds in 10 minutes without evidence of late decelerations.
- *Positive test:* Stress of uterine contraction shows repetitive persistent late decelerations with more than 50% of the uterine contractions.
- *Equivocal or suspicious:* Nonpersistent late decelerations or decelerations associated with hyperstimulation.

Nursing Management

Ascertain the woman's understanding of the CST, the reasons for the test, and the possible results before the test begins. Written consent is required in some settings. In this case, the physician/CNM is responsible for fully informing the woman about the test. Administer the CST and report the findings to the physician/CNM and the expectant woman. In some settings, the presence of the physician/CNM is required because there is a risk of initiating labor or hypertonic uterine contractions. Throughout the procedure, you will perform critical assessments and provide continual reassurance to the woman and her support person.

Amniotic Fluid Analysis

Amniocentesis is a procedure used to obtain amniotic fluid for genetic testing (early in pregnancy or between 15 and 16 weeks of pregnancy) for fetal abnormalities or to determine fetal lung maturity in the third trimester of pregnancy. During an amniocentesis, the physician scans the uterus using ultrasound to identify the fetal and placental positions and to identify adequate pockets of amniotic fluid. The skin is then cleaned with a Betadine solution. The use of a local anesthetic at the needle insertion site is optional. A 22-gauge needle is then inserted into the uterine cavity to withdraw amniotic fluid (Figure 13–7). After 15 to 20 mL of fluid has been removed, the needle is withdrawn and the site is assessed for streaming (movement of fluid), which is an indication of bleeding. The fetal heart rate and maternal vital signs are then assessed. Rh immune globulin is given to all Rh-negative women. The analysis of amniotic fluid provides valuable information about fetal status. Amniocentesis is a fairly simple procedure, although complications do occur on rare occasions (fewer than 0.5% of cases). For nursing interventions during amniocentesis, see Assisting During Amniocentesis in the *Clinical Skills Manual* `SKILLS`.

Diagnostic Uses of Amniocentesis

A number of studies can be performed on amniotic fluid. These tests can provide information about fetal health, fetal lung maturity, and genetic disorders.

EVALUATION OF FETAL HEALTH

Concentrations of certain substances in amniotic fluid provide information about the health status of the fetus. The **quadruple screen**, also called *quad screen*, is another test that can be used to screen for Down syndrome (trisomy 21), trisomy 18, and neural tube defects (NTDs). The serum test assesses for appropriate levels of alpha-fetoprotein (AFP), human chorionic gonadotropin (hCG), unconjugated estriol (UE3), and dimeric inhibin-A. The quadruple screen offers the advantage of being noninvasive but is only a screening test. The quadruple screen is less accurate and has higher false positive rates than a first-trimester combined screening test and should be offered to women for whom the first-trimester combined screening is unavailable (Kwon, Park, Kwon, et al., 2012). It is less invasive than an amniocentesis

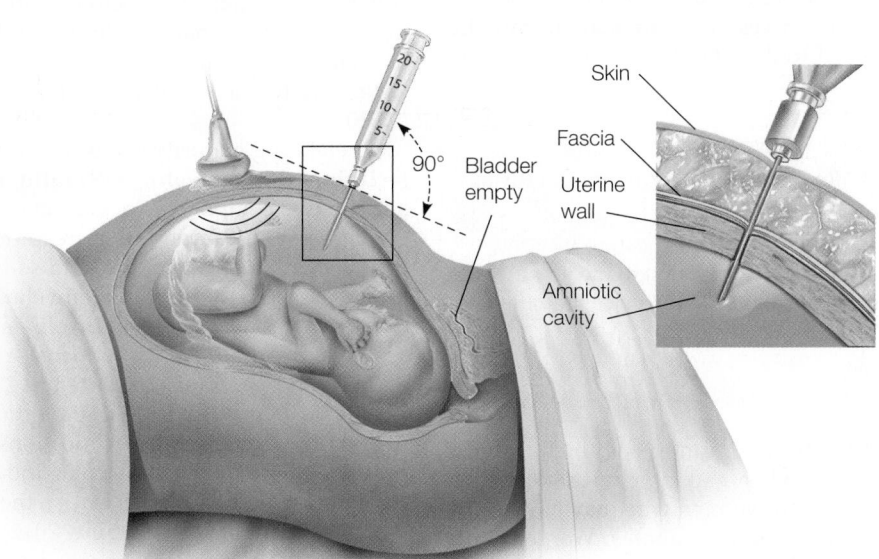

Skin
Fascia
Uterine wall
Amniotic cavity
90° Bladder empty

Figure 13–7 **Amniocentesis. The woman is usually scanned by ultrasound to determine the placenta site and to locate a pocket of amniotic fluid. As the needle is inserted, three levels of resistance are felt when the needle penetrates the skin, fascia, and uterine wall. When the needle is placed within the amniotic cavity, amniotic fluid is withdrawn.**

EVIDENCE-BASED PRACTICE | Validity of the Noninvasive Prenatal Test for the Detection of Chromosomal Abnormalities

Clinical Question
Does the Noninvasive Prenatal Test (NIPT) detect chromosomal abnormalities with a strong degree of accuracy? Which abnormalities are best detected with the NIPT?

The Evidence
Noninvasive methods for testing for fetal abnormalities reduce the risk of procedural complications for the mother and baby, and lower costs. Since becoming clinically available in 2011, the tests have been rapidly adopted. Evidence is widely available for the specificity and accuracy of these tests. One group of researchers retrieved data from more than 31,000 clients that received the NIPT, and studied the rate of true positives, false positives, and false negatives for the conditions of trisomies 21, 18, 13, and X. Another study of a statewide prenatal screening program determined how many would be accurately diagnosed in a comparison of noninvasive and invasive diagnostic tests (amniocentesis.) A third group of researchers studied more than 3400 clients to determine the relative sensitivity of the test. The samples included women who were both high- and low-risk for fetal aneuploidy. Taken together, these large-data studies support the strongest level of evidence.

The NIPT was as sensitive in the detection of chromosomal abnormalities as the invasive amniocentesis (Porrecto,

Garite, Maurel, et al., 2014). Norton, Currier, and Jeliffe-Pawlowski (2014) determined that 80% of chromosomal abnormalities were detected by NIPT; 17% were missed and were false negatives. In the large-scale report, the predictive value was 83%, with only 2 of 500 false negatives (Dar et al., 2014). Both specificity and sensitivity of the test were validated at very high rates for trisomy 21 in two of the three studies, but had less sensitivity for trisomies 18 and 13 and low sensitivity for trisomy X.

Best Practice
Mothers at high risk for chromosomal aneuploidy can be counseled that noninvasive testing is as accurate as the more invasive amniocentesis. In any case, the test will detect the abnormality at least 80% of the time, and false negatives are low. The test will be most accurate, however, for trisomy 21, and will have little accuracy for trisomy X. Mothers at risk of trisomy 21 will find the test most useful.

Clinical Reasoning
How would you construct an educational program for counseling women about their options for noninvasive prenatal testing for chromosomal abnormalities? What are the characteristics of a mother for whom the test would be most informative?

and may be used as a screening tool prior to the administration of an amniocentesis (Kwon et al., 2012). An amniocentesis is 99% accurate in diagnosing genetic abnormalities.

EVALUATION OF FETAL LUNG MATURITY

Because gestational age, birth weight, and the rate of development of organ systems do not necessarily correspond, amniotic fluid may also be analyzed to determine the maturity of the fetal lungs.

> ### Health Promotion Reducing the Rate of Preterm Births
> *Healthy People 2020* goals include reducing the rate of preterm births. Fetal lung maturity testing can reduce the number of babies born prematurely related to incorrect dating in earlier stages of pregnancy and reduce the rates of late preterm newborns.

Fetal lung maturity determination in conjunction with gestational age is important when making clinical decisions regarding the timing of birth for women who may have complications, such as preeclampsia or diabetes. Women with pregnancies that are affected by diabetes have slower fetal lung maturation than other pregnancies not complicated by diabetes.

Lecithin/Sphingomyelin (L/S) Ratio. The alveoli of the lungs are lined with a substance called **surfactant**, which is composed of phospholipids. Surfactant lowers the surface tension of the alveoli when the newborn exhales. When a newborn

with mature pulmonary function takes its first breath, a tremendously high pressure is needed to open the lungs. By lowering the alveolar surface tension, surfactant stabilizes the alveoli, and a certain amount of air always remains in the alveoli during expiration. Thus when the neonate exhales, the lungs do not collapse. A neonate born before synthesis of surfactant is complete is unable to maintain lung stability. Each breath requires the same effort as the first. This results in underinflation of the lungs and the development of respiratory distress syndrome (RDS).

Fetal lung maturity can be ascertained by determining the **lecithin/sphingomyelin (L/S) ratio**; lecithin and sphingomyelin are two components of surfactant. Early in pregnancy, the sphingomyelin concentration in amniotic fluid is greater than the concentration of lecithin, and so the L/S ratio is low (lecithin levels are low and sphingomyelin levels are high). At about 32 weeks' gestation, sphingomyelin levels begin to fall and the amount of lecithin begins to increase. By 35 weeks' gestation, an L/S ratio of 2:1 (also reported as 2.0) is usually achieved in the normal fetus. A 2:1 L/S ratio indicates that the risk of RDS is very low. Under certain conditions of stress (a physiologic problem in the mother, placenta, and/or fetus, such as hypertension or placental insufficiency), the fetal lungs mature more rapidly (Angelini & Lafontaine, 2012). Fetuses whose mothers are administered corticosteroids have an acceleration in fetal lung maturity.

PHOSPHATIDYLGLYCEROL

Phosphatidylglycerol (PG) is another phospholipid in surfactant. Phosphatidylglycerol is not present in the fetal lung fluid early in gestation. It appears when fetal lung maturity has been attained, at about 35 weeks' gestation. Because the presence of

TABLE 13–6 Fetal Lung Maturity Values

Diagnostic value: Provides information to help determine fetal lung maturity.

Results:
- An L/S ratio of 2:1 and presence of PG correlate with 35 weeks' gestation.
- An L/S ratio lower than 2:1 and/or an absence of PG may indicate underinflation of lungs and an increased risk for development of RDS.
- An LBC of over 50,000 counts/mcL is predictive of fetal lung maturity.

PG is associated with fetal lung maturity, when it is present the risk of RDS is low. PG determination is also useful in blood-contaminated specimens. Because PG is not present in blood or vaginal fluids, its presence is reliable in predicting fetal lung maturity. (See Table 13–6.)

LAMELLAR BODY COUNT.

Lamellar body counts (LBCs) are present in amniotic fluid when phosphatidylglycerol (PG) is present (Ridsdale, Lewis, Weaver, et al., 2012). When the LBC is 30,000 to 40,000 counts/mcL, probable lung maturity is assumed. The laboratory analysis for LBC is considerably less costly than the previously discussed tests and can usually be performed at the acute care facility rather than a reference laboratory (Ridsdale et al., 2012).

Future Advances in Fetal Lung Maturity Testing. Some researchers are now examining the use of Doppler ultrasound as a means of identifying fetuses whose lungs have matured by using the measurement of the fetal pulmonary artery Doppler wave acceleration time/ejection time ratio (PATET) (Schenone, Samson, Suhag, et al., 2012). Although further research is needed, research in noninvasive screening tools continues to evolve and could potentially reduce risk factors for mothers and fetuses.

SAFETY ALERT!

When an amniocentesis is being done for fetal lung maturity, continuous fetal monitoring should be performed to assess for nonreassuring fetal status.

Chorionic Villus Sampling

Chorionic villus sampling (CVS) involves obtaining a small sample of chorionic villi from the developing placenta. Chorionic villus sampling is performed in some medical centers for first-trimester diagnosis of genetic, metabolic, and deoxyribonucleic acid (DNA) studies. Chorionic villus sampling can be performed either transabdominally or transcervically. The fetal loss rate is the same regardless of the approach used, although vaginal spotting is more common with the transcervical approach (Cunningham et al., 2014).

The advantages of this procedure are early diagnosis and short waiting time for results. Whereas amniocentesis is not done until at least 16 weeks' gestation, CVS is typically performed between 10 and 12 weeks. Previous studies that evaluated the use of CVS at 9 weeks found a possible association between limb reduction birth defects and early CVS. Based on these findings, most practitioners do not recommend early CVS before 10 gestational weeks (Cunningham et al., 2014).

Risks of CVS include failure to obtain tissue, rupture of membranes, leakage of amniotic fluid, bleeding, intrauterine infection, maternal tissue contamination of the specimen, and Rh alloimmunization. Because CVS testing is performed so early in the pregnancy, it cannot detect neural tube defects. Women who desire testing for neural tube defects would need a quadruple screening at 15 to 20 weeks' gestation. Because of the risks involved, CVS testing is less commonly performed than the noninvasive testing or amniocentesis.

Nursing Management

You will assist the physician during the amniocentesis or CVS and support the woman undergoing the procedure. Although the physician has explained the procedure in advance so that the woman can give informed consent, the woman is likely to be apprehensive both about the procedure itself and about the information it may reveal. She may become anxious during the procedure and need additional emotional support. Provide support by further clarifying the physician's instructions or explanations, by relieving the woman's physical discomfort when possible, and by responding verbally and physically to the woman's need for reassurance.

Following the procedure, reiterate explanations given by the physician and provide opportunities for questions. Review the experience with the woman and present self-care measures. Typically, the woman is monitored for a short time following the procedure. Observe for contraction or uterine activity, amniotic fluid leakage, bleeding, or pain. Advise the woman of the warning signs of complications following the procedure.

Following an amniocentesis, approximately 1% of women develop complications such as amniotic fluid leakage from the puncture site or vaginal spotting. Approximately 1 in 1000 women develop infection. Needle puncture of the fetus rarely occurs during amniocentesis because of the use of ultrasound technology, which allows for continuous visualization of the fetus (Cunningham et al., 2014). Reassure the woman that although the complication rates are low, notification of her healthcare provider is necessary if any of these symptoms develop.

Clinical Tip

When explaining genetic testing options to expectant parents, inform the mother that even if a CVS shows no chromosomal abnormality, it cannot screen for neural tube defects. Women who have a normal CVS and an abnormal quadruple screen test would be offered amniocentesis. Women with risk factors for neural tube defects may want to consider amniocentesis instead of CVS because it screens for both types of disorders.

Because fetal loss occurs more commonly before 15 weeks, many practitioners theorize that the loss rates associated with CVS are higher than those associated with amniocentesis. Early amniocentesis before 15 weeks is associated with an increased risk of fetal loss when compared with performing the procedure after 15 weeks. Approximately 1 in 200 fetal losses occurs with CVS. When an amniocentesis is performed between 15 and 20 weeks, the risk of fetal loss is 1% (Corrado et al., 2012). When any invasive procedure, such as an amniocentesis or a CVS, is performed, RhoGAM should be administered to the woman if she is Rh negative to prevent alloimmunization. Documentation should be added to the medical record and provided to the woman for future reference.

Focus Your Study

- Nurses often play a key role not only in teaching families about various testing procedures, but also in providing clarity and emotional support to the woman and her family undergoing antenatal testing.

- Maternal assessment of fetal activity is very useful as a screening procedure in evaluation of fetal status.

- Ultrasound offers a valuable means of assessing intrauterine fetal growth because the growth can be followed over a period of time. It is noninvasive and painless, allows the practitioner to study the gestation serially, is nonradiating to both the woman and her fetus, and to date has shown no known harmful effects.

- Using ultrasound, the gestational sac may be detected as early as 5 or 6 weeks after the last menstrual period. Measurement of the crown–rump length in early pregnancy is most useful for accurate dating of a pregnancy. The most important and frequently used ultrasound measurements in the second trimester are biparietal diameter, head circumference, abdominal circumference, and femur length.

- First-trimester combined screening includes nuchal translucency testing and serum screening for pregnancy-associated plasma protein-A (PAPP-A) and free beta human chorionic gonadotropin (β-hCG) to determine if a fetus is at risk for trisomies 13, 18, and 21.

- Cell-free fetal DNA testing is a noninvasive maternal screening blood test that identifies trisomies 13, 18, and 21 by detecting circulating fetal DNA within the maternal serum. It detects 98.6% of fetuses affected with Down syndrome (trisomy 21).

- Doppler blood flow studies are noninvasive ultrasound screenings conducted via Doppler placed on the abdomen with the woman lying supine and is used to assess placental function and sufficiency.

- A non-stress test (NST) measures fetal heart rate (FHR) during fetal activity; FHR normally increases in response to fetal activity. The desired result is a reactive test.

- A contraction stress test (CST) provides a method for observing the response of the FHR to the stress of uterine contractions. The desired result is a negative test.

- A fetal biophysical profile (BPP) includes five fetal variables (breathing movement, body movement, tone, amniotic fluid volume, and FHR reactivity). It assesses the fetus at risk for intrauterine compromise.

- Aneuploidy screening includes nuchal translucency and PAPP-A and β-hCG or quadruple screening of AFP, hCG, diameric inhibin-A, and estriol.

- Amniocentesis can be used to obtain amniotic fluid for testing. A variety of tests are available to evaluate the presence of disease, genetic conditions, and fetal maturity.

- Percutaneous umbilical blood sampling (PUBS) is a technique used in the second and third trimesters for fetal diagnosis, assessment, and therapy.

- The lecithin/sphingomyelin (L/S) ratio of the amniotic fluid can be used to assess fetal lung maturity. The presence of phosphatidylglycerol (PG) may also provide information about fetal lung maturity.

- Lamellar body counts (LBCs) testing can be used as a predictive indicator for predicting RDS in preterm newborns.

- Chorionic villus sampling (CVS) is a procedure that obtains fetal karyotype in the first trimester. It is used to diagnose hemoglobinopathies (e.g., sickle cell anemia and alpha- and some beta-thalassemias), phenylketonuria, alpha-antitrypsin deficiency, Down syndrome, Duchenne muscular dystrophy, and factor IX deficiency.

Clinical Reasoning in Action

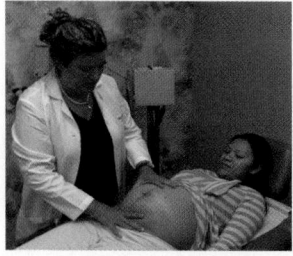

Patricia Adams is a 20-year-old, married, G2P0010 at 36 weeks' gestation with gestational diabetes. She presents to you during her prenatal visit with a complaint of decreased fetal movement for the "last day or so." Her OB history includes a 13-lb weight gain, hematocrit of 29%, diastolic BP ranging 80 to 96 mmHg, and 1+ proteinuria. A 19-week ultrasound demonstrated no fetal anatomic defects. A hemoglobin A_{1c} at 23 weeks was 5.8%. Patricia has had weekly NSTs since 28 weeks' gestation. You place Patricia on the fetal monitor for an NST. You obtain vital signs of T 97°F, P 88, R 14, BP 130/88. After 30 minutes, you observe that the fetal heart rate baseline is 160–165, variability is decreased, and repetitive variable decelerations are occurring. No contractions are noted. The fetus is very active. You notify the physician of the fetal heart rate baseline and unsatisfactory NST. The physician orders a biophysical profile (BPP) for fetal well-being. You describe and explain the biophysical profile test to Patricia.

1. How would you describe and explain the biophysical profile test?

2. To heighten Patricia's awareness of fetal movement, how would you instruct her to do a daily fetal movement record (FMR)?

3. Explain when Patricia should contact her healthcare provider.

4. Discuss the significance of fetal movement.

5. Explore factors that decrease fetal movements.

References

American College of Obstetricians & Gynecologists (ACOG). (2012). Ultrasonography in pregnancy. Noninvasive prenatal testing for fetal aneuploidy (ACOG Committee Opinion No. 545). Washington, DC: Author.

Angelini, D. J., & Lafontaine, D. (2013). *Obstetric triage and emergency care protocols.* New York, NY: Springer.

Blackburn, S. T. (2013). *Maternal, fetal, & neonatal physiology: A clinical perspective* (4th ed.). St. Louis, MO: Saunders.

Buonocore, G., Bracci, R., & Weindling, M. (2012). *Neonatology: A practical review of neonatal management.* New York, NY: Springer.

Corrado, F., Cannata, M. L., La Galia, T., Magliarditi, M., Imbruglia, L., D'anna, R., & Carlo Stella, R. (2012). Pregnancy outcome following mid-trimester amniocentesis. *Journal of Obstetrics & Gynecology, 32*(2), 117–119. doi:abs/10.3109/01443615.2011.633717

Cunningham, F. G., Leveno, K. J., Bloom, S. L., Spong, C. Y., Dashe, J. S., Hoffman, B. L., … Sheffield, J. S. (2014). *Williams obstetrics* (24th ed.). New York, NY: McGraw-Hill.

Dar, P., Curnow, K., Gross, S., Hall, M. P., Stosic, M., Demko, Z.,…Benn, P. (2014). Clinical experience and follow-up with large scale single-nucleotide polymorphism-based noninvasive prenatal aneuploidy testing. *American Journal of Obstetrics and Gynecology, 211*(527), e1–e17.

Jazayeri, A. (2012). *Macrosomia. E-medicine.* Retrieved from http://emedicine.medscape.com/article/262679-overview

Jelsema, R. (2012). In the measurement of amniotic vertical pockets, are all pockets of similar depth the same? *Journal of Ultrasound in Medicine, 31,* 666.

Kagan, K. O., Wright, D., & Nicholaides, K. H. (2015). First-trimester contingent screening for trisomies 21, 18 and 13 by fetal nuchal translucency and ductus venosus flow and maternal blood cell-free DNA testing. *Ultrasound in Obstetrics & Gynecology, 45*(1), 42–47.

King, T. L., Brucker, M. C, Kriebs, J. M., & Fahey, J.O. (2013). *Varney's midwifery* (5th ed.). New York, NY: Jones & Bartlett Learning.

Kwon, J., Park, I., Kwon, S., & Shin. J. (2012). The quadruple test for Down syndrome screening in pregnant women of advanced maternal age. *Archives of Gynecology and Obstetrics, 285*(3), 629–633. doi:10.1007/s00404-011-2052-1

Magann, E. & Ross, M.G. (2014). *Assessment of amniotic fluid volume. Up-to-date.* Retrieved from http://www.uptodate.com/contents/assessment-of-amniotic-fluid-volume

Malhotra, N., Shah, P. K., Kumar, P., & Acharya, P. (2014). *Ultrasound in Obstetrics & Gynecology.* (4th ed.). New Delhi, India: Jaypee Brothers Medical Publishers.

Malm, M. C., Lindgren, H., Rubertsson, C., Hildingsson, I., & Rådestad, I. (2014). Development of a tool to evaluate fetal movements in full-term pregnancy. *Sexual & Reproductive Healthcare, 5*(1), 31–35.

Miguelez, J., De Lourdes Brizot, M., Liao, A. W., De Carvalho, M. H. B., & Zugaib, M. (2012). Second-trimester soft markers: Relation to first-trimester nuchal translucency in unaffected pregnancies. *Ultrasound Obstetrics & Gynecology, 39,* 274–278. doi:10.1002/uog.9024

Mogra, R., Alabbad, N., & Hyett, J. (2012). Increased nuchal translucency and congenital heart disease. *Early Human Development, 88*(5), 261–267. doi:10.1016/j.earlhumdev.2012.02.009

Norton, M., Currier, B., & Jeliffe-Pawlowski, L. (2014). Rare chromosome abnormalities detected by current prenatal screening compared to expected performance using non-invasive prenatal testing (NIPT). *American Journal of Obstetrics and Gynecology, Supplement to January, 2014,* s3–s4.

Palomaki, G. E., Deciu, C., Kloza, E. M., Lambert-Messerlian, G. M., Haddow, J. E., Neveux, L. M., … Canick, J. A. (2012). DNA sequencing of maternal plasma reliably identifies trisomy 18 and trisomy 13, as well as Down syndrome: An international collaborative study. *Genetics Medicine, 14*(3), 296–305.

Porreco, R., Garite, T., Maurel, K., Marusiak, B., Ehrich, M., van den Boom, D., Deciu, C., & Bombard, A. (2014). Noninvasive prenatal screening for fetal trisomies 21, 18, 13, and the common sex chromosome aneuploidies from maternal blood using massively parallel genomic sequencing of DNA. *American Journal of Obstetrics and Gynecology, 211*(365), e1–12.

Richards, D.S. (2012). Prenatal ultrasound to detect fetal anomalies. *NeoReviews, 13*(1), e9-e19. doi:10.1542/neo.13-1-e9

Ridsdale, R., Lewis, D. F., Weaver, T. E., & Akinbi, H. T. (2012). Proteomic analysis of lamellar bodies isolated from amniotic fluid: Implications for function. *American Journal of Perinatology, 29*(4), 19–28.

Schenone, M., Samson, J., Suhag, A., Jenkins, L., & Mari, G. (2012). *A non-invasive method to predict fetal lung maturity using fetal pulmonary artery Doppler wave acceleration time/ejection time ratio.* Retrieved from http://www.eventkaddy.com/smfm2012/pdfs/363.pdf

Shafi, B. B. (2013). *Prenatal imaging findings in Down syndrome.* Retrieved from http://emedicine.medscape.com/article/402863-overview

Sonek, J., Molina, F., Hiett, A. K., & Glover, M. (2012). Prefrontal space ratio: Comparison between trisomy 21 and euploid fetuses in the second trimester. *Ultrasound in Obstetrics & Gynecology, 40*(3), 293–296. doi:10.1002/uog.11120

Tan, K. H., Smyth, R. M. D., & Wei, X. (2013). Fetal vibro-acoustic stimulation for facilitation of tests of the wellbeing of the unborn baby. Cochrane Database. CD002963. Retrieved from http://www.cochrane.org/CD002963/PREG_fetal-vibroacoustic-stimulation-for-facilitation-of-tests-of-the-wellbeing-of-the-unborn-baby

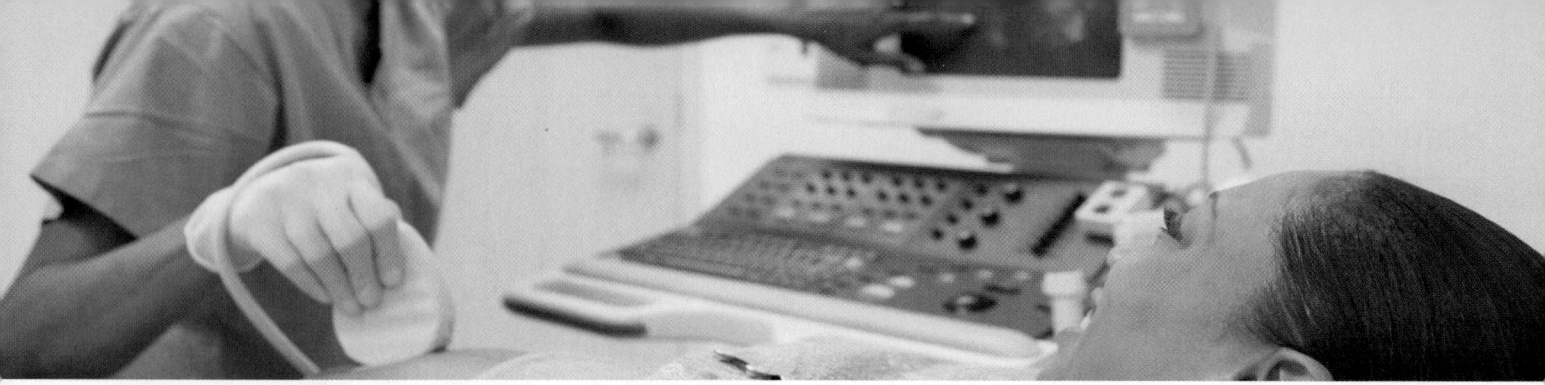

Chapter 14
Pregnancy at Risk: Pregestational Problems

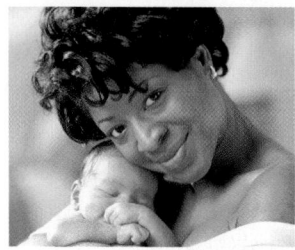

Bruce Ayres/Getty Images

I was diagnosed with type 1 diabetes when I was 16. It has taken me a while to learn how to manage it effectively, but now I am confident in my ability to maintain my blood sugar within normal limits. When my husband and I decided it was time to have a baby, I worked closely with my doctor to get myself ready for childbirth, and I have worked even harder to do the right things all during my pregnancy. I am 7 months along and doing well. I am expecting a daughter. We have decided to name her Maeve because it means "the cause of great joy" and that is what she is to us!

—Michelle, 27

⌄ Learning Outcomes

14.1 Discuss the pathology, treatment, and nursing care of pregnant women with diabetes mellitus.

14.2 Distinguish among the major types of anemia associated with pregnancy with regard to signs, treatment, implications for pregnancy, and nursing care.

14.3 Summarize the effects of alcohol and illicit drugs on the childbearing woman and her fetus/newborn.

14.4 Explain the possible implications of maternal psychologic factors and disorders in caring for the childbearing family.

14.5 Discuss AIDS, including care of the pregnant woman with HIV/AIDS, neonatal implications, ramifications for the childbearing family, and nursing care.

14.6 Describe the effects of various heart disorders on pregnancy, including their implications for nursing care.

14.7 Compare the effects of selected pregestational medical conditions on pregnancy.

Even though it is a normal process, for women with preexisting (pregestational) conditions, pregnancy may become a life-threatening event. This chapter focuses on women with pregestational medical or psychologic disorders and their possible effects on the pregnancy.

Healthy People 2020

(MICH-1.1) Reduce the rate of fetal deaths at 20 or more weeks of gestation

Care of the Woman With Diabetes Mellitus

Diabetes mellitus (DM), an endocrine disorder of carbohydrate metabolism, results from inadequate production or use of insulin. Insulin, produced by the β cells of the islets of Langerhans in the pancreas, lowers blood glucose levels by enabling glucose to move from the blood into muscle and adipose tissue cells.

Carbohydrate Metabolism in Normal Pregnancy

In early pregnancy, the rise in serum levels of estrogen, progesterone, and other hormones stimulates increased insulin production by the maternal pancreas and increased tissue response to insulin. Thus an anabolic (building-up) state exists during the first half of pregnancy, with storage of glycogen in the liver and other tissues.

In the second half of pregnancy, placental secretion of human placental lactogen (hPL) and prolactin (from the decidua), as well as elevated cortisol and glycogen levels, causes increased resistance to insulin and decreased glucose tolerance. This decreased effectiveness of insulin results in a catabolic (destructive) state during fasting periods, such as during the night or after meal absorption. Because increasing amounts of circulating maternal glucose and amino acids are diverted to the fetus, maternal fat is metabolized much more readily during fasting periods than in a nonpregnant woman. As a result of this lipolysis (maternal metabolism of fat), ketones may be present in the urine.

The delicate system of checks and balances between glucose production and glucose use is stressed by the growing fetus, who derives energy from glucose taken solely from maternal stores. This stress is known as the *diabetogenic effect of pregnancy*. Thus any preexisting disruption in carbohydrate metabolism is augmented by pregnancy, and any diabetic potential may precipitate gestational diabetes mellitus.

Pathophysiology of Diabetes Mellitus

In DM, the pancreas fails to produce insulin or does not produce enough insulin to allow necessary carbohydrate metabolism. Without adequate insulin, glucose does not enter the cells and they become energy depleted. Blood glucose levels remain high (hyperglycemia), and the cells break down their stores of fats and protein for energy. Protein breakdown results in a negative nitrogen balance; fat metabolism causes ketosis.

These pathologic developments cause the four cardinal signs and symptoms of DM:

- *Polyuria* (frequent urination) results because water is not reabsorbed by the renal tubules due to the osmotic activity of glucose.
- *Polydipsia* (excessive thirst) is caused by dehydration from polyuria.
- *Polyphagia* (excessive hunger) is caused by tissue loss and a state of starvation, which results from the inability of the cells to use the blood glucose.
- *Weight loss* (seen with marked hyperglycemia) is due to the use of fat and muscle tissue for energy.

Diagnosis of diabetes is based on the presence of clinical symptoms and laboratory tests showing elevated glucose levels in the blood, glycosuria, and ketoacidosis.

Classification

The primary classification of diabetes is based on cause and includes four main categories (American Diabetes Association [ADA], 2014):

- *Type 1 diabetes* develops because of β-cell destruction and generally results in an absolute insulin deficiency.
- *Type 2 diabetes,* the most common form, results from a combination of an insulin secretory defect and increased insulin resistance.

- *Other specific types,* of which there are eight subcategories, including, for example, genetic defects, drug-induced diabetes, and endocrine disorders.
- *Gestational diabetes mellitus.*

Gestational diabetes mellitus (GDM) is defined as any degree of glucose intolerance that has its onset or is first diagnosed during pregnancy. Diagnosis of GDM is important because even mild diabetes causes increased risk for perinatal morbidity and mortality. Furthermore, many women with GDM progress over time to overt type 2 diabetes mellitus. *Note:* Gestational diabetes mellitus is *not* a preexisting condition. It is included here, however, because many of the issues to consider in caring for a woman with GDM are similar to those involved in caring for a woman with preexisting DM.

Influence of Pregnancy on Diabetes

Pregnancy can affect diabetes significantly because the physiologic changes of pregnancy can drastically alter insulin requirements. Pregnancy may also alter the progress of vascular disease secondary to DM. Pregnancy can affect diabetes in the following ways:

- DM may be difficult to control because insulin requirements are changeable.
- During the first trimester, the need for insulin frequently decreases. Levels of hPL, an insulin antagonist, are low; fetal needs are minimal; and the woman may consume less food because of nausea and vomiting.
- Nausea and vomiting may cause dietary fluctuations and increase the risk of hypoglycemia, formerly called *insulin shock.*
- Insulin requirements begin to rise late in the first trimester as glucose use and glucose storage by the woman and fetus increase. Insulin requirements may double or quadruple by the end of pregnancy as a result of placental maturation and hPL production.
- Increased energy needs during labor may require increased insulin to balance IV glucose.
- After delivery of the placenta, insulin requirements usually decrease abruptly as a result of the loss of hPL in maternal circulation.
- A decreased renal threshold for glucose leads to a higher incidence of glycosuria.
- The risk of ketoacidosis, which may occur at lower serum glucose levels in the pregnant woman with DM than in the nonpregnant woman with diabetes, increases.
- The vascular disease that accompanies DM may progress during pregnancy.
- Hypertension may occur, contributing to vascular changes.
- Nephropathy may result from renal impairment, and retinopathy may develop (from occlusion of the microscopic blood vessels of the eye).

Influence of Diabetes on Pregnancy Outcome

The pregnancy of a woman who has diabetes carries a higher risk of complications, especially perinatal mortality and congenital anomalies. The risk can be reduced by tight metabolic control if these levels can be obtained without excessive hypoglycemia (fasting, premeal, and bedtime blood glucose levels of

60 to 99 mg/dL; peak postprandial blood glucose levels of 100 to 129 mg/dL; and HbA$_{1c}$ less than 6%) (ADA, 2014).

MATERNAL RISKS

The prognosis for the pregnant woman with gestational, type 1 or type 2 diabetes without significant vascular damage is positive. However, diabetic pregnancy still carries a higher risk of complications than normal pregnancy. In addition, the risk of developing diabetes later in life is increased in women with GDM (American College of Obstetricians and Gynecologists [ACOG], 2013).

Hydramnios, or an increase in the volume of amniotic fluid, occurs in 10% to 20% of pregnant women with diabetes. It is thought to be a result of excessive fetal urination because of fetal hyperglycemia. Premature rupture of membranes and onset of labor may occasionally be a problem with hydramnios.

Preeclampsia/eclampsia occurs more often in diabetic pregnancies than in normal pregnancies, especially when vascular changes already exist.

Hyperglycemia, due to insufficient amounts of insulin, can lead to *ketoacidosis* as a result of the increase in ketone bodies (which are acidic) released in the blood from the metabolism of fatty acids. Decreased gastric motility and the anti-insulin effects of hPL also predispose the woman to ketoacidosis. Ketoacidosis usually develops slowly but, if untreated, can lead to coma and death for mother and fetus.

Another risk to the pregnant woman with diabetes is a difficult labor (*dystocia*), caused by fetopelvic disproportion if fetal macrosomia exists.

Pregnancy can also worsen *retinopathy* in women with diabetes. However, good control of blood glucose levels lessens the impact. Hence, women with preexisting diabetes should be referred to an ophthalmologist for evaluation during pregnancy.

The pregnant woman with diabetes is also at increased risk for monilial vaginitis and urinary tract infections because of increased glycosuria, which contributes to a favorable environment for bacterial growth.

FETAL/NEONATAL RISKS

Many of the problems of the newborn result directly from high maternal plasma glucose levels. In the presence of untreated maternal ketoacidosis, the risk of fetal death increases dramatically.

The incidence of *congenital anomalies* in diabetic pregnancies is 6% to 12% and is the major cause of death of babies born to women with diabetes. Research suggests that this increased incidence is related to multiple factors including high glucose levels in early pregnancy (ACOG, 2012b). Most anomalies involve the heart, central nervous system, and skeletal system. One anomaly, *sacral agenesis*, appears almost exclusively in newborns of mothers with diabetes. In sacral agenesis, the sacrum and lumbar spine fail to develop and the lower extremities develop incompletely. Preconception counseling and strict diabetes control before conception help reduce the incidence of congenital anomalies.

Characteristically, infants of mothers with diabetes are *large for gestational age (LGA)* as a result of high levels of fetal insulin production stimulated by the high levels of glucose crossing the placenta from the mother. These elevated levels continually stimulate the fetal islets of Langerhans to produce insulin. This hyperinsulin state causes the fetus to use the available glucose, which leads to excessive growth (known as **macrosomia**) and fat deposits. If born vaginally, the macrosomic neonate is at increased risk for shoulder dystocia and traumatic birth injuries; thus, cesarean birth may be considered if birth weight is expected to exceed 4500 g (ACOG, 2013). Macrosomia can be significantly reduced by strict maternal blood glucose control.

Once the umbilical cord is cut after birth, the generous maternal blood glucose supply stops. However, continued islet cell hyperactivity leads to high insulin levels and depleted blood glucose (hypoglycemia) in 2 to 4 hours. Infants of mothers with advanced diabetes (vascular involvement) may demonstrate *intrauterine growth restriction (IUGR)*, which occurs because vascular changes in the mother decrease the efficiency of placental perfusion and the fetus is not as well sustained.

EVIDENCE-BASED PRACTICE | Best Practice Prenatal Screening for Gestational Diabetes Mellitus

Clinical Question

What are the best tests for prenatal screening for gestational onset diabetes mellitus? What is the appropriate timing of tests?

The Evidence

Gestational diabetes can have serious adverse outcomes for both mother and baby that can extend beyond the perinatal period. Appropriate and timely screening for gestational diabetes is an essential part of prenatal care. The National Guideline Clearinghouse synthesized the practice guidelines from four of the national clinical associations that guide the care gestational diabetes: The American Association of Clinical Endocrinologists (2011); the American College of Obstetricians and Gynecologists (2013); the Endocrine Society (2013); and the U.S. Preventive Services Task Force (2014). This synthesis of four primary sources of practice guidelines forms the strongest level of evidence available for practice.

The guidelines converge in two areas: pregnant women should be tested early in pregnancy (prior to 12 weeks) for undiagnosed, preexisting diabetes mellitus, and should be tested again—even if initially normal—between 24 and

28 weeks to detect emergent gestational diabetes. There does not appear to be any benefit for screening between 12 and 24 weeks if the initial tests are normal. No single test emerged as superior; a fasting plasma glucose, HbA$_{1c}$ or an untimed random plasma glucose test all functioned equally well for this purpose. All of the guidelines support postnatal screening at 6 to 12 weeks postpartum for those women who were diagnosed with gestational-onset diabetes.

Best Practice

Pregnant women should be screened for preexisting diabetes before 12 weeks' gestation, and again between 24 and 28 weeks for gestational onset of the disorder. Women who are diagnosed with gestational diabetes mellitus should be tested again 6 to 12 weeks after birth. There is no superior test, and so the least invasive and/or costly should be used.

Clinical Reasoning

What are risk factors for preexisting diabetes that might indicate screening is needed at the first prenatal visit? What are the considerations when selecting which prenatal test to use at each time period?

Respiratory distress syndrome (RDS) appears to result from high levels of fetal insulin, which inhibit some fetal enzymes necessary for surfactant production. *Polycythemia* (excessive number of red blood cells) in the newborn is mainly due to the diminished ability of glycosylated hemoglobin in the mother's blood to release oxygen. *Hyperbilirubinemia* is a direct result of the inability of immature liver enzymes to metabolize the increased bilirubin resulting from the polycythemia.

Clinical Therapy

DM occurs in about 6% to 7% of all pregnancies in the United States and of these cases, 90% are related to GDM (ACOG, 2013). Therefore, all pregnant women, regardless of risk factors, should have their risk for undiagnosed type 2 diabetes assessed at the first prenatal visit. Women at high risk (non-White, prior history of GDM or birth of an LGA neonate, marked obesity, diagnosis of polycystic ovarian syndrome, hypertension, presence of glycosuria, or a strong family history of type 2 DM) should be screened for diabetes as soon as possible.

Various screening approaches may be used. An HbA_{1c} level equal to or greater than 6.5% would be considered diagnostic, as would a fasting plasma glucose level equal to or greater than 126 mg/dL or a 2-hour plasma glucose level equal to or greater than 200 mg/dL during an oral glucose tolerance test (OGTT) (see following discussion). Women determined to have diabetes at this visit should be diagnosed as having overt diabetes and not GDM (ADA, 2014).

Two approaches to prenatal screening are currently available and performed at 24 to 28 weeks' gestation for all pregnant women not previously diagnosed with overt DM (ADA, 2014):

1. **Two-step approach** is recommended by a National Institutes of Health (NIH) Consensus Conference and ACOG (ACOG, 2013)

   - *Step 1:* Women are given nonfasting, 50-g, 1-hour OGTT. The oral glucose load can be given at any time of the day with no requirement for fasting. One hour later, plasma glucose is measured. If plasma glucose levels are elevated (equal to or greater than 140 mg/dL, depending on the laboratory used), a 100-g, 3-hour glucose test is done.

   - *Step 2:* To do the 100-g, 3-hour OGTT, the woman eats an unrestricted diet, consuming at least 150 g of carbohydrates per day for at least 3 days before her scheduled test. She then ingests 100-g oral glucose solution in the morning after an overnight fast. Plasma glucose is measured fasting and at 1, 2, and 3 hours. Gestational diabetes is diagnosed if *two or more* of the following values are met or exceeded:

Fasting	95 mg/dL
1 hour	180 mg/dL
2 hours	155 mg/dL
3 hours	140 mg/dL

2. **One-step approach** is recommended by the International Association of Diabetes and Pregnancy Study Groups (IADPSG, 2010). ADA (2015) reports that either approach—one-step or two-step—can be used.

   - In the morning, following an overnight fast, the woman ingests a 75-g oral glucose solution. Plasma glucose levels are determined fasting and at 1 and 2 hours. Gestational diabetes is diagnosed if any *one* of the following values are equaled or exceeded:

Fasting	92 mg/dL
1 hour	180 mg/dL
2 hours	153 mg/dL

LABORATORY ASSESSMENT OF LONG-TERM GLUCOSE CONTROL

Measurement of glycosylated hemoglobin levels provides information about the long-term (previous 4 to 8 weeks) control of hyperglycemia. The test measures the percentage of glycohemoglobin in the blood. Glycohemoglobin, or HbA_{1c}, is the hemoglobin to which a glucose molecule is attached. Because glycosylation is a rather slow and essentially irreversible process, the test is not reliable for screening for gestational diabetes or for close daily control. However, in women with known pregestational DM, abnormal HbA_{1c} values correlate directly with the frequency of spontaneous abortion and fetal congenital anomalies. Consequently, women with preexisting diabetes who plan to become pregnant should work to achieve HbA_{1c} levels at target levels (less than 6%) without significant hypoglycemia (ADA, 2014).

Antepartum Management of Diabetes Mellitus

To ensure an optimally healthy mother and newborn, good prenatal care using a team approach must be a top priority. The woman with gestational diabetes may find the diagnosis shocking and upsetting. She needs clear explanations about the actions she can take with regard to diet, weight gain, exercise, and the therapy that may be indicated to ensure a good outcome. The nurse-educator plays a major role in this counseling (Wong, Suwandarathne, & Russell, 2013).

The woman with pregestational diabetes needs to understand what changes she can expect during pregnancy; she should receive such teaching during preconception counseling. In addition, preconception care focuses on stringent blood glucose control prior to conception and during the first trimester. A pregnant woman with preexisting diabetes may also require referral to specialists such as an ophthalmologist or nephrologist.

DIETARY REGULATION

The pregnant woman with diabetes needs to increase her caloric intake by about 300 kcal/day. During the first trimester, the normal-weight woman generally requires about 30 kcal/kg of ideal body weight. During the second and third trimesters, she needs about 35 kcal/kg of ideal body weight. Approximately 33% to 40% of the calories should come from complex carbohydrates, 20% from protein, and 40% from fats (ACOG, 2013). The food is divided among three meals and three snacks. A bedtime snack may be indicated to prevent hypoglycemia during the night. A nutritionist should work out meal plans with the woman based on the woman's lifestyle, culture, and food preferences. The woman needs to be familiar with the use of food exchanges so she can plan her own meals. It is possible to control GDM with diet alone. Daily food records, weekly weight checks, and regular ketone testing can assist in identifying an individual's energy requirements to help avoid the need for insulin therapy (Wong et al., 2013).

GLUCOSE MONITORING

Glucose monitoring is essential to determine the need for insulin and to assess glucose control. Many physicians have the woman come in for weekly assessment of her fasting glucose levels and one or two postprandial levels. In addition, frequent self-monitoring of glucose levels is paramount in maintaining good glucose control. Self-monitoring is discussed later in the chapter.

INSULIN ADMINISTRATION

Many women with gestational diabetes need insulin to maintain normal glucose levels. Those with pregestational diabetes typically have type 1 diabetes and are already on insulin. In either case, semisynthetic human insulin or an insulin analog such as lispro or aspart should be used. Insulin is given either in multiple injections or by continuous subcutaneous infusion. Multiple injections are more common and generally produce excellent results. Many women receive a combination of intermediate and regular insulins.

A three-dose approach is often used, with a combination of intermediate-acting insulin and short-acting insulin or an analog taken before breakfast, short-acting insulin or analog at dinner, and an intermediate-acting insulin at bedtime. Some women require a four-injection approach with a small dose of a short-acting insulin or analog before lunch (Landon, Catalano, & Gabbe, 2012). Until recently, oral hypoglycemics were not generally used during pregnancy because they cross the placenta and had not been well studied. Recent research suggests that glyburide, a second-generation sulfonylurea, and metformin, a biguanide, may be safe to use in women with gestational diabetes (Caritis & Hebert, 2013; Moore, 2012).

EVALUATION OF FETAL STATUS

Information about the well-being, maturation, and size of the fetus is important for planning the course of the pregnancy and the timing of birth. See Table 14–1.

Intrapartum Management of Diabetes Mellitus

During the intrapartum period, medical therapy focuses on the following:

- *Timing of birth.* Most pregnant women with diabetes, regardless of the type, are allowed to go to full term, with spontaneous labor. Some clinicians, however, opt to induce labor in a woman at full term to avoid problems related to decreased perfusion as the placenta ages. Cesarean birth may be indicated if signs of fetal distress exist. Birth before full term may be indicated for women with diabetes who are experiencing vascular changes and worsening hypertension or if evidence of IUGR exists. To determine fetal lung maturity, the following tests may be used (O'Neill & Thorp, 2012):

Test	Lung Maturity Value
Fluorescence polarization (TDx-FLM II)	55 mg/g or greater of albumin
Lamellar body count	Greater than 32,000
Lecithin/sphingomyelin (L/S) ratio	2.0–3.5

- *Labor management.* Frequently, maternal insulin requirements decrease dramatically during labor. Consequently, maternal glucose levels are measured hourly to determine insulin need (Figure 14–1). The primary goal in controlling maternal glucose levels intrapartally is to prevent neonatal hypoglycemia (American Academy of Pediatrics [AAP] & ACOG, 2012). (Often two IV lines are used, one with a 5% dextrose solution and one with a saline solution. The saline solution is then available for piggybacking insulin or if a bolus is needed.) Because insulin clings to plastic IV bags and tubing, the tubing should be flushed with insulin before the prescribed amount is added. During the second stage of labor and the immediate postpartum period, the woman may not need additional insulin. The IV insulin is discontinued at the end of the third stage of labor.

TABLE 14–1 Fetal Surveillance by Weeks' Gestation

WEEKS' GESTATION	FETAL SURVEILLANCE
8–10	Ultrasound crown–rump measurement for estimated date of birth (EDB).
16–18 or 20	Quadruple screen for neural tube defects (maternal serum alpha-fetoprotein, hCG, unconjugated estriol, inhibin A).
18	Ultrasound confirms gestational age and diagnoses multiple pregnancy or congenital anomalies.
20–22	Fetal echocardiogram.
24	Begin ultrasounds for assessment of fetus and fetal growth.
28	Ultrasound for growth. Begin daily fetal movement counting. (See Chapter 13)
	Start weekly non-stress testing (NST). If evidence of IUGR, preeclampsia, oligohydramnios, or poorly controlled blood glucose exists, testing may begin as early as 26 weeks and may be done more often.
32	Ultrasound for growth.
32	Increase to twice weekly non-stress test (NST) or weekly biophysical profile (BPP). If the NST is nonreactive, a fetal biophysical profile or contraction stress test is performed. If the woman requires hospitalization (e.g., to control glycemia or for complications), NSTs may be done daily.
36	Ultrasound for growth.
37–39	Amniocentesis for women with poor glycemic control to document fetal pulmonary maturity prior to elective birth. Omit amniocentesis if maternal or fetal condition suggests jeopardy to either.
39–40	Birth without amniocentesis for women that have maintained good glycemic control and have excellent dating criteria.

Note: Some physicians order **fetal biophysical profiles** (ultrasound evaluation of fetal well-being in which fetal breathing movements, fetal activity, reactivity, muscle tone, and amniotic fluid volume are assessed) as part of an ongoing evaluation of fetal status.

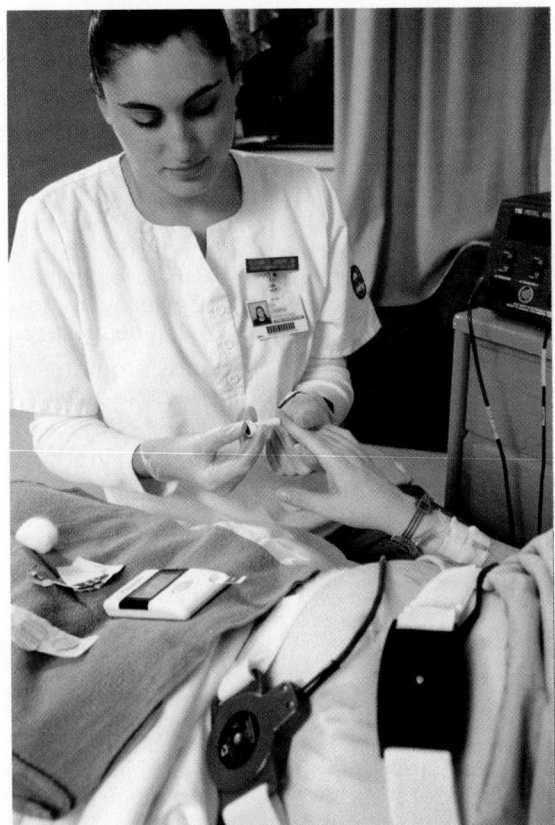

Figure 14–1 During labor the nurse closely monitors the blood glucose levels of the woman with diabetes mellitus.

Postpartum Management of Diabetes Mellitus

Generally, maternal insulin requirements fall significantly during the postpartum period because hormone levels fall after placental separation and their anti-insulin effect ceases, resulting in decreased blood glucose levels. For the first 24 hours postpartum, a woman with preexisting diabetes typically requires very little insulin and her insulin dosage is usually managed with a sliding scale. Afterward a more regular insulin dosage pattern can be reestablished based on blood glucose testing.

Women with GDM seldom need insulin during the postpartum period. Breastfeeding can be encouraged, but the nurse needs to remember that insulin requirements do decrease with breastfeeding, so a prenursing snack may be indicated (Hood, 2012). Maternal caloric needs increase during lactation to 500 to 800 kcal above prepregnant requirements, and insulin must be adjusted accordingly. Home blood glucose monitoring should continue for the woman with type 1 diabetes.

If elevated glucose levels develop, oral antihyperglycemic agents may be tried if the woman is not breastfeeding. The woman should be reassessed 6 weeks postpartum to determine whether her glucose levels are normal. If the levels are normal, she should be reassessed at a minimum of 3-year intervals (ADA, 2014).

If the newborn requires a special care nursery, the nurse should provide the parents with ongoing information, support, and encouragement to visit and be involved in the newborn's care, since establishing parent–child relationships is a high priority during the postpartum period.

The woman and her partner, if he is involved, should also receive information on family planning. Barrier methods of contraception (diaphragm, cervical cap, condom) used with a spermicide are safe, effective, economical, and the method of choice for women with insulin-dependent diabetes. The use of combined oral contraceptives (COCs) by women with diabetes is somewhat controversial. Many physicians who prescribe low-dose COCs to women with diabetes restrict them to women who have no vascular disease and do not smoke. The progesterone-only pill may also be used as may Depo-Provera. Many couples who have completed their families choose elective sterilization.

Nursing Management

For the Woman With Diabetes Mellitus or GDM

Nursing Care Plan: The Woman With Diabetes Mellitus summarizes nursing management.

Nursing Assessment and Diagnosis

Whether diabetes has been diagnosed before pregnancy occurs or the diagnosis is made during pregnancy (GDM), careful assessment of the disease process and the woman's understanding of diabetes is important. Thorough physical examination—including assessment for vascular complications of the disease, any signs of infectious conditions, and urine and blood testing for glucose—is essential on the first prenatal visit. Follow-up visits are usually scheduled twice a month during the first two trimesters and once a week during the last trimester.

Assessment provides information about the woman's ability to cope with the combined stress of pregnancy and diabetes and to follow a recommended regimen of care. Determine the woman's knowledge about diabetes and self-care before developing a teaching plan.

Nursing diagnoses that may apply to the pregnant woman with diabetes include the following (NANDA-I © 2014):

- *Overweight, Risk for,* related to imbalance between intake and available insulin
- *Injury, Risk for,* related to possible complications secondary to hypoglycemia or hyperglycemia
- *Family Processes, Interrupted,* related to the need for hospitalization secondary to DM

Planning and Implementation

For the woman with preexisting diabetes, a nurse and a physician may provide prepregnancy counseling using a team approach. Ideally, they see the couple before pregnancy so that the DM can be evaluated. The outlook for pregnancy is good if the diabetes is of recent onset without vascular complications, provided that glucose levels can be controlled.

For women with GDM, nursing care focuses heavily on client education about the condition, its implications, and its management.

COMMUNITY-BASED NURSING CARE

In many cases, women with GDM are stabilized in the hospital and necessary teaching for self-care is begun. Women with preexisting diabetes may also require hospitalization for stabilization of their diabetes. In either case, the majority of ongoing teaching and supervision of pregnant women with diabetes is then carried out by nurses in clinics, community agencies, and the women's homes.

Effective Insulin Use

Ensure that the woman and her partner understand the purpose of insulin, the types of insulin to be used, and the correct procedure for administering it. Instruct the woman's partner about insulin administration in case it becomes necessary for the partner to give it. For some highly motivated women whose glucose levels are not well controlled with multiple injections, a continuous infusion pump may improve glucose control.

Nursing Care Plan: The Woman With Diabetes Mellitus

1. Nursing Diagnosis: *Nutrition, Imbalanced, Less than Body Requirements,* **related to poor carbohydrate metabolism (NANDA-I © 2014)**

GOAL: Client will maintain adequate nutrition throughout pregnancy.

INTERVENTION	RATIONALE
• Emphasize importance of regular prenatal visits for assessment of weight gain, controlled blood sugar, fetal heart tones, urine ketones, and fundal height measurement.	• Regular follow-up and assessment of weight, blood sugar levels, fetal heart tones, urine ketones, and fundal height will promote a healthy pregnancy and outcome as well as allow for modifications in the treatment regimen if necessary.
• Coordinate care with a dietitian to assist client in meal planning and educate client on the daily caloric needs of pregnancy.	• A daily intake of high-quality foods promotes fetal growth and controls maternal glucose levels.
• Instruct client on signs and symptoms of hyperglycemia: polyphagia, nausea, hot flushes, polydipsia, polyuria, fruity breath, abdominal cramps, rapid deep breathing, headache, weakness, drowsiness, and general malaise. Instruct client on signs and symptoms of hypoglycemia: hunger, clammy skin, irritability, slurred speech, seizures, tachycardia, headache, pallor, sweating, disorientation, shakiness, blurred vision, and, if untreated, coma or convulsions.	• Maintaining a euglycemic state throughout pregnancy aids in preventing diabetic complications and promotes a positive pregnancy outcome.
• Instruct client on management of hyperglycemia and hypoglycemia.	
• Include family members in meal.	• Gives the family member a sense of involvement and an understanding of the importance of adequate nutrition in pregnancy.

EXPECTED OUTCOME: The client will maintain adequate nutrition as evidenced by adequate weight gain, normal blood sugar levels, fetal heart rate, verbalization of understanding of personal treatment regimen, and appropriate fetal growth and development during pregnancy.

2. Nursing Diagnosis: *Injury, Risk for,* **to the fetus related to possible complications associated with altered tissue perfusion secondary to maternal diagnosis of diabetes mellitus (NANDA-I © 2014)**

GOAL: Uncomplicated birth of a healthy newborn.

INTERVENTION	RATIONALE
• Assess fetal heart tones for reassuring variability and accelerations.	• Reassuring fetal heart rate variability and accelerations are interpreted as adequate placental oxygenation.
• Instruct mother on how to lie in a left recumbent position after eating and record how many fetal movements she feels in an hour.	• More than five fetal kicks in an hour are indicative of fetal well-being.
• **Collaborative:** Perform oxytocin challenge test (OCT)/contraction stress test (CST), and non-stress tests as determined by physician.	• Fetal surveillance testing assesses fetal well-being and adequate placental perfusion.
• Prepare client for frequent ultrasound assessments.	• Ultrasonography is indicated in the first trimester to confirm gestational age and then repeated regularly to evaluate fetal well-being per physician's orders.
• Prepare client for possible amniocentesis procedure.	• A sample of amniotic fluid that can be used to detect fetal lung maturity and enables medical personnel to prepare for a potential preterm birth.
• Assist physician with biophysical profile assessment.	• Helps ensure fetal well-being and a positive fetal outcome.

EXPECTED OUTCOME: The fetus will exhibit signs of adequate tissue perfusion as evidenced by positive fetal activity, reassuring fetal heart rate patterns, a biophysical profile score between 8 and 10, negative CST, L/S ratio indicating fetal lung maturity, and a reactive non-stress test.

3. Nursing Diagnosis: *Enhanced Knowledge, Readiness for,* **about the effects of blood sugar on pregnancy related to an expressed desire to maintain stable blood glucose levels (NANDA-I © 2014)**

GOAL: The client and her family will verbalize the importance of maintaining blood sugar within prescribed ranges during pregnancy.

INTERVENTION	RATIONALE
• Assess the woman's and family's cognitive level and develop a teaching strategy that will facilitate learning at that level.	• Behavior changes occur when teaching strategies are appropriate for the client and family's cognitive level.
• Teach blood glucose monitoring, insulin administration, and predicted insulin needs throughout pregnancy, and then have client and family members repeat the discussion.	• Basic understanding of the relationship between blood sugar levels and how insulin needs change throughout pregnancy will foster compliance with prescribed regimen.
• Emphasize the importance of maintaining a healthy diet and exercise program during pregnancy. Encourage client and family to develop a sample diabetic diet and exercise regimen that is appropriate for pregnancy while present in the clinic or hospital and evaluate for appropriateness.	• Involves the client and her family members in the planning of her care, and the evaluation process promotes cooperation, positive reinforcement, and a time for modifications of regimen if necessary.
• Emphasize the importance of prenatal care for the purpose of maternal and fetal surveillance.	• Frequent prenatal visits allow for modifications in regimen and promote a healthy pregnancy outcome.

EXPECTED OUTCOME: The client and family members will verbalize understanding of the effects of blood sugar fluctuations on pregnancy as evidenced by asking questions and seeking health information when necessary. The client adheres to personal treatment regimen throughout pregnancy.

4. Nursing Diagnosis: *Infection, Risk for,* **related to increased levels of glucose in urine (NANDA-I © 2014)**

GOAL: The client will have no urinary tract infections (UTIs) during pregnancy.

INTERVENTION	RATIONALE
• Encourage client to utilize preventive measures to prevent UTIs: increasing intake of water and cranberry juice, wearing cotton underwear, wiping perineum from front to back, voiding frequently, and voiding before and immediately after sexual intercourse.	• Utilizing preventive measures decreases the likelihood of client acquiring a UTI.
• Instruct client on the signs and symptoms of UTIs: urinary frequency, dysuria, cloudy urine, hematuria, lower back pain, and foul-smelling urine.	• Client will be aware of signs and symptoms of UTIs and report to physician for immediate intervention.
• **Collaborative:** Instruct client on how to obtain a clean-catch urine sample and send to laboratory for culture and sensitivity per physician's orders.	• A clean-catch urine sample will contain bacteria if a UTI is present.
• Administer prescribed antibiotic therapy and teach client about medication, adverse effects, and appropriate dosage.	• Antibiotic therapy is the appropriate treatment for a UTI. Compliance increases when a client fully understands medication regimen.
• Encourage client to drink 8–10 glasses of water each day.	• Increased fluid intake assists in flushing bacteria out of the urinary tract system.

EXPECTED OUTCOME: Client will remain free of UTIs during pregnancy as evidenced by verbalizing and complying with appropriate preventive measures, increasing fluid intake, and identifying negative urine samples during prenatal visits.

5. Nursing Diagnosis: *Anxiety* **related to unfamiliarity with diagnosis (NANDA-I © 2014)**

GOAL: The client expresses less anxiety.

INTERVENTION	RATIONALE
• Assess client's level of anxiety (mild—1, moderate—2, or severe—3) and have client verbalize causes of anxiety.	• Verbalization of anxiety provokers encourages expression of feelings and questions.
• Share information on diabetes care such as nutrition, exercise, and glucose control in a clear and concise manner.	• Accurate information gives the client a sense of control and comfort.
• Instruct client on anxiety-reducing techniques such as imagery, breathing exercises, and massage used in pregnancy.	• Gives client the tools necessary for decreasing anxiety.
• Refer client to a diabetes support group.	• A support group allows clients with similar problems to express concerns and share information with each other.

EXPECTED OUTCOME: The client demonstrates appropriate coping strategies as evidenced by utilizing resources efficiently and verbalizing feelings of anxiety and the ways to deal with them.

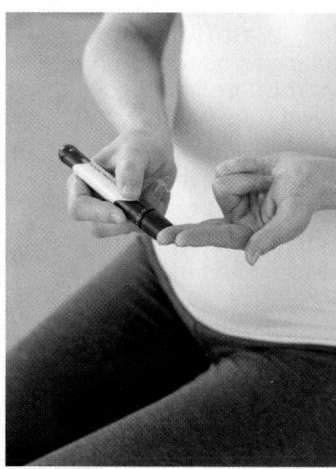

Figure 14–2 As she was taught, this pregnant woman regularly monitors her blood glucose at home.

Teach the woman how and when to monitor her blood glucose level, the desired range of blood glucose levels, and the importance of good control (Figure 14–2). Most women use a glucose meter to monitor blood sugar level because the meter is more accurate. Clients with diabetes need to keep a record of each blood sugar reading. Specific record sheets are available for this purpose.

Clinical Reasoning Glucose Intolerance

Patti Chang, a 35-year-old G3P2, is a well-educated, active Chinese American woman with no history of glucose intolerance. Her two children were born healthy at 36 weeks' gestation. She receives the usual 50-g glucose tolerance test at 26 weeks' gestation, and her plasma level is 160 mg/dL. She seems irritated and frustrated when her obstetrician tells her that it would be best to perform a 3-hour fasting glucose tolerance test. After the physician leaves the room, Patti asks you the following questions: "Will the glucose hurt my baby? What will the treatment be?"

How will you answer the questions? Why do you think Patti seems so upset?

Planned Exercise Program

Regardless of the type of diabetes, unless otherwise medically contraindicated, exercise is important for the woman's overall well-being. If she is used to a regular exercise program, encourage her to continue. Advise the woman to exercise after meals when blood sugar levels are high, to wear diabetic identification, to carry a simple sugar such as hard candy (because of the possibility of exercise-induced hypoglycemia), to monitor her blood glucose levels regularly, and to avoid injecting insulin into an extremity that will soon be used during exercise.

Clinical Tip

Have a woman with GDM who is learning to test her blood glucose do a fingerstick while you watch. For many women, actually sticking their finger can be a challenge to overcome. This also enables you to verify that correct technique is used.

If the woman has not been following a regular exercise plan, encourage her to begin gradually. Because of alterations in metabolism with exercise, the woman's blood glucose should be well controlled before she begins an exercise program. See *Health Promotion: The Pregnant Woman With Diabetes.*

Health Promotion The Pregnant Woman With Diabetes

Glucose Monitoring

Home monitoring of blood glucose levels is the most accurate and convenient method to determine insulin dose and assess control.

- Teach the woman self-monitoring techniques that are done according to a specified schedule. Women with GDM typically measure their blood glucose 4 times a day (fasting and 1 to 2 hours after meals). Women with preexisting DM should monitor their blood in the fasting state, before each meal, 1 to 2 hours after each meal, and at bedtime (ACOG, 2012b).

- Instruct the woman to regulate her insulin dosage based on blood glucose values and anticipated activity level.

- Encourage her to maintain blood glucose levels in normal ranges as follows: fasting (before eating or taking insulin), less than 95 mg/dL; 2 hours after each meal, less than 120 mg/dL (AAP/ACOG, 2012).

Review Symptoms of Hypoglycemia and Hyperglycemia

- Teach the pregnant woman with diabetes to recognize symptoms of changing glucose levels and to take appropriate action by immediately checking her capillary blood glucose level.

- If blood glucose is less than 60 mg/dL, advise her to drink one 8-oz cup of milk or 1/2 cup of orange juice, apple juice, or regular soft drink; or eat four to six pieces of hard candy; or consume 1 tablespoon of honey, brown sugar, or corn syrup. Wait 15 minutes and recheck blood glucose (Cleveland Clinic, 2012). (*Note:* Many people overtreat their symptoms by continuing to eat, but doing so can cause rebound hyperglycemia.)

- Have the woman carry a snack at all times and have other fast sources of glucose (simple carbohydrates) at hand to treat an insulin reaction when milk or juice is not available.

- Ensure that family members learn how to inject glucagon in case food does not work or is not feasible (e.g., in the presence of severe morning sickness).

Smoking

- Ensure that the woman knows that smoking has harmful effects on both the maternal vascular system and the developing fetus and thus is contraindicated for both pregnancy and diabetes.

Travel

- Insulin can be kept at room temperature while traveling. Instruct woman to keep insulin supplies with her; they should not be packed in the baggage.

- On international flights, most airlines can provide special meals if notified a few days before departure. If meals are not scheduled to be served, the woman should ensure that she has adequate food before boarding.

- Have her wear a diabetic identification bracelet or necklace and check with her physician for any instructions or advice before traveling.

Support Groups

- Many communities have diabetes support groups or education classes that are helpful to women with newly diagnosed diabetes. Refer her to them.

Cesarean Birth

- Chances for a cesarean birth increase if the pregnant woman is diabetic. Anticipate the possibility and suggest enrollment in cesarean birth preparation classes. The couple may prefer simply to discuss cesarean birth with the nurse and their obstetrician and read some books on the topic.

HOSPITAL-BASED NURSING CARE

Hospitalization may become necessary during the pregnancy to evaluate blood glucose levels and adjust insulin dosages. In such cases, monitor the woman's status and provide teaching so that she is knowledgeable about her condition and its management.

SAFETY ALERT!

Insulin is a high-risk medication that carries significant potential risks. Like all medications, nurses should use two client identifiers, administer it at the correct time, and monitor the client afterward. Nurses should have documented knowledge about insulin administration and demonstrate competency in administering, storing, and handling it and in the key assessments and findings indicated for maternity clients receiving insulin (Hurst, 2011).

During the intrapartum period, continue to monitor the woman's status, maintain her IV fluids, remain alert for signs of hypoglycemia, and provide the care indicated for any woman in labor. If a cesarean birth becomes necessary, provide appropriate care, as described in Chapter 22.

Evaluation

Expected outcomes of nursing care include the following:

- The woman is able to discuss her condition and its possible impact on her pregnancy, labor and birth, and postpartum period.
- The woman participates in developing a healthcare regimen to meet her needs and follows it throughout her pregnancy.
- The woman avoids developing hypoglycemia or hyperglycemia.
- The woman gives birth to a healthy newborn.
- The woman is able to care for her newborn.

Care of the Woman With Anemia

Anemia indicates inadequate levels of hemoglobin (Hb) in the blood. During pregnancy, *anemia* is defined as Hb less than 11 g/dL (Samuels, 2012). The common anemias of pregnancy

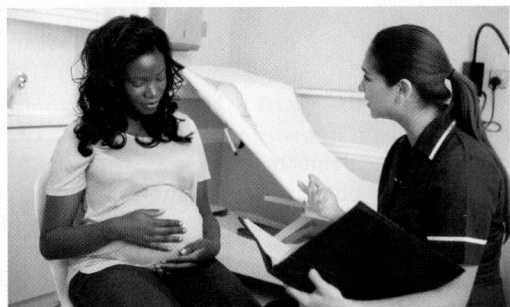

Figure 14–3 Health teaching is an important part of nursing care for the pregnant woman with sickle cell disease.

SOURCE: Monkey Business Images/Shutterstock.

are due either to insufficient Hb production related to nutritional deficiency in iron or folic acid during pregnancy or to Hb destruction in an inherited disorder such as sickle cell disease (Figure 14–3). Table 14–2 describes these common anemias.

Healthy People 2020

(MICH-15) Reduce the proportion of women of childbearing potential who have low red blood cell folate concentrations

---

Care of the Woman With Substance Abuse Problems

Substance abuse occurs when a person experiences difficulties with work, family, social relations, and health as a result of alcohol or drug use. In general, the rate of illicit drug use among pregnant women is significantly less than half the rate among nonpregnant women. Approximately 5.4% of pregnant women ages 15 to 44 report having used an illicit drug in the past month as compared to 11.4% of nonpregnant women. However, illicit drug use varies significantly by age with the highest rate among the youngest pregnant women, specifically 14.6% among females ages 15 to 17; the rate was 8.6% among those ages 18 to 25, and 3.2% among prepregnant women ages 26 to 44 (Substance Abuse and Mental Health Services Administration [SAMHSA], 2014).

Drugs that are commonly misused include tobacco, alcohol, cocaine, marijuana, amphetamines, barbiturates, hallucinogens, club drugs, heroin, and other narcotics. (Tobacco is discussed in Chapter 10 as a teratogenic substance.) Polydrug use involving multiple substances such as alcohol, tobacco, and illicit drugs is fairly common and contributes to the risks a pregnant woman faces. Table 14–3 identifies common addictive drugs and their effects on the fetus or newborn.

Healthy People 2020

(MICH 11) Increase abstinence from alcohol, cigarettes, and illicit drugs among pregnant women

---

Drug use during pregnancy, particularly in the first trimester, may have a negative effect on the health of the woman and the growth and development of the fetus. Unfortunately, prenatal drug use may be the most frequently missed diagnosis in all of maternity care. Physicians and nurses may fail to ask women about drug and alcohol use because of their own lack of knowledge, discomfort, or biases. Often substance-abusing women wait until late in pregnancy to seek health care. Moreover, the substance-abusing woman who seeks early prenatal care may not voluntarily reveal her addiction, so healthcare providers should be alert for a history or physical signs that might indicate substance abuse.

Providing effective prenatal care to chemically dependent women is often challenging for clinicians. However, pregnancy is a time when most women are receptive to caring interventions.

Clinical Tip

Keep in mind that at least 1 of 10 women in the United States, regardless of socioeconomic status or ethnic background, is currently abusing a substance. If you consider that possibility with every woman, you will ask the important questions about drug use and be alert for signs of substance abuse.

TABLE 14–2 Anemia and Pregnancy

CONDITION	BRIEF DESCRIPTION	MATERNAL IMPLICATIONS	FETAL/NEONATAL IMPLICATIONS
Iron deficiency anemia	Most common medical complication of pregnancy. Condition caused by inadequate iron intake resulting in hemoglobin (Hb) levels below 11 g/dL. To prevent this, most women are advised to take supplemental iron during pregnancy and to eat an iron-rich diet.	A pregnant woman with this anemia tires easily, is more susceptible to infection, has increased chance of preeclampsia/eclampsia and postpartum hemorrhage, and cannot tolerate even minimal blood loss during birth. Healing of episiotomy or incision may be delayed.	Risk of low birth weight, preterm birth, nonreassuring fetal status, and perinatal mortality increases in women with severe iron deficiency anemia (maternal Hb less than 6 g/dL). Fetus may be hypoxic during labor due to impaired uteroplacental oxygenation.
Sickle cell disease (also referred to as sickle cell anemia)	Recessive autosomal disease in which normal adult hemoglobin, hemoglobin A, is abnormally formed. It occurs primarily in people of African descent and occasionally in people of Southeast Asian or Mediterranean descent. The disease is characterized by sickling of the red blood cells (RBCs) in the presence of decreased oxygenation. Because the woman maintains her Hb levels by intense erythropoiesis, additional folic acid supplements (1 mg/day) are necessary. Condition may be marked by crisis with profound anemia, jaundice, high temperature, infarction, and acute pain. Crisis is treated by rehydration with intravenous fluids, administration of oxygen, antibiotics, and analgesics. The fetus is monitored throughout.	Pregnancy may aggravate sickle cell disease and bring on a vaso-occlusive crisis. Maternal mortality is rare but there is a significant risk of pyelonephritis, acute chest syndrome, and gestational hypertension (Cunningham et al., 2014). Congestive heart failure or acute renal failure may also occur. Maternal infections are treated aggressively because dehydration and fever can trigger sickling and crisis. Oxygen supplementation is used throughout labor, and IV fluids are given to maintain hydration. Fetal heart rate (FHR) is monitored closely. Antiembolism stockings may be used postpartum.	The incidence of fetal death during and immediately following an attack has decreased greatly in recent years. Prematurity and intrauterine growth restriction (IUGR) are associated with sickle cell disease. Fetal death is believed to be due to sickling attacks in the placenta (Andemariam & Browning, 2013).
Folic acid deficiency anemia	Folic acid deficiency is the most common cause of megaloblastic anemia. In the absence of folic acid, immature RBCs fail to divide, become enlarged (megaloblastic), and are fewer in number. Increased folic acid metabolism during pregnancy and lactation can result in deficiency. All women who could become pregnant should take a multivitamin containing 400 mcg daily (generally found in prenatal vitamins) before conception and through at least the first trimester of pregnancy. The condition is treated with 1 mg folate daily (see Chapter 11).	Folate deficiency is the second most common cause of anemia in pregnancy. Severe deficiency increases the risk that the mother may need a blood transfusion following birth due to anemia. She also has an increased risk of hemorrhage due to thrombocytopenia and is more susceptible to infection. Folic acid is readily available in foods such as fresh leafy green vegetables, red meat, fish, poultry, and legumes, but it is easily destroyed by overcooking or cooking with large quantities of water.	Maternal folic acid deficiency has been associated with an increased risk of neural tube defects (NTDs) such as spina bifida, meningomyelocele, and anencephaly in the newborn. Women who have already had one baby with a NTD are generally advised to take a larger dose of folic acid daily.

Substances Commonly Abused During Pregnancy

ALCOHOL

Alcohol is a central nervous system (CNS) depressant and a potent teratogen. Among pregnant women ages 15 to 44, estimates suggest that 9.4% use alcohol in a given month. This rate is significantly lower than the rate for nonpregnant women of that age (55.4%) (SAMHSA, 2014). This figure is of concern, however, because birth defects that are related to fetal alcohol exposure can occur in the first 3 to 8 weeks' gestation, often before the woman even knows she is pregnant. Alcohol use among pregnant women tends to decrease by trimester.

The effects of alcohol on the fetus may result in a group of signs known as *fetal alcohol spectrum disorders (FASD)*. FASD has characteristic physical and mental abnormalities that vary in severity (see discussion in Chapter 26). There is no final answer to how much alcohol a woman can safely drink during pregnancy. It is essential that nurses and other healthcare providers advise women about the dangers associated with drinking while pregnant (U.S. Department of Health and Human Services, 2012).

TABLE 14–3 Possible Effects of Selected Drugs of Abuse/Addiction on Fetus and Newborn

MATERNAL DRUG	EFFECT ON FETUS/NEWBORN
DEPRESSANTS	
Alcohol	Mental retardation, microcephaly, midfacial hypoplasia, cardiac anomalies, intrauterine growth restriction (IUGR), potential teratogenic effects, fetal alcohol syndrome (FAS), fetal alcohol effects (FAE).
NARCOTICS	
Heroin	Withdrawal symptoms, known as *neonatal abstinence syndrome (NAS)*, include tremors, irritability, sneezing, vomiting, fever, diarrhea, abnormal respiratory function, and possible seizures.
Methadone	With abrupt maternal termination of the drug, severe withdrawal symptoms can include preterm labor, rapid labor, abruption, nonreassuring fetal status, and meconium aspiration. Neonates may present with NAS and be small for gestational age (SGA).
BARBITURATES	
Phenobarbital	Withdrawal symptoms. Fetal growth restriction.
TRANQUILIZERS	
Diazepam (Valium)	Withdrawal symptoms.
ANTIANXIETY DRUGS	
Lithium	Congenital anomalies.
STIMULANTS	
Amphetamines	
Amphetamine sulfate (Benzedrine)	Low birth weight; withdrawal symptoms.
Cocaine	Cerebral infarctions, microcephaly, learning disabilities, poor state organization, decreased interactive behavior, CNS anomalies, cardiac anomalies, genitourinary anomalies, sudden infant death syndrome (SIDS).
Methamphetamine	SGA, low birth weight, decreased arousal, lower scores on tests of attention, verbal memory, and visual motor integration (ACOG, 2011).
Nicotine (half to one pack cigarettes/day)	Increased rate of spontaneous abortion, increased incidence of placental abruption, SGA, small head circumference, decreased length, SIDS, attention deficit hyperactivity disorder (ADHD) in school-age children.
PSYCHOTROPICS	
PCP (phencyclidine hydrochloride, "angel dust")	Withdrawal symptoms. Newborn behavioral and developmental abnormalities.
Marijuana	Possible impaired neurodevelopment in children exposed in utero; increased sensitivity to drugs of abuse; risks similar to those associated with smoking tobacco (ACOG, 2015b).

Chronic abuse of alcohol can undermine maternal health by causing malnutrition (especially folic acid and thiamine deficiencies), bone marrow suppression, increased incidence of infections, and liver disease. As a result of alcohol dependence, a woman may have withdrawal seizures in the intrapartum period as early as 12 to 48 hours after she stops drinking. Delirium tremens may occur in the postpartum period, and the newborn may suffer a withdrawal syndrome. Nurses in the maternal–newborn unit must be aware of the manifestations of alcohol abuse so they can prepare for the woman's special needs. Care includes sedation to decrease irritability and tremors, seizure precautions, intravenous (IV) fluid therapy for hydration, and preparation for an addicted newborn. Although high doses of sedatives and analgesics may be necessary for the woman, caution is advised because these medications can cause fetal depression.

Breastfeeding generally is not contraindicated, although alcohol is excreted in breast milk. Excessive alcohol consumption may intoxicate the baby and inhibit the maternal letdown reflex. Discharge planning for the alcohol-addicted mother and newborn needs to be correlated with the social service department of the hospital.

COCAINE AND CRACK

Cocaine acts at the nerve terminals to prevent the reuptake of dopamine and norepinephrine, which in turn results in vasoconstriction, tachycardia, and hypertension. Placental vasoconstriction decreases blood flow to the fetus. The onset of cocaine effects occurs rapidly, but the euphoria lasts only about 30 minutes. Euphoria and excitement are usually followed by irritability, depression, pessimism, fatigue, and a strong desire for more cocaine. This pattern often leads the user to take repeated doses to sustain the effect. Cocaine metabolites may be present in the urine of a pregnant woman for as long as 4 to 7 days after use.

Cocaine can be taken by IV injection or by snorting the powdered form. *Crack*, a form of freebase cocaine that is made up of baking soda, water, and cocaine mixed into a paste and microwaved to form a rock, can be smoked. Smoking crack leads to a quicker, more intense high because the drug is absorbed through the large surface area of the lungs.

The cocaine user is difficult to identify prenatally. Because cocaine is illegal, many women are reluctant to admit that they use it. The nurse may recognize subtle signs of cocaine use, including mood swings and appetite changes, and withdrawal symptoms such as depression, irritability, nausea, lack of motivation, and psychomotor changes.

Major adverse maternal effects of cocaine use include seizures and hallucinations, pulmonary edema, respiratory failure, and heart problems. Women who use cocaine have an increased incidence of spontaneous abortion, abruptio placentae, intrauterine growth restriction (IUGR), preterm birth, and stillbirth (Cain, Bornick, & Whiteman, 2013).

Fetal exposure to cocaine increases the risk of intrauterine growth restriction (IUGR), microcephaly, altered brain development, shorter body length, congenital anomalies, and neurobehavioral abnormalities (Niebyl & Simpson, 2012). Newborns exposed to cocaine in utero may have neurobehavioral disturbances, marked irritability, an exaggerated startle reflex, labile emotions, and an increased risk of sudden infant death syndrome (SIDS). (See Chapter 26 for further discussion.) Exposed babies are found to have more feeding difficulties than nonexposed babies. These difficulties may be related to some extent to the baby's behaviors but have also been found to be related to maternal behaviors. Hyperactivity and short attention span have been noted in toddlers prenatally exposed to opiates and older exposed children have demonstrated memory and perceptual problems (Behnke & Smith, 2013). Cocaine crosses into breast milk and may cause symptoms in the breastfeeding baby, including extreme irritability, vomiting, diarrhea, dilated pupils, and apnea. Thus women who continue to use cocaine after childbirth should avoid breastfeeding.

MARIJUANA

Marijuana is the most widely used illicit drug among women, both pregnant and nonpregnant. In reality, the impact of heavy marijuana use on pregnancy is difficult to evaluate because of the variety of social factors that may influence the impact of marijuana itself. This may change, however, now that it has been legalized in a small number of states. Smoking, whether tobacco or marijuana, poses a risk during pregnancy. Because of the risks associated with smoking, as well as the possible impact of marijuana on the neurodevelopment of children exposed in utero and their apparent increased sensitivity to drugs of abuse, ACOG (2015b) recommends that women who are considering pregnancy and pregnant women should be counseled to discontinue marijuana use.

MDMA (ECSTASY)

Methylenedioxymethamphetamine (MDMA), better known as *Ecstasy* or *Molly*, is the most commonly used of a group of drugs referred to as *club drugs*, so called because they have become popular among adolescents and young adults who frequent dance clubs and "raves." Other club drugs include flunitrazepam (Rohypnol), gamma-hydroxybutyrate (GHB), and ketamine hydrochloride. Phencyclidine (PCP) and lysergic acid diethylamine (LSD) are sometimes classified as club drugs as well.

A stimulant, MDMA is taken by mouth, usually as a tablet. It produces euphoria and feelings of empathy for others. It has been widely perceived as a "safe" drug because of a relatively low incidence of adverse reactions. However, adverse responses are very unpredictable and the incidence is growing. MDMA can cause muscle tension, involuntary teeth clenching, nausea, confusion, sleep problems, drug cravings, memory deficits, and severe anxiety. In high doses, it can lead to severe hyperthermia by interfering with the body's temperature regulation. This can lead to organ failure and even death (National Institute on Drug Abuse, 2013).

Data about the fetal and neonatal effects are sparse. Singer et al. (2012) followed a group of women who reported MDMA use during pregnancy and evaluated their infants at 1 year of age. They found that the amount of MDMA exposure during

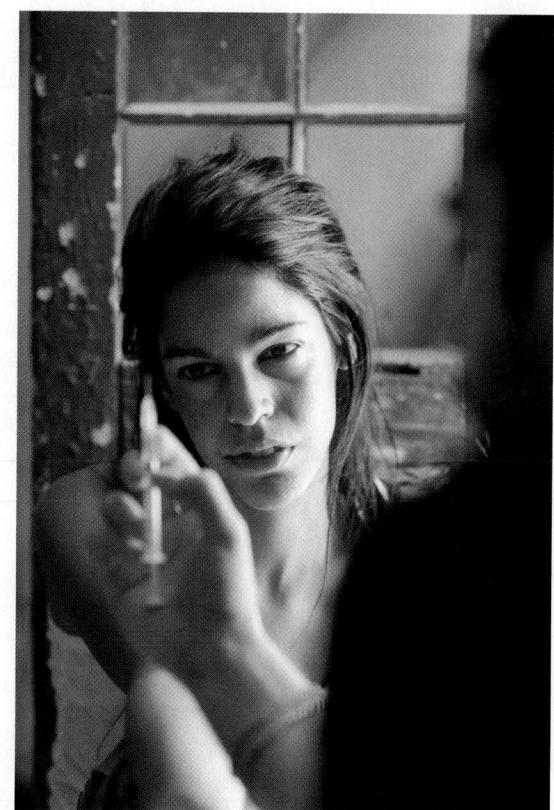

Figure 14–4 The use of illicit drugs puts the pregnant woman and her unborn child at increased risk for a variety of complications.

SOURCE: © Diego Cervo/Fotolia.

pregnancy predicted a dose-related delay on mental and motor development at 1 year of age. There appeared to be no effect on language, emotional regulation, or parenting stress.

HEROIN

Heroin is an illicit CNS depressant narcotic that alters perception and produces euphoria. It is an addictive drug that is generally administered IV (Figure 14–4). Pregnancy in women who use heroin is considered high risk because of the increased incidence in these women of poor nutrition, iron deficiency anemia, and preeclampsia. Women addicted to heroin also have a higher incidence of sexually transmitted infections because many rely on prostitution to support their drug habit.

The fetus of a woman who is addicted to heroin is at increased risk for preterm birth, IUGR, meconium aspiration, and withdrawal symptoms (neonatal abstinence syndrome [NAS]) after birth such as restlessness; shrill, high-pitched cry; irritability; fist sucking; vomiting; and seizures. Signs of withdrawal usually appear within 72 hours and may last for several days (Wang, 2014). These behaviors may interfere with successful maternal attachment and increase the risk for parenting problems or abuse in an already high-risk mother (Behnke & Smith, 2013).

Methadone is the most commonly used therapy for women dependent on opioids such as heroin. Methadone blocks withdrawal symptoms and reduces or eliminates the craving for narcotics. Dosage should be individualized at the lowest possible therapeutic level. Methadone does cross the placenta, and, consequently, newborns are at risk for NAS. However, various studies have demonstrated inconsistent long-term effects on the newborn (ACOG, 2012a). Buprenorphine, a partial opioid agonist, is an acceptable alternative because it may decrease the severity of NAS in the newborn (Niebyl & Simpson, 2012).

Clinical Therapy

A team approach to the care of the pregnant woman with substance abuse problems ensures the management necessary to provide safe labor and birth for the woman and her child.

The management of drug addiction may include hospitalization if necessary to start detoxification. "Cold turkey" withdrawal is not advisable during pregnancy because of the possible risk to the fetus. Maintenance and support therapy are best individualized to the woman's history and condition. Urine screening is also done regularly throughout pregnancy if the woman has a known or suspected substance abuse problem and should include maternal informed consent. This testing helps to identify the type and amount of drug being abused.

Nursing Management

For the Pregnant Woman With a Substance Abuse Problem

Nursing Assessment and Diagnosis

Because of the prevalence of substance abuse, it is important to screen all pregnant women for substance abuse during the health history. Several simple screening tools are available. In addition, be alert for clues in the history or appearance of the woman that suggest substance abuse. If abuse is suspected, ask direct questions, beginning with less threatening questions about use of tobacco, caffeine, and over-the-counter medications. Then progress to questions about alcohol intake and finally to questions focusing on past and current use of illegal drugs. A matter-of-fact, nonjudgmental approach is more likely to elicit honest responses.

When assessing a woman with a known substance abuse problem, focus on the woman's general health status, with specific attention to nutritional status, susceptibility to infections, and evaluation of all body systems. Also assess the woman's understanding of the impact of substance abuse on herself and on her pregnancy.

Nursing diagnoses that may apply to a woman at risk because of substance abuse include the following (NANDA-I © 2014):

- *Nutrition, Imbalanced: Less than Body Requirements,* related to inadequate food intake secondary to substance abuse
- *Infection, Risk for,* related to use of inadequately cleaned syringes and needles secondary to IV drug use
- *Health Maintenance, Ineffective,* related to a lack of information about the impact of substance abuse on the fetus

Planning and Implementation

Prevention of substance abuse during pregnancy is the ideal nursing goal and is best accomplished through education. Unfortunately, many women who abuse substances do not receive regular health care and may not seek care until they are far along in pregnancy.

Thus it is important to focus on ongoing assessment and client teaching. Consider providing information about the relationship between substance abuse and existing health problems and the implications for the woman's unborn child. Establishing a relationship of trust and support helps ensure the woman's cooperation. If possible, discuss strategies to help the woman quit (addiction treatment programs, 12-step programs, individual counseling) and suggest a referral for more in-depth assessment by a specialist.

Preparation for labor and birth should be part of prenatal planning. Nonnarcotic psychologic support and careful explanation of the labor process may help relieve the woman's fear, tension, and discomfort. If pain medication is necessary, it should not be withheld; the notion that it will contribute to further addiction is mistaken. Preferred methods of pain relief include the use of psychoprophylaxis and regional blocks, such as epidurals, or local anesthetics, such as pudendal block and local infiltration. Immediate intensive care should be available for the newborn, who is often depressed, small for gestational age (SGA), and premature. (For care of the addicted newborn, see Chapter 26.)

Evaluation

Expected outcomes of nursing care include the following:

- The woman is able to describe the impact of her substance abuse on herself and her unborn child.
- The woman gives birth to a healthy baby.
- The woman accepts a referral to social services (or another appropriate community agency) for follow-up care after discharge.

Care of the Woman With a Psychologic Disorder

The prevalence of psychologic or mental disorders among adults in the United States is 22.5% or almost one in four adults (Karg et al., 2014). **Psychologic disorders** are characterized by alterations in thinking, mood, or behavior. Although many such disorders can affect labor and birth, only the most common are discussed here. Because an in-depth discussion of psychologic disorders is beyond the scope of this text, students are encouraged to consult a mental health nursing textbook for further reference. Postpartum psychologic disorders are discussed in Chapter 30.

Maternal Implications

Depression, a common disorder that affects many pregnant women, often goes undiagnosed or untreated. Estimates suggest that 9.4% to 12.7% of pregnant women will have a major depression (Shade et al., 2011). Research findings are mixed, but women with depression may be more likely to have a preterm birth, a small-for-gestational age (SGA) newborn, or a low-birth-weight (LBW) newborn (Smith, Shao, Howell, et al., 2011).

Depression can reduce the woman's ability to concentrate or process information being provided by healthcare team members (Figure 14–5). Untreated depression can lead to inadequate self-care, poor appetite, poor weight gain, self-medication, preterm birth, and maternal suicide (Daniels, 2013). It may also lead to poor maternal–infant bonding. The labor process may feel overwhelming to a woman with depression and she may feel hopelessness about the outcome of her labor. However, she may not be able to articulate these feelings and may appear irritable or withdrawn.

Women with *bipolar disorder* experience the symptoms of depression during the depressive phase. A pregnant woman experiencing a manic episode may engage in behaviors that are dangerous to herself or her fetus including alcohol or drug use, reckless driving, driving without a seat belt, and unprotected sexual intercourse. If labor occurs during a manic phase, the woman may be hyperexcitable and exhibit poor judgment.

Anxiety disorders include a cluster of diagnoses such as panic disorder, obsessive-compulsive disorder (OCD), post-traumatic stress disorder (PTSD), general anxiety disorder, and

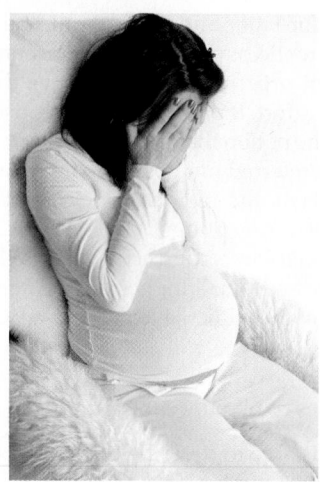

Figure 14–5 A depressed pregnant woman may be inarticulate and appear withdrawn.

SOURCE: Gladskikh Tatiana/Shutterstock.

other specific phobias. These disorders can cause a wide range of symptoms in pregnant women and laboring women. For example, women with OCD may need to repeat specific rituals as a means of coping, while women with PTSD may experience flashbacks and avoidance behaviors. Anxiety may cause the laboring woman to experience physical symptoms such as chest pain, shortness of breath, faintness, fear, or even terror. In general, laboring women with psychologic disorders tend to exhibit the behaviors characteristic of their disorders, but these behaviors may be somewhat exaggerated because of the intense emotions that are evoked in the women's memories. Women with a past history of abuse, including physical and sexual abuse, are often fearful of losing control.

Schizophrenia is the most disabling of the psychologic disorders. Women with uncontrolled schizophrenia may have difficulty managing emotions, interacting with the healthcare team, or thinking clearly. The woman's behavior may be dramatically inappropriate or she may simply be withdrawn. It is often difficult to treat schizophrenia in pregnant women because many of the medications are teratogenic and thus contraindicated. Specifically, antipsychotics can cause cardiovascular defects. These women have an increased incidence of preterm birth, low birth weight, small for gestational age, placental abnormalities, and antenatal hemorrhage.

Clinical Therapy

ACOG (2015c) recommends that clinicians use a standardized tool to screen women for depression and anxiety at least once during the prenatal period. If indicated, follow-up and treatment are essential. The goal of clinical therapy is to provide strategies that will help decrease the woman's anxiety (as well as that of her partner), keep her oriented to reality, and promote optimal functioning during pregnancy and while in labor. Pharmacologic measures such as sedatives, analgesics, or antianxiety medications are determined on an individual basis following careful assessment.

Nursing Management

For the Pregnant Woman With a Psychologic Disorder

Use therapeutic communication and sharing of information to allay anxiety for both the woman and her support person during each prenatal visit and during labor and childbirth.

Nursing Assessment and Diagnosis

Research suggests that perinatal mood and anxiety disorders are often underdetected in clinical practice unless a formal screening program is in place (Shade et al., 2011). At the first prenatal visit, begin the assessment by reviewing the woman's background. Factors such as age, marital and socioeconomic status, culture, methods of coping, support system, and understanding of the labor process contribute to the woman's psychologic response to pregnancy and birth. It is important to ask all women if they have ever been diagnosed with a psychologic disorder. If the woman has, ask her if she is currently receiving any treatment, including medications or psychotherapy. Also ask if she has ever had a psychiatric hospitalization or if she has ever had thoughts of hurting herself or others.

This same attention to detail is important when the woman goes into labor. The prenatal record should be reviewed for additional information regarding any psychiatric illnesses. During labor, assess the woman for objective cues indicating a psychologic disorder. Monotone replies and/or a flat affect may indicate depression. Women with schizophrenia may lack orientation to person, time, and place. Objective cues indicating acute anxiety or signs of a panic attack include tachycardia and hyperventilation.

As labor progresses, remain alert to the woman's verbal and nonverbal behavioral responses to the pain and anxiety. The woman who is too quiet and compliant, is disoriented, is agitated and seems uncooperative, or is experiencing acute anxiety symptoms may require further appraisal for psychologic disorders. These rare circumstances require one-on-one nursing care. A consult with a psychiatrist is often warranted.

Nursing diagnoses that may apply to the woman with a psychologic disorder include the following (NANDA-I © 2014):

- *Anxiety,* related to stress of the labor process, unfamiliar environment, and unknown caregivers
- *Fear,* related to unknown outcome of labor and invasive medical procedures
- *Coping, Ineffective,* related to increased anxiety and stress

Planning and Implementation

The primary nursing interventions center on providing support to the pregnant woman and her partner or family. During labor, families that have had the opportunity to attend prenatal classes may benefit from encouragement as they employ some of the coping techniques they have learned. If the woman begins to lose her ability to cope or her orientation to reality, assist her in regaining control and orientation by explaining where she is, why she is there, and what is currently happening; providing reassurance; decreasing stimuli; and acknowledging her fears, concerns, and symptoms.

Your ability to help the woman and her partner cope with the stress of labor is directly related to the rapport you have established with them. By employing a calm, caring, confident, nonjudgmental approach, you may be able not only to acknowledge the anxiety or other emotions the woman is feeling but also to identify the source of the distress. Once the causative factors are known, implement appropriate interventions such as offering information, comfort measures, touch, or therapeutic communication. Some women with severe psychologic disorders may have excessive symptoms during their labor and birth. Although providing emotional support is imperative, care of these women should focus on maintaining a safe environment and ensuring maternal and fetal well-being. Pharmacologic interventions may be necessary for excessive symptoms. See Chapter 30 for a discussion of medications commonly used.

Evaluation

Anticipated outcomes of nursing care include the following:

- The woman experiences a decrease in physiologic and psychologic stress and an increase in physical and psychologic comfort.
- The woman remains oriented to person, time, and place.
- The woman uses effective coping mechanisms to manage her stress and anxiety in labor.
- The woman is able to verbalize feelings about her labor.
- The woman's and her family's fears are decreased.

Care of the Woman With HIV Infection

AIDS (acquired immunodeficiency syndrome), caused by the virus known as **HIV** (human immunodeficiency virus), is one of today's major health concerns. By the end of 2013, an estimated 1,218,400 persons ages 13 or older in the United States were living with HIV/AIDS, including 156,300 who did not know they were infected (Centers for Disease Control and Prevention [CDC], 2015a). Male adults and adolescents are the largest groups of infected individuals. Of these groups, new infections occurred as follows: male-to-male sexual contact (63%), IV drug use (8%), high-risk heterosexual contact (11%), and 8% through both male-to-male sexual contact and IV drug use. Among females with HIV/AIDS, 84% were infected through high-risk heterosexual contact and 16% were infected because of IV drug use (CDC, 2015a).

Of the estimated 2,519 children under age 13 living with HIV/AIDS in the United States, 84% were exposed perinatally (CDC, 2015b). Fortunately, the incidence of new pediatric AIDS cases is declining rapidly.

Pathophysiology of HIV and AIDS

HIV-1, which causes most cases of AIDS worldwide, typically enters the body through blood, blood products, or other body fluids such as semen, vaginal fluid, and breast milk. HIV affects specific T cells, thereby decreasing the body's immune responses. This makes the affected person susceptible to opportunistic infections such as *Pneumocystis jiroveci*, which causes a severe pneumonia, candidiasis, cytomegalovirus infection, tuberculosis, and toxoplasmosis.

Once infected with the virus, the individual develops antibodies that can be detected with a reactive enzyme immunoassay (EIA) and confirmed with the Western blot test or immunofluorescence assay (IFA). A confirmed case is then categorized into one of four HIV infection stages for adults and adolescents over age 13. These stages are used for public health surveillance and not as a guide for diagnosis and therapy.

The diagnosis of AIDS is made when a person is HIV positive and has one of several specific opportunistic infections.

Maternal Risks

Recent advances and the availability of antiretroviral therapy (ART) have led women who are HIV positive and who adhere to their ART to consider pregnancy because of their increased life expectancy. If pregnancy is considered, priorities should focus on maintaining the health of the mother before, during, and after the pregnancy; preventing transmission to a potentially seronegative father; and preventing mother-to-child transmission. Reproductive assisted technology is one possibility along

with further interventions, including cesarean birth to reduce the risk of transmission to the fetus. More research is needed, however, to improve understanding of the health implications of women living with HIV (Loutfy, Sonnenberg-Schwan, Margolese, et al., 2013).

> **Developing Cultural Competence** **Variations in the Prevalence Rates of New HIV Infections**
>
> The prevalence rates per 100,000 of persons living with HIV/AIDS vary significantly among races and ethnic groups: at the end of 2012 the rates were 1011 in the Black/African American population, 347.8 in the Hispanic/Latino population, 166.4 in the Native Hawaiian/Pacific Islander population, 124.1 in the American Indian/Alaska Native population, 149.2 in the White population, and 70.5 in the Asian population (CDC, 2015b).

For women who have not had access to ART or who have not followed their plan of care, AIDS-defining symptoms that are more common in women than men include wasting syndrome, esophageal candidiasis, and herpes simplex virus disease. Kaposi sarcoma is rare in women. Non–AIDS-defining gynecologic conditions, such as vaginal *Candida* infections and cervical pathology, are prevalent among women at all stages of HIV infection.

Fetal/Neonatal Risks

HIV transmission can occur during pregnancy and through breast milk; however, it is believed that the majority of all infections occur during labor and birth. In the United States, the rate of transmission has dropped dramatically and is now less than 2% for pregnant women infected with HIV who receive prophylactic antiretroviral therapy, give birth by elective cesarean at 38 weeks before rupture of membranes, and avoid breastfeeding (Panel on Treatment of HIV-Infected Pregnant Women and Prevention of Perinatal Transmission, 2014). These decreases in transmission are dramatic and impressive.

Following birth, HIV infection in newborns should be diagnosed using HIV virologic assays as soon as possible, with initiation of antiretroviral prophylaxis immediately if the test is positive. For further discussion of the newborn who is HIV positive, see Chapter 26.

Clinical Therapy

The revised CDC HIV testing guidelines indicate that HIV screening should be emphasized as a routine part of prenatal care while continuing to ensure that the testing of pregnant women is voluntary and informed (Panel on Treatment of HIV-Infected Women, 2014). Initial testing is done using enzyme-linked immunoabsorbent assay (ELISA). If the results are positive, the Western blot test is used to confirm the diagnosis. Women who test positive should be counseled about the implications of the diagnosis for themselves and their fetus to ensure an informed reproductive choice.

All women who are infected with HIV and contemplating pregnancy should be on a maximally suppressive antiretroviral (ARV) regimen (Panel on Treatment of HIV-Infected Women, 2014). For women who have never received antiretroviral drugs, the decision as to whether to start the regimen in the first trimester or delay until after 12 weeks' gestation depends on several factors including CD4 T-lymphocyte (CD4-cell) count, HIV RNA levels, and maternal conditions such as nausea and vomiting. A combination ARV regimen may be more effective in reducing transmission if initiated in the first trimester, but benefits must be weighed against potential fetal effects of first-trimester drug exposure (CDC, 2014).

Combination ARV regimens should include a dual nucleoside reverse transcriptase inhibitor (NRTI) backbone that includes one or more NRTIs with high levels of transplacental passage (zidovudine, lamivudine, emtricitabine, tenofovir, or abacavir) (CDC, 2014).

Treatment recommendations have also been developed for the mother and baby for the intrapartum and postpartum periods. The decision about which regimen is most appropriate should be determined following discussion with the woman about the risks and benefits based on her individual HIV status.

Women with HIV infection should be evaluated and treated for other sexually transmitted infections and for conditions occurring more commonly in women with HIV, such as tuberculosis, cytomegalovirus infection, toxoplasmosis, and cervical dysplasia. Women with HIV infection with no history of hepatitis B should receive the hepatitis vaccine, which is not contraindicated prenatally, as well as the pneumococcal vaccine and an annual flu shot. In addition to routine prenatal laboratory tests, a platelet count and a complete blood count with differential should be obtained at the first prenatal visit and repeated each trimester to identify anemia, thrombocytopenia, and leukopenia, which are associated both with HIV infection and with antiviral therapy.

The woman with HIV also should be assessed regularly for serologic changes that indicate the disease is progressing. This is determined by the absolute CD4+ T-lymphocyte count, which provides the number of helper T4 cells. When the CD4+ counts fall to $200/mm^3$ or lower, opportunistic infections such as *Pneumocystis jiroveci* pneumonia are more likely to develop, and prophylaxis may need to be instituted (Panel on Treatment of HIV-Infected Women, 2014).

At each prenatal visit, women with asymptomatic HIV infection are monitored for early signs of complications, such as weight loss in the second or third trimesters or fever. The clinician inspects the mouth for signs of infections such as thrush (candidiasis) or hairy leukoplakia; the lungs are auscultated for signs of pneumonia; and the lymph nodes, the liver, and the spleen are palpated for signs of enlargement. Each trimester the woman should have a visual examination and examination of the retina to detect such complications as toxoplasmosis retinitis.

A pregnancy complicated by HIV infection, even if asymptomatic, is considered high risk, and the fetus is monitored closely. Weekly non-stress testing (NST) is begun at 32 weeks' gestation, and serial ultrasounds are done to detect IUGR. Biophysical profiles are also indicated (see Chapter 13). Invasive procedures such as amniocentesis are avoided when possible to prevent the contamination of a noninfected fetus.

Scheduled cesarean birth is indicated for women with HIV RNA levels greater than 1000 copies/mL and for women with unknown HIV RNA levels near the time of birth, whether they are on antiretroviral therapy or not. If the indication for cesarean birth is prevention of perinatal transmission of HIV, the risks to a woman should be balanced with potential benefits expected for the neonate (Panel on Treatment of HIV-Infected Women, 2014).

Women who are HIV positive are at increased risk for complications such as intrapartum or postpartum hemorrhage, postpartum infection, poor wound healing, and infections of the genitourinary tract. To prevent exposure of an uninfected neonate to HIV during labor and birth, invasive procedures such as vaginal examinations following rupture of the membranes, fetal scalp electrode monitoring, fetal scalp sampling, and vacuum extraction should be done only after carefully evaluating the risks and benefits. Thus they need careful monitoring and appropriate therapy as indicated. Following childbirth, the woman who is HIV positive should be referred to a physician knowledgeable about treating individuals with HIV infection.

Nursing Management

For the Pregnant Woman Who Is HIV Positive

Nursing Care Plan: The Woman With HIV Infection addresses nursing management.

Nursing Assessment and Diagnosis

A woman who tests positive for HIV may be asymptomatic or may present with any of the following signs or symptoms: fatigue, anemia, malaise, progressive weight loss, lymphadenopathy, diarrhea, fever, neurologic dysfunction, cell-mediated immunodeficiency, or evidence of Kaposi sarcoma (purplish, reddish brown lesions either externally or internally). If a woman tests positive for HIV or is involved in a relationship that places her at high risk, assess the woman's knowledge level about the disease, its implications for her and her fetus, and self-care measures the woman can take. Examples of nursing diagnoses that might apply to a pregnant woman who tests positive for HIV include the following (NANDA-I © 2014):

- *Health Maintenance, Ineffective,* related to lack of information about HIV/AIDS and its long-term implications for the woman and her unborn child
- *Infection, Risk for,* related to altered immunity secondary to HIV infection
- *Family Processes, Interrupted,* related to the implications of a positive HIV test in one of the family members

Planning and Implementation

COMMUNITY-BASED NURSING CARE

Women need to understand that HIV/AIDS is often a fatal disease. HIV infection can be avoided if women practice safe sex, including insisting that their partners wear a latex condom for each act of intercourse and avoiding sharing IV drug needles. Women at high risk for HIV/AIDS should be offered premarital and prepregnancy screening for HIV antibodies.

In monitoring the asymptomatic pregnant woman who is HIV positive, be alert for nonspecific symptoms such as fever, weight loss, fatigue, persistent candidiasis, diarrhea, cough, skin lesions, and behavior changes. These may be signs of developing symptomatic HIV infection. Laboratory findings such as increased viral load; decreased hemoglobin, hematocrit, and CD4+ T lymphocytes; elevated erythrocyte sedimentation rate (ESR); and abnormal complete blood count, differential, and platelets may indicate complications such as infection or progression of the disease.

Education about optimal nutrition and maintenance of wellness is important; review the information frequently with the woman. Give her information about her medication regimen during pregnancy and for her newborn after birth. See *Health Promotion: The Pregnant Woman With HIV Infection.*

HOSPITAL-BASED NURSING CARE

Protocols have been established for postexposure treatment of a healthcare worker who experiences a needlestick or exposure to the body fluids of a person with positive or unknown HIV status. The effectiveness of the therapy, usually a combined

Nursing Care Plan: The Woman With HIV Infection

1. Nursing Diagnosis: *Infection, Risk for,* related to inadequate defenses (leukopenia, suppressed inflammatory response) secondary to HIV-positive status (NANDA-I © 2014)

GOAL: Client will remain free of opportunistic infection during the course of pregnancy.

INTERVENTION	RATIONALE
• Obtain a complete health history and physical examination during first prenatal visit.	• A complete health history will help determine risk factors for the development of opportunistic infections, and a physical examination will assist in identifying any underlying problem symptoms or illnesses that may compromise the pregnancy or complicate the treatment of HIV.
• Educate the woman as to the signs and symptoms of infection.	• Early recognition of signs and symptoms of infection will allow for immediate treatment, which may decrease the severity of the infection. Signs and symptoms of infections include fever, weight loss, fatigue, persistent candidiasis, diarrhea, cough, and skin lesions (Kaposi sarcoma and hairy leukoplakia in the mouth).
• Obtain nutritional history and monitor weight gain at each prenatal visit.	• The HIV-infected woman needs to maintain optimal nutritional intake. A compromised nutritional status may affect maternal and fetal well-being. Depleted reserves of protein and iron may decrease the client's ability to fight infection, thereby making her more susceptible to opportunistic infections.
• **Collaborative:** Monitor the absolute $CD4^+$ T-lymphocyte count, erythrocyte sedimentation rate (ESR), complete blood count (CBC) with differential, and hemoglobin and hematocrit (H&H) at each prenatal visit.	• Laboratory results provide information about the woman's immune system and the potential for disease progression. Opportunistic infections are more likely to occur when the $CD4^+$ T-lymphocyte count drops below a level of $200/mm^3$. ESR can rise above 20 mm/hr with anemia and with acute and chronic inflammation. CBC with differential and platelet count helps identify anemia, thrombocytopenia, and leukopenia. H&H can also identify anemia.

EXPECTED OUTCOME: Client will remain free of opportunistic infection as evidenced by $CD4^+$ T-lymphocyte count within normal limits; no complaints of chills, fever, or sore throat; normal weight gain throughout pregnancy.

2. Nursing Diagnosis: *Health Maintenance, Ineffective,* related to a lack of information about HIV/AIDS and its long-term implications for the woman, her unborn child, and her family (NANDA-I © 2014)

GOAL: The woman and her family will verbalize the importance of following her medication regimen and of regular prenatal care.

INTERVENTION	RATIONALE
• Assess the woman's and family's level of understanding of HIV infection, its modes of transmission, and the long-term implications.	• Knowledge of the woman's (and her family's) level of understanding about her HIV infection forms a starting point for further health teaching.
• Explain the risks of mother-to-child transmission of HIV infection.	• In untreated women, the risk of transmission is 25%. That risk can be reduced to less than 2% with the availability of antiretroviral therapy, the use of cesarean birth when indicated, and formula-feeding rather than breastfeeding.
• Describe antiretroviral therapy (ART). Include the regimen prescribed, its purposes, and the procedures for taking it.	• ART therapy approaches vary based on the health status of the individual woman and whether she is currently on ART therapy. Generally, it includes oral zidovudine (ZDV) daily, IV ZDV during labor and until birth, and ZDV therapy for the baby for 6 weeks following birth.
• Discuss signs the woman should be alert for, including fever, fatigue, weight loss, cough, skin lesions, and behavior changes.	• These symptoms may indicate that the woman is developing symptomatic loss, persistent candidiasis, diarrhea, HIV infection.

EXPECTED OUTCOME: Woman will actively seek information about her condition, her treatment regimen, and her pregnancy and will cooperate with her healthcare givers.

(continued)

Nursing Care Plan: The Woman With HIV Infection (*continued*)

3. Nursing Diagnosis: *Family Processes, Dysfunctional*, related to the implications of positive maternal HIV status on fetal/neonatal well-being and long-term family functioning (NANDA-I © 2014)

GOAL: Family is able to manage stressors related to the maternal diagnosis.

INTERVENTION	RATIONALE
• Assess ability and readiness of family to learn about HIV and its long-term implications.	• Readiness is a key element in the teaching-learning process.
• Provide woman and her family with accurate, reliable information about her diagnosis, its prognosis for her and for her baby, and the immediate and long-term implications for her care.	• Fear and anxiety will lessen when the woman and her family understand her health status and the implications of the HIV diagnosis and can then plan for the future.
• Assess interactions between the woman and her family. Be alert for potentially destructive behaviors.	• If the HIV diagnosis was not expected, the couple may have to deal with issues of blame, concerns about mortality, and worries about the status of the baby. If the HIV diagnosis was known, concerns may focus on fetal/neonatal well-being. In either case, negative responses can lead to destructive behaviors.
• Assist family in realistically identifying the needs of the woman and family unit.	• Once needs are identified realistically, it is possible to plan interventions to meet the needs.
• **Collaborative:** Explore available community resources and family support systems.	• Because HIV is a long-term condition, the family may require ongoing assistance.

EXPECTED OUTCOME: Family members actively participate in the treatment plan, are involved in planning for labor and birth in light of a positive HIV status, and are able to express unresolved feelings about the diagnosis.

---

drug approach, depends on starting rapidly. Thus such exposure should be reported immediately.

SAFETY ALERT!

In 1987, the CDC stated that the increasing prevalence of HIV/AIDS and the risk of exposure faced by healthcare workers is significant enough that *precautions should be taken with all clients* (not only those with known HIV infection), especially when dealing with blood and body fluids. These precautions are called *standard precautions*.

Health Promotion **The Pregnant Woman With HIV Infection**

The psychologic implications of HIV/AIDS for the childbearing family are staggering.

- The woman is faced with the knowledge that she and her newborn, if infected, have a decreased life expectancy. If her baby is not infected, she must face the possibility that others will raise her child. She must also face the reality that she can only hope to lengthen her life by carefully following an expensive, exacting medical regimen.

- The couple must deal with the impact of the illness on the partner, who may or may not be infected, and on other children. The woman and her family may feel fearful, helpless, angry, and isolated.

- It is essential to provide complete, accurate information about the condition, transmission prevention, and ways of coping using language that is well understood by the woman and her partner.

- Ensure that the woman is referred to a comprehensive program that includes social services, psychologic support, and appropriate health care.

Evaluation

Expected outcomes of nursing care include the following:

- The woman discusses the implications of her HIV infection (or diagnosis of AIDS), its implications for her unborn child and for herself, the method of transmission, and the treatment options.

- The woman uses information about social services (or other agency referral) for follow-up assistance and counseling.

- The woman begins to verbalize her feelings about her condition and its implications for her and her family.

Care of the Woman With Heart Disease

Pregnancy results in increased cardiac output, heart rate, and blood volume. The normal heart is able to adapt to these changes without difficulty. The woman with heart disease, however, has decreased cardiac reserve, making it more difficult for her heart to handle the higher workload of pregnancy.

Cardiac disease complicates about 1% of pregnancies (Cunningham et al., 2014). The pathology found in a pregnant woman with heart disease varies with the type of disorder. The more common conditions are discussed briefly here.

Congenital heart defects have become more common in pregnant women as improved surgical techniques enable females born with heart defects to live to childbearing age. Congenital heart defects most commonly seen in pregnant women include atrial septal defect, ventricular septal defect, patent ductus arteriosus, coarctation of the aorta, and tetralogy of Fallot.

For women with congenital heart disease, the impact of pregnancy depends on the specific defect. If the heart defect has been surgically repaired and no evidence of heart disease remains, the woman may undertake pregnancy with confidence. Women with chronic cyanosis are at increased risk for complications and so are their fetuses. A few conditions such as

Eisenmenger syndrome, pulmonary hypertension, uncorrected coarctation of the aorta, severe symptomatic aortic stenosis, and Marfan syndrome in certain instances carry such great risk of complications and death that they can be considered absolute contraindications (Harris, 2011).

Rheumatic heart disease has declined rapidly in the past half century, primarily because of the availability of antibiotics for treatment. Rheumatic fever, which may develop in untreated group A β-hemolytic streptococcal infections, is an inflammatory connective tissue disease that can involve the heart, joints, central nervous system, skin, and subcutaneous tissue. When the heart is affected, mitral valve stenosis is the most common and serious lesion. Aortic valve involvement, manifested by aortic insufficiency, is the second most common problem. The tricuspid and pulmonic valves are rarely affected.

The increased blood volume of pregnancy, coupled with the pregnant woman's need for increased cardiac output, stresses the heart of a woman with mitral stenosis and increases her risk of developing congestive heart failure. Even the woman who has no symptoms at the onset of her pregnancy is at risk.

Mitral valve prolapse (MVP) is a usually asymptomatic condition commonly found in women of childbearing age. The condition is more common in women than in men and seems to run in families. In MVP, the mitral valve leaflets tend to prolapse into the left atrium during ventricular systole because the chordae tendineae that support them are long, stretched, and thin. This produces a characteristic systolic click on auscultation. In more pronounced cases of MVP, mitral valve regurgitation occurs, producing a systolic murmur.

Women with MVP usually tolerate pregnancy well. Most women require assurance that they can continue with normal activities. A few women experience symptoms—primarily palpitations, chest pain, and dyspnea—which are often due to arrhythmias. They are usually treated with propranolol hydrochloride (Inderal). Limiting caffeine intake also helps decrease palpitations.

Peripartum cardiomyopathy is a relatively rare but serious dysfunction of the left ventricle that occurs in the last month of pregnancy or the first 5 months postpartum in a woman with no previous history of heart disease. The cause is unknown, but mortality is increased with maternal age, in women who have had four or more live births, and in women of African descent (Elkayam, Jalnapurkar, & Barakat, 2012). The symptoms are similar to those of congestive heart failure: dyspnea, orthopnea, fatigue, cough, chest pain, palpitations, and edema. The condition usually presents with anemia and infection; consequently, treatment focuses on underlying abnormalities. Digitalis, diuretics, vasodilators, anticoagulants, sodium restriction, and strict bed rest are often part of the treatment. In over half of women, heart function returns to normal within 2 to 6 months with bed rest and careful monitoring (Elkayam et al., 2012). Subsequent pregnancy is strongly discouraged because the disease tends to recur during pregnancy.

Clinical Therapy

The primary goal of clinical therapy is early diagnosis and ongoing management of the woman with cardiac disease. Echocardiogram, chest x-ray, auscultation of heart sounds, and sometimes cardiac catheterization are essential for establishing the type and severity of the heart disease. The severity of the disease can also be determined by the individual's ability to perform ordinary physical activity. Table 14–4 outlines the classification of functional capacity that has been standardized by the Criteria Committee of the New York Heart Association (1994).

Women in classes I and II usually experience a normal pregnancy and have few complications, whereas those in classes III and IV are at risk for more severe complications. Because anemia

TABLE 14–4 Severity of Heart Disease by Functional Capacity

CLASS	FUNCTIONAL CAPACITY
I	Asymptomatic. No limitation of physical activity.
II	Slight limitation of physical activity. Asymptomatic at rest; symptoms occur with ordinary physical activity.
III	Marked limitation of physical activity. Comfortable at rest but symptomatic during less-than-ordinary physical activity.
IV	Inability to carry on any physical activity without discomfort. Even at rest, the person experiences symptoms of cardiac insufficiency or anginal pain; discomfort increases with any physical activity.

increases the work of the heart, it should be diagnosed early and treated if present. Infections, even if minor, also increase cardiac workload and should be treated. As pregnancy progresses, the woman's activity should be limited to minimize cardiac workload. Similarly, weight gain and sodium intake may also be restricted.

DRUG THERAPY

Besides the iron and vitamin supplements prescribed during pregnancy, the pregnant woman with heart disease may need additional drug therapy to maintain health. Antibiotic prophylaxis is not indicated for uncomplicated vaginal or cesarean birth unless infection is suspected. If the woman develops coagulation problems, the anticoagulant heparin may be used. Heparin is safest for the fetus because it does not cross the placenta (Fryearson & Adamson, 2014). The thiazide diuretics and furosemide (Lasix) may be used to treat congestive heart failure if it develops. Digitalis glycosides and common antiarrhythmic drugs may be used to treat cardiac failure and arrhythmias. These agents cross the placenta but have no reported teratogenic effect. However, they have not been adequately studied to establish their safety in pregnancy (Wilson, Shannon, & Shields, 2014).

Labor and Birth

Spontaneous natural labor with adequate pain relief is usually recommended for women in classes I and II. Special attention should be given to the prompt recognition and treatment of any signs of heart failure (Figure 14–6). Those in classes III and IV may have labor induced and may need to be hospitalized before the onset of labor for cardiac stabilization. They also require invasive cardiac monitoring during labor.

Vaginal birth with low-dose regional analgesia (epidural) is recommended with the use of forceps or vacuum assistance if necessary to limit maternal pushing. The regional analgesia helps decrease maternal cardiac output and oxygen demand by reducing pain and related maternal anxiety. Cesarean birth is used only if fetal or maternal indications exist, not on the basis of heart disease alone.

Nursing Management

For the Pregnant Woman With Heart Disease

Nursing Assessment and Diagnosis

Assess the stress of pregnancy on the heart's functioning during every antepartum visit. Note the category of functional capacity assigned to the woman; take the woman's pulse, respirations, and blood pressure; and compare the findings with the

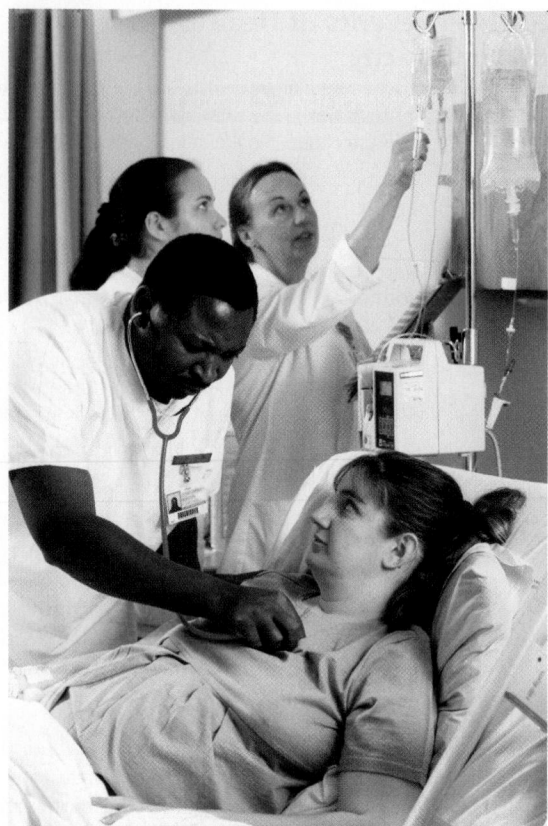

Figure 14–6 Monitoring for signs of heart failure. When a woman with heart disease begins labor, the nursing students and instructor monitor her closely for signs of congestive heart failure.

normal values expected during pregnancy. Then determine the woman's activity level, including rest, and any changes in the pulse and respirations since previous visits. Identify and evaluate other factors that would increase strain on the heart. These factors might include anemia, infection, anxiety, lack of a support system, and household and career demands.

The following signs and symptoms, if they are progressive, indicate congestive heart failure:

- Cough (frequent, with or without blood-stained sputum [hemoptysis])
- Dyspnea (progressive, on exertion)
- Edema (progressive, generalized, including extremities, face, eyelids)
- Heart murmurs (heard on auscultation)
- Palpitations
- Rales (auscultated in lung bases)
- Weight gain (related to fluid retention)

Progressiveness of the cycle is the critical factor because some of these same signs and symptoms are seen to a minor degree in a pregnancy without cardiac problems.

Nursing diagnoses that might apply to the pregnant woman with heart disease include the following (NANDA-I © 2014):

- *Cardiac Output, Decreased,* resulting in easy fatigability
- *Gas Exchange, Impaired,* related to pulmonary edema secondary to cardiac decompensation
- *Fear,* related to the effects of the maternal cardiac condition on fetal well-being

Planning and Implementation

Nursing care is directed toward maintaining a balance between cardiac reserve and cardiac workload.

ANTEPARTUM NURSING CARE

The priority of nursing action varies based on the severity of the disease process and the individual needs of the woman determined by the nursing assessment. Ensure that the woman and her family thoroughly understand her condition and its management and that they recognize signs of potential complications; this level of understanding will decrease their anxiety. Providing thorough explanations, using printed material, and giving frequent opportunities to ask questions and discuss concerns lets the woman better meet her own healthcare needs and seek assistance appropriately.

As part of health teaching, explain the purposes of the required dietary and activity changes. A diet high in iron, protein, and essential nutrients but low in sodium, with adequate calories to ensure normal weight gain, best meets the nutrition needs of the woman with cardiac disease. To help preserve her cardiac reserves, the woman may need to restrict her activities. In addition, 8 to 10 hours of sleep, with frequent daily rest periods, are essential. Because upper respiratory infections may tax the heart and lead to decompensation, the woman must avoid contact with sources of infection.

During the first half of pregnancy, the woman is seen approximately every 2 weeks to assess cardiac status. During the second half of pregnancy, the woman is seen weekly. These assessments are especially important between weeks 28 and 30, when the blood volume reaches its maximum. If symptoms of cardiac decompensation occur, prompt medical intervention is indicated to correct the cardiac problem.

INTRAPARTUM PERIOD

Labor and birth exert tremendous stress on the woman and her fetus. This stress could be fatal to the fetus of a woman with cardiac disease because the fetus may be receiving a decreased oxygen and blood supply. Thus the intrapartum care of a woman with cardiac disease is aimed at reducing physical exertion and the accompanying fatigue.

Evaluate maternal vital signs frequently to determine the woman's response to labor. A pulse rate greater than 100 beats per minute (beats/min) or respirations greater than 25 per minute may indicate the onset of cardiac decompensation and require further evaluation. Auscultate the woman's lungs frequently for evidence of rales and carefully observe for other signs that she is developing decompensation.

To ensure cardiac emptying and adequate oxygenation, encourage the laboring woman to assume either a semi-Fowler or side-lying position, with her head and shoulders elevated. Oxygen by mask, diuretics to reduce fluid retention, sedatives and analgesics, prophylactic antibiotics, and digitalis may also be used as indicated by the woman's status. Remain with the woman to support her. It is essential to keep the woman and her family informed of labor progress and management plans, collaborating with them to fulfill their wishes for the birth experience as much as possible. Maintain an atmosphere of calm to lessen the anxiety of the woman and her family.

Continuous electronic fetal monitoring provides ongoing assessment of the fetal response to labor. To prevent overexertion and the accompanying fatigue, encourage the woman to sleep and relax between contractions and give her emotional support and encouragement. Epidural anesthesia is often used to decrease exertion. During pushing, encourage the woman to use shorter, more moderate open-glottis pushing, with complete relaxation between pushes. Forceps or vacuum extraction may be used if pushing is too difficult. Monitor vital signs closely during the second stage.

POSTPARTUM PERIOD

The postpartum period is a significant time for the woman with cardiac disease. As extravascular fluid returns to the bloodstream for excretion, cardiac output and blood volume increase. This physiologic adaptation places great strain on the heart and may lead to decompensation, especially in the first 48 hours after birth.

To detect any possible problems, the woman may remain in the hospital postpartum longer than the low-risk woman. Monitor her vital signs frequently, and assess for signs of decompensation. She stays in the semi-Fowler or side-lying position, with her head and shoulders elevated, and begins a gradual, progressive activity program. Appropriate diet and stool softeners facilitate bowel movement without undue strain.

Give the woman opportunities to discuss her birth experience and help her deal with any feelings or concerns that distress her. Encourage maternal–newborn attachment by providing frequent opportunities for the mother to interact with her child.

No evidence exists that breastfeeding stresses the heart. Thus the only concern about breastfeeding for women with cardiovascular disease is related to medications the mother may be taking. These should be evaluated for the likelihood of passing into the milk or affecting lactation. Assist the breastfeeding mother to a comfortable side-lying position, with her head moderately elevated, or to a semi-Fowler position. To conserve the mother's energy, position the newborn at the breast and be available to burp the baby and reposition him or her at the other breast.

In addition to providing the normal postpartum discharge teaching, ensure that the woman and her family understand the signs of possible problems from her heart disease or other postpartum complications. Work with the woman and her family to plan an activity schedule. Visiting nurse referrals may be necessary, depending on the woman's health status.

Evaluation

Expected outcomes of nursing care include the following:

- The woman participates in developing an appropriate healthcare regimen and follows it throughout her pregnancy.
- The woman gives birth to a healthy baby.
- The woman avoids congestive heart failure, thromboembolism, and infection.
- The woman is able to identify signs and symptoms of possible postpartum complications.
- The woman is able to care effectively for her newborn.

Other Medical Conditions and Pregnancy

A woman with a preexisting medical condition needs to be aware of the possible impact of pregnancy on her condition, as well as the impact of her condition on the successful outcome of her pregnancy. Table 14–5 discusses some less common medical conditions in relation to pregnancy.

TABLE 14–5 Less Common Medical Conditions and Pregnancy

BRIEF DESCRIPTION	MATERNAL IMPLICATIONS	FETAL/NEONATAL IMPLICATIONS
ASTHMA		
Asthma, an obstructive lung condition, is the most common respiratory disease found in pregnancy, complicating approximately 8% of all pregnancies (Cossette et al., 2013). Typical symptoms include wheezing, dyspnea, and episodic coughing. A severe asthmatic attack may require hospitalization. It is managed by long-term comprehensive drug therapy to prevent airway inflammation, combined with drug treatment to manage attacks or exacerbations. Client education focuses on triggers (such as cold air, dust, smoke, exercise, food additives), methods of prevention, and treatment options.	The severity of asthma may improve, worsen, or remain unchanged during pregnancy. The mechanisms associated with these variations remain undefined; however, poor asthma control is associated with increased maternal and neonatal complications, most likely from poor adherence to the treatment regime. Maternal complications include preeclampsia, growth restriction, and preterm birth. Asthma management during labor and birth focuses on maintenance of adequate hydration and analgesia as well as continuing asthma medications.	Preeclampsia, preterm birth, low birth weight, and perinatal mortality are more common among the newborns of women who have asthma (Whitty & Dombrowski, 2012). The goal of therapy is to prevent maternal exacerbations because even a mild exacerbation can cause severe hypoxia-related complications in the fetus. If an exacerbation occurs, it should be managed in the same way as for a nonpregnant woman because the asthma drugs used are less of a threat to the fetus than a serious asthma attack.
EPILEPSY		
Chronic disorder characterized by seizures; may be idiopathic or secondary to other conditions, such as head injury, metabolic and nutritional disorders such as phenylketonuria (PKU) or vitamin B_6 deficiency, encephalitis, neoplasms, or circulatory interferences. Treated with anticonvulsants.	Vast majority of pregnancies in women with seizure disorders are uneventful and have an excellent outcome. Women with more frequent seizures before pregnancy may have exacerbations during pregnancy, but this may be related to lack of cooperation with drug regimen or sleep deprivation. During pregnancy the woman should continue to be treated with the medication that best controls her seizures. Folic acid therapy should be started prior to conception if possible. Folic acid and vitamin D are indicated throughout pregnancy (Kamyar & Varner, 2013).	Certain anticonvulsant medications are associated with increased incidence of congenital anomalies, especially cleft lip and heart defects, although the incidence has decreased in recent years. The lowest dose of a single effective medication is the goal of treatment to decrease the potential for fetal anomalies (Samuels & Niebyl, 2012). Multiple medications and valproic acid should also be avoided for women planning pregnancy when possible.

(continued)

TABLE 14–5 Less Common Medical Conditions and Pregnancy (*continued*)

BRIEF DESCRIPTION	MATERNAL IMPLICATIONS	FETAL/NEONATAL IMPLICATIONS
HEPATITIS B		
Hepatitis B, caused by the hepatitis B virus (HBV), is a major, growing health problem. Groups at risk include those from areas with a high incidence (primarily developing countries), injection drug users, prostitutes, homosexuals, those with multiple sex partners, individuals who are HIV positive, and those with occupational exposure to blood. HBV transmission is bloodborne, primarily sexually and perinatally transmitted. Because of the dramatic increase and the difficulty of vaccinating high-risk individuals before they become infected, the CDC now recommends (1) testing all pregnant women for the presence of HBsAg and prophylactic treatment for all neonates born to women who are HBsAg positive or whose status is unknown; (2) routine infant vaccination; (3) vaccination of children and adolescents through age 18 years who have not been vaccinated; and (4) vaccination of unvaccinated adults who are at risk for hepatitis B (Schillie & Murphy, 2013).	In the United States, estimates suggest 1% to 2% of the population has chronic hepatitis B (Apuzzio et al., 2012a). Hepatitis B does not usually affect the course of pregnancy. However, chronic HBV carriers have a great potential for infecting others when exposure to blood and body fluids occurs. In addition, chronic carriers may develop long-term sequelae, such as chronic liver disease and liver cancer. It is now recommended that all pregnant women be tested for the presence of HBsAg. A woman who is negative may be given the hepatitis vaccine.	Perinatal transmission most often occurs at or near the time of childbirth. In fact, women who are positive for hepatitis B surface antigen (HbsAg) have almost a 100% chance of transmitting HBV to their newborn at birth (Apuzzio et al., 2012a). More importantly, the risk of becoming a chronic carrier of the HBV is inversely related to the age of the individual at the time of initial infection. Therefore, neonates infected perinatally have the highest risk of becoming chronically infected if not treated. Routine vaccination of all neonates born to HBsAg-negative women is indicated. Babies born to HBsAg-positive mothers should receive hepatitis B immune globulin at birth or at least within the first 12 hours and should also receive the hepatitis B vaccine (Apuzzio et al., 2012b). Within 12 hours of birth, neonates born to HIV-positive women with HBV infection should be given hepatitis B immune globulin and the first dose of the HBV vaccine series. The second and third doses of vaccine should then be administered at ages 1 and 6 months, respectively (Panel on Treatment of HIV-Infected Pregnant Women, 2014).
HYPERTHYROIDISM (THYROTOXICOSIS)		
Enlarged, overactive thyroid gland; increased T_4:TBG ratio and increased basal metabolic rate (BMR). Symptoms include muscle wasting, tachycardia, excessive sweating, and exophthalmos. Treatment by antithyroid drug propylthiouracil (PTU) while monitoring free T_4 levels. Surgery used only if drug intolerance exists.	Mild hyperthyroidism is not dangerous. Increased incidence of preeclampsia and postpartum hemorrhage if not well controlled. Serious risk related to thyroid storm characterized by high fever, tachycardia, sweating, and congestive heart failure. Now occurs rarely. When diagnosed during pregnancy, may be transient or permanent.	Neonatal thyrotoxicosis is rare. Even low doses of antithyroid drug in mother may produce a mild fetal/neonatal hypothyroidism; higher dose may produce a goiter or mental deficiencies. Fetal loss not increased in euthyroid women. If untreated, rates of abortion, intrauterine death, and stillbirth increase. Breastfeeding contraindicated for women on antithyroid medication because it is excreted in the milk (may be tried by woman on low dose if neonatal T_4 levels are monitored).
HYPOTHYROIDISM		
Characterized by inadequate thyroid secretions (decreased T_4:TBG ratio), elevated TSH, lowered BMR, and enlarged thyroid gland (goiter). Iodine deficiency is the most common cause worldwide (Abel, 2011). Symptoms include lack of energy, excessive weight gain, cold intolerance, dry skin, and constipation. Treated by thyroxine replacement therapy.	Long-term replacement therapy continues; at least half of pregnant women need an increase in their thyroxine dose (Cunningham et al., 2014). Serial ultrasounds are done to monitor fetal growth; non-stress tests are not necessary in well-controlled disease but are considered beginning at 32 to 34 weeks' gestation in cases of poorly controlled disease (Abel, 2011).	If mother untreated, fetal loss is high; newborn is at risk for severe neurologic problems and congenital goiter (Sullivan, 2011). Therefore newborns are screened for T_4 level. Mild TSH elevations present little risk because TSH does not cross the placenta.
MATERNAL PHENYLKETONURIA (PKU) (HYPERPHENYLALANINEMIA)		
Inherited recessive single gene anomaly causing a deficiency of the liver enzyme needed to convert the amino acid phenylalanine to tyrosine, resulting in high serum levels of phenylalanine. Brain damage and mental retardation occur if not treated early.	Low phenylalanine diet is mandatory before conception and during pregnancy. The woman should be counseled that her children will either inherit the disease or be carriers, depending on the zygosity of the father for the disease. Treatment at a PKU center is recommended (ACOG, 2015a).	Risk to fetus if maternal treatment not begun preconception. In untreated women increased incidence of fetal mental retardation, microcephaly, congenital heart defects, and growth retardation (Prick, Hop, & Duvekot, 2012). Neonates diagnosed with PKU should begin treatment within the first week of life (ACOG, 2015a).

MULTIPLE SCLEROSIS

Neurologic disorder characterized by destruction of the myelin sheath of nerve fibers. The condition occurs primarily in young adults, more commonly in females, and is marked by periods of remission; progresses to marked physical disability in 10 to 20 years.

Exacerbation rate is reduced during the second and third trimesters but increased during the 3 months following birth. Exclusive breastfeeding for the first 2 months postpartum may be independently associated with decreased postpregnancy relapse rate, although additional studies are needed to support these preliminary findings (Houtchens, 2013).

Rest is important; help with child care should be planned. Uterine contraction strength is not diminished, but because sensation is frequently lessened, labor may be almost painless.

Some evidence for slightly increased risk of prematurity and slightly lower birth weight newborns. Risk of genetic predisposition estimated at 3% to 5%. While risk is relatively low, it is 10 times greater than for the population at large (Tsui & Martin, 2011).

RHEUMATOID ARTHRITIS

Chronic inflammatory disease believed to be caused by a genetically influenced antigen–antibody reaction. Symptoms include fatigue, low-grade fever, pain and swelling of joints, morning stiffness, pain on movement. Treated with salicylates, physical therapy, and rest. Corticosteroids used cautiously if not responsive to above.

Usually there is remission of rheumatoid arthritis symptoms during pregnancy, often with a relapse postpartum. Anemia may be present because of blood loss from salicylate therapy. Mother needs extra rest, particularly to relieve weight-bearing joints, but needs to continue range-of-motion exercises. If in remission, may stop medication during pregnancy.

Babies of women taking prednisone or prednisolone during the first trimester have a slightly increased risk of cleft palate. Its use in the later part of pregnancy increases the risk of preterm premature rupture of the membranes and small-for-gestational age newborns (Bermas, 2014).

SYSTEMIC LUPUS ERYTHEMATOSUS (SLE)

Chronic autoimmune collagen disease, characterized by exacerbations and remissions; symptoms range from characteristic rash to inflammation and pain in joints, fever, nephritis, depression, cranial nerve disorders, and peripheral neuropathies.

SLE during pregnancy needs to be actively managed with careful surveillance of blood pressure, proteinuria, and placental blood flow. SLE medications may be necessary to control exacerbations and lupus flare. Preeclampsia, prematurity, and fetal growth restriction are common complications. Women with severe disease may be counseled to avoid pregnancy (Lateef & Petri, 2013).

Increased incidence of cesarean birth, postpartum hemorrhage, and blood transfusion. Women with SLE are more likely to give birth to premature babies, smaller babies, and babies with congenital heart block (Nili, McLeod, O'Connell, et al., 2013). Neonatal lupus is characterized by a photosensitive skin rash, thrombocytopenia, neutropenia, or anemia, all of which resolve by about 6 months of age. Complete congenital heart block is the most serious complication of SLE, typically diagnosed in utero. When diagnosed, the mother is given corticosteroids that cross the placenta and decrease fetal heart inflammation. The prognosis for these newborns varies based on the extent of the cardiac damage. Live-born neonates may require a pacemaker (Akin, Baykan, Sezer, et al., 2011).

TUBERCULOSIS (TB)

Tuberculosis (TB) is a major health problem. Approximately one third of the world's population (about 1.75 billion people) carry the TB bacteria (Loto & Awowole, 2012). Worldwide TB is one of the top killers of women (CDC, 2012). Infection is caused by *Mycobacterium tuberculosis;* an inflammatory process causes destruction of lung tissue, increased sputum, and coughing. Associated primarily with poverty and malnutrition, 80% of new cases are found in developing countries primarily in Asia and Africa. In the United States, the majority of cases occur in foreign-born people. More than 75% of these individuals were born in just 15 countries (CDC, 2013). Treated with isoniazid and either ethambutol or rifampin, or both.

The incidence of pregnancy complications may be higher in women with TB. TB skin test screening is recommended for women in high-risk groups: healthcare workers; foreign-born women from countries with a high TB risk; women who have had known contact with an infectious person, those who are HIV infected, alcoholics, or illicit drug users; women living or working in homeless shelters; or prisoners and detainees (Cunningham et al., 2014). If TB is inactive due to prior treatment, isoniazid therapy is delayed until the postpartum period unless the woman is HIV positive, has close contact with a person with active TB, or has had a skin test convert to positive within the last 2 years. For those women, isoniazid is started during pregnancy (CDC, 2012). Women with active TB are treated with isoniazid, rifampin, and ethambutol during pregnancy (Cunningham et al., 2014). Extra rest and limited contact with others is required until disease becomes inactive.

Women with TB have a higher rate of spontaneous abortion, suboptimal weight gain, and preterm labor; there is also an increased incidence of neonatal mortality and low birth weight. Congenital TB is a rare complication of in utero infection but the risk of postnatal transmission to the newborn is higher (Loto & Awowole, 2012). If maternal TB is inactive, the mother may breastfeed and care for her baby. If TB is active, the newborn should not have direct contact with the mother until she is noninfectious. Isoniazid crosses the placenta, but most studies show no teratogenic effects. Rifampin crosses the placenta. Possibility of harmful effects is still being studied.

Focus Your Study

- Almost any health problem that a person can have when not pregnant can coexist with pregnancy. Some problems, such as anemias, may be exacerbated by pregnancy. Others, such as collagen disease, may go into temporary remission with pregnancy. Regardless of the health problem, careful health care is needed throughout pregnancy to improve the outcome for mother and fetus.

- The diagnosis of high-risk pregnancy can shock an expectant couple. Providing emotional support, teaching about the condition and prognosis, and educating for self-care are important nursing measures that help the client cope.

- The key point in the care of the pregnant woman with diabetes is scrupulous maternal plasma glucose control. This is best achieved by home blood glucose monitoring, multiple daily insulin injections, regular exercise, and a careful diet. To reduce incidence of congenital anomalies and other problems in the newborn, the woman should be euglycemic (have a normal blood glucose) throughout the pregnancy. Women with diabetes, even more than most other clients, need to be educated about their conditions and involved with their own care.

- Anemia indicates inadequate levels of hemoglobin (Hb) in the blood. Anemia is defined as hemoglobin less than 12 g/dL in nonpregnant women and less than 11 g/dL in pregnant and postpartum women. Iron deficiency anemia is the most common form of anemia. Other anemias include folic acid deficiency, sickle cell disease, and thalassemia.

- Substance abuse (either drugs or alcohol) not only is detrimental to the mother's health but also may have profound lasting effects on the fetus.

- HIV infection, which is transmitted via blood and body fluids, may also be transmitted transplacentally to the fetus. Currently, there is no definitive therapy for HIV/AIDS. Nurses should employ blood and body fluid precautions (standard precautions) in caring for all women to avoid potential spread of infection.

- Cardiac disease during pregnancy requires careful assessment, limitation of activity, and knowing and reporting signs of impending cardiac decompensation by both client and nurse.

- Worldwide, more women die from TB than from any other infection. Most cases are concentrated in developing countries.

Clinical Reasoning in Action

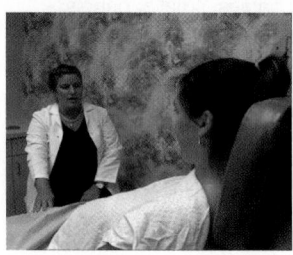

Jane Adams, a 23-year-old G3P2, at 37 weeks' gestation, presents to you in the birthing unit complaining of "vaginal pressure" but no contractions. You assess her and find that her history includes being HIV positive for 2 years, second-trimester cocaine and marijuana use, missed appointments, anemia (hematocrit 28%), and a positive syphilis serology. Jane tells you that she has other children and that they are being cared for by her mother, who has legal custody of them. You admit Jane and place her on the fetal monitor for evaluation of fetal well-being and contraction patterns. The monitor shows you that the fetal heart rate baseline is 120 to 130 with no decelerations; contractions are mild and irregular, lasting 20 to 30 seconds. You obtain vital signs of BP 130/88, temperature 97°F, P 88, R 14. A vaginal examination determines that Jane is 7 cm dilated at +1 station with intact membranes. She asks you if being HIV positive will affect her labor.

1. Discuss the prophylactic regimen for the prevention of HIV transmission to the fetus during labor.

2. Discuss the transmission of HIV to the fetus during pregnancy and birth.

3. Identify the emotional impact of HIV infection or other STIs on the woman.

4. On postpartum day 2, you inform Jane that her newborn is HIV antibody positive. How would you clarify the results?

References

Abel, D. E. (2011). Thyroid disease during pregnancy: Part 1. Thyroid function testing and hypothyroidism. *The Female Patient, 36*(1), 16–22.

Akin, M. A., Baykan, A., Sezer, S., & Gunes, T. (2011). Review of literature for the striking clinic picture seen in two infants of mothers with systemic lupus erythematosus. *Journal of Maternal–Fetal and Neonatal Medicine, 24*(8), 1022–1026.

American Academy of Pediatrics (AAP) and American College of Obstetricians and Gynecologists (ACOG). (2012). *Guidelines for perinatal care* (7th ed.). Elk Grove Village, IL: American Academy of Pediatrics.

American College of Obstetricians and Gynecologists (ACOG). (2011). *Methamphetamine abuse in women of reproductive age* (ACOG Committee Opinion No. 479). Washington, DC: Author.

American College of Obstetricians and Gynecologists (ACOG). (2012a). *Opioid abuse, dependence, and addiction in pregnancy* (ACOG Committee Opinion No. 524). Washington, DC: Author.

American College of Obstetricians and Gynecologists (ACOG). (2012b). *Pregestational diabetes mellitus* (ACOG Practice Bulletin No. 60, issued 2005, reaffirmed 2012). Washington, DC: Author.

American College of Obstetricians and Gynecologists (ACOG). (2013). *Gestational diabetes mellitus.* (ACOG Practice Bulletin No. 137). Washington, DC: Author.

American College of Obstetricians and Gynecologists (ACOG). (2015a). *Management of pregnant women with phenylketonuria.* (ACOG Committee Opinion No. 636). Washington, DC: Author.

American College of Obstetricians and Gynecologists (ACOG). (2015b). *Marijuana use during pregnancy and lactation.* (ACOG Committee Opinion No. 637). Washington, DC: Author.

American College of Obstetricians and Gynecologists (ACOG). (2015c). *Screening for perinatal depression.* (ACOG Committee Opinion No. 630). Washington, DC: Author.

American Diabetes Association (ADA). (2015). Standards of medical care in diabetes—2015. *Diabetes Care, 38*(S1), S1–90.

Andemariam B., & Browning S.L. (2013). Current management of sickle cell disease in pregnancy. *Clinics in Laboratory Medicine, 33*(2), 293–310.

Apuzzio, J., Block, J. M., Cullison, S., Cohen, C., Leong, S. L., London, W. T.,... McMahon, B. J. (2012a). Chronic hepatitis B in pregnancy: A workshop consensus statement on screening, evaluation, and management, Part 1. *The Female Patient, 37*(4), 22–27.

Apuzzio, J., Block, J. M., Cullison, S., Cohen, C., Leong, S. L., London, W. T.,... McMahon, B. J. (2012b). Chronic hepatitis B in pregnancy: A workshop consensus statement on screening, evaluation, and management, Part 2. *The Female Patient, 37*(5), 30–34.

Behnke, M., & Smith, V.C. (2013). Prenatal substance abuse: short- and long-term effects on the exposed fetus. *Pediatrics, 131*(3), e1009–e1024.

Bermas, B. (2014). Non-steroidal anti-inflammatory drugs, glucocorticoids and disease modifying antirheumatic drugs for the management of rheumatoid arthritis before and during pregnancy. *Current Opinion in Rheumatology, 26*(3), 334–340.

Cain, M. A., Bornick, P., & Whiteman, V. (2013). The maternal, fetal, and neonatal effects of cocaine exposure in pregnancy. *Clinical Obstetrics and Gynecology, 56*(1), 124–132.

Caritis, S. N., & Hebert, M. F. (2013). A pharmacologic approach to the use of glyburide in pregnancy. *Obstetrics & Gynecology, 121*(6), 1309–1312.

Centers for Disease Control and Prevention (CDC). (2012). *Global tuberculosis report 2012.* Retrieved from http://www.who.int/tb/publications/global_report/en/index.html

Centers for Disease Control (CDC). (2013). *Global tuberculosis 2013.* Retrieved from http://www.cdc.gov/tb/topic/globaltb/default.htm

Centers for Disease Control and Prevention (CDC). (2014). *Recommendations for use of antiretroviral drugs in pregnant HIV-1–infected women for maternal health and interventions to reduce perinatal HIV transmission in the United States.* Retrieved from http://aidsinfo.nih.gov/guidelines/html/3/perinatal-guidelines/0

Centers for Disease Control and Prevention (CDC). (2015a). *HIV in the United States: At a glance.* Retrieved from http://www.cdc.gov/hiv/statistics/basics/ataglance.html

Centers for Disease Control and Prevention (CDC). (2015b). *Diagnosis of HIV infection in the United States and dependent areas, 2013.* HIV Surveillance Report, Vol. 25. Retrieved from http://www.cdc.gov/hiv/library/reports/surveillance/2013/surveillance_Report_vol_25.html

Cleveland Clinic. (2012). *Gestational diabetes.* Retrieved from http://my.clevelandclinic.org/disorders/Diabetes_Gestational/hic_Gestational_Diabetes.aspx

Cossette, B., Forget, A., Beauchesne, M. F., Rey, E., Lemière, C., Larivée, P., ..., Blais, L. (2013). Impact of maternal use of asthma-controller therapy on perinatal outcomes. *Thorax, 68*(8), 724–730.

Criteria Committee of the New York Heart Association. (1994). *Nomenclature and criteria for diagnosis of diseases of the heart and great vessels* (9th ed.). Dallas, TX: American Heart Association.

Cunningham, F. G., Leveno, K. J., Bloom, S. L., Spong, C. Y., Dashe, J. S., Hoffman, B. L., ... Sheffield, J. S. (2014). *Williams obstetrics* (24th ed.). New York, NY: McGraw-Hill.

Daniels, V. (2013). Antepartum depression—screening and treatment. *International Journal of Childbirth Education, 28*(3), 67–70.

Elkayam, U., Jalnapurkar, S., & Barakat, M. (2012). Peripartum cardiomyopathy. *Cardiology Clinics, 30*(3), 435–440.

Fryearson, J., & Adamson, D. L. (2014). Heart disease in pregnancy: Ischaemic heart disease. *Best Practice & Research, Clinical Obstetrics & Gynaecology, 28*(4), 551–562.

Harris, I. S. (2011). Management of pregnancy in patients with congenital heart disease. *Progress in Cardiovascular Diseases, 53*, 305–311.

Hood, D. G. (2012). Continuous subcutaneous insulin infusion for managing diabetes. *Nursing for Women's Health, 16*(4), 310–317.

Houtchens, M. (2013). Multiple sclerosis and pregnancy. *Clinical Obstetrics and Gynecology, 56*(2), 342–349.

Hurst, H. (2011). Insulin revisited: Safety in the maternity setting. *Nursing for Women's Health, 15*(3), 244–248.

International Association of Diabetes and Pregnancy Study Groups Consensus Panel (IADPSG). (2010). International Association of Diabetes and Pregnancy Study Groups recommendations on the diagnosis and classification of hyperglycemia in pregnancy. *Diabetes Care, 33*(3), 676–683.

Kamyar, M., & Varner, M. (2013). Epilepsy in pregnancy. *Clinical Obstetrics and Gynecology, 56*(2), 330–341.

Karg, R. S., Bose, J., Batts, K. R., Forman-Hoffman, V. L., Liao, D., Hirsch, E., ... Hedden, S. L. (2014). *Past year mental disorders among adults in the United States: Results from the 2008–2012 mental health surveillance study.* Retrieved from http://www.samhsa.gov/data/sites/default/files/NSDUH-DR-N2MentalDis-2014-1/Web/NSDUH-DR-N2MentalDis-2014.htm

Landon, M. B., Catalano, P. M., & Gabbe, S. G. (2012). Diabetes mellitus complicating pregnancy. In S. G. Gabbe, J. R. Niebyl, J. L. Simpson, M. B. Landon, H. L. Galan, E. R. M. Jauniaux, & D. A. Driscoll (Eds.), *Obstetrics: Normal and problem pregnancies* (6th ed.). Philadelphia, PA: Elsevier Saunders.

Lateef, A., & Petri, M. (2013). Managing lupus patients during pregnancy. *Best Practice & Research Clinical Rheumatology, 27*(3), 435–447.

Loto, O. M., & Awowole, I. (2012). Tuberculosis in pregnancy: A review. *Journal of Pregnancy,* Article ID 379271. Retrieved from http://www.hindawi.com/journals/jp/2012/379271

Loutfy, M. R., Sonnenberg-Schwan, U., Margolese, S., & Sherr, L. (2013). A review of reproductive health research, guidelines and related gaps for women living with HIV. *AIDS Care, 25*(6), 657–666.

Moore, L. E. (2012). Gestational diabetes: Should you use oral agents? *Contemporary OB/GYN, 57*(2), 28–32.

National Institute on Drug Abuse. (2013). *DrugFacts: MDMA (Ecstasy or Molly).* Retrieved from http://www.drugabuse.gov/publications/drugfacts/mdma-ecstasy-or-molly

Niebyl, J. R., & Simpson, J. L. (2012). Drugs and environmental agents in pregnancy and lactation: Embryology, teratology, epidemiology. In S. G. Gabbe, J. R. Niebyl, J. L. Simpson, M. B. Landon, H. L. Galan, E. R. M. Jauniaux, & D. A. Driscoll (Eds.), *Obstetrics: Normal and problem pregnancies* (6th ed.). Philadelphia, PA: Elsevier Saunders.

Nili, F., McLeod, L., O'Connell, C., Sutton, E., & McMillan, D. (2013). Maternal and neonatal outcomes in pregnancies complicated by systemic lupus erythematosus: A population-based study. *Journal of Obstetrics and Gynaecology Canada, 35*(4), 323–328.

O'Neill, E., & Thorp, J. (2012). Antepartum evaluation of the fetus and fetal well-being. *Clinical Obstetrics and Gynecology, 55*(3), 722–730.

Panel on Treatment of HIV-Infected Pregnant Women and Prevention of Perinatal Transmission. (2014, March 28). *Recommendations for the use of antiretroviral drugs in pregnant HIV-1–infected women for maternal health and interventions to reduce perinatal HIV transmission in the United States* (pp. 1–117). Retrieved from http://aidsinfo.nih.gov/guidelines/html/3/perinatal-guidelines/0#

Prick, B. W., Hop, W. C. J., & Duvekot, J. J. (2012). Maternal phenylketonuria and hyperphenylalaninemia in pregnancy: Pregnancy complications and neonatal sequelae in untreated and treated pregnancies. *American Journal of Clinical Nutrition, 95*, 374–382.

Samuels, P. (2012). Hematologic complications of pregnancy. In S. G. Gabbe, J. R. Niebyl, J. L. Simpson, M. B. Landon, H. L. Galan, E. R. M. Jauniaux, & D. A. Driscoll (Eds.), *Obstetrics: Normal and problem pregnancies* (6th ed.). Philadelphia, PA: Elsevier Saunders.

Samuels, P., & Niebyl, J. R. (2012). Neurologic disorders. In S. G. Gabbe, J. R. Niebyl, J. L. Simpson, M. B. Landon, H. L. Galan, E. R. M. Jauniaux, & D. A. Driscoll (Eds.), *Obstetrics: Normal and problem pregnancies* (6th ed.). Philadelphia, PA: Elsevier Saunders.

Schillie, S.F., & Murphy, T.V. (2013). Seroprotection after recombinant hepatitis B vaccination among newborn infants: A review. *Vaccine, 31*(21), 2506–2516.

Shade, M., Miller, L., Borst, J., English, B., Valliere, J., Downs, K.,... Hare, I. (2011). Statewide innovations to improve services for women with perinatal depression. *Nursing for Women's Health, 15*(2), 127–136.

Singer, L. T., Moore, D. G., Min, M. O., Goodwin, J., Turner, J. J., Fulton, S., & Parrott, A. C. (2012). One-year outcomes of prenatal exposure to MDMA and other recreational drugs. *Pediatrics, 130*(3), 407–413.

Smith, M. V., Shao, L., Howell, H., Lin, H., & Yonkers, K. A. (2011). Perinatal depression and birth outcomes in a Healthy Start project. *Maternal–Child Nursing Journal, 15*(3), 401–409.

Substance Abuse and Mental Health Services Administration (SAMHSA). (2014). *Results from the 2013 National Survey on Drug Use and Health: Summary of National Findings* (NSDUH Series H-48, DHHS Publication No. SMA 14-4863). Rockville, MD: Substance Abuse and Mental Health Services Administration.

Sullivan, S. A. (2011). Subclinical hypothyroidism: Identification and treatment in pregnancy. *Contemporary OB/GYN, 56*(6), 46–53.

Tsui, A., & Martin, L. (2011). Multiple sclerosis and pregnancy. *Current Opinion in Obstetrics and Gynecology, 23*(6), 435–439

U.S. Department of Health and Human Services. (2012). *Healthy People 2020: Maternal, infant, and child health.* Washington, DC: U.S. Department of Health and Human Services. Retrieved from http://www.healthypeople.gov/2020/topicsobjectives2020/objectiveslist.aspx?topicid=26

Wang, M. (2014). Perinatal drug abuse and neonatal withdrawal. *eMedicine.* Retrieved from http://emedicine.medscape.com/article/978492-overview

Whitty, J. E., & Dombrowski, M. P. (2012). Respiratory diseases in pregnancy. In S. G. Gabbe, J. R. Niebyl, J. L. Simpson, M. B. Landon, H. L. Galan, E. R. M. Jauniaux, & D. A. Driscoll (Eds.), *Obstetrics: Normal and problem pregnancies* (6th ed.). Philadelphia, PA: Elsevier Saunders.

Wilson, B. A., Shannon, M. T., & Shields, K. M. (2014). *Pearson Nurse's Drug Guide 2015.* Upper Saddle River, NJ: Pearson.

Wong, V. W., Suwandarathne, H., & Russell, H. (2013). Women with pre-existing diabetes under the care of diabetes specialist prior to pregnancy: Are their outcomes better? *Australian and New Zealand Journal of Obstetrics and Gynaecology, 53*, 207–210.

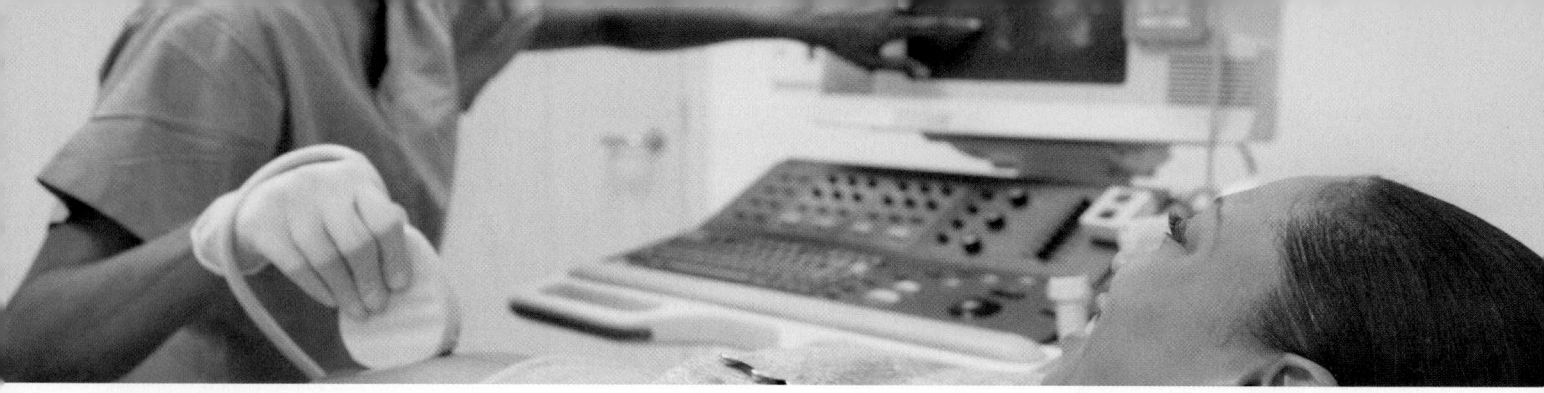

Chapter 15
Pregnancy at Risk: Gestational Onset

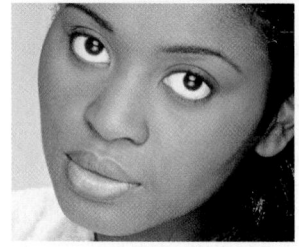

When we decided to have children we were so excited, so ready. I never expected that I would have two miscarriages. I can't tell you how hard that was to handle. Even today, with two healthy children, I remember the pain, the loss, the sense of failure, and I grieve for the children we will never know.

—Jasmine, 36

Chris Baker/Getty Images

∨ Learning Outcomes

15.1 Contrast the etiology, medical therapy, and nursing interventions for the various bleeding problems associated with pregnancy.

15.2 Discuss the medical therapy and nursing care of a woman with hyperemesis gravidarum.

15.3 Describe the maternal and fetal/neonatal risks, clinical manifestations, and nursing care of a pregnant woman with a hypertensive disorder.

15.4 Summarize the risks and implications of surgical procedures performed during pregnancy.

15.5 Relate the impact of trauma caused by an accident to the nursing care of the pregnant woman or her fetus.

15.6 Discuss the needs and care of the pregnant woman who experiences abuse.

15.7 Contrast the effects of various infections on the pregnant woman and her unborn child.

15.8 Explain the cause and prevention of hemolytic disease of the newborn secondary to Rh incompatibility.

15.9 Compare Rh incompatibility to ABO incompatibility with regard to occurrence, clinical treatment, and implications for the fetus or newborn.

In some pregnancies, problems arise that place the woman and her unborn child at risk. Regular prenatal care helps detect these complications quickly so that effective care can be provided. This chapter focuses on problems that develop during pregnancy, those with a *gestational onset*. (*Note:* Conditions such as diabetes mellitus and anemia, which may occur prior to pregnancy or develop during pregnancy, are discussed in Chapter 14.)

Care of the Woman With a Bleeding Disorder

During the first and second trimesters, the major cause of bleeding is abortion. **Abortion** is the expulsion of the fetus prior to viability, which is considered to be 20 weeks' gestation or weight of less than 500 g. Definitions of viability vary somewhat according to state reporting laws (Cunningham et al., 2014). Abortions are either *spontaneous* (occurring naturally) or *induced* (occurring as a result of medical or surgical means). **Miscarriage** is a lay term used for spontaneous abortion.

Other complications that can cause bleeding in the first half of pregnancy are ectopic pregnancy and gestational trophoblastic disease. In the second half of pregnancy, particularly in the third trimester, the two major causes of bleeding are placenta previa and abruptio placentae (see Chapter 20 for more information).

General Principles of Nursing Intervention

Spotting is relatively common during pregnancy and usually occurs following sexual intercourse or exercise because of trauma to the highly vascular cervix. However, the woman is advised to report any spotting or bleeding that occurs during pregnancy so that it can be evaluated.

It is often the nurse's responsibility to make the initial assessment of bleeding. In general, the following nursing measures are indicated:

- Monitor blood pressure and pulse frequently. The frequency is determined by the extent of the bleeding and the stability of the woman's condition.
- Observe the woman for behaviors indicative of shock, such as pallor, clammy skin, perspiration, dyspnea, or restlessness.
- Count and weigh pads to assess amount of bleeding over a given time period; save any tissue or clots expelled.
- If pregnancy is of 12 weeks' gestation or beyond, assess fetal heart tones with a Doppler.
- Prepare for intravenous (IV) therapy. There may be standing orders to begin IV therapy on clients who are bleeding.

- Prepare equipment for examination and have oxygen available.
- Collect and organize all data, including antepartum history, onset of bleeding episode, and laboratory studies (hemoglobin, hematocrit, Rh status, hormonal assays) for analysis.
- Obtain an order to type and cross-match for blood if evidence of significant blood loss exists.
- Assess coping mechanisms of the woman in crisis. Give emotional support to enhance her coping abilities by continuous, sustained presence; by clear explanation of procedures; and by communicating her status to her family. Prepare the woman for possible fetal loss. Assess her expressions of anger, denial, silence, guilt, depression, or self-blame.
- Assess the family's response to the situation.

Spontaneous Abortion (Miscarriage)

The incidence of spontaneous abortion is about 15% to 20% in clinically recognized pregnancies (Pflueger, 2013). However, advanced maternal age increases the risk significantly.

A majority of early miscarriages are related to chromosomal abnormalities. Other causes include teratogenic drugs, faulty implantation caused by abnormalities of the female reproductive tract, a weakened cervix, placental abnormalities, chronic maternal diseases, endocrine imbalances, and maternal infections. Women who use hot tubs or jacuzzis may be at increased risk for miscarriage and neural tube defects because of the hyperthermia resulting from increased core body temperature (Harms, 2012).

CLASSIFICATION

- *Threatened abortion* (Figure 15–1A). The embryo or fetus is jeopardized by unexplained bleeding, cramping, and

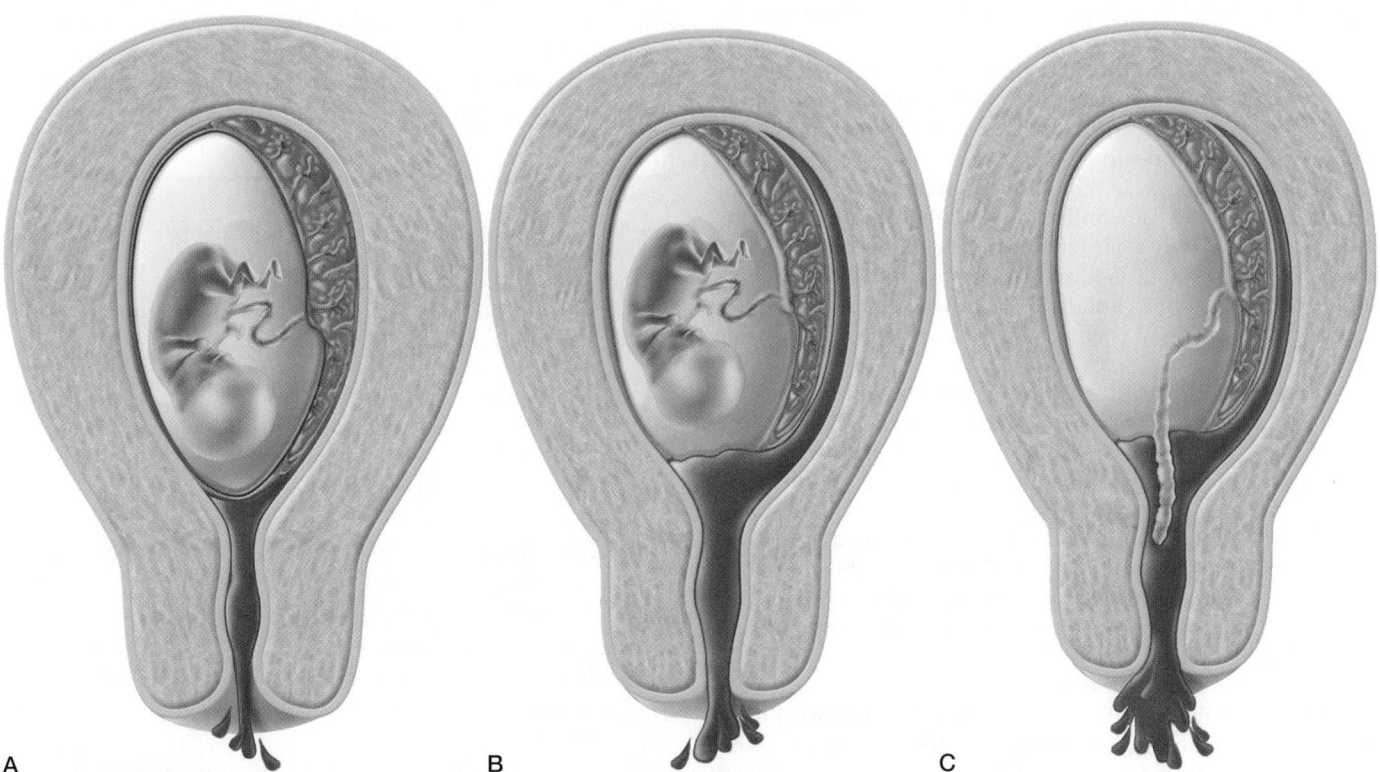

A   B   C

Figure 15–1 Types of spontaneous abortion. *A,* Threatened. The cervix is not dilated, and the placenta is still attached to the uterine wall, but some bleeding occurs. *B,* Imminent. The placenta has separated from the uterine wall, the cervix has dilated, and the amount of bleeding has increased. *C,* Incomplete. The embryo or fetus has passed out of the uterus, but the placenta remains.

backache. The cervix is closed. Bleeding may persist for days. It may be followed by partial or complete expulsion of the embryo or fetus, placenta, and membranes (sometimes called the "products of conception") or it may resolve without threatening the fetus.

- *Imminent abortion* (Figure 15–1*B*). Bleeding and cramping increase. The internal cervical os dilates. Membranes may rupture. The term *inevitable abortion* also applies.

- *Complete abortion.* All the products of conception are expelled.

- *Incomplete abortion* (Figure 15–1*C*). Some of the products of conception are retained, most often the placenta. The internal cervical os is dilated slightly.

- *Missed abortion.* The fetus dies in utero but is not expelled. Uterine growth ceases, breast changes regress, and the woman may report a brownish vaginal discharge. The cervix is closed. If the fetus is retained beyond 6 weeks, the breakdown of fetal tissues results in the release of thromboplastin, and disseminated intravascular coagulation (DIC) may develop.

- *Recurrent pregnancy loss.* Abortion occurs consecutively in three or more pregnancies. Formerly called *habitual abortion*.

- *Septic abortion.* Infection is present. It may occur with prolonged, unrecognized rupture of the membranes, pregnancy with an intrauterine device (IUD) in place, or attempts by unqualified individuals to end a pregnancy.

CLINICAL THERAPY

Pelvic cramping and backache are reliable indicators of potential spontaneous abortion. These symptoms are usually absent in bleeding caused by polyps, ruptured cervical blood vessels, or cervical erosion.

Speculum examination is done to determine the presence of cervical polyps or cervical erosion. Ultrasound scanning may detect the presence of cardiac activity and a gestational sac, or may reveal a crown-to-rump length that is small for gestational age. Laboratory determination of the human chorionic gonadotropin (hCG) level can confirm a pregnancy, but because the hCG level falls slowly after fetal death, it cannot confirm a live embryo/fetus. Serial hCG levels may be indicated to confirm a diagnosis. Hemoglobin and hematocrit levels are obtained to assess blood loss. Blood is typed and cross-matched for possible replacement needs.

The therapy prescribed for the pregnant woman with bleeding is bed rest, abstinence from coitus, and emotional support. If bleeding persists and abortion is imminent or incomplete, the woman may be hospitalized, IV therapy or blood transfusions may be started to replace fluid, and dilation and curettage (D&C) or suction evacuation is performed to remove the remainder of the products of conception. If the woman is Rh negative and not sensitized, Rh immune globulin (RhoGAM) is given within 72 hours (see discussion on Rh alloimmunization later in this chapter).

In missed abortions, the products of conception usually are expelled spontaneously. Diagnosis is based on history, pelvic examination, and a negative pregnancy test and may be confirmed by ultrasound if necessary. If this does not occur within 4 to 6 weeks after embryo or fetal death, hospitalization is necessary. If in the first trimester, D&C or suction evacuation is done. In the second trimester, labor is induced or dilation and evacuation (D&E) may be used.

Nursing Management

For the Woman Experiencing Spontaneous Abortion

Nursing Assessment and Diagnosis

Assess the woman's vital signs, amount and appearance of any bleeding, level of comfort, and general physical health. The woman's blood type and antibody status should be identified to determine the need for Rh immune globulin. If the pregnancy is 10 to 12 weeks or more, determine fetal heart rates with a Doppler. It is also important to assess the responses of the woman and her family to this crisis, their coping mechanisms, and their ability to comfort each other.

Examples of nursing diagnoses that may apply include the following (NANDA-I © 2014):

- *Pain, Acute,* related to abdominal cramping secondary to threatened abortion
- *Fluid Volume: Deficient,* related to excessive bleeding secondary to spontaneous abortion

Planning and Implementation

COMMUNITY-BASED NURSING CARE

If a woman in her first trimester of pregnancy begins cramping or spotting, she is often evaluated on an outpatient basis. Provide analgesics for pain relief if the woman's cramps are severe, and explain what is occurring throughout the process.

Feelings of shock or disbelief are normal. Couples who approached the pregnancy with joy and excitement now feel grief, sadness, and possibly anger. Because many women, even with planned pregnancies, feel some ambivalence initially, guilt is also a common emotion. These feelings may be even stronger for women who were negative about their pregnancies. The women may even believe that the miscarriage is a punishment for some wrongdoing.

Developing Cultural Competence **Individual Responses to Fetal Loss**

Remember that individual responses to fetal loss following miscarriage may vary greatly and may be influenced by ethnic or cultural norms.

- Miscarriage may be viewed in many ways. For example, it may be seen as a punishment from God, as the result of the evil eye or of a hex or curse by an enemy, or as a natural part of life.

- When grieving over a pregnancy loss, women from some cultures and ethnic groups may show their emotions freely, crying and wailing, whereas other women may hide their feelings behind a mask of stoicism.

- In some cultures the woman's partner is her primary source of support and comfort. In others, the woman turns to her mother or close female relatives for comfort.

- Avoid falling into the trap of stereotyping women according to culture. Individual responses are influenced by many factors, including the degree of assimilation into the dominant culture.

Offer psychologic support to the woman and her family by encouraging them to talk about their feelings, allowing them the privacy to grieve, and listening sympathetically to their concerns about this pregnancy and future ones. To help decrease feelings of guilt or blame, inform the woman and her family about the causes of miscarriage. If the woman has older children, she may need guidance in how to help them understand and cope with what has occurred. Refer them to other healthcare professionals for additional help as necessary.

The grieving period following a miscarriage usually lasts 6 to 24 months. Many couples can be helped during this period by an organization or support group established for parents who have lost a fetus or newborn.

HOSPITAL-BASED NURSING CARE

A woman with an incomplete or missed abortion may need a D&C or other procedure, which is typically done on an outpatient basis. Barring any complications, the woman can return home a few hours after the procedure. Monitor the woman's condition closely and provide instruction for self-care. Administer Rh immune globulin if it is indicated.

Health Promotion **After a Miscarriage**

Provide information about community resources to help the woman and her loved ones cope with the loss and advise her to:

- Report heavy or bright red vaginal bleeding, fever, chills, foul-smelling vaginal discharge, or abdominal tenderness.
- Take the full course of antibiotics if any are prescribed.
- Delay pregnancy for at least 2 months to allow sufficient time for healing.

Evaluation

Expected outcomes of nursing care include the following:

- The woman is able to explain spontaneous abortion, the treatment measures employed in her care, and long-term implications for future pregnancies.
- The woman suffers no complications.
- The woman and her partner begin verbalizing their grief and acknowledge that the grieving process lasts several months.

Ectopic Pregnancy

Ectopic pregnancy (EP) is the implantation of the fertilized ovum in a site other than the endometrial lining of the uterus. It has many causes, including tubal damage from pelvic inflammatory disease (PID), previous tubal surgery, congenital anomalies of the tube, endometriosis, previous EP, presence of an IUD, and in utero exposure to diethylstilbestrol (DES).

Ectopic pregnancy occurs in about 2% of diagnosed pregnancies. Although the incidence of EP has increased, the mortality rate in the United States has decreased to 0.5 deaths per 100,000. This decline can be credited to improved recognition of early signs and symptoms and better diagnostic methods, which allow detection before tubal rupture. Nevertheless, EP accounts for approximately 9% of maternal deaths today (Marion & Meeks, 2012).

EP occurs when the fertilized ovum is prevented or slowed in its passage through the tube and thus implants before it reaches the uterus, usually in the ampulla of the fallopian tube. *Pathophysiology Illustrated: Ectopic Pregnancy* identifies other implantation sites.

Pathophysiology Illustrated: **Ectopic Pregnancy**

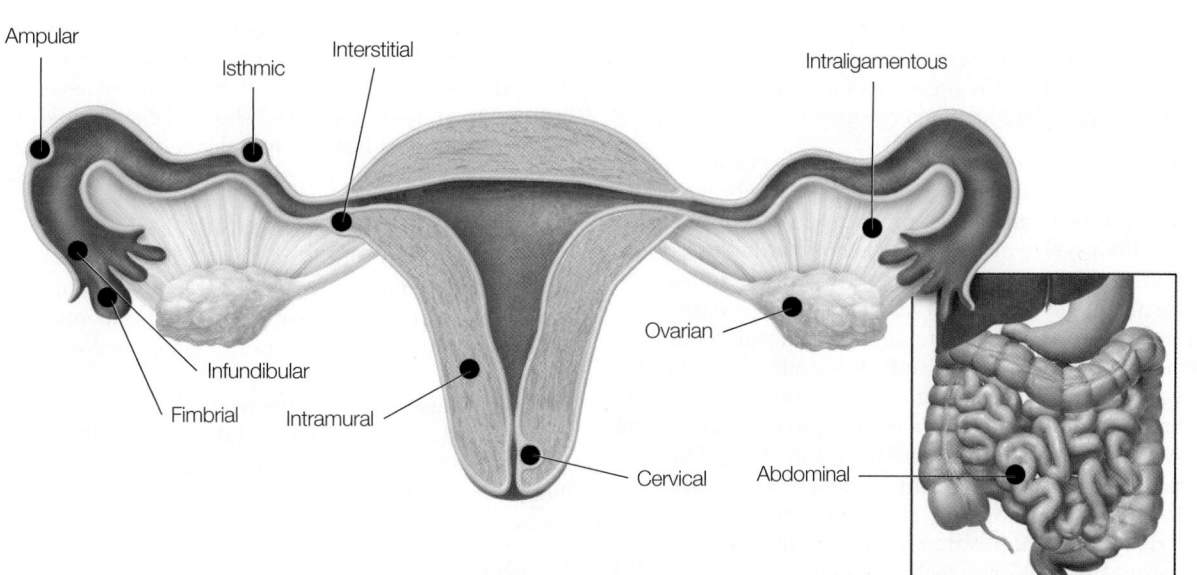

Various implantation sites in ectopic pregnancy. The most common site is within the fallopian tube, hence the name "tubal pregnancy."

Initially symptoms of pregnancy may be present, including amenorrhea, breast tenderness, and nausea. The hormone hCG is present in the blood and urine. As the pregnancy progresses, the chorionic villi grow into the tube wall or implantation site and establish a blood supply. When the embryo outgrows this space, the tube ruptures and there is bleeding into the abdominal cavity. This bleeding irritates the peritoneum, causing the characteristic symptoms of sharp, one-sided pain, syncope, and referred right shoulder pain. The woman may also have lower abdominal pain. Vaginal bleeding occurs because of fluctuations in hormone levels.

Physical examination usually reveals adnexal (area over each ovary and fallopian tube) tenderness. An adnexal mass is palpable about half the time. Bleeding is slow and chronic, and the abdomen gradually becomes rigid and very tender. With bleeding into the abdominal cavity, pelvic examination is very painful, and a mass of blood may be palpated in the lower abdomen. Laboratory tests may reveal low hemoglobin and hematocrit levels and rising leukocyte levels. In a normal pregnancy β-hCG titers double every 48 hours from 3 to 6 weeks' gestation. Ectopic pregnancies are associated with β-hCG titers that increase more slowly.

CLINICAL THERAPY

The following measures are used to establish the diagnosis of ectopic pregnancy and assess the woman's status:

- A careful assessment of menstrual history, particularly the last menstrual period (LMP), is completed.

- A pelvic examination is conducted to identify any abnormal pelvic masses and tenderness.

- Laboratory testing is completed as described previously.

- Transvaginal ultrasound is the initial test of choice to detect an intrauterine pregnancy or an adnexal mass (Jurkovic & Wilkinson, 2011). Confirming an intrauterine pregnancy nearly eliminates the diagnosis of ectopic pregnancy.

- Serial measurements of serum hCG values are taken, which should increase significantly every 2 days. Women with an ectopic pregnancy often have serial serum hCG values that increase more slowly than expected with a viable intrauterine pregnancy (Visconti & Zite, 2012).

- Laparoscopic intervention may be necessary for both diagnosis and treatment if the presence or absence of an ectopic pregnancy cannot be confirmed by other measures.

Treatment may be medical or surgical. Methotrexate is used for the woman who desires future pregnancy. The best success is obtained when the woman's ectopic pregnancy is unruptured and of 4 cm (1.6 in.) size or less, there is no fetal heart motion, and her condition is stable. In addition, the woman must have no evidence of a blood disorder or kidney or liver disease.

Methotrexate is a folic acid antagonist that interferes with the proliferation of trophoblastic cells. It is administered intramuscularly (IM) using either a single-dose or multiple-dose regimen. As an outpatient, the woman is monitored for increasing abdominal pain and β-hCG titers are determined. β-hCG titers are assessed on day 4 and day 7. If hCG levels do not decrease at least 15% from day 4 to day 7 after the initial injection, an additional dose of methotrexate is given on day 7 (Lipscomb, 2012). The multidose regimen includes methotrexate given IM and leucovorin administered orally on alternate days for up to 8 days (Visconti & Zite, 2012). This regimen is far more care intensive and is reserved for clients who present with high hCG levels.

If surgery is indicated and the woman desires future pregnancies, a laparoscopic linear salpingostomy will be performed to gently evacuate the ectopic pregnancy and preserve the tube. If the tube is ruptured or if future childbearing is not an issue, laparoscopic salpingectomy (removal of the tube) is performed, leaving the ovary in place unless it is damaged. If the woman is in shock and unstable, an abdominal incision will be made. With both medical and surgical therapies for EP, the Rh-negative nonsensitized woman is given Rh immune globulin to prevent sensitization.

Nursing Management
For the Woman With an Ectopic Pregnancy

Nursing Assessment and Diagnosis

When the woman with a suspected ectopic pregnancy is admitted to the hospital, assess the appearance and amount of vaginal bleeding and monitor vital signs for developing shock. Assess the woman's emotional state and coping abilities, and determine the couple's informational needs. Determine the woman's level of pain, which can be significant. If surgery is necessary, complete the appropriate ongoing assessments postoperatively.

Nursing diagnoses that may apply for a woman with EP include the following (NANDA-I © 2014):

- *Pain, Acute,* related to abdominal bleeding secondary to tubal rupture

- *Grieving* related to expected pregnancy loss

- *Fluid Volume: Deficient,* related to hypovolemia secondary to maternal blood loss

Planning and Implementation

COMMUNITY-BASED NURSING CARE

Women with EP are often seen initially in a clinic or office setting. Be alert to the possibility of EP if a woman presents with complaints of abdominal pain and lack of menses for 1 to 2 months. A woman receiving medical treatment using methotrexate is followed as an outpatient. Advise the woman that some abdominal pain is common following the injection, but generally it is mild and lasts only 24 to 48 hours. More severe pain might indicate treatment failure and should be evaluated. The woman should also report heavy vaginal bleeding, dizziness, or tachycardia. Stress the need to return for follow-up β-hCG testing.

HOSPITAL-BASED NURSING CARE

Once a diagnosis of EP is made and surgery is scheduled, start an IV as ordered and begin preoperative teaching. Immediately report signs of developing shock. If the woman experiences severe abdominal pain, administer analgesics and evaluate their effectiveness.

Regardless of the treatment used, the woman and her family will need emotional support during this difficult time. Their feelings and responses to this crisis are generally similar to those that occur in cases of spontaneous abortion; similar nursing actions are required.

Evaluation

Expected outcomes of nursing care include the following:

- The woman is able to explain ectopic pregnancy, treatment alternatives, and implications for future childbearing.

- The woman and her caregivers detect possible complications early and manage them successfully.
- The woman and her partner are able to begin verbalizing their loss.

Gestational Trophoblastic Disease

Gestational trophoblastic disease (GTD) is the pathologic proliferation of trophoblastic cells (the trophoblast is the outermost layer of embryonic cells). In the United States, the incidence is approximately 1 per 1000 to 1500 live births (Salani, Eisenhauer, & Copeland, 2012). It includes hydatidiform mole, invasive mole (chorioadenoma destruens), and choriocarcinoma, a form of cancer.

Hydatidiform mole (molar pregnancy) is a condition in which a proliferation of trophoblastic cells results in the formation of a placenta characterized by *hydropic* (fluid-filled) grapelike clusters. The disease results in the loss of the pregnancy and the possibility, although remote, of developing choriocarcinoma, a form of cancer, from the trophoblastic tissue.

Molar pregnancies are classified into two types, complete and partial, both of which meet the previously mentioned criteria. A *complete mole* develops from an ovum containing no maternal genetic material, an "empty egg," which is fertilized by a normal sperm. The embryo dies very early, no circulation is established, the hydropic vesicles are avascular, and no embryonic tissue is found. Choriocarcinoma seems to be more commonly associated with the complete mole (American College of Obstetricians and Gynecologists [ACOG], 2012b). *Choriocarcinoma* is invasive, malignant trophoblastic disease that is usually metastatic and can be fatal. It is discussed in more detail later.

The *partial mole* usually has a triploid karyotype (69 chromosomes). This occurs most often when a normal ovum with 23 chromosomes is fertilized by two sperm (dispermy) or by a sperm that has failed to undergo the first meiotic division and therefore contains 46 chromosomes. There may be a fetal sac or even a fetus with a heartbeat. The fetus has multiple anomalies and little chance for survival. Often, partial moles are recognized only after miscarriage, and they may go unnoticed even then.

Invasive mole (chorioadenoma destruens) is similar to a complete mole, but it involves the uterine myometrium. Treatment is the same as for complete mole.

CLINICAL THERAPY

With hydatidiform mole, the following signs may be present:

- Vaginal bleeding occurs almost universally. It is often brownish (like prune juice) because of liquefaction of the uterine clot, but it may be bright red.
- Uterine enlargement greater than expected for gestational age is a classic sign of a complete mole, which is present in about half of cases. Enlargement is due to the proliferating trophoblastic tissue and to a large amount of clotted blood.
- Hydropic vesicles (grapelike clusters) may be passed; if so, they are diagnostic (Figure 15–2). With a partial mole, the vesicles are often smaller and may not be noticed.
- Serum human chorionic gonadotropin (hCG) levels are markedly elevated because of continued secretion by the proliferating trophoblastic tissue.
- Hyperemesis gravidarum is present, probably because of the elevated hCG level.

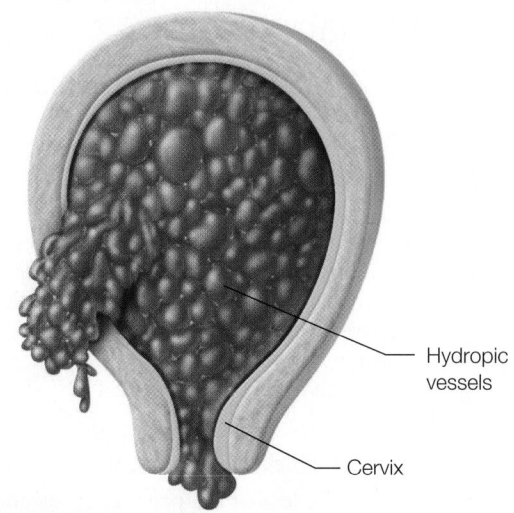

Figure 15–2 **Hydatidiform mole. A common sign is vaginal bleeding, often brownish (the characteristic "prune juice" appearance) but sometimes bright red. In this figure, some of the hydropic vessels are being passed. This occurrence is diagnostic for hydatidiform mole.**

- Anemia occurs frequently because of blood loss.
- Very low levels of maternal serum α-fetoprotein (MSAFP) are found.
- Symptoms of preeclampsia are observed before 24 weeks' gestation.
- Fetal heart tones are absent despite other signs of pregnancy.

Transvaginal ultrasound is used for diagnosis. Therapy begins with suction evacuation of the mole and curettage of the uterus to remove all fragments of the placenta. Early evacuation decreases the possibility of other complications. Rh immune globulin is administered to women with an Rh-negative blood type. If the woman is older and has completed her childbearing, or if there is excessive bleeding, hysterectomy may be the treatment of choice to reduce the risk of choriocarcinoma.

Because of the risk of choriocarcinoma, the woman treated for hydatidiform mole should receive extensive follow-up therapy. Follow-up care includes a baseline chest x-ray to detect lung metastasis and a physical examination including a pelvic examination. Approaches to ongoing monitoring vary somewhat. Typically, serum β-hCG levels are monitored weekly until negative results are obtained 3 consecutive times, then monthly for 6 to 12 months (Salani et al., 2012). The woman should avoid pregnancy during that time because the elevated hCG levels associated with pregnancy would cause confusion as to whether cancer had developed. If, after a year of monitoring, the hCG serum titers are within normal limits, a couple may be assured that a normal pregnancy can be anticipated, with a low risk of recurring hydatidiform mole.

If hCG levels plateau for 3 consecutive weeks or rise, pregnancy must be ruled out and then the woman should be evaluated for metastatic disease and treated appropriately (Salani et al., 2012). Treatment at a center specializing in GTD is advised.

Nursing Management

For the Woman With Gestational Trophoblastic Disease

Nursing Assessment and Diagnosis

Observe for symptoms of hydatidiform mole at each antepartum visit. The classic symptoms are found more frequently with the complete mole. Before evacuation the partial mole may be difficult to distinguish from a missed abortion. If a molar pregnancy is diagnosed, assess the woman's (or the couple's) understanding of the condition and its implications.

Nursing diagnoses that may apply include the following (NANDA-I © 2014):

- *Fear* related to the possible development of choriocarcinoma
- *Grieving* related to the loss of the pregnancy secondary to GTD

Planning and Implementation

COMMUNITY-BASED NURSING CARE

When a molar pregnancy is suspected, the woman needs emotional support. Answer questions about the condition and explain what ultrasound and other diagnostic procedures will entail. If a molar pregnancy is diagnosed, support the parents as they deal with their grief about the lost pregnancy and their fear about the possibility of having a serious illness (DiGiulio, Wiedaseck, & Monchek, 2012). Healthcare counselors, a member of the clergy, or a professional counselor may also be of help.

HOSPITAL-BASED NURSING CARE

When the woman is hospitalized for removal of the mole, monitor vital signs and vaginal bleeding for signs of hemorrhage. Determine the presence of abdominal pain and evaluate the woman's emotional state and coping ability. Have typed and cross-matched blood available for surgery. Administer oxytocin as ordered to keep the uterus contracted and to prevent hemorrhage. If the woman is Rh negative and not sensitized, give Rh immune globulin to prevent antibody formation.

Health Promotion **Hydatidiform Mole**
- Stress the importance of follow-up visits.
- Advise the woman to delay another pregnancy until the follow-up program has been completed.

Evaluation

Expected outcomes of nursing care include the following:

- The woman has a smooth recovery following successful evacuation of the mole.
- The woman is able to explain GTD and its treatment, follow-up, and long-term implications for pregnancy.
- The woman and her partner are able to begin talking about their grief at the loss of their anticipated child.
- The woman can discuss the importance of follow-up care and indicates her willingness to cooperate with the regimen.

Care of the Woman With Hyperemesis Gravidarum

Hyperemesis gravidarum, which is excessive vomiting during pregnancy, occurs in 0.3% to 2% of pregnancies (Nayeri, 2012). It may be mild at first, but true hyperemesis may progress to a point at which the woman not only vomits everything she swallows but also retches between meals.

Although the exact cause of hyperemesis is unclear, increased levels of human chorionic gonadotropin (hCG) may play a role. Other mechanisms that may relate to hyperemesis are displacement of the gastrointestinal tract, hypofunction of the anterior pituitary gland and adrenal cortex, abnormalities

---

EVIDENCE-BASED PRACTICE | Biologic Markers for Diagnosis of Hyperemesis Gravidarum

Clinical Question

Are there biologic markers for hyperemesis gravidarum that could help in the early detection, diagnosis, and treatment of this condition of pregnancy?

The Evidence

Nausea and vomiting are common symptoms in early pregnancy. More than half of all pregnant women will experience daily nausea in the first trimester. In up to 2% of women, though, nausea and vomiting may be so severe as to cause dehydration and weight loss that may require hospitalization. Diagnostic biomarkers could help in the early detection of hyperemesis gravidarum so that treatments can be initiated before adverse events occur. One group of clinicians conducted a systematic review of the literature to determine if there were biomarkers, and, if so, their relative usefulness in detecting either presence or severity of the condition. This type of unbiased approach to research review forms the strongest level of evidence for practice.

Historically, ketonuria has been hypothesized as a marker for the condition, but this review did not identify urinalysis for the condition as useful. Testing for human chorionic gonadotropin, thyroid hormones, estradiol, progesterone, and white blood count were inconsistently associated with the condition. Serology for *H. pylori* was predictive for hyperemesis gravidarum, and may be one marker that can identify the condition early in its onset (Niemeijer et al., 2014).

Best Practice

Early detection of hyperemesis gravidarum can enable interventions to decrease the prevalence of morbidity associated with the condition. The only test that has been shown to effectively predict the onset of the condition is serology for *H. pylori*. The test may be most useful if conducted when the first signs of protracted vomiting in pregnancy appear.

Clinical Reasoning

How would the nurse identify protracted vomiting in pregnancy, and how might it be distinguished from normal nausea and vomiting? Why might *H. pylori* be a causative agent for hyperemesis gravidarum?

of the corpus luteum, and psychologic factors. Recent studies suggest a correlation between hyperemesis and a *Helicobacter pylori* infection, a common cause of gastric and duodenal ulcers (Mansour & Nashaat, 2011; Shaban, Kandil, & Elshafei, 2014).

In severe cases, hyperemesis causes dehydration, which leads to fluid–electrolyte imbalance and alkalosis from loss of hydrochloric acid. Hypovolemia, hypotension, tachycardia, increased hematocrit and blood urea nitrogen (BUN), and decreased urine output can also occur. Dehydration may also lead to condensation of bile in the bile duct, resulting in less effective bile drainage with subsequent jaundice. If untreated, metabolic acidosis may develop. Severe potassium loss interferes with the ability of the kidneys to concentrate urine and may disrupt cardiac functioning. Starvation causes muscle wasting and severe protein and vitamin deficiencies. Fetal or embryonic death may result, and the woman may suffer irreversible metabolic changes or death. The diagnostic criteria for hyperemesis include a history of intractable vomiting in the first half of pregnancy, dehydration, ketonuria, and a weight loss of 5% of prepregnancy weight.

Clinical Therapy

The goals of treatment include control of vomiting and dehydration, restoration of electrolyte balance, and maintenance of adequate nutrition. If the woman does not respond to standard approaches to the control of nausea and vomiting in pregnancy, she may require IV fluids on an outpatient basis.

If her symptoms do not improve, hospitalization may be indicated. Initially the woman is given nothing by mouth (NPO), and IV fluids are administered. Potassium chloride is often added to the IV to prevent hypokalemia. Diclegis (a combination of doxylamine succinate and pyridoxine hydrochloride [vitamin B$_6$]) is the only U.S. Food and Drug Administration (FDA)–approved treatment of nausea and vomiting during pregnancy. It is administered daily on an empty stomach (U.S. Food and Drug Administration [FDA], 2013). If this is not effective, other pharmacologic options include promethazine (Phenergan), metoclopramide (Reglan), and ondansetron (Zofran). Typically, the woman remains NPO for 48 hours. If her condition does not improve, total parenteral nutrition may be needed. She then begins controlled oral feedings.

Nursing Management

For the Woman With Hyperemesis Gravidarum

Nursing Assessment and Diagnosis

When a woman is hospitalized for control of vomiting, assess the amount and character of any emesis, intake and output, fetal heart rate, signs of jaundice or bleeding, and her emotional state.

Nursing diagnoses that may apply include the following (NANDA-I © 2014):

- *Nutrition, Imbalanced: Less than Body Requirements,* related to persistent vomiting secondary to hyperemesis
- *Fluid Volume: Deficient,* related to severe dehydration secondary to persistent vomiting

Planning and Implementation
COMMUNITY-BASED NURSING CARE
Parenteral therapy provided at home in collaboration with a physician and a registered dietitian is sometimes used to enable the woman to remain in her home. This therapy also gives an opportunity to observe family interactions and evaluate the home environment. This assessment helps determine the pregnant woman's level of support, any significant stressors in her life, and her understanding of nutrition and self-care measures.

HOSPITAL-BASED NURSING CARE
Nursing care is supportive and directed at maintaining a relaxed, quiet environment away from food odors or offensive smells. Once oral feedings resume, food needs to be attractively served. Oral hygiene is important because the mouth is dry and may be irritated from vomitus. Monitor weight regularly. In some cases, emotional factors have appeared to play a role, although that remains controversial. Nevertheless, psychotherapy may sometimes be recommended. With proper treatment, prognosis is favorable.

Evaluation
Expected outcomes of nursing care include the following:

- The woman is able to explain hyperemesis gravidarum, its therapy, and its possible effects on her pregnancy.
- The woman's condition is corrected and complications are avoided.

Care of the Woman With a Hypertensive Disorder

Hypertension is the most common medical disorder in pregnancy, accounting for up to 15% of prenatal hospitalizations. The incidence of hypertension among pregnant women ranges from 12% to 22%, and hypertension is directly responsible for 17.6% of maternal deaths in the United States (ACOG, 2012a).

- Preeclampsia/eclampsia
- Chronic hypertension
- Chronic hypertension with superimposed preeclampsia or eclampsia
- Gestational hypertension

Healthy People 2020

(MICH-6) Reduce maternal illness and complications due to pregnancy (complications during hospitalized labor and delivery)

Preeclampsia and Eclampsia

Preeclampsia, the most common hypertensive disorder in pregnancy, is defined as an increase in blood pressure after 20 weeks' gestation accompanied by proteinuria in a previously normotensive woman. Previously, edema was included in the definition but was removed because it is such a common finding in pregnancy. However, sudden onset of severe edema warrants close evaluation to rule out preeclampsia or other pathologic processes such as renal disease.

Preeclampsia, typically categorized as mild or severe, is a progressive disorder. In its most severe form, eclampsia develops. **Eclampsia** is the occurrence of a seizure in a woman with preeclampsia who has no other cause for seizure. Eclamptic seizures may occur during the antepartum, intrapartum, or postpartum periods.

Most often preeclampsia occurs in the last 10 weeks of gestation, during labor, or in the first 48 hours after childbirth. Although birth of the fetus and removal of the placenta are the only known cure for preeclampsia, it can be controlled with early diagnosis and careful management.

PATHOPHYSIOLOGY OF PREECLAMPSIA/ECLAMPSIA

The cause of preeclampsia/eclampsia remains unknown, despite decades of research. Preeclampsia affects all the major systems of the body. The following pathophysiologic changes are associated with the disease:

- In normal pregnancy, the lowered peripheral vascular resistance and the increased maternal resistance to the pressor effects of angiotensin II result in lowered blood pressure. In preeclampsia, blood pressure begins to rise after 20 weeks' gestation, probably in response to a gradual loss of resistance to angiotensin II. This response has been linked to the ratio between the prostaglandins prostacyclin and thromboxane. Prostacyclin is a potent vasodilator that decreases blood pressure, prevents platelet aggregation, and promotes uterine blood flow. Thromboxane, produced by platelets, causes vessels to constrict and platelets to clump together. Prostacyclin is decreased in preeclampsia, allowing the potent vasoconstrictor and platelet-aggregating effects of thromboxane to dominate. These hormones are produced partially by the placenta, which helps explain the reversal of the condition when the placenta is removed and why the incidence is increased when there is a larger than normal placental mass.

- The loss of normal vasodilation of uterine arterioles and the concurrent maternal vasospasm result in decreased placental perfusion (see *Pathophysiology Illustrated: Preeclampsia*). The effect on the fetus may be growth restriction, decrease in fetal movement, and chronic hypoxia or fetal distress.

- Another theory postulates that uteroplacental ischemia acts as a trigger for preeclampsia, with other factors playing contributory roles. In the woman with preeclampsia, in addition to a reduced production of the vasoactive substance prostacyclin, there is also a decreased production of nitric oxide (NO). Nitric oxide is a potent vasodilator and important regulator of maternal blood pressure. Additionally, NO inhibits platelet aggregation and adhesion to vascular endothelium (Mao et al., 2010). NO synthesis in the placenta may play a meaningful role in maintaining a low-pressure, high-flow placental system and also may prevent intervillous thrombosis.

- In preeclampsia, normal renal perfusion is decreased. With a reduction of the glomerular filtration rate, serum levels of creatinine, BUN, and uric acid begin to rise from normal pregnant levels, while urine output decreases. Sodium is retained in increased amounts, which results in increased extracellular volume, increased sensitivity to angiotensin II, and edema. Stretching of the capillary walls of the glomerular endothelial cells allows the large protein molecules, primarily albumin, to escape in the urine, decreasing serum albumin levels. The decreased serum albumin concentration causes decreased plasma colloid osmotic pressure. This lowered pressure results in a further movement of fluid to the extracellular spaces, which also contributes to the development of edema. The decreased intravascular volume causes increased viscosity of the blood and a corresponding rise in hematocrit.

HELLP syndrome (**h**emolysis, **e**levated **l**iver enzymes, and **l**ow **p**latelet count) is sometimes associated with severe preeclampsia. Women who experience this multiple organ–failure syndrome have high morbidity and mortality rates, as do their offspring.

The hemolysis that occurs is termed *microangiopathic hemolytic anemia*. It is thought that red blood cells are fragmented during passage through small, damaged blood vessels. Elevated liver enzymes occur from blood flow that is obstructed by fibrin deposits. Hyperbilirubinemia and jaundice may also be seen. Liver distention causes epigastric pain. Thrombocytopenia (platelet count less than 100,000/mm^3) is a frequent finding

Pathophysiology Illustrated: **Preeclampsia**

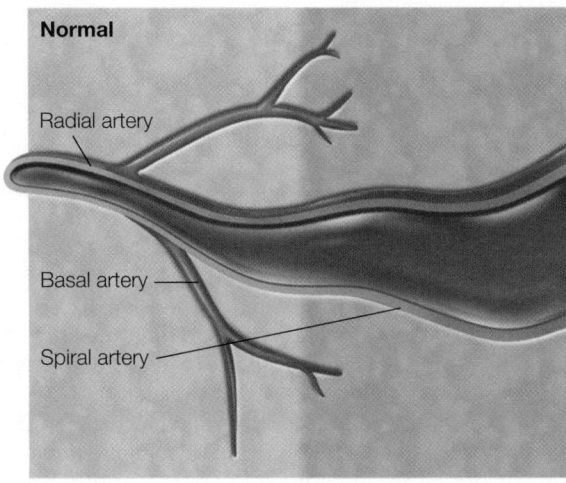

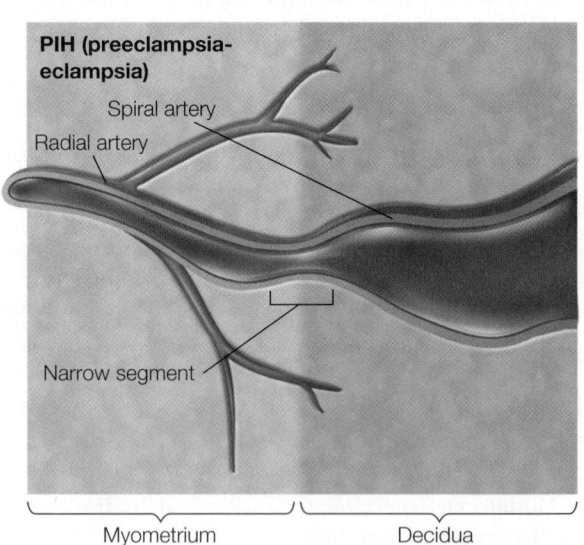

A, In a normal pregnancy, the passive quality of the spiral arteries permits increased blood flow to the placenta.
B, In preeclampsia, vasoconstriction of the myometrial segment of the spiral arteries occurs.

in preeclampsia. It occurs when platelets aggregate at the sites of vascular damage associated with vasospasm. Symptoms may include nausea, vomiting, flulike symptoms, or epigastric pain. HELLP syndrome is sometimes complicated by disseminated intravascular coagulation (DIC).

Women with HELLP syndrome are best cared for in a tertiary care center. Initially, the mother's condition should be assessed and stabilized, especially if her platelet counts are very low. The fetus is also assessed, using a non-stress test (NST) and biophysical profile (BPP). Regardless of gestational age, all women with true HELLP syndrome should give birth as expeditiously as possible.

Healthy People 2020

(MICH-5) Reduce the rate of maternal mortality

MATERNAL RISKS

Central nervous system changes associated with preeclampsia include hyperreflexia, headache, and seizures. Thrombocytopenia (platelet count less than $100,000/mm^3$) is a frequent finding in preeclampsia. The exact mechanism is not fully understood, but platelet consumption is believed to be related to endothelial damage and activation of thrombin. Women with severe preeclampsia or eclampsia are at increased risk for renal failure, abruptio placentae, DIC, ruptured liver, and pulmonary embolism.

FETAL/NEONATAL RISKS

Newborns of women with preeclampsia tend to be small for gestational age (SGA). The cause is related specifically to maternal vasospasm and hypovolemia, which result in fetal hypoxia and malnutrition. In addition, the newborn may be premature because of the necessity for early birth. At birth, the newborn may be oversedated because of medications given to the mother. The newborn may also have hypermagnesemia resulting from treatment of the woman with large doses of magnesium sulfate.

CLINICAL MANIFESTATIONS AND DIAGNOSIS

Mild Preeclampsia.   Women with mild preeclampsia may exhibit few, if any, symptoms. The blood pressure is elevated to 140/90 mmHg or higher, 1+ proteinuria may occur, and liver enzymes may be elevated minimally. Although no longer considered a diagnostic sign of preeclampsia, edema may be present.

Severe Preeclampsia.   Severe preeclampsia may develop suddenly. The following clinical signs are often present (ACOG, 2012a):

- Blood pressure of 160/110 mmHg or higher on two occasions at least 6 hours apart while the woman is on bed rest
- Proteinuria 5 g/L or higher in 24 hours or 3+ or greater on two random urine samples collected at least 4 hours apart
- Oliguria: urine output less than or equal to 500 mL in 24 hours
- Cerebral or visual disturbances
- Pulmonary edema or cyanosis
- Epigastric or right upper quadrant pain
- Impaired liver function (elevated hepatic enzymes–alanine aminotransferase [ALT] or aspartate aminotransferase [AST]) to at least twice normal
- Thrombocytopenia (less than 100,000 platelets per cubic millimeter)
- Fetal growth restriction

Other signs or symptoms that may be present include severe headache or one that persists despite analgesic therapy, blurred vision or scotomata (spots before the eyes), narrowed segments on the retinal arterioles when examined with an ophthalmoscope, retinal edema (retinas appear wet and glistening) on funduscopy, dyspnea due to pulmonary edema, moist breath sounds on auscultation, pitting edema of lower extremities while on bed rest, epigastric pain, hyperreflexia, nausea and vomiting, irritability, and emotional tension.

Eclampsia.   Eclampsia, characterized by a grand mal convulsion, may occur before labor, during labor, or early in the postpartum period. Some women experience only one seizure; others have several.

CLINICAL THERAPY

The goals of medical management are prevention of cerebral hemorrhage, convulsion, hematologic complications, and renal and hepatic diseases, and birth of an uncompromised newborn as close to term as possible.

Antepartum Management.   The clinical therapy for preeclampsia/eclampsia depends on the severity of the disease.

Home Care of Mild Preeclampsia.   For some women with mild preeclampsia, home care is an option. The woman monitors her blood pressure, weight, and urine protein daily. Weight gains of 1.4 kg (3 lb) in 24 hours or 1.8 kg (4 lb) in a 3-day period are generally a cause for concern. Remote non-stress tests (NSTs) are performed twice per week or biophysical profiles (BPPs) are done weekly. Nursing contact varies from daily to weekly, depending on physician request. Laboratory testing regularly evaluates platelet counts, uric acid and BUN, liver enzymes, and 24-hour urine specimens for creatinine clearance and total protein. It is extremely important to advise the woman to report to the physician if she develops signs of worsening preeclampsia.

Hospital Care of Mild Preeclampsia.   The woman is placed on bed rest, primarily on her left side, to decrease pressure on the vena cava, thereby increasing venous return, circulatory volume, and placental and renal perfusion. She is weighed daily and evaluated for worsening edema, persistent headache, visual changes, or epigastric pain. Urine dipstick is done daily to assess for protein; blood pressure is checked at least 4 times per day. The woman's diet should be well balanced and moderate to high in protein (80 to 100 g/day, or 1.5 g/kg/day) to replace protein lost in the urine. Sodium intake should be moderate, not to exceed 6 g/day. Excessively salty foods should be avoided, but sodium restriction and diuretics are no longer used in treating preeclampsia. Laboratory values to include CBC with platelet count, liver function tests (AST, ALT), lactic dehydrogenase (LDH), uric acid, serum creatinine, bilirubin, and 24-hour urine for protein and creatinine clearance are assessed periodically.

To achieve a safe outcome for the fetus, tests to evaluate fetal status are done more frequently as preeclampsia progresses. The following tests are used:

- Fetal movement record
- Non-stress test
- Ultrasonography at least every 3 or 4 weeks for serial determination of growth
- Biophysical profile
- Amniocentesis to determine fetal lung maturity
- Doppler velocimetry beginning at 30 to 32 weeks to screen for fetal compromise

Hospital Care of Severe Preeclampsia. In severe cases, birth may be the treatment of choice for both mother and fetus, even if the fetus is immature. Other medical therapies for severe preeclampsia include the following:

- ***Bed rest.*** Bed rest must be complete. Stimuli that may bring on a seizure should be reduced.

- ***Diet.*** A high-protein, moderate-sodium diet is given as long as the woman is alert and has no nausea or indication of impending seizure.

- ***Anticonvulsants.*** Magnesium sulfate is the treatment of choice for eclamptic seizure prevention and treatment because of its depressant action on the central nervous system.

- ***Fluid and electrolyte replacement.*** The goal of fluid intake is to achieve a balance between correcting hypovolemia and preventing circulatory overload. Fluid intake may be oral or supplemented with IV therapy. IV fluids may be started "to keep lines open" in case they are needed for drug therapy even when oral intake is adequate. Electrolytes are replaced as indicated by daily serum electrolyte levels.

- ***Corticosteroids.*** Betamethasone or dexamethasone is often administered to the woman whose fetus has an immature lung profile. Corticosteroids may also have a beneficial effect in women with HELLP syndrome.

- ***Antihypertensives.*** Antihypertensive medications are the most commonly used methods of treatment. Antihypertensive therapy is generally given for sustained systolic blood pressure of at least 160 mmHg or diastolic blood pressures of 110 mmHg or higher (ACOG, 2013). Labetalol and hydralazine are first-line medications for the treatment of acute-onset, severe hypertension in pregnancy and are generally administered by IV boluses. Labetalol should be avoided in women with asthma or heart failure (ACOG, 2015). Oral nifedipine acts rapidly and has favorable hemodynamic effects and fewer side effects than IV hydralazine. If these medications are not successful in controlling blood pressure, sodium nitroprusside may be indicated for extreme emergencies and used for the shortest amount of time possible (ACOG, 2015). Methyldopa is often used for long-term control of mild to moderate hypertension in pregnancy because it is safe and effective.

SAFETY ALERT!

Nifedipine capsules should not be used in women with known coronary artery disease, those who have had diabetes mellitus for more than 15 years, or those who are older than 45 years of age because of the risk of sudden cardiac death. In contrast, long-acting oral nifedipine has been shown to be safe and effective (Mustafa, Ahmed, Gupta, et al., 2012).

Hospital Care of Eclampsia. An eclamptic seizure requires immediate, effective treatment. A bolus of 4 to 6 g magnesium sulfate is given intravenously in 100 mL IV fluid over 20 to 30 minutes followed by 2 g/hr IV infusion (Cunningham et al., 2014). Antihypertensive agents are used to keep the diastolic blood pressure between 90 and 100 mmHg, thus avoiding a potential reduction in uteroplacental blood flow or cerebral perfusion. A sedative such as diazepam or amobarbital is used only if the seizures are not controlled by magnesium sulfate. The lungs are auscultated for pulmonary edema. The woman

is observed for circulatory and renal failure and signs of cerebral hemorrhage. Furosemide (Lasix) may be given for pulmonary edema; digitalis may be given for circulatory failure. An indwelling Foley catheter is often inserted and intake and output are monitored hourly.

The woman is assessed for signs of labor. She is also checked every 15 minutes for evidence of vaginal bleeding and abdominal rigidity, which might indicate abruptio placentae. While she is comatose, she is positioned on her side with the side rails up.`

Because of the severity of her condition, the woman is often cared for in an intensive care unit. When the condition of the woman and the fetus have been stabilized, induction of labor is considered because birth is the only known cure for preeclampsia/eclampsia. The woman and her partner should be given a careful explanation about her status and that of her unborn child and the treatment they are receiving. Plans for further treatment and for birth must be discussed with them.

Intrapartum Management. Labor may be induced by IV oxytocin when there is evidence of fetal maturity and cervical readiness. In very severe cases, cesarean birth may be necessary even if the fetus is immature.

Assessment for signs of worsening preeclampsia continues. The woman may receive IV oxytocin and magnesium sulfate simultaneously. Infusion pumps should be used, and bags and tubing must be carefully labeled.

Narcotics may be given IV for pain relief in labor. An epidural, spinal, or combined spinal-epidural can be safely administered to the woman with preeclampsia in the absence of thrombocytopenia.

Electronic fetal monitoring is used to assess fetal status continuously. Birth in the Sims or semisitting position should be considered. If the lithotomy position is used, a wedge should be placed under the right buttock to displace the uterus. The wedge should also be used if birth is by cesarean. Oxygen is administered to the woman during labor if the need is indicated by fetal response to the contractions.

A pediatrician or neonatal nurse practitioner must be available to care for the newborn at birth. This caregiver must be informed of all amounts and times of medication the woman has received during labor.

Postpartum Management. The woman with preeclampsia usually improves rapidly after giving birth, although seizures can still occur during the first 48 hours postpartum. When the hypertension is severe, the woman may continue to receive antihypertensives or magnesium sulfate postpartum.

Nursing Management

For the Woman With Preeclampsia/Eclampsia

See *Nursing Care Plan: The Woman With Preeclampsia* for information on nursing care.

Nursing Assessment and Diagnosis

Take and record the blood pressure during each antepartum visit. If the blood pressure rises, or if the normal slight decrease in blood pressure expected between 8 and 28 weeks of pregnancy does not occur, the woman should be followed closely. Also check the woman's urine for proteinuria at each visit.

If hospitalization becomes necessary, assess the following:

- ***Blood pressure.*** Assess every 1 to 4 hours, or more frequently if indicated by medication or other changes in the woman's status.

Nursing Care Plan: The Woman With Preeclampsia

1. Nursing Diagnosis: *Fluid Volume: Deficient,* **related to fluid shift from intravascular to extravascular space secondary to vasospasm (NANDA-I © 2014)**

GOAL: Client is restored to normal fluid volume levels.

INTERVENTION	RATIONALE
• Encourage woman to lie in the left lateral recumbent position.	• The left lateral recumbent position decreases pressure on the vena cava, thereby increasing venous return, circulatory volume, and placental and renal perfusion. Angiotensin II levels are decreased when there is improved renal blood flow, which helps to promote diuresis and lower blood pressure.
• Assess blood pressure every 1 to 4 hours as necessary.	• Frequent monitoring will assess for progression of the disorder and allow for early intervention to ensure maternal and fetal health and well-being.
• Monitor urine for volume and proteinuria every shift or every hour per agency protocol.	• Monitoring provides information to assess renal perfusion. Proteinuria is the last cardinal sign of preeclampsia to appear. As the disorder worsens, the capillary walls of the glomerular endothelial cells stretch, allowing protein molecules to pass into the urine. Normally, urine does not contain protein. Readings of 3+ and 4+ indicate loss of 5 g or more protein in 24 hours. Urinary output decreases when there is a reduction of the glomerular filtration rate. Urinary output that falls below 30 mL per hour or less than 700 mL in a 24-hour period should be reported.
• Assess deep tendon reflexes and clonus.	• Hyperreflexia may occur as preeclampsia worsens. Eliciting deep tendon reflexes provides information about CNS status and is also used to assess for magnesium sulfate toxicity. Reflexes are graded on a scale of 0 to 4+ using the Deep Tendon Reflex Rating Scale. A rating of 4+ is abnormal and indicates hyperreflexia. A rating of 0 or no response is also abnormal and is seen with high maternal serum magnesium levels. Clonus, an abnormal finding, is present if the foot "jerks" or taps the examiner's hand, at which time the examiner counts the number of taps or beats. The presence of clonus indicates a more pronounced hyperreflexia and is indicative of CNS irritability.
• Assess for edema.	• Edema develops as fluid shifts from the intravascular to the extravascular spaces. Edema is assessed either by weight gain (more than 3.3 lb (1.5 kg)/month in the second trimester or more than 1.1 lb (0.5 kg)/week in the third trimester) or by assessing for pitting edema (assessed by using finger pressure to a swollen area, usually the lower extremities, and grading on a scale of 1+ to 4+).
• Administer magnesium sulfate per infusion pump as ordered.	• As preeclampsia worsens, the risk of an eclamptic seizure increases. Magnesium sulfate is the treatment of choice for seizures because of its CNS depressant action. As a secondary effect, magnesium sulfate relaxes smooth muscles and may therefore decrease the blood pressure. Magnesium sulfate is contraindicated in women with myasthenia gravis.
• Assess for magnesium sulfate toxicity.	• Side effects of magnesium sulfate are dose related. Therapeutic levels are in the range of 4.8–8.4 mg/dL. As maternal serum magnesium levels increase, toxicity may occur. Signs of toxicity include decreased or absent deep tendon reflexes (DTRs), urine output below 30 mL/hr, respirations below 12, and confusion.
• Provide a balanced diet that includes 80–100 g/day or 1.5 g/kg/day of protein.	• A diet rich in protein is necessary to replace protein that is excreted in the urine.

EXPECTED OUTCOME: The signs and symptoms of preeclampsia will diminish as evidenced by decreased blood pressure, urine protein levels of zero, and a return of the DTRs to normal.

(*continued*)

Nursing Care Plan: The Woman With Preeclampsia (*continued*)

2. Nursing Diagnosis: *Injury, Risk for,* to the fetus, related to uteroplacental insufficiency secondary to vasospasm (NANDA-I © 2014)

GOAL: The fetus avoids complications related to uteroplacental insufficiency.

INTERVENTION	RATIONALE
• Instruct client to count fetal movements 3 times a day for 20 to 30 minutes.	• Fetal activity provides reassurance of fetal well-being. Decrease in fetal movement or cessation of movement may indicate fetal compromise.
• Encourage client to rest in the left lateral recumbent position.	• Lying in the left lateral recumbent position decreases pressure on the vena cava, which increases venous return, circulatory volume, and placental and renal perfusion. Blood flow to the fetus is increased, thereby reducing the risk of fetal hypoxia and malnutrition.
• **Collaborative:** Assist with serial ultrasounds.	• Maternal vasospasm and hypovolemia result from preeclampsia, which may lead to intrauterine growth restriction and oligohydramnios. Ultrasound provides assessment of fetal growth and fluid levels.
• Perform non-stress test as ordered.	• A non-stress test is performed to assess the fetal heart rate in response to fetal movement. Accelerations of fetal heart rate with fetal movement may indicate the fetus has adequate oxygenation and an intact CNS. (Refer to Chapter 13 for interpretation of NST results.)
• Describe for the woman the purposes of a biophysical profile (BPP).	• Preeclampsia or eclampsia places the woman at risk for uteroplacental insufficiency due to the loss of normal vasodilation of uterine arterioles and maternal vasospasm. This results in decreased uteroplacental perfusion, which may lead to fetal hypoxia. A BPP is one assessment tool used to evaluate fetal well-being. Providing explanation of the diagnostic test helps relieve anxiety and ensures the woman understands what the test evaluates and what the results mean.
• Assist with amniocentesis to obtain lecithin/sphingomyelin (L/S) ratio.	• Women with preeclampsia may give birth before term. Amniotic fluid may be analyzed to determine the maturity of the fetal lungs. An L/S ratio of 2:1 or greater indicates fetal lung maturity and is usually achieved by 35–36 weeks' gestation.
• Explain the purpose of Doppler flow studies.	• Doppler flow studies (umbilical velocimetry) help to assess placental function and sufficiency. Uteroplacental insufficiency is a risk for a woman with preeclampsia. If fetal growth restriction is present, Doppler velocimetry of the umbilical artery is useful for fetal surveillance.

EXPECTED OUTCOME: The fetus will have an adequate supply of oxygen and nutrients as evidenced by absence of signs of nonreassuring fetal status and fetal diagnostic test results within normal limits.

3. Nursing Diagnosis: *Health Maintenance, Ineffective,* related to deficient knowledge about new diagnosis (preeclampsia) (NANDA-I © 2014)

GOAL: The woman will describe the condition and treatment regimen.

INTERVENTION	RATIONALE
• Assess the woman and the family's understanding of preeclampsia and its implications for pregnancy.	• This assessment provides information about the woman's cognitive level and her understanding of her diagnosis. Behavioral changes occur when teaching strategies are appropriate for the woman and family's cognitive level.
• Provide information about the disease process, impact on maternal well-being, risks of progression, implications for the fetus, and dangers of eclampsia.	• Basic understanding of the condition and its implications is necessary for the woman to understand the treatment plan. A woman who shows signs of early preeclampsia often feels well and may have difficulty accepting the need to rest.
• Emphasize the importance of self-monitoring for signs that her condition is worsening and the importance of regular prenatal care for the purpose of maternal and fetal surveillance.	• The woman should be able to identify signs of disease progression, including evidence of increasing edema, decreased urine output, signs of cerebral disturbance (frontal headache, blurred vision, scotomata), epigastric or right upper quadrant pain, nausea or vomiting, and increased irritability.

EXPECTED OUTCOME: Woman will demonstrate understanding of preeclampsia and its implications as evidenced by verbalization of basic condition, signs and symptoms of progression, importance of sufficient rest in side-lying position, and need to follow prescribed diet.

- *Temperature.* Take every 4 hours, or every 2 hours if elevated or if premature rupture of the membranes (PROM) has occurred.

- *Pulse and respirations.* Determine pulse rate and respirations along with blood pressure.

- *Fetal heart rate (FHR).* Check the FHR with the blood pressure, or monitor continuously with the electronic fetal monitor if the situation indicates.

- *Urinary output.* Measure every voiding. The woman frequently has an indwelling catheter. In this case, urine output can be assessed hourly. Output should be 700 mL or greater in 24 hours, or at least 30 mL/hr.

- *Urinary protein.* Evaluate urinary protein hourly if an indwelling catheter is in place or with each voiding. Readings of 3+ or 4+ indicate loss of 5 g or more of protein in 24 hours.

- *Urine specific gravity.* Check specific gravity of the urine hourly or with each voiding. Readings over 1.040 correlate with oliguria and proteinuria.

- *Weight.* Weigh the woman daily at the same time. She should be wearing the same robe or gown and slippers. Weighing may be omitted if the woman is to maintain strict bed rest.

- *Pulmonary edema.* Observe the woman for coughing, shortness of breath, or difficulty breathing. Auscultate the lungs for moist respirations.

- *Deep tendon reflexes.* Assess the woman for evidence of hyperreflexia in the brachial, wrist, patellar, or Achilles tendons (Table 15–1). The patellar reflex is the easiest to assess (Figure 15–3). Clonus, an abnormal finding, is assessed by vigorously dorsiflexing the foot while the knee is held in a fixed position. Normally, no clonus is present. Clonus is present if the foot "jerks" or taps the examiner's hand, at which time the examiner counts the number of taps or beats and records it as such. See Assessing Deep Tendon Reflexes and Clonus in the *Clinical Skills Manual* SKILLS .

- *Placental separation.* Assess hourly for vaginal bleeding and uterine rigidity.

- *Headache.* Ask about the existence and location of any headache and its response to acetaminophen.

- *Visual disturbance.* Ask about any visual blurring or changes or scotomata. The results of the daily funduscopic examination should be recorded in the medical record.

- *Epigastric pain.* Ask about any epigastric pain. It is important to differentiate it from simple heartburn, which tends to be familiar and less intense.

- *Laboratory blood tests.* Daily tests of hematocrit to measure hemoconcentration; blood urea nitrogen (BUN), creatinine, and uric acid levels to assess kidney function; clotting studies for signs of thrombocytopenia or DIC; liver

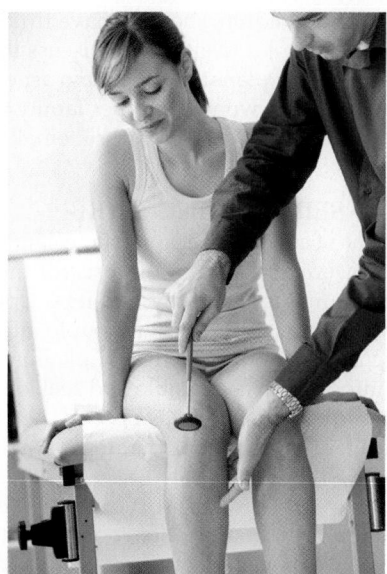

Figure 15–3 **Correct position for eliciting patellar reflex: sitting.**

SOURCE: © BSIP SA/Alamy.

enzymes; and electrolyte levels are all indicated. Magnesium levels are monitored regularly in women receiving magnesium sulfate.

- *Level of consciousness.* Observe the woman for alertness, mood changes, and any signs of impending convulsion.

- *Emotional response and level of understanding.* Carefully assess the woman's emotional response so that support and teaching can be planned accordingly.

In addition, assess the effects of any medications administered. Become familiar with the more commonly used medications and their purpose, implications, and associated untoward or toxic effects.

Examples of nursing diagnoses that might apply include the following (NANDA-I © 2014):

- *Fluid Volume: Deficient,* related to fluid shift from intravascular to extravascular space secondary to vasospasm

- *Injury, Risk for,* related to the possibility of seizure secondary to cerebral vasospasm or edema

Planning and Implementation

COMMUNITY-BASED NURSING CARE

A woman with preeclampsia may fear losing her fetus, worry about her personal relationship with her other children, and her personal and sexual relationship with her partner because of the limitations placed on her activities, be concerned about finances, and feel bored and a little resentful if she faces prolonged bed

TABLE 15–1 Deep Tendon Reflex Rating Scale

RATING	ASSESSMENT
4+	Hyperactive; very brisk, jerky, or clonic response; abnormal
3+	Brisker than average; may not be abnormal
2+	Average response; normal
1+	Diminished response; low normal
0	No response; abnormal

Health Promotion **Preeclampsia**

- The woman needs to know which symptoms are significant and should be reported at once.

- She is usually seen once or twice weekly. Explain that she may need to come in earlier than her next appointment if symptoms indicate that her condition is progressing.

rest. If she has small children, she may have trouble providing for their care. Help couples identify and discuss these concerns. Offer information and explanations if certain aspects of therapy cause difficulty. Refer the woman and her family to community resources such as support groups or homemaker services as appropriate.

HOSPITAL-BASED NURSING CARE

The development of severe preeclampsia/eclampsia is a cause for increased concern about the prognosis for the woman and her fetus. Explain medical therapy and its purpose and offer honest, hopeful information. Keep the couple informed of fetal status and discuss other concerns the couple may express. Provide as much information as possible and seek other sources of information or aid for the family as needed. Offer to contact a member of the clergy or hospital chaplain for additional support if the couple so chooses.

Maintain a quiet, low-stimulus environment for the woman. She should be in a private room in a quiet location where she can be watched closely. Limit visitors to close family members or main support persons. The woman should maintain the left lateral recumbent position most of the time, with side rails up for her protection.

Eliminate phone calls except for those that are planned because the phone ringing unexpectedly may be too jarring. To avoid a sense of isolation, however, some women find it preferable to take calls, but limit them to a certain time of day. Bright lights and sudden loud noises may precipitate seizures in the woman with severe preeclampsia.

Monitor the effectiveness of medications administered. Be alert for signs of untoward effects or developing toxic levels.

The occurrence of a convulsion is frightening to any family members who may be present, although the woman will not be able to recall it when she becomes conscious. Therefore, it is essential to offer explanations to the family members and the woman herself later.

SAFETY ALERT!

When caring for a woman with preeclampsia who is receiving IV magnesium sulfate, it is imperative to follow protocols for monitoring blood levels of magnesium. You are probably already aware of the common signs of increasing magnesium levels, such as diminished reflexes and decreased respiratory rate. However, you can also watch for some subtle clues that may suggest either the therapeutic or toxic range. When a woman's magnesium level is in the therapeutic range, she usually has some slurring of speech, awkwardness of movement, and decreased appetite. If the woman begins to have difficulty swallowing and begins to drool, she may be approaching the toxic range.

A grand mal seizure has both a tonic phase, marked by pronounced muscular contraction and rigidity, and a clonic phase, marked by alternate contraction and relaxation of the muscles, which causes the woman to thrash about wildly. When the tonic phase of the contraction begins, turn the woman to her side (if she is not already in that position) to aid circulation to the placenta. Turn her head face down to allow saliva to drain from her mouth. Attempting to insert a padded tongue blade is no longer advocated in many facilities; in others, it is used if it can be inserted without force because it may prevent injury to the woman's mouth. The side rails should be padded or a pillow put between the woman and each side rail.

After 15 to 20 seconds, the clonic phase starts. When the thrashing subsides, intensive monitoring and therapy begin. An oral airway is inserted, the woman's nasopharynx is suctioned, and oxygen is administered by nasal catheter. Fetal heart tones are monitored continuously. Monitor maternal vital signs every 5 minutes until they are stable, then every 15 minutes.

Nursing Management During Labor and Birth

Keep the woman positioned on her left side as much as possible. Carefully monitor both the woman and the fetus throughout labor. Note the progress of labor and remain alert for signs of worsening preeclampsia or its complications.

During the second stage of labor, encourage the woman to push in the side-lying position if possible. If she is unable to do so comfortably or effectively, she can be helped to a semisitting position for pushing and can then resume the lateral position between contractions. Birth is in the side-lying position or in the lithotomy position with a wedge placed under the woman's right hip. Encourage a family member or other support person to stay with the woman as much as possible. Keep the woman and her support person informed of the progress and plan of care. Whenever possible, respect their wishes concerning the birth experience.

Nursing Management During the Postpartum Period

Because the woman with preeclampsia is hypovolemic, even normal blood loss can be serious. Assess the amount of vaginal bleeding and observe the woman for signs of shock. Monitor blood pressure and pulse every 4 hours for 48 hours. Check hematocrit daily. Assess the woman for any further signs of preeclampsia. Measure intake and output. Normal postpartum diuresis helps eliminate edema and is a favorable sign.

Postpartum depression can develop after such a difficult pregnancy. To help prevent it, provide opportunities for frequent maternal–newborn contact and encourage family members to visit. The couple may have many questions, so be available for discussion. Give the couple family-planning information. Combined oral contraceptives may be used if the woman's blood pressure has returned to normal by the time they are prescribed (usually 4 to 6 weeks after birth).

Evaluation

Expected outcomes of nursing care include the following:

- The woman is able to explain preeclampsia/eclampsia, its implications for her pregnancy, the treatment regimen, and possible complications.
- The woman suffers no eclamptic seizures.
- The woman and her healthcare givers detect early evidence of increasing severity of the preeclampsia or possible complications so that treatment measures can be instituted.
- The woman gives birth to a healthy newborn.

Chronic Hypertension in Pregnancy

Chronic hypertension in pregnancy exists when the blood pressure is 140/90 mmHg or higher before pregnancy or before the 20th week of gestation (ACOG, 2013). The cause of chronic hypertension has not been determined. In most women, the disease is mild.

The woman is seen regularly for prenatal care (every 2 to 3 weeks during the first two trimesters and then weekly until birth). She is taught the importance of daily rest periods in the left lateral recumbent position and also learns to monitor her blood pressure at home. Sodium is limited to about 2.4 g/day.

Antihypertensive medication is generally used only for women with blood pressure over 160/105 mmHg or higher.

Labetalol, nifedipine, and methyldopa are the antihypertensives recommended when medication is required (ACOG, 2013).

SAFETY ALERT!
Before administering labetalol, be certain to check the woman's health history. Labetalol is contraindicated for people with bronchial asthma.

Twenty-four-hour urines, serum creatinine, uric acid, hematocrit, and ultrasound examinations are repeated at least once in the second and third trimesters.

Nursing care is directed at providing information so that the woman can meet her healthcare needs. Provide information about her diet, the need for regular rest, her medications, the need for blood pressure control, and any procedures used to monitor the well-being of her fetus.

Chronic Hypertension With Superimposed Preeclampsia

Preeclampsia may develop in women with chronic hypertension. After 20 weeks' gestation the onset of proteinuria and worsening hypertension are suggestive of superimposed preeclampsia. A rise in the serum uric acid level is helpful in identifying preeclampsia, which frequently occurs late in the second trimester or early in the third.

Gestational Hypertension

Gestational hypertension is characterized by hypertension occurring for the first time after midpregnancy without proteinuria. If preeclampsia does not develop and if the blood pressure returns to normal within 12 weeks following childbirth, the diagnosis of gestational hypertension may be assigned. If the blood pressure elevation persists after 12 weeks' postpartum, the woman is diagnosed with chronic hypertension.

Disseminated Intravascular Coagulation

Disseminated intravascular coagulation (DIC) occurs more often in pregnancies complicated by preeclampsia, abruptio placentae, intrauterine fetal demise, amniotic fluid embolism, maternal liver disease, and septic abortion. Although DIC is not considered a component of severe preeclampsia, eclampsia, or HELLP syndrome, it can occur as a complication when any of these conditions exist.

Clinical Reasoning Pregnancy Complication

Jillian Rundus is a 31-year-old G1P0 who is 35 weeks pregnant. She presents for a routine office visit with complaints of nausea and abdominal pain rating 7/10. She has had a headache and general malaise for 2 days. She denies visual changes. Upon examination, you find her to be alert and oriented and her physical examination is unremarkable with the exception of abdominal tenderness and a blood pressure of 170/110 mmHg. She has had no previous history of hypertension. Fetal heart rate ranges from 140 to 150 beats per minute.

What should the nurse do at this time?

DIC occurs when the normal clotting process is overactivated. In most instances, tissue factor entering the circulation is the primary trigger for DIC. When this occurs, there is an imbalance between the coagulation and the fibrinolytic systems. This mechanism leads to hemorrhage and shock. During these events, clots are being formed and fibrin is being deposited into the microcirculation, resulting in cell or tissue damage. This triggers further coagulation, which eventually depletes the plasma clotting factors. These fibrin clots can lead to intravascular obstruction and infarctions. In addition, the fibrinolytic system is activated, which results in the formation of fibrin-fibrinogen degradation products or fibrin split products. The release of these products decreases platelet functioning and further inhibits coagulation (Blackburn, 2013).

DIC is diagnosed when thrombocytopenia, low fibrinogen levels, and elevated fibrin split products are found in the laboratory findings. Serial platelet and serum fibrin degradation product counts are performed to monitor the mother's hematologic status. Supportive measures and reversing the causative factors are the primary interventions used to manage DIC.

Care of the Woman With a Perinatal Infection Affecting the Fetus

Fetal infection may develop at any time during pregnancy. In general, perinatal infections are most likely to cause harm when the embryo is exposed during the first trimester when organ development is occurring. Infections that occur later in pregnancy create other concerns such as growth restriction, preterm birth, and neurologic changes. (The acronym TORCH—to identify **to**xoplasmosis, **r**ubella, **c**ytomegalovirus, and **h**erpes—is occasionally used to identify the most common of these infections.) This section addresses several of the most commonly occurring viral and parasitic infections that may have an impact on the fetus if acquired during pregnancy.

Toxoplasmosis

Toxoplasmosis is caused by the protozoan *Toxoplasma gondii*. It is barely noticeable in adults, but, when contracted in pregnancy, it can profoundly affect the fetus and create long-term sequelae for affected children. The pregnant woman may contract the organism by eating raw or undercooked meat, by drinking unpasteurized goat's milk, or by contact with the feces of infected cats, either through the cat litter box or by gardening in areas frequented by cats.

FETAL/NEONATAL RISKS

The likelihood of fetal infection increases with each trimester of pregnancy, but the risk of serious impact on the fetus decreases. Thus maternal infection contracted during the first trimester is associated with the lowest incidence of fetal infection but the highest risk of severe fetal disease or death. The highest rate of fetal infection (72%) occurs when the mother contracts the infection in the third trimester, but most of these babies are born without clinical signs of infection (Duff, 2012). However, up to half of these babies will develop signs and symptoms if left untreated.

In mild cases, retinochoroiditis (inflammation of the retina and choroid of the eye) may be the only recognizable damage, and it and other manifestations may not appear until adolescence or young adulthood. Severe neonatal disorders associated with congenital infection include convulsions, coma, microcephaly, and hydrocephalus. The newborn with a severe infection may die soon after birth. Survivors are often blind, deaf, and have severe intellectual disabilities. Treatment of the mother can reduce the incidence of fetal infection and decrease the late sequelae of the infection (Duff, 2012).

CLINICAL THERAPY

Diagnosis can be made by serologic testing of antibody titers, specifically the IgG and IgM fluorescent antibody (IFA) tests. A positive IgG and negative IgM in the third trimester or any positive IgM result should be followed by confirmatory testing. The toxoplasmosis polymerase chain reaction (PCR) test of amniotic fluid is useful in diagnosing congenital toxoplasmosis. Ultrasound may be useful in detecting signs of fetal infection such as ascites, microcephaly, intracranial calcifications, and fetal growth restriction.

Pregnant women in whom maternal infection is established should receive spiramycin in the first and early second trimester and pyrimethamine/sulfadiazine and folinic acid (leucovorin) after the 18th week of pregnancy. Spiramycin is not commercially available in the United States, but it can be obtained for treatment through the Centers for Disease Control and Prevention (CDC). Newborns with congenital infection are treated with pyrimethamine, sulfadiazine, and leucovorin (Duff, 2012).

Nursing Management

For the Pregnant Woman With Toxoplasmosis

Nursing Assessment and Diagnosis

The incubation period for the disease is 10 days. The woman with acute toxoplasmosis may be asymptomatic, or she may develop myalgia, malaise, rash, splenomegaly, and enlarged posterior cervical lymph nodes. Symptoms usually disappear in a few days or weeks.

Nursing diagnoses that might apply include the following (NANDA-I © 2014):

- *Knowledge, Readiness for Enhanced,* related to a desire to understand the ways in which a pregnant woman can contract toxoplasmosis
- *Grieving* related to potential effects on baby of maternal toxoplasmosis

Planning and Implementation

During the antepartum period, discuss methods of preventing toxoplasmosis. The woman must understand the importance of avoiding poorly cooked or raw meat, especially pork, beef, lamb, and, in the Arctic region, caribou. Fruits and vegetables should be washed. She should avoid contact with the cat litter box and have someone else clean it frequently, since it takes approximately 48 hours for a cat's feces to become infectious. Stress the importance of wearing gloves when gardening and of avoiding garden areas frequented by cats.

Evaluation

Expected outcomes of nursing care include the following:

- The woman is able to discuss toxoplasmosis, its methods of transmission, the implications for her fetus, and measures she can take to avoid contracting it.
- The woman implements health measures to avoid contracting toxoplasmosis.
- The woman gives birth to a healthy newborn.

Rubella

The effects of rubella (German measles) on the fetus and newborn are great because rubella causes a chronic infection that begins in the first trimester of pregnancy and that may persist for months after birth. Fortunately, the success of the rubella vaccination program in the United States has led to a dramatic decrease in the incidence of rubella. Still, today there are pockets of unvaccinated people and cases continue to occur among babies born to women who emigrate from countries without rubella vaccination programs (American Academy of Pediatrics [AAP] & American College of Obstetricians and Gynecologists [ACOG], 2012).

FETAL/NEONATAL RISKS

The period of greatest risk for the effects of rubella on the fetus is the first trimester. Defects are rare when infection develops after 20 weeks' gestation (AAP & ACOG, 2012). The most common clinical signs of congenital infection include congenital cataracts, sensorineural deafness, and congenital heart defects, particularly patent ductus arteriosus. Other abnormalities, such as intellectual disability or cerebral palsy, may become evident in infancy. Diagnosis in the newborn can be made in the presence of these conditions and with an elevated rubella IgM antibody titer at birth. Babies born with congenital rubella syndrome are infectious and should be isolated.

CLINICAL THERAPY

The best therapy for rubella is prevention. Live attenuated vaccine is available and should be given to all children. Women of childbearing age should be tested for immunity and vaccinated if susceptible once it is established that they are not pregnant.

As part of the prenatal laboratory screen, the woman is evaluated for rubella using hemagglutination inhibition (HAI), a serology test. The presence of a 1:18 titer or greater is evidence of immunity. A titer less than 1:8 indicates susceptibility to rubella. Because the vaccine is made with attenuated virus, pregnant women are not vaccinated. However, it is considered safe for newly vaccinated children to have contact with pregnant women. Women whose titers indicate that they are susceptible to rubella should be given the rubella vaccine postpartally.

If a woman becomes infected during the first trimester, therapeutic abortion is a legally available alternative.

Nursing Management

For the Woman Who Develops Rubella During Pregnancy

Nursing Assessment and Diagnosis

The woman may be asymptomatic or may show signs of a mild infection including a maculopapular rash, lymphadenopathy, muscular achiness, and joint pain. The presence of IgM antirubella antibody is diagnostic of a recent infection. These titers remain elevated for approximately 1 month after infection.

Nursing diagnoses that may apply to the woman who develops rubella early in her pregnancy include the following (NANDA-I © 2014):

- *Coping, Ineffective,* resulting from an inability to accept the possibility of fetal anomalies secondary to maternal rubella exposure
- *Health Maintenance, Ineffective,* related to lack of knowledge about the importance of rubella immunization before becoming pregnant

Planning and Implementation

Support is vital for the couple considering abortion because of a diagnosis of rubella. Such a decision may trigger a crisis for the couple. The parents need objective data to understand the possible effects on their unborn fetus and the long-term prognosis.

Evaluation

Expected outcomes of nursing care include the following:

- The woman is able to describe the implications of rubella exposure during the first trimester of pregnancy.

- If exposure occurs in a woman who is not immune, she is able to identify her options and make a decision about continuing her pregnancy that is acceptable to her and her partner.

- The nonimmune woman receives the rubella vaccine during the early postpartum period.

- The woman gives birth to a healthy baby.

Cytomegalovirus

Cytomegalovirus (CMV) belongs to the herpesvirus group and causes both congenital and acquired infections that are referred to as cytomegalic inclusion disease (CID). This virus can be transmitted by asymptomatic women across the placenta to the fetus or by the cervical route during birth.

The virus can be found in virtually all body fluids. It can be passed between humans by any close contact, such as kissing, breastfeeding, and sexual intercourse. Asymptomatic CMV infection is particularly common in children and pregnant women. It is a chronic, persistent infection in that the individual may shed the virus continually over many years. The cervix can harbor the virus, and an ascending infection can develop after birth. Although the virus is usually innocuous in adults and children, it may be fatal to the fetus.

Accurate diagnosis in the pregnant woman is best documented by seroconversion. Identification of the virus in amniotic fluid by polymerase chain reaction (PCR) or viral culture is the most specific way of diagnosing congenital infection (Bernstein, 2012). Ultrasound findings may include fetal hydrops, growth restriction, hydramnios, cardiomegaly, and fetal ascites.

CMV is the most frequent cause of viral infection in the human fetus. Subclinical infections in the newborn can produce intellectual disability and hearing loss, sometimes not recognized for several months, or learning disabilities not seen until childhood. In children, congenital CMV is the leading cause of hearing loss (Bernstein, 2012).

For the fetus/newborn, serious long-term complications most often follow a primary maternal infection in the first half of pregnancy (Bernstein, 2012). For the fetus, this infection can result in extensive intrauterine tissue damage that leads to fetal death; to survival with microcephaly, hydrocephaly, cerebral palsy, or intellectual disability; or to survival with no damage at all. The infected newborn is often small for gestational age (SGA).

At present, no treatment exists for maternal CMV or for the congenital disease in the newborn, although a vaccine against CMV is under development and has shown promise (Anderson, 2015). Thus prevention is important. The pregnant woman should be advised to avoid areas with high concentrations of young children such as daycare centers, if possible, and to practice good handwashing techniques.

Herpes Simplex Virus

It has been estimated that one in six people between the ages of 14 and 49 (16.2%) is infected with genital herpes in the United States (Centers for Disease Control and Prevention [CDC], 2013a). Herpes simplex virus (HSV-1 or HSV-2) infection can cause painful lesions in the genital area. Lesions may also develop on the cervix. (This condition and its implications for nonpregnant women are discussed in Chapter 6.)

FETAL/NEONATAL RISKS

Primary infection poses the greatest risk to both the mother and her baby. Primary infection has been associated with spontaneous abortion, low birth weight, and preterm birth. Transmission to the fetus almost always occurs after the membranes rupture and the virus ascends or during birth through an infected birth canal. Transplacental infection is rare. The risk to the fetus varies with the route of birth and whether the lesion that is present at the time of birth is primary or recurrent. If HSV-1 or HSV-2 is acquired close to the time of labor, the risk of transmission is 30% to 50% for a vaginal birth. Exposure of the newborn to a *recurrent* lesion drops the risk of transmission to between 2% and 5% (AAP & ACOG, 2012).

The infected newborn is often asymptomatic at birth but develops symptoms of fever (or hypothermia), jaundice, seizures, and poor feeding any time after birth and up to 4 weeks of age. Approximately half of infected babies develop the characteristic vesicular skin lesions. All newborns who have neonatal herpes should be evaluated promptly and treated with acyclovir (AAP & ACOG, 2012).

CLINICAL THERAPY

The vesicular lesions of herpes have a characteristic appearance, and they rupture easily. Definitive diagnosis is made by culturing active lesions.

Women with a primary HSV infection during pregnancy can be treated with oral acyclovir or valacyclovir (CDC, 2015). Currently, there is no evidence that there are any adverse fetal effects related to exposure to any of these drugs during any trimester. For a woman with either a primary or a secondary outbreak of genital herpes during labor, or symptoms that may indicate an impending outbreak, the preferred method of childbirth is cesarean birth. Women who do not have any signs or symptoms of herpes or its prodromal symptoms at the onset of labor can give birth vaginally (CDC, 2015).

Nursing Management

For the Pregnant Woman With Herpes Simplex Virus Infection

Nursing Assessment and Diagnosis

During the initial prenatal visit, it is important to learn whether the woman or her partner has had previous herpes infections. If so, ongoing assessment is indicated as pregnancy progresses.

Nursing diagnoses that may apply include the following (NANDA-I © 2014):

- *Pain, Acute,* related to the presence of lesions secondary to herpes infection

- *Coping, Ineffective,* related to depression secondary to the risk to the fetus if herpes lesions are present at birth

Planning and Implementation

Client education about this fast-spreading disease is crucial. Inform women of the association of HSV infection with spontaneous abortion, newborn mortality and morbidity, and the possibility of cesarean birth. A woman needs to inform all healthcare providers of her infection. She should also know of the possible association of genital herpes with cervical cancer and the importance of a yearly Papanicolaou (Pap) smear.

The woman who acquired HSV infection as an adolescent may be devastated as a mature adult who wants to have a family. Counseling that allows her to express the negative feelings she may have about the infection may help. Literature may also help and is available from many public health agencies.

Evaluation

Expected outcomes of nursing care include the following:

- The woman is able to describe her infection with regard to its method of spread, therapy and comfort measures, implications for her pregnancy, and long-term implications.
- The woman gives birth to a healthy baby.

Group B Streptococcal Infection

Group B streptococcus (GBS) causes a bacterial infection found in the lower GI or urogenital tract. Women may transmit GBS to their fetus in utero or during childbirth. GBS is one of the major causes of early-onset neonatal infection. Newborns become infected in one of two ways: by vertical transmission from the mother during birth or from horizontal transmission from colonized nursing personnel or colonized babies. GBS causes severe, invasive disease in babies. In newborns, the majority of cases occur within the first week of life and are thus designated as early-onset disease. Late-onset disease occurs 1 week or more after birth.

Early-onset GBS is often characterized by signs of serious illness, including pneumonia, apnea, and shock. Late-onset GBS often manifests as meningitis or pneumonia. Long-term neurologic complications are common in both types of GBS.

Risk factors for GBS neonatal sepsis include young maternal age, African American or Hispanic race, preterm labor, maternal intrapartum fever, prolonged rupture of the membranes, previous birth of an infected baby, and GBS bacteriuria in the current pregnancy.

Guidelines for the detection and preventive treatment of newborns at risk include the following (CDC, 2010):

- All pregnant women should be screened for both vaginal and rectal GBS colonization at 35 to 37 weeks' gestation. Treatment should be based on these results, even if cultures were done earlier in pregnancy.
- Women with a positive GBS screen in late pregnancy should receive antibiotic prophylaxis at the onset of labor or the rupture of membranes.
- Women with GBS in their urine at any time during pregnancy should be treated according to guidelines for treating urinary tract infections (UTIs) during pregnancy and should receive antibiotic prophylaxis intrapartally. These women do not need vaginal and rectal cultures at 35 to 37 weeks because therapy is already indicated.
- Women who have already given birth to a newborn with invasive GBS disease should receive intrapartum antibiotic prophylaxis. Culture-based screening is not necessary for them.

- If the results of GBS screening are not known when labor begins, prophylaxis is indicated for women with any of the following risk factors: gestation less than 37 weeks, membranes ruptured 18 hours or longer, or temperature equal to or greater than 38.0°C (100.4°F).

Intrapartum antibiotic therapy is recommended as follows: initial dose of penicillin G 5 million units IV followed by 2.5 to 3 million units IV every 4 hours until childbirth. Alternatively, ampicillin may be used. In women at high risk for an anaphylactic reaction to penicillin because of marked allergy, testing is done to see if the organism is susceptible to clindamycin and erythromycin. If the organism is susceptible, clindamycin 900 mg IV every 4 hours until birth may be used. If the organism is resistant or if susceptibility testing is not done, vancomycin is administered 1 g IV every 12 hours until birth (ACOG, 2011; CDC, 2010a).

Other Infections in Pregnancy

Table 15–2 summarizes other urinary tract, vaginal, and sexually transmitted infections that contribute to risk during pregnancy. (These are described in more detail in Chapter 6.) Spontaneous abortion is frequently the result of a severe maternal infection. Some evidence links infection and prematurity. If the pregnancy is carried to term in the presence of infection, the risk of maternal and fetal morbidity and mortality increases. Thus it is essential to maternal and fetal health that infection be diagnosed and treated promptly.

> ### Clinical Reasoning Preventing Cystitis
>
> Your friend Jena Yoo, G1P0, is 6 months pregnant and mentions to you that she is developing symptoms of a bladder infection. She has had several bladder infections over the past few years and feels she has warded off others by increasing her fluid intake and drinking acidic juices. Jena tells you that she plans to use the same approach this time because she just had her prenatal appointment last week. She assures you that if symptoms persist, she will discuss it with her healthcare provider at her next prenatal visit. What advice would you give her?

Care of the Woman Requiring Surgery During Pregnancy

Although elective surgery should be delayed until the postpartum, essential surgery can generally be done during pregnancy. However, surgery poses some risks. The early second trimester is the best time to operate because there is less risk of spontaneous abortion or early labor, and the uterus is not so large as to impinge on the abdominal field.

General preoperative and postoperative care is similar for pregnant and nonpregnant women; however, special considerations must be kept in mind whenever the surgical client is pregnant. If a chest x-ray is done, the fetus should be shielded from radiation.

To prevent uterine compression of major blood vessels while the woman is supine, a wedge must be placed under the woman's right hip to tilt the uterus during both surgery and recovery. The decreased intestinal motility and delayed gastric emptying that occur in pregnancy increase the risk of vomiting when anesthetics are given and during the postoperative period.

TABLE 15–2 Infections That Put Pregnancy at Risk

CONDITION AND CAUSATIVE ORGANISM	SIGNS AND SYMPTOMS	TREATMENT	IMPLICATIONS FOR PREGNANCY
URINARY TRACT INFECTIONS (UTIs)			
Asymptomatic bacteriuria (ASB): *Escherichia, Klebsiella, Proteus* most common	Bacteria present in urine on culture with no accompanying symptoms.	Oral sulfonamides early in pregnancy, ampicillin and nitrofurantoin (Furadantin) in late pregnancy. Antibody sensitivity results will guide the selection of an appropriate antibiotic.	Women with ASB in early pregnancy may go on to develop cystitis or acute pyelonephritis by third trimester if not treated. They are also at risk for preterm labor. Oral sulfonamides taken in the last few weeks of pregnancy may lead to neonatal hyperbilirubinemia and kernicterus.
Cystitis (lower UTI): causative organisms same as for ASB	Dysuria, urgency, frequency; low-grade fever and hematuria may occur. Urine culture (clean catch) shows ↑ leukocytes. Presence of 10^5 (100,000) or more colonies bacteria/mL urine.	Same as for ASB.	If not treated, infection may ascend and lead to acute pyelonephritis.
Acute pyelonephritis: causative organisms same as for ASB	Sudden onset. Chills, high fever, flank pain. Nausea, vomiting, malaise. May have decreased urine output, severe colicky pain, dehydration. Increased diastolic BP, positive fluorescent antibody (FA) test, low creatinine clearance. Marked bacteremia in urine culture, pyuria, white blood cell (WBC) casts.	Hospitalization; IV antibiotic therapy. Other antibiotics safe during pregnancy include carbenicillin, methenamine, cephalosporins. Catheterization if output is ↓ or absent. Supportive therapy for comfort. Follow-up urine cultures are necessary.	Increased risk of preterm birth and intrauterine growth restriction (IUGR). Antibiotics used for treatment interfere with urinary estriol levels and can cause false interpretations of estriol levels during pregnancy.
VAGINAL INFECTIONS			
Vulvovaginal candidiasis (yeast infection): *Candida albicans*	Often thick, white, curdy discharge, severe itching, dysuria, dyspareunia. Diagnosis based on presence of hyphae and spores in a wet-mount preparation of vaginal secretions.	Only topical agents are recommended. Intravaginal insertion of azole preparations such as miconazole, butoconazole, or clotrimazole at bedtime for 7 days; Fluconazole is contraindicated in pregnancy (CDC, 2015).	If the infection is present at birth and the fetus is born vaginally, the fetus may contract thrush.
Bacterial vaginosis: *Gardnerella vaginalis*	Thin, watery, yellow-gray discharge with foul odor often described as "fishy." Wet-mount preparation reveals "clue cells." Application of potassium hydroxide (KOH) to a specimen of vaginal secretions produces a pronounced fishy odor.	Symptomatic pregnant women are treated with metronidazole (Flagyl) 500 mg PO BID × 7 days or metronidazole gel one applicatorful intravaginally daily × 5 days or clindamycin cream one applicatorful intravaginally at bedtime × 7 days (CDC, 2015).	CDC (2015) reports that multiple studies have failed to demonstrate a teratogenic effect from metronidazole. BV during pregnancy has been associated with premature rupture of the membranes and preterm birth.
Trichomoniasis: *Trichomonas vaginalis*	Occasionally asymptomatic. May have frothy greenish gray vaginal discharge, pruritus, urinary symptoms. Strawberry patches may be visible on vaginal walls or cervix. Wet-mount preparation of vaginal secretions shows motile flagellated trichomonads.	Single 2-g dose of metronidazole orally (CDC, 2015).	Increased risk for premature rupture of the membranes (PROM), preterm birth, and low birth weight.
SEXUALLY TRANSMITTED INFECTIONS			
Chlamydial infection: *Chlamydia trachomatis*	Women are often asymptomatic. Symptoms may include thin or purulent discharge, urinary burning and frequency, or lower abdominal pain. Lab test available to detect monoclonal antibodies specific for *Chlamydia*.	Doxycycline, ofloxacin, and levofloxacin are contraindicated during pregnancy. Thus pregnant women are treated with azithromycin or amoxicillin followed by repeat culture in 3 weeks (CDC, 2015).	Baby of woman with untreated chlamydial infection may develop newborn conjunctivitis, which can be treated with erythromycin eye ointment (but not silver nitrate). Newborn may also develop chlamydial pneumonia. May be responsible for premature labor and fetal death.

(continued)

TABLE 15–2 Infections That Put Pregnancy at Risk (*continued*)

CONDITION AND CAUSATIVE ORGANISM	SIGNS AND SYMPTOMS	TREATMENT	IMPLICATIONS FOR PREGNANCY
Syphilis: *Treponema pallidum*, a spirochete	Primary stage: chancre, slight fever, malaise. Chancre lasts about 4 weeks, then disappears. Secondary stage: occurs 6 weeks to 6 months after infection. Skin eruptions (condylomata lata); also symptoms of acute arthritis, liver enlargement, iritis, chronic sore throat with hoarseness. Diagnosed by blood tests such as VDRL, RPR, FTA, ABS. Darkfield examination for spirochetes may also be done.	For syphilis less than 1 year in duration: single dose of 2.4 million units benzathine penicillin G IM. For syphilis of more than 1 year's duration or latent syphilis of unknown duration: 2.4 million units benzathine penicillin G once a week for 3 weeks. The pregnant woman who is allergic to penicillin should be desensitized to it in the hospital and then treated with it (CDC, 2015). Sexual partners should also be screened and treated.	Syphilis can be passed transplacentally to the fetus. If untreated, one of the following can occur: second-trimester abortion, stillborn neonate at term, congenitally infected baby, uninfected live newborn.
Gonorrhea: *Neisseria gonorrhoeae*	Majority of women asymptomatic; disease often diagnosed during routine prenatal cervical culture. If symptoms are present, they may include purulent vaginal discharge, dysuria, urinary frequency, inflammation, and swelling of the vulva. Cervix may appear eroded.	Pregnant women are treated with ceftriaxone 250 mg in a single dose given IM and azithromycin 1 g orally as a single dose (CDC, 2015). All sexual partners are also treated.	Infection at time of birth may cause ophthalmia neonatorum in the newborn.
Condylomata acuminata (genital warts): caused by the human papillomavirus (HPV)	Soft, grayish pink lesions on the vulva, vagina, cervix, or anus.	Podophyllin, podofilox, sinecatechins, and imiquimod are contraindicated during pregnancy. Some caregivers recommend removing warts by surgical methods or laser because the warts can proliferate and become friable (bleed easily) during pregnancy but the results may be poor or incomplete (CDC, 2015).	Possible teratogenic effect of podophyllin. Large doses have been associated with fetal death. Cesarean birth is only indicated for women with warts that obstruct the pelvic outlet or if vaginal birth would result in significant bleeding (CDC, 2015).

Thus a nasogastric tube may be recommended before major surgery. An indwelling urinary catheter prevents bladder distention, decreases risk of injury to the bladder, and permits monitoring of output. Fetal heart rate (FHR) must be monitored electronically before, during, and after surgery.

Pregnancy causes increased secretions of the respiratory tract and engorgement of the nasal mucous membrane, often making breathing through the nose difficult. Consequently, pregnant women often need an endotracheal tube to maintain an airway during surgery. Spinal or epidural anesthesia is preferred because local anesthetics are not associated with birth defects. Caution must be exercised because this type of anesthesia may produce hypotension and respiratory apnea in the pregnant woman. Healthcare providers must guard against maternal hypoxia during surgery because uterine circulation will be decreased and fetal oxygenation can decline quickly. Blood loss is also monitored throughout the procedure and following it.

Postoperatively, encourage the woman to turn, breathe deeply, and cough regularly and to use any ventilation therapy, such as incentive spirometry, to avoid developing pneumonia. Sequential compression devices (SCDs) or support stockings during and after surgery help prevent venous stasis and the development of thrombophlebitis. Encourage leg exercises while the woman is confined to bed, and introduce ambulation as soon as possible.

Discharge teaching is very important. The woman and her family should understand what to expect regarding activity level, discomfort, diet, medications, and any special considerations. In addition, they should know the warning signs they need to report to the physician immediately.

Care of the Woman Suffering Major Trauma

Trauma complicates from 6% to 8% of pregnancies; trauma from motor vehicle crashes is the leading cause of fetal and maternal death (Mozurkewich & Pearlman, 2012). Falls and violence—including domestic violence—are the next most common causes of injury.

Late in pregnancy, when balance and coordination are affected, the woman may fall. Her protruding abdomen is vulnerable to a variety of minor injuries. The fetus is usually well protected by the amniotic fluid, which distributes the force of a blow equally in all directions, and by the muscle layers of the uterus and abdominal wall. In early pregnancy, while the uterus is still in the pelvis, it is shielded from blows by the surrounding pelvic organs, muscles, and bones.

Trauma that causes concern includes blunt trauma, penetrating abdominal injuries, and the complications of maternal shock, premature labor, and spontaneous abortion. Maternal mortality most often occurs from head trauma or hemorrhage. Uterine rupture is a rare but life-threatening complication of trauma. It may result from strong deceleration forces in an automobile crash, with or without seat belts. Traumatic separation of the placenta can occur, which causes a high rate of fetal mortality. Premature labor, often following rupture of membranes during a crash, is another serious hazard to the fetus. Premature labor can begin even if the woman is not injured. To help prevent trauma from automobile crashes, all pregnant women should wear both lap seat belts and shoulder harnesses.

Penetrating trauma most often results from gunshot wounds and stab wounds. The mother generally fares better than the fetus if the penetrating trauma involves the abdomen, as the enlarged uterus is likely to protect the mother's bowel from injury. Unfortunately, the fetal injury rate is high.

Treatment of major injuries during pregnancy focuses initially on lifesaving measures for the woman. Such measures include establishing an airway, controlling external bleeding, and administering IV fluid to alleviate shock. The woman must be kept on her left side to prevent further hypotension. Oxygen is administered. Fetal heart rate (FHR) and fetal movement are monitored. Exploratory surgery may be necessary following abdominal trauma to determine the extent of injuries. If the fetus is near term and the uterus has been damaged, cesarean birth is indicated. If the fetus is still immature, the uterus can often be repaired, and the pregnancy can continue until term.

In cases of trauma in which the mother's life is not directly threatened, fetal monitoring for a minimum of 4 hours is suggested if there are no contractions, vaginal bleeding, uterine tenderness, or leaking amniotic fluid (AAP & ACOG, 2012). Abruptio placentae may occur following a blow to the abdomen. Increased uterine irritability in the first few hours after trauma helps identify women who may be at risk for this potentially catastrophic complication.

When cardiopulmonary resuscitation (CPR) is performed on the pregnant woman late in gestation, perimortem cesarean birth is advocated if CPR is unsuccessful in the first 5 minutes. Chest compressions are less effective in the third trimester because of compression of the inferior vena cava by the gravid uterus. Cesarean birth alleviates this compression and improves resuscitation efforts in both the fetus and the mother.

Care of the Pregnant Woman Who Has Experienced Domestic Violence

Domestic violence, also called *intimate partner violence*, most often the intentional injury of a woman by her partner, frequently begins or increases during pregnancy. Estimates suggest that approximately 25% of women in the United States have experienced physical and/or sexual violence by a current or former intimate partner (Devi, 2012). Physical abuse may result in loss of pregnancy, preterm labor, low-birth-weight newborns, and fetal death. Abused women have significantly higher rates of complications such as anemia, infection, low weight gain, pelvic fracture, and placental abruption. Violence may escalate during pregnancy, and homicide by an

intimate partner is a significant cause of maternal mortality (ACOG, 2012c).

The first step toward helping the battered woman is to identify her. Asking every woman about abuse at various times during pregnancy is crucial because a woman may not disclose abuse until she knows her healthcare givers better. Screening for abuse should be done at the first prenatal visit, at least once each trimester, and then again during the postpartum period (ACOG, 2012c).

Chronic psychosomatic symptoms can be an indicator of abuse. The woman may have nonspecific or vague complaints. It is important to assess old scars around the head, chest, arms, abdomen, and genitalia. Any bruising or evidence of pain is also evaluated. Be especially alert for signs of bruising or injury to the woman's breasts, abdomen, or genitalia because these areas are common targets of violence during pregnancy. Other indicators include a decrease in eye contact; silence when the partner is in the room; and a history of nervousness, insomnia, drug overdose, or alcohol problems. Frequent visits to the emergency department and a history of accidents without understandable causes are possible indicators of abuse.

The goals of treatment are to identify the woman at risk, to increase her decision-making abilities to decrease the risk for further abuse, and to provide a safe environment for the woman and her unborn child. She needs to be aware of community resources available to her, such as emergency shelters; police, legal, and social services; and counseling. Ultimately, it is the woman's decision to either seek assistance or return to old patterns.

Because abuse often begins during pregnancy, it may be a new, unexpected experience for the woman, one she believes is an isolated incident. She needs to know that battering may continue after childbirth and may extend to the child as well. This is an important time to provide information and establish a trusted link for the woman with a healthcare professional. (For further discussion see Chapter 5.)

Care of the Woman at Risk for Rh Alloimmunization

The Rh blood group is present on the surface of erythrocytes of most of the population. When it is present, a person is said to be Rh positive. Those without the factor are Rh negative. If an Rh-negative individual is exposed to Rh-positive blood (antigen Rh[D]), an antigen–antibody response occurs, and the person forms anti-Rh agglutinin and is said to be sensitized. Subsequent exposure to Rh-positive blood can then cause a serious reaction that results in agglutination and hemolysis of red blood cells (RBCs). In the United States, about 15% to 18% of White Americans, 3% to 7% of African Americans, and 1% of Asian and Native Americans are Rh negative (Taylor, Uhlmann, Meyer, et al., 2011).

Rh alloimmunization (sensitization), also called *isoimmunization*, most often occurs when an Rh-negative woman carries an Rh-positive fetus, either to term or to termination by miscarriage or induced abortion. It can also occur if an Rh-negative nonpregnant woman receives an Rh-positive blood transfusion.

The red blood cells (RBCs) from the fetus invade the maternal circulation, thereby stimulating the production of Rh antibodies. Because this transfer of RBCs usually occurs at birth, the first child is not affected. In a subsequent

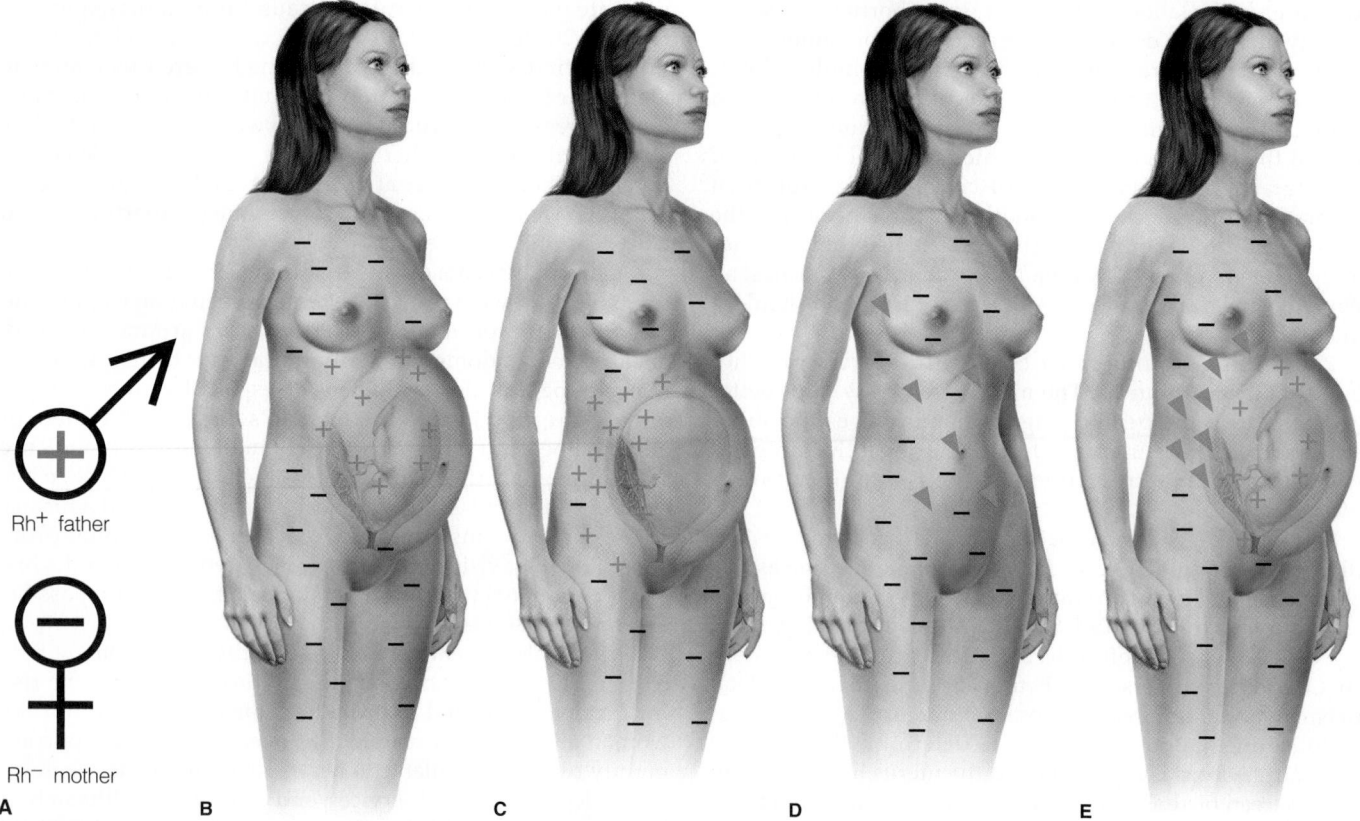

Figure 15–4 Rh alloimmunization sequence. *A*, Rh-positive father and Rh-negative mother. *B*, Pregnancy with Rh-positive fetus. Some Rh-positive blood enters the mother's bloodstream. *C*, As the placenta separates, the mother is further exposed to the Rh-positive blood. *D*, Anti–Rh-positive antibodies (triangles) are formed. *E*, In subsequent pregnancies with an Rh-positive fetus, Rh-positive red blood cells are attacked by the anti–Rh-positive maternal antibodies, causing hemolysis of the red blood cells in the fetus.

pregnancy, however, Rh antibodies cross the placenta and enter the fetal circulation, causing severe hemolysis. The destruction of fetal RBCs causes anemia in the fetus (Figure 15–4).

Healthy People 2020

(BDBS-18.4) Reduce the proportions of persons who develop adverse events due to alloimmunization among persons with hemoglobinopathies

---

Fetal-Neonatal Risks

Although maternal sensitization can now be prevented by administration of **Rh immune globulin (RhoGAM**, WinRho-SDF), the incidence of alloimmunization has increased in recent years because of the migration of Rh-negative sensitized women from countries with lower healthcare standards or limited resources to developed countries (Bettelheim et al., 2010). If treatment with Rh immune globulin is not initiated, the anemia resulting from this disorder can cause marked fetal edema, called **hydrops fetalis**. Congestive heart failure may result; marked jaundice (called *icterus gravis*), which can lead to neurologic damage (*kernicterus*), is also possible. This severe hemolytic syndrome is known as **erythroblastosis fetalis**.

SCREENING FOR Rh INCOMPATIBILITY AND SENSITIZATION

At the first prenatal visit, healthcare providers should do the following:

1. Take a history of past pregnancies, previous sensitization, abortions, blood transfusions, or children who developed jaundice or anemia during the newborn period.
2. Determine maternal blood type (ABO) and Rh factor and do a routine Rh antibody screen.
3. Identify other medical complications such as diabetes, infections, or hypertension.

An antibody screen (*indirect Coombs test*) is done to determine whether an Rh-negative woman is sensitized (has developed isoimmunity) to the Rh antigen. The test measures the number of antibodies in the maternal blood. If the pregnant woman is not sensitized, a second antibody screening test is done at 28 weeks' gestation. If the maternal antibody screen is positive, a maternal antibody titer is obtained. A woman with an elevated antibody titer should be considered sensitized and her pregnancy should be managed closely.

Clinical Therapy

ANTEPARTUM MANAGEMENT

If the antibody screen obtained at 28 weeks' gestation is negative, the woman is given an IM injection of 300 mcg Rh immune globulin as a prophylactic (preventive) measure. The Rh immune globulin provides passive antibody protection against Rh antigens. This "tricks" the body, which does not then produce antibodies of its own (active immunity). As discussed later, Rh immune globulin is also given postpartum.

If the woman is Rh negative (dd), the father of the unborn child is asked to come into the clinic or physician's office to be assessed for his Rh factor and blood type. If he is homozygous for Rh positive (DD), all his offspring will be Rh positive. If he is heterozygous (Dd), 50% of his offspring will be Rh negative and 50% heterozygous for Rh positive. If the father is Rh negative, all their children will be Rh negative, and no Rh incompatibility with the mother will occur. If the father is heterozygous or if paternity is questionable or unknown, fetal DNA testing should be done to determine the fetal Rh status. If the father is Rh negative, or if the fetus is Rh negative, no further intervention is needed (Moise, 2012).

When the woman is Rh negative and not sensitized and the father is Rh positive or unknown, Rh immune globulin is also given after each abortion (whether spontaneous or induced), ectopic pregnancy, hydatidiform mole, chorionic villus sampling (CVS), amniocentesis, placenta previa with bleeding, percutaneous umbilical blood sampling (PUBS), blunt trauma to the abdomen, external cephalic version, suspected abruption, or stillbirth.

Two primary interventions can help the fetus whose blood cells are being destroyed by maternal antibodies: early birth and intrauterine transfusion. Both carry risks. Ideally, birth should be delayed until fetal maturity is confirmed at about 36 to 37 weeks.

Ultrasound should be done at 14 to 16 weeks to determine gestational age. Ultrasound can also be used to detect ascites and subcutaneous edema, which are signs of severe fetal involvement. Other indicators of the fetal condition include an increase in fetal heart size and hydramnios.

Doppler ultrasound to measure peak systolic velocity in the middle cerebral artery (MCA-PSV) of the fetus is now the standard of care to detect fetal anemia (Taylor et al., 2011). The decreasing fetal red cell mass and concurrent decrease in blood viscosity result in an increase in fetal cardiac output and an increase in the velocity of blood flow through the middle cerebral artery, which is demonstrated by an increase in the peak systolic velocities. MCA-PSV trends over time correlate well with increasing levels of bilirubin in the amniotic fluid and should be monitored regularly starting at 15 to 18 weeks. After 35 weeks' gestation, the false-positive rate for the prediction of anemia increases (Taylor et al., 2011).

Historically, management of Rh disease was done with ΔOD (delta optical density) analysis, a test that determines the amount of bilirubin pigment found in the amniotic fluid. Normally, the concentration of bilirubin pigments in the amniotic fluid declines during pregnancy. Elevated bilirubin levels are significant. Because the amount of bilirubin found in the amniotic fluid correlates roughly with the extent of the hemolysis, the ΔOD analysis serves as an indirect predictor of the severity of the fetal anemia. It should only be used if MCA screening is not available.

Negative antibody titers can consistently identify the fetus not at risk. However, the titers cannot reliably point out the fetus in danger because titer level does not always correlate with the severity of the disease. Thus, if the maternal antibody titer is 1:16 or greater, further testing is indicated.

If MCA-PSV indicates severe fetal anemia or if fetal hydrops is present, percutaneous umbilical blood sampling (PUBS) may be performed to determine fetal hematocrit. If the hematocrit is low (generally less than 30%), the fetus is given an intrauterine blood transfusion either intravascularly through PUBS or intraperitoneally. If the fetal hematocrit is greater than 30%, the PUBS is repeated in 1 to 2 weeks (Moise & Argoti, 2012). Severely sensitized fetuses may require birth at 32 to 34 weeks.

Previously, PUBS was the only direct method of assessing the Rh status of a fetus in planning the care of a woman who is Rh negative and sensitized. Fetal Rh genotyping from maternal blood is now available and has been shown to be highly accurate (Moise & Argoti, 2012).

POSTPARTUM MANAGEMENT

The Rh-negative mother who has no antibody titer (indirect Coombs test negative, nonsensitized) and has given birth to an Rh-positive fetus (direct Coombs test negative) is given an injection of Rh immune globulin within 72 hours of childbirth so that she does not have time to produce antibodies to fetal cells that entered her bloodstream when the placenta separated. A standard dose of Rh immune globulin can prevent sensitization after exposure of up to 30 mL of Rh(D) positive blood. Rh immune globulin provides her with temporary passive immunity, which prevents the development of permanent active immunity (antibody formation).

Rh immune globulin is not given to the newborn or the father. It should not be given to a previously sensitized woman. However, sometimes after birth or an abortion, the results of the blood test do not clearly show whether the mother is already sensitized to the Rh antigen. In such cases, the Rh immune globulin is given; it will cause no harm (Table 15–3).

TABLE 15–3 Rh Alloimmunization

When trying to work through Rh problems, remember the following:

- A potential problem exists when an Rh-negative mother and an Rh-positive father conceive a child who is Rh positive.
- In this situation, the mother may become sensitized or produce antibodies to her fetus's Rh-positive blood.

The following tests are used to detect sensitization:

- Indirect Coombs test—done on the mother's blood to measure the number of Rh-positive antibodies.
- Direct Coombs test—done on the baby's blood to detect antibody-coated Rh-positive red blood cells.

Based on the results of these tests, the following may be done:

- If the mother's indirect Coombs test is negative and the baby's direct Coombs test is negative (confirming that sensitization has not occurred), the mother is given Rh immune globulin within 72 hours of birth.
- If the mother's indirect Coombs test is positive and her Rh-positive newborn has a positive direct Coombs test, Rh immune globulin is not given; in this case the baby is carefully monitored for hemolytic disease.
- It is recommended that Rh immune globulin be given at 28 weeks antenatally to decrease possible transplacental bleeding concerns.

Rh immune globulin is also administered after each abortion (spontaneous or therapeutic), antepartum hemorrhage, mismatched blood transfusion, ectopic pregnancy, amniocentesis, chorionic villi sampling (CVS), percutaneous umbilical blood sampling (PUBS), fetal cephalic version, or maternal trauma.

Nursing Management

For the Pregnant Woman With Alloimmunization

Nursing Assessment and Diagnosis

As part of the initial prenatal history, ask the mother if she knows her blood type and Rh factor. Many women are aware that they are Rh negative and that this status has implications for pregnancy. Ask the woman if she has ever received Rh immune globulin, if she has had any previous pregnancies and their outcomes, and if she knows her partner's Rh factor. If the partner is Rh negative, there is no risk to the fetus, who will also be Rh negative. If the woman does not know what Rh type she is, intervention begins after the initial laboratory data are obtained. Plan care based on the findings.

If the woman becomes sensitized during her pregnancy, nursing assessment focuses on the knowledge and coping skills of the woman and her family. After birth, review data about the Rh type of the fetus. If the newborn is Rh positive, the mother is Rh negative, and no sensitization has occurred, it is necessary to administer Rh immune globulin.

Nursing diagnoses that might apply include the following (NANDA-I © 2014):

- *Knowledge, Readiness for Enhanced*, about the purpose of Rh immune globulin related to an expressed desire to understand the treatment of Rh incompatibility.
- *Coping, Ineffective*, related to depression secondary to the development of indications of the need for fetal exchange transfusion

Planning and Implementation

During the antepartum period, explain the mechanisms involved in alloimmunization (isoimmunization) and answer any questions the woman and her partner have. It is imperative that the woman understand the importance of receiving Rh immune globulin after every miscarriage, abortion, or ectopic pregnancy. In addition, explain the purpose of the Rh immune globulin administered at 28 weeks' gestation if the woman is not sensitized.

If the woman is sensitized to the Rh factor, it poses a threat to any Rh-positive fetus she carries. Provide emotional support to the family to help the members deal with their concerns and any feelings of guilt about the baby's condition. If an intrauterine transfusion becomes necessary, provide support while also assuming responsibility as part of the healthcare team. During labor, when caring for an Rh-negative woman who has not been sensitized, ensure that the woman's blood is assessed for any antibodies and that it has also been cross-matched for Rh immune globulin. The postpartum nurse is usually responsible for administering the Rh immune globulin IM if the newborn is Rh positive. See Intramuscular Administration of Rh Immune Globulin in the *Clinical Skills Manual* SKILLS.

Evaluation

Expected outcomes of nursing care include the following:

- The woman is able to explain the process of Rh sensitization and its implications for her unborn child and for subsequent pregnancies.
- If the woman has not been sensitized, she is able to discuss the importance of receiving Rh immune globulin when necessary and cooperates with the recommended dosage schedule.
- The woman gives birth to a healthy newborn.
- If complications develop for the fetus or newborn, they are detected quickly and therapy is instituted.

Care of the Woman at Risk from ABO Incompatibility

ABO incompatibility is somewhat common but rarely causes significant hemolysis. In most cases, ABO incompatibility is limited to type O mothers with a type A or B fetus. The group B fetus of a group A mother and the group A fetus of a group B mother are only occasionally affected. Group O babies, because they have no antigenic sites on the red blood cells (RBCs), are never affected regardless of the mother's blood type. The incompatibility occurs as a result of the maternal antibodies present in her serum and interaction between the antigen sites on the fetal RBCs.

Anti-A and anti-B antibodies are naturally occurring; that is, women are naturally exposed to the A and B antigens through the foods they eat and through exposure to infection by gram-negative bacteria. As a result, some women have high serum anti-A and anti-B titers before they become pregnant. Once they become pregnant, the maternal serum anti-A and anti-B antibodies cross the placenta and produce hemolysis of the fetal red blood cells. With ABO incompatibility, the first baby is often involved, and no relationship exists between the appearance of the disease and repeated sensitization from one pregnancy to the next.

Unlike Rh incompatibility, antepartum treatment is not warranted. As part of the initial assessment, however, note whether the potential for an ABO incompatibility exists (type O mother and type A or B father). This alerts healthcare givers so that, following birth, the newborn can be assessed carefully for the development of hyperbilirubinemia. (For a discussion of hyperbilirubinemia, see Chapter 27.) Affected neonates usually have only mild anemia, and the severity of the disease demonstrated with the first-born baby is generally similar in all subsequent pregnancies.

Focus Your Study

- Several health problems associated with bleeding arise from the pregnancy itself, such as spontaneous abortion, ectopic pregnancy, and gestational trophoblastic disease. The nurse needs to be alert to early signs of these situations, to guard the woman against heavy bleeding and shock, to facilitate the medical treatment, and to provide educational and emotional support.

- Hyperemesis gravidarum, excessive vomiting during pregnancy, may cause fluid and electrolyte imbalance, dehydration, and signs of starvation in the mother and, if severe enough, death of the fetus. Treatment is aimed at controlling the vomiting, correcting fluid and electrolyte imbalance, correcting dehydration, and improving nutritional status.

- Hypertension may exist before pregnancy or, more often, may develop during pregnancy. Preeclampsia can lead to growth retardation for the fetus and, if untreated, may lead to convulsions (eclampsia) and even death for the mother and fetus. A woman's understanding of the disease process helps motivate her to maintain the required rest periods in the left lateral position.

- Therapy for severe preeclampsia usually includes bed rest, antihypertensives, anticonvulsive drugs, and careful monitoring of mother and fetus. Corticosteroids may also be indicated.

- Toxoplasmosis, rubella, cytomegalovirus, herpes, group B streptococcus (GBS) infection, and other perinatal infections all pose a grave threat to the fetus. Prevention is the best therapy. There is no known treatment for rubella or parvovirus B19, but antimicrobial drugs are available for toxoplasmosis, herpes, and GBS. A vaccine for CMV may be available in the near future.

- Universal screening for GBS is now recommended for all pregnant women at 35 to 37 weeks' gestation.

- The impact of surgery or trauma on the pregnant woman and her fetus is related to timing in the pregnancy, seriousness of the situation, and other factors influencing the situation.

- Physical violence often begins or continues during pregnancy. The nurse needs to be alert for signs of abuse, including bruising or injury to the breasts, abdomen, and genitals. The nurse should provide the woman information about violence and about community resources available to assist her.

- Rh incompatibility can exist when an Rh-negative woman and an Rh-positive partner conceive a child who is Rh positive. The use of Rh immune globulin has greatly decreased the incidence of severe sequelae due to Rh incompatibility because the drug "tricks" the body into thinking antibodies have been produced in response to the Rh antigen.

Clinical Reasoning in Action

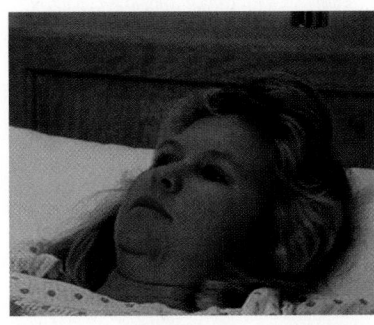

Carol Smith, a 40-year-old, single, G2P0010, presents to you at 32 weeks' gestation while you are working in the birthing unit. Her chief complaint is severe headache, nausea, and trouble seeing. She describes "blackened areas" in her visual fields bilaterally. Her prenatal record reveals long-term substance abuse, depression, and hypertension currently treated with nifedipine 60 mg by mouth once in the morning. You note that she has had two prenatal visits with this pregnancy. You determine her blood pressure to be 170/110 mmHg; deep tendon reflexes are 3+, clonus negative. She has general edema and 3+ proteinuria. You place Carol on the external fetal monitor to observe for fetal well-being and any contractions. You position her on her left side with her head elevated and use pillows for comfort.

You observe that the fetal heart rate is 143–148 beats/min with decreased variability. No fetal heart rate decelerations or accelerations are noted. The uterus is soft, and no contractions are palpated or noted on the fetal monitor.

Carol asks you why she should stay on her left side.

1. How would you explain the importance of the left side-lying position when on bed rest?

2. You administer nifedipine 10 mg sublingual and a loading dose of magnesium sulfate 4 g IV piggyback to the main IV line of Ringer lactate. What findings would indicate that Carol has therapeutic levels of magnesium?

3. What signs of magnesium toxicity should you monitor Carol for?

4. Carol asks if magnesium sulfate will affect her baby. How would you answer her?

5. Which signs of premature labor would you ask Carol to notify you of if she experiences them?

References

American Academy of Pediatrics (AAP) & American College of Obstetricians and Gynecologists (ACOG). (2012). *Guidelines for perinatal care.* Elk Grove Village, IL: Author.

American College of Obstetricians and Gynecologists (ACOG). (2011). *Prevention of early-onset group B streptococcal disease in newborns* (Committee Opinion No. 485). Washington, DC: Author.

American College of Obstetricians and Gynecologists (ACOG). (2012a). *Diagnosis and management of preeclampsia and eclampsia* (ACOG Practice Bulletin No. 33). Washington, DC: Author.

American College of Obstetricians and Gynecologists (ACOG). (2012b). *Diagnosis and treatment of gestational trophoblastic disease* (ACOG Practice Bulletin No. 53). Washington, DC: Author.

American College of Obstetricians and Gynecologists (ACOG). (2012c). *Intimate partner violence* (Committee Opinion No. 518). Washington, DC: Author.

American College of Obstetricians and Gynecologists (ACOG). (2013). Hypertension in pregnancy. Washington, DC: Author.

American College of Obstetricians and Gynecologists (ACOG). (2015). *Emergent therapy for acute-onset,* severe hypertension during pregnancy and the postpartum period (Committee Opinion No. 623. Replaces No. 514). Washington, DC: Author.

Anderson, D. E. (2015). VBI vaccines: Manufacture and purification of a third generation VLP for cytomegalovirus. Presented at the World Vaccine Congress, April 8, 2015. Retrieved from http://1o976r1jw2e culmeoxz46ig6.wpengine.netdna-cdn.com/wp-content /uploads/2015/04/VBI-Presentation-World-Vaccine -Congress-2015.pdf

Bernstein, H. B. (2012). Maternal and perinatal infection—Viral. In S. G. Gabbe, J. R. Niebyl, J. L. Simpson, M. B. Landon, H. L. Galan, E. R. M. Jauniaux, & D. A. Driscoll (Eds.), Obstetrics: Normal and problem pregnancies (6th ed.). Philadelphia, PA: Elsevier Saunders.

Bettelheim, D., Panzer, S., Reesink, H. W., Csapo, B., Pessoa, C., Guerra, F., . . . Holzgreve, W. (2010). Monitoring and treatment of anti-D in pregnancy. Vox Sanguinis: The International Journal of Transfusion Medicine, 99, 177–192.

Blackburn, S. T. (2013). Maternal, fetal, and neonatal physiology: A clinical perspective (4th ed.). St. Louis, MO: Saunders.

Centers for Disease Control and Prevention (CDC). (2010). Prevention of perinatal group B streptococcal disease: Revised guidelines from CDC, 2010. Morbidity and Mortality Weekly Report, 59 (RR10), 1–32.

Centers for Disease Control and Prevention (CDC). (2013). Genital herpes—CDC fact sheet. Retrieved from http://www.cdc.gov/std/Herpes/STDFact-Herpes.htm

Centers for Disease Control and Prevention (CDC). (2015). Sexually transmitted diseases treatment guidelines, 2015. Morbidity and Mortality Weekly Report, 64 (RR3), 1–137.

Cunningham, F. G., Leveno, K. J., Bloom, S. L., Spong, C. Y., Dashe, J. S., Hoffman, B. L., . . . Sheffield, J. S. (2014). Williams obstetrics (24th ed.). New York, NY: McGraw-Hill.

Devi, S. (2012). US guidelines for domestic violence screening spark debate. The Lancet, 379, 506.

DiGiulio, M., Wiedaseck, S., & Monchek, R. (2012). Understanding hydatidiform mole. American Journal of Maternal–Child Nursing, 37(1), 30–34.

Duff, P. (2012). Maternal and perinatal infection—Bacterial. In S. G. Gabbe, J. R. Niebyl, J. L. Simpson, M. B. Landon, H. L. Galan, E. R. M. Jauniaux, & D. A. Driscoll (Eds.), Obstetrics: Normal and problem pregnancies (6th ed.). Philadelphia, PA: Elsevier Saunders.

Harms, R. W. (2012). Is it safe to use a hot tub during pregnancy? Retrieved from http://www .mayoclinic.org/healthy-living/pregnancy-week -by-week/expert-answers/pregnancy-and-hot -tubs/faq-20057844

Jurkovic, D., & Wilkinson, H. (2011). Diagnosis and management of ectopic pregnancy. British Medical Journal, 342, d3397. doi:10.1136/bmj.d3397

Lipscomb, G. H. (2012). Medical management of ectopic pregnancy. Clinical Obstetrics and Gynecology, 55(2), 424–432.

Mansour, G. M., & Nashaat, E. H. (2011). Role of helicobacter in the pathogenesis of hyperemesis gravidarum. Archives of Gynecology and Obstetrics, 284(4), 843–847.

Mao, D., Che, J., Li, K., Han, S., Qi, Y., Wei, Z., & Lin, L. (2010). Association of homocysteine, asymmetric dimethylarginine, and nitric oxide with preeclampsia. Archives of Gynecology and Obstetrics, 282, 371–375.

Marion, L. B., & Meeks, G. R. (2012). Ectopic pregnancy: History, incidence, epidemiology, and risk factors. Clinical Obstetrics and Gynecology, 55(2), 376–386.

Moise, K. J. (2012). Red cell alloimmunization. In S. G. Gabbe, J. R. Niebyl, J. L. Simpson, M. B. Landon, H. L. Galan, E. R. M. Jauniaux, & D. A. Driscoll (Eds.), Obstetrics: Normal and problem pregnancies (6th ed.). Philadelphia, PA: Elsevier Saunders.

Moise, K. J., & Argoti, P. S. (2012). Management and prevention of red cell alloimmunization in pregnancy: A systematic review. Obstetrics & Gynecology, 5, 1132–1139.

Mozurkewich, E. L., & Pearlman, M.D. (2012). Trauma and related surgery in pregnancy. In S. G. Gabbe, J. R. Niebyl, J. L. Simpson, M. B. Landon, H. L. Galan, E. R. M. Jauniaux, & D. A. Driscoll (Eds.), Obstetrics: Normal and problem pregnancies (6th ed.). Philadelphia, PA: Elsevier Saunders.

Mustafa, R., Ahmed, S., Gupta, A., & Venuto, R. C. (2012). A comprehensive review of hypertension in pregnancy. Journal of Pregnancy, 2012, 1–20. doi:10.1155/2012/105918

Nayeri, U. A. (2012). Hyperemesis in pregnancy: Taking a tiered approach. Contemporary OB/GYN, 57(7), 22–31.

Niemeijer, M., Grooten, J., Vos, N., Bais, J., van der Post, J., Mol, B., . . . Painter, R. (2014). Diagnostic markers for hyperemesis gravidarum: A systematic review and meta-analysis. American Journal of Obstetrics and Gynecology, 211(150), e1–e15.

Pflueger, S. M.V. (2013). The cytogenics of SAB. In S.L. Gersen & M.B. Keagle (Eds.), The principles of clinical cytogenetics (3rd ed.). New York, NY: Springer.

Salani, R., Eisenhauer, E. L., & Copeland, L. J. (2012). Malignant diseases and pregnancy. In S. G. Gabbe, J. R. Niebyl, J. L. Simpson, M. B. Landon, H. L. Galan, E. R. M. Jauniaux, & D. A. Driscoll (Eds.), Obstetrics: Normal and problem pregnancies (6th ed.). Philadelphia, PA: Elsevier Saunders.

Shaban, M. M., Kandil, H. O., & Elshafei, A. H. (2014). Helicobacter pylori seropositivity in patients with hyperemesis gravidarum. The American Journal of the Medical Sciences, 347(2), 101–105.

Taylor, M., Uhlmann, R. A., Meyer, N. L., & Mari, G. (2011). Hemolytic disease: Diagnosis, counseling, and management. Contemporary OB/GYN, 56(6), 34–45.

U.S. Food and Drug Administration (FDA). (2013). FDA approves Diclegis for pregnant women experiencing nausea and Vomiting. Retrieved from http://www.fda .gov/newsevents/newsroom/pressannouncements /ucm347087.htm?source=govdelivery

Visconti, K., & Zite, N. (2012). hCG in ectopic pregnancy. Clinical Obstetrics and Gynecology, 55(2), 410–417.

Chapter 16
Processes and Stages of Labor and Birth

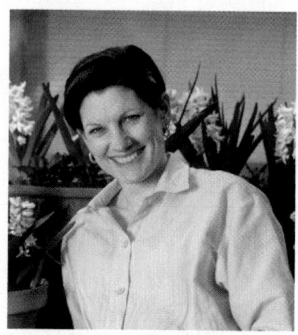

Leanne Temme/Getty Images

I think experts refer to us as a blended family. I have two sons, ages 12 and 9, from a previous marriage. They live part-time with us and part-time with their father. My husband has a 15-year-old daughter who lives with her mother. Here I am, 6 months pregnant with our first child together. It has been quite the time, getting used to the idea of a baby and trying to include our children in the pregnancy. They have all heard the heartbeat and felt the baby move. My sons are pretty blasé about it. I didn't know how Jack's daughter would respond but she has been great. Maybe this new baby will help us all grow closer together. I sure hope so.

—Letetia, 34

⌄ Learning Outcomes

16.1 Compare methods of childbirth preparation.

16.2 Describe the five critical factors that influence labor in the assessment of an expectant woman's and fetus's progress in labor and birth.

16.3 Examine an expectant woman's and fetus's response to labor based on the physiologic processes that occur during labor.

16.4 Assess for the premonitory signs of labor when caring for the expectant woman.

16.5 Differentiate between false and true labor.

16.6 Describe the physiologic and psychologic changes that occur in an expectant woman during each stage of labor in the nursing care management of the expectant woman.

16.7 Explain the maternal systemic responses to labor in the nursing care of the expectant woman.

16.8 Examine fetal responses to labor.

In the final weeks of pregnancy, both mother and baby begin to prepare for birth. The onset of labor begins a remarkable change in the relationship between the woman and her baby. In those hours and moments, the birth process may seem to carry all the power in the universe. The mother-to-be and her partner may feel stretched beyond their normal limits of concentration, purpose, endurance, and pain as they work to bring forth a precious new life.

This chapter focuses on the processes and stages of labor with a brief look at childbirth preparation methods. Subsequent chapters describe intrapartum assessment and nursing care.

Methods of Childbirth Preparation

Various types of childbirth preparation are taught in North America. Childbirth preparation classes are usually taught by certified childbirth educators. With both a theoretical and educational component, childbirth education aims to reduce anxiety while providing physiologic- and psychosocial-based education along with labor-coping techniques, including relaxation tools, such as muscle relaxation and breathing exercises.

Childbirth preparation offers several advantages. It helps a pregnant woman and her support person understand the choices in the birth setting, promotes awareness of available options, and provides tools for them to use during labor and birth. Another advantage is the satisfaction of the parents, for whom childbirth becomes a shared and profound emotional experience. In addition, each method has been shown to shorten labor. All nurses should know how these techniques differ, so that they can support each birth experience effectively. A Cochrane review recently found that women who receive continuous support during labor require less analgesia, have fewer cesarean and instrument births, and experience a shorter period of labor (Hodnett, Gates, Hofmeyr, et al., 2011). This provides additional evidenced-based practice guidance regarding the need to provide ongoing support of the woman's partner during the labor and birth process.

Programs for Preparation

Some antepartum classes, specifically oriented to preparation for labor and birth, have a name associated with a theory of pain reduction in childbirth. The most common methods are described in Table 16–1.

SAFETY ALERT!

Explain to women who are using Internet childbirth education resources that some sites may not use health professionals or experts in the childbirth field and may be written by individuals who lack formal education and training. Advise women to look for resources that are supported by licensed professionals or well-known, credible organizations.

One of the fundamental components of childbirth education is instilling confidence in the woman's ability to give birth, with contemporary models focusing on the interconnectedness of the body and spirit while (Hodnett et al., 2011). After that connection is established and understood by pregnant women, coping strategies, stress reduction, and relaxation techniques can be taught.

Another prominent organization that provides educational resources and certification for educators is the International Childbirth Education Association (ICEA) (2012), which stresses the importance of combining various techniques rather than adhering to one theoretical model. This approach provides each woman with the holistic framework to pick and choose from a variety of techniques that work best for her needs.

Body-Conditioning Exercises

Some body-conditioning exercises, such as the pelvic tilt, pelvic rock, and Kegel exercises, are taught in childbirth preparation classes. Other exercises strengthen the abdominal muscles for the expulsive phase of labor. (See Chapter 10 for a description of some recommended exercises.) Exercises aimed at adducting the legs into an extended *McRoberts position*, which is performed by flexing the mother's thighs toward her shoulders while she is lying on her back, help enable the woman to stretch her hamstring muscles, a task usually required during the second stage of labor (King, Brucker, Kriebs, et al., 2013). Many childbirth methods utilize body-conditioning exercises and encourage the practice of daily exercise to help build endurance and strength for the labor and birth process.

Relaxation Exercises

Relaxation during labor allows the woman to conserve energy and the uterine muscles to work more efficiently. Most childbirth education methods use a form of relaxation exercise as part of their philosophical basis. Without practice, it is difficult to relax the whole body in the midst of intense uterine contractions. Progressive relaxation exercises such as those taught to induce sleep can be helpful during labor.

The *touch relaxation technique* is often used as a pain relief measure in which the partner's touch enhances the woman's ability to relax or release tense muscles. During labor, the partner's touch can include light touching, stroking, or massaging as a nonverbal cue to relax. The method often combines patterned abdominal breathing with focused touch relaxation. The laboring woman learns to release tension in the specific areas or in a generalized manner when her partner touches her. The partner observes and becomes attuned to the woman's tense, tightened muscles or verbal cues that indicate discomfort. See *Teaching Highlights: Touch Relaxation Technique.*

An additional exercise is *disassociation relaxation*. The woman is taught to become familiar with the sensation of contracting and relaxing the voluntary muscle groups throughout her body. She then learns to contract a specific muscle group and relax the rest of her body. The exercise conditions the woman to relax uninvolved muscles while the uterus contracts, creating an active relaxation pattern.

See *Teaching Highlights: Visualization, Imagery, and Meditation* for other strategies to induce relaxation.

Breathing Techniques

Breathing techniques are a key element of most childbirth preparation programs. The Bradley method encourages abdomino-pelvic breathing, whereas the Kitzinger method utilizes chest breathing in collaboration with abdominal relaxation. Hypno-Birthing utilizes deep slow breathing as a center component of its philosophy. Breathing exercises help keep the mother and her unborn baby adequately oxygenated and help the mother relax and focus her attention appropriately. Breathing techniques are best taught during the final trimester of pregnancy. The nurse then supports the mother's use of breathing techniques during labor. See Chapter 18 for a discussion of breathing techniques.

TABLE 16–1 Selected Childbirth Preparation Methods

- **Lamaze** (psychoprophylactic): Dissociative relaxation, controlled muscle relaxation, and specified breathing patterns are used to promote birth as a normal process.
- **Kitzinger** (sensory-memory): Women use chest breathing, abdominal breathing, and their sensory memory to help work through the birthing process.
- **Bradley** (partner-coached childbirth): Consists of a 12-week session in which the woman works on controlled breathing and deep abdominopelvic breathing with a focus on achieving natural childbirth.
- **HypnoBirthing**: Breathing and relaxation techniques help prepare the body to work in neuromuscular harmony to make the birth process easier, safer, and more comfortable.

TEACHING HIGHLIGHTS | Touch Relaxation Technique

- The partner initially touches the woman's brow.
- The woman is encouraged to begin abdominal breathing, in which she breathes in through her nose, allowing her abdomen to rise as much as possible. The woman then breathes out through her mouth while simultaneously allowing her abdomen to fall. The partner reminds her to focus on muscle relaxation as the breath is released and to attempt to completely relax her body as she exhales.
- The partner continues gently touching the woman's brow while providing encouragement, telling her, "You are doing fine, you are releasing the tension in your forehead." After five or more breaths, the partner touches the woman's shoulders and the pattern described above is repeated.
- The partner then systematically focuses on the arms, chest, abdomen, thighs, and calves. The last instruction is for the woman to breathe in deeply and relax her entire body. The partner is advised to encourage this complete relaxation strategy at the end of each contraction to allow the woman to rest and reserve her energy between labor contractions.
- The couple should be encouraged to practice this technique prior to labor. Some couples may verbalize understanding of the technique, but actual practice should be encouraged prior to labor. This enables the woman to identify specific touch techniques that she personally finds helpful.
- Couples should be encouraged to practice the technique simulating a true labor pattern to become accustomed to the frequency needed to maintain the actual length of time and duration that will occur when the woman is in true labor. Women who regularly practice with their partners often become cued by touch alone and can begin the relaxation technique as soon as the partner touches her brow. Couples often individualize the technique to their own comfort levels and should be encouraged to make modifications that feel natural to them.

Sources: Data from Perez, P., & Hutchins, C. (2014). *The nurturing touch at birth: A labor support handbook* (3rd ed.). Johson, VT: Cutting Edge Press; Simpkin, P., & Ancheta, R. (2011). *The labor progress handbook* (3rd ed.). New York, NY: Wiley-Blackwell.

TEACHING HIGHLIGHTS | Visualization, Imagery, and Meditation

Visualization and Imagery	During pregnancy, visualization and imagery are used to induce a state of relaxation. The woman is advised to focus on a calming and relaxing image. Some women may envision a special peaceful place, while others may envision holding their baby or another pleasant event. Images can be suggested by the partner or healthcare practitioner or may be chosen by the woman herself. The partner or healthcare practitioner describes a tranquil image, such as a sparkling brook with sunshine peeking through the trees and birds singing gently in the background. During labor, this technique assists the woman with muscle relaxation and provides a positive distraction from uterine contractions, which helps conserve energy and fight fatigue.
Meditation	Meditation is a practice in which the woman remains upright in an alert position and focuses on stilling or emptying her mind. The woman focuses and repeats a particular word or sound, called a *mantra*, while attempting to reach a state of dissociation. In this state, she is detached from interacting with the environment and becomes an observer of her surroundings rather than an active participant. Mindfulness is a type of meditation that focuses on the present moment. The participant is aware of her environment and observes her thoughts and feelings without judgment. In mindfulness, the woman is encouraged to embrace the labor experience.

Preparation for Childbirth That Supports Individuality

Childbirth educators stress the value of individuality when providing information to expectant parents. The goal is to encourage women to incorporate their own natural responses into coping with the pain of labor and birth. Self-care activities that may be used include vocalization or "sounding" to relieve tension in pregnancy and labor, massage (light touch) to facilitate relaxation, use of warm water for showers or bathing during labor, visualization (imagery), relaxing music, subdued lighting, and the use of a birthing ball.

Additional ways in which the nurse can help the couple during labor and birth include the following:

- Identify the methods of childbirth preparation commonly used in your area and learn the basics of their approaches to relaxation and breathing; practice these methods so that you can support a laboring couple more effectively.

- Encourage expectant mothers and couples to make the birth a personal experience.

- Suggest the couple bring items from home that help create a more personal birthing space, such as warm socks, extra pillows or a favorite blanket, bath powder, lotion, or meaningful photos.

- Encourage the couple to listen to soothing music or watch favorite DVDs to increase personalization of the childbearing experience.

Critical Factors in Labor

Five factors are of critical importance in the process of labor and birth: the passage, the fetus, the relationship between the passage and the fetus, the physiologic forces of labor, and the psychosocial considerations. Abnormalities that affect any component of these critical forces can alter the outcome of labor and jeopardize both the expectant woman and her baby. The five factors are summarized in Table 16–2, and the first four are described in this section. Psychosocial factors are discussed in detail in Chapter 17. Labor-related complications are discussed in Chapter 21.

TABLE 16–2 Critical Factors in Labor

CRITICAL FACTORS	COMPONENTS
Birth passage	• Size of the pelvis (diameters of the pelvic inlet, midpelvis or pelvic cavity, and outlet) • Type of pelvis (gynecoid, android, anthropoid, platypelloid, or a combination) • Ability of the cervix to dilate and efface and ability of the vaginal canal and the external opening of the vagina (the introitus) to distend
Fetus	• Fetal head (size and presence of molding) • Fetal attitude (flexion or extension of the fetal body and extremities) • Fetal lie • Fetal presentation (the part of the fetal body entering the pelvis first in a single- or multiple-gestation pregnancy)
Relationship between the passage and the fetus	• Engagement of fetal presenting part • Station (location of fetal presenting part within the maternal pelvis) • Fetal position (relationship of the presenting part to one of the four quadrants of the maternal pelvis)
Physiologic forces of labor	• Frequency, duration, and intensity of uterine contractions as the fetus moves through the birth passage • Effectiveness of the maternal pushing effort • Duration of labor
Psychosocial considerations (see Chapter 17 for an in-depth discussion)	• Physical preparation for childbirth • Sociocultural values and beliefs • Previous childbirth experience(s) • Support from significant others • Emotional status

TABLE 16–3 Implications of Pelvic Type for Labor and Birth

PELVIC TYPE	PERTINENT CHARACTERISTICS	IMPLICATIONS FOR BIRTH
Gynecoid	Inlet rounded with all inlet diameters adequate Midpelvis diameters adequate with parallel side walls Outlet adequate	Favorable for vaginal birth
Android	Inlet heart-shaped, with short posterior sagittal diameter Midpelvis diameters reduced Outlet capacity reduced	Not favorable for vaginal birth Descent into pelvis is slow Fetal head enters pelvis in transverse or posterior position, with arrest of labor frequent
Anthropoid	Inlet oval in shape, with long anteroposterior diameter Midpelvis diameters adequate Outlet adequate	Favorable for vaginal birth
Platypelloid	Inlet oval in shape, with long transverse diameters Midpelvis diameters reduced Outlet capacity inadequate	Not favorable for vaginal birth Fetal head engages in transverse position Difficult descent through midpelvis Frequent delay of progress at outlet of pelvis

Note: Description of pelvic shape is exaggerated for easier comprehension.

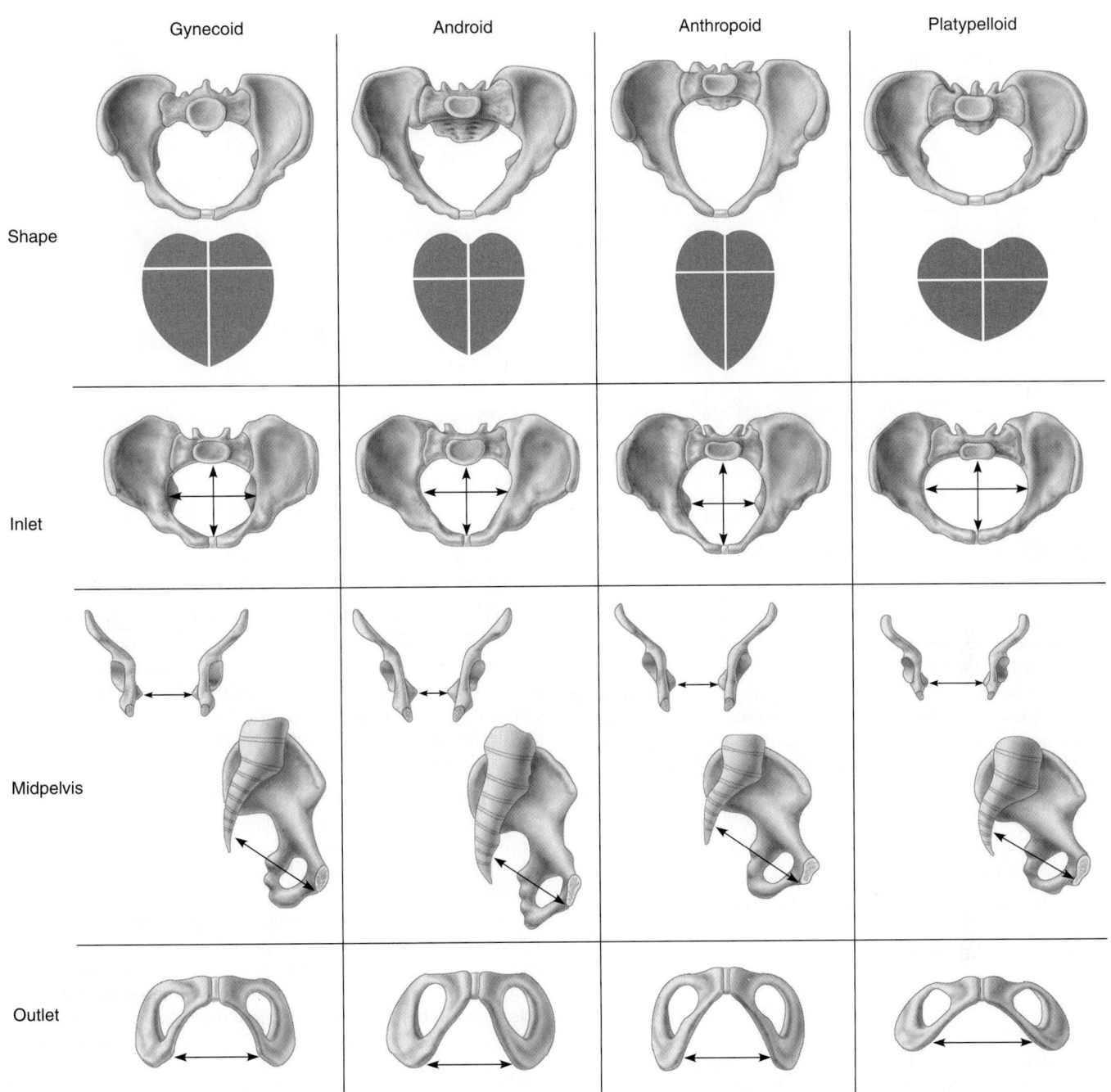

	Gynecoid	Android	Anthropoid	Platypelloid
Shape				
Inlet				
Midpelvis				
Outlet				

Figure 16–1   Comparison of Caldwell-Moloy pelvic types.

The Birth Passage

The true pelvis, which forms the bony canal through which the fetus must pass, is divided into three sections: the inlet, the pelvic cavity (midpelvis), and the outlet. (See Chapter 4 for discussion of the pelvis and Chapter 9 for assessment techniques.)

The Caldwell-Moloy classification of pelvises is widely used to differentiate bony pelvis types. The four classic types of pelvises are *gynecoid, android, anthropoid,* and *platypelloid* (Caldwell & Moloy, 1933) (Figure 16–1). The gynecoid, or female, pelvis is most common. All diameters of the gynecoid are adequate for childbirth. Implications of each type of pelvis for childbirth are summarized in Table 16–3.

The Fetus

FETAL HEAD

The fetal skull (cranium) has three major parts: the face, the base of the skull, and the vault of the cranium (roof). The bones of the face and cranial base are well fused and essentially fixed. The base of the cranium is composed of the two temporal bones, each with a sphenoid and ethmoid bone. The bones composing the vault are the two frontal bones, the two parietal bones, and the occipital bone (Figure 16–2). These bones are not fused, so this portion of the head can adjust in shape as the presenting part passes through the narrow portions of the pelvis. The cranial bones overlap under pressure of the powers of labor and the demands of the

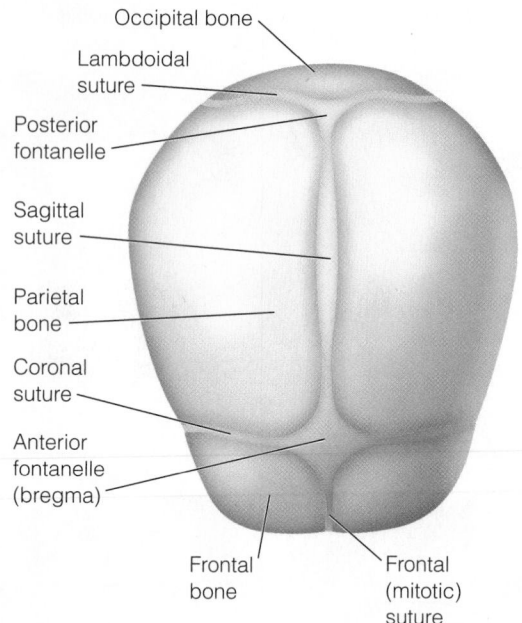

Figure 16–2 Superior view of the fetal skull.

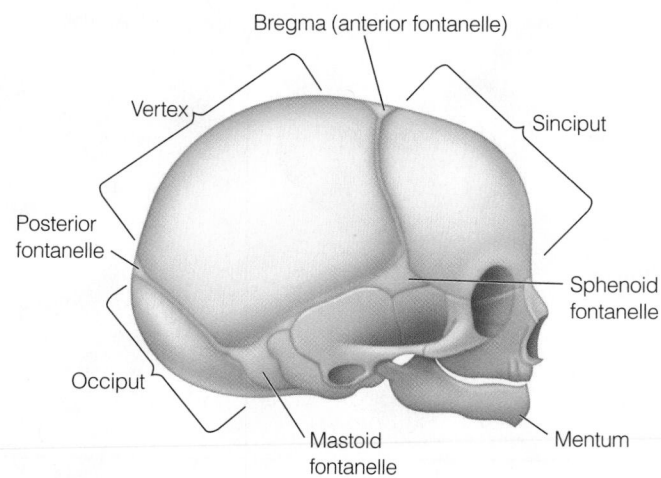

Figure 16–3 Lateral view of the fetal skull. This figure identifies the landmarks that have significance during birth.

unyielding pelvis. This overlapping is called **molding**. Once the head (the least compressible and largest part of the fetus) has been born, the birth of the rest of the body is rarely delayed.

The **sutures** of the fetal skull are membranous spaces between the cranial bones. The intersections of the cranial sutures are called **fontanelles**. These sutures allow for molding of the fetal head and help the clinician to identify the position of the fetal head during vaginal examination. The important sutures of the cranium are as follows (see Figure 16–2):

- *Frontal suture:* located between the two frontal bones; becomes the anterior continuation of the sagittal suture
- *Sagittal suture:* located between the parietal bones; divides the skull into left and right halves; runs anteroposteriorly, connecting the two fontanelles
- *Coronal sutures:* located between the frontal and parietal bones; extend transversely left and right from the anterior fontanelle
- *Lambdoidal suture:* located between the two parietal bones and the occipital bone; extends transversely left and right from the posterior fontanelle

The anterior and posterior fontanelles are clinically useful (along with the sutures) in identifying the position of the fetal head in the pelvis and in assessing the status of the newborn after birth. The anterior fontanelle is diamond shaped and measures about 2 cm by 3 cm (0.8 in. by 1.20 in.). It permits growth of the brain by remaining unossified for as long as 18 months. The posterior fontanelle is much smaller and closes within 8 to 12 weeks after birth. It is shaped like a small triangle and marks the meeting point of the sagittal suture and the lambdoidal suture.

Following are several important landmarks of the fetal skull (Figure 16–3):

- *Mentum:* fetal chin
- *Sinciput:* anterior area known as the brow
- *Bregma:* large diamond-shaped anterior fontanelle
- *Vertex:* area between the anterior and posterior fontanelles
- *Posterior fontanelle:* intersection between posterior cranial sutures

- *Occiput:* area of the fetal skull occupied by the occipital bone, beneath the posterior fontanelle

The diameters of the fetal skull vary considerably within normal limits. Some diameters shorten and others lengthen as the head is molded during labor. Fetal head diameters are measured between the various landmarks on the skull (Figure 16–4). For example, the suboccipitobregmatic diameter is the distance from the undersurface of the occiput to the center of the bregma, or anterior fontanelle.

FETAL ATTITUDE AND FETAL LIE

Fetal attitude refers to the relation of the fetal parts to one another. The normal attitude of the fetus is one of moderate flexion of the head, flexion of the arms onto the chest, and flexion of the legs onto the abdomen (Figure 16–5).

Fetal lie refers to the relationship of the cephalocaudal axis (spinal column) of the fetus to the cephalocaudal axis of the woman. The fetus may assume either a longitudinal or a transverse lie. A *longitudinal lie* occurs when the cephalocaudal axis of the fetus is parallel to the woman's spine. A *transverse lie* occurs when the cephalocaudal axis of the fetus is at a right angle to the woman's spine.

FETAL PRESENTATION

Fetal presentation is determined by fetal lie and by the body part of the fetus that enters the pelvic passage first. This portion of the fetus is referred to as the **presenting part**. Fetal presentation may be cephalic, breech, or shoulder. Cephalic presentation, in which the fetal head presents itself to the passage, occurs in approximately 97% of term births. When this presentation occurs, labor and birth are likely to proceed normally. Breech and shoulder presentations are associated with difficulties during labor, and labor does not proceed as expected; therefore, they are called **malpresentations** (see Chapter 21).

The cephalic presentation can be further classified according to the degree of flexion or extension of the fetal head (attitude):

- *Vertex presentation.* This is the most common type of presentation. The fetal head is completely flexed onto the chest, and the smallest diameter of the fetal head (suboccipitobregmatic) presents to the maternal pelvis (Figure 16–6A); the occiput is the presenting part.

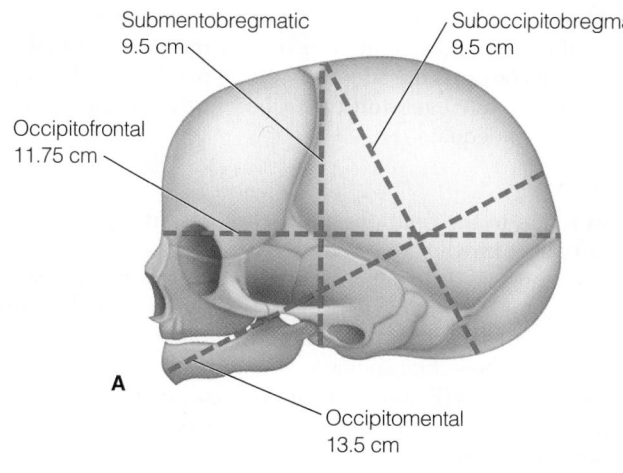

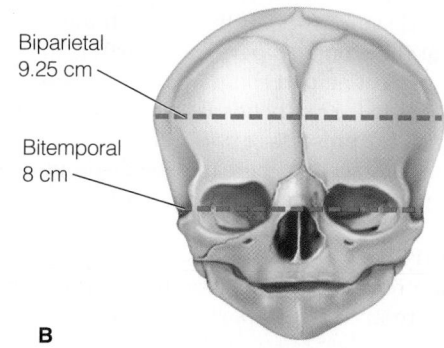

Figure 16–4 Fetal skull measurements. *A*, Typical anteroposterior diameters of the fetal skull. When the vertex of the fetus presents and the fetal head is flexed with the chin on the chest, the smallest anteroposterior diameter (suboccipitobregmatic) enters the birth canal. *B*, Transverse diameters of the fetal skull.

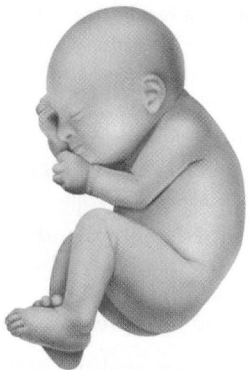

Figure 16–5 Fetal attitude. The attitude (or relationship of body parts) of this fetus is normal. The head is flexed forward, with the chin almost resting on the chest. The arms and legs are flexed.

- *Sinciput presentation* (also called *military presentation*). The fetal head is neither flexed nor extended; the occipitofrontal diameter presents to the maternal pelvis (Figure 16–6*B*); the top of the head is the presenting part.

- *Brow presentation.* The fetal head is partially extended; the occipitomental diameter, the largest anteroposterior diameter, is presented to the maternal pelvis (Figure 16–6*C*); the sinciput is the presenting part (see Figure 16–3).

- *Face presentation.* The fetal head is hyperextended (completely extended); the submentobregmatic diameter presents to the maternal pelvis (Figure 16–6*D*); the face is the presenting part.

Breech presentation is a birth in which the buttocks and/or feet are the presenting part rather than the head. It occurs in 3% to 4% of term pregnancies. These presentations are classified according to the attitude of the fetus's hips and knees. In all the following variations of the breech presentation, the sacrum is the landmark to be noted:

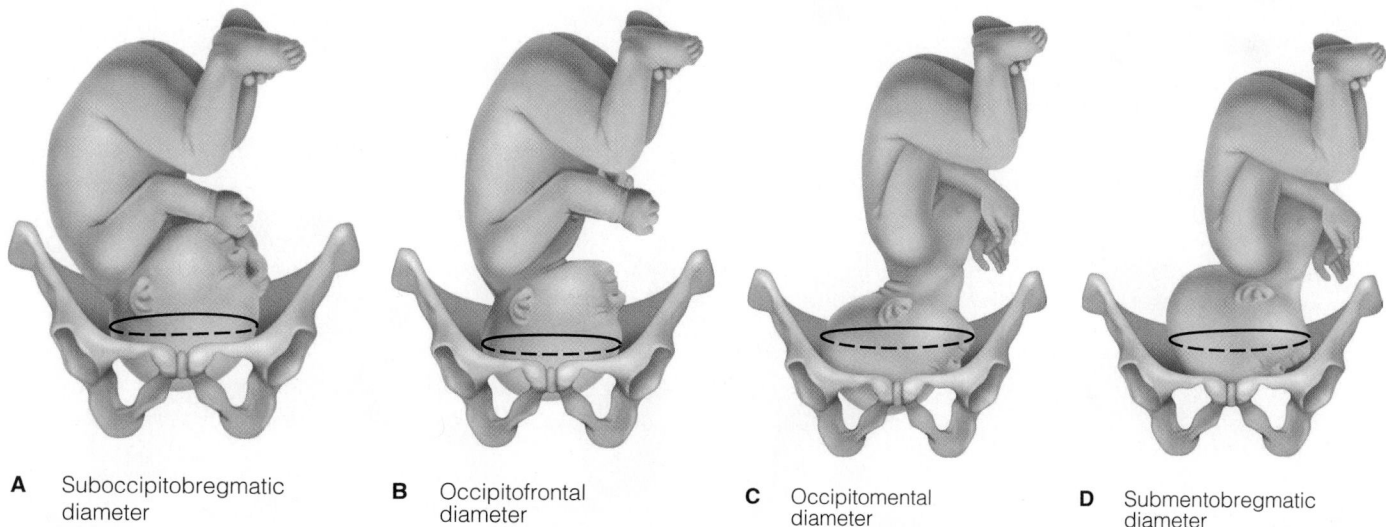

A Suboccipitobregmatic diameter

B Occipitofrontal diameter

C Occipitomental diameter

D Submentobregmatic diameter

Figure 16–6 Cephalic presentation. *A*, Vertex presentation. Complete flexion of the head allows the suboccipitobregmatic diameter to present to the pelvis. *B*, Sinciput (median vertex) presentation (also called *military presentation*) with no flexion or extension. The occipitofrontal diameter presents to the pelvis. *C*, Brow presentation. The fetal head is in complete extension, and the submentobregmatic diameter presents to the pelvis. *D*, Face presentation. The fetal head is in partial (halfway) extension. The occipitomental diameter, which is the largest diameter of the fetal head, presents to the pelvis.

- *Complete breech.* The fetal knees and hips are both flexed; the thighs are on the abdomen, and the calves are on the posterior aspect of the thighs; the buttocks and feet of the fetus present to the maternal pelvis. (See Figure 21–7C.)
- *Frank breech.* The fetal hips are flexed, and the knees are extended; the buttocks of the fetus present to the maternal pelvis. (See Figure 21–7A.)
- *Footling breech.* The fetal hips and legs are extended, and the feet of the fetus present to the maternal pelvis. (See Figure 21–7B.) In a single footling, one foot presents; in a double footling, both feet present.

A shoulder presentation is also called a *transverse lie.* Most frequently, the shoulder is the presenting part and the acromion process of the scapula is the landmark to be noted. However, the fetal arm, back, abdomen, or side may present in a transverse lie (see Chapter 21).

Relationship Between the Maternal Pelvis and Presenting Part

ENGAGEMENT

Engagement of the presenting part occurs when the largest diameter of the presenting part reaches or passes through the pelvic inlet and is at the level of the ischial spines (Figure 16–7). Engagement can be determined by vaginal examination. In primigravidas, engagement occurs approximately 2 weeks before term. Multiparas, however, may experience engagement several weeks before the onset of labor or during the process of labor. Engagement confirms the adequacy of the pelvic inlet. Engagement does not, however, indicate whether the midpelvis and outlet are also adequate.

STATION

Station refers to the relationship of the presenting part to an imaginary line drawn between the ischial spines of the maternal pelvis. In a normal pelvis, the ischial spines mark the narrowest diameter through which the fetus must pass. These spines are not sharp protrusions that harm the fetus but blunted prominences at the midpelvis. The ischial spines as a landmark have been designated as zero station (Figure 16–8). If the presenting part is higher than the ischial spines, a negative number is assigned, noting centimeters above zero station. Positive numbers indicate that the presenting part has passed the ischial spines. Station –5 is at the pelvic inlet, and station +4 is at the outlet. If the presenting part can be seen at the woman's perineum, birth is imminent. During labor the presenting part should move progressively from the negative stations to the midpelvis at zero station and into the positive stations. If the presenting part fails to descend in the presence of strong contractions, there may be disproportion between the maternal pelvis and fetal presenting part.

FETAL POSITION

Fetal position refers to the relationship of a designated landmark on the presenting fetal part to the front, sides, or back of

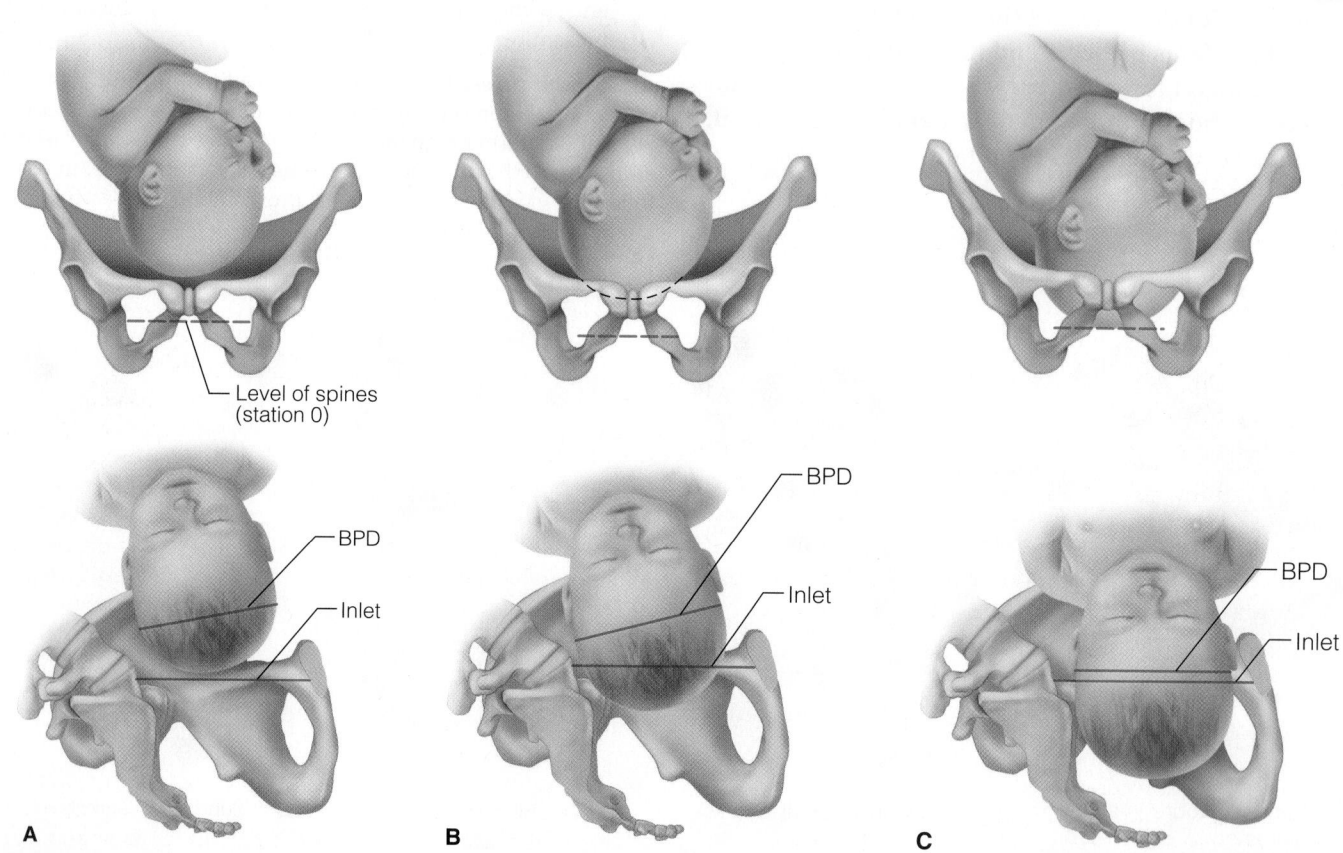

Figure 16–7 Process of engagement in cephalic presentation. *A,* Floating. The fetal head is directed down toward the pelvis but can still easily move away from the inlet. *B,* Dipping. The fetal head dips into the inlet but can be moved away by exerting pressure on the fetus. *C,* Engaged. The biparietal diameter (BPD) of the fetal head is in the inlet of the pelvis. In most instances, the presenting part (occiput) is at the level of the ischial spines (zero station).

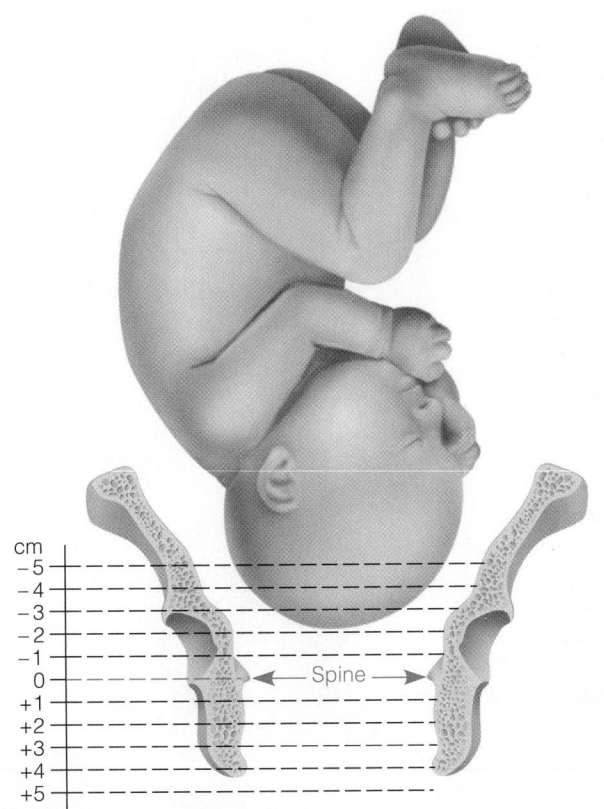

Figure 16–8 Measuring the station of the fetal head while it is descending. In this view, the station is –2/–3.

Physiologic Forces of Labor

Primary and secondary forces work together to achieve birth of the fetus, the fetal membranes, and the placenta. The *primary force* is uterine muscular contractions, which cause the complete effacement and dilatation of the cervix. The *secondary force* is the use of abdominal muscles to push during the second stage of labor. The pushing adds to the primary force after full dilatation. **Dilatation** is the process of the cervix opening during the labor process. The cervix *dilates*, or opens, from 0 to 10 cm during the first stage of labor in response to uterine contractions.

In labor, uterine contractions are rhythmic but intermittent. Between contractions a period of relaxation occurs. This allows uterine muscles to rest and provides relief for the laboring woman. It also restores uteroplacental circulation, which is important to fetal oxygenation and adequate circulation in the uterine blood vessels.

Each contraction has three phases: (1) *increment*, the building up of the contraction (the longest phase); (2) *acme*, or the peak of the contraction; and (3) *decrement*, or the letting up of the contraction. The terms *frequency, duration,* and *intensity* are used to describe uterine contractions during labor. **Frequency** refers to the time between the beginning of one contraction and the beginning of the next contraction. **Duration** is measured from the beginning of a contraction to the completion of that same contraction (Figure 16–10). **Intensity** refers to the strength of the contraction during acme. In most instances, intensity is estimated by palpating the uterine fundus during a contraction, but it may be measured directly with an intrauterine catheter. When estimating intensity by palpation, the nurse determines whether it is mild, moderate, or strong by judging the amount of indentability of the uterine wall during the acme of a contraction. If the uterine wall can be indented easily, the contraction is considered mild. Strong intensity exists when the uterine wall cannot be indented. Moderate intensity falls somewhere between. When intensity is measured with an intrauterine catheter, the normal resting pressure in the uterus (between contractions) averages 10 to 12 mmHg. During acme the intensity ranges from 25 to 40 mmHg in early labor, 50 to 70 mmHg in active labor, 70 to 90 mmHg during transition, and 70 to 100 mmHg while the woman is pushing in the second stage (Blackburn, 2013). (See Chapter 17 for further discussion of assessment techniques.)

At the beginning of labor, contractions are usually mild. As labor progresses, the duration, intensity, and frequency of contractions increase. Contractions are involuntary; the laboring woman cannot control their duration, frequency, or intensity.

After the cervix is completely dilated, the maternal abdominal muscles contract as the woman pushes. This pushing action (called *bearing down*) aids in the expulsion of the fetus and placenta. If the cervix is not completely dilated, however, bearing down can cause cervical edema (which retards dilatation), possible tearing and bruising of the cervix, and maternal exhaustion.

The duration of labor varies considerably and is related to multiple factors including fetal factors such as presentation, position, fetal weight, number of fetuses, and the station of the presenting part; maternal factors such as age, parity, maternal body weight, pain threshold, and maternal positioning during labor; uterine factors such as the intensity, frequency, and duration of contractions; and obstetric interventions such as the use of epidural anesthesia or other medications, whether the labor was induced or augmented with oxytocin (Pitocin) infusions, and whether instrument interventions such as forceps or vacuum delivery were performed (King et al., 2015).

the maternal pelvis. The landmark chosen for vertex presentations is the occiput, and the landmark for face presentations is the mentum. In breech presentations, the sacrum is the designated landmark, and the acromion process on the scapula is the landmark in shoulder presentations. If the landmark is directed toward the side of the pelvis, fetal position is designated as *transverse* rather than anterior or posterior. Three notations are used to describe fetal position:

1. Right (R) or left (L) side of the maternal pelvis

2. The landmark of the fetal presenting part: occiput (O), mentum (M), sacrum (S), or acromion process (A)

3. Anterior (A), posterior (P), or transverse (T), depending on whether the landmark is in the front, back, or side of the pelvis

These abbreviations help the healthcare team communicate the fetal position. Thus when the fetal occiput is directed toward the back and left of the birth passage, the abbreviation used is LOP (left occiput posterior). The term *dorsal* (D) is used when denoting the fetal position in a transverse lie; it refers to the fetal back. For example, RADA indicates that the acromion process of the scapula is directed toward the woman's right, and the fetus's back is anterior.

The most frequently occurring positions are illustrated in Figure 16–9. The most common fetal position is occiput anterior. When this position occurs, labor and birth are likely to proceed normally. Positions other than occiput anterior are more frequently associated with problems during labor; therefore, they are called *malpositions*. (See Chapter 21 for more information about malpositions.)

Assessment techniques to determine fetal position include inspection and palpation of the maternal abdomen and vaginal examination. They are discussed in Chapter 17.

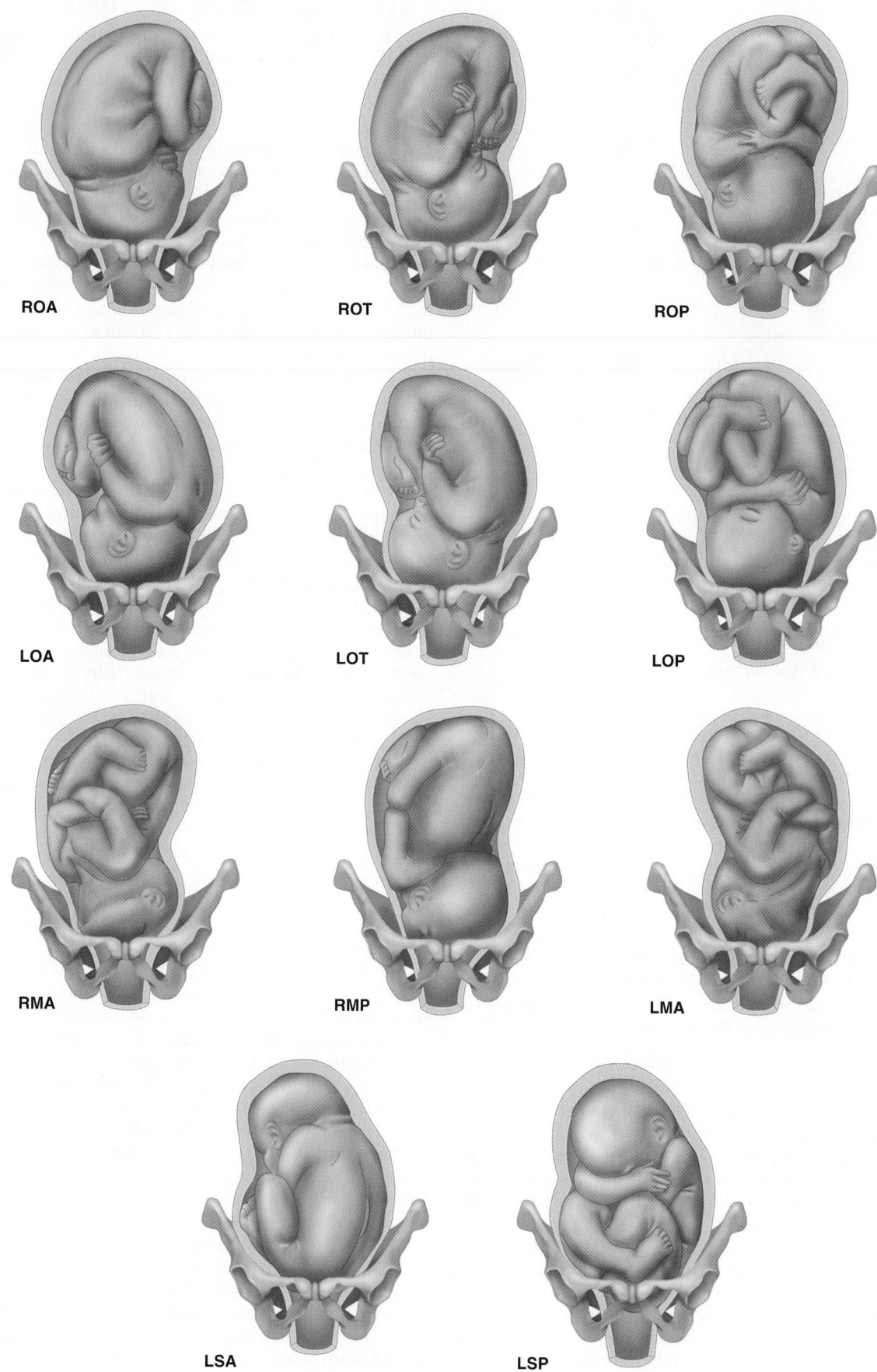

Figure 16–9 Categories of fetal presentation.

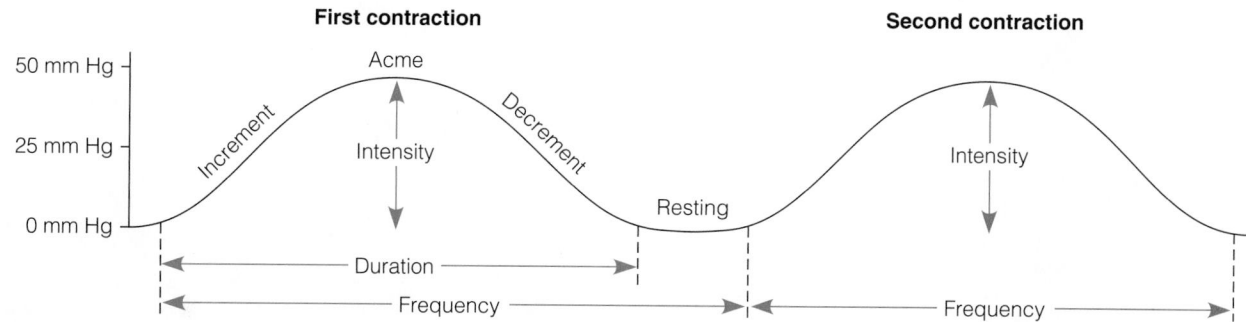

First contraction

Second contraction

50 mm Hg

Acme

25 mm Hg

Increment

Intensity

Decrement

Intensity

0 mm Hg

Resting

Duration

Frequency

Frequency

Figure 16–10 Characteristics of uterine contractions.

The Physiology of Labor

Possible Causes of Labor Onset

The process of labor usually begins between the 38th and 42nd week of gestation, when the fetus is mature and ready for birth. The exact cause of labor onset is not clearly understood. However, some important aspects have been identified:

- Progesterone relaxes smooth muscle tissue.
- Estrogen stimulates uterine muscle contractions.
- Connective tissue loosens to permit the softening, thinning, and eventual opening of the cervix (Blackburn, 2013).

Currently, researchers are focusing on the role of fetal membranes (chorion and amnion), the decidua, and the effect of progesterone withdrawal, of prostaglandin, and of corticotropin-releasing hormone in relation to labor onset (Blackburn, 2013).

PROGESTERONE WITHDRAWAL HYPOTHESIS

Progesterone, produced by the placenta, relaxes uterine smooth muscle by interfering with the conduction of impulses from one cell to the next. During pregnancy, progesterone exerts a quieting effect and the uterus generally does not have coordinated contractions. Toward the end of gestation, biochemical changes decrease the availability of progesterone to myometrial cells and may be associated with an antiprogestin that inhibits the relaxant effect but allows other progesterone actions such as lactogenesis. With the decreased availability of progesterone, estrogen is better able to stimulate contractions (Blackburn, 2013). Interestingly, progesterone administration is now used as a mechanism to prevent preterm labor and birth (Blackburn, 2013).

PROSTAGLANDIN HYPOTHESIS

Although the exact relationship between prostaglandin and the onset of labor is not yet known, the effect is clinically demonstrated by the successful induction of labor after vaginal application of prostaglandin E. Preterm labor may be stopped by using an inhibitor of prostaglandin synthesis. Oxytocin may also play a role in the process in two ways: first by direct stimulation of uterine contractions and second, indirectly, by stimulating prostaglandin production by the amnion and decidua (Blackburn, 2013).

CORTICOTROPIN-RELEASING HORMONE

Corticotropin-releasing hormone (CRH) has a possible role in labor onset. It increases throughout pregnancy, with a sharp increase at term. Plasma CRH is also increased before preterm labor, and CRH levels are elevated in multiple gestation. CRH is known to stimulate the synthesis of prostaglandin F and prostaglandin E by amnion cells (Posner, Black, Jones, et al., 2013).

Myometrial Activity

In true labor, the muscles of the upper uterine segment shorten and exert a longitudinal pull on the cervix with each contraction, causing effacement.

Effacement is the drawing up of the internal os and the cervical canal into the side walls of the uterus. The cervix changes progressively from a long, thick structure to one that is tissue-paper thin (Figure 16–11). In primigravidas, effacement usually occurs before dilatation.

The uterus elongates with each contraction, decreasing the horizontal diameter. This elongation causes a straightening of the fetal body, pressing the upper portion against the fundus and thrusting the presenting part down toward the lower uterine segment and the cervix. The pressure exerted by the fetus is called the *fetal axis pressure*. As the uterus elongates, the longitudinal muscle fibers are pulled upward over the presenting part. This action and the hydrostatic pressure of the fetal membranes cause cervical dilatation. The cervical os and cervical canal widen from less than 1 to approximately 10 cm, allowing birth of the fetus. When the cervix is completely dilated and retracted up into the lower uterine segment, it can no longer be palpated. At the same time, the round ligament pulls the fundus forward, aligning the fetus with the bony pelvis.

Musculature Changes in the Pelvic Floor

The levator ani muscle and fascia of the pelvic floor draw the rectum and vagina upward and forward with each contraction, along the curve of the pelvic floor. As the fetal head descends to the pelvic floor, the pressure of the presenting part causes the perineal structure, which was once 5 cm in thickness, to thin to less than 1 cm. The anus everts, exposing the interior rectal wall as the fetal head descends forward (Blackburn, 2013).

Premonitory Signs of Labor

Most primigravidas and many multiparas experience the following signs and symptoms of impending labor.

LIGHTENING

Lightening describes the effects that occur when the fetus begins to settle into the pelvic inlet (engagement). With fetal descent the uterus moves downward, and the fundus no longer presses on the diaphragm, which allows breathing to become

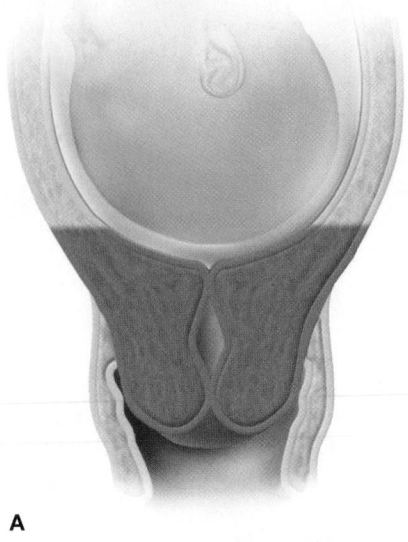

A

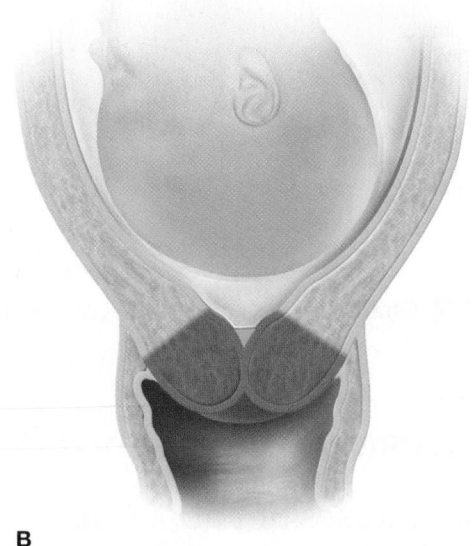

B

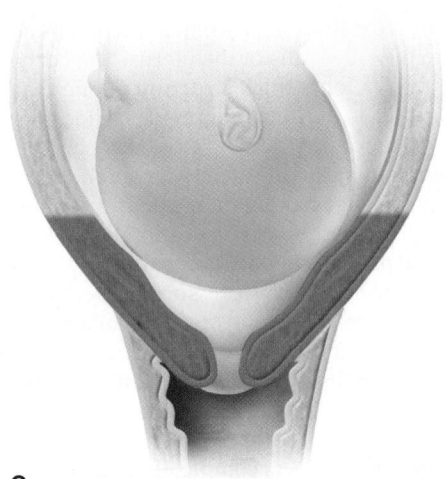

C

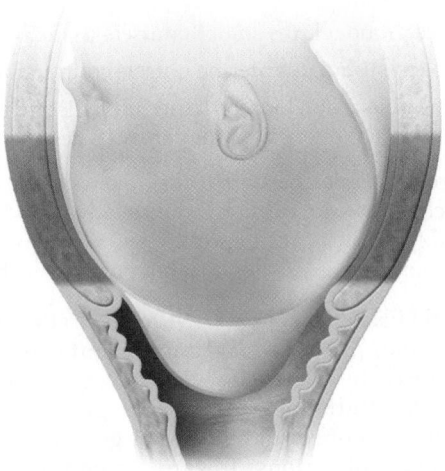

D

Figure 16–11 Effacement of the cervix in the primigravida. *A*, Beginning of labor. There is no cervical effacement or dilatation. The fetal head is cushioned by amniotic fluid. *B*, Beginning cervical effacement. As the cervix begins to efface, more amniotic fluid collects below the fetal head. *C*, Cervix about one-half effaced and slightly dilated. The increasing amount of amniotic fluid exerts hydrostatic pressure. *D*, Complete effacement and dilatation.

easier. However, with increased downward pressure of the presenting part, the woman may notice the following:

- Leg cramps or pains due to pressure on the nerves that pass through the obturator foramen in the pelvis
- Increased pelvic pressure
- Increased venous stasis, leading to edema in the lower extremities
- Increased vaginal secretions resulting from congestion of the vaginal mucous membranes

BRAXTON HICKS CONTRACTIONS

Before the onset of labor, *Braxton Hicks contractions* (the irregular, intermittent contractions that have been occurring throughout the pregnancy) may become uncomfortable. The pain seems to be focused in the abdomen and groin but may feel like the "drawing" sensations experienced by some women with

dysmenorrhea. When these contractions are strong enough for the woman to believe she is in labor, she is said to be in *false labor*. False labor is uncomfortable and may be exhausting. Since the contractions can be fairly regular, the woman has no way of knowing if they are true labor.

CERVICAL CHANGES

Considerable change occurs in the cervix during the prenatal and intrapartum period. At the beginning of pregnancy, the cervix is rigid and firm, and it must soften so it can stretch and dilate to allow the fetus passage. This softening of the cervix is called *ripening*.

As term approaches, collagen fibers in the cervix are broken down by certain enzymes. As the fibers change, their ability to bind together decreases, while the water content of the cervix increases. These changes result in a weakening and softening of the cervix.

BLOODY SHOW

During pregnancy, cervical secretions accumulate in the cervical canal to form a barrier called a *mucous plug*. With softening and effacement of the cervix, the mucous plug is often expelled, resulting in a small amount of blood loss from the exposed cervical capillaries. The resulting pink-tinged secretions are called **bloody show**. Bloody show is considered a sign that labor will begin within 24 to 48 hours. Recent intercourse or vaginal examination that includes manipulation of the cervix may also result in a blood-tinged discharge, which may be confused with bloody show.

RUPTURE OF MEMBRANES

Approximately 10% of women at term (38 through 41 weeks' gestation) experience rupture of the amniotic membranes (ROM) before the onset of labor. Rupture of membranes occurs when the amniotic sac surrounding the fetus, amniotic fluid, and placenta ruptures or is perforated and results in the expulsion of amniotic fluid from the vagina (Cunningham et al., 2014). After the membranes rupture, 90% of women give birth within 24 hours (Jazayeri, 2014). Women who are 34 weeks' gestation or more and who present with ruptured membranes without contractions are often started on an oxytocin infusion to decrease the incidence of chorioamnionitis. Women with preterm gestations of less than 34 weeks are managed conservatively provided both the mother and the fetus are stable (Jazayeri, 2014).

When the membranes rupture, the amniotic fluid may be expelled in large amounts. If engagement has not occurred, there is danger of the umbilical cord washing out with the fluid (prolapsed cord). In addition, the open pathway into the uterus increases the risk of infection. Because of these risks, when the membranes rupture, the woman is advised to call her physician/certified nurse-midwife (CNM) and proceed to the hospital or birthing center. In some instances, the fluid is expelled in small amounts and may be confused with episodes of urinary incontinence associated with urinary urgency, coughing, or sneezing. The discharge should be checked to determine its source and the appropriate action. (See Chapter 17 for assessment techniques.)

SUDDEN BURST OF ENERGY

Some women report a sudden burst of energy approximately 24 to 48 hours before labor. The cause of the energy spurt is unknown. In prenatal teaching, it is important to warn prospective mothers not to overexert themselves during this energy burst to avoid being overtired when labor begins.

Clinical Tip

Encourage expectant mothers who experience a sudden burst of energy to eat small, frequent, nutritious meals during this period, and to rest. Encourage the pregnant woman to have her spouse or partner or a friend do chores and activities that she feels are essential to complete before the baby arrives.

OTHER SIGNS

Additional premonitory signs include the following:

- Weight loss of 1 to 3 lb resulting from fluid loss and electrolyte shifts produced by changes in estrogen and progesterone levels
- Diarrhea, indigestion, or nausea and vomiting just before onset of labor

The causes of these signs are unknown.

TABLE 16–4 Comparison of True and False Labor

TRUE LABOR	FALSE LABOR
Contractions occur at regular intervals.	Contractions are irregular.
Interval between contractions gradually shortens.	Usually no change.
Contractions increase in duration and intensity.	Usually no change.
Discomfort begins in back and radiates around to abdomen.	Discomfort is usually in abdomen.
Intensity usually increases with walking.	Walking has no effect on or lessens contractions.
Cervical dilatation and effacement are progressive.	No change.

Differences Between True and False Labor

The contractions of true labor produce progressive dilatation and effacement of the cervix. They occur regularly and increase in frequency, duration, and intensity. The discomfort of true labor contractions usually starts in the back and radiates around to the abdomen. The pain is not relieved by ambulation (in fact, walking may intensify the pain).

The contractions of false labor do not produce progressive cervical effacement and dilatation. Classically, they are irregular and do not increase in frequency, duration, and intensity. The contractions may be perceived as a hardening or "balling up" without discomfort, or discomfort may occur mainly in the lower abdomen and groin. The discomfort may be relieved by ambulation, changes of position, drinking a large amount of water, or a warm shower or tub bath. Many times the only way to differentiate accurately between true and false labor is to assess effacement and dilatation. The woman must feel free to come in for accurate assessment of labor and should be counseled not to feel foolish if the labor is false. She can be reassured that false labor is common and that it often cannot be distinguished from true labor except by vaginal examination (Table 16–4).

Stages of Labor and Birth

The labor process is divided into phases and stages of labor. These represent theoretical separations in the process. A laboring woman does not usually experience distinct differences from one stage to the next.

The *first stage* begins with the onset of true labor and ends when the cervix is completely dilated to 10 cm. The *second stage* begins with complete dilatation and ends with the birth of the baby. The *third stage* begins with the birth of the baby and ends with the expulsion of the placenta. Some clinicians identify a *fourth stage*. During this stage, which lasts 1 to 4 hours after expulsion of the placenta, the uterus contracts to control bleeding at the placental site (Cunningham et al., 2014).

First Stage

The first stage of labor is divided into the *latent*, *active*, and *transition* phases. Each phase of labor is characterized by physical and psychologic changes.

LATENT PHASE

The *latent phase* starts with the beginning of regular contractions, which are usually mild. The woman feels able to cope with the discomfort. She may be relieved that labor has finally started. Although she may be anxious, she is able to recognize and express those feelings of anxiety. The woman is often talkative and smiling and is eager to talk about herself and answer questions. Excitement is high, and her partner or other support person is often as elated as she is.

Uterine contractions become established during the latent phase and increase in frequency, duration, and intensity. They may start as mild contractions lasting 30 seconds with a frequency of 10 to 30 minutes and progress to moderate ones lasting 30 to 40 seconds with a frequency of 5 to 7 minutes. As the cervix begins to dilate, it also effaces, although little or no fetal descent is evident. For a woman in her first labor (nullipara), the latent (or early) phase of the first stage of labor averages 8.6 hours but should not exceed 20 hours. The latent phase in multiparas averages 5.3 hours but should not exceed 14 hours.

At the beginning of labor, the amniotic membranes bulge through the cervix in the shape of a cone. **Spontaneous rupture of membranes (SROM)** generally occurs at the height of an intense contraction with a gush of fluid out of the vagina. In many instances, the membranes are ruptured by the physician/CNM using an instrument called an *amniohook*. This procedure is called an *amniotomy*, or **artificial rupture of membranes (AROM)**.

ACTIVE PHASE

When a woman enters the early *active phase*, her anxiety tends to increase as she senses the intensification of contractions and pain. She begins to fear a loss of control and may use a variety of coping mechanisms. Some women show decreased ability to cope and a sense of helplessness. Women who have support people and family available may feel greater satisfaction and less anxiety than those without support. During this phase the cervix dilates from about 4 to 7 cm. Fetal descent is progressive. Cervical dilatation averages 1.2 cm/hr in nulliparas and 1.5 cm/hr in multiparas.

TRANSITION PHASE

The *transition phase* is the last part of the first stage of labor. When the woman enters transition, she may show significant anxiety. She becomes acutely aware of the increasing force and intensity of the contractions. She may become restless, frequently changing position. By the time the woman enters the transition phase, she is inner directed and often tired. She may fear being left alone at the same time the support person may be feeling the need for a break. The nurse should reassure the woman that she will not be left alone. It is important to be available as relief support at this time and to keep the woman informed about where her labor support people are, if they leave the room.

During the active and transition phases, contractions become more frequent and longer in duration, and they increase in intensity. During transition, contractions have a frequency of about every 1.5 to 2.0 minutes, a duration of 60 to 90 seconds, and strong intensity. Cervical dilatation slows as it progresses from 8 to 10 cm, and the rate of fetal descent dramatically increases. The average rate of descent is 1.6 cm/hr and at least 1.0 cm/hr in nulliparas; the average rate is 5.4 cm/hr and at least 2.1 cm/hr in multiparas. The transition phase does not usually last longer than 3 hours for nulliparas or longer than 1 hour for multiparas (King et al., 2014).

As dilatation approaches 10 cm, the woman may feel increased rectal pressure and an uncontrollable desire to bear down, the amount of bloody show may increase, and the membranes may rupture (if it has not already occurred). The woman may also fear that she will be "torn open" or "split apart" by the force of the contractions. With the peak of a contraction, she may experience a sensation of pressure so great that it seems to her that her abdomen will burst open with the force. The nurse should inform the woman that what she is feeling is normal. The woman may doubt her ability to cope with labor and may become apprehensive, irritable, and withdrawn. She may be terrified of being left alone, although she does not want anyone to talk to or touch her. However, with the next contraction she may ask for verbal and physical support. Other characteristics of this phase may include the following:

- Increasing bloody show
- Hyperventilation, as the woman increases her breathing rate
- Generalized discomfort, including low backache, shaking and cramping in legs, and increased sensitivity to touch
- Increased need for partner's or nurse's presence and support
- Restlessness
- Increased apprehension and irritability
- Difficulty understanding directions
- A sense of bewilderment, frustration, and anger at the contractions
- Requests for medication
- Hiccuping, belching, nausea, or vomiting
- Beads of perspiration on the upper lip or brow
- Increasing rectal pressure and an urge to bear down

The woman in this phase is anxious to "get it over with." She may be amnesic and sleep between her frequent contractions. Her support persons may start to feel helpless and may turn to the nurse for increased help as their efforts to alleviate her discomfort seem less effective.

Second Stage

The second stage of labor begins with complete cervical dilatation and ends with birth of the baby. The second stage is usually completed within 3 hours after the cervix becomes fully dilated for primigravidas; the stage averages 15 minutes for multiparas. Contractions continue with a frequency of about every 1.5 to 2.0 minutes, duration of 60 to 90 seconds, and strong intensity. Descent of the fetal presenting part continues until it reaches the perineal floor.

Some practitioners have further subdivided the second stage into two phases including the latent/passive fetal descent stage in which the woman may initially experience the urge to push. During this time, passive fetal descent occurs in response to the uterine contractions. Nursing tasks during this phase include (Association of Women's Health, Obstetric and Neonatal Nurses [AWHONN], 2013):

- Assessing the woman's perception of the need or urge to push
- Evaluating the maternal–fetal oxygenation status to ensure adequate uteroplacental perfusion is occurring
- Assessing fetal status through recommended monitoring protocols

The second phase (within the second stage of labor) is known as the active pushing phase and occurs once the urge to push

The presence of the father during labor and at birth, although common in countries such as the United States, Canada, and Australia, is not a universal norm. Rather it is strongly influenced by cultural practices. The father is not present at the birth in many countries, including Algeria, Brazil, China, Ethiopia, and Korea. Similarly, Orthodox Jews do not allow men to attend the labor and birth (McFarland & Wehbe-Alamah, 2014).

has been established and the woman begins to actively push with her contractions. Nursing tasks during this phase include (AWHONN, 2013):

- Assessing the effectiveness of the maternal pushing efforts
- Providing encouragement and direction to obtain a more adequate pushing effort
- Assessing fetal response that occurs as maternal pushing is performed, including continued fetal assessment measures

While some women may be encouraged to begin pushing immediately after the identification of complete dilatation, others may be encouraged to delay pushing and allow for passive fetal descent, an act known as "laboring down." A recent systematic review comparing both methods of pushing did not identify any differences in maternal or fetal outcomes; however, women in the passive descent or laboring down group experienced a longer second stage of labor that resulted in a reduction of active pushing efforts (King et al., 2014). Laboring down does aid the woman who is extremely fatigued and does prevent extensive pushing efforts that may occur before the urge to push is experienced by the woman.

As the fetal head descends, the woman usually has the urge to push because of pressure of the fetal head on the sacral and obturator nerves. As she pushes, contraction of the maternal abdominal muscles exerts intra-abdominal pressure. As the fetal head continues its descent, the perineum begins to bulge, flatten, and move anteriorly. The amount of bloody show may increase. The labia begin to part with each contraction. Between contractions the fetal head appears to recede. With succeeding contractions and

maternal pushing effort, the fetal head descends farther. **Crowning** occurs when the fetal head is encircled by the external opening of the vagina (introitus), and it means birth is imminent.

The woman may feel some relief that the acute pain she felt during the transition phase is over (Table 16–5). She may also be relieved that the birth is near and she can push. Some women feel a sense of purpose that they can be actively involved. Others, particularly those without childbirth preparation, may become frightened and fight each contraction. Such behavior may be disconcerting to the woman's support persons. The woman may feel she has lost her ability to cope and become embarrassed, or she may demonstrate extreme irritability toward the staff or her supporters as she attempts to regain control over forces against which she feels helpless. Most women feel acute, increasingly severe pain and a burning sensation as the perineum distends.

SPONTANEOUS BIRTH (VERTEX PRESENTATION)
As the fetal head distends the vulva with each contraction, the perineum becomes extremely thin and the anus stretches and protrudes. With time, the head extends under the symphysis pubis and is born. When the anterior shoulder meets the underside of the symphysis pubis, a gentle push by the mother aids in the birth of the shoulders. The body then follows (see a birthing sequence in Figure 16–12). (Birth of a fetus in other than a vertex presentation is discussed in Chapter 21.)

CARDINAL MOVEMENTS OF LABOR
For the fetus to pass through the birth canal, the fetal head and body must adjust to the passage by certain positional changes. These changes, called **cardinal movements** or mechanisms of labor, are described in the order in which they occur (Figure 16–13).

Descent.   Descent occurs because of four forces: (1) pressure of the amniotic fluid, (2) direct pressure of the uterine fundus on the breech, (3) contraction of the abdominal muscles, and (4) extension and straightening of the fetal body. The head enters the inlet in the occiput transverse or oblique position because the pelvic inlet is widest from side to side. The sagittal suture is an equal distance from the maternal symphysis pubis and sacral promontory.

Flexion.   Flexion occurs as the fetal head descends and meets resistance from the soft tissues of the pelvis, the muscles of the pelvic floor, and the cervix. As a result of the resistance, the fetal chin flexes downward onto the chest.

TABLE 16–5 Characteristics of Labor

	FIRST STAGE			SECOND STAGE
	LATENT PHASE	**ACTIVE PHASE**	**TRANSITION PHASE**	**SECOND STAGE**
Nullipara	8.6 hr	4.6 hr	3.6 hr	Up to 3 hr
Multipara	5.3 hr	2.4 hr	Variable	Less than 1 hr; averages 15 min
Cervical dilatation	0–3 cm	4–7 cm	8–10 cm	
Contractions				
Frequency	Every 10–30 min, progressing to every 5–7 min	Every 2–3 min	Every 1½–2 min	Every 1½–2 min
Duration	30–40 sec	40–60 sec	60–90 sec	60–90 sec
Intensity	Begin as mild and progress to moderate; 25–40 mmHg by intrauterine pressure catheter (IUPC)	Begin as moderate and progress to strong; 50–70 mmHg by IUPC	Strong by palpation; 70–90 mmHg by IUPC	Strong by palpation; 70–100 mmHg by IUPC

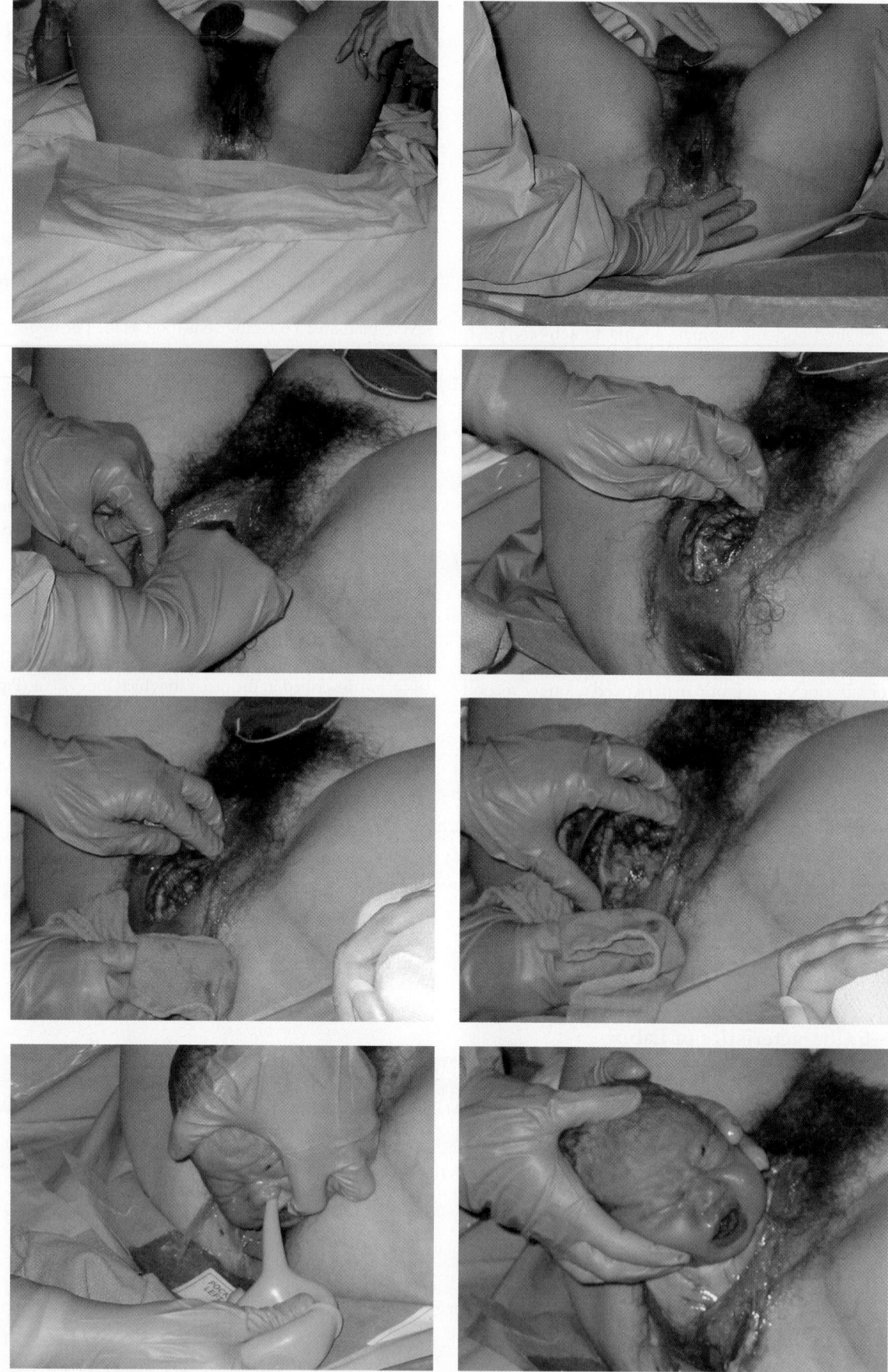

Figure 16–12 A birthing sequence.

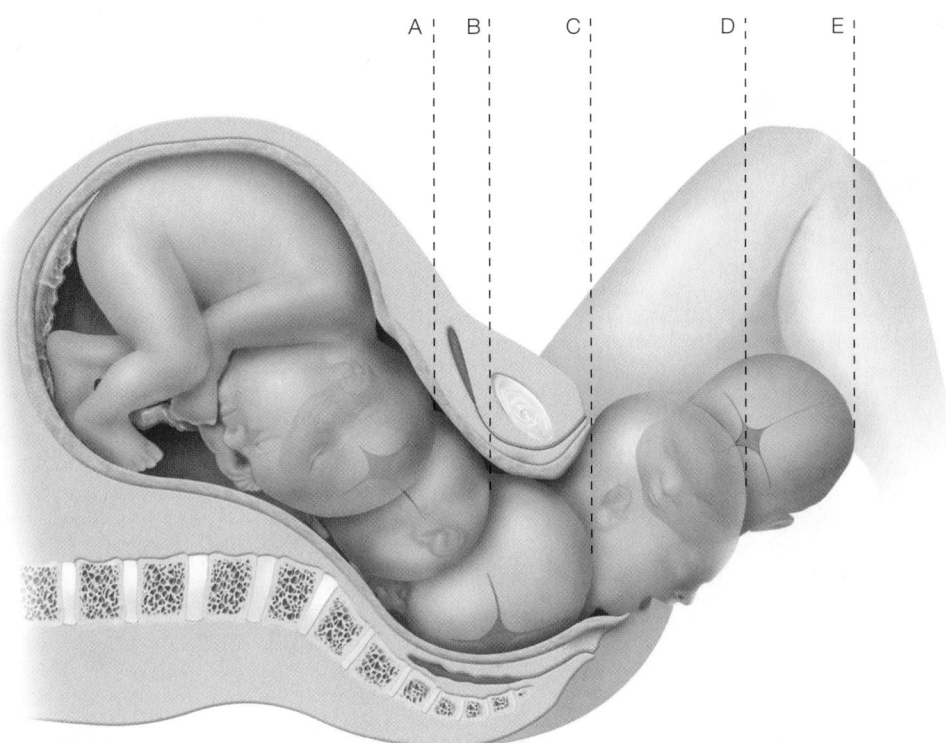

Figure 16–13 Mechanisms of labor. *A* and *B*, Descent. *C*, Internal rotation. *D*, Extension. *E*, External rotation.

Internal Rotation. The fetal head must rotate to fit the diameter of the pelvic cavity, which is widest in the anteroposterior diameter. As the occiput of the fetal head meets resistance from the levator ani muscles and their fascia, the occiput rotates—usually from left to right—and the sagittal suture aligns in the anteroposterior pelvic diameter.

Extension. The resistance of the pelvic floor, and the mechanical movement of the vulva opening anteriorly and forward, assist with extension of the fetal head as it passes under the symphysis pubis. With this positional change, the occiput, then brow and face, emerge from the vagina.

Restitution. The shoulders of the fetus enter the pelvic inlet obliquely and remain oblique when the head rotates to the anteroposterior diameter through internal rotation. Because of this rotation, the neck becomes twisted. Once the head is born and is free of pelvic resistance, the neck untwists, turning the head to one side (restitution), and aligns with the position of the back in the birth canal.

External Rotation. As the shoulders rotate to the anteroposterior position in the pelvis, the head turns farther to one side (external rotation).

Expulsion. After the external rotation, and through the pushing efforts of the laboring woman, the anterior shoulder meets the undersurface of the symphysis pubis and slips under it. As lateral flexion of the shoulder and head occurs, the anterior shoulder is born before the posterior shoulder. The body follows quickly.

Third Stage

PLACENTAL SEPARATION

After the baby is born, the uterus contracts firmly, decreasing its capacity and the surface area of placental attachment. The placenta begins to separate because of this decreased surface area. As separation occurs, bleeding results in the formation of a hematoma between the placental tissue and the remaining decidua. This hematoma speeds the separation process. The membranes are the last to separate. They are peeled off the uterine wall as the placenta descends into the vagina. Signs of placental separation usually appear about 5 minutes after the birth of the newborn. These signs are (1) a globular-shaped uterus, (2) a rise of the fundus in the abdomen, (3) a sudden gush or trickle of blood, and (4) further protrusion of the umbilical cord out of the vagina.

PLACENTAL DELIVERY

When the signs of placental separation appear, the woman may bear down to aid in placental expulsion. If this fails and the certified nurse-midwife or physician has ascertained that the fundus is firm, gentle traction may be applied to the cord while pressure is exerted on the fundus. The weight of the placenta as it is guided into the placental collection pan aids in the removal of the membranes from the uterine wall. A placenta is considered to be retained if 30 minutes have elapsed from completion of the second stage of labor.

If the placenta separates from the inside to the outer margins, it is expelled with the fetal (shiny) side presenting (Figure 16–14A). This is known as the Schultze mechanism of placental delivery or, more commonly, "shiny Schultze" (also see Figure 7–9). If the placenta separates from the outer margins inward, it rolls up and presents sideways with the maternal surface expelled first. This is known as the Duncan mechanism (see Figure 16-14B) and is commonly called "dirty Duncan" because the placental surface is rough (also see Figure 7–8). (Interventions for the third stage of labor are discussed in Chapter 18.)

Fourth Stage

The fourth stage of labor is the time, from 1 to 4 hours after birth, during which physiologic readjustment of the mother's body begins. With the birth, hemodynamic changes occur. Blood loss

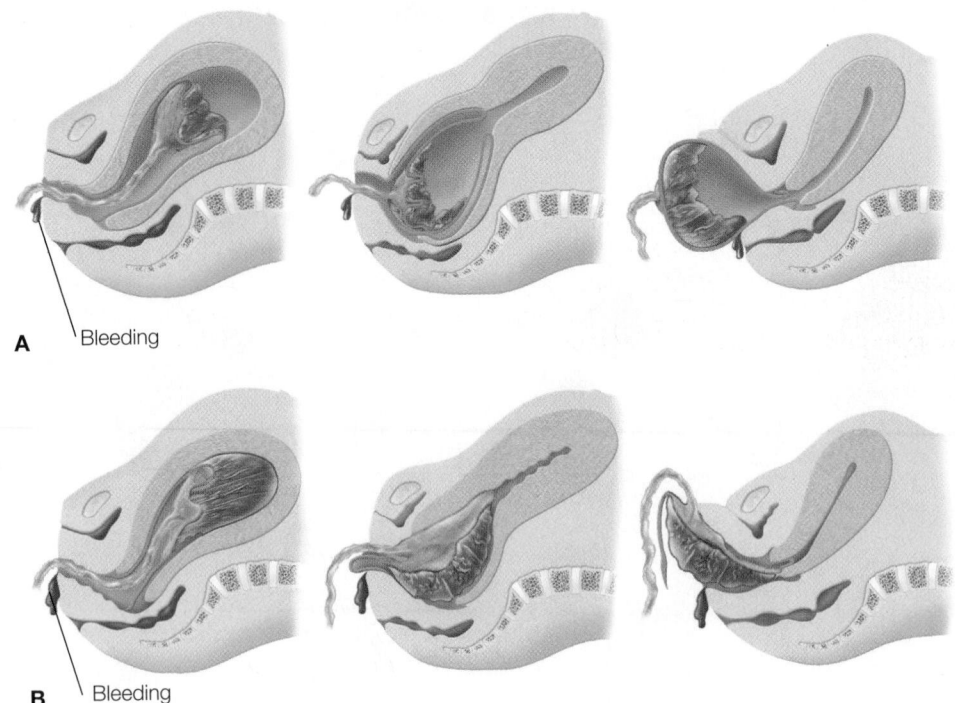

A Bleeding

B Bleeding

Figure 16–14 Placental separation and expulsion. *A*, Schultze mechanism. *B*, Duncan mechanism.

ranges from 250 to 500 mL. With this blood loss and removal of the weight of the pregnant uterus from the surrounding vessels, blood is redistributed into venous beds. This results in a moderate drop in both systolic and diastolic blood pressure, increased pulse pressure, and moderate tachycardia (Cunningham et al., 2014).

The uterus remains contracted in the midline of the abdomen. The fundus is usually midway between the symphysis pubis and umbilicus. Its contracted state constricts the vessels at the site of placental implantation. Immediately after expulsion of the placenta, the cervix is widely spread and thick.

Nausea and vomiting usually cease. The woman may be thirsty and hungry. She may experience a shaking chill, which is thought to be associated with the ending of the physical exertion of labor. The bladder is often hypotonic due to trauma during the second stage or the administration of anesthetics that decrease sensations. Hypotonic bladder can lead to urinary retention.

SAFETY ALERT!

During the fourth stage of labor, women should be assisted during their initial attempt to ambulate since dizziness and syncope can lead to falls. The woman should be advised not to hold the baby with ambulation when first attempting ambulation after the birth.

Maternal Systemic Response to Labor

The process of labor and birth affects almost all maternal physiologic systems.

Cardiovascular System

Uterine contractions and the pain, anxiety, and apprehension a laboring woman experiences stress her cardiovascular system. With each contraction, 300 to 500 mL of blood volume is forced back into the maternal circulation, which results in an increase in cardiac output of as much as 10% to 15% over the typical third-trimester levels (Blackburn, 2013). Cardiac output increases more as the laboring woman experiences pain with uterine contractions and her anxiety and apprehension increase.

Maternal position also affects cardiac output. In the supine position, cardiac output decreases, heart rate increases, and stroke volume decreases. When the woman turns to a lateral (side-lying) position, cardiac output increases (Blackburn, 2013).

BLOOD PRESSURE

As a result of increased cardiac output, blood pressure rises during uterine contractions. In the first stage, systolic pressure increases by 35 mmHg and diastolic pressure increases by about 25 mmHg. There may be further increases in the second stage during pushing (Blackburn, 2013).

Respiratory System

Oxygen demand and consumption increase when labor begins because of the presence of uterine contractions. As anxiety and pain from contractions increase, hyperventilation frequently occurs. With hyperventilation there is a fall in $PaCO_2$, and respiratory alkalosis results (Powrie, Greene, & Camann, 2012).

By the end of the first stage, most women have developed a mild metabolic acidosis compensated by respiratory alkalosis. As they push in the second stage of labor, their $PaCO_2$ levels may rise along with blood lactate levels (due to muscular activity), and mild respiratory acidosis occurs. By the time the baby is born (end of second stage), the woman has metabolic acidosis uncompensated for by respiratory alkalosis. The changes in acid–base status that occur in labor are quickly reversed in the fourth stage because of changes in women's respiratory rates. Acid–base levels return to pregnancy levels by 24 hours after birth, and to nonpregnant values a few weeks after birth (Powrie et al., 2012).

Renal System

During labor there is an increase in maternal renin, plasma renin activity, and angiotensinogen. This elevation is thought to be important in the control of uteroplacental blood flow during birth and the early postpartum period. Structurally the base of the bladder is pushed forward and upward when engagement occurs. The pressure from the presenting part may impair blood and lymph drainage from the base of the bladder, leading to edema (Cunningham et al., 2014).

Gastrointestinal System

During labor gastric motility and absorption of solid food are reduced. Gastric emptying time is prolonged, and gastric volume (amount of contents that remain in the stomach) remains increased, regardless of the time the last meal was taken. Some narcotics also delay gastric emptying time and add to the risk of aspiration if general anesthesia is used.

Immune System and Other Blood Values

The white blood cell (WBC) count increases to 25,000 to 30,000/mm³ during labor and the early postpartum period. The change in WBC count is mostly due to increased neutrophils resulting from a physiologic response to stress. The increased WBC count makes it difficult to identify an infection. Maternal blood glucose levels decrease because the body uses glucose as an energy source during contractions. Decreased blood glucose levels lead to a decrease in insulin requirements.

Pain

Pain during labor comes from a complexity of physical causes. Each woman will experience and cope with pain differently. Multiple factors affect a woman's reaction to labor pain.

CAUSES OF PAIN DURING LABOR

The pain associated with the first stage of labor is unique in that it accompanies a normal physiologic process. Even though perception of the pain of childbirth varies among women, there is a physiologic basis for discomfort during labor. Pain during the first stage of labor arises from (1) dilatation of the cervix, which is the primary source of pain; (2) stretching of the lower uterine segment; (3) pressure on adjacent structures; and (4) hypoxia of the uterine muscle cells during contraction (Blackburn, 2013). The areas of pain include the lower abdominal wall and the areas over the lower lumbar region and the upper sacrum (Figure 16–15).

During the second stage of labor, discomfort is due to (1) hypoxia of the contracting uterine muscle cells, (2) distention of the vagina and perineum, and (3) pressure on adjacent structures. The area of pain increases as shown in Figure 16–16 and Figure 16–17.

Pain during the third stage results from uterine contractions and cervical dilatation as the placenta is expelled. This stage of labor is short, and after it anesthesia is needed primarily for episiotomy repair.

FACTORS AFFECTING RESPONSE TO PAIN

Many factors affect the individual's perception of and response to pain. For example, research shows that childbirth preparation classes often reduce the need for analgesia during labor. People tend to respond to painful stimuli in the way that is acceptable in their culture. In some cultures, it is natural to communicate pain, no matter how mild, whereas members of other cultures stoically accept pain. Fatigue and sleep deprivation may also influence response to pain. The tired woman has less energy and ability to use such strategies as distraction or imagination to deal with pain. As a result she may lose her ability to cope with labor and choose analgesics or other medications to relieve the discomfort.

The woman's previous experience with pain and her anxiety level also affect her ability to manage current and future pain. Those who have had experience with pain seem more

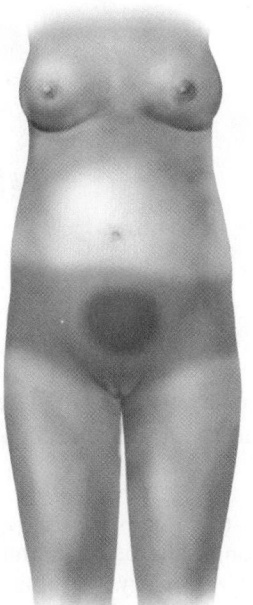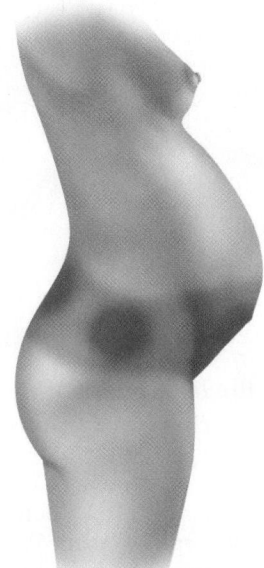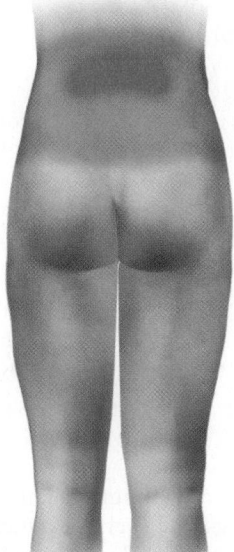

Figure 16–15 **Area of reference of labor pain during the first stage. Pain is most intense in the darkened areas.**

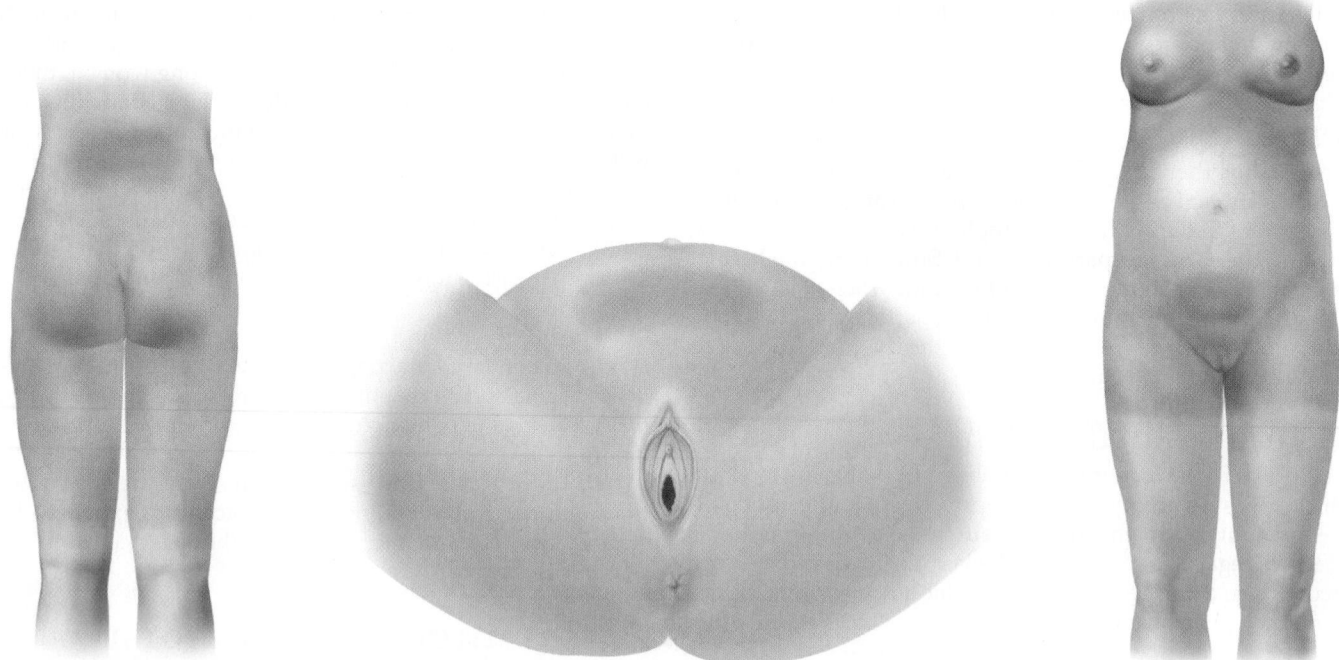

Figure 16–16 Distribution of labor pain during the later phase of the first stage and early phase of the second stage. The darkest colored areas indicate the location of the most intense pain, moderate color indicates moderate pain, and lighter color indicates mild pain. The uterine contractions, which at this stage are very strong, produce intense pain.

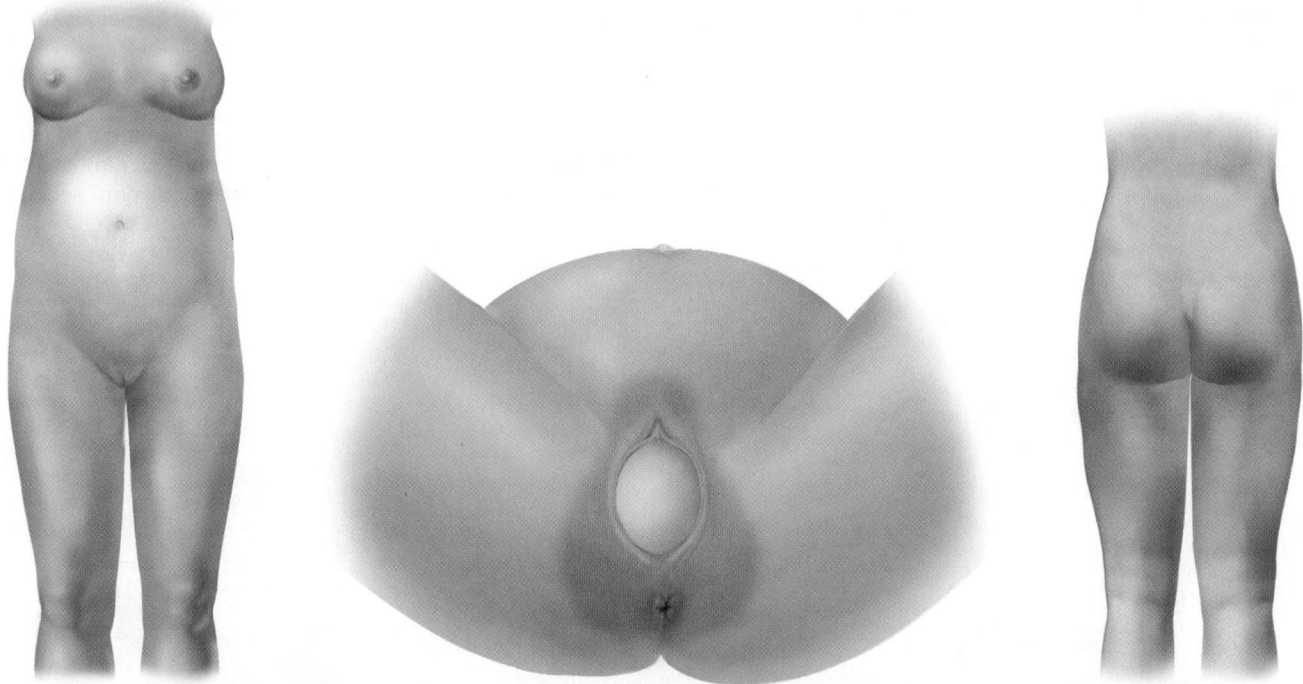

Figure 16–17 Distribution of labor pain during the later phase of the second stage and actual birth. The perineal component is the primary cause of discomfort. Uterine contractions contribute much less to the level of pain.

sensitive to painful stimuli than those who have not. Unfamiliar surroundings and events can increase anxiety, as does separation from family and loved ones. Anticipation of discomfort and questions about whether she can cope with the contractions may also increase anxiety.

Both attention and distraction influence the perception of pain. When pain sensation is the focus of attention, the perceived intensity is greater. A sensory stimulus such as a back rub can be a distraction that focuses the woman's attention on the stimulus rather than on the pain.

Fetal Response to Labor

When the fetus is healthy, the mechanical and hemodynamic changes of normal labor have no adverse effects. However, certain physiologic responses do occur:

- *Heart rate changes.* Early fetal heart rate decelerations can occur with intracranial pressures of 40 to 55 mmHg, as the head pushes against the cervix. This early deceleration is believed to be due to hypoxic depression of the central nervous system, which is under vagal control. The absence of head compression decelerations in some fetuses during labor is explained by a threshold reached more gradually in the presence of intact membranes and lack of maternal resistance. These early decelerations are harmless in a normal fetus.

- *Acid–base status in labor.* Blood flow is decreased to the fetus at the peak of each contraction, which leads to a slow decrease in pH. During the second stage of labor, as uterine contractions become longer and stronger and the woman holds her breath to push, the fetal pH decreases more rapidly. The base deficit increases, and fetal oxygen saturation drops about 10% (Blackburn, 2013).

- *Hemodynamic changes.* The adequate exchange of nutrients and gases in the fetal capillaries and intervillous spaces depends in part on the fetal blood pressure. Fetal blood pressure protects the normal fetus during the anoxic periods caused by the contracting uterus during labor. The fetal and placental reserve is usually enough to see the fetus through these anoxic periods unharmed (Blackburn, 2013).

- *Fetal sensation.* Beginning at about 37 or 38 weeks' gestation, the fetus is able to experience sensations of light, sound, and touch. The full-term fetus is able to hear music and the maternal voice. Even in utero the fetus is sensitive to light and will move away from a bright light source. The term baby is aware of pressure sensations during labor such as the touch of the healthcare provider during a vaginal examination or pressure on the head as a contraction occurs. Although the fetus may not be able to process this input, the fetus is experiencing labor as the woman labors.

Focus Your Study

- Most childbirth classes include information on body-conditioning exercises, relaxation techniques, and breathing methods.

- Labor is directly impacted by the five critical factors of labor include the birth passage, the fetus, relationship between the fetus and the pelvis, physiologic forces of labor, and psychologic factors.

- Physiologic processes that occur in labor include the presence of progesterone which causes smooth muscle relaxation; estrogen to stimulate uterine contractions, loosening of connective tissue to permit softening, thinning, and opening of the cervix; and shortening and muscles within the upper uterine segment which causes and cervix to thin and flatten.

- During labor, the fetal body is straightened as the uterus elongates with contractions causing pressure from the fetal head to facilitate cervical dilatation. Contractions also cause the rectum and vagina to draw up while the anus everts during the second stage.

- Premonitory signs of labor include lightening, Braxton Hicks contractions, cervical changes, bloody show, rupture of membranes, sudden burst of energy, slight weight loss, and gastrointestinal symptoms.

- True labor is characterized by contractions that occur at regular intervals that increase in duration and intensity. True labor contractions typically increase with activity and do not respond to resting or application of warm water. True labor continues and results in cervical changes, whereas false labor is characterized by irregular contractions that do not increase in frequency, duration or intensity, have no set patterns, may be relived through interventions such as walking, resting, or warm water application. False labor discomfort is primarily focused in the abdomen and does not result in cervical change.

- In the first stage of labor, the latent phase typically is marked by mild contractions that progressively increase in intensity and frequency and result in cervical change up to 3 cm. The active stage of labor is marked by a significant increase in contraction frequency, insanity, and duration, and results in cervical change from 4 to 7 cm. During this phase, the fetus begins to descend further down into the pelvis. In the transition phase, contractions continue to increase in intensity, duration, and frequency and the cervix dilates from 8 to 10 cm. During this phase, the woman feels rectal pressure as the fetus descends into the birth passage. Women may experience nausea and/or vomiting.

- In the second stage of labor, the cervix is completely dilated and effaced. The woman uses intra-abdominal pressure to push due to pressure of fetal head on sacral and obturator nerves. As the fetus descends, the perineum begins to bulged, flatten, and move anteriorly.

- The third stage occurs once the fetus is delivered and continues until the placenta separates and is expelled. Occasionally, mild traction of the cord is used to facilitate placenta delivery.

- The fourth stage begins immediately after the placenta delivery and is a period where significant physiologic changes occur including the redistribution of blood which results in an increased pulse and decreased blood pressure that occurs as blood shifts to the body from the uterus and the body adapts to the blood loss that has occurred. The uterus contracts during this period and is located between the symphysis pubis and the umbilicus. Women may experience a chill with shaking during this period. Urinary retention can occur as a result of anesthesia, bladder trauma, or reduced bladder tone.

- Multiple maternal systemic physiologic changes occur during labor including increased cardiac output, increase blood pressure during contractions and with maternal pushing efforts, increased oxygen demands, mild respiratory acidosis at the time of birth, increases in renin, plasma renin activity, and angiotensinogen, bladder edema, reduction in gastrointestinal functioning, increases in WBC count, and reduced glucose levels.

- Maternal pain and discomfort occur throughout labor in response to physiologic changes. In the first stage, pain occurs as the cervix dilates and lower uterine segment is stretched with contractions that results in muscle hypoxia. In the second stage, hypoxia arises as the muscles contract and

distention of the vagina, perineum, and rectal pressure occur. In third stage, pain occurs from the contractions and dilatation of the cervix that occurs when the placenta is expelled.

- In healthy fetuses, labor should cause no adverse effects. FHR changes can occur as the head pushes on the cervix. The umbilical blood flow decreases at the peak of contractions which can lead to a slight reduction in the pH. Reductions in the pH can also occur in women who hold their breath for prolonged pushing during second stage.

Clinical Reasoning in Action

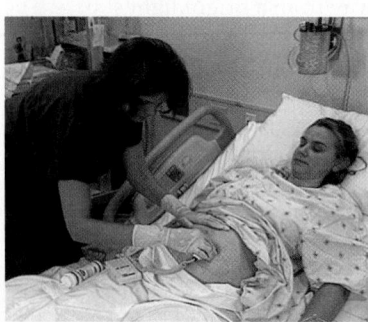

Ann Nelson, a 28-year-old, G2P0010 at 41 weeks' gestation, is admitted to the birthing unit where you are working. She is here for cervical ripening and induction of labor due to postdate pregnancy and decreased amniotic fluid volume. A review of her prenatal medical record reveals a pertinent history of infertility (clomiphene [Clomid]–induced pregnancy) and asthma (treated with inhalers on a PRN basis). The Doppler picks up a fetal heart rate of 120 beats/min. You place Ann on the electronic fetal monitor and obtain the following data: BP 126/76, T 98°F, P 82, R 16; vaginal examination reveals a 20%

effaced cervix, 1 cm dilatation in the posterior position, and vertex at –2 station. The fetal monitor shows a fetal heart rate baseline of 120 to 128 with occasional variable decelerations, accelerations to 140 with fetal activity. No contractions are noted on the monitor or palpated. Ann asks you what to expect with "cervical ripening" using prostaglandin gel.

1. Discuss the action of prostaglandin gel.
2. Ann asks you why cervical ripening and induction of labor are recommended for her and her baby. How would you best respond to her?
3. Ann asks how she will know if she is getting contractions. How would you answer her?
4. Discuss the difference between mild, moderate, and strong contractions.
5. Describe the latent phase of labor.

References

Association of Women's Health, Obstetric and Neonatal Nurses (AWHONN). (2013). *Evidence-based clinical practice guideline: Nursing care and management of the second stage of labor* (3rd ed.). Washington, DC: Author.

Blackburn, S. T. (2013). *Maternal, fetal, and neonatal physiology: A clinical perspective* (4th ed.). Philadelphia, PA: Saunders.

Caldwell, W. E., & Moloy, H. C. (1933). Anatomical variation in the female pelvis and their effect on labor with a suggested classification. *American Journal of Obstetrics and Gynecology, 26,* 479–487.

Cunningham, F. G., Leveno, K. J., Bloom, S. L., Spong, C. Y., Dashe, J. S., Hoffman, B. L., … Sheffield,

J. S. (2014). *Williams Obstetrics* (24th ed.). New York, NY: McGraw-Hill.

Hodnett, E. D., Gates, S., Hofmeyr, G. J., Sakala, C., & Weston, J. (2011). Continuous support for women during childbirth. *Cochrane Database of Systematic Reviews,* Issue 2. Art. No.: CD003766. doi:10.1002/14651858.CD003766.pub3

International Childbirth Education Association (ICEA). (2012). *ICEA philosophy statement.* Retrieved from http://www.icea.org/content/mission

Jazayeri, A. (2014). Premature rupture of membranes. *eMedicine.* Retrieved from http://emedicine .medscape.com/article/261137-overview #aw2aab6b3

King, T. K., Brucker, M. C., Kriebs, J. M., & Fahey, J. (2013). *Varney's midwifery* (5th ed.). New York, NY: Jones Bartlett Learning.

McFarland, M.R., & Wehbe-Alamah, H.B. (2014). *Leininger's culture care diversity and universality: A worldwide nursing theory* (3rd ed.). New York, NY: Jones & Bartlett.

Posner, G., Black, A., Jones, G., & Dy, J. (2013). *Oxorne Foote human labor and birth* (6th ed.). New York, NY: McGraw-Hill.

Powrie, R., Greene, M., & Camann, V. (2012). *De Swiet's medical disorders in obstetric practice* (5th ed.). New York, NY: John Wiley & Sons.

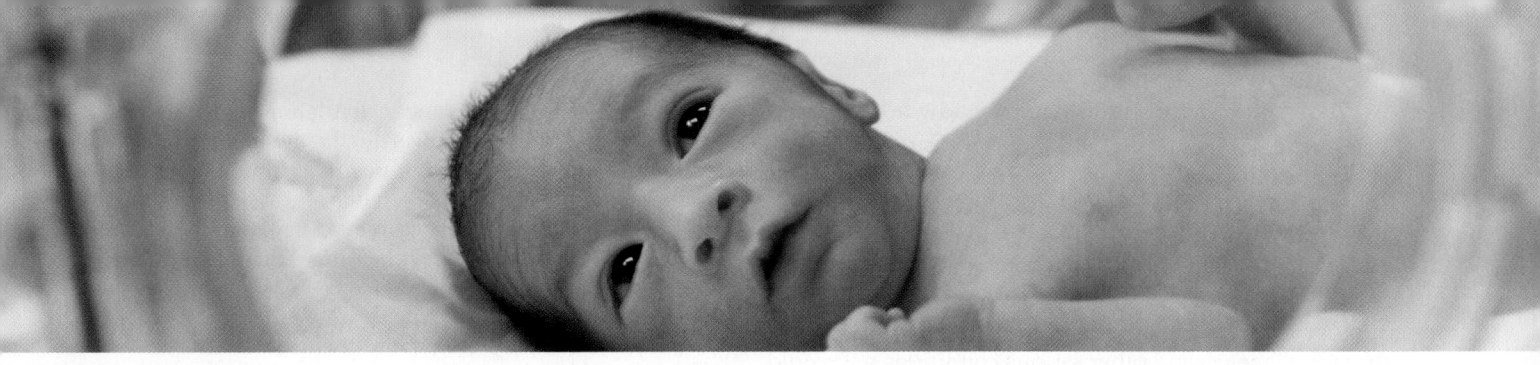

Chapter 17
Intrapartum Nursing Assessment

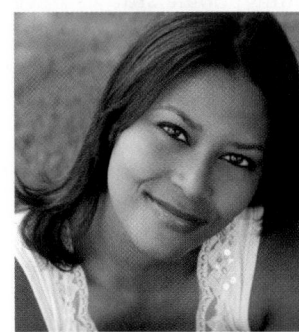

Jason Stitt/Fotolia

It was strange. After months of waiting for my baby's birth, labor took me by surprise. I wasn't quite ready to move from being pregnant to being a mother. Not that I had any choice!
—Malika, 23

∨ Learning Outcomes

17.1 Describe a maternal assessment of the laboring woman that includes the client history, high-risk screening, and physical and psychosociocultural factors.

17.2 Evaluate the progress of labor by assessing the laboring woman's contractions, cervical dilatation, and effacement.

17.3 Delineate the procedure for performing Leopold maneuvers and the information that can be obtained, including the importance of identifying accurate fetal position prior to performing a fetal heart rate assessment.

17.4 Describe the steps and frequency for performing auscultation of fetal heart rate.

17.5 Distinguish between baseline and periodic changes in fetal heart rate monitoring, and the appearance and significance of each.

17.6 Evaluate fetal heart rate tracings using a systematic approach.

17.7 Compare nonreassuring fetal heart rate patterns to appropriate nursing responses.

17.8 Explain the family's responses to electronic fetal monitoring in nursing management.

The physiologic events during labor call for many adaptations by the mother and the fetus. Thus frequent and accurate assessments are crucial. The woman's partner or chosen support person is also an integral part of the childbirth experience. Moreover, the traditional assessment techniques of observation, palpation, and auscultation are augmented by the judicious use of technology such as ultrasound and electronic monitoring. However, the technology only provides data; it is the nurse who monitors the mother and her baby.

Maternal Assessment
History

Obtain a brief oral history when the woman is admitted to the birthing area. Each agency has its own admission forms, but they usually include the following information:

- Woman's name and age
- Last menstrual period (LMP) and estimated date of birth (EDB)

- Attending physician or certified nurse-midwife (CNM)
- Personal data: blood type; Rh factor; results of serology testing; prepregnant and present weight; allergies to medications, foods, or other substances; prescribed and over-the-counter medications taken during pregnancy; and history of drug and alcohol use and smoking during the pregnancy
- History of previous illness, such as tuberculosis, heart disease, diabetes, and other serious conditions that could influence the pregnancy
- Problems in the prenatal period, such as elevated blood pressure, bleeding problems, recurrent urinary tract infections, other infections
- Pregnancy data: gravida, para, abortions, and perinatal deaths
- The method chosen for newborn feeding
- Type of prenatal education classes (childbirth education classes)
- Woman's preferences about labor and birth, such as no episiotomy, no analgesics or anesthetics, or the presence of the father or others at the birth
- Pediatrician or family practice physician
- Additional data: history of special tests such as non-stress test (NST), biophysical profile (BPP), or ultrasound; history of any preterm labor; onset of labor; amniotic fluid membrane status; and brief description of previous labor and birth
- Onset of labor
- Status of amniotic membranes (Are they intact or ruptured? If ruptured, time of rupture, color of fluid, and odor.)

PSYCHOSOCIAL CONSIDERATIONS

Assessment of psychosocial history is a critical component of intrapartum nursing assessment. The parents' psychosocial readiness, including their fears, anxieties, birth fantasies, excitement level, feelings of joy and anticipation, and level of social support, can be a critical factor in a successful birth experience. Some mothers may fear having a bowel movement during the second stage of labor and experiencing embarrassment related to this normal physiologic process. Other mothers may feel a sense of failure if they desire an unmedicated birth and then use pain medication at the actual time of labor or birth. Both the mother and father are making a transition into a new role, and both have expectations of themselves during the labor and birth experience, and as caregivers for their child and their new family. Psychosocial factors affecting labor and birth include the couple's accomplishment of the tasks of pregnancy, usual coping mechanisms in response to stressful life events, support system, preparation for childbirth, and cultural influences. Even mothers and fathers who attend childbirth preparation classes and have a solid support system can be concerned about what labor will be like, whether they will be able to perform the way they expect, whether the pain will be more than the mother expects or can cope with, and whether the father can provide helpful support. The physical and emotional stress of birth can impact a couple's responses to the labor itself.

Some women may fear the pain of contractions, whereas others welcome the opportunity to feel the birth process. Some women view the pain as threatening and associate it with a loss of control over their bodies and emotions. Other women see pain as a rite of passage into motherhood and a necessary means to an end. It is helpful for women to realize that the pain

of labor is natural. Assurances that labor is progressing normally can go a long way toward reducing anxiety and thereby reducing pain, and providing positive reinforcement that the mother is doing "a good job." In one study, empowerment and having control over one's body played key roles in determining whether a woman viewed her labor and birth positively (Nilsson, Thorsell, Hertfelt-Wahn, et al., 2013). Women who viewed their births as a positive experience were also more likely to have a sense of well-being about themselves after the experience (Nilsson et al., 2013). A wide variety of coping techniques to assist both the laboring woman and her partner are discussed in Chapters 18 and 19.

How the woman views the birth experience in hindsight may affect her mothering behaviors. It appears that any activities by the expectant woman or by healthcare providers that enhance the birth experience will be beneficial to the mother–baby connection and improve bonding. Some studies have shown that when some women are disappointed with their birth experience or have negative feelings during the third trimester, they may have some initial difficulties and be more prone to postpartum mood disorders (Nilsson et al., 2013). Psychosocial factors associated with a positive birth experience are summarized in Table 17–1.

The laboring woman's support system also influences the course of labor and birth. Some women prefer not to have a support person or family member with them. They may feel that the birth process is a private moment that they wish to reserve for themselves. However, most women choose to have significant persons (father or partner, family members, friends) with them during labor and birth. Social support tends to have a positive effect. For some families, the birth event is a celebration, and they want to create a joyful, festive atmosphere with many loved ones present. Some facilities may limit the number of family members present during labor and birth, so the nurse needs to be familiar with specific facility policies. Generally, the presence of the laboring woman's partner at the bedside provides a means to enhance communication and to demonstrate feelings of love.

Psychosocial Risk Factors. The psychosocial history is a critical component of assessment. An estimated one third of all pregnant women are exposed to some type of psychotropic medication

TABLE 17–1 Factors Associated With a Positive Birth Experience

- Motivation for the pregnancy
- Attendance at childbirth education classes
- A sense of competence or mastery
- Self-confidence and self-esteem
- Positive relationship with mate
- Perception of maintaining control during labor
- Support from mate or other person during labor
- Not being left alone in labor
- Trust in the medical and nursing staff
- Personal control of breathing patterns and comfort measures
- A physician or certified nurse-midwife who has a similar philosophy of care
- Clear information from healthcare providers regarding necessary procedures

during their pregnancies. There are growing concerns that some psychotropic medications may cause fetal and neonatal side effects, such as a shortened gestational period, short-term neonatal irritability, neurobehavioral changes, and, rarely, persistent pulmonary hypertension of the newborn. There have been reports of congenital anomalies, although no specific patterns have been noted with the exception of the use of paroxetine hydrochloride (Paxil), which is known to cause cardiac anomalies. In 2012, the American Psychological Association and the American College of Obstetricians and Gynecologists issued a joint statement indicating that these side effects cannot be attributed solely to medication administration and can also be related to the impact of depression and psychiatric illness on the pregnancies of affected mothers (Yonkers et al., 2012).

It is estimated that 10% of pregnant women meet the criteria for major depressive disorder during pregnancy and another 18% have depressive symptoms during the gestational period (Dalfen, 2014). It is also not uncommon for women to be diagnosed with other mental illnesses that may impact the labor and birth process. These may include (Davidson, 2012):

- Eating disorders
- Autism
- Learning disabilities
- Attention deficit or attention deficit hyperactivity disorder
- Anxiety
- Mood disorders

Any of these diagnoses can play a role in how the woman copes with labor and birth and should be assessed by the admitting nurse. Women with identified disorders will need ongoing assessment during the labor and birth. In addition, they are at greater risk for postpartum mood disorders and posttraumatic stress disorders (PTSDs) and warrant additional evaluation in the immediate, intermediate, and extended postpartum periods.

Because of the prevalence of intimate partner and domestic violence in our society (see Chapter 5), the nurse needs to consider the possibility that the woman may have experienced abuse at some point in her life. Many victims of domestic violence, sexual assault, or childhood abuse may have anxiety about the labor process before it begins, or the anxiety may arise during labor. Therefore, it is essential to be alert for information that may indicate abuse or a history of victimization of violence.

SAFETY ALERT!

If a woman feels unsafe in the clinical environment and fears for her safety because of past intimate partner violence, alert security and the charge nurse ahead of time to deny access to the birthing area for that partner. Antepartum assessment for domestic violence is discussed in Chapter 9.

Clinical Tip

Many nurses have difficulty asking questions about domestic violence, sexual abuse, sexual intercourse/sexual practices, and drug or alcohol use during pregnancy. However, this information is necessary to provide effective care. To create a relationship of trust with the woman, the following tips may be helpful:

- Explore your own beliefs and values.
- Use open-ended questions.
- Be receptive to the answers.
- Be accepting of others' life experiences.

Clinical Reasoning Identifying Domestic Violence

You are the birthing center nurse and you have reason to suspect that Lynn Ling, who has just been admitted in labor, may be in an abusive relationship. How could you set up an interview so that the partner would leave the room (and take any accompanying children) without feeling that you are possibly increasing the risk to the woman? What communication techniques would you use to encourage Lynn to reveal if her partner is abusive?

Intrapartum High-Risk Screening

Screening for intrapartum high-risk factors is an integral part of assessment. As the history is obtained, note the presence of any factors that may be associated with a high-risk condition. For example, the woman who reports a physical symptom such as intermittent bleeding needs further assessment to rule out abruptio placentae or placenta previa before the admission process continues. In such a case, the woman should be asked the amount of bleeding that occurred, the onset, duration, and if she needed to wear a sanitary pad. If a pad was placed, the time between pad saturation should be assessed. In cases of unknown vaginal bleeding, client teaching includes advising the woman that she should never have a vaginal examination performed if bleeding is present. It is also important to recognize the implications of a high-risk condition for the laboring woman and her fetus. For example, if there is an abnormal fetal presentation, labor may be prolonged, prolapse of the umbilical cord is more likely, and the possibility of a cesarean birth is increased.

Although physical conditions are major factors that increase risk in the intrapartum period, sociocultural variables may also increase risk; these include:

- Poverty
- Nutrition
- Degree of prenatal care received
- Cultural beliefs about pregnancy
- Communication patterns
- Social support
- Alcohol, tobacco, and drug use
- Presence of PTSD (Davidson, 2012)

Begin gathering data about sociocultural factors as the woman enters the birthing area. Observe the communication pattern between the woman and her support person or people and their responses to admission questions and initial teaching. If the woman and those supporting her do not speak English and translators are not available among the birthing unit staff, the course of labor and the ability of healthcare givers to interact and provide support and education are affected. The couple must receive information in their primary language to make informed decisions. Communication may also be affected by cultural practices such as beliefs about when to speak, who should ask questions, or whether it is acceptable to let others know about discomfort. In some countries such as Algeria, Brazil, China, and Korea, and among orthodox Jews, the father is not expected to be in the birthing area. Culturally sensitive nurses realize that this should not be interpreted as a lack of interest in the mother, the baby, or the birth itself (Spector, 2012).

Table 17–2 provides a partial list of intrapartum risk factors to keep in mind during the intrapartum assessment.

TABLE 17–2 Intrapartum High-Risk Factors

FACTOR	MATERNAL IMPLICATIONS	FETAL/NEONATAL IMPLICATIONS
Abnormal presentation	↑ Incidence of cesarean section (C/S) birth ↑ Incidence of prolonged labor	↑ Incidence of placenta previa Prematurity ↑ Risk of congenital abnormality Neonatal physical trauma ↑ Risk of intrauterine growth restriction (IUGR)
Multiple gestation	↑ Uterine distention → ↑ risk of postpartum hemorrhage ↑ Risk of C/S ↑ Risk of preterm labor	Low birth weight Prematurity ↑ Risk of congenital anomalies Twin-to-twin transfusion
Hydramnios/polyhydramnios	↑ Discomfort ↑ Dyspnea ↑ Risk of preterm labor Edema of lower extremities Increased risk of cord prolapse with artificial rupture of membranes/spontaneous rupture of membranes (AROM/SROM)	↑ Risk of esophageal or other high alimentary tract atresias ↑ Risk of CNS anomalies (myelocele)
Oligohydramnios	Maternal fear	↑ Incidence of congenital anomalies ↑ Incidence of renal lesions ↑ Risk of IUGR ↑ Risk of fetal acidosis ↑ Risk of cord compression Postmaturity
Meconium staining of amniotic fluid	Psychologic stress due to fear for baby	↑ Risk of fetal asphyxia ↑ Risk of meconium aspiration ↑ Risk of pneumonia due to aspiration of meconium
Premature rupture of membranes	↑ Risk of infection (chorioamnionitis) ↑ Risk of preterm labor ↑ Anxiety Fear for the baby Prolonged hospitalization ↑ Incidence of tocolytic therapy	↑ Perinatal morbidity Prematurity ↑ Birth weight ↑ Risk of respiratory distress syndrome Prolonged hospitalization
Induction of labor	↑ Risk of hypercontractility of uterus ↑ Risk of uterine rupture Length of labor if cervix not ready ↑ Anxiety	Prematurity if gestational age not assessed correctly Hypoxia if hyperstimulation occurs Nonreassuring fetal status can occur
Abruptio placentae	Hemorrhage Uterine atony ↑ Incidence of C/S Severe maternal abdominal pain	Fetal hypoxia/acidosis Fetal exsanguination ↑ Perinatal mortality
Placenta previa	Hemorrhage Uterine atony Increased incidence of C/S Painless vaginal bleeding	Fetal hypoxia/acidosis Fetal exsanguination Increased perinatal mortality
Failure to progress in labor	Maternal exhaustion ↑ Incidence of augmentation of labor ↑ Incidence of C/S	Fetal hypoxia/acidosis Intracranial birth injury
Precipitous labor (less than 3 hr)	Perineal, vaginal, cervical lacerations ↑ Risk of postpartum hemorrhage Maternal hematomas	Tentorial tears
Prolapse of umbilical cord	↑ Fear for baby C/S birth	Acute fetal hypoxia/acidosis

FACTOR	MATERNAL IMPLICATIONS	FETAL/NEONATAL IMPLICATIONS
Fetal heart abnormalities	↑ Fear for baby ↑ Risk of C/S, forceps, vacuum Continuous electronic monitoring and intervention in labor	Tachycardia, chronic asphyxic insult, bradycardia, acute asphyxic insult Chronic hypoxia Congenital heart block
Uterine rupture	Maternal hemorrhage Cesarean birth for hysterectomy ↑ Risk of death	Fetal anoxia Fetal hemorrhage Neonatal morbidity and mortality Fetal neurologic sequelae
Postdates (greater than 42 weeks)	↑ Anxiety ↑ Incidence of induction of labor ↑ Incidence of C/S ↑ Use of technology to monitor fetus ↑ Risk of shoulder dystocia Placental calcifications/advanced placental grading	Postmaturity syndrome ↑ Risk of fetal/neonatal mortality and morbidity ↑ Risk of antepartum fetal death ↑ Incidence or risk of large baby ↑ Risk of intrauterine growth restriction Fetal hypoxia Increased nonreassuring fetal status
Diabetes (gestational and preexisting)	↑ Risk of hydramnios ↑ Risk of hypoglycemia or hyperglycemia ↑ Risk of preeclampsia/eclampsia	↑ Risk of malpresentation ↑ Risk of macrosomia ↑ Risk of IUGR ↑ Risk of respiratory distress syndrome ↑ Risk of congenital anomalies ↑ Risk of fetal death Neonatal hypoglycemia
Preeclampsia/eclampsia	↑ Risk of seizures ↑ Risk of stroke ↑ Risk of HELLP (**h**emolysis, **e**levated **l**iver enzymes, and **l**ow **p**latelet count) syndrome and DIC (disseminated intravascular coagulation)	↑ Risk of small-for-gestational-age baby ↑ Risk of preterm birth ↑ Risk of mortality
HIV/sexually transmitted infection (STI)	↑ Risk of additional infections	↑ Risk of transplacental transmission ↑ Risk of infection during birth process or with invasive medical procedures

Intrapartum Physical and Psychosociocultural Assessment

A physical examination is part of the admission procedure and part of the ongoing care of the woman. Although the intrapartum physical assessment is not as complete and thorough as the initial prenatal physical examination (see Chapter 9), it does involve assessment of some body systems and of the actual labor process. See *Assessment Guide: Intrapartum—First Stage of Labor* later in the chapter for a framework to use when examining the laboring woman.

The physical assessment portion includes assessments performed immediately on admission as well as ongoing assessments. When labor is progressing very quickly, there may not be time for a complete nursing assessment. In that case, the critical physical assessments include significant pregnancy history, high-risk factors/problems that occurred during pregnancy, maternal vital signs, labor status, fetal status, and laboratory findings.

The cultural assessment portion provides a starting point for this increasingly important aspect of assessment. Individualized nursing care can best be planned and implemented when the values and beliefs of the laboring woman are known and honored. It is sometimes challenging to achieve a balance between cultural awareness and the risk of stereotyping because cultural responses are influenced by so many factors. Nurses are most effective when they combine an awareness of the major cultural values and beliefs of a specific group with the recognition that individual differences have an impact.

The final section of the assessment guide addresses psychosocial factors. The laboring woman's psychosocial status is an important part of the total assessment. The woman has previous ideas, knowledge, and fears about childbearing. By assessing her psychosocial status, the nurse can meet the woman's needs for information and support.

Developing Cultural Competence Use of Protective Amulets

Placing a protective amulet on the baby or in the crib is common practice among people from many countries, including Greece, Iran, Iraq, Israel, Italy, Malaysia, and Russia (Spector, 2012).

While performing the intrapartum assessment, it is crucial to follow the Centers for Disease Control and Prevention (CDC) guidelines to prevent exposure to body substances (CDC, 2011). Provide information to the woman about the precautions in a factual manner.

Methods of Evaluating Labor Progress

The nurse assesses the woman's contractions and cervical dilatation and effacement to evaluate labor progress.

CONTRACTION ASSESSMENT

Uterine contractions may be assessed by palpation or continuous electronic monitoring.

Clinical Tip

Uterine contractions are documented in frequency by the number of minutes, whereas duration is expressed in seconds.

Palpation. Assess contractions for frequency, duration, and intensity by placing one hand on the uterine fundus. Keep the hand relatively still because excessive movement may stimulate contractions or cause discomfort. Determine the frequency of the contractions by noting the time from the beginning of one contraction to the beginning of the next. If contractions begin at 7:00, 7:04, and 7:08, for example, their frequency is every 4 minutes. To determine contraction duration, note the time when tensing of the fundus is first felt (beginning of contraction) and again as relaxation occurs (end of contraction). During the acme of the contraction, intensity can be evaluated by estimating the indentability of the fundus. Assess at least three successive contractions to gain enough data to determine the contraction pattern. See Table 17–3 for a review of contraction characteristics in different phases of labor.

This is also a good time to assess the laboring woman's perception of pain. How does she describe the pain? What is her affect? Is this contraction more uncomfortable than the last one? Note and document the woman's affect and response to the contractions.

Electronic Monitoring of Contractions. Electronic monitoring of uterine contractions provides continuous data. In many birth settings, electronic monitoring is routine for high-risk clients and women having oxytocin-induced labor. Other facilities monitor all laboring women.

Electronic monitoring may be done externally with a device placed against the maternal abdomen or internally with an **intrauterine pressure catheter**. When monitoring by external means, the portion of the monitoring equipment called a *tocodynamometer*, or "toco," is positioned against the fundus of the

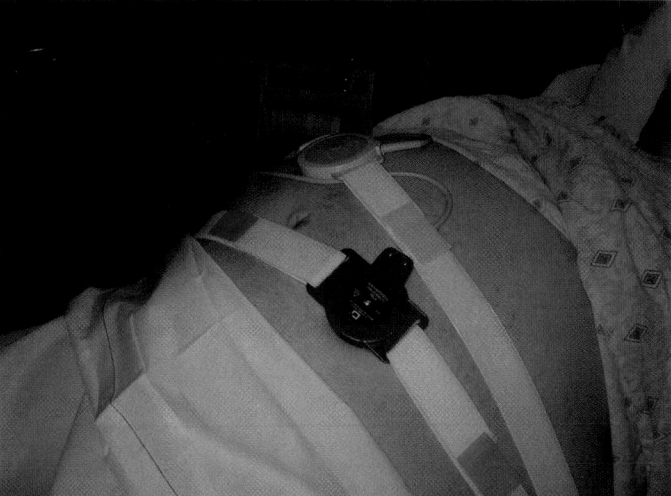

Figure 17–1 **Woman in labor with external monitor applied. The tocodynamometer placed on the uterine fundus is recording uterine contractions. The lower belt holds the ultrasonic device that monitors the fetal heart rate. The belts can be adjusted for comfort.**

SOURCE: Wilson Garcia.

uterus and held in place with an elastic belt (Figure 17–1). The toco contains a flexible disc that responds to pressure. When the uterus contracts, the fundus tightens and the change in pressure against the toco is amplified and transmitted to the electronic fetal monitor. The monitor displays the uterine contraction as a pattern on graph paper.

External monitoring provides a continuous recording of the frequency and duration of uterine contractions and is noninvasive. However, it does not accurately record the intensity of the uterine contraction, and it is difficult to obtain an accurate fetal heart rate (FHR) in some women, such as those who are very obese, those who have polyhydramnios/hydramnios (an abnormally large amount of amniotic fluid), those whose fetus is very active, and in the case of premature fetuses. In addition, the belt may bother the woman if it requires frequent readjustment when she changes position.

Internal intrauterine monitoring provides the same data and also provides accurate measurement of uterine contraction intensity (the strength of the contraction and the actual pressure within the uterus). After membranes have ruptured, the physician/CNM inserts the intrauterine pressure catheter (IUPC) into the uterine cavity and connects it by a cable to the electronic fetal monitor. In some facilities, labor and delivery nurses may obtain specialized training to perform IUPC insertions. A small micropressure device located in the tip of the catheter measures the pressure within the uterus in the resting state and during each contraction. Internal electronic monitoring is used when it is imperative to have accurate intrauterine pressure readings to evaluate the stress on the uterus.

Clinical Tip

Many experienced nurses note that when palpating a woman's uterus, mild contractions feel similar in consistency to the tip of the nose, moderate contractions feel more like the chin, and with strong contractions, there is little indentability, much like the forehead. When palpating during a contraction, compare the consistency to your nose, chin, and forehead to determine the intensity.

TABLE 17–3 Contraction and Labor Progress Characteristics

Contraction Characteristics	
Latent phase:	Every 10–30 min × 30 sec; mild, progressing to
	Every 5–7 min × 30–40 sec; moderate
Active phase:	Every 2–5 min × 40–60 sec; moderate to strong
Transition phase:	Every 1.5–2.0 min × 60–90 sec; strong
Labor Progress Characteristics	
Primipara:	At least 1.2 cm/hr dilatation
	At least 1 cm/hr descent
	Less than 2 hr in second stage
Multipara:	At least 1.5 cm/hr dilatation
	At least 2.1 cm/hr descent
	Less than 1 hr in second stage

In addition, it is important to evaluate the woman's labor status by palpating the intensity and resting tone of the uterine fundus during contractions.

Cervical Assessment

Cervical dilatation and effacement are evaluated directly by vaginal examination (see Performing an Intrapartum Vaginal Examination in the *Clinical Skills Manual* SKILLS). The vaginal examination can also provide information about membrane status, characteristics of amniotic fluid, fetal position, and station. See Figures 17–2, 17–3, and 17–4. Refer to *Assessment Guide: Intrapartum—First Stage of Labor.*

Fetal Assessment

Fetal Position and Presentation

Fetal position and presentation are determined by inspecting the woman's abdomen, palpating it, performing a vaginal examination, and auscultating fetal heart rate (FHR). Ultrasound may also be used.

INSPECTION

Observe the size and shape of the woman's abdomen. Assess the lie of the fetus by noting whether the uterus projects up and down (longitudinal lie) or left to right (transverse lie).

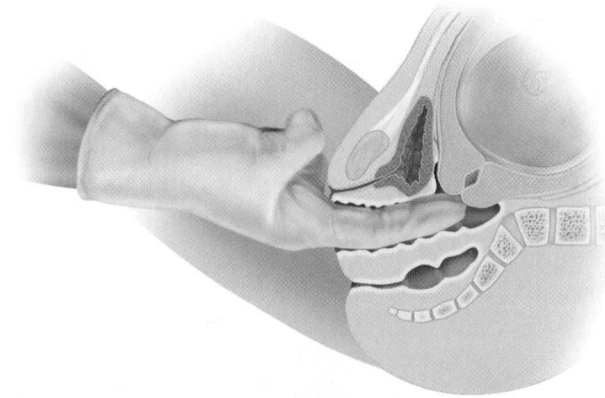

Figure 17–2 Gauging cervical dilatation. To gauge cervical dilatation, the nurse places the index and middle fingers against the cervix and determines the size of the opening. Before labor begins, the cervix is long (approximately 2.5 cm), the sides feel thick, and the cervical canal is closed, so an examining finger cannot be inserted. During labor the cervix begins to dilate, and the size of the opening progresses from 1 to 10 cm in diameter.

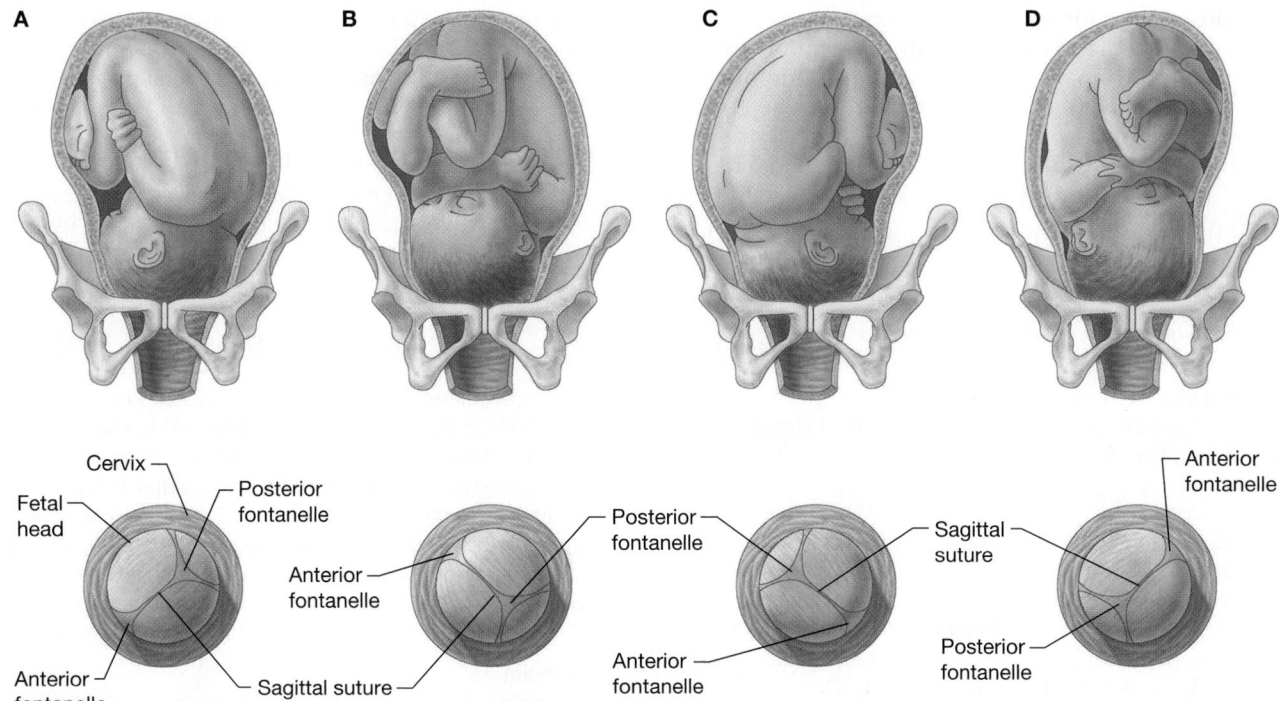

Figure 17–3 Palpating the presenting part (portion of the fetus that enters the pelvis first). *A,* Left occiput anterior (LOA). The occiput (area over the occipital bone on the posterior part of the fetal head) is in the left anterior quadrant of the woman's pelvis. When the fetus is LOA, the posterior fontanelle (located just above the occipital bone and triangular in shape) is in the upper left quadrant of the maternal pelvis. *B,* Left occiput posterior (LOP). The posterior fontanelle is in the lower left quadrant of the maternal pelvis. *C,* Right occiput anterior (ROA). The posterior fontanelle is in the upper right quadrant of the maternal pelvis. *D,* Right occiput posterior (ROP). The posterior fontanelle is in the lower right quadrant of the maternal pelvis.

Note: The anterior fontanelle is diamond shaped. Because of the roundness of the fetal head, only a portion of the anterior fontanelle can be seen in each of the views, so it appears to be triangular in shape.

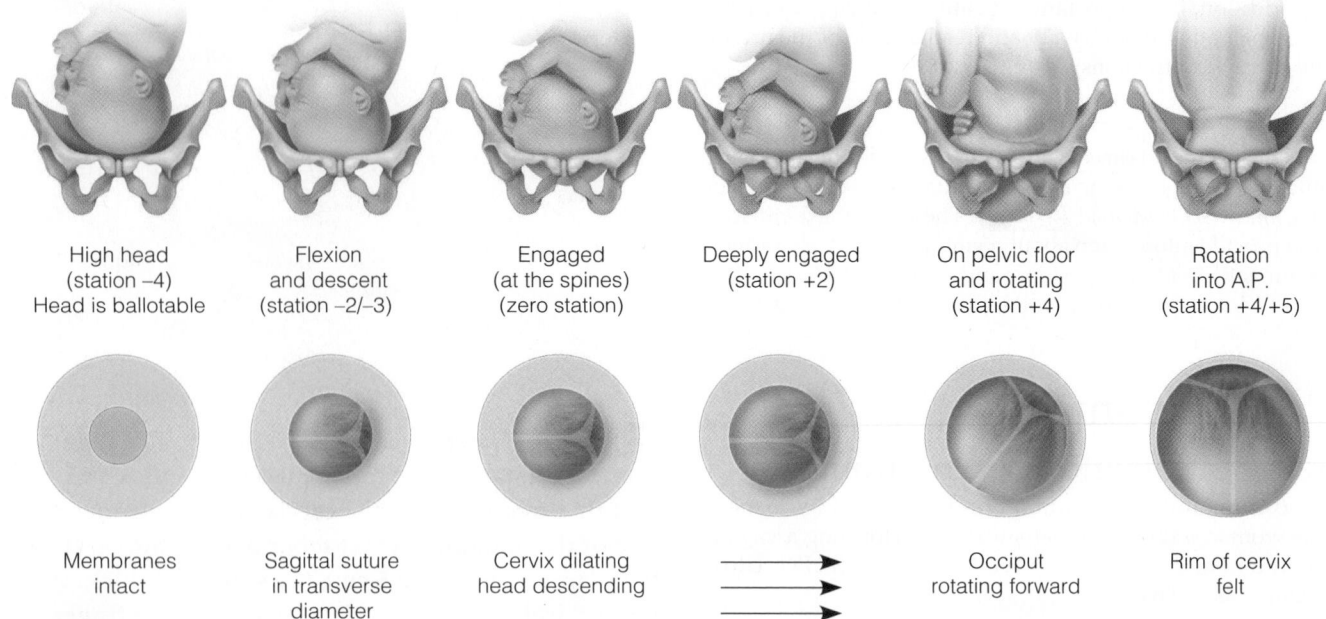

| High head (station –4) Head is ballotable | Flexion and descent (station –2/–3) | Engaged (at the spines) (zero station) | Deeply engaged (station +2) | On pelvic floor and rotating (station +4) | Rotation into A.P. (station +4/+5) |

| Membranes intact | Sagittal suture in transverse diameter | Cervix dilating head descending | | Occiput rotating forward | Rim of cervix felt |

Figure 17–4 Assessing fetal position and station. *Top:* The fetal head progressing through the pelvis. *Bottom:* The changes the nurse will detect on palpation of the occiput through the cervix while doing a vaginal examination.

PALPATION: LEOPOLD MANEUVERS

Leopold maneuvers are a systematic way to evaluate the maternal abdomen. Frequent practice increases the examiner's skill in determining fetal position by palpation. Leopold maneuvers may be difficult to perform on an obese woman or on a woman who has excessive amniotic fluid (hydramnios). Before performing Leopold maneuvers, have the woman empty her bladder and lie on her back with her feet on the bed and her knees bent. (See Figure 17–5 for technique. Also see Performing Leopold Maneuvers in the *Clinical Skills Manual* SKILLS .)

VAGINAL EXAMINATION AND ULTRASOUND

During a vaginal examination, the examiner can palpate the presenting part if the cervix is dilated. The examination also provides information about the position of the fetus and the degree of flexion of its head (in cephalic presentations). Visualization by ultrasound is used when the fetal position cannot be determined by abdominal palpation.

Auscultation of Fetal Heart Rate

The handheld Doppler ultrasound (a device that operates using ultrasound waves that transmit the sounds made by the FHR)

EVIDENCE-BASED PRACTICE | Best Practices for Fetal Heart Rate Assessment

Clinical Question
What is the most effective way to monitor fetal status in laboring women who are low risk?

The Evidence
Monitoring of the fetal heart rate is one way of assessing the well-being of the fetus during labor. The primary interest is fetal oxygenation; threats to fetal oxygenation are never higher than during labor. Electronic fetal heart rate monitoring has become widespread, even though there is little evidence that it reduces risks for low-risk mothers. Currently, nearly 97% of births in U.S. hospitals are accompanied by electronic fetal monitoring. A military nurse-researcher undertook a systematic review of the evidence to determine best practices for fetal monitoring in low-risk labor and delivery. Included in the review were the best practice bulletins of the American College of Obstetricians and Gynecologists (ACOG) and the Association for Women's Health Obstetrics, and Neonatal Nurses (AWOHNN). This type of review of practice guidelines is considered the strongest level of evidence for practice.

The recommended means of fetal monitoring in low-risk mothers is intermittent auscultation (Riffle, 2014). Using this low-technology monitoring method saves costs and results in lower rates of unnecessary assisted and surgical births. In addition, intermittent auscultation is noninvasive and requires no special equipment. Laboring mothers are free to walk, which generally enhances labor progress, and to change positions as frequently as needed to manage pain. Overall, both physiologic and psychologic outcomes were superior with intermittent auscultation.

Best Practice
Intermittent auscultation of fetal heart rate is superior to electronic fetal monitoring for low-risk mothers. This method of assuring fetal well-being is low cost, involves no special technology, and enables full mobility of the mother.

Clinical Reasoning
How can the nurse help implement this important change in practice when current practices are ingrained? What is appropriate childbirth education to empower parents to choose a low-technology option?

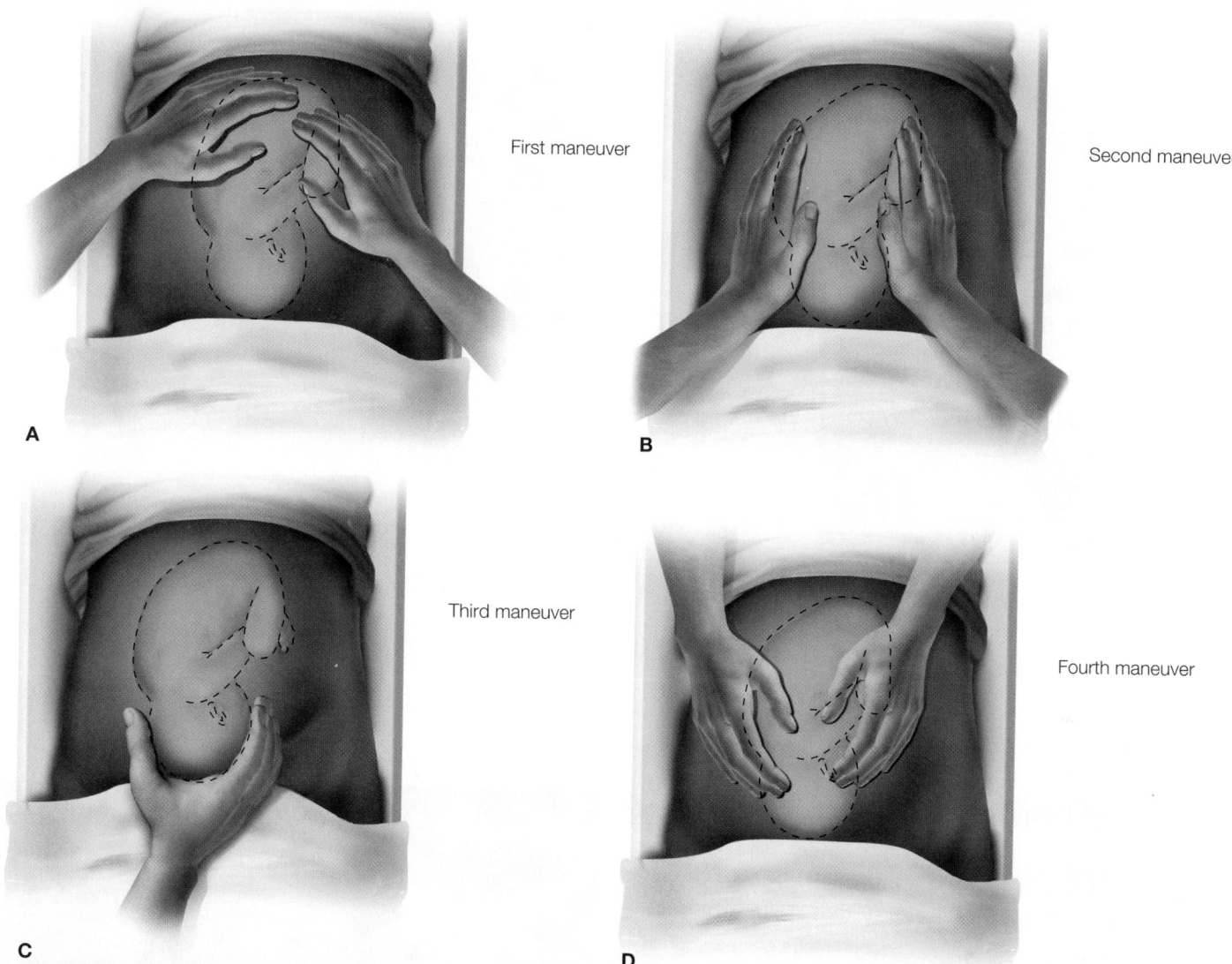

First maneuver

A

Second maneuver

B

Third maneuver

C

Fourth maneuver

D

Figure 17–5 Leopold maneuvers for determining fetal position and presentation. *A*, First maneuver: Facing the woman, palpate the upper abdomen with both hands. Note the shape, consistency, and mobility of the palpated part. The fetal head is firm and round and moves independently of the trunk. The buttock feels softer, and it moves with the trunk. *B*, Second maneuver: Moving the hands on the pelvis, palpate the abdomen with gentle but deep pressure. The fetal back, on one side of the abdomen, feels smooth, and the fetal extremities on the other side feel knobby. *C*, Third maneuver: Place one hand just above the symphysis. Note whether the part palpated feels like the fetal head or the breech and whether it is engaged. *D*, Fourth maneuver: Facing the woman's feet, place both hands on the lower abdomen and move hands gently down the sides of the uterus toward the pubis. Note the cephalic prominence or brow.

is used to auscultate the FHR between, during, and immediately after uterine contractions. Fetoscopes, which are modern combinations of both the stethoscope and the Pinard horn, can also be used to auscultate the FHR after 20 weeks. Fetoscopes are being used with decreasing frequency in modern obstetric practice, although some practitioners or clients may prefer this assessment method. Instead of listening haphazardly over the woman's abdomen for the FHR, it is useful to perform Leopold maneuvers first. Leopold maneuvers not only indicate the probable location of the FHR but also help determine the presence of multiple fetuses, fetal lie, and fetal presentation. The FHR is heard most clearly at the fetal back (Figure 17–6). Thus, in a cephalic presentation, the FHR is best heard in the

lower quadrant of the maternal abdomen. In a breech presentation, it is heard at or above the level of the maternal umbilicus. In a transverse lie, the FHR may be heard best just above or just below the umbilicus. As the presenting part descends and rotates through the pelvic structure during labor, the location of the FHR tends to descend and move toward the midline.

After the FHR is located, it is usually counted for 30 seconds and multiplied by 2 to obtain the number of beats per minute (beats/min). Check the woman's pulse against the fetal sounds. If the rates are the same, readjust the Doppler or fetoscope. Occasionally listen for a full minute, through and just after a contraction, to detect any abnormal heart rate, especially if the FHR is over 160 beats/min (tachycardia), under

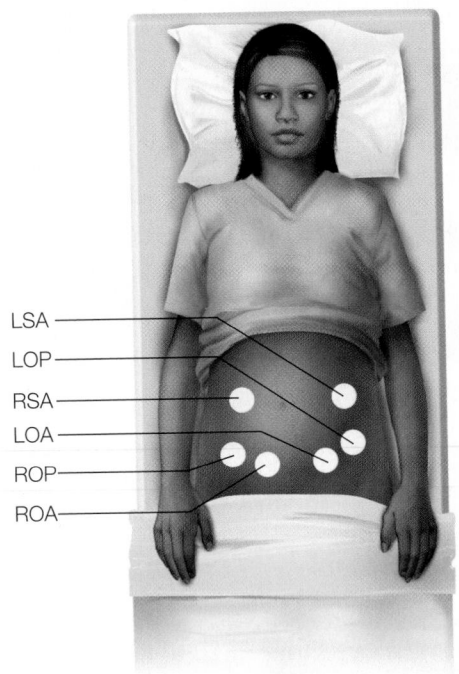

LSA
LOP
RSA
LOA
ROP
ROA

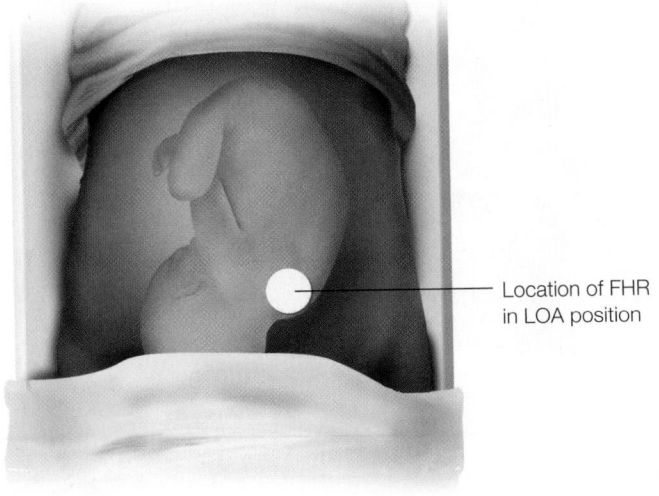

Location of FHR
in LOA position

Figure 17–6 Location of FHR in relation to the more commonly seen fetal positions.

TABLE 17–4 Frequency of Auscultation: Assessment and Documentation

LOW-RISK WOMEN	HIGH-RISK WOMEN
First stage of labor: q30min	First stage of labor: q15min
Second stage of labor: q15min	Second stage of labor: q5min

Labor Events

Assess FHR before:

- Initiation of labor-enhancing procedures (e.g., artificial rupture of membranes)
- Periods of ambulation
- Administration of medications
- Administration or initiation of analgesia or anesthesia

Assess FHR following:

- Rupture of membranes
- Recognition of abnormal uterine activity patterns, such as increased basal tone or tachysystole
- Evaluation of oxytocin (maintenance, increase, or decrease of dosage)
- Administration of medications (at time of peak action)
- Expulsion of enema
- Urinary catheterization
- Vaginal examination
- Periods of ambulation
- Evaluation of analgesia and/or anesthesia (maintenance, increase, or decrease of dosage)

Source: Adapted from American College of Obstetricians & Gynecologists. (2009, reaffirmed 2013). *Intrapartum fetal heart rate monitoring: Nomenclature, interpretation, and general management principles* (ACOG Practice Bulletin, No. 106). Washington, DC: Author.

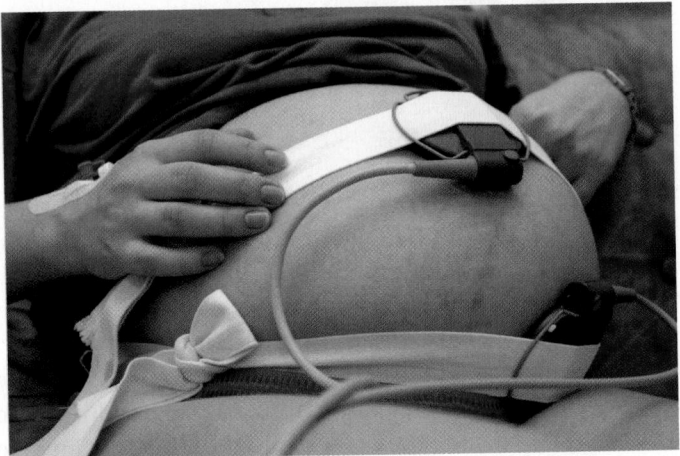

Figure 17–7 The nurse uses a Doppler to assess the fetal heart rate. Doppler monitors can be used for intermittent labor monitoring or in the outpatient or community setting.

SOURCE: © Artur Steinhagen/Fotolia.

110 beats/min (bradycardia), or irregular. If the FHR is irregular or has changed markedly from the last assessment, listen for a full minute through and immediately after a contraction. In these situations, continuous electronic fetal monitoring is warranted (Menihan & Kopel, 2014). (See Auscultating Fetal Heart Rate in the *Clinical Skills Manual* SKILLS and Table 17–4 for guidelines on how often to auscultate the FHR.) Refer to *Assessment Guide: Intrapartum—First Stage of Labor.* Figure 17–7 shows the use of a Doppler to auscultate the FHR.

Intermittent auscultation has been found to be as effective as the electronic method for fetal surveillance (American College of Obstetricians and Gynecologists [ACOG], 2014). A growing number of healthcare professionals, physicians and nurses alike, are beginning to question the widespread use of a technology that has not proven its overall worth.

Electronic Monitoring of Fetal Heart Rate

Electronic fetal monitoring (EFM) produces a continuous tracing of the FHR, which allows visual assessment of many characteristics of the FHR (see External Electronic Fetal Monitoring in the *Clinical Skills Manual* SKILLS).

INDICATIONS FOR ELECTRONIC MONITORING

If one or more of the following factors are present, the FHR and contractions are monitored by electronic fetal monitoring:

- Previous history of a stillborn (fetus dies in the uterus) at 38 or more weeks' gestation
- Presence of a complication of pregnancy (e.g., preeclampsia/eclampsia, placenta previa, abruptio placentae, multiple gestation, prolonged or premature rupture of membranes)
- Induction of labor (labor that is begun as a result of some type of intervention such as an intravenous infusion of oxytocin [Pitocin])
- Preterm labor (gestation less than 37 completed weeks)
- Decreased fetal movement
- Nonreassuring fetal status

- Meconium staining of amniotic fluid (meconium has been released into the amniotic fluid by the fetus, which may indicate a problem)
- Trial of labor after cesarean birth (TOLAC) (Menihan & Kopel, 2014). For a complete discussion of TOLAC, see Chapter 22.

METHODS OF ELECTRONIC MONITORING OF FHR

External monitoring of the fetus is usually accomplished by ultrasound. A transducer, which emits continuous sound waves, is placed on the maternal abdomen. When the transducer is placed correctly, the sound waves bounce off the fetal heart and are picked up by the electronic monitor. The actual moment-by-moment FHR is displayed graphically on a screen (Figure 17–8). In some instances, the monitor may track the maternal heart rate instead of the FHR. Avoid this error by palpating the maternal pulse or using a pulse oximeter to compare to the rate of the FHR.

Recent advances in technology have led to the development of new ambulatory methods of external monitoring. Using a telemetry system, a small, battery-operated transducer transmits signals to a receiver connected to the monitor. This system, held in place with a shoulder strap, allows the woman to ambulate, helping her to feel more comfortable and less confined during labor. In contrast, the system depicted in Figure 17–8 requires the woman to remain close to the electrical power source for the monitor.

Internal monitoring requires an internal spiral electrode. To place the spiral electrode on the fetal occiput, the amniotic membranes must be ruptured, the cervix must be dilated

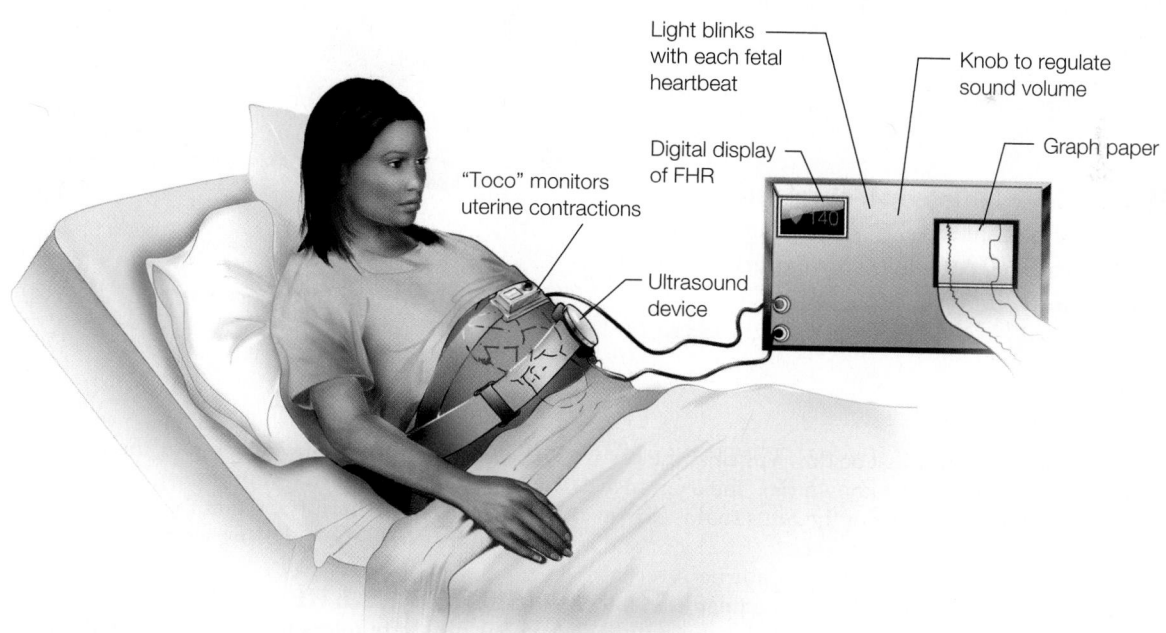

Light blinks with each fetal heartbeat

Knob to regulate sound volume

Digital display of FHR

Graph paper

"Toco" monitors uterine contractions

Ultrasound device

Figure 17–8 Electronic fetal monitoring by external technique. The tocodynamometer ("toco") is placed over the uterine fundus. The toco provides information that can be used to monitor uterine contractions. The ultrasound device is placed over the area of the fetal back. This device transmits information about the FHR. Information from both the toco and the ultrasound device is transmitted to the electronic fetal monitor. The FHR is displayed in a digital display (as a blinking light), on the special monitor paper, and audibly (by adjusting a button on the monitor). The uterine contractions are displayed on the special monitor paper as well.

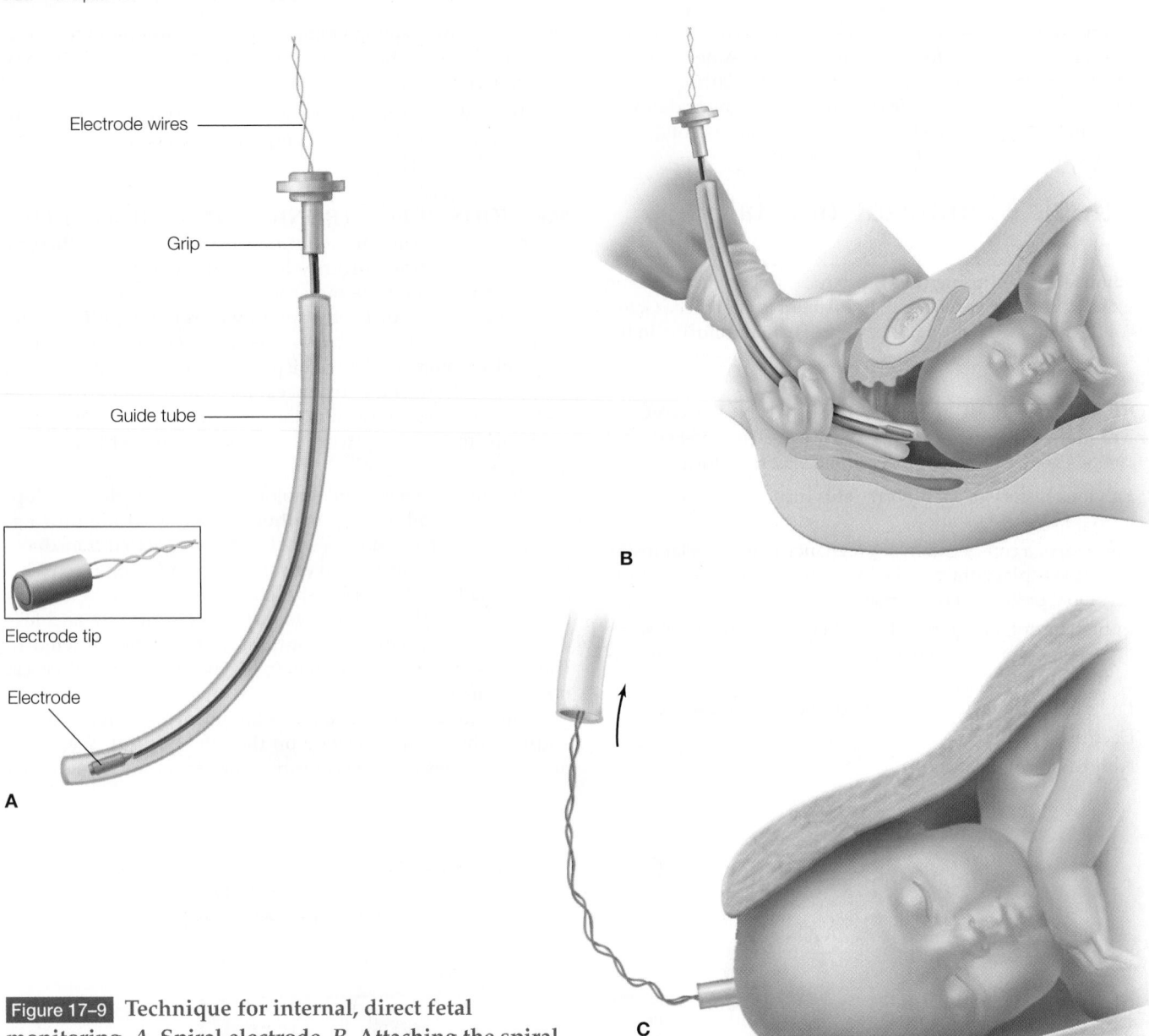

Electrode wires

Grip

Guide tube

Electrode tip

Electrode

A

B

C

Figure 17–9 Technique for internal, direct fetal monitoring. *A*, Spiral electrode. *B*, Attaching the spiral electrode to the scalp. *C*, Attached spiral electrode with the guide tube removed.

at least 2 cm, the presenting part must be down against the cervix, and the presenting part must be known (i.e., the examiner must be able to detect the actual part of the fetus that is down against the cervix). If all these factors are present, the labor and birth nurse or the physician/CNM inserts a sterile internal spiral electrode into the vagina and places it against the fetal presenting part. The spiral electrode is rotated clockwise until it is attached to the presenting part. Wires that extend from the spiral electrode are attached to a leg plate (which is placed on the woman's thigh) and then attached to the electronic fetal monitor (see Internal Electronic Fetal Monitoring: Applying a Fetal Scalp Electrode in the *Clinical Skills Manual* **SKILLS**). This method of monitoring the FHR provides more accurate continuous data than external monitoring because the signal is clearer and movement of the fetus or the woman does not interrupt

it (Figure 17–9). The FHR tracing at the top of Figure 17–10 was obtained by internal monitoring with a spiral electrode; the uterine contraction tracing at the bottom of the figure was obtained by external monitoring with a toco.

BASELINE FETAL HEART RATE

The **baseline rate** refers to the average FHR rounded to increments of 5 beats/min observed during a 10-minute period of monitoring. Normal FHR (baseline rate) ranges from 110 to 160 beats/min. This excludes periodic or episodic changes, periods of marked variability, greater than 25 beats/min. Episodic patterns are those not associated with uterine contractions, whereas periodic patterns are those associated with uterine contractions, including early, late, and variable decelerations. The duration should be at least 2 minutes (Menihan & Kopel,

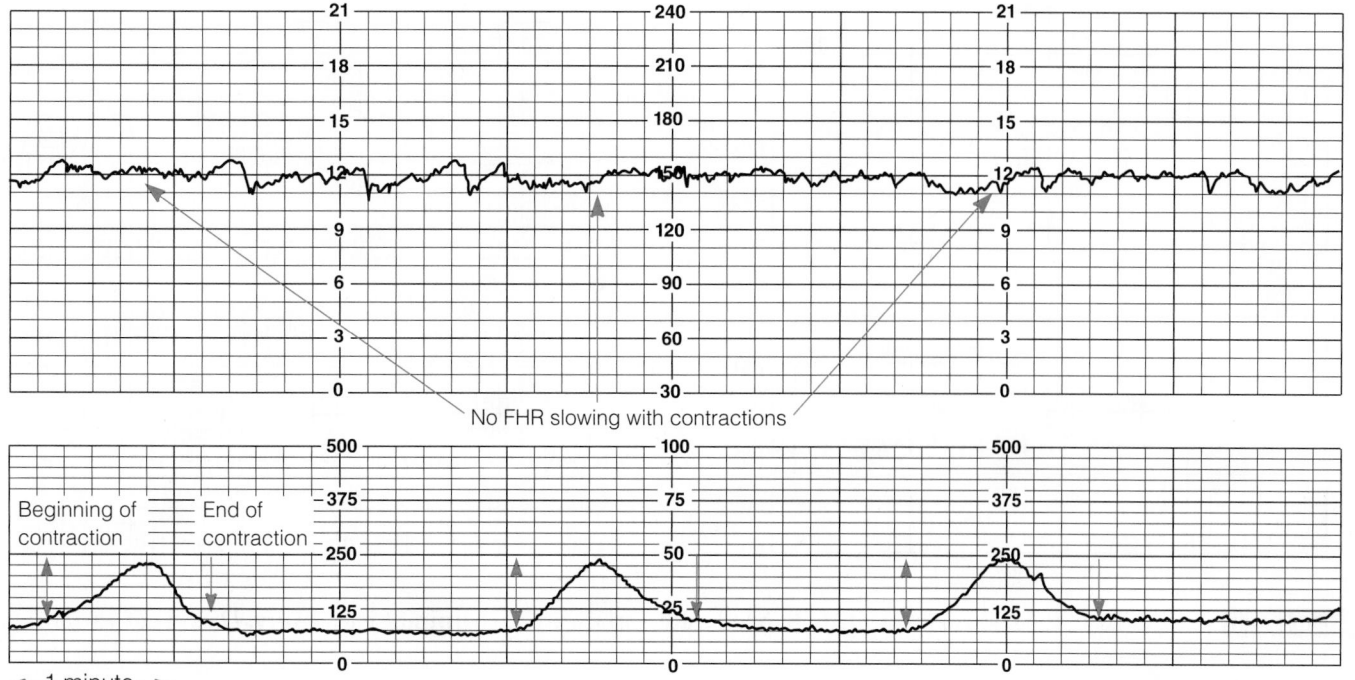

No FHR slowing with contractions

Beginning of contraction   End of contraction

◄—1 minute—►

Figure 17–10 Normal FHR pattern obtained by internal monitoring. Note normal FHR, 140 to 158 beats/min, presence of long- and short-term variability, and absence of deceleration with adequate contractions. The bottom portion depicts uterine contractions obtained by external monitoring. Each dark vertical line marks 1 minute, and each small rectangle represents 10 seconds. The contraction frequency is about every 2.5 minutes, and the duration of the contractions is 50 to 60 seconds. Arrows on the bottom of the tracing indicate beginnings of uterine contractions.

2014). There are two abnormal variations of the baseline rate: those above 160 beats/min (tachycardia) and those below 110 beats/min (bradycardia). Another change affecting the baseline is called *variability*, a change in FHR over a few seconds to a few minutes.

Fetal tachycardia is a sustained rate of 161 beats/min or above. *Marked tachycardia* is 180 beats/min or above. Causes of tachycardia include the following (Cunningham et al., 2014):

• Early fetal hypoxia, which leads to stimulation of the sympathetic system as the fetus compensates for reduced blood flow

• Maternal fever, which accelerates the metabolism of the fetus

• Maternal dehydration

• Beta-sympathomimetic drugs such as terbutaline, atropine, and isoxsuprine, which have a cardiac stimulant effect (ACOG, 2012).

• Amnionitis (fetal tachycardia may be the first sign of developing intrauterine infection)

• Maternal hyperthyroidism (thyroid-stimulating hormones may cross the placenta and stimulate FHR)

• Fetal anemia (the heart rate is increased to improve tissue perfusion)

Tachycardia is considered an ominous sign if it is accompanied by decreases in the FHR characterized as late decelerations, severe variable decelerations, or decreased variability (to be

discussed later). If tachycardia is associated with maternal fever, treatment may include antipyretics and/or antibiotics.

Fetal bradycardia is a rate less than 110 beats/min during a 10-minute period or longer. Causes of fetal bradycardia include the following (Cunningham et al., 2014):

• Late (profound) fetal hypoxia (depression of myocardial activity)

• Maternal hypotension, which results in decreased blood flow to the fetus

• Prolonged umbilical cord compression; fetal baroreceptors are activated by cord compression and this produces vagal stimulation, which results in decreased FHR

• Fetal arrhythmia, which is associated with complete heart block in the fetus

• Uterine hyperstimulation

• Abruptio placentae

• Uterine rupture

• Vagal stimulation in the second stage (since this does not involve hypoxia, the fetus can recover)

• Congenital heart block

• Maternal hypothermia

Bradycardia may be a benign or an ominous sign. If average variability exists, the bradycardia is considered benign. When bradycardia is accompanied by decreased variability and late decelerations, it is considered a sign of nonreassuring fetal status (Cunningham et al., 2014).

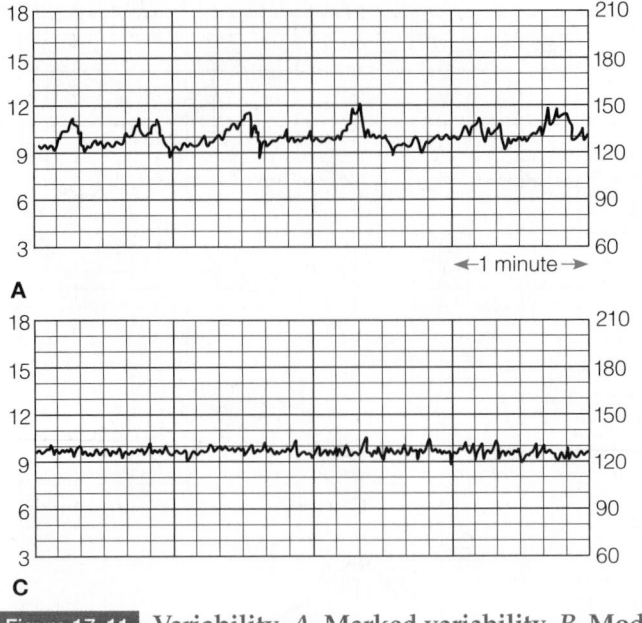
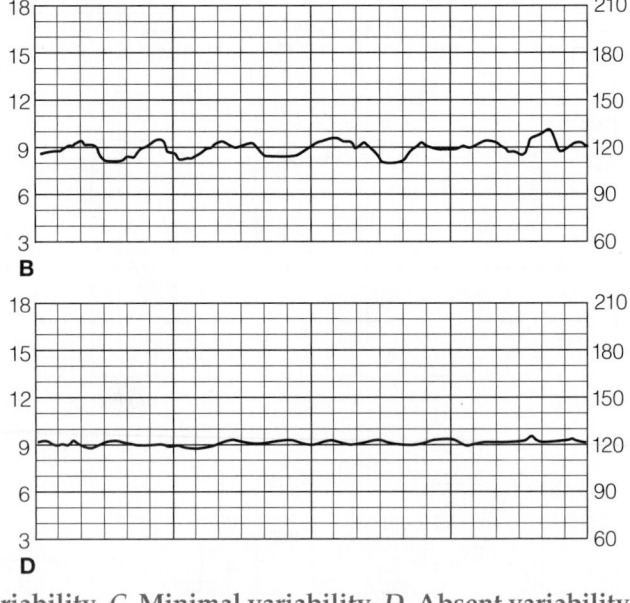

Figure 17–11 Variability. *A*, Marked variability. *B*, Moderate variability. *C*, Minimal variability. *D*, Absent variability.

BASELINE VARIABILITY

Baseline variability is a measure of the interplay (the push–pull effect) between the sympathetic and parasympathetic nervous systems over a 10-minute period. It reflects baseline fluctuations that are irregular in frequency and amplitude.

Fetal heart rate variability is defined as follows (Papadakis, McPhee, & Rabow, 2014) (see Figure 17–11):

- *Marked:* amplitude greater than 25 beats/min
- *Moderate:* amplitude 6 to 25 beats/min
- *Minimal:* amplitude detectable but 5 beats/min or less
- *Absent:* amplitude undetectable

Reduced variability is the best single predictor for determining fetal compromise (Cunningham et al., 2014). Fetal acidosis and subsequent hypoxia are highest in fetuses that have absent or minimal variability (Papadakis et al., 2014).

Causes of decreased variability include the following (Cunningham et al., 2014):

- Hypoxia and acidosis (decreased blood flow to the fetus)
- Administration of drugs such as meperidine hydrochloride (Demerol), diazepam (Valium), or hydroxyzine (Vistaril), which depress the fetal central nervous system
- Fetal sleep cycle (during fetal sleep, variability is decreased; fetal sleep cycles usually last for 20 to 40 minutes each hour)
- Fetus of less than 32 weeks' gestation (fetal neurologic control of heart rate is immature)
- Fetal anomalies affecting the heart, central nervous system, or autonomic nervous system
- Fetal dysrhythmias or fetal anomalies affecting the heart, central nervous system, or autonomic nervous system
- Previous neurologic insult
- Tachycardia

Causes of marked variability include the following (King, Brucker, Kriebs, et al., 2014):

- Early mild hypoxia (variability increases as a result of compensatory mechanism)

- Fetal stimulation or activity (stimulation of autonomic nervous system because of abdominal palpation, maternal vaginal examination, application of spiral electrode on fetal head, or acoustic stimulation)
- Fetal breathing movements
- Advancing gestational age (greater than 30 weeks' gestation)
- Stimulant medications

Absent variability that does not appear to be associated with a fetal sleep cycle or the administration of drugs is a warning sign of nonreassuring fetal status. It is especially ominous if absent or minimal variability is accompanied by late decelerations, which is explained later.

External electronic fetal monitoring is not an adequate method to assess variability. If decreased variability is noted on monitoring, application of a spiral electrode should be considered to obtain more accurate information.

ACCELERATIONS

Accelerations are transient increases in the FHR normally caused by fetal movement. When the fetus moves, the heart rate increases, just as the heart rates of adults increase during exercise. Often, accelerations accompany uterine contractions, usually due to fetal movement in response to the pressure of the contractions. Accelerations of this type are thought to be a sign of fetal well-being and adequate oxygen reserve. The accelerations with fetal movement form the basis for non-stress tests (discussed further in Chapter 13).

DECELERATIONS

Decelerations are periodic decreases in FHR from the normal baseline. They are categorized as early, late, and variable according to the time of their occurrence in the contraction cycle and their waveform (Figure 17–12). When the fetal head is compressed, cerebral blood flow is decreased, which leads to central vagal stimulation and results in early deceleration. The onset of **early deceleration** occurs before the onset of the uterine contraction. This type of deceleration is of uniform shape, is usually considered benign, and does not require intervention.

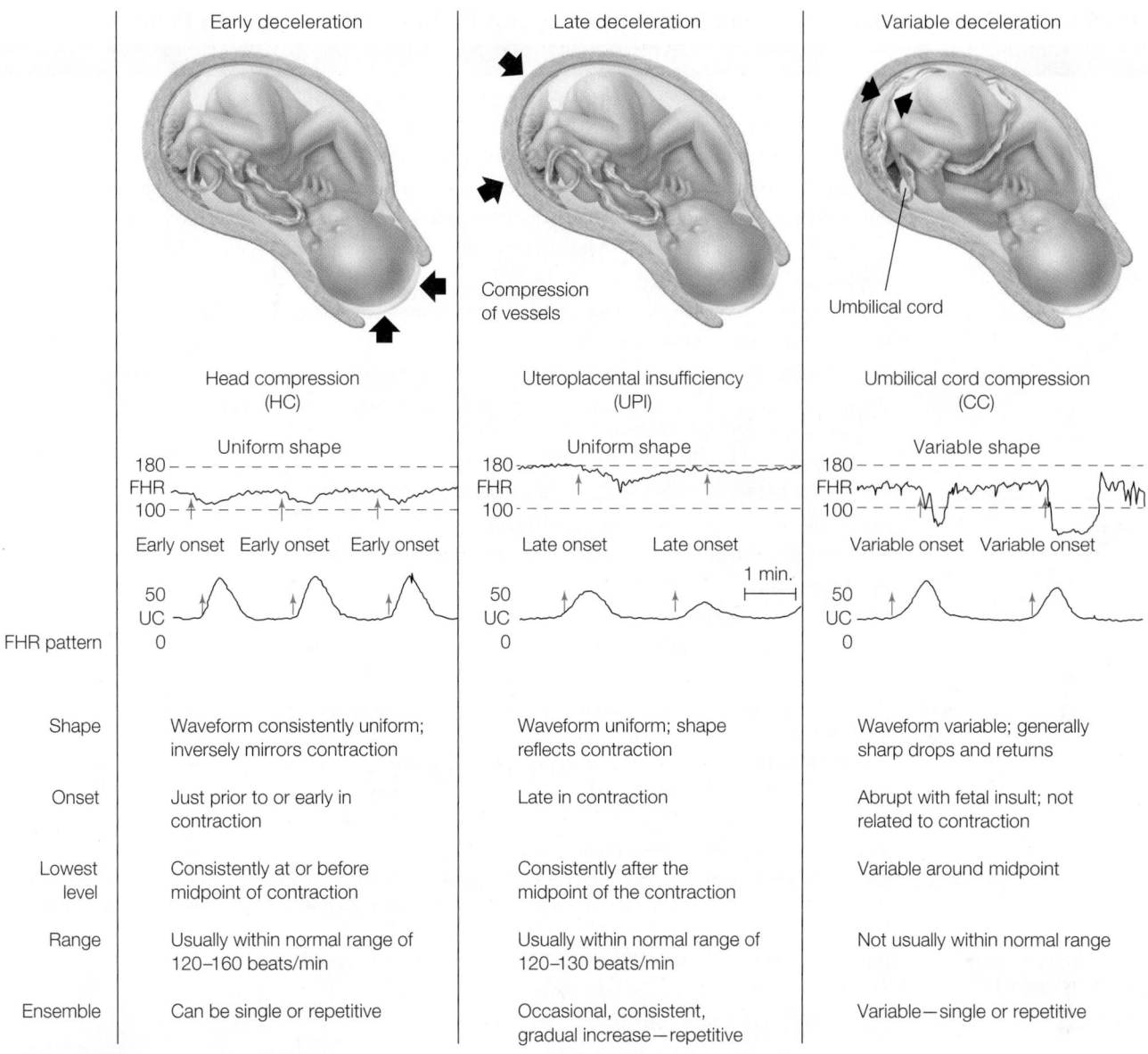

Figure 17–12 Types and characteristics of early, late, and variable decelerations.

Late deceleration is caused by uteroplacental insufficiency resulting from decreased blood flow and oxygen transfer to the fetus through the intervillous spaces during uterine contractions. The most common causes of late decelerations are maternal hypotension resulting from the administration of epidural anesthesia and uterine tachysystole associated with oxytocin infusion (Groll, 2012). The onset of the deceleration occurs after the onset of a uterine contraction and is of a uniform shape that tends to reflect associated uterine contractions. The late deceleration pattern is considered a nonreassuring sign but does not necessarily require immediate childbirth. However, if they continue and birth is not imminent, a cesarean birth may be indicated.

Variable decelerations occur if the umbilical cord becomes compressed, thus reducing blood flow between the placenta and fetus. The resulting increase in peripheral resistance in the fetal circulation causes fetal hypertension. The fetal hypertension stimulates the baroreceptors in the aortic arch and carotid sinuses, which slow the FHR. The onset of variable decelerations

varies in timing with the onset of the contraction, and the decelerations are variable in shape. This pattern requires further assessment. Nursing interventions for late and variable decelerations in FHR are presented in Table 17–5.

A *sinusoidal pattern* appears similar to a waveform. The characteristics of this pattern include absence of variability and the presence of a smooth, wavelike undulating shape. This pattern is associated with Rh alloimmunization, fetal anemia, severe fetal hypoxia, or a chronic fetal bleed. It may also occur with the administration of medications such as meperidine (Demerol) or butorphanol tartrate (Stadol). When it appears in association with medication, the pattern is usually temporary and is commonly referred to as *pseudosinusoidal* (Groll, 2012).

Decelerations are also classified based on the rate in which the FHR leaves the baseline FHR. *Episodic decelerations* occur independently of the uterine contractions and are frequently the result of external stimulations, such as vaginal examinations. *Intermittent decelerations* refer to decelerations that occur

TABLE 17–5 Guidelines for Management of Variable, Late, and Prolonged Deceleration Patterns

PATTERN	NURSING INTERVENTIONS

Variable decelerations
 	
  Isolated or occasional
 	
  Moderate
	Report findings to physician/CNM and document in medical record.
	Provide explanation to woman and partner.
	Change maternal position to one in which FHR pattern is most improved.
	Discontinue oxytocin if it is being administered and other interventions are unsuccessful.
	Perform vaginal examination to assess for prolapsed cord or change in labor progress.
	Monitor FHR continuously to assess current status and for further changes in FHR pattern.

Variable decelerations Severe and uncorrectable	Administer oxygen at 7–10 L/min. Report findings to physician/CNM and document in medical record. Provide explanation to woman and partner. Prepare for probable cesarean birth. Follow interventions listed above. Prepare for vaginal birth unless baseline variability is decreasing or FHR is progressively rising—then cesarean, forceps, or vacuum birth is indicated. Assist physician with fetal scalp sampling if ordered. Prepare for cesarean birth if scalp pH shows acidosis or downward trend.
Late decelerations	Administer oxygen by face mask at 7–10 L/min. Report findings to physician/CNM and document in medical record. Provide explanation to woman and partner. Monitor for further FHR changes. Maintain maternal position on left side. Maintain good hydration with IV fluids (normal saline or lactated Ringer). Discontinue oxytocin if it is being administered and late decelerations persist despite other interventions. Monitor maternal blood pressure and pulse for signs of hypotension; possibly increase flow rate of IV fluids to treat hypotension. Follow physician's orders for treatment for hypotension if present. Assess labor progress (dilatation and station). Assist physician with fetal blood sampling: If pH stays above 7.25, physician will continue monitoring and resample; if pH shows downward trend (between 7.25 and 7.2) or is below 7.2, prepare for birth by most expeditious means.
Late decelerations with tachycardia or decreasing variability	Report findings to physician/CNM and document in medical record. Maintain maternal position on left side. Administer oxygen by face mask at 7–10 L/min. Discontinue oxytocin if it is being administered. Assess maternal blood pressure and pulse. Increase IV fluids (normal saline or lactated Ringer solution). Assess labor progress (dilatation and station). Prepare for immediate cesarean birth. Explain plan of treatment to woman and partner. Assist physician with fetal blood sampling (if ordered).
Prolonged decelerations	Perform vaginal examination to rule out prolapsed cord or to determine progress in labor status. Change maternal position as needed to try to alleviate decelerations. Discontinue oxytocin if it is being administered. Notify physician/CNM of findings and initial interventions and document in medical record. Provide explanation to woman and partner. Increase IV fluids (normal saline or lactated Ringer solution). Administer tocolytic if hypertonus noted and ordered by physician/CNM. Anticipate normal FHR recovery following deceleration if FHR previously normal. Anticipate intervention if FHR previously abnormal or deceleration lasts more than 3 minutes.

with less than 50% of contractions and are considered recurrent if they occur with 50% or more of the contractions (Groll, 2012). Decelerations that leave the baseline for more than 2 minutes but less than 10 minutes are known as *prolonged decelerations*.

PSYCHOLOGIC REACTIONS TO ELECTRONIC MONITORING

Responses to electronic fetal monitoring can be varied and complex. Many women have little knowledge of monitoring unless they have attended a prenatal class that dealt with this subject. Some women react to electronic monitoring positively, viewing it as a reassurance that "the baby is OK." They may also feel that the monitor helps identify problems that develop in labor. Other women may have ambivalent or even negative feelings about the monitor and may feel powerless to move and react in a way that feels natural to them. They may think that the monitor is interfering with a natural process, and they do not want the intrusion. Some women may find that the equipment, wires, and sounds increase their anxiety. The discomfort of lying in one position and fear of injury to the baby are other objections.

Clinical Tip

The presence of repetitive early decelerations may be a sign of advanced dilatation or the beginning of the second stage of labor. If the monitoring strip shows recurring early decelerations, ask the laboring woman if she is experiencing any pressure. Pressure that occurs only with the contractions typically indicates advanced dilatation. Intense pressure that does not change or ease up when the contractions cease may indicate the beginning of the second stage. A vaginal examination may be performed to establish the dilatation.

Nursing Management

A key strength of technology is its ability to explain and possibly predict health patterns or problems. However, this advantage has the potential to dehumanize the nurse–client relationship. It is crucial that nurses balance technology with holistic nursing practice. Therefore, it is important to recognize that every encounter with the childbearing family offers an opportunity to provide education and empowerment to the laboring woman and her partner. Helping to provide information when needed, answering questions, and encouraging the woman to make decisions establishes a trusting nurse–client relationship.

Before using the electronic fetal monitor, explain the reason for its use and the information that it can provide. After applying the monitor, record basic information on the monitor strip. These data should include the date, client's name, physician or certified nurse-midwife's name, hospital identification number, age, gravida, para, estimated date of birth, membrane status, and maternal vital signs. As the monitor strip runs and care is provided, occurrences during labor should be recorded not only in the medical record but also on the monitor strip. This information helps the healthcare team assess current status and evaluate the tracing.

Note the following information on the tracing (Miller, Miller, & Tucker, 2012):

- Vaginal examination (dilatation, effacement, station, position)
- Amniotomy or spontaneous rupture of membranes, color and amount of amniotic fluid, presence of any odor
- Maternal vital signs
- Maternal position in bed and changes of position
- Application of spiral electrode or intrauterine pressure catheter
- Medications given
- Oxygen administration
- Maternal behaviors (emesis, coughing, hiccups)
- Fetal scalp stimulation or fetal scalp blood sampling
- Vomiting
- Pushing
- Administration of anesthesia blocks

If the monitor does not automatically add the time on the strip at specific intervals, include the time when recording any information on the strip. If more than one nurse is adding information to the monitor strip, it is essential to initial each note. The tracing is considered a legal part of the woman's medical record and is submissible as evidence in court.

The fetal monitoring strip should be reviewed regularly—at least every 30 minutes in the first stage and every 15 minutes during the second stage (King et al., 2014).

The laboring woman needs to feel that what is happening to her is the central focus. Acknowledge this need by always speaking to and looking at the woman when entering the room, before looking at the monitor.

EVALUATION OF FHR TRACINGS

With a systematic approach to evaluating FHR tracings, the nurse can make a more accurate and rapid assessment, avoid interpreting findings on the basis of inadequate or erroneous data, and easily communicate data to the woman, physician/CNM, and staff. A universal language for documentation should be used consistently within the facility to avoid errors.

Professionalism in Practice FHR and Legal Responsibilities

Nurses caring for women during childbirth are legally responsible for correctly interpreting FHR patterns, initiating appropriate nursing interventions based on those patterns, and documenting the outcomes of those interventions.

Evaluation of the electronic monitor tracing begins by looking at the uterine contraction pattern. To evaluate the contraction pattern, the nurse should do the following:

1. Determine the uterine resting tone.
2. Assess the contractions: What is the frequency? What is the duration? What is the intensity?

After evaluating the FHR tracing for the contraction pattern, the nurse may categorize the tracing according to the Three-Tier FHR Interpretation System (Table 17–6). The three-tier system for the categorization of FHR patterns is recommended by ACOG, AWHONN, and the National Institute of Child Health and Human Development (Callahan & Caughley, 2013). Categorization of the FHR tracing evaluates the fetus at that point in time; tracing patterns can and will change. A FHR tracing may move back and forth between categories depending on the clinical situation and management strategies employed.

Category I FHR tracings are normal.   They are strongly predictive of normal fetal acid–base status at the time of observation. The FHR tracings may be followed in a routine manner, and no specific action is required.

Category II FHR tracings are indeterminate.   They are not predictive of abnormal fetal acid–base status, yet there is not enough adequate evidence at present to classify these as Category I or Category III. Category II tracings require evaluation and continued surveillance and reevaluation, taking into account the entire associated clinical circumstances.

Category III FHR tracings are abnormal.   They are predictive of abnormal fetal acid–base status at the time of observation if they continue. They require prompt evaluation. Depending on the clinical situation, efforts to expeditiously resolve the abnormal

TABLE 17–6 Three-Tier Fetal Heart Rate Interpretation System

CATEGORY I	CATEGORY II	CATEGORY III
REASSURING FETAL HEART RATE (FHR) TRACINGS	**PATTERNS WARRANTING CONTINUAL ASSESSMENT**	**PATTERNS OF NONREASSURING FETAL STATUS THAT WARRANT IMMEDIATE INTERVENTION**
• Normal range FHR 110–160 beats/min • Normal FHR variability in the moderate range • Absence of variable or late decelerations • Accelerations may be present or may be absent • Early decelerations may be present or may be absent; they do not represent a nonreassuring status	• Baselines that include bradycardia with continued variability, or tachycardia • Baseline changes in variability that include minimal variability, absent variability without decelerations, or marked baseline variability • Lack of accelerations with scalp stimulation • Episodic decelerations that include recurrent variable decelerations with minimal or moderate variability, prolonged decelerations lasting >2 min but <10 min in duration, or recurrent late decelerations that maintain moderate variability • Variable deceleration patterns that include overshoots, shoulders, or slow return to baseline status	• Absent variability in baseline FHR with recurrent late decelerations, recurrent variable decelerations, and/or bradycardia • Sinusoidal FHR patterns

Source: Data from American College of Obstetricians & Gynecologists (ACOG) (2009, reaffirmed 2013). *Intrapartum fetal heart rate monitoring: Nomenclature, interpretation, and general management principles.* ACOG Practice Bulletin No. 106. Washington, DC: ACOG.

FHR pattern may include, but are not limited to, provision of maternal oxygen, change in maternal position, discontinuation of labor stimulation, and treatment of maternal hypotension. If they are not immediately corrected, acidemia will occur; therefore, birth is required via the fastest route possible.

PROVISION OF EMOTIONAL SUPPORT

It is vital to provide information to the laboring woman about the FHR pattern and the interventions, if necessary, that will help her fetus. Most women are aware that something is happening. Sharing information with them provides reassurance that a potential or actual problem is identified and that they are active participants in the interventions. Occasionally, a problem arises that requires immediate intervention. In that case, it may be helpful to say something like, "It is important for you to turn on your left side right now because the baby is having a little difficulty. I'll explain what is happening in just a few moments." This type of response lets the woman know that although an action needs to be accomplished rapidly, information will soon be provided. In the haste to act quickly, nurses and other healthcare givers must not forget that it is the woman's body and her baby.

Scalp Stimulation Test

When there is a question about fetal status, a scalp stimulation test can be used before the more invasive **fetal blood sampling**. In this test, the examiner applies pressure to the fetal scalp while doing a vaginal examination. The fetus who is not in any stress or distress responds with an acceleration of the FHR. Fetuses that fail to respond have an increased incidence of acidosis, hypoxia, and lower Apgar scores (Simkin, 2013).

Fetal vibroacoustic stimulation using a handheld artificial larynx applied to the maternal abdomen may also be used to assess fetal status. As with scalp stimulation, FHR accelerations in response are a sign of fetal well-being (King et al., 2014).

SAFETY ALERT!

If there is no fetal reaction to the scalp stimulation test and a Category II or Category III fetal heart rate tracing persists, the nurse should contact the physician/CNM to come to the woman's bedside and perform further evaluation.

Cord Blood Analysis at Birth

In some cases, when the practitioner wishes to determine if acidosis is present, a cord blood analysis will be obtained. Indications for cord blood analysis include:

- Meconium-stained amniotic fluid
- Significantly abnormal FHR patterns
- Newborn is depressed at birth
- Apgar scores are less than 7 at 5 minutes of age

The cord is clamped before the baby takes the first breath. A small amount of blood is aspirated with a syringe from one of the umbilical arteries. If the cord blood will not be analyzed immediately, a heparinized syringe should be used. Normal fetal blood pH should be above 7.25 (Blackburn, 2013). Lower levels indicate acidosis and hypoxia. Many practitioners obtain cord blood analysis to minimize medicolegal exposure.

See *Assessment Guide: Intrapartum—First Stage of Labor.*

ASSESSMENT GUIDE | Intrapartum—First Stage of Labor

Physical Assessment/ Normal Findings	Alterations and Possible Causes*	Nursing Responses to Data†
Vital Signs		
Blood pressure (BP): less than or equal to 120 systolic and 80 diastolic in adult 18 years of age or older or no more than 15–20 mmHg rise in systolic pressure over baseline BP during early pregnancy	High BP (essential hypertension, preeclampsia, renal disease, apprehension or anxiety) Low BP (supine hypotension)	Evaluate history of preexisting disorders and check for presence of other signs of preeclampsia or other hypertensive disorders. Assess for previous history of BP issues. Ensure blood pressure is being obtained with a proper cuff size because using a cuff that is too small will result in falsely abnormal elevated BP readings. Do not assess during contractions; implement measures to decrease anxiety and reassess. Turn woman on her side and recheck BP. Provide quiet environment. Have O_2 available.
Pulse: 60–100 beats per minute (beats/min)	Increased pulse rate (excitement or anxiety, cardiac disorders, early shock)	Evaluate cause, reassess to see if rate continues; report to physician.
Respirations: 12–20/minute (or pulse rate divided by 4) (may be higher during labor)	Marked tachypnea (respiratory disease), hyperventilation in transition phase Hyperventilation (anxiety)	Assess between contractions; if marked tachypnea continues, assess for signs of respiratory disease.
Pulse oximeter (if used) 95% or greater	Less than 90% (hypoxia, hypotension, hemorrhage)	Encourage slow breaths if woman is hyperventilating. Apply O_2; notify physician.
Temperature: 36.2–37.6°C (98–99.6°F)	Elevated temperature (infection, dehydration, prolonged rupture of membranes, epidural regional block)	Assess for other signs of infection or dehydration.
Weight		
25–35 lb greater than prepregnant weight	Weight gain greater than 35 lb (15.9 kg) (fluid retention, obesity, large baby, diabetes mellitus, preeclampsia), weight gain less than 15 lb (6.8 kg) (small for gestational age [SGA], substance abuse, psychosocial problems)	Assess for signs of edema. Evaluate pattern from prenatal record.
Lungs		
Normal breath sounds, clear and equal	Rales, rhonchi, friction rub (infection), pulmonary edema, asthma	Reassess; refer to physician.
Fundus		
At 40 weeks' gestation, fundus is located just below xiphoid process	Uterine size not compatible with estimated date of birth (SGA, large for gestational age [LGA], hydramnios, multiple pregnancy, placental/fetal anomalies, malpresentation)	Reevaluate history regarding pregnancy dating. Refer to physician for additional assessment.
Edema		
Nondependent/nonpitting edema	Pitting edema of face, hands, legs, abdomen, sacral area (preeclampsia)	Check deep tendon reflexes for hyperactivity; check for clonus; refer to physician.
Hydration		
Normal skin turgor, elastic	Poor skin turgor (dehydration)	Assess skin turgor; refer to physician for deviations.
Perineum		
Tissues smooth, pink color (see *Assessment Guide: Initial Prenatal Assessment* in Chapter 9)	Varicose veins of vulva, herpes lesions, genital warts	Exercise care while doing a perineal prep; note on client record need for follow-up in postpartum period; reassess after birth; refer to physician/CNM. If herpes lesions are present, do not assess the cervix if prophylaxis therapy has not been started as this increases transmission of infection.

(continued)

| ASSESSMENT GUIDE | Intrapartum—First Stage of Labor (*continued*) |

Physical Assessment/ Normal Findings	Alterations and Possible Causes*	Nursing Responses to Data†
Clear mucus; may be blood tinged with earthy or human odor	Profuse, purulent, foul-smelling drainage	Suspected gonorrhea or chorioamnionitis; report to physician/CNM; initiate care to newborn's eyes; notify neonatal nursing staff and pediatrician.
Presence of small amount of bloody show that gradually increases with further cervical dilatation	Hemorrhage	Assess BP and pulse, pallor, diaphoresis; report any marked changes. (*Note:* Gaping of vagina or anus and bulging of perineum are signs that suggest the onset of the second stage of labor.) Follow universal precautions.

Labor Status

Uterine contractions: regular pattern	Failure to establish a regular pattern, prolonged latent phase; hypertonicity; hypotonicity; dehydration	Evaluate whether woman is in true labor; ambulate if in early labor. Evaluate client status and contractile pattern. Obtain a 20-minute electronic fetal monitor (EFM) strip. Notify physician/CNM. Provide hydration.
Cervical dilatation: progressive cervical dilatation from size of fingertip to 10 cm (see Performing an Intrapartum Vaginal Examination in the *Clinical Skills Manual* SKILLS)	Rigidity of cervix (frequent cervical infections, scar tissue, failure of presenting part to descend)	Evaluate contractions, fetal engagement, position, and cervical dilatation. Inform woman of progress.
Cervical effacement: progressive thinning of cervix (see Performing an Intrapartum Vaginal Examination in the *Clinical Skills Manual* SKILLS)	Failure to efface (rigidity of cervix, failure of presenting part to engage); cervical edema (pushing effort by woman before cervix is fully dilated and effaced	Evaluate contractions, fetal engagement, and position. Notify physician/CNM if cervix is becoming edematous; work with woman to prevent pushing until cervix is completely dilated. Keep vaginal exams to a minimum.
Fetal descent: progressive descent of fetal presenting part from station –5 to +4 (see Performing an Intrapartum Vaginal Examination in the *Clinical Skills Manual* SKILLS)	Failure of descent (abnormal fetal position or presentation, macrosomic fetus, inadequate pelvic measurement)	Evaluate fetal position, presentation, and size. Evaluate maternal pelvic measurements. If descent is slow, offer birthing ball or assist with squatting position.
Membranes: may rupture before or during labor	Rupture of membranes more than 12–24 hours before onset of labor	Assess for ruptured membranes using Nitrazine test tape before doing vaginal exam. Follow universal precautions. Instruct woman with ruptured membranes to remain on bed rest if presenting part is not engaged and firmly down against the cervix. Keep vaginal exams to a minimum to prevent infection. When membranes rupture in the birth setting, *immediately assess fetal heart rate* to detect changes associated with prolapse of umbilical cord (FHR slows).
Findings on Nitrazine test tape: Membranes probably intact Yellow pH 5.0 Olive pH 5.5 Olive green pH 6.0 Membranes probably ruptured Blue-green pH 6.5 Blue-gray pH 7.0 Deep blue pH 7.5	False-positive results may be obtained if large amount of bloody show is present, previous vaginal examination has been done using lubricant, sweat or sperm is present, or tape is touched by nurse's fingers.	Assess fluid for consistency, amount, odor; assess FHR frequently. Assess fluid at regular intervals for presence of meconium staining. Follow universal precautions while assessing amniotic fluid. Reassure woman that amniotic fluid is continually produced. Teach woman that she may feel amniotic fluid trickle or gush with contractions. Change chux pads often.
Amniotic fluid clear, with earthy or human odor, no foul-smelling odor	Greenish amniotic fluid (fetal stress) Bloody fluid (abruptio placentae)	Assess FHR; do vaginal exam to evaluate for prolapsed cord; apply fetal monitor for continuous data; report to physician/CNM.
	Strong or foul odor (amnionitis)	Take woman's temperature and report to physician/CNM.

Physical Assessment/ Normal Findings	Alterations and Possible Causes*	Nursing Responses to Data†
Fetal Status		
Fetal heart rate (FHR): 110–160 beats/min	Less than 110 or greater than 160 beats/min (nonreassuring fetal status); abnormal patterns on fetal monitor: decreased variability, late decelerations, variable decelerations, absence of accelerations with fetal movement	Initiate interventions based on particular FHR pattern.
Presentation: Cephalic, 97% Breech, 3%	Face, brow, breech, or shoulder presentation	Report to physician/CNM; after presentation is confirmed as face, brow, breech, or shoulder, woman may be prepared for cesarean birth.
Position: left occiput anterior (LOA) most common	Persistent occipital posterior (OP) position; transverse arrest	Carefully monitor maternal and fetal status. Reposition mother to side-lying or hands and knees to promote rotation of fetal head.
Activity: fetal movement	Hyperactivity (may precede fetal hypoxia)	Carefully evaluate FHR; apply fetal monitor.
	Complete lack of movement (fetal distress or fetal demise)	Carefully evaluate FHR; apply fetal monitor. Report to physician/CNM.
Laboratory Evaluation		
Hematologic tests: Hemoglobin: 12–16 g/dL	Less than 11 g/dL (anemia, hemorrhage)	Evaluate woman for problems due to decreased oxygen-carrying capacity caused by lowered hemoglobin.
Complete blood count (CBC): Hematocrit: 38%–47% Red blood cell count (RBC): 4.2–5.4 million/mm³ White blood cell count (WBC): 4500–11,000/mm³, although leukocytosis to 20,000/mm³ is not unusual Platelets: 150,000–400,000/mm³	Presence of infection or blood dyscrasias, loss of blood (hemorrhage, disseminated intravascular coagulation [DIC])	Evaluate for other signs of infection or for petechiae, bruising, or unusual bleeding.
Serologic testing: Serologic test for syphilis (STS) or Venereal Disease Research Laboratory (VDRL) test: nonreactive	Positive reaction (see *Assessment Guide: Initial Prenatal Assessment* in Chapter 9)	For reactive test, notify newborn nursery and pediatrician.
Rh factor	Rh-positive fetus in Rh-negative woman	Assess prenatal record for titer levels during pregnancy. Obtain cord blood for direct Coombs test at birth.
Urinalysis		
Glucose: negative	Glycosuria (low renal threshold for glucose, diabetes mellitus)	Assess blood glucose level; test urine for ketones; ketonuria and glycosuria require further assessment of blood sugar levels.‡
Ketones: negative	Ketonuria (starvation ketosis), vomiting, hyperemesis gravidarum	
Proteins: negative	Proteinuria (urine specimen contaminated with vaginal secretions, fever, kidney disease); proteinuria of 2+ or greater found in uncontaminated urine may be a sign of ensuing pre-eclampsia	Instruct woman in collection technique; incidence of contamination from vaginal discharge is common. Report any increase in proteinuria to physician/CNM.
Red blood cells: negative	Blood in urine (calculi, cystitis, glomerulonephritis, neoplasm)	Assess collection technique (may be bloody show).
White blood cells: negative	Presence of white blood cells (infection in genitourinary tract)	Assess for signs of urinary tract infection.
Casts: none	Presence of casts (nephrotic syndrome)	

(continued)

ASSESSMENT GUIDE | Intrapartum—First Stage of Labor (continued)

Cultural Assessment§	Variations to Consider	Nursing Responses to Data†
Cultural influences determine customs and practices regarding intrapartum care.	Individual preferences may vary.	
Ask the following questions: Who would you like to remain with you during your labor and birth?	She may prefer only her partner/significant other to remain or may also want family and/or friends.	Provide support for her wishes by encouraging desired people to stay. Provide information to others (with the woman's permission) who are not in the room.
What would you like to wear during labor?	She may be more comfortable in her own clothes if permitted by facility policy.	Offer supportive materials such as chux pad if needed to protect her own clothing. Avoid subtle signals to the woman that she should not have chosen to remain in her own clothes. Have other clothing available if the woman desires. If her clothing becomes contaminated, it will be simple to place it in a plastic bag. The nurse can soak soiled clothing in cool water. The nurse needs to remember to wear disposable gloves and a plastic apron if splashing is anticipated.
What activity would you like during labor?	She may want to ambulate most of the time, stand in the shower, sit in the Jacuzzi, sit in a chair or on a stool, remain on the bed, and so forth. These activities may be impacted by facility policy.	Support the woman's wishes; provide encouragement and complete assessments in a manner so her activity and positional wishes are disturbed as little as possible.
What position would you like for the birth?	She may feel more comfortable in lithotomy with stirrups and her upper body elevated, or side-lying or sitting in birthing bed, or standing, or squatting, or on hands and knees.	Collect any supplies and equipment needed to support her in her chosen birthing position. Provide information to the coach regarding any changes that may be needed based on the chosen position.
Is there anything special you would like?	She may want the room darkened or to have curtains and windows open, music playing, a Leboyer birth (waterbirth), certain scents, her coach to cut the umbilical cord, to save a portion of the umbilical cord, to save the placenta, to videotape the birth, and so forth.	Support requests and communicate requests to any other nursing or medical personnel (so requests can continue to be supported and not questioned). If another nurse or physician does not honor the request, act as advocate for the woman by continuing to support her unless her desire is truly unsafe.
Ask the woman if she would like fluids and ask what temperature she prefers.	She may prefer clear fluids other than water (tea, clear juice). She may prefer iced, room-temperature, or warmed fluids.	Provide fluids as desired.
Observe the woman's response when privacy is difficult to maintain and her body is exposed.	Some women do not seem to mind being exposed during an exam or procedure; others feel acute discomfort.	Maintain privacy and respect the woman's sense of privacy.
		If the woman is unable to provide specific information, the nurse may draw from general information regarding cultural variation: a Southeast Asian woman may not want any family member in the room during exams or procedures. Her partner may not be involved with coaching activities during labor or birth. Muslim women may need to remain covered during the labor and birth and avoid exposure of any body part. The husband may need to be in the room but remain behind a curtain or screen so he does not view his wife at this time.
If the woman is to breastfeed, encourage her to feed her baby immediately after birth while the baby is in a more alert state.	She may want to feed her baby right away or may want to wait a little while if she feels too fatigued. However, the nurse should encourage immediate feeding when possible.	

Cultural Assessment§	Variations to Consider	Nursing Responses to Data†
Preparation for Childbirth		
Woman has some information regarding process of normal labor and birth.	Some women do not have any information regarding childbirth.	Add to present information base.
Woman has breathing and/or relaxation techniques to use during labor.	Some women do not have any method of relaxation or breathing to use, and some do not desire them.	Support breathing and relaxation techniques that client is using; provide information if needed.
Response to Labor		
Latent phase (0–3 cm): relaxed, excited, anxious for labor to be well established	May feel unable to cope with contractions because of fear, anxiety, or lack of information	Provide support and encouragement; establish trusting relationship.
Active phase (4–7 cm): becomes more intense, begins to tire	May remain quiet and without any sign of discomfort or anxiety, may insist that she is unable to continue with the birthing process	Provide support and coaching if needed.
Transitional phase (8–10 cm): feels tired, may feel unable to cope, needs frequent coaching to maintain breathing patterns		
Coping mechanisms: ability to cope with labor through utilization of support system, breathing, relaxation techniques	May feel marked anxiety and apprehension, may not have coping mechanisms that can be brought into this experience, or may be unable to use them at this time.	Support coping mechanisms if they are working for the woman; provide information and support if she exhibits anxiety or needs alternative to present coping methods.
	Survivors of sexual abuse may demonstrate fear of IVs or needles, may recoil when touched, may insist on a female healthcare giver, may be very sensitive to body fluids and cleanliness, and may be unable to labor lying down.	Encourage participation of coach or significant other if a supportive relationship seems apparent. Establish rapport and a trusting relationship. Provide information that is true and offer your presence.
Anxiety		
Some anxiety and apprehension is within normal limits	May show anxiety through rapid breathing, nervous tremors, frowning, grimacing, clenching of teeth, thrashing movements, crying, increased pulse and blood pressure.	Provide support, encouragement, and information. Teach relaxation techniques; support controlled breathing efforts. May need to provide a paper bag to breathe into if woman says her lips are tingling. Note FHR.
Sounds During Labor		
	Some women are very quiet; others moan or make a variety of noises.	Provide a supportive environment. Encourage woman to do what is right for her.
Support System		
Physical intimacy between mother and father (or mother and support person); caretaking activities such as soothing conversation, touching	Some women would prefer no contact; others may show clinging behaviors.	Encourage caretaking activities that appear to comfort the woman; encourage support to the woman; if support is limited, the nurse may take a more active role.
Support person stays in proximity	Limited interaction may come from a desire for quiet.	Encourage support person to stay close (if this seems appropriate).
Relationship between mother and father (or support person): involved interaction	The support person may seem to be detached and maintain little support, attention, or conversation.	Support interactions; if interaction is limited, the nurse may provide more information and support.
		Ensure that coach or significant other has short breaks, especially prior to transition.

*Possible causes of alterations are placed in parentheses.

†This column provides guidelines for further assessment and initial nursing intervention.

‡Glycosuria should not be discounted. The presence of glycosuria necessitates follow-up.

§These are only a few suggestions. We do not mean to imply that this is a comprehensive cultural assessment; rather, it is a tool to encourage cultural sensitivity.

Focus Your Study

- An obstetric along with high-risk screening should include vital signs, labor status, fetal status, and laboratory findings.

- A maternal assessment should include both physiologic considerations along with a cultural assessment and evaluation of psychosocial factors.

- A labor assessment should include assessment of contraction strength, frequency, and duration and a cervical assessment that includes cervical dilatation and effacement.

- Leopold maneuvers is a technique where the evaluator determines the position, presentation, and lie of the fetus by palpating the maternal abdomen in a systematic manner. The examiner palpates the abdomen gently yet firmly after the woman empties her bladder. The examiner holds one hand steady while the other hand palpates the abdomen and then switches hands. The FHR is heard most clearly over the fetal back.

- The fetal heart rate is can be assessed by a handheld Doppler or a fetoscope for intermittent monitoring. External monitoring is performed externally by an external fetal monitor or internally using an internal scalp electrode.

- Baseline fetal heart rate monitoring should be observed for 10 minutes to determine the baseline rate. Normal BL-FHR is 110 to 160, although baseline changes may include tachycardia, bradycardia, and changes in variability.

- Periodic fetal heart rate changes may include accelerations which indicate fetal well-being when they occur during a contraction or be a sign of fetal movement. Decelerations can occur for various reasons. Early decelerations are typically a sign of head compression and usually require no intervention, whereas, late decelerations are those that occur during and following the contraction or after the contraction and are related to alterations in fetal blood flow which is a nonreassuring sign.

- Variable decelerations typically occur as a result of umbilical cord compression which requires additional assessment but are usually not an indicator of fetal compromise. Sinusoidal patterns occur when there are periods of heart rate abnormalities that are often associated with Rh alloimmunization, fetal anemia, fetal hypoxia, and a chronic fetal bleed.

- Fetal heart rate tracings should be performed in a systematic manner where the uterine contraction pattern is first identified. The nurse then determines the baseline FHR, FHR variability. Presence of sinusoidal patterns or periodic changes in the FHR.

- Nonreassuring fetal patterns include severe decelerations, late decelerations of any magnitude, absence of variability and prolonged decelerations.

- Prompt interventions for nonreassuring fetal status include notifying the physician/CNM, administering oxygen to the mother, turning the mother to her left side, discontinuing oxytocin if it is being administered, continuously monitoring the FHR, and providing explanations to the mother and her partner.

- Nursing responsibilities related to EFM including explaining the use of the fetal monitor to the mother and her partner, engaging the mother directly without exclusive focus on the EFM strip, and recording pertinent data on the monitoring strip related to the woman's care and progression.

Clinical Reasoning in Action

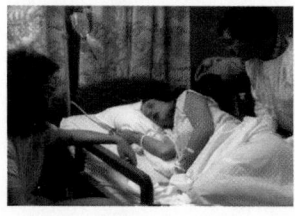

Cindy Bell, a 20-year-old gravida 2, para 1, at 40 weeks' gestation, presents to you in the birthing unit with contractions every 5 to 7 minutes. She is accompanied by her husband. Spontaneous rupture of membranes occurred 2 hours prior to admission. Cindy tells you that the fluid was colorless and clear. You orient Cindy and her family to the birthing room and perform a physical assessment, documenting that vital signs are normal. A vaginal examination demonstrates the cervix is 75% effaced, 4 cm dilated with a vertex at -1 station in the LOP position. You place Cindy on an external fetal monitor. The fetal heart rate baseline is 140 to 147 with accelerations to 156; no decelerations are noted. Contractions are 5 to 6 minutes apart, moderate intensity, and lasting 40 to 50 seconds. Cindy states she would like to stay out of bed as long as possible because lying down seems to make the contractions more painful, especially in her back.

1. Discuss the benefits of ambulation in labor.

2. Cindy would like her 5-year-old daughter to be present for the baby's birth. What would you discuss with her about the impact of having a young sibling present during labor and birth?

3. What fetal heart rate assessment will best ensure fetal well-being during the period Cindy is ambulating?

4. When a nonreassuring fetal heart pattern is detected, what remedial nursing intervention is carried out?

5. What are indications for continuous fetal monitoring in labor?

References

American College of Obstetricians and Gynecologists (ACOG). (2012). *Prevention and prediction of preterm birth.* (Practice Bulletin No. 130). Washington, DC: Author.

American College of Obstetricians and Gynecologists (ACOG) (2009, reaffirmed 2013). *Intrapartum fetal heart rate monitoring: Nomenclature, interpretation, and general management principles.* (Practice Bulletin No. 106.) Washington, DC: ACOG.

American College of Obstetricians and Gynecologists (ACOG). (2014). *Antepartum surveillance.* (Practice Bulletin No. 146.) Washington, DC: ACOG.

Blackburn, S. T. (2013). *Maternal, fetal, and neonatal physiology: A clinical perspective* (4th ed.). Philadelphia, PA: Saunders.

Callahan, T., & Caughley, A. (2013). *Blueprint in obstetrics & gynecology.* Philadelphia, PA: Lippincott, Williams, & Wilkins.

Centers for Disease Control and Prevention (CDC). (2011). Bloodborne infectious diseases: HIV/AIDS, hepatitis B, hepatitis C. Retrieved from http://www.cdc.gov/niosh/topics/bbp/universal.html

Cunningham, F. G., Leveno, K. J., Bloom, S. L., Spong, C. Y., Dashe, J. S., Hoffman, B. L., ... Sheffield, J. S. (2014). *Williams obstetrics* (24th ed.). New York, NY: McGraw-Hill.

Dalfen, A. (2014). *When baby brings the blues: Solutions for postpartum depression.* New York, NY: Collins.

Davidson, M. R. (2012). *A nurse's guide to women's mental health.* New York, NY: Springer.

Groll, C. G. (2012). *Fast facts for the L&D nurse: Labor and delivery orientation in a nutshell.* New York, NY: Springer.

King, T. K., Brucker, M. C., Kriebs, J. M., & Fahey, J. (2015). *Varney's midwifery.* (5th ed.). New York, NY: Jones Bartlett Learning.

Menihan, C. A., & Kopel, A. (2014). *Point-of-care assessment in pregnancy and women's health: Electronic fetal monitoring and sonography.* Philadelphia, PA: Lippincott, Williams, & Wilkins.

Miller, L. A., Miller, S., & Tucker, S. M. (2012). *Mosby's pocket guide to fetal monitoring: A multidisciplinary approach.* (7th ed.). St. Louis, MO: Mosby.

Nilsson, L., Thorsell, T., Hertfelt-Wahn, E., & Ekström, A. (2013). Factors influencing positive birth experiences of first-time mothers. *Nursing Research and Practice, 20(13),* 26–32. doi:10.1155/2013/349124

Papadakis, M., McPhee, S., & Rabow, M. W. (2014). *Current medical diagnosis and treatment: 2015.* Boston, MA: McGraw-Hill.

Riffle, E. (2014). Fetal heart rate assessment best practice. *International Journal of Childbirth Education, 29*(4), 55–58.

Simkin, P. (2013). *The birth partner: A complete guide for dad's, doulas, and health care professionals.* Boston, MA: Harvard Press.

Spector, R. E. (2012). *Cultural diversity in health and illness* (8th ed.). Upper Saddle River, NJ: Pearson.

Yonkers, K. A., Wisner, K. L., Stewart, D. E., Oberlander, T. F., Dell, D. L., Stotland, N.,... Lockwood, C. (2012). The management of depression during pregnancy: A report from the American Psychiatric Association and the American College of Obstetricians and Gynecologists. *FOCUS 2012, 10,* 78–89. doi:10.1176/appi.focus.10.1.78

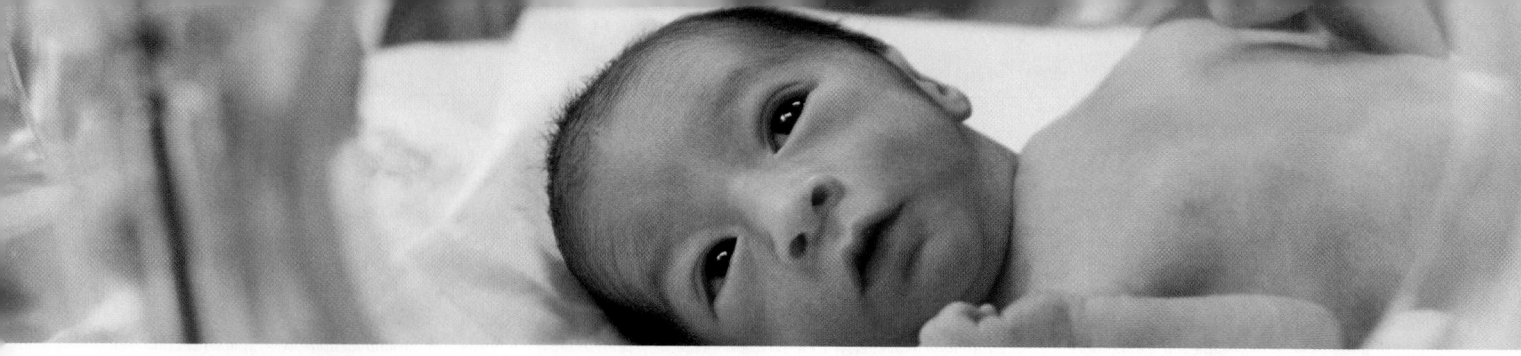

Chapter 18
The Family in Childbirth: Needs and Care

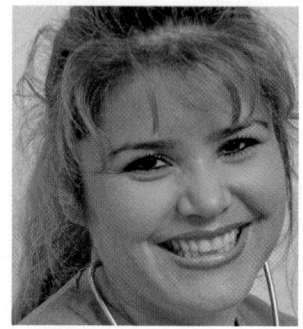

For as long as I can remember, I have been fascinated with birth. Currently, I am a labor and delivery nurse at our town's only hospital. I'm still fascinated with birth but a little nervous, too. You see, I was just admitted in early labor with my first child. Before I got here I worried that I would be a "bad" patient or that I would lose my cool. How silly I was. All that matters is that my baby is healthy and that I am able to take care of him effectively. (Yes. We know it is a boy!)

—Amanda, 31

Jonathan Nourok/PhotoEdit

Learning Outcomes

18.1 Identify admission data that should be noted when a woman is admitted to the birthing area.

18.2 Describe the nursing care of a woman and her partner/family upon admission to the birthing area.

18.3 Use assessment data to determine the nursing interventions to meet the psychologic, social, physiologic, and spiritual needs of the woman and her partner/family during each stage of labor.

18.4 Compare methods of promoting comfort during the first and second stages of labor.

18.5 Explain the immediate needs and physical assessment of the newborn following birth in the provision of nursing care.

18.6 Examine the unique needs of the adolescent during birth in the provision of nursing care.

18.7 Describe the role and responsibilities of the nurse in the management of a precipitous labor and birth.

It is time for a child to be born. The parents are about to undergo one of the most meaningful and stressful events of their lives. The adequacy of their preparation for childbirth, including the coping mechanisms, communication, and support systems that they have established, will be put to the test. Like Amanda, the childbearing woman may feel that her psychologic and physical limits are about to be challenged. These events may be even more challenging for the single woman, especially if she lacks a strong support system.

Family-centered care is a model of care based on the philosophy that the physical, sociocultural, spiritual, and economic needs of the family are combined and considered collectively when planning care for the childbearing family (Institute for Patient and Family-Centered Care, 2014). To reflect the consumer demand for family-centered care, most birthing centers now have **birthing rooms**, single rooms where the woman and her partner or family members or other support person(s) will stay for the labor, birth, recovery, and possibly the postpartum period. These rooms may be called *labor–delivery–recovery–postpartum (LDRP) rooms* or *single-room maternity care (SRMC)*.

The birthing room atmosphere is more relaxed than a traditional labor room, and families seem to feel more comfortable in it. Not having to be transferred from one area to another for birth helps the laboring woman create her own space to labor in and enhances the family's involvement. Birthing rooms usually have beds that can be adapted for birth by removing a small section near the foot. The room's decor is designed to produce a homelike atmosphere in which families can feel both safe and at ease.

The previous two chapters provided information about physiologic and psychologic changes during labor and birth and necessary nursing assessments. This chapter focuses on nursing care during labor and birth.

Healthy People 2020

(MICH–4) Reduce maternal illness and complications due to pregnancy (complications during hospitalized labor and delivery)

(MICH–6) Reduce cesarean births among low-risk (full-term, singleton, vertex presentation) women

---

Nursing Diagnoses During Labor and Birth

When devising a plan of care for the intrapartum period, the nurse can develop a general plan that encompasses the total process, from the beginning of labor through the fourth stage, or a more specific plan that identifies nursing diagnoses for each stage of labor and birth.

Examples of appropriate nursing diagnoses may include the following (NANDA-I © 2014):

- *Fear* related to uncertainty about the outcome of the birth process
- *Pain, Acute,* related to uterine contractions, cervical dilatation, and fetal descent
- *Knowledge, Readiness for Enhanced,* related to information about the fetal monitor and an expressed desire to understand equipment used
- *Family Processes, Readiness for Enhanced,* related to opportunity to incorporate newborn into the family

Nursing Management

During prenatal visits, instruct the woman to come to the birthing unit if any of the following occurs:

- Rupture of membranes (ROM)
- Regular, frequent uterine contractions (nulliparas, 5 minutes apart for 1 hour; multiparas, 6 to 8 minutes apart for 1 hour)
- Vaginal bleeding
- Decreased fetal movement

The woman in labor and her partner or support person(s) tend to be concerned about arriving at the birth center in time for the birth. Sometimes the labor is advanced and birth is imminent, but usually the woman is in early labor at admission. If time permits and the family is not familiar with what will occur during labor, provide necessary information. (See *Teaching Highlights: What to Expect During Labor.*)

The way you greet the woman and her partner influences the course of the woman's hospital stay. The sudden

---

TEACHING HIGHLIGHTS | **What to Expect During Labor**

- Describe aspects of the admission process:
  - Abbreviated history
  - Physical assessment (maternal vital signs, fetal heart rate, contraction status, status of membranes)
  - Assessment of uterine contractions (frequency, duration, intensity)
  - Orientation to surroundings
  - Introductions to other staff
  - Determination of the woman's and support person's expectations of the nurse
- Present aspects of ongoing physical care, such as when to expect assessment of maternal vital signs, fetal heart rate, and contractions.
- If an electronic fetal monitor is used, describe how it works and the information it provides. Orient the woman to sights and sounds of the monitor.
- Explain what "normal" data look like and what characteristics are being watched for.
- Be sure to note that assessments will increase as the labor progresses, especially during the transition phase, to help keep the mother and baby safe by noting any changes from the normal course.
- Explain the vaginal examination and the information it can provide.
- Review comfort techniques that may be used in labor and ascertain what the woman thinks will promote comfort.
- Review breathing techniques the woman has learned so that you can support her technique.
- Review comfort and support measures such as positioning, back rub, effleurage, touch, distraction techniques, and ambulation.
- If the woman is in early labor, offer her a tour of the birthing area.
- Have printed materials available for reference, especially for the partner or support person.
- If time permits, a brief video describing procedures may be helpful.

environmental change and the sometimes impersonal and technical aspects of admission can produce significant stress. If women and their families are greeted in a brusque, harried manner, they are less likely to look to the nurse for support. A calm, pleasant manner indicates to the woman that she is important. It helps to instill a sense of confidence in the staff's ability to provide quality care during this critical time.

Following the initial greeting, escort the woman to the birthing room and provide a quick yet thorough orientation to the facility, including the location of the restrooms, public phones, and nurse-call or emergency-call system. These simple steps can go a long way toward helping the woman and her partner feel more at ease. Explain the monitoring equipment or other unfamiliar technology and make every effort to make the environment less frightening for the laboring woman and her support person(s).

Some women prefer that their partner remain with them during the admission process, and others prefer to have the partner wait outside. While helping the woman undress and get into a hospital gown, begin to develop rapport and establish a nursing database. The experienced labor and birth nurse can obtain essential information about the woman and her pregnancy within a few minutes after admission, initiate any immediate interventions needed, and establish individualized priorities.

The woman may be facing a number of unfamiliar procedures that seem routine for healthcare providers. Remember that all women have the right to determine what happens to their bodies. The woman's informed consent should be obtained prior to any procedure that involves touching her.

If indicated, assist the woman into bed. A side-lying or semi-Fowler position rather than a supine position is most comfortable and avoids supine hypotensive syndrome (vena caval syndrome). After obtaining the essential information from the woman and her records, begin the intrapartum assessment (see Chapter 17). Once the assessment is complete, it is possible to make effective nursing decisions about care, such as the following:

- Should ambulation, bed rest, or a combination of both be encouraged?
- Is more frequent or continuous electronic fetal monitoring needed?
- What does the woman want during her labor and birth?
- Is a support person available?
- What special needs do this woman and her partner have?

Auscultate the fetal heart rate (FHR). Determine the woman's blood pressure, pulse, respirations, and oral temperature and assess contraction frequency, duration, and intensity (possibly while gathering other data). Before the vaginal examination, inform the woman about the procedure and its purpose; afterward, report the findings. If signs of advanced labor exist (frequent contractions, an urge to bear down, and so on), a vaginal examination must be done immediately. If there are signs of excessive bleeding or if the woman reports episodes of painless bleeding in the last trimester, suspect placenta previa. Do not do a vaginal examination, and notify the physician/CNM immediately.

Results of FHR assessment, uterine contraction evaluation, and the vaginal examination help determine whether the rest of the admission process can proceed at a leisurely pace or whether additional interventions are required. For example, an FHR of less than 110 beats per minute (beats/min) on auscultation indicates that a fetal monitor should be applied immediately to obtain additional data. The woman's vital signs can be assessed once the monitor is in place.

After obtaining admission data, collect a clean voided midstream urine specimen. The woman with intact membranes may collect her specimen in the bathroom. If the membranes are ruptured and the presenting part is not engaged, the woman generally remains in bed to avoid prolapse of the umbilical cord. Views vary about the wisdom of ambulation once the membranes are ruptured. The decision is generally based on history and physical findings (e.g., history of precipitous labors, indications for continuous fetal monitoring, presence of meconium), clinician orders, the woman's desires, agency policy, and safety concerns.

Use a dipstick to test the woman's urine for the presence of protein, ketones, and glucose before sending the sample to the laboratory. This procedure is especially important if edema or elevated blood pressure is noted on admission. Proteinuria of 1+ or more may be a sign of impending preeclampsia. Glycosuria (sugar in the urine) is found frequently in pregnant women because of the increased glomerular filtration rate in the proximal tubules and the inability of these tubules to increase reabsorption of glucose. However, it may also be associated with gestational diabetes, so do not discount it. Ketones can be associated with inadequate calorie intake, dehydration, vomiting, skipping meals, insulin resistance, or gestational diabetes. While the woman is collecting the urine specimen, gather the equipment needed for any procedures ordered by the physician/CNM.

Laboratory tests are done during early admission. Hemoglobin and hematocrit values help determine the oxygen-carrying capacity of the circulatory system and the woman's ability to withstand blood loss at birth. Elevation of the hematocrit may reveal hemoconcentration of blood, which occurs with edema or dehydration. A low hemoglobin, in the absence of other evidence of bleeding, suggests anemia. Blood may be typed and cross-matched if the woman is in a high-risk category. Platelets are also evaluated because low platelets can lead to bleeding problems. Additional serologic testing may be performed as indicated. HIV testing should be offered to all women who have not been previously screened (Centers for Disease Control & Prevention [CDC], 2014).

Depending on how rapidly labor is progressing, notify the physician/CNM before or after completing the admission procedures. The report should include the following information: parity, cervical dilatation and effacement, station, presenting part, status of the membranes, contraction pattern, FHR, vital signs that are not in the normal range, any significant prenatal history, the woman's birth preferences, and her reaction to labor.

Enter a nursing admission note into the computer or the medical record system. The admission note should include the reason for admission, the date and time of the woman's arrival and notification of the physician/CNM, the condition of the woman and her baby, and labor and membrane status.

Nursing Care During the First Stage of Labor

After completing the nursing assessment and diagnosis steps, a plan of care to achieve identified nursing goals should be created. For instance, if the woman and her support person did not have the opportunity to attend childbirth preparation classes, the nursing goal would be to provide desired information. To accomplish this goal, the nurse would assess the current level of the couple's understanding and then plan to provide brief explanations as labor progresses.

Integration of Family Expectations

Families come into the birth setting with basic expectations that they will not be harmed and that the labor and birth will be safe for the mother and baby. In addition, women look for the following from their nurses:

- Emotional support, which includes sustained presence of the nurse, praise, encouragement, reassurance, and companionship
- Comfort measures such as the use of touch, provision of ice chips and fluids, massage, assistance with care, and a bath or shower
- Information and advice, which includes offering information about procedures, interventions as they occur, and reports of labor progress
- Advocacy to help the woman and her partner achieve their goals, hopes, and dreams for their labor and birth experience
- Support of the partner, including encouragement, praise for his or her efforts, an opportunity for rest breaks, and role modeling

Integration of Cultural Beliefs

Knowledge of values, customs, and practices of different cultures is as important during labor as it is in the prenatal period. Without this knowledge a nurse is less likely to understand a family's behavior and may attempt to impose personal values and beliefs on them. As cultural sensitivity increases, so does the likelihood of providing high-quality care.

The following sections briefly present a few possible cultural responses to labor. General examples about any culture or belief system should be viewed as background information only. An individual example of a birthing practice will never be pertinent to all women in a given group. Within every culture, each person develops his or her own beliefs, values, and behaviors. Culture is also discussed in Chapter 2.

MODESTY

Modesty is an important consideration for women regardless of culture. However, some women may be more uncomfortable than others with the degree of exposure needed for certain procedures during labor and the birth process. Some women may be particularly uncomfortable when men are present and feel more comfortable with women; others may be uncomfortable with exposure of personal body parts regardless of the gender of the healthcare givers. The nurse should be alert to the woman's responses to examinations and procedures and provide the draping and privacy the woman needs. It is more prudent to assume that embarrassment will occur with exposure and take measures to provide privacy than to assume that it will not matter to the woman if she is exposed during procedures.

PAIN EXPRESSION

The manner in which a woman chooses to deal with the discomfort of labor varies widely. Some women seem to turn inward and remain very quiet during the whole process. They speak only to ask others to leave the room or cease conversation. Others may be very vocal, with behaviors such as counting out loud, moaning quietly, crying, or use of loud vocalization. They may also turn from side to side or change positions frequently.

In many Asian cultures, it is important for individuals to act in a way that will not bring shame on the family. Therefore, the Korean woman may not express pain outwardly for fear of shaming herself or her family. Silence is valued in Chinese society, so a woman of that heritage is usually quiet and stoic to avoid dishonoring herself or her family. Mexican women often chant the phrase "Aye yie yie" while in labor, which is actually a form of "folk lamaze." Repeating the phrase in succession several times necessitates taking long, slow, deep breaths. Thus, it is a cultural method for alleviating pain (Fontaine, 2014). European Americans demonstrate a wide variety of behaviors in response to pain, from silence to shouting. It is important to support a woman's individual expression, whatever it may be (as long as harm is not done to another), in order to enhance the birthing experience for mother, baby, and family.

Cultural Beliefs: Some Examples

It is essential to avoid stereotyping in providing care. The four examples that follow give insight into the variety of responses nurses may encounter.

Squatting during labor is common for Hmong women from Laos. They may also prefer to be active and move about. The husband is frequently present and involved in providing comfort. The woman may ask that the amniotic membranes not be ruptured until just before birth. It is thought that the escape of fluid at this time makes the birth easier. During labor the woman usually prefers only "hot" foods and warm water to drink As soon as the baby is born, the family may request that a soft-boiled egg be given to the mother to restore her energy (Spector, 2012).

Vietnamese women usually maintain self-control and may even smile throughout labor. They may prefer to walk about and to give birth in a squatting position. In labor, the woman may prefer cold beverages because pregnancy is viewed as a "hot" condition. However, during the postpartum, which is viewed as a "cold" condition, she may prefer warm liquids. The newborn is protected from praise to prevent jealousy (Fontaine, 2014).

Latina women have identified expectations of their partners during labor and birth such as wanting their partners to stay with them and to reassure them that everything will be all right. As they labor, the women want their partners to show their love and to speak using affectionate words.

Muslim women may have their husband, a female friend or relative, or a male relative with them during childbirth. If a specialist such as an anesthesiologist or neonatologist is needed, it is best to speak to the husband first and obtain his permission. Family support is important but does not preclude the importance of the nurse's presence. The woman may want to retain her head covering (*khimar*) and may prefer to wear two long-sleeved gowns to enhance modesty. It is important for a female nurse or physician/CNM to perform examinations whenever possible. After the birth Muslim fathers may call praise to Allah (*adhan*) in the newborn's right ear and clean the newborn.

Developing Cultural Competence Native American Women and Labor

Native American women typically view labor pain as natural and may use meditation, self-control, or indigenous plants or herbs, such as black cohosh, throughout their labor as well as to aid them during birth (Fontaine, 2014).

Maternity nurses can provide culturally sensitive care by first becoming acquainted with the beliefs and practices of the various cultures in their communities. In the birthing situation, the truly effective nurse supports the family's cultural practices as long as it is safe to do so.

Nursing Management

For the Woman in the First Stage of Labor

Latent Phase

As discussed in Chapter 17, it is important to assess the physical well-being of the woman and her fetus. Monitor maternal temperature every 4 hours unless the temperature is over 37.5°C (99.6°F); in such cases, take it every hour. Monitor blood pressure, pulse, and respirations every hour. If the woman's blood pressure is over 120/80 mmHg or her pulse is more than 100, notify the physician/CNM and reevaluate the blood pressure and pulse more frequently.

Palpate uterine contractions for frequency, intensity, and duration every 30 minutes. Auscultate the fetal heart rate (FHR) every 30 minutes for low-risk women and every 15 minutes for high-risk women as long as it remains between 110 and 160 beats/min and is reassuring (Miller, Miller, & Tucker, 2012). Auscultate the FHR throughout one contraction and for about 15 seconds after the contraction to ensure that there are no decelerations. If the FHR baseline is not in the 110 to 160 range or if decelerations are heard, continuous electronic monitoring is recommended. See Table 18–1 for nursing assessments during the four stages of labor.

Offer the woman fluids in the form of clear liquids or ice chips frequently, unless complications exist that may result in a cesarean birth. Some certified childbirth educators advise the woman to bring lollipops to help combat the dryness that occurs with some of the labor breathing patterns. Avoiding both liquids and solids during labor, which was once a standard of practice, is no longer deemed necessary. Evidence-based practice research and new guidelines indicate that clear fluids can be consumed throughout labor and up to 2 hours before an elective cesarean birth. Current guidelines suggest avoiding solids for 6 to 8 hours before an elective cesarean birth (American College of Obstetricians and Gynecologists [ACOG], 2009b). Eating during labor has not been associated with an increase in aspiration but some institutions continue to limit oral intake during labor (Anderson & Stone, 2013). Previously, it was believed that drinking fluids should be avoided because it can lead to vomiting caused by the decreased gastric emptying time. Foods high in fat have been associated with decreasing gastric emptying time, so they are generally avoided in labor. Although vomiting is common during the first stage of labor, many women have more energy and tolerate labor better with oral intake and have higher satisfaction with their labor and birth experience (Anderson & Stone, 2013).

TABLE 18–1 Nursing Assessments During the Stages of Labor

STAGE	MATERNAL ASSESSMENTS	FETAL ASSESSMENTS
FIRST STAGE	Blood pressure (BP), respirations each hour if in normal range.	Fetal heart rate (FHR) every 30 min for low-risk women and every 15 min for high-risk women if normal characteristics present (average variability, baseline in the 110–160 beats/min range, without late or variable decelerations).
Latent phase	Temperature every 4 hr unless over 37.5°C (99.6°F) or membranes ruptured, then every hr.	
	Uterine contractions every 30 min.	
		Note fetal activity. If electronic fetal monitor is in place, assess for reactive non-stress test (NST).
Active phase	BP, pulse, respirations every hour if in normal range.	FHR every 30 min for low-risk women and every 15 min for high-risk women if normal characteristics are present.
	Uterine contractions palpated every 15–30 min.	
Transition phase	BP, pulse, respirations every 30 min.	FHR every 30 min for low-risk women and every 15 min for high-risk women if normal characteristics are present.
	Contractions palpated at least every 15 min.	
SECOND STAGE	BP, pulse, and respirations every 5–15 min.	FHR every 15 min for low-risk women and every 5 min for high-risk women.
	Temperature every 2 hr.	
	Uterine contractions palpated continuously.	
THIRD STAGE	BP, pulse, and respirations every 5 min.	Newborn assessment at time of birth, gestational age assessment, and neurologic assessment within first hour of birth.
	Palpate uterine contractions intermittently to assess for signs of placenta separation.	
		Apgars at 1 and 5 min.
		Assess initial BP, apical pulse, respirations, and temperature.
		Assess umbilical cord for the presence of three vessels.
FOURTH STAGE	Assess maternal vital signs including temperature, BP, pulse, and respirations every 5–15 min for first hour.	Perform complete exam to include vital signs, gestational age assessment, physical examination, and neurologic reflexes once between 1 and 4 hr postbirth. After initial 8 hr, assess vitals and perform assessment every 8 hr. Skin color should be assessed every 4 hr.
	Assess fundus, lochia, perineum, laceration/episiotomy site, bladder distention, and rectum every 15 min.	

Active Phase

During the active phase, contractions have a frequency of 2 to 3 minutes, a duration of 50 to 60 seconds, and a moderate to strong intensity. Palpate contractions every 15 to 30 minutes. As the contractions become more frequent and intense, vaginal examinations assess cervical dilatation and effacement and fetal station and position. During the active phase, the cervix dilates from 4 to 7 cm, and vaginal discharge and bloody show increase. Monitor maternal blood pressure, pulse, and respirations every hour for low-risk women (unless elevated, as previously noted) and every 30 minutes for high-risk women. Auscultate the FHR every 30 minutes for low-risk women and every 15 minutes for high-risk women (Narendra, Shah, Pratap, et al., 2014).

A woman who has been ambulatory up to this point may wish to sit in a chair or on a bed. If the woman wants to lie on the bed, encourage her to assume a side-lying position, help her into a comfortable position, and place pillows to support her body. To increase comfort, offer a back rub or effleurage or place a cool cloth on the woman's forehead or across her neck. Because vaginal discharge increases, change the chux pad frequently. Washing the perineum with warm soapy water removes secretions and increases comfort. During such procedures it is essential to wear disposable gloves to avoid exposure to vaginal discharge.

If the amniotic membranes have not ruptured previously, they may do so during this phase. When the membranes rupture, immediately note the FHR on the monitor if one is being used (if the woman is not on a monitor, auscultate FHR) and then note the color, odor, and consistency of the amniotic fluid and the time of rupture. The fluid should be clear, with no odor. The presence of any frank bright red vaginal bleeding should be noted because it is not considered a normal finding. Fetal stress leads to intestinal and anal sphincter relaxation, and meconium may be released into the amniotic fluid, which turns the fluid greenish brown. Whenever meconium-stained fluid is present, apply an electronic monitor to assess the FHR continuously. Note the time of rupture because infection increases as the duration of ruptured membranes is prolonged.

Prolapse of the umbilical cord is a possible risk when membranes rupture and the fetus is not engaged, because the amniotic fluid coming through the cervix might wash the umbilical cord out through the cervix. With each contraction the cord would then become trapped between the presenting part and the maternal pelvis. The FHR is auscultated because a drop in the rate might indicate an undetected prolapsed cord. Immediate intervention is necessary to remove pressure on a prolapsed umbilical cord (see Chapter 20). (See Table 18–2 for additional deviations from the normal labor process.)

Transition

During transition the contraction frequency is every 1.5 to 2.0 minutes, duration is 60 to 90 seconds, and intensity is strong. Cervical dilatation increases from 8 to 10 cm, effacement is complete (100%), and there is usually a heavy amount of bloody show. Palpate contractions at least every 15 minutes. Sterile vaginal examinations may be done more frequently because this stage of labor usually is accompanied by rapid

TABLE 18–2 Deviations From Normal Labor Process Requiring Immediate Intervention

PROBLEM	IMMEDIATE ACTION
Woman admitted with vaginal bleeding or history of painless vaginal bleeding	Do not perform vaginal examination. Assess fetal heart rate (FHR). Evaluate amount of blood loss and initiate a pad count. Evaluate labor pattern. Notify physician/CNM immediately.
Presence of greenish or brownish amniotic fluid	Continuously monitor FHR. Evaluate dilatation of cervix and determine if umbilical cord is prolapsed. Evaluate presentation (vertex or breech). Maintain woman on complete bed rest on left side. Notify physician/CNM immediately.
Absence of FHR and fetal movement	Notify physician/CNM. Provide truthful information and emotional support to laboring couple. Remain with the couple.
Prolapse of umbilical cord	Relieve pressure on cord manually. Continuously monitor FHR; watch for changes in FHR pattern. Notify physician/CNM. Assist woman into knee-chest position or place in Trendelenburg position. Administer oxygen. Prepare for possible emergency cesarean birth.

(continued)

TABLE 18–2 Deviations From Normal Labor Process Requiring Immediate Intervention (*continued*)

PROBLEM	IMMEDIATE ACTION
Woman admitted in advanced labor; birth imminent	Prepare for immediate birth.
	Obtain critical information:
	Estimated date of birth (EDB)
	History of bleeding problems
	History of medical or obstetric problems
	Past or present use or abuse of prescription, over-the-counter (OTC), or illicit drugs
	Problems with this pregnancy
	FHR and maternal vital signs
	Whether membranes are ruptured and how long since rupture
	Blood type and Rh.
	Direct another person to contact physician/CNM.
	Do not leave woman alone.
	Provide support to couple.
	Put on gloves.

change. Take the maternal blood pressure, pulse, and respirations at least every 30 minutes, and auscultate FHR every 15 to 30 minutes.

Comfort measures are important in this phase of labor, but continual assessment is required to intervene appropriately. The woman may rapidly change from wanting a back rub and other hands-on care to wanting to be left completely alone. The support person and the nurse need to follow her cues and change interventions as needed. Because the woman is breathing more rapidly, increase her comfort by offering small spoonfuls of ice chips to moisten her mouth or offer an emollient for her dry lips. Encourage the woman to rest between contractions. If analgesics have been administered, a quiet environment enhances the quality of rest between contractions. Awaken the woman just before a contraction begins so that she can begin patterned breathing.

Some women have difficulty coping during this time and need help with their breathing. Either the support person or the nurse can breathe along with the woman during each contraction to help her maintain her pattern. It is helpful to encourage the woman and to assure her that she is doing a good job. The woman will begin to feel increased rectal pressure as the fetal presenting part moves down the birth canal. To help prevent cervical edema, encourage the woman to refrain from pushing until the cervix is completely dilated.

The end of transition and the beginning of the second stage may be indicated by a change in the woman's voice or the sounds she is making. As the fetus moves down and she feels increased pressure and a bearing-down sensation, her voice tends to deepen. A moan during a contraction takes on a more guttural quality.

Promotion of Comfort in the First Stage

The nurse's first step in planning care is to talk with the woman and her partner or support person to identify their goals. Usually, the woman or couple is concerned with discomfort, so it is helpful to identify factors that may contribute to it. These factors include uncomfortable positions, diaphoresis, continual leaking of amniotic fluid, a full bladder, a dry mouth, anxiety, and fear. Nursing interventions can minimize the effects of these factors. These interventions are described later in this section.

As the intensity of contractions increases with the progress of labor, the woman becomes less aware of the environment and may have difficulty hearing and understanding verbal instructions. The pattern of coping with labor contractions ranges from the use of highly structured breathing techniques to turning inward. Low moaning that begins deep in the throat, rocking or swaying, facial grimacing, and using loud vocalizations are all effective means of dealing with the power of labor and birth. Some women feel that making sounds helps them cope and do the work of labor, whereas others make loud sounds only as they lose their perception of control.

The most frequent physiologic manifestations of pain are increased pulse and respiratory rates, dilated pupils, increased blood pressure, and muscle tension. In labor, these reactions are transitory because the pain is intermittent. Increased muscle tension is most significant because it may impede the progress of labor. Women in labor often tighten skeletal muscles voluntarily during a contraction and remain motionless. This method of dealing with the contractions may actually increase the level of discomfort because of muscular tension, but the women may believe it is the only acceptable way to cope with the pain.

A woman generally wants touching, massage, effleurage, and other forms of physical contact during the first part of labor, but when she moves into the transition phase, she may pull away. Women may provide verbal and nonverbal signs such as crying, moaning, and beseeching the coach or nurse to hold their hand or rub their back. Some women are uncomfortable with being touched at all, regardless of the phase of labor. It is important for the nurse to confirm the woman's preferences and to meet each family on its own terms, always keeping in mind that this is their experience.

NONPHARMACOLOGIC PAIN RELIEF

The nurse can introduce the following nonpharmacologic pain relief techniques in labor to encourage maternal comfort and facilitate coping: massage, hydrotherapy, position changes, hypnosis, aromatherapy, sitting in a rocking chair/glider/birthing ball, walking, leaning against the bed or her partner, use of a transcutaneous electrical nerve stimulation (TENS) unit, visualization, relaxation techniques, the use of prayer or meditation, breathing techniques, and acupressure.

Box 18–1 Acupressure for the Laboring Woman

Acupressure is an ancient Chinese medical treatment that involves using the fingers to press key pressure points on the surface of the skin. This pressure ultimately stimulates the immune system to promote healing by triggering the release of endorphins, reducing stress through muscle relaxation, and promoting circulation. The specific acupressure point used in laboring women is the San Yin-Jiao (SP-6) acupressure point. The SP-6 acupressure point is located on the medial side of the leg, in the calf region, approximately 3 cm (1.2 in.) superior to the prominence of the inner malleus. The use of acupressure in labor has been associated with shorter labors and lower subjective and objective pain scores. Women who receive acupressure typically use less pain medication than those who do not receive acupressure (Simpkin, Bolding, Keppler, et al., 2010).

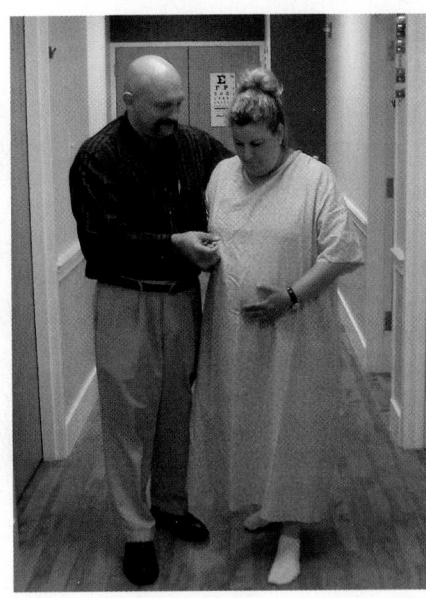

Figure 18–1 Increasing comfort and aiding in fetal descent. This woman and her partner are walking in the hospital during labor.

Many nurses readily respond to the woman's needs. As the nurse and woman or couple work together to increase comfort during contractions, a ritual of supportive measures begins to develop. The nurse watches for cues and nonverbal behaviors and asks for feedback from the woman. As labor progresses, the nurse and couple use their experience and growing rapport to change comfort measures as needed. Nursing measures used to decrease pain are discussed next.

GENERAL COMFORT

General comfort measures are of great importance during labor. By relieving minor discomforts, the nurse helps the woman optimize her ability to cope with pain. The woman can be encouraged to ambulate as long as there are no contraindications, such as vaginal bleeding or rupture of membranes before the fetus is engaged in the pelvis. Ambulation can increase comfort and aid in fetal descent (Figure 18–1).

Even if the woman prefers not to walk around, upright positions such as sitting in a rocker or leaning against a wall or bed can enhance comfort. If she stays in bed, the woman can be encouraged to assume positions that she finds comfortable (Figure 18–2). A side-lying position is generally the most advantageous for the laboring woman, although frequent position changes seem to achieve more efficient contractions. It is important to support all body parts, with the joints kept slightly flexed. For instance, when the woman is in a side-lying position, pillows may be placed against her chest and under the uppermost arm. A pillow or folded towel

---

EVIDENCE-BASED PRACTICE | Movement During Labor

Clinical Question

How does walking, moving around, and changing positions during labor affect the birth process?

The Evidence

Birth in the United States has become a high-technology venture and one of the consequences is limitation on the mother's mobility and positions. Many women remain recumbent after fetal monitoring has been initiated, if an intravenous line is inserted, or, subsequently, after administration of an epidural anesthetic. *The Journal of Perinatal Education* published a review of consensus statements of the American College of Nurse-Midwives, the Midwife Alliance of North America, and the National Association of Certified Professional Midwives regarding maternal position and movement during labor. This type of aggregation of practice guidelines forms the strongest evidence for practice.

The guidelines recommend supportive care practices that use relatively little technology and that support the normal physiologic processes of labor. Women who moved, walked, and changed position during labor reported less pain and more satisfaction with the childbirth process than women who remained

in the recumbent position in bed (Ondeck, 2014). Movement during labor actually resulted in a shorter labor, by more than an hour on average. These women also have fewer interventions during labor. Best practice means supporting the woman's natural physiologic processes without restricting movement through initiation of unnecessary intravenous lines and the use of intermittent versus continuous fetal monitoring for low-risk mothers. Despite these widely replicated findings, more than half of all laboring women remain in bed or in a recumbent position.

Best Practice

Supportive practices during labor include minimizing the use of technology so that mothers can move around, walk, and change position during labor. These women will have shorter, less painful labor and will be more satisfied with the process.

Clinical Reasoning

How can the nurse help implement this important change in practice when current practices are ingrained? What is appropriate childbirth education to empower parents to choose a low-technology option?

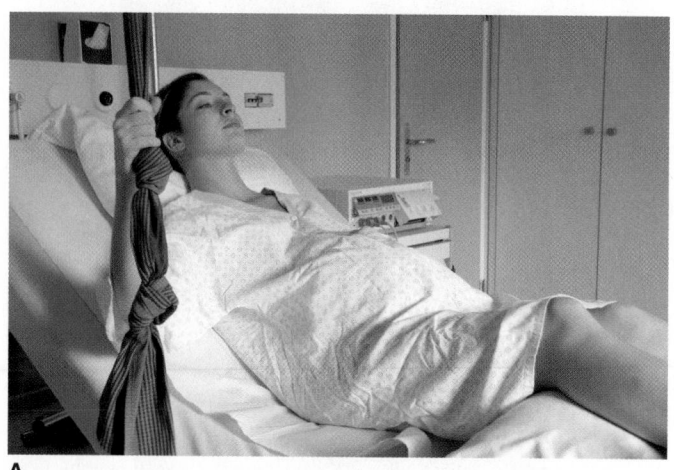
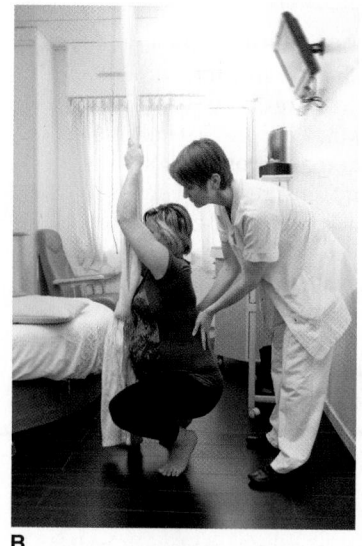
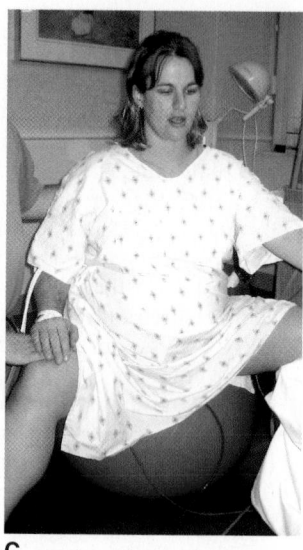

A
B
C

Figure 18–2 The laboring woman is encouraged to choose a comfortable position. *A, B*, The nurse modifies assessments and interventions as necessary. *C*, While often promoting maternal comfort during labor, the birthing ball also facilitates fetal descent and rotation and helps increase the diameter of the pelvis.

SOURCE: *A*, © olly/Fotolia. *B*, © BSIP SA/Alamy.

or blanket may be placed between her knees to support the uppermost leg and relieve tension or muscle strain. A pillow placed at the woman's midback also helps provide support. If the woman is more comfortable on her back, the head of the bed can be elevated to relieve the pressure of the uterus on the vena cava.

Pillows may be placed under each arm and under the knees to provide further support. Because a pregnant woman is at increased risk for thrombophlebitis, excessive pressure behind the knee and calf should be avoided. Pressure points should be assessed frequently.

Back rubs and frequent changes of position contribute to comfort and relaxation. Wearing socks or slippers may alleviate cold feet, just as adjusting the room's thermostat can offset excessive warmth. Attention to such details allows the woman to focus on the more important issues of giving birth.

Diaphoresis and the constant leaking of amniotic fluid can dampen the woman's gown and bed linen. Fresh, smooth, dry bed linen promotes comfort. To avoid having to change the bottom sheet following rupture of the membranes, the nurse should replace chux pads at frequent intervals (following body substance isolation precautions). Keeping the woman's perineal area as clean and dry as possible to promote comfort and to prevent infection is important.

A full bladder adds to the discomfort during a contraction and may prolong labor by interfering with the descent of the fetus. The bladder should be kept as empty as possible. Even if the woman is voiding, urine may be retained because of the pressure of the fetal presenting part. To detect a full bladder, palpate directly over the symphysis pubis. Some regional analgesia procedures contribute to the inability to void, and catheterization may be necessary. The nurse should encourage the woman to empty her bladder every 1 to 2 hours.

Clinical Tip

Support persons and family members need to be encouraged to maintain their own comfort. Because they are paying attention to the laboring woman, they may forget their own needs. It may be necessary to encourage them to take breaks, to eat and drink, and to rest. However, they may be reluctant to leave the woman unattended while they meet their own personal needs. Offer to stay with the woman during their absence. This provides reassurance that the woman will be well cared for in their absence.

HANDLING ANXIETY

A woman's anxiety as she begins labor is related to a combination of factors inherent to the process. A moderate amount of anxiety about the pain enhances the woman's ability to deal with it. In contrast, an excessive degree of anxiety decreases her ability to cope. Women who have increased anxiety about safety and their ability to cope are much more likely to describe their pain as unbearable.

To decrease anxiety not related to pain, the nurse should give information (which eases fear of the unknown), establish rapport with the couple (which helps them preserve their

Women With Special Needs Mental Health Disabilities

Women with mental health disabilities, such as posttraumatic stress disorder (PTSD), may experience flashbacks and excessive fear during labor. Supportive care with one nurse is preferred so a personal relationship and trust can be established. Labor often triggers painful flashbacks in women who have been sexually abused or sexually assaulted.

personal integrity), and express confidence in the couple's ability to work with the labor process. Remaining with the woman as much as possible conveys a caring attitude and dispels fears of abandonment. Praise for breathing, relaxation, and pushing efforts not only encourages repetition of the behavior but also decreases anxiety about the ability to cope with labor.

CLIENT TEACHING

Providing truthful information about the nature of the discomfort that will occur during labor is important. Stressing the intermittent nature and maximum duration of the contractions can be most helpful. The woman can cope with pain better when she knows that a period of relief will follow.

Clinical Tip

If a woman is experiencing severe fear or anxiety about a vaginal examination, advise her to slowly count to 10 during the examination while continually wiggling her toes. This source of distraction may lessen her fear and anxiety. It also enables the woman to have a sense of control.

Descriptions of sensations are best accompanied by information on specific comfort measures. Some women experience the urge to push during transition, when the cervix is not fully dilated and effaced. Pushing prior to complete dilatation and effacement can result in cervical edema, which in turn slows down the effacement/dilatation process, or in cervical lacerations. Panting can control this sensation (it is difficult to pant and bear down at the same time). If time permits, the nurse should explain the purpose of panting and have the woman practice before the technique is needed.

Thorough orientation and explanation of surroundings, procedures, and equipment being used also decrease anxiety, thereby reducing pain. The nurse should explain the beeps, clicks, and other strange noises and give a simplified explanation of the monitor strip, emphasizing that the use of the fetal monitor provides a way to assess the well-being of the fetus during labor. It helps to show the woman and her partner or support person how the monitor can identify the beginnings of contractions. At the onset of each contraction, the woman can be encouraged to begin her breathing technique to lessen her perception of pain.

Labor and childbirth may be a critical time for the woman with a history of childhood sexual abuse or rape. All women entering the healthcare arena need to be evaluated for a history of sexual abuse or rape. However, a woman may or may not be able to address this issue with the nurse because sharing such personal information with a stranger is difficult. It is especially important for the nurse to be alert for nonverbal cues, such as unexplained anxiety, unrelenting pain, or fear during vaginal examinations, and to be prepared to offer additional teaching and relaxation support to help offset the woman's anxiety.

SUPPORTIVE RELAXATION TECHNIQUES

Tense muscles increase resistance to the descent of the fetus and contribute to maternal fatigue. This fatigue increases pain perception and decreases the woman's ability to cope with the pain. Comfort measures, massage, water therapy using immersion in a whirlpool tub, techniques for decreasing anxiety, and client teaching can contribute to relaxation. Adequate sleep and rest are also important. The laboring woman should be encouraged to use the periods between contractions for rest and relaxation. A prolonged prodromal phase of labor may have kept her awake. Moreover, a woman beginning labor is naturally excited, making it difficult for her to sleep even if her contractions are mild and infrequent.

Distraction helps increase relaxation and ability to cope with discomfort. During early labor, conversation or activities such as light reading or playing cards or other games serve as distractions. It may be helpful to have the woman concentrate on a pleasant experience she has had in the past. Other techniques include the use of a specific visual or mental focal point, breathing techniques, counting or humming, or visualization.

Touch is another type of distraction (Figure 18–3). Although some women regard touching as an invasion of privacy or threat to their independence, many want to touch and be touched during a painful experience. Nurses can make themselves available to the woman who desires touch by placing a hand on the side of the bed within the woman's reach. The person who needs touch will reach out for contact.

Some nurses utilize **intuitive touch**, the use of physical contact with the laboring woman with the intent of helping her to slow down and regulate her breathing pattern and encouraging a reduction of anxiety and decrease of stress levels. Evidence suggests that touch induces the relaxation response, which is mediated through the neuroendocrine and sympathetic nervous systems (Konda, Vikas, Yarlagadda, 2014).

A variety of techniques can be used. These include hand-holding; stroking or patting of a woman's arm, face, or legs; placing one hand on her shoulder; putting an arm around her shoulders; and hugging. To implement intuitive touch, the nurse uses long, slow, up-and-down strokes on the woman's limbs. Special training is not needed to use this intervention; all that is needed is the intention to help regulate the breathing pattern and the willingness to use a little time to achieve this goal (Konda et al., 2014)

Mild to moderate abdominal discomfort during contractions may be relieved or lessened by effleurage. Firm pressure on the lower back or sacral area may relieve back pain associated with labor. To apply firm pressure, the nurse can place a hand or a rolled, warmed towel or blanket in the small of the woman's back. In addition to the measures just described, the

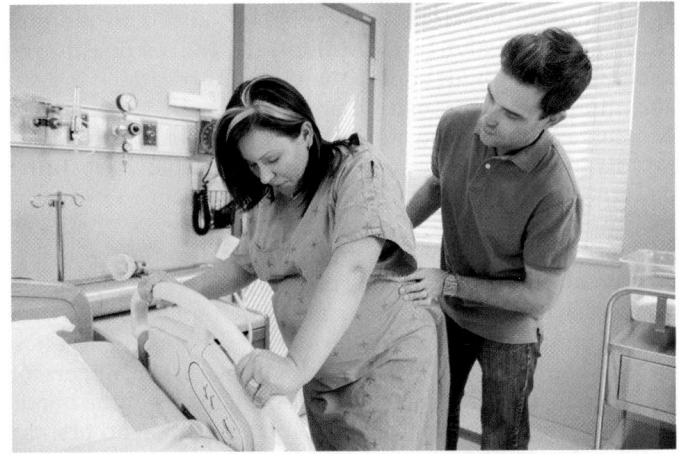

Figure 18–3 The woman's partner provides support and encouragement during labor.

SOURCE: Tyler Olson/Shutterstock.

woman's relaxation can be enhanced by providing encouragement and support for her controlled breathing techniques.

BREATHING TECHNIQUES

Breathing techniques may help the laboring woman. Used correctly they increase the woman's pain threshold, permit relaxation, enhance the woman's ability to cope with the uterine contractions, and allow the uterus to function more efficiently.

Many women learn patterned-paced breathing during childbirth preparation classes. This type of controlled breathing often has three levels. The woman tends to begin with the first level and then proceed to the next when she feels the need. Regardless of the level of breathing used, a cleansing breath begins and ends each pattern. A cleansing breath involves only the chest. It consists of inhaling through the nose and exhaling through pursed lips.

1. The first pattern may also be called slow, deep breathing or slow-paced breathing. During the breathing movements, only the chest moves. The woman inhales slowly through her nose. She moves her chest up and out during the inhalation. She exhales through pursed lips. The breathing rate is 6 to 9 breaths a minute.

2. The second pattern is called shallow or modified-paced breathing. The woman begins with a cleansing breath and at the end of the cleansing breath pushes out a short breath. She then inhales and exhales through the mouth at a rate of about 4 breaths every 5 seconds. This pattern can be altered into a more rapid rate that does not exceed 2 to 2½ breaths every second.

3. The third pattern is called pant–blow or patterned-paced breathing. It is similar to modified-paced breathing except the breathing is punctuated every few breaths by a forceful exhalation through pursed lips. A pattern of 4 breaths may be used to begin. All breaths are kept equal and rhythmic. As the contraction becomes more intense, the woman may adjust the pattern as needed to 3:1, 2:1, and finally 1:1.

If the woman has not learned a controlled breathing technique, teaching her may be difficult when she is admitted in active labor. In this instance, the nurse can teach abdominal and pant–pant–blow breathing. In abdominal breathing, the woman moves the abdominal wall upward as she inhales and downward as she exhales. This method tends to lift the abdominal wall off the contracting uterus and thus may provide some pain relief. The breathing is deep and rhythmic. As transition approaches, the woman may feel the need to breathe more rapidly. To avoid breathing too rapidly, the woman can use the pant–pant–blow breathing pattern.

Hyperventilation is the result of an imbalance of oxygen and carbon dioxide (i.e., too much carbon dioxide is exhaled, and too much oxygen remains in the body). Hyperventilation may occur when a woman breathes very rapidly over a prolonged period. The signs and symptoms of hyperventilation are tingling or numbness in the tip of the nose, lips, fingers, or toes; dizziness; spots before the eyes; or spasms of the hands or feet (carpal-pedal spasms). If hyperventilation occurs, the woman should be encouraged to slow her breathing rate and take shallow breaths. With instruction and encouragement, many women are able to change their breathing to correct the problem. It may also help to count out loud for the woman so she can pace her breathing during contractions. If the signs and symptoms continue or become more severe (i.e., they progress from numbness to spasms), the woman can breathe into a paper surgical mask or a paper bag until symptoms go away. Breathing into a mask or bag causes rebreathing of carbon dioxide. During this time, the nurse should remain with the woman to reassure her.

In some instances, analgesics or regional anesthetic blocks may be used to increase comfort and relaxation during labor. (See Chapter 19 for a discussion of pharmacologic pain management.) Table 18–3 summarizes labor progress, possible responses of the laboring woman, and support measures.

ROLE OF THE DOULA

Throughout the first stage of labor, assess and support the interactions between the woman and her support person or partner. In the absence of a partner, or when the partner wants a less active role in the support of the laboring woman, it is becoming more common for women to employ a paid care provider, often called a **doula**, who has experience in caring for laboring women. The doula typically has received special training and may even be certified. The role of the doula is to enhance the comfort and decrease the anxiety of the laboring woman. A doula can be a valuable advocate to the laboring woman and her family, as well as an asset to the labor nurse. For example, the doula might support the woman by helping identify the beginning of each contraction and encouraging her as she breathes through it.

Nursing Care During the Second Stage of Labor

The second stage is reached when the cervix is fully dilated (10 cm). The contractions continue as in the transition phase. Maternal pulse is assessed at the onset of the second stage. Blood pressure is assessed every 5 to 15 minutes, but may be done more frequently if fetal decelerations or bradycardia occur. The fetal heart rate (FHR) is assessed every 15 minutes in low-risk women and every 5 minutes in women with high-risk complications (ACOG, 2009a). Once the second stage is reached, the nurse remains with the woman continually and does not generally leave the room.

As the woman pushes during the second stage, she may make a variety of sounds. A low-pitched, grunting sound ("uhhh") usually indicates that the woman is working with the pushing. The nurse who feels comfortable with maternal sounds and stays sensitive to changes in the sounds may be able to detect if the woman is losing her ability to cope. For instance, if the woman feels afraid of the sensations produced by her pushing effort, her sound may change to a high-pitched cry or whimper. During the second stage, the woman may interpret rectal pressure as a need to move her bowels. The instinctive response is to resist and to tighten muscles rather than bear down (push). A sensation of splitting apart also occurs in the latter part of the second stage, and the woman may fear the urge to push. The woman who expects these sensations and understands that bearing down contributes to progress at this stage is more likely to do so effectively.

When the urge to bear down becomes uncontrollable and pushing begins, the nurse can help by encouraging the woman

TABLE 18–3 Normal Progress, Psychologic Characteristics, and Nursing Support During the First and Second Stages of Labor

PHASE	CERVICAL DILATATION	UTERINE CONTRACTIONS	WOMAN'S RESPONSE	SUPPORT MEASURES
Stage 1 *Latent phase*	1–3 cm	Every 10–20 min, 15–20 sec duration Mild intensity progressing to every 5–7 min, 30–40 sec duration Moderate intensity	Usually happy, talkative, and eager to be in labor. Exhibits need for independence by taking care of own bodily needs and seeking information.	Establish rapport on admission and continue to build during care. Assess information base and learning needs. Be available to consult regarding breathing technique if needed; teach breathing technique if needed and in early labor. Orient family to room, equipment, monitors, and procedures. Encourage woman and partner to participate in care as desired. Provide needed information. Assist woman into position of comfort; encourage frequent change of position; encourage ambulation during early labor. Offer fluids or ice chips. Keep couple informed of progress. Encourage woman to void every 1–2 hr. Assess need for an interest in using visualization to enhance relaxation, and teach if appropriate.
Active phase	4–7 cm	Every 2–3 min, 50–60 sec duration Moderate to strong intensity	May experience feelings of helplessness. Exhibits increased fatigue and may begin to feel restless and anxious as contractions become stronger. Expresses fear of abandonment. Becomes more dependent because she is less able to meet her needs.	Encourage woman to maintain breathing patterns. Provide quiet environment to reduce external stimuli. Provide reassurance, encouragement, support; keep couple informed of progress. Promote comfort by giving back rubs, sacral pressure, cool cloth on forehead, assistance with position changes, support with pillows, effleurage. Provide ice chips, ointment for dry mouth and lips. Encourage to void every 1–2 hr. Offer shower, whirlpool, or warm bath if available.
Transition phase	8–10 cm	Every 1.5–2 min, 60–90 sec duration Strong intensity	Tires and may exhibit increased restlessness and irritability. May feel she cannot keep up with labor process and is out of control. Exhibits physical discomforts. Fears being left alone. May fear tearing open or splitting apart with contractions.	Encourage woman to rest between contractions. If she sleeps between contractions, wake her at beginning of contraction so she can begin breathing pattern (increases feeling of control). Provide support, encouragement, and praise for efforts. Keep couple informed of progress; encourage continued participation of support persons. Promote comfort as listed earlier but recognize that many women do not want to be touched when in transition. Provide privacy. Provide ice chips, ointment for lips. Encourage to void every 1–2 hr.
Stage 2	Complete	Every 1.5–2 min	May feel out of control, helpless, panicky.	Assist woman in pushing efforts. Encourage woman to assume position of comfort. Provide encouragement and praise her efforts. Keep couple informed of progress. Provide ice chips. Maintain privacy as woman desires.

and by assisting with positioning (Figure 18–4). Most women spontaneously push very effectively in response to messages from their body. However, in some settings, sustained, forceful pushing is still advocated. In that case, when the contraction begins, the woman is told to take a cleansing breath or two, then to take a third large breath and hold it while pushing down with her abdominal muscles (called the Valsalva maneuver). A more natural approach that lets the mother wait to bear down until she feels an urge to push may shorten the pushing phase, reducing the incidence of physiologic stress in the mother and acidosis in the newborn.

A nullipara is usually prepared for birth when perineal bulging is noted. A multipara usually progresses far more quickly, so she may be prepared for the birth when the cervix is dilated 7 to 8 cm. As the birth approaches, the woman's partner or support person also prepares for the birth.

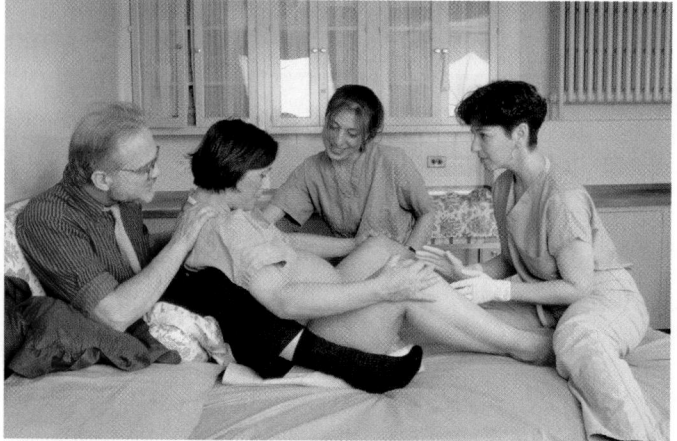

Figure 18–4 The nurse provides encouragement and support during pushing efforts.

SOURCE: Margaret Miller/Science Source.

The nurse should monitor the woman's blood pressure and the FHR between contractions, and palpate the contractions at least every 5 minutes until the birth. The nurse continues to assist the woman in her pushing efforts, keep both the woman and the coach informed of procedures and progress, and support them both throughout the birth.

Promotion of Comfort in the Second Stage

Most of the comfort measures used during the first stage remain appropriate at this time. Applying cool cloths to the face and forehead may help cool the woman involved in the intense physical exertion of pushing. The woman may feel hot and want to remove some covers. Care still needs to be taken to provide privacy even though covers are removed. The nurse should encourage the woman to rest and relax all muscles during the periods between contractions. With the support person(s), the nurse can help the woman into a pushing position with each contraction. Sips of fluids or ice chips may relieve dry mouth. Encouragement and positive reinforcement should be continually offered.

Assisting During Birth

In addition to assisting the woman and her partner, the nurse also assists the physician/CNM in preparing for the birth. The physician/CNM dons a sterile gown and gloves and may place sterile drapes over the woman's abdomen and legs. An episiotomy may be done just before the actual birth if needed. (See the discussion of episiotomy in Chapter 22.)

Shortly before the birth, the birthing room or delivery room is prepared with the equipment and materials that may be needed. Family members do not need to change into other clothing if the birth occurs in a birthing room; they don a disposable scrub suit or scrubs provided by the facility if the birth is to occur in a delivery room or surgery suite. Thorough hand washing is required of the nurses and physician/CNM. Nurses who will be in direct contact with the mother at the time of birth need to wear protective clothing such as an apron or gown with a splash apron, disposable gloves, and

eye covering. The physician/CNM also needs to wear a plastic apron or a gown with a splash apron, eye covering, and sterile gloves.

If the laboring woman is to give birth in a location other than the birthing room (such as in the case of a cesarean birth), she is moved onto her bed or a stretcher shortly before birth. To ensure the woman's safety, the side rails should be raised into a locked position. It is important that the woman not be moved from one bed to another during a contraction. During a contraction the woman feels increased discomfort and may be involved in pushing efforts. Care should be taken to preserve her privacy during the transfer. The labor bed or transfer cart must be carefully braced against the delivery table to ensure the woman's safety during the transfer.

Clinical Tip

Birth is imminent if the woman shows the following changes:

- Bulging of the perineum
- Uncontrollable urge to bear down
- Increased bloody show

Even though there are differences in the delivery room setting, the family can still be together during the birth. Family members should be encouraged to participate because the delivery room environment may seem intimidating. The family member may hesitate to continue providing support because of fear of interfering or being in the way.

MATERNAL BIRTHING POSITIONS

Until modern times, the upright posture for birth was considered normal in most societies. Women chose to squat, kneel, stand, or sit for birth. The recumbent position (lithotomy) became more usual in the Western world because of the convenience it offers in applying technology. The lithotomy position has thus become the conventional manner in which North American women give birth in hospitals. In seeking alternative positions, consumers and professionals alike are refocusing on the comfort of the laboring woman rather than on the convenience of the physician/CNM (Figure 18–5 and Table 18–4).

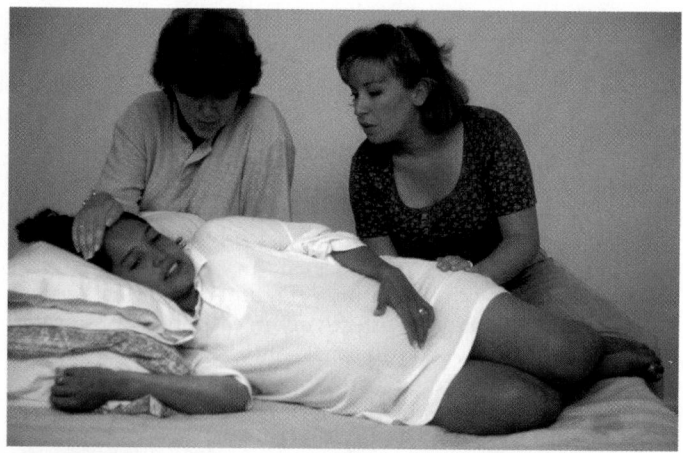

Figure 18–5 Side-lying laboring or birthing position.

SOURCE: © Angela Hampton Picture Library/Alamy.

TABLE 18–4 Comparison of Birthing Positions

POSITION	ADVANTAGES	DISADVANTAGES	NURSING ACTIONS
Sitting on birthing stool	Gravity aids descent and expulsion of baby. Does not compromise venous return from lower extremities. Woman can view birth process.	It is difficult to provide support for the woman's back.	Encourage woman to sit in a position that increases her comfort.
Semi-Fowler	Does not compromise venous return from lower extremities. Woman can view birth process.	If legs are positioned wide apart, relaxation of perineal tissues is decreased.	Assess that upper torso is evenly supported. Increase support of body by changing position of bed or using pillows as props.
Left lateral Sims	Does not compromise venous return from lower extremities. Increases perineal relaxation and decreases need for episiotomy. Appears to prevent rapid descent.	It is difficult for the woman to see the birth.	Adjust position so that the upper leg lies on the bed (scissor fashion) or is supported by the partner or on pillows.
Squatting	Size of pelvic outlet is increased. Gravity aids descent and expulsion of newborn. Second stage may be shortened.	It may be difficult to maintain balance while squatting.	Help woman maintain balance. Use a birthing bar if available.
Sitting in birthing bed	Gravity aids descent and expulsion of the fetus. Does not compromise venous return from lower extremities. Woman can view the birth process. Leg position may be changed at will.		Ensure that legs and feet have adequate support.
Hands and knees	Increases perineal relaxation and decreases need for episiotomy. Increases placental and umbilical blood flow and decreases fetal distress. Improves fetal rotation. Better able to assess the perineum. Better access to fetal nose and mouth for suctioning at birth. Facilitates birth of baby with shoulder dystocia.	Woman cannot view birth. There is decreased contact with birth attendant. Healthcare givers cannot use instruments. There may be increased maternal fatigue.	Adjust birthing bed by dropping the foot down. Supply extra pillows for increased support.

The woman is typically positioned for birth on a bed with leg supports, in a squatting position, or perhaps on her hands and knees. If a birthing bed is used, the back is elevated 30 to 60 degrees to help the woman bear down. Stirrups, if needed and used, are padded to avoid pressure. In helping the woman place her legs in the stirrups, both legs should be lifted simultaneously to avoid strain on abdominal, back, and perineal muscles. The stirrups are adjusted to fit the woman's legs. The feet are supported in the stirrup holders. The height and angle of the stirrups are adjusted so there is no pressure on the backs of the knees or the calves, which might cause discomfort and postpartum vascular problems. When stirrups are not used for the birth, the woman's legs may be placed in stirrups after the birth to enhance visibility if a perineal repair is needed.

CLEANSING THE PERINEUM

After the woman has been positioned for the birth, her vulvar and perineal areas are cleansed to increase her comfort and to remove any bloody discharge. Depending on agency protocol or on physician/CNM orders, perineal cleansing methods range from use of soapy water to aseptic technique. Once the cleansing is completed, the woman returns to the desired birthing position.

CONTINUED LABOR SUPPORT

Both the woman's partner and the nurse who has been with the woman during the labor continue to provide support during contractions. The woman is encouraged to push with each contraction and, as the fetal head emerges, is asked to take shallow breaths or to pant to prevent pushing. While supporting the head, the physician/CNM assesses whether the umbilical cord is around the fetal neck and removes it if it is, then suctions the mouth and nose with a bulb syringe. The mouth is suctioned first to prevent reflex inhalation of mucus when the nostrils are touched with the bulb syringe tip. The woman is encouraged to push again as the rest of the newborn's body is born. See the birthing sequence shown in Figure 18–6.

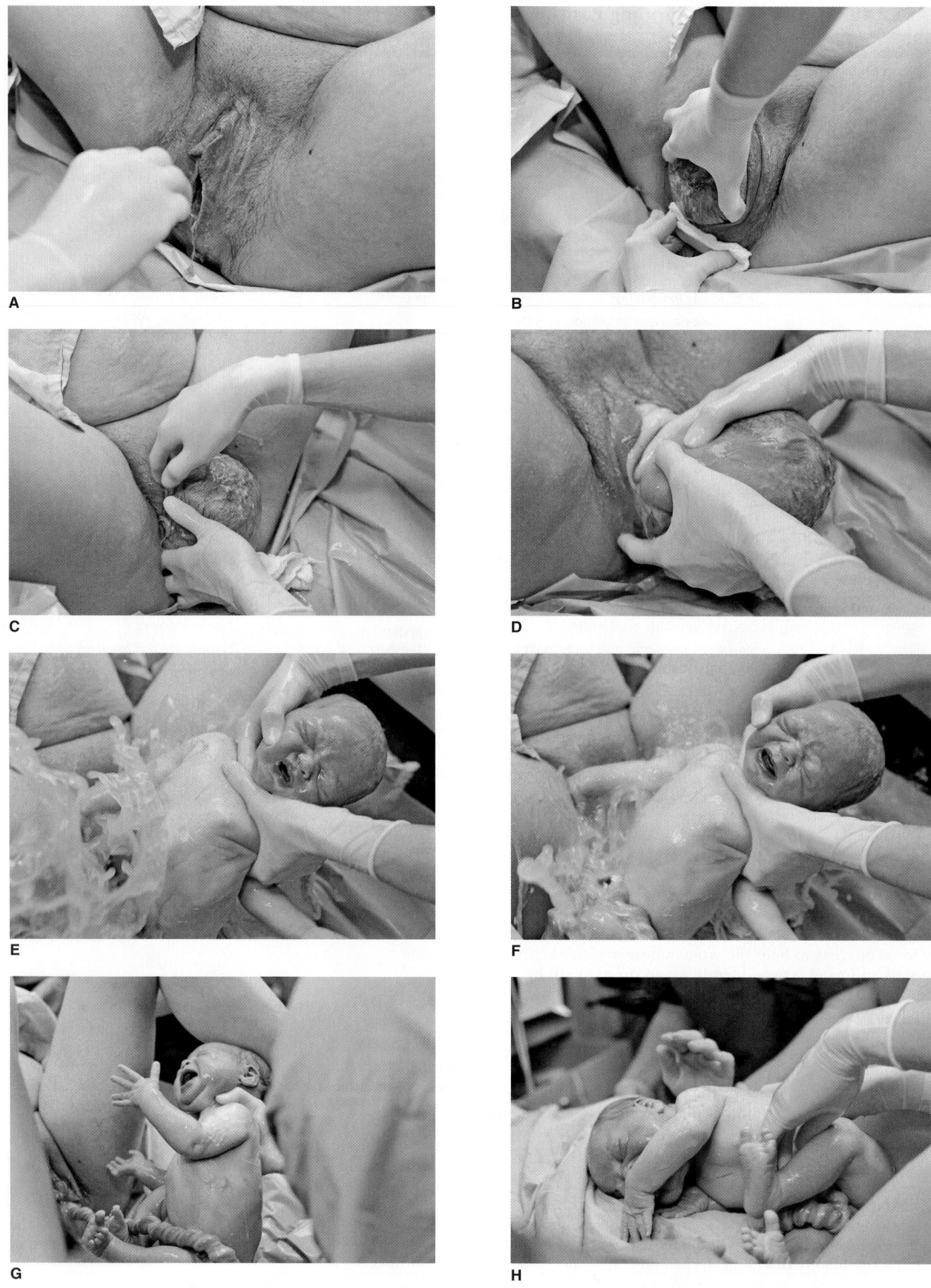

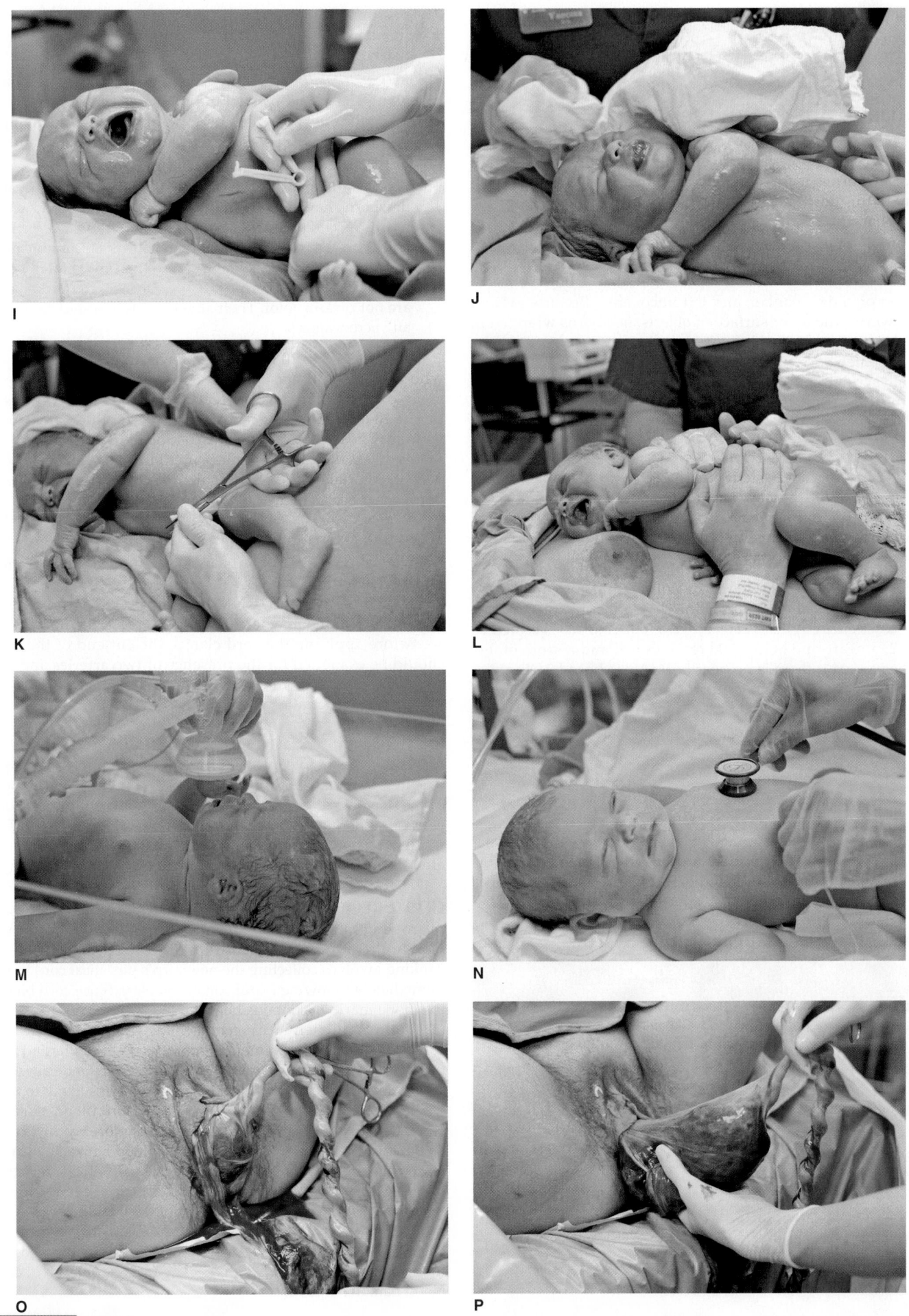

Figure 18–6 Birthing sequence.

Nursing Care During the Third and Fourth Stages of Labor

Initial Care of the Newborn

The physician/CNM places the newborn on the mother's abdomen, which promotes attachment, or in the radiant-heated unit. The newborn is maintained in a modified Trendelenburg position. In this position, gravity aids drainage of mucus from the nasopharynx and trachea. Newborns should be dried immediately and kept warm by covering them with warmed blankets or by placing them in skin-to-skin contact with their mothers. If newborns are in a radiant-heated unit, they should be dried, placed on a dry blanket, and left uncovered. Because radiant heat warms the outer surface of objects, newborns wrapped in blankets will receive no benefit from the unit.

The newborn's nose and mouth should be suctioned with a bulb syringe as needed. Most immediate care of the newborn can be done while the newborn is in the parent's arms or in the radiant-heated unit.

APGAR SCORING SYSTEM

The Apgar scoring system (Table 18–5) evaluates the physical condition of the newborn at birth. The newborn is rated 1 minute after birth and again at 5 minutes and receives a total score (**Apgar score**) ranging from 0 to 10 based on the following assessments:

1. *Heart rate* is auscultated or palpated at the junction of the umbilical cord and skin. This is the most important assessment. A heart rate above or equal to 100 is scored as 2, a heart rate below 100 receives a 1, and a score of 0 is assigned if there is no heartbeat. A newborn heart rate of less than 100 beats per minute indicates the need for immediate resuscitation.

2. *Respiratory effort* is the second most important Apgar assessment. A vigorous cry indicates adequate respirations and is scored as 2, whereas a slow, irregular respiratory effort receives a 1. Complete absence of respirations is termed *apnea* (scored 0).

3. *Muscle tone* is determined by evaluating the degree of flexion and resistance to straightening of the extremities. A normal newborn's elbows and hips are flexed, with the knees

positioned up toward the abdomen (scored as 2). Some flexion of the extremities is scored as 1, while a flaccid newborn receives a 0.

4. *Reflex irritability* is evaluated by stroking the baby's back along the spine, by flicking the soles of the feet, or by using the bulb syringe to perform oral or nasal suctioning. A cry merits a full score of 2. A grimace is 1 point, and no response is 0.

5. *Skin color* is inspected for cyanosis and pallor. Generally, newborns have blue extremities, with a pink body, which merits a score of 1. This condition is termed *acrocyanosis* and is present in many normal newborns at 1 minute after birth. A totally pink newborn scores a 2, and a totally cyanotic, pale newborn scores 0. Newborns with darker skin are not pink in color. Their skin color is assessed for pallor and acrocyanosis.

A score of 7 to 10 indicates a newborn in good condition who requires only nasopharyngeal suctioning and perhaps some oxygen near the face (called "blow-by" oxygen, see Figure 18-6*M*). If the Apgar score is below 7, resuscitative measures may be needed. (See the discussion in Chapter 26.) Apgar scores of less than 3 at 5 minutes after birth may correlate with neonatal mortality (Assunção et al., 2012). (See Assigning Newborn Apgar Scores in the *Clinical Skills Manual* SKILLS .)

CARE OF UMBILICAL CORD

Delayed cord clamping is associated with positive outcomes for the newborn and is now the preferred approach (ACOG, 2012). If the physician/CNM has not placed some type of cord clamp on the newborn's umbilical cord, the nurse does so. Before applying the cord clamp, the cut end of the cord should be examined for the presence of two arteries and one vein. The umbilical vein is the largest vessel, and the arteries are seen as smaller vessels. The nurse records the number of vessels on the birth and newborn records. The cord is clamped approximately 0.5 to 1.0 inch from the abdomen to allow room between the abdomen and clamp as the cord dries. Abdominal skin must not be clamped because this will cause necrosis of the tissue. The most common type of cord clamp is the plastic Hollister cord clamp (Figure 18–7). The Hollister clamp is removed in the nursery about 24 hours after the cord has dried.

CORD BLOOD COLLECTION FOR BANKING

A growing number of parents are arranging for cord blood banking with individual cord blood registries. Cord blood banking involves collecting the newborn's umbilical cord blood immediately following expulsion of the baby. Since cord blood, like bone marrow, contains hematopoietic stem cells, it can be used to treat numerous cancers, genetic and blood disorders, cerebral palsy, and immune disorders. Cord blood has advantages over bone marrow. It is a no-risk procedure and causes no discomfort to the newborn or mother and is less likely to trigger a potentially fatal rejection response. Cord blood can also work with a less than perfect match and is more readily available than bone marrow. Although cord blood banks have been established in the United States, universal cord blood collection does not exist. While some facilities collect volunteer donations, the majority of hospitals do not. Most of the banking performed in the United States is done by for-profit agencies where the parents pay a set fee to collect the blood and have it processed followed by an annual storage fee. The main drawback of cord blood banking is the cost.

TABLE 18–5 The Apgar Scoring System

	SCORE		
SIGN	**0**	**1**	**2**
Heart rate	Absent	Slow; less than 100 beats/min	Greater than 100 beats/min
Respiration	Absent	Slow; irregular	Good breathing with crying
Muscle tone	Flaccid	Some flexion of extremities	Active movement of extremities
Reflex response	Absent	Grimace; noticeable facial movement	Vigorous cry; coughs; sneezes; pulls away when touched
Skin color	Pale or blue	Pink body, blue extremities	Pink body and extremities

Source: Data from Apgar, V. (1966). *The newborn (Apgar) scoring system, reflections and advice.* Retrieved from http://profiles.nlm.nih.gov/ps/access/CPBBJY.pdf.

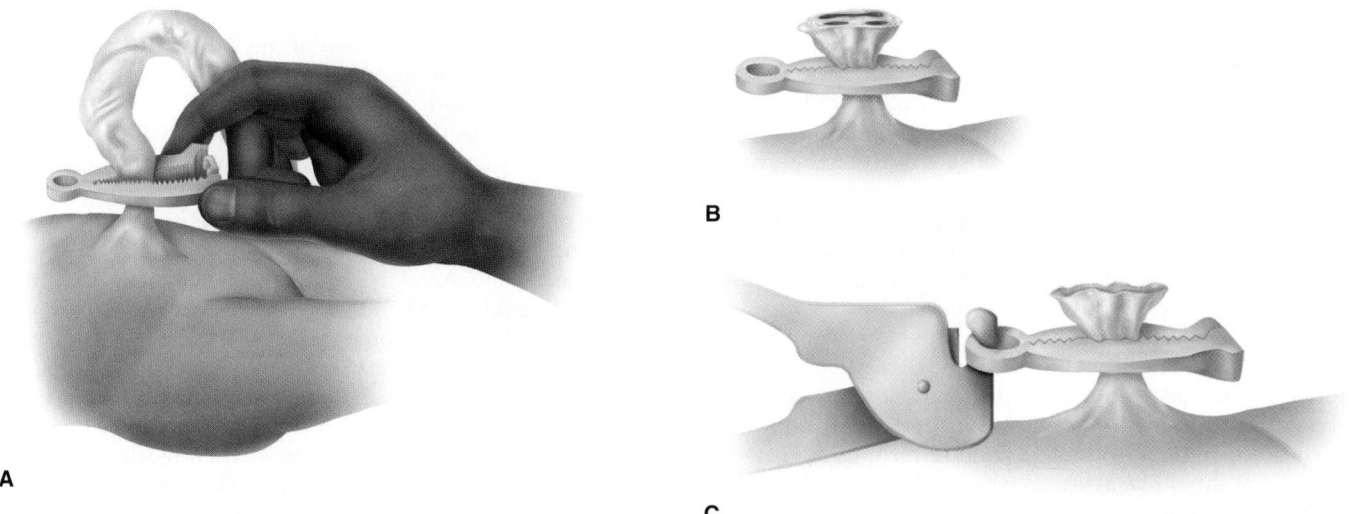

Figure 18–7 Hollister cord clamp. *A,* Clamp is positioned 0.5 to 1.0 in. from the abdomen and then secured. *B,* Cut cord. The one vein and two arteries can be seen. *C,* Plastic device for removing clamp after cord has dried. After the cord has dried, the nurse grasps the Hollister clamp on either side of the cut area and gently separates it.

Cord blood transplants can be utilized to treat a growing number of disorders. It is estimated that over 30,000 transfusions of cord blood have been performed worldwide (Ballen, Gluckman, & Boxmeyer, 2013). Although not yet regulated by the Food and Drug Administration (FDA) in the United States, other countries commonly use cord blood transplants, with the first occurring 25 years ago. With the list of treated cancers and medical complications rising that can benefit from a cord blood transplant, it is estimated that 1:5000 children will be infused with cord blood during their lifetimes (Parent's Guide to Cord Blood Foundation, 2015). Both ACOG and the American Academy of Pediatrics have issued position statements on counseling for cord blood banking. In some states, it is now mandated that practitioners disclose the cord blood options for clients that are available through private or public banks. Nurses are in a key position to discuss the advantages and disadvantages and available options with parents. While universal cord blood banking is not routinely recommended, parents who have an older child affected by a condition that may benefit from a cord blood transplant should consider cord blood banking. Recent recommendations have also been made that women at risk of giving birth prematurely should consider cord blood banking since these babies are more at risk for cerebral palsy and other neurologic injuries (Parent's Guide to Cord Blood Foundation, 2015).

Once collected, the blood is tested for infectious and genetic disorders before it is frozen. Abnormal blood results are communicated to the parents. Written consent is required for both collection and storage of cord blood, preferably upon admission or prior to the onset of labor.

These registries provide the parents with a special container for the cord blood, which they bring with them to the birth. The parents should have received directions from the registry about the storage and care of the container prior to the birth. Immediately after the newborn's umbilical cord is clamped and cut and the placenta is expelled, the physician/CNM withdraws blood from the remaining umbilical cord and the placenta and places it in the special container. The cord blood remains with the mother until it is picked up by the cord blood registry.

PHYSICAL ASSESSMENT OF THE NEWBORN

The nurse performs an abbreviated systematic physical assessment in the birthing area to detect any abnormalities (Table 18–6). (See Chapter 24 for an in-depth discussion of newborn assessment.) First, the size of the newborn and the

TABLE 18–6 Initial Newborn Evaluation

ASSESS	NORMAL FINDINGS
Respirations	Rate 36–60, irregular
	No retractions, no grunting
Apical pulse	Rate 120–160 and somewhat irregular
Temperature	Skin temp above 36.5°C (97.8°F)
Skin color	Body pink with bluish extremities
Umbilical cord	Two arteries and one vein
Gestational age	Should be 38–42 weeks to remain with parents for extended time
Sole creases	Sole creases that involve the heel

In general, expect scant amount of vernix on upper back, axilla, groin; lanugo only on upper back; ears with incurving of upper 2/3 of pinnae and thin cartilage that springs back from folding; male genitals—testes palpated in upper or lower scrotum; female genitals—labia majora larger, clitoris nearly covered

In the following situations, newborns should generally be stabilized rather than remain with parents in the birth area for an extended period of time:

- Apgar less than 8 at 1 min and less than 9 at 5 min or baby requires resuscitation measures (other than whiffs of oxygen)
- Respirations below 30 or above 60, with retractions and/or grunting
- Apical pulse below 120 or above 160 with marked irregularities
- Skin temperature below 36.5°C (97.8°F)
- Skin color pale blue or circumoral pallor
- Baby less than 38 weeks' or more than 42 weeks' gestation
- Baby very small or very large for gestational age
- Congenital anomalies involving open areas in the skin (meningomyelocele)

contour and size of the head in relationship to the rest of the body are noted. The newborn's posture and movements indicate tone and neurologic functioning.

The skin should be inspected for discoloration, presence of vernix caseosa and lanugo, and signs of trauma and desquamation (peeling of skin). Vernix caseosa is a white, cheesy substance found normally on newborns. It is absorbed within 24 hours after birth. Vernix is abundant on preterm newborns and absent on postterm newborns. Fine hair (lanugo) is often seen on preterm newborns' shoulders, foreheads, backs, and cheeks. Desquamation is seen in postterm newborns.

The nurse observes the nares (nostrils) for flaring and, as the newborn cries, inspects the palate for cleft palate. If mucus is found in the nose and mouth, it should be removed with a bulb syringe as needed. The chest is inspected for respiratory rate and the presence of retractions. If retractions are present, the newborn should be assessed for grunting or stridor. A normal respiratory rate is 30 to 60 per minute. The lungs are auscultated bilaterally for breath sounds. Absence of breath sounds on one side could mean pneumothorax. Crackles may be heard immediately after birth because a small amount of fluid may remain in the lungs; this fluid will be absorbed. Rhonchi indicate aspiration of oral secretions. If there is excessive mucus or respiratory distress, the nurse suctions the newborn with a mucus trap. (See Figure 18–8 as well as Performing Nasal Pharyngeal Suctioning in the *Clinical Skills Manual* SKILLS.) Elimination of urine or meconium should be noted and recorded on the newborn record.

NEWBORN IDENTIFICATION

The nurse places two ID bands on the newborn—one on the wrist and one on the ankle. The bands must fit snugly so they will not be lost, although caution should be used to prevent constriction. To ensure correct identification, while still in the birthing or delivery room, the mother and her partner are each given a band that matches that of the baby. The bands allow access to the newborn care areas and must not be removed until the baby is discharged.

Some facilities use newborn alarm safety devices to prevent abduction and ensure the safety of newborns in hospital settings. Umbilical cord alarms are one type of security device that are placed at the time the cord clamp is applied. The cord clamp and alarm are left in place until the mother and baby are discharged home. An alarm system that is attached to either the wrist or ankle by a band is another newborn safety device that may be utilized by some facilities (Figure 18–9). A newer option, a skin sensing tag alarm, is placed on the wrist or ankle and senses if the tag has been removed by monitoring changes in temperature that would occur if the tag were to be removed or become dislodged from the newborn. All three devices sound an alarm if the baby is removed from the hospital unit or if the device is cut or disengaged. The need for proper disinfection techniques for devices that are reused in clinical practice is imperative (Association of Perioperative Registered Nurses [AORN], 2013).

Additional hospital security measures are now commonplace in maternity settings. This includes mandating that all staff wear appropriate identification at all times. The nurse advises the parents to place the baby on the side of the bed away from the door, and to have the baby returned to the nursery whenever the mother naps or showers and no other family member is present.

Although hospital abductions are rare, they are catastrophic to the family, hospital, and community. Many abductors pose as medical personnel to gain access to the baby. Women should be advised to ask all hospital personnel for proper identification. If the mother or family feels unsure of the individual, they should immediately call on the call bell to alert the nurse and ask for other verification. If a woman is reluctant to allow a student nurse to transport her baby, the staff nurse should be asked to assist the student.

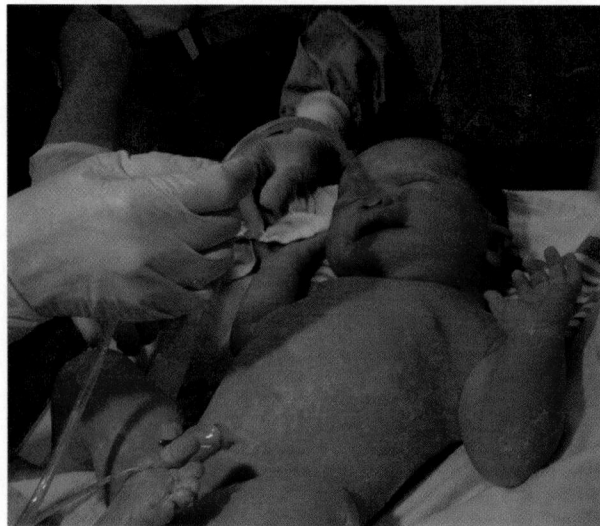

Figure 18–8 DeLee mucus trap being used to suction a newborn's mouth to remove excess secretions. One end of the suction tubing is connected to low suction, and the other end of the tubing is inserted 3 to 5 in. into the newborn's nose or mouth. Suction is applied as the tubing is pulled out. The process is repeated for as long as fluid is aspirated.

SOURCE: Wilson Garcia.

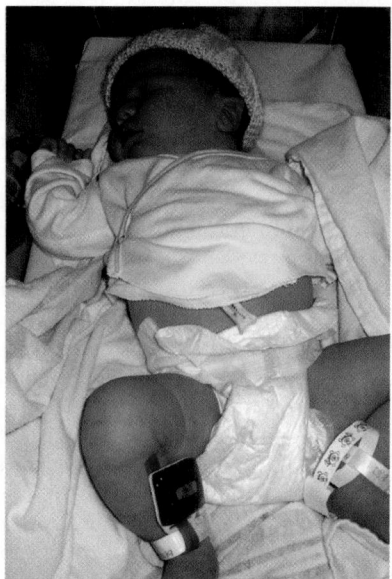

Figure 18–9 A newborn with a security device in place on one ankle.

SOURCE: Anne Garcia.

Delivery of the Placenta

After birth, the physician/CNM prepares for the delivery of the placenta (see Figure 18–6*O* and *P*). The following signs suggest placental separation:

1. The uterus rises upward in the abdomen.
2. As the placenta moves downward, the umbilical cord lengthens.
3. A sudden trickle or spurt of blood appears.
4. The shape of the uterus changes from discoid to globular.

While waiting for these signs, the nurse palpates the uterus to check for ballooning caused by uterine relaxation and subsequent bleeding into the uterine cavity. After the placenta has separated, the woman may be asked to bear down to aid delivery of the placenta.

Oxytocics are frequently given at the time of the delivery of the placenta, so the uterus will contract and bleeding will be minimized. Oxytocin (Pitocin), 10 to 20 units, may be added to an intravenous (IV) infusion, or 10 units may be given intramuscularly. Some physicians order methylergonovine maleate (Methergine), 0.2 mg administered intramuscularly, or carboprost tromethamine (Hemabate), 250 mcg/mL administered intramuscularly. In addition to administering the ordered medications, it is essential to assess and record maternal blood pressure before and after administration of oxytocics. After expulsion of the placenta, the physician/CNM inspects the placental membranes to make sure they are intact and that all cotyledons are present. If there is a defect or a part missing from the placenta, a manual uterine examination is done. On the birth record, the time of delivery of the placenta should be noted.

After the placenta is expelled, the physician/CNM inspects the vagina and cervix for lacerations and makes any necessary repairs. The episiotomy may be repaired if that has not been done previously (see Chapter 22).

Enhancing Attachment

The first few hours and even minutes after birth are an important period for the attachment of mother and baby. If this period of contact can occur during the first hour after birth, the newborn will be in the quiet state and able to interact with parents by looking at them. Newborns also turn their heads in response to a spoken voice. (For further discussion of newborn states, see Chapter 23.)

The first parent–newborn contact may be brief (a few minutes), to be followed by a more extended contact after uncomfortable procedures (expulsion of the placenta and suturing of the episiotomy) are completed. When the newborn is returned to the mother, the nurse can help her begin breastfeeding if she so desires. The baby may seek out the mother's breast, and early contact between the two can greatly affect breastfeeding success. Even if the newborn does not actively nurse, the baby can lick, taste, and smell the mother's skin. This activity by the newborn stimulates the maternal release of prolactin, which promotes the onset of lactation.

Clinical Tip

Newborn to mother skin-to-skin contact immediately following birth supports breastfeeding and bonding (Heidarzadeh, Hosseini, Ershadmanesh, et al., 2013).

Darkening the birthing room by turning out most of the lights causes newborns to open their eyes and gaze around. This in turn enhances eye-to-eye contact with the parents. (*Note:* If the physician/CNM needs a light source, the spotlight can be left on.) Treatment of the newborn's eyes may also be delayed. Many parents who establish eye contact with the newborn are content to quietly gaze at their baby. Others may show more active involvement by touching or inspecting the newborn. Some mothers talk to their babies in a high-pitched voice, which seems to be soothing to newborns. Some couples verbally express amazement and pride when they see they have produced a beautiful, healthy baby. Their verbalization enhances feelings of accomplishment and ecstasy.

Both parents need to be encouraged to do whatever they feel most comfortable doing. Some parents prefer only limited contact with the newborn immediately after birth and instead want private time together in a quiet environment. In spite of the current zeal for providing immediate attachment opportunities, nursing personnel need to be aware of parents' wishes. The desire to delay interaction with the newborn does not necessarily imply a decreased ability of the parents to bond with their newborn. (For further discussion of parent–newborn attachment, see Chapter 25.)

Nursing Management

The period of 1 to 4 hours immediately following the expulsion of the placenta, during which the mother's condition stabilizes, is often referred to as the fourth stage of labor and birth. This is actually the initial recovery period.

After childbirth, it is critical that the uterine fundus stay well contracted to clamp off uterine blood vessels at the placental site and thereby prevent hemorrhaging. Consequently, palpate the uterine fundus at frequent intervals for the first 4 hours to ensure that it remains firmly contracted. Normally, the fundus is located in the midline and at or below the umbilicus. Palpate the fundus (Figure 18–10) but do not massage it unless it is soft (boggy). When a uterus becomes boggy, pooling of blood occurs within it, causing clots. Anything left in the uterus prevents it from contracting effectively. Thus, if the uterus becomes boggy or appears to rise in the abdomen, massage the fundus until firm; then with one hand supporting the uterus at the symphysis pubis, use the other hand to exert steady pressure on the fundus to express retained clots. The uterus is very tender at this time, so all palpation and massage must be done as gently as possible.

In some women, the uterus becomes so relaxed that it cannot be found when palpation is attempted. In this case, place one hand in the midline of the abdomen at about the level of the umbilicus and begin to make kneading motions. This motion generally stimulates the uterus to contract, and it then feels like a firm, hard object. (See Assessing the Uterine Fundus Following Vaginal or Cesarean Birth in the *Clinical Skills Manual* SKILLS.)

Wash the woman's perineum with gauze squares and warmed solution and dry the area well with a towel before placing the maternity pad. If stirrups have been used, remove both of the woman's legs from the stirrups at the same time to avoid muscle strain. Encourage the woman to move her legs gently up and down in a bicycle motion. The woman remains in the same bed or is transferred to a recovery room bed. Help her don a clean gown and offer her something to drink.

During the recovery period, it is essential to monitor maternal vital signs closely. Check the maternal blood pressure at 5- to 15-minute intervals to detect any changes. Blood pressure should return to the prelabor level as a result of an increased

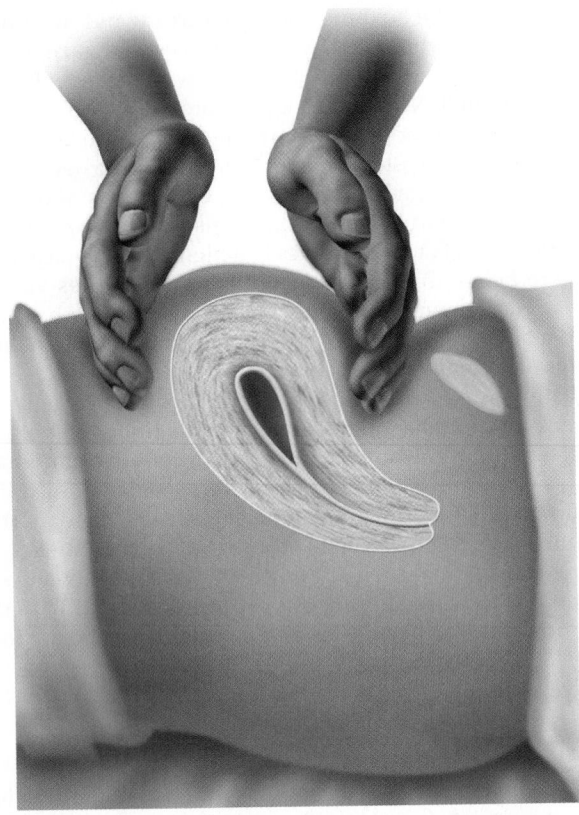

Figure 18–10 Suggested method of palpating the fundus of the uterus during the fourth stage. The left hand is placed just above the symphysis pubis, and gentle downward pressure is exerted. The right hand is cupped around the uterine fundus.

volume of blood returning to the maternal circulation from the uteroplacental shunt. Pulse rate should be slightly lower than it was during labor. Baroreceptors cause a vagal response, which slows the pulse. A rise in blood pressure may be a response to oxytocic drugs or may be caused by preeclampsia. A lowered blood pressure and a rising pulse rate may reflect blood loss. See Table 18–7.

TABLE 18–7 Maternal Adaptations Following Birth

CHARACTERISTIC	NORMAL FINDING
Blood pressure	Returns to prelabor level
Pulse	Slightly lower than in labor
Uterine fundus	In the midline at the umbilicus or 1 to 2 fingerbreadths below the umbilicus
Lochia	Red (rubra), small to moderate amount (from spotting on pads to 0.25–0.5 of pad covered in 15 min)
	Does not exceed saturation of one pad in first hour
Bladder	Nonpalpable
Perineum	Smooth, pink, without bruising or edema
Emotional state	Wide variation, including excited, exhilarated, smiling, crying, fatigued, verbal, quiet, pensive, and sleepy

Also monitor the woman's temperature. Frequently, women have tremors in the immediate postpartum period, possibly caused by a difference in internal and external body temperatures (higher temperature inside the body than outside). Another theory is that the woman is reacting to the fetal cells that have entered the maternal circulation at the placental site. A heated bath blanket placed next to the woman is helpful and can be replaced as often as the mother desires.

Inspect the bloody vaginal discharge for amount and record it as minimal, moderate, or heavy and with or without clots. This discharge, lochia rubra, should be bright red. A soaked perineal pad contains approximately 100 mL of blood. If the perineal pad becomes soaked in a 15-minute period or if blood pools under the buttocks, continuous observation is necessary. (See Evaluating Lochia in the *Clinical Skills Manual* SKILLS .) When the fundus is firm, a continuous trickle of blood may signal laceration of the vagina or cervix or an unligated vessel in the episiotomy.

If the fundus rises and displaces to the right, it is important to consider two factors:

1. As the uterus rises, the uterine contractions become less effective and increased bleeding may occur.

2. The most common cause of uterine displacement is bladder distention.

Palpate the bladder to determine whether it is distended. The bladder fills rapidly with the extra fluid volume returned from the uteroplacental circulation (and with any fluid received intravenously during labor and birth). The postpartum woman may not realize that her bladder is full because trauma to the bladder and urethra during childbirth and the use of regional anesthesia decrease bladder tone and the urge to void.

Use a variety of measures to help the mother to void. Place a warm towel across the lower abdomen or pour warm water over the perineum to relax the urinary sphincter and facilitate voiding. If the woman is unable to void, catheterization is necessary.

The perineum is inspected for edema and hematoma formation. An ice pack often reduces the swelling and alleviates the discomfort of an episiotomy.

The couple may be tired, hungry, and thirsty. Some agencies serve the couple a meal. The tired mother will probably drift off into a welcome sleep. The partner can also be encouraged to rest, since the supporting role is physically and mentally tiring. If the mother is not in a birthing room, she is usually transferred from the birthing unit to the postpartum or mother–baby area after 2 hours or more, depending on agency policy and whether the following criteria are met:

- Stable vital signs
- No bleeding
- Undistended bladder
- Firm fundus
- Sensations fully recovered from any anesthetic agent received during birth

Support of the Adolescent During Birth

As with all women, each adolescent in labor is different. The nurse can assess what each teen brings to the experience by considering the following:

- Has the adolescent received prenatal care?
- What are her attitudes and feelings about the pregnancy?

- Who will attend the birth and what is the person's relationship to her?
- What preparation has she had for the experience?
- What are her expectations and fears regarding labor and birth?
- How has her culture influenced her?
- What are her usual coping mechanisms?
- Does she plan to keep the newborn?

Adolescent females are at highest risk for pregnancy and labor complications and must be assessed carefully. Fetal well-being is established by fetal monitoring. The nurse should be especially alert for any physiologic complications of labor. The adolescent's prenatal record is carefully reviewed for risks, and she is screened for preeclampsia, cephalopelvic disproportion, anemia, drugs ingested during pregnancy, sexually transmitted infections, and size–date discrepancies.

The support role of the nurse depends on the adolescent mother's support system during labor. The adolescent may not be accompanied by someone who will stay with her during childbirth, or she may have her mother, the father of the baby, or a close friend as her labor partner. Regardless of whether the teen has a support person, it is important for the nurse to establish a trusting relationship with her. In this way, it is possible to help the teen understand what is happening to her. The adolescent given positive reinforcement for "work well done" will leave the experience with increased self-esteem despite the emotional problems that may accompany her situation. If a support person accompanies the adolescent, that person also needs encouragement and support. The nurse can explain changes in the adolescent's behavior and describe ways the support person can be of help.

The adolescent who has taken childbirth education classes is generally better prepared for labor than the adolescent who has not. However, the younger the adolescent, the less she may be able to participate actively in the process even if she has taken prenatal classes. See Figure 18–11.

The very young adolescent (age 14 and under) has fewer coping mechanisms and less experience to draw on than her older counterparts. Because her cognitive development is incomplete, the younger adolescent may have fewer problem-solving capabilities. She may be more threatened by the experience, and she may be more vulnerable to stress and discomfort.

The very young adolescent needs someone to rely on at all times during labor. She may be more childlike and dependent than older teens. Instructions and explanations should be simple and concrete. During the transition phase, the young teenager may become withdrawn and unable to express her need to be nurtured. Touch, soothing encouragement, and measures to provide comfort help her maintain control and meet her needs for dependence. During the second stage of labor, the young adolescent may feel as if she is losing control and may reach out to those around her. It is important for the nurse to remain calm and give clear, simple directions to help the teen cope with feelings of helplessness.

The middle adolescent (ages 15 to 17 years) often attempts to remain calm and unflinching during labor. Nevertheless, a caring attitude will still help her. Many older adolescents believe that they "know it all," but they may be no more prepared for childbirth than their younger counterparts. Positive reinforcement and a nonjudgmental manner will help them save face. If the adolescent has not taken childbirth preparation classes, she may require preparation and explanations. However, the older teenager's (ages 18 to 19) response to the stresses of labor is similar to that of the adult woman.

Even if the adolescent is planning to relinquish her newborn, she should be given the option of seeing and holding the baby. She may be reluctant to do this at first, but the mother's grieving process is facilitated if she sees the baby. However, seeing or holding the newborn should be the adolescent mother's choice. (See Chapter 29 for further discussion of the relinquishing mother and the adolescent parent.)

Nursing Care During Precipitous Labor and Birth

Occasionally, labor progresses so rapidly that the maternity nurse is faced with the task of managing the actual birth of the baby. The terms **precipitous labor** and **precipitous birth** are used when the labor and birth occur in 3 hours or less. The attending nurse has the primary responsibility for providing a physically and psychologically safe experience for the woman and her baby. A woman whose physician/CNM is not present may feel disappointed, frightened, abandoned, angry, and cheated. She may fear what is going to happen and feel that everything is out of her control. In working with the woman, the nurse provides support by keeping her informed about the labor progress and assuring her that the nurse will stay with her.

Clinical Tip

When birth is imminent and a physician/CNM is not present, do not take the bed apart (or "break the bed") because this increases the risk that the newborn could be dropped at the time of birth. Lower the foot of the bed slightly to create space beneath the buttocks so you are able to adequately deliver the head without the risk of a newborn fall.

If birth is imminent, the nurse must not leave the mother alone. The nurse can direct auxiliary personnel to contact the physician/CNM and retrieve the emergency birth pack ("precip pack"), which should be readily accessible to birthing rooms. A typical pack contains the following items:

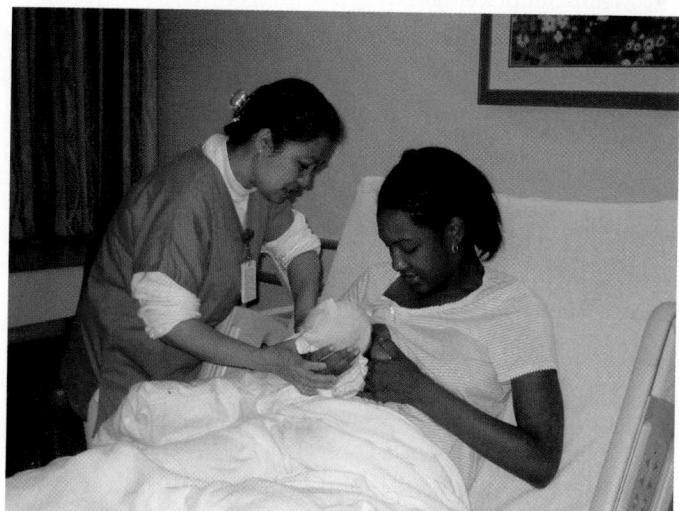

Figure 18–11 An adolescent mother receives breastfeeding assistance in the immediate postpartum period.

- A small drape that can be placed under the woman's buttocks to provide a sterile field
- A bulb syringe to clear mucus from the newborn's mouth
- Two sterile clamps (Kelly or Rochester) to clamp the umbilical cord before applying a cord clamp
- Sterile scissors to cut the umbilical cord
- A sterile umbilical cord clamp, either Hesseltine or Hollister
- A baby blanket to wrap the newborn in after birth
- A package of sterile gloves

At all times during the birth, the nurse remains calm, provides suggestions such as when to maintain a controlled breathing pattern and when to push, supports the woman's efforts, and provides reassurance.

The nurse assists in the precipitous labor and birth as follows: The woman is encouraged to assume a comfortable position. If time permits, the nurse's hands should be scrubbed with soap and water and sterile gloves donned. Sterile drapes are placed under the woman's buttocks. The nurse may place an index finger inside the lower portion of the vagina and the thumb on the outer portion of the perineum and gently massage the area to help stretch perineal tissues and prevent perineal lacerations. This procedure is called "ironing the perineum."

When the baby's head crowns, the nurse instructs the woman to pant, which decreases her urge to push. The nurse checks whether the amniotic sac is intact. If it is, the nurse tears the sac so the newborn will not breathe in amniotic fluid with the first breath.

With one hand, the nurse applies gentle pressure against the fetal head to prevent it from popping out rapidly. The nurse does not hold the head back forcibly. Rapid birth of the head may result in tears in the woman's perineal tissues. The rapid change in pressure within the fetal head may cause subdural or dural tears. The nurse supports the perineum with the other hand and allows the head to be born between contractions.

As the woman continues to pant, the nurse inserts one or two fingers along the back of the fetal head to check for the umbilical cord. If there is a nuchal cord (umbilical cord around the neck), the nurse's fingers should be bent like a fish hook in order to grasp the cord and pull it over the baby's head. It is important to check that the cord is not wrapped around the neck more than one time. If the cord is tightly looped and cannot be slipped over the baby's head, two clamps are placed on the cord, the cord is cut between the clamps, and the cord is unwound.

Immediately after birth of the head, the nurse suctions the baby's mouth, throat, and nasal passages. The nurse then places one hand on each side of the head and exerts gentle downward traction until the anterior shoulder passes under the symphysis pubis. Then gentle upward traction aids the birth of the posterior shoulder. The nurse then instructs the woman to push gently so that the rest of the body can be born quickly. As the newborn emerges, support should be provided.

The newborn is held at the level of the uterus to facilitate blood flow through the umbilical cord. The combination of amniotic fluid and vernix makes the newborn very slippery, so the nurse must be careful to avoid dropping the baby. The nose and mouth of the newborn are suctioned again, using a bulb syringe. The nurse then dries the newborn to prevent heat loss. As soon as the nurse determines that the newborn's respirations are adequate, the baby can be placed on the mother's abdomen. The newborn's head should be slightly lower than the body to aid drainage of fluid and mucus. The weight of the newborn on the mother's abdomen stimulates uterine contractions, which aid in placental separation. The umbilical cord should not be pulled. The nurse is alert for signs of placental separation (slight gush of dark blood from the vagina, lengthening of the cord, or a change in uterine shape from discoid to globular). When these signs are present, the nurse tells the mother to push so that the placenta can be delivered. The nurse inspects the placenta to determine whether it is intact.

The nurse checks the firmness of the uterus. The fundus may be gently massaged to stimulate contractions and decrease bleeding. Putting the newborn to breast also stimulates uterine contractions through release of oxytocin from the pituitary gland.

The umbilical cord may now be cut. The nurse places two sterile Kelly clamps approximately 0.5 to 1.0 inch from the newborn's abdomen. The cord is cut between the Kelly clamps with sterile scissors. The nurse places a sterile umbilical cord clamp adjacent to the clamp on the newborn's cord, between the clamp and the newborn's abdomen. The clamp must not be placed snugly against the abdomen, because the cord will dry and shrink.

The nurse cleanses the area under the mother's buttocks and inspects her perineum for lacerations. Bleeding from lacerations may be controlled by pressing a clean perineal pad against the perineum and instructing the woman to keep her thighs together.

If the physician/CNM's arrival is delayed or if the newborn is having respiratory distress, the newborn should be transported immediately to the nursery. Newborns must be properly identified before they leave the birth area. The nurse notes and places on a birth record the following information:

- Position of fetus at birth
- Presence of cord around neck or shoulder (nuchal cord)
- Time of birth
- Apgar scores at 1 and 5 minutes after birth
- Gender of newborn
- Time of expulsion of placenta
- Method of placental expulsion
- Appearance and intactness of placenta
- Mother's condition
- Any medications given to mother or newborn (per agency protocol)

Evaluation

As a result of comprehensive nursing care during the intrapartum period, the following outcomes may be anticipated:

- The mother's physical and psychologic well-being has been maintained and supported.
- The baby's physical and psychologic well-being has been protected and supported.
- The couple have had input into the birth process and have participated as much as they desired.
- The mother and her baby have had a safe birth.

Focus Your Study

- Admission data needed to develop a clinical management plan for the four stages of labor includes prenatal information and current assessments. The nurse assesses needed teaching, anticipated care that will be needed for each stage of labor, expected activity level, proposed comfort measures, elimination and nutritional needs, and the level of involvement from the family.

- Admission needs focus on orienting the woman and her family to the unit, obtaining a physical assessment, obtaining maternal vital signs and FHR, performing a labor examination that includes determining the frequency and intensity of uterine contractions, cervical dilatation and effacement, and status of the membranes. The nurse evaluates the woman's respiratory and neurologic status. Recent symptoms and an evaluation of the woman's knowledge base and support system is also assessed.

- During the first stage of labor, the nurse establishes a rapport with the woman and her support person, assesses their expectations for labor and birth, ensures privacy, and explores the woman's individual responses to pain and discomfort. Labor support should include caring for the woman's physical, emotional, social, and spiritual needs.

- In the second stage of labor, the nurse continues to ensure privacy while identifying the individuals who the mother would like present during the birth, and providing reassurance and support during the birthing process.

- Nursing care during the third and fourth stage of labor involves providing ongoing support as the woman is encouraged to hold and look at the baby. The nurse provides newborn care teaching and promotes nutritional intake for the mother.

- Comfort measures during labor focus on reducing anxiety, providing information on what to expect in labor and birth, promoting relaxation, assisting with breathing patterns, and providing education and support to the support person.

- In the first stage of labor, the nurse provides comfort measures by administering pharmacologic agents as requested and ordered, and assisting with epidural placement if the woman chooses this as a means of pain control.

- During the second stage of labor, the nurse assists with finding a comfortable position for pushing and facilitating rest and relaxation during uterine contractions.

- Immediate newborn interventions include maintaining respirations, providing warmth and preventing heat loss, prevention of infection, and ensuring the baby is properly identified immediately following birth to ensure newborn safety.

- Adolescent mothers have unique developmental needs along with basic physical needs of pregnancy that warrant additional education, support, and teaching.

- Precipitous labor and birth occurs rapidly without a physician/CNM present. The nurse attends the birth by guiding the baby through the birth canal, clamping and cutting the cord, and transferring the newborn to the nursery for assessment and care. The attending nurse assesses for placental separation and expulsion and uterine contractility.

Clinical Reasoning in Action

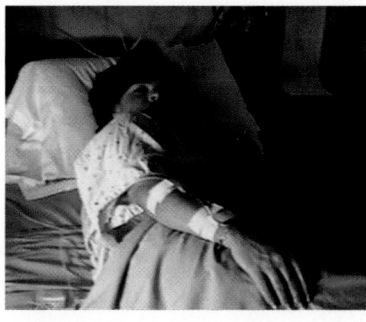

Anita Grey, a 22-year-old primigravida at 40 weeks' gestation, is admitted by you to the birthing center in labor. Anita was sent from her physician's office after being evaluated at her prenatal visit. While in the office, she was assessed to be 4 cm dilated, 100% effaced, vertex at 0 station with bulging membranes. She tells you that her husband is on his way to the birthing center and that she is anxious for him to arrive. A review of her prenatal record shows no complications affecting this pregnancy. Anita's vital signs are within normal limits. You assess the fetal heart rate and contraction pattern with the fetal monitor and observe a fetal heart rate of 140 to 150 beats/min with accelerations to 160s. Contractions are every 3 to 4 minutes × 30 seconds of moderate intensity by palpation. Anita seems to be tolerating the contractions well, but still seems anxious about her husband's arrival.

1. What steps can you take to reduce the stress and anxiety of the laboring woman and her family?

2. When you notify the physician/CNM, what pertinent information should the report contain?

3. What support measures can you give in the active phase of labor?

4. What measures can be used to decrease discomfort/pain as labor progresses?

5. What observations reflect the physiologic manifestations of pain?

References

American College of Obstetricians and Gynecologists. (ACOG). (2009a). *Intrapartum fetal heart rate monitoring: Nomenclature, interpretation, and general management principles* (ACOG Practice Bulletin No. 106). Washington, DC: Author.

American College of Obstetricians and Gynecologists (ACOG). (2009b). *Oral intake during labor* (ACOG Committee Opinion No. 441). Washington, DC: Author.

American College of Obstetricians and Gynecologists (ACOG). (2012). *Timing of umbilical cord clamping after birth* (ACOG Practice Bulletin No. 543). Washington, DC: Author.

Anderson, B. A., & Stone, S. E. (2013). Best practices in midwifery: Using the evidence to implement change. New York, NY: Springer.

Apgar, V. (1966). *The newborn (Apgar) scoring system, reflections and advice*. Retrieved from http://profiles.nlm.nih.gov/ps/access/CPBBJY.pdf

Association of Perioperative Registered Nurses (AORN). (2013). AORN Guidance Statement: reuse of single-use devices. *Perioperative Standards and Recommended Practices*. Denver, CO: AORN.

Assunção, S., Campos, J. A., Bonini, D., Ibidi, S. M., Ruano, R., & Zugaib, M. (2012). Low Apgar scores at 5 minutes in a low risk population: Maternal and obstetrical factors and postnatal outcome. *Revista da Associação Médica Brasileira, 58*(5), 587–593. Retrieved from http://www.scielo.br/scielo.php?script=sci_arttext&pid=S0104-42302012000500017&lng=en&tlng=en. 10.1590/S0104-42302012000500017

Ballen, K. K., Gluckman, E., & Broxmeyer, H. E. (2013). Umbilical cord blood transplantation: The first 25 years and beyond. *Blood, 122*(4) 491–498. doi:10.1182/blood-2013-02-453175

Centers for Disease Control and Prevention (CDC). (2014). *One test, two lives: HIV screening for prenatal care*. Retrieved from http://www.cdc.gov/Features/1Test2Lives

Fontaine, K. L. (2014). *Complementary and alternative therapies for nursing practice* (4th ed.). Upper Saddle River, NJ: Pearson.

Heidarzadeh, M., Hosseini, M., Ershadmanesh, M., & Tabari, M. G. (2013). The effect of kangaroo mother care (KMC) on breast feeding at the time of NICU discharge. *Iranian Red Crescent Medical Journal 15(4)*, 302–306. doi:10.5812/ircmj.2160

Institute for Patient and Family-Centered Care. (2014). *Family-centered care*. Retrieved from http://www.ipfcc.org/faq.html

Konda, A., Vikas, R., Yarlagadda, P. (2014). An intuitive multi-touch surface and gesture based interaction for video surveillance systems. *International Journal of Future Computer and Communication, 3*(3), 197–201.

Miller, L. A., Miller, S., & Tucker, S. M. (2012). Mosby's pocket guide to fetal monitoring: A multidisciplinary approach. (7th ed.). St. Louis, MO: Mosby.

Narendra, M., Shah, P. K., Pratap, K., & Prashap, A. (2014). *Ultrasound in obstetrics & gynecology*. (4th ed.). Pradesh, India: Jaypee Brothers Medical.

Ondeck, M. (2014). Healthy birth practice #2: Walk, move around, and change positions throughout labor. *The Journal of Perinatal Education, 23*(4), 188–193.

Parent's Guide to Cord Blood Foundation. (2015). *Odds of use*. Retrieved from http://parentsguidecordblood.org/odds.php

Simpkin, P., Bolding, A., Keppler, A., & Durham, J. (2010). *Pregnancy, childbirth, and the newborn: The complete guide* (4th ed.). Hopkins, MN: Meadowbrooke.

Spector, R. E. (2012). *Cultural diversity in health and illness* (8th ed.). Upper Saddle River, NJ: Pearson.

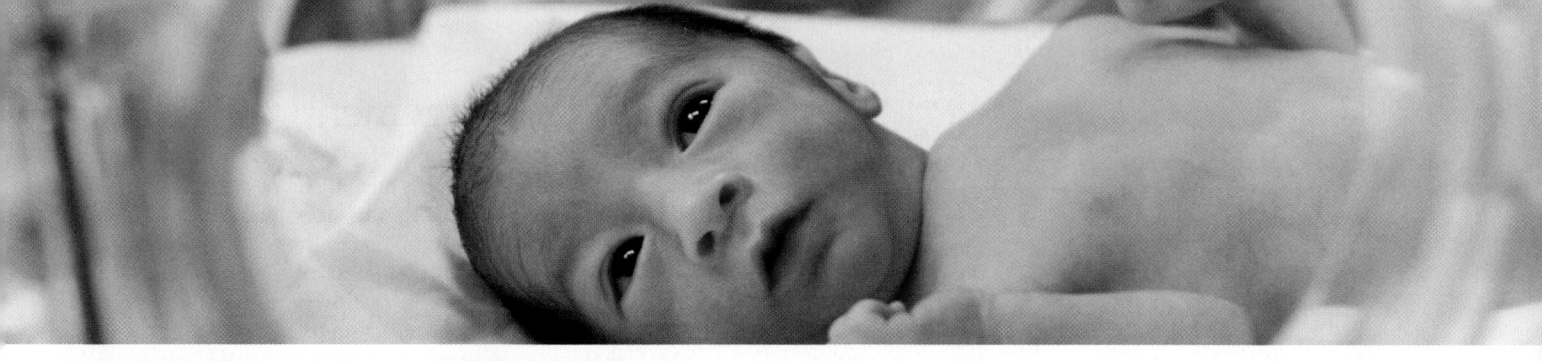

Chapter 19
Pharmacologic Pain Management

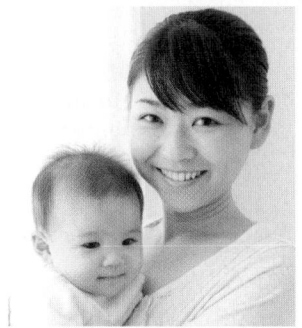

We had attended our classes and practiced through the last few weeks, but I was not ready for the amount of discomfort that I felt during my labor. I've always been able to handle pain much better, but this pain was very different. I had hoped to go through all of labor and birth without medications, but we had talked about it and I knew that if I felt I needed something, it would be all right. My nurse was also helpful and supportive of my decision. She helped me feel that I was making a good decision and that I wasn't failing somehow.

—Kyung-aie, 36

taka/Fotolia

∨ Learning Outcomes

19.1 Describe the use, administration, dose, onset of action, and adverse effects of systemic drugs to promote pain relief during the nursing management of the woman in labor and her fetus.

19.2 Compare the major types of regional analgesia and anesthesia, including area affected, advantages, disadvantages, techniques, and nursing management of the laboring woman and her fetus.

19.3 Explain the possible complications of regional anesthesia in nursing management of the laboring woman and her fetus.

19.4 Describe the nursing management for the laboring woman and her fetus related to general anesthesia.

19.5 Describe the major complications of general anesthesia during labor in nursing management of the woman in labor and her fetus.

Childbearing women experience varying levels of pain and other demanding sensations during labor and birth. As discussed in Chapter 18, nursing interventions directed toward pain relief begin with psychologic measures such as providing information, support, and encouragement. Measures to promote physical comfort include back rubs, showers, whirlpool baths, and the application of cool cloths. Some laboring women need no further interventions.

For other women, the progression of labor brings increasing pain that interferes with their ability to cope. These women may elect to use pharmacologic agents such as systemic medications, regional nerve blocks (epidural, spinal, or combined epidural-spinal), and local anesthetic blocks (pudendal and perineal) to decrease discomfort, increase relaxation, and reestablish their ability to participate more effectively in the labor and birth experience. The methods are not all mutually exclusive,

and any of them may be used in combination with nonpharmacologic comfort measures. The use of general anesthesia has very limited use in modern obstetrics. It is occasionally used during emergency cesarean births, although this trend continues to decrease because of the associated adverse maternal and fetal effects.

Although systemic analgesics and regional anesthetic blocks may affect the fetus, so do the laboring woman's pain and stress. During labor, maternal respirations and oxygen consumption increase, and this decreases the amount of oxygen available to the fetus. In addition, the pain and stress can lead to metabolic acidosis and the release of catecholamines, which cause maternal blood vessels to constrict, lessening oxygen and nutrient supply to the fetus (Blackburn, 2013).

There is a good deal of peer pressure on expectant parents to have the "ideal" birth experience. They may plan a natural childbirth, in which case the need for analgesia may make them feel inadequate and guilty. The nurse has a special role in helping a woman and her partner or support person accept alterations in their original plan and recognize the unique qualities of their birth experience. Reassurance that accepting analgesia for discomfort is not a failure can help maintain the woman's self-esteem. The emphasis should be on achieving a healthy, satisfying outcome for the family. Evidence has shown that women who have continuous one-to-one support during labor were more likely to have a spontaneous vaginal birth, less likely to require analgesia, and less likely to report dissatisfaction with their childbirth experience (Anderson & Stone, 2013). Also, the American College of Obstetricians and Gynecologists has concluded that a woman's request is sufficient justification for pain relief during labor (Anderson & Stone, 2013).

Systemic Medications

Note that this discussion of obstetric analgesia and anesthesia applies only to a healthy woman and fetus. Pain relief during labor and birth for women with high-risk conditions, such as preterm labor, preeclampsia, blood disorders, asthma, obstructive sleep apnea, substance abuse issues, or diabetes mellitus, requires skilled decision making, close observation, and awareness of all the potential threats to both the woman and her baby (Wong, 2014). Few conditions warrant a contraindication to systemic medications. However, women with myasthenia gravis should not be given systemic medications and instead are better candidates for epidural anesthesia (Wong, 2014). The goal of pharmacologic analgesia during labor is to provide maximum pain relief at minimum risk for the mother and fetus. To reach this goal, clinicians must consider a number of factors, including the following:

- All systemic medications used for pain relief during labor cross the placental barrier by simple diffusion, but some medications cross more readily than others.
- Medication action in the body depends on the rate at which the substance is metabolized by liver enzymes and excreted by the kidneys.
- High medication doses may remain in the fetus for long periods because fetal liver enzymes and kidney excretion are inadequate for metabolizing analgesic agents.

Clinical Reasoning Anesthesia During Labor

Luisa Silva, a 33-year-old G1P0, is 32 weeks pregnant. She is trying to decide whether she should accept any analgesia during her labor. She has finished childbirth education classes and wants an unmedicated labor and birth. She says, "I want to do this on my own, but I'm afraid it may be too much. Will it be OK if I need to take something?" What will you tell her?

Nursing Management

Analgesic medications provide pain relief for the laboring woman but also affect the fetus and the labor process. Pain medication given too early may prolong labor and depress the fetus; if given too late, it is of minimal use to the woman and may lead to respiratory depression in the newborn. The mother and fetus should be assessed and the contraction pattern evaluated before administering prescribed systemic medications.

Maternal assessment parameters include the following:

- The woman is willing to receive medication after being advised about the risks and benefits of the medication.
- Maternal vital signs are stable.
- Contraindications (such as specific medication allergy, respiratory compromise, myasthenia gravis, or current medication dependence) are not present.

Fetal assessment parameters include:

- The fetal heart rate (FHR) baseline is between 110 and 160 beats per minute, and no late decelerations or nonreassuring FHR patterns are present.
- Variability is present.
- The fetus exhibits normal movement, and accelerations are present with fetal movement.
- The fetus is term.

Assessment of labor includes:

- Documentation of the contraction pattern
- The cervical status, including cervical position, consistency, effacement, dilatation, and station

Before administering the medication, once again ascertain whether the woman has a history of any medication reactions or allergies and provide information about the medication. (See *Teaching Highlights: What Women Need to Know About Pain-Relief Medications.*) Maternal vital signs, FHR, contraction pattern, and pain level should be assessed and documented before administering any pain medication. After giving the medication, record the medication name, dose, route, and site, as well as the woman's blood pressure (BP) and pulse, within the electronic medical record (EMR). If the woman is alone, side rails should be raised to provide safety. Assess the FHR for possible adverse effects of the medication. After the medication has been administered, document the woman's pain level, the effectiveness of the medication, and any adverse effects if they occurred.

When an analgesic medication is administered by intramuscular or subcutaneous route, it takes a few minutes for the effect to be felt. Continue with other supportive measures to enhance comfort, such as ensuring a quiet environment, providing a back rub or cool cloth, assisting with relaxation and

---

TEACHING HIGHLIGHTS | What Women Need to Know About Pain-Relief Medications

Before receiving medications, the woman should understand the following:

- Type of medication administered
- Route of administration
- Expected effects of medication
- Implications for fetus or newborn
- Safety measures needed (e.g., remain in bed with side rails up)

visualization exercises, or providing therapeutic touch until the woman feels the effect of the medication. Often, continued reassurance and verbal praise have a calming effect. When the medication begins to take effect, the woman may sleep between contractions. This short period of rest helps her relax and can restore her energy. When the physician/certified nurse midwife (CNM) orders an intravenous route, the effect of the medication will be felt within a few minutes, so if any change of position is necessary or if the woman needs to void, suggest that the woman complete these activities before receiving the medication. Some women may be so uncomfortable that they do not want anything except the medication. In this case, administering the medication first would be more helpful for the women.

Opioid Analgesics

Opioid analgesic agents that are injected into the circulation have their primary action at sites in the brain, activating the neurons that descend to the spinal cord. The opioid analgesics used in early labor are given in either intermittent doses or, less commonly, by patient-controlled administration. It is unclear if these medications work by providing an analgesic effect or by inducing sedation; however, the medications do have a quieting effect that reduces pain for the laboring woman (Anderson & Stone, 2013). See Table 19–1 for information about analgesics used in labor. Opioid analgesics should be used with caution with women with a history of substance abuse (Wong, 2014).

BUTORPHANOL TARTRATE (STADOL) AND NALBUPHINE HYDROCHLORIDE (NUBAIN)

Butorphanol tartrate (Stadol) is a synthetic agonist–antagonist opioid analgesic agent. The medication has been proven to be effective in reducing pain intensity in laboring women. Respiratory depression of both the mother and fetus or newborn can occur if given late in the first stage of labor but can be reversed with naloxone (Narcan).

The most common side effect associated with butorphanol (Stadol) is drowsiness. Dizziness, fainting, and hypotension can also occur (Wilson, Shannon, & Shields, 2014). Urinary retention following administration of butorphanol is not common but does occur. Therefore, the nurse should be alert for bladder

TABLE 19–1 Analgesics Used in Labor

DRUG/CLASS	DOSAGE, ROUTE, FREQUENCY	COMMON SIDE EFFECTS	LIFE-THREATENING REACTIONS	CONTRAINDICATIONS
Stadol (butorphanol tartrate): CNS agent, analgesic, narcotic agonist/antagonist	IM 1–2 mg every 4 hr IV 0.5–2 mg every 4 hr; rapid onset; peak: 30–60 min; duration 3–4 hr Intranasal: 1 mg (1 puff) may repeat in 90 sec (max. dose every 3–4 hr)	Sedation; sweaty, clammy skin; nausea and vomiting	Respiratory depression	Narcotic dependency, breastfeeding, women with chronic hypertension or preeclampsia
Nubain (nalbuphine hydrochloride): CNS agent analgesic, narcotic agonist	10–20 mg every 3–6 hr PRN subcutaneous IM/IV	Sedation, dizziness, fainting, hypotension, hypertension	Respiratory depression	Hypersensitivity to the drug
Demerol (meperidine hydrochloride): CNS agent, analgesic, narcotic agonist	IV 2.5–15 mg every 4 hr	Pruritus, dizziness, sedation, nausea, constipation	Respiratory depression, convulsions, cardiovascular collapse, cardiac arrest, respiratory depression in newborn, bronchoconstriction, neonatal neurotoxicity	Hypersensitivity to the drug, convulsive disorders, breastfeeding, undiagnosed acute abdomen
Fentanyl (Sublimaze): Short-acting opiate agonist, analgesic	50–100 mcg every 2 hr IV/IM IV give over 1–2 min; immediate onset; peak 30–60 min, duration limited to 30–60 min IM onset 7–15 min	Bradycardia, hypotension, nausea, vomiting, and respiratory depression	Muscle rigidity, especially in the respiratory muscles	Women with opioid dependency

distention when a woman has received butorphanol for analgesia during labor, has IV fluids infusing, and receives regional anesthesia for the birth. Butorphanol needs to be protected from light and stored at room temperature (Wilson et al., 2014).

Butorphanol is contraindicated in women taking monoamine oxidase inhibitors (MAOIs) for depression (Wilson et al., 2014).

SAFETY ALERT!

Because the most common side effect of butorphanol tartrate (Stadol) is drowsiness, the mother should be advised to remain in bed with side rails up to prevent falls or injuries after administration of the medication.

Like butorphanol, nalbuphine hydrochloride (Nubain) is a synthetic agonist–antagonist opioid analgesic and may precipitate medication withdrawal if the woman is physically dependent on opioids. It also crosses the placenta to the fetus and can cause a nonreassuring fetal heart rate and neonatal respiratory depression. In the birth setting, nalbuphine may be given directly into the tubing of a running IV infusion, and 10 mg should be administered over 3 to 5 minutes (Wilson et al., 2014). Both nalbuphine and butorphanol can have a ceiling effect where the pain reduction qualities do not increase, but the side effects increase. Nalbuphine is often the medication of choice because it is associated with less nausea and vomiting and a lower incidence of respiratory depression. Nalbuphine is also associated with increased maternal sedation, which allows the mother an opportunity to rest between contractions.

FENTANYL (SUBLIMAZE)

Fentanyl is a short-acting opiate that has been used during labor to relieve pain and induce sedation. Fentanyl is 50 to 100 times more potent than morphine. Fentanyl has less neonatal neurobehavioral depression than meperidine hydrochloride (Demerol) because it does not cross the placenta. However, neonatal depression can still occur, although at much lower rates when compared with meperidine. Fentanyl results in less sedation, nausea, vomiting, and pruritus compared with meperidine. See Table 19–1.

SAFETY ALERT!

Fentanyl has a variety of drug interactions that should be evaluated prior to administration, including CNS depressants; antipsychotics; anxiolytics; certain antihistamines such as diphenhydramine (Benadryl) and hydroxyzine (Vistaril); barbiturates; tricyclic antidepressants; high levels of alcohol; and skeletal muscle relaxants, such as cyclobenzaprine (Flexeril) and baclofen (Lioresal). Cimetidine (Tagamet) has been associated with confusion, disorientation, and seizures when given concurrently with fentanyl (Chestnut et al., 2014).

Additive Medications

The use of additive medications can decrease anxiety and increase the effectiveness of analgesics when given simultaneously. These medications, which are classified as tranquilizers, have no specific properties that decrease pain; however, they do work well to provide relief without increasing unwanted side effects. This enhancement enables the woman to receive a smaller dose of the opioid being administered. These medications can also be used to manage the unpleasant side effects,

such as nausea or vomiting, associated with the administration of opioid analgesics.

Commonly used analgesic medications include promethazine (Phenergan), hydroxyzine (Vistaril), propiomazine (Largon), and promazine (Sparine). The main side effect is sedation, which may be helpful in promoting rest in women who have had a prolonged labor or who have had little sleep; however, the effect may be undesirable to other women.

Opiate Antagonist: Naloxone (Narcan)

Because naloxone is an antagonist with little or no agonistic effect, it exhibits little pharmacologic activity in the absence of opioids. Naloxone can be used to reverse the mild respiratory depression that follows administration of small doses of opiates such as fentanyl and meperidine, as well as butorphanol tartrate and nalbuphine hydrochloride. Naloxone is the medication of choice when the depressant is unknown because it will cause no further depression (Wilson et al., 2014). An initial dose of 0.4 to 2.0 mg may be administered intravenously to the laboring woman. If the woman is nonresponsive, the medication can be readministered every 2 to 3 minutes. The nurse should be prepared to provide basic airway management, including the chin-lift/jaw-thrust maneuver, and initiation of respirations through a bag-valve-mask device when the woman is not immediately responsive and respiratory depression is occurring. It is typically administered to mothers who have received opioids within 4 hours of the birth (Wilson et al., 2014). When naloxone is given, other resuscitative measures may be indicated, and trained personnel should be readily available. The duration of the medication's effect is shorter than that of the analgesic medication for which it is acting as an antagonist, so the nurse must be alert to the return of respiratory depression and the need for repeated doses. Naloxone should not be given to women with known or suspected opiate dependency because it may precipitate severe withdrawal (Wilson et al., 2014). Naloxone may be given to the newborn if needed after birth. The newborn dose is 0.1 mg/kg and may need to be repeated if respiratory effort remains abnormal.

Regional Anesthesia and Analgesia

Regional anesthesia is the temporary loss of sensation produced by injecting an anesthetic agent (called a *local*) into direct contact with nervous tissue. Loss of sensation happens because the local agents stabilize the cell membrane, which prevents initiation and transmission of nerve impulses. The regional anesthetic blocks most commonly used in childbirth include the epidural, spinal, and combined epidural-spinal blocks. Epidural blocks may be used for analgesia during labor and vaginal birth and for anesthesia during cesarean birth.

An epidural relieves pain associated with the first stage of labor by blocking the sensory nerves supplying the uterus. Pain associated with the second stage of labor and with birth can be alleviated with epidural, combined epidural-spinal, and pudendal blocks (see Figure 19–1).

Until recently, the same anesthetic agents used for regional epidurals were also used to produce **regional analgesia** (pain relief to a body region) during labor. This practice was problematic because the anesthetic agents used alter the transmission of impulses to the bladder, making voiding difficult. The agents also interfere with blood pressure stability and leg movement.

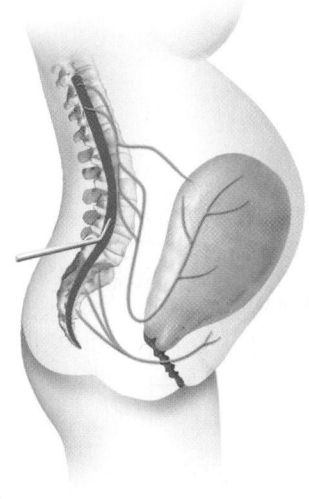
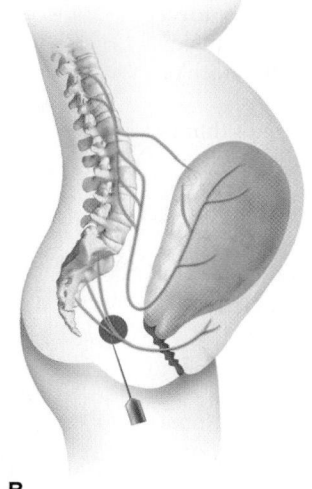
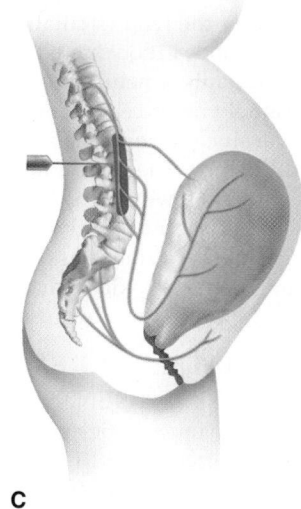

A B C

Figure 19-1 Schematic diagram showing pain pathways and sites of interruption. *A*, Lumbar sympathetic (spinal) block: relief of uterine pain only. *B*, Pudendal block: relief of perineal pain. *C*, Lumbar epidural block: dark area demonstrates peridural (epidural) space and nerves affected, and the gray tube represents a continuous plastic catheter.

The descent of the fetus is slowed and an increased risk of severe perineal lacerations occurs in primigravida women, more commonly when epidural anesthesia is used (Loewenberg-Weisband, Grisaru-Granovsky, Ioscovich, et al., 2014). In current practice, regional analgesia is now obtained by injecting an opioid such as fentanyl along with only a small amount of anesthetic agent. New medication combinations relieve the woman's pain while minimizing the side effects associated with a reduction in the urge to push (Anderson & Stone, 2013).

The intrathecal injection of opioids results in another type of regional analgesia. In this case, the opioid is injected into the subarachnoid space. It is important for the anesthesia provider to provide a test dose before giving the entire dose to determine that the catheter is correctly placed. Fentanyl citrate and preservative-free morphine are the most commonly used medications. This typically results in more effective pain relief over the subsequent 24 hours after birth, although the incidence of nausea, pruritus, and urticaria may be increased in some women (Chestnut et al., 2014).

Nursing care during administration of regional analgesia is directed toward helping the woman void before administration, assisting her with positioning during and after the procedure, monitoring and assessing vital signs and respiratory status, monitoring analgesic effect, and determining fetal well-being. Reassurance and thorough explanations help decrease anxiety and fear. Additional measures may be needed to address pruritus, nausea and vomiting, and urinary retention.

As with other procedures, the woman needs to know how the block is given, the expected effect on her and the fetus, advantages and disadvantages, and possible complications. Many women discuss possible anesthetic blocks with their healthcare provider at some point in the pregnancy. If they have not, it is important to give them an opportunity to ask questions and obtain information before receiving the block while in labor.

Anesthetic Agents for Regional Blocks

Local anesthetic agents block the conduction of nerve impulses from the periphery to the central nervous system by preventing the propagation of an action potential from the source of pain

(Chestnut et al., 2014). The types of nerve fibers are differentially sensitive to the various anesthetic agents. In general, the smaller the fiber, the more sensitive it is to local agents. For example, it is possible to block the small C and A delta fibers, which transmit pain and temperature, without blocking the larger A alpha, A beta, and A gamma fibers, which continue to maintain a sense of pressure, muscle tone, position sense, and motor function.

Absorption of local anesthetics depends primarily on the vascularity of the area of injection. The agents themselves contribute to increased blood flow by causing vasodilation. High concentrations of medications cause greater vasodilation. Good maternal physical condition or a high metabolic rate aids absorption. Malnutrition, dehydration, electrolyte imbalance, and cardiovascular and pulmonary problems increase the potential for toxic effects. The pH of tissues affects the rate of absorption, which has implications for fetal complications such as acidosis. The addition of vasoconstrictors such as epinephrine delays absorption and prolongs the anesthetic effect because vasoconstrictors decrease uteroplacental blood flow. The breakdown of local anesthetics in the body is accomplished by the liver and plasma esterase, and the resulting substance is eliminated by the kidneys. It is important to use the weakest concentration and the smallest amount necessary to produce the desired results.

Types of Local Anesthetic Agents

Two types of local anesthetic agents are currently available: esters and amides. The ester type includes procaine hydrochloride (Novocain), chloroprocaine hydrochloride (Nesacaine), and tetracaine hydrochloride (Pontocaine). Esters are rapidly metabolized; therefore, toxic maternal levels are not as likely to be reached, and placental transfer to the fetus is prevented. Ester-linked agents have a higher incidence of allergic reactions when compared with amides. However, they do not appear to have a higher incidence of fetal effects (Chestnut et al., 2014).

Amide types include lidocaine hydrochloride (Xylocaine), mepivacaine hydrochloride (Carbocaine), and bupivacaine hydrochloride (Marcaine). Amide types are more powerful and longer acting agents. They readily cross the placenta, can be measured in the fetal circulation, and affect the fetus for a prolonged period. Lidocaine has been associated with major neurologic and minor neurologic toxicity; therefore, the dose of lidocaine should not exceed 75 mg.

Ropivacaine (Naropin) is a new-generation amide that is also used in labor. The pain relief effects are similar to those of other amides. However, the blockade effect is slightly lower than other amides, thus increasing the rates of vaginal births and decreasing instrument-assisted births. Levobupivacaine (Chirocaine) has less toxicity than ropivacaine and is safer in longer surgical procedures because it has decreased toxicity.

ADVERSE MATERNAL REACTIONS TO ANESTHETIC AGENTS

Reactions to local anesthetic agents range from mild symptoms to cardiovascular collapse. Mild reactions include palpitations, tinnitus, apprehension, confusion, and a metallic taste in the mouth. Moderate reactions include more severe degrees of mild symptoms plus nausea and vomiting, hypotension, and muscle twitching, which may progress to convulsions. Severe reactions are sudden loss of consciousness, coma, severe hypotension, bradycardia, respiratory depression, and cardiac arrest. Anesthetic agents should not be used unless an intravenous line is in place.

The preferred treatment for a mild toxic reaction is administration of oxygen and IV injection of a short-acting barbiturate to diminish anxiety.

NEONATAL NEUROBEHAVIORAL EFFECTS OF ANESTHESIA AND ANALGESIA

Many studies have focused on the neurobehavioral effects on the newborn of pharmacologic agents used during labor and birth. Although analgesic and anesthetic agents may alter the behavioral and adaptive function of the newborn, physiologic factors such as hunger, degree of hydration, and time within the sleep–wake cycle may also exert an influence. In one study, women who had received epidural anesthesia had higher rates of breastfeeding cessation at 1 month postpartum than women who did not receive epidural anesthesia, even when other variables were controlled for within the study (Dozier et al., 2012). Note that more neurologic impairment occurs in the newborn resulting from the normal birth process than from epidural complications.

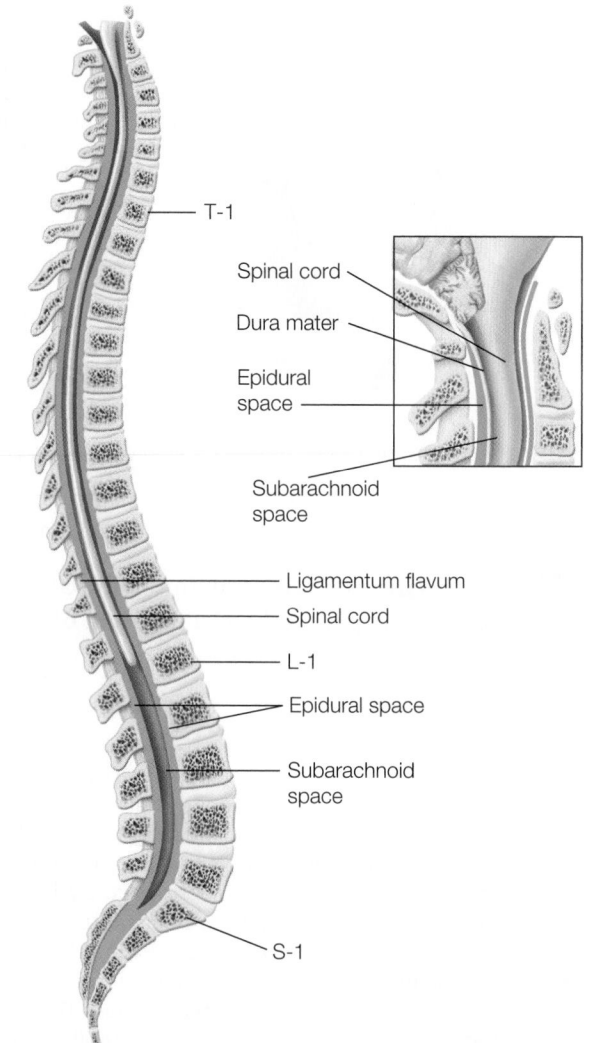

Figure 19–2 **The epidural space lies between the dura mater and the ligamentum flavum, extending from the base of the skull to the end of the sacral canal.**

Epidural Block

A lumbar **epidural block** involves injection of an anesthetic agent into the epidural space to provide pain relief throughout labor. The epidural space, a potential space between the dura mater and the ligamentum flavum, is accessed through the lumbar area (Figure 19–2). The epidural is most frequently used as a continuous block to provide analgesia and anesthesia from active labor through episiotomy repair (Figure 19–3).

Epidurals have become a relatively common method of analgesia and anesthesia during labor and birth in the United States. It is estimated that 61% of all women in the United States receive an epidural during their labor. Non-Hispanic White women had the highest rates of epidural use (68.8%) followed by non-Hispanic Black women (62.1%). Native American women used epidural anesthesia the least (42.1%). Epidural use decreases with maternal age (Osterman & Martin, 2011). An epidural can be given as soon as active labor is established.

As the childbearing population is becoming older, many pregnant women have various high-risk medical conditions. Some of these conditions create additional risk factors for the woman undergoing epidural anesthesia. Risk factors that warrant increased observation include maternal obesity, asthma,

---

Box 19-1 **Acupressure and Manual and Electrical Stimulation as a Means to Reduce Epidural Use for Labor Pain**

Acupressure with the addition of manual or electrical stimulation can reduce the risk of receiving epidural anesthesia in labor (Vixner et al., 2014). The acupressure point for labor and birth is found in the webbing between the thumb and index finger. This point should never be stimulated during pregnancy because it stimulates uterine contractions. The mother places her right thumb on the back of her left hand and her right index finger on the front of the left hand at the acupressure point. She can rub the point to stimulate labor and squeeze the point to decrease labor pain. Another acupressure point is found between the inner ankle bone and the Achilles tendon. Squeezing for 1 minute on each ankle reduces labor pain. Electrical stimulation of these sites can also be used. While these methods did not show a reduction in labor pain itself, it did reduce epidural use.

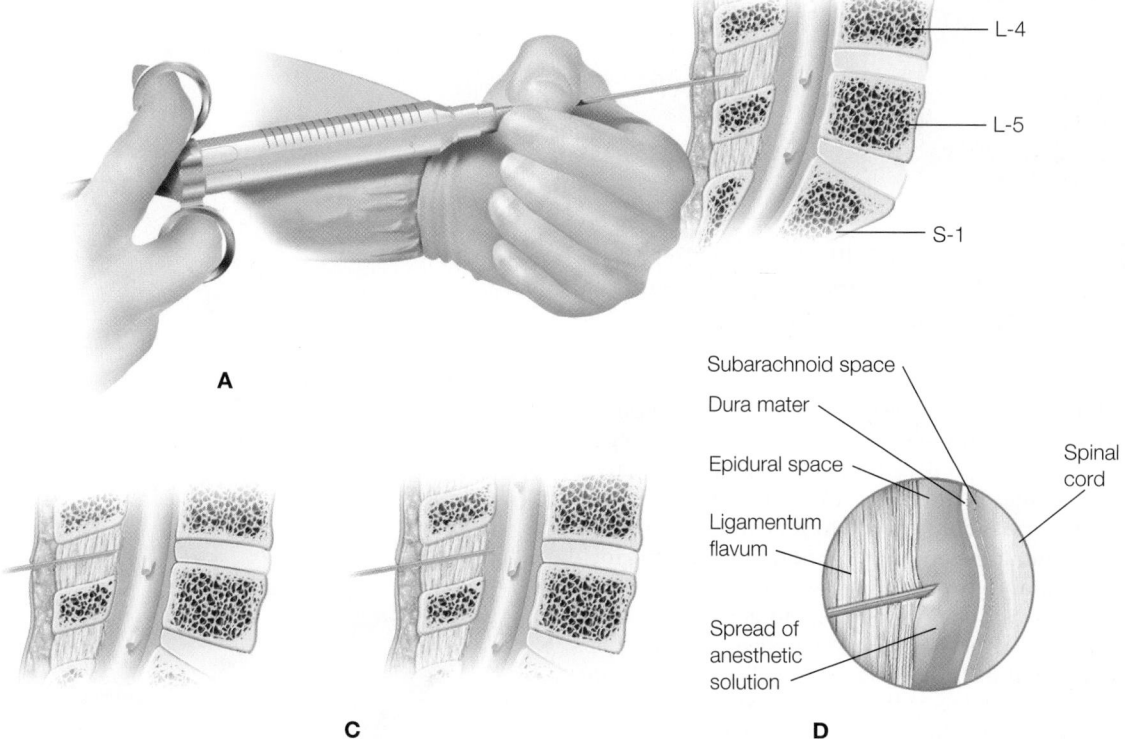

Figure 19–3 Technique for lumbar epidural block. *A*, Proper position for insertion. *B*, Needle in the ligamentum flavum. *C*, Tip of needle in epidural space. *D*, Force of injection pushing dura away from tip of needle.

obstructive sleep apnea, cardiac disease, coagulopathy, spinal cord injuries, substance abuse, and women with a history of liver disease (Wong, 2014).

ADVANTAGES

The epidural block relieves discomfort during labor and birth, and the woman is fully awake and a part of the birth process. Epidural anesthesia results in fewer adverse fetal effects when compared with intravenous analgesia or general anesthesia. It can also allow the woman to rest and regain strength before she needs to push during the second stage. The continuous epidural allows different blocking for each stage of labor, so that the fetus is able to descend and rotate in the maternal pelvis; many times the woman's urge to bear down is preserved. Epidurals that combine anesthesia and an opioid agent are often effective in providing postoperative pain relief for longer periods of time.

Opioids are used with epidural blocks for labor. Some of the agents used include morphine and fentanyl (Chestnut et al., 2014). When only opioids are used epidurally, rather than in combination with another type of agent, the amount of pain relief is not as effective, especially toward the end of labor; therefore, a combination of opioids and a low dose of local anesthesia is given (Chestnut et al., 2014).

DISADVANTAGES

The most common complication of an epidural block is maternal hypotension, which is generally prevented by administering intravenous fluid before epidural placement, left uterine displacement, and maternal positioning on her side. In some instances, labor progress and fetal descent may be slowed, and pushing efforts in the second stage may be less effective because of a decrease in sensation. There appears to be an increase in forceps or vacuum use related to epidural

anesthesia (King, Brucker, & Krebs, 2013). Delay in return of bladder sensation may result in urinary retention and the need for catheterization during labor and in the fourth stage (King et al., 2013). Low back pain can also occur after an epidural and is usually more common in women who underwent vaginal deliveries. Women with a history of prepregnancy back pain or back surgery tend to have less relief with an epidural (Wong, 2014). Typically, epidurals do not cause chronic low back pain, although the woman can have soreness at the insertion site for a few days.

CONTRAINDICATIONS

The absolute contraindications for epidural block are client refusal, infection at the site of the needle puncture, maternal problems with blood coagulation (coagulopathies), raised intracranial pressure, specific medication allergy to the agent being used, and hypovolemic shock (King et al., 2013).

Nursing Management

Assessment of the woman's knowledge level about an epidural block is essential. Before providing information, determine the woman's current knowledge and evaluate factors related to learning, such as primary language spoken, ability to hear and interpret information, and the presence of anxiety. Although the nurse is an integral person in providing information, the anesthesia provider is the essential person to provide information and to obtain written informed consent.

In preparation for the epidural, encourage the woman to empty her bladder because the block may interfere with her ability to void. Assess the woman's pain level, maternal blood pressure, pulse, respirations, and FHR to determine that normal parameters are present and to establish a baseline. Continuous electronic fetal monitoring to assess fetal status and frequent

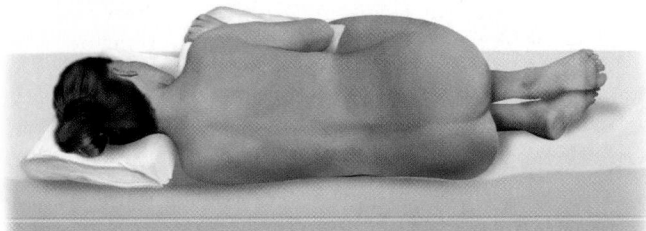

Figure 19–4 Correct maternal positioning. The back is straight and vertical, the shoulders are square, and the upper leg is prevented from rolling forward.

monitoring of maternal blood pressure and pulse for hypotension are essential. An intravenous infusion is usually begun with an 18-gauge plastic indwelling catheter. A large-gauge catheter is used so that IV fluids can be administered quickly if hypotension occurs. A bolus of 500 to 1000 mL of IV fluid is given before beginning the epidural block to decrease the incidence of hypotension.

Either of two positions can be used to achieve epidural placement: side-lying or sitting. The side-lying position is less commonly used, but if the side-lying position is used, assist the woman to move to the edge of the bed, where the mattress is firmer and provides more support. Support the woman's head with a small pillow so it remains in alignment with the spine. A pillow may also be placed in front of her chest to provide support for her upper arm. Her back needs to remain straight, with the shoulders square. Her legs are bent and her knees kept together so that the upper hip does not roll forward and cause the spine to twist (Figure 19–4).

The block may also be given with the woman in a sitting position, with her back flexed and her feet supported on a stool (Figure 19–5). Advise the woman to push her back toward the anesthesia provider. Typically, the nurse stands directly in front of the woman with hands placed on the woman's shoulders. The woman is encouraged to arch her back and push back toward the analgesia provider. After positioning, continue to provide support and try to ensure that the woman does not move during the procedure. After the needle and catheter are placed, assist the woman into a reclining position.

Clinical Tip

Advise the woman to identify when uterine contractions are occurring. Tell her that the nurse monitors contractions and will notify the anesthesia provider when a contraction is starting. Reassure her that the anesthesiologist will administer the injection between contractions when she is comfortable. Provide encouragement and reposition the woman as needed after a contraction occurs, since it is common for the woman to slouch during intense uterine contractions.

Assess maternal vital signs frequently per protocol until the block wears off. Blood pressure can be monitored by a mechanical blood pressure device or directly by you. Record vital signs on the fetal monitor strip and/or on the client record. Encourage the woman to maintain a side-lying position to maximize uteroplacental blood flow and to change her position (from side to side) frequently to increase circulation, promote comfort, and avoid a one-sided block. Assess the woman's ability to lift her legs and her level of sensation every 30 minutes to monitor the effects of the nerve block.

Assess the woman's bladder for distention at frequent intervals because the epidural block decreases the urge to urinate.

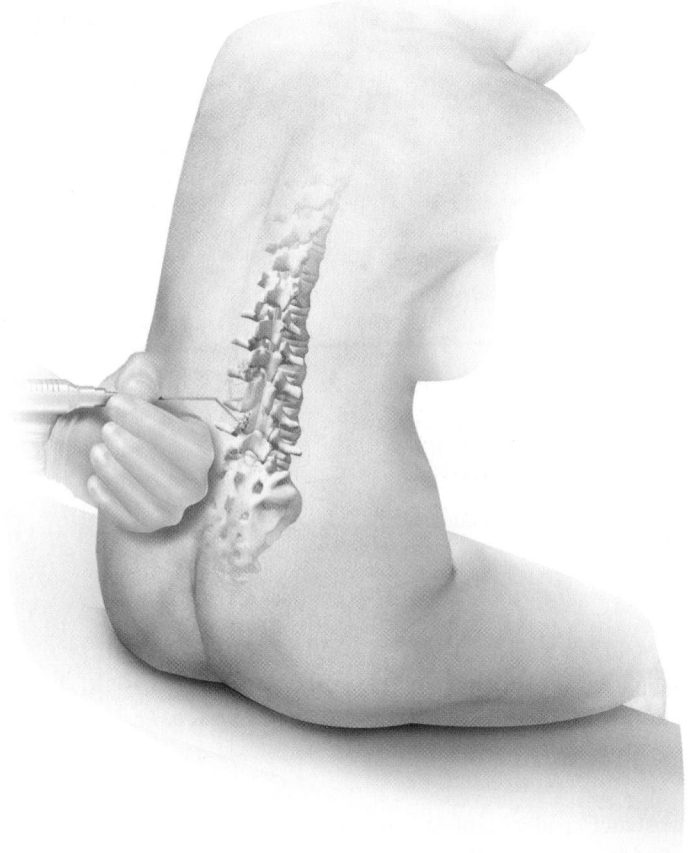

Figure 19–5 Correct sitting position for woman having an epidural anesthesia block: shoulders rolled forward and back exposed for needle insertion.

During the second stage of labor, the woman with an epidural block may need assistance with pushing. You may need to tell the woman when contractions begin and give extra assistance by holding her legs during pushing efforts. The woman's legs need to be protected from pressure applied to them while sensation is diminished. If the woman has little or no control of her legs, stirrups may be needed to avoid injury.

The most common side effect of epidural regional block is hypotension. The risk can be minimized by a preload fluid bolus of crystalloid solution (Gabbe et al., 2012). If hypotension occurs, increase the IV flow rate (to increase intravascular volume and raise the blood pressure), ensure or verify left uterine displacement (to increase circulation), and administer oxygen (to improve oxygenation). If blood pressure is not restored in 1 to 2 minutes, ephedrine 5 to 10 mg IV is administered (Gabbe et al., 2012). After ephedrine is administered, the blood pressure is continually monitored and the maternal and fetal responses are recorded.

The epidural may cause elevation of maternal temperature (pyrexia). Pyrexia may be confused with maternal infection and frequently results in additional testing of the newborn to rule out infection (Gabbe et al., 2012).

Headache (which may occur with spinal blocks) is not a side effect of epidural anesthesia because the dura mater of the spinal canal has not been penetrated and there is no leakage of spinal fluid. Motor control of the legs is weak but not totally absent after birth. Return of complete sensation and the ability to control the legs are essential before ambulation is attempted. Recovery may take several hours, depending on the anesthetic agent and the dose given.

To assess sensation, touch various parts of the woman's legs and abdomen bilaterally to determine if the touch can be felt. Evaluate motor control by asking the woman to raise her knees, to lift her feet (one at a time) off the bed, or to dorsiflex her foot. Even though assessments may indicate that sensation and motor control have returned, be ready to support the woman's weight as she stands and quickly return her to bed if motor control is inadequate. In addition, blood pressure assessments will help to determine the safety of ambulation. Assess blood pressure while the woman is lying down, then sitting in the bed. As long as blood pressure values remain stable (no evidence of orthostatic hypotension), a standing blood pressure is assessed. To maintain safety, it is advisable to have additional assistance when the woman stands for the first time. See Assisting With and Caring for the Woman With an Epidural During Labor in the *Clinical Skills Manual* SKILLS.

Women With Special Needs Spinal Cord Injury

Women with a spinal cord injury may be prone to autonomic dysreflexia, the most significant medical complication, especially when their injury is above T5 through T6 level. This condition is attributed to a loss of hypothalamic control of sympathetic spinal reflexes and occurs in clients with viable spinal cord segments distal to the level of injury. Epidural anesthesia is recommended as a means to decrease autonomic dysreflexia and should be introduced early in labor to reduce the incidence of this complication.

Continuous Epidural Infusion

Epidural anesthesia may be given with a continuous infusion pump. Some of the benefits include good to excellent analgesia, infrequent nausea, minimal sedation, decreased anxiety, earlier mobilization, retained cough reflex, decreased risk of deep vein thrombosis, decreased myocardial oxygen demand, and ease of administration. A continuous infusion reduces the use of bolus dosages, which may provide intermittent pain control.

Ease of administration does not imply lack of need for close observation. Malfunctioning equipment with subsequent overdose is always a possibility. Fortunately, infusion pumps designed specifically for use in epidural anesthesia have safety factors incorporated. Continuous epidural infusions should be administered with the same precautions used for intermittent injections.

Some of the potential problems of epidural infusions include breakthrough pain, sedation, nausea and vomiting, pruritus, and hypotension. Breakthrough pain may occur at any time during the epidural infusion but usually occurs when the infusion rate of the agent is below the recommended therapeutic rate. It may also occur when the infusion pump rate is altered or the integrity of the epidural line is broken. When breakthrough pain occurs, the nurse checks the integrity of the epidural infusion line and notifies the analgesia provider. There may be standing orders for treatment of breakthrough pain, but it is best to inform the analgesia provider of any problems that occur. Often, breakthrough pain can be corrected with a bolus dose of medication. In rare circumstances, the epidural itself may need to be replaced.

Some women may experience *hot spots*, or areas of incomplete anesthesia coverage. Nursing interventions include position changes. If the hot spot becomes too uncomfortable, an anesthesia provider can administer additional medication. In some cases, the epidural will need to be replaced.

General sedation and resulting respiratory depression may occur from the systemic effect of the epidural agents as they are absorbed into the circulation. The respiratory rate, along with the quality of respirations, should be assessed no less frequently than every 15 to 30 minutes. The nurse should notify the anesthetist of any significant decreases in respiratory rate or respiratory pattern change. If the respiratory rate decreases below 12 respirations per minute, naloxone may be given to counteract the effect of the anesthetic agent; typically respirations then return to a normal rate.

Nausea and vomiting can occur at any time during or after epidural infusion. The nurse should give an antiemetic if one is ordered and notify the analgesia provider. The nausea and vomiting can make the woman very uncomfortable, and the infusion rate of the epidural may need to be decreased or terminated to alleviate this discomfort. Nausea and vomiting can sometimes occur as a result of transition rather than as a direct side effect of the epidural infusion.

Pruritus (itching and rash) may occur at any time during the epidural infusion. It usually appears first on the face, neck, or torso and is usually the result of the agent in the epidural infusion. Treatment generally involves administration of diphenhydramine hydrochloride (Benadryl). If no standing order exists, the nurse notifies the anesthetist and identifies the problem. The epidural infusion may need to be decreased or terminated.

Hypotension may occur from hypovolemia or from the effect of the epidural. Treatment involves administering oxygen by mask, administering a bolus of crystalloid fluid, and notifying the anesthetist. Usually standing orders for treatment of hypotension are graded in terms of the degree of hypotension. The epidural infusion may have to be terminated and the woman placed in the Trendelenburg position.

Epidural Opioid Analgesia After Birth

To provide analgesia for approximately 24 hours after the birth, the analgesia provider may inject an opioid, such as morphine sulfate (Duramorph) or fentanyl (Sublimaze), into the epidural space immediately after the birth. The analgesic effect begins approximately 30 to 60 minutes after the injection. The side effects include pruritus, nausea and vomiting, and urinary retention (Wilson et al., 2014). The onset seems to occur early, and it resolves within 14 to 16 hours after the birth.

Spinal Block

In a **spinal block**, a local anesthetic agent is injected directly into the spinal fluid in the spinal canal to provide anesthesia for cesarean birth and occasionally for vaginal birth. This technique involves passing through the epidural space and dura mater and injecting the medication directly into the cerebral spinal fluid. The technique of administration varies depending on whether the spinal block is being given for a cesarean or vaginal birth (Figure 19–6).

ADVANTAGES

The advantages of spinal block are immediate onset of anesthesia, relative ease of administration, a need for smaller medication volume, and maternal compartmentalization of

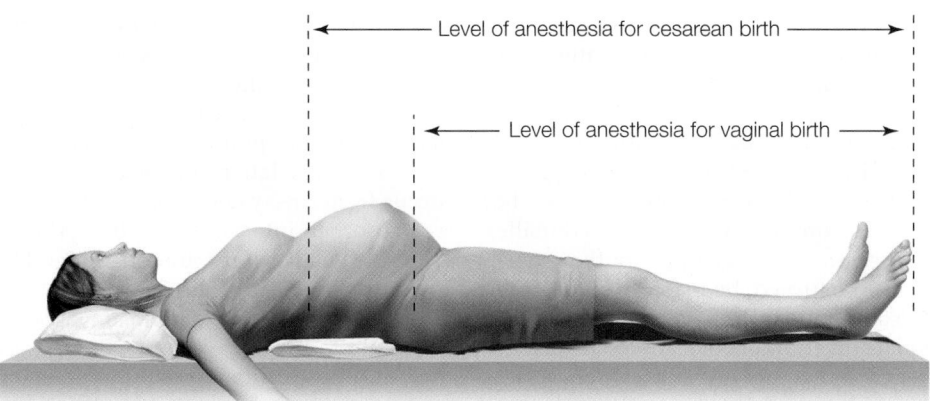

Level of anesthesia for cesarean birth

Level of anesthesia for vaginal birth

Figure 19–6 Levels of spinal anesthesia for vaginal and cesarean births.

the medication. This approach is favored when an emergency cesarean birth is rapidly needed and anesthesia is immediately warranted.

DISADVANTAGES

The primary disadvantage of spinal block is blockade of sympathetic nerve fibers, resulting in a high incidence of hypotension; maternal hypotension may lead to alterations in the fetal heart rate and fetal hypoxia. In addition, uterine tone is maintained, which makes intrauterine manipulation difficult.

CONTRAINDICATIONS

Contraindications for spinal block include severe hypovolemia, infection over the puncture site, sepsis, coagulation problems, and client refusal (Suresh, Segal, Preston, et al., 2013).

Nursing Management

If an intravenous infusion is not already in place, it is started with a 16- to 18-gauge plastic catheter. A bolus of 500 to 1000 mL is infused rapidly. Assess maternal vital signs, pain level, and the FHR to establish a baseline and then position the woman in a sitting (or a side-lying) position. The woman sits on the side of the bed or operating room table and places her feet on a stool. She places her arms between her knees or up around your shoulders, places her head to her chest, and arches her back to widen the intervertebral spaces. Support the woman in this position and palpate the uterus to identify the beginning of uterine contractions (if labor is present). The analgesia provider injects the anesthetic agent between contractions. If the anesthetic agent is injected during a contraction, the level of anesthesia obtained is higher and may compromise respirations.

The woman remains in a sitting position for 30 seconds and then returns to a lying position, with a rolled towel or blanket under her right hip to displace the uterus from the vena cava. Monitor maternal blood pressure and pulse frequently per protocol or physician's order. The blood pressure is also reassessed when the woman is moved after birth because movement may lower blood pressure.

If the spinal block is being used during vaginal birth, monitor uterine contractions and instruct the woman to bear down during a contraction. The block may reduce the woman's ability to push, although the new combinations of medications tend to decrease this side effect. Sometimes, the birth may be assisted with forceps or vacuum extractor (see Chapter 22).

After birth, the temporary motor paralysis of the woman's legs continues. Exercise caution when moving the woman from the birthing bed (or operating room table) to protect her from

injury. The woman remains in bed for 6 to 12 hours following the block; she may not regain sensation and control of her bladder for 8 to 12 hours and may need to be catheterized. An indwelling bladder catheter is usually inserted before surgery for women undergoing cesarean birth.

The epidural or spinal catheter is removed by either you or an analgesia provider. Remove the tape used to secure the block. Then grasp the catheter between your fingers and slowly remove with gentle traction. Inspect the catheter to ensure the tip did not break off. Place a bandage or gauze and tape over the site. It is not unusual for a small amount of bleeding to occur initially upon removal. Continuous bleeding warrants a call to the anesthesia provider. Document removal of the catheter and any adverse effects.

Combined Spinal-Epidural Block

Spinal anesthesia may be combined with an epidural block. The combined spinal-epidural (CSE) block can be used for labor analgesia and for cesarean birth. The anesthetic and analgesic agents used differ according to the purpose of the CSE block. A CSE is accomplished by inserting an epidural needle into the epidural space. A narrow-gauge atraumatic (24- to 27-gauge pencil point) needle is inserted through the epidural needle, through the dura, and into the cerebral spinal fluid. A small amount of local anesthetic agent, opioid, or both is injected, and the atraumatic needle is withdrawn. An epidural catheter is then threaded through the epidural needle and into the epidural space. The epidural needle is removed, and the epidural catheter is secured.

An advantage of CSE block is that the spinal (intrathecal) anesthetic and/or analgesic agent has a faster onset than medications that are injected into the epidural space. Most medications are used in low dose, so spinal analgesia may be given in early labor to assist in alleviating labor pain. The epidural is activated when active labor begins. Another advantage of a CSE block is that laboring women can ambulate after the CSE is placed.

SAFETY ALERT!
Advise women with a CSE in place always to have assistance during ambulation to prevent falls.

Pudendal Block

A **pudendal block**, administered by a transvaginal method, intercepts signals to the pudendal nerve (Figure 19–7). The pudendal block provides perineal anesthesia for the latter part

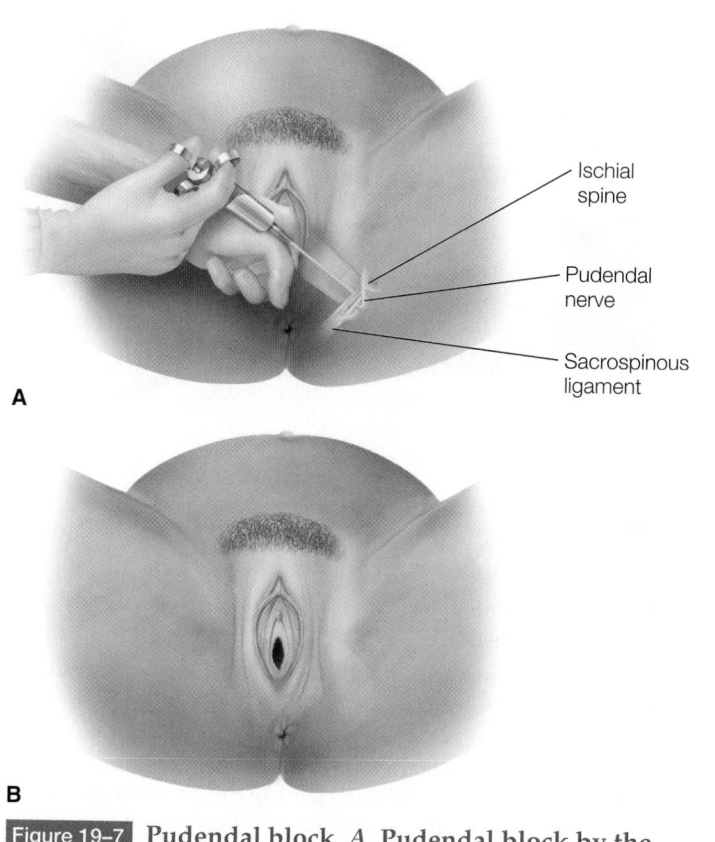

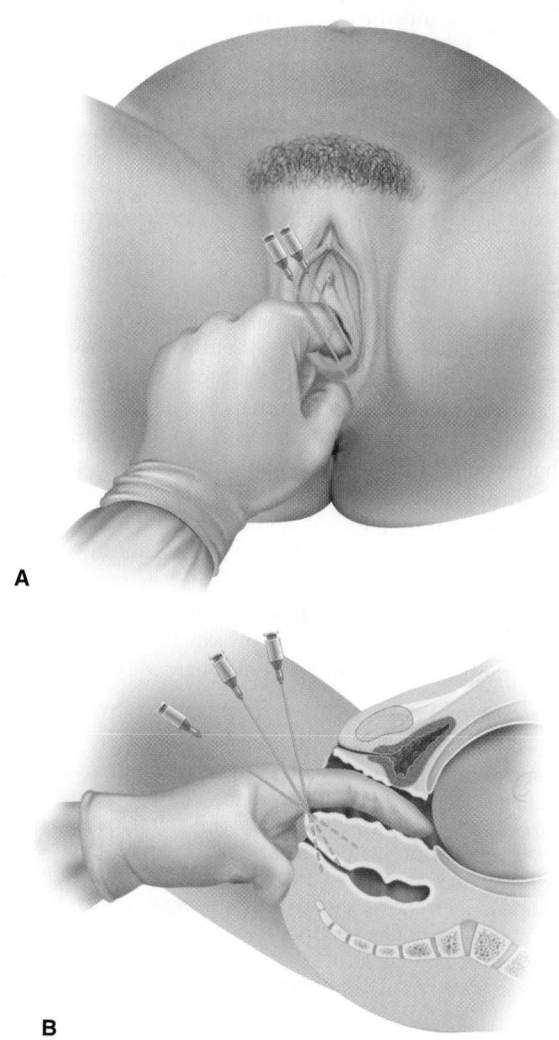

Figure 19–7 Pudendal block. *A*, Pudendal block by the transvaginal approach. *B*, Area of perineum affected by pudendal block.

Figure 19–8 Local infiltration anesthesia. *A*, Technique of local infiltration for episiotomy and repair. *B*, Technique of local infiltration showing fan pattern for the fascial planes.

of the first stage of labor, the second stage, birth, and episiotomy repair. The pudendal block relieves the pain of perineal distention and typically relieves pain in the lower vagina, vulva, and perineum but not the discomfort of uterine contractions (King et al., 2013).

Advantages of the pudendal block are ease of administration and absence of maternal hypotension. It also may be used to decrease the discomfort of low forceps or vacuum-assisted birth. Because a pudendal block does not alter maternal vital signs or FHR, additional assessments are not necessary. The nurse explains the procedure and answers any questions.

The disadvantages of the pudendal block include possible broad ligament hematoma, perforation of the rectum, and trauma to the sciatic nerve. A moderate dose of anesthetic agent has minimal ill effects on the course of labor, but the urge to push may decrease.

Local Infiltration Anesthesia

Local infiltration anesthesia is accomplished by injecting an anesthetic agent into the intracutaneous, subcutaneous, and intramuscular areas of the perineum (Figure 19–8). It is generally used at the time of birth, both in preparation for an episiotomy, if one is needed, and for the episiotomy repair. Women who have followed some type of prepared childbirth method and want minimal analgesia and anesthesia usually do not object to local anesthesia for the episiotomy or laceration repair. The administration procedure is technically uncomplicated and is practically free from complications.

A disadvantage of local infiltration is that large amounts of local anesthetic must be used to infuse the tissues. Although any local anesthetic may be used, chloroprocaine hydrochloride

(Nesacaine), lidocaine hydrochloride (Xylocaine), tetracaine hydrochloride (Pontocaine), and mepivacaine hydrochloride (Carbocaine) are the agents of choice because of their capacity for diffusion. Because local anesthetic agents have no effect on maternal vital signs or FHR, additional assessments are unnecessary.

General Anesthesia

Occasionally, **general anesthesia** (induced unconsciousness) may be needed for cesarean birth. The method used to achieve general anesthesia is usually a combination of intravenous injection and inhalation of anesthetic agents. Maternal complications include difficulty in maternal intubation resulting in increased incidence of vomiting and aspiration, increased blood loss because of uterine relaxation, and possible difficulty remembering events in the early postpartum period (Gabbe et al., 2012).

A common fetal complication is fetal depression. The depression in the fetus is directly proportional to the depth and duration of the anesthesia. Babies born to mothers who have received general anesthesia have lower 1-minute Apgar scores and a higher incidence of metabolic acidosis than those who are given regional anesthesia for an emergency cesarean birth (Vanita, Kajal, Babita, et al., 2011). General anesthesia is not advocated when the fetus is considered to be at high risk, particularly in preterm birth.

Nitrous oxide is an inhaled anesthesia agent that has been used in the United Kingdom for decades as an option for pain control in laboring women. Its use is beginning to gain acceptance in the United States and will likely increase in the future.

Nursing Management

Because pregnancy results in decreased gastric motility, and the onset of labor halts the process almost entirely, food eaten hours earlier may remain undigested in the stomach. It is important to find out when the laboring woman last ate and record this information on the client's medical record and anesthesia record. Even when food and fluids have been withheld, the gastric juice produced during fasting is highly acidic and can cause chemical pneumonitis if aspirated. Prophylactic antacid therapy to reduce the acidic content of the stomach before general anesthesia is common practice. A nonparticulate antacid (such as sodium citrate/citric acid), H2-receptor antagonists (such as cimetidine [Tagamet] or famotidine [Pepcid]), or the use of prokinetic medications (such as metoclopramide), may also help empty gastric contents.

Clinical Tip

Some women may wake from general anesthesia with an awareness of events that occurred during a cesarean birth. A small number of women experience unpleasant thoughts or nightmares as a result. If a woman expresses anxiety or states she has unpleasant memories of the birth, the nurse should encourage her to discuss her feelings and the experiences she remembers. The analgesia provider and physician should be notified so they can establish a therapeutic dialogue with the woman. Some women may have to be referred for counseling to prevent or treat posttraumatic stress disorder.

Before induction of anesthesia, place a wedge under the woman's right hip to displace the uterus and prevent vena caval compression in the supine position. The woman should also be preoxygenated with 3 to 5 minutes of 100% oxygen.

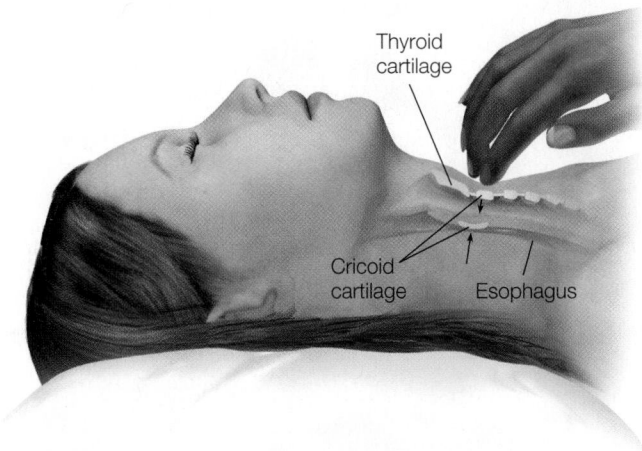

Figure 19–9 Cricoid pressure technique. Proper position for fingers in applying cricoid pressure until a cuffed endotracheal tube is placed by the analgesia provider or certified nurse-anesthetist. The cricoid cartilage is depressed 2 to 3 cm posteriorly so that the esophagus is occluded.

Intravenous fluids are started so that access to the intravascular system is immediately available. During the preparation, counsel the woman on what to expect and explain that the baby will have limited exposure to the anesthetic agents.

During the process of rapid induction of anesthesia, apply cricoid pressure to occlude the esophagus and prevent possible aspiration; the esophagus is occluded by applying 1 to 2 kg before the loss of consciousness and increasing that to 2 to 4 kg after the induction of anesthesia. The amount of pressure applied is critical because too much pressure can result in difficulty in performing a successful intubation. Too little pressure can result in aspiration. Cricoid pressure is maintained until the anesthesia provider has placed the endotracheal tube and indicates that the pressure can be released. Figure 19–9 shows the appropriate technique.

Focus Your Study

- The goal of systemic analgesia is to provide maximum pain relief with minimum risk to the mother and fetus after cervical dilatation has occurred and maternal and fetal vital signs are stable.

- Systemic drug administration may cause fetal respiratory depression at birth if given too late in labor. Naloxone (Narcan) should be available at birth to treat respiratory depression in the newborn.

- Epidural anesthesia is an injectable anesthetic agent whose administration requires a preload intravenous bolus with a crystalloid solution that then results in little to no sensation below the uterus.

- Because of the numbness caused by epidural anesthesia, reduced pushing during the second stage and inability to urinate may occur. Urinary catheterization may be needed to facilitate bladder emptying as a result of a reduction in sensation.

- Women receiving epidural anesthesia require frequent blood pressure monitoring along with monitoring when a position change occurs to detect hypotension, a side effect that can lead to fetal hypoxia. Evaluation of motor and sensory sensation is also required.

- Continuous epidural anesthesia provides effective pain relief and is usually associated with less nausea and a greater ability to cough, although it is sometimes associated with breakthrough pain, sedation, itching, hypotension, and respiratory depression.

- Spinal blocks utilize a local anesthetic agent that is injected directly into the spinal column resulting in immediate onset, thus making the level of anesthesia dependent on the level of administration. Spinal anesthesia can be administered higher for cesarean birth or lower for vaginal birth.

- The use of spinal anesthesia requires frequent blood pressure monitoring since hypotension can occur which can lead to fetal hypoxia. The woman's legs must be protected for 8 to 12 hours after birth because of decreased movement and reduced sensation.

- Women receiving spinal anesthesia typically have an indwelling urinary catheter because of decreased bladder sensation and tone.

- A pudendal block uses a local anesthesia at the end of labor that is directly injected into the pudendal nerve to produce anesthesia to the lower vagina, vulva, and perineum without having any effect on the labor or the fetus.

- Pudendal blocks can be associated with several complications including hematoma, perforation of the rectum, and trauma to the sciatic nerve.

- Local infiltration anesthesia is typically injected in laboring women prior to birth if an episiotomy is anticipated or for the repair of a laceration or episiotomy after birth.

- Local infiltration requires large amounts of anesthetic and only provides pain relief at the site of insertion; it has no maternal or fetal side effects.

- Regional anesthesia, either spinal or epidural, is associated with maternal hypotension, bladder distention, less ability to effectively push in second stage, higher perineal laceration rates, and possible neurologic damage.

- While spinal anesthesia can result in a severe headache, epidural anesthesia can result in an elevated maternal temperature.

- General anesthesia for obstetric use is rare; however, its use necessitates a variety of interventions including obtaining a history of last oral consumption; administering prescribed medications, such as antacids; placing a wedge under the mother's right hip; providing oxygen prior to the start of surgery; ensuring patent intravenous access; and possible assistance to the anesthesia provider in applying cricoid pressure during endotracheal tube placement.

- General anesthesia can result in fetal depression, uterine relaxation, vomiting, and aspiration.

Clinical Reasoning in Action

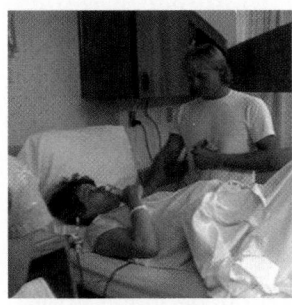

Sandra, a 26-year-old G1P0, is in active labor when she presents to you at the birthing center. She has been in labor for 5 hours and is clearly tired and seems to be having difficulty coping with the pain. Her contractions are occurring every 2 to 4 minutes, lasting 50 to 60 seconds, and are moderate to strong in intensity. You assess the fetal heart rate of 120 to 130 beats/min with early decelerations; moderate variability is present. Sandra's vital signs are stable and her laboratory results are within normal limits. She is requesting an epidural analgesia

for pain control. A vaginal examination demonstrates the cervix is 100% effaced, 6 cm dilated with the vertex at 0 station in the left occiput transverse (LOT) position. You notify the physician of Sandra's wish for pain relief and labor progress. You review the client's record for written consent for regional analgesia and assist the anesthesia provider with the procedure.

1. Discuss the advantages of regional analgesia.
2. Describe the nursing responsibility during the administration of regional analgesia.
3. Discuss the side effects of regional analgesia.
4. What are the absolute contraindications for an epidural block?
5. How do you assist Sandra with the second stage of labor when she cannot feel her contractions?

References

Anderson, B. A., & Stone, S. E. (2013). *Best practices in midwifery: Using the evidence to implement care*. New York, NY: Springer Publishing Company.

Blackburn, S. T. (2013). *Maternal, fetal, & neonatal physiology*. (4th ed.). Maryland Heights, MO: Elsevier.

Chestnut, D. H., Wong, C. A., Tsen, L. C., Kee, W. D. N., Beilin, Y., & Mhyre, J. (2014). *Chestnut's obstetric anesthesia: Principles & practice: Expert consult*. Philadelphia, PA: Saunders.

Dozier, A. M., Howard, C. R., Brownell, E. A., Wissler, R. N., Glanz, J. C., Ternullo, S. R., ... Laurence, R. A. (2012). Labor epidural anesthesia, obstetrical factors, and breastfeeding cessation. *Maternal and Child Health Journal*, 17(4), 689–698. doi:10.1007/s10995-012-1045-4

Gabbe, S. G., Niebyl, J. R., Galan, H., Jauniaux, E. R. M., Landon, M., Simpson, J. L., & Driscoll, D. (2012).

Obstetrics: Normal & problem pregnancies (6th ed.). Philadelphia, PA: Saunders.

King, T., Brucker, M., & Krebs, J. (2013). *Varney's midwifery* (5th ed.). Boston, MA: Jones & Bartlett.

Loewenberg-Weisband, Y., Grisaru-Granovsky, S., Ioscovich, A., Samueloff, A., & Calderon-Margalit, R. (2014). Epidural analgesia and severe perineal tears: A literature review and large cohort study. *Journal of Maternal-Fetal and Neonatal Medicine*, 27(17). doi:10.3109/14767058.2014.889113.

Osterman, M. J. K., & Martin, J. A. (2011). Epidural and spinal anesthesia use during labor: 27-state reporting area, 2008. *National Vital Statistics Reports*, 59(5), 1–14.

Suresh, M. S., Segal, B. S., Preston, R. L., Fernando, C., & Mason, L. (2013). *Shnider & Levinson's anesthesia for obstetrics* (5th ed.). Philadelphia, PA: Lippincott, Williams, & Wilkins.

Vanita, A., Kajal, J., Babita, G., Jaswinder, K., & Saurabh, D. (2011). Best neonatal outcome following emergency cesarean delivery in nonreassuring fetal heart rate: General or a low-dose spinal anesthesia. *Journal of Obstetric Anaesthesia and Critical Care*, 1(2), 67–72.

Vixner, L., Schytt, E., Stener-Victorin, E., Waldenstrom, U., Pettersson, H., & Martensson, L. B. (2014). Acupuncture with manual and electrical stimulation for labour pain: A longitudinal randomised controlled trial. *BMC Complementary and Alternative Medicine*, 14, 187. doi:10.1186/1472-6882-14-187

Wilson, B. A., Shannon, M. T., & Shields, K. L. (Eds.). (2015). *Pearson's nurse's drug guide: 2016*. Upper Saddle River, NJ: Prentice Hall.

Wong, C. (2014). Anesthesia in high-risk obstetrics. *Global Library of Women's Medicine*. doi 10.3843/glowm.10217

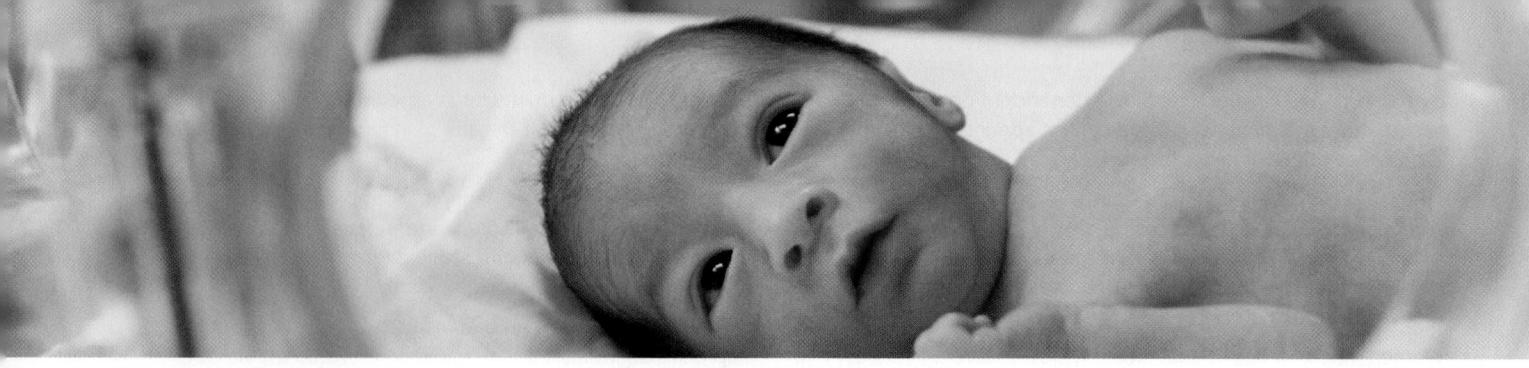

Chapter 20
Childbirth at Risk: Prelabor and Intrapartum Complications

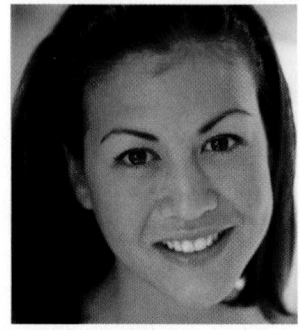

When I learned that we were going to have twins I was stunned. How would we ever manage? Our daughters were born 2 weeks early but both weighed over 5 pounds and did well. The early days were far from easy, especially breastfeeding. I was always tired, and it seemed that at least one of the girls was always awake. But they shared a room and after a while they got on the same schedule. That made things easier. They are 2 years old now and such amazing little people. Marcel and I feel that we are blessed with double joy!

—Monique, 31

Ryan McVay/Getty Images

∨ Learning Outcomes

20.1 Explain the possible causes, risk factors, and clinical therapy for premature rupture of the membranes or preterm labor in determining the nursing management of the woman and her fetus/newborn.

20.2 Compare placenta previa and abruptio placentae, including implications for the mother and fetus, as well as nursing care.

20.3 Explain cervical insufficiency and describe its clinical therapy.

20.4 Explain the maternal and fetal/neonatal implications and the clinical therapy in determining the nursing management of the woman with multiple gestation.

20.5 Compare the identification, maternal and fetal/neonatal implications, clinical therapy, and nursing management of the woman with hydramnios and oligohydramnios.

After the first trimester, the majority of pregnancies progress smoothly to term. In some cases, however, complications can occur before the onset of labor that significantly impact the outcome of pregnancy. This chapter presents content related to the most common of these conditions. Labor-related complications are discussed in Chapter 21.

Care of the Woman With Premature Rupture of Membranes

Premature rupture of membranes (PROM) is spontaneous rupture of the membranes before the onset of labor. PROM affects approximately 8% to 10% of all pregnancies.

Preterm PROM (PPROM), which affects approximately 2% to 4% of all pregnancies, is the rupture of membranes occurring before 37 weeks' gestation (Jazayeri, 2014). Although the exact cause is unknown, PPROM and PROM are associated with:

- Infection
- Previous history of PPROM/PROM
- Hydramnios
- Multiple pregnancy
- Urinary tract infection (UTI)
- Amniocentesis
- Placenta previa
- Abruptio placentae
- Trauma
- Cervical insufficiency
- History of laser conization or loop electrosurgical excision procedure (LEEP)
- Bleeding during pregnancy
- Maternal genital tract anomalies
- Reduced mean platelet volume in the first trimester (Ekin, Gezer, Kulhan, et al., 2014)

Maternal risk is related to infection, specifically *chorioamnionitis* (intra-amniotic infection resulting from bacterial invasion before birth). In addition, abruptio placentae occurs more frequently in women with PROM. Other rare complications include retained placenta and hemorrhage, maternal sepsis, and maternal death.

Fetal/neonatal implications include:

- Risk of respiratory distress syndrome (with PPROM)
- Fetal sepsis caused by ascending pathogens
- Malpresentation
- Prolapse of the umbilical cord
- Nonreassuring fetal heart rate tracings
- Compression of the umbilical cord related to oligohydramnios
- Premature birth
- Increased perinatal morbidity and mortality

PROM that occurs at term is associated with favorable outcomes. Gestations from 32 to 36 weeks generally have favorable outcomes, although there may be some complications caused by prematurity. In general, neonates born before 32 weeks have some complications, including respiratory distress syndrome (RDS), necrotizing enterocolitis, intraventricular hemorrhage, and sepsis. The earlier the gestational age, the greater the likelihood of neonatal complications (Hanna & Kiefer, 2012).

Clinical Therapy

A sterile speculum examination is done to detect the presence of amniotic fluid in the vagina. If fluid is not obviously pooling, information can be gained by using Nitrazine paper, which turns deep blue when amniotic fluid is present. Because certain bacterial pathogens can also result in a positive Nitrazine test, a microscopic examination (ferning test) should be used to confirm a rupture. It is considered a definitive test. Digital examination increases the risk of infection and is not recommended until a management plan has been determined.

EVIDENCE-BASED PRACTICE | Antibiotics for Premature Rupture of Membranes

Clinical Question
Should antibiotics be used to prevent infection after premature rupture of membranes?

The Evidence
Premature rupture of membranes is linked to a higher risk of infection for the mother and potential morbidity for the baby. However, antibiotics carry the risks of potential maternal anaphylaxis and bacterial resistance and should not be used unless evidence supports clear benefit for both mother and neonate. Two Cochrane Reviews were conducted on the use of antibiotics for PROM; one review focused on pregnancies that were near term (37+ weeks) and the other focused on preterm (less than 37 weeks). Cochrane Reviews are systematic reviews of randomized trials that are highly structured and peer reviewed. These reviews form the strongest level of evidence for practice.

No clear benefit was determined for mothers or babies for the administration of antibiotics when the pregnancy was near term (Wojcieszek, Stock, & Flenady, 2014). These studies encompassed nearly 3000 women and demonstrated that there was a higher surgical birth rate in those women who were administered antibiotics without clear demonstrated benefit for

mother or child. The reverse was true for PROM in pregnancies of less than 37 weeks' duration. These mothers had a lower rate of infection, a longer pregnancy, and better neonatal outcomes (Kenyon, Boulvain, & Neilson, 2013). The risk of perinatal death was not affected by the administration of antibiotics in either group. No clear direction was given for the specific antibiotic that was best, although one—co-amoxiclav—should be avoided because it was associated with subsequent necrotizing enterocolitis in neonates.

Best Practice
The use of antibiotics for treatment of PROM depends on the term of the pregnancy. They are not helpful for those women whose pregnancy has passed 37 weeks and no clear benefit emerges. For women with pregnancies of less than 37 weeks' duration, both maternal and neonatal outcomes are improved when antibiotics are administered.

Clinical Reasoning
What education can be provided to the parents to support using a full round of antibiotics for early PROMs? What side effects should the nurse observe for when administering antibiotics to these women?

Fetal well-being is assessed through a fetal heart rate (FHR) tracing or biophysical profile (BPP). In addition, the gestational age of the fetus is calculated to develop a management plan. The gestational age of the fetus and the presence or absence of infection determine the direction of treatment for PROM. If maternal signs and symptoms of infection are evident, antibiotic therapy (usually by intravenous infusion) is begun immediately, and the fetus is born vaginally or by cesarean regardless of the gestational age. Prophylactic antibiotics are often administered for the first 48 hours while awaiting culture results. Upon admission to the nursery, the newborn is assessed for sepsis and placed on antibiotics. (Chapter 27 provides further information about the newborn with sepsis.)

Management of PPROM in the absence of infection and gestation of less than 37 weeks is usually conservative. The woman is hospitalized on bed rest. On admission, complete blood cell count (CBC), C-reactive protein, and urinalysis are obtained, as are cultures, including chlamydia, gonorrhea, and group B streptococcus. An ultrasound is done to determine gestational age, amniotic fluid level, and fetal well-being. Continuous electronic fetal monitoring may be ordered at the beginning of treatment but usually is discontinued after a few hours unless the fetus is estimated to be very low birth weight (VLBW) or if the tracing is of concern. Regular non-stress tests (NSTs) or biophysical profiles are used to monitor fetal well-being. (These tests are discussed in Chapter 13.) Maternal blood pressure, pulse, temperature, and FHR are assessed every 4 hours. Regular laboratory evaluations are done to detect maternal infection. Vaginal examinations are avoided to decrease the chance of infection. As the gestation approaches 34 weeks, fetal lung maturity studies are indicated (see Chapter 13).

Maternal corticosteroid administration promotes fetal lung maturity and helps to prevent respiratory distress syndrome and other complications. Currently, a single course of corticosteroids is recommended. Repeat courses of corticosteroids should not be routinely used because they have not been shown to improve neonatal outcomes and are associated with an increased incidence of chorioamnionitis (Gyamfi-Bannerman et al., 2012). Research has not yet determined whether a repeat dose at 30 to 32 weeks may help stimulate alveoli that were not formed when the initial dose was given (Gyamfi-Bannerman et al., 2012). Administration of corticosteroids to late preterm newborns has not been shown to produce clinical benefits (Gyamfi-Bannerman et al., 2012).

The use of magnesium sulfate is now a standard of care and is administered to women with premature rupture of membranes occurring between 23 6/7 and 31 6/7 weeks' gestation. Magnesium sulfate is administered for its neuroprotective benefits, which has resulted in a reduction of cerebral palsy in newborns who received the drug regimen prior to birth. The loading dose is 4 to 6 g, which is then followed by 2 g/hr for at least 12 hours or until birth occurs. If birth does not occur within 24 hours, the medication is stopped. Indications to resume additional doses include progression to preterm labor (American College of Obstetricians and Gynecologists [ACOG], 2012).

Healthy People 2020

(MICH-1.5) Reduce the rate of postneonatal deaths (between 28 days and 1 year)

(MICH-8.1) Reduce low birth weight (LBW)

(MICH-8.2) Reduce very low birth weight (VLBW)

Health Promotion Reducing Risk of Infection During Pregnancy

Pregnant women should avoid all individuals with a history of recent infection, rashlike illness, fever, or unknown illnesses to reduce their risk of acquiring infection during pregnancy.

Nursing Management
For the Woman With Premature Rupture of Membranes

Nursing Assessment and Diagnosis

Perform a careful assessment that includes the following:

- Determine the duration of the rupture of the membranes.
- Ask the woman when her membranes ruptured and when labor began.
- Determine gestational age to prepare for the possibility of a preterm birth.
- Observe the mother for signs and symptoms of infection, especially by reviewing her white blood cell (WBC) count, temperature, pulse rate, and the character of her amniotic fluid.
- Assess for maternal fever and hydration status.
- Assess the coping abilities of the woman and her partner, specifically if a preterm birth is anticipated.
- Determine if the woman and her partner have attended childbirth education classes.

Nursing diagnoses that may apply to a woman with PROM include the following (NANDA-I © 2014):

- *Gas Exchange, Impaired,* in the fetus related to compression of the umbilical cord secondary to prolapse of the cord
- *Coping, Ineffective,* related to unknown outcome of the pregnancy
- *Anxiety,* related to unknown birth outcomes
- *Childbearing Process, Risk for Ineffective,* related to potential preterm birth and maternal infection

Planning and Implementation

Nursing actions should focus on the woman, her partner, and the fetus:

- Monitor for and report signs of infection to the physician or certified nurse-midwife (CNM).
- Evaluate uterine activity and fetal response to the labor, but vaginal examinations are not done unless absolutely necessary because this increases the risk of infection.
- Encourage the woman to rest on her side to promote optimal uteroplacental perfusion. Use comfort measures to help promote rest and relaxation.
- Ensure that hydration is maintained, particularly if the woman's temperature is elevated.

Education is another important aspect of nursing care. The woman and her partner, if he or she is involved, need to understand the implications of PROM and all treatment methods. It is important to address side effects and alternative treatments. The couple needs to know that although the membranes are ruptured, amniotic fluid continues to be produced.

| TEACHING HIGHLIGHTS | Explaining Amniotic Membranes |

To help a laboring woman and her family understand how the amniotic membranes provide protection, use a color chart that shows a side view of the fetus in the uterus with the membranes intact. Ask them to visualize what would happen if the membranes rupture. They will be able to see that pathogens have direct access to the uterus, increasing the risk of infection. They will also see that, when the membranes rupture and the fluid escapes, the cord could "wash out" with the fluid and become trapped between the pelvis and fetal head, causing cord compression.

Providing psychologic support for the couple is critical:

- Help reduce anxiety by listening empathetically, relaying accurate information, and providing explanations of procedures.

- Prepare the couple for a cesarean birth, a preterm newborn, and the possibility of fetal or newborn demise as may be necessary.

- Initiate consultation with the neonatologist or pediatric healthcare provider to give the woman and her partner an opportunity to ask questions if a preterm birth is anticipated.

Evaluation

Expected outcomes of nursing care include the following:

- The woman's risk of infection and of cord prolapse decrease.

- The couple is able to discuss the implications of PROM and all treatments and alternative treatments.

- The couple verbalizes understanding that they did not cause the event.

- The pregnancy is maintained without trauma to the mother or fetus.

Care of the Woman at Risk Because of Preterm Labor

Labor that occurs between 20 and 36 completed weeks of pregnancy is called **preterm labor (PTL)**. (Postterm labor is discussed in Chapter 21.) Prematurity continues to be the number one perinatal and neonatal problem in the United States, with 11.4% of all live births occurring prematurely (March of Dimes, 2015). This statistic has improved over the last several years. Slight improvement was noted in women who smoke, uninsured women, and in later preterm births (March of Dimes, 2015). Native American women continue to have the highest rates of preterm birth (March of Dimes, 2015). Often, PTL is related to multiple risk factors; only rarely is there a single cause. Table 20–1 presents a list of risk factors for spontaneous preterm labor.

Maternal implications of PTL include psychologic stress related to the baby's condition and physiologic stress related to medical treatment for preterm labor.

Fetal/neonatal implications include increased morbidity and mortality, especially caused by respiratory distress syndrome (RDS), increased risk of trauma during birth, and

TABLE 20–1 Risk Factors for Spontaneous Preterm Labor

Abdominal surgery during second or third trimester	Abdominal trauma
Abortion, first trimester—more than two	Abortion—second trimester
Age (less than 17 or over 35 years)	Anemia
Bacterial vaginosis, *Escherichia coli* (ascending intrauterine infection)	Bleeding after 12 weeks
Cervical cerclage in situ	Cervical insufficiency
Cervical shortening/1 cm	Cervix dilated/1 cm at 32 weeks
Cigarettes—more than 10/day	Clotting disorders
Diethylstilbestrol (DES) exposure	Diabetes
Domestic violence	Febrile illness
Fetal abnormality	Foreign body (e.g., intrauterine device [IUD])
History of cone biopsy	History of pyelonephritis or other maternal infection
Hydramnios	Hypertension (preeclampsia, gestational hypertension, chronic hypertension)
In vitro fertilization (singleton or multiple gestation)	
Low socioeconomic status	Low maternal weight
Non-White race	Multiple gestation
Periodontal disease	Obesity
Prenatal care: inadequate or none	Poor weight gain
Previous preterm labor with term birth	Previous preterm birth
Sexually transmitted infection (STI) (trichomoniasis, chlamydial infection)	Prolonged standing or lifting
Stress	Social support, lack of
Time between pregnancies—less than 6–9 months	Substance abuse
Uterine irritability	Uterine anomaly
	Uteroplacental ischemia

maturational deficiencies (fat storage, heat regulation, immaturity of organ systems).

Clinical Therapy

All women should receive education on the risk for PTL and be taught to recognize its symptoms. If any symptoms are present, women should be told to notify their physician/CNM immediately. Prompt diagnosis is necessary to stop preterm labor before it progresses to the point where intervention is ineffective. Women at increased risk of PTL should be evaluated for signs and symptoms at each prenatal visit.

SAFETY ALERT!

Because of the risk of adverse maternal and fetal outcomes, labor is not interrupted if one or more of the following conditions are present: severe preeclampsia or eclampsia, chorioamnionitis, hemorrhage, maternal cardiac disease, poorly controlled diabetes mellitus or thyrotoxicosis, maternal bleeding with hemodynamic instability, maternal contraindications to tocolytics (agent specific), severe abruptio placentae, fetal anomalies incompatible with life, fetal death, nonreassuring fetal status, or fetal maturity.

Tocolysis is the use of medications in an attempt to stop labor. Drugs currently used as tocolytics include the β-adrenergic agonists (also called β-mimetics), cyclooxygenase (prostaglandin synthetase) inhibitors, and calcium channel blockers such as nifedipine (Procardia). Because of adverse fetal effects, the use of cyclooxygenase (prostaglandin synthetase) inhibitors are rarely used because they may cause neonatal adverse effects, oligohydramnios, and constriction of the ductus arteriosus (Simhan & Caritis, 2015). The β-mimetics terbutaline sulfate (Brethine) and magnesium sulfate were once the most widely used tocolytics but are now commonly being replaced with calcium channel blockers, such as nifedipine. Nifedipine has potential side effects as well, including the following (Wilson, Shannon, & Shields, 2015):

- Lightheadedness or dizziness
- Flushing sensation
- Headache
- Weakness
- Nausea
- Gastrointestinal upset

Other possible side effects are rare but may include muscle cramps, tremor, peripheral edema, nervousness, palpitations, respiratory symptoms, and nasal congestion (Wilson et al., 2015).

Although tocolytic drugs suppress uterine contractions and allow pregnancy to continue, they may cause maternal side effects; the most serious is maternal pulmonary edema. While reducing the dose and duration of therapy sometimes reduces the side effects, long-term use of terbutaline sulfate (Brethine) is no longer considered the standard of care. Because of risk of maternal morbidity, other medications are commonly used for long-term management.

Side effects of β-adrenergic agonists (also called β-mimetics) may include:

- Maternal peripheral vasodilatation resulting in hypotension
- Maternal tachycardia
- Fetal tachycardia

- Maternal hypoglycemia
- Fetal hypoglycemia
- Maternal cardiac dysrhythmia
- Maternal pulmonary edema

The selection of magnesium sulfate, calcium channel blockers, or β-mimetics also depends on the experience of the healthcare providers. Although some practitioners use a cocktail approach, using various drugs concurrently, there are no established guidelines or procedures for combination use. Detailed research trials that examine the effectiveness of a multipharmacologic approach are needed. Some drugs should not be concurrently used, such as magnesium sulfate and nifedipine (Procardia). In current practice, magnesium sulfate is no longer recommended for preterm labor but is recommended for neuroprotection of the preterm fetus.

If the provider is administering magnesium sulfate for neuroprotection, the dosage is 4–6 g in 100 mL of IV fluid followed by 2 g/hr for 12 hours or until birth occurs. If the preterm labor is stopped, additional administration should be given if preterm labor begins again and if additional cervical change has been documented. The protocol includes administration up to 24 hours if birth has not occurred prior to that time (ACOG, 2012).

Health Promotion **Risk Factors for Preterm Labor**

Women should discontinue all use of alcohol, tobacco, and drugs. They are risk factors for preterm labor and birth.

Side effects with the loading dose may include:

- Flushing; feeling warm
- Headache
- Nystagmus
- Nausea
- Dizziness
- Lethargy; sluggishness
- Pulmonary edema

Fetal side effects may include hypotonia and lethargy that persists for 1 or 2 days following birth. Respiratory depression in the newborn can also occur (ACOG, 2014).

One calcium channel blocker, nifedipine (Procardia), is becoming increasingly popular in treating preterm labor because it is easily administered orally or sublingually and has few serious maternal side effects. It decreases smooth muscle contractions by blocking the slow calcium channels at the cell surface. The most common side effects are related to arterial vasodilation and include hypotension, tachycardia, facial flushing, and headache. Nifedipine may be coadministered with the β-mimetics.

SAFETY ALERT!

Nifedipine should *not* be used with magnesium because both drugs block calcium and simultaneous administration has been implicated in serious maternal side effects related to low calcium levels.

TEACHING HIGHLIGHTS | Preterm Labor

- Describe the dangers of preterm labor, especially the risk of prematurity in the neonate, and all the potential problems.
- Explain that many of the early symptoms of labor, such as backache and increased bloody show, may be subtle initially.
- Summarize self-care measures (see Table 20–2) the woman can take to prevent preterm labor.
- Teach the woman how to palpate for uterine contractions. Demonstrate and ask for a return demonstration.

Progesterone supplementation is another form of treatment that has been an effective management tool in reducing preterm births in women with a history of at least one preterm birth at less than 34 gestational weeks. Use of progesterone is considered appropriate in singleton pregnancies when there is a past history of PROM or PTL in a previous pregnancy and may be considered in women with a shortened cervical length. It is not routinely administered to women who are asymptomatic with a multiple gestation (Norwitz & Caughey, 2011). The use of hydroxyprogesterone caproate (Makena) injection was approved by the Food and Drug Administration (FDA) in 2011 as a weekly injection, beginning between 16 and 21 weeks. It is used to prevent preterm labor in women with a history of at least one preterm birth. Hydroxyprogesterone caproate is not indicated for women with a multiple gestation (FDA, 2011).

The use of magnesium sulfate treatment has been used for neuroprotection in women with preterm newborns and has been found to offer protection against the development of cerebral palsy (discussed previously in PPROM section). When magnesium sulfate is given, it should be administered following strict hospital policy because it warrants intensive maternal and fetal monitoring (ACOG, 2012).

Corticosteroids (typically betamethasone or dexamethasone) should be administered antenatally to any women at risk for preterm birth because of their beneficial effect on preventing neonatal respiratory distress syndrome (RDS), intraventricular hemorrhage (IVH), necrotizing enterocolitis (NEC), and neonatal mortality (ACOG, 2014). Women who are candidates for tocolysis are candidates for antenatal corticosteroids, regardless of fetal gender, race, or availability of surfactant therapy for the newborn, especially between 24 and 34 weeks' gestation. Betamethasone is primarily used and should be administered in two intramuscular doses. When dexamethasone is used, four doses are given.

Nursing Management

For the Woman With Preterm Labor

Nursing Assessment and Diagnosis

During the antepartum period, identify the woman at risk for preterm labor by noting the presence of risk factors. During the intrapartum period, assess the progress of labor and the physiologic impact of labor on the mother and fetus.

Nursing diagnoses that may apply to the woman with preterm labor include the following (NANDA-I © 2014):

- *Fear* related to risk of early labor and birth
- *Coping, Ineffective,* related to need for constant attention to pregnancy
- *Pain, Acute,* related to uterine contractions

Planning and Implementation

COMMUNITY-BASED NURSING CARE

Once the woman at risk for preterm labor has been identified, she needs to be taught about the importance of recognizing the onset of labor (see *Teaching Highlights: Preterm Labor*).

Periodic telephone calls by a home care nurse are also a common part of care. During these phone visits it is important to assess the symptoms of preterm labor and to review fetal movement counting, as well as assessing the woman's emotional state. Perinatal depression occurs in a significant number of women and is more common in women with pregnancy complications. A formal screening tool should be used to assess depression. Women with a history of depression are at a greater risk for preterm birth (Davidson, 2012). Provide information about support groups and other community resources for women at risk for preterm birth.

Teaching the woman to be aware of the signs and symptoms of preterm labor is a primary objective. She should be alert for the following:

- Uterine contractions that occur every 10 minutes or less, with or without pain
- Mild menstrual-like cramps felt low in the abdomen
- Constant or intermittent feelings of pelvic pressure that feel like the baby pressing down
- Rupture of membranes
- Constant or intermittent low, dull backache
- A change in the vaginal discharge (an increase in amount, a change to more clear and watery, or a pinkish tinge)
- Abdominal cramping with or without diarrhea

Teach the woman to evaluate contraction activity once or twice a day. She does so by lying down tilted to one side with a pillow behind her back for support. The woman places her fingertips on the fundus of the uterus, which is above the umbilicus (navel). She checks for contractions (hardening or tightening in the uterus) for about 1 hour. It is important for the pregnant woman to know that uterine contractions occur occasionally throughout the pregnancy. However, if they occur every 10 minutes for 1 hour, the cervix could begin to dilate, and labor could ensue.

Ensure that the woman knows when to report signs and symptoms. If contractions occur every 10 minutes (or more frequently) for 1 hour, if any of the other signs and symptoms are present for 1 hour, or if clear fluid begins leaking from the vagina, the woman should telephone her physician/CNM, clinic, or hospital birthing unit and make arrangements to be checked for ongoing labor. Healthcare givers need to be aware that the woman's call must be taken seriously. When a woman is at risk for preterm labor, she may have many episodes of contractions and other signs or symptoms. If she is treated positively, she will feel freer to report problems as they arise.

TABLE 20–2 Self-Care Measures to Prevent Preterm Labor

- Rest two or three times a day lying on your left side.
- Drink 2–3 qt of water or fluid each day. Avoid caffeine drinks. Filling a quart container and drinking from it will eliminate the need to keep track of numerous glasses of fluid.
- Empty your bladder at least every 2 hr during waking hours.
- Avoid lifting heavy objects. If small children are in the home, work out alternatives for picking them up, such as sitting on a chair and having them climb on your lap.
- Avoid prenatal breast preparation such as nipple rolling or rubbing nipples with a towel. This is not meant to discourage breastfeeding but to avoid the potential increase in uterine irritability.
- Pace necessary activities to avoid overexertion.
- Curtail or eliminate sexual activity that involves nipple stimulation or leads to orgasm.
- Find pleasurable ways to help compensate for limitations of activities and boost the spirits.
- Try to focus on 1 day or 1 week at a time rather than on longer periods of time.
- If on bed rest, get dressed each day and rest on a couch rather than becoming isolated in the bedroom.

Source: Prepared in consultation with the Prematurity Prevention Program at the University of Washington Medical Center.

Preventive self-care measures are also important. You have a vital role in communicating the self-care measures described in Table 20–2.

HOSPITAL-BASED NURSING CARE

Supportive nursing care is important to the woman in preterm labor during hospitalization. This care consists of promoting bed rest, monitoring vital signs (especially blood pressure and respirations), measuring intake and output, and continuous monitoring of fetal heart rate (FHR) and uterine contractions. Place the woman on her left side to facilitate maternal–fetal circulation. Keep vaginal examinations to a minimum. If medications are being used, administer them and monitor the mother and fetus for any adverse effects.

Whether preterm labor is arrested or proceeds, the woman and her partner, if involved, experience intense psychologic stress. The primary aim of the nurse is to decrease the anxiety level associated with the risk of having a preterm newborn by providing emotional support. It is important to recognize the stress of prolonged bed rest and lack of sexual contact and to help the couple find satisfactory ways of dealing with those stresses. With empathetic communication, it is possible to assist the woman and her partner to express their feelings, which commonly include guilt and anxiety, thereby helping them identify and implement coping mechanisms. Keep them informed about the labor progress, the treatment regimen, and the status of the fetus. In the event of imminent vaginal or cesarean birth, the woman or couple should be offered brief but ongoing explanations to prepare them for the actual birth process and the events following the birth. Arrange for consultations with the neonatologist or pediatrician to assist the woman and her partner in anticipating potential neonatal complications and risks for the newborn.

Evaluation

Expected outcomes of nursing care include the following:

- The woman is able to discuss the cause, identification, and treatment of preterm labor.

- The woman states that she feels comfortable in her ability to cope with her situation and has resources available to her.
- The woman can describe appropriate self-care measures and can identify characteristics that need to be reported to her caregiver.
- The woman successfully gives birth to a healthy baby.

Healthy People 2020

(MICH-9.1) Reduce total preterm births

(MICH-9.2) Reduce late preterm or live births at 34 to 36 weeks of gestation

(MICH-9.3) Reduce live births at 32 to 33 weeks of gestation

(MICH-9.4) Reduce very preterm or live births at less than 32 weeks of gestation

Care of the Woman at Risk Because of Bleeding During Pregnancy

Bleeding during pregnancy always requires assessment. The most common causes of bleeding during the first and second trimesters (i.e., spontaneous abortion, ectopic pregnancy, and gestational trophoblastic disease) are addressed in Chapter 15. The three most clinically significant causes of bleeding in the second half of pregnancy, placenta previa and abruptio placentae, as well as cervical insufficiency, are discussed here. Other placental problems are addressed in Chapter 21. Bleeding that occurs after 12 gestational weeks increases the risk of pregnancy complications such as preterm birth. Bleeding during pregnancy decreases uterine perfusion and reduces fetal oxygenation, which can result in nonreassuring fetal status.

Placenta Previa

In **placenta previa**, the placenta is implanted in the lower uterine segment rather than the upper portion of the uterus. This implantation may be on a portion of the lower segment or over the internal cervical os. As the lower uterine segment contracts and dilates in the later weeks of pregnancy, the placental villi are torn from the uterine wall, exposing the uterine sinuses at the placental site. Bleeding begins, but because its amount depends on the number of sinuses exposed, initially it may be either scanty or profuse. Placenta previa is categorized (Figure 20–1) as being (Cunningham et al., 2014):

- *Low lying:* The placenta is implanted in the lower uterine segment in proximity to but not covering the os.
- *Partial:* The internal os is partially covered.
- *Marginal:* The edge of the placenta is covered.
- *Complete:* The internal os is completely covered.

The cause of placenta previa is unknown. Statistically, it occurs in 0.3% to 0.5% of all women in the United States (Joy, 2015). Women of African descent and Asian women may be at higher risk, although there is conflicting research in this area. Women who have undergone a prior cesarean birth are at higher risk for placenta previa. The risk further increases the numbers of cesarean births. Advanced maternal age has been identified as a risk factor with increased risk being directly correlated to increases in maternal age (Joy, 2015).

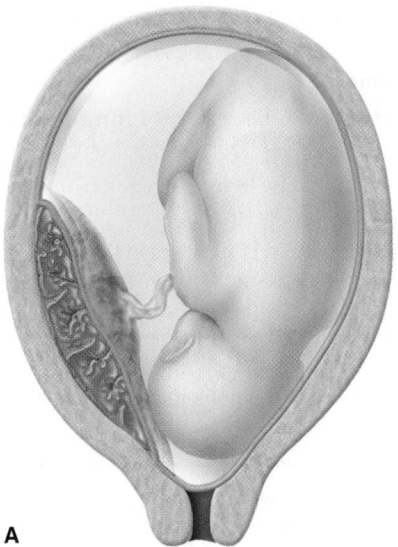
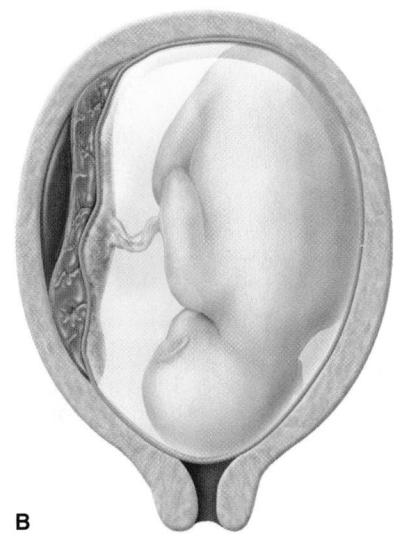
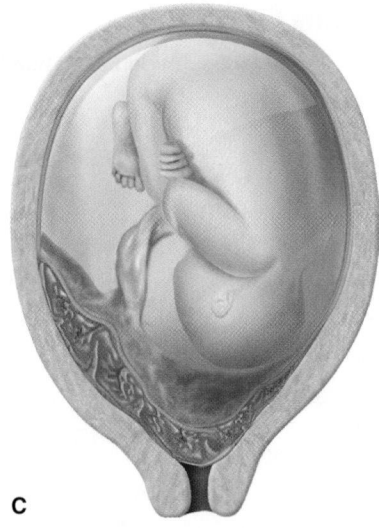

A   B   C

Figure 20–1 Classification of placenta previa. *A*, Low-lying placental implantation. *B*, Marginal placenta previa. *C*, Complete placenta previa.

FETAL/NEONATAL IMPLICATIONS

The prognosis for the fetus depends on the extent of placenta previa. In cases of a marginal previa or a low-lying placenta, the woman may be allowed to labor. Changes in the fetal heart rate (FHR) and meconium staining of the amniotic fluid may be apparent. In a profuse bleeding episode, the fetus is compromised and suffers some hypoxia. FHR monitoring is imperative when the woman is admitted, particularly if a vaginal birth is anticipated because the presenting part of the fetus may obstruct the flow of blood from the placenta or umbilical cord. If nonreassuring fetal status occurs, cesarean birth is indicated. Women who are diagnosed with a complete or partial previa will undergo a cesarean birth because the risk of intrapartum hemorrhage is high. After birth, blood sampling should be done to determine whether the intrauterine bleeding episodes of the woman have caused anemia in the newborn.

CLINICAL THERAPY

The goal of medical care is to identify the cause of bleeding and to provide treatment that will ensure birth of a mature newborn. Indirect diagnosis is made by localizing the placenta through tests that require no vaginal examination, such as a transabdominal ultrasound scan. Until placenta previa is ruled out, vaginal examinations should never be performed on a woman with bleeding because the examiner's fingers could perforate the placenta if cervical dilatation has occurred. Once placenta previa is ruled out, a vaginal examination can be performed with a speculum to determine the cause of bleeding (such as cervical lesions).

The differential diagnosis of placental or cervical bleeding takes careful consideration. Partial separation of the placenta may also present with painless bleeding, and true placenta previa may not demonstrate overt bleeding until labor begins, thus confusing the diagnosis.

Care of the woman with painless late-gestational bleeding depends on (1) the week of gestation during which the first bleeding episode occurs and (2) the amount of bleeding. If the pregnancy is less than 37 weeks' gestation, expectant management is used to delay birth until about 37 weeks' gestation to allow the fetus time to mature. Expectant management involves the following:

1. Providing bed rest with bathroom privileges as long as the woman is not bleeding
2. Performing no vaginal examinations
3. Monitoring blood loss, pain, and uterine contractility
4. Evaluating FHR with an external fetal monitor
5. Monitoring maternal vital signs
6. Performing a complete laboratory evaluation: hemoglobin, hematocrit, Rh factor, and urinalysis
7. Providing intravenous fluid (lactated Ringer solution)
8. Having 2 units of cross-matched blood available for transfusion

If frequent, recurrent, or profuse bleeding persists, or if fetal well-being appears threatened, a cesarean birth may be needed. See Table 20–3 for assessment and management of placenta previa.

Nursing Management

For the Woman With Placenta Previa

Nursing Assessment and Diagnosis

Assessment of the woman with placenta previa must be ongoing to prevent or treat complications that are potentially lethal to the mother and fetus. Painless, bright-red vaginal bleeding is the most accurate diagnostic sign of placenta previa. If this sign develops during the last 3 months of pregnancy, placenta previa should always be considered until ruled out by ultrasound examination. The first bleeding episode is generally scanty. If no vaginal examinations are performed, it often subsides spontaneously. However, each subsequent hemorrhage is more profuse.

The uterus remains soft; if labor begins, it relaxes fully between contractions. The FHR usually remains stable unless profuse hemorrhage and maternal shock occur. As a result of the placement of the placenta, the fetal presenting part is often unengaged, and transverse lie is common.

TABLE 20–3 Assessment and Management of Placenta Previa

Gestation Less Than 37 Weeks	
Assessment	**Management/Action**
Bleeding stopped	Bed rest
No uterine contractions	Vital signs every 4 hr
No abdominal pain	Provide IV fluids
Non-stress test (NST) reactive	Type and cross-match blood
	Monitor client closely
Assessment	**Management/Action**
Bleeding begins again	Cesarean birth
or	
Labor has begun	
or	
Maternal vital signs decline	
or	
Fetal status is nonreassuring	
Assessment	**Management/Action**
Complete previa	Cesarean birth
Gestation More Than 37 Weeks	
Assessment	**Management/Action**
Bleeding minimal or stopped	Induction of labor possible if:
Reassuring fetal status	Low-lying or marginal previa
	Cervix is ripe
	Cephalic presentation
	Fetal head down in pelvis
Assessment	**Management/Action**
Bleeding continues	Cesarean birth
or	
Complete previa	

Source: Data from Posner, G., & Black, A. (2013). Oxorne & Foote human labor and birth. (6th ed.). Philadelphia, PA: McGraw-Hill.

It is important to assess blood loss, pain, and uterine contractility both subjectively and objectively. Maternal vital signs and the results of blood and urine tests provide additional data about the woman's condition. Evaluate the FHR with continuous external fetal monitoring. Observe and verify the family's ability to cope with the anxiety associated with an unknown outcome.

Nursing diagnoses that may apply include the following (NANDA-I © 2014):

- *Fluid Volume: Deficient,* related to hypovolemia secondary to excessive blood loss
- *Gas Exchange, Impaired,* of the fetus related to decreased blood volume and maternal hypotension
- *Anxiety* related to concern for own personal status and the baby's safety

Planning and Implementation

Monitor the woman and her fetus to determine the status of the bleeding and the responses of the mother and baby. Do the following tasks:

- Take vital signs.
- Record intake and output.

- Perform ongoing continuous fetal monitoring.
- Perform ongoing continuous uterine activity monitoring with external tocodynamometer.
- Prepare a whole-blood setup to be ready for intravenous infusion.
- Establish a patent intravenous line before caregivers undertake any invasive procedures.
- Monitor maternal vital signs every 15 minutes in the absence of hemorrhage and every 5 minutes with active hemorrhage.

Clinical Tip

The amount of bleeding from the vagina is not a reliable guide to the degree of placental separation.

Provision of emotional support for the family is an important nursing care goal. During active bleeding, the assessments and management are directed toward physical support. However, emotional aspects need to be addressed simultaneously. Explain the assessments and treatment measures needed. Provide time for questions, and act as an advocate in obtaining information for the family. Emotional support can also be offered by staying with the family and using touch.

Promotion of neonatal physiologic adaptation is another important nursing responsibility. Check the newborn's hemoglobin, cell volume, and erythrocyte count immediately and then monitor them closely. The newborn may require oxygen, administration of blood, and admission into a special-care nursery.

Evaluation

Anticipated outcomes of nursing care include the following:

- The cause of hemorrhage is recognized promptly and corrective measures are taken.
- The woman's vital signs remain in the normal range.
- Any other complications are recognized and treated early.
- The family understands what has happened and the implications and associated problems of placenta previa.
- The woman and her baby have a safe labor and birth.

Abruptio Placentae

Abruptio placentae is the premature separation of a normally implanted placenta from the uterine wall. Premature separation, the leading cause of perinatal mortality, is considered a catastrophic event because of the severity of the resulting hemorrhage. The incidence of abruptio placentae is 0.5% to 1.0% of all pregnancies, but it accounts for 10% to 15% of all perinatal deaths (Cunningham et al., 2014)

The cause of abruptio placentae is largely unknown. Placental abruption occurs when the placenta separates from the uterine wall. While placental abruption typically presents as painful vaginal bleeding, concealed bleeding can also occur. The nurse needs to assess for placental abruption in any woman who complains of intense ongoing uterine pain. Risk factors associated with placental abruption include maternal age over 35 or under 20 years, increased parity, cigarette smoking, alcohol use, cocaine abuse, trauma, retroplacental fibromyoma, post-amniocentesis complication, maternal hypertension, rapid uterine decompression associated with hydramnios and multiple gestation, preterm premature rupture of membranes (PPROM), uterine

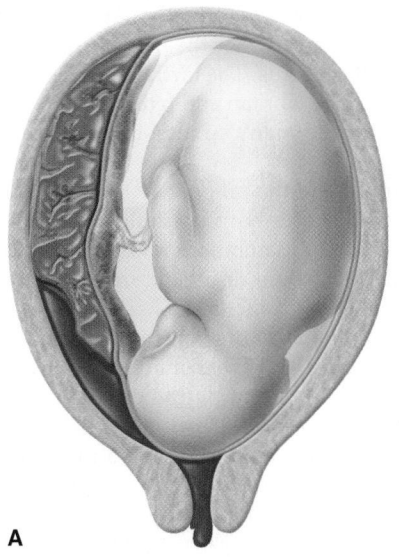 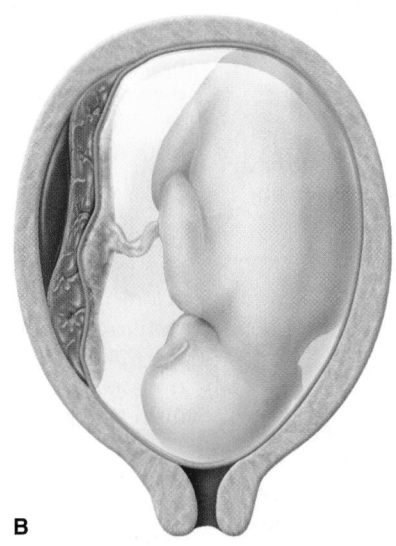 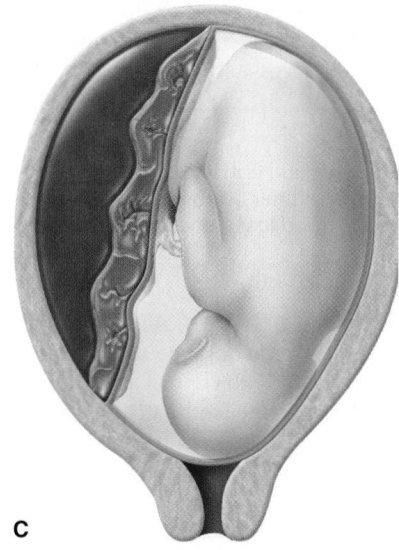

A   B   C

Figure 20–2 Abruptio placentae. *A*, Marginal abruption with external hemorrhage. *B*, Central abruption with concealed hemorrhage. *C*, Complete separation.

malformations or fibroids, placental anomalies, short umbilical cord, subchorionic hematoma, elevated second-trimester maternal serum alpha-fetoprotein, previous abruption, and inherited thrombophilia (Cunningham et al., 2014).

Abruptio placentae is subdivided into three types (Figure 20–2):

- *Marginal.* The placenta separates at its edges, the blood passes between the fetal membranes and the uterine wall, and the blood escapes vaginally (also called *marginal sinus rupture*).

- *Central.* The placenta separates centrally, and the blood is trapped between the placenta and the uterine wall. Entrapment of the blood results in concealed bleeding.

- *Complete.* Massive vaginal bleeding is seen in the presence of total separation.

Abruptio placentae may also be graded according to the severity of clinical and laboratory findings as follows (Deering, 2014):

Grade 1 (Mild): Mild separation with slight vaginal bleeding. Fetal heart rate (FHR) pattern and maternal blood pressure unaffected. Accounts for 40% of abruptions.

Grade 2 (Moderate): Partial abruption with moderate bleeding. Significant uterine irritability is present. Maternal pulse may be elevated, although blood pressure is stable. Signs of fetal compromise evident in FHR. Accounts for 45% of abruptions.

Grade 3 (Severe): Large or complete separation with moderate to severe bleeding. Maternal shock and painful uterine contractions present. Fetal death common. Accounts for about 15% of abruptions.

The signs and symptoms of placental abruption are listed in Table 20–4. In severe cases of central abruptio placentae, the blood invades the myometrial tissues between the muscle fibers. This occurrence accounts for the uterine irritability that is a significant sign of abruptio placentae. If hemorrhage continues, eventually the uterus turns entirely blue because the

TABLE 20–4 Differential Signs and Symptoms of Placenta Previa and Abruptio Placentae

	PLACENTA PREVIA	ABRUPTIO PLACENTAE
Onset	Quiet and sneaky	Sudden and stormy
Bleeding	External	External or concealed
Color of blood	Bright red	Dark venous
Anemia	Equal to blood loss	Greater than apparent blood loss
Shock	Equal to blood loss	Greater than apparent blood loss
Preeclampsia/eclampsia	Absent	May be present
Pain	Only labor	Usually severe and steady
Uterine tenderness	Absent	Present
Uterine tone	Soft and relaxed	Firm to stony hard
Uterine contour	Normal	May enlarge and change shape
Fetal heart tones	Usually present	Present or absent
Engagement	Absent	May be present
Presentation	May be abnormal	No relationship

Source: Data from Posner, G., & Black, A. (2013). *Oxorn & Foote human labor and birth* (6th ed.). Philadelphia, PA: McGraw-Hill.

muscle fibers are filled with blood. After birth the uterus contracts poorly. This condition is known as a *Couvelaire uterus* and frequently necessitates hysterectomy.

Clinical Tip

When assessing a woman for vaginal bleeding, make sure to have the woman lift her bottom completely off the bed so you can observe for blood loss beneath the buttocks.

MATERNAL IMPLICATIONS

As a result of the damage to the uterine wall and the retroplacental clotting with central abruption, large amounts of thromboplastin are released into the maternal blood supply. This thromboplastin in turn triggers the development of disseminated intravascular coagulation (DIC) and resultant hypofibrinogenemia. Fibrinogen levels, which are ordinarily elevated in pregnancy, may drop in minutes to the point at which blood will no longer coagulate.

Maternal mortality is now uncommon, although maternal morbidity still occurs (Cunningham et al., 2014). Postpartum problems depend in large part on the severity of the intrapartum bleeding, coagulation defects (DIC), hypofibrinogenemia, and time between separation and birth. Moderate to severe hemorrhage results in hemorrhagic shock, which may prove fatal to the mother if it is not rapidly reversed. In the postpartum period, women with this disorder are at risk for hemorrhage and renal failure caused by shock, vascular spasm, intravascular clotting, or a combination of these factors.

FETAL/NEONATAL IMPLICATIONS

Perinatal mortality associated with abruptio placentae is about 25% (Cunningham et al., 2014). In severe cases, in which most of the placenta has separated, the infant mortality rate is near 100%. In less severe separation, fetal outcome depends on the level of maturity and the length of time to birth. The most serious complications in the newborn arise from preterm labor, anemia, and hypoxia. If fetal hypoxia progresses unchecked, irreversible brain damage or fetal demise may result. Thorough assessment and prompt action on the part of the healthcare team can improve both fetal and maternal outcomes.

CLINICAL THERAPY

Disseminated intravascular coagulation (DIC) is a complex pathologic activation of coagulation (blood clotting) mechanisms that can sometimes occur as a complication in pregnancy. In DIC, small clots are formed within blood vessels that consume coagulation proteins and platelets. When this pathologic process occurs, abnormal coagulation and abnormal bleeding result in various systems, including in the skin (e.g., where a needle puncture occurred), gastrointestinal, and respiratory systems. Incisions may also bleed. This cascade of events leads to microclots that disrupt normal blood flow to major organs and can lead to organ failure. DIC is extremely serious and accounts for 25% of maternal deaths (Ramin & Ramin, 2012).

Because of the risk of DIC, evaluating the results of coagulation tests is imperative. In DIC, fibrinogen levels and platelet counts usually decrease; prothrombin times and partial thromboplastin times are normal to prolonged. If the values are not markedly abnormal, serial testing may be helpful in establishing an abnormal trend indicative of coagulopathy. Another test determines levels of fibrin-degradation products; these values rise with DIC.

After establishing the diagnosis, immediate priorities are maintaining the cardiovascular status of the mother and developing a plan for the birth of the fetus. The birth method selected depends on the condition of the woman and fetus and the speed at which the birth will occur; in many circumstances, cesarean birth will be the safest option.

If the separation is mild and the pregnancy is late preterm, labor may be induced and the fetus born vaginally with as little trauma as possible. If rupture of membranes and oxytocin infusion by pump do not initiate labor, a cesarean birth is required. A long delay would raise the risk of increased hemorrhage, with resulting hypofibrinogenemia. Supportive actions to decrease the risk of DIC include typing and cross-matching for blood transfusions (at least 3 units), evaluating the clotting mechanism, and providing intravenous fluids.

In cases of moderate to severe placental separation, a cesarean birth is done after treatment of hypofibrinogenemia by intravenous infusion of cryoprecipitate or fresh-frozen plasma. Vaginal birth is impossible with a Couvelaire uterus because the uterus would not contract properly in labor, and a hysterectomy is often needed.

The hypovolemia that accompanies severe abruptio placentae is life threatening and must be combated with whole blood. If the fetus is alive but experiencing stress, emergency cesarean birth is the method of choice. With a stillborn fetus, vaginal birth is preferable if bleeding has stabilized, unless maternal shock from hemorrhage is uncontrollable. Intravenous fluids are administered. Central venous pressure (CVP) monitoring may be needed to evaluate intravenous fluid replacement. An absolute level is not as important as the response to fluid replacement. CVP is evaluated hourly, and the results are communicated to the physician. Elevations of CVP may indicate fluid overload and pulmonary edema. Laboratory testing is ordered to provide ongoing data regarding hemoglobin, hematocrit, and coagulation status. The hematocrit is maintained at 30% through the administration of packed red blood cells or whole blood (Cunningham et al., 2014). Measures are taken to stimulate labor to effect a vaginal birth, if possible. An amniotomy may be performed, and oxytocin is given. Progressive dilatation and effacement usually occur.

Nursing Management

Any woman who presents with intense uterine pain and tenderness should be assessed for placental abruption. Although not typical, it is important to note that the amount of bleeding is not always associated with the degree of separation. The degree of separation can only be confirmed with an ultrasound examination. Ensure that bedside ultrasound equipment is readily available if possible. Vaginal examinations are contraindicated and should not be performed by the nurse. Evaluation by the healthcare provider may include a vaginal examination once placenta previa has been ruled out. In women without evidence of imminent birth, anticipate a probable cesarean birth.

Electronic monitoring of the uterine contractions and resting tone between contractions provides information about the labor pattern and effectiveness of the oxytocin induction. Because uterine resting tone is frequently increased with abruptio placentae, it must be evaluated frequently for further increase. Abdominal girth measurements may be ordered hourly and are obtained by placing a tape measure around the maternal abdomen at the level of the umbilicus. Another method of evaluating uterine size, which increases as more bleeding occurs at the site of abruption, involves placing a mark at the top of the uterine fundus; the distance from the symphysis pubis to the mark may

Nursing Care Plan: Hemorrhage in the Third Trimester

1. Nursing Diagnosis: *Fluid Volume: Deficient, Risk for,* **related to excessive vascular loss during pregnancy (NANDA-I © 2014)**

GOAL: Woman will not experience significant fluid volume deficit during the third trimester of pregnancy.

INTERVENTION	RATIONALE
• Monitor vital signs: i.e., temperature—normal range is 96.8°–100.4°F (36°–38°C), pulse—normal is 60–90, respirations—normal is 12–22, blood pressure (BP)—normal range is 110/70 to 135/85, central venous pressure—normal range is 5–10 mmHg. Compare present BP with woman's baseline BP. Note pulse pressure.	• Any deviations in a woman's baseline vital signs could indicate intravascular fluctuations.
• Weigh pads and chux. If the woman has bathroom privileges, instruct her on initiating pad counts. Teach the woman how to weigh pads and chux, with each gram equal to approximately 1 mL of blood loss.	• The combination of weighing and counting pads and chux assists medical personnel in determining the woman's blood loss.
• Report amount of blood loss within a specific period (e.g., 50 mL of bright-red blood on pad in 20 min).	
• Monitor urinary output hourly and measure urine specific gravity (normal: 1.010–1.025).	• A decrease in urinary output (less than 30 mL/hr) and an increase in specific gravity suggest dehydration and a need for an increase in fluid intake.
• Palpate bilateral peripheral pulses (normal: equal and strong) and note capillary refill (normal: less than 3 sec). Also, assess skin color and temperature (normal: pink, warm, dry, and intact).	• Helps determine signs of circulatory loss or hypovolemic shock, which include weak pulses, capillary refill greater than 3 sec, skin color that is cyanotic or pallor, and skin temperature that is cool and clammy.
• Assess mental status at frequent intervals.	• Excessive blood loss can lead to changes in mentation.
• Assess the woman for signs and symptoms of disseminated intravascular coagulation.	• Provides vital information on maternal status.
• Instruct the woman on the importance of strict bed rest and avoidance of any sexual activity that involves nipple stimulation or that might lead to orgasm.	• Bleeding may cease with limited activity. Pressure on the abdomen and orgasms can stimulate uterine activity, thereby causing bleeding. Nipple stimulation may result in uterine contractions, as can orgasm.
• Monitor fetal status and uterine activity by continuous fetal monitoring.	• May determine the origin of bleeding and fetal well-being.
• **Collaborative:** Collect and review blood work: complete blood count (CBC), type and cross-match, Rh titer, fibrinogen levels, platelet count, activated partial thromboplastin time (APTT), prothrombin time (PT), and human chorionic gonadotropin (hCG) levels.	• Determines blood loss and need for intervention if blood work is abnormal.
• Administer appropriate isotonic IV solutions and blood products (e.g., plasma expanders, whole blood, serum albumin, or packed red blood cells) as ordered by the physician.	• Reverses shock symptoms by increasing blood volume.
• Insert Foley catheter.	• Close monitoring of urinary output will aid in determining adequate renal perfusion.

EXPECTED OUTCOME: The woman will show signs of adequate fluid volume during pregnancy as evidenced by vital signs within normal limits, capillary refill in less than 3 sec, adequate sensorium, and urine output greater than 30 mL/hr.

2. Nursing Diagnosis: *Tissue Perfusion: Peripheral, Ineffective,* **(uteroplacental) related to hypovolemia secondary to excessive maternal blood loss (NANDA-I © 2014)**

GOAL: The fetus will have no evidence of hypoxia during pregnancy.

INTERVENTION	RATIONALE
• Assess maternal vital signs.	• Closely monitoring maternal physiologic status and circulatory status will assist in determining if an episode of bleeding has occurred and allow for interventions to protect maternal and fetal well-being.

(continued)

Nursing Care Plan: Hemorrhage in the Third Trimester (*continued*)

• Monitor fetal heart tones continuously, assessing for variability, accelerations, and decelerations, and record.	• Continuous electronic fetal monitoring will aid in detecting signs of fetal hypoxia and allow time for appropriate intervention.
• Assess fundal height.	• Determines an approximate gestational age.
• Assess labor progression by determining cervical dilatation and effacement if contractions are present.	• This provides information on maternal labor status.
• **Collaborative:** Perform scalp stimulation to assess fetal accelerations.	• FHR acceleration is considered 15 beats above the baseline lasting for 15 sec and is indicative of fetal well-being.
• Assess amniotic fluid for meconium.	• Impaired gas exchange relaxes fetal intestinal motility, causing expulsion of meconium into amniotic fluid.
• Assist the physician during ultrasonography and amniocentesis for lecithin/sphingomyelin (L/S) ratio sample.	• Determines viability and alerts appropriate medical personnel of fetal age if birth is imminent.

EXPECTED OUTCOME: Fetus will demonstrate adequate tissue perfusion as evidenced by fetal heart tones that remain within 110–160 beats/min, long-term variability and short-term variability present, positive periodic changes (no variable or late decelerations), and fetal scalp blood pH greater than 7.25.

3. Nursing Diagnosis: *Fear/Anxiety* related to personal and fetal well-being secondary to third-trimester hemorrhage (NANDA-I © 2014)

GOAL: The woman will verbalize a decrease in fear and anxiety.

INTERVENTION	RATIONALE
• Maintain frequent contact with the woman and family members.	• Establishes trust with the woman and her family members, so they will not feel alone or abandoned.
• Provide the woman with accurate, reliable information concerning diagnosis and prognosis.	• Fear and anxiety will lessen when the woman is informed of health status and is allowed to make decisions based on present situation.

EXPECTED OUTCOME: The woman will actively seek information about diagnosis and prognosis.

• Allow the woman and family members to verbalize the origin of fears.	• Recognizing the origin of fear gives the woman and her family the appropriate tool to begin the process of developing coping strategies for dealing with the fears.
• Explain all procedures in an easy-to-understand, nonthreatening manner, and allow the woman and family members to ask questions.	• Accurate information prepares the woman and family members for the impending procedures, thereby reducing fear of the unknown.

EXPECTED OUTCOME: The woman and her family members develop appropriate coping strategies that decrease fear and anxiety.

---

then be measured hourly. Overdistention of the uterus can lead to a ruptured uterus, another life-threatening complication. See *Nursing Care Plan: Hemorrhage in the Third Trimester.*

Clinical Tip

When faced with an emergent situation, tell the woman she needs to follow your instructions quickly and that you will explain what is happening as soon as possible once you take the necessary measures to ensure that she and the baby are safely cared for.

Care of the Woman With Cervical Insufficiency

Cervical insufficiency is painless dilatation of the cervix without contractions due to a structural or functional defect of the cervix. The woman is usually unaware of contractions and presents with advanced effacement and dilatation and, possibly, bulging membranes.

The origin of cervical insufficiency is multifactorial.

1. *Congenital factors/structural defect.* May be found in women exposed to diethylstilbestrol (DES) or those with a bicornuate uterus. Additionally, may be related to a structural defect in tensile strength at the cervicoisthmic junction of the cervix. Women with collagen disorders (Ehlers-Danlos syndrome) are also at risk (Norwitz, 2014).

2. *Acquired factors.* May be related to inflammation, infection, subclinical uterine activity, cervical trauma, cone biopsy, late second-trimester elective abortions, hemorrhage, or increased uterine volume (as with a multiple gestation). Loop electrosurgical excision procedure (LEEP) of the cervix has been found to significantly increase the risk of preterm births (Norwitz, 2014).

A woman's obstetric history may give her healthcare provider an indication of increased risk for cervical insufficiency.

Factors include multiple gestations, repetitive second-trimester losses, previous preterm birth, progressively earlier births with each subsequent pregnancy, short labors, previous elective abortion or cervical manipulation, DES exposure, or other uterine anomaly. These women will benefit from close surveillance of cervical length with transvaginal ultrasound beginning between 16 and 24 weeks' gestation. Cervical effacement occurs from the internal os out and can be seen on ultrasound as "funneling." Alteration is apparent in a transvaginal scan when fundal pressure is applied or the woman assumes a standing position. In addition, women at risk for cervical insufficiency need to be informed early in pregnancy of warning signs of impending birth, such as lower back pain, pelvic pressure, and changes in vaginal discharge.

Transvaginal ultrasound measurements of cervical length between 16 and 28 weeks' gestation identify groups at risk for preterm birth. Success rates measured by prevention of preterm birth due to the placement of a cervical cerclage are directly related to the degree of cervical shortening that has occurred prior to the procedure (Norwitz, 2014). Women with a greater than 33-mm cervical length are at low risk for preterm birth, whereas women with a cervical length less than 15 mm have a 60% chance of preterm birth within the following 7-day period (Norwitz, 2014). Fetal fibronectin (fFn) testing is another means to determine if preterm birth may occur, and screening can be conducted between 22 and 34 weeks in women with intact amniotic membranes and cervical dilatation less than 3 cm. Women with a positive fFn test along with ultrasonic evidence of a cervical length of less than 30 mm are at a far greater risk of preterm birth (Norwitz, 2014).

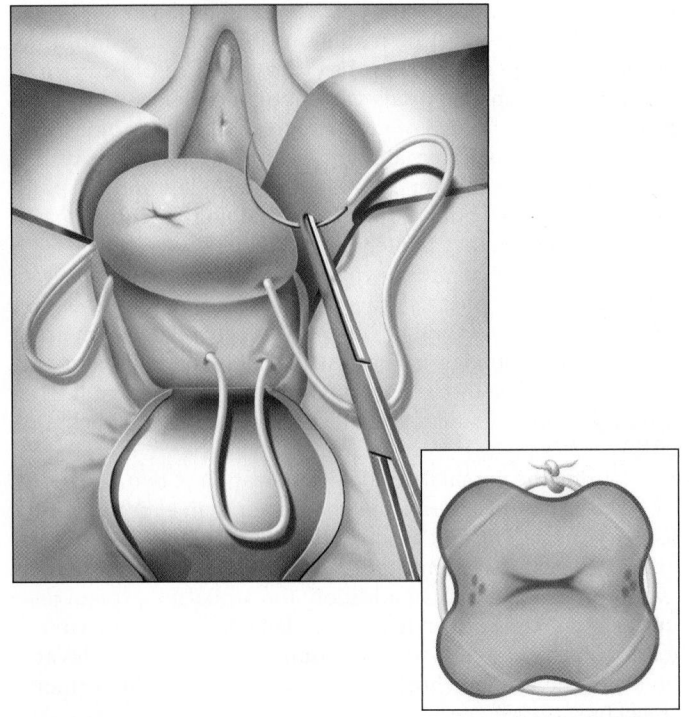

Figure 20–3 A cerclage, or purse-string suture, is inserted in the cervix to prevent preterm cervical dilatation and pregnancy loss. After placement, the string is tightened and secured anteriorly.

Clinical Tip

Care should be taken when performing a transvaginal ultrasound for cervical length, as excessive pressure on the vaginal probe or a full maternal bladder are associated with falsely long measurements.

Progesterone supplements are indicated for women beginning as early as 16 weeks' gestation when cervical shortening has occurred and there is a history of a previous preterm birth. Supplementation should continue until 36 weeks. In women with no previous preterm birth, cervical length less than 20 mm is also an indication for progesterone supplementation.

Other medical therapies that have been used include serial cervical ultrasound assessments, bed rest, antibiotics, anti-inflammatory drugs, and cervical pessary placement (Cunningham et al., 2014).

Cerclage Procedures

A **cerclage** is a surgical procedure in which a stitch is placed in the cervix to prevent a spontaneous abortion or premature birth (Norwitz, 2014). (See Figure 20–3.) Surgical options include the various types of cerclage procedures. An elective cervical cerclage may be placed late in the first trimester or early in the second trimester with an 80% to 90% success rate in preventing fetal loss and premature labor and birth. A cerclage placed for emergent reasons, when dilatation and effacement have already occurred, is successful in 40% to 60% of cases (Cunningham et al., 2014). Cervical cerclage has been established as an effective preterm birth measure in women with a shortened cervix and a previous preterm birth but is not routinely recommended in women without a preterm birth or in women with multiple gestations (Norwitz, 2014).

An abdominal cerclage is rarely performed and is used in women who have either failed two or more previous transvaginal cerclages or in whom a transvaginal cerclage is technically impossible to perform because of extreme shortening, scarring, or laceration of the cervix (Norwitz, 2014). Transabdominal cerclage placement requires a laparotomy for placement and removal and typically results in a cesarean section birth (Norwitz, 2014).

In cases in which cervical dilatation is discovered unexpectedly, an attempt may be made to "rescue" the pregnancy by placing a cerclage after cervical dilatation is advanced. In some instances, decompression of a bulging amniotic sac must be accomplished immediately before the cerclage placement. In this situation, a preoperative evaluation for infection, ruptured membranes, and uterine activity may be prudent. Tocolytics (drugs that stop labor), broad-spectrum antibiotics, and anti-inflammatory agents are given perioperatively and for ongoing treatment. Exposure of the amniotic membranes increases the chance of cerclage failure when compared with an elective placement of a cerclage.

An uncomplicated elective cerclage may be done on an outpatient basis or the woman may be hospitalized and discharged after 24 to 48 hours. An emergency cerclage, however, requires hospitalization for 5 to 7 days or longer. After 37 completed weeks of gestation, the suture may be cut and vaginal birth permitted, or the suture may be left in place and a cesarean birth performed to avoid repeating the procedure in subsequent pregnancies.

Care of the Woman With Multiple Gestation

In part because of advances in infertility treatments, the incidence of twins in the United States has increased by 65% since 1980 (Blackburn, 2013). In 2012, the rate of twins was 33.1 per 1000 births (Martin, Hamilton, Osterman, et al., 2013).

Multifetal births account for only 3% of all births in the United States (Blackburn, 2013). Triplet and higher order multiples occur in 124.4 per 100,000 births (Martin et al., 2013). The incidence of spontaneous twins varies but is highest among African Americans, women of greater age and parity, women with a family history of fraternal twins, and women who are tall and overweight. The incidence is low in the Asian and Hispanic populations (Blackburn, 2013). The physiology of multiple gestation is discussed in Chapter 7.

Twins that occur from two separate ova are called *dizygotic* (two zygotes), or *fraternal*, twins. The fetuses may be the same sex or different sexes and are no more closely related genetically than any other siblings. In contrast, 33% of twins are *monozygotic*, or *identical*, twins; they develop from one fertilized ovum. They are genetically identical and always the same sex (Blackburn, 2013).

During the prenatal period, visualization of two gestational sacs at 5 to 6 weeks, fundal height greater than expected for the length of gestation, and auscultation of heart rates that differ by at least 10 beats per minute are the most likely clues to multiple-gestation pregnancies. In addition, the alpha-fetoprotein level on the quadruple screen is usually elevated, and many women experience severe nausea and vomiting (caused by elevated levels of the human chorionic gonadotropin [hCG] hormone) (Blackburn, 2013).

Maternal Implications

During her pregnancy, the woman may experience physical discomfort such as shortness of breath, dyspnea on exertion, backaches and musculoskeletal disorders, and pedal edema. Other associated problems include (Blackburn, 2013):

- Urinary tract infections
- Threatened abortion
- Anemia
- Gestational hypertension
- Preeclampsia/eclampsia
- Preterm labor and birth
- Premature rupture of membranes
- Thromboembolism
- Placenta previa
- Placental abruption
- Placental disorders

Complications during labor include abnormal fetal presentations, uterine dysfunction, prolapsed cord, and hemorrhage at birth or shortly after (Blackburn, 2013).

Fetal/Neonatal Implications

The perinatal mortality rate is approximately 3 times greater for twins than for a single fetus, although the mortality rate for triplets and higher-order multiple births is 4 times higher (Blackburn, 2013). The perinatal mortality rate for monoamniotic siblings has been estimated to be as high as 10% to 32% (Blackburn, 2013). Fetal problems include decreased intrauterine growth rate for each fetus, increased incidence of fetal anomalies, increased risk of prematurity and its associated problems, abnormal presentations, increase in cord accidents, and an increase in cerebral palsy (Blackburn, 2013). Twins are more likely to have long-term disabilities when compared with children who were singleton births. Primiparous women who

are pregnant with twins have higher rates of complications and prematurity than multiparous women (Blackburn, 2013). Multifetal pregnancies that are conceived spontaneously have better outcomes than those achieved with assisted reproductive technology. Even singleton births achieved with assisted technology have a higher incidence of adverse outcomes, specifically increased incidences of newborns with cerebral palsy (Blackburn, 2013).

Clinical Therapy

Once the presence of twins has been detected, preventing and treating problems that infringe on the development and birth of normal fetuses is the most significant clinical goal. Prenatal visits are more frequent for women with twins than for those with one fetus. Women with multiple-gestation pregnancies need to understand the nutritional implications of multiple fetuses, the assessment of fetal activity, the signs of preterm labor, and the danger signs of pregnancy.

If the initial ultrasound scan performed at 18 to 20 weeks' gestation is normal and no risk factors are identified, serial ultrasounds performed every 3 to 4 weeks are used to assess the growth of each fetus. Monochorionic diamniotic placentation is considered a significant risk factor that occurs when the zygote separates to form two yolk sacs but the zygotes share a single chorion and a single placenta. These pregnancies require the use of ultrasound to monitor fetal growth. Ultrasounds are performed every 2 to 3 weeks to detect possible twin-to-twin transfusion syndrome (Cunningham et al., 2014). Twin-to-twin transfusion occurs in 15% to 30% of such pregnancies and results in abnormal placental vascular anastomoses, in which one twin receives more perfusion, nutrients, and oxygenation than the other twin. This typically is identified by growth discrepancies between the two fetuses and often necessitates preterm birth via cesarean (Cunningham et al., 2014).

A systematic review of studies of hospitalization and bed rest for multiple pregnancy showed insufficient evidence to support routine bed rest (Cunningham et al., 2014). More recent strategies include work leave, lifestyle modifications, and avoidance of sexual activity, although well-designed controlled studies supporting the use of these interventions is lacking in the current literature.

Third-trimester testing usually begins at 32 to 34 weeks' gestation and may include a non-stress test (NST) or biophysical profile (BPP). A reactive NST is associated with good fetal outcome if birth occurs within 1 week of the testing. The NST is done every 3 to 7 days until birth or until results become nonreactive. The BPP is also accurate in assessing fetal status with twin pregnancies. A biophysical profile of 8 or better for each fetus is considered reassuring, and weekly or biweekly BPPs and NSTs continue until birth.

Intrapartum management requires careful attention to maternal and fetal status. The mother should have an IV with a large-bore needle in place. Anesthesia and cross-matched blood should be readily available. The twins are monitored by continuous dual electronic fetal monitoring.

The decision about method of birth, which depends on a variety of factors, may not be made until labor occurs. The presence of maternal complications such as placenta previa, abruptio placentae, or severe preeclampsia usually indicates the need for cesarean birth. Fetal factors such as severe intrauterine growth restriction (IUGR), preterm birth, fetal anomalies, non-reassuring fetal status, and unfavorable fetal position or presentation also require cesarean birth.

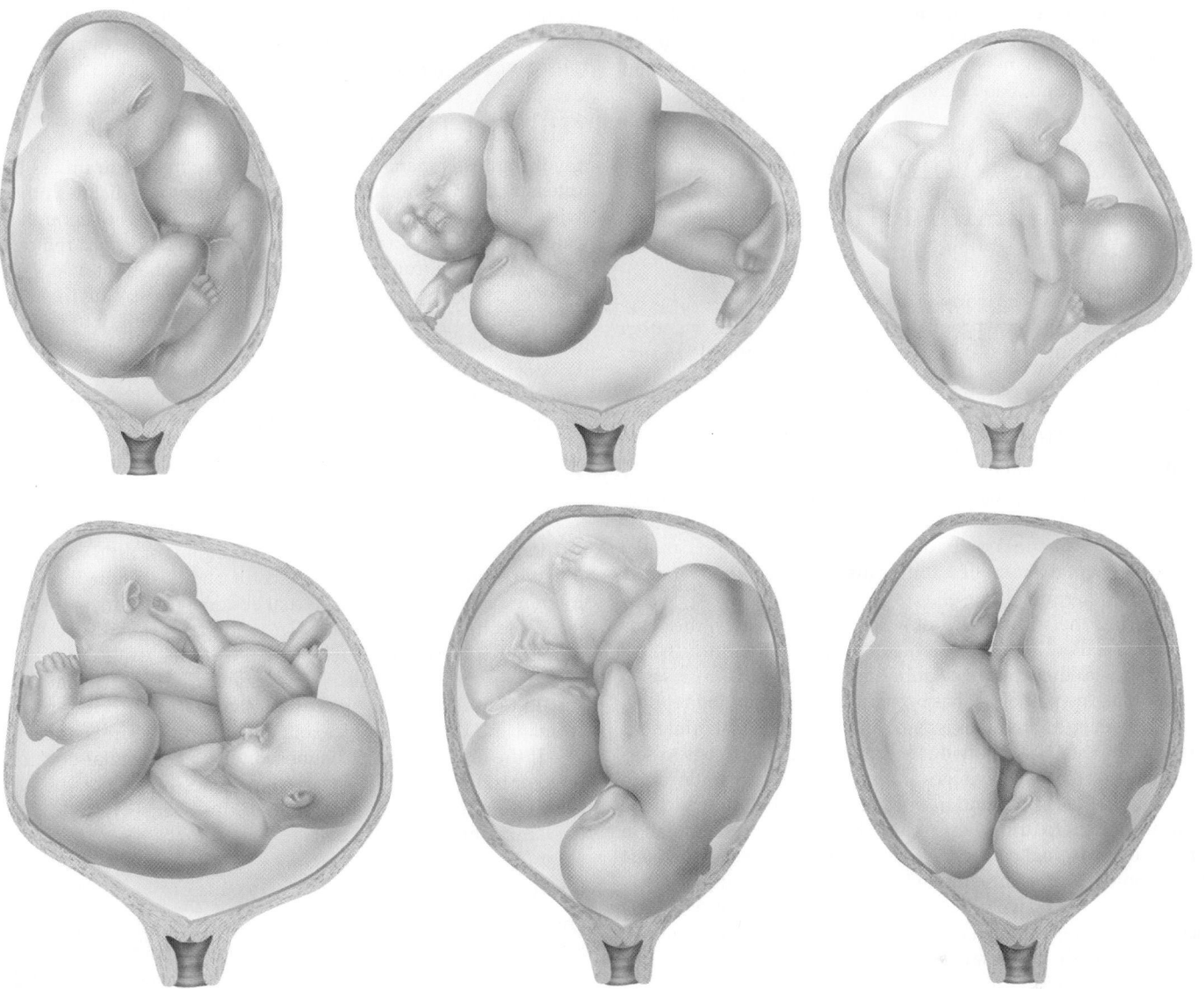

Figure 20–4 Twins may be in any of these presentations while in utero.

Any combination of presentations and positions can occur with multiple births. Figure 20–4 shows some possible presentations of twins. When the presenting fetus is in a nonvertex position, cesarean birth is indicated.

Nursing Management

For the Woman With Multiple Gestation

Community-Based Nursing Care

During pregnancy the woman may need counseling about diet and daily activities. Help her plan meals to meet her increased needs. Nutritional requirements vary somewhat based on the mother's prepregnancy weight and the estimated weight of the twins. A daily intake of 3500 kcal (minimum) and 175 g protein is recommended for a woman with normal-weight twins, although an intake of 4000 kcal and 200 g of protein is recommended if the twins are underweight. A prenatal vitamin and 1 mg of folic acid should also be taken daily. A total weight gain of 40 to 45 lb (18.8 to 20.45 kg), with a 24-lb (11-kg) gain by 24 weeks, is recommended for women with multiple-gestation pregnancy (Cunningham et al., 2014).

Counseling about daily activities may include encouraging the woman to plan frequent rest periods during the day. The rest period is most effective if the woman rests in a side-lying position (which increases uteroplacental blood flow) and elevates her lower legs and feet to reduce edema. Back discomfort may be relieved by pelvic rocking, maintaining good posture, consistent use of a pregnancy belt to support the abdomen and lower back, and using good body mechanics when lifting objects and moving about.

Hospital-Based Nursing Care

During labor the fetal heart rates (FHRs) of the siblings are monitored continuously by an electronic fetal monitor (EFM). Electronic monitoring equipment now makes it possible to monitor the fetuses simultaneously. They are monitored throughout labor and vaginal birth or up to the time of abdominal incision if a cesarean is done. Most multiple gestations are now delivered via cesarean birth.

After birth, prepare to receive two or more newborns instead of one. This means duplicating everything, including resuscitation equipment, radiant warmers, and newborn identification papers and bracelets. Additional staff members should be available for newborn resuscitation, monitoring, and newborn care. Special precautions should be taken to ensure correct identification of the newborns. The first born is usually tagged Baby A; the second, Baby B; and so on.

Care of the Woman With Abnormal Amniotic Fluid Volume

Amniotic fluid serves many important functions during pregnancy. However, some pregnancies are complicated by either an excessive amount of amniotic fluid or a reduced amount of fluid.

Hydramnios

Hydramnios (also called *polyhydramnios*) is defined as amniotic fluid volume greater than 2000 mL. Hydramios occurs in about 1% of all pregnancies (Cunningham et al., 2014). The exact cause of hydramnios is unknown; however, it may occur in cases of major congenital anomalies. It may also be idiopathic in nature without a determined cause.

During the second half of a normal pregnancy, the fetus begins to swallow and inspire amniotic fluid and to urinate, which contributes to the amount of amniotic fluid present. In cases of hydramnios, no pathology has been found in the amniotic epithelium. However, hydramnios is associated with fetal malformations that affect the fetal swallowing mechanism and neurologic disorders in which the fetal meninges are exposed in the amniotic cavity. This condition is also found in cases of anencephaly, in which the fetus is thought to urinate excessively because of overstimulation of the cerebrospinal centers. When monozygotic twins manifest hydramnios, it is because the twin with the increased blood volume urinates excessively. Because the weight of the placenta has been found to be increased in some cases of hydramnios, increased functioning of the placental tissue may be a factor.

There are two types of hydramnios: chronic and acute. In the chronic type, the fluid volume gradually increases and is a problem of the third trimester. Most cases are of this variety. In acute cases, the volume increases rapidly over a period of a few days. The acute type is usually diagnosed between 20 and 24 weeks' gestation.

MATERNAL IMPLICATIONS

When the amount of amniotic fluid is over 3000 mL, the woman experiences shortness of breath and edema in the lower extremities from compression of the vena cava. Milder forms of hydramnios occur more frequently and are associated with minimal symptoms. Hydramnios is associated with maternal disorders such as diabetes and Rh sensitization and with multiple-gestation pregnancies. It can also occur as a result of infections such as syphilis, toxoplasmosis, cytomegalovirus, herpes, and rubella.

If the amniotic fluid is removed rapidly before birth, abruptio placentae can result from too sudden a change in the size of the uterus. Because of overdistention of uterine muscles, uterine dysfunction can occur in the intrapartum period, and the incidence of postpartum hemorrhage increases.

FETAL/NEONATAL IMPLICATIONS

Fetal malformations and preterm birth are common with hydramnios; thus the perinatal mortality rate is fairly high. Prolapsed cord can occur when the membranes rupture, creating a further complication for the fetus. The incidence of malpresentations also increases. In addition, the incidence of preterm labor and cesarean birth is significantly increased in pregnancies complicated by hydramnios.

Clinical Therapy

Hydramnios is managed with supportive treatment unless the intensity of the woman's distress and symptoms dictates otherwise. If the accumulation of amniotic fluid is severe enough to cause maternal dyspnea and pain, hospitalization and removal of the excessive fluid are required. Fluid can be removed vaginally or by amniocentesis. The dangers of performing the technique vaginally are prolapsed cord and the inability to remove the fluid slowly. If amniocentesis is performed, it should be done with the aid of sonography to prevent inadvertent damage to the fetus and placenta. In addition, the fluid should be removed slowly to prevent abruption.

Nursing Management

Suspect hydramnios when the fundal height increases out of proportion to the gestational age. As the amount of fluid increases, it may be difficult to palpate the fetus and auscultate the FHR. In more severe cases, the maternal abdomen appears extremely tense and tight on inspection. On sonography, large spaces can be identified between the fetus and the uterine wall.

When amniocentesis is performed, it is vital to maintain sterile technique to prevent infection. Offer support to the woman and her partner by explaining the procedure to them.

If the fetus has been diagnosed with a congenital defect in utero or is born with a defect, the family needs psychologic support. Often the nurse collaborates with social services to offer the family this additional help.

Oligohydramnios

Oligohydramnios is defined as a less-than-normal amount of amniotic fluid (approximately 500 mL is considered normal). This condition affects 1% to 3% of all pregnancies (Zheng, 2012). Oligohydramnios is diagnosed when the largest vertical pocket of amniotic fluid visible on ultrasound examination is 5 cm (2 in.) or less (Cunningham et al., 2014).

The exact cause of this condition is unknown. It is found in cases of postmaturity; maternal hypertensive disorders, with intrauterine growth restriction (IUGR) secondary to placental insufficiency; and in fetal conditions associated with major renal malformations, including renal aplasia with dysplastic kidneys and obstructive lesions of the lower urinary tract. If oligohydramnios occurs in the first part of pregnancy, there is a danger of fetal adhesions (one part of the fetus may adhere to another part).

Health Promotion **Oligohydramnios**

Because oligohydramnios is often associated with hypertensive complications and hyperglycemia, women should be carefully assessed for these risk factors at the initial prenatal visit. Obese women have a higher incidence of these risk factors and should strive to maintain a healthy weight gain during pregnancy. Healthy dietary practices, regular exercise, monitoring for blood pressure and glucose level abnormalities are all practices that can help reduce risk factors for oligohydramnios.

MATERNAL IMPLICATIONS

When oligohydramnios exists, labor can be dysfunctional, and progress is slow. The woman should be monitored for hypertensive disorders.

FETAL/NEONATAL IMPLICATIONS

During the gestational period, fetal skin and skeletal abnormalities may occur because fetal movement is impaired as a result of reduced amniotic fluid volume. Because there is less fluid available for the fetus to use during fetal breathing movements, pulmonary hypoplasia may develop. During the labor and birth, oligohydramnios reduces the cushioning effect for the umbilical cord, and cord compression is more likely to occur. Decreased amniotic fluid also contributes to fetal head compression.

SAFETY ALERT!

Oligohydramnios increases the risk for an adverse fetal event; therefore, women should be counseled to perform fetal movement assessments regularly. Any reduction or lack of fetal movement should be immediately reported to the healthcare practitioner for further evaluation.

Clinical Therapy

During the antepartum period oligohydramnios may be suspected when the uterus does not increase in size according to the dates, the fetus is easily palpated and outlined by the examiner, and the fetus is not ballottable. The fetus can be assessed by biophysical profiles, non-stress tests, and serial ultrasounds.

As soon as the fetus is term, induction is typically scheduled because the fetus is at an increased risk for intrauterine fetal demise. During labor, the fetus is monitored by continuous EFM to detect cord compression, which is indicated by variable decelerations. Some clinicians advocate the use of an *amnioinfusion* (a transcervical instillation of 250 mL of warmed sterile saline, followed by a continuous infusion rate of 100 to 200 mL/hr) after membranes have ruptured to decrease the frequency and severity of variable decelerations in the FHR during labor. In order for an amnioinfusion to be performed, an intrauterine pressure catheter must be in place. The fluid is administered in a blood warmer to maintain a constant temperature. It is imperative to monitor for expulsion of the fluid to prevent overdistention of the uterus. The infusion of saline provides more fluid for the umbilical cord to float in and thereby lessens or prevents cord compression. See Chapter 22 for more information about amnioinfusion.

Nursing Management

Continuous electronic fetal monitoring is an important part of the assessment during the labor and birth. Evaluate the EFM tracing for the presence of variable decelerations or other nonreassuring signs (such as increasing or decreasing baseline, decreased variability, presence of late decelerations). If variable decelerations are noted, change the woman's position (to relieve pressure on the umbilical cord), and notify the physician/CNM. If the tracing is not reassuring, a cesarean birth is performed. After the birth, the newborn is evaluated for signs of congenital anomalies, pulmonary hypoplasia, and postmaturity.

Focus Your Study

- Premature rupture of membranes (PROM) occurs when the amniotic membranes rupture prior to the onset of labor. Preterm premature rupture of membranes (PPROM) occurs when the fetus is premature and may be caused by infection, multiple pregnancy, bleeding during pregnancy, trauma, a variety of other factors, or have an unknown etiology.

- Nursing interventions related to PROM and PPROM include prevention of infection by limiting vaginal examinations and changing the bed pads frequently. Close fetal monitoring and assessing for uterine contractions is also warranted.

- Preterm labor may be treated with tocolytics, betamethasone to promote fetal lung maturation, magnesium sulfate to provide neuroprotection, and monitoring for progression of labor.

- Placenta previa occurs when the placenta implants in the lower segment of the uterus. It may partially or completely cover the cervical os. With placenta previa, bleeding occurs as the cervix begins to dilate and may be mild to severe depending on how much of the placenta covers the cervical os.

- Fetal implications of placenta previa may include hypoxia, anemia, or both from a bleeding episode.

- Nurses should assess for blood loss, pain, and uterine contractions; however, vaginal examinations are contraindicated since they can worsen bleeding.

- Abruptio placentae occurs when the placenta prematurely separates from the uterine wall and can cause severe hemorrhage, maternal or fetal death, and maternal clotting disorders. Nursing interventions include assessing uterine tone and measuring abdominal girth.

- Cervical insufficiency is the premature dilatation of the cervix; it is the most common cause of second-trimester abortion. Assessments typically include transvaginal ultrasound imaging for cervical length, fetal fibronectin testing, and assessing for cervical dilatation. Treatment may include progesterone supplementation and surgical cerclage placement.

- Women with a multiple gestation have a higher incidence of complications and require assessments of each fetus, frequent monitoring and education for preterm labor, and intermittent rest periods. During labor, equipment and staff should be available to receive each baby upon birth.

- Hydramios occurs when the amniotic fluid exceeds 2000 mL and may be associated with fetal swallowing and neurologic disorders, maternal infection, Rh sensitization, multiple gestation, and maternal diabetes. Women may experience shortness of breath and edema in the lower extremities.

- Hydramnios that exceeds 3000 mL of amniotic fluid may require an amniocentesis, which requires monitoring for

complications and providing support if a fetal anomaly is identified.

- Oligohydramnios occurs when amniotic fluid is reduced and may occur when fetal renal anomalies exist, when placental insufficiency is present, or in postmature fetuses.

Clinical Reasoning in Action

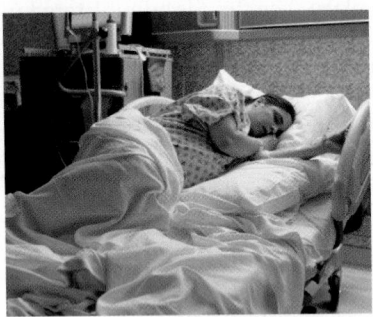

SOURCE: Eric Fowke/Alamy.

Monique Waleski, a 34-year-old G1P0, at 32 weeks' gestation, contacts her physician's office because she has been experiencing labor contractions that have gradually increased in frequency. She reports that she has been having about eight contractions an hour for the past 2 hours. She is instructed to meet her physician at the birthing unit for further evaluation.

At the birthing unit, a vaginal examination reveals that Monique's cervix is dilated 3 cm and 80% effaced. Contractions continue to occur every 7 to 8 minutes. Her fFN test is positive. She is

diagnosed with preterm labor. You position her on her left side and start an IV infusion.

Her physician tells Monique that she wants to begin tocolysis using magnesium sulfate and then prescribes 2 doses of betamethasone. You explain to Monique and her partner that you will be giving her the magnesium sulfate by infusion pump and the betamethasone by IM injection once a day today and tomorrow. She asks you about the two medications, including their specific purposes.

1. Explain the concept of tocolysis and the purpose of magnesium sulfate.

2. Describe the concept of a loading dose and maintenance dose.

3. How will you know if Monique is developing toxic levels of magnesium?

4. Describe the role of corticosteroids used during preterm labor.

References

American College of Obstetricians and Gynecologists (ACOG). (2012). *Magnesium sulfate administration for neonatal neuroprotection: Patient selection and protocol.* Washington, DC: Author.

American College of Obstetricians and Gynecologists (ACOG). (2014). *ACOG Practice Advisory on use of antenatal corticosteroids.* Washington, DC: Author.

Blackburn, S. T. (2013). *Maternal, fetal, and neonatal physiology: A clinical perspective* (4th ed.). Philadelphia, PA: Saunders.

Cunningham, F. G., Leveno, K. J., Bloom, S. L., Spong, C. Y., Dashe, J. S., Hoffman, B. L., . . . , Sheffield, J. S. (2014). *Williams obstetrics* (24th ed.). New York, NY: McGraw-Hill.

Davidson, M. R. (2012). *Nurse's guide to women's mental health.* New York, NY: Springer.

Deering, S. H. (2014). Abruptio placentae. *eMedicine.* Retrieved from http://emedicine.medscape.com /article/252810-overview#a0101

Ekin A., Gezer C., Kulhan G., Avci, M. E., & Taner, C. E. (2014). Can platelet count and mean platelet volume during the first trimester of pregnancy predict preterm premature rupture of membranes? *Journal of Obstetric & Gynaecological Research, 4*(12), 293–297.

Food and Drug Administration (FDA). (2011). *FDA approves drug to reduce risk of preterm birth in at-risk pregnant women.* Retrieved from http://www.fda.gov /NewsEvents/Newsroom/PressAnnouncements /ucm242234.htm?sms_ss=email&at _xt=4d50034cbfa7fa33%2C0

Gyamfi-Bannerman, C., Gilbert, S., Landon, M. B., Spong, C. Y., Rouse, D. J., Varner, M. W., . . . Mercer, B. M.;

for the Eunice Kennedy Shriver National Institute of Child Health and Human Development (NICHD) Maternal-Fetal Medicine Units (MFMU) Network. (2012). Effect of antenatal corticosteroids on respiratory morbidity in singletons after late-preterm birth. *Obstetrics & Gynecology, 119*(3), 555–559. doi:10.1097/AOG.0b013e31824758f6

Hanna, N., & Kiefer, D. (2012). A translational view of biomarkers in preterm labor. *American Journal of Reproductive Immunology, 67*(4), 268–272. doi:10.1111/j.1600-0897.2012.01112.x

Jazayeri, A. (2014). Premature rupture of membranes *.Medscape.* Retrieved from http://emedicine .medscape.com/article/261137-overview

Joy, S. (2015). Placenta previa. *Medscape.* Retrieved from http://emedicine.medscape.com /article/262063-overview#a0156

Kenyon, S., Boulvain, M., & Neilson, J. (2013). Antibiotics for preterm rupture of membranes. *Cochrane Database of Systematic Reviews.* Issue 12, Art. No.: CD001058.

March of Dimes. (2015). *March of Dimes premature birth report card.* Retrieved from http://www .marchofdimes.org/mission/prematurity-reportcard .aspx#

Martin, J. A., Hamilton, B. E., Osterman, M. J. K., Curtain, S. C., & Matthews, T. J. (2013). Births: Final data for 2012. *National Vital Statistics Reports, 62*(9), 1–87.

Norwitz, E. R. (2014). *Cervical insufficiency treatment and management.* Retrieved from http://emedicine.medscape.com/article/1979914 -treatment#showall

Norwitz, E. R., & Caughey, A. B. (2011). Progesterone supplementation and the prevention of preterm birth. *Reviews in Obstetrics and Gynecology, 4*(2), 60–72.

Posner, G., & Black, A. (2013). Oxorne & Foote human labor and birth. (6th ed.). Philadelphia, PA: McGraw-Hill.

Ramin, S., & Ramin, K. (2012). *Disseminated intravascular coagulation during pregnancy.* Retrieved from http://www.uptodate.com/contents/disseminated- intravascular-coagulation-during-pregnancy

Ross, M. G. (2013). *Preterm labor.* Retrieved from http:// emedicine.medscape.com/article/260998 -overview#aw2aab6b4

Simhan, H., & Caritis, S. (2015). *Inhibition of acute preterm labor. Up-to-date.* Retrieved from http://www .uptodate.com/contents/inhibition-of-acute -preterm-labor

U.S. Department of Health and Human Services. (2011). *Healthy People 2020: Improving the health of Americans.* Retrieved from www.healthypeople .gov

Wilson, B. A., Shannon, M. T., & Shields, K. L. (Eds.). (2015). *Pearson's nurse's drug guide: 2016.* Upper Saddle River, NJ: Prentice Hall.

Wojcieszek, A., Stock, O., & Flenady, V. (2014). Antibiotics for prelabour rupture of membranes at or near term. *Cochrane Database of Systematic Reviews.* Issue 10. Art. No.: CD001807.

Zheng, T. (2012). *Comprehensive handbook of obstetrics and gynecology* (2nd ed.). Phoenix, AZ: Phoenix Medical Press.

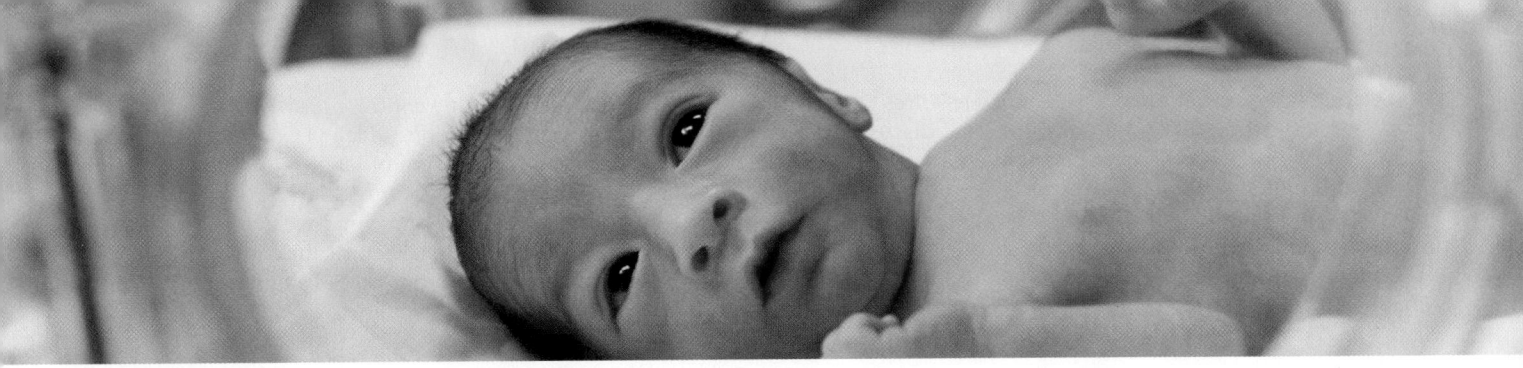

Chapter 21
Childbirth at Risk: Labor-Related Complications

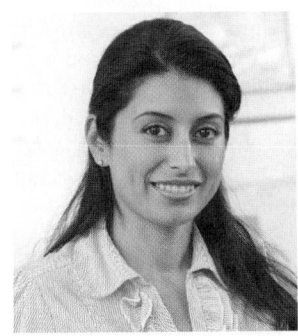

We arrived at the birthing unit with such wonderful plans for the birth of our first baby. I was able to do my breathing with the assistance of my husband and the nurse. Then suddenly my baby's heart rate dropped. It lasted for about 20 seconds but it felt like a lifetime. The nurse helped me to my side, and just stayed with us while we waited and watched the fetal monitor. There were no further problems, but I will never forget that moment.

—Yolanda, 26

Monkey Business/Fotolia

Learning Outcomes

21.1 Compare tachysystolic and hypotonic labor patterns, including the risks, clinical therapy, and nursing management.

21.2 Describe the risks and clinical therapy in determining the nursing management of postterm pregnancy on the childbearing family.

21.3 Relate the various types of fetal malposition and malpresentation to the nursing management for each.

21.4 Explain the identification, risks, and clinical therapy in determining the nursing management of the woman and fetus at risk for fetal macrosomia.

21.5 Relate the maternal implications, clinical therapy, prenatal history, and conditions that may be associated with nonreassuring fetal status to the nursing management of the mother and fetus.

21.6 Describe the nursing management of the mother and fetus with a prolapsed umbilical cord.

21.7 Summarize the identification, maternal and fetal/neonatal implications, clinical therapy, and nursing management of the woman with amniotic fluid embolism (anaphylactoid syndrome of pregnancy).

21.8 Explain the types, maternal and fetal/neonatal implications, and clinical therapy in determining the nursing management of the woman with cephalopelvic disproportion.

21.9 Identify common complications of the third and fourth stages of labor.

21.10 Explain the etiology, diagnosis, and phases of grief in determining the nursing management of the family experiencing perinatal loss.

Successful completion of a pregnancy requires the harmonious functioning of the critical factors discussed in the *Critical Factors in Labor* section in Chapter 16: the birth passage, the fetus, the relationship between the passage and the fetus, and the forces of labor. Disruptions in any of these components may cause dystocia (abnormal or difficult labor). The most common of these disruptions are discussed in this chapter.

Care of the Woman With Dystocia Related to Dysfunctional Uterine Contractions

The onset of labor is a time that often triggers emotions that may include excitement, relief, fear, anxiety, and anticipation. Normal labor patterns may be irregular initially but eventually result in regular contractions that increase in frequency, duration, and intensity as labor progresses. Most women develop a contraction pattern that follows these characteristics that lead to a normal progression of labor and subsequent birth. Chapter 17 provides an overview of labor assessment.

Dystocia, or difficult labor, may be caused by a wide variety of problems, the most common of which is dysfunctional (or uncoordinated) uterine contractions. These uncoordinated contractions result in a prolonged labor. Contractions that result in a more normal progression of labor tend to be moderate to strong when palpated and occur regularly (two to four contractions in 10 minutes in early labor and four to five per 10 minutes in later phases). Dysfunctional contractions are typically irregular in strength, timing, or both. These irregular uterine contractions often arrest cervical dilatation.

Tachysystolic Labor Patterns

A normal contraction pattern is shown in Figure 21–1*A*. A tachysystolic labor pattern refers to a pattern of "more than five contractions in 10 minutes, averaged over a 30-minute window, contractions lasting 2 minutes or more, contractions of normal duration occurring within 1 minute of each other or no resting tone between contractions. Contractions occurring six or more times in 10 minutes, lasting longer than 2 minutes, or increasing resting tone is greater than 20 mg per mmHg with an IUPC" (intrauterine pressure catheter) (American College of Obstetricians and Gynecologists [ACOG], 2011, p. 12). The term is specifically connected with the contraction pattern and often results in fetal heart rate (FHR) changes. The presence or absence of FHR decelerations should be documented. This pattern is commonly associated with induced or augmented labors but can also occur in spontaneous labor.

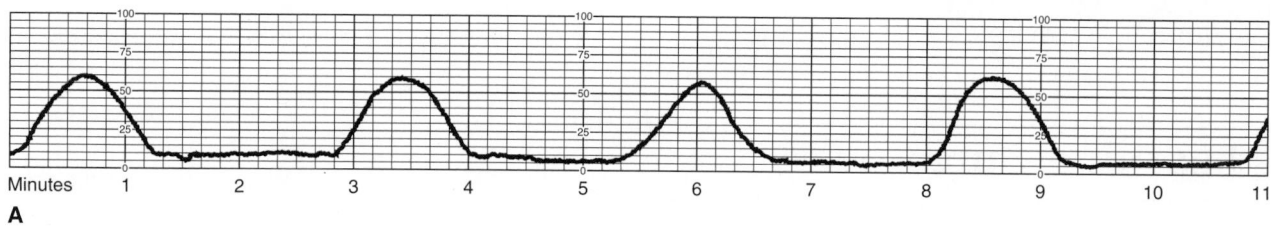

A

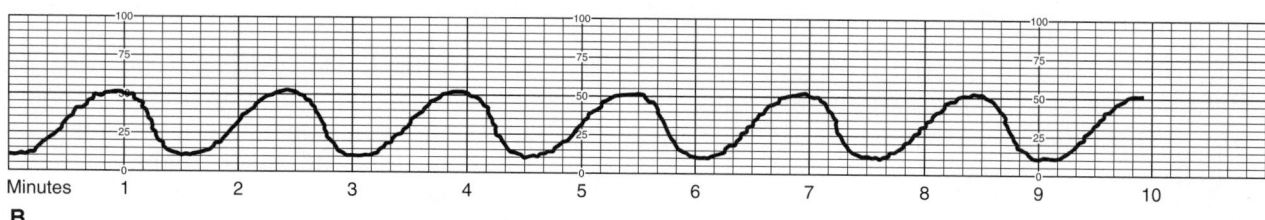

B

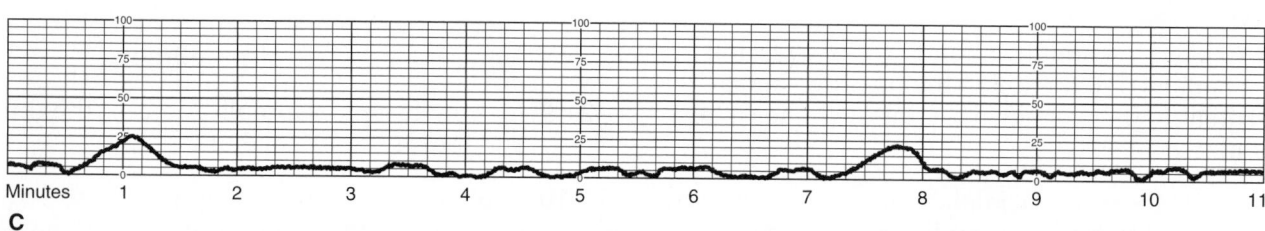

C

Figure 21–1 Comparison of labor patterns. *A*, Normal uterine contraction pattern. In this example, contraction frequency is every 3 minutes; duration is 60 seconds. The baseline resting tone is below 10 mmHg. *B*, Tachysystolic uterine contraction pattern. Note that the contraction frequency is every 1.5 minutes, duration is 90.0 seconds. The baseline resting tone is 10 mmHg. *C*, Hypotonic uterine contraction pattern. In this example, the contraction frequency is every 7 minutes (with some uterine activity between contractions), duration is 50 seconds, and intensity increases approximately 25 mmHg during contractions.

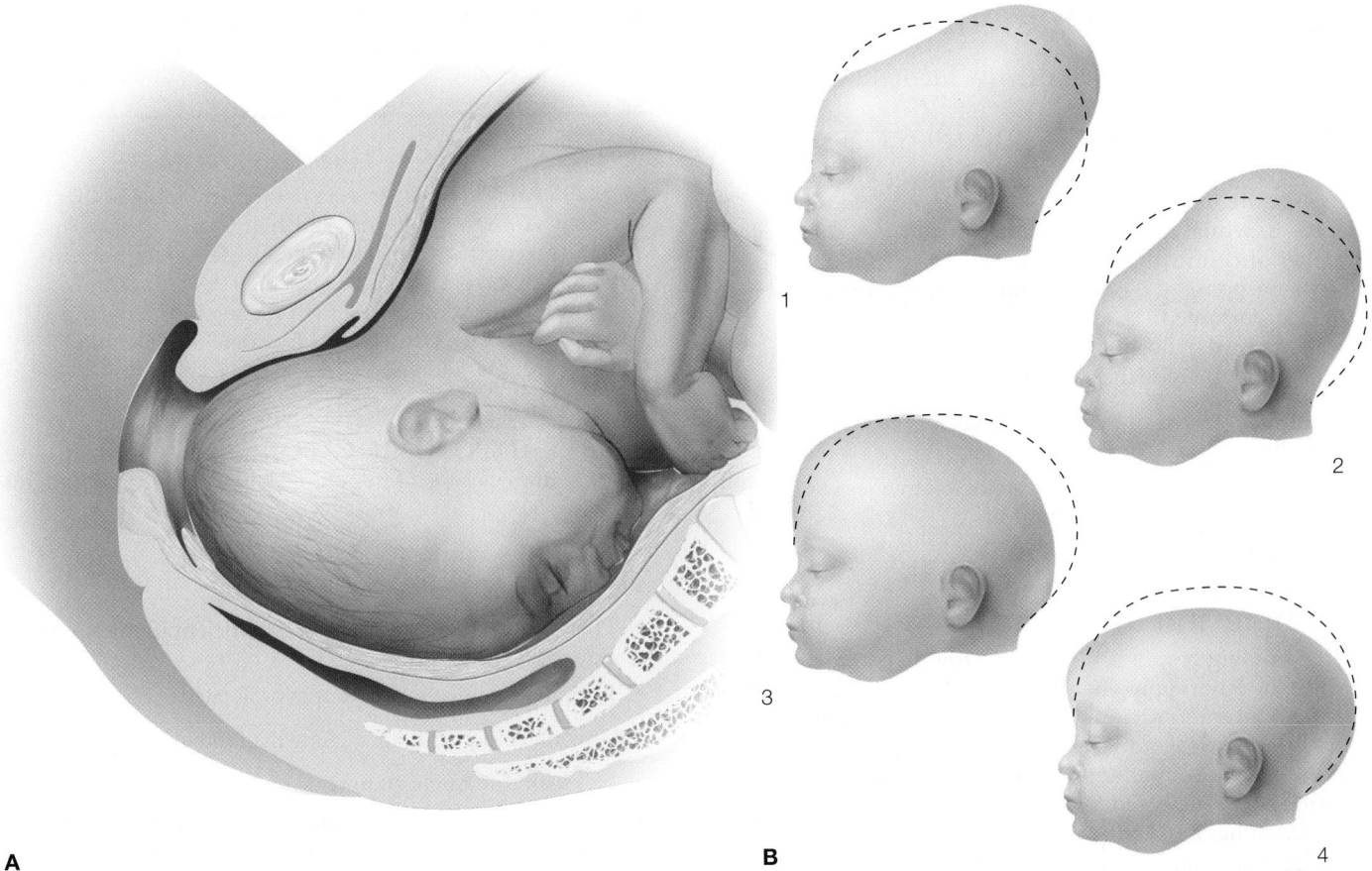

A   **B**

> **Figure 21–2** Effects of labor on the fetal head. *A,* Caput succedaneum formation. The presenting portion of the scalp area is encircled by the cervix during labor, causing swelling of the soft tissue. *B,* Molding of the fetal head in cephalic presentations: (1) occiput anterior, (2) occiput posterior, (3) brow, (4) face.

RISKS OF TACHYSYSTOLIC LABOR

Maternal risks of tachysystolic labor include the following:

- Increased discomfort due to uterine muscle cell anoxia
- Fatigue as the pattern continues
- Stress on coping abilities
- Dehydration and increased incidence of infection if labor is prolonged
- Placental abruption

Fetal/neonatal risks include the following:

- Nonreassuring fetal status because contractions and increased uterine tone interfere with the uteroplacental exchange of gases and nutrients
- Prolonged pressure on the fetal head, which may result in cephalohematoma, caput succedaneum, or excessive molding (Figure 21–2)

CLINICAL THERAPY

In 2008, the National Institute of Child Health and Human Development (NICHD), along with ACOG and the Society for Maternal–Fetal Medicine, revised fetal monitoring guidelines to better interpret and document fetal heart rate patterns. The guidelines provide practitioners with more concrete criteria and determine more effective management strategies.

Management of tachysystolic labor with nonreassuring fetal heart rate patterns includes discontinuing oxytocin (if being administered), turning mother to left lateral position, giving an IV bolus of 250 to 300 mL of lactated Ringer solution, applying oxygen via facemask at 8 to 10 L/min, and, if ordered, administering terbutaline 0.25 mg.

Regardless of the interventions taken, tachysystole should be reported to the physician/CNM along with the nursing actions that have been performed. When tachysystole occurs with normal FHR patterns, maternal repositioning to either the right or left side should be performed, and a fluid bolus of 250 to 300 mL of lactated Ringer solution should be administered. If contractions continue at greater than five contractions in 10 minutes, the oxytocin infusion should be decreased by half. If after 10 minutes, excessive contractions continue, the oxytocin infusion should be stopped completely. Terbutaline 0.25 mg should be on hand for any woman experiencing tachysystole. If the tachysystole resolves within 20 to 30 minutes of discontinuation, oxytocin can be restarted at half the last given rate. Longer periods of cessation of tachysystole of 35 to 45 minutes require the oxytocin infusion to be restarted at the 2 milliunits per minute rate with continuous monitoring to ensure reoccurrence does not develop (ACOG, 2011).

Clinical Tip

To determine whether the fetal heart rate (FHR) is reassuring, look for the following: baseline FHR of 110 to 160 beats/min, presence of variability, spontaneous accelerations, and absence of decelerations. In order to effectively determine if a FHR is reassuring, a category should be assigned. The absence of recurrent variables or late or prolonged decelerations are also indicative of a reassuring FHR tracing.

Nursing Management

For the Woman Experiencing Tachysystolic Labor

Nursing Assessment and Diagnosis

As part of the labor assessment, evaluate the relationship between the intensity of the pain being experienced and the degree to which the cervix is dilating and effacing. Note the number of contractions that occur within a 10-minute period and the response of the FHR. Continuous electronic fetal monitoring is warranted.

Nursing diagnoses that may apply to the woman in tachysystolic labor include the following (NANDA-I © 2014):

- *Fatigue* related to inability to relax and rest secondary to a tachysystolic labor pattern
- *Coping, Ineffective*, related to ineffectiveness of breathing techniques to relieve discomfort
- *Anxiety* related to possible nonreassuring fetal heart tone

Planning and Implementation

A key nursing responsibility is to provide comfort and support to the laboring woman and her partner and to keep them informed of interventions being administered along with the rationale for each intervention. The woman experiencing a tachysystolic labor pattern will probably be very uncomfortable because of the increased force of contractions. Her anxiety level and that of her partner may be high. Work to reduce the woman's discomfort and promote a more effective labor pattern.

Nursing interventions include position changes, therapeutic touch, and visualization, as well as comfort measures such as mouth care, change of linens, effleurage, and relaxation exercises. The use of tub baths or a warm shower can help promote comfort and uterine relaxation; however, continuous fetal monitoring must be maintained. If sedation is ordered, ensure that the environment is conducive to relaxation. The labor partner may also need assistance in helping the woman cope. A calm, understanding approach offers the woman and her partner further support. Providing information about the cause of the tachysystolic labor pattern and assuring the woman that she is not overreacting to the situation are important nursing actions.

Client education is key for the woman experiencing tachysystolic labor. She needs information about the dysfunctional labor pattern and the possible implications for her and her baby. Information will help relieve anxiety and thereby increase relaxation and comfort. Explain treatment options and offer opportunities to ask questions. Have all needed equipment on hand, including terbutaline, should it need to be administered.

Evaluation

Expected outcomes of nursing care include the following:

- The woman has increased comfort and decreased anxiety.
- The woman and her partner are able to cope with the labor.
- The woman experiences a more effective labor pattern.

Hypotonic Labor Patterns

A hypotonic labor pattern usually develops in the active phase of labor, after labor has been well established. Hypotonic labor is characterized by fewer than two to three contractions in a 10-minute period (see Figure 21–1C). Hypotonic labor may occur when the uterus is overstretched from a twin gestation or in the presence of a large fetus, hydramnios, or grand multiparity. Bladder or bowel distention and cephalopelvic disproportion (CPD) may also be associated with this pattern.

> **Clinical Reasoning** Fetal Heart Rate Tracing
>
> A fetal heart rate (FHR) tracing demonstrates the following: baseline heart rate of 140 with variability of 6 to 10 beats/min. When you compare the FHR with the uterine contractions, you note that there is a slowing of the FHR at the time of the contraction and that the FHR tracing looks like the contraction curve, but it is upside down. Based on this tracing, what would you do?

RISKS OF HYPOTONIC LABOR

Maternal implications of hypotonic labor patterns include the following risks:

- Maternal exhaustion
- Stress on coping abilities
- Postpartum hemorrhage from insufficient uterine contractions following birth
- Intrauterine infection if labor is prolonged

Fetal/neonatal implications include the following:

- Nonreassuring fetal status due to prolonged labor pattern
- Fetal sepsis from pathogens that ascend from the birth canal in the presence of ruptured membranes

CLINICAL THERAPY

The goals of clinical therapy are to improve the quality of the uterine contractions and to ensure a safe outcome for the woman and her baby. Uterine contractions can be stimulated in several ways, including the use of oxytocin (Pitocin), amniotomy, stimulation of the nipples, or a combination of these methods, which cause the release of oxytocin. Before initiating treatment for hypotonic labor, the physician/CNM validates the adequacy of pelvic measurements and completes tests to establish gestational age if fetal maturity is in question. After CPD, fetal malpresentation, and fetal immaturity have been ruled out, oxytocin may be given intravenously (IV) via an infusion pump to improve the quality of uterine contractions. Intravenous fluid is useful to maintain adequate hydration and prevent maternal exhaustion. Amniotomy is sometimes used to stimulate the labor process. The application of an electric breast pump or manual stimulation of the nipples may help strengthen uterine contractions, and is an excellent starting point for women who want an unmedicated birth.

Some physicians support the use of *active management of labor* (AMOL), a process whereby labor is managed from the beginning with amniotomy, timed cervical examinations are performed, and augmentation of labor with IV administration of oxytocin (Pitocin) is begun if a specified level of progress is not met. Supporters of AMOL contend that it is a preventive treatment that reduces the chance for protracted labor and decreases the cesarean birth rate. Opponents argue that the use of AMOL increases the incidence of infection (because of frequent vaginal examinations), necessitates the use of additional interventions, and increases the incidence of instrument-assisted births (King, Brucker, Kriebs, et al., 2013).

An improvement in the quality of uterine contractions is demonstrated by noticeable progress in the labor. If the labor pattern does not become effective or if other complications develop, further interventions, including cesarean birth, may be necessary.

Nursing Management

For the Woman Experiencing Hypotonic Labor

Nursing Assessment and Diagnosis

Assessment of contractions (for frequency, intensity, and duration), maternal vital signs, and FHR provides data to evaluate maternal–fetal status. Also be alert for signs and symptoms of infection and dehydration. Because of the stress associated with a prolonged labor, observe the woman and her partner's success in implementing coping mechanisms.

Nursing diagnoses that may apply to the woman in hypotonic labor include the following (NANDA-I © 2014):

- *Pain, Acute*, related to uterine contractions secondary to dysfunctional labor
- *Coping, Ineffective*, related to unanticipated discomfort and slow progress in labor
- *Fatigue* related to prolonged labor and discomfort

Planning and Implementation

Nursing measures to promote maternal–fetal physical well-being include frequent monitoring of contractions, maternal vital signs, and FHR. If amniotic membranes are ruptured, assess for the presence of meconium, which makes close observation of fetal status more critical because it often indicates that the fetus is experiencing some form of stress. An intake and output record provides a way of determining maternal hydration or dehydration. Encourage the woman to void every 2 hours, and check her bladder for distention. Because labor may be prolonged, continue to monitor the woman for signs of infection (elevated temperature, chills, foul-smelling amniotic fluid, and fetal tachycardia). Vaginal examinations should be kept to a minimum to decrease the risk of introducing an infection.

The couple experiencing a hypotonic labor pattern requires emotional support. Help them cope with the frustration of a lengthy labor process. Combine a warm, caring approach with techniques to reduce anxiety and discomfort.

The teaching plan needs to include information about the dysfunctional labor process and implications for the mother and baby. Disadvantages of and alternatives to treatment also need to be discussed and understood.

Evaluation

Expected outcomes of nursing care include the following:

- The woman maintains comfort during labor.
- The woman understands the type of labor pattern that is occurring and the treatment plan.

Care of the Woman With Postterm Pregnancy

A **postterm pregnancy** is one that extends more than 294 days or 42 weeks past the first day of the last menstrual period (LMP). In 2013, the American College of Obstetricians and Gynecologists revised terminology related to pregnancy duration. The following terminology was adopted.

- *Extremely preterm:* birth occurring at or before 25 weeks of pregnancy
- *Very preterm:*, birth occurring at less than 32 weeks of pregnancy

- *Moderately preterm:* birth occurring between 32 and 34 weeks of pregnancy
- *Late preterm:*, birth occurring between 34 and 36 weeks of pregnancy
- *Full-term*: birth occurring between 39 weeks 0 days and 40 weeks and 6 days
- *Late-term:* birth that occurs between 41 weeks 0 days and 41 weeks 6 days
- *Postterm:* birth that occurs beyond 42 weeks 0 days

Postterm birth is distinct from a *postdate* pregnancy, which means that the pregnancy has gone beyond the estimated date of birth (EDB) at 40 weeks. The incidence of postdate pregnancy ranges from 7% to 12% but only 4% of pregnancies last longer than 43 weeks (Caughley, 2013). The cause of true postterm pregnancy is unknown, but it seems to occur more frequently in primigravidas, women with a history of prolonged pregnancy, and in the presence of fetal anencephaly or placental sulfatase deficiency (Caughley, 2013). Women who have experienced a previous postterm pregnancy have a 30% to 40% incidence of postterm pregnancy in subsequent pregnancies (Caughley, 2013).

Risks of Prolonged Pregnancy

Maternal risks associated with prolonged pregnancy include the following (Caughley, 2013):

- Probable labor induction
- Increased risk for large-for-gestational-age (LGA) newborn and resultant perineal trauma
- Increased incidence of forceps-assisted, vacuum-assisted, or cesarean birth
- Increased psychologic stress as the due date passes and concern for the baby increases
- Increased risk of infection

Fetal risks include the following (Caughley, 2013):

- Decreased perfusion from the placenta
- Oligohydramnios (decreased amount of amniotic fluid), which increases the risk of cord compression
- Meconium aspiration (aspiration of meconium-stained amniotic fluid by the fetus at the time of birth), which is more likely if oligohydramnios and thick meconium are present
- Low 5-minute Apgar score

Some fetuses continue to grow beyond the 42nd week of pregnancy and can be excessively large at birth (macrosomia). In other cases, the intrauterine environment becomes unfavorable for growth, uteroplacental insufficiency occurs, and at birth the neonate has lost muscle mass and subcutaneous fat. This is known as *dysmaturity syndrome*. The macrosomic fetus is at risk for birth trauma, whereas the small-for-gestational-age (SGA) fetus is at risk for nonreassuring fetal status during labor because there is often associated oligohydramnios (Caughley, 2013).

Clinical Therapy

In managing prolonged pregnancy, some caregivers prefer induction at 41 weeks; others advocate expectant management by doing a non-stress test (NST) and biophysical profile (BPP) (especially the amniotic fluid volume portion of the BPP— the amniotic fluid index) 2 to 3 times a week to evaluate fetal well-being (Caughley, 2013). If the fetal assessment tests indicate a problem, interventions are begun to accomplish the birth.

Nursing Management

For the Woman With Postterm Pregnancy

Nursing Assessment and Diagnosis

When the woman is admitted into the birthing area, ongoing assessments of fetal well-being begin as soon as the postterm condition has been verified. Identify reassuring FHR characteristics and evaluate for the presence of nonreassuring patterns, such as nonperiodic variable decelerations, so that corrective actions can be taken. When the amniotic membranes rupture, assess the fluid for meconium. In addition, assess the woman's knowledge about the condition, implications for her baby, risks, and possible interventions.

Nursing diagnoses that may apply to the woman with postterm pregnancy include the following (NANDA-I © 2014):

- *Fear* related to the unknown outcome for the baby
- *Coping, Ineffective*, related to anxiety about the status of the baby
- *Anxiety* related to potential unknown maternal and fetal outcomes

Planning and Implementation

COMMUNITY-BASED NURSING CARE
If the woman has not been assessing fetal movement every day, teach her how to do so. It is vital to stress the importance of

identifying inadequate fetal movement and immediately contacting her healthcare provider. (See the *Fetal Activity Monitoring* section in Chapter 13 for further discussion of techniques to detect fetal movement.)

Client education about the postterm pregnancy is another important nursing responsibility. Address the implications and associated risks for the baby, as well as possible treatment plans. The woman and her partner need opportunities to ask questions and clarify information.

HOSPITAL-BASED NURSING CARE
Promoting fetal well-being requires careful assessment of the response of the fetus during labor. If oligohydramnios exists, obtain a continuous FHR tracing and evaluate it frequently. Variable decelerations are often associated with oligohydramnios because the decreased amount of fluid may allow compression of the umbilical cord. When oligohydramnios is present, an amnioinfusion is sometimes performed to increase the fluid in the uterine cavity. If an amnioinfusion is used, be alert for potential cord prolapse. (Amnioinfusion is discussed in detail in Chapter 22.) When preterm premature rupture of fetal membranes (PPROM) is present, the risk of prolapsed umbilical cord can also occur. If the fetus is macrosomic, carefully assess labor progress (contraction characteristics, progressive cervical dilatation, and fetal descent).

Emotional support is a key nursing intervention for women with pregnancies that extend past their due dates. Women experiencing postterm pregnancy frequently feel increased stress and anxiety and have difficulty coping. Encouragement, support, and recognition of the woman's anxiety are helpful strategies.

Evaluation

Expected outcomes of nursing care include the following:

- The woman has knowledge about the postterm pregnancy.
- The woman and her partner feel supported and able to cope with the postterm pregnancy.
- Fetal status is maintained, any abnormalities are quickly identified, and supportive measures are initiated.

Care of the Woman and Fetus at Risk Because of Fetal Malposition

Persistent occiput posterior (POP) position is the most common fetal malposition and occurs when the fetus does not rotate but is born in the occiput posterior (OP) position. (See Figure 16–9 to review fetal presentations.) This position may be normal in women with small pelvises. It may also be related to poor contractions, abnormal flexion of the head, inadequate maternal pushing efforts usually related to epidural anesthesia, or a large fetus. Labor may be prolonged; however, most POP fetuses are born without the aid of forceps.

Risks of Fetal Malposition

Maternal risks related to the POP position include the following:

- Risk of third- or fourth-degree perineal lacerations during birth
- Risk of extension of a midline episiotomy

Fetal implications do not include an increased mortality risk unless labor is prolonged or additional interventions such as forceps-assisted, vacuum-assisted, or cesarean birth are required.

Clinical Therapy

Clinical treatment focuses on close monitoring of maternal and fetal status and labor progress to determine whether vaginal or cesarean birth is the safer method. A cesarean birth is chosen if maternal or fetal problems make a vaginal birth unwise or if cephalopelvic disproportion (CPD) is present. The majority of POP fetuses are born vaginally, either spontaneously or with the assistance of forceps. The forceps can be used to assist in the birth of the fetus while it is still in the occiput posterior position or to rotate the occiput to an anterior position (called Scanzoni maneuver). (See Chapter 22 for further discussion of forceps use.)

Women With Special Needs **Autonomic Dysreflexia**

Autonomic dysreflexia is a rare complication that can occur in women with a spinal cord injury. It is caused by overstimulation of the nerve pathways and is characterized by paroxysmal hypertension, intense throbbing headaches, profuse perspiration, nasal stuffiness, anxiety, and skin flushing. Cognitive impairment may also occur. The condition is life threatening and requires prompt intervention and immediate evaluation from the obstetrician and anesthesiologist.

Nursing Management

For the Laboring Woman With the Fetus in Persistent Occiput Posterior Position

Nursing Assessment and Diagnosis

Signs and symptoms of a POP position include complaints of intense back pain by the laboring woman, a dysfunctional labor pattern, hypotonic labor (the fetal head does not put adequate pressure on the cervix), arrest of dilatation, or arrest of fetal descent. The back pain is caused by the fetal occiput compressing the sacral nerves. Further assessment may reveal a depression in the maternal abdomen above the symphysis. FHR is typically heard far laterally on the abdomen. On vaginal examination, the physician/CNM finds the wide, diamond-shaped anterior fontanelle in the anterior portion of the pelvis. This fontanelle may be difficult to feel because of molding of the fetal head.

Nursing diagnoses that may apply to women with POP-positioned fetuses include the following (NANDA-I © 2014):

- *Pain, Acute*, related to back discomfort secondary to the OP position
- *Coping, Ineffective*, related to unanticipated discomfort and slow progress in labor

PLANNING AND IMPLEMENTATION

Changing maternal posture has been used for many years to enhance rotation of OP or occiput transverse (OT) to occiput anterior (OA). A number of position changes may be tried. For instance, the woman may be asked to lie on one side and then asked to move to the other side as the fetus begins to rotate. This side-lying position may promote rotation; it also enables the support person to apply counterpressure on the sacral area to decrease discomfort. A knee–chest position provides a downward slant to the vaginal canal, directing the fetal head downward on descent. A hands-and-knees position is often effective in rotating the fetus. In addition to maintaining a hands-and-knees position on the bed, the woman may try pelvic rocking, and the support person may firmly stroke the abdomen. The stroking begins over the fetal back and swings around to the other side of the abdomen. After the fetus has rotated, the woman lies in a Sims position on the side opposite the fetal back.

Evaluation

Expected outcomes of nursing care include the following:

- The woman's discomfort is decreased.
- The coping abilities of the woman and her partner are strengthened.

Care of the Woman and Fetus at Risk Because of Fetal Malpresentation

In a normal presentation, the occiput is the presenting part (Figure 21–3A). *Fetal malpresentations* include brow, face, breech, shoulder (transverse lie), and compound presentation.

Brow Presentation

In a *brow presentation*, the forehead of the fetus becomes the presenting part. In the *sinciput (military) presentation*, the fetal head is between flexion and extension (Figure 21–3B), whereas in the

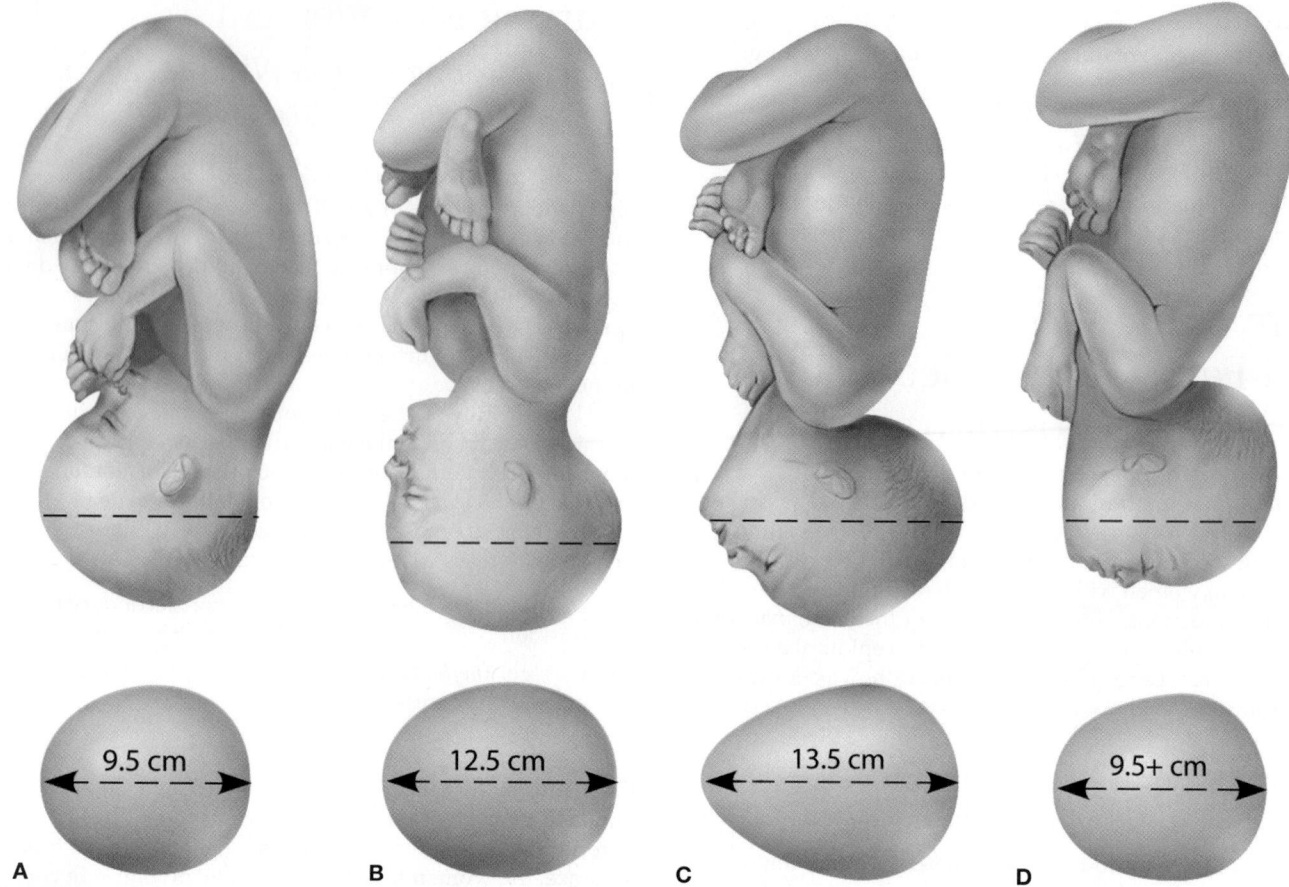

A   **B**   **C**   **D**

Figure 21–3 Types of cephalic presentations. *A*, The occiput is the presenting part because the head is flexed and the fetal chin is against the chest. The largest anteroposterior (AP) diameter that presents and passes through the pelvis is approximately 9.5 cm (3.2 in.). *B*, Sinciput (military) presentation. The head is neither flexed nor extended. The presenting AP diameter is approximately 12.5 cm (4.9 in.). *C*, Brow (occipitomental) presentation. The largest diameter of the fetal head (approximately 13.5 cm [5.3 in.]) presents in this situation. *D*, Face presentation. The AP diameter is 9.5 cm (3.2 in.).

occipitomental presentation, the fetal head enters the birth canal with the widest diameter of the head (approximately 13.5 cm [5.4 in.]) foremost (Figure 21–3C).

The brow presentation occurs more often in multiparas than in nulliparas and is thought to be due to lax abdominal and pelvic musculature. Many brow presentations spontaneously convert to face or occipital presentations. Brow presentations are the least common types of abnormal presentations.

RISKS OF BROW PRESENTATION
Maternal implications of brow presentation include increased risk of the following:

- Longer labor due to ineffective contractions and slow or arrested fetal descent
- Cesarean birth if brow presentation persists

Fetal/neonatal risks include increased mortality because of cerebral and neck compression and damage to the trachea and larynx. In addition, facial edema, bruising, and exaggerated molding of the newborn's head may be observed.

CLINICAL THERAPY
If a brow presentation fails to convert to occipital or face presentation, cesarean birth is indicated in most cases (King et al., 2013). If a vaginal birth is attempted, the woman is closely monitored for cephalopelvic disproportion (CPD), facial edema,

and nonreassuring fetal status. Attempts to convert brow presentations manually or through the use of forceps or vacuum are contraindicated, as is the use of oxytocin. The use of oxytocin can result in dystocia. Scalp electrodes should not be placed when the fetus is in a brow presentation (King et al., 2013).

Nursing Management
For the Laboring Woman With the Fetus in Brow Presentation

Nursing Assessment and Diagnosis
A brow presentation can be detected on vaginal examination by palpation of the diamond-shaped anterior fontanelle on one side and orbital ridges and root of the nose on the other side.

Nursing diagnoses that may apply to a woman with a brow presentation include the following (NANDA-I © 2014):

- *Knowledge, Deficient*, related to lack of information about the possible maternal–fetal effects of brow presentation
- *Injury, Risk for*, to the fetus related to pressure on fetal structures secondary to brow presentation
- *Fear* related to sudden need for cesarean birth if conversion does not occur

Evaluation

Expected outcomes of nursing care include the following:

- The woman and her partner understand the implications and associated problems of brow presentation.
- The mother and her baby have a safe labor and birth.

Face Presentation

In a face presentation, the face of the fetus is the presenting part (Figure 21–3D and Figure 21–4). The fetal head is hyperextended even more than in the brow presentation. Face presentation occurs most frequently in multiparas, in preterm birth, and in the presence of anencephaly. The incidence of face presentation is about 1 in 600 births.

Planning and Implementation

Closely observe the woman for labor problems and the fetus for signs of hypoxia as evidenced by late decelerations and bradycardia. Provide emotional support to the family. Explain the fetal position to the woman and her support person or interpret what the physician/CNM has told them. Stay close at hand to reassure the couple, inform them of any changes, and assist them with labor-coping techniques. In face and brow presentations, the newborn's face may be edematous. The couple may need help in beginning the attachment process because of the newborn's facial appearance. After the baby is inspected for any abnormalities, you and the pediatrician can assure the couple that the facial edema is only temporary and will subside in 3 or 4 days and that the molding will be much less visible in a few days (even though completion of the process takes several weeks).

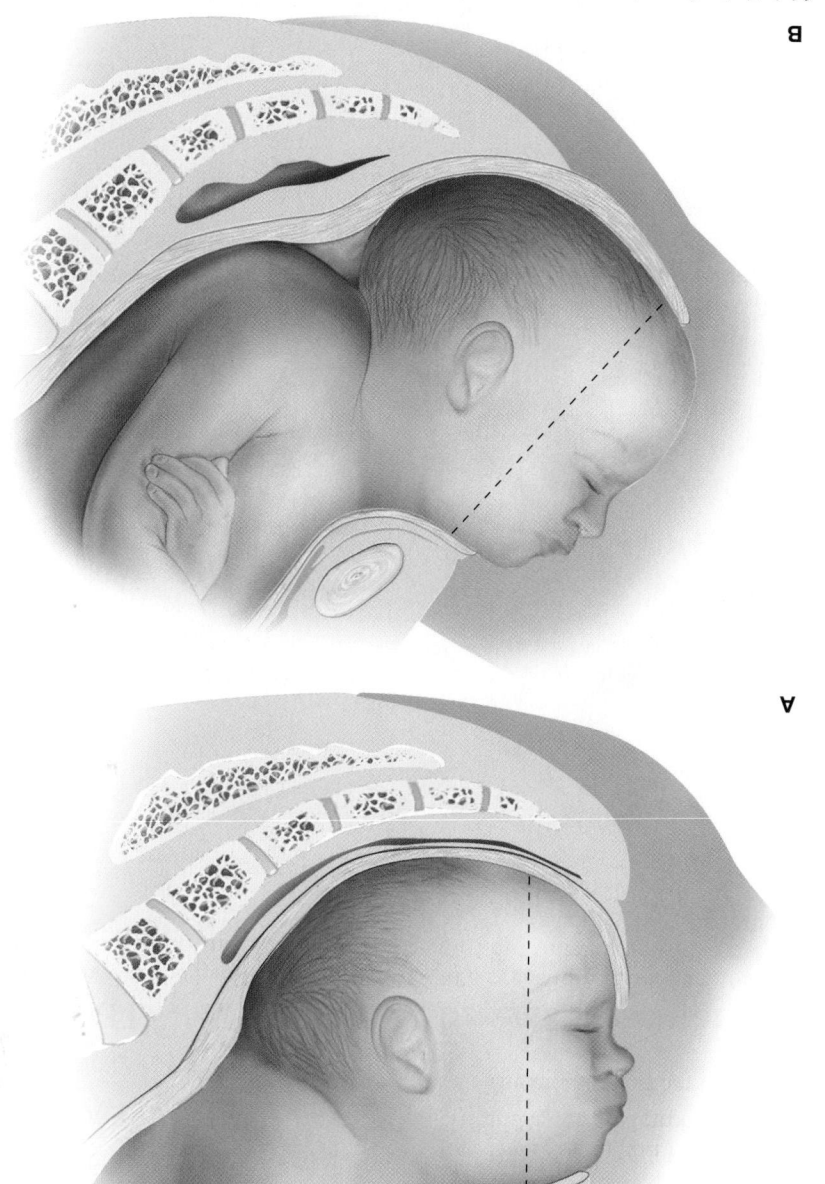

Figure 21–4 ■ Mechanism of birth in face (mentoanterior) position. A, The submentobregmatic diameter at the outlet. B, The fetal head is born by the movement of flexion.

RISKS OF FACE PRESENTATION

Maternal risks related to face presentation include the following:

- Increased risk of CPD and prolonged labor
- Increased risk of infection (with prolonged labor)
- Cesarean birth if fetal chin is posterior (mentum posterior)

Fetal/neonatal risks include the following:

- Cephalohematoma
- Edema of the face and throat if the fetal chin is anterior (mentum anterior)
- Pronounced molding of the head
- Nonreassuring fetal status

CLINICAL THERAPY

A vaginal birth may be anticipated if no CPD is present, the chin (mentum) is anterior, and the labor pattern is effective, and the fetal status is reassuring. Many mentum posterior presentations spontaneously convert to anterior in the late stages of labor. If the mentum remains posterior, a vaginal birth is not possible and a cesarean birth is necessary (Figure 21–5).

Nursing Management

For the Laboring Woman With the Fetus in Face Presentation

Nursing Assessment and Diagnosis

When performing Leopold maneuvers, the back of the fetus is difficult to outline with a face presentation, and a deep furrow can be palpated between the hard occiput and the fetal back (Figure 21–6). Fetal heart tones are audible on the side where the fetal feet are palpated. It may be difficult to determine by vaginal examination whether a breech or face is presenting, especially if facial edema is already present. During the vaginal examination, palpation of the saddle of the nose and the gums should be attempted. When assessing engagement, remember that the face has to be deep within the pelvis before the biparietal diameters have entered the inlet.

Nursing diagnoses that may apply to the woman with a fetus in face presentation include the following (NANDA-I © 2014):

- *Fear* related to unknown outcome of the labor and a possible instrument-assisted or cesarean birth
- *Injury, Risk for,* to the newborn's face related to edema secondary to the birth process

Planning and Implementation

Nursing interventions are the same as those indicated for the brow presentation.

Evaluation

Expected outcomes of nursing care include the following:

- The woman and her partner understand the implications and associated problems of face presentation.
- The mother and her baby have a safe labor and birth.

Breech Presentation

In a breech presentation, the fetal head is not the presenting part but rather is found in the fundus of the uterus. The exact

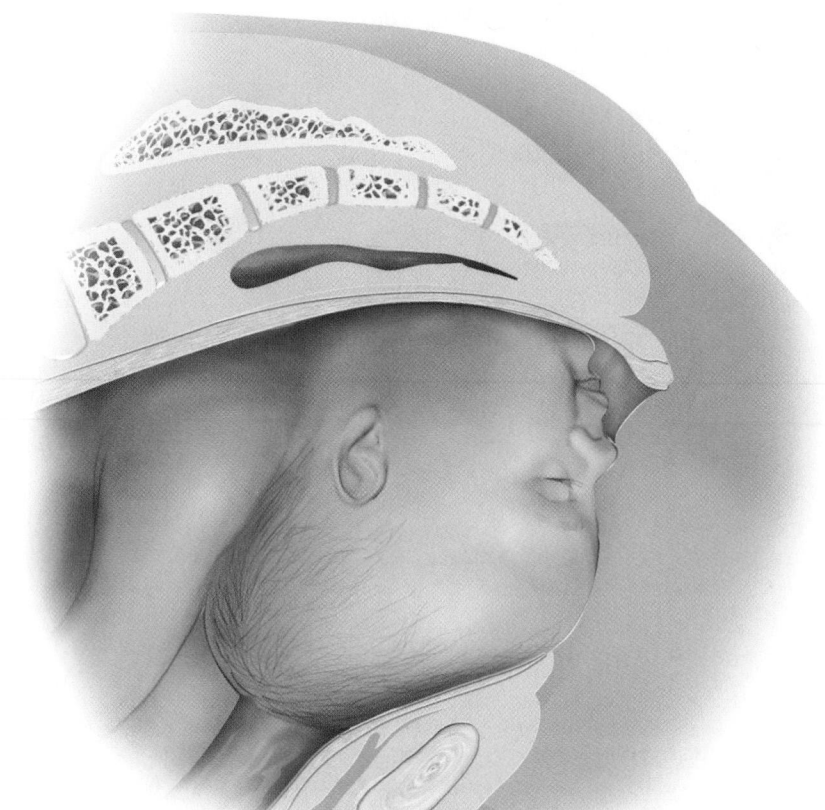

Figure 21–5 Face presentation. Mechanism of birth in mentoposterior position. Fetal head is unable to extend farther. The face becomes impacted.

permit palpation of facial features of the fetus.

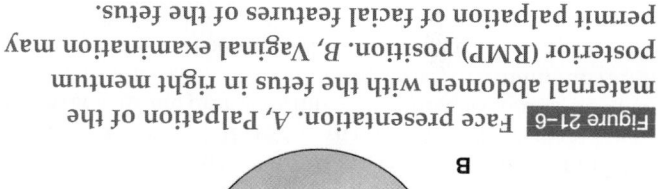

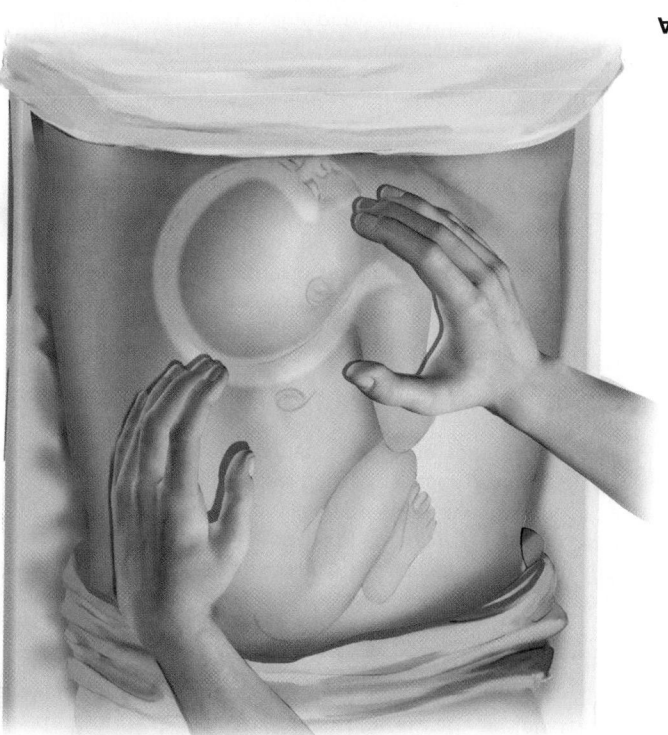

Figure 21–6 Face presentation. A, Palpation of the maternal abdomen with the fetus in right mentum posterior (RMP) position. B, Vaginal examination may permit palpation of facial features of the fetus.

cause of breech presentation (Figure 21–7) is unknown. This malpresentation occurs in about 3% to 4% of labors and is frequently associated with preterm birth, placenta previa, hydramnios, multiple gestation, uterine anomalies (such as bicornuate uterus), and fetal anomalies (especially anencephaly and hydrocephaly) (Cunningham et al., 2014).

RISKS OF BREECH PRESENTATION

The maternal implication of breech presentation is a likelihood of cesarean birth. Fetal/neonatal implications include the following (Cunningham et al., 2014):

- Higher perinatal morbidity and mortality rates
- Increased risk of prolapsed cord, especially in incomplete breeches because space is available between the cervix and presenting part
- Increased risk of cervical cord injuries caused by hyperextension of the fetal head during vaginal birth
- Increased risk of asphyxia and nonreassuring fetal status
- Increased risk of birth trauma (especially of the head) during either vaginal or cesarean breech birth

CLINICAL THERAPY

Current clinical therapy is directed toward converting the breech presentation to a cephalic presentation prior to the beginning of labor. Some physicians attempt an external cephalic version (ECV) at 36 to 38 weeks' gestation as long as the woman is not in labor. (See Chapter 22 for discussion of external version.) ACOG (2012) recommends a planned cesarean birth for the fetus in a breech presentation because of the significant increase in complications associated with breech vaginal births.

Nursing Management

For the Laboring Woman With the Fetus in Breech Presentation

Nursing Assessment and Diagnosis

Frequently, it is the nurse who first recognizes a breech presentation. On palpation, the firm fetal head is felt in the uterine fundus and the wider sacrum in the lower part of the abdomen.

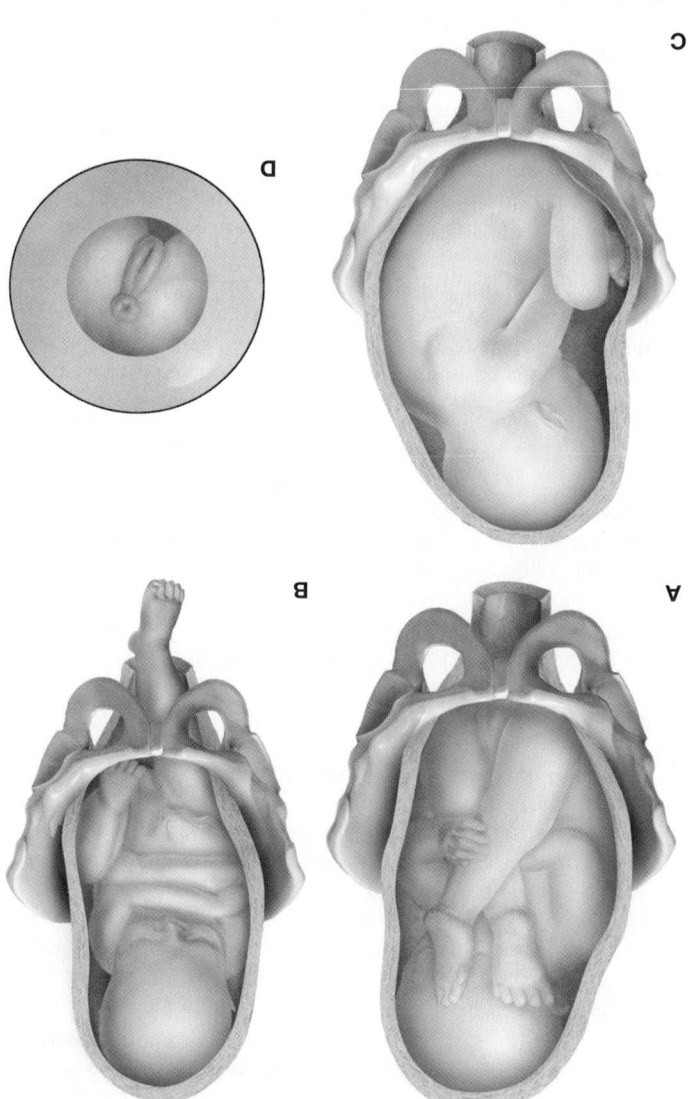

Figure 21–7 Breech presentation. A, Frank breech. B, Incomplete (footling) breech. C, Complete breech in left sacral anterior (LSA) position. D, On vaginal examination the nurse may feel the anal sphincter. The tissue of the fetal buttocks feels soft.

setup. You may be asked to assist the physician if forceps are needed for the birth. Few physicians are adequately trained in managing a breech vaginal birth.

SAFETY ALERT!
Some breech vaginal births occur spontaneously. It is of great importance to have an attending physician at the beside and to inform the charge nurse so the operating room can be set up. The neonatal response team should also be in attendance. If a physician with breech vaginal birth experience is readily available, the charge nurse should request assistance from that healthcare provider.

When a planned vaginal breech birth occurs, the operating room is equipped with a "double setup" in place. If difficulties arise with the birth, the room is already prepared for a cesarean so the procedure can be performed quickly. A neonatal response team or provider should be present in case adverse fetal effects arise. If the family and physician/CNM decide on a cesarean birth, provide assistance as with any cesarean birth.

Evaluation
Expected outcomes of nursing care include the following:
• The woman and her partner understand the implications and associated problems of breech presentation.
• Major complications are recognized early and corrective measures are instituted.
• The mother and baby have a safe labor and birth.

Transverse Lie (Shoulder Presentation) of a Single Fetus
A transverse lie occurs in approximately 1 in 300 term births (Cunningham et al., 2014). Maternal conditions associated with a transverse lie are grand multiparity with relaxed uterine muscles, preterm fetus, abnormal uterus, excessive amniotic fluid, placenta previa, and contracted pelvis (Figure 21-8).

CLINICAL THERAPY
The management of shoulder presentation depends on the gestational age. If discovered before term, the management is expectant (watchful) because some fetuses may change presentation without intervention. When a shoulder presentation is still evident at 37 completed weeks of gestation, an external cephalic version (ECV) attempt (followed, if successful, by induction of labor) is recommended because the associated risk of prolapsed cord is significant. Intrapartum ECV is often successful in early labor and can reduce the need for cesarean birth. If it is unsuccessful, cesarean birth is indicated.

Nursing Management
A transverse lie can be identified by inspection and palpation of the abdomen, by auscultation of the FHR, and by vaginal examination. On inspection, the woman's abdomen appears widest from side to side as a result of the long axis of the fetus's body lying parallel to the ground and across the mother's uterus.

On palpation, no fetal part is felt in the fundal portion of the uterus or above the symphysis. The head may be palpated on one side and the breech on the other. Fetal heart rate is usually auscultated just below the midline of the umbilicus. If a

---

Box 21-1 Moxibustion to Promote Version in Breech Presentations

Traditional Chinese medicine uses the herb mugwort in the form of moxa to promote version in a breech presentation. Moxa is a system of treatment, often combined with acupuncture, in which an herb is dried, rolled into cones (like incense cones), and placed on certain meridian points of the body. The moxa is then lit and allowed to burn close to the skin; hence the "bustion" component of the name. The heat and pungency of mugwort stimulate the point, and it is believed that the energy moves through the body and increases fetal activity.

The meridian point that is used in moxibustion to promote version in breech presentation is acupoint BL 67, located beside the outer corner of the fifth toenail. Treatment may take from 7 days to 2 weeks. There is limited evidence suggesting that moxibustion is an effective modality in managing breech presentations; however, when combined with acupuncture and postural techniques (knee–chest position), the incidence of version increases (Coyle, Smith, & Peat, 2012).

If the sacrum has not descended, ballottement causes the entire fetal body to move. Furthermore, fetal heart rate (FHR) is usually auscultated above the umbilicus. Passage of meconium into the amniotic fluid due to compression of the fetus's intestinal tract is common.

If membranes are ruptured, be particularly alert for a prolapsed umbilical cord, especially in footling breeches because there is space between the cervix and presenting part through which the cord can slip. If the baby is small and the membranes rupture, the danger is even greater. The risk of a prolapsed umbilical cord is one reason any woman with ruptured membranes should not ambulate until a full assessment, including vaginal examination, has been performed.

Nursing diagnoses that may apply to a woman with a breech presentation include the following (NANDA-I © 2014):
• *Gas Exchange, Impaired*, in the fetus related to interruption in umbilical blood flow secondary to compression of the cord
• *Knowledge, Deficient*, related to lack of information about the implications and associated complications of breech presentation for the mother and fetus
• *Injury, Risk for*, related to unintended breech vaginal birth

Planning and Implementation
During labor, promote maternal–fetal well-being by frequently assessing fetal and maternal status. Because the fetus is at increased risk for prolapse of the cord, agency protocols may call for continuous fetal monitoring. If the head is not completely engaged, continuous monitoring is warranted and the woman should maintain complete bed rest. Provide teaching and information about the breech presentation and the nursing care needed.

Most physicians perform cesarean births because of the increased fetal risks associated with breech vaginal birth. Vaginal birth is more common in multiparous women with a proven pelvis (prior birth of a normal or large fetus without difficulty). Assist with the vaginal birth by including Piper forceps (used to guide the after-coming fetal head) in the birth table

Care of the Woman and Fetus at Risk for Macrosomia

Fetal **macrosomia** is defined as a birth weight of more than 4500 g (9.9 lb) (Cunningham et al., 2014). (*Note:* Some sources say 4000 g [8.8 lb].) The condition is more common with prepregnancy maternal obesity, excessive maternal weight gain, grand multiparity, prior history of macrosomia, a male fetus, maternal diabetes, prolonged gestation, and in women of Hispanic ethnic background (Posner, Dy, Black, et al., 2013). Macrosomia is also more common in fetuses who have erythroblastosis fetalis (Posner et al., 2013).

Risks of Macrosomia

Maternal implications of macrosomia include increased risk of the following:

- Cephalopelvic disproportion (CPD)
- Dysfunctional labor and prolonged labor
- Soft-tissue laceration during vaginal birth
- Postpartum hemorrhage
- Third- and fourth-degree lacerations or extension of episiotomy if performed

Fetal/neonatal implications include increased risk of the following:

- Meconium aspiration
- Asphyxia
- Shoulder dystocia, in which, after birth of the head, the anterior shoulder fails to deliver either spontaneously or with gentle traction (unresolved shoulder dystocia can lead to fetal death)
- Upper brachial plexus injury and fractured clavicles
- Hypoglycemia, polycythemia, and hyperbilirubinemia

Clinical Therapy

The occurrence of maternal and fetal problems associated with excessively large babies may be lessened somewhat by identifying macrosomia before the onset of labor. If a large fetus is suspected, the maternal pelvis should be evaluated carefully. Fetal size can be estimated by palpating the crown-to-rump length of the fetus in utero and by ultrasound or x-ray pelvimetry. Studies indicate that palpation and ultrasound provide equally effective assessments of fetal weight. When the uterus appears excessively large, hydramnios, an oversized fetus, or multiple gestation must be considered as the possible cause.

When fetal weight is estimated to be 4500 g (9.9 lb) or more, a cesarean birth is usually planned. For diabetic women with macrosomia and fetal weight greater than or equal to 4000 g (8.8 lb), a cesarean is also indicated. The best method of birth for an estimated fetal weight of 4000 to 4500 g (8.8 to 9.9 lb) is debatable. The discussion centers primarily on the incidence of shoulder dystocia during vaginal birth and the difficulty in accurately estimating the fetal weight. Unexpected shoulder dystocia during vaginal birth can be a grave problem. Shoulder dystocia is marked by the presence of a "turtle sign," in which the fetal head emerges and then quickly retracts as the shoulder becomes wedged beneath the public bone.

SAFETY ALERT!

As an emergency measure, the physician/CNM may ask the nurse to assist the woman into the McRoberts maneuver (sharp flexion of the thighs toward the hips and abdomen) or to apply gentle suprapubic pressure in an attempt to aid in the birth of the fetal shoulders. Fundal pressure should never be used because it can further wedge the anterior shoulder under the symphysis pubis.

Nursing Management

Assist in identifying women who are at risk for carrying a large fetus and those who exhibit signs of macrosomia. Because these women are prime candidates for dystocia and its complications, frequently assess the fetal heart rate (FHR) for indications of

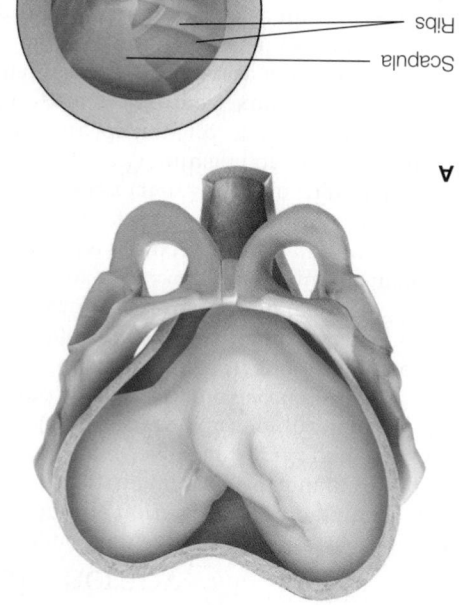

Figure 21-8 **A,** Transverse lie. Shoulder presentation. **B,** On vaginal examination the nurse may feel the acromion process as the fetal presenting part.

Acromion process
Humerus
Ribs
Scapula

A

B

presenting part is palpated on vaginal examination, it is the ridged thorax or possibly an arm compressed against the chest. Assist in the interpretation of the fetal presentation and provide information and support to the couple. Assess maternal and fetal status frequently, and prepare the woman for a cesarean birth (see Chapter 22).

Clinical Tip

If a fetus converts to a transverse lie later in the pregnancy, the woman may report greater ease of breathing, a reduction of heartburn, and less pressure on her bladder.

Compound Presentation

A compound presentation is one in which there are two presenting parts, such as the occiput and fetal hand or the complete breech and fetal hand. Most compound presentations resolve themselves spontaneously, but others require additional manipulation at birth.

nonreassuring fetal status and evaluate the rates of cervical dilatation and fetal descent.

Apply the fetal monitor for continuous fetal evaluation. Early decelerations (caused by fetal head compression) could mean size disproportion at the bony inlet. Report any sign of labor dysfunction or nonreassuring fetal status to the physician/CNM immediately. Lack of fetal descent is another indicator that should alert the nurse to the possibility that the baby is too large for a vaginal birth.

Provide support for the laboring woman and her partner and information about the implications of macrosomia and possible associated problems. During the birth, continue to provide support and encouragement to the woman or the couple.

Inspect macrosomic newborns after birth for cephalohematoma, Erb palsy, and fractured clavicles, and inform the nursery staff of any problems so that the newborn can be closely monitored for cerebral, neurologic, and motor problems.

In a woman with a macrosomic fetus, the uterus has been stretched farther than it would have been with an average-sized fetus. Blood glucose monitoring of the fetus is recommended since macrosomia is often associated with gestational diabetes. The overstretching may lead to contractile problems during labor or after birth. After birth, the overstretched uterus may not contract well (uterine atony) and will feel boggy (soft). In this case, uterine hemorrhage is likely. The fundus of the uterus is massaged to stimulate contraction; IV or IM oxytocin (Pitocin) may be needed.

SAFETY ALERT!

Methergine is sometimes prescribed for women with ongoing uterine atony and can aid in reducing postpartum hemorrhage. Methergine is contraindicated in women with any type of hypertensive disorder. Monitor the blood pressure closely prior to administration. Monitor maternal vital signs closely for deviations suggestive of shock.

Care of the Woman and Fetus in the Presence of Nonreassuring Fetal Status

When the oxygen supply is insufficient to meet the physiologic needs of the fetus, a nonreassuring fetal status may result. This status may be transient or chronic, and may be prompted by a variety of factors. The most common are cord compression and uteroplacental insufficiency, possibly caused by preexisting maternal or fetal disease or placental abnormalities. If the resulting hypoxia persists and metabolic acidosis occurs, the situation could cause permanent damage to or be life threatening for the fetus.

Maternal Implications

Indications of nonreassuring fetal status greatly increase the psychologic stress of a laboring woman and her family members. Professional staff members may become so involved in assessing fetal status and initiating corrective measures that they fail to provide the woman and her partner with explanations and emotional support. It is imperative to offer both. In many instances, if birth is not imminent, the woman must undergo cesarean birth. This method of birth may be a source of fear and frustration, too, if the couple prepared for a shared vaginal birth experience.

Clinical Therapy

The most common initial signs of nonreassuring fetal status are variations from the normal heart rate pattern and decreased fetal movement. Meconium-stained amniotic fluid and the presence of ominous fetal heart rate (FHR) patterns such as persistent late decelerations (regardless of the depth of deceleration), persistent and severe variable decelerations (especially if the return to baseline is prolonged), and prolonged decelerations are signs of nonreassuring fetal status. When these patterns are detected, corrective measures used **intrauterine resuscitation** to optimize the oxygen exchange within the maternal–fetal circulation should be started without delay.

Treatment of maternal hypotension involves having the woman turn to a left lateral position (right lateral position may also be tried), beginning an IV infusion or increasing the flow rate if an infusion is already in place, or, if cord prolapse is suspected, having the woman assume a knee–chest position. Position changes that result in an increase in the fetal heart rate should be maintained. Perform a vaginal examination to attempt to detect a prolapsed cord. Decrease uterine activity by discontinuing IV oxytocin (Pitocin) administration or administering a tocolytic agent (such as terbutaline) to decrease contraction frequency and intensity. Administer oxygen to the woman via facial mask.

Healthcare givers can obtain additional information about the condition of the fetus by fetal scalp blood sampling, fetal scalp stimulation, or fetal acoustic stimulation (see the *Fetal Acoustic and Vibroacoustic Stimulation Tests* section in Chapter 13). See Table 21–1 for management of nonreassuring fetal status.

TABLE 21–1 Management of Nonreassuring Fetal Status

- Recognize pattern changes that are indicative of nonreassuring fetal status such as:
- Deep, repetitive variable decelerations
- Prolonged decelerations
- Ongoing late decelerations
- Begin intrauterine resuscitation measures:
- Change maternal position.
- Correct maternal hypotension.
- Discontinue oxytocin (Pitocin).
- Administer medications, such as terbutaline, to decrease uterine activity.
- Increase intravenous fluid rate or begin IV immediately if not already established.
- Assess for prolapsed cord via vaginal examination.
- If abnormal patterns resolve, continue with continuous electronic fetal monitoring.
- If abnormal patterns do not resolve and vaginal birth is imminent, proceed with vaginal birth as quickly as possible.
- If birth not imminent and bradycardia persists, or if a scalp pH level is less than 7.20, a cesarean birth is indicated.
- If these tests are reassuring, cautious assessments can continue every 15 minutes until birth occurs.
- If testing becomes nonreassuring, a cesarean should be performed.

Care of the Woman and Fetus With a Prolapsed Umbilical Cord

A **prolapsed umbilical cord** results when the umbilical cord precedes the fetal presenting part. When this occurs, pressure is placed on the umbilical cord as it is trapped between the presenting part and the maternal pelvis. Consequently, the vessels carrying blood to and from the fetus are compressed (Figure 21–9). Prolapse of the cord may occur with rupture of the membranes if the presenting part is not well engaged in the pelvis.

Risks of Prolapsed Umbilical Cord

Although a prolapsed cord does not directly precipitate physical alterations in the woman, her immediate concern for the baby creates enormous stress. The woman may need to deal with some unusual interventions, a cesarean birth, and, in some circumstances, the death of her baby.

For the fetus, compression of the cord results in decreased blood flow and leads to nonreassuring fetal status. If labor is under way, the cord is compressed further with each contraction. If the pressure on the cord is not relieved, the fetus will die.

Clinical Therapy

Preventing prolapse of the cord is the preferred medical approach. A laboring woman with a confirmed rupture of membranes will be kept in the Trendelenburg position until the fetal head is well engaged and the risk of a prolapse is significantly decreased. If a prolapse occurs, relieving the compression on the cord is critical to fetal outcome. The medical and nursing team must work together to facilitate birth.

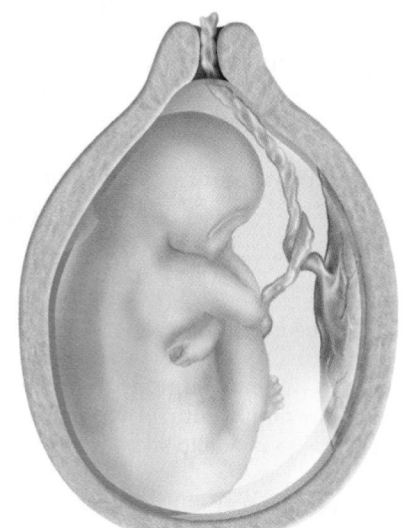

Figure 21–9 Prolapse of the umbilical cord.

Nursing Management

Review the woman's prenatal history and note the presence of any conditions (such as preeclampsia, diabetes, renal disease, or intrauterine growth restriction [IUGR]) that may be associated with decreased uteroplacental–fetal blood flow. When the membranes rupture, assess the FHR immediately and note the characteristics of the amniotic fluid. As labor progresses, be especially alert to suspicious changes in the FHR. At all times, encourage and support maternal positioning that maximizes uteroplacental–fetal blood flow.

Bed rest is indicated for all laboring women with a history of ruptured membranes until engagement with no cord prolapse has been documented. Furthermore, with spontaneous rupture of membranes or amniotomy, the fetal heart rate (FHR) should be auscultated for at least a full minute and at the beginning and end of contractions for several contractions. If fetal bradycardia is detected on auscultation, perform a vaginal examination to rule out cord prolapse. In the presence of cord prolapse, electronic monitor tracings show severe, moderate, or prolonged variable decelerations with baseline bradycardia.

If a loop of cord is discovered, the examiner's gloved fingers must remain in the vagina to provide firm pressure on the fetal head (to relieve compression) until the physician/CNM arrives. This is a lifesaving measure. Give the mother oxygen via face mask, and monitor the FHR to determine whether the cord compression is adequately relieved.

The force of gravity can be employed to relieve umbilical cord compression. The nurse can instruct the woman to assume the knee–chest position (Figure 21–10) or can adjust the bed to the Trendelenburg position, and transport the woman to the delivery or operating room in this position. The cord may be occultly prolapsed with an actual loop extending into the vagina or lying alongside the presenting part. It may be pulsating strongly or so weakly that it is difficult to determine upon palpation of the cord whether the fetus is alive.

Nursing Management

Because there are few outward signs of cord prolapse, each pregnant woman is advised to call her physician/CNM when the membranes rupture and to go to the office, clinic, or birthing facility. Perform a sterile vaginal examination to determine if there is danger of cord prolapse. If the presenting part is well engaged, the risk of cord prolapse is minimal, and the woman may ambulate as desired. If the presenting part is not well engaged, bed rest is recommended to prevent cord prolapse.

Because cord prolapse can be associated with fetal death, some physicians/CNMs insist that bed rest be maintained after rupture of membranes regardless of fetal engagement. This can lead to conflict if the laboring woman and her partner do not hold the same opinions. Ease this situation by helping the physician/CNM and the couple to communicate.

During labor any alteration of the FHR or the presence of meconium in the amniotic fluid indicates the need to assess for cord prolapse. Vaginal birth is possible with prolapsed cord if the cervix is completely dilated and pelvic measurements are adequate. If these conditions are not present, cesarean birth is the method of choice. (See Care of the Woman With Prolapsed Cord in the Clinical Skills Manual SKILLS.)

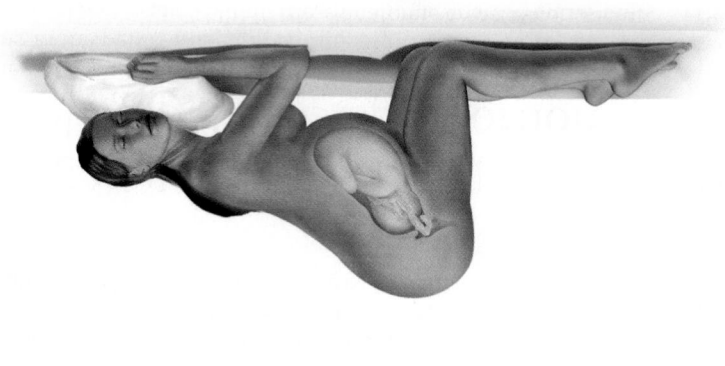

Figure 21–10 Knee–chest position is used to relieve cord compression during cord prolapse emergency.

Care of the Woman and Fetus at Risk Owing to Anaphylactoid Syndrome of Pregnancy

In the presence of a small tear in the amnion or chorion high in the uterus, a small amount of amniotic fluid may leak into the chorionic plate and enter the maternal system as an **amniotic fluid embolism**, a condition called **anaphylactoid syndrome of pregnancy**. The fluid can also enter at areas of placental separation or cervical tears. Under pressure from the contracting uterus, the fluid is driven into the maternal circulation and then the maternal lungs. The more debris in the amniotic fluid (such as meconium), the greater the maternal problems. This condition, although rare, can be catastrophic. Risk factors associated with it include a tumultuous labor, placental abruption, trauma, induction of labor, eclampsia, operative vaginal birth, cesarean birth, and multiple gestation, among other things (Blackburn, 2013).

Maternal Implications

The woman with an amniotic fluid embolism experiences sudden onset of respiratory distress, circulatory collapse, acute hemorrhage, and cor pulmonale (failure of the right ventricle) as the embolism blocks the vessels of the lungs. She exhibits dyspnea and cyanosis leading to hemorrhagic shock and coma and may develop seizures. Birth must be facilitated immediately to obtain a live fetus.

Clinical Therapy

Any woman exhibiting chest pain, dyspnea, cyanosis, frothy sputum, tachycardia, hypotension, and massive hemorrhage requires the cooperation of every member of the healthcare team if her life is to be saved. Medical interventions are supportive. Recovery is contingent on return of the mother's cardiovascular and respiratory stability. If necessary, a cesarean birth is performed.

Nursing Management

In the absence of the physician/CNM, administer oxygen under positive pressure until medical help arrives. An intravenous line is quickly established. If respiratory and cardiac arrest occur, initiate cardiopulmonary resuscitation (CPR) immediately.

Ready the equipment necessary for blood transfusion and for the insertion of the CVP line. As the blood volume is replaced, using fresh whole blood to provide clotting factors, the CVP must be monitored frequently. In the presence of cor pulmonale, fluid overload could easily occur.

Care of the Woman With Cephalopelvic Disproportion

The birth passage includes the maternal bony pelvis, beginning at the pelvic inlet and ending at the pelvic outlet, and the maternal soft tissues within these anatomic areas. A contracture (narrowed diameter) in any of the described areas can result in **cephalopelvic disproportion (CPD)** if the fetus is larger than the pelvic diameters. Abnormal fetal presentations and positions occur in CPD as the fetus moves to accommodate its passage through the maternal pelvis.

The gynecoid and anthropoid pelvic types are usually adequate for vertex birth, but the android and platypelloid types are predisposed to CPD. Certain combinations of types also can result in pelvic diameters inadequate for vertex birth. (See Chapter 16 for a description of pelvic types and their implications for childbirth.)

Although rare, CPD can also occur as a result of trauma or fracture of the pelvis. A complete health history that identifies a past fracture warrants a more extensive pelvic examination to determine abnormalities that may have occurred as a result of trauma.

> **Women With Special Needs Cephalopelvic Disproportion**
>
> Women with certain birth defects are prone to CPD, making a cesarean birth the only choice for birth. Women with dwarfism have platypelloid pelvises which are not compatible with vaginal birth. The physician caring for a woman with dwarfism should consult with another physician with experience in performing cesarean births on this population because some women's pelvic anatomy may have slight deviations.

Types of Contractures

The pelvic inlet is contracted if the shortest anterior–posterior diameter is less than 10 cm (3.7 in.) or the greatest transverse diameter is less than 12 cm (4.7 in.). The anterior–posterior diameter may be approximated by measuring the diagonal conjugate, which in the contracted inlet is less than 11.5 cm (4.5 in.). Clinical pelvimetry measurements are used to determine the smallest anterior–posterior diameter through which the fetal head must pass. X-ray pelvimetry can also be a method to identify pelvic deviations but is not routinely used in pregnant women.

The treatment goal is to allow the natural forces of labor to push the biparietal diameter of the fetal head beyond the potential interspinous obstruction. Although forceps may be used, they cause difficulty because pulling on the head destroys flexion, and the space is further diminished. A bulging perineum and crowning indicate that the obstruction has been passed.

An interischial tuberous diameter of less than 8 cm (3.15 in.) constitutes an outlet contracture. Outlet and midpelvic contractures frequently occur simultaneously. Whether vaginal birth can occur depends on the woman's interischial tuberous diameters and the fetal posteriosagittal diameter.

Risks of Cephalopelvic Disproportion

When CPD is present, the mother experiences prolonged labor. Membrane rupture can result from the force of the unequally distributed contractions being exerted on the fetal membranes. In obstructed labor, in which the fetus cannot descend, uterine rupture can occur. With delayed descent, necrosis of maternal soft tissues can result from pressure exerted by the fetal head. Eventually, necrosis can cause fistulas from the vagina to other nearby structures. Difficult, forceps-assisted births can also result in damage to maternal soft tissue.

If the membranes rupture and the fetal head has not entered the inlet, there is a danger of cord prolapse. Excessive molding of the fetal head can result. Traumatic, forceps-assisted birth can damage the fetal skull and central nervous system.

Clinical Therapy

Fetopelvic relationships can be assessed by comparing pelvic measurements obtained by a manual examination before labor and by computed tomography (CT) or magnetic resonance imaging (MRI). An estimated weight of the fetus is obtained by ultrasound measurements.

When the pelvic diameters are borderline or questionable, a *trial of labor* (TOL) may be advised. In this process, the woman continues to labor, and careful, frequent assessments of cervical dilatation and fetal descent are made. As long as there is continued progress, the TOL continues. If progress ceases, the decision for a cesarean birth is made.

Nursing Management

The adequacy of the maternal pelvis for a vaginal birth should be assessed both during and before labor. During the intrapartum assessment, the size of the fetus and its presentation, position, and lie must also be considered. (See Chapter 17 for intrapartum assessment techniques.)

Suspect CPD when labor is prolonged, cervical dilatation and effacement are slow, lack of fetal descent is noted, and engagement of the presenting part is delayed. The couple may need support in coping with the stresses of this complicated labor. Keep the couple informed of what is happening and explain the procedures being used. This knowledge reassures the couple that measures are being taken to resolve the problem.

Nursing actions during the TOL are similar to care during any labor except that cervical dilatation and fetal descent are assessed more frequently. Both contractions and the fetus should be monitored continuously. Report any signs of nonreassuring fetal status to the physician/CNM immediately.

The mother may be positioned in a variety of ways to increase the pelvic diameters. Sitting or squatting increases the outlet diameters and may be effective when there is failure of, or slow, fetal descent. Changing from one side to the other or maintaining a hands-and-knees position may assist the fetus in the occiput posterior position to change to an occiput anterior position. The mother may instinctively want to assume one of these positions. If not, the nurse can encourage a change of position.

Care of the Woman With a Complication of the Third or Fourth Stage of Labor

Common complications of the third and fourth stages of labor include retained placenta, lacerations, and placenta accreta.

Retained Placenta

Retention of the placenta beyond 30 minutes after birth is termed **retained placenta**. It occurs in 1 in 100 to 1 in 200 vaginal births (Benirschke, Burton, & Baergen, 2012). Risk factors for placental retention include previous history of retained placenta, prior uterine surgery, maternal age more than 35, placenta, labor induction, and grand multiparity (Davidson, 2013). Bleeding as a result of a retained placenta can be excessive. If placental expulsion does not occur, the physician/CNM attempts to remove the placenta manually. In women who do not have an epidural in place, intravenous sedation may be required because of the discomfort caused by the procedure. Failure to retrieve the placenta via manual removal usually necessitates surgical removal by curettage. If the woman does not have an epidural in place, the procedure can be performed under general anesthesia. Retained placenta may be a symptom of an accreta, increta, or percreta (to be discussed shortly).

Lacerations

Lacerations of the cervix or vagina may be indicated when bright-red vaginal bleeding persists in the presence of a well-contracted uterus. The incidence of lacerations is higher when the childbearing woman is young or a nullipara, has an epidural, has forceps-assisted birth and an episiotomy, and has not done perineal massage or preparation during pregnancy. Vaginal and perineal lacerations are often categorized in terms of degree, as follows:

- **First-degree laceration** is limited to the fourchette, perineal skin, and vaginal mucous membrane.
- **Second-degree laceration** involves the perineal skin, vaginal mucous membrane, underlying fascia, and muscles of the perineal body; it may extend upward on one or both sides of the vagina.
- **Third-degree laceration** extends through the perineal skin, vaginal mucous membranes, and perineal body and involves the anal sphincter; it may extend up the anterior wall of the rectum.
- **Fourth-degree laceration** is the same as third-degree but extends through the rectal mucosa to the lumen of the rectum; it may be called a third-degree laceration with a rectal wall extension.

Placenta Accreta

The chorionic villi attach directly to the myometrium of the uterus in **placenta accreta**. Two other types of placental adherence are **placenta increta**, in which the myometrium is invaded, and **placenta percreta**, in which the myometrium is penetrated. The adherence itself may be total, partial, or focal, depending on the amount of placental involvement. The incidence of placenta accreta is 1 in 533 births (Posner et al., 2013). It is the most common type, accounting for almost three-fourths of adherent placentas.

The primary complication with placenta accreta is maternal hemorrhage and failure of the placenta to separate following birth of the baby. An abdominal hysterectomy may be necessary depending on the amount and depth of involvement.

Care of the Woman and Fetus With Placental Problems

The most common types of placental problems—placenta previa and abruptio placentae—are discussed in Chapter 20. Other problems of the placenta are presented in Table 21–2.

TABLE 21-2 Placental and Umbilical Cord Variations

PLACENTAL VARIATION	MATERNAL IMPLICATIONS	FETAL/NEONATAL IMPLICATIONS
SUCCENTURIATE PLACENTA		
One or more accessory lobes of fetal villi will develop on the placenta.	Postpartum hemorrhage from retained lobe	None, as long as all parts of the placenta remain attached until after birth of the fetus
CIRCUMVALLATE PLACENTA		
A double fold of chorion and amnion form a ring around the umbilical cord, on the fetal side of the placenta.	Increased incidence of late abortion, antepartum hemorrhage, and preterm labor	Intrauterine growth restriction, prematurity, fetal death
BATTLEDORE PLACENTA		
The umbilical cord is inserted at or near the placental margin.	Increased incidence of preterm labor and bleeding	Prematurity, nonreassuring fetal status
VELAMENTOUS INSERTION OF THE UMBILICAL CORD		
The vessels of the umbilical cord divide some distance from the placenta in the placental membranes.	Hemorrhage if one of the vessels is torn	Nonreassuring fetal status, hemorrhage

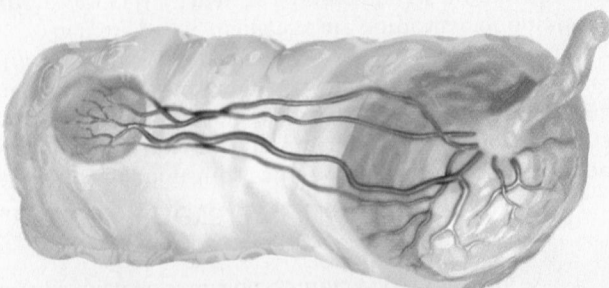

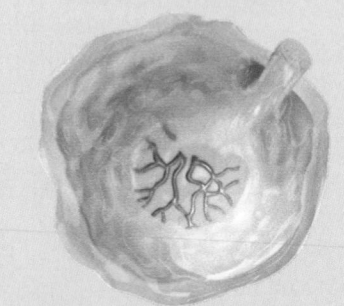

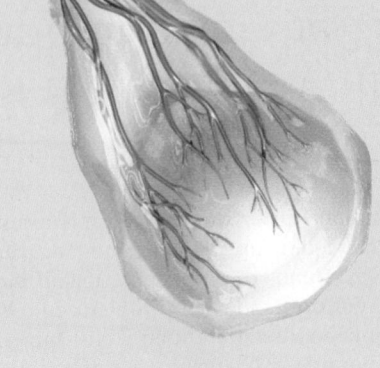

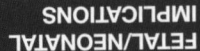

Care of the Family

Experiencing Perinatal Loss

Perinatal loss is death of a fetus or neonate from the time of conception through the end of the newborn period 28 days after birth. Spontaneous abortion (miscarriage) in the antepartum period is discussed in Chapter 15; this section discusses intrauterine fetal death (IUFD) after 20 weeks' gestation, often referred to as *stillbirth* or *fetal demise.*

Common Causes of Perinatal Loss

Antepartum fetal deaths, although infrequent, account for about half of all perinatal mortality in the United States. About 70% to 90% of all stillbirths occur before the onset of labor, with more than half occurring between 20 and 28 weeks' gestation (Davidson, 2013). In the United States, the fetal death rate is 6.05 fetal births per 1000 births (Child Health USA, 2013). The fetal death rate in the United States has dramatically declined by 20% since 1990. Fetal death is more common in African American women followed by Native Americans/Native Alaskans (Child Health USA, 2013).

The cause of fetal death may be unknown, or it may be related to fetal factors such as chromosomal disorders, birth defects, exposure to teratogens, infections, or complications of multiple gestation or fetal growth restriction; maternal factors such as chronic hypertension, preeclampsia or eclampsia, diabetes, advanced maternal age, Rh incompatibility, uterine rupture, or ascending maternal infection; or placental factors such as placenta previa, abruptio placentae, or a cord accident. In 25% of fetal deaths, the cause remains unknown even after autopsy (Davidson, 2013).

Perinatal loss in industrialized countries has declined in recent years as early diagnosis of congenital anomalies and advances in genetic testing techniques have increased the use of elective termination. Fetal death occurs more frequently in monochorionic twins and in pregnancies conceived by assisted reproductive technologies (Davidson, 2013). Certain genetic testing procedures such as amniocentesis and chorionic villus sampling (CVS) can actually cause fetal loss.

In industrialized countries, maternal obesity, advanced maternal age, maternal smoking, maternal substance abuse, primiparity, small-for-gestational-age (SGA) fetuses, abruptions, maternal hypertension, and diabetes are the most common etiologies of stillbirth (Davidson, 2013). In developing countries, infection plays a significant role in fetal deaths. Ascending bacterial organisms include *Escherichia coli*, group B streptococci, and *Ureaplasma urealyticum*. These infections can occur either before or after the membranes have ruptured, resulting in fetal demise. Viral causes of fetal demise include parvovirus and coxsackievirus. *Toxoplasma gondii, Listeria monocytogenes,* and the organisms that cause leptospirosis, Q fever, and Lyme disease have also been identified as causative factors for stillbirth. Untreated syphilis is associated with a high stillborn rate as are malaria infections when contracted for the first time by the mother during pregnancy (Davidson, 2013). These infections carry a much higher morbidity and mortality rate in developing countries.

Certain maternal conditions can also be associated with higher rates of fetal death. Past maternal exposure to certain bacterial and viral antigens can produce an autoimmune response that can result in fetal death (Blackburn, 2013). Women with acquired and immune thrombophilia have higher rates of miscarriage and fetal demise than those without hematologic alterations (Blackburn, 2013).

Maternal Physiologic Implications

Prolonged retention of the dead fetus may lead to the development of disseminated intravascular coagulation (DIC), also called *consumption coagulopathy,* in the mother. After the release of thromboplastin from the degenerating fetal tissues into the maternal bloodstream, the extrinsic clotting system is activated, triggering the formation of multiple tiny blood clots. Fibrinogen and factors V and VII are subsequently depleted, and the woman begins to display symptoms of DIC. Fibrinogen levels begin a linear descent 3 to 4 weeks after the death of the fetus and continue to decrease in the absence of appropriate medical intervention.

Besides DIC, other adverse outcomes can occur if the onset of labor and subsequent birth are delayed. Women with prolonged retention of a dead fetus are more prone to infection. A resulting infection can cause endometritis or sepsis. The longer the pregnancy continues, the higher the incidence of maternal infection.

Although immediate induction is routinely performed, there may be situations in which induction is delayed, such as maternal refusal or the presence of a multiple gestation. In these cases, fibrinogen levels are monitored weekly or biweekly to recognize and prevent progressive coagulopathy from occurring (Hanan, Al-Kadri, & Tamim, 2012).

Clinical Therapy

When fetal death has occurred, abdominal x-ray examination may reveal a Spalding sign, an overriding of the fetal cranial bones. In addition, maternal estriol levels fall. Diagnosis of intrauterine fetal death (IUFD) is confirmed by absence of heart action on ultrasound. Without medical intervention, most women have spontaneous labor within 2 weeks of fetal death. The once common practice of waiting for the onset of labor has largely been abandoned in recent years since the risks of complications increase with delaying the birth. Prompt birth also increases the ability to identify the cause of death.

In modern practice, most women with a diagnosed fetal demise are given the option of waiting a few days or scheduling an induction procedure immediately. Most women will elect for an induction within a day or two of the final diagnosis. The mode of induction is dependent on the gestational age of the fetus, the readiness of the cervix, and previous mode of birth. In women who have had a previous cesarean birth, a repeat cesarean may be performed since the use of oxytocin (Pitocin) or prostaglandin agents can increase the risk of a uterine rupture.

The treatment of choice for fetal demise is now misoprostol. Women with a favorable cervix may be given oxytocin. Misoprostol may be given orally or vaginally. Higher vaginal doses are associated with shorter labors. Misoprostol use in women with a previous cesarean section warrants close monitoring. The use of misoprostol should only be given in facilities with adequate emergency resources in place (Bracken et al., 2013).

Postbirth Evaluation

Identifying the causative factor of fetal loss assists many families in progressing through the grieving process. Information obtained from a postmortem examination or postmortem studies can provide vital information related to the cause of the fetal death, the possibility for reoccurrence, and closure for the couple. The types of studies and tests performed depend on the parents' past history, medical history, and preferences for the depth of testing desired. Chromosomal studies should be considered

Phases of Grief

Grief is an individual's total response to a loss, including physical symptoms, thoughts, feelings, functional limitations, and spiritual reactions. It may be manifested by certain behaviors and rituals of *mourning*, such as weeping or visiting a gravesite, which help the person experience, accept, and adjust to the loss. The period of adjustment to loss is known as *bereavement*. (*Note:* Grief as it relates to the birth of an at-risk newborn is discussed in Chapter 30.)

The behaviors that couples exhibit while mourning may be associated with the five stages of grieving described in *On Death and Dying* (Kübler-Ross, 1969). Often, the first stage is *denial* of the death of the fetus. Even when the initial healthcare provider suspects fetal demise, the couple is hoping that a second opinion may be different. Some couples may not be convinced of the death until they see and hold the stillborn baby after birth. The second stage is *anger*, resulting from feelings of loss, loneliness, and perhaps guilt. The anger may be projected at significant others and healthcare team members, or it may be absent when the death is sudden and unexpected. The mother may attempt to identify a specific event that caused the death and may blame herself. *Bargaining*, the third stage, may or may not be present, depending on the couple's preparation for the death of the fetus. If the death is unanticipated, the couple may not have time for bargaining. When the death is expected, such as in the case of a known lethal congenital anomaly, bargaining is more commonly seen. It is marked by the couple making mental trade-offs in exchange for the fetus being healthy. In the fourth stage, *depression* is evidenced by preoccupation, weeping, and withdrawal. Changing hormonal levels in the first 24 to 48 hours after birth may compound the depression and associated grief.

The final stage, *acceptance*, surfaces when resolution occurs. This stage is highly individualized and may take months to years to complete.

Clinical Tip

No matter who you are or how much nursing experience you have, when an expectant family is in pain because of their loss, it can be difficult to know the right thing to say. A good start is to say, "I'm so sorry, I don't know what to say." The nurse can play a therapeutic role by sitting quietly with the mother, holding her hand, and speaking of the beauty of the baby's fingers, toes, and hair, and other specific characteristics of the baby.

if the couple has a history of other second- or third-trimester losses or if either parent has a suspected balanced translocation or mosaic chromosomal pattern (Davidson, 2013).

If an intra-amniotic infection is the suspected cause, cultures of both the placenta and the fetus should be obtained. If specific infections are being considered, both IgM and IgG antibodies should be drawn to determine if an acute infectious process has occurred.

All stillborn babies should have a careful visual inspection at the time of birth for obvious defects or abnormalities. The placenta and membranes should also be closely examined, and the placenta should be sent to pathology for further testing. The umbilical cord should be inspected for true knots, a velamentous insertion, lack of Wharton jelly, or a short cord to determine if a cord accident was the cause. If a specific cause is suspected, blood tests and x-rays can be performed. An autopsy is the best mechanism to determine the cause of death; however, in the event that the parents decline an autopsy, magnetic resonance imaging (MRI) can also provide detailed information (Blackburn, 2013).

Most practitioners perform a CBC and antibody screen upon admission. Because diabetes is a causative factor, a random or postpartum glucose level can be obtained to rule out this cause. Additional maternal factors that can also be evaluated are listed in Table 21-3.

TABLE 21-3 Tests to Determine Cause of Fetal Loss

FETAL TESTING	MATERNAL TESTING
Fetal blood tests and x-rays	Diabetes testing
Autopsy or MRI	CBC with platelet count
Placental studies	Kleihauer-Betke test
Chromosomal studies (if indicated)	Abnormal antibody testing (lupus anticoagulant, anticardiolipin antibodies)
	Thyroid-stimulating hormone (TSH) levels
	Infectious disease testing (rubella, syphilis, malaria, toxoplasmosis, cytomegalovirus)
	Hereditary thrombophilia testing
	Toxicology testing

Maternal Death

Maternal death is defined by the World Health Organization (WHO) (2012) as "the death of a woman while pregnant or within 42 days of termination of pregnancy, irrespective of the duration and the site of the pregnancy, from any cause related to or aggravated by the pregnancy or its management, but not from accidental or incidental causes." The most common causes of maternal death are hemorrhage, hypertensive disorders, embolism, infection, and preexisting chronic conditions, such as diabetes and cardiovascular disease. Obesity is also becoming a significant factor in maternal deaths because of the medical conditions that result (Centers for Disease Control & Prevention [CDC], 2014). The national maternal mortality rate was 18.5 deaths per 100,000 live births, reaching the highest rate it has seen in 25 years (Kassenbaum et al., 2014). In 2013, maternal deaths in the United States mostly occurred in women of advanced maternal age and typically occurred in the intrapartum or postpartum period (Kassenbaum et al., 2014). However, the number of maternal deaths is not decreasing, and the death of even one mother on a perinatal unit can be a devastating experience for all involved. The United States is the only developed country in the world whose maternal death rates continue to increase.

For the husband, or father of the child, the death of his partner is shocking (even if she had previous medical problems) and traumatic. There is an even deeper shock presenting, here, in that the death is surrounding an expectedly joyous event, a birth. The grieving process is complicated by a number of factors (such as caring for the newborn while grieving his partner) and is too comprehensive a topic for this text. What is important for nurses caring for the father and/or other family members is to recognize that initial grief reactions may be extremely intense. As long as no one is violating the foundational principles of grief reaction (i.e., not hurting themselves, others, or personal property), the father and family should be fully supported through this initial time with all support available to them and their facility in which the nurse is practicing. Interactions should be brief and direct, such as offering tissues and straightforward condolences (e.g., "I'm so sorry this is happening to you"). As with all losses, it is important to resist offering explanations or platitudes. There are no adequate explanations and platitudes and, in most cases, prove harmful.

For the staff, a maternal death on the perinatal unit can be traumatic as well. When a death occurs on any unit, there are individual as well as group reactions to the event (Blood & Cacciatore, 2014). The individual nurses involved may experience feelings of shock, sadness, anger, guilt, and other grief-associated reactions. The unit as a whole may experience feelings of inadequacy, anger, guilt, confusion, and depression. For the nurses directly involved, the father and family must still be cared for and for everyone on the unit, nursing care continues.

It is important for management in these situations to step in and provide an opportunity for the staff to express their feelings in a safe environment. Intervention for the staff could include professional debriefing or, where professional assistance is not available, simply calling a staff meeting to allow the nurses to work through some of the emotions while supporting one another (Blood & Cacciatore, 2014). The most important thing for nurses to remember is to take care of their own grief reactions and allow time for personal healing. Focusing on the positive aspects of the situation where they exist (such as personal kindness shown to the mother before the death, or to the family in the aftermath) is an important step in the healing process as well as reflecting objectively on those things out of one's personal control (the mother's underlying medical issues or unforeseen complications). The idea, as with the loss of a baby, is to eventually memorialize the event with a balanced perspective, recognizing where personal effectiveness as well as limitations exists and learning to live with them, both personally and professionally.

Nursing Management

For the Family Experiencing Perinatal Death

Nursing Assessment and Diagnosis

Cessation of fetal movement reported by the mother to the nurse is frequently the first indication of fetal death. It is followed by a gradual decrease in the signs and symptoms of pregnancy. Fetal heart tones are absent, and fetal movement is no longer palpable. Once fetal demise has been established, assess the family members' ability to adapt to their loss. Open communication between the mother, her partner, and the healthcare team members contributes to a realistic understanding of the medical condition and its associated treatments. Discuss prior experiences the family has had and what they feel were their perceived coping abilities at that time. Identifying the family's social supports and resources is also important.

Perinatal loss may also occur in the intrapartum period as a result of an intrapartum complication, such as an unresolved shoulder dystocia, prolapsed umbilical cord, abruptio placentae, or other complication. In such emergency situations, healthcare team members often focus on the physical needs of the mother and an attempt to save the fetus's life. Commonly, the family is not informed that a perinatal death has occurred until the baby is born. Thus the parents are faced with the sudden and completely unanticipated death of their baby. The most common reaction is protest or disbelief.

Although the physician/CNM informs the family of the death, the nurse continues one-on-one care with the family, providing both physical and emotional support throughout this crucial period. Assist the family members in the grief process and explore their immediate wishes for viewing and holding their deceased child.

Nursing diagnoses that may apply include the following (NANDA-I © 2014):

- *Grieving* related to imminent loss of a child
- *Coping: Family, Compromised,* related to the death of a child/unresolved feelings regarding perinatal loss
- *Hopelessness* related to sudden, unexpected fetal loss
- *Spiritual Distress, Risk for,* related to intense suffering secondary to unexpected fetal loss

Planning and Implementation

Most facilities have an established protocol to follow in the event of perinatal death. The protocol typically provides a holistic focus for family-centered nursing care. It is important for the entire healthcare team to be notified so collaborative care can be initiated. When fetal death has been confirmed before admission, the entire staff on the unit is informed so they can avoid making inappropriate remarks. Many facilities have a symbol, such as a card with a leaf, heart, or cluster of flowers, that is placed on the mother's door so all staff members are aware of the loss (Figure 21-11). Postmortem bereavement photography is a growing trend that has been embraced by many parents and healthcare providers who have been involved in fetal loss. In a study by Blood and Cacciatore (2014), 92 of 104 families requested postmortem photography when offered. After discharge, 11 families expressed regret they did not obtain postmortem photographs of their stillborn baby. The need for sensitivity and open dialogue is essential for families facing the perinatal death.

PREPARING THE FAMILY FOR THE BIRTH

On arrival at the facility, the couple with a known or suspected fetal demise should immediately be placed in a private room. When possible, the woman should be in a room that is farthest away from other laboring women. Take care not to leave the couple in the waiting room with other expectant parents or visitors waiting for news from other women in labor.

The couple should be allowed to remain together as much as they wish. Provide privacy and maintain a supportive environment. Give the couple complete information about what to expect and what will happen. Encourage and

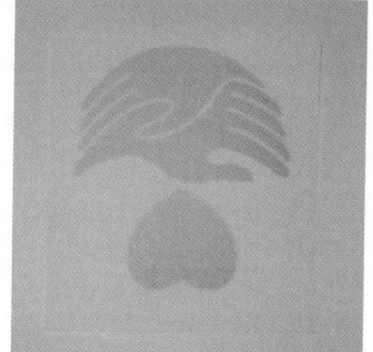

Figure 21-11 Door card.
SOURCE: Share Pregnancy & Infant Loss Support, Inc.

answer questions. Stay with the couple so they do not feel alone and isolated; however, continuously assess cues from the couple. Some couples may want to be alone. Some couples may want outside support, such as family members or friends, to be present during the labor. Facilitate the couple's wishes.

When possible, the same nurse should provide care for the couple so a therapeutic relationship can be established. As the relationship develops, provide solace by listening to the couple without offering ongoing commentary. Also provide ongoing opportunities for the couple to ask questions. It is not uncommon for the family to ask the same questions repeatedly as part of the initial grief process. Provide clear explanations and straightforward answers.

Consider cultural factors in providing care. Although not everyone from a given culture responds to loss in the same way, responses to fetal death are often influenced by cultural and personal beliefs. Similarly, responses to loss may be influenced by spiritual beliefs. In considering religious practices, it is prudent simply to ask the family how they can best be helped to meet their religious needs. Some families may desire to see a spiritual adviser. If so, offer to contact the hospital chaplain or another cleric for them. It is important to let the family process their own beliefs and feelings about the meaning, purpose, and significance of the life and death of their baby.

If a grief counselor is available, arrange an initial interaction with the couple if they are willing. A social worker is commonly involved. Coordinate members of the collaborative care team so a comprehensive plan of care can be initiated.

Explain details of the plan of care and allow the family to ask questions and make decisions for their labor and birth preferences. Review the availability of anesthesia and analgesia. The woman typically can have pain medication whenever she desires. Facilitate the participation of the woman and her partner in the labor and birth process.

Remember that, in contrast to a typical birth experience, the birth of a stillborn baby marks both the beginning and the end. It is imperative that the couple and family have all wishes and preferences respected. However, the family may have difficulty making decisions during this period. Assist the couple to explore their feelings and help them to make decisions about who is present and what rituals will occur during and following the birth. Examples of birth preferences include the following:

- Use of music, dimmed lighting, or other environmental preferences
- Laboring or birthing in a specific position
- Having the baby placed on the mother's chest immediately after birth
- Allowing the father to cut the umbilical cord
- Presence of other family members or friends at the birth

Sometimes couples worry that others may view their preferences as "strange" or "wrong." Reassure the family that it is their experience and that there are no right or wrong feelings or wishes.

The couple may have waves of overwhelming grief, disbelief, or sadness. Encourage the couple to experience the grief that they feel. It is not uncommon for one partner to attempt to put on a "brave front," feeling that by showing grief he or she will make the other partner feel worse. It is also not uncommon for partners to have intense feelings that they are unable to share. Encourage partners to express their emotions freely to the extent they are able. Help them understand that they may each experience different feelings.

SUPPORTING THE FAMILY IN VIEWING THE STILLBORN BABY

Advocates of seeing the stillborn baby believe that viewing assists in dispelling denial and enables the couple to progress to the next step in the grieving process. If they choose to see their stillborn baby, prepare the couple for what they will see by saying, "She is going to feel cold," "He is going to be blue," or other appropriate statements. If the parents have shared with you the name they had chosen for their baby, use that name in discussing the baby, for example, "Jessie's face is bruised." Another common practice is to wrap the baby in a blanket or apply a hat to cover birth defects. This allows the parents an opportunity to view the baby before seeing the birth defect. Most parents will eventually remove the covering to inspect the baby; however, applying a covering allows them time to adjust to the appearance at their own pace.

Some families will hold their babies for a short time before returning them to the nurse, whereas others will wish to spend a great deal of time with their babies. Allow the baby to remain with the family for as long as the family desires. Some parents may elect to bathe or dress their stillborn babies; support them in their choice. A couple may want other family members, friends, or their other children to see the baby. Act as an advocate to ensure that the family's wishes are respected.

Developing Cultural Competence | Grief Responses and Interactions

- Cultures that are stoic in nature can be difficult to assist. Stoicism may stem from family or cultural background, shock, or denial. It is important to ascertain the underlying reason so that appropriate interventions, where warranted, can occur (Doka & Davidson, 2014).
- In male-dominant cultures, mothers experiencing perinatal loss may tend to focus on their "failure" as a woman to successfully reproduce. Reassure these women (while respecting cultural beliefs) that nothing they did or did not do affected the outcome. A reiteration of known medical causes may be helpful (Doka & Davidson, 2014).
- In cultures in which the extended family is the couple's main source of support, it is important to allow as much interaction with family members as possible. In cultures where privacy is valued above all, help the family limit visitors if that is their preference (Doka & Davidson, 2014).
- Avoidance is not therapeutic. If you are not certain what the family needs, simply ask them how you can help to accommodate their wishes. Families appreciate an honest and caring attitude.

Women With Special Needs | Intellectual Disability

For the woman with an intellectual disability, understanding of the cause and process of neonatal death may be difficult owing to cognitive abilities and grief responses. A grief counselor should be on hand and one-to-one support is warranted. Self-blame may be more common in these women, and reassurance, education, and support are imperative.

PROVIDING DISCHARGE CARE

Most facilities prepare a remembrance box or package for the family to take home. This typically consists of a photograph taken of the baby or the family, a card with the baby's footprints, a crib card, identification band, a lock of hair, and possibly a blanket or clothing worn by the baby. In the event that the couple declines the package, it is common for the hospital to retain these items for a specific period in case they change their minds.

After the birth, give the couple the option of an early discharge (as early as 6 to 8 hours after the birth). Facility protocol will dictate where mothers are transferred after a perinatal loss. Some hospitals have the women remain on the birthing unit; others give the mother the option of choosing a postpartum room or one on a medical unit. If the mother is transferred to a postpartum room, select a room for her that is far away from other rooms and the newborn nursery. It is imperative that all staff members, as well as student nurses, be notified of the mother's status.

Include information on the grief process in discharge information (Figure 21–12). Prepare the couple to return home by stressing that others may not know what to say, and that even loved ones may make inappropriate comments because they do not know how to respond to grief and loss. This can prepare the couple for the reactions of others. If there are siblings, each will usually progress through age-appropriate grieving. Provide the parents with information about normal mourning reactions, both psychologic and physiologic.

When caring for a family suffering from a perinatal loss, it is important to remember that the nurse experiences many of the same grief reactions as the parents of a stillborn baby. It is important to have colleagues and family members available for counseling and support.

FACILITATING THE FAMILY'S GRIEF WORK

The parents of a stillborn baby suffer a devastating experience that precipitates an intense emotional trauma. During pregnancy the couple has already begun the attachment process, which now must be ended through the grieving process. Facilitating the family's grief work is thus a critical nursing intervention—one that requires skill, sensitivity, and compassion.

Following discharge, some families may need closure of the intrapartum event in order to continue their grief work. A consultation can be scheduled with the practitioner who cared for them during the pregnancy and birth. Families may also wish to read the results of tests performed during the intrapartum

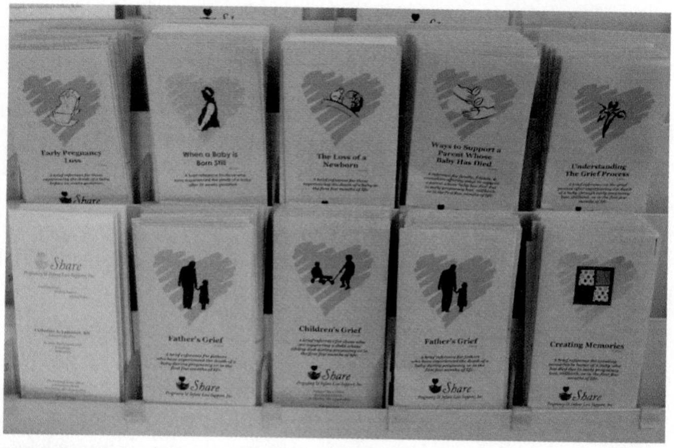

Figure 21-12 Bereavement literature.

SOURCE: Share Pregnancy & Infant Loss Support, Inc.

period and the autopsy report. Provide a copy of the medical record to the couple and encourage them to ask questions, express their feelings, and ask for clarification.

Families are routinely referred for counseling services after a perinatal loss has occurred. A counselor who specializes in perinatal issues can provide expertise and assist the couple in their grieving. Partners should be allowed to verbalize fears and concerns about future pregnancies. When appropriate, also provide referrals to genetic counselors, religious support persons, and social service agencies.

Besides referral information, the woman should receive scheduled, follow-up phone calls to assess the family's functioning and their progress with grief work. Use these follow-up phone calls to provide pertinent information and identify additional resources for the family.

As the grief process ensues, encourage families to implement cultural, religious, or social customs that will assist them in grieving and mourning. Advise the family that certain upcoming milestones, such as holidays, future birthdays, baby showers, Mother's Day, Father's Day, and other social events may trigger their grief. The family can better cope with these events if they are adequately prepared.

REFERRING THE FAMILY TO COMMUNITY SERVICES

Although most facilities have an established protocol for families experiencing perinatal loss, more comprehensive intervention programs are being established in communities to assist these families. Community support groups that focus on perinatal loss can provide an important support network and resources. Specialized groups, such as those focused on early pregnancy loss, stillbirth, and perinatal loss associated with specific congenital anomalies, allow families the opportunity to interact with peers who have lost babies under similar circumstances. Provide the group name, contact person (if possible), and phone number. Various books written by mothers who have lost children are available in bookstores and are valuable resources for grieving parents.

Internet technology has allowed large numbers of individuals to share information and to participate in online support groups. Internet resources can be effective for all families and may be the only resources available for families in rural, underserved areas.

Specialized community outreach programs are another resource that can provide assistance to grieving families; some provide early counseling to parents whose fetus has a known lethal congenital anomaly. In perinatal hospice programs, parents are given the opportunity to explore options, such as elective termination or waiting for the onset of spontaneous labor or a medically induced labor. For families wishing to continue their pregnancies, the program typically assigns a multidisciplinary team who provides compassionate care, ongoing counseling, referral to support groups, and spiritual guidance (Perinatal Hospice, 2014).

CARE OF THE COUPLE WHO HAS EXPERIENCED LOSS IN A PREVIOUS PREGNANCY

Couples who have had previous perinatal loss typically enter a subsequent pregnancy with conflicting feelings and may experience ambivalence, fear, and anxiety. Many times, their past experience is relived when another pregnancy occurs. Some couples conceive soon after a loss, while others wait years. Some couples enter a subsequent pregnancy with grief work largely completed, while others are still experiencing unresolved grief.

The nurse caring for a couple who has had a previous loss needs to be kind, compassionate, and patient. Couples need specific information and clear explanations of all prenatal information. Make referrals to genetic counselors when appropriate. Some couples may wish to have a consultation with a perinatologist. If unresolved grief issues are present or the family experiences extreme anxiety, counseling may be beneficial.

Interventions to decrease anxiety can help the couple tremendously. At the first visit, an early ultrasound can be performed to verify the presence of the fetal heart. In early pregnancy, women may be fearful when first-trimester pregnancy symptoms begin to resolve. It may be helpful for these women to come in for weekly visits for a period of time simply to hear the fetal heartbeat. This intervention may continue to be helpful until the woman begins to feel fetal movement. Throughout the pregnancy, the office or clinic nurse can play a key role by providing reassurance and answering questions that the woman may have.

Women with a previous loss typically receive additional antepartum testing throughout the pregnancy. Ultrasounds can be used to provide reassurance and assess fetal growth and development, placental functioning, and cord variations. Non-stress testing and biophysical profiles can be performed weekly after 32 weeks to ensure fetal well-being. Fetal kick counts should be initiated at 28 weeks and continue until the birth occurs. Women with a previous loss should give birth at their expected date of birth or when the pregnancy is at term and should not go over their due date, since placental functioning can decline in postdate pregnancies.

Evaluation

Expected outcomes of nursing care for the family experiencing perinatal loss include the following:

- Family members express their feelings about the death of their baby.
- Family members participate in the decision making regarding preferences for the labor, birth, and the immediate postpartum period.
- Family members participate in the decision of whether to see their baby and other decisions about the baby.
- The family has resources available for continued support.
- Family members know the community resources available and have names and phone numbers to use if they choose.
- The family is moving into and through the grieving process.

Focus Your Study

- Tachysystolic labor patterns are characterized by frequent but inefficient uterine contractions that fail to result in effacement or dilatation. With this pattern, there is a prolonged latent phase that results in maternal fatigue and stress and prolonged fetal head compression. Interventions include sedation, pain medication, bed rest, and hydration.

- Hypotonic labor patterns are characterized by less than two or three contractions in a 10-minute period during the active phase of labor and can also result in maternal fatigue and alterations in maternal coping strategies. Risks of hypotonic labor include prolonged labor, infection, postpartum hemorrhage, sepsis, and dehydration. Nursing interventions are aimed at performing pelvimetry to rule out cephalopelvic disproportion (CPD), monitoring for symptoms of infection, providing comfort measures and ongoing fetal assessment. Oxytocin (Pitocin) induction or labor stimulation may be ordered.

- Postterm pregnancy occurs when the pregnancy extends beyond 42 weeks. Common fetal complications may include oligohydramnios, meconium aspiration, decreased placental perfusion, macrosomia, and small for gestational age. Common interventions include labor induction and vacuum-assisted birth or cesarean birth.

- Fetal malpositions and malpresentations may include occiput posterior position, brow, face, breech, or transverse lie. Abnormal fetal malpositions and malpresentations can prolong labor, increase the use of vacuum or forceps use, cause fetal injury if a vaginal birth is attempted, or necessitate a cesarean birth.

- Fetal macrosomia is identified by Leopold maneuvers, ultrasound, and clinical pelvimetry. Close monitoring is warranted for complications such as labor dysfunction, and nonreassuring fetal status. Neonates born vaginally are at risk for cephalohematoma, Erb palsy, and fractured clavicles. Nursing interventions should focus on treatment of hemorrhage, including fundal massage.

- Cephalopelvic disproportion (CPD) occurs when the presenting part encounters difficulty maneuvering through the pelvis, which typically results in prolonged labor. Although some types of CPD can be delivered vaginally, in most cases, a cesarean birth is performed. Woman may increase the pelvic diameter during labor by squatting, sitting, rolling from side to side, or maintaining a knee–chest position.

- Anaphylactoid syndrome of pregnancy is a rare potentially fatal obstetric complication that occurs when a small tear in the chorion or amnion high in the uterus, which may allow amniotic fluid to enter the maternal circulatory system either during or shortly after birth. Symptoms commonly include respiratory arrest and hemorrhage. CPR and transfusion is performed until the woman is stabilized.

- Detection of a prolapsed umbilical cord is made by performing a vaginal exam. If a prolapsed cord is found, the nurse should have the woman maintain a knee–chest position while providing pressure against the presenting part to maintain umbilical cord blood flow as much as possible. Prompt notification of the physician/CNM is warranted because prompt birth is mandated.

- Nonreassuring fetal status requires intrauterine resuscitation measures that include placing the woman in a left lateral position, administering oxygen, discontinuing oxytocin (if in use), and notification of the obstetric care provider.

- The most common third- and fourth-stage complications include retained placenta, lacerations, and placenta accreta. Retained placenta beyond 30 minutes requires a manual removal of the placenta. Lacerations are repaired after birth and typically do not cause complications. Placenta accreta may result in an inability to remove the placenta and can result in hemorrhage and possible hysterectomy.

- Fetal loss can occur owing to multiple factors, including maternal factors, fetal factors, and placental factors. Families need extensive support when a fetal or maternal loss occurs. A grief counselor should be utilized to provide additional support for the nursing and medical staff.

Clinical Reasoning in Action

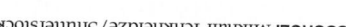

June Dice, a 25-year-old G3P1011, is admitted to you in labor and delivery at 38 weeks with a moderate amount of dark-red vaginal bleeding. June's prenatal history is significant for late prenatal care (20 weeks' gestation by ultrasound) and cocaine abuse. An ultrasound is done upon admission that demonstrates a marginal placental abruption. You place June on the fetal monitor and observe a fetal heart rate baseline of 146 to 155 with accelerations to 166 with fetal movement. There are occasional mild variable decelerations with a quick return to baseline. Contraction pattern is interpreted as an irritable uterus. An intravenous infusion with Ringer lactate is started with a #18 intracath. June's vital signs are within normal limits. Her hematocrit is 29%. You assist the physician with a vaginal examination to rupture membranes and insert a fetal scalp electrode and intrauterine pressure catheter. A small amount of light yellow-green amniotic fluid is observed. The examination shows June is 4 cm dilated, 50% effaced, vertex at −1 station. You follow protocol and start an oxytocin-induction/augmentation. June is asking why oxytocin is needed.

SOURCE: Mikhail Tchkheidze/Shutterstock.

1. Explain the goal of labor induction/augmentation in response to June's question.
2. Explain potential risk factors associated with oxytocin induction of labor.
3. You observe a nonreassuring fetal heart rate of 144 to 150 beats/min with decreased variability, and persistent late decelerations with each contraction. What interventions would you immediately take?
4. What supportive actions are taken to decrease the risk of hypofibrinogenemia?
5. What complications might be present in the newborn at birth?

References

American College of Obstetricians & Gynecologists. (2011). Optimizing protocols in obstetrics: Induction of labor. ACOG. Washington DC.

American College of Obstetricians and Gynecologists. (2012). Mode of term singleton breech delivery (ACOG Committee Opinion No. 340). Washington, DC: Author.

American College of Obstetricians and Gynecologists. (2014). Practice bulletin: Management of late-term and postterm pregnancies. Clinical Management Guidelines for Obstetrician-Gynecologists, 124(2), Part 1, 390–395.

Beníschke, K., Burton, G., & Baergen, R. (2012). Involution of implantation site: Retained placenta. Pathology of the Human Placenta, 241–248. doi:10.1007/978-3-642-23941-0_10

Blackburn, S. T. (2013). Maternal, fetal, & neonatal physiology: A clinical perspective (4th ed.). St. Louis, MO: Saunders.

Blood, C., & Cacciatore, J. (2014). Best practice in bereavement photography after perinatal death. BMC Psychology, 2:15. doi:10.1186/2050-7283-2-15

Bracken, H., Ngoc, N. N., Banks, E., Blumenthal, P., Derman, R., Patel, A., ... Winkoff, B. (2013). Misoprostol for treatment of intrauterine fetal death at 14–28 weeks of pregnancy. American Journal of Obstetrics and Gynecology, 208(1), S62–S63. doi:10.1016/j.contraception.2013.11.014

Caughey, A. B. (2013). Postterm pregnancy. eMedicine. Retrieved from http://emedicine.medscape.com/article/261369-overview#aw2aab6bb

Centers for Disease Control & Prevention (CDC). (2014). Pregnancy complications. Retrieved from http://www.cdc.gov/reproductivehealth/maternalinfanthealth/pregcomplications.htm

Child Health USA. (2013). Fetal mortality. Retrieved from http://mchb.hrsa.gov/chusa13/perinatal-health-status-indicators/p/fetal-mortality.html

Coyle, M. E., Smith, C. A., & Peat, B. (2012). Cephalic version by moxibustion for breech presentation. Cochrane Database of Systematic Reviews, Issue 5. Art. No.: CD003928. doi:10.1002/14651858.CD003928.pub3

Cunningham, F. G., Leveno, K. J., Bloom, S. L., Spong, C. Y., Dashe, J. S., Hoffman, B. L., ... Sheffield, J. S. (2014). Williams obstetrics (24th.). New York,

Davidson, M. R. (2013). Fast facts for the antepartum and postpartum nurse: A nursing orientation and care guide in a nutshell. New York, NY: Springer.

Doka, K. J., & Davidson, J. D. (2014). Living with grief: Who we are, how we grieve. Philadelphia, PA: Hospice Foundation of America.

Hanan, M., Al-Kadri, F., & Tamim, H. (2012). Factors contributing to intra-uterine fetal death. Archives of Gynecology and Obstetrics. doi:10.1007/s00404-012-2426-z

Kassebaum, N. J., Villa, A., Coggeshell, M. A., Shack-elford, K. A., Steiner, C., Heuton, K. R., ... Lozano, R. (2014). Global, regional, and national levels and causes of maternal mortality during 1990–2013: A systematic analysis for the Global Burden of Disease Study 2013. The Lancet, 384, (9947), 980–1004. doi: http://dx.doi.org/10.1016/S0140-6736(14)60696-6

King, T. L., Brucker, M. C., Kriebs, J. M., & Fahey, J. O. (2013). Varney's midwifery (6th ed.). New York, NY: Jones & Bartlett Learning.

Kübler-Ross, E. (1969). On death and dying. New York, NY: Macmillan.

Perinatal Hospice. (2014). Perinatal hospice and palliative care. Retrieved from http://www.perinatalhospice.org/perinatal_hospices.html

Posner, G. D., Dy, J., Black, A. V., & Jones, G. D. (2013). Oxorn-Foote human labor and birth (6th ed.). New York, NY: McGraw-Hill.

World Health Organization. (2012). Maternal mortality. Retrieved from http://www.who.int/mediacentre/factsheets/fs348/en/index.html

Chapter 22
Birth-Related Procedures

With our first baby, all of a sudden I had to have a cesarean. Everything happened so fast but our son was OK, and that's all that mattered. With our second baby, I wanted to try a vaginal birth. Even though I wanted to, I was afraid. I don't know what I would have done without my nurse. She stayed with me the whole time and kept giving me support. She explained what was happening and gave encouragement. I felt safe. I had a beautiful baby girl after 8 hours of labor.

—Marianne, 22

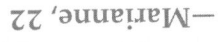
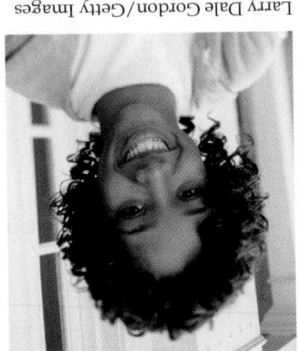

Larry Dale Gordon/Getty Images

∨ Learning Outcomes

22.1 Explain the methods, purpose, and contraindications of external and podalic versions that determine nursing management.

22.2 Describe the use of amniotomy in the nursing management of the woman and fetus.

22.3 Compare the methods for inducing labor, explaining their advantages and disadvantages in determining the nursing management of women during labor induction.

22.4 Describe the measures to prevent episiotomy, the types of episiotomy performed, and the associated nursing management.

22.5 Explain the indications and maternal and neo-natal risks that impact nursing management during forceps-assisted birth.

22.6 Describe the use of and risk of vacuum extraction to assist birth.

22.7 Explain the indications for cesarean birth, impact on the family unit, preparation and teaching needs, and associated nursing management.

22.8 Examine the risks, guidelines, and nursing management of the woman undergoing trial of labor after cesarean.

M ost births occur without the need for operative obstetric intervention. However, in some instances, procedures are necessary to maintain the safety of the woman and the fetus. The most common of these procedures are version, amniotomy, amnioinfusion, cervical ripening, induction of labor, episiotomy, forceps- or vacuum-assisted birth, and vaginal birth following a previous cesarean birth. Generally, women are aware of the possible need for an obstetric procedure during their labor and birth. However, some women expect to have a "natural" experience and feel disappointed, angry, or even guilty when an unanticipated procedure is needed. This conflict between expectation and the need for intervention presents a challenge to maternity nurses. The nurse provides information regarding any procedure to help the woman and her partner understand what is proposed, the anticipated benefits and possible risks, and any alternatives.

Care of the Woman During Version

Version, or turning the fetus, is a procedure used to change the fetal presentation by abdominal or intrauterine manipulation. The most common type of version is external cephalic

version (ECV), in which the fetus is changed from a breech to a cephalic presentation by external manipulation of the maternal abdomen (Figure 22–1). A less common type of version, called **podalic version**, is used only with the second fetus during a vaginal twin birth and only if the twin does not descend readily or if the heart rate is nonreassuring. The use of podalic versions is declining as more women with a second twin in a nonvertex presentation are counseled to undergo a cesarean birth (Rosman et al., 2015). The success rates of ECV in singleton pregnancies averages approximately 50% with ranges from 35% to 86%; however, the procedure is attempted on only about 50% to 60% of women (Rosman et al., 2015).

Criteria for External Cephalic Version

If breech or shoulder presentation (transverse lie) is detected in the later weeks of pregnancy, an external cephalic version may be attempted. Before the ECV is begun, an ultrasound is used to locate the placenta and to confirm fetal presentation. The following criteria should be met before performing external version:

- The pregnancy is at 36 or more weeks of gestation. A version may result in complications that require immediate birth by cesarean (American College of Obstetrics and Gynecology [ACOG], 2014).
- A non-stress test (NST), obtained immediately before performing the version, is reactive. A reactive NST indicates fetal well-being.
- The fetal breech is not engaged. Once the presenting part is engaged, it is difficult—if not impossible—to do a version.

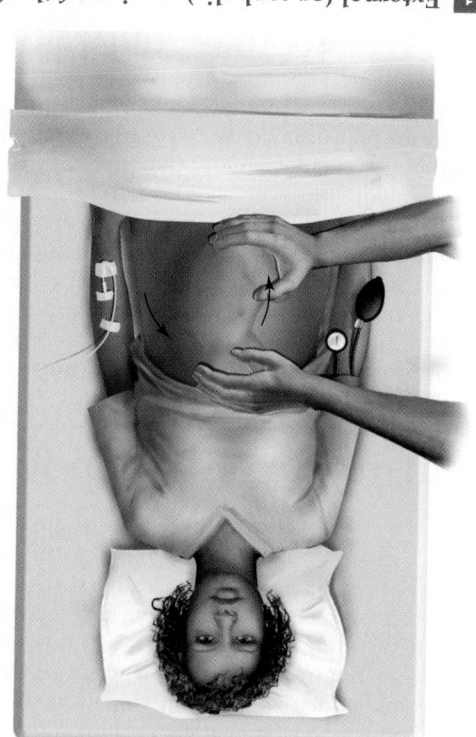

Figure 22–1 External (or cephalic) version of the fetus. A new technique involves applying pressure to the fetal head and buttocks so that the fetus completes a "backward flip" or "forward roll."

Contraindications for External Version

Contraindications include the following:

- Maternal problems, such as uterine anomalies, uncontrolled preeclampsia, or third-trimester bleeding
- Complications of pregnancy, such as rupture of membranes, oligohydramnios, hydramnios, or placenta previa or vasa previa
- Previous cesarean birth or other significant uterine surgery
- Multiple gestations
- Nonreassuring fetal heart rate (FHR) or other evidence of uteroplacental insufficiency
- Fetal abnormalities, such as intrauterine growth restriction (IUGR) or nuchal cord

Before the external version procedure begins, an intravenous line may be established to administer medications in case of difficulty. The woman may receive terbutaline subcutaneously to relax the uterus. Some physicians may also order regional anesthesia for the procedure. Both tocolytics and regional anesthesia have been associated with higher success rates and fewer cesarean births (ACOG, 2014). Ultrasound is frequently used to provide information about the fetal position. The version is discontinued in the presence of severe maternal pain or significant fetal bradycardia or decelerations.

Nursing Management

On admission, begin a thorough assessment by verifying that there are no contraindications to the version procedure. Obtain maternal vital signs and a reactive NST. This initial assessment period provides an ideal time for educating the woman and her partner and for addressing their concerns. They can be encouraged to express their understanding and expectations of the procedure. At the same time, the possibility of failure of the ECV and slight risk of cesarean birth if the FHR becomes nonreassuring can be discussed. Explain what will occur in either of these circumstances to better prepare the woman and her partner if intervention becomes necessary. Although the physician is ultimately responsible for obtaining informed consent, it is also the nurse's role to ensure that the woman understands the procedure and has the opportunity to ask questions and voice her concerns or fears.

SAFETY ALERT!

External cephalic version is considered a safe procedure but should be performed only when there is the ability to provide a cesarean delivery if necessary (Davidson, 2013).

Clinical Tip

Because the ECV procedure can be uncomfortable, encourage the woman to take slow, deep breaths. Using distraction and speaking in a calm, reassuring voice can help decrease fear and anxiety.

Place an intravenous (IV) line before beginning the procedure to maintain IV access in case of a complication. Throughout the procedure, continue to monitor maternal blood pressure, pulse, and comfort level frequently (because the mother may experience pain during the procedure). Fetal well-being is ascertained before, intermittently during, and for (at least) 30 minutes following the procedure, using electronic fetal monitoring (EFM), ultrasound, or

Care of the Woman During Amniotomy

Amniotomy is the artificial rupture of the amniotic membranes (AROM). It is probably the most common invasive procedure in obstetrics. Because the amniotomy requires that an instrument, called an *amnihook*, be inserted through the cervix, at least 2 cm (0.8 in.) of cervical dilatation is required. Some clinicians may also perform amniotomy by inserting a fetal scalp electrode on the fetal head as a means to rupture membranes.

SAFETY ALERT!
The fetal head should be engaged prior to rupturing the membranes to prevent a possible prolapsed umbilical cord, a situation in which the umbilical cord slips through the cervical opening ahead of the presenting part. This constitutes an obstetric emergency and can be avoided by using strict criteria before an amniotomy is performed. (For a discussion of umbilical cord prolapse, see Chapter 21.)

Amniotomy has been used as a means to shorten labor. A recent study that examined amniotomy and the length of labor did show a reduction in the first stage of labor, which in turn resulted in a shortage of time needed for oxytocin (Pitocin) induction, fewer cesarean births, and no increases in maternal fever (Gagnon-Gervais et al., 2012). Amniotomy can also be used at any time during the first stage to augment labor (accelerate the progress). Amniotomy is more effective in multiparous women. This is because the cervix is more pliable. Amniotomy manipulates both hormones and mechanical factors to stimulate labor. Upon rupturing the membranes, natural prostaglandins are released that stimulate uterine contractions. The escape of amniotic fluid allows the presenting part to descend and place direct pressure on the cervix, thus resulting in an acceleration of dilatation.

Amniotomy may also be done during labor to apply an internal fetal heart monitoring electrode to the scalp or to insert an intrauterine pressure catheter. In addition, amniotomy allows assessment of the color and composition of amniotic fluid.

AROM Procedure

While performing a vaginal examination, the physician/certified nurse-midwife (CNM) introduces an amnihook into the vagina and makes a small tear in the amniotic membrane, which allows amniotic fluid to escape.

Nursing Management

Explain the AROM procedure to the woman and then assess fetal presentation, position, and station because amniotomy is usually delayed until engagement has occurred. Ask the woman to assume a semireclining position and drape her to provide privacy. The fetal heart rate (FHR) is assessed just before and immediately after the amniotomy, and the two FHR assessments are compared. If there are marked changes, check for prolapse of the cord. The amniotic fluid is inspected for amount, color, odor, and the presence of meconium or blood. While wearing disposable gloves, cleanse and dry the woman's perineal area and change the underpads as needed. Because there is now an open pathway for organisms to ascend into the uterus, the number of vaginal examinations must be kept to a minimum to reduce the chance of introducing an infection. In addition, monitor the woman's temperature a minimum of every 2 hours. Provide information regarding the expected effects of the amniotomy. It is important for the woman to know that amniotic fluid is constantly produced because some women may worry that they will experience a "dry birth." See Assisting with Amniotomy in the *Clinical Skills Manual* SKILLS.

both. Also assess maternal–fetal response to the tocolytic. Provide aftercare instructions, which may include maternal monitoring for contractions and fetal movement (fetal kick counts).

Care of the Woman During Amnioinfusion

Amnioinfusion (AI) is a technique by which warmed, sterile normal saline or Ringer lactate solution is introduced into the uterus through an intrauterine pressure catheter (IUPC). Amnioinfusion can be used intrapartally to increase the volume of fluid in cases of oligohydramnios, in which cord compression causes fetal heart rate (FHR) deceleration and nonreassuring fetal status. It provides an extra cushion of fluid that relieves pressure on the umbilical cord and promotes increased perfusion to the fetus. Amnioinfusion may also be indicated for preterm labor with premature rupture of membranes.

Nursing Management

The nurse is often the first person to detect changes in FHR associated with cord compression. When cord compression is suspected, the immediate intervention is to assist the laboring woman to another position. If this intervention is not successful in restoring the FHR, an amnioinfusion may be considered.

Clinical Tip

Before the AROM procedure, place several layers of disposable pads under the woman's buttocks and a folded towel between her legs. The towel readily absorbs the fluid released during the procedure and prevents soiling of the bed linens. After the procedure, remove the towel as well as all layers of absorbent pads that have been soiled. To increase the woman's comfort, place several clean absorbent pads under her buttocks because amniotic fluid will continue to leak from the vagina.

Help administer the AI, assess the woman's vital signs and contraction status, and monitor the fetal heart rate by continuous electronic fetal monitoring (EFM). It is important to provide ongoing information to the laboring woman and her partner and to answer questions as they arise. Comfort measures and positioning are vital because the woman is now on bed rest. Frequent changing of disposable underpads and perineal care are also needed because of the constant leakage of fluid from the vagina. Ensure that fluids that are infused into the uterus are being adequately expelled. Fluid expulsion is evaluated by counting sanitary pads and visual observation during perineal care.

Care of the Woman During Cervical Ripening

Cervical ripening is softening and effacing of the cervix. It may be used for the pregnant woman who is at term or late preterm when there is a medical or obstetric indication for induction of labor. In general, cervical ripening agents are used when the cervix is unfavorable for induction. Bishop (1964) developed a prelabor scoring system that is helpful in predicting the potential

TABLE 22-1 Prelabor Status Evaluation Scoring System

FACTOR	ASSIGNED VALUE: BISHOP SCORE			
	0	1	2	3
Cervical dilatation	Closed	1–2 cm	3–4 cm	5 cm or more
Cervical effacement	0%–30%	40%–50%	60%–70%	80% or more
Fetal station	–3	–2	–1, 0	+1, or lower
Cervical consistency	Firm	Moderate	Soft	
Cervical position	Posterior	Midposition	Anterior	

Source: Data from Bishop, E. H. (1964). Pelvic scoring for elective inductions. *Obstetrics & Gynecology, 24,* 266.

success of induction (Table 22–1). Components evaluated are cervical dilatation, effacement, consistency, and position, as well as the station of the fetal presenting part. A score of 0, 1, 2, or 3 is given to each assessed characteristic. The higher the total score for all the criteria, the more likely it is that labor will occur. The lower the total score, the higher the failure rate. A favorable cervix is the most important criterion for a successful induction (Posner, Black, & Jones, 2013). The presence of a cervix that is anterior, soft, 50% effaced, and dilated at least 2 cm (0.8 in.), with the fetal head at 1 to +1 station or lower (Bishop score of 8 or 9), is favorable for successful induction (Posner et al., 2013). If the cervix is unfavorable, a method of cervical ripening may be tried.

Pharmacologic methods of cervical ripening include the use of prostaglandin (PG) agents (Prepidil, Cervidil) and misoprostol (Cytotec), which is a synthetic PGE_1 analogue. The use of prostaglandin agents became popular when Prepidil gel, which contains 0.5 mg dinoprostone, a prostaglandin E_2 (PGE_2) agent, was first used to induce women with an unfavorable cervix. It is placed either intracervically or intravaginally. Prostaglandin agents placed intravaginally are superior to intracervical placement (ACOG, 2013a). Most facilities are now using newer agents such as dinoprostone (Cervidil) or misoprostol (Cytotec) for labor induction.

Dinoprostone (Cervidil)

Dinoprostone (Cervidil) is packaged as a 2-cm (0.8-in.) square vaginal insert that resembles a thin piece of cardboard. It releases 10 mg of dinoprostone at a rate of 0.3 mg/hr over 12 hours. In recent studies, women being induced with Cervidil had less pain than women who had received prostaglandin gel, resulting in improved physical and emotional well-being of the mother (Stephenson, Hawkins, Powers, et al., 2014).

Cervidil has been associated with cervical ripening, reducing the length of labor, and lowering the requirements for oxytocin (Pitocin) during labor induction (ACOG, 2013a). Prostaglandin agents are typically used when labor induction is indicated, but not emergent, such as maternal gestational diabetes, postdates, or large-for-gestational-age (LGA) fetuses who warrant birth occurring in the near future. For example, a woman who is over 41 weeks of gestation but has a very unfavorable cervix may be given prostaglandin gel to ripen her cervix before an oxytocin induction is scheduled.

Clinical Tip

Advise the woman that prostaglandin agents commonly cause uterine stimulation after insertion. Review the signs of labor that warrant further assessment after discharge home. Teach the woman the difference between common reactions to the prostaglandin agents (such as cramping, uterine irritability, and gel leakage) and the true signs of labor (strong regular contractions, rupture of membranes) before she leaves the hospital.

Misoprostol (Cytotec)

Misoprostol (Cytotec) is a synthetic PGE_1 analogue that some healthcare agencies use to ripen the cervix and induce labor. It is available as a tablet and can be administered using several routes including the following: oral, vaginal, rectal, sublingual, or buccal. Although the last two routes are effective, they are rarely used. The rectal route is primarily used when attempting to control postpartum hemorrhaging (Stephenson et al., 2014). While practitioners may opt to administer the medication using different routes, a Cochrane review found that the rectal and vaginal routes are more commonly associated with uterine tachysystolic patterns, and that the oral route is just as effective in producing cervical ripening while reducing the duration of oxytocin (Pitocin) infusion (Cunningham et al., 2014). Studies also provide evidence that using dosages of 25 mcg at intervals of 4 hours or more is associated with a lower incidence of tachysystole (Cunningham et al., 2014). Although conflicting research findings can be confusing, it is important to note that misoprostol is delivered via various routes and yields successful results.

Since the 1990s, misoprostol (Cytotec) has been contraindicated for inducing labor in women who have had a previous cesarean birth or have a scar on their uterus (ACOG, 2013a). Although quite rare, misoprostol has also been associated with uterine rupture in women who have no previous scar on their uterus (Cunningham et al., 2014). Other risk factors for uterine rupture include a high-dose regimen (100 mcg or higher), advanced gestational age, and five or more previous pregnancies (Cunningham et al., 2014). After a careful review of the literature and current studies, ACOG (2013a) issued the following recommended guidelines for misoprostol administration:

- Use only during the third trimester for cervical ripening or labor induction.
- One-fourth tablet or 25 mcg should be the initial dosage.
- Recurrent administration should not exceed dosing intervals of more than 3 to 6 hours.
- Oxytocin (Pitocin) should not be administered less than 4 hours after the last misoprostol (Cytotec) dose.
- Continuous fetal and uterine monitoring should be performed in a hospital setting.

Absolute contraindications for the use of misoprostol include the following:

- Presence of uterine contractions 3 times in 10 minutes
- Significant maternal asthma
- History of previous cesarean birth or other uterine scar
- Bleeding during the pregnancy
- Presence of placenta previa
- Fetal tachycardia, nonreassuring fetal heart rate tracing, meconium passage

Nursing Management

Physicians/CNMs and birthing room nurses who have had special education and training may administer cervical ripening agents. Provide the woman and her support person(s) information about the procedure, and answer any questions they may have. Assess baseline maternal vital signs, and apply an electronic fetal monitor (EFM). The EFM tracing should indicate minimal or absent uterine activity, a reassuring fetal heart rate (FHR) pattern, and a reactive non-stress test (NST). If uterine contractions are not occurring regularly, the ripening agent is inserted into the vagina. If prescribed, misoprostol (Cytotec) is administered every 3 to 6 hours until adequate cervical change occurs (ACOG, 2013a). Instruct the woman to lie supine with a right hip wedge for a specified time (usually at least 1 hour). The woman can then assume any comfortable position. As discussed previously, monitor the woman for uterine hyperstimulation and FHR abnormalities (changes in baseline rate, variability, presence of decelerations) for at least 2 hours following insertion. The insert should be removed immediately if uterine hyperstimulation or nonreassuring fetal status occurs. A beta-adrenergic agent should also be administered if hyperstimulation occurs (Forrest Pharmaceuticals, 2015).

Care of the Woman During Labor Induction

ACOG defines **labor induction** as the stimulation of uterine contractions before the spontaneous onset of labor, with or without ruptured amniotic membranes, for the purpose of accomplishing birth. Induction may be indicated in the presence of the following (Cunningham et al., 2014):

- Diabetes mellitus
- Preeclampsia/eclampsia
- Premature rupture of membranes (PROM) with established fetal maturity
- Chorioamnionitis
- Postterm gestation, especially in association with oligohydramnios
- Intrauterine fetal demise (IUFD)
- Intrauterine fetal growth restriction (IUGR)
- Alloimmunization
- Nonreassuring antepartum testing

Relative indications include chronic hypertension, systemic lupus erythematosus, gestational diabetes, hypercoagulation disorders, cholestasis of pregnancy, polyhydramnios, fetal anomalies requiring specialized neonatal care, logistical factors (risk of rapid birth, distance from hospital, psychologic factors, advanced cervical dilatation), and previous stillbirth (Cunningham et al., 2014). With the new definitions of term pregnancy, inductions prior to 39 weeks should be avoided whenever possible owing to fetal maturity issues (ACOG, 2014).

Healthy People 2020

(MICH-6) Reduce maternal illness and complications due to pregnancy (complications during hospitalized labor and delivery)

All contraindications to spontaneous labor and vaginal birth are contraindications to the induction of labor. Maternal contraindications include but are not limited to the following (Cunningham et al., 2014):

- Client refusal
- Placenta previa or vasa previa
- Floating fetal presenting part
- Prior uterine incision that would preclude a trial of labor
- Active genital herpes infection
- Umbilical cord prolapse
- Acute severe nonreassuring fetal status
- Absolute cephalopelvic disproportion

Relative contraindications include cervical carcinoma; malpresentation, such as breech; and funic presentation. A **funic presentation** is when the umbilical cord is interposed between the cervix and the presenting part. It can be located by clinical evaluation or by ultrasound (Cunningham et al., 2014).

Labor Readiness

Before attempting an induction, assess fetal maturity and cervical readiness to ensure that both the woman and fetus are ready for the onset of labor. In recent years, more specific definitions of term pregnancy have evolved. Women who have completed 39 weeks are considered term. A woman with a pregnancy less than 39 completed weeks is considered preterm and should not undergo an elective induction. Inductions that are medically indicated may have to be performed prior to this if significant maternal or fetal risk factors are present. Some organizations no longer support elective induction of labor for any reason, stating the risks far outweigh any benefits (Association of Women's Health, Obstetric, & Neonatal Nurses [AWHONN], 2013).

SAFETY ALERT!
Elected inductions prior to 39 completed weeks or in women with inaccurate or unsure dating are at risk for a variety of adverse fetal outcomes including stressors on the fetus, respiratory distress syndrome (RDS), longer separation from the mother, interrupted bonding, and less breastfeeding, which increases the risk of childhood obesity and chronic illness. Additionally, when complications occur, newborns are more likely to be admitted to the neonatal intensive care unit (NICU) and have longer hospital stays and more hospital readmissions. Maternal risks associated with induction of labor include increased risk of postpartum hemorrhages, which increases the risk for blood transfusions, hysterectomy, placenta implantation abnormalities in future pregnancies, a longer hospital stay, more hospital readmissions, and, in the worst case scenario, death (AWHONN, 2014).

FETAL MATURITY

The gestational age of the fetus is best evaluated by accurate maternal menstrual dating and early ultrasounds. Women who begin prenatal care later in the pregnancy with unsure dating should not be induced because it is possible that the gestational age is less than 39 completed weeks, which is considered preterm. These women have to be evaluated on a case-by-case basis when medical necessity warrants induction of labor. Amniotic fluid studies also provide valuable information in assessing fetal lung maturity (see Chapter 13).

CERVICAL READINESS

The findings on vaginal examination help determine whether cervical changes favorable for induction have occurred. The use of Bishop scoring (previously discussed) provides an appropriate assessment to determine if a woman can move forward with an induction or if cervical ripening agents are needed.

Methods of Inducing Labor

When the cervix is favorable, the most frequently used methods of induction are amniotomy (discussed previously), stripping the amniotic membranes, mechanical dilatation with intracervical catheter, intravenous oxytocin (Pitocin) infusion, and complementary methods.

STRIPPING THE MEMBRANES

A nonpharmacologic method of induction frequently used by physicians/CNMs is stripping (or sweeping) the amniotic membranes. The practitioner inserts a gloved finger into the internal os and rotates it 360 degrees twice, separating the amniotic membranes that are lying against the lower uterine segment. This is thought to release prostaglandins that stimulate uterine contractions. The procedure is usually uncomfortable and can result in cramping, uterine contractions, and vaginal bleeding.

MECHANICAL DILATATION WITH INTRACERVICAL CATHETER

An intracervical catheter is sometimes used to facilitate mechanical dilatation of the cervix when the cervix is unfavorable or a low Bishop score has been established. When first used in obstetrics, Foley catheters were placed within the cervix and the balloon was inflated to facilitate mechanical dilatation of the cervix. This method has been shown to be effective in stretching the cervix without increasing the incidence of infection and without causing fetal tachysystole, which can occur with the use of prostaglandin agents (Davidson, 2013). The disadvantages include difficulty with placement and failure to maintain placement. Women are limited in their ability to ambulate postinsertion because of the risk of displacement. Mechanical dilatation is sometimes performed with weighted, double-ballooned catheters, which have been shown to decrease the first stage of labor (Lutgendorf, Johnson, Terpstra, et al., 2012). Some practitioners may also combine intracervical balloon dilatation with prostaglandin agents to shorten the first stage of labor (Posner et al., 2013).

OXYTOCIN (PITOCIN) INFUSION

Administration of oxytocin (Pitocin) is effective for initiating uterine contractions to induce labor and may also be used to enhance ineffective contractions (labor augmentation). A primary line of 1000 mL of electrolyte solution (e.g., lactated Ringer solution) is started intravenously. Ten units of oxytocin is added to a secondary line of intravenous (IV) fluid so the resulting mixture will contain 10 milliunits/mL of oxytocin (1 milliunit/min, or 6 mL/hr), and the prescribed dose can be calculated easily. After the primary infusion is started, the oxytocin solution is piggybacked into the primary tubing port closest to the catheter insertion. The infusion is then administered using an infusion pump to control the flow rate precisely. The rate of infusion is based on physician/CNM protocol and careful assessment of the contraction pattern. The goal for induction is to achieve stable contractions every 2 to 3 minutes that last 40 to 60 seconds. The uterus should relax to full baseline resting tone between each contraction. Progress is determined by changes in the effacement and dilatation of the cervix and station of the presenting part.

Oxytocin (Pitocin) induction is not without some associated risks, including hyperstimulation of the uterus, resulting in uterine contractions that are too frequent or too intense, with an increased resting tone. Hypertonic contractions may lead to decreased placental perfusion and nonreassuring fetal status. Excess oxytocin concentrations can result in maternal hypertension, tachysystolic labor patterns, uterine rupture, placental abruption, rapid labor and birth, decrease in placental functioning, and water intoxication. Fetal effects may include fetal hypoxia, nonreassuring fetal status, hyperbilirubinemia, trauma from rapid birth, and fetal bradycardia (Wilson, Shannon, & Shields, 2015).

Nursing Management

While the use of oxytocin (Pitocin) is common in obstetric practice, it is important to follow guidelines to ensure safe administration. Oxytocin is contraindicated in some women (Table 22–2). Prior to administration and with each increase in dosage, perform the following:

- Assess FHR; frequency, duration, and intensity of uterine contractions and presence of decelerations, accelerations, and uterine resting tone every 15 minutes and before each increase in the oxytocin infusion rate.
- Record client activities (such as change of position, vomiting), procedures done (amniotomy, sterile vaginal examination), and administration of analgesic agents to allow for interpretation and evaluation of tracing.
- Assess cervical dilatation as needed.

Continually assess for adverse maternal and fetal effects, including nonreassuring fetal status (bradycardia, late or deep and repetitive variable decelerations); uterine contractions that occur more than every 2 minutes; contractions that exceed a duration of more than 60 seconds; or insufficient relaxation of the uterus between contractions or a steady increase in resting tone is noted (ACOG, 2013a).

Nursing management of adverse effects begins by discontinuing the IV oxytocin infusion, opening up the primary solution for immediate infusion, turning woman to side, and if nonreassuring fetal status is present, administering oxygen by tight face mask at 8 to 10 L/min. Instruct another staff member to notify the physician/CNM. Maintain an intake and output record.

Protocols for oxytocin (Pitocin) administration vary depending on the setting and individualized policies. The maximum rate is 40 milliunits/min (ACOG, 2013a). When indicated, the maximum dose is generally between 16 and 40 milliunits/min. Decrease oxytocin by similar increments once labor has progressed to

---

TABLE 22–2 Maternal Contraindications for Oxytocin (Pitocin) Administration

- Severe preeclampsia/eclampsia
- Predisposition to uterine rupture (in nullipara over 35 years of age, multigravida 4 or more, overdistention of the uterus, previous major surgery of the cervix or uterus)
- Cephalopelvic disproportion
- Malpresentation or malposition of the fetus
- Cord prolapse
- More than one previous cesarean birth
- Preterm baby
- Rigid, unripe cervix
- Total placenta previa
- Presence of nonreassuring fetal status

5 to 6 cm dilatation. During administration, maternal vital signs, including blood pressure, heart rate, and oxygen saturation, are monitored every 15 minutes.

0.5 milliunit/min = 3 mL/hr	8 milliunits/min = 48 mL/hr
1.0 milliunit/min = 6 mL/hr	10 milliunits/min = 60 mL/hr
1.5 milliunits/min = 9 mL/hr	12 milliunits/min = 72 mL/hr
2 milliunits/min = 12 mL/hr	15 milliunits/min = 90 mL/hr
4 milliunits/min = 24 mL/hr	18 milliunits/min = 108 mL/hr
6 milliunits/min = 36 mL/hr	20 milliunits/min = 120 mL/hr

SAFETY ALERT!

Prior to increasing an oxytocin (Pitocin) infusion, maternal vital signs, FHR, fetal tracing category, and the contraction frequency, duration, and intensity should be assessed. Institutions may vary with the protocol used; however, oxytocin dosage should not exceed 40 units in 1000 mL. Oxytocin dosing is dictated by the maternal and fetal responses and the contractions and cervical dilatation responses, thus requiring continuous maternal, fetal, and contraction monitoring. It is imperative to know the concentration of oxytocin in milliunits per minute to prevent accidental overdosage.

Clinical Reasoning Determining Infusion Rate

You are a birthing center nurse caring for Wendy Johnson, G2P1, during a oxytocin (Pitocin) infusion to induce her labor. Wendy has been receiving the medication via infusion pump for 4 hours and currently is receiving 6 milliunits/min (36 mL/hr). You have just completed your assessments and found the following: BP 120/80, pulse 80, respirations 16; contractions every 3 minutes lasting 60 seconds and of strong intensity; the FHR baseline is 144 to 150 with average variability; and cervical dilatation is 6 cm (2.4 in.). Will you continue the same infusion rate, increase the rate, or decrease the rate?

COMPLEMENTARY METHODS

Although not frequently presented in medical (allopathic) or nursing texts, a variety of more natural, noninvasive methods of inducing labor can be effective. These methods include sexual intercourse; self or partner nipple or breast stimulation; the use of herbs, castor oil, or enemas; and acupuncture. Many CNMs and their clients desire a less medical approach to birth and want to use natural methods when possible. The cautions and contraindications for these natural methods are the same as those for medical induction of labor. It is also important to understand that some of them may not have undergone scientific research as rigorous as that used for pharmacologic agents.

Sexual intercourse is a logical method of inducing cervical ripening and uterine contractions; female orgasm stimulates contractions, and male ejaculate is a rich source of prostaglandins. Penetration during intercourse can also stimulate the lower uterine segment and cause uterine contractions. In addition, breast and nipple stimulation, which are often part of lovemaking, cause the production of endogenous oxytocin, which in turn stimulates the uterus to contract (Davidson, 2013).

Herbal preparations and other homeopathic solutions have not been scientifically studied to the same extent as other natural methods. The healthcare giver needs a thorough personal knowledge or ongoing consultation with a homeopathic physician to safely recommend the use of these approaches during late pregnancy. Some herbal products, such as blue cohosh, have been found to cause complications and should not be routinely recommended during pregnancy (Posner et al., 2013).

Ingesting castor oil has been used for many years, but it has not been well studied as a method of labor induction. The mechanism of action is not understood. A Cochrane review found that no clinical effectiveness could be established, and that all women who ingested castor oil experienced nausea, indicating that such recommendations lack evidence-based guidelines and should not be routinely recommended. While harmful effects have not been identified, success rates in stimulation of labor have not been supported (Rakel, 2012).

Acupuncture and acupressure have been used for centuries in Eastern medicine as a means for inducing labor or preventing postdate pregnancies, although the number of carefully researched studies in this area is limited. Women who receive acupressure and acupuncture are less likely to need labor induction than women who do not receive these therapies (Rakel, 2012).

Nursing Management

Aspects to address during client teaching about induction of labor include the purpose, the procedure itself, nursing care that will be provided, assessments, comfort measures, and a review of breathing techniques that may be used during labor. Regardless of the induction method used, close observation and accurate, ongoing assessments are mandatory to provide safe, optimal care for both woman and fetus. A qualified clinician should be readily accessible to manage any complications that may occur.

As contractions are established, perform vaginal examinations to evaluate cervical dilatation, effacement, and station. The frequency of vaginal examinations primarily depends on the woman's parity, comfort level, and strength of her contractions. If evaluating the need for analgesia, perform a vaginal examination to avoid giving the medication too early and increasing the risk of prolonging labor. This examination also helps identify advanced dilatation and imminent birth.

Oxytocin (Pitocin) induction protocols recommend obtaining baseline data (maternal temperature, pulse, respirations, blood pressure), a 20- to 30-minute electronic fetal monitor (EFM) recording demonstrating a reassuring fetal heart rate (FHR), a reactive non-stress test (NST), and the contraction status before starting an induction. Use a fetal monitor to provide continuous data.

Before each increase of the oxytocin (Pitocin) infusion rate, assess the following:

- Maternal blood pressure, pulse, respirations, temperature, and pain level
- Contraction status including frequency, duration, intensity, and resting tone
- FHR baseline, variability, and reactivity, noting the presence of accelerations, any decelerations, or bradycardia

---

SAFETY ALERT!

Women receiving oxytocin (Pitocin) warrant ongoing assessment every 15 minutes and need closer ongoing observation when oxytocin levels are increased. If the nurse cannot adequately monitor the woman immediately following a dosage increase, it is advisable to wait to increase the medication until careful monitoring capabilities are available.

Explain the induction or augmentation procedure to the woman and answer any questions the family may have. An informative orientation provides the woman with a sense of control, participation in active decision making, and decreases anxiety. Women should be offered as much autonomy as possible and should be offered telemetry units when available, which enable ambulation, sitting in a rocking chair, use of a birthing ball, or the option to use the shower or bathtub. *Nursing Care Plan: For Induction of Labor* provides nursing interventions for women undergoing oxytocin (Pitocin) induction.

Nursing Care Plan: For Induction of Labor

1. Nursing Diagnosis: *Injury, Risk for,* **related to tachysystole of uterus caused by induction of labor (NANDA-I © 2014)**

GOAL: Progression of labor without difficulty or complications

INTERVENTION	RATIONALE
• Obtain a baseline for maternal blood pressure, pulse, respirations, temperature, and pain level.	• Oxytocin (Pitocin) induction can affect the cardiovascular system. Blood pressure may initially be decreased. If the induction is prolonged the blood pressure (BP) may increase by 30%. Respirations can become elevated because of pain sensation, anxiety, or physiologic causes. Temperature is obtained to monitor for infection. The pain level is assessed continuously to determine if pain medication is warranted or changes in vital signs are caused by maternal discomfort.
• Place client on external fetal monitor for 20 min to obtain a baseline for fetal heart rate (FHR) and variability.	• Assesses for fetal well-being. Normal FHR ranges from 110 to 160 beats/min. Variability measuring three to five fluctuations in 1 minute is documented as average. Continuous electronic fetal monitoring (EFM) is performed during an oxytocin induction.
• Perform non-stress test.	• A non-stress test is performed to assess the fetal heart rate in response to fetal movement. Accelerations of FHR with fetal movement may indicate the fetus has adequate oxygenation and an intact central nervous system. A reactive non-stress test indicates there were at least two accelerations of 15 beats/min above baseline, lasting 15 sec in a 20-min period.
• Insert IV line and begin primary infusion with 1000 mL of electrolyte solution.	• An electrolyte solution such as lactated Ringer is used for the primary solution. A primary IV allows continuous intravenous access and fluid infusion in the event the oxytocin drip needs to be discontinued.
• Piggyback oxytocin solution into primary IV tubing, via pump, in the port closest to the IV insertion site.	• Oxytocin is mixed in 1000 mL of an electrolyte solution (usually 5% dextrose in lactated Ringer solution) and piggybacked to main IV line. A pump is used to ensure dosage accuracy.
• Begin oxytocin infusion per agency protocol.	• The rate to be used is determined by physician/CNM orders or agency protocol.
• Monitor infusion pump and connections.	• This ensures adequate dosing. Early identification of problems with the infusion site, the piggyback connection, or flow rate will minimize effects on uterine contractions and FHR. If a problem is found, correct and restart infusion at the beginning dose.
• Monitor and evaluate maternal BP and pulse before each increase in the oxytocin infusion rate.	• Prolonged inductions may increase the blood pressure by 30%. The oxytocin infusion rate should not be advanced if maternal hypertension or hypotension is present or if there are any radical changes in pulse rate.
• Evaluate urine output.	• There is an antidiuretic effect with dosages of oxytocin above 20 milliunits/min. This level decreases free water exchange in the kidneys, therefore markedly decreasing urine output.
• Evaluate and document FHR before each increase in oxytocin infusion rate.	• During oxytocin infusion, FHR should range between 110 and 160 beats/min. Tachysystole of the maternal uterus may cause nonreassuring fetal status. Fetal bradycardia may occur along with a decrease in variability, leading to fetal hypoxia. Fetal tachycardia may also occur. If persistent fetal bradycardia or fetal tachycardia occurs, the oxytocin is discontinued.

(continued)

Nursing Care Plan: For Induction of Labor (*continued*)

- Evaluate and document contraction pattern before each increase of the oxytocin infusion rate.

- Increase oxytocin infusion dosage until adequate contractions are achieved or the maximum dose per agency protocol is reached.

- Evaluate contraction frequency, duration, and intensity before increasing the infusion rate. Discontinue oxytocin infusion and infuse primary solution if signs of tachysystole of the uterus are detected.

- Initiate treatment measures to reverse the effects of oxytocin infusion if fetal tachycardia or bradycardia occurs.

- Contractions every 2–3 min, lasting 40–60 sec with moderate intensity, are considered adequate. Cervical dilatation progresses an average of 1.2 cm/hr to 1.5 cm/hr (0.5 in./hr to 0.6 in./hr) during the active phase of labor.

- Oxytocin may be increased every 20–40 min until an adequate contraction pattern is achieved.

- Signs of tachysystole include contraction frequency more than 2 min, duration exceeding 60 sec, and increased resting tone. Tachysystole of the uterus puts the client at risk for abruptio placentae and uterine rupture.

- When the FHR falls outside the normal range (110–160 beats/min), treatment measures should be initiated. To reverse the effects of oxytocin, immediately discontinue oxytocin, infuse primary solution, administer oxygen by tight face mask at 8–10 L/min, place client in side-lying position, and notify physician/CNM.

EXPECTED OUTCOME: Contractions will increase in frequency, duration, and intensity. An increase in cervical dilatation, effacement, and intensity will be achieved. The uterus will remain soft between contractions.

USE OF OXYTOCIN (PITOCIN) IN FOURTH STAGE

Oxytocin (Pitocin) is sometimes used after the expulsion of the placenta to decrease uterine bleeding. Bleeding can also be reduced by initiating early breastfeeding, which promotes the release of oxytocin and increase uterine contractility (AWHONN, 2015). Oxytocin can be given intramuscularly or intravenously in the postpartum period after maternal vital signs have been assessed. If bleeding is well controlled, oxytocin is typically discontinued after a short period of time.

Care of the Woman During an Episiotomy

An **episiotomy** is a surgical incision of the perineal body to enlarge the outlet. It is the second most common procedure in maternal–child care and has long been thought to minimize the risk of lacerations of the perineum and the overstretching of perineal tissues. However, episiotomy may actually increase the risk of fourth-degree perineal lacerations (Posner et al., 2013). Although very common, the routine use of episiotomy has been seriously questioned for several years. Research suggests that (1) rather than protecting the perineum from lacerations, the presence of an episiotomy makes it more likely that the woman will have anal sphincter tears and (2) perineal lacerations heal more quickly than deep perineal tears (King, Brucker, Kriebs, et al., 2013). In clinical practice, research has shown that the incidence of major perineal trauma (extension to or through the anal sphincter) is more likely to happen if a midline episiotomy is done (Davidson, 2013). Women with previous episiotomies were more likely to have a repeat episiotomy or a spontaneous laceration when compared with those women who had a spontaneous laceration without the use of episiotomy during their first pregnancies (Lurie, Kedar, Boaz, et al., 2012). Additional complications associated with episiotomy are blood loss, infection, pain, and perineal discomfort that may continue for days or weeks past birth, including painful intercourse (Lurie et al., 2012).

Developing Cultural Competence Participating in Childbirth Decisions

Although many North American women have specific beliefs and expectations for childbirth, other cultural or religious groups may not verbalize specific requests or ideas for their labor experience. Some women from various cultures typically do not express their preferences but instead depend on their healthcare practitioner to make decisions regarding procedures that may be indicated. They typically view healthcare providers as authority figures and participate less in their own healthcare decision making (Selin, 2012).

Factors That Predispose Women to Episiotomy

Overall, factors that place a woman at increased risk for episiotomy are primigravid status, large or macrosomic fetus, occiput–posterior position, use of forceps or vacuum extractor, and shoulder dystocia. Other factors that may be mitigated by nurses and physicians/CNMs include the following:

- Use of lithotomy and other recumbent positions (cause excessive and uneven stretching of the perineum)

- Encouraging or requiring sustained breath holding during second-stage pushing (causes excessive and rapid perineal stretching, can adversely affect blood flow in mother and fetus, and requires woman to be responsive to healthcare givers' directions rather than to her own urges to push spontaneously)

- Arbitrary time limit placed by the physician/CNM on the length of the second stage

Preventive Measures

These general tips help reduce the incidence of routine episiotomies:

- Perineal massage during pregnancy for nulliparous women

- Natural pushing during labor, and avoiding the lithotomy position or pulling back on legs (which tightens the perineum)
- Side-lying position for pushing, which helps slow birth and diminish tears
- Warm or hot compresses on the perineum and firm counterpressure
- Encouraging a gradual expulsion of the neonate at the time of birth by encouraging the mother to "push, take a breath, push, take a breath" thereby easing the baby out slowly
- Avoiding immediate pushing after epidural placement

Episiotomy Procedure

The two types of episiotomy in current practice are midline and mediolateral (Figure 22–2). Just before birth, when approximately 3 to 4 cm (1.2 to 1.6 in.) of the fetal head is visible during a contraction, the episiotomy is performed using sharp scissors with rounded points. The *midline incision* begins at the bottom center of the perineal body and extends straight down the midline to the fibers of the rectal sphincter. The *mediolateral incision* begins in the midline of the posterior fourchette and extends at a 45-degree angle downward to the right or left. The mediolateral episiotomy is seldom used and is typically reserved for severe cases when a large incision is made

in emergent situations, such as a prolapsed umbilical cord or undiagnosed breech birth.

The episiotomy is usually performed with regional or local anesthesia but may be done without anesthesia in emergency situations. It is generally proposed that as crowning occurs, the distention of the tissues causes numbing. Repair of the episiotomy (episiorrhaphy) and any lacerations is completed either during the period between birth of the newborn and expulsion of the placenta or after expulsion of the placenta. Adequate anesthesia must be given for the repair. Many practitioners prefer to wait until the placenta has been delivered in case complications occur and manual exploration of the uterus is indicated.

Clinical Tip

Although it is no longer recommended, some practitioners continue routinely to perform episiotomy. Therefore, nurses should provide information about episiotomy and encourage women to talk to their practitioner about the incidence of its use within the practice. Encourage women who are opposed to an episiotomy to discuss their objection to the procedure with their healthcare provider at a prenatal visit before the onset of labor. Advise women that episiotomies are sometimes indicated, such as in cases of severe fetal nonreassuring status, macrosomia, instrument-assisted births, or an unresolving shoulder dystocia.

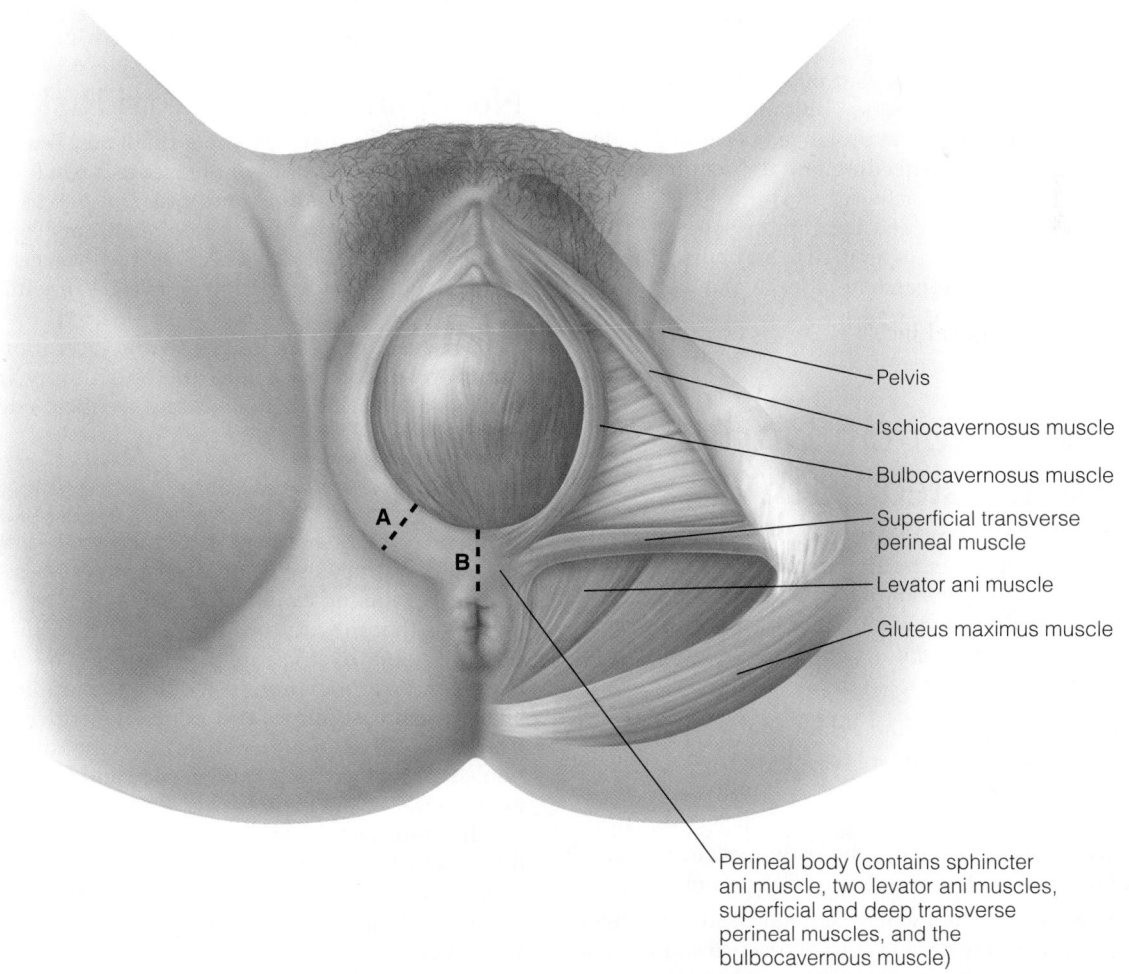

Pelvis

Ischiocavernosus muscle

Bulbocavernosus muscle

Superficial transverse perineal muscle

Levator ani muscle

Gluteus maximus muscle

Perineal body (contains sphincter ani muscle, two levator ani muscles, superficial and deep transverse perineal muscles, and the bulbocavernous muscle)

Figure 22–2 **The two common types of episiotomies are midline and mediolateral.** *A,* **Right mediolateral.** *B,* **Midline.**

Nursing Management

The woman needs to be supported during the episiotomy and the repair because she may feel some pressure or pulling or tugging sensations. If anesthesia is inadequate, she may feel pain. Placing a hand on the woman's shoulder and talking with her can provide comfort and distraction from the repair process. If the woman is having more discomfort than she can handle, act as an advocate in communicating the woman's needs to the physician/CNM. At all times, the woman needs to be the one who decides whether the amount of discomfort she is experiencing is tolerable. She should never be told, "This doesn't hurt." She is the person experiencing the discomfort, and her evaluation needs to be respected.

Record the type of episiotomy on the birth record. Include this information in a report to subsequent healthcare givers so that adequate assessments can be made and relief measures can be instituted.

Comfort measures may begin immediately after birth with the application of an ice pack to the perineum. For optimal effect, the ice pack should be applied for 20 to 30 minutes and removed for at least 20 minutes before being reapplied. Assess the perineal tissues frequently to prevent injury from the ice pack. Inspect the episiotomy site every 15 minutes during the first hour after the birth for redness, swelling, tenderness, bruising, and hematomas. To adequately assess the episiotomy site, have the woman roll onto her side with the head of the bed in the lowered position. Lift the woman's top leg and inspect the suture line carefully. Instruct the mother in postpartum care, such as perineal hygiene, self-care, and comfort measures. (See further discussion on nursing care after episiotomy in Chapter 29.)

It is important to recognize that perineal pain continues for a period of time, and it may be significant. Do not discount this pain. Women who experience prolonged perineal pain tend to have problems with breastfeeding and depression and are reluctant to reestablish sexual activity.

Nursing advocacy is needed to promote selective rather than routine episiotomy. It is imperative to stay current regarding new information and research in order to maintain current practice standards.

Care of the Woman During Forceps-Assisted Birth

Forceps are surgical instruments designed to assist in the birth of a fetus by providing either traction or the means to rotate the fetal head to an occiput-anterior position. In medical literature and practice, **forceps-assisted birth** is also known as *instrumental delivery* or *operative vaginal delivery*. Three categories of forceps application exist:

1. Outlet forceps are applied when the fetal skull has reached the perineum, the fetal scalp is visible, and the sagittal suture is not more than 45 degrees from the midline.

2. Low forceps are applied when the leading edge (presenting part) of the fetal skull is at a station of +2 or more.

3. Midforceps are applied when the fetal head is engaged. Midforceps are rarely used in clinical practice and are associated with higher adverse outcomes.

Indications for Forceps-Assisted Birth

Forceps may be indicated in the presence of any condition that threatens the mother or fetus and that can be relieved by birth. Conditions that put the woman at risk include heart disease, pulmonary edema, infection, and exhaustion. Fetal conditions include premature placental separation and nonreassuring fetal status. Forceps may be used to shorten the second stage of labor and assist the woman's pushing effort. They may also be used when regional anesthesia has affected the woman's motor innervation and she cannot push effectively.

Before forceps are used, the following conditions must be met (Cunningham et al., 2014):

- The cervix must be completely dilated and the exact position and station of the fetal head known.

- Membranes must be ruptured to allow a firm grasp on the fetal head, which must be engaged and in vertex or face presentation.

- The type of pelvis should be known because certain pelvic types do not permit rotation.

- The maternal bladder should be empty and adequate anesthesia given.

- No degree of cephalopelvic disproportion can be present.

- The operator must have the knowledge to perform the procedure.

- Maternal anesthesia is available.

- Adequate staff is available with the ability to perform a cesarean birth if indicated.

- Maternal consent has been obtained.

Neonatal and Maternal Risks

Some newborns may develop a small area of ecchymosis and/or edema along the sides of the face as a result of forceps application. Facial lacerations and brachial plexus can also occur. Caput succedaneum or cephalohematoma (with subsequent hyperbilirubinemia) may occur, as may transient facial paralysis. Although rare, cerebral hemorrhages, fractures, brain damage, and fetal death have also been reported.

Maternal risks include possible lacerations of the birth canal; extensions of a midline episiotomy into the anus; increased bleeding, bruising, and perineal edema; and anal incontinence.

Nursing Management

Using ongoing assessment, note the variables that are associated with an increased rate of instrument-assisted or operative birth. Nursing care measures can then be directed toward variables that may reduce the incidence of these factors. For example, labor dystocia may be corrected by changing maternal position, ambulation, use of breast/nipple stimulation or an electric breast pump, and frequent bladder emptying. Fetal heart rate (FHR) abnormalities may be improved by position changes, increased fluid intake, and/or adequate oxygen exchange.

If a forceps-assisted birth is required, explain the procedure briefly to the woman. With adequate regional anesthesia the woman should feel only pressure during the procedure. Ensure that adequate anesthesia is provided by alerting the physician if the woman experiences discomfort or pain. Encourage the woman to use breathing techniques that help prevent her from pushing during

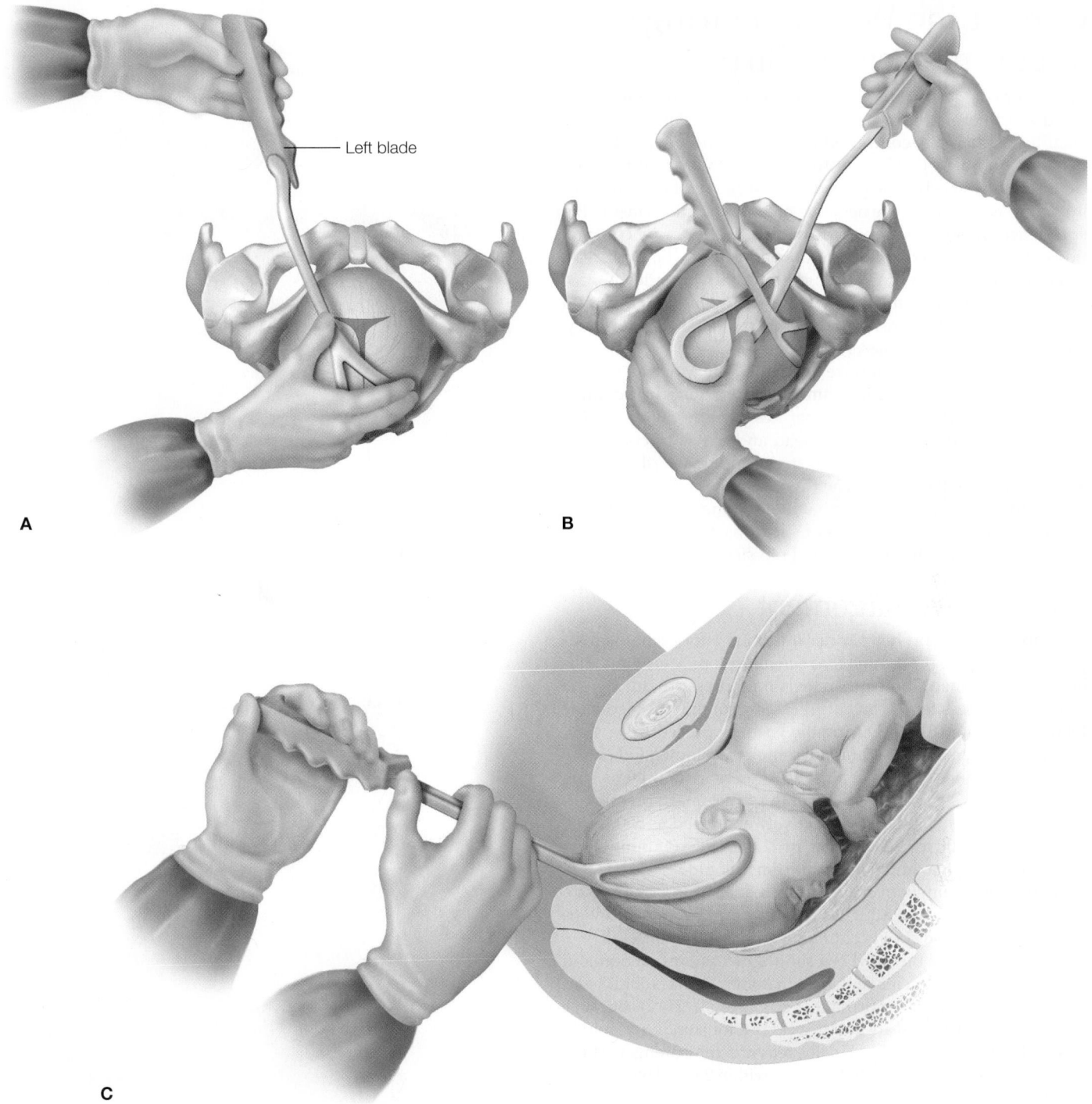

Left blade

A

B

C

Figure 22–3 Application of forceps in occiput-anterior (OA) position. *A*, The left blade is inserted along the left side wall of the pelvis over the parietal bone. *B*, The right blade is inserted along the right side wall of the pelvis over the parietal bone. *C*, With correct placement of the blades, the handles lock easily. During uterine contractions, traction is applied to the forceps in a downward and outward direction to follow the birth canal.

application of the forceps (Figure 22–3). Monitor contractions and advise the physician when one is present. With each contraction the physician provides traction on the forceps as the woman pushes. Reinforce to the woman that she needs to push while traction is being applied, explaining that the combined efforts help with expulsion of the fetus. It is not uncommon to observe mild fetal bradycardia as traction is being applied to the forceps. This bradycardia results from head compression and is transient.

Immediately following birth, assess the newborn for facial edema, bruising, caput succedaneum, cephalohematoma, and any signs of cerebral edema. In the fourth stage, assess the woman for perineal swelling, bruising, hematoma, excessive bleeding, and hemorrhage. In the postpartum period, it is important to assess for signs of infection if lacerations occurred during the procedure. Provide an opportunity for the woman to ask questions and reiterate explanations as needed.

Care of the Woman During Vacuum-Assisted Birth

Vacuum-assisted birth is an obstetric procedure used to facilitate the birth of a fetus by applying suction to the fetal head. The vacuum extractor is composed of a soft suction cup attached to a suction bottle (pump) by tubing. The suction cup, which comes in various sizes, is placed against the fetal occiput, and the pump is used to create negative pressure (suction) inside the cup. Traction is applied in coordination with uterine contractions, descent occurs, and the fetal head is born (Figure 22–4). General recommendations include that there should be progressive descent with the first two pulls and that the procedure should be limited to prevent cephalohematomas, brain injury, and fetal death (Edgar, Baskett, Young, et al., 2012).

Two types of vacuums are available. The Mityvac is used in settings where a sterile instrument is not required. The nurse typically holds the pump and operates it while the physician applies the vacuum to the fetal head and exerts traction. The Kiwi vacuum can be used in both sterile and nonsterile settings and is much smaller in size. The Kiwi vacuum is also associated with a lower incidence of cephalohematoma and caput (chignon). The availability and use of vacuums may be dependent on what the facility has in stock and physician preference.

Nursing Management

Keep the woman and her partner informed about what is happening during the procedure. If adequate regional anesthesia has been administered, the woman feels only pressure during the procedure. Assess fetal heart rate (FHR) by continuous electronic fetal monitoring (EFM). During the vacuum procedure, a slow incremental increase in vacuum pressure is recommended before applying traction, starting at a negative pressure and increasing gradually at 0.2 kg/cm² every 2 minutes to achieve a pressure of approximately 0.8 kg/cm² (alternatively expressed as 500 to 600 mmHg, 500 to 600 torr, 23.6 in Hg, or 11.6 lb/in.²) (Cunningham et al., 2014). The maximum allowable time should not exceed 8 to 10 minutes (Cunningham et al., 2014). Frequent pop-offs are associated with failure and a higher rate of complications and warrant reconsideration about continuing with the attempt.

Assessment of the newborn should include inspection and continued observation for cephalohematomas, intracerebral hemorrhage, and retinal hemorrhages (Edgar et al., 2012). Because babies born via vacuum are at increased risk for jaundice, carefully assess the baby's skin color. Finally, reassure the parents that the caput on the baby's head will disappear within 2 to 3 days.

Care of the Family During Cesarean Birth

Cesarean birth, the birth of the baby through an abdominal and uterine incision, is one of the oldest surgical procedures known. Until the 20th century, cesarean procedures were primarily used in an attempt to save the fetus of a dying woman. As the maternal and perinatal morbidity and mortality rates associated with cesarean birth steadily decreased throughout the 20th century, the proportion of cesarean births increased. Beginning in the early 1970s, the cesarean birth rate rose steadily for almost two decades. However, in 1989, in an effort to control healthcare costs, the number of cesarean births began to decline. In 2013, the rate of cesarean births performed in the United States was 32.8% (ACOG, 2013b). Canada's cesarean section rate is also at

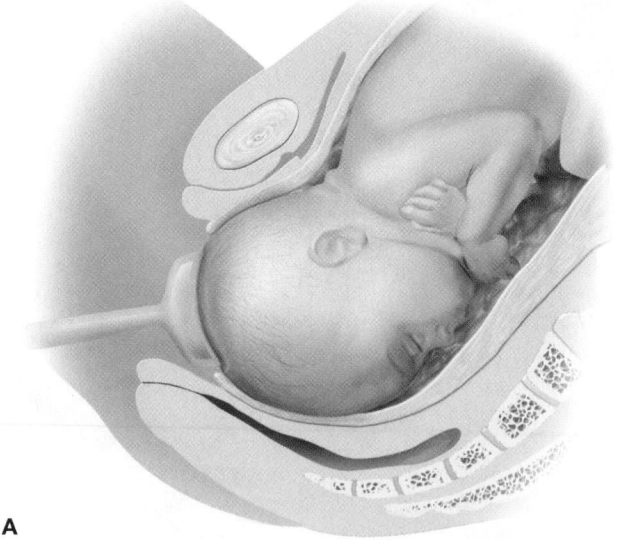

A

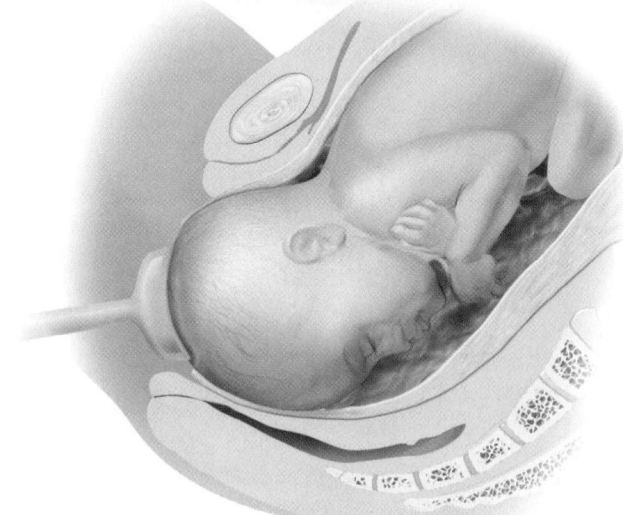

B

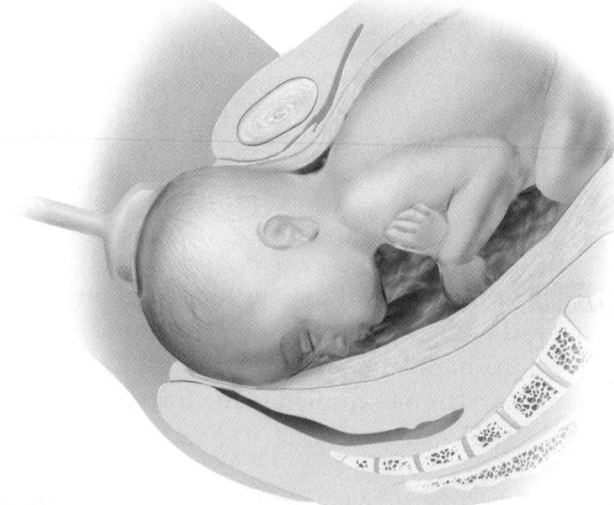

C

Figure 22–4 Vacuum extractor traction. *A*, The cup is placed on the fetal occiput, creating suction. Traction is applied in a downward and outward direction. *B*, Traction continues in a downward direction as the fetal head begins to emerge from the vagina. *C*, Traction is maintained to lift the fetal head out of the vagina.

an all-time high at 26% (Women's Health Data Directory, 2012). While cesarean births have decreased by 5% at 38 weeks, they have increased by over 4% after 39 weeks owing to changes in considerations of new term birth definitions, thus changing the data (ACOG, 2013b).

Cesarean birth rates differ dramatically around the globe. It is estimated that more than 18.5 million cesarean births are performed annually (World Health Organization [WHO], 2015). Cesarean birth is the least common in the Sub-Saharan African countries with rates averaging 0.3%. However, in these areas, many women do not have access to cesarean births, which leads to the world's highest maternal and infant morbidity (WHO, 2015). The cesarean birth rate in East Asia, the Caribbean, and Latin America continues to rise. Brazil (45.9%) and the Dominican Republic (41.9%) have the highest cesarean birth rates in the world (WHO, 2015). Other countries with cesarean rates over 30% include China, United States, Mexico, Argentina, Italy, Australia, Chile, Paraguay, Cuba, Portugal, Uruguay, Iran, and South Korea (WHO, 2015). Countries with low cesarean birth rates include Iceland (15.6%), Qatar (15.9%), Belgium (15.9%), Poland (16.1%), and Finland (16.3%) (WHO, 2015). Overall, the incidence of cesarean birth has continued to increase around the world.

The increasing rate in the United States is linked to a rise in repeat cesarean births fueled by concerns regarding the risk of uterine rupture with a vaginal birth after a previous cesarean birth. There is also an increase in requests from women for cesarean births so that they can avoid the pain of labor and vaginal birth. The trend increased further when some medical literature stated that vaginal births could result in pelvic floor damage during the birth process, although the majority of pelvic floor injuries are associated with operative vaginal births (King et al., 2013). There is also an emerging trend to "schedule" birth into busy routines to meet specific needs of the parents, such as coordinating work projects, arranging for babysitting of older children, or arranging for relatives who live in other geographic locations to travel to be present for the birth itself.

During the past few years, there has been a rise in the number of nulliparous women requesting cesarean births. This trend has led to further increases in the cesarean birth rate. Although cesarean birth on request is associated with a reduction in maternal hemorrhage risk, it is also associated with increases in neonatal respiratory problems, longer hospitalizations, and an increase in complications in subsequent pregnancies, including placental implantation problems and uterine rupture (King et al., 2013). Therefore, cesarean birth without medical indications should not be recommended for women desiring several children, for women less than 39 gestational weeks, or when pregnancy dating is unknown or may be inaccurate. It should also not be motivated by the possibility of the lack of an anesthesiologist at a later time in an institution (Posner et al., 2013). In some developing countries, such as Nigeria, cesarean by request is viewed as a guarantee that a woman will deliver a live baby and will avoid labor pains (Okonkwo, Ojengbede, Morhason-Bello, et al., 2012).

Many other factors have contributed to the rise in the cesarean birth rate and need to be considered in any discussion about decreasing the rate. These factors include an increased use of epidural anesthesia, maternal age over 35, failed inductions, decline in vaginal breech deliveries, decreases in operative vaginal deliveries, increased repeat cesarean rates, reduced vaginal birth after cesarean birth rates, increased physician scheduling of cesarean births for personal convenience, policy statements from professional organizations encouraging cesarean birth, political pressure from malpractice insurance carriers who attempt to dictate practice standards, and fear of litigation (AWHONN, 2014).

Indications for Cesarean Birth

Commonly accepted indications for cesarean birth include complete placenta previa, cephalopelvic disproportion, placental abruption, active genital herpes, umbilical cord prolapse, failure to progress in labor, nonreassuring fetal status, previous classic incision on the uterus (either previous cesarean birth or myomectomy), more than one previous cesarean birth, benign and malignant tumors that obstruct the birth canal, and cervical cerclage.

Certain maternal medical conditions are contraindications to a vaginal birth and warrant a cesarean birth. These include cardiac disorders; severe maternal respiratory disease; central nervous system disorders that increase intracranial pressure; mechanical vaginal obstruction, such as an ovarian mass or lower uterine segment fibroids; HIV infection in the mother; and severe mental illness that results in an altered state of consciousness (Society for Maternal–Fetal Medicine, 2012). Other indications that are now commonly associated with cesarean birth include breech presentation, previous cesarean birth, major congenital anomalies, and severe Rh alloimmunization. However, note that in some of these circumstances, the babies may be able to be delivered vaginally.

Maternal Mortality and Morbidity

Cesarean births have a higher maternal mortality rate than vaginal births. For every 100,000 who give birth via a successful trial of labor after cesarean (TOLAC), 4 maternal deaths will occur compared to 13 deaths that will occur as a result of an elective repeat cesarean delivery (ERCD) (National Institutes of Health Consensus Development Conference Panel, 2015). Perinatal morbidity is often associated with infection, hypertensive disorders, reaction to anesthesia, blood clots, and bleeding problems (Goldenberg, McClure, & Kamath, 2012).

In addition to the complications associated with cesarean birth, there are also risks that increase maternal mortality and morbidity in subsequent pregnancies. Women who have previously given birth via cesarean have a 0.39% risk of uterine rupture in subsequent pregnancies (Nahum, 2015). Women who have had a previous cesarean birth have an increased risk of bleeding problems, placenta previa, abruptio placentae, fetal demise, and neonatal respiratory distress. In addition, there is an increased use of oxygen administration in fetuses whose mothers have previously given birth via cesarean (Nahum, 2015).

Healthy People 2020

(MICH-7.1) Reduce cesarean births among low-risk (full-term, singleton, and vertex presentation) women

(MICH 7.2) Reduce cesarean birth among low-risk women giving birth with a prior cesarean birth

---

Skin Incisions

The skin incision for a cesarean birth is either transverse (Pfannenstiel) or vertical and is not indicative of the type of incision made into the uterus. The transverse incision (Figure 22–5) is made across the lowest and narrowest part of the abdomen. Because the incision is made just below the pubic hairline, it is almost invisible after healing. The limitation of this type of skin incision is that it does not allow for extension of the incision if needed. This incision is used when time permits (e.g., with failure to progress and stable fetal and maternal status) because it usually requires more time to make and repair.

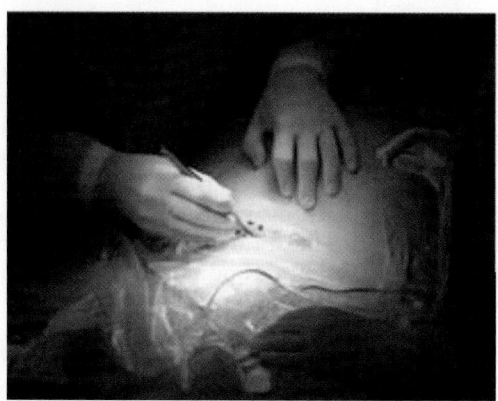

Figure 22–5 Transverse skin incision for a cesarean birth.

SOURCE: Wilson Garcia.

The vertical incision, which is rarely used in current obstetric practice, is made between the navel and the symphysis pubis. This type of incision is quicker and is therefore preferred in cases of nonreassuring fetal status when rapid birth is indicated, with preterm or macrosomic neonates, or when the woman is significantly obese (Cunningham et al., 2014). Time factors, client preference, previous vertical skin incision, or physician preference determines the type of skin incision.

Uterine Incisions

The type of uterine incision depends on the need for the cesarean birth. The choice of incision affects the woman's opportunity for a subsequent vaginal birth and her risks of a ruptured uterine scar with a subsequent pregnancy.

The two major locations of uterine incisions are in the lower uterine segment and in the upper segment of the uterine corpus. The most common lower uterine segment incision is a transverse incision (Figure 22–6). Another incision, the classic vertical incision, which is made into the upper uterine segment, was the method of choice for many years but is almost never performed in modern obstetrics. More blood loss results, and it is more difficult to repair. Most important, it carries an increased risk of uterine rupture with subsequent pregnancy, labor, and birth because the upper uterine segment is the most contractile portion of the uterus. See Table 22–3 for the advantages and disadvantages of the three types of uterine incisions.

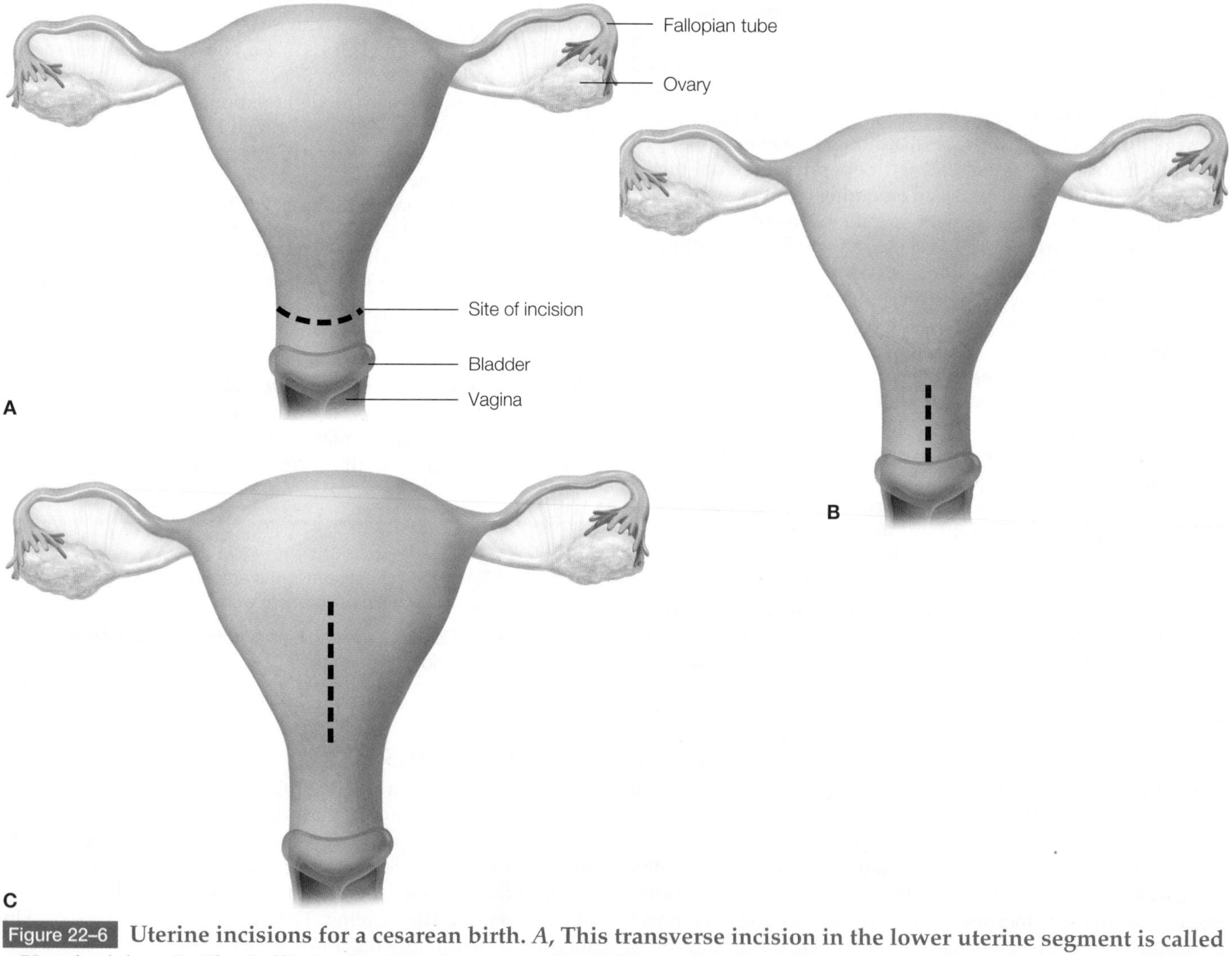

A

Fallopian tube

Ovary

Site of incision

Bladder

Vagina

B

C

Figure 22–6 Uterine incisions for a cesarean birth. *A*, This transverse incision in the lower uterine segment is called a Kerr incision. *B*, The Sellheim incision is a vertical incision in the lower uterine segment. *C*, This view illustrates the classic uterine incision that is done in the body (corpus) of the uterus. The classic incision was commonly done in the past and is associated with increased risk of uterine rupture in subsequent pregnancies and labor.

TABLE 22–3 Types of Uterine Incisions for Cesarean Birth

LOWER UTERINE SEGMENT TRANSVERSE INCISION (KERR) (MOST COMMONLY USED)

ADVANTAGES	DISADVANTAGES
Less blood loss because it is the thinnest part of the uterus	Takes longer to make a transverse incision and complete the repair
Easier to repair	Size of incision is limited because of the presence of major vessels on either side of the uterus
Requires minimal dissection of the bladder from underlying myometrium	Can extend laterally into the uterine vessels
Less chance of adherence of bowel or omentum to the incision line	Incision may stretch and become a thin sheath, causing problems in subsequent labors
Area is less likely to rupture during subsequent pregnancies	

LOWER UTERINE SEGMENT VERTICAL INCISION (SELLHEIM)

ADVANTAGES	DISADVANTAGES
Preferred for:	Incision may extend into the cervix
Multiple gestation	Extensive dissection of the bladder
Placenta previa	Controlling bleeding and closure can be difficult
Nonreassuring fetal status	Carries a high risk of rupture with subsequent labor
Abnormal presentation	Future births need to be cesarean
Preterm and macrosomic fetuses	

UPPER UTERINE SEGMENT VERTICAL INCISION (CLASSIC)

ADVANTAGES	DISADVANTAGES
None; now used infrequently	Heavy blood loss
	Difficult to repair
	Increased risk of uterine rupture with subsequent pregnancy

Source: Data from Cunningham, F. G., Leveno, K. J., Bloom, S. L., Spong, C.Y., Dashe, J. S., Hoffman, B. L., . . . Sheffield, J. S. (2014). *Williams obstetrics* (24th ed.). NewYork, NY: McGraw-Hill Medical.

Developing Cultural Competence Translating Operative Reports

Women from other countries who have had a previous cesarean birth typically have a vertical skin incision; however, the skin incision does not provide data on the type of uterine incision that was performed. Obtain an operative report if possible. Operative reports in other languages need to be translated by personnel familiar with medical terminology. If an operative report cannot be obtained, which is common, provide the woman with a thorough explanation regarding the need for a repeat cesarean.

Analgesia and Anesthesia

There is no perfect anesthesia for cesarean birth. Each has its advantages, disadvantages, possible risks, and side effects. Goals for analgesia and anesthesia administration include safety, comfort, and emotional satisfaction for the client. (For a discussion of analgesia and anesthesia, see Chapter 19.) In contemporary practice, the use of epidurals or spinal anesthesia has increased to the point that they are almost exclusively used during cesarean birth. General anesthesia is rarely used and is associated with increased maternal and neonatal complications.

Women With Special Needs Dwarfism in Childbearing Women

There are over 200 types of dwarfism that may impact childbearing women. Women with dwarfism are at risk for alterations in ambulation as the center of gravity changes. In addition, owing to their pelvic bone anatomy, these women are unable to have a vaginal birth. Women with dwarfism should be scheduled for an elective cesarean birth at 39 gestational weeks. Should spontaneous labor occur prior to the surgery date, they should be advised to proceed directly to the birthing facility for a cesarean birth.

Nursing Management

For the Woman Having a Cesarean Birth

Preparation for Cesarean Birth

Because one of every four births is a cesarean, preparation for this possibility should be an integral part of all prenatal education. Pregnant women and their partners should be encouraged to discuss the possibility of a cesarean birth with their physicians/CNMs and at the same time discuss their specific needs and desires under those circumstances. Their preferences may include the following:

- Participating in the choice of anesthetic
- Father or partner being present during the procedures and/or birth
- Father or partner being present in the recovery or postpartum room
- Video recording and/or taking pictures of the birth as allowed by facility (many facilities now forbid video recording)
- Delayed instillation of eye drops to promote eye contact between parent and newborn in the first hours after birth
- Physical contact or holding the newborn while in the operating and/or recovery room (by the father/partner if the mother cannot hold the baby)
- Breastfeeding in the recovery area within the first hour of birth

Information that couples need about cesarean birth includes the following:

- What preparatory procedures to expect
- Description or viewing of the birthing room
- Types of anesthesia for birth and analgesia available postpartum
- Sensations that may be experienced
- Roles of significant others

- Interaction with newborn
- Immediate recovery phase
- Postpartum phase

Preparing the woman and her family for birth involves more than the procedures of establishing an intravenous line, instilling a urinary indwelling catheter, and performing an abdominal prep. As discussed previously, good communication skills are essential for preparing the woman and her support person. Use therapeutic touch and direct eye contact (if culturally acceptable and possible) to assist the woman in maintaining a sense of control and to lessen anxiety.

If the cesarean birth is scheduled and not an emergency, there is ample time for preoperative teaching. Relay this information in a birth-oriented rather than surgery-oriented context. This provides an opportunity for the woman to express her concerns, ask questions, and develop a relationship with you.

In preparation for surgery, the woman is given nothing by mouth. To reduce the likelihood of serious pulmonary damage if gastric contents are aspirated, antacids may be administered within 30 minutes of surgery. If epidural anesthesia is used, you may assist with the procedure, monitor the woman's blood pressure and response, and continue electronic fetal monitoring (EFM). Perform an abdominal and perineal prep, insert an indwelling catheter to prevent bladder distention, and start an intravenous line with a large-bore needle to permit blood administration if it becomes necessary. Order preoperative medication, notify the pediatrician, and prepare to receive the new baby. Ensure that the radiant warmer is working and that resuscitation equipment is available.

Clinical Tip

Women undergoing elective cesarean birth can be taught many aspects of postoperative teaching before their birth experience. Important components of client education that can be emphasized before birth include dealing with postoperative discomfort, splinting the incision to decrease pain, frequent deep breathing and coughing, and the importance of early ambulation. Women who receive this information before the birth are more apt to remember it when it is reviewed in the early postpartum period.

Assist in positioning the woman on the operating table. Fetal heart rate (FHR) is assessed before surgery and during preparation because fetal hypoxia can result from the supine position. The operating room table is adjusted so it slants slightly to one side or a hip wedge (folded blanket or towels) is placed under the woman's right hip to tip the uterus slightly and reduce compression of blood vessels. The uterus should be displaced 15 degrees from the midline. This helps relieve the pressure of the heavy uterus on the vena cava and lessens the incidence of vena cava compression and maternal supine hypotension. The suction should be in working order and the urine collection bag should be positioned under the operating table to obtain proper drainage. Auscultation or EFM of the fetal heart rate is continued until immediately before the procedure. A last-minute check is done to ensure that the fetal scalp electrode has been removed if the fetus was internally monitored.

Continue to provide reassurance and describe the various procedures being performed along with their rationales to ease anxiety and give the woman a sense of control.

Preparation for Elective Birth After Cesarean Birth

When a couple is anticipating an elective birth after cesarean (EBAC), they have a general understanding of what will occur, which can help them make informed choices about their birth experience. Couples who have had previous negative experiences need an opportunity to describe what they felt. Encourage them to identify what they would like to do differently and to list options that would make the experience more positive. Those who have already had positive experiences need reassurance that their needs and desires will be met in a similar manner and should be allowed to discuss any fears or anxieties. For women who previously labored and then had an unexpected cesarean birth, the experience may be perceived as negative. Positive aspects that can be emphasized include participation in selecting the birth date, lack of fatigue related to labor, ability to prepare and make arrangements for other children, and ability of other family members or friends to be present at the hospital during or immediately after birth if desired by the couple.

Preparation for Emergency Cesarean Birth

When the need for a cesarean birth emerges suddenly, the period preceding surgery must be used to its greatest advantage. It is imperative that healthcare givers use their most effective communication skills in supporting the couple. Describe what the couple may anticipate during the next few hours. Asking the couple, "What questions or concerns do you have about the decision?" gives them an opportunity for clarification. Prepare the woman in stages, giving her information and the rationales for interventions before beginning any procedure. It is essential to tell the woman (1) what is going to happen, (2) why it is being done, and (3) what sensations she may experience. This allows the woman to be informed and to consent to the procedure, which gives her a sense of control and reduces her feelings of helplessness.

Supporting the Father or Partner

Every effort should be made to include the father or partner in the birth experience. When attending the cesarean birth, the father/partner wears protective coverings similar to those worn by others in the operating suite. A stool can be placed beside the woman's head so that he or she can sit nearby to provide physical touch, visual contact, and verbal reassurance.

To promote the participation of the father/partner who chooses not to be in the operating suite, you can do the following:

1. Allow the father/partner to be nearby, where he can hear the newborn's first cry.
2. Allow the father/partner to hold the newborn near the head of the mother to facilitate early parental bonding.
3. Encourage the father/partner to carry or accompany the newborn to the nursery for the initial assessment.
4. Involve the father/partner in postpartum care in the recovery room.

Some facilities have policies that prohibit a support person from being in the operating room if the woman requires general anesthesia or if an emergency birth is being performed. In these situations, the support person should receive a thorough explanation of what is happening and why, be advised when the staff will return to provide information, know the expected length of time for the procedure, and be reassured that the mother is receiving the care she and the baby need. Because this exclusion is stressful for family members, staff should try to provide information as soon as possible after providing emergency care to the mother. Having another staff member check in on the family and provide updates and reassurance often helps decrease the family's anxiety.

Immediate Postnatal Recovery Period

After birth assess the Apgar score and complete the same initial assessment and identification procedures used for vaginal births. Identification bands must be placed on the newborn and the mother (as well as the father or support person, if present) before removing the baby from the operating room. Every effort should be made to assist the parents in bonding with their newborn. If the mother is awake, one of her arms can be freed to enable her to touch and stroke the baby. The newborn may be placed on the mother's chest or held in an en face position. If physical contact is not possible, provide a running narrative so the mother knows what is happening with her baby. Assist the anesthesiologist or nurse anesthetist with raising the mother's head so she can see her baby immediately after birth. The parents can be encouraged to talk to the baby, and the father can hold the baby until she or he is taken to the nursery.

Assess the mother's vital signs every 5 minutes until they are stable, then every 15 minutes for 2 hours, then every 4 hours until she is discharged to the postpartum unit. Remain with the woman until she is stable.

Evaluate the dressing and perineal pad every 15 minutes for at least an hour. The fundus should be gently palpated to determine whether it is remaining firm; it may be palpated by placing a hand to support the incision. Intravenous oxytocin (Pitocin) is usually administered to promote the contractility of the uterine musculature. If the woman has been under general anesthesia, she should be positioned on her side to facilitate drainage of secretions, turned, and assisted with coughing and deep breathing every 2 hours for at least 24 hours. If she has received a spinal or epidural anesthetic, the level of anesthesia is checked every 15 minutes until full sensation has returned. It is important to monitor intake and output and to observe the urine for a bloody tinge, which could mean surgical trauma to the bladder. The physician prescribes medication to relieve the mother's pain and nausea, and it is administered as needed.

Clinical Tip

Promote bonding by allowing the mother to hold or nurse the newborn during this time period. If the baby has been moved to a separate area, such as the nursery, encourage maternal participation by allowing the support person to visit the baby and report back to the mother. The support person can take digital pictures or bring back the blanket that was used to wrap up the baby immediately after the birth. Offering frequent updates, such as, "Your baby's doing just fine," provide reassurance to the mother if separation is needed.

Care of the Woman Undergoing Trial of Labor After Cesarean (TOLAC) and Vaginal Birth After Cesarean (VBAC)

In the late 1990s, there was an increasing trend to have a trial of labor and attempt **vaginal birth after cesarean (VBAC)**, now also known as a **trial of labor after cesarean (TOLAC)**, in cases of nonrecurring indications for a cesarean (such as umbilical cord prolapse, breech, placenta previa, or nonreassuring fetal status). This trend was influenced by consumer demand and studies that supported VBAC as a viable alternative to repeat cesarean.

In current practice, TOLAC should be performed in facilities where there is immediate access to perform an emergency cesarean birth if medically indicated. This requires in-house anesthesia and in-house, round-the-clock obstetric services. In facilities that cannot meet these criteria, the availability of TOLAC may be limited and require women who desire a TOLAC to travel to larger hospital facilities.

Between 1970 and 2007, media reports identifying risks of VBAC introduced extensive debate regarding its safety. At the same time, trends in counseling women to have an elective repeat cesarean birth are driving cesarean births to an all-time high in the United States. Although TOLAC is associated with a higher risk of uterine rupture, the overall maternal mortality rates are higher for women undergoing an elective repeat cesarean delivery (ERCD), which prompted revision of protocols to determine which groups of women could safely have a TOLAC.

The ACOG (2013b) guidelines update states that the following aspects are encouraging when considering a TOLAC:

- A woman with one or two previous cesarean births and a low transverse uterine incision
- A clinically adequate pelvis based on clinical pelvimetry or prior vaginal birth
- A woman with one previous cesarean birth with an undocumented uterine scar unless there is a high suspicion there was a classic incision performed previously
- Absence of other uterine scars or history of previous uterine rupture

The most common risks associated with failed TOLAC births are maternal hemorrhage, infection, operative injury, thromboembolism, hysterectomy, and death (ACOG, 2013b). Complications associated with uterine rupture include hemorrhage, uterine scar separation or uterine rupture, hysterectomy, surgical injuries, neonatal death, and neurologic complications (see Chapter 20). The incidence of uterine rupture is 0.5% to 0.9% of all trials of labors when the mother has had a previous cesarean birth. The incidence of uterine rupture is directly correlated with the type of uterine incision the woman has obtained in a previous birth. Low transverse incisions have the lowest risk, whereas classic and vertical incisions carry a higher risk of uterine rupture (ACOG, 2013b). Women who go into spontaneous labor have a much lower incidence of uterine rupture (0.4%) compared with women who undergo oxytocin (Pitocin) induction (0.9% to 1.1%) (ACOG, 2013b). Prostaglandin agents should not be used in women attempting a TOLAC because of the increased risk of uterine rupture. The incidence of uterine rupture in women who receive a prostaglandin agent is as high as 1.4 per 100 (ACOG, 2013b).

Conservative policies, such as awaiting spontaneous labor, avoiding prostaglandin agents, and avoiding elective inductions, can assist in reducing the incidence of uterine rupture. Women with an unfavorable cervix who are in need of an induction for medical indications may be treated with a transcervical catheter to initiate mechanical dilatation; however, research findings are inconsistent, with one study finding a slightly higher incidence of uterine rupture compared to spontaneous labor (ACOG, 2013b).

Women who have a successful TOLAC have lower incidences of infection, less blood loss, fewer blood transfusions, and shorter hospital stays. Healthcare costs are considerably lower for women who have a TOLAC than for those who have a repeat cesarean birth (ACOG, 2013b). After a woman had one successful VBAC, the risks of neonatal and maternal complications were low in subsequent attempts. In general, 60% to 80% of women who undergo a TOLAC have a successful VBAC.

Research shows a close correlation between maternal weight and success for TOLAC (ACOG, 2013c). In one study that examined obese and morbidly obese women, the TOLAC success rate was only 2.3%, although the neonatal death rate rose significantly as a mother's body mass index (BMI) rose (Belogolovkin et al., 2012). Although ACOG does not provide specific guidelines on obesity as a contraindication to TOLAC, all factors should be presented to the woman so she can make an informed choice related to her intended birth options. Women with a BMI more than 30 should receive an anesthesia consult upon admission to the labor and delivery unit.

Nursing Management

The nursing care of a woman undergoing TOLAC varies according to institutional protocols. Generally, a saline lock is inserted for IV access if needed or an intravenous infusion of fluids is started, continuous electronic fetal monitoring (EFM) is used, and clear fluids may be taken. A woman at higher risk may require additional precautionary measures, such as internal monitoring after the membranes have ruptured. Take care to ensure that the woman and her partner feel safe but not unduly restricted by the TOLAC status. When available, telemetry monitors can be utilized so mothers can ambulate within the hallways and take tub baths and showers.

Supportive and comfort measures are very important. The woman may be excited about this opportunity to experience labor and vaginal birth, or she may be hesitant and frightened about the possibility of complications. The presence of the nurse is important in providing information and encouragement for the laboring woman and her partner.

Focus Your Study

- External cephalic versions are done after 36 weeks to change a nonvertex presentation to a vertex presentation. External pressure is applied to the maternal abdomen to facilitate a change in presentation when the fetal part is not engaged.

- A non-stress test (NST) should be performed prior to an external cephalic version (ECV), and tocolytics medications should be administered to promote uterine relaxation.

- Podalic versions are performed to turn a second twin into the correct position for a vaginal birth when the twin does not descend spontaneously or when nonreassuring fetal heart tones are present.

- An amniotomy (artificial rupture of the amniotic membranes) is performed to induce or augment labor or when internal monitoring is required for the mother or fetus. After an amniotomy is performed, it is important to check the FHR, color of the amniotic fluid, and presence of any odor. Complications may include infection and umbilical cord prolapse.

- Induction of labor occurs when a medical complication results in the need for birth to occur or when postdates occur. Means of labor induction include cervical ripening agents, stripping the membranes manually, mechanical dilatation, and oxytocin (Pitocin) infusion. The administration of pharmacologic intervention increases the risk of tachysystole and nonreassuring fetal status.

- The routine use of episiotomies is now contraindicated in contemporary obstetric practice. Episiotomies may be either midline or medilateral. Prevention of episiotomy includes natural pushing, side-lying position; avoidance of the lithotomy position or pulling back on legs, and avoiding immediate pushing

after epidural placement. Encouraging a gradual expulsion of the neonate by doing controlled breathing pattern during second stage also reduces the incidence of episiotomies and lacerations.

- After birth, an ice pack should be placed on the perineum. Nursing management includes frequent inspection and teaching the new mother proper perineal hygiene measures.

- Forceps birth is indicated to shorten the second stage of labor due to maternal exhaustion, presence of nonreassuring fetal status, premature separation of the placenta, and certain medical conditions, when pushing is contraindicated, such as certain cardiac conditions.

- The use of forceps may be associated with newborn bruising, facial edema, facial lacerations, cephalohematoma, and transient facial paralysis, and with maternal vaginal lacerations, increased bleeding, bruising, and perineal edema.

- Vacuum extraction births can be associated with perineal lacerations, fetal jaundice, and cephalohematoma.

- Indications for cesarean birth include nonreassuring fetal status, lack of labor progression, maternal infection, pelvic size disproportion, placenta previa, maternal complications, and elective repeat cesarean birth. Nursing care should include preoperative teaching, and postoperative care including fundal checks, incision care, intake and output monitoring, assessment of bowel and bladder functioning, and pain management.

- Trial of labor after cesarean is considered a safe alternative for most women. Maternal and fetal risk factors should be evaluated prior to a TOLAC and immediate cesarean birth facilities should be available. TOLAC requires certain criteria be met to ensure maternal and fetal safety.

Clinical Reasoning in Action

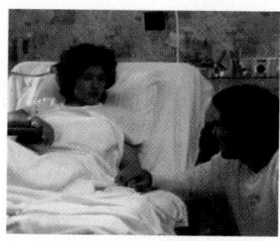

Betsy Jones, a 28-year-old G1P0 at 39 weeks' gestation, and her husband present to you in the labor suite for an external cephalic version procedure by her obstetrician. You introduce yourself and review her prenatal record for any significant risk factors or contraindications to the version procedure. Her prenatal record is significant in that the fetus has been in a persistent frank breech position. You encourage Betsy and her husband to express their understanding and expectations of the procedure. You discuss certain criteria to be met prior to the procedure and obtain vital signs as follows: T 98.8°F, P 88, R 14, BP 110/80,

urine screening negative for sugar, albumin, and ketones. You place Betsy on the external electronic fetal monitor, which demonstrates a fetal heart rate baseline of 140 to 152 with long-term variability. There are no contractions observed by the monitor or Betsy. After explaining how to record fetal movement on the monitor, you proceed with an NST.

1. Explain the contraindications to the version procedure.
2. Discuss the criteria that should be met prior to performing external version.
3. How would you explain to Betsy and her husband what to expect during the version procedure?
4. What support would you give Betsy during the procedure?
5. Explain postversion discharge teaching.

References

American College of Obstetricians and Gynecologists (ACOG). (2013a). *Induction of labor* (ACOG Practice Bulletin No. 107). Washington, DC: Author.

American College of Obstetricians and Gynecologists (ACOG). (2013b). *Vaginal birth after previous cesarean delivery* (Practice Bulletin No. 115). Washington, DC: Author.

American College of Obstetricians and Gynecologists (ACOG). (2013c). *Obesity in pregnancy* (Committee Opinion No. 549). Washington, DC: Author.

American College of Obstetricians and Gynecologists (ACOG). (2014). *External cephalic version.* (ACOG Practice Bulletin No. 13). Washington, DC: Author.

Association of Women's Health, Obstetric, & Neonatal Nurses. (AWHONN). (2013). AWHONN Position Statement: Non-medically indicated induction and augmentation of labor. *Journal of Obstetric, Gynecologic & Neonatal Nursing, 43*(5), 678–681. doi:10.1111/1552-6909.12499

Association of Women's Health, Obstetrical, and Neonatal Nurses. (AWHONN). (2014). AWWHONN recommends reducing preventable harm to moms and babies by eliminating overuse of labor induction. News Release: September 23, 2014. Retrieved from https://www.awhonn.org/awhonn/content.do?name=07_PressRoom/7B7_Sept23-Labor-Induction-Overuse.htm

Association of Women's Health, Obstetric, & Neonatal Nurses. (AWHONN). (2015). AWHONN Position Statement: Breastfeeding. *Journal of Obstetric, Gynecologic & Neonatal Nursing, 44*(1), 145–150. doi:10.1111/1552-6909.12530

Belogolovkin, V., Crisan, L., Lynch, O., Weldeselasse, H., August, E. M., Alio, A. P., & Salihu, H. M. (2012). Neonatal outcomes of successful VBAC among obese and super-obese mothers. *Journal of Maternal–Fetal and Neonatal Medicine, 25*(6), 714–718. doi:10.3109/14767058.2011.596594

Bishop, E. H. (1964). Pelvic scoring for elective inductions. *Obstetrics and Gynecology, 24*, 266.

Cunningham, F. G., Leveno, K. J., Bloom, S. L., Spong, C. Y., Dashe, J. S., Hoffman, B. L., … Sheffield, J. S.

(2014). *Williams obstetrics* (24th ed.). New York, NY: McGraw-Hill.

Davidson, M. R. (2013). *Fast facts for the antepartum and postpartum nurse: An orientation in a nut shell.* New York, NY: Springer.

Edgar, D. C., Baskett, T. F., Young, D. C., & O'Connell, T. M. (2012). Neonatal outcome following failed Kiwi OmniCup vacuum extraction. *Journal of Obstetrics & Gynaecology in Canada, 34*(7), 620–625.

Forrest Pharmaceuticals. (2015). *Cervidil dinoprostone 10 mg vaginal insert.* St. Louis, MO: Author.

Gagnon-Gervais, K., Bujold, E., Iglesias, M., Duperron, L., Masse, A., Mayrand, M., … Audibert, F. (2012). Early versus late amniotomy for labour induction: A randomized controlled trial. *Journal of Maternal–Fetal and Neonatal Medicine, 25*(11), 2326–2329. doi:10.3109/14767058.2012.695819

Goldenberg, R. L., McClure, E. M., & Kamath, B. D. (2012). Intrapartum perinatal mortality. *Indian Pediatrics, 49*(3), 187–190. doi:10.1007/s13312-012-0050-4

King, T. L., Brucker, M. C, Kriebs, J. M., & Fahey, J.O. (2013). *Varney's midwifery* (5th ed.). New York, NY: Jones & Bartlett Learning.

Lurie, S., Kedar, D., Boaz, M., Golan, A., & Sadan, O. (2012). Need for episiotomy in a subsequent delivery following previous delivery with episiotomy. *Archives of Gynecology and Obstetrics.* doi:10.1007/s00404-012-2551-8

Lutgendorf, M. A., Johnson, A., Terpstra, E. R., Snider, T. C., & Magann, E. F. (2012). Extra-amniotic balloon for preinduction cervical ripening: a randomized comparison of weighted traction versus unweighted. *Journal of Maternal–Fetal and Neonatal Medicine, 25*(6), 581–586. doi:10.3109/14767058.2011.587063

Nahum, G. G. (2015). *Uterine rupture in pregnancy.* Retrieved from http://reference.medscape.com/article/275854-overview#aw2aab6b5

National Institutes of Health Consensus Development Conference Panel. (2015). National Institutes of Health Consensus Development conference state-

ment: Vaginal birth after cesarean: *Obstetrics & Gynecology, 115*(6), 1279.

Okonkwo, N. S., Ojengbede, O. A., Morhason-Bello, I. O., & Adedokun, B. O. (2012). Maternal demand for cesarean section: Perception and willingness to request by Nigerian antenatal clients. *International Journal of Women's Health, 4*, 141–148. doi:10.2147/IJWH.S10325

Posner, G., Black, A., & Jones, G. (2013). *Oxorn-Foote labor and birth* (6th ed.). Philadelphia, PA: McGraw-Hill.

Rakel, D. (2012). *Integrative medicine* (3rd ed.). Philadelphia, PA: Elsevier.

Rosman, A. N., Vlemmix, F., Beuckens, A., Rijnders, M. E., Opmeer, B. C., Mol, B. W. J., … Fleuren, M. A. (2014). Facilitators and barriers to external cephalic version for breech presentation at term among health care providers in the Netherlands: a quantitative analysis. *Midwifery, 30*(3), e145–e150.

Selin, H. (2012). *Childbirth across cultures: Ideas and practices of pregnancy, childbirth and the postpartum.* Rotterdam, Netherlands: Springer.

Society for Maternal–Fetal Medicine. (2012). *High-risk pregnancy care, research, and education for over 35 years.* Retrieved from https://www.smfm.org/attachedfiles/SMFMMonograph3.1.pdf

Stephenson, M. L., Hawkins, J. S., Powers, B. L., & Wing, D. A. (2014). Misoprostol vaginal insert for induction of labor: A delivery system with accurate dosing and rapid discontinuation. *Women's Health, 10*(1), 29–36. doi:10.2217/whe.13.49

Wilson, B. A., Shannon, M. T., & Shields, K. M. (Eds.). (2015). *Nursing drug guide: 2016.* Upper Saddle River, NJ: Pearson.

Women's Health Data Directory. (2012). *Cesarean section.* Retrieved from http://www.womenshealthdata.ca/category.aspx?catid=108&rt=3

World Health Organization (WHO). (2015). *The global numbers and costs of additionally needed and unnecessary caesarean sections performed per year: Overuse as a barrier to universal coverage* (World Health Report, Background Paper No. 30). Retrieved from http://www.who.int/healthsystems/topics/financing/healthreport/30C-sectioncosts.pdf

Chapter 23

The Physiologic Responses of the Newborn to Birth

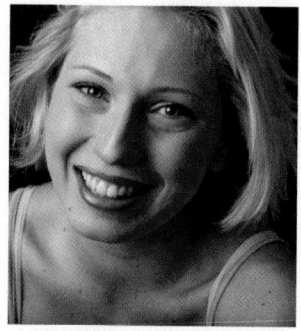

I remember clearly when they held him up for us to see and my husband and I cried and laughed and it was so amazing. He was 9 1/2 pounds and was so beautiful. Even though my labor was long, his Apgars were good.

—Crystal, 26

Scott T. Baxter/Getty Images

⌄ Learning Outcomes

23.1 Summarize the cardiopulmonary changes that must occur for the newborn to successfully transition to extrauterine life.

23.2 Identify the differences in fetal and adult hemoglobin and why this is important in the transition to extrauterine life.

23.3 Relate the process of thermogenesis in the newborn and the major mechanisms of heat loss to the challenge of maintaining newborn thermal stability.

23.4 Identify the reasons a newborn may develop jaundice and nursing interventions to decrease the probability of jaundice.

23.5 Delineate the functional abilities of the newborn's gastrointestinal tract and liver.

23.6 Relate the development of the newborn's kidneys to the newborn's ability to maintain fluid and electrolyte balance.

23.7 Describe basic newborn immunologic responses.

23.8 Explain the physiologic and behavioral characteristics of newborn neurologic function, patterns of behavior during the periods of reactivity, and possible nursing interventions.

23.9 Describe the normal sensory-perceptual abilities and behavioral states seen in the newborn period and the associated nursing care.

The newborn period is the time from birth through the 28th day of life. During this period, the newborn adjusts from intrauterine to extrauterine life. This transition from fetus to newborn is the most complex physiologic adaptation that occurs in the human experience and involves virtually every organ system of the body (Graves & Haley, 2013). The nurse needs to be knowledgeable about a newborn's normal physiologic and behavioral adaptations and to recognize alterations from normal. The first 6 hours of life, in which the newborn stabilizes respiratory and circulatory functions, are called **neonatal transition**.

Respiratory Adaptations

To begin life as a separate being, the baby must immediately establish respiratory functioning and ventilation. Adequate gas exchange in conjunction with marked circulatory changes are radical and rapid changes crucial to successful transition to extrauterine life.

Fetal Lung Development

The respiratory system is in an ongoing state of development during fetal life, and lung development continues into early childhood. During the first 20 weeks' gestation, development is limited to the differentiation of pulmonary, vascular, and lymphatic structures. From 20 to 24 weeks, alveolar ducts begin to appear, followed by primitive alveoli at 24 to 28 weeks. During this time, the alveolar epithelial cells begin to differentiate into type I cells (structures necessary for gas exchange) and type II cells (structures that provide for the synthesis and storage of surfactant).

Surfactant, a lipoprotein that coats the inner surfaces of the alveoli, is composed of surface-active phospholipids (lecithin and sphingomyelin), which are critical for alveolar stability.

At 28 to 32 weeks of gestation, the number of type II cells increases, and surfactant is produced within them. Surfactant production peaks at about 35 weeks of gestation and remains high until term, paralleling late fetal lung development. At this time, the lungs are structurally developed enough to maintain good lung expansion and adequate exchange of gases at birth. The newborn born before the lecithin/sphingomyelin (L/S) ratio is 2:1 will have varying degrees of respiratory distress. (See discussion of L/S ratio and respiratory distress syndrome in Chapter 27.)

During intrauterine development, the lungs are filled with fetal lung fluid produced by the pulmonary epithelium, which stretches the lung tissue and stimulates growth of alveoli. Production and maintenance of a normal volume of fetal lung fluid are essential for normal lung growth (Fraser, 2014). Through intermittent fetal breathing movements, the fetus practices respiration, develops the chest wall muscles and the diaphragm, as well as regulates lung fluid volume.

Fetal Circulation

In utero, the placenta is the organ of gas exchange. The low vascular resistance of the placenta and the high vascular resistance of the fluid-filled lungs result in shunts characteristic of fetal circulation. From the placenta, highly oxygenated blood (oxygen saturation of 65% to 70%) flows through the umbilical vein. A small amount of blood perfuses the liver, with the majority of blood volume flowing through the inferior vena cava and to the right atrium. Because of intracardiac streaming, blood is preferentially directed from the right atrium across the **foramen ovale (FO)** (an opening in the septum between the atria) into the left atrium, the left ventricle, and the ascending aorta (Fraser, 2014). This results in better oxygenated fetal blood directed to the myocardium and fetal brain.

A smaller volume of blood enters the right ventricle and is pumped through the pulmonary artery. Because pulmonary vascular resistance is very high due to the fluid-filled fetal lungs, more than 60% of right ventricular output bypasses the lung and flows through the **ductus arteriosus (DA)** (a tubular connection between the pulmonary artery and descending aorta) into the descending aorta (Fraser, 2014). This mixing of well-oxygenated and poorly oxygenated blood results in an

TABLE 23–1 Fetal and Neonatal Circulation

SYSTEM	FETAL	NEONATAL
Pulmonary blood vessels	Constricted, with very little blood flow; lungs not expanded	Vasodilation and increased blood flow; lungs expanded; increased oxygen stimulates vasodilation.
Systemic blood vessels	Dilated, with low resistance; blood mostly in placenta	Arterial pressure rises because of loss of placenta; increased systemic blood volume and resistance.
Ductus arteriosus	Large, with no tone; blood flow from pulmonary artery to aorta	Reversal of blood flow; now from aorta to pulmonary artery because of increased left atrial pressure. Ductus is sensitive to increased oxygen and body chemicals and begins to constrict.
Foramen ovale	Patent, with increased blood flow from right atrium to left atrium	Increased pressure in left atrium attempts to reverse blood flow and shuts one-way valve.

oxygen saturation of 45% in the blood that perfuses the lower part of the body. Vascular resistance of the placenta is low; approximately 50% of the combined ventricular cardiac output flows through the umbilical arteries to the placenta, where it releases carbon dioxide and waste products and collects oxygen and nutrients (Graves & Haley, 2013). Therefore, in fetal circulation, the right and left ventricles function together, in parallel, rather than sequentially (one after the other), to perfuse the fetal body and the placenta. See Table 23–1.

Cardiopulmonary Adaptation

Marked changes occur in the cardiopulmonary system at birth. During late gestation, lung fluid secretion decreases. The onset of labor stimulates the production of catecholamines and other hormones, causing fetal pulmonary epithelial cells to begin reabsorption of fluid from the alveolar spaces (Fraser, 2014). With birth, the change in the sensory environment from the warm, dark womb to the brightly lighted, cold delivery room is an important stimulus for the initiation of breathing (Van Woudenberg, Wills, & Rubarth, 2012). The cold stimulates skin sensory receptors, and the newborn responds with rhythmic respirations. A number of physical and sensory influences help to sustain respiration after birth. They include the numerous tactile, auditory, visual, and painful stimuli of birth and the normal handling after delivery. Joint movement results in enhanced proprioceptor stimulation to the respiratory center. Thoroughly drying and then placing the baby in skin-to-skin contact with the mother provides stimulation in a comforting way, as well as decreases heat loss.

The neonate's first breaths of air initiate a sequence of events that empties the airways of fluid, establishes volume and function of the newborn's lungs, and causes fetal circulation to convert to neonatal circulation. The initial first breaths generate

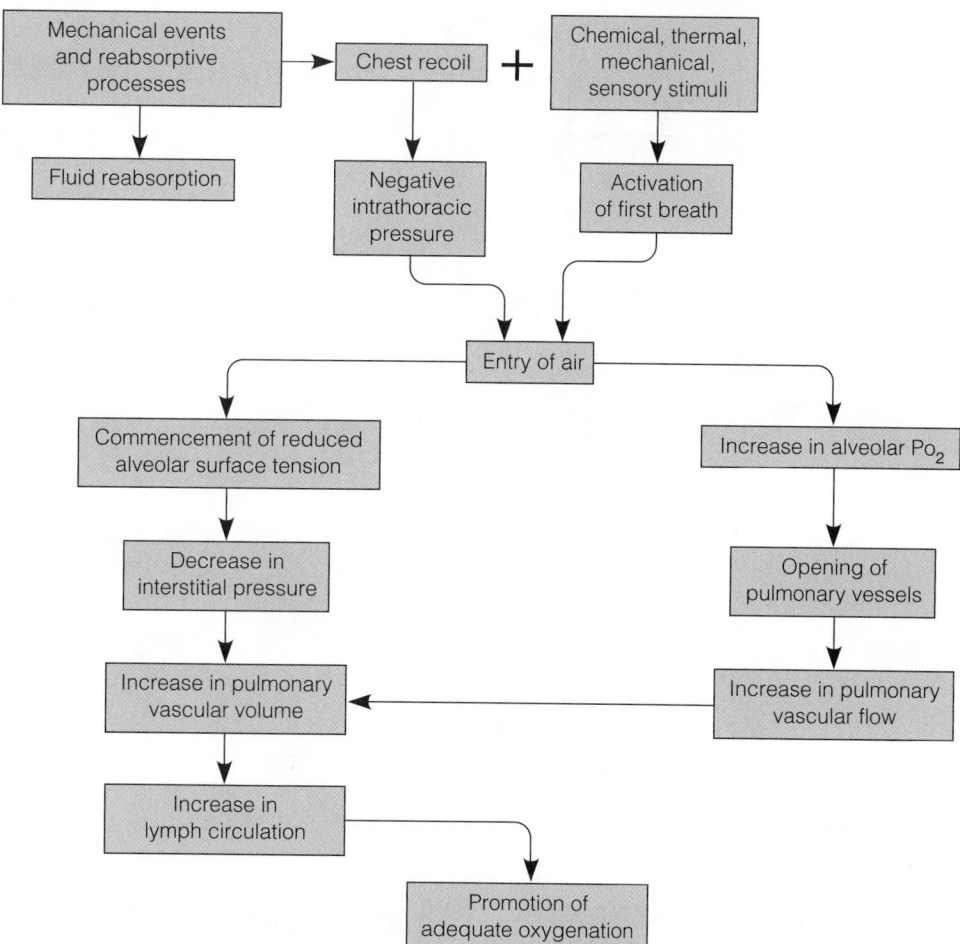

Figure 23–1 Initiation of respiration in the newborn.

a high negative pressure, driving fluid from the lungs and filling the alveoli with air. As the lungs expand and are exposed to higher concentrations of oxygen (room air), pulmonary vascular resistance falls, causing pulmonary vasodilation and increased blood flow to the lungs. Figure 23–1 summarizes the initiation of respiration.

When the umbilical cord is clamped, the low-resistance placenta is excluded from circulation; cessation of blood flow through the umbilical vein facilitates collapse of the *ductus venosus (DV)*, and the systemic vascular resistance increases. Thus the fetal pulmonary to systemic pressure relationships are reversed, and systemic pressure becomes greater than pulmonary pressure. These pressure changes cause the foramen ovale to close. As pressure in the pulmonary artery decreases and pressure in the aorta increases, the shunt across the ductus arteriosus reverses to left to right and constricts, leading to closure in the first few days of life. This closure of fetal shunts establishes the serial arterial–venous circulation indicative of neonatal circulation. See Figure 23–2.

In summary, the four major cardiopulmonary actions of **cardiopulmonary adaptation** (Figure 23–3) are as follows:

1. *Increased systemic vascular resistance and decreased pulmonary vascular resistance.* With the loss of the low-resistance placenta, systemic vascular resistance increases, resulting in greater systemic pressure. At the same time, lung expansion and exposure to high oxygen concentrations increase pulmonary blood flow and dilate pulmonary blood vessels. The combination of vasodilation and

increased pulmonary blood flow decreases pulmonary vascular resistance. As the pulmonary vascular beds open, the systemic vascular pressure increases, enhancing perfusion of the other body systems.

2. *Closure of the foramen ovale.* Closure of the foramen ovale is a function of changing arterial pressures. In utero, pressure is greater in the right atrium, and the foramen ovale is open after birth, shunting blood from the right atrium to the left. The decreased pulmonary vascular resistance and the decreased umbilical venous return to the right atrium also cause a decrease in right atrial pressure. The pressure gradients across the atria are now reversed, with left atrial pressure greater; this causes the foramen ovale to functionally close 1 to 2 hours after birth. Anatomic closure of the foramen ovale occurs within 30 months (Graves & Haley, 2013).

3. *Closure of the ductus arteriosus.* Initial elevation of the systemic vascular pressure above the pulmonary vascular pressure increases pulmonary blood flow by reversing the flow through the ductus arteriosus. Blood now flows from the aorta into the pulmonary artery. An increase in blood PO_2 triggers the ductus arteriosus to constrict. In utero, the placenta produces prostaglandin E_2 (PGE_2), which causes ductus vasodilation. With the loss of the placenta and increased pulmonary blood flow, PGE_2 levels drop, leaving the active constriction by PO_2 unopposed. Functional closure of the ductus arteriosus in the well newborn starts within 18 hours after birth; fibrosis or anatomic closure occurs within 2 to 3 weeks after birth (Fraser, 2014).

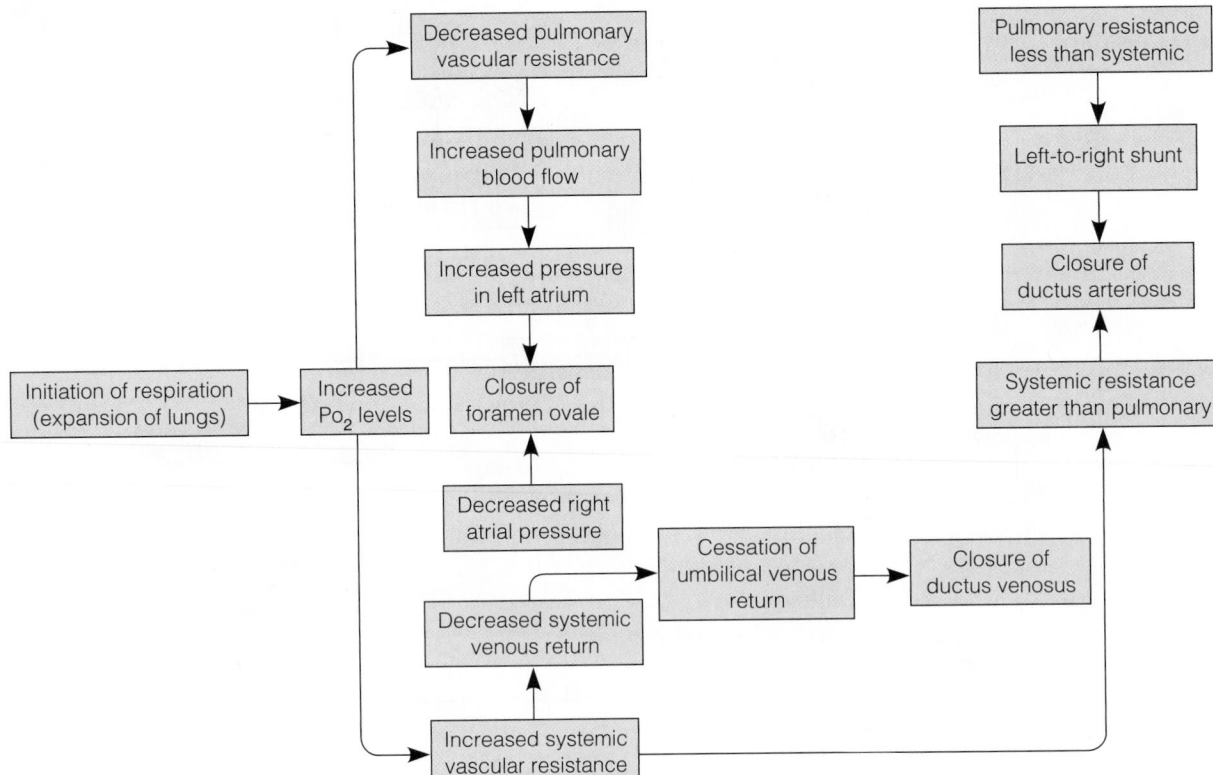

Figure 23–2 **Transitional circulation: Conversion from fetal to neonatal circulation.**

4. ***Closure of the ductus venosus.*** Closure of the ductus venosus is related to mechanical pressure changes that result from severing the cord, redistribution of blood, and cardiac output. Closure of the ductus venosus forces perfusion of the liver. Fibrosis or anatomic closure of the ductus venosus occurs within 2 months, at which time it becomes known as the ligamentum venosum.

Maintaining Respiratory Function

The ability of the lung to maintain oxygenation and ventilation (the exchange of oxygen and carbon dioxide) is influenced by such factors as *lung compliance* and *airway resistance*. Lung compliance is influenced by the elastic recoil of the lung tissue and by anatomic differences in the newborn. The newborn has a relatively large heart and mediastinal structures that reduce available lung space. Also, the newborn chest is equipped with weak intercostal muscles, a rigid rib cage with horizontal ribs, and a high diaphragm that restricts the space available for lung expansion. The large abdomen further encroaches on the diaphragm to decrease lung space. Another factor that limits ventilation is airway resistance, which depends on the radius length and number of airways. Airway resistance is increased in the newborn when compared with adults.

Characteristics of Newborn Respiration

The normal newborn respiratory rate is 30 to 60 breaths per minute. Initial respirations may be largely diaphragmatic, shallow, and irregular in depth and rhythm. The abdomen's movements are synchronous with chest movements. Breathing patterns in newborns can be irregular and variable. Periodic breathing is common in preterm newborns, but can also be seen in term babies. **Periodic breathing** is defined as "pauses in respiratory movements that last for up to 20 seconds alternating with breathing" (Blackburn, 2013). Periodic breathing is rarely associated with changes in skin color or heart rate, and it has no prognostic significance. Tactile or other senses stimulate the respiratory center and convert periodic breathing patterns to normal breathing patterns during neonatal transition. With deep sleep, the pattern is reasonably regular. Periodic breathing occurs with rapid eye movement (REM) sleep, and grossly irregular breathing is evident with motor activity, sucking, and crying. Cessation of breathing lasting more than 20 seconds is defined as *apnea* and is abnormal in term newborns. Apnea may or may not be associated with changes in skin color or heart rate (a drop below 100 beats per minute [beats/min]). Apnea always needs to be further evaluated.

Newborns tend to be obligatory nose breathers because the nasal route is the primary route of air entry. This is because of the high position of the epiglottis and the position of the soft palate (Blackburn, 2013). Newborns need to breathe through their noses in order to feed without choking. Although many term newborns can breathe orally, with nasal occlusion, nasal obstructions can cause respiratory distress. Therefore, it is important to keep the nose and throat clear. Immediately after birth, and for about the next 2 hours, respiratory rates of 60 to 70 breaths per minute are normal. Acrocyanosis is normal

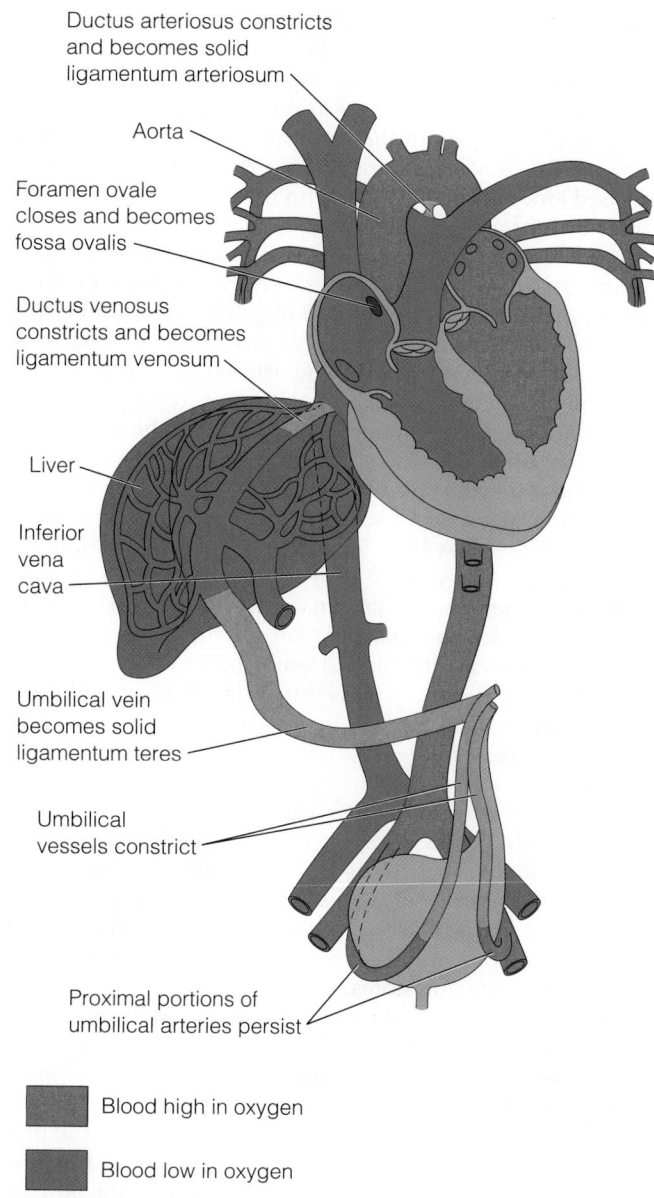

Ductus arteriosus constricts and becomes solid ligamentum arteriosum

Aorta

Foramen ovale closes and becomes fossa ovalis

Ductus venosus constricts and becomes ligamentum venosum

Liver

Inferior vena cava

Umbilical vein becomes solid ligamentum teres

Umbilical vessels constrict

Proximal portions of umbilical arteries persist

Blood high in oxygen

Blood low in oxygen

Figure 23–3 Major changes that occur in the newborn's circulatory system.

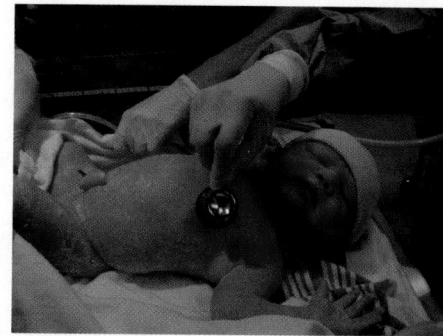

Figure 23–4 Apical pulse rates should be obtained by auscultation for a full minute, preferably when the newborn is asleep.

SOURCE: Wilson Garcia.

awake states. In the full-term newborn, the heart rate may drop to 80 to 100 beats per minute during deep sleep (Van Woudenberg et al., 2012).

Apical pulse rates should be obtained by auscultation for a full minute, preferably when the newborn is asleep (Figure 23–4). The heart rate should be evaluated for abnormal rhythms or beats. Peripheral pulses of all extremities should also be evaluated to detect any inequalities or unusual characteristics. While radial pulses are readily found, peripheral pedal pulses may be difficult to palpate in the newborn. Additionally, brachial and femoral pulses are usually easily palpated in the well newborn.

BLOOD PRESSURE

Blood pressure (BP) tends to be highest immediately after birth and then descends to its lowest level at about 3 hours of age. By days 4 to 6, the blood pressure rises and plateaus at a level approximately the same as the initial level. Blood pressure is sensitive to the changes in blood volume that occur in the transition to newborn circulation (Figure 23–5). Peripheral perfusion pressure is a particularly sensitive indicator of the newborn's ability to compensate for alterations in blood volume before changes in blood pressure.

Blood pressure values during the first 12 hours of life vary with the birth weight and gestational age. Crying may cause

for the first 24 hours. If respirations drop below 30 or exceed 60 per minute when the newborn is at rest, or if retractions, cyanosis, or nasal flaring and expiratory grunting occur, the clinician should be notified. Any increased use of the intercostal muscles (retractions) may indicate respiratory distress. (See Chapter 27 and Table 27–1 for signs of respiratory distress.) Some institutions do allow the pulse oxygen to remain low for several minutes after birth because it takes approximately 8 minutes on average for pulse oxygen saturations to rise above 90% (Raab & Kelly, 2013).

Characteristics of Cardiac Function

HEART RATE

Shortly after the first cry and the start of changes in cardiopulmonary circulation, the newborn heart rate can accelerate to 180 beats per minute. The average resting heart rate in the first week of life is 110 to 160 beats per minute in a healthy, full-term newborn but may vary significantly during deep sleep or active

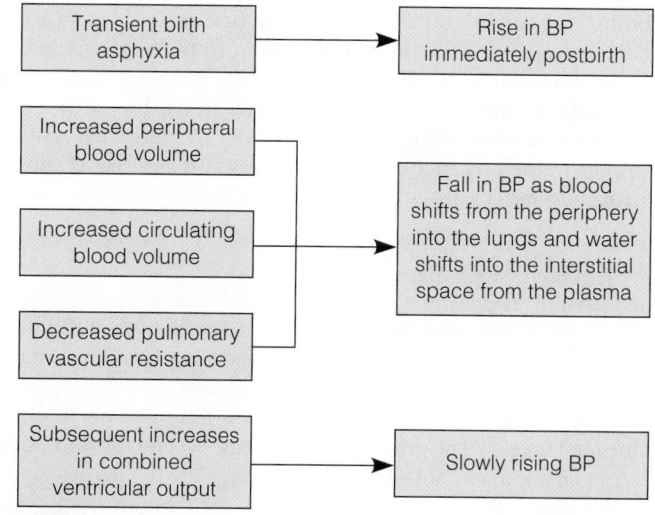

Transient birth asphyxia	Rise in BP immediately postbirth
Increased peripheral blood volume	
Increased circulating blood volume	Fall in BP as blood shifts from the periphery into the lungs and water shifts into the interstitial space from the plasma
Decreased pulmonary vascular resistance	
Subsequent increases in combined ventricular output	Slowly rising BP

Figure 23–5 Response of blood pressure (BP) to changes in neonatal blood volume.

an elevation in both the systolic and diastolic blood pressure; thus accuracy is more likely in the quiet newborn. Capillary refill should be less than 3 seconds when the skin is blanched. The average mean blood pressure is 31 to 61 mmHg in full-term resting newborns over 3 kg (6.6 lb) during the first 12 hours of life (Glomella, 2013). In the preterm newborn, the average mean blood pressure varies according to weight and degree of illness. Blood pressure in the lower extremities is usually higher than that in the upper extremities.

HEART MURMURS

Murmurs are produced by turbulent blood flow. In newborns, 90% of all murmurs are transient and not associated with anomalies.

Cardiac murmurs are often present in the initial newborn period as transition from fetal to neonatal circulation occurs. These murmurs heard in the transition period (the first 48 hours of life) should be followed up (Blackburn, 2013). Such murmurs usually involve incomplete closure of the ductus arteriosus or foramen ovale. Soft murmurs may be heard as the pulmonary branch arteries increase their blood flow from 7% to 50% of the combined ventricular output during transition, causing a physiologic peripheral pulmonary stenosis. Clicks may normally be heard at the lower left sternal border as the great vessels dilate to accommodate systolic blood flow in the first few hours of life. Because of the current practice of early discharge, murmurs associated with ventricular septal defect and patent ductus arteriosus are not often picked up until the first well-baby checkup at 4 to 6 weeks of age. Hearing a murmur is often the most common means of recognizing cardiac disease.

CARDIAC WORKLOAD

Before birth, the right ventricle does approximately two thirds of the cardiac work, resulting in increased size and thickness of the right ventricle at birth. After birth, the left ventricle has a significantly greater increase in volume load than the right ventricle, and it needs to progressively increase in size and thickness. This may explain why right-sided heart defects are better tolerated than left-sided ones and why left-sided heart defects rapidly become symptomatic after birth.

Hematopoietic System

Birth brings dramatic changes in circulation and oxygenation, which affect hematopoiesis. The mean hemoglobin level in cord blood at term is 17 g/dL (Glomella, 2013). Normally, the hemoglobin and hematocrit values rise in the first several hours after birth because of the movement of plasma from intravascular to the extravascular space. By 3 to 5 days after birth, nucleated red blood cells are normally no longer found in the blood of term or preterm newborns, but may be present in marked elevated numbers in the presence of hemolysis or hypoxic stress (Diab & Luchtman-Jones, 2015).

Oxygen Transport

The transportation of oxygen to the peripheral tissues depends on the type of hemoglobin in the red blood cells. In the fetus and newborn, a variety of hemoglobins exist, the most significant being fetal hemoglobin (HbF) and adult hemoglobin (HbA). Approximately 70% to 90% of the hemoglobin in the fetus and newborn is of the fetal variety. The greatest difference between HbF and HbA relates to the transport of and release of oxygen to the tissues.

Because HbF has a greater affinity for oxygen than does HbA, the oxygen saturation in the newborn's blood is greater than in the adult's, but the amount of oxygen released to the tissues is less. Because of this high concentration of oxygen in the blood with HbF, hypoxia in the newborn is particularly difficult to recognize. Clinical manifestations of cyanosis do not appear until low blood levels of oxygen are present.

Fetal blood flowing through the umbilical vein in utero is 65% to 70% oxygen saturated; this relative hypoxia causes increased amounts of erythropoietin to be secreted, resulting in active erythropoiesis (an increase in nucleated red blood cells and reticulocytes). Erythropoiesis is regulated by the hormone erythropoietin, which is produced in the kidneys. Levels of erythropoietin rise in response to hypoxia and anemia, causing an increase in production of red blood cells. After birth, the increases in oxygen saturation and arterial oxygen levels shut down the production of erythropoietin temporarily. Normally, the hemoglobin and hematocrit values rise in the first several hours after birth because of the movement of plasma from intravascular to extravascular space. The fetal hemoglobin concentration in blood decreases after birth by approximately 3% per week and is less than 5% to 8% of total hemoglobin by 6 months of age (Bagwell, 2014). This initial decline in hemoglobin creates a phenomenon known as **physiologic anemia of the newborn**. The newborn usually tolerates this physiologic state without any clinical difficulties. Hemoglobin values fall, mainly from a decrease in red cell mass rather than from the dilutional effect of increasing plasma volume. The fact that red cell survival is lower in newborns than in adults, and that red cell production is less, also contributes to this anemia. Neonatal RBCs have a lifespan of 60 to 70 days, approximately one half to two thirds of an adult's RBC lifespan (Bagwell, 2014). Erythropoiesis resumes normally when levels of erythropoietin rise in response to low hemoglobin levels and tissue oxygen needs (Bagwell, 2014). Once erythropoiesis resumes, iron stores will be used to produce new RBCs. Most babies require supplemental iron to maintain adequate iron stores.

By 3 to 5 days after birth, nucleated red blood cells are normally no longer found in the blood of term or preterm newborns, but may be present in markedly elevated numbers in the presence of hemolysis or hypoxic stress. The absolute number of neutrophils in the blood of the neonate is greater than that found in older children, while the absolute number of lymphocytes is equivalent to that in older children. The platelet count of the newborn is comparable to adult values. A number of maternally administered pharmacologic agents have been implicated in hematologic abnormalities of the fetus or newborn. Therefore, obtaining an accurate maternal history, including medications, is important.

Blood volume is approximately 85 mL/kg of body weight for a term newborn (Diab & Luchtman-Jones, 2015). For example, a 3.6 kg (8 lb) newborn has a blood volume of 306 mL. Blood volume varies based on the amount of placental transfusion received during the delivery of the placenta prior to cord clamping, as well as other factors, including the following:

1. *Gestational age.* There appears to be a positive association between gestational age, RBC numbers, and hemoglobin concentration.

2. *Prenatal and/or perinatal hemorrhage.* Significant prenatal or perinatal bleeding decreases the hematocrit level and causes hypovolemia.

3. *The site of the blood sample.* Hemoglobin and hematocrit levels are significantly higher in capillary blood than in venous blood. Sluggish peripheral blood flow creates RBC stasis, thereby increasing RBC concentration in the capillaries. Consequently, blood samples taken from venous blood sites are more accurate than those from capillary sites.

Delayed Cord Clamping

In utero, the fetus's blood flows through the umbilical cord to and from the fetus and the placenta, bringing oxygen and nutrition to the fetus from the mother's blood. If the umbilical cord is left unclamped for a short period of time after birth, some of the blood from the placenta passes to the newborn (this is called *placental transfusion*) to increase the neonate's blood volume and improve blood flow to the newborn's organs (Katheria, Truong, Cousins, et al., 2015). For many years, the standard of care has included immediate clamping of the umbilical cord at birth. The World Health Organization was the first to recommend delayed cord clamping as a standard for all babies at birth. Although many randomized control trials of term and preterm newborns have evaluated the benefits and risks of immediate umbilical cord clamping versus delayed umbilical cord clamping, generally defined as umbilical cord clamping performed 30 to 60 seconds after birth, the ideal timing for umbilical cord clamping has not yet been established and continues to be a subject of controversy and debate (American College of Obstetricians and Gynecologists [ACOG], 2014).

Physiologic studies in term newborns have demonstrated that placental blood is rapidly transferred into the newborn via the uninterrupted umbilical cord in a stepwise fashion over the initial seconds after birth. Approximately 80 mL of blood is transferred by 1 minute after birth, reaching approximately 100 mL at 3 minutes after birth (ACOG, 2014). Providing newborns with additional blood through delayed umbilical cord clamping may facilitate transition from fetal to neonatal circulation (Katheria et al., 2015). Reviews of multiple clinical trials found that delayed umbilical cord clamping had both positive and negative effects on neonatal outcomes. Newborns in the delayed umbilical cord clamping group had significantly higher levels of hemoglobin compared with newborns in the immediate umbilical cord clamping group. Newborns in the delayed umbilical cord clamping group also had higher ferritin levels until 6 months of age and fewer suffered from iron deficiency anemia (Raju, 2013). However, a significant increase was noted in the need for phototherapy for jaundice in the delayed umbilical cord clamping group.

The benefits of delayed umbilical cord clamping for the preterm newborn are much more compelling. Clinical trials in preterm babies found that delaying umbilical cord clamping was associated with fewer newborns who required blood transfusion for anemia and/or low blood pressure. Also, a significant reduction in the incidence of intraventricular hemorrhage and less risk of necrotizing enterocolitis (a severe infection in the bowel) were found in neonates in the delayed umbilical cord clamping group (ACOG, 2014; Katheria et al., 2015). These effects may be related to an improvement in the circulating neonatal blood volume and better control of blood pressure following placental transfusion. However, there are some legitimate arguments for clamping the umbilical cord soon after birth. Maternal emergency and concern that delayed umbilical cord clamping could hinder the timely initiation of resuscitation for the asphyxiated newborn or one with cardiopulmonary failure are valid reasons for immediate umbilical cord clamping (Raju, 2013).

Coagulation

The platelet count of the newborn is comparable to adult values; however, the newborn may have transient diminished platelet function. Transient neonatal thrombocytopenia may occur in babies born to mothers with severe hypertension or HELLP syndrome (hemolysis, elevated liver enzymes, and low platelet count) (see Chapter 15 for a discussion of HELLP syndrome) and in babies born to mothers who have idiopathic isoimmune thrombocytopenia. Coagulation factors II, VII, IX, and X (synthesized in the liver) require vitamin K for the final steps of synthesis. The absence of intestinal flora needed to synthesize vitamin K in the newborn gut results in a quick decrease of these clotting factors after birth. These clotting factors then slowly increase, but do not approach adult levels until 9 months of age or later (Bagwell, 2014). This decrease may be lessened by administration of vitamin K, effectively preventing early occurring hemorrhagic disease of the newborn. Although newborn bleeding problems are rare, an injection of vitamin K (AquaMEPHYTON) is given prophylactically on the day of birth. (Hemorrhagic disease of the newborn is discussed in more depth in Chapter 26.) See Table 23–2 for normal electrolyte, blood, and blood gas values of the normal term newborn.

Leukocytosis is a normal finding, because the stress of birth stimulates increased production of neutrophils during the first

TABLE 23–2 Normal Term Newborn Cord Blood and Cord Blood Gas Values

LABORATORY DATA	NORMAL RANGE
Cord Blood Values	
Hemoglobin	14–20 g/dL
Hematocrit	43%–63%
WBC	10,000–30,000/mm³
WBC differential	
Neutrophils	40%–80%
Lymphocytes	20%–40%
Monocytes	3%–10%
Platelets	150,000–350,000/mm³
Reticulocytes	3%–7%
Sodium	127–144 mEq/L
Potassium	3.4–9.9 mEq/L
Chloride	103–111 mEq/L
Bicarbonate	18–23 mEq/L
Carbon dioxide	13–27 mmol/L
Calcium	8.2–111 mg/dL
Glucose	45–96 mg/dL
Total protein	4.8–7.3 g/dL
Cord Blood Gas Values	
Venous Blood Gas	
pH	7.25–7.35
PO_2	2–32 mmHg
PCO_2	40–50 mmHg
Base Excess	± 0–5
HCO_3	22
Arterial Blood Gas	
pH	7.14–7.4
PO_2	16–20 mmHg
PCO_2	32–68 mmHg
Base Excess	± 0–10
HCO_3	15–26.8

Source: Data from Fanaroff, A. A., & Martin, R. J. (Eds.). (2015). *Neonatal-perinatal medicine* (10th ed.). St. Louis, MO: Mosby.

few days of life. Neutrophils then decrease to 35% of the total leukocyte count by 2 weeks of age. Lymphocytes play a role in antibody formation and eventually become the predominant type of leukocyte and the total white blood cell count falls.

Temperature Regulation

Temperature regulation is the maintenance of thermal balance by the loss of heat to the environment at a rate equal to heat production. Newborns are *homeothermic*; they attempt to stabilize their internal (core) body temperatures within a narrow range in spite of significant temperature variations in their environment. Thermoregulation in the newborn is closely related to the rate of metabolism and oxygen consumption. Within a specific environmental temperature range, called the **neutral thermal environment (NTE)** zone, the rates of oxygen consumption and metabolism are minimal, and internal body temperature is maintained because of thermal balance (Blackburn, 2013). Thus the normal newborn requires higher environmental temperatures to maintain a thermoneutral environment than adults.

Several newborn characteristics affect the establishment of thermal stability:

- Heat transfer from neonatal organs to skin surface is increased compared to adults because of the neonate's decreased subcutaneous fat and large body surface to weight ratio.

- Neonates rely on nonshivering thermogenesis for heat production via metabolism of brown adipose tissue.

- Blood vessels in the newborn are closer to the skin than those of an adult. Therefore, the circulating blood is influenced by changes in environmental temperature and in turn influences the hypothalamic temperature-regulating center.

- The flexed posture of the term newborn decreases the surface area exposed to the environment, thereby reducing heat loss.

- Preterm newborns have increased heat loss via evaporation because of increased total body water and thin skin.

A table listing neutral thermal environmental temperatures gives a recommended temperature range depending on the weight and age of the newborn (see *Thermoregulation of the Newborn*, in the *Clinical Skills Manual* SKILLS). Generally speaking, the smaller newborns in each weight group will require a temperature in the higher portion of the temperature range. Within each time range, the younger the baby, the higher the temperature required. For example, the preterm or small-for-gestational-age (SGA) newborn has less adipose tissue and is hypoflexed, and therefore requires higher environmental temperatures to achieve a neutral thermal environment. Larger, well-insulated newborns may be able to cope with lower environmental temperatures. If the environmental temperature falls below the lower limits of the NTE, the newborn responds with increased oxygen consumption and metabolism, which results in greater heat production. Prolonged exposure to the cold may result in depleted glycogen stores and acidosis. Oxygen consumption also increases if the environmental temperature is above the NTE.

Heat Loss

A newborn is at a distinct disadvantage in maintaining a normal temperature. With a large body surface in relation to mass and a limited amount of insulating subcutaneous fat, the full-term newborn loses about 4 times the heat of an adult. The newborn's poor thermal stability is primarily because of excessive heat loss rather than impaired heat production. Because of the risk of hypothermia and possible cold stress, minimizing heat loss in the newborn after birth is essential (see Chapter 27 for nursing management).

Two major routes of heat loss are from the internal core of the body to the body surface and from the external surface to the environment. Usually, the core temperature is higher than the skin temperature, resulting in continuous transfer or conduction of heat to the surface. The greater the difference in temperature between core and skin, the more rapidly heat transfers. The transfer is accomplished through an increase in oxygen consumption, depletion of glycogen stores, and metabolization of brown fat. Heat loss from the body surface to the environment takes place in four ways—by convection, radiation, evaporation, and conduction (Figure 23–6).

- **Convection** is the loss of heat from the warm body surface to the cooler air currents. Air-conditioned rooms, air currents with a temperature below the newborn's skin temperature, oxygen by mask, and removal from an incubator for procedures increase convective heat loss in the newborn. The amount of heat transferred depends on the velocity of the moving air, the temperature difference between the air and the newborn's skin, and the proportion of body surface area exposed.

- **Radiation** losses occur when heat transfers from the heated body surface to cooler surfaces and objects not in direct contact with the body. The walls of a room or of an incubator are potential causes of heat loss by radiation, even if the ambient temperature of the incubator is within the thermal neutral range for that newborn. Placing cold objects (such as ice for blood gases) onto the incubator or near the newborn in the radiant warmer will increase radiant losses.

- **Evaporation** is the loss of heat incurred when water is converted to a vapor. The newborn is particularly prone to lose heat by evaporation immediately after birth (when the baby is wet with amniotic fluid) and during baths; thus, drying the newborn is critical. Evaporation accounts for 25% of heat loss immediately after delivery (Blackburn, 2013). Evaporation also occurs from expired air from the respiratory tract. Radiant warming beds and bank phototherapy lights accentuate evaporative loss.

- **Conduction** is the loss of heat to a cooler surface by direct skin contact. Chilled hands, cool scales, cold examination tables, and cold stethoscopes can cause loss of heat by conduction. Even if objects are warmed to the incubator temperature, the temperature difference between the newborn's core temperature and the ambient temperature may be significant. This difference results in heat transfer.

Once the newborn has been dried after birth, the highest losses of heat generally result from radiation and convection. The newborn can respond to the cooler environmental temperature with adequate peripheral vasoconstriction, but this mechanism is not entirely effective because of the minimal amount of fat insulation present, the large body surface, and ongoing thermal conduction. Because of these factors, minimizing the baby's heat loss and preventing hypothermia are imperative. Most hospitalized newborns are weighed daily. Placing unclothed newborns on a cold scale can induce heat loss. Therefore, the undressed newborn should be examined in a warm environment with an external heat source such as a radiant warmer. (See Chapter 27 for nursing measures to prevent hypothermia.)

Bath time is when many newborns experience cold stress. To minimize the risk, always bathe newborns in a warm room, gather all supplies prior to beginning the bath, and prewarm soaps or shampoos. Dry with warmed blankets and dress immediately. The newborn's head accounts for a large portion of body surface area and has great capacity for heat loss, so placing a hat on the baby is an effective way to minimize heat loss. Placing the newborn skin-to-skin with the mother after bathing is a good way to help rewarm and maintain body temperature.

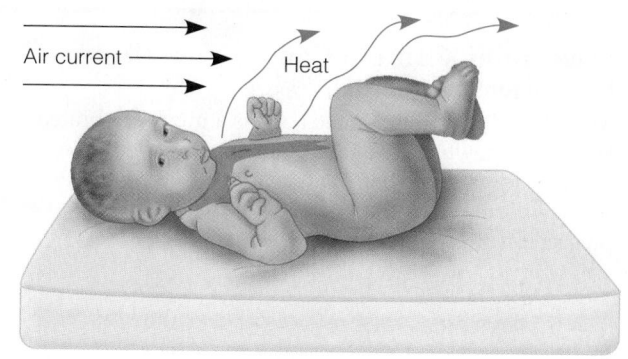

A. Convection

Heat Production (Thermogenesis)

When exposed to a cool environment, the newborn requires additional heat. The newborn has several physiologic mechanisms that increase heat production, or **thermogenesis**. These mechanisms include increased basal metabolic rate, muscular activity, and chemical thermogenesis (also called *nonshivering thermogenesis [NST]*).

NST is an important mechanism of heat production unique to the newborn. It occurs when skin receptors perceive a drop in the environmental temperature and, in response, transmit sensations to stimulate the sympathetic nervous system. NST uses the newborn's stores of **brown adipose tissue (BAT)** (also called *brown fat*) to provide heat. It increases in the fetus at about 25 to 26 weeks' gestation and continues to increase until 3 to 5 weeks after the birth of a term newborn, unless the fat is depleted by cold stress (Blackburn, 2013). Brown fat is deposited in the midscapular area, around the neck, and in the axillas, with deeper placement around the trachea, esophagus, abdominal aorta, kidneys, and adrenal glands (see the shaded areas in Figure 23–6). BAT receives its name from the dark color caused by its enriched blood supply, dense cellular content, and abundant nerve endings. These characteristics of brown fat cells promote rapid metabolism, heat generation, and heat transfer to the peripheral circulation. The large numbers of brown fat cells increase the speed with which triglycerides are metabolized to produce heat but cause increased oxygen consumption and caloric output in the already compromised newborn.

Shivering, a form of muscular activity common in the cold adult, is rarely seen in the newborn. If the newborn shivers, it means the newborn's metabolic rate has already doubled. The extra muscular activity does little to produce needed heat.

An increase in metabolism as a result of hypothermia results in an increase in oxygen consumption. A decrease in the environmental temperature of 2°C, from 33° to 31°C (91.4° to 87.8°F), is a drop sufficient to double the oxygen consumption of a term newborn. Keeping the normal newborn warm promotes normal oxygen requirements, whereas chilling can cause the newborn to show signs of respiratory distress.

When exposed to cold, the normal term newborn is usually able to cope with the increase in oxygen requirements, but the preterm newborn may be unable to increase ventilation to the necessary level of oxygen consumption. (See Chapter 27 for a discussion of cold stress.) Because oxidation of fatty acids depends on the availability of oxygen, glucose, and adenosine triphosphate (ATP), the newborn's ability to generate heat can be altered by pathologic events such as hypoxia, acidosis, and hypoglycemia or by medication that blocks the release of norepinephrine. The effect of certain drugs such as meperidine (Demerol) may also prevent metabolism of brown fat. Newborn hypothermia prolongs as well as potentiates the effects of many analgesic and anesthetic drugs in the newborn.

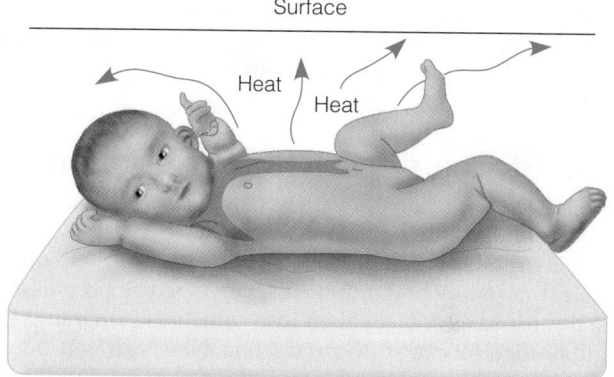

B. Radiation

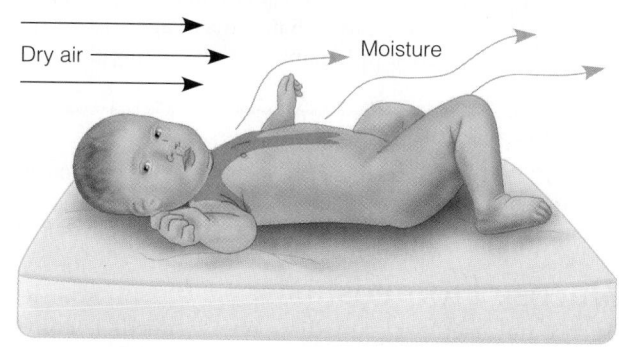

C. Evaporation

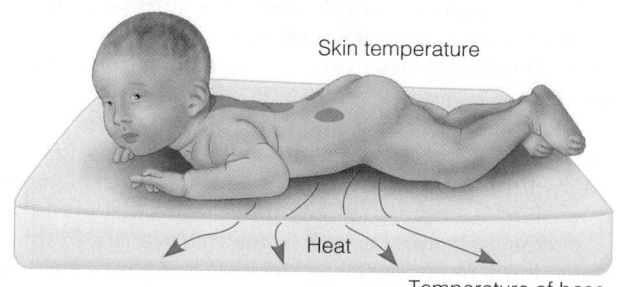

D. Conduction

Figure 23–6 Methods of heat loss. *A*, Convection. *B*, Radiation. *C*, Evaporation. *D*, Conduction. The distribution of brown adipose tissue (brown fat) in the newborn is shown in the shaded areas.

Hepatic Adaptations

The liver performs many essential functions, including the production of bile, regulation of plasma proteins and glucose, and
the biotransformation of drugs and toxins. The neonate has less
than 20% of the hepatocytes that are present in the adult liver,
and liver growth continues after birth until it reaches its mature
size.

Iron Storage and RBC Production

Iron is an essential micronutrient that plays a significant role in
critical cellular functions in all organ systems. The serum iron
level in umbilical cord blood is elevated compared to maternal
levels (Diab & Luchtman-Jones, 2015). As red blood cells (RBCs)
are destroyed after birth, their iron content is stored in the liver
until needed for new RBC production. Newborn iron stores are
determined by total body hemoglobin content and length of
gestation. The term newborn has about 270 mg of iron at birth,
and about 140 to 170 mg of this amount is in the hemoglobin. If
the mother's iron intake has been adequate, enough iron will be
stored to last until the infant is 5 months of age. See Chapter 32
for discussion of iron supplementation after 6 months of age.

Healthy People 2020

> (NWS-21) Reduce iron deficiency among young children and
> females of childbearing age

Glucose Homeostasis

Glucose not used for immediate energy needs is converted
to glycogen and stored in the liver, heart, and skeletal muscles as glycogen. During fasting, glycogen is broken down to
reform glucose and released by the liver. Fetal glucose levels
are approximately 80% of the mother's glucose level. Glycogen storage for postnatal energy needs begins early in gestation, with most glycogen stores accumulating during the third
trimester.

After umbilical cord clamping, the neonate's blood glucose level falls, reaching a nadir at about 1 to 2 hours of age.
In these first hours after birth, the neonatal brain metabolizes
the newborn's abundant stores of lactate, so that even though
the glucose concentration may be low, the neonatal brain is not
energy deficient. By secreting glucagon and suppressing insulin release, the newborn gradually mobilizes glucose to meet
energy needs. Thus, even if a healthy term baby is not fed soon
after birth, blood glucose levels rise at 3 to 4 hours of age (Cloherty, Eichenwald, Hansen, et al., 2012). However, hepatic glycogen is rapidly depleted if feeding is not established early. The
nurse may assess the glucose level on admission if risk factors
are present or per agency protocol (see *Care of the Newborn With
Hypoglycemia* in Chapter 27).

Conjugation of Bilirubin

Conjugation, or the changing of bilirubin into an excretable
form, is the conversion of the yellow lipid-soluble pigment
(unconjugated, indirect) into water-soluble pigment (excretable,
direct). Unconjugated bilirubin is fat soluble, has a propensity
for fatty tissues, is not in an excretable form, and is a potential toxin. **Total bilirubin** is the sum of conjugated (direct) and
unconjugated (indirect) bilirubin.

Fetal unconjugated bilirubin crosses the placenta to be
excreted, so the fetus does not need to conjugate bilirubin. Total
bilirubin at birth is usually less than 3 mg/dL unless an abnormal hemolytic process has been present in utero. After birth,
the newborn's liver must begin to conjugate bilirubin. This
produces a normal rise in serum bilirubin levels in the first few
days of life.

The bilirubin formed after RBCs are destroyed is transported
in the blood bound to albumin. The bilirubin is transferred into the
hepatocytes and bound to intracellular proteins. These proteins
determine the amount of bilirubin held in a liver cell for processing and consequently determine the amount of bilirubin uptake
into the liver. The activity of uridine-diphosphoglucuronosyl
transferase (UDPGT) enzyme results in the attachment of unconjugated bilirubin to glucuronic acid (product of liver glycogen),
producing conjugated (direct) bilirubin. Direct bilirubin is excreted
into the tiny bile ducts, then into the common duct and duodenum.
The conjugated bilirubin then progresses down the intestines,
where bacteria transform it into urobilinogen (urine bilirubin) and
stercobilinogen. Stercobilinogen is not reabsorbed but is excreted as
a yellow-brown pigment in the stools.

Even after the bilirubin has been conjugated and bound, it
can be changed back to unconjugated bilirubin via the enterohepatic circulation. In the intestines, β-D-glucuronidase enzyme
acts to split off (deconjugate) the bilirubin from glucuronic acid
if it has not first been acted on by gut bacteria to produce urobilinogen; the free bilirubin is reabsorbed through the intestinal
wall and brought back to the liver via portal vein circulation.
This recycling of the bilirubin and decreased ability to clear bilirubin from the system are prevalent in babies with very high
β-D-glucuronidase activity levels, those who are exclusively
breastfed, and those with delayed bacterial colonization of the
gut (such as with the use of antibiotics) and further increases
the newborn's susceptibility to jaundice (Figure 23–7).

The newborn liver has relatively less glucuronyl transferase activity in the first few weeks of life than an adult liver. This
reduction in hepatic activity, along with a relatively large bilirubin load, decreases the liver's ability to conjugate bilirubin and
increases susceptibility to jaundice. Jaundice (icterus) is the yellowish coloration of the skin and sclera caused by the presence
of bilirubin in elevated concentrations. *Hyperbilirubinemia* is an
elevated total serum bilirubin level. Abnormal values differ by
gestational age, days of life, and presence of risk factors.

Physiologic Jaundice

Physiologic jaundice (nonpathologic unconjugated hyperbilirubinemia) develops in more than 60% of term newborns and
80% of preterm neonates and is visible when the serum bilirubin concentration is greater than 6 to 7 mg/dL (Blackburn, 2013).
Usually, bilirubin levels increase soon after birth because of
increased bilirubin production and/or delayed bilirubin elimination, as well as by a unique neonatal phenomenon of enterohepatic recirculation of bilirubin. However, by the end of the first
week of life, the bilirubin levels decline. Peak bilirubin levels
are reached between days 3 and 5 in the full-term newborn and

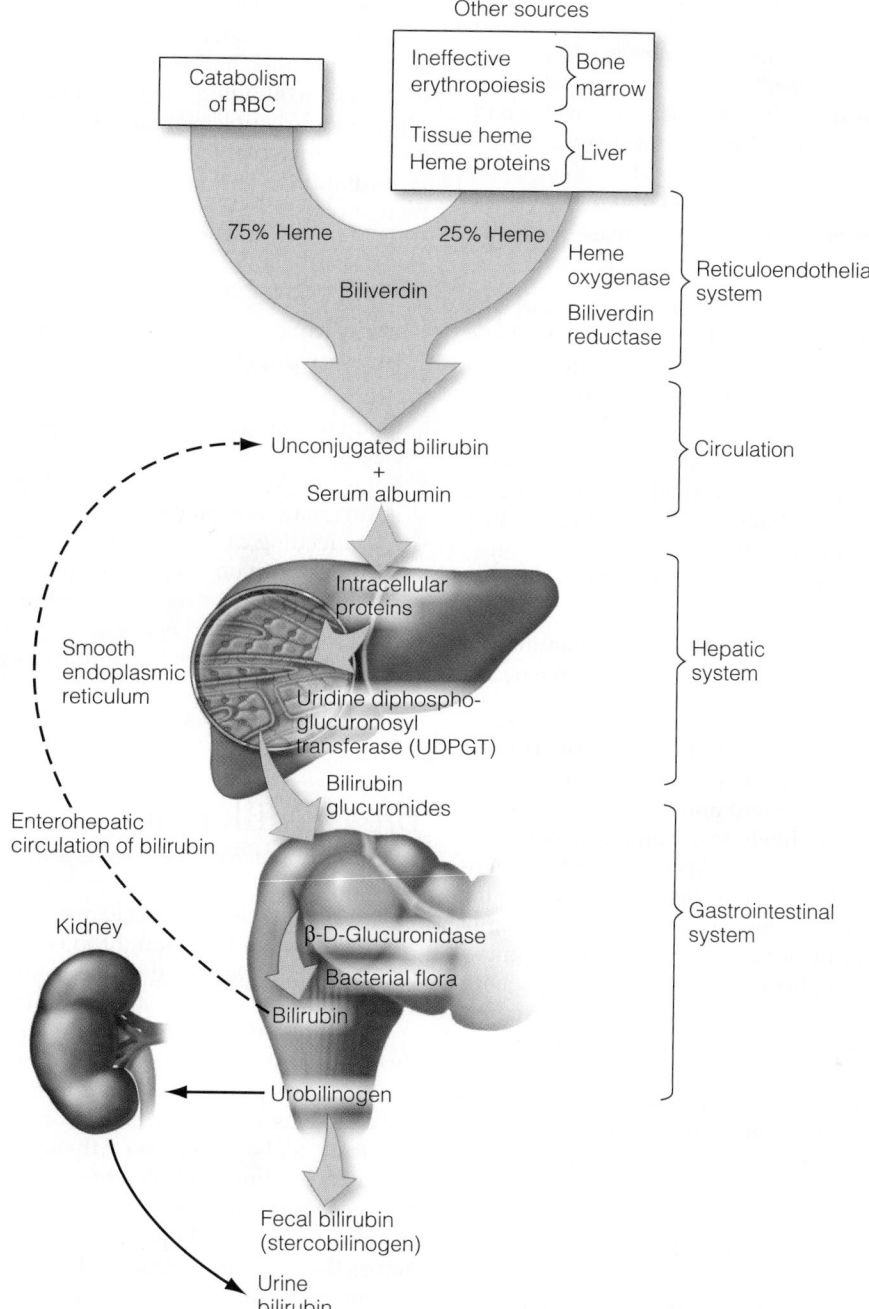

Figure 23–7 Conjugation of bilirubin in newborns.

between days 5 and 7 in the preterm newborn. This condition does not have a pathologic basis, but rather is a normal biologic response of the newborn. Note that these values are established for European and American White newborns. Chinese, Japanese, Korean, and Native American newborns have considerably higher bilirubin levels that are not as apparent and that persist for longer periods with no apparent ill effects (Blackburn, 2013).

Because of the shorter lifespan of fetal RBCs, newborns have a 2 to 3 times greater production or breakdown of bilirubin. Bruising from the delivery process can also increase the amount of bilirubin to be handled by the liver. The low volume and inadequate caloric intake of the newborn's initial feedings increase reabsorption of bilirubin and are further aggravated by decreased gastrointestinal activity characteristic of the early postnatal period (Bhutani, Vilms, & Hamerman-Johnson, 2010). Enterohepatic recirculation of bilirubin is the deconjugation and

reabsorption of bilirubin that occurs in the bowel. The signs of physiologic jaundice appear *after* the first 24 hours postnatally. This differentiates physiologic jaundice from pathologic jaundice (see Chapter 27), which is clinically seen at birth or within the first 24 hours of postnatal life.

In some newborns, the rise of bilirubin continues or accelerates. Thus, unmonitored and untreated severe hyperbilirubinemia may progress to excessive levels that are associated with bilirubin neurotoxicity (kernicterus). All newborns should be routinely monitored for the development of jaundice, and nurseries should have protocols for the assessment of jaundice. Jaundice can be detected by blanching the skin with digital pressure on the forehead, midsternum, or knee to reveal the underlying color of the skin (Bhutani et al., 2010). The newborn develops jaundice in cephalocaudal progression, which means that jaundice is first seen in the face and then travels down the trunk.

SAFETY ALERT!
Universal screening for hyperbilirubinemia and not visual inspection alone is necessary for early identification of elevated bilirubin levels in newborns. (Association of Women's Health, Obstetric and Neonatal Nurses [AWHONN], Clinical Position Statement, 2005, reaffirmed 2009).

Several newborn care procedures will decrease the probability of high bilirubin levels.

- Maintain the newborn's skin temperature at 36.5°C (97.8°F) or above; cold stress results in acidosis. Acidosis decreases available serum albumin-binding sites, weakens albumin-binding powers, and causes elevated unconjugated bilirubin levels.

- Monitor stool for amount and characteristics. Bilirubin is eliminated in the feces; inadequate stooling may result in reabsorption and recycling of bilirubin. Early breastfeeding should be encouraged because the laxative effect of colostrum increases excretion of meconium and transitional stool.

- Encourage early feedings to promote intestinal elimination and bacterial colonization and provide caloric intake necessary for hepatic binding proteins to form.

However, absence of jaundice is not an indication of absence of hyperbilirubinemia. Therefore, screening using hour-specific bilirubin measurement and clinical risk factors can identify neonates who are likely to develop severe hyperbilirubinemia. Predischarge bilirubin screening identifies neonates with bilirubin levels higher than the 75th percentile for age in hours. Clinical risk factors for severe hyperbilirubinemia include exclusive and insufficient breast milk feedings, family history of neonatal jaundice, bruising, assisted delivery with vacuum or forceps, cephalohematoma, Asian ethnicity, maternal age (more than 25 years), male gender, and gestational age. (See Chapter 27 for more information.)

If jaundice becomes apparent, nursing care is directed toward keeping the newborn well hydrated and promoting intestinal elimination. (For specific nursing management and therapies, see *Nursing Care Plan: The Newborn With Hyperbilirubinemia* in Chapter 27.)

Physiologic jaundice may upset parents; provide emotional support and thorough explanation of the condition. If the baby is placed under phototherapy, a few additional days of hospitalization may be required, which may also upset parents. Encourage them to meet the emotional needs of their newborn by continuing to feed, hold, and caress the newborn. If the mother is discharged, encourage the parents to return for feedings and to telephone or visit when possible. In many instances, the mother, especially if she is breastfeeding, may elect to remain hospitalized with her newborn; the nurse should support this decision. If insurance limitations make this unrealistic, it may be possible to find an empty room for the discharged mother and her family to use while visiting the newborn. As an alternative to continued hospitalization, the newborn may be treated with home phototherapy. (See section on phototherapy in Chapter 27 for more information.)

Breastfeeding Jaundice

Breastfeeding is implicated in jaundice in some newborns. *Breastfeeding jaundice* occurs in the first days of life in 12.9% of breastfeeding newborns having a bilirubin level greater than 12 mg/dL (Glomella, 2013). It is related to inadequate fluid intake with some element of dehydration and not with any abnormality in milk composition (Hardy, D'Agata, & McGrath, 2016). Prevention and treatment of early breastfeeding jaundice includes encouraging frequent (every 2 to 3 hours) breastfeeding, avoiding supplementation in nondehydrated newborns, and accessing maternal lactation counseling. Breastfeeding jaundice is self-limiting; it peaks around day 3 as enteral intake increases, then resolves.

Developing Cultural Competence Interpreting Illness Through Cultural Beliefs

Cultural beliefs lead mothers to interpret illness within their cultural framework, especially when left without clear and understood explanations (Lauderdale, 2012). For example, some Latina women believe that showing strong maternal emotions during pregnancy and during breastfeeding can be detrimental. They blame jaundice in their newborn on *bili* associated with anger. Such maternal reactions can be lessened by careful explanations to the mothers about the diagnosis, prognosis, duration, and management options for jaundice, and the possibility for recurrence.

Breast Milk Jaundice

Breast milk jaundice occurs in approximately 2% to 4% of term newborns with an onset of 4 to 7 days of life (Riley, Spencer, & Prater, 2014). The exact mechanism of true breast milk jaundice is unknown, but it is thought to be due to unidentified factors in breast milk interfering with bilirubin metabolism causing an exaggerated physiologic jaundice (Cloherty et al., 2012).

In contrast to breastfeeding jaundice, breast milk jaundice is related to milk composition promoting increased bilirubin reabsorption from the intestine. Some women's breast milk contains several times the normal concentration of certain free fatty acids. These free fatty acids may compete with bilirubin for binding sites on albumin and inhibit the conjugation of bilirubin or increase lipase activity, which disrupts the RBC membrane. Increased lipase activity enhances absorption of bile across the gastrointestinal tract membrane, thereby increasing the enterohepatic circulation of bilirubin.

Newborns with breastmilk jaundice appear well, and at present development of kernicterus (toxic levels of bilirubin in the brain) has not been documented. Temporary cessation of breastfeeding may be advised if bilirubin reaches presumed toxic levels of approximately 20 mg/dL or if the interruption is necessary to establish the cause of the hyperbilirubinemia. Total serum bilirubin levels may reach 12 to 20 mg/dL and persist up to 2 months. In cases of breast milk jaundice, within 24 to 36 hours after breastfeeding is discontinued the newborn's serum bilirubin levels begin to fall dramatically. With resumption of breastfeeding, the bilirubin concentration may have a slight rise of 2 to 3 mg/dL, with a subsequent decline (Table 23–3).

Clinical Tip

Encourage and support mothers who desire to breastfeed their newborns. Assist and instruct them on how to pump and express milk during the interrupted breastfeeding period. Reassure them that nothing is wrong with their milk or mothering abilities.

TABLE 23–3 Factors in Physiologic, Breast Milk, and Breastfeeding Jaundice

Physiologic Jaundice

- Physiologic jaundice occurs after the first 24 hours of life.
- During the first week of life, bilirubin should not exceed 13 mg/dL. Some pediatricians allow levels up to 15 mg/dL.
- Bilirubin levels peak at 3–5 days in term newborns.

Breast Milk Jaundice

- Bilirubin levels begin to rise after the first week of life when mature breast milk comes in.
- A peak of 5–10 mg/dL is reached at 2–3 weeks of age.
- It may be necessary to interrupt breastfeeding for a short period when bilirubin reaches 20 mg/dL.

Breastfeeding Jaundice

- Bilirubin levels rise after the first 24 hours of age.
- Levels peak on the third or fourth day of life and decline through the first month to normal levels.
- The incidence can be decreased by increasing the number of breastfeeding episodes to 8–12 in 24 hours.

Gastrointestinal Adaptations

By 36 to 38 weeks' gestation, the gastrointestinal system is adequately mature, with enzymatic activity and the ability to transport nutrients.

Digestion and Absorption

Birth represents a dramatic change of nutrition from a fetal diet rich in carbohydrates and poor in fat to a neonatal diet rich in fat and poor in carbohydrates. As soon as lactation is initiated, the newborn receives a high-fat, low-carbohydrate diet because colostrum and the initial milk are rich in fat and poor in lactose.

The full-term newborn has sufficient intestinal and pancreatic enzymes to digest most simple carbohydrates, proteins, and fats. The carbohydrates requiring digestion in the newborn are usually disaccharides (lactose, maltose, sucrose), which are split into monosaccharides (galactose, fructose, and glucose) by the enzymes of the intestinal mucosa. Lactose is the primary carbohydrate in the breastfeeding newborn and is generally easily digested and well absorbed. The only enzyme lacking is pancreatic amylase, which remains relatively deficient during the first few months of life. Newborns have trouble digesting starches (changing more complex carbohydrates into maltose) so they should not eat solids until after the first 6 months of life.

Although proteins require more digestion than carbohydrates, they are well digested and absorbed from the newborn intestine. The newborn digests and absorbs fats less efficiently because of the minimal activity of the pancreatic enzyme lipase. The newborn excretes about 10% to 20% of the dietary fat intake compared with 10% for the adult. The newborn absorbs the fat in breast milk more completely than the fat in cows' milk because breast milk consists of more medium-chain triglycerides and contains lipase. (See Chapter 25 for further discussion of newborn nutrition.) Following intestinal absorption, nutrients are delivered to the liver by the portal blood and directly delivered to the peripheral tissues (Lalles, 2012).

Healthy People 2020

(MICH-21) Increase the proportion of infants who are breastfed

The fetal gastrointestinal tract is sterile. Microbes begin to establish as soon as the newborn's oral mucosa is exposed to the environment. The gastrointestinal microbiota is important in the development of immune tolerance to allergens. The mode of delivery sets the pattern of gastrointestinal tract colonization. Babies born by vaginal delivery become colonized by microbes present in the birth canal and mother's gastrointestinal tract, whereas babies born by cesarean section are initially colonized by skin flora (Sim et al., 2012). The establishment and type of feeding are major factors influencing the composition of gastrointestinal tract microbes. Formula-fed infants have elevated levels of the bacteria *Clostridia* and *Bacteroides*, while the microbiota of the breastfed infant has abundant *Bifidobacteria* due to natural prebiotics in human breast milk (Sim et al., 2012). Breast milk confers significant anti-infective benefits.

By birth, the newborn has experienced swallowing, gastric emptying, and intestinal propulsion. In utero, fetal swallowing is accompanied by gastric emptying and peristalsis of the fetal intestinal tract. By the end of gestation, peristalsis becomes much more active in preparation for extrauterine life. Fetal peristalsis is also stimulated by hypoxia, causing the expulsion of meconium into the amniotic fluid in postterm fetuses.

Air enters the stomach immediately after birth. The small intestine is filled with air within 2 to 12 hours and the large bowel within 24 hours. The salivary glands are immature at birth, and the newborn produces little saliva until about 3 months of age. The newborn's stomach can hold 50 to 60 mL. It empties intermittently, starting within a few minutes of the beginning of a feeding and ending 2 to 4 hours after feeding. Bowel sounds are present within the first 30 to 60 minutes of birth, and the newborn can successfully feed during this time. The newborn's gastric pH becomes less acidic about a week after birth and remains less acidic than that of adults for the next 2 to 3 months.

The cardiac sphincter is immature, as is neural control of the stomach, so some regurgitation may be noted in the neonatal period. Continuous vomiting or regurgitation should be monitored closely and reported promptly, as it may be indicative of a more serious problem. Bilious vomiting is abnormal and must be evaluated thoroughly because it might represent a condition that warrants prompt surgical intervention.

Adequate digestion and absorption are essential for newborn growth and development. If optimal nutritional support is available, postnatal growth should parallel intrauterine growth; that is, after 30 weeks' gestation, the fetus gains 30.0 g (1.05 oz) per day and adds 1.2 cm (0.5 in.) to body length daily. To gain weight at the intrauterine rate, the term newborn requires 120 cal/kg/day. After birth, caloric intake is often insufficient for weight gain until the newborn is 5 to 10 days old. During this time, there may be a weight loss of 5% to 10% in term newborns. A shift of intracellular water to extracellular space and insensible water loss accounts for the weight loss; thus failure to lose weight when caloric intake is inadequate may indicate fluid retention.

Clinical Reasoning **Newborn Weight Loss**

Jonathon Sykes is a 5-day-old term male newborn who has returned to the hospital for a lactation visit. Jonathon's birth weight was 3260 g (7 lb, 3 oz) and his current weight is 2963 g (6 lb, 8.5 oz). The lactation nurse is worried about this weight loss, and shares her concerns with Jonathon's mother. What would you tell Jonathon's mother about his weight loss since birth? What are other questions you might ask Jonathon's mother about his intake and output habits? Based on his birth weight, what is the appropriate number of kilocalories that Jonathon needs to take in?

Elimination

Term newborns usually pass meconium within 24 hours of life and almost always within 48 hours. **Meconium** is formed in utero from the amniotic fluid and its constituents, intestinal secretions, and shed mucosal cells. It is recognized by its thick, tarry black or dark green appearance. Transitional (thin brown to green) stools consisting of part meconium and part fecal material are passed for the next day or two, and then the stools become entirely fecal. Generally, the stools of a breastfed newborn are pale yellow (but may be pasty green); they are more liquid and more frequent than those of formula-fed newborns, whose stools are paler and often the consistency of peanut butter (see Figure 25–24). Frequency of bowel movement varies but ranges from one every 2 to 3 days to as many as 10 daily. Mothers should be counseled that the newborn is not constipated as long as the bowel movement remains soft. Table 23–4 summarizes the newborn's physiologic adaptation to extrauterine life.

Urinary Tract Adaptations

Kidney Development and Function

In utero, the placenta is the organ responsible for fluid and electrolyte homeostasis. After birth, the kidney assumes the role of regulation. The kidney is structurally developed with a full complement of functioning nephrons by 34 to 36 weeks of gestation.

Glomerular filtration occurs as blood passes through the capillaries and plasma is filtered through the glomerular capillary walls. Filtrate is collected in the Bowman space and the tubules, where composition is modified until it is excreted as urine. Glomerular filtration rate (GFR) doubles in the first 2 weeks of life in term neonates to 30 to 40 mL/minute (Parker, 2014). The neonate's ability to dilute urine is fully developed, but concentrating ability is limited (Parker, 2014). A major function of the kidney is to maintain osmolality of extracellular fluid within the narrow range compatible with optimal cellular function. The ability to concentrate urine fully is attained by 3 months of age. Feeding practices may affect the osmolarity of the urine but have limited effect on concentration of the urine.

Characteristics of Newborn Urinary Function

Many newborns void immediately after birth, and the voiding frequently goes unnoticed. Among normal newborns, 90% void by 24 hours after birth and 99% void by 48 hours after birth (Cloherty et al., 2012). A newborn who has not voided by 48 hours should be assessed for adequacy of fluid intake, bladder distention, restlessness, and symptoms of pain. The appropriate clinical personnel should be notified if indicated.

The initial bladder volume is 6 to 44 mL of urine. Unless edema is present, normal urinary output is often limited, and the voidings are scanty until fluid intake increases. (The fluid of edema is eliminated by the kidneys, so newborns with edema have a much higher urinary output.) The first 2 days postnatally, the newborn voids two to six times daily, with a urine output of 15 mL/kg/day. The newborn subsequently voids 5 to 25 times every 24 hours, with a volume of 25 mL/kg/day. Observation and documentation of adequate output are a component of transitional care.

Following the first voiding, the newborn's urine frequently appears cloudy (because of mucus content) and has a high specific gravity, which decreases as fluid intake increases. Occasionally, pink stains ("brick dust spots") appear on the diaper. These are caused by urates and are innocuous. Blood may occasionally be observed on the diapers of female newborns. This *pseudomenstruation* is related to the withdrawal of maternal hormones. Males may have bloody spotting from a circumcision if performed. In the absence of apparent causes for bleeding, the clinician should be notified. During early infancy, normal urine is straw colored and almost odorless, although odor occurs when certain drugs are given, metabolic disorders exist, or infection is present. Table 23–5 contains urinalysis values for the normal newborn.

Immunologic Adaptations

Neonatal defense against infections in utero or after delivery is dependent on maternal immunity because neonates lack immunologic memory and often have slower capacities to develop immune responses (Futata, Fusaro, de Brito, et al., 2012). Maternal–fetal infection transmission (transplacental, perinatal, postnatal) is a major cause of morbidity and mortality in newborns. Also limitations in the newborn's inflammatory response result in failure to recognize, localize, and destroy invasive bacteria and viruses. Thus the signs and symptoms of infection are often subtle and nonspecific in the newborn. The newborn also has a poor hypothalamic response to pyrogens; therefore, fever is not a reliable indicator of infection. In the neonatal period, hypothermia is a more reliable sign of infection. (Futata et al., 2012).

Components of the immune system include both nonspecific mechanisms and specific immune responses. Nonspecific immune mechanisms include phagocytosis, inflammatory response, complement, and coagulation. These nonspecific immune mechanisms function without prior exposure, can be

---

TABLE 23–4 Physiologic Adaptations to Extrauterine Life

- Periodic breathing may be present.

- Desired axillary temperature of 36.5° to 37.5°C (97.7°–99.5°F) stabilizes 4–6 hr after birth for term newborn (Cloherty et al., 2012).

- Desired blood glucose level reaches 60–70 mg/dL by third postnatal day.

- Stools progress from (for detailed discussion see Chapter 25):

  - Meconium (thick, tarry, black; meconium plug may be expelled)

  - Transitional stools (thin, brown to green)

  - Breastfed newborns (yellow-gold, soft or mushy)

  - Formula-fed newborns (pale yellow, formed, and pasty)

TABLE 23–5 Newborn Urinalysis Values

Protein less than 5–10 mg/dL
WBC less than 2–3/hpf
RBC 0
Casts 0
Bacteria 0
Color pale yellow

identified early in gestation, and reach functional development at 32 to 33 weeks' gestation.

The specific immune responses consist of cell-mediated (T cell) and humoral (B cell) systems. The maturation of specific immune responses begins in utero at about 7 to 12 weeks' gestation. The newborn's immune system has a decreased ability to develop effective antibody responses. Humoral immunity is a specific antibody-mediated response that functions most effectively if there has been recent exposure.

Of the three major types of immunoglobulins that are primarily involved in immunity—IgG, IgA, and IgM—only IgG crosses the placenta. The pregnant woman forms antibodies in response to illness or immunization. This process is called **active acquired immunity**. When IgG antibodies are transferred to the fetus in utero, **passive acquired immunity** results because the fetus does not produce the antibodies itself. IgG antibodies are very active against bacterial toxins.

Because the maternal IgG is transferred primarily during the third trimester, preterm newborns (especially those born before 34 weeks' gestation) may be more susceptible to infection. In general, newborns have immunity to tetanus, diphtheria, smallpox, measles, mumps, poliomyelitis, and a variety of other bacterial and viral diseases. The period of resistance varies: Immunity against common viral infections such as measles may last 4 to 8 months, whereas immunity to certain bacteria may disappear within 4 to 8 weeks.

IgM antibodies are produced in response to blood group antigens, gram-negative enteric organisms, and some viruses in the expectant mother. Because IgM does not normally cross the placenta, most or all of it is produced by the fetus beginning at 10 to 15 weeks' gestation. Elevated levels of IgM at birth may indicate placental leaks or, more commonly, antigenic stimulation in utero. Consequently, elevations suggest that the newborn was exposed to an intrauterine infection such as syphilis or TORCH syndrome (toxoplasmosis, rubella, cytomegalovirus, herpesvirus hominis type 2 infection). (For further discussion, see Chapter 15.) The lack of available maternal IgM in the newborn also accounts for the susceptibility to gram-negative enteric organisms such as *Escherichia coli*.

IgA immunoglobulins appear to provide protection mainly on secreting surfaces such as the respiratory tract, gastrointestinal tract, and eyes. Serum IgA does not cross the placenta and is not normally produced by the fetus in utero. Colostrum, the forerunner of breast milk, is very high in the secretory form of IgA. Consequently, it may be of significance in providing some passive immunity to the newborn of a breastfeeding mother.

It is customary to begin the majority of routine immunizations at 2 months of age so that the infant can develop active acquired immunity. Some immunizations for specific viruses (such as hepatitis B) are even given the first day after birth. (See discussion of newborn immunization in Chapter 25.)

Neurologic Adaptation

The newborn's brain is about one quarter the size of an adult's, and myelination of nerve fibers is incomplete. Unlike the cardiovascular and respiratory systems, which undergo tremendous changes at birth, the nervous system is minimally influenced by the actual birth process. Because many biochemical and histologic changes have yet to occur in the newborn's brain, the postnatal period is considered a time of risk with regard to the development of the brain and nervous system. For neurologic development—including development of intellect—to proceed, the brain and other nervous system structures must mature in an orderly, unhampered fashion. (For discussion of cranial nerves, see Chapter 24.)

Intrauterine Environment Influence on Newborn Behavior

Newborns respond to and interact with the environment in a predictable pattern of behavior that is somewhat shaped by their intrauterine experience. This intrauterine experience is affected by intrinsic factors such as maternal nutrition and external factors such as the mother's physical environment. Depending on the newborn's temperament, neonatal behavioral responses to different stresses vary. Some newborns react quietly to stimulation, others become overreactive and tense, and some may exhibit a combination of the two.

Factors such as exposure to intense auditory stimuli in utero can eventually be manifested in the behavior of the newborn. For example, the fetal heart rate (FHR) initially increases when the pregnant woman is exposed to auditory stimuli, but repetition of the stimuli leads to decreased FHR. Thus the newborn who was exposed to intense noise during fetal life is significantly less reactive to loud sounds postnatally.

Characteristics of Newborn Neurologic Function

Normal newborns are usually in a position of partially flexed extremities with the legs near the abdomen. When awake, the newborn may exhibit purposeless, uncoordinated bilateral movements of the extremities. The organization and quality of the newborn's motor activity are influenced by a number of factors, including the following (Brazelton & Nugent, 2011):

- Sleep-alert states
- Presence of environmental stimuli, such as heat, light, cold, and noise
- Conditions causing a chemical imbalance, such as hypoglycemia
- Hydration status
- State of health
- Recovery from the stress of labor and birth

The newborn's body growth progresses in a cephalocaudal (head-to-toe), proximal–distal fashion. The newborn is somewhat hypertonic; that is, there is resistance to extending the elbow and knee joints. Muscle tone should be symmetric. Diminished muscle tone and flaccidity may indicate neurologic dysfunction.

Reflexes, including the Moro, grasping, Babinski, rooting, and sucking reflexes, are characteristic of neurologic integrity. (For discussion of reflexes, see Chapter 24.) Complex behavioral patterns reflect the newborn's neurologic maturation and integration. A newborn who can bring a hand to the mouth may be demonstrating motor coordination as well as a self-quieting technique, thus increasing the complexity of the behavioral response. **Self-quieting ability** is the ability of newborns to use their own resources to quiet and comfort themselves.

Habituation is the newborn's ability to process and respond to complex stimulation. For example, when a bright light is flashed into the newborn's eyes, the initial response is blinking, constriction of the pupil, and perhaps a slight startle reaction. However, with repeated stimulation, the newborn's responses gradually diminish and disappear. The capacity to ignore repetitive disturbing stimuli is a defense mechanism readily allowing the newborn to shut out overwhelming and disturbing stimuli. Sensory abilities include visual, auditory, olfactory, taste, and tactile capacities.

Periods of Reactivity

The newborn usually shows a predictable pattern of behavior during the first several hours after birth, characterized by two **periods of reactivity** separated by a sleep phase.

FIRST PERIOD OF REACTIVITY

The first period of reactivity lasts approximately 30 minutes after birth. During this period the newborn is awake and active and may appear hungry and have a strong sucking reflex. This is the natural and best opportunity to initiate breastfeeding if the mother has chosen it. Bursts of random, diffuse movements alternating with relative immobility may occur. Respirations are rapid, as high as 80 breaths per minute, and there may be retraction of the chest, transient flaring of the nares, and grunting. The heart rate is rapid, and the rhythm may be irregular. Bowel sounds are usually absent.

PERIOD OF INACTIVITY TO SLEEP PHASE

After approximately half an hour the newborn's activity gradually diminishes, and the heart rate and respirations decrease as the newborn enters the sleep phase. The sleep phase may last from a few minutes to 2 to 4 hours. During this period, the newborn will be difficult to awaken and will show no interest in sucking. Bowel sounds become audible, and cardiac and respiratory rates return to baseline values.

SECOND PERIOD OF REACTIVITY

During the second period of reactivity, the newborn is again awake and alert. This period lasts 4 to 6 hours in the normal newborn. Physiologic responses are variable during this stage. The heart and respiratory rates increase; however, the nurse must be alert for apneic periods, which may cause a drop in the heart rate and oxygen level (desaturation). The newborn is stimulated to continue breathing during such times. The newborn may develop rapid color changes and become mildly cyanotic or mottled during these fluctuations. Production of respiratory and gastric mucus increases, and the newborn responds by gagging, choking, and regurgitating.

SAFETY ALERT!

Because babies are often unable to handle oral secretions effectively enough to protect their airway, parents must be instructed in the proper use of the bulb syringe. The bulb syringe used correctly creates mild suction for removal of oral and nasal secretions. Overuse or vigorous use of the bulb syringe causes unnecessary trauma and inflammation of the small nasal airways resulting in swelling and partial airway obstruction. See Performing Nasal Pharyngeal Suctioning, in the *Clinical Skills Manual* SKILLS.

Continued close observation and intervention may be required to maintain a clear airway during this period of reactivity. The gastrointestinal tract becomes more active. The newborn often passes the first meconium stool and may also have an initial voiding. The newborn will indicate readiness for feeding by such behaviors as sucking, rooting, and swallowing. If feeding was not initiated in the first period of reactivity, it is done at this time. (See Chapter 25 for further discussion of this first feeding.)

Behavioral States of the Newborn

The behavior of the newborn can be divided into three categories: the sleep state, the transitional state, and the alert state (McGrath & Vittner, 2015). These postnatal behavioral states are similar to those that have been identified during pregnancy. Subcategories are identified under each major category.

SLEEP STATES

The sleep states are as follows:

1. *Deep or quiet sleep.* Deep or quiet sleep is characterized by closed eyes with no eye movements; regular, even breathing; and jerky motions or startles at regular intervals. Behavioral responses to external stimuli are likely to be delayed. Startles are rapidly suppressed, and changes in state are not likely to occur. Heart rate may range from 100 to 120 beats per minute.

2. *Active or light sleep (rapid eye movement [REM] sleep).* The baby has irregular respirations; eyes closed, with REM; irregular sucking motions; minimal activity; and irregular but smooth movement of the extremities. Environmental and internal stimuli may initiate a startle reaction and a change of state.

Newborn sleep cycles have been recognized and defined according to duration. The length of the sleep cycle depends on the age of the newborn. At term, REM active sleep and quiet sleep occur in intervals of 50 to 60 minutes (Gardner, Goldson, & Hernandez, 2016). About 45% to 50% of the newborn's total sleep is active sleep, 35% to 45% is quiet sleep, and 10% is transitional between these two periods. Growth hormone secretion depends on regular sleep patterns. Any disturbance of the sleep–wake cycle can result in irregular spikes of growth hormone. REM sleep stimulates the highest peaks of growth hormone and the growth of the neural system. Over time, the newborn's sleep–wake patterns become diurnal; that is, the newborn sleeps at night and stays awake during the day. (See *Assessment of Neurologic Status* in Chapter 24 for a short discussion of Brazelton's assessment of newborn states.)

ALERT STATES

In the first 30 to 60 minutes after birth, many newborns display a quiet alert state, characteristic of the first period of reactivity (Figure 23–8). Nurses should use these alert states to encourage bonding and breastfeeding. These periods of alertness tend to be short the first 2 days after birth to allow the baby to recover from the birth process. Subsequent alert states are of choice or of necessity. Increasing choice of wakefulness by the newborn

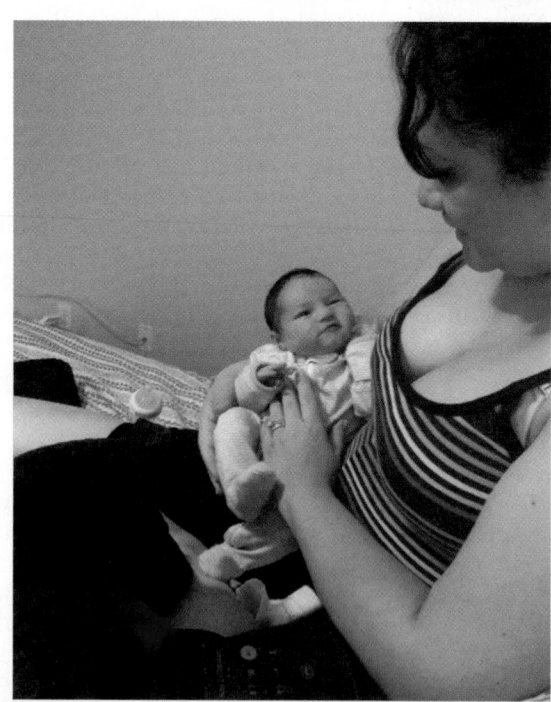

Figure 23–8 **Mother and baby gaze at each other. This quiet alert state is the optimal state for interaction.**

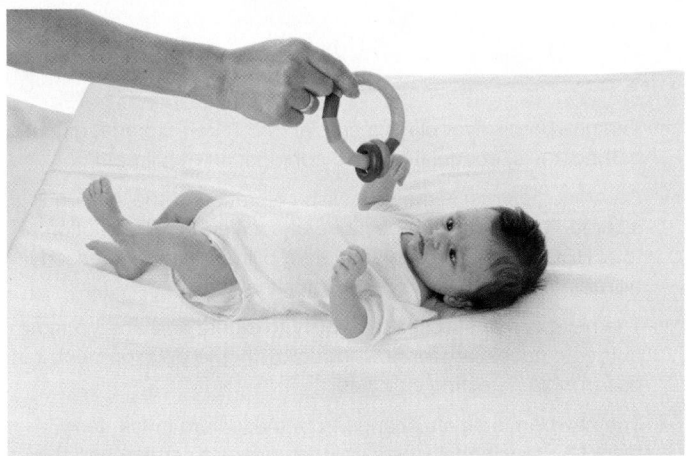

Figure 23–9 **Newborn in active alert state turning his head to follow an object.**

indicates a maturing capacity to achieve and maintain consciousness. Heat, cold, and hunger are but a few of the stimuli that can cause wakefulness by necessity. Once the disturbing stimuli are removed, the newborn tends to fall back asleep.

The following are subcategories of the alert state (McGrath & Vittner, 2015).

1. *Drowsiness.* The behaviors common to the drowsy state are open or closed eyes; fluttering eyelids; semidozing appearance; and slow, regular movements of the extremities. Mild startles may be noted from time to time. Although the reaction to a sensory stimulus is delayed, a change of state often results.

2. *Quiet alert.* In the wide-awake state, the newborn is alert and follows and fixates on attractive objects, faces, or auditory stimuli. Motor activity is minimal, and the response to external stimuli is delayed.

3. *Active alert.* In the active alert awake state, the newborn's eyes are open and motor activity is quite intense, with thrusting movements of the extremities. Environmental stimuli increase startles or motor activity, but individual reactions are difficult to distinguish because of the generally high activity level (Figure 23–9).

4. *Crying.* Intense crying is accompanied by jerky motor movements. Crying serves several purposes for the newborn. It may be a distraction from disturbing stimuli such as hunger and pain. Fussiness often allows the newborn to discharge energy and reorganize behavior. Most important, crying elicits an appropriate response of help from the parents.

Sensory Capacities of the Newborn

VISUAL CAPACITY

Orientation is the newborn's ability to notice, to follow, and to fixate on appealing and attractive complex visual stimuli. The newborn prefers the human face and eyes and bright shiny objects. As the face or object comes into the line of vision, the newborn responds with bright, wide eyes, still limbs, and fixed staring. This intense visual involvement may last several minutes, during which time the newborn is able to follow the stimulus from side to side. The newborn uses this sensory capacity to become familiar with family, friends, and surroundings.

AUDITORY CAPACITY

The newborn responds to auditory stimulation with a definite, organized behavior repertoire. During all interactions, care providers should observe the neonate's response to sound. The stimulus used to assess auditory response should be selected to match the state of the newborn. A rattle is appropriate for light sleep, a voice for an awake state, and a clap for deep sleep. As the newborn hears the sound, the cardiac rate rises, and a minimal startle reflex may be seen. If the sound is appealing, the newborn will become alert and search for the site of the auditory stimulus. Newborns prefer the sound of the human voice to nonhuman sounds. The newborn's hearing should be evaluated prior to discharge. (See Chapter 25 for discussion of newborn hearing screening tests.)

Healthy People 2020

(ENT-VSL-1) Increase the proportion of newborns who are screened for hearing loss by no later than age 1 month, have audiologic evaluation by age 3 months, and are enrolled in appropriate intervention services no later than age 6 months

---

OLFACTORY CAPACITY

Newborns can select their mother by smell and are apparently able to select people by smell (Lehtonen, 2015). Newborns are able to distinguish their mothers' breast pads from those of other mothers at just 1 week postnatally and will preferentially turn toward the smell of the mother.

TASTE AND SUCKING

The newborn responds differently to varying tastes and can distinguish between sweet and sour at 3 days of age. Sugar, for example, increases sucking. While breastfeeding, the newborn sucks in bursts, with frequent regular pauses. The bottle-fed newborn tends to suck at a regular rate, with infrequent pauses.

When awake and hungry, the newborn displays rapid searching motions in response to the rooting reflex. Once feeding begins, the newborn establishes a sucking pattern according to the method of feeding. Finger sucking is seen in utero as well as after birth. The newborn frequently uses nonnutritive sucking as a self-quieting activity, which assists in the development of self-regulation.

TACTILE CAPACITY

The newborn is very sensitive to being touched, cuddled, and held. Often a mother's first response to an upset or crying newborn is touching or holding. Swaddling, placing a hand on the abdomen, or holding the arms to prevent a startle reflex are other methods of soothing the newborn. The quieted newborn is then able to attend to and interact with the environment. Touch is also used to rouse a drowsy newborn, making the baby more alert for feeding.

TEACHING HIGHLIGHTS | Newborn/Infant Crying

While the mother and newborn are in the hospital, the nurse has a perfect opportunity to teach parents techniques to deal with newborn/infant crying and fussiness. It is important for parents and caregivers to know that for the first several months crying is the only means of communication available to the baby and usually signifies unmet needs.

Focus Your Study

- Newborn respiration is initiated primarily by chemical, mechanical, and reabsorptive processes associated with thermal and sensory stimulation.

- The production of surfactant is crucial to keeping the lungs expanded during expiration by reducing alveolar surface tension.

- Onset of respirations stimulates cardiovascular changes: Air enters the lungs; oxygen content rises in alveoli and stimulates relaxation of pulmonary arteries. This leads to a decrease in pulmonary vascular resistance, which allows complete vascular flow to the lungs. With increased oxygenated pulmonary blood flow and loss of the placenta, systemic blood flow increases and the foramen ovale and ductus arteriosus begin to close.

- The newborn is an obligatory nose breather. Respirations move from being primarily shallow, irregular, and diaphragmatic to synchronous abdominal and chest breathing.

- Normal respiratory rate is 30 to 60 breaths per minute.

- The status of the cardiopulmonary system may be measured by evaluating the heart rate, blood pressure, and presence or absence of murmurs. The normal heart rate is 80 to 160 beats/min.

- Oxygen transport in the newborn is significantly affected by the presence of greater amounts of HbF (fetal hemoglobin) than HbA (adult hemoglobin). HbF holds oxygen more efficiently but releases it to the body tissues only at low PO_2 levels.

- Newborn blood values are affected by: Gestational age, prenatal and/or perinatal hemorrhage, site of the blood drawing, and timing of the clamping of the umbilical cord.

- Thermoregulation in the newborn is closely related to the rate of metabolism and oxygen consumption

- Evaporation is the primary heat loss mechanism in newborns who are wet from amniotic fluid or a bath. In addition, excessive heat loss occurs from radiation and convection because of the newborn's larger surface area compared with weight and from thermal conduction because of the marked difference between core temperature and skin temperature.

- The primary source for heat production in the cold-stressed newborn is brown adipose tissue.

- By secreting glucagon and suppressing insulin release, the newborn gradually mobilizes glucose to meet energy needs.

- The newborn's liver plays a crucial role in iron storage, glucose homeostasis, coagulation, and conjugation of bilirubin

- Jaundice (icterus) is the yellowish coloration of the skin and sclerae. It may develop because of accelerated destruction of fetal RBCs, impaired conjugation of bilirubin, and increased bilirubin reabsorption from the intestinal tract.

- The newborn possesses the ability to digest and absorb most nutrients necessary for newborn growth and development, but has trouble digesting starches.

- The newborn's stools change from meconium (thick, tarry, black) to transitional stools (thinner, brown to green) and then to the distinct forms for either breastfed newborns (yellow-gold, soft, or mushy) or formula-fed newborns (pale yellow, formed, and pasty). Most newborns pass their first stool within 24 to 48 hours of birth.

- The newborn's kidneys are characterized by a decreased rate of glomerular flow, limited tubular reabsorption, limited excretion of solutes, and limited ability to concentrate urine. Most newborns void within 24 hours of birth.

- The immune system in the newborn is not fully activated until it begins to produce its own immunity at about 4 weeks of age. The newborn does possess some immunologic abilities and has passive immunity from the mother, lasting from 4 weeks to 8 months.

- Neurologic functioning in the newborn is evident from the newborn's interaction with the environment, presence of synchronized motor activity, and well-developed sensory capacities.

- The first period of reactivity lasts for 30 minutes after birth. The newborn is alert and hungry at this time, making this a natural opportunity to promote attachment.

- The second period of reactivity requires close monitoring by the nurse because apnea, decreased heart rate, gagging, choking, and regurgitation are likely to occur and require nursing intervention.

- Behavioral states in the newborn can be divided into sleep states and alert states.

- Sensory and perceptual development proceeds in a specific order: tactile/vestibular, olfactory/gustatory, and auditory/visual.

- Some of the behavioral capabilities of the newborn that assist in adaptation to extrauterine life include self-quieting ability and habitation.

Clinical Reasoning in Action

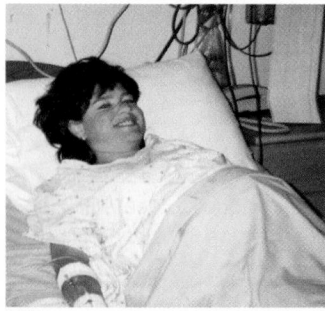

Sandra Dee, a 21-year-old, G1P0, at 36 weeks' gestation, has been in labor for the last 12 hours and is fully dilated with caput visible on the perineum. The fetal heart rate is 148 to 152 with early deceleration down to 142 with contraction and pushing. Her contractions are 4 to 5 minutes apart and of good quality. Sandra's mother and sister are present for the birth. Her prenatal record shows no significant pregnancy problems or complications, and her vital signs have been stable within normal limits. Sandra has received 2 doses of Stadol for a total of 2 mg IV for pain relief during her labor. The last dose was given 2 hours ago. You assist with the vaginal birth of a live baby without an episiotomy. You observe the sex and time as the midwife places the newborn girl on the mother's abdomen, suctions out the baby's mouth and nose, and proceeds to clamp the cord. You dry and stimulate the newborn to breathe, remove the wet blanket and replace it with a dry one, and place the baby skin-to-skin on the mother's chest. You assess the need for resuscitation. The baby has a lusty cry spontaneously less than 30 seconds after birth. You palpate the cord, obtaining a heart rate of 120, and observe that the baby's chest and face are pink, and the legs and arms are flexed with open fists.

1. Explain the changes that must occur in the newborn's cardiopulmonary system at birth.

2. What criteria do you look for when you assess the newborn for adequate cardiopulmonary adaptation at birth?

3. What steps do you take to maintain a neutral thermal environment at birth?

4. Sandra plans to breastfeed. When would you initiate the first feeding?

5. Discuss nursing actions that can decrease the probability of high bilirubin levels in the newborn.

References

American College of Obstetricians and Gynecologists (ACOG). (2012, reaffirmed 2014). Timing of umbilical cord clamping after birth. *Committee on Obstetric Practice, 120*(6).

Association of Women's Health, Obstetric and Neonatal Nurses (AWHONN). (2005, reaffirmed 2009). *Clinical position statement: Universal screening for hyperbilirubinemia.* Washington, DC: Author.

Bagwell, G. A. (2014). Hematologic system. In C. Kenner & J. W. Lott (Eds.), *Comprehensive neonatal nursing care* (5th ed., pp. 334–375). New York, NY: Springer.

Bhutani, V. K., Vilms, R. J., & Hamerman-Johnson, L. (2010). Universal bilirubin screening for severe neonatal hyperbilirubinemia. *Journal of Perinatology, 30,* S6–S15.

Blackburn, S. T. (2013). *Maternal, fetal, & neonatal physiology: A clinical perspective* (4th ed.). St. Louis, MO: Saunders.

Brazelton, T. B., & Nugent, J. K. (2011). *The neonatal behavioral assessment scale* (4th ed.). London, England: MacKeith.

Cloherty, J. R., Eichenwald, E. C., Hansen, A. R., & Stark, A. R. (2012). *Manual of neonatal care* (7th ed.). Philadelphia, PA: Lippincott Williams & Wilkins.

Diab, Y., & Luchtman-Jones, L., (2015). The blood and hematopoietic system. In R. J. Martin, A. A. Fanaroff, & M. C. Walsh (Eds.), *Fanaroff & Martin's neonatal-perinatal medicine* (10th ed., pp. 1294–1343). St. Louis, MO: Elsevier Mosby.

Fraser, D. (2014). Newborn adaptation to extrauterine life. In K. R. Simpson & P. A. Creehan (Eds.). *Perinatal nursing* (4th ed., pp.581–596). Philadelphia, PA: Lippincott Williams & Wilkins

Futata, E. A., Fusaro, A. E., de Brito, C. A., & Sato, M. N. (2012). The neonatal immune system: Immunomodulation of infections in early life. *Expert Reviews: Anti-Infective Therapies 10*(3), 289–298.

Gardner, S. L., Goldson, E., & Hernandez, J. A. (2016). The neonate and the environment: Impact on development. In S. L. Gardner, B. S. Carter, M. Enzman-Hines, & J. A. Hernandez (Eds.), *Merenstein & Gardner's handbook of neonatal intensive care* (8th ed., pp. 262–314). St. Louis, MO: Mosby.

Glomella, T. L. (Ed.). (2013). *Neonatology: Management, procedures, on-call problems, diseases, and drugs* (7th ed.). New York, NY: McGraw-Hill Education.

Graves, B. W., & Haley, M. M. (2013). Newborn transition. *Journal of Midwifery & Women's Health. 58* (6), 662–670.

Hardy, W., D'Agata, A., & McGrath, J. M. (2016). The infant at risk. In S. Mattson & J. E. Smith (Eds.), *Core curriculum for maternal-newborn nursing* (5th ed., pp. 363–416). St. Louis, MO: Saunders.

Katheria, A. C., Truong, G., Cousins, L., Oshiro, B., & Finer, N. N. (2015). Umbilical cord milking versus delayed cord clamping in preterm infants. *Pediatrics 136* (1), 61–69. doi:10.1542/peds.2015-0368.

Lalles, J. P. (2012). Long term effects of pre- and early postnatal nutrition and environment on the gut. *Journal of Animal Science, 90,* 421–429.

Lauderdale, J. (2012). Transcultural perspectives in childbearing. In M. M. Andrews & J. S. Boyle (Eds.), *Transcultural concepts in nursing care* (6th ed., pp. 91–122). Philadelphia, PA: Wolters Kluwer/Lippincott Williams & Wilkins.

Lehtonen, L. (2015). Assessment and optimization of neurobehavioral development in preterm infant. In R. J. Martin, A. A. Fanaroff, & M. C. Walsh (Eds.), *Fanaroff & Martin's neonatal-perinatal medicine* (10th ed., pp. 1001–1017). St. Louis, MO: Elsevier Mosby.

McGrath, J. M., & Vittner, D. (2015). Behavioral assessment. In E. P. Tappero & M. E. Honeyfield (Eds.), *Physical assessment of the newborn* (5th ed., pp. 193–219). Petaluma, CA: NICU INK

Parker, L. A. (2014). Genitourinary system. In C. Kenner & J. W. Lott (Eds.), *Comprehensive neonatal nursing care* (5th ed., pp. 472–507). New York, NY: Springer.

Raab, E. L., & Kelly, L. K. (2013). Normal newborn assessment & care. In A. H. Decherney, L. Nathan, N. Laufer, & A. S. Roman (Eds.), *Current diagnosis & treatment: Obstetrics & gynecology* (11th ed., pp. 181–189). New York, NY: McGraw-Hill.

Raju, T. N. (2013). Timing of umbilical cord clamping after birth for optimizing placental transfusion. *Current Opinions in Pediatrics, 25,* 180–187.

Riley, C., Spencer, B., & Prater, L. S. (2014). Normal term newborn. In C. Kenner & J. W. Lott (Eds.), *Comprehensive neonatal nursing care* (5th ed., pp. 113–132). New York, NY: Springer.

Sim, K., Powell, E., Shaw, A. G., McClure, Z., Bangham, M., & Kroll, J. S. (2012). The neonatal gastrointestinal microbiota: The foundation of future health? *Archives of Diseases of Children: Fetal Neonatal Edition, 98*(4), F362–F364.

Van Woudenberg, C. D., Wills, C. A., & Rubarth, L. B. (2012). Newborn transition to extrauterine life. *Neonatal Network, 31*(5), 317–322.

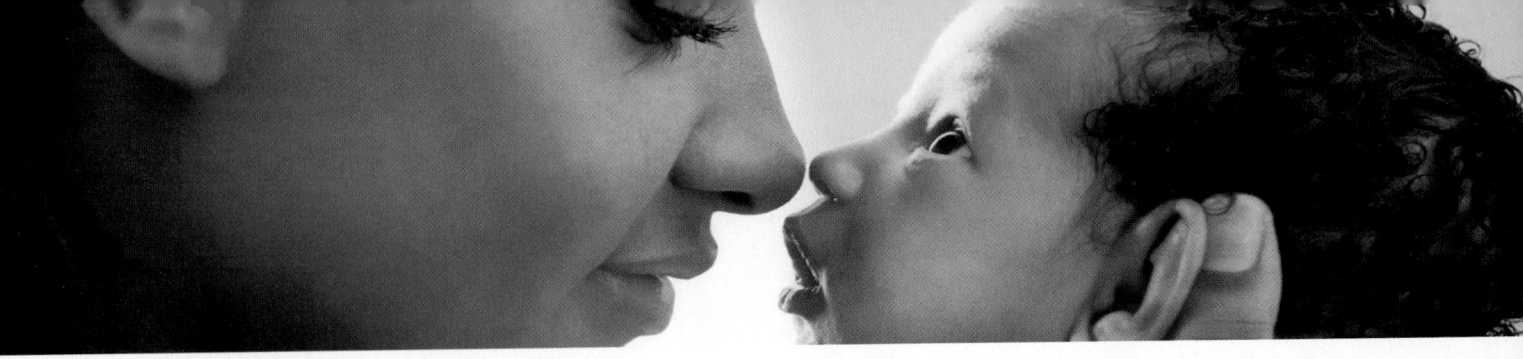

Chapter 24
Nursing Assessment of the Newborn

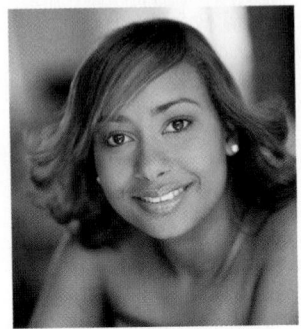

Like most parents, when I held my son for the first time, I checked that all his fingers and toes were present. Then he looked at me with wide, bright, serious eyes and began my introduction to his unique personality.

—Leah, 23

Radius Images/Alamy

⌄ Learning Outcomes

24.1 Describe the physical and neuromuscular maturity characteristics assessed to determine the gestational age of the newborn.

24.2 Summarize the components of a systematic physical assessment of the newborn and the significance of normal variations and abnormal findings.

24.3 Describe the components of a neurologic assessment.

24.4 Describe the neurologic/neuromuscular characteristics of the newborn.

24.5 Identify the reflexes that may be present at birth.

24.6 Correlate normal behavioral characteristics of the newborn with variations that may be present.

24.7 Describe how to use the assessment procedure and results of the newborn physical and the neurologic and behavioral assessments to teach and involve the parents in their baby's care and to allay their concerns.

Newborns communicate their needs primarily by behavior. Because nurses are the most consistent professional observers of the newborn, they can translate this behavior into information about a newborn's condition and respond with appropriate nursing interventions. This chapter focuses on the assessment of the newborn and the interpretation of these findings.

Newborn assessment is a continuous process designed to evaluate development and adjustments to extrauterine life. In the birth setting, the Apgar scoring procedure and careful observation form the basis of assessment and are correlated with information such as the following:

- Maternal prenatal history
- Birthing history

- Maternal analgesia and anesthesia
- Complications of labor or birth
- Treatment instituted immediately after birth, in conjunction with determination of clinical gestational age
- Consideration of the classification of newborns by weight and gestational age and by neonatal mortality risk
- Physical examination of the newborn

The nurse incorporates data from these sources with the assessment findings during the first 1 to 4 hours after birth to formulate a plan for nursing intervention.

The various newborn assessments and the data obtained from them are valuable only to the degree to which they are shared with the parents. The parents must be included in the assessment process from the moment of their child's birth. The *Apgar* score and its meaning should be explained immediately to the family (see Chapter 18 for a discussion of the Apgar score). As soon as possible, the parents should take part in the physical and behavioral assessments as well.

The nurse encourages the parents to identify the unique behavioral characteristics of their newborn and to learn nurturing activities. Attachment is promoted when parents have an opportunity to explore their newborn in private, identifying individual physical and behavioral characteristics. The nurse's supportive responses to parents' questions and observations are essential throughout the assessment process. The newborn physical examination is the beginning of newborn health surveillance and health education for the newborn's family that continues into the community setting.

Timing of Newborn Assessments

During the first 24 hours of life, the newborn makes the critical transition from intrauterine to extrauterine life. The risk of mortality and morbidity is statistically high during this period. Assessment of the newborn is essential to ensure that the transition proceeds successfully.

There are major time frames for assessments of newborns while they are in the birth facility.

- *Delivery room disposition.* The first assessment is done in the birthing area immediately after birth to determine the need for resuscitation or other interventions. The stable newborn should stay with the family after birth to initiate early attachment. The newborn with complications is usually taken to the special nursery for further evaluation and intervention.

- *Nursery or couplet care admission examination.* A second assessment may be done by the nursery nurse as part of routine admission procedures. During this assessment, the nurse carries out a brief physical examination to estimate gestational age and evaluate the newborn's adaptation to extrauterine life. No later than 2 hours after birth, the admitting nursery nurse should evaluate the newborn's status and any problems that place the newborn at risk.

- *Before discharge examination.* A certified nurse-midwife (CNM), physician, or nurse practitioner will carry out an examination similar to the well-baby admission examination. This includes a behavioral assessment and additional information from the baby's stay in the birthing unit to assess if the newborn is ready for routine care at home. A complete physical examination is done to detect any emerging or potential problems. When the birthing center stay is short, a combination admission-discharge examination is appropriate.

This chapter presents the procedures for estimating gestational age and performing the complete physical examination and behavioral assessment. Chapter 18 discusses the immediate postbirth assessment. Chapter 25 describes the brief assessment performed during the first 4 hours of life.

Estimation of Gestational Age

The nurse must establish the newborn's gestational age in the first 4 hours after birth so that careful attention can be given to age-related problems. Traditionally, a newborn's gestational age was determined from the date of the pregnant woman's last menstrual period. However, this method was accurate only 75% to 85% of the time. Because of the problems that develop with the preterm newborn or the newborn whose weight is inappropriate for gestational age, a more accurate system was developed to postnatally evaluate the newborn. Once learned, the procedure can be done in a few minutes.

SAFETY ALERT!

It is essential that the nurse wear gloves when assessing the newborn in these early hours after birth and before the first bath until amniotic fluid, vaginal secretions, and blood on the skin are removed.

Clinical **gestational age assessment tools** have two components: (1) external physical characteristics and (2) neurologic or neuromuscular development. Physical characteristics generally include the following:

- Sole creases
- Amount of breast tissue
- Amount of lanugo
- Cartilaginous development of the ear
- Testicular descent and scrotal rugae in the male
- Labial development in the female

These objective clinical criteria are not influenced by labor and birth and do not change significantly within the first 12 hours after birth.

The neurologic examination facilitates assessment of functional or physiologic maturation in addition to physical development. However, the newborn's nervous system is unstable during the first 24 hours of life, therefore neurologic evaluation findings based on reflexes or assessments dependent on the higher brain centers may not be reliable. If the neurologic findings drastically deviate from the gestational age derived by evaluation of external characteristics, a second assessment is done in 24 hours.

The neurologic assessment components (excluding reflexes) can aid in assessing the gestational age of newborns of less than 34 weeks' gestation. Between 26 and 34 weeks, neurologic changes are significant, whereas significant physical changes are less evident. Ballard et al. (1991) developed the *estimation of gestational age by maturity rating*, a simplified version of the well-researched *Dubowitz tool*. The Ballard tool omits some of the neuromuscular tone assessments, which are difficult to assess in very ill newborns or those on respirators, and leg recoil. In the Ballard tool, each physical and neuromuscular finding is given a value, and the total score is matched to a gestational age. The maximum score on the Ballard tool is 50, which corresponds to a gestational age of 44 weeks.

For example, on completion of a gestational assessment of a 1-hour-old newborn, the nurse gives a score of 3 to all the physical characteristics, for a total of 18, and gives a score of 3 to all neuromuscular assessments, for a total of 18. The physical characteristics score of 18 is added to the neurologic score of 18 for a total score of 36, which correlates with 38+ weeks' gestation. Because all newborns vary slightly in the development of physical characteristics and maturation of neurologic function, scores usually vary instead of all being 3, as in this example.

Postnatal gestational age assessment tools can overestimate preterm newborns of less than 28 weeks' gestational age and underestimate postterm or more than 43 weeks' gestation newborns. Ballard et al. (1991) in the **New Ballard Score (NBS)** added criteria for more accurate assessment of the gestational age of newborns between 20 and 28 weeks' gestation and less than 1500 g (3.3 lb). They suggest that the assessments should be made within 12 hours of birth to optimize accuracy, especially in newborns of less than 26 weeks' gestational age. Also, the Ballard assessment may be overstimulating to newborns of less than 27 weeks' gestation (Cavaliere & Sansoucie, 2014). Some maternal conditions, such as preeclampsia, diabetes, and maternal analgesia and anesthesia, may affect certain gestational assessment components and warrant further evaluation. Maternal diabetes, although it appears to accelerate fetal physical growth, seems to retard maturation. Maternal hypertension states, which retard fetal physical growth, seem to speed maturation.

Newborns of women with preeclampsia on magnesium sulfate may have a poor correlation with the neuromuscular criteria involving active muscle tone and edema. Maternal analgesia and anesthesia may cause respiratory depression in the newborn. Babies with respiratory distress syndrome (RDS) tend to be flaccid and edematous and to assume a "froglike" posture (see Chapter 27 for a discussion of RDS). These characteristics affect the scoring of the neuromuscular components of the assessment tool used. The NBS gestational age assessment tool will be used throughout the chapter to demonstrate the assessment of the physical and neuromuscular criteria associated with gestational age.

Assessment of Physical Maturity Characteristics

The nurse first evaluates observable characteristics without disturbing the baby. Selected physical characteristics common to the Dubowitz and Ballard gestational assessment tools are presented here in the order in which they might be most effectively evaluated:

1. *Resting posture*, although a neuromuscular component, should be assessed as the baby lies undisturbed on a flat surface (Figure 24–1).

2. *Skin* in the preterm newborn appears thin and transparent, with veins prominent over the abdomen early in gestation. As the newborn approaches term, the skin appears opaque because of increased subcutaneous tissue. Disappearance of the protective vernix caseosa promotes skin desquamation; this is commonly seen in postmature newborns (more than 42 weeks' gestational age) and those showing signs of placental insufficiency; see Chapter 26 for a discussion of postmature newborns).

3. *Lanugo*, a fine hair covering, decreases as gestational age increases. The amount of **lanugo** is greatest at 28 to 30 weeks and then disappears, first from the face and then from the trunk and extremities. It is most abundant over the back (particularly between the scapulae), although it will be noted over the face, legs, and arms (Figure 24–2).

4. *Sole (plantar) creases* are reliable indicators of gestational age in the first 12 hours of life. Later, the skin of the foot begins drying, and superficial creases appear. Development of sole creases begins at the top (anterior) portion of the sole and, as gestation progresses, proceeds to the heel (Figure 24–3). Peeling may also occur. Plantar creases vary with race. In newborns of African descent, plantar creases may be less developed at term.

5. The nurse inspects the *areolae* and gently palpates the *breast bud tissue* by applying the forefinger and middle finger to the breast area and measuring the tissue between them in centimeters or millimeters (Figure 24–4). At term gestation, the tissue measures between 0.5 and 1.0 cm (5 and 10 mm).

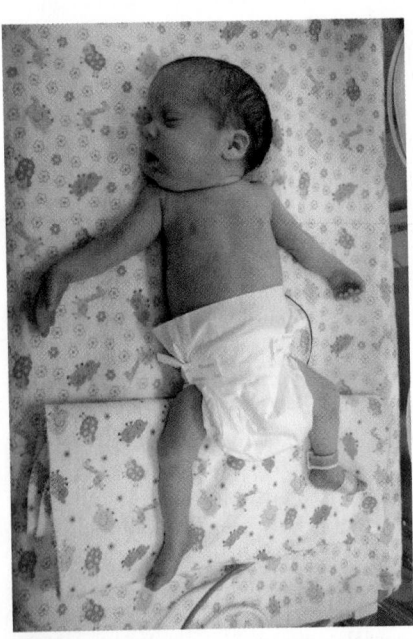 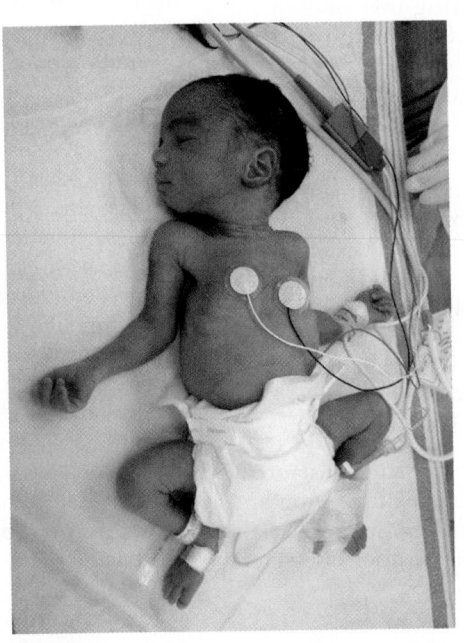 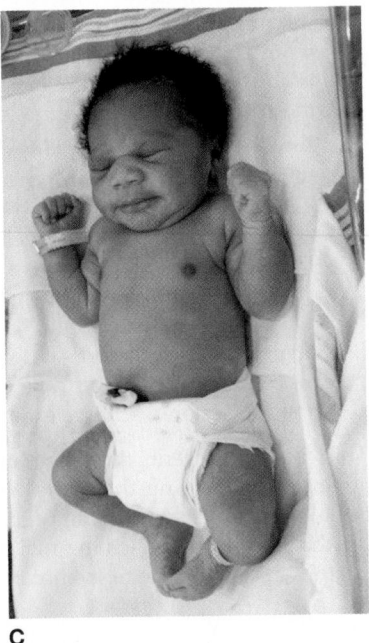

A   B   C

Figure 24–1 Resting posture. *A*, Newborn exhibits beginning of flexion of the thigh. The gestational age is approximately 31 weeks. Note the extension of the upper extremities. Score 1 or 2. *B*, Newborn exhibits stronger flexion of the arms, hips, and thighs. The gestational age is approximately 35 weeks. Score 3. *C*, The full-term newborn exhibits hypertonic flexion of all extremities. Score 4.

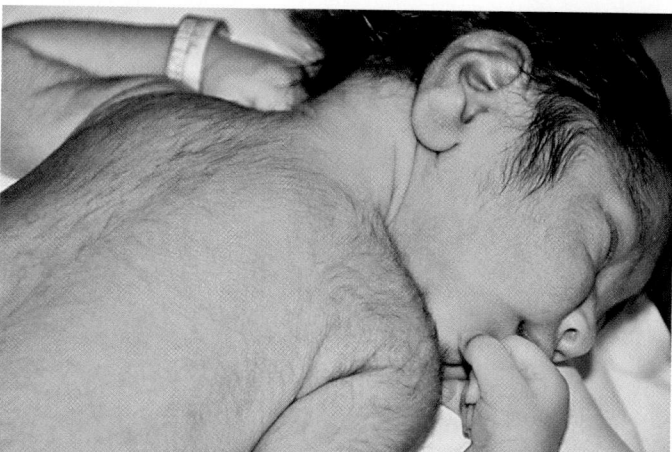

Figure 24–2 Lanugo.

SOURCE: Vanessa Howell, RN, MSN.

During the assessment, the nipple should not be grasped firmly because skin and subcutaneous tissue will prevent accurate estimation of size. The nurse must do this procedure gently to avoid causing trauma to the breast tissue.

As gestation progresses, the breast bud tissue mass and areolae enlarge. However, a large breast tissue mass can occur as a result of specific conditions other than advanced gestational age or the effects of maternal hormones on the baby. In the large-for-gestational-age (LGA) newborn, a diabetic mother's accelerated development of breast tissue is a reflection of subcutaneous fat deposits. Small-for-gestational-age (SGA) (asymmetric) term or postterm newborns may have used subcutaneous fat (which would have been deposited as breast tissue) to survive in utero; as a result, their lack of breast tissue may

indicate a gestational age of 34 to 35 weeks, even though other factors indicate a term or postterm newborn (Cloherty, Eichenwald, Hansen, et al., 2012).

6. *Ear form and cartilage distribution* develop with gestational age. The cartilage gives the ear its shape and substance (Figure 24–5). In a newborn of less than 34 weeks' gestation, the ear is relatively shapeless and flat; it has little cartilage, so the ear folds over on itself and remains folded. By approximately 36 weeks' gestation, some cartilage and incurving of the upper pinna are present, and the pinna springs back slowly when folded. (The nurse tests this response by holding the top and bottom of the pinna together with the forefinger and thumb and then releasing them or by folding the pinna of the ear forward against the side of the head, releasing it, and observing the response.) By term, the newborn's pinna is firm, stands away from the head, and springs back quickly from the folding.

7. *Male genitals* are evaluated for size of the scrotal sac, presence of rugae (wrinkles and ridges in the scrotum), and descent of the testes (Figure 24–6). Before 36 weeks, the scrotum has few rugae, and the testes are palpable in the inguinal canal. By 36 to 38 weeks, the testes are in the upper scrotum, and rugae have developed over the anterior portion of the scrotum. By term, the testes are generally in the lower scrotum, which is pendulous and covered with rugae.

8. The appearance of the *female genitals* depends in part on subcutaneous fat deposition and therefore relates to fetal nutritional status (Figure 24–7). The clitoris varies in size, and occasionally is so swollen that it is difficult to identify the sex of the newborn. This swelling may be caused by adrenogenital syndrome, which causes the adrenals to secrete excessive amounts of androgen and other hormones. At 30 to 32 weeks' gestation, the clitoris is prominent, and the labia majora are small and widely separated. As gestational

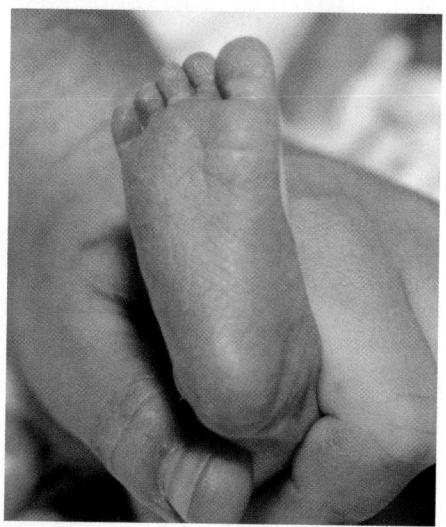 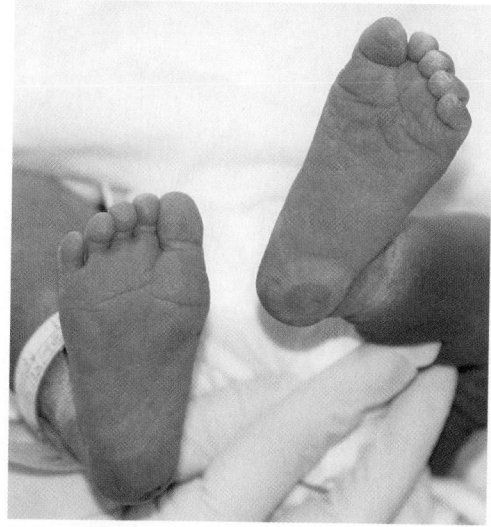 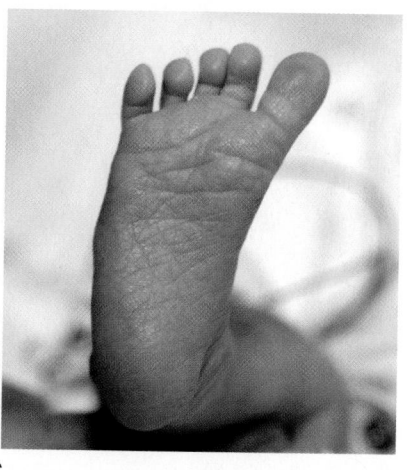

A B C

Figure 24–3 Sole creases. *A*, Newborn has a few sole creases on the anterior portion of the foot. Note the slick heel. Score 2. The gestational age is approximately 35 weeks. *B*, Newborn has a deeper network of sole creases on the anterior two thirds of the sole. Note the slick heel. Score 3. The gestational age is approximately 37 weeks. *C*, The full-term newborn has deep sole creases down to and including the heel as the skin loses fluid and dries after birth. Score 4. Sole (plantar) creases can be seen even in preterm newborns.

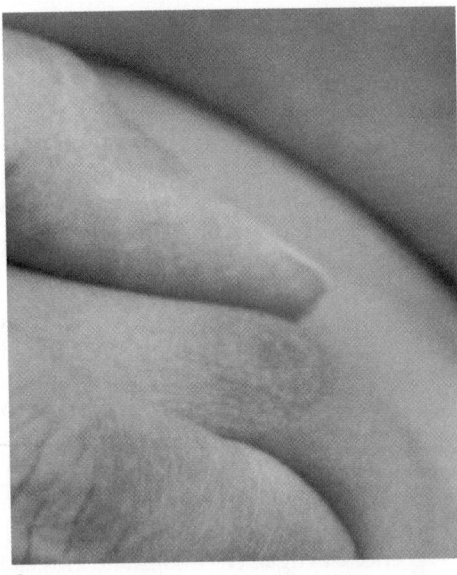
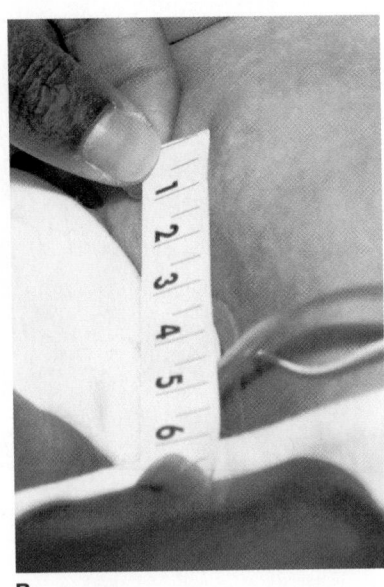

A   **B**

Figure 24–4 Breast tissue. *A*, Newborn has a visible raised area greater than 0.75 cm (0.3 in.) diameter. Score 3. The gestational age is 38 weeks. *B*, Gently compress the tissue between the middle and index fingers and measure the tissue in centimeters or millimeters. Absence of or decreased breast tissue often indicates a premature or small-for-gestational-age (SGA) newborn.

age increases, the labia majora increase in size. At 36 to 40 weeks, they nearly cover the clitoris. At 40 weeks and beyond, the labia majora cover the labia minora and clitoris.

Other physical characteristics assessed by some gestational age scoring tools include the following:

1. *Vernix* covers the preterm newborn. The postterm newborn has no vernix. After noting vernix distribution, the birthing area nurse (wearing gloves) dries the newborn

to prevent evaporative heat loss, thus disturbing the vernix and potentially altering this gestational age criterion. The birthing area nurse must communicate to the neonatal nurse the amount of vernix and the areas of vernix coverage.

2. *Hair* of the preterm newborn has the consistency of matted wool or fur and lies in bunches rather than in the silky, single strands of the term newborn's hair.

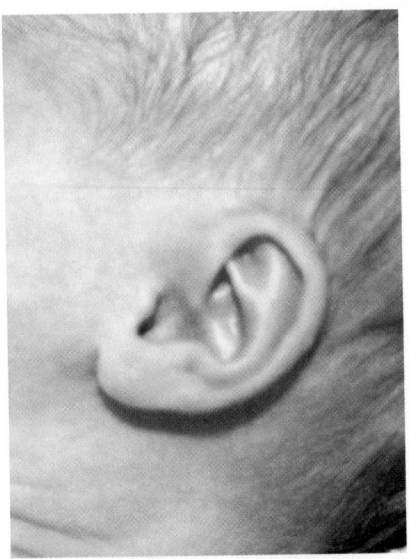
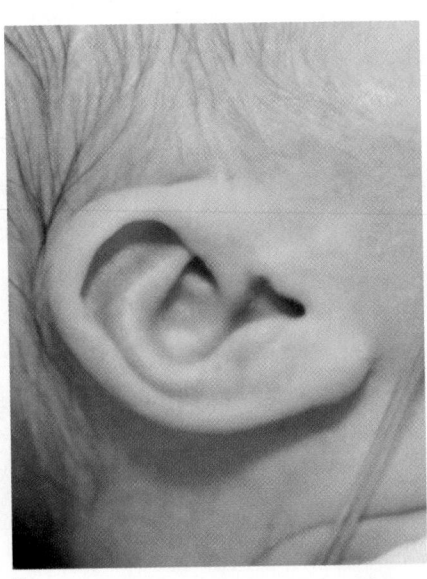
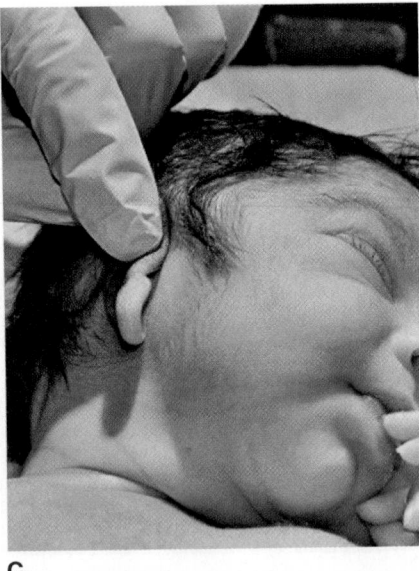

A   **B**   **C**

Figure 24–5 Ear form and cartilage. *A*, The ear of the newborn at approximately 36 weeks' gestation shows incurving of the upper two thirds of the pinna. Score 2. *B*, Newborn at term shows well-defined incurving of the entire pinna. Score 3. *C*, The pinna is folded toward the face and released. If the auricle stays in the position in which it is pressed or returns slowly to its original position, it usually means the gestational age is less than 38 weeks.

SOURCE: *C*. Jo Engle, RN, MSN, NNP-BC and Vanessa Howell, RN, MSN.

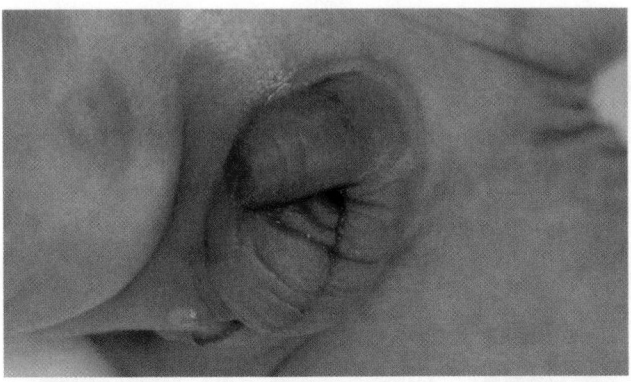

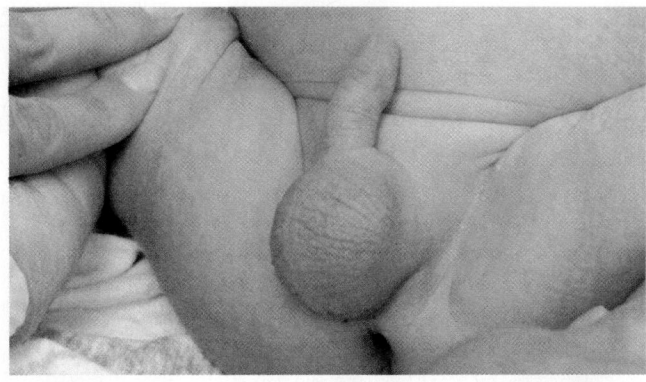

A   **B**

Figure 24–6 Male genitals. *A*, Preterm newborn's testes are not within the scrotum. The scrotal surface has few rugae. Score 2. *B*, Term newborn's testes are generally fully descended. The entire surface of the scrotum is covered by rugae. Score 3.

3. *Skull firmness* increases as the fetus matures. In a term newborn, the bones are hard, and the sutures are not easily displaced. The nurse should not attempt to displace the sutures forcibly.

4. *Nails* appear and cover the nail bed at about 20 weeks' gestation. Nails extending beyond the fingertips may indicate a postterm newborn.

Assessment of Neuromuscular Maturity Characteristics

The central nervous system of the fetus matures at a fairly constant rate. Tests have been designed to evaluate neurologic status as manifested by development of neuromuscular tone. One significant neuromuscular change is that muscle tone progresses from extensor tone to flexor tone and from the lower to the upper extremities as the neurologic system matures in a *caudocephalad* (tail-to-head) progression. The neuromuscular

evaluation requires more manipulation and disturbances than the physical evaluation of the newborn. The neuromuscular evaluation is best performed when the newborn has stabilized.

1. The *square window sign* is elicited by gently flexing the newborn's hand toward the ventral forearm until resistance is felt. The angle formed at the wrist is measured (Figure 24–8).

2. *Recoil* is a test of flexion development. Because flexion first develops in the lower extremities, recoil is first tested in the legs. Place the newborn on the back on a flat surface. With a hand on the newborn's knees, the nurse places the baby's legs in flexion, then extends them parallel to each other and flat on the surface. The response to this maneuver is recoil of the newborn's legs. According to gestational age, they may not move or they may return slowly or quickly to the flexed position. Preterm newborns have less muscle tone than term newborns, so preterm newborns have less recoil.

   Test arm recoil by flexion at the elbow and extension of the arms at the newborn's side. While the baby is in the

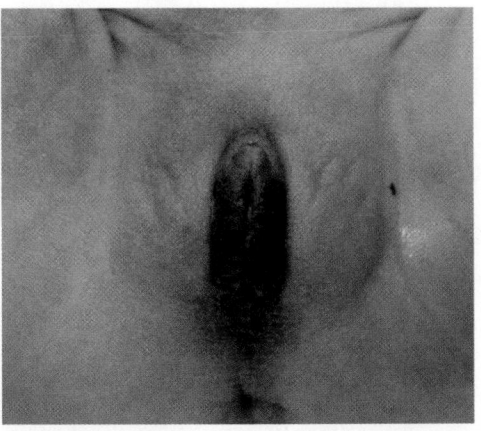

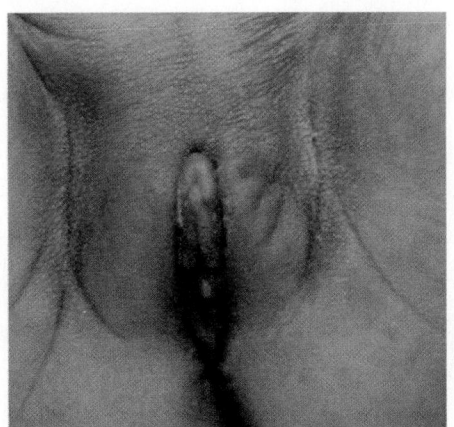

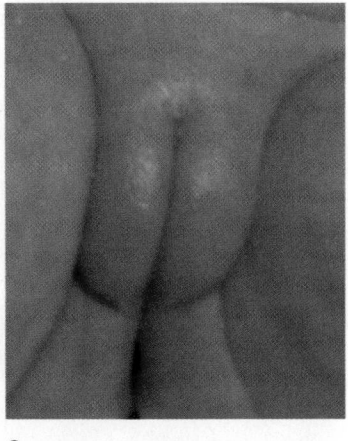

A   **B**   **C**

Figure 24–7 Female genitals. *A*, Newborn has a prominent clitoris. The labia majora are widely separated, and the labia minora, viewed laterally, would protrude beyond the labia majora. Score 1. The gestational age is 30 to 36 weeks. *B*, The clitoris is still visible. The labia minora are now covered by the larger labia majora. Score 2. The gestational age is 36 to 40 weeks. *C*, The term newborn has well-developed, large labia majora that cover both the clitoris and labia minora. Score 3. The labia minora is often dark in some ethnic and racial groups of newborns.

SOURCE: *C.* Christine Mescolotto.

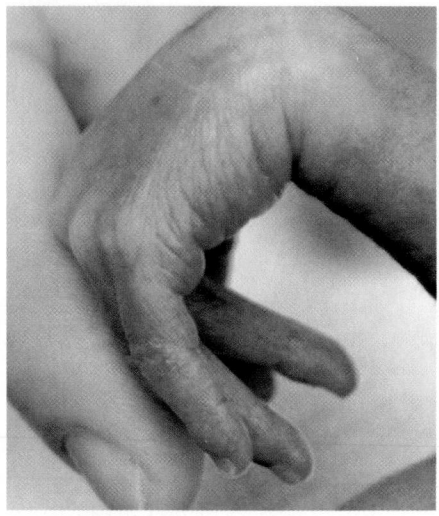 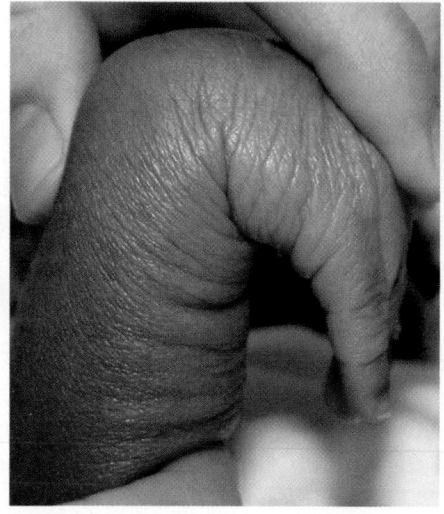 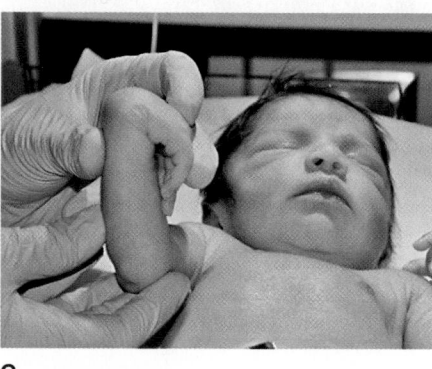

A   **B**   **C**

Figure 24–8   Square window sign. *A*, This angle is 90 degrees and suggests an immature newborn of 28 to 32 weeks' gestation. Score 0. *B*, A 30- to 40-degree angle is commonly found in newborns from 38 to 40 weeks' gestation. Score 2 to 3. *C*, A 0- to 15-degree angle occurs in newborns from 40 to 42 weeks' gestation. Score 4.

SOURCE: *C*. Vanessa Howell, RN, MSN.

supine position, the nurse completely flexes both elbows, holds them in this position for 5 seconds, extends the arms at the baby's side, and releases them. On release, the elbows of a full-term newborn form an angle of less than 90 degrees and rapidly recoil back to a flexed position. The elbows of a preterm newborn have slower recoil time and form an angle greater than 90 degrees. Arm recoil is also slower in healthy but fatigued newborns after birth; therefore, arm recoil is best elicited after the first hour of birth, when the baby has had time to recover from the stress of the birth. The deep sleep state also decreases the arm recoil response. Assessment of arm recoil should be bilateral to rule out brachial palsy.

3. The *popliteal angle* (degree of knee flexion) is determined with the newborn flat on the back. The thigh is flexed on the abdomen and chest, and the nurse places the index finger of the other hand behind the newborn's ankle to extend the lower leg until resistance is met. The angle formed is then measured. Results vary from no resistance in the very immature newborn to an 80-degree angle in the term newborn.

4. The *scarf sign* is elicited by placing the newborn supine and drawing an arm across the chest toward the newborn's opposite shoulder until resistance is met. The location of the elbow is then noted in relation to the midline of the chest (Figure 24–9). A preterm newborn's elbow will cross the midline of the chest, whereas a full-term newborn's elbow will not cross midline.

5. The *heel-to-ear extension* is performed by placing the newborn in a supine position and then gently drawing the foot

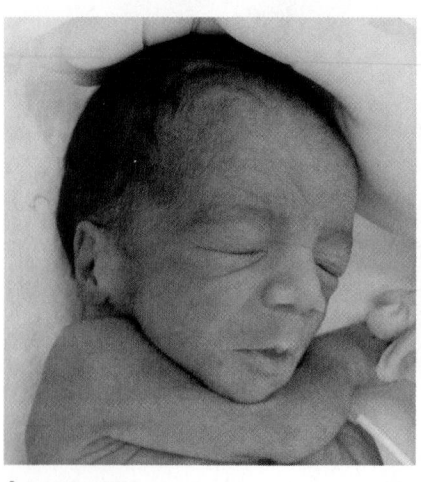 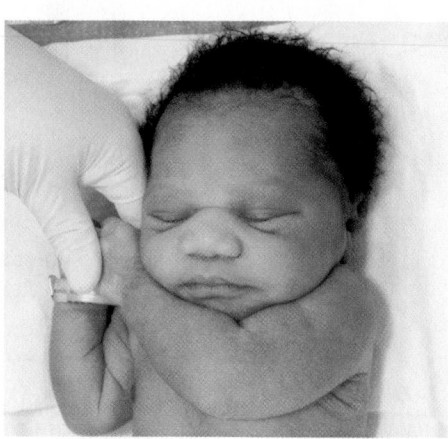 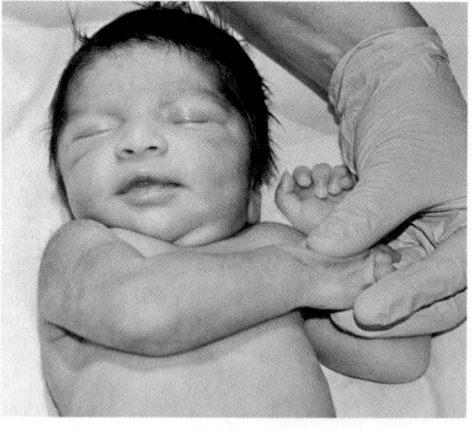

A   **B**   **C**

Figure 24–9   Scarf sign. *A*, No resistance is noted until after 30 weeks' gestation. The elbow can be readily moved past the midline. Score 1. *B*, The elbow is at midline at 36 to 40 weeks' gestation. Score 2. *C*, Beyond 40 weeks' gestation, the elbow will not reach the midline. Score 4.

SOURCE: *C*. Vanessa Howell, RN, MSN.

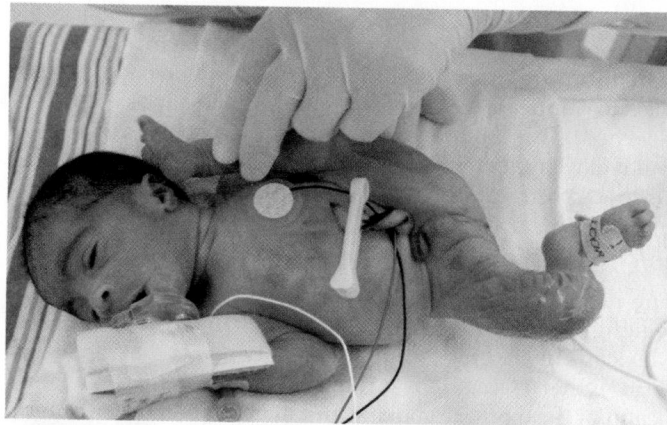

Figure 24–10 Heel to ear. No resistance. Leg fully extended. Score 0.

toward the ear on the same side until resistance is felt. The nurse should allow the knee to bend during the test. It is important to hold the buttocks down to keep from rolling the baby. Both the proximity of foot to ear and the degree of knee extension are assessed. A preterm, immature newborn's leg will remain straight and the foot will go to the ear or beyond (Figure 24–10). With advancing gestational age, the newborn demonstrates increasing resistance to this maneuver. Maneuvers involving the lower extremities of newborns who had frank breech presentations should be delayed to allow for resolution of leg positioning.

6. *Ankle dorsiflexion* is determined by flexing the ankle on the shin. The nurse uses a thumb to push on the sole of the newborn's foot while the fingers support the back of the leg. Then the angle formed by the foot and the interior leg is measured (Figure 24–11). Intrauterine position and congenital deformities can influence this sign.

7. *Head lag* (neck flexor) is measured by pulling the newborn to a sitting position and noting the degree of head lag. Total

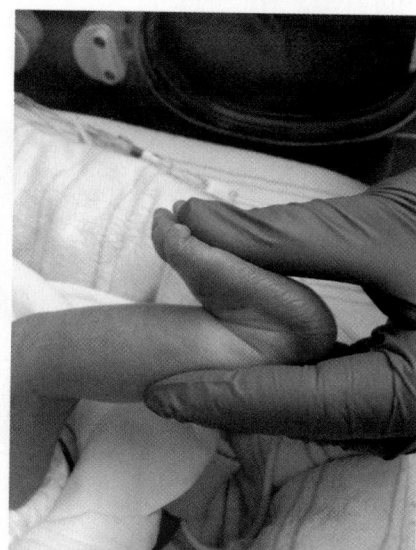

Figure 24–11 Ankle dorsiflexion. A 45-degree angle indicates 32 to 36 weeks' gestation.

SOURCE: Carol Harrigan, RNC, MSN, NNP-BC.

lag is common in newborns up to 34 weeks' gestation. Full-term newborns can support their heads momentarily.

8. *Ventral suspension* (horizontal position) is evaluated by holding the newborn prone on the nurse's hand. The position of the head and back and the degree of flexion in the arms and legs are noted. Some flexion of arms and legs indicates 36 to 38 weeks' gestation; fully flexed extremities, with head and back even, are characteristic of a term newborn.

9. *Major reflexes* such as *sucking, rooting, grasping, Moro, tonic neck,* and others are evaluated during the newborn examination. These reflexes are discussed later in the chapter.

A supplementary method for estimating gestational age (done by the healthcare provider or nurse practitioner) is to view the vascular network of the cornea with an ophthalmoscope. The nurse may need to delay administration of prophylactic eye ointment in preterm newborns until after this vascular eye examination is done. The amount of vascularity present over the surface of the lens assists in identifying newborns of 27 through 34 weeks' gestational age.

When the gestational age determination and birth weight are considered together, the newborn can be identified as one whose growth is:

- *Small for gestational age (SGA)* (below the 10th percentile)
- *Appropriate for gestational age (AGA)* (between the 10th and 90th percentile)
- *Large for gestational age (LGA)* (above the 90th percentile)

This determination (Figure 24–12) enables the nurse to anticipate possible physiologic problems. This growth

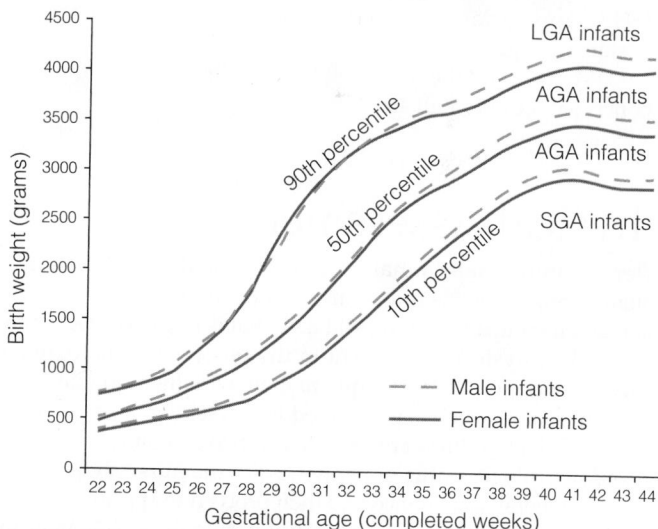

Figure 24–12 Select reference percentiles for birth weight at each gestational age from 22 to 44 completed weeks for male and female singleton infants: 10th, 50th, and 90th percentiles. Data from 3,423,215 male and 3,267,502 female infants in the 1999–2000 U.S. Natality datasets.

SOURCE: Oken, E., Kleinman, K. P., Rich-Edwards, J., & Gillman, M. W. (2003). A nearly continuous measure of birth weight for gestational age using a United States national reference. *BMC Pediatrics, 3,* 6. Retrieved from http://www .biomedcentral.com/1471-2431/3/6 © 2003 Oken et al.; licensee BioMed Central Ltd. This is an open access article: verbatim copying and redistribution of this article are permitted in all media for any purpose, provided this notice is preserved along with the article's original URL.

information is used in conjunction with a complete physical examination to establish a plan of care appropriate for the individual newborn. For example, an SGA or LGA newborn often requires frequent glucose monitoring and early feedings. (See Chapter 26 for a more complete discussion of these categories and the potential problems associated with them.)

Healthy People 2020
> (MICH–8) Reduce low birth weight (LBW) and very low birth weight (VLBW)

Clinical Reasoning Determining Gestational Age

A nurse has completed the gestational assessment on newborn Travis Bell who weighs 3000 g (6.6 lb) and is 48 cm (18.9 in.) long with a head circumference of 33 cm (13 in.). His Apgar scores were 8 at 1 minute and 9 at 5 minutes. Other assessment data include skin dry and cracking with pale areas and rare veins, no lanugo, sole creases covering the entire sole, raised areola 3 mm (0.125 in.), well-curved pinna soft with ready recoil, and testes descended with moderate rugae. Reflex data include square window at 0 degree, arm recoil 100 degree, popliteal angle 100 degree, scarf sign yield elbow will not reach midline, heel to ear 90 degree, and posture fully flexed. The parents express concerns over his small size.

What are the newborn's physical maturity score and neuromuscular maturity score?

Interpret the newborn's combined scores of neuromuscular and physical maturity.

Determine if the newborn is small for gestational age (SGA), appropriate for gestational age (AGA), or large for gestational age (LGA).

What should the nurse tell the parents regarding their concern over his small size?

Physical Assessment

After the initial determination of gestational age and related potential problems, the nurse carries out a more extensive physical assessment in a warm, well-lit area that is free of drafts. Completing the physical assessment in the presence of the parents provides an opportunity to acquaint them with their unique newborn. The examination is performed in a systematic, head-to-toe manner, and all findings are recorded. When assessing the physical and neurologic status of the newborn, the nurse should first consider general appearance and then proceed to specific areas.

Assessment Guide: Newborn Physical Assessment (see later in the chapter) outlines how to systematically assess the newborn. Normal findings, alterations, and related causes are presented and correlated with suggested nursing responses. The findings are typical for a full-term newborn.

General Appearance

The newborn's head is disproportionately large for the body. The neck looks short because the chin rests on the chest. Newborns have a prominent abdomen, sloping shoulders, narrow hips, and rounded chests. The center of the baby's body is the umbilicus rather than the symphysis pubis as in the adult. The body appears long and the extremities short.

Newborns tend to stay in a flexed position similar to the one maintained in utero and will offer resistance when the extremities are straightened. This flexed position contributes to the short appearance of the extremities. The hands are tightly clenched. After a breech birth, the feet are usually dorsiflexed, and it may take several weeks for the baby to assume the typical newborn posture.

Weight and Measurements

The normal full-term White newborn has an average birth weight of 3405 g (7 lb, 8 oz). Newborns of African, Asian, or Mexican American descent are usually somewhat smaller at term. Other factors that influence weight are age, size, and health of the mother (smoking and malnutrition decrease birth weight). After the first week, and for the first 6 months, the newborn's weight increases about 198 g (7 oz) weekly.

Approximately 70% to 75% of the newborn's body weight is water. During the initial newborn period (the first 3 or 4 days), term newborns have a physiologic weight loss of about 5% to 10% because of fluid shifts. This weight loss may reach 15% for preterm newborns. Large babies also tend to lose more weight because of greater fluid loss in proportion to birth weight. If weight loss is greater than 10%, clinical reappraisal is indicated. Factors contributing to weight loss include insufficient fluid intake resulting from delayed breastfeeding or a slow adjustment to the formula, increased volume of meconium excreted, urination, and dehydration or consistent chilling (because of nonshivering thermogenesis).

The length of the normal newborn is difficult to measure because the legs are flexed and tensed. To measure length, the nurse should place newborns flat on their backs with their legs extended as much as possible (Figure 24–13). The average length is 50 cm (20 in.), and the range is 46 to 56 cm (18 to 22 in.). The newborn will grow approximately 2.5 cm (1 in.) a month for the next 6 months. This is the period of most rapid growth.

At birth, the newborn's head is one fourth the size of an adult's head. The circumference (biparietal diameter) of the newborn's head is 32 to 37 cm (12.5 to 14.5 in.). For accurate measurement, the nurse places the tape over the most prominent part of the occiput and brings it just above the eyebrows (Figure 24–14A). The circumference of the newborn's head is approximately 2 cm (0.8 in.) greater than the circumference of the newborn's chest at birth, and will remain in this proportion

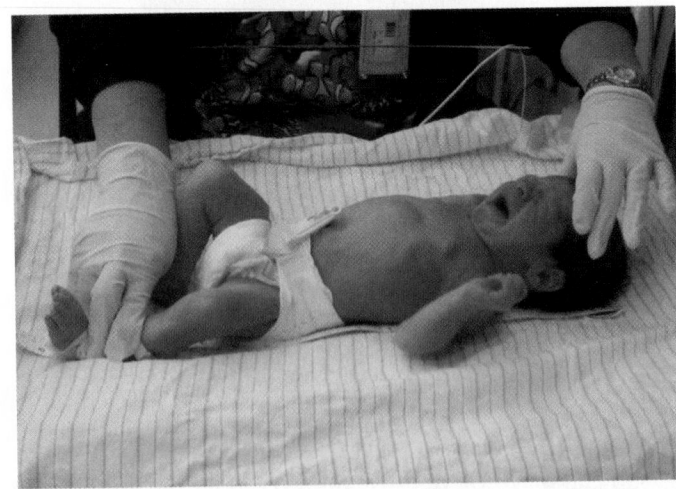

Figure 24–13 **Measuring the length of the newborn.**
SOURCE: Vanessa Howell, RNC, MSN.

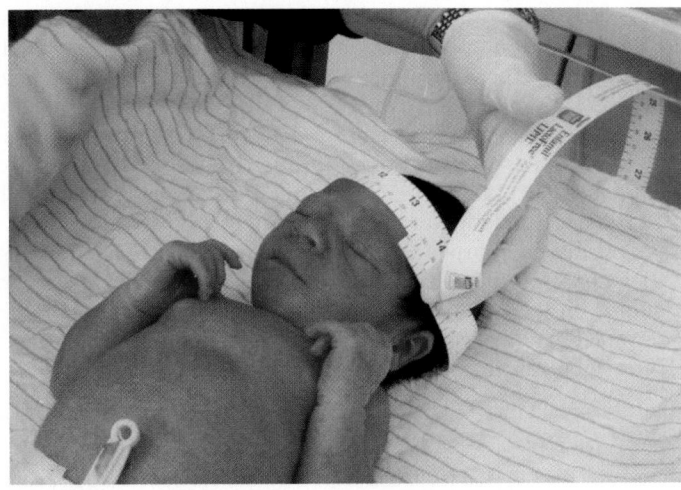

A

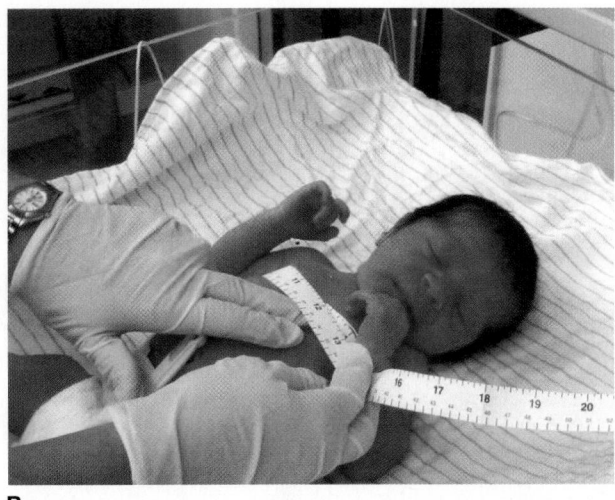

B

Figure 24–14 *A*, Measuring the head circumference of the newborn. *B*, Measuring the chest circumference of the newborn.

SOURCE: Vanessa Howell, RNC, MSN.

for the next few months. (Factors that alter this measurement are discussed in the section titled "Head" later in this chapter.) It is best to take another head circumference on the second day if the newborn experienced significant head molding or developed a caput from the birth process.

The average circumference of the chest is 32 cm (12.5 in.) and ranges from 30 to 35 cm (12 to 14 in.). Chest measurements are taken with the tape measure placed at the lower edge of the scapulae and brought around anteriorly, directly over the nipple line (Figure 24–14*B*). The abdominal circumference, or girth, may also be measured at this time by placing the tape around the newborn's abdomen at the level of the umbilicus, with the bottom edge of the tape at the top edge of the umbilicus (Table 24–1).

Temperature

Initial assessment of the newborn's temperature is critical. In utero, the temperature of the fetus is about the same as, or slightly higher than, the expectant mother's temperature. When babies enter the outside world, their temperature can suddenly drop as a result of exposure to cold drafts and the skin's heat loss mechanisms.

If no heat conservation measures are started, the normal term newborn's deep body temperature falls 0.1°C (0.2°F) per minute; skin temperature drops 0.3°C (0.5°F) per minute. Skin temperature markedly decreases within 10 minutes after exposure to room air. The temperature should stabilize within 8 to 12 hours. Temperature is monitored at least every 30 minutes

until the newborn's status has remained stable for 2 hours (American Academy of Pediatrics [AAP] Committee on Fetus and Newborn & American College of Obstetricians and Gynecologists [ACOG], 2012).

Thereafter, the nurse should assess temperature at least once every 8 hours, or according to institutional policy. In newborns who have been exposed to group B hemolytic streptococcus, more frequent temperature monitoring may be required (see Chapter 23 for a discussion of the physiology of temperature regulation).

Temperature can be assessed by the axillary skin method, a continuous skin probe, or via the rectal route. Axillary temperature reflects body (core) temperature and the body's compensatory response to the thermal environment. In preterm and term newborns, there is less than 0.1°C (0.2°F) difference between temperatures at the two sites and the axillary method is preferred. If the axillary method is used, the thermometer must remain in place at least 3 minutes, unless an electronic thermometer is used. Axillary temperature ranges from 36.5° to 37.2°C (97.7° to 99.0°F). Keep in mind that axillary temperatures can be misleading because the friction caused by apposition of the inner arm skin and upper chest wall and the nearness of brown fat to the probe may elevate the temperature (Figure 24–15).

Skin temperature is measured most accurately by means of continuous skin probe, especially for small newborns or newborns maintained in incubators or under radiant warmers. Normal skin temperature is 36.0° to 36.5°C (96.8° to 97.8°F).

TABLE 24–1 Newborn Measurements

MEASUREMENT	AVERAGE	RANGE	GROWTH
Weight (Weight is influenced by a variety of factors, and maternal age and size. Physiologic weight loss 5% to 10% for term newborns, up to 15% for preterm newborns.)	3405 g (7 lb, 8 oz)	2500–4000 g (5 lb, 8 oz–8 lb, 13 oz)	198 g (7 oz) per week for first 6 months
Length	50 cm (20 in.)	46–56 cm (18–22 in.)	2.5 cm (1 in.) per month for first 6 months
Head circumference (Approximately 2 cm [0.8 in.] larger than chest circumference)	33–35 cm (13–14 in.)	32.0–37.0 cm (12.5–14.5 in.)	
Chest circumference	32.0 cm (12.5 in.)	30–35 cm (12–14 in.)	

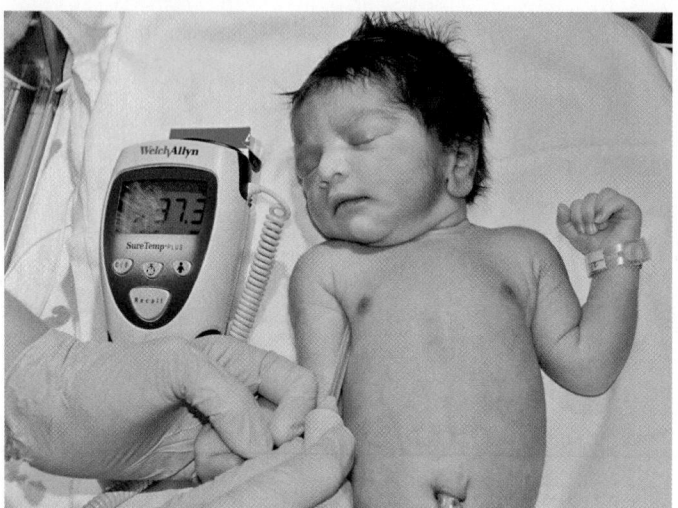

Figure 24–15 Axillary temperature measurement. The thermometer should remain in place for 3 minutes. The newborn's arm should be tightly but gently pressed against the thermometer and the newborn's side, as illustrated.

SOURCE: Vanessa Howell, RN, MSN.

Continuous assessment of skin temperature allows time for initiation of interventions before a more serious fall in core temperature occurs (Figure 24–16).

Rectal temperature is assumed to be the closest approximation to core temperature, but the accuracy of this method depends on the depth to which the thermometer is inserted. Normal rectal temperature is 36.6° to 37.2°C (97.8° to 99.0°F). The rectal route is *not* recommended as a routine method unless done with a digital or electronic thermometer (American Academy of Pediatrics, 2013).

Temperature instability, a deviation of more than 1°C (2°F) from one reading to the next, or a subnormal temperature may indicate an infection. In contrast to an elevated temperature in older children, an increased temperature in a newborn

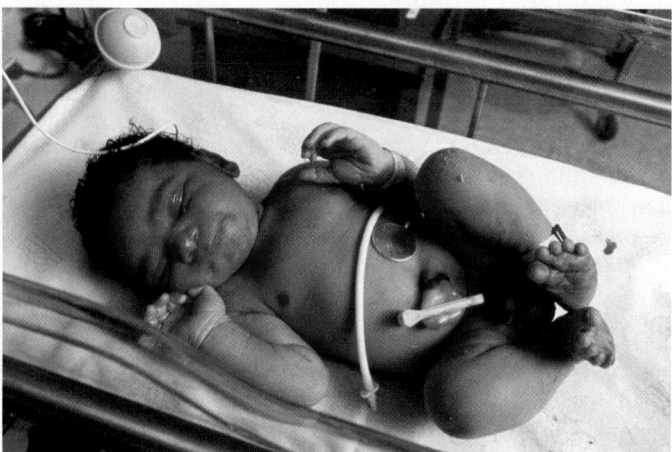

Figure 24–16 Temperature monitoring for the newborn. A skin thermal sensor is placed on the newborn's abdomen, upper thigh, or arm and secured with porous tape or a foil-covered foam pad.

SOURCE: Tom McCarthy/PhotoEdit, Inc.

may indicate a reaction to too many coverings, too hot a room, or dehydration. Dehydration, which tends to increase body temperature, occurs in newborns whose feedings have been delayed for any reason. Newborns may respond to overheating (a temperature greater than 37.5°C [99.5°F]) by increased restlessness and eventually by perspiration after 35 to 40 minutes of exposure (Blackburn, 2013). The perspiration appears initially on the head and face and then on the chest.

Many newborns initially cannot perspire, so they increase their respiratory and heart rates, which increases oxygen consumption. Whether the initial temperature is elevated or subnormal the newborn must have a stable temperature per agency protocol prior to leaving the nursery.

Healthy People 2020

(MICH–1.8) Reduce the rate of infant deaths from sudden infant death syndrome (SIDS)

Clinical Tip

Measuring weight and height often aggravates newborns and may alter their vital signs. For better accuracy, take the newborn's vital signs before weighing and measuring. In addition, assess the respiratory rate and heart rate before taking the temperature.

Skin Characteristics

Although the newborn's skin color varies with genetic background, all healthy newborns have a pink tinge to their skin. The ruddy hue results from increased red blood cell concentrations in the blood vessels and limited subcutaneous fat deposits.

Skin pigmentation is slight in the newborn period, so color changes may be seen even in darker-skinned babies. White newborns often have a pink-tinged or ruddy skin tone a few hours after birth, and African American newborns may have a reddish brown to pale pink with yellow or red-tinged skin color. Hispanic and Asian newborns range from a pink or rosy red to olive or yellow skin tone (Cloherty et al., 2012). Skin pigmentation deepens over time; therefore, variations in skin color indicating illness are more difficult to evaluate in African American and Asian newborns (Cloherty et al., 2012). A newborn who is cyanotic at rest and pink only with crying may have *choanal atresia* (congenital blockage of the passageway between the nose and pharynx). If crying increases the cyanosis, heart or lung problems should be suspected. Very pale newborns may be anemic or have hypovolemia (low blood pressure) and should be evaluated for these problems.

Acrocyanosis (bluish discoloration of the hands and feet) may be present in the first 2 to 6 hours after birth but can be normal for up to 24 hours (Figure 24–17). This condition is caused by poor peripheral circulation, which results in vasomotor

---

Developing Cultural Competence Keeping Newborns Warm

In the Latino culture and others, parents may be overly concerned about keeping their newborn warm. Parents should be informed that overdressing babies while they are sleeping is related to a higher risk of sudden infant death syndrome (SIDS) and that bundling them excessively can be uncomfortable and lead to heat rash.

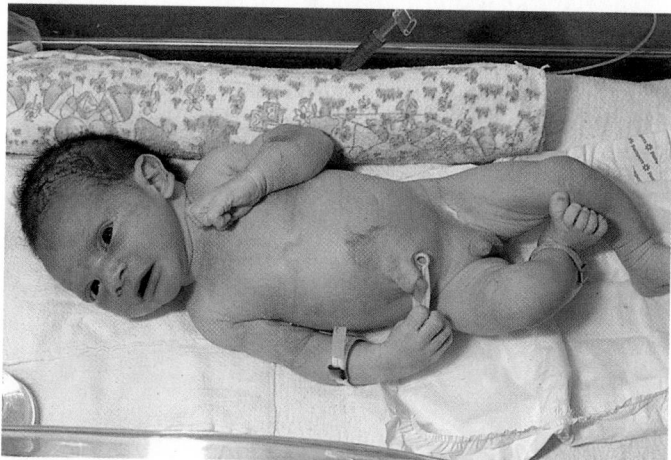

Figure 24–17 Acrocyanosis.

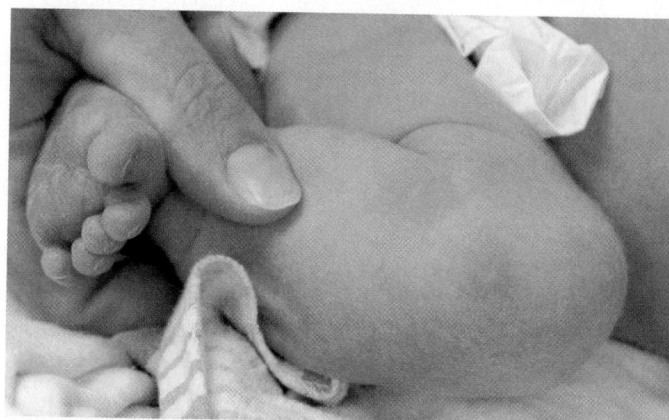

Figure 24–18 Erythema toxicum on leg.

instability and capillary stasis, especially when the baby is exposed to cold. Therefore, blue hands and nails are a poor indicator of decreased oxygenation in a newborn. If the central circulation is adequate, the blood supply should return quickly (2 to 3 seconds) to the extremity after the skin is blanched with a finger. The nurse assesses the face and mucous membranes for pinkness that reflects adequate oxygenation. Further oxygenation assessment is needed if there are signs of respiratory distress. Pulse oximetry can be obtained.

Mottling (lacy pattern of dilated blood vessels under the skin) occurs as a result of general circulation fluctuations. It may last several hours to several weeks or may come and go periodically. Mottling may be related to chilling or prolonged apnea, sepsis, or hypothyroidism.

The **Harlequin sign** (clown) color change is occasionally noted: A deep red color develops over one side of the newborn's body while the other side remains pale, so that the skin resembles a clown's suit. This color change results from a vasomotor disturbance in which blood vessels on one side dilate while the vessels on the other side constrict (Glomella, 2013). It usually lasts from 1 to 20 minutes. Affected newborns may have single or multiple episodes, but they are transient and clinically insignificant. The nurse should document each occurrence.

Jaundice (yellowish discoloration of skin and mucous membranes) is first detectable on the face (where skin overlies cartilage) and the mucous membranes of the mouth; it has a head-to-toe progression and regresses in the opposite direction (Cloherty et al., 2012). Jaundice is evaluated by blanching the tip of the nose, the forehead, the sternum, or the gum line. This procedure must be carried out in appropriate lighting. If jaundice is present, the area will appear yellowish immediately after blanching. Another area to assess for jaundice is the sclera.

Jaundice must be evaluated and its cause determined immediately to prevent possible serious sequelae. The jaundice may be related to immature liver function, hematomas, or poor feeding. It also may be caused by blood incompatibility, oxytocin (Pitocin) augmentation or induction, or a severe hemolysis process. Any jaundice noted before 24 hours of age should be reported to the physician or nurse practitioner. Breastfeeding is a possible cause of late-onset jaundice.

Erythema toxicum is an eruption of lesions in the area surrounding a hair follicle that are firm, vary in size from 1 to 3 mm, and consist of a white or pale yellow papule or pustule with an erythematous base. It is often called "newborn rash" or "flea bite" dermatitis. The rash may appear suddenly, usually over the trunk and diaper area, and is frequently widespread (Figure 24–18). The lesions do not appear on the palms of the hands or the soles of the feet. The peak incidence is at 24 to 48 hours of life. The condition rarely presents at birth or after 5 days of life. The cause is unknown, and no treatment is necessary. Some clinicians believe it may be caused by irritation from clothing. The lesions disappear in a few hours or days. If a maculopapular rash appears, a smear of the aspirated papule will show numerous eosinophils on staining; no bacteria will be cultured.

Milia, which are exposed sebaceous glands, appear as raised white spots on the face, especially across the nose (Figure 24–19). No treatment is necessary because they will clear spontaneously within the first month. Newborns of African heritage have a similar condition called *transient neonatal pustular melanosis*.

Skin turgor is assessed to determine hydration status, the need to initiate early feedings, and the presence of any infectious processes. The usual place to assess skin turgor is over the abdomen, forearm, or thigh. Skin should be elastic and should return rapidly to its original shape.

Vernix caseosa, a whitish, cheeselike substance, covers the fetus while in utero and lubricates the skin of the newborn. The skin of the term or postterm newborn has less vernix and is frequently dry. Peeling is common, especially on the hands and feet, in the postterm newborn.

Forceps marks may be present after a vaginal birth. The newborn may have reddened areas over the cheeks and jaws. It is important to reassure the parents that these marks will

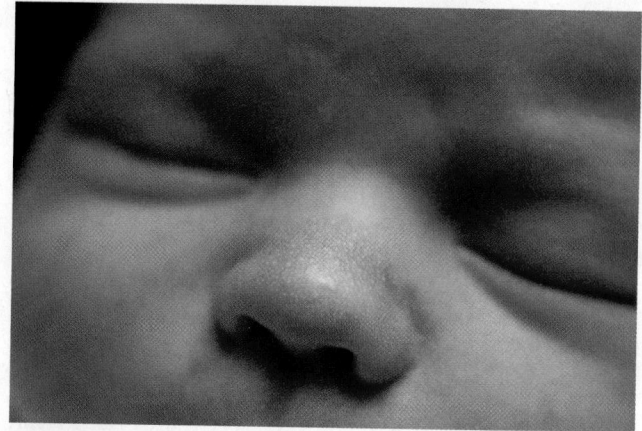

Figure 24–19 Facial milia over bridge of nose.

SOURCE: © Jack Sullivan/Alamy.

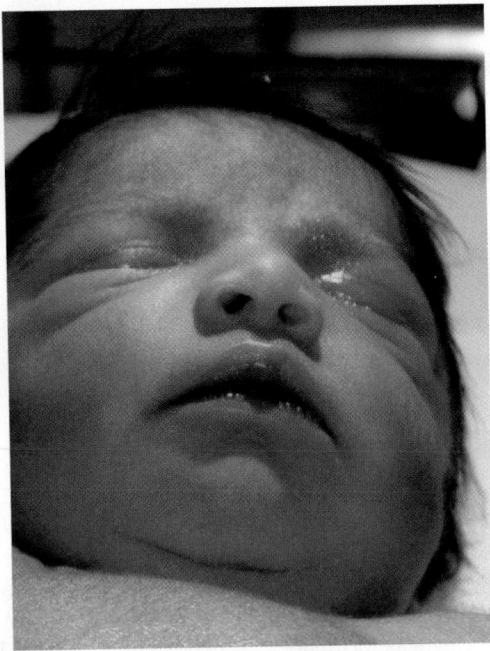

Figure 24–20 Sucking blister in middle of upper lip.

SOURCE: Vanessa Howell, RN, MSN.

disappear, usually within 1 or 2 days. Transient facial paralysis resulting from the forceps pressure is a rare complication. Vacuum extractor suction marks (abrasions or ecchymosis) on the vertex of the scalp may be seen when vacuum extractors are used to assist with the birth (Gleason & Devaskar, 2012). These are benign and do not indicate any underlying brain lesions.

Sucking blisters (vesicles or bullae) may appear on the lips, fingers, or hands of newborns as a result of vigorous sucking, either in utero or after birth. These sucking blisters (Figure 24–20) may be intact or ruptured and require no treatment.

Birthmarks

Telangiectatic nevi (stork bites) appear as pale pink or red spots and are frequently found on the eyelids, nose, lower occipital bone, and nape of the neck (Figure 24–21). These

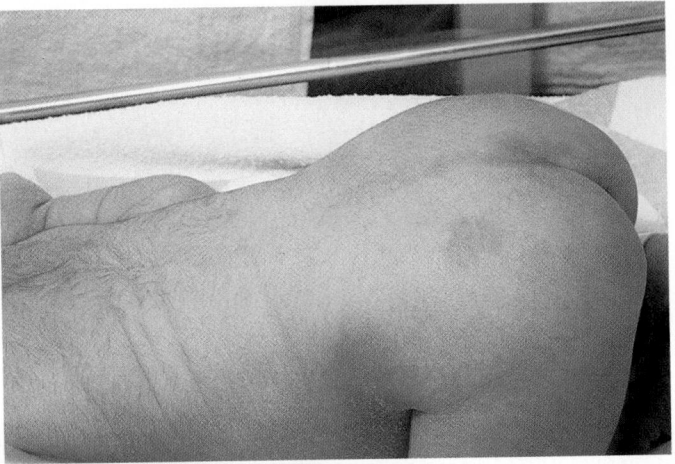

Figure 24–22 Mongolian blue spots.

lesions are common in newborns with light complexions and are more noticeable during periods of crying. These areas have no clinical significance and usually fade by the second birthday.

Congenital dermal melanocytes, also called *Mongolian blue spots*, are macular areas of bluish black or gray-blue pigmentation usually on the dorsal area and the buttocks but may be anywhere on the body (Figure 24–22). They are common in newborns of Asian, Hispanic, and African descent and other dark-skin races and can be seen in 1% to 9% of Whites. They gradually fade during the first or second year of life. They may be mistaken for bruises and should be documented in the newborn's medical record.

Nevus flammeus (port-wine stain) is a capillary angioma directly below the epidermis. It is a nonelevated, sharply demarcated, red-to-purple area of dense capillaries (Figure 24–23). In newborns of African descent, it may appear as a purple-black stain. The size and shape vary, but it commonly appears on the face. It does not grow in size, does not fade with time, and does not blanch as a rule. The birthmark may be concealed by using an opaque cosmetic cream. If convulsions and other neurologic problems accompany the nevus flammeus, the clinical picture is suggestive of *Sturge-Weber syndrome*, with involvement of

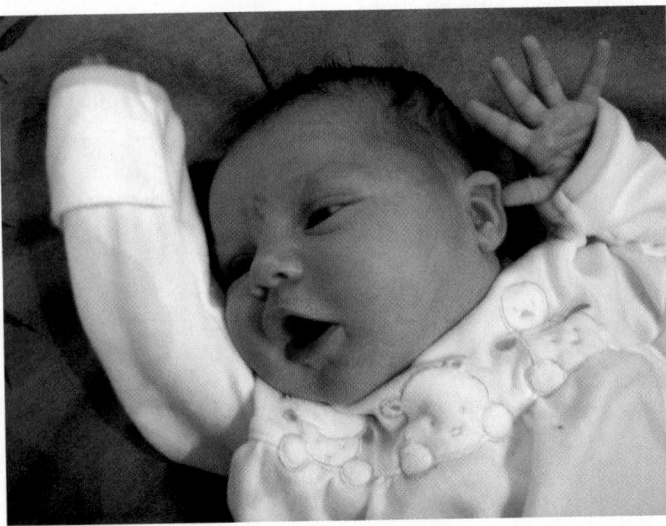

Figure 24–21 Stork bites over left eyelid and near right eyebrow.

SOURCE: Anne Garcia.

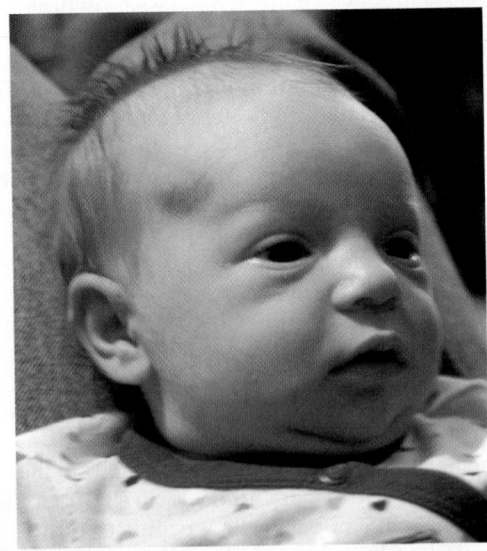

Figure 24–23 Port-wine stain over temple area.

the fifth cranial nerve (the ophthalmic branch of the trigeminal nerve).

Nevus vasculosus (strawberry mark) is a capillary hemangioma. It consists of newly formed and enlarged capillaries in the dermal and subdermal layers. It is a raised, clearly delineated, dark red, rough-surfaced birthmark commonly found in the head region. Such marks usually grow (often rapidly) starting during the second or third week of life and may not reach their fullest size until about 6 months (Witt, 2015). They begin to shrink and start to resolve spontaneously several weeks to months after they reach peak growth. A pale purple or gray spot on the surface of the hemangioma signals the start of resolution. The best cosmetic effect is achieved when the lesions are allowed to resolve spontaneously.

Head

The newborn's head is large (approximately one fourth of the body size), with soft, pliable cranial skull bones. For most term newborns, the occipital-frontal circumference (OFC) is 32 cm to 37 cm (12.6 in. to 14.6 in.). The head may appear asymmetric in the newborn of a vertex birth. This asymmetry, called **molding**, is caused by the overriding of the cranial bones during labor and birth (Figure 24–24). The degree of molding varies with the amount and length of pressure exerted on the head. Within a few days after birth, the overriding usually diminishes and the suture lines become palpable; therefore, a second measurement is indicated a few days after birth. Any extreme differences in head size may indicate *microcephaly* (abnormally small head) or *hydrocephalus* (an abnormal buildup of fluid in the brain) and can result in an enlarged head. Variations in the shape, size, or appearance of the head measurements may be caused by *craniosynostosis* (premature closure of the cranial sutures), which will need to be corrected through surgery to allow brain growth, and *plagiocephaly* (asymmetry caused by pressure on the fetal head during gestation) (Johnson, 2015).

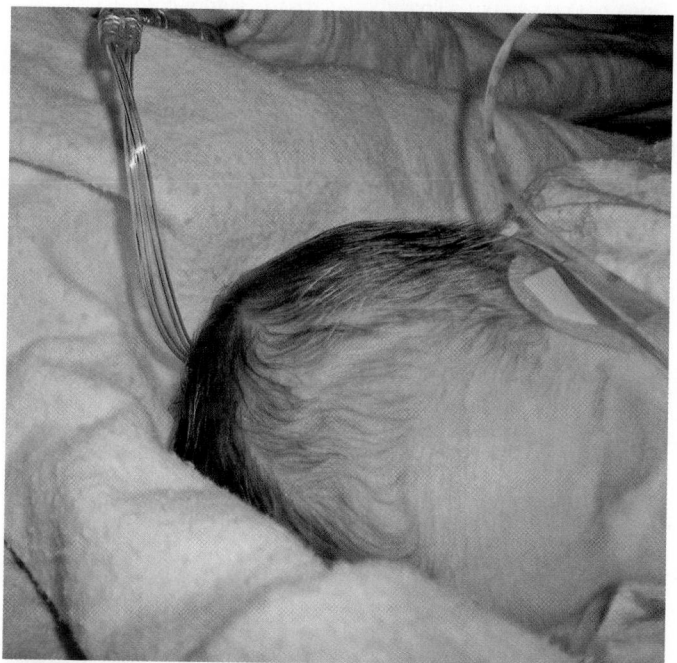

Figure 24–24 **Overlapped cranial bones produce a visible ridge in a premature newborn. Easily visible overlapping does not occur often in term newborns.**
SOURCE: Vanessa Howell, RN, MSN.

Two *fontanels* ("soft spots") may be palpated on the newborn's head. Fontanels, which are openings at the juncture of the cranial bones, can be measured with the fingers. Accurate measurement necessitates that the examiner's finger be measured in centimeters. The assessment should be carried out with the newborn in a sitting position and not crying. The *diamond-shaped anterior fontanel* is approximately 3 to 4 cm (1.2 to 1.6 in.) long by 2 to 3 cm (0.79 to 1.2 in.) wide. It is located at the juncture of the frontal and parietal bones. The *posterior fontanel*, smaller and triangular, is formed by the parietal bones and the occipital bone and is 0.5 by 1.0 cm (0.20 to 0.39 in.). Because of molding, the fontanels are smaller immediately after birth than several days later. The anterior fontanel closes within 18 months, whereas the posterior fontanel closes within 8 to 12 weeks.

The fontanels are a useful indicator of the newborn's condition. The anterior fontanel may swell when the newborn cries or passes a stool or may pulsate with the heartbeat, which is normal. A bulging fontanelle usually signifies increased intracranial pressure, and a depressed fontanelle indicates dehydration. The sutures between the cranial bones should be palpated for the amount of overlapping. In newborns whose growth has been restricted, the sutures may be wider than normal, and the fontanels may also be larger because of impaired growth of the cranial bones. In addition to inspecting the newborn's head for degree of molding and size, the nurse should evaluate it for soft-tissue edema and bruising.

Cephalohematoma

Cephalohematoma is a collection of blood resulting from ruptured blood vessels between the surface of a cranial bone (usually parietal) and the periosteal membrane (Figure 24–25). The scalp in these areas feels loose and slightly edematous. These areas emerge as defined hematomas between the first and second day. Although external pressure may cause the mass to fluctuate, it does not increase in size when the newborn cries. Cephalohematomas may be unilateral or bilateral and do not cross suture lines. They are relatively common in vertex births and may disappear within 2 weeks to 3 months. They may be associated with physiologic jaundice because extra red blood cells are being destroyed within the cephalohematoma. A large cephalohematoma can lead to anemia and hypotension.

Caput Succedaneum

Caput succedaneum is a localized, easily identifiable, soft area of the scalp, generally resulting from a long and difficult labor or vacuum extraction (Figure 24–26). The sustained pressure of the presenting part against the cervix results in compression of local blood vessels, and venous return is slowed. Slowed venous return causes an increase in tissue fluids, an edematous swelling, and occasional bleeding under the periosteum. The caput may vary from a small area to a severely elongated head. The

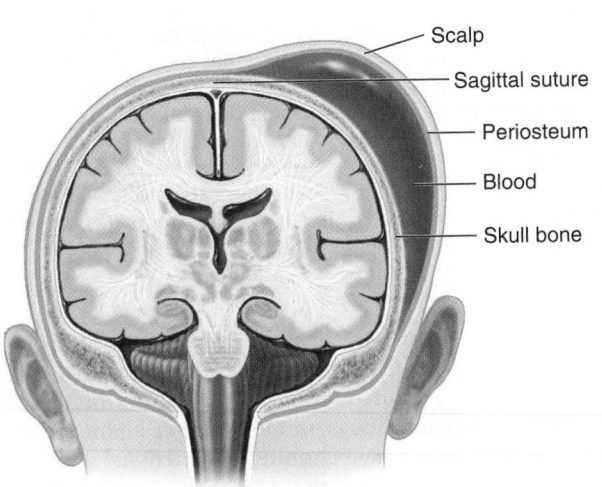

A

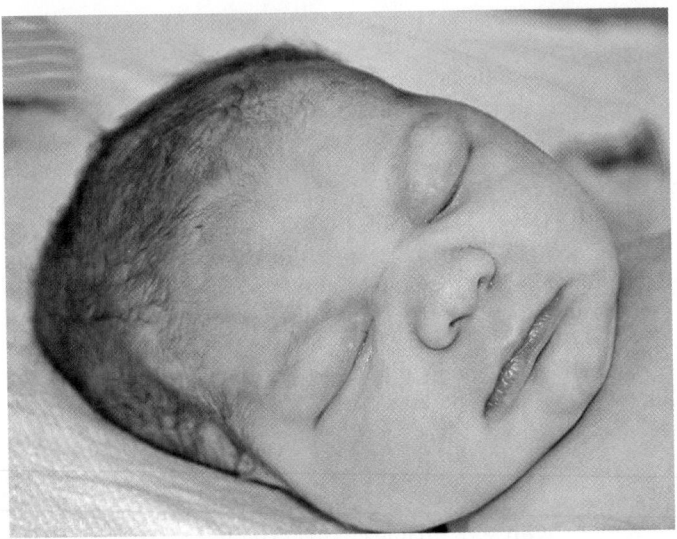

B

Figure 24–25 *A*, Cephalohematoma is a collection of blood between the surface of a cranial bone and the periosteal membrane. *B*, This is a cephalohematoma over the right parietal bone.

SOURCE: Vanessa Howell, RN, MSN.

fluid in the caput is reabsorbed within 12 hours to a few days after birth. Caputs resulting from vacuum extractors are sharply outlined, circular areas up to 2 cm (0.8 in.) thick. They disappear more slowly than naturally occurring edema. See Table 24–2.

Hair

The term newborn's hair is smooth with texture variations depending on ethnic background. Scalp hair is usually high over the eyebrows. Assessment of the newborn's hair characteristics such as color, quantity, texture, hairlines, direction of growth, and hair whorls can identify genetic, metabolic, and neurologic disorders (Johnson, 2015). For example, coarse, brittle, and dry hair may indicate hypothyroidism.

Face

The newborn's face is well designed to help the newborn suckle. Sucking (fat) pads are located in the cheeks, and a labial

TABLE 24–2 Comparison of Cephalohematoma and Caput Succedaneum

CEPHALOHEMATOMA	CAPUT SUCCEDANEUM
Collection of blood between cranial (usually parietal) bone and periosteal membrane	Collection of fluid, edematous swelling of the scalp
Caused by subperiosteal hemorrhage	Caused by pressure of the fetal head against the cervix during labor, which decreases blood flow to the area and results in edema
Does not cross suture lines	Crosses suture lines
Appears on first and second day, increases in size for 2–3 days	Present at birth or shortly thereafter, does not increase in size
Disappears after 2–3 weeks or may take months	Reabsorbed within 12 hr or a few days after birth

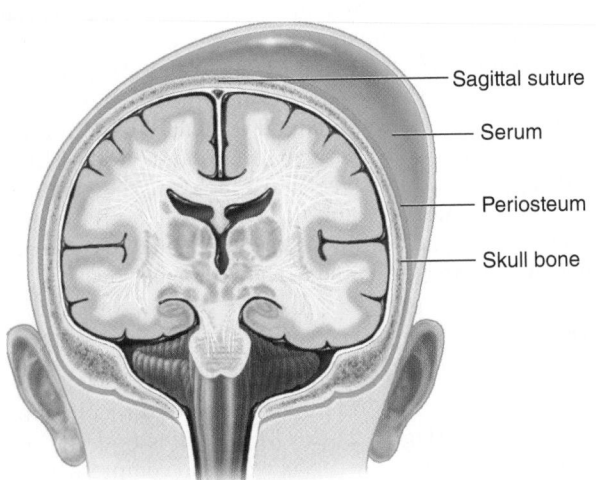

A

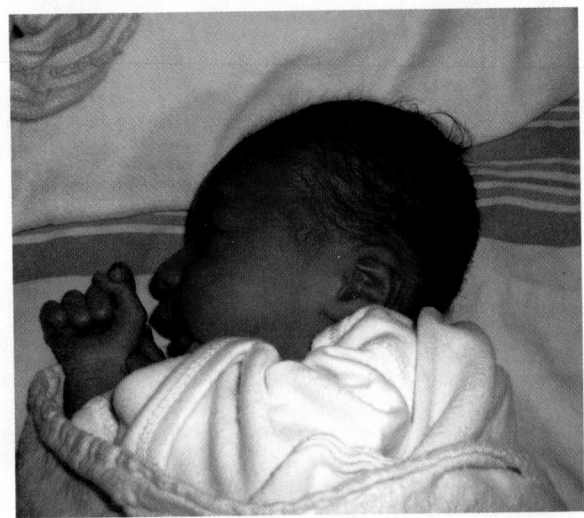

B

Figure 24–26 *A*, Caput succedaneum is a collection of fluid (serum) under the scalp. *B*, Newborn with caput succedaneum.

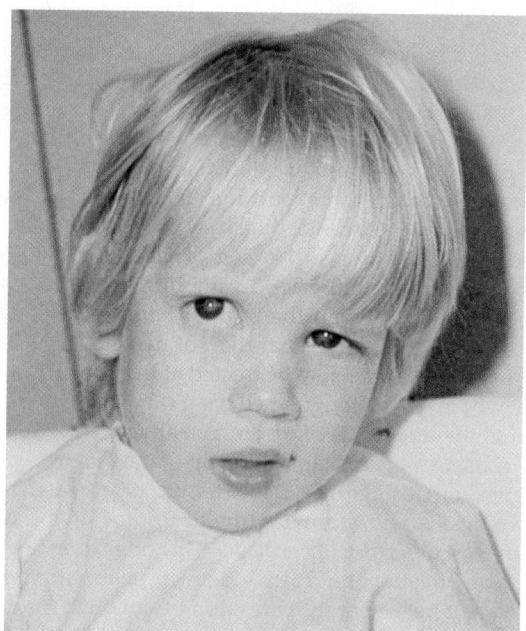

Figure 24–27 Facial paralysis. Paralysis of the left side of the face from injury to the left facial nerve.

SOURCE: Science Source.

tubercle (sucking callus) is frequently found in the center of the upper lip. The chin is recessed, and the nose is flattened. The lips are sensitive to touch, and the sucking reflex is easily initiated. Symmetry of the eyes, nose, and ears is evaluated. See *Assessment Guide: Newborn Physical Assessment* for deviations in symmetry and variations in size, shape, and spacing of facial features. Facial movement symmetry should be assessed to determine the presence of facial palsy. Facial paralysis appears when the newborn cries; the affected side is immobile, and the palpebral (eyelid) fissure widens (Figure 24–27). Paralysis may result from forceps-assisted birth or pressure on the facial nerve from the maternal pelvis during birth. Facial paralysis usually disappears within a few days to 3 weeks, although in some cases it may be permanent.

Eyes

The eyes of the newborn of northern European descent are a blue–gray or slate blue–gray color. Dark-skin newborns tend to have dark eyes at birth. Scleral color tends to be bluish white because of its relative thinness. A blue sclera is associated with osteogenesis imperfecta. The infant's eye color is usually established at approximately 3 months, although it may change any time up to 1 year.

The eyes should be checked for size, equality of pupil size, reaction of pupils to light, blink reflex to light, and edema and inflammation of the eyelids. The eyelids are usually edematous during the first few days of life because of the pressure associated with birth.

Erythromycin and tetracycline (in some agencies) are used prophylactically instead of silver nitrate and usually do not cause chemical irritation of the eye (see Chapter 25). The instillation of silver nitrate drops in the newborn's eyes may cause edema, and **chemical conjunctivitis** may appear a few hours after instillation, but it disappears in 1 to 2 days (Cloherty et al., 2012). If infectious conjunctivitis exists, the newborn has the same purulent (greenish yellow) discharge exudate as in chemical conjunctivitis, but it is caused by gonococci, *Chlamydia*, staphylococci, or a variety of gram-negative bacteria. It requires treatment with ophthalmic antibiotics. Onset is usually after the second day. Edema of the orbits or eyelids may persist for several days until the newborn's kidneys can evacuate the fluid.

Small **subconjunctival hemorrhages** appear in about 10% of newborns and are commonly found on the sclera. These hemorrhages are caused by the changes in vascular tension or ocular pressure during birth. They will remain for a few weeks and are of no pathologic significance. Parents need reassurance that the newborn is not bleeding from within the eye and that vision will not be impaired.

The newborn may demonstrate transient strabismus caused by poor neuromuscular control of eye muscles (Figure 24–28). It gradually regresses in 3 to 4 months. The "doll's eye" phenomenon is also present for about 10 days after birth. As the newborn's head position is changed to the left and then to the right, the eyes move to the opposite direction. "Doll's eye" results from underdeveloped integration of head-eye coordination.

The nurse should observe the newborn's pupils for opacities or whiteness and for the absence of a normal red retinal reflex. Red retinal reflex is a red-orange flash of color observed when an ophthalmoscope light reflects off the retina. In a newborn with dark skin color, the retina may appear paler or more grayish. The color of the red reflex can also be abnormal with retinoblastoma. Absence of red reflex occurs with cataracts. Congenital cataracts should be suspected in newborns of mothers with a history of rubella, cytomegalic inclusion disease, or syphilis. Brushfield spots (black or white spots on the periphery of the iris) can be associated with trisomy 21 (Johnson, 2015).

The cry of the newborn is commonly tearless because the lacrimal structures are immature at birth and are not usually fully functional until the second month of life. However, some babies produce tears during the newborn period.

Poor oculomotor coordination and absence of accommodation limit visual abilities, but newborns have peripheral vision, can fixate on objects near (20.3 cm to 25.4 cm [8 in. to 10 in.]) and in front of their face for short periods, can accommodate to large objects (7.6 cm [3 in.] tall by 7.6 cm [3 in.] wide), and can seek out high-contrast geometric shapes. Newborns can perceive faces, shapes, and colors and begin to show visual preferences early. Newborns generally blink in response to bright lights, to a tap on the bridge of the nose (glabellar reflex), or to a light touch

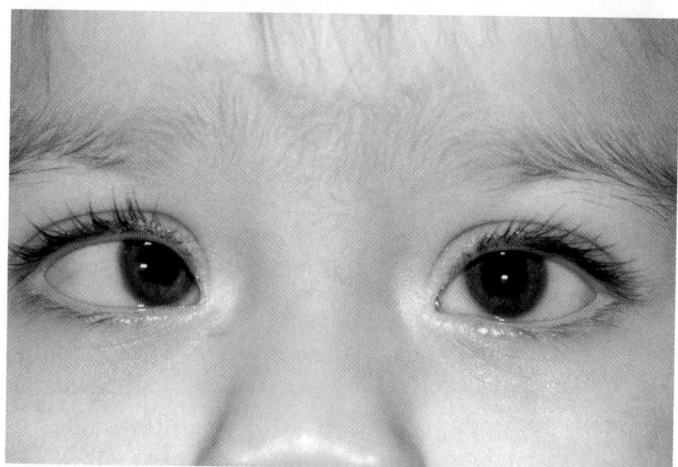

Figure 24–28 Transient strabismus in the newborn may be due to poor neuromuscular control.

SOURCE: Biophoto Associates/Science Source.

on the eyelids. Pupillary light reflex is also present. Examination of the eye is best accomplished by rocking the newborn from an upright position to the horizontal a few times or by other methods, such as diminishing overhead lights, which elicit an opened-eye response.

Nose

The newborn's nose is small and narrow. Infants are characteristically nose breathers for the first few months of life and generally remove obstructions by sneezing. Nasal patency is ensured if the newborn breathes easily with the mouth closed. If respiratory difficulty occurs, the nurse checks for choanal atresia (congenital blockage of the passageway between the nose and pharynx). This can be done by observing the newborn feeding or by gently occluding each of the nares (Caveliere & Sansoucie, 2014).

The newborn has the ability to smell after the nasal passages are cleared of amniotic fluid and mucus. Newborns demonstrate this ability by the search for milk. They turn their heads toward a milk source, whether bottle or breast. Newborns react to strong odors, such as alcohol, by turning their heads away or blinking.

Mouth

The lips of the newborn should be pink, and a touch on the lips should produce sucking motions. Saliva is normally scant. The taste buds develop before birth, and the newborn can easily discriminate between sweet and bitter flavors.

The easiest way to examine the mouth completely is to stimulate newborns to cry such as by gently depressing the tongue, thereby causing them to open the mouth fully. It is extremely important to examine the entire mouth to check for a cleft palate, which can be present even in the absence of a cleft lip. The examiner moves an unpowdered, gloved index finger along the hard and soft palates to feel for any openings (Figure 24–29). Occasionally, an examination of the gums will reveal *precocious teeth* over the area where the lower central incisor will erupt. If they

appear loose, they should be removed to prevent aspiration. Gray-white lesions (inclusion cysts) on the gums may be confused with teeth. On the hard palate and gum margins, **Epstein pearls**, small glistening white specks (keratin-containing cysts) that feel hard to the touch, are often present. They usually disappear in a few weeks and are of no significance. **Thrush** may appear as white patches that look like milk curds adhering to the mucous membranes, and bleeding may occur when patches are removed. Thrush is caused by *Candida albicans*, often acquired from an infected vaginal tract during birth, antibiotic use, or poor hand washing when the mother handles her newborn. Thrush is treated with a preparation of nystatin (Mycostatin). The mother may also need to be treated at the same time.

A newborn who is tongue-tied has a ridge of frenulum tissue attached to the underside of the tongue at varying lengths from its base, causing a heart shape at the tip of the tongue. "Clipping the tongue," or cutting the ridge of tissue, is not usually recommended unless the newborn has trouble feeding. In this case, the physician would perform a *frenotomy*. This ridge does not usually affect speech or eating, but cutting does create an entry for infection. Transient nerve paralysis resulting from birth trauma may be manifested by asymmetric mouth movements when the newborn cries or by difficulty with sucking and feeding.

Ears

The ears of the newborn are soft and pliable and should recoil readily when folded and released. In the normal newborn, the top of the ear (pinna) should be parallel to the outer and inner canthus of the eye. The ears should be inspected for shape, size, firmness of cartilage, and position. *Low-set ears* are characteristic of many syndromes and may indicate chromosomal abnormalities (especially trisomies 13 and 18), intellectual disability, and internal organ abnormalities, especially bilateral renal agenesis as a result of embryologic developmental deviations (Figure 24–30). *Preauricular skin tags* may be present just in front of the ear. Visualization of the tympanic membrane is not usually done soon after birth because blood and vernix block the ear canal.

Following the first cry, the newborn's hearing becomes acute as mucus from the middle ears is absorbed, the eustachian tubes become aerated, and the tympanic membranes become visible. The newborn's hearing initially can be evaluated by noting the baby's response to loud or moderately loud noises that are not accompanied by vibrations. The sleeping newborn should stir or awaken in response to nearby sounds. (This is not a very accurate test, but it may alert the examiner to a possible problem.) The newborn can discriminate the individual characteristics of the human voice and is especially sensitive to sound

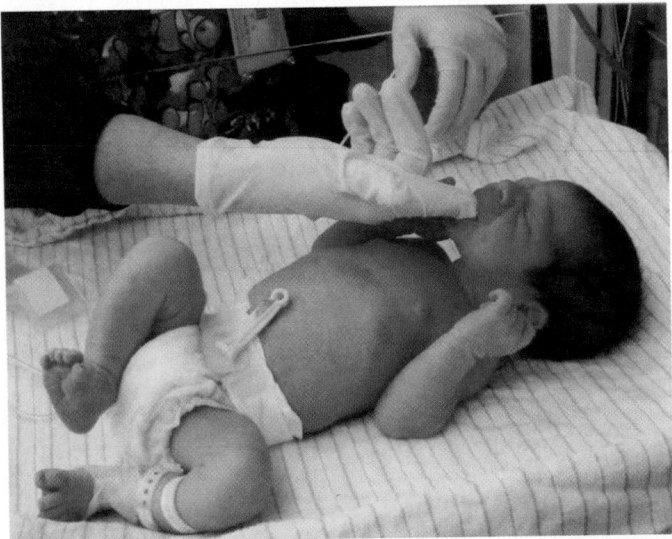

Figure 24–29 The nurse inserts a gloved index finger into the newborn's mouth and feels for any openings along the hard and soft palates. *Note:* Gloves or a finger cot are always worn to examine the palate.

SOURCE: Vanessa Howell, RNC, MSN.

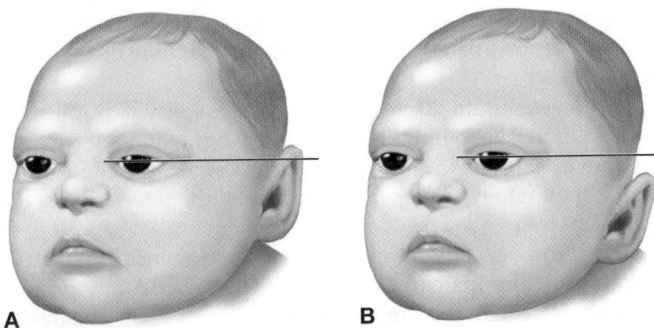

A   **B**

Figure 24–30 The position of the external ear may be assessed by drawing a line across the inner and outer canthus of the eye to the insertion of the ear. *A*, Normal position. *B*, True low-set position.

levels within the normal conversational range. The newborn in a noisy nursery may habituate to the sounds and not stir unless the sound is sudden or much louder than usual. The AAP has endorsed universal newborn hearing screening (UNHS) before discharge from the birthing unit as the standard of care (AAP & ACOG, 2012; Johnson, 2015). See Chapter 25 for discussion of newborn hearing screening.

Neck

A short neck, creased with skin folds, is characteristic of the normal newborn. Because muscle tone is not well developed, the neck cannot support the full weight of the head, which rotates freely. The head lags considerably when the newborn is pulled from a supine to a sitting position, but the prone newborn is able to raise the head slightly. The neck is palpated for masses and the presence of lymph nodes and is inspected for webbing. Adequacy of range-of-motion and neck muscle function is determined by moving the head while supporting the newborn to prevent injury. Injury to the sternocleidomastoid muscle (congenital torticollis) must be considered in the presence of neck rigidity.

The nurse evaluates the clavicles for evidence of fractures, which occasionally occur during difficult births or in newborns with broad shoulders. The normal clavicle is straight. If fractured, a lump and a grating sensation (crepitus) during movements may be palpated along the course of the side of the break. The nurse also elicits the Moro reflex (see Table 24–4) to evaluate bilateral equal movement of the arms. If the clavicle is fractured, the response will be demonstrated only on the unaffected side.

Chest

The thorax is cylindric and symmetric at birth, and the ribs are flexible. The general appearance of the chest should be assessed. A protrusion at the lower end of the sternum, called the *xiphoid cartilage*, is frequently seen. It is under the skin and will become less apparent after several weeks as adipose tissue accumulates.

Engorged breasts occur frequently in both male and female newborns. This condition, which occurs by the third day, is a result of maternal hormonal influences and may last up to 2 weeks (Figure 24–31). A whitish secretion from the nipples may also be noted. The newborn's breast should not be massaged or squeezed because this may cause a breast abscess. Supernumerary nipples are occasionally noted below and medial to the true nipples. These harmless pink or brown (in dark-skin newborns) spots vary in size and do not contain glandular tissue. Accessory nipples can be differentiated from pigmented nevi (moles) by placing the fingertips alongside the accessory nipple and pulling the adjacent tissue laterally. The accessory nipple will appear dimpled.

Clinical Tip

Vital sign assessments are most accurate if the newborn is at rest, so measure pulse and respirations first if the baby is quiet. To soothe a crying baby, try placing your moistened gloved finger in the baby's mouth, and then complete your assessment while the baby suckles.

Cry

The newborn's cry should be strong, lusty, and of medium pitch. A high-pitched, shrill cry is abnormal and may indicate neurologic disorders or hypoglycemia. Periods of crying usually vary

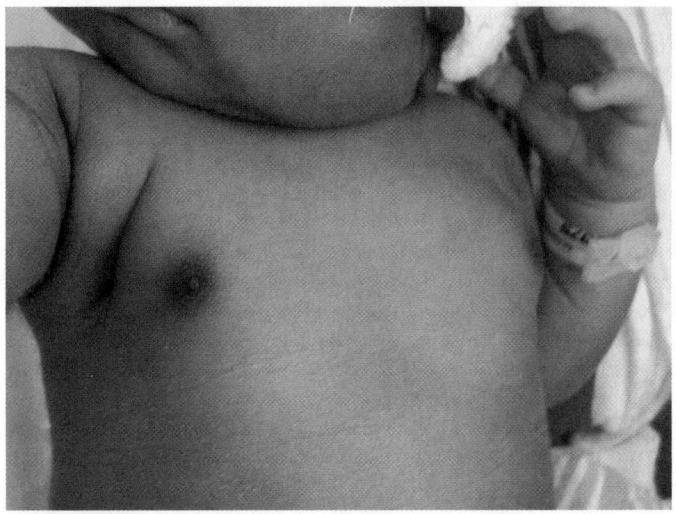

Figure 24–31   **Breast hypertrophy.**

in length after consoling measures are used. Babies' cries are an important method of communication and alert caregivers to changes in their condition and needs (see Chapter 30).

Respiration

Normal breathing for a term newborn is 30 to 60 respirations per minute and is predominantly diaphragmatic, with associated rising and falling of the abdomen during inspiration and expiration. The nurse should note any signs of respiratory distress, nasal flaring, intercostal or xiphoid retraction, expiratory grunt or sigh, seesaw respirations, or tachypnea (greater than 60 breaths per minute). Hyperextension (chest appears high) or hypoextension (chest appears low) of the anteroposterior diameter of the chest should also be noted. Both the anterior and posterior chest are auscultated. Some breath sounds are heard best when the newborn is crying, but localizing and identifying breath sounds is difficult in the newborn. Upper airway noises and bowel sounds can be heard over the chest wall, making auscultation difficult. Because sounds may be transmitted from the unaffected lung to the affected lung, the absence of breath sounds may not be diagnosed. Air entry may be noisy in the first couple of hours until lung fluid resolves, especially after cesarean births. Brief periods of periodic breathing occur, but no color or heart rate changes occur in healthy, term newborns. Sepsis should be suspected in full-term newborns experiencing apneic episodes.

Heart

Heart rates can be as rapid as 180 beats per minute (beats/min) in newborns and fluctuate a great deal, especially if the baby moves or is startled. The normal range is 110 to 160 beats/min. The heart is examined for rate and rhythm, position of the apical impulse, and heart sound intensity. Dysrhythmias should be evaluated by the physician.

The pulse rate is variable and is influenced by physical activity, crying, state of wakefulness, and body temperature. Auscultation is performed over the entire heart region (precordium), below the left axilla, and below the scapula. Apical pulse rates are obtained by auscultation for a full minute, preferably when the newborn is asleep.

The placement of the heart in the chest should be determined when the newborn is in a quiet state. The heart is relatively large at birth and is located mid to left chest and high in the chest, with its apex somewhere between the fourth and fifth intercostal space.

A shift of heart tones in the mediastinal area to either side may indicate pneumothorax, dextrocardia (heart placement on the right side of the chest), or a diaphragmatic hernia. The experienced nurse can detect these and many other problems early with a stethoscope. Auscultate heart sounds using both the bell and diaphragm of the stethoscope. Normally, the heartbeat has a "toc tic" sound. A slur or slushing sound (usually after the first sound) may indicate a *murmur.* Although 90% of all murmurs are transient and are considered normal, they should be monitored closely by a physician. Many murmurs are secondary to closing of patent ductus arteriosus or patent foramen ovale, which should close 1 to 2 days after birth. (See Chapters 26 and 47 for discussions of congenital heart defects in the infant and child.)

Peripheral pulses (brachial, femoral, pedal) are also evaluated to detect any lags or unusual characteristics. Brachial pulses are palpated bilaterally for equality and compared with the femoral pulses. Femoral pulses are palpated by applying gentle pressure with the middle finger over the femoral canal (Figure 24–32). Decreased or absent femoral pulses may indicate coarctation of the aorta or hypovolemia and require additional evaluation. A wide difference in blood pressure between the upper and lower extremities also indicates coarctation of the aorta.

The measurement of blood pressure is best accomplished by using a noninvasive blood pressure device (Figure 24–33). If a blood pressure cuff is used, the newborn's extremities must be immobilized during the assessment, and the cuff should cover two thirds of the upper arm or upper leg. Movement, crying, and inappropriate cuff size can give inaccurate measurements of the blood pressure.

Blood pressure may not be measured routinely on healthy newborns, but it is essential for newborns who are having distress, are premature, or are suspected of having a critical cardiac anomaly, renal disease, or clinical signs of hypotension (Vargo, 2015). Newborns who have birth asphyxia and are on ventilators have significantly lower systolic and diastolic blood pressures than healthy newborns. If a cardiac anomaly is suspected, blood pressure is measured in all four extremities (Table 24–3). At birth, systolic values usually range from 70 to 50 mmHg and diastolic values from 45 to 30 mmHg. By the tenth day of life, blood pressure rises to 90/50 mmHg.

Clinical Tip

If possible, obtain blood pressure measurement during quiet sleep or sleep state. Place the cuff on the arm or leg and give the newborn time to quiet. Obtain an average of two to three measurements when making clinical decisions. Follow mean blood pressure to monitor changes, as it is less likely to be erroneous. Noninvasive blood pressure may overestimate blood pressure in very-low-birth-weight newborns.

Abdomen

The nurse can learn a great deal about the newborn's abdomen without disturbing the baby. The abdomen should be cylindric, protrude slightly, and move with respiration. A certain amount

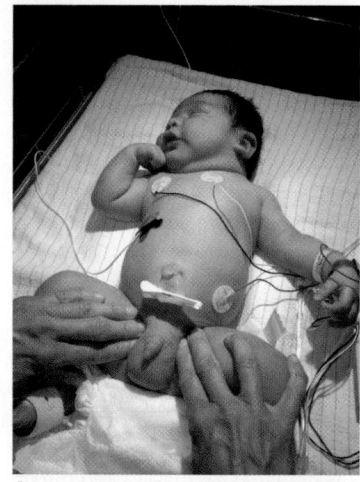

A

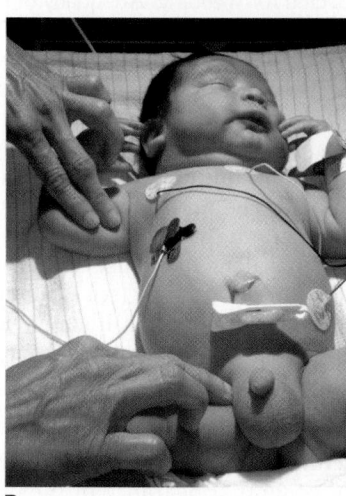

B

Figure 24–32 *A,* Bilaterally palpate the femoral arteries for rate and intensity of the pulses. Press fingertip gently at the groin as shown. *B,* Compare the femoral pulses to the brachial pulses by palpating the pulses simultaneously for comparison of rate and intensity.

SOURCE: Carol Harrigan, RNC, MSN, NNP.

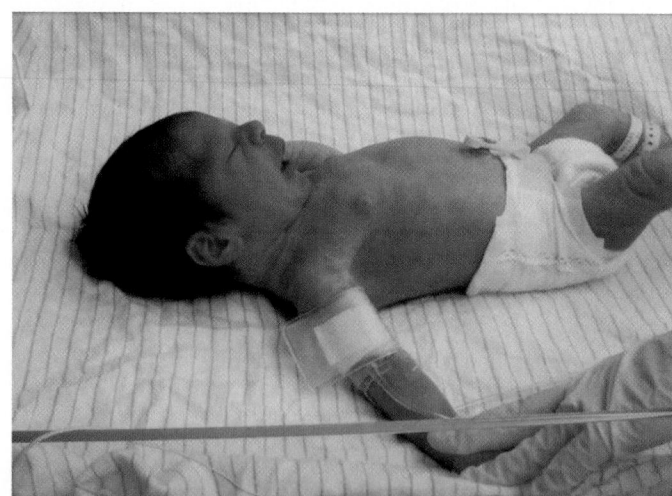

Figure 24–33 Blood pressure measurement using the Dinamap and Doppler devices. The cuff can be applied to either the newborn's upper arm or the thigh.

SOURCE: Vanessa Howell, RNC, MSN.

TABLE 24–3 Newborn Vital Signs

PULSE
110–160 beats/min

During sleep as low as 80 beats/min; if crying, up to 180 beats/min (Glomella, 2013)

Apical pulse counted for 1 full minute

RESPIRATIONS
30–60 respirations/minute

Predominantly diaphragmatic but synchronous with abdominal movements

Respirations counted for 1 full minute

BLOOD PRESSURE
70–50/45–30 mmHg at birth

90/50 mmHg at day 10

TEMPERATURE
Normal range: 36.5°–37.5°C (97.7°–99.4°F)

Axillary: 36.4°–37.2°C (97.5°–99°F)

Skin: 36°–36.5°C (96.8°–97.7°F)

Rectal: 36.6°–37.2°C (97.8°–99°F)

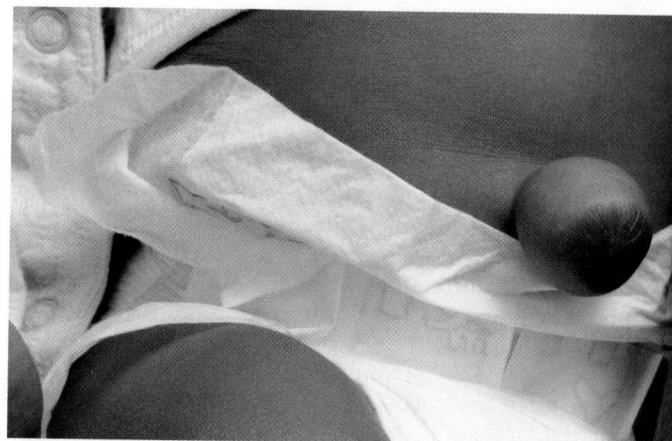

Figure 24–34 Umbilical hernia.

cord hernia and associated patent omphalomesenteric duct (Figure 24–34). Umbilical hernias are more common in infants of African American descent than in White infants (Goodwin, 2015). Umbilical hernias usually close spontaneously by 2 years of age.

Developing Cultural Competence Native Americans and Umbilical Cord Care

In the Woodland Indian tribe, upon birth, the umbilical cord is tied and a small piece is saved. This section of the umbilical cord is sewn into a deerskin diamond-shaped pocket. The pocket is hung over the infant's crib to provide protection for the infant.

of laxness of the abdominal muscles is normal. A scaphoid (hollow-shaped) appearance suggests the absence of abdominal contents, often seen in diaphragmatic hernias. No cyanosis should be present, and few if any blood vessels should be apparent to the eye. There should be no gross distention or bulging. The more distended the abdomen, the tighter the skin becomes, with engorged vessels appearing. Distention is the first sign of many gastrointestinal abnormalities.

Before palpation of the abdomen, the nurse should auscultate for the presence or absence of bowel sounds in all four quadrants. Bowel sounds may be present by 1 hour after birth. Palpation can cause a transient decrease in bowel sounds intensity.

Abdominal palpation should be done systematically. The nurse palpates each of the four abdominal quadrants and moves in a clockwise direction until all four quadrants have been palpated for softness, tenderness, and the presence of masses. The nurse should place one hand under the back for support during palpation.

Umbilical Cord

Initially, the umbilical cord is white and gelatinous in appearance, with the two umbilical arteries and one umbilical vein readily apparent. Because a single umbilical artery is frequently associated with congenital anomalies, the nurse should count the vessels during the newborn assessment. The cord begins drying within 1 or 2 hours of birth and is shriveled and blackened by the second or third day. (Care of the umbilical cord is discussed in Chapter 25.)

Cord bleeding is abnormal and may result from tension on the cord or clamp. Foul-smelling drainage is also abnormal and is generally caused by infection, which requires immediate treatment to prevent septicemia. Serous or serosanguineous drainage that continues after the cord falls off may indicate a granuloma. If the newborn has a patent urachus (abnormal connection between the umbilicus and bladder), moistness or draining urine may be apparent at the base of the cord. Another umbilical cord anomaly that can occur is umbilical

Genitals

FEMALE NEWBORNS
Examine the labia majora, labia minora, and clitoris and note the size of each as appropriate for gestational age. A vaginal tag or hymenal tag is often evident and will usually disappear in a few weeks. During the first week of life, the female newborn may have a vaginal discharge composed of thick, whitish mucus. This discharge, which can become tinged with blood, is called **pseudomenstruation** and is caused by the withdrawal of maternal hormones. *Smegma*, a white, cheeselike substance, is often present between the labia. Removing it may traumatize tender tissue.

MALE NEWBORNS
The nurse inspects the penis to determine whether the urinary orifice is correctly positioned. *Hypospadias* occurs when the urinary meatus is located on the ventral surface of the penis, whereas in *epispadias,* the meatus is on the dorsal surface of the glans. Hypospadias occurs most commonly among people of Western European descent. *Phimosis* is a condition in which the opening of the foreskin (prepuce) is small and the foreskin cannot be pulled back over the glans at all. This condition may interfere with urination, so the adequacy of the urinary stream should be evaluated.

The scrotum is inspected for size and symmetry. Scrotal color variations are especially prominent in African American, Indian, and Hispanic newborns (Cloherty et al., 2012). The scrotum should be palpated to verify the presence of both testes and to rule out *cryptorchidism* (failure of testes to descend). The testes are palpated separately between the thumb and forefinger, with the thumb and forefinger of the other hand placed together over the inguinal canal. Scrotal edema and discoloration are common in breech births. *Hydrocele* (a collection of fluid surrounding the testes in the scrotum) is common in newborns and should be identified. It usually resolves without intervention. The presence of a discolored or dusky scrotum and solid testis should raise the suspicion of testicular torsion, which should be reported immediately.

Anus

The anal area is inspected to verify that it is patent and has no fissure. Imperforate anus and rectal atresia may be ruled out by observation. Digital examination, if necessary, is done by a physician or nurse practitioner. The nurse also notes the passage of the first meconium stool. Atresia of the gastrointestinal tract or meconium ileus with resultant obstruction must be considered if the newborn does not pass meconium in the first 24 hours of life.

Extremities

Extremities are examined for gross deformities, extra digits or webbing, clubfoot, and range-of-motion. Normal newborn extremities appear short, are generally flexible, and move symmetrically.

ARMS AND HANDS

Nails extend beyond the fingertips in term newborns. The nurse should count fingers and toes. *Polydactyly* is the presence of extra digits on either the hands or the feet. *Syndactyly* refers to fusion (webbing) of fingers or toes, which can be hereditary or associated with trisomy 21 (Down syndrome). The hands are inspected for normal palmar creases. A single palmar crease is frequently present in children with trisomy 21.

Brachial palsy, paralysis of portions of the arm, results from trauma to the brachial plexus during a difficult birth. It occurs commonly when strong traction is exerted on the head of the newborn in an attempt to deliver a shoulder lodged behind the symphysis pubis in the presence of shoulder dystocia. Brachial palsy may also occur during a breech birth if an arm becomes trapped over the head and traction is exerted.

The portion of the arm affected is determined by the nerves damaged. **Erb-Duchenne paralysis (Erb palsy)** involves damage to the upper arm (fifth and sixth cervical nerves) and is the most common type. Injury to the eighth cervical and first thoracic nerve roots and the *lower portion* of the plexus produces the relatively rare lower arm injury. The *whole-arm type* results from damage to the entire plexus.

With Erb-Duchenne paralysis, the newborn's arm lies limply at the side. The elbow is held in extension, with the forearm pronated. The newborn is unable to elevate the arm, and the Moro reflex cannot be elicited on the affected side. Lower arm injury causes paralysis of the hand and wrist; complete paralysis of the limb occurs with the whole-arm type.

The degree of nerve damage, which results from the trauma and hemorrhage within the nerve sheath, determines recovery. Complete recovery occurs within a few months with minimal trauma. Moderate trauma may result in partial paralysis. Recovery is unlikely with severe trauma, and muscle wasting may develop.

LEGS AND FEET

The legs of the newborn should be of equal length and with symmetric skin folds. However, they may assume a fetal posture, similar to the position in utero, and it may take several days for the legs and feet to relax into a normal position. The nurse should assess for asymmetry of inner thigh folds, limited hip abduction, and the Allis sign (an indication of fracture in the neck of the femur in which a finger easily sinks into the relaxed fascia between the great trochanter and the iliac crest) (Figure 24–35A). To further evaluate hip dislocation or hip instability, the Ortolani and Barlow maneuvers are performed. The nurse (or more commonly, the physician or nurse practitioner) performs the **Barlow maneuver** (Figure 24–35B, C) to rule out the possibility of developmental dysplastic hip, also called *congenital hip dysplasia* (hip dislocatability). The examiner grasps and adducts the newborn's thigh and applies gentle downward pressure. Dislocation can be felt as the femoral head slips out of the acetabulum.

The **Ortolani maneuver** (Figure 24–35D) should be performed with the newborn relaxed and quiet on a firm surface. With hips and knees flexed at a 90-degree angle, the examiner grasps the newborn's thigh with the middle finger over the greater trochanter and lifts the thigh to bring the femoral head from its posterior position toward the acetabulum. With gentle abduction of the thigh, the femoral head is returned to the acetabulum and the examiner feels a sense of reduction or a "clunk" as the femoral head returns, confirming the diagnosis of an unstable or dislocatable hip.

Examine the feet for evidence of a talipes deformity (clubfoot). Intrauterine position frequently causes the feet to appear to turn inward (Figure 24–36); this is termed a *"positional" clubfoot*. If the feet can easily be returned to the midline by manipulation, no treatment is indicated and the nurse teaches range-of-motion exercises to the family. Further evaluation is indicated when the foot will not turn to a midline position or align readily. This is considered the most severe type of "true clubfoot," or talipes equinovarus.

Back

With the newborn prone, examine the back. The spine should appear straight and flat because the lumbar and sacral curves do not develop until the newborn begins to sit. The base of the spine is examined for a dermal sinus. A nevus pilosus ("hairy nerve") is occasionally found at the base of the spine in newborns. It is significant because it is frequently associated with spina bifida. A pilonidal dimple should be reported to the healthcare provider to ascertain that there is no connection to the spinal canal.

Assessment of Neurologic Status

The neurologic examination should begin with a period of observation, noting the general physical characteristics and behaviors of the newborn. Important behaviors to assess are the *state of alertness, resting posture, cry,* and *quality of muscle tone and motor activity*.

The usual position of the newborn is with partially flexed extremities, with the legs abducted to the abdomen. When awake, the newborn may exhibit purposeless, uncoordinated

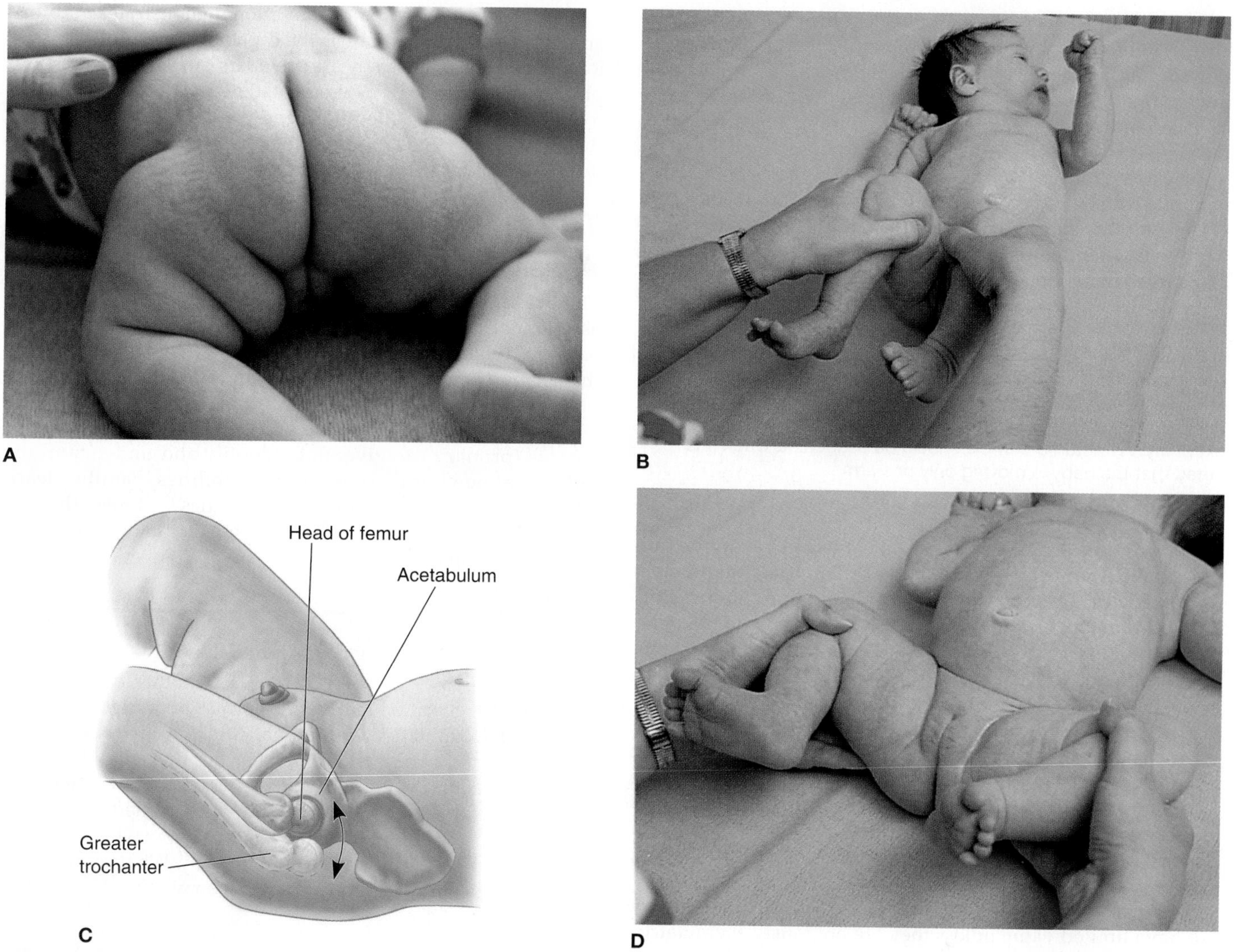

Figure 24–35 *A,* The asymmetry of gluteal and thigh fat folds seen in newborn with left developmental dysplasia of the hip. *B,* The Barlow (dislocation) maneuver. Baby's thigh is grasped and adducted (placed together) with gentle downward pressure. *C,* Dislocation is palpable as the femoral head slips out of the acetabulum. *D,* The Ortolani maneuver puts downward pressure on the hip and then inward rotation. If the hip is dislocated, this maneuver will force the femoral head back into the acetabular rim with a noticeable "clunk."

Head of femur
Acetabulum
Greater trochanter

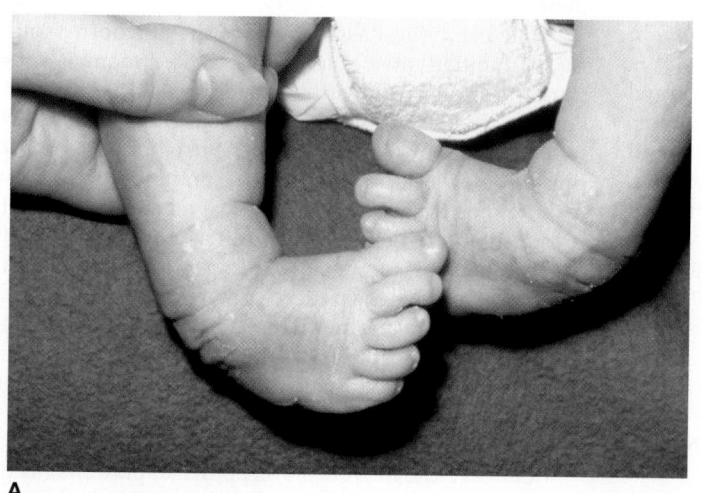
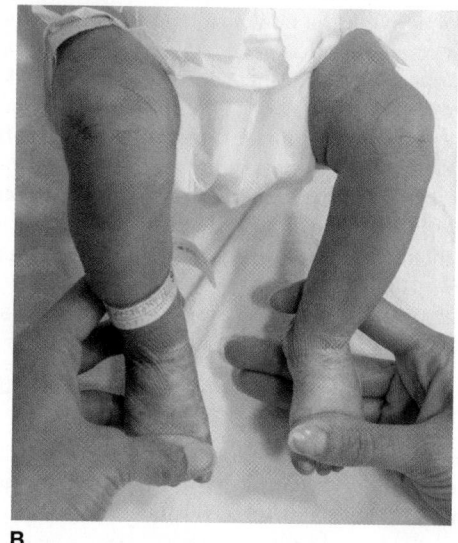

Figure 24–36 *A,* Bilateral talipes equinovarus (clubfoot). *B,* To determine the presence of clubfoot, the nurse moves the foot to the midline. Resistance indicates true clubfoot.

SOURCE: *A.* Jim Stevenson/Science Source.

bilateral movements of the extremities. If these movements are absent, minimal, or obviously asymmetric, neurologic dysfunction should be suspected. Eye movements are observable during the first few days of life. An alert newborn is able to fixate on faces and brightly colored objects. Shining a bright light in the newborn's eyes elicits the blinking response.

Evaluate muscle tone by moving various parts of the body while the head of the newborn is in a neutral position. The newborn is somewhat hypertonic; that is, there should be resistance to extending the elbow and knee joints. Muscle tone should be symmetric. Diminished muscle tone and flaccidity require further evaluation.

Clinical Tip

Always examine more closely any newborn who is reluctant to move an extremity. Fractures are often asymptomatic in the newborn. Paralytic injuries are characterized by immobility of an extremity. A fractured clavicle should be suspected when it is noted that the baby is moving only one arm.

Tremors or jitteriness (tremor-like movements) in the full-term newborn must be evaluated to differentiate the tremors from seizures. Tremors may also be related to hypoglycemia, hypocalcemia, or substance withdrawal. Environmental stimuli may initiate tremors. Jitteriness may be distinguished from tonic-clonic seizure activity because it usually can be stopped by the newborn's sucking on the extremity or by the nurse holding or flexing the involved extremity. A fine jumping of the muscle is likely to be a central nervous system (CNS) disorder and requires further evaluation. Newborn seizures may consist of no more than chewing or swallowing movements, deviations of the eyes, rigidity, or flaccidity because of CNS immaturity. In contrast to tremors, seizures are not usually initiated by stimuli, and cannot be stopped by holding.

Specific deep tendon reflexes can be elicited in the newborn but have limited value unless they are obviously asymmetric. The knee jerk is typically brisk; a normal ankle clonus may involve three or four beats. Plantar flexion is present.

The immature CNS of the newborn is characterized by a variety of reflexes. Because the newborn's movements are uncoordinated, methods of communication are limited, and control of body functions is restricted, the reflexes serve a variety of purposes. Some aid in feeding (rooting, sucking) and may not be very active if the newborn has eaten recently, and some stimulate human interaction (grasping). In addition, newborns can blink, gag, yawn, cough, sneeze, and draw back from pain (protective reflexes). They can even move a little on their own. When placed on their stomachs, they push up and try to crawl (prone crawl). Absence or a variance in the response requires motor function by a specialist. Absence of the *plantar grasp* and *Galant (truncal) incurvation* reflexes requires neurologic evaluation. The most common reflexes found in the normal newborn are shown in Table 24–4.

The nurse uses the following steps to assess CNS integration:

1. Insert a gloved finger into the newborn's mouth to elicit a sucking reflex.

2. As soon as the newborn is sucking vigorously, assess hearing and vision responses by noting changes in sucking in the presence of a light, a rattle, and a voice.

3. The newborn should respond to such stimuli with a brief cessation of sucking, followed by continuous sucking with repetitious stimulation.

This CNS integration examination demonstrates auditory and visual integrity as well as the capability of complex behavioral interactions. As healthcare providers carry out the newborn physical and neurologic assessment, they are always on the alert to recognize possible alterations and possible injuries related to the birth process that require further investigation and intervention. (See Table 24–5 for potential types of birth trauma.)

The Brazelton Neonatal Behavioral Assessment Scale

The **Brazelton Neonatal Behavioral Assessment Scale** is an assessment tool used to identify the newborn's repertoire of behavioral responses to the environment and also documents the newborn's neurologic adequacy and capabilities. (For complete discussion of all test items and maneuvers, see Nugent, 2013.) It provides a way for the nurse, in conjunction with the parents (primary caregivers), to identify and understand the individual newborn's states and capabilities. Families learn which responses, interventions, or activities best meet the special needs of their newborn, and this understanding fosters positive attachment experiences.

Clinical Reasoning Newborn Behavior

Maria Reyes, a 19-year-old G2 (now P2) mother, delivered a 40 weeks' gestation female newborn 24 hours ago. The newborn examination was normal. Mrs. Reyes says she has noticed that the baby cries more than her first child did and seems to require holding for longer periods of time after feeding before "quieting down." She is concerned that she is doing something wrong and wants to know when her newborn will start to act like her first baby. What should you discuss with her about newborn behavior?

Because the first few days after birth are a period of behavioral disorganization, the complete assessment should be done on the third day after birth. The nurse should make every effort to elicit the best response. This may be accomplished by repeating tests at different times or by testing during situations that facilitate the best possible response, such as when the parents are holding, cuddling, rocking, or singing to their baby.

The behavioral assessment of the newborn should be carried out initially in a quiet, dimly lighted room, if possible. The nurse first determines the newborn's state of consciousness because scoring and introduction of the test items are correlated with the sleep or waking state. The newborn's state depends on physiologic variables, such as the amount of time from the last feeding, positioning, environmental temperature, health status, presence of such external stimuli as noises and bright lights, and the wake–sleep cycle. An important characteristic of the newborn period is the pattern of states, as well as the transitions from one state to another. The pattern of states is a predictor of the newborn's receptivity and ability to respond to stimuli in a cognitive manner. Babies learn best in a quiet, alert state and in an environment that is supportive and protective and that provides appropriate stimuli.

Observe the newborn's sleep–wake patterns (as discussed in Chapter 23), including the rapidity with which the newborn moves from one state to another, the ability to be consoled, and the ability to diminish the impact of disturbing stimuli. The

TABLE 24–4 Common Newborn Reflexes

Tonic neck reflex (fencer position). Elicited when the newborn is supine and the head is turned to one side. In response, the extremities on the same side straighten, whereas on the opposite side they flex. This reflex may not be seen during the early newborn period, but once it appears it persists until about the third month.

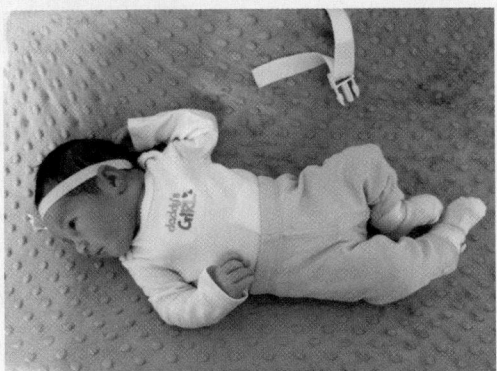

Tonic neck reflex.
SOURCE: Craig London.

Moro reflex. Elicited when the newborn is startled by a loud noise or lifted slightly above the crib and then suddenly lowered. In response, the newborn straightens arms and hands outward while the knees flex. Slowly the arms return to the chest, as in an embrace. The fingers spread, forming a C, and the newborn may cry. This reflex may persist until about 6 months of age.

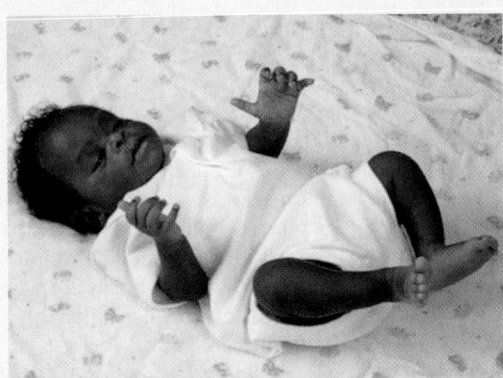

Moro reflex.

Stepping reflex. When held upright with one foot touching a flat surface, the newborn puts one foot in front of the other and "walks." This reflex is more pronounced at birth and is lost in 4–8 weeks.

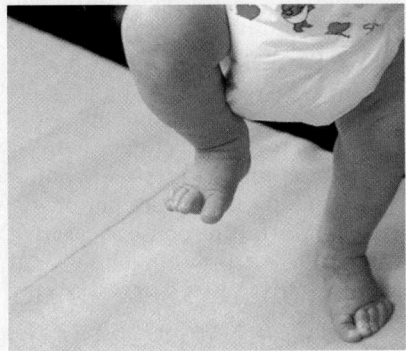

Stepping reflex.

Palmar grasping reflex. Elicited by stimulating the newborn's palm with a finger or object; the newborn grasps and holds the object or finger firmly enough to be lifted momentarily from the crib.

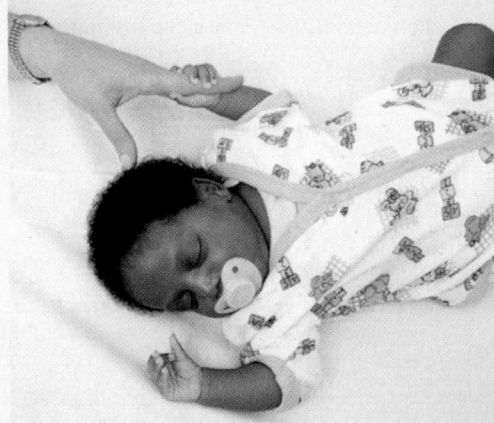

Palmar grasping reflex.

Rooting reflex. Elicited when the side of the newborn's mouth or cheek is touched. In response, the newborn turns toward that side and opens the lips to suck (if not fed recently).

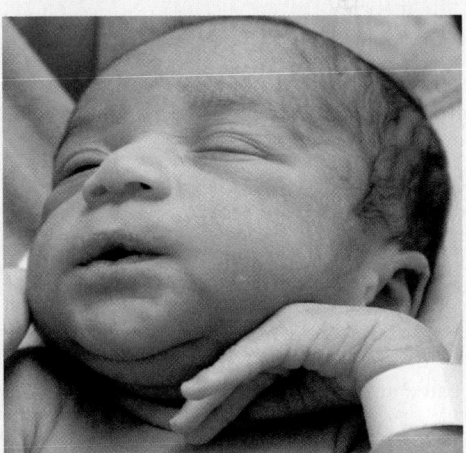

Rooting reflex.

Sucking reflex. Elicited when an object is placed in the newborn's mouth or anything touches the lips. Newborns suck even while sleeping; this is called *nonnutritive sucking*, and it can have a quieting effect on the baby. Disappears by 12 months.

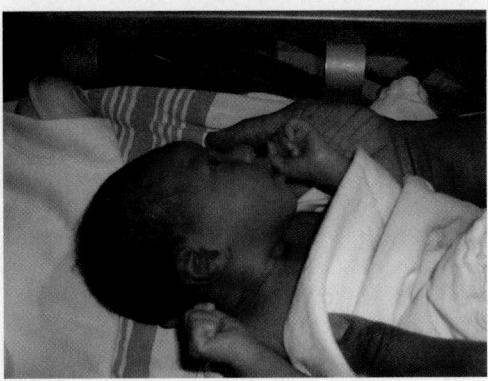

Sucking reflex.

TABLE 24–5 Potential Types of Birth Trauma

CLASSIFICATION	EXAMPLES*
Soft-tissue injuries	Lacerations, abrasions, bruising, fat necrosis
Skull injuries	Cephalohematoma, *fractures
Scalp laceration/abscess	Fetal scalp electrode
Intracranial hemorrhage	Subdural, subarachnoid
Eye injuries	*Subconjunctival and retinal hemorrhages
Bone fractures	Clavicle, *facial bones, humerus, femur
Nasal injuries	Dislocation, *fractures
Dislocations	Hips
Cranial nerve injuries	Facial nerve, *brachial plexus, *phrenic nerve, recurrent laryngeal nerve (vocal cord paralysis), Horner syndrome

*Most common birth injuries seen in newborns.

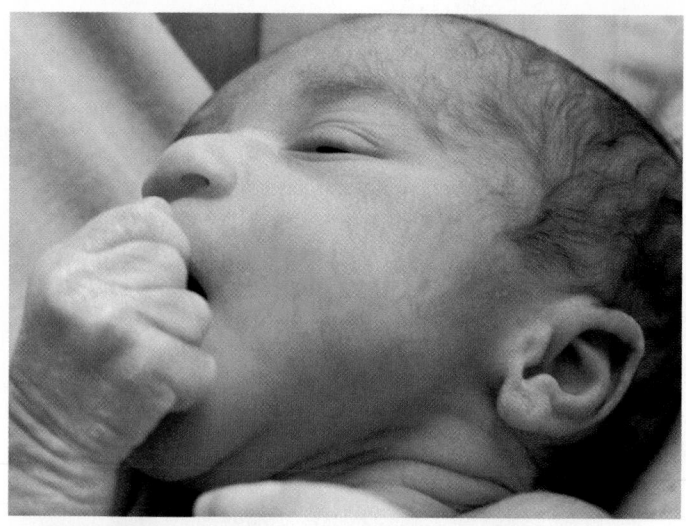

Figure 24–37 The newborn can bring hand to mouth as a self-soothing activity.

following questions may provide the nurse with a framework for assessment:

- Does the newborn's response style and ability to adapt to stimuli indicate a need for parental interventions that will alert the newborn to the environment so that the baby can grow socially and cognitively?
- Are parental interventions necessary to lessen the outside stimuli, as in the case of the baby who responds to sensory input with intensity?
- Can the newborn control the amount of sensory input that will be experienced?

The behaviors, and the sleep–wake states in which they are assessed, are categorized as follows:

- *Habituation.* The nurse assesses the newborn's ability to diminish or shut down innate responses to specific repeated stimuli, such as a rattle, bell, light, or pinprick.
- *Orientation to inanimate and animate visual and auditory assessment stimuli.* The nurse observes how often and where the newborn attends to auditory and visual stimuli. Orientation to the environment is determined by an ability to respond to clues given by others and by a natural ability to fix on and follow a visual object horizontally and vertically. This capacity and parental appreciation of it are important for positive communication between newborn and parents; the parents' visual (*en face*) and auditory (soft, continuous voice) presence stimulates their newborn to orient to them. Inability or lack of response may indicate visual or auditory problems. It is important for parents to know that their newborn can turn to voices soon after birth or by 3 days of age and can become alert at different times with a varying degree of intensity in response to sounds.
- *Motor activity.* Several components are evaluated. Motor tone of the newborn is assessed in the most characteristic state of responsiveness. This summary assessment includes overall use of tone as the newborn responds to being handled—whether during spontaneous activity, prone placement, or horizontal holding—and overall assessment of body tone as the newborn reacts to all stimuli.

- *Variations.* Frequency of alert states, state changes, color changes (throughout all states as examination progresses), activity, and peaks of excitement are assessed.
- *Self-quieting activity.* This assessment is based on how often, how quickly, and how effectively newborns can use their resources to quiet and console themselves when upset or distressed. Considered in this assessment are such self-consolatory activities as putting hand to mouth, sucking on a fist or the tongue, and attuning to an object or sound (Figure 24–37). The newborn's need for outside consolation must also be considered (e.g., seeing a face; being rocked, held, or dressed; using a pacifier; being swaddled).

  Newborns who are neurologically impaired are unable to use self-quieting activities and require more frequent comforting from caregivers when stimulated. For example, drug-positive newborns often exhibit abnormal sleep and feeding patterns and irritability. Swaddling newborns is a way to provide comfort and security. Swaddling also helps the newborn organize and control body movements and behaviors. Blanket swaddling should be loose and should allow the baby easy hand to mouth access to promote self-soothing abilities. Tight swaddling, "straitjacket" techniques with arms at sides, is not comforting and may further agitate the baby.

- *Cuddliness or social behaviors.* This area encompasses the newborn's need for, and response to, being held. Also considered is how often the newborn smiles. These behaviors influence the parents' self-esteem and feelings of acceptance or rejection. Cuddling also appears to be an indicator of personality. Cuddlers appear to enjoy, accept, and seek physical contact; are easier to placate; sleep more; and form earlier and more intense attachments. Noncuddlers are active and restless, have accelerated motor development, and are intolerant of physical restraint. Smiling, even as a grimace reflex, greatly influences parent–newborn feedback. Parents identify this response as positive.

Newborn Physical Assessment Guide

Review the *Assessment Guide: Newborn Physical Assessment* for systematically assessing the newborn. Normal findings, alterations, and related causes are presented and correlated with suggested nursing responses. The findings are typical for a full-term newborn.

ASSESSMENT GUIDE | Newborn Physical Assessment

Physical Assessment/Normal Findings	Alterations and Possible Causes*	Nursing Responses to Data†
Vital Signs		
Blood pressure (BP): At birth: 70–50/ 45–30 mmHg	Low BP (hypovolemia, shock)	Monitor BP in all cases of distress, prematurity, or suspected anomaly.
Day 10: 90/50 mmHg (may be unable to measure diastolic pressure with standard sphygmomanometer)		Low BP: Refer to physician immediately so measures to improve circulation are begun.
Pulse: 110–160 beats/min (if in deep asleep, as low as 70 beats/min; if crying, up to 180 beats/min)	Weak pulse (decreased cardiac output)	Assess skin perfusion by blanching (capillary refill test—normal less than 3 sec).
	Bradycardia (severe asphyxia)	Correlate finding with BP assessments; refer to physician.
	Tachycardia (over 160 beats/min at rest) (infection, CNS problems, arrhythmia, stress, hypovolemia)	Carry out neurologic and thermoregulation assessments.
		Check BP and hematocrit (Hct).
Respirations: 30–60 breaths/min	Tachypnea (pneumonia, respiratory distress syndrome [RDS])	Identify sleep–wake state; correlate with respiratory pattern.
Synchronization of chest and abdominal movements	Rapid, shallow breathing (hypermagnesemia caused by large milligram doses given to mothers with preeclampsia)	Evaluate for all signs of respiratory distress; report findings to physician.
Diaphragmatic and abdominal breathing	Respirations below 30 breaths/min (maternal anesthesia or analgesia)	
Transient tachypnea	Expiratory grunting, subcostal and substernal retractions; flaring of nares (respiratory distress); apnea (cold stress, respiratory disorder)	Evaluate for cold stress. Report findings to physician/neonatal nurse practitioner.
Crying: Strong and lusty Moderate tone and pitch	High-pitched, shrill (neurologic disorder, hypoglycemia)	Discuss newborn's use of cry for communication. Assess and record abnormal cries.
Cries vary in length from 3–7 min after consoling measures are used	Weak or absent (CNS disorder, laryngeal problem)	Reduce environmental noises.
	Inconsolable crying (GI discomforts, feeding intolerances)	
Temperature: Axilla 36.4°–37.2°C (97.5°–99°F)	Elevated temperature (room too warm, too much clothing or covers, dehydration, sepsis, brain damage)	Notify physician or nurse practitioner of elevation or drop.
	Subnormal temperature (brainstem involvement, cold, sepsis)	Counsel parents on possible causes of elevated or low temperatures, appropriate home care measures, and when to call physician.
Heavier newborns tend to have higher body temperatures	Swings of more than 2°F from one reading to the next or subnormal temperature (infection)	Teach parents how to take rectal and/or axillary temperature; assess parents' information regarding use of thermometer; provide teaching as needed.
Weight: 2500–4000 g (5 lb, 8 oz–8 lb, 13 oz)	Less than 2748 g (less than 6 lb) = SGA or preterm newborn	Plot weight and gestational age on growth chart to identify high-risk newborns.
	Greater than 4050 g (greater than 9 lb) = LGA or infant of diabetic mother (IDM)	Ascertain body build of parents. Counsel parents regarding appropriate caloric intake.
Within first 3–4 days, normal weight loss of 5%–10%	Loss greater than 15% (low fluid intake, loss of meconium and urine, feeding difficulties, diabetes insipidus)	Notify physician of net losses or gains.
Large babies tend to lose more because of greater fluid loss in proportion to birth weight except infants of diabetic mothers		Calculate fluid intake and losses from all sources (insensible water loss, radiant warmers, and phototherapy lights). Daily weights and before discharge.

(continued)

ASSESSMENT GUIDE | Newborn Physical Assessment (*continued*)

Physical Assessment/Normal Findings	Alterations and Possible Causes*	Nursing Responses to Data†
Length: 46–56 cm (18–22 in.) Grows 10 cm (3 in.) during first 3 months	Less than 45 cm (17.7 in.) (congenital dwarf) Short/long bones proximally (achondroplasia) Short/long bones distally (Ellis–van Creveld syndrome)	Assess for other signs of dwarfism. Determine other signs of skeletal system adequacy. Plot progress at subsequent well-baby visits.
Posture		
Body usually flexed, hands may be tightly clenched, neck appears short as chin rests on chest	Only extension noted, inability to move from midline (trauma, hypoxia, immaturity)	Record spontaneity of motor activity and symmetry of movements.
In breech presentations, feet are usually dorsiflexed	Constant motion (maternal caffeine intake or drug withdrawal)	If parents express concern about newborn's movement patterns, reassure and evaluate further if appropriate.
Skin		
Color: Color consistent with genetic background	Pallor of face, conjunctiva (anemia, hypothermia, anoxia)	Discuss with parents common skin color variations to allay fears. Skin color can vary widely in newborns of African descent.
Newborns of European descent: pink-tinged or ruddy color over face, trunk, extremities	Beefy red (hypoglycemia, immature vasomotor reflexes, polycythemia)	Document extent and time of occurrence of color change.
Newborns of African descent or Native American: reddish brown to pale pink with yellow or red tinge		
Newborns of Asian descent: pink or rosy red to yellow, olive tinge		
Common variations: acrocyanosis, circumoral cyanosis, Mongolian spots, or harlequin color change	Meconium staining (nonreassuring fetal status) Jaundice (hemolytic reaction from blood incompatibility within first 24 hr, sepsis)	Obtain hemoglobin (Hgb) and Hct values, obtain bilirubin levels. Assess for respiratory difficulty. Differentiate between physiologic and pathologic jaundice.
Mottled when undressed	Cyanosis (choanal atresia, CNS damage or trauma, respiratory or cardiac problem, cold stress)	Assess degree of (central or peripheral) cyanosis and possible causes; refer to physician.
Minor bruising: over buttocks in breech presentation and over eyes and forehead in facial presentations		Discuss with parents cause and course of minor bruising related to labor and birth.
Texture: Smooth, soft, flexible, may have dry, peeling hands and feet	Generalized cracked or peeling skin (SGA or postterm; blood incompatibility; metabolic, kidney dysfunction)	Report to physician.
	Seborrheic dermatitis (cradle cap) Absence of vernix (postmature)\ Yellow vernix (meconium staining)	Instruct parents to shampoo the scalp and anterior fontanel areas daily with mild soap or baby shampoo; rinse well; avoid use of oil.
Turgor: Elastic, returns to normal shape after pinching	Maintains tent shape (dehydration)	Assess for other signs and symptoms of dehydration.
Pigmentation: Clear; milia across bridge of nose, forehead, or chin will disappear within a few weeks		Advise parents not to pinch or prick these pimple-like areas.
Café-au-lait spots (one or two)	Six or more (neurologic disorder such as von Recklinghausen disease, cutaneous neurofibromatosis)	If there are six or more café-au-lait spots, refer for genetic and neurologic consult.
Congenital dermal melanocytosis (Mongolian blue spots) common over dorsal area and buttocks in dark-skin newborns		Assure parents of normalcy of this pigmentation; it will fade in first year or 2.
Erythema toxicum	Impetigo (group A β-hemolytic streptococcus or *Staphylococcus aureus* infection)	If impetigo occurs, instruct parents about hand washing and linen precautions during home care.

Physical Assessment/Normal Findings	Alterations and Possible Causes*	Nursing Responses to Data†
Telangiectatic nevi	Hemangiomas: Nevus flammeus (port-wine stain) Nevus vascularis (strawberry hemangioma) Cavernous hemangiomas	Collaborate with physician. Counsel parents about birthmark's progression to allay misconceptions. Record size and shape of hemangiomas. Refer for follow-up at well-baby clinic.
Rashes	Rashes (infection)	Assess location and type of rash (macular, papular, vesicular). Obtain history of onset, prenatal history, and related signs and symptoms.
Petechiae of head or neck (breech presentation, cord around neck)	Generalized petechiae (clotting abnormalities)	Determine cause; advise parents if further health care is needed.
Head		
General appearance, size, movement Round, symmetric, and moves easily from left to right and up and down; soft and pliable	Asymmetric, flattened occiput on either side of the head (plagiocephaly) Head held at angle (torticollis) Unable to move head side to side (neurologic trauma)	Instruct parents to change newborn's positions frequently when awake. When awake, needs to spend "tummy time" and should be placed supine for sleep per "safe to sleep" guidelines. Determine adequacy of all neurologic signs.
Circumference 32–37 cm (12.5–14.5 in.); 2 cm (0.8 in.) greater than chest circumference; head one fourth of body size	Extreme differences in size may be micro-encephaly (Cornelia de Lange syndrome, cytomegalic inclusion disease [CID], rubella, toxoplasmosis, chromosomal abnormalities), hydrocephalus (meningomyelocele, achondroplasia), anencephaly (neural tube defect) Head is 3 cm (1.2 in.) or more larger than chest circumference (preterm, hydrocephalus)	Measure circumference from occiput to frontal area using metal or paper tape. Measure chest circumference using metal or paper tape and compare to head circumference. Record measurements on growth chart. Reevaluate at well-baby visits.
Common variations: Molding: Breech and cesarean newborns' heads are round and well shaped	Cephalohematoma (trauma during birth, may persist up to 3 months) Caput succedaneum (long labor and birth; disappears in 1 week)	Evaluate neurologic response. Observe for hyperbilirubinemia. Check Hct. Reassure parents regarding common manifestations caused by birth process and when they should disappear.
Fontanels: Palpation of juncture of cranial bones	Overlapping of anterior fontanel (malnourished or preterm newborn)	Discuss normal closure times with parents and care of "soft spots" to allay misconceptions.
Anterior fontanel: 3–4 cm (1.2–1.6 in.) long by 2–3 cm (0.8–1.2 in.) wide, diamond shaped	Premature closure of sutures (craniosynostosis)	Refer to physician.
Posterior fontanel: 1–2 cm (0.4–0.8 in.) at birth, triangle shaped	Late closure (hydrocephalus)	Observe for signs and symptoms of hydrocephalus.
Slight pulsation	Moderate to severe pulsation (vascular problems)	Refer to physician.
Moderate bulging noted with crying, stooling, or pulsations with heartbeat	Constant bulging (increased intracranial pressure, meningitis) Sunken (dehydration)	Evaluate neurologic status. Evaluate hydration status. Report to physician.
Hair		
Texture: Smooth with fine texture variations (Note: Variations depend on ethnic background.)	Coarse, brittle, dry hair (hypothyroidism) White forelock (Waardenburg syndrome)	Instruct parents regarding routine care of hair and scalp.
Distribution: Scalp hair high over eyebrows (Spanish, Mexican hairline begins mid-forehead and extends down back of neck.)	Low forehead and posterior hairlines may indicate chromosomal disorders	Assess for other signs of chromosomal aberrations. Refer to physician.
Face		
Symmetric movement of all facial features, normal hairline, eyebrows and eyelashes present		Assess and record symmetry of all parts, shape, regularity of features, sameness or differences in features.

(continued)

ASSESSMENT GUIDE | Newborn Physical Assessment (*continued*)

Physical Assessment/Normal Findings	Alterations and Possible Causes*	Nursing Responses to Data†
Spacing of features: Eyes at same level, nostrils equal size, cheeks full, and sucking pads present	Eyes wide apart—ocular hypertelorism (Apert syndrome, cri du chat, Turner syndrome)	Observe for other signs and symptoms indicative of disease states or chromosomal aberrations.
Lips equal on both sides of midline	Abnormal face (Down syndrome, cretinism, gargoylism)	
Chin recedes when compared with other bones of face	Abnormally small jaw—micrognathia (Pierre Robin syndrome, Treacher Collins syndrome)	Maintain airway; do not position supine. Initiate surgical consultation and referral.
Movement: Makes facial grimaces	Inability to suck, grimace, and close eyelids (cranial nerve injury)	Initiate neurologic assessment and consultation.
Symmetric when resting and crying	Asymmetry (paralysis of facial cranial nerve)	Assess and record symmetry of all parts, shape, regularity of features, and sameness or differences in features.
Eyes		
General placement and appearance: Bright and clear; even placement; slight nystagmus (involuntary cyclic eye movements)	Gross nystagmus (damage to third, fourth, and sixth cranial nerves)	
Concomitant strabismus	Constant and fixed strabismus	Reassure parents that strabismus is considered normal up to 6 months.
Move in all directions	Lack of pigmentation (albinism)	Discuss with parents any necessary eye precautions.
Blue or slate blue–gray	Brushfield spots may indicate Down syndrome (a light or white speckling of the outer two thirds of the iris)	Assess for other signs of Down syndrome.
Brown color at birth in dark-skin newborns		Discuss with parents that permanent eye color is usually established by 3 months of age.
Eyelids: Position: above pupils but within iris, no drooping	Elevation of (hydrocephalus) or retraction of upper lid (hyperthyroidism)	Assess for signs of hydrocephalus and hyperthyroidism.
	"Sunset sign" lid elevation and downward gaze (hydrocephalus), ptosis (congenital or paralysis of oculomotor muscle)	Evaluate interference with vision in subsequent well-baby visits.
Eyes on parallel plane	Upward slant in non-Asians (Down syndrome)	Assess for other signs of Down syndrome.
Epicanthal folds in Asians and 20% of newborns of northern European descent	Epicanthal folds (Down syndrome, cri du chat syndrome)	
Movement: Blink reflex in response to light stimulus	Blink absent (CNS injury, cranial nerve damage)	Evaluate neurologic status. Refer to physician.
Eyes open wide in dimly lighted room		
Inspection: Edematous for first few days of life, resulting from birth; no lumps or redness	Purulent drainage (infection); infectious conjunctivitis (gonococcus, chlamydia, staphylococcus, or gram-negative organisms)	Initiate good hand washing. Refer to physician. Evaluate newborn for seborrheic dermatitis; scales can be removed easily.
	Marginal blepharitis (lid edges red, crusted, scaly)	
Cornea: Clear	Ulceration (herpes infection); large cornea or corneas of unequal size (congenital glaucoma)	Refer to ophthalmologist.
Corneal reflex present	Clouding, opacity of lens (cataract)	Assess for other manifestations of congenital herpes; institute nursing care measures.
Sclera: May appear bluish in newborn, then white; slightly brownish color frequent in newborns of African descent	True blue sclera (osteogenesis imperfecta)	Refer to physician.
Pupils: Pupils equal in size, round, and react to light by accommodation	Anisocoria—unequal pupils (CNS damage)	Refer for neurologic examination.
	Dilation or constriction (intracranial) damage, retinoblastoma, glaucoma; pupils nonreactive to light or accommodation (brain injury)	

Physical Assessment/Normal Findings	Alterations and Possible Causes*	Nursing Responses to Data†
Slight nystagmus in newborn who has not learned to focus	Nystagmus (labyrinthine disturbance, CNS disorder)	
Pupil light reflex demonstrated at birth or by 3 weeks of age		
Conjunctiva: Chemical conjunctivitis	Pale color (anemia)	Obtain Hct and Hgb. Reassure parents that chemical conjunctivitis will subside in 1–2 days and subconjunctival hemorrhage disappears in a few weeks.
Subconjunctival hemorrhage		
Palpebral conjunctiva (red but not hyperemic)	Inflammation or edema (infection, blocked tear duct)	
Vision: 20/200	Cataracts (congenital infection)	Record any questions about visual acuity, and initiate follow-up evaluation at first well-baby checkup.
Tracks moving object to midline		
Fixed focus on objects at a distance of about 10–20 in. (3.8–6.7 cm); may be difficult to evaluate in newborn		
Prefers faces, geometric designs, and black and white to colors		
Lashes and lacrimal glands: Presence of lashes (lashes may be absent in preterm newborns)	No lashes on inner two thirds of lid (Treacher Collins syndrome); bushy lashes (Hurler syndrome); long lashes (Cornelia de Lange syndrome)	
Cry commonly tearless	Excessive tearing (plugged lacrimal duct, natal narcotic withdrawal), glaucoma	Demonstrate to parents how to milk blocked tear duct.
		Refer to ophthalmologist if tearing is excessive before third month of life.
Nose		
Appearance of external nasal aspects: May appear flattened as a result of birth process	Continued flat or broad bridge of nose (trisomy 21)	Arrange consultation with specialist. May be normal racial variation—Asian or African ancestry.
Small and narrow in midline, even placement in relationship to eyes and mouth	Low bridge of nose, beaklike nose (Apert syndrome, Treacher Collins syndrome) Upturned (Cornelia de Lange syndrome)	Initiate evaluation of chromosomal abnormalities.
Patent nares bilaterally (nose breathers)	Blockage of nares (mucus and/or secretions), choanal atresia	Inspect for obstruction of nares.
Sneezing common to clear nasal passages	Flaring nares (respiratory distress)	Maintain oral airway until surgical correction is made.
Responds to odors, may smell breast milk	No response to stimulating odors	Inspect for obstruction of nares.
Mouth		
Function of facial, hypoglossal, glossopharyngeal, and vagus nerves: Symmetry of movement and strength	Mouth draws to one side (transient seventh cranial nerve paralysis due to pressure in utero or trauma during birth, congenital paralysis)	Initiate neurologic consultation.
	Fishlike shape (Treacher Collins syndrome)	Administer artificial tears if eye on affected side of face is unable to close.
Presence of gag, swallowing, coordinated with sucking reflexes;	Suppressed or absent reflexes	Evaluate other neurologic functions of these nerves.
Adequate salivation		
Palate (soft and hard): Hard palate dome-shaped	High-steepled palate (Treacher Collins syndrome), bifid uvula (congenital anomaly)	Assess for other congenital anomalies.
Uvula midline with symmetric movement of soft palate		
Palate intact, sucks well when stimulated	Clefts in either hard or soft palate (polygenic disorder)	Initiate a surgical consultation referral.
Epithelial (Epstein) pearls appear on mucosa		Assure parents that these are normal and will disappear at 2 or 3 months of age.

(continued)

ASSESSMENT GUIDE | Newborn Physical Assessment (*continued*)

Physical Assessment/Normal Findings	Alterations and Possible Causes*	Nursing Responses to Data†
Esophagus patent, some drooling common in newborn	Excessive drooling or bubbling (esophageal atresia)	Test for patency of esophagus.
Tongue: Free moving in all directions, midline	Tongue-tied	Further assess neurologic functions.
	Lack of movement or asymmetric movement (neurologic damage)	Test reflex elevation of tongue when depressed with tongue blade.
	Fasciculations (fine tremors)	
	Spinal muscular atrophy	
Pink color, smooth to rough texture, noncoated	Deviations from midline (cranial nerve damage).	Check for signs of weakness or deviation.
	White cheesy coating (thrush)	Differentiate between thrush and milk curds by wiping patches; if white patches don't come off easily, it is thrush.
	Tongue has deep ridges	Reassure parents that tongue pattern may change from day to day.
Tongue proportional to mouth	Large tongue with short frenulum (cretinism, trisomy 21, other syndromes)	Evaluate in well-baby clinic to assess development delays. Initiate referrals.
Ears		
External ear: Without lesions, cysts, or nodules	Nodules, cysts, or sinus tracts in front of ear	Evaluate characteristics of lesions.
	Adherent earlobes	
	Low-set ears (genetic anomaly or syndrome)	Counsel parents to clean external ear with washcloth only; discourage use of cotton-tip applicators.
	Preauricular skin tags	Refer to physician for ligation.
Hearing: Eustachian tubes are cleared with first cry	Presence of one or more risk factors	Assess history of risk factors for hearing loss.
Attends to sounds; sudden or loud noise elicits Moro reflex	No response to sound stimuli (deafness)	Test for Moro reflex.
Neck		
Appearance: Short, straight, creased with skin folds	Abnormally short neck (Turner syndrome)	Report findings to physician.
	Arching or inability to flex neck (meningitis, congenital anomaly)	
Posterior neck lacks loose extra folds of skin	Webbing of neck (Turner syndrome, trisomy 21, trisomy 18)	Assess for other signs of these syndromes.
Clavicles: Straight and intact	Knot or lump on clavicle (fracture during difficult birth)	Obtain detailed labor and birth history; apply figure-8 bandage.
		Consider oral analgesics.
Moro reflex elicitable	Unilateral Moro reflex response on unaffected side (fracture of clavicle, brachial palsy, Erb-Duchenne paralysis)	Collaborate with physician.
Symmetric shoulders	Hypoplasia	
Chest		
Appearance and size: Circumference: 32.5 cm (12.8 in.), 1–2 cm (0.4–0.8 in.) less than head		Measure at level of nipples after exhalation.
Wider than it is long		
Normal shape without depressed or prominent sternum	Funnel chest (congenital or associated with Marfan syndrome)	Determine adequacy of other respiratory and circulatory signs.
Lower end of sternum (xiphoid cartilage) may be protruding; is less apparent after several weeks	Continued protrusion of xiphoid cartilage (Marfan syndrome, "pigeon chest")	Assess for other signs and symptoms of various syndromes.
Sternum 8 cm (3.1 in.) long	Barrel chest	

Physical Assessment/Normal Findings	Alterations and Possible Causes*	Nursing Responses to Data†
Expansion and retraction: Bilateral expansion	Unequal chest expansion (pneumonia, pneumothorax, respiratory distress)	Assess respiratory effort regularity, flaring of nares, difficulty on both inspiration and expiration.
No intercostal, subcostal, or supra-costal retractions	Retractions (respiratory distress)	
	Seesaw respirations (respiratory distress)	
Auscultation: Breath sounds are louder in babies than adults because there is less subcutaneous tissue to muffle transmission	Decreased breath sounds (decreased respiratory activity, atelectasis, pneumothorax)	Obtain transillumination. Record findings and consult physician.
Chest and axillae clear on crying	Increased breath sounds (resolving pneumonia or in cesarean births)	Perform assessment and report to physician any positive findings.
Bronchial breath sounds (heard where trachea and bronchi closest to chest wall, above sternum and between scapulae):		
Bronchial sounds bilaterally	Adventitious or abnormal sounds (respiratory disease or distress)	Evaluate color for pallor or cyanosis. Report to physician.
Air entry clear		
Rales may indicate normal newborn atelectasis		
Cough reflex absent at birth, appears in 2 or more days		
Breasts: Flat with symmetric nipples	Lack of breast tissue (preterm or SGA)	
Breast tissue diameter 5 cm (2 in.) or more at term	Discharge	Evaluate for infection.
Distance between nipples 8 cm (3.1 in.)		
Breast engorgement occurs on third day of life; liquid discharge may be expressed in term newborns	Enlargement	Reassure parents of normality of breast engorgement.
	Breast abscesses	
	Supernumerary nipples	No intervention is necessary.
	Dark-colored nipples	
Heart		
Auscultation: Location: lies horizontally, with left border extending to left of midclavicle		
Regular rhythm and rate	Arrhythmia (anoxia), tachycardia, bradycardia	Refer all arrhythmias and gallop rhythms. Initiate cardiac evaluation.
Determination of point of maximal impulse (PMI)	Malpositioning (enlargement, abnormal placement, pneumothorax, dextrocardia, diaphragmatic hernia)	
Functional murmurs	Location of murmurs (possible congenital cardiac anomaly)	Evaluate murmur: location, timing, and duration; observe for accompanying cardiac pathology symptoms; ascertain family history.
No thrills		
Horizontal groove at diaphragm shows flaring of rib cage to mild degree	Marked rib flaring (vitamin D deficiency)	Initiate cardiopulmonary evaluation; assess pulses and blood pressures in all four extremities for equality and quality.
	Inadequacy of respiratory movement	
Abdomen		
Appearance: Cylindric with some protrusion, appears large in relation to pelvis, some laxness of abdominal muscles	Distention, shiny abdomen with engorged vessels (gastrointestinal abnormalities, infection, congenital megacolon)	Examine abdomen thoroughly for mass or organomegaly. Measure abdominal girth.
No cyanosis, few vessels seen	Scaphoid abdominal appearance (diaphragmatic hernia)	Report deviations of abdominal size.
Diastasis recti—common in newborns of African descent		
	Increased or decreased peristalsis (duodenal stenosis, small bowel obstruction)	Assess other signs and symptoms of obstruction.
	Localized flank bulging (enlarged kidneys, ascites, or absent abdominal muscles)	Refer to physician.

(continued)

ASSESSMENT GUIDE | Newborn Physical Assessment (*continued*)

Physical Assessment/Normal Findings	Alterations and Possible Causes*	Nursing Responses to Data†
Umbilicus: No protrusion of umbilicus (protrusion of umbilicus common in newborns of African descent) Bluish white color	Umbilical hernia Patent urachus (congenital malformation)	Measure umbilical hernia by palpating the opening and record; it should close by 1 year of age; if not, refer to physician.
	Omphalocele (covered defect) Gastroschisis (uncovered defect)	Cover omphalocele and gastroschisis with sterile, moist dressing or plastic sterile bag.
Cutis navel (umbilical cord projects), granulation tissue present in navel	Redness or exudate around cord (infection) Yellow discoloration (hemolytic disease, meconium staining)	Instruct parents on cord care and hygiene.
Two arteries and one vein apparent	Single umbilical artery (congenital anomalies)	Refer anomalies to physician.
Begins drying 1–2 hr after birth No bleeding	Discharge or oozing of blood from the cord	
Auscultation of all four quadrants: Soft bowel sounds heard shortly after birth every 10–30 sec	Bowel sounds in chest (diaphragmatic hernia) Absence of bowel sounds Hyperperistalsis (intestinal obstruction)	Collaborate with physician. Assess for other signs of dehydration or infection.
Femoral pulses: Palpable, equal bilateral	Absent or diminished femoral pulses (coarctation of aorta)	Monitor blood pressure in upper and lower extremities.
Inguinal area: No bulges along inguinal area	Inguinal hernia	Initiate referral.
No inguinal lymph nodes felt		Continue follow-up in well-baby clinic.
Bladder: Percusses 1–4 cm (0.4–1.6 in.) above symphysis	Failure to void within 24–48 hr after birth	Check whether baby voided at birth.
Should void within 24 hr after birth; if not, at time of birth	Exposure of bladder mucosa (exstrophy of bladder)	
Urine—inoffensive, mild odor	Foul odor (infection)	Obtain urine specimen if infection is suspected. Consult with clinician.
Genitals Gender clearly delineated	Ambiguous genitals	Refer for genetic consultation.
Male **Penis:** Slender in appearance, about 2.5 cm (1 in.) long, 1 cm (0.4 in.) wide at birth.	Micropenis (congenital anomaly) Meatal atresia	Observe and record first voiding.
Normal urinary orifice, urethral meatus at tip of penis	Hypospadias, epispadias	Collaborate with physician in presence of abnormality. Delay circumcision.
Noninflamed urethral opening	Urethritis (infection)	Palpate for enlarged inguinal lymph nodes and record painful urination.
Foreskin adheres to glans	Ulceration of meatal opening (infection, inflammation)	Evaluate whether ulcer is because of diaper rash; counsel regarding care.
Uncircumcised foreskin tight for 2–3 months	Phimosis—if still tight after 3 months	Instruct parents on how to care for uncircumcised penis.
Circumcised		Teach parents how to care for circumcision.
Erectile tissue present		
Scrotum: Skin loose and hanging or tight and small; extensive rugae and normal size.	Large scrotum containing fluid (hydrocele)	Shine a light through scrotum (transilluminate) to verify diagnosis.
Normal skin color	Minimal rugae, small scrotum	Assess for prematurity.
Scrotal discoloration common in breech	Red, shiny scrotal skin (orchitis)	
Testes: Descended by birth; not consistently found in scrotum	Undescended testes (cryptorchidism)	If testes cannot be felt in scrotum, gently palpate femoral, inguinal, perineal, and abdominal areas for presence.
Testes size 1.5–2.0 cm (0.6–0.8 in.) at birth	Enlarged testes (tumor) Small testes (Klinefelter syndrome or adrenal hyperplasia)	Refer and collaborate with physician for further diagnostic studies.

Physical Assessment/Normal Findings	Alterations and Possible Causes*	Nursing Responses to Data†
Female		
Mons: Normal skin color, area pigmented in dark-skin newborns		
Labia majora cover labia minora in term and postterm newborns; symmetric size appropriate for gestational age	Hematoma, lesions (trauma)	Evaluate for recent trauma.
	Labia minora prominent	Assess for prematurity.
Clitoris: Normally large in newborn	Hypertrophy (hermaphroditism)	Refer for genetic workup.
Edema and bruising in breech birth		
Vagina: Urinary meatus and vaginal orifice visible (0.5 cm [0.2 in.] circumference)	Inflammation; erythema and discharge (urethritis)	Collect urine specimen for laboratory examination.
Vaginal tag or hymenal tag disappears in a few weeks	Congenital absence of vagina	Refer to physician.
Discharge; smegma under labia	Foul-smelling discharge (infection)	Collect data and further evaluate reason for discharge.
Bloody or mucoid discharge	Excessive vaginal bleeding (blood coagulation defect)	
Buttocks and Anus		
Buttocks symmetric	Pilonidal dimple	Examine for possible sinus. Instruct parents about cleansing this area.
Anus patent and passage of meconium within 24–48 hr after birth	Imperforate anus, rectal atresia (congenital gastrointestinal defect)	Evaluate extent of problems. Initiate surgical consultation.
No fissures, tears, or skin tags	Fissures	Perform digital examination to ascertain patency if patency uncertain.
Extremities and Trunk		
Short and generally flexed, extremities move symmetrically through range-of-motion but lack full extension	Unilateral or absence of movement (spinal cord involvement)	Review birth record to assess possible cause.
	Fetal position continued or limp (anoxia)	
All joints move spontaneously; good muscle tone, of flexor type, birth to 2 months	Spasticity when newborn begins using extensors (cerebral palsy)	Collaborate with physician.
Arms: Equal in length	Brachial palsy (difficult birth)	Report to clinician.
Bilateral movement	Erb-Duchenne paralysis	
Flexed when quiet	Muscle weakness, fractured clavicle	
	Absence of limb or change of size (phocomelia, amelia)	
Hands: Normal number of fingers	Polydactyly (Ellis–van Creveld syndrome)	Report to clinician.
	Syndactyly—one limb (developmental anomaly)	
	Syndactyly—both limbs (genetic component)	
Normal palmar crease	Single palmar crease (Down syndrome)	Refer for genetic workup.
Normal size hands	Short fingers and broad hand (Hurler syndrome)	
Nails present and extend beyond fingertips in term newborn	Cyanosis and clubbing (cardiac anomalies)	Evaluate for history of distress in utero.
	Nails long or yellow stained (postterm)	Carry out cardiac and respiratory assessments.
		Check pulse oximetry.
Spine: C-shaped spine	Spina bifida occulta (nevus pilosus)	Evaluate extent of neurologic damage; initiate care of spinal opening.
Flat and straight when prone	Dermal sinus	
Slight lumbar lordosis	Myelomeningocele	
Easily flexed and intact when palpated	Head lag, limp, floppy trunk (neurologic problems)	
At least half of back devoid of lanugo		

(continued)

ASSESSMENT GUIDE | Newborn Physical Assessment (*continued*)

Physical Assessment/Normal Findings	Alterations and Possible Causes*	Nursing Responses to Data†
Full-term newborns in ventral suspension should hold head at 45-degree angle, back straight		Elicit reflex to assess degree of involvement.
Hips: No sign of instability	Sensation of abnormal movement, jerk, or snap of hip dislocation	Physician or nurse practitioner examines all newborns for dislocated hip before discharge from birthing center.
Hips abduct to more than 60 degrees	Limited abduction (developmental dysplasia of hip)	If this is suspected, refer to orthopedist for further evaluation. Reassess at well-baby visits.
Inguinal and buttock skin creases: Symmetric inguinal and buttock creases	Asymmetry (dislocated hips)	Refer to orthopedist for evaluation. Counsel parents regarding symptoms of concern, and discuss therapy.
Legs: Legs equal in length	Shortened leg (dislocated hips)	Refer to orthopedist for evaluation.
Legs shorter than arms at birth	Lack of leg movement (fractures, spinal defects)	Counsel parents regarding symptoms of concern, and discuss therapy.
Feet: Foot is in straight line	Talipes equinovarus (true clubfoot)	Discuss differences between positional and true clubfoot with parents.
		Teach parents passive manipulation of foot.
Positional clubfoot—based on position in utero		Refer to orthopedist if not corrected by 3 months of age.
Fat pads and creases on soles of feet	Incomplete sole creases in first 24 hours of life (premature)	
Talipes planus (flat feet) normal under 3 years of age		Reassure parents that flat feet are normal in infants.
Neuromuscular		
Motor function: Symmetric movement and strength in all extremities	Limp, flaccid, or hypertonic (CNS disorders, infection, dehydration, fracture)	Appraise newborn's posture and motor functions by observing activities and motor characteristics.
May be jerky or have brief twitchings	Tremors (hypoglycemia, hypocalcemia, infection, neurologic damage)	Evaluate for electrolyte imbalance, hypoglycemia, and neurologic functioning.
Head lag not over 45 degrees	Delayed or abnormal development (preterm, neurologic involvement)	
Neck control adequate to maintain head erect briefly	Asymmetry of tone or strength (neurologic damage)	Refer for genetic evaluation.

*Possible causes of alterations are identified in parentheses.
†This column provides guidelines for further assessment and initial nursing interventions.

Focus Your Study

- A perinatal history, determination of gestational age, physical examination, and behavioral assessment form the basis for complete newborn assessment.

- The common physical characteristics included in the gestational age assessment are skin, lanugo, sole (plantar) creases, breast tissue and size, ear form and cartilage, and genitals.

- The neuromuscular components of gestational age scoring tools are usually posture, square window sign, popliteal angle, arm recoil, heel-to-ear extension, and scarf sign.

- By assessing the physical and neuromuscular components specified in a gestational age tool, the nurse can determine the gestational age of the newborn.

- After determining the gestational age of the newborn, the nurse can assess how the baby will make the transition to extrauterine life and can anticipate potential physiologic problems.

- The nurse identifies the newborn as small for gestational age (SGA), appropriate for gestational age (AGA), or large for gestational age (LGA) and prioritizes individual needs.

- Normal ranges for vital signs assessed in newborns are heart rate of 110 to 160 beats per minute; respiratory rate of 30 to 60 respirations per minute; axillary temperature of 36.5° to 37.2°C (97.7° to 99°F); skin temperature of 36° to 36.5°C (96.8° to 97.8°F); rectal temperature of 36.6° to 37.2°C (97.8° to 99°F); and blood pressure of 70/45 to 50/30 mmHg (at birth).

- Normal newborn measurements include weight from 2500 to 4000 g (5 lb, 8 oz to 8 lb, 13 oz), with weight dependent on maternal size and age; length from 48 to 52 cm (18 to 22 in.); and head circumference from 32 to 37 cm (12.5 to 14.5 in.). Head circumference is approximately 2 cm (0.8 in.) larger than the chest circumference.

- The newborn should have a head that appears large for its body; and has a prominent abdomen, sloping shoulders, narrow hips, and rounded chest. The body appears long and the extremities short. Newborns tend to stay in a flexed position and will resist straightening of the extremities. Hands remain clenched

- Neurologic assessment characteristics are: State of alertness, resting position, muscle tone, cry, and motor activity. Neuromuscular assessment characteristics are: Symmetric movements and strength of all extremities, head lag less than 45 degrees and ability to hold head erect briefly.

- Commonly elicited newborn reflexes are tonic neck, Moro, palmar grasping, rooting, sucking, and blink.

- Newborn behavioral abilities include habituation, orientation to visual and auditory stimuli, motor activity, cuddliness, and self-quieting activity. Behaviorally, the newborn will sleep the majority of the time and wake for feeding. The baby should be easily consoled when upset.

- An important role of the nurse during the physical and behavioral assessments of the newborn is to teach parents about their newborn and involve them in their baby's care. This facilitates the parents' identification of their newborn's uniqueness and allays their concerns.

Clinical Reasoning in Action

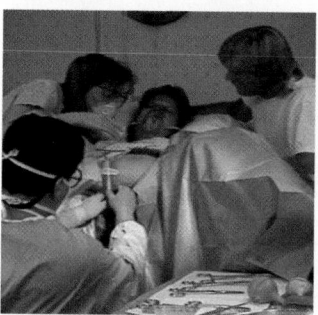

Susan Pine, a 21-year-old G2, now P1011, delivers a 39 2/7-weeks' gestation female newborn. The vaginal birth is assisted with a vacuum extractor. The prenatal record is significant for an increase of maternal blood pressure to 140/90 mmHg on the day of birth. Susan is treated with magnesium sulfate during her labor and has an epidural analgesia for the pain of labor. The baby's Apgar is 8 and 9 at 1 and 5 minutes, and she has been admitted to the newborn nursery. The newborn's admission examination is normal except for a 2-cm (0.8-in.) round caput succedaneum. Now, 8 hours later, the baby's condition is stable and she needs to be bottle-fed. You take her to her mother's room where you observe that Susan does not reach out to take her from you. She seems unsure when handling her baby. Susan asks you about the swelling on her baby's head and wonders if it will ever go away.

1. How would you explain the cause of Susan's baby's caput succedaneum?

2. Compare the difference between a cephalohematoma and caput succedaneum.

3. Explore with Susan her baby's reflexes and state of alertness.

4. Susan asks you how she will know what her baby needs. How would you respond?

References

American Academy of Pediatrics. (2013). *How to take a child's temperature.* Retrieved from http://www.healthychildren.org/English/health-issues/conditions/fever/Pages/How-to-Take-a-Childs-Temperature.aspx

American Academy of Pediatrics (AAP) Committee on Fetus and Newborn & American College of Obstetricians and Gynecologists (ACOG) Committee on Obstetrics. (2012). *Guidelines for perinatal care* (7th ed.). Evanston, IL: Author.

Ballard, J. L., Khoury, J. C., Wedig, K., Wang, L., Eilers-Walsman, B. L., & Lipp, R. (1991). New Ballard score, expanded to include extremely premature infants. *Journal of Pediatrics, 119*(3), 417–423.

Blackburn, S. T. (2013). *Maternal, fetal, neonatal physiology: A clinical perspective* (4th ed.). London, UK: MacKeith.

Cavaliere, T. A. & Sansoucie, D. A. (2014). Assessment of the newborn and infant. In C. Kenner & J. W. Lott (Eds.). *Comprehensive neonatal nursing care.*(5th ed., pp. 71–112). New York, NY: Springer.

Cloherty, J. P., Eichenwald, E. C., Hansen, A. R., & Stark, A. R. (2012). *Manual of neonatal care* (7th ed.). Philadelphia, PA: Lippincott Williams & Wilkins.

Gleason, C. A., & Devaskar, S. U. (2012). *Avery's diseases of the newborn.* (9th ed.) St. Louis, MO: Elsevier Saunders.

Glomella, T. L. (Ed.) (2013). *Neonatology: Management, procedures, on-call problems, diseases, and drugs* (7th ed.). New York, NY: McGraw-Hill Education.

Goodwin, M. (2015). Abdomen assessment. In E. P. Tappero & M. E. Honeyfield (Eds.), *Physical assessment of the newborn.* (5th ed., pp. 111–120). Petaluma, CA: NICU Ink.

Johnson, P. (2015). Head, eyes, ears, nose, mouth, and neck assessment. In E. P. Tappero & M. E. Honeyfield (Eds.), *Physical assessment of the newborn.* (5th ed., pp. 61–78). Petaluma, CA: NICU Ink.

Nugent, J. K. (2013). The competent newborn and the neonatal behavioral assessment scale: T. Berry Brazelton's legacy. *Journal of Child and Adolescent Psychiatric Nursing 26*(3), 173–179.

Vargo, L. (2015). Cardiovascular assessment. In E. P. Tappero & M. E. Honeyfield (Eds.), *Physical assessment of the newborn.* (5th ed., pp. 93–110). Petaluma, CA: NICU Ink.

Witt, C. (2015). Skin assessment. In E. P. Tappero & M. E. Honeyfield (Eds.), *Physical assessment of the newborn.* (5th ed., pp. 45–60). Petaluma, CA: NICU Ink.

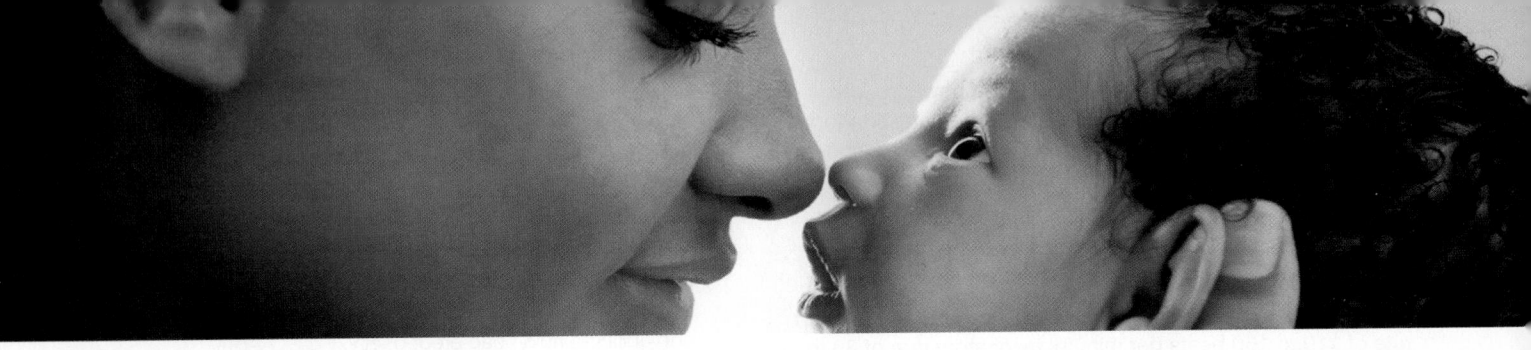

Chapter 25
The Normal Newborn: Needs, Care, and Feeding

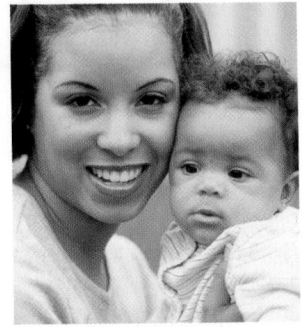

When our daughter was laid in my arms right after birth she was so delicate. I had not dared to hope that we would be blessed with a girl because there were so few girls in my husband's family. Our 2-year-old niece was the first girl in 107 years, so I had pretty much decided that another boy would be just fine. But here she was, right here in my arms.

—Catherine, 32

Stockbyte/Getty Images

⌄ Learning Outcomes

25.1 Summarize essential information to be obtained about a newborn's birth experience and immediate postnatal period.

25.2 Explain how the physiologic and behavioral responses of the newborn during the first 4 hours after birth (admission and transitional period) determine the nursing care of the newborn.

25.3 Identify activities that should be included in a daily care plan for a normal newborn.

25.4 Explain the advantages and disadvantages of breastfeeding and formula-feeding in determining the nursing care of both mother/family and newborn.

25.5 Formulate guidelines for helping both breast- and formula-feeding mothers to feed their newborns successfully in hospital and community-based settings.

25.6 Describe the influence of cultural values on newborn care, especially feeding practices.

25.7 Identify the safety needs of the newborn in the birthing unit and at home

25.8 Describe the common concerns of families regarding their newborn.

25.9 Identify opportunities to individualize parent teaching and enhance each parent's abilities and confidence while providing newborn care in the birthing unit.

At the moment of birth, numerous physiologic adaptations begin to take place in the newborn's body. Because of these dramatic changes, newborns require close observation to determine how smoothly they are making the transition to extrauterine life. Newborns also require specific care that enhances their chances of making the transition successfully.

The two broad goals of nursing care during this period are the following:

1. Promote the physical well-being of the newborn by providing comprehensive care to the newborn while in the mother–baby unit.

2. Support the establishment of a well-functioning family unit by teaching family members how to care for their new baby and support their efforts so that they feel confident and competent.

Thus the nurse must be knowledgeable about necessary family adjustments as well as the health care needs of the newborn. It is important that the family return home confident, knowing that they have the support, information, and skills to care for their newborn. Equally important is the need for each member of the family to begin a unique relationship with the newborn. The cultural and social expectations of individual families and communities affect the ways in which normal newborn care is carried out.

The previous two chapters presented an informational database of the physiologic and behavioral changes occurring in the newborn and the pertinent nursing assessments that are needed. This chapter discusses nursing management while the newborn is in the birthing unit and feeding methods for the full-term, healthy newborn.

Admission and the First 4 Hours of Life

Immediately after birth, the baby is formally admitted to the healthcare facility.

Nursing Management

For the Newborn During Admission and the First 4 Hours of Life

Nursing Assessment and Diagnosis

Before the birth, review the prenatal record of the mother for information concerning possible risk factors for the baby. These include infectious disease screening results, drug or alcohol use by the mother, gestational diabetes, and any other data determined to be of use in anticipating the needs of the newborn. In addition, review the birth record for prolonged rupture of membranes, instrument or vacuum delivery, use of narcotic analgesia, presence of meconium, and any other data that may impact the newborn's ability to successfully transition to the extrauterine environment.

During the first hours after birth, a preliminary physical examination will be conducted, including an assessment of the newborn's physiologic adaptations. In many birthing units, the nurse performs and documents the initial head-to-toe physical assessment during the first hour of transition. The nurse is responsible for notifying the healthcare provider of any deviations from normal. A complete physical examination is also performed later by the healthcare provider—within the first 24 hours after birth and within 24 hours before discharge. This can be accomplished with one physical examination (see Chapter 24) (American Academy of Pediatrics [AAP] & American College of Obstetricians and Gynecologists [ACOG], 2012).

Nursing diagnoses are based on an analysis of the assessment findings. Physiologic alterations of the newborn form the basis of many nursing diagnoses, as does the family members' incorporation of them in caring for their newborn. Nursing diagnoses that may apply to newborns include the following (NANDA-I © 2014):

- *Airway Clearance, Ineffective*, related to presence of mucus and retained lung fluid
- *Body Temperature: Imbalanced, Risk for*, related to evaporative, radiant, conductive, and convective heat losses
- *Pain, Acute*, related to heel sticks for glucose or hematocrit tests, vitamin K injection, or hepatitis B immunization

As discussed in Chapter 23, the newborn's physiologic adaptation to extrauterine life occurs rapidly and all body systems are affected. Therefore, many of these nursing diagnoses and associated interventions must be identified and implemented in a very short period of time.

Planning and Implementation

INITIATING ADMISSION PROCEDURES

If the initial assessment, which must be performed within 2 hours after birth, indicates that the newborn is not at risk physiologically, you can perform many of the routine admission procedures in the presence of the parents in the birthing area. Some care measures indicated by the assessment findings may be performed by you or by the family members under your guidance in an effort to educate and support the family. Other interventions may be delayed until the newborn has been transferred to an observational nursery.

First check and confirm the newborn's identification with the mother's identification and then obtain and record all significant information. The essential data to be recorded on the newborn's medical record are as follows:

1. *Condition of the newborn.* Pertinent information includes the newborn's Apgar scores at 1 and 5 minutes, any resuscitative measures required in the birthing area, physical examination, vital signs, voidings, and passing of meconium. Complications to be noted are excessive mucus, delayed spontaneous respirations or responsiveness, abnormal number of cord vessels, and obvious physical abnormalities.

2. *Labor and birth record.* A copy of the labor and birth record should be placed in the newborn's medical record or be accessible on the computer. The record contains the significant data about the birth—for example, duration, course, and status of mother and fetus throughout labor and birth and any analgesia or anesthesia administered to the mother. Take particular care to note any variation or difficulties, such as prolonged rupture of membranes, abnormal fetal position, presence or absence of meconium-stained amniotic fluid, signs of nonreassuring fetal heart rate during labor, nuchal cord (cord around the newborn's neck at birth), precipitous birth, use of forceps or vacuum extraction assisted device, maternal analgesics and anesthesia received within 1 hour before birth, and administration of antibiotics during labor.

3. *Antepartum history.* Preexisting maternal conditions or any maternal problems that may have compromised the fetus in utero, such as preeclampsia, spotting, illness, recent infections (evidence of chorioamnionitis), blood type, rubella status, serology results, hepatitis B screen results, colonization with group B streptococci, recent exposure to infectious disease, HIV status, or a history of maternal substance abuse, are of immediate concern in newborn assessment. The medical record should also include information about maternal age, estimated date of birth (EDB), previous pregnancies, and presence of any congenital anomalies. An HIV serology test should be encouraged and performed according to state law (AAP & ACOG, 2012).

4. *Parent–newborn interaction information.* Note the parents' interactions with their newborn and their desires regarding care, such as rooming in, circumcision, and the type of feeding. Information about other children in the home, available support systems, interactional patterns within each family unit, situations that compromise lactation

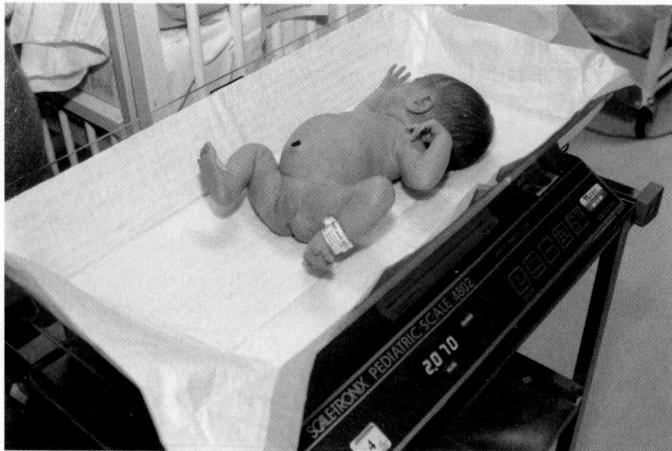

Figure 25–1 **Weighing of newborn: The scale is cleaned and balanced before each weighing, with the protective pad in place.**

(breast surgery, previous lactation failure), and any high-risk circumstances (adolescent mother, domestic violence, history of child abuse) helps in providing comprehensive care (AAP & ACOG, 2012).

As part of the admission procedure, weigh the newborn in both kilograms and pounds and ounces. In the United States, parents understand weight best when it is stated in pounds and ounces. Clean, cover, and set the scale to zero each time a newborn is weighed to prevent cross-infection. Remove all clothing and blankets for accurate weight and do the weighing under a warmer light to avoid heat loss from conduction (Figure 25–1).

Measure the newborn, recording the measurements in both centimeters and inches. The three routine measurements are length, head circumference, and chest circumference. In some facilities, abdominal girth may also be measured (see Table 24–1). Rapidly assess the baby's color, muscle tone, alertness, and general state. Remember that the first period of reactivity may have concluded, and the baby may be in the sleep-inactive phase, which makes the newborn hard to arouse. Do basic assessments for estimating gestational age and complete the physical assessment (see *Assessment Guide: Newborn Physical Assessment* in Chapter 24).

In addition to obtaining vital signs, perform a hematocrit and blood glucose evaluation on at-risk newborns or as clinically indicated (such as for small-for-gestational-age [SGA] or large-for-gestational-age [LGA] newborns, or if the newborn is jittery). These procedures may be done on admission or within the first 2 hours after birth (AAP & ACOG, 2012). (See Performing a Capillary Puncture, in the *Clinical Skills Manual* SKILLS.)

MAINTAINING A CLEAR AIRWAY AND STABLE VITAL SIGNS

Be sure that free flow oxygen is readily available. Place the newborn in a supine position (or side position, if the baby has copious secretions). If necessary, use a bulb syringe or DeLee wall suction (see Chapter 18 and Figure 18–8; also see Performing Nasal Pharyngeal Suctioning in the *Clinical Skills Manual* SKILLS) to remove mucus from the stomach to help prevent possible aspiration. When possible, this procedure should be delayed for 10 to 15 minutes after birth to reduce the potential for severe vasovagal reflex apnea.

In the absence of any newborn distress, continue with the admission by taking the newborn's vital signs (see Table 24–3). The initial temperature is taken by the axillary method. A wider range of normal exists for axillary temperature, specifically 36.4° to 37.2°C (97.5° to 99.0°F).

Once the initial temperature is taken, monitor the core temperature either by obtaining axillary temperatures at intervals or by placing a skin sensor on the newborn for continuous reading. The vital signs for a healthy term newborn should be monitored at least every 30 minutes until the newborn's condition has remained stable for 2 hours (AAP & ACOG, 2012). The newborn's respirations may be irregular, yet still be normal. Brief periods of apnea, lasting only 5 to 10 seconds with no color or heart rate changes, are considered normal. The normal pulse range is 110 to 160 beats per minute (beats/min), and the normal respiratory range is 30 to 60 respirations per minute. See Thermoregulation of the Newborn in the *Clinical Skills Manual* SKILLS.

MAINTAINING A NEUTRAL THERMAL ENVIRONMENT

A neutral thermal environment is essential to minimize the newborn's need for increased oxygen consumption and use of calories to maintain body heat in the optimal range of 36.4° to 37.2°C (97.5° to 99.0°F). If the newborn becomes hypothermic, the body's response can lead to metabolic acidosis, hypoxia, and shock.

A neutral thermal environment is best achieved by performing the newborn assessment and interventions with the newborn unclothed and under a radiant warmer. The radiant warmer's thermostat is controlled by the thermal skin sensor taped to the newborn's abdomen, upper thigh, or arm and can give a reading closely correlated with the mean body temperature (see Figure 24–16). The sensor indicates when the newborn's temperature exceeds or falls below the acceptable temperature range. Be aware that leaning over the newborn may block the radiant heat waves from reaching the newborn (Blackburn, 2013)

Clinical Tip
A snug cap can be fashioned from a piece of stockinette to help reduce heat loss from the head.

In light of early discharge practices (12 to 48 hours), healthy term newborns can be safely bathed immediately after the admission assessment is completed. The Association of Women's Health, Obstetrics and Neonatal Nurses (AWHONN) (2013) recommends washing off only the blood and fluid with the first bath and massaging the vernix into the skin. The baby is bathed while still under the radiant warmer; bathing may be done in the parents' room and by the parents. Bathing the newborn offers an excellent opportunity for teaching and welcoming parents' involvement in the care of their newborn. If there is any doubt regarding the baby's condition, a sponge bath may be given when the baby's temperature is normal and vital signs are stable (about 2 to 4 hours after birth), when the baby's condition dictates, or when the parents wish to give the first bath.

Recheck the newborn's temperature after the bath and, if it is stable, dress the baby in a shirt, diaper, and cap; wrap the baby and place in an open crib at room temperature. If the newborn's axillary temperature is below 36.5°C (97.7°F), return the newborn to the radiant warmer or place skin-to-skin with the mother to rewarm and promote early bonding and breastfeeding. The rewarming process should be gradual to prevent hyperthermia.

TABLE 25-1 Maintenance of Stable Newborn Temperature

Take action to help the newborn maintain a stable temperature:

- Keep the newborn's clothing and bedding dry.
- Double-wrap the newborn and put on a stocking cap.
- Use the radiant warmer during procedures.
- Reduce the newborn's exposure to drafts.
- Warm objects that will be in contact with the newborn (e.g., stethoscope, blankets).
- Encourage the mother to snuggle with the newborn under blankets or to breastfeed the newborn with a cap and a light cover on.

(See Chapter 24 for information about temperature assessment and instability and Table 25–1.)

PREVENTING VITAMIN K DEFICIENCY BLEEDING

A prophylactic injection of phytonadione vitamin K_1 (Aqua-MEPHYTON) is recommended to prevent vitamin K deficiency bleeding (VKDB) and hemorrhage, which can occur because of low prothrombin levels in the first few days of life. The potential for hemorrhage is considered to result from the absence of gut bacterial flora, which influences the production of vitamin K_1 in the newborn (see section on *Coagulation* in Chapter 23 for further discussion). Current recommendations underscore the need for treatment in newborns who are exclusively breast-fed (Blackburn, 2013). Vitamin K injection can be delayed up to 6 hours after birth (Marcewicz, 2014). It is often given in the labor and delivery unit before transfer to the newborn nursery.

A one-time-only prophylactic dose of 0.5 to 1.0 mg is given intramuscularly in the middle third of the vastus lateralis muscle, located in the lateral aspect of the thigh (Figure 25–2). Before injecting, thoroughly clean the newborn's skin site for the injection with a small alcohol swab. Use a 25-gauge, 5/8-in. needle for the injection. (Figure 25–3). If the mother received anticoagulants during pregnancy, an additional dose may be ordered by the health-care provider and is given 6 to 8 hours after the first injection.

Neonatal side effects can be pain and edema at the injection site. Allergic reactions, such as rash and urticaria, may also occur. Nursing consideration should include:

- Protect drug from light.
- Give vitamin K_1 before circumcision procedure.
- Observe for signs of local inflammation.
- Observe for bleeding (usually occurs on second or third day). Bleeding may be seen as generalized ecchymoses or bleeding from umbilical cord, circumcision site, nose, or gastrointestinal tract. Results of serial prothrombin time (PT) and international normalized ratio (INR) should be assessed.

PREVENTING EYE INFECTION

Another nursing responsibility is administering the legally required prophylactic eye treatment for *Neisseria gonorrhoeae*, which may have infected the newborn of an infected mother during the birth process. A variety of topical agents appear to be equally effective. Ophthalmic ointments that are used include 0.5% erythromycin (Ilotycin Ophthalmic), 1% tetracycline, or per agency protocol. All are also effective against *Chlamydia*, which has a higher incidence rate of infection than gonorrhea.

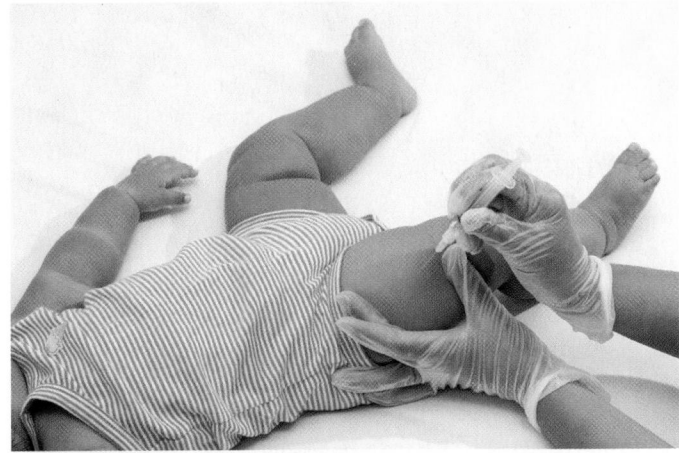

Figure 25–2 **Procedure for vitamin K injection. Cleanse area thoroughly with alcohol swab and allow skin to dry. Bunch the tissue of the upper outer thigh (vastus lateralis muscle) and quickly insert a 25-gauge, 5/8-in. needle at a 90-degree angle to the thigh. Slowly inject the solution to distribute the medication evenly and minimize the baby's discomfort. Remove the needle and gently massage the site with an alcohol swab.**

SOURCE: © Marlon Lopez/Shutterstock.

Successful eye prophylaxis requires that the medication be instilled into the lower conjunctival sac of each eye (Figure 25–4). After administration, gently close the eye and manipulate to ensure the spread of ointment (Wilson, Shannon, & Shields, 2015). It is instilled only once in each eye (AAP & ACOG, 2012). The ointment may be administered in the birthing area or, alternatively, 1 hour later in the nursery so that eye contact between newborn and parent is facilitated and the bonding process immediately after birth is not interrupted.

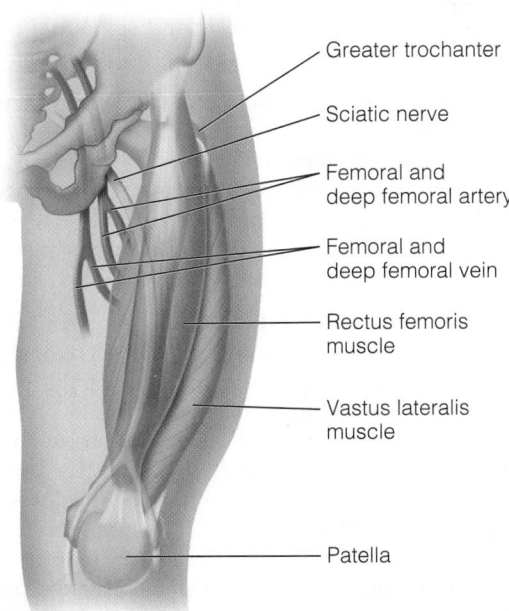

Greater trochanter
Sciatic nerve
Femoral and deep femoral artery
Femoral and deep femoral vein
Rectus femoris muscle
Vastus lateralis muscle
Patella

Figure 25–3 Injection site. The middle third of the vastus lateralis muscle is the preferred site for intramuscular injection in the newborn.

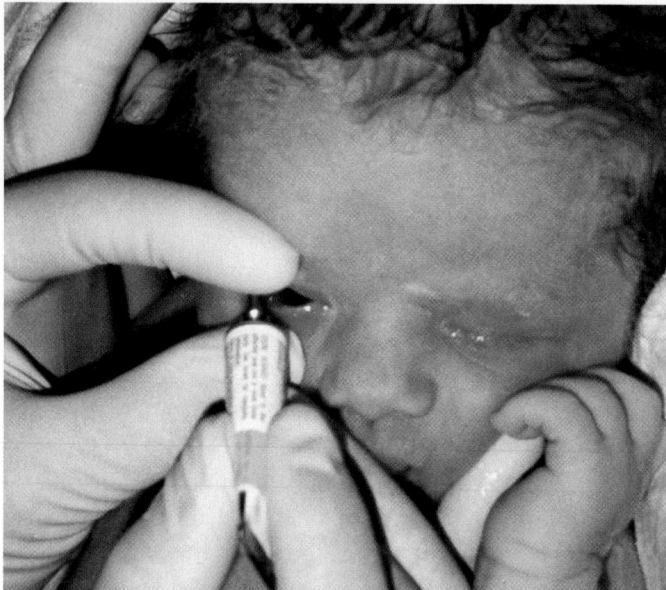

Figure 25–4 **Ophthalmic ointment. Retract the lower eyelid outward to instill a 0.25-in. (1 cm)–long strand of ointment from a single-dose tube along the lower conjunctival surface. Make sure that the tip of the tube does not touch the eye.**

Nursing considerations include the following:

- Use standard precautions before instillation to prevent introduction of bacteria if the baby has not been bathed yet.

- Do not irrigate the eyes after instillation. Use a new tube or single-use container for ophthalmic ointment administration shortly after birth. Excess ointment may be wiped away after 1 minute.

- Observe for hypersensitivity.

- Teach parents about the need for eye prophylaxis. Educate parents regarding side effects and signs that need to be reported to the healthcare provider.

Eye prophylaxis medications can cause chemical conjunctivitis, which gives the newborn some discomfort and may interfere with the ability to focus on the parents' faces. The resulting edema, inflammation, and discharge may cause concern if the parents have not been informed that the side effects will clear in 24 to 48 hours and that this prophylactic eye treatment is necessary for the newborn's well-being.

EARLY ASSESSMENT OF NEONATAL DISTRESS

During the first 24 hours of life, be constantly alert for signs of distress. If the newborn is with the parents during this period, take extra care to teach them how to maintain their newborn's temperature, recognize the hallmarks of newborn distress, and respond immediately to signs of respiratory problems. The parents must learn to observe the newborn for changes in color or activity, grunting or "sighing" sounds with breathing, rapid breathing with chest retractions, or facial grimacing. Their interventions include nasal and oral suctioning with a bulb syringe, positioning, and vigorous fingertip stroking of the newborn's spine to stimulate respiratory activity if necessary. You must be available immediately if the newborn develops distress (Table 25–2).

A common cause of neonatal distress is early-onset group B streptococcal (GBS) disease. Infected mothers transmit GBS

TABLE 25–2 Signs of Newborn Distress

- Respiratory changes
  - Increased respiratory rate (more than 60/minute) or difficult respirations
  - Grunting
  - Sternal, substernal, intercostal retractions
  - Nasal flaring
  - Excessive mucus
- Color change
  - Cyanosis (central: skin, lips, tongue)
  - Pallor
  - Mottling
  - Plethora (ruddy skin)
- Abdominal distention or mass
- Vomiting of bile-stained material
- Absence of meconium elimination within 48 hours of birth
- Absence of urine elimination more than 24 hours after birth (AAP & ACOG, 2012)
- Temperature instability (hypothermia or hyperthermia)
- Jitteriness, irritability, or abnormal movements
- Difficult to waken, lethargy, or hypotonicity
- Weight change greater than 10% loss of weight from birthweight

Source: Data from AAP & ACOG (2012).

Clinical Reasoning Early Respiratory Efforts

You overhear Mr. Johannson speaking to his mother on the phone. He is telling her about the "cute little grunting noises" his 30-minute-old baby makes. The newborn is in the room with the mother. What is your best course of action?

---

infection to their babies during labor and birth; thus it is recommended that at-risk mothers receive intrapartum antimicrobial prophylaxis (IAP) for GBS disease. All newborns of mothers identified as at risk should be assessed and observed for signs and symptoms of sepsis (see Chapter 15 for discussion of maternal care and Chapter 27 for discussion of newborn care).

FACILITATING EARLY PARENT–NEWBORN ATTACHMENT

To facilitate **parent–newborn attachment**, eye-to-eye contact between the parents and their newborn is extremely important during the early hours after birth when the newborn is in the first period of reactivity. The newborn is alert during this time, the eyes are wide open, and the baby often makes direct eye contact with human faces within optimal range for visual acuity (7 to 8 in.). It is theorized that this eye contact is an important foundation in establishing attachment in human relationships (Klaus & Klaus, 1985). Consequently, administration of the prophylactic eye medication is often delayed, but no more than 1 hour, to provide an opportunity for a period of eye contact between parents and their newborn, thus facilitating the attachment process (AAP & ACOG, 2012). Parents who cannot be with their newborns in this first period because of maternal or neonatal distress may need reassurance that the bonding process can proceed normally as soon as both mother and baby are stable.

Another situation that can facilitate attachment is the interactive bath. While bathing their newborn for the first time, parents attend closely to their baby's behavior. In this way, the newborn becomes an active participant and parents are drawn into an interaction with their newborn. During this time, you may interpret the newborn's behavior for the parents, model ways to respond to the behavior, and support parental strategies for doing so.

> **Professionalism in Practice** Skin-To-Skin Contact
>
> Many hospital units remove newborns from their mother following birth to allow convenient assessment and performance of procedures by hospital staff despite the preponderance of evidence that supports immediate skin-to-skin contact (SSC) between mother (or father) and the newborn. Nurses are the professionals most often at the mother's bedside; they have the power and an obligation to serve as leaders and change agents by promoting clinical practices that are supported by research evidence.

Evaluation

When evaluating the nursing care provided during the period immediately after birth, the nurse may anticipate the following outcomes:

- The newborn's adaptation to extrauterine life is successful as demonstrated by all vitals within acceptable parameters.
- The newborn's physiologic and psychologic integrity is supported.
- Positive interactions between parent and newborn will be supported.

The Newborn Following Transition

Once a healthy newborn has demonstrated successful adaptation to extrauterine life, the newborn needs appropriate observations for the first 6 to 12 hours after birth and the remainder of the stay in the birthing facility.

Nursing Management

For the Newborn Following Transition

Nursing Assessment and Diagnosis

Examples of nursing diagnoses that may apply during daily care of the newborn include the following (NANDA-I © 2014):

- *Breathing Pattern, Ineffective*, related to periodic breathing
- *Nutrition, Imbalanced: Less than Body Requirements*, related to limited nutritional and fluid intake and increased caloric expenditure
- *Urinary Elimination, Impaired*, related to meatal edema secondary to circumcision
- *Infection, Risk for*, related to umbilical cord healing, circumcision site, immature immune system, or potential birth trauma (forceps or vacuum extraction birth)

- *Knowledge, Readiness for Enhanced*, related to information about basic newborn care, male circumcision, and breast-feeding and/or formula-feeding
- *Family Processes, Readiness for Enhanced*, related to integration of newborn into family or demands of newborn care and feeding

> **Clinical Reasoning** Newborn Breathing Difficulties
>
> Aisha Khan gave birth to a healthy girl 2 hours ago; she calls you to her room. She sounds frightened and says her baby cannot breathe. You find Aisha cradling her newborn in her arms. The baby is mildly cyanotic, is waving her arms, and has mucus coming from her nose and mouth. What would you do?

Planning and Implementation

MAINTAINING CARDIOPULMONARY FUNCTION

Assess vital signs every 6 to 8 hours or more, depending on the newborn's status. The newborn should be placed on the back (supine) for sleeping. A bulb syringe is kept within easy reach should the newborn need oral-nasal suctioning. If the newborn has respiratory difficulty, clear the airway. Vigorous fingertip stroking of the baby's spine will frequently stimulate respiratory activity. A cardiorespiratory monitor can be used on newborns that are not being observed at all times and are at risk for decreased respiratory or cardiac function. Indicators of risk are pallor, cyanosis, ruddy color, apnea, and other signs of instability. Changes in skin color may indicate the need for closer assessment of temperature, cardiopulmonary status, hematocrit, glucose, and bilirubin levels.

MAINTAINING A NEUTRAL THERMAL ENVIRONMENT

Make every effort to maintain the newborn's temperature within the normal range by continuing interventions started in the first 4-hour period. A newborn whose temperature falls below optimal level uses calories to maintain body heat rather than for growth. Chilling also decreases the affinity of serum albumin for bilirubin, thereby increasing the likelihood of newborn jaundice. In addition, it increases oxygen use and may cause respiratory distress. An overheated newborn will increase activity and respiratory rate in an attempt to cool the body. Both measures deplete caloric reserves, and the increased respiratory rate leads to increased insensible fluid loss (Blackburn, 2013).

> **Clinical Reasoning** Maintaining the Newborn's Temperature
>
> John Fredricks, the father of a newborn less than a day old, has the baby lying supine and wearing only a diaper. When you suggest that the baby may need more covering, he responds: "He doesn't like all that stuff on. After all, he's been naked until now."
>
> What actions and teaching are appropriate in this situation?

PROMOTING ADEQUATE HYDRATION AND NUTRITIONAL STATUS

Record caloric and fluid intake and enhance adequate hydration by maintaining a neutral thermal environment and offering early and frequent feedings. Early feedings promote gastric emptying and increase peristalsis, thereby decreasing the potential for hyperbilirubinemia by decreasing the amount of time fecal material is in contact with enzyme β-glucuronidase in the small intestine. This enzyme frees the bilirubin from the feces, allowing it to be reabsorbed into the vascular system (see Chapter 27 for a detailed discussion of hyperbilirubinemia).

Record voiding and stooling patterns. The first voiding should occur within 24 hours and the first passage of stool within 48 hours. When these do not occur, continue the normal observation routine while assessing for abdominal distention, bowel sounds, hydration, fluid intake, and temperature stability.

Newborns should be weighed at the same time each day for accurate comparisons and should be kept warm during the weighing. A weight loss of up to 10% for term newborns is considered within normal limits during the first week of life (Cloherty, Eichenwald, Hansen, et al., 2012). This weight loss is the result of limited intake, loss of excess extracellular fluid, and passage of meconium. Tell the parents about the expected weight loss, the reason for it, and the expectations for regaining the birth weight. Birth weight is usually regained by 2 weeks if feedings are adequate.

Excessive handling can cause an increase in the newborn's metabolic rate and caloric use and cause fatigue. Be alert to the newborn's subtle cues of fatigue, including a decrease in muscle tension and activity in the extremities and neck, as well as loss of eye contact, which may be manifested by fluttering or closure of the eyelids. Quickly cease stimulation when signs of fatigue appear. Demonstrate to parents the need to be aware of newborn cues and to wait for periods of alertness for contact and stimulation. Assess the woman's comfort and latching-on techniques if she is breastfeeding, or assess the bottle-feeding techniques. Breastfeeding and formula-feeding the newborn are discussed in detail later in this chapter.

PROMOTING SKIN INTEGRITY

Newborn skin care, including bathing, is important for the health and appearance of the individual newborn and for infection control within the nursery. Ongoing skin care involves cleansing the buttock and perianal areas with fresh water and cotton or a mild soap and water with diaper changes. If commercial baby wipes are used, those without alcohol should be selected. Perfumed and latex-free wipes are also available.

The umbilical cord is assessed for signs of bleeding or infection. Removal of the cord clamp within 24 to 48 hours of birth reduces the chance of tension injury to the area. Keeping the umbilical stump clean and allowing it to air dry without the routine application of topical agents can reduce the chance for infection (AWHONN, 2013) (Figure 25–5). See Umbilical Cord Clamp: Application, Care, and Removal in the *Clinical Skills Manual* SKILLS .

Many types of routine cord care are practiced, including the use of air-drying, triple dye, an antimicrobial agent such as bacitracin, or application of 70% alcohol to the cord stump, but should not be encouraged (AWHONN, 2013). These practices are largely based on tradition rather than evidence-based findings. The skin absorption and toxicity of triple-dye agents

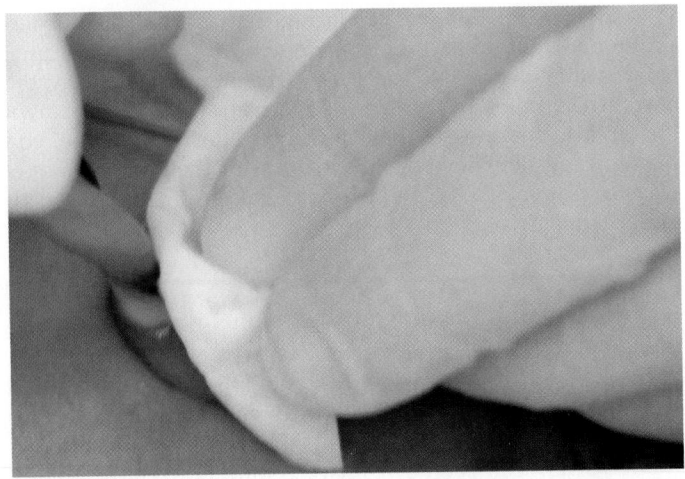

Figure 25–5 Routine umbilical cord care. The umbilical cord base is carefully cleansed.

in newborns have not been carefully studied. No single method of umbilical cord care has been proven to be superior in preventing umbilical cord colonization of microorganisms and infection (omphalitis) (AWHONN, 2013). Folding the diaper down to avoid covering the cord stump can prevent contamination of the area and promote drying. Cord care per agency policy is your responsibility. The cord should look dark and dry up before falling off (Figure 25–6). It is also your responsibility to instruct parents in caring for the cord and observing for signs and symptoms of infection after discharge, such as foul smell, redness and greenish yellow drainage, localized heat and tenderness, or bright red bleeding or if the area remains unhealed 2 to 3 days after the cord stump has sloughed off.

PROMOTING SAFETY

The threat of newborn abduction requires that hospitals have active programs to prevent such an event (Fraser, 2014). Be aware of these policies and follow them rigorously. Informing parents of their role in this process is part of a comprehensive safety plan.

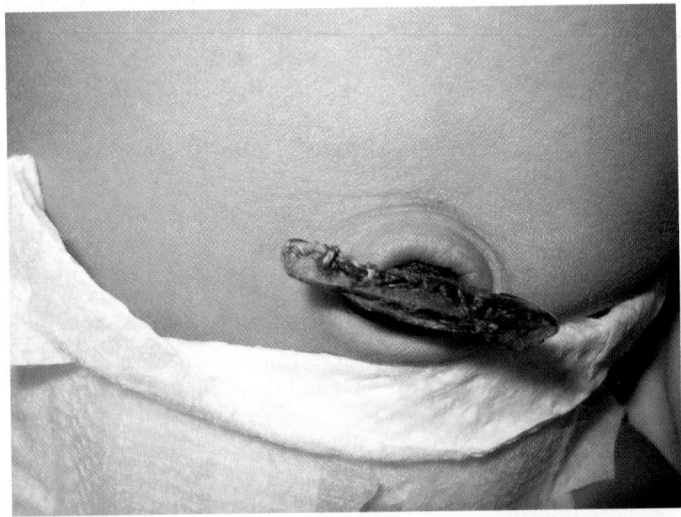

Figure 25–6 The umbilical cord looks dark and dries up prior to falling off.

Parental measures to prevent abduction and promote newborn safety include the following:

Security

- Check that identification bands are in place as the parents care for their baby and, if missing, ask that they be replaced immediately.
- If an electronically tagged band is used, keep the newborn within the bounds of the system and notify the staff if the band becomes loose or comes off (see Figure 18-9).
- Allow only people with proper birthing unit identification to remove the baby from the room. If parents do not know the staff person, they should call the nurse for assistance.
- Report the presence of any suspicious people on the birthing unit.

Safety

- Never leave the newborn alone in the room. If parents walk in the halls or take a shower, they should have a family member watch the newborn, or they should return the newborn to the nursery.
- Never lift the newborn if feeling weak, faint, or unsteady on one's feet. Instead, the parent should call for assistance.
- Always keep an eye and hand on the newborn when out of the crib because babies can fall from beds and other surfaces if left alone.
- Protect from infection, even though newborns do possess some immunity. All caregivers should practice good hand washing before and after giving care. Parents should ask visitors to leave if they have any of the following: cold, diarrhea, discharge from sores, or contagious disease. Security monitoring devices should be sterilized after use to prevent transmission of infection.

PREVENTING COMPLICATIONS

Newborns are at continued risk for the complications of hemorrhage, late-onset cardiac symptoms, and infection. Pallor may be an early sign of hemorrhage and must be reported to the healthcare provider. The newborn is placed on a cardiorespiratory monitor to permit continuous assessment. Several newborn conditions put newborns at risk for hemorrhage. Cyanosis that is not relieved by oxygen administration requires emergency intervention, may indicate a congenital cardiac condition or shock, and requires ongoing assessment.

It is recommended that nursing staff gown and glove when handling a newborn until the first bath to avoid contamination by blood and amniotic fluids. Infection in the nursery is best prevented by requiring that all personnel who have direct contact with newborns scrub for 2 to 3 minutes from the fingertips up to and including the elbows at the beginning of each shift. The hands must also be washed with soap and rubbed vigorously for 15 seconds, or a topical antimicrobial applied, before and after contact with every newborn and after touching any soiled surface such as the floor or one's hair or face. Instruct parents to practice good hand washing and/or use of an antiseptic hand cleaner before touching the newborn. Emphasize that anyone holding the baby should practice good hand washing, even after the family returns home. In some clinical settings, family members are asked to wear gowns (preferably disposable) over their street clothes during their contact with newborns. These are good opportunities to reinforce the efficacy of hand washing in preventing the spread of infection.

Jaundice occurs in most newborns. Most jaundice is benign, but because of the potential toxicity of bilirubin, newborns must be monitored to identify those who might develop severe hyperbilirubinemia and, in rare cases, acute bilirubin encephalopathy or kernicterus (see Chapter 27 for more detailed discussion) (AAP & ACOG, 2012). Current recommendations include obtaining a total serum bilirubin level in any newborn who is visibly jaundiced in the first 24 hours of life, and obtaining either a serum or transcutaneous bilirubin level before discharge. Nomograms for evaluating risk factors based on bilirubin levels and age of baby are available (see Chapter 23).

CIRCUMCISION

Circumcision is a surgical procedure in which the prepuce, an epithelial layer covering the tip of the penis, is separated from the glans penis and excised. This permits exposure of the glans for easier cleaning.

Scientific evidence demonstrates that the preventive health benefits of elective circumcision of newborn males outweigh the risks of this procedure (Healthy Children, 2015g). However, the 2012 AAP policy statement reaffirmed that it does not recommend *routine* circumcision but acknowledges that medical indications for circumcision still exist (AAP, 2012a).

Circumcision *should not be performed* if the newborn is premature or compromised, has a known bleeding problem, or is born with a genitourinary defect such as hypospadias or epispadias, which may necessitate the use of the foreskin in future surgical repairs.

Parents will need to weigh medical information in the context of their own religious, ethical, and cultural beliefs and practices, as it is the parents who must ultimately decide whether circumcision is in the best interests of their child (Healthy Children, 2015g). To ensure informed consent, parents should be informed during the prenatal period about possible long-term medical effects of circumcision and noncircumcision. Parents must be knowledgeable about the potential risks and outcomes of circumcision. Hemorrhage, infection, difficulty in voiding, separation of the edges of the circumcision, discomfort, and restlessness are early potential problems (Cloherty et al., 2012). You can allay parents' anxiety by sharing information and allowing them to express their concerns.

Circumcision Care

The procedure is performed when the newborn is well stabilized and has received an initial physical examination by a healthcare provider. Before a circumcision, ensure that the healthcare provider has explained the procedure, determine whether the parents have any further questions about the procedure, and verify that the circumcision permit is signed. As with any surgical procedure, the newborn's identification band should be checked to verify his identity before the procedure begins. Gather the equipment and prepare the newborn by removing the diaper and placing him on a padded circumcision board or some other type of restraint, but restraining only the legs. These restraint measures along with the application of warm blankets to the upper body increase comfort during the procedure. In Jewish circumcision ceremonies, the baby is held by the father or godfather and given wine before the procedure.

A variety of devices (Gomco clamp, Plastibell, Mogen clamp) are used for circumcision (Figures 25–7 and 25–8), and all produce minimal bleeding. Therefore, make special note of newborns with a family history of bleeding disorders or with mothers who took anticoagulants, including aspirin, prenatally. During the procedure, assess the newborn's response.

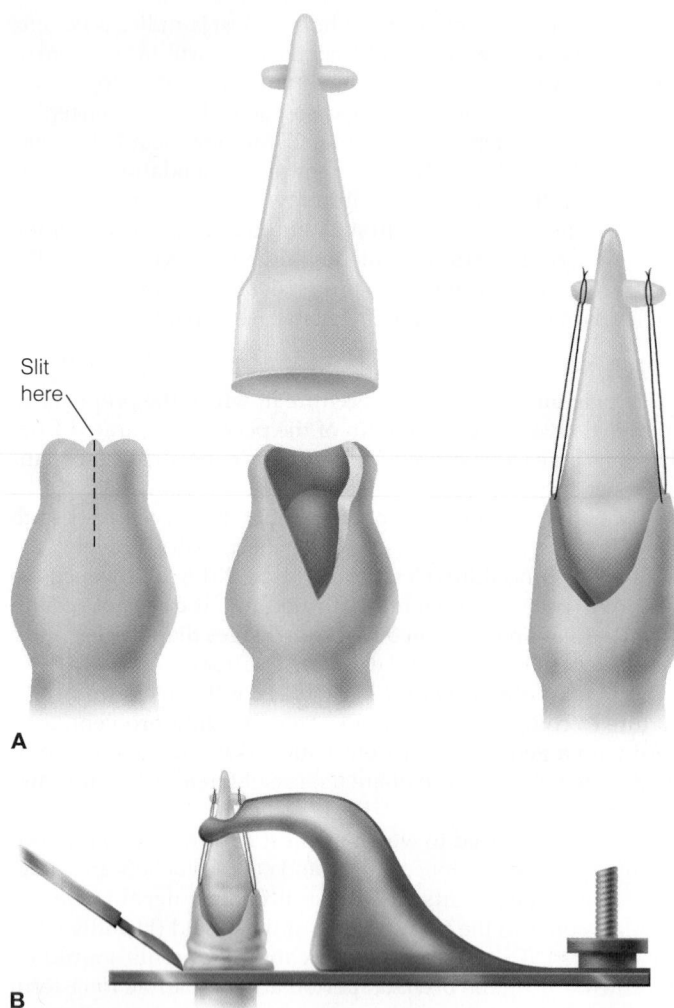

Slit here

A

B

Figure 25–7 Circumcision using the Yellen or Gomco clamp. *A*, The prepuce is drawn over the cone, and *B*, the clamp is applied. Pressure is maintained for 3 to 4 minutes, and then excess prepuce is cut away.

One important consideration is pain experienced by the newborn. The 2012 AAP policy recommends that acceptable methods of analgesia (dorsal penile nerve block [DPNB], subcutaneous ring block, and eutectic mixture of local anesthetics [EMLA] cream) be used during circumcision to decrease procedural pain (Cloherty et al., 2012). The DPNB and subcutaneous ring block are the most effective options. The use of sucrose pacifiers has also been studied. Indications are that a combination of methods is most effective in reducing pain during circumcision (AAP & ACOG, 2012).

During the procedure, provide comfort measures such as swaddling, lightly stroking the newborn's head, providing a pacifier for nonnutritive sucking, and talking to him. Following the circumcision, the newborn should be held and comforted by you or a family member. Be alert to any behavioral cues that these measures are overstimulating the newborn instead of comforting him. Such cues include turning away of the head, increased generalized body movement, skin color changes, hyperalertness, and hiccuping. See Assisting with Circumcision and Providing Circumcision Care in the *Clinical Skills* SKILLS Manual.

Ideally, assess the circumcision every 30 minutes for at least 2 hours following the procedure. It is important to observe the first voiding after a circumcision to evaluate for urinary obstruction related to penile injury or edema.

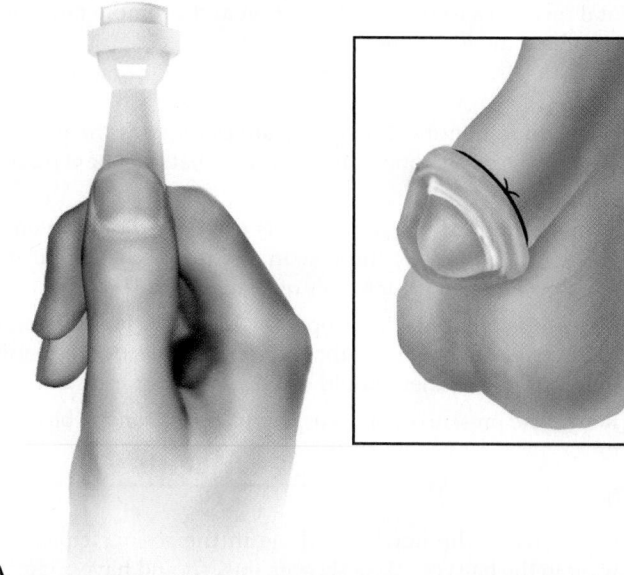

A

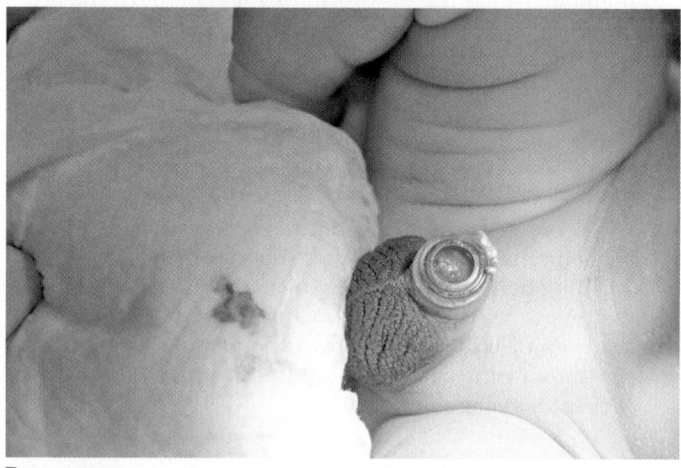

B

Figure 25–8 Circumcision using the Plastibell. *A*, The bell is fitted over the glans. A suture is tied around the bell's rim and the excess prepuce is cut away. The plastic rim remains in place for 3 to 4 days until healing occurs. The bell may be allowed to fall off; it is removed if still in place after 8 days. *B*, Plastibell.

SOURCE: *B*, Vanessa Howell, RN, MSN.

If the Plastibell is used, provide information to the parents about normal appearance and how to observe for infection. Inform them that the Plastibell should fall off within 8 days. If it remains on after 8 days, they should consult with the newborn's healthcare provider. Though no ointments or creams should be used while the bell remains, application of petroleum ointment may protect granulation tissue afterward (AWHONN, 2013).

CARE OF THE UNCIRCUMCISED NEWBORN

Teach the parents of an uncircumcised male baby about good hygienic practices. Tell them that the foreskin and glans are two similar layers of cells that separate from each other. The separation process begins prenatally and is normally completed between 3 to 5 years of age. In the process of separation, sterile sloughed cells build up between the layers. This buildup looks similar to the smegma secreted after puberty, and it is harmless.

Health Promotion Newborn Circumcision Care

Teach family members how to assess for unusual bleeding, how to respond if it is present, and how to care for the newly circumcised penis. Parents of newborns circumcised with a method other than Plastibell should receive the following information:

- Clean with warm water with each diaper change.

- Apply petroleum ointment for the next few diaper changes to help prevent further bleeding and to protect the healing tissue afterward (Figure 25–9).

- If bleeding does occur, apply light pressure with a sterile gauze pad to stop the bleeding within a short time. If this is not effective, contact the healthcare provider immediately, or take the newborn to the healthcare provider.

- The glans normally has granulation tissue (a yellowish film) on it during healing. Continued application of a petroleum ointment (or ointment suggested by the healthcare provider) can help protect the granulation tissue that forms as the glans heals.

- Report to the healthcare provider any signs or symptoms of infection, such as increasing swelling, pus drainage, and cessation of urination.

- When diapering, ensure that the diaper is not too loose to cause rubbing with movement, or too tight to cause pain.

- If the newborn's healthcare provider recommends oral analgesics, follow instructions for proper measuring and administration.

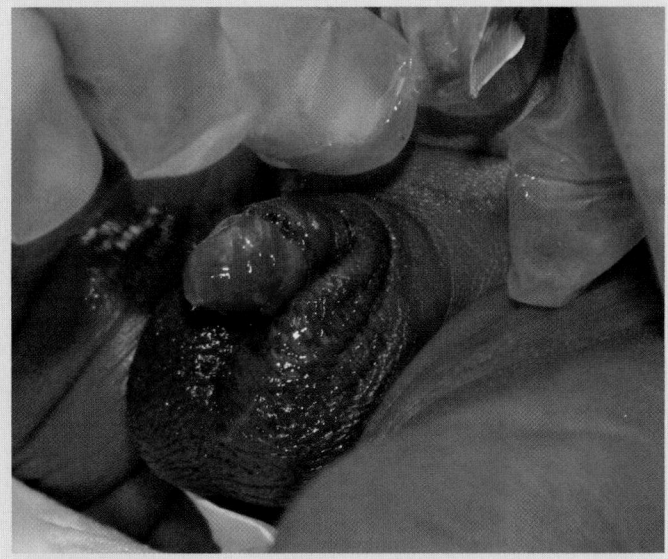

Figure 25–9 Following circumcision, petroleum ointment may be applied to the site for the next few diaper changes.

Occasionally, during the daily bath, the parent can gently test for retraction. If retraction has occurred, daily gentle washing of the glans with soap and water is sufficient to maintain adequate cleanliness. The parents should teach the child to incorporate this practice into his daily self-care activities. Most uncircumcised males have no difficulty doing so.

ENHANCING PARENT–NEWBORN ATTACHMENT

Encourage parent–newborn attachment by involving all family members with the new member of the family. (For specific interventions see Chapters 18 and 29 and *Teaching Highlights: What Parents Need to Know About Enhancing Attachment*.) Discuss waking activities such as talking with the newborn while making eye contact, holding the newborn in an upright position (sitting or standing), gently bending the newborn back and forth while grasping under the knees and supporting the head and back with the other hand, or gently rubbing the newborn's hands and feet. Quieting activities may include swaddling or bundling the baby to increase a sense of security; using slow, calming movements; and talking softly, singing, or humming to the newborn. See Box 25–1 for a discussion of infant massage.

Caring for newborns in the birthing setting and fostering parent–newborn attachment means that the nurse will have contact with parents from a wide variety of racial, religious, and cultural backgrounds. Although it may not be possible to be conversant with all cultures, the nurse can demonstrate cultural competence with both colleagues and parents. The nurse must be sensitive to the cultural beliefs and values of the family and be aware of cultural variations in newborn care such as naming the newborn, giving compliments about the newborn, and using good luck charms (see *Developing Cultural Competence: Examples of Cultural Beliefs and Practices Regarding Baby Care*).

TEACHING HIGHLIGHTS | What Parents Need to Know About Enhancing Attachment

- Information on the periods of reactivity, expected newborn responses, and normal newborn physical characteristics.
- The gradual developmental nature of the bonding process and the reciprocal interactive nature of the process.
- The newborn's capabilities for interaction such as nonverbal communication abilities. Nonverbal communications include movement, gaze, touch, facial expressions, and vocalizations—including crying. Eye contact is considered one of the cardinal factors in developing newborn–parent attachment and will be integrated with touching and vocal behaviors.
- Touching, including stroking, patting, massaging, and kissing, will progress to interactive touch between parent and baby; parents need to assimilate these and other comforting behaviors (talking, singing, swaddling, rocking) into daily routines with their baby.
- The newborn's behaviors will change as the baby matures, and it is important for parents to be consistent in response to their baby's cues and needs.
- Information about pamphlets, videos, and support groups in the community.

Box 25–1 Infant Massage

Infant massage is a common childcare practice in many parts of the world, especially Africa and Asia, and has recently gained attention in the United States. Parents can be taught to use infant massage as a method to facilitate the bonding process and to reduce the stress and pain associated with teething, constipation, inoculations, and colic. Infant massage not only induces relaxation for the baby but also provides a calming and "feel-good" interaction for the parents, which fosters the development of warm, positive relationships.

Evaluation

When evaluating the nursing care provided during the newborn period, the nurse may anticipate the following outcomes:

- The baby's physiologic and psychologic integrity is supported by maintaining stable vital signs and interactions based on normal newborn behaviors.
- The newborn feeding pattern will be satisfactorily established.
- The parents express understanding of the bonding process and display attachment behaviors.

Developing Cultural Competence Baby Naming in Kenya

In Kenya, the naming of a child is an important event. Names are commonly selected to mirror important or current events. For example, a baby who is born while traveling may be given a name that means "wanderer" or "traveler." Other names may be chosen after a relative who is among the "living-dead" (deceased). It is believed that this results in a partial reincarnation of that relative, especially if the child has characteristics in common with that individual. It is also believed there is a connection between newborns and the spirit world.

In some parts of the country, the name is chosen when the baby is crying. Different names of the living or dead are called, and if the baby stops crying when a particular name is called, that becomes the baby's given name. In some areas, the name is given on the third day and is marked by a celebration with feasting and rejoicing. On the fourth day, the father of the baby commonly hangs an iron necklace on the baby's neck. It is at this time that the baby is considered a full human being and the connection with the spirit world is lost.

Developing Cultural Competence Examples of Cultural Beliefs and Practices Regarding Baby Care*

Umbilical Cord

- People of Latin American or Filipino cultural background may use an abdominal binder or bellyband to protect against dirt, injury, and umbilical hernia. They may also apply oils to the stump of the cord or tape metal to the umbilicus to ward off evil spirits (D'Avanzo & Geissler, 2008).
- People of northern European ancestry may expect a sterile cutting of the cord at birth. They may allow the stump to air-dry and discard the cord once it falls off.
- Chinese and some Latin American parents cauterize the stump with a hot flame, hot coal, or the like (Smith, 2009).
- In Kenya and Iran, women may express colostrum onto the cord stump (Smith, 2009).
- In Ecuador, the cord stump is left long in girls to prevent a small uterus and problems with childbirth (Smith, 2009).

Parent–Infant Contact

- People of Asian ancestry may pick up the baby as soon as it cries, or they may carry the baby at all times.
- Several native North American nations' people, notably the Navajos, may use cradle boards, so the baby can be with family, even during work, and feel secure (Woodring & Andrews, 2012).
- The Muslim father traditionally calls praise to Allah in the newborn's right ear and cleans the baby after birth.

Circumcision

- People of Muslim and Jewish ancestry practice circumcision as a religious ritual.
- Many natives of Africa and Australia practice circumcision as a puberty rite.
- Native Americans and people of Asian and Latin American cultures rarely perform circumcision (Lipson & Dibble, 2008).
- According to 2006 global estimates, about 30% of males are circumcised (World Health Organization [WHO], 2008).

Health and Illness

- Some people from Latin American cultural backgrounds may believe that touching the face or head of a baby when admiring it will ward off the "evil eye." They also may not cut the baby's nails to avoid nearsightedness and instead put mittens on the baby's hands to prevent scratching. They also may believe that fat babies are healthy (Woodring & Andrews, 2012).
- Some people of Asian heritage may not allow anyone to touch the baby's head without asking permission.
- Some Orthodox Jews believe that saying the baby's name before the formal naming ceremony will harm the baby.
- Asians and Haitians may delay naming their babies until after the confinement month (D'Avanzo & Geissler, 2008).
- Some people of Vietnamese ancestry believe that cutting a baby's hair or nails will cause illness.

*Note: The information given here is meant only to provide examples of the behaviors that may be found within certain cultures. Not all members of a culture practice the behaviors described.

Newborn Feeding

Early nutrition has a significant impact on the present and future health and well-being of the baby because this is a period of rapid growth and brain development. Good nutrition fosters physical growth and helps maintain a healthy immune system. In addition, feeding is an important component of newborn socialization that promotes cognitive and emotional development.

The newborn's diet must supply all the nutrients required by the body in the proper quantities to meet the newborn's rapid rate of physical and neurologic growth and development. A newborn's diet should provide adequate hydration and sufficient calories and must include protein, carbohydrates, fat, vitamins, and minerals. Exclusive breast milk and/or iron-fortified 20-calorie/ounce formula are sufficient as sole sources of nutrition to meet the dietary needs of the baby from birth up to 6 months of age. Complementary solid foods are introduced in the second half of the first year, and the infant continues to receive breast milk and/or formula until at least 12 months of age (AAP, 2012b). See Chapter 32 for a discussion of infant nutrition.

Choice of Feeding: Breast Versus Formula

Feeding their newborn is an exciting, satisfying, but often worrisome task for parents. Meeting this essential need of their new baby helps parents strengthen their attachment to their baby and fosters their self-images as nurturers and providers, yet carries great responsibility. Whether a woman chooses to breastfeed or formula-feed, she can adequately meet her baby's needs. As questions about feeding arise, the nurse works with the woman to help her develop skill in her chosen method. In every interaction, it is the nurse's responsibility to support the parents and promote the family's sense of confidence.

The mother usually decides to breastfeed or formula-feed by the sixth month of pregnancy and often even before conception. However, she may not make her final decision until admission to the birth center. The decision is often influenced by relatives, especially the baby's father and maternal grandmother (Janke, 2014), by friends, and by social customs rather than being based on knowledge about the nutritional and psychologic needs of the mother and her newborn.

Once the parents have made an informed choice of feeding method, the nurse's primary responsibilities are to support the family's decision and to help the family achieve a positive result. No woman should be made to feel either inadequate or superior because of her choice in feeding. There are advantages and disadvantages to breastfeeding and bottle-feeding, but positive bonds in parent–newborn relationships can be developed with either method.

Breastfeeding
Breast Milk Production

The female breast is divided into 15 to 20 lobes, separated from one another by fat and connective tissue, and interspersed with blood vessels, lymphatic vessels, and nerves. These lobes are subdivided into connected lobules composed of small units

---

EVIDENCE-BASED PRACTICE | Increasing Breastfeeding Rates

Clinical Question

Is telephone consultation effective in increasing breastfeeding rates, especially among low-income and underserved mothers?

The Evidence

Despite widespread evidence about the benefits of breastfeeding for both mother and baby, breastfeeding rates remain relatively low. National data show that less than half of babies born in the United States are fed any breast milk at 6 months of age, and only 16% of babies at this age are exclusively breastfed. Babies who are breastfed have stronger immune systems, lower risk of allergies, fewer dental caries, and reduced incidence of sudden infant death syndrome. Support for breastfeeding is an important perinatal effort. This researcher undertook a systematic review of the literature to determine evidence-based strategies for enhancing breastfeeding that could be delivered efficiently and with low cost via telephone consultation. The studies reviewed included samples of more than 500 mothers. This type of structured review of randomized trials forms the strongest evidence for practice.

An effective strategy for low-income and underserved mothers used scheduled telephone support provided by lactation consultants. Weekly telephone consultation for the first 3 postnatal months was effective in increasing breastfeeding rates and duration (Flannery, 2014). Monthly telephone consultation from 3 to 6 months was effective in sustaining the effect. The types of telephone consultation that were most effective were anticipatory guidance, education, and empowerment.

The review also reported that the use of a lactation consultant was desirable but not imperative; peer counseling and support was effective in encouraging mothers to breastfeed for a longer duration. Services provided by either group increased breastfeeding rates by 27% to 34%. Women in these studies reported that the credentials of the counselors were not as important as their approach; mothers wanted counseling from someone they trusted, who entered into a dialogue rather than a lecture, and who offered information that was not confusing or conflicting. The advantage of telephone consultation was the lack of geographic boundaries; one of the studies in the review focused exclusively on rural mothers and found the effects were similar to those women who had access to urban services.

Best Practice

Telephone consultation that involves supportive communication, an authentic dialogue, and accurate information provided routinely during the postnatal period can increase the rate and duration of breastfeeding. This type of consultation is effective for low income and rural mothers as well as those in urban areas.

Clinical Reasoning

Describe an example of the ways in which breastfeeding counseling can be provided so that it is perceived as trustworthy and part of two-way communication. What are some of the barriers to breastfeeding that could be addressed with this intervention?

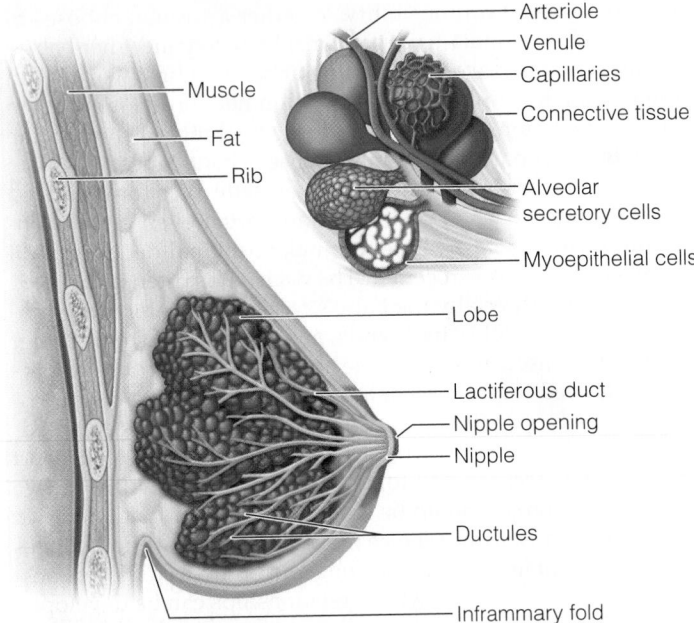

Labels: Muscle, Fat, Rib, Arteriole, Venule, Capillaries, Connective tissue, Alveolar secretory cells, Myoepithelial cells, Lobe, Lactiferous duct, Nipple opening, Nipple, Ductules, Inframmary fold

Figure 25–10 Anatomy of the breast.

called *alveoli* where milk is synthesized by the alveolar secretory epithelium. The lobules have a system of lactiferous ducts that join larger ducts and eventually open onto the nipple surface. Mothers are often surprised to see milk coming out of multiple nipple pores when they express their milk. See Figure 25–10 to view the anatomy of the breast.

> **Health Promotion** *Healthy People 2020* **Objectives for Exclusive Breastfeeding**
> The goals of the *Healthy People 2020* national health promotion and disease prevention program state that at least 82% of all mothers will initiate breastfeeding, at least 61% will continue to breastfeed until their infants are 6 months old, and at least 34% will continue to breastfeed until their infants are 12 months old. The *Healthy People 2020* objective for exclusive breastfeeding at 3 months is 46%; the current rate is 33.6%. The *Healthy People 2020* objective for exclusive breastfeeding at 6 months is 26%; the current rate is 14.1% (U.S. Breastfeeding Committee, 2011). It is the healthcare provider's responsibility to provide the parents with accurate information about the distinct advantages of breastfeeding to the mother and baby.

Physiologic and Endocrine Control of Lactogenesis

During pregnancy, increased levels of estrogen stimulate breast duct proliferation and development, and elevated progesterone levels promote the development of lobules and alveoli in preparation for lactation. Prolactin levels rise from approximately 10 ng/mL prepregnancy to 200 ng/mL at term. However, lactation is suppressed during pregnancy by elevated progesterone levels secreted by the placenta. Once the placenta is expelled at birth, progesterone levels fall and the inhibition is removed, triggering milk production. This occurs whether the mother has breast stimulation or not. However, if by the third or fourth day breast stimulation is not occurring, prolactin levels begin to drop.

Initially, lactation is under endocrine control. The hormone **prolactin** is released from the anterior pituitary in response to breast stimulation from suckling or the use of a breast pump. Prolactin levels double each time the baby suckles at the breast regardless of the age of the baby or duration of lactation. Prolactin stimulates the milk-secreting cells in the alveoli to produce milk, then rapidly drops back to baseline. If more than approximately 3 hours occur between stimulation, prolactin levels begin to drop below baseline. To reverse the overall decline in prolactin level, the mother can be encouraged to stimulate her breasts more frequently (e.g., every 1.5 to 2 hours). Mothers should be strongly encouraged to stimulate their breasts frequently if their newborns are not effective feeders or if they are separated from their babies. Prolactin receptors are established during the first 2 weeks postpartum in response to frequency of breast stimulation (Walker, 2016). Inadequate development of prolactin receptors during this time is likely to negatively impact the mother's long-term milk volume. By 2 weeks (14 days) postpartum, prolactin levels will be back to prepregnancy levels and milk production will cease if stimulation of the breasts by breastfeeding or pumping does not occur (Walker, 2016).

The milk that flows from the breast at the start of a feeding or pumping session is called **foremilk**. The foremilk is watery milk high in protein and lactose and low in fat (1% to 2%). This milk has trickled down from the alveoli between feedings to fill the lactiferous ducts. It is low-fat milk because the fat globules made in the alveoli stick to each other and to the walls of the alveoli and do not trickle down.

In addition to prolactin release, stretching of the nipple and compression of the areola signal the hypothalamus to trigger the posterior pituitary gland to release oxytocin. **Oxytocin** acts on the myoepithelial cells surrounding the alveoli in the breast tissue to contract, ejecting milk, including the fat globules present, into the ducts. This process is called the milk ejection reflex, better known in lay terms as the **letdown reflex** or *letdown response*. The average initial letdown response occurs about 2 minutes after a baby begins to suckle, and there will be 4 to 10 letdown responses during a feeding session. The milk that flows during letdown is called hindmilk. **Hindmilk** is rich in fat (can exceed 10%) and therefore high in calories. In a sample of expressed breast milk, the average total fat concentration is about 4% and the total caloric content is about 20 calories/ounce.

By 6 months of breastfeeding, prolactin levels are only 5 to 10 ng/mL, yet milk production continues. A whey protein called *feedback inhibitor of lactation (FIL)* has been identified as influencing milk production through a negative feedback loop. FIL is present in breast milk and functions to decrease milk production. The more milk that remains in the breast for a longer period of time, the more milk production is decreased. On the other hand, the more often the breasts are emptied, the lower the level of FIL and the faster milk is produced. This mechanism of regulating milk at the local level is called *autocrine control*. This process is key to understanding how a mother maintains or loses her milk supply (Blackburn, 2013).

A number of factors can delay or impair lactogenesis. Maternal factors include cesarean birth, primiparity, long duration of stage 1 or stage 2 of labor, postpartum hemorrhage, type 1 diabetes, untreated hypothyroidism, obesity, polycystic ovary syndrome, retained placenta fragments, vitamin B_6 deficiency, history of previous breast surgery, insufficient glandular breast tissue, and significant stress (Janke, 2014). Other factors that can interfere with breastfeeding include smoking and use of alcohol, as well as some prescription and over-the-counter medications (e.g., antihistamines, combined birth control pills). One of the most important factors that influences breast milk production and the success of breastfeeding is the regular emptying of the breast. Therefore, mothers who opt to give their baby a bottle—and who do not pump to replace the feeding—are putting breastfeeding success in jeopardy.

STAGES OF HUMAN MILK

During the establishment of lactation there are three stages of human milk: colostrum, transitional milk, and mature milk.

Colostrum is the initial milk that begins to be secreted during midpregnancy and is immediately available to the baby at birth. The volume of colostrum is small, and this encourages the newborn to nurse frequently, helping to stimulate milk production. No supplementation with other fluids is necessary unless there is a medical indication. Colostrum is a thick, creamy yellowish fluid with concentrated amounts of protein, fat-soluble vitamins, and minerals, and it has lower amounts of fat and lactose compared with mature milk. It also contains antioxidants and high levels of lactoferrin and secretory IgA. It promotes the establishment of *Lactobacillus bifidus* flora in the digestive tract, which helps to protect the newborn from disease and illness. Colostrum also has a laxative effect on the newborn, which helps the baby pass meconium stools, which in turn helps decrease hyperbilirubinemia.

The onset of copious milk secretion begins between 32 and 96 hours postpartum. For most women this is observed on day 3. Laypeople refer to this as the milk "coming in," and it is called **transitional milk**. Transitional milk has qualities intermediate to colostrum and mature milk but may look indistinguishable from colostrum. It is still light yellow in color but is more copious than colostrum and contains more fat, lactose, water-soluble vitamins, and calories. See Figure 25–11 to view a picture of transitional milk. By day 5, most mothers are producing about 16 oz/day (Riordan, 2016).

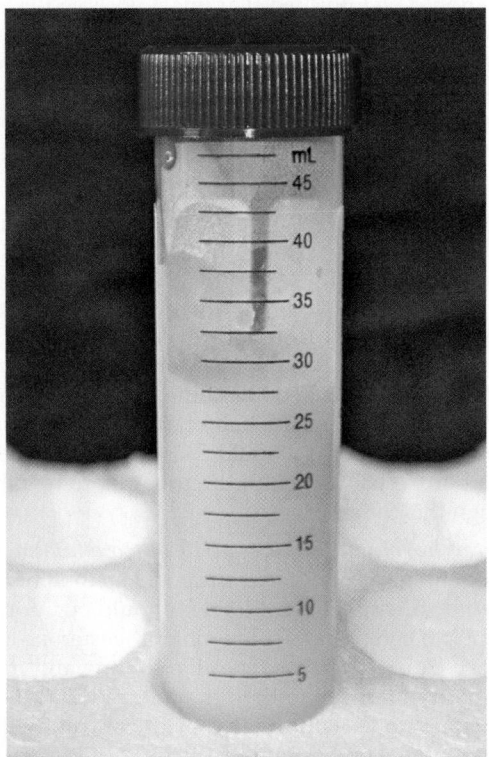

Figure 25–11 **Transitional human milk.**

SOURCE: Brigitte Hall, RNC, MSN, IBCLC.

Mature milk is white or slightly blue-tinged in color. It is present by 2 weeks postpartum and continues thereafter until lactation ceases. Mature milk contains about 13% solids (carbohydrates, proteins, and fats) and 87% water. Although mature human milk appears similar to skim cow's milk and may cause mothers to question whether their milk is "rich enough," mothers should be reassured that this is the normal appearance of mature human milk and that it provides the baby with all the necessary nutrients. Although gradual changes in composition do occur continuously over periods of weeks to accommodate the needs of the growing baby, in general, the composition of mature milk is fairly consistent with the exception of the fat content as noted previously. Milk production continues to increase slowly over the first month. By 6 months postpartum a mother produces about 27 oz (800 mL) per day (Blackburn, 2013).

Advantages of Breast Milk

In their breastfeeding policy statement, the American Academy of Pediatrics recommends exclusive breastfeeding as the preferred feeding for all babies, with a few exceptions, for the first 6 months and continued breastfeeding during the introduction of solids until the infant is 12 months old or older, as desired (AAP, 2012b). There is overwhelming scientific evidence that shows that breastfeeding provides newborns and infants with specific nutritional, immunologic, and psychosocial advantages over formula-feeding (AAP & ACOG, 2012b).

NUTRITIONAL ADVANTAGES

Human milk provides optimum nutrition for the human baby because it is species specific. The macronutrients such as protein, fat, and carbohydrates (lactose) are synthesized by the mother in the alveoli of the breasts by specialized secretory cells. Micronutrient elements such as vitamins and minerals derive from the circulating maternal plasma. There are more than 200 distinct components in breast milk, with more remaining to be identified (Riordan, 2016).

Additional health advantages for breastfed babies include reduced risk of developing type 1 or type 2 diabetes mellitus, lymphoma, leukemia, Hodgkin disease, obesity, hypercholesterolemia, and asthma. There are health benefits to the breastfeeding mother as well; when breastfeeding is initiated immediately after delivery, there is decreased risk for postpartum bleeding and more rapid uterine involution. Research has also shown that breastfeeding offers a protective function against premenopausal breast cancer and ovarian cancer and may be associated with a decrease in type 2 diabetes, rheumatoid arthritis, and hypertension (Healthy Children, 2015a).

IMMUNOLOGIC ADVANTAGES

The immunologic advantages of breast milk include varying degrees of protection from respiratory tract and gastrointestinal tract infections, necrotizing enterocolitis, urinary tract infections, otitis media, bacterial meningitis, bacteremia, and allergies (Healthy Children, 2015b). Transplacental passage of maternal immunoglobulin gradually diminishes over the first 6 months of life until the infant can begin to produce immunoglobulins. Human milk–derived immunologic protection helps supplement this protection.

Secretory IgA, an immunoglobulin present in colostrum and breast milk, has antiviral, antibacterial, and antigenic-inhibiting properties, specifically across mucosal surfaces such as the intestinal tract. Secretory IgA plays a role in decreasing the permeability of the small intestine to help prevent large protein molecules from triggering an allergic response. Other constituents of colostrum and breast milk that act to inhibit the growth of bacteria or viruses are *Lactobacillus bifidus*, lysozymes, lactoperoxidase, lactoferrin, transferrin, and various immunoglobulins.

All babies should receive vaccination following a schedule as recommended by the Centers for Disease Control and Prevention (CDC) (CDC, 2015b). The current vaccination schedule can be viewed online at the CDC website for Breastfeeding Resources (CDC, 2015b). (See Chapter 43 for discussion of immunizations.) Mothers may worry that their antibodies will inactivate the live poliovirus. But breastfeeding does not adversely affect immunization and is not a contraindication for any vaccine. Some mothers also wonder if it is safe for them to receive vaccinations while breastfeeding. Mothers should be reassured that most vaccines can safely be taken during the lactation period (Sachs & AAP Committee on Drugs, 2013).

Healthy People 2020

(MICH-21) Increase the proportion of infants who are ever breastfed

---

PSYCHOSOCIAL BENEFITS OF BREASTFEEDING

The psychosocial advantages of breastfeeding include increased self-esteem, enhanced bonding, and a decrease in stress for the mother and baby.

A mother's self-esteem is increased in knowing that she has provided the perfect food for her baby and provided protection with her own antibodies. For many mothers, breastfeeding takes effort, understanding, and an emotional commitment to endure the demands of this lifestyle choice. The mother's sense of accomplishment in being able to satisfy her baby's needs for nourishment and comfort can be a tremendous source of personal satisfaction. Also, breastfeeding can provide the baby with a fresh, clean, naturally warm source of nutrition. Women who breastfeed, by its nature, have close contact with their babies. Newborns are very responsive to touch, and it is vital for the baby's emotional well-being. The tactile stimulation associated with breastfeeding can communicate warmth, closeness, comfort, and the opportunity to learn each other's behavioral cues and needs. From the release of prolactin and oxytocin while breastfeeding, mothers may feel more affectionate toward their newborns, have improved letdown response, and breastfeed more frequently and for longer periods of time (Healthy Children, 2015a). See Table 25–3 for a comparison of breastfeeding and formula-feeding.

POTENTIAL DISADVANTAGES TO BREASTFEEDING

The following is a list of sometimes cited potential disadvantages to breastfeeding:

- *Pain with breastfeeding.* Breastfeeding is a natural process but requires a certain knowledge base that formerly was passed along from generation to generation. With the decline in the extended family structure, this source of knowledge and assistance is often missing for the new mother. Nipple tenderness is the most common source of discomfort and is usually related to improper positioning and/or not obtaining a proper attachment of the baby on the breast. Pain can also be related to engorgement or infection. Breastfeeding with proper technique should not hurt, and these mothers should be encouraged to seek assistance from a knowledgeable person skilled in lactation.

- *Leaking milk.* Some women will leak milk when their breasts are full and it is nearly time to breastfeed again or whenever they experience let-down, which can be triggered by hearing, seeing, or even thinking of their babies. If this causes concern to the mother, she can be instructed on how to apply gentle pressure directly over her nipple for a minute or so to stop the leaking momentarily. The mother can wear nursing pads inside her bra (with instructions to change wet pads frequently). Mothers should be given reassurance that this problem diminishes over time.

- *Embarrassment.* Some mothers feel uncomfortable about breastfeeding because they are modest or may feel embarrassed because our society views breasts as sexual objects and/or an unfriendly social environment makes it difficult to breastfeed in public. This is not an easy issue to overcome. Some mothers will feel more confident after learning how to breastfeed discreetly while in public.

- *Stress.* Many mothers feel a lot of stress juggling work or school and the demands of home life. Some mothers cite this reason for wanting to wean. There are options to suggest for this concern. Mothers can learn about "double pumping" to save time. A double electric breast pump allows the mother to pump both breasts simultaneously, which cuts the pumping time in half. If a mother struggles to keep up her milk supply, she can try taking an herbal supplement to give her milk supply a boost, unless contraindicated for her. Finally, it is still preferable to decrease the frequency of pumping rather than quitting altogether, if that makes things more manageable for the mother. Babies who get some breast milk are still receiving more of the benefits of breast milk than babies who do not receive any breast milk.

- *Unequal feeding responsibilities/fathers left out.* Some parents want feedings to be a shared responsibility. The parents should be informed that it is advisable for the father to wait to bottle-feed the baby with expressed breast milk until after the milk supply and breastfeeding are established, generally when their baby is about 3 to 4 weeks old. In the meantime, encourage the father to be supportive of the breastfeeding mother, to have a lot of skin-to-skin contact with his baby, and to share the responsibilities of all other aspects of baby care (e.g., bathing, dressing, diapering, burping, rocking).

- *Diet restriction.* Some mothers think that they have to give up eating certain foods when they breastfeed. This is generally not true. Most mothers can still eat all the foods they are accustomed to eating. Mothers do need to restrict alcohol intake and keep caffeine to a minimum. In the uncommon case where a baby has intolerance or allergy symptoms, the mother should consult with a lactation consultant or the baby's healthcare provider to help her work through this complication.

- *Limited hormonal birth control options.* Some mothers think that they cannot use a hormonal method of birth control while breastfeeding. Mothers should be informed that using birth control pills containing progesterone and estrogen can cause a decrease in milk volume and may affect the quality of breast milk. It is preferred that the mother who wants to use a hormonal birth control method consider using the progestin-only pill (e.g., Micronor, Nor-QD, Aygestin, or Norlutate); receive Depo-Provera, a progestin-only injection administered every 90 days; or have a progestin-only implant. Although progestin-only hormonal birth

TABLE 25–3 Comparison of Breastfeeding and Formula-Feeding

BREASTFEEDING	FORMULA (IRON-ENRICHED)-FEEDING
NUTRITION	
Species specific. An ideal balance of nutrients, efficiently absorbed. High bioavailability of iron leaves less iron for bacterial growth, cell injury.	Derived from bovine milk and/or plant sources. Lower bioavailability of nutrients requires higher concentrations in milk. Additives may cause intolerance.
Higher levels of essential fatty acids, lactose, cystine, and cholesterol, necessary for brain and nerve growth.	Still missing numerous ingredients. Formulas do not contain cholesterol. Soy and hydrolysate formulas do not contain lactose. Docosahexaenoic acid (DHA) and arachidonic acid (ARA) now added.
Composition varies according to gestational age and stage of lactation, meeting changing nutritional needs.	Nutritional value not varied. Nutritional adequacy depends on proper preparation/dilution.
Long-term decreased incidence of diabetes, cancer, obesity, asthma.	
Contains unsaturated fats.	Contains saturated fats.
Babies determine the volume of milk consumed.	Parents or healthcare provider determine the volume consumed. Overfeeding may occur if caregiver is determined that baby empty bottle.
Frequency of feeding is determined by baby's cues. May feed more frequently as milk digestion is faster.	Frequency of feeding is determined by baby's cues. May feed less frequently as milk digestion is slower.
IMMUNOLOGIC PROPERTIES	
Contains immunoglobulins, enzymes, and leukocytes that protect against pathogens. Nutrients promote growth of *Lactobacillus*, protective bacteria. Lower rates of urinary tract infections, otitis media, and other infectious diseases.	No anti-infective properties. Formula is linked to an increased incidence of gastrointestinal and respiratory tract infections.
Anti-infective properties present in the milk permit longer storage duration.	Potential for bacterial contamination exists during preparation and storage.
Breast milk is hypoallergenic, with minimal risk of protein allergy/intolerance.	Cow's milk protein allergy relatively common.
MATERNAL HEALTH	
Faster return to pre-pregnancy weight.	Provides nutrition when breast milk not available because of maternal illness, medication/drug use, or lactation failure (breast surgery, endocrine disease).
Breastfeeding associated with lower risk of breast, ovarian cancer.	
PSYCHOSOCIAL ASPECTS	
Skin-to-skin contact enhances bonding.	Both parents can participate in positive parent–baby interaction during feeding.
Hormones of lactation promote maternal feelings and sense of well-being.	Father can assume feeding responsibilities.
The value system of modern society can create barriers to successful breastfeeding.	
Some mothers may feel ashamed or embarrassed.	
Breastfeeding after returning to work may be difficult.	
COST	
Healthy diet for mother.	Hypoallergenic formula is more expensive than standard formula. Cost approximately $1400/year.
Savings for infant medical costs: approximately $400 average in first year of life.	Ancillary costs: bottles or bottle liners, nipples, cleaning costs.
Ancillary costs: nursing pads, nursing bras.	Refrigeration is needed if preparing more than one bottle at a time.
A breast pump may be needed.	
Refrigeration is necessary for storing expressed milk.	
CONVENIENCE	
Milk is always the perfect temperature. No preparation time is needed.	Formula must be purchased commercially. Preparation is time consuming. Less convenient for traveling or for night feedings.
The mother must be available to feed or will need to provide expressed milk to be given in her absence.	Mother need not be present—anyone can feed the baby.
If she misses a feeding, the mother must express milk to maintain lactation.	
The mother may experience slight discomfort in the early days of lactation.	

control is compatible with lactation, it is recommended that the mother wait 6 weeks before taking the hormonal medication to ensure a good milk supply (AAP, 2012b). Mothers can be reassured that barrier methods of birth control and natural family planning do not interfere with lactation at all and are good options to consider as well.

- *Vaginal dryness associated with breastfeeding.* Some mothers experience vaginal dryness related to a low level of estrogen while lactating. This is only a temporary side effect. A water-based lubricant such as K-Y jelly or Astroglide can be used during intercourse until the woman weans and estrogen levels increase again.

MEDICATIONS

Mothers can be reassured that most prescription and over-the-counter medications are safe for the breastfeeding baby. Medications taken by the breastfeeding mother may penetrate human milk to some degree. This is the primary reason that mothers cite for discontinuing breastfeeding. Having a basic understanding of the kinetics of drug entry into human milk, as well as factors influencing its availability to the baby (bioavailability) may help the nursing mother to continue safely breastfeeding her baby.

It should be noted that (1) most drugs penetrate into human milk, (2) almost all medications appear in only small amounts in human milk (usually less than 1% of the maternal dosage), and (3) very few drugs are contraindicated for breastfeeding women (Briggs & Freeman, 2015; Hale, 2014; Sachs & AAP Committee on Drugs, 2013).

The healthcare provider should consider the following when prescribing a medication (Sachs & AAP Committee on Drugs, 2013):

- Mother's need for the medication
- Drug's potential effect on milk production
- Amount of drug excreted into the milk
- Extent of oral absorption of the drug by the baby
- Drug's potential adverse effects to the baby
- Baby's age and health

The properties of a drug influence its passage into breast milk, as does the amount of the drug taken, the frequency and route of administration, and the timing of the dose in relationship to infant feeding. The drug's effects are influenced by the baby's age, the feeding frequency, the volume of milk taken, and the degree of absorption through the gastrointestinal tract. LactMed is a database that has current data on individual medications.

SAFETY ALERT!
The mother should be advised to inform her healthcare provider and her baby's healthcare provider that she is breastfeeding when a drug is prescribed for her.

Five adjustments should be made when administering drugs to a nursing mother to decrease the effects of the medication on the baby (Blackburn, 2013):

1. Avoid long-acting forms of drugs. The infant may have difficulty metabolizing and excreting them, and accumulation may be a problem.
2. Consider absorption rates and peak blood levels in scheduling the administration of the drugs. Less of the drug

crosses into the milk if the baby is fed before the mother is given the oral medication.
3. Use preparations that can be given at longer intervals (once versus 3 to 4 times per day).
4. Select the drug that shows the least tendency to pass into breast milk when alternatives are available.
5. Use single-symptom drugs versus multisymptom drugs (e.g., a decongestant for allergy rather than a multisymptom drug, especially because liquid forms may contain alcohol).

CONTRAINDICATIONS

In some instances breastfeeding is or may be contraindicated:

- Mother is HIV positive or has AIDS and is counseled against breastfeeding, except in countries where the risk of neonatal death from diarrhea and other disease (excluding AIDS) is high (Janke, 2014).
- Mother has active, untreated tuberculosis, has varicella, is HTLV1-positive (human T-cell leukemia virus type 1), or has another illness, on a case-by-case basis.
- Mother has active herpes on her breast—the baby may still feed on the unaffected side only until the lesion has healed.
- Mother uses illicit drugs (e.g., cocaine, heroin) or is an alcoholic; however, AAP (2012b) allows breastfeeding when the mother is taking methadone as part of a drug withdrawal program.
- Mother smokes, posing health risks to herself and potential secondhand exposure risks to her baby. Research shows that smoking by breastfeeding mothers can significantly alter babies' sleep–wake cycles, causing them to sleep less, and also affects milk flavor. Maternal smoking can result in breast milk concentrations of nicotine of 1.5 to 3.0 times the maternal plasma concentration. However, babies who receive breast milk from mothers who smoke are healthier than babies who receive formula and live in a household with smokers. Mothers who smoke cigarettes can breastfeed. To minimize effects on the baby, mothers should time their smoking to immediately *after* breastfeeding and should not smoke in the same room as the baby (AAP & ACOG, 2012). Smoking has been associated with an increase in respiratory infections and allergies as well as being a considerable risk factor for low milk supply and poor weight gain in the baby (AAP, 2012b)
- Mother takes specific medications (e.g., radioactive isotopes, antimetabolites chemotherapy drugs). A mother with a diagnosis of breast cancer should not breastfeed so that she can begin treatment immediately (Janke, 2014).
- Baby has galactosemia.

POTENTIAL PROBLEMS IN BREASTFEEDING

Because mothers are discharged from the birthing unit before breastfeeding is well established, they are frequently alone when they encounter changes in the breastfeeding process. Many women stop nursing if the situations they encounter seem to pose problems. Nurses can offer anticipatory guidance regarding common breastfeeding phenomena and provide resources such as seeking help from a lactation specialist and contact information for lactation support groups for the woman's use after discharge. (See Chapter 29 for a detailed discussion of self-care measures the nurse can suggest to a woman with a breastfeeding problem after discharge from the birthing unit.)

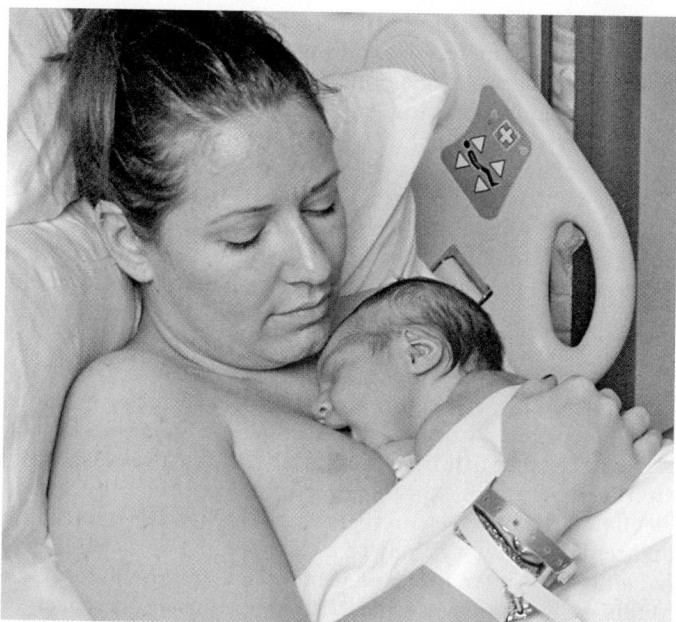

Figure 25–12 **Mother and newborn skin-to-skin.**

SOURCE: Brigitte Hall, RNC, MSN, IBCLC.

Timing of Newborn Feedings

The timing of newborn feedings is ideally determined by physiologic and behavioral cues rather than a set schedule.

INITIATING THE FIRST FEEDING

If there are no complications at the birth and the mother is not overly sedated, the newborn may be placed on the mother's chest after birth. This skin-to-skin contact after birth helps the baby maintain body temperature, helps with self-regulation, increases maternal oxytocin levels, helps the mother to notice subtle feeding cues, and promotes bonding (Figure 25–12).

The timing of the first feeding varies depending on whether the newborn is to be breastfed or formula-fed and whether there were any complications during pregnancy or birth, such as maternal diabetes or intrauterine growth restriction (IUGR). Mothers who choose to breastfeed their newborns should be encouraged to put the baby to the breast during the first period of reactivity. This practice should be encouraged because successful, long-term breastfeeding during infancy appears to be related to beginning breast feedings in the first few hours of life. Sleep–wake states affect feeding behavior and need to be considered when evaluating the newborn's sucking ability.

Throughout the first 2 hours after birth, but especially during the first hour of life, the newborn is usually alert and ready to breastfeed. This first feeding should not be forced. Some babies are content just licking the nipple or nuzzling up against the breast initially. Early breastfeeding can enhance maternal–newborn bonding and facilitate release of oxytocin, which helps contract the uterus, expelling the placenta and decreasing the risk of postpartum hemorrhage.

Early feedings benefit the newborn because they enhance maternal–newborn attachment; stimulate peristalsis, helping to eliminate the by-products of bilirubin conjugation (which decreases the risk of jaundice); help prevent hypoglycemia; promote the passage of meconium; provide the immunologic protection of colostrum; and begin to stimulate further maternal milk production, helping prevent later feeding difficulties.

If the mother plans to bottle-feed, she and her newborn can still enjoy skin-to-skin contact initially. Formula-feedings are not typically initiated in the birthing room. Bottle-fed newborns are offered formula as soon as they show an interest or feeding cues or per agency policy. For both breastfed and formula-fed babies, early feeding enhances maternal–newborn attachment and stimulates peristalsis, helping to eliminate the by-products of bilirubin conjugation (which decreases the risk of jaundice).

Assessment of the newborn's physiologic status is a primary and ongoing concern to the nurse throughout the first feeding. Extreme fatigue coupled with tachypnea, dusky color, and diaphoresis while feeding is most likely symptomatic for respiratory and/or cardiac problems or, rarely, esophageal anomalies (see Chapter 26). Findings associated with esophageal anomalies include maternal polyhydramnios and increased oral mucus in the newborn.

Although the nurse is always on the alert for any complications, keep in mind that it is not unusual for healthy newborns to regurgitate a small amount of mucus, fluid, or milk shortly after feeding or to develop hiccups. Most babies have "wet burps" at some point and virtually all have some degree of reflux. Holding the baby upright on the parent's chest for 15 to 20 minutes after a feeding and not placing the baby in a car seat or swing (which increases abdominal pressure) for that time can help decrease the incidence of reflux. Once the newborn is tolerating feeding, the baby's normal position after feeding is on the back.

ESTABLISHING A FEEDING PATTERN

An "on-demand" feeding program facilitates each baby's own rhythm and helps a new mother establish lactation. Unrestricted feedings are best accomplished by hospitals that provide mother-baby rooming-in practices on a 24-hour basis. When the father is able to room in with the mother and new baby, it allows both parents to participate and learn how to care for their newborn; this has been shown to be important in the development of the family relationship. Having the father room in also allows the mother with a cesarean delivery to keep her baby at the bedside. When mothers and babies are not separated after birth, mothers and fathers are better able to respond to their babies' needs more quickly than the nursery staff may be able to, resulting in less newborn crying, natural feeding intervals, and an adequate number of feedings in a 24-hour period.

Following the initial alert period (approximately the first 2 hours after birth), the newborn typically falls into a deep sleep for several hours. Mothers should be encouraged to rest during this time too. Upon awakening, the newborn will likely want to nurse frequently, alternating between relatively short periods of light sleep and quiet wakefulness. As wakefulness and interest in nursing increase, the newborn will often cluster 5 to 10 feeding episodes over 2 to 3 hours (Riordan, 2016). The mother may misinterpret "cluster feedings" in the first few days of life to mean that her baby is not satisfied because she is not producing enough milk. The nurse should take this opportunity to reinforce the mother's perception that the baby wants additional milk, but point out that cluster feeding is a normal and necessary pattern to stimulate the mother's milk production. Formula supplementation is not indicated and will actually delay milk production.

Some healthy newborns are uninterested in nursing and just want to sleep for the first few days after birth. This pattern is noted in babies whose mothers have had a difficult labor, a prolonged pushing stage during delivery, or medication (especially multiple dosing) for labor pain or for a cesarean birth.

Late-preterm newborns (babies born between 34 0/7 to 36 6/7 weeks' gestation) also tend to be very sleepy for the first few days, much more so than full-term newborns (Spong, 2013). In addition, male babies who have undergone a circumcision procedure often become very sleepy after surgery. These sleepy babies are at risk of losing an excessive amount of weight, becoming dehydrated, and developing exaggerated jaundice in just a few days after birth. In addition, the mother may develop pathologic engorgement if her baby does not wake up to breast-feed frequently and effectively during this time.

To avoid these complications, parents can be taught techniques to wake their sleepy baby whenever the baby shows signs of being in the light state-of-sleep cycle. With a little help, the baby may be gently aroused to breastfeed. One method is to remove the baby's blanket and clothing so that the baby is wearing only a diaper and T-shirt. Babies feed better when they are not bundled, and they can actually achieve a better attachment without the bulk of extra clothing and blankets in the way. If the room is too cool for the newborn to feed in just a diaper and T-shirt, have the mother apply a blanket over the top of her baby *after* the baby has attached to the breast. Another technique is to undo and check the baby's diaper. Sitting the baby in a burping position and gently "walking" fingers along the back will usually arouse the baby. Parents should also be encouraged to talk or sing to their baby while trying these techniques to further arouse their baby from sleep.

If the newborn falls asleep after the first few suckles, encourage the mother to use tactile stimulation while the baby is still attached to the breast. The mother can also be encouraged to use breast compression or breast massage while the baby is breastfeeding to keep milk trickling into the baby's mouth until the mother is stimulated to release her milk. If this is not sufficient to keep the newborn actively feeding, suggest that the mother remove the baby from the breast momentarily and try to burp the baby. The baby may not actually burp but the burping technique may help wake the baby.

A newborn's feeding pattern may change again when the mother's breasts become fuller. Mothers' breasts begin to look and feel noticeably heavier between the second and fourth day postpartum. When milk production has noticeably increased, the cluster feeding pattern ceases until the newborn has the first growth spurt at about 2 weeks of age. Now a baby generally feeds every 1.5 to 3 hours around the clock, about 8 to 12 feedings per day. Feeding intervals are counted from the time of the start of one feeding to the start of the next feeding. During this engorgement phase of lactation, some babies may struggle initially with latch-on, especially if the mother allows greater than 3 hours to lapse between feedings. If the newborn is not breastfeeding often or effectively enough to soften the breasts, then the breasts may become quite firm and the mother's nipple may become less pliable and this can lead to a shallow latch attachment and sore nipples. If this occurs, the mother can try to express some milk to soften her areola before latching her baby. When her baby breast-feeds on this fuller than usual breast, it is not uncommon for the baby to only want to feed on just the one side. This feeding pattern usually does not last long either. Within days the baby will be back to feeding at both breasts again.

Formula-fed newborns generally sleep longer at a stretch and awaken to feed every 3 to 4 hours, typically feeding only 6 to 8 times per day. To compensate for sleeping longer between feedings, formula-fed babies feed a larger volume at each feeding. It will be awhile before the baby sleeps through the night.

Regardless of whether a mother is breastfeeding or formula-feeding her baby, many parents are distressed by their newborn's erratic feeding pattern. Parents need to be informed about normal infant feeding and sleeping patterns and be aware that these patterns vary among babies and change over days, weeks, and months according to the baby's growth and development. In the beginning, the "average" newborn sleeps a total of 16 hours a day. Newborns wake to feed and generally fall back to sleep within an hour.

Satiety behaviors are the same for formula-fed babies as for breastfed babies. These behaviors include longer pauses toward the end of the feeding and noticeable total body relaxation (the baby lies limp with hands down at the side and unclenched). The baby may also release the mother's nipple or the bottle nipple, and may fall asleep. If a baby is satiated and content following feedings, is meeting daily output expectations, and is gaining weight as expected, then feedings are going well.

On the other hand, if a breastfeeding baby awakens shortly after feeding and is exhibiting feeding cues, this baby should be offered the breast again regardless of when the last feeding occurred. The newborn may be cluster feeding or may not have fed efficiently at the previous feeding. Pacifier use in response to this early waking is especially inappropriate. The pacifier needlessly postpones the feeding, which is indicated based on hunger cues and can have a negative consequence for the mother's milk supply and the newborn's weight. The American Academy of Pediatrics recommends waiting to introduce a pacifier in the breastfeeding newborn until breastfeeding is well established; generally when the baby is 3 to 4 weeks old. A formula-feeding baby can be offered a pacifier any time after birth, which is thought to help reduce the risk for sudden infant death syndrome (SIDS) (Healthy Children, 2015e).

SAFETY ALERT!
Parents should be instructed never to put honey or corn syrup on their baby's pacifier to encourage the baby to accept it. Honey and possibly corn syrup may be contaminated with *Clostridium botulinum*, a bacterium that causes infantile botulism. Botulism is rare, but when it occurs, it causes serious illness.

Both breastfed and formula-fed babies experience growth spurts at certain times and require increased feeding. The breast-feeding mother may meet these increased demands by nursing more frequently to increase her milk supply. It takes about 72 hours for the milk supply to increase adequately to meet the new demand. A slight increase in feedings meets the formula-fed baby's needs. Once the formula-feeding baby appears satiated, the baby should not be forced to continue to feed in order to the finish the bottle.

Nourishing her newborn is a major concern of the new mother. Her feelings of success or failure may influence her self-concept as she assumes her maternal role. With proper instruction, support, and encouragement from professionals, breastfeeding becomes a source of pleasure and satisfaction to both the parents and baby.

Cultural Considerations in Newborn Feeding

Healthcare providers can learn about an individual client's cultural background by engaging in discussions with the client and asking questions in a sensitive and respectful way. This provides opportunity to validate healthy practices and to exert a positive influence on other matters. An occasion for this kind of dialogue might arise during interactions with a new mother who may have misconceptions about breastfeeding. For example, if a new mother says she heard that getting upset or angry will spoil her milk, you can point out that this belief likely stems from the correct observation that breastfeeding babies can sense maternal tension (which also may delay letdown) and may therefore act fussy as well, appearing to behave as if they were getting "spoiled milk." Then reassure the mother that there is no evidence that the milk composition itself is changed. This will allow you to focus on the real issues of bonding and relaxation technique. Simply understanding what is really going on may help the mother to be more relaxed.

Whenever possible, it is best to have a female, nonfamily member translator present to interpret for a mother. For Muslim women, it is culturally unacceptable for them to speak about intimate matters in front of their families. Therefore, it would be inappropriate to ask the new mother's husband or her children to be her interpreter. Even among those who speak English, language barriers and miscommunications still exist due in part to words having different meanings to people of different cultures. It is important to give enough explanation to ensure that the mother clearly understands the information provided. These are but a few of the numerous cultural influences related to feeding. (See *Developing Cultural Competence: Breastfeeding in Other Cultures.*) When nurses are faced with a baby care practice different from the ones to which they are accustomed, they need to evaluate the effect of the practice. Different practices are not necessarily inferior. The nurse should intervene only if the practice is actually harmful to the mother or baby.

Professionalism in Practice Breastfeeding Promotion Legislation

It is important to be a patient advocate and be involved in legislative initiatives on the national and local level. The Breastfeeding Promotion Act of 2009 was enacted into law on March 23, 2010, and acts to protect breastfeeding in the workplace by providing five provisions. These include

Title I: Amending the Civil Rights Act of 1964 to protect lactating women from being fired or discriminated against in the workplace.

Title II: Giving tax incentives to businesses that establish a private space in the workplace for their employees to breastfeed or express their milk. Employers can also receive tax credits for supplying breastfeeding equipment and providing lactation consultation services for their employees.

Title III: Establishing set standards for breast pumps to ensure that they are safe and effective.

Title IV: Expanding the Internal Revenue Code definition of "medical care" to include breastfeeding equipment and lactation services as tax-deductible for families.

Title V: Requiring employers with 50 or more employees to provide lactating employees break time and a private area to express their milk.

In addition, the U. S. Department of Labor (2011) enacted the Fair Labor Standards Act: Break Time for Nursing Mothers provision.

Breastfeeding in public is another frequently expressed concern that can create a barrier to achieving *Healthy People 2020* breastfeeding goals. Although people agree that breastfeeding is the most natural and healthy way to feed a baby, mothers feel conflicted because in the United States breast exposure is often viewed in a sexual context, and this may lead to disapproval of attempts to breastfeed in public. Public places are incorporating "mother rooms" to provide a comfortable, private area for the nursing mother. There is no state that prohibits breastfeeding in a public place, and currently 49 states, the District of Columbia, and the Virgin Islands have created laws that specify that a woman is permitted to breastfeed in any location in which she is authorized to be (National Conference of State Legislatures, 2015). Mothers may also be taught how to breastfeed discreetly in public. This is often taught at breastfeeding classes or mother-to-mother support group meetings. See Figure 25–13 to observe a mother discreetly breastfeeding. Some mothers may prefer a baby blanket or shawl to drape over their chests, which will provide more coverage. Finally, mothers who prefer not to breastfeed even discreetly in public can be encouraged to at least pump their breasts and feed the expressed milk in a bottle so they have the option of getting out of the house.

Breastfeeding Technique

BREASTFEEDING POSITIONS AND LATCHING ON

Breastfeeding is not instinctive, it is learned. It is a natural process, but it takes "know-how." Ideally, each breastfeeding mother should have a breastfeeding evaluation to determine any knowledge deficits, acknowledge any concerns, provide instructions, and assist with breastfeeding.

Positioning.   There are many breastfeeding positions, but only the four classic breastfeeding positions will be discussed here: (1) modified cradle position, (2) cradle position, (3) football (or clutch) hold position, and (4) side-lying position (Figures 25–14 through 25–17). After a mother has fed using one position, encourage her to try a different position when she offers her second breast. Alternating positions facilitates drainage of the breasts and changes the pressure points on the breast. This will provide

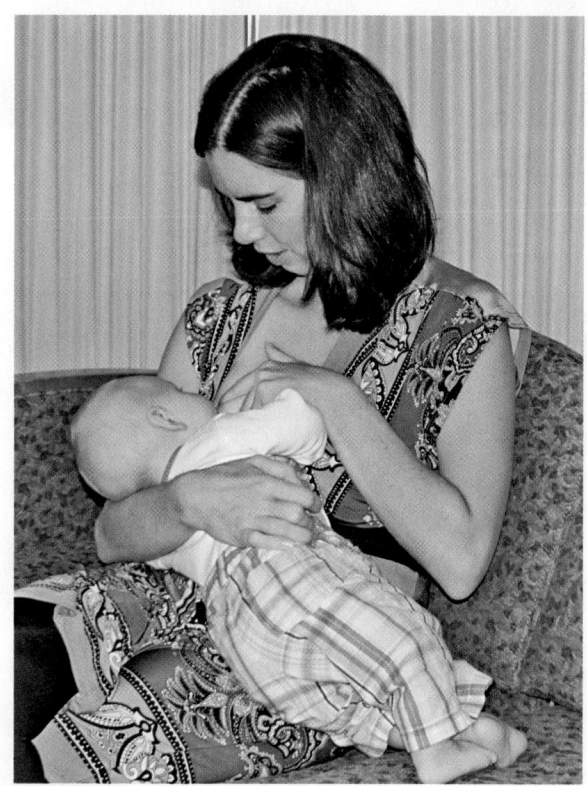

Figure 25–13 **Breastfeeding discreetly.**

SOURCE: Brigitte Hall, RNC, MSN, IBCLC.

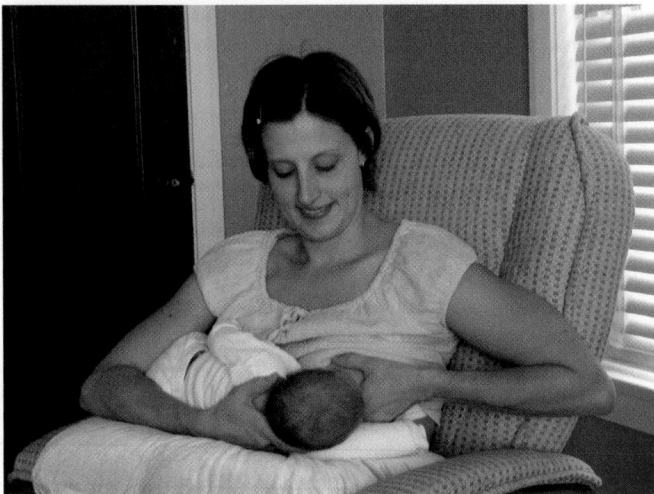

Figure 25–14   Modified cradle position.

SOURCE: Brigitte Hall, RNC, MSN, IBCLC.

- Have the mother sit comfortably in upright position using good body alignment. Use pillows for support (may use Boppy, body pillow, or standard bed pillows). Lap pillow should help bring the baby up to breast level so the mother does not lean over baby.
- Place the baby on the mother's lap and turn the baby's entire body toward the mother (the baby is in side-lying position). Position the baby's body so that the baby's nose lines up to the nipple. Maintain the baby's body in a horizontal alignment.
- To feed at left breast, the mother supports the baby's head with her right hand at nape of the baby's neck (allow head to slightly lag back); the mother's right thumb by the baby's left ear, and right forefinger near the baby's right ear.
- With the mother's free left hand, she can offer her left breast.

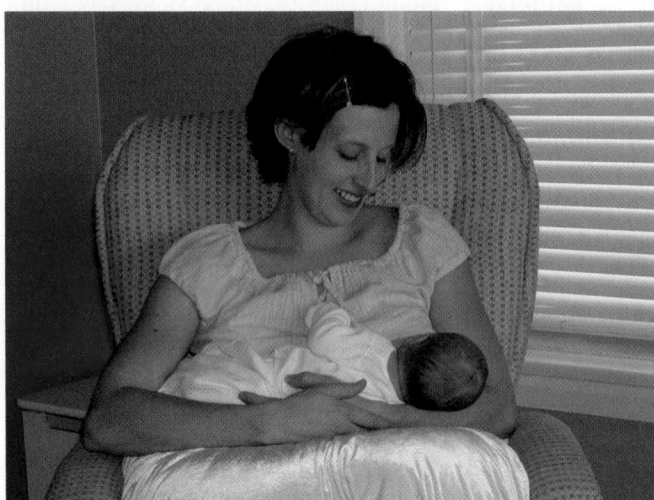

Figure 25–15   Cradle position.

SOURCE: Brigitte Hall, RNC, MSN, IBCLC.

- Have the mother sit comfortably in upright position using good body alignment. Use pillows for support (may use Boppy, body pillow, or standard bed pillows). Lap pillow should help bring the baby up to breast level so the mother does not lean over the baby.
- Place the baby on the mother's lap and turn the baby's entire body toward the mother (the baby is in side-lying position). Position the baby's body so that the baby's nose lines up to the nipple. Maintain the baby's body in a horizontal alignment.
- If feeding from the left breast, have the mother cradle the baby's head near the crook of her left arm while supporting her baby's body with her left forearm.
- With the mother's free right hand, she can offer her left breast.

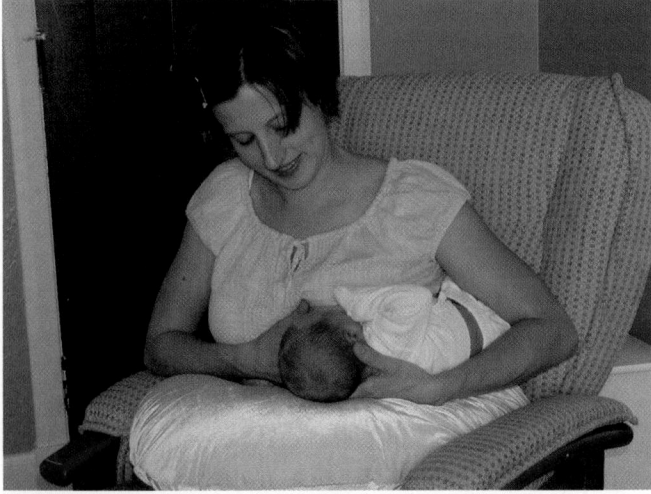

Figure 25–16   Football hold position.

SOURCE: Brigitte Hall, RNC, MSN, IBCLC.

- Have the mother sit comfortably and use pillows to raise the baby's body to breast level. If using a Boppy and the Boppy is in "normal" position on the mother's lap, turn it counterclockwise slightly (if feeding at left breast) to provide extended support for the baby's body resting along the mother's left side and near the back of the mother's chair.
- If feeding at left breast, place the baby on the left side of the mother's body, heading the baby into position feet first. The baby's bottom should rest on the pillow near the mother's left elbow.
- Turn the baby slightly on her side so that she faces the breast.
- The mother's left arm clutches the baby's body close to the mother's body. The baby's body should feel securely tucked in under the mother's left arm.
- Have the mother support the baby's head with her left hand. With the mother's free right hand, she can offer her breast. (Good position for the mother with C-section.)

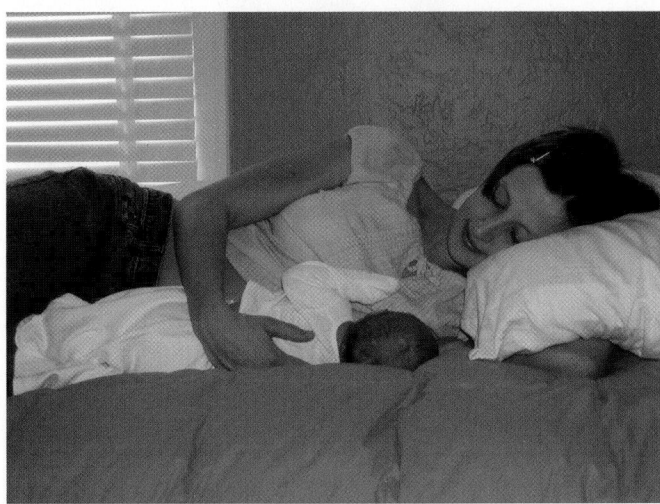

Figure 25–17 **Side-lying position.**

SOURCE: Brigitte Hall, RNC, MSN, IBCLC.

- Have the mother rest comfortably lying on her side (left side for this demonstration). Use pillows to support the mother's head and back, and provide support for the mother's hips by placing a pillow between her bent knees.
- Place the baby in side-lying position next to the mother's body. The baby's body should face the mother's body. The baby's nose should line up to the mother's nipple. Place a roll behind the baby's back, if desired.
- With the mother's free right hand, she can offer her left breast. After the baby is securely attached, mom can rest her right hand anywhere that is comfortable for her.

some relief to the mother with sore nipples. In addition to the classic positions, "laid-back" breastfeeding is being advocated. This concept is based on biologic nursing (BN), a mother-centered approach, and purports that women can find the best position for themselves because breastfeeding initiation is intrinsic for both mother and baby (La Leche League International, 2013).

Latching On. It is important to have the mother and baby positioned properly in order to achieve an optimal attachment. If, for example, the baby is lying flat on the back (supine position) to feed, then the baby can obtain only a shallow latch (not attached far back onto the areola). The baby's shoulder becomes an obstacle putting distance between the baby's mouth and the mother's breast. Anything that contributes to a shallow latch is going to cause sore nipples and other complications. The baby could have a short lingual frenulum (tongue-tied) and not be able to properly cup the breast, resulting in painful, cracked nipples and poor

milk transfer. Nipple trauma, although relatively common, is not normal. (See Chapter 29 for a discussion of breastfeeding with inverted or flat nipples.)

The baby needs to attach the lips onto the breast or, more accurately, far back onto the areola, not on the nipple. If the baby attaches just to the nipple, the mother will have sore nipples and pain may inhibit the letdown reflex. To obtain a deep latch, the mother needs to be taught how to elicit the newborn's rooting reflex, stimulating the baby to open the mouth as widely as possible (like a big yawn). Once the baby does this, the mother should quickly but gently draw her baby in toward her. During the first few days of life, the newborn typically only opens the mouth widely for a second or so, and then begins to close the mouth again. If the mother misses her chance to get her baby latched on, she needs to simply start over again.

Figures 25–18 through 25–23 demonstrate various positions and techniques used in latching on.

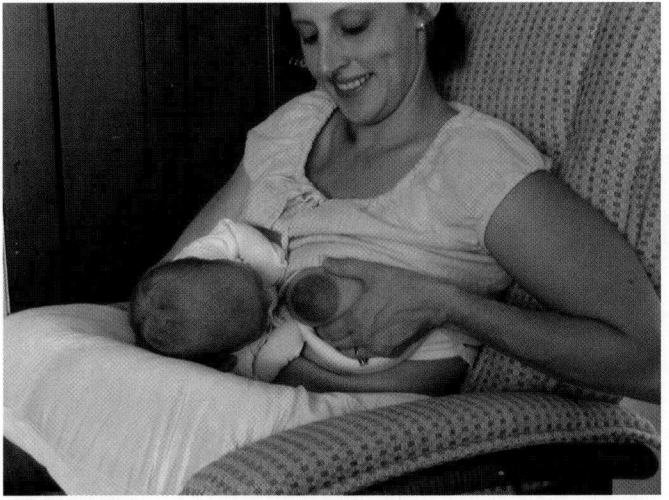

Figure 25–18 **C-hold hand position.**

SOURCE: Brigitte Hall, RNC, MSN, IBCLC.

To be ready to draw the baby's mouth onto the mother's breast, as soon as the baby opens her mouth widely enough, the mother needs to have her hand supporting her breast in the ready position. She can use various hand holds, but she needs to keep her fingers well behind the areola. One such hand position is called the "C-hold." In this hold, the thumb is placed on top of the breast near 12:00 position and the other four fingers are placed on the underside of the breast near the 6:00 position (depends on mother's hand size and length of fingers). The key point is to keep the fingers at least 1½ inches back from the base of the nipple as the fingers support the breast. Mothers are not often aware of where they place their fingers especially on the underside of the breast. If the fingers are too far forward (too close to the nipple), then the baby cannot grasp a large amount of areola in her mouth and this results in a "shallow" latch. A shallow latch is associated with nipple pain and ineffective drainage of the breast.

An alternate hand hold not shown is a "U-hold" hand position. The thumb and forefinger are near the 3 and 9 position on the breast again with fingers at least 1½ inches back from the base of the nipple; the body of the hand rests on the lower portion of the breast. Using this hand hold, the mother's arm position is down at her side rather than sticking outward as it is when supporting the breast using the C-hold position.

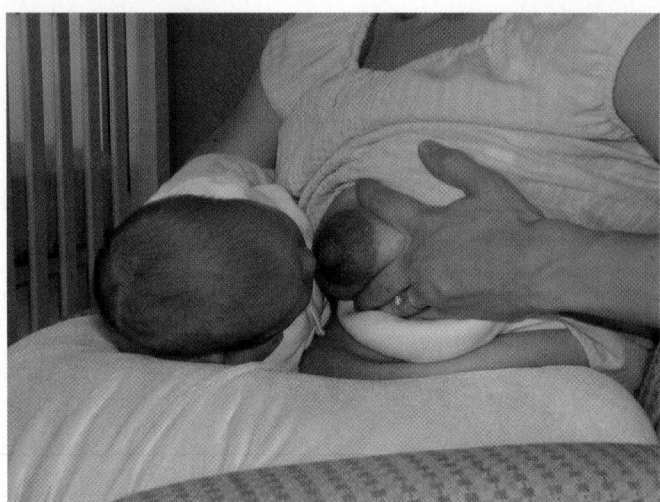

The scissor hold is often discouraged because mothers (especially mothers with small hands) have a difficult time keeping their fingers off the areola or at least 1½ inches back from the base of the areola. Here, the mother is able to support her breast well without letting her fingers encroach onto the areola.

The mother should be instructed to gently support the breast and not press too deeply, which can obstruct the flow of milk through the ducts.

Figure 25–19 Scissor hold hand position.

SOURCE: Brigitte Hall, RNC, MSN, IBCLC.

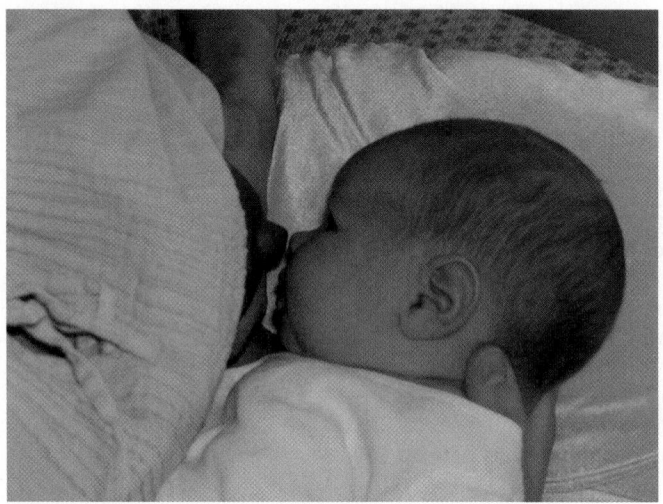

Before eliciting the rooting reflex, it is important to have the baby in good alignment. When the baby opens his mouth to latch on, the goal is to achieve a deep, asymmetric latch attachment. The goal is not to center the nipple in the baby's mouth. The rationale for this is to optimize oral-motor function. The jaw is a hinge joint. The upper jaw is immobile; the lower jaw compresses the breast. The breast is efficiently drained if more areola is drawn into the baby's mouth from the inferior aspect of the breast and a smaller amount drawn in from the superior aspect of the areola. Aligning the baby to the mother with baby's nose facing mother's nipple permits the jaw to be in a lower position. The next step is to let the baby drop his head back (head in "sniff position"), so that the baby leads into the breast with the chin.

Figure 25–20 Nose to nipple.

SOURCE: Brigitte Hall, RNC, MSN, IBCLC.

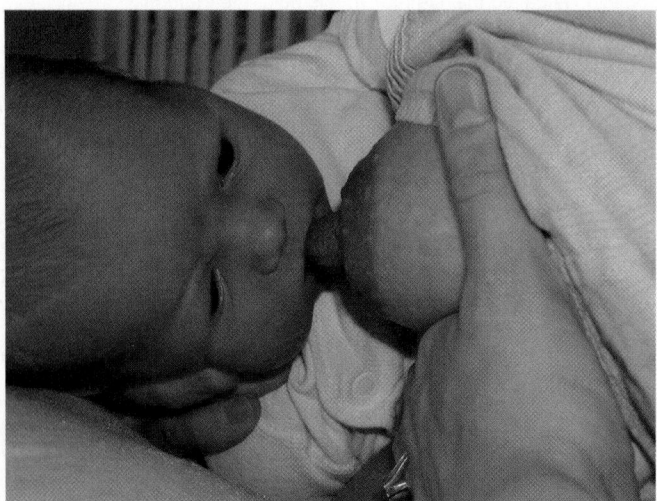

To trigger the rooting reflex, teach the mother to use her nipple to stroke downward in a vertical motion across the middle of baby's lower lip. Initially, the baby may respond by licking or smacking. This is a normal response to the stimulus. Encourage the mother to keep stimulating the baby's lower lip until the baby finally opens the mouth widely. If the baby is not responding at all, then the baby is probably too sleepy and may need help waking up. After trying wake up techniques, the baby may be ready to try breastfeeding again.

Figure 25–21 Initial attempt to elicit the rooting reflex.

SOURCE: Brigitte Hall, RNC, MSN, IBCLC.

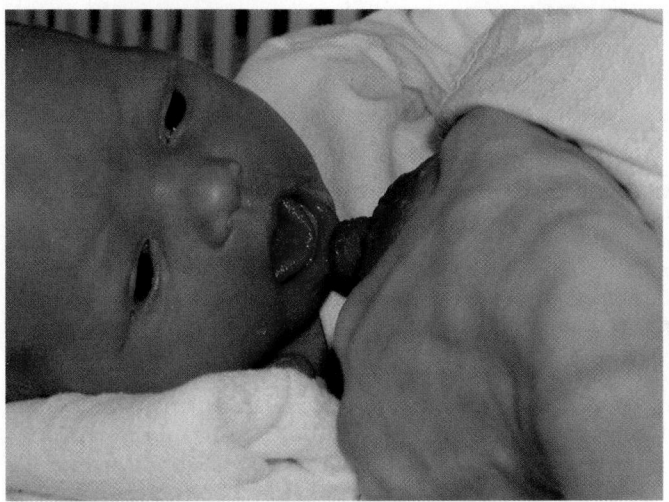

Figure 25–22 Continued attempt to elicit rooting reflex.

SOURCE: Brigitte Hall, RNC, MSN, IBCLC.

Teach the mother to be patient and wait for the newborn's mouth to gape open as widely as possible. Here the baby needs to open the mouth even wider before the mother draws her baby toward the breast. The mother should be encouraged to continue stroking the baby's lip until the baby opens the mouth wider.

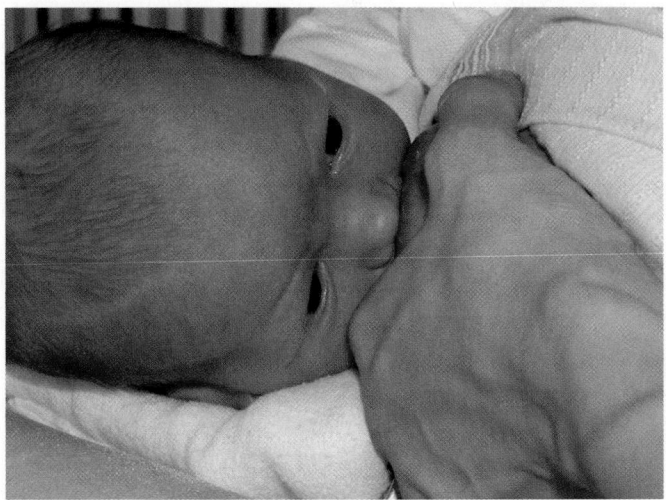

Figure 25–23 Baby is latched on.

SOURCE: Brigitte Hall, RNC, MSN, IBCLC.

Once the baby has latched onto the breast, the mother should check that the baby is latched-on properly. The baby's chin should be embedded into the mother's breast and the nose should be very close but not actually touching the breast. The nose should be centered. If the mother feels a little pinch on her areola, she can slowly release the hand supporting her breast so she can have a free hand to attempt to move her baby's jaw gently downward. To do this maneuver, the mother needs to place the thumb or forefinger of her free hand (the hand that just released the breast) on the baby's lower jaw (there is a horizontal groove to use as leverage—the groove on the baby's chin is parallel with the baby's lips). With gentle downward pressure the mother should feel relief of any persistent tenderness. This procedure opens the jaw wider and it also helps to roll out the baby's lower lip that may have been inadvertently drawn into the baby's mouth. As the baby begins to suckle, there should be no dimpling of the cheeks and no smacking or clicking noises.

Clinical Tip

As you assist new mothers with breastfeeding, it is important to create a relaxed environment and approach to breastfeeding. Encourage the mother to get into a comfortable position, well supported with pillows. Remind her to bring the baby to her breast rather than leaning forward to the baby.

BREASTFEEDING ASSESSMENT

During the birthing unit stay, the nurse must carefully monitor the progress of the breastfeeding pair. A systematic assessment of several breastfeeding episodes provides the opportunity to teach the new mother about lactation and the breastfeeding process, provide anticipatory guidance, and evaluate the need for follow-up care after discharge. Criteria for evaluating a breastfeeding session include maternal and newborn cues, latch-on, position, letdown, nipple condition, newborn response, and maternal response. The literature provides various tools to guide the assessment and documentation of the breastfeeding efforts, such as the LATCH Scoring Table.

BREASTFEEDING EFFICIENCY

The mother should be taught to observe the newborn for effective, active breastfeeding. The baby should have a rhythmic suckling pattern (the slight pause between jaw compressions on the breast permits the mouth to fill with milk before swallowing). To note if the jaw compressions are strong enough, the mother should observe or feel if there is movement at the bilateral temporomandibular joints located in front of the baby's ears.

The baby should maintain a rhythmic feeding pattern with only brief pauses (lasting only seconds, not minutes) between spurts of active feeding, with the feeding session typically lasting for 10 to 20 minutes on the first breast. The baby may feed only a few minutes on the second breast or not at all, so the mother should alternate the first breast at the next feeding. The mother should visually observe for swallowing and later, as her milk is abundant, she will hear the baby's swallows. Discourage the mother from watching the clock to determine when the baby needs to switch breast sides but rather encourage her to watch the newborn's feeding pattern to note when active feeding ceases. When satiated, the newborn will either pull away from the breast or fall asleep. The baby will be extremely relaxed at

Developing Cultural Competence Breastfeeding in Other Cultures

Among traditional societies around the world, weaning from the breast occurs when a child is between 2 and 4 years of age. Some people of African ancestry may wean their babies after they begin to walk.

Some women of Asian heritage may breastfeed their babies for the first 1 to 2 years of life. Many women of Cambodian heritage practice breastfeeding on demand without restriction, or, if formula-feeding, provide a "comfort bottle" in between feedings (Lipson & Dibble, 2008).

Chinese women go through a 30-day period of home confinement ("doing the month" [*zuo yue zij*] following delivery, during which they are not permitted to bathe or wash their hair (Callister, 2014). This is a centuries-old tradition to nurture the mother back to her prenatal state and intended to keep her body warm to ward off *fong* (flatulence) and other future health ailments. A *Pui Yuet* (companion) is hired to provide total care for the mother and newborn. The Pui Yuet will cook traditional confinement foods daily (provide "heating foods" and avoid "cooling foods"). Most foods must be cooked in sesame oil and old ginger. The mother drinks hot herbal tea with her meals and is not permitted to drink any water because it is thought to cause water retention (Callister, 2014).

Muslim women generally breastfeed until their children are 2 years of age. This is encouraged in the Koran. Although Muslim women do not breastfeed in public, they will breastfeed in front of family members and relatives as long as the breast is not exposed (Ott, Al-Khadhuri, & Al-Junaibi, 2003).

People of Iranian heritage may breastfeed female babies longer than male babies.

Some Asians, Cambodian, Hispanics, Eastern Europeans, and Native Americans may delay breastfeeding because they believe colostrum is "bad" (Callister, 2014; Wambach, 2016). Haitian mothers may believe that "strong emotions" spoil breast milk, and that thick breast milk causes skin rashes and thin milk results in diarrhea (Callister, 2014).

To increase breastmilk production, Ethiopian women eat a special diet of milk and warm oat and honey gruel, Arab women eat lentil soup, and Korean women eat a special seaweed soup with beef broth (Callister, 2014; Purnell, 2013).

the end of the feeding and will sleep until the next feeding is due (at least an hour). As the baby matures, the feeding intervals will lengthen.

Clinical Tip

With a sleepy baby, unwrap the baby, encourage lots of skin-to-skin contact between the mother and baby, and have the mother rest with her baby near her breast so that the baby can feel and smell the breast. Encourage the mother to watch for feeding cues, such as hand-to-mouth activity, fluttering eyelids, vocalization (but not necessarily crying), and mouthing activities.

Another indicator of breastfeeding efficiency is softening of the mother's breasts, although this is not a reliable indicator in the first few days postpartum while breast milk volume is low. Within a week, however, this is a good indicator of milk transfer.

The newborn who feeds well will have a characteristic output. See Figure 25–24 for breastfeeding intake and output expectations. The newborn should also have the characteristic weight loss followed by weight gain pattern discussed earlier in this chapter.

In situations where there is a question regarding milk transfer effectiveness, it can be most reliably measured by obtaining prebreastfeeding and postbreastfeeding weight checks using an accurate infant scale. The difference in preweights and postweights is the amount of milk (each gram increase reflects 1 mL) transferred to the baby and may be useful in assessing breastfeeding efficiency and maternal milk volume.

Women With Special Needs Breastfeeding Assistance

For the woman with upper extremity impairment, breastfeeding may require assistance from a partner or care provider should she chose to breastfeed. Women with limited arm strength or manual dexterity may require wrist supports to maintain a proper latch-on. These women are also more prone to nipple soreness, cracking, and bleeding because when the baby slips off the nipple, it may be more difficult to reattach the baby properly. A lactation consultation should be performed with all women with upper extremity limitations.

TEACHING HIGHLIGHTS | Successful Breastfeeding Evaluation

A baby is probably getting enough milk if:

- The baby is nursing at least 8 times in 24 hours.
- In a quiet room, the mother can hear her baby swallow while nursing, once her milk supply has become abundant.
- The mother's breasts appear to soften after breastfeeding.
- The number of wet diapers increases daily by a minimum of one additional diaper until the fifth day after birth; after day 5, the baby should have six to eight wet diapers daily.
- The baby's stools are beginning to lighten in color by the third day after birth, or have changed to yellow no later than day 5.

Note: Offering a supplemental bottle is not a reliable indicator because most newborns will take a few ounces even if they are getting enough breast milk.

- Newborns should breastfeed 8 to 12 times per day and should appear relaxed after feeding.
- Colostrum is all that a newborn needs in the first few days of life in most cases.
- It is normal for a newborn to lose up to 7% of birth weight in the first few days; however, up to 10% weight loss is tolerated if the mother's breasts are full, the baby is observed to breastfeed well and is not dehydrated.
- Newborns should gain 10 grams/kg/day after the mother's milk supply is abundant (about day 4 of life).
- Newborns should be back to their birth weight by 2 weeks of age.
- Newborn's stool should change in color, consistency, and frequency during the first few days of life. The photo images noted below depict stool color progression. Some babies progress faster to yellow milk stools, as early as day 3.

Day 1

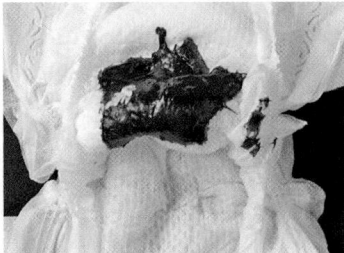

Minimum Output

On day 1, the newborn should produce at least one wet diaper and one meconium stool by 24 hours of age.

Note the pinkish-red "brick dust" appearance on the diaper. The uric acid crystals produced by the kidneys is associated with concentrated urine. A red flag is raised if their presence is continued beyond day 2 or 3 of life.

Day 2

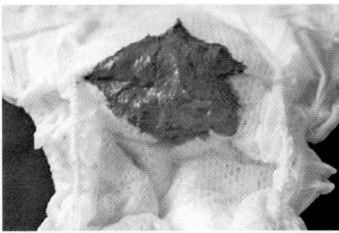

On day 2, the newborn should produce at least two wet diapers and two early transitional stools in a 24-hour period by 48 hours of age.

Day 3

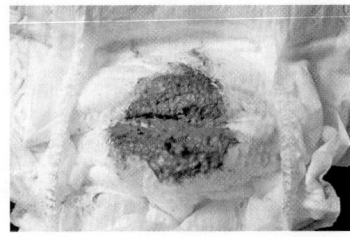

On day 3, the newborn should produce at least three wet diapers and three transitional stools in a 24-hour period by 72 hours of age.

When a mother's milk supply is abundant on day 2, some babies will have transitioned to yellow milk stools as early as day 3.

Day 4

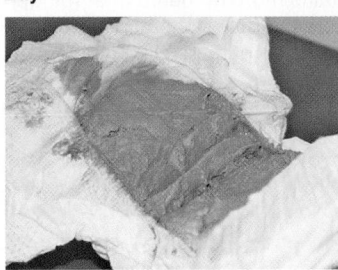

On day 4, the newborn should produce at least four wet diapers and three to four yellow-green transitional stools or yellow milk stools in a 24-hour period by 96 hours of age.

Day 5

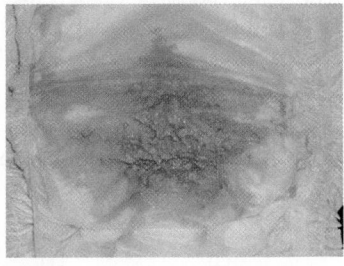

On day 5, the newborn should produce at least five wet diapers and three to four yellow milk stools per day; the stools are typically explosive and have a curdy or seedy appearance.

Hereafter, breastfeeding newborns will consistently produce at least six well-saturated wet diapers per day. These babies will typically continue to produce at least three to four yellow milk stools daily, but may have up to 10 stools per day until they are about a month old. Infants 4 weeks or older may suddenly decrease their stool frequency, even skipping days.

Figure 25–24 **Breastfeeding intake and output expectations.**

SOURCE: Brigitte Hall, RNC, MSN, IBCLC.

BOTTLE-FEEDING BREAST MILK

There are a number of reasons for bottle-feeding breast milk. The nurse should evaluate the indications in order to recommend the best technique for the mother and her particular need.

Hand Expression. Some mothers prefer to hand express their milk rather than use a breast pump, and many find that in the immediate postpartum period hand expression of milk may be a more effective method of removing drops of colostrum than using an electric breast pump. Nurses should teach all mothers the skill of hand expressing breast milk, as it is possible the mother will find herself in a situation without a breast pump and need to relieve herself from engorgement.

To facilitate hand expressing breast milk, the mother should be sure her breasts are clean (avoid using soap on nipples), her hands are washed, and she has taken a few minutes to relax and gently massage her breasts before beginning. She should be sitting up straight or leaning slightly forward (a pillow behind the back is helpful), because gravity aids in the flow of milk.

To help the mother hand express breast milk, have the mother follow steps 1 through 4 of the pumping instructions provided in Table 25–4. The mother can then use the Marmet technique of hand expression (Box 25–2). It is important that the mother take care to place her hands exactly as directed. She should take care not to traumatize her breasts or nipples. Hand expression should not be painful. Most mothers will need assistance in learning this technique initially. Reassure the mother that this skill is learned; with practice, she can become an expert at hand expression.

Pump. Although hand expression can be efficient, many mothers will choose to use a mechanical breast pump to express their milk. Not all breast pumps are of the same quality, even within the same category (see Figures 25–27, 25–28, and 25–29 and Table 25–5). Pumps generally cycle from low to high suction at a frequency similar to that of a breastfeeding infant (about 45 to 60 cycles per minute). However, differences in the quality of the pump motor or the presence or absence of controls over suction pressure mean that some pumps will generate inadequate

---

TABLE 25–4 Pumping Instructions and Storage Guidelines

1. Once a day rinse the breasts with water while bathing or showering. Avoid applying soap directly on the nipples.
2. Wash hands well with soap and water before preparing to pump.
3. Take a few minutes to massage the breasts and relax. Do some slow, deep breathing and think about or look at a picture of your baby. Being relaxed is very important for releasing milk from the breasts. (Stress can inhibit or delay let-down because stress hormones, such as cortisol and epinephrine, can block receptors for let-down.)
4. Sit up straight or lean slightly forward. A pillow placed behind your back may facilitate the slightly tilted forward posture, as gravity aids in the flow of milk from the breasts.
5. For single-sided pumping, pump each breast for 10 to 20 minutes. Some mothers find that they empty their breasts more efficiently if they switch back and forth from one breast to the other as the milk flow diminishes, until they have stimulated each breast for 15 to 20 minutes. The entire pumping session will last 30 to 40 minutes.
6. Pump the expressed milk preferably into glass or plastic bottles. Mothers of healthy babies may also use bottle bags or liners intended for human milk collection and storage; however, note that up to 60% of secretory IgA (SIgA) is lost when milk is stored in these kinds of containers for 48 hours because of the attraction of the antibodies to the polyethylene material used in making the bottle bags/liners (Riordan, 2016). Because of the loss of antibodies that can occur with bottle bags or liners, mothers of preemies and fragile babies should especially avoid using these kinds of storage containers. Do not fill milk storage containers more than 3/4 full because milk expands during freezing.
7. Feed *freshly* expressed breast milk whenever there is a need to give a supplement, when possible. Reserve the stored milk for times when fresh milk is not available (e.g., when separated from baby). Fresh breast milk retains more nutrients than refrigerated or frozen milk, although these are still preferred over formula. Expressed human milk may be stored in the refrigerator for up to 8 days, but if intended to be frozen, this should be done within 48 hours of initial refrigeration. Avoid placing human milk in the freezer door or on the bottom of a self-defrosting freezer because the temperature fluctuates more in those areas.
8. Store expressed human milk in volumes the baby is likely to consume at a single feeding or in a volume the baby will consume in a day.
9. Human milk should never be thawed in a microwave oven or placed in a pan and warmed up on the stove. These methods may cause the milk to warm up too hot (and unevenly) and can burn a baby as well as cause heat-sensitive nutrients to be destroyed. Frozen milk can be thawed safely using one of two methods:
    • For a quick thaw, remove the container of frozen milk from the freezer, place the container in a bowl in the sink, and run warm water over it for no longer than 15 minutes. Take care not to immerse the container in water because water may leach into the container of milk, possibly contaminating it and diluting it.
    • For a slow thaw overnight, take the frozen container of milk from the freezer the day before or several hours before it is needed and let it defrost in the refrigerator (not on the kitchen counter) over several hours. The time it takes to defrost depends on the volume in the container. Note that breast milk that has been sitting for a while will normally separate. See Figure 25–25 to view breast milk that has separated. To remix it, simply swirl the bottle (avoid vigorous shaking) until the milk is evenly mixed. Make certain that the fat that clings to the wall of the container has mixed into the milk. If the volume in the bottle is more than can be used in one feeding, pour only the amount needed into a clean bottle, and put the rest of the milk immediately back in the refrigerator. Place the feeding bottle in a bowl in the sink and run warm water over it for no longer than 15 minutes. The bottle should remain fairly upright, and the water level in the bowl should remain below the lid of the bottle or milk container to prevent water from inadvertently entering the bottle.
10. Previously frozen thawed breast milk is good in the refrigerator for 24 hours only. It must be used in that time frame or discarded. Thawed milk should never be refrozen.
11. Check the temperature of the milk before feeding it. Babies will drink milk when the milk temperature is between room temperature and body temperature (roughly 65 to 100 degrees).
12. Any milk left over from a feeding should be discarded within an hour of starting the feeding. The reason for this is because saliva "back washes" into the bottle while nipple feeding, and the saliva contains bacteria that can multiply and potentially make a baby sick.

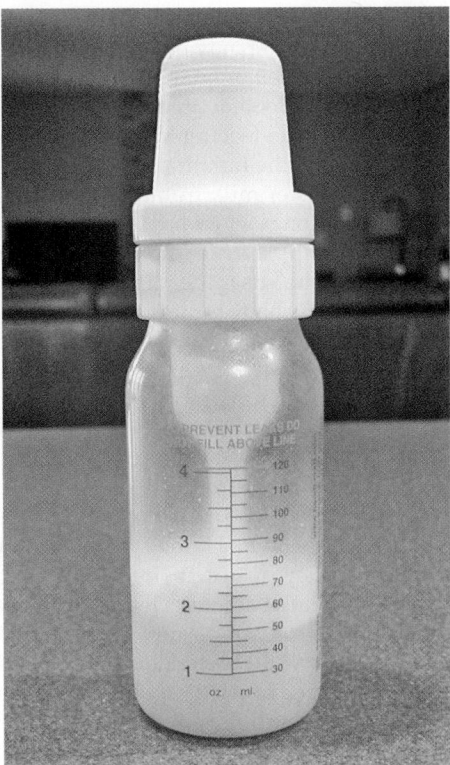

Figure 25–25 **Expressed breast milk that has separated.**

SOURCE: Brigitte Hall, RNC, MSN, IBCLC.

pressure or cycle too slowly to be effective, whereas others may exert too high a suction that can cause injury. Breast flange size, proper fit, and comfort are other variables to consider. Some good-quality pumps have multiple flange sizes available to accommodate the various nipple sizes of mothers. Excessive rubbing of the mother's nipple in the flange tunnel can cause discomfort and result in a decreased volume expressed. The nurse should refer the mother to a lactation consultant or other person knowledgeable regarding different breast pumps.

Storing Human Breast Milk.   There are different guidelines for storage of expressed breast milk (EBM) depending on whether

---

Box 25–2 The Marmet Technique

1. The mother will position her thumb at the 12:00 position on the top edge of the areola (about 1.0 to 1.5 in. back from the tip of her nipple) and her forefinger and middle fingerpads at the 6:00 position on the bottom edge of the areola (about 1.0 to 1.5 inches from the tip of her nipple). If positioned correctly, a line between the thumb and fingers will cross the nipple (see Figure 25–26).

2. Next, the mother will stretch her areola back toward her chest wall without lifting her fingers off her breast.

3. Now she should roll her thumb and fingers simultaneously forward. This action compresses the ducts beneath the areola and stimulates the breast to empty both manually and by triggering the letdown reflex.

4. The mother should repeat the sequence multiple times to completely drain her breasts. She should try to maintain a steady rhythm, cycling 45 to 60 times/ minute. It is also more effective if the mother repositions her fingers to other positions on the same breast (e.g., 3:00 and 9:00, 1:00, and 7:00) when the milk flow slows.

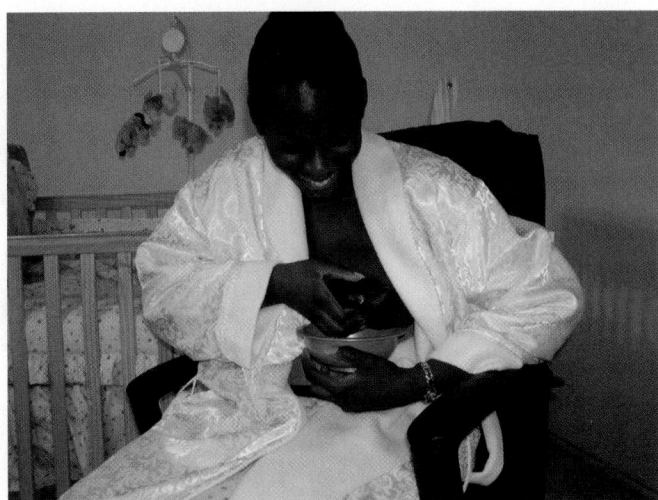

Figure 25–26 **Hand expression of breast milk.**

SOURCE: Brigitte Hall, RNC, MSN, IBCLC.

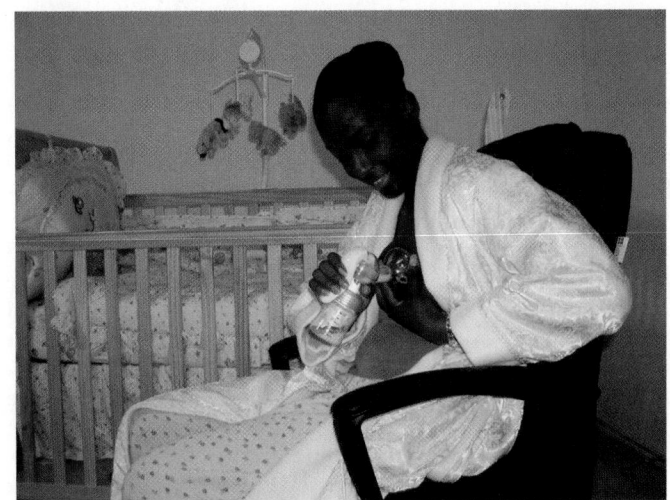

Figure 25–27 **Manual breast pump.**

SOURCE: Brigitte Hall, RNC, MSN, IBCLC.

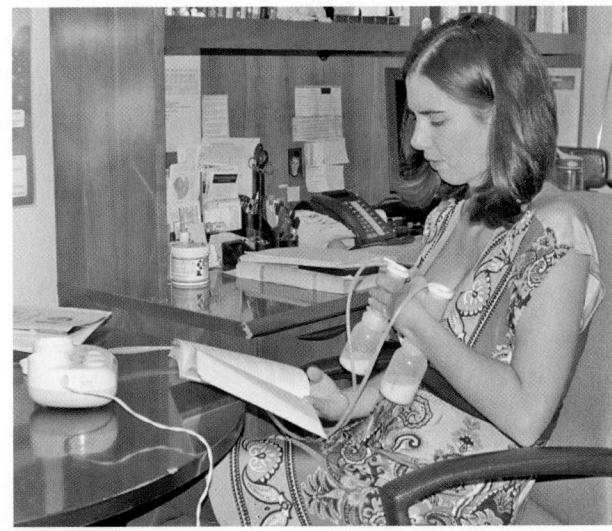

Figure 25–28 **Individual double electric breast pump.**

SOURCE: Brigitte Hall, RNC, MSN, IBCLC.

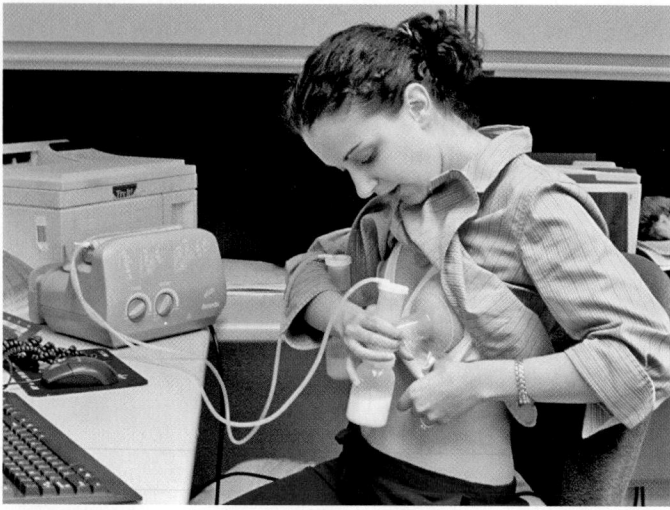

Figure 25–29 | Hospital-grade multiuser breast pump.

SOURCE: Brigitte Hall, RNC, MSN, IBCLC.

the baby is a healthy full-term baby or a premature or sick baby in the hospital. The guidelines in Table 25–6 (which also includes storage guidelines for formula) are intended as a resource for the mother of a healthy, full-term baby.

SUPPLEMENTARY FORMULA-FEEDING FOR BREASTFED NEWBORNS

Supplementary formula-feedings for the breastfeeding newborn are not routinely recommended. Supplementation should only be given when medically indicated (Janke, 2014). Routine supplements are unnecessary in the early days after birth, and bottle-feeding may cause the newborn to develop an incorrect sucking pattern or may cause the baby to refuse the breast altogether (Riordan, 2016). Early supplementation with formula may contribute to a delay in early maternal milk production, may result in maternal engorgement after the mother's milk production has increased, and may possibly sensitize an at-risk newborn for milk-protein allergy. These types of problems have been implicated in early breastfeeding terminations (Mercer et al., 2010).

A newborn's refusal to breastfeed after receiving bottles in the early postdelivery period may be related to a phenomenon referred to as *nipple confusion* or, more accurately termed, *nipple preference*. This potential problem occurs because the techniques for breastfeeding and bottle-feeding are different. In breastfeeding, the baby has to open the mouth very wide in order to latch onto the breast. To transfer milk from the mother's breast the baby has to extend the tongue forward, cupping the nipple and drawing the mother's nipple deep into the mouth until the teat reaches the "comfort zone" near the junction of the baby's hard and soft palates. After the baby creates suction from the tongue and cheeks and seals the latch with the lips, then the baby rhythmically compresses the breast with the jaw while the tongue moves in an undulating motion to move fluid toward the pharynx before swallowing, all in coordination with breathing. On average, it takes a couple of minutes before the breastfeeding mother's milk flow increases during let-down. With bottle-feeding, the baby keeps the tongue retracted and uses the tip of the tongue to block the flow of milk, which otherwise drips continuously by gravity even when suction is not applied. The bottle-feeding baby merely needs to create suction with the mouth on the bottle nipple and the fluid easily flows.

At times, there are valid medical indications for supplementing a breastfeeding newborn in the early postpartum period. When supplementation is indicated, the first choice is to use the mother's own milk (fresh, previously expressed, or frozen/thawed). If maternal milk is not available, pasteurized donor milk is the next choice, and then formula (Jones, 2013). Supplementation can be administered using various methods based on the particular situation, parental preference, and agency policy.

Formula-Feeding

With more attention being placed on promoting and assisting breastfeeding mothers, the teaching needs of the mother who is formula-feeding may inadvertently get overlooked. Nurses may assume that families can simply follow the formula preparation instructions on the formula containers. Parents need teaching, counseling, and support. Parents need to learn about the feeding pattern for a formula-feeding baby, the intake and output

TABLE 25-5 Types of Breast Pumps and Indications for Use

INDICATION	MANUAL BREAST PUMP (FIGURE 25–27)	SMALL BATTERY/ ELECTRIC BREAST PUMP	INDIVIDUAL DOUBLE ELECTRIC BREAST PUMP (FIGURE 25–28)	HOSPITAL-GRADE MULTIUSER DOUBLE ELECTRIC BREAST PUMP (FIGURE 25–29)
A missed feeding	■	◊		
An evening out	■	◊		
Working part-time	■	◊		
Convenience—occasional use	■	◊		
Working full-time			*	*
Premature/hospitalized baby				*
Low milk supply				*
Sore nipples/engorgement			*	*
Latch-on problems/infection			■	*
Drawing out flattish nipples	■	◊	*	*

■ Good ◊ Better * Best

Source: Adapted from the *Medela Breastfeeding Information Guide Tips and Products.* (2010). Table: Which Breast Pump Is Best for You? (p. 9). McHenry, IL: Medela, Inc.

TABLE 25–6 Storage Guidelines for Human Milk and Formula

MILK	ENVIRONMENT	TIME UNTIL DISCARD
Human milk or formula, opened/reconstituted	Being fed	Finish feed within 1 hr
Fresh human milk	Room temperature 72°–79°F (22.2°–26.0°C)	4 hr
Fresh human milk	Room temperature 66°–72°F (18.8°–22.2°C)	6–10 hr
Fresh human milk	Cooler w/ frozen ice packs 59°F (15°C)	24 hr
Formula, opened/reconstituted	Room temperature	2 hr
Thawed human milk	Refrigerator	24 hr
Formula, opened/reconstituted	Refrigerator	24–48 hr (see label)
Fresh human milk	Refrigerator	8 days
Formula powder, opened can	Room temperature	1 month
Fresh human milk	Freezer	3–4 months
Formula/powder in sealed container	Avoid excessive heat	Printed expiration date
Thawed human milk	Freezer	Do not refreeze
Formula	Freezer	Do not freeze

Sources: Data from Human Milk Banking Association of North America (HMBANA). (2011). *Best practice for expressing, storing and handling human milk in hospitals, homes and child care settings* (3rd ed.). Raleigh, NC: Author; Mead-Johnson Nutritionals. (2012). *Pediatric products handbook.* New York, NY: Bristol-Myers Squibb Company; Ross Products Division. (2014). *Pediatric nutritionals product guide.* Columbus, OH: Abbott Laboratories.

expectations, the recommended type of formula for their baby, how to prepare and store formula, what equipment they will need, feeding technique, and safety precautions. (See Table 25–4.)

Formula-Feeding Guidelines and Technique

Commercial formulas are available in three forms: powder, concentrate, and ready-to-feed. There are situations in which one formula may be better to use than another, but in general, convenience and cost usually influence the parents' decision.

- *Powdered formula* is the least expensive type of formula. This formula can be made up one bottle at a time, or multiple bottles can be prepared, but they must be used within 24 to 48 hours. Standard powdered formula is made by adding one level scoop of powdered formula to 60 mL (2 oz) of water. Powdered formulas are not sterile. Powdered formula is made from pasteurized liquid that is then freeze-spray dried into a powder; contamination with microorganisms can occur in the final stages of production. Preparation of any baby formula, but especially powdered formulas, requires careful handling to avoid contamination with microorganisms.

- *Formula concentrate* is more expensive than powder but is not as expensive as ready-to-feed formula. Formula concentrate is commercially sterile. This formula must be diluted with an equal part of water. By adding boiled water that has been cooled, sterility can be maintained.

- *Ready-to-feed* formula is the easiest to use because it does not require any mixing; however, this convenience comes at a cost—it is the most expensive formula. It is indicated for use when adequate water is not available, when the baby is immunocompromised and requires commercially sterile (pasteurized) formula, when an inexperienced babysitter will be feeding the baby, and for convenience.

Whatever the type of formula chosen, the nurse should underscore the importance of proper preparation and prompt refrigeration. Parents will need to be briefed on safety precautions during formula preparation. A primary concern is proper mixing to reconstitute formula. Parents need clear instructions to avoid unintentional harm to their baby. Parents should be instructed to follow the directions on the formula container label precisely as written. They should know that adding too much water during preparation dilutes the nutrients and caloric density. This contributes to undernourishment, insufficient weight gain, and possibly water intoxication, which can cause hyponatremia and seizures. Not adding enough water concentrates nutrients and calories and can tax a baby's immature kidneys and digestive system as well as cause dehydration. See Table 25–6 for storage guidelines for formula.

Recommended sanitary precautions and additional safety precautions are shown in Box 25–3.

Parents also need guidance about what kind of water to use to reconstitute formula (see Table 25–7 to review types of water sources) and should discuss with their baby's healthcare provider whether to boil the water before use. If boiling is used, parents need to be instructed to heat the water until it reaches a rolling boil, to continue to let the water boil for 1 to 2 minutes, and, most importantly, to allow the water to cool before using it to reconstitute the formula. Parents should also be instructed not to let the water boil down to a low level in the pan because this can cause minerals in the water to become concentrated.

Use of distilled bottle water and filtered tap water raises concerns with regard to fluoride. The American Academy of Pediatrics recommends that no fluoride supplements be given to a baby before 6 months of age (AAP & ACOG, 2012). Parents should be encouraged to read the labels on bottled water to see if fluoride has been added and to determine if the water source is suitable depending on the baby's age (Table 25–7).

BOTTLES AND NIPPLES

Parents often have questions about the kind of bottles and nipples to purchase. Many newly designed bottles are marketed to lessen air intake while a baby feeds. There is not a particular bottle design that is best for all babies. A key point to emphasize to the families is feeding technique. Parents should try to avoid situations in which a baby is crying for a prolonged time. Crying results in increased ingestion of air even before

Box 25–3 Sanitary Precautions and Safety Precautions for Baby Formula

- Check the expiration date on the formula container.
- Ensure good hand washing before preparing formula; never dip into the can without clean hands.
- Clean bottles, nipples, rings, discs, and bottle caps.
  a. Washing in a dishwasher when available (small items and heat-sensitive items on top rack secured in a basket), or
  b. Boiling briefly (1 to 2 minutes) in a pot of water, or
  c. Cleaning using a microwave sterilization kit, or
  d. Cleaning using very warm soapy water and a nipple and bottle brush.
- Inspect and replace bottle nipples as soon as they show wear; worn nipples can break apart and can become a choking hazard.
- Wash the top of the formula container before piercing the lid.
- Shake the liquid formulas well before pouring off the desired amount.
- Shake prepared milk that has been sitting in the refrigerator before feeding.
- Allow tap water to run for 1 minute before obtaining water to use for mixing—this helps clear any lead standing in the pipes. Also, always use cold tap water, as warm water tends to contain higher levels of lead.
- Use only the scoop supplied in the can of formula when formula preparation instructions call for a "scoop" of powdered formula. A scoop should not be "packed" and should be leveled off (e.g., with the back of a knife).
- Do not add anything else to the bottle, except under direction of the baby's healthcare provider.
- Milk in a bottle should be warmed by placing the bottle in a bowl of warm tap water for no longer than 15 minutes. Do not fill the bowl with water higher than the rim of the bottle. (Babies can take cold formula but most young babies will prefer it warm.)
- Allow freshly prepared (unused) formula to sit out at room temperature for no longer than 2 hours; use an insulated pack to transport formula. Milk left over in the bottle after a feeding should be discarded.
- In warm weather, transport reconstituted formula or concentrate from an open can in an insulated pack with frozen gel packs.
- Travel with water and formula separated—carry premeasured water bottles and bottles with premeasured amounts of powdered formula, or carry premeasured commercially prepared formula packets, or have the can of formula available.
- Holding the baby during feeding (even when the infant can hold the bottle) promotes bonding and prevents supine feedings.
- Do not allow the baby to formula-feed in a supine position because this increases the risk of otitis media and dental caries in the older infant.
- Never prop a bottle—this is a choking hazard.
- Allow babies to take what they want AND to stop when they want. Overfeeding can lead to obesity.

TABLE 25–7 Water Sources

TYPE	DESCRIPTION
Distilled water	Minerals and most other impurities have been removed. It will not contain any fluoride. An acceptable water source for reconstituting formula.
Filtered tap water	Some minerals and impurities removed during filtration, including fluoride. This is an acceptable water source for reconstituting formula.
Natural mineral water	Comes from protected groundwater and by law cannot be treated. Naturally contains high levels of minerals and sodium and so is not suitable for babies or for reconstituting formula.
Spring water	Comes from a single nonpolluted groundwater source, but unlike natural mineral water, it can be further treated. Because there is no regulation requiring the mineral content to be printed on the bottle label, it is best to avoid this water source for reconstituting formula.
Tap water	Water from the municipal water supply, and regulated by drinking water regulations. It is treated and considered safe for use in reconstituting formula.
Well water	Needs to be tested before use. Higher risk of nitrate poisoning. Untested water is not recommended for use in reconstituting formula.

the baby has started feeding. Babies who are very hungry also gulp more air. For these situations, instruct the parents to burp their baby frequently to prevent a large emesis (Figure 25–30 and Figure 25–31). The parent may even want to attempt to pat the baby's back briefly before starting the feeding to calm a crying baby and possibly burp as well. Another tip to avoid excessive ingestion of air is to have the parent hold the baby cradled in the arms while bottle-feeding, and tilting the bottle at a 45-degree angle in order for fluid to cover the nipple. This prevents the baby from sucking in air and

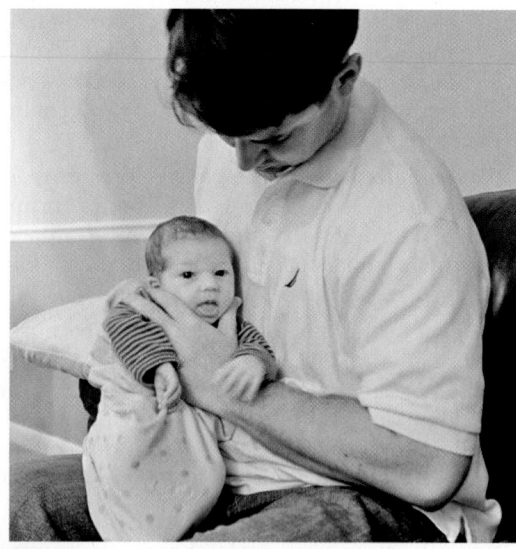

Figure 25–30 Burping baby sitting up on lap.

SOURCE: Brigitte Hall, RNC, MSN, IBCLC.

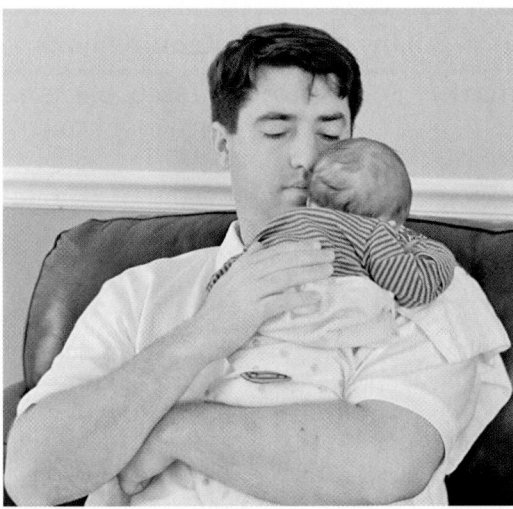

Figure 25–31 Burping baby over the shoulder.
SOURCE: Brigitte Hall, RNC, MSN, IBCLC.

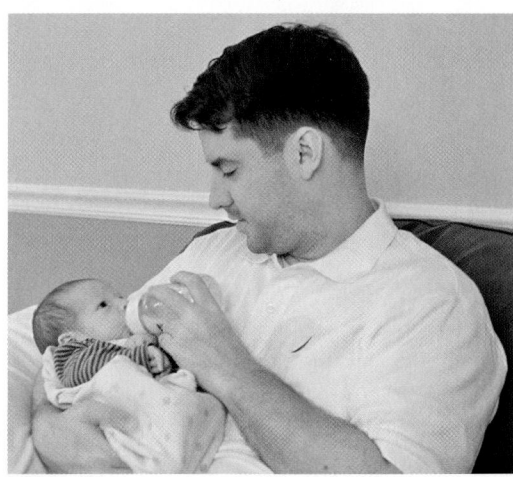

Figure 25–32 Bottle-feeding.
SOURCE: Brigitte Hall, RNC, MSN, IBCLC.

swallowing it. The vented bottle design eliminates the negative effects of a vacuum and channels air through an internal vent system above the milk avoiding air bubbles in the milk. See Figure 25–32 to view a baby bottle-feeding.

Parents will want to consider a slow-flow nipple for all newborns and for older breastfeeding infants learning to formula-feed—over time, the infant will graduate to medium-flow and high-flow nipples. Nipples come in different shapes. Generally, nipple shape plays a greater importance for breastfeeding babies receiving expressed breast milk or supplemental formula in a bottle. Breastfed babies transition best going from breast to bottle and back to breast again when using a bottle nipple that has a relatively wide base (to help maintain a wide open latch) and a medium to long nipple length. Another variable to consider is nipple construction. Nipples are generally made from either rubber or silicone. Families with a history of sensitivity to latex are advised to use silicone nipples. Silicone nipples also have less of an odor, which may be an issue for some babies who are breastfed.

To know if a newborn is bottle-feeding well, the nurse needs to observe a bottle-feeding session. Parents should be informed that if the baby is sucking effectively, the parents should observe bubbles rising in the fluid of standard bottles. (If a family is using vented bottles or bottles with liners that retract as fluid is removed, bubbles will not be detected.) No bubbles will be observed if the parent unintentionally places the bottle nipple under the baby's tongue, preventing the baby from sucking effectively. Some newborns, especially premature newborns, raise the tongue to the roof of the mouth, and so it is sometimes a challenge to place the nipple on top of the tongue. Babies who persistently leak milk from the side of the mouth may be getting fluid too quickly. The nurse could suggest using a slower flowing nipple. If symptoms persist, the newborn should have an oral evaluation. The baby could have a short lingual frenulum (tongue-tied) and not be able to properly cup the tongue under the nipple and channel fluid to the back of the throat, or may have an oral-motor dysfunction and need speech therapy or occupational therapy evaluation.

There has been a growing concern regarding specific chemicals used in the manufacture of plastic baby bottles, the material used in lining formula cans, and soft plastics such as bisphenol-A

(BPA) that could leach from polycarbonate plastic used in the manufacture of some baby bottles and transfer into the baby's milk (U.S. Food and Drug Administration [USFDA], 2013).

SAFETY ALERT!
Parents need to be instructed to read product labels to see if the merchandise they are purchasing is free of these potentially harmful chemicals. If product labels do not explicitly state that they are free of these chemicals, then it cannot be assumed they are BPA-free, PVC-free, lead-free, and phthalates-free.

If parents cannot afford to purchase new BPA-free bottles, then encourage them to limit heating the bottles (avoid using the dishwasher and bottle warmers) and throw out old bottles with scratches. The harmful chemicals are leached most when the plastic is heated or damaged.

Involving Fathers

Our traditional view of the family following the birth of a child places most of the attention on the mother and newborn, oftentimes leaving the father out. Nurses need to recognize this and make every effort to speak to both parents when entering the mother's room. Fathers play a vital role in the family by providing support to the mother and care for their newborn. If a mother has chosen not to breastfeed, the father can be involved with bottle-feedings from the start. However, if the mother is breastfeeding, it is important to ask the father to wait to introduce a bottle until the mother's milk supply and breastfeeding are well established. The father can be encouraged to assist with breastfeeding in the meantime. He can help the mother get in position and help tweak the baby's latch if the mother complains of any discomfort. The father can also massage the mother's breasts during breastfeeding to help stimulate the sleepy baby to feed better and to relieve any engorgement.

The father can help with other aspects too. He can help burp the baby, change diapers, and bathe and comfort the baby. The father can also provide skin-to-skin contact that enhances bonding, provides comfort to the newborn, and calms the baby down before offering the breast. One strategy is to have the

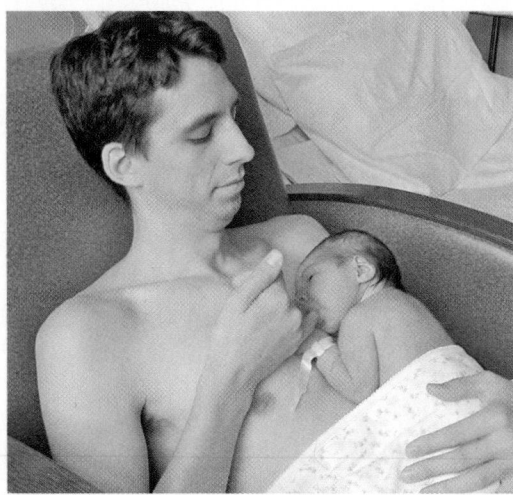

Figure 25–33 Father and newborn skin-to-skin.

SOURCE: Brigitte Hall, RNC, MSN, IBCLC.

father hold the baby vertically on his chest and let the baby suck on a clean finger for a minute or so (see Figure 25–33). These are just a few ways to involve the father after the birth of the baby. These interactions promote father–mother–newborn bonding and are important for paternal role development.

Promotion of Successful Newborn Breastfeeding

With the trend toward earlier discharge from the birthing center, there is limited time for inpatient education. Teaching moments, when they occur, may not be optimal because of the distraction of visitors and the mother's being sleep deprived, uncomfortable, or under the effects of an analgesic. It is important that parents receive verbal and written instructions and community resource information to which they can later refer. (See Chapter 29 for a complete discussion of self-care measures the nurse can suggest to a woman with a breastfeeding problem after discharge from the birthing center.)

To promote a supportive hospital environment for breastfeeding, the Baby-Friendly Hospital Initiative recognizes hospitals and birthing centers that offer optimal lactation services and comply with the 10 steps outlined in Table 25–8. Baby-Friendly status is not easy to achieve. One obstacle to achieving Baby-Friendly status, among many, is having to agree not to accept free or low-cost formula. As of July 2015, there were approximately 288 hospitals in the United States with the Baby-Friendly designation, according to an update on the Baby-Friendly Hospital Initiative USA website (Baby-Friendly Hospital Initiative USA, 2015).

Preparation for Discharge

Although the adjustment to parenting is a normal process, going home presents a critical transition for the family. The parents become the primary caregivers for the newborn and must provide a nurturing environment in which the emotional and physical needs of the newborn can be met. Nursing interventions focus on promoting health and preventing possible problems.

TABLE 25–8 Baby-Friendly Requirements

BABY-FRIENDLY 10 STEPS TO SUCCESSFUL BREASTFEEDING

- Have a written breastfeeding policy that is routinely communicated to all healthcare staff.
- Train all healthcare staff in skills necessary to implement this policy.
- Inform all pregnant women about the benefits and management of breastfeeding.
- Help mothers initiate breastfeeding within 1 hour of birth.
- Show mothers how to breastfeed and maintain lactation, even if they should be separated from their newborns.
- Give newborns no food or drink other than breast milk, unless medically indicated.
- Practice rooming in—that is, allow mothers and newborns to remain together 24 hours a day.
- Encourage breastfeeding on demand.
- Give no artificial teats or pacifiers (also called dummies or soothers) to breastfeeding newborns.
- Foster the establishment of breastfeeding support groups and refer mothers to them on discharge from the hospital or clinic.

Source: World Health Organization/United Nations Children's Emergency Fund (WHO/UNICEF). (2010). *U.S. committee for UNICEF interim program in the United States to promote the Baby-Friendly ten steps to successful breastfeeding.* Washington, DC: Government Printing Office.

Nursing Management

For the Newborn in Preparation for Discharge

Nursing Assessment and Diagnosis

When preparing for discharge, assess whether parents have realistic expectations of the newborn's behavior and the depth of their knowledge in caring for their newborn.

Nursing diagnoses that may apply to the newborn's family include the following (NANDA-I © 2014):

- *Parenting, Readiness for Enhanced*, related to appropriate behavioral expectations for the newborn
- *Family Processes, Readiness for Enhanced*, related to integration of newborn into family unit or demands of newborn care and feeding.

Planning and Implementation

PARENT TEACHING

To meet the parent's need for information, the nurse who is responsible for the care of the mother and newborn should assume the primary responsibility for parent education. Nearly every contact with the parents presents an opportunity for sharing information that can facilitate their sense of competence in newborn care. You will need to recognize and respect the many good ways of providing safe care. Unless their care methods are harmful to the newborn, the parents' methods of giving care should be reinforced rather than contradicted.

The information that follows is provided to increase your knowledge of newborn care and can also be used to meet parents' needs for information. If they are new parents, gently teach them by example and provide instructions geared to their needs and previous knowledge about the various aspects of newborn care.

Observe how parents interact with their newborn during feeding and caregiving activities. Even during a short stay, there are opportunities to provide information and observe whether

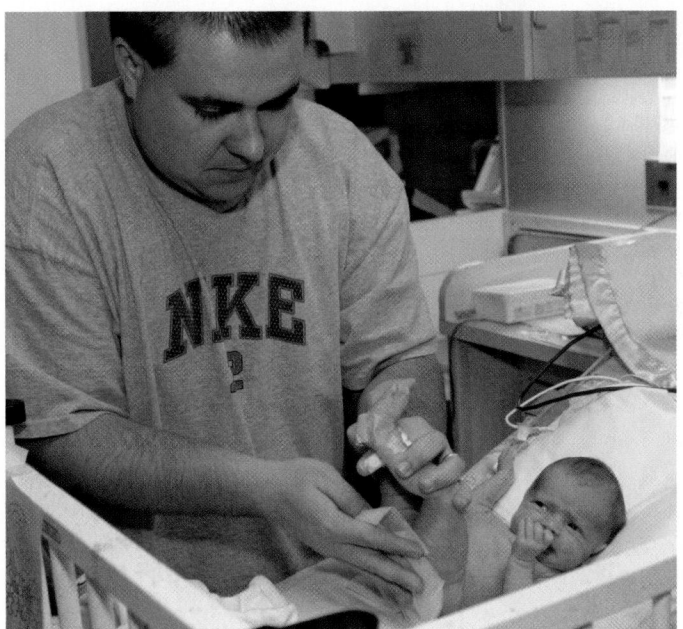

Figure 25–34 A father demonstrates competence and confidence in diapering his newborn daughter.

Clinical Reasoning Newborn Vaginal Drainage

You are caring for Sarah Feldstein, who had her first child, a daughter, about 4 hours ago. She appears visibly upset when changing her baby's diaper and says she thinks something is wrong because her daughter has tissue protruding from her vagina and some bleeding in her diaper. What would you do?

newborn's legs and then gently lifting upward. This technique provides security and support for the head (which the newborn is unable to support until 3 or 4 months of age).

You must be an excellent role model for families in the area of safety. Safety topics include proper positioning of the newborn on the back to sleep and correct use of the bulb syringe. The baby should never be left alone anywhere but in the crib. Remind the mother that while she and her newborn are together in the birthing unit, she should never leave her baby alone for security reasons and because newborns spit up frequently the first day or two after birth. Other newborn safety measures are discussed in detail in Chapter 29.

Women With Special Needs Teaching Infant Care Practices

The woman with a developmental disability may need to be shown how to carry out certain infant care practices and need repeated demonstrations and additional explanations. Teaching should be based on the woman's level of understanding with teaching methods customized for her individualized learning needs. Demonstration by the nurse with a return demonstration is an effective tool to ensure the skill is understood and done correctly.

Demonstrating a bath (see Chapter 29), cord care, and temperature assessment is the best way to provide information on these topics to parents.

Demonstrate and review the taking of axillary or tympanic temperatures and discourage the use of mercury thermometers. It is important that families understand the differences and know how to select a thermometer. The newborn's temperature needs to be taken only when signs of illness are present. Advise parents to call their healthcare provider immediately if they observe any signs of illness.

Nasal and Oral Suctioning

Most newborns are obligatory nose breathers for the first months of life. They generally maintain air passage patency by coughing or sneezing. However, during the first few days of life the newborn has increased mucus, and gentle suctioning with a bulb syringe may be indicated but only in cases of obvious obstruction. The newborn's mouth should be suctioned first so that there is nothing to aspirate if the newborn gasps when the nose is suctioned (AAP & ACOG, 2012). Demonstrate the use of the bulb syringe in the mouth and nose and have the parents do a return demonstration. The parents should repeat this demonstration of suctioning and cleansing the bulb before discharge so they feel confident in performing the procedure. Care should be taken to apply only gentle suction to prevent nasal bleeding.

To suction the newborn, the bulb syringe is compressed before the tip is placed in the nostril. Take care not to occlude the

the parents are comfortable with changing the diapers of, wrapping, handling, and feeding their newborn (Figure 25–34). Do both parents get involved in the newborn's care? Is the mother depending on someone else to help her at home? Does the mother give reasons (e.g., "I'm too tired," "My stitches hurt," or "I'll learn later") for not wanting to be involved in her baby's care? As the family provides care, enhance parental confidence by giving them positive feedback. If the parents encounter problems, express confidence in their abilities to master the new skill or information, suggest alternatives, and serve as a role model. All these factors need to be considered when evaluating the educational needs of the parents. Providing mother-baby care and home care instruction on the night shift assists with education needs for early discharge parents.

One-to-one teaching while you are in the mother's room is the most effective educational method rated as such by both first-time and experienced postpartum parents. With shorter stays, most teaching unfortunately tends to focus on newborn feeding and immediate physical care needs of the mother, with limited anticipatory guidance provided in other areas. To address this deficit, see *Teaching Highlights: What to Tell Parents About Infant Care,* which includes a broad range of information important to share with new parents.

Clinical Tip

For clients who are hearing impaired, videotapes with information in both spoken and signed formats are most helpful. Birthing centers should have handouts available for families who do not speak English and for the birthing center that does not have interpreters (not family members) or language interpreter phones.

General Instructions for Newborn Care

One of the first concerns of anyone who has not had the experience of picking up a baby is how to do it correctly. The newborn is easily picked up by sliding one hand under the neck and shoulders and the other hand under the buttocks or between the

TEACHING HIGHLIGHTS	What to Tell Parents About Newborn Care

Immediate Safety Measures for the Newborn

- Watch for excessive mucus: use a bulb syringe to remove mucus.
- Have baby sleep on the back in a crib or in someone's arms.

Voiding and Stool Characteristics and Patterns

- Urine is straw to amber color without foul smell. Small amounts of uric acid crystals are normal in first days of life (may be mistaken by parents as blood in diaper because of reddish "brick dust" appearance).
- At least 6 to 10 wet diapers a day after the first few days of life.
- Normal progression of stool changes: (1) meconium (thick, tarry, dark green); (2) transitional stools (thin, brown to green); (3a) breastfed newborn: yellow gold, soft or mushy stools; (3b) formula-fed newborn: pale yellow, formed and pasty stools.
- Only one to two stools a day for formula-fed baby.
- Six to 10 small, loose yellow stools per day or only one stool every few days after breastfeeding is well established (after about 1 month).
- Wash hands with clean water before and after care.
- Keep the cord dry and exposed to air or loosely covered with clean clothes. (If cultural custom demands binding of the abdomen, a sanitary method such as the use of a clean piece of gauze can be recommended.)
- Clean the cord and skin around the base with a cotton swab or cotton ball. Clean two to three times a day or with each diaper change. Touching the cord, applying unclean substances to it, and applying bandages should be avoided. Do not give tub baths until the cord falls off in 7 to 14 days.
- Fold diapers below the umbilical cord to air-dry the cord (contact with wet or soiled diapers slows the drying process and increases the possibility of infection).
- Check the cord each day for any odor, oozing of greenish yellow material, or reddened areas around the cord. Expect tenderness around the cord and darkening and shriveling of the cord. Report to the healthcare provider any signs of infection.
- Normal changes in cord: The cord should look dark and dry up before falling off. A small drop of blood may present when the cord falls off.
- Never pull the cord or attempt to loosen it.

Care Required for Circumcision and Uncircumcised Newborns

Circumcision Care

- Squeeze water over the circumcision site once a day.
- Rinse the area off with warm water and pat dry.
- Apply a small amount of petroleum jelly (unless a Plastibell is in place) with each diaper change.
- Fasten a diaper over the penis snugly enough so that it does not move and rub the tender glans.
- Because the glans is sensitive, avoid placing baby on the stomach for the first day after the procedure.
- Check for any foul-smelling drainage or bleeding at least once a day.
- Let the Plastibell fall off by itself (about 8 days after circumcision). It should not be pulled off.
- Light, sticky, yellow drainage (part of healing process) may form over the head of the penis.

Uncircumcised Care

- Clean the uncircumcised penis with water during diaper changes and with bath.
- Do not force the foreskin back over the penis; foreskin will retract normally over time (may take 3 to 5 years).

Techniques for Waking and Quieting Newborns

Waking Baby

- Loosen clothing, change diaper.
- Hand-express milk onto baby's lips.
- Talk with baby while making eye contact.
- Hold baby in upright position (sitting or standing).
- Have baby do sit-ups (gently and rhythmically bend baby back and forth while grasping the baby under the knees and supporting baby's head and back with your other hand).
- Play patty-cake with baby.
- Stimulate the rooting reflex (brush one cheek with a hand or nipple).
- Increase skin contact (gently rub hands and feet).

Quieting Baby

- Check for a soiled diaper.
- Hold swaddled baby upright against midchest, supporting the bottom and back of head. Baby can hear heartbeat, feel warmth, and hear your softly spoken words or calming sounds.
- Use slow, calming movements with baby.
- Softly talk, sing, or hum to baby.

Signs of Illness

See Table 25–9: When Parents Should Call Their Healthcare Provider.

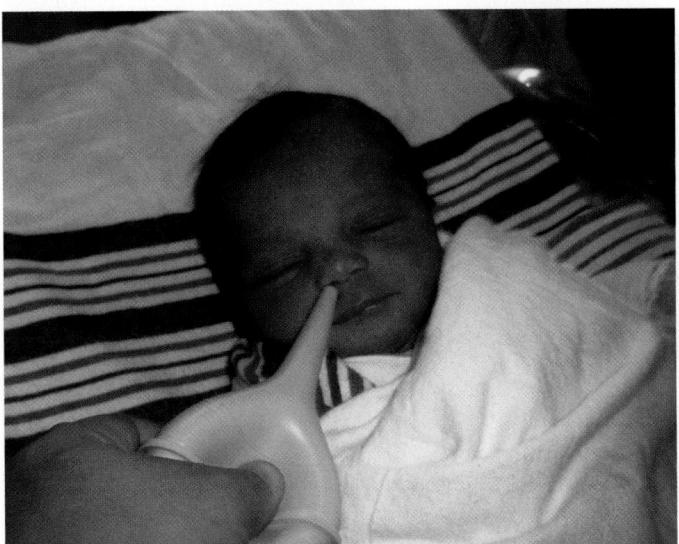

Figure 25–35 Nasal and oral suctioning. The bulb is compressed, the tip is placed in either the mouth or the nose, and the bulb is released.

passageway. The bulb is permitted to reexpand slowly by releasing the compression on the bulb (Figure 25–35). The bulb syringe is removed from the nostril, and drainage is then compressed out of the bulb and onto a tissue. The bulb syringe may also be used in the mouth if the newborn is spitting up and unable to handle the excess secretions. The bulb is compressed, the tip of the bulb syringe is placed about 1 in. to one side of the newborn's mouth, and compression is released. This draws up the excess secretions. The procedure is repeated on the other side of the mouth. The roof of the mouth and the back of the throat are avoided because suction in these areas might stimulate the gag reflex.

The bulb syringe should be washed in warm, soapy water and rinsed in warm water daily and as needed after use. Rinsing with a half-strength white vinegar solution followed by clear water may help to extend the useful life of the bulb syringe by inhibiting bacterial growth. A bulb syringe should always be kept near the newborn. New parents who are inexperienced with babies may fear that the baby will choke and are relieved to know how to take action if such an event occurs. They should be advised to turn the newborn's head to the side or hold the newborn with the head down as soon as there is any indication of gagging or vomiting and to use the bulb syringe as needed. See Performing Nasal Pharyngeal Suctioning in the *Clinical Skills* SKILLS Manual.

Some newborns may have transient edema of the nasal mucosa following suctioning of the airway after birth. Demonstrate the use of normal saline to loosen secretions, and instruct parents in the gentle and moderate use of the bulb syringe to avoid further irritation of the mucous membranes. If parents will be using humidifiers at home, instruct them to follow the manufacturer's cleaning instructions carefully so that molds, spores, and bacteria from a dirty humidifier do not enter the baby's environment.

SAFETY ALERT!
You will find that left-handed people tend to hold the baby over their right shoulder, and right-handed people do the opposite. This keeps the dominant hand free. However, most health personnel wear their name tags on the left side. To avoid scratching the baby's face, wear your name tag on the same side as your dominant hand.

Sleep and Activity

The National Institute of Child Health and Human Development and the American Academy of Pediatrics recommend that healthy term babies be placed on their backs to sleep. Teach parents the importance of following "Safe to Sleep Guidelines" to reduce the incidence of sudden infant death syndrome (SIDS) (Healthy Children, 2015e). No evidence exists that newborns need to be placed on their sides initially because of copious or thick secretions. Placing babies on their backs in the newborn period serves to educate parents regarding infant positioning. Studies indicate that parents position their babies in the same positions they observe in the hospital setting, so nurses must demonstrate this behavior to reduce the risk of SIDS. If exceptions are warranted, these should be explained to families so they do not misinterpret what they observe. The placement of babies in a prone position during supervised wakeful play sessions or "tummy time" should be encouraged as well (Healthy Children, 2015e, f). Regular periods of tummy time enhances a baby's gross motor skills and upper body strength and reduces the incidence of positional plagiocephaly. Also encourage parents to hold their babies and not allow them to remain in infant carriers for prolonged periods of time.

Healthy People 2020

(MICH-21) Increase the proportion of infants who are put to sleep on their backs

---

Perhaps nothing is more individual to each baby than the sleep–activity cycle. It is important to recognize the individual variations of each newborn and to assist parents as they develop sensitivity to their baby's communication signals and rhythms of activity and sleep. See Chapter 23 for a detailed discussion of sleep–wake activity.

Car Safety Considerations

Half of the children killed or injured in automobile crashes could have been protected by the use of federally approved car seats. Newborns must go home from the birthing unit in a car seat adapted to fit them (Figure 25–36). Babies should never be placed in the front seat of a car equipped with a passenger-side airbag. The car seat should be positioned to face the rear of the car until the baby is 2 years old, or until they reach maximum height and weight for their seat (Healthy Children, 2015c). Ensure that all parents are knowledgeable about the benefits of child safety seat use and proper installation. Encourage parents to have their infant safety seats checked by local groups trained specifically for that purpose. The Seat Check Initiative provides locations and information about child safety seats.

NEWBORN SCREENING AND IMMUNIZATION PROGRAMS

Before the newborn and mother are discharged from the birthing unit, inform the parents about **newborn screening tests** and tell them when to return to the birthing center or clinic if further tests are needed. Newborn screening tests include the following:

- Blood spot screening, which allows for diagnosis of many disorders that might otherwise go unidentified and untreated in children. The number of disorders screened differs slightly from state to state.
- Hearing screening
- Hyperbilirubinemia screening
- Critical congenital heart disease screening

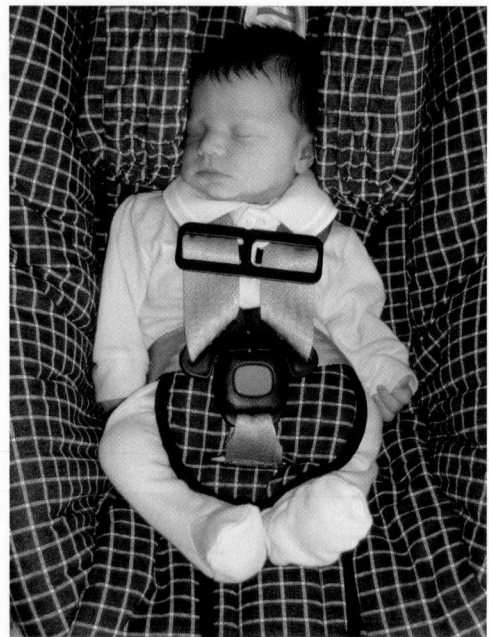

Figure 25–36 An infant car restraint such as this one should be used from birth to about 24 months of age.

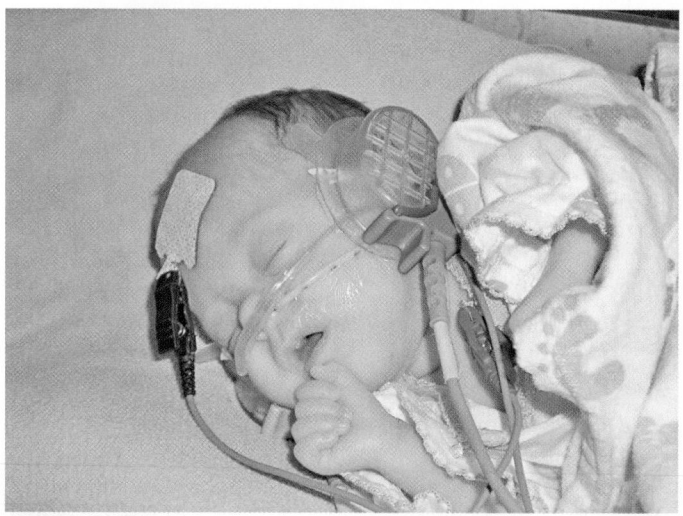

Figure 25–37 Newborn hearing screen.

SOURCE: Vanessa Howell, RN, MSN.

For information on the specific disorders tested for in your state, you can visit the website of the National Newborn Screening and Genetic Resource Center (Genetics Home Reference, 2015). It is the responsibility of the nursing staff to see that these screening tests are completed by the time of discharge and that the parents understand the need for follow-up tests where indicated (AAP, 2011).

Hearing loss is found in 1 to 3 per 1000 babies in the normal newborn population (CDC, 2015a). Hearing screenings before discharge are now conducted in all 50 states. The recommended initial newborn hearing screening should be accomplished before discharge from the birthing unit with appropriate follow-up if the newborn fails to pass the initial screen in all hospitals providing obstetric services.

Sometimes newborns fail to pass these tests for reasons other than hearing loss. Amniotic fluid in the ear canals is a frequent cause of suboptimal test results. In these cases, babies are retested in a week or two. The current goal is to screen all babies by 1 month of age, confirm hearing loss with audiologic examination by 3 months of age, and treat with comprehensive early intervention services (CDC, 2015a). Typically, screening programs use a two-stage screening approach (otoacoustic emissions [OAE] repeated twice, OAE followed by auditory brainstem response [ABR], or automated ABR repeated twice). Families need to be educated about appropriate interpretation of screening test results and appropriate steps for follow-up (Figure 25–37) (Healthy Children, 2015d).

Immunization programs against the hepatitis B virus during the newborn period and infancy are in place in many states, at least 20 countries, and high-incidence areas such as American Samoa. Universal vaccination of babies is recommended. Parents need to be advised whether their birthing center provides newborn hepatitis vaccination so that an adequate follow-up program can be set in motion (AAP & ACOG, 2012). Recombinant hepatitis B vaccine (Engerix-B, Recombivax HB) is used as a prophylactic treatment against all subtypes of hepatitis B virus. It provides passive immunization for newborns of HBsAg-negative and HBsAg-positive mothers. Hepatitis B can be transmitted across the placenta, but most newborns are infected during birth.

The vaccine is produced from baker's yeast and plasmid containing the HBsAg gene. Hepatitis B (thimerosal-free) vaccine contains more than 95% HBsAg protein and is an inactivated (noninfective) product. Babies of HBsAg-positive mothers should concurrently receive 0.5 mL of hepatitis B immunoglobulin (HBIG) prophylaxis at separate injection sites (CDC, 2015b; Wilson et al., 2015). The dosing schedule is dependent on the mother's status as seen below:

- The first dose of 0.5 mL (10 mcg) is given intramuscularly into the anterolateral thigh within 12 hours of birth for babies born to HBsAg-positive mothers. The second dose of vaccine is given at least 1 month after the first dose and followed by a final dose at least 4 months after the first dose and at least 3 months after the second dose, but not before 6 months of age (CDC, 2015b).

- Babies born to HBsAg-negative mothers receive their first dose of vaccine at birth, the second dose at 1 to 2 months, and the third dose at 6 to 18 months (AAP & ACOG, 2012). Hepatitis B immunoglobulin is administered within 72 hours.

- Babies whose mother's HBsAg status is unknown should receive the same doses of vaccine as babies born to HBsAg-positive mothers.

The only common side effect is soreness at the injection site. Occasionally, there is erythema, swelling, warmth, and induration at the injection site, irritability, or a low-grade fever (37.7°C [99.8°F]). Nursing considerations include:

- The vaccine should be used as supplied. Do not dilute. Shake well.

- Do not inject intravenously or intradermally.

- Monitor for adverse reactions. Monitor temperature closely.

- Have epinephrine available to treat possible allergic reactions.

- Responsiveness to the vaccine is age dependent. Preterm newborns weighing less than 1000 g (2.2 lb) have lower seroconversion rates. Consider delaying the first dose until the newborn is term postconceptual age (PCA) or use a 4-dose schedule.

Teach the family all necessary caregiving methods before discharge. A checklist may be helpful to determine whether the teaching has been completed and to verify the parents' knowledge on leaving the birthing unit (Figure 25–38). Review all areas for understanding or answer outstanding questions with the mother and father, without rushing, and take time to resolve all queries. Any concerns of yours or the parents are noted.

NEWBORN CARE TEACHING CHECKLIST

Please read the *New Baby* booklet and view the film before completing this checklist. In the **Need Teaching** column, check off the areas in which you would like further instruction, advice, or demonstration.

	Need Teaching	Teaching Done	Nurse's Initials/Date
Breastfeeding			
Positioning			
Latching on			
Removing baby from nipple			
Let-down reflex			
Supply and demand concept			
How often and for how long			
Knowing if baby is getting enough			
Supplementing			
Expressing milk by hand			
Going back to work while breastfeeding			
Formula Feeding			
Feeding baby a bottle			
Cleaning bottles and nipples			
Choosing a formula			
Preparing formula			
Demand feeding			
Baby Care			
Positioning baby after feeding			
Burping			
Bathing			
Caring for circumcision/genital/umbilical area			
Taking baby's temperature—when to call the doctor			
Using a bulb syringe			
Elimination—what to expect			
Checking for signs of jaundice			
Caring for skin, rashes, milia			
Comforting crying baby			
Signs that baby is sick			
Positioning in crib (Safe to Sleep)			
Safety			
Baby is choking or gagging—what to do			
Shaken baby syndrome			
Newborn screening tests and immunizations			
Using infant car seat			

Other Concerns:

Language spoken by mother:

_____

Was an interpreter used?

_____

I understand the teaching instructions given on the specified topics and have no further questions.

Nurse's signature(s):

_____

_____
Mother's Signature

_____

Date:_____

_____

Date:_____

Figure 25–38 A newborn care teaching checklist is completed before discharge.

TABLE 25-9 When Parents Should Call Their Healthcare Provider

- Temperature above 38.0°C (100.4°F) axillary or below 36.6°C (97.8°F) axillary
- Continual rise in temperature
- More than one episode of forceful vomiting or frequent vomiting over a 6-hr period
- Refusal of two feedings in a row
- Lethargy (listlessness), difficulty in awakening baby
- Cyanosis (bluish discoloration of skin) with or without a feeding
- Absence of breathing longer than 20 sec
- Inconsolable baby (quieting techniques are not effective) or continuous high-pitched cry
- Discharge or bleeding from umbilical cord, circumcision, or any opening (except vaginal mucus or pseudomenstruation)
- Two consecutive green, watery stools or black stools or increased frequency of stools
- No wet diapers for 18 to 24 hr or fewer than six to eight wet diapers per day after 4 days of age
- Development of eye drainage
- Yellowing of skin (jaundice)

COMMUNITY-BASED NURSING CARE

Discuss with parents ways to meet their newborn's needs, ensure safety, and appreciate the newborn's unique characteristics and behaviors. By assisting parents in establishing links with their community-based healthcare provider, you can get the new family off to a good start. Parents also need to know the signs of illness, how to reach the healthcare provider or after-hours clinic, and the importance of follow-up after discharge (Table 25–9). Parents should also check with their healthcare provider for advice about over-the-counter medications to be kept in the medicine cabinet.

The family should have the healthcare provider's phone number, address, and any specific instructions. Having the birthing unit or nursery phone number is also reassuring to a newborn's family. Encourage them to call with questions. Follow-up calls lend added support by providing another opportunity for parents to have their questions answered.

The follow-up newborn examination should be within 48 hours of discharge. When the family is unable to visit their healthcare provider within that time period, a home visit should be done. The home visit focuses on normal newborn care, assessment for hyperbilirubinemia (jaundice), extreme weight loss, feeding problems, and knowledge related to newborn care and feeding within the family unit.

Routine well-baby visits should be scheduled with the clinic or healthcare provider. Regardless of the type of follow-up services available in the community, you must contribute to the newborn's health by stressing the importance of routine care and by helping families who have no follow-up plans to connect to local resources for care. (For a detailed discussion of home care, see Chapter 29.)

Evaluation

When evaluating the nursing care provided in preparation for discharge, the following outcomes may be anticipated:

- The parents demonstrate safe techniques in caring for their newborn.
- Parents verbalize developmentally appropriate behavioral expectations of their newborn and knowledge of community-based newborn follow-up care.

Focus Your Study

- The overall goal of newborn nursing care is to provide comprehensive care while promoting the establishment of a well-functioning family unit.
- The period immediately following birth, during which adaptation to extrauterine life occurs, requires close monitoring to identify any deviations from normal.
- Nursing goals during the first hours after birth (admission and transitional period) are to maintain a clear airway and stable vital signs, maintain a neutral thermal environment, prevent hemorrhage and infection, early assessment of neonatal distress, initiate oral feedings, and facilitate attachment.
- The newborn is routinely given prophylactic vitamin K to prevent possible hemorrhagic disease of the newborn.
- Prophylactic eye treatment for *Neisseria gonorrhoeae* is legally required on all newborns.
- Nursing goals in daily newborn care include maintaining cardiopulmonary function, maintaining a neutral thermal environment, promoting adequate hydration and nutrition, preventing complications, promoting safety, and enhancing attachment and family knowledge of child care.
- Following a circumcision, the newborn must be observed closely for signs of bleeding, inability to void, and signs of infection.
- A weight loss of more than 10% is excessive and requires an evaluation and follow-up. Newborns should be back to their birth weight by 10 to 14 days of age. Generally, infants double their birth weight by 5 months, triple their birth weight by 1 year of age, and quadruple their birth weight by 2 years.
- The American Academy of Pediatrics (AAP) recommends exclusive breastfeeding for the first 6 months and continued breastfeeding until the infant is 1 year old or older.
- Human milk has immunologic and nutritional properties that make it the optimal food for the first year of life.

- Mature human milk and standard commercially prepared formulas provide 20 kcal/oz.

- Neither cow's milk nor soy milk should be given to babies before 1 year of age. The use of skim milk or low-fat cow's milk is not recommended for children under 2 years old.

- Most maternal medications are transmitted through human milk to some degree, but few are actually contraindicated.

- Signs indicating a newborn's readiness to feed include hand-to-mouth movements, rooting, smacking, fussing, and crying (a late-feeding cue).

- The nurse must be sensitive to cultural beliefs and values of the family and be aware of cultural variation regarding infant feeding practices.

- Breastfeeding mothers should be taught to use proper positioning and latch-on technique. The mother should be advised to alternate feeding positions periodically to promote efficient drainage of all the ducts in the breast.

- During the first few days after birth, the minimum output expectations for an exclusively breastfeeding newborn are the following: one wet/one stool on day 1; two wets/two stools on day 2; three wets/three to four stools on day 3; four wets/three to four stools on day 4; five wets/three to four stools on day 5. Thereafter, an exclusively breastfeeding newborn has a minimum of six to eight wet diapers and three to four yellow milk stools each day, generally during the first month of life.

- Newborns' stools start as black and sticky at birth and transition to yellow, curdy, or seedy by day 5, or sooner.

- The formula-feeding mother may need help learning about the types of formulas and how to prepare and store formula. Like the breastfeeding mother, she will benefit from understanding feeding cues and proper technique for feeding her baby.

- Essential daily care includes assessing vital signs, weight, overall color, intake, output, umbilical cord and circumcision, newborn nutrition, parent education, and attachment.

- Individual birthing units should practice safety measures to prevent abductions and provide information to parents regarding their role in this area and in general newborn safety measures.

- Signs of illness in newborns include temperature above 38.0°C (100.4°F) axillary or below 36.6°C (97.8°F) axillary, more than one episode of forceful vomiting, refusal of two feedings in a row, lethargy, cyanosis with or without a feeding, and absence of breathing for longer than 20 seconds.

- Newborn blood spot screening may be done on all newborns in the first 1 to 3 days. Hearing screening and critical congenital heart disease screening may be completed before discharge.

Clinical Reasoning in Action

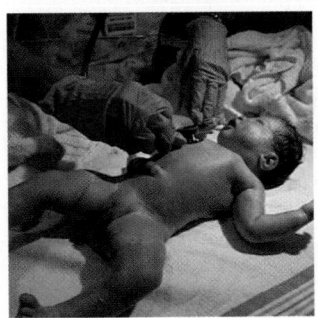

Alice Fine, age 32, G1, now P1001, spontaneously delivers a 7.25-lb baby girl over a median episiotomy. The baby's Apgars are 7 and 9 at 1 and 5 minutes. The baby is suctioned, stimulated, and given free-flow oxygen at birth. As the nurse on duty, you admit baby Fine to the newborn nursery, place her under a radiant heater, and perform a newborn assessment. You obtain the vital signs of temperature 97°F, heart rate 128, respiration 55. A physical examination demonstrates no abnormalities, and you note that there were no significant problems with the pregnancy, the mother's blood type is A+, and she plans to bottle-feed. You monitor the baby until her vital signs are stable and then take her to the mother's room for her first bottle-feeding at 60 minutes old.

1. How would you review measures to promote the safety of the newborn from abduction?

2. How would you explain the technique to suction the newborn with a bulb syringe?

3. Describe the care of the newborn's cord.

4. How would you review bottle-feeding with the mother?

References

American Academy of Pediatrics (AAP). (2011). Strategies for implementing screening for critical congenital heart disease. *Pediatrics, 2011*(128), e1259. doi:10.1542/peds.2011-1317

American Academy of Pediatrics (AAP). (2012a). Circumcision policy statement. *Pediatrics, 130*, 585. doi:10.1542/peds.2012-1989

American Academy of Pediatrics (AAP). (2012b). Policy statement: Breastfeeding and the use of human milk. *Pediatrics, 129(3)*, e827–841.

American Academy of Pediatrics (AAP) Committee on Fetus and Newborn & American College of Obstetricians and Gynecologists (ACOG) Committee on Obstetrics. (2012). *Guidelines for perinatal care* (7th ed.). Evanston, IL: Author.

Association of Women's Health, Obstetrics and Neonatal Nurses (AWHONN). (2013). *Neonatal skin care: Evidence based clinical practice guideline* (3rd ed.). Washington, DC: AWHONN.

Baby-Friendly Hospital Initiative USA. (2014). *Implementing the UNICEF/WHO baby-friendly hospital initiative in the U.S.* Retrieved from https://www.babyfriendlyusa.org/find-facilities

Blackburn, S. T. (2013). *Maternal, fetal, & neonatal physiology: A clinical perspective* (4th ed.). St. Louis, MO: Saunders.

Briggs, G. G., & Freeman, R. K. (2015). *Drugs in pregnancy and lactation: A reference guide to fetal and neonatal risk* (10th ed.). Philadelphia, PA: Wolters Kluwer Health

Callister, L. C. (2014). Integrating cultural beliefs and practices when caring for childbearing women and families. In K. R. Simpson & P. A. Creehan (Eds.), *Perinatal nursing* (3rd ed., pp. 29–57). Philadelphia, PA: Lippincott Williams & Wilkins.

Centers for Disease Control and Prevention (CDC) (2015a). *Hearing loss in newborn: Screening and diagnosis.* Retrieved from http://www.cdc.gov/ncbddd/hearingloss/screening.html

Centers for Disease Control and Prevention (CDC) Advisory Committee on Immunization Practices. (2015b). *Recommended childhood and adolescent immunization schedule, United States 2015.* Retrieved from http://www.cdc.gov/vaccines/schedules/hcp/child-adolescent.html

Cloherty, J. P., Eichenwald, E. C., Hansen, A. R., & Stark, A. R. (2012). *Manual for neonatal care* (7th ed.). Philadelphia, PA: Lippincott Williams & Wilkins.

D'Avanzo, C. E., & Geissler, E. M. (2008). *Pocket guide to cultural assessment* (4th ed.). St. Louis, MO: Mosby.

Flannery, V. (2014). Increasing breastfeeding rates: Evidence-based strategies. *International Journal of Childbirth Education, 29*(4), 59–62.

Fraser, D. (2014). Newborn adaptation to extrauterine life. In K. R. Simpson & P. A. Creehan (Eds.). *Perinatal Nursing* (4th ed., pp. 581–596). Philadelphia, PA: Lippincott Williams & Wilkins.

Genetics Home Reference. (2015). *Newborn screening.* Retrieved from http://www.ghr.nlm.nih.gov/nbs

Hale, T. W. (2014). *Medications and mothers' milk* (16th ed.). Amarillo, TX: Pharmasoft.

Healthy Children. (2015a). *Benefits of breastfeeding for mom.* Retrieved from http://www.healthychildren.org/English/ages-stages/baby/breastfeeding/Pages/Benefits-of-Breastfeeding-for-Mom.aspx

Healthy Children. (2015b). *Breastfeeding benefits your baby's immune system.* Retrieved from http://www.healthychildren.org/English/ages-stages/baby/breastfeeding/Pages/Breastfeeding-Benefits-Your-Baby%27s-Immune-System.aspx

Healthy Children. (2015c). *Car seats: Information for families for 2014.* Retrieved from http://www.healthychildren.org/English/news/Pages/AAP-Updates-Recommendations-on-Car-Seats.aspx http://www.healthychildren.org/English/news/Pages/AAP-Updates-Recommendations-on-Car-Seats.aspx

Healthy Children. (2015d). *Purpose of newborn hearing screening.* Retrieved from http://www.healthychildren.org/English/ages-stages/baby/Pages/Purpose-of-Newborn-Hearing-Screening.aspx

Healthy Children). (2015e). *Reduce the risk of SIDS.* Retrieved from http://www.healthychildren.org/English/ages-stages/baby/sleep/Pages/Preventing-SIDS.aspx

Healthy Children (2015f). *Sleep position: Why back is best.* Retrieved from http://www.healthychildren.org/English/ages-stages/baby/sleep/Pages/Sleep-Position-Why-Back-is-Best.aspx

Healthy Children. (2015g). *Where we stand: Circumcision.* Retrieved from http://www.healthychildren.org/English/ages-stages/prenatal/decisions-to-make/Pages/Where-We-Stand-Circumcision.aspx

Human Milk Banking Association of North America (HMBANA). (2011). *Best practice for expressing, storing and handling human milk in hospitals, homes and child care settings* (3rd ed.). Raleigh, NC: Author.

Janke, J. (2014). Newborn nutrition. In K. R. Simpson & P. A. Creehan (Eds.), *Perinatal nursing* (4th ed., pp. 626–661). Philadelphia, PA: Lippincott Williams & Wilkins.

Jones, F. (2016). Donor milk banking. In J. Riordan and K. Wambach (Eds.), *Breastfeeding and human lactation* (5th ed. pp. 523–548). Boston, MA: Jones & Bartlett.

Klaus, M., & Klaus, P. (1985). *The amazing newborn.* Menlo Park, CA: Addison-Wesley.

La Leche League International. (2013). *How do I position my baby to breastfeed?* Retrieved from http://www.llli.org/faq/positioning.html

Lipson, J. G., & Dibble, S. L. (2008). *Culture & clinical care* (7th ed.). San Francisco, CA: The Regents, University of California.

Marcewicz, L. (2014). Late vitamin K deficiency bleeding in infants: Are we seeing a re-emergence? *Medscape.* Jan. 27, 2014.

Mead-Johnson Nutritionals. (2012). *Pediatric products handbook.* New York, NY: Bristol-Myers Squibb Company. Retrieved from http://www.meadjohnson.com/pediatrics/us-en/sites/hcp-usa/files/LB6-complete-5-12.pdf

Mercer, A. M., Teasley, S. L., Hopkinson, J., McPherson, D. M., Simon, S. D., & Hall, R. T. (2010). Evaluation of a breastfeeding assessment score in a diverse population. *Journal of Human Lactation, 26*(1), 42–48.

National Conference of State Legislatures. (2015). *Breastfeeding laws.* Retrieved from http://www.ncsl.org/GoogleResults.aspx?q=breastfeeding%20law

Ott, B. B., Al-Khadhuri, J., & Al-Junaibi, S. (2003). Preventing ethical dilemmas: Understanding Islamic health care practices. *Pediatric Nursing, 29*(3), 227–230.

Purnell, L. P. (2013). *Transcultural health care: A culturally competent approach* (4th ed.). Philadelphia, PA: F. A. Davis

Riordan, J. (2016). The biological specificity of breastmilk. In J. Riordan and K. Wambach (Eds.), *Breastfeeding and human lactation* (5th ed. pp. 121–169). Boston, MA: Jones & Bartlett.

Sachs, H. C., & American Academy of Pediatrics (AAP) Committee on Drugs. (2013). Transfer of drugs and therapeutics into human breast milk: An update on selected topics. *Pediatrics, 132*(3), e796–809.

Smith, C. K. (2009). Some traditional umbilical cord practices cord care practices in developing countries. Retrieved from www.midwiferytoday.com

Spong, C. Y. (2013). Defining "term" pregnancy: Recommendations from the defining " term" pregnancy workgroup. J*ournal of the American Medical Association, 309,* 2445–2446.

U.S. Breastfeeding Committee. (2011). *Healthy People 2020: Breastfeeding objectives.* Retrieved from http://www.usbreastfeeding.org/LegislationPolicy/FederalPolicies/HealthyPeople2020BreastfeedingObjectives/tabid/120/Default.aspx

U.S. Department of Labor. (2011). *Section 7(r) of the Fair Labor Standards Act—Break Time for Nursing Mothers Provision.* Retrieved from http://www.dol.gov/whd/nursingmothers/Sec7rFLSA_btnm.htm

U.S. Food and Drug Administration (FDA). (2013). *Bisphenol A (BPA).* Retrieved from http://www.niehs.nih.gov/health/topics/agents/sya-bpa/index.cfm

Walker, M. (2016). Breast pumps and other technologies. In J. Riordan and K. Wambach (Eds.), *Breastfeeding and human lactation* (5th ed. pp. 419–466). Boston, MA: Jones & Bartlett

Wambach, K. (2016).The cultural context of breastfeeding. In J. Riordan and K. Wambach (Eds.), *Breastfeeding and human lactation* (5th ed. pp. 895–913). Boston, MA: Jones & Bartlett.

Wilson, B. A., Shannon, M. T., & Shields, K. M. (2015). *Pearson nurse's drug guide 2015.* Upper Saddle River, NJ: Pearson Education.

Woodring, B. C., & Andrews, M. M. (2012). Transcultural perspectives in the nursing care of children and adolescents. In M. M. Andrews & J. S. Boyle (Eds.), *Transcultural concepts in nursing care* (6th ed., pp. 123–156). Philadelphia, PA: Lippincott.

World Health Organization (WHO). (2008). Male *circumcision information package.* Retrieved from http://www.who.int/hiv/pub/malecircumcision/infopack/en/index.html

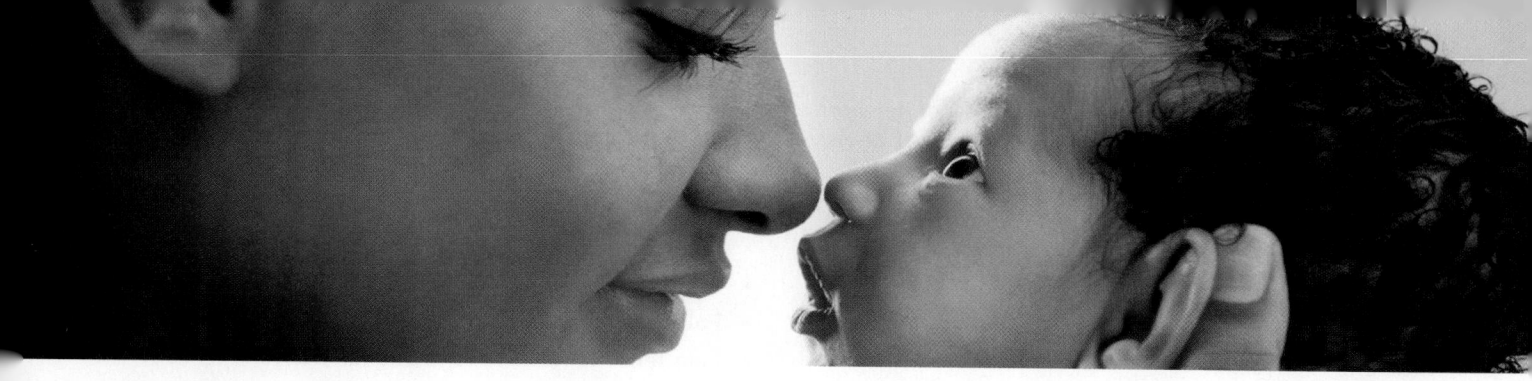

Chapter 26

The Newborn at Risk: Conditions Present at Birth

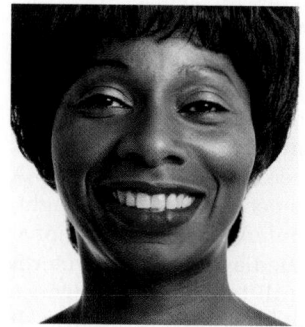

Digital Vision/Getty Images

There is an initial flurry of activity when my baby is taken into the NICU. Now my entire universe, everything that I am, constricts down to focus on our little one. She hardly dents this world, a withery face that shows a kind of infinitely pained acceptance, breath and heartbeat almost nothing, and a pose that moves to rest, resisting nothing. I look at my small daughter with eyes naked with amazement and unsure joy.

—Jontelle, 42

▽ Learning Outcomes

26.1 Explain the factors present at birth that indicate an at-risk newborn.

26.2 Compare the underlying etiologies of the physiologic complications of small-for-gestational-age (SGA) newborns and preterm appropriate-for-gestational-age (Pr AGA) newborns and the nursing management for each.

26.3 Explain the impact of maternal diabetes mellitus on the newborn.

26.4 Compare the characteristics and potential complications that influence nursing management of the postterm newborn and the newborn with postmaturity syndrome.

26.5 Discuss the physiologic and behavioral characteristics of the preterm newborn that predispose each body system to various complications and

that are used in developing a plan of care that includes nutritional management.

26.6 Summarize the nursing assessments of and initial interventions for a newborn with selected congenital anomalies.

26.7 Explain the special care needed by an alcohol- or drug-exposed newborn.

26.8 Relate the consequences of maternal HIV/AIDS to the nursing management of newborns at risk for HIV/AIDS in the neonatal period and the issues for their caregivers.

26.9 Identify the physical examination findings during the early newborn period that would make the nurse suspect a congenital cardiac defect or congestive heart failure.

Many levels of nursery care have evolved in response to increasing knowledge about at-risk newborns. Along with the newborn's parents, the nurse is an important caregiver in all these settings. As a member of the collaborative healthcare team, the nurse is a technically competent professional who contributes the high-touch human care necessary in the high-tech perinatal environment.

In addition to the availability of a high level of newborn care, various other factors influence the outcome of at-risk newborns, including the following:

- Birth weight
- Gestational age
- Intrauterine growth pattern
- Type and length of newborn illness
- Environmental factors
- Maternal factors
- Maternal–newborn separation

Identification of At-Risk Newborns

An at-risk newborn is one susceptible to illness (morbidity) or even death (mortality) because of dysmaturity, immaturity, physical disorders, or complications during or after birth. In most cases, the newborn is the product of a pregnancy involving one or more predictable risk factors, including the following:

- Low socioeconomic level of the mother
- Limited access to health care or no prenatal care
- Exposure to environmental dangers, such as toxic chemicals and illicit drugs
- Preexisting maternal conditions such as heart disease, diabetes, hypertension, hyperthyroidism, and renal disease
- Maternal factors such as age and parity
- Medical conditions related to pregnancy and their associated complications
- Pregnancy complications such as abruptio placentae, placenta previa, oligohydramnios, preterm labor, premature rupture of membranes, preeclampsia, and uterine rupture.

Various risk factors and their specific effects on the pregnancy outcome are listed in Table 9–1. Because these factors and the perinatal risks associated with them are known, the birth of at-risk newborns can often be anticipated. The pregnancy can be closely monitored, treatment can be started as necessary, and arrangements can be made for birth to occur at a facility with appropriate resources to care for both mother and baby.

Whether or not prenatal assessment indicates that the fetus is at risk, the course of labor and birth and the baby's ability to withstand the stress of labor cannot be predicted. Thus, the nurse's use of electronic fetal heart monitoring or fetal heart auscultation by Doppler plays a significant role in detecting stress or distress in the fetus. Immediately after birth the Apgar score is a helpful tool for identifying the at-risk newborn, but it is not the only indicator of possible long-term outcomes.

The newborn classification and neonatal mortality risk chart is another useful tool for identifying newborns at risk. Before this classification tool was developed, birth weight of less than 2500 g (5.5 lb) was the sole criterion for determining immaturity. Clinicians then recognized that a newborn could weigh more than 2500 g and still be immature. Conversely, a newborn weighing less than 2500 g might be functionally at term or beyond. Thus birth weight and gestational age together are now the criteria used to assess neonatal maturity and mortality risk.

According to the newborn classification and neonatal mortality risk chart, gestation (postmenstrual age) is divided as follows (American College of Obstetricians and Gynecologists [ACOG] & Society for Maternal-Fetal Medicine [SMFM], 2013; Spong, 2013):

- Preterm: less than or equal to 36 weeks, 6 days
- Late preterm: 34 weeks, 0 days to 36 weeks, 6 days
- Early Term: 37 weeks, 0 days through 38 weeks, 6 days
- Full Term: 39 weeks, 0 days through 40 weeks, 6 days
- Late Term: 41 weeks, 0 days through 6 days
- Postterm: 42 weeks, 0 days and beyond

Late preterm is a new classification that refers to subgroups of newborns between 34 weeks, 0 days' and 36 weeks, 6 days' gestation. Late-preterm newborns have demonstrated increased incidences of morbidity and length of stay when compared to full-term babies (Cloherty, Eichenwald, Hansen, et al., 2012). (See Chapter 29 for a discussion of the long-term needs of late-preterm newborns.) Morbidities associated with prematurity continue into early term gestation and are compounded by socioeconomic status (Ruth, Roos, Hildes-Ripstein, et al., 2013).

Large-for-gestational-age (LGA) newborns are those who plot above the 90th percentile curve on intrauterine growth curves. Appropriate-for-gestational-age (AGA) newborns are those that plot between the 10th percentile and 90th percentile growth curves. **Small-for-gestational-age (SGA)** newborns are those that plot below the 10th percentile growth curve. A newborn is assigned to a category depending on birth weight, length, occipital–frontal head circumference, and gestational age. For example, a newborn classified as *Pr SGA* is preterm and small-for-gestational-age. The full-term newborn whose weight is appropriate for gestational age is classified *F AGA*. It is important to note that intrauterine growth charts are influenced by altitude and the ethnicity of the newborn population used to create the chart. Also, the assigned newborn classification may vary according to the intrauterine growth curve chart used; therefore, the chart used should correlate with the characteristics of the patient population.

Neonatal mortality risk is the baby's chance of death within the newborn period—that is, within the first 28 days of life. Seventy-five percent of all neonatal deaths occur within the first week, with the highest rates occurring during the first day of life. The neonatal mortality risk decreases as both gestational age and birth weight increase. Newborns who are Pr SGA have the highest neonatal mortality risk. The previously high mortality rates for LGA newborns have decreased at most perinatal centers because of improved management of diabetes in pregnancy and recognition of potential complications of LGA newborns.

Neonatal morbidity can be anticipated based on birth weight and gestational age. The neonatal morbidity by birth weight and gestational age tool assists in determining the needs of particular newborns for special observation and care. For example, a newborn of 2000 g (4.4 lb) at 40 weeks' gestation should be carefully assessed for evidence of neonatal distress, hypoglycemia, congenital anomalies, congenital infection, and polycythemia.

Identifying the nursing care needs of the at-risk newborn depends on minute-to-minute observations of the changes in the newborn's physiologic status. The organization of nursing care must be directed toward the following:

- Decreasing physiologically stressful situations
- Observing constantly for subtle signs of change in clinical condition
- Interpreting laboratory data and coordinating interventions

- Conserving the newborn's energy for healing and growth
- Providing for developmental stimulation and maintenance of sleep cycles
- Assisting the family in developing attachment behaviors
- Involving the family in planning and providing care

Care of the Small-for-Gestational-Age/Intrauterine Growth Restriction Newborn

Currently, newborns are considered small-for-gestational-age (SGA) when they are less than the 10th percentile for birth weight; very small-for-gestational-age is when they are 2 standard deviations below the population norm or less than the third percentile (Rozance & Rosenberg, 2012) (Figure 26–1). When possible, the birth weight charts that are used to assign the SGA classification to a newborn should be based on the local population into which the newborn is born. A SGA newborn may be preterm, term, or postterm. An undergrown newborn may be also said to have **intrauterine growth restriction (IUGR)**, which describes the pregnancy circumstance of advanced gestation and decreased growth potential of the fetus. This classification of abnormal growth is also enhanced by looking at growth potential by adjusting birth weight reference limits for first-trimester maternal height, birth order, and fetal neonatal sex.

SGA newborns are commonly seen with mothers who smoke or have high blood pressure, causing these babies to have an increased incidence of perinatal asphyxia and perinatal mortality when compared with AGA newborns (ACOG, 2013). The incidence of polycythemia and hypoglycemia is also higher in this group of newborns.

Factors Contributing to IUGR

IUGR may be caused by maternal, placental, or fetal factors and may not be apparent antenatally. Intrauterine growth is linear (follows expected growth line) in the normal pregnancy from approximately 28 to 38 weeks' gestation. After 38 weeks, growth is variable, depending on the growth potential of the fetus and placental function. The most common causes of growth restriction are as follows:

- *Maternal factors.* Primiparity, grand multiparity, multiple-gestation pregnancy (twins and higher-order multiples), lack of prenatal care, age extremes (less than 16 years or more than 40 years), and low socioeconomic status (which can result in inadequate health care, inadequate education, and inadequate living conditions) affect IUGR (Cloherty et al., 2012). Before the third trimester, the nutritional supply to the fetus far exceeds its needs. Only in the third trimester are maternal malnutrition and drug abuse limiting factors in fetal growth.

- *Maternal disease.* Maternal heart disease, substance abuse (drugs, tobacco, alcohol), sickle cell disease, phenylketonuria (PKU), lupus erythematosus, and asymptomatic pyelonephritis are associated with SGA and IUGR. Complications associated with preeclampsia, chronic hypertensive vascular disease, and advanced diabetes mellitus can diminish blood flow to the uterus, thereby decreasing oxygen delivery to the fetus and minimizing organ growth.

- *Environmental factors.* High altitude, exposure to x-rays, excessive exercise, work-related exposure to toxins, hyperthermia, and maternal use of drugs that have teratogenic effects, such as nicotine, alcohol, antimetabolites, marijuana, anticonvulsants, opioids, amphetamines, heroin, and cocaine, affect fetal growth (Cloherty et al., 2012; Mari & Tate, 2013; Resnik & Creasy, 2014).

- *Placental factors.* Placental conditions such as small placenta, infarcted areas, single umbilical artery, placenta previa, reverse end-diastolic blood flow, or inherited coagulopathy disease causing thrombosis may affect circulation to the fetus, which becomes more deficient with increasing gestational age (Geary, 2013).

- *Fetal factors.* Congenital infections such as TORCH infections (*t*oxoplasmosis, *o*ther agents, *r*ubella, *c*ytomegalovirus, *h*erpes simplex virus), syphilis congenital malformations, discordant twins, sex of the fetus (female fetuses tend to be smaller), chromosomal syndromes (trisomies 13, 18, 21), two-vessel umbilical cord, and inborn errors of metabolism can predispose a fetus to fetal growth disturbances.

Identifying fetuses with IUGR is the first step in detecting common disorders associated with affected newborns. The perinatal history of maternal conditions, early dating of pregnancy by first-trimester ultrasound measurements, antepartum testing (non-stress test, contraction stress test, biophysical profile; for more information on these tests, see Chapter 13), Doppler velocimetry of placenta, gestational age assessment, and the physical and neurologic assessment of the newborn are important methods (Cloherty et al., 2012; Mari & Tate, 2013).

Clinical Tip

In assessing a growth-restricted newborn resulting from unexplained maternal etiology (e.g., hypertension, placental insufficiency), an in utero viral infection may be the cause.

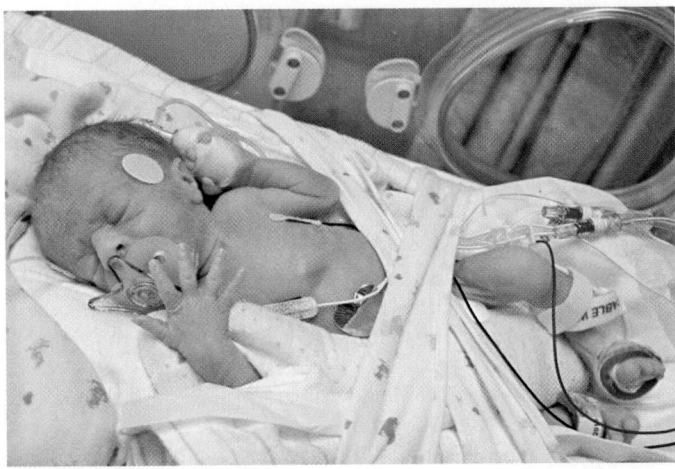

Figure 26–1 **Thirty-one-week gestational age, SGA 2-day-old baby girl.**

SOURCE: Carol Harrigan, RN, MSN, NNP-BC.

Patterns of IUGR

Intrauterine growth occurs by an increase in both cell number and cell size. If insult occurs early during the critical period of organ development in the fetus, fewer new cells are formed, organs are small, and organ weight is subnormal. In contrast, growth failure that begins later in pregnancy does not affect the total number of cells, only their size. The organs are normal, but their size is diminished. There are two clinical pictures of IUGR newborns, symmetric and asymmetric.

- *Symmetric (proportional) IUGR.* Caused by long-term maternal conditions (such as chronic hypertension, severe malnutrition, chronic intrauterine viral infection, substance abuse [drugs, alcohol, tobacco], anemia) or fetal genetic abnormalities (Resnik & Creasy, 2014). Symmetric IUGR can be noted by ultrasound in the first half of the second trimester. In symmetric IUGR there is chronic, prolonged restriction of growth in the size of organs, weight, length, and, especially, head circumference.

- *Asymmetric (disproportional) IUGR.* Associated with an acute compromise of uteroplacental blood flow. Some associated causes are placental infarcts, preeclampsia, and poor weight gain in pregnancy. The growth restriction is usually not evident before the third trimester because, although weight is decreased, length and head circumference (used as a growth indicator) remain appropriate for that gestational age. In these babies, head growth is usually spared. After 36 weeks' gestation, the abdominal circumference of a normal fetus becomes larger than the head circumference. In asymmetric IUGR, the head circumference remains larger than the abdominal circumference. Thus measuring only the biparietal diameter on ultrasound will not reveal asymmetric IUGR. An early indicator of asymmetric IUGR is a decrease in the growth rate of the abdominal circumference, reflecting subnormal liver growth, a reduction in glycogen stores, and a scarcity of subcutaneous fat (Gleason & Devaskar, 2012). Birth weight is below the 10th percentile, whereas head circumference and/or length may be between the 10th and 90th percentiles. Asymmetric SGA newborns related to IUGR are particularly at risk for asphyxia, pulmonary hemorrhage, hypocalcemia, and hypoglycemia.

Despite growth restriction, physiologic maturity develops according to gestational age. The term SGA newborn's chances for survival are better than those of the preterm AGA newborn because of organ maturity, although this newborn still faces many potential difficulties.

Common Complications of the SGA/IUGR Newborn

The complications occurring most frequently in the SGA/IUGR newborn include the following:

- *Fetal hypoxia (impaired oxygenation).* The SGA/IUGR newborn suffers chronically lower-than-normal oxygen levels in utero, which leaves little reserve to withstand the demands of normal labor and birth. Thus perinatal asphyxia and its potential systemic problems can occur. Cesarean birth may be necessary because of worsening fetal compromise and intolerance to labor.

- *Aspiration syndrome.* In utero hypoxia can cause the fetus to gasp during birth, resulting in aspiration of amniotic fluid into the lower airways. It can also lead to relaxation of the anal sphincter and passage of meconium. This may result in aspiration of the meconium in utero or with the first breaths after birth.

- *Hypothermia.* Diminished subcutaneous fat (used for survival in utero), depletion of brown fat in utero, and a large surface area decrease the IUGR newborn's ability to conserve heat. The flexed position assumed by the term SGA newborn diminishes the effect of surface area.

- *Hypoglycemia.* An increase in metabolic rate in response to heat loss and poor hepatic glycogen stores causes hypoglycemia. In addition, the newborn is compromised by inadequate supplies of enzymes to activate gluconeogenesis (conversion of nonglucogen sources such as fatty acids and proteins to glucose). Excessive sensitivity to insulin resulting in hyperinsulinism may contribute to hypoglycemia.

- *Polycythemia.* The number of red blood cells is increased (central hematocrit greater than 65%) in the SGA/IUGR newborn. This finding is considered a physiologic response to in utero chronic hypoxic stress. Polycythemia may contribute to hypoglycemia and hyperviscosity.

Newborns who have significant SGA/IUGR tend to have a poor prognosis, especially when born before 37 weeks' gestation. Factors contributing to poor outcome include the following:

- *Congenital malformations.* Congenital malformations occur in 5% of SGA/IUGR newborns (Cloherty et al., 2012). The more severe the IUGR, the greater the chance for malformation as a result of impaired mitotic activity and cellular hypoplasia.

- *Intrauterine infections.* When fetuses are exposed to intrauterine infections such as rubella and cytomegalovirus (CMV), they are profoundly affected by direct invasion of the brain and other vital organs by the offending virus.

- *Continued growth difficulties.* SGA newborns tend to be shorter than newborns of the same gestational age. Asymmetric IUGR newborns can be expected to catch up in weight and approach their inherited growth potential when given an optimal environment.

- *Cognitive difficulties.* Often, SGA/IUGR newborns can exhibit subsequent learning disabilities. The disabilities are characterized by attention deficit hyperactivity disorder (ADHD), attention deficit disorder (ADD), and poor fine motor coordination (writing and drawing) (Glomella, 2013).

CLINICAL THERAPY
The goal of medical therapy for SGA/IUGR newborns is early recognition and implementation of the medical management of potential problems.

Nursing Management
For the SGA/IUGR Newborn

Nursing Assessment and Diagnosis
The nurse is responsible for assessing gestational age and identifying signs of potential complications associated with SGA newborns. All body parts of the symmetric IUGR baby are in proportion (the head does not appear overly large or excessively long in relation to the other body parts), but they are below normal size for the baby's gestational age. These newborns are generally vigorous.

The asymmetric IUGR newborn appears long, thin, and emaciated, with loss of subcutaneous fat tissue and muscle mass. The baby may have loose skinfolds; dry, desquamating skin; and a thin and often meconium-stained cord. The head appears relatively large (although it approaches normal size) because the chest size and abdominal girth are decreased. The baby may have a vigorous cry and appear alert and wide-eyed.

Nursing diagnoses that may apply to the SGA newborn include those listed in *Nursing Care Plan: The Small-for-Gestational-Age Newborn* and the following (NANDA-I © 2014):

- *Hypothermia* related to decreased subcutaneous fat
- *Nutrition, Imbalanced: Less than Body Requirements* related to SGA's increased metabolic rate
- *Tissue Perfusion: Peripheral, Ineffective,* related to polycythemia and increased blood viscosity
- *Parenting, Risk for Impaired,* related to prolonged separation of newborn from parents secondary to illness and prolonged hospital stay

Planning and Implementation

HOSPITAL-BASED NURSING CARE

Hypoglycemia, the most common metabolic complication of SGA/IUGR, produces such sequelae as CNS abnormalities and neurodevelopmental disabilities (intellectual disability). Conditions such as asphyxia, hyperviscosity, and cold stress may also affect the baby's outcome. Meticulous attention to physiologic parameters is essential for immediate nursing management and reduction of long-term disorders. (See *Nursing Care Plan: The Small-for-Gestational-Age Newborn.*)

COMMUNITY-BASED NURSING CARE

The long-term needs of the SGA/IUGR newborn include careful follow-up evaluation of patterns of growth and possible disabilities that may later interfere with learning or motor functioning. Long-term follow-up care is essential for infants with congenital malformations, congenital infections, and obvious sequelae from physiologic problems. Parents of the SGA/IUGR newborn need support, because a positive atmosphere can enhance the baby's growth potential and the child's ultimate outcome.

Evaluation

Expected outcomes of nursing care include the following:

- The SGA/IUGR newborn is free from respiratory compromise.
- The SGA/IUGR newborn maintains a stable temperature.
- The SGA/IUGR newborn is free from hypoglycemic episodes and maintains glucose homeostasis.
- The SGA/IUGR newborn gains weight and takes breast or formula feedings without developing physiologic distress or fatigue.
- The parents verbalize their concerns about their baby's health problems and understand the rationale behind management of their newborn.

Care of the Large-for-Gestational-Age (LGA) Newborn

A newborn whose birth weight is at or above the 90th percentile on the intrauterine growth curve (at any week of gestation) is considered large-for-gestational-age (LGA). Some AGA newborns have been incorrectly categorized as LGA because of miscalculation of the date of conception caused by postconceptual bleeding. Careful gestational age assessment is essential to identify the potential needs and problems of these babies.

The best known condition associated with excessive fetal growth is maternal diabetes; however, only a small fraction of large newborns are born to diabetic mothers. The cause of the majority of cases of LGA newborns is unclear, but certain factors or situations have been found to correlate with their birth (Cloherty et al., 2012; Hay, 2012):

- It is estimated that 3% to 10% of all pregnancies are complicated by diabetes, with 60% of these women having gestational diabetes and 33% having insulin-dependent (type 1) diabetes.
- The increased size, called *macrosomia*, of a LGA infant of a diabetic mother (IDM) is directly proportional to high, unstable maternal glucose concentrations.
- Multiparous women have 2 to 3 times the number of LGA babies as primigravidas.
- Hispanic mothers tend to have larger babies.
- Male newborns are typically larger than female newborns.
- Babies with erythroblastosis fetalis, Beckwith-Wiedemann syndrome (a genetic condition associated with macroglossia, omphalocele, and newborn hypoglycemia and hyperinsulinemia), or transposition of the great vessels are usually large.

The increase in the LGA newborn's body size is characteristically proportional, although head circumference and body length are in the upper limits of intrauterine growth. The exception to this rule is the infant of a diabetic mother (IDM), whose body weight is higher, usually greater than 4 kg (9.7 lb), but whose length and head circumference may be in the normal range. Macrosomic newborns have poor motor skills and have difficulty regulating behavioral states. LGA newborns tend to be more difficult to arouse to a quiet alert state.

Common Complications of the LGA Newborn

Complications of the LGA newborn can include the following:

- *Birth trauma caused by cephalopelvic disproportion (CPD).* Often, LGA newborns have a biparietal diameter greater than 10 cm (4 in.) or are associated with a maternal fundal height measurement greater than 42 cm (16 in.) without the presence of polyhydramnios. The major complication of being macrosomic is birth injury to the head, upper body, and nerves following a vaginal birth; other complications include birth asphyxia, shoulder dystocia, fractured clavicles, fractured humerus, brachial plexus palsy, facial paralysis, phrenic nerve palsy, depressed skull fractures, cephalohematoma, and intracranial hemorrhage.
- *Complications of hypoglycemia, polycythemia, and hyperviscosity.* These disorders are most often seen in IDMs, newborns with erythroblastosis fetalis, or newborns with Beckwith-Wiedemann syndrome.

Nursing Management

The perinatal history, in conjunction with ultrasonic measurement of fetal skull (biparietal diameter) and gestational age testing, is important in identifying an at-risk LGA newborn. Essential components of the nursing assessment are monitoring vital signs, screening for hypoglycemia and polycythemia, and observing for signs and symptoms related to birth trauma.

Nursing Care Plan: For the Small-for-Gestational-Age Newborn

1. Nursing Diagnosis: *Gas Exchange, Impaired,* related to amniotic fluid or meconium aspiration (NANDA-I © 2014)

GOAL: The newborn's respiratory rate and effort will be within normal limits, with no periods of apnea or evidence of worsening distress.

INTERVENTION	RATIONALE
• Obtain maternal prenatal, labor, and delivery records.	• Provides information and clues of potential fetal stress that may have occurred during the antepartum and intrapartum period. In addition, the delivery record will provide information concerning the newborn's respiratory status at birth, such as the Apgar score.
• Maintain airway patency through judicious airway suctioning.	• Respiratory distress in small-for-gestational-age (SGA) newborns is due to in utero hypoxia and aspiration of amniotic fluid or meconium-stained fluid.
• Observe for worsening signs of respiratory distress such as generalized cyanosis, increasing retractions, grunting, and nasal flaring (as evidenced by Silverman respiratory index), sustained tachypnea, apnea episodes, inequality of breath sounds, presence of rales and rhonchi.	
• Monitor and maintain adequate axillary body temperature (36.4°–37.2°C [97.5°–99.0°F]) to avoid increased oxygen consumption.	• Temperature elevation may cause metabolic rate and oxygen needs to increase when associated with meconium aspiration.
• Administer supplemental oxygen or other interventions (e.g., high-flow nasal cannula, nasal continuous positive airway pressure [CPAP], intubation with mechanical ventilation) per order for management of symptoms related to respiratory distress. (See Chapter 27 for nursing care and treatment of meconium aspiration and neonate resuscitation.)	• Provides healthcare personnel with information on cardiac and pulmonary status.
• Implement treatment plan for respiratory distress.	
• Monitor glucose levels.	• Respiratory distress increases consumption of glucose.
• *Collaborative:* Obtain blood gas (ABG or CBG) and pulse oximetry parameters, chest x-ray per healthcare provider orders.	
• Monitor newborn's cardiopulmonary status, pulse oximetry readings, and blood gas values.	• Oxygen demands increase with meconium aspiration. Obtaining serial blood gases and chest x-ray will provide medical personnel with baseline information of newborn's respiratory status, and effective medical interventions can be initiated.

EXPECTED OUTCOMES: The newborn will maintain adequate respiratory gas exchange as evidenced by respirations of 30–60/min with pulse oximetry and blood gases within normal limits and will show no signs and symptoms of respiratory distress.

2. Nursing Diagnosis: *Thermoregulation, Ineffective,* secondary to decreased subcutaneous fat (NANDA-I © 2014)

GOAL: The newborn's temperature will be stable and maintained within normal limits.

INTERVENTION	RATIONALE
• Provide neutral thermal environment (NTE) range for newborn based on postnatal weight.	• Neutral thermal environment charts used for preterm newborns are not reliable for weight of SGA newborns.
• Place a skin probe to maintain newborn's temperature at 36.0°–36.5°C (96.8°–97.8°F)	• A neutral thermal environment requires minimal oxygen consumption to maintain a normal core temperature.

- Obtain axillary temperatures and compare with registered skin probe temperature. If discrepancy exists, evaluate potential cause.
- Adjust and monitor incubator or radiant warmer to maintain set skin temperature, using the servo-control mode.
- Minimize heat losses and prevent cold stress by:
  1. Warming and humidifying oxygen without blowing over face to avoid increasing oxygen consumption
  2. Keeping skin dry, especially immediately following delivery
  3. Keeping incubators, radiant warmers, and open cribs away from windows and cold external walls and out of drafts
  4. Avoiding placing newborn on cold surrounding objects such as metal treatment tables, cold x-ray plates, and scales
  5. Using radiant warmers during procedures
  6. Wrapping the baby in blankets and covering the head with a hat.
- Observe for consequences of cold stress: hypoglycemia, hypoxia, lethargy, pallor, metabolic acidosis (for further discussion see Chapter 27)

- Discrepancies between axillary and skin probe monitor temperatures may be due to mechanical causes or the burning of brown fat.

- Physical principles of heat loss effects include:
  1. Evaporation—loss of heat from baby by water evaporation from the skin, especially seen immediately after birth
  2. Convection—loss of heat from baby to the surrounding air
  3. Conduction—loss of heat from baby to the surface in which the baby is in direct contact with
  4. Radiation—loss of heat from baby to cooler, surrounding surfaces (not in direct contact)

- Hypothermia is a potential problem for an SGA newborn because:
  1. SGA newborn has decreased brown fat stores available for thermogenesis, because they have been used in utero for survival.
  2. SGA newborn has poor insulation due to minimal subcutaneous tissues, because they have been used in utero for survival.

EXPECTED OUTCOMES: The newborn will not exhibit consequences of hypothermia as evidenced by skin temperature maintenance of 36.0°–36.5°C (96.8°–97.8°F) and axillary temperature maintenance of 36.4°–37.2°C (97.5°–99.0°F).

---

3. **Nursing Diagnosis:** *Injury, Risk for,* **related to decreased glycogen stores and impaired gluconeogenesis (NANDA-I © 2014)**

GOAL: Newborn will have a normal blood glucose level.

INTERVENTION	RATIONALE
• Monitor blood glucose levels per SGA protocol and report values less than 40 mg/dL. (The exact definition of hypoglycemia varies in the literature; it is best to follow your hospital's guidelines.)	• Combined with depletion of glycogen stores, impaired gluconeogenesis predisposes SGA newborns to profound hypoglycemia within first few hours of life.
• Observe, record, and report symptoms of hypoglycemia: irritability, cyanosis, lethargy, hypotonia, poor feeding, temperature instability, tremors, jitteriness, seizure activity, and apnea.	• Target glucose screen >40 mg/dL prior to routine feedings (Armentrout, 2015).
• Initiate feeding schedule for SGA newborns after screening for blood glucose level and symptoms of hypoglycemia per hospital protocol.	• Frequent monitoring of heel stick glucose assists in identifying decreased glucose levels.
• Provide glucose intake either through early enteral feeding (before 1 hr) and/or by intravenous (IV) per healthcare provider order.	• Provision of glucose through early feedings (begin within first hour of age) assists in maintaining glucose levels within the defined parameters. Always treat symptomatic hypoglycemia with IV glucose.

(See further discussion of hypoglycemia in Chapter 27.)

EXPECTED OUTCOMES: The newborn will not exhibit signs and symptoms of hypoglycemia as evidenced by a euglycemic state and blood glucose greater than 45 mg/dL.

(continued)

Nursing Care Plan: For the Small-for-Gestational-Age Newborn *(continued)*

4. Nursing Diagnosis: *Nutrition, Imbalanced: Less than Body Requirements,* **related to increased metabolic needs in the newborn (NANDA-I © 2014)**

GOAL: Newborn will show positive growth as evidenced by increased serial measurements of weight, length, and occipital–fontal circumference (OFC).

INTERVENTION	RATIONALE
• Assess suck, swallow, and breathe reflexes.	• Sterile water or breast milk may be used to test gag and swallow reflex because it causes fewer pulmonary complications in the presence of gastrointestinal tract abnormalities and/or aspiration of feeding.
• Assess for a nondistended, soft abdomen with active bowel sounds.	• Prevents feeding problems and assists in determining the best method of feeding for newborn and feeding readiness (Jones, 2012).
• Initiate oral feeding per protocol at 1 hr of age; use expressed breast milk, if available, or commercially prepared formula based on hospital protocol.	• SGA newborns require more calories/kg for growth than appropriate-for-gestational-age (AGA) newborns because of increased metabolic activity and oxygen consumption secondary to increased percentage of body weight made up by visceral organs.
	• Human milk is preferred for feeding term, preterm, and sick newborns.
• Supplement oral feedings with IV intake per orders.	• Small, frequent feedings of high-calorie formula are used because of limited gastric capacity and decreased gastric emptying.
• Advance to concentrated formulas that supply more calories in less volume, such as 22 or 24 cal/oz.	
• Promote growth by providing caloric intake of 110–140 cal/kg/day in small amounts.	• Growth is evaluated by increase in weight (about 15–30 g/day), length, and OFC.
• Observe, record, and report signs of feeding intolerance or fatigue occurring during breast-feeding or bottle-feedings.	• Decrease in exhaustion is an important consideration in feeding SGA newborn; gavage tube feeding may need to be initiated.
	• SGA newborns with in utero reversed or absent end-diastolic blood flow are at high risk for developing necrotizing enterocolitis (NEC) (Geary, 2013).
	• Adequate nutritional intake promotes growth and prevents such complications as metabolic catabolism and hypoglycemia.
• Supplement gavage or nipple-feedings with IV therapy per healthcare provider order until oral intake is sufficient to support growth.	• Gavage feedings require less energy expenditure on the part of the newborn.
• Establish a nipple-feeding program that is begun slowly and progresses slowly, such as nipple-feed once per day, nipple-feed once per shift, progressing to nipple-feed every other feeding.	• Cue-based feedings (based on engagement and hunger cues) allows the newborn to become an active participant in the feeding process (Newland, L'Huillier, & Petrey, 2013).
• Initiate breastfeeding attempts when newborn shows readiness.	
• Monitor daily weight with anticipation of small amount of weight loss when nipple-feedings start.	• Nipple-feeding, an active rather than passive intake of nutrition, requires energy expenditure and burning of calories by newborn.
• Weekly OFC and length measurements plotted on growth charts.	• Head circumference is an indicator for brain growth, at the rate of 0.5 cm/week.

EXPECTED OUTCOMES: The newborn will maintain consistent weight gain pattern as evidenced by less than 2%/day weight loss and tolerates enteral feedings.

5. Nursing Diagnosis: *Parenting, Impaired*, related to lack of knowledge of infant care and prolonged separation of newborn and parents secondary to illness and prolonged hospitalization (NANDA-I © 2014)

GOAL: Parents will bond with their baby and have realistic expectations about their baby. Parents are comfortable taking newborn home. They are able to demonstrate normal infant care and assessments of possible complications and know when to return for follow-up.

INTERVENTION	RATIONALE
• Support emotionally the psychologic well-being of family, including positive parent–newborn attachment and sensory stimulation of newborn.	• Parent–newborn attachment begins in first few hours or days following birth. SGA newborns may experience prolonged periods of separation from their parents, which necessitates intervention to ensure parent–newborn attachment.
• Include parents in determining newborn's plan of care and encourage their participation. Encourage parents to visit frequently. Provide opportunities for parents to touch, hold, talk to, and care for baby. Determine the type and amount of appropriate sensory stimulation and implement sensory stimulation program.	• Facilitating kangaroo care allows the baby to be placed skin-to-skin with a parent, which contributes to the overall health and growth of the baby as well as providing crucial involvement by the parents (Ludington-Hoe, 2013).
• Prepare for discharge by instructing parents in such areas as feeding techniques, formula preparation, and breastfeeding; bathing, diapering, and hygiene; temperature monitoring; administration of vitamins; care of complications and preventing exposure to infections; normal elimination patterns, normal reflexes and activity, and how to promote normal growth and development without being overprotective; returning for continued medical care; and availability of community resources if indicated.	• Parents should receive the same postpartum teaching as any parent taking a newborn home. • Parents need to understand the changes to expect in color of the newborn's stool and number of bowel movements plus odor from formula-feeding or breastfeeding to avoid unnecessary concern. SGA newborns usually do not require referral to community agencies such as visiting nurse associations unless there is a specific problem requiring assistance.

EXPECTED OUTCOMES: The parent will demonstrate ability to perform basic infant care tasks as evidenced by exhibiting appropriate attachment behaviors (e.g., talking to and holding the baby) and feeding and bathing the baby.

Address parental concerns about the visual signs of birth trauma and the potential for continuation of the overweight pattern. Help parents learn to arouse and console their newborn and facilitate attachment behaviors. Mothers of LGA newborns with facial or head bruising may be reluctant to interact with their newborns because they fear hurting their babies. The nursing care involved in the complications associated with LGA newborns is similar to the care needed by the IDM and is discussed in the next section.

Care of the Infant of a Diabetic Mother

The **infant of a diabetic mother (IDM)** is considered at risk and requires close observation during the first few hours to the first few days of life. Mothers with severe diabetes or diabetes of long duration associated with vascular complications may give birth to small-for-gestational-age (SGA) or premature newborns. The typical IDM, when the diabetes is poorly controlled or gestational, is large-for-gestational-age (LGA). The newborn is macrosomic, ruddy in color, and has excessive adipose (fat) tissue (Figure 26–2). The umbilical cord is thick and the placenta is large. There is a higher incidence of macrosomic babies born

to certain ethnic groups (Native Americans, Mexican Americans, African Americans, Pacific Islanders).

IDMs have decreased total body water, particularly in the extracellular spaces, and are therefore not edematous. Their excessive weight is because of increased weight of the visceral organs, cardiomegaly (hypertrophy), and increased body fat. The only organ not affected is the brain.

The excessive fetal growth of the IDM is caused by exposure to high levels of maternal glucose, which readily crosses the placenta. The fetus responds to these high glucose levels with increased insulin production and hyperplasia of the pancreatic beta cells. The main action of the insulin is to facilitate the entry of glucose into muscle and fat cells. Once in the cells, glucose is converted to glycogen and stored. Insulin also inhibits the breakdown of fat to free fatty acids, thereby maintaining lipid synthesis; increases the uptake of amino acids; and promotes protein synthesis. Insulin is an important regulator of fetal metabolism and has a "growth hormone" effect that results in increased linear growth. IDMs may be obese as children and adolescents (Moore, Hauguel-DeMouzon, & Catalano, 2014).

Common Complications of the IDM

Although IDMs are usually large, they have immature physiologic functions and exhibit many of the problems of the preterm

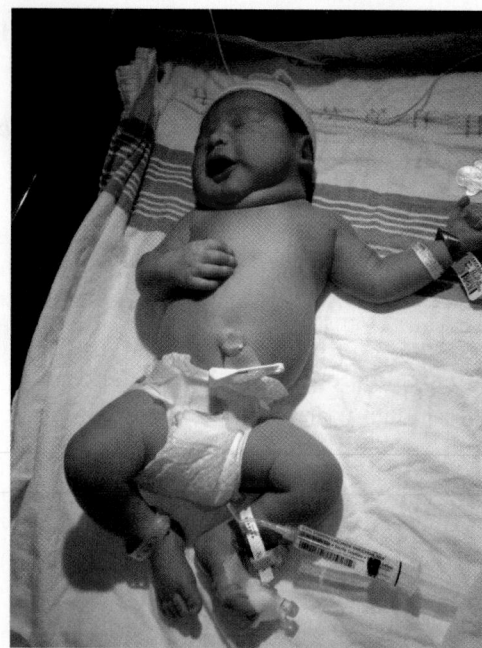

Figure 26–2 Macrosomic newborn of an undiagnosed gestational diabetic mother born at 35 weeks' gestation weighing 3775 g (8.3 lb). Note the peripheral IV in his foot placed to give a D₁₀W bolus.

SOURCE: Carol Harrigan, RN, MSN, NNP-BC.

(premature) newborn. The complications most often seen in an IDM are as follows:

- *Low glucose concentrations.* Hypoglycemia, defined as a blood sugar less than 40 mg/dL or per agency thresholds, occurs transiently in the immediate newborn period for all newborns, but sooner and with increased frequency and to lower levels in IDMs (Moore et al., 2014). Once the fetus is delivered and the maternal glucose supply is severed, the IDM continues to produce high levels of insulin, which deplete the newborn's blood glucose within hours after birth. IDMs also have less ability to release glucagon and catecholamines, which normally stimulate glucagon breakdown and glucose release. The incidence of hypoglycemia in IDMs varies according to the degree of success in controlling the maternal diabetes, the maternal blood sugar level at the time of birth, the length of labor, the class of maternal diabetes, and early versus late feedings of the newborn (Daley, 2014). Signs and symptoms of hypoglycemia, which may present within minutes to hours following delivery, include tremors, cyanosis, apnea, temperature instability, poor feeding, and hypotonia. Seizures may occur in severe cases.

- *Hypocalcemia.* Hypocalcemia is defined as a serum calcium of less than 7 mg/dL. Tremors are the obvious clinical sign of hypocalcemia. They may be caused by the increased incidence of prematurity in IDMs and by the stresses of a difficult pregnancy, labor, and birth. Diabetic women tend to have decreased serum magnesium levels at term secondary to increased urinary calcium excretion, which causes secondary hypoparathyroidism in their babies. Other factors may include vitamin D antagonism, which results from elevated cortisol levels, hypophosphatemia from tissue catabolism, and decreased serum magnesium levels. Treatment is rarely necessary

- *Hyperbilirubinemia.* This condition may be seen at 48 to 72 hours after birth. It may be caused by slightly decreased extracellular fluid volume, which increases the hematocrit level. This elevation facilitates an increase in red blood cell breakdown, thereby increasing bilirubin levels. The presence of hepatic immaturity may impair bilirubin conjugation. Enclosed hemorrhages resulting from complicated vaginal birth may also cause hyperbilirubinemia.

- *Birth trauma.* Because most IDMs are macrosomic, trauma may occur during labor and birth resulting in shoulder dystocia, brachial plexus injuries, subdural hemorrhage, cephalohematoma, and asphyxia.

- *Polycythemia.* Fetal hyperglycemia and hyperinsulinism result in increased oxygen consumption, which can lead to fetal hypoxia (Raab & Kelly, 2013). Glycohemoglobin (HbA₁c) binds to oxygen, decreasing the oxygen available to the fetal tissues. This tissue hypoxia stimulates increased erythropoietin production, which increases both the hematocrit level and the potential for hyperbilirubinemia. See Chapter 14 for discussion of HbA₁c.

- *Respiratory distress syndrome (RDS).* This complication occurs especially in newborns of diabetic mothers who are not well controlled (Moore et al., 2014). Insulin antagonizes the cortisol-induced stimulation of lecithin synthesis that is necessary for lung maturation. Therefore, IDMs may have less mature lungs than expected for their gestational age. There is also a decrease in the phospholipid phosphatidylglycerol (PG), which stabilizes surfactant. The insufficiency of PG increases the incidence of RDS. Therefore, it is important to test for the presence of PG in the amniotic fluid before birth.

  RDS does not appear to be a problem for infants born of diabetic mothers who have decreased placental perfusion; instead, the stresses of poor uterine blood supply may lead to increased production of steroids, which accelerates lung maturation. IDMs may also have a delay in closure of the ductus arteriosus and decreases in postnatal pulmonary artery pressure (Hay, 2012).

- *Congenital birth defects.* These may include congenital heart defects (transposition of the great vessels, ventricular septal defect, patent ductus arteriosus), small left colon syndrome, renal anomalies, neural tube defects, and sacral agenesis (caudal regression) (Cloherty et al., 2012). Early close control of maternal glucose levels before and during pregnancy decreases the risk of birth defects. See Chapter 14 for more information.

Clinical Therapy

Prenatal management is directed toward controlling maternal glucose levels, which minimizes the common complications of IDMs. Because the onset of hypoglycemia occurs between 1 and 3 hours after birth in IDMs (with a spontaneous rise to normal levels by 4 to 6 hours), blood glucose determinations should be done on cord blood or by heelstick hourly during the first 4 hours after birth and then at 4-hour intervals until the risk period (about 48 hours) has passed or per agency protocol (Figure 26–3).

IDMs whose serum glucose level falls below 40 mg/dL should have early feedings with formula or breast milk (colostrum). If normal glucose levels cannot be maintained with oral feedings, an intravenous (IV) infusion of glucose will be necessary. (See Chapter 27 for detailed discussion of hypoglycemia in the newborn.)

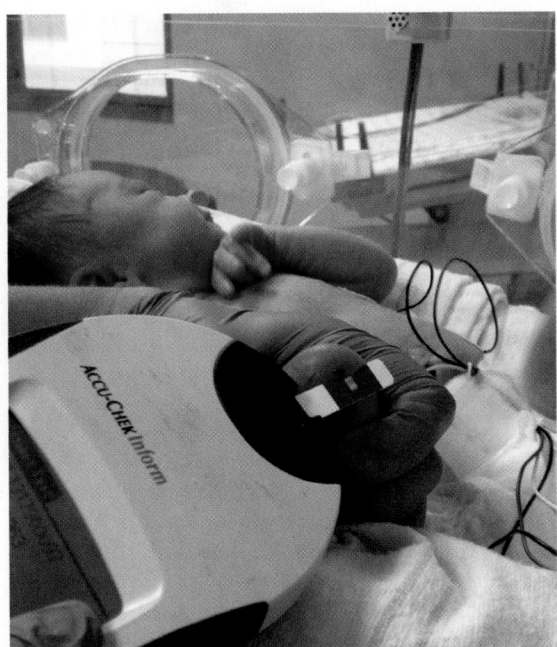

Figure 26–3 Nurse obtaining a bedside blood glucose.
SOURCE: Carol Harrigan, RN,MSN, NNP-BC.

Nursing Management

For the Infant of a Diabetic Mother (IDM)

Nursing Assessment and Diagnosis

Do not be lulled into thinking that a big baby is a mature baby. In almost every case, because of the newborn's large size, the IDM will appear older than gestational age scoring indicates. Consider both the gestational age and whether the baby is AGA or LGA in planning and providing safe care. In caring for the IDM, assess for signs of respiratory distress, hyperbilirubinemia, birth trauma, and congenital anomalies.

SAFETY ALERT!

When infusing either a $D_{10}W$ bolus or a constant infusion, be careful not to administer too much glucose too fast in order to prevent hyperglycemic-induced insulin secretion. When beginning IV fluids on a symptomatic IDM, it is best to start an IV glucose infusion at 4 to 6 mg/kg/min to avoid rebound hypoglycemia (Armentrout, 2015).

Nursing diagnoses that may apply to IDMs include the following (NANDA-I © 2014):

- *Nutrition, Imbalanced: Less than Body Requirements,* related to increased glucose metabolism secondary to hyperinsulinemia
- *Gas Exchange, Impaired,* related to respiratory distress secondary to impaired production of surfactant
- *Tissue Perfusion: Peripheral, Ineffective,* secondary to polycythemia related to increased synthesis of erythropoietin, chronic intrauterine hypoxia, and increased metabolic rate
- *Injury, Risk for,* related to trauma during vaginal delivery due to macrosomia
- *Tissue Integrity, Impaired,* related to poor maternal metabolic control
- *Family Processes, Interrupted,* related to the illness of the baby

Planning and Implementation

Nursing care of the IDM is directed toward early detection and ongoing monitoring of hypoglycemia (by performing glucose tests) and polycythemia (by obtaining central hematocrits), RDS, and hyperbilirubinemia. (These conditions are presented in Chapter 27.) Assess for signs of birth trauma and congenital anomalies.

Parent teaching is directed toward preventing macrosomia and the resulting fetal/neonatal problems by instituting early and ongoing diabetic control. Advise parents that with early identification and care, most IDMs' neonatal problems have no significant sequelae.

Evaluation

Expected outcomes of nursing care include the following:

- The IDM's respiratory distress and metabolic problems are minimized.
- The parents understand the effects of maternal diabetes on the baby's health and preventive steps they can initiate to decrease its impact on subsequent pregnancies.
- The parents verbalize their concerns about their baby's health problems and understand the rationale behind management of their newborn.

Care of the Postterm Newborn

The **postterm newborn** is any newborn born after 42 completed weeks of gestation. Postterm or prolonged pregnancy occurs in approximately 7% of all pregnancies (Bowers, 2014). The cause of postterm pregnancy is not completely understood, but several factors are known to be associated with it. (See Chapter 20 for a discussion of maternal factors.) Many pregnancies classified as prolonged are thought to be a result of inaccurate estimates of date of birth (EDB). Postterm pregnancy is more common in Australian, Greek, and Italian ethnic groups.

Most babies born as a result of prolonged pregnancy are of normal size and health; some continue growing and are over 4000 g (8.8 lb) at birth, which supports the contention that the postterm fetus can remain well nourished. Potential intrapartum problems for these healthy but large fetuses are cephalopelvic disproportion (CPD) and shoulder dystocia. (See Chapter 21 for discussion of the necessary assessments and interventions.)

Common Complications of the Newborn With Postmaturity Syndrome

The term **postmaturity** applies only to the newborn who is born after 42 completed weeks of gestation and also demonstrates characteristics of *postmaturity syndrome*. Postterm newborns have begun to lose weight but usually have a normal length and head circumference (Cloherty et al., 2012).

The characteristics of postmature newborns are primarily caused by a combination of advanced gestational age, placental aging and decreased placental function, and continued exposure to amniotic fluid. The truly postmature newborn is at high risk for morbidity and has a mortality rate 2 to 3 times greater than that of term newborns. Although today the percentages are extremely low, the majority of postmature fetal deaths occur during labor because the fetus uses up necessary body reserves.

The following are common disorders of the postmature newborn:

- Hypoglycemia, from nutritional deprivation and depleted glycogen stores

- Meconium aspiration in response to in utero hypoxia as the stress of labor begins. The presence of oligohydramnios increases the danger of aspirating thick meconium. Severe meconium aspiration syndrome increases the baby's chance of developing persistent pulmonary hypertension, pneumothorax, and chemical pneumonitis.

- Polycythemia caused by increased production of red blood cells (RBCs) in response to hypoxia

- Congenital anomalies of unknown cause

- Seizure activity because of hypoxic insult

- Cold stress because of loss or poor development of subcutaneous fat

Clinical Therapy

The aim of antenatal management is to differentiate the fetus who has postmaturity syndrome from the fetus who at birth is large, well nourished, alert, and tolerating the prolonged (postterm) pregnancy. Antenatal tests that are done to evaluate fetal status and determine obstetric management and their use in postterm pregnancy are discussed in more depth in Chapters 14 and 20. If the amniotic fluid is meconium stained, an amnioinfusion may be done during labor. This procedure dilutes the meconium by directly infusing either normal saline or Ringer lactate into the uterus, decreasing the risk of meconium aspiration syndrome. (For detailed discussion of clinical management and care of the newborn at risk for meconium aspiration, see Chapter 27.)

Hypoglycemia is monitored by serial glucose determinations per agency protocols. The baby may be placed on glucose infusions or given early feedings if respiratory distress is not present, but these measures must be instituted with caution because of the frequency of asphyxia in the first 24 hours. Postmature newborns are often voracious eaters.

For the small-for-gestational-age (SGA) newborn who is postmature, peripheral and central hematocrits are tested to determine the presence of polycythemia. Fluid resuscitation can be initiated. In extreme cases, a partial exchange transfusion may be necessary to prevent polycythemia and adverse sequelae such as hyperviscosity. Oxygen is provided for respiratory distress. In addition, temperature instability and excessive loss of heat can result from decreased liver glycogen stores. (See Chapter 27 for thermoregulation techniques.)

Nursing Management

For the Newborn With Postmaturity Syndrome

Nursing Assessment and Diagnosis

The newborn with postmaturity syndrome appears alert. This wide-eyed, alert appearance is not necessarily a positive sign because it may indicate chronic intrauterine hypoxia. The baby typically has dry, cracking, parchment-like skin without vernix or lanugo (Figure 26–4). Fingernails are long, and scalp hair is profuse. The newborn's body appears long and thin. The wasting involves depletion of previously stored subcutaneous

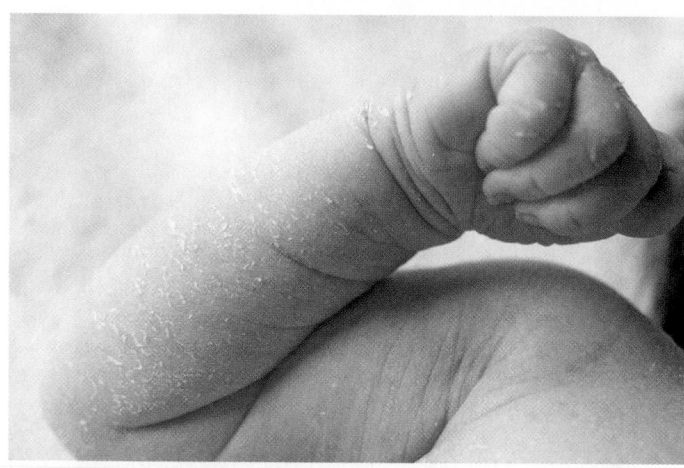

Figure 26–4 The skin of the postterm newborn exhibits deep cracking and peeling of skin.

SOURCE: Paolo Koch/Science Source.

tissue, causing the skin to be loose. Fat layers are almost nonexistent.

Postmature newborns frequently have meconium staining, which colors the nails, skin, and umbilical cord. The varying shades (yellow to green) of meconium staining can give some clue as to whether the expulsion of meconium in utero was a recent or chronic problem. Green coloring indicates a more recent event.

Nursing diagnoses that may apply to the postmature newborn include the following (NANDA-I © 2014):

- *Hypothermia* related to decreased liver glycogen and brown fat stores

- *Nutrition, Imbalanced: Less than Body Requirements,* related to increased use of glucose secondary to in utero stress and decreased placental perfusion

- *Gas Exchange, Impaired,* related to airway obstruction from meconium aspiration

- *Tissue Perfusion: Peripheral, Ineffective,* related to increased blood viscosity caused by polycythemia

PLANNING AND IMPLEMENTATION

Nursing care of the postmature newborn is directed toward early detection and ongoing monitoring of hypothermia (by regulating thermoregulation), hypoglycemia (by performing glucose tests), polycythemia (by obtaining central hematocrits), and meconium aspiration and RDS (by monitoring cardiopulmonary status). (These conditions are discussed in Chapter 27.)

Encourage parents to express their feelings and fears about the newborn's condition and potential long-term problems. Give careful explanations of procedures, include the parents in the development of care plans for their baby, and encourage follow-up care as needed.

Evaluation

Expected outcomes of nursing care include the following:

- The postterm newborn establishes effective respiratory function.

- The postmature baby is free of metabolic alterations (hypoglycemia) and maintains a stable temperature.

The Newborn at Risk: Conditions Present at Birth

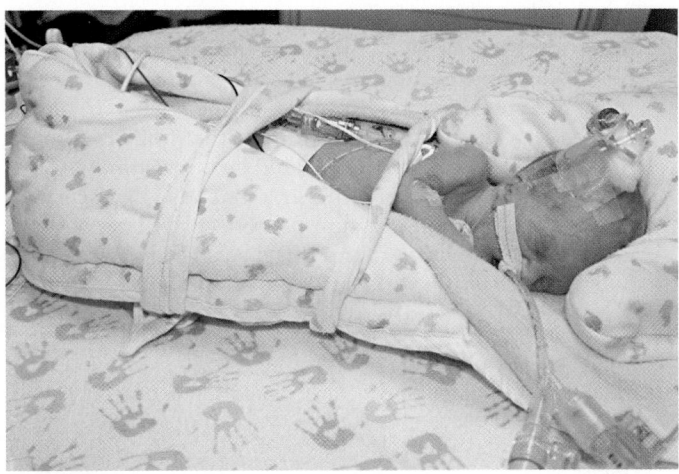

Figure 26–5 A 6-day-old, 26-week gestational age, 960-g (2-lb) preterm newborn.

SOURCE: Carol Harrigan, RN, MSN, NNP-BC.

Care of the Preterm (Premature) Newborn

A **preterm newborn** is any baby born at 37 or fewer weeks' gestation (ACOG & Society for Maternal-Fetal Medicine (SMFM), 2013; Spong, 2013) (Figure 26–5). With the help of modern technology, babies are surviving at younger gestational ages, but not without significant morbidity. The incidence of all preterm births in the United States in 2011 was approximately 11.7%, dropping for the fifth consecutive year, with the largest decline seen among babies born at 34 to 36 weeks' gestation (Brooks, 2013; Lynch, Dezen, & Brown, 2012). The United States still has the highest rate of preterm birth of any industrialized country, which costs businesses about 12 times as much as uncomplicated healthy births (Brooks, 2013). The rise in multiple birth rates has markedly influenced overall rates of low-birth-weight (LBW) newborns. Prematurity and LBW are common in single adolescents and women. (See Chapter 20 for a discussion of preterm labor.)

The major problem of the preterm newborn is the variable immaturity of all systems. The degree of immaturity depends on the length of gestation. Because of immaturity, the premature newborn is ill equipped to smoothly traverse the complex, interconnected pathways from intrauterine to extrauterine life.

Alteration in Respiratory and Cardiac Physiology

The preterm newborn is at risk for respiratory problems because the lungs are not fully mature and not fully ready to take over the process of gas exchange until 37 to 38 weeks' gestation. Critical factors in the development of respiratory distress syndrome (RDS) include the following:

1. The preterm newborn is unable to produce adequate amounts of surfactant. (See Chapter 23 for a discussion of respiratory adaptation and development.) Inadequate surfactant lessens compliance (ability of the lung to fill with air easily), thereby increasing the inspiratory pressure needed to expand the lungs with air. This progressive atelectasis leads to an inability to develop a functional residual capacity (FRC), causing an ineffective exchange of oxygen and

carbon dioxide. As a result, the baby becomes hypoxic, pulmonary blood flow is inefficient, and the preterm newborn's available energy is depleted.

2. The muscular coat of pulmonary blood vessels is incompletely developed. Consequently, the pulmonary arterioles do not constrict as well in response to decreased oxygen levels. This lowered pulmonary vascular resistance leads to left-to-right shunting of blood through the ductus arteriosus, which increases the blood flow back into the lungs.

3. Normally, the ductus arteriosus responds to increasing oxygen levels and prostaglandin E levels by vasoconstriction; in the preterm newborn who is more susceptible to hypoxia, the ductus may remain open. A patent ductus increases the blood volume to the lungs, causing pulmonary congestion, increased respiratory effort, carbon dioxide retention, and bounding femoral pulses.

The common complications of the cardiopulmonary system in preterm newborns are discussed later in this chapter and in Chapter 27.

Alterations in Thermoregulation

Heat loss is a major problem in preterm newborns. Two factors limiting heat production are the decreased availability of glycogen in the liver and the amount of brown fat available for heat production, both of which appear in the third trimester. Because the muscle mass is small in preterm newborns and muscular activity is diminished (they are unable to shiver), heat production is further limited.

Five physiologic and anatomic factors increase heat loss in the preterm newborn:

1. The preterm baby has a higher ratio of body surface to body weight. This means that the baby's ability to produce heat (based on body weight) is much less than the potential for losing heat (based on surface area). The loss of heat in a preterm newborn weighing 1500 g (3.3 lb) is 5 times greater per unit of body weight than in an adult.

2. The preterm baby has very little subcutaneous fat, which is the human body's insulation. Without adequate insulation, heat is easily conducted from the core of the body (warmer temperature) to the surface of the body (cooler temperature). Heat is lost from the body as the blood vessels, which lie close to the skin surface in the preterm newborn transport blood from the body core to the subcutaneous tissues.

3. The preterm baby has thinner, more permeable skin than the term baby. This increased permeability contributes to a greater insensible water loss as well as to heat loss.

4. Flexion of the extremities decreases the amount of surface area exposed to the environment. Extension of the extremities in the hypotonic "frog" position increases the surface area exposed to the environment and thus increases heat loss. The gestational age of the baby influences the amount of flexion, from completely hypotonic and extended at 28 weeks to strong flexion displayed by 36 weeks.

5. The preterm baby has a decreased ability to vasoconstrict superficial blood vessels and conserve heat in the body core.

In summary, gestational age is directly proportional to the ability to maintain thermoregulation; thus the more preterm the newborn, the less able the baby is to maintain heat balance. The goal is to prevent heat loss by providing a neutral thermal environment (NTE), whereby the metabolic rate and oxygen consumption are kept at a minimum. Using a servo-control skin probe is one of the most important considerations in nursing management of the preterm newborn. Other nursing interventions assisting in the thermoregulation of the preterm newborn include increasing the delivery room temperature, loosely covering the baby with polyethylene wrap, placing the baby in a plastic bag from feet to shoulders, and placing the baby on a chemical mattress. Cold stress, with its accompanying severe complications, needs to be minimized and ultimately prevented to lessen morbidity and mortality of the preterm newborn (see Chapter 27).

Alteration in Gastrointestinal Physiology

Maturation of the digestive and absorptive process is more variable, however, and occurs later in gestation. As a result of gastrointestinal (GI) immaturity, the preterm newborn has the following ingestion, digestive, and absorption problems (Ditzenberger, 2015):

- A marked danger of aspiration and its associated complications because of the baby's poorly developed gag reflex, incompetent esophageal cardiac sphincter, and poor sucking and swallowing reflexes.
- Difficulty in meeting high caloric and fluid needs for growth because of small stomach capacity.
- Limited ability to convert certain essential amino acids to nonessential amino acids. Certain amino acids, such as histidine, taurine, and cysteine, are essential to the preterm newborn but not to the term newborn.
- Inability to handle the increased osmolarity of formula protein because of kidney immaturity. The preterm newborn requires a higher concentration of whey protein than of casein.
- Difficulty absorbing saturated fats because of decreased bile salts and pancreatic lipase. Severe illness of the newborn may also prevent intake of adequate nutrients.
- Difficulty with lactose digestion initially because processes may not be fully functional during the first few days of a preterm newborn's life. The preterm newborn can digest and absorb most simple sugars.
- Deficiency of calcium and phosphorus may exist because two thirds of these minerals are deposited in the last trimester. Rickets and significant bone demineralization caused by deficiency of calcium and phosphorus, which are deposited primarily in the last trimester, are also problems.
- Increased basal metabolic rate and increased oxygen requirements caused by fatigue associated with sucking.
- Feeding intolerance and necrotizing enterocolitis (NEC) as a result of diminished blood flow and tissue perfusion to the intestinal tract because of a combination of contributing factors including prematurity, formula feeding, bacterial colonization, and hypoxemia/ischemia events (Bradshaw, 2015).

Alteration in Renal Physiology

Specific characteristics of the preterm newborn that pose clinical problems in the management of fluid and electrolyte balance include the following:

- The glomerular filtration rate (GFR) is directly related to lower gestational age and increases steadily after 34 weeks'

postconceptual age (PCA). The GFR is also decreased in the presence of diseases or conditions that decrease the renal blood flow and perfusion, such as severe respiratory distress, hypotension, and asphyxia. Preterm newborns usually have some urine output during the first 24 hours of life. By day 3, urine output should be approximately 1 to 3 mL/kg/hr. Anuria and oliguria may also be observed. A low systolic blood pressure can reflect any diseases that decrease cardiac output and affect renal blood flow. Systolic blood pressure varies with gestational age and PCA.

Clinical Tip
A gradual decline in urine may be associated with a drop in the newborn's blood pressure.

- The preterm newborn's kidneys are limited in their ability to concentrate urine or to excrete excess amounts of fluid because of a blunted response to antidiuretic hormone (ADH). This means that if excess fluid is administered, the baby is at risk for fluid retention and overhydration. If too little is administered, the baby will become dehydrated because of the inability to retain adequate fluid.
- The preterm kidneys begin excreting glucose (glycosuria) at a lower serum glucose level than that of the term newborn. Therefore, glycosuria with hyperglycemia can lead to osmotic diuresis and polyuria.
- The kidney's buffering capacity is reduced, predisposing the baby to metabolic acidosis. Bicarbonate is excreted at a lower serum level, and acid is excreted more slowly. Therefore, after periods of hypoxia or insult, the preterm newborn's kidneys require a longer time to excrete the lactic acid that accumulates.
- The immaturity of the renal system affects the preterm newborn's ability to excrete drugs. Because excretion time is longer, many drugs are given over longer intervals (e.g., every 24 hours instead of every 12 hours). Urine output must be carefully monitored when the baby is receiving nephrotoxic drugs such as gentamicin and vancomycin. In the event that urine output is poor, drugs can become toxic in the baby much more quickly than in the adult.

Alteration in Immunologic Physiology

The preterm newborn has an increased susceptibility to infections acquired in utero that may have precipitated preterm labor and birth. However, all preterm newborns have immature specific and nonspecific immunity.

In utero, the fetus receives passive immunity against a variety of infections from maternal IgG immunoglobulins, which cross the placenta. Because most of this immunity is acquired in the last trimester of pregnancy, the preterm newborn has few antibodies at birth. These provide less protection and become depleted earlier than in a full-term newborn. This may be a contributing factor in the higher incidence of recurrent bacterial infection during the first year of life as well as in the immediate neonatal period. (See *Care of the Newborn With Infection* in Chapter 27.)

The other immunoglobulin significant for the preterm newborn is secretory IgA, which does not cross the placenta but is found in breast milk. Breast milk's secretory IgA provides immunity to the mucosal surfaces of the GI tract, protecting the newborn from enteric infections such as those caused by *Escherichia coli* and *Shigella*.

Another altered defense against infection in the preterm newborn is the skin surface. In very small babies, the skin is easily excoriated, and this factor, coupled with many invasive procedures, places the baby at great risk for nosocomial infections. It is vital to use good hand hygiene techniques in the care of these babies to prevent unnecessary infection.

SAFETY ALERT!

The sudden onset of apnea and bradycardia, coupled with metabolic acidosis in an otherwise healthy, growing premature newborn, may be suggestive of bacterial sepsis, especially if a central line is present.

Alteration in Neurologic Physiology

Because the period of most rapid brain growth and development occurs during the third trimester of pregnancy, the closer to term a baby is born, the better the neurologic prognosis. A common interruption of neurologic development in the preterm newborn is caused by intraventricular hemorrhage (IVH).

Hydrocephalus may develop as a consequence of an IVH caused by an obstruction at the cerebral aqueduct (Scher, 2013).

Alteration in Reactivity Periods and Behavioral States

The newborn's response to extrauterine life is characterized by two periods of reactivity (see Chapter 23). However, the preterm newborn's periods of reactivity are delayed. In the very ill baby, these periods of reactivity may not be observed at all because the baby may be hypotonic and unreactive for several days after birth. In general, stable preterm newborns do not demonstrate the same behavioral states as term newborns. Preterm newborns tend to be more disorganized in their sleep–wake cycles and are unable to attend as well to the human face and objects in the environment. Neurologically, their responses (sucking, muscle tone, states of arousal) are weaker than full-term newborns' responses.

The more knowledge parents have about the meaning of their baby's responses and behavior cues, the better prepared they will be to meet their newborn's needs and to form a positive attachment with their child. See discussion of developmental care for the preterm newborn later in this section.

EVIDENCE-BASED PRACTICE | Improving Outcomes for Late Preterm Newborns

Clinical Question

What interventions support the best outcomes for late preterm babies (neonates born between 34 weeks 0 days and 36 weeks 6 days gestation)?

The Evidence

In 2006, the National Institutes of Health recommended using the term *late preterm* to describe those babies born between 34 0/7 and 36 6/7 weeks of gestation. While these neonates are often considered *near term*, this reference underestimates the risks to this population. Nearly 10% of all births fall into this classification, and the newborns have a higher rate of hypothermia, respiratory complications, feeding difficulty, extended lengths of stay, and infant mortality. It is now recognized that this group of newborns requires careful perinatal monitoring, customized feeding plans, consideration of neurologic development, and close follow up after they go home (Baker, 2015a). An interprofessional team of nurses from labor and delivery, neonatal ICU, and postpartum care collaborated on a systematic review of the literature to develop an evidence-based practice guideline for this group of at-risk babies. This type of structured review based on randomized trials and culminating in a practice guideline forms the strongest level of evidence.

Best practice focuses on appropriate monitoring and prevention of complications. Late preterm newborns—or babies weighing less than 2000 g (4.4 lb)—should be admitted to a neonatal ICU for at least 24 hours of observation and monitoring. Babies born between 35 and 36 weeks of gestation should

be monitored for signs of respiratory distress, particularly those with a birth Apgar of 4 or less. Newborns of greater than 36 weeks' gestation can be moved to the mother/baby unit unless clinically unstable. These babies should be admitted to a specialty care unit if they have persistent oxygen requirements, any evidence of apnea, an inability to take adequate feeding, respiratory distress, or inability to regulate body temperature (Baker, 2015b). If admitted to a specialty care unit, these babies should have frequent measurement of vital signs, an external heat source until body temperature stabilizes, blood glucose on admission and then every 8 hours, and routine feeding when the respiratory rate is below 60. Transfer to the mother/baby unit should occur only when all criteria are met to facilitate mother/baby interaction, achieve adequate nutritional intake, and breathe without distress.

Best Practice

Late preterm newborns have an elevated risk of complications, and should be treated as at-risk neonates. Close monitoring of respiratory condition, feeding behavior, neurologic status, and blood glucose is needed to recognize signs of distress and other complications. Babies can be transferred to routine care when they are stable and able to feed adequately.

Clinical Reasoning

What assessments should the nurse include to be sure that the baby is stable and can be cared for by the mother? What will be included in the discharge teaching plan for these mothers?

Management of Nutrition and Fluid Requirements

Early feedings are extremely valuable for the premature newborn in maintaining normal metabolism and lowering the possibility of such complications as hypoglycemia, hyperbilirubinemia, hyperkalemia, osteopenia of prematurity, and other digestive system problems.

NUTRITIONAL REQUIREMENTS

Oral (enteral) caloric intake necessary for growth in an uncompromised healthy preterm newborn is 110 to 140 kcal/kg/day and should be begun as soon as clinically possible (Blackburn, 2013). Early feedings are associated with improved glucose homeostasis, immune functions, and weight gain patterns, ultimately resulting in early discharge home. Human milk is preferred for feeding the preterm newborn with significant benefits for the mother, baby, family, and society (O'Hare, Wood, & Fiske, 2013). Human donor milk is an available option to the high-risk newborn whose mother in unable to produce sufficient amounts of milk. To meet the high caloric needs of the growing premature baby, breast milk may be fortified or special preterm formulas may be used.

Whether breast milk or formula is used, feeding protocols are established based on the baby's weight and estimated stomach capacity. Initial formula-feedings are gradually increased as the baby tolerates them.

In addition to a higher calorie and protein formula, preterm newborns should receive supplemental multivitamins, including vitamins A, D, and E, iron, and trace minerals. A diet high in polyunsaturated fats (which preterm newborns tolerate best) increases the requirement for vitamin E. Preterm formulas also need to contain medium-chain triglycerides (MCT) and additional amino acids such as cysteine, as well as calcium, phosphorus, and vitamin D supplements to increase mineralization of bones.

Nutritional intake is considered adequate when there is consistent weight gain of 20 to 30 g/day. Initially, no weight gain may be noted for several days, but total weight loss should not exceed 15% of the total birth weight or more than 1% to 2% per day. Some institutions add the criteria of head circumference growth and increase in body length of 1 cm (0.4 in.) per week, once the newborn is stable.

METHODS OF FEEDING

The preterm newborn is fed by various methods depending on the baby's gestational age, health and physical condition, and neurologic status. The three most common oral feeding methods are bottle, breast, and gavage.

Bottle-Feeding. Preterm newborns who have a coordinated as well as rhythmic suck–swallow–breathing pattern are usually between 32 and 34 weeks' postconception age and may be fed by bottle. Oral readiness to feed is best described by the following engagement and hunger cues (Newland et al., 2013):

- Bringing hands to the mouth
- Being alert
- Exhibiting fussiness
- Sucking on fingers or pacifier
- Exhibiting rooting behavior
- Showing relaxed facial expression and good tone

To avoid excessive expenditure of energy, a soft, yellow, single-hole nipple is usually used (milk flow is less rapid). The baby is fed in a semisitting or side-lying position and burped

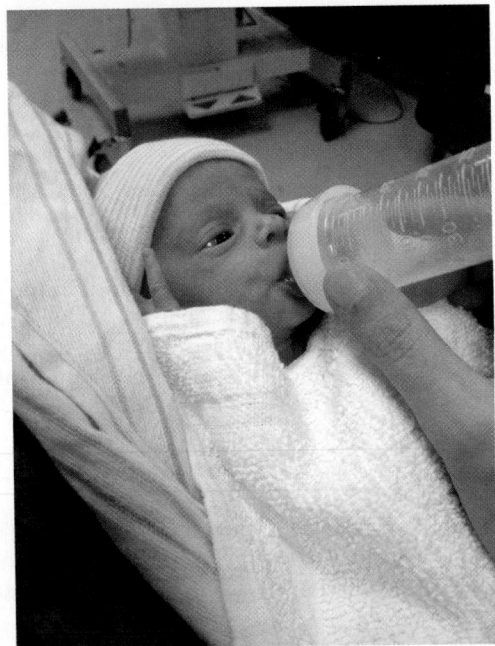

Figure 26–6 Mother bottle-feeding her premature newborn with expressed breast milk.

SOURCE: Carol Harrigan, RN, MSN, NNP-BC.

gently after each 0.5 to 1.0 oz. The feeding should take no longer than 15 to 20 minutes (nippling requires more energy than other methods). Premature newborns who are progressing from gavage-feedings to bottle-feeding should start with one session of bottle-feeding a day and slowly increase the number of times a day a bottle is given until the baby tolerates all feedings from a bottle (Figure 26–6).

Sucking may be affected by age, asphyxia, sepsis, intraventricular hemorrhage, or other neurologic insult. Before initiating nipple-feeding, the nurse observes for signs of stress, such as tachypnea (more than 60 respirations per minute), respiratory distress, or hypothermia, which may increase the risk of aspiration. During the feeding the nurse observes the baby for signs of feeding difficulty (tachypnea, cyanosis, bradycardia, lethargy, uncoordinated suck and swallow). Difficulty in bottle-feeding is often associated with a milk bolus that is too large for the newborn's oral cavity and can lead to aspiration. Demand feeding protocols, based on the baby's hunger cues, should be considered for a growing premature newborn only when there is sufficient caloric intake to promote consistent weight gain (Newland et al., 2013). See Table 26–1.

Clinical Tip

The more preterm the baby is at birth, the longer it will take to reach the maturational state required to be successful at oral feedings.

Breastfeeding. Mothers who wish to breastfeed their preterm newborns are given the opportunity to put the baby to the breast as soon as the baby has demonstrated a coordinated suck and swallow reflex, is showing consistent weight gain, and can control body temperature outside of the incubator, regardless of weight. Preterm newborns tolerate breastfeeding with higher transcutaneous oxygen pressures and better maintenance of body temperature than during bottle-feeding. Besides breast milk's many benefits for the baby, it allows the mother to contribute actively to the baby's

TABLE 26–1 Cue-Based Feeding Readiness Scales

FEEDING								
Readiness								
Quality								
Caregiver								
Time								
Quantity								
Nipple (circle breast or write nipple color)	Breast Nipple color	Breast Nipple color	Breast Nipple color	Breast Nipple color	Breast Nipple color	Breast Nipple color	Breast Nipple color	Breast Nipple color
Initial								

Readiness

Breastfeed (Bottle)

SCORE	DESCRIPTION
1	Drowsy, alert, or fussy prior to care. Rooting and/or hands to mouth/takes pacifier. Good tone.
2	Drowsy or alert once handled. Some rooting or takes pacifier. Adequate tone.

Breastfeed (No bottle)

SCORE	DESCRIPTION
3	Briefly alert with care. No hunger behaviors. No change in tone.
4	Sleeping throughout care. No hunger cues. No change in tone.

Gavage only

SCORE	DESCRIPTION
5	Needs increased O_2 with care. Apnea/bradycardia (A/B) with care. Tachypnea over baseline with care.

Caregiver Techniques

SCORE	DESCRIPTION
A	Side-lying position
B	External pacing
C	Adding or increasing O_2 during feed
D	Imposed breaks
E	Stimulation for/recovery from A/B
F	Frequent burping
G	Nipple change
H	Other (specify)

Quality Breastfeeding

SCORE	DESCRIPTION
1	Latched well with a strong coordinated suck for >15 min.
2	Latched well with a strong coordinated suck initially, but fatigues with progression. Active suck for 8–15 min.
3	Difficulty maintaining a strong, consistent latch. May be able to nurse intermittently but active for only <15 min.
4	Latch is weak/inconsistent, with a frequent need to relatch. Limited effort with inconsistent pattern. May be considered nonnutritional breastfeeding (NNBF).
5	Unable to latch to breast and achieve suck–swallow-breathe pattern. May have difficulty arousing to a state conducive to breastfeeding. Could result in frequent or significant A/B's and/or tachypnea significantly above baseline with feeding.

Quality Bottle

SCORE	DESCRIPTION
1	Nipples with a strong coordinated suck throughout feed.
2	Nipples with a strong coordinated suck initially, but fatigues with progression.
3	Nipples with consistent suck, but difficulty coordination swallow; some loss of liquid or difficulty pacing. Benefits from external pacing.
4	Nipples with a weak/inconsistent suck. Little to no rhythm. May require some rest breaks.
5	Disorganized; unable to coordinate suck–swallow–breathe pattern despite packing. May result in frequent or significant A/Bs or large amounts of liquid loss and or tachypnea significantly above baseline with feeding.
6	Dysfunctional; abnormal or deviant oral motor patterns evidenced by inability to extract fluid from nipple.

Sources: Data from Baylor University Medical Center, Dallas, Texas; Ludwig, S. M., & Weitzman, K. A. (2007). Changing feeding documentation to reflect infant-driven feeding practice. *Newborn and Infant Nursing Reviews, 7,* 155–160.

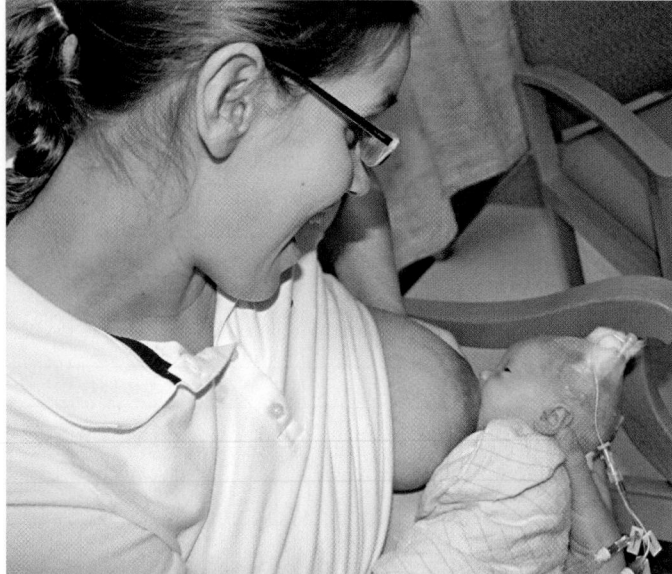

Figure 26–7 This mother is breastfeeding her premature newborn.

SOURCE: Carol Harrigan, RN, MSN, NNP-BC.

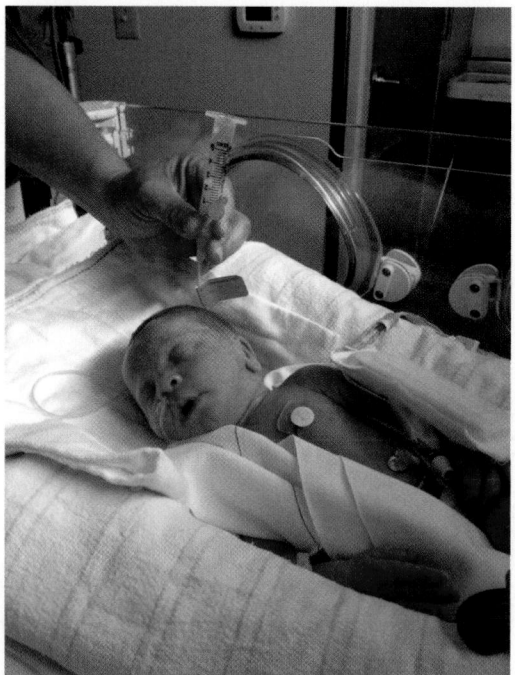

Figure 26–8 Gavage feeding a preterm newborn, flowing in by gravity.

SOURCE: Carol Harrigan, RN, MSN, NNP-BC.

well-being (Figure 26–7). The nurse should encourage mothers to breastfeed if they choose to do so. It is important to be aware of the advantages of breastfeeding, as well as the possible disadvantages of breast milk as the sole source of food for the preterm newborn. (For an in-depth discussion of breastfeeding, see Chapter 25.)

By initiating skin-to-skin holding of premature newborns in the early intensive care phase, mothers can significantly increase milk volume, thereby overcoming lactation problems. Many mothers of preterm babies seem to find the football hold position (see Figure 25–16) the most convenient breastfeeding position. Feeding may take up to 45 minutes, and babies should be burped as they alternate breasts. The length of feeding time is monitored so that the preterm newborn does not expend too many calories.

The nurse should coordinate a flexible feeding schedule so babies can nurse during alert times and be allowed to set their own pace. Feedings should be on demand, but a maximum number of hours between feedings should be set. The mother begins with one feeding at the breast and then gradually increases the number of times during the day that the baby breastfeeds. Even if the baby cannot be put to the breast, mothers can pump their breasts, and the breast milk can be given via gavage. Use of the double-pumping system produces higher levels of prolactin than sequential pumping of the breasts. When breastfeeding is not possible because the baby is too small or too weak to suck at the breast, an option for the mother may be to express her breast milk into a cup. The milk touches the baby's lips and is lapped by the protruding motions of the tongue.

Gavage Feeding. The gavage feeding method is used with preterm newborns (less than 34 weeks' gestation) who lack or have a poorly coordinated suck and swallow reflex or are ill and ventilator dependent. Gavage feeding (see Administering a Gavage/Tube Feeding in the *Clinical Skills Manual* SKILLS) may be used as an adjunct to nipple-feeding if the baby tires easily or as an alternative if a newborn is losing weight because of the energy expenditure required for nippling. Gavage feedings are administered by the intermittent bolus or continuous drip method (Figure 26–8). Currently, there are no conclusive studies supporting one method over

the other. In common practice, bolus feedings are usually initiated, but if intolerance occurs, then the feedings are changed to infuse on a pump over a set amount of time (e.g., over an hour) or continuously. Gavage feeding is not without its consequences, including gastroesophageal reflux (GER), which can lead to significant emesis, food refusal, dysphagia, oral eversion, and aspiration (Jones, 2012).

Early initiation of minimal enteral nutrition (MEN) via gavage is now advocated as a supplement to parenteral nutrition. MEN refers to small-volume feedings of formula or human milk (usually less than 24 mL/kg/day) that are designed to "prime" the intestinal tract, thereby stimulating many of its hormonal and enzymatic functions (Cloherty et al., 2012). Benefits of early feeding (as early as 24 to 72 hours of life) include the following:

- No increase in the incidence of necrotizing enterocolitis
- Fewer days on total parenteral nutrition (TPN), thereby decreasing the incidence of cholestatic jaundice
- Increased weight gain
- Increased muscle maturation of the gut as well as muscle growth
- Increased gut peristalsis and gut hormone levels, which can lead to improved feeding tolerance
- Shorter time required to reach full-volume enteral feedings
- Lower risk of osteopenia
- Possible decrease in the total number of hospital days in the NICU

SAFETY ALERT!

Orogastric gavage catheter placement is preferable to nasogastric because most newborns are obligatory nose breathers. If nasogastric is used, a #5 French catheter should be used to minimize airway obstruction.

FLUID REQUIREMENTS

The calculation of fluid requirements must take into account the newborn's weight and postnatal age. Recommendations for fluid therapy in the preterm newborn are approximately 80 to 100 mL/kg/day for day 1, 100 to 120 mL/kg/day for day 2, and 120 to 150 mL/kg/day by day 3 of life. These amounts may be increased up to 180 mL/kg/day if the baby is extremely premature, receiving phototherapy, or under a radiant warmer, facilitating an increase in insensible water losses. If the baby is not hydrated properly, excessive insensible water loss can lead to hypernatremia, hyperkalemia, hypovolemia, hypotension, and oliguria. Fluid losses can be minimized through the use of heat shields and added humidification in the incubator. Daily weights, and sometimes twice-a-day weights, are the best indicator of fluid status in the preterm newborn. The expected weight loss during the first 5 to 6 days of life in a preterm baby is 15% to 20% of birth weight (Cloherty et al., 2012).

Common Complications of Preterm Newborns and Their Clinical Management

The goals of medical and nursing care are to meet the preterm newborn's growth and development needs and to anticipate and manage the complications associated with prematurity. The most common complications associated with prematurity are as follows:

1. *Apnea of prematurity.* Apnea of prematurity refers to cessation of breathing for 20 seconds or longer or for less than 20 seconds when associated with cyanosis, pallor, and bradycardia. Apnea is a common problem in the preterm newborn less than 36 weeks, presenting between day 2 and day 7 of life. The etiology of apnea is multifactorial but is thought to be primarily a result of neuronal immaturity, a factor that contributes to the preterm newborn's irregular breathing patterns (central apnea). Obstructive apnea can occur when there is cessation of airflow associated with blockage of the upper airway (small airway diameter, increased pharyngeal secretions, altered body alignment and positioning). Gastroesophageal reflux (GER) is defined as a movement of gastric contents into the lower esophagus caused by poor esophageal sphincter tone, causing laryngospasm, which leads to bradycardia and apnea. Apnea of prematurity is then a diagnosis of exclusion.

2. *Patent ductus arteriosus (PDA).* The ductus arteriosus fails to close because of decreased pulmonary arteriole musculature and hypoxemia. Symptomatic PDA is often seen around the time when premature newborns are recovering from RDS. Patent ductus arteriosus often prolongs the course of illness in a preterm newborn and leads to chronic pulmonary dysfunction.

Clinical Tip

A growing premature newborn showing clinical signs of worsening respiratory status (e.g., increased oxygen needs, increased ventilatory settings), acidosis, and hypotension may be exhibiting signs and symptoms of a patent ductus arteriosus (PDA).

---

3. *Respiratory distress syndrome (RDS).* Respiratory distress results from inadequate surfactant production.

4. *Intraventricular hemorrhage (IVH).* Intraventricular hemorrhage is the most common type of intracranial hemorrhage in small preterm newborns, especially those weighing less than 1500 g (3.3 lb) or of less than 34 weeks' gestation. Up to 34 weeks' gestation, the preterm baby's brain ventricles are lined by the germinal matrix, which is highly susceptible to hypoxic events such as respiratory distress, birth trauma, and birth asphyxia. The germinal matrix is highly vascular, and these blood vessels rupture in the presence of hypoxia (Scher, 2013).

Other common problems of preterm newborns such as NEC were briefly discussed in the earlier physiologic sections. (For in-depth discussions of RDS, hyperbilirubinemia, hypoglycemia, anemia of prematurity, and sepsis, see Chapter 27.)

SAFETY ALERT!

An extremely premature, low-birth-weight newborn who presents with a sudden drop in hemoglobin along with the onset of severe metabolic acidosis, a "waxy" color, and hypotension may have experienced an intraventricular hemorrhage.

Long-Term Needs and Outcome

The care of preterm newborns and their families does not stop on discharge from the nursery. Within the first year of life, low-birth-weight preterm infants face higher mortality rates than term infants. Causes of death include sudden infant death syndrome (SIDS)—which occurs about 5 times more frequently in the preterm infant—respiratory infections, and neurologic defects. Morbidity is also much higher among preterm infants, with those weighing less than 1500 g (3.3 lb) at birth at highest risk for long-term complications.

The most common long-term needs observed in preterm infants include the following:

- *Retinopathy of prematurity (ROP).* Premature newborns are particularly susceptible to characteristic retinal changes, known as ROP, which can result in visual impairment. The disease is now viewed as multifactorial in origin. Increased survival of very-low-birth-weight (VLBW) babies may be the most important factor in the increased incidence of ROP.

SAFETY ALERT!

According to AAP (2013), all newborns with a birth weight of less than or equal to 1500 g (3.3 lb) or gestational age of 30 weeks or less and selected newborns with a birth weight between 1500 and 2000 g (3.3 and 4.4 lb) or gestational age of more than 30 weeks with an unstable clinical course should have a retinal screening examination (see Figure 26–9).

- *Bronchopulmonary dysplasia (BPD).* Long-term lung disease is a result of damage to the alveolar epithelium secondary to positive pressure respiratory therapy and high oxygen concentration. These infants have long-term dependence on oxygen therapy and an increased incidence of respiratory infection during their first few years of life.

- *Neurologic problems.* The most common neurologic defects include cerebral palsy, hydrocephalus, seizure disorders, lower IQ, and learning disabilities. However, the socioeconomic climate and family support systems are extremely important influences on the child's ultimate school performance in the absence of major neurologic defects. Families can be reminded that risk does not equal injury, injury does not equal damage, and description of damage does not allow a precise prediction about recovery or outcome.

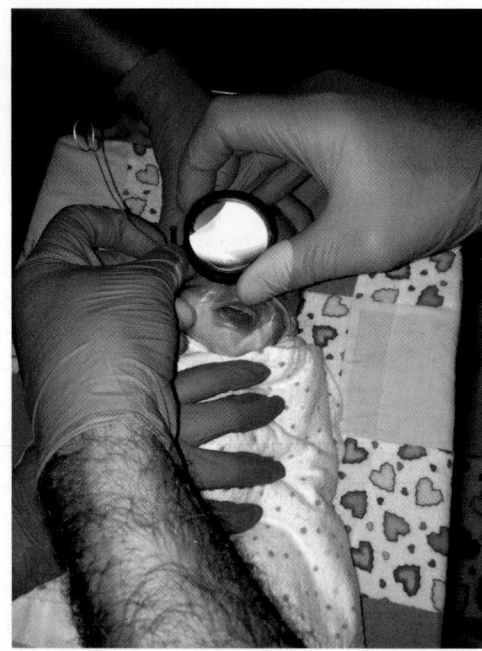

Figure 26–9 A pediatric ophthalmologist performing an eye examination on a preterm newborn screening for ROP.

SOURCE: Carol Harrigan, RN, MSN, NNP-BC.

- *Auditory problems.* Preterm babies should have a formal audiologic exam before discharge and at 3 to 6 months (corrected age). Tests currently used to measure hearing functions of the newborn are the evoked otoacoustic emissions (EOAE) or the automated auditory brain response (AABR) test (Figure 26–10). Any baby with repeated abnormal results should be referred to speech/language specialists.

Healthy People 2020

(ENT-VSL-1.1) Increase the proportion of newborns who are screened for hearing loss no later than age 1 month

---

- *Speech problems.* The most frequently observed speech defects involve delayed development of receptive and expressive ability that may persist into the school-age years.

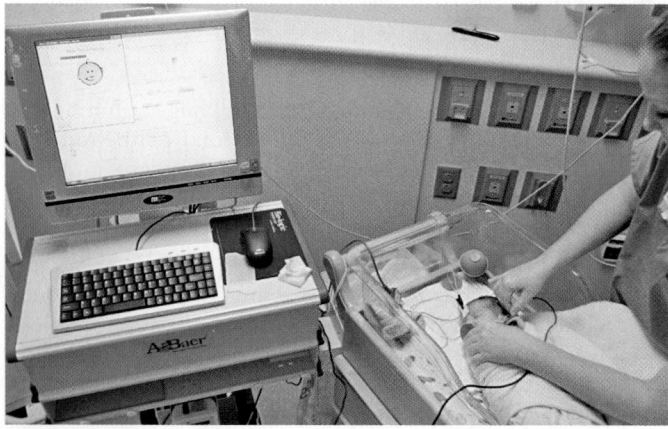

Figure 26–10 Preterm newborns should have a formal hearing test prior to discharge.

SOURCE: Carol Harrigan, RN, MSN, NNP-BC.

When evaluating the newborn's abilities and disabilities, parents must understand that developmental progress must be evaluated based on chronologic age from the expected date of birth, not from the actual date of birth (corrected age). In addition, the parents need the consistent support of healthcare professionals in the long-term management of their babies. Many new and ongoing concerns arise as the high-risk infant grows and develops; the goal is to promote the highest quality of life possible.

Nursing Management

For the Preterm Newborn

Nursing Assessment and Diagnosis

Assess the physical characteristics and gestational age of the preterm newborn accurately to anticipate the special needs and problems of the baby. Physical characteristics vary greatly depending on gestational age, but the following characteristics are frequently present:

- *Color.* Usually pink or ruddy but may be acrocyanotic (cyanosis, jaundice, or pallor are abnormal and should be noted)
- *Skin.* Reddened, translucent, blood vessels readily apparent, lack of subcutaneous fat
- *Lanugo.* Plentiful, widely distributed
- *Head size.* Appears large in relation to body
- *Skull.* Bones pliable, fontanelle smooth and flat, sutures approximated or overriding
- *Ears.* Minimal cartilage, pliable, folded over
- *Nails.* Soft, short
- *Genitals.* Male: Nonrugated, small scrotum; testes may or may not be descended, or found in the inguinal canals. Female: Prominent clitoris and labia minora
- *Posture.* Flaccid, froglike position
- *Cry.* Weak, feeble
- *Reflexes.* Poor suck, swallow, and gag; incomplete Moro
- *Activity.* Jerky, generalized movements (not seizure related), decreased tone

Determining gestational age in preterm newborns requires knowledge and experience in administering gestational assessment tools. The tool used should be specific, reliable, and valid.

Nursing diagnoses that may apply to the preterm newborn include the following (NANDA-I © 2014):

- *Gas Exchange, Impaired,* related to immature pulmonary vasculature and inadequate surfactant production
- *Breathing Pattern, Ineffective,* related to immature central nervous system
- *Nutrition, Imbalanced: Less than Body Requirements,* related to weak suck and swallow reflexes and decreased ability to absorb nutrients
- *Thermoregulation, Ineffective,* related to hypothermia secondary to decreased glycogen and brown fat stores
- *Fluid Volume, Deficient,* related to high insensible water losses and inability of kidneys to concentrate urine
- *Infection, Risk for,* related to lack of passive immunity and immature immune defenses due to preterm birth
- *Family Processes, Dysfunctional,* related to anger or guilt at having given birth to a premature baby

Planning and Implementation

MAINTENANCE OF RESPIRATORY FUNCTION

Preterm newborns have an increased danger of respiratory obstruction because their bronchi and trachea are so narrow that mucus can obstruct the airway. Maintain patency through judicious suctioning, but only on an as-needed basis.

Positioning can also affect respiratory function. If the baby is in the supine position, slightly elevate the head to maintain the airway, being careful to avoid hyperextension of the neck because the trachea will collapse. Also, because the newborn has weak neck muscles and cannot control head movement, ensure that this head position is maintained by placing a small roll under the shoulders. The prone position splints the chest wall and decreases the amount of respiratory effort used to move the chest wall, and it thus facilitates chest expansion and improves air entry and oxygenation. However, this position has become controversial, as it has been attributed to sudden infant death syndrome (SIDS); therefore be sure to explain to the parents why sleep positioning is different during the acute phase of the premature baby's illness. Weak or absent cough or gag reflexes increase the chance of aspiration in the premature newborn. Ensure that the baby's position facilitates drainage of mucus or regurgitated formula.

Healthy People 2020

(MICU-20) Increase the proportion of infants who are put to sleep on their back

---

Monitor heart and respiratory rates with cardiorespiratory monitors and observe the newborn to identify alterations in cardiopulmonary status. Signs of respiratory distress include the following:

- Cyanosis (serious sign when generalized)
- Tachypnea (sustained respiratory rate greater than 60/minute after first 4 hours of life)
- Retractions
- Expiratory grunting
- Nasal flaring
- Apneic episodes
- Presence of rales or rhonchi on auscultation
- Diminished air entry

If respiratory distress occurs, administer oxygen per healthcare provider order to relieve hypoxemia. If hypoxemia is not treated immediately, it may result in patent ductus arteriosus or metabolic acidosis. If oxygen is administered to the newborn, monitor the oxygen concentration with a pulse oximeter. Periodic arterial blood gas sampling to monitor oxygen concentration in the baby's blood is essential because hyperoxemia may lead to ROP.

Be sure to consider respiratory function before initiation of feedings as well as during feeding to prevent aspiration as well as increased energy expenditure and oxygen consumption.

MAINTENANCE OF NEUTRAL THERMAL ENVIRONMENT

Providing a neutral thermal environment minimizes the oxygen consumption required to maintain a normal core temperature; it also prevents cold stress and facilitates growth by decreasing the calories needed to maintain body temperature. The preterm newborn's immature central nervous system, as well as small brown fat stores, provides poor temperature control. A small baby (less than 1200 g [2.6 lb]) can lose 80 kcal/kg/day through radiation of body heat. Implement all the usual thermoregulation measures discussed in Chapters 25 and 27.

In addition, to minimize heat loss and temperature instability for preterm and LBW newborns, do the following:

1. Allow skin-to-skin contact (SSC) between mother and newborn to maintain warmth and faster security (see *kangaroo care*, described later).

2. Warm and humidify oxygen to minimize evaporative heat loss and decrease oxygen consumption.

3. Place the preterm baby in a double-walled incubator to avoid radiative heat losses. Some institutions care for preterm newborns under radiant warmers, piping in humidity (swamping) and covering the babies' bodies with polyethylene plastic wrap. Do not use Plexiglas shields on radiant warmer beds because they block the infrared heat.

4. Avoid placing the baby on cold surfaces such as metal treatment tables and cold x-ray plates (conductive heat loss). Pad cold surfaces with diapers and use radiant warmers during procedures, place the preterm newborn on prewarmed mattresses, and warm hands before handling the baby to prevent heat transfer via conduction.

5. Use warmed ambient humidity within the incubator. Humidity can decrease insensible and transdermal water loss because of evaporative heat loss (Lund et al., 2013). However, humidity should only be started once the newborn's temperature is within normal limits.

6. Keep the skin dry (evaporative heat loss) and place a cap on the baby's head. The head makes up 25% of the total body size.

7. Keep radiant warmers, incubators, and cribs away from windows and cold external walls (radiative heat loss) and out of drafts (conductive heat loss).

8. Open incubator portholes and doors only when necessary, and use plastic sleeves on portholes to decrease convective heat loss.

9. Use a skin probe to monitor the baby's skin temperature. Correlate ambient temperatures with the skin probe in the incubator using the servocontrol rather than the manual mode. The temperature should be 36° to 37°C (96.8° to 98.6°F). Temperature fluctuations indicate hypothermia or hyperthermia. Be careful not to place skin temperature probes over bony prominences, areas of brown fat, poorly vasoreactive areas such as extremities, or excoriated areas.

10. Warm formula or stored breast milk before feeding.

11. Use reflector patch over the skin temperature probe when using a radiant warmer bed so that the probe does not sense the higher infrared temperature as the baby's skin temperature and therefore decrease the heater output.

Once preterm newborns are medically stable, they can be clothed with a double-thickness cap, cotton shirt, and diaper, and, if possible, swaddled in a blanket. Familiarize yourself with the individual institution's protocol for weaning preterm newborns from an incubator to a crib.

MAINTENANCE OF FLUID AND ELECTROLYTE STATUS

Keep the newborn hydrated by providing adequate intake based on weight, gestational age, chronologic age, and volume of sensible and insensible water losses. Adequate fluid intake should compensate for increased insensible losses and the amount needed for renal excretion of metabolic products. Insensible water losses can be minimized by providing high ambient humidity, humidifying oxygen, using heat shields, covering the skin with plastic wrap, and placing the baby in a double-walled incubator.

Evaluate the hydration status of the baby by assessing and recording signs of dehydration. Identify signs of overhydration by observing the newborn for edema or excessive weight gain and by comparing urine output with fluid intake.

Weigh the preterm newborn at least once daily at the same time each day. *Weight change is one of the most sensitive indicators of fluid balance.* Weighing diapers is also important for accurate input and output measurements (1 mL = 1 g). A comparison of intake and output measurements over an 8- or 24-hour period provides important information about renal function and fluid balance. Assessment of patterns and whether they show a net gain or loss over several days is also essential to fluid management. Monitor blood serum levels and pH to evaluate for electrolyte imbalances.

Accurate hourly intake calculations are needed when administering intravenous fluids. Because the preterm newborn is unable to excrete excess fluid, it is essential to maintain the correct amount of IV fluid to prevent overload. Accuracy can be ensured by using neonatal or pediatric infusion pumps. Urine-specific gravity and pH are obtained periodically. Hydration is considered adequate when the urine output is 1 to 3 mL/kg/hr.

SAFETY ALERT!

To prevent electrolyte imbalance and dehydration, take care to give the correct intravenous (IV) solutions, as well as the correct volumes and concentrations of formulas.

PROVISION OF ADEQUATE NUTRITION AND PREVENTION OF FATIGUE DURING FEEDING

The feeding method depends on the preterm newborn's feeding abilities and health status. Both nipple and gavage methods are initially supplemented with intravenous therapy until oral intake is sufficient to support growth. Early, small-volume enteral feedings called *minimal enteral nutrition via gavage* have proved to be of benefit to the very-low-birth-weight newborn (see section on Methods of Feeding earlier in the chapter). Formula or breast milk (with or without fortifiers to increase caloric content) is incorporated into the feedings slowly. This is done to avoid overtaxing the digestive capacity of the preterm newborn.

Before each feeding, measure abdominal girth and auscultate the abdomen to determine the presence and quality of bowel sounds. Such assessments permit early detection of abdominal distention, visible bowel loops, and decreased peristaltic activity, which may indicate NEC or paralytic ileus. Check for residual formula in the stomach before feeding when the newborn is fed by gavage. This procedure also can be performed when the nipple-fed newborn presents with abdominal distention. The presence of increasing residual formula is an indication of intolerance to the type or amount of feeding or the increase in amount of feeding. Carefully watch for other signs of feeding intolerance including guaiac-positive stools (occult blood in stools), lactose in the stools (reducing substance in the stools), emesis, loose stools, and temperature instability. Preterm newborns who are ill or who fatigue easily with nipple-feedings are usually fed by gavage. The baby is essentially passive with these methods, thus conserving energy and calories. As the

baby matures, gavage feedings are replaced with nipple- (breast or formula) feedings to assist in strengthening the sucking reflex and in meeting oral and emotional needs. Signs that indicate readiness for oral feedings are a strong gag reflex, presence of nonnutritive sucking, and rooting behavior. Both low-birth-weight and preterm newborns nipple-feed more effectively in a quiet state. Establish a gradual nipple-feeding program, such as one nipple-feeding per day, then one nipple-feeding per shift, and then a nipple-feeding every other feeding. Daily weights are monitored because often there is a small weight loss when nipple-feedings are started secondary to energy expenditure for nippling. After feedings, place the baby on the right side (with support to maintain this position) or on the abdomen. These positions facilitate gastric emptying and decrease the chance of aspiration if regurgitation occurs. Gastroesophageal reflux is not uncommon in preterm newborns. Long-term gavage feeding may create nipple aversion that will require developmental occupational therapy interventions.

Involve the parents in feeding their preterm baby (Figure 26–11). This is essential to the development of attachment between parents and baby. In addition, it increases parental knowledge about the care of their newborn and helps them cope with the situation.

PREVENTION OF INFECTION

The nurse bears the responsibility for minimizing the preterm newborn's exposure to pathogenic organisms. The preterm newborn is susceptible to infection because of an immature immune system and thin and permeable skin. Invasive procedures, techniques such as umbilical catheterization and mechanical ventilation, and prolonged hospitalization place the baby at greater risk for infection.

Strict hand hygiene and use of separate equipment for each baby help minimize the preterm newborn's exposure to infectious agents. Most nurseries have adopted the Centers for Disease Control and Prevention (CDC) standard precautions of isolating every baby and the Joint Commission requirement

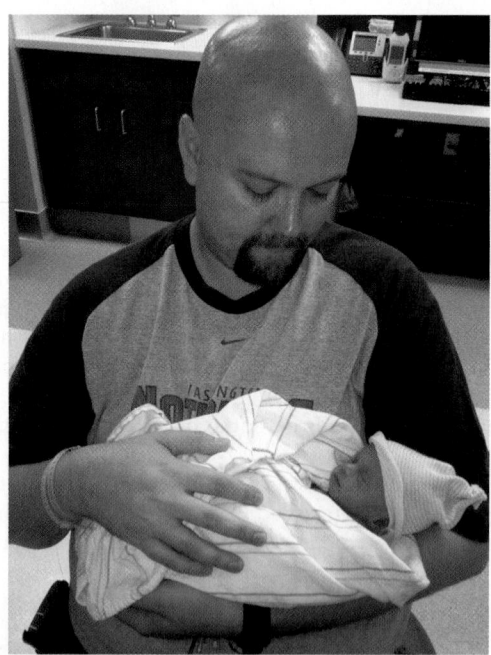

Figure 26–11 Promotion of attachment between father and his premature twin daughter.

SOURCE: Carol Harrigan, RN, MSN, NNP-BC.

that staff members have short-trimmed nails and no artificial nails. Staff members are required to complete a 2- to 3-minute scrub using iodine-containing antibacterial solutions, which inhibit growth of gram-positive cocci and gram-negative rod organisms. Other specific nursing interventions include limiting visitors, requiring visitors to wash their hands, maintaining strict aseptic practices when changing IV tubing and solutions (IV solutions and tubing should be changed every 24 hours or per agency protocols), administering parenteral fluids, and assisting with sterile procedures. Incubators and radiant warmers should be changed weekly. To prevent pressure-area breakdown, change the baby's position regularly, do range-of-motion exercises, and use water-bed pillows or an air mattress. To avoid skin tears, a protective transparent covering can be applied over vulnerable joints; however, this method is used sparingly (Blackburn, 2013). Cleansing for sterile procedures should be done with a Betadine solution and then removed with sterile water following completion of the procedure. Use water-activated gel electrodes and hydrogel skin probe covers, which both use as little adhesive as possible to decrease tissue damage. Chemical skin preps and tape may cause skin trauma and should be avoided as much as possible.

Clinical Tip

By 10 to 14 days of life, the skin integrity of the preterm newborn becomes mature and similar to that of a full-term newborn.

If infection (sepsis) occurs in the preterm newborn, you may be the first to identify its subtle clinical signs, such as lethargy and increased episodes of apnea and bradycardia. Inform the clinician of the findings immediately and implement the treatment plan per clinician orders in the presence of infection. (For specific nursing care required for the newborn with an infection, see Chapter 27.)

PROMOTION OF PARENT–NEWBORN ATTACHMENT

Preterm newborns can be separated from their parents for prolonged periods after illness or complications that are detected in the first few hours or days following birth. The resultant interruption in parent–newborn bonding necessitates intervention to ensure successful attachment.

Take measures to promote positive parental feelings toward the preterm newborn. Photographs of the baby can be given to parents to have at home or to the mother if she is in a different hospital or too ill to come to the nursery and visit. Place the baby's first name on the incubator as soon as it is known to help the parents feel that their baby is a unique and special person. Provide a weekly card with the baby's footprint, weight, and length. You also can give parents the telephone number of the nursery or intensive care unit and the names of staff members so that they have access to information about their baby at any time of the day or night. Encourage visits from siblings and grandparents to foster attachment, paying close attention to visiting policies and guidelines of the NICU.

Early involvement in the care of and decisions about their baby provides the parents with realistic expectations for their baby. The unique personality characteristics of the baby and the parents influence the bonding and contribute to the interactive process for the family. By observing the newborn's patterns of behavior and responses, especially sleep–wake states, you can teach parents optimal times for interacting with their baby. Parents need education to develop caregiving skills and to understand the premature baby's behavioral characteristics.

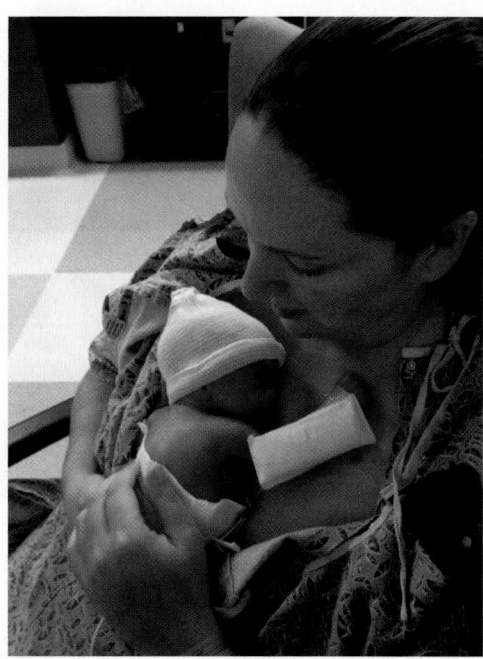

Figure 26–12 Kangaroo (skin-to-skin) care facilitates a closeness and attachment between mother and her premature baby.

SOURCE: Carol Harrigan, RN, MSN, NNP-BC.

Encourage their daily participation (if possible), as well as early and frequent visits.

Skin-to-skin holding (kangaroo care) helps parents feel close to their small newborn (Figure 26–12). *Skin-to-skin care (SSC)* is defined as the practice of holding babies skin-to-skin next to their parents. The baby is usually naked, except for a diaper, and placed on the mother's or father's bare chest. They are then both covered with a blanket. Benefits of skin-to-skin care as a developmental intervention include the following (Ludington-Hoe, 2013):

- Improved oxygenation as evidenced by an increase in transcutaneous oxygen levels
- Enhanced temperature regulation
- Decline in the episodes of apnea and bradycardia
- Increased periods of quiet sleep
- Stabilization of vital signs
- Positive interaction between parent and baby, which enhances attachment and bonding
- Increased growth parameters
- Early discharge

Limitations to skin-to-skin care may be due to staff uneasiness when moving the newborn while attached to multiple IV lines, monitor leads, and respiratory equipment. The restricted confines of the nursery may be another limiting factor to safely maneuver, position, and hold the baby.

With the parents, plan nursing care around the times when the baby is alert and best able to attend. The more knowledge parents have about the meaning of their newborn's responses, behaviors, and cues for interaction, the better prepared they will be to meet their newborn's needs and form a positive attachment with their child. Parental involvement in difficult care decisions is essential and discussed in greater detail in Chapter 27.

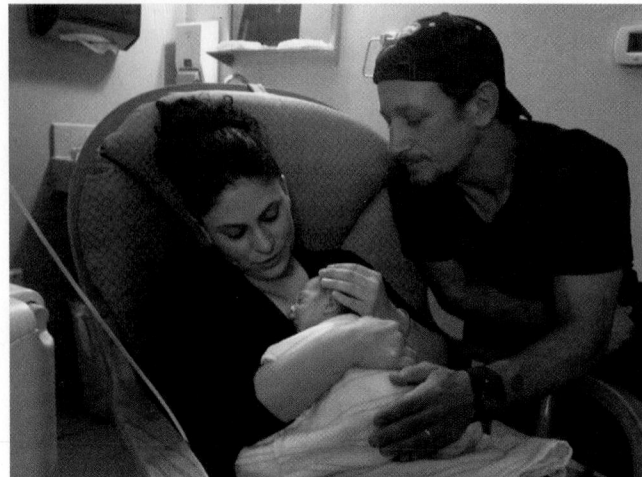

Figure 26–13 **Family bonding occurs when parents have opportunities to spend time with their newborn.**

SOURCE: Carol Harrigan, RN, MSN, NNP-BC.

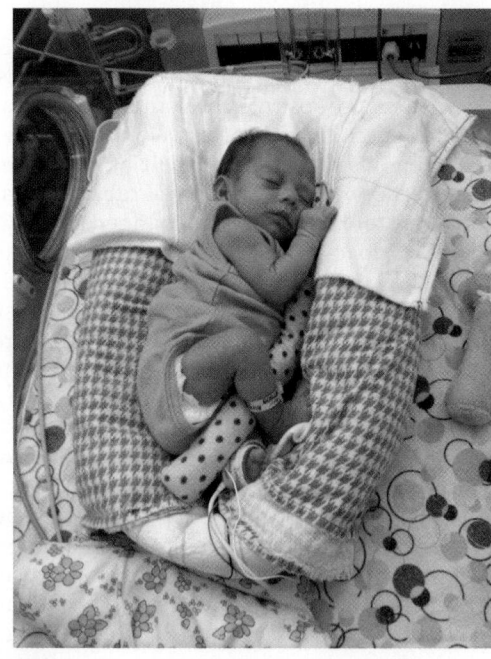

Figure 26–14 **A 3-week-old, 31 weeks' gestational age newborn is nested and developmentally positioned. Hand-to-mouth behavior facilitates self-consoling and soothing activities.**

SOURCE: Carol Harrigan, RN, MSN, NNP-BC.

Some parents may progress easily to touching and cuddling their baby; however, others will not. Parents need to know that their feelings are normal and that the progression of acquaintanceship can be slow. Rooming-in or "nesting" can provide another opportunity for the stable preterm newborn and family to get acquainted; it offers both privacy and readily available help (Figure 26–13).

PROMOTION OF DEVELOPMENTALLY SUPPORTIVE CARE

Prolonged separation and the NICU environment necessitate individualized baby sensory stimulation programs. Determine the appropriate type and amount of visual, tactile, and auditory stimulation.

Some preterm newborns are not developmentally able to deal with more than one sensory input at a time. The Assessment of Preterm Infant Behavior (APIB) scale identifies individual preterm newborn behaviors according to five areas of development (Als, Butler, & Costa, 2005). The preterm baby's behavioral reactions to stimulation are observed, and developmental interventions are then based on reducing detrimental environmental stimuli to the lowest possible level and providing appropriate opportunities for development (Blackburn, 2013).

Providing developmentally supportive, as well as family-centered, care has been proven to improve the outcomes of the critically ill newborn. The NICU environment contains many detrimental stimuli that you can help reduce. Noise levels can be lowered by replacing alarms with lights or silencing alarms quickly and keeping conversations away from the baby's bedside. Dimmer switches should be used to shield the baby's eyes from bright lights, and blankets may be placed over the top portion of the incubator. Dimming the lights may encourage babies to open their eyes and be more responsive to their parents. Nursing care should be planned to decrease the number of times the baby is disturbed. Signs (e.g., "Quiet Please") can be placed near the bedside to allow the baby some periods of uninterrupted sleep (Blackburn, 2013). Some other suggested developmentally supportive interventions include the following:

- Facilitate handling by using containment measures when turning or moving the newborn or doing procedures such as suctioning. Use the hands to hold the baby's arms and legs flexed close to the midline of the body. This helps stabilize the baby's motor and physiologic subsystems during stressful activities.

- Touch the baby gently and avoid sudden postural changes.

- Promote self-consoling and soothing activities, such as placing blanket rolls or approved manufactured devices next to the baby's sides and against the feet to provide "nesting." Swaddle the baby to maintain extremities in a flexed position while ensuring that the hands can reach the face. This permits the baby to do hand-to-mouth activities (Figure 26–14). Also provide self-consoling objects for the baby to grasp (e.g., a piece of blanket, oxygen tubing, a finger) during caregiving.

- Simulate the kinesthetic advantages of the intrauterine environment by using sheepskin and approved water beds. Water bed and pillow use has been reported to improve sleep, decrease motor activity, and lead to more mature motor behavior, fewer state changes, and a decreased heart rate.

- Provide opportunities for nonnutritive sucking with a pacifier. This improves transcutaneous oxygen saturation; decreases body movements; improves sleep, especially after feedings; and increases weight gain.

As NICUs become more and more developmentally supportive, complementary care has become an adjunct to that nurturing environment. This holistic approach in caring for the low-birth-weight newborn attempts not only to mimic the intrauterine environment, but also to foster parent–newborn bonding by simultaneously caring for the body, spirit, and mind. See Box 26–1.

PREPARATION FOR HOME CARE

Parents are often anxious when their premature newborn is transferred out of the NICU or is discharged home. Parents of preterm babies should receive the same postpartum teaching as

Box 26–1 Complementary Care in the NICU

- *Aromatherapy* is the use of scent to alter mood or behavior to produce a calming and sedating effect. There is an enhanced bonding process between mothers and newborns associated with the natural body odor emitted from the mother (Kassity-Krich & Jones, 2014). Aromatherapy is utilized in the NICU by placing an article of clothing belonging to the mother next to the newborn to produce a soothing and consoling effect on the baby in her absence. Researchers are also investigating other aromatherapies, including peppermint as a respiratory stimulant, chamomile as a method to regulate sleep–wake cycles, Brazilian guava for its analgesic effects, and lavender sitz baths for management of diaper rash.

- *Music therapy* as a noninvasive auditory stimulus has been shown to be advantageous in the premature newborn. The music used in NICUs includes primarily lullabies and soft acoustical pieces that are pleasant, soothing, and calming. Such music has been shown to effect newborn physiologic responses, such as improving oxygenation and increasing weight gain. It also has behavioral effects, leading to enhanced parental bonding and increased intervals of nonnutritive sucking periods. Language development is also enhanced if the music is live and sung by the mother or another female, which is preferential to the baby. However, the overall noise level in the NICU needs to be considered before including any extra auditory stimulation, including music therapy (Kassity-Krich & Jones, 2014).

- *Infant massage* and *gentle human touch (GHT)* have been practiced for many centuries. The types of stimulation include massage with stroking, gentle touch without stroking, and therapeutic touch or "hands-on" containment. Practitioners report such physiologic benefits as stimulating blood and lymphatic flow, promoting weight gain in premature babies, regulating sleep patterns, and many emotional and behavioral benefits. Massage demonstrates compassion while increasing the parent's empathy and understanding of the baby. It helps parents learn to interpret their baby's behavioral cues such as facial expression, various crying patterns, and other body language. At the same time, it helps babies learn about their various body parts and boundaries and feel how they integrate into the whole. *Therapeutic touch* reduces motor activity and energy expenditure by the baby and also promotes comfort.

any parent taking a new baby home. Prior to discharge, encourage the parents to spend time caring directly for their baby. This familiarizes them with their baby's behavior patterns and helps them establish realistic expectations about the baby. Some hospitals have a special room near the nursery where a mother can spend the night and "nest" with her baby before discharge.

Discharge instruction includes breastfeeding and formula-feeding techniques, formula preparation, and vitamin administration. If the mother wishes to breastfeed, teach her to pump her breasts to keep the milk flowing and provide milk even before discharge. Give information on bathing, diapering, hygiene, and normal elimination patterns and prepare the parents to expect changes in the color of the baby's stool, number of bowel movements, and timing of elimination if the baby is switched from formula to breast milk. This information can prevent unnecessary concern by the parents.

Discuss normal growth and development patterns, reflexes, and activity for preterm newborns. In these discussions, emphasize ways to promote bonding behaviors and deal with newborn crying. Care of the preterm newborn with complications, feeding problems, prevention of infections, and recognizing signs of a sick baby and the need for continued medical follow-up are other key issues. Family-care conferences with the collaborative care team involved in the care of the preterm newborn are often helpful just prior to discharge.

Families with preterm newborns usually do not need to be referred to community agencies, such as visiting nurse assistance. Referral may be necessary if the baby has severe congenital abnormalities, feeding problems, or complications with infections or respiratory problems, or if the parents seem unable to cope with an at-risk baby. Parents of preterm babies can benefit from meeting with others in a similar situation to share common experiences and concerns. Refer parents to support groups sponsored by the hospital or by others in the community and make connections for parents with early education intervention centers.

Preterm and low-birth-weight (LBW) babies are at greater risk of increased morbidity from vaccine-preventable diseases. Stable preterm babies show consistently high rates of seroconversion following the first dose of hepatitis B vaccine even when the first dose is given as early as 1 month after birth (American Academy of Pediatrics [AAP] Committee on Fetus and Newborn & American College of Obstetricians and Gynecologists [ACOG] Committee on Obstetrics, 2012). The medically stable preterm baby and LBW baby should receive full doses of diphtheria, tetanus, acellular pertussis, *Haemophilus influenzae* type b (Hib), hepatitis B, poliovirus, rotovirus, and pneumococcal conjugate vaccines (PCV) at a chronologic age consistent with the schedule recommended for full-term babies. The influenza vaccine should be administered at 6 months of age before the beginning of and during the influenza season. The vaccine for immunoprophylaxis against respiratory syncytial virus (RSV) is given to those high-risk newborns prior to discharge from the NICU and monthly thereafter during local RSV season.

Evaluation

Expected outcomes of nursing care include the following:

- The preterm newborn is free of respiratory distress and establishes effective respiratory function.

- The preterm newborn gains weight and shows no signs of fatigue or aspiration during feedings.

- The preterm newborn demonstrates a serial head circumference growth rate of 1 cm (0.4 in.) per week.

- The parents are able to verbalize their anger and guilt feelings about the birth of a preterm baby and show attachment behavior such as frequent visits and growing confidence in their participatory care activities.

Care of the Newborn With Congenital Anomalies

The birth of a baby with a congenital defect places both newborn and family at risk. Many congenital anomalies can be life threatening if not corrected within hours after birth; others are very visible and cause families emotional distress. Table 26–2 identifies common anomalies and their early management and nursing

TABLE 26–2 Congenital Anomalies: Identification and Care in the Newborn Period

CONGENITAL ANOMALY	NURSING ASSESSMENTS	NURSING GOALS AND INTERVENTIONS
CONGENITAL HYDRO-CEPHALUS (progressive ventricular enlargement due to a malformation and obstruction in the flow of the *cerebrospinal fluid* [CSF] pathways)	Enlarged or full fontanelles Split or widened sutures "Setting sun" eyes Head circumference greater than 90% on growth chart Visibly distended scalp veins Behavioral state changes; may become increasingly irritable or lethargic	Assess presence of hydrocephalus: Measure and plot initial occipital–frontal circumference (OFC) measurement; then measure daily. Check fontanelle for bulging and sutures for widening. Obtain neurosurgery consult. Assist with imaging studies, to include cranial ultrasound, CT scan, and MRI. Maintain skin integrity: Change position frequently. Use gel pillow under head. Postoperatively, position head off operative site, watch for signs of infection.
CHOANAL ATRESIA (unilateral or bilateral bony occlusion of posterior nares)	Respiratory distress (cyanosis and retractions at rest) Noisy respirations Difficulty breathing during feeding (obligatory nose breathers) Obstruction by thick mucus	Assess patency of nares: Listen for breath sounds while holding baby's mouth closed and alternately compressing each nostril. Assist with passing a catheter through each naris to confirm diagnosis. Obtain ENT consult. Maintain respiratory function: Assist with taping airway in mouth to prevent respiratory distress. Position with head elevated to improve air exchange.
CLEFT LIP (unilateral or bilateral visible defect) 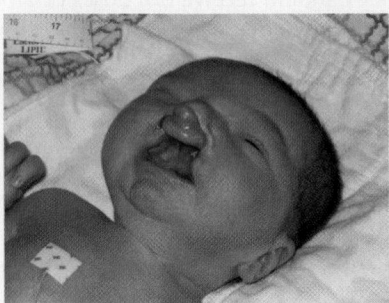 Bilateral cleft lip with cleft abnormality involving both hard and soft palates. **SOURCE:** Carol Harrigan, RN, MSN, NNP-BC.	May involve upper lip only or may involve external nares, nasal cartilage, nasal septum, and alveolar process Flattening or depression of midfacial contour	Provide nutrition: Feed with special nipple and bottle. Burp frequently (increased tendency to swallow air and reflex vomiting). Obtain craniofacial/ENT consult. Clean cleft with sterile water (to prevent crusting on cleft before repair). Support parental coping: Assist parents with grief over loss of idealized baby. Encourage verbalization of their feelings about visible defect.
CLEFT PALATE (fissure connecting oral and nasal cavity)	May involve uvula and soft palate May extend forward to nostril involving hard palate and maxillary alveolar ridge Difficulty in sucking Expulsion of formula through nose	Prevent aspiration/infection: Place in side-lying position to facilitate drainage. Obtain craniofacial/ENT consult. Feed in upright position (to prevent formula from flowing back into nasal passages, to aid swallowing and discourage aspiration). Provide nutrition: Feed with special nipple and bottle. Formula may escape through the nose, which is common (nasal regurgitation). Burp after each ounce (tend to swallow large amounts of air). Plot weight gain patterns to assess adequacy of diet. Provide parental support: Refer parents to community agencies, support groups, and speech pathologists. Encourage verbalization of frustrations because feeding process is long and frustrating. Praise all parental efforts. Encourage parents to seek prompt treatment for upper respiratory infection (URI) and teach them ways to decrease URI.

CONGENITAL ANOMALY	NURSING ASSESSMENTS	NURSING GOALS AND INTERVENTIONS
TRACHEOESOPHAGEAL FISTULA (lower esophageal segment connects to the lower trachea with upper esophageal segment ending blindly [atresia])	History of maternal polyhydramnios Excessive oral secretions Constant drooling Abdominal distention beginning soon after birth Periodic choking and cyanotic episodes Immediate regurgitation when feeding Aspiration of pharyngeal contents into trachea. Signs/symptoms: tachypnea, retractions, rhonchi, decreased breath sounds, cyanotic spells Reflux of gastric contents into trachea leading to aspiration pneumonia Inability to pass nasogastric tube (will not pass beyond 10–15 cm from nares)	Maintain respiratory status and prevent aspiration. Withhold feeding until esophageal patency is determined by chest radiograph Obtain a surgical consult. Place an indwelling Replogle tube attached to low intermittent suction to control saliva and mucus (to prevent aspiration pneumonia) in esophageal pouch. Elevate head of bed 20–40 degrees (to prevent reflux of gastric contents). Keep baby calm (crying causes air to pass through fistula and to distend intestines, causing compression of the diaphragm and respiratory embarrassment). Maintain fluid and electrolyte balance. Begin broad-spectrum antibiotics secondary to risk of aspiration pneumonia. Give fluids to replace esophageal drainage and maintain hydration. Provide parent education: Explain staged repair—primary or staged—provision of gastrostomy, ligation of fistula, repair of atresia. Keep parents informed; clarify and reinforce healthcare provider's explanations regarding malformation, surgical repair, preoperative and postoperative care, and prognosis.

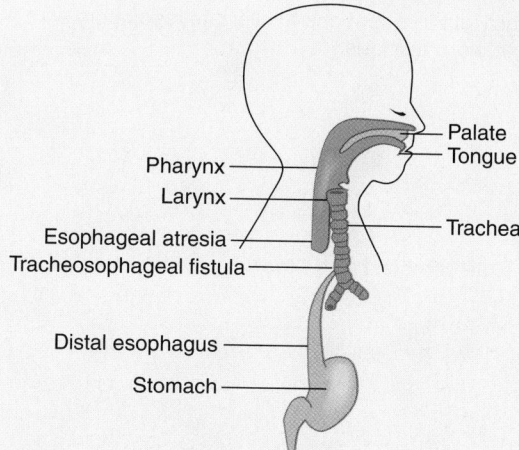

The most frequently seen type of congenital tracheoesophageal fistula with esophageal atresia.

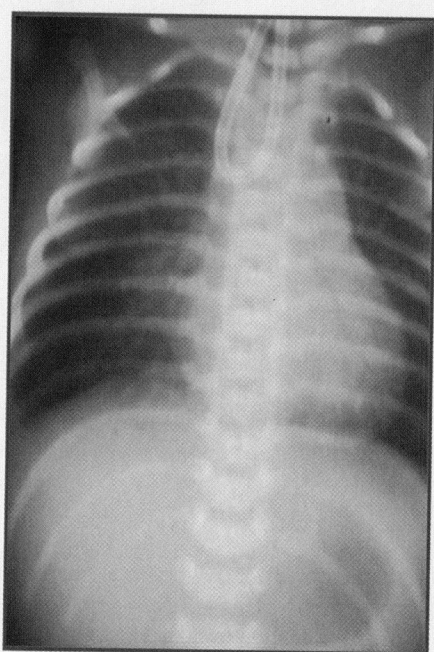

TEF with esophageal atresia. Note coiled NG tube and large stomach bubble.
SOURCE: Carol Harrigan, RN, MSN, NNP-BC.

(continued)

TABLE 26–2 Congenital Anomalies: Identification and Care in the Newborn Period (*continued*)

CONGENITAL ANOMALY	NURSING ASSESSMENTS	NURSING GOALS AND INTERVENTIONS
DIAPHRAGMATIC HERNIA (portion of intestines in the thoracic cavity through abnormal opening in diaphragm, occurring commonly on the left side)	Difficulty initiating respirations secondary to hypoplastic lung on affected side, compression of lung on contralateral side Gasping respirations with nasal flaring and chest retractions Barrel chest and scaphoid abdomen Asymmetric chest expansion Breath sounds may be diminished or absent, usually on affected side Heart sounds displaced to contralateral side Bowel sounds may be heard in thoracic cavity	Nurse should never ventilate with bag and mask O_2 because the stomach and intestines will become air-filled and distended, further compressing the lungs. Obtain chest radiograph to confirm diagnosis. Obtain a surgical consult. Maintain respiratory status: Administer oxygen, prepare for intubation and ventilation (considered a respiratory emergency). Initiate gastric decompression by placing an indwelling Replogle tube attached to low intermittent suction. Place in high semi-Fowler position (to use gravity to keep abdominal organs' pressure off diaphragm). Turn onto affected side to allow unaffected lung expansion. Carry out interventions to alleviate respiratory and metabolic acidosis.

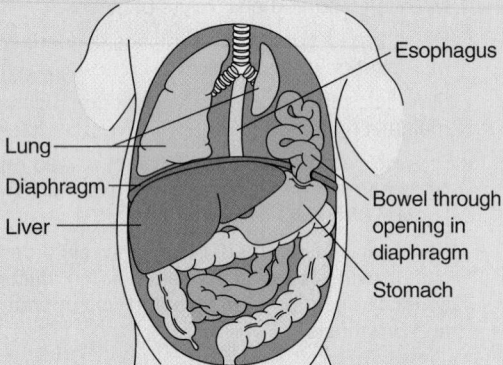

Esophagus

Lung

Diaphragm

Liver

Bowel through opening in diaphragm

Stomach

Diaphragmatic hernia. Note compression of the lung by the intestine on the affected side.

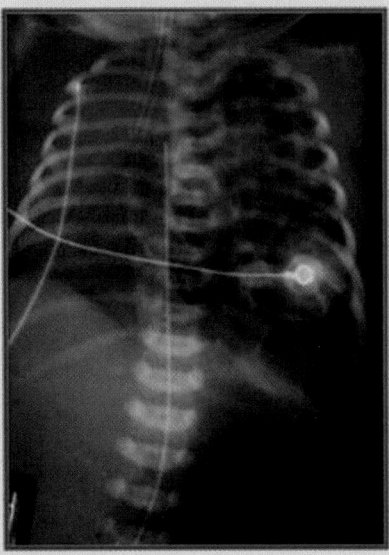

Diaphragmatic hernia. Note bowel gas pattern in the upper left chest with a shift in the mediastinum to the right.
SOURCE: Carol Harrigan, RN, MSN, NNP-BC.

| **OMPHALOCELE** (herniation of abdominal contents into base of umbilical cord) | Encased in a protective, transparent membrane | Maintain hydration and temperature.

Place newborn in sterile bag up to and covering defect.

Obtain surgical consult.

Initiate gastric decompression by insertion of an indwelling Replogle tube attached to low suction (to prevent distention of lower bowel and impairment of blood flow).

Position to prevent trauma to defect.

Administer broad-spectrum antibiotics to prevent infection. |

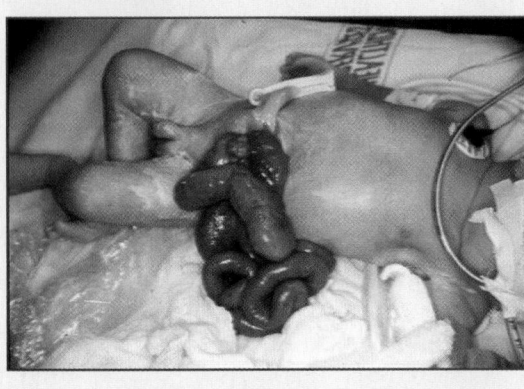

Newborn with omphalocele.
SOURCE: Carol Harrigan, RN, MSN, NNP-BC.

CONGENITAL ANOMALY	NURSING ASSESSMENTS	NURSING GOALS AND INTERVENTIONS
GASTROSCHISIS (full-thickness defect in abdominal wall allowing viscera outside the body to the right of an intact umbilical cord)	No protective covering Intestines exposed to the caustic amniotic fluid Associated with intestinal atresia, malrotation Large amount of evaporative fluid losses from exposed bowel	Maintain hydration and temperature. Provide normal saline for hypovolemia/fluid resuscitation. Place newborn in sterile bag up to axilla in a side-lying position to prevent trauma of the bowel. *Do not cover defect with wet saline gauze.* Obtain surgical consult. Initiate gastric decompression by insertion of an indwelling Replogle tube attached to low suction; measure and replace gastric output. Administer broad-spectrum antibiotics to prevent infection of exposed bowel.

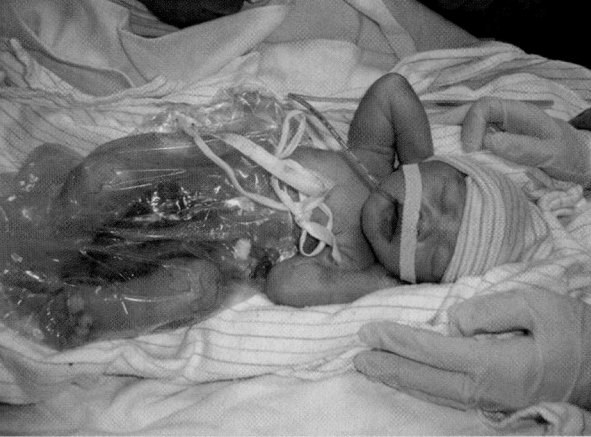

Term newborn with gastroschisis. Note the externalized loops of bowel visible through the bag.
SOURCE: Carol Harrigan, RN, MSN, NNP-BC.

PRUNE BELLY SYNDROME (congenital absence of one or more layers of abdominal muscles)	Oligohydramnios leading to pulmonary hypoplasia common Deficiency of the abdominal wall musculature causing the abdomen to be shapeless Skin hangs loosely and is wrinkled in appearance Associated with urinary abnormalities (urethral obstruction, renal dysplasia) In boys, cryptorchidism is common; rarely occurs in girls	Maintain respiratory status: May need to be immediately intubated and ventilated. Obtain surgical and urology consult. Prevent trauma and infection. Administer broad-spectrum antibiotics. Place a urinary catheter and monitor urinary output. Carry out interventions to alleviate respiratory and metabolic acidosis. Keep parents updated and informed about prognosis.

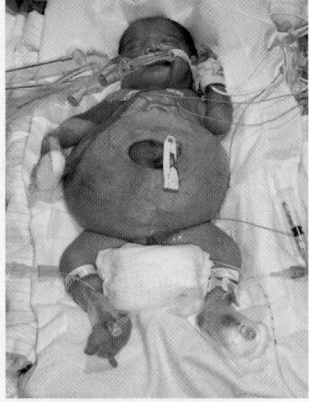

Prune belly syndrome.
SOURCE: Carol Harrigan, RN, MSN, NNP-BC.

(continued)

TABLE 26–2 Congenital Anomalies: Identification and Care in the Newborn Period (*continued*)

CONGENITAL ANOMALY	NURSING ASSESSMENTS	NURSING GOALS AND INTERVENTIONS
MYELOMENINGOCELE (saclike cyst containing meninges, spinal cord, and nerve roots in thoracic and/or lumbar area)	Myelomeningocele directly connects to sub-arachnoid space so hydrocephalus often associated No response or varying response to sensation below level of defect May have constant dribbling of urine Incontinence or retention of stool Anal wink may or may not be present	Prevent trauma and infection. Position on abdomen or on side and restrain (to prevent pressure and trauma to sac). Obtain neurosurgery and urology consult. Meticulously clean buttocks and genitals after each void and stool (to prevent contamination and infection of sac). Cover with protective plastic wrap over sac (to prevent trauma, rupture and drying). *Do not cover defect with wet saline gauze.* Administer broad-spectrum antibiotics to prevent infection. Observe sac for oozing of fluid. Credé bladder (apply downward pressure on bladder with thumbs, moving urine toward the urethra) as ordered to prevent urinary stasis. Assess amount of sensation and movement below defect. Obtain baseline occipital–frontal circumference (OFC) measurements; then measure head circumference daily (to detect hydrocephalus). Check fontanelle for fullness and bulging.
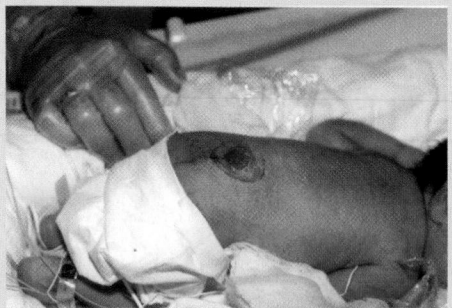 Newborn with lumbar myelomeningocele. **SOURCE:** Carol Harrigan, RN, MSN, NNP-BC.		
IMPERFORATE ANUS (absence of anal opening, may or may not have a fistula connection Boy: fistula between rectum and urinary tract, scrotum, penis, perineum Girl: fistula between rectum and vagina or perineum)	Inability to visualize rectal opening No meconium is passed Meconium passed through fistula or malpositioned anus Gradual abdominal distension if no fistula present	Inspect perineal area for presence of fistula. Initiate gastric decompression by insertion of an indwelling Replogle tube attached to low suction if no fistula present; measure and replace gastric output. Maintain fluid balance. Obtain surgical consult.
CONGENITAL DISLOCATED HIP AND CLUBFOOT	See discussion in Chapter 24	

care in the newborn period. When one congenital anomaly is found, healthcare providers should look for others, particularly in body systems that develop at the same time during gestation.

Care of the Infant of a Substance-Abusing Mother

Substance abuse during pregnancy is often undiagnosed and underestimated, putting the pregnant woman at high risk for maternal and fetal morbidity as well as significant neonatal withdrawal. Tetratogenicity, poor maternal nutrition, poor placental perfusion, and placental insufficiency leading to growth restriction in the fetus are common obstetric concerns for the substance-abusing mother. The drug use of the substance-abusing mother may vary from infrequent, recreational use to daily use due to psychologic and physiologic addiction. An **infant of a substance-abusing mother (ISAM)** may be exposed to a number of licit and illicit drugs singularly or in combination (see Table 26–3). Identification of these intrauterine drug-exposed newborns becomes essential not only to anticipate problems in the delivery room and in the nursery but also to recognize those babies at risk for long-term neurodevelopmental sequelae following discharge.

Healthy People 2020

(MICH-11) Increase abstinence from alcohol, cigarettes, and illicit drugs among pregnant women

---

Alcohol Dependence

Fetal alcohol syndrome (FAS), a leading cause of preventable, nongenetic intellectual disability, includes a group of physical, behavioral, and cognitive abnormalities frequently found in babies exposed to alcohol in utero. It is estimated that complete FAS occurs in up to 1 to 4 per 1000 live births annually in some United States and Western European populations (Chambers & Scialli, 2014). FAS rates are higher among Native Americans, Alaska natives, African Americans, and women of low socioeconomic status.

A new set of guidelines for diagnosis and referral of babies and children with FAS has been developed. Currently, the term **fetal alcohol spectrum disorder (FASD)** has been used to include all categories of prenatal alcohol exposure, including FAS. The diagnostic categories for FASD take into consideration the various clinical manifestations of FAS, the social and family environment, and, if available, the maternal alcohol history. Five diagnostic categories are used to describe effects of alcohol exposure:

TABLE 26–3 Common Drugs of Abuse

OPIOIDS/OPIATES	CNS STIMULANTS	CNS DEPRESSANTS/SEDATIVES	HALLUCINOGENS
Codeine	Amphetamines	Alcohol	Inhalants
Darvon	Cocaine	Barbiturates	LSD
Demerol	Methamphetamines	Benzodiazepines	Solvents and aerosols (glue, gasoline, paint, cleaning solutions)
Fentanyl	Nicotine	Chloral Hydrate	
Heroin	Phencyclidines	Cannabinoids (marijuana)	
Hydrocodone (Lortab, Vicodin)	Ritalin		
Hydromorphone (Dilaudid)			
Methadone			
Morphine			
Oxycodone (Percocet, OxyContin)			

1. FAS with a confirmed history of maternal alcohol intake.

2. FAS with phenotypic features but no confirmed history of maternal alcohol intake.

3. Partial FAS with confirmed history of maternal alcohol intake, some facial abnormalities, and one of the following: CNS abnormalities, growth restriction, or behavioral or cognitive disabilities.

4. Alcohol-related birth defects (ARBD) are usually determined only by a positive maternal drinking history. They present with one or more birth defects including malformations and dysplasias of the heart, bone, kidney, vision, or hearing systems and do not exhibit the classic facial dysmorphology of the FAS baby (Chambers & Scialli, 2014).

5. Alcohol-related neurodevelopmental disorder (ARND) causes CNS neurodevelopmental abnormalities and complex behavior and cognitive abnormalities. ARBD and ARND can occur together.

Although it has been known that ethanol freely crosses the placenta to the fetus, it is now known that its by-products are equally responsible for the damage. There is also strong evidence that the amount of alcohol ingested is directly responsible for the neurodevelopment outcomes of these babies; heavy alcohol use is defined as binge drinking 1 or 2 times per week and consumption of six standard drinks per occasion (Chambers & Scialli, 2014). Often, the consumption of alcohol occurs during conception, when critical fetal organogenesis is most adversely affected. (Chapter 14 discusses alcohol abuse in pregnancy.) The effects of other substances often combined with alcohol, such as nicotine, diazepam (Valium), marijuana, and caffeine, as well as poor diet, enhance the likelihood of FAS.

LONG-TERM COMPLICATIONS FOR THE BABY WITH FASD

Because of the failure-to-thrive appearance, many FASD babies are often evaluated for deficiencies in organic and inorganic amino acids. These babies have a delay in oral feeding development but have a normal progression of oral motor function. Many babies with FASD nurse poorly and have persistent vomiting until 6 to 7 months of age. They have difficulty adjusting to solid foods and show little spontaneous interest in food.

CNS dysfunctions are the most common and serious problem associated with FASD. Hypertonicity and increased placidity are seen in these babies. They also have a decreased ability to block out repetitive stimuli. Children exhibiting FASD can be severely intellectually disabled. These children show impulsivity, cognitive impairment, and speech and language abnormalities indicative of CNS involvement. As they progress through the adolescent years, they change from very thin and underweight children to those who are overweight and often obese. Short stature and microcephaly persist.

Nursing Management

For the Newborn With Fetal Alcohol Spectrum Disorder (FASD)

Nursing Assessment and Diagnosis

Newborns with FASD show the following characteristics:

- *Abnormal structural development and CNS dysfunction.* These include irritability, hypotonia, microcephaly, and hyperactivity and cognitive disability in childhood.

- *Growth deficiencies.* The growth of babies with FASD is often restricted in regard to weight, length, and head circumference. These babies continue to show a persistent postnatal growth deficiency, with head circumference and linear growth most affected.

- *Distinctive facial abnormalities.* These include short palpebral fissures; epicanthal folds; broad nasal bridge; flattened midfacies; short, upturned, or beaklike nose; micrognathia (abnormally small lower jaw); hypoplastic maxilla; thin upper lip or vermilion border; and smooth philtrum (groove on upper lip) (Cloherty et al., 2012). Figure 31-4 shows a child with FASD.

- *Associated anomalies.* Abnormalities affecting the heart (primarily septal and valvular defects), eyes (optic nerve hypoplasia), ears (conductive and sensorineural hearing loss), kidneys, and skeleton (especially involving joints, such as congenital dislocated hips) systems are often noted.

An alcohol-exposed newborn in the first week of life may show symptoms that include sleeplessness, excessive arousal states, inconsolable crying, abnormal reflexes, hyperactivity with little ability to maintain alertness and attentiveness to environment, jitteriness, abdominal distention, and exaggerated mouthing behaviors such as hyperactive rooting and increased nonnutritive sucking. Seizures may be common. These symptoms commonly persist throughout the first month of life but may continue longer. Alcohol dependence in the newborn and infant is physiologic, not psychologic. Signs and symptoms of withdrawal often appear within 3 to 12 hours and can last up to 18 months (Wang, 2014). Seizures after the neonatal period are rare.

Nursing diagnoses that may apply to the FASD newborn include the following (NANDA-I © 2014):

- *Nutrition, Imbalanced: Less than Body Requirements,* related to decreased food intake and hyperirritability
- *Infant Behavior: Disorganized,* related to central nervous system involvement secondary to maternal alcohol use
- *Coping, Ineffective,* related to dysfunctional family dynamics and substance-dependent mother

Planning and Implementation

HOSPITAL-BASED NURSING CARE

Nursing care of the FASD newborn is aimed at avoiding heat loss, providing adequate nutrition, and reducing environmental stimuli. The FASD baby is most comfortable in a quiet, dimly lit environment. Because of their feeding problems, these newborns require extra time and patience during feedings. It is important to provide consistency in the staff working with the baby and parents and to keep personnel and visitors to a minimum at any one time.

Inform the alcohol-dependent mother that breastfeeding is not contraindicated but that excessive alcohol consumption may intoxicate the newborn and inhibit the letdown reflex. Monitor the newborn's vital signs closely and observe for evidence of seizure activity and respiratory distress.

COMMUNITY-BASED NURSING CARE

Babies affected by maternal alcohol abuse are also at risk psychologically. Restlessness, sleeplessness, agitation, resistance to cuddling or holding, and frequent crying can be frustrating to parents because their efforts to relieve the distress are unrewarded. Feeding difficulties can also result in frustrations for the caregiver and digestive upsets for the baby. Frustration may cause the parents to punish the baby or result in the unconscious desire to stay away from the baby. Either outcome may create an unstable family environment and result in failure to thrive.

Focus on providing support for the parents and reinforcing positive parenting activity. Before discharge, give parents opportunities to provide baby care so that they can feel confident in their interpretations of their baby's cues and ability to meet the baby's needs. It is essential to refer the family to social services and visiting nurse or public health nurse associations. Follow-up care and teaching can strengthen the parents' skill and coping abilities and help them create a stable, healthy environment for their family. The baby with FASD should be involved in intervention programs that monitor the child's developmental progress, health, and home environment.

Evaluation

Expected outcomes of nursing care include the following:

- The FASD newborn is able to tolerate feedings and gain weight.

- The FASD newborn's hyperirritability or seizures are controlled, and the baby has suffered no physical injuries.
- The parents are able to identify the special needs of their newborn and accept outside assistance as needed.

Opiate Dependency

Patterns of abuse of opiates, including heroin, morphine, codeine, and prescription narcotics, in childbearing women have increased in the last several years (Prasad, 2014).(See section on *Substances Commonly Abused During Pregnancy* in Chapter 14 for more discussion of maternal substance abuse.)

Twenty-one to 94% of newborns with intrauterine opiate exposure are predisposed to a number of physical and neurodevelopmental complications associated with withdrawal (Pritham, Paul, & Hayes, 2012). Of those newborns, 46% to 78% will likely go on to require pharmocologic intervention for neonatal withdrawal requiring extended hospital stay (Pritham et al., 2012). Almost all opioid drugs readily cross the placenta and enter the fetal circulation, resulting in problems in the fetus in utero or in the newborn following delivery. Because opioid receptors are primarily in the CNS and GI tract, the signs and symptoms reflect CNS irritability, autonomic irritability, and GI dysfunction (Wang, 2014). The effects of polydrug use on the newborn must always be taken into consideration.

The greatest risks to the fetus of the drug-abusing mother are as follows:

- *Intrauterine asphyxia.* Asphyxia is often a direct result of fetal withdrawal secondary to maternal withdrawal. Fetal withdrawal is accompanied by hyperactivity, with increased oxygen consumption. Insufficiency of oxygen can lead to fetal asphyxia. Moreover, women addicted to narcotics tend to have a higher incidence of preeclampsia, abruptio placentae, and placenta previa, resulting in placental insufficiency and fetal asphyxia.
- *Intrauterine infection.* Sexually transmitted infections (syphilis, gonorrhea, HPV, chlamydia), HIV, and hepatitis are often connected with the pregnant addict's lifestyle. In addition, intravenous drug abuse can predispose the mother to many infections including cellulitis, endocarditis, and chorioamnionitis (Cunningham et al., 2014). Such infections can involve the fetus.
- *Intrauterine growth restriction (IUGR).* There is a high correlation between substance abuse and poor maternal nutrition. In addition, diminished placental function has been evident as an additional cause for compromised fetal growth including weight and occipital–frontal circumference (OFC). This in turn contributes to the increase risk for stillbirths (Cunningham et al., 2014). Surveillance during the antenatal period, to include serial fetal ultrasounds, fundal height measurements, Doppler velometry readings, biophysical profiles, and non-stress tests (NSTs), will assist in diagnosing IUGR in the substance-abusing mother.
- *Low Apgar scores.* Low scores may be related to the intrauterine asphyxia or the medication the woman received during labor. The use of a narcotic antagonist (nalorphine or naloxone) to reverse respiratory depression is contraindicated because it may precipitate acute withdrawal in the newborn.

Common Complications of the Drug-Exposed Newborn

The newborn of a woman who abused drugs during her pregnancy is predisposed to the following problems:

- *Respiratory distress.* The heroin-addicted newborn frequently suffers respiratory stress, mainly meconium-aspiration pneumonia and transient tachypnea. Meconium aspiration is usually secondary to increased oxygen consumption and activity experienced by the fetus during intrauterine withdrawal. Transient tachypnea may develop secondary to the inhibitory effects of narcotics on the reflex responsible for clearing the lungs. Respiratory distress syndrome (RDS), however, occurs less often in heroin-addicted newborns, even in those who are premature, because they have tissue oxygen–unloading capabilities comparable to those of a 6-week-old term infant. In addition, heroin stimulates production of glucocorticoids via the anterior pituitary.

- *Neonatal jaundice.* Newborns of methadone-addicted women may develop jaundice because of prematurity. By contrast, babies of mothers addicted to heroin or cocaine have a lower incidence of hyperbilirubinemia because these substances contribute to early maturity of the liver.

- *Congenital anomalies and growth restriction.* Babies of cocaine-addicted mothers exhibit congenital malformations involving bony skull defects, such as microencephaly, and symmetric intrauterine growth restriction (IUGR), cardiac defects, and genitourinary defects. In addition, there is a higher incidence of sudden death syndrome (SIDS). Babies exposed to methamphetamines during gestation may show a higher incidence of cleft lip and palate, cardiac anomalies, microcephaly, and low birth weight (LBW) (Blackburn, 2013). However, congenital anomalies are rare.

- *Behavioral abnormalities.* Babies exposed to cocaine have poor state organization. They exhibit decreased interactive behaviors when tested with the Brazelton Neonatal Behavioral Assessment Scale. These babies also have difficulty moving through the various sleep and wake states and have problems attending to and actively engaging in auditory and visual stimuli.

- *Withdrawal.* The most significant postnatal problem of the drug-exposed newborn is opiate withdrawal (usually from heroin or methadone). The onset of the withdrawal manifestations often begins within the first 24 to 48 hours of life; effects can be seen for as long as 21 days (Wang, 2014) See Table 26–4 for the clinical manifestations of newborn withdrawal.

During the first 2 years of life, many cocaine-exposed infants demonstrate susceptibility to behavior lability and the inability to express strong feelings such as pleasure, anger, or distress, or even a strong reaction to being separated from their parents. As a result, these infants have poor social interaction skills, cannot habitate to external stimuli, become easily overstimulated, and have difficulty sleeping. Cocaine-exposed infants are at higher risk for motor development problems, delays in expressive language skills, and feeding difficulties because of swallowing problems (Blackburn, 2013). Behavioral state control is poorly developed in drug-exposed infants, who tend to rapidly progress from sleep to the awake state of crying without a smooth transition from one state to the next. These infants also have a higher incidence of gastrointestinal and respiratory illnesses related not to drug exposure but to the mother's lack of education regarding proper infant care, feeding, and hygiene. After birth, the baby born to a drug-dependent mother may also be subject to neglect, abuse, or both.

TABLE 26–4 Clinical Manifestations of Newborn Withdrawal

Central Nervous System Signs	Autonomic Signs
• High-pitched cry	• Stuffy nose, sneezing
• Hyperirritability, difficult to console, restlessness	• Yawning
• Increased muscle tone	• Mottled
• Exaggerated reflexes	• Tachypnea (greater than 60 breaths/minute when quiet)
• Tremors, myoclonic jerks	• Sweating
• Seizures	• Hyperthermia
• Sneezing, hiccups, yawning	**Cutaneous Signs**
• Short, unquiet sleep	• Excoriated buttocks, knees, elbows
Gastrointestinal Signs	• Facial scratches
• Disorganized, vigorous suck	• Pressure-point abrasions
• Excessive sucking	
• Vomiting	
• Poor weight gain	
• Sensitive gag reflex	
• Diarrhea	
• Poor feeding (less than 15 mL on first day of life; takes longer than 30 minutes per feeding)	

CLINICAL THERAPY

For optimal fetal and neonatal outcome, the heroin-addicted woman should receive complete prenatal care as early as possible to reduce maternal morbidity and mortality rates and to promote fetal stability and growth (Prasad, 2014). Methadone maintenance programs have been the standard treatment for mothers who are addicted to heroin to combat the cravings and to prevent withdrawal. For those women dependent on narcotics, it is not recommended that they be withdrawn completely while pregnant because this induces fetal withdrawal with poor newborn outcomes.

Newborn treatment may include management of complications; serologic tests for syphilis, HIV, and hepatitis B; urine drug screen and meconium analysis; and social service referral. Screening of meconium provides a more comprehensive and accurate indication of exposure over a longer gestational period than does screening of neonatal urine (and is comparable to umbilical cord tissue samples (Wang, 2014). Neonatal hair should be used in conjunction with urine and meconium analysis.

Pharmacologic management for opiate withdrawal may include oral morphine sulfate solution, paregoric, tincture of opium, oral methadone, phenobarbital (adjunct therapy) clonidine (adjunct therapy), and diazepam. In addition, the use of the mother's expressed breast milk or breastfeeding by women who are in methadone-maintenance programs has been beneficial for substance-exposed babies in decreasing the need for lengthy neonatal abstinence syndrome (NAS) treatment (Wang, 2014). Nutritional support is important in light of the increase in energy expenditure that withdrawal may entail.

Nursing Management

For the Substance-Exposed Newborn

Nursing Assessment and Diagnosis

Early identification of the newborn needing clinical or pharmacologic interventions decreases the incidence of neonatal mortality and morbidity. The identification of substance-exposed newborns is determined primarily by clinical indicators in the prenatal period including maternal presentation, history of substance use or abuse, medical history, or toxicology results. During the newborn period, nursing assessment focuses on the following:

- Discovering the mother's last drug intake and dosage level. Women may be reluctant to disclose this information; therefore, a nonjudgmental interview technique is essential (AAP & ACOG, 2012).

- Assessing for congenital malformations and the complications related to intrauterine withdrawal such as SGA, asphyxia, meconium aspiration, and prematurity.

- Identifying the signs and symptoms of newborn withdrawal or neonatal abstinence syndrome (see Table 26–5).

Although many of the signs and symptoms of drug withdrawal are similar to those seen with hypoglycemia and hypocalcemia, drug-exposed babies have glucose and calcium values within normal limits.

Neonatal abstinence syndrome (NAS) includes both physiologic and behavioral responses. The severity of withdrawal can be assessed by a scoring system based on observations

TABLE 26–5 Neonatal Abstinence Syndrome Signs and Symptoms

Central Nervous System Disturbances

Cry	• Continuous high-pitched cry
	• Excessive high-pitched cry
Sleep	• Sleeps less than 3 hr after feeding
	• Sleeps less than 2 hr after feeding
	• Sleeps less than 1 hr after feeding
Moro reflex	• Markedly hyperactive Moro reflex
	• Hyperactive Moro reflex
Tremors	• Moderate-severe tremors undisturbed
	• Mild tremors undisturbed
	• Moderate-severe tremors disturbed
	• Mild tremors disturbed
Convulsions	• Generalized convulsions
	• Myoclonic jerks
	• Increased muscle tone
	• Excoriation (specific area)

Metabolic Disturbances

Thermo-regulation	• Sweating
	• Fever over 101.0°F (38.4°C and higher)
	• Fever, under 101°F (99.0°–100.8°F/37.2°–38.2°C)

Vasomotor Disturbances

	• Frequent yawning (more than 3–4 times/interval)
	• Mottling of the skin
	• Nasal stuffiness
	• Sneezing (more than 3–4 times/interval)

Respiratory Disturbances

Respiration	• Nasal flaring
	• Respiratory rate more than 60/min with retractions
	• Respiratory rate more than 60/min

Gastrointestinal Disturbances

Feeding	• Poor feeding
	• Excessive sucking
Vomiting	• Projectile vomiting
	• Regurgitation
Stooling	• Watery stools
	• Loose stools

Note:
- Signs and symptoms are listed in descending order of severity for each subgroup.
- Signs/symptoms are scored 1–5, with 5 being the most severe using a neonatal abstinence score sheet
- The newborn should be evaluated every 4 hours and a daily weight noted.

Source: Data from Finnegan, L. P. Neonatal abstinence syndrome. In N. Nelson (Ed.), *Current Therapy in Neonatal-Perinatal Medicine*, (2nd ed.), 1990, Ontario, CA: B.C. Decker; Zahorodny, W., Rom, C., Whitney, W., Giddens, S., Samuel, M., Maichuk, G., & Marshall, R. (1998). The neonatal withdrawal inventory: A simplified score of newborn withdrawal. *Developmental and Behavioral Pediatrics*, 19(2), 89–93. doi:10.1097/00004703-199804000.

and measurement of the responses to neonatal abstinence such as the Finnegan scale. It evaluates the newborn every 4 hours on 31 potentially life-threatening signs, which are given a score from 1 to 5 (Table 26–5). A newer option, the Neonatal Withdrawal Inventory (NWI), is another tool that evaluates and scores seven prominent signs of withdrawal; each sign is given a predetermined weight of 1 to 4, with the highest total score of 19 (Zahorodny et al., 1998). Both NAS scoring tools help to guide the need for pharmacologic intervention; pharmacologic treatment is warranted for three consecutive Finnegan or NWI scores greater than 8. Many hospitals have modified existing scales and have created a scoring system of their own.

Nursing diagnoses that may apply to drug-dependent newborns include the ones in the nursing care plan as well as the following (NANDA-I © 2014):

- *Breathing Pattern, Ineffective,* related to meconium aspiration syndrome due to fetal stress and hypoxia
- *Skin Integrity, Impaired,* related to constant activity, diarrhea
- *Sleep Pattern, Disturbed,* related to CNS excitation secondary to drug withdrawal
- *Parenting, Impaired,* related to hyperirritable behavior of the baby and lack of knowledge of infant care

Planning and Implementation

HOSPITAL-BASED NURSING CARE

Care of the drug-dependent newborn is based on reducing withdrawal symptoms and promoting adequate respiration, temperature, and nutrition. See *Nursing Care Plan: The Newborn of a Substance-Abusing Mother* for specific nursing measures. Some general nursing care measures include the following:

- Perform neonatal abstinence scoring per hospital protocol.
- Monitor temperature for hypothermia.
- Monitor pulse and respirations carefully every 15 minutes and pulse oximetry until stable.
- Provide small, frequent feedings, especially in the presence of vomiting, regurgitation, and diarrhea.
- Position on the right side-lying or in semi-Fowler to avoid possible aspiration of vomitus or secretions.
- Monitor weight-gain pattern daily to assess the need for increased calorie content of formula.
- Administer medications as ordered, such as oral morphine elixir, methadone, and deodorized tincture of opium (DTO). A sedative, such as phenobarbital, is usually used in combination with an opioid, as it does not control any of the GI symptoms associated with NAS (Wang, 2014).
- Monitor frequency of diarrhea and vomiting and weigh baby every 8 hours during withdrawal.
- Swaddle with hands near mouth to minimize injury and achieve more organized behavioral state. (Offer a pacifier for nonnutritive, excessive sucking [Figure 26–16]. Gentle, vertical rocking can be successful in calming a baby who is out of control.)
- Protect baby's face and extremities from excoriation by using mittens, as well as soft sheets or sheepskin. Apply protective skin emollient to the groin area with each diaper change
- Place the newborn in a quiet, dimly lit area of the nursery

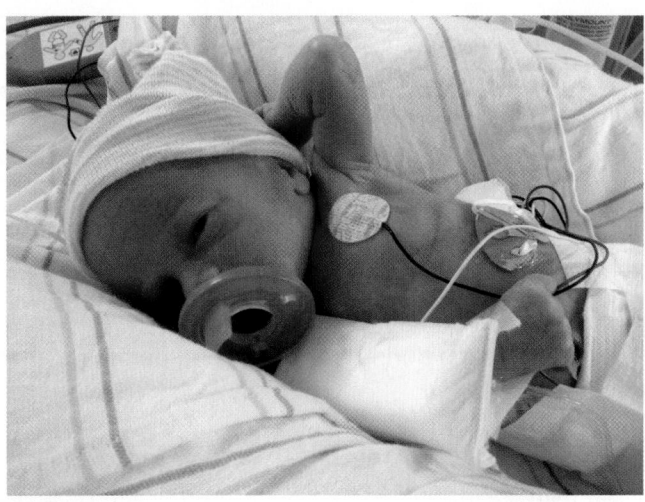

Figure 26–15 Nonnutritive sucking on a pacifier has a calming effect on the preterm newborn and also facilitates readiness to bottle-feed.

SOURCE: Carol Harrigan, RN, MSN, NNP-BC.

COMMUNITY-BASED NURSING CARE

Parents need assistance to prepare for what they can expect for the first few months at home. At the time of discharge, instruct the mother to anticipate mild jitteriness and irritability in the newborn, which may persist from 6 days to 8 weeks, depending on the initial severity of the withdrawal (Blackburn, 2013). Babies with neonatal abstinence syndrome are at significantly higher risk for sudden infant death syndrome (SIDS) when the mother used heroin, cocaine, or opiates. The baby should sleep supine, and home apnea monitoring should be implemented. Help the mother learn feeding techniques, comforting measures, how to recognize newborn cues, and appropriate parenting responses. Counsel parents regarding available resources, such as support groups, as well as signs and symptoms that indicate the need for further care. Ongoing evaluation is necessary because of the potential for long-term problems. Follow up on missed appointments in order to bring parents back into the healthcare system, thereby improving parent and baby outcomes and promoting a positive, interactive environment after birth (AAP & ACOG, 2012).

Evaluation

Expected outcomes of nursing care include the following:

- The newborn tolerates feedings, gains weight, and has a decreased incidence of diarrhea.
- The parents learn innovative ways to comfort their newborn.
- The parents are able to cope with their frustrations and begin to use outside resources as needed.

Newborns of Mothers Who Are Tobacco Dependent

Despite increased knowledge about the dangers to the fetus and newborn, 22.5% of women continue to smoke during pregnancy (Barron, 2014). The common consequence of tobacco use is addiction to nicotine. Most smokers report true enjoyment, associated with a sense of relaxation during stress, especially with the first cigarette of the day.

Nursing Care Plan: The Newborn of a Substance-Abusing Mother

1. Nursing Diagnosis: *Infant Behavior: Disorganized, Risk for,* **related to perinatal substance abuse (NANDA-I © 2014)**

GOAL: The newborn will be free of signs and symptoms of central nervous system (CNS) effects from maternal substance abuse.

INTERVENTION	RATIONALE
• Obtain prenatal records and question the mother about history of drug use. Include type of drug or drugs used, duration, time and amount of last dose taken during pregnancy and during labor and delivery.	• Confirms what drugs, if any, were abused during pregnancy. If enrolled in a methadone-maintenance program, neonatal abstinence syndrome (NAS) withdrawal will be more significant and predictable. • Noting the mother's last drug ingestion will provide the medical staff with an approximate time frame to expect the newborn to exhibit withdrawal symptoms.
• Obtain meconium drug screen using newborn's first stool.	• Confirms what drugs, if any, were abused during pregnancy. Indications to test a newborn: history of drug abuse, no prenatal care, unexplained placental abruption, changes in behavioral state of newborn.
• Assess newborn for signs and symptoms of withdrawal (e.g., high-pitched shrill cry, sneezing, vomiting, diarrhea, hypertonicity, restlessness, and wakefulness) using neonatal abstinence scoring tool per hospital guidelines.	• The average symptoms of withdrawal occur 72 hr after birth; however, symptoms may appear as early as 6–24 hr after birth.
• Provide a quiet, calm, darkened environment. Swaddle baby tightly and place in a side-lying or prone position.	• Providing a quiet environment decreases stimuli, therefore reducing CNS symptoms.
• Carefully plan tests and/or treatments to avoid excessive stimuli.	• Planning care promotes rest and reduces external stimuli.
• Use soothing techniques such as rocking, cuddling, soft music, and soft tones when speaking.	• These activities promote comfort, security, and newborn bonding.
• Administer appropriate medications as ordered by healthcare provider. Monitor efficacy of these medications as evidenced by a decrease in NAS scores.	• These medications aid the baby in minimizing symptoms related to withdrawal.

EXPECTED OUTCOMES: Newborn will have no signs and symptoms of CNS effects of maternal substance abuse as evidenced by reduced hyperactivity, irritability, normal sleep–wake pattern, no jitteriness, and no seizure activity.

2. Nursing Diagnosis: *Airway Clearance, Ineffective,* **related to suppression of respiratory system (NANDA-I © 2014)**

GOAL: Newborn will be free of signs and symptoms of respiratory distress after birth.

INTERVENTION	RATIONALE
• Obtain maternal prenatal, labor, and birth records.	• Provides information about fetal stress that may have occurred during the prenatal or intrapartum period. In addition, the birth record will provide information concerning the baby's respiratory status at birth, for example, the Apgar score.
• Assess newborn's respiratory rate and effort, skin color, heart rate, presence or absence of cough reflex, and symptoms of respiratory distress.	• Maternal narcotic consumption may depress the cough reflex and respiratory center of the newborn after birth. Symptoms such as cyanosis, tachycardia, grunting, retractions, and nasal flaring may indicate hypoxia.
• Position baby in a side-lying or semi-Fowler position.	• Prevents aspiration.
• Monitor baby for temperature elevation.	• Temperature elevation may cause metabolic rate and oxygen needs to increase when associated with CNS stimulation.

- **Collaborative:** Obtain arterial blood gas (ABG) and chest radiograph as ordered by healthcare provider.

- Monitor baby's cardiac status and pulmonary status using electrocardiogram (ECG) and pulse oximetry.

- Oxygen demands increase with drug withdrawal. Obtaining an ABG and chest radiograph will provide healthcare personnel baseline information on newborn's respiratory status, and effective medical interventions can be initiated.

- Provides healthcare personnel with cardiac and pulmonary status.

EXPECTED OUTCOMES: The newborn will maintain adequate respiratory effort as evidenced by respirations of 30–60/min; no signs of retractions, grunting, or cyanosis; arterial blood gas values within normal range; and normal pulse oximetry saturations for gestational age.

---

3. **Nursing Diagnosis:** *Nutrition, Imbalanced: Less than Body Requirements,* related to vomiting and diarrhea, uncoordinated suck and swallow reflex, and hypertonia secondary to withdrawal (NANDA-I © 2014)

GOAL: The newborn will maintain a consistent weight gain pattern.

INTERVENTION	RATIONALE
• Review gestational age assessment.	
• Assess baby's sucking and swallowing reflexes.	
• Monitor regurgitation, vomiting, diarrhea.	• Gastrointestinal (GI) hypermobility, irritation, and CNS stimulation can increase nutritional needs.
• Use bulb syringe judiciously before feedings if newborn is having problems with nasal stuffiness and congestion.	• Allows newborn to breathe easier by ridding the nasal passages of excessive mucus.
• Initiate appropriate feedings per healthcare provider orders (e.g., nipple and/or gavage); may need supplemental IV fluids.	• Oral feeding may be difficult because of CNS hyperactivity and GI hypermobility.
• Provide small frequent feedings of a high-calorie formula.	• Facilitates nutritional intake because small-for-gestational-age (SGA) newborns require 110–140 kcal/kg/day for adequate nutrition.
• Position baby on right side after feedings.	• Prevents regurgitation and promotes gastric emptying.
• Monitor baby's weight and document on graph.	• Identifies abnormalities in weight gain/loss and allows for early intervention when necessary.
• Offer pacifier between feedings for nonnutritive sucking.	• Nonnutritive sucking allows for sucking practice, management of pain, and self-consoling behaviors.

EXPECTED OUTCOMES: The newborn will tolerate feedings and maintain consistent weight gain pattern evidenced by no regurgitation or aspiration of feedings and adequate weight gain according to weight graph.

---

4. **Nursing Diagnosis:** *Parenting, Risk for Impaired,* related to lack of knowledge of infant care (NANDA-I © 2014)

GOAL: The parent will demonstrate ability to independently provide care for the newborn.

INTERVENTION	RATIONALE
• Assess mother's desire to learn baby care tasks as well as evaluate her present physical and emotional stability.	• Provides knowledge of mother's ability to care for baby.
• Instruct mother on coping strategies (e.g., exercise, listening to music, and discussing concerns openly) to manage stressful situations.	• Gives mother the tools to handle stress, thereby decreasing the chances of exhibiting abusive behavior.
• Assess mother's insight into her own chemical dependency.	• Assistance in enrollment into a chemical dependency program may be necessary before mother can independently care for baby.

(continued)

Nursing Care Plan: The Newborn of a Substance-Abusing Mother (*continued*)

- Instruct mother on signs and symptoms of withdrawal and treatment interventions.

- Offer a night of "nesting in" with newborn before discharge.

- Encourage mother and family members to perform basic baby care tasks.

- Initiate social service consult.

- Assists the mother in understanding baby's behaviors and gives her the tools to intervene without feeling anxious.

- Assists parents to care for baby by themselves, but with nursing support nearby.

- Facilitates attachment and increases parenting competence.

EXPECTED OUTCOMES: The parent will demonstrate ability to perform basic baby care tasks as evidenced by exhibiting appropriate attachment behaviors (e.g., talking to and holding baby), and feeding and bathing baby.

RISKS OF TOBACCO TO THE FETUS AND NEWBORN

Preconceptual cigarette smoking has been found to decrease fertility. Fortunately, the reduction in fertility is reversible if the woman stops smoking. Smoking during pregnancy has been associated with spontaneous abortion, placenta previa, and abruptio placentae.

The most studied compound found in cigarette smoking that can adversely affect the intrauterine environment is carbon monoxide. Carbon monoxide binds hemoglobin to form carboxyhemoglobin, which reduces the oxygen-carrying capacity of the blood. Oxygen molecules are then displaced, thus lowering fetal oxygen levels and impairing tissue oxygenation; consequently, the fetus can experience intrauterine hypoxia and ischemia. This chronic hypoxia causes the fetus to produce more red blood cells to increase available oxygen-carrying sites, resulting in polycythemia/ hyperviscosity, which can further impair placental blood flow. Mothers who smoke during pregnancy are more likely to have intrauterine growth restriction (IUGR) newborns and premature newborns. These babies typically weigh 150 to 250 g (0.3 to 0.5 lb) less than babies of nonsmokers (Cloherty et al., 2012). The nicotine in cigarettes acts as a neuroteratogen that interferes with fetal development, specifically the developing nervous system. Additional risks to the fetus and newborn of the mother who smokes include the following (Barron, 2014):

- *Intrauterine growth restriction and/or prematurity* secondary to cigarette metabolites crossing the placenta, displacing oxygen from hemoglobin, and impairing tissue oxygenation

- *Intrauterine distress* presenting as meconium staining and low Apgar scores

- *Neonatal neurobehavioral abnormalities* such as impaired habituation, orientation, consolability, orientation to sound

- *Hypertonia* or *hypotonia, increase in tremors, increased Moro reflex*

- *Signs of nicotine toxicity* (tachycardia, irritability, poor feeding)

- *Sudden infant death syndrome (SIDS)*

CLINICAL THERAPY

Inquiry into tobacco and smoke exposure should be a routine part of the prenatal history. Preconception and prenatal counseling about the effects of cigarette smoking on pregnancy and the fetus should occur. An estimated 5% reduction in perinatal mortality would occur if smoking during pregnancy were eliminated (AAP & ACOG, 2012). Mothers should be counseled that eliminating or reducing smoking even late in pregnancy can improve fetal growth. The use of nicotine patches (instead of smoking) reduces the absorption of nicotine and thereby may increase the birth weight of the fetus. See section on *Tobacco* in Chapter 10 for further discussion of prenatal smoking cessation and other intervention programs.

Cotinine, a metabolite of nicotine, has been found in fetal body fluids. There is also a positive correlation between the number of cigarettes smoked per day and the concentration of cotinine in maternal urine. Other factors that influence fetal and maternal serum cotinine concentrations are nicotine content of the cigarette and the time elapsed between the last cigarette smoked and the sampling. These findings indicate that cotinine may be used as a marker of maternal–fetal tobacco exposure during pregnancy (Prasad & Jones, 2014).

Nursing Management

Newborns of mothers who are tobacco dependent may be screened with the NICU Network Neurobehavioral Scale (NNNS) to assess their neurologic, behavioral, and stress/abstinence neurobehavioral function.

The potential for long-term respiratory problems such as asthma, as well as cognitive and receptive language delays that may persist into school age, should be evaluated.

Care of the Newborn Exposed to HIV/AIDS

Approximately 33.3 million people around the world live with HIV (Greenfield, 2013). In the United States, the CDC estimates that each year 215 to 370 babies with HIV infections are born (Glomella, 2013). Preventative strategies, including prenatal testing, antiretroviral therapy, viral load measurements, and scheduled cesarean sections, have reduced the risk of maternal–child transmission of HIV to approximately 1% to 2% (CDC, 2014). Most HIV transmissions during the perinatal and newborn periods occur across the placenta, across the amniotic membranes, or through breast milk or contaminated blood (Greenfield, 2013). The risk of vertical transmission in mothers not receiving an antiretroviral (ARV) drug regimen such as oral zidovudine (AZT) during gestation is 25% to 40% in the United States (Greenfield, 2013). Pregnant women should be universally tested (with patient notification) for HIV infection as part of the routine battery of prenatal laboratory tests unless they decline the test (i.e., opt-out approach) as permitted by local and state regulation. Refusal of testing should be documented. For further discussion of maternal and fetal HIV/AIDS, see Chapter 14. Some babies infected by maternal–fetal transmission suffer from severe immunodeficiency, with HIV disease progressing more rapidly during the first year of life.

Early identification of babies with or at risk for HIV/AIDS is essential during the newborn period in addition to a consultation with a pediatric HIV specialist. Currently available HIV serologic tests (enzyme-linked immunosorbent assay [ELISA] and Western blot test) cannot distinguish between maternal and infant antibodies; therefore, they are inappropriate for babies up to 18 months of age. It may take up to 18 months for infected babies to form their own antibodies to HIV (Greenfield, 2013). The preferred test for diagnosis of HIV infection in newborns is the bDNA polymerase chain reaction (PCR) assay and HIV RNA assays (Smith & Carley, 2014). A positive result by 48 hours of age suggests in utero transmission, thus allowing early identification and treatment. If testing is performed at birth, umbilical cord blood should not be used, as it may be contaminated with maternal blood, leading to a false positive result. A repeat, confirmatory HIV DNA PCR is done at 14 to 21 days, 1 to 2 months, and 4 to 6 months postnatally (Smith & Carley, 2014).

For newborns, AZT is started prophylactically 2 mg/kg/dose PO every 6 hours beginning as soon after birth as possible and continuing for 6 weeks; dosing for preterm babies is 2 mg/kg/dose PO every 12 hours for the first 2 weeks, then three times a day for the next 4 weeks. If the HIV DNA PCR is positive, the National Institutes of Health (NIH) recommends changing to combination antiretroviral therapy; this has been shown to decrease the rate of servoconversion of babies born to mothers infected with HIV (Davis & Yawetz, 2012). Breastfeeding in developed countries should be avoided with an HIV-positive mother as transmission of the HIV virus to the newborn in breast milk is well documented (Davis & Yawetz, 2012). A baseline complete blood count (CBC) with differential and platelets is obtained as anemia is one of the side effects of AZT therapy (Smith & Carley, 2014).

Clinical Reasoning Newborn With Possible HIV

Mrs. Jean Corrigan, a 23-year-old G1P1 positive for HIV, has just given birth to a 7 lb, 1 oz baby girl. As she watches you assessing her daughter in the birthing room, she asks why you are wearing gloves and whether her daughter will have to be in isolation. What will your response be?

Nursing Management

Many newborns exposed to HIV/AIDS are premature or small-for-gestational age (SGA), or both, and show evidence of failure to thrive during neonatal and infant periods. They can show signs and symptoms of disease within days of birth. Signs that may be seen in the early infancy period include enlarged spleen and liver, swollen glands, recurrent respiratory infections, rhinorrhea, interstitial pneumonia (rarely seen in adults), recurrent GI (diarrhea and weight loss) and urinary system infections, persistent or recurrent oral candidiasis infections, and loss of achieved developmental milestones (McLean, 2014). There is also a high risk of acquiring *Pneumocystis jirovecii* pneumonia. Opportunistic diseases such as gram-negative sepsis and problems associated with prematurity are the primary causes of mortality in HIV-infected babies.

Nursing care of the newborn exposed to HIV/AIDS includes all the care normally given to any newborn in a nursery. In addition, include care for a newborn suspected of having a bloodborne infection, as with hepatitis B.

SAFETY ALERT!

Standard precautions should be used when caring for the newborn immediately after birth until all maternal blood is removed and when obtaining blood samples via vein puncture or heelstick. The blood of all newborns must be considered potentially infectious because the status of the baby's blood is often not known until after the baby is discharged. For further discussion of the infant with HIV/AIDS, see *Immunodeficiency Disorders* in Chapter 48.

Health Promotion Preventing Infection

Most institutions recommend that their healthcare providers wear gloves during all diaper changes, especially in the presence of diarrhea, because blood may be in the stool and should be considered part of standard precautions (AAP & ACOG, 2012). There is a window of time before seroconversion occurs when the baby is still considered infectious. See Table 26–6 for some general issues for all nurses and healthcare providers of newborns at risk for HIV/AIDS. In addition, provide for comfort; keep the newborn well nourished and protected from opportunistic infections; administer good skin care to prevent skin rashes; and facilitate growth, development, and attachment.

Care of the Newborn With a Congenital Heart Defect

Congenital heart defects (CHD), the most common congenital defect, occur in approximately 8 to 12 per 1000 live births (depending on severity of the structural defects). Of those, 7.4% of all infant deaths are related to CHD, with a small percentage being undiagnosed until autopsy (Frank, Bradshaw, Beekman, et al., 2013). Of the cardiac lesions associated with death during the first 2 weeks of life, the most common are coarctation of the aorta, aortic valve stenosis, interrupted aortic arch, hypoplastic left heart syndrome, truncus arteriosus, and critical pulmonary stenosis. Coincidently, only 25% of all cardiac lesions are identified on a prenatal ultrasound. Some babies go home with their parents before their heart defect is detected. These babies with *critical congenital heart disease (CCHD)* are at risk for serious complications within the first few days or weeks of life and often require emergency care. It is crucial for the nurse to have comprehensive knowledge of congenital heart disease and perform a thorough cardiac assessment to detect deviations from normal and to initiate interventions prior to hospital discharge following birth.

Healthy People 2020

(MICH-1.7) Reduce the rate of infant deaths related to birth defects (congenital heart defects)

Overview of Congenital Heart Defects

In the majority of cases of congenital heart malformations, the cause is multifactorial with no specific trigger. Other factors that might influence development of congenital heart malformation can be classified as environmental or genetic. Infections of the pregnant woman, such as rubella, cytomegalovirus, coxsackievirus B, and influenza, have been implicated. Steroids,

TABLE 26–6 Issues for Caregivers of Newborns at Risk for HIV/AIDS

Resuscitation	For suctioning use a bulb syringe, mucus extractor, or meconium aspirator with wall suction on low setting. Use masks, goggles, and gloves.
Admission care	To remove blood from baby's skin, give warm water–mild soap bath using gloves as soon as possible after admission.
Hand hygiene	Thorough hand hygiene is indicated before and after caring for baby. Hands must be washed immediately if contaminated with blood or body fluids. Wash hands after removal of gloves.
Gloves	Gloves are indicated when touching blood or other high-risk fluids. Gloves should also be worn when handling newborns before and during their initial baths, cord care, eye prophylactics, and vitamin K administration.
Mask, goggle, and gown	Not routinely needed unless coming in contact with placenta or the blood and amniotic fluid on the skin of the newborn.
Needles and syringes	Used needles should not be recapped or bent; they should be disposed of in a puncture-resistant plastic container belonging specifically to that baby. After the newborn is discharged, the container is discarded.
Specimens	Blood and other specimens should be double bagged and/or sealed in an impervious container and labeled according to agency protocol.
Equipment and linen	Articles contaminated with blood or body fluids should be discarded or bagged according to isolation or agency protocol.
Body fluid spills	Blood and body fluid spills should be cleaned promptly with a solution of 5.25% sodium hypochlorite (household bleach) diluted 1:10 with water. Apply for at least 30 sec, then wipe after the minimum contact time.
Education and support	Provide education and psychologic support for family and staff. Nurses and healthcare providers who avoid contact with a baby at risk or who overdress in unnecessary isolation garb subtly exacerbate an already difficult family situation. Information resources include the National AIDS Hotline (1-800-342-2437) and HIV/AIDS Treatment Enforcement Service website.
Exempted personnel	Immunologically compromised staff (pregnant women may be included in this group) and possibly infectious staff members should not care for these babies.

Sources: Data from Krist, A. H., & Crawford-Faucher, A. (2002). Management of newborns exposed to maternal HIV infection. *American Family Physician, 65*(10), 2049–2056; Smith, J. R., & Carley, A. (2014). Common neonatal complications. In K. R. Simpson & P. A. Creehan (Eds.), *AWHONN's perinatal nursing* (4th ed., pp. 662–698). Philadelphia, PA: Lippincott Williams & Wilkins.

alcohol, lithium, and some anticonvulsants have been shown to cause malformations of the heart. Seasonal spraying of pesticides has also been linked to an increase in congenital heart defects. Clinicians are also beginning to see cardiac defects in babies of mothers with phenylketonuria (PKU), an amino acid disorder, who do not follow their diets. Babies with Down syndrome, Turner syndrome, and Holt-Oram syndrome, as well as trisomy 13 and trisomy 18, frequently have heart lesions. Increased incidence and risk of recurrence of specific defects occur in families.

The most common cardiac defects seen in the first 6 days of life are left ventricular outflow obstructions (mitral stenosis, aortic stenosis or atresia), hypoplastic left heart, coarctation of the aorta, patent ductus arteriosus (PDA, the most common defect in premature babies), transposition of the great vessels, tetralogy of Fallot, and large ventricular septal defect or atrial septal defects. Many cardiac defects may not manifest themselves until after discharge from the birthing unit.

Nursing Management

The primary goal of the neonatal nurse is to identify cardiac defects early and initiate referral to the healthcare provider. The three most common manifestations of cardiac defect are cyanosis, detectable heart murmur, and congestive heart failure signs (tachycardia, tachypnea, diaphoresis, hepatomegaly,

cardiomegaly). See Chapter 47 for a detailed discussion of the clinical manifestations and medical–surgical management of these specific cardiac defects. Initial repair of heart defects in the newborn period is becoming more commonplace. The NICU staff is now involved in both the preoperative and postoperative care of newborns. The benefits for the cardiac newborn of being cared for by NICU staff include the staff's knowledge of neonatal anatomy and physiology, experience in supporting the family, and an awareness of the newborn's developmental needs.

After the baby is stabilized, decisions are made about ongoing care. The parents need careful and complete explanations and the opportunity to take part in decision making. They also require ongoing emotional support. Families with a baby born with any congenital anomaly also need genetic counseling about future conception. Parents need opportunities to verbalize their concerns about their baby's health maintenance and their understanding of the rationale for follow-up care.

Clinical Tip

When cyanosis occurs in an otherwise healthy 12- to 24-hour-old newborn displaying no respiratory distress and is not resolved with oxygen, think about cardiac issues, especially a ductal-dependent lesion (termed *happy tachypnea*).

Focus Your Study

- Early identification of potential high-risk fetuses through assessment of preconception, prenatal, and intrapartum factors such as maternal low socioeconomic level, environmental dangers, maternal age and parity, preexisting maternal conditions, and pregnancy complications facilitates strategically timed nursing observations and interventions.

- High-risk newborns, whether they are premature, small-for-gestational age (SGA), large-for-gestational-age (LGA), postterm, or infants of a diabetic or substance-abusing mother, have many similar problems, although their problems are based on different physiologic processes.

- SGA newborns are associated with perinatal asphyxia and resulting meconium aspiration syndrome, hypothermia, hypoglycemia, hypocalcemia, polycythemia, congenital anomalies, and intrauterine infections. Long-term problems include continued growth and learning difficulties.

- LGA newborns are at risk for birth trauma as a result of cephalopelvic disproportion (CPD), meconium aspiration syndrome, hypoglycemia, polycythemia, and hyperviscosity.

- Infants of diabetic mothers (IDMs) are at risk for hypoglycemia, hypocalcemia, hyperbilirubinemia, polycythemia, and respiratory distress due to delayed maturation of their lungs.

- Postterm newborns often encounter intrapartum problems such as cephalopelvic disproportion (CPD), shoulder dystocia, and birth traumas, hypoglycemia, polycythemia, meconium aspiration, cold stress, and possible seizure activity.

- The common problems of the preterm newborn are results of the baby's immature body systems including respiratory distress syndrome (RDS), patent ductus arteriosus (PDA), hypothermia and cold stress, feeding difficulties and necrotizing enterocolitis (NEC), marked insensible water loss and loss of buffering agents through the kidneys, infection, anemia of prematurity, apnea and intraventricular hemorrhage (IVH), retinopathy of prematurity, and behavioral state disorganization. Long-term needs and problems include chronic lung disease,

speech defects, sensorineural hearing loss, and neurologic sequelae.

- Newborns of alcohol-dependent mothers are at risk for alterations in physical characteristics and the long-term complications of the central nervous system (CNS) dysfunction, including lower IQ, hyperactivity, language abnormalities, and congenital anomalies.

- Newborns of drug-dependent mothers experience drug withdrawal as well as respiratory distress, jaundice, congenital anomalies, and behavioral abnormalities. With early recognition and intervention, the potential long-term physiologic, neurodevelopmental, and emotional consequences of these difficulties can be avoided or at least lessened in severity.

- Newborns of mothers with HIV/AIDS require early recognition and treatment so that the physiologic and emotional consequences may be lessened in severity and Centers for Disease Control and Prevention (CDC) guidelines implemented.

- Cardiac defects are a significant cause of morbidity and mortality in the newborn period. Early identification and nursing and medical care of newborns with cardiac defects are essential to the improved outcome of these babies. Care is directed toward lessening the workload of the heart and decreasing oxygen and energy consumption.

- The nursing care of the newborn with special problems involves understanding normal physiology, the pathophysiology of the disease process, clinical manifestations, and supportive or corrective therapies. Only with this theoretical background can the nurse make appropriate observations concerning responses to therapy and development of complications.

- The nurse facilitates interdisciplinary communication with the parents. Parents of at-risk newborns need support from nurses and healthcare providers to understand the special needs of their baby and feel confident in their ability to care for their baby at home.

Clinical Reasoning in Action

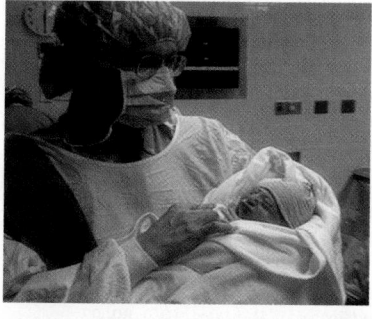

As the nurse on duty, you are caring for baby Jonathan, a 38-week IDM male born by repeat cesarean birth to a 32-year-old G3 now P3 mother. Jonathan's Apgar scores are 7 and 9 at 1 and 5 minutes. At 2 hours of age, the baby has an elevated respiratory rate of 100 to 110, heart rate of 165 with Grade II/VI intermittent machinery murmur, and mild cyanosis. He is now receiving 30% oxygen and has a respiratory rate of 70 to 80. The baby's clinical course, chest x-ray, and laboratory results are all consistent with transient tachypnea of the newborn and patent ductus arteriosus.

The mother calls you to ask about how her baby is doing. She tells you that her last child was born at 30 weeks and had to be hospitalized for 6 weeks. She says, "I really tried to do it right this time," and asks you if this baby will have the same respiratory problem.

1. What should you tell the mother?
2. What can you do to facilitate mother–baby attachment?
3. Discuss the emotional response of parents to the birth of an ill or at-risk baby.
4. Discuss the four psychologic tasks essential for coping with the stress of an at-risk newborn and providing a basis for the maternal–baby relationship.
5. Baby Jonathan is being discharged tomorrow. Review the elements of discharge and home care instructions.

References

Als, H., Butler, S., & Kosta, S. (2005). The assessment of preterm infant's behavior (APIB): Furthering the understanding and measurement of neurodevelopmental competence in preterm and full-term infants. *Mental Retardation and Developmental Disabilities Research Reviews, 11*(1), 94–102. doi:10.1002/mrdd.20053

American Academy of Pediatrics (AAP) & American College of Obstetricians and Gynecologists (ACOG). (2012). *Guidelines for perinatal care* (7th ed.). Elk Grove Village, IL: Author.

American College of Obstetricians and Gynecologists (ACOG). (2013). Practice bulletin Number 134: Fetal growth restriction. *Obstetrics & Gynecology, 121,* 1122–1133.

American College of Obstetricians and Gynecologists (ACOG) & Society for Maternal-Fetal Medicine. (2013). Committee opinion No. 579: Definition of term pregnancy. *Obstetrics &Gynecology, 122,* 1139–1140.

Armentrout, D. (2015). Glucose management. In M. Terese Verklan & M. Walden (Eds.), Core curriculum for neonatal intensive care nursing (5th ed. pp. 162–171). St. Louis, MO: Saunders.

Baker, B. (2015a). Evidence-based practice to improve outcomes for late preterm infants. *Journal of Obstetric, Gynecologic & Neonatal Nursing (JOGNN), 44*(1), 127–134.

Baker, B. (2015b). Improving outcomes for late preterm infants and their mothers. *Journal of Obstetric, Gynecologic & Neonatal Nursing (JOGNN), 44*(1), 100–101.

Barron, M. L. (2014). Antenatal care. In K. R. Simpson & P. A. Creehan (Eds.), *AWHONN's perinatal nursing* (4th ed., pp. 89–121). Philadelphia, PA: Lippincott Williams & Wilkins.

Blackburn, S. (2013). *Maternal, fetal, & neonatal physiology: A clinical perspective* (4th ed.). Philadelphia, PA: Saunders.

Bowers, B. (2014). Prenatal, intrapartal, and postnatal risk factors. In C. Kenner & J. W. Lott (Eds.), *Comprehensive neonatal nursing care* (5th ed. pp. 28–54). New York, NY: Springer.

Bradshaw, W. T. (2015). Gastrointestinal disorders. In M. Terese Verklan & M. Walden (Eds.), *Core curriculum for neonatal intensive care nursing* (5th ed. pp. 583–631). St. Louis, MO: Saunders.

Brooks, M. (2013). *US preterm birth rate drops to 15-year low, but more to go.* Retrieved from http://www.medscape.com/viewarticle/813632

Centers for Disease Control and Prevention (CDC). (2014). *HIV among pregnant women, infants, and children.* Retrieved from http://www.cdc.gov/hiv/risk/gender/pregnantwomen/facts/

Chambers, C., & Scialli, A. R. (2014). Teratogenesis and environmental exposure. In R. K. Creasy & R. Resnik (Eds.), *Maternal-fetal medicine: Principles and practice* (7th ed., pp. 465–472). Philadelphia, PA: Saunders.

Cloherty, J. R., Eichenwald, E. C., Hansen, A. R., & Stark, A. R. (2012). *Manual of neonatal care.* Philadelphia, PA: Lippincott Williams & Wilkins.

Cunningham, F. G., Leveno, K. J., Bloom, S. L., Spong, C. Y., Dashe, J. S., Hoffman, B. L., ... & Sheffield, J. S.(2014). *Williams obstetrics* (24th ed.). New York, NY: McGraw-Hill.

Daley, J. M. (2014). Diabetes in pregnancy. In K. R. Simpson & P. A. Creehan (Eds.), *AWHONN's perinatal nursing* (4th ed., pp. 203–223). Philadelphia, PA: Lippincott Williams & Wilkins.

Davis, J. A., & Yawetz, S. (2012). Management of HIV in the pregnant woman. *Clinical Obstetrics and Gynecology, 55*(2), 531–540. doi:10.1097/GRF.0b013e31824f3ae1

Ditzenberger, G. R. (2015). Nutritional management. In M. Terese Verklan & M. Walden (Eds.), *Core curriculum for neonatal intensive care nursing* (5th ed. pp. 172–196). St. Louis, MO: Saunders.

Frank, L. H., Bradshaw, E., Beekman, R., Mahle, W. T., & Martin, G. R. (2013). Critical congenital heart disease screening using pulse oximetry. *Journal of Pediatrics 162*(3), 445–453.

Geary, E. (2013). Risk of necrotizing enterocolitis and feeding interventions for preterm infants with abnormal umbilical artery doppler. *Neonatal Network, 32*(1), 5–14.

Gleason, C. A., & Devaskar, S. U. (2012). *Avery's diseases of the newborn* (9th ed.) St. Louis, MO: Elsevier Saunders.

Glomella, T. L. (Ed.) (2013). *Neonatology: Management, procedures, on-call problems, diseases, and drugs* (7th ed.). New York, NY: McGraw-Hill Education.

Greenfield, R. A. (2013). *Pediatric HIV infection.* Retrieved from http://emedicine.medscape.com/article/965086-overview?src=wnl_ref_prc_peds&uac

Hay, W. W. (2012). Care of the infant of the diabetic mother. *Current Diabetes Report, 12*(1), 4–15. doi:10.1007/s11892-011-0243-6

Jones, L. R. (2012). Oral feeding readiness in the neonatal intensive care unit. *Neonatal Network, 31*(3), 148–155.

Kassity-Kritch, N. A., & Jones, J. E. (2014). Complementary and integrative therapies. In C. Kenner & J. W. Lott (Eds.), *Comprehensive neonatal nursing care* (5th ed. pp. 773–782). New York, NY: Springer.

Ludington-Hoe, S. M. (2013) Kangaroo care as a neonatal therapy. *NAINR, 13*(2), 73–75.

Lund, C. H., Brandon, D., Holden, A. C., Kuller, J., Hill, C. M. (2013). Neonatal skin care: Evidence-based clinical practice guidelines (3rd ed.). Washington, DC, AWHONN.

Lynch, E., Dezen, T., & Brown, N. (2012). *U. S. preterm birth rate shows five-year improvement.* Retrieved from http://www.marchofdimes.com/news/united-states-preterm-birth-rate-shows-five-year-improvement.aspx

Mari, G., & Tate, D. L. (2013). *Detection and surveillance of IUGR.* Retrieved from http://contemporaryobgyn.modernmedicine.com/print/374473

McLean, K. R. (2014). Emerging infections. In C. Kenner & J. W. Lott (Eds.), *Comprehensive neonatal nursing care* (5th ed. pp. 619–639). New York, NY: Springer.

Moore, T. R., Hauguel-DeMouzon, S., & Catalano, P. (2014). Diabetes in pregnancy. In R. K. Creasy & R. Resnik (Eds.), *Maternal-fetal medicine: Principles and practice* (7th ed., pp. 988–1021). Philadelphia, PA: Saunders.

Newland, L., L'Huillier, M. W., & Petrey, B. (2013). Implementation of cue-based feeding in a level III NICU. *Neonatal Network, 32*(2), 132–137.

O'Hare, E. M., Wood, A., & Fiske, E. (2013). Human milk banking. *Neonatal Network, 32*(3), 175–183.

Prasad, M. (2014). *When opiate abuse complicates pregnancy.* Retrieved from http://contemporaryobgyn.modernmedicine.com/print/379353

Prasad, M. R., & Jones, H. E. (2014). Substance abuse in pregnancy. In R. K. Creasy & R. Resnik (Eds.), *Maternal-fetal medicine: Principles and practice* (7th ed., pp. 1132–1145). Philadelphia, PA: Saunders.

Pritham, U. A., Paul, J. A., & Hayes, M. J. (2012). Opioid dependency in pregnancy and length of stay for neonatal abstinence syndrome. *Journal of Obstetric, Gynecologic, and Neonatal Nursing (JOGNN), 41*(2), 180–189.

Raab, E. L., & Kelly, L. K. (2013). Neonatal resuscitation. In A. H. Decheneny, L. Nathan, N. Laufer, & A. S. Roman (Eds.), *Current diagnosis & treatment: Obstetrics & gynecology* (11th ed., pp. 369–388). New York, NY: McGraw-Hill/Lange.

Resnik, R., & Creasy, R. K. (2014). Intrauterine growth restriction. In R. K. Creasy & R. Resnik (Eds.), *Maternal-fetal medicine: Principles and practice* (7th ed., pp. 743–755). Philadelphia, PA: Saunders.

Rozance, P. J., & Rosenberg, A. A. (2012). The neonate. In S. G. Gabbe, J. R Niebyl, J. L. Simpson, M. B. Landon, H. L. Galan, E. R. M. Jauniaux, & D. A. Driscoll (Eds.), *Obstetrics: Normal and problem pregnancies* (6th ed., pp. 481–516). St. Louis, MO: Elsevier.

Ruth, C. A., Roos, N., Hildes-Ripstein, E., & Brownell, M. (2013). The influence of gestational age and socioeconomic status on neonatal outcomes in late preterm and early term gestation: A population based study. *BioMed Central Pregnancy & Childbirth. 12*(1), 62. doi: 10.1186/1471-2393-12-62

Scher, M. S. (2013). Brain disorders of the fetus and neonate. In A. A. Fanaroff & J. M. Fanaroff (Eds.), *Klaus & Fanaroff's care of the high-risk neonate* (6th ed., pp. 476–524). Philadelphia, PA: Elsevier.

Smith, J. R., & Carley, A. (2014). Common neonatal complications. In K. R. Simpson & P. A. Creehan (Eds.), *AWHONN's perinatal nursing* (4th ed., pp. 662–698). Philadelphia, PA: Lippincott Williams & Wilkins.

Spong, C. Y. (2013). Defining "term" pregnancy: Recommendations from the defining "term" pregnancy workgroup. *JAMA, 309,* 2445–2446.

Wang, M. (2014). Perinatal drug abuse and neonatal drug withdrawal. Retrieved from http://emedicine.medscape.com/article/978492

Zahorodny, W., Rom, C., Whitney, W., Giddens, S., Samuel, M., Maichuk, G., & Marshall, R. (1998). The neonatal withdrawal inventory: A simplified score of newborn withdrawal. *Developmental and Behavioral Pediatrics, 19*(2), 89–93. doi:10.1097/00004703-199804000-00004

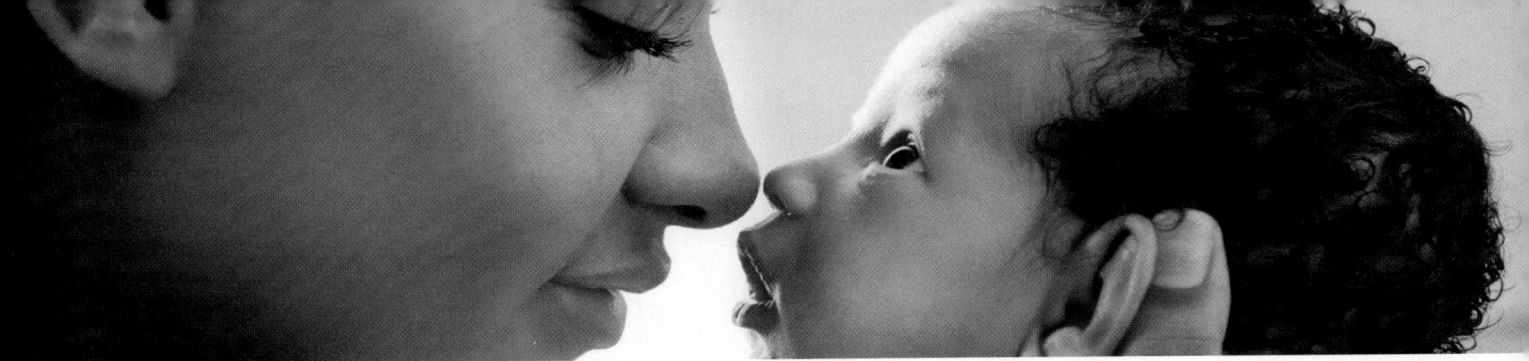

Chapter 27
The Newborn at Risk: Birth-Related Stressors

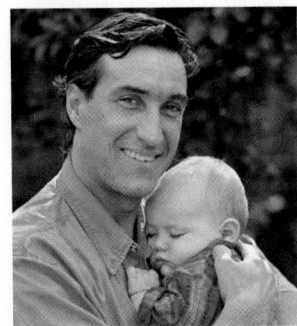

We watched him breathe every precious breath. He was covered with wires and tubes. The rhythmic tides of his sleeping and feeding spaciously measured his days and nights. We kept watch. He was special to us and we would say over and over, "Daddy and Mommy are here and we love you."

—**Alan and Claudia, parents of a baby with respiratory distress syndrome**

Leanne Temme/Getty Images

∨ Learning Outcomes

27.1 Discuss how to identify newborns in need of resuscitation and the appropriate method of resuscitation based on prenatal/labor record and observable physiologic indicators.

27.2 Differentiate, based on clinical manifestations, among the various types of respiratory distress (respiratory distress syndrome, transient tachypnea of the newborn, and meconium aspiration syndrome) in the newborn and their related nursing management.

27.3 Discuss selected types of metabolic abnormalities (including cold stress and hypoglycemia), their effects on the newborn, and the nursing implications.

27.4 Differentiate between physiologic and pathologic jaundice according to timing of onset (in hours), cause, possible sequelae, and specific management.

27.5 Explain how Rh incompatibility or ABO incompatibility can lead to the development of hyperbilirubinemia.

27.6 Identify nursing responsibilities and rationale in caring for the newborn receiving phototherapy.

27.7 Describe the causes and nursing management of newborns with anemia.

27.8 Describe the nursing assessments that would lead the nurse to suspect newborn sepsis and the nursing management of the newborn with an infection.

27.9 Relate the consequences of maternally transmitted infections, such as maternal syphilis, gonorrhea, Herpesviridae family (HSV or CMV), and chlamydia, to the nursing management of babies in the neonatal period.

27.10 Describe the interventions to facilitate parental attachment and meet the special initial and long-term needs of parents of at-risk newborns.

arked homeostatic changes occur during the newborn's transition from fetal to neonatal life. Because the most rapid anatomic and physiologic changes occur in the cardiopulmonary system, most major problems of the newborn are usually related to this system. These problems include asphyxia, respiratory distress syndrome (RDS), cold stress, jaundice, hemolytic disease, and anemia. Ideally, most problems are anticipated and identified prenatally. Some treatment may be initiated in this period, whereas other intervention measures are begun at or immediately after birth.

Care of the Newborn at Risk From Asphyxia

Perinatal asphyxia occurs in 1% to 1.5% of live births, and the incidence increases as the gestational age decreases (Cloherty, Eichenwald, & Stark, 2012; Pappas & Robey, 2015). Neonatal asphyxia results in circulatory, respiratory, and biochemical changes. Circulatory patterns that accompany asphyxia indicate an inability of the newborn to make the transition to extrauterine circulation—in effect, a return to fetal circulatory patterns, with the majority of the blood bypassing the lungs, thus failing to become oxygenated. Failure of lung expansion and establishment of respiration rapidly produces serious biochemical changes, including hypoxemia (decreased oxygen in the blood), metabolic acidosis (increased acidity of blood reflected by low pH), and hypercarbia (excess levels of carbon dioxide in the blood) (Cloherty et al., 2012).

These biochemical changes produce the following results:

- Pulmonary vasoconstriction and high pulmonary vascular resistance in relation to the lower systemic vascular resistance (following birth the pulmonary vascular resistance should be markedly lower than the systemic vascular resistance)

- Hypoperfusion of the lungs

- A large right-to-left shunt (from the right side of the heart to the left side of the heart) through the ductus arteriosus, bypassing the lungs and impeding oxygenation of the blood

As right atrial pressure exceeds left atrial pressure, the foramen ovale reopens, and blood flows from right to left (Cloherty et al., 2012). See Chapter 23 for a review of normal newborn cardiopulmonary adaptation.

However, the most serious biochemical abnormality is a change from aerobic to anaerobic metabolism in the presence of hypoxia. This change results in the buildup of lactate, which combines with hydrogen to form lactic acid, and the development of metabolic acidosis. Lactic acidosis can develop after prolonged tissue hypoxia (oxygen starvation) as active cells rely on anaerobic metabolism.

Simultaneous respiratory acidosis may also occur because of a rapid increase in carbon dioxide (PCO_2) during asphyxia. In response to hypoxia and anaerobic metabolism, the amounts of free fatty acids (FFAs) and glycerol in the blood increase. Glycogen stores are also mobilized to provide a continuous glucose source for the brain. Hepatic and cardiac stores of glycogen may be used up rapidly during an asphyxial incident.

The newborn is supplied with several protective mechanisms against hypoxic insults. These include:

- Relatively immature brain

- Resting metabolic rate lower than that of adults

- Ability to mobilize substances within the body for anaerobic metabolism and to use energy more efficiently

- Intact circulatory system able to redistribute lactate and hydrogen ions in tissues still being perfused

Severe prolonged hypoxia overcomes these protective mechanisms, resulting in brain damage or death of the newborn. The newborn suffering apnea requires immediate resuscitative efforts. The need for resuscitation can be anticipated if specific risk factors are present during the pregnancy or labor and birth period.

Risk Factors Predisposing to Asphyxia

The need for resuscitation may be anticipated if the mother demonstrates the antepartum and intrapartum risk factors described in Tables 9–1 and 17–2.

Fetal/neonatal risk factors are as follows (American Academy of Pediatrics [AAP] & American Heart Association [AHA], 2011; Gomella, 2013):

- Nonreassuring fetal heart rate (FHR) pattern/sustained bradycardia

- Impairment of maternal oxygenation (maternal asthma/cardiac disease)

- Anything affecting blood flow through the placenta

- Significant intrapartum bleeding

- Difficult birth, prolonged labor

- Fetal scalp/capillary blood sample acidosis pH less than 7.2

- Narcotic use in labor

- History of meconium in amniotic fluid

- Prematurity

- Male baby

- Small-for-gestational age (SGA) or macrosomia

- Infant of a diabetic mother (IDM)

- Multiple births

- Structural lung abnormality/oligohydramnios (congenital diaphragmatic hernia, lung hypoplasia)

- Congenital heart disease

- Anemia: isoimmunization, fetal-maternal hemorrhage, parvovirus

Risk factors are not always apparent prenatally. Particular attention must be paid to all at-risk pregnancies during the intrapartum period. Certain aspects of labor and birth challenge the oxygen supply to the fetus, and often the at-risk fetus has less tolerance to the stress of labor (indicated by decelerations, a fixed baseline heart rate, or lack of variability of the FHR) and birth (AAP & AHA, 2011).

Clinical Therapy

The initial goal of clinical management is to identify the fetus at risk for asphyxia, so that resuscitative efforts can begin at birth.

Fetal biophysical assessment (see Chapter 13), combined with monitoring of fetal pH, FHR, and fetal oximeter if available during the intrapartum period, may help identify the presence of nonreassuring fetal status. If nonreassuring fetal status is present, appropriate measures can be taken to deliver the fetus immediately, before major damage occurs, and to treat the asphyxiated newborn.

The stress of labor causes an intermittent decrease in exchange of gases in the placental intervillous space, which causes the fall in pH and fetal metabolic acidosis. The acidosis is primarily metabolic. During labor, a fetal pH of

- 7.25 or higher is considered normal (nonacidemia)
- 7.20 or less is considered an ominous sign of intrauterine asphyxia (acidemia)
- Less than 7 is considered pathologic acidemia (Cloherty et al., 2012).

However, low fetal pH without associated hypoxia can be caused by maternal acidosis secondary to prolonged labor, dehydration, and maternal lactate production.

Assessment of the newborn's need for resuscitation begins at the time of birth by assessing skin color, heart rate, and respirations/respiratory effort of the newborn. The nurse should note the time of the first gasp, first cry, and onset of sustained respirations in order of occurrence. The Apgar score (see Chapter 18 for discussion of the Apgar score) may be helpful in describing the status of the newborn at birth and subsequent adaptation to the extrauterine environment, but should not be used to determine whether certain steps need to be taken during resuscitation. The Apgar can serve as a measure of the neonate's response to effective resuscitation and clinical status (Pappas & Robey, 2015). If indicated, resuscitation should be started before the 1-minute Apgar score is calculated. An assisted Apgar scoring system is recommended by the AAP Committee on the Fetus and Newborn, which documents the assistance the newborn is receiving at the time his or her score is assigned (American Academy of Pediatrics [AAP] & American College of Obstetricians and Gynecologists [ACOG], 2012). The Apgar score at 1 minute tends to relate to intrapartum depression, an ischemic or hypoxic event in utero, and subsequent scores relate to adequacy of resuscitative efforts (Rubarth, 2012). Retrospective Apgar scores are likely to be assigned when stabilizing critically ill newborns. A score of less than 7 at 5 minutes following birth requires that additional scores be assigned every 5 minutes up to 20 minutes (AAP & AHA, 2011).

Resuscitative efforts are required by 10% of all newborns to begin breathing, 3% require positive pressure ventilation, and 1% of all newborns require more extensive resuscitative efforts (AAP & AHA, 2011; Sawyer, Laubach, Hudak, et al., 2013; Trevisanuto et al., 2013). Identification of newborns who may require resuscitation is accomplished by carrying out a rapid assessment of four characteristics by asking the following questions:

1. What is the gestational age?
2. Is the amniotic fluid clear of meconium and evidence of infection?
3. How many babies are expected?
4. Are there any other risk factors?

Following birth, these three questions need to be posed:

1. Is the baby term?
2. Is the baby breathing and crying?
3. Does the baby have good muscle tone?

If the answers to these questions are "yes," then the baby does not need resuscitation and should not be separated from the mother. If the answer to *any* of the previous questions is "no," then the baby should receive resuscitative assistance (AAP & AHA, 2011). The baby should receive one or more of the following categories of action:

- Initial steps in stabilization (warming, positioning, clearing the airway as necessary, drying, stimulating, and repositioning)
- Oxygen administration with continuous monitoring of the pulse oximeter, preferably on the right hand or wrist because it will be measuring the amount of oxygen available to the brain (Bagwell, 2014b)
- Positive pressure ventilation
- Chest compressions
- Administration of epinephrine, volume expansion, or both (AAP & AHA, 2011; AAP & ACOG, 2012)

SAFETY ALERT!

In the birthing room, exposure to blood or other body fluids is inevitable. Standard precautions must be practiced by wearing caps, goggles or glasses, gloves, and impervious gowns until the cord is cut and the newborn is dried and wrapped (Cloherty et al., 2012).

Resuscitation Management

After the first few breaths, the nurse places the newborn in a level "sniff" position (the head is tilted just far enough back so that the baby appears to be sniffing the air with the nose pointed upward) under a radiant heat source and dries the baby quickly with warm blankets to maintain abdominal skin temperature at about 36.5° to 37.0°C (97.7° to 98.6°F). The stable newborn may be placed on the mother's chest or abdomen "skin-to-skin" as another heat source. If assessment indicates that further assistance and formal resuscitation are necessary, the baby continues in the radiant warmer in a position that facilitates easy access by healthcare providers (Gleason & Devaskar, 2012).

Breathing is established by employing the simplest form of resuscitative measures initially, with progression to more complicated methods, as required. For example:

1. Position and clear airway as necessary. Simple stimulation is provided by rubbing the back with a blanket or towel, while simultaneously drying the baby.

2. If respirations have not been initiated or are inadequate (gasping or occasional respirations), the lungs must be inflated with positive pressure (Niermeyer, Clarke, & Hernandez, 2016). The proper sized mask is positioned securely on the face (over the nose and mouth, avoiding the eyes) with the baby's head in a *sniffing* or neutral position (Figure 27–1). Hyperextension of the baby's neck will obstruct the trachea and must be avoided. An airtight connection is made between the baby's face and the mask (thus allowing the flow inflating bag to inflate). The lungs are inflated rhythmically by squeezing the bag.

All devices utilized for ventilation of newborns during resuscitation should have a pressure gauge/manometer in place. These devices include the following:

- Self-inflating bag
- Flow inflating/anesthesia bag
- T-Piece resuscitator (AAP & AHA, 2011; Bagwell, 2014b)

Supplemental oxygen is not utilized when initiating resuscitation on a term newborn. The amount of oxygen administered is titrated from 21% (room air) to 100% based on clinical assessment of the preterm newborn (Saugstad

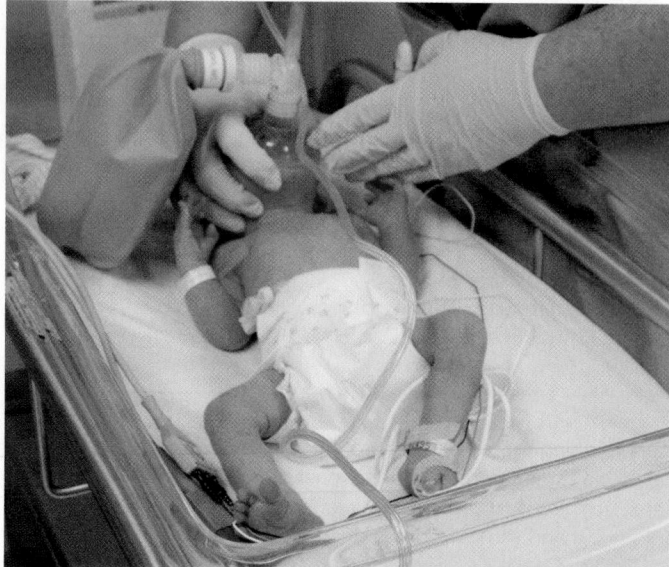

Figure 27–1 Demonstration of resuscitation of a newborn with bag and mask. Note that the mask covers the nose and mouth, and the head is in a neutral position. The resuscitating bag is placed to the side of the baby so that chest movement can be seen.

et al., 2014; Trevisanuto et al., 2013). Oxygen is a medication, and it is only administered in the presence of central cyanosis or when the pulse oximeter readings are less than expected for the age of the newborn. Too much oxygen can actually cause long-term detrimental outcomes (Sabir, Jary, Tooley, et al., 2012). Oxygen saturation of the neonate in utero is approximately 60%, and it typically increases to greater than 90% during the first 10 minutes following birth. An anesthesia bag with an attached manometer or modified self-inflating bag and adequate liter flow of 5 to 10 L/min is utilized for neonatal resuscitation (AAP & AHA, 2011).

3. Chest movement is observed for proper ventilation. Air entry and heart rate (HR) are checked by auscultation; HR may be quickly checked by palpating the base of the umbilical cord stump and counting the pulsations for 6 seconds and then multiplying by 10. Manual resuscitation is coordinated with any voluntary efforts. During positive pressure ventilation, squeeze the resuscitation bag just enough to improve HR, color, and muscle tone, at a rate of 40 to 60 breaths per minute. Pressure should be adequate to move the chest wall. The pressure gauge (manometer) must be in place to avoid over distention of the newborn's lungs and other problems such as pneumothorax or abdominal distention. An inspiratory pressure of approximately 20 cmH$_2$O should be adequate to start. Increasing the pressure to 30 cmH$_2$O or greater is occasionally necessary if there is no improvement in heart rate, color, and muscle tone; however, the amount of pressure should never exceed 40 cmH$_2$O (AAP & AHA, 2011; Bagwell, 2014b). If ventilation is adequate, the chest moves symmetrically with each inspiration, bilateral breath sounds are audible, and the lips and mucous membranes become pink. Distention of the stomach is controlled by inserting a nasogastric tube for decompression.

4. Endotracheal intubation may be needed. However, most newborns, except for very-low-birth-weight (VLBW) (less than 1500 g [3.3 lb]) babies, can be effectively resuscitated by bag-and-mask ventilation. An increasing HR and CO$_2$ detection are the primary methods for confirming endotracheal tube placement.

Once breathing has been established, the HR should increase to over 100 beats per minute. If the HR is absent or the HR remains less than 60 beats per minute after 30 seconds of effective positive pressure with oxygen concentration of 21% to 100% to elicit an oxygen saturation of 60% to 65% at 1 minute and 85% to 95% at 10 minutes of age, external cardiac massage (chest compression) is begun (AAP & AHA, 2011).

SAFETY ALERT!

Establishing effective ventilation is the highest priority in neonatal resuscitation. Do not start chest compressions without first establishing effective ventilation (as evidenced by audible bilateral breath sounds and chest movement) (AAP & AHA, 2011).

Chest compressions are started immediately if there is no detectable heartbeat. The procedure for performing chest compression is as follows:

1. The baby is positioned properly on a firm surface.
2. The resuscitator stands at the foot or head of the baby and the examiner places both thumbs over the lower third of the sternum (just below an imaginary line drawn between the nipples) with the fingers wrapped around and supporting the back (Figure 27–2A). Alternatively, the examiner can use two fingers instead of the thumbs (Figure 27–2B). The two-thumb method is preferred because it may provide better coronary perfusion pressure and a more consistent and controlled depth of compression; however, it makes access to the umbilical cord for medication administration more difficult (AAP & AHA, 2011).
3. The sternum is depressed to sufficient depth to generate a palpable pulse or approximately one third of the anterior–posterior depth of the chest at a rate of 90 beats per minute (AAP & AHA, 2011). Use a 3:1 ratio of heartbeat to assisted ventilation, 90 chest compressions: 30 breaths per minute (AAP & AHA, 2011; Hemway, Christman, & Perlman, 2013).

SAFETY ALERT!

Remember to say, "One and two and three and breathe, and one and two and three and breathe" out loud and demonstrate with finger movements so all members of the resuscitation team are aware of where they are in the cycle. There are 5 cycles in 10 seconds.

Drugs that should be available in the birthing area include those needed in the treatment of shock and cardiac arrest. Oxygen is the "drug" used most often because of its effectiveness in ventilation. After 30 seconds of ventilation and coordinated cardiac compression, the newborn's cardiopulmonary status is reassessed by palpating the umbilical cord for a pulse. If the newborn has not responded with spontaneous respirations and an HR above 60 beats/min, resuscitative medications are necessary (AAP & AHA, 2011; Cloherty et al., 2012; Gomella, 2013). The most accessible route for administering medications is the umbilical vein (intravenous [IV]). When the HR remains below 60 beats/min, despite 30 seconds of assisted ventilation followed by another 30 seconds of coordinated chest compression,

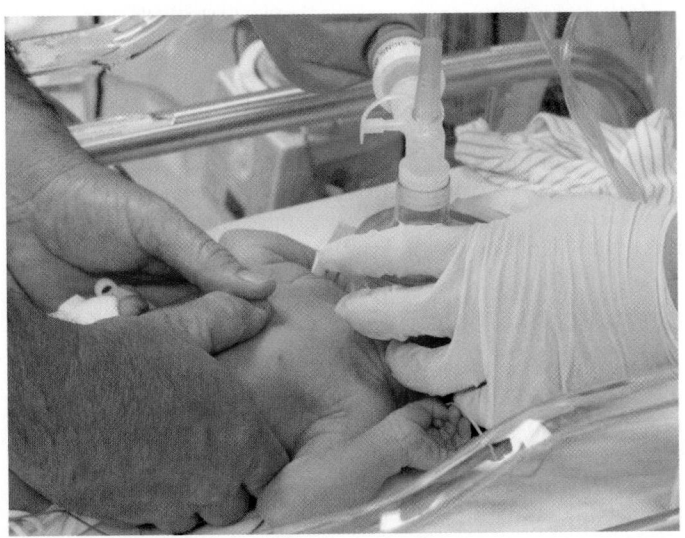
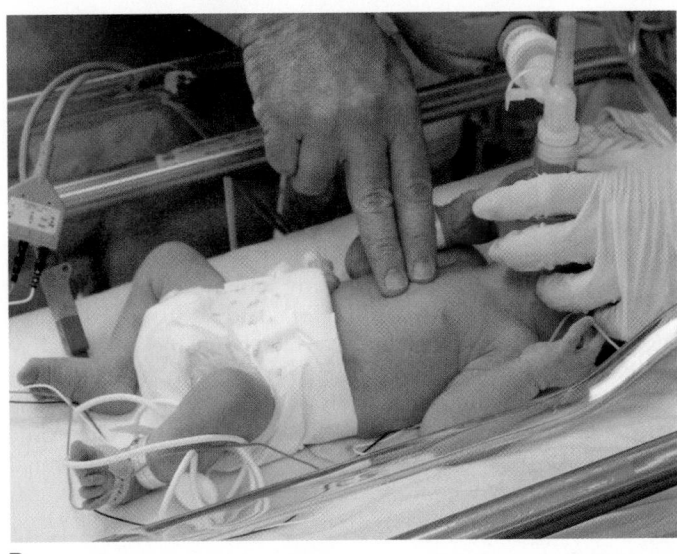

A   **B**

Figure 27–2 **External cardiac massage. The lower third of the sternum is compressed with two fingertips or thumbs at a rate of 90 beats per minute.** *A*, **In the thumb method, the fingers support the baby's back and both thumbs compress the sternum.** *B*, **In the two-fingers method, the tips of two fingers of one hand compress the sternum, and the other hand or a firm surface supports the baby's back.**

epinephrine, a cardiac stimulant, is indicated. If persistent bradycardia is present, epinephrine (0.1 to 0.3 mL/kg of a 1:10,000 solution [0.1 mg/mL]) is given through the umbilical vein catheter as rapidly as possible. Endotracheal administration may be considered while IV access is being established. When epinephrine is administered by endotracheal tube, consider a higher dose (0.5 to .01 mL/kg) (AAP & AHA, 2011; Bagwell, 2014b; Gomella, 2013; Sawyer et al., 2013). Naloxone hydrochloride (0.1 mg/kg), a narcotic antagonist, is used to reverse known iatrogenic narcotic depression; however, it is not currently recommended to be given during initial resuscitation if adequate ventilation is available (AAP & AHA, 2011; Gomella, 2013).

If shock develops because of hypovolemia (e.g., low blood pressure [BP], pallor, or poor peripheral perfusion), the baby may be given a volume expander such as normal saline (0.9 NaCl solution) in a dose of 10 mL/kg via umbilical vein route. If there is a known fetal hemorrhage or fetal anemia, whole blood (O Rh-negative cross-matched against the mother's blood) and packed red blood cells (RBCs) given over a 5- to 10-minute period can be used for volume expansion and treatment of hypovolemic shock.

Nursing Management

For the Newborn Needing Resuscitation

Nursing Assessment and Diagnosis

Communication between the obstetric office or clinic and the birthing area nurse helps in the identification of newborns who may be in need of resuscitation. When the woman arrives in the birthing area, you should have the prenatal/antepartum record and should note any contributory prenatal history factors and assess present fetal status. As labor progresses, nursing assessments include ongoing monitoring of fetal heartbeat and its response to contractions, assisting with fetal scalp blood

sampling (if available), and observing for the presence of meconium in the amniotic fluid, when ruptured, to help identify possible fetal asphyxia. In addition, alert the interdisciplinary resuscitation team and the practitioner responsible for the care of the newborn of any potential high-risk laboring women.

Nursing diagnoses that may apply to the newborn with asphyxia and the newborn's parents include (NANDA-I © 2014):

- *Breathing Pattern, Ineffective,* related to lack of spontaneous respirations at birth secondary to in utero asphyxia
- *Cardiac Output, Decreased,* related to impaired oxygenation
- *Coping: Family, Compromised,* related to baby's lack of spontaneous respirations at birth and parents' fear of losing their newborn

Planning and Implementation

HOSPITAL-BASED NURSING CARE

Following identification of possible high-risk situations, the next step in effective resuscitation is assembling the necessary equipment and ensuring proper functioning.

Check and maintain equipment to ensure its reliability before an emergency arises. The equipment must be cleaned or replaced and restocked immediately after each use and rechecked before every birth. Inspect all equipment—bag and mask, pressure manometer, oxygen and flow meter, pulse oximeter, laryngoscope bulb/battery, and suction machine—for damaged or nonfunctioning parts before a birth or when setting up an admission bed. A systematic check of the emergency cart and equipment is a routine responsibility of each shift. It is desirable to assemble equipment for pH and blood gas determination as well.

During resuscitation it is essential that the baby is kept warm. Dry the newborn quickly with prewarmed towels or blankets and put a hat on the baby to prevent evaporative heat loss, and then place the baby under a prewarmed radiant warmer with servo-control set at 36.5°C (97.7°F). The radiant warmer provides an overhead radiant heat source (a thermostatic mechanism that is secured to the baby's abdomen, over a solid organ like the liver, triggers the radiant warmer to turn on or off to maintain a constant temperature). An open bed is necessary for easy access to the newborn.

Training and knowledge about resuscitation are vital to personnel in the birth setting for both normal and high-risk births. Neonatal Resuscitation Program (NRP) certification is renewed every 2 years for personnel working with newborns. Resuscitation is at least a two-person effort, and additional support should be called for as needed. One member of the collaborative care team must have the skill to perform airway management, line placement, and ventilation (AAP & ACOG, 2012). The resuscitative efforts are recorded in the newborn's electronic health record (EHR) so that all members of the interprofessional healthcare team will have access to this information.

Healthy People 2020

(MICH-1.2) Decrease fetal and infant deaths during perinatal period (28 weeks of gestation to 7 days after birth)

(MICH-1.4) Decrease neonatal deaths (within the first 28 days of life)

(MICH-33) Increase the proportion of very-low-birth-weight (VLBW) infants born at Level III hospitals or subspecialty perinatal centers

---

PARENT TEACHING

Family members may be present during resuscitation in the birthing room and in the neonatal ICU (NICU), but the procedure can be particularly distressing for the parents. If the need for resuscitation is anticipated, assure the parents that an interprofessional healthcare team will be present at the birth specifically for their newborn. Advise the parents that a support person will be available for them also. As soon as the baby's condition has been stabilized, a member of the collaborative care team needs to discuss the baby's condition with the parents. The parents may have many fears about the reasons for resuscitation and the condition of their baby following the resuscitation (White, 2012).

Evaluation

Expected outcomes of nursing care include the following:

- The newborn requiring resuscitation is promptly identified, and intervention is started early.
- The newborn's metabolic and physiologic processes are stabilized, and recovery is proceeding without complications.
- The parents can verbalize the reason for resuscitation and what was done to resuscitate their newborn.
- The parents can verbalize their fears about the resuscitation process and potential implications for their baby's future.

Care of the Newborn With Respiratory Distress

Respiratory distress syndrome (RDS) is an inappropriate respiratory adaptation to extrauterine life. The nurse caring for a baby with respiratory distress needs to understand the normal pulmonary and circulatory physiology (see Chapter 23), the pathophysiology of the disease process, clinical manifestations, and supportive and corrective therapies. Only with this knowledge can the nurse make appropriate observations about responses to therapy and development of complications. The newborn communicates needs only by behavior or physiologic parameters that must be interpreted by the NICU nurse. The neonatal nurse interprets this behavior as clues about the individual baby's condition. This section discusses respiratory distress syndrome, transient tachypnea of the newborn, and meconium aspiration syndrome.

Respiratory Distress Syndrome

Respiratory distress syndrome (RDS), also referred to as *hyaline membrane disease (HMD)*, is the result of inadequate production of pulmonary surfactant, a substance produced in the lungs that keeps alveoli from collapsing on expiration (Smith & Carley, 2014). The syndrome occurs more frequently in premature White babies than in babies of African descent and almost twice as often in boys as in girls (Cloherty et al., 2012)

All the factors precipitating the pathologic changes of RDS have not been determined, but the main factors associated with its development include:

- *Prematurity.* All preterm newborns—no matter their size—and especially infants of diabetic mothers (IDMs) are at risk for RDS. The incidence of RDS increases with the degree of prematurity, with most deaths occurring in newborns weighing less than 1500 g (3.3 lb). The maternal and fetal factors resulting in preterm labor and birth, complications of pregnancy, indications for cesarean birth, and familial tendency are all associated with RDS.

- *Surfactant deficiency disease.* Normal pulmonary adaptation requires adequate surfactant, a lipoprotein that coats the inner surface of the alveoli. Surfactant provides alveolar stability by decreasing the alveoli's surface tension and tendency for collapse. Surfactant is produced by type II alveolar cells starting at about 24 weeks' gestation. In the normal or mature newborn lung, it is continuously synthesized, oxidized during breathing, and replenished. Adequate surfactant levels lead to better lung compliance and permit breathing with less work. RDS is due to alterations in surfactant quantity, composition, function, or production (Van Woudenberg, Wills, & Rubarth, 2012).

Development of RDS indicates a failure to synthesize surfactant, which is required to maintain alveolar stability (see section on *Cardiopulmonary Adaptation* in Chapter 23). Upon expiration, this instability increases atelectasis, which causes hypoxia and acidosis because of the lack of gas exchange (Smith & Carley, 2014; Van Woudenberg et al., 2012). These conditions further inhibit surfactant production and cause pulmonary vasoconstriction. The resulting lung instability causes the biochemical problems of hypoxemia (decreased PO_2), hypercarbia (increased PCO_2), and acidemia (decreased pH), primarily metabolic, which further increase pulmonary vasoconstriction and hypoperfusion; alveolar endothelial and epithelial damage; and subsequent protein-rich interstitial and alveolar edema. The cycle of events of RDS leading to eventual respiratory failure is diagrammed in *Pathophysiology Illustrated.*

Because of these pathophysiologic conditions, the newborn must expend increasing amounts of energy to reopen the collapsed alveoli with every breath, so that each breath becomes more difficult than the last. The progressive expiratory atelectasis upsets the physiologic homeostasis of the pulmonary and cardiovascular systems and prevents adequate gas exchange. Breathing

Pathophysiology Illustrated: **Respiratory Distress Syndrome (RDS)**

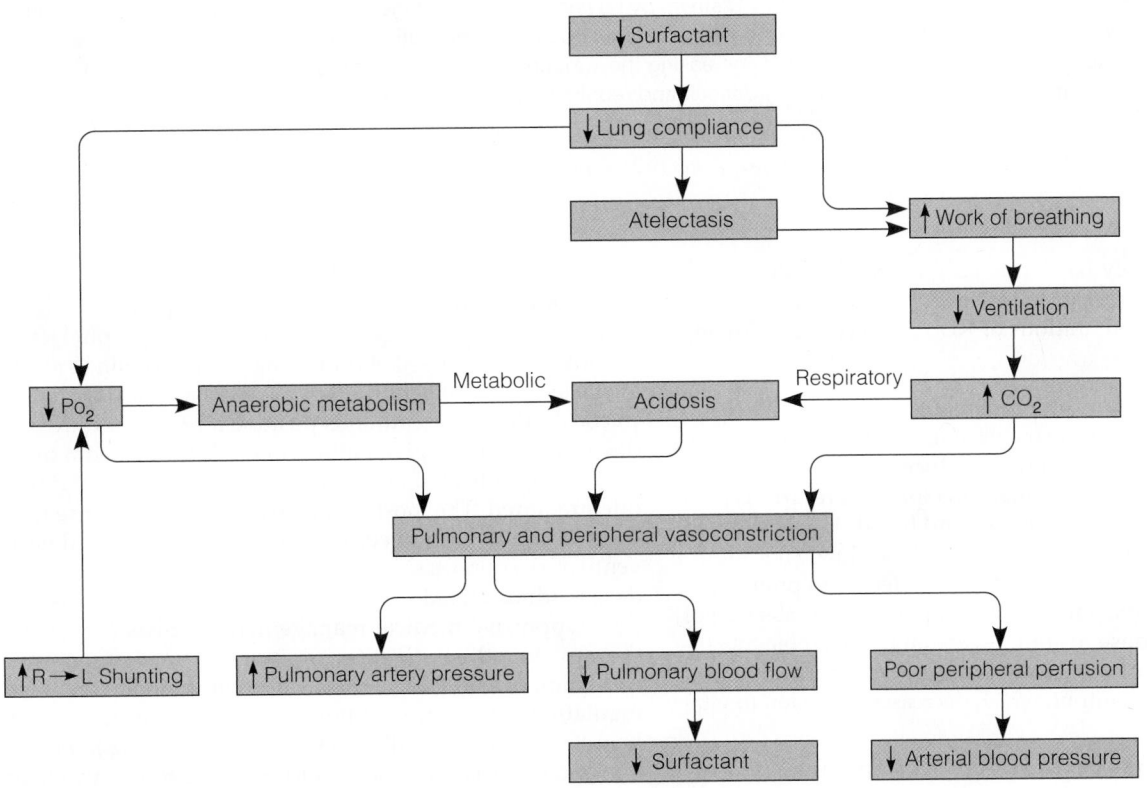

Cycle of events of RDS leading to eventual respiratory failure.

SOURCE: Modified from Gluck, L., & Kulovich, M. V. (1973). Fetal lung development. *Pediatric Clinics of North America, 20,* 375.

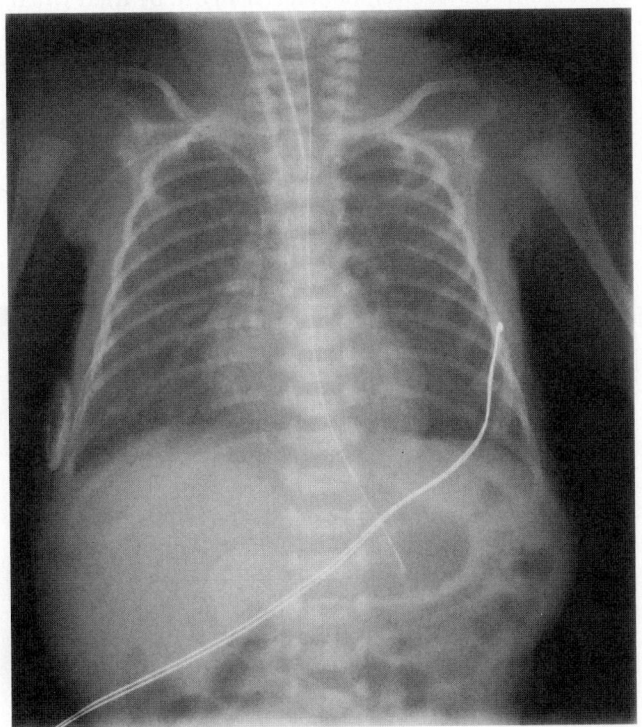

RDS chest x-ray. Chest radiograph of respiratory distress syndrome characterized by a reticulogranular pattern with areas of microatelectasis of uniform opacity and air bronchograms.

SOURCE: Carol Harrigan, RN, MSN, NNP-BC.

becomes progressively harder as lung compliance decreases, which makes it more difficult to inflate the lungs and breathe.

The physiologic alterations of RDS produce the following complications:

- *Hypoxia.* As a result of hypoxia, the pulmonary vasculature constricts, pulmonary vascular resistance increases, and pulmonary blood flow is reduced. Increased pulmonary vascular resistance may precipitate a return to fetal circulation as the ductus opens and blood flow is shunted around the lungs in a right-to-left blood flow. This shunting increases the hypoxia and further decreases pulmonary perfusion. Hypoxia also causes impairment or absence of metabolic response to cold; reversion to anaerobic metabolism, resulting in lactate accumulation (acidosis); and impaired cardiac output, which decreases perfusion to vital organs.

- *Respiratory acidosis.* Increased PCO_2 and decreased pH are results of alveolar hypoventilation. A persistent rise in PCO_2 is a poor prognostic sign of pulmonary function and adequacy because the increased PCO_2 and decreased pH are results of alveolar hypoventilation.

- *Metabolic acidosis.* Because of the lack of oxygen at the cellular level, the newborn begins anaerobic metabolism with an increase in lactate levels and a resulting base deficit (loss of bicarbonate). As the lactate levels increase, the pH decreases in an attempt to maintain acid–base homeostasis.

The classic radiologic picture of RDS is diffuse bilateral reticulogranular (ground glass appearance) density, with portions of the air-filled tracheobronchial tree (air bronchogram) outlined by the opaque ("white-out") lungs with widespread atelectasis, potentially obliterating the heart borders (Cloherty et al., 2012). See *Pathophysiology Illustrated: Respiratory Distress Syndrome (RDS)*. The progression of x-ray findings parallels the pattern of resolution, which usually occurs in 7 to 10 days, and the time of surfactant reappearance, unless surfactant replacement therapy has been used (Blackburn, 2013). Echocardiography is a valuable tool in diagnosing vascular shunts that move blood either away from or toward the lungs.

CLINICAL THERAPY

The primary goal of prenatal management is to prevent preterm birth through early assessment of fetal lung maturity, aggressive treatment of preterm labor, and administration of glucocorticoids to enhance fetal lung development (see Chapter 15). Antenatal steroids reduce the incidence and severity of RDS and improve survivability of the 24 to 34 weeks' gestation and very-low-birth-weight newborn (less than 1250 g [2.75 lb]) (Cloherty et al., 2012).

Postnatal surfactant replacement therapy, given as prophylaxis or rescue treatment, is available for babies to decrease the severity of RDS in low-birth-weight newborns (Polin, Carlo, & Committee on the Fetus and Newborn, 2014). Babies born at less than 30 weeks' gestation who receive prophylactic surfactant show increased chronic lung disease (Polin et al., 2014). Surfactant replacement therapy is delivered through an endotracheal tube or a continuous positive airway pressure (CPAP) device and may be given either in the birthing room or in the nursery, as indicated by the severity of RDS. Repeat doses are often required. The most frequently reported response to treatment is rapidly improved oxygenation and decreased need for ventilatory support, sometimes occurring quite quickly after the dose is administered.

Supportive medical management consists of ventilatory therapy, blood gas monitoring, pulse oximetry monitoring, correction of acid–base imbalance, environmental temperature regulation, adequate nutrition, and protection from infection. Ventilatory therapy is directed toward preventing hypoventilation and hypoxia. Mild cases of RDS may require only increased humidified oxygen concentrations. Use of CPAP may be required in moderately afflicted newborns. Babies with severe cases of RDS require mechanical ventilatory assistance from a respirator (Figure 27–3) (Fanaroff & Fanaroff, 2013).

High-frequency ventilation (HFV) can be tried when conventional ventilator therapy is not successful, and it sometimes can be the primary mode of ventilation to minimize lung injury in very small and/or sick babies (Gomella, 2013). In some institutions, morphine or fentanyl is used for its analgesic and sedative effects.

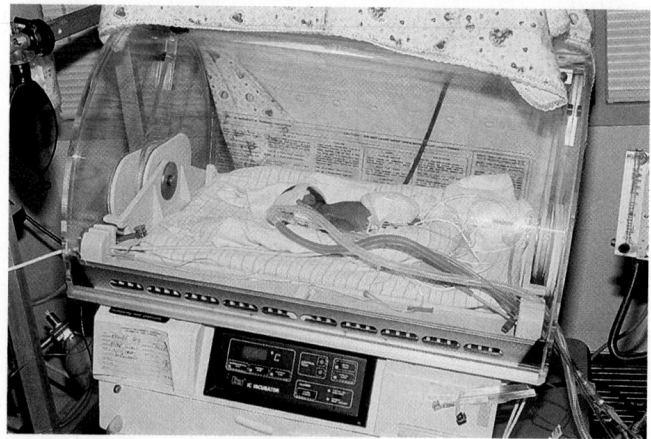

Figure 27–3 Mechanical ventilatory assistance. One-day-old, 27 weeks' gestational age, 1450-g (3-lb) baby on respirator and in isolette.

SOURCE: Carol Harrigan, RN, MSN, NNP-BC.

Clinical Tip

In babies with respiratory distress syndrome (RDS) who are on ventilators, increased urination/diuresis (determined by weighing diapers) may be an early clue that the baby's condition is improving (usually in the second to fourth day). As fluid moves out of the lungs into the bloodstream, alveoli open, and kidney perfusion increases; this results in increased voiding. At this point, the nurse must monitor chest expansion closely. If chest expansion is increasing, pulmonary compliance is improving and ventilator settings may have to be decreased, sometimes quite soon after surfactant dosing. Too high a ventilator setting may "blow the lungs," resulting in pneumothorax. If diuresis does not occur, it is a sign that *bronchopulmonary dysplasia (BPD)*, also called *chronic lung disease of prematurity (CLD)*, may be developing (Cloherty et al., 2012).

Nursing Management

Look for characteristics of RDS such as increasing cyanosis, tachypnea (greater than 60 respirations per minute), grunting respirations, nasal flaring, significant retractions, and apnea. Table 27–1 reviews clinical findings associated with respiratory distress in general. The Silverman-Anderson index is a tool that evaluates signs of respiratory distress and may be used in the birthing area.

Based on clinical parameters, a neonatal nurse implements therapeutic approaches to provide the newborn with respiratory distress with a very supportive environment (Figure 27–4) that includes maintaining thermoregulation to decrease respiratory effort and decrease infection secondary to invasive procedures and using standard precautions. (See *Nursing Care Plan: The Newborn With Respiratory Distress Syndrome.*) Newborns with

TABLE 27–1 Clinical Assessments Associated With Respiratory Distress

CLINICAL PICTURE	SIGNIFICANCE
SKIN COLOR	
Pallor or mottling	These represent poor peripheral circulation caused by systemic hypotension and vasoconstriction and pooling of independent areas (usually in conjunction with severe hypoxia).
Cyanosis (bluish tint)	Depending on hemoglobin concentration, peripheral circulation, intensity and quality of viewing light, and acuity of observer's color vision, this is frankly visible in advanced hypoxia. Central cyanosis is most easily detected by examination of mucous membranes and tongue.
Jaundice (yellow discoloration of skin and mucous membranes caused by presence of unconjugated [indirect] bilirubin)	Metabolic alterations (acidosis, hypercarbia, asphyxia) of respiratory distress predispose a newborn to dissociation of bilirubin from albumin-binding sites and deposition in the skin and central nervous system.
Edema (presents as slick, shiny taut skin)	This is characteristic of preterm newborns because their total protein concentration is low, with a decrease in colloidal osmotic pressure and transudation of fluid. Edema of hands and feet is frequently seen within first 24 hours and resolved by fifth day in babies with severe RDS.
RESPIRATORY SYSTEM	
Tachypnea (normal respiratory rate 30–60/min, sustained, elevated respiratory rate 60+/min)	Increased respiratory rate is the easiest detectable sign of respiratory distress after birth. Because of the premature newborn's very compliant chest wall, it is more energy efficient to increase the respiratory rate than the depth of respirations. This compensatory mechanism attempts to increase respiratory dead space to maintain alveolar ventilation and gas exchange in the face of an increase in mechanical resistance. As a decompensatory mechanism it increases workload and energy output by increasing respiratory rate, which causes increased metabolic demand for oxygen and thus increases alveolar ventilation on an already overstressed system.
Apnea (episode of nonbreathing for more than 20 sec; periodic breathing, a common "normal" occurrence in preterm newborns, is defined as apnea of 5–10 sec alternating with 10–15 sec of ventilation) that is sometimes quite rapid	This poor prognostic sign indicates cardiorespiratory disease, CNS disease, metabolic alterations, intracranial hemorrhage, sepsis, or immaturity. Physiologic alterations include decreased oxygen saturation, respiratory acidosis, and bradycardia.
CHEST	
Chest movement	Inspection of the thoracic cage includes shape, size, and symmetry of movement. Respiratory movements should be symmetric and diaphragmatic; asymmetry such as seesaw-like movements reflects pathology (pneumothorax, diaphragmatic hernia). Increased anteroposterior diameter indicates air trapping (meconium aspiration syndrome).
Labored respirations indicate severity of retractions (see below), grunting, and nasal flaring, which are signs of labored respirations	Indicates marked increase in the work of breathing.
Retractions (inward pulling of soft parts of the chest cage—suprasternal [above the sternum], substernal, intercostals [between the ribs]—at inspiration)	These reflect the significant increase in negative intrathoracic pressure necessary to inflate stiff, noncompliant lungs. Newborns attempt to increase lung compliance by using accessory muscles. Lung expansion markedly decreases. Seesaw respirations are seen when the chest flattens with inspiration and the abdomen bulges. Retractions increase the work of breathing and O_2 need. As a result, assisted ventilation may be necessary because of exhaustion.
Nasal flaring (inspiratory dilation of nostrils)	This compensatory mechanism attempts to lessen the resistance of the narrow nasal passage.

(continued)

TABLE 27–1 Clinical Assessments Associated With Respiratory Distress (*continued*)

CLINICAL PICTURE	SIGNIFICANCE
Expiratory grunt (Valsalva maneuver in which the baby exhales against a partially closed glottis, thus producing an audible moan)	This increases intrapulmonary pressure, which decreases or prevents atelectasis, thus improving oxygenation and alveolar ventilation. It allows more time for the passage of oxygen into the circulatory system. Intubation should not be attempted unless the baby's condition is rapidly deteriorating, because it prevents this maneuver and allows the alveoli to collapse.
Rhythmic body movement with labored respirations (chin tug, head bobbing, retractions of anal area)	This is a result of using abdominal and other respiratory accessory muscles during prolonged forced respirations.
Auscultation of chest reveals decreased air exchange, with harsh breath sounds or fine inspiratory rales; rhonchi may be present	Decrease in breath sounds and distant quality may indicate interstitial or intrapleural air or fluid.
CARDIOVASCULAR SYSTEM	
Continuous systolic murmur may be audible	Patent ductus arteriosus is a common occurrence with hypoxia, pulmonary vasoconstriction, right-to-left shunting, and congestive heart failure.
Heart rate usually within normal limits (fixed heart rate may occur with a rate of 110–120 beats/min)	A fixed heart rate indicates a decrease in vagal control.
Point of maximal impulse usually located at fourth to fifth intercostal space, left sternal border	Displacement may reflect dextrocardia, pneumothorax, or diaphragmatic hernia.
HYPOTHERMIA	
	This is inadequate functioning of metabolic processes that require oxygen to produce necessary body heat.
MUSCLE TONE	
Flaccid, hypotonic, unresponsive to stimuli Hypertonia and/or seizure activity	These may indicate deterioration in the newborn's condition and possible CNS damage caused by hypoxia, acidemia, or hemorrhage.

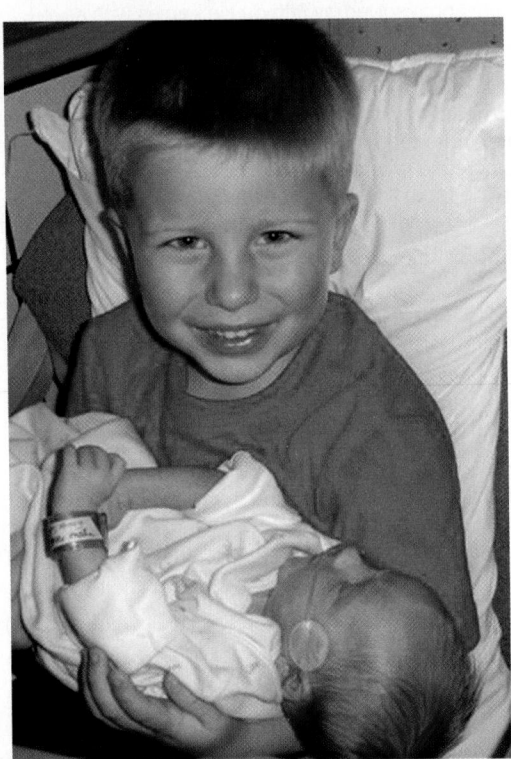

Figure 27–4 **This baby born at 36 weeks' gestational age had severe RDS. He has ongoing oxygen needs provided by a nasal cannula but still can be held by his proud big brother.**

SOURCE: Lisa Smith-Pedersen, RNC, MSN, NNP-BC.

severe respiratory distress are cared for in NICUs by nurses with advanced knowledge and training. Nursing interventions and criteria for instituting mechanical ventilation depend on institutional protocol. Noninvasive oxygen monitoring provides real-time trend information that is particularly useful in babies showing frequent swings in PaO_2 and oxygen saturation. Use of these methods (pulse oximetry, transcutaneous oxygen monitor) can also reduce the frequency of blood gas sampling. Methods of noninvasive oxygen monitoring and nursing interventions are included in Table 27–2. (The nursing care of babies on ventilators or with umbilical artery catheters is not discussed here.) Ventilatory assistance with high-frequency ventilators shows positive results.

Transient Tachypnea of the Newborn

Some newborns, primarily large-for-gestational-age (LGA), term and late preterm babies, may develop progressive respiratory distress that clinically can resemble RDS. Other risk factors include maternal diabetes and asthma, male sex of the fetus, macrosomia (possibly related to maternal diabetes), and cesarean section delivery, without especially elective spontaneous labor. Some term babies with progressively worsening respiratory distress may benefit from exogenous surfactant (Gardner, Himes, & Nyp, 2016). Typically, supplemental oxygen of less than 40% will alleviate the hypoxia (Cloherty et al., 2012; Fanaroff & Fanaroff, 2013). They may have had intrauterine or intrapartum asphyxia due to maternal oversedation or poor uterine perfusion, maternal bleeding, prolapsed cord, or breech presentation. The newborn then fails to clear the airway of lung fluid, mucus, and other debris or an excess of fluid in the lungs due to aspiration of amniotic or tracheal fluid (Gomella, 2013). Transient tachypnea of the newborn (TTN) is also more prevalent in cesarean birth

TABLE 27–2 Oxygen Monitors

TYPE	FUNCTION AND RATIONALE	NURSING INTERVENTIONS
PULSE OXIMETRY—SpO$_2$		
Estimates beat-to-beat arterial oxygen saturation.	Calibration is automatic.	Understand and use oxyhemoglobin dissociation curve.
Microprocessor measures saturation by the absorption of red and infrared light as it passes through tissue.	Less dependent on perfusion than TcPO$_2$ and TcPCO$_2$; however, functions poorly if peripheral perfusion is decreased because of low cardiac output.	Monitor trends over time and correlate with arterial blood gases.
		Check disposable sensor at least q8h.
Changes in absorption related to blood pulsation through vessel determine saturation and pulse rate.	Much more rapid response time than TcPO$_2$—offers real-time readings.	
	Can be located on extremity, digit, or palm of hand, leaving chest free; not affected by skin characteristics.	
	Requires understanding of oxyhemoglobin dissociation curve.	
	Pulse oximeter reading of 88% to 93% reflects a PaO$_2$ of 50–80 mmHg (Cloherty et al., 2012).	
	Extreme sensitivity to movement; decreases if average of 7th or 14th beat is selected rather than beat to beat.	
	Poor correlation with extreme hyperoxia.	
TRANSCUTANEOUS OXYGEN MONITOR—TcPO$_2$		
Measures oxygen diffusion across the skin.	When transcutaneous monitors are properly calibrated and electrodes are appropriately positioned, they will provide reliable, continuous, noninvasive measurements of PO$_2$, PCO$_2$, and oxygen saturation.	Use TcPO$_2$ to monitor trends of oxygenation with routine nursing care procedures.
Clark electrode is heated to 43.0°C (109.4°F) (preterm) or 44.0°C (111.2°F) (term) to warm the skin beneath the electrode and promote diffusion of oxygen across the skin surface. PO$_2$ is measured when oxygen diffuses across the capillary membrane, skin, and electrode membrane (Cloherty et al., 2012).	Readings vary when skin perfusion is decreased.	Clean electrode surface to remove electrolyte deposits; change solution and membrane once a week.
	Reliable as trend monitor.	Allow machine to stabilize before drawing arterial gases; note reading when gases are drawn and use values to correlate.
	Frequent calibration necessary to overcome mechanical drift.	Ensure airtight seal between skin surface and electrode; place electrodes on clean, dry skin on upper chest, abdomen, or inner aspect of thigh; avoid bony prominences.
	Following membrane change, machine must "warm up" 1 hr prior to initial calibration; otherwise, after turning it on, it must equilibrate for 30 min prior to calibration.	
	When placed on baby, values will be low until skin is heated; approximately 15 min required to stabilize.	
	Second-degree burns are rare but can occur if electrodes remain in place too long.	Change skin site and recalibrate at least every 4 hr inspect skin for burns; if burns occur, use lowest temperature setting and change position of electrode more frequently.
	Decreased correlations noted with older babies (related to skin thickness), with babies with low cardiac output (decreased skin perfusion), and with hyperoxic babies.	
	The adhesive that attaches the electrode may abrade the fragile skin of the preterm baby.	Adhesive discs may be cut to a smaller size, or skin prep may be used under the adhesive circle only; allow membrane to touch skin surface at center.
	May be used for both preductal and postductal monitoring of oxygenation for observations of shunting.	

newborns who have not had the *thoracic squeeze* that occurs during vaginal birth and removes some of the lung fluid.

Usually, the newborn experiences little or no difficulty at the onset of breathing. However, shortly after birth, expiratory grunting, flaring of the nares, subcostal retractions, desaturation, and mild cyanosis may be noted in the newborn breathing room air (Gardner et al., 2016). Air will become trapped, and an increase in the anterior/posterior diameter of the chest will be observed. Tachypnea is usually present by 6 hours of age, with respiratory rates consistently greater than

60 breaths per minute (breaths/min), and possibly reaching 80 to 100 breaths/min and higher, with a requirement of oxygen. Mild respiratory and metabolic acidosis may be present within the first 6 hours. These clinical signs usually improve within 12 to 24 hours. In mild TTN, the signs can improve within 24 hours but may continue for 48 to 72 hours when more severe and possibly last up to 1 week (Cloherty et al., 2012).

CLINICAL THERAPY

Initial x-ray findings may be identical to those showing RDS within the first 3 hours. However, radiographs of babies with transient tachypnea usually reveal a generalized overexpansion of the lungs (hyperaeration of alveoli), which is identifiable principally by flattened contours of the diaphragm. Dense streaks (increased vascularity) radiate from the hilar region and represent engorgement of the lymphatic vessels, which clear alveolar fluid on initiation of air breathing. Within 48 hours, the chest x-ray examination is generally normal with the exception of perihilar markings, which may remain visible for 3 to 7 days because of remaining fluid in the periarterial tissue (Fanaroff & Fanaroff, 2013; Gomella, 2013).

Clinical Reasoning Transient Tachypnea of the Newborn

You are caring for baby girl, Linn, who is a 39-week, AGA female born by repeat cesarean birth to a 34-year-old G3, now P3, mother. Baby Linn's Apgar scores were 7 at 1 minute and 9 at 5 minutes. At 2 hours of age, you note an elevated respiratory rate of 70 to 80 and mild cyanosis. The baby is now receiving 30% oxygen and has a respiratory rate of 100 to 120. The baby's clinical course, chest x-ray examination, and laboratory work are all consistent with transient tachypnea of the newborn. Linn's mother calls you to ask about her baby. She tells you that her last child was born at 30 weeks' gestation, had respiratory distress syndrome requiring ventilator support, and was hospitalized for 6 weeks. She asks you, "Is this the same respiratory distress?" What will you tell her?

Supplemental oxygen, usually under an oxygen hood, may be required to correct the hypoxemia (Cloherty et al., 2012) (Figure 27–5). Fluid and electrolyte requirements should be met intravenously during the acute phase of the disease. Oral feedings are contraindicated because of rapid respiratory rates and the subsequent risk of aspiration.

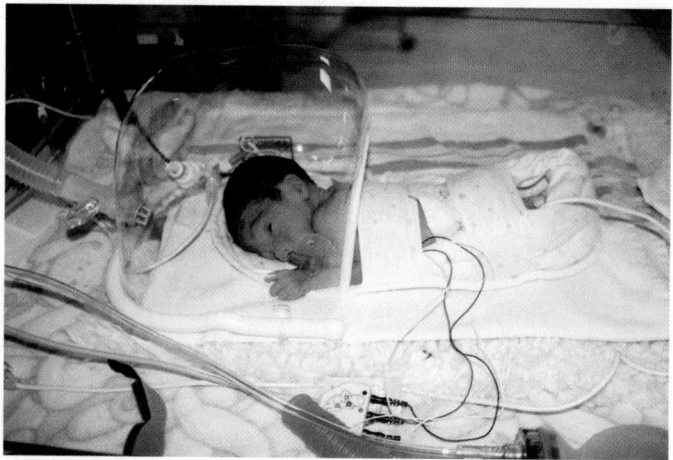

Figure 27–5 **Premature newborn under oxygen hood. Baby is nested and has a nonnutritive sucking pacifier.**
SOURCE: Lisa Smith-Pedersen, RNC, MSN, NNP-BC.

When hypoxemia is severe and tachypnea continues, persistent pulmonary hypertension must be considered and treatment measures initiated. If pneumonia or sepsis is suspected initially, antibiotics may be administered prophylactically.

Nursing Management

For nursing actions, see *Nursing Care Plan: The Newborn With Respiratory Distress Syndrome.*

The Newborn With Meconium Aspiration Syndrome

Because the body's physiologic response to asphyxia is increased intestinal peristalsis, relaxation of the anal sphincter and the presence of meconium in the amniotic fluid indicates that the fetus may be suffering from asphyxia, either in the immediate period during labor or perhaps some time in the recent past (Marks, 2012). However, if the fetus is in a breech position, the presence of meconium in the amniotic fluid does not necessarily indicate asphyxia.

Approximately 8% to 20% of all live-born, late-preterm, near or term newborns are born through meconium-stained amniotic fluid (MSAF) (Swarnam, Soraisham, & Sivanandan, 2012). Of the newborns born through MSAF, one third develop **meconium aspiration syndrome (MAS)** (Marks, 2012; Swarnam et al., 2012). This fluid may be aspirated into the tracheobronchial tree by the fetus in utero or during the first few breaths taken by the newborn.

Presence of meconium in the lungs produces the following:

- Mechanical obstruction of airways: ball-valve action (air is allowed in but not exhaled), so that alveoli over distend; with oxygen and carbon dioxide trapping and hyperinflation, air leaks such as pneumothorax are common.

- Chemical pneumonitis leading to the possible development of secondary bacterial pneumonias.

- Inactivation of natural surfactant (Fanaroff & Fanaroff, 2013; Gomella, 2013).

CLINICAL MANIFESTATIONS OF MAS

Clinical manifestations of MAS include:

- Fetal hypoxia in utero a few days or a few minutes before birth, indicated by a sudden increase in fetal activity followed by diminished activity, slowing of fetal heart rate (FHR) or weak and irregular heartbeat, loss of beat-to-beat variability, and meconium staining of amniotic fluid or particulate meconium

- Presence of signs of distress or depression at birth, such as pallor, cyanosis, apnea, slow heartbeat, and low Apgar scores (below 6) at 1 and 5 minutes

After the initial resuscitation, the severity of the ongoing clinical symptoms correlates with the extent of aspiration. Many newborns require mechanical ventilation at birth because of immediate signs of distress (generalized cyanosis, tachypnea, and severe retractions). An overdistended, barrel-shaped chest with increased anteroposterior diameter is common. Auscultation reveals diminished air movement, with prominent rales and rhonchi. Abdominal palpation may reveal a displaced liver caused by diaphragmatic depression resulting from the overexpansion of the lungs. Yellowish/pale green staining of the skin, nails, and umbilical cord is usually present, especially if the incident occurred sometime before birth (Fanaroff & Fanaroff, 2013).

The MAS chest x-ray film reveals asymmetric, coarse, patchy densities and possible hyperinflation (9 to 11 rib expansion), which

Nursing Care Plan: For the Newborn With Respiratory Distress Syndrome

1. Nursing Diagnosis: *Breathing Pattern, Ineffective*, **related to immature lung development or inadequate lung surfactant (NANDA-I © 2014)**

GOAL: The newborn will maintain an effective breathing pattern.

INTERVENTION	RATIONALE
• Review maternal birth records, noting medications given to mother before birth and the baby's condition at birth such as Apgar scores and resuscitative measures.	• Several drugs suppress respiratory function in the newborn.
• Initiate cardiac and respiratory monitoring and calibrate these monitors every 8 hours or per unit protocol.	• Close monitoring detects periodic apneic spells and allows for medical intervention if necessary.
• Monitor baby's respiratory rate and rhythm, pulse, blood pressure, and activity.	• Increases in respiratory rate and pulse and alteration in rhythm and blood pressure may indicate respiratory distress.
• Assess skin color; note signs of cyanosis, duskiness, and pallor.	• Any changes in the normal skin color may indicate a physiologic change occurring.
• Clear baby's airway by suctioning PRN with bulb syringe.	• Opens airway by clearing mucus and allows maximum respiratory effort.
• Administer warmed, humidified oxygen by oxygen hood and monitor the oxygen concentrations every 30 minutes.	• Prevents mucosal dryness and maintains an even level of oxygen administration.
• Do not allow oxyhood to touch baby's face; maintain a stable oxygen concentration by increasing and decreasing oxygen by 5% to 10% increments.	• Allowing oxyhood to touch baby's face may cause apnea by stimulating the facial nerve.
• **Collaborative:** Obtain arterial blood gases (ABGs) per healthcare provider/NNP orders.	• Obtaining ABGs is essential in managing a baby receiving oxygen. Suctioning may cause a discrepancy in ABG readings and should be avoided.
1. Maintain constant O_2 concentration for 15–30 min before sample is obtained.	
2. Avoid stimulating baby for 15 min before obtaining sample.	
3. Avoid suctioning baby before obtaining sample.	
4. Obtain sample in heparinized tuberculin syringe and maintain the temperature of the sample.	
5. Assess the patency of the arterial line to prevent clot formation, and then replace blood used to clear line.	
6. Flush line with 2 mL heparinized solution before restarting flow of IV fluids.	
7. Monitor transcutaneous pulse oximeter continuously or hourly and record. Rotate sensor site every 3–4 hr.	
• Assess baby's need for mechanical ventilation: apnea present, hypoxia (PaO_2 less than 50 mmHg), hypercapnia ($PaCO_2$ greater than 60 mmHg), respiratory acidosis (pH less than 7.2).	• Mechanical ventilation improves oxygenation and ventilation, resulting in rise in PaO_2 and decrease in $PaCO_2$.
• Administer mechanical ventilation per hospital protocol.	• Continuous positive airway pressure (CPAP) or positive end-expiratory pressure (PEEP) can be administered by nasal prongs, nasopharyngeal or oral intubation.

EXPECTED OUTCOMES: The newborn will maintain an effective breathing pattern as evidenced by respirations of 30–60 breaths/min, arterial blood gases are within normal range, baby is free of signs of retractions or nasal flaring, and blood pH is 7.35–7.45.

2. Nursing Diagnosis: *Thermoregulation, Ineffective,* **related to increased respiratory effort (NANDA-I © 2014)**

GOAL: The newborn will exhibit no signs of hypothermia.

INTERVENTION	RATIONALE
• Review maternal prenatal and intrapartum records. Note any medications mother received during these times.	• Medications such as meperidine (Demerol) and magnesium sulfate used by the mother during the prenatal or intrapartum periods significantly interfere with the baby's ability to retain heat.

(continued)

Nursing Care Plan: For the Newborn With Respiratory Distress Syndrome (continued)

INTERVENTION	RATIONALE
• Assess baby's temperature frequently. Place servo-probe on baby's skin over a solid organ.	• Hypothermia leads to pulmonary vasoconstriction because of the increase in oxygen consumption. Cold stress leads to increased oxygen needs; consequently, brown fat is used to maintain body temperature.
• Observe for signs of increased oxygen consumption and metabolic acidosis.	• Hypoxia and acidosis further depress surfactant production.
• Warm and humidify all inspired gases and record temperature of delivered gases.	• Cold air/oxygen blown in face of newborn is stimulus for consumption of oxygen and glucose and increased metabolic rate.
• Use radiant warmers or incubators with servo controls and open cribs with appropriate clothing.	• Maintains neutral thermal environment.
• Note signs and symptoms of respiratory distress, including tachypnea, apnea, cyanosis, acrocyanosis, bradycardia, lethargy, weak cry, and hypotonia.	• These signs can predispose the baby to metabolic acidosis.

EXPECTED OUTCOMES: The newborn will not exhibit signs and symptoms of hypothermia as evidenced by temperature maintenance of 97.7°–99.1°F (36.5°–37.3°c) and no signs and symptoms of respiratory distress.

3. Nursing Diagnosis: *Nutrition, Imbalanced: Less than Body Requirements,* related to increased metabolic needs in the newborn (NANDA-I © 2014)

GOAL: Newborn will gain weight in a normal curve.

INTERVENTION	RATIONALE
• Assess suck, swallow, gag, and cough reflexes.	• Prevents feeding problems and assists in determining the best individualized method of feeding for baby.
• Assess respiratory status of baby. If any problems are noted, notify healthcare provider/NNP.	• In the presence of respiratory distress avoid oral fluids and initiate parenteral nutrition per healthcare provider/NNP orders.
• Monitor IV rates per infusion pump (starting at 80 mL/kg/day) as ordered by healthcare provider/NNP.	• Allows for close monitoring of fluid intake.
• Record hourly intake and output (I&O) and daily weights.	• IV fluids are administered to replace sensible and insensible water loss, as well as evaporative water loss secondary to respiratory distress. Monitoring I&O will prevent circulatory system overload that can lead to pulmonary edema and cardiac problems.
• Provide total parenteral nutrition (TPN) when indicated.	• TPN is used as nutritional alternative if bowel sounds are not present and/or baby remains in acute distress.
• Advance, based on tolerance, from IV to gastrointestinal (GI) feedings. Gavage or nipple feedings are used, and IV is used as supplement (discontinued when oral intake is sufficient).	• If IV is discontinued before oral intake is established, baby will not receive adequate calories. • Formula or breast milk stimulates GI hormones necessary for a functional absorptive GI tract. • Avoid complications associated with nutrition by IV route only.
• Provide adequate caloric intake: consider amount of intake, type of formula, route of administration, and need for supplementation of intake by other routes.	• Calories are essential to prevent catabolism of body proteins and metabolic acidosis due to starvation or inadequate caloric intake.
• Assess infusion site for signs and symptoms of infection, including erythema, edema, and drainage with a foul odor.	• Appropriate intervention can be initiated when signs and symptoms of infection are detected early. Treatment may avoid infection and sepsis in the baby.

EXPECTED OUTCOMES: The newborn will maintain steady weight gain as evidenced by no more than 2%/day weight loss, tolerates oral feedings, and urine output of 1–3 mL/kg/hr.

4. Nursing Diagnosis: *Fluid Volume: Imbalanced, Risk for,* related to increased insensible water losses (NANDA-I © 2014)

GOAL: The newborn will not exhibit signs of dehydration and will display appropriate weight gain.

INTERVENTION	RATIONALE
• Observe for weight fluctuations by obtaining daily weights.	• Fluctuations in weight may indicate water imbalance or inadequate caloric intake.
• Document cumulative balances of intake (IV fluid administration and feedings) and output (urine collection bags, weighing or counting diapers) hourly.	• Balanced fluid intake and output suggest homeostasis.

- Obtain urinalysis; monitor closely specific gravity and nitrites.
- Monitor vital signs including blood pressure, pulse, temperature, and mean arterial pressure (MAP).
- Assess baby for signs of dehydration (i.e., poor skin turgor, pale mucous membranes, and sunken anterior fontanelle).
- Assess IV site for signs of infection (erythema and edema) and infiltration.
- **Collaborative:** Obtain labs for hematocrit (Hct), serum calcium, serum magnesium, serum potassium, blood urea nitrogen (BUN), creatinine, and uric acid levels.
- Administer fluids, blood products, and electrolytes as ordered by healthcare provider/NNP.

- Specific gravity greater than 1.013 and nitrites present in the urine are indicative of not enough fluid intake.
- A MAP of less than 20 mmHg may indicate hypotension.

- Detecting signs and symptoms of dehydration early in the newborn is important because early interventions are vital to prevent further damage.
- If signs and symptoms of infection are noted, intervention is necessary and IV site should be changed.
- Determines necessity for TPN administration.

- Replaces low nutrient stores and treats anemia if present.

EXPECTED OUTCOMES: The newborn will be free of signs and symptoms of dehydration as evidenced by intake equaling output, urine specific gravity in normal range, and a weight gain of at least 20–30 g/day.

EVIDENCE-BASED PRACTICE | Antibiotics for Meconium-Stained Amniotic Fluid in Labor

Clinical Question
Are antibiotics effective for preventing maternal and neonatal infections when amniotic fluid is meconium stained?

The Evidence
Meconium-stained amniotic fluid (MSAF) increases the risk of maternal and neonatal infections. Pregnant women with MSAF are more likely to develop inflammation of the fetal membranes caused by bacteria (chorioamnionitis). These mothers are also at higher risk of postpartum endometritis, and their babies are at higher risk of neonatal sepsis. Fetal stress may trigger gasping in the fetus, which results in aspiration of the meconium-stained fluid and can cause a host of respiratory difficulties. These investigators conducted a systematic review to determine if the administration of antibiotics could reduce the incidence of maternal infections and neonatal sepsis and other consequences of respiratory compromise. The review, published in the rigorous *Cochrane Database of Systematic Reviews*, is a highly structured review of randomized trials and forms the strongest evidence for practice.

The only antibiotic tested was ampicillin-sulbactam, and it appeared to have no effect on the rate of neonatal sepsis and subsequent neonatal intensive care admission. There was also no measurable effect on maternal endometritis rates. However, there was a significant decrease in the rate of chorioamnionitis,

reducing the mothers' risk of this condition by about a third (Siriwachirachai, Sangkomkamhang, Lumbiganon, et al., 2014). The investigators noted that the evidence that the antibiotic had no effect was weaker for the neonates, as there was a relatively small sample, and a large effect would have been needed to draw a conclusion that it was completely ineffective. In addition, only one antibiotic was tested. However, the effect on maternal infection was so strong that its use is recommended, and no adverse effects were observed in either mother or baby when this antibiotic was used. Additional research with a range of antibiotics is warranted to discover if other antibiotics may be effective in preventing neonatal complications of MSAF.

Best Practice
Antibiotics should be administered to mothers with meconium-stained amniotic fluid to reduce the risk of chorioamnionitis. The drug has no measurable adverse effects and has been shown to be safe for both mother and baby.

Clinical Reasoning
Why might an antibiotic be effective for prevention of maternal infections and not for the neonate? What client teaching is needed for the mother with meconium-stained amniotic fluid in terms of her self-care and care of the neonate?

---

may predispose the newborn to air leak syndrome such as pneumothorax or pneumomediastinum (Fanaroff & Fanaroff, 2013).

CLINICAL THERAPY
The combined efforts of the maternity and pediatric team are needed to prevent MAS. Previously, the most effective form of preventive management was intrapartum suctioning after the head of the newborn was delivered but the shoulders and chest were still in the birth canal. Current evidence does not support this practice, as routine intrapartum oropharyngeal and nasopharyngeal suctioning does not prevent or alter the course of MAS (AAP & ACOG, 2012; Fanaroff & Fanaroff, 2013).

If the newborn is vigorous, even if there is meconium-stained amniotic fluid, no subsequent special resuscitation such

as tracheal suctioning is indicated. Injury to the vocal cords is also more likely to occur during attempts to intubate a vigorous newborn.

If the newborn has absent or depressed respirations, heart rate less than 100 beats per minute, or poor muscle tone, direct tracheal suctioning with a DeLee device attached to low-pressure wall suction by a specially trained healthcare provider is recommended. The glottis is visualized and the trachea suctioned to remove meconium or other aspirated material from beneath the glottis to decrease the possibility of human immunodeficiency virus (HIV) transmission.

Further resuscitative efforts are undertaken as indicated, following the same principles of clinical therapy used for asphyxia (discussed earlier in this chapter). Resuscitated newborns should be transferred immediately to the nursery for closer observation. The baby should be maintained in a neutral thermal environment and tactile stimulation should be minimized. An umbilical arterial line may be used for direct monitoring of arterial blood pressures, as well as blood sampling for pH and blood gases. An umbilical venous catheter may be placed for infusion of IV fluids, blood, or medications.

Treatment usually involves delivery of high levels of oxygen and high-pressure ventilation. High pressures may be needed to cause sufficient expiratory expansion of obstructed terminal airways or to stabilize airways that are weakened by inflammation so that the most distal atelectatic (collapsed) alveoli are ventilated. Naturally occurring surfactant may be inactivated by the presence of meconium and the subsequent inflammatory response that occurs. Surfactant replacement therapy is most effective when given as a prophylactic measure. Providing exogenous surfactant possibly decreases mortality (Swarnam et al., 2012; Walsh, Daigle, DiBlasi, et al., 2013). Systemic blood pressure and pulmonary blood flow must be maintained. Dopamine or dobutamine, or both, may be used to maintain systemic blood pressure.

Newborns with respiratory failure who are not responding to conventional ventilator therapy may require treatment with high-frequency ventilation and/or nitric oxide therapy or extracorporeal membrane oxygenation (ECMO) if baby is greater than 1.8 kg (4.0 lb) and 34 weeks estimated gestational age (EGA) (Fanaroff & Fanaroff, 2013; Gomella, 2013). Inhaled nitric oxide has proven successful for newborns with meconium aspiration, pneumonia, and PPHN who are not responding to traditional treatment modalities, and it avoids the need for ECMO.

Nursing Management

For the Newborn With Meconium Aspiration Syndrome

Nursing Assessment and Diagnosis

During the intrapartum period observe for signs of fetal hypoxia and meconium staining of amniotic fluid. At birth, assess the newborn for signs of distress. During the ongoing assessment of the newborn, carefully observe for complications such as pulmonary air leaks, PPHN, hypotension and poor cardiac output, inadequate renal function, cerebral and pulmonary edema, sepsis secondary to bacterial pneumonia, and any signs of intestinal necrosis from ischemia.

Nursing diagnoses that may apply to the newborn with MAS and the newborn's parents include the following (NANDA-I © 2014):

- *Gas Exchange, Impaired,* related to aspiration of meconium and amniotic fluid during birth
- *Nutrition, Imbalanced: Less than Body Requirements,* related to respiratory distress and increased energy requirements
- *Coping: Family, Compromised,* related to life-threatening illness in term newborn

Planning and Implementation

HOSPITAL-BASED NURSING CARE
Initial interventions are aimed at early identification of meconium aspiration. When significant aspiration occurs, therapy is supportive with the primary goals of maintaining appropriate gas exchange and

minimizing complications. Nursing interventions after resuscitation should include maintaining adequate oxygenation and ventilation, regulating temperature, performing glucose testing by glucometer to check for hypoglycemia, monitoring calcium levels, observing IV fluid administration, calculating necessary fluids (which may be restricted in the first 48 to 72 hours because of cerebral edema), providing caloric requirements with total parenteral nutrition (TPN), and monitoring IV antibiotic therapy.

Evaluation
Expected outcomes of nursing care include the following:

- The newborn at risk for MAS is promptly identified and early intervention is initiated.
- The newborn is free of respiratory distress and metabolic alterations.
- The parents verbalize their concerns about their baby's health problem and survival and understand the rationale behind the management of their newborn.

Care of the Newborn With Cold Stress

Cold stress is excessive heat loss resulting in the use of compensatory mechanisms (such as increased respirations and nonshivering thermogenesis/use of brown fat stores) to maintain core body temperature close to 37.0°C (98.6°F) (Cloherty et al., 2012). Heat loss that results in cold stress occurs in the newborn through the mechanisms of evaporation, convection, conduction, and radiation. (See Chapter 23 for types of thermoregulation.) Heat loss at birth that leads to cold stress can play a significant role in the severity of respiratory distress syndrome (RDS) and the ultimate outcome for the baby. Both preterm and small-for-gestational-age (SGA) newborns are at increased risk for cold stress because they have decreased adipose tissue, brown fat stores, and glycogen available for metabolism (Fanaroff & Fanaroff, 2013).

As discussed in Chapter 23, the newborn's major source of heat production in nonshivering thermogenesis (NST) is brown fat metabolism. The ability of a newborn to respond to cold stress by NST is impaired in the presence of several conditions:

- Hypoxemia (PO_2 less than 50 torr)
- Intracranial hemorrhage or any central nervous system (CNS) abnormality
- Hypoglycemia (blood glucose level less than 40 mg/dL)

When these conditions occur, the baby's temperature should be monitored more closely and the neutral thermal environment conscientiously maintained. You must recognize these conditions and treat them as soon as possible. The metabolic consequences of cold stress, caused by activation of the sympathetic nervous system, can be devastating and potentially fatal to a newborn. Oxygen requirements increase; even before noting a change in temperature, glucose use increases; acids are released into the bloodstream; and surfactant production decreases (Fanaroff & Fanaroff, 2013). The effects are graphically depicted in Figure 27–6.

Nursing Management

The amount of heat lost by a newborn depends to a large extent on the actions of the nurse or caregiver. Prevention of hypothermia

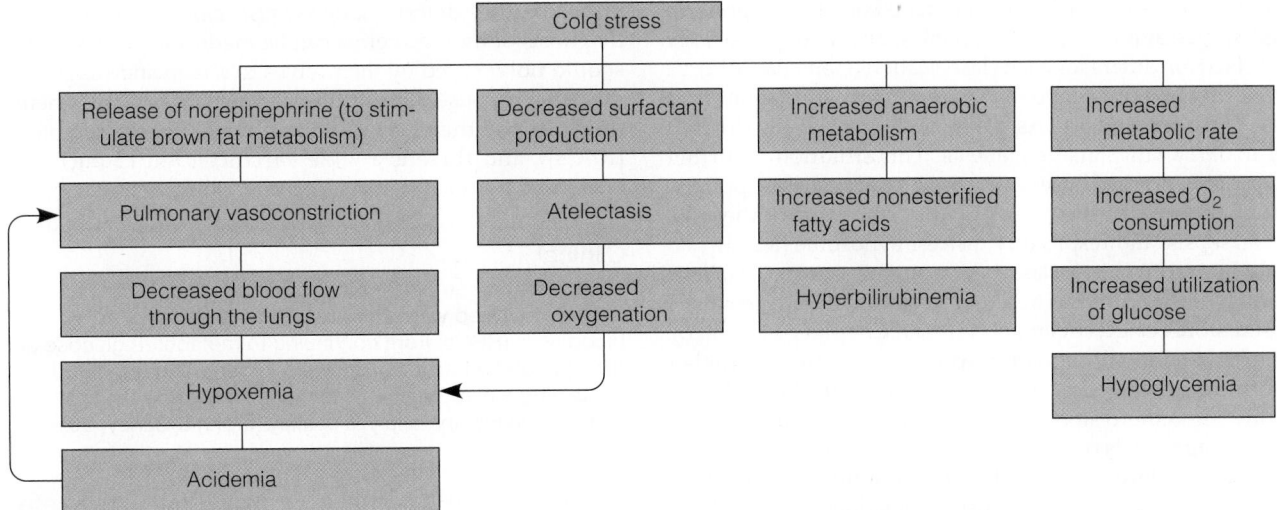

Figure 27–6 Cold stress chain of events. The hypothermic, or cold-stressed, newborn attempts to compensate by conserving heat and increasing heat production. These physiologic compensatory mechanisms initiate a series of metabolic events that results in hypoxemia and altered surfactant production, metabolic acidosis, hypoglycemia, and hyperbilirubinemia.

is especially critical in the very-low-birth-weight (VLBW) newborn. Placing the VLBW newborn in a polyethylene wrapping or the use of a chemically activated warming mattress immediately following birth can decrease the postnatal fall in temperature that normally occurs (Gardner & Hernandez, 2016). Using noncotton head coverings can significantly decrease heat loss after childbirth because the head makes up a large percentage of the surface area of the neonate. Convective, radiant, and evaporative heat loss can all be reduced. Swaddling and nesting maintain flexion, which reduces exposed surface area and thus convective and radiant losses.

Observe the baby for signs of cold stress. These include increased movements and respirations, decreased skin temperature and peripheral perfusion, development of hypoglycemia, and, possibly, development of metabolic acidosis.

Vasoconstriction is the initial response to cold stress; because it initially decreases skin temperature, monitor and assess skin temperature instead of rectal temperature. A decrease in rectal (core) temperature means that the newborn has long-standing cold stress. By monitoring skin temperature, possible decrease will become apparent before the baby's core temperature is affected.

If a decrease in skin temperature is noted, determine whether hypoglycemia is present. Hypoglycemia is a result of the metabolic effects of cold stress and is suggested by glucometer values below 40 to 50 mg/dL, tremors, irritability or lethargy, apnea, or seizure activity.

If hypothermia occurs, the following nursing interventions should be initiated (Gomella, 2013):

- Maintain a neutral thermal environment (NTE); adjust based on the gestational age and postnatal age.
- Warm the newborn slowly, because rapid temperature elevation may cause hypotension and apnea.
- Increase the air temperature in hourly increments of 1.0°C (33.8°F) until the baby's temperature is stable.
- Monitor temperature every 15 to 30 minutes to determine whether the newborn's temperature is increasing, assessing the temperature with the use of skin, axillary (most

commonly utilized method), or infrared (IR) thermometers (Smith, Alcock, & Usher, 2013).

- Remove plastic wrap, caps, and heat shields while rewarming the baby so that cool air as well as warm air is not trapped.
- Warm IV fluids before infusion.
- Initiate efforts to block heat loss by evaporation, radiation, convection, and conduction.
- Maintain the newborn in NTE.

Assess for the presence of anaerobic metabolism and initiate interventions for the resulting metabolic acidosis. Attempts to burn brown fat increase oxygen consumption, lactic acid levels, and metabolic acidosis. Hypoglycemia may be reversed by adequate glucose intake, as described in the following section.

Care of the Newborn With Hypoglycemia

Hypoglycemia, low blood sugar, can affect 1 to 3 newborns per 1000 live births, and up to 15% of them are born growth restricted (Harris, Weston, & Harding, 2012; Smith & Carley, 2014). An operational threshold for intervention in newborn hypoglycemia is a plasma glucose concentration of less than 40 to 45 mg/dL at any time in any newborn. It requires follow-up glucose measurement to document normal values (AAP & ACOG, 2012; Cloherty et al., 2012; Fanaroff & Fanaroff, 2013; Riley, Spencer, & Prater, 2014). Within the first hours to days of life, normal asymptomatic newborns may have a transient glucose level in the 30s (mg/dL) that will increase either spontaneously or with feedings. Plasma glucose values less than 20 to 25 mg/dL should be treated with parenteral glucose $D_{10}W$, regardless of the age or gestation, to raise plasma glucose to greater than 45 mg/dL. There is no absolute threshold that can be applied to all babies. Glucose concentrations must be looked at in conjunction with risk assessment and clinical manifestations.

Hypoglycemia is the most common metabolic disorder occurring in infants of diabetic mothers (IDM), small-for-gestational-age (SGA) babies, the smaller of twins, babies born to mothers with preeclampsia, male babies, and preterm average-for-gestational-age (AGA) babies. The pathophysiology of hypoglycemia differs for each classification (Gomella, 2013).

Preterm newborns have not been in utero a sufficient time to store glycogen and fat. As a result, they have a decreased ability to carry out gluconeogenesis. This situation is further aggravated by increased use of glucose by the tissues (especially the brain and heart) during stress and illness (hypothermia, asphyxia, sepsis, and respiratory distress syndrome [RDS]).

Newborns of White's classes A through C or type 1 diabetic mothers (women with diagnosed or gestational diabetes) have increased stores of glycogen and fat (see Chapters 14 and 26). Circulating insulin and insulin responsiveness are also higher when compared with other newborns. Because the high glucose loads present in utero stop at birth, and the newborn continues to produce high levels of insulin from their pancreatic beta cells, the newborn experiences rapid and profound hypoglycemia (Gomella, 2013). Babies with recurrent episodes of hypoglycemia may have long-term neurologic deficits (Harris et al., 2012).

The SGA newborn has used up glycogen and fat stores because of intrauterine malnutrition and has a blunted hepatic enzymatic response with which to produce and use glucose. Any newborn stressed at birth from asphyxia or cold also quickly uses up available glucose stores and becomes hypoglycemic. Epidural anesthesia may alter maternal–fetal glucose homeostasis, resulting in hypoglycemia.

Clinical Therapy

The goal of management includes early identification of hypoglycemia through observation and screening of newborns at risk (Fanaroff & Fanaroff, 2013; Gomella, 2013; Harris et al., 2012). The newborn may be asymptomatic, or any of the following may occur:

- Lethargy, sleepiness, and limpness
- Poor feeding, poor/inadequate sucking reflex, vomiting
- Hypothermia or temperature instability
- Pallor, cyanosis
- Apnea, irregular respirations, respiratory distress, cyanosis, tachypnea
- Hypotonia, possible loss of swallowing reflex
- Tremors, jerkiness, jitteriness, seizure activity, irritability, eye rolling
- High-pitched cry
- Exaggerated Moro reflex
- Temperature instability

Universal blood glucose screening before clinical signs develop is not recommended by the AAP (Committee on the Fetus and Newborn & Adamkin, 2011). Aggressive treatment is recommended after a single low blood glucose value if the newborn shows any of these symptoms. In at-risk babies, routine screening should be done frequently during the first hours of life and then whenever any of the noted clinical manifestations appears or at 1- to 4-hour intervals until the risk period has passed.

Hypoglycemia may also be defined as a *glucose oxidase reagent strip with reflectance meter* below 40 mg/dL, but only when corroborated with laboratory blood glucose (see Performing a Capillary Puncture in the *Clinical Skills Manual* SKILLS). Point-of-care testing (POCT) methods use whole blood, an enzymatic reagent strip, and a reflectance meter or color chart. Bedside glucose oxidase strip tests can screen for hypoglycemia,

but laboratory determinations *must confirm* the results before a diagnosis of hypoglycemia can be made. Glucose reagent strips should not be used by themselves to screen and diagnose hypoglycemia because their results depend on the baby's hematocrit (they react to the glucose in the plasma, not the red blood cells [RBCs]), and there is a wide variance (5 to 15 mg/dL) when compared with laboratory determinations.

Clinical Tip

Venous blood samples for the laboratory should be placed on ice and analyzed within 30 minutes of drawing to prevent the red blood cells (RBCs) from continuing to metabolize glucose and giving a falsely low reading. Avoid transporting the blood in tubes containing a glycolytic inhibitor such as fluoride. Transport blood samples on ice and analyze quickly (Smith & Carley, 2014).

Blood glucose sampling techniques can significantly affect the accuracy of the blood glucose value. It is important to note that whole blood glucose concentrations are 10% to 15% lower than plasma glucose concentration (Cloherty et al., 2012). The higher the hematocrit, the greater the difference between whole blood and plasma values. Also, venous blood glucose concentrations are approximately 15% to 19% lower than arterial blood glucose concentrations because the tissues extract some glucose before the blood enters the venous system. Newer point-of-care techniques, such as using a glucose oxidase analyzer or an optical bedside glucose analyzer, are more reliable for bedside screening but must also be validated with laboratory chemical analysis.

Adequate caloric intake is important. Early breastfeeding or formula-feeding is one of the major preventive approaches. If early feeding or intravenous (IV) glucose is started to meet the recommended fluid and caloric needs, the blood glucose is likely to remain above the hypoglycemic level. During the first hours after birth, asymptomatic newborns may be given oral glucose contained in formula or breast milk (glucose water should not be used because it causes a rapid increase in glucose followed by an abrupt decrease), and then another plasma glucose measurement is obtained within 30 to 60 minutes after feeding.

IV infusions of a dextrose solution D_5W to $D_{10}W$ (5% to 10%) begun immediately after birth should prevent hypoglycemia. Plasma glucose levels are obtained when the parenteral infusion is started. However, in the very small AGA or SGA newborn, infusions of 10% dextrose solution may cause hyperglycemia to develop, requiring an alteration in the glucose concentration. An IV glucose solution should be calculated based on body weight of the baby and fluid requirements and correlated with blood glucose tests to determine adequacy of the infusion treatment.

In more severe cases of hypoglycemia, glucagon or corticosteroids may be administered. It is thought that steroids enhance gluconeogenesis from noncarbohydrate protein sources (Gomella, 2013; Smith & Carley, 2014).

Nursing Management

For the Newborn With Hypoglycemia

Nursing Assessment and Diagnosis

The objectives of nursing assessment are to identify newborns at risk and to screen symptomatic babies. For newborns diagnosed with hypoglycemia, assessment is ongoing and includes careful monitoring of glucose values. Glucose strips, urine dipstick, and urine volume tests (monitor only if above 1 to 3 mL/kg/hr) may be evaluated frequently for osmotic diuresis and glycosuria.

Nursing diagnoses that may apply to the newborn with hypoglycemia include the following (NANDA-I © 2014):

- *Nutrition, Imbalanced: Less than Body Requirements*, related to increased glucose use secondary to physiologic stress
- *Breathing Pattern, Ineffective*, related to tachypnea and apnea
- *Pain, Acute*, related to frequent heel sticks secondary to glucose monitoring

Planning and Implementation

Monitor all at-risk groups within 30 to 60 minutes after birth and before feedings or whenever there are abnormal signs. Monitor the IDM within 30 minutes of birth. Once an at-risk newborn's blood sugar level is stable, glucose testing every 2 to 4 hours (or per agency protocol), or before feedings, adequately monitors glucose levels. See Figures 27–7 and 27–8.

The method of feeding greatly influences glucose and energy requirements; thus careful calculation of glucose requirements and attention to glucose monitoring are required during the transition from IV to oral feedings. Titration of IV glucose may be required until the newborn is able to take adequate amounts of formula or breast milk to maintain a normal blood sugar level. Enteral feedings are increased to maintain adequate glucose and caloric intake and also normal blood glucose levels. Titrate by decreasing the concentration of parenteral glucose gradually to 5% (D_5W), and then reducing the rate of infusion (mg/kg/min), and slowly discontinuing it over 4 to 6 hours. Enteral feeds are increased to maintain an adequate glucose and caloric intake and maintain normal blood glucose levels.

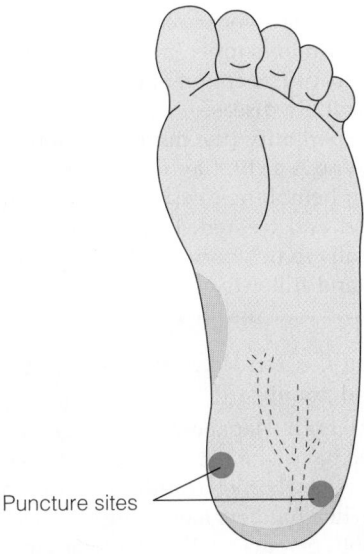

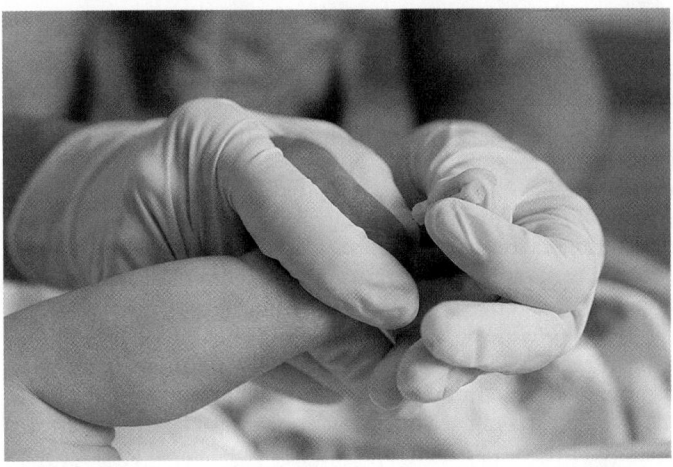

Figure 27–8 Heelstick. With a quick, piercing motion, puncture the lateral heel with a micro lancet. Be careful not to puncture too deeply.

PAIN RELIEF IN THE NICU

The newborn relies on the nurse's observational, assessment, and interventional skills for prompt, safe, and effective pain relief. It is vital to assist babies to cope with and recover from necessary painful clinical procedures. A variety of nonpharmacologic pain prevention and relief techniques have been shown to be effective in reducing pain from minor procedures in newborns.

Any unnecessary stimuli (i.e., noise, visual, tactile, and vestibular) of the newborn should be avoided, if possible. Developmental care, which includes limiting environmental stimuli, lateral positioning, the use of supportive bedding, and attention to behavioral cues, assists the newborn to cope with painful procedures (Gomella, 2013; Walden, 2014).

Containment with swaddling or facilitated tucking (holding the arms and legs in a flexed position) is effective in reducing excessive immature motor responses. Swaddling also may provide comfort through other senses, such as thermal, tactile, and proprioceptive senses. Breastfeeding and skin-to-skin contact/kangaroo care with the mother during the painful procedure may help to relieve pain (Gomella, 2013; Walden, 2014).

Nonnutritive sucking (NNS) refers to the provision of a pacifier into the baby's mouth to promote sucking without the provision of breast milk or formula for nutrition. NNS is thought to produce analgesia through stimulation of orotactile and mechanoreceptors when the pacifier is placed into the baby's mouth. Allowing nonnutritive sucking with a pacifier aids in the reduction of procedural pain and stress (Gomella, 2013; Walden, 2014).

A wide range of oral sucrose doses has been used for procedural pain relief (heelsticks, venipuncture, IM injections), and while no optimal dose has been established, a solution of 24% sucrose solution is agreed upon (Walden, 2014). The sweetness of the sucrose, a disaccharide, elevates the pain threshold through endogenous opioid release in the CNS and produces a calming effect (Gomella, 2013; Walden, 2014).

Evaluation

Expected outcomes of nursing care include the following:

- The newborn at risk for hypoglycemia is identified, and prompt intervention is started.
- The newborn's glucose level is stabilized, and recovery is proceeding without sequelae.

Puncture sites

Figure 27–7 Potential puncture sites for heelsticks. Avoid gray-shaded areas to prevent injury to arteries and nerves in the foot and the important longitudinally oriented fat pad of the heel, which in later years could impede walking if injured.

Care of the Newborn With Jaundice

The most common abnormal physical finding in newborns is jaundice (*icterus neonatorum*). Some degree of newborn jaundice, resulting from elevated unconjugated bilirubinemia, with total serum bilirubin levels greater than 5mg/dL, occurs in up to 80% of healthy newborns in the first 7 days following birth (Bhutani et al., 2013; Gomella, 2013; Turnbull & Petty, 2012). **Jaundice** is a yellowish coloration of the skin and sclerae of the eyes that develops from the deposit of yellow pigment bilirubin in lipid-/fat-containing tissues. Fetal unconjugated bilirubin is normally cleared by the placenta in utero, so total bilirubin at birth is usually less than 3 mg/L unless an abnormal hemolytic process has been present. Postnatally, the baby must conjugate bilirubin (convert a lipid-soluble pigment into a water-soluble pigment that can be excreted) in the liver.

The rate and amount of conjugation of bilirubin depend on the rate of hemolysis, the bilirubin load, the maturity of the liver, and the presence of albumin-binding sites. See Chapter 23 for discussion of conjugation of bilirubin. A normal, healthy, full-term newborn's liver is usually mature enough and produces enough glucuronyl transferase that the total serum bilirubin concentration does not reach a pathologic level. The diagnosis of pathologic jaundice is given to newborns who exhibit jaundice within the first 24 hours of life, have a total serum bilirubin concentration increase of greater than 0.2 mg/dL/hr, surpass the 95th percentile on the nomogram for age in hours, or have persistent visible jaundice after 1 week of age in term newborns or after 2 weeks in preterm newborns (Casey, 2013; Turnbull & Petty, 2012).

Pathophysiology of Hyperbilirubinemia

Serum albumin-binding sites are usually sufficient to conjugate enough bilirubin to meet the normal demands of the newborn. However, certain conditions such as fetal or neonatal asphyxia and neonatal drugs such as indomethacin can decrease the binding affinity of bilirubin to albumin because acidosis impairs the capacity of albumin to hold bilirubin. Hypothermia and hypoglycemia release free fatty acids that dislocate bilirubin from albumin. Maternal medications such as sulfa drugs and salicylates compete with bilirubin for these sites. Finally, premature newborns have less albumin available for binding with bilirubin. Neurotoxicity is possible because unconjugated bilirubin has a high affinity for extravascular tissue, such as fatty tissue (subcutaneous tissue) and cerebral tissue.

Bilirubin not bound to albumin can cross the blood–brain barrier, damage cells of the CNS, and produce kernicterus or **acute bilirubin encephalopathy (ABE)**. **Kernicterus** (meaning "yellow nucleus") refers to the deposition of indirect or unconjugated bilirubin in the basal ganglia of the brain and to the permanent neurologic sequelae of untreated **hyperbilirubinemia** (elevation of bilirubin level) (Cloherty et al., 2012). The incidence is 0.5 to 2 per 100,000 live births (Maisels, 2012).

The classic acute bilirubin encephalopathy of kernicterus most commonly found with Rh and ABO blood group incompatibility is less common today because of aggressive treatment with phototherapy and exchange transfusions. Kernicterus cases are reappearing as a result of early discharge and the increased incidence of dehydration (as a result of discharge before the mother's milk is established). Unfortunately, current therapy cannot distinguish all babies who are at risk. It is recommended that *all* newborns be screened for bilirubin level prior to leaving the hospital using total serum bilirubin (TSB) or transcutaneous bilirubin (TcB). It is also advised to record information on gestation, birth weight, bilirubin/albumin ratios, and risk factors on the electronic health record (EHR) (Maisels & Watchko, 2012).

Causes of Hyperbilirubinemia

A primary cause of hyperbilirubinemia is **hemolytic disease of the newborn**. All pregnant women who are Rh negative or who have blood type O (possible ABO blood incompatibility) should be asked about outcomes of any previous pregnancies and history of blood transfusion. Prenatal amniocentesis with spectrophotographic examination may be indicated in some cases. Cord blood from newborns is evaluated for bilirubin level, which normally does not exceed 5 mg/dL. Newborns of Rh-negative and O blood type mothers are carefully assessed for appearance of jaundice and levels of serum bilirubin.

Alloimmune hemolytic disease, also known as **erythroblastosis fetalis**, occurs when an Rh-negative mother is pregnant with an Rh-positive fetus and maternal antibodies cross the placenta. Maternal antibodies enter the fetal circulation, then attach to and destroy the fetal RBCs. The fetal system responds by increasing RBC production. Jaundice, anemia, and compensatory erythropoiesis result. A marked increase in immature RBCs (erythroblasts) also occurs, hence the designation erythroblastosis fetalis. Because of the widespread use of Rh immune globulin (RhoGAM), the incidence of erythroblastosis fetalis has dropped dramatically (Turnbull & Petty, 2012).

Hydrops fetalis, the most severe form of erythroblastosis fetalis, occurs when maternal antibodies attach to the Rh site on the fetal RBCs, making them susceptible to destruction; severe anemia and multiorgan system failure result. Cardiomegaly with severe cardiac decompensation and hepatosplenomegaly occurs. Severe generalized massive edema (anasarca) and generalized fluid effusion into the pleural cavity (hydrothorax), pericardial sac, and peritoneal cavity (ascites) develop. Jaundice is not present until the newborn period because the bilirubin pigments are excreted through the placenta into the maternal circulation. The hydropic hemolytic disease process is also characterized by hyperplasia of the pancreatic islets, which predisposes the newborn to neonatal hypoglycemia similar to that of IDMs. These babies have increased bleeding tendencies because of associated thrombocytopenia and hypoxic damage to the capillaries. Hydrops is a frequent cause of intrauterine death among babies with Rh disease.

ABO incompatibility (the mother is blood type O and the baby is blood type A or B) may result in jaundice, although it rarely results in hemolytic disease severe enough to be clinically diagnosed and treated. Hepatosplenomegaly may be found occasionally in newborns with ABO incompatibility, but hydrops fetalis and stillbirth are rare.

Developing Cultural Competence Ethnic Variations and Jaundice

East Asian newborns (Japanese, Chinese, and Filipino ethnic groups) have a higher occurrence of hyperbilirubinemia than White newborns. In addition, babies with Asian fathers and White mothers have a higher incidence of jaundice than if both parents are White. Other ethnic groups at risk for increased bilirubinemia are Navajo, Eskimo, and Sioux Native American newborns; Greek newborns; Sephardic-Jewish newborns; Asian ancestry newborns; and some Hispanic newborns. The incidence is lower in African Americans (Gomella, 2013).

During pregnancy, predisposing maternal conditions include hereditary spherocytosis, diabetes, intrauterine infections, gram-negative bacilli infections that stimulate production of maternal alloimmune antibodies, drug ingestion (such as sulfas, salicylates, novobiocin, and diazepam), and oxytocin administration. Early prenatal identification of the fetus at risk for Rh or ABO incompatibility allows prompt treatment. (See Chapter 20 for discussion of in utero management of this condition.)

The prognosis for a newborn with hyperbilirubinemia depends on the extent of the hemolytic process and the underlying cause. Severe hemolytic disease may result in fetal or early neonatal death from the effects of anemia—cardiac decompensation, edema, ascites, and hydrothorax. Hyperbilirubinemia may lead to kernicterus if not aggressively treated. The initial symptoms requiring acute intervention of an exchange transfusion are poor tone, lethargy, and/or feeding/sucking issues (Kamath-Rayne, Thio, Deacon, et al., 2016). Continuing worsening progression includes neurologic damage, which may cause death, cerebral palsy, cognitive impairment, or hearing loss/ nerve deafness, or, to a lesser degree, perceptual impairment, delayed speech development, hyperactivity, muscle incoordination, or learning difficulties (Kamath-Rayne et al., 2016). Intravenous gamma globulin (IVIG) may be used with newborns suffering from isoimmune hemolytic disease, 1 g/kg over 4 hours and repeated in 12 hours if required (Gomella, 2013).

Clinical Therapy

LABORATORY AND DIAGNOSTIC ASSESSMENTS

The best treatment for hemolytic disease is prevention by early recognition of prenatal risk factors such as Rh and ABO incompatibility (see Chapter 15 for discussion of in utero management of this condition), and attention to certain neonatal clinical conditions. Neonatal hyperbilirubinemia can be considered pathologic and requires further investigation if any of the following criteria are met (Bhutani, Johnson, & Keren, 2004; Gomella, 2013):

1. Clinically evident jaundice appears before 24 hours of life or if jaundice seems excessive for the newborn's age in hours.

2. Serum bilirubin concentration rises by more than 0.2 mg/ dL per hour.

3. Symptoms of primary illness

4. Total serum bilirubin concentration exceeds the 95th percentile on a nomogram.

5. Conjugated bilirubin concentrations are greater than 2 mg/dL or more than 20% of the total serum bilirubin concentration.

6. Clinical jaundice persists for more than 8 days in a term newborn and 14 days in a premature newborn (Cloherty et al., 2012).

Initial diagnostic procedures are aimed at differentiating jaundice resulting from increased bilirubin production, impaired conjugation or excretion, increased intestinal reabsorption, or a combination of these factors.

Transcutaneous bilirubin (TcB) measurements are a noninvasive method of assessing bilirubin levels and may be used for predischarge risk assessment (Figure 27–9). A TcB can be performed quickly and painlessly, and repeated measures are easily obtained. TcB can quantify the amount of bilirubin pigment in the newborn's skin. Nurses need to measure bilirubin levels to confirm the presence, absence, or suspicion of jaundice.

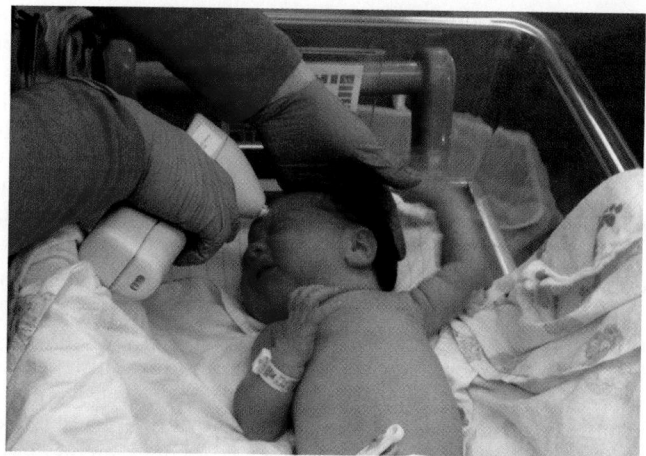

Figure 27–9 **A newborn being screened with a transcutaneous bilirubinometer.**

SOURCE: Lisa Smith-Pedersen, RN, MSN, NNP-BC.

However, it is important to remember that total serum bilirubin levels remain the standard of care for confirmation or diagnosis of hyperbilirubinemia (Maisels & Watchko, 2012).

Because of the shorter life span of red blood cells in the newborn, a significant bilirubin load is produced. When bilirubin breaks down, carbon monoxide (CO) is released. This production of CO is being investigated as a marker in the study of bilirubin production. Measuring end-tidal CO (ETCO) has been shown to provide results similar to those of laboratory bilirubin; however, devices to measure CO are not widely available.

Essential laboratory evaluations are Coombs test, serum bilirubin levels (direct and total), hemoglobin, reticulocyte percentage, white cell count, and positive smear for cellular morphology.

Clinical Tip

The transcutaneous bilirubinometer (TcB) is a screening product that can be utilized on newborns prior to discharge, at any time during hospitalization, or at a follow-up visit at the pediatrician's office. The benefits are that it is a noninvasive screening tool and it can be done on all newborns except for those receiving phototherapy. Any elevated results need to be verified with a total serum bilirubin level (TsB). Results are found to be within 2 to 3 mg/dL of the TsB. Depending on the manufacturer, the recommendation is to test on the forehead or the sternum of the neonate (Bosschaart et al., 2012; Maisels, 2012; Mantagou et al., 2012; Wolff, Schinasi, Lavelle, et al., 2012).

The Coombs (direct antiglobulin test [DAT]) test is performed to determine whether jaundice is because of Rh or ABO incompatibility. The indirect Coombs test measures the amount of Rh-positive antibodies in the mother's blood. Rh-positive red blood cells are added to the maternal blood sample. If the mother's serum contains antibodies, the Rh-positive red blood cells will agglutinate (clump) when rabbit immune antiglobulin is added, which is a positive test result. The direct Coombs test reveals the presence of antibody-coated (sensitized) Rh-positive red blood cells in the newborn. Rabbit immune antiglobulin is added to the specimen of neonatal blood cells. If the neonatal red blood cells agglutinate, they have been coated with maternal antibodies, a positive result.

If the hemolytic process is caused by Rh sensitization, laboratory findings reveal the following: (1) an Rh-positive newborn with a positive Coombs test; (2) increased erythropoiesis with many immature circulating red blood cells (nucleated blastocysts); (3) anemia, in most cases; (4) elevated levels (5 mg/dL or more) of bilirubin in cord blood; and (5) a reduction in albumin-binding capacity. Maternal data may include an elevated anti-Rh titer and spectrophotometric evidence of a fetal hemolytic process.

If the hemolytic process is caused by ABO incompatibility, laboratory findings reveal an increase in reticulocytes. The resulting anemia is usually not significant during the newborn period and is rare later on. The direct Coombs test may be negative or mildly positive, whereas the indirect Coombs test may be strongly positive. Babies with a positive direct Coombs test have increased incidence of jaundice, with bilirubin levels in excess of 10 mg/dL. Increased numbers of spherocytes (spherical, plump, mature erythrocytes) are seen on a peripheral blood smear. Increased numbers of spherocytes are not seen on blood smears from babies with Rh disease.

THERAPEUTIC MANAGEMENT

Whatever the cause of hyperbilirubinemia, management of these newborns is directed toward alleviating anemia, removing maternal antibodies and sensitized erythrocytes, increasing serum albumin levels, reducing serum bilirubin levels, and minimizing the consequences of hyperbilirubinemia. Early discharge of newborns from birthing centers has significantly influenced the diagnosis and management of neonatal jaundice, increasing the emphasis on outpatient and home care management.

If hemolytic disease is present, it may be treated with phototherapy, exchange transfusion, and drug therapy. When determining the appropriate management of hyperbilirubinemia caused by hemolytic disease, the three relevant variables are the newborn's (1) serum bilirubin level, (2) birth weight, and (3) age in hours. If a newborn has hemolysis with an unconjugated bilirubin level of 14 mg/dL, weighs less than 2500 g (5.5 lb) (birth weight), and is 24 hours old or less, an exchange transfusion may be the best management. However, if that same newborn is over 24 hours of age, which is past the time during which an increase in bilirubin would occur because of pathologic causes, phototherapy may be the treatment of choice to prevent the possible complication of kernicterus.

PHOTOTHERAPY

Phototherapy is the exposure of the newborn to high-intensity light. It may be used alone or in conjunction with exchange transfusion to reduce serum bilirubin levels. Exposure of the newborn to high-intensity light (a bank of fluorescent light bulbs, LEDs [light-emitting diodes], or bulbs in the blue-light spectrum) decreases serum bilirubin levels in the skin by facilitating biliary excretion of unconjugated bilirubin. Phototherapy decreases serum bilirubin levels by changing bilirubin from the non–water-soluble (lipophilic) form to water-soluble by-products that can then be excreted via urine and bile.

Photoisomerization occurs when the natural form of bilirubin is exposed to light at a certain wavelength and the bilirubin is converted to a less toxic form. The new isomer, photobilirubin, is created rapidly but is quite unstable. The photobilirubin is bound to albumin, transported to the liver, and incorporated into bile. If it is not quickly eliminated from the bowel, it can convert back to its original form and return to the bloodstream. In addition, the photodegradation breakdown products formed when light oxidizes bilirubin can be excreted in the urine.

Phototherapy is a primary intervention that is used more for the prevention of hyperbilirubinemia to halt bilirubin levels from climbing dangerously high. The decision to start phototherapy is based on two factors: gestational age and age in hours. Phototherapy is most effective in the first 24 to 48 hours of usage; frequently, the light can be discontinued during or immediately after this time frame. Phototherapy does not alter the underlying cause of jaundice, and hemolysis may continue to produce anemia. Many researchers have recommended initiating phototherapy "prophylactically" in the first 24 hours of life in high-risk, very-low-birth-weight (VLBW), or severely bruised newborns. The risk category of newborns requiring follow-up or intervention for hyperbilirubinemia is evaluated by plotting their serum bilirubin level and age in hours on a nomogram. Phototherapy is not benign; especially in the preterm neonate, it has been attributed to destruction of platelets, hemolysis, and prolonged patency of the fetal ductus arteriosus (Hintz et al., 2011).

Clinical Tip

When excreted, the newborn's urine will be much darker in color/appearance because of the excreted higher conjugated bilirubin content.

Phototherapy can be provided by conventional banks of phototherapy lights, a fiberoptic blanket attached to a halogen light source around the trunk of the newborn, LEDs, or a combination of these delivery methods. Conventional banks of phototherapy lights are the most effective source available but can mask cyanosis and causes dizziness and nausea in the staff. Levels should continue to decline when phototherapy covers a wider surface area. If a drop in bilirubin levels is not reached, then an exchange transfusion should be considered. Most phototherapy units will provide this level of irradiance 45 to 50 cm (18 to 20 in.) below the lamps. The nurse can use a photometer to measure and maintain desired irradiance levels. The nurse keeps track of the number of hours each lamp is used so that each can be replaced before its effectiveness is lost (Bhutani & Committee on the Fetus and Newborn, 2011). Disadvantages of lights are that they create a difficult work environment and can distort a baby's color.

With the fiberoptic blanket, the light stays on at all times, and the newborn is accessible for care, feeding, and diaper changes; greater surface area is exposed and there are no thermoregulation issues. The eyes are not covered. Fluid and weight loss are not complications of this system. Furthermore, it makes the baby accessible to the parents and is less alarming to parents than standard phototherapy. Many institutions and pediatricians use fiberoptic blankets for home care. A combination of a fiberoptic light source in the mattress under the baby and a standard light source above may also be used. This is termed *intensive phototherapy*. Intensive phototherapy should reduce the total serum bilirubin (TSB) by 1 to 2 mg/dL within 4 to 8 hours. Levels should continue to decline when phototherapy covers a wider surface area. If a drop in bilirubin levels is not reached, then an exchange transfusion should be considered. The nurse uses a photometer to measure and maintain desired irradiance levels.

EXCHANGE TRANSFUSION

Exchange transfusion is the withdrawal and replacement of the newborn's blood with donor blood. It is used to treat anemia with red blood cells that are susceptible to maternal antibodies, to remove sensitized red blood cells that would soon be lysed, to remove serum bilirubin, to provide bilirubin-free albumin, and to increase the binding sites for bilirubin. Concerns about exchange transfusion are related to the use of blood products and associated potential for HIV infection and hepatitis. If the TSB is at or approaching the exchange level, blood should be sent for immediate typing and cross-matching. Blood for exchange transfusion is modified whole blood (red cells and plasma) cross-matched against the mother and compatible with the baby.

Nursing Management

For the Newborn With Jaundice

Nursing Assessment and Diagnosis

Assessment is aimed at identifying prenatal and perinatal factors that predispose the newborn to the development of jaundice and at recognizing the jaundice as soon as it is apparent. Significant hyperbilirubinemia in the neonatal population is often due to a multitude of causes, including a genetic basis. Clinically, ABO incompatibility presents as jaundice and occasionally as hepatosplenomegaly. Fetal hydrops or erythroblastosis is rare (see Chapter 15). Hemolytic disease of the newborn is suspected if one or more of the following are evident:

- The placenta is enlarged.
- The newborn is edematous, with pleural and pericardial effusion plus ascites.
- Pallor or jaundice is noted during the first 24 to 36 hours.
- Hemolytic anemia is diagnosed.
- The spleen and liver are enlarged.

Carefully note changes in behavior and observe for evidence of bleeding. If laboratory tests indicate elevated bilirubin levels, check the newborn for jaundice about every 2 hours and record observations.

To check for jaundice in lighter skinned babies, blanch the skin over a bony prominence (forehead, sternum) by pressing firmly with the thumb. After pressure is released, if jaundice is present, the area appears yellow before normal color returns. Check oral mucosa and the posterior portion of the hard palate and conjunctival sacs for yellow pigmentation in darker skinned babies. Jaundice progresses in a cephalocaudal direction from the face to the trunk and then to the lower extremities. The overall progression of jaundice should be noted. Assessment in daylight gives the best results, because pink walls and surroundings may mask yellowish tints, and yellow light makes differentiation of jaundice difficult. Record and report the time at onset of jaundice. If jaundice appears, careful observation of the increase in depth of color and of the newborn's behavior is mandatory.

Assess the newborn's behavior for neurologic signs associated with hyperbilirubinemia, which are rare but may include hypotonia, diminished reflexes, lethargy, or seizures.

Nursing diagnoses that may apply to care of a newborn with jaundice include the diagnoses in the nursing care plan and the following (NANDA-I © 2014):

- *Injury, Risk for,* related to use of phototherapy
- *Fluid Volume: Deficient, Risk for,* related to insensible water loss and frequent loose stools.
- *Neurovascular Dysfunction: Peripheral, Risk for,* related to neurologic damage secondary to kernicterus
- *Parenting, Risk for Impaired,* related to deficient knowledge of infant care and prolonged separation of baby and parents secondary to illness

Planning and Implementation

HOSPITAL-BASED NURSING CARE

Hospital-based care is described in *Nursing Care Plan: For the Newborn With Hyperbilirubinemia.*

Phototherapy success is measured every 12 hours or daily by serum bilirubin levels (more frequently if there is hemolysis or a higher level before initiation of phototherapy). The phototherapy lights must be turned off while drawing blood for serum bilirubin levels. Because it is not known whether phototherapy injures the delicate eye structures, particularly the retina, apply eye patches over the newborn's closed eyes during exposure to banks of phototherapy lights (see Figure 27–10 and Newborn Receiving Phototherapy in the *Clinical Skills Manual* SKILLS). Discontinue conventional phototherapy and remove the eye patches at least once per shift to assess the eyes for the presence of conjunctivitis. Also remove eye patches to allow eye contact during feeding (for social stimulation) or when parents are visiting (to promote parental attachment).

Most phototherapy units will provide this level of irradiance 6 to 12 μW/cm^2/nm below the lamps for conventional phototherapy and greater than 25 to 30 μW/cm^2/nm for intensive phototherapy (Gomella, 2013; Vandborg, Hansen, Greisen, et al., 2012). A photometer can be used to measure and maintain desired irradiance levels. Disadvantages of lights are that they create a difficult work environment and can distort a baby's color. Be careful about using ointments under bilirubin lights because they may cause burns.

Some parents may feel guilty about their baby's condition and think they have caused the problem. Under stress, parents may not be able to understand the healthcare provider's first explanations. Expect the parents to need explanations repeated and clarified and that they may need help voicing their questions and fears. Eye and tactile contact with the baby is encouraged. Coach parents when they visit with the baby. After the mother's discharge, keep parents informed of their baby's condition and encourage them to return to the hospital or to telephone at any time so that they can be fully involved in the care of their baby. Tell parents that they can expect a rebound of 1 to 2 mg/dL after discontinuation of phototherapy and that a follow-up bilirubin test may be done (Cloherty et al., 2012).

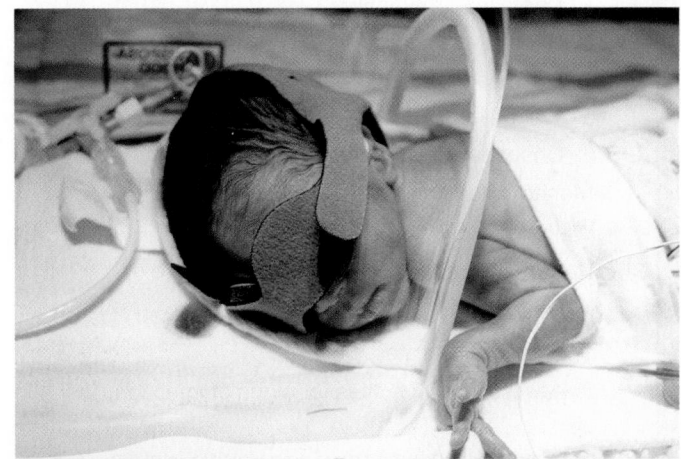

Figure 27–10 Newborn receiving phototherapy. The phototherapy light is positioned over the incubator. Bilateral eye patches are always used during photo light therapy to protect the baby's eyes.

SOURCE: Lisa Smith-Pedersen, RNC, MSN, NNP-BC.

Nursing Care Plan: For the Newborn With Hyperbilirubinemia

1. Nursing Diagnosis: *Tissue Integrity, Impaired,* **related to predisposing factors associated with hyperbilirubinemia (NANDA-I © 2014)**

GOAL: Newborns at risk for jaundice and early signs of jaundice will be identified.

INTERVENTION	RATIONALE
• Evaluate baby's history for predisposing factors for hyperbilirubinemia.	• Early identification of risk factors enables the nurse to monitor babies for early signs of hyperbilirubinemia. Acidosis, hypoxia, and hypothermia increase the risk of hyperbilirubinemia at lower bilirubin levels.
• Observe color of amniotic fluid at time of rupture of membranes.	• Amber-colored amniotic fluid indicates hyperbilirubinemia.
• Assess baby for developing jaundice in daylight if possible.	• Early detection is affected by nursery environment. Artificial lights (with pink tint) may mask beginning of jaundice.
1. Observe sclera.	1. Most visible sign of hyperbilirubinemia is jaundice noted in skin, sclera, or oral mucosa. Onset is first seen on face and then progresses down the trunk.
2. Observe skin color and assess by blanching.	2. Blanching the skin leaves a yellow color to the skin immediately after pressure is released.
3. Check oral mucosa, posterior portion of hard palate, and conjunctival sacs for yellow pigmentation in dark-skinned newborns.	3. Underlying pigment of dark-skinned babies may normally appear yellow.
• Report jaundice occurring within 24 hours of birth.	

EXPECTED OUTCOMES: Newborn's jaundice is identified early.

2. Nursing Diagnosis: *Fluid Volume: Imbalanced, Risk for,* **related to phototherapy (NANDA-I © 2014)**

GOAL: The newborn will not exhibit signs of dehydration and will display appropriate weight gain.

INTERVENTION	RATIONALE
• Offer feedings every 2–3 hr.	• Adequate hydration increases peristalsis and excretion of bilirubin.
• Breastfeed on demand with no supplementation unless excessive weight loss or increasing total serum bilirubin (TSB) with adequate feeding.	
• Provide 25% extra fluid intake.	• Replace fluid losses due to watery stools, if under phototherapy.
• Assess for dehydration:	• Phototherapy treatment may cause liquid stools and increased insensible water loss, which increases risk of dehydration.
1. Poor skin turgor	
2. Depressed fontanelles	
3. Sunken eyes	
4. Decreased urine output	
5. Weight loss	
6. Changes in electrolytes	
• Monitor intake and output (I&O).	
• Weigh daily.	
• Report signs of dehydration.	
• Administer IV fluids:	
1. Monitor flow rates.	• Prevents fluid overload.
2. Assess insertion sites for signs of infection.	• IV fluids may be used if baby is dehydrated or in presence of other complications. IV may be started if exchange transfusion is to be done.

EXPECTED OUTCOMES: Newborn will have good skin turgor, clear amber urine output of 1–3 mL/kg/hr, six to eight wet diapers/day, and will maintain weight.

3. Nursing Diagnosis: *Injury, Risk for,* **related to use of phototherapy (NANDA-I © 2014)**

GOAL: Newborn will not have any corneal irritation/drainage, skin breakdown, or major fluctuations in temperature.

INTERVENTION	RATIONALE
• Cover baby's eyes with eye patches while under photo-therapy lights. Cover testes/penis in male babies.	• Protects retina from damage due to high intensity light and testes from damage from heat.
• Make certain that eyelids are closed before applying eye patches.	• Prevents corneal abrasions.
• Remove baby from under phototherapy and remove eye patches during feedings.	• Provides visual stimulation and facilitates attachment behaviors.
• Inspect eyes each shift for conjunctivitis, drainage, and corneal abrasions due to irritation from eye patches.	• Prevents or facilitates prompt treatment of purulent conjunctivitis.
• Administer thorough perianal cleansing with each stool or change of perianal protective covering.	• Frequent stooling increases risk of skin breakdown. Prevents infection.
• Provide minimal coverage—only of diaper area.	• Provides maximal exposure. Shielded areas become more jaundiced, so maximum exposure is essential.
• Avoid the use of oily applications on the skin.	• Prevents superficial burns to skin.
• Reposition baby every 2 hr.	• Provides equal exposure of all skin areas and prevents pressure areas.
• Observe for bronzing of skin.	• Bronzing is related to use of phototherapy with increased direct bilirubin levels or liver damage; may last for 2–4 months.
• Place Plexiglas shield between baby and light.	• Hypothermia and hyperthermia are common complications of phototherapy.
• Monitor baby's skin and core temperature frequently until temperature is stable.	• Hypothermia results from exposure to lights, subsequent radiation, and convection losses.
• Check axillary temperature with readings on servo-controlled unit on incubator.	• Hyperthermia may result from the increased environmental heat.
• Regulate incubator temperature as needed.	• Additional heat from phototherapy lights frequently causes a rise in the baby's and incubator's temperatures.
	• Fluctuations in temperature may occur in response to radiation and convection.

EXPECTED OUTCOMES: Newborn's eyes are protected, skin is intact, and baby maintains a stable temperature.

---

4. Nursing Diagnosis: *Parenting, Risk for Impaired,* **related to deficient knowledge of infant care and prolonged separation of newborn and parents secondary to illness (NANDA-I © 2014)**

GOALS: Parents will bond with newborn and have realistic expectations about their baby. Parents are comfortable taking their baby home. They are able to demonstrate normal infant care and assessments of possible complications, and they know when to return for follow-up.

INTERVENTION	RATIONALE
• Encourage parents to provide tactile stimulation during feeding and diaper changes.	• Newborn has normal needs for tactile stimulation.
	• Presence of equipment may discourage parents from interacting with newborn.
• Encourage cuddling and eye contact during feedings.	• Provides opportunity for parents to bond with their newborn.
• Offer suggestions to comfort restless baby:	• Provides comfort and decreases sensory deprivation.
• Nesting when beneath bili lights	
• Talking softly and singing quietly to baby	
• Taped music or tape recording of evening activities from home	
• Rhythmic patting of buttocks	
• Firm, nonstroking touch, assisting with control of extremities	
• Pacifier for nonnutritive sucking	
• Encourage family/friend support of mother/parents (i.e., meals, rest, child care for siblings, allow expressions of concerns/feelings).	• Decreases strain on mother/parents by assisting with other responsibilities and allows for additional time with newborn for bonding and care.
• Evaluate additional psychosocial needs.	• Parents may not understand what is happening or why.

(continued)

Nursing Care Plan: For the Newborn With Hyperbilirubinemia (*continued*)

- Discuss rationale for treatment and possible side effects of phototherapy with family (stool changes, increased fluid loss, possible temp instability, slight lethargy, rash, altered sleep–wake patterns).
- Instruct family on baby's care while undergoing phototherapy:
  - Safety precautions—bili mask (to protect eyes), incubator door closed and latched, covering genitalia per policy.
  - Skin care, cord care, circumcision care as appropriate.
  - Lab draws, rationale I&O.
- Encourage parent/significant other/sibling involvement in baby's care as possible.
- Give explanation of equipment being used and changes in bilirubin levels. Allow parents an opportunity to ask questions; reinforce or clarify information as needed.
- Evaluate family's understanding of information.
- As necessary, review role of pumping breasts and offering formula for limited time.

- Assist mother to pump her breasts to maintain milk supply.

- Healthcare provider preference of treatment modalities may vary. Parents may not understand why their newborn is not receiving a treatment that another with the same condition is receiving.

- The etiology of breast milk jaundice remains uncertain. The serum bilirubin levels begin to fall within 48 hr after discontinuation of breastfeeding. Opinion of healthcare providers varies regarding the need for discontinuing breastfeeding.
- If breastfeeding is temporarily discontinued, assess mother's knowledge of pumping her breasts in regular increments (q 2–3 hr), and provide information and support as needed.

EXPECTED OUTCOMES: The parent will demonstrate ability to perform basic infant care tasks as evidenced by exhibiting appropriate attachment behaviors (e.g., talking to and holding baby), feeding baby, and caring for baby under home bili therapy.

Parents verbalize understanding of rationale and possible side effects from phototherapy; parents/family demonstrate safety precautions when caring for baby; parents getting meals and rest and verbalize support given.

Clinical Tip

If the area of jaundice around the eyes begins to disappear, it is probable that the eye patches are allowing light to enter and better eye protection is needed.

While the mother is still hospitalized, phototherapy can also be carried out in the parents' room if the only problem is hyperbilirubinemia and the parents agree to do the following:

- Keep the baby in the room for 24 hours a day.
- Take emergency action (e.g., for choking) if necessary.
- Complete instruction checklists.
- Sign a consent form per agency protocol.

Give the instructions to the parents but also continue to monitor the baby's temperature, activity, intake & output (I&O), and positioning of eye patches (if conventional light banks are used) at regular intervals.

COMMUNITY-BASED NURSING CARE

Some studies have shown that the early discharge of newborns and their mothers comes with an increase in hospital readmissions and an elevated risk of pathologic hyperbilirubinemia. Home phototherapy use is recommended only if the bilirubin level is plotted on the nomogram and found to be in the "optional phototherapy" range. Any newborn with a level in the higher range should be hospitalized for continual phototherapy and serum bilirubin levels closely monitored on a regular schedule.

Jaundice and its phototherapy treatment can be very disturbing to parents and may generate feelings of guilt and fear. The parents' perception of and/or misconceptions about jaundice can affect parent-baby interactions. Explain the causes of jaundice and emphasize that it is usually a transient problem and one to which all newborns must adapt after birth. Reassurance and support are vital especially for the breastfeeding mother, who may question her ability to adequately nourish her newborn.

It is essential that the impact of cultural beliefs be considered. Some Latina women believe that showing strong maternal emotions during pregnancy and breastfeeding can be detrimental. *Bilis* associated with anger may be blamed by some Latina women for jaundice.

If the baby is to receive phototherapy at home, teach the parents to record the baby's temperature, weight, fluid I&O, stools, and feedings and to use the phototherapy equipment. In addition, if phototherapy lights are being used, parents must agree that the baby will be exposed to the lights for long periods of time; that they will hold the baby for only short periods for feedings, comforting, and cleansing of the perineal area; and that the room temperature will be regulated to minimize heat loss. Fiber-optic phototherapy blankets eliminate the need for eye patches, decrease heat loss because the baby is clothed, and provide more opportunities for interaction between the baby and parents (Figure 27–11). The best method of home phototherapy depends on the cause of the hyperbilirubinemia and the rate of progression

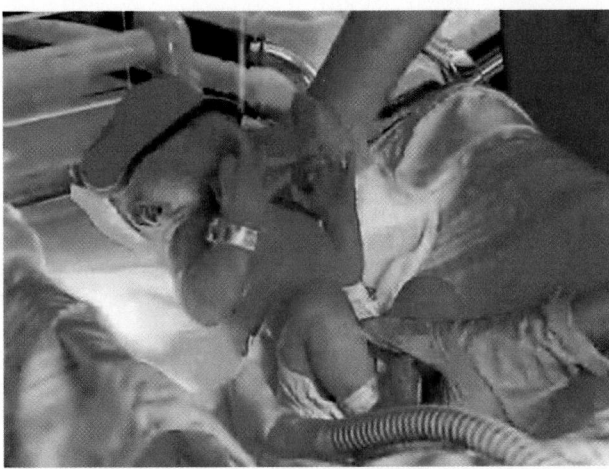

Figure 27–11 Newborn on fiberoptic "bili" mattress and under phototherapy lights. A combination of fiberoptic light source mattress and standard phototherapy light source above may also be used. *Note:* The color is distorted because of the reflection of the bili light mattress.

of the jaundice. Ongoing monitoring of bilirubin levels is essential with home phototherapy and can be carried out in the home, in the follow-up clinic, or in the clinician's office.

Clinical Reasoning Suspected Hyperbilirubinemia

Baby boy Martin is a term newborn born by vaginal delivery with vacuum assist. His mother has blood type O positive, and baby Martin has blood type A positive. The baby has a normal complete blood count (CBC) with a hematocrit of 60%. While performing a physical examination on baby Martin on day 2 of life, the nurse notes that he has a large cephalohematoma, an enlarged liver on palpation (hepatomegaly), and is clinically jaundiced. The nurse suspects that baby Martin has hyperbilirubinemia and discusses her findings with the healthcare provider, who orders a total bilirubin level be drawn. The results show a level of 16 mg/dL at 39 hours of age. The decision is made to start this baby on phototherapy treatment.

What risk factors and clinical findings does this baby have that predispose him to hyperbilirubinemia? How would the nurse explain baby Martin's hyperbilirubinemia and subsequent treatment and nursing care to his mother?

Evaluation

Expected outcomes of nursing care include the following:

- The newborn at risk for development of hyperbilirubinemia is identified, and action is taken to minimize the potential impact of hyperbilirubinemia.

- The baby does not have any corneal irritation or drainage, skin breakdown, or major fluctuations in temperature.

- Parents understand the rationale for, goal of, and expected outcome of therapy.

- Parents verbalize concerns about their baby's condition and identify how they can facilitate their baby's improvement.

Care of the Newborn With Anemia

Neonatal anemia is often difficult to recognize by clinical evaluation alone. The hemoglobin concentration in greater than 34 weeks gestational age and full-term newborns is 14 to 20 g/dL (Gomella, 2013). Newborns with central hemoglobin values of less than 11 mg/dL (term) and 7 to 9 g/dL (preterm), at their lowest point at 8 to 12 weeks of age for term-born babies, and 4 to 8 weeks of age for preterm babies, are usually considered anemic (Arcara & Tschudy, 2012; Gomella, 2013).

Blood loss (hypovolemia) can also occur in utero from placental bleeding (placenta previa or abruptio placentae). Intrapartum blood loss may be fetomaternal, fetofetal, or the result of umbilical cord bleeding. Birth trauma to abdominal organs (adrenal hemorrhage) or the cranium (subgaleal bleed) may produce significant blood loss, and cerebral bleeding may occur because of hypoxia, hypercapnia, and reperfusion injury (Gomella, 2013).

Excessive hemolysis of red blood cells is usually a result of blood group incompatibilities but may be caused by infections. The most common cause of impaired RBC production is a genetically transmitted deficiency in glucose-6-phosphate dehydrogenase (G-6-PD). Anemia and jaundice are the presenting signs (Gomella, 2013).

A condition known as **physiologic anemia of infancy** exists as a result of the normal gradual drop in hemoglobin; theoretically, the bone marrow stops production of RBCs in response to higher oxygen levels resulting from initiation of breathing, reaching the lowest point, or nadir, by 2 to 3 months of age for term-born and 3 to 6 or 4 to 8 weeks of age for preterm-born babies. At that point, the bone marrow begins production of RBCs again, and the anemia disappears (Arcara & Tschudy, 2012; Taylor & Kennedy, 2013).

The preterm baby's hemoglobin reaches a nadir sooner than does a term newborn's because a preterm baby's red blood cell survival time is shorter than that of a term newborn. This difference is a result of several factors: the preterm baby's rapid growth rate, decreased iron stores, and an inadequate production of erythropoietin (EPO). Iatrogenic causes occur more in preterm babies as their condition requires more laboratory assessment (Taylor & Kennedy, 2013).

Clinical Therapy

Hematologic problems can be anticipated based on the pregnancy history and clinical manifestations. The age at which anemia is first noted is also of diagnostic value. Clinically, light-skinned anemic babies are very pale in the absence of other symptoms of shock and usually have abnormally low red blood cell counts. In acute blood loss, symptoms of shock such as pallor, low arterial blood pressure, and a decreasing hematocrit value may be present.

The initial laboratory workup should include determination of the following:

- Hemoglobin and hematocrit measurements
- Reticulocyte count
- Examination of peripheral blood smear
- Direct Coombs test of newborn's blood
- Examination of maternal blood smear for fetal erythrocytes (Kleihauer-Betke test)
- Bilirubin levels (in hemolytic disease)

Mild or chronic anemia in a baby may be treated adequately with iron supplements alone or with iron-fortified formulas. Folate and vitamin E may have to be supplemented depending on the type of formula ingested (Bagwell, 2014a). In severe cases of anemia, transfusions with O-negative or typed and cross-matched packed red cells are the preferred method of treatment.

Management of anemia of prematurity includes treating the causative factor (e.g., antibiotics/antivirals used for infection, steroid therapy for disorders of erythrocyte production) and supplemental iron. Blood transfusions (dedicated units of blood) are kept to a minimum.

Use of recombinant human erythropoietin (rEPO) in preterm neonates can be beneficial in decreasing blood transfusions by stimulating the baby's own red blood cell production (Gomella, 2013; Ohls, Roohi, Peceny, et al., 2012).

Nursing Management

Assess the newborn for symptoms of anemia (pallor). If the blood loss is acute, the baby may exhibit the following signs of shock:

- Capillary filling time greater than 3 seconds
- Decreased pulses
- Tachycardia
- Low blood pressure

Signs of compromise include the following:

- Poor weight gain
- Tachycardia
- Tachypnea
- Apneic episodes

The baby should be placed on constant cardiac and respiratory monitoring. Promptly report any symptoms indicating anemia or shock. Continued observations will be necessary to identify physiologic anemia as the preterm newborn grows. Try to prevent iron deficiency by limiting phlebotomy losses and recording it in tenths of a milliliter. The total blood removed is assessed and replaced by transfusion when necessary or by starting iron therapy at 2 weeks postnatal age. For long-term management, see section on *Normocytic Anemia* in Chapter 49.

Care of the Newborn With Infection

Newborns up to 1 month of age are particularly susceptible to infection, referred to as **sepsis neonatorum**, caused by organisms that do not typically cause significant disease in older children. Once any infection occurs in the newborn, it can spread rapidly through the bloodstream, regardless of its primary site. The incidence of *early-onset neonatal sepsis (EONS)* is 2.2 per 1000 live births (Gomella, 2013). EONS, seen in the first 7 days of life, is caused primarily by vertical transmission of maternal organisms, commonly group B streptococcus (Polin & the Committee on the Fetus and Newborn, 2012). *Escherichia coli* was found to be the most commonly causative agent; however, there is no standard prophylactic treatment (Bondi et al., 2013; Johnson, 2012). Late-onset sepsis occurs between the second week and third month of age.

Nosocomial infections are infections acquired while a baby is in the neonatal intensive care unit (NICU) that usually are caused by organisms introduced during procedures or on equipment required to save the life of the neonate (Polin, Denson, Brady, et al., 2012). Methicillin-resistant *Staphylococcus aureus* (MRSA) and *Candida*, which cause 10% of late-onset

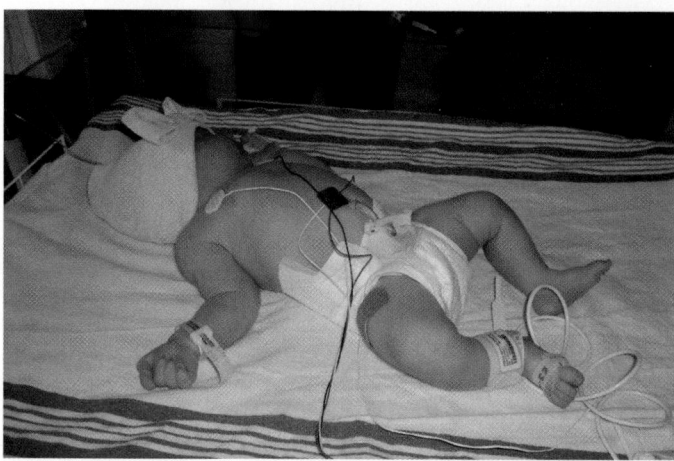

Figure 27–12 **Term newborn with suspected sepsis.**

SOURCE: Valentina Mescolotto.

sepsis, are two of the most common pathogens causing hospital-acquired infections in the NICU population (Johnson, 2012). The general debilitation and underlying illness often associated with prematurity necessitate invasive procedures such as umbilical catheterization, intubation, resuscitation, ventilatory support, monitoring, parenteral alimentation (especially lipid emulsions), and prior broad-spectrum antibiotic therapy.

However, even full-term newborns are susceptible because their immunologic systems are immature. Their immune systems lack the complex factors involved in effective phagocytosis and the ability to localize infection or to respond with a well-defined, recognizable inflammatory response. In addition, all newborns lack IgM immunoglobin, which is necessary to protect against bacteria, because it does not cross the placenta (refer to Chapter 23 for immunologic adaptations in the newborn period). Figure 27–12 shows a term newborn with suspected sepsis.

Healthy People 2020

(HAI-1) Reduce central line–associated bloodstream infections (CLABSI)

(HAI-2) Reduce invasive healthcare-associated methicillin-resistant *Staphylococcus aureus* (MRSA) infections

Most nosocomial infections in the NICU present as bacteremia/sepsis, urinary tract infections, meningitis, or pneumonia. Maternal antepartum infections such as rubella, toxoplasmosis, cytomegalic inclusion disease, and herpes may cause congenital infections and resulting disorders in the newborn. Intrapartum maternal infections, such as amnionitis, are sources of neonatal infection (see Chapter 15 for more detailed information). Passage through the birth canal and contact with the vaginal flora (β-hemolytic streptococci, herpes, *Listeria*, gonococci) expose the baby to infection (Table 27–3). With infection anywhere in the fetus or newborn, the adjacent tissues or organs are easily penetrated, and the blood–brain barrier is ineffective. Septicemia is more common in males, except for infections caused by group B β-hemolytic streptococcus.

Gram-negative organisms (especially *E. coli, Enterobacter cloacae, Serratia marcescens, Pseudomonas aeruginosa,* and *Klebsiella pneumoniae*) account for 15% to 20% of late-onset sepsis, and the gram-positive organism β-hemolytic streptococcus is the most common causative agent. *Pseudomonas* is a common contaminant of ventilatory support and oxygen therapy equipment.

TABLE 27–3 Maternally Transmitted Newborn Infections

INFECTION	NURSING ASSESSMENT	NURSING PLAN AND IMPLEMENTATION
GROUP B STREPTOCOCCUS		
1%–2% colonized, with 1 in 10 developing disease. Early onset—usually within hours of birth or within first week. Late onset—1 week to 3 months.	Severe respiratory distress (grunting and cyanosis). May become apneic or demonstrate symptoms of shock. Meconium-stained amniotic fluid seen at birth.	Early assessment of clinical signs necessary. Assist with x-ray examination—shows aspiration pneumonia or respiratory distress syndrome. Immediately obtain blood, gastric aspirate, external ear canal, and nasopharynx cultures. Administer antibiotics, usually aqueous penicillin or ampicillin combined with gentamicin, as soon as cultures are obtained. Early assessment and intervention are essential to survival.
CONGENITAL SYPHILIS		
Spirochetes cross placenta after 16th–18th week of gestation. The more recent the maternal infection, the greater the likelihood of transmission. Most are asymptomatic at birth but develop symptoms within first 3 months of life.	Check perinatal history for positive maternal serology. Assess baby for: Elevated cord serum IgM and FTA-ABS (fluorescent treponemal antibody absorbed) IgM Rhinitis (snuffles) Fissures on mouth corners and excoriated upper lip Red rash around mouth and anus Copper-colored rash over face, palms, and soles Irritability, generalized edema, particularly over joints; bone lesions; painful extremities, hepatosplenomegaly, jaundice, congenital cataracts, small for gestational age (SGA), and failure to thrive	Refer to evaluate for blindness, deafness, learning or behavioral problems. Initiate standard precautions until baby has been on antibiotics for at least 24 hr. Administer penicillin. Provide emotional support for parents because of their feelings about mode of transmission and potential long-term sequelae.
GONORRHEA		
Approximately 30%–35% of newborns born vaginally to infected mothers acquire the infection.	Assess for: Ophthalmia neonatorum (conjunctivitis) Purulent discharge and corneal ulcerations Neonatal sepsis with temperature instability, poor feeding response, and/or hypotonia, jaundice	Administer ophthalmic antibiotic ointment or penicillin. If positive maternal test, single-dose systemic antibiotic therapy (AAP & ACOG, 2012). Make a follow-up referral to evaluate any loss of vision.
HERPES TYPE 2		
Usually transmitted during vaginal birth; a few cases of in utero transmission have been reported.	Check perinatal history for active herpes genital lesions. Small cluster vesicular skin lesions over all the body about 6 to 9 days of life. Disseminated form—disseminated intravascular coagulation (DIC), pneumonia, hepatitis with jaundice, hepatosplenomegaly, and neurologic abnormalities. Without skin lesions, assess for fever or subnormal temperature, respiratory congestion, tachypnea, and tachycardia.	Carry out careful hand washing and contact precautions (gown and glove isolation with linen precautions) (AAP & ACOG, 2012). Obtain throat, conjunctiva, cerebral spinal fluid (CSF), blood, urine, rectal, and lesion cultures to identify herpes virus type 2 antibodies in serum IgM fraction. Cultures positive in 24–48 hr. Administer intravenous acyclovir (Zovirax). Make a follow-up referral to evaluate potential sequelae of microcephaly, spasticity, seizures, deafness, or blindness. Encourage parental rooming-in and touching of the newborn. Show parents appropriate hand hygiene procedures and precautions to be used at home if mother's lesions are active.
CYTOMEGALOVIRUS (CMV)		
Most common cause of congenital infection in the United States—approximately 1% of all newborns (AAP & ACOG, 2012). Transmission occurs in utero or during labor, or may happen postnatally through breast milk.	Congenital CMV disease, including intrauterine growth restriction, jaundice, hepatosplenomegaly, petechiae or purpura (blueberry muffin spots), thrombocytopenia, and pneumonia. Central nervous system (CNS) manifestations are very common and include lethargy and poor feeding, hypertonia or hypotonia, microcephaly, intracranial calcifications, chorioretinitis, and sensorineural deafness.	Diagnosis of congenital CMV infection is established by isolating virus from urine, saliva, or tissue obtained during the first 3 weeks of life. All babies in whom the diagnosis is suspected should have a viral culture performed; a CT scan of the brain is particularly important to document the extent of CNS involvement; eye exam and hearing test; close long-term follow-up evaluating for developmental effects.

(continued)

TABLE 27–3 Maternally Transmitted Newborn Infections (*continued*)

INFECTION	NURSING ASSESSMENT	NURSING PLAN AND IMPLEMENTATION
ORAL CANDIDAL INFECTION (THRUSH)		
Acquired during passage through birth canal.	Assess newborn's buccal mucosa, tongue, gums, and inside the cheeks for white plaques (seen at 5–7 days of age). Check diaper area for bright-red, well-demarcated eruptions. Assess for thrush periodically when newborn is on long-term antibiotic therapy.	Differentiate white plaque areas from milk curds by using cotton tip applicator (if it is thrush, removal of white areas causes raw, bleeding areas). Maintain cleanliness of hands, linen, clothing, diapers, and feeding apparatus. Instruct breastfeeding mothers on treating their nipples with nystatin. Administer nystatin swabbed on oral lesions 1 hr after feeding or nystatin instilled in baby's oral cavity and on mucosa. Swab skin lesions with topical nystatin.
CHLAMYDIA TRACHOMATIS		
Acquired during passage through birth canal.	Assess for perinatal history of preterm birth. Symptomatic newborns present with pneumonia. Chlamydial conjunctivitis presents with inflammation, yellow discharge, and eyelid swelling 5–14 days after birth. Assess for chronic follicular conjunctivitis (corneal neovascularization and conjunctival scarring).	Instillation of prophylactic ophthalmic erythromycin is controversial (AAP & ACOG, 2012). Treat chlamydial conjunctivitis or pneumonia with oral erythromycin for 14 days. Monitor for hypertrophic pyloric stenosis. Initiate follow-up referral for eye complications and late development of pneumonia at 4–11 weeks postnatally.

Gram-positive bacteria, especially coagulase-negative (CoNS) *Staphylococcus epidermidis* and *Staphylococcus aureus*, which combined cause 60% to 70% of infections, are common pathogens in nosocomial bacteremias, pneumonias, and urinary tract infections (Gomella, 2013; Johnson, 2012).

Protection of the newborn from infections starts prenatally and continues throughout pregnancy and birth. Prenatal prevention should include maternal screening for sexually transmitted infection and monitoring of rubella titers in women who test negative. Intrapartumly, sterile technique is essential. Viral cultures are the definitive tests but take time to get results. Visual examination of the lesions is often reported on the labor and birth record to identify a woman with herpes. Placenta and amniotic fluid cultures are obtained if amnionitis is suspected. Local eye treatment with an antibiotic ophthalmic ointment is given to all newborns to prevent damage from gonococcal (occurring 3 days following birth) and possibly chlamydial (occurring 7 to 10 days after birth) infections. Prophylactic antibiotic therapy for asymptomatic women who test positive for group B streptococcus (GBS) during the intrapartum period helps prevent EOS. There has been a decrease in clinical neonatal sepsis rates because of the use of prenatal prophylactic antibiotic therapy (Lukacs & Schrag, 2012; Smith & Carley, 2014).

Clinical Therapy

Newborns with a history of possible exposure to infection in utero (e.g., premature rupture of membranes [PROM] more than 24 hours before birth or questionable maternal history of infection, maternal fever, chorioamnionitis, or high-risk behavior [such as multiple sexual partners or illicit drug use]) should have cultures taken as soon after birth as possible. Cultures are obtained before antibiotic therapy is begun (Bennett, 2013; Polin & Committee on the Fetus and Newborn, 2012).

1. Anaerobic and aerobic blood culture is taken from a peripheral site rather than an umbilical vessel because catheters have yielded false-positive results because of contamination. The skin is prepared by cleaning with a unit-specified antiseptic solution and allowed to dry; the specimen is obtained with a sterile needle/syringe. Correct sterile technique will lessen the likelihood of contamination.

Health Promotion **Preventing Newborn Infections**
The following measures will help to prevent newborn infections.

During the prenatal period:

- Conduct maternal screening for sexually transmitted infections.
- Monitor rubella titers in women who test negative.

During the intrapartum period:

- Sterile technique is essential.
- Visual exam of any lesions should be reported on the labor and birth record to identify a woman with herpes.
- Placenta and amniotic fluid cultures are obtained if amnionitis is suspected.
- Prenatal prophylactic antibiotic therapy for asymptomatic women who test positive for GBS helps prevent early-onset sepsis and has shown a decrease in clinical neonatal sepsis rates (Lukacs & Schrag, 2012; Smith & Carley, 2014).

During the postpartum period:

- Local eye treatment with an antibiotic ophthalmic ointment is given to all newborns to prevent damage from gonococcal infections (occurring 3 days following birth) and the possibility of chlamydial infection (occurring 7 to 10 days after birth).

2. Spinal fluid culture is done following a spinal tap/lumbar puncture if there are concerns about central nervous system (CNS) symptoms/pathology. The fluid can be analyzed for culture and Gram stain as well as for viral presence.

3. The specimen for urine culture is best obtained by a suprapubic bladder aspiration or sterile catheterization (Gomella, 2013).

4. Skin cultures are taken of any lesions or drainage from lesions or reddened areas.

5. Tracheal aspirate cultures, if intubated, may be obtained.

Other laboratory investigations include a complete blood count, C-reactive protein (CRP), procalcitonin (PCT), chest x-ray examination, serology, and gram stains of cerebrospinal fluid, urine, skin exudate, and umbilicus. White blood cell (WBC) count with differential may indicate the presence or absence of sepsis. A level of 30,000 to 40,000 mm³ WBC may be normal in the first 24 hours of life, whereas low WBC (less than 5000 to 7500/mm³) may be indicative of sepsis. A low neutrophil count and high band (immature white cells) count indicate that an infection is present. Stomach aspirate should be sent for culture and smear if a gonococcal infection or amnionitis is suspected. CRP, an acute-phase reactant protein synthesized in response to inflammation, may or may not be elevated initially. Other inflammatory responses may cause an elevation in the CRP, so it should not be used as the only indicator of infection (Smith & Carley, 2014). The CRP may be helpful in watching for improvement once antibiotic therapy is initiated. PCT is most diagnostic in late-onset septicemia (LOS) as it rises in the first 48 hours (Bennett, 2013; Gomella, 2013).

Serum IgM levels are elevated (normal level less than 20 mg/dL) in response to transplacental infections (Blackburn, 2013). If available, counterimmunoelectrophoresis tests for specific bacterial antigens are performed. In the future repetitive sequence-based polymerase chain reactions (rep-PCRs) will be used to identify specific infectious organisms within hours instead of days (Cloherty et al., 2012). Evidence of congenital infections may be seen on skull x-ray films for cerebral calcifications (cytomegalovirus, toxoplasmosis), on bone x-ray films (syphilis, cytomegalovirus), and in serum-specific IgM levels (rubella). Cytomegalovirus infection is best diagnosed by urine culture.

Because neonatal infection causes high mortality, therapy is instituted before results of the septic workup are obtained. A combination of two broad-spectrum antibiotics, such as ampicillin and gentamicin, is given in large doses but only until a culture with sensitivities is obtained.

After the pathogen and its sensitivities are determined, appropriate specific antibiotic therapy is begun. Rotating aminoglycosides has been suggested to prevent development of resistance. Use of cephalosporins and, in particular, cefotaxime has emerged as an alternative to aminoglycoside therapy in the treatment of neonatal infections for infants 1 to 3 months of age (Bennett, 2013). For newborns under 1 month of age, third-generation cephalosporins are not currently recommended as single-agent therapy (Bennett, 2013).

Duration of therapy varies from 7 to 14 days (Table 27–4). If cultures are negative and symptoms subside, antibiotics may be

TABLE 27–4 Neonatal Sepsis Antibiotic/Antiviral Therapy

DRUG	DOSE (MG/KG) TOTAL DAILY DOSE	SCHEDULE FOR DIVIDED DOSES	ROUTE	COMMENTS
Acyclovir (Zovirax)	20 mg/kg	q 8 hr	IV	Length of treatment is 14 days for skin/eye/mouth (SEM) or 21 days for CNS and disseminated disease: herpes.
Ampicillin	50 to 100 mg/kg	q 12 hr* q 8 hr† q 6 hr**	IM or IV	Effective against gram-positive microorganisms, *Listeria*, and most *Escherichia coli* strains. Higher doses indicated for meningitis. Used with aminoglycoside for synergy.
Cefotaxime (Claforan)	50 mg/kg/dose 100–150 mg/kg/day	q 12 hr* q 8 hr q 6 hr**	IM or IV	Active against most major pathogens in babies; effective against aminoglycoside-resistant organisms; achieves cerebrospinal fluid (CSF) bactericidal activity; lack of ototoxicity and nephrotoxicity; wide therapeutic index (levels not required); resistant organisms can develop rapidly if used extensively; ineffective against *Pseudomonas*, *Listeria*.
Gentamicin	2.5–3 mg/kg 5–7.5 mg/kg/day 4–5 mg/kg/dose (first week of life)	q 24–48 hr‡ ***	IM or IV	Effective against gram-negative rods and staphylococci; may be used instead of kanamycin against penicillin-resistant staphylococci and *E. coli* strains and *Pseudomonas aeruginosa*. May cause neurotoxicity, ototoxicity, and nephrotoxicity. Need to follow serum levels. Must never be given as IV push. Must be given over at least 30–60 min. In presence of oliguria or anuria, dose must be decreased or discontinued. In babies less than 1000 g or 29 weeks, lower dosage 2.5–3 mg/kg/day. Monitor serum levels before administration of second dose.
	4–5 mg/kg/dose (first week of life)	q 24–48 hr		Peak 5–12 mcg/mL Trough 0.5–1 mcg/mL
Vancomycin	10–20 mg/kg 30 mg/kg/day	q 12–24 hr*‡ q 8 hr†	IV	Effective for methicillin-resistant strains (*Staphylococcus epidermidis*); must be administered by slow intravenous infusion to avoid prolonged cutaneous eruption. For smaller newborns, less than 1200 g (2.6 lb), less than 29 weeks, smaller dosages and longer intervals between doses. Nephrotoxic, especially in combination with aminoglycosides. Slow IV infusion over at least 60 min. Peak 25–40 mcg/mL Trough 5–10 mcg/mL

*Up to 7 days of age.

** ≥45 weeks postmenstrual age.

†Greater than 7 days of age.

‡Dependent on gestational age.

***Dependent on postnatal age.

discontinued after 2 days/48 hours of negative blood cultures. A normal CRP at 48 hours also supports discontinuing antibiotics if blood cultures are negative. Supportive physiologic care may be required to maintain respiratory, hemodynamic, nutritional, and metabolic homeostasis.

Nursing Management
For the Newborn With Infection

Nursing Assessment and Diagnosis

Symptoms of infection are most often noticed by the nurse during daily care of the newborn. The baby may deteriorate rapidly in the first 12 to 24 hours after birth if β-hemolytic streptococcal infection is present, with signs and symptoms mimicking RDS. In other cases, the onset of sepsis may be gradual, with more subtle signs and symptoms. The most common signs that may be observed include the following:

- Subtle behavioral changes—the newborn "isn't doing well," the mother states. "Something isn't right with my baby." The baby is often lethargic or irritable (especially after the first 24 hours), hypotonic, and hypotensive. Color changes may include pallor, duskiness, cyanosis, or a "shocky" appearance. The skin may be cool and clammy.
- Temperature instability, manifested most commonly by hypothermia (recognized by a decrease in skin temperature) or, rarely in newborns, hyperthermia (elevation of skin temperature), necessitates a corresponding increase or decrease in incubator temperature to maintain a neutral thermal environment.
- Feeding intolerance is evidenced by a decrease in total intake, an increase in residuals if nasogastric (NG) tube feeding is used, abdominal distention, vomiting, poor sucking, lack of interest in feeding, and diarrhea.
- Hyperbilirubinemia, petechial hemorrhages, hepatosplenomegaly.
- Tachycardia initially, followed by spells of apnea/bradycardia.

Signs and symptoms may suggest CNS disease (jitteriness, tremors, seizure activity). A differential diagnosis is necessary because of the similarity of symptoms to other more specific conditions.

Nursing diagnoses that may apply to the newborn with sepsis neonatorum and the family include the following (NANDA-I © 2014):

- *Infection, Risk for,* related to newborn's immature immunologic system
- *Fluid Volume: Deficient,* related to feeding intolerance
- *Coping: Family, Compromised,* related to present illness resulting in prolonged hospital stay for the newborn

Planning and Implementation

In the nursery, environmental control and prevention of acquired infection are the responsibilities of the neonatal nurse. An infected newborn can be isolated effectively in an isolette and receive close observation. It is important to promote strict hand washing technique for all who enter the nursery, including nursing colleagues; healthcare providers; laboratory, x-ray, and respiratory therapists; and parents. Visits by unnecessary personnel should be discouraged. Be prepared to assist in the aseptic collection of specimens for laboratory investigations. Scrupulous care of equipment—changing and cleaning of incubators at least every 3 to 7 days, removing and sterilizing wet equipment every 24 hours, preventing cross use of linen and equipment, cleaning sinkside equipment such as soap containers periodically, and taking special care with the open radiant warmers (access without prior hand washing is much more likely than with the closed incubator)—will prevent contamination.

PROVISION OF ANTIBIOTIC THERAPY
Administer antibiotics as ordered by the nurse practitioner or healthcare provider. It is your responsibility to be knowledgeable about the following:

- The proper dose to be administered, based on the weight of the newborn and desired peak and trough levels
- The appropriate route of administration, because some antibiotics cannot be given intravenously
- Admixture incompatibilities, because some antibiotics are precipitated by intravenous solutions or by other antibiotics
- Side effects and toxicity

For term newborns being treated for infections, neonatal home infusion of antibiotics should be considered as a viable alternative to continued hospitalization. The infusion of antibiotics at home by skilled RNs facilitates parent–newborn bonding while meeting the baby's ongoing healthcare needs.

PROVISION OF SUPPORTIVE CARE
In addition to antibiotic therapy, physiologic supportive care is essential in caring for a septic newborn. The following care measures should be carried out:

- Observe for resolution of symptoms or development of other symptoms of sepsis.
- Maintain neutral thermal environment with accurate regulation of humidity and oxygen administration.
- Provide respiratory support: administer oxygen, use pulse oximetry, observe and monitor respiratory effort.
- Provide cardiovascular support: observe and monitor pulse and blood pressure; observe for hyperbilirubinemia, anemia, and hemorrhagic symptoms.
- Provide adequate calories, because oral feedings may be discontinued due to increased mucus, abdominal distention, vomiting, and aspiration.
- Provide fluids and electrolytes to maintain homeostasis; monitor weight changes, urine output, and urine specific gravity.
- Observe for the development of hypoglycemia, hyperglycemia, acidosis, hyponatremia, and hypocalcemia.

Restricting parental visits has not been shown to have any effect on the rate of infection and may be harmful for the newborn's psychologic development. With instruction and guidance, both parents should be allowed to handle the baby and participate in daily care. Support of the parents is crucial. They need to be informed of the newborn's prognosis as treatment continues and to be involved in care as much as possible. They also need to understand how infection is transmitted.

Evaluation

Expected outcomes of nursing care include the following:

- The risks for development of sepsis are identified early, and immediate action is taken to minimize the development of the illness.

- Appropriate use of aseptic technique protects the newborn from further exposure to illness.
- The baby's symptoms are relieved, and the infection is treated.
- The parents verbalize concerns about their baby's illness and understand the rationale behind the management of their newborn.

Care of the Family With Birth of an At-Risk Newborn

The birth of a preterm or ill baby or a newborn with a congenital anomaly is a serious crisis for a family (Sweet & Mannix, 2012). Throughout the pregnancy, both parents, together and separately, have felt excitement, experienced thoughts of acceptance, and pictured what their baby would look like. Both parents have wished for a perfect baby and feared an unhealthy one. Each parent and family member must accept and adjust when the fantasized fears become reality (Zimmerman & Bauersachs, 2012).

Parental Responses

Family members have acute grief reactions to the loss of the idealized baby they have envisioned. In a preterm birth, the mother is denied the last few weeks of pregnancy that seem to prepare her psychologically for the stress of birth and the attachment process. Attachment at this time is fragile, and interruption of the process by separation can affect the future mother–child relationship (Discenza, 2012b; Sweet & Mannix, 2012). Parents express grief as shock and disbelief, denial of reality, anger toward self and others, guilt, blame, and concern for the future. Self-esteem and feelings of self-worth are jeopardized (Walker, 2013).

Feelings of guilt and failure often plague mothers of preterm newborns. Guilt fantasies may lead her to wonder what she might have done to cause the early labor. She might ask herself questions such as, "Why did labor start?" "What did I do (or not do)?" "Was it because I had sexual intercourse with my husband (a week, 3 days, a day) ago?" "Was it because I carried three loads of laundry up from the basement?" "Am I being punished for something done in the past—even in childhood?"

The period of waiting between suspicion and confirmation of abnormality or dysfunction is a very anxious one for parents because it is difficult, if not impossible, to begin attachment to the baby if the newborn's future is questionable. During the waiting period, parents need support and acknowledgment that this is an anxious time. They must be kept informed about tests and efforts to gather additional data, as well as efforts to improve their baby's outcome (Sweet & Mannix, 2012). It is helpful to tell both parents about the problem at the same time, with the baby present. An honest discussion of the problem and anticipatory management at the earliest possible time by health professionals help the parents (1) maintain trust in the healthcare provider and nurse, (2) appreciate the reality of the situation by dispelling fantasy and misconception, (3) begin the grieving process, and (4) mobilize internal and external support.

Nurses need to be aware that anger is a universal response by parents to a preterm birth. It is best that the parents direct it outward because holding it in check requires great energy, which is then diverted away from grieving and physical recovery from pregnancy and giving birth. Anger may be directed at the healthcare provider and/or nurse, at the food, at nursing care, or at hospital regulations and routines (Discenza, 2012b). Parents rarely show anger with the baby; such responses can precipitate guilt feelings. Perceived maternal stress may be lessened and the mother empowered if information is provided regarding preterm behavioral cues. This empowers the mother and allows her to better care for her child. The mother of a preterm baby who has to spend time in a neonatal intensive care unit (NICU) suffers from psychologic distress similar to posttraumatic stress disorder (PTSD). The nurse working with a mother in the NICU setting has the opportunity to encourage maternal competence and confidence, both during and after hospitalization, by teaching interpretation of her baby's behavioral cues, prompting maternal care of the baby while in the NICU, and facilitating expression of her feelings (for more detailed discussion of PTSD see Chapter 30). The father also may suffer from depression both before and after the birth of the child, adding to the discord in the family unit and compounding the perceived stress experienced by the mother.

Solnit and Stark (1961) postulated that grief and mourning of the loss of the loved object—the idealized child—mark parental reactions to a baby with abnormalities. *Grief work,* the emotional reaction to significant loss, must occur before adequate attachment to the actual baby is possible. Parental detachment precedes parental attachment. The parents must first grieve the loss of the wished-for perfect child, and then must adopt the imperfect child as the new love object.

Some degree of postpartum depression occurs in new mothers up to 15% of the time, and rates can be as high as 32% to 63% in mothers with babies in the NICU. Maternal depression can have a negative impact on attachment with the newborn (Bicking & Moore, 2012). Other members of the family also may suffer from depressive symptoms (Sweet & Mannix, 2012). Although reactions and steps of attachment are altered by the birth of these babies, a healthy parent–child relationship can occur.

Developmental Consequences

The baby who is born prematurely, is ill, or has a malformation or disorder is at risk for emotional, intellectual, and cognitive developmental delays. The risk is directly proportional to the seriousness of the problem and the length of treatment. Necessary physical separation of family and newborn and the tremendous emotional and financial burdens may adversely affect the parent–child relationship. The recent trend to involve the parents with their newborn early, repeatedly, and over protracted periods of time has done much to facilitate positive parent–child relationships (Bicking & Moore, 2012).

Parents must have a clear picture of the reality of the handicap and the types of developmental hurdles ahead. Unexpected behaviors and responses from the baby because of the defect or disorder can be upsetting and frightening. The demands of care for the child and disputes regarding management of behavior stress family relationships. The entire interprofessional healthcare team may need to pool their resources and expertise to help parents of children born with problems or disorders so that both parents and children can thrive. Involving the parents in rounds can be a valuable tool to enhance their feelings of inclusion in the care and decision-making process of their NICU baby (Graci, 2013).

Nursing Management
For the Family of an At-Risk Newborn

Nursing Assessment and Diagnosis

A concurrent illness of the mother or other family members or other concurrent stress (lack of health insurance, loss of job, age of parents) may change the family response to the baby. Feelings of apprehension, guilt, failure, and grief that are verbally or nonverbally expressed are important aspects of the nursing history. These observations enable all professionals to be aware of the parental state, coping behaviors, and readiness for attachment, bonding, and caretaking. Appropriate nursing assessments during interviewing and relating to the family include the following:

- *Level of understanding.* Observations concerning the family's ability to assimilate information given and to ask appropriate questions; the need for constant repetition of information.
- *Behavioral responses.* Appropriateness of behavior in relation to information given; lack of response; flat affect.
- *Difficulties with communication.* Deafness (reads lips only); blindness; dysphasia; understanding only a non-English language.
- *Paternal and maternal education level.* Parents who are unable to read or write; parents with eighth-grade–level education; parents with a graduate-level degree or healthcare background.

Documentation of such information, gathered through continuing contact and development of a therapeutic family relationship, allows all professionals to understand and use the nursing history to provide continuous individualized care.

A record of visits, caretaking procedures, affect (in relating to the newborn), and telephone calls indicates the level or lack of parental attachment. Serial observations, rather than just isolated observations that cause concern, must be obtained. Grant (1978) developed a conceptual framework depicting adaptive and maladaptive responses to parenting of a preterm or less-than-perfect baby (Table 27–5).

If a pattern of distancing behaviors evolves, institute appropriate intervention. Follow-up studies have found that a statistically significant number of preterm, sick, and congenitally defective babies suffer from failure to thrive, battering, or other disorders of parenting. Early detection and intervention may prevent these aberrations in parenting behaviors from leading to irreparable damage or death.

Nursing diagnoses that may apply to the family of a newborn at risk include the following (NANDA-I © 2014):

- *Grieving, Complicated,* related to loss of idealized newborn
- *Fear* related to emotional involvement with an at-risk newborn
- *Parenting, Impaired,* related to impaired bonding secondary to feelings of inadequacy about caretaking activities

TABLE 27–5 Adaptive and Nonadaptive Parental Responses to a Newborn's Health Crisis

Parental tasks at this time include the following:

- Understanding the newborn's medical condition and needs
- Adapting to the NICU environment
- Assuming the main caretaking role
- Taking responsibility for the baby after discharge
- Coping with the death of the baby

ADAPTIVE RESPONSES	NONADAPTIVE RESPONSES
• Frequent visits to baby and calls to the unit	• Failure to visit baby or communicate with unit
• Emotional involvement with baby	• Emotional withdrawal from baby
• Positive interaction with baby during hospitalization	• Lack of interaction with baby during hospitalization
• Eagerness to assume caretaking during baby's hospitalization	• Resistance to providing care of the baby during hospitalization
• Increasing sense of parental competence	• Lack of a sense of parental competence
• Growing attachment to baby	• Failure to achieve attachment to baby
• Realistic interpretation of medical information	• Inability to understand or accept medical information
• Acceptance of baby's condition	• Unhealthy preoccupation with baby's condition
• Understanding of the causes of baby's condition	• Blaming others for baby's condition
• Eagerness to assume total responsibility for baby	• Fear of going home with baby
• Realistic understanding of baby's needs at discharge	• Negative view of baby and his or her needs at discharge
• Open discussion of concerns and needs to staff and family	• Inability to discuss needs and concerns with staff and family
• Fair and realistic expectations of staff	• Distrustful and hostile attitude toward staff

POSITIVE OUTCOME	NEGATIVE OUTCOME
• Healthy parent–child relationship	• Poor parent–child relationship
• Marital and family equilibrium is maintained	• Failure to thrive
	• Vulnerable child syndrome
	• Marital and family equilibrium is compromised

Source: Data from Grant, P. (1978). *Family & community health.* Philadelphia, PA: Lippincott Williams & Wilkins.

Planning and Implementation

HOSPITAL-BASED NURSING CARE

In their sensitive and vulnerable state, parents are acutely perceptive about others' responses and reactions (particularly nonverbal) to the newborn. Parents can be expected to identify with the responses of others. Therefore, it is imperative that medical and nursing staff be fully aware of the parents' feelings and come to terms with their own feelings so that they are comfortable and at ease with the baby and the grieving family.

Nurses may feel uncomfortable, not knowing what to say to parents, or may fear confronting their own feelings as well as those of the parents. Each nurse must work out personal reactions with instructors, peers, clergy, parents, or significant others. It is helpful to have a stockpile of therapeutic questions and statements to initiate meaningful dialog with parents. Opening statements can be as follows:

"You must be wondering what could have caused this."

"Are you thinking that you (or someone else) may have done something?"

"How can I help?"

"Are you wondering how you are going to manage?"

Avoid statements such as:

"It could have been worse."

"It's God's will."

"You have other children."

"You are still young and can have more."

"I understand how you feel."

Always remember that this baby and this situation are important now.

Support of Parents for Initial Viewing of the Newborn

Before parents see their newborn, prepare them for the visit. It is important to present a positive, realistic attitude regarding the baby. An overly negative, fatalistic attitude further alienates the parents from their newborn and retards attachment behaviors. Instead of beginning to bond with their baby, the parents will anticipate their loss and the process of grieving. Once started, this process is very difficult to reverse.

All babies exhibit strengths as well as deficiencies; prepare the parents to see both the deviations and the normal aspects of their baby. You may say, "Your baby is small, about the length of my two hands. She weighs 2 lb, 3 oz, but is very active and cries when we disturb her. She is having some difficulty breathing, but is breathing without assistance and is in only 35% oxygen and room air is 21%." Many NICUs have booklets for parents to read before entering the units. Through explanations and pictures, the parents are better prepared to deal with the feelings they may experience when they see their newborn for the first time (Figure 27–13). Describe the equipment being used for the at-risk newborn and its purpose before the parents enter the intensive care unit.

Upon entering the unit, parents may be overwhelmed by the sounds of monitors, alarms, and respirators, as well as by the unfamiliar language and "foreign" atmosphere. Preparing the parents by having familiar healthcare providers accompany them to the unit can be reassuring. The primary nurse and healthcare provider caring for the newborn need to be with the parents when they first visit their baby. Parental reactions vary, but initially there is usually an element of shock. Providing chairs and time to regain composure assists

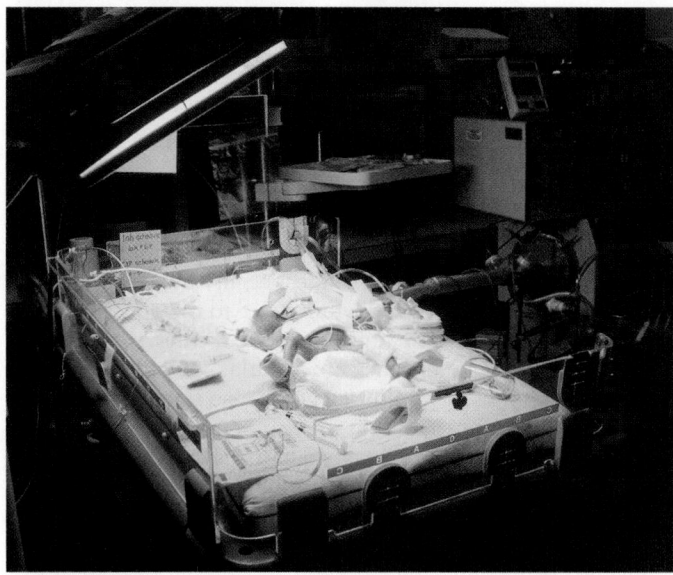

Figure 27–13 **This 25 weeks' gestational age baby with respiratory distress syndrome may be frightening for her parents to see for the first time because of the technology that is attached to her.**

SOURCE: Lisa Smith-Pedersen, RNC, MSN, NNP-BC.

the parents. Slow, complete, and simple explanations—first about the baby and then about the equipment—allay fear and anxiety.

Concern about the baby's physical appearance is common yet may remain unvoiced. Parents may express concerns such as, "He looks so small and red—like a drowned rat." "Why do her genitals look so abnormal?" and "Will that awful-looking mouth [cleft lip and palate] ever be normal?" Anticipate and address such questions. Use of pictures, such as of a baby after cleft lip repair, may be reassuring to doubting parents. Knowledge of the development of a "normal" preterm baby allows you to make reassuring statements such as, "The baby's skin may look very red and transparent with lots of visible veins, but it is normal for her maturity. As she grows, subcutaneous fat will be laid down, and these superficial veins will become less visible."

The nursing staff sets the tone of the NICU. Nurses foster the development of a safe, trusting environment by viewing the parents as essential caregivers, not as visitors or nuisances in the unit. It is important to provide parents privacy when needed and easy access to staff and facilities. An uncrowded and welcoming atmosphere lets parents know "You are welcome here." However, even in crowded physical surroundings, nurses can convey an attitude of openness and trust.

A trusting relationship is essential for collaborative efforts in caring for the baby. Work toward therapeutically using your own responses to relate to the parents on a one-to-one basis. Each individual has different needs, different ways of adapting to crisis, and different means of support. Use techniques that are real and spontaneous to them and avoid words or actions that are foreign to them. Gauge your interventions so that they match the parents' pace and needs.

Implementation of family-centered care, a team approach with healthcare professionals and the family, in which the parents, grandparents, and older siblings are vital members of the team, is important to bonding and the development of the family unit (Chinchilla, 2012). Show concern and support by planning time to spend with the parents, by being psychologically as well as physically present, by encouraging open discussion and grieving, by repetitious explanations (as necessary), by providing privacy as needed, and by encouraging contact with the newborn. Identifying and clarifying feelings and fears decrease distortions in perception, thinking, and feeling. Invest the baby with value in the eyes of the parents by providing meticulous care to the newborn, talk and coo (especially in the face-to-face position) while holding or providing care to the newborn, refer to the baby by gender or name, and relate the newborn's activities ("He took a whole ounce of formula," "She took hold of the blanket and just wouldn't let go"). Also note the "normal" characteristics and capabilities of each newborn as well as the newborn's needs. Learn the baby's name and refer to the baby by name. When the baby is physiologically stable and of an appropriate weight, allowing the baby to be dressed in clothes has been determined to aid the mother in perceiving the baby as a "person" or "actual baby."

Facilitation of Attachment if Neonatal Transport Occurs

Transport to a regional referral center some distance from the parents' community may be necessary. It is essential that the mother see and touch her newborn before the baby is transported. Bringing the mother to the nursery or taking the baby in a warmed transport incubator to the mother's bedside will allow her to see the baby before transportation to the center. When the baby reaches the referral center, a staff member should call the parents with information about the baby's condition during transport, safe arrival at the center, and present condition.

Support of parents, with explanations from the professional staff, is crucial. Occasionally, the mother may be unable to see the newborn before transport, for example, if she is still under general anesthesia or experiencing postpartum complications such as shock, hemorrhage, or seizures. In these cases, take a photograph of the baby to give to the mother and provide an explanation of the baby's condition and problems and a detailed description of the baby's characteristics. An additional photograph is also helpful for the father to share with siblings or the extended family. With the increased attention to improved fetal outcome, prenatal maternal transports, rather than neonatal transports, are occurring more frequently. This practice gives the mother of an at-risk newborn the opportunity to visit and care for her baby during the early postpartum period.

Promotion of Touching and Parental Caretaking

Parents visiting a preterm, small-for-gestational-age (SGA), or sick newborn may need several visits to become comfortable and confident in their ability to touch the baby without injuring her or him. Barriers such as incubators, incisions, monitor electrodes, and tubes may delay the mother's development of comfort in touching the newborn.

Klaus and Kennell (1982) have demonstrated a significant difference in the amount of eye contact and touching behaviors of mothers of normal newborns and mothers of preterm newborns. Whereas mothers of normal newborns progress within minutes to palm contact of the baby's trunk, mothers of preterm babies are slower to progress from fingertip to palm contact and from the extremities to the trunk. The progression to palm contact with the baby's trunk may take several visits to the nursery.

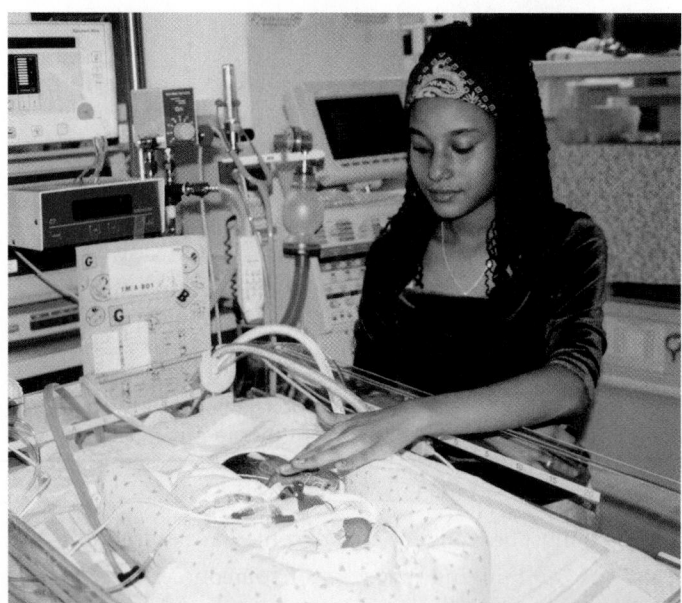

Figure 27–14 Beginnings of attachment. Mother of this 26-week-gestational-age 600-g (1.3-lb) newborn begins attachment through fingertip touch.

SOURCE: Lisa Smith-Pedersen, RNC, MSN, NNP-BC.

Use support, reassurance, and encouragement to help the mother develop positive feelings about her ability and importance to her baby. Touching facilitates "getting to know" the baby and thus establishes a bond with the baby. Touching and seeing the baby help the mother realize the "normals" and potential of her baby (Figure 27–14).

Encourage parents to meet their newborn's need for stimulation. Stroking, rocking, cuddling, singing, and talking should be an integral part of the parents' caretaking responsibilities when tolerated by their baby. Bonding can be facilitated by encouraging parents to visit and become involved in their baby's care (Figure 27–15). Skin-to-skin contact (kangaroo care), usually between the mother, father, or surrogate (another

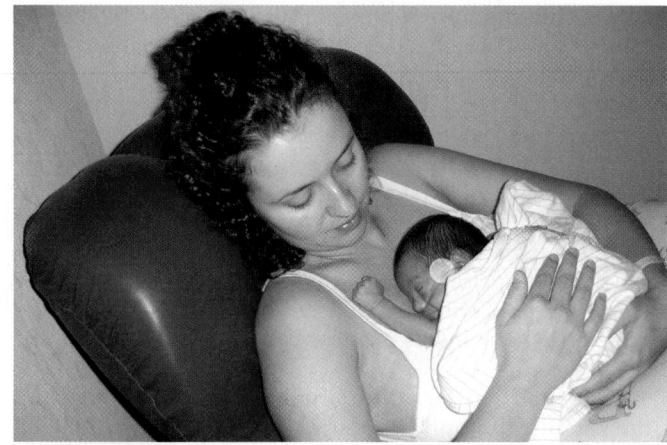

Figure 27–15 Facilitating bonding. This mother of a 31-week-gestational-age newborn with respiratory distress syndrome is spending time with her baby and meeting the baby's need for cuddling.

SOURCE: Lisa Smith-Pedersen, RNC, MSN, NNP-BC.

person instead of the parents) and the neonate, was first introduced over 40 years ago. It is now utilized to enhance bonding and impacts positively in both the behavior and physiology of the newborn (Discenza, 2012a; Ludington-Hoe, 2011). Something as simple as softly reading a book to the baby can help during this time (Walker, 2013). When visiting is impossible, the parents should feel free to phone whenever they wish to receive information about their baby. Showing a warm, receptive attitude provides support. Facilitate parenting by personalizing a baby to the parents, by referring to the baby by name, or relating personal behavioral characteristics. Statements such as, "Jenny loves her pacifier," help make the newborn seem individual and unique.

The variety of equipment needed for life support is hardly conducive to anxiety-free caretaking by the parents. However, even the sickest baby may be cared for, if only in a small way, by the parents. Demonstration and explanation, followed by support of the parents in initial caretaking behaviors, positively reinforce parents' sense of success (Zimmerman & Bauersachs, 2012). Changing their baby's diaper, providing skin or oral care, or helping the nurse turn the baby may at first provoke anxiety, but the parents will become more comfortable and confident in caretaking and feel satisfied by the baby's reactions and their ability "to do something" (Skene, Franck, Curtis, et al., 2012). By complimenting the parents' competence in caretaking, you also increase their self-esteem, which has received recent "blows" of guilt and failure. *Never give the parents a task that they might not be able to accomplish.* Cues that the parents are ready to become involved with the newborn's care include their reference to the baby by name and their questioning as to the amount of feeding taken, sleeping patterns, appearance today, and the like. Simple inclusion of the parents in providing comfort care for their baby is an early step in transferring care from the medical staff to the parents (Skene et al., 2012).

Often parents of high-risk newborns have ambivalent feelings toward the nurse. These feelings may take the form of criticism of the care of the baby, manipulation of staff, or personal guilt. You should accept this behavior, but continue to remind the parents that it is okay and natural to feel disappointment, a sense of failure, helplessness, or anger about the birth. The overprotectiveness and overoptimism are defense mechanisms. To deny the negative feelings only entrenches them further, delays their resolution, and delays realistic planning. Instead of fostering (by silence), you need to intervene appropriately to enhance parent–newborn attachment. Learn to deal with ambivalent feelings that contribute to a competitive atmosphere. For example, avoid making unfavorable comparisons between the baby's responses to parental and nursing caretaking. Verbalizations that improve parental self-esteem are essential and easily shared. You can point out that, in addition to physiologic use, breast milk is important because of the emotional investment of the mother. Pumping, storing, labeling, and delivering quantities of breast milk is a time-consuming "labor of love" for mothers. Positive remarks about breast milk reinforce the maternal behavior of caretaking and providing for her baby: "Breast milk is something that only you can give your baby," "You really have brought a lot of milk today," "Look how rich this breast milk is," or "Even small amounts of milk are important, and look how rich it is."

If the newborn begins to gain weight while being fed breast milk, it is important to point this correlation out to the mother. Advise parents that initial weight loss with beginning nipple feedings is common because of the increased energy expended when the baby begins active rather than passive nutritional intake.

During a quiet time it may help to encourage the parents to talk about their hopes and fears and to facilitate their involvement in parent groups. Encourage parents to provide care for their newborn even if the baby is very sick and likely to die. Detachment is easier after attachment because the parents are comforted by the knowledge that they did all they could for their child while the baby was alive.

Facilitation of Family Adjustment During Crisis

During crisis, it is difficult to maintain interpersonal relationships. Yet in a newborn intensive care area, the parents are expected to relate to many different care providers. It is important that parents have as few professionals as possible relaying information to them. A primary nurse should coordinate care and provide continuity for parents. Care providers are individuals and thus will use different terms, inflections, and attitudes. These subtle differences are monumental to parents and may confuse, confound, and produce anxiety. The transfer of the baby from the NICU to a step-down unit or transport back to the home hospital provokes parental anxiety because they must now deal with new healthcare professionals. The nurse not only functions as a liaison between the parents and the various healthcare professionals interacting with the newborn and parents but also offers clarification, explanation, interpretation of information, and support to the parents (Chinchilla, 2012).

Encourage parents to deal with the crisis with help from their support system. The support system attempts to meet the emotional needs and to provide support for the family members in crisis and stress situations. Biologic kinship is not the only valid criterion for a support system; an emotional kinship is the most important factor. In our mobile society of isolated nuclear families, the support system may be a next-door neighbor, a best friend, or perhaps a schoolmate. Search out the significant others in the lives of the parents and help them understand the problems so that they can be a constant parental support.

The impact of the crisis on the family is individual and varied. To institute appropriate interventions, view the birth of any baby (normal newborn, preterm newborn, baby with congenital anomaly) as defined by the family. It is important to encourage open intrafamily communication. Discourage the family from keeping secrets from one another, especially between spouses/partners, because secrets undermine the trust of relationships. Well-meaning rationales such as, "I want to protect her," "I don't want him to worry about it," and so on can be destructive to open communication and to the basic element of a relationship—trust.

The needs of siblings should not be overlooked. Siblings have been looking forward to the new baby, and they, too, suffer a degree of loss. Young children may react with hostility and older ones with shame at the birth of a baby with an anomaly. Both reactions may make siblings feel guilty. Parents, who may be preoccupied with working through their own feelings, often cannot give the other children the attention and support they need. Sometimes another child becomes the focus of family tension. Anxiety thus directed can take the form of finding fault or of overconcern. This is a form of denial; the parents cannot face the real worry—the baby at risk. After observing and assessing the situation, ensure that another family member or friend steps in to support the siblings of the affected baby.

Parents from minority cultures must deal with language barriers and cultural differences that can make feelings of isolation and uncertainty more acute. Healthcare providers have the professional responsibility to be aware of the cultural needs of all clients and to ensure those needs are met. Feelings of isolation and uncertainty influence not only the parent's emotional responses to the ill newborn, but also their utilization of services and interaction with health professionals. Hospital cultural interpreter programs can assist families with interactions with staff, as well as provide translation during family meetings, collaborative care family conferences, and parent support groups.

Families with children in the NICU may become friends and support one another. To encourage the development of these friendships and to provide support, many units have established parent groups. The core of the groups consists of parents whose babies were once in the intensive care unit. Most groups make contact with families within a day or two of the newborn's admission to the unit, through either phone calls or visits to the hospital. Early one-on-one parent contacts are more effective than discussion groups in helping families work through their feelings. This personalized method gives the grieving parents an opportunity to express personal feelings about the pregnancy, labor, and birth and their "different from expected" baby with others who have experienced the same feelings and with whom they can identify.

COMMUNITY-BASED NURSING CARE

Predischarge planning begins once the newborn's condition becomes stable and it seems likely the newborn will survive. These medically fragile babies remain vulnerable for several years (Holditch-Davis, Miles, Burchinal, et al., 2011). Discharge preparation and care conferences should involve a collaborative care team approach. The NICU nursing staff is the fulcrum for aiding in the transition of high-risk newborns from the intensive care unit to the home. Effective open communication with the families during the entire discharge planning phase of care empowers the families to assume the role of primary caregiver for their children. Adequate predischarge teaching helps parents transform any feelings of inadequacy they may have into feelings of self-assurance and attachment.

SAFETY ALERT!

The high incidence of prematurity and low birth weight (LBW) in multiple-birth babies and the corresponding risks for sudden infant death syndrome (SIDS) should be considered. As with all families at discharge, parents of multiples should be taught SIDS risk-reduction practices, which include supine positioning, babies sleeping in parents' room, firm bedding surface, no loose coverings/items, and no barriers between babies.

Provide home care instructions in an optimal environment for parental learning. Learning should take place over time, to avoid bombarding the parents with instructions in the day or hour before discharge. Parents often enjoy performing minimal caretaking tasks, with gradual expansion of their role. Many NICUs provide facilities for parents to room in with their newborns for a few days before discharge. This allows parents a degree of independence in the care of their baby with the security of nursing help nearby. This practice is particularly helpful for anxious parents, parents who have not had the opportunity to spend extended time with their baby, or parents who will be giving complex physical care at home, such as gastrostomy feeding and medication administration (Lopez, Anderson, & Feutchinger, 2012; Schlittenhart, Smart, Miller, et al., 2012). According to Lopez et al. (2012), parents of NICU graduates do not feel adequately prepared for the transition from the NICU to home with their babies. Teaching that occurs with daily

interaction of the NICU staff is not always perceived by the family as adequate, and the stress levels of the family while in the NICU can be a barrier to a learning environment.

Families interact with staff while gradually transitioning to sole caretakers of their medically complex high-risk newborn. When discharging a medically fragile baby to home, schedule a predischarge home visit by a public health nurse or home health agency. This discharge visit evaluates the home for any possible issues that may complicate the parents' ability to care for their at-risk newborn, especially if there are multiple monitoring equipment needs.

The basic elements of discharge and home care instruction are as follows:

- Teach the parents routine well-baby care, such as bathing, taking a temperature, preparing formula, and breastfeeding.

- Help parents learn to do special procedures as needed by the newborn, such as gavage or gastrostomy feedings, tracheostomy or enterostomy care, medication administration, CPR, and operation of the apnea monitor. Before discharge, the parents should be as comfortable as possible with these tasks and should demonstrate independence. Written tools and instructions are useful for parents to refer to once they are home with the baby, but they should not replace actual participation in the baby's care.

- Make sure that all applicable screening (metabolic, vision, hearing) tests, immunizations, and respiratory syncytial virus (RSV) prophylaxis are done before discharge and that all records are given to the primary care provider and parents.

- Refer parents to community health and support organizations. The Visiting Nurse Association, public health nurses, or social services can assist the parents in the stressful transition from hospital to home by providing the necessary home teaching and support. Some NICUs have their own parent support groups to help bridge the gap between hospital and home care. Parents can also find support from a variety of community organizations, such as mothers-of-twins groups, March of Dimes Birth Defects Foundation, services for children with disabilities, and teen mother and child programs. Each community has numerous agencies capable of assisting the family in adapting emotionally, physically, and financially to the chronically ill baby. Be familiar with community resources and help the parents identify which agencies may benefit them.

- Help parents recognize the growth and development needs of their baby. A development program begun in the hospital can be continued at home, or parents may be referred to an infant development program in the community.

- Arrange medical follow-up care before discharge. The baby will need to be followed up by a family pediatrician, a well-baby clinic, or a specialty clinic. The first appointment should be made before the baby is discharged from the hospital.

- Evaluate the need for special equipment for infant care (such as a respirator, oxygen, apnea monitor, feeding pump) in the home. Any equipment or supplies should be placed in the home before the baby's discharge.

- Ensure that a medical home for continuing medical care for the baby has been identified and a plan for transfer of information and care has been completed as needed.

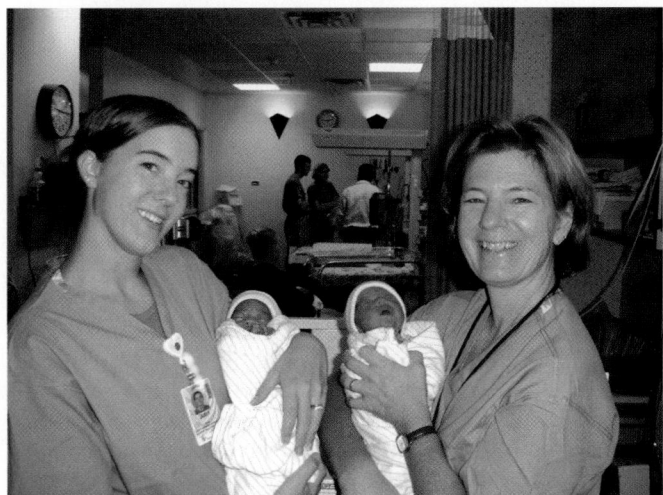

Figure 27–16 Discharge day. These 33 weeks' gestational age twins are being held by staff in the NICU on the happy day of discharge. This is what is so rewarding about working in the NICU: healthy babies going home to their families.

SOURCE: Lisa Smith-Pedersen, RNC, MSN, NNP-BC.

- Arrange for neonatal hospice for parents of the medically fragile baby as needed.

- Further evaluation after the baby has gone home is useful in determining whether the crisis has been resolved satisfactorily. The parents are usually given the intensive care nursery's telephone number to call for support and advice. The ability to contact the NICU, perhaps even utilizing video conferencing, can be an effective method of support following discharge (Lopez et al., 2012). The staff can follow up each family with visits or telephone calls at intervals for several weeks to assess and evaluate the baby's (and parents') progress (Figure 27–16).

Evaluation

Expected outcomes of nursing care include the following:

- The parents are able to verbalize their feelings of grief and loss.

- The parents verbalize their concerns about their newborn's health problems, care needs, and potential outcome.

- The parents are able to participate in their newborn's care and show attachment behaviors.

Considerations for the Nurse Who Works With At-Risk Newborns

The birth of a baby with a problem is a traumatic event with the potential for either disruption or growth, or both, of the involved family. NICU staff nurses may never see the long-term results of the specialized sensitive care they give to parents and their newborns. Their only immediate evidence of effective care may be the beginning resolution of parental grief; or discharge of a recovered, thriving baby to the care of happy parents; and the beginning of reintegration of family life.

Nurses cannot provide support unless they themselves are supported. Working in an emotional environment of "lots of living and lots of dying" takes its toll on staff. NICUs are among the most stressful areas in health care for patients, families, and nurses. Nurses bear most of the stress and largely determine the atmosphere of the NICU. The nurse's ability to cope with stress is the key to creating an emotionally healthy environment and a positive working atmosphere. The emotional needs and feelings of the staff must be recognized and dealt with so that the staff can support the parents. An environment of openness to feelings and support in dealing with their human needs and emotions is essential for the staff.

As caregivers, nurses may be unaware of their need to grieve for their own losses in the NICU. Nurses must also go through the grief work that parents experience. Techniques such as group meetings, individual support, and primary care nursing may assist in maintaining staff mental health. Reunions in some nurseries are beneficial for the families and healthcare providers so they are able to see the children after discharge.

Focus Your Study

- The sick newborn—whether preterm, term, or postterm—must be managed within narrow physiologic parameters. These parameters (respiratory, cardiovascular, and thermal regulation) will maintain physiologic homeostasis and prevent introduction of iatrogenic stress to the already stressed baby.

- The nursing care of the newborn with special problems involves understanding normal physiology, the pathophysiology of the disease process, clinical manifestations, and supportive or corrective therapies. Only with this theoretical background can the nurse make appropriate observations concerning responses to therapy and development of complications.

- Asphyxia results in significant circulatory, respiratory, and biochemical changes in the newborn that make the successful transition to extrauterine life difficult. Asphyxia requires early identification and resuscitative management. Newborns needing resuscitation have a weak cry, poor respiratory effort and retractions at birth

- Resuscitation methods include:

  - Stimulation by rubbing the newborn's back. (Done initially to all newborns.)

  - Use of positive pressure to inflate the lungs. (Used if respirations are inadequate or have not been initiated.)

- Endotracheal intubation. (Used immediately for severely premature newborns, newborns with known congenital anomalies, and newborns who do not respond to stimulation or bag and mask.)

- Medications: Naloxone (Narcan) may be used to reverse effects of narcotics given to mother prior to birth.

- Newborn conditions that commonly present with respiratory distress and require oxygen and ventilatory assistance are:

  - Respiratory distress syndrome (RDS) is a lack of sufficient surfactant that causes labored respirations and increased work at breathing. It is seen most frequently in premature newborns. Nursing care involves administration of surfactant, close assessment, and supportive care if mechanical ventilation is needed.

  - Transient tachypnea of the newborn usually results from excess fluid in the lungs. Newborn breathes normally at birth, but develops symptoms of respiratory distress by 4 to 6 hours of age. Nursing care involves initiating oxygen therapy and restricting oral feedings until respiratory status improves.

  - Meconium aspiration syndrome (MAS) shows signs and symptoms of respiratory distress beginning at birth. Care depends on the amount of meconium that is aspirated and the activity level of the newborn. If baby is vigorous even in presence of meconium—no subsequent special resuscitation. If baby has absent or depressed respirations, HR less than 100 beats per minute, or poor muscle tone—direct tracheal suctioning by specially trained personnel.

  - After initial suctioning and/or resuscitation efforts, nursing care involves ongoing assessment for signs and symptoms of respiratory distress and supportive care of the baby requiring mechanical ventilation or ECMO.

- Cold stress sets up the chain of physiologic events of hypoglycemia, pulmonary vasoconstriction, hyperbilirubinemia, respiratory distress, and metabolic acidosis.

- Nurses are responsible for early assessment and detection and initiation of treatment for hypoglycemia. Nursing interventions include: keeping the baby warm during any transport; observe for any subtle signs of hypoglycemia; have baby go to breast or feed early in neonatal period; and assess blood glucose frequently.

- Physiologic jaundice occurs in 50% of all newborns; appears after 24 hours of age, is not visible after 10 days of age and may require phototherapy. Pathologic jaundice is usually caused by ABO or Rh incompatibility; may be present within 24 hours of birth; treatment begins with phototherapy, but may progress to exchange transfusions. Untreated hyperbilirubinemia (due to either type of jaundice) may result in neurotoxicity.

- In Rh incompatibility: Maternal antibodies enter the fetal circulation, then attach to and destroy fetal red blood cells; fetal system produces more RBCs and hyperbilirubinemia, anemia, and jaundice result. In ABO incompatibility the mother is type O and baby is type A or B and it is less severe than Rh incompatibility.

- Nursing responsibilities for the newborn receiving phototherapy include: expose maximum amount of skin surface for optimal therapeutic results; apply eye patches while banks of phototherapy lights are in progress; assess eyes for signs/symptoms of conjunctivitis per agency protocol; frequently monitor temperature; offer baby breast milk or formula frequently to assist in excretion of bilirubin. Additionally, keep parents informed of need for phototherapy and encourage them to hold and care for baby while undergoing phototherapy.

- Anemia (decreased amount of red blood cell volume) in newborns results from prenatal blood loss, birth trauma, infection, or blood group incompatibility. Anemia places the newborn at risk for alterations in blood flow and the oxygen-carrying capacity of the blood.

- Nursing assessment of the septic newborn involves identifying very subtle clinical signs that are also seen in other clinical disease states such as: lethargy or irritability, pallor or duskiness, hypothermia, feeding intolerance, hyperbilirubinemia. and tachycardia, bradycardia, or apneic spells. The nursing care includes: obtain cultures before antibiotic therapy starts; carry out laboratory sepsis workup; and administer antibiotics as prescribed. Also provide supportive care to include NTE, respiratory and cardiovascular support, nutrition, monitor fluid and electrolyte homeostasis, and observe for complications.

- All newborns receive eye prophylaxis with ophthalmic antibiotic because of the possibility of transmission of gonorrhea or chlamydia during the birth process. Maternal syphilis requires that the baby be isolated from other newborns and receive antibiotics at birth. Maternal herpes virus infection requires administration of IV antiviral medications in the immediate newborn period as well as multiple cultures (skin, spinal fluid) for presence of herpes virus.

- The nurse is the facilitator for interprofessional communication with the parents, identifying their level of understanding of their newborn's care and their need for emotional support. Initially, the parents need to understand the baby's problem, including expected treatments.

- The nurse needs to prepare and facilitate the parents' viewing of the newborn by promoting touching and parental participation in care of the baby. Ensure parents understand routine well-baby care, normal growth and development of infants, and have referrals for normal infant screening procedures

- Parents should have medical follow-up arranged and referral for any special equipment required at home and understand how to perform any special procedures needed to care for the baby.

- Parents of at-risk newborns need support from nurses and healthcare providers to facilitate their adjustment to the special needs of their baby and to feel comfortable in an overwhelming and unfamiliar environment.

Clinical Reasoning in Action

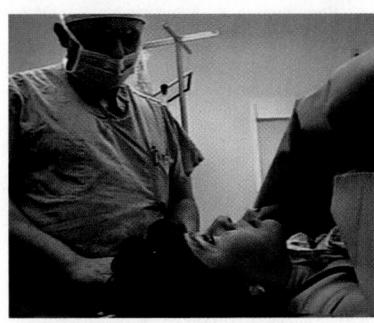

Rebecca Prince, age 21, G2 now P2, gives birth to a 5 lb baby at 38 weeks' gestation by primary cesarean birth for nonreassuring fetal status. The baby's Apgars are 7 and 9 at 1 and 5 minutes. The baby is suctioned and given titrated oxygen at birth with the pulse oximeter monitored and then is admitted to the newborn nursery for transitional care and does well. You are the nurse caring for baby Prince at 36 hours old. You review the newborn's record and note that the baby's blood type is A+ and his mother is O+. Rebecca wants to breastfeed. You are performing a shift assessment on baby Prince when you observe that the baby has a unilateral cephalohematoma and is lethargic. You blanch the skin over the sternum and observe a yellow discoloration of the skin. Laboratory tests reveal a serum bilirubin level of 12 mg/dL, hematocrit 55%, a mildly positive direct Coombs test, and a positive indirect Coombs test. Baby Prince is diagnosed with hyperbilirubinemia secondary to ABO incompatibility and cephalohematoma. You provide phototherapy by fiberoptic blanket around the trunk of the baby and take him to his mother's room.

1. How would you explain the purpose of phototherapy to the mother?
2. Plot the bilirubin on the hour-specific nomogram to assess the zone.
3. Explain the follow-up laboratory testing required and when it will be required.
4. Describe the care the mother can give to the newborn.
5. Discuss the advantage of fiberoptic blanket phototherapy for the newborn.

References

American Academy of Pediatrics (AAP) & American Heart Association (AHA). (2011). *Textbook of neonatal resuscitation* (6th ed.). Elk Grove Village, IL: American Academy of Pediatrics & American Heart Association.

American Academy of Pediatrics (AAP), Committee on the Fetus and Newborn, & American College of Obstetricians and Gynecologists (ACOG), Committee on Obstetric Practice. (2012). *Guidelines for perinatal care* (7th ed.). Elk Grove Village, IL: Author.

Arcara, K., & Tschudy, M. (2012). *The Harriet Lane handbook: Mobile medicine series, expert consult: Online* (19th ed.). New York, NY: Elsevier Health Sciences.

Bagwell, G. A. (2014a). Hematologic system. In C. Kenner & J. W. Lott (Eds.), *Comprehensive neonatal nursing care* (5th ed., pp. 334–375). New York, NY: Springer.

Bagwell, G. A. (2014b). Resuscitation and stabilization of the newborn and infant. In C. Kenner & J. W. Lott (Eds.), *Comprehensive neonatal nursing care* (5th ed., pp. 55–70). New York, NY: Springer.

Bennett, N. J. (2013). Bacteremia. *Medscape reference: Drugs, diseases & procedures*. Retrieved from http://emedicine.medscape.com/article/961169-overview

Bhutani, V. K., & Committee on the Fetus and Newborn. (2011). Phototherapy to prevent severe neonatal hyperbilirubinemia in the newborn infant 35 or more weeks of gestation. *Pediatrics 128*, e1046–1052. doi:10.1542/peds.2011-1494

Bhutani, V. K., Johnson, L. H., & Keren, R. (2004). Diagnosis and management of hyperbilirubinemia in the term neonate: For a safer first week. *Pediatric Clinics of North America, 51*(4), 843–861.

Bhutani, V. K., Stark, A. R., Lazzeroni, L. C., Poland, R., Gourley, G. R., Kazmierczak, S., ... Stevenson, D. K. (2013). Predischarge screening for severe neonatal hyperbilirubinemia identifies infants who need phototherapy. *The Journal of Pediatrics, 162*, 477–482.

Bicking, C., & Moore, G. A. (2012). Maternal perinatal depression in the neonatal intensive care unit: The role of the neonatal nurse. *Neonatal Network, 31*(5), 295–304.

Blackburn, S. T. (2013). *Maternal, fetal, & neonatal physiology: A clinical perspective* (4th ed.). St. Louis, MO: Saunders.

Bondi, E., Evans, R., Mischler, M., Benel-Stenzel, M., Horstmann, S., Lee, V., ... Gigliotti, F. (2013). Epidemiology of bacteremia in febrile infants in the United States. *Pediatrics, 132*(6), 990–996.

Bosschaart, N., Kok, J. H., Newsum, A. M., Ouweneel, D. M., Mentink, R., van Leeuwen, T. G., & Aalders, M. C. G. (2012). Limitations and opportunities of transcutaneous bilirubin measurements. *Pediatrics, 129*(4), 689–694.

Casey, G. (2013). Jaundice: An excess of bilirubin. *Kai Tiaki Nursing New Zealand, 19*(1), 20–24.

Chinchilla, M. K. (2012). Patient family-centered care: A bedside RN's perspective. *Neonatal Network, 31*(5), 341–344.

Cloherty, J. P., Eichenwald, E. C., Hansen, A. R., & Stark, A. R. (2012). *Manual of neonatal care* (7th ed.). Philadelphia, PA: Lippincott Williams & Wilkins

Committee on the Fetus and Newborn & Adamkin, D. H. (2011). Clinical report: Postnatal glucose homoeostasis in late-preterm and term infants. *Pediatrics, 127*(3), 575–579.

Discenza, D. (2012a). Kangaroo care: Worth the time and effort. *Neonatal Network, 31*(3), 189.

Discenza, D. (2012b). Preemie parent frustration: Dealing with insensitive comments. *Neonatal Network, 31*(1), 52–53.

Fanaroff, A. A., & Fanaroff, J. M. (2013). *Klaus and Fanaroff's care of the high-risk neonate* (6th ed.). Philadelphia, PA: Elsevier Saunders.

Gardner, S. L., Enzman-Himes, M. & Nyp, M. (2016). Respiratory diseases. In S. L. Gardner, B. S. Carter, M. Enzman-Hines, & J. A. Hernandez (Eds.), *Merenstein & Gardner's handbook of neonatal intensive care* (8th ed., pp. 565–648). St. Louis. MO: Mosby Elsevier.

Gardner, S. L. & Hernandez, J. (2016). Heat balance. In S. L. Gardner, B. S. Carter, M. Enzman-Hines, & J. A. Hernandez (Eds.), *Merenstein & Gardner's handbook of neonatal intensive care* (8th ed., pp. 105–125). St. Louis. MO: Mosby Elsevier.

Gleason, C. A., & Devaskar, S. U. (2012). *Avery's diseases of the newborn* (9th ed.) St. Louis, MO: Elsevier Saunders.

Gomella, T. L. (2013). *Neonatology: Management, procedures, on-call problems, diseases, and drugs* (7th ed.). New York, NY: Lange McGraw-Hill.

Graci, A. (2013). A rounding system to enhance patient, parent, and neonatal nurse interactions and promote patient safety. *Journal of Obstetric, Gynecological, and Neonatal Nursing (JOGNN), 42*, 239–242.

Grant, P. (1978). Psychological needs of families of high risk infants. *Family and Community Health, 1*(3), 91–102.

Harris, D. L., Weston, P. J., & Harding, J. E. (2012). Incidence of neonatal hypoglycemia in babies identified as at risk. *The Journal of Pediatrics, 161*, 787–791.

Hemway, R. J., Christman, C., & Perlman, J. (2013). The 3:1 is superior to a 15:2 ratio in a newborn manikin model in terms of quality of chest compressions and number of ventilations. *Arch Dis Child Fetal Neonatal Ed, 98*(1), F42–45.

Hintz, S. R., Stevenson, D. K., Yao, Q., Wong, R. J., Das, A., Van Meurs, K. P., ... Higgins, R. D. (2011). Is phototherapy exposure associated with better or worse outcomes in 501- to 1000-g-birthweight infants? *Acta Paediatrica, 100*, 960–965. doi:10.1111/j.1651-2227.02175x

Holditch-Davis, D., Miles, M. S., Burchinal, M. R., & Goldman, B. D. (2011). Maternal role attainment with medically fragile infants: Part 2. Relationship to the quality of parenting. *Research in Nursing Health, 34*(1), 35–48. doi:10.1002/nur.20418

Johnson, P. J. (2012). Antibiotic resistance in the NICU. *Neonatal Network, 31*(2), 109–114.

Kamath-Rayne, B. D., Thio, E. H., Deacon, J., & Hernandez J. J. (2016). Neonatal hyperbilirubinemia. In S. L. Gardner, B. S. Carter, M. Enzman-Hines, & J. A. Hernandez (Eds.), *Merenstein & Gardner's handbook of neonatal intensive care* (8th ed., pp. 511–536). St. Louis. MO: Mosby Elsevier.

Klaus, M. H., & Kennell, J. H. (1982). *Maternal-infant bonding* (2nd ed.). St. Louis, MO: Mosby.

Lopez, G. L., Anderson, K. H., & Feutchinger, J. (2012). Transition of premature infants from hospital to home life. *Neonatal Network, 31*(4), 207–214.

Ludington-Hoe, S. M. (2011). Thirty years of kangaroo care science and practice. *Neonatal Network, 30*(5), 357–362.

Lukacs, S. L., & Schrag, S. J. (2012). Clinical sepsis in neonates and young infants, United States, 1988–2006. *The Journal of Pediatrics, 160*, 960–965.

Maisels, M. J. (2012). Noninvasive measurements of bilirubin. *Pediatrics, 129*(4), 779–781.

Maisels, M. J., & Watchko, J. F. (2012). Treatment of hyperbilirubinemia. In G. Buonocore, R. Bracci, & M. Weindling (Eds.), *Neonatology: A practical approach to neonatal management* (pp. 629–640). Milan, Italy: Springer-Verlag.

Mantagou, L., Fouzas, S., Skylogianni, E., Giannakopoulos, I., Karatza, A., & Varvarigou, A. (2012). Trends in transcutaneous bilirubin in neonates who develop significant hyperbilirubinemia. *Pediatrics, 130*, e898–e904.

Marks, M. (2012). Evidence-based midwifery: The case against newborn suctioning. *Midwifery Today (Summer 2012)*, 21–22.

Niermeyer, S., Clarke, S. B., & Hernandez J. J. (2016). Delivery room care. In S. L. Gardner, B. S. Carter, M. Enzman-Hines, & J. A. Hernandez (Eds.), *Merenstein & Gardner's handbook of neonatal intensive care* (8th ed., pp. 47–70). St. Louis. MO: Mosby.

Ohls, R. K., Roohi, M., Peceny, H. M., Schrader, R., & Bierer, R. (2012). A randomized, masked study of weekly erythropoietin dosing in preterm infants. *The Journal of Pediatrics, 160*, 790–795.

Pappas, B. E. & Robey, D. L. (2015). Neonatal delivery room resuscitation. In M. T. Verklan & M. Walden (Eds.), *Core curriculum for neonatal intensive care nursing.* (5th ed. pp. 77–94). MO, St. Louis, MO: Saunders.

Polin, R. A., & the Committee on the Fetus and Newborn. (2012). Management of neonates with suspected or proven early-onset bacterial sepsis. *Pediatrics, 129*, 1006–1015.

Polin, R. A., Carlo, W. A., & the Committee on the Fetus and Newborn. (2014). Surfactant replacement therapy for preterm and term neonates with respiratory distress. *Pediatrics, 133*(1), 156–163. doi:10.1542/peds.2013-3443

Polin, R. A., Denson, S., Brady, M. T., & the Committee on the Fetus and Newborn and Committee on Infectious Diseases. (2012). Strategies for prevention of health care-associated infections in the NICU. *Pediatrics, 129*(4), e1085–e1093.

Riley, C., Spencer, B., & Prater, L. S. (2014). Normal term newborn. In C. Kenner & J. W. Lott (Eds.), *Comprehensive neonatal nursing care* (5th ed., pp. 113–132). New York, NY: Springer.

Rubarth, L. (2012). The Apgar score: Simple yet complex. *Neonatal Network, 31*(2), 169–176.

Sabir, H., Jary, S., Tooley, J., Liu, X., & Thoresen, M. (2012). Increased inspired oxygen in the first hours of life is associated with adverse outcome in newborns treated for perinatal asphyxia with therapeutic hypothermia. *The Journal of Pediatrics, 161*, 409–416.

Saugstad, O. D., Aune, D. Aguar, M., Kapadia, V., Finer, N. & Vento, M., (2014). Systematic review and meta-analysis of optimal initial fraction of oxygen levels in the delivery room at ≤ weeks. *Acta Paediatrica 103*(7), 744.

Sawyer, T., Laubach, V. A., Hudak, J., Yamamura, K., & Pocrnich, A. (2013). Improvements in teamwork during neonatal resuscitation after interprofessional Team STEPPS training, *Neonatal Network, 32*(1), 26–33. doi:10.1891/0730-0832.32.1.26

Schlittenhart, J. M., Smart, D., Miller, K., & Severtson, B. (2012). Preparing parents for NICU discharge: An evidence-based teaching tool. *Nursing for Women's Health, 15*(6), 486–494.

Siriwachirachai, T., Sangkomkamhang, U., Lumbiganon, P., & Laopaiboon, M. (2014). Antibiotics for meconium-stained amniotic fluid in labour for preventing maternal and neonatal infections. *Cochrane Database of Systematic Reviews*, Issue 11. Art. No. CD007772.

Skene, C., Franck, L., Curtis, P., & Gerrish, K. (2012). Parental involvement in neonatal comfort care. *Journal of Obstetric, Gynecological, and Neonatal Nursing (JOGNN), 41*, 786–797.

Smith, J., Alcock, G., & Usher, K. (2013). Temperature measurement in the preterm and term neonate: A review of the literature. *Neonatal Network, 32*(1), 16–25.

Smith, J. R., & Carley, A. (2014). Common neonatal complications. In K. R. Simpson & P. C. Creehan (Eds.), *AWHONN perinatal nursing* (4th ed., pp. 662–698). Philadelphia, PA: Wolter Kluwer.

Solnit, A., & Stark, M. (1961). Mourning and the birth of a defective child. *Psychoanalytic Study of the Child, 16*, 505.

Swarnam, K., Soraisham, A. S., & Sivanandan, S. (2012). Advances in the management of meconium aspiration syndrome. *International Journal of Pediatrics* 2012. doi: 10:1155/2012/359571

Sweet, L., & Mannix, T. (2012). Identification of parental stressors in a Australian neonatal intensive care unit. *Neonatal, Paediatric and Child Health Nursing, 15*(2), 8–16.

Taylor, T. A., & Kennedy, K. A. (2013). Randomized trial of iron supplementation versus routine iron intake in VLBW infants. *Pediatrics, 131*(2), e433–e438.

Trevisanuto, D., Cengio, V. D., Doglioni, N., Cavallin, F., Zanardo, V., Parotto, M., & Weiner, G. (2013). Oxygen delivery using a neonatal self-inflating resuscitation bag: Effect of oxygen flow. *Pediatrics, 131*, e1144–e1149.

Turnbull, V., & Petty, J. (2012). Early inset jaundice in the newborn: Understanding the ongoing care of mother and baby. *British Journal of Midwifery, 20*(9), 615–622.

Van Woudenberg, C. D., Wills, C. A., & Rubarth, L. B. (2012). Newborn transition to extrauterine life. *Neonatal Network, 31*(5), 317–322.

Vandborg, P. K., Hansen, B. M., Greisen, G., & Ebbesen, F. (2012). Dose-response relationship of phototherapy for hyperbilirubinemia. *Pediatrics, 130*, e352–e357.

Walden, M. (2014). Pain in the newborn and infant. In C. Kenner & J. W. Lott (Eds.), *Comprehensive neonatal nursing care* (5th ed., pp. 571–587). New York, NY: Springer.

Walker, L. J. (2013). Bonding with books: The parent-infant connection in the neonatal intensive care unit. *Neonatal Network, 32*(2), 104–109.

Walsh, B. K., Daigle, B., DiBlasi, R. M., & Restrepo, R. D. (2013). AARC clinical practice guideline. Surfactant replacement therapy: 2013. *Respiratory Care, 58*(2), 367–375.

White, A. L. (2012). Parents vs. neonatal resuscitation team: Who should decide? *The Kansas Nurse, 87*(3), 17–19.

Wolff, M., Schinasi, D. A., Lavelle, J., Boorstein, N., & Zorc, J. J. (2012). Management of neonates with hyperbilirubinemia: Improving timelines of care using a clinical pathway. *Pediatrics, 130*, e1688–e1694.

Zimmerman, K., & Bauersachs, C. (2012). Empowering NICU parents. *International Journal of Childbirth Education, 27* (1), 50–53.

Chapter 28
Postpartum Adaptation and Nursing Assessment

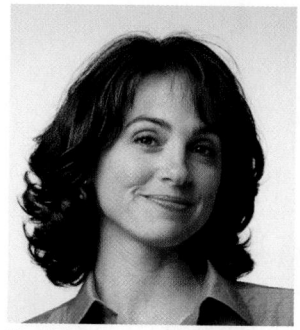

I acutely felt the fatigue and sense of loss of the relationship with my baby that I had during pregnancy. But then the wonderful part happened with the reuniting with my new daughter. Holding her, having her latch on to my breast to get nourishment, and her looking into my eyes to say "Hello, Mom."

—Susan, 34

Kevin Peterson/Getty Images

Learning Outcomes

28.1 Describe the basic physiologic changes that occur in the postpartum period as a woman's body returns to its prepregnant state.

28.2 Describe the psychologic adjustments that normally occur during the postpartum period.

28.3 Describe the physiologic and psychologic components of a systematic postpartum assessment.

28.4 Describe the common concerns of the mother that are considered in a postpartum assessment.

28.5 Examine the physical and developmental tasks that the mother must accomplish during the postpartum period.

28.6 Relate how the nursing assessment of early attachment incorporates factors that influence development of a positive parent–infant attachment.

During the **puerperium**, or postpartum period, the woman readjusts, physically and psychologically, from pregnancy and birth. The period begins immediately after birth and continues for approximately 6 weeks, or until the body has returned to a near nonpregnant, or prepregnant, state.

This chapter describes the physiologic and psychologic changes that occur postpartum and the basic aspects of a thorough postpartum assessment.

Postpartum Physical Adaptations

Comprehensive nursing assessment is based on a sound understanding of the normal anatomic and physiologic processes of the puerperium. These processes involve the reproductive organs and other major body systems.

Reproductive System

INVOLUTION OF THE UTERUS

The term **involution** is used to describe the rapid reduction in size and the return of the uterus to a nonpregnant state. Following separation of the placenta, the decidua of the uterus is irregular, jagged, and varied in thickness. The spongy layer of the decidua is cast off as lochia, and the basal layer of the decidua remains in the uterus to become differentiated into two layers within the first 48 to 72 hours after birth. The outermost layer becomes necrotic and is sloughed off in the lochia. The layer closest to the myometrium contains the fundi of the uterine endometrial glands, and these glands lay the foundation for the new endometrium. Except at the placenta site, this process is completed in approximately 3 weeks. The placental site can take up to 6 weeks to be completely healed (Cunningham et al., 2014; Pessel & Tsai, 2013). Bleeding from the larger uterine vessels of the placental site is controlled by compression of the retracted uterine muscle fibers. The clotted blood is gradually absorbed by the body. Some of these vessels are eventually obliterated and replaced by new vessels with smaller lumens.

The placental site heals by a process of exfoliation and growth of endometrial tissue. This occurs with upward endometrial growth in the decidua basalis under the placental site, with simultaneous growth of endometrial tissue from the margins of the site. The infarcted superficial tissue then becomes necrotic and is sloughed off (Blackburn, 2013). Exfoliation is a very important aspect of involution; if healing of the placental site leaves a fibrous scar, the area available for future implantation is limited, as is the number of possible pregnancies.

With the dramatic decrease in the levels of circulating estrogen and progesterone following placental separation, the uterine cells atrophy, and the hyperplasia of pregnancy begins to reverse. Proteolytic enzymes are released, and macrophages migrate to the uterus to promote autolysis (self-digestion) (James, 2014). Protein material in the uterine wall is broken down and absorbed. Factors that enhance involution include an uncomplicated labor and birth, complete expulsion of the placenta or membranes, breastfeeding, manual removal of the placenta during a cesarean birth, and early ambulation. Factors that slow uterine involution and the rationale for each factor are listed in Table 28–1.

CHANGES IN FUNDAL POSITION

The **fundus** (top portion of the uterus) is situated in the midline midway between the symphysis pubis and the umbilicus (Figure 28–1). Immediately following the birth of the placenta, the uterus contracts to the size of a large grapefruit. The walls of the contracted uterus are in proximity, and the uterine blood vessels are firmly compressed by the myometrium. Within 6 to 12 hours after birth, the fundus of the uterus rises to the level of the umbilicus because of blood and clots that remain within the uterus and changes in support of the uterus by the ligaments. A fundus that is above the umbilicus and boggy (feels soft and

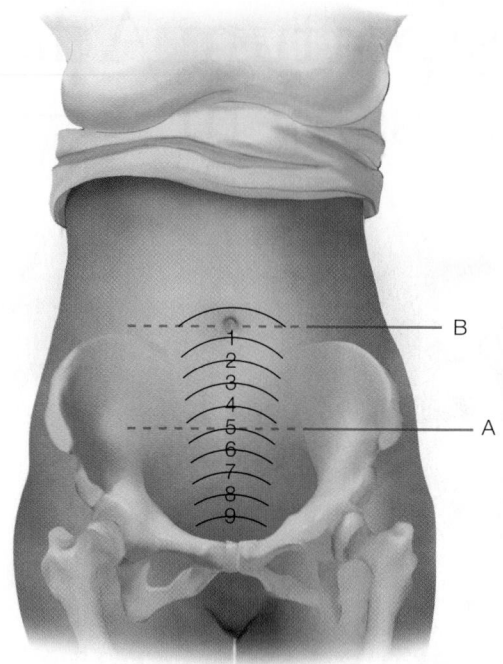

Figure 28–1 Involution of the uterus. *A,* Immediately after delivery of the placenta, the top of the fundus is in the midline and approximately halfway between the symphysis pubis and the umbilicus. About 6 to 12 hours after birth, the fundus is at the level of the umbilicus. *B,* The height of the fundus then decreases about one finger-breadth (approximately 1 cm) each day.

TABLE 28–1 Factors That Slow Uterine Involution

FACTOR	RATIONALE
Prolonged labor	Muscles relax because of prolonged time of contraction during labor.
Anesthesia	Muscle relaxation results in a "boggy uterus."
Difficult birth	The uterus is manipulated excessively causing muscle fatigue.
Grand multiparity	Repeated distention of uterus during pregnancy and labor leads to muscle stretching, diminished tone, and muscle relaxation.
Full bladder	As the uterus is pushed up and usually to the right, pressure on it interferes with effective uterine contraction.
Incomplete expulsion of placenta or membranes	The presence of even small amounts of tissue interferes with the ability of the uterus to remain firmly contracted.
Infection	Inflammation interferes with the uterine muscle's ability to contract effectively.
Overdistention of uterus	Overstretching of uterine muscles with conditions such as multiple gestation, polyhydramnios, or a very large baby may set the stage for slower uterine involution.

spongy rather than firm and well contracted) is associated with excessive uterine bleeding. As blood collects and forms clots within the uterus, the fundus rises; firm contractions of the uterus are interrupted, causing a **boggy uterus (uterine atony)**.

When the fundus is higher than expected on palpation and is not in the midline (usually deviated to the right), distention of the bladder should be suspected; the bladder should be emptied immediately and the fundal height remeasured (Figure 28–2). If the woman is unable to void, in-and-out catheterization of the bladder may be required. In the immediate postpartum period, many women may not be aware of a full bladder. Because the uterine ligaments are still stretched, a full bladder can move the uterus. By the end of the puerperium these ligaments have regained their nonpregnant length and tension.

After birth, the top of the fundus remains at the level of the umbilicus for about half a day. On the first postpartum day (first day following birth), the top of the fundus is located about 1 cm (0.4 in.) below the umbilicus. On day 3 after delivery, the fundus is 3 cm (1.18 in.) below the umbilicus (James, 2014). The top of the fundus descends approximately 1 cm (one finger-breadth [width of index, second, or third finger]) per day, until it descends into the pelvis on the 10th day. By 6 to 8 weeks, the uterus weighs 60 grams (2 oz) (Whitmer, 2016).

If the mother is breastfeeding, the release of endogenous oxytocin from the posterior pituitary in response to suckling hastens involution of the uterus. Barring complications, such as infection or retained placental fragments, the uterus approaches its prepregnant size and location by 5 to 6 weeks. In women who had an oversized uterus during the pregnancy (because of hydramnios, birth of a large-for-gestational-age [LGA] baby, or multiple gestation), the time frame for an immediate uterine involution process is lengthened (Blackburn, 2013). If intrauterine infection is present, in addition to foul-smelling lochia

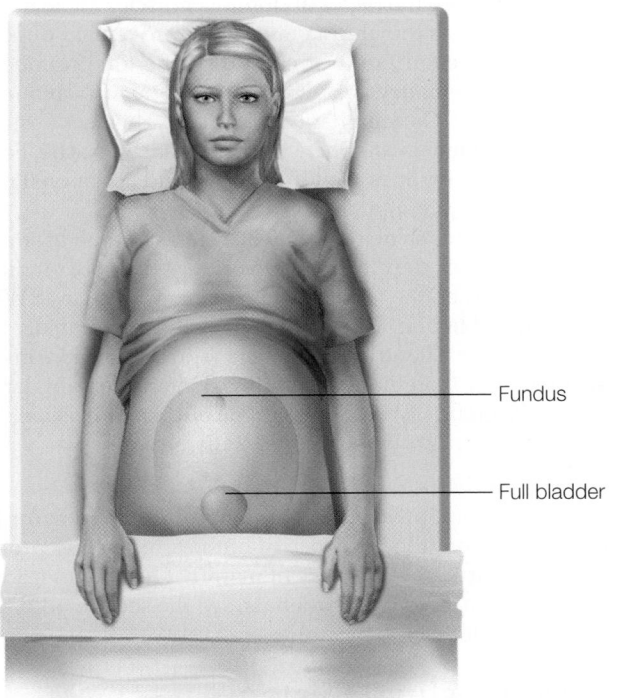

Figure 28–2 Displacement and deviation of the uterus. The uterus becomes displaced and deviated to the right when the bladder is full.

— Fundus

— Full bladder

or vaginal discharge, the uterine fundus descends much more slowly. When infection is suspected, other clinical signs such as fever and tachycardia in addition to delay in involution must be assessed. Any slowing of descent is called **subinvolution** (for further discussion of subinvolution, see Chapter 30).

LOCHIA

The uterus rids itself of the debris remaining after birth through a discharge called **lochia**, which is classified according to its appearance and contents. **Lochia rubra** is dark red. It occurs for the first 2 to 3 days and contains epithelial cells, erythrocytes, leukocytes, shreds of decidua, and occasionally fetal meconium, lanugo, and vernix caseosa. Clotting is often the result of pooling of blood in the upper portion of the vagina. A few small clots (no larger than a nickel) are common, particularly in the first few days after birth. However, lochia should not contain large (plum-size) clots; if it does, the cause should be investigated without delay. **Lochia serosa** is a pinkish color. It follows from about day 3 until day 10. Lochia serosa is composed of serous exudate (hence, the name), shreds of degenerating decidua, erythrocytes, leukocytes, cervical mucus, and numerous microorganisms (Blackburn, 2013). The red blood cell (RBC) component decreases gradually, and a creamy or yellowish discharge persists for an additional week or 2. This final discharge, termed **lochia alba** (from the Latin word for "white") is composed primarily of leukocytes, decidual cells, epithelial cells, fat, cervical mucus, cholesterol crystals, and bacteria.

Recent studies examining lochia patterns have found that the lochia rubra phase lasts longer than generally assumed, and that it varies according to breastfeeding practice and parity (Blackburn, 2013). Variation in the duration of lochia discharge is not uncommon; however, the trend should be toward a lighter amount of flow and a lighter color of discharge. When the lochia flow stops, the cervix is considered closed, and chances of infection ascending from the vagina to the uterus decrease.

Like menstrual discharge, lochia flow has a musty, stale odor that is not offensive. Microorganisms are always present in the vaginal lochia, and by the second day following birth, the uterus is contaminated with the vaginal bacteria. It is thought that an infection does not develop because the organisms involved are relatively nonvirulent. Any foul smell to the lochia or used peripad suggests infection and the need for prompt additional assessment for uterine tenderness and fever.

The total average volume of lochia is about 225 mL, and the daily volume gradually decreases (Blackburn, 2013). Discharge is greater in the morning because of pooling in the vagina and uterus while the mother lies sleeping. The amount of lochia may also be increased by exertion or breastfeeding. Multiparous women usually have more lochia than first-time mothers. Women who undergo a cesarean birth typically have less lochia than women who give birth vaginally (Blackburn, 2013).

Evaluation of lochia is necessary not only to determine the presence of hemorrhage but also to assess uterine involution. The type, amount, and consistency of lochia determines the stage of healing of the placental site, and a progressive change from bright red at birth to dark red to pink to white or clear discharge should be observed. Persistent discharge of lochia rubra or a return to lochia rubra indicates subinvolution or late postpartum hemorrhage (see Chapter 30).

The nurse should exercise caution when evaluating bleeding immediately after birth. The continuous seepage of blood is consistent with cervical or vaginal lacerations and may be effectively diagnosed when the bleeding is evaluated in conjunction with the consistency of the uterus. Lacerations should be suspected if the uterus is firm and of expected size and if no clots are expressed.

CERVICAL CHANGES

Following birth, the cervix is flabby, formless, and may appear bruised. The lateral aspects of the external os are frequently lacerated during the birth process (Cunningham et al., 2014). The external os is markedly irregular and closes slowly. It admits two fingers for a few days following birth, but by the end of the first week, it admits only a fingertip.

The shape of the external os is permanently changed by the first childbearing. The characteristic dimple-like os of the nullipara changes to the transverse slit (fish-mouth) os of the multipara (Pessel & Tsai, 2013). After significant cervical laceration or several lacerations, the cervix may appear lopsided. Because of the slight change in the size of the cervix, a diaphragm or cervical cap will need to be refitted if the woman is using one of these methods of contraception.

VAGINAL CHANGES

Following birth, the vagina appears edematous and gaping and may be bruised. Small superficial lacerations may be evident, and the rugae are obliterated. The apparent bruising is caused by pelvic congestion and trauma and will quickly disappear. The hymen, torn and jagged, heals irregularly, leaving small tags called carunculae myrtiformes.

Clinical Reasoning Variation in Fundus Status

You have completed your assessment of Patty Clark, a 24-year-old, G2P2 woman who is 24 hours past childbirth. The fundus is just above the umbilicus and slightly to the right. Lochia rubra is present, and a pad is soaked every 2 hours. What would you do?

The size of the vagina decreases and rugae return within 3 to 4 weeks (Blackburn, 2013; James, 2014). This facilitates the gradual return to smaller, although not nulliparous, dimensions. By 6 weeks, the nonlactating woman's vagina usually appears normal. The lactating woman is in a hypoestrogenic state because of ovarian suppression, and her vaginal mucosa may be pale and without rugae; the effects of the lowered estrogen level may lead to dyspareunia (painful intercourse), which may be reduced by the addition of a water-soluble personal lubricant. Tone and contractility of the vaginal orifice may be improved by perineal tightening exercises such as Kegel exercises (see Chapter 10), which may begin soon after birth. The labia majora and labia minora are more flaccid in the woman who has borne a child than in the nullipara woman.

PERINEAL CHANGES

During the early postpartum period, the soft tissue in and around the perineum may appear edematous, with some bruising. If an episiotomy or a laceration is present, the edges should be drawn together. Occasionally, ecchymosis occurs, and this may delay healing. Initial healing of the episiotomy or laceration occurs in 2 to 3 weeks after the birth, although complete healing may take up to 4 to 6 months (Blackburn, 2013). Perineal discomfort may be present during this time.

RECURRENCE OF OVULATION AND MENSTRUATION

The return of ovulation and menstruation varies for each postpartum woman. Menstruation generally returns as soon as 7 weeks in 70% and by 12 weeks in all nonlactating mothers or as late as 3 years in 70% of breastfeeding mothers (Pessel & Tsai, 2013). The return of ovulation is directly associated with a rise in the serum progesterone level. In nonlactating mothers, the average time to first ovulation can occur within 70 to 75 days, with a mean time of 6 months in lactating women (Pessel & Tsai, 2013).

The return of ovulation and menstruation in breastfeeding mothers is usually prolonged and is associated with the length of time the woman breastfeeds and whether formula supplements are used. If a mother breastfeeds for less than 1 month, the return of menstruation and ovulation is similar to that of the nonbreastfeeding mother. In women who exclusively breastfeed, menstruation is usually delayed for at least 3 months. Suckling by the infant typically results in alterations in the gonadotropin-releasing hormone (GnRH) production, which is thought to be the cause of amenorrhea (Blackburn, 2013). Although exclusive breastfeeding helps to reduce the risk of pregnancy for the first 6 months after birth, it should be relied on only temporarily and if it meets the observed criteria for the lactational amenorrhea method (LAM). Furthermore, because ovulation precedes menstruation and women often supplement breastfeeding with bottles and pacifiers, breastfeeding is not considered a reliable means of contraception.

Abdomen

The uterine ligaments (notably the round and broad ligaments) are stretched and require the length of the puerperium to recover. Although the stretched abdominal wall appears loose and flabby, it responds to exercise within 2 to 3 months. **Diastasis recti abdominis**, a separation of the abdominal muscle, may occur with pregnancy, especially in women with poor abdominal muscle tone (Figure 28–3). If diastasis occurs, part of the abdominal wall has no muscular support but is formed only by skin, subcutaneous fat, fascia, and peritoneum. This may be especially pronounced in women who have undergone a cesarean section because the rectus abdominis muscles are manually separated to access the uterine muscle. Improvement depends on the physical condition of the mother, the total number of pregnancies, pregnancy spacing, and the type and amount of physical exercise (Cunningham et al., 2014). This may result in a pendulous abdomen and increased maternal backache. Fortunately, diastasis responds well to exercise, and abdominal muscle tone can improve significantly.

The striae (stretch marks), which occur as a result of stretching and rupture of the elastic fibers of the skin, take on different colors based on the mother's skin color. The striae of White mothers are red to purple at the time of birth and gradually fade to silver or white. The striae of mothers with darker skin, in contrast, are darker than the surrounding skin and remain darker. These marks gradually fade after a time but remain visible.

Lactation

During pregnancy, breast development in preparation for lactation results from the influence of both estrogen and progesterone. After birth, the interplay of maternal hormones leads to milk production. (For further details, see the section on *Breastfeeding* in Chapter 25.)

Gastrointestinal System

Hunger following birth is common, and the mother may enjoy eating a light meal. Frequently, she is quite thirsty and will drink large amounts of fluid. Drinking fluids helps replace fluids lost during labor, in the urine, and through perspiration.

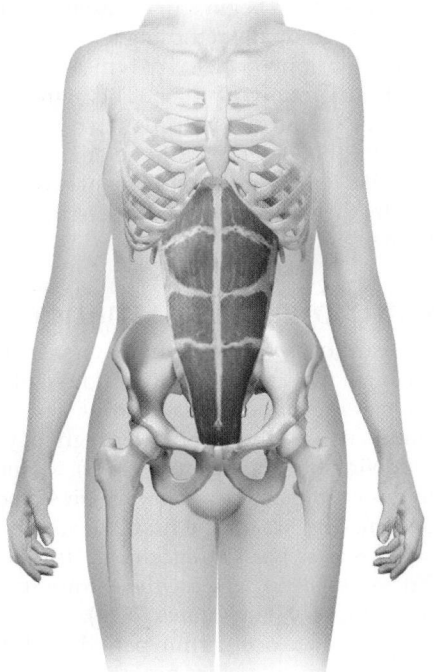 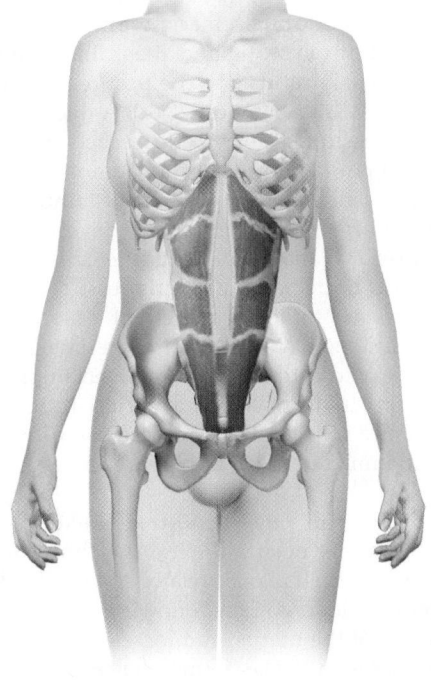

Normal location of rectus
muscles of the abdomen

Diastasis recti: separation
of the rectus muscles

Figure 28–3 Diastasis recti abdominis, which involves a separation of the abdominal musculature, commonly occurs after pregnancy.

The bowels tend to be sluggish following birth because of the lingering effects of progesterone, decreased abdominal muscle tone, and bowel evacuation associated with the labor and birth process (Whitmer, 2016). Women who have had an episiotomy, lacerations, or hemorrhoids may tend to delay elimination for fear of increasing their pain or because they believe their stitches will be torn if they bear down. In refusing or delaying the bowel movement, the woman may cause increased constipation and more pain when bowel elimination finally occurs. Pain medications and narcotics also can contribute to constipation and sluggish bowels.

The woman with a cesarean birth may receive clear liquids shortly after surgery; once bowel sounds are present, her diet is quickly advanced to solid food. In addition, the woman may experience some initial discomfort from flatulence, which is relieved by early ambulation and use of antiflatulent medications. Chamomile tea and peppermint tea may also be helpful in reducing discomfort from flatulence. It may take a few days for the bowel to regain its tone, especially if general anesthesia was used. The woman who has had a cesarean or a difficult birth may benefit from stool softeners.

Urinary Tract

The postpartum woman has an increased bladder capacity, swelling and bruising of the tissue around the urethra, decreased sensitivity to fluid pressure, and a decreased sensation of bladder filling. Consequently, she is at risk for overdistention, incomplete bladder emptying, and a buildup of residual urine. Women who have had an anesthetic block have inhibited neural functioning of the bladder and are more susceptible to bladder distention, difficulty voiding, and bladder infections.

In addition, immediate postpartum use of oxytocin to facilitate uterine contractions following expulsion of the placenta has an antidiuretic effect. Following cessation of the oxytocin, the woman will experience rapid bladder filling.

Urinary output increases during the early postpartum period (first 12 to 24 hours) because of *puerperal diuresis*. The kidneys must eliminate an estimated 2000 to 3000 mL of extracellular fluid with the normal pregnancy, which causes rapid filling of the bladder (Blackburn, 2013). Thus adequate bladder elimination is an immediate concern. Women with preeclampsia, chronic hypertension, and diabetes experience greater fluid retention than other women, and postpartum diuresis is increased accordingly.

If urine stasis exists, chances for urinary tract infection increase because of bacteriuria and the presence of dilated ureters and renal pelvises, which persist for about 6 weeks after birth. A full bladder may also increase the tendency of the uterus to relax by displacing the uterus and interfering with its contractility, leading to hemorrhage. In the absence of infection, the dilated ureters and renal pelvises return to prepregnant size by the end of the sixth week.

Vital Signs

During the postpartum period, with the exception of the first 24 hours, the woman should be afebrile. A maternal temperature of up to 38.0°C (100.4°F) may occur after childbirth as a result of the exertion and dehydration of labor. An increase in temperature to between 37.8° and 39.0°C (100.0° to 102.2°F) may also occur during the first 24 hours after the mother's milk comes in (Cunningham et al., 2014). However, in women not meeting these criteria, infection must be considered in the presence of an increased temperature (see discussion in Chapter 30).

Immediately following childbirth, many women experience a transient rise in both systolic and diastolic blood pressure, which spontaneously returns to the prepregnancy baseline during the next few days (James, 2014). A decrease may indicate physiologic readjustment to decreased intrapelvic pressure, or it may be related to uterine hemorrhage. Orthostatic hypotension, as indicated by feelings of faintness or dizziness immediately after standing up, can develop in the first 48 hours as a result of abdominal engorgement that may occur after birth. A low or decreasing blood pressure may reflect hypovolemia secondary to hemorrhage, but it is a late sign. Blood pressure elevations may result from excessive use of oxytocin or vasopressor medications. Because preeclampsia can persist into or occur first in the postpartum period, routine evaluation of blood pressure is needed. If a woman complains of headache, hypertension must be ruled out before analgesics are administered.

Puerperal bradycardia with rates of 50 to 70 beats per minute (beats/min) commonly occurs during the first 6 to 10 days of the postpartum period. It may be related to decreased cardiac effort, the decreased blood volume following placental separation and contraction of the uterus, and increased stroke volume. A pulse rate greater than 100 beats/min may be indicative of hypovolemia, infection, fear, or pain and requires further assessment (Whitmer, 2016).

Blood Values

Blood values should return to the prepregnant state by the end of the postpartum period. Pregnancy-associated activation of coagulation factors may continue for variable amounts of time after birth. This condition, in conjunction with trauma, immobility, or sepsis, predisposes the woman to the development of thromboembolism. The incidence of thromboembolism is reduced by early mobilization.

Nonpathologic leukocytosis often occurs during labor and in the immediate postpartum period, with white blood cell (WBC) counts of 25,000 to 30,000/mm^3. WBC values typically return to normal levels by the end of the first postpartum week. Leukocytosis combined with the normal increase in erythrocyte sedimentation rate (ESR) may obscure the diagnosis of acute infection at this time (James, 2014).

Hemoglobin and hematocrit levels may be difficult to interpret in the first 2 days after birth because of the changing blood volume. This loss in blood in the first 24 hours accounts for half of the red blood cell (RBC) volume gained during the course of the pregnancy. Blood loss averages 200 to 500 mL with a vaginal birth and nearly 1000 mL with a cesarean birth (Pessel & Tsai, 2013). Lochia constitutes less than 25% of this blood loss. As extracellular fluid is excreted, hemoconcentration occurs, with a concomitant rise in hematocrit. A drop in values indicates an abnormal blood loss. The following is a convenient rule to remember: A 2- to 3- percentage point drop in hematocrit equals a blood loss of 500 mL (James, 2014). After 3 to 4 days, mobilization of interstitial fluid leads to a slight increase in plasma volume. This hemodilution leads to a decrease in hemoglobin, hematocrit, and plasma protein by the end of the first postpartum week. Decreases in plasma volume reach nonpregnant levels by 4 to 6 weeks postpartum (Blackburn, 2013).

Platelet levels typically fall as a result of placental separation. They then begin to increase by the third to fourth postpartum day, gradually returning to normal by the sixth postpartum week. Fibrinolytic activity typically returns to normal during the hours following birth. The hemostatic system as a whole reaches its normal prepregnant status by 3 to 4 weeks postpartum; however, the diameter of deep veins can take up to 6 weeks to return to prepregnant levels (Blackburn, 2013). This is why there is a prolonged risk of thromboembolism in the first 6 weeks following birth.

Cardiovascular Changes

The cardiovascular system undergoes dramatic changes during the birth that can result in cardiovascular instability because of an increase in the cardiac output. The cardiac output typically stabilizes and returns to prepregnancy levels within an hour following birth (Blackburn, 2013). Maternal hypervolemia acts to protect the mother from excessive blood loss. Cardiac output declines by 30% in the first 2 weeks and reaches normal levels by 6 to 12 weeks (Blackburn, 2013). Diuresis in the first 2 to 5 days assists to decrease the extracellular fluid and results in a weight loss of 3 kg (James, 2014). Failure of diuresis to occur in the immediate postpartum period can lead to pulmonary edema and subsequent cardiac problems. This is seen more commonly in women with a history of preeclampsia or preexisting cardiac problems (James, 2014).

Neurologic and Immunologic Changes

Neurologic problems and disorders can predispose women to higher rates of morbidity and mortality during pregnancy and in the postpartum period. Headaches are the most common neurologic symptoms encountered by postpartum women. Headaches can result from fluid shifts in the first week after birth, leakage of cerebrospinal fluid into the extradural space during spinal anesthesia, pregnancy-induced hypertension, fluid and electrolyte imbalance, preeclampsia, or stress (James, 2014). It is estimated that up to 40% of postpartum women develop headaches within the first week following birth when estrogen drops precipitously (James, 2014; Lim, Evangelou & Jurgens, 2014). There may be an increased incidence in headache if the woman had spinal or epidural anesthesia. Migraine headaches, although less frequent during pregnancy, tend to resume in the postpartum period. Migraine headaches usually reoccur in the first week following birth (Nicholson, 2014). Women with epilepsy are 9 times more likely to have a seizure during labor or in the first 24 hours after birth than during pregnancy (Samuels & Niebyl, 2012). The postpartum woman with epilepsy is more likely to be diagnosed with depression and referral to a therapist or support group should be made (Klein, 2012). The physiologic changes of pregnancy that may have required increasing antiepileptic drug (AED) dosage are now removed, and retitration of the AEDs is required to prevent toxicity. Women with multiple sclerosis (MS) and Guillain-Barré syndrome are more likely to have symptoms in the postpartum period than during pregnancy (Nicholson, 2014; Samuels & Niebyl, 2012). Myasthenia gravis (autoimmune disease) affects the neuromuscular junctions. The increase in symptoms during pregnancy is variable; however, the first month of pregnancy and the first month of the postpartum period are the most critical (Kalayjian, Goodwin, & Lee, 2013).

Weight Loss

An initial weight loss of about 10 to 12 lb (4.5 to 5.4 kg) occurs as a result of the birth of the baby, delivery of the placenta, and loss of amniotic fluid. Diuresis accounts for the loss of an additional 5 lb (2.27 kg) during the early puerperium. By the sixth to eighth week after birth, many women have returned to approximately their prepregnant weight if they gained the average 25 to 30 lb (11.4 to 13.6 kg). For others, a return to prepregnant weight may take longer. Women often express concern about the slow pace of their postpartum weight loss. Multiparas tend to be more positive than primiparas, probably because the multipara's previous experience has prepared her for the fact that the body does not immediately return to a prepregnant state.

Postpartum Chill

Frequently, the mother experiences intense tremors that resemble shivering from a chill immediately after birth. Several theories have been offered to explain this shivering: It is the result of the sudden release of pressure on the pelvic nerves after birth, a response to a fetus-to-mother transfusion that occurred during placental separation, a reaction to maternal epinephrine production during labor and birth, or a reaction to epidural anesthesia. If not followed by fever, this chill is of no clinical concern, but it is uncomfortable for the woman. The nurse can increase the woman's comfort by covering her with a warmed blanket and reassuring her that the shivering is a common, self-limiting situation. If she allows herself to go with the shaking, the shivering will last only a short time. Some women may also find a warm beverage helpful. Later in the puerperium, chill and fever indicate infection and require further evaluation.

Postpartum Diaphoresis

The elimination of excess fluid and waste products via the skin during the puerperium produces increased perspiration. Diaphoretic (sweating) episodes frequently occur at night, and the woman may awaken drenched with perspiration. This perspiration is not significant clinically, but the mother should be protected from chilling.

Afterpains

Afterpains are more common in multiparas than in primiparas and are caused by intermittent uterine contractions. Although the uterus of the primipara usually remains consistently contracted, the lost tone of the multiparous uterus results in alternate contraction and relaxation. This phenomenon also occurs if the uterus has been markedly distended, as with a multiple-gestation pregnancy or polyhydramnios, or if clots or placental fragments were retained. These afterpains may cause the mother severe discomfort for 2 to 3 days after birth. The administration of oxytocic agents stimulates uterine contraction and increases the discomfort of the afterpains. Because endogenous oxytocin is released when the baby suckles, breastfeeding also increases the frequency and severity of the afterpains. Lysine, an essential amino acid, has been identified as a supplement that decreases the incidence of pain following an episiotomy. The recommended adult dosage is 12 mg/kg of body weight per day. It is also present in dietary sources, including meat, cheese, fish, eggs, soybeans, and nuts.

A warm water bottle placed against the lower abdomen may reduce the discomfort of afterpains. In addition, the breastfeeding mother may find it helpful to take a mild analgesic agent approximately 1 hour before feeding her baby. The nurse can assure the nursing mother that the prescribed analgesics are not harmful to the newborn and help improve the quality of the breastfeeding experience. An analgesic is also helpful at bedtime if the afterpains interfere with the mother's rest.

Postpartum Psychologic Adaptations

The postpartum period is a time of readjustment and adaptation for the entire childbearing family, but especially for the mother. The woman experiences a variety of responses as she adjusts to a new family member, postpartum discomforts, changes in her body image, and the reality that she is no longer pregnant.

Taking-In and Taking-Hold

Initially after birth during the *taking-in* period, the woman tends to be passive and somewhat dependent. She follows suggestions, hesitates to make decisions, and is still rather preoccupied with her needs (Rubin, 1984). She may have a great need to talk about her perceptions of her labor and birth. This helps her work through the process, sort out the reality from her fantasized experience, and clarify anything that she did not understand. Food and sleep are major needs.

By the second or third day after birth, the new mother is often ready to resume control of her body, her mothering, and her life in general. Rubin (1984) labeled this the *taking-hold* period. If she is breastfeeding, she may worry about her technique or the quality of her milk. If her baby spits up after a feeding, she may view it as a personal failure. She may also feel demoralized by the fact that the nurse or an older family member handles her baby proficiently while she feels unsure and tentative. She requires assurance that she is doing well as a mother. Today's mothers seem to be more independent and adjust more rapidly, exhibiting behaviors of "taking-in" and "taking-hold" in shorter time periods than those previously identified.

Becoming a Mother (BAM)

Maternal role attainment (MRA) is the process by which a woman learns mothering behaviors and becomes comfortable with her identity as a mother. As the mother grows to know her baby and forms a relationship, the mother's maternal identity gradually and systematically evolves and she "binds in" to the infant (Rubin, 1984). In most cases, maternal role attainment occurs within 3 to 10 months after birth.

Mercer proposed replacing the term *maternal role attainment* with the term **becoming a mother (BAM)**. She stated that BAM "more accurately encompasses the dynamic transformation and evolution of a woman's persona than does MRA, and the term MRA should be discontinued" (Mercer, 2004, p. 226). BAM more accurately reflects the transition process of becoming a mother that changes throughout the maternal–child relationship.

Postpartum nurses need to be aware of the long-term adjustments and stresses that the childbearing family faces as its members adjust to new and different roles. Nursing interventions that foster the process of becoming a mother include the following categories:

- Instructing for newborn/infant caregiving
- Building awareness of and responsiveness to newborn/infant interactive capabilities
- Promoting maternal–infant attachment
- Preparing the women for the maternal social role preparation
- Encouraging interactive therapeutic nurse–client relationships

Maternal/social role preparation and interactive therapeutic nurse–client relationships have a greater impact on the progress of becoming a mother than formal teaching.

Professionalism in Practice   Enhancing Patient-Centered Care

Mercer (2006) emphasized the importance of individualized dialogue between the mother and the nurse, which involves "a mutual identification by the mother and the nurse of the mother's needs and the available resources among the mother's family and friends, her community, and the larger society. With the mother's input about her preferences for available assistance. . . . Appropriate referrals may be made" (p. 650). Professional nurses who follow Mercer's recommendations enhance the process of a mother and engage in patient-centered care.

Postpartum Blues

The **postpartum blues** consist of a transient period of depression that occurs during the first few days of the puerperium. It may be manifested by mood swings, anger, weepiness, anorexia, difficulty sleeping, and a feeling of being letdown. This mood change frequently occurs while the woman is still hospitalized, but it may occur at home as well. Changing hormone levels are certainly a factor; psychologic adjustments, an unsupportive environment, and insecurity also have been identified as potential causes. In addition, fatigue, discomfort, and overstimulation may play a role. Postpartum pain is found after both vaginal and cesarean births and has been shown to be associated with postpartum depression (Ding, Wang, Qu, et al., 2014). Managing acute postpartum pain supports the new mother's ability to emotionally attach and care for her baby.

Nurses should take cultural and ethnic influences into account when assessing for the signs of postpartum depression (PPD). In a Pregnancy Risk Assessment Monitoring System survey, women of Asian/Pacific Islander descent had more than 3 times the rate of PPD than their White counterparts and were more likely to be diagnosed with PPD after the birth of a female baby (Liu & Tronick, 2013). Gestational diabetes was a risk factor for PPD among African American women. Some characteristics, such as the baby's gender, are not commonly thought of as predictors for depression, but are predictive in specific ethnic groups. Across all the ethnic groups, prenatal depression is a strong predictor of PPD and assessment for signs of depression both before and after the birth is best practice.

EVIDENCE-BASED PRACTICE | Psychosocial and Psychologic Interventions for Preventing Postpartum Depression

Clinical Question

What kinds of psychosocial and psychologic interventions may be helpful in the prevention of postpartum depression?

The Evidence

There is substantial evidence identifying the risk factors for the development of postpartum depression. It has been theorized that these risk factors could serve as the basis for designing psychosocial and psychologic interventions that could be offered during pregnancy and the immediate postpartum period to prevent the occurrence of this serious condition. Two researchers conducted a systematic review to first discover if these types of interventions are effective preventive measures. A secondary goal of the review was to determine the specific aspects of these interventions that were effective, such as professionally versus lay-based interventions; individually based versus group-based interventions; effects of interventions on onset and duration of depression; and relationship of treatment and specific risk factors. This review was structured and peer reviewed and published in the rigorous *Cochrane Database of Systematic Reviews*, which forms the strongest level of evidence. Twenty-eight studies with samples totaling almost 17,000 women were represented in this review.

Women who received psychosocial and/or psychologic interventions were considerably less likely to experience postpartum depression (Dennis & Dowswell, 2014). The most promising interventions were the provision of intensive, individualized postpartum home visits provided by nurses or nurse-midwives. These women had nearly half the rate of postpartum depression as women without this support. Peer-provided telephone support by lay women was also successful, as was interpersonal psychotherapy provided by professional counselors. Using risk factors to identify mothers who were most likely to develop postpartum depression aided in its prevention.

Best Practice

Psychosocial and psychologic interventions are clearly effective in preventing postpartum depression. Mothers should be assessed for risk factors and interventions should be applied accordingly. These interventions can be provided through professionally based home visits or psychotherapy, or by lay peers via telephone consultation.

Clinical Reasoning

What are some of the prenatal risk factors that might help identify women who should receive interventions for prevention of postpartum depression? What might be the major components of a psychosocial or psychologic intervention?

Postpartum blues usually resolve naturally within 10 to 14 days, but if they persist or symptoms worsen, the woman may need evaluation for postpartum depression (see Chapter 30 for an in-depth discussion of postpartum depression and psychosis). Ideally, a depression assessment should be completed each trimester to update a pregnant woman's risk status for postpartum depression). If not done previously, the nurse assesses the woman for predisposing factors during labor and the postpartum stay. Several depression scales are available for assessing postpartum depression (see Chapter 30 for further discussion).

Importance of Social Support

After the birth of a baby, a woman and her partner may find that family relationships become increasingly important. The attention that their baby receives from family members is a source of satisfaction to the new parents. In many cases, the ties to the woman's family become especially good. New fathers may report that their relationships with their in-laws become far more positive and supportive. However, the increased family interaction can be a source of stress, especially for new mothers, who tend to have more contact with the families.

Developing Cultural Competence Middle Eastern Initial Postpartum Experience

In many countries in the Middle East that follow a patriarchal system, the new mother and her baby stay with the husband's family following the birth. Frequent visits from the woman's family are discouraged and may even be viewed as burdensome by the husband's family. Typically, only women visit the new mother during the postpartum period. For the birth of the first baby, the wife's parents are expected to purchase all of the baby's supplies and clothing.

The new parents may also have increasing contact with other parents of small children while contact with coworkers declines. Of great concern are women and their partners who have no families or friends with whom to form social networks. Isolation at a time when women feel an increased need for support can result in tremendous stress and is often a contributing factor in situations of postpartum depression, child neglect, or abuse. New mother support groups are helpful for women who lack a social support system. Postpartum doulas are professionals trained to help the new mother after the birth of the baby. As a "mother's helper," postpartum doula services are tailored to help the new mother feel as rested as possible and well-nourished and to keep her household in good order so that she can focus her energy on her new baby.

Development of Family Attachment

Some parents may lack any experience with babies and may feel overwhelmed by the newborn. Bonding is a series of steps in which the mother, father, and baby develop relationships.

Maternal–Newborn Attachment Behavior

A mother's first interaction with her newborn is influenced by many factors, including her involvement with her family of origin, her relationships, the stability of her home environment, the communication patterns she developed, and the degree of nurturing she received as a child. These factors have shaped the person she has become. The following personal characteristics are also important.

- *Level of trust.* What level of trust has this mother developed in response to her life experiences? What is her philosophy of childrearing? Will she be able to treat her baby as a unique individual with changing needs that should be met as much as possible?
- *Level of self-esteem.* How much does she value herself as a woman and as a mother? Does she feel generally able to cope with the adjustments of life?
- *Capacity for enjoying herself.* Is the mother able to find pleasure in everyday activities and human relationships?
- *Adequacy of knowledge about childbearing and childrearing.* What beliefs about the course of pregnancy, the capabilities of newborns, previous experiences with infants/children, and the nature of her emotions may influence her behavior at first contact with her newborn and later?
- *Prevailing mood or usual feeling tone.* Is the woman predominantly content, angry, depressed, or anxious? Is she sensitive to her own feelings and those of others? Will she be able to accept her own needs and to obtain support in meeting them?
- *Reactions to the present pregnancy.* Was the pregnancy planned? Did it go smoothly? Were there ongoing life events that enhanced her pregnancy or depleted her reserves of energy? How have other life roles changed because of her pregnancy and motherhood?

By the time of birth, each mother has developed an emotional orientation of some kind to the baby based on these factors.

Professionalism in Practice Promoting Skin-to-Skin Contact

Many hospital units remove newborns from their mother following birth to allow convenient assessment and performance of procedures by hospital staff despite a preponderance of evidence that supports immediate skin-to-skin contact (SSC) between mother (or father) and the newborn. Nurses are the professionals most often at the client's bedside; they have the power and an obligation to serve as leaders and change agents by promoting clinical practices that are supported by research evidence.

INITIAL MATERNAL ATTACHMENT BEHAVIOR

After labor and birth, a new mother will demonstrate a fairly regular pattern of maternal behaviors as she continues to familiarize herself with her newborn. In a progression of touching activities, the mother proceeds from fingertip exploration of the newborn's extremities toward palmar contact with larger body areas and finally to enfolding the baby with the whole hand and arm. The time taken to accomplish these steps varies from minutes to days. The mother increases the proportion of time spent in the *en face* position (Figure 28–4). She arranges herself or the newborn so that she has direct face-to-face and eye-to-eye contact. There is an intense interest in having the baby's eyes open. When the newborn's eyes are open, the mother characteristically greets and talks in high-pitched tones to her baby.

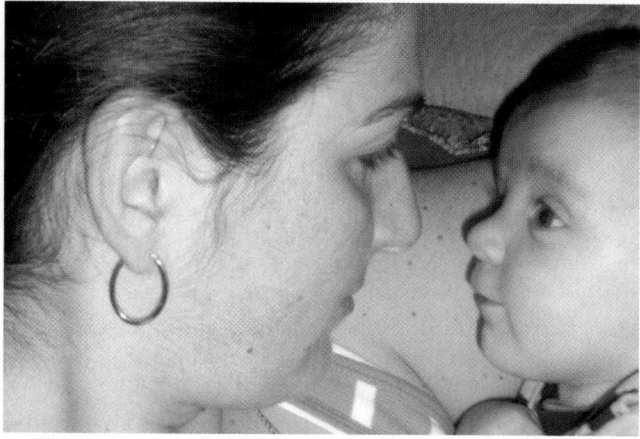

Figure 28–4 The mother has direct face-to-face and eye-to-eye contact in the *en face* position.

SOURCE: Joanna and Christopher Allen.

In most instances, the mother relies heavily on her senses of sight, touch, and hearing in getting to know what her baby is really like. She tends also to respond verbally to any sounds emitted by the newborn, such as cries, coughs, sneezes, and grunts. The sense of smell may be involved as well.

While interacting with her newborn, the mother may be experiencing shock, disbelief, or denial. She may state, "I can't believe she's finally here" or "I feel like he is a stranger." On the other hand, feelings of connectedness between the newborn and the rest of the family can be expressed in positive or negative terms: "She's got your cute nose, Daddy" or "Oh, no! He looks just like Matthew, and he was an impossible baby." A mother's facial expressions or the frequency and content of her questions may demonstrate concerns about the newborn's general condition or normality, especially if her pregnancy was complicated or if a previous baby was not healthy.

During the first few days after her baby's birth, the new mother applies herself to the task of getting to know her baby. This is termed the *acquaintance phase*. If the newborn gives clear behavioral cues about needs, the baby's responses to mothering will be predictable, which will make the mother feel effective and competent. Other behaviors that make a baby more attractive to caretakers are smiling, grasping a finger, nursing eagerly, and being easy to console.

During this time the newborn is also becoming acquainted. Within a few days after birth, newborns show signs of recognizing recurrent situations and responding to changes in routine. To the extent that their mother is their world, it can be said that they are actively acquainting themselves with her.

During the *phase of mutual regulation*, mother and newborn seek to determine the degree of control each partner in their relationship will exert. In this phase of adjustment, a balance is sought between the needs of the mother and the needs of the baby. The most important consideration is that each should obtain a good measure of enjoyment from the interaction. During this phase, negative maternal feelings are likely to surface or intensify. Because "everyone knows that mothers love their babies," these negative feelings often go unexpressed and are allowed to build up. If they are expressed, the response of friends, relatives, or healthcare providers is often to deny the feelings to the mother: "You don't mean that." Some negative feelings are normal in the first few days after birth, and the nurse should be supportive when the mother vocalizes these feelings.

When mutual regulation arrives at the point where both mother and baby primarily enjoy each other's company, reciprocity has been achieved. **Reciprocity** is an interactional cycle that occurs simultaneously between mother and baby. It involves mutual cuing behaviors, expectancy, rhythmicity, and synchrony. The mother develops a new relationship with an individual who has a unique character and evokes a response entirely different from the fantasy response of pregnancy. When reciprocity is synchronous, the interaction between mother and baby is mutually gratifying and is sought and initiated by both partners (Feldman, 2012).

Clinical Tip

Newborns are sometimes taken from their parents immediately after birth and placed in a special care or intensive care nursery. This separation can interfere with the normal attachment process. If this occurs, parents should be brought to the nursery as soon as possible to interact with their babies, and should be allowed to hold and care for their babies as much as possible. If the newborn is in an incubator and cannot be held, encourage the parents to stroke the baby's hand, foot, or cheek. Provide reassurance that this will not hurt the baby and is in fact beneficial.

Father–Newborn Interactions

In Western cultures, commitment to family-centered maternity care has fostered interest in understanding the feelings and experiences of the new father. Evidence suggests that the father has a strong attraction to his newborn, and that the feelings he experiences are similar to the mother's feelings of attachment (Figure 28–5). The characteristic sense of absorption, preoccupation, and interest in the baby demonstrated by fathers during early contact is termed **engrossment**. Differences

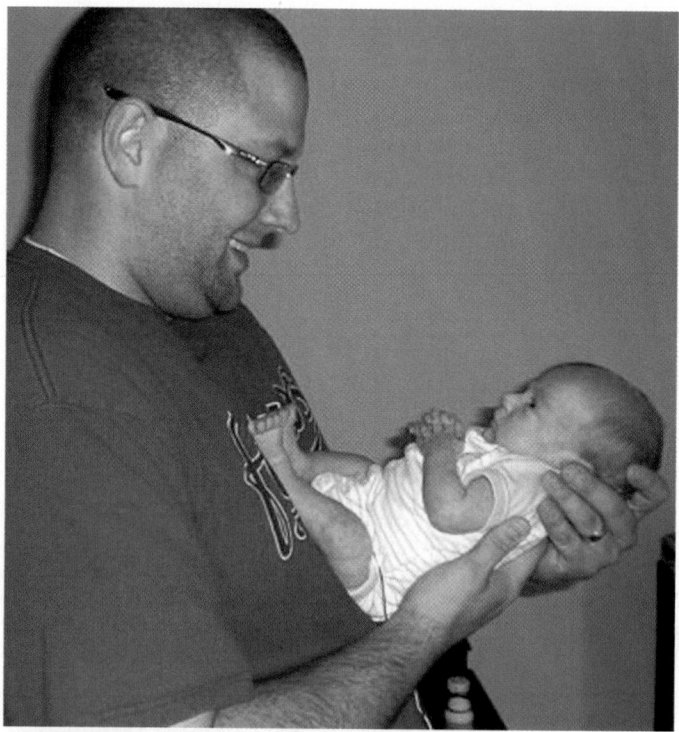

Figure 28–5 The father experiences strong feelings of attraction during engrossment.

SOURCE: Joanna and Christopher Allen.

in involvement still exist among fathers in Western culture and may be influenced by factors other than culture (e.g., previous experience with paternal role or exposure to male/father role models).

Developing Cultural Competence **Muslim Paternal Attachment**

In some cultures, there may be little involvement of the father in newborn care. In the Muslim culture, for example, emphasis on childrearing and infant care activities is on the mother and extended female family members. Nurses need to be aware of cultural differences when evaluating a father's interaction with his newborn.

Siblings and Others

Babies are capable of maintaining a number of strong attachments without loss of quality. These attachments may include siblings, grandparents, aunts, and uncles. The social setting and personality of the individual seem to be significant factors in the development of multiple attachments. Birth centers are especially geared toward the inclusion of the family in the birth process. In the hospital setting, the advent of open visiting hours and rooming-in permits siblings and others to participate in the attachment process.

Cultural Influences in the Postpartum Period

Whereas Western culture places primary emphasis on the events of birth, many other cultures place greater emphasis on the postpartum period. For women not of the dominant American culture, the new mother's culture and personal values influence her beliefs about her postpartum care. Her expectations about food, fluids, rest, hygiene, medications, relief measures, support, and counsel—as well as other aspects of her life—will be influenced by the beliefs and values of her family and cultural group. Sometimes, a new mother's wishes will differ from the expectations of the healthcare provider or nurse. (See Chapter 2 for an in-depth discussion of cultural factors.)

All nurses belong to their particular ethnoculture and also share in the culture of health care. As a part of the healthcare cultural group, nurses implement practices that support their general beliefs, such as offering food in the recovery period following birth, providing iced fluids, expecting the woman to ambulate as soon as possible, and assuming the woman will want to shower and perhaps wash her hair soon after birth. It is important for nurses to recognize that they are approaching their client's care from their own perspective and that, to individualize care for each mother, they need to assess the woman's preferences, her level of acculturation and assimilation to Western culture, her linguistic abilities, and her educational level (Callister, 2014; Lauderdale, 2012). In addition, the nurse should have the mother exercise her choices when possible and support those choices, with the help of cultural awareness and a sound knowledge base.

The woman of European heritage may expect to eat a full meal and have large amounts of iced fluids after the birth, in the belief that the food restores energy and the fluids help replace fluid lost during the labor. She may want to ambulate shortly after the birth, shower, wash her hair, and put on a fresh gown. She may expect a short stay in the hospital and may or may not

be interested in educational classes. Women of the Islamic faith may have specific modesty requirements; the woman must be completely covered, with only her feet and hands exposed, and no man, other than the husband or a family member, may be alone with her (Lauderdale, 2012).

Some cultures emphasize certain postpartum routines or rituals for mother and baby that are designed to restore the hot–cold balance of the body. Some women of Hispanic, African, and Asian cultures may avoid cold after birth. This prohibition includes cold air, wind, and all water (even if heated). On the other hand, some women of traditional Mexican descent may avoid eating "hot" foods such as pork just after the birth of a baby (considered a "hot" experience). It is important to note that each individual or cultural group may define hot and cold conditions and foods differently. The nurse should ask each woman what she can eat and what foods she thinks would be helpful for healing. The nurse may encourage family members to bring preferred foods and drinks for the mother.

In many cultures, the extended family plays an essential role during the puerperium. The grandmother is often the primary helper to the mother and newborn. She brings wisdom and experience, allowing the new mother time to rest and giving her ready access to someone who can help with problems and concerns as they arise. African American mothers often model their mothering skills after their older female relatives. In addition, these same older female relatives frequently provide child care as needed (Purnell, 2013).

It is important to ensure access of all family members to the mother and newborn. Visiting hours may be waived to allow family members or authority figures access to the mother and newborn. These practices show respect and foster a blending of old and new behaviors to meet the goals of all concerned (Purnell, 2013).

Developing Cultural Competence **Caring for the Orthodox Jewish Couple**

The orthodox Jewish couple's beliefs and practices are strictly adhered to in their dress, communication, dietary practices, and activities of daily living in the postpartum time. The nurse should assist the woman in maintaining her modesty in her dress and keeping her hair covered at all times. For the first 7 days after delivery, the woman will be given special treatment and will be cared for by family members. Jewish clients may request a kosher diet. Some traditional Jewish couples avoid physical contact while the woman is experiencing any vaginal discharge; unfortunately, the man following this custom may be viewed as being unsupportive by the staff during the postpartum period. Resting after childbirth is considered crucial for the first 6 weeks. The woman will breastfeed her newborn. The baby will not be named nor will the newborn boy be circumcised until a later date after discharge from the hospital. The Sabbath is sacred and begins at sundown on Friday evening and ends after dark on Saturday. During this time neither the man nor the woman will use electricity, travel, or write. They will not tear or cut anything. So if the woman is in the hospital during the Sabbath, the nurse should be sensitive to the fact that any forms that may need to be signed will have to be signed before or after the Sabbath. For example, the orthodox woman will need the nurse to adjust an electric bed, turn off/on lights, tear pieces of toilet paper for her to use, etc. The woman will not leave the hospital and travel home until after the Sabbath (Lauderdale, 2012).

Postpartum Nursing Assessment

Comprehensive care is based on a thorough assessment that identifies individual needs or potential problems.

Risk Factors

Ongoing assessment and client education during the puerperium is designed to meet the needs of the childbearing family and to detect and treat possible complications. Table 28–2 identifies factors that may place the new mother at risk during the postpartum period. The nurse uses this knowledge during the assessment and is particularly alert for possible complications associated with identified risk factors.

Physical Assessment

The nurse should remember several principles when preparing for and completing the assessment of the postpartum woman:

- Select a time that will provide the most accurate data. Palpating the fundus when the woman has a full bladder, for example, may give false information about the progress of involution. Ask the woman to void before assessment.

- Consider the client's need for possible premedication before any painful assessment such as fundal massage.

- Provide an explanation of the purpose of regular assessment to the woman.

- Ensure that the woman is relaxed before starting; perform the procedures as gently as possible to avoid unnecessary discomfort.

- Document and report the results as clearly as possible.

- Take appropriate precautions to prevent exposure to body fluids.

While performing the physical assessment, the nurse should also be teaching the woman. For example, when assessing the breasts of a lactating woman, the nurse can discuss breast care, breast milk production, the letdown reflex, and breast self-examination. A new mother may be very receptive to instruction on postpartum abdominal tightening exercises when the nurse assesses the woman's fundal height and diastasis. The assessment provides an excellent time to provide information about the body's postpartum physical and anatomic changes as well as danger signs to report. See *Teaching Highlights: Common Postpartum Concerns.* Because the time new mothers spend in the postpartum unit is limited, nurses need to use every available opportunity for client education about self-care. To assist nurses in recognizing these opportunities, examples of client teaching during the assessment are provided throughout the following discussion.

VITAL SIGNS

Many nurses begin by assessing vital signs because the findings are more accurate when they are obtained with the woman at rest. In addition, establishing whether the vital signs are within the expected normal range will assist the nurse in determining if other assessments are needed. For instance, if the temperature is elevated, the nurse considers the time since birth and gathers information to determine whether the woman is dehydrated or whether an infection is developing.

Temperature elevations (less than 38.0°C [100.4°F]) caused by normal processes should last for only 24 hours.

TABLE 28–2 Postpartum High-Risk Factors

FACTOR	MATERNAL IMPLICATION
Preeclampsia	↑ Blood pressure
	↑ CNS irritability
	↑ Need for bed rest → ↑ risk thrombophlebitis
Diabetes	Need for insulin regulation
	Episodes of hypoglycemia or hyperglycemia
	↓ Healing
Cardiac disease	↑ Maternal exhaustion
Cesarean birth	↑ Healing needs
	↑ Pain from incision
	↑ Risk of infection
	↑ Length of hospitalization
	Exacerbation of carpal tunnel syndrome
Overdistention of uterus (multiple gestation, hydramnios)	↑ Risk of hemorrhage
	↑ Risk of thrombophlebitis (C/S risk)
	↑ Risk of anemia
	↑ Risk of breastfeeding problems (C/S risk)
	↑ Stretching of abdominal muscles
	↑ Incidence and severity of afterpains
Abruptio placentae, placenta previa	Hemorrhage → anemia
	↓ Uterine contractility after birth → ↑ infection risk
Precipitous labor (less than 3 hr)	↑ Risk of lacerations to birth canal → hemorrhage
Prolonged labor (greater than 24 hr)	Exhaustion
	↑ Risk of hemorrhage
	Nutritional and fluid depletion
	↑ Bladder atony and/or trauma
	↑ Pain and bruising from prolonged time in stirrups
Difficult birth	Exhaustion
	↑ Risk of perineal lacerations
	↑ Risk of hematomas
	↑ Risk of hemorrhage → anemia
Extended period of time in stirrups at birth	↑ Risk of thrombophlebitis
Retained placenta	↑ Risk of hemorrhage
	↑ Risk of infection

The nurse evaluates any elevation of temperature in light of associated signs and symptoms and carefully reviews the woman's history to identify other factors, such as premature rupture of membranes (PROM) or prolonged labor, which might increase the incidence of infection in the genital tract.

TEACHING HIGHLIGHTS | Common Postpartum Concerns

Several postpartum occurrences cause special concern for mothers. The nurse will frequently be asked about the following events.

Source of Concern	Explanation
Gush of blood that sometimes occurs when she first arises	Results from normal pooling of blood in the vagina when the woman lies down to rest or sleep. Gravity causes blood to flow out when she stands.
Passing clots	Blood pools at the top of the vagina and forms clots that are passed upon rising or sitting on the toilet.
Night sweats	Normal physiologic occurrence that results as the body attempts to eliminate excess fluids that were present during pregnancy. May be aggravated by a plastic mattress pad.
Afterpains	More common in multiparas. Caused by contraction and relaxation of uterus. Increased by oxytocin, breastfeeding. Relieved with mild analgesics and time.
"Large stomach" after birth and failure to lose all weight gained during pregnancy	The baby, amniotic fluid, and placenta account for only a portion of the weight gained during pregnancy. The remainder takes approximately 6 weeks to lose. Abdomen also appears large because of decreased muscle tone. Postpartum exercises will help.

Alterations in vital signs may indicate complications, so the nurse assesses them at regular intervals. After an immediate, transient rise after birth, the blood pressure should remain stable. The pulse often shows a characteristic slowness that is no cause for alarm. Pulse rates return to prepregnant norms very quickly unless complications arise.

SAFETY ALERT!
During the first few hours after birth, the woman may have some orthostatic hypotension. This will cause her to have a lower blood pressure (BP) reading in a sitting position. For the most accurate reading use manual BP cuffs and measure the woman's BP with her in the same position each time, preferably lying on her back with her arm at her side. Because of the propensity for hypotension, the nurse should assist the mother the first few times she attempts to ambulate after childbirth.

The nurse informs the woman of her vital signs and provides information about the normal changes in blood pressure and pulse. This may present an opportunity to determine whether the mother knows how to assess her own and her baby's temperature, how to read a thermometer, and how to select a thermometer from the wide variety now available.

AUSCULTATION OF LUNGS
The breath sounds should be clear. Women who have been treated for preterm labor or preeclampsia are at higher risk for pulmonary edema. (See *Care of the Woman With a Hypertensive Disorder* in Chapter 15 for further discussion.)

BREASTS
Before examining the breasts, the nurse dons gloves and then assesses the fit and support provided by the woman's bra and, if appropriate, offers information about how to select a supportive bra. A properly fitting bra supports the breasts and helps maintain breast shape by limiting stretching of supporting ligaments and connective tissue. If the mother is breastfeeding, the straps of the bra should be cloth, not elastic (because cloth has less stretch and provides more support), and easily adjustable. The back should be wide and have at least three rows of hooks

to adjust for fit. Traditional nursing bras have a fixed inner cup and a separate half cup that can be unhooked for breastfeeding while the cup continues to support the breast. Purchasing a nursing bra one size larger than the prepregnant size will usually result in a good fit because the breasts increase in size with milk production.

Clinical Tip
An easy way to remember the components specific to the postpartum examination is to remember the term BUBBLEHE: B–breast, U–uterus, B–bladder, B–bowel, L–lochia, E–episiotomy/laceration/edema, H–Homans/hemorrhoids, E–emotional. Some agencies include a final R (BUBBLEHER) to represent RhoGAM and rubella immunizations (see Chapter 29 for further discussion).

The nurse can then ask the woman to remove her bra so the breasts can be examined. The nurse notes the size and shape of the breasts and any abnormalities, reddened or hot areas, or engorgement. The breasts are lightly palpated for softness, slight firmness associated with filling, firmness associated with engorgement, warmth, and tenderness. The nipples are assessed for fissures, cracks, soreness, and inversion. The nurse teaches the woman the characteristics of the breast and explains how to recognize problems such as fissures and cracks in the nipples.

The nonbreastfeeding mother is assessed for evidence of breast discomfort, and relief measures are instituted if necessary. (See discussion of lactation suppression in the nonbreastfeeding mother in Chapter 29.) Breast assessment findings for a nonbreastfeeding woman may be recorded as follows: "Breasts soft, filling, no evidence of nipple tenderness or cracking, nipples everted."

ABDOMEN AND FUNDUS
Before examination of the abdomen, the woman should void. This practice ensures that a full bladder is not displacing the uterus or causing any uterine atony; if atony is present, other causes (such as uterine relaxation associated with a regional block, overstretched uterus, or distended bladder) must be investigated.

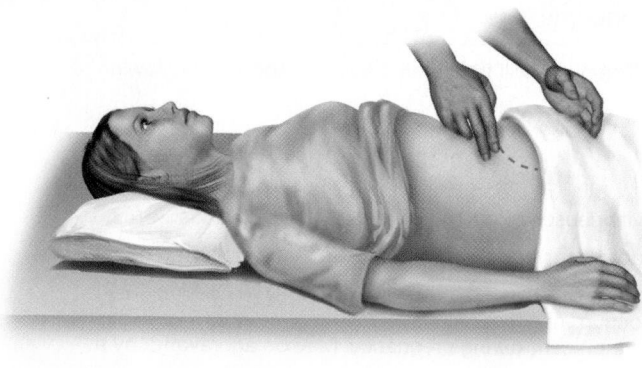

Figure 28–6 **Measurement of descent of fundus for the woman with a vaginal birth. The fundus is located two fingerbreadths below the umbilicus.**

Clinical Tip

Gloves may be put on before assessing the abdomen and fundus and must be worn when you are ready to assess the perineum and lochia.

The nurse determines the relationship of the fundus to the umbilicus and also assesses the firmness of the fundus. The top of the fundus is measured in finger breadths above, below, or at the umbilicus (Figure 28–6). See Assessing the Status of the Uterine Fundus After Vaginal or Cesarean Birth in the *Clinical Skills Manual* SKILLS. The nurse notes whether the fundus is in the midline or displaced to either side of the abdomen. If not midline, the uterus position should be located. The most common cause of displacement is a full bladder; this finding requires further assessment. If the fundus is in midline but higher than expected, it is usually associated with clots within the uterus. The nurse should then record the results of the assessment.

Clinical Tip

During postpartum assessment, a firm uterus typically feels like a grapefruit because the muscles are well contracted. If the uterus loses its ability to contract and begins to relax, it is called *boggy*. A boggy uterus feels softer, like a sponge, or may become so relaxed that you cannot feel it at all. If the uterus is boggy but you can still feel it, massage it until it becomes firm. If you cannot feel it at all, place the side of one hand just above the woman's symphysis pubis to provide stability. Then place the other hand at the level of the umbilicus. (The fundus may have risen to this level because it is relaxed and filling with blood.) Press deeply into the abdomen and massage in a circular motion. You will usually feel the uterus begin to firm up under your hand. If you do not, move your hand slightly lower on the abdomen, and repeat the process.

In the woman who has had a cesarean birth, the abdominal incision is extremely tender. The nurse should palpate the fundus with extreme care and inspect the abdominal incision for signs of healing, such as approximation (edges of incision appear "glued" together), bleeding, and any signs of infection, including drainage, foul odor, or redness. The nurse should document whether internal sutures, Steri-Strips, or staples are intact. The nurse can also review characteristics of normal healing, incision care, and discuss signs of infection.

Clinical Tip

Assessing the status of the uterine fundus may be uncomfortable. In addition to explaining the importance of the assessment to the mother, you can show her how to perform frequent light massage of the fundus herself to promote uterine involution. She may be delighted to be able to feel the difference between where the fundus is now and where the top of the uterus was just prior to delivery. Involving her in her own care encourages her participation. In addition, having her massage her own uterus may lessen bleeding and reduce the need for more thorough massage.

LOCHIA

The nurse then evaluates the lochia, including character, amount, odor, and the presence of clots. During the first 1 to 3 days, the lochia should be rubra. A few small clots are normal and occur as a result of blood pooling in the vagina. However, the passage of numerous or large clots is abnormal, and the cause should be investigated immediately. After 2 to 3 days, the lochia flow becomes serosa.

Lochia should never exceed a moderate amount, such as that needed to partially saturate perineal pads daily, with an average of six. However, because this number is influenced by an individual woman's pad-changing practices, as well as the absorbency of the pad, the nurse needs to question her about the length of time the current pad has been in use, whether the amount is normal compared with her typical menstrual period, and whether any clots were passed before this examination, such as during voiding. If heavy bleeding is reported but not seen, the nurse asks the woman to put on a clean perineal pad and then reassesses the woman's pad in 1 hour (Figure 28–7). See Evaluating Lochia in the *Clinical Skills Manual* SKILLS.

SAFETY ALERT!

If blood loss exceeds the guidelines given in this chapter, weigh the perineal pads and the chux pads to estimate the blood loss more accurately. Typically, 1 g = 1 mL blood. Because blood can pool below the woman on the absorbent pad make sure you elevate the buttocks as part of your assessment.

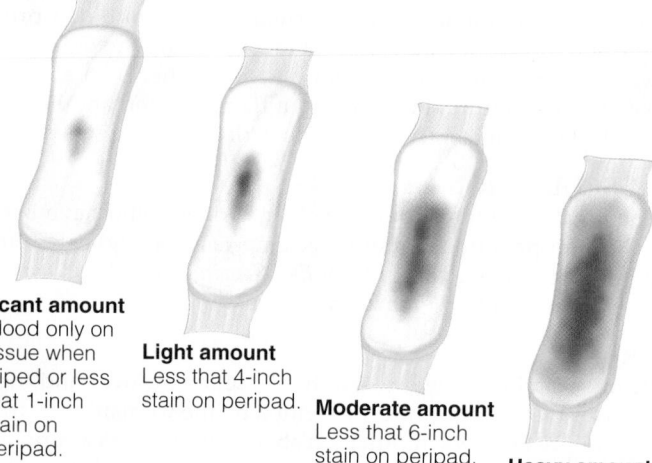

Scant amount
Blood only on tissue when wiped or less that 1-inch stain on peripad.

Light amount
Less that 4-inch stain on peripad.

Moderate amount
Less that 6-inch stain on peripad.

Heavy amount
Saturated peripad within 1 hour.

Figure 28–7 **Suggested guideline for assessing lochia volume.**

TABLE 28–3 Changes in Lochia That Cause Concern

CHANGE	POSSIBLE PROBLEM	NURSING ACTION
Presence of clots	Inadequate uterine contractions that allow bleeding from vessels at the placental site	Assess location and firmness of fundus. Assess voiding pattern. Record and report findings.
Persistent lochia rubra	Inadequate uterine contractions; retained placental fragments; infection; undetected cervical laceration	Assess location and firmness of fundus. Assess activity pattern. Assess for signs of infection. Record and report findings.

Clots and heavy bleeding may be caused by uterine relaxation (atony), retained placental fragments, or rarely, an unknown cervical laceration (seen as heavy bleeding but with firm fundus), that may require further assessment (Table 28–3). Because of the evacuation of the uterine cavity during cesarean birth, women with such surgery usually have less lochia after the first 24 hours than mothers who give birth vaginally. If the woman is at increased risk for bleeding, or is actually experiencing heavy flow of lochia rubra, her blood pressure, pulse, and uterus need to be assessed frequently, and the healthcare provider may prescribe oxytocin (Pitocin), methylergonovine maleate (Methergine), or misoprostol (Cytotec).

The odor of the lochia is inoffensive and never foul. If a foul odor is present, so is an infection. When using narrative nursing notes, document the amount of lochia first, followed by character. For example:

- Lochia: moderate rubra
- Lochia: small rubra/serosa

Clinical Tip

The parity, length of time since delivery, method of delivery, size of baby/gestation (and other factors that could cause hyperextension of the uterus such as multiple gestation, polyhydramnios, and large-for-gestational age) must be considered when deciding whether the amount and color of the lochia is appropriate.

PERINEUM

The perineum is inspected with the woman lying in a Sims position. The nurse lifts the buttock to expose the perineum and anus.

If an episiotomy was done or a laceration required suturing, the nurse assesses the wound. To evaluate the state of healing, the nurse inspects the wound for **r**edness, **e**dema, **e**cchymosis, **d**ischarge/drainage, and **a**pproximation (REEDA scale). After 24 hours, some edema may still be present, but the skin edges should be well approximated so that gentle pressure does not separate them. Gentle palpation should elicit minimal tenderness, and there should be no hardened areas suggesting infection. Ecchymosis interferes with normal healing, as does infection. Foul odors associated with drainage indicate infection. Hematomas sometimes occur, although these are considered abnormal.

The nurse next assesses whether hemorrhoids are present around the anus (Figure 28–8). If present, they are assessed for size, number, and pain or tenderness. (See Postpartum Perineal Assessment in the *Clinical Skills Manual* SKILLS .)

During the assessment, the nurse talks with the woman to determine the effectiveness of comfort measures that have been used. The nurse provides teaching about the episiotomy or perineal laceration. Some women do not thoroughly understand what and where an episiotomy is, and they may believe that the stitches must be removed as with other types of surgery. Frequently, when women fear that the stitches must be removed manually, they are afraid to ask about them. While explaining the findings of the assessment, the nurse provides information about the episiotomy, its location, and the signs that are being

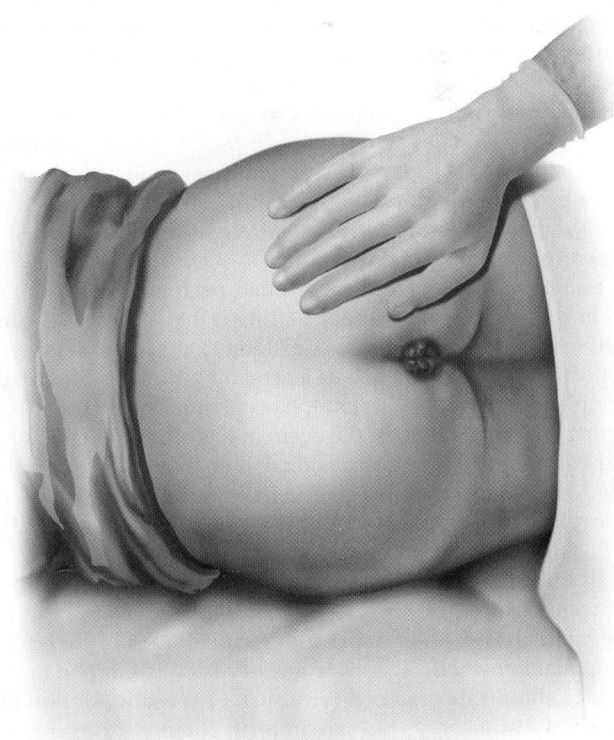

Figure 28–8 Intact perineum with hemorrhoids.

assessed. In addition, the nurse can add that the sutures are special and will dissolve slowly over the next few weeks as the tissues heal. By the time the sutures are dissolved, the tissues are strong and the incision edges will not separate. This is also an opportunity to teach comfort measures that may be used and reinforce the need to consult with the healthcare provider before using over-the-counter (OTC) medications/supplements if breastfeeding (see section on *Relief of Perineal Discomfort* in Chapter 29).

Clinical Tip

In evaluating the perineum, use the REEDA scale as a quick re-minder of what to assess. Specifically:

R = redness

E = edema or swelling

E = ecchymosis or bruising

D = discharge/drainage

A = approximation (how well the edges of an incision—the episi-otomy—or a repaired laceration seem to be holding together)

An example of documenting a perineal assessment might read: "Midline episiotomy; no edema, tenderness, or ecchy-mosis present. Skin edges well approximated" or, if a perineal laceration repair, "Skin edges intact, no edema, tenderness, or ecchymosis, pain meds helpful. Woman reports sitz bath and astringent wipes or pain relief measures are controlling discomfort."

LOWER EXTREMITIES

Postpartum women are at increased risk for *thrombophlebitis*, thrombus formation, and inflammation involving the leg vein (see Chapter 30 for a discussion of thrombophlebitis). If throm-bophlebitis occurs, the most likely site will be the women's legs. To assess for thrombophlebitis, the nurse should have the woman stretch her legs out with the knees slightly flexed and the legs relaxed. The nurse then grasps the woman's foot and sharply dorsiflexes it. The second leg is assessed in the same way. No discomfort or pain should be present. If pain is elic-ited, the nurse notifies the healthcare provider that the woman has a positive Homans sign (Figure 28–9). The pain is caused by inflammation of the vessel. The nurse also evaluates the legs for edema by comparing both legs because usually only one leg is involved. Any areas of redness, tenderness, and increased skin temperature are also noted.

Some facilities have discontinued performing a Homans sign in the nursing assessment, stating it is not diagnostic and could lead to emboli if a clot is dislodged during assessment. Supporters advocate its use as a screening tool, and there are no published reports of an emboli occurring as a result of per-forming a Homans sign. In the event of a positive Homans sign, diagnosis is made by compression or duplex ultrasonography. Low-dose heparin therapy is used in postpartum women who do develop a deep venous thrombosis (Cunningham et al., 2014; James, 2014).

Early ambulation is an important aspect in the prevention of thrombophlebitis. Most women are able to be up shortly after birth or once they have fully recovered from the effects of regional anesthetic agents, if one has been used. The moth-er's legs should be assessed for return of sensation following regional anesthesia. The cesarean birth client requires range-of-motion exercises until she is ambulating more freely. If the mother is unable to get up soon after delivery, sequential com-pression devices may be used.

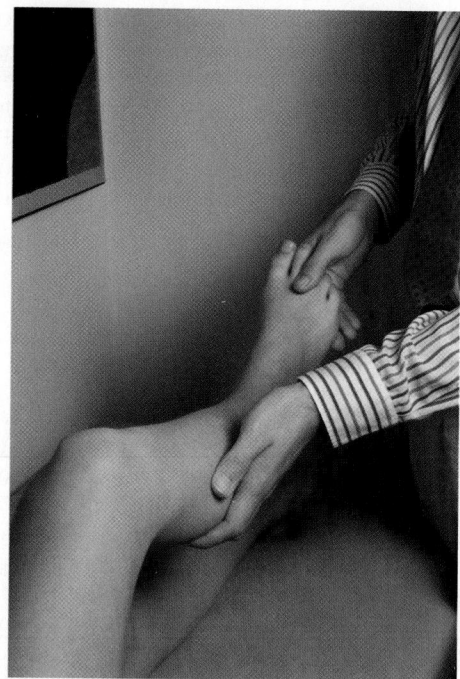

Figure 28–9 **Homans sign. With the woman's knee flexed, the nurse dorsiflexes the foot. Pain in the foot or leg is a positive Homans sign.**

SOURCE: © Image Source/Getty Images.

Client teaching associated with assessment of the lower extremities focuses on the signs and symptoms of thrombophle-bitis. In addition, the nurse may review self-care measures to promote circulation and measures to prevent thrombophlebitis, such as leg exercises that may be performed in bed, dorsiflexion on an hourly basis while on bed rest, ambulation, and avoiding pressure behind the knees and crossing the legs.

The nurse records the results of the assessment on a flow-sheet or a summary nursing note. If tenderness and warmth have been noted, they might be recorded as follows: "Tender-ness, warmth, slight edema, and slight redness noted on pos-terior aspect of left calf—positive Homans. Woman advised to avoid pressure to this area; lower leg elevated and moist heat applied per agency protocol. Call placed to Dr. Garcia to report findings."

ELIMINATION

During the hours after birth, the nurse carefully monitors a new mother's bladder status. A boggy uterus, a displaced uterus, or a palpable bladder are signs of bladder distention and require nursing intervention.

The postpartum woman can quickly show signs of bladder distention, possibly as soon as 1 to 2 hours after childbirth. This distention results because of normal postpartum diuresis. The nurse should assess the bladder for distention until the woman demonstrates complete emptying of the bladder with each voiding. The nurse may employ techniques to facilitate voiding, such as helping the woman out of bed to void or pouring warm water on the vulva, running water in the sink, and encouraging the woman to relax and take deep breaths. The healthcare pro-vider will order catheterization when the bladder is distended and the woman cannot void, when she is voiding small amounts (less than 100 mL) frequently, or when no voiding has occurred in 8 hours. Although many healthcare providers write orders stating that the woman can be catheterized in 8 hours if she has not voided, the nurse needs to assess the bladder and any voiding pattern frequently before the end of the 8-hour period. Some women require catheterization sooner. The mother who has had a cesarean birth may have an indwelling catheter inserted prophylactically. The same assessments should be made in evaluating bladder emptying once the catheter has been removed.

The nurse elicits information from the woman about the adequacy of her fluid intake, whether she feels she is emptying her bladder completely when she voids, and any signs of urinary tract infection (UTI) she may be experiencing.

In the same way, the nurse obtains information about the new mother's intestinal elimination and any concerns she may have about it. Many mothers fear that the first bowel movement will be painful and possibly even damaging if an episiotomy has been done. Often, women have defecated during labor or childbirth; therefore, bowel movements normally return within 2 to 3 days after a vaginal childbirth. Stool softeners may be ordered to increase bulk and moisture in the fecal material and to allow more comfortable and complete evacuation. Constipation should be avoided to prevent pressure on sutures and increased discomfort. To enhance bowel elimination and help the woman reestablish her normal bowel pattern, the nurse can encourage ambulation, increased fluid intake (up to 2000 mL/day or more), and additional fresh fruits and roughage in her diet.

During the assessment, the nurse may provide information about postpartum diuresis and explain why the woman may be emptying her bladder so frequently. Information about the need for additional fluid intake, with suggestions of specific amounts, may be helpful. The woman should drink at least eight 8-oz glasses of water or juice daily in addition to other fluids. Breastfeeding mothers will have a higher requirement. The nurse discusses with the woman signs of urinary retention and overflow voiding and may review symptoms of UTI if it seems an appropriate moment for teaching. The nurse can also review methods of assisting bowel elimination and provide opportunities for the woman to ask questions.

REST AND SLEEP STATUS

Physical fatigue often affects other adjustments and functions of the new mother. The mother requires energy to make the psychologic adjustments to a new baby and to a new role. Fatigue is often a highly significant factor in a new mother's apparent disinterest in her newborn. Frequently, the woman is so tired from a long labor and birth that everything seems to be an effort. To avoid inadvertently classifying a very tired mother as one with a potential attachment problem, the nurse should do a psychologic assessment on more than one occasion. After a nap the new mother is often far more receptive to her baby and her surroundings. During the postpartum assessment, the nurse evaluates the amount of rest a new mother is getting. If the woman reports difficulty sleeping at night, the nurse should try to determine the cause. If it is simply the strange environment, a warm drink and back rub may prove helpful. Appropriate nursing measures are indicated if the woman is bothered by normal postpartum discomforts such as afterpains, diaphoresis, or episiotomy or hemorrhoidal pain. The impact of rooming-in on the mother's ability to rest should be assessed. See Chapter 29 for more detailed discussion of comfort/pain relief measures.

The nurse should encourage a daily rest period and schedule hospital activities to allow time for napping. The nurse can also provide information about the fatigue a new mother experiences, strategies to promote rest/sleep at home, and the impact it can have on a woman's emotions and sense of control.

Developing Cultural Competence Rest, Seclusion, and Dietary Restraint in Non-Western Cultures

Rest, seclusion, and dietary restraint practices in many traditional non-Western cultures (African, traditional Mexican, Chinese, Japanese, South Asian groups) are designed to assist the woman and her baby during postpartum vulnerable periods. The period of postpartum vulnerability and seclusion varies between 7 and 40 days. In Ghana, new mothers are relieved from all chores, told to abstain from sex, and not allowed to leave the home (Holtz & Grisdale, 2012; Lauderdale, 2012). Seclusion practices and decreased activity are designed to decrease the influence of spirits or of spreading evil and misfortune. The time of seclusion coincides with the period of lochial flow or postpartum bleeding.

NUTRITIONAL STATUS

As a part of the nutritional assessment, the nurse can provide teaching about the nutritional needs of the woman during the postpartum period. See the postpartum nutrition discussion in Chapter 11. Visiting the mother during mealtime provides an opportunity for unobtrusive nutritional assessment and counseling.

During pregnancy the daily recommended dietary allowances call for increased amounts of calories, protein, and most vitamins and minerals. After birth, the nonbreastfeeding mother should be advised about the need to reduce her caloric intake by about 300 kcal daily and to return to prepregnancy levels for other nutrients. The breastfeeding mother should increase her daily caloric intake by about 200 kcal over the pregnancy requirements, or a total of 500 kcal over the prepregnant requirement. New mothers are advised that it is common practice to prescribe iron supplements for 3 months after birth. The hemoglobin and hematocrit values are then checked at the postpartum visit to detect any anemia.

Basic discussion often proves helpful, followed by referral as needed. In all cases, literature on nutrition should be provided, so that the woman will have a source of information after discharge. The nurse should inform the dietitian of any mother who is a vegetarian, has food allergies or lactose intolerance, or whose cultural or religious beliefs require specific foods. Appropriate meals can then be prepared for her. Many women, especially those who gained more than the recommended number of pounds during their pregnancies, are interested in losing weight after birth. The dietitian can design weight-reduction diets to meet nutritional needs and food preferences. The nurse may also refer women with unusual eating habits or numerous questions about good nutrition to the dietitian. As part of a nutritional assessment, the nurse can provide teaching about the nutritional needs of the woman during the postpartum period.

Psychologic Assessment

During the first several postpartum weeks, the woman must accomplish certain physical, psychologic, and developmental tasks:

- Restoring physical condition
- Developing competence in caring for and meeting the needs of her baby
- Establishing a relationship with her new baby

- Adapting to altered lifestyles and family structure resulting from the addition of a new member

Adequate assessment of the mother's psychologic adjustment is an integral part of postpartum evaluation. Some new mothers have little or no experience with newborns and may feel totally overwhelmed. They may show these feelings by asking questions and reading all available material or by becoming passive and quiet because they simply cannot deal with their feelings of inadequacy. Unless a nurse questions the woman about her plans and previous experience in a supportive, nonjudgmental way, the nurse might conclude that the woman is disinterested, withdrawn, or depressed. Clues indicating adjustment difficulties include excessive continued fatigue, marked depression, excessive preoccupation with physical status or discomfort, evidence of low self-esteem, lack of support systems, marital problems, inability to care for or nurture the newborn, and current family crises (illness or unemployment). These characteristics frequently indicate a potential for maladaptive parenting, which may lead to child abuse or neglect (physical, emotional, intellectual) and cannot be ignored. Referrals to public health nurses or other available community resources may provide greatly needed assistance and alleviate potentially dangerous situations.

ASSESSMENT OF EARLY ATTACHMENT

The beginnings of parent–newborn attachment may be observed in the first few hours after birth. Continued assessments may occur during the postpartum stay and during home visits after discharge. A nurse in any of the postpartum settings should note progress toward attachment. The assessment should include both parents when possible; however, in this section, these behaviors focus primarily on the mother's attachment process. As discussed previously, research shows that fathers experience similar attachment feelings to those experienced by mothers. The following questions can be addressed in the course of nurse–client interaction:

- Is the mother attracted to her newborn? To what extent does she seek face-to-face contact and eye contact? Has she progressed from fingertip touch, to palmar contact, to enfolding the baby close to her own body? Is attraction increasing or decreasing? If the mother does not exhibit increasing attraction, why not? Do the reasons lie primarily within her, with the baby, or with the environment?

- Is the mother inclined to nurture her baby? Is she progressing in her interactions with her baby?

- Does the mother act consistently? If not, is the source of unpredictability within her or her baby?

- Is her mothering consistently carried out? Does she seek information and evaluate it objectively? Does she develop solutions based on adequate knowledge of valid data? Does she evaluate the effectiveness of her maternal care and adjust appropriately?

- Is she sensitive to the newborn's needs as they arise? How quickly does she interpret her baby's behavior and react to cues? Does she seem happy and satisfied with the baby's responses to her efforts? Is she pleased with feeding behaviors? How much of this ability and willingness to respond is related to the baby's nature and how much to her own?

- Does she seem pleased with her baby's appearance and gender? Does she experience pleasure when interacting with her baby? What interferes with the enjoyment? Does she speak to the baby frequently and affectionately? Does she call the baby by name? Does she point out family traits or characteristics she sees in the newborn?

- Are there any cultural factors that might modify the mother's response? For instance, is it customary for the grandmother to assume most of the childcare responsibilities while the mother recovers from childbirth?

When the nurse has addressed these questions and assembled the facts, the nurse's intuition and knowledge should combine to answer three more questions: Is there a problem in attachment? What is the problem? What is its source? The nurse can then devise a creative approach to the problem as it presents itself in the context of a unique, developing mother–baby relationship. See *Assessment Guide: Postpartum—First 24 Hours After Birth.*

Discharge Assessment and Follow-Up

The final discharge assessment should include a physical examination and appropriate discharge teaching that includes both maternal and newborn care guidelines. The optimal time for a home visit or follow-up phone call is 3 to 4 days after birth; this provides opportunities for further assessment of mothers and their newborns and teaching. (See *Assessment Guide: Postpartum—First Home Visit and Anticipated Progress at 6 Weeks* in Chapter 29.)

Women With Special Needs Modifications for Mobility Disorders

For the woman with a mobility disorder, specialized equipment will be needed in order for her to care for the baby. Modifications should include a lower crib and changing table height, arrangement of care supplies in an area she can adequately reach, and space in the nursery or designated infant sleep location for a wheelchair or walker to move easily, if used.

During this time period, infections, poor feeding, excessive weight loss, jaundice, and other problems become apparent (James, 2014). The follow-up phone call is often initiated by a nurse from the postpartum unit of the agency where the mother gave birth. It is made soon after discharge and is designed to provide assessment and, if necessary, care; to reinforce knowledge and provide additional teaching; and to make referrals if indicated. Alternatively, a follow-up phone call from a nurse from the healthcare provider's office can provide new mothers with a source of support and an opportunity to ask questions. Women who appear to be having adjustment problems should be scheduled for an appointment for further evaluation.

In ideal situations, a family approach involving the father, newborn, and other siblings permits a total evaluation and provides an opportunity for all family members to ask questions and express concerns. In addition, a family approach can sometimes enable the nurse to identify disturbed family patterns more readily and suggest, or even institute, therapeutic measures to prevent future problems of neglect or abuse.

ASSESSMENT GUIDE | Postpartum—First 24 Hours After Birth

Physical Assessment/Normal Findings	Alterations and Possible Causes*	Nursing Responses to Data**
Vital Signs		
Blood pressure (BP): Should remain consistent with baseline BP during pregnancy.	High BP (preeclampsia, essential hypertension, renal disease, anxiety).	Evaluate history of preexisting disorders and check for other signs of preeclampsia (proteinuria).
	Drop in BP (may be normal; uterine hemorrhage).	Assess for other signs of hemorrhage ($\uparrow$ pulse, cool clammy skin).
Pulse: 60–100 beats/minute. May be bradycardia of 50–70 beats/min.	Tachycardia (difficult labor and birth, hemorrhage).	Evaluate for other signs of hemorrhage ($\downarrow$ BP, cool clammy skin).
Respirations: 12–20/min.	Marked tachypnea (respiratory disease).	Assess for other signs of respiratory disease.
Temperature: 36.6°–38.0°C (98.0° –100.4°F).	After first 24 hr temperature of 38.0°C (100.4°F) or above suggests infection.	Assess for other signs of infection; notify healthcare provider/CNM.
Breasts		
General appearance: Smooth, even pigmentation; changes of pregnancy still apparent; one may appear larger.	Reddened area (mastitis).	Assess further for signs of infection.
Palpation: Depending on postpartum day, may be soft, filling, full, or engorged.	Palpable mass (caked breast, mastitis). Engorgement (venous stasis). Tenderness, heat, edema (engorgement, caked breast, mastitis).	Assess for other signs of infection: If blocked duct, consider heat, massage, position change for breastfeeding. Assess for further signs. Report mastitis to healthcare provider/CNM.
Nipples: Supple, pigmented, intact; become erect when stimulated.	Fissures, cracks, soreness (problems with breastfeeding), not erectile with stimulation (inverted nipples).	Reassess technique; recommend appropriate interventions.
Lungs		
Sounds: clear to bases bilaterally.	Diminished (fluid overload, asthma, pulmonary embolus, pulmonary edema).	Assess for other signs of respiratory distress.
Abdomen		
Musculature: Abdomen may be soft, have a "doughy" texture; rectus muscle intact.	Separation in musculature (diastasis recti abdominis).	Evaluate size of diastasis; teach appropriate exercises for decreasing the separation.
Fundus: Firm, midline; following expected process of involution.	Boggy (full bladder, uterine bleeding).	Massage until firm; assess bladder and have woman void if needed; attempt to express clots when firm. If bogginess remains or recurs, report to healthcare provider.
May be tender when palpated. Cesarean section incision dressing; dry and intact.	Constant tenderness (infection). Moderate to large amount of blood or serosanguineous drainage on dressing.	Assess for evidence of endometritis. Assess for hemorrhage. Reinforce dressing and notify healthcare provider/CNM.
Lochia		
Scant to moderate amount, earthy odor; no clots.	Large amount, clots (hemorrhage). Foul-smelling lochia (infection).	Assess for firmness, express additional clots; begin peripad count. Assess for other signs of infection; report to healthcare provider/CNM.
Normal progression: First 1–3 days: rubra.	Failure to progress normally or return to rubra from serosa (subinvolution).	Report to healthcare provider/CNM.
Following rubra: Days 3–10: serosa (alba seldom seen in hospital).		
Perineum		
Slight edema and bruising in intact perineum.	Marked fullness, bruising, pain (vulvar hematoma).	Assess size; apply ice glove or ice pack; report to healthcare provider/CNM.

(continued)

ASSESSMENT GUIDE | Postpartum—First 24 Hours After Birth (*continued*)

Physical Assessment/Normal Findings	Alterations and Possible Causes*	Nursing Responses to Data**
Episiotomy: No redness, edema, ecchymosis, or discharge; edges well approximated.	Redness, edema, ecchymosis, discharge, or gaping stitches (infection).	Encourage sitz baths; review perineal care, appropriate wiping techniques.
Hemorrhoids: None present; if present, should be small and nontender.	Full, tender, inflamed hemorrhoids.	Encourage sitz baths, side-lying position; Tucks pads, anesthetic ointments, manual replacement of hemorrhoids, stool softeners, increased fluid intake.
Costovertebral Angle (CVA) Tenderness		
None.	Present (kidney infection).	Assess for other symptoms of urinary tract infection (UTI); obtain clean-catch urine specimen; report to healthcare provider/CNM.
Lower Extremities		
No pain with palpation; negative Homans sign.	Positive findings (thrombophlebitis).	Report to healthcare provider/CNM.
Elimination		
Urinary output: Voiding in sufficient quantities at least every 4–6 hr; bladder not palpable.	Inability to void (urinary retention). Symptoms of urgency, frequency, dysuria (UTI).	Employ nursing interventions to promote voiding; if not successful, obtain order for catheterization. Report symptoms of UTI to healthcare provider.
Bowel elimination: Should have normal bowel movement by second or third day after birth.	Inability to pass feces (constipation caused by fear of pain from episiotomy, hemorrhoids, perineal trauma).	Encourage fluids, ambulation, roughage in diet; sitz baths to promote healing of perineum; obtain order for stool softener.

Cultural Assessment†	Variations to Consider	Nursing Responses to Data**
Determine customs and practices regarding postpartum care. Ask the mother whether she would like fluids, and ask what temperature she prefers.	Individual preference may include room-temperature or warmed fluids rather than iced drinks.	Provide for specific request if possible. If woman is unable to provide specific information, the nurse may draw from general information regarding cultural variation.
Ask the mother what foods or fluids she would like.	Special foods or fluids to hasten healing after childbirth.	Mexican women may want food and fluids that restore hot–cold balance to the body. Women of European background may ask for iced fluids.
Ask the mother whether she would prefer to be alone during breastfeeding.	Some women may be hesitant to have someone with them when their breast is exposed.	Provide privacy as desired by mother.

Psychologic Adaptation		
During first 24 hr: Passive; preoccupied with own needs; may talk about her labor and birth experience; may be talkative, elated, or very quiet.	Very quiet and passive; sleeps frequently (fatigue from long labor; feelings of disappointment about some aspect of the experience; may be following cultural expectation).	Provide opportunities for adequate rest; provide nutritious meals and snacks that are consistent with what the woman desires to eat and drink; provide opportunities to discuss birth experience in nonjudgmental atmosphere if the woman desires to do so.
Usually by 12 hr: Beginning to assume responsibility; some women eager to learn; easily feels overwhelmed.	Excessive weepiness, mood swings, pronounced irritability (postpartum blues; feelings of inadequacy; culturally proscribed behavior).	Explain postpartum blues; provide supportive atmosphere; determine support available for mother; consider referral for evidence of profound depression.
Attachment		
En face position; holds baby close; cuddles and soothes; calls by name; identifies characteristics of family members in baby; may be awkward in providing care.	Continued expressions of disappointment in gender, appearance of baby; refusal to care for baby; derogatory comments; lack of bonding behaviors (difficulty in attachment, following expectations of cultural/ethnic group).	Provide reinforcement and support for infant caretaking behaviors; maintain nonjudgmental approach and gather more information if caretaking behaviors are not evident.

Cultural Assessment†	Variations to Consider	Nursing Responses to Data**
Initially may express disappointment over gender or appearance of baby but within 1–2 days demonstrates attachment behaviors.		

Client Education

Has basic understanding of self-care activities and infant care needs; can identify signs of complications that should be reported.	Unable to demonstrate basic self-care and infant care activities (knowledge deficit; postpartum blues; following prescribed cultural behavior and will be cared for by grandmother or other family member).	Identify predominant learning style. Determine whether woman understands English and provide interpreter if needed; provide reinforcement of information through conversation and through written material (remember that some women and their families may not be able to understand written materials because of language difficulties or inability to read); provide information regarding infant care skills that are culturally consistent; give woman opportunity to express her feelings; consider social service home referral for women who have no family or other support, are unable to take in information about self-care and infant care, and demonstrate no caretaking activities.

*Possible causes of alterations are identified in parentheses.
**This column provides guidelines for further assessment and initial nursing actions.
†These are only a few suggestions. It is not our intent to imply this is a comprehensive cultural assessment.

Focus Your Study

- The uterus involutes rapidly, primarily through a reduction in cell size.

- Involution is assessed by measuring fundal height. The fundus is at the level of the umbilicus within a few hours after birth and should decrease by approximately one fingerbreadth per day.

- The placental site heals by a process of exfoliation, so no scar formation occurs.

- Lochia progresses from rubra to serosa to alba and is assessed in terms of type, quantity, and characteristics.

- The abdomen may have decreased muscle tone (flabby consistency) initially. The nurse should assess for diastasis recti abdominis, separation of the rectus abdominis muscles.

- Constipation may develop postpartum because of decreased tone in the abdominal muscles, limited diet, and denial of the urge to defecate because of fear of pain.

- Decreased bladder sensitivity, increased capacity, and postpartum diuresis may lead to problems with bladder elimination. Frequent assessment and prompt intervention are indicated. A fundus that is boggy but does not respond to massage, is higher than expected, or deviates to the side usually indicates a full bladder.

- Postpartum, a healthy woman should be normotensive and afebrile. Bradycardia is common.

- The white blood cell (WBC) count is often elevated postpartum. Activation of clotting factors predisposes the woman to thrombus formation.

- Psychologic adaptations of the postpartum woman are traditionally described as "taking in" and "taking hold" on her journey to maternal role attainment.

- Postpartum blues is a common occurrence, and ways to prevent and cope with it should be discussed not only with the mother but also with her significant other(s). Signs of postpartum depression should be discussed as well.

- In consideration of the client's background, the nurse should recognize and respect cultural variations and individual preferences.

- Postpartum assessment should be completed in a systematic way, usually head to toe, and should include assessment of rest and sleep, nutrition, and attachment. The assessment provides opportunities for informal client teaching.

- In the weeks following birth, the woman's physical condition returns to a nonpregnant state, and she gains competence in caregiving and confidence in herself as a parent.

Clinical Reasoning in Action

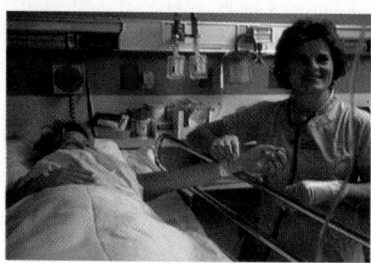

Janet Burns, a 25-year-old G3P3, is 2 hours past a low forceps vaginal birth with a right medial lateral episiotomy of a live 8-lb baby boy. You obtain vital signs of BP 118/70, T 98.8°F, P 76, R 14. You observe the fundus is +1 fingerbreadth above the umbilicus and slightly to the right. Her episiotomy is slightly ecchymotic and well approximated without edema or discharge. Ice has been applied to the episiotomy for the last 20 minutes. Lochia rubra is present and a pad was saturated in 90 minutes.

Janet has an intravenous of Ringer lactate with 10 units of oxytocin (Pitocin) infusing at 100 mL/hr in her lower left arm and is complaining of moderate abdominal cramping. Janet's baby is sleeping peacefully in the bassinet next to her bed. She tells you that she is very tired and requests some pain medication so she can sleep for a while.

1. What nursing assessment is of immediate concern?
2. Discuss care of her episiotomy and perineum.
3. What other self-care measures could you advise?
4. Discuss postpartum occurrences that may cause special concern for the mother.
5. Janet expressed concern about her episiotomy healing. What information can you offer?

References

Blackburn, S. T. (2013). *Maternal, fetal, & neonatal physiology: A clinical perspective* (3rd ed.). St. Louis, MO: Saunders.

Callister, L. C. (2014). Integrating cultural beliefs and practices when caring for childbearing women and families. In K. R. Simpson & P. A. Creehan (Eds.), *Perinatal nursing* (4th ed., pp. 41–64). Philadelphia, PA: Lippincott Williams & Wilkins.

Cunningham, F. G., Leveno, K. J., Bloom, S. L., Spong, C. Y., Dashe, J. S., Hoffman, B. L., ... Sheffield, J. S. (2014). *Williams obstetrics* (24th ed.). New York, NY: McGraw-Hill.

Dennis, C. & Dowswell, T. (2013). Psychosocial and psychological interventions for preventing postpartum depression. *Cochrane Database of Systematic Reviews*, Issue 2. Art. No.:CD001134.

Ding, T., Wang, D., Qu, Y., Chen, Q., & Zhu, S. (2014). Epidural labor analgesia is associated with a decreased risk of postpartum depression: A prospective cohort study. *Anesthesia & Analgesia 119*(2), 383–92.

Feldman, R. (2012). Parent-infant synchrony: A biobehavioral model of mutual influences in the formation of affiliative bonds. *Monographs of the Society for Research in Child Development, 77*(2), 42–51.

Holtz, C., & Grisdale, S. (2012). Global health in reproduction and infants. In C. Holtz (Ed.), *Global health care: Issues and policies* (2nd ed.). Boston, MA: Jones & Bartlett.

James, D. C. (2014). Postpartum care. In K. R. Simpson & P. A. Creehan (Eds.), *Perinatal nursing* (4th ed., p. 530). Philadelphia, PA: Lippincott Williams & Wilkins.

Kalayjian, L., Goodwin, T. M., & Lee, R. H. (2013). Nervous system & autoimmune disorders in pregnancy. In A. H. Decherney, L. Nathan, T. M. Goodwin, N. Laufer, & A. Roman (Eds.), *Current diagnosis and treatment: Obstetrics & gynecology* (11th ed., pp. 533–542). Boston, MA: McGraw-Hill.

Klein, A. (2012). The postpartum period in women with epilepsy. *Neurologic Clinics, 30*(3), 867–875.

Lauderdale, J. (2012). Transcultural perspectives in childbearing. In M. M. Andrews & J. S. Boyle (Eds.), *Transcultural concepts in nursing care* (6th ed., pp. 91–122). Philadelphia, PA: Lippincott Williams & Wilkins.

Lim, S. Y., Evangelou, N., & Jurgens, S. (2014). Postpartum headache: Diagnostic considerations. *Practical Neurology, 14*(2), 92–99.

Liu, C., & Tronick, E. (2013). Rates and predictors of postpartum depression by race and ethnicity: Results from the 2004 to 2007 New York City PRAMS Survey (Pregnancy Risk Assessment Monitoring System.) *Maternal Child Health, 17*, 1599–1610.

Mercer, R. T. (2004). Becoming a mother versus maternal role attainment. *Journal of Nursing Scholarship, 36*(3), 226–232.

Mercer, R. T. (2006). Nursing support of the process of becoming a mother. JOGNN: *Journal of Obstetric, Gynecologic, & Neonatal Nursing, 35*(5), 649–651. doi:10.1111/J.1552-6909.2006.00086.x

Nicholson, T. B. (2014). Neurological disorders. In R. G. Jordan, J. L. Engstrom, J. A. Marfell, & C. L. Farley (Eds.), *Prenatal and postnatal care: A woman-centered approach* (1st ed., pp. 570–579). Ames, IA: Wiley Blackwell.

Pessel, C., & Tsai, M. C. (2013). The normal puerperium. In A. H. DeCherney, L. Nathan, N., & A. S. Roman (Eds.), *Current diagnosis & treatment: Obstetrics & gynecology* (11th ed., pp. 190–213). New York, NY: McGraw-Hill.

Purnell, L. D. (2013). *Transcultural health care: A culturally competent approach* (4th ed.). Philadelphia, PA: F. A. Davis.

Rubin, R. (1984). *Maternal identity and the maternal experience*. New York, NY: Springer.

Samuels, P., & Niebyl, J. R. (2012). Neurologic disorders. In S. G. Gabbe, J. R. Niebyl, & J. L. Simpson (Eds.), *Obstetrics: Normal and problem pregnancies* (6th ed.). Philadelphia, PA: Churchill Livingstone Elsevier.

Whitmer, T. (2016). Physical and psychologic changes after childbirth. In S. Mattson & J. E. Smith (Eds.), *Core curriculum for maternal-newborn nursing* (6th ed., pp. 297–313). Philadelphia, PA: Association of Women's Health, Obstetric and Neonatal Nurses /Elsevier

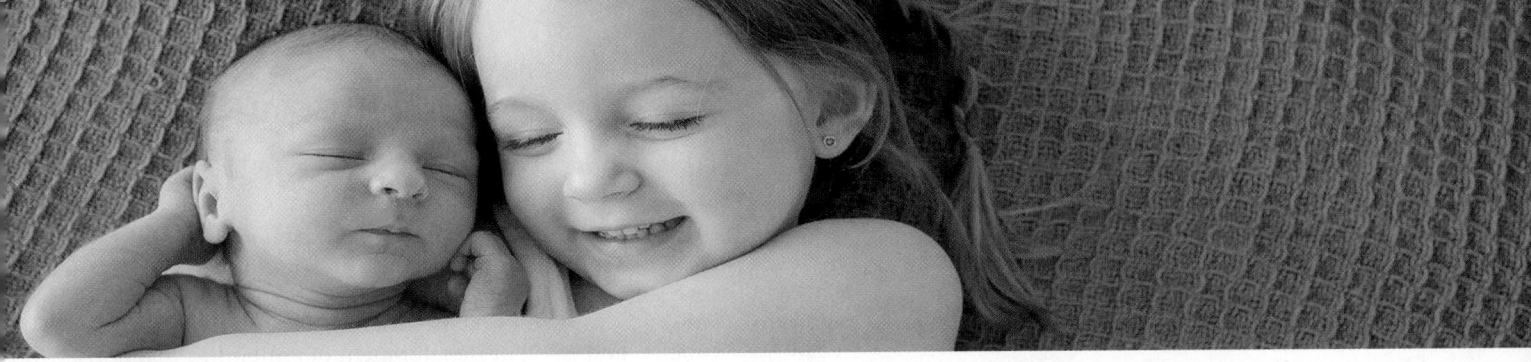

Chapter 29
The Postpartum Family: Early Care Needs and Home Care

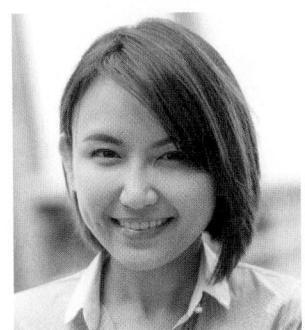

More than anything else that happened after my baby was born, I was surprised by the fatigue I felt. In the first few weeks, I spent every minute that my baby slept cleaning, doing laundry, and the like. Then, during my checkup, the nurse-midwife told me that I had to rest when my baby slept. What a difference that made. Suddenly I was less overwhelmed and more able to enjoy being a mother.

—Mai Ling, 26

alice_photo/Fotolia

⌄ Learning Outcomes

29.1 Formulate nursing diagnoses and nursing care based on the findings of the normal postpartum assessment and teaching needs.

29.2 Describe appropriate nursing interventions to promote postpartum maternal comfort, rest, and well-being.

29.3 Explain factors that affect postpartum family wellness in the provision of nursing care and client teaching.

29.4 Compare the postpartum nursing needs of the woman who experienced a cesarean birth with the needs of a woman who gave birth vaginally.

29.5 Examine the nursing needs of the childbearing adolescent during the postpartum period.

29.6 Describe possible approaches to sensitive, holistic nursing care for the woman who relinquishes her newborn.

29.7 Explain the specific postpartum needs for women with obesity, developmental disabilities, or history of sexual abuse.

29.8 Identify postpartum teaching needs that should be modified to provide sensitive care to meet the needs of lesbian mothers.

29.9 Identify teaching topics related to postpartum discharge.

29.10 Identify the main purposes and components of home visits during the postpartum period.

29.11 Summarize actions a nurse should take to ensure personal safety as well as fostering a caring relationship during a home visit.

29.12 Describe maternal and family assessment and anticipated progress after birth.

29.13 Delineate interventions to address the common concerns of breastfeeding mothers following discharge.

29.14 Describe the assessment and care of the newborn during postpartum home care.

A thorough discussion of postpartum adaptation and nursing assessment was provided in Chapter 28. This chapter describes how the nurse can use the remaining steps of the nursing management process effectively to plan and provide care. Specific nursing responses to the mother's physical needs and the family's psychosocial needs are described at length.

Nursing Care During the Early Postpartum Period

For most postpartum women, physical recovery goes smoothly and is considered a healthy process. Because of this perception, healthcare providers too often assume that the woman and her family have no real needs and that no care plan is needed. Nothing could be further from the truth. Every member of the family has needs, although the needs may not be obvious, especially if they are psychologic or educational.

Nursing Diagnoses

The postpartum family's needs, which should be identified during assessment, are the basis for developing nursing diagnoses. Many nurses have suggested that nursing diagnoses are difficult to make in a wellness setting because of their emphasis on "problems." Nurses involved in the effort to formulate standardized diagnoses recognize this difficulty and continue working to develop nursing diagnoses that are more congruent with wellness settings.

Many agencies that use nursing diagnoses prefer to use only the NANDA diagnoses. Consequently, physiologic alterations form the basis of many postpartum diagnoses. Examples of such diagnoses include (NANDA-I © 2014):

- *Breastfeeding, Ineffective,* related to postpartum pain from a cesarean birth or maternal fatigue
- *Constipation* related to fear of tearing stitches or pain
- *Pain, Acute,* related to perineal trauma secondary to episiotomy or birth

  Diagnoses related to family coping or instructional needs are also used frequently. Examples of these diagnoses include (NANDA-I © 2014):

- *Knowledge, Readiness for Enhanced,* about infant care related to an expressed desire to improve parenting skills
- *Anxiety* related to self and infant care secondary to lack of knowledge of appropriate care practices
- *Coping: Family, Readiness for Enhanced,* related to successful adjustment to new baby
- *Health Management, Readiness for Enhanced,* related to desire to obtain optimal health in the postpartum period

Nursing Plan and Implementation

An important component of postpartum nursing care is client teaching, which must be individualized to the learning capability and readiness of the parent(s). As part of the teaching role, the nurse discusses desired outcomes and goals with the mother and family members as soon as possible following the birth. Interventions can then be designed to achieve optimal health promotion. Strategies for promoting effective learning are discussed shortly, and specific teaching content is provided throughout the rest of this chapter. Home care visits and phone contacts help ensure that new parents have the necessary skills and resources to care for their baby.

Promotion of Maternal Comfort and Well-Being

The nurse can promote and restore maternal physical well-being by monitoring uterine status, vital signs, cardiovascular status, elimination patterns, nutritional needs, sleep and rest, and learning needs. Some women also require medication to relieve pain, treat anemia, provide immunity to rubella, and prevent development of antibodies in a nonsensitized Rh-negative woman. Most postpartum women need nursing interventions to promote their comfort and relieve stress. During the postpartum period, ongoing assessments are warranted to assess the physiologic changes that have occurred and ensure that adequate return to a nonpregnant state is occurring. After birth, the examination of the uterine status, lochia, and episiotomy is performed every 15 minutes for 1 hour, then every 30 minutes × 2, then every hour × 2, then every 4 hours × 2, and then every 8 hours until the woman is discharged home.

Postpartum Examination

A complete assessment for the postpartum woman should include assessing the breasts, uterus, bowels, bladder, lochia, episiotomy, hemorrhoids, and emotional status. The mnemonic BUBBLEHE provides the nurse with a means to memorize these components of a postpartum assessment. Table 29–1 provides the normal and abnormal findings that can be identified in the postpartum period and interventions for routine care.

Occasionally, medications are needed to promote uterine contractions. These include oxytocin, discussed in Chapter 22, and methylergonovine maleate (Methergine). The nurse also monitors the amount, consistency, color, and odor of the lochia on an ongoing basis. Continued assessment is warranted during the first 24 hours because early postpartum hemorrhage typically occurs in the 24 hours after birth and is most commonly related to uterine atony (the top portion of the uterus is soft and spongy rather than firm and well contracted) (Lowe, 2012). Table 29–2 describes the position of the uterine fundus following birth. See Chapter 30 for treatment of uterine atony.

Relief of Perineal Discomfort

Before selecting a method to help relieve perineal discomfort, the nurse needs to assess the perineum to determine the degree of edema and other problems. It is also important to ask the woman if she believes any special measures will be particularly effective and to offer her choices when possible. The nurse uses disposable gloves while applying all relief measures and washes hands before and after using the gloves. At all times it is essential for the nurse to remember hygienic practices, such as moving from the front of the perineum (area of the symphysis pubis) to the back (area around the anus). Avoiding contamination between the anal area and the urethral/vaginal area is vital to the prevention of infection.

PERINEAL CARE

Perineal care after each elimination cleanses the perineum, prevents infection, and helps promote comfort. The woman should be instructed to wash her hands before and after changing peri-pads or performing pericare. The nurse demonstrates how to cleanse the perineum and assists the woman as necessary. Many agencies provide peri-bottles that the woman can use to squirt

TABLE 29-1 BUBBLEHE Mnemonic for Postpartum Examination

AREA TO BE ASSESSED	NORMAL FINDINGS	ABNORMAL FINDINGS	INTERVENTIONS FOR ROUTINE CARE
Breasts	Soft or filling No cracking or bleeding from nipples Nipples erect with stimulation Colostrum present	Nipples flat or inverted Unable to obtain erect nipples with feeding or use of breast pump Reddened, tender area warm to touch (possible mastitis or engorgement) Cracked, bleeding nipples (possible trauma from breast-feeding, fissure, infection)	Advise use of a supportive bra. Suggest that breast shells be worn for flat or inverted nipples. Obtain an order for a lactation consult as needed. Note that cracking and bleeding are most commonly related to improper positioning with feeding. Contact healthcare provider immediately if symptoms of infection are present.
Uterus	Fundus firm, midline, position dependent on time since birth but should be at or below umbilicus (see Table 29–2)	Uterus boggy, soft, shifted to the right or not midline, position above umbilicus (possible full bladder, subinvolution) Excessive tenderness with palpation (possible endometritis)	Teach woman to monitor her uterus for firmness. Advise frequent voiding to reduce incidence of bleeding. Suggest use of ibuprofen for any afterbirth pains. Inform woman that breastfeeding aids with involution process. For heavier than expected bleeding, try uterine massage.
Bowels	Abdomen soft, nondistended Normal bowel sounds in all quadrants Passing flatus Bowel movements occur without difficulty	Abdomen distended with discomfort noted No flatus Constipation, reduced bowel sounds	Encourage ambulation, fluids, diet high in fiber, stool softeners. Enema may be needed. Note that women with third- or fourth-degree lacerations need stool softeners.
Bladder	Nondistended, nonpalpable on exam Adequate voiding Urine clear yellow (may contain lochia)	Distended Unable to void or inadequate voiding pattern that does not fully empty bladder	Encourage frequent voiding. Measure first three voids after birth to ensure adequate bladder emptying.
Lochia	Lochia rubra immediately after birth until 3 days Lochia serosa from 3–10 days Lochia alba after that Scant to moderate amount with earthy odor	Heavy amount Clotting Foul smelling Persistent lochia rubra that does not change to serosa	Teach that perineal hygiene includes frequent voiding and cleaning self from front to back. Instruct on consistent use of a "peri-bottle" while lochia present. Provide sitz bath if ordered.
Episiotomy	Episiotomy or perineum with mild edema Laceration or episiotomy should be intact and well approximated	Excessive edema Bruising Hematoma Discharge Sutures not well approximated or loose	Apply ice to perineum for 20 min on then 20 min off for first 24 hr. Give local perineal medication preparations. Provide sitz baths after first 24 hr. Review perineal hygiene measures.
Hemorrhoids	Rectum intact Hemorrhoids may be present but are small and nontender	Full Tender Inflamed	Teach client about helpful topical agents: witch hazel pads, anesthetic ointments or creams. Try manual replacement of hemorrhoids. Increase fluids and fiber. Encourage sitz baths and side-lying position.
Emotional status	Adequate maternal–newborn attachment is observed Verbalization on proper care of baby Some anxiety is normal	Lack of interest in newborn Lack of expected maternal–newborn attachment behaviors Excessive worrying Depression	Provide education on infant care practice, postpartum needs. Explore support system availability. Refer to support groups and new mother groups. Encourage frequent rest periods. Review baby blues and signs of postpartum depression.

TABLE 29–2 Position of the Uterine Fundus Following Birth

TIME	POSITION OF FUNDUS
Immediately after birth	Top of fundus is in the midline about midway between the symphysis pubis and umbilicus.
6–12 hr after birth	Top of fundus is in the midline and at the level of the umbilicus.
1 day after birth	Top of fundus is in the midline and 1 finger-breadth below the umbilicus.
Second day after birth and thereafter	Top of fundus remains in the midline and descends about 1 fingerbreadth per day.

warm tap water over her perineum following elimination. To cleanse her perineum, the woman should use moist antiseptic towelettes or toilet paper in a blotting (patting) motion and should be taught to start at the front and proceed toward the back to prevent contamination from the anal area.

Many women have never used perineal pads and will need teaching and assistance in using them during the postpartum period. To prevent contamination, the perineal pad should be applied from front to back (place the front portion against the perineum first) and changed when saturation occurs or after each perineal cleansing. The woman is advised to hold the pad on the sides to prevent contamination. The pad needs to be placed snugly against the perineum but should not produce pressure. If the pad is worn too loosely, it may rub back and forth, irritating perineal tissues and causing contamination between the anal and vaginal areas. The pad should be changed after urination and defecation. Women should be advised to cleanse the perineal area with soap and water at least 1 time per day in addition to using the peri-bottle after each void or pad change (Brincat, Crosby, McLeod, et al., 2015). Advise the woman that the pad should be changed at least 4 times per day to prevent contamination from bacteria (Brincat et al., 2015). Women should be advised that perineal pain is common and will decrease gradually each day. Most women note complete resolution within 8 weeks of birth (Brincat et al., 2015). (For information regarding the care of the perineum following an episiotomy, see *Teaching Highlights: Episiotomy Care.*)

ICE PACK

If an episiotomy is done at the time of birth, an ice pack is generally applied to the perineum to reduce edema and provide numbing of the tissues, which promotes comfort. In some agencies, chemical ice bags are used. These are usually activated by folding both ends toward the middle. The nurse can create inexpensive ice bags by filling a disposable glove with ice chips or crushed ice and then taping the top of the glove closed. To protect the perineum from burns caused by contact with such an ice pack, the glove needs to be rinsed under running water to remove any powder and then wrapped in an absorbent towel or washcloth before placing it against the perineum. To attain the maximum effect of this cold treatment, a pattern of applying the ice pack for approximately 20 minutes and then removing it for about 10 minutes should be followed during the first 2 hours to reduce edema. Usually, ice packs are needed for the first 24 hours to reduce pain (Brincat et al., 2015). The nurse provides information about the purpose of the ice pack, as well as anticipated effects, benefits, and possible problems, and explains how to prepare an ice pack for home use if edema is present and early discharge is planned.

SITZ BATH

The warmth of the water in a sitz bath provides comfort, decreases pain, and promotes circulation to the tissues, which promotes healing and reduces the incidence of infection (Figure 29–1). In some facilities, the use of the sitz bath has declined and is reserved only for women who have third- and fourth-degree lacerations (see Chapter 30 for discussion of lacerations of the genital tract), whereas in other facilities, it is offered to all women who have edema or a laceration following birth. Sitz baths may be ordered 3 times a day (TID) and as needed (PRN). The nurse prepares the sitz bath by cleaning the equipment and adding water at 38.9° to 40.6°C (102° to 105°F). The woman is encouraged to remain in the sitz bath for about 20 minutes. It is important for the woman to have a clean, unused towel to pat dry her perineum after the sitz bath and to have a clean perineal pad to apply. Care needs to be taken during the first sitz bath because the moist heat may cause the woman to faint. The nurse places a call bell well within reach and asks the woman to use it if she feels dizzy or lightheaded or develops difficulty hearing. The nurse also checks on the woman at frequent intervals.

Cool sitz baths have been used because they are effective in reducing perineal edema and reducing the response of nerve endings that cause perineal discomfort (Brincat et al., 2015). In administering a cool sitz bath, have the woman start with the water at room temperature and add ice according to the woman's comfort. Some women may prefer a warm sitz bath and achieve greater comfort levels from warmed water so personal preference should be valued.

The nurse provides information about the purpose and use of the sitz bath; anticipated effects, benefits, and possible problems; and safety measures to prevent overheating, scalds, chills,

---

TEACHING HIGHLIGHTS | **Episiotomy Care**

- Describe the process of wound healing.
- Discuss the risks of contamination of the episiotomy by bacteria from the anal area.
- Describe techniques that are used to keep the episiotomy clean and promote healing:
  - Sitz bath
  - Use of peri-bottle following each voiding or defecation
  - Pad change following each elimination and at regular intervals
  - Ice pack or ice-filled glove to perineum immediately following childbirth
  - Judicious use of analgesics or topical anesthetics
  - Tightening buttocks before sitting
- Identify signs of episiotomy infection (redness, edema, drainage, incomplete approximation of the edges).
- Advise the woman to contact her healthcare provider if signs of infection develop.

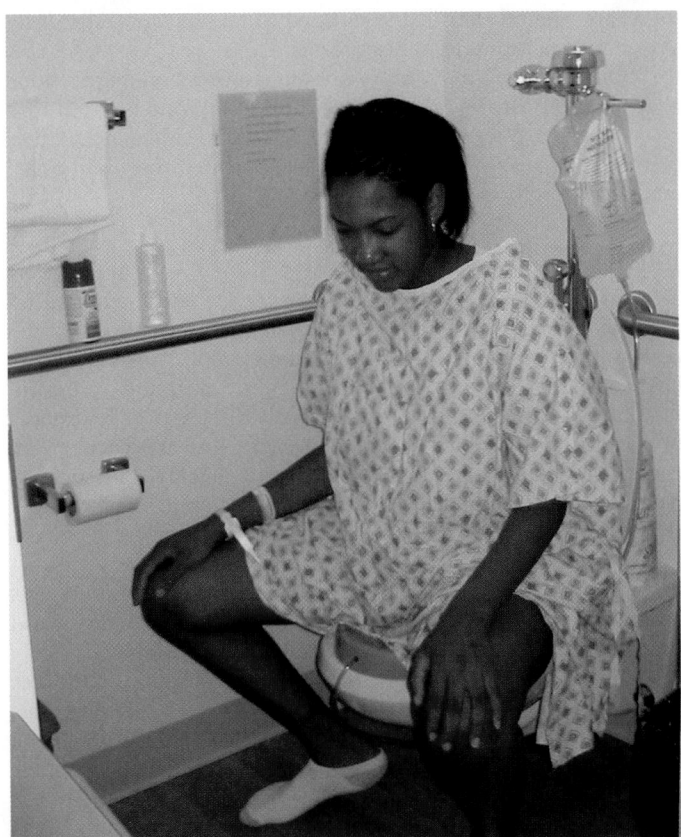

Figure 29–1 **A sitz bath promotes healing and provides relief from perineal discomfort during the initial weeks following birth.**

or injury from fainting or slipping while getting into or out of the tub. Home use of sitz baths may be recommended for the woman with an extensive episiotomy. The woman may use a portable sitz bath or her bathtub. It is important for the nurse to emphasize that in using a bathtub, the woman should draw only 4 to 6 in. of water, assess the temperature, and use the water only for the sitz and not for bathing. If the woman takes a sitz bath, she should release the water, have a helper clean the tub, and draw new water before bathing to prevent infection.

TOPICAL AGENTS

Topical anesthetics such as Dermoplast aerosol spray and Americaine spray may be used to relieve perineal discomfort. The woman is advised to apply the anesthetic after a sitz bath or perineal care. Witch hazel compresses may be used to relieve perineal discomfort and edema. Nupercainal ointment or Tucks (witch hazel pads) may be ordered for relief of both hemorrhoidal and perineal pain. The nurse should emphasize the need for the woman to wash her hands before and after using the topical treatments.

The nurse provides information about the anesthetic spray or topical agent. The woman needs to understand the purpose, use, anticipated effects and benefits, and possible problems associated with the product. The nurse can combine a demonstration of application with teaching. A return demonstration is a useful method of evaluating the woman's understanding.

Relief of Hemorrhoidal Discomfort

Some mothers experience hemorrhoidal pain after giving birth (see Figure 28–8). Relief measures include the use of sitz baths, topical anesthetic ointments, rectal suppositories, or witch hazel pads applied directly to the anal area. The woman may be taught to digitally replace external hemorrhoids in her rectum. Handwashing to prevent contamination to the vagina is essential. She may also find it helpful to maintain a side-lying position when possible and to avoid prolonged sitting. The mother is encouraged to maintain an adequate fluid intake, and stool softeners are administered to ensure greater comfort with bowel movements. Mothers should be advised to avoid straining with bowel movements because this can increase the severity and discomfort associated with hemorrhoids. The hemorrhoids usually disappear a few weeks after birth if the woman did not have them before her pregnancy.

Relief of Afterpains

Afterpains are the result of intermittent uterine contractions. A primipara may not experience afterpains because her uterus is able to maintain a contracted state. However, multiparous women and those who have had a multiple-gestation pregnancy or hydramnios frequently experience discomfort from afterpains as the uterus contracts intermittently. Breastfeeding women are also more likely to experience afterpains than formula-feeding women because of the release of oxytocin when the baby suckles.

The nurse can suggest that the woman lie prone, with a small pillow under her lower abdomen, and explain that the discomfort may feel intensified for about 5 minutes but then diminishes greatly if not completely. The prone position applies pressure to the uterus and therefore stimulates contractions. When the uterus maintains a constant contraction, the afterpains cease. Additional nursing interventions include a sitz bath (for warmth), positioning, ambulation, or administration of an analgesic agent. For breastfeeding mothers, an analgesic administered 30 minutes to an hour before nursing helps promote comfort and enhances maternal–newborn interaction (see Table 29–6).

The nurse provides information about the cause of afterpains and methods to decrease discomfort. The nurse explains any medications that are ordered, including their expected effect, benefits, and possible side effects, and any special considerations such as the possibility of dizziness or sleepiness with particular medications.

Relief of Discomfort From Immobility and Muscle Strain

Discomfort may be caused by immobility. The woman who has been in stirrups or has pulled back on her legs for an extended period of time may experience muscular aches from such

---

TEACHING HIGHLIGHTS | Self-Evaluation of the Perineum

After the mother completes the sitz bath, teach her to inspect the perineal area for burns (that could be related to using water that is too hot), edema, and approximation by using a handheld mirror. If the mother routinely inspects the area, she will be aware of changes that may indicate an infection, such as redness, poor approximation, drainage, or odor.

extreme positioning. It is not unusual for women to experience joint pain and muscular pain in both arms and legs, depending on the effort they exerted during the second stage of labor.

Early ambulation is encouraged to help reduce the incidence of complications such as constipation and thrombophlebitis. It also helps promote a feeling of general well-being. The nurse provides information about ambulation and the importance of monitoring any signs of dizziness or weakness. Assist the woman the first few times she gets up during the postpartum period. Fatigue, effects of medications, loss of blood, and lack of food intake may cause feelings of dizziness or faintness when the woman stands up. Because this may be a problem during the woman's first shower, the nurse should remain in the room, check the woman frequently, and have a chair close by in case she becomes faint. During this first shower the nurse instructs the woman in the use of the emergency call button in the bathroom; she is advised that, if she becomes faint during a future shower, she should sit down and press the call button for assistance immediately.

Relief of Discomfort From Postpartum Diaphoresis

Postpartum diaphoresis (excessive perspiration) may cause discomfort for new mothers. The nurse can offer a fresh, dry gown and change bed linens to enhance the mother's comfort. Some women may feel refreshed by a shower. For women experiencing hot flashes as a result of changing hormones, a cool shower may be preferable over a warm or hot shower. It is necessary to consider cultural practices and realize that some Hispanic and Asian women prefer to delay showering. Nurses can offer these women a warm or cool washcloth to increase comfort. The nurse provides information about the normal physiologic changes that cause diaphoresis and methods to increase comfort.

Because diaphoresis may also increase thirst, the nurse can offer fluids as the woman desires. Again, the nurse needs to ask the woman about her preferred beverage. Women of western European background may prefer iced drinks, whereas Asian women may prefer hot tea or water at room temperature. It is important to ascertain the woman's wishes rather than operate from one's own values or cultural beliefs.

Suppression of Lactation in the Nonbreastfeeding Mother

For the woman who chooses not to breastfeed, lactation may be suppressed by mechanical inhibition. Although signs of engorgement do not usually appear until the second or third postpartum day, engorgement is best prevented by beginning mechanical methods of lactation suppression as soon as possible after birth. Ideally, this involves having the woman begin wearing a supportive, well-fitting bra within 6 hours after birth. A tight-fitting sports bra may be preferred by some women. The bra is worn continuously until lactation is suppressed (usually about 5 to 7 days) and is removed only for showers. The bra provides support and eases the discomfort that can occur with tension on the breasts because of fullness. Ice packs should be applied over the axillary area of each breast for 20 minutes 4 times daily. This practice should begin soon after birth. In addition, ice is useful in relieving discomfort if engorgement occurs.

The mother is advised to avoid any stimulation of her breasts by her baby, herself, breast pumps, or her sexual partner until the sensation of fullness has passed (usually about 5 to 7 days). Such stimulation increases milk production and delays the suppression process. Heat is avoided for the same reason;

therefore, the mother is encouraged to let shower water flow over her back rather than her breasts.

Some mothers may inquire about suppression medications used in the past for nonnursing mothers. Women should be informed that, because of concerns related to side effects, these medications are no longer used. Mechanical, rather than pharmacologic, methods are now employed.

Relief of Emotional Stress

The birth of a child, with the changes in role and the increased responsibilities it produces, is a time of emotional stress for the new mother. During the early postpartum period, the mother may be emotionally labile, and mood swings and tearfulness are common. Initially the mother may repeatedly discuss her experiences of labor and birth. This allows the mother to integrate her experiences. If she believes that she did not cope well with labor, she may have feelings of inadequacy and may benefit from reassurance that she did well. Some women feel that they did not have any perception of time during the labor and birth and want to know how long it really lasted, or they may not remember the entire experience. In this case, it is helpful for the nurse to talk with the woman and provide the information that she is missing and desires.

During this time the new mother must also adjust to the loss of her fantasized child and accept the child she has borne. This task may be more difficult if the child is not of the desired sex or has birth defects (see Chapter 26). Women who deliver prematurely may experience guilt or have feelings of inadequacy. Immediately after the birth (the taking-in period) the mother is focused on bodily concerns and may not be fully ready to learn about personal and infant care. Following the initial dependent period, the mother becomes very concerned about her ability to be a successful parent (the taking-hold period). During this time the mother requires reassurance that she is effective. She also tends to be receptive to teaching and demonstration designed to assist her in mothering successfully. The depression, weepiness, and "let-down feeling" that characterize the postpartum blues are often a surprise for the new mother. She requires reassurance that these feelings are normal, an explanation of why they occur, and a supportive environment that permits her to cry without feeling guilty.

Promotion of Maternal Rest and Activity

Following childbirth some women feel exhausted and in need of rest. Other women may be euphoric and full of psychic energy, ready to relive and recount the experience of birth repeatedly. The nurse can provide a period for airing of feelings and then encourage a period of rest. Nurses also promote rest by organizing their activities to avoid frequent interruptions for the woman.

Relief of Fatigue

Physical fatigue often affects other adjustments and functions of the new mother. For example, fatigue can reduce milk flow, thereby increasing problems with establishing breastfeeding. Energy is also needed to make the psychologic adjustments to a new baby and to assume new roles. It is helpful for the new mother to know that fatigue may persist for several weeks or even months. Persistent fatigue is especially common when mothers attempt to perform activities while the baby is napping instead of resting themselves. The nurse teaches women that this practice can lead to chronic fatigue and should be avoided. Mothers who have other children may feel overwhelmed with trying to meet the needs of their other child(ren). Severe ongoing fatigue can also be a symptom of a thyroid disorder and should be evaluated by a clinician. Although most new mothers feel tired, if they have perceived the pregnancy and birth as a natural process, they tend to view themselves as healthy and well. Fatigue can also be a symptom of postpartum depression and should be discussed with the healthcare provider if symptoms continue or are accompanied by other signs of depression.

Specific groups of mothers are at a higher risk for postpartum fatigue. These include mothers of multiples, mothers with hospitalized newborns who must make multiple trips to the hospital to visit their babies, mothers of babies with birth defects or special needs, mothers who lack social support, and mothers who return to work before the advised 6-week time period. A mother who has been on extended bed rest during the pregnancy may also be more at risk for fatigue. Because many families are now geographically separated and may be unable to come and spend time with the mother and new baby, fatigue may also be more common in these women when the mother is left to care for herself and baby in the early postpartum period.

Developing Cultural Competence Postpartum Recuperation

Most mothers view the postpartum period as a time for recuperation. In many non-Western cultures, the 40 days following a birth are a time of recovery when female relatives or friends assist the new mother in her daily activities (Zerwekh & Garneau, 2014). In northern Africa, for example, the 40-day period after birth is considered a time of transition for the mother. The mother and baby are not separated during this time. This practice is known to prevent postpartum psychosis and facilitate bonding (Zerwekh & Garneau, 2014). This is also the custom in India, where it is believed by some that the mother and new baby need protection from evil spirits as well as from exposure to illness because they are both considered vulnerable during this time period (Zerwekh & Garneau, 2014).

In Mexico, this period is briefer, lasting only 20 days. During the first 7 days, nonhousehold members are not permitted to visit or enter the home. The mother gradually increases activity after the first week. The end of the postpartum period is marked by a *sobada*, a massage performed by the midwife on the 20th day after birth (Zerwekh & Garneau, 2014).

Women With Special Needs Mental Illness

Women with a history of mental illness are at an increased risk for postpartum mood and anxiety disorders. Risks increase with lack of sleep, and these women should be counseled to take frequent naps and avoid sleep deprivation.

Resumption of Activity

Ambulation and activity may gradually increase after birth. The new mother should avoid heavy lifting, excessive stair climbing, and strenuous activity. One or two daily naps are essential and are most easily achieved if the mother sleeps when her baby does. Women with older children often find it difficult to get adequate rest because they want to spend time with their older children when the baby is napping. The woman should

be cautioned that fatigue and exhaustion can become a vicious cycle and should be avoided. Assistance in the household can help prevent this and can enable the mother to spend special time with older children while others take over household tasks.

By the second week at home, the woman may resume light housekeeping. Although it is customary to delay returning to work for 6 weeks, most women are physically able to resume practically all activities by 4 to 5 weeks. In some cases, if bleeding returns, it is often a sign that the mother is overdoing her activities and should decrease some activity. Delaying the return to work until after the final postpartum examination minimizes the possibility of problems.

Postpartum Exercises

The woman should be encouraged to begin simple exercises while in the birthing unit and to continue them at home. Kegel exercises should be reviewed and begun while the woman is still in the hospital (see Chapter 10 and Figure 10–12). She is advised that increased lochia or pain means she should reevaluate her activity and make necessary alterations. Most agencies provide a booklet describing suggested postpartum exercises. (Exercise routines vary for women undergoing cesarean birth or tubal ligation after childbirth.)

Exercise during the postpartum period has several health benefits for new mothers. Exercise can help maintain insulin and high-density lipoprotein (HDL) cholesterol levels, as well as improve aerobic fitness. The postpartum woman is more likely to have positive views of her well-being, more self-esteem, and less fatigue if she continues to do stretching and her own pattern of exercise after she is home. The addition of pelvic floor exercises can also decrease such problems as urinary leakage or incontinence. Exercise also helps facilitate postpartum weight loss, reduces stress, and provides the mother with needed time alone.

Sexual Activity and Contraception

Typically, postpartum couples resume sexual intercourse once the episiotomy is healed and the lochial flow has stopped (Leeman & Rogers, 2012). Because this usually occurs by the end of the third week, before the 6-week check, it is important that the woman and her partner have information about what to expect. The nurse may inform the couple that, because the vaginal vault is "dry" (lacking estrogen), some form of water-soluble lubrication such as K-Y jelly or Astroglide may be necessary during intercourse. The female-superior and side-lying coital positions may be preferable because they allow the woman to control the depth of penile penetration. Couples should be counseled that intercourse may be uncomfortable for the woman for some time and that patience is imperative.

Breastfeeding couples should be forewarned that during orgasm milk may spurt from the nipples because of the release of oxytocin. Some couples find this spurt pleasurable or amusing, but others choose to have the woman wear a bra during sexual activity. Nursing the baby before lovemaking reduces the chance of milk release (Leeman & Rogers, 2012).

Other factors may inhibit satisfactory sexual experiences: the baby's crying may "spoil the mood," the woman's changed body may seem unattractive to her or her partner, maternal sleep deprivation may reduce the woman's desire, and the woman's physiologic response to sexual stimulation may be altered because of hormonal changes. By 3 months postpartum, many couples have returned to prepregnant levels of sexual interest and activity; however, this is highly variable. It is not abnormal for women, especially when breastfeeding, to experience decreased libido for several months (Leeman &

| TEACHING HIGHLIGHTS | Resumption of Sexual Activity After Childbirth |

- Delay intercourse until no lochia is present because lochia indicates that healing is not yet complete.
- Tenderness of the vagina and perineum may cause discomfort. The partner may test the woman's level of comfort by slipping a lubricated finger inside her vagina. The female-superior and side-lying positions may be preferable because they let the woman control the depth of penetration of the penis.
- Vaginal dryness may occur because the vagina is "hormone poor." Discomfort as a result of dryness can be avoided by using a water-soluble lubricant.
- Based on the amount of breast engorgement and tenderness present, the partner may need to avoid breast stimulation during foreplay or use a very gentle approach.
- Escape of milk during sexual activity can be minimized by breastfeeding immediately beforehand.
- Fatigue and the new baby's schedule may have a negative impact on the woman's feelings of desire. Napping when the baby sleeps helps decrease fatigue. However, fatigue may be a reality couples need to accept during the early postpartum months.
- Contraception is important even during the early postpartum period. The woman's body needs adequate time to heal and recover from the stress of pregnancy and childbirth. Couples opposed to contraception may choose abstinence at this time.

Rogers, 2012). Decreased libido can be associated with hormonal changes, fatigue, stress, and lack of time because of family and work demands.

With anticipatory guidance during the prenatal and postpartum periods, the couple can be forewarned of potential temporary problems. Anticipatory guidance is enhanced if the couple can discuss their feelings and reactions as they are experienced. (See *Teaching Highlights: Resumption of Sexual Activity After Childbirth*.)

Information on contraception is often provided as part of discharge teaching if it is permissible within the healthcare agency. The nurse can also be an important resource for the woman and her partner during postpartum follow-up. Couples typically choose to use contraception to control the number of children they will have or to determine the spacing of future children. However, some religious-based hospital facilities prohibit nurses and other healthcare providers from discussing contraception. If the nurse is discussing birth control, it is important to emphasize that in choosing a specific method, consistency of use is essential. The nurse needs to identify the advantages, disadvantages, risks, and contraindications of the various methods to help the couple, or the single mother, make an informed choice about the most practical and compatible method. (For a more detailed discussion of contraceptive methods, see Chapter 5.) Breastfeeding women are commonly concerned that a contraceptive method will interfere with their ability to breastfeed. Breastfeeding women should be given available options and choose the method that best fits their lifestyle, financial situation, and personal preference.

Pharmacologic Interventions

Pharmacologic preparations, including pain medications, vaccinations (rubella and Tdap), and Rh immune globulin, are frequently administered in the postpartum period. For complete pharmacologic interventions used in the postpartum period, consult a drug guide. Vaccinations that should be administered in the immediate postpartum period are included in Table 29–3.

Promotion of Effective Parent Learning

Meeting the educational needs of the new mother and her family is a primary challenge facing the postpartum nurse. Each woman's educational needs vary based on her age, background,

educational level, experience, and expectations. However, because the mother spends only a brief period of time in the postpartum area, identifying and addressing individual instructional needs can be difficult. Effective education provides the childbearing family with sufficient knowledge to meet many of their own health needs and to seek assistance if necessary.

The nurse first assesses the learning needs of the new mother through observation, sensitivity to nonverbal cues, and tactfully phrased questions. For example, "What plans have you made for handling things when you get home?" may elicit a response of several words and may provide the opportunity for some information sharing and guidance. Some agencies also use checklists of common concerns for new mothers. The woman can check the concerns that are of interest to her.

Teaching during the postpartum period is a continuous process in which the nurse takes opportunities throughout interactions with the new parents to identify learning opportunities and offer teaching interventions. The nurse can also plan and implement teaching in a logical, nonthreatening way based on knowledge and respect of the family's cultural values and beliefs. Unless the nurse believes a culturally related activity would be harmful, it can be supported and encouraged.

Nurses need to consider the mother's physical and psychosocial needs when conducting postpartum teaching. Initially, women may be exhausted from the birth experience and their concentration may be impaired. Later, the new mother may be preoccupied with visitors and phone calls. Information should be delivered a little at a time and repeated to make sure that the parents understand what the nurse has discussed with them. Repetition is a valuable tool in the postpartum environment. In addition, many women are discharged during the first 48 hours after birth, making postpartum education difficult. When performing teaching sessions, the father's schedule must also be considered. If the father returns to work during the immediate postpartum period, he may be more likely to attend teaching sessions scheduled in the late afternoon or early evening (Figure 29–2). In some cultures, such as the Hispanic culture, female relatives often assist the new mother and baby. It is important to include any care providers in the teaching session.

Postpartum units use a variety of instructional methods, including handouts, formal classes, videotapes, and individual interaction. Printed materials are helpful for new mothers to consult if questions arise at home. Some facilities offer a hotline service that new mothers can call with questions or concerns. As the cultural diversity in the United States continues to grow, the need for culturally sensitive information is imperative.

TABLE 29–3 Vaccinations for Postpartum Administration

RUBELLA VIRUS VACCINE, LIVE (MERUVAX 2)

Dose/Route:

Single-dose vial, inject subcutaneously in outer aspect of the upper arm.

Indication:

Stimulate active immunity against rubella virus. Rubella titer of less than 1:10 or antibody negative on enzyme-linked immunosorbent assay (ELISA) test.

Adverse Effects:

Burning or stinging at the injection site; about 2–4 weeks later may have rash, malaise, sore throat, or headache.

Nursing Implications:

Obtain informed consent. Determine whether woman has sensitivity to neomycin (vaccine contains neomycin); is immunosuppressed, or has received blood transfusions (not to be administered within 3 months of blood transfusion, plasma transfusion, or serum immune globulin). To be given at discharge.

Client Teaching:

Name of drug, expected effect, possible adverse effects, possible comfort measures to use if adverse effects occur; rubella titer will be assessed in about 3 months. Instruct woman to AVOID PREGNANCY for 30 days following vaccination. Provide information regarding contraceptives and their use.

Nursing Diagnoses (NANDA-I © 2014) Related to Drug Therapy:

Knowledge, Deficient, regarding drug therapy

Self-Health Management, Readiness for Enhanced, related to information about postpartum contraception regarding an expressed desire to avoid pregnancy following rubella vaccination

Pain related to rash and malaise

TDAP (REDUCED DIPHTHERIA TOXOID AND ACELLULAR PERTUSSIS)

Dose/Route:

Single-dose vial, inject subcutaneously in outer aspect of the upper arm.

Indication:

Any woman who is nonimmune and has not received the vaccination during pregnancy should be vaccinated in the postpartum period.

Adverse Effects:

Soreness, redness or swelling at injection site, fever, headache, nausea, vomiting, diarrhea, stomach upset, swelling of the entire arm (rare)

Nursing Implications:

Confirm criteria for administration are present. Inject entire contents of vial. Advise woman of potential adverse reactions.

Client Teaching:

Name of drug, expected action, possible side effects; report soreness at injection site to nurse; advise primary care provider of any vaccinations received in the postpartum period.

Nursing Diagnoses (NANDA-I © 2014) Related to Drug Therapy:

Self-Health Management, Readiness for Enhanced, related to information about need for updated immunizations to reduce the incidence of contracting and spreading disease

Pain related to soreness at injection site

RHOGAM (RH IMMUNE GLOBULIN SPECIFIC FOR D ANTIGEN)

Dose/Route:

Postpartum: One vial IM within 72 hr of birth. *Antepartum:* One vial microdose RhoGAM IM at 28 weeks in Rh-negative women; after amniocentesis, spontaneous or therapeutic abortion, or ectopic pregnancy.

Indication:

Prevention of sensitization to the Rh factor in Rh-negative women and to prevent hemolytic disease in the newborn in subsequent pregnancies (see Chapter 15). Mother must be Rh negative, not previously sensitized to Rh factor. Baby must be Rh positive, direct antiglobulin negative.

Adverse Effects:

Soreness at injection site.

Nursing Implications:

Confirm criteria for administration are present. Ensure correct vial is used for the client (each vial is cross-matched to the specific woman and must be carefully checked). Inject entire contents of vial.

Client Teaching:

Name of drug, expected action, possible side effects; report soreness at injection site to nurse; woman should carry information regarding Rh status and dates of RhoGAM injections with her at all times; explain use of RhoGAM with subsequent pregnancies.

Nursing Diagnoses (NANDA-I © 2014) Related to Drug Therapy:

Self-Health Management, Readiness for Enhanced, related to information about future need for Rh immune globulin regarding an expressed desire to understand the long-term implications of her Rh-negative status

Pain related to soreness at injection site

Along with culturally diverse material, teaching aids should be presented in the woman's native language when possible. Written materials should be available and translators or language lines should be utilized. Many clients are now accustomed to using the Internet and may prefer to use online support groups and access educational materials found online. As technology expands, the nurse must remain current with the changing technology and the resources it creates. Evaluation of learning may also take several forms: return demonstrations, question-and-answer sessions, and even formal evaluation tools. Follow-up phone calls after discharge provide additional evaluative information and continue the helping process for the family.

Teaching content should include information on role changes and psychologic adjustments as well as skills. Risk factors and signs of postpartum depression should be reviewed with all women. Information is also essential for women with

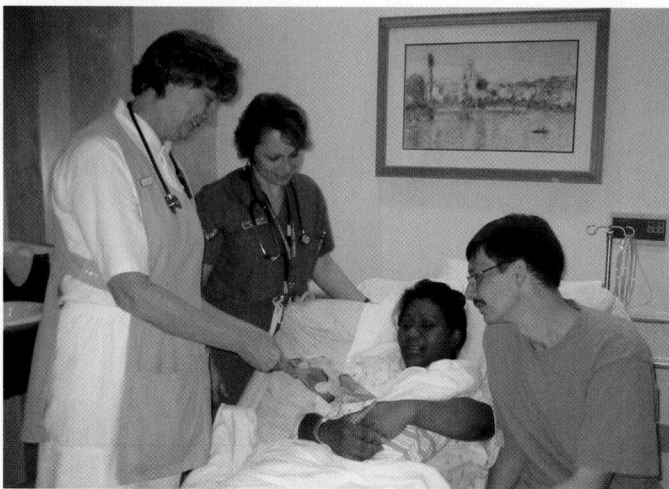

Figure 29-2 Postpartum teaching. The nurse provides educational information to both parents.

specialized educational needs such as the mother who has had a cesarean birth, the parents of twins, the parents of a baby with congenital anomalies, parents with other young children, and parents with a child that will require long-term hospitalization. Because more and more women with disabilities are now having children, they may require additional support and education. Anticipatory guidance can help prepare parents for the many changes they will experience with a new family member.

Promotion of Family Wellness

A positive maternity experience is likely to have a positive effect on the entire family. The family that receives appropriate information and has adequate time to interact with its newest member in a supportive environment will feel more comfortable and secure at home.

Today, most facilities support *family-centered care* that is focused on keeping the mother and baby together as much as the mother desires. This type of care is called **mother–baby care**, or **couplet care**, and provides increased opportunities for parent–child interactions because the newborn shares the mother's room and they are cared for together. Mother–baby care provides the mother with time to bond with her baby and to learn to care for her baby in a supportive environment. It is especially conducive to a hunger-demand feeding schedule for both breastfeeding and formula-feeding babies. This arrangement also allows the father, siblings, grandparents, and others to participate in the care of the new baby. Women who give birth in a facility that offers mother–baby care are often more satisfied with their postpartum experience than women who are cared for under different care models. Contemporary practice advocates a "rooming-in" model of care where the mother and newborn remain together as much as possible.

Mother–baby unit policies must be flexible enough to permit the mother to return the baby to the nursery if she finds it necessary because of fatigue or physical discomfort. Some mother–baby units also return the newborns to a central nursery at night so the mothers can get more rest.

Reactions of Siblings

Mother–baby care provides excellent opportunities for family bonds to grow when the mother, father/partner, newborn, and siblings begin functioning as a family unit immediately after the birth. When mother–baby care is not available, liberal sibling

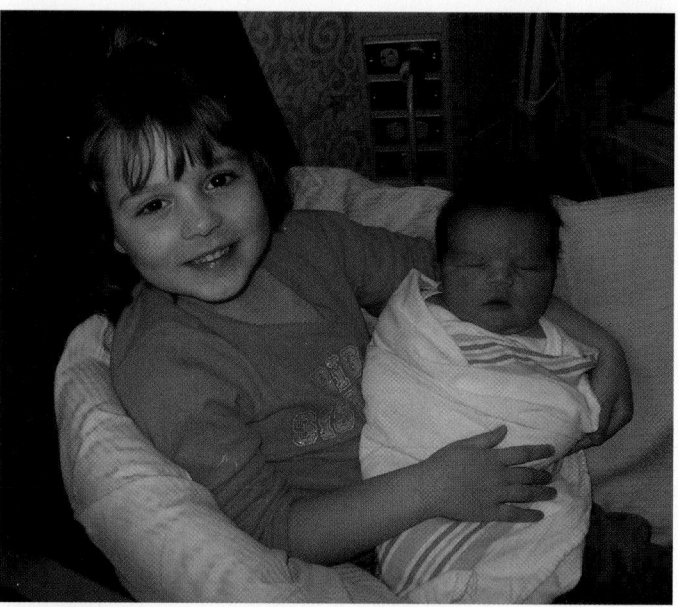

Figure 29-3 Siblings and the newborn. The sister of this newborn becomes acquainted with the new family member during a nursing assessment.
SOURCE: Wilson Garcia.

visitation policies can help meet the family's needs. A visit to the mother–baby unit reassures children that their mother is well and still loves them. It also provides an opportunity for the children to become familiar with the new baby. For the mother, the pangs of separation are lessened as she interacts with her children and introduces them to the newest family member (Figure 29–3). Even babies who require intensive care nursery admissions should be allowed to have sibling visits whenever possible. Although preventing preemies and other newborns who require intensive care services from infection is a valid concern, policies that involve taking the sibling's temperature before each visit and documenting the sibling's health status can provide a safeguard that still promotes family bonding. Some of these babies may be hospitalized for weeks or months. Sibling visitation allows the early incorporation of the baby into the family unit for siblings.

Clinical Tip
Because siblings may feel left out with the addition of a new family member, provide positive feedback to promote attachment. For example, pointing out to the older child that "Carlos is looking at you," or asking, "Do you think he knows you're his big sister?" can help make siblings feel accepted and valued. Also identify ways in which siblings can help the new mother, for example, by bringing her a cup of water or singing the baby a favorite lullaby.

Teach parents that, although they may have prepared their children for the presence of a new brother or sister, the actual arrival of the baby in the home requires some adjustments. Although it may be more chaotic for the parents, allowing the children to come to the hospital to pick up mom and the new baby can signify their importance in the family process. If small children are waiting at home, it is helpful if the father carries the baby inside. This practice keeps the mother's arms free to hug and touch her older children. Many mothers bring a doll home with them for an older child. Caring for the doll alongside the mother or father helps the child to identify with the parents. This identification helps decrease anger and the need to regress to gain attention.

Parents may also provide supervised times when older children can hold the new baby and perhaps even help with a feeding or diapering. Many parents may have concerns about the children "hurting" the new baby, but with proper supervision, the siblings are more likely to develop an attachment to their new sibling. The other children feel a sense of accomplishment and learn tenderness and caring. The nurse also suggests that parents spend one-to-one quality time with each of their older children each day. This may require some careful planning, but it confirms the parents' continuing love for the other children and promotes siblings' acceptance of the newborn.

Promotion of Parent–Newborn Attachment During the Postpartum Period

Nursing interventions to enhance the quality of parent–newborn attachment should be designed to promote feelings of well-being, comfort, and satisfaction. Although many new mothers lack experience and feel overwhelmed with their babies, certain groups of women are at higher risk for alterations in parent–infant attachment. These include women who are unemployed, single, living in poverty, or have a previous history of mental health issues, parents with developmental disabilities, parents with substance abuse issues, low-birth-weight babies, and firstborn babies (Michigan Department of Community Health, 2015). Other factors such as a baby's temperament and genetic factors may also impact parent–infant bonding (Michigan Department of Community Health, 2015). These mothers warrant additional assessment and support from the nurse to ensure proper bonding is taking place.

Following are some suggestions for ways the nurse can promote parent–newborn attachment during the postpartum stay:

- Determine the parenting style and goals of the baby's mother and father/partner and adapt them when possible in planning nursing care for the family. This includes giving the parents choices about their initial time with their new baby.

- Provide time and as much privacy as possible for the new family to become acquainted. Allow siblings to visit throughout the postpartum stay if requested by the parents.

- Arrange the healthcare setting so that the individual nurse–client relationship can be developed. A primary nurse can develop rapport and assess the mother's strengths and needs.

- Use anticipatory guidance to prepare the parents for expected problems of adjustment. Model appropriate behaviors based on the baby's cues and behaviors.

- Include parents in any nursing intervention, planning, and evaluation. Give choices when possible.

- Initiate and support measures to alleviate fatigue in the parents.

- Help parents identify, understand, and accept both positive and negative feelings related to the overall parenting experience.

- Support and assist parents in determining the personality and unique needs of their baby.

The beginnings of parent–newborn attachment may be observed in the first few hours after birth (see Chapter 25 for a discussion of early attachment behaviors). Continued assessments may occur during the postpartum stay (Chapter 28 discusses the development of family attachment) and during home visits after discharge. As the nurse assesses attachment, it is important to remember that cultural values, beliefs, and practices will direct the childcare activities and self-care practices.

Nursing Care Following Cesarean Birth

After a cesarean birth the new mother has postpartum needs similar to those of women who have given birth vaginally. Because she has undergone major abdominal surgery, however, the woman's nursing care needs are also similar to those of other surgical clients.

Promotion of Maternal Physical Well-Being After Cesarean Birth

The chances of pulmonary infection are increased because of immobility after the use of narcotics and sedatives and because of the altered immune response in postoperative clients. Therefore, the woman is encouraged to cough and deep breathe every 2 to 4 hours while awake until she is ambulating frequently. Leg exercises are also encouraged every 2 hours until the woman is ambulating. These exercises increase circulation, help prevent thrombophlebitis, and also aid intestinal motility by tightening abdominal muscles. For women who are not ambulatory, a sequential compression device (SCD) system may be ordered to increase circulation and prevent deep vein thrombosis.

Early ambulation, eating a low roughage diet shortly after birth, and breastfeeding soon after birth all enhance the recovery of the mother and decrease complications in the postoperative period. Even though a cesarean birth is an operative procedure, most women giving birth are relatively healthy and therefore are less likely to experience postoperative complications when compared with other surgical clients.

> **Health Promotion** **Reducing Cesarean Births**
> *Healthy People 2020* objectives (U.S. Department of Health and Human Services [USDHHS], 2015) include reducing the number of cesarean births in low-risk women. Nurses can explain to women that even though a cesarean birth was performed for this birth, a trial of labor after cesarean (TOLAC) may be a viable option in the future.

The nurse monitors and manages the woman's pain experience during the postpartum period. Sources of pain include incisional pain, gas pain, referred shoulder pain, periodic uterine contractions (afterbirth pains), discomfort related to breastfeeding, and pain from voiding, defecation, or constipation.

Nursing interventions are oriented toward preventing or alleviating pain or helping the woman cope with pain. The nurse should undertake the following measures:

- Administer analgesics as needed, especially during the first 24 to 72 hours after childbirth. Use of analgesics relieves the woman's pain and enables her to be more mobile and active. Some facilities administer ibuprofen on a continuous basis in the early postpartum period to decrease swelling, reduce pain, and decrease the need for, or frequency of, narcotic agents. Women who have undergone a cesarean birth may receive a morphine sulfate injection

(Duramorph) via the epidural or spinal anesthesia catheter, which provides 16 to 24 hours of pain relief.

- Promote comfort through proper positioning, frequent position changes, massage, back rubs, oral care, and the reduction of noxious stimuli such as noise and unpleasant odors.

- Encourage visits by significant others, including the newborn and older children. These visits distract the woman from the painful sensations and help reduce her fear and anxiety.

- Encourage the use of breathing, relaxation, guided imagery, and distraction (e.g., stimulation of cutaneous tissue) techniques taught in childbirth preparation class.

Epidural analgesia administered just after the cesarean birth is an effective method of pain relief for most women in the first 24 hours following birth.

In some geographic areas, certain pain relief techniques continue to be used, although the frequency of their use is decreasing. These techniques include the following:

- Patient-controlled analgesia (PCA) may be used in cases when the woman is given a bolus of analgesia, usually morphine or fentanyl, at the beginning of therapy and is then able to administer smaller, more frequent doses on demand for pain control.

- Continuous epidural infusion (CEI) technique, in which the epidural catheter is left in place following the cesarean birth and medication is continually administered via an electric pump that is controlled by the client.

- Continuous peripheral nerve block that delivers a local anesthetic through a tiny catheter that is positioned directly into the wound site and connected to an external balloon that allows medication to be delivered at a steady rate for up to 5 days after the birth and creates a numbing effect at the incision site.

- General anesthetic is the least desired form of anesthesia because of the multiple maternal and fetal side effects it produces, which may include difficulty with resuming a normal diet resulting in abdominal distention, nausea, vomiting, flatus pain, or bloating.

Sometimes women who have had a cesarean birth have other discomforts that can be relieved with pharmacologic interventions. The nurse assesses the woman for other symptoms, such as nausea, itching (which is typically related to the morphine used in the epidural), and headache. If the woman is experiencing nausea, an antiemetic can be administered. Itching can also be relieved with pharmacologic interventions. Nonsteroidal anti-inflammatory drugs (NSAIDs) are effective in managing headaches and other body aches.

The nurse can minimize discomfort and promote satisfaction as the mother assumes the activities of her new role. Instruction and assistance in assuming comfortable positions when holding or breastfeeding the baby will do much to increase the mother's sense of competence and comfort. The woman should be taught to splint her incision when she ambulates to decrease pulling on the incision and the discomfort created by contraction of the abdominal muscles.

Other measures are aimed at other needs that are unique to the woman who has had an operative birth. These include (Fowles, Cheng, & Mills, 2012):

- Assessing the consistency of the abdomen. Women with a firm, distended abdomen may be having difficulty passing flatus or stool.

- Assessment of the intravenous (IV) site, flow rate, and patency of the IV tubing.

- Monitoring the condition of surgical dressings or the incision site using the REEDA scale (redness, edema, ecchymosis, discharge, and approximation of the suture line) along with skin temperature at and around the incision line.

The cesarean birth mother usually does extremely well postoperatively. Most women are ambulating by the day after the surgery. Usually by the second postpartum day the woman can shower, which seems to provide a mental as well as physical lift. Most women are discharged by the third day after birth.

Promotion of Parent–Newborn Interaction After Cesarean Birth

Many factors associated with cesarean birth may hinder successful and frequent parent–newborn interaction. These factors include the physical condition of the mother and newborn and maternal reactions to stress, anesthesia, and medications. The father or significant other may be concerned about the mother and preoccupied with her condition, resulting in less interaction with the newborn. The mother and her baby may be separated after birth because of birthing unit routines, prematurity, or neonatal complications or a birth defect. A healthy baby born by uncomplicated cesarean is no more fragile than one born vaginally.

In some cases, signs of depression, anger, or withdrawal may indicate a grief response to the loss of the fantasized birth experience. Fathers as well as mothers may experience feelings of "missing out," guilt, or even jealousy toward another couple who had a vaginal birth. The couple who have experienced a cesarean birth may need the opportunity to tell their story repeatedly to work through these feelings. The nurse can provide factual information about their situation and support the couple's effective coping behaviors. The nurse should acknowledge their feelings while emphasizing the importance of a healthy birth outcome. Enhanced communication during the labor, birth, and in the immediate period after birth, along with specific teaching related to issues regarding a cesarean birth, is associated with less maternal distress and improved satisfaction with the birth experience (Nilsson, Lundgren, Karlström, et al., 2012). It is also important to remember that some women may feel more comfortable with a cesarean birth and may have requested a primary or repeat cesarean birth.

Clinical Reasoning Repeat Cesarean

You walk into her room and find Dana Sullivan, a 29-year-old G2P2, crying 48 hours after a repeat cesarean birth. She states, "I'm not ready to go home. With my first baby they made me go home after 2 days. Can they make me go home so early again?"

What therapeutic nursing questions would you ask Dana to assess her reluctance to go home?

During the initial taking-in phase, the new parents are processing their new role and may be nurturing themselves and each other. This is normal and expected. By the second or third day, the cesarean birth mother moves into the "taking-hold" period and is usually receptive to learning how to care for herself and her baby. During this period, the focus shifts from the mother and father/partner to the baby. Vulnerability can occur during this period and the parents may feel overwhelmed. The need for nursing intervention to guide the new parents is essential. Special emphasis should be given to home management. The nurse can encourage the mother to let others assume responsibility for housekeeping and cooking. Fatigue not only prolongs recovery but also interferes with breastfeeding and mother–newborn interaction, increases the risk of prolonged postpartum blues, and leads to feelings of being overwhelmed.

The presence of the father or partner during the birth process positively influences the woman's perception of the birth event. The father's/partner's presence reduces the woman's fears, enhances her sense of control, and enables the couple to share feelings and respond to each other with touch and eye contact. Later, they have the opportunity to relive the experience and fill in any gaps or missing pieces. The presence of the father/partner is especially valuable if the mother has had general anesthesia. The father/partner can take pictures, hold the baby, and foster the discovery process by directing the mother's attention to the details of the newborn. Sometimes, during the taking-hold phase, the father/partner can feel neglected or excluded. This will soon pass as the letting-go stage begins. During this transition, the family incorporates the baby into the family unit and other family members, such as grandparents and siblings, get to know the baby and be included in the new family routine.

The baby born by cesarean is typically removed from the operating room before the mother is able to hold the newborn. Separation of the family unit is not medically necessary unless the baby needs to be stabilized or there is a complication occurring in the operating room. The practice is typically historical in nature. Agencies that embrace family-centered care can advocate to keep the mother–baby couple together as much as possible. The nurse can play a crucial role in facilitating interaction by encouraging the father/partner or support person to stand beside the warmer and interact with the baby. Often, the baby can be given to the father/partner or support person to hold. The baby can be held close to the mother and placed against her cheek so direct eye contact can occur. The nurse can also arrange for the newborn to stay with the parents in the recovery area in the immediate postoperative period. This gives the family time to interact when the baby is in an alert state.

Often new parents perceive the parenting role as an extension of the childbearing role. Inability to fulfill expected childbearing behavior (vaginal birth) may lead to parental feelings of role failure and frustration. If the parents' attitude is more positive than negative, successful resolution of subsequent stressful events is more likely. The nurse can help families alter their negative definitions of cesarean birth and bolster and encourage positive perceptions.

Nursing Care of the Postpartum Adolescent

The adolescent mother may have special postpartum needs, depending on her level of maturity and her support system. The nurse needs to assess maternal–newborn interaction, roles of support people, plans for discharge, knowledge of childrearing, and plans for follow-up care. It is imperative that a community health service contact the adolescent shortly after discharge.

Contraception counseling is an important part of teaching. *Healthy People 2020* objectives (USDHHS, 2015) include using contraception as a means of pregnancy planning. The incidence of repeat pregnancies during adolescence is high. The younger the adolescent, the more likely she is to become pregnant again. Nurses should be aware of the state laws that govern their jurisdictions in order to determine if providing contraception without parental consent is allowed. In states where adolescents can obtain birth control without parental consent, it is often more comfortable for the adolescent to address these issues without others present. (Chapter 12 discusses adolescent pregnancy in depth.) Adolescents may encounter obstacles when attempting to obtain contraceptives. These may include embarrassment about discussing the topic; concerns about confidentiality, such as not wanting their parents to know or having to give permission; and lack of knowledge regarding available methods (Cherry & Dillon, 2014). Nurses can play a key role in overcoming these obstacles by providing teaching and referrals that address these barriers.

The nurse has many opportunities for teaching the adolescent about her newborn in the postpartum unit. Because the nurse is a role model, the manner in which she handles the newborn greatly influences the young mother. If he is present, the father should be included in as much of the teaching as possible. If the grandparents are going to take an active role in caring for the infant, they should also be included in teaching *if* desired by the new mother.

As with older parents, a newborn examination done at the bedside gives adolescents information about their baby's health and shows possible positions for handling the baby. The nurse can also use this time to provide information about newborn and infant behavior. Parents who have some idea of what to expect from their baby are less frustrated with the newborn's behavior.

The adolescent mother appreciates positive feedback about her newborn and her developing maternal responses. Praise and encouragement will increase her confidence and self-esteem. Young mothers with low self-esteem, family conflict, and few social supports are more likely to encounter postpartum depression (Cherry & Dillon, 2014). Careful assessment of these factors should be made during the postpartum period so appropriate referrals can be provided before discharge.

Group classes for adolescent mothers should include information about infant care skills, such as taking the baby's temperature, clearing the nose and mouth, monitoring growth and development, feeding the baby, providing well-baby care, and identifying danger signals in the ill newborn. These classes can also address unique needs of teen mothers, such as peer relationships, added responsibilities, and goal setting.

Ideally, teenage mothers should visit adolescent clinics for assessment of themselves and their child for several years after birth. In this way, the adolescent's enrollment in classes on parenting, need for vocational guidance, and school attendance can be supported and followed closely. School systems' classes for young mothers are an excellent way of helping adolescents finish school and learn how to parent at the same time. Some public high schools have on-site childcare centers to assist with childcare needs and to provide an opportunity for adolescents to learn important child development principles and childcare tasks.

Nursing Care of the Woman Who Relinquishes Her Baby

Women who choose to give their babies up for adoption typically are single, White, never-married adolescents. It is much less common in Black and Hispanic cultures to consider adoption. Less than 1% of all births in the United States result in an adoption (Center for American Progress, 2015). The majority of young women who relinquish their children have higher education and income levels, higher future educational/career goals, are emotionally unready for parenthood, and experience disapproval from parents or partners who reject the idea of the young mother raising the baby. Other women are affected by substance abuse issues or issues involved in court proceedings that have terminated or altered parental rights because of incarceration or past abuse issues.

SAFETY ALERT!

The Infant Safe Haven Acts were enacted to protect newborns from death caused by abandonment; to provide a means for a mother to place her baby up for adoption anonymously; and to ensure that relinquished babies are left with safe providers who can care for them and provide medical services. The relinquishing mother is protected from prosecution for neglect or abandonment under the law (Child Welfare Information Gateway, 2012). Discharge teaching should include this information to all mothers.

Surrogacy

Surrogacy is also becoming more common in the United States, resulting in relinquishment agreements that may not show up in the adoption statistics. Even though the mother has entered a legal agreement to give up the child she is carrying, she still faces grief issues. The mother who chooses to let her child be adopted usually experiences intense ambivalence. Several factors contribute to this ambivalence. First, there are social pressures against giving up one's child. Additionally, the woman has usually made considerable adjustments in her lifestyle to carry and give birth to this child, and may be unaware of the growing bond between her and her child. Her attachment feelings may peak upon seeing her baby. At the same time, she may not have told friends and relatives about the pregnancy and so may lack a support system to help her work through her feelings and support her decision making. After childbirth, the mother needs to complete a grieving process to work through her loss and its accompanying grief, loneliness, guilt, and other feelings.

Nursing Interventions

The nurse focuses on assisting the mother with grief, which occurs as part of the relinquishment process. Mothers who relinquish their babies often experience disenfranchised grief, that is, grief that is unrecognized or not socially accepted. When the relinquishing mother is admitted to the birthing unit, the nurse should be informed about the mother's decision to relinquish the baby and facilitate any special requests for the birth and encourage the woman to express her emotions. After the birth, the mother should have access to the baby while she decides how much, if any, interaction she wants with the newborn. Seeing the newborn often aids the grieving process and provides an opportunity for the birth mother to say goodbye. Modern adoptions afford the birth mother with multiple choices, such as meeting and interviewing perspective parents, the option to have contact after the adoption, limited visitation, and open adoption practices. Some mothers may continue to receive narrative updates and photos of their children.

Postpartum nursing care also includes arranging ongoing care for the relinquishing mother. Some mothers may request an early discharge or a transfer to another medical unit. When possible, the nurse supports these requests.

Postpartum Care for Special Populations

Nursing Care of the Postpartum Woman With Obesity

As obesity increases in the United States, the postpartum nurse will care for a growing number of mothers who are obese or morbidly obese. The woman with obesity has needs similar to those of other postpartum women, but she needs special attention to prevent injury, respiratory complications, thromboembolic disease, and infection, for which she is at high risk.

The nurse should carefully assess the woman for airway obstruction and hypoxia, particularly if she received opioids. Ambulation should be encouraged as soon as possible to prevent pneumonia. The use of sequential compression devices (SCDs) and early ambulation is essential to the prevention of deep vein thrombosis, especially if the woman had a cesarean birth. If mechanical vacuum devices are used to facilitate drainage from her incision following a cesarean birth, the woman should be educated about them. The mother should demonstrate how to visualize, clean, and completely dry her incision prior to discharge. The use of a mirror may be helpful. She needs to recognize and promptly report signs of infection or dehiscence of her surgical incision or episiotomy repair.

SAFETY ALERT!

The nurse needs to utilize adequate personnel and appropriate assistive devices to maintain safety for both the woman who is obese and staff members during position changes, transport, and ambulation. Additionally, the new mother may need extra supervision and assistance when breastfeeding her baby to ensure newborn safety.

Nursing Care of the Postpartum Lesbian Mother

Although the literature regarding gay and lesbian families is growing, much of it is focused on options for conception, challenges experienced by gay parents, and legal issues. As contemporary legislation evolves and same-sex marriage legality is increasingly common, new legal issues surrounding childbearing will likely arise. Some states are examining changing legal practices regarding adoption and birth certificate options to allow both spouses to be listed on birth certificates. Little has been published about the labor, delivery, and postpartum experiences of lesbian mothers. Spidsberg and Sørlie (2012) examined lesbian couples and found that lesbian couples have a unique and different bond compared to heterosexual couples. In general, most lesbian partners often feel more at ease in the delivery room than many fathers. The nonpregnant partner often assumes a co-mothering role in the family unit. The main needs of lesbian couples identified in Spidsberg and Sørlie's qualitative study were to have an open relationship with healthcare providers who were accepting of their differences and to be able to build a rapport between the nurse and the couple.

Clinical Question

How is the experience of conception, pregnancy, and birth different for lesbian mothers?

The Evidence

Societal definitions of "family" have changed substantially and a larger number of lesbian committed couples are opting for one partner to undergo physiologic birth. The 2000 census revealed more than 300,000 self-reported lesbian families, of which more than a third were raising biologic children. While research has shown that the desire and motivation to have children among lesbian couples is quite similar to those in heterosexual relationships, little is known about the experience of conception, pregnancy, and birth as it applies to this population. These researchers conducted an in-depth qualitative study to understand the reactions of lesbian couples to the normal processes of conception, birth, and parenting. More than 120 hours of interviews and observation were included in this integrative study. While quantitative model-testing will make this evidence stronger for practice, the large sample size and extended contact make this good evidence for practice.

These mothers felt differently about the conception, pregnancy, and birth process than mothers from more traditional families. This sense of "differentness" permeated the entire experience. Several themes illustrated their sense of being different. The woman who elected to be the biologic mother often felt "normal" about the pregnancy, while the nonbiologic mother had strong legal and biologic concerns. This sense of uncertainty about legal rights was an ongoing concern for the woman who elected not to carry the pregnancy. These women also were concerned about losing their relationship, and therefore custody, since the rights of lesbian mothers have not been clearly established. The nonbiologic mother often felt incomplete and inadequate as a parent, and there was little support because the population of lesbian mothers is often hidden and not publicly acknowledged (Wojnar & Katzenmeyer, 2014). A surprising finding was that the condition of postpartum depression affected both biologic and nonbiologic parents in these relationships.

Best Practice

Lesbian couples have unique needs during conception, pregnancy, and birth. Sensitivity to the special conditions surrounding these pregnancies is needed to reassure the mothers of their adequacy as parents and to ease their concerns. Finding support for these women can help them deal with the uncertainty and demands of motherhood.

Clinical Reasoning

How can the nurse provide support to lesbian mothers so that they have an optimal pregnancy and birth experience? How might these mothers find support systems that can ease their concerns?

Nurses need to examine their own feelings about how they perceive alternative families and be mindful of their nonverbal expressions when interacting with these families (Spidsberg & Sørlie, 2012).

The nurse should maintain an attitude that is respectful, caring, and open to sexual diversity when working with all clients. Lesbian partners, regardless of marital status, should be given the same rights and care that heterosexual couples receive in the acute care setting. Providing quality client-centered care for any postpartum woman involves acknowledging, welcoming, and involving her intimate partner in care and decision making. The nurse should be aware that standardized postpartum instructions, particularly those related to intercourse and contraception, will need to be individualized and amended.

Nursing Care of the Postpartum Mother With a Developmental Disability

The postpartum time period is one of great growth in the maternal mothering role. New mothers are faced with various challenges and different learning opportunities. Women with developmental or intellectual disabilities are at particular risk during this time period. Material should be presented to them in an easy-to-understand format. Peer mentors are often helpful role models for these women. Teaching should be conducted at a level that is achievable for the individual woman. A needs assessment should be performed to determine what needs the mother and new family may have. Community and private resources should be available to make the transition to the postpartum period as flawless as possible.

Nursing Care of the Postpartum Mother With a History of Sexual Abuse

Women who have been sexually abused tend to have more anxiety and stress related to hospital procedures, interactions with unfamiliar staff, and being touched in general. The postpartum woman who has a history of sexual abuse may have difficulty establishing trust and may feel uncomfortable when private demonstrations are being performed. The nurse should treat the woman with respect by providing draping whenever possible. Speaking to the woman in private protects her fragile emotions from being observed by others. Support groups may offer the mother with a history of sexual abuse a safe haven to share her experiences and the impact they have on her mothering.

Preparation for Discharge

In preparation for discharge, the nurse evaluates the mother's and newborn's progress toward identified outcomes and provides discharge teaching.

Discharge Criteria

Ideally, preparation for discharge begins the moment a woman is admitted to the birthing unit. Before discharge, the nurse assesses the mother's physical and psychologic condition, the newborn's adjustment to extrauterine life, the family's overall adjustment, and the need for outside resources. Nursing efforts should be directed toward assessing the parents' knowledge, expectations, and beliefs and then providing anticipatory guidance and teaching accordingly. Because teaching is one of the primary responsibilities of the postpartum nurse, many agencies have elaborate teaching programs and videos. The nurse should spend time with the parents to determine if they have any last-minute questions. In general, the following criteria should be assessed and met before discharge:

- Normal vital signs
- Appropriate involution of the uterus
- Appropriate amount of lochia without evidence of infection
- Knowledge of signs of infection
- Episiotomy or laceration well approximated with a decrease in edema or bruising
- Ability to perform pericare and apply medications to perineal or anal area if ordered
- Ability to void and pass flatus (some facilities' criteria may include having a bowel movement before discharge)
- Ability to take fluids and foods without difficulty
- Ability to care for self and newborn
- Has received rubella vaccine, Tdap, or RhoGAM if indicated (see Table 29–3)

Additional outcomes for the cesarean birth mother include the following:

- States in own words the reason for the cesarean birth
- Maintains desired pain control
- Maintains moderate mobility level

Ensuring that the woman has met the criteria before discharge decreases the incidence of complications or readmission in the postpartum period.

Discharge Teaching

In general, discharge teaching includes at least the following information and maternal activities:

1. Review of literature and videos the woman has received or viewed that explains recommended postpartum exercises, the need for adequate rest, the need to avoid overexertion initially, and the recommendation to abstain from sexual intercourse until lochia has ceased. (If the family desires information about birth control methods, the nurse can provide such information at this time.)

2. Information geared to the specific nutritional needs of breastfeeding or formula-feeding mothers. (If the mother has been receiving vitamins and/or iron supplements, the nurse encourages her to continue until the first postpartum examination.) Demonstrates proper breastfeeding techniques and breast care or describes formula preparation, formula-feeding techniques, and nonlactating breast care.

3. How to provide basic care for the baby; when to anticipate that the cord will fall off; when the baby can have a tub bath; when the baby will need her or his first immunizations; and so on. (Parents should also be comfortable feeding and handling the baby, and should practice basic principles of safety, including the need to use a car seat when the baby is in a car.) See more detailed discussion later in the home care section.

4. Procedure for obtaining copies of her baby's birth certificate.

5. When to schedule the first appointment for her postpartum examination and for her newborn's first well-baby examination.

6. Signs of possible complications (see Table 29–4) and encouragement for the woman to contact her caregiver if she develops any of them. Signs and symptoms that indicate possible problems in the baby and who the parents should contact about them.

7. Information on local agencies and/or support groups, such as La Leche League, Mothers of Twins, adolescent groups, or new mother support groups, that might be of particular assistance to the family. Displays appropriate interaction with baby. Identifies the symptoms of postpartum depression and available resources.

8. Phone number of the mother–baby unit or information hotline and encouragement to call if she has any questions or concerns. Plans for home care visits so that the parents know when to expect the visit and what it entails.

The nurse can also use this final opportunity to reassure the couple of their ability to be successful parents. The nurse can stress the baby's need to feel loved and secure and urge parents to talk to each other and work together to solve any problems that arise.

Considerations for Follow-Up Care

In 1998, the Newborns' and Mothers' Health Protection Act went into effect. This federal law ensures that all insurance companies cover a 48-hour stay for vaginal deliveries and a 96-hour stay for women who have undergone a cesarean birth (U.S. Department of Labor, 2009). In consideration of the risks associated with voluntary early discharge, more than half of all U.S. states have passed legislation mandating a home visit if the family was discharged before 48 hours.

Early discharges have implications for the mother, including the risk of postpartum hemorrhage and difficulties with breastfeeding. In addition, opportunities for the mother to become comfortable with her new baby may be compromised. The risk of postpartum depression commonly occurs in the first month following the birth. Women who receive some type of

TABLE 29–4 When to Contact the Primary Healthcare Provider

After discharge, a woman should contact her healthcare provider if any of the following develop:

- Sudden, persistent, or spiking fever
- Change in the character of the lochia—foul smell, return to bright-red bleeding, excessive amount, passage of large clots
- Pain at the site of a laceration, episiotomy, or abdominal incision
- Evidence of wound infection including redness, swelling, severe or worsening pain, or foul-smelling discharge
- Evidence of mastitis, such as breast tenderness, reddened areas, malaise
- Evidence of thrombophlebitis, such as calf pain, tenderness, redness
- Evidence of urinary tract infection, such as urgency, frequency, burning on urination
- Continued severe or incapacitating postpartum depression
- Inability to care for self or baby for any physical or psychologic reason

follow-up assessment from a nurse experience less depression than those who do not receive postpartum follow-up (Surkan, Gottlieb, McCormick, et al., 2012). In addition, extended family members who live at a distance and have agreed to assist the new family in the first few weeks after birth may not have arrived yet. Furthermore, in the first 24 hours after childbirth, the mother may be too tired or may not be ready emotionally to participate in learning activities. In all cases of early discharge, a home visit by an experienced postpartum nurse can be invaluable.

These early discharges present a challenge to nurses because the time available for nursing assessments and client teaching is greatly reduced. In addition, many conditions in the newborn, such as jaundice, ductal-dependent cardiac lesions, and gastrointestinal obstructions, may take longer than 2 days to develop, and identification of these problems depends on a skilled, experienced professional (American Academy of Pediatrics [AAP] Committee on Fetus and Newborn, 2014). Other experts contend that breastfeeding may not be well established before 48 hours and discharge before this time can lead to increased rates of dehydration and poor breastfeeding outcomes (AAP Committee on Fetus and Newborn, 2014).

The need for follow-up postpartum care is essential. Most women who had a vaginal birth are seen at 6 weeks while women who had a cesarean birth are evaluated at the 2-week visit. *Healthy People 2020* objectives (USDHHS, 2015) include increasing the number of women who receive medical care at a 6-week-postpartum visit.

Women with a history of a previous psychiatric disorder or a family history of postpartum mood and anxiety disorders should receive postpartum depression (PPD) screening prior to the 6-week check-up. Women with bipolar disorder are at risk for both PPD and postpartum psychosis and warrant close observation, especially in the first weeks after birth. See Chapter 30 for an in-depth discussion.

Special emphasis has also been placed on the needs of the **late preterm newborn**, born between 34 and 37 weeks (Association of Women's Health, Obstetric and Neonatal Nurses [AWHONN], 2014). Late preterm babies are at a greater risk for increases in mortality and morbidity because they are physically not mature and are more prone to have physiologic and metabolic complications (AWHONN, 2014). Readmissions for infection and jaundice are more common in later preterm babies than in term babies (AWHONN, 2014). The American Academy of Pediatrics (AAP) has identified specific risk factors in late preterm babies that increase the likelihood of readmission and neonatal mortality. These include being first born, breastfeeding at the time of discharge, having a mother who has had labor and childbirth complications, having public insurance as your source of payment, and being an Asian/Pacific Islander (Barfield & Lee, 2012). Special attention by the home health nurse is warranted for these newborns to ensure a proper home transition and to identify possible early complications (AWHONN, 2014).

Following discharge, various services are available in most communities to meet the needs of the postpartum family. The goal is to help ensure that all family members have the opportunity to meet healthcare needs, regardless of their resources. Some types of follow-up care include telephone follow-up and home visits.

TELEPHONE FOLLOW-UP

Telephone follow-up is offered to families before discharge, and a mutually agreed-on time is set for the call. Typically the call is made within 3 days after discharge or earlier if desired, lasts about 20 minutes, and is goal directed. To perform effective telephone assessment, the nurse must be able to listen skillfully, ask open-ended questions, and project an attitude of caring. If the assessment reveals any signs of a postpartum complication, the nurse refers the woman to her healthcare provider for further evaluation. The plan of care developed and implemented during a telephone conversation is limited to supportive counseling, teaching, and referral.

It is also fairly common for a home care nurse to make a telephone follow-up call to a family a few days after a home visit to provide additional information, address questions or areas of confusion, and make referrals if indicated. The mother may have multiple questions and is generally at a high level of learning readiness. Some women may prefer a telephone-based follow-up because it requires less preparation and time than a home visit. PPD screening should be performed at this time.

In addition to these scheduled follow-up telephone calls, nurses in birthing, newborn, and postpartum units, as well as clinic nurses, often receive phone calls from postpartum families seeking advice or care. These calls must be triaged immediately. Calls with urgent or life-threatening implications should be referred appropriately, either by initiating an immediate call to the practitioner or, in rare circumstances, calling 9-1-1.

Finally, many communities have established 24-hour help lines for new parents to call when they have questions or need support. In areas where help lines are not available, parents may be directed to call the birthing center. In either case, the nurse provides the number so that it is readily accessible for the family.

HOME VISIT

If the mother, family, and healthcare provider have chosen discharge earlier than 48 hours after vaginal birth, in some states the mother may request a total of three home visits. The home setting provides an opportunity for the nurse and family to interact in a more relaxed environment in which the family has control. In some instances, the challenges of assessing and enhancing self-care and infant care may be unique in the home, and the nurse will have many opportunities to exercise critical thinking to develop creative options with the family. The nurse should explain that, unlike community health visits, only one or two home visits are typically planned and spaced out over the next week, and long-term follow-up by the postpartum nurse is not anticipated. Occasionally, the nurse may schedule additional home visits based on the findings of the first home visit and the follow-up phone call.

Evaluation

Anticipated outcomes of comprehensive postpartum nursing care of the family include the following:

- The mother is reasonably comfortable and has learned pain relief measures.
- The mother is rested and understands how to add more activity over the next few days and weeks.
- The mother's physiologic and psychologic well-being have been supported.
- The mother verbalizes her understanding of self-care measures.
- The new parents demonstrate how to care for their baby.
- The new parents have had opportunities to form attachment with their baby.
- Follow-up care contacts have been initiated as needed.

Considerations for the Home Visit

Before the home visit, the nurse (who is experienced in postpartum maternal and newborn care) prepares by identifying the purpose of the home visit and gathering needed materials and equipment. A personal contact while the woman is still in the birth setting or a previsit telephone call is used to arrange the appointment with the woman and her family. During the previsit contact, it is important for the nurse to clearly identify the purpose and goals of the visit and to begin establishing rapport.

Purpose and Timing of the Home Visit

Postpartum home care is focused more on assessment, teaching, facilitating learning, and counseling than on physical care. First, it provides an opportunity to assess the status of the mother and baby for signs of any complications. The established guidelines for discharge of the mother and baby mean the nurse can expect certain levels of health and wellness. However, because the status of the mother and newborn can change, the nurse should stay alert for deviations from the norm and identify conditions that may warrant further medical evaluation or rehospitalization. The nurse can also complete follow-up blood work if needed.

In addition, the nurse assesses adaptation of the family to the new baby and adjustment of any siblings. The nurse also assesses the parents' skill in bathing, dressing, handling, and comforting their newborn, and the appropriateness and safety of the home environment.

Another purpose of the home visit is to ascertain current informational needs and to offer requested information in a more relaxed setting. Postpartum home care provides opportunities for enhancing self- and infant-care techniques initially presented in the birth setting. Many times, questions and concerns arise at home that were not identified in the hospital.

In addition, the nurse answers questions about breastfeeding, provides support and encouragement, and addresses the need for referrals to clinics, classes, or postpartum support groups.

Mental health screening in the postpartum period should focus on assessing the new mother for postpartum mood and anxiety disorders. The nurse should obtain a birth history to determine if the mother perceives a traumatic birth experience. Postpartum onset of depression, anxiety, and posttraumatic stress disorder may occur. Postpartum psychosis is an uncommon disorder but represents a medical emergency that requires immediate hospitalization and treatment by specialty care providers.

Maintaining Safety

In the past, nurses were perceived as a mainstay of communities and could move in most settings without fear or concern for safety. Today, some communities are not safe for visiting nurses. It is important for the nurse to follow basic safety rules when conducting a home visit, including the following:

- Know the specific address and ask for directions during the previsit contact. If the area is not familiar, trace out the route on a map or use an Internet program to provide directions before leaving for the visit and take a map along. Even with a global positioning system (GPS), some areas may not be included or found within the system, so always have a backup plan in place.
- Carry a fully charged cellular phone and a working flashlight, especially for night visits.
- Notify an instructor or supervisor when leaving for a visit and check in as soon as the visit is completed.

Many agencies that provide home care services have established violence prevention programs to help ensure safety. Nurses in the community need to be aware of their environment and alert to environmental cues, whether overt or subtle. In addition, the following recommendations are important:

- Investigate the neighborhood prior to leaving car.
- Avoid walking in crowded, violent areas.
- In high-risk areas, visit the family during the day. Inform the family of your arrival time and ask them to call a supervisor if you do not arrive after 15 minutes.
- Park in well lit, populated areas with car windows and doors locked.
- Before leaving for the visit, lock personal belongings in the trunk of the car, out of sight.
- Wear clothing and identification consistent with agency policy. Wear a name tag identifying you as a nurse and carry identification.
- Avoid wearing expensive jewelry or pins of a religious or political nature that might be seen as offensive.
- Use appropriate personal body language that does not exhibit fear, aggression, or anger.
- Observe all family members' body language during the visit and be prepared to terminate the visit quickly if you feel discomfort.
- Be alert for signs that a person is becoming enraged (reddened neck and/or face, clenched fists, pacing). If any family member is violent, or if drug or alcohol abuse is occurring, leave the home and report the incident to your supervisor.
- Leave the home immediately in a non-confrontational manner if any weapon or illegal substances are visible.
- If a situation arises that feels unsafe, or a "gut feeling" tells you something is not right, terminate the visit immediately.

SAFETY ALERT!

If the visit is in an area that seems unsafe, it may be wise for two nurses to go together. Nurses should avoid entering areas where violence is in progress. In such cases, they should return to the car and contact the police or dial 9-1-1. Most people are more comfortable in familiar neighborhoods and have some hesitation when entering homes in other residential areas. First home visits may feel uncomfortable because they are unfamiliar, but with experience comfort increases.

Fostering a Caring Relationship With the Family

Although the nurse in the birthing center strives to enhance family autonomy and control, the atmosphere of the institutional environment may cause the new mother and family to feel disempowered. It is important for the professional nurse

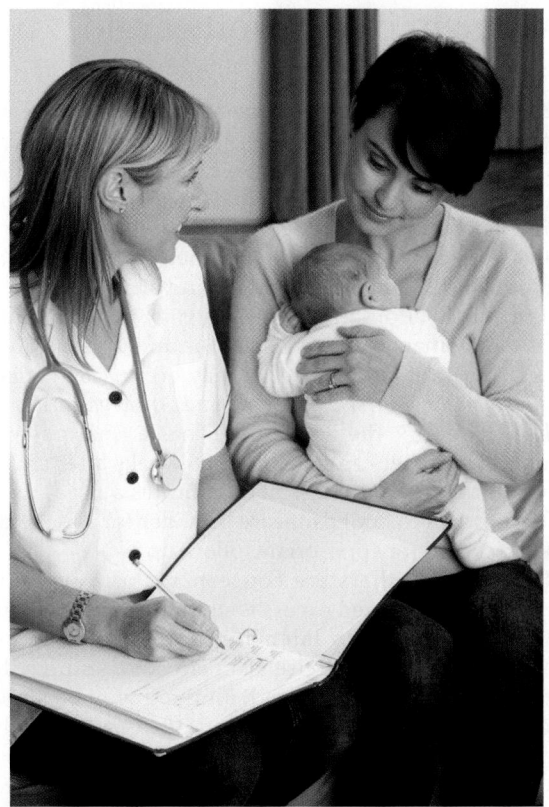

Figure 29–4 Nurse providing care and teaching to new mother and baby at the home visit.

SOURCE: Monkey Business Images/Shutterstock.

When the door is answered, the nurse should make an introduction and confirm that the location is correct. If a place to sit is not indicated, the nurse may inquire, "Where is the best place to sit so that we can talk for a while?" In some families, offering refreshments may be an important aspect of welcoming a visitor. In this case, it is beneficial to the relationship for the nurse to accept the refreshment graciously. Many cultures have strong ties to certain foods and beverages during the postpartum period. Accepting the food or beverage conveys acceptance of cultural norms. It is helpful for the nurse to be familiar with various cultural norms and traditions (Spector, 2012).

The maternal psychologic assessment focuses on attachment, adjustment to the parental role, sibling adjustment, the mother's perception of her new role and coping, and educational needs.

In ideal situations, a family approach involving the presence of the father and any siblings provides an opportunity to observe family interactions and opportunities for all family members to ask questions and express concerns. In addition,

to recognize that the parameters of the home visit are different. In the home, the family members have control of their environment and the nurse is an invited visitor (Figure 29–4). The nurse can rely on the same characteristics of a caring relationship that have been integral to hospital-based practice—regard for clients, genuineness, empathy, and establishment of trust and rapport—when providing care in the home setting (Table 29–5). Evidence of these characteristics forms the foundation for a caring relationship.

Professionalism in Practice Reporting Unsanitary Conditions in the Home

As healthcare professionals, nurses are required to report infant neglect or abuse. When practicing in private homes, the nurse will be exposed to a wide range of home management practices with regards to aesthetics and sanitation. For example, the nurse will need to distinguish a home that is simply messy from a home that is unsanitary. It is important to develop rapport with the parents and to provide education as needed when sanitation issues are present. In certain cases, a follow-up visit is warranted. In cases of extreme filth or severe pest infestations, the nurse will need to use critical thinking skills to determine whether the most vulnerable client—the baby—is at risk for injury. If that is the case, the nurse should notify the appropriate authorities and follow the home care agency plan for such contingencies. If in doubt, the nurse should call upon resource persons and supervisors for assistance.

TABLE 29–5 Fostering a Caring Relationship

DEMONSTRATED GOAL	APPROACHES TO ACHIEVE GOAL
Regard	Introduce yourself to the family. Call the family members by their surnames until you have been invited to use the given or a less formal name.
	Ask to be introduced to other members of the family who are present. Allow the mother or spokesperson to assume this role. Remember, in some cultures, it may be a male figure or a mother figure who assumes the primary role. Use active listening. Maintain objectiveness.
	Ask permission before sitting.
Genuineness	Mean what you say. Make sure that your verbal and nonverbal messages are congruent.
	Be nonjudgmental. Do not make assumptions about individuals or settings.
	Always strive to demonstrate caring behaviors.
	Be prepared for the visit, honestly answer questions and provide information, and be truthful. If you do not know the answer to a question, tell the client you will find the information and report back.
Empathy	Listen to the mother and family "where they are" without judgment. Be attentive to what the birthing experience is for them so that you will understand from their perspective.
	Remember that empathy denotes understanding, not sympathy.
Trust and rapport	Do what you say you will do.
	Be prepared for the visit and be on time.
	Follow-up on any areas that are needed.

any questionable family interaction pattern such as one suggestive of abuse or neglect may be evident and further referral could be considered if needed.

Home Care: The Mother and Family

During the first home visit, the nurse completes a physical assessment of the mother and a psychosocial assessment of the family. Teaching for self-care is commonly required for new mothers, especially breastfeeding mothers with nipple soreness, engorgement, and other concerns. Family teaching related to resumption of sexual activity and contraception may also be required.

Developing Cultural Competence Role of **Extended Family**

In some cultures, extended family members such as grandmothers and aunts play a major role in the care of the postpartum woman and her family. Sometimes, these family members take full responsibility for running the household throughout the postpartum period. In other families, they concentrate entirely on the mother's or newborn's care. When culturally appropriate, include these extended family members in postpartum education sessions.

Assessment of the Mother and Family

Before performing the physical assessment, the nurse should ensure the mother's privacy. The physical assessment focuses on maternal physical adaptation, which is assessed by focusing on vital signs, breasts, abdominal musculature, elimination patterns, reproductive tract, and laboratory values. The nurse also talks with the mother about her diet, fatigue level, ability to rest and sleep, pain management, and signs of postpartum complications. In addition, for breastfeeding mothers, the nurse assesses the woman's feeding technique and presents information about possible problems that may occur. (See *Assessment Guide: Postpartum—First Home Visit and Anticipated Progress at 6 Weeks*.) Generally, the new mother has a final postpartum examination with her caregiver about 6 weeks after childbirth. However, if the nurse's assessment indicates a need, the nurse refers the woman to her healthcare provider for care before the 6-week check and for appropriate follow-up.

Many new mothers are concerned about weight loss. Women who have gained excess weight during the pregnancy are at risk for obesity in later life. Counseling the mother about proper diet and exercise is an effective strategy to lose weight in the postpartum period. Nursing women should be counseled that extreme weight loss strategies are not advised, but that healthy food choices and exercise can aid in weight reduction. There are also weight loss programs designed specifically for nursing mothers that can offer counseling, group support, and monitoring in the postpartum period.

ASSESSMENT GUIDE | Postpartum—First Home Visit and Anticipated Progress at 6 Weeks

Physical Assessment/Normal Findings	Alterations and Possible Causes[*]	Nursing Responses to Data[†]
Vital Signs		
Blood pressure: return to normal prepregnant level	Elevated blood pressure (anxiety, essential hypertension, renal disease), preeclampsia (can occur postpartum)	Review history, evaluate normal baseline; refer to healthcare provider if necessary.
Pulse: 60–100 beats/min (or prepregnant normal rate)	Increased pulse rate, tachycardia, chest pain (excitement, anxiety, cardiac disorders)	Count pulse for full minute, note irregularities; marked tachycardia or beat irregularities require additional assessment and possible healthcare provider referral.
Respirations: 12–20/min	Marked tachypnea or abnormal patterns (respiratory disorders)	Evaluate for respiratory disease; refer to healthcare provider
Temperature: 36.6°–37.6°C (98°–99.6°F).	Increased temperature (infection)	Assess for signs and symptoms of infection or disease state.
Weight		
2 days: possible weight loss of 12–20+ lb	Minimal weight loss (fluid retention, preeclampsia)	Evaluate for fluid retention, edema, deep tendon reflexes, and blood pressure elevation.
6 weeks: returning to normal prepregnant weight	Retained weight (excessive caloric intake)	Determine amount of daily exercise. Provide dietary teaching. Refer to dietitian if necessary for additional dietary counseling.
	Extreme weight loss (excessive dieting, inadequate caloric intake)	Discuss appropriate diets, refer to dietitian for additional counseling if necessary.

Physical Assessment/Normal Findings	Alterations and Possible Causes*	Nursing Responses to Data†
Breasts		
Nonbreastfeeding: 2 days: may have mild to moderate tenderness; small amount of milk may be expressed 6 weeks: soft, with no tenderness; return to prepregnant size	Some engorgement (incomplete suppression of lactation) Redness; marked tenderness (mastitis) Palpable mass (tumor)	Engorgement may be seen in nonbreastfeeding mothers. Advise client to wear a supportive, well-fitted bra; avoid very warm showers; avoid pumping or any stimulation of breasts; use ice packs for comfort; evaluate for signs and symptoms of mastitis (rare in nonbreastfeeding mothers). Par-cooked cabbage leaves can be placed against the breast to relieve engorgement.
Breastfeeding: full, with prominent nipples; lactation established	Cracked, fissured nipples (feeding problems) Redness, marked tenderness, or even abscess formation (mastitis) Palpable mass (full milk duct, tumor)	Counsel about nipple care. Observe infant feeding. Evaluate client condition, evidence of fever, redness, or tender area, refer to healthcare provider for initiation of antibiotic therapy, if indicated. Opinion varies as to value of breast examination for breastfeeding mothers; some feel a breastfeeding mother should examine her breasts monthly, after feeding, when breasts are empty; if palpable mass is felt, refer to physician for further evaluation. For breast inflammation instruct the mother to: 1. Keep breast empty by frequent feeding. 2. Rest when possible. 3. Take prescribed pain relief medication. 4. Force fluids. 5. Take antibiotics if ordered. If symptoms are accompanied by fever, flulike symptoms, or redness, instruct woman to call her healthcare provider and take an analgesic.
Abdominal Musculature		
2 days: improved firmness, although "bread dough" consistency is not unusual, especially in multipara; striae pink and obvious	Marked relaxation of muscles	Evaluate exercise level; provide information on appropriate exercise program.
Cesarean incision healing	Use the REEDA scoring system: redness, ecchymosis, edema, discharge from incision site, and approximation.	Evaluate for infection; refer to healthcare provider if necessary.
6 weeks: muscle tone continues to improve; striae may be beginning to fade, may not achieve a silvery appearance for several more weeks; linea nigra fading	Assess for tenderness and pain.	
Elimination Pattern		
Urinary tract: return to prepregnant urinary elimination routine	Urinary incontinence, especially when lifting, coughing, laughing, and so on (urethral trauma, cystocele)	Assess for cystocele; instruct in appropriate muscle tightening exercises; refer to healthcare provider.
	Pain or burning when voiding, urgency and/or frequency, pus, blood, or white blood cells (WBC) in urine, pathogenic organisms in culture (urinary tract infection)	Evaluate for urinary tract infection; obtain clean-catch urine; refer to healthcare provider for treatment if indicated.
Routine urinalysis within normal limits (proteinuria disappeared)	Sugar or ketone in urine—may be some lactose present in urine of breastfeeding mothers (diabetes)	Evaluate diet; assess for signs and symptoms of diabetes; refer to healthcare provider.

(continued)

ASSESSMENT GUIDE | Postpartum—First Home Visit and Anticipated Progress at 6 Weeks (*continued*)

Physical Assessment/Normal Findings	Alterations and Possible Causes*	Nursing Responses to Data†
Bowel habits: 2 days: May be some discomfort with defecation, especially if client had severe hemorrhoids or third- or fourth-degree extension	Severe constipation or pain when defecating (trauma or hemorrhoids)	Discuss dietary patterns; encourage fluids and high-fiber diet, adequate roughage. Counsel on the effects of medications. Continue use of stool softener if necessary to prevent pain associated with straining; continue sitz baths, periods of rest for severe hemorrhoids; assess healing of episiotomy and/or lacerations; severe constipation may require administration of laxatives, stool softeners, and an enema if not contraindicated (check with healthcare provider).
6 weeks: return to normal prepregnancy bowel elimination	Marked constipation (inadequate fluid/fiber intake)	See previous discussed interventions.
	Fecal incontinence or constipation (rectocele)	Assess for evidence of rectocele; instruct in muscle tightening exercises; refer to healthcare provider.
Reproductive Tract		
Lochia: 2 days: lochia rubra or lochia serosa, scant amounts, fleshy odor	Excessive amounts and/or large clots (nonfirm uterus), foul odor (infection), passing tissue (possible retained placenta)	Assess for evidence of infection and/or failure of the uterus to decrease in size; refer to healthcare provider.
6 weeks: no lochia, or return to normal menstruation pattern	See above	See above.
Fundus and perineum: 2 days: Fundus is at least 2 fingerbreadths below the umbilicus; uterine muscles still somewhat lax; introitus of vagina lacks tone—gapes when intra-abdominal pressure is increased by coughing or straining	Uterus not decreasing in size appropriately (infection)	Assess fundus for firmness and/or signs of infection; refer to healthcare provider if indicated.
Episiotomy and/or lacerations healing; no signs of infection; may have some bruising and tenderness	Evidence of redness, severe pain, poor tissue approximation in episiotomy and/or laceration (wound infection)	Utilize cool or warm sitz baths, topical medications.
6 weeks: uterus almost returned to prepregnant size with almost completely restored muscle tone	Continued flow of lochia, failure to decrease appropriately in size (subinvolution)	Assess for evidence of subinvolution and/or infection; refer to physician for further evaluation and treatment if necessary.
Hemoglobin and Hematocrit Levels		
6 weeks: hemoglobin (Hb) 12 g/dL; hematocrit (Hct) 37% ± 5%	Hb less than 12 g/dL; Hct 32% (anemia)	Assess nutritional status, assess for signs or symptoms of anemia, begin (or continue) supplemental iron; for marked anemia (Hb less than or equal to 9 g/dL) additional assessment and/or healthcare provider referral may be necessary.
Attachment		
Bonding process demonstrated by soothing, cuddling, and talking to baby; appropriate feeding techniques; eye-to-eye contact; calling baby by name.	Failure to bond demonstrated by lack of behaviors associated with bonding process, calling baby by nickname that promotes ridicule, inadequate weight gain, baby is dirty, hygienic measures are not being maintained, severe diaper rash, failure to obtain adequate supplies to provide infant care (malattachment).	Provide counseling; talk with the woman about her feelings regarding the baby; provide support for the caretaking activities that are being performed; refer to public health nurse for continued home visits; refer if abuse or neglect is suspected.

Physical Assessment/Normal Findings	Alterations and Possible Causes*	Nursing Responses to Data†
Parent interacts with baby and provides soothing, caretaking activities.	Parent is unable to respond to the baby's needs (inability to recognize needs, inadequate education and support, fear, family stress).	Provide support for caretaking activities observed; provide information regarding caretaking activities, such as responding to crying of the baby; methods of wrapping the baby; methods of soothing the baby such as swaddling, rocking; increasing stimuli by singing to the baby or decreasing stimuli by putting the baby to rest in quiet room; methods of holding the baby; differences in the cry. Identify support system such as friends, neighbors; provide information regarding community resources and support groups.
Parents express feelings of comfort and success with the parent role.	Evidence is seen of stress and anxiety (difficulty moving into or dealing with the parent role).	Provide support and encouragement; provide information regarding progression into parent role and assist parents in talking through their feelings; refer to community resources and support groups.
Woman is in the informal or personal stage of maternal role attainment.	Woman is still greatly influenced by others, has not developed an image or style of her own (woman remains in the anticipatory stage).	Provide role modeling for the woman in working through problem solving with the baby; provide encouragement as she thinks through decisions and develops her sense of problem solving; encourage her to make decisions regarding infant care.
Adjustment to Parental Role		
Parents are coping with new roles in terms of division of labor, financial status, communication, readjustment of sexual relations, and adjusting to new daily tasks.	Inability to adjust to new roles (immaturity, inadequate education and preparation, ineffective communication patterns, inadequate support, current family crisis).	Provide counseling; refer to parent groups.
Education		
Mother understands self-care measures.	Knowledge of self-care is inadequate (inadequate education).	Provide education and counseling.
Parents are knowledgeable regarding infant care.	Knowledge of infant care is inadequate (inadequate education).	
Siblings are adjusting to new baby.	Sibling rivalry is excessive.	
Parents have a method of contraception.	Birth control method has not been chosen.	

*Possible causes of alterations are identified in parentheses.
†This column provides guidelines for further assessment and initial nursing intervention.

Breastfeeding Concerns Following Discharge

Because mothers are discharged from the birthing unit before breastfeeding is well established, they are frequently alone when they encounter changes in the breastfeeding process. Many women stop nursing if the situations they encounter seem problematic. For this reason, the nurse providing a home visit is in a unique position to positively impact the duration and success of breastfeeding (Kronborg, Vaeth, & Kristensen, 2012). Table 29–6 summarizes self-care measures the nurse can suggest to a woman with a breastfeeding problem.

Regardless of feeding method (newborn feeding is discussed in detail in Chapter 25), it is important for the nurse to assess the newborn's fluid and nutritional intake. As part of the physical assessment, the newborn's nude weight is determined. If the weight loss since birth is 10% or more, the nurse assesses the baby for signs of dehydration such as loose skin with decreased skin turgor, dry mucous membranes, sunken anterior fontanelle, and decreased frequency and amount of voiding and stooling. Risk factors for suboptimal breastfeeding include maternal obesity, primiparity, young maternal age, use of formula supplementation, use of pacifiers, cesarean birth, second stage of labor greater than 1 hour, low birth weight, breastfeeding difficulty, and flat or inverted nipples (Chapman & Pérez-Escamilla, 2012).

TABLE 29–6 Common Breastfeeding Problems and Remedies

PROBLEM	POSSIBLE CAUSE	REMEDIES
NIPPLES NOT GRASPABLE	Flat or inverted nipples	• Use Hoffman technique to break adhesions. • Wear breast shells to encourage nipples to protrude. • Grasp nipples and roll gently between the fingers to increase protractility. • Form the nipple before breastfeeding by hand shaping, ice, or wearing nipple shells a half-hour before feeding. • Use a breast pump to draw nipples out so that the mother can then put the baby to the breast.
	Engorged breasts	• Treat engorgement by feeding the baby more frequently. • A hand or electric pump or manual emptying of the breast can be done if the baby in unable to grasp the nipple.
	Large breasts	• Support breast with opposite hand, or use rolled towel under breast to bring nipple to the level of baby's mouth. • Avoid having the nipple pointing downward because this makes latch-on more difficult. • Use C-hold to make nipple accessible to baby.
ENGORGEMENT	Missed or infrequent feedings	• Breastfeed frequently (every 1.5 hr). • Massage and hand express or pump to empty breasts completely when feedings are missed or when a full feeling develops in breasts and baby is not available or willing to feed. • Avoid excessive stimulation or pumping between feedings because this will increase milk production. • Place warm compresses on breast just before feeding to soften breast. • Use cold applications between feedings to slow milk production (frozen bagged vegetables, ice packs, and par-cooked cabbage leaves) (Arora, Vatsa, & Dadhwal, 2008).
	Breasts not emptied at feedings	• Massage breasts and use warm cloths before feedings. • Breastfeed long enough to empty breasts (10–15 min on each side at each feeding). • If baby will not feed long enough to empty breasts, hand express or pump after feeding.
	Inadequate let-down	• Use relaxation techniques, massage, and warm compresses before breastfeeding. • Relax in warm shower with water running from back over shoulders and breasts, hand expressing to relieve fullness. • Use hand or electric pump before placing baby on breast to encourage let-down. • Listen to soothing music; use visualization or breathing techniques. • If caused by anxiety, try to eliminate the source of tension.
	Baby sleepy or not eager to feed	• Use rousing techniques (e.g., hold baby upright, unwrap blanket, change diaper). • Preexpress milk onto nipple or baby's lips to entice baby. • Avoid use of bottles of water or formula; these will decrease baby's willingness to suckle.
INADEQUATE LET-DOWN	Let-down not well established	• Give the baby ample time at the breast (at least 15 min per side) to allow for let-down and complete emptying. • Breastfeed in a quiet spot away from distractions. • Massage breasts and apply warm compresses before breastfeeding. • Drink juice, water, or tea (no caffeine) before and during breastfeeding. • Condition let-down by setting up a routine for beginning feedings. • Use relaxation, visualization, and breathing techniques. • Stimulate the nipple manually before breastfeeding. • Concentrate thought on the baby and milk flow; turn on a faucet so that the sound of running water helps stimulate let-down. • Take a warm shower before feedings. • Use breast pump to stimulate the let-down. • Avoid waiting to put baby to breast until the baby is famished because this may increase maternal anxiety. • Assess for maternal pain, cold temperature, or anxiety before feeding.

PROBLEM	POSSIBLE CAUSE	REMEDIES
	Mother overtired or overextended	• Nap or rest when the baby rests. • Limit distractions, limit visitors, focus on personal needs. • Lie down to breastfeed. • Simplify daily chores; set priorities.
	Mother tense, pressured	• Identify the causes of tensions and eliminate or minimize them. • Decrease fatigue. • Have others assist with other household duties or tasks. • Use relaxation, visualization, and breathing exercises to promote relaxation and comfort.
	Mother caught in cycle of little milk, worry, less milk	• Try all of the actions listed above. • Counsel mother that most women do produce enough milk. • Have baby weighed to ensure adequate weight gain, which is a reflection of milk supply. • Encourage frequent, uninterrupted feedings. • Consult a lactation consultant as needed.
CRACKED NIPPLES	All causes of sore nipples carried to extreme	• Refer to all actions for sore nipples. • Ensure baby is properly positioned. • Feed baby more frequently. • Avoid soaps, perfumes, or other cleaning products that can dry out nipples and predispose them to cracking. • Express milk after feeding and rub into nipple allowing it to air dry. • Use emollients or lanolin as directed by healthcare provider/lactation consultant. • Consult doctor about using ibuprofen (Motrin), acetaminophen (Tylenol), or other painkiller. • Improve nutritional status, increasing protein, vitamin C, zinc.
	Local infection (baby with staphylococcus or other organism may have infected mother's nipples)	• Refer to healthcare provider.
PLUGGED DUCTS	Poor positioning	• Try a variety of positions for complete emptying. • Alternate positions so that different areas of the nipple have different compression pressure. • Avoid incomplete emptying of breast. • Breastfeed at least 10 min per side after let-down. • Alternate breastfeeding positions. • If baby does not empty breasts, pump or express milk after feedings.
	External pressure on breast	• Use larger-size bra, insert bra extender, or go braless. • Wear a sports bra instead of a traditional bra. • Use nursing bra instead of pulling up conventional bra to breastfeed to avoid pressure on ducts. • Avoid bunching up sweater or nightgown under arm during breastfeeding.
SORE NIPPLES	Poor positioning	• Alternate breastfeeding positions throughout the day. • Bring the baby close to feed so the baby does not pull on the breast. • Place the nipple and some of the areola in the baby's mouth. • Check to ensure the baby is put on and off the breast properly. • Check to ensure the nipple is back far enough in the baby's mouth. • Hold the baby closely during feeding so the nipple is not constantly being pulled. • Ensure that baby's shoulder, hip, and knees are all properly aligned and facing the mother.
	Baby chewing or nuzzling onto nipple	• Form the nipple for the baby. • Set up a pattern of getting the baby onto the breast using the rooting reflex.

(continued)

TABLE 29–6 Common Breastfeeding Problems and Remedies (*continued*)

PROBLEM	POSSIBLE CAUSE	REMEDIES
	Baby sucking on end of nipple	• Ensure the nipple is way back in the baby's mouth by getting the baby properly onto the breast. • Check for an inverted nipple. • Check for engorgement. • If baby is initially placed incorrectly on the end of the nipple, break the suction using a fish hook motion with your index finger and reposition baby on nipple properly. • Do not allow baby to nurse on end of nipple; reposition immediately.
	Baby chewing his or her way off the nipple (nipple being pulled out of baby's mouth at end of feeding)	• Remove the baby from the breast by placing a finger between the baby's gums to ensure suction is broken. • End feeding when the baby's suckling slows, before the baby has a chance to chew on the nipple.
	Baby overly eager to nurse	• Breastfeed more often. • Preexpress milk to hasten let-down, avoiding vigorous suckling.
	Dry colostrum or milk causing nipple to stick to bra or breast pads	• Moisten bra or pads before taking off so as not to remove keratin. • Ensure that nipples are dry before replacing bra or clothing against nipples.
	Nipples not allowed to dry	• Remove plastic liners from milk pads. • Air dry breast completely after nursing. • Change nursing pads frequently. • Switch to cotton nursing pads.
	Nipple skin not resistant to stress	• Improve diet, especially adding fresh fruits and vegetables and vitamin supplements. • Eliminate or decrease use of sugary foods, alcohol, caffeine, cigarettes. • Check use of cleansing or drying agents.
	Natural oils removed or keratin layers broken down by drying agents (soap, alcohol, shampoo, deodorant)	• Eliminate irritants. • Wash breasts with water only.

NIPPLE SORENESS

Some discomfort often occurs initially with breastfeeding; it peaks between days 3 and 6 and then recedes. Breastfeeding difficulty and nipple soreness are often causes for women to discontinue breastfeeding. The nurse should counsel the mother not to switch to formula feeding or delay feedings because these measures cause engorgement and more soreness (Wambach & Riordan, 2014). Discomfort that lasts throughout the feeding or past the first week demands attention.

The baby's position at the breast is a critical factor in nipple soreness. The mother's hand should be off the areola, and the baby should be facing the mother's chest, with ear, shoulder, and hip aligned (see Figure 25-16). Because the area of greatest stress to the nipple is in line with the newborn's chin and nose, nipple soreness may be decreased by encouraging the mother to rotate positions when feeding the baby. Changing positions alters the focus of greatest stress and promotes more complete breast emptying.

Nipple soreness may also develop if the baby has faulty sucking habits. Nipples may have injured tips that are bruised, scabbed, or blistered from the nipple entering the baby's mouth at an upward angle and rubbing against the roof of the mouth or from poor latch-on (Wambach & Riordan, 2014). Soreness may also result from continuous negative pressure if the baby falls asleep with the breast in the mouth.

Chewed nipples, which result from improper positioning, are cracked or tender at or near the base. In these cases, the baby's jaws close only on the nipple instead of on the areola, or the baby's mouth is not opened wide enough or has slipped down to the nipple from the areola as a result of engorgement. Soreness on the underside of the nipple is caused by the baby nursing with the bottom lip tucked in rather than out, causing a friction burn. In such cases, even vigorous sucking produces little milk because the milk sinuses under the areola are not compressed. This situation results in a frustrated baby and marked soreness for the mother. The problem is overcome by manipulating the baby's bottom lip with a fingertip before beginning the feeding, positioning the baby with as much areola as possible in the mouth, and rotating the baby's positions at the breast.

Nipple soreness is especially pronounced during the first few minutes of a feeding. If the mother is not expecting this discomfort, she may become discouraged and quickly stop. The let-down reflex may take a few minutes to activate, and it may not occur if the mother stops nursing too quickly. The baby is unsatisfied, and the possibility of breast engorgement increases.

Nipple soreness can also result from the vigorous feeding of an overeager baby. Thus the mother may find it helpful to nurse more frequently. Again, promoting let-down just before feeding may help. Other self-care measures include applying ice to the nipples and areola for a few minutes before feeding to

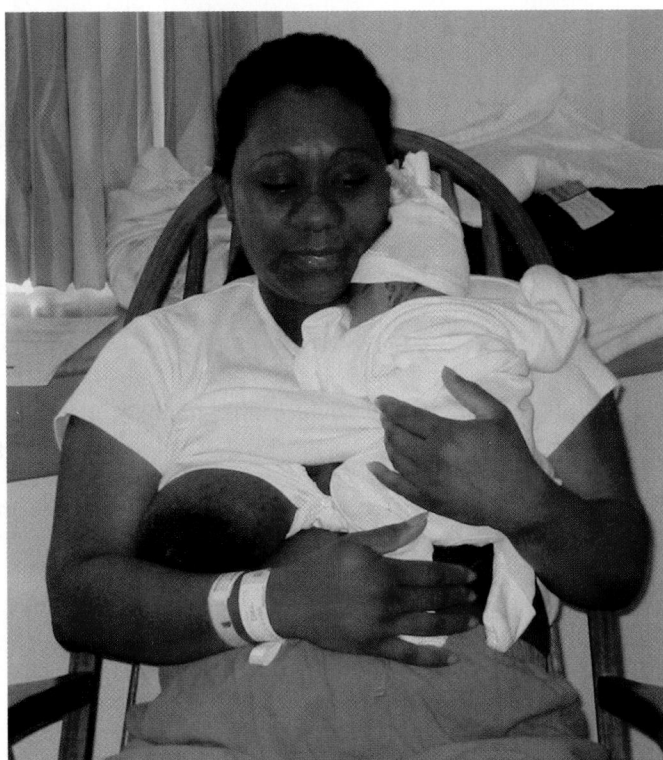

Figure 29–5 **Mothers with sore nipples can leave bra flaps down after feedings to promote air drying and prevent chapping.**

promote nipple erectness and numb the tissue initially. To promote dryness, the mother may leave her bra flaps down for a few minutes after feeding (Figure 29–5) or expose her nipples to sunlight or ultraviolet light for 30 seconds at first, gradually increasing to 3 minutes. Drying the nipples with a hair dryer on a low-heat setting also facilitates drying and promotes healing (Wambach & Riordan &, 2014). The use of petroleum-based products such as Vaseline, A & D, cocoa butter, and baby oil to lubricate the nipples is discouraged because the petroleum interferes with skin respiration and may prolong soreness. Because of the risk of allergic reactions, Massé cream (risk of peanut allergy) is discouraged. In addition, products that are washed off before breastfeeding are avoided because of the irritation that washing produces. During bathing, mothers should be advised only to rinse their nipples with water and to avoid soap because this can dry the nipple and lead to soreness.

Current research as to the effectiveness of nipple lubricants is inconclusive. Thus many lactation experts recommend that the mother's own milk be applied to the nipples and allowed to air dry. Breast milk is high in fat, fights infection, and will not irritate the nipples. Moreover, it is readily available at no cost to the mother. For some women with very dry or severely sore nipples, hypoallergenic medical-grade anhydrous lanolin cream or peppermint gel may help prevent or aid in healing cracked nipples. This product poses a low risk of allergy because the alcohols that contribute to the allergic response have been removed.

If the woman finds that her bra or clothing rubs against her nipples and adds to her discomfort, she may insert shells into her bra. Medela Shells relieve friction and promote air circulation. Breast shields may be an effective aid for preterm babies who have a reduced ability to latch on. If a woman uses breast pads inside her bra to keep milk from leaking onto her clothes,

she should change the pads frequently so the nipples remain dry. Some women may be sensitive to the plastic liner within the disposable pad, so the plastic can be removed or they can be encouraged to try cotton pads.

Box 29–1 Remedies for Nipple Soreness

Older remedies for nipple soreness are receiving renewed acceptance. For instance, tea bags may be moistened in warm water and applied to the nipples. The tannic acid seems to help toughen the nipples, and the warmth is soothing and promotes healing. Tannic acid also has anti-inflammatory properties that can help relieve discomfort. Other therapies have included warm compresses and heat applications (Strong, 2011).

Clinical Tip

If the mother continually has soreness because of a delay in let-down, encourage her to massage the breast in a circular pattern and apply warm compresses just before each breastfeeding session. These activities encourage let-down, increasing the chance that it will occur at the same time that the baby is placed on the breast.

If nipple soreness persists, the woman should be advised to consult a certified lactation consultant to determine the etiology of the soreness. Nipple dermatitis, which causes swollen, reddened, burning nipples, is most commonly caused by thrush or by allergic response to breast cream preparations. If the nipple soreness has a sudden onset and is accompanied by burning or itching, shooting pains through the breast, and a deep pink coloration of the nipple, it may be caused by a thrush infection transmitted from the baby to the mother. White patches or streaks in the baby's mouth indicate a need for treatment of the mouth and nipple infection. The infection can be treated with a variety of antifungal preparations and does not preclude breastfeeding. It is important for both the mother and the baby to receive treatment to prevent cross-transfer of the fungus (*Candida albicans*).

CRACKED NIPPLES

When a breastfeeding mother complains of soreness, the nurse carefully examines the nipples for fissures or cracks and observes the mother during breastfeeding to see whether the baby is correctly positioned at the breast. If the positioning is correct and cracks exist, interventions are necessary. All the interventions described for sore nipples may be used. It may also help the mother to begin nursing on the breast that is less sore. This approach allows the let-down reflex to occur in the affected breast and permits the baby to do more vigorous sucking on the less tender breast, which decreases trauma to the cracked nipple. For the mother's comfort, analgesics may be taken approximately 1 hour before nursing.

BREAST ENGORGEMENT

A distinction exists between breast fullness and engorgement. All lactating women experience a transitional fullness at first, initially caused by venous congestion and later caused by accumulating milk. However, this fullness generally lasts only 24 hours, the breasts remain soft enough for the newborn to suckle, and there is no pain. Engorged breasts are hard, painful, and warm and appear taut and shiny. The consistency is like gravel.

The baby should suckle for an average of 15 minutes per feeding and should feed at least 8 to 12 times in 24 hours (Wambach & Riordan, 2014). If the baby is unable to nurse more frequently, the mother may express some milk manually or with a pump, taking care to avoid traumatizing the breast tissue. As previously noted, warm compresses before nursing stimulate let-down and soften the breast so that the baby can grasp the areola more easily. Cool compresses after nursing can help slow refilling of the breasts and provide comfort to the mother. Ice packs may also be used as a comfort measure. The mother should wear a well-fitted nursing bra 24 hours a day to support the breasts and prevent discomfort from tension.

PLUGGED DUCTS

Some mothers experience plugging of one or more ducts, especially in conjunction with or following engorgement. When breast milk pools within a duct and then dries, it forms a white, hardened plug that is typically visible at the outlet of the duct at the nipple surface. Because milk accumulates behind a plugged duct, women also experience an area of fullness, tenderness, and/or lumpiness in the associated region of the breast.

Self-care measures include the use of heat and massage. The nurse can encourage the mother to massage her breasts from her chest wall forward to the nipple while standing in a warm shower or following the application of moist heat to the breast. Warm compresses can be used and changed as temperature requires. The mother should then nurse her baby starting on the unaffected breast if the plugged breast is tender. Some lactation consultants advocate starting on the affected side because the more vigorous sucking may help dislodge the plug. A breast pump may also be effective in unplugging the duct.

Prevention of plugged ducts involves frequent nursing and the use of a variety of positions to ensure complete emptying. Some mothers discover that pressure from a shoulder strap on a purse, their infant sling, or a car seat belt causes recurring plugged ducts in the compressed area. Repositioning the device may help prevent plugged ducts in these women. Prevention and prompt correction of plugged ducts is important because a plugged duct could lead to mastitis (inflammation of the breast) (mastitis is discussed in detail in Chapter 30).

EFFECTS OF ALCOHOL AND MEDICATIONS

Mothers may ask the home care nurse about the use of alcohol and medications when breastfeeding. According to the Association of Reproductive Health Professionals (ARHP) (2013) multiple considerations should be considered when advising the mother on alcohol use:

- Alcohol consumption among breastfeeding women should be limited to occasional use after breastfeeding is well established.
- Breastfeeding mothers should not consume alcohol for at least 3 to 4 hours before nursing
- Mothers who do occasionally drink while lactating should be advised to consume the alcohol after breastfeeding rather than shortly before a feeding in order to minimize the amount the baby receives.
- Alcohol consumption can reduce milk supply by 23%.
- Heavy alcohol intake can be associated with impaired motor development, altered sleep patterns, decreased milk intake, and unsafe parental care. Mothers with alcoholism who consume large quantities of alcohol daily should be advised not to breastfeed.

It has long been recognized that medications taken by the breastfeeding mother may penetrate breast milk to some degree. But we now have a better understanding of the kinetics of drug entry into breast milk, as well as factors influencing its bioavailability to the nursing baby. This is important, because use of medication has been identified as a barrier to breastfeeding and a major reason women cite for discontinuing it (Wambach & Riordan, 2014). Note that (1) most drugs pass into breast milk, (2) almost all medications appear in only small amounts in human milk (usually less than 1% of the maternal dosage), and (3) very few drugs are contraindicated for breastfeeding women (Briggs, Freeman, & Yaffe, 2012). The properties of a drug influence its passage into breast milk, as does the amount of the drug taken, the frequency and route of administration, and the timing of the dose in relationship to infant feeding. The drug's effects are influenced by the baby's age, the feeding frequency, the volume of milk taken, and the degree of absorption through the gastrointestinal tract. If the medication is not compatible with breastfeeding but is needed for only a short time, the mother can use a breast pump to maintain lactation and discard the milk.

SAFETY ALERT!

The mother should be advised to inform her healthcare provider and her baby's healthcare provider that she is breastfeeding when a drug is prescribed for her.

BREASTFEEDING AND THE WORKING MOTHER

The best preparation for maintaining lactation after returning to work is frequent, unlimited breastfeeding. Even when well planned, the first day back to work may be fraught with emotional and physical distress. Anticipatory guidance from the nurse may facilitate the transition from maternity leave to work. The earlier the breastfeeding mother returns to work, the more often she will need to pump her breasts to express the breast milk. Because milk production follows the principle of supply and demand, if breasts are not pumped, the milk supply will decrease.

Healthy People 2020

(MICH 22) Increase the proportion of employers that have worksite lactation support programs

---

Clinical Reasoning Difficulties With Breastfeeding

Ann Nyembe calls you from home in tears on her third postpartum day. She states breastfeeding was going well in the hospital but now her breasts are swollen, hard, and very painful, and her baby is refusing to suckle. Ann expresses some disappointment that "the breastfeeding didn't work" because she truly believes that breastfeeding is best for babies, and she enjoyed her breastfeeding experience in the hospital, especially breastfeeding the baby immediately after birth. But she also states she has been crying all day and can no longer tolerate her painful breasts. In addition, she says the baby "seems happier" with the bottle. What actions can the nurse recommend to Ann to increase the likelihood she will continue breastfeeding and to decrease her discomfort?

"As part of the Affordable Care Act enacted in 2010, the Fair Labor Standards Act was amended to require employers to provide reasonable break time and a private place for nursing mothers to express milk while at work" (USD-HHS, 2011, p. 51). Many working mothers, particularly lower-income employees, may not be aware of their right to continue breastfeeding after they return to work. The professional nurse can advocate for clients by informing and encouraging them to discuss breastfeeding and the law with their employers.

An electric breast pump and double collection system are considered the optimal means of milk expression. However, this is not the only method; mechanical means may not suit some women. Sometimes, a mother has a flexible schedule and can return home or have the baby brought to her to nurse at lunch time. If this is not possible, the baby may be fed expressed milk via bottle or spoon. (For proper storage of breast milk, see section on *Bottle-Feeding Breast Milk* in Chapter 25.) The mother should wait until lactation is well established before introducing the bottle. Most babies adjust to the bottle within 7 to 10 days.

To maintain a milk supply, the working mother must pay special attention to her fluid intake. She can ensure adequate intake by drinking extra fluid at each break and when possible during the day. It is also helpful to nurse more on weekends, nurse during the night, eat a nutritionally sound diet, and continue manual expression or pumping when not nursing.

Night nursing presents a dilemma: It may help a working mother maintain her milk supply, but it may also contribute to fatigue. Some women choose to have the baby sleep nearby so that breastfeeding is more easily accomplished; other women find it difficult to sleep soundly when the baby is close by. For the mother who works long hours or has a rigid work schedule, the best alternative may be to limit breastfeeding to morning and evening feedings, with supplemental feedings at other times. This choice allows her to maintain a close relationship with the baby and provides some of the unique benefits of breast milk.

MATERNAL CONCERNS ABOUT BREASTFEEDING

Table 29–7 summarizes concerns new mothers may have about breastfeeding and ways the nurse can respond.

Clinical Tip

Babies with special needs sometimes benefit from a longer duration of breastfeeding. Babies who are prone to allergies, gastrointestinal reflux, or impaired motility of the gastrointestinal tract may receive benefits from continued breastfeeding that their mothers may be unaware of. These women should be counseled to discuss weaning with their pediatricians or infant specialists before weaning because the benefits of breastfeeding may influence their choice of timing regarding weaning (see Chapter 32 for a discussion of weaning).

TABLE 29–7 Maternal Concerns About Breastfeeding

CONCERN	RESPONSE
Pain	Breastfeeding with proper technique should not hurt. Instruct the mother on proper technique and if she still has difficulty encourage her to seek assistance from a lactation specialist.
Leaking milk	Instruct the mother on how to apply gentle pressure directly over her nipple for a minute or so to gradually stop the leaking. The use of nursing pads (with instructions to change wet pads frequently), wearing printed tops that camouflage small leaks, and reassurance that the problem lessens with time may help alleviate this problem.
Embarrassment	An unfriendly social environment may make it difficult to breastfeed in public. Classes and support groups can teach the mother how to breastfeed discreetly while in public, such as draping a blanket or shawl over her chest to provide more coverage.
Father feels left out	Inform the parents that it is advisable for the father to wait to bottle-feed the baby with expressed breast milk until after breastfeeding is established. In the meantime, encourage the father to be supportive of the breastfeeding mother, to have a lot of skin-to-skin contact with his baby, and to share the responsibilities of all other aspects of infant care (e. g., bathing, dressing, diapering, burping, rocking).
Limited hormonal birth control options	Using birth control pills containing progesterone and estrogen can cause a decrease in milk volume and may affect the quality of breast milk. It is preferred that the mother who wants to use a hormonal birth control method consider using the progestin-only minipill (i.e., Nicronor, Nor-QD, Aygestin, or Norlutate); receive Depo-Provera, a progestin-only injection administered every 90 days; or have a progestin-only implant. Although progestin-only hormonal birth control is compatible with lactation, it should not be started at the time of discharge. It is recommended that the mother wait 6 weeks before taking the hormonal medication to ensure a good milk supply. Mothers can be reassured that barrier methods of birth control and natural family planning do not interfere with lactation at all and are good options to consider as well.
Vaginal dryness	Give reassurance that this is only a temporary side effect of a low level of estrogen while lactating. A water-based lubricant such as K-Y jelly or Astroglide can be used during intercourse until the mother weans and estrogen levels increase again.

Home Care: The Newborn

In the home, a newborn physical examination is performed as described in Chapter 24. The nurse also assesses and reinforces knowledge related to infant care as detailed in the following paragraphs.

Handling and Positioning

The nurse demonstrates methods of positioning and handling the newborn as needed. As the family members provide care, the nurse can instill confidence by giving them positive feedback. If a family member encounters problems, the nurse can suggest alternatives and serve as a role model.

When holding the newborn, one of the following positions can be used (Figure 29–6). The *cradle hold* is frequently used during feeding. It provides a sense of warmth and closeness, permits eye contact, frees one of the adult's hands, and provides security because the cradling protects the newborn's body. Extra security is provided by gripping the baby's thigh with the hand while the arm supports the newborn's body. This grip is important to use when the baby is being carried. The *upright position* provides security and a sense of closeness and is ideal for burping the baby. One hand should support the neck and shoulders, while the other hand holds the buttocks or is placed between the newborn's legs. The newborn may also be held upright in a cloth sling carrier that gently holds the baby against the parent's chest and frees the hands for other tasks. The *football hold* frees one of the caregiver's hands and permits eye contact. This hold is ideal for shampooing, carrying, or breastfeeding. It frees the caregiver to talk on the telephone, answer the door, or do the myriad tasks that await attention at this busy time.

The baby's position should be changed periodically throughout the early months of life, because skull bones are soft, and permanently flattened areas may develop if the newborn consistently lies in one position. The awake newborn is frequently positioned on the side with the dependent arm forward to provide support and to prevent rolling. The side-lying position aids drainage of mucus and allows air to circulate around the cord. It is also comfortable for the newly circumcised male. After feeding, the newborn may be placed on the right side to aid digestion and to prevent aspiration of regurgitated feedings; this position also makes it easier to expel air bubbles from the stomach.

Although the side-lying position is appropriate when the baby is awake and under observation, babies should always sleep on their backs (Figure 29–7). The American Academy of Pediatrics has recommended sleeping in nonprone positions since 1992 to reduce the risk of sudden infant death syndrome (SIDS). *Healthy People 2020* goals (USDHHS, 2015) are aimed at increasing the number of babies who are placed on their backs for sleep. Since the initiation of the "Safe to Sleep" campaign, there has been an increase in malformation of the skull caused by a decrease in **tummy time** (prone positioning while the baby is awake). The syndrome is also known as *deformational plagiocephaly*, or positional plagiocephaly. These babies commonly have a flat spot on their skull, usually on the back or side, that is caused by continued placement in the same position. Babies who are not placed on their stomachs while awake at least 3 times daily are at risk for this skull malformation. Often, these malformations will resolve on their own by 1 year of age, but sometimes infants need to wear a specially fitted helmet to correct the malformation (Flannery, Looman, & Kemper, 2012).

Healthy People 2020

(MICH-20) Increase the proportion of infants who are put to sleep on their backs

---

Tummy time is important for all babies because it assists them with learning developmentally appropriate skills; builds muscle strength for their shoulders, neck, and back; and

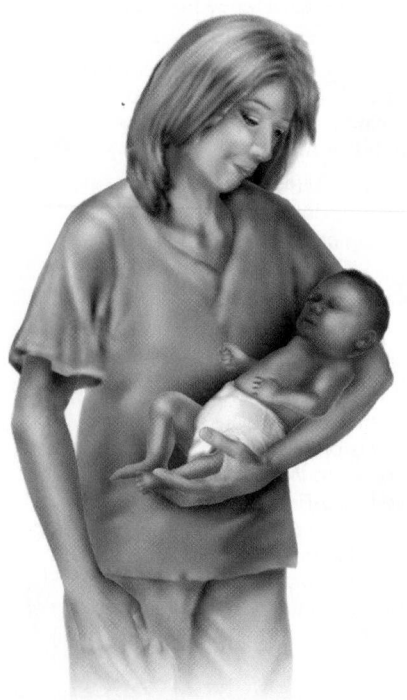
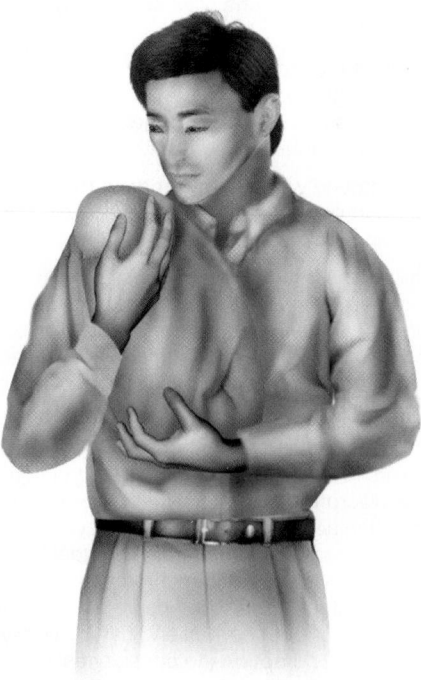
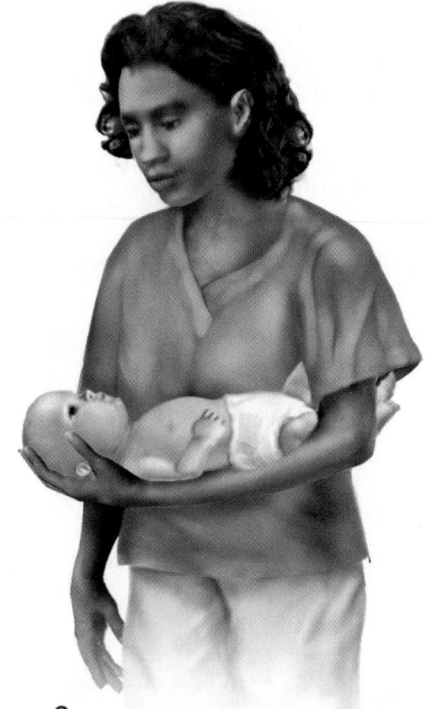

A **B** **C**

Figure 29–6 Various positions for holding a baby. *A,* Cradle hold. *B,* Upright position. *C,* Football hold.

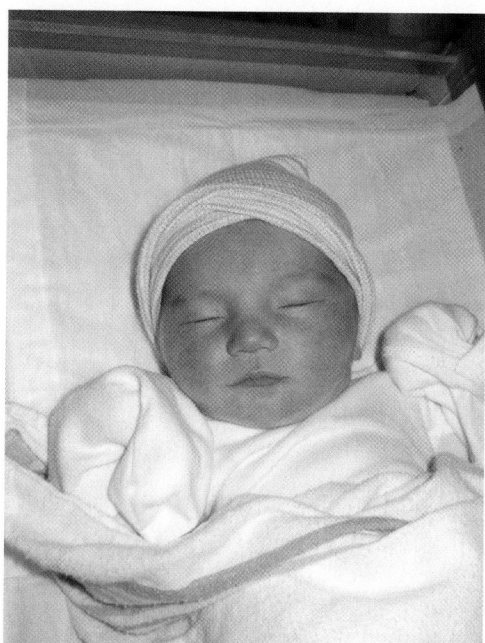

Figure 29–7 Babies should be placed on their backs when sleeping.

prevents deformational plagiocephaly (Flannery et al., 2012). Babies should be placed on their tummies only when they are under direct supervision of a parent or adult.

Professionalism in Practice Professional Nurse Endorsement of Safe to Sleep Guidelines

In addition to the recommendations for the home sleep environment, the AAP (2011) included guidelines that apply to healthcare providers and other professionals.

- Healthcare providers and other professionals should endorse the guidelines designed to prevent SUID (sudden unexpected infant death) and SIDS beginning at birth.

- Manufacturers should follow the guidelines in all marketing and advertising.

- The campaign should expand beyond SIDS reduction to the promotion of an overall safe sleep environment.

Bathing

An actual bath demonstration is the best way for the nurse to provide information about bathing to parents. Because excess bathing and the use of soap remove natural skin oils and dry out the newborn's sensitive skin, bathing should be done every other day or twice a week. Sponge baths are recommended for the first 2 weeks or until the umbilical cord completely falls off and the umbilicus has healed. Some agencies use a tub bath for the bath demonstration. See Initial Newborn Bath, in the *Clinical Skills Manual* SKILLS .

At home, bath supplies can be kept in a plastic bag or some type of container to eliminate the necessity of hunting for them each time. For the baby's tub, the family may want to use a plastic dishpan, a clean kitchen or bathroom sink, or a large bowl. If using a sink, care should be taken to keep the baby away from faucets from which accidental burns could occur. Expensive baby tubs are not necessary, but some prefer to purchase them.

Before starting, if no one else is at home, the parent may want to take the phone off the hook and put a sign on the door to prevent being disturbed. Having someone home during the first few baths will be helpful because that person can get forgotten items, attend to interruptions, and provide moral support. The room should be warm and free of drafts.

SPONGE BATHS

After the supplies are gathered, the tub (or any of the containers mentioned) is filled with water that is warm to the touch. Even though the newborn will not be placed in the tub, the bath giver carefully tests the water temperature with an elbow or forearm. Families may also choose to purchase a thermometer to help them determine when the bath water is at approximately 37.8°C (100.0°F) and safe to use. An unperfumed, mild soap such as Castile or Neutrogena should be used and kept on a soap dish or paper towel, not added to the water. Before the bath, the newborn should be wrapped in a blanket, with a T-shirt and diaper on, to keep the baby warm and secure.

To start the bath, the adult wraps a washcloth once around the index finger and wets it with water. *Soap is not used on the face.* Each eye is gently wiped from inner to outer corner. This direction prevents the potential for clogging the tear duct at the inner corner, where the eye naturally drains. A different portion of the washcloth is used for each eye to prevent cross contamination. Cotton balls can also be used for this purpose, a new one for each eye. Some swelling and drainage may be present the first few days after birth because of eye prophylaxis.

The bath giver washes the ears next by wrapping the washcloth once around an index finger and gently cleaning the external ear and behind the ear. Cotton swabs are never used in the ear canal because it is possible to put the swab too far into the ear and damage the ear drum. In addition, the swab may push any discharge farther down into the ear canal. The caregiver then wipes the remainder of the baby's face. Many babies start to cry at this point. The face should be washed every day and the mouth and chin wiped off after each feeding.

The neck is washed carefully but thoroughly with the washcloth. Soap may now be used. Formula or breast milk and lint collect in the skin folds of the neck, so it may be helpful to sit the newborn up, supporting the neck and shoulders with one hand while washing the neck with the other hand.

Next, the bath giver unwraps the blanket, removes the T-shirt, and wets the chest, back, and arms with the washcloth. The bath giver may then lather the hands with soap and wash the baby's chest, back, and arms. The umbilical cord should be kept clean and dry. Wetting the cord is avoided, if possible, because it delays drying. The proximity of the umbilical vessels makes the cord a possible entry area for infection. See Chapter 25 for care of the umbilical cord and signs and symptoms of problems. Soap is rinsed off with the wet washcloth, and the upper part of the body is dried with a towel or blanket. The newborn's upper body is then wrapped with a clean, dry blanket to prevent a chill.

The bath giver then unwraps the newborn's legs, wets them with the washcloth, and lathers, rinses, and dries them well. If the newborn has dry skin, a small amount of unscented lotion or ointment (petroleum jelly or A & D ointment) may be used. Ointments are thought to be better than lotions for dry, cracked feet and hands. Baby oil is not recommended because it clogs skin pores. Powders are not currently recommended. Families should be warned that baby powder can cause serious respiratory problems if inhaled. If parents want to use powder, they should be advised to use one that is talc free. The powder should be shaken into the hand and then placed on the newborn rather than shaken directly onto the baby.

The genital area is cleansed with soap and water daily and with water after each wet or dirty diaper. Girls are washed from the front of the genital area toward the anus to prevent fecal contamination of the urethra and thus the bladder. Newborn girls often have a thick, white mucous discharge or a slight bloody discharge from the vaginal area. This discharge is normal for the first 1 to 2 weeks after birth and should be wiped off with a damp cloth during diaper changes. The labia should be wiped, but the inner labial folds should not be aggressively cleaned.

Parents of uncircumcised boys should cleanse the penis daily. Even minimal retraction of the foreskin is not advised (see in-depth discussion of care of uncircumcised male babies in Chapter 25). Boys who have been circumcised also need daily gentle cleansing. Squeeze warm water over the baby's penis, letting the warm water run over the circumcision site. The area is rinsed off with warm water and lightly patted dry. A small amount of petroleum jelly, A & D ointment, or bactericidal ointment may be put on the circumcised area until the healing is complete, but excessive amounts may block the meatus and should be avoided. It is important to avoid using ointments if a Plastibell is in place because use of ointments may cause the Plastibell ring to slip off the penis too early. The Plastibell usually falls off within 5 to 8 days.

It is important to cleanse the diaper area with each diaper change to prevent diaper rash. Although this cleansing is done on a routine basis, a diaper rash may occasionally occur. Baby powder or cornstarch is not recommended for diaper rash. Baby powder may cake with urine and irritate the perineal area; cornstarch may promote fungal infection. Ointments that provide a barrier, such as zinc oxide, A & D ointment, and petroleum jelly, are effective for diaper rash. If the ointment does not help the rash, families using single-use (disposable) diapers should try another brand. If they use cloth diapers, a different detergent or fabric softener, more thorough rinsing, and hanging them in the sun to dry may alleviate the problem. If the rash persists, parents should discuss the problem with their healthcare provider because it may be caused by a fungal infection.

The last step in bathing is washing the hair (a step some suggest doing first). The newborn is swaddled in a dry blanket, leaving only the head exposed, and held in the football hold with the head tilted slightly downward to prevent water from running into the eyes. Water should be brought to the head by a cupped hand. The baby should never be placed under running water because extreme changes in temperature can lead to burns. The hair is moistened and lathered with a small amount of mild shampoo. A very soft brush may be used to massage the shampoo over the entire head, including the fontanelles. The hair is then rinsed and toweled dry. Oils or lotions are not used on the newborn's head unless there is evidence of cradle cap. Moistening the scaly area with lotion or mineral oil half an hour or more before shampooing softens the crusts or scales and makes it easier to remove them with a soft brush during the shampoo.

TUB BATHS

The baby may be put in a small tub after the cord has fallen off and, for boys, when the circumcision site is healed (approximately 2 weeks) (Figure 29–8). Newborns usually enjoy a tub bath more than a sponge bath, although some cry during either type. Only 3 or 4 inches of water are needed in the tub. To prevent slipping, a washcloth is placed in the bottom of the tub or sink. Some parents choose to bring the newborn into the tub with them.

The baby's face is washed in the same manner as for a sponge bath. The parent then places the newborn in the tub using the cradle hold and grasping the distal thigh. The neck is

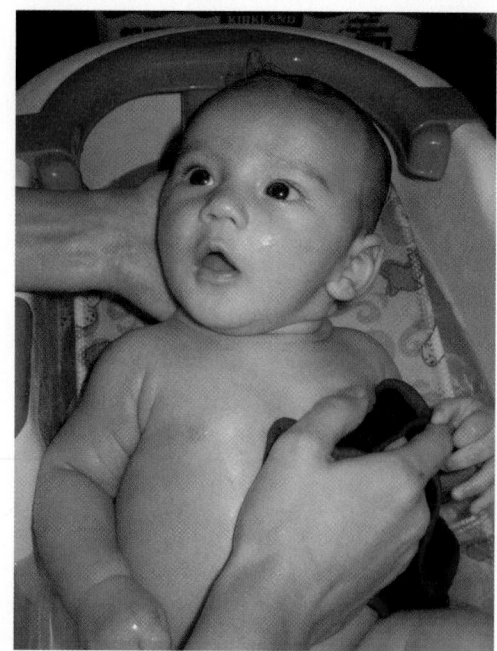

Figure 29–8   **When bathing the newborn, the caregiver must support the head. Wet babies are very slippery.**

supported by the parent's elbow in the cradle position. An alternative hold is to support the newborn's head and neck with the forearm while grasping the distal shoulder and arm.

Because wet newborns are slippery, some parents pull a cotton sock (with holes cut out for the fingers) over their supporting arm to provide a "nonskid" surface. The newborn's body may be washed with a soapy washcloth or hand. To wash the back, the bath giver places the noncradling hand on the newborn's chest with the thumb under the newborn's arm closest to the adult. Gently tipping the newborn forward onto the supporting hand frees the cradling arm to wash the back. After the bath, the newborn is lifted out of the tub in the cradle position, dried well, and wrapped in a dry blanket. The hair is then washed in the same way as for a sponge bath.

Nail Care

The nails of the newborn are seldom cut in the birthing center. During the first days of life, the nails may adhere to the skin of the fingers, and cutting is contraindicated. Within a week the nails separate from the skin and frequently break off. If the nails are long or if the newborn is scratching his or her face, the nails may be trimmed. Trimming is most easily done while the baby is asleep. Nails should be cut straight across using adult cuticle scissors or blunt-ended infant cuticle scissors. Nails may also be filed.

Dressing the Newborn

Newborns need to wear a T-shirt, diaper (diaper cover or plastic pants if using cloth diapers), and a sleeper. On a fairly cool day, they should be wrapped in a light blanket while being fed. Newborns should be covered with a blanket in air-conditioned buildings. The blanket should be unwrapped or removed when inside a warm building. At home, the amount of clothing the newborn wears is determined by the temperature. Families who maintain their home at 15.5° to 18.3°C (60° to 65°F) should dress the baby more warmly than those who maintain a temperature of 21.1° to 23.9°C (70° to 75°F).

Newborns should wear head coverings outdoors to protect their sensitive ears from drafts. A blanket can be wrapped around the baby, leaving one corner free to place over the head while outdoors or in crowds for added protection. The nurse must advise families about the ease with which a newborn's skin can burn when exposed to the sun. To prevent sunburn, the newborn should remain shaded, wear a light layer of clothing, and avoid being directly exposed to sun during peak hours between 10 a.m. and 4 p.m.

Diaper shapes vary and are subject to personal preference (Figure 29–9). Prefolded and disposable diapers are usually rectangular. Cloth diapers may also be triangular or kite folded. Extra material is placed in front for boys and toward the back for girls to increase absorbency. Cloth diapers, some of which now use Velcro and highly absorbent materials, have been used more frequently in recent years because of the environmental concerns related to disposable diapers.

Baby clothing should be laundered separately with a mild soap or detergent. Cloth diapers may be presoaked before washing. All clothing should be rinsed twice to remove soap and residue and to decrease the possibility of rash. Some newborns may not tolerate clothing treated with fabric softeners added to the washer or dryer.

Temperature Assessment

As the nurse prepares to teach parents about taking their baby's temperature, it is important to provide opportunities for discussion and demonstration. Families often need a review of how to take the baby's temperature and when to call their primary healthcare provider.

The nurse discusses the different types of thermometers available for home use. It is important that parents understand the differences and how to select the appropriate one. Tympanic membrane (ear) thermometers use infrared temperature scanning techniques to determine the baby's temperature. Infrared forehead thermometers are also available and are commonly used in some facilities. Other parents elect to use a digital thermometer. The nurse reviews the correct procedure for using the chosen thermometer.

Parents need to take the newborn's temperature only when signs of illness are present. They should call their healthcare provider immediately if the temperature exceeds 38.4°C (101.0°F) rectally or 38.0°C (100.4°F) axillary. In premature babies, a low temperature may be a sign of infection; therefore,

if the temperature is below 36.1°C (97.0°F) rectally or 36.6°C (97.8°F) axillary, the pediatrician should be notified.

Parents should discuss management of flu, colds, teething, constipation, diarrhea, gas discomfort, and other common ailments with their clinician before they occur. When analgesic or antipyretic medication is needed, clinicians frequently recommend acetaminophen or ibuprofen drops. Parents should not give any form of aspirin for an illness unless specifically directed to do so by their healthcare provider; use of aspirin in viral illnesses has been linked to Reye syndrome in children.

Clinical Tip

Healthcare facilities no longer use glass thermometers because of the risks associated with resulting mercury spillage should one break. Parents should be advised not to use mercury thermometers and should be encouraged to discard them at a hazardous materials site specific to mercury thermometers. Before teaching families about temperature taking, you might find it helpful to visit a local pharmacy and review the types of thermometers available, the costs of the most commonly used methods, and the instructions provided. This will enable you to answer questions accurately when you work with parents or caregivers.

Stools and Urine

The appearance and frequency of a newborn's stools can cause concern for parents. The nurse prepares them by discussing and showing pictures of meconium stools and transitional stools and by describing the difference between breast milk and formula stools. Although babies develops their own stooling patterns, parents can expect the following (see Figure 25–24):

- Breastfed newborns may have 6 to 10 small, semiliquid, yellow stools per day by the 3rd or 2nd day, when milk production is established, unless the mother is having problems with her milk supply. Once breastfeeding is well established, usually by 1 month, the baby may have only one stool every few days because of the increased digestibility of breast milk. However, they may still have several daily. Constipation is unlikely to occur in newborns receiving only breast milk. Infrequent stooling in the first few weeks may indicate inadequate milk intake.

- Formula-fed babies may have only one or two stools a day; they are more formed and yellow or yellow-brown.

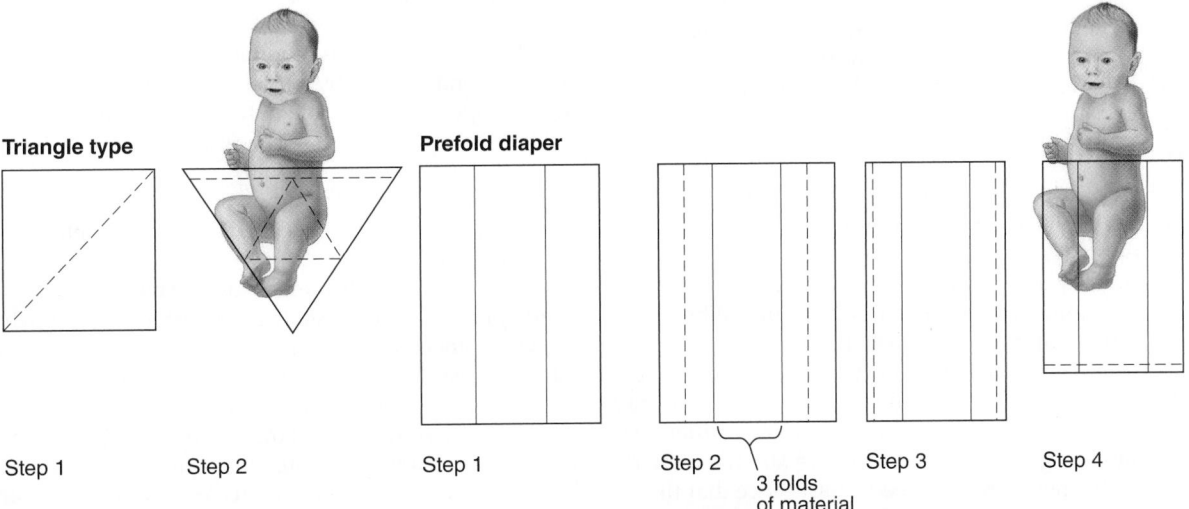

Triangle type   **Prefold diaper**

Step 1   Step 2   Step 1   Step 2   Step 3   Step 4

3 folds of material

Figure 29–9 Two basic cloth diaper shapes. Dotted lines indicate folds.

The parents may also be shown pictures of a constipated stool (small, pellet-like) and diarrhea (loose, green, or perhaps blood tinged). Families should understand that a green color is common in transitional stools, so that transitional stools are not confused with diarrhea during the first week of a newborn's life. Constipation may indicate that the newborn needs additional fluid intake. Parents may try offering additional water in an attempt to reverse the constipation. Parents should be counseled that each baby develops a personal stooling pattern, and some babies may not pass a stool daily. As long as the baby appears comfortable and is not in distress, this can be normal for that baby and is not a cause for concern.

Babies normally void 5 to 8 times per day. Fewer than six to eight wet diapers a day may indicate that the newborn needs more fluids. Frequency of voiding is easy to assess with cloth diapers. Parents who use superabsorbent single-use disposable diapers may have difficulty determining voiding patterns because the surface of the diaper feels dry. The liquid pools inside the filling of the diaper.

Clinical Tip

If parents using disposable diapers are unable to determine if the diaper is wet, advise them to tear off the top layer of the diaper and examine the cotton batting beneath the absorbent layer. It is easier for parents to see urine saturation and a change of color on this portion of the diaper in order to determine if the baby has voided.

Sleep and Activity

The newborn demonstrates several different sleep–wake states after the initial periods of reactivity described in Chapter 23. Six newborn sleep–wake states have been identified (see Table 29–8). It is not uncommon for a newborn to sleep almost continuously for the first 2 to 3 days following birth, awakening only for feedings every few hours. Indeed, it is not uncommon to have difficulty feeding the newborn during the first 24 to 48 hours because of this deep sleep. Some newborns bypass this stage and require only 12 to 16 hours of sleep. The parents need to know that this pattern is normal.

Infants typically do not sleep through the night until they are at least 3 months of age or weigh 12 to 13 lb (5443 to 5897 g). Some infants sleep through the night as early as 8 weeks, whereas others do not sleep through the night until 6 months of age or beyond. It is estimated that two thirds of infants sleep through the night by the age of 6 months. Although newborns typically sleep up to 16 hours per day, they do so in short time intervals. Some parents may be tempted to try home remedies, such as giving babies cereal in their bottles or other additives that are said to assist their children in sleeping through the night. Parents should be counseled that these remedies are not recommended.

Crying

For the newborn, crying is the only means of expressing needs vocally. Families learn to distinguish different tones and qualities of the newborn's cry. The amount of crying is highly individual. Some cry as little as 15 to 30 minutes in 24 hours, and others cry as long as 2 hours every 24 hours. When crying continues after causes such as discomfort and hunger are eliminated, the newborn may be comforted by swaddling or by rocking and other reassuring activities. There is some indication that newborns who are held more tend to be calmer and cry less when not being held. Some parents are afraid that holding may "spoil" the newborn and need reassurance that this is not the case. Picking babies up when they cry teaches them that adults are responsive to them. This helps build a sense of trust

in humankind. Excessive crying should be noted and assessed, taking other factors into consideration. After the first 2 or 3 days, newborns settle into individual patterns.

Coping with prolonged crying may be a challenge for new parents, who may respond by withdrawing their affection from the newborn, providing routine care and feeding, but not becoming emotionally attached. Other parents may respond by neglecting, abandoning, or even hitting or shaking their newborn. Parents need to understand the serious, even life-threatening consequences of such behavior. For example, a neglected or abandoned newborn can quickly become dehydrated, and hitting can cause internal hemorrhage, bruising, and fractures. Shaking can cause brain hemorrhage, spinal cord injury, retinal hemorrhage or detachment, long-term developmental problems, intellectual disability, or even death. This collection of symptoms that are caused by vigorously shaking a baby is known as **shaken baby injuries**, or *shaken baby syndrome*, and is a form of abusive head trauma (AHT) and inflicted traumatic brain injury (ITBI). Shaken baby syndrome is also sometimes referred to as *intentional injuries*.

An educational program devised by the National Center on Shaken Baby Syndrome called "The Period of PURPLE Crying" uses a three-pronged approach that aims to educate adults on the normality of crying for many babies during the first few months of life. The program includes (1) parental education prior to discharge home about infant crying patterns, coping strategies, and the hazards of shaking, (2) family support and education during home visits by nurses and in the clinic with providers, and (3) a public media campaign designed to alter the culture of adult response to a well but crying baby. The acronym PURPLE derives from the character of the crying that some healthy infants experience between 2 and 4 months of age:

- **P**: Peak of crying
- **U**: Unexpected
- **R**: Resists soothing
- **P**: Painlike face
- **L**: Long lasting
- **E**: Evening and late afternoon (Stout, 2014)

Stout (2014) described implementation of The Period of Purple Crying programs that may be helpful for nurses who want to pursue this interprofessional approach in their communities. More information on this program is available online from the National Center on Shaken Baby Syndrome. (For more information on child abuse, see Chapters 42 and 55.)

To increase parents' coping abilities, suggest that they initially respond to the baby's crying by checking for hunger, a wet or soiled diaper, excessive cold or heat, restrictive or chafing clothing or blankets, or other comfort concerns. If these are not present, suggest holding or rocking the baby as previously discussed. Other calming measures include burping the baby (which provides repetitive tactile stimulation and disperses air bubbles), placing the baby in a mechanized infant swing, or taking the baby for a ride in a stroller or car. Some babies are soothed by white noise such as the sound of a dryer or the static on an untuned radio, whereas others are soothed when bound "papoose style" on the mother's or father's chest, swaddled, bathed, or massaged.

Crying can also be associated with gastrointestinal upset in babies. The parents should discuss concerns with the physician or nurse practitioner to ensure the crying is not associated with a physical cause, such as acid reflux, ear infections, or other physical conditions. In addition, it is not uncommon for babies to cry after feedings because of pain from a buildup of air bubbles in the stomach and an inability to pass flatus. Some practitioners recommend simethicone after each feeding to decrease the incidence of flatus pain. Placing the baby in a prone position across the lap while burping the baby can also aid in passing flatus.

Safety Considerations

Newborns should not have pillows, blankets, bumper pads, or stuffed animals in the crib while they sleep; these items could cause suffocation. Mattresses should fit snugly in a crib to prevent entrapment and suffocation, and the crib should be inspected regularly to determine whether it is in safe working order. Crib slats should be no more than 2 3/8 in. apart. Parents can be encouraged to attend infant cardiopulmonary resuscitation (CPR) classes, especially if there is a family history of SIDS or the baby requires special care.

Many families, especially breastfeeding families, practice **cosleeping**, in which the baby sleeps with the mother or both parents during the night. The American Academy of Pediatrics and other recent research does not recommend cosleeping because it is considered a risk factor for SIDS (Blair, 2015). However, some families and cultures may still participate in this practice and thus warrant appropriate teaching measures.

Cosleeping families should be counseled to follow these safety guidelines:

- Place the baby on a firm mattress, never on comforters, pillows, or a waterbed.

- Never sleep with your baby if you have been using drugs or have become intoxicated.

- Ensure that the baby is protected from rolling off the bed or becoming entrapped in bed rails or a space between the frame and the mattress.

- As with crib sleeping, remove all decorative pillows, stuffed animals, toys, or blankets that could impair the baby's breathing. Do not cover the baby with blankets, sheets, or down comforters.

- Make sure the baby is sleeping on the back.

- Ensure plenty of ventilation to the baby.

- Avoid overdressing the baby because the parent's body heat will reduce the need for excess clothing.

- Never smoke in bed with the baby. Family members should smoke outdoors and not in the household with the baby.

- If additional children are sleeping in the bed, make sure they are not sleeping directly next to the baby.

Clinical Tip

Advise parents that if they become frustrated with a crying baby, they should put the baby in the crib or in a safe location and allow themselves time to calm down. Sometimes going outside the door, counting to 10, doing deep breathing, or calling a friend can help. Remind parents that crying never hurts a baby, but shaking can seriously injure the baby. Reassure parents that all new parents have times when they feel frustrated and do not know what to do. This is a normal part of parenting a newborn.

The AAP and forensic researchers recommend that the safest place for the baby to sleep is in the parents' room with the baby in a crib in proximity to the parents for the first 6 months of life. The use of pacifiers has also been associated with a reduction in SIDS deaths (Blair, 2015).

Smoking poses multiple risks to the newborn and any older children living in the household. Infants living in a household with a smoker have a higher rate of hospital admissions during the first year of life. They are more prone to ear infections, asthma, allergies, and other respiratory problems (see Chapter 46).

Smoking also creates a fire hazard within the household. Smoking is the primary cause of household fires in the United States. The incidence of such fires increases dramatically when other intoxicating agents are ingested, such as alcohol or drugs. Parents should be counseled to smoke outdoors; use large, heavy ashtrays to avoid tipping; ensure that all cigarette butts are properly extinguished; and never smoke in bed.

Healthy People 2020

(MICH-18) Reduce postpartum relapse of smoking among women who quit smoking during pregnancy

---

Postpartum Classes and Support Groups

Services for families range from educational, such as classes on nutrition, exercise, infant care, and parenting, to specific healthcare programs, such as well-baby checks, immunization clinics, family-planning services, new mother support groups, and more.

Postpartum classes are becoming more common as caregivers recognize the continuing needs of the childbearing family. In many instances, classes are prepared to meet the specific needs of a variety of families so that, for example, single mothers and adolescent mothers can attend class with peers. A series of structured classes may focus on topics such as parenting, postpartum exercise, or nutrition, or there may be loosely structured group sessions that address mothers' concerns as they arise. Such classes offer chances for the new mother to socialize, share her concerns, and receive encouragement. Because baby-sitting arrangements may be difficult or expensive, it is desirable to provide child care for newborns and siblings; in some instances, babies may remain with mothers during the class.

Many communities offer support groups through birthing centers, hospitals, or other facilities. La Leche League, an excellent support group for breastfeeding mothers, typically meets monthly and is open to all pregnant and breastfeeding mothers of newborns, infants, and toddlers. The Women, Infants, and Children (WIC) Supplemental Nutrition Program may have a lactation consultant on staff or may have a contract with a lactation consultant in private practice in the community. Some military facilities provide lactation services to their service members and dependents. It is very helpful to have a handout listing available services.

Women who have children with special needs may need additional support. Referring them to peer counselors or support groups is an effective way to help them find both support and information.

Many parents today look to the Internet for information on parenting and newborn care. Nurses have an opportunity to assist parents in evaluating the reliability of the information they find. Criteria that suggest that Internet information is reliable and of high quality include affiliation with a university medical or nursing school or a government agency; inclusion of authors' credentials, education, board certification, and affiliations; referencing of information; currency of information; similarity of information when compared with other sources; and easy accessibility.

TABLE 29–8 Newborn Sleep and Awake States*

NEWBORN STATES	PHYSICAL CHARACTERISTICS	BODY ACTIVITY	EYE MOVEMENTS
SLEEP STATES			
Quiet sleep (also known as deep sleep)	Anabolic, restorative sleep, increased cell mitosis and replication, lowered oxygen consumption, release of growth hormone.	Typically still, may occasionally startle or twitch.	None.
Active sleep (also known as light sleep or rapid eye movement [REM] state)	Processing and recording information. Often linked to learning. Is the highest proportion of sleep and precedes awakening.	Some body movements.	Rapid eye movement (REM), closed eyelids may flutter.
AWAKE STATES			
Drowsy (also known as semi-dozing)	May return to sleep or awaken further.	Smooth movements with variable activity level. May experience mild startles intermittently.	Eyes may open and close. May appear heavy lidded, or eyes may appear like slits.
Quiet alert	Attentive to environment, focus attention on stimuli.	Minimal.	Eyes bright and wide.
Active alert	Baby's eyes are open, not as bright as in quiet alert. More body activity than in a quiet alert state.	Smooth movements may be interspersed with mild startles from time to time.	Eyes open with a gazed, dull appearance.
Crying	Communication tool, response to unpleasant stimuli from environment or internal stimuli. Characterized by intense crying for more than 15 sec.	Increased motor activity, skin color changes to darkened appearance, red, or ruddy.	Eyes may be tightly closed or open.

FACIAL MOVEMENTS	BREATHING PATTERN	RESPONSES	CAREGIVER IMPLICATIONS
None or may have occasional sucking movements.	Slow and regular.	Only intense or disturbing stimuli will arouse baby, threshold to stimuli is high.	Difficult to arouse for feedings. Teach parents to time feedings when baby is in a more responsive state. Baby may arouse slightly if an attempt is made to awaken but typically returns to the quiet sleep state.
May smile or make fussing or crying noises.	Irregular.	More responsive to internal stimuli (hunger) and external stimuli (such as being picked up by caregiver). When stimulated may arouse, return to quiet sleep, or remain in active sleep.	Inexperienced care providers may attempt to feed when baby makes normal crying sounds.
May have no facial movements and appear still, or may have some facial movements.	Irregular.	Usually reacts to stimuli but may be slowed. May change to other states such as quiet alert, active alert, or crying.	To stimulate baby, provide verbal, sight, or oral stimulation. If left alone, baby may return to a sleep state.
Attentive appearance.	Regular.	Most attentive, focus attention on stimuli.	In the first hours after birth, may experience intense alertness before going into a long sleeping period. This state increases in intensity as the baby becomes older. Providing stimuli will help maintain a quiet alert or active alert state. Baby provides pleasure and positive feedback to care providers. Good time to feed baby.
May be still with or without facial movements.	Irregular.	Reacts to stimuli with delayed responses to stimuli, or may change to quiet alert or crying state.	Baby may be fussy and become sensitive to stimuli, may become more and more active and start crying. If fatigue or caregiver interventions disturb this state, baby may return to a drowsy or sleep state.
Grimaces.	More irregular than in other states.	Very responsive to internal or external unpleasant stimuli.	Indicates that the baby's limits have been reached. May be able to console self and return to an alert or sleep state, or may need intervention from caregiver.

*A state is a group of characteristic behaviors and physiologic changes that occur together in a regular pattern.

Source: Healthy Children, (2013). Ages & stages. Retrieved from http://www.healthychildren.org/English/ages-stages/baby/Pages/States-of-Consciousness-in-Newborns.aspx

Focus Your Study

- Postpartum and newborn care should include nursing diagnoses that focus on the normal course for postpartum care and facilitate optimal health promotion. Goals should be collaboratively agreed upon by the nurse and the family.

- Appropriate nursing interventions in the postpartum period include promotion and restoration of maternal physical well-being which is facilitated by monitoring uterine status, vital signs, cardiovascular status, elimination patterns, nutritional needs, sleep and rest, and support and educational needs. Prevention of sleep deprivation and gradual return to activities should be encouraged. Exercises specific to postpartum needs promotes health benefit for the mother.

- Pharmacologic needs may include medications to promote comfort, treat anemia, provide immunity to rubella and Tdap, and prevent development of antigens (in the nonsensitized Rh-negative woman).

- Promotion of family wellness focuses on integration of the siblings and assisting in forming bonds with their new sibling, expectations for the couple to resume sexual activity, the need for contraception, and helping to establish and role model parent–newborn attachment.

- Postpartum assessments include basic assessment parameters for the mother regardless of the mode of birth. Assessments include a basic physical examination inclusive of fundal checks, breast examination, perineal evaluation, lochia assessment, and assessment of the bowel and bladder.

- Women undergoing a cesarean birth also require assessment of their incision and bowel sounds. The woman should also be encouraged to turn, cough, and deep breath and ambulate as early as possible. Women undergoing a surgical birth require more pain medication and fatigue easier because of the stress of surgery.

- Adolescent mothers have varying needs. The nurse should evaluate the adolescent mother in terms of her level of maturity, available support systems, cultural back ground, and existing knowledge, and then plan care accordingly.

- The mother who decides to relinquish her baby needs emotional support. She should be able to decide whether to see and hold her baby, and any special requests regarding the birth should be honored. Physical care is provided and early discharge is sometimes requested and should be honored if the mother is medically stable.

- Women with obesity need special attention to prevent injury, respiratory complications, thromboembolic disease, and infection.

- Women with developmental disabilities should be presented with educational materials that are in an easy-to-understand format. Teaching should be conducted at a level that is achievable for the individual.

- Women with a history of sexual abuse tend to have more anxiety and stress related to hospital procedures, interactions with unfamiliar staff, and being touched in general. Treat the woman with respect by providing draping and speaking to her in private. Support groups may be helpful.

- Lesbian and gay families should be treated with respect and a caring approach. Nurses may need to customize their care management and teaching, since contraceptive education is not needed. Many same-sex couples are legally married. Regardless of marital status, partners/spouses should be treated the same as heterosexual couples.

- Discharge teaching should focus on physical care, care needs of the mother and baby, appropriate follow-up care, and community resources. Written and verbal communication should be provided in the family's native language.

- Home visits should focus on physical assessment of mother and baby, screening for postpartum mood and anxiety disorders, adaptation and adjustment of the family to the new baby, and assessment of informational needs. The nurse provides educational information and answers questions while addressing any concerns of the new family.

- Home health nurses need to ensure personal safety through adequate preparation before, during, and after the home visit. Home visits center on building a caring trusting relationship with the family.

- During the home visit, nurses should expect maternal physical findings that reflect normal recovery such as normal vital signs; reduction in weight; breasts and nipples without cracks, fissures, or other signs of injury or breastfeeding difficulty; healing incision for women who have undergone a cesarean birth; normal bowel and bladder functioning (with full return to prepregnant state by 4 to 6 weeks postpartum); reduction of lochia; and reduction in uterine size.

- The family assessment should reveal appropriate demonstration of bonding, an increase level of comfort in providing newborn care, appropriate sibling adjustment, and adjustment to the parent role. Contraception should be addressed during the visit.

- It is not unusual for breastfeeding mothers to experience nipple soreness, cracked nipples, engorgement, and plugged ducts. Mothers should be encouraged to nurse often, change positions while nursing, and ensure a complete latch-on. Milk should be expressed after each feeding, and rubbed onto the nipples, which are then left to air dry.

- Newborn home care should include baby's weight, length, heart rate, head circumference, and any signs of jaundice; feeding concerns or problems; reinforcement of correct techniques for holding and bathing the baby; and proper monitoring of temperature assessment, stool and urine, sleep and activity, crying, and safety considerations. The nurse should reinforce the need for newborn screening and necessary immunizations.

Clinical Reasoning in Action

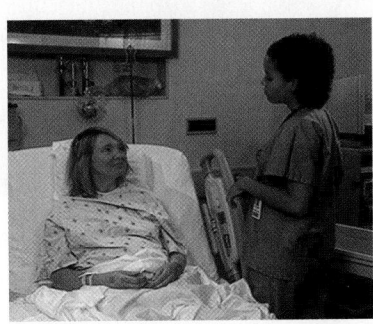

Wendy Callahan, a 31-year-old G3P2, gave birth to an 8.5-lb baby boy by primary cesarean birth for failure to progress. The baby's Apgar scores were 9 and 9 at 1 and 5 minutes. The baby was admitted to the newborn nursery for transitional observation. Wendy was transferred to the postpartum unit, where you assume her care. You introduce yourself and orient her to the room, call bell, and safety measures. You perform an initial assessment, with all findings within normal limits. Wendy tells you she is very tired and would like to rest while her baby is in the nursery. Her husband and family have left the hospital after spending time with her in the recovery room but will return later. She admits she is disappointed that she could not give birth vaginally even though she pushed for 2 hours. She says, "This baby was just too big."

1. How would you discuss with Wendy the need for frequent assessments after birth?
2. Explain "maternity blues" or "baby blues."
3. Explore activities to minimize maternity blues.
4. Discuss concerns of a woman experiencing her second pregnancy.
5. Discuss behaviors that inhibit paternal attachment.

References

American Academy of Pediatrics (AAP) Committee on Fetus and Newborn. (2011). SIDS and other sleep-related infant deaths: Expansion of recommendations for a safe infant sleeping environment. *Pediatrics, 128*, 1341–1347. doi:10.1542/peds.2011-2285

American Academy of Pediatrics (AAP) Committee on Fetus and Newborn. (2014). Hospital stay for healthy term newborns. Washington, DC: Author.

Association of Reproductive Health Professionals (ARHP). (2013). Postpartum counseling. Retrieved from http://www.arhp.org/publications-and-resources /quick-reference-guide-for-clinicians/postpartum -counseling/diet

Association of Women's Health, Obstetric and Neonatal Nurses (AWHONN). (2014). *Assessment and care of the late preterm infant. Evidence-based clinical practice guideline.* Washington, DC: Author.

Barfield, W. D., & Lee, K. G. (2012). *Late preterm infants.* Retrieved from http://www.uptodate.com/contents/ late-preterm-infants

Blair, P. S. (2015). Co-sleeping and suffocation. *Forensic Science, Medicine, and Pathology, 11*(2), 1–2.

Briggs, G. G., Freeman, R. K., & Yaffe, S. J. (2012). *Drugs in pregnancy and lactation: A reference guide to fetal and neonatal risk* (9th ed.). Baltimore, MD: Lippincott Williams & Wilkins.

Brincat, C., Crosby, E., McLeod, A., & Fenner, D. E. (2015). Experiences during the first four years of a postpartum perineal clinic in the USA. *International Journal of Gynecology & Obstetrics, 128*(1), 68–71.

Center for American Progress. (2015). *The adoption option.* Retrieved from http://www.americanprogress. org/issues/women/report/2010/10/18/8460/the -adoption-option

Chapman, D. J., & Pérez-Escamilla, R. (2012). Breastfeeding among minority women: Moving from risk factors to interventions. *Advances in Nutrition, 3*(1), 95–104.

Cherry, A., & Dillon, M. (2014). *International handbook of adolescent pregnancy: Medical, psychosocial, and public health responses.* New York, NY: Springer.

Child Welfare Information Gateway. (2012). *Infant safe haven laws: Summary of state laws.* Retrieved from http://www.childwelfare.gov/systemwide/laws _policies/statutes/safehaven.cfm

Flannery, A. B., Looman, W. S., & Kemper, K. (2012). Evidence-based care of the child with deformational plagiocephaly, Part II: Management. *Pediatric Health Care, 26*(5), 320–331.

Fowles, E. R., Cheng, H. R., & Mills, S. (2012). Postpartum health promotion interventions: A systematic review. *Nursing Research, 61*(4), 269–282. doi:10.1097/NNR.0b013e3182556d29

Kronborg, H., Vaeth, M., & Kristensen, I. (2012). The effect of early postpartum home visits by health visitors: A natural experiment. *Public Health Nurse, 29*(4), 289–301.

Leeman, L. M., & Rogers, R. G. (2012). Sex after childbirth: Postpartum sexual function. *Obstetrics & Gynecology, 119*(3), 647–655. doi:10.1097/ AOG.0b013e3182479611

Lowe, N. K. (2012). The persistent problem of postpartum hemorrhage. *Journal of Obstetric, Gynecologic, & Neonatal Nursing, 41*(4), 459–460. doi:10.1111/ j.1552-6909.2012.01397.x

Michigan Department of Community Health. (2015). *Infant mental health.* Retrieved from http://michigan. gov/mdch/0,4612,7-132-2941_4868_7145 -14659–,00.html

Nilsson, C., Lundgren, I., Karlström, A., & Hildingsson, I. (2012). Self-reported fear of childbirth and its association with women's birth experience and mode of delivery: A longitudinal population-based study. *Women and Birth: Journal of the Australian College of Midwives, 25*(3), 114–121.

Spector, R. E. (2012). *Cultural diversity in health and illness* (8th ed.). Upper Saddle River, NJ: Prentice Hall Health.

Spidsberg, B. D., & Sørlie, V. (2012). An expression of love—midwives' experiences in the encounter with lesbian women and their partners. *Journal of Advanced Nursing, 68*(4), 796–805. doi:10.1111 /j.1365-2648.2011.05780.x

Stout, J. R. (2014). *Evaluating an evidence-based prevention program delivered by primary-care providers and in-home nurse visits: The period of purple crying: an abusive head-trauma prevention program* (Doctoral dissertation, North Dakota State University).

Strong, G. D. (2011). Provider management and support for breastfeeding pain. *Journal of Obstetric, Gynecologic, and Neonatal Nursing, 40*(6), 753–764.

Surkan, P. J., Gottlieb, B. R., McCormick, M. C., Hunt, A., & Peterson, K. E. (2012). Impact of a health promotion intervention on maternal depressive symptoms at 15 months postpartum. *Maternal and Child Health Journal, 16*(1), 139–148.

U.S. Department of Health and Human Services (USD-HHS). (2011). *The surgeon general's call to action to support breastfeeding.* Washington, DC: U.S. Department of Health and Human Services, Office of the Surgeon General. Retrieved from http://www. surgeongeneral.gov/library/calls/breastfeeding/callto-actiontosupportbreastfeeding.pdf

U.S. Department of Health and Human Services (US-DHHS). (2015). *Healthy People 2020: Topics and objectives.* Retrieved from http://www.healthypeople. gov/2020/ topicsobjectives2020/default.aspx

U.S. Department of Labor. (2009). Fact sheet: Newborn & mother's health protection act. Retrieved from http:// www.dol.gov/ebsa/newsroom/fsnmhafs.html

Wambach, K., & Riordan, J. (2014). Breastfeeding and human lactation. (5th ed.). Boston, MA: Jones & Bartlett.

Wojnar, D., & Katzenmeyer, A. (2014). Experiences of preconception, pregnancy, and new motherhood for lesbian nonbiological mothers. *Journal of Obstetrical, Gynecological, and Neonatal Nursing (JOGNN), 43*(1), 50–60.

Zerwekh, J., & Garneau, A. Z. (2014). *Nursing today: Transition and trends* (8th ed.) Philadelphia, PA: Saunders.

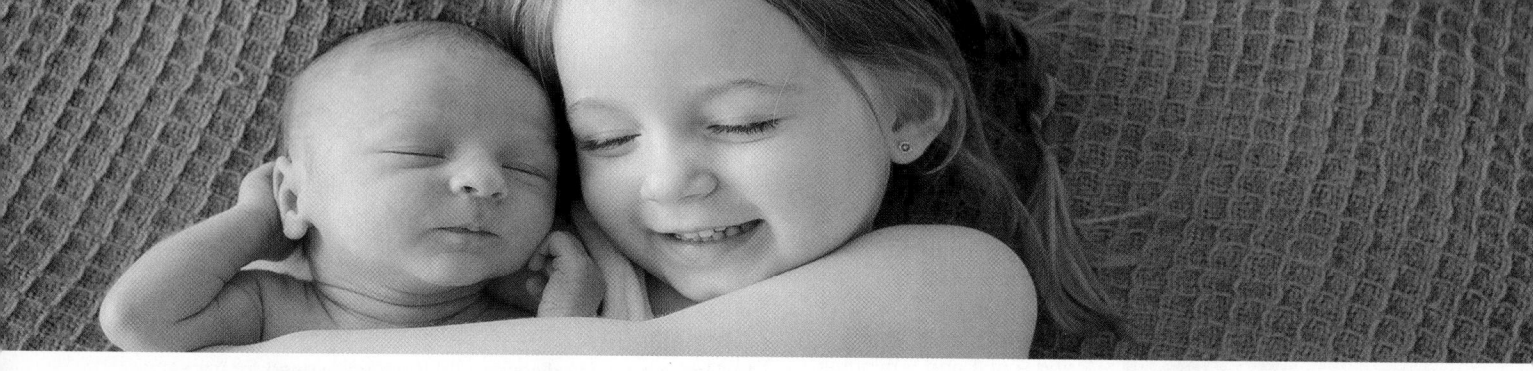

Chapter 30
The Postpartum Family at Risk

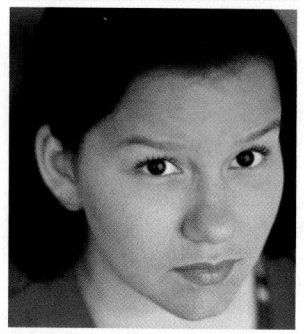

Ryan McVay/Getty Images

We are surviving. Maybe just. I was told that babies ate at six-ten-two-six-ten-two, but no one said that he would eat at five-seven-nine-eleven or so it seems. I am either getting ready to feed him or just finished feeding and changing him. But I love him without bounds. I feel a need to protect him from ever being hurt or wounded. During that first week, when I was tired and recovering from the emergency cesarean, I was afraid that I would not be able to shelter and help this young son grow up.

—Kate, 34

Learning Outcomes

30.1 Identify the causes, contributing factors, signs and symptoms, clinical therapy, and nursing interventions for early and late postpartum hemorrhage.

30.2 Explain the causes, contributing factors, signs and symptoms, clinical therapy, and nursing interventions for reproductive tract infection.

30.3 Develop a nursing care plan that reflects knowledge of etiology, pathophysiology, clinical therapy, and nursing and preventive

management for the woman experiencing urinary tract infection, lactation mastitis, or a postpartum psychiatric disorder.

30.4 Identify the causes, contributing factors, signs and symptoms, clinical therapy, and nursing interventions for postpartum thromboembolic disease.

30.5 Evaluate the woman's knowledge of healthcare promotion measures and signs of postpartum complications to be reported to the primary care provider.

The postpartum period is typically viewed as a smooth, uneventful transition time—and often it is, even with the challenges of new parenthood and the integration of a new person into the family. However, it is important for the nurse to be aware of physical or emotional complications that may develop postpartum. The nurse should teach the family the signs of postpartum complications, findings to report to the healthcare provider/certified nurse-midwife (CNM), and preventive measures, if available.

Early postpartum discharge challenges the nurse to impart anticipatory information about normal postpartum recovery and self-care for the mother and her newborn, as well as be vigilant about recognizing when things go wrong. Postpartum complications can be life threatening to the mother and require immediate collaborative management. These complications

sometimes necessitate readmission of the woman to the hospital, thereby disrupting the family and adding concerns not only about her health but also about the way in which infant care will be managed. The most common complications of the postpartum period are hemorrhage, infection, thromboembolic disease, and postpartum psychiatric disorders. These complications are the major focus of this chapter.

Healthy People 2020

(MICH-5) Reduce the rate of maternal mortality to 11.4 maternal deaths per 100,000 live births

(MICH-6) Reduce maternal illness and complications due to pregnancy (complications during hospitalized labor and delivery) to 28.0%

Care of the Woman With Postpartum Hemorrhage

Hemorrhage in the postpartum period is described as either early (immediate or primary) or late (delayed or secondary). **Early (primary) postpartum hemorrhage** occurs in the first 24 hours after childbirth and is the more common of the two. **Late (secondary) postpartum hemorrhage** occurs from 24 hours to 6 weeks after birth. Postpartum hemorrhage (PPH) continues to be a cause of significant maternal mortality and morbidity, although there has been a decrease in the Western world over recent years. The decrease in mortality and morbidity has been attributed to better management of uterine atony, the primary cause of PPH. However, cases of PPH due to uterine rupture and placenta accreta are on the rise—a direct consequence of the increasing rate of cesarean births (Sosa, 2014). Worldwide, PPH is the leading cause of pregnancy-related deaths, and it is estimated that 140,000 women die from postpartum hemorrhage every year, approximately one sixth of them in the United States (Poggi, 2013).

The traditional definition of postpartum hemorrhage has been a blood loss of greater than 500 mL following childbirth. However, that definition is currently being questioned because careful quantification indicates that the average blood loss in a vaginal birth is actually greater than 500 mL, the average blood loss after a cesarean childbirth exceeds 1000 mL, and the average blood loss is more than 1500 mL during repeat cesarean birth (Harvey & Dildy, 2013). Clinically, PPH can be defined as a drop in maternal hematocrit levels of 10% or more from predelivery baseline or excessive bleeding that causes hemodynamic instability or the need for a blood transfusion (Sosa, 2014).

Clinical estimates of blood loss tend to underestimate actual loss by up to 50% (Cunningham et al., 2014). Clinical estimation of blood loss at childbirth is difficult because blood mixes with amniotic fluid and is obscured as it oozes onto sterile drapes or is sponged away. As the amount of blood loss increases, as in the case of hemorrhage, estimates are likely to be even less accurate than with normal childbirth. Moreover, postpartum hemorrhage may occur intra-abdominally, into the broad ligament, or into hematomas arising from genital tract trauma, wherein the blood loss is concealed. Given the increased blood volume of pregnancy, the clinical signs of hemorrhage—such as increasing pulse, decreased blood pressure, and decreasing urinary output—do not appear until as much as 1000 to 2000 mL or 10% or more of the woman's hematocrit has been lost (Robbins, Martin, & Wilson, 2014).

SAFETY ALERT!

To meet the standard of care in cases of postpartum hemorrhage, rapid response systems are needed in every obstetric setting that will enable nurses to respond quickly to independently implement certain actions based on evidence-based protocols, similar to a call for coding someone experiencing a cardiac arrest. This multidisciplinary team approach helps to organize roles and prioritize care to stabilize the patient in a timely manner, thus averting massive hemorrhage.

Early (Primary) Postpartum Hemorrhage

At term, blood volume and cardiac output have increased so that 20% of cardiac output, or 750 to 1000 mL per minute, perfuses the pregnant uterus, supporting the developing fetus

(Sosa, 2014). When the placenta separates from the uterine wall, the many uterine vessels that have carried blood to and from the placenta are severed abruptly. The normal mechanism for hemostasis after delivery of the placenta is contraction of the interlacing uterine muscles to occlude the open sinuses that previously brought blood into the placenta. Absence of prompt and sustained uterine contractions (uterine atony) can result in significant blood loss. Other causes of postpartum hemorrhage include laceration of the genital tract; episiotomy; retained placental fragments; vulvar, vaginal, or subperitoneal hematomas; uterine inversion; uterine rupture; problems of placental implantation; and coagulation disorders.

UTERINE ATONY

Uterine atony (relaxation of the uterus) is the leading cause of early postpartum hemorrhage, accounting for over 50% of PPH cases (Poggi, 2013). Although uterine atony can occur after any childbirth, its contributing factors include the following (Cunningham et al., 2014; Poggi, 2013; Sosa, 2014):

- Overdistention of the uterus caused by multiple gestation, hydramnios, or a large baby (macrosomia)
- Dysfunctional or prolonged labor, which indicates that the uterus is contracting abnormally
- Oxytocin augmentation or induction of labor
- Grand multiparity, because stretched uterine musculature contracts less vigorously
- Use of anesthesia (especially halothane) or other drugs, such as magnesium sulfate, calcium channel blockers such as nifedipine, or tocolytics, any of which cause the uterus to relax
- Prolonged third stage of labor—more than 30 minutes
- Preeclampsia
- Asian or Hispanic heritage
- Operative birth (includes vacuum extraction or forceps-assisted births)
- Retained placental fragments
- Placenta previa or accreta
- Obesity (Wetta et al., 2013)

Hemorrhage from uterine atony may be slow and steady rather than sudden and massive. The blood may escape the vagina or collect in the uterus, where it is evident as large clots. The uterine cavity may distend with up to 1000 mL or more of blood, although the perineal pad and linen protectors remain suspiciously dry. A treacherous feature of postpartum hemorrhage is that maternal vital signs may not change until significant blood loss has occurred because of the increased blood volume associated with pregnancy.

SAFETY ALERT!

It is critical to remember that a woman with no identifiable risk factors may hemorrhage after childbirth as well.

The woman and her partner may wish to have some private time engaging with the newborn when he or she is appropriately warm and ready for an early visit. But postpartum women must be assessed at frequent intervals, especially in the initial hours after delivery of the placenta when most deaths from hemorrhage occur.

Ideally, PPH is prevented, beginning with adequate prenatal care, good nutrition, avoidance of traumatic procedures, risk assessment, early recognition, and management of complications as they arise. Review of maternal records for risk factors will help nurses to plan assessment timelines to maximize early identification and management of excessive bleeding. A prior history of PPH increases the woman's risk by double in a subsequent pregnancy (Oberg, Hernandez-Diaz, Palmsten, et al., 2014).

There is evidence that active management of the third stage of labor through administration of an oxytocic drug after delivery, controlled traction on the umbilical cord, and uterine massage after birth could prevent half of the cases of postpartum hemorrhage (Poggi, 2013). Any woman at risk should be typed and cross-matched for blood transfusion.

Clinical Therapy. The goals of medical management of PPH are to stop the hemorrhage, correct hypovolemia, and treat the underlying cause. After expulsion of the placenta, the fundus is palpated to ensure that it is firmly contracted. If it is not firm, gentle fundal massage is performed until the uterus contracts. Fundal massage is uncomfortable for the woman who has not received regional anesthesia; she will need an explanation for why this procedure is necessary and support as massage is initiated. Clinical guidelines schedule vital signs and assessment of fundal contractility and lochia at regular intervals (see Chapters 28 and 29). When excessive bleeding continues despite external uterine massage, the healthcare provider may elect to do a bimanual massage (Figure 30–1A). Bimanual massage compresses the body of the uterus from below while the abdominal hand massages the fundus from above.

If uterine massage is not effective, uterine stimulants (uterotonic agents) will be administered to contract the atonic musculature. Oxytocin, ergotamine, prostaglandin analog, and misoprostol are most often used (Thorp & Laughton, 2014). See *Medications Used to Treat: Uterine Stimulants Used to Prevent and Manage Uterine Atony* for a summary of critical nursing information about the use of uterine stimulants to control bleeding. The need for IV fluid replacement and blood transfusion is determined on the basis of hemoglobin and hematocrit results as well as coagulation studies.

Conservative management includes uterine stimulants to contract the atonic musculature. Oxytocin, ergotamine, and prostaglandin are most often used. Misoprostol, best known to the obstetric community for its use in labor induction, is being used to prevent and treat uterine atony after failed attempts to control bleeding with oxytocics. Sublingual misoprostol (800 micrograms) has been found to be as effective as oxytocin (40 units/L) (Poggi, 2013). When conservative measures do not successfully control bleeding, surgical intervention is required. In order of increasing invasiveness, surgical procedures include uterine balloon tamponade (Cunningham et al., 2014; Poggi, 2013), selective radiographic-guided pelvic arterial embolization (Robbins et al., 2014; Rouse, 2013), uterine suturing techniques (Ayadi, Robinson, Geller, et al., 2013), ligation of the uterine or hypogastric arteries, and, as a last resort, hysterectomy, which clearly ends childbearing (Harvey & Dildy, 2013).

LACERATIONS OF THE GENITAL TRACT

Early postpartum hemorrhage is associated with lacerations of the perineum, vagina, or cervix. Several factors predispose women to higher risk of reproductive tract lacerations:

- Nulliparity
- Epidural anesthesia
- Precipitous childbirth (less than 3 hours)
- Forceps- or vacuum-assisted birth
- Macrosomia
- Use of oxytocin

EVIDENCE-BASED PRACTICE | Treatment for Postpartum Hemorrhage

Clinical Question

What treatment reduces the risk of maternal mortality from postpartum hemorrhage?

The Evidence

After birth, the blood vessels in a woman's uterus contract, clamping blood flow and limiting bleeding after the placenta has detached. Without strong contraction of the blood vessels, hemorrhage can occur; this condition is one of the top five causes of maternal mortality in both developed and developing nations. Treatment for postpartum hemorrhage is essential to save the mother's life, yet the drug that has been proven effective for this purpose (oxytocin) requires refrigeration and is not useful in developing countries. These researchers studied the effectiveness of alternative drugs and procedures as compared to oxytocin by conducting a systematic review of randomized trials. Interventions included prostaglandins (such as misoprostol), blood-clotting agents (such as tranexamic acid), surgical techniques to ligate the uterine artery, and radiologic interventions that assisted in blocking the main artery by using gel foams. This structured guideline, published in the rigorously reviewed *Cochrane Database of Systematic Reviews*, forms the strongest level of evidence. This review included 10 randomized controlled trials involving more than 4000 women.

Overall, none of the treatments worked as well as oxytocin. The prostaglandin misoprostol was moderately successful in stopping hemorrhage, although it was not as effective as oxytocin (Mousa, Blum, Senoun, et al., 2014). Neither compression nor surgical methods were as effective as oxytocin. These treatments and misoprostol caused more side effects than did oxytocin when used as a first-line therapy for the treatment of primary postpartum hemorrhage. Using misoprostol as an adjunct treatment with oxytocin showed no additional benefit. However, misoprostol does not need refrigeration, and in developing nations or areas without adequate medication storage, it does confer some protection against mortality from hemorrhage.

Best Practice

Oxytocin is the best and first-line treatment for postpartum hemorrhage. It is more effective and has fewer side effects than misoprostol or surgical/radiologic procedures. However, oxytocin requires refrigeration, so in some developing countries, misoprostol confers some protection against maternal mortality and does not require special storage.

Clinical Reasoning

What are some creative ways for refrigerating oxytocin when standard refrigeration is unavailable? What are ways to estimate blood loss so that interventions can be applied in a timely way?

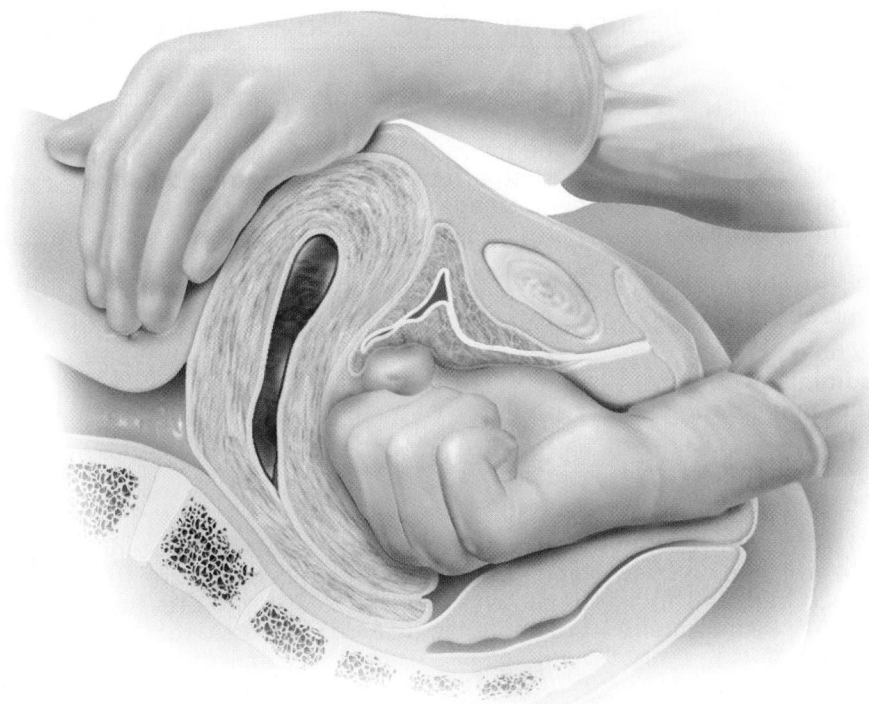

A

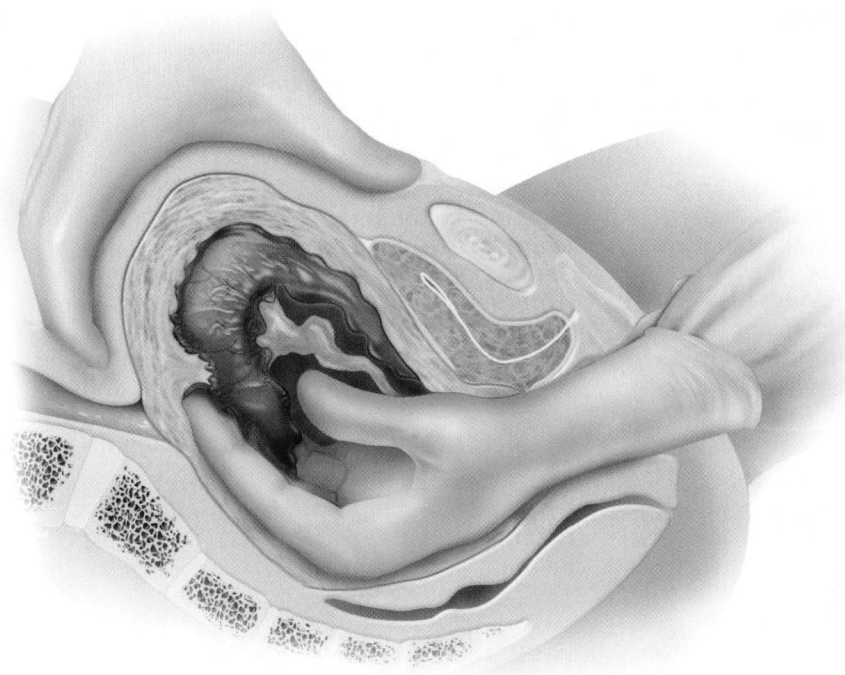

B

Figure 30–1 *A*, Manual compression of the uterus and massage with the abdominal hand usually will effectively control hemorrhage from uterine atony. *B*, Manual removal of placenta. The fingers are alternately abducted, adducted, and advanced until the placenta is completely detached. Both procedures are performed only by the healthcare provider.

Genital tract lacerations should be suspected when vaginal bleeding persists in the presence of a firmly contracted uterus. The nurse who suspects a laceration should notify the clinician so that the laceration can be immediately sutured to control the hemorrhage and restore the integrity of the reproductive tract. The woman may be moved to a delivery or surgical area for access to special lighting to facilitate treatment.

Episiotomy is an often underappreciated source of postpartum blood loss because of slow, steady bleeding, especially if it was done early in the birth process. To fully assess the episiotomy site, the nurse must position the woman on her side. (See discussion of episiotomy in Chapter 22.)

Medications Used to Treat: Uterine Stimulants Used to Prevent and Manage Uterine Atony

DRUG	DOSING INFORMATION	CONTRAINDICATIONS	EXPECTED EFFECTS	SIDE EFFECTS
Oxytocin (Pitocin, Syntocinon)	IV use: 10–40 units in 500–1000 mL crystalloid fluid at 50 milliunits/min administration rate. Onset: immediate. Duration: 1 hr. **IV bolus administration not recommended.** IM use: 10 units. Onset: 3–5 min. Duration: 2–3 hr.	None for use in postpartum hemorrhage. Avoid undiluted rapid IV infusion, which causes hypotension.	Rhythmic uterine contractions that help to prevent or reverse postpartum hemorrhage caused by uterine atony.	Uterine hyperstimulation, mild transient hypertension, water intoxication rare in postpartum use.
Methylergonovine maleate (Methergine)	IM use: 0.2 mg every 2–4 hr. Onset: 2–5 min. Duration: 3 hr (for 5 dose maximum). PO use: 0.2 mg every 4 hr (for 6 doses). Onset: 7 to 15 min. Duration: 3 hr (for 1 week). **IV administration not recommended—can cause dangerous hypertension and stroke.**	Women with labile or high blood pressure or known sensitivity to drug, cardiac disease, and Raynaud disease. Use with caution during lactation.	Sustained uterine contractions that help to prevent or reverse postpartum hemorrhage caused by uterine atony; management of postpartum subinvolution.	Hypertension, dizziness, headache, flushing/ hot flashes, tinnitus, nausea and vomiting, palpitations, chest pain. Overdose or hypersensitivity is recognized by seizures; tingling and numbness of fingers and toes.
Prostaglandin (PGF$_{2a}$, Carboprost tromethamine [Hemabate], Prostin/15M)	IM use: 0.25 mg repeated every 15–90 min, up to 8 doses max. Healthcare provider may elect to administer by direct intramyometrial injection.	Women with active cardiovascular, renal, liver disease, or asthma or with known hypersensitivity to drug.	Control of refractory cases of postpartum hemorrhage caused by uterine atony; generally used after failed attempts at control of hemorrhage with oxytocic agents.	Nausea, vomiting, diarrhea, headache, flushing, bradycardia, bronchospasm, wheezing, cough, chills, fever.
Dinoprostone (Prostin E$_2$)	Vaginal or rectal suppository 20 mg every 2 hr. Stored in frozen form—must be thawed to room temperature.	Avoid if woman is hypotensive or has asthma or acute inflammatory disease.	Stimulate uterine contractions	Fever is common and occurs within 15–45 min of insertion; bleeding, abdominal cramps, nausea and vomiting.
Misoprostol (Cytotec)	800–1000 micrograms rectally. Rapid effects, contractions within minutes.	History of allergies to prostaglandins.	Used to prevent and treat uterine atony after failed attempts to control bleeding with oxytocics.	Diarrhea, abdominal pain, headache

NURSING IMPLICATIONS WITH UTERINE STIMULANTS

- Note expected duration of action of drug being administered and take care to recheck fundus at that time for adequate tone.

- When the drug is ineffective and the fundus remains atonic (boggy or uncontracted) and bleeding continues, massage the fundus. If massage fails to cause sustained contraction, consider the status of the urinary bladder. If uterine tone is not restored after the bladder is empty and fundal massage has been performed, notify the healthcare provider immediately.

- Monitor woman for signs of known side effects of the drug; report to healthcare provider if side effects occur.

- Remind the woman and her support person that uterine cramping is an expected result of these drugs and that medication is available for discomfort. Administer analgesic medications as needed for pain relief. Provide nonpharmacologic comfort measures. If analgesic medication ordered is insufficient for pain relief, notify the healthcare provider.

- Provide information to the woman and her family regarding the importance of not smoking during Methergine administration (nicotine from cigarettes leads to constricted vessels and may lead to hypertension) and signs of toxicity.

When Prostaglandin Is Used

- Check temperature every 1–2 hr. Administer antipyretic medication as ordered for prostaglandin-induced fever.

- Auscultate breath sounds frequently for signs of adverse respiratory effects.

- Assess for nausea, vomiting, and diarrhea. Administer antiemetic and antidiarrheal medications as ordered. (In some settings, women are premedicated with these drugs.)

Sources: Data from Robbins, K. S., Martin, S. R., & Wilson, W. C. (2014). Intensive care considerations for the critically ill parturient. In R. K. Creasy & R. Resnik (Eds.), *Maternal–fetal medicine: Principles and practice* (7th ed., pp. 1182–1214). Philadelphia, PA: Saunders; Sosa, M. E. (2014). Bleeding in pregnancy. In K. R. Simpson & P. A. Creehan (Eds.), *AWHONN's perinatal nursing* (4th ed., pp. 143–162). Philadelphia, PA: Lippincott Williams & Wilkins.

RETAINED PLACENTAL FRAGMENTS

Retained placental fragments may be a cause of early postpartum hemorrhage and are also the most common cause of late hemorrhage. Retention of fragments is usually attributable to partial separation of the placenta during massage of the fundus before spontaneous placental separation. Therefore, this practice should be avoided.

SAFETY ALERT!

Postpartum nurses are wise to appreciate that most deaths from postpartum hemorrhage are not caused by catastrophic bleeding episodes but by ineffective management of slow, steady blood loss.

Following birth, the placenta should always be inspected for intactness and for evidence of missing fragments or cotyledons on the maternal side and for vessels that transverse to the edge of the placenta outward along the membranes of the fetal side, which may indicate succenturiate placenta and a retained lobe. Uterine exploration may be required to remove missing fragments (Figure 30–1*B*). This cause should be immediately suspected if bleeding persists and no lacerations are noted. Sonography may be used to diagnose retained placental fragments. Curettage, formerly standard treatment, is now thought by some to traumatize the implantation site, thereby increasing bleeding and the potential for uterine adhesions. However, it may be necessitated by the degree of hemorrhage (Poggi, 2013).

VULVAR, VAGINAL, AND PELVIC HEMATOMAS

Hematomas occur as a result of injury to a blood vessel from birth trauma, often without noticeable trauma to the superficial tissue, or from inadequate hemostasis at the site of repair of an incision or laceration. The soft tissue in the area offers no resistance, and hematomas containing 250 to 500 mL of blood may develop rapidly. Signs and symptoms vary somewhat with the type of hematoma. Hematomas may be vulvar (involving branches of the pudendal artery), vaginal (especially in the area of the ischial spines), vulvovaginal, or subperitoneal. The latter are rare; however, they are the most dangerous because of the large amount of blood loss that can occur without clinical symptoms until the woman becomes hemodynamically unstable. Subperitoneal hematomas involve the uterine artery branches or vessels in the broad ligaments and require laparotomy for surgical correction.

Risk factors for hematomas include preeclampsia, use of pudendal anesthesia, first full-term birth, precipitous labor, prolonged second stage of labor, macrosomia, forceps- or vacuum-assisted births, and history of vulvar varicosities (Distefano et al., 2013). Hematomas less than 3 cm (1.2 in.) in size and nonexpanding are managed expectantly with ice packs and analgesia. Small hematomas usually resolve over several days. For larger hematomas and those that expand, surgical management is usually required. The hematoma is evacuated using incision and drainage. The bleeding vessel is ligated, and the wound closed, with or without vaginal packing. A temporary indwelling urinary catheter may be necessary because voiding may be impossible with packing in place (Francois & Foley, 2012).

The hematoma site is an ideal medium for the growth of flora normally present in the genital tract. Consequently, broad-spectrum antibiotics are usually ordered to prevent infection or abscess.

UTERINE INVERSION

Uterine inversion—a prolapse of the fundus to or through the cervix so that the uterus is, in effect, turned inside out after birth—is a rare but life-threatening cause of postpartum hemorrhage. Although not always preventable, uterine inversion is often associated with factors such as fundal implantation or abnormal adherence of the placenta, weakness of the uterine musculature, uterine relaxation secondary to anesthesia or drugs such as magnesium sulfate, and excess traction on the umbilical cord or vigorous manual removal of the placenta. Most cases of uterine inversion are managed by immediate repositioning of the uterus within the pelvis by the healthcare provider under intravenous tocolysis or general anesthesia (Robbins et al., 2014).

Late (Secondary) Postpartum Hemorrhage

Although early postpartum hemorrhage usually occurs within hours after birth, delayed hemorrhage generally occurs within 1 to 2 weeks after childbirth, most frequently as a result of **subinvolution** (failure to return to normal size) of the placental site or retention of placental fragments. Blood loss at this time may be excessive but rarely poses the same risk as that from immediate postpartum hemorrhage. Late postpartum hemorrhage is much less common but can be extremely stressful for the woman and her family who are at home by this time.

The site of placental implantation is always the last area of the uterus to regenerate after childbirth. In the case of subinvolution, adjacent endometrium and the decidua basalis fail to regenerate to cover the placental site. Faulty implantation in the less vascular lower uterine segment, retention of placental tissue, or infection may contribute to subinvolution. With subinvolution, the postpartum fundal height is greater than expected. In addition, lochia flow often fails to progress from rubra to serosa to alba normally. Lochia rubra that persists longer than 2 weeks postpartum is highly suggestive of subinvolution, although studies show there is a great variability in normal lochia patterns (Fletcher, Grotegut, & James, 2012). Some women report scant brown lochia or irregular heavy bleeding. Leukorrhea, backache, and foul-smelling lochia may occur if infection is a cause. There may be a history of heavy early postpartum bleeding or difficulty with expulsion of the placenta. When portions of the placenta have been retained in the uterus, bleeding continues because normal uterine contractions that constrict the bleeding site are prohibited. Presence of placental tissue within the uterus can be confirmed by pelvic ultrasound.

Subinvolution is most commonly diagnosed during the routine postpartum examination at 4 to 6 weeks. The woman may relate a history of irregular or excessive bleeding or describe the symptoms listed previously. An enlarged, softer-than-normal uterus palpated bimanually is an objective indication of subinvolution. Treatment includes oral administration of methylergonovine maleate (Methergine) 0.2 mg every 4 hours for 24 to 48 hours (see *Medications Used to Treat: Uterine Stimulants Used to Prevent and Manage Uterine Atony*). When uterine infection is present, antibiotics are also administered. If retained placenta is suspected or other treatment is ineffective, curettage may be indicated (Poggi, 2013).

Nursing Management

For the Woman at Risk for Postpartum Hemorrhage

Nursing Assessment and Diagnosis

Careful and ongoing assessment of the woman during labor and birth and evaluation of her prenatal history will help identify factors that put her at risk for postpartum hemorrhage. Following birth, assess periodically for evidence of vaginal bleeding. Regularly and frequently assess fundal height and uterine tone or contractility; such assessments will alert you to the possible development or recurrence of hemorrhage. Monitor the bladder for evidence of increasing distention. Immediate intervention can sometimes help to prevent excessive bleeding that occurs when a full bladder displaces the uterus and interferes with contractility. This assessment can be done visually, by pad counts, or by weighing the perineal pads. In cases of excessive bleeding, be alert for signs of impending hypovolemic shock and the development of coagulation problems, such as disseminated intravascular coagulation (DIC) (see Chapter 15 for a discussion of DIC).

For all complaints of perineal pain, examine the perineal area for signs of hematomas: ecchymosis, edema, tenseness of tissue overlying the hematoma, a fluctuant mass bulging at the introitus, and extreme tenderness to palpation. Estimating the size on first assessment of the perineum will enable you to better identify increases in size and the potential blood loss. Notify the healthcare provider if a hematoma is suspected. Decrease the risk of vulvar or vaginal hematoma by applying an ice pack to the woman's perineum during the first hour after birth and intermittently thereafter for the next 8 to 12 hours. If a small hematoma develops despite preventive measures, a sitz bath after the first 12 hours will aid fluid absorption once bleeding has stopped and will promote comfort, as will the judicious use of analgesic agents. Close monitoring of the woman who has had excessive bleeding is important during sitz baths to ensure safety. In cases of excessive bleeding, be alert for signs of impending hypovolemic shock. Frequent noninvasive monitoring should continue: heart rate, blood pressure, auscultation of heart sounds and breath sounds, oxygen saturation, skin turgor, color, temperature, color and moisture of mucous membranes, capillary refill, level of consciousness, and urinary output, possibly with Foley catheter/urometer, and electrocardiogram (ECG) readings.

Development of a rapid response team is a patient safety initiative. When obstetric postpartum hemorrhage occurs, the interprofessional perinatal rapid response team needs to work collaboratively to treat the underlying cause, manage the blood loss, and lessen the risk to the mother (ACOG Committee on Patient Safety and Quality Improvement, 2014; James, 2014)).

Nursing diagnoses that may apply to a woman experiencing postpartum hemorrhage include the following (NANDA-I © 2014):

- *Fluid Volume: Deficient*, related to blood loss secondary to uterine atony, lacerations, or retained placental fragments

- *Tissue Perfusion: Peripheral, Risk for Ineffective*, related to hypovolemia

- *Bleeding, Risk for*, related to lack of information about signs of delayed postpartum hemorrhage

Planning and Implementation

HOSPITAL-BASED NURSING CARE

Upon detection of a soft, boggy uterus, massage it until firm. If the uterus is not contracting well and appears larger than anticipated, you may express clots during fundal massage. Once clots have been expressed, the uterus tends to contract more effectively. Overly aggressive massage should be avoided so as not to injure the vessels in the broad ligaments or cause reactive relaxation of the musculature

---

Clinical Tip

A boggy uterus indicates that the uterus is not well contracted. This results in increased uterine bleeding, which may remain in the uterus and form clots or may result in increased flow. To assess the amount of blood loss, you must first massage the uterus until it is firm and then express clots. Even though the woman may have a firm uterus, significant bleeding can occur from causes other than uterine atony. To accurately determine the amount of blood loss, it is not sufficient to assess only the peri-pad. You should also ask the woman to turn on her side so you can assess underneath her for pooling of blood.

If the woman seems to have a slow, steady, free flow of blood, do pad counts and if possible begin to weigh the perineal pads (1 mL = 1 g) (Harvey & Dildy, 2013). Monitor the woman's vital signs every 15 minutes, or more frequently if indicated (James, 2014). If the fundus is displaced upward or to one side because of a full bladder, encourage the woman to empty her bladder—or catheterize her if she is unable to void—to allow for efficient uterine contractions. Excessive bleeding or uterine atony despite fundal massage necessitates prompt notification to the healthcare provider.

When there are risk factors for postpartum hemorrhage, or frequent fundal massage has been necessary to sustain uterine contractions, maintain any vascular access (IV) started during labor and anticipate the need for a second IV in case additional fluids, medications, or blood is necessary. If blood has been cross-matched earlier, check that blood is available in the blood bank.

As the woman's blood volume becomes depleted, positioning her with her legs elevated to 30 degrees facilitates venous return and promotes oxygenation. Unlike the Trendelenberg position used in the past for those in shock, this position does not impede breathing or cardiac function and promotes cerebral circulation. Supplemental oxygen may be necessary to keep peripheral tissues oxygenated when blood is shunted to protect vital organs like the brain and kidneys. See Box 30–1: Nursing Actions During Postpartum Hemorrhage.

FLUID REPLACEMENT AND TRANSFUSION

A prominent role of the nurse during PPH is the administration of crystalloid fluids (normal saline and lactated Ringer solution) or of blood and blood products. Typically, lost intravascular volume is replaced initially with rapid administration of warmed crystalloid solutions, in a 3 mL solution per 1 mL of estimated blood lost ratio (Francois & Foley, 2012). With rapid attempts to replace depleted blood volume, you must carefully monitor the woman for evidence of fluid overload.

When blood loss is significant and vital signs become unstable, crystalloid fluid replacement can no longer compensate for the loss, and transfusion of blood products becomes necessary. When blood products are transfused, watch for transfusion reactions and respond promptly according to hospital procedures.

Box 30–1 Nursing Actions During Postpartum Hemorrhage

- Call for help. Initiate response team as per hospital protocol.
- Massage uterus until firm.
- Administer prescribed medications.
- Ensure large-bore (14-, 16-, or 18-gauge) needle IV access (consider starting a second line).
- Replace volume with normal saline or lactated Ringer solution.
- Apply pulse oximeter and administer oxygen according to agency protocol.
- Insert a Foley catheter to empty the bladder and accurately measure output.
- Maintain accurate intake and output measurements.
- Assess blood loss; weigh peri-pads or Chux dressing for objective estimate of blood loss.
- Monitor pulse and blood pressure every 15 minutes or more often as indicated.
- Assess for shock.
- Elevate the legs to a 20- to 30-degree angle to increase venous return.
- Draw blood for CBC, type and cross-match, coagulation studies, and blood chemistry.
- Notify blood bank that transfusion may be necessary; administer blood products as ordered.
- Continuous electrocardiogram (ECG) monitoring may be indicated for hypotension, continuous bleeding, tachycardia, or shock.
- Prepare for additional interventions such as uterine tamponade, exploratory laparotomy, or uterine artery embolization.
- Anticipate pain management needs for fundal massage and uterotonic medications.
- Provide emotional support for the woman and her family.

Sources: Data from James, D. C. (2014). Postpartum care. In K. R. Simpson & P. A. Creehan (Eds.), *AWHONN's perinatal nursing* (4th ed., pp. 553–555); American College of Obstetrics & Gynecology. (2006). ACOG Practice Bulletin: Clinical management guidelines for obstetrician-gynecologists #76. *Obstetrics & Gynecology, 108*(4), 1039–1046.

Keeping the woman as comfortable as possible with perineal care and frequent changes of disposable pads is important, but her position cannot be allowed to compromise venous return or oxygenation. She will be kept NPO in case surgery is needed, so oral care is important for comfort. There are many interruptions when the patient is experiencing a complication, so you will need to seek opportunities to promote rest whenever possible. Any intervention to help with maternal–newborn bonding in the interval of separation is of great value to the woman—photographs or videotapes of the newborn, direct reports from the nursery staff, and brief visits to the room if her condition allows. Encourage the father to visit the newborn and bring information to the mother.

Clearly, the care of the woman experiencing postpartum hemorrhage depends on good nursing assessment and prompt reporting of nonreassuring findings to the healthcare provider. However, direct treatment methods require the collaboration of a healthcare provider and, in some cases, radiographic or surgical staff. You will become an important liaison between these departments, keeping the necessary individuals apprised of the woman's status. For example, if additional transfusions of whole blood or blood products are anticipated, you will need to keep the hospital laboratory informed to facilitate timely response. Care may well include the preprocedural preparation of the woman for surgery or for procedures such as arterial embolization performed by a radiologist.

After a postpartum hemorrhage, evaluate the woman for signs of anemia, such as fatigue, pallor, headache, thirst, and orthostatic changes in pulse or blood pressure (BP), and review the results of all hematocrit determinations. All medical interventions, IV infusions, blood transfusions, oxygen therapy, and medications such as uterine stimulants are monitored as necessary and evaluated for effectiveness. Urinary output should be monitored to determine adequacy of fluid replacement and renal perfusion, with amounts less than 30 mL/hr being reported to the healthcare provider (Sosa, 2014).

Help the woman plan activities so that adequate rest is possible. The woman who is experiencing anemia and fatigue related to hemorrhage may need assistance with self-care and progressive ambulation for several days. When she is able to be out of bed to shower, use of a shower chair permits independence while providing a measure of safety in case the woman experiences weakness or dizziness.

SAFETY ALERT!
The emergency call light should be easily accessible whenever nurses have left the bedside, even temporarily.

The mother may find it difficult to care for her baby because of the fatigue associated with blood loss. Try to find ways to promote maternal–newborn attachment while accommodating the mother's health needs. The mother may require additional assistance in caring for her baby. If she has intravenous lines in place, even carrying the newborn may be awkward. For the mother who feels compelled to do as much as possible, you may also need to give the mother "permission" to return her baby to the nursery so she can have adequate periods of uninterrupted rest.

If the father of the baby or the woman's partner is involved in the birth experience, including that person in the plan of care is a productive strategy. This person can support the mother's recovery by helping to meet her physical needs while encouraging her to rest. The mother is likely to feel less concern over her limited opportunities for the newborn's care if she can witness the father/partner interacting with and caring for the newborn. The extent to which the father/partner becomes involved with the care of the mother and baby must be carefully balanced with the need to be rested for the extra responsibilities the support person will assume when the mother and newborn child are discharged from the hospital.

SAFETY ALERT!
Good hand hygiene using standard precautions throughout the hospitalization and emphasizing proper hand hygiene for home care is important to minimize risk of postpartum infection.

COMMUNITY-BASED NURSING CARE

For most postpartum women, routine discharge instructions include advice such as, "You take care of the baby, and let someone else care for you, the family, and the household." Because of her fatigue and weakened condition, the woman who experienced postpartum hemorrhage may be unable even to care

Health Promotion **Preventing Postpartum Bleeding**
The woman and her family or other support persons should receive clear, preferably written, explanations of the normal postpartum course, including changes in the lochia and fundus and signs of abnormal bleeding. Instructions for the prevention of bleeding should include fundal massage, ways to assess the fundal height and consistency, and inspection of any episiotomy and lacerations, if present. The woman should receive instruction in perineal care (see discussion on perineal care in Chapter 29). The mother and her family are advised to contact her healthcare provider if any of the signs of postpartum hemorrhage occur (Table 30–1). If iron supplementation is ordered, instructions for proper dosage should be provided along with client teaching to enhance absorption and avoid constipation and nausea. The Western herb shepherd's purse can be used in tea or tincture form to help control postpartum bleeding. Yarrow is often used with shepherd's purse as a homeostatic agent. Cinnamon and cayenne have also been used. Always report bleeding to a healthcare provider.

for her newborn unassisted. The caregivers at home need clear, concise explanations of her condition and needs for recovery. For example, all should understand the woman's need to rest and to be given extra time to rest after any necessary activity. They should also be told that anemia is associated with postpartum depression so that they can be vigilant for and promptly report any change in the woman's affect (Albacar et al., 2011).

To ensure her safety, advise the woman to rise slowly to minimize the likelihood of orthostatic hypotension. Until she regains strength, she should be seated when holding the newborn.

The person who assumes responsibility for grocery shopping and meal preparation needs advice about the importance of including foods high in iron in the daily menus. Having the woman indicate her preferences from a list of such foods will promote cooperation with the diet. Also explain the rationale for continuing medications containing iron and remind the woman that vitamin C–containing fluids maximize absorption of iron, and tea or milk products prevent absorption (Albacar et al., 2011).

The woman should continue to count perineal pads for several days so that she can recognize any recurring problems with excessive blood loss (hypovolemia). The debilitated condition and anemia associated with hemorrhage increase the woman's

---

TABLE 30–1 Signs of Postpartum Hemorrhage

- Excessive or bright-red bleeding (saturation of more than one pad per hour)
- A boggy fundus that does not respond to massage
- Abnormal clots
- High temperature
- Any unusual pelvic discomfort or backache
- Persistent bleeding in the presence of a firmly contracted uterus
- Rise in the level of the fundus of the uterus
- Increased pulse or decreased BP
- Hematoma formation or bulging/shiny skin in the perineal area
- Decreased level of consciousness

Clinical Reasoning Postpartum Hemorrhage

Betsy Lambert is a primigravida who had a spontaneous vaginal delivery at 09:41 today. An overview of her history reveals the following: 23 years old, married, G1P0 on admission to Labor Unit. Pregnancy normal. Rh positive. No drug allergies. Labs on admission to L&D normal with exception of hemoglobin 11 g and hematocrit 32%. Labor: 13 hours. Estimated blood loss: 450 mL. Delivered female (7 lb 7 oz) spontaneously after epidural anesthesia. Apgar 9/10. Newborn examination was within normal limits and routine newborn orders were implemented. Day shift reports firm fundus; voided 210 mL around 1100; vital signs stable. Baby visited and breastfed briefly with help from lactation nurse. Ate lunch and had Tylenol #3 at 1300 for perineal pain. Has been sleeping for long intervals.

You find Mrs. Lambert still dozing but awaken her for examination and note the following: BP 112/60, HR 116, R 20, T 100. Breasts—soft, nontender, wearing support bra. Uterus—fundus firm and 2 cm below umbilicus slightly left of midline. Bladder—possibly slightly distended but she feels no urge to void. Lochia—the two perineal pads and blue absorbent underpads are covered with bright red blood. Perineum—covered with blood, as are thighs. Some of the blood has dried on the skin. Slight edema noted—midline episiotomy intact. Ice pack in place but ice melted. Homans sign—negative. Emotional status—reports her husband went home to rest and will be back at dinnertime. Talks with excitement about first attempt to nurse baby. Asks for something cold to drink. The patient cannot remember when she was last checked for bleeding. You don gloves and wash her perineum gently and her thighs and change all her pads so you can better assess her degree of bleeding. An IV is in place with 10 units of oxytocin (Pitocin) (100 mL is left in the IV bag).

You return, as promised, in 15 minutes to reevaluate her lochia and find that her perineal pads are again covered in blood. Based on your assessments and Mrs. Lambert's laboratory findings, what actions will you take first? If one of your anticipated actions is to inform the healthcare provider, what specific information will you report and what management should you anticipate initially? What follow-up care will you anticipate performing during the remainder of your shift?

risk of puerperal infection. She and her caregivers should use good hand hygiene technique and minimize exposure to infection in the home. Give the woman's caregivers a list of the signs of infection and ensure that they understand the importance of alerting the healthcare provider immediately if signs occur.

In addition to meeting the woman's physical needs, you will need to assess the couple's coping strategies and resources for dealing with the impending crisis. Providing realistic information, offering to call those in their support network, and exploring effective coping strategies can be of immeasurable value as the couple tries to maintain a sense of balance in this difficult situation. A sense of emergency often accompanies late postpartum hemorrhage. Because it commonly occurs 1 to 2 weeks after birth, the couple is generally at home, involved in the day-to-day activities demanded by their new roles, when the unexpected, excessive bleeding begins. Quick decisions about childcare arrangements must often be made so that the

mother can return to the hospital. Both mother and father are likely to be alarmed by the excessive bleeding and concerned about her prognosis. There may be additional worries about separation from the newborn, especially when the mother is breastfeeding. The father may find himself torn between the needs of the mother and those of the newborn. Ideally, arrangements can be made to minimize separation of the family members.

Evaluation

Expected outcomes of nursing care include the following:

- Signs of postpartum hemorrhage are detected quickly and managed effectively.
- Maternal–newborn attachment is maintained successfully.
- The woman is able to identify abnormal changes that might occur following discharge and understands the importance of notifying her caregiver if they develop.

Care of the Woman With a Reproductive Tract Infection or Wound Infection

Puerperal infection is an infection of the reproductive tract associated with childbirth that occurs any time up to 6 weeks postpartum. The most common postpartum infection is endometritis (metritis), which is infection limited to the uterine lining. Indeed, the cause of postpartum fever is presumed to be metritis until proven otherwise. However, infection can spread by way of the lymphatic and circulatory systems to become a progressive disease resulting in parametrial cellulitis and **peritonitis** (infection involving the peritoneal cavity). Other causes of postpartum fever should be considered: respiratory complications such as atelectasis or pneumonia, acute pyelonephritis, thrombophlebitis, or breast engorgement, which rarely lasts more than 24 hours (Duff, 2014).

Maternal death from sepsis is increasing in countries with an advanced healthcare system (Acosta et al., 2014).Although the death rate from postpartum infection is low in the United States, infection accounts for 11% of pregnancy-related deaths. Uterine infections are relatively uncommon following uncomplicated vaginal births, but they continue to be a major source of morbidity for women who give birth by cesarean section. Routine antibiotic prophylaxis for cesarean childbirth in conjunction with aseptic technique, fewer traumatic operative births, a better understanding of labor dystocia, improved surgical intervention, and a population that is generally at less risk from malnutrition and chronic debilitative disease have contributed to a reduction in overall postpartum morbidity and mortality

The standard definition of **puerperal morbidity**, established by the Joint Committee on Maternal Welfare, is *a temperature of 38°C (100.4°F) or higher, with the temperature occurring on any 2 of the first 10 postpartum days, exclusive of the first 24 hours, and when taken by mouth by standard technique at least four times a day.* During today's short obstetric hospital stays, the temperature is measured every 6 hours in most settings, consistent with the definition for puerperal morbidity. However, serious infections can occur in the first 24 hours or may cause only persistent low-grade temperatures. Therefore, careful assessment of all postpartum women with elevated temperatures is essential.

The vagina and cervix of approximately 70% of all healthy pregnant women contain pathogenic bacteria that, alone or in combination, are sufficiently virulent to cause excessive infection. Although the uterus is considered a sterile cavity before rupture of the fetal membranes, bacterial contamination of amniotic fluid with membranes still intact at term is more common than previously believed and may contribute to premature labor.

Following rupture of membranes and during labor, contamination of the uterine cavity by vaginal or cervical bacteria can easily occur. Other factors must also be present for infection to occur such as the change to an alkaline pH of the vagina postpartum that favors growth of aerobes.

Because shortened inpatient stays are the norm in maternity care, women will likely be discharged following childbirth before clinical signs of puerperal infection are evident. According to Bianco, Roccia, Pileggi, et al. (2013), 84% of postpartum infections manifest after hospital discharge. Consequently, perinatal nurses are challenged to analyze the woman's history and clinical course for risk assessment and to recognize the early subtle signs of infection so that discharge may be delayed as needed. Before discharge, the nurse advises the woman about preventive measures, including scrupulous hand hygiene, and signs of infection. Nurses should educate the client and her family about the risk of infection and how to recognize and respond appropriately should it occur.

Postpartum Endometritis

Postpartum endometritis (metritis), an inflammation of the endometrium portion of the uterine lining occurring any time up to 6 weeks postpartum, may occur in 30% to 35% of those who give birth by cesarean after an extended period of labor and ruptured membranes (Duff, 2014).

Postpartum infection from vaginal delivery primarily affects the placental implantation site, the decidua, and adjacent myometrium. Bacteria that colonize the cervix and vagina gain access to the amniotic fluid during labor and postpartum and begin to invade devitalized tissue (the lower uterine segment, lacerations, and incisions). The same pathogenesis, polymicrobial proliferation and tissue invasion, is associated with cesarean delivery, but surgical trauma, additional devitalization of tissue, blood and serum accumulation, and foreign bodies (sutures, staples) provide additional favorable anaerobic bacterial conditions. For highly indigent populations, the risk remains high (Poggi, 2013). See Table 30–2 for a list of common causative organisms.

TABLE 30–2 Common Causative Organisms in Metritis

AEROBES	ANAEROBES
• Group A, B, D streptococci	• *Peptostreptococcus*
• *Enterococcus*	• *Clostridium* species
• *Staphylococcus* species	• *Bacteroides* species
• *Escherichia coli*	• *Chlamydia trachomatis*
• *Klebsiella pneumonia*	• Genital mycoplasma
• *Proteus mirabilis*	
• *Gardnerella vaginalis*	
• *Neisseria gonorrhoeae*	

Sources: Data from Duff, P. (2014). Maternal and fetal infectious disorders. In R. K. Creasy & R. Resnik (Eds.), *Maternal–fetal medicine: Principles and practice* (7th ed., pp. 823–851). Philadelphia, PA: Saunders; Poggi, S. B. H. (2013). Postpartum hemorrhage & the abnormal puerperium. In A. H. DeCherney, L. Nathan, & A. S. Roman (Eds.), *Current diagnosis & treatment: Obstetrics & gynecology* (11th ed., pp. 349–368). New York, NY: McGraw-Hill.

Clinical findings of metritis in the initial 24 to 36 hours postpartum tend to be related to group B streptococcus (GBS). Late-onset postpartum endometritis/metritis is most commonly associated with genital mycoplasmas and *Chlamydia trachomatis* (Duff, 2014).

Risk factors for postpartum uterine infection include the following:

- Cesarean birth is the single most significant risk, especially when it occurs after an extended labor with ruptured membranes. The incidence of infection can be as high as 35% without antibiotic prophylaxis and 10% or less with prophylactic coverage (Duff, 2014).
- Prolonged premature rupture of the amniotic membranes (PPROM).
- Prolonged labor preceding cesarean birth.
- Multiple vaginal examinations during labor.
- Compromised health status (low socioeconomic status, anemia, obesity, smoking, use of illicit drugs or alcohol, poor nutritional state).
- Use of fetal scalp electrode or intrauterine pressure catheter for internal monitoring during labor.
- Obstetric trauma—episiotomy, laceration of perineum, vagina, or cervix.
- Chorioamnionitis—infection of placenta, chorion, and amnion.
- Preexisting bacterial vaginosis or *Chlamydia trachomatis* infection.
- Instrument-assisted childbirth—vacuum or forceps.
- Manual removal of the placenta or uterine exploration after delivery.
- Retained placental fragments.
- Lapses in aseptic technique by surgical staff.
- Diabetes mellitus.
- Immunocompromised status.

Assessment findings consistent with endometritis are foul-smelling lochia, fever (usually between 38.3°C [101.0°F] and 40°C [104°F]), uterine tenderness on palpation, lower abdominal pain, tachycardia, and chills (James, 2014).

Prophylactic antibiotics during cesarean section decreases the incidence of endometritis by as much as 60%, particularly after prolonged labor or ruptured membranes. Traditionally, antibiotics are given to the mother during surgery after the umbilical cord is cut, thus avoiding difficulties in evaluating the baby for sepsis should the baby develop symptoms of infection. More recent evidence supports the administration of antibiotics 30 to 60 minutes prior to surgery, with no increase in neonatal infection (Duff, 2014).

Pelvic Cellulitis (Parametritis)

Pelvic cellulitis (parametritis) is infection involving the connective tissue of the broad ligament or, in more severe forms, the connective tissue of all the pelvic structures. The infection generally ascends upward in the pelvis by way of the lymphatics in the uterine wall, but may also occur if pathogenic organisms invade a cervical laceration that extends upward into the connective tissue of the broad ligament—a direct pathway into the pelvis. Infection involving the peritoneal cavity is peritonitis. A pelvic abscess is most commonly found as a palpable mass in the uterine ligaments, the cul-de-sac of Douglas, and the subdiaphragmatic space. Parametritis may be a secondary result of pelvic vein thrombophlebitis. This condition occurs when the clot, usually in the right ovarian vein, becomes infected and the wall of the vein breaks down from necrosis, spilling the infection into the connective tissues of the pelvis.

A woman suffering from parametritis may demonstrate a variety of symptoms, including marked high temperature (38.9° to 40°C [102° to 104°F]), chills, malaise, lethargy, abdominal pain, subinvolution of the uterus, tachycardia, and local and referred rebound tenderness (Poggi, 2013). If peritonitis develops, the woman becomes acutely ill, with severe pain, marked anxiety, high fever, rapid and shallow respirations, pronounced tachycardia, excessive thirst, abdominal distention, nausea, and vomiting.

Perineal Wound Infections

Given the degree of bacterial contamination that occurs with normal vaginal birth, it is surprising that more women do not have infections of the episiotomy or repaired lacerations of the perineum, vagina, or vulva. Good aseptic technique is the likely rationale. When perineal wound infection occurs, it is recognized by the classic signs: redness, warmth, edema, purulent drainage, and, later, gaping of the wound that had previously been well approximated. Local pain may be severe.

Cesarean Wound Infections

After cesarean delivery, wound infection is most often associated with concurrent endometritis. The wound is typically red, indurated, tender at the margins, and draining purulent exudate. Some women have cellulitis without actual purulent drainage. Clinical examination is usually sufficient for diagnosis, but culture of the exudate should be routinely done since community-acquired methicillin-resistant *Staphylococcus aureus* (CA-MRSA) infections are possible (Cunningham et al., 2014).

Clinical Therapy

The infection site and causative organism are diagnosed by careful history and complete physical examination, blood tests, aerobic and anaerobic endometrial cultures (although cultures may be of limited value because multiple organisms are usually present), and urinalysis to rule out urinary tract infection (UTI).

Localized wound infection is treated with broad-spectrum antibiotics, sitz baths, and analgesics as necessary for pain relief. Wounds with evidence of pus or serosanguineous effusion or an infected stitch site are opened and drained completely. Once the incision and drainage (I&D) of the wound is complete, it should be irrigated with warm saline 2 to 3 times daily and a clean dressing should be applied. It is then allowed to heal by secondary intention (Duff, 2014). Alternatively, it may be packed with saline dampened gauze and repacked 2 to 3 times daily and covered with clean gauze using aseptic technique. This allows removal of necrotic debris when packing is removed. Antibiotics with coverage against *Staphyloccus aureus* should be given. Antibiotics are typically continued until the wound base is clean and any signs of cellulitis have resolved.

Endometritis is treated with intravenous antibiotics, such as cephalosporins or penicillins. Women generally improve within 2 days of initiating antibiotics, which are continued until the patient has been afebrile and asymptomatic for 24 hours. If fever continues at 48 hours after antibiotic therapy, an additional workup is necessary to check for refractory pelvic infection.

Parametritis and peritonitis are treated with aggressive IV therapy. Broad-spectrum antibiotics effective against the most common causative organisms are chosen initially until the results of culture and sensitivity reports are available. If multiple organisms are present, the approach to antibiotic therapy is continued unless no improvement is observed; then the antibiotic is changed. With appropriate antibiotic coverage, improvement should occur within a few days. Antibiotics are generally continued until the woman is afebrile and asymptomatic for 24 hours (Duff, 2014).

Approximately 90% to 95% of women with postpartum infection respond quickly to antibiotic therapy or drainage of abscesses and are associated with complete recovery and no long-term sequelae (Duff, 2014).

Nursing Management

For the Postpartum Woman With Puerperal Infection

Nursing Assessment and Diagnosis

Inspect the woman's perineum every 8 to 12 hours for signs of early infection. The REEDA scale helps in remembering to consider *r*edness, *e*dema, *e*cchymosis, *d*ischarge, and *a*pproximation. Immediately report any degree of induration (hardening) to the clinician.

Note and report the presence of fever, malaise, abdominal pain, foul-smelling lochia, larger than expected uterus, tachycardia, and other signs of infection so that treatment can begin. The white blood cell (WBC) count, a usual objective measure of infection, cannot be used reliably because of the normal increase in WBCs during the postpartum period; a WBC count of 14,000 to 16,000 mm^3 is not an unusual finding. However, an increase in WBC level of more than 30% in a 6-hour period is indicative of infection.

Nursing diagnoses that may apply to the woman with a puerperal infection include the following (NANDA-I © 2014):

- *Injury, Risk for*, related to the spread of infection
- *Pain* related to the presence of infection
- *Parenting, Risk for Impaired*, related to delayed parent–newborn attachment secondary to malaise and other symptoms of infection

Planning and Implementation

HOSPITAL-BASED NURSING CARE

Careful attention to standard precautions and aseptic techniques during labor, birth, and postpartum is essential. As the nurse caring for a woman during the postpartum period, you are responsible for teaching her self-care measures that are helpful in preventing infection. If the woman has a draining wound or purulent lochia, it is especially important that those in contact with soiled items and linens practice good hand hygiene. Provide clear, concise instructions about wound care and how to discard soiled dressings appropriately to safeguard the woman and her caregivers.

If the woman is seriously ill, ongoing assessment of urine-specific gravity, as well as intake and output, is necessary. It is also necessary to carefully administer antibiotics as ordered and regulate the intravenous fluid rate. Ongoing assessment of the woman's condition is vital to detect subtle changes in her health status. Address the woman's comfort needs related to hygiene, positioning, oral hygiene, and pain relief.

Promoting maternal–newborn attachment can be difficult with the acutely ill woman. You can provide pictures of the baby and keep the mother informed of the baby's well-being. Mementos, such as a footprint, a note written by the father "from the baby," or a videotape of the baby can be comforting to the mother during their separation. If she feels up to it, the new mother will also benefit from brief visits with her newborn.

Generally, breastfeeding is not contraindicated with postpartum infections. However, if the mother is seriously ill and is unable to nurse the baby, lactation should be supported with frequent pumping as tolerated. The partner of a seriously ill woman will be concerned about her condition and torn about spending time with her or with their newborn. Because maternal–newborn bonding may be compromised, father–newborn bonding can be especially important. See *Nursing Care Plan: The Woman With a Puerperal Perineal Wound Infection* for specific nursing care measures.

Nursing Care Plan: The Woman With a Puerperal Perineal Wound Infection

1. Nursing Diagnosis: *Infection, Risk for,* related to traumatized tissues (NANDA-I © 2014)

GOAL: The woman will be free of complications associated with infection.

INTERVENTION	RATIONALE
• Encourage the woman, staff, and family members to adhere to a strict hand hygiene policy.	• Hand hygiene kills bacteria and prevents cross-contamination.
• Review the woman's prenatal, intrapartum, and postpartum records for underlying problems that could contribute to poor wound healing or increased risk for spread of infection.	• Identifying underlying problems gives the caregiver an opportunity to initiate preventive measures that will promote healthy wound healing and stop the spread of infection.
• Monitor blood pressure, pulse, respiration, and temperature.	• Obtain baseline data; signs and symptoms of septic shock produce a decrease in blood pressure and an increase in respirations. Temperature increase of 38.0°C (100.4°F) or greater on any 2 days after the first 24 hr indicates infection.
• Instruct the woman on proper perineal care including wiping perineum from front to back after voiding, washing the perineum after voiding and defecating, and changing peri-pads frequently.	• Proper perineal care techniques enhance good hygiene and assist in removing urine and fecal contaminants from perineum. Changing peri-pads frequently decreases skin contact with a moist medium that favors bacterial growth.
• Encourage a well-balanced diet with adequate protein, calories, and vitamin C.	• Protein and vitamin C are essential nutrients for tissue healing and repair.
• Continue prenatal vitamins and iron as ordered	
• Encourage the woman to consume 2000 mL of fluid a day.	• Maintains hydration and increases circulating volume. Dilutes organisms that are eliminated with voiding.
• Encourage use of the sitz bath, Surgigator, or the perineal light 2 to 4 times a day for at least 10–15 min.	• Moist or dry heat to the perineum increases localized blood flow, promotes healing, and provides comfort.
• Encourage early ambulation.	• Enhances circulation and drainage of lochia.
• Assess and report signs and symptoms of infection in perineum including redness, erythema, edema, discharge, approximation of wound edges (REEDA), and pain.	• Identifying signs and symptoms of infection early allows for prompt treatment and healing.
• **Collaborative:** Obtain lab work as ordered by the healthcare provider including culture and sensitivity, complete blood count (CBC) with differential, and white blood cell (WBC) count.	• Identifies abnormal lab values for early intervention. In addition, identifies infection and its causative organism for appropriate antibiotic treatment.
• Administer antibiotic therapy as ordered by the healthcare provider.	• Fights infection and helps prevent ascension of organisms into further tissue.
• Promote wound drainage by assisting healthcare provider in opening the wound if necessary. Also, if the wound is greater than 2–3 cm (0.8–1.2 in.), pack with iodoform gauze.	• Iodoform gauze is used to maintain patency of wound opening. This promotes drainage and prevents abscesses from developing.
• Report signs and symptoms of severe infections: foul-smelling lochia, uterine subinvolution, uterine tenderness, severe lower abdominal pain, elevated temperature, elevated WBC count, general malaise, chills, lethargy, tachycardia, nausea and vomiting, and abdominal rigidity.	• Reporting signs and symptoms of severe infections early allows for initiation of appropriate therapy by the healthcare provider and prevents further spread of the invading pathogen.

EXPECTED OUTCOME: The woman will be free of complications associated with infection as evidenced by practicing behaviors that prevent the spread of infection and promote timely wound healing.

2. Nursing Diagnosis: *Pain, Acute,* related to the infection process (NANDA-I © 2014)

GOAL: The woman will be free of pain or have a level of relief that is acceptable.

INTERVENTION	RATIONALE
• Assess pain location and intensity; have the woman describe on a scale from 1 (mild) to 10 (severe). Assess nonverbal signs of pain, including facial grimacing and agitation.	• Assesses the need for pain management and evaluates interventions already implemented.
• Encourage the woman to discuss anxiety and fears.	• Reduces anxiety/fear and may decrease the woman's perception of pain.
• Encourage frequent rest periods and decrease disturbing environmental stimuli.	• Frequent rest periods will conserve woman's energy. Excessive environmental stimuli may increase woman's pain perception.
• Promote relaxation by encouraging diversionary activities including radio/television, reading, guided imagery, deep breathing techniques, massage, visualization, and meditation.	• Promotes relaxation and refocuses woman's attention away from the intensity of pain.
• **Collaborative:** Administer analgesics as ordered by the healthcare provider, evaluating the response to the analgesic and any adverse effects in a timely manner.	• Relieves pain and interrupts the pain, fear, tension cycle to facilitate relaxation.

EXPECTED OUTCOME: Woman is free of pain or has an acceptable level of pain as evidenced by verbalization of pain relief and the exhibition of a relaxed demeanor.

---

3. Nursing Diagnosis: *Parenting, Risk for Impaired,* related to pain secondary to maternal infection and/or separation from newborn to minimize exposure (NANDA-I © 2014)

GOAL: Mother will have no problems bonding with newborn and assuming responsibility for the care of the baby with assistance and later independently.

INTERVENTION	RATIONALE
• Provide quality time for mother and baby contact.	• Aids in the bonding process.
• Encourage the partner or family members to give the woman videos and pictures of the baby if the mother's condition requires separation from the baby.	• Promotes bonding and gives the mother reassurance that the baby is being cared for.
• Encourage the partner and family members to become involved with the care of the newborn and verbalize interaction to the mother.	• Allows the mother to feel as though she is involved in the care of the baby.
• Encourage the mother to feed (breast or bottle) baby if her condition is stable. If the mother is unable to breastfeed, encourage and assist her in pumping her breasts to maintain milk production.	• Hands-on participation in the baby's care gives mother a positive outlook.
• Assess maternal support systems.	• As the mother is recovering, she will need assistance in household organization and personal care.
• **Collaborative:** Offer referrals to home health services, doula services, lactation services, and/or support groups.	• Ensures the woman's well-being and identifies problems that may require intervention.

EXPECTED OUTCOME: Mother will bond with the newborn as evidenced by exhibiting appropriate attachment behaviors when interacting with baby, providing care to self and baby, and verbalization of understanding of the parenting role.

Community-Based Nursing Care

The woman with a puerperal infection needs assistance when she is discharged from the hospital. If the family cannot provide this home assistance, a referral to home care services is needed. Home care services should be contacted as soon as puerperal infection is diagnosed so that a nurse can meet with the woman for a family and home assessment and development of a home care plan.

Instruct the family in the care of a newborn, including feeding, bathing, cord care, immunizations, and significant observations that should be reported. A well-baby appointment should be scheduled. The woman who wishes to breast-feed when her condition allows can maintain lactation by pumping her breasts regularly. Instruct the breastfeeding mother receiving antibiotics to inspect the baby's mouth for signs of thrush and to report the finding to the healthcare provider.

Instruct the mother regarding activity, rest, medications, diet, and signs and symptoms of complications. She should also be scheduled for a return medical visit. She needs to know the importance of taking the entire course of prescribed antibiotics even though she may begin to feel better before the bottle is empty. She also needs to be informed about the importance of pelvic rest; that is, she should not use tampons or douches nor have intercourse until she has been examined by the healthcare provider and told it is safe to resume those activities.

Evaluation

Expected outcomes of nursing care include the following:

- The infection is quickly identified and treated successfully, without further complications.
- The woman understands the infection and the purpose of therapy; she cooperates with ongoing antibiotic therapy after discharge.
- Maternal–newborn attachment is maintained.

Care of the Woman With a Urinary Tract Infection

The postpartum woman is at increased risk of developing a urinary tract infection (UTI) caused by normal postpartum diuresis, increased bladder capacity, decreased bladder sensitivity from stretching or trauma, and possible inhibited neural control of the bladder following the use of general or regional anesthesia and contamination from catheterization. The number of catheterizations performed during labor has increased. It is essential that the mother empty the bladder completely with each voiding.

Overdistention of the Bladder

Overdistention occurs postpartum when the woman is unable to empty her bladder, usually because of trauma or the effects of anesthesia. Women who have not sufficiently recovered from the effects of anesthesia cannot void spontaneously, and catheterization is necessary. After the effects of regional anesthesia have worn off, if the woman cannot void, post-partum urinary retention is highly indicative of UTI (Poggi, 2013). Other risk factors for urinary retention after childbirth include nulliparity, instrumental childbirth, and prolonged labor (Pessel & Tsai, 2013).

CLINICAL THERAPY

Overdistention in the early postpartum period is often managed by draining the bladder with a straight catheter as a one-time measure. If the overdistention recurs or is diagnosed later in the postpartum period, an indwelling catheter is generally ordered for 24 hours. An alternative urinary retention protocol involves bladder ultrasound scans with intervention based on the amount of urine volume.

Nursing Management

For the Postpartum Woman With a Urinary Tract Infection

Nursing Assessment and Diagnosis

The overdistended bladder appears as a large mass, reaching sometimes to the umbilicus and displacing the uterine fundus upward. Increased vaginal bleeding occurs, the fundus is boggy, and the woman may complain of cramping as the uterus attempts to contract. Some women also experience backache and restlessness.

Nursing diagnoses that may apply when a woman has difficulties with overdistention of the bladder include the following (NANDA-I © 2014):

- *Infection, Risk for*, related to urinary stasis secondary to overdistention
- *Urinary Retention* related to decreased bladder sensitivity and normal postpartum diuresis

Planning and Implementation

Diligent monitoring of the bladder during the recovery period and preventive health measures greatly reduce the chances for overdistention of the bladder. Encourage the mother to void spontaneously and help her use the toilet, if possible, or the bedpan, if she has received conductive anesthesia. This will help prevent overdistention in most cases. Help the woman to a normal position for voiding (i.e., sitting with the legs and feet lower than the trunk) and provide privacy to encourage voiding. The woman should receive medication for whatever pain she may be having before she attempts to void because pain may cause a reflex spasm of the urethra. Applying perineal ice packs after childbirth helps minimize edema, which may interfere with voiding. Pouring warm water over the perineum or having the woman void in the sitz bath may also be effective. Some women note that hearing running water nearby, blowing bubbles through a straw into a glass of water, or voiding onto a bedpan into which a few drops of tincture of peppermint have been added helps stimulate voiding.

If catheterization becomes necessary, careful, meticulous aseptic technique is employed during catheter insertion. The vagina and vulva are traumatized to some degree by vaginal birth, and edema is common. This edema may obscure the urinary meatus; therefore, be extremely careful when cleansing the vulva and inserting the catheter. It is imperative to discard a catheter that has inadvertently been introduced into the vagina and thus contaminated. Catheterization is an uncomfortable procedure because of the postpartum trauma and edema of the tissue, so be careful and gentle not only when inserting the catheter but also when handling and cleaning the perineal area.

If the amount of urine drained from the bladder reaches 800 mL, the catheter is clamped and taped firmly to the woman's leg. Take the woman's vital signs before and after the procedure and note the woman's responses. After an hour, the catheter may be unclamped and placed on gravity drainage. This technique protects the bladder and prevents rapid intra-abdominal decompression (James, 2014). When the indwelling catheter is removed, a urine specimen is often sent to the laboratory. The tip of the catheter is also removed and may be sent for culture.

Evaluation

Expected outcomes of nursing care include the following:

- The woman voids adequately to meet the demands of the increased fluid shifts during the postpartum period.
- The woman does not develop infection caused by stasis of urine.
- The woman actively incorporates self-care measures to decrease bladder overdistention.

Cystitis (Lower Urinary Tract Infection)

Retention of residual urine, bacteria introduced at the time of catheterization, and a bladder traumatized by birth combine to provide an excellent environment for the development of cystitis. *Escherichia coli* has been demonstrated to be the causative agent in most cases of postpartum cystitis and pyelonephritis (in both lower and upper UTI). *Klebsiella pneumoniae* and *Proteus* species are significant pathogens, especially in women with histories of recurrent UTIs (Poggi, 2013). Generally, the infection ascends the urinary tract from the urethra to the bladder and then to the kidneys because vesicoureteral reflux (backward flow of urine) forces contaminated urine into the renal pelvis.

CLINICAL THERAPY

When cystitis is suspected, a clean-catch midstream urine sample is obtained for microscopic examination, culture, and sensitivity tests. The specimen may require collection by the nurse with the woman on a bedpan because few postpartum women can collect a true midstream, clean-catch specimen without contaminating the specimen with lochia. A catheterized specimen is avoided when possible because of the increased risk of infection. When the bacterial concentration is greater than 100,000 colonies of the same organism per milliliter of fresh urine, infection is generally present. Counts between 10,000 and 100,000 suggest infection, particularly if clinical symptoms are noted.

In the clinical setting, antibiotic therapy is often initiated before culture and sensitivity reports are available. Frequently used antibiotics include a preparation of trimethoprim-sulfamethoxazole double strength (Bactrim DS, Septra DS), one of the short-acting sulfonamides, nitrofurantoin (Macrodantin), and in the case of sulfa allergy, ampicillin or amoxicillin–clavulanic acid (Augmentin). The antibiotic is changed later if indicated by the results of the sensitivity report. Antispasmodics or urinary analgesic agents, such as phenazopyridine hydrochloride (Pyridium), may be given to relieve discomfort.

Nursing Management
For the Postpartum Woman With Cystitis

Nursing Assessment and Diagnosis

Encourage women to void every 2 to 4 hours to prevent urinary stasis and to report any sensations of incomplete emptying of the bladder or dysuria. Symptoms of cystitis often appear 2 to 3 days after childbirth and may include frequency, urgency, dysuria, and nocturia. Gross hematuria may be noted but high fever and systemic symptoms are not expected.

When a UTI progresses to pyelonephritis, systemic symptoms usually occur, and the woman becomes acutely ill. Symptoms include chills, high fever, flank pain (unilateral or bilateral), nausea, and vomiting, in addition to the signs of lower UTI. Costovertebral angle tenderness on palpation may be noted on exam but is not required for diagnosis. Clean-catch urine specimens show large numbers of white blood cells and are positive for infection (bacterial growth more than 100,000 colony forming/mL of urine) (James, 2014).

Nursing diagnoses that may apply if a woman develops postpartum cystitis include the following (NANDA-I © 2014):

- *Pain, Acute*, with voiding related to dysuria secondary to infection
- *Health Management, Ineffective*, related to need for information about self-care measures to prevent UTI

Planning and Implementation

Screening for asymptomatic bacteriuria in pregnancy should be routine. Encourage frequent emptying of the bladder during labor and postpartum to prevent overdistention and trauma to the bladder. Catheterization technique and nursing actions to prevent overdistention (previously discussed) also apply. The woman with pyelonephritis must understand the importance of follow-up care after discharge to prevent recurrence or further complications.

Health Promotion Avoiding Postpartum UTIs

Advise the postpartum woman to continue good perineal hygiene after discharge. Also advise the woman to maintain a good fluid intake (at least eight to ten 8-oz glasses daily), especially of water, and to empty her bladder whenever she feels the urge to void, but at least every 2 to 4 hours while awake. Once sexual intercourse is resumed, the new mother should void before (to prevent bladder trauma) and following intercourse (to wash contaminants from the vicinity of the urinary meatus). Wearing underwear with a cotton crotch to facilitate air circulation also reduces the risk of UTI. Acidification of the urine is thought to aid in preventing and managing UTI. Therefore, advise the woman to avoid carbonated beverages, coffee, citrus fruits, tomatoes, and chocolate, which increase the alkalinity of urine, and to drink low-sugar juices such as cranberry, plum, apricot, and prune and take vitamin C, which increase the acidity of urine (Zaccardi, 2013).

Evaluation

Expected outcomes of nursing care include the following:

- The woman identifies the signs of UTI and her condition is treated successfully.
- The woman incorporates self-care measures to prevent the recurrence of UTI as part of her personal hygiene routine.
- The woman cooperates with any long-term therapy or follow-up.
- Maternal–newborn attachment is maintained and the woman is able to care for her newborn effectively.

Care of the Woman With Mastitis

Mastitis is an infection of the interlobular connective tissue in the breast that occurs primarily in lactating women. (Chapter 29 discusses the breastfeeding difficulties of the woman with mastitis.) Onset is usually between 2 and 8 weeks postpartum or any other time that nursing frequency decreases. It ranges in severity from local inflammation to abscess and septicemia. The incidence of mastitis is estimated to be as high as 33% in breastfeeding mothers and less than 1% in nonlactating mothers (Jahanfar, Ng, & Teng, 2013).

The usual causative organisms are *Staphylococcus aureus, Haemophilus parainfluenzae, H. influenzae, Escherichia coli,* and *Streptococcus* species (Poggi, 2013). Infectious mastitis is a very serious infection, with fever, chills, headache, flulike muscle aches and malaise, and a warm, reddened, painful area of the breast, often wedge shaped because of the connective tissue septal divisions of the breast (James, 2014) (Figure 30–2).

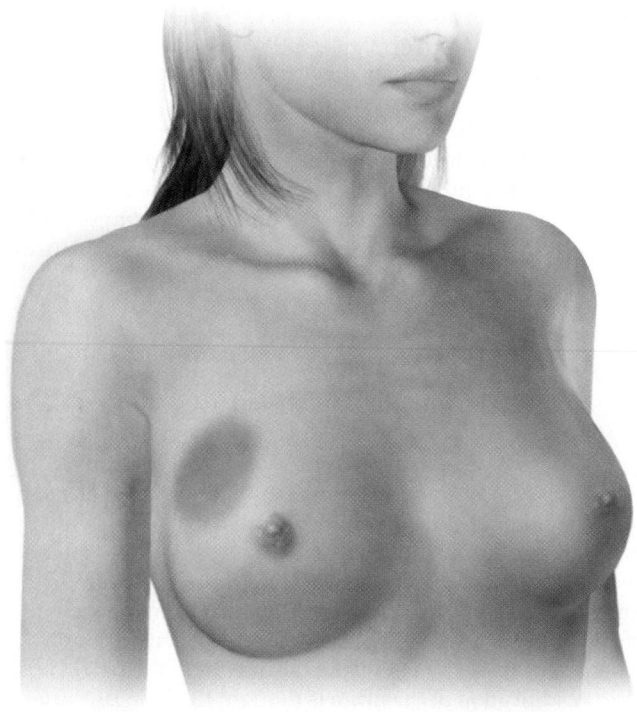

Figure 30–2 Mastitis. Erythema and swelling are present in the upper outer quadrant of the breast. Axillary lymph nodes are often enlarged and tender. The segmental anatomy of the breast accounts for the demarcated, often V-shaped wedge of inflammation.

The infection usually begins when bacteria invade the breast tissue after it has been traumatized in some way (see the factors commonly associated with mastitis in Table 30–3). Milk serves as a favorable medium for the invasive bacteria; thus, milk stasis is another risk factor. The most common sources of pathogenic organisms are the baby's nose and throat, although other sources include the hands of the mother or birthing unit personnel and the woman's circulating blood. Babies of women with mastitis generally remain well unless the causative organism is Candida albicans.

When *Candida albicans* is the causative organism of mastitis, entering the breast through a small fissure or abrasion on the nipple, the baby will often have thrush, a candidal infection of the mouth. There may be a history of a recent course of antibiotics in the woman. Signs include late-onset nipple pain and burning pain of the nipple/areola, followed by stabbing pain of the breast during and between feedings (Lawrence & Lawrence, 2014). Eventually, the skin of the affected breast becomes pink, shiny, flaking, and pruritic. Women may notice a yeasty odor to their milk. Unless the mother and her newborn are treated for *Candida*, recolonization will occur when breastfeeding is resumed.

TABLE 30–3 Factors Associated With Development of Mastitis

MILK STASIS
Failure to change the baby's position to allow emptying all lobes
Failure to alternate breasts at feedings
Poor suck
Poor let-down
ACTIONS THAT PROMOTE ACCESS/MULTIPLICATION OF BACTERIA
Poor hand hygiene technique
Improper breast hygiene
Failure to air dry breasts after breastfeeding
Use of plastic-lined breast pads that trap moisture against nipple
BREAST/NIPPLE TRAUMA
Incorrect positioning for breastfeeding
Poor latch-on
Failure to rotate position on nipple
Incorrect or aggressive pumping technique
Cracked nipples
OBSTRUCTION OF DUCTS
Restrictive clothing
Constricting bra
Underwire bra
CHANGE IN NUMBER OF FEEDINGS/FAILURE TO EMPTY BREASTS
Attempted weaning
Missed feeding
Prolonged sleeping, including sleeping through night
Favoring side of nipple soreness
LOWERED MATERNAL DEFENSES
Fatigue
Stress

Clinical Therapy

The diagnosis of mastitis is usually made based on clinical signs and symptoms. Culture and sensitivity of the breast milk may be done in some cases where the patient does not respond to antibiotics or has a severe, unusual, or recurring case of mastitis (Wambach, 2016). If a culture of the breast milk is ordered, it is more reliable with a midstream-type collection process. The nipple is washed first; then the first 3 mL of breast milk is manually expressed and discarded, after which the actual specimen is collected.

Treatment of mastitis primarily includes frequent and complete emptying of the breasts, as well as antibiotic coverage. Supportive measures such as rest, increased fluid intake (at least 2.0 to 2.5 L/day), a supportive bra, local application of warm, moist heat or ice packs, and analgesics should also be implemented (James, 2014). Nonsteroidal anti-inflammatory agents are recommended to treat both fever and inflammation. The preferred antibiotics are usually penicillinase-resistant penicillins, such as dicloxacillin 500 mg every 6 hours orally or, with history of mild milk allergy, a cephalosporin such as cephalexin 500 mg every 6 hours orally (Duff, 2014). The woman should continue to breastfeed; in fact, regular drainage of both breasts actually helps by preventing milk stasis and abscess formation, and there is virtually no risk to the newborn. If there has been no change in symptomatology in 48 hours, modification of the antibiotic therapy will be considered. There have been increasing cases of methicillin-resistant *Staphylococcus aureus* mastitis (MRSA). When a woman does not respond to first-line antibiotics, MRSA should be considered and a breast milk culture and antibiotic sensitivity should be ordered (Wambach, 2016).

Candidal infections can be especially stubborn. Initial treatment generally involves antifungal creams or ointments once or twice daily, as well as treating the baby with oral nystatin for a full 2 weeks (Lawrence & Lawrence, 2014). Another treatment option is oral fluconazole (Diflucan), which is excreted in breast milk but is not considered to be toxic to the baby and can be used if other agents fail (Lawrence & Lawrence, 2014). Women should be instructed to cleanse their nipples with warm water and allow air drying before application of the antifungal medication (Lawrence & Lawrence, 2014).

Probiotics are a category of dietary supplements consisting of beneficial microorganisms (*pro* means "for" and *biotic* means "life" versus *antibiotic*, which literally means "against life"). Probiotics compete with disease-causing microorganisms in the gastrointestinal tract. When antibiotics are taken, they kill many of the beneficial bacteria that exist naturally in the digestive tract. Supplementing with probiotics after a course of antibiotics is frequently prescribed by nutritionists and complementary practitioners. Commonly used probiotics include *Lactobacillus acidophilus* and *Bifidobacterium bifidum;* other species of *Lactobacillus* and *Bifidobacterium* have been shown to be effective in such conditions as diarrhea and vaginal infections. *Bifidobacterium* also competes against *Candida albicans*. Probiotics can be taken in the form of powder, capsules, and suppositories, or in fermented milk products such as yogurt or kefir.

Other complementary therapies used for mastitis include belladonna, acupuncture, oxytocin nasal spray to improve milk ejection, a traditional Chinese herb known as extracts of *Fructus gleditsiae*, application of cabbage leaves over the affected area to relieve engorgement, and application of a solution of bacteriocin nisin to nipple and areola to treat staphylococcal mastitis (Wambach, 2016).

Abscess formation is a complication of mastitis, resulting from delayed treatment, treatment failure, or abrupt weaning of the baby. Abscesses are usually in the upper outer quadrants of the breast and will show a localized area of erythema, exquisite tenderness, and induration. Breast abscess may require incision and drainage. Breastfeeding can usually continue on the affected breast, as long as the incision is well away from the areola. The baby can continue to nurse on the unaffected breast (Walker, 2014) .

Improved outcome, a decreased duration of symptoms, and decreased incidence of a breast abscess result if the breasts continue to be emptied by either breastfeeding or pumping. Thus continued breastfeeding is recommended in the process of mastitis. The plan of care should include contacting the woman within 24 hours of initiation of treatment to ensure that symptoms are subsiding.

Nursing Management
For the Postpartum Woman With Mastitis

Nursing Assessment and Diagnosis

Each day assess the mother's breast consistency, skin color, surface temperature, nipple condition, and presence of pain to detect early signs of problems that may predispose her to mastitis. Observe the mother breastfeeding her baby to ensure proper technique (see Chapter 25). Consultation with a lactation specialist can be of great value, especially for first-time mothers.

If an infection develops, assess for contributing factors such as cracked nipples, poor hygiene, engorgement, supplemental feedings, change in routine or infant feeding pattern, abrupt weaning, and lack of proper breast support so that these factors can be corrected as part of the treatment plan.

Nursing diagnoses that may apply to the woman with mastitis include the following (NANDA-I © 2014):

- *Trauma, Risk for*, related to lack of information about appropriate breastfeeding practices
- *Breastfeeding, Ineffective*, related to pain secondary to development of mastitis

Planning and Implementation

Preventing mastitis is far simpler than treating it. Ideally, mothers are instructed in proper breastfeeding technique prenatally. Assist the mother to breastfeed soon after childbirth and review correct technique. Comanagement of breastfeeding between the nurse and a certified lactation specialist is often possible. Encourage new mothers, even those not breastfeeding, to wear a good supportive bra at all times to prevent milk stasis, especially in the lower lobes, and to change breast pads frequently (James, 2014).

Meticulous hand hygiene by the breastfeeding mother and all personnel is the primary measure in preventing epidemic nursery infections and subsequent maternal mastitis. Prompt attention to mothers who have blocked milk ducts eliminates stagnant milk as a growth medium for bacteria. If the mother finds that one area of her breast feels distended, she can rotate the position of her baby for nursing, manually express milk remaining in the breast after feeding (usually necessary only if the baby is not sucking well), or massage the caked area toward the nipple as the baby nurses. Mothers who develop mastitis can apply warm, moist compresses to the affected area before and during breastfeeding. Encourage the mother to breastfeed frequently, starting with the unaffected breast until let-down occurs in the affected breast, then switching to the affected breast until it is emptied completely. After nursing, the mother can leave a small amount of milk on each nipple to prevent cracking, allow nipples to air dry, and apply cold packs to reduce pain and edema (James, 2014). Early identification of and intervention for sore nipples are also essential, as is prompt assessment of the breastfeeding mother's breast when thrush is discovered in her newborn's mouth. For a detailed discussion of breastfeeding problems, see section on Breastfeeding Concerns Following Discharge in Chapter 29.

DISCHARGE PLANNING AND HOME CARE TEACHING

Make sure the woman is aware of the importance of regular, complete emptying of the breasts to prevent engorgement and stasis. She should also understand the role of let-down in successful breastfeeding, correct positioning of the baby on the nipple, proper latch-on, and the principle of supply and demand. If the mother is taking antibiotics, she needs to understand the importance of completing the full course of antibiotics, even if the infection seems to clear quickly. Babies tolerate the small amount of antibiotics in breast milk without difficulty. Breastfeeding mothers who are returning to work outside the home need information on how to do so successfully. Because mastitis tends to develop after discharge, it is important to include information about signs and symptoms in the discharge teaching and printed materials (Table 30–4). All flulike symptoms should be considered a sign of mastitis until proven otherwise. If symptoms develop, the woman should contact her healthcare provider immediately because prompt treatment helps to prevent abscess formation.

COMMUNITY-BASED NURSING CARE

Because symptoms seldom occur before the second to fourth week postpartum, birthing unit nurses often are not fully aware of how uncomfortable and acutely ill the woman can be. The home care nurse who suspects mastitis on the basis of assessment findings should refer the woman to her healthcare provider.

If the mother feels too ill to breastfeed or develops an abscess that prevents nursing, help the mother obtain a breast pump to help her maintain lactation and provide opportunities for demonstration and return demonstration of pumping. Assist the mother in dealing with her feelings about temporarily being unable to breastfeed. Referral to a lactation consultant or the La Leche League can be invaluable to the woman's physical and emotional adjustment to mastitis.

Evaluation

Expected outcomes of nursing care include the following:

- The woman is aware of the signs and symptoms of mastitis.
- The woman reports the mastitis signs and symptoms early and is treated successfully.
- The woman resumes breastfeeding if she chooses.
- The woman understands self-care measures she can employ to prevent the recurrence of the mastitis.

Care of the Woman With Postpartum Thromboembolic Disease

Thromboembolic disease may occur during the antepartum, but it is generally considered a postpartum complication. *Venous thrombosis* refers to blood clot (thrombus formation) at an area of impeded blood flow in a superficial or deep vein, usually in the legs. When the thrombus is formed in response to inflammation in the vein wall, it is termed **thrombophlebitis**. Pulmonary embolism, a rare, life-threatening condition, occurs when thrombi formed in the deep leg veins are carried to the pulmonary artery, obstructing pulmonary blood flow to one or both lungs.

Three major causes of thromboembolic disease, often referred to as the *Virchow triad,* are hypercoagulability of blood, venous stasis, and injury to the epithelium of the blood vessel. Changes in the woman's coagulation system in pregnancy contribute to hypercoagulability and compression of the common iliac vein by the gravid uterus, which leads to venous stasis (Witcher & Hamner, 2013). These factors increase the risk of thromboembolic disease in pregnant and postpartum women approximately 2 to 6 times. In contrast, deep vein thrombosis (DVT), which is more serious, occurs most commonly in postpartum women between postpartum days 10 and 20.

Risk factors associated with increased risk of thromboembolic disease include the following:

- Cesarean birth
- Immobility (prolonged)
- Obesity
- Cigarette smoking
- Previous thromboembolic disease or strong family history

TABLE 30–4 Symptoms of Engorgement, Plugged Duct, and Mastitis

ONSET	LOCATION	HEAT/SWELLING	TEMPERATURE	PAIN	GENERAL SYMPTOMS
ENGORGEMENT					
Gradual; postpartum	Entire breast	Breast is hot and swollen	Less than 38.4°C (101.1°F)	Entire breast	None
PLUGGED DUCT					
Gradual; after feedings	One side of breast	Little or no heat; there may be swelling	Less than 38.4°C (101.1°F)	Mild pain on affected side	None
MASTITIS					
Sudden; usually after about 10 days	Generally one side of breast	Swelling on affected side; skin is red and hot	Greater than 38.4°C (101.1°F)	Intense pain on affected side	Similar to flu

Source: Data from Lawrence, R. A., & Lawrence, R. M. (2014). *Breastfeeding: A guide for the medical profession* (8th ed.). Philadelphia, PA: Elsevier Mosby.

- Trauma to extremity (can include injury from incorrect positioning or prolonged interval in stirrups during labor)
- Varicose veins
- Diabetes mellitus
- Advanced maternal age
- Multiparity
- Anemia
- Malignancy
- Inherited coagulation pathway deficiency
- Protein C & S deficiency

Factors contributing directly to the development of thromboembolic disease postpartum include (1) increased amounts of certain blood-clotting factors; (2) postpartum thrombocytosis (increased quantity of circulating platelets and their increased adhesiveness); (3) release of thromboplastin substances from the tissue of the decidua, placenta, and fetal membranes; and (4) increased amounts of fibrinolysis inhibitors. Women are at risk for thromboembolic disease during the childbearing period especially during labor and the postpartum period. Attention should be given to nursing measures that might prevent or deal with this complication (Table 30–5).

Superficial Leg Vein Disease

Superficial thrombophlebitis is far more common postpartum than during pregnancy. Often the clot involves one of the saphenous veins. This disorder is more common in women with pre-existing varices (enlarged veins), although it is not limited to these women. They may also occur as a sequelae to IV catheterization. Symptoms usually become apparent about postpartum day 3 or 4 and include tenderness in a portion of the vein, some local heat and redness, normal temperature or low-grade fever, and occasionally slight elevation of the pulse. A tender palpable cord may be noted along a portion of the veins. Treatment involves application of local heat, elevation of the affected limb, bed rest, analgesics, and the use of elastic support hose (James, 2014). Anticoagulants are usually not necessary unless complications develop. Pulmonary embolism is extremely rare.

Women With Special Needs Lupus

Women with lupus have a higher incidence of thromboembolic disease and need close observation for the development of deep vein thrombosis (DVT) and pulmonary embolism (PE). Early ambulation and frequent leg exercises should be encouraged. Symptoms of thromboembolic disease should be reviewed. Hormonal contraceptives that contain estrogen are contraindicated in these women.

Deep Vein Thrombosis

Deep vein thrombosis (DVT) is more frequently seen in women with a history of thrombosis. Obstetric complications, such as hydramnios, preeclampsia, and operative birth, are also associated with an increased incidence. After a clinical diagnosis of DVT, a woman's risk in a subsequent pregnancy increases.

Clinical manifestations may include edema of the ankle and leg and an initial low-grade fever often followed by high temperature and chills. Other findings include tenderness or pain, a palpable cord, changes in limb color, and difference in limb circumference of more than 2 cm (0.8 in.). Depending on the vein involved, the woman may complain of pain in the popliteal and lateral tibial areas (popliteal vein), pain in the entire lower leg and foot (anterior and posterior tibial veins), inguinal tenderness (femoral vein), or pain in the lower abdomen (iliofemoral vein). The Homans sign (Figure 28–9) may or may not be positive. Most DVTs occur in the left leg. Because of reflex arterial spasm, sometimes the limb is pale and cool to the touch and peripheral pulses may be diminished or difficult to palpate. These signs and symptoms have less than 50% specificity, however, and diagnosis of DVT is usually confirmed by compression ultrasound and D-dimer assays (Leung & Lockwood , 2014).

Clinical Therapy

Treatment of acute DVT or pulmonary embolus involves the immediate administration of anticoagulants. Unfractionated heparin or low molecular weight heparin (LMWH) are the drugs

TABLE 30–5 Measures to Decrease Risk of Thromboembolic Disease in Childbearing Women

ANTEPARTUM MEASURES	INTRAPARTUM MEASURES	POSTPARTUM MEASURES
• Advise woman to avoid sedentary lifestyle and to exercise as possible (walking is ideal). • Advise to quit smoking. • Teach to avoid prolonged standing or sitting in one position or sitting with legs crossed. • Encourage elevation of legs when sitting. • Teach to avoid tight knee-high hose or other constrictive garments. • Encourage to take frequent breaks during long car trips to walk around and while working if she sits most of the day, thereby preventing prolonged venous stasis.	• Encourage ambulation unless contraindicated in early labor; later, encourage leg exercises. • Do not gatch bed or use pillows under knees. • Pad stirrups to prevent pressure on popliteal vessels. • Ensure correct positioning in stirrups to minimize pressure on the popliteal area. • Limit time in stirrups as much as possible because trauma is a factor. • After cesarean birth, initiate leg/foot exercises as soon as possible (in recovery) to promote venous return. • Use antiembolism stockings for women at risk for DVT.	• Encourage early ambulation. • For patients on bed rest, advise or assist with turning and leg exercises every 2 hr (woman may be encouraged to rotate ankles and to "write baby's name in the air with her toes"). • Encourage fluids to avoid dehydration. • Advise no smoking. • Use antiembolism stockings with those at risk, including after cesarean birth. • Advise against prolonged sitting and crossing of legs. • Encourage elevation of legs while sitting.

of choice. An example of a possible regimen is a subcutaneous injection of Enoxaparin 1 mg/kg twice daily (Witcher & Hamner, 2013). Heparin therapy is continued until the international normalized ratio (INR) with oral warfarin is achieved at 2 to 3. An advantage of LMWH is a safe profile and dosing not reliant on monitoring the activated partial thromboplastin time (aPTT) at a laboratory. Maintenance with warfarin sodium (Coumadin) is started at 1 to 5 days. In some cases thrombolytics (streptokinase or urokinase) or an embolectomy may be used. Strict bed rest and elevation of the affected leg are required, and analgesics are given as necessary to relieve discomfort. In most cases, thrombectomy (surgical removal of the clot) is not necessary.

Once the symptoms have subsided (usually in several days), the woman may begin walking while wearing elastic support stockings. The woman will continue on warfarin sodium (Coumadin) for several weeks postpartum or up to 3 months or more depending on the circumstances of the thrombolic event (Witcher & Hamner, 2013). While taking warfarin sodium, prothrombin times are assessed periodically to maintain correct dosage levels. Periodic assessment for signs of bleeding is essential, including those for hematuria and fecal occult blood. In those who cannot be given anticoagulants or have had a venous thromboembolism (VTE) event despite full anticoagulation, a vena cava filtering device may be considered (American College of Obstetrics & Gynecology [ACOG], 2011; Cunningham et al., 2014). To prevent recurrence in subsequent pregnancies, prophylactic treatment will be considered.

Clinical Reasoning Postpartum Leg Pain

Wanda Sugiyama, G1P1, had a cesarean birth after a prolonged labor and failure to progress. As she is walking in the hallway with her husband, you notice that Wanda is limping slightly, and you comment on that observation. Wanda responds that she is having pain in her right lower leg. She says, "Maybe I pulled a muscle during labor." What would you do?

Nursing Management

For the Postpartum Woman With Thromboembolic Disease

Nursing Assessment and Diagnosis

Carefully assess the woman's history for factors predisposing her to development of thrombosis or thrombophlebitis. In addition, as part of regular postpartum assessment, be alert to any complaints of pain in the legs, inguinal area, or lower abdomen because such pain may indicate deep vein thrombosis (DVT). Also assess the woman's legs for evidence of edema, temperature change, or pain with palpation.

Nursing diagnoses that may apply to a postpartum woman with a thrombotic disease include the following (NANDA-I © 2014):

- *Tissue Perfusion: Peripheral, Ineffective*, related to obstructed venous return
- *Pain, Acute*, related to tissue hypoxia and edema secondary to vascular obstruction
- *Knowledge, Deficient*, related to self-care after discharge on anticoagulant therapy

Planning and Implementation

HOSPITAL-BASED NURSING CARE

Women are at risk for thromboembolic disease during the childbearing period especially during labor and the postpartum period. Attention should be given to nursing measures that might prevent or deal with this complication (refer to Table 30–5).

Once DVT is diagnosed, maintain the heparin therapy, provide appropriate comfort measures, and monitor the woman closely for signs of pulmonary embolism. Assess for evidence of bleeding related to heparin and keep the antagonist for heparin, protamine sulfate, readily available. Remind the woman to mention her history of thrombosis or thrombophlebitis to her healthcare provider during subsequent pregnancies so that preventive measures can be instituted early (James, 2014). See *Nursing Care Plan: The Woman With Thromboembolic Disease.*

Women discharged on warfarin sodium (Coumadin) should be taught about the drug and safety factors associated with its use. See *Teaching Highlights: What the Postpartum Woman Taking Warfarin Needs to Know.*

COMMUNITY-BASED NURSING CARE

Because the mother with postpartum thromboembolic disease will depend on others for much of her initial home care, it is helpful for the father of the newborn to be involved in preparations for discharge. Provide ample time to answer questions and clarify instructions, verbally and in writing. It is especially important to assess the couple's plans to ensure complete bed rest for the mother. They might explore ways for her to maintain bed rest and still spend quality time with her newborn and any other children. For example, young children can sit on the bed for storytelling or play quiet games, and the newborn's crib can be placed next to the mother's bed.

The father/partner may be assuming multiple roles in these circumstances—household manager, parent, worker, and caregiver. Fatigue is inevitable. There may also be financial concerns as a result of prolonged health care or his extended time away from work to care for the family. Many concerns will not surface until the couple actually returns home and fully comprehends the reality of their situation. For that reason, it is valuable to provide them with an accessible resource person and to plan telephone or home visit follow-up care.

Signs of postpartum thrombophlebitis may not occur until after discharge from the birthing unit. Consequently all couples must be taught to recognize its signs and symptoms and appreciate the importance of reporting them immediately and not massaging the affected leg. If signs and symptoms occur after discharge, a short readmission may be required. In that case every effort is made to allow mother, father, and newborn to remain together.

After DVT, some women continue to have leg pain, edema, and dermatitis of the affected extremity for prolonged periods caused by a residual venous abnormality. This situation can significantly affect quality of life. Continuing use of compression stockings can help prevent the complication of DVT.

Evaluation

Expected outcomes of nursing care include the following:

- The woman seeks treatment for her thrombophlebitis early and is managed successfully, without further complications.
- At discharge the woman is able to explain the purpose, dosage regimen, and necessary precautions associated with any prescribed medications such as anticoagulants.

Nursing Care Plan: The Woman With Thromboembolic Disease

1. **Nursing Diagnosis:** *Tissue Perfusion: Peripheral, Ineffective,* **related to interruption of venous blood flow secondary to complications of labor and birth (NANDA-I © 2014)**

GOAL: The woman's presenting signs and symptoms are relieved.

INTERVENTION	RATIONALE
• Assess, record, and report signs of thrombophlebitis.	• Early detection of developing thrombophlebitis permits prompt treatment. As the thrombus increases in size, signs of obstruction also increase.
• Assess leg for edema, peripheral pulse, temperature, color, and tenderness every 8 hours. Initially note presence of palpable cord. Homans sign may be assessed, but is only positive in less than 50% of patients with a DVT (James, 2014).	• Edema/swelling, diminished or absent peripheral pulse, pallor, cool skin temperature, and tenderness are symptoms of deep vein thrombosis (DVT) and indicate dysfunction of peripheral circulation in the lower extremities. Measure circumference of lower leg to monitor for swelling. Peripheral pulses in both legs should be palpated for pulse rate and pulse strength to allow for comparison. A lower extremity cool to the touch may be due to reflex arterial spasm.
• Maintain bed rest during the acute phase.	• Bed rest is ordered to decrease the possibility that a portion of the clot will dislodge and result in pulmonary embolism.
• Provide warm, moist soaks as ordered.	• Warmth promotes blood flow to affected area.
• Maintain limb in elevated position.	• Elevation of affected limb promotes venous return and helps decrease edema.
• Initiate progressive ambulation following the acute phase and provide properly fitting compression stockings before ambulation. These should be properly measured.	• Elastic compression stockings or "TEDs" help prevent pooling of venous blood in lower extremities. Stockings should be carefully measured according to guidelines to ensure proper pressure gradient and avoid "garter-like" roll at top.
	• Woman may begin to ambulate within a few days when symptoms subside.
• **Collaborative:** Administer unfractionated heparin as ordered, by continuous intravenous drip, heparin lock, or subcutaneously, or administer low molecular weight heparin (LMWH) subcutaneously as ordered including:	• Heparin does not dissolve blood clot but is administered to prevent further clotting and improve tissue perfusion. It is safe for breast-feeding mothers because heparin is not excreted in breast milk.
1. Monitor IV or heparin lock site (if in use) for patency, signs of infiltration, or signs of infection.	
2. Obtain international normalized ratio (INR) and partial thromboplastin time (PTT) per healthcare provider order and review before administering heparin.	
3. Observe for signs of anticoagulant overdose with resultant bleeding including:	
a. Hematuria	
b. Epistaxis	
c. Ecchymosis or petechiae	
d. Bleeding gums	
4. Provide protamine sulfate, per healthcare provider order, to combat bleeding problems related to heparin overdose.	• Protamine sulfate is a heparin antagonist, given intravenously, which is almost immediately effective in counteracting bleeding complications caused by heparin overdose.
5. Monitor and report any signs of pulmonary embolism.	• Pulmonary embolism is a major complication of DVT/thrombophlebitis.

(continued)

Nursing Care Plan: The Woman With Thromboembolic Disease (*continued*)

6. Initiate or support any emergency treatment.

• Signs and symptoms may occur suddenly and require immediate emergency treatment; prognosis is related to size and location of embolism.

7. Obtain prothrombin time (PT) and review before beginning warfarin. Repeat periodically per healthcare provider order.

• PT is the test most commonly used to monitor the blood of women receiving warfarin.

EXPECTED OUTCOME: Woman will have increased venous return from lower leg as evidenced by decreased edema in lower leg, negative Homans sign, and no pain or tenderness in lower leg.

2. Nursing Diagnosis: *Pain, Acute*, related to tissue hypoxia and edema secondary to vascular obstruction (NANDA-I © 2014)

GOAL: Woman will obtain relief of pain or experience level of pain that is acceptable.

INTERVENTION	RATIONALE
• Administer analgesics per healthcare provider order. Notify healthcare provider if pain is not relieved.	• Analgesics act to relieve pain and enable the woman to rest. Aspirin or ibuprofen products are contraindicated because they inhibit platelet adhesiveness. Acetaminophen may be ordered by the healthcare provider.
• Observe or report disruptive effects of pain on emotions and behavior.	• Once pain decreases, woman is more likely to ambulate, which will help increase venous return and decrease edema.
• Provide supportive nursing comfort measures such as backrubs, provision of quiet time for sleep, diversional activities, or imagery.	

EXPECTED OUTCOME: Woman will have reduction in pain as evidenced by a pain level less than 5 at all times.

3. Nursing Diagnosis: *Parenting, Risk for Impaired*, related to decreased maternal-newborn interaction secondary to bed rest and IVs (NANDA-I © 2014)

GOAL: Woman will demonstrate evidence of positive physical and social interaction with newborn.

INTERVENTION	RATIONALE
• Maintain mother–newborn attachment when mother is on bed rest:	• Maternal–newborn attachment is enhanced by frequent contact and opportunities to interact.
1. Provide frequent contacts for mother and baby; modified rooming-in if possible by having the crib placed close to the mother's bed and nurse checks often to help mother lift or move baby.	
2. Encourage mother to continue feeding baby.	

EXPECTED OUTCOME: Woman will develop attachment bonds as evidenced by physical interactions: good eye contact, touching the baby, holding baby close, attempting to comfort baby, and kissing baby, and social interactions: calling baby by name, making positive comments about baby, asking questions about baby, asking questions about baby care, and talking to baby.

4. Nursing Diagnosis: *Family Processes, Interrupted*, related to illness of family member (NANDA-I © 2014)

GOAL: Woman and her family will cope effectively with her illness.

INTERVENTION	RATIONALE
• Encourage woman to express her concerns to her partner. Assist couple in planning ways to manage while woman is hospitalized and after her discharge.	• Illness of any family member impacts the entire family. This is especially true when the family situation is such that the mother is the primary nurturer and she is absent. Family members attempt to continue their own roles while also assuming the tasks of the missing mother. This can result in crisis.

- Encourage partner or support person to bring other children to the hospital to visit mother and meet new sibling.
- Encourage partner or support person to bring in family pictures and notes from other children. Encourage phone calls.
- Contact social services if indicated to obtain additional assistance for family if needed.

EXPECTED OUTCOMES: Woman expresses assurance that her family misses her but is coping effectively as evidenced by:

- Family visits woman frequently.
- Woman and family verbalize plan for division of family tasks while the woman is hospitalized and understanding of potential needs of woman once released from hospital.

---

5. Nursing Diagnosis: *Bleeding, Risk for,* related to lack of information about DVT/thrombophlebitis, its treatment, preventive measures, and the medication warfarin sodium (Coumadin) (NANDA-I © 2014).

GOAL: Woman will understand her condition, its treatment, safety during treatment, and long-term implications.

INTERVENTION	RATIONALE
• Provide information (both verbal and written supplements) about the woman's condition, its treatment regimen, the importance of compliance, and safety factors. Provide contact information that the woman can access 24/7.	• Such discussion is essential to help the woman understand the condition, her medication, and its implications. She must have a clear understanding to be able to provide effective self-care.
• Discuss ways of avoiding circulatory stasis such as avoiding prolonged standing, sitting, crossing legs, and wearing restrictive clothing.	• Prolonged sitting, standing, and crossing legs should be avoided, as these activities decrease venous return.
• Review need to wear support stockings and to plan for rest periods with legs elevated.	
• In the presence of DVT, discuss the following:	
1. The use of warfarin, its side effects, possible interactions with other medications, and the need to have dosage assessed through periodic checks of the prothrombin time.	• Patient placed on warfarin (Coumadin) therapy for 2–6 months at home.
2. Signs of bleeding, which may be associated with warfarin sodium and need to be reported immediately, include the following: hematuria, epistaxis, ecchymosis, bleeding gums, and rectal bleeding.	
3. Monitor menstrual flow: bleeding may be heavier.	
4. Review need for woman to eat a consistent amount of leafy green vegetables (lettuce, cabbage, brussels sprouts, broccoli) every day.	• These foods are high in vitamin K and will affect balance between dose of warfarin and prothrombin.
5. Instruct the woman to report any bleeding that continues more than 10 minutes.	
6. Instruct the woman to do the following:	
a. Routinely inspect the body for bruising.	
b. Carry medical alert card indicating she is on anticoagulant therapy.	
c. Use electric razor to avoid scratching skin.	
d. Use soft-bristle toothbrush.	
e. Avoid binge alcohol intake or keep at minimum.	
f. Avoid taking certain herbs such as ginger, garlic, and ginkgo and any other drugs that can prolong PT without checking with the healthcare provider.	

(continued)

Nursing Care Plan: The Woman With Thromboembolic Disease (*continued*)

g. Note that stools may change color to pink, red, or black as a result of anticoagulant use.

h. Advise all health providers, including dentists, that she is taking anticoagulants.

EXPECTED OUTCOMES: Woman has health promotion knowledge as evidenced by:

- Woman verbalizes understanding of ways to avoid circulatory stasis, need to wear supportive stockings, medications dosage and side effects, and the importance of a balanced diet.
- Woman verbalizes understanding of signs and symptoms of bleeding that need to be reported to healthcare provider.

TEACHING HIGHLIGHTS | What the Postpartum Woman Taking Warfarin Needs to Know

- Warfarin is compatible with breastfeeding (Hale & Rowe, 2014).
- Foods high in vitamin K lessen warfarin's effectiveness, thus you will need to strive for consistent daily intake so that accurate dosage of the drug can be achieved. If intake of vitamin K decreases significantly, there is a risk of bleeding.
- Foods high in vitamin K include cauliflower, soybean and canola oil, mayonnaise, broccoli, green and black tea, peppers, spinach, collard and other leafy greens. Many multivitamins contain vitamin K; you may take them but, again, should do so consistently.
- Cranberry juice increases the effects of warfarin and, if desired, should be consumed in moderation and with consistency.
- Binge alcohol use inhibits warfarin metabolism; an occasional alcoholic beverage does not affect coagulation adversely.
- Several herbals affect the efficacy of warfarin sodium; for example, garlic, ginger, and ginkgo prolong prothrombin time (PT) and should be avoided.
- Vitamin C doses up to 500 mg per day and vitamin E doses up to 400 international units per day are considered safe; higher doses can affect coagulation.
- Certain medications such as aspirin and other nonsteroidal anti-inflammatory drugs increase anticoagulant activity and should be avoided.
- Be alert for signs of bleeding, such as bleeding gums, epistaxis, petechiae or ecchymosis, and evidence of blood in the urine or stool.
- Check for possible medication interaction with warfarin before taking any other medication.
- Be cautious about using sharp objects such as knives or razor blades to avoid injury.
- Avoid risky behaviors that could contribute to falls.
- Wear protective gloves during gardening or heavy housework and always wear shoes to keep hands and feet safe from injury.
- Carry a MedicAlert card or wear a bracelet stating that you are taking warfarin in case of emergency.
- Inform all healthcare providers (including dentists) that you are taking anticoagulants and to have vitamin K available in case of bleeding.
- Bleeding should be reported if it fails to stop within 10 minutes.
- Keep scheduled appointments for PT assessment to guide dosing.
- Consider utilizing point-of-care testing, which decreases the inconvenience of going to the laboratory. Home self-testing involves a single capillary fingerstick (CoaguChek, ProTime, Avocet) to test thromboplastin-mediated clotting expressed as PT or INR. The therapeutic range of INR is 2–3, and the risk of bleeding increases significantly when the INR is 3 or greater (Leung & Lockwood, 2014).

- The woman can discuss the self-care measures and ongoing therapies (such as need for rest and the use of elastic stockings) that are indicated.
- The woman has bonded successfully with her newborn and is able to care for her baby effectively.

Care of the Woman With a Postpartum Psychiatric Disorder

Types of Postpartum Psychiatric Disorders

The classification of postpartum psychiatric disorders is a subject of some controversy. The *Diagnostic and Statistical Manual of Mental Disorders (DSM-5)* (American Psychiatric Association [APA],

2013) contains a peripartum onset specifier to the mood disorder diagnostic category of psychiatric disorders. It is proposed that postpartum psychiatric disorders be considered one diagnosable syndrome with three subclasses: (1) adjustment reaction with depressed mood, (2) postpartum mood episodes with psychotic features, and (3) peripartum major mood episodes (also known as postpartum depression). The incidence, etiology, symptoms, treatment, and prognosis vary with each subclass.

ADJUSTMENT REACTION WITH DEPRESSED MOOD

Adjustment reaction with depressed mood is also known as **postpartum blues** or as *maternal blues* or *baby blues*. It occurs in as many as 85% of mothers and is characterized by mild depression interspersed with happier feelings (Pessel & Tsai, 2013). The condition is more severe in primiparas than in multiparas and seems related to the rapid alteration of estrogen, progesterone, and prolactin levels after birth, challenges of new motherhood, fatigue, and lifestyle adjustments. New mothers experiencing postpartum blues commonly report feeling overwhelmed, unable to cope, fatigued, anxious, irritable, and oversensitive. A key feature is episodic tearfulness and rapid mood shifts, often without an identifiable reason. Not uncommonly, when asked why she is crying, this woman responds that she does not know. Cunningham et al. (2014) identifies several factors that contribute to the "blues":

- Emotional letdown that follows labor and childbirth
- Physical discomfort typical in the early postpartum
- Fatigue
- Anxiety about caring for the newborn after discharge
- Severe PMS (premenstrual syndrome)
- Depression during pregnancy or previous depression unrelated to pregnancy

Validating the existence of this phenomenon, labeling it as a real but normal adjustment reaction, and providing reassurance can offer a measure of relief. Assistance with self-care and infant care, rest, good nutrition, information, and family support aid recovery. Helping the new mother anticipate a transient emotional letdown after discharge is important guidance from the nurse, as is talking with her about her view of "the perfect mother." Trying to achieve that image can contribute to fatigue and exacerbate the letdown feeling. The partner should be encouraged to watch for and report signs that the new mother is not returning to a more normal mood but slipping into a deeper depression or that happier times are no longer interspersed with the blues.

PERIPARTUM MAJOR MOOD EPISODES

Peripartum major mood episodes, also known as **postpartum depression (PPD)**, is clinical depression, categorized by the *Diagnostic and Statistical Manual of Mental Disorders* (DSM-5) as Major Depressive Disorder with Peripartum Onset (APA, 2013). Postpartum depression has been shown to occur in 10% to 20% of all postpartum women across several studies (APA, 2013).

Risk factors for postpartum depression include the following:

- History of major depression
- Depression during pregnancy
- History of postpartum depression or bipolar illness (recurrence rates are ≥ 20%)
- Stressful life events
- Primiparity
- Ambivalence about maintaining the pregnancy
- Occurrence of postpartum blues
- Lack of social support
- Lack of a stable and supportive relationship with parents (especially her father, as a child) or partner
- The woman's dissatisfaction with herself, including body image problems and eating disorders
- Complications of delivery
- Loss of newborn
- Age (adolescence increases risk)

Although it may occur at any time during the first postpartum year, the periods of greatest risk occur around the fourth week, just before the initiation of menses, and upon weaning. It is not always associated with depression during pregnancy, although gestational depression is a strong predictor of PPD.

Women with postpartum depression are at risk for suicide, most prominently as they enter or exit the deeply depressed state. In a deep depression, the woman is unlikely to be able to plan and carry out suicide. For that reason, signs of improvement in depression should be celebrated with some caution. Whereas the woman with postpartum psychosis may attempt suicide because of illogical thought processes, the woman with major depression attempts suicide because her suffering is so great that dying seems a more favorable option than continuing to live in such pain. She may also attempt suicide to save her newborn from some perceived or real threat—including the possibility that she herself might harm the baby. The risk of suicide is greater in those who have attempted suicide previously, have a specific plan, and can access the means or weapon identified within the plan. The more specific the plan, the greater the probability of an attempt.

For women considered to be at high risk, telephone follow-up after delivery or an earlier clinic appointment than 6 weeks may be helpful. Nurses in the pediatrician's office assisting with well-child visits have an excellent opportunity to screen women for PPD (Liberto, 2012). Community health nurses who are seeing other members of the family or parish nurses who know new mothers in their congregation can observe for evidence of depression. The Postpartum Depression Screening Scale (PDSS) and the Edinburgh Postnatal Depression Scale (EPDS) are useful and validated for screening for postpartum depression.

The woman's safety, and that of her child(ren), is a priority. Inquiring about suicidal ideas and assessment for thoughts and feelings toward the baby, hallucinations and delusions, and impulsiveness that might put the baby and siblings at risk is critical. The woman and her family need information about the illness and its expected course, including the risk of recurrence, as well as comprehensive information about the treatment plan. They need opportunities to clarify misconceptions about mental illness and to have answers to questions. Referral to local or online support groups may be helpful.

Treatment for PPD is most successful with a combination of individual or group psychotherapy and antidepressants (Burt & Stein, 2013). The expected outcomes for mild to moderate depression treated with antidepressants and psychotherapy are good; recurrence rates are increased after each episode of depression. The serotonin reuptake inhibitors (SSRIs) are used most often, as well as tricyclic antidepressants. Monoamine oxidase inhibitors (MAOIs) are rarely used in the treatment of PPD because these drugs have a high profile of interacting with other medications. Women typically continue antidepressants for 1 year after symptoms abate.

All current antidepressant agents are excreted into breast milk. However, most SSRIs and tricyclic antidepressants are considered safe with breastfeeding. Because of its prolonged half-life, fluoxetine (Prozac) is usually not recommended for nursing mothers as a first choice (Hale & Rowe, 2014). Healthcare providers need to educate their breastfeeding postpartum clients who need antidepressants about the different alternatives and help them to balance the risks and benefits with the safety profiles. The final decision about continuing to breastfeed and to take antidepressants is the informed woman's. To help in making the decision, she and her significant other need to be helped to consider how she will respond without pharmacologic therapy and how unmedicated depression will affect the maternal-infant relationship and the infant's well-being and development. An invaluable online resource for prescribers with current information on drug safety and toxic effects during pregnancy and lactation is the LactMed Database.

Electroconvulsive therapy (ECT) is used as a more rapid treatment for those with severe depression or mania, for those who are unresponsive to other treatment, or for those who are at high risk of suicide. Antidepressants may take 2 to 3 weeks to become effective. ECT results often become noticeable within 1 week (Kellner et al., 2012).

POSTPARTUM MOOD EPISODES WITH PSYCHOTIC FEATURES

The most serious of postpartum psychiatric disorders is **postpartum mood episodes with psychotic features**, also called **postpartum psychosis**. Although relatively rare (1 to 2 in 1000), this disorder gains considerable national attention in the media and is considered an emergency, given the risk of infanticide or suicide. Symptoms usually become evident within the first few days after birth. Clinical features progress rapidly and include the following (Burt & Stein, 2013):

- Sleep disturbances—the woman is unable to sleep, even when her baby is sleeping
- Depersonalization—seeming unaware of or distant from the immediate environment and individuals within it
- Confusion; irrational or disorganized thinking; bizarre behaviors
- Hallucinations; delusions
- Psychomotor disturbances—stupor or agitated state sometimes with rapid and incoherent speech

Significant risk factors include previous postpartum psychosis and/or a history of bipolar disorder. Family history of postpartum psychosis and bipolar disorder have also been found to increase the risk (Burt & Stein, 2013).

Women With Special Needs Bipolar Disorder

Women with a history of bipolar disorder have a 100 times higher risk of developing postpartum psychosis. A complete assessment should include administering a postpartum depression scale and assessing the woman for symptoms that would be considered atypical and may be an indicator of psychosis. The woman and her support persons should be educated about symptoms that warrant immediate medical intervention.

The woman with a psychosis experiences delusions and/or visual, auditory, or tactile hallucinations. In some women, these symptoms support her perceptions that the baby should not be allowed to live or that she should commit suicide. For example, she may believe that her newborn is evil, is some form of "changeling," and will harm her or others or she may believe that her newborn would be "better off dead" than living in such an evil world. She may contemplate suicide because she believes that her child would be better off without a mother than with her as such a "terrible, crazy mother." Illogical thinking or evidence of bonding difficulties may serve as cues to infanticide and suicide risk; however, this assessment is often challenging because of periods of lucidity seen in some psychotic women. Nurses in various clinical settings who come in contact with this woman may note that the child has been neglected or the woman is practicing unsafe behaviors because of the woman's cognitive impairment.

For example, a pediatric nurse noticed that one of her clients placed her newborn across the room at the edge of the narrow examination table while she paced back and forth across the room, muttering to herself, appearing not to notice the baby. This same woman came to her appointment during heavy snow with both her baby and herself underdressed for warmth.

Provisions for safety of the woman and baby are paramount. This woman needs immediate referral to psychiatric care, usually requiring admission to an inpatient psychiatric hospital. Continued assessment of her symptomatology, safety, and functional capacity is a major nursing role in the setting. An initial history, physical examination, and laboratory work will help to rule out an organic cause of acute psychosis.

A dilemma exists for breastfeeding women for whom lithium or psychotropic medication is being considered. Because babies have immature hepatic and renal systems and a more permeable blood–brain barrier, they may be vulnerable to side effects, especially when younger than 2 months of age, premature, or exposed to these medications in utero. With the exception of lithium (which is rated a category 5 [use with caution] by the American Academy of Pediatrics), the amount of psychotropic drugs excreted into breast milk appears to be modest and not to compromise growth and development (Rowe, Baker, & Hale, 2014). Parents of a baby need to be educated to consider these factors in making a decision about the use of psychotropic medications: (1) severity of symptoms and their effect on the baby if medications are not used; (2) benefits of breastfeeding to the baby; (3) potential risks to the baby if psychotropics are used; and (4) preferences of the woman. If psychotropics are prescribed, the lowest dose possible of monotherapy should be used, and the baby should be monitored carefully by a pediatrician for difficulty being aroused from sleep, rigidity, tremors, irritability, poor hydration, and poor feeding with failure to gain weight (Rowe et al., 2014)

POSTTRAUMATIC STRESS DISORDER

Many women envision their own labor and delivery unfolding in a particular way and may experience angst if their labor reality fails to match their expectations. Labor and birth situations that go awry, including those associated with complications, may cause **posttraumatic stress disorder (PTSD)** (also called *posttraumatic stress syndrome [PTSS]*), which the APA's *Diagnostic and Statistical Manual of Mental Disorders (DSM-5)* (2013) describes as "the development of characteristic symptoms following exposure to one or more traumatic events." Traumatic events during childbirth may include emergency cesarean sections, surgery or medical interventions without adequate anesthesia, or the loss of a baby.

Vossbeck-Elsebusch, Freisfeld and Ehring (2014) found that 1% to 6% of postpartum women meet the diagnostic criteria for PTSD. At particular risk for PTSD are women who have histories of prior trauma and/or prior psychiatric histories and women who undergo emergency cesarean sections (Whitmer, 2016). For this woman, the facts of the labor and birth have become distorted, perhaps because of pain or change in consciousness related to medications she received. Perhaps she underwent an emergency cesarean delivery or her baby had a serious physical anomaly. Perhaps her labor coach could not make the trip to the hospital in time for the birth or she experienced a postpartum hemorrhage. Her perceptions of what occurred and the actions of those involved frequently are far different from the reality, perhaps even seeming delusional.

Clinical features of PTSD include feeling numb, seeming dazed and unaware of her environment, intrusive thoughts and flashbacks to the threatening event, difficulty thinking, difficulty sleeping, irritability, and avoidance of others and reminders of the traumatic event. These signs and symptoms may not be evident until after the woman has left the birth setting. Distress associated with the original traumatic event can recur at anniversaries, and some women are hesitant to consider future pregnancies because of this birth trauma (Beck & Watson, 2010).

Based on the qualitative research and the work of others related to traumatic birth experiences, Beck and Watson (2010) suggest the following implications for nursing care:

1. Intervene, whenever possible, to prevent traumatic birth experiences.
2. Provide technically competent, concerned care for the woman and family.
3. Assess for anxiety and fears on admission to labor and provide information to dispel myths.
4. Debrief the woman and family after a stressful traumatic childbirth experience.
5. Visit the woman during her hospitalization to assess for evidence of signs of early trauma.

Women should be asked to tell their birth story, to compare and contrast the actual experience with their birth plan or prior visions of the special day, and to tell what went well for them and what part, if any, of the experience was unexpected, troublesome, disappointing, or distressing.

Nurses who work in childbirth settings should appreciate that a woman they are admitting at any point in time may have previously had a traumatic birth. That woman will need sensitive healthcare providers who provide additional support and information and follow the birth plan to the extent possible. Subsequent childbirth following a traumatic birth experience provides a woman an opportunity to heal, and nurses have the responsibility to help these women to "reclaim their bodies and complete their journey to motherhood" (Beck & Watson, 2010).

Clinical Therapy

Women with a history of postpartum psychosis or depression or other risk factors should be referred to a mental health professional for counseling and biweekly visits between the second and sixth week postpartum for evaluation. Medication, individual or group psychotherapy, and practical assistance with child care and other demands of daily life are common treatment measures for both disorders; however, the specific therapies used may vary. It is important for the nurse to realize that many of the drugs used in treating postpartum psychiatric conditions are contraindicated in breastfeeding women.

Treatment of postpartum psychosis is directed at the specific type of psychotic symptoms displayed and may include lithium, antipsychotics, or electroconvulsive therapy in combination with psychotherapy, removal of the baby, and social support.

Support groups are successful adjuncts to the previously discussed treatments. Within a support group of postpartum women and their partners, a couple may feel consolation that they are not alone in their experience. Moreover, the group provides a forum for exchanging information about postpartum depression, learning stress reduction measures, and experiencing renewed self-esteem and support. The most effective support groups provide for safe child care to facilitate attendance. If a support group is not available locally, the woman and her family may be encouraged to contact Depression After Delivery (DAD), now a national web-based support network that provides education and volunteers, or Postpartum Support International. The Mills Depression and Anxiety Symptom-Feeling Checklist is also available online.

Nursing Management

For the Postpartum Woman With a Psychiatric Disorder

Nursing Assessment and Diagnosis

Assessment for factors predisposing a woman to postpartum depression or psychosis should begin prenatally and continue during her labor and postpartum stay. Questions designed to detect problems can be included as part of the routine prenatal history interview or questionnaire. Answers to open-ended questions can be telling: What has been your greatest surprise about motherhood? Your greatest disappointment? Biggest concern? Biggest challenge? Or how does being a mother compare to what you had envisioned? Women with a personal or family history of psychiatric disease, particularly postpartum depression or psychosis, need prenatal instructions on the signs and symptoms of depression and may need additional emotional support.

New mothers and their families expect a challenging adjustment period after bringing home a new baby; they may not realize that their experiences are outside the norm. There is general anticipation that motherhood will be a happy occasion; a woman may not be able to admit her unhappiness out of shame or embarrassment that she is somehow different as a mother. The woman might be concerned that telling someone, even a professional, about her symptoms makes her sound "crazy" and that her baby might be taken away (Logsdon, Tomasulo, Eckert, et al., 2012). One woman reported that she wanted help and sensed she needed it, but did not know which doctor to call. "I had only been home for 3 weeks and my postpartum clinic visit was 3 weeks away when I started feeling so desperate. Should I call my OB? The pediatrician had seen the baby in the hospital nursery but we hadn't visited him yet and, besides, I'm not his patient—I'm an adult. My family doctor doesn't see pregnancy-related problems, so who do I call?"

Several screening tools are available for assessing postpartum depression. The routine use of a screening tool in a matter-of-fact approach significantly increases the diagnosis because the woman does not feel singled out. The Edinburgh Postnatal Depression Scale (EPDS) is likely the most widely used screening tool for postpartum depression in large populations of women. The tool has been validated, computerized, and used in telephone screening. Recent studies looked at the use of an interactive voice response system that delivered an automated version of the EPDS via telephone. Results suggested that the use of automated telephone screening may be a useful adjunct to office-based screening for postpartum depression (Kim et al., 2012). Mothers who score above 12 on the EPDS are likely to be suffering from postpartum depression. Another tool is Beck's (2002) revised Postpartum Depression Predictors Inventory (PDPI–Revised) (Table 30–6). This tool is also a practical and simple screening checklist to use during routine care with all postpartum women to identify

TABLE 30–6 Postpartum Depression Predictors Inventory (PDPI)—Revised and Guide Questions for Its Use

DURING PREGNANCY		
MARITAL STATUS	**CHECK ONE**	
1. Single	❏	
2. Married/cohabitating	❏	
3. Separated	❏	
4. Divorced	❏	
5. Widowed	❏	
6. Partnered	❏	
SOCIOECONOMIC STATUS		
Low	❏	
Middle	❏	
High	❏	
SELF-ESTEEM	**Yes**	**No**
Do you feel good about yourself as a person?	❏	❏
Do you feel worthwhile?	❏	❏
Do you feel you have a number of good qualities as a person?	❏	❏
PRENATAL DEPRESSION		
1. Have you felt depressed during your pregnancy?	❏	❏
If yes, when and how long have you been feeling this way?		
If yes, how mild or severe would you consider your depression?		
PRENATAL ANXIETY		
1. Have you been feeling anxious during your pregnancy?	❏	❏
If yes, how long have you been feeling this way?		
UNPLANNED/UNWANTED PREGNANCY		
Was the pregnancy planned?	❏	❏
Is the pregnancy unwanted?	❏	❏
HISTORY OF PREVIOUS DEPRESSION		
1. Before this pregnancy, have you ever been depressed?	❏	❏
If yes, when did you experience this depression?		
If yes, have you been under a healthcare provider's care for this past depression?	❏	❏
If yes, did the healthcare provider prescribe any medication for your depression?	❏	❏
SOCIAL SUPPORT		
1. Do you feel you receive adequate emotional support from your partner?	❏	❏
2. Do you feel you receive adequate instrumental support from your partner (e.g., help with household chores or babysitting)?	❏	❏
3. Do you feel you can rely on your partner when you need help?	❏	❏
4. Do you feel you can confide in your partner? (Repeat same questions for family and again for friends.)	❏	❏
MARITAL SATISFACTION		
1. Are you satisfied with your marriage (or living arrangement)?	❏	❏
2. Are you currently experiencing any marital problems?	❏	❏
3. Are things going well between you and your partner?	❏	❏
LIFE STRESS		
1. Are you currently experiencing any stressful events in your life such as:		
Financial problems?	❏	❏
Marital problems?	❏	❏

	Yes	No
Death in the family?	❏	❏
Serious illness in the family?	❏	❏
Moving?	❏	❏
Unemployment?	❏	❏
Job change?	❏	❏

AFTER DELIVERY, ADD THE FOLLOWING ITEMS

CHILDCARE STRESS

	Yes	No
1. Is your baby experiencing any health problems?	❏	❏
2. Are you having problems with your baby feeding?	❏	❏
3. Are you having problems with your baby sleeping?	❏	❏

INFANT TEMPERAMENT

1. Would you consider your baby irritable or fussy?	❏	❏
2. Does your baby cry a lot?	❏	❏
3. Is your baby difficult to console or soothe?	❏	❏

MATERNITY BLUES

1. Did you experience a brief period of tearfulness and mood swings during the first week after delivery?	❏	❏

COMMENTS:

Source: Beck, C. T. (2002). Revision of the Postpartum Predictors Inventory. *Journal of Obstetric, Gynecologic, and Neonatal Nursing, 30*(4), 394–402 (Table 2 on PDPI, pp. 399–400). Washington, DC: AWHONN. © 2002 by the Association of Women's Health, Obstetric and Neonatal Nurses. All rights reserved.

those who might be experiencing postpartum depression so that early management might be initiated. The Postpartum Depression Screening Scale (PDSS) is another widely used and validated tool and has the highest sensitivity. No matter what approach used to assess for postpartum depression, enabling the woman's voice to be heard about her feelings of maternal role transition and how she is adjusting in this vulnerable time is of inestimable value. Listening to her story provides a critical emic (insider's) view of her circumstances as opposed to an etic (outsider's) view.

In providing daily care, observe the woman for objective signs of depression—anxiety, irritability, poor concentration, forgetfulness, sleep difficulties, appetite change, fatigue, and tearfulness—and listen for statements indicating feelings of failure and self-accusation. Severity and duration of symptoms should be noted. Report as soon as possible for further evaluation any behaviors and/or verbalizations that are bizarre or seem to indicate a potential for violence against herself or others, including the baby. Be aware that many normal physiologic changes of the puerperium are similar to symptoms of depression (lack of sexual interest, appetite change, fatigue). It is essential that observations be as specific and as objective as possible and that they are carefully documented.

Beck (2008) found that anxiety was a prominent feature of illness for some women, and suggested that women be assessed for their level of anxiety, particularly regarding infant care. Because of the strong association between interrupted sleep and postpartum depression and the finding that severe fatigue was an excellent predictor of postpartum depression, assessing fatigue level at least 2 weeks' postpartum by telephone may be helpful in predicting depression risk early. Restorative sleep improves one's ability to cope and make decisions, thereby producing a sense of better self-control.

A central challenge for nursing is identifying women at risk of suicide. Family members of the depressed woman should also be alert to signals that she may be intent on self-harm; advise them that threats should always be taken seriously. Tell family members to be especially vigilant for suicide when the woman seems to be feeling better.

If a woman admits that she has thought of hurting herself, assessment of the risk that she will follow through is imperative. The mnemonic **SAL** is useful for risk assessment:

- Is there a *Specific* plan with a designated time?
- Is there an *Accessible* weapon or other means?
- How *Lethal* is the method identified in the plan?

A specific plan that identifies a highly lethal method that is immediately accessible is evidence of very high risk of suicide. Immediate intervention is critical; emergency psychiatric hospitalization is likely necessary. Those considered a threat to themselves or others may be admitted to involuntary hospitalization for a minimum of 48 hours until further evaluation is complete.

Family members of the depressed woman should also be alert to signals that she may be intent on self-harm; they must be advised that threats should always be taken seriously. Clues to suicide that might be noted by family are comments such as, "I don't deserve to live," "Life is no longer worth living," or "You won't have to worry about me for long." Someone who is considering suicide may also telephone or write family or friends to say good-bye or give away prized possessions. Family members should be told to be especially vigilant for suicide when the woman seems to be feeling better.

Possible nursing diagnoses that may apply to a woman with a postpartum psychiatric disorder include the following (NANDA-I © 2014):

- *Coping, Ineffective*, related to postpartum depression
- *Parenting, Risk for Impaired*, related to postpartum mental illness
- *Violence, Self-Directed, Risk for*, related to possible suicide
- *Violence, Other-Directed, Risk for*, related to violence directed at newborn and other children related to depression

Planning and Implementation

Nurses working in antepartum settings or teaching childbirth classes play indispensable roles in helping prospective parents appreciate the lifestyle changes and role demands associated with parenthood. Offer realistic information and anticipatory guidance and debunk myths about the perfect mother or perfect newborn to help prevent postpartum depression. Social support teaching guides are available for nurses to help postpartum women explore their needs for postpartum support.

Alert the mother, spouse/partner, and other family members to the possibility of postpartum blues in the early days after birth and reassure them of the short-term nature of the condition. Describe the symptoms of postpartum depression and encourage the mother to call her healthcare provider if symptoms become severe, if they fail to subside quickly, or if at any time she feels she is unable to function. Encouraging the mother to plan how she will manage at home and providing concrete suggestions on how to cope will aid in her adjustment to motherhood. *Teaching Highlights: Primary Prevention Strategies for Postpartum Depression* provides suggestions that serve as important prevention measures for postpartum depression.

Information, emotional support, and assistance in providing or obtaining care for the baby may be needed. Assist family members by identifying community resources, making referrals to public health nursing services and social services, and providing a list of telephone numbers as well as emergency services that they may need. Postpartum follow-up is especially important, as well as visits from a psychiatric home health nurse.

COMMUNITY-BASED NURSING CARE

Home visits, especially for early discharge families, are invaluable in fostering positive adjustments for the new family. Telephone follow-up at 2 to 3 weeks postpartum to ask whether the mother is experiencing difficulties is also helpful. Monitoring for signs of depression or performing a brief screening at well-baby follow-ups also can be valuable for early identification and timely intervention.

Depression does appear to interfere with optimal mothering; there is less interaction between mother and child, more mood and cognitive development problems, and more visits to the doctor in these children. A diagnosis of postpartum depression or other psychiatric disorder will pose major problems for the family, especially the father/partner. The symptoms of these disorders are difficult to witness and may be harder to understand than physical problems such as hemorrhage and infection. The father/partner may feel hurt by the new mother's hostility, worry that she is becoming insane, or be baffled by her mood swings and lack of concern about herself, the newborn, or household responsibilities. Certainly, there is cause for concern about how the newborn and any other children are being affected. Very real practical matters—running the household; managing the children, including the totally dependent newborn; and caring for the mother—may be added to his usual routines and work responsibilities. It is not surprising that, even in the most supportive families, relationships may suffer in

---

TEACHING HIGHLIGHTS | Primary Prevention Strategies for Postpartum Depression

1. Celebrate childbirth but appreciate that it is a life-changing transition that can be stressful—at times it can seem overwhelming. Share your feelings with each other and/or others.
2. Consider keeping a journal in which you write down feelings. Not only is it emotionally cathartic, it provides a great memory book.
3. Appreciate that you do not have to know everything to be a good parent—it is okay to seek advice during this transition.
4. Connect with others who are parents—use them as a support and information network.
5. Set a daily schedule and follow it even if you do not feel like it. Structuring activity helps counteract the inertia that comes with feeling sad or unsettled.
6. Prioritize daily tasks. Decide what must be done and what can wait. Try to get one major thing done every day. Remember, you do not always have to look like a magazine fashion model.
7. Remember that you do not have to entertain or care for everyone who drops by. Doing something for someone else, however, often tends to make you feel better.
8. If people volunteer to help you with tasks or baby care, take them up on it. While your volunteer is in action, do something pleasurable or get some rest.
9. Maintain outside interests. Plan some time every day—even if it's just 15 minutes—to do something exclusively for "you" that is pleasurable.
10. Eat a healthful diet. Limit alcohol. Quit smoking. Get some exercise. (All of these can positively affect the immune system.)
11. Get as much sleep as possible. Rest whenever you can, such as when the baby is napping. If you have other young children, bring them onto your bed to read or play quietly while you lie down.
12. Limit major changes (moves, job changes, etc.) the first year insofar as possible.
13. Spend time with others.
14. If things get overwhelming, and you feel yourself slipping into depression, reach out to someone for help.
15. Attend a local postpartum support group if one is available. Consider also an international program such as Postpartum Support International.

response to these circumstances. It is often the father/partner or another close family member who in desperation makes contact with the healthcare agency. This is especially difficult when the mother is reluctant to admit she is suffering emotional difficulty or is too ill to recognize her own needs.

The integration of the newborn into the family and care of the newborn and other children can be further compromised by concurrent postpartum depression in the father/partner. With both parents having depressive symptoms, the newborn and other children are further at risk.

Evaluation

Expected outcomes of nursing care include the following:

- The woman's signs of depression are identified and she receives therapy quickly.
- The newborn is cared for effectively by the father or another support person until the mother is able to provide care.
- The mother and newborn will remain safe.
- The newborn is integrated into the family.

Focus Your Study

- Nursing assessment and intervention play a large role in preventing postpartum complications.
- The main causes of early postpartum hemorrhage and the appropriate nursing interventions include:
  - Uterine atony: perform fundal massage and check for clots.
  - Laceration of vagina and cervix (suspect if mother is bleeding heavily in presence of firmly contracted fundus): contact healthcare provider to suture the laceration.
  - Retained placental fragments (suspect if patient is bleeding, fundus is firm and no lacerations are present): thoroughly inspect placenta.
  - General assessment includes fundus for signs of bogginess, perineal pads for excessive vaginal bleeding and for normal changes in lochia progression.
- Late postpartum hemorrhage most often originates from retained placental fragments, and usually occurs 1 to 2 weeks after birth; although not usually as catastrophic as early hemorrhage, it may require readmission. The appropriate nursing interventions include: provide mother with discharge instructions, including information about possible complications.
- Thorough nursing history for causes and contributing factors for reproductive tract infection such as: C-section, prolonged labor preceding C-section, prolonged premature rupture of the amniotic membranes, oxytocin induction of labor, chorioamnionitis, and obstetric trauma such as: episiotomy; laceration of perineum, vagina, or cervix; and multiple vaginal exams. The most common postpartum infection is metritis, which is limited to the uterine cavity.
- To prevent postpartum reproductive tract infections, the nurse will:
  - Assess patient in general and incisions for signs of infection such as: temperature of 38.0°C (100.4°F) or higher, with temperature occurring on any 2 of the first 10 postpartum days, exclusive of the first 24 hours; foul, bloody discharge from vagina or incision; uterine tenderness; chills, malaise, lethargy, subinvolution of the uterus; lack of wound healing (REEDA).
  - Implement standard precautions; aseptic technique during labor, birth, and postpartum period.
  - Use good hand hygiene techniques to prevent transmission of infective material and provide clear instructions about wound care.
  - Administer antibiotics.
  - Address comfort needs related to hygiene, positioning, oral hygiene, and pain.

- A postpartum woman is at increased risk for developing urinary tract problems because of normal postpartum diuresis, increased bladder capacity, decreased bladder sensitivity from stretching or trauma, and possibly inhibited neural control of the bladder following the use of anesthetic agents. The nurse needs to assess for burning during urination, avoid urinary catheterization when possible and encourage the woman to void frequently.
- Mastitis is an inflammation of the breast primarily seen in breastfeeding women. Symptoms such as cracking of the nipples, plugged ducts, and redness and pain in the breast seldom occur before the fourth postpartum week. It is important to teach mother proper latching-on techniques and breast care. Continuation of breastfeeding is recommended as part of the treatment plan.
- Thromboembolic disease originating in the veins of the leg, thigh, or pelvis may occur antepartum or postpartum and carries with it the potential for creating a life-threatening pulmonary embolus. Nursing assessments of all body systems include frequent vital signs and peripheral pulses assessments, checking CMS, and assessment for Homans sign each shift. Thrombophlebitis signs and symptoms include pain and swelling in the lower extremities and localized heat and redness. To prevent thromboembolic disease, the nurse will assess lower extremities for signs of thrombophlebitis, encourage early ambulation, and assess for pulmonary embolus.
- Although many different types of psychiatric problems may be encountered in the postpartum period, postpartum blues is the most common. Postpartum blues episodes (feelings of overwhelming sadness and lack of desire to care for newborn) occur frequently in the week after birth, are associated with hormonal fluctuations, and are typically transient.
- Risk factors for postpartum depression should be screened for routinely during pregnancy and the postpartum period. Nurses should be alert to the risk of suicide and infanticide in cases of severe postpartum depression or psychosis.
- Telephone calls and home visits are effective measures for extending comprehensive care into the home setting of the postpartum family at risk. Support groups in which child care is available also can be an invaluable community service by professional nurses.

Clinical Reasoning in Action

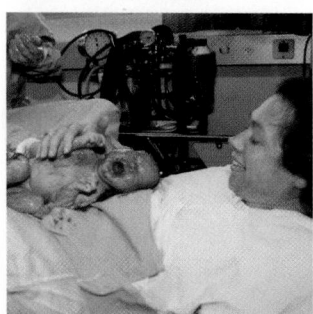

Betty Jones, a 32-year-old G4P2012, is admitted to the postpartum unit after the precipitous birth of a preterm (35 weeks' gestation) 4-lb baby girl followed by a postpartum tubal ligation. Betty's vital signs and postpartum assessment are within normal limits. She has an abdominal dressing that is dry and intact and she is able to void. Her IV with 10 units of oxytocin (Pitocin) is infusing well in her lower left arm. She admits to 3 on a pain scale of 10. Betty admits to active use of crack cocaine throughout her pregnancy, and smoked it most recently 5 hours before she gave birth. She is HIV positive with a CD4 count of 726 cells/mm^3 and was treated with zidovudine during the pregnancy, labor, and birth. She also has a history of genital herpes and was treated for chlamydial infection during the pregnancy. Her newborn has been admitted to the special care nursery because of her preterm status. Betty anticipates her baby will be taken into foster care when discharged from the nursery. Wishing to establish as much of a relationship with her baby as possible before that happens, she asks if she can breastfeed the baby while she is in the hospital.

1. What is your response to Betty's request to breastfeed her baby?

2. Over the course of the first postpartum day, Betty appears lethargic and spends most of her time sleeping. After her evening visitors leave, you observe that she is highly energetic and excitable. Would urine testing be useful to help determine if Betty has used cocaine this evening?

3. Betty wishes for an early discharge from the hospital. What physical criteria must be met before leaving the hospital?

4. Discuss when she should contact her healthcare provider after her discharge for follow-up.

References

Acosta, C. D., Kurinczuk, J. J., Lucas, D. N., Tuffnell, D. J., Sellers, S., & Knight, M. (2014) Severe maternal sepsis in the UK, 2011–2012: A national case-control study. Retrieved from http://www.Plosmedicine.org/article/info%3Adoi%2F10.1371%2Fjournal.pmed.1001672

Albacar, G., Sans, T., Martín-Santos, R., García-Esteve, L., Guillamat, R., Sanjuan, J., … Vilella, E. (2011). An association between plasma ferritin concentrations measured 48h after delivery and postpartum depression. *Journal of Affective Disorders, 131*(1–3), 136–142. doi:10.1016/j.jad.2010.11.00

American College of Obstetrics & Gynecology (ACOG). (2011). Thromboembolism in pregnancy. Practice Bulletin No. 123. *Obstetrics & Gynecology, 118,* 718–29.

American College of Obstetrics & Gynecology (ACOG) Committee on Patient Safety and Quality Improvement (2014). Preparing for clinical emergencies in obstetrics and gynecology. Committee Opinion No. 590. *Obstetrics & Gynecology, 123,* 722–725.

American Psychiatric Association (APA). (2013). *Diagnostic and statistical manual of mental disorders: DSM-5* (5th ed.). Arlington, VA: Author.

Ayadi, A. M., Robinson, N., Geller, S., & Miller, S. (2013). Advances in the treatment of postpartum hemorrhage. *Expert Review of Obstetrics & Gynecology, 8*(6), 525–537.

Beck, C. T. (2002). Revision of the postpartum depression predictors inventory. *Journal of Obstetric, Gynecologic, and Neonatal Nursing (JOGNN), 31*(4), 394–402.

Beck, C. T. (2008). *Postpartum mood and anxiety disorders: Case studies, research, and nursing care* (Practice Bulletin) (2nd ed.). Washington, DC: AWHONN.

Beck, C., & Watson, S. (2010). Subsequent childbirth after a previous traumatic birth. *Nursing Research, 59*(4), 241–249. doi:10.1097/NNR.0b013e3181e501fd

Bianco, A., Roccia, S., A., Pileggi, C., & Pavia, M. (2013). Postdischarge surveillance following delivery: The incidence of infections and associated factors. *American Journal of Infection Control, 41*(6), 549–553. doi:10.1016/j.ajic.2012.06.011

Burt, V. K., & Stein, K. (2013). Treatment of women. In R.E. Hales, S.C. Yudofsky, & L.W. Roberts (Eds.), *The American Psychiatric Publishing textbook of psychiatry* (6th ed.). Arlington, VA: American Psychiatric Publishing.

Cunningham, F. G., Leveno, K. J., Bloom, S. L., Spong, C. Y., Dashe, J. S., Hoffman, B. L., … Sheffield, J. S. (2014). *Williams obstetrics* (24th ed.). New York, NY: McGraw-Hill.

Distefano, M., Casarella, L., Amoroso, S., Di Stasi, C., Scambia, G., & Tropeano, G. (2013). Selective arterial embolization as a first-line treatment for postpartum hematomas. *Obstetrics & Gynecology, 121*(2 Pt 2 Suppl 1), 443–447. doi:10.1097/AOG.0b013e31827d90e1

Duff, P. (2014). Maternal and fetal infectious disorders. In R. K. Creasy & R. Resnik (Eds.), *Maternal–fetal medicine: Principles and practice* (7th ed., pp. 802–851). Philadelphia, PA: Saunders.

Fletcher, S., Grotegut, C. A., & James, A. H. (2012). Lochia patterns among normal women: A systematic review. *Journal of Women's Health (15409996), 21*(12), 1290–1294. doi:10.1089/jwh.2012.3668

Francois, K. E., & Foley, M. R. (2012). Antepartum and postpartum hemorrhage. In S. G. Gabbe, J. R. Niebyl, J. L. Simpson, M. B. Landon, H. L. Galan, E. R. Jauniaux, & D. A. Driscoll (Eds.), *Obstetrics: Normal and problem pregnancies.* (6th ed.). Philadelphia, PA: Saunders.

Hale, T. W., & Rowe, H. E. (2014). *Medications & mothers' milk 2014.* (16th ed.). Plano, TX: Hale Publishing..

Harvey, C. J., & Dildy, G. A. (2013). Obstetric hemorrhage. In N. H. Troiano, C. J. Harvey, & B. F. Chez (Eds.), *AWHONN's high-risk & critical care obstetrics* (3rd ed., pp. 246–273). Philadelphia, PA: Lippincott.

Jahanfar, S., Ng, C. J., & Teng, C. L. (2013). Antibiotics for mastitis in breastfeeding women. *Cochrane Database of Systematic Reviews,* Issue 2. Art. No.: CD005458. doi: 10.1002/14651858.CD005458.pub3.

James, D. C. (2014). Postpartum care. In K. R. Simpson & P. A. Creehan (Eds.), *AWHONN's perinatal nursing* (4th ed., pp. 530–580). Philadelphia, PA: Lippincott Williams & Wilkins.

Kellner, C., Greenberg, R., Murrough, J., Bryson, E., Briggs, M., & Pasculli, R. (2012). ECT in treatment-resistant depression. *American Journal of Psychiatry, 169*(12), 1238–1244. doi:10.1176/appi.ajp.2012.12050648

Kim, H. G., Geppert, J., Quan, T., Bracha, Y., Lupo, V., & Cutts, D. B. (2012). Screening for postpartum depression among low-income women using an interactive voice response system. *Maternal and Child Health Journal, 16*(4), 921–928. doi:10.1007/s10995-011-0817-6

Lawrence, R. M., & Lawrence, R. A. (2014). The breast and the physiology of lactation. In R. K. Creasy & R. Resnik (Eds.), *Maternal–fetal medicine: Principles and practice* (7th ed., pp. 112–130). Philadelphia, PA: Saunders.

Liberto, T. L. (2012). Screening for depression and help-seeking in postpartum women during well-baby pediatric visits: An integrated review. *Journal of Pediatric Healthcare, 26*(2), 109–117. doi:10.1016/j.pedhc.2010.06.012

Leung, A. N., & Lockwood, C. J. (2014). Thromboembolic disease in pregnancy. In R. K. Creasy & R. Resnik (Eds.), *Maternal–fetal medicine: Principles and practice* (7th ed., pp. 906–916). Philadelphia, PA: Saunders.

Logsdon, M., Tomasulo, R., Eckert, D., Beck, C., & Lee, C. (2012). Identification of mothers at risk for postpartum depression by hospital-based perinatal nurses. *MCN: The American Journal of Maternal Child Nursing, 37*(4), 218–225. doi:10.1097 /NMC.0b013e318251078b

Mousa, H., Blum, J., Senoun, G., Shakur, H., & Alfirevic, Z. (2014). Treatment for primary postpartum haemorrhage. *Cochrane Database of Systematic Reviews,* Issue 2. Art. No.: CD003249.

Oberg, A., Hernandez-Diaz, S., Palmsten, K., Almqvist, C., & Bateman, B. (2014). Patterns of recurrence of postpartum hemorrhage in a large population-based cohort. *American Journal of Obstetrics and Gynecology, 210*(229), e1–e8.

Pessel, C., & Tsai, M. C. (2013). The normal puerperium. In A. H. DeCherney, L. Nathan, N. Laufer, & A. S. Roman (Eds.), *Current diagnosis & treatment: Obstetrics & gynecology* (11th ed., pp. 190–213). New York, NY: McGraw-Hill.

Poggi, S. B. (2013). Postpartum hemorrhage and abnormal puerperium. In A. H. DeCherney, L. Nathan, N. Laufer, & A. S. Roman (Eds.), *Current diagnosis & treatment: Obstetrics & gynecology* (11th ed., pp. 349–368). New York, NY: McGraw- Hill.

Robbins, K. S., Martin, S. R., & Wilson, W. C. (2014). Intensive care considerations for the critically ill parturient. In R. K. Creasy & R. Resnik (Eds.), *Maternal–fetal medicine: Principles and practice* (7th ed., pp. 1182–1214). Philadelphia, PA: Saunders.

Rouse, D. J., (2013). What is new in postpartum hemorrhage? *Obstetrics & Gynecology, 122,* 693–694. doi:10.1097/AOG.0b013e3182a2c357

Rowe, H., Baker, T. E. C., & Hale, T. W. (2016). Drug therapy and breastfeeding. In K. Wambach & J. Riordan (Eds.), *Breastfeeding and human lactation* (5th ed., pp. 171–206). Burlington, MA: Jones & Bartlett Learning.

Sosa, M. E. (2014). Bleeding in pregnancy. In K. R. Simpson & P. A. Creehan (Eds.), *AWHONN's perinatal nursing* (4th ed., pp. 143–162). Philadelphia, PA: Lippincott Williams & Wilkins.

Thorp, J. M., & Laughton, S. K. (2014). Clinical aspects of normal and abnormal labor. In R. K. Creasy & R. Resnik (Eds.), *Maternal–fetal medicine: Principles and practice* (7th ed., pp. 673–706). Philadelphia, PA: Saunders

Vossbeck-Elsebusch, A. N., Freisfeld, C. & Ehring, T. (2014). Predictors of posttraumatic stress symptoms following childbirth. *BMC Psychiatry, 14,* 200. doi:10.1186/1471-244X-14-200

Walker, M. (2014). Common breastfeeding problems. In R. G. Jordan, J. L. Engstrom, J. A. Marfell, & C. L. Farley (Eds.), *Prenatal and postnatal care: A woman-centered approach.* (pp.499–513). Ames, IA: John Wiley & Sons.

Wambach, K. (2016) Breast-related problems. In K. Wambach & J. Riordan (Eds.), *Breastfeeding and human lactation,* (5th ed., pp. 319–357). Burlington, MA: Jones & Bartlett Learning.

Wetta, L. A., Szchowski, J. M., Seals, S., Mancuso, M. S., Biggo, J. R., & Tita, A. T. N., (2013) Risk factors for uterine atony/postpartum hemorrhage requiring treatment after vaginal delivery. *American Journal of Obstetrics and Gynecology, 209*(51), e1–6.

Whitmer, T. (2016). Physical and psychologic changes after childbirth. In S. Mattson & J. E. Smith (Eds.), *Core curriculum for maternal-newborn nursing* (6th ed., pp. 297–313). Philadelphia, PA: Association of Women's Health, Obstetric and Neonatal Nurses /Elsevier.

Witcher, P. M., & Hamner, L. (2013). Venous thromboembolism in pregnancy. In N. H. Troiano, C. J. Harvey, & B. F. Chez (Eds.), *AWHONN's high-risk & critical care obstetrics* (3rd ed., pp. 285–301). Philadelphia, PA: Lippincott.

Zaccardi, J. E. (2013). Managing urinary tract infections in women. *Clinical Advisor for Nurse Practitioners, 16*(2), 24–32.

Chapter 31
Growth and Development

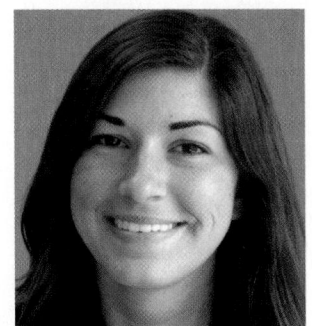

We want to help our adopted daughter Irena grow into a healthy and special child. She had challenges in her short life in Romania that we can only imagine. We worry about how we can help her grow and develop.

—Mother of Irena, 2 years old

∨ Learning Outcomes

31.1 Describe the major theories of development as formulated by Freud, Erikson, Piaget, Kohlberg, social learning theorists, and behaviorists.

31.2 Recognize risks to developmental progression and factors that protect against those risks.

31.3 Plan nursing interventions for children that are appropriate for each child's developmental state based on theoretical frameworks.

31.4 Explain contemporary developmental approaches such as temperament theory, ecologic theory, and the resilience framework.

31.5 Identify major developmental milestones for infants, toddlers, preschoolers, school-age children, and adolescents.

31.6 Synthesize information from several theoretical approaches to plan assessments of the child's physical growth and developmental milestones.

31.7 Describe the role of play in the growth and development of children.

31.8 Use data collected during developmental assessments to implement activities that promote development of children and adolescents.

C hildren develop as they interact with their surroundings. They learn skills at different ages, but the order in which they learn them is universal. Development is affected by factors such as nutrition and cultural practices, as well as the social situation in the country or neighborhood. While each child will develop in a unique manner influenced by genetic makeup, life experiences, and the interactions among these factors, certain principles of development assist parents and the nurse in fostering positive adaptations for the child.

This chapter covers general principles of growth and development and explores several theories related to childhood development, as well as their nursing applications. Each age group, from infancy through adolescence, is described in detail. Developmental milestones, physical and cognitive characteristics, play

patterns, and communication strategies are presented, as are conditions that interfere with usual developmental progression. The information provided helps guide developmentally appropriate care for children in each age group and in a variety of situations. These concepts can be applied when caring for all children, including those in special situations.

Principles of Growth and Development

It is essential to understand the concepts of growth and development when learning to care for children. A skilled pediatric nurse integrates knowledge of physical growth and psychosocial development into each child healthcare encounter. **Growth** refers to an increase in physical size. Growth represents quantitative changes such as height, weight, blood pressure, and number of words in the child's vocabulary. **Development** refers to a qualitative increase in capability or function. Developmental skills, such as the ability to sit without support or to throw a ball overhand, unfold in a complex manner influenced by the relationship between the child's innate capabilities and the stimuli and support provided in the environment. The quantitative and qualitative changes in body organ functioning, ability to communicate, and performance of motor skills develop over time and are key components in the process of planning pediatric health care.

Each child displays a unique maturational pattern during the process of development. Although the exact age at which skills emerge differs, the sequence or order of skill performance is uniform among children. Skill development proceeds according to two processes: from the head downward; and from the center of the body outward.

- **Cephalocaudal development** (Figure 31–1) proceeds from the head downward through the body and toward the feet. For example, at birth an infant's head is much larger proportionately than the trunk or extremities. Similarly, infants learn to hold up their heads before sitting and to sit before standing. Skills such as walking that involve the legs and feet develop last in infancy.

- **Proximodistal development** (see Figure 31–1) proceeds from the center of the body outward toward the extremities. For example, infants are first able to control the trunk, then the arms; only later are fine motor movements of the fingers possible. As the child grows, both physical and cognitive skills differentiate from general to more specific

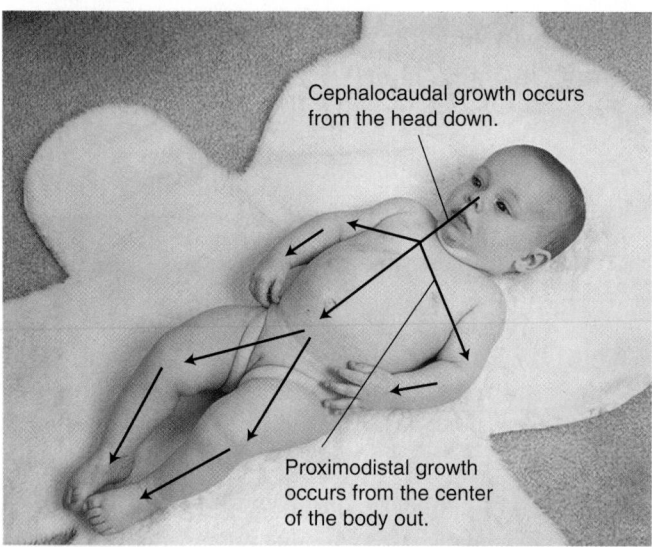

Cephalocaudal growth occurs from the head down.

Proximodistal growth occurs from the center of the body out.

Figure 31–1 Cephalocaudal and proximodistal development. **In normal cephalocaudal growth, the child gains control of the head and neck before the trunk and limbs. In normal proximodistal growth, the child controls arm movements before hand movements. For example, the child reaches for objects before being able to grasp them. Children gain control of their hands before their fingers, that is, they can hold things with the entire hand before they can pick something up with just their fingers.**

skills. Pediatric nurses use these concepts of predictable and sequential developmental direction to analyze the infant's and child's present state and to partner with parents to plan ways to encourage and support the next emerging developmental abilities.

During the childhood years, extraordinary changes occur in all aspects of development. Physical size, motor skills, cognitive ability, language, sensory ability, and psychosocial patterns all undergo major transformations. Nurses study normal patterns of development to identify children who demonstrate unexpected developmental findings. These assessments can guide the nurse in planning interventions for the child and family, such as referring the child for a diagnostic evaluation or rehabilitation, or teaching the parents how to provide adequate stimulation for the child. Nurses use **anticipatory guidance** to predict upcoming developmental tasks or needs of a child and to perform appropriate teaching related to them. When development is proceeding normally, the nurse uses his or her knowledge of these normal patterns to provide approaches based on the child's cognitive and language ability, to offer appropriate toys and activities during illness, and to respond therapeutically during interactions with the child. See Chapters 34 to 36 for specific application of developmental surveillance into health promotion visits. For situations with special challenges, such as in adoptions, additional interventions may be needed (see *Growth and Development*).

Growth and Development

About 15% of annual adoptions in the United States, or over 7000, are international adoptions. China, South Korea, Russia, Ethiopia, Uganda, Ukraine, and Haiti are among the most common countries of origin for orphans being adopted in the United States (U.S. Department of State, 2015). While all adoptions can be stressful for the new parents and child, international adoptions pose a unique set of circumstances that influence the child's development.

Parents need to protect themselves and others from infectious diseases when traveling to bring home a child from another country. They should consult their local health district and healthcare providers for a list of recommended immunizations for the country they are visiting. They should also obtain a list of medications and supplies to carry for themselves and the child, such as antidiarrheal medicine, decongestants, analgesics, bandages, and hand sanitizer (Children's Hospital of Philadelphia, 2012).

Parents require counseling to learn about cultural practices, language, and other differences they may encounter. Once they bring the child home, they will need support as the child grows to integrate the child's history and culture into their family. The moment when the child meets an adoptive parent may be seen as joyous by the parent but can be traumatic for the young child, who is being separated from familiar adults. Parents need preparation for establishing trust with the child (Children's Hospital of Philadelphia, 2012).

The adopted child should be examined once home for length, weight, and head circumference. If growth is delayed, continued monitoring and dietary interventions will be needed. The psychosocially based problem of avoidant/restrictive food intake disorder (formerly called eating disorder of infancy and childhood or failure to thrive) should also be considered. (See Chapter 32 for a thorough discussion of this condition.) Parasitic infection and chronic diseases are possible causes of continuing growth abnormalities. Perform developmental screening to provide a baseline for future developmental observations. Frequent physical and psychosocial assessments will be needed, and teaching is provided for parents to enhance development.

While a primary purpose of understanding and monitoring development is to be able to apply anticipatory guidance so that parents and nurses can provide the child with appropriate toys and experiences, there is also a very important link between safety and development. Developmental knowledge provides information about the major illness and accident risks for each age group as well as preventive techniques. For example, a 6-month-old child should never be left alone on a high surface, preschoolers must be carefully monitored while playing, and teenagers must demonstrate responsibility before being allowed to drive. As you read this chapter, try to identify the physical, cognitive, and social reasons that guide the safety precautions to be taken with children of various ages.

Major Theories of Development

Child development is a complex process. Many theorists have attempted to organize their observations of behavior into a description of principles or a set of stages. Each theory focuses on a particular facet of development. Most developmental theorists separate children into age groups by common characteristics (Table 31–1).

Freud's Theory of Psychosexual Development

THEORETICAL FRAMEWORK
Sigmund Freud (1856–1939) was a physician in Vienna, Austria. His work with adults experiencing a variety of neurologic disorders led him to develop an approach called *psychoanalysis*, which explored the driving forces of the unconscious mind. These psychoanalytic techniques led Freud to believe that early childhood experiences form the unconscious motivation for actions in later life. He believed that sexual energy is centered

TABLE 31–1 Developmental Age Groups

DEVELOPMENTAL STAGE	AGE GROUP	CHARACTERISTICS
Infancy	Birth to 12 months	Includes infants or babies up to 1 year of age, who all require a high level of care in daily activities.
Toddlerhood	1–3 years	Characterized by increased motor ability and independent behavior.
Preschool	3–6 years	The preschooler refines gross and fine motor ability and language skills and often participates in a preschool learning program.
School age	6–12 years	Begins with entry into a school system and is characterized by growing intellectual skills, physical ability, and independence.
Adolescence	12–18 years	Begins with entry into the teen years. Mature cognitive thought, formation of identity, and influence of peers are important characteristics of adolescence.

TABLE 31–2 Common Defense Mechanisms Used by Children

DEFENSE MECHANISM	DEFINITION	EXAMPLE
Regression	Return to an earlier behavior	A child who has been previously toilet trained becomes incontinent when a new infant is born into the family.
Repression	Involuntary forgetting of uncomfortable situations	An abused child cannot consciously recall episodes of abuse.
Rationalization	An attempt to make unacceptable feelings acceptable	A child explains hitting another because "he took my toy."
Fantasy	A creation of the mind to help deal with unacceptable fear	A hospitalized child who is weak pretends to be Superman.

in specific parts of the body at certain ages. Unresolved conflict and unmet needs at a certain stage lead to a fixation of development at that stage (Dunn & Craig, 2013).

Freud viewed the personality as a structure with three parts: The *id* is the basic sexual energy that is present at birth and drives the individual to seek pleasure; the *ego* is the realistic part of the person, which develops during infancy and searches for acceptable methods of meeting impulses; and the *superego* is the moral/ethical system, which develops in childhood and contains a set of values and a conscience (Dunn & Craig, 2013). The ego diverts impulses and protects itself from excess anxiety by use of **defense mechanisms**, including regression to earlier stages and repression or forgetting of painful experiences such as child abuse (Table 31–2).

Clinical Reasoning International Adoption Counseling
Michael and Alyssa had tried for several years to have a biologic child. After an unsuccessful in vitro fertilization, they decided to try to adopt a child. They explored opportunities with adoption agencies and learned that international adoption would be possible for them. They adopted 2-year-old Irena from Romania several months ago. Irena appears small for her age, but she seems to be thriving in her new environment. She is learning to say a few English words and is responding appropriately to care and interactions.

Despite thorough investigation of Michael and Alyssa by the adoption agency, they received only scant information about Irena's history. They were told that she was left at an orphanage by her birth mother when she was about 7 months old; the birth mother stated that the pregnancy and birth were normal. According to reports, the birth mother had decided to relinquish the child because she had two older children to care for and her husband had left home nearly a year before and had not been heard from since.

How can you work with Michael and Alyssa to ensure special attention to Irena's growth and healthcare needs, such as physical growth, language, and social skills? Consider both assessment and planned interventions.

What will Irena's cultural needs be as she grows older? How can Michael and Alyssa prepare to tell her about her adoption and background someday?

STAGES

Oral (Birth to 1 Year). The infant derives pleasure largely from the mouth, with sucking and eating as primary desires.

Anal (1 to 3 Years). The young child's pleasure is centered in the anal area, with control over body secretions as a prime force in behavior.

Phallic (3 to 6 Years). Sexual energy becomes centered in the genitalia as the child works out relationships with parents of the same and opposite sexes.

Latency (6 to 12 Years). Sexual energy is at rest in the passage between earlier stages and adolescence.

Genital (12 Years to Adulthood). Mature sexuality is achieved as physical growth is completed and relationships with others occur.

NURSING APPLICATION

Freud emphasized the importance of meeting the needs of each stage in order to move successfully into future developmental stages. The crisis of illness can interfere with normal developmental processes and add challenges for the nurse striving to meet an ill child's needs. For example, the importance of sucking in infancy guides the nurse to provide a pacifier for the infant who cannot have oral fluids. The preschool child's concern about sexuality guides the nurse to provide privacy and clear explanations during any procedures involving the genital area. It may be necessary to teach parents that masturbation by the young child is normal and to help parents deal with it through distraction or refocusing. The adolescent's focus on relationships suggests that the nurse should include questions about significant friends during history taking. Table 31–3 summarizes techniques the nurse can use to apply these theoretical concepts to the care of children.

Erikson's Theory of Psychosocial Development

THEORETICAL FRAMEWORK

Erik Erikson (1902–1994) studied Freud's theory of psychoanalysis under Freud's daughter, Anna. He later established his own developmental theory, which describes psychosocial stages during eight periods of human life. Five of Erikson's eight stages apply to children and are described below. For each stage, Erikson identified a crisis, that is, a particular challenge that exists for healthy personality development to occur (Erikson, 1963, 1968). The word "crisis" in this context refers to normal maturational social needs rather than to a single critical event. Each developmental crisis has two possible outcomes. When needs are met, the consequence is healthy and the individual moves on to future stages with particular strengths. When needs are not met, an unhealthy outcome occurs that will influence future social relationships.

STAGES

Trust Versus Mistrust (Birth to 1 Year). The task of the first year of life is to establish trust in the people providing care. Trust is fostered by provision of food, clean clothing, touch, and comfort. If basic needs are not met, the infant will eventually learn to mistrust others.

Autonomy Versus Shame and Doubt (1 to 3 Years). The toddler's sense of autonomy or independence is shown by controlling body excretions, saying no when asked to do

something, and directing motor activity and play. Children who are consistently criticized for expressions of autonomy or for lack of control—for example, during toilet training—will develop a sense of shame about themselves and doubt in their abilities.

Initiative Versus Guilt (3 to 6 Years). The young child initiates new activities and considers new ideas. This interest in exploring the world creates a child who is involved and busy. Constant criticism, on the other hand, leads to feelings of guilt and a lack of purpose.

Industry Versus Inferiority (6 to 12 Years). The middle years of childhood are characterized by development of new interests and by involvement in activities. The child takes pride in accomplishments in sports, school, home, and community. If the child cannot accomplish what is expected, however, the result will be a sense of inferiority.

Identity Versus Role Confusion (12 to 18 Years). In adolescence, as the body matures and thought processes become more complex, a new sense of identity, or self, is established. The self, family, peer group, and community are all examined and redefined. The adolescent who is unable to establish a meaningful definition of self will experience confusion in one or more roles of life.

NURSING APPLICATION

Erikson's theory is directly applicable to the nursing care of children. Health promotion and health maintenance visits in the community provide opportunities for helping caregivers meet children's needs. Parents benefit from learning what the child's developmental tasks are at each stage and from discussing ideas about how to encourage healthy psychosocial development. Such discussions also may highlight parental concerns and provide a forum for reassurance about normal developmental characteristics, such as a child who does not follow through on each activity as a preschooler or tries different hairstyles each month as an adolescent.

The child's usual support from family, peers, and others is interrupted by hospitalization. The challenge of hospitalization also adds a situational crisis to the normal developmental crisis a child is experiencing. Although the nurse may meet many of the hospitalized child's needs, continued parental involvement is necessary both during and after hospitalization to ensure progression through expected developmental stages (see Table 31–3).

Piaget's Theory of Cognitive Development

THEORETICAL FRAMEWORK

Jean Piaget (1896–1980) was a Swiss scientist who wrote detailed observations of the behavior of his own and other children. Based on these observations, Piaget formulated a theory of cognitive (or intellectual) development. He believed that the child's view of the world is influenced largely by age and maturational ability. Given nurturing experiences, the child's ability to think matures naturally (Ginsberg & Opper, 1988; Piaget, 1972). The child incorporates new experiences via **assimilation** and changes to deal with these experiences by the process of **accommodation**. An example of assimilation occurs when the infant uses reflexes to suck on objects that touch the lips. With more experience the infant accommodates to learn that not all objects are pleasant to suck and cognitive structures change to integrate and learn from the experiences.

TABLE 31–3 Nursing Applications of Theories of Freud, Erikson, and Piaget

AGE GROUP	THEORIST/DEVELOPMENTAL STAGE	CHARACTERISTICS OF STAGE	NURSING APPLICATIONS
Infant (birth to 1 year)	Freud: Oral stage	The baby obtains pleasure and comfort through the mouth.	When a baby is not able to take foods or fluids, offer a pacifier if not contraindicated. After painful procedures, offer a baby a bottle or pacifier or have the mother breastfeed.
	Erikson: Trust versus mistrust stage	The baby establishes a sense of trust when basic needs are met.	Hold the hospitalized baby often. Offer comfort after painful procedures. Meet the baby's needs for food and hygiene. Encourage parents to room in. Manage pain effectively with use of pain medications and other measures.
	Piaget: Sensorimotor stage	The baby learns from movement and sensory input.	Use crib mobiles, manipulative toys, wall murals, and bright colors to provide interesting stimuli and comfort. Use toys to distract the baby during procedures and assessments.
Toddler (1–3 years)	Freud: Anal stage	The child derives gratification from control over body excretions.	Ask about toilet training and the child's rituals and words for elimination during admission history. Continue child's normal patterns of elimination in the hospital. Do not begin toilet training during illness or hospitalization. Accept regression in toileting during illness or hospitalization. Have potty chairs available in hospital and childcare centers.
	Erikson: Autonomy versus shame and doubt stage	The child is increasingly independent in many spheres of life.	Allow self-feeding opportunities. Encourage child to remove and put on own clothes, brush teeth, or assist with hygiene. (A) If immobilization for a procedure is necessary, proceed quickly, providing explanations and comfort.
	Piaget: Sensorimotor stage (end); preoperational stage (beginning)	The child shows increasing curiosity and explorative behavior. Language skills improve.	Ensure safe surroundings to allow opportunities to manipulate objects. Name objects and give simple explanations.
Preschooler (3–6 years)	Freud: Phallic stage	The child initially identifies with the parent of the opposite sex but by the end of this stage identifies with the same-sex parent.	Be alert for children who appear more comfortable with male or female nurses, and attempt to accommodate them. Encourage parental involvement in care. Plan for playtime and offer a variety of materials from which to choose.
	Erikson: Initiative versus guilt stage	The child likes to initiate play activities.	Offer medical equipment for play to lessen anxiety about strange objects. (B) Assess children's concerns as expressed through their drawings. Accept the child's choices and expressions of feelings.

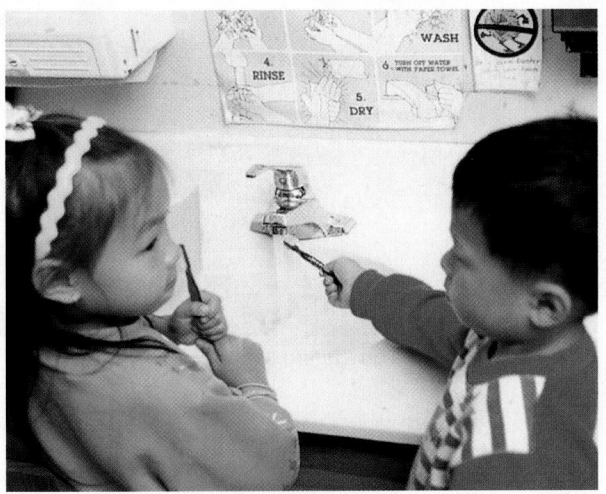

A

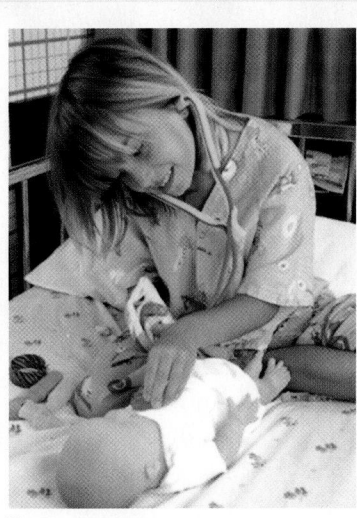

B

(continued)

TABLE 31–3 Nursing Applications of Theories of Freud, Erikson, and Piaget (*continued*)

AGE GROUP	THEORIST/DEVELOPMENTAL STAGE	CHARACTERISTICS OF STAGE	NURSING APPLICATIONS
	Piaget: Preoperational stage	The child is increasingly verbal but has some limitations in thought processes. Causality is often confused, so the child may feel responsible for causing an illness.	Offer explanations about all procedures and treatments. Clearly explain that the child is not responsible for causing an illness in self or family member.
School age (6–12 years)	Freud: Latency stage	The child places importance on privacy and understanding the body.	Provide gowns, covers, and underwear. Knock on door before entering. Explain treatments and procedures.
	Erikson: Industry versus inferiority stage	The child gains a sense of self-worth from involvement in activities.	Encourage the child to continue schoolwork while hospitalized. Encourage the child to bring favorite pastimes to the hospital. (*C*) Help the child adjust to limitations on favorite activities.
	Piaget: Concrete operational stage	The child is capable of mature thought when allowed to manipulate and see objects.	Give clear instructions about details of treatment. Show the child equipment that will be used in treatment.
Adolescent (12–18 years)	Freud: Genital stage	The adolescent's focus is on genital function and relationships.	Ensure access to gynecologic care for adolescent females and testicular examinations for adolescent males. Provide information on sexuality. Ensure privacy during health care. Have brochures and videos available for teaching about sexuality.
	Erikson: Identity versus role confusion stage	The adolescent's search for self-identity leads to independence from parents and reliance on peers.	Provide a separate recreation room for teens who are hospitalized. (*D*) Take health history and perform examinations without parents present. Introduce adolescent to other teens with same health problem.
	Piaget: Formal operational stage	The adolescent is capable of mature, abstract thought.	Give clear and complete information about health care and treatments. Offer both written and verbal instructions. Continue to provide education about the disease to the adolescent with a chronic illness, as mature thought now leads to greater understanding.

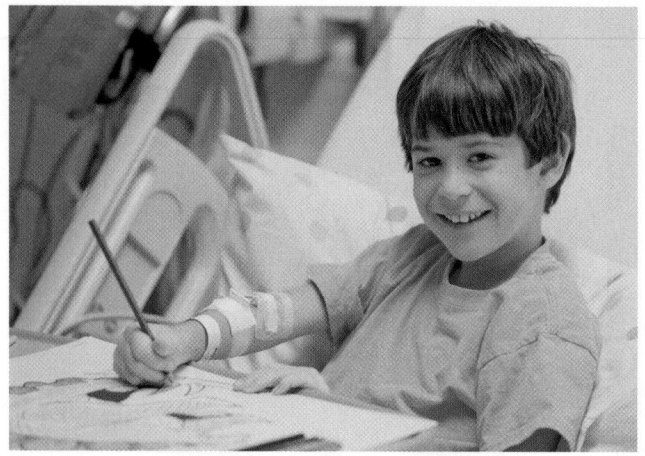

C iStock/Getty Images

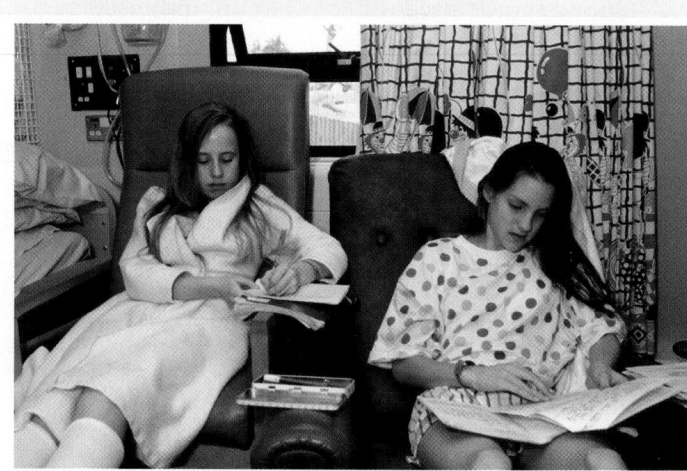

D Photofusion Picture Library/Alamy

STAGES

Sensorimotor (Birth to 2 Years).
Infants learn about the world by input obtained through the senses and by their motor activity. Six substages are characteristic of this stage.

Use of Reflexes (Birth to 1 Month).
The infant begins life with a set of reflexes such as sucking, rooting, and grasping. By using these reflexes, the infant receives stimulation via touch, sound, smell, and vision. The reflexes thus pave the way for the first learning to occur.

Primary Circular Reactions (1 to 4 Months).
Once the infant responds reflexively, the pleasure gained from that response causes repetition of the behavior. For example, if a toy grasped reflexively makes noise and is interesting to look at, the infant will grasp it again.

Secondary Circular Reactions (4 to 8 Months).
Awareness of the environment grows as the infant begins to connect cause and effect. The sounds of bottle preparation will lead to excited behavior. If an object is partially hidden, the infant will attempt to uncover and retrieve it.

Coordination of Secondary Schemes (8 to 12 Months).
Intentional behavior is observed as the infant uses learned behavior to obtain objects, create sounds, or engage in other pleasurable activities. **Object permanence** (the knowledge that something continues to exist even when out of sight) begins when the infant remembers where a hidden object is likely to be found; it is no longer "out of sight, out of mind." However, the concept of object permanence is not fully developed. The infant knows the parent well, objects to new people, and seems very worried when the parent leaves. Other caretakers may be rejected because the infant does not understand that the parent will return. This phase of "stranger anxiety" is quite common and heralds the infant's growing recognition of and desire to be cared for by the parent.

Tertiary Circular Reactions (12 to 18 Months).
Curiosity, experimentation, and exploration dominate as the toddler tries out actions to learn results. At this age, children turn objects in every direction, place them in their mouths, use them for banging, and insert them in containers as they explore their qualities and uses.

Mental Combinations (18 to 24 Months).
Language provides a new tool for the toddler to use in understanding the world. Language enables the child to think about events and objects before or after they occur. Object permanence is now fully developed as the child actively searches for objects in various locations and out of view. The child who has had successful separations from the parents followed by their return, such as hours spent in another's home or childcare center, begins to understand that the missing parent will return.

Preoperational (2 to 7 Years).
The young child thinks by using words as symbols, but logic is not well developed. Two substages characterize this stage.

Preconceptual Substage.
During the preconceptual substage (2 to 4 years), vocabulary and comprehension increase greatly but the child is egocentric (i.e., unable to see things from the perspective of another).

Intuitive Substage.
In the intuitive substage (4 to 7 years), the child relies on transductive reasoning (drawing conclusions from one general fact to another). For example, when a child disobeys a parent and then falls and breaks an arm that same day, the child may ascribe the broken arm to bad behavior.

Cause-and-effect relationships are often unrealistic or a result of magical thinking (the belief that events occur because of thoughts or wishes).

Additional characteristics noted in the thought of preschoolers include *centration*, or the ability to consider only one aspect of a situation at a time, and *animism*, or giving life to inanimate objects because they move, make noise, or have certain other qualities.

Concrete Operational (7 to 11 Years).
Transductive reasoning has given way to a more accurate understanding of cause and effect. The child can reason quite well if concrete objects are used in teaching or experimentation. The concept of conservation (that matter does not change when its form is altered) is learned at this age.

Formal Operational (11 Years to Adulthood).
Fully mature intellectual thought has now been attained. The adolescent can think abstractly about objects or concepts and consider different alternatives or outcomes.

NURSING APPLICATION
Piaget's theory is essential to pediatric nursing. The nurse must understand a child's thought processes in order to design stimulating activities and meaningful, appropriate teaching plans. What activities could be planned for a hospitalized child based on his or her expected cognitive level? How can cognitive development be encouraged in a school-age child receiving home health services? Understanding a child's concept of time suggests how far in advance to prepare that child for procedures. Similarly, decisions about offering manipulative toys, reading stories, drawing pictures, or giving the child reading material to explain healthcare measures depend on the child's cognitive stage of development (see Table 31–3).

Kohlberg's Theory of Moral Development

THEORETICAL FRAMEWORK
Lawrence Kohlberg (1927–1987) was a German theorist who used Piaget's cognitive theory as a basis for his theory of moral development. He presented stories involving moral dilemmas to children and adults and asked them to solve the dilemmas. Kohlberg then analyzed the motives they expressed when making decisions about the best course to take. Based on the explanations given, Kohlberg established three levels of moral reasoning. Although he provided age guidelines, he stated that they are approximate and that many people never reach the highest (postconventional) stage of development (Santrock, 2012).

STAGES

Preconventional (4 to 7 Years).
Decisions are based on the desire to please others and to avoid punishment.

Conventional (7 to 12 Years).
Conscience, or an internal set of standards, becomes important. Rules are important and must be followed to please other people and "be good."

Postconventional (12 Years and Older).
The individual has internalized ethical standards on which to base decisions. Social responsibility is recognized. The value in each of two differing moral approaches can be considered and a decision made.

NURSING APPLICATION
Decision making is required in many areas of health care. Children can be assisted to make decisions about health care and to

consider alternatives when available. Keep in mind that young children may agree to participate in research simply because they want to comply with adults and appear cooperative. Guidelines for child participation in research are available (see Chapter 1).

Parents can be provided with information so that they can assist their children in moral judgments. Encourage talking with a child or adolescent about how a particular decision was made. Parents can then add information and help the child learn to integrate more factors into decision making. Talking about the process is important in helping children progress to higher moral development stages. Focusing on the feelings of others, using positive discipline techniques, and clearly identifying positive and negative behaviors are important.

Social Learning Theory

THEORETICAL FRAMEWORK
Originally from Canada, psychologist Albert Bandura (1925–) has conducted research at Stanford University for many years. He believes that children learn attitudes, beliefs, customs, and values through their social contacts with adults and other children. Children imitate (or model) the behavior they see; if the behavior is positively reinforced, they tend to repeat it. The external environment and the child's internal processes are key elements in social learning theory (Bandura, 1986, 1997a).

Bandura believes that an important determinant of behavior is self-efficacy, or the expectation that someone can produce a desired outcome. For example, if adolescents believe they can avoid use of drugs or alcohol, they are more likely to do so. A child who has confidence in his or her ability to exercise regularly or lose weight has a greater chance of success with these behavior changes. Parents who have confidence in their ability to care adequately for their infants are more likely to do so (Bandura, 1997b). See *Evidence-Based Practice: Concept of Self-Efficacy* for further examples of application of the concept of self-efficacy.

NURSING APPLICATION
The importance of modeling behavior can readily be applied in health care. Children are more likely to cooperate if they see adults or other children performing a task willingly. A frightened child may watch another child perform vision screening or have blood drawn and then decide to allow the procedure to take place. Contact with positive role models is useful when teaching children and adolescents self-care for chronic diseases such as diabetes. Give positive reinforcement for desired performance.

Nurses can use the concept of self-efficacy to increase the chance of success with lifestyle behavior changes. For example, encouraging youth who are trying to quit smoking, providing them with role models, and pointing out parental successes with their children all demonstrate methods of fostering self-efficacy.

Behaviorism

THEORETICAL FRAMEWORK
John Watson (1878–1958) was an American scientist who applied the research of animal behaviorists like Pavlov and Skinner to children. Pavlov and, later, Skinner worked with animals, presenting a stimulus such as food and pairing it with another stimulus such as a ringing bell. Eventually the animal being fed began to salivate when the bell rang. As Skinner and, then, Watson began to apply these concepts to children, they showed that behaviors can be elicited by positive reinforcement, such as a

---

EVIDENCE-BASED PRACTICE | Concept of Self-Efficacy

Clinical Question
How can nurses use the concept of self-efficacy when planning interventions for children and families?

The Evidence
Parental self-efficacy is the belief that parents can manage a range of tasks and situations in caring for their children. Higher self-efficacy scores in parents were predictive of greater success in treatment of young children who were overweight (Davies, Terhorts, Nakonechny, et al., 2014). The authors of this literature review also established an Internet site to provide information and enhance self-efficacy in parents regarding healthy lifestyles for children (Davies et al., 2014).

Mothers who have a greater degree of self-efficacy about ability to breastfeed are significantly more likely to begin and to continue breastfeeding. A Breastfeeding Self-Efficacy Scale has been developed to identify risk and protective factors that influence the self-efficacy of new mothers. Evaluating breastfeeding self-efficacy in Hispanic women was able to inform the topics for teaching that would best promote breastfeeding (Joshi, Trout, Aguirre, et al., 2014).

An intervention with over 1000 students in grades 5 and 6 was effective in increasing youth self-efficacy regarding television viewing time and decreasing television viewing time (Salmon et al., 2011).

Best Practice
In addition to providing information about health behaviors, nurses need to integrate methods to increase self-efficacy in teaching projects with families. Assessments should be designed to identify self-efficacy of parents and children around health topics of interest. When planning interventions to encourage health behaviors in children and adolescents, assess the youth's beliefs that the new behaviors are important and that they can be adopted. Include interventions that demonstrate that others have adopted the health behaviors and plan approaches to enhance the child's belief in ability to change.

Clinical Reasoning
Plan a teaching project about the importance of physical activity and healthy eating for presentation to a group of 12-year-olds. What approaches will enhance the self-efficacy of the children? How would interventions to enhance self-efficacy differ for young elementary school children from those in middle or high school? What theoretical approaches discussed earlier in this chapter help you to understand the cognitive abilities of children at various ages and suggest ways to influence their self-efficacy?

food treat, or extinguished by negative reinforcement, such as scolding or withdrawal of attention. Watson believed that he could make a child into anyone he desired—from a professional to a thief or beggar—simply by reinforcing behavior in certain ways (Santrock, 2012).

NURSING APPLICATION

Behaviorism has been criticized for being simplistic and for its denial of people's inherent capacity to respond willfully to events in the environment. However, this theory does have some use in health care. When particular behaviors are desired, healthcare providers can establish positive reinforcement to encourage these behaviors. Using behavioral techniques, nurses may influence the behavior of children by giving a sticker to a child after a physical examination or blood draw. Parents often use reinforcement in toilet training and other skills learned in childhood.

Ecologic Theory

THEORETICAL FRAMEWORK

There is controversy among theorists concerning the relative importance of heredity versus environment—or nature versus nurture—in human development. **Nature** refers to the genetic or hereditary capability of an individual. **Nurture** refers to the effects of the environment on a person's performance (Figure 31–2). Piaget believed in the importance of internal cognitive structures that unfold at their appointed times, given any environment that provides basic opportunities. He emphasized the strength of nature. The behaviorist John Watson, on the other hand, believed that behaviors are primarily shaped by environmental responses; he thus stressed the predominance of nurture. Contemporary developmental theories increasingly recognize the interaction of nature and nurture in determining the child's development.

Urie Bronfenbrenner (1917–2005), a professor at Cornell University, formulated the ecologic theory of development to explain the unique relationship of the child with all of life's experiences or systems (Bronfenbrenner, 1986, 2005;

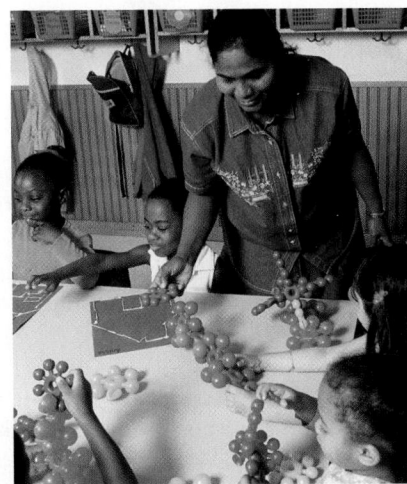

Figure 31–2 **An example of nurturing. Children exposed to pleasant stimulation and who are supported by an adult will develop and refine their skills faster. Group activities such as these provide an opportunity for both motor skill and psychosocial development. Can you identify which skills are being developed?**

Bronfenbrenner, McClelland, Ceci, et al., 1996). **Ecologic theory** emphasizes the presence of mutual interactions between the child and these various settings or systems. Neither nature nor nurture is considered of more importance. Bronfenbrenner believed each child brings a unique set of genes—as well as specific attributes such as age, gender, health, and other characteristics—to his or her interactions with the environment. The child then interacts in many settings at different levels or systems (Figure 31–3).

LEVELS/SYSTEMS

Microsystem. This level is defined as the daily, consistent, close relationships such as home, child care, school, friends, and neighbors. For the child with a chronic illness requiring regular care, the healthcare providers may even be part of the microsystem. In the ecologic model, the child influences each of the settings in the microsystem, in addition to being influenced by them, with reciprocal interactions.

Mesosystem. This level includes relationships of microsystems with one another. For example, two microsystems for most children are the home and the school. The relationships between these microsystems are shown by parents' involvement in their children's school. This involvement, in turn, influences the effects of the home and school settings on the children.

Exosystem. This level is composed of those settings that influence the child even though the child is not in close daily contact with the system. Examples include the parents' jobs and the governing board of the local school district. Although the child may not go to the parents' workplaces, the child can be influenced by policies related to health care, sick leave, inflexible work hours, overtime, or travel, or even by the mood of the boss (through its impact on the parent). Likewise, when a local school board votes to ban certain books or to finance a field trip, the child is influenced by these decisions; the child, in turn, can help establish an atmosphere that will guide future school board decisions.

Macrosystem. This level includes the beliefs, values, and behaviors expressed in the child's environment. Culture is a powerful influence in the macrosystem, as is the political system. For instance, a democratic system creates different beliefs, values, and even eating practices than an anarchic system.

Chronosystem. This final level brings the perspective of time to the previous settings. The time period during which the child grows up influences views of health and illness. For example, the experiences of children with influenza in the 19th versus the 20th century were quite different. The age of the parent, child, and other family members also influences views of health.

NURSING APPLICATION

Nurses use ecologic theory when they assess the child's settings to identify influences on development. Table 31–4 provides an assessment tool based on this theory. Interventions are planned to enhance the strengths of the child's settings and to improve on areas that are not supportive.

Temperament Theory

THEORETICAL FRAMEWORK

In contrast to behaviorists such as Watson or maturational theorists such as Piaget, Stella Chess and Alexander Thomas recognize the innate qualities of personality that each individual brings to the events of daily life. They, like Bronfenbrenner, believe the

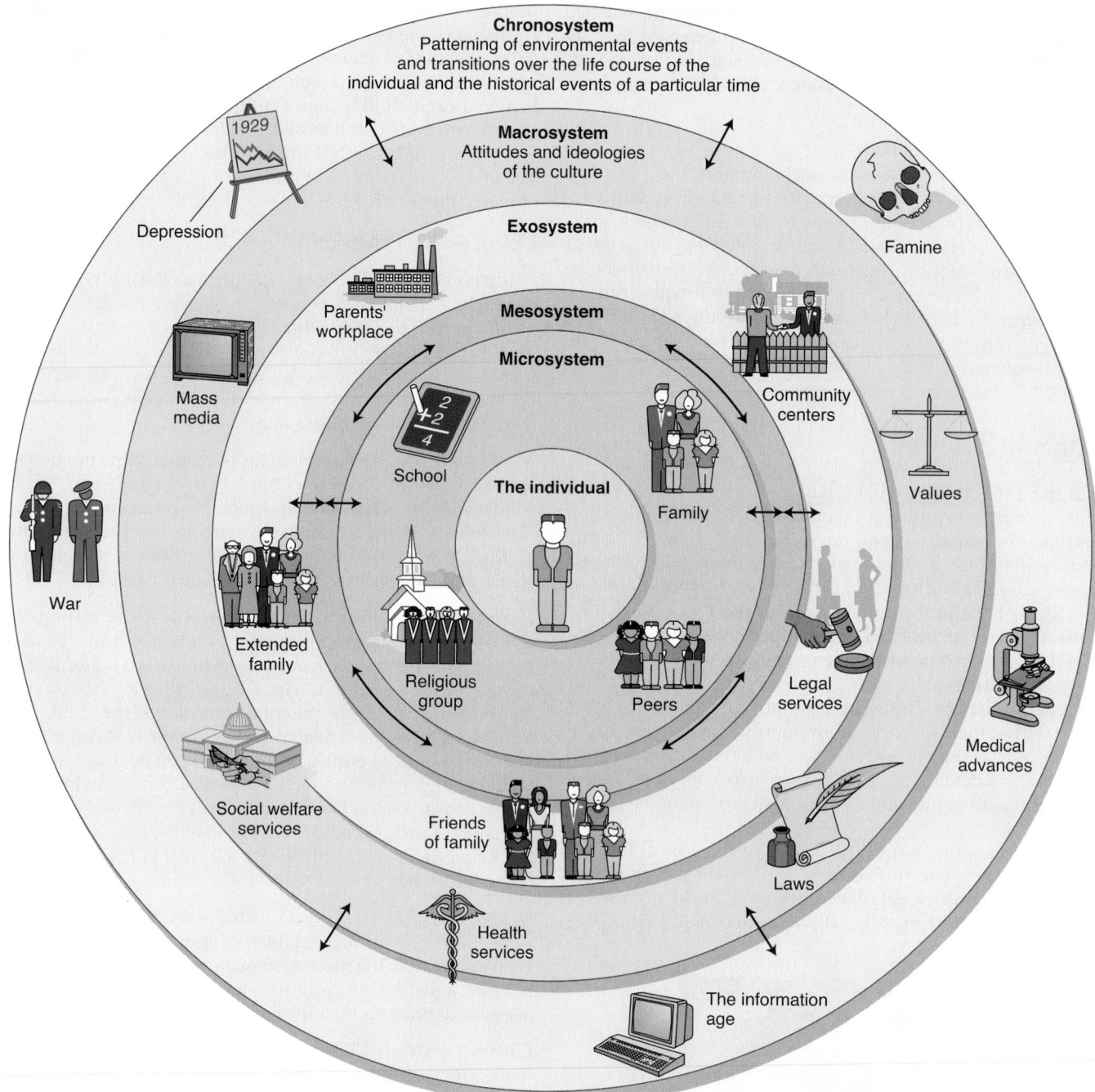

Figure 31–3 Bronfenbrenner's ecologic theory of development views the individual as interacting within five levels or systems.

SOURCE: Data from Santrock, J. W. (2007). *Life-span development.* Madison, WI: Brown & Benchmark. Based on Bronfenbrenner's (1979, 1986) works in Contexts of child rearing: Problems and prospects. *American Psychologist, 34,* 844–850; Ecology of the family as a context for human development: Research perspectives. *Developmental Psychology, 22,* 723–742.

child is an individual who both influences and is influenced by the environment. However, Chess and Thomas focus on one specific aspect of development—the wide spectrum of behaviors possible in children—identifying nine parameters of response to daily events (Table 31–5). Their theory is based on a research study entitled the New York Longitudinal Study, which began with infants in 1956 and has continued into the adulthood of these participating individuals. By careful observations of responses to life events, Chess and Thomas identified characteristics of personality that provide the basis for the study on temperament. Infants

generally display clusters of responses, which are classified into three major personality types (Table 31–6). Although most children do not demonstrate all behaviors described for a particular type, they usually show a grouping indicative of one personality type (Chess & Thomas, 1995, 1996, 1999).

Recent research demonstrates that personality characteristics displayed during infancy are often consistent with those seen later in life. Predicting future characteristics is not possible, however, because of the complex and dynamic interaction of personality traits and environmental reactions.

TABLE 31–4 Assessment of Ecologic Systems in Childhood—Bronfenbrenner

MICROSYSTEMS	MESOSYSTEMS	EXOSYSTEMS	MACROSYSTEMS	CHRONOSYSTEMS
Parents	Parents' involvement in child care or school	Community centers	Cultural group membership	Child's and parents' ages
Significant others in close contact	Parents' involvement in community	Local political influences	Beliefs and values of group	Period in historic time
Childcare arrangements	Parents' relationships with significant others (e.g., grandparents, care providers)	Parents' work	Political structure	
School		Parents' friends and activities		
Neighborhood contacts		Social services		
Clubs		Health care		
Friends, peers	Influences of religious community (e.g., church, synagogue, mosque) or parents and school	Libraries		
Religious community (e.g., churches, synagogues, mosques)				

TABLE 31–5 Nine Parameters of Personality

PARAMETER	DESCRIPTION	SCORING
1. Activity level	The degree of motion during eating, playing, sleeping, bathing.	Scored as high, medium, or low
2. Rhythmicity	The regularity of schedule maintained for sleep, hunger, elimination.	Scored as regular, variable, or irregular
3. Approach or withdrawal	The response to a new stimulus such as a food, activity, or person.	Scored as approachable, variable, or withdrawn
4. Adaptability	The degree of adaptation to new situations.	Scored as adaptive, variable, or nonadaptive
5. Threshold of responsiveness	The intensity of stimulation needed to elicit a response to sensory input, objects in the environment, or people.	Scored as high, medium, or low
6. Intensity of reaction	The degree of response to situations.	Scored as positive, variable, or negative
7. Quality of mood	The predominant mood during daily activity and in response to stimuli.	Scored as positive, variable, or negative
8. Distractibility	The ability of environmental stimuli to interfere with the child's activity.	Scored as distractible, variable, or nondistractible
9. Attention span and persistence	The amount of time devoted to activities (compared with other children of the same age) and the degree of ability to stick with an activity in spite of obstacles.	Scored as persistent, variable, or nonpersistent

Source: Data from Chess, S., & Thomas, A. (1996). *Temperament: Theory and practice*. Philadelphia, PA: Brunner/Mazel, Publishers.

Many other researchers have expanded the work of Chess and Thomas, developing assessment tools for temperament types. The concept of "goodness of fit" is an outgrowth of this theory. Goodness of fit refers to whether parents' expectations of their child's behavior are consistent with the child's temperament type. There is a "good fit" when the properties of the environment are in accord with the child's capabilities, characteristics, and style of behavior, and when the people in the environment know how to best support the child (The Center for Parenting Education, 2014). For example, an infant who is very active and reacts strongly to verbal stimuli may be unable to sleep well when placed in a room with older siblings. A child who is slow to warm up may not perform well in the first few months at a new school, much to the parents' disappointment. When parents understand a child's temperament characteristics, they are better able to shape the environment to meet the child's needs.

NURSING APPLICATION

The concept of personality type or temperament is a useful one for nurses. Nurses can assess the temperament of young children and alter the environment to meet their needs. This may involve moving a hospitalized child to a single room to ensure adequate rest if the child is easily stimulated, or allowing a shy child time to become accustomed to new surroundings and equipment before beginning procedures or treatments.

Parents are often relieved to learn about temperament characteristics. They learn to appreciate their children's qualities and to adapt the environment to meet the children's needs. A burden of guilt can also be lifted from parents who feel that they are responsible for their child's actions. Parents may be taught ways to enhance goodness of fit between the child's personality and the environment (Chess & Thomas, 1999) (Table 31–7).

TABLE 31–6 Patterns of Temperament

PATTERN	DESCRIPTION	% OF N.Y. LONGITUDINAL STUDY PARTICIPANTS
The "easy" child	Generally moderate in activity Shows regularity in patterns of eating, sleeping, and elimination Usually positive in mood Adapts to new situations when subjected to new stimuli Able to accept rules Works well with others	Approximately 40%
The "difficult" child	Displays irregular schedules for eating, sleeping, and elimination Adapts slowly to new situations and persons Displays a predominantly negative mood Intense reactions to the environment common	Approximately 10%
The "slow-to-warm-up" child	Initial withdrawal, followed by gradual, quiet, slow interaction with the environment Adapts slowly to new situations Mild reactions to environment	Approximately 15%
Mixed	Some of each personality type's characteristics apparent	Approximately 35%

Source: Chess, S., & Thomas, A. (1995). *Temperament in clinical practice.* New York, NY: Guilford Press.

TABLE 31–7 Ways to Improve Goodness of Fit Between Parents and Child

CHILD'S BEHAVIOR	PARENTS' ADAPTATIONS
Extremely active	Plan periods of active play several times a day. Have restful periods before bedtime to foster sleep.
Shy	Allow time to adapt at own pace to new people and situations.
Easily stimulated	Have quiet room for sleeping for an infant. Have quiet room for homework for a school-age child.
Short attention span	Provide projects that can be completed in a short period. Gradually encourage longer periods at activities.

Resiliency Theory

THEORETICAL FRAMEWORK

Why do some children coming from similar backgrounds have such different behavioral outcomes? The resiliency theory examines the individual's characteristics as well as the interaction of these characteristics with the environment. **Resilience** is the ability to function with healthy responses even when faced with significant stress and adversity (Benard, 2014; Henderson, Benard, & Sharp-Light, 2007). In this model, the individual or family members experience a crisis that provides a source of stress, and the family interprets or deals with the crisis based on resources available. Families and individuals have **protective factors**, which are characteristics that provide strength and assistance in dealing with crises, and **risk factors**, which are characteristics that promote or contribute to their challenges (Cairns, Yap, Pilkington, et al., 2014). Risk and protective factors can be identified in children, in their families, and in their communities. (See Chapter 42 for further description of the interplay of social and environmental factors with individual characteristics.) A crisis for a young child might be a transfer to a new childcare provider. Protective factors could involve past positive experiences with new people, an "easy" temperament, and the new childcare provider's awareness of adaptation needs of young children to new experiences. Risk factors for a similar child might be repeated moves to new childcare providers, limited close relationships with adults, and a "slow-to-warm-up" temperament.

Once confronted by a stress or crisis, the child and family first experience the **adjustment phase**, characterized by disorganization and unsuccessful attempts at meeting the crisis. In the **adaptation phase**, the child and family meet the challenge and use resources to deal with the crisis. Adaptation may lead to increasing resilience as well when the child and family learn about new resources and inner strengths and develop the ability to deal more effectively with future crises. Components and examples are described in Table 31–8.

NURSING APPLICATION

Nurses gather information about the individual characteristics, prior life experiences, and environmental factors that act as protective and risk factors for children. Table 31–9 lists questions that can be helpful as the nurse gathers information from a child or family members. Nurses then use concepts of resiliency theory in planning interventions for children and families. Nursing strategies can target risk factors, such as encouraging gun safety in families with firearms, and by teaching about use of gun trigger locks and locked gun cabinets. In addition, protective factors can be emphasized, such as encouraging holding and verbalization to parents of infants to provide an environment that allows for trust establishment and speech development.

Influences on Development

Both nature and nurture are important in determining individual patterns of development. The interaction of these two forces can explain differences in time frames for acquisition of developmental skills, personality variations between identical twins, and other unique characteristics of individuals. Genetic

TABLE 31–8 Components of Intervention in the Resiliency Wheel

COMPONENT	EXAMPLE OF INTERVENTIONS
Provide caring and support.	Listen to concerns. Provide information based on developmental level.
Set and communicate high expectations.	Express confidence in child's ability to succeed. Provide youth and families with resources.
Provide opportunities for meaningful participation.	Facilitate the youth's problem solving about ways to improve situations.
Increase prosocial bonding.	Assist youth to work with others on positive, purposeful activities. Facilitate community participation.
Set and communicate high expectations.	Communicate rules and establish routines. Assist families in setting clear expectations for behaviors and consequences.
Teach life skills.	Encourage communication of thoughts and feelings. Facilitate critical thinking and problem solving skills.

Source: Adapted from Resiliency in Action. (2014). *The resiliency wheel*. Retrieved from http://www.resiliency.com/free-articles-resources/crisis-response-and-the-resiliency-wheel/

TABLE 31–9 Assessment Questions to Determine Resilience Capability

CATEGORY	QUESTIONS
To determine risk factors, ask:	• Describe the event that occurred and what it has been like for your family. • What other stressors do you have in your family right now? • Are there financial worries? • Are there things you think and worry about late at night? • Describe your job, your friends. • What is a typical day like? • Describe your neighborhood. • Do you have friends, people to call in emergencies?
To determine protective factors, ask:	• What gives you strength? • How do you deal with this stress? • What do you think you do well in your family? • Who do you call when you need help? • Do you have a computer? Internet access? • Are you religious? Spiritual? • Do you exercise regularly? • How do you spend free time?

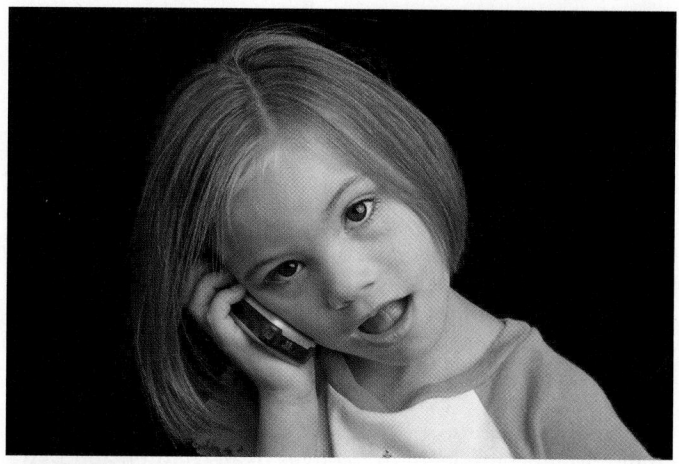

Figure 31–4 **A child with fetal alcohol syndrome.**

SOURCE: Rick's Photography/Shutterstock.

and environmental factors interact and contribute to individual differences in rates and outcomes of child development.

Genetic inheritance plays an important part in the child's potential and the unfolding of developmental milestones. See Chapter 3 for a description of chromosomes and genes. Every chromosome carries many genes that determine physical characteristics, intellectual potential, personality type, and other traits. Children are born with the potential for certain features; however, their interaction with the environment influences how and to what extent particular traits are manifested.

Some Asian cultures calculate age from the time of conception. This practice acknowledges the profound influence of the prenatal period. The mother's nutrition and general state of health play a part in pregnancy outcome. Poor nutrition can lead to small infants and infants with compromised neurologic performance, slow development, or impaired immune status with resultant high disease rates. Low maternal stores of iron can result in anemia in the infant (American Academy of Pediatrics, 2013). Maternal smoking is associated with low-birth-weight infants. Ingestion of alcoholic beverages, including beer and wine, during pregnancy may lead to fetal alcohol syndrome (Figure 31–4). Illicit drug use by the mother may result in neonatal addiction, convulsions, hyperirritability, poor social responsiveness, and other neurologic disturbances.

Even prescription or over-the-counter drugs may adversely affect the fetus. This was brought to general attention with the drug thalidomide, which was commonly used in Europe to treat nausea during the 1950s. This drug resulted in the birth of infants with limb abnormalities to women who used the drug during pregnancy. Differences in physiology related to gastric emptying, renal clearance, drug distribution, and other factors contribute to variations in pharmacokinetics during pregnancy. Drugs can cause teratogenesis (abnormal development of the fetus) or mutagenesis (permanent changes in the fetus's genetic material). See Chapter 10 for a description of the Food and Drug Administration's (FDA's) established risk categories for drugs in pregnancy.

Some maternal illnesses are harmful to the developing fetus. An example is rubella (German measles), which is rarely a serious disease for adults but can cause deafness, vision defects, heart defects, and intellectual disability in the fetus if it is acquired by a pregnant woman. A fetus can also acquire diseases such as acquired immunodeficiency syndrome (AIDS)/human immunodeficiency virus (HIV) infection or hepatitis B from the mother.

Radiation, chemicals, and other environmental hazards may adversely affect a fetus when the mother is exposed to any of these influences during her pregnancy. The best outcomes for infants occur when mothers eat well; exercise regularly; seek early prenatal care; refrain from use of drugs, alcohol, tobacco, and excessive caffeine; and follow general principles of good health.

As we have seen, both nature and nurture are important in determining individual patterns of development. These two forces interact in unique ways in each individual, explaining differences in time frames for acquisition of developmental skills among children, personality variations between identical twins, and other unique characteristics of individuals. An environmental factor that is extremely important in the development of children is the profile of family characteristics. The family is an important component in the lives of all children and plays an essential role in fostering the development of youth. A significant concept in families is that of parenting. How children are parented interacts with their individual characteristics to influence risk and protective factors, personality characteristics, and developmental outcomes. The families into which children are born influence them profoundly. Children are supported in different ways and acquire different worldviews depending on such factors as whether one or both parents work, how many siblings are present, and whether an extended family is close by. Note should be made of variations in family structure such as single parent, homosexual parents, extended family, and stepparents. Foster parenting and movement of children into a number of foster homes during childhood influences self-esteem and the ability to perform at potential. How might a nontraditional "family" setting, such as an adoptive or foster home, influence a child's development?

development of the children in these groups. Foods commonly eaten vary among people with different cultural backgrounds and influence the incidence of health problems such as cardiovascular disease in these groups. The Native American practice of carrying infants on boards often delays walking when measured against the norm for walking on some developmental tests. Children who are carried by straddling the mother's hips or back for extended periods have a low incidence of developmental dysplasia of the hip since this keeps their hips in an abducted position. It is important for nurses to take cultural practices into account when performing developmental screening; some tests may not be culturally sensitive and can inaccurately label a child as delayed when the pattern of development is simply different in the group, perhaps due to childrearing practices in the family. In addition, certain ethnic or racial groups are more prone to develop certain diseases due to genetic variations. Examples include Hispanics, who have a high incidence of diabetes; African Americans, who more commonly have sickle cell disease; and Northern European Americans, who have a higher incidence of phenylketonuria.

All cultural groups have rules regarding patterns of social interaction. Schedules of language acquisition are determined by the number of languages spoken and the amount of speech in the home. The particular social roles assumed by men and women in the culture affect school activities and ultimately career choices. Attitudes toward touching and other methods of encouraging developmental skills vary among cultures. Chapter 37 includes further descriptions of other factors that influence child development such as school and child care, community services, and additional community and family factors.

Professionalism in Practice Foster Care

On a given day, about 400,000 U.S. children are in foster care, with the average time in such care being nearly 2 years (U.S. Department of Health and Human Services, 2013). Each state is responsible for establishing the standards of education, environmental provision, and other factors of foster homes. The Office of Data, Analysis, Research and Evaluation of the ACYF maintains information about foster care in the United States through the Adoption and Foster Care Analysis and Reporting System (AFCARS). The Foster Care Independence Act of 1999 fosters youth who are who are becoming too old for the foster care system to achieve self-sufficiency. The U.S. Education and Training Voucher Program helps youth to obtain college or vocational training at a free or reduced cost.

Nurses should recognize that children who are in foster care may have experienced family situations that were challenging or traumatic, and can be dealing with new living situations. Carefully assess the stress, adaptation, and risk and protective factors in children who are living in foster homes. Evaluate proximity to siblings and other family members as well as expectations for return to the primary family or adoption options. Support foster families so that they can provide the care needed for their foster children.

Infant (Birth to 1 Year)

Imagine the experience of tripling body weight in 1 year, or becoming proficient in understanding fundamental words in a new language and even speaking a few. These and many more accomplishments take place in the first year of life. Starting the year as a mainly reflexive creature, the infant can walk and communicate by the year's end. Never again in life is development so rapid and profound.

Physical Growth and Development

The first year of life is one of rapid change for the infant. The birth weight usually doubles by about 5 months and triples by the end of the first year (Figure 31–5). Height increases by about a foot during this year. Teeth begin to erupt at about 6 months, and by the end of the first year, the infant has six to eight deciduous teeth (see Chapter 34). Physical growth is closely associated with type and quality of feeding. (See Chapter 32 for a discussion of nutrition in infancy.)

Body organs and systems, although not fully mature at 1 year, function differently than they did at birth. Kidney and liver maturation helps the 1-year-old excrete drugs or other toxic substances more readily than in the first weeks of life. The changing body proportions mirror changes in developing internal organs. Maturation of the nervous system is demonstrated by increased control over body movements with growing differentiation from general to specific skills, thus enabling the infant to sit, stand, and walk. Sensory function also increases as the infant begins to discriminate visual images, sounds, and tastes (Table 31–10).

Another factor that influences child development is that of culture. The traditional customs of the many cultural groups represented in North American society influence the

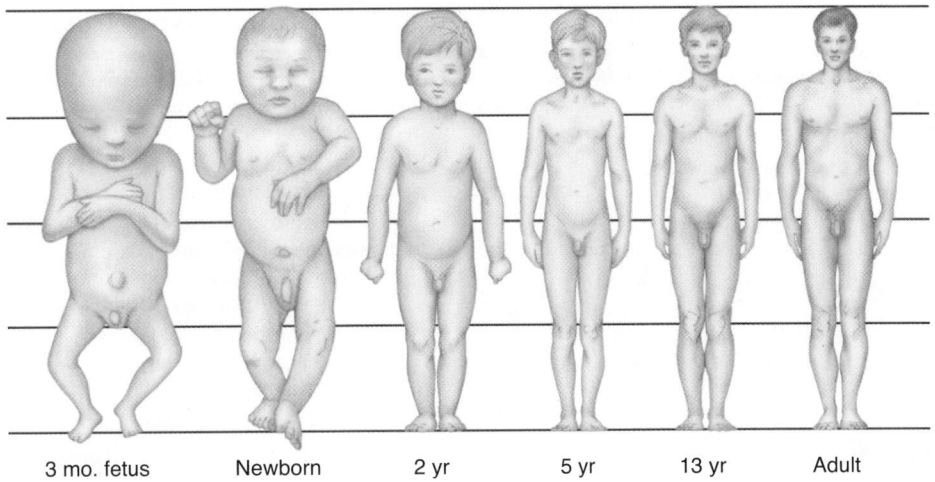

3 mo. fetus Newborn 2 yr 5 yr 13 yr Adult

Figure 31–5 Body proportions at various ages.

Cognitive Development

The brain continues to increase in complexity during the first year. Most of the growth involves maturation of cells, with only a small increase in number of cells. This growth of the brain is accompanied by development of its functions. One only has to compare the behavior of an infant shortly after birth with that of a 1-year-old to understand the incredible maturation of brain function. The newborn's eyes widen in response to sound; the 1-year-old turns to the sound and recognizes its significance. The 2-month-old cries and coos; the 1-year-old says a few words and understands many more. The 6-week-old grasps a rattle for the first time; the 1-year-old reaches for toys and feeds self.

The infant's behaviors provide clues about thought processes. Piaget's work outlines the infant's actions in a set of

TABLE 31–10 Physical Growth and Development Milestones During Infancy

AGE	PHYSICAL GROWTH	FINE MOTOR ABILITY	GROSS MOTOR ABILITY	SENSORY ABILITY
Birth to 1 month	Gains 140–200 g (5–7 oz)/week Grows 1.5 cm (1/2 in.) in first month Head circumference increases 1.5 cm (1/2 in.)/month	Holds hand in fist (A) Draws arms and legs to body when crying	Inborn reflexes such as startle and rooting are predominant activity May lift head briefly if prone (B) Alerts to high-pitched voices Comforts with touch (C)	Prefers to look at faces and black-and-white geometric designs Follows objects in line of vision (D)

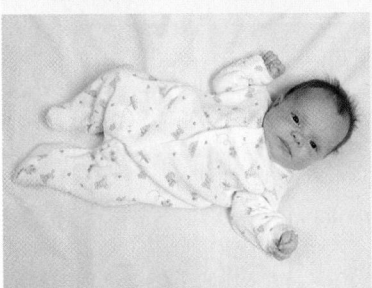

A Holds hand in fist

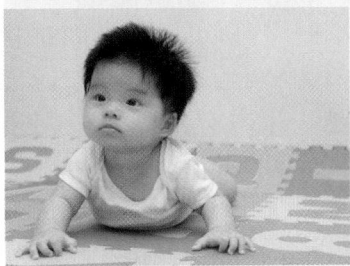

B May lift head

Kenishirotie/Shutterstock

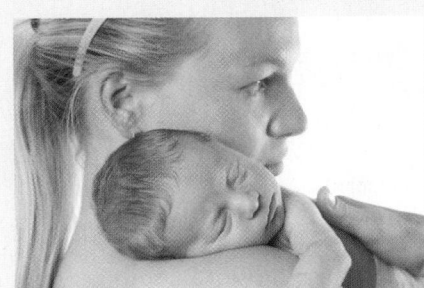

C Comforts with touch

Dora Zett/Shutterstock

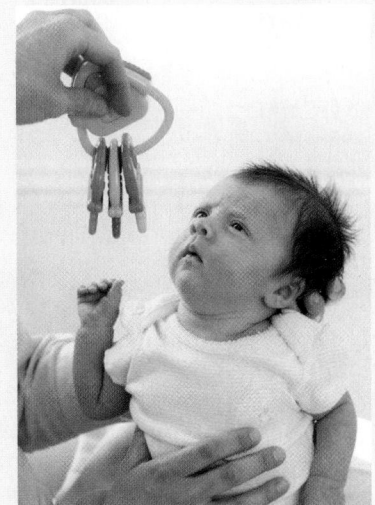

D Follows objects

Vanessa Davis/DK Images

(continued)

TABLE 31–10 Physical Growth and Development Milestones During Infancy (*continued*)

AGE	PHYSICAL GROWTH	FINE MOTOR ABILITY	GROSS MOTOR ABILITY	SENSORY ABILITY
2–4 months	Gains 140–200 g (5–7 oz)/week Grows 1.5 cm (1/2 in.)/month Head circumference increases 1.5 cm (1/2 in.)/month Posterior fontanelle closes Ingests 120 mL/kg/24 hr (2 oz/lb/24 hr)	Holds rattle and other objects when placed in hand (*E*) Looks at and plays with own fingers Brings hands to midline	Moro reflex fading in strength Can turn from side to back and then return (*F*) Decrease in head lag when pulled to sitting position; sits with head held in midline with some bobbing When prone, holds head and supports weight on forearms (*G*)	Follows objects 180 degrees Turns head to look for voices and sounds

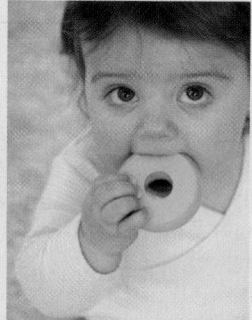

E Holds rattle and other objects

Vanessa Davis/DK Images

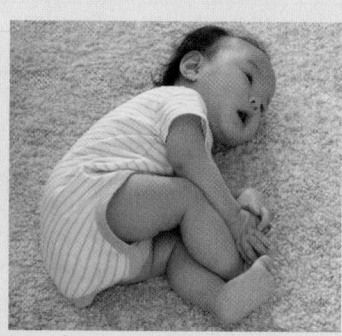

F Can turn from side to back

Vanessa Davis/DK Images

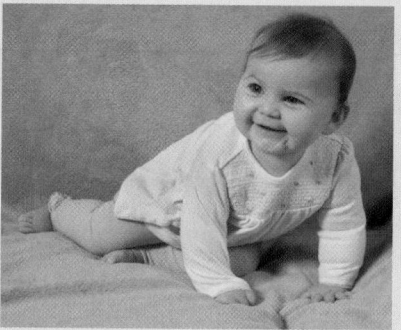

G Holds head up and supports weight with arms

AGE	PHYSICAL GROWTH	FINE MOTOR ABILITY	GROSS MOTOR ABILITY	SENSORY ABILITY
4–6 months	Gains 140–200 g (5–7 oz)/week Doubles birth weight at 5–6 months Grows 1.5 cm (1/2 in.)/month Head circumference increases 1.5 cm (1/2 in.)/month Teeth may begin erupting by 6 months Ingests 100 mL/kg/24 hr (1 1/2 oz/lb/24 hr)	Grasps rattles and other objects at will; drops them to pick up another offered object (*H*) Mouths objects Holds feet and pulls to mouth Holds bottle Grasps with whole hand (palmar grasp) Manipulates objects (*I*)	Head held steady when sitting No head lag when pulled to sitting Turns from abdomen to back by 4 months and then back to abdomen by 6 months When held standing supports much of own weight (*J*)	Examines complex visual images Watches the course of a falling object

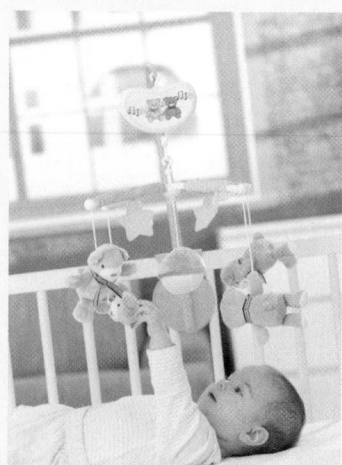

H Grasps objects at will

StockLite/Shutterstock

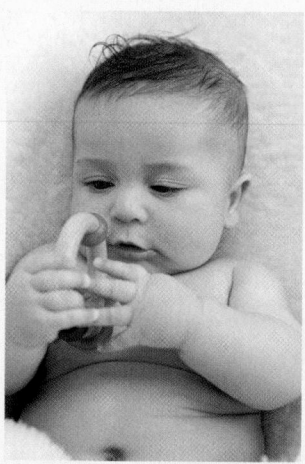

I Manipulates objects

Vanessa Davis/DK Images

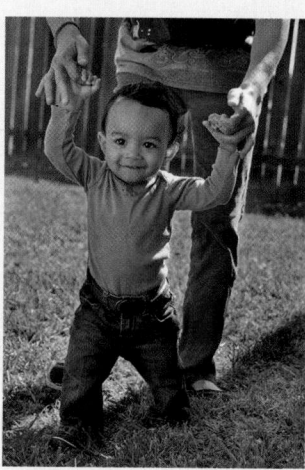

J Supports most of weight when held standing

AGE	PHYSICAL GROWTH	FINE MOTOR ABILITY	GROSS MOTOR ABILITY	SENSORY ABILITY
6–8 months	Gains 85–140 g (3–5 oz)/week Grows 1 cm (3/8 in.)/month Growth rate slower than first 6 months	Bangs objects held in hands Transfers objects from one hand to the other Beginning pincer grasp at times	Most inborn reflexes extinguished Sits alone steadily without support by 8 months (K) Likes to bounce on legs when held in standing position	Responds readily to sounds Recognizes own name and responds by looking and smiling Enjoys small and complex objects at play

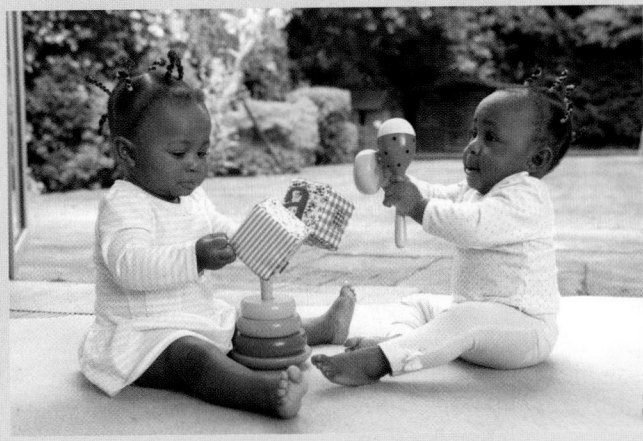

K Sits alone without support

Ruth Jenkinson/DK Images

AGE	PHYSICAL GROWTH	FINE MOTOR ABILITY	GROSS MOTOR ABILITY	SENSORY ABILITY
8–10 months	Gains 85–140 g (3–5 oz)/week Grows 1 cm (3/8 in.)/month	Picks up small objects (L) Uses pincer grasp well (M)	Crawls or pulls whole body along floor by arms (N) Creeps by using hands and knees to keep trunk off floor Pulls self to standing and sitting by 10 months Recovers balance when sitting	Understands words such as "no" and "cracker" May say one word in addition to "mama" and "dada"

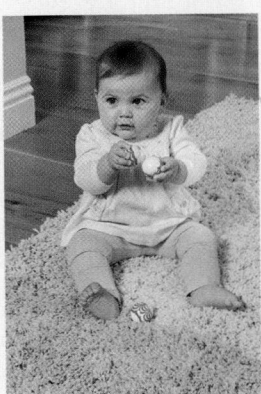

L Picks up small objects

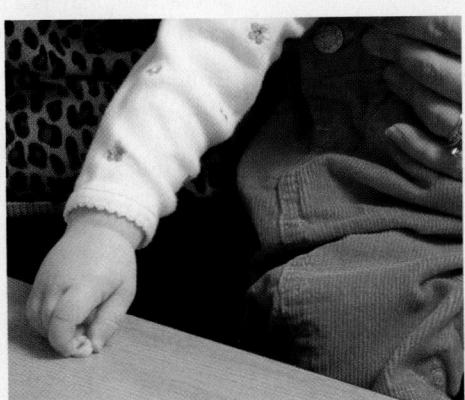

M Uses pincer grasp well

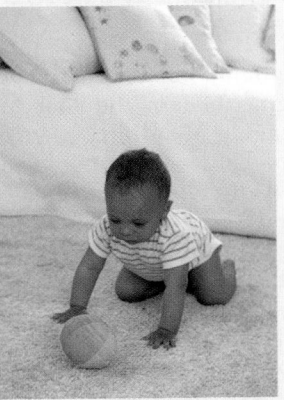

N Crawls or pulls body by arms

Vanessa Davis/DK Images

(continued)

TABLE 31–10 Physical Growth and Development Milestones During Infancy (*continued*)

AGE	PHYSICAL GROWTH	FINE MOTOR ABILITY	GROSS MOTOR ABILITY	SENSORY ABILITY
10–12 months	Gains 85–140 g (3–5 oz)/week Grows 1 cm (3/8 in.)/month Head circumference equals chest circumference Triples birth weight by 1 year	May hold crayon or pencil and make mark on paper Places objects into containers through holes (*O*)	Stands alone (*P*) Walks holding onto furniture Sits down from standing (*Q*)	Plays peek-a-boo and patty cake

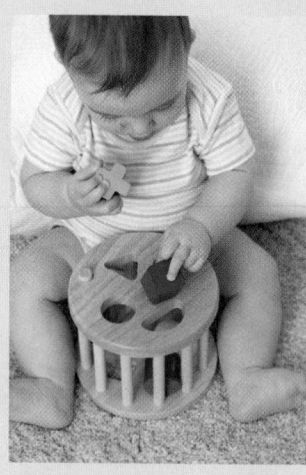

O Places objects in container through holes

Vanessa Davis/DK Images

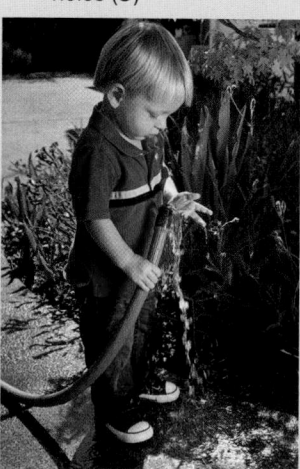

P Stands alone

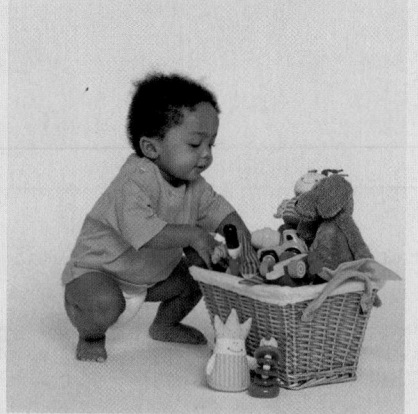

Q Sits down from standing

Victoria Blackie/DK Images

rapidly progressing changes in the first year of life. The infant receives stimulation through sight, sound, and feeling, which the maturing brain interprets. This input from the environment interacts with internal cognitive abilities to enhance cognitive functioning.

Psychosocial Development

PLAY

An 8-month-old infant is sitting on the floor, grasping blocks and banging them on the floor. Infants spend much of their time engaging in **solitary play**, or playing by themselves. When a parent walks by, the infant laughs and waves hands and feet wildly. Physical capabilities enable the infant to move toward and reach out for objects of interest. Cognitive ability is reflected in manipulation of blocks to create different sounds. Social interaction enhances play. The presence of a parent or other person increases interest in surroundings and teaches the infant different ways to play.

The play of infants begins in a reflexive manner. When an infant moves extremities or grasps objects, the foundations of play are established. The feel and sound of these activities give pleasure to the infant, who gradually performs them purposefully. For example, when a parent places a rattle in the hand of a 6-week-old infant, the infant grasps it reflexively. As the hands move randomly, the rattle makes an enjoyable sound. The infant learns to move the rattle to create the sound and then finally to grasp the rattle at will to play with it.

The next phase of infant play focuses on manipulative behavior. The infant examines toys closely, looking at them, touching them, and placing them in the mouth. The infant learns a great deal about texture, qualities of objects, and all aspects of the surroundings. At the same time, interaction with others becomes an important part of play. The social nature of play is obvious as the infant plays with other children and adults.

Toward the end of the first year, the infant's ability to move in space enlarges the sphere of play (Table 31–11). The infant who has begun crawling or walking can get to new places, find new toys, discover forgotten objects, or seek out other people for interaction. Play is a reflection of every aspect of development, as well as a method for enhancing learning and maturation.

PERSONALITY AND TEMPERAMENT

Why does one infant frequently awaken at night crying while another sleeps for 8 to 10 hours undisturbed? Why does one infant smile much of the time and react positively to interactions while another is withdrawn with unfamiliar people and frequently frowns and cries? Such differences in responses to the environment are believed to be inborn characteristics of temperament. Infants are born with a tendency to react in certain ways to noise and to interact differently with people. They may display varying degrees of regularity in activities of eating and sleeping, and manifest a capacity for concentrating on tasks for different amounts of time.

Nursing assessment identifies personality characteristics of the infant that the nurse can share with the parents. With this information the parents can appreciate more fully the uniqueness of their infant and design experiences to meet the infant's needs. Parents can learn to modify the environment to promote adaptation. For example, an infant who does not adapt easily to new situations may cry, withdraw, or develop another way of coping when adjusting to new people or places. Parents might be advised to use one or two babysitters rather than engaging new sitters frequently. If the infant is easily distracted when eating, parents can feed the infant in a quiet setting to encourage a focus on eating. Although the infant's temperament is unchanged, the ability to fit with the environment is enhanced.

TABLE 31–11 Psychosocial Development During Infancy

AGE	PLAY AND TOYS	COMMUNICATION
Birth–3 months	Prefers visual stimuli of mobiles, black-and-white patterns, mirrors Auditory stimuli are music boxes, tape players, soft voices Responds to rocking and cuddling Moves legs and arms while adult sings and talks Likes varying stimuli—different rooms, sounds, visual images	Coos Babbles Cries
3–6 months	Prefers noise-making objects that are easily grasped like rattles Enjoys stuffed animals and soft toys with contrasting colors	Vocalizes during play and with familiar people Laughs
6–9 months	Likes teething toys Increasingly desires social interaction with adults and other children Soft toys that can be manipulated and mouthed are favorites	Cries less Squeals and makes pleasure sounds Babbles multisyllabically (mamamamama) Increases vowel and consonant sounds Links syllables together Uses speechlike rhythm when vocalizing with others
9–12 months	Enjoys large blocks, toys that pop apart and go back together, nesting cups and other objects Laughs at surprise toys like jack-in-the-box Plays interactive games like peek-a-boo Uses push-and-pull toys	Understands "no" and other simple commands Says "dada" and "mama" to identify parents Learns one or two other words Receptive speech surpasses expressive speech

See Chapter 34 for further application of this information to health promotion of the infant.

COMMUNICATION

Even at a few weeks of age, infants communicate and engage in two-way interaction. Comfort is expressed by soft sounds, cuddling, and eye contact. The infant displays discomfort by thrashing the extremities, arching the back, and crying vigorously. From these rudimentary skills, communication ability continues to develop until the infant speaks several words at the end of the first year of life (Table 31–11).

Nurses assess communication to identify possible abnormalities or developmental delays. Infants understand (receptive speech) more words than they can speak (expressive speech). Abnormalities may be caused by a hearing deficit, developmental delay, or lack of verbal stimulation from caretakers. Children in families with multiple languages speak in each language.

Nursing interventions focus on providing a stimulating environment. Encourage parents to speak to infants and teach words. Hospital nurses should include the infant's known words when providing care.

Growth and Development
Strategies for communicating with infants include the following:

- Hold for feedings.
- Hold, rock, and talk to infant often.
- Talk and sing frequently during care.
- Tell names of objects.
- Use high-pitched voice with newborns.
- When the infant is upset, swaddle and hold securely.

Toddler (1 to 3 Years)

Toddlerhood is sometimes called the first adolescence. An infant only months before, the child from 1 to 3 years is now displaying independence and negativism. Pride in newfound accomplishments emerges.

Physical Growth and Development

The rate of growth slows during the second year of life. Parents may become concerned because the child has a limited food intake. They may need reassurance that this is normal. (See Chapter 32 for further discussion of nutrition in toddlerhood.)

By age 2 years, the birth weight has usually quadrupled and the child is about one half of the adult height. Body proportions begin to change, with the legs longer and the head smaller in proportion to body size than during infancy (see Figure 31–5). The toddler has a pot-bellied appearance and stands with feet apart to provide a wide base of support. By approximately 33 months, eruption of deciduous teeth is complete, with 20 teeth being present.

Gross motor activity develops rapidly (Table 31–12) as the toddler progresses from walking to running, kicking, and riding a Big Wheel tricycle (Figure 31–6). As physical maturation occurs, the toddler develops the ability to control elimination patterns (see *Growth and Development* and *Developing Cultural Competence: Childrearing Practices*).

TABLE 31–12 Physical Growth and Development Milestones During Toddlerhood

AGE	PHYSICAL GROWTH	FINE MOTOR ABILITY	GROSS MOTOR ABILITY	SENSORY ABILITY
1–2 years	Gains 227 g (8 oz) or more per month Grows 9–12 cm (3.5–5 in.) during this year Anterior fontanelle closes	By end of second year, builds a tower of four blocks (*A*) Scribbles on paper (*B*) Can undress self (*C*) Throws a ball	Runs Shows growing ability to walk and finally walks with ease Walks up and down stairs a few months after learning to walk with ease (*E*) Likes push-and-pull toys (*F*)	Visual acuity 20/50
2–3 years	Gains 1.4–2.3 kg (3–5 lb)/year Grows 5–6.5 cm (2–2.5 in.)/year	Draws a circle and other rudimentary forms Learns to pour Learning to dress self (*D*)	Jumps Kicks ball Throws ball overhand	

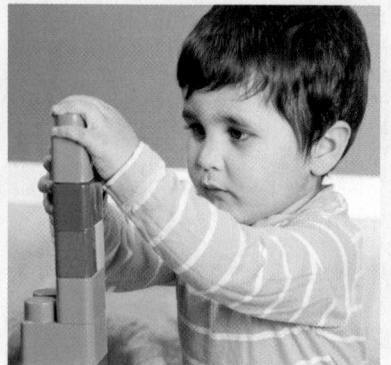

A Builds tower of four blocks

Fernando Cortes/Shutterstock

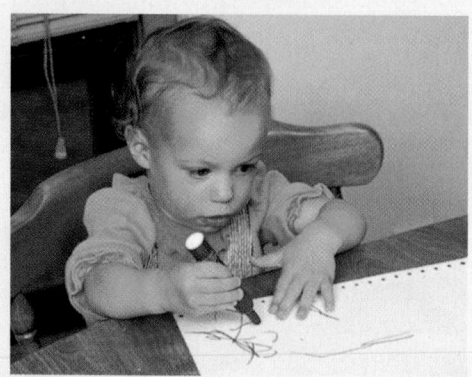

B Scribbles on paper

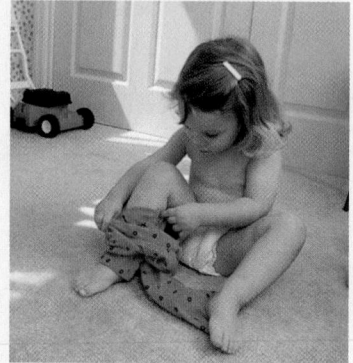

C Can undress self

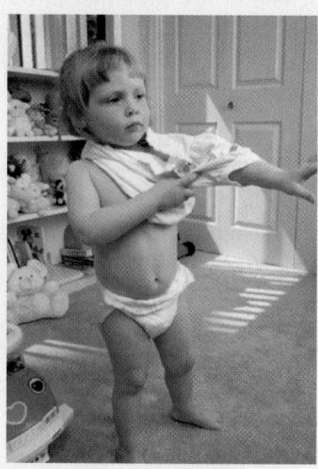

D Learning to dress self

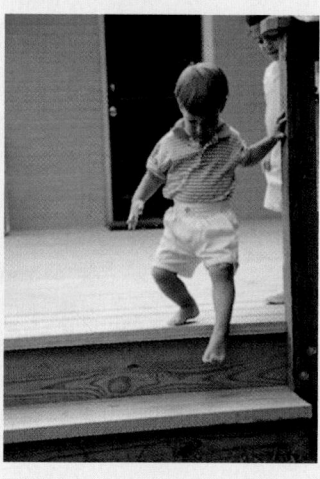

E Walks up and down stairs

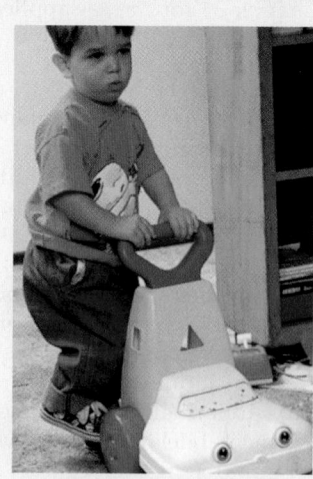

F Likes push-and-pull toys

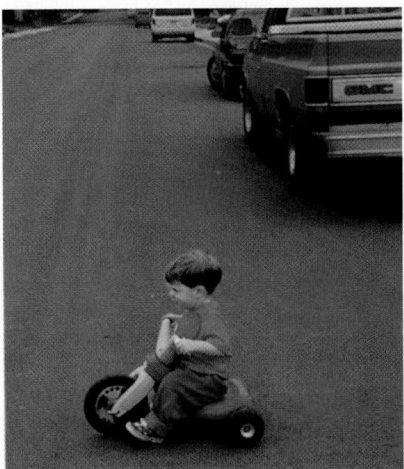

Figure 31–6 Gross motor activity. This toddler has learned to ride a Big Wheel, which he is doing right into the street. Toddlers must be closely watched to prevent injury.

Growth and Development

Strategies for toilet training include the following:

- When are children ready to learn toileting?
- Are parents responsible for the differences in ages at which toilet training is accomplished?
- Does toilet training provide clues to a child's intellectual ability?

We know that children are not ready for toilet training until several developmental capabilities exist: to stand and walk well, to pull pants up and down, to recognize the need to eliminate and then to be able to wait until they are in the bathroom. Once this readiness is apparent, the child can be given a small potty chair and the procedure explained.

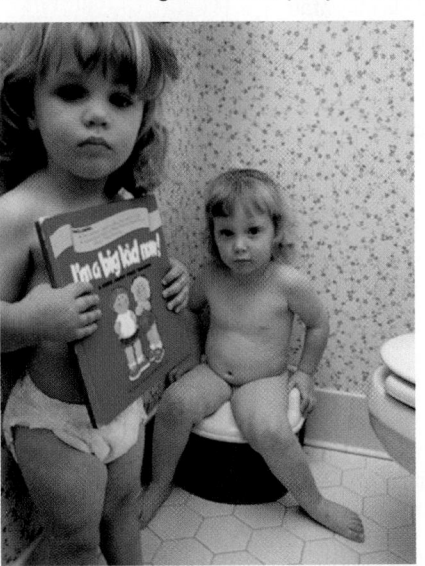

Children often prefer their own chairs on the floor to using a large toilet. The child should be placed on the chair at regular intervals for a few moments and can be given a reward or praise for successes. If the child seems not to understand or does not wish to cooperate, it is best to wait a few weeks and then try again. Just as all of development is subject to individual timetables, toilet training occurs with considerable variability from one child to another. Identify for parents the developmental characteristics of their child and encourage them to appreciate without anxiety the unfolding of skills. These timetables are not predictive of future development.

The child who is ill or hospitalized or has other stress often regresses in toilet-training activities. It is best to quietly reinstitute attempts at training after the trauma. Potty chairs should be available on pediatric units and toileting habits identified during initial assessment so that regular routines can be followed and the child's usual words for elimination can be used.

Cognitive Development

During the toddler years, the child moves from the sensorimotor to the preoperational stage of development. The early use of language awakens in the 1-year-old the ability to think about objects or people when they are absent. Object permanence is well developed.

At about 2 years of age, the increasing use of words as symbols enables the toddler to use preoperational thought. Rudimentary problem solving, creative thought, and an understanding of cause-and-effect relationships are now possible.

Psychosocial Development

PLAY

Many changes in play patterns occur between infancy and toddlerhood. For example, developing motor skills enable toddlers to bang pegs into a pounding board with a hammer. The social nature of toddler play is also readily seen. Toddlers find the company of other children pleasurable, even though socially interactive play may not occur. Two toddlers tend to play with similar objects side by side, occasionally trading toys and words. This is called **parallel play**. This playtime with other children helps toddlers develop social skills. Toddlers engage in play activities they have seen at home, such as pounding with a hammer and talking on the phone. This imitative behavior teaches them new actions and skills.

Physical skills are manifested in play as toddlers push and pull objects, climb in and out and up and down, run, ride a Big Wheel, turn the pages of books, and scribble with a pen. Both gross motor and fine motor abilities are enhanced during this age period.

Cognitive understanding enables the toddler to manipulate objects and learn about their qualities. Stacking blocks and placing rings on a building tower teach spatial relationships and other lessons that provide a foundation for future learning. Various kinds of play objects should be provided for the toddler to meet play needs. These play needs can easily be met whether the child is hospitalized or at home (Table 31–13).

PERSONALITY AND TEMPERAMENT

The toddler retains most of the temperamental characteristics identified during infancy but may demonstrate some changes. The normal developmental progression of toddlerhood also plays a part in responses. For example, the infant who previously responded positively to stimuli, such as a new babysitter, may appear more negative in toddlerhood. The increasing independence characteristic of this age is shown by the toddler's use of the word "no." The parent and child constantly adapt their responses to each other and learn anew how to communicate with each other.

COMMUNICATION

Because of the phenomenal growth of language skills during the toddler period, adults should communicate frequently with

TABLE 31–13 Psychosocial Development During Toddlerhood

AGE		PLAY AND TOYS	COMMUNICATION
1–3 years	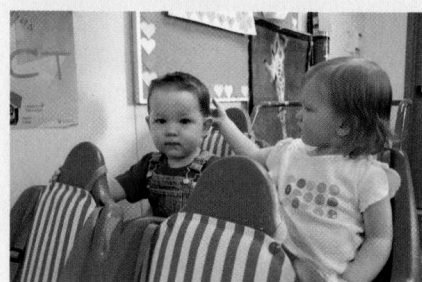	Refines fine motor skills by use of cloth books, large pencil and paper, wooden puzzles Facilitates imitative behavior by playing kitchen, grocery shopping, toy telephone Learns gross motor activities by riding Big Wheel tricycle, playing with soft ball and bat, molding water and sand, tossing ball or bean bag Cognitive skills develop with exposure to educational television shows, music, stories, and books	Increasingly enjoys talking Exponential growth of vocabulary, especially when spoken and read to Needs to release stress by pounding board, frequent gross motor activities, and occasional temper tantrums Likes contact with other children and learns interpersonal skills

children in this age group. Toddlers imitate words and speech intonations, as well as the social interactions they observe.

At the beginning of toddlerhood, the child may use four to six words in addition to "mama" and "dada." Receptive speech (the ability to understand words) far outpaces expressive speech. By the end of toddlerhood, however, the 3-year-old has a vocabulary of almost 1000 words and uses short sentences.

Communication occurs in many ways, some of which are nonverbal. Toddler communication includes pointing, pulling an adult over to a room or object, and speaking in expressive jargon. **Expressive jargon** is using unintelligible words with normal speech intonations as if truly communicating in words. Another communication method occurs when the toddler cries, pounds feet, displays a temper tantrum, or uses other means to illustrate dismay. These powerful communication methods can upset parents, who often need suggestions for handling them. It is best to verbalize the feelings shown by the toddler, for example, by saying, "You must be very upset that you cannot have that candy. When you stop crying you can come out of your room," and then ignore further negative behavior. The toddler's search for autonomy and independence creates a need for such behavior. Sometimes an upset toddler responds well to holding, rocking, and stroking.

Growth and Development

Strategies for communicating with toddlers include the following:

- Give short, clear instructions.
- Do not give choices if none exist. For example, do not ask "Do you want to take your medicine now?" but rather say "What juice do you want after you take your medicine—apple or orange?"
- Offer a choice of two alternatives when possible.
- Approach positively and slowly, allowing time for the toddler to adjust.
- Tell toddler what you are doing, and say the names of objects.

Parents and nurses can promote a toddler's communication by speaking frequently, naming objects, explaining procedures in simple terms, expressing feelings that the toddler seems to be displaying, and encouraging speech. The toddler from a bilingual home is at an optimal age to learn two languages. If the parents do not speak English, the toddler will benefit from a daycare experience in which the providers do, so that the child can learn both languages.

The nurse who understands the communication skills of toddlers is able to assess expressive and receptive language and communicate effectively, thereby promoting positive healthcare experiences for these children (Table 31–14).

TABLE 31–14 Communicating With a Toddler

Procedures such as drawing blood can be frightening for a toddler. Effective communication minimizes the trauma caused by such procedures:

- Avoid telling toddlers about the procedure too far in advance. They do not have an understanding of time and can become quite anxious.
- Use simple terminology. "We need to get a little blood from your arm. It will help us to find out if you are getting better." If the parent is willing, say, "Your mom will hold your arm still so we can do it quickly."
- Allow the toddler to cry. Acknowledge that it must be frightening and that you understand.
- Perform the procedure in a treatment room so that the toddler's bed and room are a safe haven.
- Be sure the toddler is restrained, with the joints above and below the procedure immobilized.
- Use a Band-Aid to cover up the site. This can reassure the toddler that the body is still intact.
- Allow the toddler to choose a reward such as a sticker after the procedure.
- Praise the toddler for cooperation and acknowledge that you know this was difficult.
- Comfort the toddler by rocking, offering a favorite drink, playing music, and holding. If parents are present, they can offer the comfort needed.

Preschool Child (3 to 6 Years)

The preschool years are a time of new initiative and independence. Most children are in a childcare center or school for part of the day and learn a great deal from this social contact. Language skills are well developed, and the child is able to understand and speak clearly. Endless projects characterize the world of busy preschoolers. They may work with play dough to form animals, then cut out and paste paper, then draw and color.

Physical Growth and Development

Preschoolers grow slowly and steadily, with most growth taking place in the long bones of the arms and legs. The short, chubby toddler gradually gives way to a slender, long-legged preschooler (Table 31–15).

TABLE 31–15 Physical Growth and Development Milestones During the Preschool Years

PHYSICAL GROWTH

Gains 1.5–2.5 kg (3–5 lb)/year Grows 4–6 cm (1 1/2–2 1/2 in.)/year

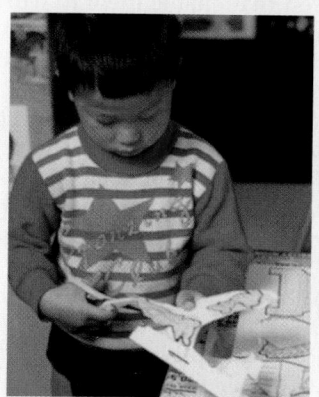

A Uses scissors

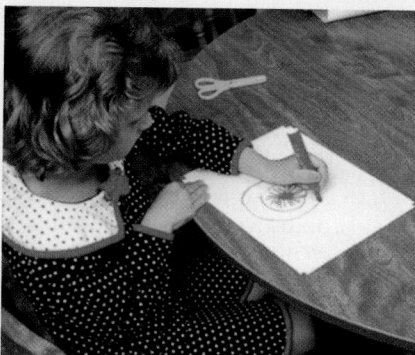

B Draws circle, square, cross

FINE MOTOR ABILITY

Uses scissors (*A*)

Draws circle, square, cross (*B*)

Draws at least a six-part person

Enjoys art projects such as pasting, stringing beads, using clay

Learns to tie shoes at end of preschool years (*C*)

Buttons clothes (*D*)

Brushes teeth (*E*)

Uses spoon, fork, knife

Eats three meals with snacks

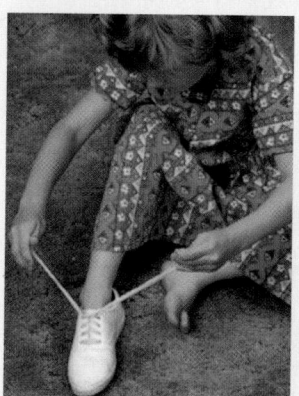

C Ties shoes

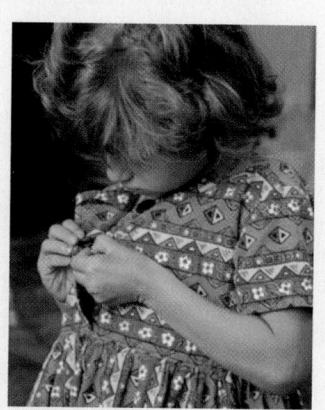

D Buttons clothes

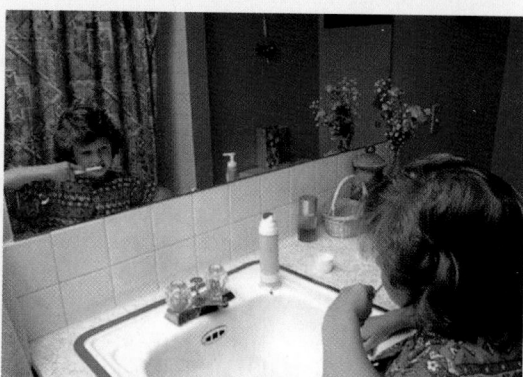

E Brushes teeth

GROSS MOTOR ABILITY

Throws a ball overhand

Climbs well (*F*)

Rides bicycle (*G*)

SENSORY ABILITY

Visual acuity continues to improve

Can focus on and learn letters and numbers (*H*)

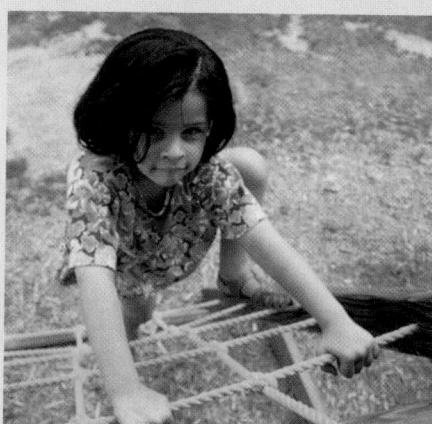

F Climbs well

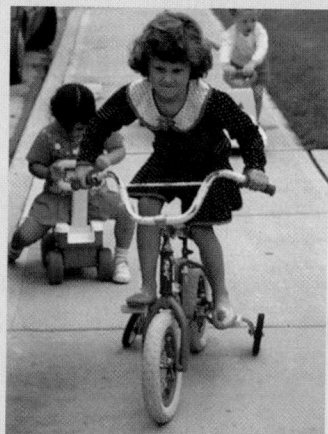

G Rides bicycle or bicycle with training wheels

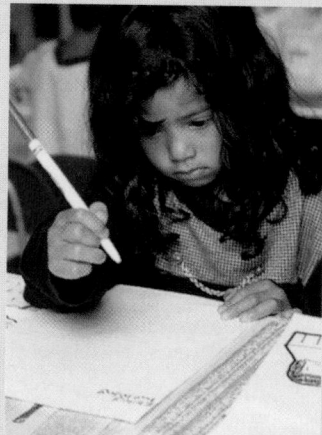

H Learns letters and numbers

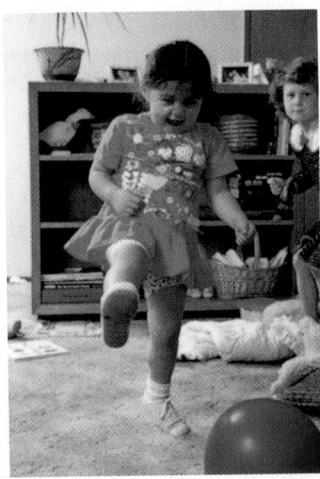

Development of physical skills in preschoolers. Preschoolers continue to develop advanced skills such as kicking a ball without falling down.

Physical skills continue to develop (Figure 31–7). The preschooler runs with ease, holds a bat, and throws balls of various types. Writing ability increases, and the preschooler enjoys drawing and learning to write a few letters.

The preschool period is a good time to encourage good dental habits. Children can begin to brush their own teeth with parental supervision and help to reach all tooth surfaces. Parents should floss children's teeth, give fluoride as prescribed if the water supply is not fluoridated, and schedule the first dental visit so the child can become accustomed to the routine of periodic dental care.

Cognitive Development

The preschooler exhibits characteristics of preoperational thought. Symbols or words are used to represent objects and people, enabling the young child to think about them. This is a milestone in intellectual development; however, the preschooler still has some limitations in thought (Table 31–16).

Psychosocial Development

PLAY

The preschooler has begun playing in a new way. Toddlers simply play side by side with friends, each engaging in his or her own activities, but preschoolers interact with others during play. For example, one child cuts out colored paper while her friend glues it on paper in a design. This new type of interaction is called **associative play** (Figure 31–8). The child life therapist in hospital settings recognizes the therapeutic value of play in planning activities for children that enable them to work through feelings about procedures and separation, as well as facilitating the normal developmental need for interaction with other children.

In addition to this social dimension of play, other aspects of play also differ. The preschooler enjoys large motor activities such as swinging, riding a tricycle, and throwing a ball. Increasing manual dexterity is demonstrated in greater complexity of drawings and manipulation of blocks and modeling. These changes necessitate planning of playtime to include appropriate activities. Preschool programs and child life departments in hospitals help meet this important need.

Materials provided for play can be simple but should guide activities in which the child engages. Since fine motor activities are popular, paper, pens, scissors, glue, and a variety of other such objects should be available. The child can use them to create important images such as pictures of people, hospital beds, or friends. A collection of dolls, furniture, and clothing can be

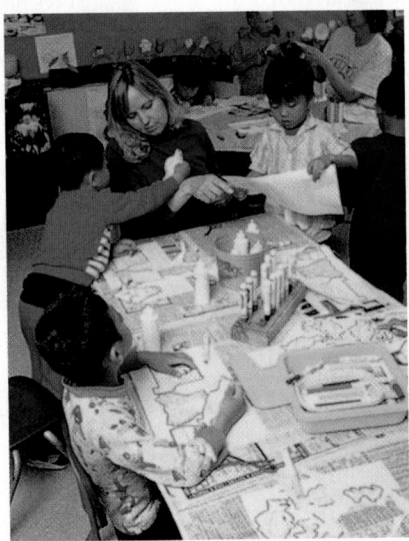

These preschoolers are participating in associative play, which means they can interact. One child is cutting out shapes, and the other is gluing them in place.

TABLE 31–16 Characteristics of Preoperational Thought

CHARACTERISTIC	DEFINITION	EXAMPLE
Egocentrism	Ability to see things only from one's own point of view	The child who cannot understand why parents may need to leave the hospital for work when the child wishes them to be present
Transductive reasoning	Connecting two events in a cause-and-effect relationship simply because they occur together in time	A child who, awakening after surgery and feeling pain, notices the intravenous infusion and believes that it is causing the pain
Centration	Focusing on only one particular aspect of a situation	The child who is concerned about breathing through an anesthesia mask and will not listen to any other aspects of preoperative teaching
Animism	Giving lifelike qualities to nonliving things	The child who views a monitoring machine as alive because it beeps

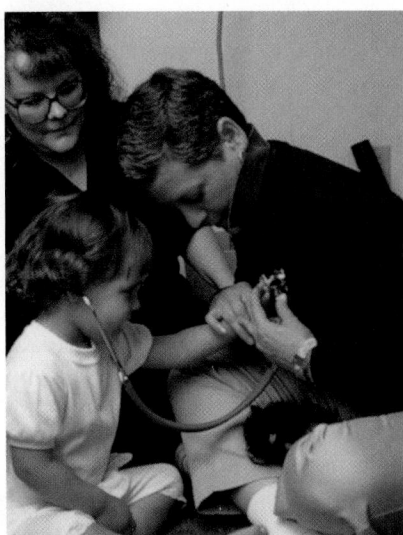

Figure 31–9 Jasmine is participating in dramatic play with a nurse while her mother looks on. In dramatic play, the child uses props to play out the drama of human life. It can be an excellent way for a nurse to assess the developmental level of children while talking to them. Notice that the child and the nurse are on the floor at the same level and the atmosphere is informal. Why is it important to be at the same level as the child?

manipulated to represent parents and children, nurses and physicians, teachers, or other significant people. Because fantasy life is so powerful at this age, the preschooler readily uses props to engage in **dramatic play**, that is, the living out of the drama of human life (Figure 31–9).

The nurse can use playtime to assess the preschool child's developmental level, knowledge about health care, and emotions related to healthcare experiences. Observations about objects chosen for play, content of dramatic play, and pictures drawn can provide important assessment data. The nurse can also use play periods to teach the child about healthcare procedures and offer an outlet for expression of emotions (Table 31–17).

PERSONALITY AND TEMPERAMENT
Characteristics of personality observed in infancy tend to persist over time. The preschooler may need assistance as these characteristics are expressed in the new situations of preschool or nursery school. An excessively active child, for example, will need gentle, consistent handling to adjust to the structure of a classroom. Encourage parents to visit preschool programs to choose the one that would best foster growth in their child. Some preschoolers enjoy the structured learning of a program that focuses on cognitive skills, whereas others are happier and more open to learning in a small group that provides much time for free play. Nurses can help parents to identify their child's personality or temperament characteristics and to find the best environment for growth.

COMMUNICATION
Language skills blossom during the preschool years. The vocabulary grows to over 2000 words, and children speak in complete sentences of several words and use all parts of speech. They practice these newfound language skills by endlessly talking and asking questions.

Growth and Development
Strategies for communicating with preschoolers include the following:

- Allow time for child to integrate explanations.
- Verbalize frequently to the child.
- Use drawings and stories to explain care.
- Use accurate names for body functions.
- Allow choices.

The sophisticated speech of preschoolers mirrors the development occurring in their minds and helps them to learn about the world around them. However, this speech can be quite deceptive. Although preschoolers use many words, their grasp of meaning is usually literal and may not match that of adults. These literal interpretations have important implications for healthcare providers. For example, the preschooler who is told she will be "put to sleep" for surgery may think of a pet recently euthanized; the child who is told that a dye will be injected for a diagnostic test may think he is going to die; mention of "a little stick" in the arm can cause images of tree branches rather than of a simple immunization.

The child may also have difficulty focusing on the content of a conversation. The preschooler is egocentric and may be unable to move from individual thoughts to those the nurse is proposing in a teaching situation.

TABLE 31–17 Psychosocial Development During the Preschool Years

AGE	PLAY AND TOYS	COMMUNICATION
3–6 years	Associative play is facilitated by simple games, puzzles, nursery rhymes, songs	All parts of speech are developed and used, occasionally incorrectly
	Dramatic play is fostered by dolls and doll clothes, play houses and hospitals, dress-up clothes, puppets	Communicates with a widening array of people
	Stress is relieved by pens, paper, glue, scissors	Play with other children is a favorite activity
	Cognitive growth is fostered by educational television shows, music, stories, and books	Health professionals can: • Verbalize and explain procedures to children • Use drawings and stories to explain care • Use accurate names for body functions • Allow the child to talk, ask questions, and make choices

Concrete visual aids such as pictures of a child undergoing the same procedure or a book to read together enhance teaching by meeting the child's developmental needs. Handling medical equipment such as intravenous bags and stethoscopes increases interest and helps the child to focus. Teaching may have to be done in several short sessions rather than one long session.

School-Age Child (6 to 12 Years)

Errol, 10 years old, arrives home from school shortly after 3 P.M. each day. He immediately calls his friends and goes to visit one of them. They are building models of cars and collecting baseball cards. Endless hours are spent on these projects and on discussions of events at school that day (Figure 31–10).

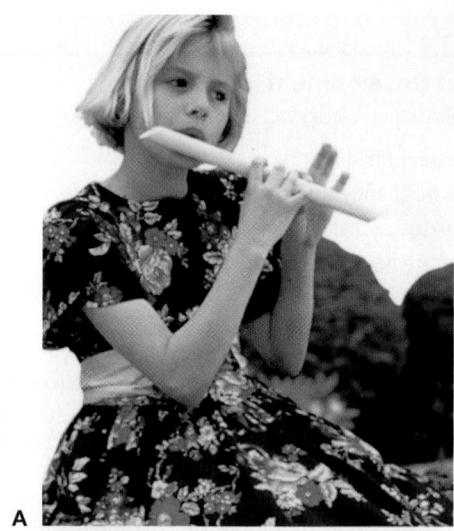

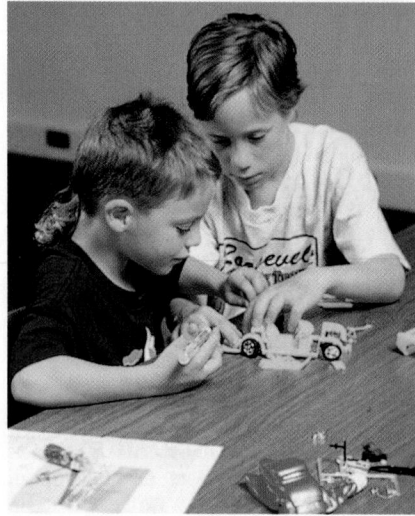

Figure 31-10 *A,* School-age children may take part in activities that require practice. This is a consideration when children are hospitalized and unable to practice or perform. Why? *B,* School-age children enjoy spending time with others the same age on projects and discussing the activities of the day. This is an important consideration when they are in an acute care setting. When you are in the clinical setting, look for examples of this type of interaction taking place.

Nine-year-old Karen practices soccer two afternoons a week and plays in games each weekend. She also is learning to play the flute and spends her free time at home practicing. Although practice time is not her favorite part of music, Karen enjoys the performances and wants to play well in front of her friends and teacher. Her parents now allow her to ride her bike unaccompanied to the store or to a friend's house.

These two school-age children demonstrate common characteristics of their age group. They are in a stage of industry in which it is important to the child to perform useful work. Meaningful activities take on great importance and are usually carried out in the company of peers. A sense of achievement in these activities is important to develop self-esteem and to prevent a sense of inferiority or poor self-worth.

Physical Growth and Development

School age is the last period in which girls and boys are close in size and body proportions. As the long bones continue to grow, leg length increases (see Figure 31–5). Fat gives way to muscle, and the child appears leaner. Jaw proportions change as the first deciduous tooth is lost at 6 years and permanent teeth begin to erupt. Body organs and the immune system mature, resulting in fewer illnesses among school-age children. Medications are less likely to cause serious side effects, since they can be metabolized more easily. The urinary system can adjust to changes in fluid status. Physical skills are also refined as children begin to play sports, and fine motor skills are well developed through school activities (Table 31–18 and Figure 31–11).

Although it is commonly believed that the start of adolescence (age 12 years) heralds a growth spurt, the rapid increases in size commonly occur during the school-age period. Girls may begin a growth spurt by 9 or 10 years and boys a year or so later. Nutritional needs increase dramatically with this spurt.

The loss of the first deciduous teeth and the eruption of permanent teeth usually occur at about age 6 years, or at the beginning of the school-age period. Of the 30 permanent teeth, 22 to 26 erupt by age 12 years and the remaining molars follow during the teenage years. The school-age child should be closely monitored to ensure that brushing and flossing are adequate, that fluoride is taken if the water supply is not fluoridated, that dental care is obtained to provide for examination of teeth and alignment, and that loose teeth are identified before surgery or other events that may lead to loss of a tooth.

Cognitive Development

The child enters the stage of concrete operational thought at about 7 years. This stage enables school-age children to consider alternative solutions and solve problems. However, school-age children continue to rely on concrete experiences and materials to form their thought content.

During the school-age years, the child learns the concept of **conservation** (that matter is not changed when its form is altered). At earlier ages a child believes that when water is poured from a short, wide glass into a tall, thin glass, there is more water in the taller glass. The school-age child recognizes that although it may look like the taller glass holds more water, the quantity is the same. The concept of conservation is helpful when the nurse explains medical treatments. The school-age child understands that an incision will heal, that a cast will be removed, and that an arm will look the same as before once the intravenous infusion is removed.

TABLE 31–18 Physical Growth and Development Milestones During the School-Age Years

PHYSICAL GROWTH	FINE MOTOR ABILITY	GROSS MOTOR ABILITY	SENSORY ABILITY
Gains 1.4–2.2 kg (3–5 lb)/year	Enjoys craft projects	Rides two-wheeler (A)	Can read
Grows 4–6 cm (1 1/2–2 1/2 in.)/year	Plays card and board games	Jumps rope (B) Roller skates or ice skates	Able to concentrate for longer periods on activities by filtering out surrounding sounds (C)

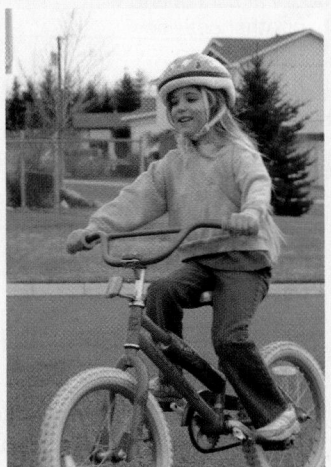

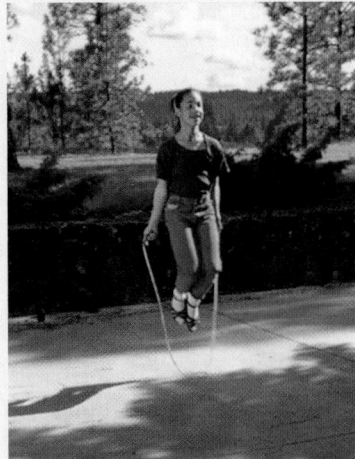

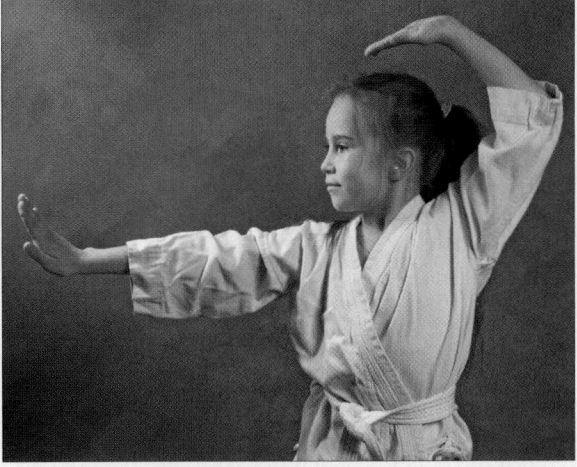

A Rides two-wheeler **B** Jumps rope **C** Concentrates on activities for longer periods
Shutterstock

Psychosocial Development

PLAY

When the preschool teacher tries to organize a game of baseball, both the teacher and the children become frustrated. Not only are the children physically unable to hold a bat and hit a ball, but they seem to have no understanding of the rules of the game and do not want to wait for their turn at bat. By 6 years of age, however, children have acquired the physical ability to hold the bat properly and may occasionally hit the ball. School-age children also understand that everyone has a role—the pitcher, the catcher, the batter, the outfielders. They cooperate with one another to form a team, are eager to learn the rules of the game, and want to ensure that these rules are followed exactly (Table 31–19).

The characteristics of play exhibited by the school-age child are cooperation with others and the ability to play a part in order to contribute to a unified whole. This type of play is called **cooperative play**. The concrete nature of cognitive thought leads to a reliance on rules to provide structure and security. Children have an increasing desire to spend much of playtime with friends, which demonstrates the social component of play. Play is an extremely important method of learning and living for the school-age child. Active physical play has decreased in recent years as television viewing and playing of computer games have increased, leading to poor nutritional status and a high rate of overweight among children. See Chapter 32 for further discussion of nutrition and physical activity in children.

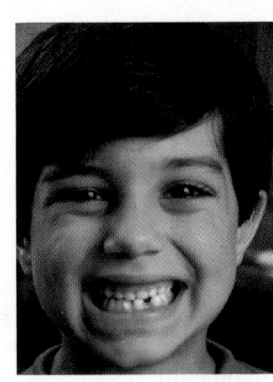

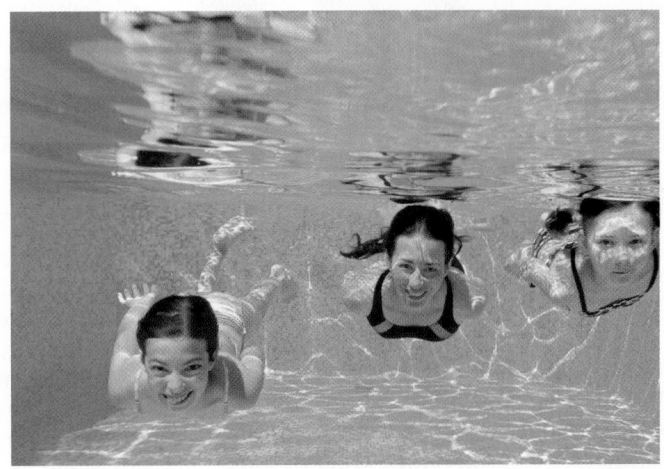

Figure 31–11 School-age children's physical development. *Left*, Front teeth are lost around age 6 years. The family may have rituals associated with the loss of teeth that could affect the child's behavior if he loses a tooth while in the hospital. *Right*, School-age girls and boys enjoy participating in sports. They begin to lose fat while developing their muscles, so they appear leaner than at earlier ages.

TABLE 31–19 Psychosocial Development During the School-Age Years

AGE	ACTIVITIES	COMMUNICATION
6–12 years 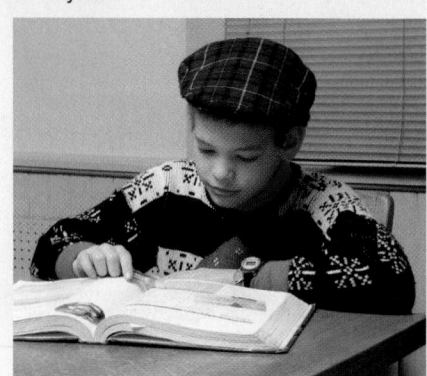	Gross motor development is fostered by ball sports, skating, dance lessons, water and snow skiing/boarding, biking A sense of industry is fostered by playing a musical instrument, gathering collections, starting hobbies, playing board and video games Cognitive growth is facilitated by reading, crafts, word puzzles, schoolwork	Mature use of language Ability to converse and discuss topics for increasing lengths of time Spends many hours at school and with friends in sports or other activities Health professionals can: • Assess child's knowledge before teaching • Allow the child to select rewards following procedures • Teach techniques such as counting or visualization to manage difficult situations • Include both parent and child in healthcare decisions

When a child is hospitalized, the separation from playmates can lead to feelings of sadness and purposelessness. School-age children often feel better when placed in multibed units with other children. Games can be devised even when children are wheelchair bound (Figure 31–12). Normal, rewarding parts of play should be integrated into care. Friends should be encouraged to visit or call a hospitalized child. Discharge planning for the child who has had a cast or brace applied should address the activities the child can engage in and those the child must avoid. Reinforce the importance of playing games with friends.

PERSONALITY AND TEMPERAMENT

The enduring aspects of temperament continue to be manifested during the school years. The child classified as "difficult" at an earlier age may now have trouble in the classroom. Advise parents to provide a quiet setting for homework and to reward the child for concentration. For example, after homework is completed, the child can watch a television show. Creative efforts and alternative methods of learning should be valued. Encourage parents to see their children as individuals who may not all learn in the same way. The "slow-to-warm-up" child may need encouragement to try new activities and to share experiences with others, while the "easy" child will readily adapt to new schools, people, and experiences.

COMMUNICATION

During the school-age years, the child should learn how to correct any lingering pronunciation or grammatical errors. Vocabulary increases, and the child is taught about parts of speech in school. School-age children enjoy writing and can be encouraged to keep a journal of their experiences while in the hospital as a method of dealing with anxiety. It is uncommon for school-age children to understand words as literally as preschoolers.

Growth and Development

Strategies for communicating with school-age children include the following:

• Provide concrete examples of pictures or materials to accompany verbal descriptions.
• Assess knowledge before planning teaching.
• Allow child to select rewards following procedures.
• Teach techniques such as counting or visualization to manage difficult situations.
• Include child in discussions and history with parent.
• Be honest in explanations and all communications.

Figure 31–12 **The nurse can help the hospitalized school-age child and family accept and adjust to new circumstances. Encouraging the child in a wheelchair to participate in group activities can help build confidence in physical skills. Good self-esteem, goal attainment, personal satisfaction, and general health are the continued benefits.**

SEXUALITY

While children become aware of sexual differences between genders during preschool years, they deal much more consciously with sexuality as school-age children. As children mature physically, they need information about their body changes so that they can develop a healthy self-image and an understanding of the relationships between their bodies and sexuality. Children become interested in sexual issues and are often exposed to erroneous information on television shows, in magazines, or from friends and siblings. Schools and families need to find opportunities to teach school-age children factual information about sex and to foster healthy concepts of self and others. It is advisable to ask occasional questions about sexual issues to learn how much the child knows and to provide correct information when answers demonstrate confusion. Both friends and the media are common sources of erroneous ideas. Appropriate and inappropriate touch should be discussed, with lists of trusted people who can be approached (teachers, clergy, school counselors, family members, neighbors) to discuss any episodes with which the child feels uncomfortable. Even these trusted people can be implicated in inappropriate episodes, so encourage the child to go to more than one person, an important approach if the child is uncomfortable about a relationship with any individual.

Adolescent (12 to 18 Years)

Adolescence is a time of passage signaling the end of childhood and the beginning of adulthood. Although adolescents differ in behaviors and accomplishments, they are in a period of identity formation. If a healthy identity and sense of self-worth are not developed in this period, role confusion and purposeless struggling will ensue. The adolescents encountered in nursing practice represent various degrees of identity formation, and each will offer unique challenges.

Physical Growth and Development

The physical changes ending in **puberty**, or sexual maturity, begin near the end of the school-age period. The prepubescent period is marked by a growth spurt at an average age of 10 years for girls and 13 years for boys. The increase in height and weight is generally remarkable and is completed in 2 to 3 years (Table 31–20). The growth spurt in girls is accompanied by an increase in breast size and growth of pubic hair. Menstruation occurs last and signals achievement of puberty. In boys, the growth spurt is accompanied by growth in size of the penis and testes and by growth of pubic hair. Deepening of the voice and growth of facial hair occur later, at the time of puberty. See Chapter 33 for a description of the pubertal stages.

During adolescence children grow stronger and more muscular and establish characteristic male and female patterns of fat distribution. The apocrine and eccrine glands mature, leading to increased sweating and a distinct odor to perspiration. All body organs are now fully mature, enabling the adolescent to take adult doses of medications.

The adolescent must adapt to a rapidly changing body for several years. Height, weight, and body proportions increase. Such changes occur with great variability so an adolescent may be at different points of maturation than peers. These physical changes, hormonal variations, and differences in timing offer challenges to identity formation. The adolescent must incorporate the new body, its functions, and retain a healthy sense of self in relationship to peers. The formation of self-identity is a psychologic process but is necessarily closely connected with the bodily changes occurring.

Cognitive Development

Adolescence marks the beginning of Piaget's last stage of cognitive development, the stage of formal operational thought. The adolescent no longer depends on concrete experiences as the basis of thought but develops the ability to reason abstractly. Such concepts as justice, truth, beauty, and power can be understood. The adolescent revels in this newfound ability and spends a great deal of time thinking, reading, and talking about abstract concepts.

The ability to think and act independently leads many adolescents to rebel against parental authority and experiment with risky behaviors. Through these actions, adolescents seek to establish their own identity and values.

Psychosocial Development

ACTIVITIES
Maturity leads to new activities. Adolescents may drive, ride buses, or bike independently. They are less dependent on parents for transportation and spend more time with friends.

TABLE 31–20 Physical Growth and Development Milestones During Adolescence

PHYSICAL GROWTH	FINE MOTOR ABILITY	GROSS MOTOR ABILITY	SENSORY ABILITY
Variation in age of growth spurt During growth spurt, girls gain 7–25 kg (15–55 lb) and grow 2.5–20 cm (2–8 in.); boys gain approximately 7–29.5 kg (15–65 lb) and grow 11–30 cm (4 1/2–12 in.)	Skills are well developed (A)	New sports activities attempted and muscle development continues (B) Some lack of coordination common during growth spurt	Fully developed

A Fine motor skills are well developed

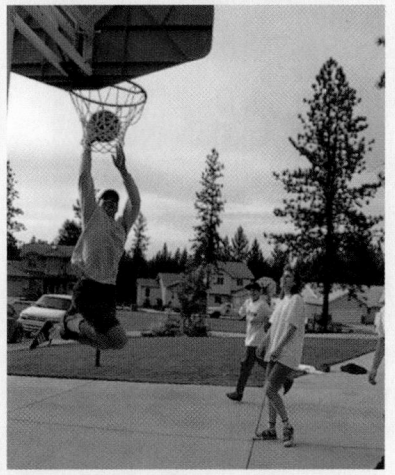

B New sports activities attempted

TABLE 31–21 Psychosocial Development During Adolescence

AGE	ACTIVITIES	COMMUNICATION
12–18 years 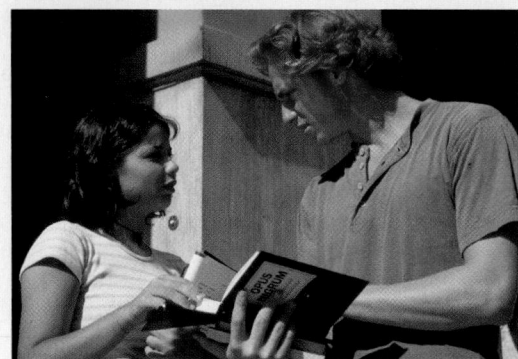	Sports—ball games, gymnastics, water and snow skiing/boarding, swimming, school sports School activities—drama, yearbook, class office, club participation Quiet activities—reading, schoolwork, television, computer, video games, music	Increasing communication and time with peer group—movies, dances, driving, eating out, attending sports events Applying abstract thought and analysis in conversations at home and school

Activities include participation in sports and extracurricular school activities, as well as "hanging out" and attending movies or concerts with friends (Table 31–21). The peer group becomes the focus of activities (Figure 31–13), regardless of the teen's interests. Peers are important in establishing identity and providing meaning. Although same-sex interactions dominate,

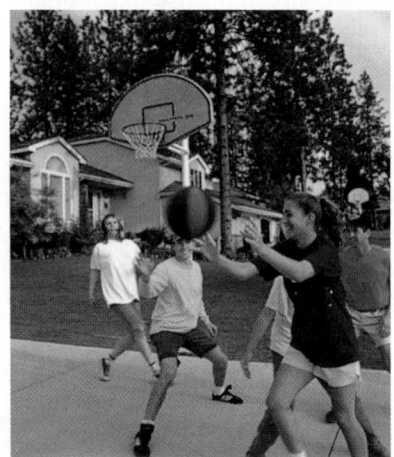

A

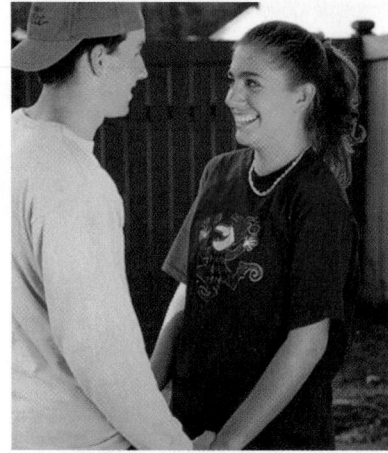

B

Figure 31–13 Peer group activities in adolescence. Social interaction between children of same and opposite sex is as important inside the acute care setting as it is outside. *A,* Teenagers enjoy playing together. *B,* Emotional relationships form during adolescence.

boy–girl relationships are more common than at earlier stages. Adolescents thus participate in and learn from social interactions fundamental to adult relationships.

PERSONALITY AND TEMPERAMENT

Characteristics of temperament manifested during childhood usually remain stable in the teenage years. For instance, the adolescent who was a calm, scheduled infant and child often demonstrates initiative to regulate study times and other routines. Similarly, the adolescent who was an easily stimulated infant may now have a messy room, a harried schedule with assignments always completed late, and an interest in many activities. It is also common for an adolescent who was an easy child to become more difficult because of the psychologic changes of adolescence and the need to assert independence.

As during the child's earlier ages, the nurse's role may be to inform parents of different personality types and to help them support the teen's uniqueness while providing necessary structure and feedback. Nurses can help parents understand their teen's personality type and work with the adolescent to meet expectations set by teachers and others in authority.

COMMUNICATION

The adolescent uses and understands all parts of speech. Colloquialisms and slang are commonly used with the peer group. The adolescent often studies a foreign language in school, having the ability to understand and analyze grammar and sentence structure.

The adolescent increasingly leaves the home base and establishes close ties with peers. These relationships become the basis for identity formation. There is generally a period of stress or crisis before a strong identity can emerge. The adolescent may try out new roles by learning a new sport or other skills, experimenting with drugs or alcohol, wearing different styles of clothing, or trying other activities. It is important to provide positive role models and a variety of experiences to help the adolescent make wise choices.

Adolescents also have a need to leave the past, to be different, and to change from former patterns to establish their own identities. Rules that are repeated constantly and dogmatically will probably be broken in the adolescent's quest for self-identity. This poses difficulties when the adolescent has a health problem, such as diabetes, or a heart problem that requires ongoing care. Introducing the adolescent to other teens who manage the same problem appropriately is usually more successful than telling the adolescent what to do.

Ensure privacy during the taking of health histories or interventions with teens. Even if a parent is present for part of a history or examination, the adolescent should be given the opportunity to relay information or ask questions alone with the healthcare provider. Give the adolescent a choice of whether to have a parent present during an examination or while care is provided. Most information shared by an adolescent is confidential. Some states mandate disclosure of certain information to parents, such as an adolescent's desire for an abortion. In these cases, the adolescent should be informed of what will be disclosed to the parent.

Setting up teen rooms (recreation rooms for use only by adolescents) or separate adolescent units in hospitals can provide necessary peer support during hospitalization. Most adolescents are not pleased when placed on a unit or in a room with young children. Choices should be allowed whenever possible. These might include preference for evening or morning bathing, the type of clothes to wear while hospitalized, timing of treatments, and who should be allowed to visit and for how long. Use of negotiations and agreements with adolescents may increase compliance. Firmness, gentleness, choices, and respect must all be balanced during care of adolescent clients.

Growth and Development

Strategies for communicating with adolescents include the following:

- Provide written as well as verbal explanations.
- Direct history and explanations to teen alone; then include parent.
- Allow for safe exploration of topics by suggesting that teen is similar to other teens. ("Many teens with diabetes have questions about how to eat foods they and their friends like and still stay within their diet needs. How about you?")
- Arrange meetings for discussions with other teens.

SEXUALITY

With maturation of the body and increased secretion of hormones, the adolescent achieves sexual maturity. This complex process involves a growing interest in sexuality and romantic or sexual relationships, an interplay of the forces of society and family, and identity formation. The early adolescent progresses from dances and other social events with members of the opposite sex; the late adolescent is mature sexually and may have regular sexual encounters. Nearly one half of all high-school students in the United States have had intercourse, and 34% had intercourse in the previous 3 months. However, 59% of youths did not use a condom at their last sexual encounter, putting this age group at high risk of acquiring sexually transmitted infections (Kann et al., 2014).

Teenagers need information about their bodies and emerging sexuality. To make informed decisions about their behavior, teenagers should understand the interests and forces they experience. Including sex education in school classes and healthcare encounters is important. Information on how to prevent sexually transmitted infections (STIs) is given, with most school districts now providing some teaching on AIDS. Far more common risks to teens, however, are diseases such as gonorrhea and herpes. Health histories should include questions on sexual activity, STIs, and birth control use and understanding. Most hospitals routinely perform pregnancy screening on adolescent girls before elective procedures.

Adolescents benefit from clear information about sexuality, an opportunity to develop relationships with adolescents in various settings, an open atmosphere at home and school where problems and issues can be discussed, and previous experience in problem solving and self-decision making. Sexual issues should be among topics that adolescents can discuss openly in a variety of settings. Alternatives and support for their decisions should be available.

Some adolescents identify with a sexual minority group such as lesbian, gay, bisexual, or transgender. They are at particular risk of being stigmatized and harassed by other youth or adults. They are more likely to suffer a variety of problems, such as isolation, rejection by family and friends, violence, and suicide, and to take sexual risks (Steever, Francis, Gordon, et al., 2014). Nurses are instrumental in helping these youth by providing information for them and their parents, integrating sexual minority content into school sexual curricula, and providing referrals for health care and social care when needed. See Chapter 42 for further information about the health issues related to homosexuality and other sexual minority practices.

Focus Your Study

- Development unfolds in a predictable pattern, but at different rates dependent on the particular characteristics and experiences of each child.

- Major theories of development encompass the psychosexual (Freud), psychosocial (Erikson), cognitive (Piaget), moral (Kohlberg), social learning (Bandura), and behavioral (Skinner and Watson) components of individuals.

- The ecologic theory of Bronfenbrenner and the temperament theory of Chess and Thomas emphasize the interactions of the individual with the environment.

- Resiliency theory examines risk and protective factors that hinder or help children and families when dealing with developmental and life crises.

- The newborn period begins at birth and ends at about 1 month and is characterized by adaptation to extrauterine life. Infancy spans 1 month to 1 year and is marked by rapid physical growth, mastery of basic fine and gross motor skills, and emerging cognitive and language skills.

- Toddlers range in age from 1 to 3 years and become increasingly mobile and communicative. Preschool years range from

3 to 6 and are marked by increasing social skills, coordination, and language mastery.

- School age spans the years from 6 to 12, and puberty occurs from 9 to 12 years, marked by a growth spurt and sexual maturation. Adolescence begins at 12 years and lasts through the teen years, with physical, emotional, cognitive, and social maturation.

- The nurse assesses development at each stage and provides anticipatory guidance and other interventions to foster optimal development.

Clinical Reasoning in Action

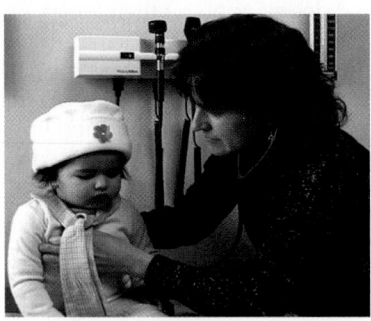

You encounter a 12-month-old child, Julia, while working in the developmental clinic. Her mother tells you that their family practice physician had concerns that Julia might have a developmental delay. She was a full-term baby and there were no complications throughout her mother's pregnancy or delivery. Julia's mother tells you that she has a generally shy and slow-to-warm-up temperament. She makes little eye contact with you and prefers to sit on her mother's lap and cling to her arms if a stranger gets close. She is able to pick up small objects, babble, crawl, and use her pincer grasp. She is not able to walk, hold a crayon, or speak any words. Julia clearly has a developmental delay.

1. What are some examples of toys you can suggest to Julia's parents based on her developmental level (not based on her age)?

2. What are some examples of hazards you can advise Julia's parents about avoiding based on her developmental level?

3. What is a suggestion you can give the parents about dealing with a child like Julia who has a shy or slow-to-warm-up temperament?

References

American Academy of Pediatrics. (2013). *Pediatric nutrition handbook* (7th ed.). Elk Grove Village, IL: Author.

Bandura, A. (1986). *Social foundations of thought and actions: A social cognitive theory.* Englewood Cliffs, NJ: Prentice Hall.

Bandura, A. (1997a). *Self efficacy in changing societies.* New York, NY: Cambridge University Press.

Bandura, A. (1997b). *Self efficacy: The exercise of control.* New York, NY: Freeman.

Benard, B. (2014). *The foundations of the resiliency framework.* Retrieved from http://www.resiliency .com/free-articles-resources/the-foundations-of-the -resiliency-framework/

Bronfenbrenner, U. (1986). Ecology of the family as a context for human development: Research perspectives. *Developmental Psychology, 22,* 723–742.

Bronfenbrenner, U. (Ed.). (2005). *Making human beings human: Bioecological perspectives on human development.* Thousand Oaks, CA: Sage.

Bronfenbrenner, U., McClelland, P. D., Ceci, S. J., Moen, P., & Wethington, E. (1996). *The state of Americans.* New York, NY: Free Press.

Cairns, K. E., Yap, M. B., Pilkington, D., & Jorm, A. F. (2014). Risk and protective factors for depression that adolescents can modify: A systematic review and meta-analysis of longitudinal studies. *Journal of Affective Disorders, 169C,* 61–75. doi: 10.1016/j .jad.2014.08.006

The Center for Parenting Education. (2014). *Temperament: Understanding "goodness of fit."* Retrieved from http://centerforparentingeducation.org/library -of-articles/child-development/unique-child-equation /temperament/understanding-goodness-of-fit/

Chess, S., & Thomas, A. (1995). *Temperament in clinical practice.* New York, NY: Guilford Press.

Chess, S., & Thomas, A. (1996). *Temperament: Theory and practice.* Philadelphia, PA: Brunner/Mazel, Publishers.

Chess, S., & Thomas, A. (1999). *Goodness of fit: Clinical applications from infancy through adult life.* Philadelphia, PA: Brunner/Mazel, Publishers.

Children's Hospital of Philadelphia. (2012). *International adoption health program.* Retrieved from http://www .chop.edu/service/adoption/health-considerations

Davies, J. A., Terhorts, L., Nakonechny, A. J., Skukla, N., & Saadawi, G. E. (2014). The development and effectiveness of a health information website designed to improve parents' self-efficacy in managing risk for obesity in preschoolers. *Journal for Specialists in Pediatric Nursing.* doi: 10.1111/jspn.12086

Dunn, W. L., & Craig, G. J. (2013). *Understanding human development* (3rd ed.). Upper Saddle River, NJ: Pearson Education.

Erikson, E. (1963). *Childhood and society.* New York, NY: Norton.

Erikson, E. (1968). *Identity: Youth and crisis.* New York, NY: Norton.

Ginsberg, H., & Opper, S. (1988). *Piaget's theory of intellectual development* (3rd ed.). Paramus, NJ: Prentice Hall.

Henderson, N., Benard, B., & Sharp-Light, M. (2007). *Resiliency in action.* Ojai, CA: Resiliency in Action.

Joshi, A., Trout, K. E., Aguirre, T., & Wilhelm. S. (2014). Exploration of factors influencing initiation and continuation of breastfeeding among Hispanic women living in rural settings: A multi-methods study. *Rural Remote Health, 14,* 2955.

Kann, L., Kinchen, S., Shanklin, S. L., Flint, K. H., Hawkins, J., Harris, W. A., . . . Zaza, S. (2014). Youth Risk Behavior Surveillance—2013. *Morbidity and Mortality Weekly Report SS, 63*(4), 1–172.

Piaget, J. (1972). *The child's conception of the world.* Totowa, NJ: Littlefield, Adams.

Salmon, J., Jorna, M., Hume, C., Arundell, L., Dhahine, J., Tienstra, J., & Crawford, C. (2011). A translational research intervention to reduce screen behaviours and promote physical activity among children: Switch-2-Activity. *Health Promotion International, 26,* 311–321.

Santrock, J. (2012). *Life-span development* (14th ed.). Boston, MA: McGraw-Hill.

Steever, J., Francis, J., Gordon, L. P., & Lee, J. (2014). Sexual minority youth. *Primary Care, 42,* 651–669.

U.S. Department of State. (2015). *Intercountry adoption.* Retrieved from http://travel.state.gov/content /adoptionsabroad/en/about-us/statistics.html

U.S. Department of Health and Human Services. (2013). *Recent demographic trends in foster care. Data brief 2013-1.* Retrieved from http://www.acf.hhs .gov/sites/default/files/cb/data_brief_foster_care _trends1.pdf

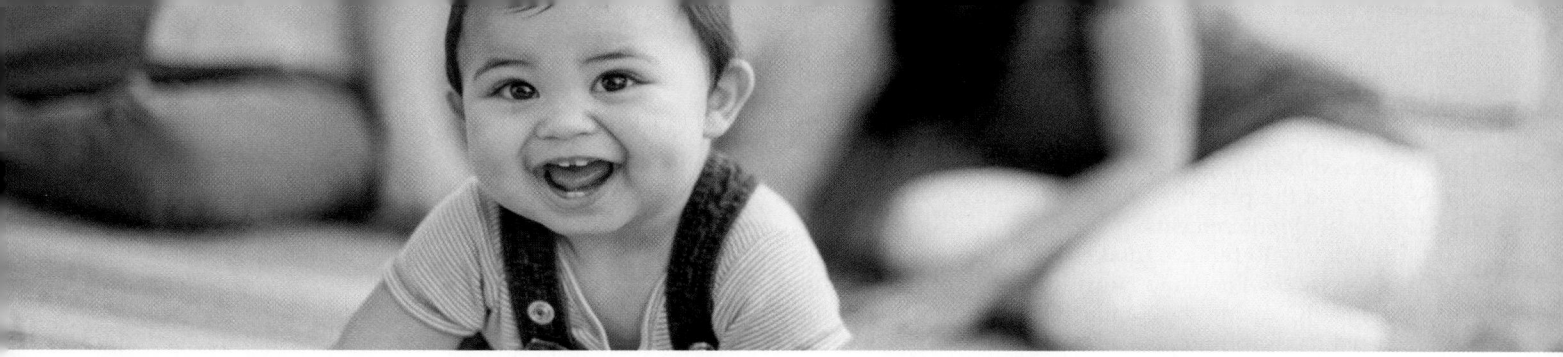

Chapter 32
Infant, Child, and Adolescent Nutrition

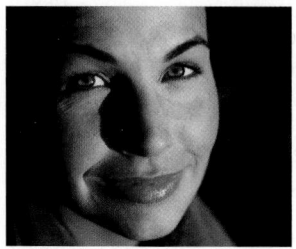

It is exciting to see Joey progressing into the school setting. Being with children his age will really help him develop in many ways. We're just worried because he needs to get only foods he can chew and swallow so he does not choke. He also needs his tube feedings during school to be sure he gets enough energy to do well.

—Mother of Joey, 11 years old

Ryan McVay/Getty Images

Learning Outcomes

32.1 Discuss major nutritional concepts pertaining to the growth and development of children.

32.2 Describe and plan nursing interventions to meet nutritional needs for all age groups from infancy through adolescence.

32.3 Integrate methods of nutritional assessment into nursing care of infants, children, and adolescents.

32.4 Identify and explain common nutritional problems of children.

32.5 Develop nursing interventions for children with nutritional disorders.

Adequate nutrition is an essential component of growth and development. The child's nutritional status begins before birth and is related to the mother's nutritional state. All children must be assessed for nutritional status, followed by teaching or other interventions to enhance health. Nurses are instrumental in giving parents information about normal nutritional needs of infants, children, and adolescents. Common techniques to assess nutrition, such as measuring growth and monitoring hematocrit, provide needed information about whether intake of nutrients is adequate.

All children and their parents can benefit from information about nutritional needs, but some children have additional concerns that must be considered. The nurse recognizes the special requirements of children with conditions such as feeding disorders, food allergies, cystic fibrosis, cerebral palsy, or diabetes. Nutrition monitoring is provided throughout childhood so that dietary counseling can be integrated with other teaching to promote development. How can the nurse bridge the various settings in which children's nutritional needs are met? These might include the home, childcare settings, schools, and hospitals. How can the nurse help the family prepare for meeting the nutritional needs of a child who has special needs during car or plane travel?

Some children have unique nutritional needs due to their social environments. Parents may not be knowledgeable about the nutritional requirements of children. Perhaps the family is vegetarian and needs extra help to ensure intake of essential nutrients. If finances are limited, the family may need resources such as food stamps, food banks, or budget planning. The nurse considers the high rate of childhood obesity and common nutritional deficits when applying concepts of health promotion with families. Whatever the nurse's setting, knowledge of nutrition must be integrated within nursing care.

General Nutrition Concepts

Nutrition refers to taking in food and assimilating it metabolically for use by the body. It is an essential component of life and therefore an important body of knowledge to consider in discussions of child growth and development. The body requires a wide array of nutrients. **Macronutrients**, or the major building blocks of the body, are carbohydrates, protein, and fat. Vitamins and minerals are **micronutrients**, or substances needed in small quantities for healthy body functioning. The need for nutrients is dependent on activity level, state of health, and the presence of disease or other stress-related and age-related requirements.

The **Dietary Reference Intakes (DRIs)** are a set of values established by the Food and Nutrition Board of the Institute of Medicine (IOM) and the National Academy of Science that can be used to assess and plan intake for individuals of different ages (Institute of Medicine, 2011). They commonly include the Estimated Average Requirement, or EAR (intake needed to meet requirements of 50% of the population); Recommended Dietary Allowance, or RDA (intake needed to meet requirements of 97% to 98% of the population); Adequate Intake, or AI (used when data to support EAR are not available); and Upper Intake, or UI (maximum level unlikely to pose health risk). Although the DRI approach is used in the United States, other countries have developed their own approaches to dietary standards. For example, Canada uses Adequate Intake and Reference Nutrient Intake, while the United Kingdom uses Recommended Daily Nutrient Intakes. The aims of these standards are to provide a method to evaluate individual and population diets and to plan nutrition programs and education. DRIs are generally specific to males and females in several age categories. See Appendix F for a list of DRIs for children and adolescents.

Although the DRIs provide useful information when evaluating diets, their use can be time consuming. What "quick check" can provide feedback about the daily diets of children? The nurse should be familiar with the U.S. MyPlate food guide and hang posters that illustrate its healthy choices in schools, clinics, and hospitals. It is a fast way to examine children's intakes for 1 day and evaluate whether they meet most requirements. Instead of calculating amounts of nutrients ingested, the MyPlate program focuses on categories of foods, which readily reflects the actual intake. The numbers of servings from various categories stay constant throughout childhood, while the serving sizes increase as the child gets older. See Figure 32–1 for MyPlate, and consult the U.S. Department of Agriculture (USDA) website for ethnic/cultural food guides for vegetarians and those from various ethnic groups, such as Hispanic and Native American.

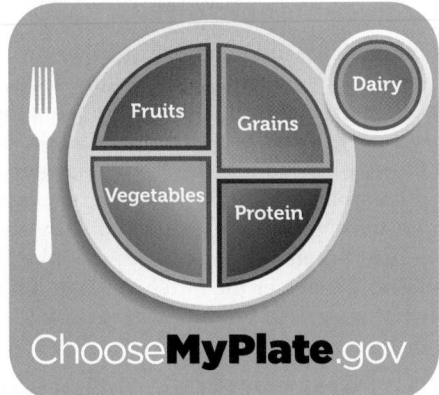

Figure 32–1 The U.S. MyPlate food guide is used to provide teaching about amounts of foods recommended for daily intake.

SOURCE: From U.S. Department of Agriculture and U.S. Department of Health and Human Services. (2011). Retrieved from http://www.choosemyplate.gov

Nutritional Needs

Nutritional needs evolve during all of infancy and childhood. They support growth and development and influence the progression of the child along the developmental path. Nutritional intake helps to maintain the health of the child and fosters a state of maximal potential or health promotion. Specific needs during each developmental stage are discussed in this section. A detailed description of breastfeeding and bottlefeeding for the newborn can be found in Chapter 25, while additional pertinent information about infant nutrition is discussed below.

Infancy

FLUID AND MACRONUTRIENTS

Fluid requirements during the neonatal period are high (140 to 160 mL/kg/day) because of the newborn's decreased ability to concentrate urine and increased overall metabolic rate. Although the infant's total body water content is high (75% to 80%) compared with an adult (60%), the infant has an increased surface area to mass ratio and decreased renal absorptive capacity that makes the infant more susceptible to dehydration from insufficient fluid intake or increased fluid loss caused by diarrhea, vomiting, or another source of fluid loss. Parents and caretakers should be aware of the signs of dehydration. See Chapter 44 for further information about fluid needs in infancy.

The basal metabolic rate (BMR) refers to the energy needed for thermoregulation, cardiorespiratory function, cellular activity, and growth. A newborn requires 100 to 115 kcal/kg/day at 1 month. In breast milk, the primary carbohydrate is lactose. In addition to providing energy, lactose also functions to enhance the absorption of calcium, magnesium, and zinc. Human milk also contains other carbohydrates such as glucosamines and nitrogen-containing oligosaccharides. Glucosamines are one of the building blocks for connective tissues. Oligosaccharides promote the growth of *Lactobacillus bifidus*, which promotes an intestinal acidic environment that is hostile to harmful bacteria, making it difficult for them to thrive (Lawrence & Lawrence, 2011).

Infants receive approximately 50% of their calories from fat. Fats also help the body absorb the fat-soluble vitamins A, D, E, and K. Fats are a precursor of prostaglandins and other hormones. Fatty acids are a key component to brain development. Their derivatives, docosahexaenoic acid (DHA) and arachidonic acid (ARA), are long-chain polyunsaturated fatty acids (LCPUFAs) needed for myelination of the spinal cord and other nerves, and for development of visual acuity and cognitive and behavioral functions (Cloherty, Eichenwald, & Stark, 2012).

Approximately 98% of human milk fat is in the form of triglycerides, and a small amount is from cholesterol. Cholesterol levels in breast milk may also stimulate the production of enzymes that lead to more efficient metabolism of cholesterol, thereby reducing its harmful long-term effects on the cardiovascular system.

Fat content is the most variable component in breast milk, ranging from 30 to 50 g/L. It is influenced by maternal parity, duration of pregnancy, the stage of lactation, diurnal regulation, and changes in fat content even during a single feeding. Multiparous mothers produce milk with a lower content of fatty acids than primiparous women. Mothers of preterm infants have a greater concentration of LCPUFAs in their milk compared with mothers of term infants. By receiving this preterm breast milk, preterm infants receive the increased concentrations of DHA and ARA intended for their growth (Lawrence & Lawrence, 2011).

Phospholipids and cholesterol levels are higher in colostrum compared with mature milk, although overall fat content is higher in mature breast milk compared with colostrum. Fat content is generally higher in the evening and lower in the early morning. Within a single feeding session, an infant initially receives the low-fat foremilk before receiving the higher calorie, high-fat hindmilk. Finally, the fat content of breast milk is also affected by maternal diet and maternal fat stores. Mothers on low-fat diets have increased production of medium-chain fatty acids (C6–C10), and mothers with high levels of body fat produce breast milk with a higher fat content (Lawrence & Lawrence, 2011).

The fats in milk-based formulas are modified in an attempt to parallel the fat profile of breast milk by removing the butterfat from cow's milk and adding vegetable oils. The different blends of fats all provide a fatty acid profile that is similar to breast milk in terms of amount of saturated, monounsaturated, and polyunsaturated fats present. Since 2002, infant formulas have been supplemented with DHA and ARA. However, breast milk also contains 167 other fatty acids of uncertain function that are absent from formula (Cloherty et al., 2012).

Proteins are the building blocks for muscle and organ structure. They are key to the body's metabolic processes including energy metabolism, cell signaling, growth, and immune function. Milk proteins are often grouped into casein and whey proteins. Whey protein is the predominant dietary protein in human milk. During digestion this type of protein creates soft curds that are easily and quickly broken down. Because of this, breastfeeding babies digest their meals in 90 minutes and need to feed often, receiving about 8 to 12 feedings per day. Casein is the major phosphoprotein found in milk. Cow's milk contains a high amount of casein (a low ratio of whey to casein— approximately 20:80) compared with mature human milk (60:40 whey:casein). Because of its tendency to form curds, milk with high amounts of casein is less easily digested. Cow's milk–based formulas are usually modified to get closer to the whey:casein ratio of human milk.

MICRONUTRIENTS

The fat-soluble vitamins (vitamins A, D, E, and K) are found in both cow's milk–based formula and breast milk. After absorption via the lymphatic system, vitamins enter the blood and are transported to the various tissues. Excessive amounts of fat-soluble vitamins may result in toxicity, and there is general agreement that no routine fat-soluble vitamin supplementation is needed with the exception of vitamin D. See *Teaching Highlights: Supplements for Breastfed Babies* for recommendations regarding vitamin D and other nutrients.

The vitamin B complex and vitamin C are water-soluble vitamins that pass readily from serum to breast milk. However, mothers who follow a strict vegetarian or macrobiotic diet may have insufficient vitamin B_{12} in their milk. In that case, the exclusively breastfed infant should receive vitamin B_{12} supplementation. Formula is fortified with adequate amounts of the water-soluble vitamins to meet the DRIs. Unlike fat-soluble vitamins, any excess

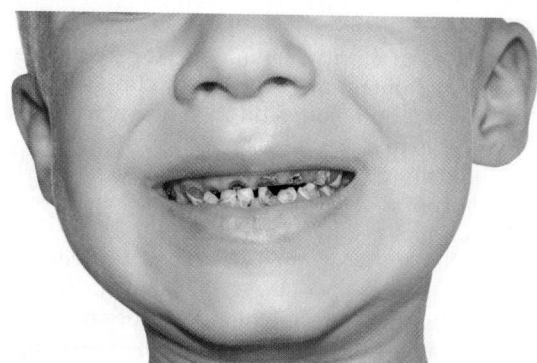

Figure 32–2 Early childhood caries. This child has had major tooth decay related to sleeping as an infant and toddler while sucking bottles of juice and milk.

SOURCE: Everst/Alamy.

water-soluble vitamins ingested are simply excreted and the threat of toxicity is low (Lawrence & Lawrence, 2011).

Both human milk and infant formulas contain several major and trace minerals to satisfy the needs of the growing infant. The mineral content of breast milk does not appear to be influenced by maternal diet.

DENTAL HEALTH

Early childhood caries, the presence of one or more decayed, lost, or filled tooth surfaces in a primary tooth from birth to 6 years of age, can occur when a young child is allowed to breast-feed or drink from a bottle for long periods, especially when sleeping (AAP Committee on Nutrition, 2013; Colak, Dulgergil, Dalli, et al., 2013) (Figure 32–2). The milk, juice, or other fluid pools around the upper anterior teeth, salivary flow decreases, and acid buffering is decreased, resulting in tooth decay. Nurses should teach parents to avoid putting the child to bed with a bottle and encourage pacifier use or a bottle of water instead. The child should not walk around with a bottle during the day. Mothers who breastfeed should also be cautioned to limit feeding to specific times rather than letting the infant breastfeed every few minutes (sometimes done when infant and mother co-sleep) so that milk will not pool in the mouth during sleep. When sleepy, the infant does not swallow well and the milk is in constant contact with the teeth where milk sugars can decay erupting teeth.

Parents can be taught beginning dental care for the infant, which includes wiping the teeth off daily once they erupt with a piece of moist gauze or a small infant toothbrush. Some pediatric dentists like to see the child for a first dental visit at about 1 year of age, while others wait until the child is older. The nurse should encourage the parents to select and establish contact with a dental provider when the child is nearing the end of infancy.

TEACHING HIGHLIGHTS | Supplements for Breastfed Babies

1. Each baby receives a vitamin K injection after birth to promote adequate blood clotting. After that, no further vitamin K is needed since children manufacture this vitamin in the gut once they begin eating.
2. Vitamin D is recommended at a minimum of 400 International Units/day for all infants (American Academy of Pediatrics [AAP] Section on Breastfeeding, 2012).
3. Iron is not needed unless the infant is not eating food containing iron by 4 to 6 months. The baby may need an iron source earlier if the mother was anemic during pregnancy or while breastfeeding.
4. Fluoride 0.25 mg is given after 6 months of age if water is not fluoridated to a level of 0.6 part per million (ppm), or if the baby is not drinking any water (American Association of Pediatric Dentistry, 2014).

WEANING

Weaning is the term used when infants stop breastfeeding or bottlefeeding and obtain most liquids by cup. At about 8 to 9 months, a cup should be offered to the infant with assistance being provided so that learning about drinking from a cup can begin. By about 1 year of age, infants are usually able to drink most liquids from a cup with a lid, so bottles can be slowly withdrawn and replaced by cups.

The decision to wean the baby from the breast may be made for a variety of reasons, including family or cultural pressures, changes in the home situation, pressure from the woman's partner, or a personal opinion about when weaning should occur. Some infants wean themselves spontaneously despite the wishes of the mother. For the woman who is comfortable with breastfeeding and well informed about the process, the appropriate time to wean her infant will become evident if she is sensitive to the child's cues, such as increased interest in other foods and decreased frequency of feeding (Centers for Disease Control and Prevention [CDC], 2011a). The infant who is weaned before 12 months should be given iron-fortified infant formula rather than cow's milk.

Healthy People 2020

(MICH-21) Increase the proportion of infants who are breastfed
- Ever: target 81.9%
- At 6 months: target 60.6%
- Exclusively through 3 months: target 46.2%
- Exclusively through 6 months: target 25.5%

If weaning is timed to respond to the child's cues, and if the mother is comfortable with the timing, it can be accomplished with less difficulty than if the process begins before mother and child are ready emotionally. Nevertheless, weaning is a time of emotional separation for mother and baby; it may be difficult for them to give up the closeness of their nursing sessions. The nurse who understands this possibility can help the mother see that her infant is growing up and plan other comforting, consoling, and play activities to replace breastfeeding. A gradual approach is the easiest and most comforting way to wean the child from breastfeeding.

During weaning, the mother should substitute one cup feeding or bottlefeeding for one breastfeeding session over a few days to a week so that her breasts gradually produce less milk. Eliminating the breastfeedings associated with meals first facilitates the mother's ability to wean the infant because satiation with food lessens the desire for milk. Over a period of several weeks she can substitute more cup feedings or bottlefeedings for breastfeedings. The slow method of weaning prevents breast engorgement, allows infants to alter their eating methods at their own rates, and provides time for psychologic adjustment.

INTRODUCTION OF COMPLEMENTARY FOODS

When should other foods be added to the infant's diet? Although some parents add other foods when the infant is only days or weeks old, and such practices are often culturally derived, it is best to take cues from the infant's developmental milestones. The American Academy of Pediatrics recommends introducing complementary foods at about 6 months (AAP, 2014a). At this age, the extrusion reflex (or tongue thrust) decreases and the infant can sit well with support. The infant is also developing the ability to appreciate texture and swallow

TABLE 32–1 Introduction of Solid Foods in Infancy

RECOMMENDATION	RATIONALE
Introduce rice or other single-grain baby cereal at about 6 months.	Single grains are easy to digest and have low allergenic potential, and baby preparations contain iron.
Introduce fruits or vegetables at 6–8 months. Some healthcare providers recommend vegetable introduction before fruits.	Fruits and vegetables provide needed vitamins. Vegetables are not as sweet as fruits; introducing them first may enhance acceptability to the infant.
Introduce meats at 8–10 months.	Meats are harder to digest, have high protein load, and should not be fed until close to 1 year of age.
Use single-food prepared baby foods rather than combination meals.	Combination meals usually contain more sugar, salt, and fillers.
Introduce one new food at a time, waiting at least 3–4 days to introduce another. Delay feeding eggs, strawberries, wheat, corn, fish, and nut products until close to 2–3 years of age.	If a food allergy or intolerance develops, it will be easy to identify. The foods listed are those most commonly associated with food allergies.
Avoid carrots, beets, squash, beans, and spinach (especially if prepared at home) before 6 months of age. Have well water evaluated for nitrates (the recommended level is less than 10 mg/L).	Nitrates in these foods and in water near agricultural runoff can be converted to nitrite by young infants, causing methemoglobinemia. Commercial baby foods are adjusted for nitrates, so levels are lower than in foods prepared in the home.
Infants can be fed mashed portions of table foods such as peas, corn, rice, and potatoes.	This is a less expensive alternative to jars of commercially prepared baby food; it allows parents of various cultural groups to feed ethnic foods to infants.
Avoid adding sugar, salt, and spices when preparing baby foods at home.	Infants need not become accustomed to these flavors; they may get too much sodium from salt or develop gastric distress from some spices.
Avoid honey until at least 1 year of age.	Infants cannot detoxify *Clostridium botulinum* spores sometimes present in honey and can develop botulism.

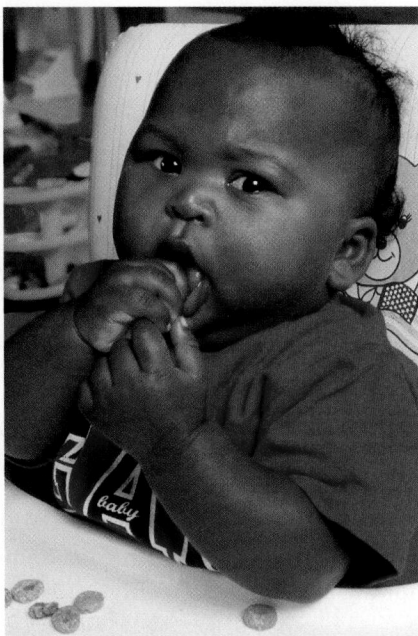

Figure 32–3 Introducing finger foods. The baby who has developed the ability to grasp with thumb and forefinger should receive some foods that can be held in the hand.

TABLE 32–2 Infant Nutritional Patterns

AGE	PATTERN
Birth–1 month	• Eats every 2–3 h, breast or bottle • 2–3 oz (60–90 mL) per feeding
2–4 months	• Has coordinated suck–swallow • Eats every 3–4 h • 3–4 oz (90–120 mL) per feeding
4–6 months	• Begins baby food, usually rice cereal, 2–3 T, twice daily • Consumes breast milk or formula 4 or more times daily • 4–5 oz (100–150 mL) per feeding
6–8 months	• Eats baby food such as rice cereal, fruits, and vegetables, 2–5 T, 3 times daily • Consumes breast milk or formula 4 times daily • 6–8 oz (160–225 mL) per feeding
8–10 months	• Enjoys soft finger foods 3 times daily • Consumes breast milk or formula 4 times daily • 6 oz (160 mL) per feeding • Uses cup with lid
10–12 months	• Eats most soft table foods with family 3 times daily • Uses cup with or without lid • Attempts to feed self with spoon though spills often • Consumes breast milk or formula 4 times daily • 6–8 oz (160–225 mL) per feeding

nonliquid foods and can indicate desire for food or turn away when full. At 6 to 12 months, complementary foods are offered in addition to the intake of breast milk or formula rather than replacing that essential nutrient (AAP, 2014a) (see Table 32–1).

The first complementary food added to the infant's diet is often rice or other single-grain cereal. The advantages of introducing cereal first is that it provides iron at an age when the infant's prenatal iron stores begin to decrease, it seldom causes allergy, and it is easy to digest. A tablespoon or two is fed to the infant once or twice daily just before formula or breastfeeding. The infant may appear to spit out food at first because of normal back-and-forth tongue movement. Parents should not interpret this early feeding behavior as indicating dislike for the food. With a little practice the infant becomes adept at spoon feeding.

Once the infant eats 1/4 cup of food twice daily, usually at 6 to 8 months of age, vegetables or fruits can be introduced, at a rate of one new food every several days (Table 32–1). By 8 to 10 months of age, most fruits and vegetables have been introduced and strained meats or other protein (e.g., tofu, cheese, mashed cooked beans) can be added to the infant's diet. Finger foods are introduced during the second half of the first year as the infant's palmar and then finger grasp develops and as teeth begin to erupt (Figure 32–3). Infants enjoy toast, O-shaped cereal, finely sliced meats, cheese, yogurt, tofu, and small pieces of cooked, softened vegetables. Certain foods are associated with choking and should be avoided.

SAFETY ALERT!
Advise parents to use caution when providing finger foods to the infant. Hard foods and some soft and malleable ones slip easily into the throat and may cause choking. Avoid hot dogs, hard vegetables, candy, and chunks of peanut butter. Infants and other young children should always be supervised while eating. Be sure parents are familiar with techniques for airway obstruction removal and have emergency numbers clearly listed on their phones.

Certain foods are more commonly associated with development of food allergies, and avoiding them in infancy may decrease allergy incidence. Typically, recommendations for infants at risk due to family history of allergy are to delay feeding of cow's milk until 1 year, eggs until 2 years, and peanuts, nuts, fish, and shellfish until 3 years (AAP, 2014a). However, a recent study found that children at risk of peanut allergy due to manifestation of food allergy in infancy or a family history of allergy have a lowered risk of having peanut allergy at age 5 years if they consume peanuts frequently within the first year of life (Du Toit et al., 2015). When infants have allergies to some foods or have a family history of allergy, refer them for current management to a pediatrician and/or an immunologist.

As food and juice intake increase, formula-feedings or breastfeedings decrease in amount and frequency (Table 32–2). If breastfeeding is not chosen, or if supplemental feedings are provided, only iron-fortified infant formula should be used during the first year of life. Cow's milk (including evaporated milk) can lead to bleeding and anemia (see sections on iron and anemia in this chapter), can interfere with absorption of some nutrients, and has a high solute load, which immature kidneys can have difficulty excreting. Iron-fortified formula should always be used when the infant under 12 months drinks formula. When breastfed babies are not eating foods with iron by 6 months, supplemental iron may need to be added. Careful dietary assessment and discussion of intake by the nurse at health visits helps the practitioner decide if supplemental iron is needed.

Parents who want to make baby foods at home can be encouraged and instructed to do so. Some commercially prepared foods have unnecessary additives such as salt, sugar, and food starch, and they may be costly for some families. Parents can easily blend fruits and vegetables the family is eating without adding salt, sugar, or seasoning. Prepared foods should be used promptly and stored in the refrigerator between feedings. Foods can also be placed into ice cube trays and frozen; a cube or two can be defrosted at mealtime. Nurses should caution parents to avoid certain home-prepared vegetables and not to use honey in foods for infants as it can lead to infant botulism because infants cannot detoxify the *Clostridium botulinum* spores sometimes present in honey (see Table 32–1). If foods or fluids are microwaved, they should be shaken, stirred, and checked for temperature so that hot areas in the food do not burn the infant.

Toddlerhood

Why do parents of toddlers frequently become concerned about the small amount of food their children eat? Why do toddlers seem to survive and even thrive with minimal food intake? The toddler often displays the phenomenon of **physiologic anorexia**, which occurs when the extremely high metabolic demands of infancy slow to keep pace with the more moderate growth rate of toddlerhood. Although it can appear that the toddler eats nothing at times, intake over days or a week is generally sufficient and balanced enough to meet the body's demands for nutrients and energy.

Parents often need knowledge about the types of foods that constitute a healthy diet. The nurse can offer fresh food alternatives with lower sodium content to replace hot dogs, microwave meals, or fast foods by providing information about easy preparation of sliced meats, cheese, tofu, fruits, and vegetables. Healthy snacks for young children include yogurt, cheese, milk, slices of bread with peanut butter, thinly sliced fruits, and soft vegetables.

Healthy People 2020

(NWS-19) Reduce consumption of sodium in the population aged 2 years and older

---

Parents should be advised to offer a variety of nutritious foods several times daily (three meals and two snacks) and let the toddler make choices from the foods offered. They should offer foods only at mealtimes and have the child sit in a high chair or on a special seat at the table to eat (Figure 32–4). Small portions are most appealing to the toddler. A general guideline for food quantity at a meal is one tablespoon of each food per year of age.

The toddler should drink 16 to 24 oz (1/2 to 3/4 L) of milk daily; whole milk is recommended from 1 to 2 years, and after 2 years of age 2% is appropriate. Parents should be cautioned against giving the toddler more than a quart (1 L) of milk daily since this interferes with the desire to eat other foods, leading to dietary deficiencies. Recall that the child should not be put to bed with a bottle or allowed to carry a bottle of milk or juice around during the day on account of the risk of early childhood caries (see earlier discussion). In addition, parents should be advised to use only 100% fruit juice and to limit consumption of this juice to 4 to 6 oz daily for children ages 1 to 6 years to decrease the likelihood of becoming overweight, developing dental caries, or experiencing abdominal discomfort (AAP, 2011). Unpasteurized juice should never be used since it may contain pathogens particularly harmful to young children. Drinking water and eating whole fruits, which provide fiber, are healthier alternatives. Avoid more than one meal weekly from a fast-food restaurant because such meals generally are high in fat and sugar and low in fiber.

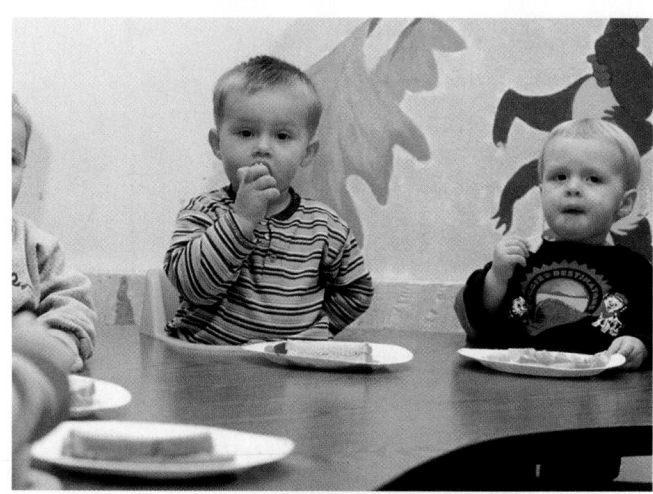

Figure 32–4 **Fostering healthy eating habits. Toddlers should sit at a table or in a high chair to eat to minimize the chance of choking and to foster positive eating patterns.**

Growth and Development

Toddlers generally eat three meals and two to three snacks daily. Toddlers can drink 2% milk or "follow-up" formula, starting at 2 years of age. Follow-up formula contains less fat than infant formula, and some parents prefer its convenience, although it is not necessary; 2% milk is appropriate to use at that age. Cups are recommended, and bottle use should be discontinued. Drinks should be consumed at mealtimes and for snacks while sitting at a table; carrying cups during the day while playing or at other activities is not recommended. The child is learning to use utensils but may prefer fingers, and still needs small serving sizes.

Learning how to eat with others is an important task of toddlerhood. The toddler displays characteristic autonomy or independence during mealtime. Advise parents to provide opportunities for self-feeding of food with fingers and utensils and to allow some simple choices, such as type of liquid or cup to use. Young children should eat at a table with others, not be allowed to run and play while eating, and eat at specified meal and snack times. Toddlers should be taught to brush teeth after each meal, and care providers should offer assistance and supervision. A dental visit should occur during toddlerhood.

Because social skills are developing, the hospitalized toddler may eat better if allowed to have meals with parents or other hospitalized children. See Chapter 39 for further suggestions about management of nutrition in hospitalized children.

Preschool

The diet of the preschooler is similar to that of the toddler, but mealtime is now a more social event. Preschoolers like the company of others while they eat, and they enjoy helping with food preparation and table setting (Figure 32–5). Involving them in these tasks can provide a forum for teaching about nutritious foods and principles of preparation, such as the need for refrigeration, safety around stoves, and cleanliness. Visits to fast-food restaurants should be limited to about once weekly, and parents can use the opportunity to assist the child in making wise choices of nutritionally adequate foods in that setting.

Although the rate of growth is slow and steady during the preschool years, the child may have periods of **food jags** (eating

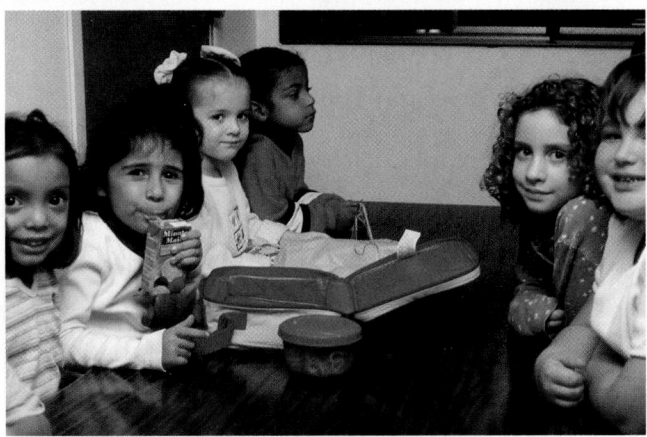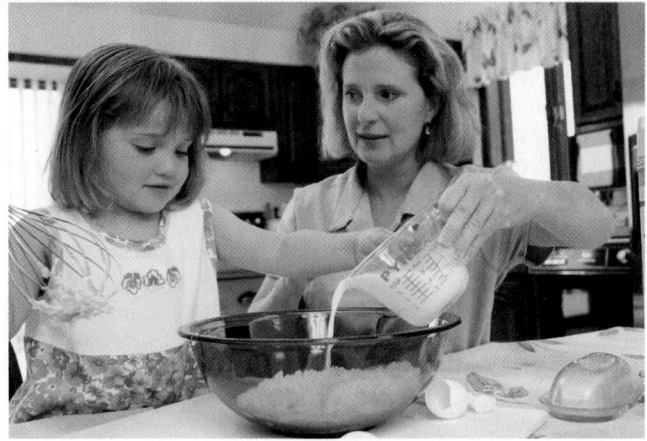

Figure 32–5 **Preschoolers learn food habits by eating with others. Engaging them in food preparation enhances knowledge of food and promotes intake at meals.**

only a few foods for several days or weeks) and greater or lesser intake. Parents should be advised to assess food intake over a 1- or 2-week period rather than at each meal to obtain a more accurate impression of total intake. Food jags can be handled by providing the desired food along with other foods to foster choice. The child who chooses not to eat at snack time or meal-time should not be given other foods in between. The child will become hungry and get accustomed to eating when food is provided. Three meals and two or three snacks daily are the norm. Fruit juice should be limited to 8 to 12 oz daily, and begin teaching the "5-a-day" program that supports having five servings of fruits/vegetables each day.

The preschool period is a good time to continue encouraging good dental habits. Children can begin to brush their own teeth with parental supervision and help to reach all tooth surfaces. Fluoride supplements should be used when the water supply is not fluoridated (fluoride concentration below 0.7 mg/L) (U.S. Department of Health and Human Services, 2015). If the child has not yet visited a dentist, the first dental visit should be scheduled so the child can become accustomed to the routine of dental care.

School Age

The school-age years are a period of gradual growth when energy requirements remain at a steady level, although at some point during these years most children experience a preadolescent growth spurt. Girls may begin a growth spurt by 10 or 11 years, and boys a year or so later. Nutritional needs increase dramatically with this spurt, with large numbers of calories and increased amounts of other nutrients being required (see Appendix F for Dietary Reference Intakes).

School-age children are increasingly responsible for preparing snacks, lunches, and even some other meals. These years are a good time to teach children how to choose nutritious foods and plan a well-balanced meal. Because school-age children operate at the concrete level of cognitive thought, nutrition teaching is best presented by using pictures, samples of foods, videotapes, handouts, and hands-on experience.

School-age children often prefer the types of food eaten at home and may be resistant to new food items. A hospitalized child may refuse to eat, slowing the recuperative process. Nurses should encourage family members to bring favorite foods from home that meet nutritional requirements. This can be especially helpful when the hospital serves food only from the dominant cultural group. A child accustomed to a diet of rice, tofu, and vegetables may not enjoy a hospital meal of hamburger and fries. By school-age, food has become strongly associated with social interaction, so it is beneficial to have children eat together or to invite family members to take the child off the unit to eat or to bring in food from home and eat with the child. Many hospitals allow children to plan a pizza night or sponsor other events to encourage eating in a social atmosphere.

Most children consume at least one meal daily in school. While children may bring lunches to school, most participate in school lunch programs, and perhaps school breakfast programs. Nurses should become familiar with the policies of school districts in their areas for providing foods, snacks, and reduced-price food to students in need. During the past decade, many school systems in the United States have allowed vending machines for carbonated sweetened beverages and snacks to be installed in public schools. Part of the profits from these machines has enabled revenue-strapped school districts to enhance their incomes. However, schools are increasingly challenged about the presence of the machines, especially in light of the growing problem of overweight among youth. Some school districts have now limited the number of machines or the hours during which they can be used by students, and some have removed all sweetened beverages from vending machines. Nurses are able to provide information for districts about the problems of obesity and the need for healthy foods for youth. Nurses are also involved in planning for nutritional maintenance when children have special needs in the school setting, such as diet or tube feedings.

Healthy People 2020

(NWS-14) Increase the contribution of fruits to the diets of the population aged 2 years and older

(NWS-15) Increase the variety and contribution of vegetables to the diets of the population aged 2 years and older

---

The loss of the first deciduous teeth and the eruption of permanent teeth usually occur at about 6 years, or at the beginning of the school-age period. Of the 32 permanent teeth, 22 to 26 erupt by age 12 years, and the remaining molars follow in the teenage years. See Chapter 33 for the typical sequence of tooth eruption and Chapter 35 for dental care needs during childhood. The school-age child should be closely monitored to ensure that brushing and flossing are adequate, that fluoride is taken if the fluoride concentration in the water supply is below 0.7 mg/L, that dental care is obtained to provide for examination of teeth and alignment, and that loose teeth are identified before surgery or sports participation.

Adolescence

Most adolescents need well over 2000 calories daily to support the growth spurt, and some adolescent boys require nearly 3000 or more calories daily. When teenagers are active in a variety of sports, these requirements increase further. Because adolescents prepare much of their own food and often eat with friends, they need to be taught about good nutrition. Developing a diet that includes a large number of calories, meets vitamin and mineral requirements, and is acceptable to the teen may be a challenge.

The pregnant adolescent has even more challenging nutrient requirements. See Chapter 11 for details about needs during pregnancy. An adolescent who is hospitalized and does not like the hospital lunch might ask a friend who visits to bring a soft drink and chips; however, the teen may be receptive to offers of juice and pizza, a more nutritious meal. Small improvements should be viewed positively because they may lead to further changes. See *Evidence-Based Practice: Adolescents and Nutritional Choices.*

Fast food represents a significant intake for many adolescents. It is commonly high in fat, calories, and sodium while being low in essential nutrients such as calcium, folic acid, riboflavin, vitamins A and C, and fiber. Many schools are redesigning cafeterias and food programs to entice more teens to eat at school rather than nearby fast-food restaurants. Adding fruits and salads and allowing choices can enhance the quality of food intake. School nurses play a vital role in helping to tailor a healthy school nutrition program and teaching teens about the healthiest choices at their favorite fast-food restaurants.

Peer group influence is important to teens, so group sessions in which adolescents eat lunch together can provide a forum for influencing food habits. What other methods might encourage positive nutritional habits among teens?

Nutritional Assessment

What is the best indication that a child's nutrition is adequate? Which data collection methods provide the most accurate information about a child's dietary intake? The nurse plays an important role in assessing the diets of children and in seeking additional evaluation from dietitians and nutritionists in complex situations.

Physical and Behavioral Measurement

GROWTH MEASUREMENT

A common method of evaluating the adequacy of diet is measurement of growth. **Anthropometric measurement** is the term used to refer to assessment of various parts of the body. Anthropometry of young children commonly includes weight, length, and head circumference. Standing height is substituted for length once the child can stand. Head circumference, also known as *occipital-frontal circumference (OFC)*, is measured during infancy and into early years when there are growth concerns. Additional measurements that may be included in special circumstances include chest circumference, mid-upper arm circumference, and skinfold measurement at sites such as triceps, abdomen, and subscapular regions. Grids are available for each measurement and assist in providing a thorough nutritional assessment when weight and height are abnormally high or low. The accompanying *Clinical Skills Manual* SKILLS presents techniques for accurate measurement of weight, length, height, chest circumference, and head circumference.

After collecting the measurements, the nurse plots them on the appropriate standardized growth curves for weight, length to height, head circumference, and body mass index (Figure 32–6). **Body mass index (BMI)** is a calculation based on the child's

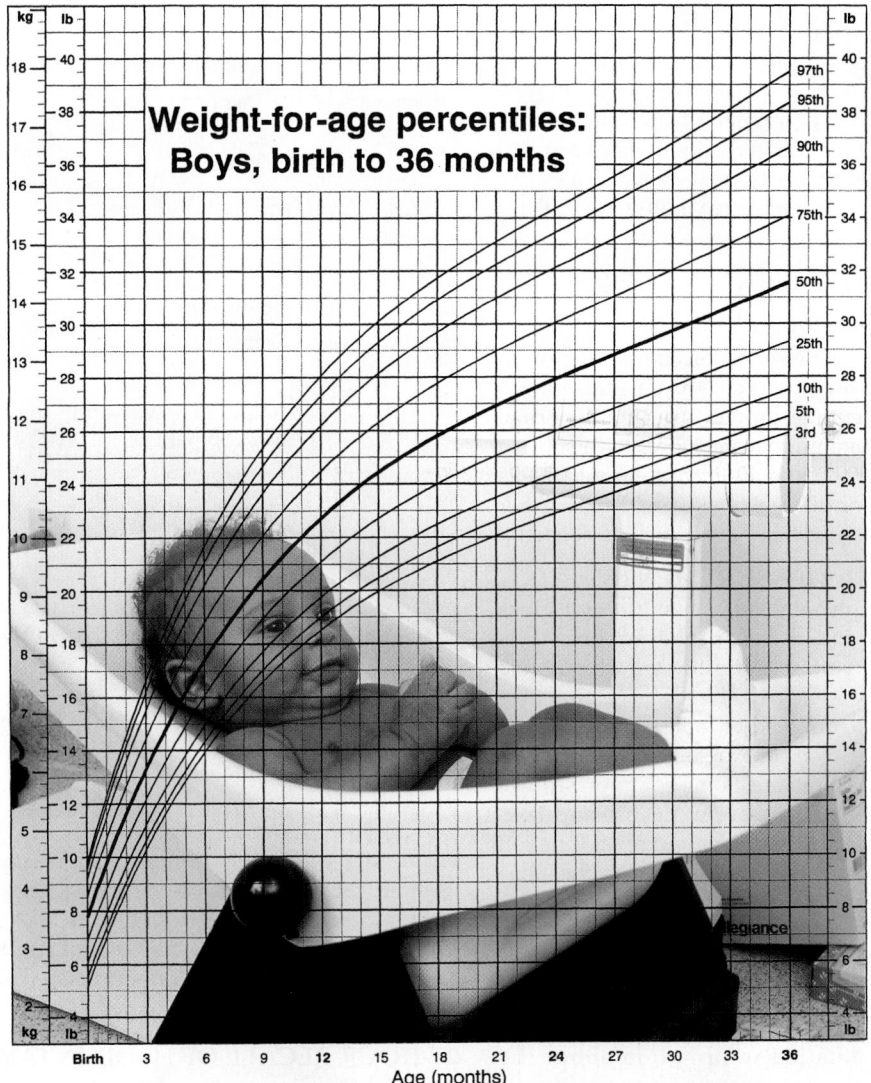

Figure 32–6 Plotting measurements on the growth curve. The nurse accurately measures the child and then places height and weight on appropriate growth grids for the child's age and gender.

weight and height, or length, and is calculated as kilograms of weight per square meter of height. This is a useful calculation for determining if the child's height and weight are in proportion and identifies which percentile the child falls in for each measurement. Children normally fall between the 10th and 90th percentiles. A measurement below the 10th percentile, especially for BMI, may indicate undernutrition, while one over the 90th percentile can indicate overnutrition. However, it is important to look at the differences between measurements. An infant in the 90th percentile for length, weight, and head circumference is proportional and may be a naturally large baby. On the other hand, a child who is consistently in the 10th percentile for all measurements, but is growing steadily and is at a normal development level, may simply be a small child. Much cultural and individual variation exists in size. See Appendix C for standardized growth curves by gender and age for infants, children, and adolescents. Visit the Centers for Disease Control and Prevention (CDC) website (www.cdc.gov) to find specialized growth grids for children with conditions such as Down syndrome.

Developing Cultural Competence Growth Patterns Among Immigrant Children

The revised growth grids now in use were standardized using a cross section of the U.S. population. However, children from some other countries or cultures may fall outside of these curves. For example, new immigrants or adoptees may be in lower percentiles and may "catch up" over several months or years. Children of immigrants from developing countries tend to be larger than their parents. Even when small, children should follow normal growth patterns. For example, a child who remains at the 10th or 25th percentile for height but continues to grow slowly does not fall to a lower percentile.

The nurse should plot measurements on the same growth curve with earlier percentiles for the child. When measurements follow the same percentile over time, growth is generally normal for the child and nutrition is likely adequate. However, a sudden or sustained change in percentile may indicate a chronic disorder, emotional difficulty, or a nutritional intake problem. Further assessment of physical status and dietary intake will be needed.

ADDITIONAL PHYSICAL MEASUREMENTS

Many observations from the physical assessment provide clues to nutritional status. Dietary intake can affect every body system, and a combination of certain symptoms may suggest specific nutritional problems. Some common physical manifestations of nutritional status are outlined in Table 32–3.

Laboratory measurements can provide useful information when nutritional status is questionable. Some common studies include hematocrit and hemoglobin, serum glucose and fasting insulin, lipids and lipoproteins, and liver and renal function studies. Adding some further measurements such as chest circumference and skinfolds (measurement of fat at certain body sites such as triceps, scapular, and abdominal areas) may also be useful (Lee & Nieman, 2013).

Dietary Intake

The nurse should obtain detailed information about the child's dietary intake when there is a potential for nutritional deficiency due to disease, knowledge deficit, or socioeconomic status. The mother's dietary intake during pregnancy

TABLE 32–3 Clinical Manifestations of Dietary Deficiencies/Excesses

NUTRIENT	DEFICIENCY MANIFESTATION	EXCESS MANIFESTATION
Vitamin A	Night blindness Skin dryness and scaling	Headache Drowsiness Hepatomegaly Vomiting and diarrhea
Vitamin C	Abnormal hair (coiled shape) Skin abnormalities (dermatitis and lesions) Purpura Bleeding gums Joint tenderness Sudden heart failure	Usually none—excess is excreted in urine
Vitamin D	Rib deformity Bowed legs Bone and joint pain Muscle weakness Periodontal disease Increased rates of respiratory and skin infections/irritation	Drowsiness
B vitamins	Weakness Decreased deep tendon reflexes Dermatitis	Usually none—excess is excreted in urine
Protein	Hepatomegaly Edema Scant, depigmented hair	Kidney failure
Carbohydrate	Emaciation Decreased energy Retarded growth and development	Overweight
Iron	Lethargy Slowed growth and developmental progression Pallor	Vomiting, diarrhea, abdominal pain Pallor Cyanosis Drowsiness Shock

may provide information about the child's nutritional state and it can be assessed for pertinent information. After the information is collected, the dietary intake should be compared to the recommended levels for a child of that age and gender (see Figure 32–1 for the U.S. MyPlate food guide; see Appendix F for Recommended Dietary Allowances). The 24-hour recall of intake, a food frequency questionnaire, and a dietary screening history (Tables 32–4 and 32–5) provide a good overview of the infant's or child's intake and eating patterns. A food diary provides precise information about the child's food intake.

24-HOUR RECALL OF FOOD INTAKE

The 24-hour diet recall is frequently used to assess the adequacy of the diet. People can generally remember their intake in the past day so results are fairly accurate, it is easy to

TABLE 32–4 Dietary Screening History for Infants

Overview Questions

What was the infant's birth weight?

At what age did the birth weight double and triple?

Was the infant premature?

Does the infant have any feeding problems such as difficulty sucking and swallowing, spitting up, fatigue, or fussiness?

If Infant Is Breastfed

How long does the baby nurse at each breast?

What is the usual schedule for breastfeeding?

Does the baby also take any milk or formula? Amount and frequency? What type?

If Infant Is Formula-Fed

What formula is used? Is it iron fortified?

How is it prepared?

Do you hold or prop the bottle for feedings?

How much formula is taken at each feeding?

How many bottles are taken each day?

Does the baby take a bottle to bed for naps or nighttime? What is in the bottle?

If Infant Is Fed Other Foods

At what age did the baby start eating other foods?

Cereal	Finger foods
Fruit/juices	Meats
Vegetables	Other protein sources

Do you use commercial baby food or make your own?

Does the baby eat any table foods?

How often does the baby take solid foods?

How is the baby's appetite?

Do you have any concerns about the baby's feeding habits?

Does the baby take a vitamin supplement? Fluoride?

Have there been any allergic reactions to foods? Which ones?

Does the baby spit up frequently?

Have there been any rashes?

What types of stools does the baby have? Frequency? Consistency?

TABLE 32–5 Dietary Screening History for Children

What types of food or beverage does the child especially like?

What foods or beverages does the child dislike?

What is the child's typical eating schedule? Meals and snacks?

Does the child eat with the family or at separate times?

Where does the child eat each meal?

Who prepares the food for the family?

What methods of cooking are used? Baking? Frying? Broiling? Grilling?

What ethnic foods are commonly eaten?

Does the family eat in a restaurant frequently? What type?

What type of food does the child usually order?

Is the child on a special diet?

Does the child need to be fed, feed himself or herself, need assistance eating, or need any adaptive devices for eating?

What is the child's appetite like?

Does the child take any vitamin supplements (iron, fluoride)?

Does the child have any allergies? What types of symptoms?

What types of regular exercise does the child get?

Are there any concerns about the child's eating habits?

- Additives used, such as condiments, table salt, spices, milk to mix formula
- Food preparation methods, including adding fats to cook, removal or retention of fats on meats
- Vitamins and supplements, types and doses
- Whether the intake is typical (in situations such as illness or vacation, intake may be different than usual)

Once the 24-hour recall is obtained, the nurse needs to analyze the intake by first doing a quick check to compare servings of various food types with the U.S. MyPlate food guide, as described earlier (see also Figure 32–1). Next the nurse should do a detailed analysis to compute calories, carbohydrate, protein, and fat intake and compare them to recommended amounts. All major vitamins and minerals are also computed

gather the data and analyze results, and only a few minutes are needed. The nurse should ask the parent or child to list all foods eaten during the past 24 hours (Figure 32–7). It is usually helpful to ask for a description of activities in the last day, then start with the most recent event and move backwards, integrating food intake into the daily schedule. For example, the nurse might begin by saying, "You mentioned you got up early to come to the clinic today. What did Sam eat at home before you left? Did he have a snack as you traveled here or after you arrived?" While asking about the foods eaten, the nurse should inquire specifically about the following:

- All meals and snacks
- Amounts of each food item consumed (having various size measuring cups, bowls, and plates available so accurate amounts can be indicated is helpful)
- Types of specific foods used, such as whole milk versus nonfat or 2%, brand names of cereals, specific types of margarine or butter

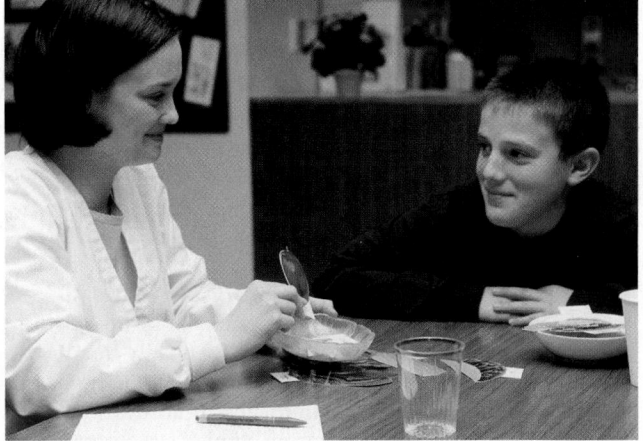

Figure 32–7 The 24-hour diet recall. The nurse is interviewing a child about foods eaten in the last day. Note the models of food and dishes for accurate assessment of serving sizes.

and comparisons made to the DRIs. This computation may be done by hand, using a book of nutrients in common foods, or it may be done on the computer. Several computer programs are available, and the federal government has a website that provides intake levels and comparisons to the RDAs. It may be useful to compute a personal 24-hour recall or that of a child in the clinical setting with the Healthy Eating Index.

FOOD FREQUENCY QUESTIONNAIRE

Food frequency questionnaires are available that can be easily administered to parents or children. Usually, they ask about how often certain types of foods are eaten in a specified period such as a week. Long questionnaires can evaluate a total diet, while short ones focus on specific items such as fruit and vegetable intake. A short questionnaire about milk intake or fruit and vegetable intake may be helpful before planning a teaching project on nutrition to a class of school-age children. Knowing their usual intake of a food item can provide helpful information for planning the project.

DIETARY SCREENING HISTORY

The nurse should ask the parent about the infant's or child's eating habits using the questions listed in Tables 32–4 and 32–5. Responses provide information about the family's eating habits and food beliefs beyond that collected on a 24-hour dietary recall or food frequency questionnaire.

FOOD DIARY

Parents are asked to keep a food diary when the child has a nutrition problem or disorder that requires dietary management, such as malnutrition, obesity, or diabetes. All meals and snacks, with food preparation method and quantities eaten over a 1- to 7-day period, are recorded. Eating patterns change significantly for holidays or family gatherings, so parents should be asked to select typical days for the food diary or to record specific events affecting food intake. Including 1 weekday and 1 weekend day may be helpful. Parents need to be reminded of all the places children might have eaten, such as the childcare center, school, friends' houses, or neighbors. Food diaries can provide a great deal of helpful information, but they take time and motivation to complete well (Lee & Nieman, 2013). The nurse should be sure instructions are complete and that the form has a place to record amounts, preparation, events occurring, and where food was eaten. The nurse or parent may need to obtain the school lunch menu and talk with the school lunch personnel to add accurate school intake. The nurse completes the nutritional assessment indicated for a child and may consult with or refer the family to a dietitian or nutritionist for additional assessment and teaching.

Developing Cultural Competence Dietary Intake Varies Among Cultures

Each culture has eating practices that influence dietary intake. It is important to understand the foods commonly eaten by each cultural group and their contribution to the total nutrition of the child. Depending on the populations nurses work with, they may need to ask about intake of freshly caught fish or wild game such as pheasants and elk. Home-prepared sausages and cheese may be part of diets. Berries and garden produce might be eaten. Foods from ethnic markets may include spices, dried mushrooms, and other products. Some groups do not eat meat or specific types of meats. Using open-ended questions when gathering data will increase the likelihood of obtaining an accurate evaluation of diet.

TABLE 32–6 Food Insecurity Screening

1. Does your household ever run out of money to buy food to make a meal?
2. Do you or members of your household ever eat less than you feel you should because there is not enough money for food?
3. Do you or members of your household ever cut the size of meals or skip meals because there is not enough money for food?
4. Do your children ever eat less than you feel they should because there is not enough money for food?
5. Do you ever cut the size of your children's meals or do they skip meals because there is not enough money for food?
6. Do your children ever say they are hungry because there is not enough food in the house?
7. Do you ever rely on a limited number of foods to feed your children because you are running out of money to buy foods for a meal?
8. Do any of your children ever go to bed hungry because there is not enough money to buy food?

Scoring: 5–8 yes responses = hungry; 1–4 yes responses = risk of hunger. From Washington State Department of Health.

Common Nutritional Concerns

Childhood Hunger

Although most Americans live in a land of plenty, significant numbers of children periodically experience hunger. **Food security** is access at all times to enough nourishment for an active, healthy life. In contrast, **food insecurity** indicates an inability to acquire or consume adequate quality or quantity of foods in socially acceptable ways, or the uncertainty that one will be able to do so; at least 10% of U.S. children live in households that periodically experience food insecurity (USDA, 2013a).

The major cause of hunger in children is poverty, and since, on average, more than one in five children are poor, their families may be unable to provide sustainable nutrition at all times (Children's Defense Fund, 2014). Many single-income families have a head of household moving into the workforce, so incomes are often not sufficient to provide for family food needs (see Chapter 1 for a description of Temporary Assistance for Needy Families). Families may be ineligible for food assistance programs even though they cannot afford enough food for all their members. Children with special nutritional needs are at particular risk since it may be more costly to buy and prepare formula or foods for a child with allergies, diabetes, or an immune disorder.

Children with insufficient dietary intake are at risk for a wide array of health problems. They may become anemic; have a high rate of infectious disease due to a lowered immune response; have slowed developmental maturation, delayed or stunted physical growth, and learning disorders; and be at greater risk of overweight, cardiovascular disease, and diabetes in adulthood (Children's Defense Fund, 2014). Subsequently, the national and individual cost of childhood hunger is great.

Nurses are well positioned to evaluate families for food insecurity in a variety of hospital, clinic, school, and home settings. In addition to the assessment of the individual child's nutritional status, further questions can determine families with potential problems. Nurses should administer a screening tool to identify risk in families (Table 32–6). Most parents go without food themselves in order to feed their children, so food insecurity may not have directly affected all children. However, anxiety over providing food can be very stressful for families, and diet quality deteriorates as insecurity increases. If families have experienced food insecurity or may be likely to at some time, nurses should be sure to provide them with access to community agencies and programs that can help. What resources are available locally to help families with food insecurity?

Overweight and Obesity

The current incidence of overweight children in the United States is epidemic and is associated with a wide array of health problems, such as type 2 diabetes, stroke, gallbladder disease, arthritis, cardiovascular disease, sleep disturbances, hypertension, dyslipidemia, respiratory problems, certain cancers, interference with physical activity, social stigma, discrimination, depression, and low self-esteem (CDC, 2014a). A historic high of 17% of children and adolescents are at or above the 95th percentile for BMI (obese) and about the same amount fall from the 85th to 94th percentiles for BMI (overweight), designating about one third of U.S. youth as being overweight or obese (CDC, 2014a).

Many reasons are cited for the increase in overweight children. The number of calories consumed is not increasing, but children tend to exercise less, particularly in daily life. They infrequently walk or ride bikes either because of the convenience of driving or because of unsafe neighborhoods. Television viewing is very high among youth; movies, Internet, computer games, social networking, and cell phones are further examples of media commonly used by youth. U.S. children spend, on average, over 7 hours daily on such media (National Heart, Lung and Blood Institute, 2013). Inactive pursuits do not require high caloric energy, leading to an imbalance in intake and demand for calories. Additionally, television viewing is often accompanied by ingestion of high-calorie foods and subjects children to food marketing of unhealthy foods.

The percentage of calories from fat consumed in the United States is among the highest in the world. Although no more than 25% to 35% of calories should come from total dietary fat, and no more than 10% from saturated fat, about 35% of calories consumed in the United States are supplied by fat and over 11% by saturated fat (U.S. Department of Health and Human Services [USDHHS], 2011). Most fats should be supplied from polyunsaturated and monounsaturated fatty acids, but current diets contain low amounts of those fats and high amounts of trans-fatty acids (USDHHS, 2011). The high rate of dietary fat is related to the amount of fast food consumed, and influenced by snacking as well.

Goals of nursing management are to prevent new cases of overweight, identify children who are overweight, and to support youth and families to establish healthy lifestyles that promote weight loss and maintenance of recommended weight. Perform assessment of height, weight, and BMI. Measure blood pressure and determine whether it is within normal limits. Evaluate amount of screen/social activities, sedentary behavior, and physical activity levels. When prevention and behavioral changes have not been successful, some adolescents will have bariatric surgery. Guidelines have been established for adolescents that consider age, physical maturity, BMI, and comorbidities (Brei & Mudd, 2014).

Nurses can help parents and children build good nutritional and exercise habits throughout life, thus decreasing the incidence of overweight and its attendant health risks. Children under 2 years of age should have no exposure to screen activities. Parents should be advised that screen activities by children older than age 2 should be limited to a maximum of 2 hours daily, and that a television, video games, or other screens should not be placed in children's bedrooms (AAP, 2014b). Daily exercise routines of 30 to 60 minutes can be included in the schedules of most families. Aim to meet the current recommendation of 60 minutes daily for children with some activity including muscle strengthening and flexibility. Also, nurses should teach about the MyPlate food guide and its integration into a healthy life. Healthy snacks include fruits, vegetables, grains, and nuts. "Super sizing" fast foods and eating out often should be avoided.

Risks for poor health often cluster together in individuals and families. Nurses need to be alert for situations in which parents are overweight and children have elevated blood pressure, exercise infrequently, or are in upper percentiles for weight, BMI, or skinfold measurements. Be alert for early menarche, which can help identify overweight girls who need intervention for obesity prevention. The presence of risk factors necessitates further dietary and risk assessment so that a management plan can be implemented. See resources such as "Helping Your Overweight Child" and "Take Charge of Your Health: A Teenager's Guide to Better Health" (http://win.niddk.nih.gov/publications).

Consult the *Nursing Care Plan* in this chapter for further interventions appropriate for the child who is overweight.

Nursing Care Plan The Child Who Is Overweight

1. Nursing Diagnosis: *Obesity* **related to excessive intake in comparison to metabolic needs (NANDA-I © 2014)**

GOAL: The child will demonstrate adequate intake of all nutrients without excessive energy intake.

INTERVENTION	RATIONALE
• Perform thorough nutritional assessment of child.	• Assessment assists in identification of dietary risks and strengths as well as health conditions related to nutrition.
• Share results of assessment with child and family by showing weight, height, and body mass index grids.	• Many families do not consider their child overweight. Concrete information about the child's size in comparison with recommendations assists in establishing the importance of weight management.
• Assess access to sufficient nutritious foods for the family at all times.	• Food insecurity promotes inadequate intake alternating with excess intake of high-calorie foods.
• Identify with the child and family 2–3 target areas to begin weight management. Examples might include: • Having fast food only once weekly • Switching to low-fat dairy products • Keeping two more fresh fruits and vegetables in the house and two less snack foods	• Changing dietary patterns drastically is difficult and may lead to giving up the attempt at weight management. Partnering with the family to set goals enhances chances of success.
• Integrate nutrition information into each visit. Examples of topics include: • Dietary requirements for age group • Effects of simple sugar and fat intake on weight • Beneficial effects of fruits, vegetables, whole grains, and nonfat dairy • Reading food labels • Healthy choices in fast-food restaurants • Calculation of fat content of foods	• Nutrition information is best learned in an ongoing program.
• Use growth grids to help child and family establish a weight reduction or maintenance goal.	• Goals motivate families to achieve desired health behaviors. The goal for a young child may be weight maintenance so that as the child grows in height, the correct proportion is reached, while weight reduction may be needed for older children or youth who are very obese.

EXPECTED OUTCOME: Child meets all dietary requirements while achieving weight and body mass index goal.

2. Nursing Diagnosis: *Coping: Family, Readiness for Enhanced,* **related to need to foster health of family member (NANDA-I © 2014)**

GOAL: The family will assist child to manage stressors and to develop new strategies to support weight control goals.

INTERVENTION	RATIONALE
• Include key family members in some of the counseling sessions with the child who is overweight.	• Key members of the family are those who purchase foods, provide support for the child, and participate in decisions about health.
• Encourage the family to eat together at least once daily if possible or to increase number of meals eaten together weekly.	• The family is an important support system in weight loss programs. Eating as a family or in a social situation can provide a chance to promote healthy foods; intake is generally lower fat and calorie than when eating alone.
• Seek a resource for the child to be monitored about twice monthly; this may be a healthcare provider office, nutritionist, school nurse, or other person.	• The resource provides opportunity to monitor the child's progress and to offer support, additional information, and problem-solving techniques.

EXPECTED OUTCOME: Child expresses satisfaction with family understanding and support of weight.

3. Nursing Diagnosis: *Activity Intolerance* related to sedentary lifestyle (NANDA-I © 2014)

GOAL: The child will demonstrate activity tolerance by adequate oxygenation, respiratory effort, and ability to speak during brisk walking, biking, or other activity.

INTERVENTION	RATIONALE
• Establish daily exercise routine beginning with 15–30 minutes daily of walking.	• Starting with brief amounts of exercise makes the child feel comfortable and enhances potential for success.
• Gradually increase activity over 1–2 months until 60 minutes of daily exercise is maintained.	• Gradual increase as the cardiovascular and respiratory systems adapt is generally comfortable for children; 60 minutes of moderate activity daily is recommended for children.
• Use activities enjoyed by the child and suggest options as necessary; refer the family to community resources such as swimming pools, organized sports, and biking groups.	• Activities the child enjoys will be more likely to remain in usual activity patterns; exercising with others in groups increases motivation.
• Have families plan at least 1–2 activities they can do together weekly.	• This fosters family relationships and provides support and motivation for the child.
• Limit screen activities to a maximum of 2 hours daily. • Have child keep a log of hours of television, video games, computer, and other similar activities. Tell child never to snack while doing screen activities.	• Increased use of screen activities is related to poor dietary habits and increased sedentary behaviors and excess weight.

• Ask about use of tobacco in children in fifth grade or higher.
  • Inquire about exposure to environmental tobacco smoke at all ages.
  • Perform teaching to discourage tobacco use or offer cessation programs as needed.
	• Most adults who smoke began the habit in childhood; middle school years are the most common age for smoking initiation.
	  • Smoking by others in the household can be harmful to children.
	  • Smoking decreases respiratory reserves and worsens several cardiovascular disease risks.

EXPECTED OUTCOME: Child demonstrates ability to engage in moderate activity for 60 minutes with minimal respiratory discomfort.

4. Nursing Diagnosis: *Self-Esteem, Chronic Low,* related to weight (NANDA-I © 2014)

GOAL: The child expresses positive perception of self-worth and confidence in ability to deal with issues related to weight.

INTERVENTION	RATIONALE
• Facilitate development of a positive outlook by exposing child to others who have been successful with weight loss.	• Increases motivation and feelings of self-efficacy.
• Praise child for weight loss, weight maintenance, increased physical activity, and other achievements. • Help the child establish rewards for meeting goals, such as purchase of new clothing.	• Enhances judgment of self-worth and pride in accomplishments.
• Partner with parents so that they understand the value of praise and never label the child using derogatory words such as "fat."	• Family members are usually the most intimate support system for the child.

EXPECTED OUTCOME: Child speaks positively about accomplishments in weight control management.

Developing Cultural Competence Overweight **Causes Health Disparities Among Certain Groups**

Overweight is more common among some ethnic and socioeconomic groups. Lack of knowledge about foods and physical activity, limited access to fresh produce and safe places to exercise, and easy access to increasing numbers of fast foods may all constitute risk factors. Lower income, and Hispanic, African American, or Native American ethnic identity are all associated with higher incidence of overweight, especially among women. National goals to eliminate health disparities in income and ethnic groups have been set (USDHHS, 2011).

Food Safety

In the United States, about 48 million people (1 in 6) contract foodborne illnesses every year. Some cases are quite mild, whereas others can be very severe. About 128,000 people are hospitalized, and about 3000 die from these illnesses (CDC, 2014b). Children are at greater risk of severe illness and death from food and water because of their immature gastrointestinal and immune systems. Children who are immunocompromised are at even greater risk. Among the most common pathogens are *Campylobacter, Salmonella, Vibrio, Shigella, Cryptosporidium, Listeria, Yersinia,* and *Escherichia coli* (CDC, 2011b, 2014c). Worldwide, over 3 million people die of illness related to unsafe drinking water each year, and most of those deaths are among children.

Foodborne illness transmission is associated with food preparation and storage practices, lack of adequate training of retail employees about foods and hygiene, and increasing amounts and types of foods being imported from other countries. Some examples of contaminated foods in the past few years include undercooked hamburger meat, cross-contamination of salad bar items from meats, unpasteurized apple cider, green onions, raw spinach, prepackaged salad and delicatessen meat, berries, and sprouts. While most infected persons experience acute diarrhea, some can develop complications such as hemolytic uremic syndrome (Chapter 52) or thrombocytic purpura (Chapter 49). Health personnel should integrate teaching regularly so that families can decrease risks of foodborne illness. Recommend that families avoid consumption of unpasteurized milk, raw or undercooked oysters, raw or undercooked eggs, raw or undercooked ground beef, and undercooked poultry (CDC, 2011b). Check the information regarding outbreaks at www.foodsafety.org.

Food may carry products other than microorganisms that can be harmful. An example is mercury, which may be concentrated in certain types of fish. This metal can cause harm to the developing nervous system of fetuses, infants, and young children when consumed regularly. The U.S. Food and Drug Administration (FDA) and Environmental Protection Agency (EPA) note that fish are an important part of a healthy diet, but that certain recommendations should be followed to lower the risk of experiencing mercury's detrimental effects. Women who may become pregnant, are pregnant or breastfeeding, and young children should:

- Eliminate shellfish, shark, swordfish, king mackerel, and tilefish from the diet.
- Eat 8 to 12 oz (two average meals) a week of a variety of low-mercury fish, such as shrimp, canned light tuna, salmon, pollock, and catfish. Albacore or white tuna has more mercury than light tuna, so limit white tuna to one meal weekly. (Children should have two to three servings per week of low-mercury fish in amounts appropriate for their age and caloric needs.)

Check for local advisories about the safety of fish caught in local waters. (U.S. Food and Drug Administration, 2014).

Common Dietary Deficiencies

Dietary deficiencies can occur in children and some are common in selected populations. While children can have deficits in nearly any nutrient, a number of nutrient deficits are more common in childhood. Limitations in the food supply or patterns of dietary intake cause most deficiencies, while children with certain disease processes, such as metabolic diseases, may have difficulty absorbing or using nutrients ingested. (See Chapter 53 for a discussion of inborn errors of metabolism.) The nutrient deficiencies of a population are a result of genetic factors, characteristics of the food supply, and intake patterns of particular groups.

Developing Cultural Competence Vitamin A Deficiency

Vitamin A deficiency is common in developing countries. The vitamin is found in liver, dairy products, and fish. Provitamin A sources are yellow and dark green vegetables. The vitamin is fat soluble and stored in the liver. When deficient, children develop night blindness, vision loss, and high rates of infection. Public health efforts have been directed at identifying populations of children with low vitamin A status and providing the vitamin in capsule form or in commonly ingested foods.

IRON

Newborns have a store of iron obtained from their mothers in the uterus if the maternal nutritional state was satisfactory and the baby was of normal gestational age. Breast milk contains little iron, but the iron it does contain has high bioavailability. However, by 4 to 6 months of age, the baby's iron stores begin to decrease and a dietary source of iron must be added for the infant. Enriched rice cereal is commonly used to meet these initial iron needs. In babies who do not have adequate stores or do not take in enough iron, **anemia**, or a reduction in the number of red blood cells, can result (Figure 32–8). Feeding cow's milk during infancy can also cause anemia by irritating the gut and leading to small but consistent loss of blood from the gastrointestinal tract; cow's milk should not be fed in the first year of life. When formulas are used, they should be iron fortified to

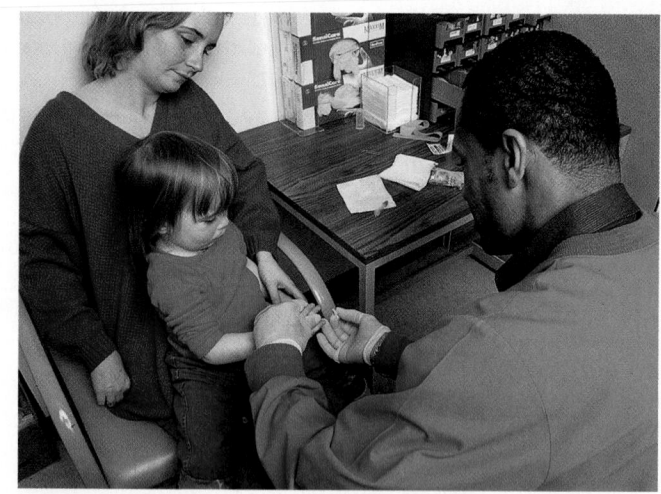

Figure 32–8 Screening for anemia. Most Head Start centers participate in screening programs to identify children at risk for anemia.

help avoid iron-deficiency anemia. Iron-fortified infant cereals are a good source of the mineral.

Adolescent females comprise another group commonly deficient in iron. Their deficiency is related to loss of blood in menses, metabolic need of the growth spurt, and poor dietary balance due to sporadic dieting. Further discussion of the symptoms and treatment of iron-deficiency anemia can be found in Chapter 49. Encourage intake of good iron sources such as meats, eggs, dried fruits, and iron-fortified cereal. Instruct families on safe iron administration, and ensure follow-up evaluations of iron levels when nutritional supplements are administered.

CALCIUM

Calcium is an essential nutrient for bone development during childhood and adolescence. An increased intake of soda pop and fruit juices is related to a decrease in calcium intake, especially among adolescents. During the adolescent growth spurt, almost 40% of the adult bone mass is accumulated, and by age 18 years for females and age 20 years for males, 90% of peak bone mass is achieved (National Institute of Arthritis and Musculoskeletal and Skin Diseases, 2012). Inadequate intake puts the person at risk for osteoporosis later in life since it is not possible to make up for earlier deficits. Although genetic variables account for some of the influence on adult bone mass, increasing calcium intake has been shown to promote bone formation. While the recommended daily intake for adolescents is 1300 mg, the average intake for young males is 870 to 1260 mg and for females is only 750 to 960 mg (only half of the recommended level) (National Institutes of Health, 2013). Nurses should encourage foods such as milk and milk products, egg yolks, grains, legumes, nuts, and fruit juice with added calcium.

Adolescents at highest risk for impaired bone development include female athletes and others who diet excessively to maintain slimness. Teens who exercise excessively may manifest the "female athlete triad" of disordered eating that leads to excessive thinness, excessive exercise, and amenorrhea. A high rate of fractures and osteomalacia can result, in addition to an extreme risk of osteoporosis in adulthood (Ackerman & Misra, 2011). Asking about menstrual patterns as well as exercise and diet can be combined with physical measurements of height and weight to obtain pertinent information about the teen athlete. See the discussion of the eating disorders anorexia nervosa and bulimia nervosa later in this chapter.

VITAMIN D

Vitamin D is needed for bone mineralization. Vitamin D deficiencies were once believed to be rare; however, an increase in cases of vitamin D–deficient rickets has recently been observed. Although vitamin D can be synthesized in the skin upon exposure to sunlight, the amount of sunlight needed for manufacture is variable and determined by the amount of skin exposed, the color of the skin, the latitude, and time of the year (Wagner, Greer, Section on Breastfeeding, et al., 2008). Owing to this variability and the small amount of vitamin D in breast milk, it is now recommended that all infants from birth to 6 months receive a minimum intake of 400 International Units daily. All persons 6 months and older should receive 600 International Units daily (Ross, Taylor, Yaktine, et al., 2011). This vitamin is needed to enhance absorption of calcium, so a lack of vitamin D can contribute to calcium deficiency as well. When rickets is suspected, laboratory studies should include 25-OH vitamin D (20–29 ng/mL indicates insufficiency of vitamin D, and below 20 ng/mL is a deficiency state), serum calcium, phosphorus, alkaline phosphatase, creatinine, electrolytes, parathyroid hormone, and hematocrit. Radiographs of extremities should be taken (American Association for Clinical Chemistry, 2014). Encourage

parents to discuss vitamin D intake with the healthcare provider at health promotion visits so proper intake can be ensured.

FOLIC ACID

Epidemiologic evidence has linked increasing maternal folic acid (the most common form of folate in the human body) intake with decreased incidence of neural tube defects such as spina bifida in offspring. Folate levels are low among adolescents, putting them at particular risk of birth defects when they have babies (AAP Committee on Nutrition, 2013). The FDA approved fortification of cereals and breads with folate to decrease the population risk of related congenital anomalies. All women ages 15 to 45 years should consume 0.4 mg of folic acid daily, and pregnant women should consume 0.6 mg. In addition to cereals and breads, other good sources of folate include spinach, avocado, green leafy vegetables, beans and peas, liver, and fruits such as oranges and grapefruits.

PROTEIN-ENERGY MALNUTRITION

Although the micronutrient deficiencies described previously are the most common problems in developed countries, macronutrient deficiencies are the most common nutritional problems worldwide. While kwashiorkor indicates protein deficiency, and marasmus is a lack of energy-producing calories, both deficiencies often occur together and are referred to as protein-energy malnutrition (PEM). Protein deficiency manifests with edema, leading to the large abdomens and rounded faces seen in severely malnourished children. Other symptoms include scant, depigmented hair, skin changes, and decreased serum proteins. It can occur following severe diarrhea or other infection in susceptible children. Caloric deficiency results in emaciation, decreased energy levels, and retarded development (see Table 32–3). PEM may occur when a child is weaned in order for the mother to provide breast milk to a new baby. Adoptees and immigrants to developed countries sometimes manifest with at least mild PEM, so careful nutritional assessment is needed to provide adequate nutrition.

Celiac Disease

Celiac disease, or gluten-sensitive enteropathy, is a chronic malabsorption syndrome. About 1 in 133 persons have celiac disease. It is more common among members of the same family and in children with Down syndrome or Turner syndrome (National Institute of Diabetes and Digestive and Kidney Disease [NIDDK], 2012).

Celiac disease is an immunologic disorder characterized by intolerance for gluten, a protein found in wheat, barley, rye, and oats. Inability to digest glutenin and gliadin (protein fractions) results in the accumulation of the amino acid glutamine, which is toxic to mucosal cells in the intestine. Damage to the villi ultimately impairs the absorptive process in the small intestine.

In the early stages, celiac disease affects fat absorption, resulting in excretion of large quantities of fat in the stools (steatorrhea). Stools are greasy, foul smelling, frothy, and excessive. As changes in the villi continue, the absorption of protein, carbohydrates, calcium, iron, folate, and vitamins A, D, E, K, and B_{12} becomes impaired.

Symptoms usually occur when solid foods containing gluten are introduced to the child's diet (generally between 6 months to 2 years of age), although celiac disease is sometimes first diagnosed in adulthood. The classic features of celiac disease in infancy include chronic diarrhea, growth impairment, and abdominal distention. The child also demonstrates poor appetite, lack of energy, and muscle wasting with hypotonia. Atypical features are present in children diagnosed with delayed-onset celiac disease around 5 to 7 years of age. Symptoms include nausea, vomiting, recurrent abdominal pain, bloating, tooth enamel defects, and aphthous ulcers (Rashid, Zarkadas, Anca, et al., 2011). Other symptoms may include delayed growth, iron deficiency, and abnormal liver function tests.

Diagnosis is confirmed through measurement of fecal fat content, duodenal biopsy, and improvement with removal of gluten products from the diet. Serum screening tests for immunoglobulin (IgA) antiendomysial antibodies and IgA antitissue transglutaminase antibodies are commonly used in the diagnosis of celiac disease (Garcia-Manzanares & Lucendo, 2011; NIDDK, 2012).

Management of celiac disease involves total exclusion of gluten from the diet. This gluten-free diet is a lifetime treatment. Barley, wheat, and rye are completely eliminated; oat products are sometimes tolerated. Symptoms generally improve within a few days to weeks. Supplementation with fat-soluble vitamins, vitamin B_{12}, folic acid, calcium, and iron may be needed depending on the results of serum testing (Daitch & Epperson, 2011).

The intestinal villi return to normal in about 6 months. Growth should improve steadily, and height and weight should reach normal range within 1 year.

Nursing Management

Nursing care focuses on supporting the parents in maintaining a gluten-free diet for the child. Thoroughly explain the disease process to the parents. Emphasize the necessity of following a gluten-free diet. Help parents to understand that celiac disease requires lifelong dietary modifications that should not be discontinued when the child is symptom-free. Discontinuation of the diet places the child at risk for growth retardation and the development of gastrointestinal cancers in adulthood. All children with celiac disease should be seen by a dietitian several times during childhood. Nutritional assessment and continued teaching to maintain a gluten-free diet take place at these visits. Dietary management is made difficult by hidden gluten in many prepared foods, such as chocolate candy, prepared meats, ice cream, soups, condiments, and food starch.

An infant or toddler's diet is easily monitored at home. When the child enters school, however, ensuring adherence to dietary restrictions becomes more difficult. In addition to easily identified gluten-based foods, such as bread, cake, doughnuts, cookies, and crackers, the child must also avoid processed foods that contain gluten as a filler. School-age children and adolescents are often tempted to eat these foods, especially when among peers. Emphasize the need for compliance while meeting the child's developmental needs.

The child's special dietary needs can place a financial burden on the family. Parents need to purchase prepared rice or corn flour products or make their own bread and bakery products. Advise parents that getting a dietary prescription enables them to deduct the cost of these ingredients and commercially prepared products as a medical expense.

Because the entire family must adapt to the diet, parents and siblings need support and management skills. For information and support, refer parents and children to several organizations, including the American Celiac Society, the Celiac Sprue Association/United States of America, and the Gluten Intolerance Group.

Expected outcomes of nursing care include the following:

- The child maintains adequate nutrition to support growth and development needs.
- The child achieves growth and developmental milestones appropriate for age.
- The child and family understand the dietary restrictions and appropriately plan meals.

Feeding and Eating Disorders

Deficiencies in food intake related to available nutrients and safety of the food supply were discussed in the previous section. In addition to these issues of availability, nutrient intake is affected by psychologic issues of individuals as well. Disorders of food intake span the entire developmental spectrum and can affect pregnant women, young children, and adolescents. Some of the most common feeding and eating disorders are discussed in the following sections.

COLIC

Colic is a feeding disorder of infants characterized by paroxysmal abdominal pain and severe crying. The crying generally lasts at least 3 hours and occurs on at least 3 days per week. Crying episodes peak around 6 weeks of age and generally resolve by 3 to 4 months of age (Holt, Wooldridge, Story, et al., 2011). The etiology of colic is unknown. Proposed causes include feeding too rapidly and swallowing large amounts of air.

Characteristically, the infant cries loudly and continuously, often for several hours. The infant's face may become flushed. The abdomen is distended and tense. Often the infant draws up the legs and clenches the hands. Episodes occur at the same time each day, usually in the late afternoon or early evening. Crying may stop only when the child is completely exhausted or after passage of flatus or stool.

The symptoms initially may resemble intestinal obstruction or peritoneal infection. These conditions must be ruled out along with sensitivity to formula. Treatment is supportive; no general medical consensus exists on effective treatments or interventions for colic. Some healthcare providers recommend medications such as simethicone (Mylicon) drops. Some recommend formula change to a soy formula or an elemental formula such as Pregestimil.

Nursing care requires a thorough history of the infant's diet and daily schedule and the events surrounding episodes of colicky behavior. Assessment of the infant's feeding patterns and diet includes type, frequency, and amount of feeding (if breastfeeding, maternal diet history) and frequency of burping. Inquire about onset, duration, and characteristics of cry during colic episodes. Ask the parents what measures are used to relieve crying and their effectiveness.

When possible, observe the feeding method. Parents of infants with colic are often tired and frustrated. They require frequent reassurance that they are not to blame for the infant's condition. Suggest ways of alleviating some of the infant's symptoms and discomfort. These include using a front-carrying sling, swaddling, playing soothing music, using a pacifier, or giving a warm bath or massage of the abdomen. The breastfeeding mother should avoid gas-producing foods and the infant should be burped frequently during feedings. An important consideration is the significant impact of colic on families. Colic can place extreme stress and fatigue on the family, so active support and counseling for the mother and other family members is important.

PICA

Pica is an eating disorder characterized by ingestion of nonfood items or food items consumed in abnormal quantities or forms. Examples of ingested items include starch, peeling paint, paper, soil components, flour, and coffee grounds. Clinical manifestations include zinc and iron deficiencies as well as symptoms of lead or other heavy metal poisoning (see Chapter 42) if these substances are contained in peeling paint or other ingested material. Pica most commonly manifests in pregnancy when women have abnormal cravings for nonfood products, and this can seriously impair the developing fetus (see Chapter 11 for more information). Some children also ingest abnormal amounts of nonfood items and fail to take in adequate nutrients from food. Treatment for children involves removing access to the substances, ensuring an adequate and nutritious diet, and treating any dietary deficiencies noted.

AVOIDANT/RESTRICTIVE FOOD INTAKE DISORDER (FORMERLY CALLED FEEDING DISORDER OF INFANCY AND EARLY CHILDHOOD OR FAILURE TO THRIVE)

Avoidant/restrictive food intake disorder describes a syndrome in which infants or young children fail to eat enough food to meet requirements for nutrition or energy (American Psychiatric Association [APA], 2013). This disorder accounts for 5% to 10% of pediatric hospitalizations in children under 1 year of age, and many more children are managed in community settings (Kliegman, Stanton, St. Geme, et al.,, 2011).

Etiology and Pathophysiology. Some disease states can contribute to poor intake, such as congenital AIDS (see Chapter 48), inborn errors of metabolism (see Chapter 53), congenital heart defect (see Chapter 47), neurologic disease (see Chapter 54), and esophageal reflux (see Chapter 51). However, avoidant/restrictive food intake disorder is not attributable to a medical or mental disorder (APA, 2013).

Infants and children whose parents or caretakers experience poverty, depression, substance abuse, intellectual disability, or psychosis are at risk for this disorder. Parents may be socially and emotionally isolated, or may lack knowledge of infant nutritional and nurturing needs. A reciprocal interaction pattern may exist in which the parent does not offer enough food or is not responsive to the infant's hunger cues, and the infant is irritable, not soothed, and does not give clear cues about hunger. Parental neglect is a contributor to the condition. Preterm and small-for-gestational-age babies more commonly have eating disorders (Kliegman et al., 2011).

Clinical Manifestations. The characteristics of this food intake disorder are persistent failure to eat adequately with no weight gain or with weight loss in an infant or child that is not

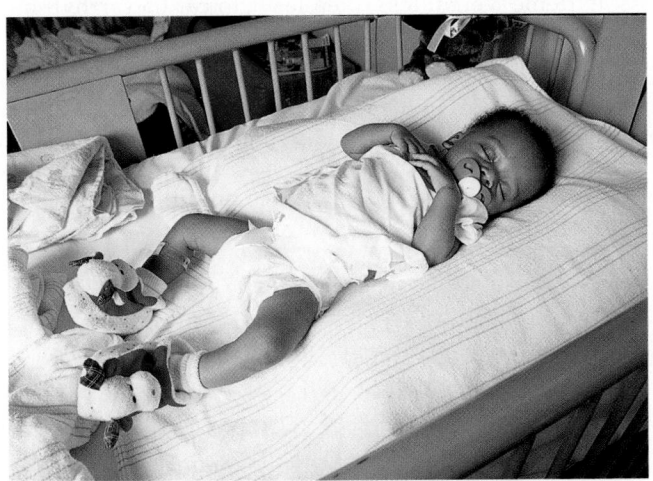

Figure 32–9 Avoidant/restrictive food intake disorder (formerly feeding disorder of infancy and childhood or failure to thrive). Infants with food intake disorder may not look severely malnourished, but they fall well below the expected weight and height norms for their age. This infant, who appears to be about 4 months old, is actually 8 months old. He has been hospitalized for food intake disorder.

associated with other medical conditions or mental disorders, and is not caused by lack of or unavailability of food. Weight is generally below the 5th percentile, and weight-for-length is less than 80% of ideal weight (Kliegman et al., 2011). Infants with food intake disorder refuse food, may have erratic sleep patterns, are irritable and difficult to soothe, and are often developmentally delayed (Figure 32–9).

Clinical Therapy. A thorough history and physical examination are needed to rule out any chronic physical illness. The infant or child may be hospitalized so that healthcare providers can establish a routine for feeding and sleeping. The goals of treatment are to provide adequate caloric and nutritional intake, promote normal growth and development, and assist parents in developing feeding routines and responding to the infant's cues of physical and psychologic hunger. Interprofessional teams that include nutrition teaching, home visits, parenting skills information, and other support are most successful (Cole & Lanham, 2011).

Nursing Management

For the Child With Avoidant/Restrictive Food Intake Disorder

Nursing Assessment and Diagnosis

Nursing assessment of the child is essential for establishing the best intervention plan for a child with food intake disorder. Documenting accurate weight and height each time any child is seen for health care provides an important record of growth patterns over time. This helps identify the child with an eating food intake disorder. The child's activity level, developmental milestones, and interaction patterns provide important information. When feeding the child, observe how the child indicates hunger or satiety, the ability of the child to be soothed, and general interaction patterns such as eye contact, touch, and "cuddliness."

Ask parents about stresses in their lives; these may prevent appropriate interaction with the child. Asking about the pregnancy and birth can elicit information about early disturbances in the child–parent relationship. Are there other children in the family, and, if so, do they have eating problems? Observe the child and parent behaviors while they feed the child; cues given by each person and interactional modes such as rocking, singing, talking, and body postures are important.

Some of the nursing diagnoses pertinent for the young child with an eating food intake disorder include the following (NANDA-I © 2014):

- *Nutrition, Imbalanced: Less than Body Requirements* related to inability to ingest proper amounts of food
- *Development: Delayed, Risk for,* related to inadequate food intake
- *Parenting, Risk for Impaired,* related to lack of knowledge about the child's nutritional needs
- *Fatigue* related to malnutrition

Planning and Implementation

Nursing care centers on performing a thorough history and physical assessment, observing parent–child interactions during feeding times, and providing necessary teaching to enable parents to respond appropriately to their child's needs. The child is often hospitalized initially and evaluated for potential organic causes while staff members feed the child. Tube feedings may be needed temporarily until normal intake can be ensured. Accurate weights, nutritional assessments, and developmental evaluation should be done to see if the child grows more normally. Additional diagnostic tests may be carried out at this time to rule out organic causes of poor growth.

Once a diagnosis of nonorganic food intake disorder is confirmed, parents become involved in feeding the child. Observations of feeding and continued careful physical assessments are needed. Carefully record the child's intake at each meal or feeding. Teach parents how to understand and respond to the child's cues of hunger and satiety. Teach them to hold, rock, and touch the infant during feedings and establish eye contact with infants and older children.

Developing Cultural Competence Height and Weight Growth Standards

Each child should maintain a height and weight growth pattern similar to the population standard. Asian American children may normally be below the 5th percentile on growth charts and not have an eating food intake disorder. Suspect a food intake disorder when the infant or child falls 1 standard deviation below the prior achieved growth curve and either fails to gain weight or loses weight over several months.

Upon discharge, referral to an agency that can continue monitoring of the home situation is needed. This provides an opportunity to observe feeding during a home visit and evaluate stresses and behavior patterns among family members. Frequent growth measurement and development must be ensured so the child is adequately nourished. Parents may need referral to community resources to help them manage stressful situations in their lives and to enhance their parenting skills.

Evaluation

Expected outcomes of nursing care include the following:

- Adequate growth and normal development of the infant is achieved.
- An improved parent–child relationship is established.

ANOREXIA NERVOSA

Anorexia nervosa is a potentially life-threatening eating disorder that occurs primarily in teenage girls and young women. An estimated 3% of adolescents in the United States are affected by anorexia nervosa or a related eating disorder, with females affected nearly three times more than males (National Institute of Mental Health [NIMH], 2011). The typical client is White and from a middle-class to upper-middle-class family. Age at onset varies from 8 years onward, with 19 years as the most common age at onset (NIMH, 2011).

Etiology and Pathophysiology.

Many causes are believed to contribute to the onset of anorexia. Cultural overemphasis on thinness may contribute to the excessive concern with dieting, body image, and fear of becoming fat that is experienced by many adolescents. Chemical changes have been found in the brain and blood of individuals with anorexia, leading to theories about a biologic cause. Often a significant life stress, loss, or change precedes the onset of anorexia. Stress hormones are commonly elevated in adolescents with anorexia, and immune system function may be disturbed.

Many experts view family issues as contributory to anorexia. Intrafamilial conflicts and dysfunctional family patterns may occur when parents are overly controlling and perfectionistic. The adolescent's eating behaviors may be an attempt to exercise independence and resolve internal psychologic conflicts.

The adolescent may engage in lengthy and vigorous exercise (up to 4 hours daily) to prevent weight gain. Laxatives or diuretics may be used to induce weight loss. As the disorder progresses, the adolescent perceives the ever-thinner body as becoming more beautiful. Youths may share weight loss techniques with friends who are anorectic and search out Internet sites that are positive about anorexia. The body responds to the abnormal eating behaviors as if starvation were occurring. Leukopenia, electrolyte imbalance, and hypoglycemia develop as a result of PEM. Once the body mass decreases below a critical level, menstruation ceases.

The adolescent who has anorexia and becomes pregnant is at risk for disturbances in prenatal care and outcomes as well as potential harm to the baby. See Chapter 11 for further information about eating disorders in pregnancy.

Clinical Manifestations.

Adolescents with anorexia are characterized by extreme weight loss accompanied by a preoccupation with weight and food, excessive compulsive exercising, peculiar patterns of eating and handling food, and distorted body image. They may prepare elaborate meals for others but eat only low-calorie foods. Characteristically, the fear of becoming fat does not decrease with continued weight loss. Accompanying signs and symptoms of depression, crying spells, feelings of isolation and loneliness, and suicidal thoughts and feelings are common. The disorder is often associated with mental illness such as obsessive-compulsive disorder, anxiety disorders (see Chapter 55), and history of abuse.

Physical findings include cold intolerance, dizziness, constipation, abdominal discomfort, bloating, irregular menses, and malnutrition (Figure 32–10). Hypothalamic suppression can lead to disturbances of gynecologic function, osteoporosis, decreased bone density, and fractures. Lanugo (fine, downy body hair) may be present. Fluid and electrolyte imbalances, especially potassium imbalances, are common. The child or adolescent is usually energetic despite significant weight loss. Extreme weight loss often leads to cardiac arrhythmias (bradycardia).

Clinical Therapy.

Diagnosis is based on a comprehensive history, physical examination revealing characteristic clinical manifestations, and the criteria listed in Table 32–7. Diagnostic tests commonly include hematocrit and hemoglobin, serum electrolytes, and serum vitamins and vitamin precursors. Bone

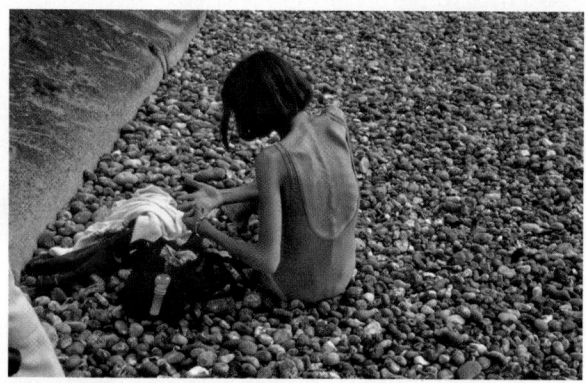

Figure 32–10 Anorexia nervosa. Note the loss of subcutaneous tissue in the back, arms, and pelvis.

SOURCE: Sally and Richard Greenhill/Alamy.

TABLE 32–7 DSM-5 Diagnostic Criteria for Anorexia Nervosa

A. Restriction of energy intake relative to requirements, leading to a significantly low body weight in the context of age, sex, developmental trajectory, and physical health. *Significantly low weight* is defined as a weight that is less than minimally normal or, for children and adolescents, less than that minimally expected.

B. Intense fear of gaining weight or of becoming fat, or persistent behavior that interferes with weight gain, even though at a significantly low weight.

C. Disturbance in the way in which one's body weight or shape is experienced, undue influence of body weight or shape on self-evaluation, or persistent lack of recognition of the seriousness of the current low body weight.

Specify whether:

- *Restricting type:* During the last 3 months, the individual has not engaged in recurrent episodes of binge eating or purging behavior (i.e., self-induced vomiting or the misuse of laxatives, diuretics, or enemas). This subtype describes presentations in which weight loss is accomplished primarily through dieting, fasting, and/or excessive exercise.
- *Binge-eating/purging type:* During the last 3 months, the individual has engaged in recurrent episodes of binge eating or purging behavior (i.e., self-induced vomiting or the misuse of laxatives, diuretics, or enemas).

Specify if:

- *In partial remission:* After full criteria for anorexia nervosa were previously met, Criterion A (low body weight) has not been met for a sustained period, but either Criterion B (intense fear of gaining weight or becoming fat or behavior that interferes with weight gain) or Criterion C (disturbances in self-perception of weight and shape) is still met.
- *In full remission:* After full criteria for anorexia nervosa were previously met, none of the criteria have been met for a sustained period of time.

Specify current severity:

The minimum level of severity is based, for adults, on current body mass index (BMI) (see below) or, for children and adolescents, on BMI percentile. The ranges below are derived from World Health Organization categories for thinness in adults; for children and adolescents, corresponding BMI percentiles should be used. The level of severity may be increased to reflect clinical symptoms, the degree of functional disability, and the need for supervision.

- *Mild:* BMI ≥ 17 kg/m^2
- *Moderate:* BMI 16–16.99 kg/m^2
- *Severe:* BMI 15–15.99 kg/m^2
- *Extreme:* BMI < 15 kg/m^2

Source: Used with permission from American Psychiatric Association. (2013). *Diagnostic and statistical manual of mental disorders* (5th ed.). Washington, DC: Author. Copyright © 2013 American Psychiatric Association.

density examination for females with lengthy amenorrhea is recommended (Mehler, Cleary, & Gaudiani, 2011).

The goals of treatment are to restore a healthy weight, address the psychologic issues associated with the condition, and reduce behaviors that lead to inadequate intake and relapse (NIMH, 2011). A firm focus is placed on reaching a targeted weight with a gradual weight gain of 2 to 3 lb/week in those hospitalized or 0.5 to 1 lb/week in outpatient care (Agency for Healthcare Research and Quality, 2014). Enteral feedings or total parenteral nutrition (TPN) may be necessary to replace lost fluid, protein, and nutrients, although the adolescent often perceives these feedings as a punitive measure.

Individual treatment and family therapy are used to address dysfunctional family patterns and assist the family to accept and deal with the adolescent as an independent and less-than-perfect individual (Brewerton & Costin, 2011; Lock, 2011). Family involvement is crucial to effect a lasting change in the adolescent. Nurses, psychologists, family therapists, and dietitians commonly partner to plan and implement therapy.

Long-term outpatient treatment, in either an individual or a group setting, is frequently necessary. Counseling that engages self-help techniques may be continued for 2 to 3 years to ensure that weight gain and self-image are maintained. Antidepressant drugs such as imipramine (Tofranil) or desipramine (Norpramin) may be prescribed for coexisting conditions such as depression, anxiety, or obsessive-compulsive disorders. However, they are not generally useful in the primary treatment of the disorder (Flament, Bissada, & Spettique, 2011).

Indications for hospitalization include loss of 25% to 30% of body weight or being at 85% or less of healthy weight, fluid and electrolyte imbalances, cardiac arrhythmias, hypotension, or the need to provide a more intense period of therapy if outpatient treatment fails to produce improvement. Behavior modification techniques are used extensively in combination with counseling and other methods in the care of the hospitalized adolescent with anorexia.

Nursing Management
For the Child With Anorexia Nervosa

Nursing Assessment and Diagnosis

Obtain a thorough individual and family history. Ask about usual eating patterns, daily caloric intake, exercise patterns, and menstrual history. Ask about medication use; include prescription, nonprescription, and herbal products. Is there a family history of eating disorders? Assess for signs of malnutrition. Obtain height and weight measurements and compare with norms for the general population. Because the client with anorexia often wears layers of clothes when being weighed, strive to obtain an accurate measurement. Mid–upper arm circumference, skinfold thickness, waist-to-hip ratio, and body composition measurement may all be obtained (Mattar, Godart, Melchior, et al., 2011).

Nursing diagnoses for the adolescent with anorexia nervosa include the following (NANDA-I © 2014):

- ***Nutrition, Imbalanced: Less than Body Requirements*** related to inadequate food intake
- ***Fluid Volume: Deficient, Risk for,*** related to inadequate fluid intake or fluid volume loss from overuse of laxatives and diuretics
- ***Body Temperature, Imbalanced, Risk for,*** related to excessive weight loss and absence of subcutaneous fat
- ***Constipation*** related to inadequate food intake and overuse of laxatives
- ***Body Image, Disturbed,*** related to distorted perception of body size and shape
- ***Self-Esteem, Chronic Low,*** related to dysfunctional family dynamics
- ***Coping: Family, Compromised,*** related to parental tendency to be overly controlling and perfectionistic

Planning and Implementation

Nursing care centers on meeting nutritional and fluid needs, preventing complications, administering medications, supporting psychologic interventions, and providing referral to appropriate resources. Specific treatment measures vary depending on physical complications, length and degree of illness, emotional symptoms accompanying the disorder, and family dynamics. Resistance to treatment is common, and nurses who care for adolescents with anorexia must deal with their own feelings of frustration and anger.

PROVIDE PSYCHOLOGIC SUPPORT

Care for the adolescent with anorexia necessarily includes psychologic support as an important component. The nurse will refer the family to a specialist who can counsel and recommend further treatment. Families of a youth with anorexia should be involved in support groups and should also receive information about the condition and the youth's plan of care. The adolescent is often treated with individual counseling and encouragement to participate is needed. Interventions that improve self-concept and lead to a realistic body image are needed. They may include encouragement for participation in sports, praise for participation in the treatment plan, and immediate referral for relapses as treatment progresses.

MEET NUTRITIONAL AND FLUID NEEDS

Monitor nutritional and fluid intake, encourage consumption of food, and observe eating behaviors at mealtime. Elimination patterns may be altered as a result of increased intake during hospitalization. Monitor for possible problems, including abdominal distention, constipation, or diarrhea. Daily monitoring of serum electrolytes is necessary.

If TPN is administered, watch for complications such as circulatory overload, hyperglycemia, or hypoglycemia. Use strict aseptic technique when changing tubing or dressings.

ADMINISTER MEDICATIONS

Monitor vital signs if the adolescent is receiving antidepressants. Watch for signs of hypertension and tachycardia. Administer medications after meals because it helps to prevent gastric irritation. Be alert for substance abuse. People with anorexia often use excessive laxatives or products such as ephedra (also known as ma huang) to induce weight loss. Changes in the central nervous system, vital signs, and other findings may indicate over-the-counter or herbal drug use.

PROVIDE REFERRAL TO APPROPRIATE RESOURCES

Refer parents and other family members to the American Anorexia and Bulimia Association, National Eating Disorders Organization, and National Association of Anorexia Nervosa & Associated Disorders for further information about the disorder and a list of support groups in their area.

Evaluation

Expected outcomes for nursing care include recommended level of weight gain, maintenance of adequate fluid volume and balanced electrolytes, maintenance of normal blood pressure and heart rhythm, beginning of positive sense of self-esteem, intake of nutritionally balanced diet, and use of psychologic counseling to understand the disorder.

BULIMIA NERVOSA

Bulimia nervosa is an eating disorder characterized by **binge eating** (a compulsion to consume large quantities of food in a short period of time). Usually the episodes of bingeing are followed by various methods of weight control (purging), such as self-induced vomiting, large doses of laxatives or diuretics, or a combination of methods. Persons are overly concerned with body shape and weight (APA, 2013). Bulimia affects 1% of the general population, with prevalence in young women about 3 times that in men (NIMH, 2011). Like anorexia, it affects adolescent and young adult females more commonly than males. The disorder usually begins in middle to late adolescence at an average age of 20 years.

Etiology and Pathophysiology. Causes of bulimia nervosa are similar to those of anorexia nervosa: sensitivity to social pressure for thinness, body image difficulties, and long-standing dysfunctional family patterns. Families may be chaotic and distant rather than overinvolved as seen in the person with anorexia. Many individuals with bulimia experience depression. It is not clear whether the depression is a cause or a result of the individual's inability to control the bingeing and purging cycles. An adolescent with bulimia often binges after any stressful event.

Bingeing usually occurs in secret for several hours until the individual is stopped by abdominal discomfort, by another person, or by vomiting. At first, the episodes of binge eating are pleasurable. Immediately following the binge episode, however, feelings of guilt, shame, anger, depression, and fear of loss of control and weight gain arise. As these feelings intensify, the adolescent with bulimia becomes increasingly anxious. This usually initiates the purge behaviors.

Purging eliminates the discomfort from bloating and also prevents weight gain. This relieves the feelings of depression and guilt, but only temporarily. Adolescents with bulimia commonly practice the binge–purge cycle many times a day, losing their ability to respond to normal cues of hunger and satiety.

Clinical Manifestations. Bulimia is often a "silent" disorder since it is easily concealed from healthcare providers and families. Only about 6% of those with the condition are believed to receive treatment. Adolescents with bulimia are preoccupied with body shape, size, and weight. They may appear overweight or thin and usually report a wide range of average body weight over the years. Physical findings depend on the degree of purging, starvation, dehydration, and electrolyte disturbance. Erosion of tooth enamel, increased dental caries, and gum recession, which result from vomiting of gastric acids, are common findings. Vomiting-induced calluses may be seen on the back of an affected individual's hand. Abdominal distention is often seen. Esophageal tears and esophagitis may also occur.

Clinical Therapy. A comprehensive history is necessary because most adolescents with bulimia appear normal in weight or only slightly underweight. Diagnostic tests include hematocrit, hemoglobin, and serum electrolytes; they may identify signs of altered electrolyte and hematologic status. Lowered potassium levels are related to repetitive vomiting since gastric contents have a high potassium level. The diagnosis is confirmed by the presence of specific criteria (Table 32–8).

Treatment includes management of physiologic problems and cognitive-behavior therapy. Medications, such as fluoxetine 60 mg/day for adolescents, may be prescribed (Hay & Claudino, 2011). Management involves a variety of healthcare providers such as physicians, nurses, and therapists. Behavior modification focuses on modifying the dysfunctional eating patterns and restoring normal patterns. Until the episodes of bingeing and purging are under control, feelings of discouragement

TABLE 32–8 DSM-5 Diagnostic Criteria for Bulimia Nervosa

A. Recurrent episodes of binge eating. An episode of binge eating is characterized by both of the following:
  - Eating, in a discrete period of time (e.g., within any 2-hour period), an amount of food that is definitely larger than what most individuals would eat in a similar period of time under similar circumstances.
  - A sense of lack of control over eating during the episode (e.g., a feeling that one cannot stop eating or control what or how much one is eating).

B. Recurrent inappropriate compensatory behaviors in order to prevent weight gain, such as self-induced vomiting; misuse of laxatives, diuretics, or other medications; fasting; or excessive exercise.

C. The binge eating and inappropriate compensatory behaviors both occur, on average, at least once a week for 3 months.

D. Self-evaluation is unduly influenced by body shape and weight.

E. The disturbance does not occur exclusively during episodes of anorexia nervosa.

Specify if:

- *In partial remission:* After full criteria for bulimia nervosa were previously met, some, but not all, of the criteria have been met for a sustained period of time.
- *In full remission:* After full criteria for bulimia nervosa were previously met, none of the criteria have been met for a sustained period of time.

Specify current severity:

The minimum level of severity is based on the frequency of inappropriate compensatory behaviors (see below). The level of severity may be increased to reflect other symptoms and the degree of functional disability.

- *Mild:* An average of 1–3 episodes of inappropriate compensatory behaviors per week.
- *Moderate:* An average of 4–7 episodes of inappropriate compensatory behaviors per week.
- *Severe:* An average of 8–13 episodes of inappropriate compensatory behaviors per week.
- *Extreme:* An average of 14 or more episodes of inappropriate compensatory behaviors per week.

Source: Used with permission from American Psychiatric Association. (2013). *Diagnostic and statistical manual of mental disorders (5th ed.).* Washington, DC: Author. Copyright © 2013 American Psychiatric Association.

and hopelessness prevail. Thus the focus early in treatment is on initiating an immediate behavioral change. Once initial interventions have been successful, group therapy sessions work well for people with anorexia or bulimia. Specific treatment measures may include the following:

- Educating the adolescent about good nutrition (including food choices and caloric content)
- Encouraging the adolescent to keep a log or food journal and assisting the adolescent to make connections between emotional states, stress, and the impulse to binge or purge
- Setting up a daily dietary routine of three meals and three snacks a day (using the same foods for each meal and snack every day to change misconceptions about the weight-gaining potential of certain foods and to decrease anxiety about what food must be eaten at the next meal)

Once these initial measures have been taken, the underlying psychosocial issues are explored. The goals of therapy are to provide the adolescent with bulimia with adaptive coping skills and to improve self-esteem.

Most adolescents with bulimia do not require hospitalization. Serious abnormalities in fluid and electrolyte levels caused by uncontrollable cycles of bingeing and vomiting, accompanied by depression or suicidal activity, are indications of the need for hospitalization. The prognosis is good with long-term therapy.

Nursing Management

For the Child With Bulimia Nervosa

Nursing Assessment and Diagnosis

Obtain a thorough individual and family history, including daily dietary intake and weight fluctuations. Inquire about problems such as abdominal pain or distention, which may indicate an abnormal eating or elimination pattern. Assess the oral mucosa for signs of damage to tooth enamel caused by purging; examine hands for evidence of vomiting-induced calluses.

Following are nursing diagnoses that may be appropriate for the adolescent with bulimia nervosa (NANDA-I © 2014):

- *Nutrition, Imbalanced: Less than Body Requirements* related to disordered food intake
- *Fluid Volume, Deficient, Risk for,* related to fluid volume loss
- *Tissue Integrity, Impaired,* related to chemical effects of vomited gastric acids on mucous membranes
- *Knowledge, Deficient (Adolescent),* related to health risks of excessive use of laxatives and diuretics
- *Anxiety* related to discomfort with weight and eating patterns
- *Self-Esteem, Chronic Low,* related to dysfunctional family dynamics
- *Coping, Ineffective,* related to life stressors

Planning and Implementation

Nursing care includes monitoring nutritional intake and elimination patterns, preventing complications, and providing appropriate referrals.

During hospitalization the client should keep a food diary. Be alert to the adolescent who hides, gives away, or discards food from the tray or who exits to use the bathroom after meals. The adolescent should be monitored for at least 30 minutes after meals by remaining in a central area in the company of the nurse or other responsible individuals. Withdrawal from laxatives and diuretics is managed with careful observation for alterations in fluid and electrolyte status. Cardiac monitoring may be necessary if potassium levels are seriously altered. Esophageal tearing or esophagitis is treated to promote mucosal healing. Medications such as antidepressants may be administered. Encourage continuation of group and other therapy sessions.

Adolescents with bulimia and their families can be referred to organizations such as those listed earlier in the section on anorexia for assistance and information about the disorder.

Evaluation

Expected outcomes for nursing care for the adolescent with bulimia include healthy mucous membranes and skin, adequate intake of fluids and food, balanced food intake, maintenance of normal weight, adequate support and healthy psychologic balance, and absence of bingeing and purging.

Food Reactions

Food reaction encompasses any adverse reaction to foods or substances ingested in foods. The most common food reaction is **food intolerance**, an abnormal physiologic response to a food that is not immunoglobulin E (IgE)–mediated. Examples include indigestion or flatulence upon eating certain foods, a sweating reaction to some spices, rhinitis, and hives with urticaria (Mansoor & Sharma, 2011). See the discussion of lactose intolerance that follows. Milk and grain products are common causes of food intolerance. Chemical additives, antibiotics, preservatives, and food colorings also can cause food-sensitivity reactions.

The most serious type of reaction is **food allergy**, an IgE-mediated reaction that is potentially systemic, characteristically rapid in onset, and may be manifested as swelling of the lips, mouth, uvula or glottis, generalized urticaria, and in severe reactions, anaphylaxis. Food allergies are the most common cause of anaphylaxis and are more prevalent in children with a family history of allergic reactions to various substances and foods (**atopy**). The foods that most commonly cause allergy are fish, shellfish, peanuts, tree nuts, eggs, soy, wheat, corn, strawberries, and cow's milk products. About 0.6% of children have an allergy to peanuts, and the incidence has increased in the past two decades (National Institute of Allergy and Infectious Diseases [NIAID], 2011). A majority of the 150 deaths from food allergies that occur annually in the United States are due to peanut allergy.

Children who have both food allergy and asthma are most at risk of death from anaphylaxis due to a food allergy. Allergic individuals need to be aware of hidden substances in prepared foods. For example, the child allergic to nuts will experience a reaction to a food if nut extracts are used in its preparation. Note that certain foods can cause either allergy or intolerance so accurate diagnosis is needed. An example is cow's milk, which can cause an allergy with IgE-mediated systemic reaction, or an intolerance from gastrointestinal response to milk proteins (diarrhea, vomiting, abdominal pain) as a result of lack of the enzyme lactase in the gastrointestinal tract.

Delayed hypersensitivity reactions are attributed to digestive products of food and require a thorough diet history over several days to identify the offending food. These reactions are more difficult to diagnose, since the reaction can occur up to 24 hours after ingestion of the food. There may also be biphasic reactions that occur 1 to 30 hours after an initial anaphylaxis. Such reactions can be severe and life threatening. Therefore, every child with a food allergy who ingests the allergen should be promptly treated with epinephrine and transported to an emergency facility for further management and monitoring.

Diagnostic tests to identify suspected food allergies include measurement of serum IgE levels, scratch tests, and the **radioallergosorbent test (RAST)**, in which radioimmunoassay measures IgE antibodies to specific allergens. (See Chapter 48 for further information about these tests.) In cases of past allergic response, the food is absolutely avoided. In food intolerance, a diet diary is kept, noting date, type of foods eaten, and reaction, if any. Foods should be eaten singly for several days to determine whether they cause a reaction.

Treatment consists of eliminating the offending foods from the child's diet. Collaborative care involving the child, parents, school, and healthcare providers is needed to ensure that the child with food allergies does not get exposed to the offending allergen, and that all children with food reactions can avoid contact with foods to which they are allergic or intolerant. When the child is exposed

to the food, epinephrine should be administered and transport to a treatment center should be immediate. Treatment in the hospital may include additional measures as needed such as bronchodilators, antihistamines, and oxygen therapy (NIAID, 2011).

Nursing Management

Prevention is the first step. Instruct parents of infants to introduce new foods at a rate of not more than one new food every 3 to 5 days. If food intolerance is noted, the causative food can be easily identified. Discuss any changes in diet or preparation of formula. Reassure parents that the child's symptoms will disappear when the offending foods are removed from the diet.

Be alert for skin, respiratory, and other characteristic manifestations of food allergy in children. Immediately call 9-1-1 for care. All such cases should be referred to an allergist for diagnosis. If an allergy is identified, help the family to identify and remove the offending foods. Emphasize the importance of reading food labels for hidden foods that can trigger an allergic response. The child, family, school, and other settings should be prepared at all times for immediate response to food allergy.

SAFETY ALERT!

Children with food allergies should wear an alert bracelet and carry emergency medication such as an EpiPen. Nurses in schools and offices must instruct families, schoolteachers, and others about the child's allergy and what to do in case of accidental ingestion of the food product. Assist them to set up prevention and emergency treatment plans.

Refer the family to the Food Allergy Network. Recognize that food allergies can be stressful for children and families, as they worry about exposure in daily life.

The child with food intolerance needs to avoid the food to ensure comfort and an absence of the annoying symptoms associated with it. Although, unlike with an allergic reaction, intolerance is not life threatening, the family needs to learn about hidden sources of the food product so that it can be avoided and alternative foods can be suggested for their use.

Lactose Intolerance

Lactose intolerance is the inability to digest lactose, a disaccharide found in milk and other dairy products. It results from a congenital or acquired deficiency of the enzyme lactase. Congenital lactase deficiency of infancy is a rare disorder. Lactose intolerance is considered a biologic norm, occurring in 50% to 100% of African Americans, Native Americans, Asian Americans, and Hispanics, and only 15% of White Americans (National Dairy Council, 2011).

Abdominal pain, flatulence, and diarrhea occur shortly after birth when the infant is unable to hydrolyze lactose. Diarrhea develops rapidly after the child ingests milk and milk products. Some children are able to tolerate small ingestions of lactose but have symptoms when larger amounts are consumed. Incidence of lactose intolerance increases with advancing age throughout childhood.

Diagnosis is based on a thorough history and a hydrogen breath test, which measures the amount of hydrogen left after fermentation of unabsorbed carbohydrates. Implementing a lactose-free diet for a period of time may eliminate the symptoms, thus confirming the diagnosis. Treatment for infants includes switching to lactose-free formula. For older children, eliminating lactose-containing foods is recommended. Lactase enzyme tablets can be added to milk or sprinkled on foods to aid digestion.

Nursing Management

Nursing care is primarily supportive. Carefully explain dietary modifications to parents and discuss alternative sources of calcium. Discuss the need for supplementation of calcium and vitamin D to prevent deficiencies. Teach families how to read food labels to find hidden sources of lactose. For example, milk solids may be found in breads, cakes, candies, salad dressings, margarine, and processed food. Suggest lactase tablets for children who want to eat some dairy products.

Nutritional Support

Sports Nutrition and Ergogenic Agents

Regular physical activity should be encouraged for all children, with at least 60 minutes of activity recommended daily. However, during vigorous or prolonged exercise, or during hot weather, child and adolescent athletes may have special nutritional needs. A well-balanced diet, reflective of recommended foods, is needed. A wide variety of fresh fruits and vegetables, grains, and complex carbohydrates usually provides for adequate caloric intake. When the child is hungry, extra calories should come from the food groups listed here rather than from increased intake of fat. When the child or teen is very active, sports bars or drinks can provide the additional needed calories in a nutritionally balanced manner. As always, the height, weight, and BMI percentiles are the best assurance that the child is growing adequately over time. Adequate energy to perform the sport as well as be attentive and productive at school and for other activities should also be considered.

Water should be increased during activity both to minimize chance of dehydration and also to maximize performance. About 1 hour before vigorous exercise, the child should drink 1 to 2 glasses (8 to 16 oz) of water and should repeat the same amount of fluid just before the exercise begins. Young children may not feel thirsty and should be encouraged to drink 13 mL/kg during activity and exercise with rest periods every 15 to 20 minutes (Rowland, 2011). Water is usually the best replacement, but during extended exercise, sports drinks may be a good alternative for some of the fluid intake. Frequent or excessive intake of caloric sports drinks and those with caffeine should be discouraged (AAP Committee on Nutrition and the Council on Sports Medicine and Fitness, 2011). Additional water is needed for the first 2 hours after activity. Weight loss of 1 lb indicates a loss of about 1/2 quart of fluid, and weight loss of 1% of body weight can influence performance. The nurse should be sure the child takes in fluid to replace all losses.

Some common nutrients that may be deficient in all teens, but even more often in the athlete, are calcium and iron. The increased blood volume common in the well-conditioned person necessitates greater intake. Calcium-rich foods such as milk products and dark green vegetables, and iron-rich foods such as meats and grains, can guard against deficiencies. While many adolescents believe that they need extra protein during athletic season, most Americans eat adequate protein to meet even the increased needs of sports. On the other hand, the vegetarian child or adolescent may need help to plan a diet with adequate protein.

Many teens take a wide variety of dietary supplements, believing that they act as **ergogenic aids**, or products that enhance performance during sports by influencing energy, alertness, or body composition. Most of the claims of these products are unproven, and their safety has not usually been investigated, especially in the young. Effects on youth whose bodies are still developing are particularly unknown and the risks are high for permanent interference with some normal growth patterns. Offer guidance and help the family and teen investigate claims before choosing to use a product. If youths use supplements, they should be instructed about doses, desired effects, and potential side effects. Some sports and coaches may encourage small size and dieting, or encourage use of dietary supplements to increase weight and muscle. Children and adolescents in activities such as ballet, wrestling, track or running, and horse racing may have health risks associated with inconsistent or inadequate intake.

Approximately 3.2% of U.S. high school students (4.0% of males and 2.2% of females) report taking illegal anabolic steroids; up to 8.8% in some communities report use (CDC, 2014d). These products can have a wide array of side effects. They may stop growth of long bones, lead to endocrine imbalance, and cause increased tendon rupture. They are also illegal in sporting events. Andro and DHEA are steroidal hormones used by some athletes. They can cause masculinization of females, disruption of glucose balance, insulin sensitivity, dyslipidemia, decrease in potential height, bone and joint abnormalities, and aggressive behavior (O'Malley, 2013).

Some common amino acid nutritional supplements include creatine, carnitine, and glutamine. Although the side effects of these substances are minimal, their possible enhancement of performance is temporary and outcomes of long-term use are unknown. Increasing protein intake to meet needs during periods of high activity is a better alternative. Creatine has been studied more than most supplements; it is made by the body and is present in many protein sources. Supplemental creatine increases the creatine level in muscle and may help to increase performance in short bursts of activity, while not affecting endurance sports. The increase in muscle mass that can occur is actually due to water and is lost quickly when the supplement is discontinued.

Minerals such as chromium, iron, and calcium are used by some youths. Ask about the athlete's social group and whether ergogenic aids are used; this is a strong predictor of their adoption and is reason for additional counseling. The nurse should ask careful and sensitive questions such as, "Many athletes take supplements to aid in performance in sports. What supplements do you take or are you considering?" Information should be provided to enhance the youth's understanding of nutrition and sports performance. Generally, a balanced diet with adequate carbohydrate, protein, and fat will meet the needs of most athletes and lead to maximal sport performance. School nurses can work with physical education teachers and coaches to plan appropriate programs for youth to prevent use of ergogenic aids.

Herbs, Probiotics, and Prebiotics

Many families use food products to promote health and treat diseases. These include herbal products that may be acquired from health food stores or the Internet. Herbs are not tested nor regulated by the government, so amounts of ingredients are often not known. Ask families about what herbal products they use regularly or to treat disease. Learn about the herbs and any research that has been conducted with children.

Another type of food product is a **probiotic**, a food supplement containing a live microorganism that alters the balance of gut microflora, thereby providing a health benefit. Common probiotics include *Lactobacillus* and *Bifidobacterium*, which are commonly found in the human gastrointestinal tract, are enhanced by eating yogurt with live cultures, and may be helpful in treating diarrhea or atopic dermatitis. Daily intake of pasteurized yogurt with live cultures can safely be encouraged for children.

A **prebiotic** is a nondigestible food ingredient that can stimulate growth or activity of probiotic bacteria (Mitsuoka, 2014). For example, oligosaccharides enhance proliferation of the beneficial *Bifidobacterium*.

Inquire about the family's treatment of common childhood disorders. Include questions about food and nutritional supplements at all well-child visits. Provide information for the family as needed.

Health-Related Conditions

Many health conditions influence the child's nutritional state. Conversely, the child's nutritional state can influence the state of health. See *Pathophysiology Illustrated* for examples of some common conditions that influence nutritional needs. These conditions are discussed in various chapters throughout the text. Discuss with classmates how to adjust normal nutritional assessment and teaching due to the presence of a healthcare concern. Which conditions influence absorption of nutrients? Which cause changes in nutritional intake requirements? Some children benefit from special dietary aids, such as eating utensils and cups that are easy to grasp. Therapists can evaluate and make recommendations about devices that can assist the child at meals.

Vegetarianism

Some families choose to eat vegetarian diets and can be helped and encouraged in their endeavors. Several variations in intake occur. **Vegetarians** eat no poultry, meat, or fish. **Lacto-ovovegetarians** eat eggs and dairy products, whereas **lactovegetarians** eat dairy products but not eggs. In contrast, **vegans** are strict vegetarians and eat no animal products. When someone says he or she is vegetarian, it is best if the nurse asks specific questions about what the individual will and will not eat.

The vegetarian diet is healthy, easy to follow, and may even provide extra health benefits (Academy of Nutrition and Dietetics, 2013). Some deficiencies may exist; assessment and planning can ensure that they do not develop. Vegans should be sure to include adequate dietary vitamins D and B_{12}, zinc, iron, calories, protein, and fat. Completing a 24-hour diet recall for pregnant or lactating women and vegetarian children, with analysis for RDAs, can be helpful. The nurse should be sure to routinely assess growth and other nutritional measures, as well as provide ideas of various foods to meet nutritional needs and perform other general nutritional teaching. When a vegetarian child is hospitalized, the nurse should plan with the nutrition department and the child's family to meet intake needs.

Growth and Development

When a pregnant teen follows a vegetarian diet, she needs additional help to encourage adequate nutrition. A 24-hour or 2-day diet diary helps identify nutritional needs. Consider additional pregnancy needs for energy, protein, omega-3 fatty acids, iron, vitamin D, and calcium; note that vitamin B_{12} is recommended as a supplement. Use the vegetarian food guide available through the Academy of Nutrition and Dietetics.

Enteral Therapy

Enteral therapy is a form of nutritional support provided when a child cannot take in enough food orally to sustain health. Since it is the closest form of nutritional support to the natural method of eating, it has the least untoward effects and greatest rate of success. Some children who use enteral therapy are those with cerebral palsy or other neurologic conditions that lead to weakness of the throat and mouth, those with neoplasm or immune dysfunction, and those in acute states of recovery from accidents or illness (Figure 32–11).

Although a tube can be inserted into the nasal opening and placed through the esophagus into the stomach (nasogastric

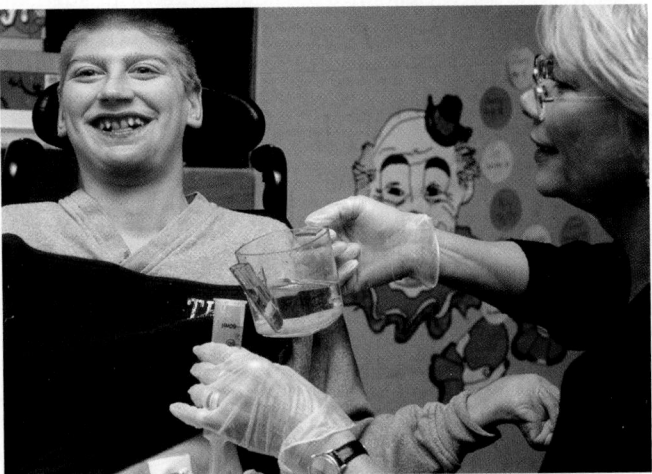

Figure 32–11 Enteral therapy. This child has returned to school following surgery. He has difficulty chewing and swallowing food due to cerebral palsy. The school nurse has taught his teacher how to safely administer some enteral feedings during school hours.

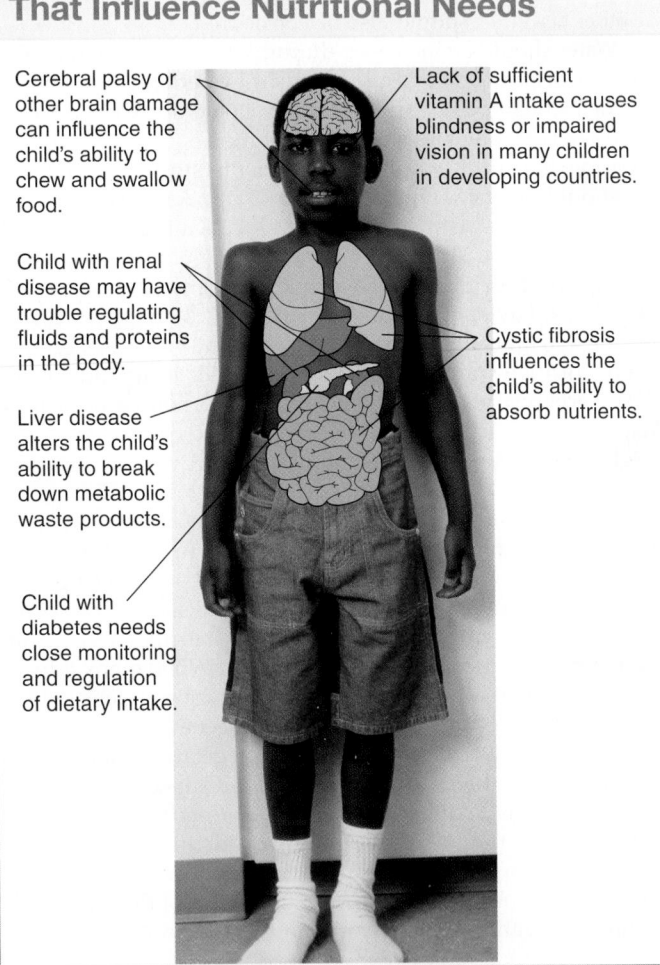

Pathophysiology Illustrated: **Conditions That Influence Nutritional Needs**

Cerebral palsy or other brain damage can influence the child's ability to chew and swallow food.

Lack of sufficient vitamin A intake causes blindness or impaired vision in many children in developing countries.

Child with renal disease may have trouble regulating fluids and proteins in the body.

Cystic fibrosis influences the child's ability to absorb nutrients.

Liver disease alters the child's ability to break down metabolic waste products.

Child with diabetes needs close monitoring and regulation of dietary intake.

tube), a tube surgically placed into the stomach through an abdominal opening, a jejunal or gastric tube, is preferred for long-term use. As long as the child can absorb and use nutrients, enteral therapy can be successful in providing calories and essential nutrients. Commercially prepared formulas are available, and specially formulated solutions can be adapted for children with specific dietary needs. Nursing care includes care of the gastrostomy tube and entry site to prevent infection and skin breakdown. Ensure that a nasogastric tube is correctly placed before each tube feeding. For both nasogastric and gastric feedings, an empty syringe is often used to check residuals or the amount of fluid not absorbed since the previous feeding. Teach families enteral feeding techniques when they will perform the process at home and arrange for periodic evaluation of technique. Perform regular nutritional assessments. See Chapter 51 for suggestions on management of nursing care during tube feedings. See the accompanying *Clinical Skills Manual* SKILLS .

Total Parenteral Nutrition (TPN)

Total parenteral nutrition (TPN) makes it possible to provide intravenous nutritional support for people who cannot eat or are unable to absorb nutrients from the intestinal tract in a normal manner and are at risk of severe malnutrition. Examples of children who benefit from this method of nutrition are those with congenital malformation of the gastrointestinal tract, brain injury, or severe burns; it may also be used for support after bone marrow transplant, sepsis, or other critical conditions.

A catheter is inserted so that a sterile nutrition solution is infused directly into the bloodstream. A central venous catheter is used to promote safe infusion. Fluids usually contain glucose; electrolytes such as sodium, potassium, calcium, magnesium, phosphate, and chloride; vitamins; and proteins. Lipid emulsions are another type of TPN used in some children. Meticulous care is needed, whether in the hospital or at home, to ensure safe TPN infusion and treatment. The nurse performs initial assessment, ongoing evaluation, and monitoring of treatment; verifies the solution type and rate of administration; ensures that solution storage recommendations are followed; and administers the solutions in the hospital or other settings. See the *Clinical Skills Manual* SKILLS for the protocols for TPN management.

Clinical Reasoning The Child With Special Nutritional Needs

Joey was diagnosed with cerebral palsy early in life. He is now 11 years old and has recently been enrolled in school. Part of the healthcare plan being implemented in the school involves fostering a positive nutritional state. Joey has limited ability to swallow, related to muscle weakness of cerebral palsy, and is therefore unable to ingest enough calories by mouth to ensure his optimal growth and development. Joey had a feeding tube inserted into his stomach at an early age and receives some of his nutrition by this method.

The school nurse has met with Joey's parents and his home health nurse to learn about the amount and type of tube feedings he receives, as well as the texture of oral feedings he can manage. The nurse will plan the feeding schedule at school to facilitate adequate nutrition in that setting. In addition, careful ongoing nutritional assessment will be needed to evaluate if Joey is getting the calories and other nutrients he needs for growth and development. The school nurse is also educating the classroom teachers and other school personnel about Joey's unique nutritional requirements.

How will you organize Joey's care and educate teachers and other staff if you are the case manager for his integration within the school system?

Focus Your Study

- Adequate nutritional intake is necessary for the normal growth and development of children.

- Children with medical or psychosocial conditions require additional nutritional support.

- Dietary intake patterns vary throughout childhood. As the child grows, the child is able to metabolize different types of food and gain greater gross and fine motor control.

- Nutritional assessment is an essential part of nursing care and may involve approaches such as growth measurement and intake records.

- Common nutrition concerns in childhood include hunger, overweight, foodborne illness, celiac disease, and dietary deficiencies.

- The child with avoidant/restrictive food intake disorder requires comprehensive assessment and ongoing management to foster parent–child interaction and adequate nutritional intake.

- The most common eating disorders of adolescents are anorexia nervosa and bulimia nervosa.

- A combination of behavioral management, counseling, and medication is often used in treatment programs for eating disorders.

- Food allergy represents a life-threatening condition for children, whereas food intolerance can lead to uncomfortable but non-life-threatening symptoms.

- Children engaging in sports, and those who eat vegetarian diets, may need guidance to meet nutrition needs.

- Some children require alternative feeding methods, such as enteral and parenteral feedings.

Clinical Reasoning in Action

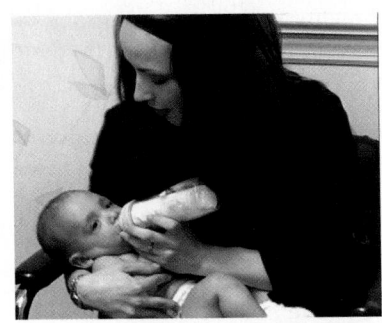

A mother is seeing the pediatric nurse practitioner you are working with for her son Jonathan's 3-month, well-baby checkup at the local community health clinic. The baby is in the 90th percentile for weight and in the 50th percentile for length and is fed Similac formula with iron. According to the medical history, Jonathan had respiratory syncytial virus (RSV) when he was 1 month old and there are smokers in the house (see Chapter 46 for more information on RSV). The nurse practitioner has asked you to educate the mother about feeding her 3-month-old baby. The mother has raised concerns that the baby is not sleeping through the night, and the baby's grandmother has suggested adding cereal to his bottle at night to help him sleep. Jonathan has met all developmental milestones and has not yet developed teeth.

1. What type of advice can you give the mother about adding cereal to the bottle?
2. Why is rice cereal recommended as the first food to introduce when Jonathan is able to start solid foods?
3. What is the reason only iron-fortified formula or breast milk is recommended the entire first year of life for Jonathan rather than cow's milk?
4. Based on Jonathan's length and weight percentiles on the growth chart, his mother wonders if he should be put on a "diet." What would be the appropriate response to her concern?

References

Academy of Nutrition and Dietetics. (2013). *Vegetarianism: The facts*. Retrieved from http://www.eatright.org/Public/content.aspx?id=6442478107&terms=vegetarian%20diet

Ackerman, K. E., & Misra, M. (2011). Bone health and the female athlete triad in adolescent athletes. *Physician Sportsmedicine, 39*, 131–141.

Agency for Healthcare Research and Quality. (2014). *Practice guideline for treatment of persons with eating disorders*. Retrieved from http://www.guideline.gov/content.aspx?id=9318

American Academy of Pediatrics (AAP). (2011). *Fruit juice and your child's diet*. Retrieved from http://www.healthychildren.org

American Academy of Pediatrics (AAP) Committee on Nutrition and the Council on Sports Medicine and Fitness. (2011). Clinical report—Sports drink and energy drinks for children and adolescents: Are they appropriate? *Pediatrics.* doi:10.1542/peds.2011-0965

American Academy of Pediatrics (AAP) Section on Breastfeeding. (2012). Breastfeeding and the use of human milk. *Pediatrics, 129*, e827–e841.

American Academy of Pediatrics (AAP) Committee on Nutrition. (2013). *Pediatric nutrition handbook* (7th ed.). Elk Grove Village, IL: American Academy of Pediatrics.

American Academy of Pediatrics (AAP). (2014a). *Switching to solid foods*. Retrieved from http://www.healthychildren.org/English/ages-stages/baby/feeding-nutrition/Pages/Switching-To-Solid-Foods.aspx

American Academy of Pediatrics (AAP). (2014b). *Where we stand: TV viewing time*. Retrieved from http://www.healthychildren.org/English/family-life/Media/Pages/Where-We-Stand-TV-Viewing-Time.aspx

American Association for Clinical Chemistry. (2014). *The ABC's of pediatric laboratory medicine—R is for Rickets*. Retrieved from https://www.aacc.org/members/divisions/pediatrics/Newsletter/2013/summer_2013/Pages/story3.aspx#

American Association of Pediatric Dentistry. (2014). *Guidelines for fluoride therapy*. Retrieved from http://www.aapd.org/media/Policies_Guidelines/G_fluoridetherapy.pdf

American Psychiatric Association (APA). (2013). *The diagnostic and statistical manual of mental disorders* (5th ed.) (DSM-5). Arlington, VA: Author.

Bindler, R. C., Goetz, S., Butkus, S. N., Power, T. G., Ullrich-French, S., & Steele, M. (2012). The process of curriculum development and implementation for an adolescent health project in middle schools. *Journal of School Nursing, 28*, 13–23.

Brei, M. N., & Mudd, S. (2014). Current guidelines for weight loss surgery in adolescents. *Journal of Pediatric Health Care, 28*, 288–294.

Brewerton, T. D., & Costin, C. (2011). Long-term outcome of residential treatment for anorexia nervosa and bulimia nervosa. *Eating Disorders, 19*, 132–144.

Centers for Disease Control and Prevention (CDC). (2011a). *Breastfeeding among U.S. children born 1999–2007* (CDC National Immunization Survey). Retrieved from http://www.cdc.ov/breastfeeding/data/NIS_data

Centers for Disease Control and Prevention (CDC). (2011b). *2011 estimates of foodborne illness in the United States*. Retrieved from http://www.cdc.gov/Features/dsFoodborneEstimates

Centers for Disease Control and Prevention (CDC). (2014a). *Childhood obesity facts*. Retrieved from www.cdc.gov/obesity/data/childhood.html

Centers for Disease Control and Prevention (CDC). (2014b). *Estimates of foodborne illness in the United States*. Retrieved from http://www.cdc.gov/foodborneburden/index.html

Centers for Disease Control and Prevention (CDC). (2014c). *Trends in foodborne illness in the United States*. Retrieved from http://www.cdc.gov/foodborneburden/trends-in-foodborne-illness.html

Centers for Disease Control and Prevention (CDC). (2014d). Youth risk behavior surveillance—United States, 2013. *Morbidity and Mortality Weekly Report, 63*(SS-4), 1–172.

Children's Defense Fund. (2014). *The state of America's children*. Washington, DC: Author. Retrieved from www.childrensdefense.org/child-research-data-publications/state-of-americas-children/

Cloherty, J. P., Eichenwald, E. C., & Stark, A. R. (2012). *Manual for neonatal care* (7th ed.). Philadelphia, PA: Lippincott Williams & Wilkins.

Colak, H., Dulgergil, C. T., Dalli, M., & Hamidi, M. M. (2013). Early childhood caries updates: A review of causes, diagnoses, and treatments. *Journal of Natural Science, Biology and Medicine, 4*, 29–38.

Cole, S. Z., & Lanham, J. S. (2011). Failure to thrive: An update. *American Family Physician, 83*, 829–834.

Daitch, L., & Epperson, J. N. (2011). Celiac disease. *Clinician Reviews, 21*(4), 49–55.

Du Toit, G., Roberts, G., Sayre, P. H., Bahnson, H. T., Radulovic, S., Santos, A. F., . . . LEAP Study Team. (2015). Randomized trial of peanut consumption in infants at risk for peanut allergy. *New England Journal of Medicine, 372*, 803–813.

Flament, M. F., Bissada, H., & Spettique, W. (2011). Evidence-based pharmacotherapy of eating disorders. *International Journal of Neuropsychopharmacology, 15*, 189–207.

Garcia-Manzanares, A., & Lucendo, A. J. (2011). Nutritional and dietary aspects of celiac disease. *Nutrition in Clinical Practice, 26*, 163–173.

Hay, P. J., & Claudino, A. M. (2011). Clinical psychopharmacology of eating disorders: A research update. *International Journal of Neuropsychopharmacology, 15*, 209–222.

Holt, K., Wooldridge, N., Story, M., & Sofka, D. (2011). *Bright futures nutrition* (3rd ed.). Elk Grove Village, IL: American Academy of Pediatrics.

Institute of Medicine. (2011). *Dietary reference intakes: Calcium and vitamin D*. Washington, DC: National Academies Press.

Kliegman, R. M., Stanton, B., St. Geme, J., Schor, N., & Behrman, R. E. (2011). *Nelson's textbook of pediatrics* (19th ed.). Philadelphia, PA: Elsevier Saunders.

Lawrence, R. A., & Lawrence, R. M. (2011). *Breastfeeding: A guide for the medical profession* (7th ed.). Philadelphia, PA: Mosby.

Lee, R. D., & Nieman, D. C. (2013). *Nutrition assessment* (6th ed.). Boston, MA: McGraw-Hill.

Lock, J. (2011). Evaluation of family treatment models for eating disorders. *Current Opinion in Psychiatry, 24*, 274–279.

Mansoor, D. K., & Sharma, H. P. (2011). Clinical presentations of food allergy. *Pediatric Clinics of North America, 58*, 315–326.

Mattar, L., Godart, N., Melchior, J. C., & Pichard, C. (2011). Anorexia nervosa and nutrition assessment: Contribution of body composition measurements. *Nutrition Research Reviews*, *24*, 39–45.

Mehler, P. S., Cleary, B. S., & Gaudiani, J. L. (2011). Osteoporosis in anorexia nervosa. *Eating Disorders*, *19*, 194–202.

Mitsuoka, T. (2014). Development of functional foods. *Bioscience of Microbiota, Food and Health*, *33*, 117–128.

National Dairy Council. (2011). *Lactose intolerance among different ethnic groups*. Retrieved from http://www.nationaldairycouncil.org/SiteCollection-Documents/LI%20and%20Minorites_FINALIZED.pdf

National Heart, Lung and Blood Institute. (2013). *Reduce screen time*. Retrieved from http://www.nhlbi.nih.gov/health/educational/wecan/reduce-screen-time/

National Institute of Allergy and Infectious Diseases (NIAID). (2011). *Guidelines for diagnosis and management of food allergy in the United States*. Washington, DC: U.S. Department of Health and Human Services.

National Institute of Arthritis and Musculoskeletal and Skin Diseases. (2012). *Osteoporosis: Peak bone mass in women*. Retrieved from http://www.niams.nih.gov/Health_Info/Bone/Osteoporosis/bone_mass.asp

National Institute of Diabetes and Digestive and Kidney Diseases (NIDDK). (2012). *Celiac disease*. Retrieved from http://digestive.niddk.nih.gov/ddiseases/pubs/celiac

National Institute of Mental Health (NIMH). (2011). *What are eating disorders?* Retrieved from http://www.nimh.nih.gov/health/publications/eating-disorders/index.shtml

National Institutes of Health. (2013). *Calcium*. Retrieved from http://ods.od.nih.gov/factsheets/Calcium-HealthProfessional/

O'Malley, P. A. (2013). The drive to win and never grow old: the risks of anabolic steroid abuse and update for the clinical nurse specialist. *Clinical Nurse Specialist*, *27*, 117–120.

Rashid, M., Zarkadas, M., Anca, A., & Limeback, H. (2011). Oral manifestations of celiac disease: A clinical guide for dentists. *Journal of the Canadian Dental Association*, *77*, b39.

Ross, A. C., Taylor, C. L., Yaktine, A. L., & Del Valle, H. B. (Eds.). (2011). *Dietary reference intakes for calcium and vitamin D*. Washington, DC: Institute of Medicine.

Rowland, T. (2011). Fluid replacement requirements for child athletes. *Sports Medicine*, *41*, 279–288.

Siega-Riz, A. M., El Ghormli, L., Mobley, C., Gillis, B., Stadler, D., Hartstein, J., . . . HEALTHY Study Group. (2011). The effects of the HEALTHY study intervention on middle school student dietary intakes. *International Journal of Behavioral Nutrition and Physical Activity*, *8*, 7.

U.S. Department of Agriculture (USDA). (2013a). *Household food security in the United States in 2012*. Retrieved from www.ers.usda.gov/media/1183204/err-155-report-summary.pdf

U.S. Department of Agriculture (USDA). (2013b). *National school lunch program*. Retrieved from http://www.fns.usda.gov/sites/default/files/NSLPFactSheet.pdf

U.S. Department of Agriculture (USDA). (2014). *Local school wellness policy*. Retrieved from http://www.fns.usda.gov/tn/local-school-wellness-policy

U.S. Department of Health and Human Services (USDHHS). (2011). *Healthy People 2020*. Retrieved from http:// healthypeople.gov/2020/topicsobjectives2020/pdfs/ nutritionandweight.pdf

U.S. Department of Health and Human Services (USDHHS). (2015). *U.S. public health service recommendation for fluoride concentration in drinking water for the prevention of dental caries*. Retrieved from http://www.publichealthreports.org/documents/PHS_2015_Fluoride_Guidelines.pdf

U.S. Food and Drug Administration. (2014). *Fish: What pregnant women and parents should know*. Retrieved from http://www.fda.gov/food/foodborneillnesscontaminants/metals/ucm393070.htm

Vaczy, E., Seaman, B., Peterson-Sweeney, K., & Hondorf, C. (2011). Passport to health: An innovative tool to enhance healthy lifestyle choices. *Journal of Pediatric Health Care*, *25*, 31–37.

Wagner, C. L., Greer, F. R., Section on Breastfeeding, & Committee on Nutrition (2008). Prevention of rickets and vitamin D deficiency in infants, children, and adolescents. *Pediatrics*, *122*, 1142–1152.

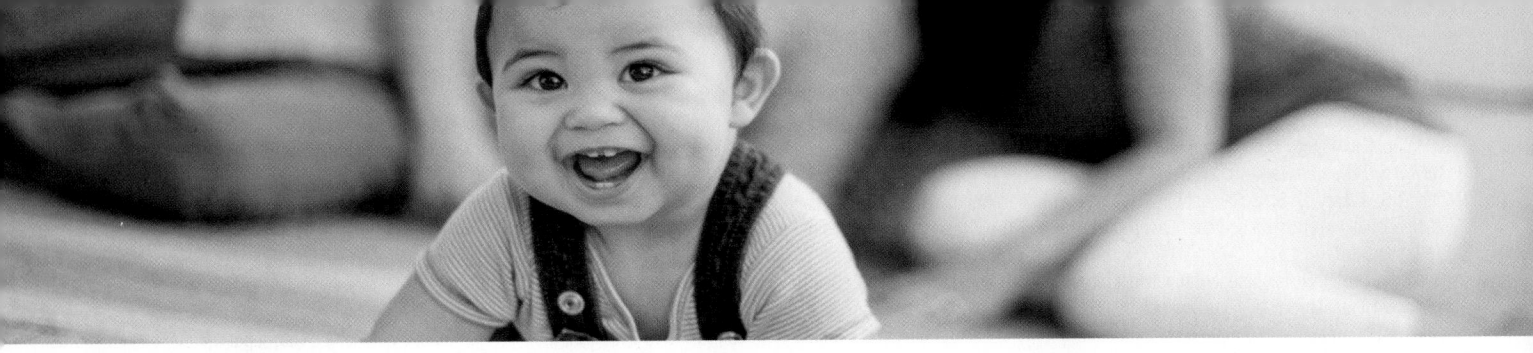

Chapter 33
Pediatric Assessment

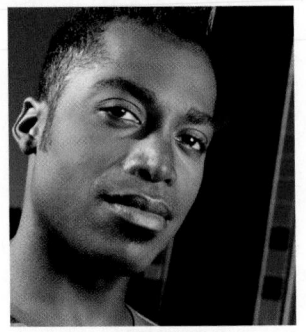

I was scared when we brought Colby to the hospital. He looked helpless, afraid, and sick. The nurses and doctors took over when we got to the hospital, and I felt better because they seemed to know what to do.

—Father of Colby, 6 months old

Ryan McVay/Getty Images

⌄ Learning Outcomes

33.1 Describe the elements of a health history for infants and children of different ages.

33.2 Apply communication strategies to improve the quality of historical data collected.

33.3 Demonstrate strategies to gain cooperation of a young child for assessment.

33.4 Describe the differences in sequence of the physical assessment for infants, children, and adolescents.

33.5 Modify physical assessment techniques for the age and developmental stage of the child.

33.6 List five normal variations in pediatric physical findings (such as breast budding in a girl) found during a physical assessment.

33.7 Evaluate the growth pattern of an infant or child.

33.8 Distinguish between expected and unexpected physical signs to identify at least five signs that require urgent nursing intervention.

How do examination techniques vary by the age of the child? How does the nurse encourage infants and toddlers to cooperate with the examination? This chapter provides an overview of pediatric assessment, including history taking and examination techniques geared to the unique needs of pediatric clients. Strategies for obtaining the child's history are presented first. The remainder of the chapter then outlines a systematic process for physical examination of the pediatric client.

Anatomic and Physiologic Characteristics of Infants and Children

Children and infants are not only smaller than adults; they also have very different physiology. Knowledge of pediatric anatomic and physiologic differences will aid in recognizing

normal variations found during the physical examination. It also assists with understanding the different physiologic responses children have to illness and injury. The illustration in *As Children Grow: Children Are Not Just Small Adults* provides an overview of important anatomic and physiologic differences between children and adults.

Obtaining the Child's History

Communication Strategies

The health history interview is a very personal conversation with a parent, caretaker, or adolescent during which private concerns and feelings are shared. Try to ensure that both parties clearly understand the information exchange and use effective communication with the parent or the child. Effective communication is difficult to accomplish because parents and children

As Children Grow: **Children Are Not Just Small Adults**

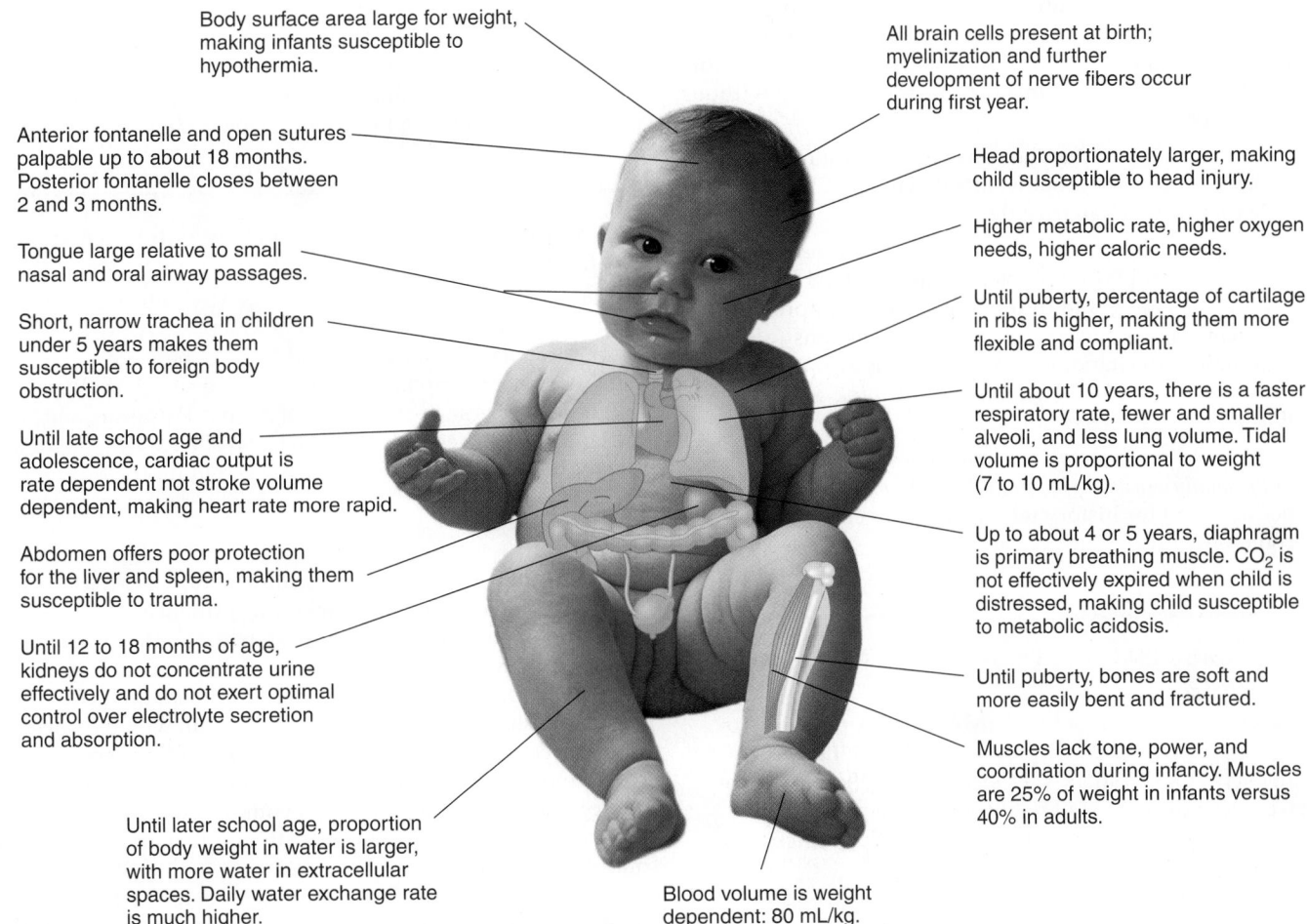

Body surface area large for weight, making infants susceptible to hypothermia.

Anterior fontanelle and open sutures palpable up to about 18 months. Posterior fontanelle closes between 2 and 3 months.

Tongue large relative to small nasal and oral airway passages.

Short, narrow trachea in children under 5 years makes them susceptible to foreign body obstruction.

Until late school age and adolescence, cardiac output is rate dependent not stroke volume dependent, making heart rate more rapid.

Abdomen offers poor protection for the liver and spleen, making them susceptible to trauma.

Until 12 to 18 months of age, kidneys do not concentrate urine effectively and do not exert optimal control over electrolyte secretion and absorption.

Until later school age, proportion of body weight in water is larger, with more water in extracellular spaces. Daily water exchange rate is much higher.

All brain cells present at birth; myelinization and further development of nerve fibers occur during first year.

Head proportionately larger, making child susceptible to head injury.

Higher metabolic rate, higher oxygen needs, higher caloric needs.

Until puberty, percentage of cartilage in ribs is higher, making them more flexible and compliant.

Until about 10 years, there is a faster respiratory rate, fewer and smaller alveoli, and less lung volume. Tidal volume is proportional to weight (7 to 10 mL/kg).

Up to about 4 or 5 years, diaphragm is primary breathing muscle. CO_2 is not effectively expired when child is distressed, making child susceptible to metabolic acidosis.

Until puberty, bones are soft and more easily bent and fractured.

Muscles lack tone, power, and coordination during infancy. Muscles are 25% of weight in infants versus 40% in adults.

Blood volume is weight dependent: 80 mL/kg.

Children are not just small adults. There are important anatomic and physiologic differences between children and adults that will change based on a child's growth and development.

may not always correctly interpret what the nurse says, just as the nurse may not understand completely what the parent or child says. People's interpretation of information is based on their life experiences, culture, and education.

STRATEGIES TO BUILD RAPPORT WITH THE FAMILY

When obtaining the nursing history, make sure the parents understand the purpose of the interview and how the information will be used for the child's benefit. To develop rapport, demonstrate interest in and concern for the child and family during the interview. This rapport forms the foundation for the collaborative relationship between the nurse and parent that will lead to the best nursing care for the child. The following strategies help to establish rapport with the child's family during the nursing history:

- *Introduce yourself* (name, title or position, and role in caring for the child). To demonstrate respect, ask all family members present what name they prefer you to use when talking with them.

- *Explain the purpose of the interview* and why the nursing history is different from the information collected by other health professionals. For example, "Nurses use this information to plan nursing care best suited for your child."

- *Provide privacy* and remove as many distractions as possible during the interview. If the client's room does not offer privacy, attempt to find a vacant room or lounge to interview the child and parent. Assure the parents and the child that the information provided is protected under the Health Insurance Portability and Accountability Act (HIPAA), a federal law that requires written consent before personal health information can be shared with healthcare providers outside the facility.

- *Direct the focus of the interview* with open-ended questions. Open-ended questions are useful to initiate the interview, develop a rapport, and understand the parent's perceptions of the child's problem. For example, "What problems led to Roberto's admission to the hospital?" Use close-ended questions or directing statements to clarify information or to obtain detailed information. For example, "How high was Tommy's fever this morning?"

- *Ask one question at a time* so that the parent or child understands what piece of information is desired and so that it is clear which question the parent is answering. "Does any member of your family have diabetes, heart disease, or sickle cell disease?" is a multiple question. Ask about each disease separately to ensure the most accurate response.

- *Involve the child in the interview* by asking age-appropriate questions. Young children can be asked, "What is your doll's name?" or "Where does it hurt?" Demonstrating an interest in the child initiates development of rapport with both child and parents. Ask older children and teens questions about their illness or injury. Offer them an opportunity to discuss their major concerns privately without parents present.

- *Be honest with the child* when answering questions or when giving information about what will happen. Children need to learn that they can trust their nurse.

- *Choose the language style best understood by the parent and child*. Commonly used phrases or medical terms may have different meanings to different people. To improve communication, ask the parents or child questions to ensure that their understanding of a phrase or term is correct. For example, "You used the term *hyperactivity*. Tell me what this behavior means to you."

- *Use an interpreter to improve communication when not fluent in the family's primary language*. Avoid using a family member or friend for history taking to ensure client and family confidentiality.

Developing Cultural Competence Phrasing Your Questions

Some cultural groups, particularly Asians, try to anticipate the answers you want to hear, or say yes even if they do not understand the question. This is done in an effort to please you or as an expression of politeness. Remember to use open-ended questions or phrase your questions in a neutral manner.

CAREFUL LISTENING

Complete attention is necessary to "hear" and accurately interpret information the parents and child give during the nursing history. While carefully listening to the information provided, pay attention to how it is expressed, and observe behavior during the interaction.

- Does the parent hesitate or avoid answering certain questions?

- Pay attention to the parent's attitude or tone of voice when the child's problems are discussed. Determine if it is consistent with the seriousness of the child's problem. The tone of voice can reveal anxiety, anger, or lack of concern.

- Be alert to any underlying themes. For example, the parent who talks about the child's diagnosis, but repeatedly refers to the impact of the illness on the family's finances or on meeting the needs of other family members, is requesting that these issues be addressed.

- Observe the parent's *nonverbal* behavior (posture, gestures, body movements, eye contact, and facial expression) for consistency with the words and tone of voice used. Is the parent interested in and appropriately concerned about the child's condition? Behaviors such as sitting up straight, making eye contact, and appearing apprehensive reflect appropriate concern for the child. Physical withdrawal, failure to make eye contact, or a happy expression could be inconsistent with the child's serious condition.

Subtle nonverbal and verbal cues may indicate that the parent has not provided complete information about the child's problem. Observe for behaviors such as avoiding eye contact, change in voice pitch, or hesitation when responding to a question. Be supportive and ask clarifying questions to encourage further description or the expression of information that is difficult for the parent or child to share. For example, "It sounds like that was a very difficult experience. How did Lily react?"

Developing Cultural Competence Interaction Patterns

Prolonged eye contact may be avoided by some cultural groups, such as persons of Native American, African American, Hindu, Japanese, and Chinese heritage, because it is considered impolite, aggressive, or a sign of disrespect. Other cultures such as persons of Arabic, European, and Russian heritage seek eye contact, and some may look for a response or impact regarding what is said (Purnell, 2014).

Encourage parents to share information, even if it is private or sensitive, especially when it influences nursing care planning. Often parents avoid sharing some information because they want to make a good impression, or they do not understand the value of the missing information. If parents hesitate to share information, briefly explain why the question was asked—for example, to make their child's hospital experience more pleasant or to begin planning for the child's discharge and home care. Silence is common in some Asian and Native American groups as they attempt to form responses to questions.

In some cases, the parent may become too agitated, upset, or angry to continue responding to questions. When the information is not needed immediately, move on to another portion of the history to determine whether the parent is able to respond to other questions. Depending on the emotional status of the parent, it may be appropriate to collect the remaining information later.

Data to Be Collected

Nurses collect and organize health, medical, and personal-social history to plan a child's nursing care. The health status, psychosocial, and developmental data are organized to help develop the nursing diagnoses and the nursing care plan.

CLIENT INFORMATION

Obtain the child's name and nickname, age, sex, and ethnic origin. The child's birth date, race, religion, address, and phone number can be obtained from the admission form. Ask the parent for an emergency contact address and phone number, as well as a work phone number. Record the name of the person providing the client history and that person's relationship to the client.

PHYSIOLOGIC DATA

Collect information about the child's health problems and diseases chronologically in a format similar to the traditional medical history.

Chief Concern. Identify the child's primary problem or reason for hospital admission or visit to a healthcare setting, and document it using the parent's or child's exact words.

TABLE 33–1 History of Present Illness or Injury

CHARACTERISTIC	DEFINING VARIABLES
Onset	Sudden or gradual, previous episodes, date and time began
Type of symptom	Pain, itching, cough, vomiting, runny nose, diarrhea, rash, etc.
Location	Generalized or localized—be anatomically precise
Duration	Continuous or episodic symptoms, length of episodes
Severity	Effect on daily activities (e.g., interrupted sleep, decreased appetite, unable to attend school)
Influencing factors	What relieves or worsens symptoms, what precipitated the problem, recent exposure to infection or allergen
Past evaluation for the problem	Laboratory studies and diagnostic procedures, physician's office or hospital where done, results of past examinations
Previous and current treatment	Prescribed and over-the-counter drugs used, complementary therapies (e.g., heat, ice, rest), response to treatments

TABLE 33–2 Birth History

Prenatal condition	• Mother's age, health during pregnancy, prenatal care, weight gained, special diet, use of alcohol or drugs, expected date of birth • Details of illnesses, radiograph or sonogram findings, hospitalizations, medications, complications, and their timing during pregnancy • Prior obstetric history
Intrapartum— description of birth	• Site of birth (hospital, home, birthing center) • Labor induced or spontaneous, time of rupture of membranes, length of labor, color of amniotic fluid, complications • Vaginal or cesarean birth, forceps or suction used, vertex or breech position • Length of pregnancy (weeks), single or multiple birth
Condition of baby at birth	• Birth weight, Apgar score, cried immediately • Need for incubator, resuscitation, oxygen, ventilator • Any abnormalities detected, meconium staining
Postnatal condition	• Difficulties in the nursery—feeding, respiratory problems, jaundice, cyanosis, rashes, seizures • Length of hospital stay, special nursery, home with mother • Breastfed or bottlefed, weight lost/ gained in hospital • Medical care needed in first week—readmission to hospital

History of Present Illness or Injury. Obtain a detailed description of the current health problem that includes the characteristics in Table 33–1. Each problem is described separately.

Past History. This more detailed description of the child's prior health problems includes all major past illnesses and injuries. Identify all major illnesses, including common communicable diseases. Identify major injuries, their cause or mechanism, and their severity. Obtain information about each prior surgery, its purpose, and if the surgery required overnight hospitalization. For all hospitalizations, identify the reason and length of stay. Identify the circumstances for any prior transfusion (blood, blood products, or immune globulin), type of transfusion, and reaction. Obtain information about each specific diagnosis, treatment, outcome, complication or residual problem, and the child's reaction to the event. Use the guidelines in Table 33–2 to obtain a *birth history* when the child's present problem may be related to problems during the pregnancy, birth, and newborn care.

Current Health Status. Obtain a detailed description of each aspect of the child's typical health status.

- *Health maintenance*—child's primary healthcare provider, dentist, and other healthcare providers, timing of last visit to each.
- *Medications*—prescribed and over-the-counter medications (oral, topical, injectable) used daily or frequently for fever, colds, coughs, and rashes. Ask about the use of herbs, plants, teas, or other complementary therapies.
- *Allergies*—to food, medication, animals, insect bites, or other exposures, and the type of reaction (e.g., respiratory difficulty, rash, hives, itching).
- *Immunizations*—review dates immunizations were received. Ask about any unexpected reactions. Inquire about the reason

if not up-to-date. (See Chapter 43 for the recommended immunization schedule.)

- *Safety measures used*—car restraint system, window guards, medication storage, sports protective gear, smoke detectors, bicycle helmet, firearm storage, water safety, and others.
- *Activities and exercise*—usual play and/or sports activities; physical mobility and limitations, adaptive equipment used.
- *Nutrition*—formula-fed or breastfed; if breastfed, for how long, type and amount of daily formula and other liquid intake; when solid foods were introduced; enrollment in the Special Supplemental Nutrition Program for Women, Infants, and Children (WIC). Contrast the child's food intake to the appropriate amount for age and weight (see Chapter 32).
- *Sleep*—infant sleep position, length and timing of naps and nighttime sleep; nightmares or night terrors, snoring, other sleep disturbances; where the child sleeps; bedtime rituals.

TABLE 33–3 Familial or Hereditary Diseases

Infectious diseases	Tuberculosis, HIV, hepatitis, herpes
Heart disease	Heart defects, myocardial infarctions, hypertension, dyslipidemia, sudden childhood deaths
Allergic disorders	Eczema, hay fever
Eye disorders	Glaucoma, cataracts, vision loss
Ear disorders	Hearing loss, unusual shape or position of ears
Hematologic disorders	Sickle cell disease, thalassemia, glucose-6-phosphate dehydrogenase (G6PD) deficiency, hemophilia
Respiratory disorders	Cystic fibrosis, asthma
Cancer	Retinoblastoma, cancer with early age of onset
Endocrine disorders	Diabetes mellitus types 1 and 2, hypothyroidism, hyperthyroidism, Turner syndrome
Brain disorders	Intellectual disability, epilepsy, psychiatric disorders
Musculoskeletal disorders	Muscular dystrophy, scoliosis, spina bifida
Gastrointestinal disorders	Pyloric stenosis, ulcers, colitis, celiac disease, polycystic kidneys
Metabolic disorders	Phenylketonuria, galactosemia, maple syrup urine disease, Tay-Sachs disease, Gaucher disease
Problem pregnancies	Repeated miscarriages, stillbirths
Learning problems	Attention deficit disorder, Down syndrome, fragile X syndrome

Familial and Hereditary Diseases. Collect data about hereditary diseases and other significant health conditions for three generations of family members, including the parents, grandparents, aunts, uncles, cousins, child, and siblings, using information listed in Table 33–3. Collect information about the health status of each parent. Record information in either a family genogram or pedigree (see Chapter 3) or a narrative format.

Review of Systems. Collect a comprehensive overview of the child's health during the review of systems using the guidelines from Table 33–4. Additional signs and symptoms associated with the child's condition may be identified, as well as other problems with no direct relationship to the child's health problem that could potentially impact nursing care or home care. For example, asking about allergies may reveal a latex allergy that requires the use of nonlatex supplies and preparation for allergic reactions. For each problem, obtain the treatment, outcomes, residual problems, and age at time of onset.

PSYCHOSOCIAL DATA

Obtain information about family composition to establish a socioeconomic and sociologic context for planning the child's care in the hospital, community, and at home.

- *Family composition*—family members living in the home, their relationship to the child, marital status of parents or other family structure, and people helping to care for the child
- *Financial resources*—household members employed, family income, healthcare resources (e.g., private insurance, Medicaid, Child Health Insurance Program [CHIP]), and other resources (Supplemental Nutrition Assistance Program [SNAP], Temporary Assistance for Needy Families [TANF], or WIC)
- *Home environment*—housing description (condition, potential lead exposure, safe play area); city or well water; sanitation; and availability of electricity, heat, and refrigeration
- *Community environment*—neighborhood description; safety, playgrounds, transportation, and access to shopping; school or childcare arrangements
- *Family or lifestyle changes*—for example, recent unemployment, relocations, or divorce; how the child and family members have coped

Newborns. The psychosocial history for parents of newborns should focus on readiness to care for the newborn at home. Inquire about support for the parent in the initial postpartum period, safe transport, and a home environment that provides heat, refrigeration, and safe water supplies.

Children. Information about the child's daily routines, psychosocial data, and other living patterns should focus on issues that have an impact on the quality of daily living (Table 33–5).

Adolescents. The psychosocial history for adolescents should focus on critical areas in their lives that may contribute to a less than optimal environment for normal growth and development. Key topics that should be addressed are included in the HEEADSSS screening tool (Brown, 2011):

- **Home environment**
- **Education and employment**
- **Eating**
- **Activities**
- **Drugs (substance abuse)**
- **Sexuality**
- **Suicidal thoughts**
- **Safety, savagery (exposure to violence)**

DEVELOPMENTAL STATUS

Information about the child's motor, cognitive, language, and social development will help to plan nursing care. Ask the parent about the child's developmental milestones and current fine and gross motor skills. Obtain the age at which the child first used words appropriately and the current words used or language ability. Actual assessment of the child with a parent questionnaire may also be used to collect this information. For children in school, ask about academic performance to assess cognitive development. Ask the parent about the child's manner of interaction with other children, family members, and strangers. For adolescents, ask about school performance and activities indicating development of independence and autonomy. (See Chapter 31 for developmental assessment guidelines.)

TABLE 33–4 Review of Systems

BODY SYSTEMS	SAMPLES OF ISSUES TO IDENTIFY
General	General growth pattern, overall health status, ability to keep up with other children or tires easily with feeding or activity, fever, sleep patterns
	Allergies, type of reaction (hives, rash, respiratory difficulty, swelling, nausea), seasonal or with each exposure
Skin and lymph	Rashes, dry skin, itching, changes in skin color or texture, new lesions, tendency for bruising, swollen or tender lymph glands
Hair and nails	Hair loss, changes in color or texture, use of dye or chemicals on hair
	Abnormalities of nail growth or color
Head	Headaches, concern about size of head
Eyes	Vision problems, squinting, crossed eyes, lazy eye, wears glasses; eye infections, redness, tearing, burning, rubbing, swelling eyelids
Ears	Ear infections, frequent discharge from ears, or tubes in ears
	Hearing loss (no response to loud noises or questions, inattentiveness, date of last hearing test), hearing aids or cochlear implant
Nose and sinuses	Nosebleeds, nasal congestion, colds with runny nose, seasonal symptoms, sinus pain or infections
	Nasal obstruction, difficulty breathing, snoring at night
Mouth and throat	Mouth breathing, difficulty swallowing, lesions, sore throats, streptococcal infections, mouth odor
	Tooth eruption, cavities, braces, orthodontic devices
	Voice change, hoarseness, speech problems
Cardiac and hematologic	Heart murmur, anemia, hypertension, cyanosis, edema, rheumatic fever, chest pain, bruises easily, easily tires with exercise
Chest and respiratory	Trouble breathing, choking episodes, cough, wheezing, cyanosis; exposure to tuberculosis, bronchiolitis, bronchitis, other infections
Gastrointestinal	Bowel movements, frequency, color, consistency, discomfort; constipation or diarrhea; abdominal pain; bleeding from rectum; flatulence
	Usual appetite, nausea or vomiting
Urinary	Frequency, urgency, dysuria, foul-smelling urine, dribbling, strength of urinary stream, undescended testicles
	Toilet trained—age when day and night dryness attained, enuresis
Reproductive	For pubescent children
Female	Menses onset, amount, duration, frequency, discomfort, problems; vaginal discharge, breast development
Male	Puberty onset, emissions, erections, pain or discharge from penis, swelling or pain in testicles
Both	Sexual activity, use of contraception, sexually transmitted infections
Musculoskeletal	Weakness, clumsiness, poor coordination, balance, tremors, abnormal gait, painful muscles or joints, swelling or redness of joints, fractures
Neurologic	Seizures, fainting spells, dizziness, numbness, brain injury or concussion; problems with articulation
	Memory or learning problems, attention span, hyperactivity

Developmental Approach to the Examination

The sequence and approach to the examination vary by age, but the techniques are the same for all ages (Table 33–6). Provide a comfortable atmosphere for the examination with privacy so that modesty is respected. Explain the procedures as you begin to perform them. In young children, a foot-to-head sequence is often used so that the least distressing parts of the examination are completed first. In older cooperative children, the head-to-toe approach is generally used. Experienced examiners often vary the sequence, such as by auscultating the lungs, heart, and abdomen when an infant or toddler is asleep or quiet.

NEWBORNS AND INFANTS UNDER 6 MONTHS OF AGE

Infants are among the easiest children to examine because they do not resist the examination procedure. Keep the parent

TABLE 33–5 Daily Living Patterns

Role relationships	• Family relationships/alterations in family process • Social and peer relationships and interactions, child care, preschool, school, clubs, sports groups
Self-perception/self-concept	• Personal identity and role identity • Self-esteem, body image, presence of nonvisible disorder such as a brain injury
Coping/stress tolerance	• Temperament, coping behaviors • Discipline methods used • Any substance abuse
Values and beliefs	• Part of a spiritual group or faith community • Any foods, drinks, or medical interventions prohibited according to spiritual beliefs, special food preparation • Personal values/beliefs
Home care provided for child's condition	• Resources needed/available, respite care available • Knowledge and skills of parents, other family members
Sensory/perceptual problems	• Adaptations to daily living for any sensory loss (vision, hearing, cognitive, or motor)

TABLE 33–6 Examination Techniques

TECHNIQUE	DESCRIPTION
Inspection	Purposeful observation of the child's physical features and behaviors during the entire physical examination. Physical feature characteristics include size, shape, color, movement, position, and location. Adequate lighting is essential. Detection of odors is also a part of the inspection.
Palpation	Use of touch to identify characteristics of the skin, internal organs, and masses. Characteristics include texture, moistness, tenderness, temperature, position, shape, consistency, and mobility of masses and organs. The palmar surface of the fingers and the fingertip pads are used for determining position, size, consistency, and masses. The ulnar surface of the hand is best for detecting vibrations.
Auscultation	Listening to sounds produced by the airway, lungs, stomach, heart, and blood vessels to identify their characteristics. Auscultation is usually performed with a stethoscope to enhance the sounds heard in the chest and abdomen. Speech is also assessed during auscultation.
Percussion	Striking the surface of the body, either directly or indirectly, to set up vibrations that reveal the density of underlying tissues and borders of internal organs in the chest and abdomen. As the density of the tissue increases, the percussion tone becomes quieter. The tone over air is the loudest, and the tone over solid areas is soft.

Note: Standard precautions are used during the physical examination. Perform good hand hygiene before contact with the child and wear gloves for any contact with mucous membranes and body fluids.

present to provide comfort and security for the infant during the examination by feeding, using a pacifier, cuddling, or changing the diaper to keep the infant calm and quiet. Distraction such as rocking or clicking noises may help when the infant begins to get distressed. Observe the infant for general level of activity, overall mood, and responsiveness to handling.

Be flexible with the sequence of the examination, taking advantage of times when the infant is quiet or asleep to auscultate lung, heart, and abdominal sounds. If the infant continues to be quiet or can be quieted with a pacifier, palpate the abdomen while the muscles are relaxed. The remainder of the examination can proceed in a head-to-toe sequence. Portions of the examination that may disturb the infant, such as the examination of the hips, should be performed last.

INFANTS OVER 6 MONTHS OF AGE

Because of developing separation and stranger anxiety, it is often best to examine the infant and toddler on the parent's lap and then held against the parent's chest for some steps, such as the ear examination (Figure 33–1). The infant will not object to having clothing removed, but make sure the room is warm for the infant's comfort. Observe the infant's general level of activity, mood, and responsiveness to handling by the parent.

Smile and talk soothingly to the infant during the procedure. Use toys to distract the older infant. Use a pacifier or bottle to quiet the child when necessary. Because the infant may be

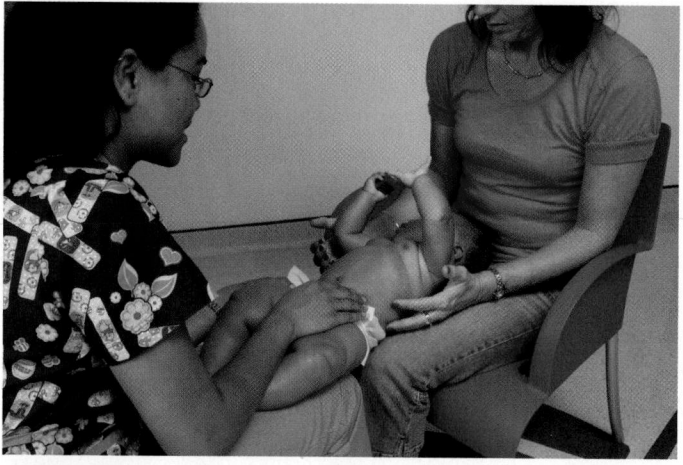

Figure 33–1 Infants and toddlers are often fearful of separation from the parent. With the legs of the nurse and mother put together knee-to-knee, this infant has a surface to lie on that facilitates cooperation for the abdominal examination.

fearful of being touched by a stranger, begin with the feet and hands before moving to the trunk. However, take advantage of opportunities to listen to heart, lung, and abdominal sounds when the infant is sleeping or quiet.

TODDLERS

Toddlers may be active, curious, shy, cautious, or slow to warm up. Because of stranger anxiety, keep toddlers with their parents, often examining them on the parent's lap. For invasive procedures (ear and mouth examination) the parent can hold the child close to the chest with legs between the parent's legs. Attempt to reduce the child's anxiety by demonstrating the use of instruments on the parent or security object. The cranial nerve assessment or developmental assessment can be used as a method to gain cooperation for other procedures.

Avoid asking the child if you can perform a part of the examination because the typical response will be "no." Rather, tell the child what you will do at each step of the examination, using a confident voice that expects cooperation. When a choice is possible, let the child have some control. For example, let the toddler choose which ear to examine first or to stand or sit for a certain part of the examination. Much of the neurologic and musculoskeletal assessment is performed by observing the child play and walk around in the examining room. Begin the examination by touching the feet and then moving gradually toward the body and head. Use instruments to examine the ears, eyes, and mouth last as they often cause anxiety.

PRESCHOOLERS

Assess the willingness of the child to be separated from the parent. Younger children may prefer to be examined on the parent's lap, while older children will be comfortable on the examining table. Most children are willing to undress, but leave the underpants on until conducting the genital examination. Most preschoolers are cooperative during the physical examination. Some children will prefer to have the head, eyes, ears, and mouth examined first while others will prefer to postpone them to the end.

Allow the child to touch and play with the equipment. Give simple explanations about the assessment procedures, and offer choice when there is one during the examination. Use distraction to gain cooperation during the examination, such as asking the child to count, name colors, or talk about a favorite activity. Give positive feedback when the child cooperates.

SCHOOL-AGE CHILDREN

School-age children willingly cooperate and want to be helpful during the examination, so have them sit on the examining table. Anticipate the development of modesty in school-age children and offer a patient gown to cover the underwear. Let the older school-age child determine if the examination will be conducted in privacy or with the parent or siblings present.

A head-to-toe sequence can be used in this age group. Demonstrate how the instruments are used and let the child handle them if they wish. During the examination, explain what you are doing and why. Offer as many choices as possible to help the child feel empowered. The examination is a good opportunity to teach the child about how the body works, such as letting the child listen to heart and breath sounds.

ADOLESCENTS

Protect the adolescent's modesty by providing a private place to undress and put on the patient gown, and then during the examination by covering the parts of the body not being assessed. Examine the adolescent in the head-to-toe sequence as used for adults. Perform the examination without parent or siblings unless the adolescent specifically requests the parent's presence, but provide a chaperone (preferably the same gender as the client) when the parent or accompanying adult is not present. See *Professionalism in Practice: Using Chaperones to Examine Adolescents.*

Adolescents often have a lot of concerns regarding their developing bodies. When appropriate, provide reassurance about the normal progression of secondary sexual characteristic development and what further changes to expect.

Professionalism in Practice Using Chaperones to Examine Adolescents

A chaperone (same gender as the client), such as a nurse or patient-care technician rather than a family member, should be provided when examining a female adolescent's breasts and during the anorectal and genital examination of both boys and girls. However, the use of a chaperone should be a shared decision between the examiner and the adolescent client (American Academy of Pediatrics Committee on Practice and Ambulatory Medicine, 2011). Hospitals and health clinics often have policies regarding the use of chaperones with pediatric clients for physical examinations as well as diagnostic or treatment procedures to guide nurses on when a chaperone should be used and how this should be documented.

General Appraisal

The examination begins upon first meeting the child (Figure 33–2). Observe the child's general appearance and behavior. The child should appear well nourished and well developed. Infants and young children are often fearful and seek reassurance from their parents. Is the child encouraged to speak? Is the child appropriately reassured or supported by the parent? The child should feel secure with the parent and perceive permission to interact with the nurse.

Measure the infant's weight, length, and head circumference. (See the *Clinical Skills Manual* SKILLS .) After the child is 2 years of age and can stand, measure the child's height rather than

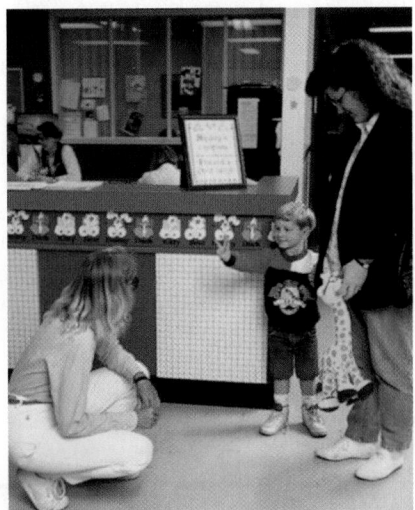

Figure 33–2 Examination of the child begins during the first contact. Observe the behavior of the child and the tone the parent uses when talking with the child. Does the child appear well nourished? Does the child appear secure with the parent?

length. Accurate measurement is important as medication dosages and fluids are based on weight. Growth measurements are then plotted on growth charts throughout childhood to assure health or to identify the impact of disease on the child. (See the growth charts for all ages of boys and girls in Appendix C.)

Once the weight and height of children have been measured, calculate the body mass index (BMI) (see Chapter 32). The BMI is a formula used to assess total body fat and nutritional status. For children, it helps determine if their height and weight are proportional for their age. Visit the Centers for Disease Control and Prevention website and enter the child's height and weight for an automatic calculation of the BMI. A BMI for age under the 5th percentile indicates the child is underweight. The child is at risk for overweight when the BMI for age is greater than the 85th percentile, and the child is overweight when the BMI is greater than the 95th percentile.

Take the child's temperature, heart rate, respiratory rate, and blood pressure (see the *Clinical Skills Manual* SKILLS).

Assessing Skin and Hair Characteristics

Examination of the skin requires good lighting to detect variations in skin color and to identify lesions. Daylight is preferred when available. Rather than inspecting the entire skin surface of the child at one time, examine the skin simultaneously with other body systems as each region of the body is exposed. Follow standard precautions by wearing gloves when palpating mucous membranes, open wounds, and lesions.

Inspection of the Skin

SKIN COLOR
The color of the child's skin usually has an even distribution. Check for color variations—such as increased or decreased pigmentation, pallor, mottling, bruises, erythema, cyanosis, or jaundice—that may be associated with local or generalized conditions. Some variations in skin color are common and normal, such as freckles found in the White population and hyperpigmented patches (Mongolian spots) usually found on the sacral region in infants with dark skin (see Figure 24–22). (See Chapter 24 for more information on newborn skin.)

Ecchymosis or bruising is common on the forehead, knees, shins, and lower arms as children stumble and fall. Bruises are uncommon in infants who are not yet walking, unless they have a bleeding disorder condition (Anderst, Carpenter, Abshire, et al., 2013). Bruises found on other parts of the child's body, especially in various stages of healing, should raise a suspicion of child abuse (see Chapter 42). Bruises go through several skin color changes (red, purple, black, blue, yellow, green, and brown) as the body breaks down hemoglobin and blood cells over several days before returning to normal skin color. Note any tattoos or body piercings.

Developing Cultural Competence Skin Tone **Differences**

The palms of the hands and soles of the feet are often lighter than the rest of the skin surface in darker-skinned children. In addition, their lips may appear slightly bluish.

When a skin color abnormality is suspected, inspect the buccal mucosa and tongue to confirm the color change. This is important in darker-skinned children because the mucous membranes are usually pink, regardless of skin color. Press the gums lightly for 1 to 2 seconds. Any residual color, such as that seen in jaundice or cyanosis, is more easily detected in blanched skin. Generalized cyanosis is associated with respiratory and cardiac disorders. Jaundice is associated with liver disorders.

Palpation of the Skin
Lightly touch or stroke the skin surface to palpate the skin and to evaluate the following characteristics:

- *Temperature*—normally feels cool to the touch when the wrist or dorsum of the hand is placed against the child's skin. Excessively warm skin may indicate the presence of fever or inflammation, whereas abnormally cool skin may be a sign of shock or cold exposure.

- *Texture*—expect soft, smooth skin over the entire body. Identify any areas of roughness, thickening, or **induration** (area of extra firmness with a distinct border). Abnormalities in texture are associated with endocrine disorders, chronic irritation, and inflammation.

- *Moistness*—normally dry to the touch, but may feel slightly damp when the child has been exercising or crying. Excessive sweating without exertion is associated with a fever or with an uncorrected congenital heart defect.

- *Resilience*—taut, elastic, and mobile because of the balanced distribution of intracellular and extracellular fluids. To evaluate skin turgor, pinch a small amount of skin on the abdomen between the thumb and forefinger, release the skin, and watch the speed of recoil (Figure 33–3). Skin that is elastic rapidly returns to its previous contour and is expected. Skin that tents or feels doughy takes longer to resume its original contour and is commonly associated with dehydration.

If **edema**, an accumulation of excess fluid in the interstitial spaces, is present, the skin feels doughy or boggy. To test for the degree of edema present, press for 5 seconds against a bone beneath the area of puffy skin, release the pressure, and observe how rapidly the indentation disappears. If the indentation disappears rapidly, the edema is "nonpitting." Slow disappearance

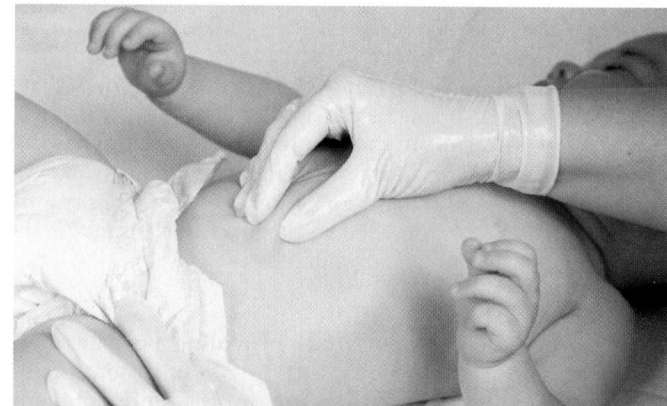

Figure 33–3 Tenting of the skin is associated with poor skin turgor. Assess skin turgor on the abdomen, forearm, or thigh. Skin with elasticity and normal turgor will return to a flat position quickly.

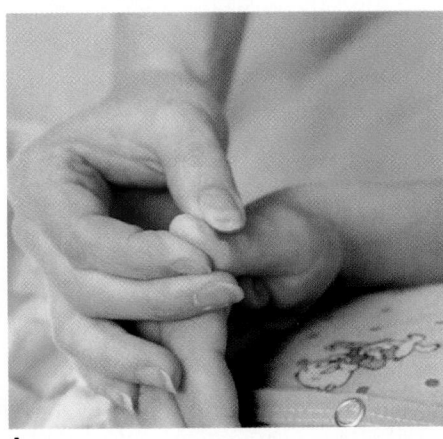

A

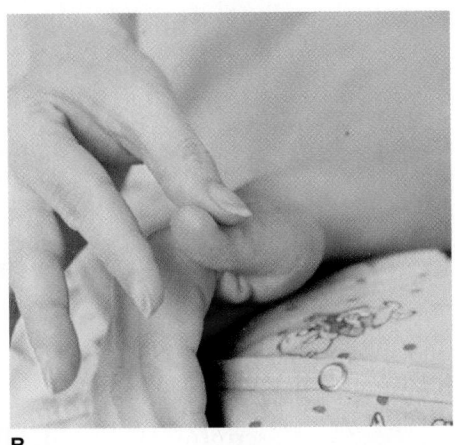

B

Figure 33–4 **Capillary refill technique.** *A,* **Press against the palmar tip of a finger, toe, or over a bony surface (e.g., jaw) for 2 to 3 seconds until the skin is blanched.** *B,* **Quickly release the pressure and count the number of seconds it takes for the color or blood to return to the veins. A capillary refill time of greater than 2 seconds could be related to dehydration, shock, or constriction around a limb such as a tight bandage or cast.**

of the indentation indicates "pitting" edema, which is commonly associated with kidney or heart disorders.

Capillary Refill Time

One technique to evaluate the adequacy of tissue *perfusion* (oxygen circulating to the tissues) is the capillary refill time (Figure 33–4*A* and *B*). The capillary refill time is normally less than 2 seconds. When the time is prolonged, assess the child for dehydration, hypovolemic shock, or a physical constriction such as a cast or bandage that is too tight.

Skin Lesions

Skin lesions usually indicate an abnormal skin condition. Characteristics such as location, size, type of lesion, pattern, and discharge, if present, provide clues about the cause of the condition. Inspect and palpate the isolated or generalized skin color abnormalities, elevations, lesions, or injuries to describe all characteristics present.

Primary lesions (such as macules, papules, and vesicles) are often the skin's initial response to injury or infection.

Hyperpigmented patches (Mongolian spots) and freckles are normal findings also classified as primary lesions (see the illustrations in *Pathophysiology Illustrated: Common Primary Skin Lesions and Associated Conditions*). Secondary lesions (such as scars, ulcers, and fissures) are the result of irritation, infection, and delayed healing of primary lesions (see Table 57–1).

Primary lesions often appear in common patterns that help distinguish between lesions.

- *Annular*—circular, begins in center and spreads to periphery (e.g., ringworm); when annular lesions run together they are polycyclic
- *Linear*—in a row or stripe (e.g., poison ivy)
- *Herpetiform*—grouped or clustered (e.g., herpes, chickenpox)
- *Reticulated*—networked or lacelike (e.g., parvovirus B19)

Inspection of the Hair

Inspect the scalp hair for color, distribution, and cleanliness. The hair shafts should be evenly colored, shiny, and either curly or straight. Variation in hair color not caused by bleaching or coloring may be associated with a nutritional deficiency. Normally, hair is distributed evenly over the scalp. Investigate areas of hair loss. Hair loss in a child may result from tight braids or skin lesions such as ringworm. (See Chapter 57 for information about fungal infections.) Notice any unusual hair growth patterns. An unusually low hairline on the neck or forehead may be associated with a congenital disorder such as hypothyroidism.

Children are frequently exposed to head lice. Inspect the individual hair shafts for small nits (lice eggs) that adhere to the hair (see Chapter 57). None should be present.

Observe the distribution of body hair as other skin surfaces are exposed during examination. Fine hair covers most areas of the body. Body hair in unexpected places should be noted. For example, a tuft of hair at the base of the spine often indicates a spinal defect.

Note the age at which pubic and axillary hair develops in the child. Pubic hair begins to develop in children between 8 and 12 years of age, and axillary hair develops about 6 months later (see Figures 33–29 and 33–30). Facial hair is noted in boys shortly after axillary hair develops. Development at an unusually young age is associated with precocious puberty.

Palpation of the Hair

Palpate the hair shafts for texture. Hair should feel soft or silky with fine or thick shafts. Endocrine conditions such as hypothyroidism may result in coarse, brittle hair. Part the hair in various spots over the head to inspect and palpate the scalp for crusting or other lesions. If lesions are present, describe them using the characteristics presented in *Pathophysiology Illustrated*.

Developing Cultural Competence Hair Characteristics

Hair varies by genetic origin. Children of African origin often have curly, wavy, or coiled hair that breaks easily. Children of Asian origin have hair that is coarse and straight. White children have hair with fine to medium coarseness that is straight or wavy.

Pathophysiology Illustrated: Common Primary Skin Lesions and Associated Conditions

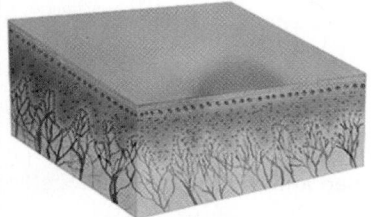

Lesion name: Macule

Description: Flat, nonpalpable, diameter less than 1 cm (½ in.)

Example: Freckle, rubella, rubeola, petechiae

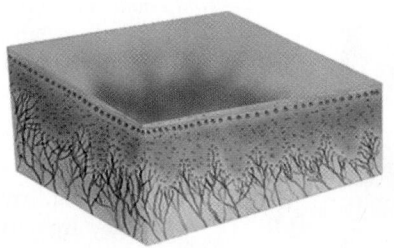

Lesion name: Patch

Description: Macule, diameter greater than 1 cm (½ in.)

Example: Vitiligo, hyperpigmented patch (Mongolian spot)

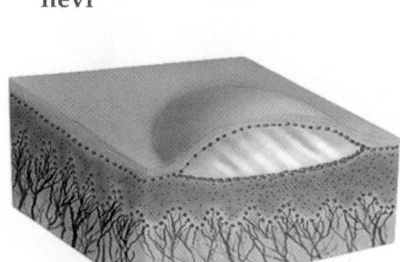

Lesion name: Papule

Description: Elevated, firm, diameter less than 1 cm (½ in.)

Example: Warts, pigmented nevi

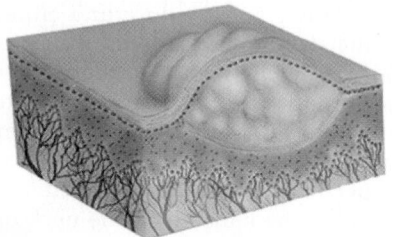

Lesion name: Tumor

Description: Elevated, solid, diameter greater than 2 cm (1 in.)

Example: Neoplasm, hemangioma

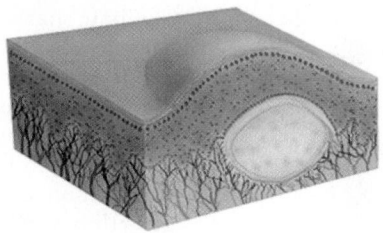

Lesion name: Nodule

Description: Elevated, firm, deeper in dermis than papule, diameter 1 to 2 cm (½ to 1 in.)

Example: Erythema nodosum

Lesion name: Vesicle

Description: Elevated, filled with fluid, diameter less than 1 cm (½ in.)

Example: Early chickenpox, herpes simplex

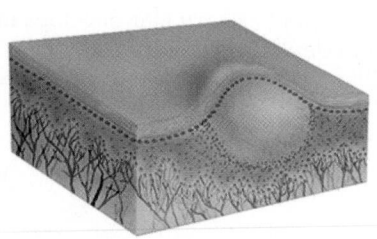

Lesion name: Pustule

Description: Vesicle filled with purulent fluid

Example: Impetigo, acne

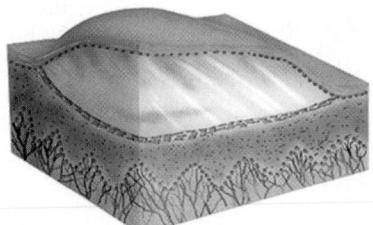

Lesion name: Bulla

Description: Vesicle diameter greater than 1 cm (½ in.)

Example: Burn blister

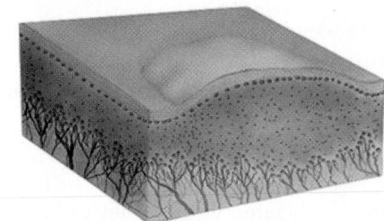

Lesion name: Wheal

Description: Irregular elevated solid area of edematous skin

Example: Urticaria, insect bite

Assessing the Head for Skull Characteristics and Facial Features

Inspection of the Head and Face

During early childhood the skull's sutures expand to allow for brain growth. Infants and young children normally have a rounded skull with a prominent occipital area. The shape of the head changes during childhood, and the occipital area becomes less prominent. An abnormal skull shape can result from premature closure of the sutures.

Clinical Tip

Children who were low-birth-weight infants often have a flat, elongated skull because the soft skull bones were flattened by the weight of the head early in infancy. Head flattening is also associated with the back-lying sleep positions in infants.

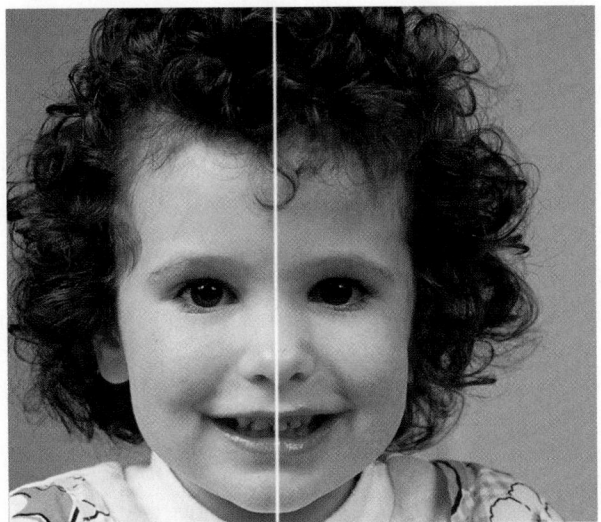

Figure 33–5 To inspect the face for symmetry, draw an imaginary line down the middle of the face over the nose and compare the features on each side. Significant asymmetry may be caused by paralysis of cranial nerve V or VII, in utero positioning, or swelling from infection, allergy, or trauma.

The head circumference of infants and young children is routinely measured until 2 years of age to ensure that adequate growth for brain development has occurred. The *Clinical Skills Manual* **SKILLS** describes the proper technique. A larger-than-normal head is associated with hydrocephalus, and a smaller-than-normal head suggests microcephaly.

Inspect the child's face for symmetry when the child is resting, smiling, talking, and crying (Figure 33–5). Significant asymmetry may result from paralysis of trigeminal or facial nerves (cranial nerves V or VII), in utero positioning, and swelling from infection, allergy, or trauma.

Next inspect the face for unusual facial features such as coarseness, wide eye spacing, or disproportionate size. Tremors, tics, and twitching of facial muscles are often associated with seizures.

Palpation of the Skull

Palpate the skull in infants and young children to assess the sutures and fontanelles and to detect soft bones (see *As Children Grow: Sutures*).

SUTURES

Use your fingerpads to palpate each suture line. The edge of each bone in the suture line can be felt, but normally there is no separation of the two bones. If additional bone edges are felt, a skull fracture may be present.

FONTANELLES

At the intersection of the sutures, palpate the anterior and posterior fontanelles. The fontanelle should feel flat and firm inside the bony edges. The anterior fontanelle is normally smaller than 5 cm (2 in.) in diameter at 6 months of age and then becomes progressively smaller. It closes between 12 and 18 months of age. The posterior fontanelle closes between 2 and 3 months of age.

A tense fontanelle, bulging above the margin of the skull when the child is sitting quietly, is an indication of increased

As Children Grow: **Sutures**

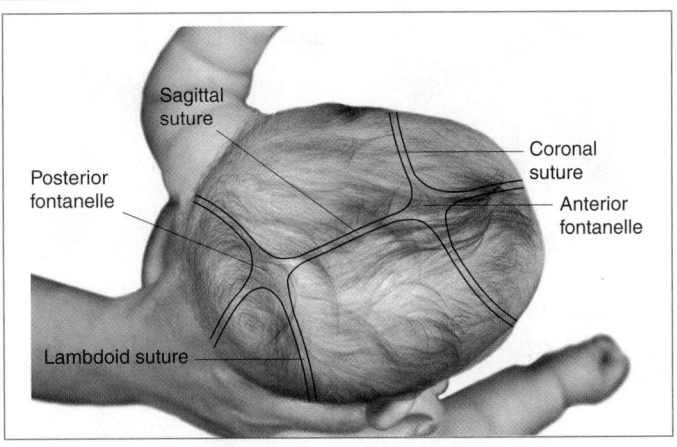

The sutures are fibrous connections between bones of the skull that have not yet ossified. The fontanelles are formed at the intersection of these sutures where bone has not yet formed. Fontanelles are covered by tough membranous tissue that protects the brain. The posterior fontanelle closes between 2 and 3 months. The anterior fontanelle and sutures are palpable up to the age of 18 months. The suture lines of the skull are seldom palpated after 2 years of age. After that time the sutures rarely separate.

> **Developing Cultural Competence** Touching the Head
>
> The head is a sacred part of the body to some Southeast Asians. Ask for permission before touching the infant's head to palpate the sutures and fontanelles (Purnell, 2014, p. 412). When a Hispanic child is examined, however, many families consider not touching the head bad luck.

intracranial pressure. A soft fontanelle, sunken below the margin of the skull, is associated with dehydration.

Assessing Eye Structures, Function, and Vision

Equipment needed for this examination includes an ophthalmoscope, vision chart, penlight, small toy, and an index card or paper cup.

Inspection of the External Eye Structures

Inspect the external eye structures, including the eyeballs, eyelids, and eye muscles. Test the function of cranial nerves II, III, IV, and VI, which innervate the eye structures.

EYE SIZE AND SPACING

Inspect the eyes and surrounding tissues simultaneously when examining facial features (Figure 33–6). The eyes should be the same size but not unusually large or small. Observe for eye

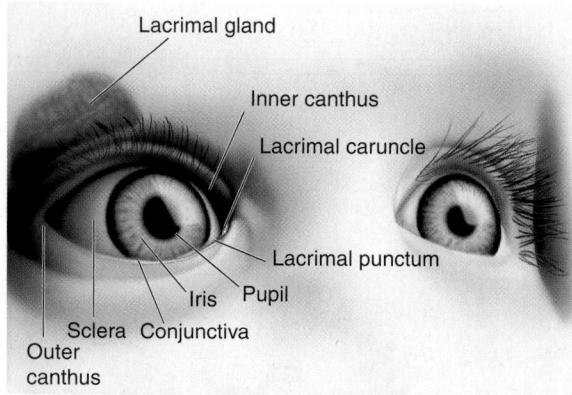

Figure 33–6 **External structures of the eye. Notice that the light reflex is at the same location on each eye.**

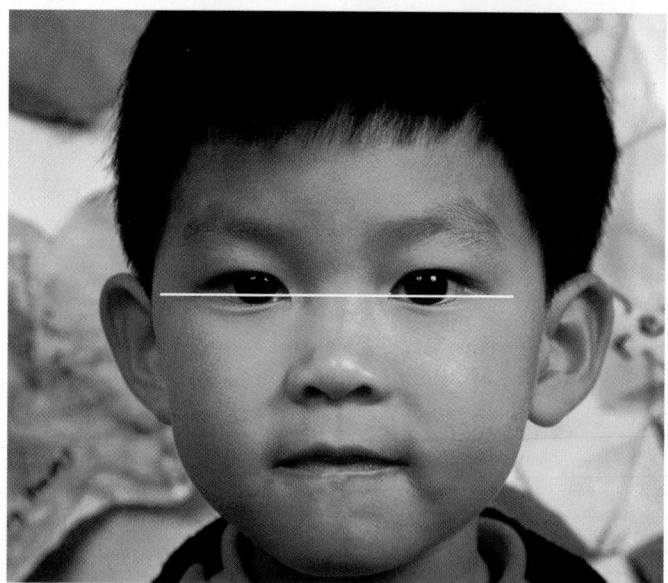

Figure 33–7 **To identify the palpebral slant, draw an imaginary line across the medial canthi and extend it to each side of the face. When the imaginary line crosses the lateral canthi, the palpebral fissures are horizontal and no slant is present. When the lateral canthi fall above the line, the eyes have an upward slant. A downward slant is present when the lateral canthi fall below the line. Look at Figures 33–6, 33–8, and 33–10. Which type of eye slant do these children have? Are epicanthal folds present?**

bulging, which can be identified by retracted eyelids, or for a sunken appearance. Bulging may be associated with a tumor, and a sunken appearance may reflect dehydration.

Next inspect the eyes to see if they are appropriately distanced from each other. The distance between the inner canthi of the eyes should equal the distance between the inner and outer canthi of the child's eye (Hummel, 2011). **Hypertelorism**, or widely spaced eyes, can be a normal variation in children.

EYELIDS AND EYELASHES

Inspect the eyelids for color, size, position, mobility, and condition of the eyelashes. Eyelids should be the same color as surrounding facial skin and free of swelling or inflammation along the edges. Sebaceous glands that look like yellow striations are often present near the hair follicles. Eyelashes curl away from the eye to prevent irritation of the conjunctivae.

Inspect the conjunctivae lining the eyelids by pulling down the lower lid and then everting (rolling upward) the upper lid. The conjunctivae should be pink and glossy. No redness or excess tearing should be present.

When the eyes are open, inspect the level at which the upper and lower lids cross the eye. Each lid normally covers part of the iris but not any portion of the pupil. The lids should also close completely over the iris and cornea. *Ptosis*, drooping of the lid over the pupil, is often associated with injury to the oculomotor nerve, cranial nerve III. *Sunset sign*, in which the sclera is seen persistently between the upper lid and the iris, may indicate hydrocephalus or increased intracranial pressure.

Inspect the eyes for the palpebral slant (Figure 33–7). The eyelids of most people open horizontally. An upward slant is a normal finding in Asian children; however, children with Down syndrome also often have an upward slant (Figure 33–8). A downward slant is seen in some children as a normal variation. Children of Asian descent often have an extra fold of skin, known as the **epicanthal fold**, covering all or part of the lacrimal caruncle on the nasal side of the eye.

EYE COLOR

Inspect the color of each sclera, iris, and bulbar conjunctiva. The sclera is normally white or ivory in darker-skinned children. Sclerae of another color suggest the presence of an underlying disease. For example, yellow sclerae indicate jaundice. Typically, the iris is blue or light colored at birth and becomes pigmented within 6 months. Different colored irises are rare and may be associated with a tumor, injury, or genetic syndrome (Olitsky,

Hug, Plummer, et al., 2016). Inspect the iris for the presence of *Brushfield spots*, white specks in a linear pattern around the iris circumference, which are often associated with Down syndrome. The bulbar conjunctivae, which cover the sclera to the

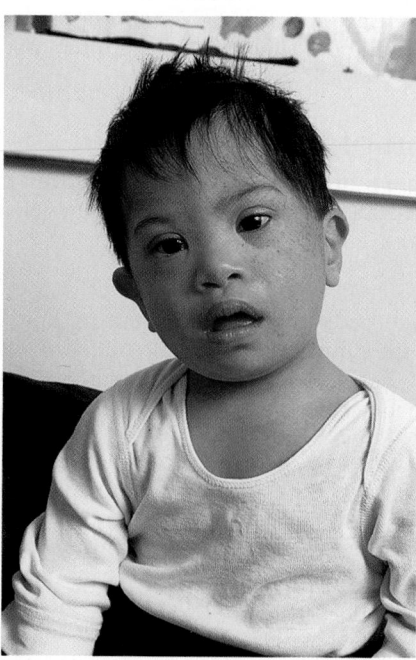

Figure 33–8 **The eyes of this boy with Down syndrome show an upward slant.**

edge of the cornea, are normally clear. Redness can indicate eyestrain, allergies, or irritation.

PUPILS

Inspect the size and shape of the pupils. Normally, the pupils are round, clear, and equal in size. Some children have a **coloboma**, which is a keyhole-shaped pupil caused by a notch in the iris. This sign can indicate that the child has other congenital anomalies.

To test the pupillary response to light, shine a bright light into one eye. A brisk constriction of both the pupil exposed to direct light and the other pupil (consensual response) is a normal finding.

To test pupillary response to accommodation, ask the child to look first at a near object (e.g., a toy) and then at a distant object (e.g., a picture on the wall). The expected response is pupil constriction with near objects and pupil dilation with distant objects. These procedures test cranial nerve II.

ASSESSMENT OF THE EYE MUSCLES

It is important to detect *strabismus*, a muscle imbalance that makes the eyes look crossed, which can cause vision impairment if uncorrected. Use the following procedures to detect a muscle imbalance:

- *Extraocular movements.* Seat the child at eye level to evaluate the extraocular movements. Hold a toy or penlight 30 cm (12 in.) from the child's eyes and move it through the six cardinal fields of gaze. Make sure the child's eyes move rather than the head. Both eyes should move together, tracking the object. This procedure tests the oculomotor, trochlear, and abducens nerves (cranial nerves III, IV, and VI, respectively) (Figure 33–9).

- *Corneal light reflex.* To test the corneal light reflex, shine a light on the child's nose, midway between the eyes. Identify the location where the light is reflected on the cornea of each eye. The light reflection is normally symmetric, at the same spot on each cornea (see Figure 33–6). An asymmetric

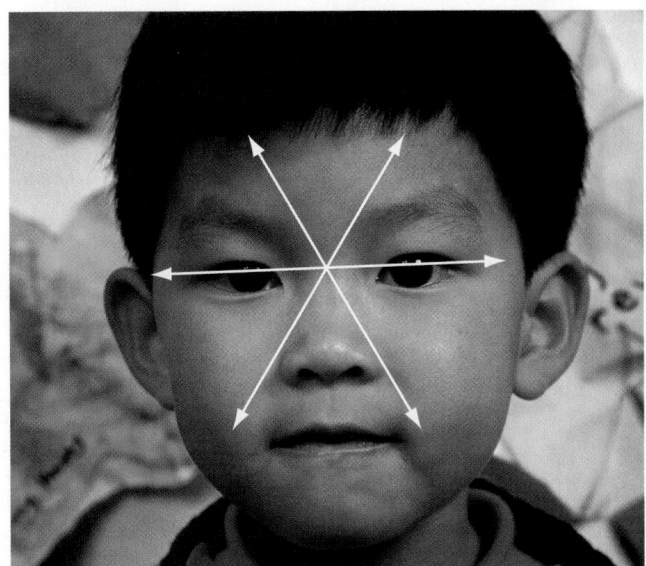

Figure 33–9 To assess extraocular movements have the child sit at your eye level. Hold a toy or penlight about 30 cm (12 in.) from the child's eyes and move it through the six cardinal fields of gaze. Both eyes should move together, tracking the object. This procedure tests cranial nerves III, IV, and VI.

corneal light reflex after 6 months of age indicates a muscle imbalance.

- *Cover–uncover test.* This test can be used only for older, cooperative children, starting at about 5 years of age. See Figure 33–10 for the technique. Perform the procedure for both eyes. Because the eyes work together, no obvious movement of either eye is expected. Eye movement indicates a muscle imbalance.

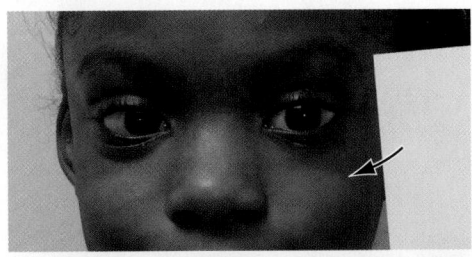

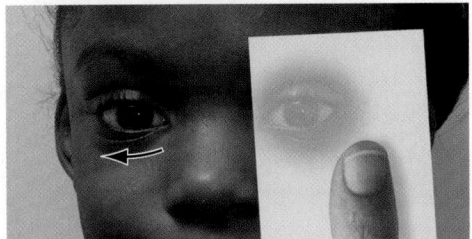

A Right, uncovered eye is weaker.

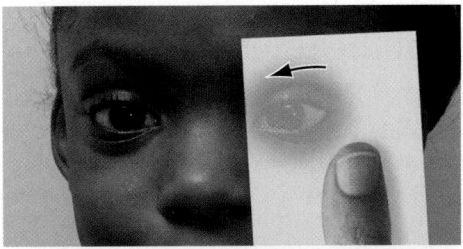

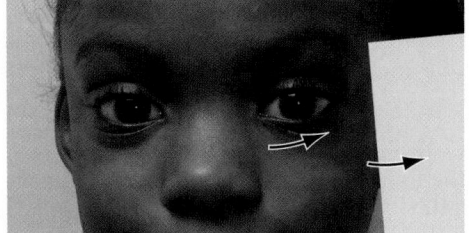

B Left, covered eye is weaker.

Figure 33–10 Cover–uncover test. With the child at your eye level, ask the child to look at a picture on the wall. *A*, Cover one eye with an index card or paper cup and simultaneously watch for any movement of the uncovered eye. If the uncovered eye jumps to fixate on the picture, it has a muscle weakness. *B*, Remove the cover from the eye and simultaneously watch the eye that was covered for any movement to fixate on the picture. If the eye has a muscle weakness, it drifts to a relaxed position once covered.

Vision Assessment

Because vision is such an important sense for learning, assessment is essential to detect any serious problems. Vision is evaluated using an age-appropriate vision test, but no simple method exists. Photo screening or an autorefractor may be used to assess vision in some preschool and school-age children. See the *Clinical Skills Manual* SKILLS .

INFANTS AND TODDLERS

When the infant's eyes are open, test the blink reflex by moving your hand quickly toward the infant's eyes. A quick blink is the normal response. An absent blink reflex can indicate that the infant is blind.

To test an infant's ability to visually track an object, hold a light or toy about 15 cm (6 in.) from the infant's eyes. When the infant has fixated on or is staring at the object, move it slowly to each side. Refer the infant who does not follow the object with the eyes and by moving the head. Once an infant has developed skills to reach for and then pick up objects, observe play behavior to evaluate vision. Children under 3 years of age should be able to easily find and pick up small pieces of food.

STANDARDIZED VISION CHARTS

Standardized vision charts can be used to test vision when the child can understand directions and cooperate, usually at about 3 or 4 years of age. The HOTV, Snellen E, and Picture charts are used to test visual acuity of preschool-age children just as the Snellen Letter chart is used for school-age children and adolescents. For all screening tools used to test far vision, make sure the child is the appropriate distance from the chart, usually 10 or 20 feet. Cover one eye so each eye is evaluated separately before testing them together. See the *Clinical Skills Manual* SKILLS for the use of these charts. Vision develops during early childhood. Refer children who fail photoscreening and those who do not correctly identify most images with each eye on the standardized vision chart 20/50 line for 3-year-olds, 20/40 line for 4-year-olds, and 20/32 line for 5-year-olds (American Association for Pediatric Ophthalmology and Strabismus, 2014).

Inspection of the Internal Eye Structures

The funduscopic examination with an ophthalmoscope allows the structures of the internal eye—the retina, optic disc, arteries and veins, and macula—to be examined. This examination is most often performed by experienced examiners. To assist the examiner, darken the room so the child's pupils dilate. Encourage cooperation by explaining the procedure to the child. Have a picture on the wall or have the parent or assistant hold a toy for the child to stare at so that the child's eye will remain open.

RED REFLEX

A penlight or the light of an ophthalmoscope can be used to assess the **red reflex**, the orange-red glow of the vascular retina as the light travels through the cornea, aqueous humor, lens, and vitreous humor to the retina. Shine the light at both eyes from a distance of 45 cm (18 in.). The red reflexes should be an orange-red glow that is symmetric and uniform in shape and color. Black spots or opacities within the red reflex are abnormal and may indicate congenital cataracts, hemorrhage, or corneal scars. A white reflex is associated with a tumor or retinoblastoma (see Chapter 50).

Assessing the Ear Structures and Hearing

Equipment needed for this examination includes an otoscope, noisemakers (bell, rattle, tissue paper), and a 500- to 1000-Hz tuning fork.

Inspection of the External Ear Structures

The position and characteristics of the *pinna*, the external ear, are inspected as a continuation of the head and eye examination. See Figure 33–11 to determine if the pinna is considered "low set," which is often associated with congenital renal disorders.

Inspect the pinna for any malformation. The pinna should be completely formed, with an open auditory canal. Next, inspect the tissue around the pinna for abnormalities. A pit or hole in front of the auditory canal may indicate the presence of a sinus. If the one pinna protrudes outward, there may be swelling behind the ear, a sign of infection in the mastoid process of the temporal bone of the skull.

Inspect the external auditory canal for any discharge. A foul-smelling, purulent discharge may indicate the presence of a foreign body or an infection in the external canal. Clear fluid or a blood-tinged discharge may indicate a cerebrospinal fluid leak associated with a basilar skull fracture.

Inspection of the Tympanic Membrane

Examination of the tympanic membrane is important in infants and young children because they are prone to otitis media, a middle ear infection. To examine the auditory canal and tympanic membrane, use an otoscope, an instrument with a magnifying lens, bright light, and speculum. Choose the largest ear speculum that fits into the auditory canal to form a seal for testing the movement of the tympanic membrane and to reduce the risk for injury to the auditory canal if the child moves suddenly.

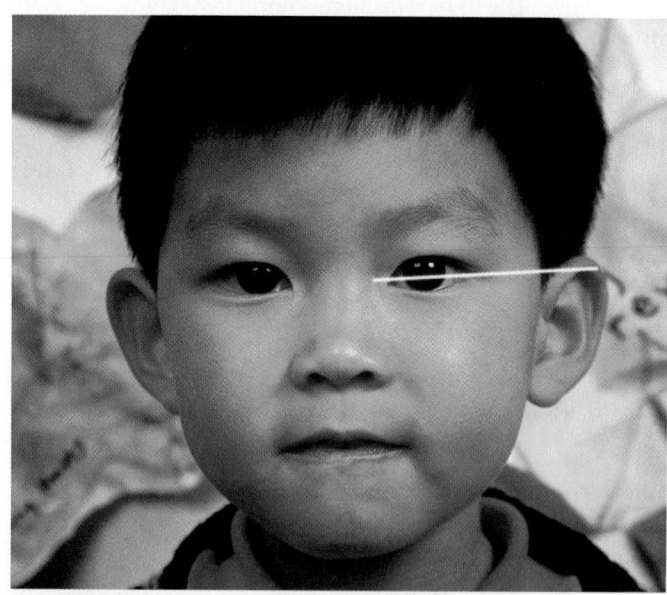

Figure 33–11 To evaluate the placement of the external ears, draw an imaginary line through the medial and lateral canthi of the eye toward the ear. This line normally passes through the upper portion of the pinna. The pinna is considered "low set" when the top lies completely below the imaginary line. Low-set ears are often associated with renal disorders.

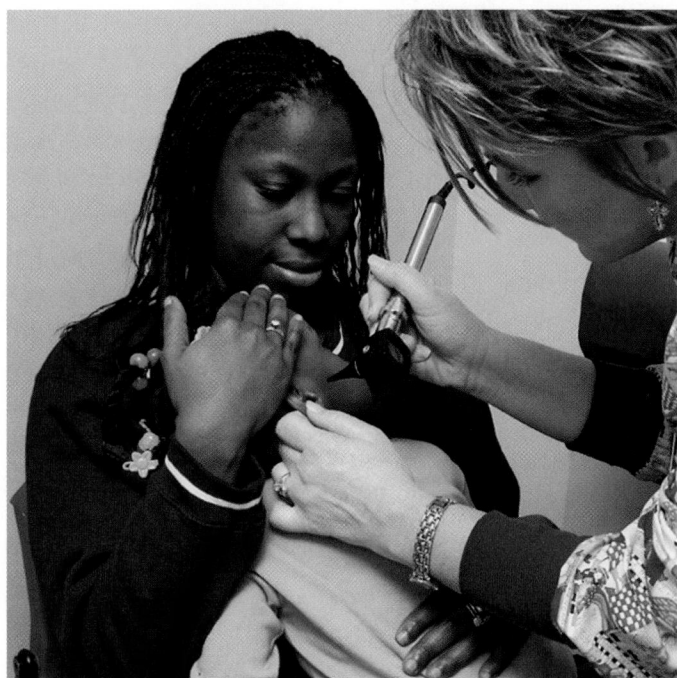

Figure 33–12 Inspecting the tympanic membrane. To restrain an uncooperative child, place the child on the parent's lap with the child's head and chest held firmly against the parent's chest. Keep your hands free to hold the otoscope and position the external ear.

Toddlers and young children often resist having their ears inspected with the otoscope because of past painful experiences, so postpone this until the end of the assessment for this age group. Use simple explanations to prepare the child. Let the child play with the otoscope or demonstrate how it is used on the parent or a doll. Figure 33–12 illustrates one method of human restraint for an uncooperative toddler or preschool child. See the *Clinical Skills Manual* SKILLS.

To begin using the otoscope, hold the handle in the palm of your hand closest to the child's face. If using a pneumatic squeeze bulb, hold it between your index finger and the otoscope handle. When the child is cooperative, rest the back of your hand holding the otoscope against the child's head to stabilize it. Your other hand is used to pull the pinna back and either up or down, whichever position straightens the auditory canal and provides the best view of the tympanic membrane (Figure 33–13).

Slowly insert the speculum into the auditory canal, inspecting the walls for signs of irritation, discharge, or a foreign body. The walls of the auditory canal are normally pink, and some cerumen is present. Children often put beads, peas, or other small objects into their ears. If the auditory canal is obstructed by cerumen or a foreign body, warm water irrigation can be used to clean the canal.

SAFETY ALERT!
Never irrigate the ear canal if any discharge is present in the auditory canal, as the tympanic membrane may be ruptured. Water could enter the middle ear and potentially worsen the infection.

The tympanic membrane, which separates the outer ear from the middle ear, is usually pearly gray and translucent. It reflects light, and the bones (ossicles) in the middle ear are normally visible (Figure 33–14). When the auditory canal is sealed

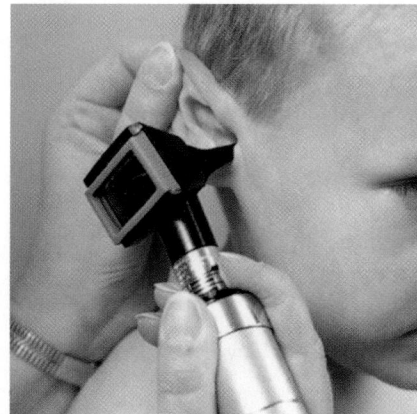

Figure 33–13 To straighten the auditory canal, pull the pinna back and up for children over 3 years of age. Pull the pinna down and back for children under 3 years of age.

and the pneumatic attachment is squeezed and released, the tympanic membrane normally moves in and out in response to the positive and negative pressure applied. Table 33–7 lists the abnormal findings during examination of the tympanic membranes. See Figures 45–4 and 45–5 for the tympanic membrane appearance when acute otitis media and otitis media with effusion are present.

Hearing Assessment

Hearing evaluation is important in children of all ages because hearing is essential for normal speech development and learning. Hearing loss may occur at any time during early childhood as the result of birth trauma, frequent otitis media, meningitis, or antibiotics that damage cranial nerve VIII. Hearing loss may also be associated with congenital anomalies and genetic syndromes. The hearing of newborns is evaluated at birth, and hearing is evaluated throughout childhood.

Evaluate hearing by observing the child's responses to various auditory stimuli using age-appropriate methods. Use hearing and speech articulation milestones as an initial hearing screen. When a hearing deficiency is suspected as a result of screening, refer the child for audiometry or tympanometry. *Audiometry* is a screening procedure using air conduction that measures hearing for pure-tone frequencies and loudness. The high- and low-pitch sounds are presented through earphones and are used to test different sound frequencies and the loudness needed to hear each sound. Hearing loss is determined when the child needs higher-than-normal decibels (louder sound) to hear a tone. *Tympanometry* is a test to estimate the pressure in the middle ear, and it is an indirect measure of tympanic membrane movement. See the *Clinical Skills Manual* SKILLS.

INFANTS AND TODDLERS
Select noisemakers with different frequencies that will attract the child's attention, such as a rattle, bell, and tissue paper. Ask the parent or an assistant to entertain the infant with a quiet toy, such as a teddy bear. Stand behind the infant, about 60 cm (2 feet) away from the infant's ear but outside the infant's field of vision, and make a soft sound with the noisemaker. Have the parent or assistant observe the child for any of the following responses when the noisemaker is used: widening the eyes, briefly stopping all activity to listen, or turning the head toward the sound. Repeat the test in the other ear and with the other noisemakers.

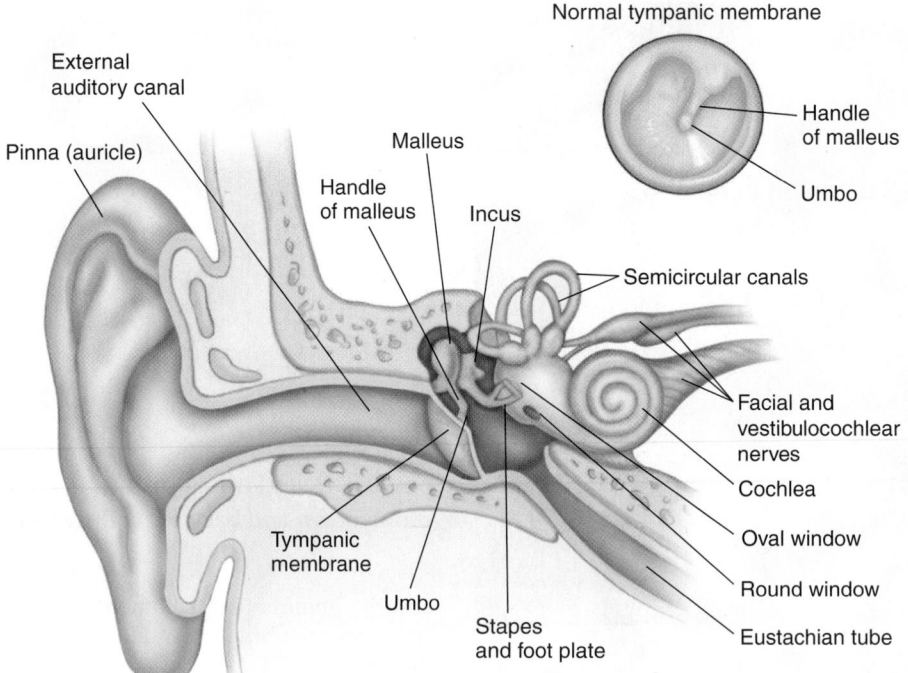

Figure 33–14 The tympanic membrane normally has a triangular light reflex with the base on the nasal side pointing toward the center. The bony landmarks, the umbo and handle of malleus, are seen through the tympanic membrane.

Growth and Development Indicators of Hearing Loss

Infant:

- No startle reaction to loud noises.
- Does not turn toward sounds by 4 months of age.
- Babbles as a young infant but does not keep babbling or develop speech sounds after 6 months of age.

Young child:

- No speech by 2 years of age.
- Inability to follow age-appropriate directions, such as "Bring me the block."
- Speech sounds are not distinct at appropriate ages.

PRESCHOOL AND OLDER CHILDREN

Use whispered words to evaluate the hearing of children over 3 years of age. Position your head about 30 cm (12 in.) away from the child's ear, but out of the range of vision so the child cannot read your lips. Use words easily recognized by the child, such as *Mickey Mouse*, *hot dog*, and *popsicle*, and ask the child to repeat the words. Repeat the test with different words in the opposite ear. The child should correctly repeat the whispered words. If the child will not repeat the whispered words, use a whisper to ask the child to point to different body parts or objects. Remember to stay out of the child's line of sight so lip reading is not possible. The child should point to the correct body part each time.

BONE AND AIR CONDUCTION OF SOUND

A tuning fork may be used to evaluate the hearing of school-age children who can follow directions. Hold the stem and lightly

TABLE 33–7 Unexpected Findings on Examination of the Tympanic Membrane and Their Associated Conditions

CHARACTERISTICS	TYMPANIC MEMBRANE UNEXPECTED FINDINGS	ASSOCIATED CONDITIONS
Color	Redness	Infection in middle ear
	Slight redness	Prolonged crying
	Amber	Serous fluid in middle ear
	Deep red or blue	Blood in middle ear
Light reflex	Absent	Bulging tympanic membrane, infection in middle ear
	Distorted, loss of triangular shape	Retracted tympanic membrane, serous fluid in middle ear
Bony landmarks	Extra prominent	Retracted tympanic membrane, serous fluid in middle ear
Movement	No movement	Infection or fluid in middle ear
	Excessive movement	Healed perforation

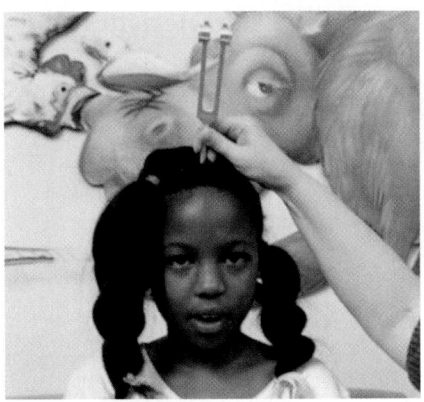 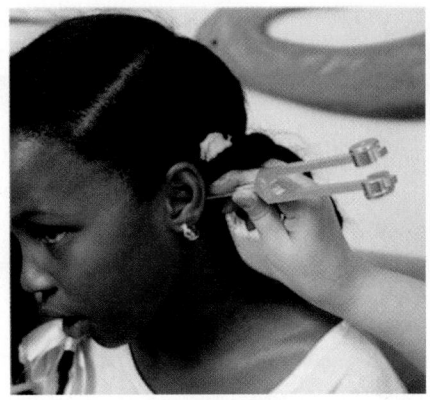 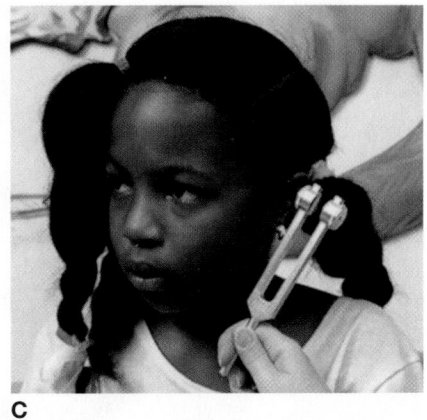

A B C

Figure 33–15 Testing bone and air conduction. *A,* Weber test. Place vibrating tuning fork on midline of the child's head. *B,* Rinne test, step 1. Place vibrating tuning fork on mastoid process. *C,* Rinne test, step 2. Reposition still vibrating tines between 2.5 and 5.0 cm (1 and 2 in.) from ear.

tap the tines of the tuning fork to begin the vibration. Avoid touching the vibrating tines, which will dampen the sound. Test bone conduction by placing the handle of the tuning fork on the child's skull. Test air conduction by holding the vibrating tines close to the child's ear (Figure 33–15).

- *Weber test:* Place the vibrating tuning fork on top of the child's skull in the midline. Ask the child if the sound is heard better in one ear or in both ears equally. The sound should be heard equally in both ears. If the sound is heard better in one ear (lateralized to affected ear), conductive hearing loss may be present.
- *Rinne test:* Place the vibrating tuning fork handle on the mastoid process behind an ear. Ask the child to say when the sound is no longer heard. Immediately move the tuning fork, holding the vibrating tines about 2.5 to 5 cm (1 to 2 in.) from the same ear. Again, ask the child to say when the sound is no longer heard. The child normally hears the air-conducted sound twice as long as the bone-conducted sound. Repeat the Rinne test on the other ear. When the sound is heard longer by bone conduction than air conduction, the affected ear may have conductive hearing loss. When sound is heard longer by air conduction than bone conduction, but less than twice as long, the affected ear may have sensorineural hearing loss.

Assessing the Nose and Sinuses for Airway Patency and Discharge

An otoscope with a nasal speculum or a penlight is needed for this examination.

Inspection of the External Nose

Examine the external nose characteristics and placement on the face during the assessment of the facial features. Inspect the external nose for size, shape, symmetry, midline placement on the face, and for the presence of unusual characteristics. For example, a crease across the nose between the cartilage and bone is often caused when an allergic child uses a hand to rub an itchy nose upward. **Nasal flaring**, widening of the nares

with breathing, is a sign of respiratory distress and should not be present.

The nose should be proportional in size to other facial features, have symmetric nasolabial folds, and be positioned in the middle of the face. Asymmetry of the nasolabial folds may be associated with injury to the facial nerve (cranial nerve VII). A flattened nasal bridge is the expected finding in Asian and Black children but may also be seen in children with Down syndrome. A saddle-shaped nose is associated with congenital defects such as cleft palate.

Palpation of the External Nose

When a deformity is noted, gently palpate the nose to detect any pain or break in contour. No tenderness or masses are expected. Pain and a contour deviation are usually the result of trauma.

NASAL PATENCY

The child's airway must be patent to ensure adequate oxygenation. To test for nasal patency, occlude one nostril and observe the child's effort to breathe through the open nostril with the mouth closed. Repeat on the other nostril. Breathing should be noiseless and effortless.

If the child struggles to breathe, a nasal obstruction may be present. Nasal obstruction may be caused by a foreign body, congenital defect, dry mucus, discharge, polyp, or trauma. Young children commonly place objects up their noses, and unilateral nasal flaring is a sign of such an obstruction.

Growth and Development

Newborns and infants under 6 months of age will not automatically open their mouths to breathe when their nose is occluded, such as by mucus.

Assessment of Smell

The olfactory nerve (cranial nerve I) can be tested in school-age children and adolescents, but it is rarely done. When testing smell, choose scents the child will easily recognize such as orange, chocolate, peanut butter, and mint. When the child's eyes are closed, occlude one nostril and hold the scent under the nose. Ask the child to take a deep sniff and identify the scent. Alternate odors between the nares. The child can normally identify common scents.

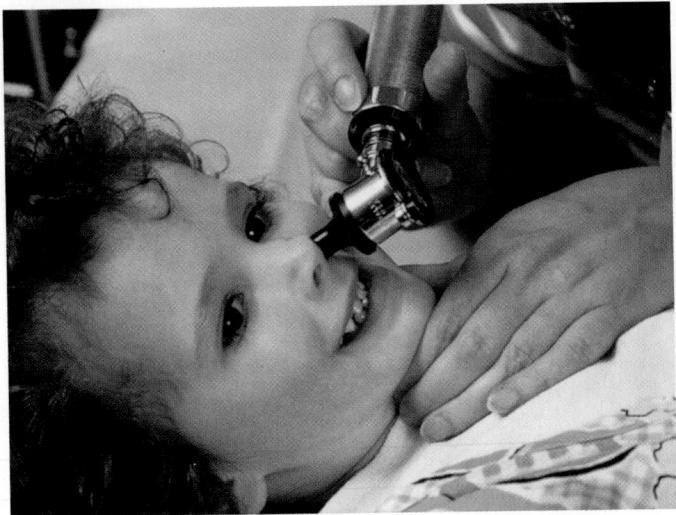

Figure 33–16 Technique for examining the nose. For infants and young children, push the tip of the nose upward and shine the light at the end of the nose. The nasal speculum of the otoscope can be used in older children. Avoid touching the septum of the nose with the speculum to prevent injury.

Inspection of the Internal Nose

Inspect the internal nose for color of the mucous membranes and the presence of any discharge, swelling, lesions, or other abnormalities. Use a bright light, such as an otoscope light or penlight. See Figure 33–16.

MUCOUS MEMBRANES AND NASAL SEPTUM

The mucous membranes should be dark pink and glistening. A film of clear discharge may also be present. Turbinates, if visible,

TABLE 33–8 Nasal Discharge Characteristics and Associated Conditions

DISCHARGE DESCRIPTION	ASSOCIATED CONDITION
Watery	
Clear, bilateral	Allergy
Serous, unilateral	Spinal fluid from a basilar skull fracture
Mucoid or purulent	
Bilateral	Upper respiratory infection
Unilateral	Foreign body
Bloody	Nosebleed, trauma

should be the same color as the mucous membranes and have a firm consistency. When the turbinates are pale or bluish gray, the child may have allergies. A polyp, a rounded mass projecting from the turbinate, is also associated with allergies.

The nasal septum should be straight without perforations, bleeding, or crusting. Crusting will be noted over the site of a nosebleed.

DISCHARGE

Observe for the presence of nasal discharge, noting if it is unilateral or bilateral. Nasal discharge is not a normal finding unless the child is crying. Discharge may be watery, mucoid, purulent, or bloody. Table 33–8 lists conditions associated with nasal discharge.

Inspection of the Sinuses

The sinuses are air-filled spaces that develop during childhood. See the illustration in *As Children Grow: Sinus Development*. Inspect the face for any puffiness and swelling around one or both eyes; normally, neither is present. To palpate over the maxillary sinuses, press up under both zygomatic arches with the

As Children Grow: **Sinus Development**

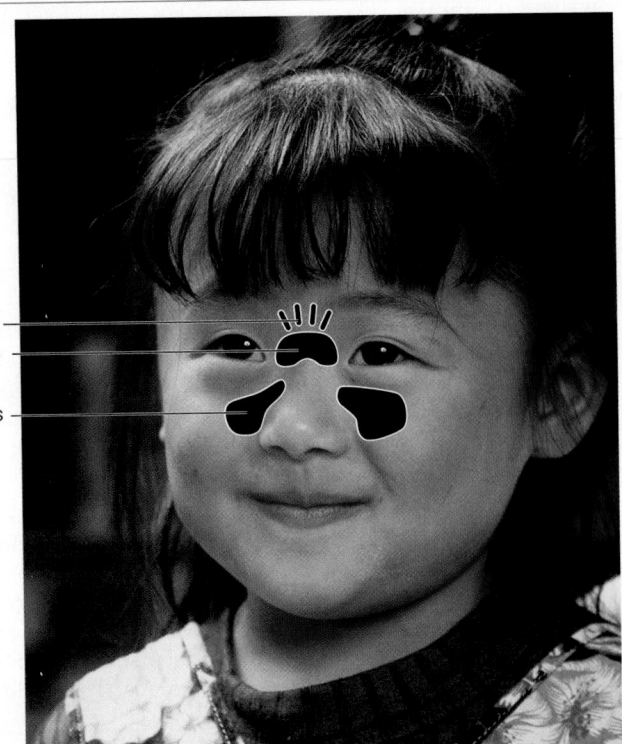

Ethmoid sinuses
Sphenoid sinus
Maxillary sinuses

The ethmoid sinuses are present at birth and air filled. The maxillary sinuses are present at birth and become air filled by 4 years of age. The sphenoid sinuses are present by 5 years of age. The frontal sinuses form at about 7 to 8 years of age and are completely developed by adolescence (Pappas & Hendly, 2016).

thumbs. To palpate the ethmoid sinuses, press up against the bone above both eyes with the thumbs. No swelling or tenderness is expected. Tenderness may indicate sinusitis. Sinus infections can occasionally occur in young children.

Assessing the Mouth and Throat for Color, Function, and Signs of Abnormal Conditions

Equipment needed to examine the mouth and throat includes a tongue blade and penlight. Wear gloves when examining the mouth.

Inspection of the Mouth

Young children often need coaxing and simple explanations before they will cooperate with the mouth and throat examination. Most children readily show their teeth. If the child resists by clenching the teeth, gently separate them with a tongue blade. Mouth structures for inspection are illustrated in Figure 33–17.

LIPS

Inspect the lips for color, shape, symmetry, moisture, and lesions. The lips are normally symmetric without drying, cracking, or other lesions. Lip color is normally pink in White children and more bluish in darker-skinned children. Pale, cyanotic, or cherry-red lips indicate poor tissue perfusion caused by various conditions. Note any clefts or edema.

SAFETY ALERT!

Avoid examining the mouth if there are signs of respiratory distress, high fever, drooling, and intense apprehension. These may be signs of epiglottitis. Inspecting the mouth may trigger a total airway obstruction. (See Table 46–3 for more information.)

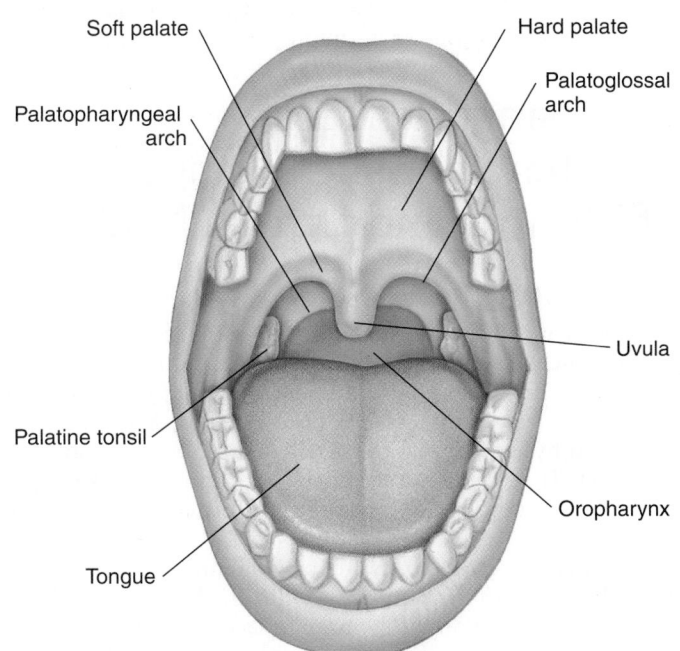

Soft palate

Palatopharyngeal arch

Palatine tonsil

Tongue

Hard palate

Palatoglossal arch

Uvula

Oropharynx

Figure 33–17 The structures of the mouth.

TEETH

Inspect and count the child's teeth. The timing of tooth eruption is often genetically determined, but it occurs in a regular sequence. See Figure 33–18 for the typical sequence of tooth eruption for both deciduous and permanent teeth.

Inspect the condition of the teeth, look for loose teeth, and note any spaces where teeth are missing. Note any dental care, braces, or orthodontic appliances. Compare empty tooth spaces with the child's developmental stage of tooth eruption. Once the permanent teeth have erupted, none should be missing. Teeth are normally white, without a flattened, mottled, or pitted appearance. Discolorations on the crown of a tooth may indicate caries. Discolorations on the tooth surface may be associated with some medications or excessive fluoride intake.

MOUTH ODORS

During inspection of the teeth, be alert to any abnormal odors that may indicate problems such as diabetic ketoacidosis, infection, or poor hygiene. Be alert for alcohol odors in older children that could signal substance abuse.

GUMS AND BUCCAL MUCOSA

Inspect the gums for color and adherence to the teeth. The gums are normally pink, with a stippled or dotted appearance. Use a tongue blade to help visualize the gums around the upper and lower molars. No raised or receding gum areas should be apparent around the teeth. When inflammation, swelling, or bleeding is observed, palpate the gums to detect tenderness. Inflammation and tenderness are associated with infection and poor nutrition. Hyperplasia may be associated with some medications, such as phenytoin.

Inspect the mucous membrane lining the cheeks for color and moisture. The mucous membrane is usually pink, but patches of hyperpigmentation are commonly seen in darker-skinned children. The *Stensen duct*, the parotid gland opening, is opposite the upper second molar bilaterally. Normally pink, the duct opening becomes red when the child is infected with mumps. Small pink sucking pads can be present in infants. No areas of redness, swelling, or ulcerative lesions should be present.

TONGUE

Inspect the tongue for color, moistness, size, tremors, and lesions. The child's tongue is normally pink and moist, without a coating, and it fits easily into the mouth. A protuberant tongue is associated with various genetic conditions, such as Down syndrome. A pattern of gray, irregular borders that form a design (geographic tongue) is often normal, but it may be associated with fever, allergies, or drug reactions. Tremors are abnormal. A white adherent coating on an infant's tongue may be caused by thrush, a *Candida* infection (see Chapter 57).

Observe the mobility of the tongue by asking the child to touch the gums above the upper teeth with the tongue. This tongue movement is adequate to enunciate all speech sounds clearly. Ask the child to stick out the tongue and lift it so the underside of the tongue and the floor of the mouth can be inspected.

PALATE

Inspect the hard and soft palates to detect any clefts or masses or an unusually high arch. The palate is normally pink, dome shaped, and has no cleft. The uvula hangs freely from the soft palate. A high-arched palate can be associated with sucking difficulties in young infants.

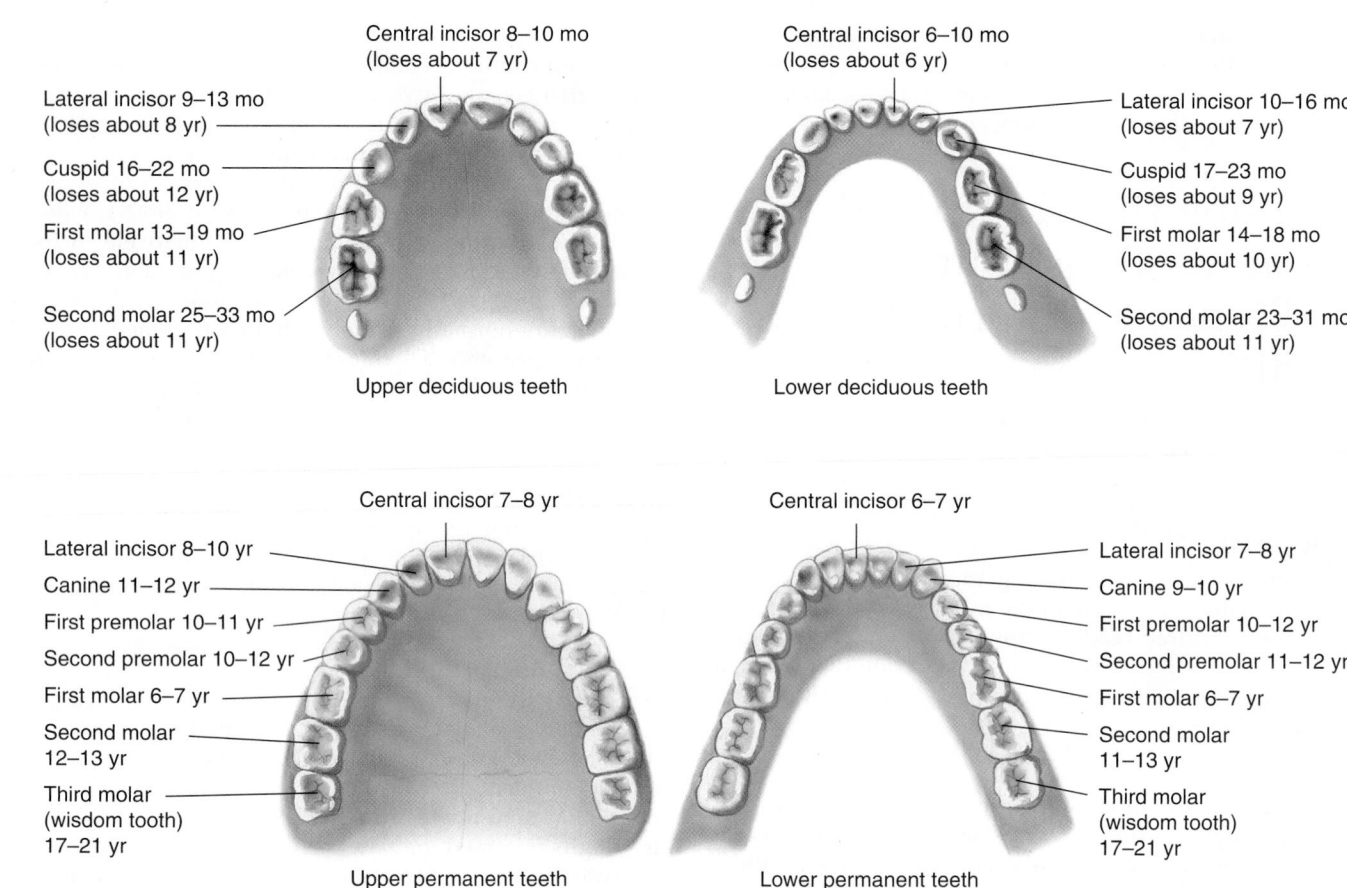

Figure 33–18 Usual ages and sequence of tooth eruption for both deciduous and permanent teeth. The bottom deciduous teeth are shed before upper teeth, and bottom permanent teeth erupt first as well.

Palpation of the Mouth Structures

Using gloves, palpate any masses seen in the mouth to determine their characteristics, such as size, shape, firmness, and tenderness. No masses should be found.

To assess the tongue's strength, while simultaneously testing the hypoglossal nerve (cranial nerve XII), place your index finger against the child's cheek and ask the child to push against your finger with the tongue. Some pressure against the finger is normally felt.

To palpate the palate, insert your gloved little finger, with the finger pad upward, into the mouth. While the infant sucks against your finger, palpate the entire palate. This procedure also tests the strength of the sucking reflex, innervated by the hypoglossal nerve (cranial nerve XII). No clefts should be palpated.

Inspection of the Throat

Use a flashlight to inspect the throat for color, swelling, lesions, and the condition of the tonsils. Ask the child to open the mouth wide and stick out the tongue. Use a tongue blade, if needed, to visualize the posterior pharynx. Moistening the tongue blade may decrease the child's tendency to gag. The throat is normally pink without lesions, drainage, or swelling. The epiglottis lies behind the tongue and is normally pink like the rest of the buccal mucosa. Swelling or bulging in the posterior pharynx may be associated with a peritonsillar abscess (see Chapter 45).

During childhood the tonsils are large in proportion to the size of the pharynx because lymphoid tissue grows fastest in early childhood. The tonsils should be pink without exudate, but crypts (fissures) may be present as a result of prior infections. The size of the tonsils can be graded as indicated in the *Pathophysiology Illustrated: Tonsil Size With Infection* diagram.

When using a tongue blade to see the throat and tonsils, the gag reflex may be triggered. A symmetric rising movement of the uvula should be observed as the child gags. The gag reflex is not often specifically tested in children.

Assessing the Neck for Characteristics, Range of Motion, and Lymph Nodes

Inspection of the Neck

Inspect the neck for size, symmetry, swelling, and any abnormalities such as *webbing*, an extra fold of skin on each side of the neck. A short neck with skinfolds is normal for infants. The neck is normally symmetric without swelling. Swelling may be caused by local infections such as mumps or a congenital defect. The neck lengthens between 3 and 4 years of age. Webbing is commonly associated with Turner syndrome (see Chapter 53).

Infants develop head control by 2 months of age when the infant has enough neck strength to lift the head up and look around when lying on the stomach. A lack of head control can result from neurologic injury, such as an anoxic episode.

Pathophysiology Illustrated: **Tonsil Size With Infection**

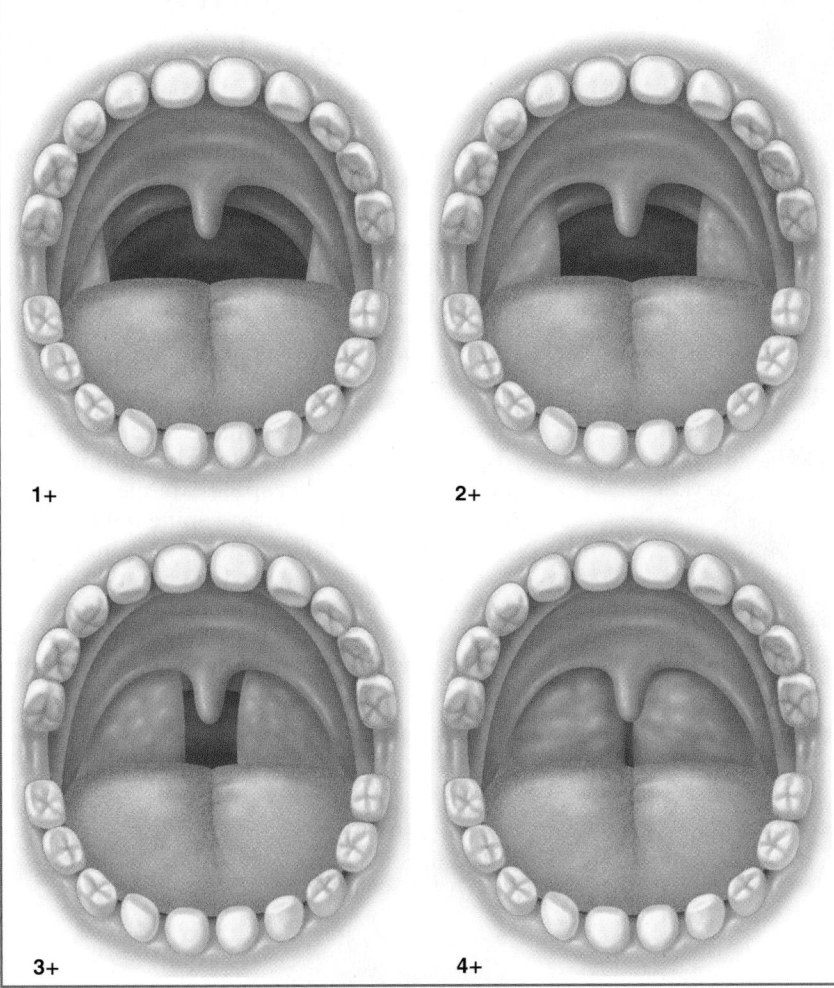

1+

2+

3+

4+

Tonsil size can be graded from 1+ to 4+ in relation to how much of the airway is obstructed. Tonsil size of 1+ and 2+ is normal. Tonsil size of 3+ is common with infections such as strep throat. Tonsils that "kiss" or nearly touch each other (4+) significantly reduce the size of the airway.

Palpation of the Neck

Face the child and use your finger pads to simultaneously palpate both sides of the neck for lymph nodes, as well as the trachea and thyroid.

LYMPH NODES

To palpate the lymph nodes, slide your finger pads gently over the lymph node chains in the head and neck. One sequence is to palpate the lymph nodes in the occipital area, around the ears, under the jaw, and then the cervical chain in the neck (Figure 33–19). Firm, clearly defined, nontender, movable lymph nodes up to 1 cm (½ in.) in diameter are common in young children. Enlarged, firm, warm, tender lymph nodes indicate a local infection.

TRACHEA

To palpate the trachea, place your thumb and forefinger on each side of the trachea near the chin and slowly slide down the trachea to determine its position and to detect the presence of any masses. The trachea is normally in the midline of the neck. It is difficult to palpate in children less than 3 years of age because of their short necks. Any shift to the right or left of midline may indicate a tumor or a collapsed lung.

THYROID

As the fingers slide over the trachea in the lower neck, attempt to feel the isthmus of the thyroid, a band of glandular tissue crossing over the trachea. The lobes of the thyroid wrap behind the trachea and are normally covered by the sternocleidomastoid muscle. Because of the anatomic position of the thyroid, its lobes are not usually palpable in the child unless they are enlarged.

Range of Motion Assessment

To test the neck's range of motion, ask the child to touch the chin to each shoulder and to the chest and then to look at the ceiling. Move a light or toy in all four directions when assessing infants. Children should freely move the neck and head in all four directions without pain.

When the child is unable to move the head voluntarily in all directions, passively move the child's neck through the expected range of motion. Limited horizontal range of motion may be a sign of **torticollis**, persistent head tilting. Torticollis results from a birth injury to the sternocleidomastoid muscle or from unilateral vision or hearing impairment. Pain with flexion of the neck toward the chest (Brudzinski sign) may indicate meningitis (see Chapter 54).

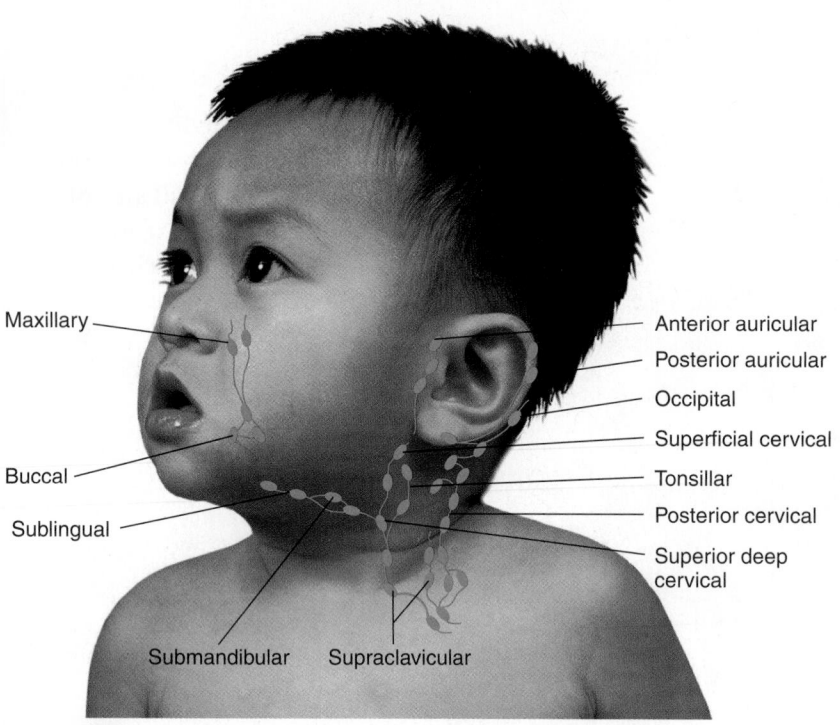

Figure 33–19 Palpate for enlarged lymph nodes in front of and behind the ears, under the jaw, in the occipital area, and in the cervical chain of the neck.

Maxillary
Buccal
Sublingual
Submandibular
Supraclavicular
Anterior auricular
Posterior auricular
Occipital
Superficial cervical
Tonsillar
Posterior cervical
Superior deep cervical

Assessing the Chest for Shape, Movement, Respiratory Effort, and Lung Function

Examination of the chest includes the following procedures: inspecting the size and shape of the chest, palpating chest movement that occurs during respiration, observing the effort of breathing, and auscultating breath sounds. A stethoscope is needed.

Inspection of the Chest

The chest skeleton provides most of the landmarks used to describe the location of findings during examination of the chest, lungs, and heart. The intercostal spaces are the horizontal markers. The sternum and spine are the vertical landmarks. When both a horizontal and a vertical landmark are used, the location of findings can be precisely described on the right or left side of the child's chest (Figures 33–20 and 33–21). The distance between the finding and the

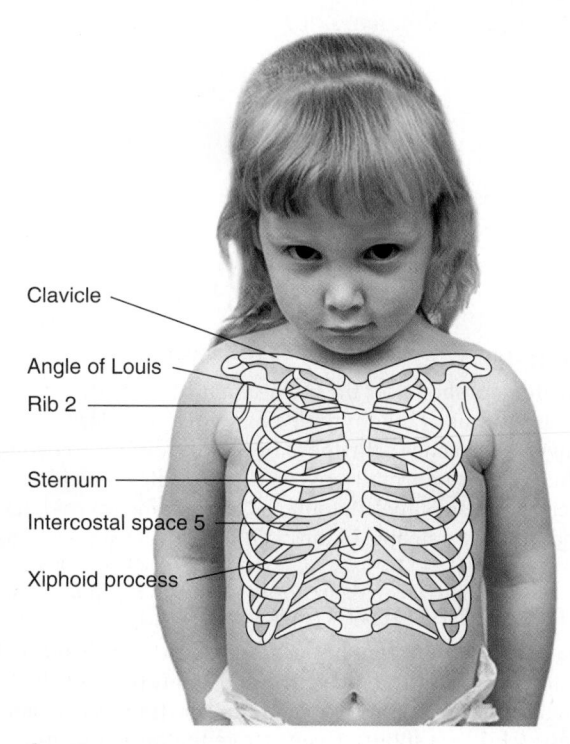

Clavicle
Angle of Louis
Rib 2
Sternum
Intercostal space 5
Xiphoid process

A

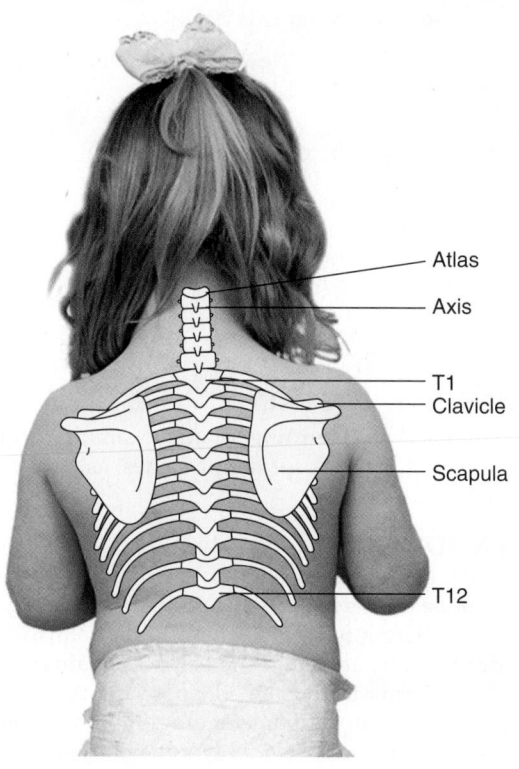

Atlas
Axis
T1
Clavicle
Scapula
T12

B

Figure 33–20 Ribs and intercostal spaces are the horizontal landmarks used to describe the location of chest findings. *A,* To determine the rib number on the anterior chest, palpate down from the top of the sternum until a horizontal ridge, the angle of Louis, is felt. Directly to the right and left of that ridge is the second rib. The second intercostal space is immediately below the second rib. Ribs 3–12 and the corresponding intercostal spaces can be counted as the fingers move toward the abdomen. *B,* To determine the rib number on the posterior chest, find the protruding spinal process of the seventh cervical vertebra at the shoulder level. The next spinal process belongs to the first thoracic vertebra, which attaches to the first rib.

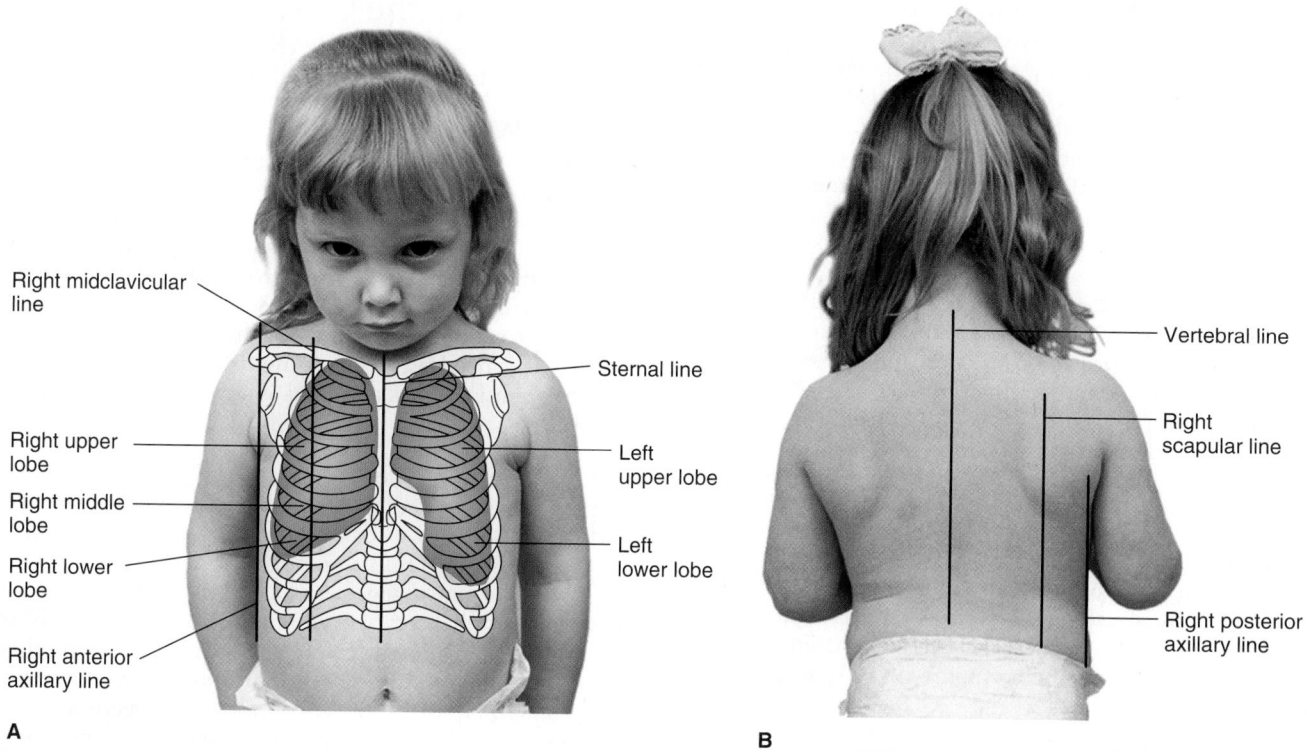

Right midclavicular line

Sternal line

Right upper lobe

Left upper lobe

Right middle lobe

Right lower lobe

Left lower lobe

Right anterior axillary line

Vertebral line

Right scapular line

Right posterior axillary line

A

B

Figure 33–21 The sternum and spine are the vertical landmarks used to describe the anatomic location of findings. Imaginary vertical lines, parallel to the midsternal and spinal lines, are used to further describe the location of findings. The midclavicular line is through the middle of the clavicle. The midaxillary line is through the middle of the axilla. The scapular line is through the bottom angle of the scapula. *A*, Anterior vertical landmarks. *B*, Posterior vertical landmarks.

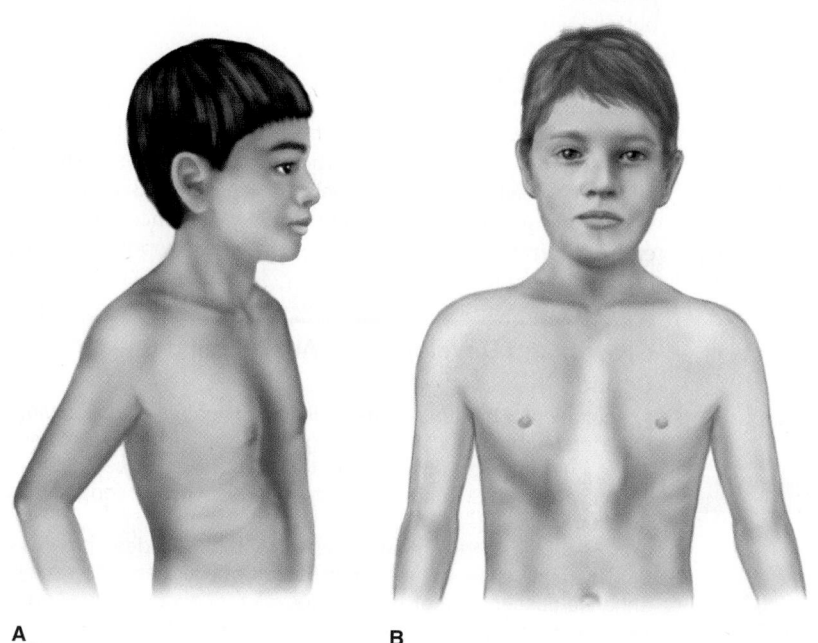

A

B

Figure 33–22 Abnormal chest shape. *A*, Pectus carinatum (funnel chest) in which the lower portion of the sternum is depressed, decreasing the anteroposterior diameter. *B*, Pectus excavatum (pigeon chest) in which the sternum protrudes, increasing the anteroposterior diameter.

center of the sternum (midsternal line) or the midspinal line can be measured with a ruler.

Position the child on the parent's lap or on the examining table with all clothing above the waist removed to inspect the chest. The thoracic muscles and subcutaneous tissue are less developed in children than in adolescents and adults, so the chest wall is thinner and the rib cage is more prominent unless obesity is present.

SHAPE OF THE CHEST

Inspect the chest for any irregularities in shape. In infants, the chest is rounded with the anteroposterior diameter approximately equal to the lateral diameter. By 2 years of age, the chest becomes more oval with growth, and the lateral diameter is greater than the anteroposterior diameter. If a child over 2 years of age has a rounded chest, a chronic obstructive lung condition such as asthma or cystic fibrosis may be present.

An abnormal chest shape may result from structural deformities, such as pectus carinatum and pectus excavatum (Figure 33–22). Scoliosis, curvature of the spine, causes a lateral deviation of the chest (see Chapter 56). A shield-shaped chest, unusually broad with widely spaced nipples, may be associated with Turner syndrome (see Chapter 53).

CHEST MOVEMENT AND RESPIRATORY EFFORT

The diaphragm is the primary muscle used for ventilation by infants and young children. As the thoracic muscles develop, they become the primary ventilation muscles. Chest movement with breathing is normally symmetric bilaterally. On inspiration, the chest and abdomen should rise simultaneously and fall on expiration. The chest movement of infants and young children is less pronounced than the abdominal movement. Asymmetric chest rise is associated with a collapsed lung.

The thoracic muscles serve as accessory respiratory muscles in infants and young children. When the child has a condition that causes a partial airway obstruction, the accessory muscles are used for inspiration and retractions are seen. **Retractions**, visible depression of tissue between the ribs of the chest wall with each inspiration, indicate an increased work of breathing and often respiratory distress (see *Pathophysiology Illustrated: Retraction Sites* in Chapter 46).

RESPIRATORY RATE

Because infants and young children use the diaphragm as the primary breathing muscle, observe or feel the rise and fall of the abdomen to count the respiratory rate in children under age 6 years. Table 33–9 gives the normal respiratory rates for each age group.

Growth and Development Respiratory Rate

Infants and children have a faster respiratory rate than adults because of their higher metabolic rate and oxygen requirement. Young children are also unable to increase the depth of respirations because the intercostal muscles are inadequately developed to lift the chest wall and increase intrathoracic volume (Chameides, Samson, Schexnayder, et al., 2011, p. 42).

To get the most accurate reading of a young infant's respiratory rate, wait until the baby is sleeping or resting quietly. Use the stethoscope to auscultate the rate or place your hand on the abdomen. Count the number of breaths for an entire minute because newborns and young infants can have irregular respirations.

Tachypnea, an increased respiratory rate, occurs in response to excitement, fear, respiratory distress, fever, and other conditions that increase oxygen needs. A sustained respiratory rate higher than normal for age is an important sign of respiratory distress. The child is at risk for developing hypoxemia if treatment is not started. An abnormally slow respiratory rate occurs in response to respiratory failure.

TABLE 33–9 Normal Respiratory Rate Ranges by Age

AGE	RESPIRATORY RATE PER MINUTE
Newborn	30–55
1 year	25–40
3 years	20–30
6 years	16–22
10 years	16–20
17 years	12–20

Palpation of the Chest

Palpation is used to evaluate chest movement, respiratory effort, deformities of the chest wall, and tactile fremitus.

CHEST WALL

To palpate the chest motion with respiration, place your palms and outspread fingers on each side of the child's chest. Confirm the bilateral symmetry of chest motion. Use your finger pads to palpate any depressions, bulges, or unusual chest wall shape that might indicate abnormal findings such as tenderness, cysts, other growths, crepitus, or fractures. None should be found. **Crepitus**, a crinkly sensation palpated on the chest surface, is caused by air escaping into the subcutaneous tissues. It often indicates a serious injury to the upper or lower airway.

TACTILE FREMITUS

To palpate **tactile fremitus**, vibrations produced by crying and talking, place the palms of your hands on each side of the chest. Ask the child to repeat a series of words or numbers, such as *puppy dog*, *kitty cat*, or *ice cream*. As the child repeats the words, move your hands systematically over the anterior and posterior chest, comparing the quality of vibrations side to side. The vibration or tingling sensation is normally palpated over the entire chest. Decreased sensations indicate that air is trapped in the lungs, as occurs with asthma.

Auscultation of the Chest

Auscultate the chest with a stethoscope to assess the quality and characteristics of breath sounds, to identify abnormal breath sounds, and to evaluate vocal resonance. Use an infant or pediatric stethoscope when available to help localize any unexpected breath sounds. Use the stethoscope diaphragm because it transmits the high-pitched breath sounds better.

BREATH SOUNDS

Evaluate the quality and characteristics of breath sounds over the entire chest, comparing sounds between the sides. Select a routine sequence for auscultating the entire chest so assessment of all lobes of the lungs will be consistently performed. Figure 33–23 shows one suggested chest auscultation sequence. Listen to an entire inspiratory and expiratory phase at each spot on the chest before moving to the next site.

Growth and Development Auscultating Breath Sounds

Auscultation of breath sounds is difficult when an infant is crying. If the infant continues to cry after giving a pacifier, bottle, or toy, all is not lost. At the end of each cry the infant takes a deep breath, which you can use to assess breath sounds, vocal resonance, and tactile fremitus.

Encourage toddlers and preschoolers to take deep breaths by blowing a pinwheel or piece of tissue off of your hand. This may enhance auscultation of subtle wheezes that occur at the end of expiration.

When trying to encourage the child to breathe normally while auscultating the chest, use suggestive language to increase cooperation: "You certainly are good at breathing slowly. Have you been practicing?" The child will often deepen and slow the breathing pattern as you praise the effort.

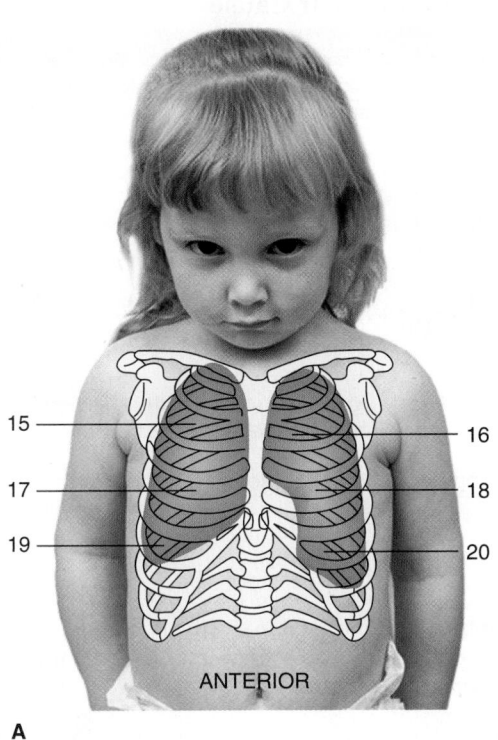
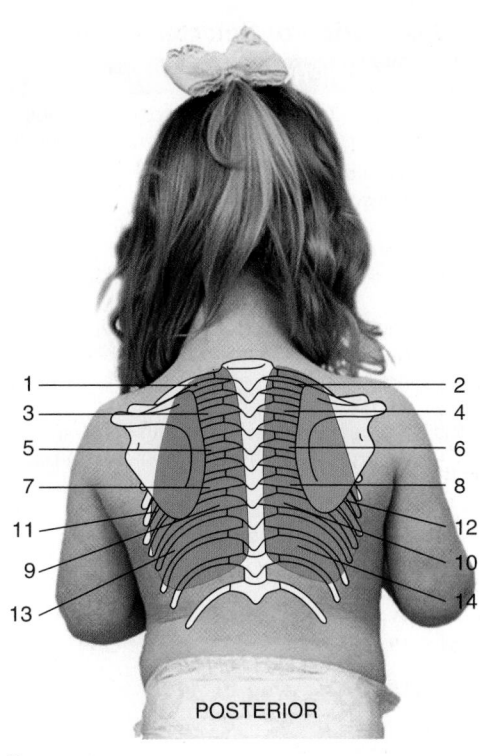

A   **B**

Figure 33–23   One sequence for auscultation of the chest.

Three types of normal breath sounds are usually heard when the chest is auscultated.

- *Vesicular breath sounds* are low-pitched, swishing, soft, short expiratory sounds usually heard in older children but not in infants and young children.
- *Bronchovesicular breath sounds* are medium-pitched, hollow, blowing sounds heard equally on inspiration and expiration in all age groups.
- *Bronchial/tracheal breath sounds* are hollow and higher pitched than vesicular breath sounds.

Breath sounds normally have equal intensity, pitch, and rhythm bilaterally. Absent or diminished breath sounds may indicate a pneumothorax or airway obstruction.

Clinical Tip

Infants and young children have a thin chest wall because of immature muscle development. The breath sounds of one lung are heard over the entire chest. It takes practice to accurately identify absent or diminished breath sounds in infants and young children. Because the distance between the lungs is greatest at the apices and midaxillary areas in young children, these sites are best for identifying absent or diminished breath sounds. Carefully auscultate, comparing the quality of breath sounds heard bilaterally.

VOCAL RESONANCE

Auscultate to evaluate **vocal resonance**, the transmission of voice sounds through the chest. Have the child repeat a series of words, such as *apple*, *banana*, and *cereal*. Use the stethoscope to auscultate the chest, comparing the quality of sounds from side to side and over the entire chest. Voice sounds, with words and syllables muffled and indistinct, are normally heard throughout the chest.

If voice sounds are absent or more muffled than usual, an airway obstruction condition such as asthma may be present. If voice sounds are more distinct, louder, or clearer, a lung consolidation condition such as pneumonia may be present.

ABNORMAL BREATH SOUNDS

Abnormal breath sounds, also called adventitious sounds, generally indicate disease. Examples of abnormal breath sounds are crackles, rhonchi (sonorous wheezing), and sibilant **wheezing** (a noise resulting from the passage of air through mucus or fluids in a narrowed lower airway). To further assess abnormal breath sounds, identify the following:

- Location; for example, side of body and lung lobe(s)
- Presence during part or entire phase of inspiration or expiration
- Change in character or disappearance when the child coughs or changes position

It takes practice to routinely identify these adventitious sounds. Table 33–10 describes adventitious sounds.

ABNORMAL VOICE SOUNDS

Observe the quality of the voice and other audible sounds. A cough is a reflexive clearing of the airway associated with a respiratory infection. Hoarseness is associated with inflammation of the larynx.

Percussion of the Chest

Percussion of the chest may be performed by an experienced examiner to assess the resonance of the lungs and size of underlying organs, such as the heart. Radiographic examination is commonly used for this evaluation.

TABLE 33–10 Description of Selected Adventitious Sounds and Their Cause

TYPE	DESCRIPTION	CAUSE
Fine crackles	High-pitched, discrete, noncontinuous sound heard at end of inspiration; does not clear with coughing (*Rub pieces of hair together beside your ear to duplicate the sound.*)	Air passing through watery secretions in the smaller airways (alveoli and bronchioles)
Coarse crackles	Loud, lower pitched, more moist or bubbly sound heard during inspiration; does not clear by coughing	Air passing through thicker secretions in the airway
Sibilant wheezing	Higher pitched, musical, squeaking, or hissing noise usually heard continuously during inspiration or expiration, but generally louder on expiration; does not clear with coughing	Air passing through mucus or fluids in a narrowed lower airway (bronchioles) as with asthma
Rhonchi (sonorous wheezing)	Coarse, low-pitched sound like a snore, heard during inspiration or expiration; may clear with coughing	Air passing through thick secretions that partially obstruct the larger bronchi and trachea
Stridor	High-pitched, piercing sound most often heard during inspiration without a stethoscope	Whistling sound as air passes through a narrowed trachea and larynx, associated with croup

Clinical Reasoning **Assessing a Child With Bronchiolitis**

Aliyah, 6 months old, is brought by her mother and father to the emergency department. She is an emergency admission from the local pediatrician's office with a diagnosis of bronchiolitis. As Aliyah's nurse, you are responsible for assessing her condition after she arrives on the pediatric nursing unit.

What procedures are used to perform a physical examination on a 6-month-old? Identify all the components of the physical assessment used to detect signs of respiratory difficulty.

Assessing the Breasts

Inspection of the Breasts

The nipples of prepubertal boys and girls are symmetrically located near the midclavicular line at the fourth to sixth ribs. The areolae are normally round and more darkly pigmented than the surrounding skin. Inspect the anterior chest for other dark spots that may indicate *supernumerary nipples*, small, undeveloped nipples and areolae that may be mistaken for moles. Their presence may be associated with congenital renal or cardiac anomalies.

See the section later in this chapter for a discussion of breast development with puberty.

Palpation of the Breasts

Boys and girls have no palpable breast tissue before puberty. Palpate the developing breasts of adolescent girls for abnormal masses or hard nodules. With the girl lying down, use a concentric or vertical stripe pattern covering all areas of each breast, including the axilla, areola, and the nipple. Gently squeeze the nipples for discharge. Breast tissue normally feels dense, firm, and elastic. Any mass needs further evaluation.

During adolescence, the majority of boys have *gynecomastia*, unilateral or bilateral breast enlargement. It is often most noticeable around 14 years of age and commonly disappears by the time of full sexual maturity. Palpate the tissue to differentiate actual breast tissue from fatty tissue in the pectoral area, and to detect any masses.

Assessing the Heart for Heart Sounds and Function

A stethoscope and sphygmomanometer are needed to assess the heart.

Inspection of the Precordium

Begin the heart examination by inspecting the anterior chest (precordium). Place the child in a reclining or semi-Fowler position, either on the parent's lap or on the examining table. Inspect the shape and symmetry of the anterior chest from the front and side views. Asymmetry and bulging of the left side of the chest wall may indicate an enlarged heart. Observe for any chest movement associated with the heart's contraction. A *heave*, an obvious lifting of the chest wall during contraction, may indicate an enlarged heart.

Palpation of the Precordium

Lightly place the surface of your fingers together on the chest wall to systematically palpate the precordium for any pulsations, heaves, or vibrations. Palpating with minimal pressure increases the chance of detecting abnormal findings.

The **apical impulse**, the point of maximum intensity, is located where the left ventricle taps the chest wall during contraction. The apical impulse is sometimes seen on the anterior chest wall of thin children, but it is normally felt as a slight tap against one fingertip. Use the topographic landmarks of the chest to describe its location (see Figures 33–20 and 33–21).

Growth and Development

The location of the apical impulse changes as the child's rib cage grows. In children under 7 years old, it is located in the fourth intercostal space just medial to the left midclavicular line. In children over 7 years old, it is located in the fifth intercostal space at the left midclavicular line.

TABLE 33–11 Normal Heart Rates for Children of Different Ages

AGE	HEART RATE RANGE (BEATS/MIN)	AVERAGE HEART RATE (BEATS/MIN)
Newborns	100–170	120
Infants to 2 years	80–130	110
2–6 years	70–120	100
6–10 years	70–110	90
10–16 years	60–100	85

Any other sensation palpated is usually abnormal. A *lift* is the sensation of the heart lifting up against the chest wall. It may be associated with an enlarged heart or a heart contracting with extra force. A **thrill** is a vibration that may feel like a cat's purr. It is caused by turbulent blood flow from a defective heart valve and a heart murmur. If present, the thrill is palpated in the right or left second intercostal space. To describe the thrill location, use the topographic landmarks of the chest (see Figures 33–20 and 33–21) and estimate the diameter of the thrill palpated.

Heart Rate and Rhythm

The apical heart rate can be counted at the site of the apical impulse either by palpation or by auscultation. Count the apical rate for 1 minute in infants and in children who have an irregular rhythm. The brachial or radial pulse rate should be the same as the auscultated apical heart rate. Table 33–11 gives normal heart rates in children of different ages.

Clinical Tip

The child's heart rate varies with age, decreasing as the child grows older. The heart rate also increases in response to exercise, excitement, anxiety, and fever. Such stresses increase the child's metabolic rate, creating a simultaneous need for more oxygen. Children respond to the need for more oxygen by increasing their heart rate, a response called *sinus tachycardia*.

Listen carefully to the heart rate rhythm. Children often have a normal cycle of irregular rhythm associated with respiration called *sinus arrhythmia* in which the child's heart rate is faster on inspiration and slower on expiration. When any rhythm irregularity is detected, ask the child to take a breath and hold it while you listen to the heart rate. The rhythm should become regular during inspiration and expiration. Other rhythm irregularities are abnormal (see Chapter 47).

Auscultation of the Heart

Auscultation is also used to assess the characteristics of the heart sounds and to detect abnormal heart sounds. Use the bell of the stethoscope to detect these lower pitched sounds.

Auscultate the heart with the child first when sitting and then reclining. This will help detect differences in heart sounds caused by a change in the child's position or by a change in the position of the heart near the chest wall. If differences in heart sounds are detected with a position change, place the child in the left lateral recumbent position and auscultate again.

IDENTIFYING HEART SOUNDS

Heart sounds result from the closure of the valves and any vibration or turbulence of blood produced by that valve closure.

Two primary sounds, S_1 and S_2, are heard when the chest is auscultated.

- S_1, the first heart sound, is produced by closure of the tricuspid and mitral valves at the beginning of ventricular contraction. The two valves close almost simultaneously to prevent the back flow of blood into the atria.
- S_2, the second heart sound, is produced by the closure of the aortic and pulmonic valves. Once blood has reached the pulmonic and aortic arteries, the valves close to prevent back flow into the ventricles.

Clinical Tip

To distinguish between S_1 and S_2 heart sounds in each listening area, palpate the carotid pulse while auscultating the heart. The heart sound heard simultaneously with the pulsation is S_1.

Sound is easily transmitted in liquid, and it travels best in the direction of blood flow. Auscultate heart sounds at specific areas on the chest wall in the direction of blood flow, just beyond the valve (Figure 33–24). The sounds produced by the heart valves or blood turbulence are heard throughout the chest in thin infants and children. Both S_1 and S_2 can be heard in all listening areas.

Auscultate heart sounds for quality (distinct versus muffled) and intensity (loud versus soft). First, distinguish between S_1 and S_2 in each listening area. Heart sounds are usually distinct and crisp in children because of their thin chest wall. Muffled or indistinct sounds may indicate a heart defect or congestive heart failure. Document the area where heart sounds are heard the best. Table 33–12 and Figure 33–24 review the location where each sound is normally best heard for assessment of quality and intensity. If an extra heart sound is heard (e.g., a murmur), auscultate the heart in the sitting, reclining, and left lateral recumbent positions to detect any differences associated with position change.

SPLITTING OF THE HEART SOUNDS

After distinguishing the first and second heart sounds, try to detect a split S_2. When the child takes a deep breath more blood returns to the right ventricle than the left ventricle, causing the pulmonic valve to close a fraction of a second later than the aortic valve; this is called *physiologic splitting*. Auscultate over the pulmonic area while the child breathes normally and then while the child takes a deep breath. The S_2 splitting may be heard after a deep breath, and then with regular breathing, it is heard as

TABLE 33–12 Listening Sites for Auscultation of the Quality and Intensity of Heart Sounds

HEART SOUND	SITES WHERE BEST HEARD	SITES WHERE HEARD SOFTLY
S_1	Apex of the heart Tricuspid area Mitral area	Base of the heart Aortic area Pulmonic area
S_2	Base of the heart Aortic area Pulmonic area	Apex of the heart Tricuspid area Mitral area
Physiologic splitting	Pulmonic area	
S_3	Mitral area	

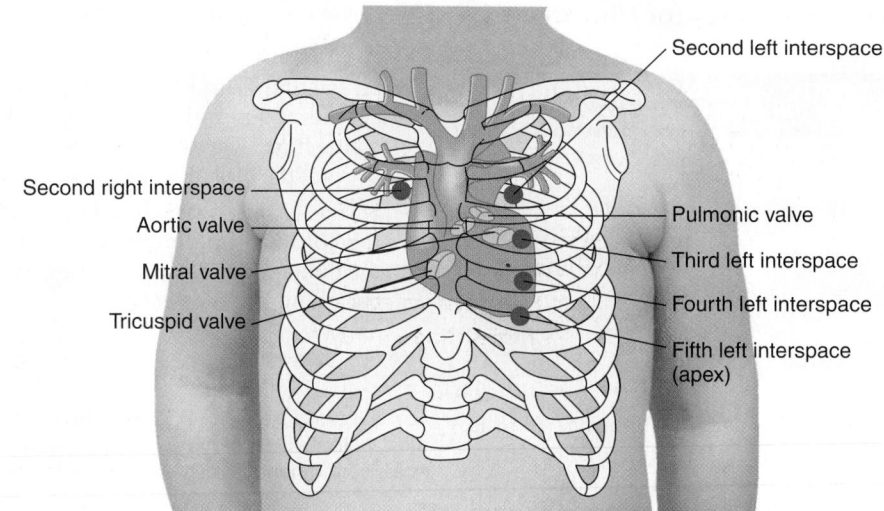

Figure 33–24 Remember that sound travels in the direction of blood flow when auscultating heart sounds. Rather than listen for heart sounds over each heart valve, auscultate heart sounds at specific areas on the chest wall away from the valve itself. These areas are named for the valve producing the sound. *Aortic*: second right intercostal space near the sternum. *Pulmonic*: second left intercostal space near the sternum. *Tricuspid*: fifth right or left intercostal space near the sternum. *Mitral* (apical): in infants—third or fourth intercostal space, just left of the left midclavicular line; in children—fifth intercostal space at the left midclavicular line.

a single sound. If S_2 splitting does not vary with normal and deep respirations, it is called *fixed splitting*, which is an abnormal finding associated with an atrial septal defect in the heart.

EXTRA HEART SOUNDS

A third heart sound, S_3, is occasionally heard in children as a normal finding. The S_3 heart sound is caused when blood rushes through the mitral valve and splashes into the left ventricle. It is heard in diastole, just after S_2. It is distinguished from a split S_2 because it is louder in the mitral area than in the pulmonic area.

Murmurs, or abnormal heart sounds, are sometimes auscultated. These sounds are produced by blood passing through a defective valve, great vessel, or other heart structure. Some murmurs are benign or innocent, whereas others may indicate a congenital heart defect. Consult an experienced examiner to distinguish between murmurs.

It takes practice to hear murmurs in children. Often, murmurs must be very loud to be detected. For softer murmurs, normal heart sounds must be distinguished before an extra sound is recognized. When a murmur is detected, define the characteristics of the extra sound, including:

- *Intensity.* How loud is it? Can a thrill also be palpated? (See *Clinical Tip.*)
- *Location.* Where is the murmur the loudest? Identify the listening area and precise topographic landmarks. Is the child sitting or lying down? Do the murmur characteristics change when the child changes position?
- *Radiation or transmission.* Is the sound transmitted over a larger than expected area of the chest, to the axilla, or to the back?
- *Timing.* Is the murmur heard best after S_1 or S_2? Is it heard during the entire phase between S_1 and S_2?
- *Quality.* Describe what the murmur sounds like—for example, machine-like, musical, or blowing.

VENOUS HUM

A venous hum is caused by turbulent blood flow in the internal jugular veins. Auscultate over the supraclavicular fossa above the middle of the clavicle or over the upper anterior chest with the bell of the stethoscope. A venous hum is heard as a continuous low-pitched hum throughout the cardiac cycle. It is heard louder during diastole and does not change with respirations. It may be quieted when the child turns the neck, lies down, or when the jugular vein is occluded. A venous hum may be associated with anemia, but it has no pathologic significance.

Completing the Heart Examination

A complete assessment of heart function also includes palpating the pulses, measuring the blood pressure, and evaluating signs from other systems.

PALPATION OF THE PULSES

Palpate the characteristics of the pulses in the extremities to assess the circulation. The technique and sites for palpating the pulse are the same as those used for adults. Evaluate the pulsation for rate, regularity of rhythm, and strength in each extremity and compare your findings bilaterally. Palpate the femoral pulses, which should be as strong as the brachial pulsations. A weaker femoral pulse is associated with coarctation of the aorta.

Growth and Development

Infants have a low systolic blood pressure, and detecting the distal pulses is often difficult. Use the brachial artery in the arms and the popliteal or femoral artery in the legs to evaluate the pulses. The radial and distal tibial pulses are normally palpated easily in older children.

BLOOD PRESSURE

To assess the blood pressure, wait until the child has been seated and quiet for 3 to 5 minutes. To obtain the most accurate reading, select an appropriately sized cuff for the extremity selected. Use the right arm when possible, as this arm was used for development of blood pressure standards. See the *Clinical Skills Manual* SKILLS for the technique for obtaining the blood pressure in children.

With the cuff snugly wrapped around the arm, hold the arm with the antecubital fossa at the level of the heart. Use the bell of the stethoscope to hear softer Korotkoff sounds. The systolic reading is the onset of Korotkoff sounds. The diastolic reading is the fifth Korotkoff sound (Lande, 2016).

Measure the blood pressure twice and average the two readings. Compare the systolic and diastolic readings with the standard blood pressure values by age, gender, and height percentile in Appendix D. A blood pressure value at the 50th percentile for the child's age, gender, and height percentile is considered the midpoint of the normal blood pressure range. A systolic or diastolic reading at or above the 95th percentile indicates hypertension.

For any child with a potential heart condition, obtain a blood pressure reading in both an arm and a leg and compare the readings. The blood pressure in the leg should be 10 to 20 mmHg higher than the arm reading (Bernstein, 2016). If the reading in the leg is lower than that in the arm, coarctation of the aorta may be present.

OTHER SIGNS

Skin color, capillary refill, and respiratory effort are additional elements of a complete heart examination. Cyanosis is most commonly associated with a congenital heart defect in children. A capillary refill time of greater than 2 seconds indicates poor perfusion of the tissues. Signs of respiratory distress (tachypnea, flaring, and retractions) may be associated with the child's attempts to compensate for hypoxemia caused by a congenital heart defect.

Assessing the Abdomen for Shape, Bowel Sounds, and Underlying Organs

The location of underlying organs and structures of the abdomen must be considered when the abdomen is examined. The abdomen is commonly divided by imaginary lines into quadrants for the purpose of identifying underlying structures (Figure 33–25). A stethoscope is needed to examine the abdomen. Perform inspection and auscultation before palpation and percussion because touching the abdomen may change the characteristics of bowel sounds.

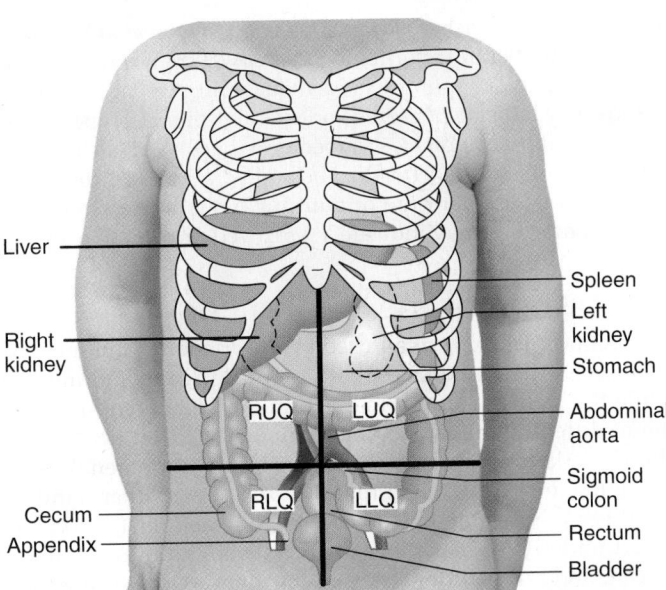

Figure 33–25 **Topographic landmarks of the abdomen. The abdomen is commonly divided by imaginary lines into quadrants for the purpose of identifying underlying structures.**

Inspection of the Abdomen

Begin the examination of the abdomen by inspecting the shape and contour, condition of the umbilicus and rectus muscle, and abdominal movement. Inspect the shape of the abdomen from the front and side with good lighting to identify an abnormal contour. The child's abdomen is normally symmetric and rounded or flat when the child is supine. A scaphoid or sunken abdomen is abnormal and may indicate dehydration.

See Chapter 24 for guidelines to assess the newborn's umbilical stump. After the stump falls off, inspect the umbilicus for continued drainage, which may indicate an infection or a granuloma. Inspect the umbilicus in infants and toddlers because these children often have an *umbilical hernia*, a protrusion of abdominal contents through an open umbilical muscle ring.

Inspect the abdominal wall for any depression or bulging at midline above or below the umbilicus, indicating separation of the rectus abdominis muscles. The depression may be up to 5 cm (2 in.) wide. Measure the width of the separation to monitor change over time. As abdominal muscle strength develops, the separation usually becomes less prominent. However, the splitting may persist if congenital muscle weakness is present.

ABDOMINAL MOVEMENT

Infants and children up to 6 years of age breathe with the diaphragm. The abdomen rises simultaneously with the chest during inspiration and falls with expiration. Other abdominal movements such as peristaltic waves are abnormal. **Peristaltic waves** are visible rhythmic contractions of the intestinal wall smooth muscle, which moves food through the digestive tract. Their presence generally indicates an intestinal obstruction, such as pyloric stenosis (see Chapter 51).

Auscultation of the Abdomen

To evaluate bowel sounds, auscultate the abdomen with the diaphragm of the stethoscope. Bowel sounds normally occur every 10 to 30 seconds. They have a high-pitched, tinkling, metallic quality. Loud gurgling (borborygmi) is heard when the child is hungry. Listen in each quadrant long enough to hear at least one bowel sound. Before determining that bowel sounds are absent, auscultate at least 5 minutes in each quadrant. Absence of bowel sounds may indicate peritonitis or a paralytic ileus. Hyperactive bowel sounds may indicate gastroenteritis or a bowel obstruction.

Next, auscultate over the abdominal aorta and the renal arteries for a vascular hum or murmur. No murmur should be heard. A murmur may indicate a narrowed or defective artery.

Percussion of the Abdomen

Indirect percussion is often used by experienced examiners to evaluate borders and sizes of abdominal organs and masses while the child is supine. To perform indirect percussion, lay the middle finger of your nondominant hand on the child's abdomen, keeping your other fingers off the abdomen. With a springlike motion, use the fingertip from your other hand to tap the finger resting on the abdomen. Listen for the tone to detect underlying structures. Dullness is found over the liver, spleen, and full bladder. Tympany is found over the stomach or the intestines when an obstruction is present. Tympany may be found over areas beyond the stomach in infants because of air swallowing. A resonant tone may be heard over other areas.

Palpation of the Abdomen

Both light and deep palpation are used to examine the abdominal organs and to detect any masses. *Light palpation* is used to evaluate the tenseness of the abdomen (how soft or hard it is), the liver, the presence of any tenderness or masses, and any defects in the abdominal wall. *Deep palpation* is used to detect masses, define their shape and consistency, and identify abdominal tenderness.

Perform the abdominal examination when the child is calm and cooperative to get the best assessment. To begin palpation, position the child supine with knees flexed. Stand beside the child and place your warmed fingertips across the child's abdomen. Organs and other masses are more easily palpated when the abdominal wall is relaxed. Watch the child's face during palpation for signs of pain (e.g., a grimace or constriction of the pupils).

Growth and Development Abdominal Assessment

Infants and toddlers often feel more secure for the abdominal assessment when lying supine across both the parent's and the examiner's laps. A bottle, pacifier, or toy may distract the child and improve cooperation for the examination.

When examining the child, use suggestive words to help the child relax the abdomen. "How soft will your tummy get when my hand feels it? Does it get softer than this? Yes. See, it softens as you breathe out. Will it also be softer here?" The child learns to relax the abdomen and is challenged to do it better.

When a child is ticklish, use a firm touch and do not pretend to tickle the child at any point in the examination. Alternatively, put the child's hand on the abdomen and place your hand over the child's. Let your fingertips slide over to touch the abdomen. The child has a sense of being in control, and you may be able to palpate directly.

Older children may need distraction, especially when abdominal tenderness and guarding are present. Have the child perform a task that requires some concentration, such as pressing the hands together or pulling locked hands apart.

LIGHT PALPATION

For light palpation, use a superficial, gentle touch that slightly depresses the abdomen. Usually, the abdomen feels soft and no tenderness is detected. Palpate any bulging along the abdominal wall, especially along the rectus muscle and umbilical ring, which could indicate a hernia. If an umbilical hernia is present, measure the diameter of the muscular ring rather than the protrusion. The muscle ring normally becomes smaller and closes by 4 years of age.

Locate and lightly palpate the lower liver edge. Place the fingerpads in the right midclavicular line at the level of the umbilicus and move the fingers closer to the costal margin with each expiration. As the liver edge descends with inspiration, a flat, narrow ridge is usually felt. The liver edge is normally palpated 2 to 3 cm (about 1 in.) below the right costal margin in infants and toddlers, but it may not be palpated in older children. If the liver edge is more than 3 cm (a little over 1 in.) below the right costal margin, the liver is enlarged, possibly due to congestive heart failure or hepatic disease.

DEEP PALPATION

To perform deep palpation, press the fingers of one hand (for small children) or two hands (for older children) more deeply into the abdomen. Because the abdominal muscles are most relaxed when the child takes a deep breath, ask the child to take regular deep breaths when palpating each area of the abdomen.

The spleen tip may be felt at the left costal margin in the midclavicular line when the child takes a deep breath. The spleen is enlarged if it is easily palpated below the left costal margin. The kidneys are in a deep layer of abdominal muscles and intestines, and they are rarely palpated except in newborns. A tubular mass commonly palpated in the lower left or right quadrant is often an intestine filled with feces. A distended bladder is often palpated as a firm, central, dome-shaped mass above the symphysis pubis in young children.

SAFETY ALERT!

If an enlarged kidney or unexpected mass is detected during abdominal palpation, do not continue to palpate the kidney. Notify the primary healthcare provider immediately. The mass could be a Wilms tumor.

Assessment of the Inguinal Area

The inguinal area is inspected and palpated during the abdominal examination to detect enlarged lymph nodes or masses. The femoral pulse, a part of the heart examination, may be assessed simultaneously with the abdominal examination.

Inspect the inguinal area for any change in contour, comparing sides. A small bulging noted over the femoral canal in girls may be associated with a femoral hernia. A bulging in the inguinal area in boys may be associated with an inguinal hernia.

Palpate the inguinal area for lymph nodes and other masses. Small lymph nodes, less than 1 cm (½ in.) in diameter, are often present in the inguinal area because of minor injuries on the legs. Any tenderness, heat, or inflammation in these palpated lymph nodes could be associated with a local infection.

Assessing the Genital and Perineal Areas for External Structural Abnormalities

Nurses may perform an external genital examination or assist another healthcare provider. In younger children, the genital and perineal examination is performed immediately after assessment of the abdomen. Gloves, lubricant, and a penlight are needed for the examination.

Examination of the genitalia and perineal area can cause stress in children because they sense their privacy has been invaded. To make young children feel more secure, position them on the parent's lap with their legs spread apart. Children can also be positioned on the examining table with their knees flexed and the legs spread apart like a frog.

Clinical Tip

Preschool-age children are often taught that strangers are not permitted to touch their "private parts." When a child this age actively resists examination of the genital area, ask the parent to tell the child you have permission to look at and touch these parts of the body. You may wish to reinforce the teaching by saying the nurse or doctor can look only when the parent is in the room.

Some children develop modesty during the preschool period. Briefly explain what you need to examine and why. Then calmly and efficiently examine the child.

Inspection of the Female External Genitalia

Inspect the external genitalia of girls for color, size, and symmetry of the mons pubis, labia, urethra, and vaginal opening (Figure 33–26). Simultaneously look for any abnormal findings such as swelling, inflammation, masses, lacerations, or discharge.

Inspect the mons pubis for pubic hair and its characteristics. See Figure 33–29 for guidelines to assess the stage of pubic hair development.

The labia minora are usually thin and pale in preadolescent girls but become dark pink and moist after puberty. In young infants, the labia minora may be fused and cover the structures in the vestibule. If fused, the adhesions should be separated by another health professional.

Use the thumb and forefinger of one gloved hand to separate the labia minora to inspect the structures in the vestibule. No lesions or signs of inflammation are expected around the urethral or vaginal opening. Redness and **excoriation** (scratches

and abrasions of the skin) are often associated with an irritant such as bubble bath. The hymen is just inside the vaginal opening. In preadolescents, it is usually a thin membrane with a crescent-shaped opening. The vaginal opening is usually about 1 cm (½ in.) in adolescents when the hymen is intact. Sexually active adolescents may have a vaginal opening with irregular edges.

Preadolescent girls do not normally have a vaginal discharge. Adolescents often have a clear discharge without a foul odor. Menses generally begin approximately 2 years after breast bud development. A foul-smelling discharge in preschool-age children may be associated with a foreign body. Various organisms may cause a vaginal infection in older children.

SAFETY ALERT!

Signs of sexual abuse in young children include bruising or swelling of the vulva, foul-smelling vaginal discharge, enlarged opening of the vagina, and rash or sores in the perineal area (see Chapter 42).

An internal vaginal examination and palpation of the female genitalia by an experienced health professional is indicated when abnormal findings such as a vaginal discharge or trauma to the external structures is noted.

Inspection of the Male Genitalia

Inspect the male genitalia for the structural and pubertal development of the penis, scrotum, and testicles. Have boys sit with their legs crossed in front of them. This position puts pressure on the abdominal wall to push the testicles into the scrotum. See Figure 33–30 for guidelines to assess the staging of pubic hair and external genital development.

PENIS

Inspect the penis for size, foreskin, hygiene, and position of the urethral meatus. The length of the nonerect penis in the newborn is normally 2 to 3 cm (about 1 in.). The penis enlarges in length and breadth during childhood and puberty. The penis is normally straight. A downward bowing of the penis may be caused by a **chordee**, a fibrous band of tissue associated with hypospadias.

When the penis is circumcised, the glans penis is exposed, and it is normally clean and smooth without inflammation or ulceration. The urethral meatus is a slit-shaped opening near the tip of the glans. No discharge should be present. If the penis is not circumcised, a foreskin opening large enough for a good urinary stream is normal even when the foreskin does not fully retract, which is a common finding in boys between 3 and 6 years of age. To inspect the glans penis of an uncircumcised boy, the foreskin is gently retracted by the child, parent, or examiner. Avoid forcible retraction of the foreskin to prevent damage to the tissues and the formation of adhesions between the foreskin and glans. Evaluate the degree of foreskin retraction and the meatal location and size. It is usually possible to visualize the meatus.

Location of the urethral meatus at another site on the penis is abnormal, indicating hypospadias or epispadias (see Chapter 52). A round, pinpoint urethral meatus may indicate meatal stenosis. *Phimosis* is the presence of an abnormal ring of tissue distal to the glans that prevents retraction of the foreskin to allow visualization of the meatus. Erythema and edema of the glans (*balanitis*) may result from an infection or trauma.

Inspect the urinary stream. The stream is normally strong without dribbling.

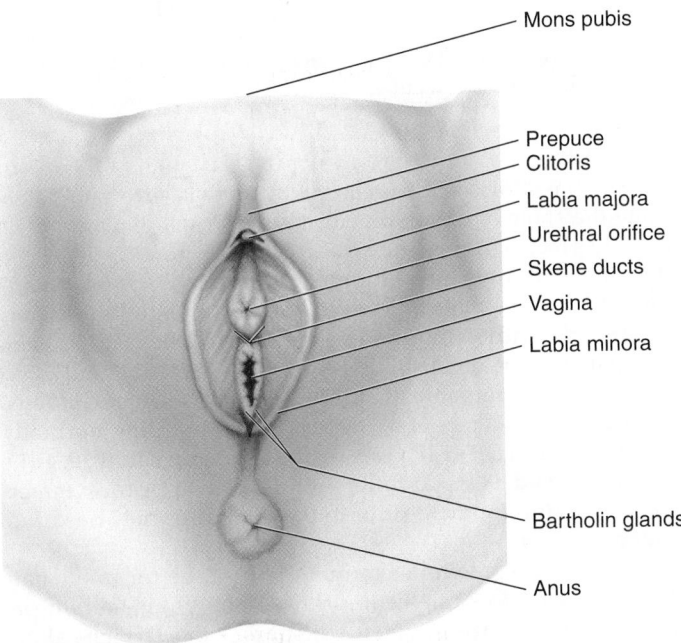

— Mons pubis

— Prepuce
— Clitoris
— Labia majora
— Urethral orifice
— Skene ducts
— Vagina
— Labia minora

— Bartholin glands

— Anus

Figure 33–26 **Anatomic structures of the female genital and perineal area.**

SCROTUM

Inspect the scrotum for size, symmetry, presence of the testicles, and any abnormalities. The scrotum is normally loose and pendulous with *rugae* (wrinkles). The scrotum of infants often appears large in comparison to the penis. A small, undeveloped scrotum that has no rugae indicates undescended testicles. Enlargement or swelling of the scrotum is abnormal. It may indicate an inguinal hernia, hydrocele, torsion of the spermatic cord, or testicular inflammation. A deep cleft in the scrotum may indicate ambiguous genitalia.

Palpation of the Male Genitalia

Palpate the shaft of the penis for nodules and masses. None should be present.

Palpate the scrotum for the presence of the testicles. Make sure your hands are warm to avoid stimulating the cremasteric reflex that causes the testicles to retract. Place your index finger and thumb over the inguinal canal on the side palpated. This keeps the testicle from retracting into the abdomen (Figure 33–27). Gently palpate each testicle. The testicles are normally smooth and equal in size. They are approximately 1 to 1.5 cm (½ in.) in diameter until puberty, when they increase in size. A hard, enlarged, painless testicle may indicate a tumor.

If a testicle is not palpated in the scrotum, an experienced examiner palpates the inguinal canal for the presence of the testicle and may try to move the testicle to the scrotum to palpate its size and shape. The testicle is descendable when it can be moved into the scrotum. An undescended testicle is one that will not move out of the inguinal canal or one that cannot be palpated. An experienced examiner also palpates the length of the spermatic cord between the thumb and forefinger from the testicle to the inguinal canal. It normally feels solid and smooth. No tenderness is expected.

When bulging or swelling of the scrotum is present, an experienced examiner palpates the scrotum to identify the characteristics of the mass and whether it is unilateral or bilateral. If the mass pushes back through the external inguinal

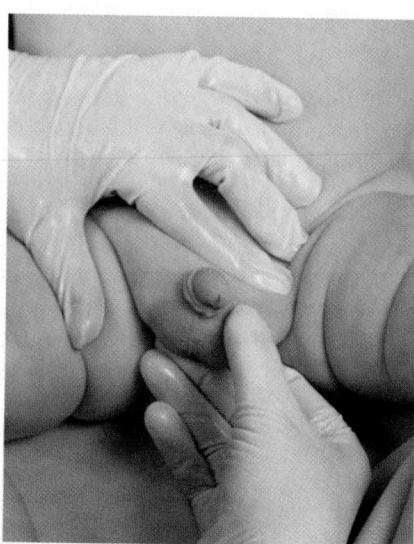

Figure 33–27 When palpating the scrotum for descended testicles and spermatic cords, place the index finger over the inguinal canal to keep the testicle in the scrotum. Gently palpate the testicle with only enough pressure to detect the size and shape.

ring, it is a reducible inguinal hernia rather than incarcerated. A bright penlight under the scrotum is used to see if a red glow is seen (transillumination), indicating a hydrocele rather than a hernia.

Anus and Rectum

When the child is supine or prone, inspect the anus for sphincter control and any abnormal findings such as inflammation, fissures, or lesions. The external sphincter is usually closed. Inflammation and scratch marks around the anus may be associated with pinworms. A protrusion from the rectum may be associated with a rectal wall prolapse or a hemorrhoid.

Lightly touching the anal opening should stimulate an anal contraction or "wink." Absence of a contraction may indicate the presence of a lower spinal cord lesion. Passage of meconium by newborns indicates a patent anus.

Only an experienced examiner should perform a rectal examination. It is indicated for symptoms of intra-abdominal, rectal, bowel, or stool abnormalities. To assist the examiner and to reduce the child's anxiety, distract the child with an age-appropriate toy or discussion. Let the child know that the lubricant might feel cold. As the examiner's finger is positioned, help the child to relax the sphincter by "pushing out the poop."

Assessing Pubertal Development and Sexual Maturation

The age when secondary sexual characteristics appear can vary with race and ethnicity, environmental conditions, geographic location, and nutrition. For example, in the United States, Black girls and boys have an earlier onset of secondary sexual characteristics than non-Hispanic White and Hispanic girls and boys (Herman-Giddens et al., 2012). A higher body mass index appears to contribute to earlier development of puberty in girls, but not in boys (Biro et al., 2013). If no pubertal changes are seen by age 13 years in girls or 14 years in boys, further evaluation is needed (Loomba-Albrecht & Styne, 2012).

Girls

Inspect the adolescent's breasts while she is sitting to determine the stage of development. Breast development in girls usually precedes other pubertal changes. Figure 33–28 shows the stages of breast development. *Thelarche*, or breast budding, is the first stage of pubertal development in the majority of girls, indicating breast stage 2. Breast tissue is seen and palpated below a slightly enlarging areola (1 cm [½ in.] in diameter of palpable glandular tissue) (Herman-Giddens, Bourdony, Dowshen, et al., 2011). Breast budding normally occurs between 8 and 10 years of age (Biro et al., 2013). A girl's breasts often develop at different rates and appear asymmetric. Breast development prior to 6 years of age may need further evaluation.

During the genital examination, observe for pubic hair development. Preadolescent girls have no pubic hair. Initial pubic hair is lightly pigmented, sparse, and straight along the labia majora. Figure 33–29 illustrates the normal stages of female pubic hair development. Breast development usually precedes pubic hair development. The presence of pubic hair follows testicular enlargement about 2 years later in genitalia Tanner stage 3 (Herman-Giddens et al., 2012). The pubic hair becomes darker, dense, and curly, extending over the pubic area in a diamond pattern by the completion of puberty. The mean age for completing pubertal development for boys (stage 5) in the United States is 15 years of age (Herman-Giddens et al., 2012). Stages of pubic hair and external genital development follow a standard pattern, as seen in Figure 33–30.

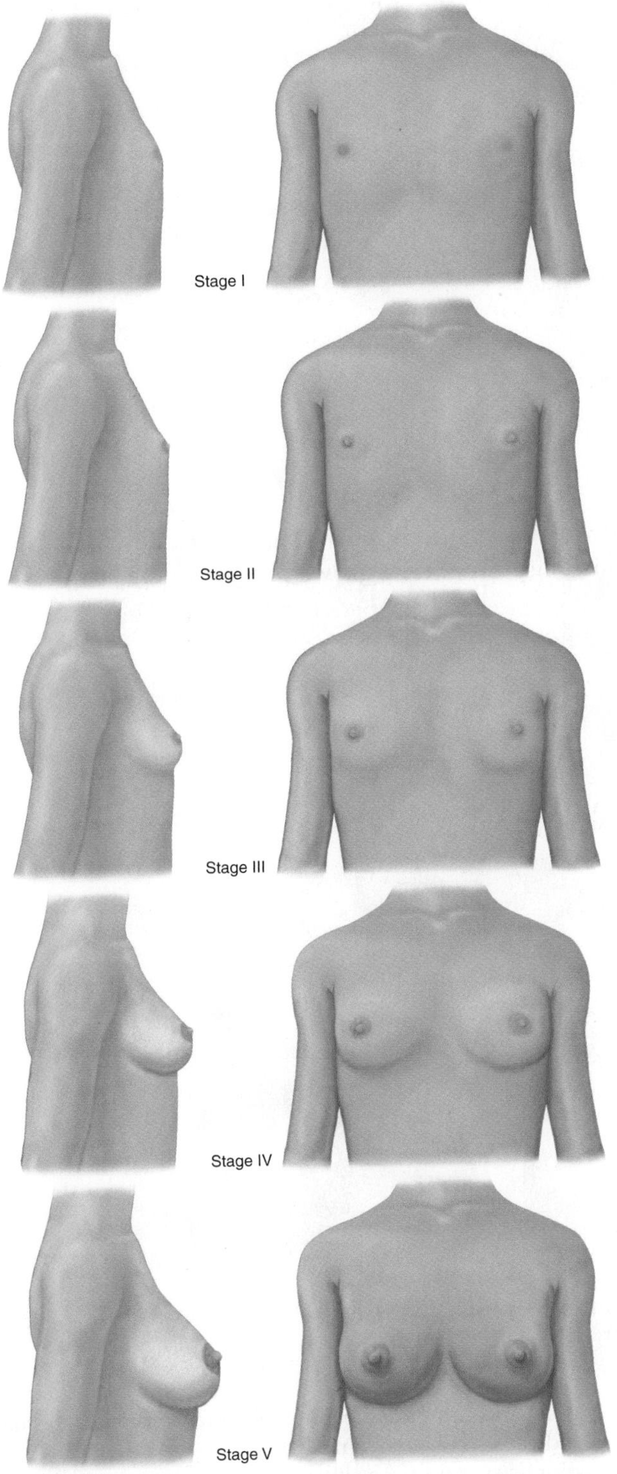

Sexual Maturity Timeline

The sexual maturity rating (SMR) is an average of the breast and pubic hair development stages in girls and of the genital and pubic hair stages in boys. The rating is a number between 2 and 5, as stage 1 is prepubertal. The SMR is then related to other physiologic events that happen during puberty. Compare the stage of the child's secondary sexual characteristics with information in Table 33–13.

Figure 33–28 **Normal stages of breast development.**

before 8 years of age is unusual and may indicate premature pubertal development. The progression of puberty changes often takes 5 years to reach maturity.

Boys

Initial signs of pubertal development in boys are enlargement of the testicles and thinning of the scrotum at a mean age of 9 to 10 years of age, depending on ethnicity. Straight, downy pubic hair first appears at the base of the penis at a mean age of 10 to 11.5 years, depending on ethnicity. Penis enlargement generally

TABLE 33–13 Sexual Maturity Timeline

GENDER AND DEVELOPMENT CATEGORIES	TIME SPAN AND PHYSIOLOGIC CHANGES
Girls	
Breast development	Over 4 to 4.5 years, proceeding from stages 2 to 5
Pubic hair development	Over 4 to 4.5 years, usually initiated after breast development
Onset of menstruation	At about breast stage 4 (see Figure 33–28), 1 year after peak height velocity
Growth spurt	Height velocity begins increasing about 6 months before breast budding. Peak height velocity occurs between breast and pubic hair stages 3 and 4 (see Figures 33–28 and 33–29)
Boys	
Genital (penis and testes) development	Over 4.5 years, proceeding from stages 2 to 5; testicular development precedes growth of the penis (see Figure 33–30)
Pubic hair development	Over 3.5 years
Facial and axillary hair	Begins about 2 years after pubic hair development begins
Voice change	Greatest change between genital stages 3 and 4
Onset of ejaculation	At about genital stage 3
Growth spurt	Over 4 to 5 years, greatest height velocity is in the first 2 to 3 years with peak height velocity between genital and pubic hair stages 3 and 4 (see Figure 33–30)

Source: Data from Herman-Giddens, M. E., Bourdony, C. J., Dowshen, S. A., & Reiter, E. O. 2011). *Assessment of sexual maturity stages in girls and boys.* Elk Grove Village, IL: American Academy of Pediatrics; Susman, E. J., Houts, R. M., Steinberg, L., Belsky, J., Cauffman, E., De Hart, G., . . . Eunice Kennedy Shriver NICHD Early Child Care Research Network. (2010). Longitudinal development of secondary sexual characteristics in girls and boys between ages 9½ and 15½ years. *Archives of Pediatric and Adolescent Medicine, 164*(2), 166–173; Hochberg, Z., & Belsky, J. (2013). Evo-devo of human adolescence: Beyond disease models of early puberty. *BMC Medicine, 11,* 113. doi:10.1186/1741-7015-11-113.

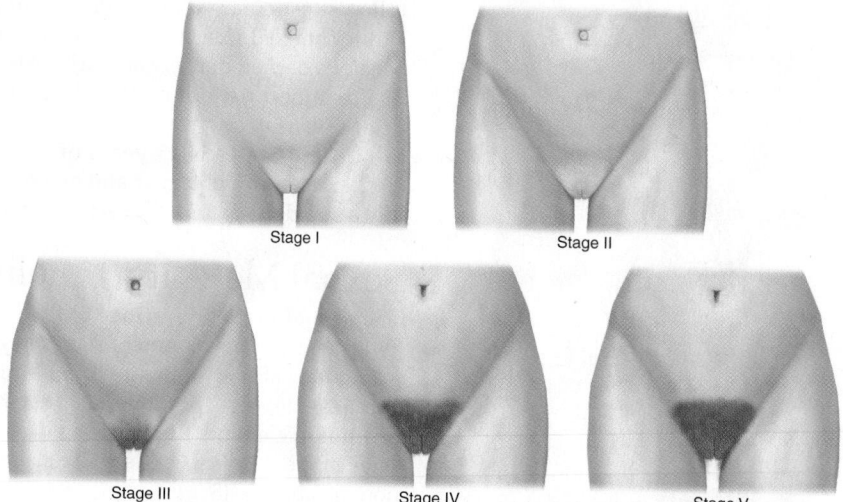

Figure 33–29 The stages of female pubic hair development with sexual maturation. In stage 2, soft downy hair along the labia majora is an indication that sexual maturation is beginning. Hair grows progressively coarse and curly as development proceeds.

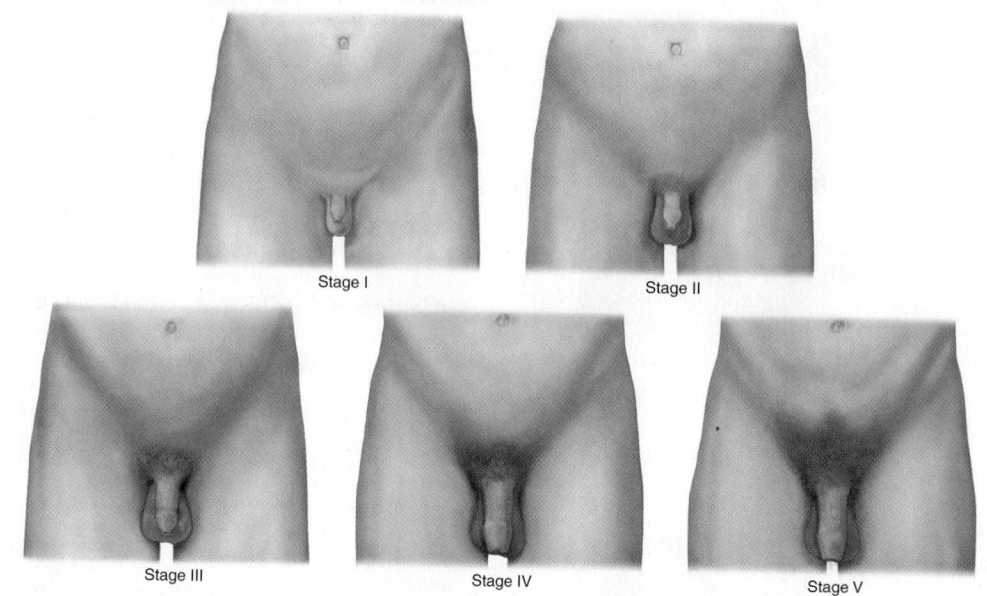

Figure 33–30 The stages of male pubic hair and external genital development with sexual maturation.

Assessing the Musculoskeletal System for Bone and Joint Structure, Movement, and Muscle Strength

Inspection of the Bones, Muscles, and Joints

Inspect and compare the arms and then the legs for differences in alignment, contour, skinfolds, length, and deformities. The extremities normally have equal length, circumference, and numbers of skinfolds bilaterally. Extra skinfolds and a larger circumference may indicate a shorter extremity.

Inspect and compare the joints bilaterally for size, discoloration, and ease of voluntary movement. Joints are normally the same color as surrounding skin, with no sign of swelling. Children should voluntarily flex and extend joints during normal activities without pain. Redness, swelling, and pain with movement may indicate injury or infection.

Palpation of the Bones, Muscles, and Joints

Palpate the bones and muscles in each extremity for muscle tone, masses, or tenderness. Muscles normally feel firm, and bony masses are not normally present. Doughy muscles may indicate poor muscle tone. Rigid muscles, or hypertonia, may be associated with an active seizure or cerebral palsy. A mass over a long bone may indicate a recent fracture or a bone tumor.

Palpate each joint and surrounding muscles to detect any swelling, masses, heat, or tenderness. None is expected when the joint is palpated. Tenderness, heat, swelling, and redness can result from injury or a chronic joint inflammation such as juvenile idiopathic arthritis.

Range of Motion and Muscle Strength Assessment

RANGE OF MOTION

Observe the child during typical play activities, such as reaching for objects, climbing, and walking, to assess range of motion of all major joints. Children spontaneously move their joints through the full normal range of motion with play activities when no pain is present. Limited range of motion may indicate injury, inflammation of a joint, or a muscle abnormality.

When a joint is suspected of having limited active range of motion, perform passive range of motion. Flex and extend, abduct and adduct, or rotate the affected joint cautiously to avoid causing extra pain. Full range of motion without pain is normal. Limitations in movement may indicate injury, inflammation, or malformation. Increased passive range of motion may indicate muscle weakness.

MUSCLE STRENGTH

Observe the child's ability to climb onto an examining table, throw a ball, clap hands together, or move around on the bed. The child's ability to perform age-appropriate play activities indicates good muscle tone and strength. Attainment of age-appropriate motor development is another indicator of good muscle strength (Table 33–14).

To assess the strength of specific muscles in the extremities, engage the child in some games. Compare muscle strength bilaterally to identify muscle weakness. For example, the child squeezes the examiner's fingers tightly with each hand; pushes against and pulls the examiner's hands with the hands, lower legs, and feet; and resists extension of a flexed elbow or knee. Children normally have good muscle strength bilaterally. Unilateral muscle weakness may be associated with a nerve injury. Bilateral muscle weakness may result from a congenital

TABLE 33–14 Selected Gross Motor Milestones for Age

GROSS MOTOR MILESTONES	AVERAGE AGE ATTAINED (MONTHS)
If prone, pushes up on elbows	4
Rolls over in both directions	6
Gets to sitting position and sits without support	9
Creeps or crawls	9
Pulls self to standing position	12
Takes a few steps walking alone	12
May walk up steps	18
Climbs on furniture without help	24
Rides tricycle	36

Source: Data from Centers for Disease Control and Prevention. (2014). *Developmental milestones.* Retrieved from http://www.cdc.gov/ncbddd/actearly/milestones/index.html

TABLE 33–15 Normal Development of Posture and Spinal Curves

AGE	POSTURE AND SPINAL CURVES
2–3 months	Holds head erect when held upright; thoracic kyphosis when sitting
6–8 months	Sits without support; spine is straight
10–15 months	Walks independently; straight spine
Toddler	Protruding abdomen; lumbar lordosis
School-age child	Height of shoulders and hips is level; balanced thoracic convex and lumbar concave curves

disorder such as Down syndrome. Asymmetric weakness may be associated with conditions such as cerebral palsy.

When generalized muscle weakness is suspected in a preschool- or school-age child, ask the child to stand up from the supine position. Children are normally able to rise to a standing position without using their arms as levers. Children who push their body upright using their arms and hands may have generalized muscle weakness, known as a positive *Gowers sign*. This may indicate muscular dystrophy (see Chapter 56).

Posture and Spinal Alignment

POSTURE

Inspect the child's posture when standing from a front, side, and back view. The shoulders and hips are normally level. The head is held erect without a tilt, and the shoulder contour is symmetric. After beginning to walk, young children often have a pot-bellied stance because of lumbar lordosis. The spine has normal thoracic convex and lumbar concave curves after 6 years of age. Table 33–15 describes normal posture and spinal curvature development.

SPINAL ALIGNMENT

Assess the school-age child and adolescent for **scoliosis**, a lateral spine curvature. Stand behind the child, observing the height of the shoulders and hips (Figure 33–31). Ask the child to bend forward slowly at the waist, with the head and arms toward the floor. No lateral curve should be present in either position. The ribs normally stay flat bilaterally. The lumbar concave curve should flatten with forward flexion (Figure 33–32). A lateral curve to the spine or a one-sided rib hump is an indication of scoliosis (see Chapter 56).

Inspection of the Upper Extremities

The alignment of the arms is normally straight, with a minimal angle at the elbows, where the bones articulate.

Count the fingers. Extra finger digits (*polydactyly*) or webbed fingers (*syndactyly*) are abnormal. Inspect the creases on the palmar surface of each hand (Figure 33–33). Multiple creases across the palm are normal.

Inspect the nails for size, shape, and color. Nails are normally convex, smooth, and pink. **Clubbing**, widening of the nail bed with an increased angle between the proximal nail fold and nail, is abnormal (see Figure 47–3 in Chapter 47). Clubbing is associated with chronic respiratory and cardiac conditions.

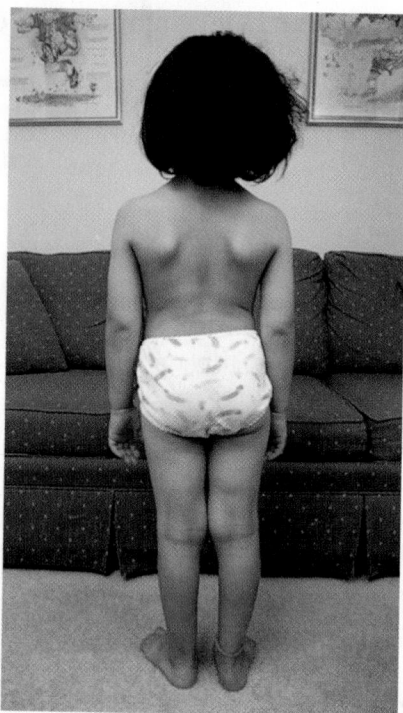

Figure 33–31 When evaluating spinal alignment, look at the level of the iliac crests and shoulders to see if they are level. Are creases at the waist similar or more prominent on one side? What signs does this child have? This child may have scoliosis.

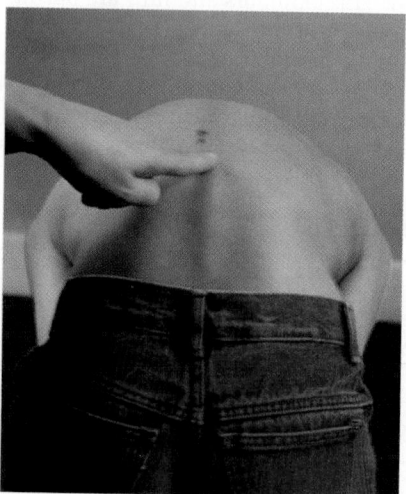

Figure 33–32 To inspect the spine for scoliosis ask the child to slowly bend forward at the waist with arms extended toward the floor. Run your forefinger down the spinal processes, palpating each vertebra for a change in alignment. A lateral curve to the spine or a one-sided rib hump is an indication of scoliosis.

Inspection of the Lower Extremities

Assess the hips of newborns and young infants for dislocation or subluxation. First inspect and compare the number of skinfolds on the upper legs. An uneven number of skinfolds may indicate a hip dislocation or difference in leg length. Then

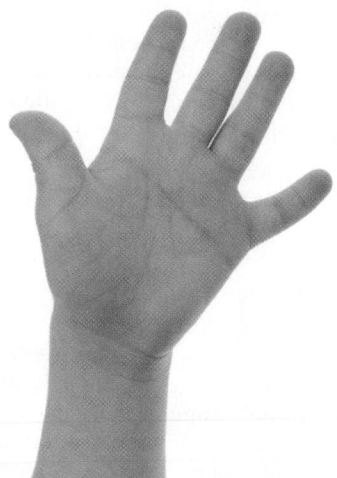

Figure 33–33 Transverse crease on palmar surface of the hand is associated with Down syndrome.

SOURCE: EVAfotografie/Getty Images.

check for the Allis sign, a difference in knee height symmetry (Figure 33–34). The Ortolani-Barlow maneuver is used to assess an infant's hips for dislocation or subluxation during the first year of life. (See Figure 24–36.)

View the child from behind and observe as the child stands on one leg and then the other. The iliac crests should stay level. If the iliac crest on the lifted leg appears lower, the hip abductor muscles on the weight-bearing side are weak, known as the *Trendelenburg sign*.

LEGS AND FEET

Inspect the alignment of the legs with the child standing. After a child is 4 years of age, the alignment of the long bones is expected to be straight at the knees and ankles. The alignment of the lower extremities in infants and toddlers changes as bones straighten with weight bearing. To evaluate the toddler with bowlegs, have the child stand on a firm surface. Measure the distance between the knees when the child's ankles are together. No more than 1.5 in. (3.5 cm) between the knees is normal. See Figure 33–35 for assessment of knock-knees.

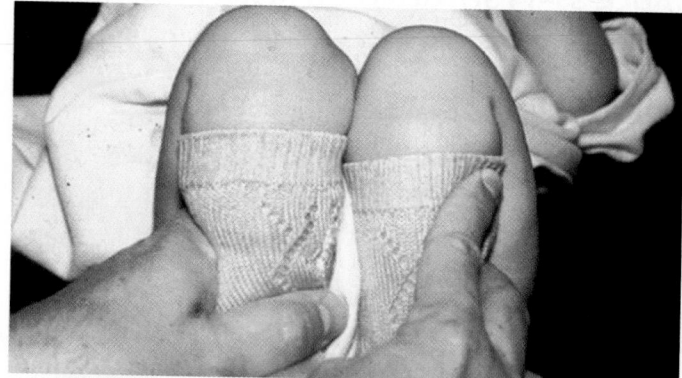

Figure 33–34 To check knee height symmetry flex the infant's hips and knees so the heels are as close to the buttocks as possible. Place the feet flat on the examining table. The knees are usually the same height. A difference in knee height (Allis sign), as seen here, is an indicator of hip dislocation.

SOURCE: Used with permission International Hip Dysplasia Institute.

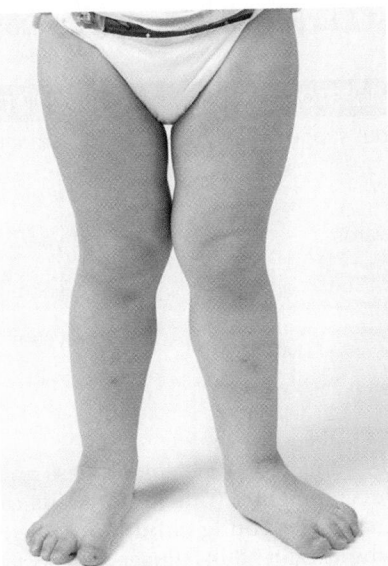

Figure 33–35 To evaluate the child with knock-knees, have the child stand on a firm surface. Measure the distance between the ankles when the child stands with the knees together. The normal distance is not more than 2 in. (5 cm) between the ankles.

Growth and Development Leg Alignment

Infants are often born with a twisting of the tibia caused by positioning in utero (tibial torsion). The infant's toes turn in as a result of the tibial torsion. Toddlers go through a skeletal alignment sequence of bowlegs (genu varum) and knock-knees (genu valgum) before the legs assume a straight alignment.

Inspect the feet for alignment, the presence of all toes, and any deformities. The weight-bearing line of the feet is usually in alignment with the legs. Many newborns have a flexible forefoot inversion (*metatarsus adductus*) that results from uterine positioning. Any fixed deformity is abnormal.

Inspect the feet for the presence of an arch when the child is standing. Children up to 3 years of age normally have a fat pad over the arch, giving the appearance of flat feet. Older children normally have a longitudinal arch. The arch is usually seen when the child stands on tiptoe or is sitting. Inspect the nails of the feet as for the hands.

Assessing the Nervous System

The nervous system is assessed for cognitive function, balance, coordination, cranial nerve function, sensation, and reflexes. Equipment needed for this examination includes a reflex hammer, cotton balls, a penlight, and tongue blades.

Clinical Tip

The neurologic examination provides an opportunity to develop rapport with the child. Many of the procedures can be presented as games that young children enjoy. You can assess cognitive function by how well the child follows directions for tests of strength and coordination. As the assessment proceeds, the child develops trust and may be more cooperative with examination of other body systems.

Cognitive Function

Observe the child's behavior, facial expressions, gestures, communication skills, activity level, and level of consciousness to assess cognitive functioning. Match the neurologic examination to the child's stage of development. For example, cognitive function is evaluated much differently in infants than in older children because infants cannot use words to communicate.

BEHAVIOR

The alertness of infants and children is indicated by their behavior. Infants and toddlers are curious but seek the security of the parent either by clinging or by making frequent eye contact. Older children are often anxious and watch the examiner's actions. Lack of interest in assessment or treatment procedures may indicate a serious illness. Excessive activity or an unusually short attention span may be associated with an attention deficit hyperactivity disorder.

COMMUNICATION SKILLS

Speech, language development, and social skills provide good clues to cognitive functioning. Listen to speech articulation and words used, comparing the child's performance with standards of social development and expected language development for age (Table 33–16). Toddlers can normally follow simple directions such as, "Show me your mouth." By 3 years of age, the child's speech should be easily understood. Delay in language and social skill development may be associated with cognitive disability or hearing loss.

MEMORY

Immediate, recent, and remote memory can be tested in children starting at approximately 4 years of age. Immediate memory can be tested by asking the child to repeat a series of words or numbers, such as the names of favorite characters from a book, television show, or movie. Children can remember more words or numbers with age: three words or numbers at age 4 years, four words or numbers at age 5 years, and five words or numbers at age 6 years.

TABLE 33–16 Expected Language Development for Age

LANGUAGE MILESTONES	AGE ATTAINED
Babbles speechlike sounds, including *p*, *b*, and *m*	4–6 months
Has 1–2 words like *mama*, *dada*, *bye-bye*	12 months
Increases words each month; two-word combinations (e.g., "Where baby?" and "Want cookie")	1–2 years
Two- to three-word sentences to ask for things or talk about things; large vocabulary; speech understood by family members	2–3 years
Sentences may have four or more words; speech understood by most people	3–4 years
Says most sounds correctly except a few like *l*, *s*, *r*, *v*, *z*, *ch*, *sh*, *th*; tells stories and uses same grammar as rest of family	4–5 years

Source: Data from American Speech and Language Association. (2014). *How does your child hear and talk?* Retrieved from http://www.asha.org/public/speech/development/chart.htm

To evaluate recent memory, ask the child to repeat and then remember a special name or object (e.g., Cinderella or hamburger). Then 5 to 10 minutes later during the examination, have the child recall the name or object. To evaluate remote memory, ask the child to repeat his or her address or birth date or a nursery rhyme. By 5 or 6 years of age, children are normally able to recall this information without difficulty.

LEVEL OF CONSCIOUSNESS

When approaching the infant or child, observe his or her level of consciousness and activity, including facial expressions, gestures, and interaction. Children are normally alert, and sleeping children arouse easily. The child who cannot be awakened is unconscious. A lowered level of consciousness may be associated with a number of neurologic conditions such as a brain injury, seizure, infection, or brain tumor.

Cerebellar Function

Observe the young child at play to assess coordination and balance. Development of fine motor skills in infants and preschool children provides clues to cerebellar function.

BALANCE

Observe the child's balance during play activities such as walking, standing on one foot, and hopping. See Table 33–17 for expected balance milestones for age. The Romberg procedure can also be used to test balance in children over 3 years of age (Figure 33–36). Once balance and other motor skills are attained, children do not normally stumble or fall when tested. Poor balance may indicate cerebellar dysfunction or an inner ear disturbance.

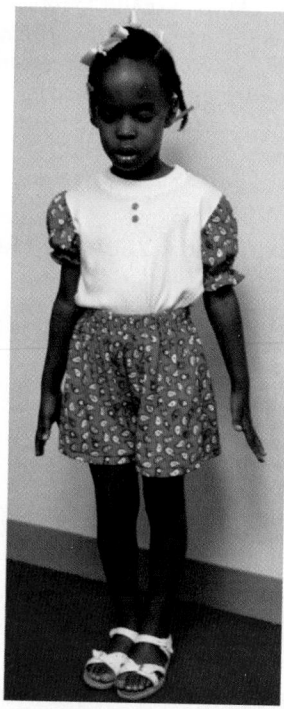

Figure 33–36 Use the Romberg procedure to evaluate balance. Ask the child to stand with feet together and eyes closed. Protect the child from falling by standing close. Preschool-age children may extend their arms to maintain balance, but older children can normally stand with their arms at their sides.

TABLE 33–17 Expected Balance Development for Age

BALANCE MILESTONES	AGE ATTAINED
Stands without support briefly	12 months
Walks alone well	15 months
Walks backwards	2 years
Balances on 1 foot momentarily	3 years
Hops on 1 foot	4 years

COORDINATION

Tests of coordination assess the smoothness and accuracy of movement. Development of fine motor skills can be used to assess coordination in young children (Table 33–18). After 6 years of age, the tests for adults (finger-to-nose, finger-to-finger, heel-to-shin, and alternating motion) can be used (Figure 33–37). Jerky movements or inaccurate pointing (past pointing) indicate poor coordination, which can be associated with delayed development or a cerebellar lesion.

GAIT

A normal gait requires intact bones and joints, muscle strength, coordination, and balance. Inspect the walking child from both the front and rear views. The iliac crests are normally level during walking, and no limp is expected. Toddlers beginning to walk have a wide-based gait and limited balance, and eventually gain more balance and a more narrow-based gait.

A limp may indicate injury or joint disease. Staggering or falling may indicate cerebellar ataxia. *Scissoring*, in which the thighs tend to cross forward over each other with each step, may be associated with cerebral palsy or other spastic conditions.

Cranial Nerve Function

To assess the cranial nerves in infants and young children, modify the procedures used to assess school-age children and adults (Table 33–19). Abnormalities of cranial nerves may be associated with compression due to an injury, tumor, or infection in the brain.

TABLE 33–18 Expected Fine Motor Development for Age

FINE MOTOR MILESTONES	AVERAGE AGE ATTAINED (MONTHS)
Reaches for a toy with one hand	4
Transfers objects between hands, brings objects to mouth	6
Thumb finger grasp to pick up small objects	9
Bangs items together, releases toy without help	12
Uses spoon to feed self	18
Builds tower of four or more blocks	24

Source: Data from Centers for Disease Control and Prevention. (2014). *Developmental milestones.* Retrieved from http://www.cdc.gov/ncbddd/actearly/milestones/index.html

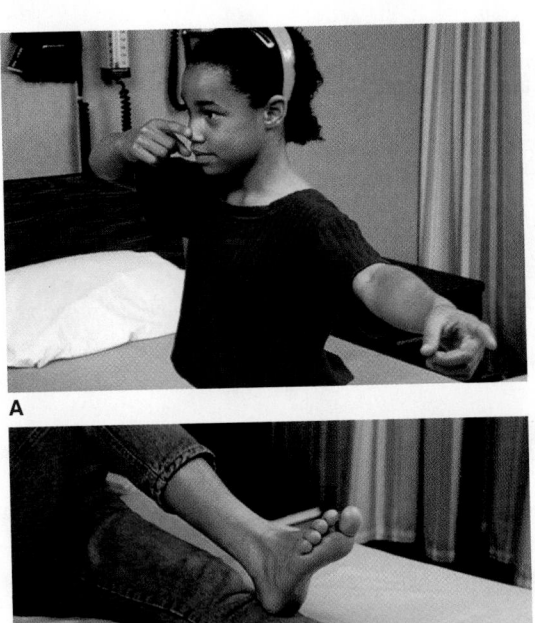

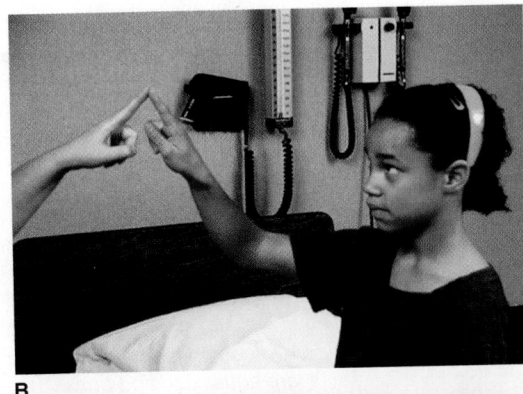

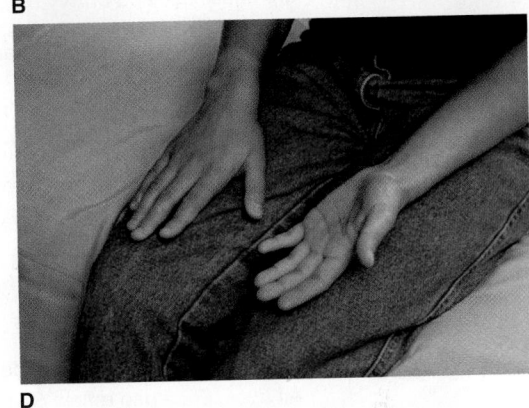

Figure 33–37 Tests of coordination. *A, Finger-to-nose test.* Ask the child to close the eyes and touch the nose, alternating the index fingers of the hands. *B, Finger-to-finger test.* Ask the child to alternately touch his or her nose and your index finger with his or her index finger. Move your hand to several positions within the child's reach to test pointing accuracy. Repeat the test with the child's other hand. *C, Heel-to-shin test.* Ask the child to rub his or her leg from the knee to the ankle with the heel of the other foot. Repeat the test with the other foot. This test is normally performed without hesitation or inappropriate placement of the foot. *D, Rapid alternating motion test.* Ask the child to rapidly rotate his or her wrist so the palm and dorsum of the hand alternately pat the thigh. Repeat the test with the other hand. Hesitating movements are abnormal. Mirroring movements of the hand not being tested indicate a delay in coordination skill refinement.

Sensory Function

To assess sensory function, compare the responses of the body to various types of stimulation. Bilateral equal responses are normal. Loss of sensation may indicate a brain or spinal cord lesion. Withdrawal responses to painful procedures indicate normal sensory function in an infant.

To test *superficial tactile sensation*, stroke the skin on the lower leg or arm with a cotton ball or a finger while the child's eyes are closed. Cooperative children over 2 years of age can normally point to the location touched.

To test *superficial pain sensation*, ask the child to close the eyes, and touch the child in various places on each arm and leg. Alternate the sharp and dull ends of a broken tongue blade or a paper clip. Children over 4 years of age can normally distinguish between a sharp and dull sensation each time. To improve the child's accuracy with the test, let the child practice describing the difference between the sharp and dull stimulations.

An inability to identify superficial touch and pain sensations may indicate sensory loss. Identify the extent of sensory loss, such as all areas below the knee. Other sensory function tests (temperature, vibratory, deep pressure pain, and position

sense) are performed when sensory loss is found. Refer to other texts for a description of these procedures.

Common Newborn Reflexes

Evaluate the movement and posture of newborns and young infants by the Moro, palmar grasp, plantar grasp, placing, stepping, and tonic neck newborn reflexes. These reflexes appear and disappear at expected intervals in the first few months of life as the central nervous system develops. Movements are normally equal bilaterally. An asymmetric response may indicate a serious neurologic problem on the less responsive side. (See Table 24–4, *Common Newborn Reflexes,* for more information.)

Superficial and Deep Tendon Reflexes

Evaluate the superficial and deep tendon reflexes to assess the function of specific segments of the spine.

SUPERFICIAL REFLEXES

Assess superficial reflexes by stroking a specific area of the body. The plantar reflex, testing spine levels L4 to S2, is routinely

TABLE 33–19 Age-Specific Procedures for Assessment of Cranial Nerves in Infants and Children

CRANIAL NERVE[a]	ASSESSMENT PROCEDURE AND NORMAL FINDINGS[b]
I Olfactory	Infant: Not tested.
	Child: Not routinely tested. Give familiar odors to child to sniff, one naris at a time. *Identifies odors such as orange, peanut butter, and chocolate.*
II Optic	Infant: Shine a bright light in eyes. *A quick blink reflex and dorsal head flexion indicate light perception.*
	Child: Test vision and visual fields if cooperative. *Visual acuity appropriate for age.*
(III Oculomotor) (IV Trochlear) (VI Abducens)	Infant: Shine a penlight at the eyes and move it side to side. *Focuses on and tracks the light to each side.*
	Child: Move an object through the six cardinal points of gaze. *Tracks object through all fields of gaze.*
	All ages: Inspect eyelids for drooping. Inspect pupillary response to light. *Eyelids do not droop and pupils are equal size and briskly respond to light.*
V Trigeminal	Infant: Stimulate the rooting and sucking reflex. *Turns head toward stimulation at side of mouth and sucking has good strength and pattern.*
	Child: Observe the child chewing a cracker. Touch forehead and cheeks with cotton ball when eyes are closed. *Bilateral jaw strength is good. Child points to location touched by cotton ball.*
VII Facial	All ages: Observe facial expressions when crying, smiling, frowning, etc. *Facial features stay symmetric bilaterally.*
VIII Acoustic	Infant: Produce a loud sound near the head. *Blinks in response to sound, moves head toward sound or freezes position.*
	Child: Whisper words and ask for them to be repeated. *Repeats words correctly.*
(IX Glossopharyngeal) (X Vagus)	Infant: Observe swallowing during feeding. *Good swallowing pattern.*
	All ages: Elicit gag reflex. *Gags with stimulation.*
XI Spinal accessory	Infant: Not tested.
	Child: Ask child to raise the shoulders and turn the head side to side against resistance. *Good strength in neck and shoulders.*
XII Hypoglossal	Infant: Observe feeding. *Sucking and swallowing are coordinated.*
	Child: Tell the child to stick out the tongue. Listen to speech. *Tongue is midline with no tremors. Words are clearly articulated.*

[a]Bracketed nerves are tested together.
[b]Italic text indicates normal findings.

evaluated in children (Figure 33–38). The cremasteric reflex is assessed in boys by stroking the inner thigh of each leg. The testicle and scrotum on the stroked side normally rise.

DEEP TENDON REFLEXES

To assess the deep tendon reflexes, tap a tendon near specific joints with a reflex hammer (or with the index finger for infants), comparing responses bilaterally. Inspect for movement in the associated joint and palpate the strength of the expected muscle contraction. The numeric scoring of deep tendon reflexes is as follows:

Grade	Response Interpretation
0	No response
1+	Slow, minimal response
2+	Expected response, active
3+	More active or pronounced than expected
4+	Hyperactive, clonus may be present

Table 33–20 provides guidelines for assessment of the biceps, triceps, brachioradialis, patellar, and Achilles deep tendon reflexes. The best response to deep tendon reflex testing is

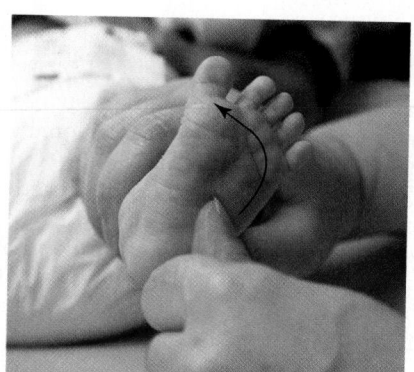

Figure 33–38 To assess the plantar reflex, stroke the bottom of the infant's or child's foot in the direction of the arrow. Watch the toes for plantar flexion or the *Babinski response*, fanning, and dorsiflexion of the big toe (as seen here). The Babinski response is normal in children under 2 years of age. Plantar flexion of the toes is the normal response in older children. A Babinski response in children over 2 years of age can indicate neurologic disease.

TABLE 33–20 Assessment of Deep Tendon Reflexes and the Associated Spinal Segment Tested

DEEP TENDON REFLEX	TECHNIQUE AND NORMAL FINDINGS*	SPINE SEGMENT TESTED
Biceps 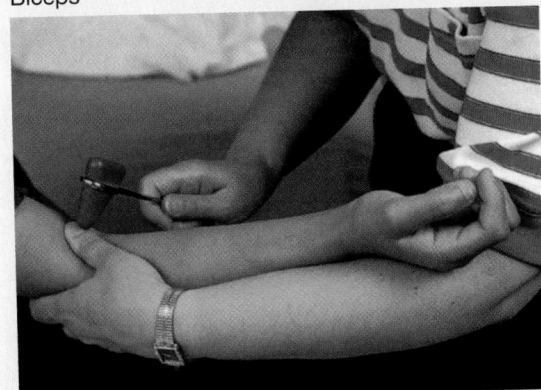	Flex the child's arm at the elbow, and place your thumb over the biceps tendon in the antecubital fossa. Tap your thumb. *Elbow flexes as the biceps muscle contracts.*	C5 and C6
Triceps 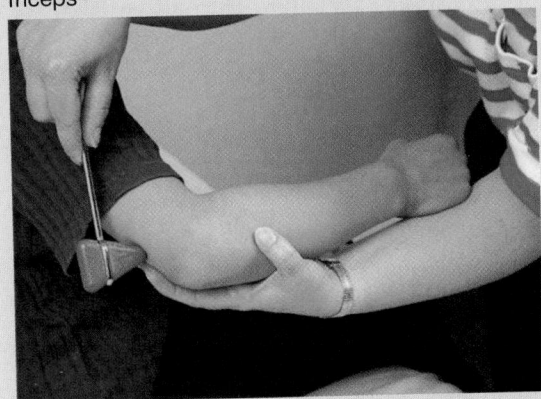	With the child's arm flexed, tap the triceps tendon above the elbow. *Elbow extends as the triceps muscle contracts.*	C6, C7, and C8
Brachioradialis 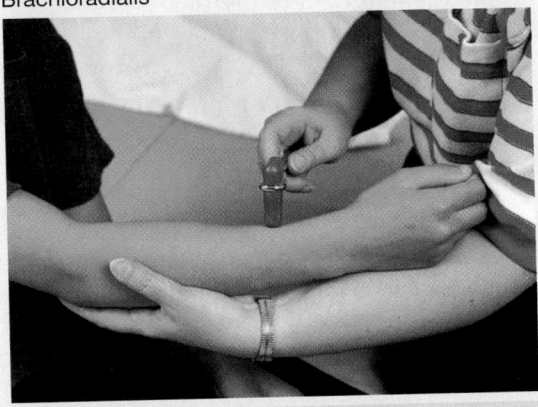	Lay the child's arm with the thumb upright over your arm. Tap the brachioradial tendon 2.5 cm (1 in.) above the wrist. *Forearm pronates (palm facing downward) and elbow flexes.*	C5 and C6
Patellar 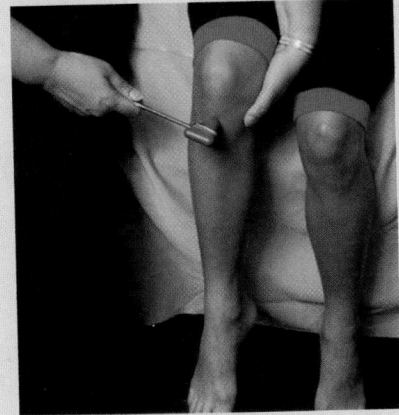	Flex the child's knees, and when the legs are relaxed, tap the patellar tendon just below the knee. *Knee extends (knee jerk) as the quadriceps muscle contracts.*	L2, L3, and L4

(continued)

TABLE 33–20 Assessment of Deep Tendon Reflexes and the Associated Spinal Segment Tested (*continued*)

DEEP TENDON REFLEX	TECHNIQUE AND NORMAL FINDINGS*	SPINE SEGMENT TESTED
Achilles 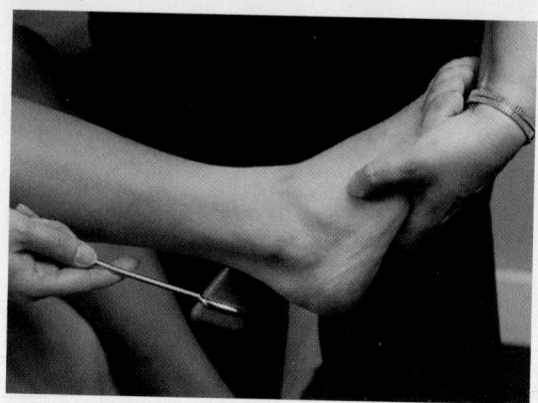	While the child's legs are flexed, support the foot and tap the Achilles tendon. *Plantar flexion (ankle jerk) as the gastrocnemius muscle contracts.*	S1 and S2

*Italic text indicates normal findings.

achieved when the child is relaxed or distracted. Making the child focus on another set of muscles may provide a more accurate response. When testing the reflexes on the lower legs, have the child press the hands together or try to pull them apart when gripped together. Responses are normally symmetric bilaterally. The absence of a response is associated with decreased muscle tone and strength. Hyperactive responses are associated with muscle spasticity.

Performing an Intermittent Examination

In a hospital setting after a more comprehensive physical examination at time of admission, the nurse performs a focused assessment to monitor the child's status at intervals appropriate for the child's condition. This assessment includes a general health status overview and a more focused review of the body systems or body regions affected by the child's condition. Findings are compared with prior assessments to determine a change that would indicate a need for a more comprehensive assessment.

The general health status overview for all children includes the following:

- Alertness, responsiveness, or ability to interact
- Cardiorespiratory status—color, ease of breathing, vital signs
- Comfort level or pain score
- Movement of extremities
- Behavior—age appropriateness
- Skin—color, temperature, resilience, swelling
- Fluid and food intake
- Bowel function and urinary output
- Focused assessment of the body systems or body regions affected by child's condition and response to treatment (e.g., respiratory infection, surgery, wound)

If findings during this focused assessment reveal differences from a prior assessment, a more thorough assessment is needed.

Analyzing Data From the Physical Examination

Once the physical examination has been completed, group any abnormal findings for each system with those of other systems. Use clinical judgment to identify common patterns of physiologic responses associated with health conditions. Individual abnormal physiologic responses are also the basis of many nursing diagnoses. Be sure to record all findings from the physical assessment legibly, in detail, and in the format approved by your institution.

Focus Your Study

- The elements of a health history include the chief concern, details about the present illness or injury, past health history, current health status, psychosocial and developmental data, family history, and review of systems. A birth history may be collected for infants.

- Communication strategies that may improve the quality of health information collected include the following: introducing yourself and explaining the purpose of the interview, providing privacy and confidentiality, using open-ended questions, and asking one question at a time. Ask the child questions when appropriate. Seek feedback to confirm your understanding of information provided.

- Several strategies may help improve the cooperation of the young child for the physical examination, such as allowing the child to stay on the parent's lap, providing an opportunity for the child to hold and inspect any equipment before it is used, and making a game out of tests for muscle strength, coordination, and developmental assessment.

- The sequence for performing a physical examination varies by the age of the child.
  - For infants and toddlers, perform procedures in a feet-to-head sequence to postpone the ear and throat examination that cause anxiety until the end. Take advantage of opportunities to listen to the lungs, heart, and abdomen when the infant is quiet or sleeping.
  - A head-to-feet sequence can be used for all other ages; however, the genital examination may be saved to the end.

- Special assessment techniques used for infants and toddlers include measuring the head circumference, palpating the fontanelles, using toys to assess vision and hearing, and keeping the child on the parent's lap.

- Examination modifications for preschoolers include using easily recognized names or words to assess hearing and memory, using play and games to assess muscle strength and coordination, and asking the child to show the teeth to begin assessment of the mouth.

- Adolescents should be asked their preference for having a parent present during the examination, and pubertal development should be assessed.

- Examples of normal variations found when examining children include hyperpigmented patches (Mongolian spots), epicanthal folds of the eyes, sucking pads in the mouth of an infant, breath sounds heard over the entire chest, a rounded chest in infants, abdominal movement with breathing, bowlegs and knock-knees, and pubertal changes.

- Evaluating the growth pattern of a child involves accurate measurements of infant length, child height, weight, and head circumference and then plotting the measurements on the appropriate growth curve for age. The child's percentile of growth for each measurement is then compared to prior measurements. The body mass index is used to determine if the child's weight is appropriate for height.

- Examples of unexpected physical examination findings that require urgent nursing intervention include altered level of consciousness, bradycardia, tachypnea, pain, signs of dehydration, stridor, retractions, and cyanosis.

Clinical Reasoning in Action

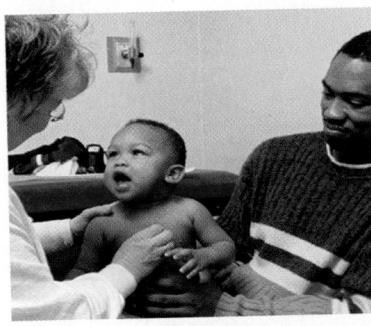

It is a relatively calm night in the children's hospital emergency department when a 6-month-old infant named Colby is brought in by emergency personnel from an automobile crash. Colby was buckled in his infant rear-facing car safety seat, riding with his parents when another car rear-ended them. The parents were not hurt and did not need to go to the hospital. The father immediately called 911 on his cell phone after the crash. When the ambulance arrived at the emergency department, the EMT gave you this report. Colby was alert and quiet in his father's arms when the ambulance arrived on the scene, and he did not have any obvious signs of injury. Colby and his father were brought to the hospital to make sure Colby did not sustain any injuries from the crash. His vital signs are as follows: temperature—98.9°F, respirations—32, pulse—110, and blood pressure—85/39. Colby is in no apparent distress. His pupils are equal, round, and reactive to light. His anterior fontanelle is flat, and he has equal movements of extremities. His breath sounds are clear and equal bilaterally. His heart sounds have a regular rate and rhythm without murmur. He voided around 2 hours ago, before the accident.

1. The fontanelles are an important body part to examine in infants and toddlers. In the scenario with Colby, it can give an indication of increased intracranial pressure related to a brain injury. Describe the placement of the fontanelles, and when they are expected to close and no longer be palpated. Why is the head more likely to sustain injury in an infant like Colby versus an adult?

2. After reviewing the scenario, what can you tell the parents about Colby's vital signs at this time? What is the difference between adult vital signs and Colby's vital signs?

3. What observations are made to check Colby's mental status?

4. If a heart murmur were to be found on examination of Colby, what would be the five ways to describe it?

References

American Academy of Pediatrics Committee on Practice and Ambulatory Medicine. (2011). Use of chaperones during the physical examination of the pediatric patient. *Pediatrics, 127*(5), 991–993.

American Association for Pediatric Ophthalmology and Strabismus. (2014). *Vision screening recommendations*. Retrieved from http://www.aapos.org/terms/conditions/131

American Speech and Language Association. (2014). *How does your child hear and talk?* Retrieved from http://www.asha.org/public/speech/development/chart.htm

Anderst, J. D., Carpenter, S. L., Abshire, T. C., & the Section on Hematology/Oncology and Committee on Child Abuse and Neglect. (2013). Evaluation for bleeding disorders in suspected child abuse. *Pediatrics, 131*(4), e1314–1322.

Bernstein, D. (2016). Coarctation of the aorta. In R. M. Kliegman, B. F. Stanton, J. W. St. Geme, & N. F. Schor (Eds.), *Nelson textbook of pediatrics* (20th ed., pp. 2205–2207). Philadelphia, PA: Elsevier.

Biro, F. M., Greenspan, L. C., Galvez, M. P., Pinney, S. M., Teitelbaum, S., Windham, G. C., . . . Wolff, M. S. (2013). Onset of breast development in a longitudinal cohort. *Pediatrics, 132*(5), 1–9.

Brown, N. (2011). Adolescent medicine. In M. M. Tschudy & K. M. Arcara (Eds.), *The Harriet Lane handbook* (19th ed., pp. 118–135). St. Louis, MO: Elsevier.

Centers for Disease Control and Prevention. (2014). *Developmental milestones*. Retrieved from http://www.cdc.gov/ncbddd/actearly/milestones/index.html

Chameides, L., Samson, R. A., Schexnayder, S. M., & Hazinski, M. F. (Eds.). (2011). *Pediatric advanced life support: Provider manual*. Dallas, TX: American Heart Association.

Herman-Giddens, M. E., Bourdony, C. J., Dowshen, S. A., & Reiter, E. O. (2011). *Assessment of sexual maturity stages in girls and boys.* Elk Grove Village, IL: American Academy of Pediatrics.

Herman-Giddens, M. E., Steffes, J., Harris, D., Slora, E., Hussey, M., Dowshen, S. A., . . . Reiter, E. O. (2012). Secondary sexual characteristics in boys: Data from the Pediatric Research in Office Settings Network. *Pediatrics, 130*(5), e1058–e1068.

Hochberg, Z., & Belsky, J. (2013). Evo-devo of human adolescence: beyond disease models of early puberty. *BMC Medicine, 11,* 113. doi:10.1186/1741-7015-11-113

Hummel, P. (2011). Newborn assessment. In E. M. Chiocca (Ed.), *Advanced pediatric assessment* (pp. 199–229).

Philadelphia, PA: Wolters Kluwer Lippincott Williams & Wilkins.

Lande, M. B. (2016). Systemic hypertension. In R. M. Kliegman, B. F. Stanton, J. W. St. Geme, & N. F. Schor (Eds.), *Nelson textbook of pediatrics* (20th ed., pp. 2294–2303). Philadelphia, PA: Elsevier.

Loomba-Albrecht, L. A., & Styne, D. M. (2012). The physiology of puberty and its disorders. *Pediatric Annals, 41*(4), e73–e80. doi: 10.3928/00904481-20120307-08

Olitsky, S. E., Hug, D., Plummer, L. S., Stahl, E. D., Ariss, M. M., & Lindquist, T. P. (2016). Abnormalities of pupil and iris. In R. M. Kliegman, B. F. Stanton, J. W. St. Geme, & N. F. Schor (Eds.), *Nelson textbook of pediatrics* (20th ed., pp. 3023–3026). Philadelphia, PA: Elsevier.

Pappas, D. E., & Hendly, J. O. (2016). Sinusitis. In R. M. Kliegman, B. F. Stanton, J. W. St. Geme, & N. F. Schor (Eds.), *Nelson textbook of pediatrics* (20th ed., pp. 2014–2017). Philadelphia, PA: Elsevier.

Purnell, L. D. (2014). *Guide to culturally competent care* (3rd ed.). Philadelphia, PA: F. A. Davis.

Susman, E. J., Houts, R. M., Steinberg, L., Belsky, J., Cauffman, E., De Hart, G., . . . Eunice Kennedy Shriver NICHD Early Child Care Research Network. (2010). Longitudinal development of secondary sexual characteristics in girls and boys between ages 9½ and 15½ years. *Archives of Pediatric and Adolescent Medicine, 164*(2), 166–173.

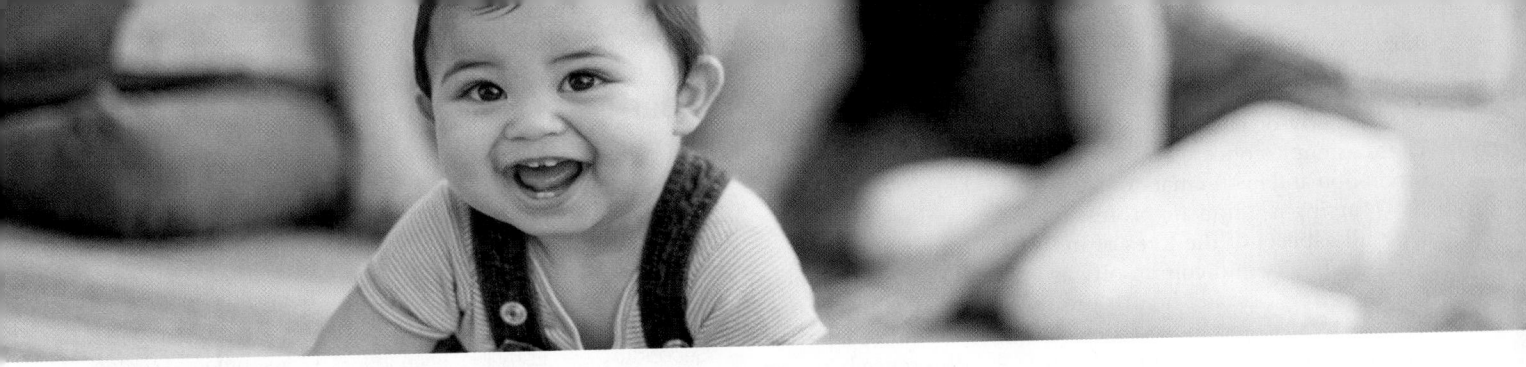

Chapter 34
Health Promotion and Maintenance: General Concepts, the Newborn, and the Infant

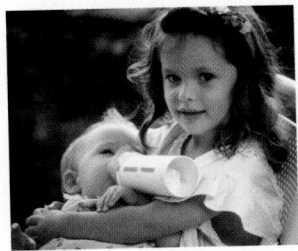

Roger Charity/Getty Images

Mommy was really glad to go see the nurse today. She brought our baby and me. Grandma said that they would give us a card that would help us buy food. I'm glad because I'm tired of eating peanut butter. Mommy said we could get some milk and juice, and even some chicken.

—Melody, age 4, sister of 7-month-old Amanda

Learning Outcomes

34.1 Define health promotion and health maintenance.

34.2 Describe how health promotion and health maintenance are facilitated by partnering with families during health supervision visits.

34.3 Describe the components of a health supervision visit.

34.4 Apply the preventive care schedule for screenings and health assessment.

34.5 Analyze the nurse's role in providing health promotion and health maintenance for the newborn and infant.

34.6 Perform the general observations made of infants and their families as they come to the pediatric healthcare home for health supervision visits.

34.7 Synthesize the areas of assessment and intervention for health supervision visits of newborns and infants: growth and developmental surveillance, nutrition, physical activity, oral health, mental and spiritual health, family and social relations, disease prevention strategies, and injury prevention strategies.

34.8 Plan health promotion and health maintenance strategies employed during health supervision visits of newborns and infants.

34.9 Recognize the importance of family in newborn and infant health care, and include family assessment and collaboration in each health supervision visit.

A major goal of *Healthy People 2020* is to help individuals attain long, healthy lives free of preventable disease, disability, injury, and premature death across all life stages (U.S. Department of Health and Human Services, 2011). The concepts of health promotion and health maintenance provide for nursing interventions that contribute to meeting these goals. Many students in health professions begin their studies with a strong interest in the care of ill individuals. However, as time progresses, they learn that "well" people also care. They need teaching to improve diet, reduce stress, and obtain

851

immunizations. They may seek information about how to exercise properly or ensure a safe environment for their children. These examples of care and teaching are components of health promotion and health maintenance.

Nursing is a holistic profession that examines and works with all aspects of the lives of individuals, and has a strong focus on family and community as well. Nurses are uniquely positioned to provide health promotion and health maintenance activities, and indeed these activities should be a part of each encounter with families. What is the difference between health promotion and health maintenance? When should nurses engage in activities that focus on health? How are these activities integrated into health supervision visits for the infant and young child? How do nurses partner with other healthcare professionals to offer comprehensive health services in settings accessible to parents and young children? How can nurses help children and their families to maximize length and quality of life? These are some of the questions that will be explored in this chapter, with specific activities that target families with newborns, infants, and young children.

General Concepts

To understand health promotion and health maintenance, it is important to develop a definition of health. The World Health Organization (WHO) defines **health** as a state of complete physical, mental, and social well-being and not merely the absence of disease and infirmity (WHO, 2010). Others view the quality of "complete well-being" as impossible to attain, and therefore have further developed the concept to apply to persons with health challenges as well as those who are "healthy." Health in this expanded view is dynamic, changing, and unfolding; it is the realization of a state of actualization or potential (Pender, Murdaugh, & Parsons, 2015). This basic human right is necessary for the development of societies, so social determinants of health status are increasingly the focus of research and public policy.

Health promotion refers to activities that increase well-being and enhance wellness or health (Pender et al., 2015). These activities lead to actualization of positive health potential for all individuals, including those with chronic or acute conditions, as well as persons whose social experiences puts them at risk for poor health. Examples include providing information and resources in order to:

- Enhance good nutrition at each developmental stage
- Integrate physical activity into the child's daily events
- Provide adequate housing
- Promote oral health
- Foster positive personality development

Health promotion is concerned with development of strategies that seek to foster conditions that allow populations to be healthy and to make healthy choices (WHO, 2011). Nurses engage in health promotion by partnering with children and families to promote family strengths in the areas of lifestyles, social development, coping, and family interactions. They also provide **anticipatory guidance** for families because they understand the child's upcoming developmental stages, and they teach families how to provide an environment that helps children achieve the milestones of each stage. This concept is explored more fully later in this chapter. Some nurses become involved in public policy forums in their communities in order to improve the social determinants of health, such as access to care, nutritious foods, and safe environments.

TABLE 34–1 Levels of Preventive Health Maintenance Activities

LEVEL	DESCRIPTION	EXAMPLES OF NURSING ACTIONS
Primary prevention	Activities that decrease opportunity for illness or injury	Giving immunizations Teaching about car safety seats
Secondary prevention	Early identification and treatment of a condition to lessen its severity	Developmental screening Vision and hearing screening
Tertiary prevention	Reduction in the consequences of a disease or condition with aim of restoring optimal function	Rehabilitation activities for child after a car crash

Source: Data from Centers for Disease Control and Prevention (CDC). (2013). *The concept of prevention.* Retrieved from http://www.cdc.gov/arthritis/temp/pilots-201208/pilot1/online/arthritis-challenge/03-Prevention/concept.htm

Health maintenance (or health protection) refers to activities that preserve an individual's present state of health and that prevent disease or injury occurrence. Examples of these activities include conducting developmental screening or surveillance to identify early deviations from normal development, providing immunizations to prevent illnesses, and teaching about common childhood safety hazards. Health maintenance activities are commonly preventive, and terminology common to community or public health nursing explains the levels and aims of preventive actions. Prevention levels are identified as primary prevention, secondary prevention, and tertiary prevention (Table 34–1).

While it is clear that health promotion and health maintenance activities are closely linked and often overlap, there are some differences. Health maintenance focuses on known potential health risks and seeks to prevent them or to identify them early so that intervention can occur. Health promotion looks at the strengths and goals of individuals, families, and populations, and seeks to use them to assist in reaching higher levels of wellness. It involves partnerships with the family as health goals are set, and with other health professionals and resources to provide for meeting a family's goals. Nurses apply both health promotion and health maintenance concepts when providing health care, recognizing that the concepts overlap. Health promotion and health maintenance are integrated into healthcare visits for children, with the care provider applying both knowledge of health maintenance concepts and adding information the family has identified that will assist in increasing health or wellness (health promotion). These activities commonly take place at "well-child" or health supervision visits.

Health supervision for children is the provision of services that focus on disease and injury prevention (health maintenance), growth and developmental surveillance, and health promotion at key intervals during the child's life. What health promotion and health maintenance activities are parts of health supervision visits? How can these activities be integrated into all settings where care is provided for children? What are the recommended times for health visits to occur and what care is provided at certain times? How can health supervision visits be organized to accomplish the goals of the family and health professionals? In this chapter and the following two chapters, we discuss the integration of health supervision in various settings, recommended schedules for health supervision visits, and partnering with families to achieve health goals and promote child development.

All children need a medical home, where accessible, continuous, and coordinated health supervision is provided during the developmental years. *Accessibility* refers to both financial and geographic access; *continuous* indicates that the care is ongoing with consistent care providers; *coordination* refers to the need for communication among health professionals to provide for the needs of the child. A medical home or **pediatric healthcare home** is therefore the site where comprehensive, family-centered, culturally effective, and compassionate health care is provided by a pediatric healthcare professional focused on the overall well-being of children and families (American Academy of Pediatrics, 2014). When a family has an established partnership with a healthcare provider, family-centered health services can be provided based on the family's risks and protective factors. These services may be provided in physicians' offices, community health clinics, the home, schools, childcare centers, shelters, or mobile vans (Figure 34–1). Coordination of care among these entities promotes the concept of a medical neighborhood that includes all components of care, with seamless flow of health information (Taylor, Lake, Nysenbaum, et al., 2011). The U.S. Department of Health and Human Services, the American Academy of Pediatrics (AAP), and the American Medical Association have developed national guidelines for preventive healthcare services for infants, children, and adolescents. The National Association of Pediatric Nurse Practitioners (NAPNAP) supports the list of comprehensive services of a pediatric healthcare home identified by the AAP (AAP, 2014).

Healthy People 2020

(MICH-30.1) Increase the proportion of children who have access to a medical home

- While 57.5% of children under age 18 years had an established medical home in 2007, the objective of 63.3% of children with such access is the present goal (U.S. Department of Health and Human Services, 2011).

The health supervision visit is individualized to the family and child. Standardized screenings and examinations are included, and time is provided for the family's specific concerns and questions about the child's health and development. Nurses play an integral part in these comprehensive visits, and they partner with other healthcare providers to accomplish health supervision.

A tracking system in the pediatric healthcare home site helps to identify appropriate health supervision activities for each child at every visit. Most often, computers are used to list appropriate topics for visits at specific ages. If a child misses a visit, the family can be contacted by phone, text, or e-mail, and encouraged to come in for the recommended care. A family may be called if their child is lacking some immunizations. Recognizing that not all families get into the healthcare home for each recommended visit, every health encounter, including an episodic illness visit or care for a chronic illness, is a potential time to complete health promotion and health maintenance activities. For example, immunizations may sometimes be given during a visit for an acute condition such as otitis media (ear infection) if the child has missed a prior health supervision visit. Even when children are seen in hospitals, emergency departments, or other settings, it is important to ask about their pediatric healthcare home and when the last visit occurred. Identify children who need basic health supervision services and provide them or refer to other settings for meeting these needs at another time.

Nurses play an important role in managing health supervision visits. Depending on the setting, the nurse may provide all services or support other healthcare providers by obtaining an updated health history, screening for diseases and other conditions, conducting a developmental assessment, and providing immunizations, anticipatory guidance, and health education. Nurses in all settings are instrumental in identifying children who need health supervision and are not obtaining recommended care (Figure 34–2).

While health supervision visits can address many health-related topics, there is generally a limited time in which to engage a child or family. The nurse needs to direct the

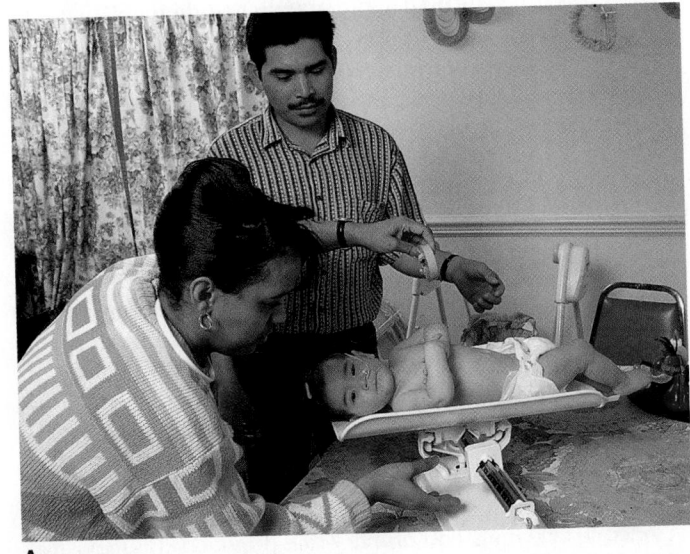

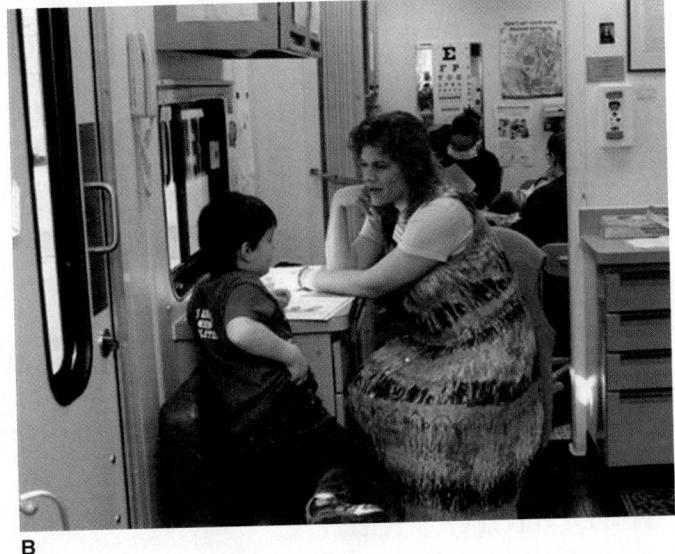

A   **B**

Figure 34–1 Delivery of health promotion services. *A,* A nurse is providing a health supervision visit in the child's home after discharge from the hospital for an acute illness. *B,* A nurse is providing information to a child visiting a mobile healthcare van.

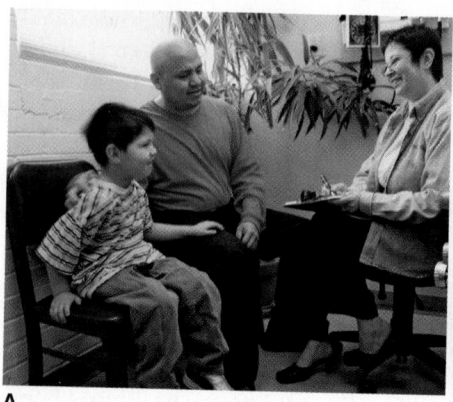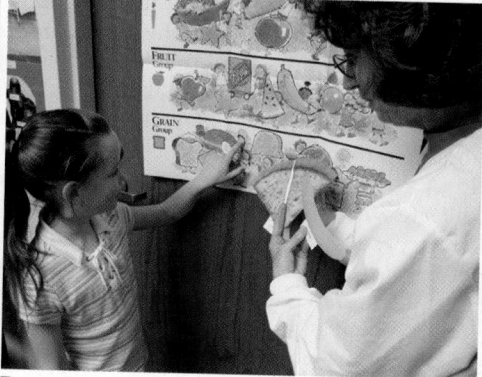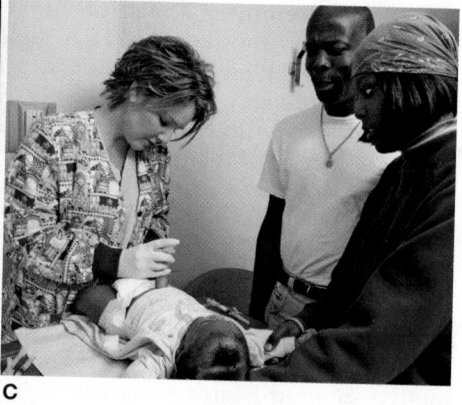

A   B   C

Figure 34–2 Identifying children who need health care. The nurse plays many roles in providing health promotion and health maintenance for children. *A,* Data are collected from the time a nurse calls the child and family to the examination room and during the history-taking phase. The nurse asks questions while observing the child's behaviors and the relationship between parent and child. The nurse also performs screening tests, including blood pressure, tuberculosis, vision and hearing, and developmental screening. *B,* Interventions that include teaching may take place. *C,* A nurse may administer immunizations as parents watch and assist by holding the child. Nurses also play important roles in teaching families information to enhance health.

encounters and have some ideas for pertinent agendas. *Bright Futures* booklets provide guidance about how the nurse can manage health supervision visits. Six concepts should be integrated into care (Hagan, Shaw, & Duncan, 2008):

1. The healthcare provider *builds effective partnerships* with the family. A **partnership** is a relationship in which participants join together to ensure healthcare delivery in a way that recognizes the critical roles and contributions of each partner in promoting health and preventing illness. The partners in child health include the child, family, health professionals, and the community.

2. The nurse *fosters family-centered communication* by showing interest in the child and family, and effectively conveying information and understanding.

3. The nurse *focuses on health promotion and health maintenance topics during visits*, recognizing that families may not initiate these discussions.

4. The nurse *manages time well* to enable health promotion topics to be addressed during visits. This includes reviewing the child's health record and selecting topics pertinent to the child's age and the family's situation.

5. The nurse *educates the family during "teachable moments."* Large teaching plans are not always needed; children and families often learn best when presented with small bits of information based on the parent's questions or the nurse's observations.

6. The nurse *becomes an advocate for child health issues.* When an issue arises while caring for a child, seek additional data from various sources, talk with others, and strategize how the problem could be solved.

Components of Health Promotion/Health Maintenance Visits

The nurse identifies and addresses pertinent topics for health promotion and health maintenance during health supervision visits. Nurses also apply their knowledge of areas that need to

be addressed with an infant or child of a particular age, and then make general observations of the child and family to identify additional topics for discussion. While categories to consider vary depending on the age of the child, the family's particular needs, and community resources, there are some common topics that generally require attention. Often, nurses start with the topics suggested for the child's age, integrating general observations as the visit progresses and further identifying assessment areas needed in particular situations. The American Academy of Pediatrics and other organizations review and make recommendations for the screening and health assessments to be included at each age.

Professionalism in Practice   Schedule for Preventive Health Services

The Recommendations for Preventive Health Care, for the child from the prenatal visit of the mother through age 21 years, were updated in 2014 and published in the journal *Pediatrics* (American Academy of Pediatrics Committee on Practice and Ambulatory Medicine, Bright Futures Periodicity Schedule Workgroup, 2014). The Patient Protection and Affordable Care Act requires the coverage of these recommendations. Some changes in the 2014 schedule include addition of congenital heart disease screening of all newborns; alcohol, drug, and depression screenings; expansion of cholesterol screening; anemia identification; and HIV screening in adolescents.

The nurse should be aware of the screening guidelines and integrate these recommendations into health supervision visits and other child healthcare settings. Screening tools for specific age groups should be readily accessible and provided to the family and primary care providers during visits. Plans should be in place for further evaluation and referral as necessary when screenings result in abnormal findings. The integration of recommended screenings and follow-up should be carefully documented in the child's record.

Pediatric nurses make *general observations* of infants and their families whenever they encounter them. Nurses who are observant during the health supervision visit have many opportunities for assessing the family. These general observations begin when the family is called in and welcomed by the nurse to the facility. They continue as the infant or child is weighed and measured, and throughout the visit. Nurses observe the physical contact between the child and other family members, the developmental tasks displayed by the child, and parental level of stress or ease in conducting childcare activities.

Growth and developmental surveillance provides important clues about the child's condition and environment. The child's height, weight, and body mass index are calculated at each health supervision visit, and results are placed on percentile charts (see Chapters 31 and 32 for more information). Parents are given the information in written form and it is interpreted for them if needed. A thorough physical assessment is performed to ensure the child is growing as expected and has no abnormal or unexplained physical findings (see Chapter 33). **Developmental surveillance** is a flexible, continuous process of skilled observations that provides data about the child's capabilities, allows for early identification of any neurologic problems, and helps to verify that the home environment is stimulating. Early development is important to later health, and it must be evaluated consistently and systematically during healthcare visits (Centers for Disease Control and Prevention [CDC], 2014a). Information may be collected from several sources—for instance, a questionnaire that the parent completes, questions asked during the interview, or observation of the child during the visit. Parents can also be interviewed to identify any developmental concerns they may have about the child or adolescent. When talking with parents, review physical, social, and communication milestones for infants, young children, older children, or adolescents. Detailed milestones for each age group are found in Chapter 31. Standardized developmental questionnaires are effective for developmental surveillance of most children, especially when time for health supervision visits is limited. Screening tests should be administered at the 9-, 18-, and the 24- or 30-month visits (CDC, 2014a; Lipkin, 2011). When performing developmental monitoring with standardized screening tools, nurses make sure all directions are followed by:

- Choosing the proper test for the child's age and desired information
- Reading directions thoroughly or using specific training tools available
- Practicing as needed until proficient with the test
- Calculating the infant's or child's age correctly, especially if premature
- Attempting to develop rapport with the infant or child to get the best performance
- Following directions for administration of items; in some cases, parents can be asked if a child demonstrates specific skills at home, especially if the child is not willing to perform an item during testing
- Noting the behavior and cooperativeness of the child during the screening process
- Analyzing the findings using the test instructions to make the correct interpretation

Failure to perform an item on a screening tool does not mean the child has failed the test (see *Developing Cultural Competence: English as a Second Language and Developmental Testing*).

The child should be reevaluated at a future visit. Schedule the appointment at a time of day when the child is awake and rested. Provide parents with guidance on specific methods for stimulating the child. Failure of multiple items is of greatest concern. Follow the guidelines of the particular developmental screening test for referral to further diagnostic developmental assessment.

Developing Cultural Competence English as a Second Language and Developmental Testing

Children who have recently come from other countries and even some born in this country who live in families from minority ethnic groups may have difficulty with some items on developmental screening tests. For example, children who are not skilled in the English language may not understand some instructions or be able to answer questions about definitions of words. When parents do not speak English as a primary language and the examiner uses English, common terms might be misinterpreted. Parents might not understand what is meant if you ask, "Does your baby have a mobile over the crib at home?" or "Is she starting to be afraid of strangers?" How can you be alert for language differences and become sensitive to miscommunication?

Nutrition evaluation is a vital part of each health supervision visit. It makes important contributions to general health and fosters growth and development. Include observations and screening relevant to nutritional intake at each health supervision visit. Eating proper foods for age and activity ensures that children have the energy for proper growth, physical activity, cognition, and immune function. Nutrition is closely linked to both health promotion and health maintenance. See Chapter 32 for detailed nutritional assessments for each age group. Find out what questions parents have about feeding their children. Use the information gathered to provide both health promotion and health maintenance interventions.

Physical activity provides many physical and psychologic health benefits. However, there is a growing disparity between recommendations and reality among most children. Research by the Centers for Disease Control and Prevention (CDC) identified that 15.2% of children from 9th to 12th grades report no free-time physical activity, while 47% had recommended activity 5 days/week and only 27% met the recommendation 7 days/week (CDC, 2014b). When schools do not offer daily physical education, many children have no regular activity. Participation in physical activity declines as youth get older, and females are considerably less active than males (CDC, 2014b). Inquire about activities the child prefers and amount of time for activity during the day. As the child grows older, include questions about sedentary activities such as number of hours spent watching television or playing computer games. Inquire if the child plays sports at school or in the community. Ask about activities in a typical day to measure amount of activity. Once the nurse gathers data about physical activity, interventions are implemented to enhance activity patterns.

Although *oral health* may seem to require the knowledge of a specialist, it has many implications that relate to general health care. Oral health is important because teeth assist in language development, impacted or infected teeth lead to systemic illness, and teeth are related to positive self-image formation. Dental caries is the most common chronic disease of children.

Many youth in the United States are affected by tooth decay and pain that interfere with activities of daily living such as eating, sleeping, attending school, and speaking (CDC, 2011a, 2011b). The nurse applies health promotion to dental health by teaching about oral care and access to dental visits. Health maintenance activities relate to prevention of caries and illness related to dental disease.

Developing Cultural Competence Unmet Dental Needs

About 6% of U.S. children have unmet dental needs, but 7% of children from families living in poverty have such needs (Child Trends, 2013). In addition, Hispanic children, children with disabilities, children with parents who have a low educational level, or those without health insurance are also more likely to have unmet dental needs (Child Trends, 2013). All children in the Medicaid program are eligible for dental coverage through the Early and Periodic Screening, Diagnostic, and Treatment (EPSDT) program. Private and public clinics in many communities provide low-cost or free care for families with limited financial resources. Many families do not realize their children could receive these services. Find out what resources are available in your state and community, and refer as needed. See Chapter 1 for further description of programs mentioned here.

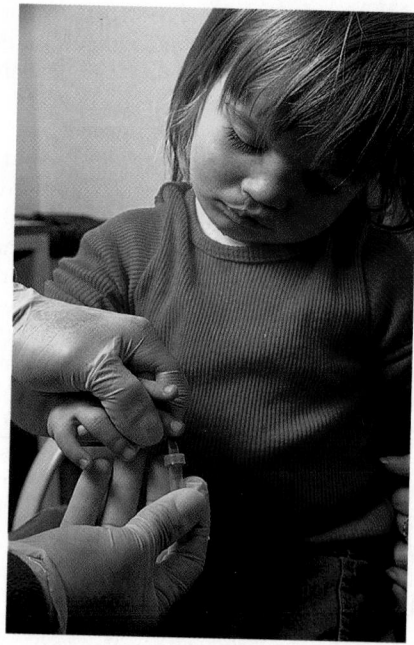

Figure 34–3 Blood screening test. This young child is having a blood screening test to detect iron deficiency anemia. Children are often screened for adequate levels of iron in later infancy and during toddlerhood.

Mental and spiritual health are important concepts to address in health promotion and health maintenance visits. Parents can be encouraged to keep a record of mental health issues to bring to health supervision visits. This helps them understand that the healthcare professional is willing to partner with them to assist in dealing with mental health. Suggest topics such as child and parental mood, child temperament, stresses and ways that family members manage stress, or sleep patterns. Make notes in the record as a reminder of questions to ask at the next visit. The child and family are both observed for appropriateness of affect and mood. Be alert for signs of depression, stress, anxiety, and child abuse or neglect. The nurse establishes both health promotion and health maintenance goals related to child and family mental health. Health promotion goals relate to adequate resources to meet family challenges and protective factors such as involvement in extended family and the community. Teaching stress reduction techniques such as meditation, relaxation, and imagery, as well as providing resources for yoga or other techniques, is helpful. Health maintenance goals relate to prevention of mental health problems. Examples include providing resources when domestic violence occurs, or referring cases of suspected child abuse or neglect. The **spiritual dimension** is a connection with a greater power than that in the self, and guides a person to strive for life purpose, joy, peace, and fulfillment (Pender et al., 2015). For some, spiritual health may be fostered by membership in a faith-based group; for others, it may be feeling part of a society with a purpose of greater good, or setting goals for the future. Ask about the family's meaningful activities. Provide links to faith-based groups as needed.

The *relationships* that a child establishes with others begin at birth. The first and most important set of relationships develops with the family. The mother, father, siblings, and perhaps extended family are the contexts in which the baby learns to relate with others. With growth, the world widens to encompass other children, friends of the family, peers, school, and the larger community network. Analyzing the child's relationships at all ages provides important clues to social interactions. From the moment the family is called in from a waiting area, be alert for clues to family interactions. Likewise, other social interactions are important to evaluate. Does the young infant interact in an age-appropriate manner with the healthcare provider or other children in the area? Ask the parents questions about family and social interactions. Once assessment has taken place, establish goals and interventions related to family and social relationships.

Disease prevention strategies focus mainly on health maintenance, or prevention of disease. Some health disruptions can be detected early and treatment for the condition can begin. **Screening** is a procedure used to detect the possible presence of a health condition before symptoms are apparent. It is usually conducted on large groups of individuals at risk for a condition and represents the secondary level of prevention (Figure 34–3). Most screening tests are not diagnostic by themselves but are followed by further diagnostic tests if the screening result is positive. Once a screening test identifies the existence of a health condition, early intervention can begin, with the goal of reducing the severity or complications of the condition (secondary prevention). Another way to prevent diseases is to immunize children against common communicable diseases (primary prevention). See Chapter 43 for the complete list of childhood immunizations and schedules for administration.

Most childhood mortality and hospitalization is related to injury (CDC, 2012) (see Chapter 1 for more information). Therefore, it is important for the nurse to integrate *injury prevention* strategies in all health supervision visits. The family is constantly challenged to maintain a safe environment as the child grows older, reaches more advanced developmental levels, is exposed to a widening world outside of the family, and has less supervision. Safety teaching should be integrated with developmental progression. Asking parents to bring their questions about safety to each visit can be a good starting point for discussion. The nurse considers knowledge about the age of the child and information from the health supervision visit to plan health maintenance interventions related to injury. Teaching is performed, resources are made available, and parents and children who have experienced injury are invited to present their experiences.

Many other topics might be discussed during health supervision visits. They may relate to either health maintenance activities designed to preserve health, or health promotion activities designed to enhance or improve the state of wellness. Topics include extended family members and their role in the child's life, cultural variations or inclusion, or development of moral values and ethical behaviors.

Health Promotion and Maintenance of the Newborn and Infant

The month following delivery is a time of huge transition for the new mother and her family. Not only is the mother coping with hormonal shifts and a **postpartum** (after giving birth) body, but roles and relationships are also changing. The role of the nurse is to assess knowledge about self-care and newborn care, teach health promotion and maintenance activities, promote parental confidence in newborn caregiving, and facilitate a partnership among healthcare professionals and the family.

Infancy is a major life transition for the baby and parents. The infant accomplishes phenomenal physical growth and many developmental milestones while the family adapts to the addition of a new member and establishes new goals for each of its existing members. Infant health supervision visits are very important to support the health of the baby and the family unit. These visits begin after the newborn period, at about 1 month of age. This is the time when parents establish an ongoing partnership with a healthcare provider. A "medical home" or "pediatric healthcare home" is identified to serve the baby's health needs. The goals of health supervision visits are to identify and address the health promotion and health maintenance needs of the infant.

Facilitating breastfeeding, helping parents to understand their newborn's and infant's temperament, and employing strategies to ensure adequate sleep by the baby and parents are examples of health promotion activities. Health maintenance activities focus on disease and injury prevention. Some examples of these interventions include administering immunizations and teaching about infant car seats.

An established relationship with a healthcare provider and agency is important so that trust develops and the family will feel comfortable about turning to the professionals for information and guidance as the baby grows. Nurses play a vital role in welcoming new families into office and clinic settings, establishing rapport, and applying principles of communication so that trust and positive partnerships develop between providers and families. Infancy is a time when the child grows in physical, psychologic, and cognitive ways; health supervision visits play a key role in fostering healthy growth and development. When should the infant be seen for health supervision visits? What are key components of these visits? How can the nurse best assess and intervene to ensure the infant's health and safety? These are some of the questions that will be answered in this section of the chapter.

Early Contacts With the Family

Most obstetric healthcare providers encourage the expectant mother to choose her newborn's healthcare provider prior to the baby's birth (see *Clinical Reasoning: Choosing the Newborn's Healthcare Provider*). Pediatric healthcare providers usually welcome a short office visit, sometimes at no charge, to allow the expectant mother and healthcare provider to assess their compatibility prior to initiating the healthcare provider relationship. Many pediatric healthcare providers provide written information to expectant parents, explaining their professional philosophy of care as well as information about services.

> ### Clinical Reasoning Choosing the Newborn's Healthcare Provider
> Parents are encouraged to visit the pediatric healthcare home before the baby is born. This will help the parents decide if the healthcare provider offers the type of care they want for their infant. Prepare a list of questions that parents could ask during a visit to the provider they are interested in interviewing. Be sure this list addresses the availability of healthcare providers, frequency of well-child supervision, cost and insurance information, and other pertinent topics.

Health promotion and maintenance for the newborn begin during the stay in the hospital or birthing center (see Chapters 25, 26, and 27). On discharge, referral may be indicated to a lactation consultant or follow-up healthcare visit. The hospital length of stay for a healthy mother and newborn after term delivery is short, approximately 48 hours for a vaginal birth and 72 to 96 hours for an uncomplicated cesarean birth. Discharge of the mother and baby should only occur after appropriate growth is confirmed and a thorough physical examination shows normal results. There should be time to identify any problems and to make certain that the family can care for the newborn at home, and ideally the mother and newborn should be discharged together (AAP, 2011a; AAP, n.d.). For newborns discharged between 48 and 72 hours of age, the first follow-up healthcare visit should occur by 5 days of age. The purpose of this visit is to ensure that the newborn is continuing to progress normally and that no previously undiscovered problems have surfaced. At this initial contact, the nurse promotes maternal confidence in caregiving and offers education and anticipatory guidance. Careful assessments are made for hyperbilirubinemia, feeding problems, or other abnormalities. Further visits are established as needed from 5 days to 1 month; the first scheduled health supervision of infancy is at 1 month of age.

Health promotion and maintenance for infancy occur in a series of health supervision visits during the first year of life. Schedules vary among facilities, but a common pattern includes visits at about 1 month, 2 months, 4 months, 6 months, 9 months, and 1 year of age. In addition, most children have some episodic illnesses such as gastrointestinal illness or otitis media and visit the facility at other times for treatment of these illnesses. A few children have chronic or serious healthcare problems during the first year, and have extensive contact with the healthcare home and other services.

During these first visits, assess the family for protective factors and risks. Protective factors might include knowledge level of infant needs, support from family and friends, and the mother's good health and nutritional state during pregnancy. Risk factors could include limited financial resources, lack of preparation for the baby, and illness or other stress among family members. Ask about how the family traveled to the visit, and if convenient times and transportation are available. Lack of access during

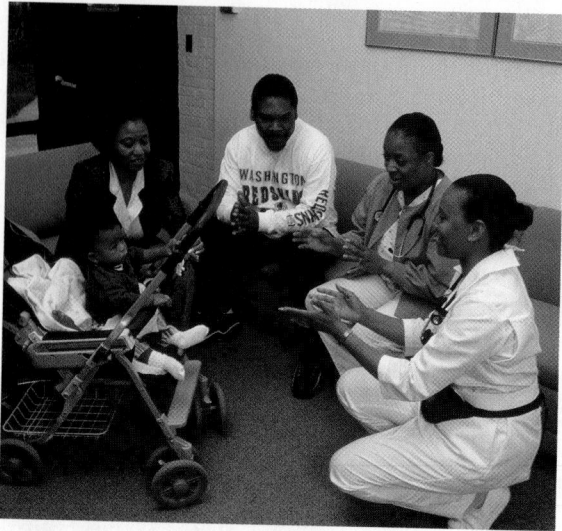

Figure 34–4 General observations. The nurse begins assessment of the infant's family when they are seen in the waiting room and called in for care. What observations can you make of the infant's general appearance? Developmental accomplishments? Interaction of parents with the baby?

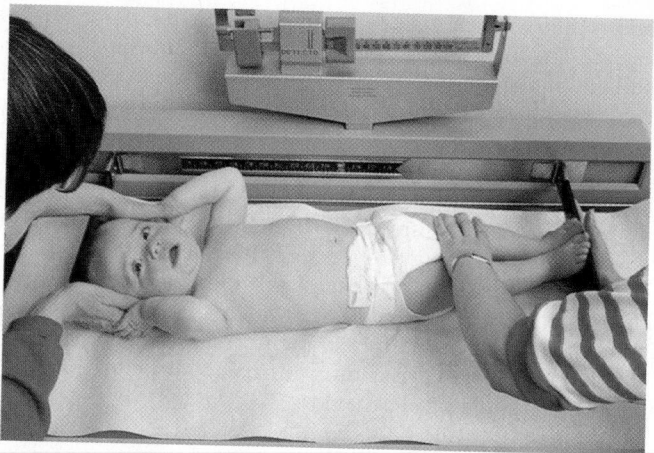

Figure 34–5 Measuring physical growth. Weighing and measuring length during health supervision visits provides important information about the child's nutrition and general development. This young infant was measured and then while the parents dressed the child the nurse placed the findings on the growth grid.

times the family is not at work and other health system barriers sometimes interfere with attendance at health supervision visits. Knowledge of risk factors will shape the nursing interventions during the first health supervision in infancy. The nurse applies health promotion principles by building on strengths and fosters health maintenance by intervening to minimize risks.

General Observations

When the family comes to the clinic or office for care with a newborn or infant, general observations should begin at first contact (Figure 34–4). Welcome the family warmly to the facility and comment on the baby. Ask how the family is doing with the baby and how the adjustment is going. Be alert for signs of fatigue or depression in the parents, as these can occur when caring for an infant and can interfere with bonding and positive transition. Look for clues about cultural orientation. The nurse gathers information in order to assess the needs of the family, to invite discussion, to validate positive parenting efforts, and to promote partnership between the family and the healthcare team. Upon entering the examination room, it is helpful to explain the plans for the visit, such as,

> I will weigh and measure Sarah now and show you how she is growing. Then I'll ask a few questions about her eating, sleeping, and other things. Then the nurse practitioner will be in to do Sarah's physical examination. Do you have any questions as we start? Will you undress Sarah now so we can weigh her accurately?

Growth and Developmental Surveillance

Assessment of growth and development begins at birth and continues in newborn and infant health promotion and maintenance visits. (See Chapter 31 for important background/theoretical information about growth and development.) Note the posture, flexion, reflexes, and physical attributes that help evaluate gestational age. Physical growth and meeting

of developmental milestones provide important information about infants. The baby is measured for accurate length, weight, and head circumference (Figure 34–5). (See the *Clinical Skills Manual* SKILLS and Chapter 33 for detailed information about the physical examination.) The measurements should be placed on growth grids and interpreted. Parents enjoy seeing how the baby is progressing and are usually eager to learn about the child's weight gain and growth percentiles. Be alert for an infant who demonstrates a change in percentile range. For example, if the baby was in the 75th percentile for length and weight at birth, but has fallen to below the 50th percentile for weight, additional assessment of the baby's feedings is needed. Likewise, if the head circumference is much lower or higher than the length and weight percentiles, further neurologic and developmental assessment should be done.

Growth measurement is followed by a physical assessment. The nurse may complete parts of the assessment, with the remainder performed by the physician, nurse practitioner, or other primary care provider. The assessment evaluates each body system, with particular attention being paid to the heart, skin, musculoskeletal system, abdomen, and neurologic status. See Chapter 24 for assessment of the newborn and Chapter 33 for a thorough discussion of physical assessment throughout infancy and childhood.

Developmental surveillance is integrated into each infant healthcare visit by observing developmental milestones in the infant. (See Chapter 31 for a summary of milestones expected at different ages.) When there is no opportunity to observe a skill directly, ask parents about whether the infant performs the skill (see *Developing Cultural Competence: Cultural Influences on Developmental Tests*). In addition to direct observation, parents are usually requested to fill in a form that asks questions about common developmental tasks. Review the results and determine if additional questions should be asked. Signs of **developmental delay**—a delay in mastering functions, such as motor coordination and behavioral skills—in a full-term infant usually merit immediate investigation by a pediatrician, pediatric developmental specialist, pediatric neurologist, or a multidisciplinary team of professionals. Parents require additional emotional support, clear and honest communication, and resources to cope with the stress of this situation.

The nurse establishes health promotion and maintenance interventions related to growth and development assessment data. Anticipatory guidance related to development is a major component of health promotion. The nurse anticipates the next milestones the infant will be meeting, and recommends ways for the parents to support the infant in progression. Some health promotion activities include:

- Teach about introducing foods that will foster growth.
- Encourage use of toys and activities that will assist in meeting the next developmental milestones.
- Demonstrate gross and fine motor skills that the infant has achieved.
- Demonstrate to parents how the child will focus on their faces and mimic their vocal sounds.

Other interventions are focused on health maintenance or disease and injury prevention. Safety hazards and ways to avoid them are discussed, and parents are given brochures, website addresses, or videotapes to enhance injury prevention information. Can you outline additional health promotion and health maintenance interventions that relate to the newborn's and infant's growth and development?

Nutrition

The importance of nutrition during the newborn period and the first year of life cannot be overemphasized. Babies will triple their birth weight by 1 year of age and therefore have a great need for nutritional balance. From the first sips of breast milk or formula as a newborn, to eating the family meal at 1 year of age, the fast progression of nutritional intake patterns is obvious. See Chapter 25 for details about the importance of breastfeeding and Chapter 32 for a thorough description of nutritional needs for the infant.

During each visit the nurse seeks to learn what the baby is eating, and whether the family has any questions or concerns related to intake (Holt, Wooldridge, Story, et al., 2011). Open-ended questions are a good way to begin, with more specific questions inserted after the parent's perceptions are known. Breastfeeding is encouraged and supported during the newborn and infancy periods, and information about safe formula feeding is provided when the family has chosen that method of feeding. Once the baby is in the second half of the first year, food patterns of the family become more important. Consider childcare settings as well.

Observations from other portions of the visit can provide clues about additional questions to ask. If an infant has not gained weight as expected and has fallen into a lower weight percentile, more specific analysis of intake is needed. Ask for a recall of the baby's intake in the previous day. When the baby does not meet developmental milestones on schedule or is lethargic, intake may be inadequate for age. In these cases, support may be needed to ensure adequate intake; a thorough description of feeding may be the first step in analyzing the problem and planning interventions. When the child's ability to take in nutrients or the parent's ability to feed the baby is questioned, an observation of a feeding might take place, either at the healthcare setting or during a home visit.

Additional nutritional assessment measures are used at certain points in the first year. A hematocrit or hemoglobin is generally performed between 9 and 12 months of age. Lead screening may be needed in certain population groups (see Chapter 42 for more information). Food security screening can be used when appropriate (see Chapter 32) (AAP Committee on Nutrition, 2013). Each visit includes nutritional teaching about important items. The topics for discussion vary according to age group. See Table 34–2 for suggested teaching topics at specific ages. Desired outcomes for nutrition in infancy include adequate growth, normal nutritional assessment findings, and knowledge by parents of the nutritional needs of the infant.

Physical Activity

Muscle development begins early in fetal life. The flexed position of the newborn demonstrates development of the flexor muscles and relaxation of the extensor muscles. This flexed position protects the newborn, conserves energy by reducing movement, and reduces heat loss. During the first month of life, the newborn gradually "unfolds" and the body straightens. Movements begin to change from reflexive to purposeful.

Physical activity is needed for adequate development of fine and gross motor skills in infancy. Unlike other times of life, the focus is on providing only the opportunities for activity, without a need to focus on motivation. As long as infants are meeting developmental milestones and have a stimulating environment that provides opportunity for fine and gross motor activity, they will use their motor skills, thus enhancing their performance. Time should be provided each day for the infant to reach for objects, freely exercise legs and arms, and increasingly use head control.

Playing with parents or others and being surrounded by toys and other stimulating items will encourage motor behavior in all body parts. Ask the parents for a description of the infant's typical day and listen for these types of play periods. While infants should sleep on their backs, they need supervised play periods when they are awake that are spent on their stomachs. This encourages developmental skills and lessens flattening of the back of the head from excessive positioning on back (Kadey & Roane, 2012). Observe the physical skills of the infant (see Chapter 31) for motor developmental norms, ask questions about play periods provided, and compose a list of the family protective factors and risk factors in this area. Table 34–3 lists some risk and protective factors related to physical activity of newborns and infants.

Based on the results of assessment and using the concept of anticipatory guidance, the nurse plans appropriate teaching for health promotion. Health maintenance deals with prevention of physical development delays. Examples of nursing activities are teaching parents to allow the arms and legs of infants to be outside of covers for some period each day to enhance movement, and

TABLE 34–2 Nutrition Teaching for Health Promotion and Health Maintenance Visits

AGE	NUTRITION TEACHING	
Newborn	Support breastfeeding efforts. Teach correct formula types and preparation if used. Teach burping and rate of feeding information.	Encourage families to view feedings as social interactions; emphasize importance of holding the newborn and not propping bottles.
1 month	Continue teaching listed above. Offer support for breastfeeding and reinforce that breast milk is the only intake needed by infants at this age.	
2 months	Continue teaching listed above. Review fluid needs of infants. Reinforce food safety for partially used bottles of breast milk or formula. Use warm water for heating bottles rather than microwave to avoid burning.	Warn against feeding honey in the first year of life due to risk of botulism. Begin daily cleaning of infant gums. Provide information about any supplements needed (e.g., iron for premature infant; continuation of 400 International Units/day of vitamin D for all infants).
4 months	Continue teaching listed above. Discuss introduction of first foods between 4 and 6 months, and surveillance for symptoms of allergy or intolerance.	Discuss changing food patterns such as increasing amounts and decreasing numbers of daily milk feedings.
6 months	Continue teaching listed above. Reinforce proper introduction of new foods, to include rice cereal, vegetables, and fruits. Discuss any unusual food reactions observed. Introduce cup for drinking. Introduce soft finger foods.	Serve juice only in a cup and limit to no more than 6 oz daily. Caution about common choking foods and items. Provide information about fluoride supplement if water supply is not fluoridated.
9 months	Continue teaching listed above. If mother does not continue to breastfeed, teach family to use iron-fortified formula for the first year of life. Encourage self-feeding of finger foods, integrating common foods for the family.	Introduce source of protein such as tofu, cheese, mashed beans, and slivers of meats.
12 months	Continue teaching listed above. Support mother who wishes to continue breastfeeding beyond 1 year of age.	Encourage cups for all feedings other than breast.

suggesting toys that encourage attention and movement, such as mobiles and music boxes. The nurse evaluates the success of interventions by the child's progression in physical activity milestones at each health supervision visit. Adequate parental understanding of the importance of physical activity and the means of supporting the child's activities is an important outcome of care.

Oral Health

The first teeth begin to erupt about midway during infancy. Two front teeth are common at about 6 months of age. However, even before this, parents lay the foundation for good oral health. The mother's intake during pregnancy and breastfeeding is essential to ensuring adequate availability of calcium and other nutrients that will be used as the infant's teeth develop. The nurse in child health supervision settings ensures that the infant has adequate intake of these nutrients via breastfeeding and other foods. A dietary recall of the mother's intake, as well as the infant's, is one way of assessing for nutrients. When the water supply is not fluoridated, inquire about use of fluoride drops.

Help the family establish healthy dental habits. The parents should wipe the infant's gums with soft moist gauze once or twice

TABLE 34–3 Risk and Protective Factors Regarding Physical Activity in the Newborn and Infancy Periods

RISK FACTORS	PROTECTIVE FACTORS
• Premature birth • Delayed developmental milestones • Limited stimulation by family or other care providers • Lack of knowledge by family about infant's physical activity needs • Limited community resources for families with infants	• Meets developmental milestones at expected ages • Has contact with parents, siblings, and others for significant time each day • A supportive environment with room to play safely; stimulating surroundings • Physically active family • Family knowledge about infant's physical activity needs • Community programs that promote physical activity in infants and information for families

Source: Data from Hagan, J. F., Shaw, J. S., & Duncan, P. M. (Eds.). (2008). *Bright futures: Guidelines for health supervision of infants, children, and adolescents* (3rd ed.). Elk Grove Village, IL: American Academy of Pediatrics.

daily. This helps to clean residues of food from the gums and gets the infant accustomed to having something wiping the gums, a practice that may assist when toothbrushing begins. Families are also cautioned to avoid having the infant breastfeed when sleeping, to avoid use of bottles in bed, and not to allow the infant to drink at will from a bottle during the day. These practices are linked to **early childhood caries** (see Chapter 32) and can lead to tooth decay. Nurses assess for the presence of teeth and whether patterns are similar to those expected (see Chapter 33 for additional information). It is wise to ask if the infant has had any difficulty with teeth eruption. Many infants have increased crying and disrupted sleep when teething. Suggest comfort measures such as offering cool beverages and safe "teething toys" for the infant. The American Academy of Pediatric Dentistry (AAPD) recommends an oral examination within 6 months of the eruption of the first tooth and no later than 12 months of age. They recommend that the parents establish a "dental home" by that time to ensure ongoing oral care for the child (AAPD, 2013).

Mental and Spiritual Health

The infant's mental health is related to early experiences, inborn characteristics such as temperament and resilience, and relationships with caregivers. The first year of life provides many opportunities for the infant to develop positive mental health; interventions during this important period can enhance the child's future mental status.

One way to evaluate mental health is to look carefully at the growth and development surveillance data that were described earlier. Children who feel secure and have nurturing environments usually grow as expected and perform milestones at usual times. Slow growth and delayed development are sometimes related to feeding disorders of infancy and early childhood (see Chapter 32). In these cases, a disturbed relationship with the primary caregiver influences the psychologic state of the infant and results in decreased food intake. Another way to assess mental health is to observe the child and parent interacting. Does the parent hold the newborn securely and does the infant cuddle and settle into the parent's arms? (See Figure 34–6.) Is there eye contact between parent and infant? Does the parent appear comfortable in holding and comforting the newborn? These interactions indicate bonding or positive attachment.

During the first year, the infant learns to identify the primary caregivers; beginning at about 6 months of age, infants may cry or protest when a person other than a familiar caregiver holds them. This is called **stranger anxiety** and indicates expected attachment to parents. Similarly, infants in the second half of the first year of life may exhibit **separation anxiety** by inconsolable crying and other signs of distress when parents are not present. These behaviors are normal, demonstrate healthy attachment to primary caregivers, and indicate mental health. Help parents to recognize them as expected occurrences. Provide ideas of how to deal with this behavior. The parents can remain in sight and talk to the baby during health supervision examinations. They should be encouraged to hold and comfort the baby after painful procedures like immunizations. Once the infant has experienced that the parent leaves and returns, security in the care of others can emerge.

Another important indication of infant mental health is the ability to comfort oneself. **Self-regulation** is the process of dealing with feelings, learning to soothe self, and focusing on activities for increasing periods of time. Newborns learn how to comfort and calm themselves. Ask parents if the newborn or infant sucks a finger, softly rocks, or otherwise comforts self when distressed. Some infants prefer to be alone and quiet when

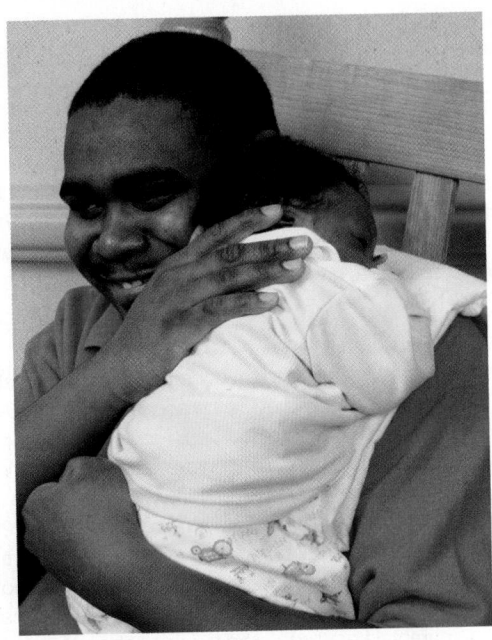

Figure 34–6 Assessing mental health. Interactions between the parent and infant provide clues to mental health. Do the adult and child appear comfortable with each other? Is eye contact and vocalization present? Are their bodies soft and relaxed or tense?

tired or distressed; others calm better when held, rocked, or placed in an infant swing. Help the parents to identify and reinforce the baby's methods of self-soothing, and teach swaddling and rocking techniques. Self-regulation is needed by the baby when learning to go to sleep while tired and agitated. Nurses use health promotion principles to teach about sleep patterns in infants, and implement health maintenance when partnering with families to deal with problem sleep behaviors that lead to infant and parent fatigue (see *As Children Grow: Infant Sleep Patterns* and *Evidence-Based Practice: Infant Sleep*).

As Children Grow: **Infant Sleep Patterns**

- In the first 6 months, infants sleep from 14 to 18 hours each day.
- The number of night awakenings varies for infants and may even vary from night to night.
- Nurses can teach parents that variability in sleep patterns is common, and not usually the result of changes in the infant's daily schedule.
- From 6 to 12 months, infants generally sleep 12 to 14 hours daily, with longer sleep periods at night and accompanied by one to three naps daily.
- Parents can be encouraged to settle on a nighttime routine for the infant, such as a short quiet playtime, bath, breastfeeding, or bottlefeeding with decreased lighting and soothing music.

Source: Data from Middlemiss, W., Yuare, R., & Huey, E. L. (2014). Translating evidence-based knowledge about sleep into practice. *Journal of the American Association of Nurse Practitioners*. doi: 10.1002/2327-6924.12159

EVIDENCE-BASED PRACTICE | Infant Sleep

Clinical Question

Many babies have limited sleeping periods during the night, and their night awakenings disturb parents' sleep. Parents may have busy days and be unable to nap and, hence, possibly not be able to perform at a safe and productive level during the day. Parental stress and depression are associated with frequent child awakenings. What strategies are needed to assist them in supporting the infant's sleep?

The Evidence

Sleep of the infant is an important concern for many parents, but there is little research-based evidence about what strategies really improve infant sleep. A study of 314 twin pairs found that most sleep disturbances in early childhood are linked to environmental factors, and thus behavioral interventions with parents are suggested for altering infant sleep patterns (Brescianini et al., 2011). Consistent with these findings, a study evaluating 170 parents for knowledge of child sleep found that most parents could not answer the majority of questions correctly. The researchers suggested that evaluating parental knowledge and teaching about developmental progression of sleep patterns should occur during health visits

(Schreck & Richdale, 2011). A cross-cultural study found that parents from predominantly Asian countries were more likely to identify sleep disturbance in their children than those from countries with a majority of White parents. These findings suggest that information is needed about cultural differences in sleep expectations of parents (Sadeh, Mindell, & Rivera, 2011).

Best Practice

This evidence-based practice provides implications for nursing care. Ask parents of young newborns to record the infant sleep patterns. As the infant nears 3 to 4 months of age, patterns should demonstrate few night wakenings and feedings. Teach parents about how to minimize stimulation and interaction at night. Provide opportunities to review results at future health supervision visits, or offer telephone or other support to parents.

Clinical Reasoning

What reasons might working parents have for responding eagerly and interacting with an infant who awakens at night? Do you think there are other reasons why infants awake at night? What clues help you to decide if an infant sleep problem exists?

The newborn enters a family with spiritual strengths and limitations. The nurse assesses the family and provides additional resources when needed. Although the infant is not mature enough to understand the family's spiritual framework, the atmosphere in the family that relates to nurturing, valuing children, providing a safe and secure environment, and recognizing mental balance is conveyed readily to the infant. The infant's social and psychologic health are closely related to these factors. Assess the family's meaningful activities and practices and engagement in faith-based practices. Ask if they have needs or desires for referrals in the community such as to an organized religious body or other meaningful activities.

Many of the nurse's interventions are aimed at healthy mental health development in the infant. Health promotion activities focus on teaching parents the needs of infants for security and interaction. Suggest healthy sleep patterns starting with the newborn visit and explain how they can be achieved. Teach self-regulation skills so that the parents can help the infant become quiet and calm. Health maintenance seeks to identify infants with disruptions in mental health status, often manifested by growth or interaction abnormalities. When the infant has disturbed sleep patterns or difficulty calming self when upset, or the parents do not interpret infant cues related to hunger or discomfort, the nurse plans interventions to help prevent further problems. An expected outcome for these activities is the reestablishment of expected growth and development and age-appropriate interactions of the infant with others.

Relationships

Family adaptation to a new baby begins in pregnancy, and evidence of initial family adaptation to pregnancy may be predictive of future parental coping (Hagan et al., 2008). Upon birth, the family is the primary site where the infant learns to interact with other people. Therefore, family dynamics must be examined during health supervision visits. Strengths and needs of the family are identified during psychosocial screening. Some factors in the mental health of the parents directly affect the

atmosphere in the home, and the resulting health of the newborn and infant. Depression in parents or other family members is an important condition that has the potential to influence the infant's health. (See Chapter 30 for information about risks in the postpartum family.) Interactions with parents who are depressed will be altered; caretaking, both physical and emotional, can be impaired. Another challenge to the mental health of families and the infants in these families is that of domestic violence, a situation in which parents or adult care providers commit violent acts toward one another. Child abuse or maltreatment is another risk that occurs in some families with infants. This problem is a serious issue that causes disturbed mental status in the baby. See Chapter 42 for a detailed description of child abuse and its effect on infants and older children. Suspected child abuse must be reported to legal authorities in order to protect children.

The infant's social interactions both within and outside the family display unbelievable growth in the first year. The role of the nurse related to infant social interactions in health supervision visits is to evaluate the social skills of the infant, learn what parents have noticed about the baby's temperament and how it fits with their lives, and make suggestions for positive social development. Desired outcomes for the infant include establishment of close relationships with parents and other family members, a stimulating home environment that is responsive to the baby's temperament, and developmental progression in social interactions.

Disease Prevention Strategies

Disease prevention in the newborn period includes metabolic screening, hearing screening, eye examination, immunization, prevention of environmental smoke exposure, sudden infant death syndrome (SIDS) risk reduction, formula safety, minimizing exposure to disease, and hand hygiene for the family.

Infants are prone to many infectious diseases, especially once passive immunity from the mother wanes at about 6 months of age (see Chapters 43 and 48). Recommended immunizations are administered on schedule to provide protection from some diseases. Recommended immunizations for newborn and infancy are listed in Table 34–4. Further details on immunizations can be found in Chapter 43. Instruct parents about upcoming immunizations and when the infant should be seen again. Be sure the parent understands the risks and benefits of each immunization. Answer their questions truthfully, and have resources on hand such as brochures and videotapes for interested parents.

During each health supervision visit in infancy, the nurse performs recommended screenings and counsels the parents about why such screenings are important. Vision and hearing screenings are consistently performed. Screenings for anemia and lead poisoning are added at particular times or with certain groups. Families with certain genetic diseases such as sickle cell disease or cystic fibrosis may choose to have screening for the infant so that supportive care can begin early if the child has the disease. Parents benefit from teaching about common diseases and conditions of young children and measures for their prevention. Ask about secondhand smoke (environmental tobacco smoke) and encourage smoking parents to quit. Teach parents to put infants to sleep on their backs to assist in lowering the chance of SIDS (see Chapter 46 for a thorough discussion of SIDS). Be sure parents have a phone number to call when they have questions about conditions or whether the baby should be seen by the healthcare provider (see *Teaching Highlights: When to Contact the Healthcare Provider*). Evaluate the family's ability to understand verbal and written instructions. Desired outcomes for disease prevention strategies include adequate management of health problems, integration of immunization and other preventive measures into care of the infant, and family understanding of preventive measures recommended for infants.

Injury Prevention Strategies

New parents are sometimes unaware of sources of potential injury for the newborn. Some aspects of injury prevention are pertinent to the newborn's immediate care and other topics promote discussion and provide opportunities for anticipatory guidance during all of infancy. In the immediate newborn period, the nurse should assess the parents' knowledge of injury prevention strategies, and promote healthy and safe behaviors. Injury prevention strategies include proper and consistent use of an infant car seat and strategies to prevent falls, burns, choking, drowning, and suffocation.

TABLE 34–4 Routine Immunizations Recommended During Newborn and Infancy Periods

IMMUNIZATION	AGE RECOMMENDED
Hepatitis B	At birth (1st dose) 1–2 months (2nd dose) 6–18 months (3rd dose)
Hepatitis A	12 months (1st dose) 18 months or at least 6 months after 1st dose (2nd dose)
Diphtheria, tetanus, pertussis	2, 4, and 6 months (3 doses)
Rotavirus	2 and 4 months (2 doses) **OR** 2, 4, and 6 months (3 doses) (The requirement of 2 or 3 doses is related to which of the two available vaccines is used.)
Haemophilus influenzae type b	2, 4, and 6 months (3 doses; 3rd dose is not needed if PRP-OMP [Pedvax HIB or Comvax] is used for primary series)
Inactivated poliovirus	2, 4, and 6–18 months (3 doses)
Pneumococcal	2, 4, and 6 months (3 doses)
Influenza	Annually from 6 months

During the first year of life, injury becomes an increasingly common cause of mortality. Strategies must be included in every health supervision visit to lower the risk of injury. Nurses should never assume that parents understand how to insert an infant car seat correctly or what types of toys and foods can lead to choking. Know the most common hazards at each age and teach parents methods of avoiding them (Tables 34–5 and 34–6).

Begin the conversation by asking parents what safety hazards they are aware of in the child's environment. Use this information as the starting point for discussion. Give positive feedback for their awareness of hazards and measures they have taken to prevent them. Consider using a home assessment survey that assists parents in identifying hazards that may be present in their homes. When infants visit friends, relatives, or neighbors, they may be exposed to other hazardous situations.

TEACHING HIGHLIGHTS	When to Contact the Healthcare Provider

Instruct parents to contact a healthcare provider if the child has:
- Axillary temperature ≥99.3°F (37.4°C) (Identify for the provider the technique used for temperature measurement, such as axillary, forehead, oral, rectal, or ear, so adequate evaluation can be made.)
- Seizure
- Skin rash, purplish spots, petechiae
- Change in activity or behavior that makes the parent uncomfortable
- Unusual irritability, lethargy
- Failure to eat
- Vomiting
- Diarrhea
- Dehydration
- Cough

Data from Hagan, J. G., Shaw, J. S., & Duncan, P. M. (Eds.). (2008). *Bright futures: Guidelines for health supervision of infants, children, and adolescents* (3rd ed.). Elk Grove Village, IL: American Academy of Pediatrics.

TABLE 34–5 Injury Prevention in Infancy

HAZARD	DEVELOPMENT CHARACTERISTICS	PREVENTIVE MEASURES
Falls	Mobility increases in first year of life, progressing from squirming movements to crawling, rolling, and standing.	Do not leave the newborn or infant unsecured in infant seat, even in newborn period. Do not place on high surfaces such as tables or beds unless holding child. *(A)* Once mobile by crawling, keep doors to stairways closed or use gates. Standing walkers have led to many injuries and are not recommended.
Burns	Infant is dependent on caretakers for environmental control. The second half of the first year is marked by crawling and increased mobility. Objects are explored by touching and placing in mouth.	Check temperature of bath water and food/liquids for drinking. Cover electrical outlets. Supervise infant so that play with electrical cords cannot occur.
Motor vehicle crashes	Infant is dependent on caretakers for placement in car. On impact with another motor vehicle, an infant held on a lap acts as a missile.	Use only approved restraint systems (according to federal motor vehicle safety standards). The seat must be used for every trip, even if very short. The seat must be properly buckled to the car's lap belt system. *(B)*
Drowning	Infant cannot swim and is unable to lift head.	Never leave a newborn or infant alone in a bath of even 2.5 cm (1 in.) of water. Supervise when in water even when a life preserver is worn. Supervision should be provided by adults, not older children. Flotation devices such as arm inflatables are not certified life preservers.
Poisoning	Newborns and infants are dependent on caretakers to keep harmful substances out of reach.	Keep medicines out of reach. Teach proper dosage and administration of medicines to parents. Cleaning products and other harmful substances should not be stored where the infant can reach them. Remove plants from play areas. Have poison control center number by telephone.
Choking	The second half of infancy is marked by exploratory reaching and mouthing of objects. Infant explores objects by placing them in the mouth. *(C)*	Avoid foods that commonly cause choking. Keep small toys away from infants, especially toys labeled "not intended for use by those under 3 years."
Suffocation	The newborn and young infant have minimal head control and may be unable to move if vomiting or having difficulty breathing.	Position newborn and infant on back for sleep. *(D)* Do not place pillows, stuffed toys, bumpers, blankets, or other objects in the crib (AAP, 2011b). Do not use plastic in crib. Avoid latex balloons. Cosleeping with the parent is discouraged because of the danger of suffocation. Sleep with the baby near but not in the parental bed.
Strangulation	Infant is able to get head into railings or crib slats but cannot remove it.	Be sure older cribs have slats spaced 6 cm (2⅜ in.) or less apart. The mattress must fit tightly against the crib rails.

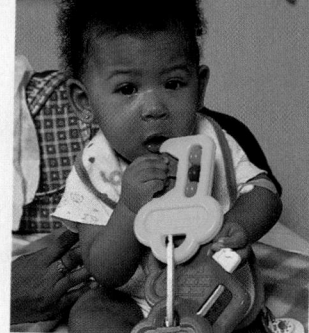

A Never leave infant unsecured or on high surface.

B Always use approved restraint system. Place infant in rear-facing seat in back seat of car.

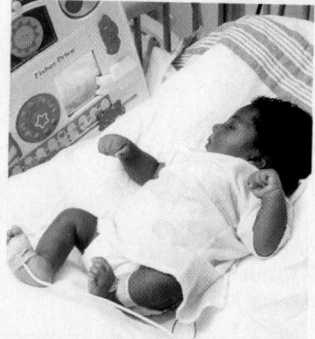

C Explores objects with mouth.

D Place infant on back for sleeping; keep toys clear.

TABLE 34–6 Injury Prevention Topics by Age

AGE	INJURY PREVENTION TEACHING TOPICS	
Birth–1 month	Use car safety seat approved for the newborn or infant; install as directed in rear-facing direction in the back seat. Put baby to sleep on back. Avoid loose bedding and toys in crib; avoid clothes and blankets with loose strings and do not tie a pacifier around the neck or with a string. Avoid tobacco use in the environment. Provide adult supervision of the baby at all times by trusted individuals. Test bath water temperature and never leave the baby alone in the bath.	Never place baby on high object such as counter, table, or bed; always keep one hand on the baby during activities like diaper changes to prevent falling. Wash hands correctly and often. Avoid contact with persons with communicable diseases. Have smoke alarms and avoid fire hazards. Learn infant CPR and airway obstruction removal. Never shake the baby. Have plans for emergency care.
2 months	Follow the above. Use only recommended playpens or cribs and keep sides up. Avoid moldy environments. Keep baby toys cleaned.	Avoid exposure to direct sunlight for the baby. Keep sharp and small objects out of baby's environment. Keep hot water heater lower than 120°F (49°C). Review emergency plan with all care providers.
4 months	Follow the above. Get all poisonous substances out of baby's view and reach; install locks to keep them inaccessible.	Do not use latex balloons or plastic bags near the baby.
6 months	Follow the above. Use only a car seat approved for the weight of the child and always use the seat in rear-facing position in the back seat. Empty containers of water immediately after use; be sure pools or other bodies of water are locked and not accessible to baby. Use sunscreen, hat, and long sleeves when baby is in the sun. Keep heavy and sharp objects out of reach; check that all poisons are locked away including in homes visited; keep pet food and cosmetics out of reach.	Do not drink hot liquids or eat soup while holding the baby. Have poison control number by phones and programmed into cell phones. Be alert for dangers of hot curling irons and other appliances. Have electrical cords out of reach and not hanging down. Have home and environment checked for lead hazards. Lower infant crib mattress if still in upper position. Install gates and guards on stairs and windows. Never use an infant walker.
9 months	Follow the above. Crawl on the floor and look for hazards at baby's eye level. Pad sharp corners on tables and other furniture.	Watch for tables, chairs, and other devices the baby may use for climbing to unsafe places.
12 months	Follow the above. Keep the infant in a rear-facing car seat until 2 years of age; place in back seat and never in front seat with a passenger air bag; have installation checked for safety. Start teaching the child to wash hands frequently, demonstrating and washing with the child. Provide own personal items such as clothing and blankets to childcare providers; wash often. Change batteries in home smoke alarms and check system.	Turn handles to back of stove; use back rather than front burners; watch for hot liquids. Check care provider setting for safety hazards. Remember that responsible adults should always supervise your infant, not other children. Peruse home once again for hazards now that the child is more active, climbing, and walking. Check playgrounds for hazards and always supervise the child in a playground.

Source: Data from Hagan, J. G., Shaw, J. S., & Duncan, P. M. (Eds.). (2008). *Bright futures: Guidelines for health supervision of infants, children, and adolescents* (3rd ed.). Elk Grove Village, IL: American Academy of Pediatrics.

Grandparents may not have a home that is "baby-proofed" and the infant could have access to electrical cords, machinery, medicines, or other hazards. Help the parents to evaluate the childcare home or center. Focus on car safety since this is a frequent cause of injury for infants. Provide brochures and other types of information about recommendations. Refer every family for a car seat examination at a certified examination center. Provide resources for car seats if the family is not able to afford one. Discuss other possible safety hazards such as extensions on the parent's bicycle and use of baby strollers in areas where cars are present.

Nursing Management

For the Health Promotion and Maintenance of the Newborn and Infant

Nursing Assessment and Diagnosis

The nurse working in clinics, offices, and other settings that offer primary care for newborns and infants should be skillful in assessing health promotion and health maintenance. The infant's growth, developmental level, general physical health, and mental/social health are assessed. Family interactions and other settings where the infant spends time are evaluated for risks and protective factors that influence the child's development. Assess the health of siblings and patterns of integrating the infant into the rest of the family. Particular attention is directed at assessment of risk for diseases and injuries. The data-gathering phase always provides parents with the opportunity to ask questions and relay concerns. Further assessment may need to be directed at these areas.

Based on the assessment data, the nurse establishes nursing diagnoses that become the basis for nursing interventions. Both areas of strength and need are included; often the family's strengths can be used to further promote health. Nursing diagnoses established during a health supervision visit of an infant might include the following (NANDA-I © 2014):

- *Breastfeeding, Readiness for Enhanced*, related to the mother's confidence and knowledge

- *Breastfeeding, Interrupted*, related to the mother's resumption of employment outside the home

- *Coping: Family, Compromised*, related to recent role changes

- *Attachment, Risk for Impaired (Parent/Child)*, related to anxiety associated with parenting role

- *Sleep Pattern, Disturbed (Infant)*, related to frequently changing sleep routines and cycles

- *Skin Integrity, Impaired (Infant)*, related to developmental factors

- *Infection, Risk for (Infant)*, related to inadequate acquired immunity

- *Injury, Risk for (Infant)*, related to design of environment

- *Development: Delayed, Risk for*, related to parental substance abuse

Planning and Implementation

The nurse plays a vital role in successful health promotion and health maintenance activities. The newborn period is essential for building a relationship between parents and healthcare professionals that sets the stage for the months and years to come. Explain to the parents what procedures are being performed and their purpose. Encourage them to ask questions and share their perceptions of the infant's personality, development, and other traits. This will enhance their understanding that health care involves a partnership between them and the care providers. It will lead to trust that promotes their ability to share concerns honestly. The first year of the baby's life is a key time for establishing a trusting relationship with health professionals.

Recognize the importance of data provided by simple assessments such as length and weight. Analyze all findings to learn if the child is developing as expected. Much of the visit is spent in teaching parents about topics such as safety measures, providing anticipatory guidance related to development, assisting with integration of the newborn into the family, and relaying resources for support of the family in the community, on the Internet, or in other areas. Parenting classes, childcare facilities, and family planning resources are examples of common parental needs. Perform recommended physical and developmental assessment, administer screening tests, and give immunizations. Be sure parents understand the need for tests and treatments, and relay the results of tests to them.

Nurses who work in hospitals, emergency services, and other facilities are an important link in health supervision. Ask where and how often the child is seen for care. Check immunization schedules to be sure they are up-to-date. When the child is not being seen regularly, find out if the family does not know the importance of these visits or lacks resources to obtain the necessary care. Refer them to resources as needed so that they can identify a pediatric healthcare home. Some agencies that provide health supervision are equipped to perform home visits on a regular basis or in case of special need. When nurses make regular home visits to families with many risk factors, health outcomes are improved. Seeing the family in the natural setting enables the nurse to tailor interventions to the specific situation. Nutrition, safety, and other teaching is more effective when it matches the family's needs. For example, showing how to set up a stimulating environment with safe materials, even if toys are limited, is an effective nursing strategy. Ensure that home visits are performed whenever appropriate and available either through the pediatric healthcare home or other community agency.

Before the family leaves the facility, be sure they have the next appointment scheduled. Summarize content of the present visit, emphasizing the family's strengths and the baby's newly acquired developmental skills. Sensitively list any areas that require work in the coming weeks, such as baby-proofing the home or encouraging the infant to reach for objects. Provide a journal or notebook in which the parents can record the infant's development and write down questions to ask during future visits. Suggest possible topics for the parents to think about, and provide books, brochures, and other printed material.

Evaluation

Expected outcomes of nursing care for the infant and family in health promotion and health maintenance include the following:

- Parents state common safety hazards at the infant's present and upcoming ages.

- The newborn and infant demonstrate normal patterns of growth and progression in developmental milestones.

- The newborn and infant remain free of disease and injury.

- The newborn and infant are well adjusted, showing positive response to the environment and interactions with significant others.

Focus Your Study

- Health is a dynamic state of physical, mental, and social well-being and is the objective of health promotion and health maintenance activities.

- Health supervision visits are healthcare encounters designed to provide assessment, screening, developmental surveillance, immunizations, and health information.

- Health supervision visits include general observations, as well as growth and development, nutrition, physical activity, oral health, mental health, spiritual, and relationship surveillance.

- Partners in providing health supervision are the child, family, health professionals, and community.

- Health promotion and health maintenance interventions are essential components of all child health care, even during periods of acute or chronic illness.

- The first contact between the infant's pediatric healthcare home and the parents should ideally occur prior to birth.

- A trusting relationship between the family and the healthcare provider fosters a partnership that is influential in promoting the development of the infant.

- The nurse establishes diagnoses based on a thorough assessment of the child and family during healthcare visits.

- The nurse and family collaboratively establish goals for the infant, and the nurse plans interventions to meet these goals.

Clinical Reasoning in Action

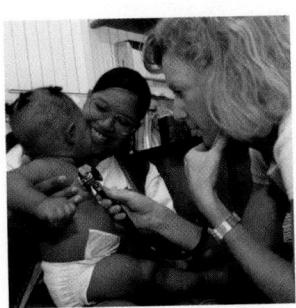

SOURCE: Steven Rubin/The Image Works.

Sahil is a 6-month-old boy who is brought to the clinic by his mother, Clarisse, and his grandmother, who just moved into the home to help Clarisse. Sahil's father recently needed to leave the country on a prolonged work assignment. Clarisse is very nervous about being the main adult responsible for Sahil since her husband's departure. As you assess Sahil, you find that he is smiling readily, is able to sit on his own with little support, and has length and weight at the 50th percentiles. His mother told you that she is breastfeeding and has been feeding Sahil some table food such as rice and tofu. She has returned to work so the grandmother will provide care during the day while Clarisse is at work. You review the immunization record and find that several immunizations are due at today's visit.

1. As Clarisse returns to work, Sahil will likely be consuming less breast milk and have more table foods and formula added to the diet. What questions will you ask Clarisse and Sahil's grandmother to evaluate their knowledge of dietary recommendations for infants? Compose a teaching plan that is appropriate for integration of increasing types of food into the diet of a 6-month-old child.

2. What immunizations are generally needed for 6-month-old infants? When should Sahil return for his next immunizations?

3. You have identified that Clarisse needs support and socialization with other young mothers. How will you locate community resources that are helpful to young families? Decide what parenting information would be helpful to build Clarisse's confidence in caring for Sahil without her husband present. Suggest some ways that she, Sahil, and the father can communicate with each other regularly.

4. The major health problem for infants is related to safety hazards. Sahil is becoming more mobile and curious. Write a teaching plan that includes topics and specific teaching requirements at his age.

References

American Academy of Pediatric Dentistry (AAPD). (2013). *Policy on the dental home* (pp. 24–25). AAPD Reference Manual. Chicago, IL: Author.

American Academy of Pediatrics (AAP). (2011a). *Where we stand: Newborn discharge from hospital.* Retrieved from http://www.healthychildren.org/English/ages-stages/prenatal/delivery-beyond/pages

American Academy of Pediatrics (AAP). (2011b). SIDS and other sleep-related infant deaths: Expansion of recommendations for a safe infant sleeping environment. *Pediatrics, 128,* e1341–e1367.

American Academy of Pediatrics (AAP). (2014). *Agenda for children: Medical home.* Retrieved from http://www.aap.org/en-us/about-the-aap/aap-facts/AAP-Agenda-for-Children-Strategic-Plan/Pages/AAP-Agenda-for-Children-Strategic-Plan-Medical-Home.aspx

American Academy of Pediatrics (AAP). (n.d.). *Appropriate newborn hospital stays.* Retrieved from http://www.aap.org/en-us/about-the-aap/aap-press-room/aap-press-room-media-center/Pages/Appropriate-Newborn-Hospital-Stays.aspx

American Academy of Pediatrics (AAP) Committee on Nutrition. (2013). *Pediatric nutrition handbook* (7th ed.). Elk Grove Village, IL: Author.

American Academy of Pediatrics Committee on Practice and Ambulatory Medicine, Bright Futures Periodicity Schedule Workgroup. (2014). 2014 Recommendations for pediatric preventive health care. *Pediatrics, 133,* 568–570.

Brescianini, S., Volzone, A., Fagnani, C., Patriarca, B., Grimaldi, V., Lanni, R., . . . Stazi, J. A. (2011). Genetic and environmental factors shape infant sleep patterns: A study of 18-month-old twins. *Pediatrics, 127,* e1296. doi:10.1542/peds.2010-0858

Centers for Disease Control and Prevention (CDC). (2011a). *Caries experience and untreated tooth decay.* Retrieved from http://apps.nccd.cdc.gov/nohss/IndicatorV.asp?Indicator=2,3

Centers for Disease Control and Prevention (CDC). (2011b). *Oral health.* Retrieved from http://www.cdc.gov/chronicdisease/resources/publications/AAG/doh.htm

Centers for Disease Control and Prevention (CDC). (2012). *Causes of death by age group.* Retrieved from http://www.cdc.gov/injury/wisqars/pdf/leading_causes_of_death_by_age_group_2011-a.pdf and http://www.cdc.gov/injury/wisqars/pdf/leading_cause_of_nonfatal_injury_2012-a.pdf

Centers for Disease Control and Prevention (CDC). (2013). *The concept of prevention.* Retrieved from http://www.cdc.gov/arthritis/temp/pilots-201208/pilot1/online/arthritis-challenge/03-Prevention/concept.htm

Centers for Disease Control and Prevention (CDC). (2014a). *Developmental monitoring and screening.* Retrieved from http://www.cdc.gov/ncbddd/childdevelopment/screening.html

Centers for Disease Control and Prevention (CDC). (2014b). Youth risk behavior surveillance—United States, 2013. *Morbidity and Mortality Weekly Report*, *63*(SS-4), 1–172.

Child Trends. (2013). *Unmet dental needs.* Retrieved from http://www.childtrends.org/?indicators=unmet -dental-needs

Hagan, J. G., Shaw, J. S., & Duncan, P. M. (Eds.). (2008). *Bright futures: Guidelines for health supervision of infants, children, and adolescents* (3rd ed.). Elk Grove Village, IL: American Academy of Pediatrics.

Holt, K., Wooldridge, N., Story, M., & Sofka, D. (Eds.). (2011). *Bright futures: Nutrition* (3rd ed.). Elk Grove Village, IL: American Academy of Pediatrics.

Kadey, H. J., & Roane, H. S. (2012). Effects of access to a stimulating object on infant behavior during tummy time. *Journal of Applied Behavior Analysis*, *45*, 395–399.

Lipkin, P. H. (2011). Developmental and behavioral surveillance and screening within the medical home.

In R. G. Voight (Ed.), *Developmental and behavioral pediatrics* (pp. 69–92). Elk Grove Village, IL: American Academy of Pediatrics.

Middlemiss, W., Yuare, R., & Huey, E. L. (2014). Translating evidence-based knowledge about sleep into practice. *Journal of the American Association of Nurse Practitioners.* doi: 10.1002/2327-6924 .12159

Pender, N. J., Murdaugh, C. L., & Parsons, M. A. (2015). *Health promotion in nursing practice* (7th ed.). Upper Saddle River, NJ: Pearson Prentice Hall.

Sadeh, A., Mindell, J., & Rivera, L. (2011). "My child has a sleep problem": A cross-cultural comparison of parental definitions. *Sleep Medicine*, *12*(5), 478–482.

Schreck, K. A., & Richdale, A. L. (2011). Knowledge of childhood sleep: A possible variable in under or misdiagnosis of childhood sleep problems. *Journal of Sleep Research*, *20*, 589–597. doi:10.1111 /j.1365-2869.2011.00922.x

Taylor, E. F., Lake, T., Nysenbaum, J., Peterson, G., & Meyers, D. (2011). *Coordinating care in the medical neighborhood: Critical components and available mechanisms.* White Paper (Prepared by Mathematica Policy Research under Contract No. HHSA290200900019I T02). AHRQ Publication No. 11-0064. Rockville, MD: Agency for Healthcare Research and Quality.

U.S. Department of Health and Human Services. (2011). *Healthy People 2020. The vision, mission, and goals of Healthy People 2020.* Retrieved from http://www .healthypeople.gov/2020/Consortium/HP2020 Framework.pdf

World Health Organization (WHO). (2010). *Health promotion.* Retrieved from http://www.who.int/topics /health_promotion/en

World Health Organization (WHO). (2011). *Health promotion: 7th global conference on health promotion.* Retrieved from http://www.who.int/healthpromotion /conferences/7gchp/en

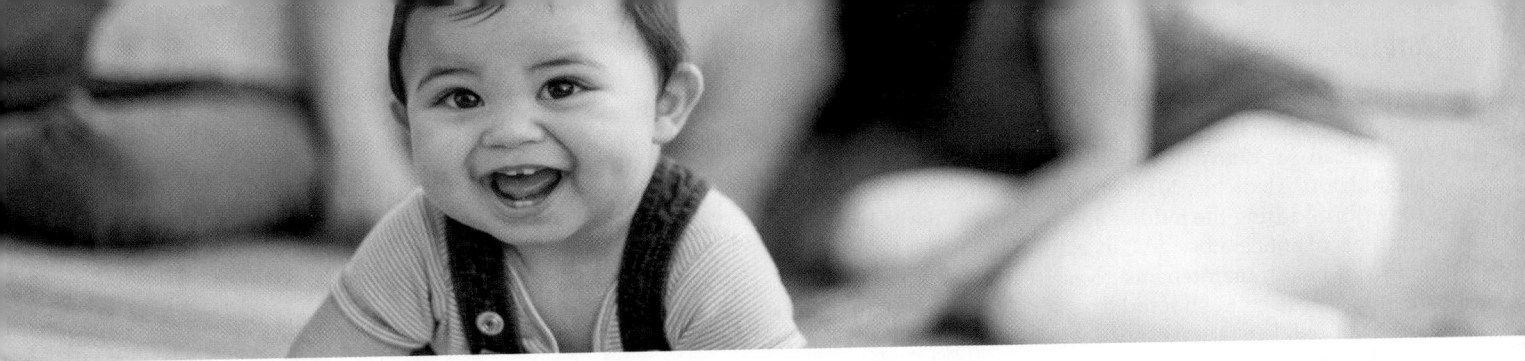

Chapter 35
Health Promotion and Maintenance: The Toddler and the Preschooler

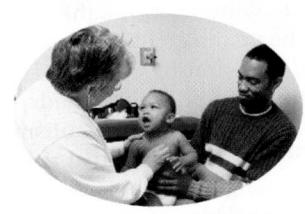

Clarence is such a happy baby, but he is so active. We get exhausted in the evenings after we have worked all day and he needs such close supervision not to fall down stairs or hurt himself. How do parents like us have time to work, take care of our home, and spend time with their toddler?

—Sonia, mother of 15-month-old Clarence

Learning Outcomes

35.1 Describe the areas of assessment and intervention for health supervision visits for toddler and preschool children: growth and developmental surveillance, nutrition, physical activity, oral health, mental and spiritual health, family and social relations, disease prevention strategies, and injury prevention strategies.

35.2 State components of self-concept for preschool children.

35.3 Plan health promotion and health maintenance strategies employed during health supervision visits of toddlers and preschoolers.

35.4 Discuss the importance of family in child health care, and include family assessment in each health supervision visit.

35.5 Integrate pertinent mental health care into health supervision visits for toddlers and preschoolers.

35.6 Examine data about the family and other social relationships to prioritize interventions and to maintain health of toddlers and preschoolers.

Health Promotion and Maintenance: The Toddler and Preschooler

The years following infancy are challenging for parents as the child grows and acquires new developmental skills. The child progresses from the first tentative steps and words at a year of age through the "terrible twos" of toddlerhood and into preschool age when over half of children attend some type of education program, have developed effective verbal communication, and acquire many gross and fine motor skills (Child Trends, 2012). Toddler and preschool ages are often grouped as "young childhood" since the family remains the primary system within which the child interacts. Healthcare providers address common health concerns such as nutrition, sleep, and growing independence. Facing consistent changes in development, parents rely on the "pediatric healthcare home" ("medical home") for advice and information. Regular health visits are recommended at 12, 15, 18, 24, and 30 months and at about 3, 4, and 5 years of age. The Recommendations for Preventive Pediatric

Health Care published by the Committee on Practice and Ambulatory Medicine, Bright Futures Periodicity Schedule Workgroup (American Academy of Pediatrics Committee on Practice and Ambulatory Medicine, 2014) provide guidance for the screenings to perform during the toddler and preschool ages. Nurses apply concepts of anticipatory guidance during visits for health promotion and health maintenance to assist parents in the transitions they face. The child should have an established "dental home" as well. Dental visits are generally recommended twice annually.

Health supervision of young children applies:

1. *Assessment*, including screening tests, evaluations, and observations
2. *Education*, including anticipatory guidance about coming developmental tasks
3. *Intervention*, including parent counseling, home visits when appropriate, and scheduling of future visits
4. *Care coordination* among resources serving the family

General Observations

The relationship with the family should be established as a partnership in care of the child. If, however, the family is new to this healthcare home, reach out to welcome family members warmly and express interest in them as individuals and parents. Families may feel uncomfortable in healthcare settings, and it is important to establish positive rapport so they will be able to ask questions and bring up concerns about the child.

While calling the toddler in from the waiting room, it is amazing that this young child is now able to walk in, even if needing some parental guidance. Watch for the child's desire for independence or signs of continuing reliance on the parent. By preschool age, the child is totally independent in walking and usually engages in conversations easily. After welcoming the preschool child warmly, assess the child's social skills and motor activities. Direct greetings or questions to the child to evaluate stranger anxiety and ability to understand simple commands or questions. What verbal skills are observed? Observe the child's general appearance, nutrition, and state of health.

Health supervision visits are adapted for older toddlers and preschoolers to include observations of parental discipline and interaction style. Does the parent respond to the child's questions? Were age-appropriate toys or activities brought to the visit to help occupy the child while waiting? Is the child alert and observant of the environment?

Growth and Developmental Surveillance

An essential assessment integrated into the visit is measurement of growth. Weight and length are measured and compared to expected patterns of growth. Once the child can stand upright to be measured, sometime between 2 and 3 years of age, charts for standing height rather than recumbent length are used. Body mass index (BMI) is first calculated at 2 years of age and provides information about the relationship of height and weight (see Chapter 32 for additional information). Head circumference is usually measured until 2 years of age. (Consult growth grids in Appendix C.)

Growth continues to be a primary way of evaluating the child's nutritional status. It may also provide clues about conditions that have not yet been evaluated such as endocrine, cardiac, or other disorders. Depending on the results of growth measurements, the nurse may gather additional data. For a child under the 5th percentile for weight or BMI, detailed

recording of nutritional intake should begin. Laboratory studies such as hematocrit and hemoglobin can be performed. Patterns of family growth can be examined. What size are the parents and siblings? Ask if the child has had any illness or hospitalization. For children above the 85th percentile for BMI, detailed dietary intake and physical activity history should be taken.

The physical assessment is performed, with some parts conducted by the nurse and others by the primary care provider such as a physician or nurse practitioner. See Chapter 33 for a thorough discussion of physical examination. The order of the examination and the approaches to the child are particularly important at this age. Leave intrusive procedures such as ear and eye examinations and visualization of genitalia until the end of the examination. Integrate techniques such as allowing the child to play with the stethoscope, asking the child to "blow out" the light from the otoscope, or having the child make a game of pushing the legs against the examiner to measure symmetry of strength (Figure 35–1). Preschoolers are generally interested in their bodies, and teaching about parts of the examination is helpful. During the physical examination, ask the parents pertinent questions. Consider the young child's expected developmental milestones (see information in Chapter 31) and ask questions related to these milestones. Recommended screenings include blood pressure, vision and hearing, autism (at 18 and 24 months; see Chapter 55), and, for the child at risk, hematocrit, hemoglobin, and lead screening (see Chapter 42).

Nurses generally have in-depth knowledge of child development through growth and development courses and pediatric nursing curricula, and are thus well positioned to address parental concerns related to child development. Development is the key organizing principle of early childhood health care. Developmental screening and services should be integrated within health care, childcare, and school settings to include the multiple sites common for young children. (Refer to Chapter 31 for expected milestones at each stage.) Developmental surveillance is integrated throughout the healthcare visit as you observe the child's fine motor, gross motor, language, and social/emotional skills. Developmental screening or testing is also performed; inquire if the child has had developmental testing done at a childcare agency or another site. Ideal screening tools include input from the family in addition to observations by the healthcare provider. Screening tools currently recommended for young children are listed in Table 35–1. See *Evidence-Based Practice: Fetal Alcohol Spectrum Disorders.*

TABLE 35–1 Developmental Screening Tools for Young Children

TOOL	UPPER AGE
Ages and Stages Questionnaire	66 months
Brigance Screens	1st grade
Developmental Assessment of Young Children, 2nd edition	5 years
Early Screening Profiles	7 years
FirstSTEP	6 years
Parents' Evaluation of Developmental Status	8 years
Survey of Well-Being of Young Children	5 years

Source: Adapted from Child Trends. (2014). *Early childhood developmental screening: A compendium of measures for children ages birth to five.* Retrieved from http://www.acf.hhs.gov/programs/ecd /watch-me-thrive

EVIDENCE-BASED PRACTICE | Fetal Alcohol Spectrum Disorders

Clinical Question

Alcohol ingestion by the pregnant woman can result in birth defects called *fetal alcohol spectrum disorders (FASD)*, ranging from fetal alcohol syndrome to fetal alcohol effects. Children may have characteristic facial and other physical abnormalities, or they may appear normal but have learning and behavioral difficulties. Early identification of these disorders can prevent one of the primary causes of developmental delay in children. (See Chapter 55 for further information.) What is the nursing role in prevention of FASD, evaluation of young children for the problem, and becoming knowledgeable about community resources for families when a child exhibits FASD?

The Evidence

In a study of First Steps program (designed to provide pregnancy guidance for women at high risk), retrospective analysis of participants demonstrated significant improvement in alcohol abstinence by participants (Rasmussen et al., 2012). However, in spite of prevention efforts, alcohol exposure during pregnancy occurs and can result in serious consequences for young children. A recent meta-analysis found that prenatal alcohol exposure of the fetus was significantly associated with gross motor deficits in children, particularly in balance, coordination, and ball skills (Lucas et al., 2014). Therefore, motor coordination evaluation is critical in young children so that early identification of problems associated with FASD can result in treatment. In a study with practicing nurses and student nurses, student nurses were found to lack knowledge

related to binge drinking, facial abnormalities associated with FASD, and diagnosis of the disorder (Zoorob, Durkin, Gonzalez, et al., 2014).

Best Practice

Preventive programs with women at high risk of alcohol ingestion during pregnancy can be helpful to decrease consumption and therefore lower risk of FASD occurrence. In addition, when working with toddlers and preschoolers, the nurse must integrate physical assessment for physical signs of fetal alcohol exposure, as well as developmental screening and, particularly, gross motor performance. Children who have difficulty in this area should be referred for further developmental testing. Student nurses should become familiar with both the physical features present in some children with FASD and the developmental/social behavioral components (see Chapter 55). This is an example of the importance of thorough knowledge of development and comprehensive observations and screening during the physical examination.

Clinical Reasoning

How can you ask questions sensitively to determine use of alcohol and knowledge of FASD among pregnant women? Describe the gross motor skills you expect to see in toddlers and preschoolers and areas that might concern you about their abilities. What resources are present in your community to support the toddler or preschooler who manifests fetal alcohol syndrome disorder?

Topics pertinent for inquiry and anticipatory guidance at health supervision visits of young children include sleep patterns, discipline techniques, toilet training, learning and reading practices, communication, and parental issues and questions. Many children, especially by preschool age, are attending a childcare center (Child Trends, 2012). Ask about the experience and whether developmental skills are a focus of activity. Ask if the parent is pleased with the childcare experience or needs further resources. Guidelines for evaluating childcare settings are available through the National Resource Center for Health and Safety in Child Care and Early Education (2013).

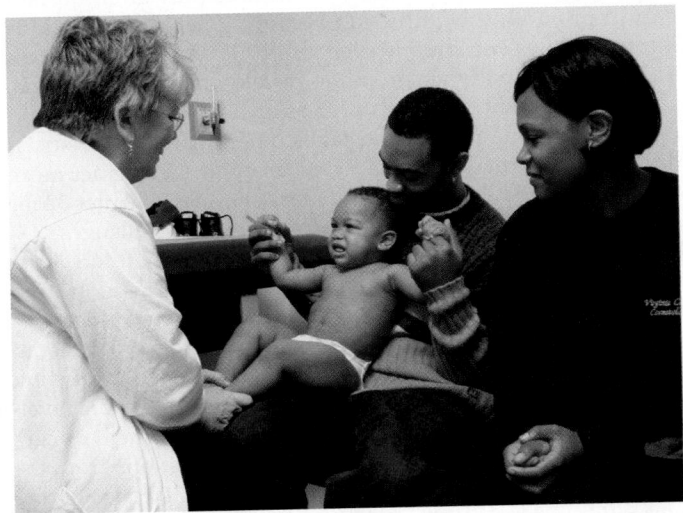

A

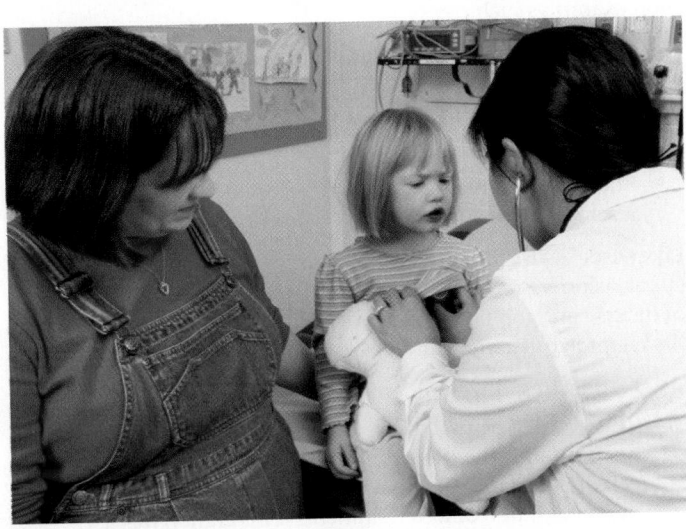

B

Figure 35–1 Examining the toddler or preschooler. The approach to examination of the toddler or preschooler is important in order to elicit cooperation. *A,* The toddler may accept parts of the examination best when seated on the parent's lap as shown in this photo of a boy with his father. *B,* The preschooler likes the opportunity to touch and become comfortable with equipment used or, in this case, holds a doll that receives the same examinations as the child.

TABLE 35–2 Nutrition Teaching for Health Promotion and Health Maintenance Visits

AGE (YEARS)	NUTRITION TEACHING	
1	Support mother who continues to breastfeed.	Provide food and water safety guidelines (see Chapter 32).
	Wean child from bottle by substituting cup.	Be sure all major food groups have been introduced.
	If beginning to use cow's milk, use whole milk (may change to 2% at 2 years of age).	Limit high-fat and high-sugar foods.
	Limit juice to 4–6 oz daily; offer water several times daily; use plain water and avoid flavored water or sugared/electrolyte drinks.	Review amounts of food commonly consumed and frequency of feedings.
	Encourage safety measures—use high chair with strap, secure child and use caution in grocery carts, do not allow foods to be eaten in car.	Review use of fluoride if water supply is not fluoridated.
	Provide information on choking and airway obstruction removal training.	
2	Ask if the mother is still breastfeeding and support the decision to continue or to wean child, as she desires.	Teach parents methods for dealing with temper tantrums over food—make food available at meal and snack times only, do not force intake, offer a variety of foods.
	Encourage total removal of bottle if still in use.	Teach that child may have days of very low intake due to slowing growth rate.
	Ensure that all foods common to family have been offered.	
	Offer child-sized eating utensils.	
	Child can change to low-fat or skim milk if family desires.	
	Limit milk to 2–3 servings daily.	
3	Most children are weaned from breastfeeding and drink 1% or 2% milk.	Recognize importance of social nature of eating; expect child to sit for a short period at meals with family.
	Teach normal intake and decreasing number of snacks.	Meals and snacks should not be eaten while watching television.
	Engage child in food preparation and pouring liquids from small pitcher.	
	Recognize that food jags (periods when only 1 or 2 foods are eaten) are common.	
4	Encourage involving child in snack selection and preparation.	Alter intake as appropriate depending on weight and BMI.
	Start to teach food groups and importance of nutrition for the body.	Dairy products consumed should all be low or reduced fat.

Health promotion growth and development issues for toddlers and preschoolers are addressed at each visit. Some common examples include:

- Explaining growth patterns and what is expected in the months ahead

- Providing toys that encourage development of the coming developmental milestones

- Showing parents the child's developmental progression on a screening tool

Likewise, health maintenance activities are included in health supervision visits, with the primary purpose being prevention of disease and injury. Specific examples are included throughout the chapter, but some general areas addressed are:

- Connecting developmental skills with risks for injury such as drowning and motor vehicle crashes

- Recognizing the possibility of exposure to infectious diseases as the child begins a childcare experience and addressing recognition of and treatments for common diseases

Expected outcomes for the child include normal growth and development patterns for motor, language, and social/emotional skills; parental knowledge of stimulating activities for the child; awareness of the family about risks to growth and development; and healthy body systems for the child.

Nutrition

The child's nutritional status continues to play an important part in promoting health and preventing health disruptions during toddler and preschooler years. Good nutrition fosters normal growth patterns, promotes developmental progression, and helps prevent disorders such as anemia, tooth decay, and immune dysfunction. Eating takes on an increasingly social dimension during early childhood as children interact more with adults and other children at mealtimes. See Chapter 32 for further information about nutritional needs and challenges.

For toddlers, questions for the family focus on introduction of foods, the child's eating patterns, and transition from breast or bottle to other liquids. The toddler often consumes small amounts of foods, and parents consequently worry about the change in appetite. Showing them that the child is growing normally can help allay their anxiety about this common developmental variation. Preschoolers interact with others during food preparation and meal consumption. Questions from the nurse should focus on the child's likes and dislikes for particular foods, behavior at the table, and establishment of healthy family eating patterns. Ask how often the family eats out, especially at fast-food restaurants. When parents are busy and older siblings are in activities, both toddlers and preschoolers may be eating foods such as french fries or milk shakes several times weekly. Suggest alternative approaches to the busy lifestyle, such as bringing fresh fruit slices along when an older sibling is at a sporting event, keeping a cooler in the car to maintain cool items, and limiting fast-food meals to no more than one or two weekly. Obtain nutritional information about common fast-food options in your community and share these with parents. Assist them to make healthy choices when eating out. Encourage the family to set times when they all eat together, even if only a few times weekly. If children help with preparations for this family meal, and then eat together, nutritional knowledge and intake can be positively enhanced. When the child is in a childcare center or home, encourage the parents to find out what food is provided for the child in that setting.

During the toddler and preschool years, children are gaining much more independence about food choices and patterns of eating. At the same time, their eating patterns depend mainly on the family, so assessment should involve the entire family unit (see *Developing Cultural Competence: Family Nutrition*). Parents can benefit from receiving information about nutrition for young children (Table 35–2).

Developing Cultural Competence Family Nutrition

Each family integrates their own cultural backgrounds and past experiences into food preparation and choices. Ask what foods are common in the child's cultural group and help the family learn when to introduce each food. For example, rice may be a first food for an Asian baby rather than rice cereal. Be sure the child also takes in adequate iron sources in the first foods offered. Tofu or bean paste may be a common protein source in some diets. A Native American child may eat fish or wild game, along with berries and roots. Ask and learn about each family's cultural patterns. Learn what you can about cultural groups in your community. Encourage the family to offer the young child their usual foods, as long as they meet needs for requirements, are prepared with minimal salt and seasoning, and are soft enough to avoid choking. Perform diet recalls and analyses to check for any specific teaching needs in all families.

Health promotion interventions include actions such as supporting breastfeeding for young toddlers and being sure preschoolers have a role in selecting foods for healthy snacks. Parental education is influential in shaping their young child's diet and should be integrated into all visits (Holt, Wooldridge, Story, et al., 2011). Important health promotion teaching includes the concept of "5 a day," or ensuring five servings of fruits and vegetables in the daily diet (American Academy of Pediatrics [AAP] Committee on Nutrition, 2013). Likewise, "3 a day of dairy" encourages families to provide at least three servings of dairy for children every day. Nurses and parents partner together to ensure that the young child establishes healthy eating habits at home and in other daily settings. Health maintenance activities focus primarily on disease and injury prevention, with examples of feeding practices that do not include common choking foods, and limiting daily fruit juice intake to prevent dental caries and excessive caloric intake. Desired outcomes related to nutrition include meeting normal growth and development milestones, maintaining a recommended weight, expanding understanding of healthy food patterns, and preventing nutrition-related disorders.

Physical Activity

The toddler and preschooler consistently show gains in fine and gross motor abilities. They walk and run independently and often engage in physical activity in school and other settings. They commonly visit parks, swim, attend childcare centers, and help with some household tasks. These activities are important, both because they assist the child to continue to develop motor skills and because they limit the amount of time spent in sedentary behavior. The toddler and preschool years are an important time for setting the habits for physical activity during all of childhood.

During toddler years the main emphasis is on providing experiences that encourage further motor development. The child needs to walk, run, hop, push and pull objects, and throw balls. Motor activity is a major component in all playtimes, and activities should engage the child's large and small muscle groups. The National Association for Sport and Physical Education (NASPE) has established recommendations for toddlers and preschoolers: a minimum of 60 minutes per day of unstructured physical activity, a minimum of 60 minutes per day of structured physical activity, and a maximum of 60 minutes of sedentary behavior at any one time exclusive of sleep (Beets, Bornstein, Dowda, et al., 2011; Centers for Disease Control and Prevention [CDC], 2011) (Figure 35–2).

By the preschool years, coordination develops quickly. Physical activity is important for all children, including those with developmental disabilities. The preschooler learns to balance, walk on one foot, skip, and throw and catch with greater accuracy. **Kinesthesia**, or the sense of one's body position and movement, develops during these years. Eye–hand coordination improves at the same time that visual acuity matures. The social component plays an important role as children learn to engage in games and activities cooperatively with others.

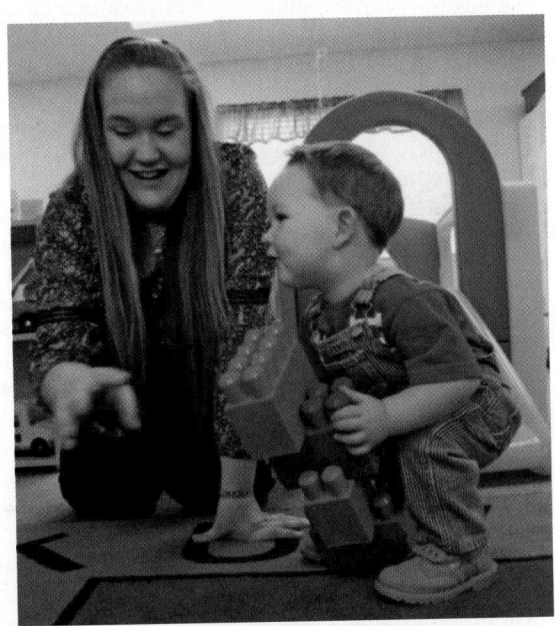

Figure 35–2 This toddler enjoys motor activity that uses large muscle groups. The preschooler spends much of playtime in activities that lead to coordination of both small and large muscle mass. List several physical activities that you can suggest for the parents of children in each of these age groups.

TABLE 35–3 Risk and Protective Factors Regarding Physical Activity in Toddlerhood and Preschool

RISK FACTORS	PROTECTIVE FACTORS
• Developmental delay • Slow development of social skills	• Expected developmental progression
• Limited stimulation by family or other care providers • Limited social time with other children • Long work hours by parents	• Easily engages socially with others • Regular contact with other young children
• Reluctance to try new physical activity • Limited access to balls, slides, balance beams, tricycles, and other materials that foster physical activity • Adequate safety gear for activities is not available	• Eagerness to try new physical activity • Access to balls, slides, balance beams, tricycles, and other materials that foster physical activity • Adequate safety gear that properly fits child is available
• Parents who have little physical activity on a daily basis • Lack of knowledge by family about child's physical activity needs	• Family members engage in daily physical activity • Family members spend time in physical activity with child • Family understands motor developmental milestones and importance of physical activity in childhood
• Television or other screen activities are engaged in for more than 2 hr daily	• Television and other screen activities are limited to no more than 2 hr daily
• Limited community resources for child care and physical activity • Unsafe neighborhood and lack of lawns, parks, and other facilities	• Neighborhood contains access to child care that integrates physical activity • Neighborhood is safe, and contains lawns, parks, and other facilities

The nurse applies the concept of resilience by identifying both risk and protective factors related to physical activity (Table 35–3). The assessment becomes the basis for nursing interventions, both to reinforce positive physical activity and to make recommendations for changes where needed.

Both children and adults are commonly overweight and sedentary in today's society, so emphasis on physical activity should be a part of each health supervision visit. Nurses and parents are partners in planning activities for the young child; patterns set in motion at this early age will continue into the rest of childhood and into adulthood (Simmonds et al., 2015). Suggestions for the family may include setting guidelines to limit television and other screen activities to a maximum of 2 hours daily in order to facilitate adequate physical activity time. Children should not have television and computers in their bedrooms because use of such media can disturb sleep, and children learn best from play rather than media exposure (AAP Council on Communications and Media, 2013). Health promotion teaching imparts to parents the benefits of activity, such as a healthy immune and cardiovascular system, positive self-concept of the child, and the child's learning of important motor skills. Health maintenance teaching focuses on disease prevention, such as avoidance of overweight, and injury prevention, with use of protective gear for sports.

Expected outcomes of health promotion and health supervision related to physical activity are daily inclusion of at least 60 minutes of activity into life patterns, normal developmental progression of the musculoskeletal system, growth in coordination, and appropriate balance between dietary intake and physical activity so that normal weight is maintained.

Oral Health

The early childhood years play an important part in the child's future oral health, and yet dental care remains one of the most preventable and common unmet healthcare needs for children in developed countries. About 28% of children from 2 to 5 years have had dental caries, and 21% have untreated dental caries (National Institute of Dental and Craniofacial Research, 2014). **Early childhood caries (ECC)** is defined as one or more decayed, missing, or filled tooth surfaces in a child 71 months of age or younger (AAP Committee on Nutrition, 2013; Colak, Dulgergil, Dalli, et al., 2013). (See Chapter 31 for further information.) This condition is promoted by inadequate preventive care, which can include diet, brushing, feeding habits, and lack of dental care. ECC is serious because young children with the condition are more likely to have continuing dental problems that can influence speech, cause pain, and delay development. Teaching prevention at an early age is key to preventing the problem.

The nurse assists the family to ensure oral health for the young child. By 1 year of age, the child should have made a first visit to the dentist. The child should have an established dental home for regular care and recommendations (American Academy of Pediatric Dentistry [AAPD] Council on Clinical Affairs, 2013). By about 2 years of age, the toddler has a full set of 20 primary teeth, called **deciduous teeth**, that will be lost during childhood, beginning at about 6 years. Evaluate these teeth for condition and number. They help to maintain space for the permanent teeth, foster positive eating habits, and are needed for language development. Inquire about how the family cleans the teeth and, if the child has any dental decay, ask them to demonstrate their daily care. At the end of preschool, the first of the deciduous teeth are lost, an important developmental event for most children.

By 2 to 4 years of age, young children have discontinued using pacifiers and thumbsucking. These habits are harmful when permanent teeth begin erupting at about 6 years (American Dental Association [ADA], 2011). Parents should be instructed gradually to remove the pacifier by 1 to 2 years of age. Many young children continue to thumbsuck, which is a comforting and reassuring habit. Usually, the child who is 2 to 4 years old is ready to discontinue thumbsucking, and parents can promote this process by praising the child for not sucking, helping the child to find alternative sources of comfort such as rubbing a blanket, putting a sock on the hand at nap or nighttime to serve as a reminder not to suck, and working with the preschooler to identify the reward when no thumbsucking is seen for a week or more (ADA, 2011).

Based on the results of the assessment of the child's teeth, observation of language skills, and answers to questions directed at parents, plan interventions that will foster maintenance of oral health, thus preventing dental disease. (See Chapter 45 for emergency treatment of dental injury.) These may include referral to low-cost dental clinics, provision of toothbrush and toothpaste, demonstration to the parents and young child about proper brushing technique, and teaching about limiting sweet snacks and drinks. A dental visit will assist in identifying children at moderate or high risk of dental caries; for these children, a "smear" of fluoridated toothpaste should be used for brushing, and in 2- to 5-year-olds, a pea-size amount of fluoridated toothpaste can be used. For other children, nonfluoridated toothpaste is used (American Academy of Pediatric Dentistry [AAPD], 2014). Remember to positively reinforce health promotion practices such as good oral hygiene for toddlers and preschoolers who brush, visit the dentist, and are careful to limit intake of sweets. Desired outcomes for oral health are eruption of a normal set of deciduous teeth, regular dental care, nutrition and hygiene practices that foster dental health, and knowledge of child and parent about oral health.

Mental and Spiritual Health

The family plays a key role in fostering a positive self-image and setting the stage for the young child's mental health. As the family is called in for the visit, begin an assessment of the family's methods of influencing mental health. Observe communication and interactions in the family and the child's ability to interact with healthcare providers. Ask for a description of a typical day or what the child has recently begun to do. The child's sense of self and mental status are related to new accomplishments. Inquire about toilet training, tooth brushing, choosing clothes and getting dressed, using crayons, or other developmental tasks.

Toddlers and preschoolers use **self-regulation** (the ability to soothe and comfort the self) to control anger, excessive desires for objects or foods, and other nonsocial behaviors. To assist the child in developing the ability to control and regulate self, parents often use discipline techniques. Ask about how the parent deals with the child who is having a temper tantrum or showing other undesirable behaviors. Reinforce positive ways of helping the child set limits for self and make suggestions when parents need assistance (see *Teaching Highlights: Positive Discipline*). The goal of discipline is to help the child develop a sense of right and wrong, and to learn acceptable ways of dealing with other people.

Adequate sleep and rest are needed for children to master self-regulation. Most toddlers have established regular sleeping patterns with occasional night awakenings. They sleep about 10 to 12 hours at night with one or two daytime naps. Parents have usually learned to establish clear routines such as reading a story, back rubbing, and then leaving the child alone. Occasionally, parents who work during the day may feel guilty about putting the child to sleep. Help them to spend quality time with the child after arriving home, and then to establish clear sleeping expectations. Transitional objects such as blankets or toys are important for the toddler and can be used during childcare experiences to provide comfort and help maintain normal routines. Some families prefer to have children sleep in

---

TEACHING HIGHLIGHTS | Positive Discipline

First, provide structure that enhances the possibility of desirable behaviors:

- Limit rules to those that are essential. It will be easier to enforce a few important rules than many that are nonessential.
- Provide an environment where the child is mainly free to explore safely in order to avoid constant cautions. For example, have adequate play space for toddlers with limited fragile glassware in the usual daily environment. It is easier for the toddler to learn not to touch a few objects when adequate objects are provided for play.
- Spend time interacting with the child several times each day. Praise positive behaviors frequently. Preschoolers often like to have charts with stars to record picking up toys, helping a parent, and other positive behaviors. Once a certain number of stars is reached, a reward, such as stickers or an outing with the parent, is earned.

When the child shows undesirable behaviors:

- Use distraction as the first approach and praise the child for selecting the new activity suggested by the parent.
- Tell the child one time that the behavior is unsatisfactory and what will happen if the behavior persists.
- Separate the child from a setting in which behavior is undesirable. Place the child in "time-out," a separate place that is safe. Toddlers can be placed in a playpen or crib, while preschoolers are told to sit on a chair. One minute of time-out per year of age is a good length of time. Once time-out is over, provide a positive activity and move the child directly toward the activity.

When undesirable behaviors include other people, such as biting or hitting:

- Tell the child clearly that it is not okay to hurt another person. Encourage and role model proper language to explain feelings.
- Separate the child immediately from the situation and use time-out.
- If there are repeated episodes, be sure the child is getting adequate sleep and food, has opportunities for active play that releases energy, and has positive attention from many people in the environment. Be sensitive to stresses such as a recent trauma or a new sibling.
- Encourage the child to "use words" instead of hitting or biting. Until able to do so on their own, parents can model this behavior. "You feel like saying, 'I am really upset that you took my toy away.' Let's use words instead of hitting so your sister knows that."

the bed with parents. Advise against this pattern, but if this is the parents' decision, be sure they are aware of safety hazards such as suffocation in excessive bedding, injury related to falling between headboard and frame, parental smoking that could lead to a fire, or parental deep sleeping or alcohol and drug use that can lead to such sound sleep that it is possible to roll onto and suffocate the child.

The preschooler sleeps about 9 to 11 hours and may have one or no naps each day. Some quiet playtime can be beneficial even for the preschooler who does not nap. At this age, some children begin to awaken at night and may need some assistance in falling back to sleep. **Nightmares** are frightening dreams that awaken the child, who is often crying and upset. Parents can reassure the child, rub the child's back, provide some repeat of a bedtime routine such as reading a story, and then allow the child to settle into sleep again. It is not advisable to bring children to the parental bed since they may start to awaken at night in order to continue this practice. **Night terrors** (or sleep terrors) are characterized by a child who cries out, appears frightened, and has tachycardia and tachypnea. However, in contrast to nightmares, the child having a night terror is not fully awake and may appear disoriented (Mayo Clinic, 2014). Parents should quietly talk to and comfort the child, allowing the child to return to sleep. The child has no recollection of these events the next morning.

The toddler gains more independence in many aspects of life such as mobility and speech. The control over toileting is another milestone that signals greater independence and can lead to a sense of self-control. Ask parents if the toddler has shown interest in toilet training and how they intend to work with the child to attain control over bowel and bladder. (See Chapter 31 for further discussion about toilet training.) Preschoolers are generally well trained for bowel and bladder with only occasional accidents. These should be treated with understanding rather than blame in order for healthy self-concept to develop.

Preschoolers have a growing awareness of gender and sexuality issues. They may ask questions about kissing, love, or their genitals. These questions should be truthfully answered, leaving the child with a positive sense of sexuality. Some exploration of genitals may occur, and children should be told simply that it is something that should occur in private, and then be offered other activities to engage them when with other people.

The family's spiritual orientation takes on additional meaning for the toddler and preschooler. They can participate in the family's faith-based practices, which enlarge their microsystem influences to include that of the religious group, thus reinforcing the child's learning about right and wrong. The nurse assesses the family's faith-based or spiritual beliefs and provides support for the family's approach, whether it is in established religious organizations or in the family's other meaningful activities (Pender, Murdaugh, & Parsons, 2015).

Health promotion activities focus on development of a healthy self-concept in the toddler and young child by helping parents to set up successful play experiences, to praise the child for successes, to use effective limit-setting techniques, and to realize and appreciate the child's unique characteristics. Health maintenance seeks to avoid the poor self-image that can occur with constant criticism or expectations not in alignment with the toddler's or preschooler's developmental capabilities. Further examples of the family interactions that can influence the child's self-concept are provided in the following section on relationships.

Desired outcomes for the child related to mental and spiritual health include emergence of a positive self-esteem, ability to self-regulate behaviors, emergence of methods to handle daily stressors, and normal developmental progression in tasks such as toilet training and sleep.

Relationships

Family members are part of the microsystem for the toddler and preschooler and, as such, form a vital part of the child's environment. Families with members who handle stress well and have healthy lifestyle patterns offer security for the young child. When parents are stressed or depressed, the mental status of all family members can be affected. Ask how things are going for the family in general. Inquire about siblings and whether there are any issues of concern that might influence the toddler or preschooler. Illness or behavior problems in a sibling can decrease the parent's ability to deal with other children. The focus on a sibling in need can be confusing to a toddler or preschooler. Be alert for signs of child abuse and for substance abuse in family members (refer to Chapter 42). Have the parents become separated or divorced? Is there a new stepparent?

During questions and observations, the nurse identifies family risk and protective factors. Reinforce strengths and provide services and referrals to deal with risks. Some strengths include the following:

- The family spends time together each day.
- Parents are proud of the child's accomplishments and knowledgeable about developmental progression.
- Childcare center personnel and family members interact regularly to plan consistent approaches for the toddler and preschooler.
- The teen mother of a toddler is enrolled in a high school continuation program with a childcare component.

Examples of risks to mental health include the following:

- Mother has been diagnosed with depression.
- Family member in home uses street drugs.
- Child awakens with night terrors.
- Child was recently in a serious motor vehicle crash.
- Teen mother is estranged from own family and has few goals and resources.

Toddlers continue to grow in social abilities, while preschoolers demonstrate large strides in socializing with others. Expect that most toddlers will enjoy playing with other children, although they play "side by side" in a parallel manner and not cooperatively. They also engage in play with adults for short periods, such as throwing a ball. However, preschoolers begin to engage in activities that involve other children directly in cooperative play. They play "house" where one child plays the mother and another the child. They engage in simple games where each plays a separate role. Their interactions with adults display similar maturity as they take on tasks such as setting the table for dinner or picking up books from the floor. Social skills involve getting along with others. Young children exhibit maturing skill in language development, a primary medium for social exchange. From just a few words at 1 year, the child has progressed to stating three-word sentences by 3 years of age. While all parts of speech are not in place, young children certainly have the ability to make needs and thoughts known. Assessment of language skills provides a mirror into this important means of socializing.

Successful social skills involve separating from the parent at times. During toddlerhood, most children spend some time away from parents. Initially they may be fearful and display crying, but gradually they learn to adapt to the new person and place. Preschoolers need to begin developing relationships with other adults and children in order to adapt to the school setting at about 5 years of age. Ask how many people the child has contact with each week and how they manage separation from the parent. Encourage parents to see separation as a skill the child is learning rather than something that is guilt producing for them. When they leave the child in a secure setting, they should hug, provide a favorite object, and leave. Short periods initially will teach the child that the parent can be trusted to return.

Expected outcomes of health promotion and health maintenance activities with young children include appropriate social skills with parents, siblings, and other children and adults; successful management of temperament characteristics; adjustment to time away from the home; and improving language/communication skills.

Disease Prevention Strategies

Toddlers and preschoolers commonly have 6 to 10 upper respiratory infections annually, so teaching good hygiene is a helpful preventive measure (Lucille Packard Children's Hospital, 2012). Some immunizations are given during this age period in order to complete a basic series. For the child who has not had all immunizations, extra visits to catch them up to recommended levels might be needed. At the end of the preschool period, a complete review of the immunization record is done so that any needed immunizations are administered before school entry. See Table 35–4 for immunizations recommended during toddlerhood and preschool (additional immunizations may be needed for children at high risk for certain diseases). Toddlers and preschoolers should be screened for health problems during health supervision visits, such as asthma, obesity, or other issues manifested by a review of body systems. Earlier visits may have failed to identify a problem on account of the child's young age, so areas such as vision, hearing, and developmental milestones are always included.

Recognize that the environment is a powerful influence on the health of children. Ask if parents or others in the home smoke. Discourage this practice and describe the health implications for the child. Is the neighborhood generally safe? Is there toxicity exposure from air, water, or other mediums? Ask about lead exposure in the home (see Chapter 42 for more information). How much television and other screen time is common in the home? Older siblings who allow the preschooler to play violent video games or watch many hours of inappropriate television can affect the mental health of the young child. Do parents watch the evening news, even when it involves violence, in front of young children? Do they discuss television shows with the child?

Ask if the child has had any diseases, whether common ones such as a middle ear infection, or less common ones such as a serious respiratory infection. Has the child been diagnosed with a chronic disorder such as cystic fibrosis or hemophilia? How has that affected his or her general health and family functioning?

Desired outcomes for disease prevention include integration of a healthy lifestyle into the family's daily life, prompt treatment of acute diseases, and individualization of all health supervision topics for the child with a chronic condition or special healthcare need.

TABLE 35–4 Routine Immunizations Recommended During Toddlerhood and Preschool Age

IMMUNIZATION	AGE RECOMMENDED
Hepatitis B	6–18 months: Administer dose #3 if series not completed during infancy (usually doses #1 and #2 are administered in early infancy, with dose #3 from 6–18 months of age)
Hepatitis A	Series of 2 doses with first at 12 months and second at least 6 months later
Diphtheria, tetanus, acellular pertussis (DTaP)	15–18 months (#4) (first 3 administered in infancy) 4–6 years (#5)
Haemophilus influenzae type b	12–15 months (#4 or will be #3 for PRP-OMP type that requires only 3 doses for whole series) (first doses administered in infancy)
Inactivated poliovirus	4–6 years (#4) (first 3 doses administered in infancy)
Measles, mumps, rubella	12–15 months (#1)
Varicella	12–18 months (#1) 4–6 years (#2)
Pneumococcal	12–15 months (#4)
Influenza	Annually

Note: Schedule may need to be adapted if child did not receive all recommended immunizations during infancy. See Chapter 43 and the CDC and AAP websites for further information.

Injury Prevention Strategies

Injuries remain a common healthcare problem for children during the toddler and preschooler years. Toddlers' and preschoolers' mobility, physical skills, and lack of understanding of the presence of hazards put them at particular risk. In addition, children are sometimes left to play alone for short periods, and toddlers and preschoolers can quickly get into dangerous situations. Every healthcare visit needs to include an assessment of risks and teaching to prevent injuries. Tables 35–5 and 35–6 list injury hazards and his or her prevention during these age periods.

Ask parents what they think the most common hazards are for the age of the child, and add other hazards to their awareness. Car safety always needs reinforcing as the types of seats recommended change as the child matures. Children should be in a rear-facing car seat in the back seat until at least age 2 years, and preferably until 4 years or when the child has reached the top height or weight limit allowed by the car seat manufacturer. Once the child has reached the highest height and weight allowed by the rear-facing seat, a forward-facing car seat with a harness should be placed in the back seat. Once the child has outgrown the recommendations for height and weight for the forward-facing car seat, a booster seat in the back seat is recommended (AAP, 2014).

TABLE 35–5 Injury Prevention in Toddlerhood

	HAZARD	DEVELOPMENTAL CHARACTERISTICS	PREVENTIVE MEASURES
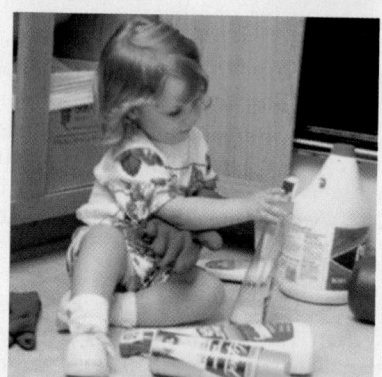	Falls	Gross motor skills improve: Toddler is able to move chairs to counters and can climb up ladders.	Supervise toddler closely. Provide safe climbing toys. Begin to teach acceptable places for climbing.
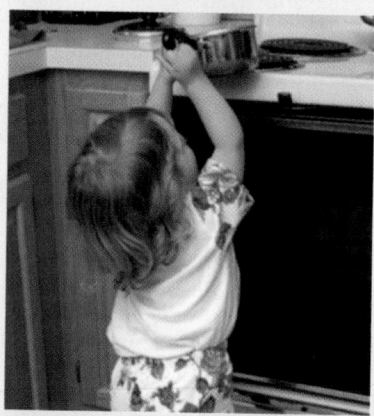	Poisoning	Gross motor skills enable toddler to climb onto chairs and then cabinets. Medicines, cosmetics, and other poisonous substances are easily reached.	Keep medicines and other poisonous material locked away. Use child-resistant containers and cupboard closures. Post the Poison Control Center number (1-800-222-1222) by telephone and tape it on cell phones and program the cell phone with the number.
	Burns	Toddler is tall enough to reach stove top. Toddler can walk to fireplace and may reach into fire. Electrical cords may be placed in mouth.	Keep pot handles turned inward on stove. Do not burn fires without close supervision. Use a fire screen in fireplaces. Supervise child during play and keep electrical cords, power strips, and other hazards out of reach or covered securely.
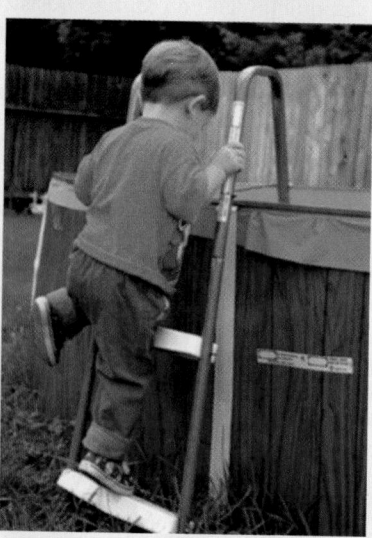	Drowning	Toddler can walk onto docks or pool decks. Toddler may stand on or climb seats on boat. Toddler may fall into buckets, toilets, and fish tanks and be unable to get top of body out.	Supervise any child near water. Swimming classes do not protect a toddler from drowning. Use child-resistant pool covers. Use approved child life jackets near water and on boats. Empty buckets when not in use.
	Motor vehicle crashes	Toddler may be able to undo seat belt, may resist using car seat, demonstrating characteristic negativism and autonomy.	Use approved safety seat only; toddler is not large enough to use car seat belts. Insist on safety seat use for all trips and position seat in rear seat of car. Verify that child is belted in properly before starting car. Keep the child in a rear-facing seat until at least 2 years of age and preferably longer, until achieving the highest weight or height recommended for the seat by the manufacturer; then a forward-facing car seat with harness should be used in the back seat.

TABLE 35–6 Injury Prevention in the Preschool Years

	HAZARD	DEVELOPMENTAL CHARACTERISTICS	PREVENTIVE MEASURES
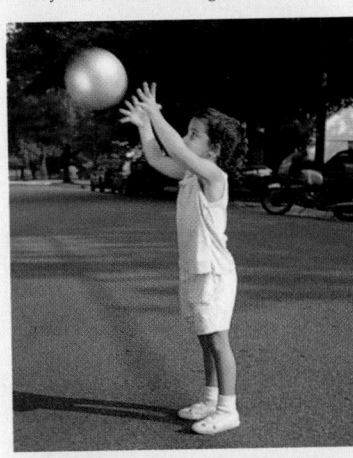 Ruth Jenkinson/DK Images	Motor vehicle crashes	By about 4–5 years, the child independently gets into car and puts on seat belt. Child may forget to belt up or may do so incorrectly.	Verify that child is belted in properly before starting car. Keep the child in a rear-facing seat secured in the back seat until at least 2 years of age and preferably longer, until achieving the highest weight or height recommended for the seat by the manufacturer. Forward-facing seats with harness placed in the back seat are used next. Once the child has outgrown the car seat, a booster seat is used in the back seat.
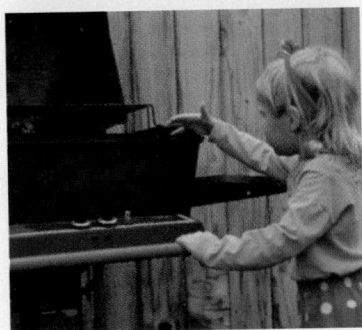	Motor vehicle and pedestrian accidents	Preschooler may play outside alone or with friends. Preschooler is unable to judge speed of moving car and assumes driver knows that he or she is present.	Teach child never to go into road. A safe, preferably enclosed, play yard is recommended. The child should be supervised by adults at all times.
	Drowning	Preschooler who has had swimming lessons may choose to go into a lake or pool.	Teach child never to go into water without an adult. Provide supervision whenever child is near water.
	Burns	Preschooler can understand the hazards of fire.	Teach child to stop, drop, and roll if clothes are on fire. Practice escapes from home are useful. A visit to a fire station can reinforce learning. Teach child how to call 9-1-1.
	Needlesticks in hospital and home	Preschooler can ambulate and is interested in new objects.	Keep needles out of reach. Remove from hospital unit immediately after use. Instruct families on safe disposal if a family member uses needles at home (e.g., a family member with diabetes).
	Electrical injury in hospital and home	Preschooler is mobile and may trip over cords and equipment or may choose to examine them.	Avoid use of electrical cords if possible. Keep equipment out of major traffic areas. Cover any electrical outlets not being used for equipment. Monitor child closely.

Recommend that parents have their car seat checked by a child safety seat inspector (Figure 35–3). Give them the addresses of the closest inspection stations. These can be located by going through the National Highway Traffic Safety Administration (2014) (www.nhtsa.dot.gov). Check your particular state laws regulating car safety seats for children.

Other common and serious safety hazards are falls and drowning. In addition to providing general guidelines about safety, these most common injuries should be directly addressed. Children often fall down stairs, from counters where they have been placed or crawled, and from grocery carts. Drowning episodes occur when toddlers and preschoolers are not watched every moment while in the bathtub, near a pool or spa, at a lake or ocean, or when they fall from boats without personal flotation devices on. While all young children should begin to take swimming lessons, this does not guarantee their

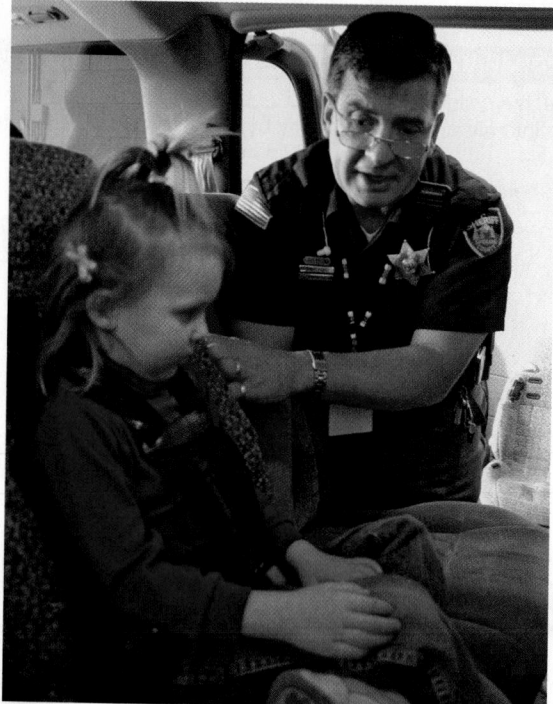

Figure 35–3 This police officer is certified to examine car seats for children and make recommendations for parents. He is examining a preschooler in a booster seat for proper fit, alignment, and installation. Many car seats are improperly installed or not the proper type for a specific age/size of child, so centers that check seats provide an important service.

safety around water. The AAP (2013) recommends swimming lessons for all children by age 4 years and for children from 1 to 4 years if lessons are available and the parents believe the child is ready for lessons. Children also play with balls, and may follow them as they roll or are thrown into the street. Nursing interventions concentrate on relaying to parents the severity of the risk of falls, drowning, and other hazards for children. Teach them to be aware of the dangers and to avoid them, both at home and in other settings. Refer them to classes on first aid and cardiopulmonary resuscitation.

The child spends more time away from the parent than during earlier developmental stages. Childcare situations should provide the same supervision the child receives at home. Help parents to ask questions and feel confident in safety at other settings. For example, while parents may be cautious about gun safety at home, few of them inquire if a home the child is visiting has guns and how they are stored.

Preschool is a time when teaching can become directed both to the parents and to their children. Preschoolers are receptive to practicing street crossing and tricycle/bicycle riding skills. It may be helpful to have a place in the clinic or office where they can be taught basic skills such as hand washing or street crossing. Consider the time of year, climate, and geographic location and teach appropriately. Spring is often a good time to teach bicycle and water safety, while winter hazards may include teaching about the hazards of wood stoves or other heating devices. See Table 35–7 for further information about toddler and preschooler hazards and safety teaching needed.

SAFETY ALERT!
Young children die each year when they are left confined in parked vehicles and suffer heatstroke. Occasionally, children gain access to a vehicle and accidentally lock themselves inside. In most cases, however, parents leave a child unattended, either forgetting the child is in the car, or remembering but underestimating the danger of heat effects. Nurses can be effective in instructing families to keep cars locked so young children cannot gain access, and to never leave a child in a parked car, either in or out of a car seat, even for a few moments, no matter what the outside temperature (Safe Kids, 2014).

Desired outcomes for the child are integration of safe practices into car restraints and other daily activities, progression through toddlerhood and preschool with no serious injuries, prompt care for minor injuries, and understanding by child, parent, and other care providers of the common safety hazards at this age.

Nursing Management

For the Health Promotion and Maintenance of the Toddler and Preschooler

Nursing Assessment and Diagnosis

Nurses partner with other healthcare professionals such as physicians, nurse practitioners, and speech therapists to assess health promotion and health maintenance status of young children. The toddler and preschool years are characterized by much developmental progression, and strategies need to be constantly adapted to meet the particular needs of the child and family. It is important to realize that the parents are partners in the care of the child and that every health supervision visit should address their questions and concerns. Their observations of the child are an invaluable part of the process. As preschoolers become more verbal, they become partners with others in the healthcare team. Ask preschoolers what they want to learn, what questions they have about staying well, and other pertinent questions.

Toddlers and preschoolers are examined for growth, physical health status, and mental/social characteristics. Development is an area that many pediatricians feel ill prepared to address but which parents commonly want addressed. Additionally, developmental surveillance must occur at every healthcare visit, with standardized screening at 9, 18, and 24 to 30 months. Nurses are adept at describing normal developmental milestones, evaluating the progression of children, and using anticipatory guidance to address parental developmental concerns.

Based on a thorough assessment, the nurse will establish nursing diagnoses that are appropriate for the young child and family. Potential nursing diagnoses established during a health supervision of a toddler or preschooler might include the following (NANDA-I © 2014):

- *Anxiety* related to change of environment (new care provider)
- *Role Conflict, Parental,* related to lack of support from significant others
- *Development: Delayed, Risk for,* related to lead exposure
- *Sleep Deprivation* related to nightmares and night terrors
- *Knowledge, Readiness for Enhanced,* related to parental desire for safety information
- *Skin Integrity, Impaired,* related to hyperthermia (sunburn)

TABLE 35–7 Disease and Injury Prevention Topics by Age

AGE	INJURY PREVENTION TEACHING TOPICS	
15 months	Wash adult and toddler hands frequently.	Have poison control number by phones and taped onto and programmed into cell phones.
	Clean toys with soap and water regularly.	Be alert for dangers of hot curling irons and other appliances.
	Provide child's own bedding for childcare setting and wash weekly.	Have electrical cords out of reach and not hanging down.
	Use forward-facing car safety seat if child is 20 lb; install correctly and have installation checked; place in back seat and never in front seat with a passenger air bag.	Keep water temperature no higher than 120°–125°F (49°–52°C).
	Empty containers of water immediately after use; be sure pools or other bodies of water are locked and not accessible.	Have home environment checked for lead hazards; arrange for blood lead level testing when appropriate (see Chapter 42).
	Use sunscreen, hat, and long sleeves in the sun.	Secure the child in shopping carts.
	Keep heavy and sharp objects out of reach; check that all poisons are locked away, including in homes visited; keep pet food and cosmetics out of reach.	Do not let child have access to alcoholic drinks.
		Remember that responsible adults should always supervise your child, not other children.
		Know CPR, airway obstruction removal, and other first aid.
18 months	Follow the above.	Use a helmet on the child when taking the child on the back of a bicycle.
	Bolt heavy objects securely to the wall to prevent them from being pulled down (such as bookcases and televisions).	Check batteries in home smoke alarms, CO or radon monitors, and check system monthly; change batteries on a scheduled basis as recommended by manufacturer.
	Be cautious of the toddler near machinery in the yard, such as lawn mowers and farm equipment.	Ask care providers about discipline methods; do not allow corporal punishment.
2–3 years	Follow the above.	Teach how to cross streets.
	When the child is 40 lb, switch to a belt-positioning booster seat, using vehicle lap and shoulder belt; continue to place booster seat in rear seat of the car.	Provide a helmet for riding tricycles.
		Check playgrounds for safety hazards and hard surfaces under equipment; ensure cushioned surface.
	Teach hand hygiene after toileting and other activities.	
	Clean potty chair thoroughly.	
	Keep guns unloaded and locked away in a different locked place than ammunition; have trigger locks installed.	
3–4 years	Follow the above.	Know CPR, airway obstruction removal, and other first aid for the child who has become a preschooler.
	Do not let child play unsupervised.	
4–5 years	Follow the above.	Teach safety around strangers (never go with a stranger; find a trusted person such as a parent or police).
	Continue teaching safety skills to the child.	
	Continue supervising when near streets or water sources.	

Source: Data from Hagan, J. F., Shaw, J. S., & Duncan, P. M. (Eds.). (2008). *Bright futures: Guidelines for health supervision of infants, children, and adolescents* (3rd ed.). Elk Grove Village, IL: American Academy of Pediatrics.

Planning and Implementation

Based on the nursing diagnoses, the nurse works with other partners to plan strategies to meet the needs of the family. Explain that assessment questions are asked to provide a picture of the child that can be helpful in partnering with parents to plan health care. Reinforce the importance of the family coming to health supervision visits with their own list of issues. See *Clinical Reasoning: Families Who Miss Scheduled Healthcare Visits*. Work with other healthcare professionals to be sure all needs of a particular child and family are addressed.

Some teaching takes place as the examination occurs. Explain the height and weight measurements and their meaning. Relate them to questions about dietary intake and family food patterns. During the physical examination, insert information about common infections such as otitis media (middle ear infection) and share immunization information.

Clinical Reasoning Families Who Miss Scheduled Healthcare Visits

Clarence, described in this chapter's opening scenario, is being seen at 15 months of age. He missed his 12-month visit and was last seen at 9 months. How can you ask the parents about the reasons they may have missed the 12-month visit? What immunizations must be "caught up" now that some were missed? (See Chapter 43 for immunization schedules.) What components of developmental surveillance are particularly important for you to perform at this visit?

If the family has been reluctant to ask questions, reflect on the child's development. "Many children have trouble sleeping through the night; is that the case for Cassandra? What helps her to sleep? What is it like at her bedtime?" Developmental areas such as sleep, discipline, toilet training, and expected developmental milestones should be addressed. If the parents were provided in an earlier visit with a journal to record observations and questions, ask if they have brought it with them.

Health promotion activities are emphasized during the visit. Health promotion related to physical activity includes teaching about toys that encourage activity, such as balls, music, push toys, and tricycles. Review nutritional intake and encourage introduction of new foods, healthy snack and meal choices, and positive eating for busy families. Emphasize the importance of play to healthy child development. Provide ideas for incorporating free playtime each day. Apply concepts of anticipatory guidance as you address the child's approaching developmental progression. If the child will soon be toilet trained, provide information about possible approaches. If the child is learning to swim or has access to water, reinforce safety precautions near water. For the child going to a new childcare center, provide the parents with a list of questions they can ask the care provider, and tips to assist in the transition to a new setting.

Health maintenance activities are added to the visit as you give immunizations and screen for tuberculosis, lead screening, or problems with language, vision, or hearing. Provide instruction on use of nonprescription medications, including use of acetaminophen after immunizations. Precautions, safe dosing, and checking with the healthcare provider should be addressed. The focus of these activities is to prevent disease or to find it early before serious consequences arise. Whenever you find information that may indicate a problem, be sure to refer the child to the primary care provider, such as the physician or nurse practitioner. You may even recommend that another specialist, such as a speech pathologist or dentist, see the child. Other health maintenance activities that must be part of each visit with a toddler or preschooler involve teaching about common hazards and how to avoid them. Emergency care in case of injury is also helpful information for parents, so first aid classes can be recommended. Ask about daycare, preschool, or kindergarten attendance or future plans.

Healthy People 2020

(V-1) Increase the proportion of preschool children aged 5 years and under who receive vision screening

- While only 40% of preschool children receive vision screening presently, a goal of 44% has been set. Nurses should ensure that all preschool children receive vision screening in childcare centers and at health supervision visits.

(V-2) Reduce blindness and visual impairment in children and adolescents aged 17 years and under

- While 28% of children are blind or visually impaired, when more children are screened in their early years, less than 25% of children should experience visual impairment.

SAFETY ALERT!

Nearly 2000 children are injured annually by falls related to baby gates. Those under 2 years more commonly push over an expandable gate and fall down stairs with the gate. Child over 2 years may climb the gate or open it and thus fall down stairs, often sustaining soft tissue injuries. Ask parents if their homes have stairs. If so, what type of protection is available for the child? Is an expandable gate used? If so, would the parents be able to change to one that is installed into the wall studs? Can a preschooler climb the gate? If so, it is safer to remove the gate and supervise the child more closely (Cheng, Fletcher, Roberts, et al., 2014).

Conclude the visit with some words of praise about both the parent's and child's accomplishments. Schedule the date for the next visit. List any resources helpful to the family, including the clinic/office contact information and emergency services.

TEACHING HIGHLIGHTS | Toy and Playground Safety

Play is essential to the physical and cognitive growth of toddlers and preschoolers. However, toys can present hazards for young children, and parents need guidelines to follow when selecting toys. These include (Safe Kids, 2011b):

- Select toys intended for the age of the child, as indicated on the label. Some toys have small parts or can break into small parts, and should not be given to children younger than 3 years. They should not be too heavy for the child to manipulate them appropriately. Toys with strings, straps, or cords longer than 7 in. pose strangulation hazards.
- Assemble toys as directed and check them frequently for breakage; remove all packing materials before providing toys for the child.
- Do not use older repainted toys unless certain that paint used contained no lead.
- Select cloth toys that are nonflammable, flame resistant, or flame retardant. Avoid electrical and battery-powered toys in children younger than 8 years.
- Do not allow latex balloons and especially noninflated balloons to be used as toys.

Playgrounds provide a location for healthy development of children, but can also be responsible for child injuries. Home playgrounds are the sites of most playground injuries. Falls, strangulation, and head impacts are examples of frequent playground injuries. Some tips can be provided to parents (Safe Kids, 2011a):

- Surfaces should be composed of soft and loose material such as mulch or fine sand. The surface should be 12 in. deep and extend 6 ft around equipment.
- Equipment should not allow the child to be more than 5 ft off the surface.
- Strangulation poses a high risk so be sure to remove ties, ribbons, drawstrings, and other hanging items from clothing and play areas.
- Ensure that the equipment is intended for the age of the child. Separate playgrounds for young and older children are recommended.
- Consult the U.S. Consumer Product Safety Commission for playground equipment standards. Inspect equipment regularly.
- Always supervise the young child on a playground at all times.

Evaluation

Parents should be asked occasionally to evaluate the care they are receiving at the health promotion and health maintenance site. Use these comments to monitor and adjust procedures as needed. The expected outcomes for nursing care of the toddler and preschooler include the following:

- The child demonstrates normal patterns of growth and progression in developmental milestones.
- The child remains free of disease and injury.
- Parents relay satisfaction with the pediatric healthcare home.
- The child manifests positive physical, social, and emotional adjustment.

Focus Your Study

- General observations of physical ability and social interactions are made as the toddler and preschooler appear for the healthcare visit.

- Questions about growth and information related to physical health are integrated during the physical examination.

- The examination should include all areas on the American Academy of Pediatrics Recommendations for Preventive Pediatric Health Care, with the approaches adapted to the young child.

- Developmental surveillance is integrated within each health promotion/health maintenance visit, and an appropriate developmental screening test is used.

- Toddlers and preschoolers gradually take on mature eating patterns; assessment of nutritional status involves growth, oral health and teeth, foods eaten, and family food patterns.

- Physical ability progresses steadily in young children; opportunities for daily active periods are necessary for healthy growth.

- Early years are essential to development of a positive sense of self, positive social interactions with others, and healthy lifestyle behaviors.

- Immunizations are administered to prevent infectious disease, and safety hazards are addressed at each healthcare visit, with suggestions provided to avoid disease and injury.

Clinical Reasoning in Action

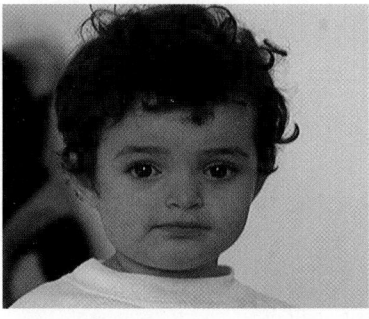

Quinton and his mother have come into the office for his 2-year-old well-child checkup. During the visit you learn that his mother stays home with him during the day and his father often works overtime. His only significant medical history incident was when he had stitches placed in his forehead for falling on the edge of a table when he was 15 months old. There is a family history of attention deficit disorder and Crohn disease. His height is in the 75th percentile, weight is in the 50th percentile, and body mass index is between the 25th and 50th percentiles. His temperature is 98.9°F (37°C) and his pulse is 80. He is described by his parents as a picky eater and tends to eat the same foods frequently. They also say he tends to eat well on some days and other days will hardly eat anything. On the days he is not eating well, his mother will often resort to giving him soda or a sugary snack just so he is "getting something." Quinton sleeps about 7 hours per night, and his mother usually ends up sleeping with him because he continues to fight going to sleep after being put to bed. He does not have a regular bedtime or rest routine and he usually naps in the car during the day. His mother tells you that her only break during the day when she is at home with Quinton is when he is watching television in his bedroom, so he often watches 2 to 4 hours per day. Quinton has a soft stool every day and has not showed any interest in potty training at this time. He is developmentally able to go up and down stairs, kick a ball, scribble on paper, and is able to speak in three- to four-word sentences. During the visit at the office, it is obvious his parents have difficulty controlling him and frequently make threats and offer bribes to get him to behave properly. He starts screaming and kicking when his parents set limits on his behavior in the office, and his parents say they are frequently exhausted and do not know what to do about his high energy level. They also are concerned because they feel like the discipline methods they have been using are not working, and he is getting into so many things in the home that they are concerned he may hurt himself. They have used spanking and time-outs, but they do not seem to improve his behavior. They think he may have some type of medical condition like attention deficit disorder considering it does run in their family.

1. At 2 years of age, a consistent routine will help a toddler behave more appropriately. What are some of the things you can tell Quinton's parents regarding his sleep and nutrition habits to help establish a better routine?

2. How can you advise Quinton's parents about positive approaches to disciplining him?

3. How can you advise Quinton's parents about disciplining him when it is needed?

4. What are some suggestions you can give Quinton's parents about handling his temper tantrums?

References

American Academy of Pediatric Dentistry (AAPD). (2014). *Guideline on infant oral health care (2012)*. Retrieved from http://www.aapd.org/assets/1/7/G_Infant OralHealthCare.pdf#xml=http://pr- http://www.aapd .org/media/Policies_Guidelines/G_InfantOralHealthCare .pdf

American Academy of Pediatric Dentistry (AAPD) Council on Clinical Affairs. (2013). *Policy on the dental home* (pp. 24–25). AAPD Reference Manual. Chicago, IL: Author.

American Academy of Pediatrics (AAP). (2013). *Water safety and young children*. Retrieved from http:// www.healthychildren.org/English/safety-prevention /at-play/Pages/Water-Safety-And-Young-Children.aspx

American Academy of Pediatrics (AAP). (2014). *Car seats: Information for families for 2014*. Retrieved from http://www.healthychildren.org/English /safety-prevention/on-the-go/Pages/Car-Safety -Seats-Information-for-Families.aspx

American Academy of Pediatrics (AAP) Committee on Nutrition. (2013). *Pediatric nutrition handbook* (7th ed.). Elk Grove Village, IL: Author.

American Academy of Pediatrics (AAP) Committee on Practice and Ambulatory Medicine, Bright Futures Periodicity Schedule Workgroup. (2014). 2014 Recommendations for pediatric preventive health care. *Pediatrics, 133,* 568–570.

American Academy of Pediatrics (AAP) Council on Communications and Media. (2013). Children, adolescents, and the media. *Pediatrics, 132,* 958–961.

American Dental Association (ADA). (2011). *Thumbsucking*. Retrieved from http://www.ada.org/2977.aspx

Beets, M. W., Bornstein, D., Dowda, M., & Pate, R. R. (2011). Compliance with national guidelines for physical activity in U.S. preschoolers: Measurement and interpretation. *Pediatrics, 127*(4), 658–664.

Centers for Disease Control and Prevention (CDC). (2011). *How much physical activity do children need?* Retrieved from http://www.cdc.gov/physicalactivity /everyone/guidelines/children/html

Cheng, Y. W., Fletcher, E. N., Roberts, K. J., & McKenzie, L. B. (2014). Baby gate-related injuries among children in the United States, 1990–2010. *Academic Pediatrics, 14,* 256–261.

Child Trends. (2012). *Early childhood program enrollment*. Retrieved from http://www.childtrendsdatabank .org/?q=node/280

Child Trends. (2014). *Early childhood developmental screening: A compendium of measures for children ages birth to five*. Retrieved from http://www.acf.hhs .gov/programs/ecd/watch-me-thrive

Colak, H., Dulgergil, C. T., Dalli, M., & Hamidi, M. M. (2013). Early childhood caries updates: A review of causes, diagnoses, and treatments. *Journal of Natural Science, Biology and Medicine, 4,* 29–38.

Hagan, J. F., Shaw, J. S., & Duncan, P. M. (2008). *Bright futures: Guidelines for health supervision of infants, children, and adolescents* (3rd ed.). Elk Grove Village, IL: American Academy of Pediatrics.

Holt, K., Wooldridge, N., Story, M., & Sofka, D. (2011). *Bright futures: Nutrition* (3rd ed.). Elk Grove Village, IL: American Academy of Pediatrics.

Lucas, B. R., Latimer, J., Pinto, R. Z., Ferreira, M. L., Doney, R. Lau, M., . . . Elliot, E. J. (2014). Gross motor deficits in children prenatally exposed to alcohol: A meta-analysis. *Pediatrics, 134,* e192–e209.

Lucille Packard Children's Hospital. (2012). *Upper respiratory infection*. Retrieved from http://www.lpch.org /DiseaseHealthInfo/HealthLibrary/respire/uricold.html

Mayo Clinic. (2014). *Sleep terrors (night terrors)*. Retrieved from http://www.mayoclinic.org/diseases-conditions /night-terrors/basics/risk-factors/con-20032552

National Highway Traffic Safety Administration. (2014). *How to find the right car seat*. Retrieved from http://www.safercar.gov/parents/Car-Seat-Safety .htm

National Institute of Dental and Craniofacial Research. (2014). *Dental caries (tooth decay) in children (age 2 to 11)*. Retrieved from http://www.nidcr.nih.gov /DataStatistics/FindDataByTopic/DentalCaries /DentalCariesChildren2to11.htm

National Resource Center for Health and Safety in Child Care and Early Education. (2013). *Stepping stones* (3rd ed.). Retrieved from http://nrckids.org/CFOC3 /index.html

Pender, N. J., Murdaugh, C. L., & Parsons, M. A. (2015). *Health promotion in nursing practice* (7th ed.). Upper Saddle River, NJ: Pearson Prentice Hall.

Rasmussen, C., Kully-Martens, K., Denys, K., Badry, D., Henneveld, D., Wyper, K., & Grant T. (2012). The effectiveness of a community-based intervention program for women at-risk for giving birth to a child with Fetal Alcohol Spectrum Disorder (FASD). *Community Mental Health Journal, 48,* 12–21.

Safe Kids. (2011a). *Playground safety fact sheet*. Retrieved from http://www.safekids.org/our-work/research /fact-sheets/playground-safety-fact-sheet.html

Safe Kids. (2011b). *Preventing injuries: At home, at play, and on the way*. Retrieved from http://www.safekids .org/our-work/research/fact-sheets/toy-safety -fact-sheet.html

Safe Kids. (2014). *Heatstroke*. Retrieved from http://www .safekids.org/heatstroke

Simmonds, M., Burch, J., Llewellyn, A., Griffiths, C., Yang, H., Owen, C., . . . Woolacott, N. (2015). The use of measures of obesity in childhood for predicting obesity and the development of obesity-related disease in adulthood: A systematic review and meta-analysis. *Health Technology Assessment, 19,* 1–336.

U.S. Department of Health and Human Services. (2011). *Healthy People 2020*. Retrieved from http://healthy -people.gov/2020/topicsobjectives2020/pdfs /nutritionandweight.pdf

Zoorob, R. J., Durkin, K. M., Gonzalez, S. J., & Adams, S. (2014). Training nurses and nursing students about prevention, diagnosis, and treatment of fetal alcohol spectrum disorders. *Nurse Education in Practice, 14,* 338–344.

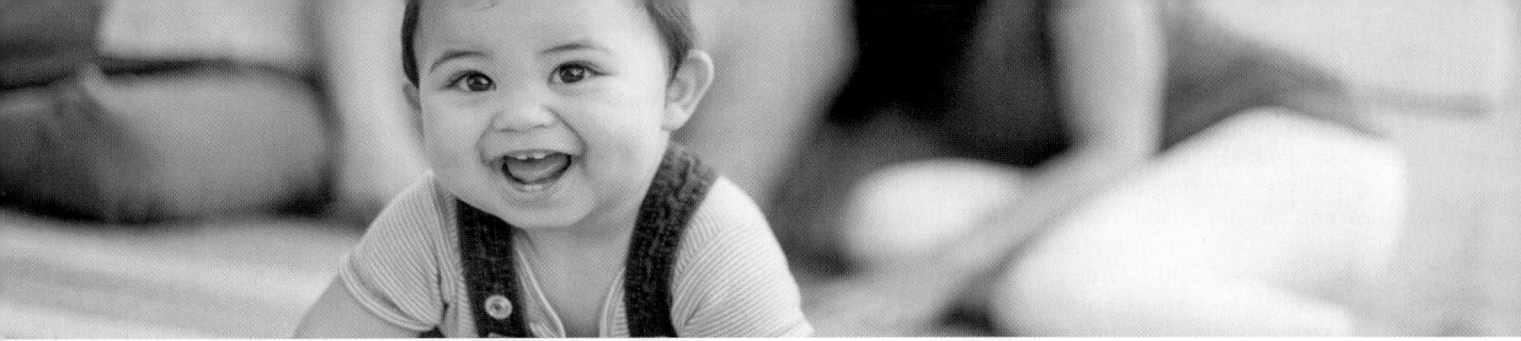

Chapter 36

Health Promotion and Maintenance: The School-Age Child and the Adolescent

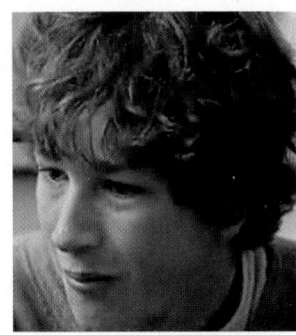

I know I should not be using chewing tobacco, but a lot of my friends use it, and I want to fit in with them. I would like to quit, but I really don't know how.

—Jeremy, 16 years old

⌄ Learning Outcomes

36.1 Identify the major health concerns of the school-age and adolescent years.

36.2 Describe the general observations made of school-age children, adolescents, and families as they come to the "pediatric healthcare home" for health supervision visits.

36.3 Apply communication skills in interactions with school-age children and adolescents.

36.4 Apply assessment skills to plan data-gathering methods for nutrition, physical activity, oral health, and mental health status of youth.

36.5 Synthesize data from history and examination of the school-age child and adolescent with knowledge of development to plan interventions appropriate during health supervision visits.

36.6 Plan with school-age children and adolescents to help them integrate activities to promote health and to prevent disease and injury.

Health Promotion and Maintenance: The School-Age Child

The older childhood years span the time when most children enter kindergarten at about 5 years of age and progress until adolescence begins at about 12 to 13 years of age. Even though health promotion and health maintenance remain important during this time, less frequent visits to the pediatric healthcare home are recommended. In addition, most children are relatively healthy and need few immunizations, which may lead to only sporadic visits for care. Whenever older school-age children are seen in health care, even for illness or emergency care, it is wise to ask when the last "well-child" or health supervision visit was scheduled. Encourage the parents to make an appointment if the child is due for a visit. Visits are generally recommended at about 5 years of age, when most children are going to kindergarten, and then at 6, 7, 8, 9, 10, 11, and 12 years of age. The visits during this time will focus on monitoring physical and developmental changes, establishing good health habits related to important issues such as nutrition, physical activity, and mental health; learning the importance of avoiding tobacco, alcohol, and drugs; ensuring success in school, family, and extracurricular activities; and fostering good decision-making and problem-solving skills.

General Observations

The first school-age health supervision visit usually occurs just before entry into kindergarten. During this visit the child has a thorough examination to be certain that physical development is normal, developmental milestones have been met for fine and gross motor skills, school readiness is displayed in social skills and language, and final sets of basic immunizations are completed. The child is often excited about the visit because it is associated with beginning school; some anxiety is often felt, as it may be the first time the child is aware of getting "shots." As with earlier visits, the nurse's observations begin as the child is called in for the visit. It is wise to speak to the child first, introducing yourself and welcoming the child and parents to the office or clinic. Many children of this age actively participate in conversations, making teaching and gathering data easy. For children who are quiet or look to the parents, allow more time for them to get to know the healthcare provider, directing most initial questions to parents. This may be the first visit where the child is old enough to be a partner in the healthcare visit. Establishing positive rapport with the child will be more likely to enhance efforts designed to teach about health. At the same time, family-centered care, or a partnership to include decision making jointly by the family and the healthcare provider, is important for school-age health (Kuo et al., 2011).

Notice whether the child brought a book, toy, or some other object to the visit. How are the parents interacting with the child? What types of speech tones are used? Is there mutual respect or are parents and child ignoring each other or having disagreements? The child should walk with symmetry and ease of movement, follow instructions about where to go and taking off shoes for weighing, and demonstrate clear language skills with parent or healthcare personnel.

By the time children come for visits at age 6 to 8 years, they are expected to be increasingly active in sports, school activities, music, or other interests. Look for clues about their interests as they arrive. Did they bring books or an electronic device? What are the reading topics or favorite types of music? Ask what they are doing during the summer or about their two favorite after-school activities. Have them describe a typical day to obtain clues about their life.

Some children do not commonly come to clinics, offices, or other settings for health supervision visits. School nurses or nurse practitioners in school-based clinics sometimes offer health promotion/health maintenance activities in the school setting. A major focus of school nurses is making the environment conducive to health for groups of children. School nurses may:

- Offer some parts of examination to individual children, such as growth and developmental surveillance.
- Conduct health screenings, such as vision, hearing, lipids, or scoliosis.

- Work with food service personnel and administration to improve meal and snack quality and minimize unhealthy choices in vending machines.
- Work with teachers to integrate concepts such as physical activity and self-esteem into classroom activities.

The nurse often links children with healthcare needs to other community services.

During health supervision visits, watch the parents' responses as children answer questions. Be alert for the parent who interrupts the child or constantly "corrects" what is said. Comments by the parent should involve praise of the child or looking to the child for opinions on certain topics. This indicates that a partnership is developing in the family and that family members work together and value each other. Also direct some questions to the parents. Ask if they came with specific questions or concerns that should be addressed. If the child has an individualized education or health plan (see Chapter 37), ask if the parent brought a copy, if the plan is still appropriate, or if it needs updating; facilitate a meeting with the school district about the plan if indicated. Allow the parent an opportunity to meet with the physician, nurse practitioner, or other professional in a private place and without the child present if desired. Be alert for family dynamics that can influence mental health status. Ask if there have been any important changes in the family and how they have influenced the child. During conversations, be alert for reports of separation; divorce; remarriages; ill parents, siblings, or grandparents; recent or upcoming moves; parent job changes; substance abuse; incarceration of family members; custody disputes; or other issues. Integrate a family history of diseases into the examination. Such topics can be followed up with further questions, as described later in the mental health section, to learn how they influence the child.

Growth and Developmental Surveillance

When the child first comes into the health supervision site, take height and weight measurements. Be sure to have the child remove shoes and coats. Ask the child and parents if they know the child's current height and weight, and if they have any questions. Plot the percentiles for these measurements, calculate body mass index (BMI) and its percentile, and explain the meaning of these findings later in the visit. Recognize that children do not grow uniformly; they have periods of slow growth followed by fast spurts. Similar to earlier ages, watch for children who have changed channels on a growth grid, and for those above the 85th percentile or below the 5th percentile for BMI, and gather additional nutritional data in these cases (see Chapter 32).

School-age children have begun to learn about their bodies, and so they should be active participants in the physical examination. Explain what you are doing and why. Carry out a head-to-toe examination, paying particular attention to systems and skills that influence performance in school, such as vision, hearing, muscular strength, and coordination. See Chapter 33 for detailed information about the physical examination. Remember to provide feedback about the findings; families appreciate knowing that the child's vision is normal and strength is well developed. Tell them what findings are normal as well as areas that may need more assessment or intervention. Inquire about the child's sleep patterns. During the examination, ask for a description of any illnesses the child has had. Children of school age are generally healthy, with only a few upper respiratory infections or other minor illnesses annually. Unusual complaints may indicate a need for further testing, as discussed in the disease prevention section later in this chapter. Specific screenings for school-age visits include vision, hearing, hematocrit/hemoglobin, and lipid screening (10-year visit recommended for lipids) (American Academy of Pediatrics Committee on Practice and Ambulatory Medicine, 2014).

School-age children frequently have minor injuries. These might include falls from bicycles, skin rashes from exposure to plants on a hiking trip, bruises from a ball sport, and other minor mishaps. Be alert for more serious problems that may indicate a need for additional detailed data gathering and teaching (see the injury prevention section later in this chapter for examples).

Developmental surveillance continues to be an important part of the examination for school-age children. Some milestones can be observed during the visit, while other information is obtained by report of parent and child. This information is combined with reports about school and other activities in order to establish that the child is developing as expected.

Desired outcomes for growth and developmental surveillance include normal progression with developmental tasks, absence of physical and psychosocial abnormalities or trauma, and integration of safe practices into daily life.

Nutrition

Key concepts related to nutrition in school-age children are independence and formation of habits that influence the future. First, children are increasingly independent in food choices. They usually have strong likes and dislikes for certain foods. They may arrive home from school each day to an empty house and prepare their own snacks. During school, they choose what to eat from the school lunch, or the sack lunch sent by family. They may have access to vending machines or sales of snacks during school hours. While independence in food choices is growing, the child is greatly influenced in those choices by friends and the media. Foods that may be rejected often include fresh vegetables and fruits, since they get little media attention, and friends may not prefer them.

At a time when the child chooses many of the foods in the daily diet, habits are being formed that will affect nutrition and health in general in the years to come. Good choices will help to promote health—to maintain weight at a recommended level, provide nutrients for adequate growth and activity, and prevent onset of some chronic diseases. Conversely, poor choices can lead to overweight and its accompanying problems, lack of adequate calcium and resultant osteoporosis, eating disorders, or lack of energy for brain growth and optimal performance in school. The patterns established during this period are often influential in later nutritional status. Knowledge about foods, family participation in good nutritional practices, and access to healthy foods can all be enhanced by nursing intervention during this critical formative period.

Continue to perform height and weight measurements, body mass index calculations, and examination of percentiles for growth grid measurements. Slow, steady growth is the norm during the early school-age years; it will be followed by a growth spurt when the child nears puberty.

During the visit, observations provide information about nutritional status. What is the condition of the nails, skin, and hair? What is the energy level and reported physical activity? Does the child look lean or overweight? As the child nears

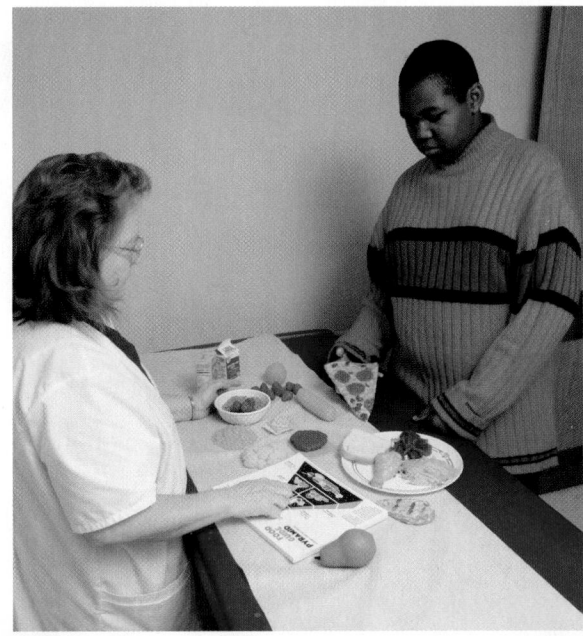

Figure 36–1 This school-age child is receiving teaching from the nurse about food choices. What benefit do the food models provide in this situation? What other teaching techniques can you suggest?

puberty, there may be an increase in fat stores as a preparation for the pubertal growth spurt. Integrate some questions for the parent and child into the visit that provide clues about diet. While observing the child and family and asking dietary questions, list risks and protective factors related to nutrition. Examples of protective factors include adequate access to nutritious foods, a family garden, and weight and height within normal limits; risk factors may include inadequate access to nutritious foods, excess intake of calories during television viewing, and lack of vegetables in the daily diet. Reinforce the positive practices of the family and inform the child of how food choices relate to energy level, school performance, and general health. Risk factors become the basis for teaching and planning with the family for necessary change. It is difficult to tackle several nutritional changes at one time, so concentrate on those most needing attention, and on those the family agrees are important. Provide information about healthy snacks to keep at home, ways to improve calcium intake, the importance of getting at least five fruit/vegetable servings daily, limitation of soda pop to one serving daily, and the importance of family meals (Figure 36–1). Desired outcomes for health maintenance include absence of overweight and other potential chronic diseases, adequate intake of all nutrients, and increasing child and family knowledge about nutrition.

Physical Activity

Just as food choices during the school-age years are likely to influence the child's future nutrition, physical activity during these years is often crucial to development of lifelong exercise habits. During these years, the child who is physically active continues to refine skills such as eye–hand coordination, muscular strength, agility, and speed. Some children become skilled at ball sports such as basketball, football, soccer, or baseball. Others focus on gymnastics, wrestling, horseback riding, or hockey (Figure 36–2). Some do not like team or organized sports

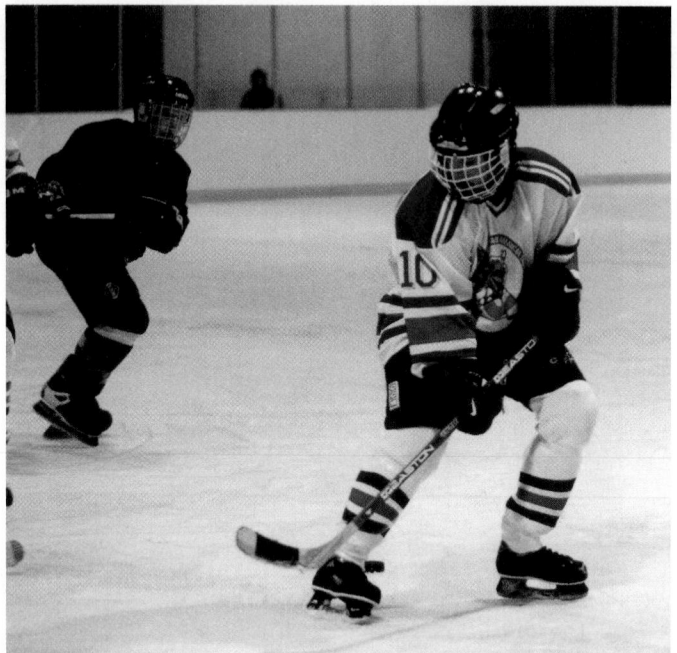

Figure 36–2 Everyone needs to be physically active. Some children participate in school sports. Others, such as these boys playing hockey, choose a sport that is available in the community. Other children prefer to walk, ride a bike, or engage in other more solitary activities. Determine what is enjoyable for a particular child and provide assistance in integrating desired activity into daily routines.

but choose rollerblading, skateboarding, skiing, or biking. Whatever the interest, it is important that children identify some physical activity and continue to develop motor skills. The benefits include socialization, positive sense of accomplishment and self-esteem, weight control, and increasing physical ability (Figure 36–3). Children who do not have an activity of importance often fall behind their peers in agility and skill, making future attempts at an activity very difficult and less likely to be successful.

As in earlier periods in life, the nurse lists risk and protective factors related to school-age physical activity (Table 36–1). Families are often significant in promoting physical activity for children. Find out what the parents do for physical activity and how often. Do they attend a sports club after work or does the child see them engaging in exercise? Most families can include some walking, yard work, or other activity that is done together in order to engage the child. Do they walk to a neighbor's house or a nearby store rather than driving? Do they always take elevators, or choose the stairs in buildings? What is the activity level of siblings? When older siblings are involved in sports, the younger child often is encouraged to develop skills in the same sport.

The child spends much of the day in school, and so this setting is important to consider. In an effort to conserve financial resources, some schools have decreased physical education (PE) programs. Children may not have regular PE classes, and there may be few standards of performance. In addition, many states and provinces have established tests and standards for performance in certain cognitive areas. In an attempt to increase teaching time to meet standards, some schools have cut out recess and other breaks. Some schools are located in unsafe areas and outside recreation is not advisable.

It is unrealistic to expect children to sit for long periods without physical activity, and such practice reinforces the poor

TABLE 36–1 Risk and Protective Factors Regarding Physical Activity in School-Age Children

RISK FACTORS	PROTECTIVE FACTORS
• Developmental delay and special needs	• Expected developmental skill level
• Limited role modeling of daily physical activity by parents and other family members	• Parents exercise daily and exercise with the child some of this time in a setting the child can see • Parents set expectation that everyone in family will choose a physical activity and engage in it regularly
• Limited facilities in the neighborhood to encourage activity, such as parks, skateboard facilities, rinks, ball courts	• Neighborhood provides access to parks, skateboard facilities, rinks, ball courts, and other facilities
• Inadequate financial resources to join clubs or pay for organized sports	• Family has adequate financial resources to pay for health club or organized sports
• Safety gear for activities chosen is not available due to cost, or child is reluctant to use the gear	• Recommended safety gear that properly fits child is available • The child understands importance of safety gear and accepts using such equipment
• School cuts to physical education programs and recess	• Schools provide physical education each day with a variety of offerings; student gets to choose and set goals for some activities • Schools schedule recess or physical activity breaks twice daily
• School tryouts for sports that eliminate all but the best players in certain sports	• Sports teams are leveled so that all students desiring to play a particular sport, such as soccer, are able to do so
• Reluctance to try new activity	• Willing to try new activities
• Worry about competence and physical appearance	• Feels self-confident in ability and physical appearance • Sets goals for learning physical skills
• Television viewing or other screen activities for more than 2 hr daily	• Television viewing and other screen activities are limited to no more than 2 hr daily

Source: Data from Hagan, J. F., Shaw, J. S., & Duncan, P. M. (Eds.). (2008). *Bright futures: Guidelines for health supervision of infants, children, and adolescents* (3rd ed.). Elk Grove Village, IL: American Academy of Pediatrics.

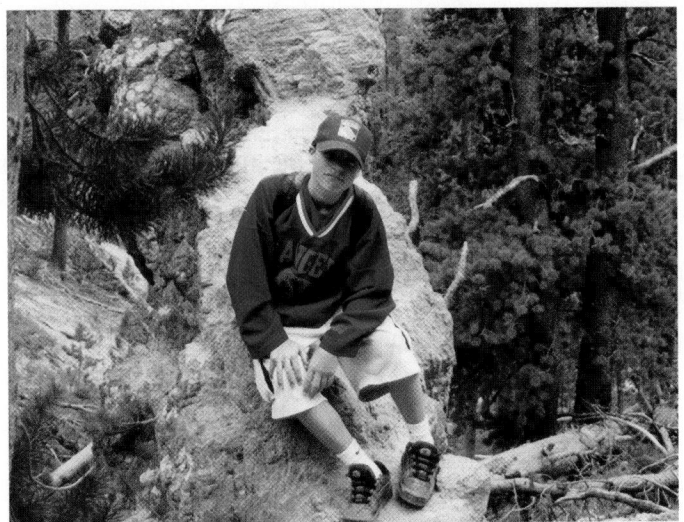

Figure 36–3 Benefits of physical activity. School-age children often enjoy hikes with family, clubs, or other groups. What are the physical and mental health benefits from this activity?

habits of inadequate exercise among children. Schools that offer a variety of activities, including intramural (rather than only organized competitive) sports, are more likely to encourage a wide variety of children to be active. At least half of the recommended 60 minutes of daily vigorous physical activity should be provided in school, along with an adequate amount of unstructured playtime during recess (Centers for Disease Control and Prevention [CDC], 2011a). Nurses are influential members of school committees and can encourage the integration of activity in the school day. They may be able to serve on a school or community committee, informing other committee members of the benefits of exercise to enhance cognitive performance and general health. Teachers and school administrators can be supplied with models of successful school activity programs. Nurses can often be influential in finding community volunteers to work with teams of students. Student nurses, physical education students, senior citizens, and others in the community may be able to help young children play baseball, tennis, or soccer. Other volunteers may teach stretching or warm-up activities. Community partners such as businesses may provide protective gear or uniforms for school sports, especially if the business name can be displayed. In addition, schools can offer alternative activities that some children might prefer to traditional organized sports.

It is essential to consider physical activity for the child who has special healthcare needs. It may be difficult for schools to plan an activity for the child with cerebral palsy, visual impairment, or developmental delay. Search for other community resources and help the family to access them. There may be programs for children to ride horses, swim, ski, and engage in other physical activities. Search out the Special Olympics for children with disabilities. Imagine the thrill that awaits a child who has rarely moved quickly when riding a sled or sliding on skis.

To summarize, health promotion activities for the nurse include teaching about activities that parents can do with their children, becoming active in fostering physical education programs in schools, acting as a positive role model, and helping interested children to partner with community resources for activity. Health maintenance outcomes include encouragement for use of safety gear and correct techniques to prevent injury from sport participation.

Oral Health

Many changes occur in the mouth during the school-age years, necessitating periodic examination. At about 6 years of age, most children lose a tooth, usually in the front. Following that, all 20 of the deciduous or primary teeth will be lost, and the permanent teeth will simultaneously begin to erupt. See Chapter 33 for the schedule of deciduous tooth loss and permanent tooth eruption. In addition, the jaw line elongates and teeth move into new positions. Periodic dental visits focus on both the placement of teeth and oral hygiene.

During the health promotion visit, examine the teeth. Look to see how many deciduous and permanent teeth are present. Describe the child's oral hygiene. Ask how often the child brushes, flosses, and visits the dentist. The child should have learned how to brush and floss during preschool years and now be performing the skills independently. If dental caries or poor oral hygiene is apparent, ask the child to demonstrate brushing and flossing. Reinforce the need for brushing twice daily and flossing once daily. Provide toothpaste and toothbrushes as gifts during health supervision visits. Local dentists will often provide these supplies to encourage oral hygiene.

Dental visits are recommended every 6 months. If the child is not visiting on that schedule, ask if finances or transportation is an issue, if the family needs a referral to a dentist, or if there is some other reason. If caries or malocclusion is present, stress the need for a dental appointment soon. Inquire about use of fluoride if the water supply is not fluoridated. Ask if the child has had sealants applied to the permanent teeth; most dentists believe these will help to prevent future caries (American Academy of Pediatric Dentistry [AAPD], 2012). Offer to help parents locate resources to assist with dental care expenses if needed. State and community programs are often available to assist families, and nurses should search out resources in their own communities and regions.

Many children have a high intake of sugared foods and snacks. If this is apparent from the nutritional assessment, discuss the importance of limiting these foods and brushing after their consumption. Frequent brushing is needed when the child has braces. Ask how they are caring for the braces and what the orthodontist has recommended.

The nurse's health promotion activities include positive reinforcement of good hygiene habits, and health maintenance involves teaching about the need for improved care and limiting food that furthers the formation of caries. Desired outcomes include recommended oral hygiene, attendance at recommended dental visits, and absence of dental caries.

Clinical Reasoning Dental Health

The family of 7-year-old Mario just moved to your city. You learn in a healthcare visit that Mario has never been to a dentist. You notice that several of his teeth are decayed. He has started to lose his primary teeth and has two permanent teeth in place. A dietary recall demonstrates that he drinks two to three sweetened beverages daily and likes to eat candy whenever possible.

Describe the daily dental hygiene that Mario should be practicing. Plan a teaching session for Mario and his parents. What other cues will you look for in his dietary recall in order to identify risk and protective factors for oral health? How will you locate resources in the community to recommend for the family so that Mario can receive dental care?

Mental and Spiritual Health

SELF-ESTEEM AND SELF-CONCEPT

The school-age years are marked by the emergence of new cognitive skills and the development of self-esteem. **Self-esteem** reflects feelings of self-worth or value. **Self-concept** refers to evaluations of the self in certain specific areas, such as those related to academic achievement, athletic ability, physical appearance, and social interactions (Santrock, 2012). A child with a positive self-concept feels competent, is able to meet challenges, and applies lessons from successes and failures. Specific facets of self-concept include **body image**, the idea that one forms about one's body, and **sexuality**, the person's view of self as a sexual being. Together, self-concept and self-esteem include all of the cognitive, emotional, spiritual, sexual, and physical aspects of the individual.

The child who believes in his or her ability to face good times and bad has a lowered chance of mental illness such as depression, eating disorder, and anxiety. Parents are encouraged to evaluate and help to build the child's sense of self-esteem (see *Teaching Highlights: Evaluating and Fostering Self-Esteem*).

Many of the areas discussed already in this chapter provide clues to the child's self-concept. Does the child take part in sports or other physical activities? Such activity may reflect a positive self-concept and body image. However, if the child is forced to do these sports by parents and feels inadequate in their performance, these activities may promote a negative self-concept and body image. Ask about children's activities and how they feel about them. Do they enjoy them? How do they rate their performance?

Is the child increasingly independent and responsible for self? Success in achieving developmental milestones leads to a positive sense of self-esteem in the child. Parents are encouraged to evaluate and help to build the child's sense of self-esteem. A low sense of self-esteem is noted when the child states a disinterest in exercise, school clubs, and family activities. This can lead to loneliness, depression, and mental health problems such as eating disorders. When these feelings are noted during a health supervision visit, the nurse should recommend that the child see a counselor at school or another setting, and should recommend that parents be included in the sessions so that they can best help the child.

It is obvious that the family plays a critical part in the child's developing self-esteem and mental health. To understand the child, it is necessary to ask questions about and explore dynamics in the family. Several protective factors have been identified for families (U.S. Department of Health and Human Services, 2011):

- Nurturing bonds and attachment are formed.
- Parents have knowledge about parenting skills and child development.
- Parents demonstrate resilience by recognizing their own stress and enhancing their problem-solving abilities.
- Parents have a wide array of support systems to provide social connections.
- Caregivers are available who provide resources to meet basic needs, such as finances, housing, and food.

School-age children continue to develop their abilities to self-regulate activities and responses to situations. At this age, the abilities to solve problems and assume more responsibility for self are important. Encourage parents to discuss issues with the child and to seek solutions together when appropriate. The child assumes more responsibility for assisting with meal preparation and home chores, coming home alone after school, and caring for younger siblings. Encourage the parents to praise the child for assuming more family responsibilities and recognize that the child will need some guidance when taking on new tasks.

TEACHING HIGHLIGHTS | Evaluating and Fostering Self-Esteem

Parents play an important part in fostering a child's self-esteem. The nurse can ask them to evaluate the child and provide suggestions about positive actions.

Evaluation Questions	Positive Actions
What does your child do well?	Build on the child's strengths and talents; affectionately point out the child's abilities.
How does your child respond to failure?	Assist children to assess their own performance; help them to see lessons that mistakes can teach.
Does your child have close friends?	Arrange structured playtimes such as going to a movie or cooking with a friend.
How does your child respond to new challenges?	Give the child responsibilities at home; encourage your child to try new experiences; help the child feel a sense of control over outcomes.
How does your own personality compare to your child's?	Recognize differences in style; appreciate the unique qualities of each child; tailor expectations to the child and not to self or other children.
Are you setting reasonable and attainable expectations for your child?	Be a positive role model; establish goals for behaviors together.

Source: Data from KidsHealth. (2011). *Developing your child's self-esteem*. Retrieved from http://kidshealth.org/parent/emotions/feelings/self_esteem.html

Ask about and observe the family's relationships. Evaluate the effect of family interactions on the child. Model respectful interchanges by listening carefully to the child, as well as the parent. Gently speak directly to the child if parents answer for the child or seem to put the child down. Provide brochures and examples of ways to show children their importance. Encourage both parents to come to child healthcare visits and support the involvement of both parents in childrearing. Ask about family stressors such as job changes, financial concerns, illness, substance abuse, and domestic violence. About one half of marriages end in divorce, so be prepared to offer suggestions to deal with this situation. Ask about and identify risk factors and protective factors. The child's strengths are used to assist the family functioning and will, in turn, give the child a sense of accomplishment. Some examples include the following:

- A child who is able to act independently can be given responsibility for parts of the home or family function, such as planning the menu for dinner two evenings weekly, caring for a family pet, or completing household chores.

- A creative child can be given the task of planning book readings and other activities for a younger sibling.

- A child with a talent for design can be asked to set the table for dinner guests.

SEXUALITY AND SEXUALITY EDUCATION

The school-age child is developing a sense of body image and sexuality. Be aware of the child's appearance and dress. Some children may have poor posture, display a sense of insecurity, and seem uncomfortable with themselves. Others may dress as if they were much older, seem sophisticated, and are clearly assuming the role identification with their gender group. Ask the parents in a private setting what observations they have about the child's body image and sexuality. Inquire about friends in whom the child seems romantically or sexually interested, and whether the parent has concerns.

Questions related to sexuality will emerge during school years. They should be answered truthfully and fully. Even children who do not ask questions usually need information related to sexuality education. They may get information in school beginning in about fourth grade, but often still have misconceptions about the bodies of men and women, sexual intercourse, how babies are born, and other topics. Suggest that parents read books with their children that deal with these issues at a level children understand. If books are available at home, children will be likely to look at them and ask questions. They should be in the home from third grade on since many young girls have body changes as early as 9 or 10 years of age (see Chapter 33). This can often put both the parent and child at ease and open the door to discussion. Parents should be advised to talk with teachers to learn what is presented in school and be able to supplement and clarify this information. Having discussions at a young age will help lead to further discussion as the child gets older. Nurses often perform sexuality education in schools or work with school districts in establishing policies regarding sexuality education plans. Help the parents plan to discuss appropriate and inappropriate touch so that the child understands and states those who can help in situations that lead to discomfort. (See Chapter 42 for a thorough discussion of child abuse.)

Suggest to parents that computers and other media provide information that can confuse children. Encourage them to watch movies with their children, engage in frank discussions related to sexuality observed, and answer questions truthfully. Children generally learn about topics such as sexual intercourse, homosexuality, and childbirth from school discussions and the media. It is better to learn from parents than from friends or the media. A few moments alone with parents and the child separately at healthcare visits may help to identify the concerns of each related to sexuality.

By approximately 9 to 12 years (fourth to sixth grades), most girls have started to have prepubertal body changes and have had their first menses. This is another opening for discussions about mature bodies of men and women and the transformation from childhood to greater maturity. Boys mature about 2 years later than girls. Without an event such as menstruation, parents may be less likely to start discussions with male children. Suggest that parents consciously begin conversations with boys periodically to explain changes they see in themselves and their peers. See Chapter 33 for further discussion of the body changes seen in the prepubertal period and during puberty.

SLEEP

Sleep is important for children because it helps provide the energy they will need to perform well in school and other activities. They generally take charge of bedtime routines with reminders about the time to go to sleep, and they sleep through the night. Sleep time varies from 8 to 12 hours, depending on child and activity level. Busy schedules may interrupt this pattern, leading to irritability, lack of concentration, or even hyperactive behavior. Help children and families plan for healthy practices of **sleep hygiene**, or behaviors that foster a regular and sufficient sleep pattern, as well as daytime alertness (Mayo Clinic, 2013).

Sleepwalking and sleep talking sometimes occur at this age, but usually decrease as the child nears adolescence. Children who have stress at home, such as parental fighting, ill family members, or inadequate food or shelter, may not get enough sleep and fall asleep at school. Ask children if they fall asleep in class, and seek additional information about family stressors. This can lead to interventions such as recommending family counseling or referring to resources to obtain better housing or more stable food sources.

SCHOOL

School is a major microsystem that influences the lives of children and plays a role in self-concept and mental health formation. The child is usually ready for kindergarten when (Hagan, Shaw, & Duncan, 2008):

- Communication and cognitive skills are sufficient to support learning.

- The child can successfully separate from parents.

- Experiences with other children show ability to make friends and regulate own behavior.

- The child can follow rules and directions.

Help parents learn ways that they can facilitate a healthy transition to school, such as ensuring good sleep and eating routines, reading with the child, showing interest in school activities, and finding a space in the home for the child's school-related work.

When examining a school-age child, ask for a description of a best friend. If the child is unable to provide this, isolation may be occurring. Inquire about what the three best and three worst things are about school. Children with low self-concepts often have trouble talking about and evaluating school. Find

Nurses should inquire about the sleep patterns and amount of sleep that children receive. Ask if they are frequently tired or have trouble sleeping. Some simple behaviors help to promote sleep and are referred to as sleep hygiene. They include (Mayo Clinic, 2013):
- Go to bed and get up at approximately the same time each day, including weekends.
- Follow a bedtime routine to prepare for sleep.
- Recognize that we do not "make up" sleep that is "lost" by sleeping in.
- Avoid caffeine, including tea, coffee, and carbonated beverages, for several hours before sleep.
- Gradually slow down activity about an hour or two before bedtime.
- Do not watch television, play games, text on the phone, or conduct other activities in the sleep location.
- Avoid naps in the late afternoon or evening.
- Darken the room for sleep.

out where the child attends school, if the area is generally safe, and how the child gets to school. Encourage the parents to meet the child's teachers, to become active in school activities, and to be available to solve problems with school personnel when needed. Partner with the parents and child when interventions are needed. An office nurse may contact a school nurse when the child needs support in the school environment. This may occur if the child has become ill and missed school, has family stressors, does not get along well with a teacher, or has a condition such as attention deficit disorder. Identify the risk and protective factors in the school environment and plan interventions to support the child when risks are present.

EVALUATING MENTAL HEALTH AND SPIRITUAL HEALTH

Certain mental health disorders are commonly seen during the school years. One example is anxiety problems that result in worries, fears, physical symptoms, stress, and sleep disorders without significantly impairing daily functioning. However, some anxiety disorders affect functioning and have more striking characteristics such as clinging, abdominal pain and headache, and refusal to attend school. Posttraumatic stress syndrome and depression may also be seen. See Chapter 55 for further description of these disorders. Anxiety disorder, posttraumatic stress, and depression should be referred to a mental health specialist for treatment. However, all children worry at times, and this type of anxiety can be helped by learning coping skills and relaxation techniques.

Spiritual health is the ability to develop a spiritual nature, including awareness of a life purpose or meaning, a sustaining power during times of stress, a feeling of harmony with the universe, and a sense of fulfillment (Pender, Murdaugh, & Parsons, 2015). School age is a time when children learn more about the people and the world around them, and begin to find their place in that world. Connection with faith-based groups assists some children and families in defining the purpose of life, while others may do so through social activity or a strong moral sense of responsibility. Ask children what brings happiness, how they help other people, or if they are members of a church, synagogue, or mosque. If families seem to have little purpose, parents are withdrawn or depressed, or the child has difficulty answering questions about meaningful activities, suggest methods of engagement in the community. Strategies might include providing contacts at local religious events, posting flyers about community events designed to bring unity to various cultural groups, or suggesting services needing volunteers

in the community. Families who spend time together and find meaning in supporting each other nurture the spiritual health of their members. Suggest that every family plan a "family night" weekly when they play games, talk, eat, or engage in other activities together.

The nurse has an important role in fostering the mental and spiritual health of school-age children. Health promotion fosters the strengths of families and children, leading to healthy self-concept and positive self-esteem. Health maintenance seeks to prevent mental health disruptions. Be alert for risk factors in families since they represent the need for intervention. Expected outcomes for health promotion and health maintenance activities with school-age children include formation of a positive sense of self-esteem and healthy body image, use of coping skills to deal with stress, sleep patterns that meet needs for rest, and a growing purpose and meaning in life.

Relationships

Although the school-age child is gradually moving away from the family as the center of life, the family remains an important anchor. Ask about siblings, grandparents, and other extended family members. Sometimes these persons assist in the child's formation of a self-concept. Peers are increasingly important to the school-age child's self-identity. School age is a time of cooperative engagement with others. All children need to learn how to make and maintain friendships and work with others on projects and in recreation.

Inquire about the child's friends and activities at school. In private, ask parents if they are comfortable with the child's selection of friends. Find out if the parents facilitate friendships by allowing other children to come to the home and providing transportation as needed. When the child experiences a risk factor such as a move to a new town or school, role-play how to meet new children and how to make friends. If the child feels like an outcast or outsider among peers at school, explore how the family can create a safe and secure place for the child through extracurricular activities with children who have similar interests. When children are home schooled, the family should encourage social events and contacts after usual school hours.

Since peers are important to the school-age child, the child may feel pressure to appear like others, to fit in, and to do what others encourage. Although such pressures are often associated with teen years, they usually begin earlier, at least by 8 or 9 years of age. Ask children what kinds of things their friends try to get them to do that they know they should not do, or if friends have tried to get them to smoke. Middle school years are the most common age for beginning to smoke, so always ask if the child has tried smoking, being careful to do this when the parent is not present and the child is more likely to be honest. When parents are not in the room they may also tell you about other activities, such as playing with guns, trying alcohol or other substances, or other risky behavior. It is best to ask children what they do in these situations, what they want to do, and who they can talk to about these events. Offer information about the risks connected with behaviors that are described, and suggest people such as parents, teachers, counselors, or clergy who are possible resources. If the child's health is at risk, be sure to report the activity to the physician or other healthcare provider so that it can be pursued and the child's safety can be assured. Activities such as playing with firearms or visiting a friend whose parents are making methamphetamine, for example, place children in extreme danger.

Parents often need guidance to help them in setting limits for their school-age children. The child is becoming more independent but unacceptable behaviors must still be managed by successful discipline techniques. Some guidelines that can help families include talking calmly about behaviors that are unacceptable, using techniques such as natural consequences or withholding privileges, modeling, and suggesting stress relief such as physical activity (American Academy of Pediatrics [AAP], 2011a).

School age is often a time when children first experience violence in relationships with others. Some children are bullied, while others are the bullies. Anger and aggression can occur, and children may engage in violence with each other. Ask children to describe when they last had a disagreement with someone and how the problem was solved. Suggest people who can help, such as school nurses, teachers, and counselors, and be sure that children feel safe in schools, neighborhoods, and homes. Ask parents how they resolve arguments between children at home and what help they need to help children learn problem-solving skills. Find out what policies the local schools have to assist in decreasing harassment of and by children. Become active on school committees that help children learn how to solve problems peacefully and how to respond to episodes of violence. See Chapter 42 for further discussion of violence in children and a detailed discussion of bullying.

The child's temperament (see Chapter 31) still plays a part in response to situations and the ability to self-regulate. The "difficult" child may have trouble getting to sleep or being quiet in the classroom. Have parents plan more physical activity for this child. Teach the child that bedtime routines are helpful and that sitting near the front of the class can help with concentration. The "slow to warm up" child may need ideas about what to say when meeting new people. Parents can help the child prepare for a new school by visiting the school with the child, talking about it, and meeting with the teacher so that a warm welcome can occur. The "easy" child is usually adaptable in most situations and is regular in activities. However, this child may object when other children interrupt, fail to take turns, or otherwise "break the rules" of behavior. They might need help to understand differences in temperament in order to be more tolerant of classmates and their behaviors. Often nurses in schools address the issue of individual differences by speaking with classes or small groups of children.

The nurse takes an active role in promoting the child's health by anticipating developmental issues and preparing the parents and child to deal with them. Health maintenance outcomes include prevention of problems such as bullying.

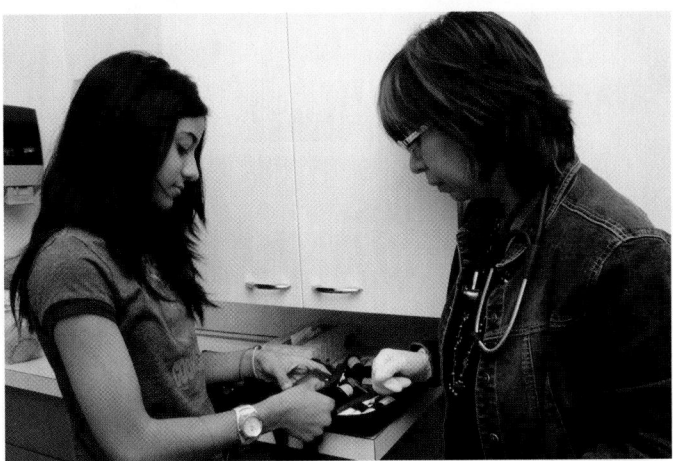

Figure 36–4 **School nurse's role in managing health problems. A student with diabetes is showing the school nurse how she programs her insulin pump. The nurse has partnered with nurses in the endocrinology office to learn about the type of pump the student is using. Such collaboration contributes to the monitoring and management of diabetes.**

Disease Prevention Strategies

School-age children are generally healthy. The immune system is mature (see Chapter 48), personal hygiene practices are more developed than at earlier ages, and immunizations are usually complete. Engage school-age children in active pursuit of their own health. Teach strategies that can enhance the prevention of diseases. Nurses in offices and schools can teach children how to wash hands effectively, how respiratory infections are transmitted, what can cause gastrointestinal illness, and how to best manage their own health problems (Figure 36–4). Ask children in your settings what topics are of most interest to them and be prepared to suggest common areas of concern such as safety, skin care, athletics, and illnesses. Children can understand the connection between eating well and avoiding illness, maintaining normal weight and preventing type 2 diabetes, avoiding smoking to prevent cancer and other respiratory diseases, maintaining oral hygiene to promote oral health, and exercising to prevent hypertension.

School-age children are in the concrete stage of intellectual development, according to Piaget (see Chapter 31). This means that teaching is most effective when opportunities are provided to touch, feel, and otherwise become actively engaged in learning. When teaching about smoking, provide models of lungs and have the students breathe through a straw to demonstrate the effects of airway narrowing. These concrete activities will teach them concepts better than simple lecture or reading (Figure 36–5). Concepts of health promotion tend to be abstract since they deal with supporting one's highest potential for wellness. Thus it becomes even more important to provide concrete methods of learning.

Immunizations are generally up-to-date for school-age children. However, some children may have missed earlier doses because of illness or missed healthcare visits. Evaluate the immunization record to be sure it meets all recommendations. The most common immunization needs at this time include the following:

- Hepatitis B (whole series or a missed third dose)
- Hepatitis A (two doses if not previously administered)

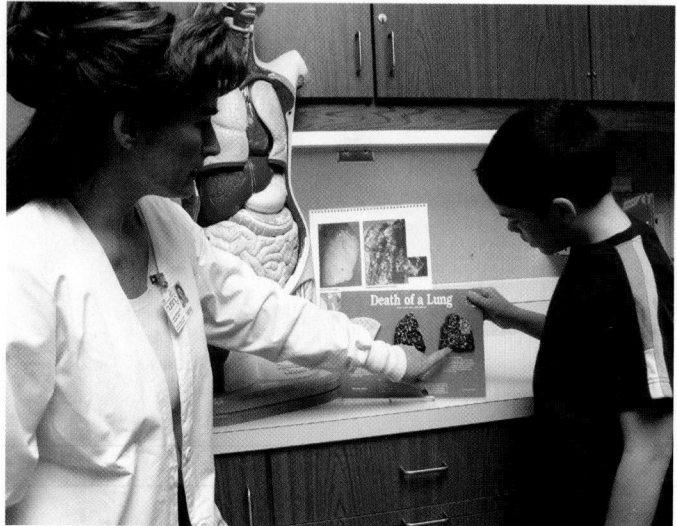

Figure 36–5 Concrete experiences for health teaching. This boy is learning about the effects of smoking on the body through the concrete experience of examining a model of the lungs. Why does this type of hands-on technique help school-age children to learn concepts?

- Poliomyelitis, and measles-mumps-rubella (if booster doses of each were not given prior to school entry)
- Tetanus-diphtheria-acellular pertussis (Tdap) at the 11- to 12-year visit
- Varicella if not given earlier and the child has not had the disease
- Human papillomavirus (HPV) three-dose series at 9 years or older
- Meningococcal conjugate vaccine at 11 years with booster at 16 years
- Influenza annually
- Certain vaccines for children at high risk, such as meningococcal and pneumococcal (see Chapter 43 for further information on immunizations)

Screenings for health risks should occur during the visit. These include hearing and vision screening, blood pressure monitoring, tuberculin skin test, and, in some cases, screening for hyperlipidemia and lead exposure (American Academy of Pediatrics Committee on Practice and Ambulatory Medicine, 2014). Unusual complaints may indicate a need for further testing. Examples include the following:

- Pain other than brief discomfort after an injury
- Headaches
- Bruising
- Lack of coordination
- Repeated infections
- Decreasing vision or hearing
- Problems or changes in school performance or behavior

Children who have an identified health problem or developmental disability may have additional needs for screening and for interventions to assist with health maintenance. For example, the child with cystic fibrosis will need information to reduce the risk of respiratory infection, and the child with

diabetes may need additional blood studies. The child who has difficulty reading will need alternative approaches to teaching correct hand hygiene; demonstration with explanation may be the best approach.

Inquire about any medications the child takes, including vitamins, fluoride, and nonprescription medications. Some families use complementary therapy for common conditions such as respiratory infections or gastrointestinal complaints. Complementary therapy is quite common in families where children have chronic conditions such as attention deficit hyperactivity disorder, autism, and skin conditions (Ben-Arye et al., 2011).

Parents should receive explanations about the screening tests performed and the results obtained. Inform them about vision and hearing results. Send home or call about results of blood tests when available. Be sure they understand the findings and have resources to assist in preventing or treating the specific disease in their children. Have them call with questions about health problems the child develops, and provide information about lowering risks of diseases. Be sure that families know when to keep children home from school (elevated temperature, active vomiting or diarrhea, coughing up brown or green mucus). Assist schools in setting guidelines for management of infectious diseases in that setting. Contact the local county and state health department for infectious disease guidelines for schools. Desired outcomes for the school-age child include prevention of infectious diseases, prompt treatment for acute infections, and careful management of existing health conditions in order to maximize health potential.

Injury Prevention Strategies

Injuries are a common cause of morbidity and mortality among school-age children, and each health maintenance encounter should include injury prevention strategies. Children of this age have more independence and may be harmed by activities they engage in without adults present, such as playing with fire or firearms. They participate in many sports and other physical activities and may sustain related injuries. Some children unfortunately suffer from harm due to physical abuse or other forms of violence (see Chapter 42).

Many common injuries are preventable with simple use of protective gear and the following safety guidelines. About 7% to 8% of youth rarely or never wear seat belts in automobiles, and in some states, up to 16% do not use seat belts (CDC, 2014). Certain groups of children are more at risk than others of not taking protective measures. Many children ride bicycles, but only a fraction of them use helmets. Strategies to make helmet use more attractive and to ensure correct wearing of helmets are needed (see *Evidence-Based Practice: Bicycle Helmet Effectiveness and Use*).

Identify youth engaging in risky activities and teach them safe practices. Join with schools and community groups to establish education programs. Provide information about adequate conditioning for sports in order to decrease chance of overuse injury. Each visit should contain basic history questions related to injury prevention. Pursue topics that appear to indicate problems. Once information has been collected during the visit, plan two or three health maintenance topics that seem most important for injury prevention in the family. When there is a history of injury in the child, partner with the family to plan ways to avoid repeated harm. Table 36–2 lists some common injury hazards during the school years, and Table 36–3 offers suggestions for injury prevention teaching.

EVIDENCE-BASED PRACTICE | Bicycle Helmet Effectiveness and Use

Clinical Question
About 800 people die of bicycle-related injuries annually in the United States and there are over 500,000 emergency room visits for bicycle injuries, 60% of which are in children. Youth from 15 to 24 years old have the highest rate of bicycle injuries (CDC, 2013). Although helmets can reduce injury, many times they are not worn or are worn incorrectly. What are the factors that foster helmet use, and how can nurses contribute to efforts for use of bicycle helmets?

The Evidence
Wearing bicycle helmets is associated with higher household incomes, living in a state with a bicycle helmet law, younger ages, and having health insurance (Devoe, Tillotson, Wallace, et al., 2012). Bicycle helmets are often the wrong size or incorrectly adjusted so that they fit children improperly (Thai, McIntosh, & Pang, 2014).

Best Practice
Nurses should provide information about helmet use for bicycles and other vehicles. Engage children at community events and in schools. Inquire about helmet use at every healthcare visit. Reinforce proper fit and maintenance of helmets.

Clinical Reasoning
Where will you find information about helmet safety? What educational programs are available in your schools and communities? Are helmets made available for families that might not be able to buy them? How do you determine if a child is wearing a helmet correctly? Plan educational materials and programs for children who bicycle, ride skateboards, or use scooters.

TABLE 36–2 Injury Prevention in the School-Age Years

	HAZARD	DEVELOPMENTAL CHARACTERISTICS	PREVENTIVE MEASURES
	Motor vehicle/pedestrian/biking crashes	Child plays outside; may follow ball into road; rides two-wheeler.	Teach child safe outside play, especially near streets. Reinforce use of bike helmet. Teach biking safety rules and provide safe places for riding.
	Firearms	Child may have been shown location of guns; is interested in showing them to friends.	Teach child never to touch guns without parent present. Guns should be kept unloaded and locked away. Guns and ammunition should be stored in different locations. Be sure guns have trigger locks.
	Burns	Child may perform experiments with flames or toxic substances.	Teach child what to do in case of fire or if toxic substances touch skin or eyes. Reinforce teaching about 9-1-1.
	Assault	Child may be left alone after school and may walk, bike, or take public transportation alone.	Provide telephone numbers of people to contact in case of an emergency or if child feels lonely. Leave child alone for brief periods initially, and evaluate child's success in managing time. Teach child not to accept rides from, talk to, or open doors to strangers. Teach child how to answer the phone.

TABLE 36–3 Injury Prevention Topics by Age

AGE (YEARS)	INJURY PREVENTION TEACHING TOPICS	
5–8	Use a booster seat, properly positioned in the back seat of the car; once large enough for the vehicle seat belt, use both lap and shoulder belts.	Teach safety with strangers.
	Never place a child in the front seat of a car with a passenger air bag. Restrain all children younger than 13 years in the rear seat.	Provide a list of people a child can approach if feeling threatened by touch or other experience.
	Be sure the child knows how to swim and works on these skills regularly.	Choose care providers carefully; occasionally pick up child earlier than expected; ask about policies regarding discipline and do not leave child with someone who uses corporal punishment.
	Protect the child with sunscreen when outside.	Be sure the child knows emergency numbers, names, and plans.
	Check smoke alarms and keep them functioning properly.	Review carefully any hazardous event that has occurred with the child and summarize what was done correctly and how response could be improved.
	Have an escape plan in case of fire in the home.	
	Keep poisons, electrical appliances, and fire starters locked.	Limit screen time to 2 hr daily; do not allow violent games or viewing.
	Keep firearms unloaded and locked; store ammunition in a separate locked location; have trigger locks installed on guns; keep dangerous knives locked.	Review behavior with strangers regularly such as not getting in cars and not engaging in phone or Internet conversations.
	Provide protective gear for bicycling and other activities and insist that it be worn.	
	Teach safety precautions for bicycling and other activities.	
8–10	Use car booster seat until child sits upright against back seat with bent knees over edge of seat; insist on use of lap and shoulder belts.	Do not allow child to operate power tools or machinery.
	Do not place child in front seat of car with a passenger air bag.	Continue to reinforce other teaching described above, include child more fully, and expand responsibility to the child with increasing age.
10–12	Continue to reinforce teaching described above.	Avoid high noise levels such as when listening to music through earphones.
	Parents and child should attend class on cardiopulmonary resuscitation and airway obstruction removal.	

Source: Data from Hagan, J. F., Shaw, J. S., & Duncan, P. M. (Eds.). (2008). *Bright futures: Guidelines for health supervision of infants, children, and adolescents* (3rd ed.). Elk Grove Village, IL: American Academy of Pediatrics.

Developing Cultural Competence Use of Safety Protection

There are marked differences in behaviors that influence unintentional injuries. Although about 8% of children rarely or never wear a seat belt in the car, Black males are most at risk, with almost 12% not using seat belts. In addition, 88% of youth who ride bicycles rarely or never wear a bicycle helmet, but the rates vary, with 94% of Black and 92% of Hispanic youth not wearing helmets, while 86% of White youth do not wear bicycle helmets (CDC, 2013, 2014). How will you inquire about seat belt and bicycle helmet use in an open-ended manner during health promotion visits? Consider asking these questions:

- Where do you sit when you ride in the car?
- Who do you usually ride with?
- Do you drive? If so, how often do you text or hold and talk on your phone while you drive?
- Are there seat belts? How often do you use them?
- Do you ride a bike?
- Do you have a bicycle helmet? How often do you wear the helmet?

Plan strategies to include all children and families, especially those at high risk of not using seat belts or bicycle helmets.

Nursing Management

For the Health Promotion and Maintenance of the School-Age Child

Nursing Assessment and Diagnosis

Assessment of health promotion and health maintenance topics occurs in many settings with school-age children. They may be seen in offices, clinics, or other settings designed to provide such care. They may come for episodic care for a fracture or infection when health promotion and health maintenance can be easily integrated. They may be seen in the home or neighborhood center, and are frequently encountered by nurses in schools. Opportunities for assessment and intervention should be used whenever they occur. The individual child is examined, and the family, friends, school, and community are addressed. In addition, these visits provide an opportunity to identify early and intervene for health-related problems that emerge or become apparent in school age.

Assessment can be considered on two levels with school-age children. Individual children may be assessed for height and weight, for immunization status, and for use of protective gear during sports. Populations of children may also be assessed since school age is the first time that large numbers of children are together in certain settings. The findings from such assessments will become the basis of an **individualized approach** or a **population-based approach** to health promotion and health maintenance. For example, nurses commonly measure height and weight, calculate body mass index (BMI) for *individual* children seen in a clinic, share results with the family, and address appropriate teaching about weight control and nutritious intake. In other settings, nurses may measure a *classroom* of children and use the collective data to plan appropriate interventions. If 40% of children in a school are classified as overweight by BMI percentile, much emphasis should be placed on teaching about dietary intake, physical activity, and the relationship of recommended weight levels to chronic disease risk. However, if only a small number of children are overweight, interventions may not be as extensive about this topic.

Nurses perform assessment of growth in school-age children, look for achievement of developmental tasks, assess physical and mental health, and assess social characteristics. Based on the assessment of the individual child or populations of children, nursing diagnoses for children and families are established. Possible nursing diagnoses include the following (NANDA-I © 2014):

- *Development: Delayed, Risk for,* related to abuse
- *Parenting, Impaired,* related to lack of knowledge about child health maintenance
- *Sleep Deprivation* related to sleep terrors
- *Violence: Other-Directed, Risk for,* related to history of witnessing family violence
- *Loneliness, Risk for,* related to long periods alone after school

Planning and Implementation

The nurse is instrumental in planning interventions to promote and maintain health in school-age children. These interventions may take place in offices, homes, or clinics with an individual child, or in schools and other community settings with groups of children.

When working with individuals, summarize the strengths and needs identified during the visit, and ask the child and family if they concur. Plan together with them to provide the needed information for topics developed during the visit. Be sure to emphasize those areas where the family excels. For example, positively reinforce use of car seat belts (see *Teaching Highlights: Car Safety for the School-Age Child*), use of protective sports gear, and being current with immunizations. Summarize the next expected developmental tasks, such as increasing independence and growing self-responsibility for choosing snacks and television shows. Then provide anticipatory guidance to assist with the child's growing independence. As peers are becoming more important, always focus some discussion on maintaining healthy social relationships through school peers, religious or community events, and sibling contacts.

Most families welcome a combination of discussion and reading material or pertinent websites for later exploration. Provide telephone numbers of resources for questions and community contacts. Tell the parents when the next health promotion/maintenance visit is recommended. If working with school children for episodic care, ask when the last health maintenance visit occurred. If a child is seen for health care after a bicycling accident, the family may be receptive to teaching about safety precautions. When the child is exposed to skin injuries, a review of the last tetanus booster may reevaluate health maintenance needs. Use every opportunity to work with individual children and insert appropriate health promotion/health maintenance topics.

When working with groups of children, health promotion focuses on known needs, interests, and risk areas. Nurses in school settings have used a variety of creative approaches to promote the health of youth. Nurses in schools can set up a program to train students in health topics; these students then become peer coaches or health advocates in working with other students. Another activity is evaluating the components of school health programs and making recommendations for additions as needed. In school settings, nurses have used a variety of creative approaches to promote the health of youth. Nurses in this setting can establish programs to train students in health topics; these students then become coaches or health advocates who can work with other students, especially those of younger ages. Nurses may also evaluate components of school health programs and offer recommendations for additions as needed. Bulletin boards, community newspapers, television, and community group membership may all be as effective as teaching in school classrooms. Stress reduction teaching should be provided on group and individual levels. Nurses can teach or assist in development of progressive relaxation, deep breathing, biofeedback, yoga, or meditation. Interventions will be most effective if they begin with an understanding of the population served.

Evaluation

Seek evaluation from parents during visits for care. Were their questions answered? Do they know where to turn for advice? Do they know when the child should be seen again for health promotion/maintenance?

TEACHING HIGHLIGHTS | Car Safety for the School-Age Child

Even though parents may have been diligent about car seat and seat belt use when children were younger, guidelines change and they need teaching about current requirements for the school-age child.

Recommendations include the following:

- The child should be kept in a rear-facing seat as long as possible. Generally, by 4 years of age, the child has outgrown the rear-facing seat and should be in a forward-facing car seat with a harness in the back seat. This type of seat is recommended for children 4–7 years of age.
- Once the child outgrows the largest height and weight recommended by the manufacturer for the forward-facing seat (usually by 8 years of age), a booster seat is used in the back seat.
- Once the child is large enough for the regular seat belt, the lap belt must lie snugly across the upper thighs and the shoulder belt should be snug across the shoulder and chest.
- Keep all children in the back seat until 13 years of age; this is the safest location for them in the car (American Academy of Pediatrics, 2011b, 2014; National Highway Traffic Safety Administration, 2012).

The expected outcomes for nursing care of individual school-age children include the following:

- The child demonstrates normal patterns of growth and development.
- The child, family, and community provide a supportive and nurturing environment for the child.
- The child shows growing independence in directing own health promotion activities.

Expected outcomes of nursing care for groups of children include the following:

- The children identify lifestyle decisions that influence their health status.
- The school and community offer resources that help to lessen risk factors related to health and disease/injury prevention.

Health Promotion and Maintenance: The Adolescent

Adolescents are often seen only sporadically for health care, even though visits are recommended annually. They are usually healthy, may not need immunizations, and consequently do not often come for health care, although annual visits are recommended (American Academy of Pediatrics Committee on Practice and Ambulatory Medicine, 2014). If adolescents seek care for a minor illness, birth control, or a sports examination, the visit should be viewed as a health supervision opportunity.

Professionalism in Practice **Adolescent Healthcare International Guidelines**

The World Health Organization (WHO) realizes that adolescents are neither young children, nor young adults, and therefore have unique healthcare needs. The WHO made several recommendations for adolescent health care (WHO, 2014):

- Adolescent care should evolve from being "adolescent friendly" to "adolescent responsive" in order to be meaningful to youth.
- Universal healthcare coverage should be available for all adolescents.
- E-health, m-health (electronic and mobile, respectively), and in-school delivery of care should be offered for adolescents.
- An adolescent-competent workforce should be trained.

Nurses play a role in establishing adolescent-responsive health care in schools, community centers, and via electronic venues. A full range of services can be developed, with input from adolescents themselves about their needs and delivery choices. All nurses working with adolescents must have a thorough understanding of development, best approaches, and common healthcare needs.

While all components of the usual visit may not be performed, at least those parts most important are inserted into care. If time is limited, the nurse has to decide which topics to address during a healthcare visit. It is advisable to start with the topic of most interest to the teen and then to include injury prevention teaching, since injury is the greatest risk to teens. Health promotion topics such as dietary and exercise habits could be discussed.

Lifestyle behaviors are responsible for most of the preventable diseases, and all typically have origins in adolescent years, including sedentary lifestyle, unhealthy diet, tobacco and other substance use, and risk taking. Mental health assessment and teaching are other areas of prime importance. If the teen is at immediate risk, such as considering suicide in response to depression, this must be dealt with immediately by collaborating with a mental health specialist.

What general principles can guide programs to promote health in adolescents? Some researchers have analyzed theory application and approaches of programs, and others have suggested key elements of programs (see *Clinical Reasoning: Applying Theory to Plan for Adolescent Health*). Programs assist adolescents in taking on health promotion behaviors by fostering a sense of competence, promoting decision making, and increasing motivation for change toward healthy behaviors (Pender et al., 2015). When establishing youth programs, whether with individual adolescents or with groups, the nurse includes evaluation of the effectiveness of the plan, and uses methods to expand and sustain successful approaches.

Clinical Reasoning **Applying Theory to Plan for Adolescent Health**

Several theories guide healthcare professionals in establishing health promotion programs for adolescents. These theories provide an organized approach to planning and suggest the strategies that will be most successful, based on the person's motivation and developmental age (Pender et al., 2015). One such theory that is commonly used in adolescent care is the social cognitive theory.

This theory was developed by Albert Bandura, whose work is described in Chapter 31, and is frequently used in health research (Bandura, 1986, 1997a, 1997b; Connor, George, Gullo, et al., 2011; Davies, Terhorst, Nakonechny, et al., 2014). The key components of his theory involve **self-efficacy** (the person's belief in the ability to perform a behavior) and **outcome expectancy** (what the person expects to get from performing a certain behavior). Learning a new behavior occurs through **modeling**, or imitating the behavior of someone else. Bandura believes that individuals make decisions about health behaviors based on thoughts about the consequences and outcomes of those behaviors. The person's characteristics, such as self-efficacy and outcome expectancy, interact with the external environment and the behavioral choices available. All of these components together determine health behaviors, and all can be influenced to promote health.

When seeking to promote physical activity behaviors in youth, essential components include the following:

- Encourage the youth to believe they can perform the activity (self-efficacy).
- Point out the positive aspects of the behavior (outcome expectancy).
- Show the youth how to do the activity (modeling).
- Provide a physical setting and opportunity for performing the behavior (environment).
- Allow trial and error, choice in time, and extent of activity (behavioral choices).

Compose a teaching plan to encourage increased physical activity for a teen, using all components of the social cognitive theory. List the outcome measures or goals for the teaching, the interventions, and methods of evaluation.

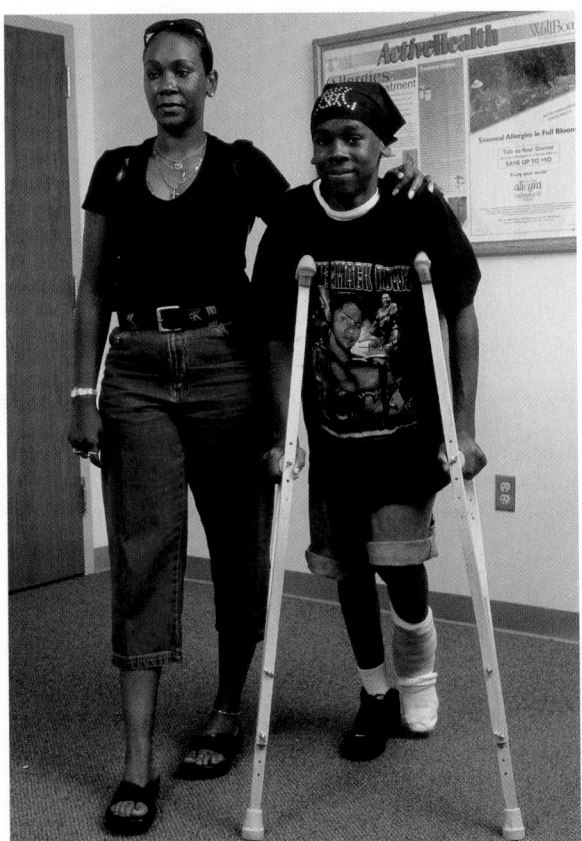

Figure 36–6 **Healthcare visit with a teen. Parents often accompany teens with a healthcare problem when they come in for the examination. Provide an opportunity to see both the teen and parent privately and integrate general health promotion and health maintenance into the visit. What questions can you ask this teen? What teaching might be needed?**

General Observations

The beginning of the visit with an adolescent can be an important time to gather information, just as it is with younger children. However, the observations you make will relate to the adolescent's more advanced stage of development.

Ideally the facility has a waiting area that is designed for adolescents. Teens often dislike waiting for health care with either young children or older adults. Teen waiting areas are popular because they provide a special place, thereby relaying that the adolescent is important, and can use video kiosks and other contemporary methods to impart health information while the teen waits (Figure 36–6). As you call the adolescent back for care, observe if parents or friends are present, or if the teen is alone. Young adolescents often come with parents to the facility, and parents often then wait in the waiting room during the examination. If the young adolescent comes in for a special problem, such as a skin lesion or other health concern, the parent may accompany the adolescent into the examination room. If someone comes with the teen, it may be necessary to provide some private time by asking the other person to wait outside for a moment. Reassure parents that there will be time to talk with them about any of their concerns and questions, and provide them with an opportunity to ask questions and obtain information.

Some teens are comfortable in healthcare settings and actively engage in conversation, while others are nervous and will need more explanations and reassurance during the first steps of measurement and blood pressure. By adolescence, boys and girls should be assuming more of a partnership role in their own health care. As the visit begins, greet adolescents warmly, ask what concerns and questions they have, and ask for their opinions and reactions throughout the visit. This will show that their thoughts are important and that they play an important role in guiding the healthcare visits. When adolescents are visiting the same office or clinic that they came to during childhood, they usually know and feel comfortable with the care providers. If the setting is new to them, explain procedures and introduce personnel so they feel more at ease.

Growth and Developmental Surveillance

Adolescence spans several years, and growth and developmental issues vary throughout the period. For young adolescents, or those from about 12 to 13 years of age, growth measurement remains important. These youth are still growing, and use of percentile grids continues to be an important part of care. Growth should remain in the same percentile channel as during childhood, with girls reaching nearly adult height at this age, and boys still continuing to grow. As always, be alert for youth who have either increased or decreased percentiles, or are above the 85th percentile or below the 5th percentile for body mass index (BMI). They will need additional assessment of nutritional intake and physical activity.

By middle (14 to 16 years) and late adolescence (17 to 19 years), adult growth is nearly achieved, earlier for girls than boys. While measurement continues to be performed, nurses assess the BMI carefully to be sure the height and weight indicate appropriate intake and exercise. Overweight at this age is likely to continue into adulthood, particularly if parents are overweight, so early intervention will be needed to decrease this potential. Other youth may have eating disorders and should be referred to a specialist for care. Children from homes without sufficient financial resources may be hungry and lack adequate food of high quality (known as *food insecurity*). Parents who were eligible for the Special Supplemental Nutrition Program for Women, Infants, and Children (WIC) services when children were younger may not receive them once the child is an adolescent, so the increasing dietary intake needs of their teens cannot be met. If an adolescent is thin and has little energy, consider this possibility; administer a food security questionnaire such as the one provided by the U.S. Department of Agriculture (www.ers.usda.gov). Even the child who is overweight may live in a family with insufficient resources since foods with high fat and caloric content are often less expensive than those with greater nutrient value. For example, a "dollar menu" at a fast-food restaurant meets hunger needs faster and with less expense than a home-prepared meal of fresh fruits, vegetables, and grains. In addition, people who have experienced periods of hunger from inadequate food resources may overeat when food is available, a pattern that promotes weight gain (see Chapter 32).

Few options exist for measuring the developmental competence of adolescents, but observations and questions during care provide information about the meeting of developmental milestones. Key tasks for adolescents involve separating from the parents and establishing positive relationships with peers. The young teen may come to an appointment with a parent and still rely on that parent to answer some questions during the examination. However, middle and late teens should be increasingly able to come alone, answer questions themselves, and assume responsibility for healthcare decisions. Offer older teens the option of coming into the room alone, stating, "Your mom can wait here and we can come and get her later. Does that sound all right?" During time with the adolescent, ask questions to learn about peer interactions and activities.

The adolescent may receive a physical examination from a nurse practitioner or a physician. See Chapter 33 for components of the examination. Some particular parts of the examination to include for teens are scoliosis screening, sexual maturity rating (Tanner stages), breast examination, testicular examination, testing for sexually transmitted infections (among those sexually active), pelvic examination, and Pap smear (for sexually active females), hematocrit/hemoglobin for anemia when risk assessment warrants, hearing and vision screening when needed, annual blood pressure, lipid screening for those with family history of early heart disease or other risk factors, and tuberculosis screening for those in high-risk areas (American Academy of Pediatrics Committee on Practice and Ambulatory Medicine, 2014).

Most adolescents do not want their parents present during the examination, but occasionally will want a parent present for something like a first pelvic examination or a blood draw. Ask them their wishes in a confidential setting so they can freely make the choice. They also may choose to have a same-gender healthcare provider complete the genitourinary examination. Expected outcomes of care include screening and early identification for common health problems, normal patterns of growth, and meeting of developmental milestones.

Nutrition

The young adolescent needs a well-balanced diet to support the growth of this period, and the late adolescent requires intake that supports physical activity and provides nutrients for metabolism and to promote the immune system. While nutritional intake is important, teens often do not eat well. They may be busy and do not want to plan meals, they like to eat foods that are popular with other teens (so high fat and sugar intake can be common), they may be dieting to achieve weight loss, and some do not have enough financial resources to access healthy foods.

Combine the information from measurement of the adolescent with the answers to questions about diet to identify possible areas for intervention. Find out what questions the teen has about foods, diet, maintaining desired weight, and topics such as vegetarianism or supplements to enhance athletic performance. See Chapter 32 for further detail about these special nutritional topics. Health promotion plans focus on practices that lead to healthy growth and development. They may include teaching about:

- Getting five fruits and vegetables daily
- Including whole-grain products to replace refined products whenever possible
- The importance of eating three meals each day, including breakfast and lunch
- Eating together as a family several times weekly, which enhances quality food intake
- How to plan menus and prepare foods for balanced intake

Health maintenance plans center on those practices that prevent disease, including:

- Limiting refined sugar and high-fat intake (such as soft drinks and fried foods) to maintain weight at recommended level

- Including two to three servings of dairy products daily to enhance bone formation and decrease chance of osteoporosis as an adult
- Using resources for treatment of eating disorders if they are identified

While much of nutrition teaching should be aimed directly at the adolescent, parents are also included. They can be effective contributors to healthy intake by providing plenty of fruits and vegetables for snacks, having foods attractively prepared and ready for consumption when the teen is hungry, planning several meals together as a family each week, encouraging milk or other forms of calcium intake, and setting a good example for food intake. Help parents to identify the youth with an eating disorder and provide resources for intervention in these cases. Consider as well the teen with a baby. The adolescent who is pregnant or breastfeeding has even more need for nutritional teaching and may need financial resources to access sufficient food (see Chapter 11). How can the nurse combine in the teaching plan the growth and developmental needs of an adolescent with those of her new baby?

Physical Activity

Many adolescents suffer from the effects of inadequate physical activity. As children get older and enter the teenage years, physical activity decreases, particularly in girls. Sixty minutes daily of moderate or vigorous activity is recommended for teens, but 15% do not get this level of exercise even 1 day a week, and 53% do not achieve this activity 5 out of 7 days of the week (CDC, 2014). The percentage is lower among some groups, such as females, Blacks, and Hispanics, with wide state variation (CDC, 2014). At a time when teens are not very active as a group, physical education requirements in school are also decreasing. Only 24% of 12th-grade male and 16% of 12th-grade female students regularly attend a physical education class (CDC, 2014). Physical activity levels must therefore be assessed at each health supervision visit or in other contacts with adolescents. Apply resilience theory as discussed in Chapter 31, and assess youth, family, and community for risk and protective factors regarding physical activity (Table 36–4).

Some youth have established regular physical activity programs, and their behaviors should be encouraged (Figure 36–7). Be alert for adolescents who exercise but have other health problems. Some athletes try to eat very little to remain a certain weight for wrestling, running, or other sports. Integrate nutritional teaching that includes the importance of adequate intake for sports performance. Other athletes use nutritional supplements to enhance performance. While most are not harmful, few have proven benefits and their cost is not warranted. Some may actually be harmful to adolescents, such as prolonged use of creatinine and any use of steroids.

Some youth have very little physical activity and feel incompetent in performing many sports. Work with them to find at least one thing they can do on a daily basis—walking their dog in the neighborhood, riding a bike to the store, using stairs instead of elevators when possible, parking on the far side of the school lot and walking farther, swimming at a club their parents belong to or at a local YMCA or YWCA, or saving money to take lessons for something they have always dreamed of doing, such as horseback riding or golf. The community health nurse can form interest groups at schools and community centers that provide an outlet for adolescents who cannot "make the team" for school sports. Encourage parents and adolescents to set goals together to integrate some physical activity daily.

TABLE 36–4 Risk and Protective Factors Regarding Physical Activity in Adolescence

RISK FACTORS	PROTECTIVE FACTORS
• Lives in rural or other isolated setting with little opportunity for contact with other teens • Lives in urban area that is unsafe or provides little opportunity for outside physical activity • Presence of neighborhood hazards and unsafe areas • Lack of neighborhood programs for physical activity promotion	• Has opportunities for participation in physical activity at home, at school, and in the community • School provides daily physical education classes • Neighborhood and community provide physical activity options • Has many friends living close who participate in physical activity • Public policies maintain parks, green spaces, biking trails, playgrounds
• Has a developmental disability that impairs physical movement	• Programs are available for adolescents with developmental disabilities or other healthcare needs
• Does not like physical activity	• Likes physical activity
• Has a pattern and history of low activity levels • Is overweight • Does not feel competent in most sports	• Has exercised during all of childhood, often with parents
• Limited financial resources to pay registration fees or buy protective gear for sports	• Availability of financial and other resources for sports gear and protective equipment
• Family members who have little physical activity • Parents who are not active in school sports and committees • Parents who do not like physical activity and have had low levels while their teen was growing up • Parents who have little time or facilities for exercise, or always exercise at a club—out of view of their family	• Parents participate in regular physical activity and encourage the adolescent to do so also • Youth and parents agree to a limit of 2 hours daily of screen time
• Lack of youth and parent knowledge about physical activity needs and benefits	• Knowledgeable about benefits of activity; committed to maintaining exercise patterns

Source: Data from Hagan, J. F., Shaw, J. S., & Duncan, P. M. (Eds.). (2008). *Bright futures: Guidelines for health supervision of infants, children, and adolescents* (3rd ed.). Elk Grove Village, IL: American Academy of Pediatrics.

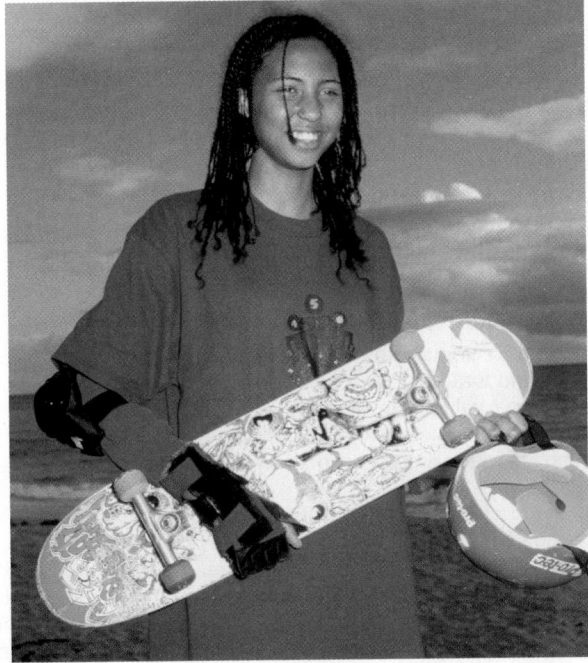

Figure 36–7 **Teen use of safety measures. This teen girl is an avid "boarder." How can you encourage and praise her for this activity? What clues do you have that she is using adequate safety measures?**

What risk and protective factors for physical activity exist in your community? Go to www.activelivingbydesign.org to examine the positive effect community planning can have on its members' exercise levels.

The nurse's activities for health promotion concentrate on teaching the health and mental benefits of physical activity such as increased energy, weight control, and a feeling of control and success. Health maintenance focuses on viewing physical activity as a method to prevent disease such as cardiovascular disease and diabetes. Youth who have family members with these diseases or meet adults who have them are more likely to understand the importance of their own activity. Desired outcomes include maintenance of weight within recommended level, daily exercise of 60 minutes, and establishment of lifetime exercise routines.

Oral Health

Continued dental care during the adolescent years can ensure oral health. The recommendations remain the same as those for young children. The adolescent should floss daily, brush twice daily with a small amount of fluoridated toothpaste, and visit a dental care provider every 6 months. By about 14 years of age, those adolescents who do not have fluoridated water and have been taking fluoride can stop this supplement. Even the molars have been formed by that age so fluoride tablets are no longer needed. Continue to examine the condition of the teeth and the number of erupted permanent teeth present. Be alert for any unusual growths and ulcers in the mouth and refer for care as needed.

Unavailability of dental insurance for the adolescent is a potential concern. The teen whose family does not have dental insurance needs referrals for care to affordable resources. Dental specialists clean off plaque that has formed, apply sealants to erupting molars, examine the teeth for caries, and perform restorative care. Certain groups are more at risk for inadequate dental care (see *Developing Cultural Competence: Dental Care*).

When working with these populations, nurses can question access to care and make recommendations that foster regular checkups.

Developing Cultural Competence Dental Care

Analysis of several national surveys, such as the National Center for Health Statistics and the National Health Interview Survey, shows marked disparity in oral health. The major factor in disparity of dental care is lack of dental insurance. While 42% of youth from families without insurance did not have a dental visit in the previous year and 27% of them had unmet dental needs, only 11% of youth from families with insurance lacked a previous year visit and only 4% had unmet dental needs. People without dental insurance commonly are poor and are more often from Hispanic and immigrant groups (Child Trends, 2013).

When working with adolescent populations from groups at high risk for lack of dental coverage or high incidence of caries, include dental assessment in health supervision visits, and have resources for care readily available to carry out referrals as needed. The Affordable Care Act provides for two dental visits annually, so assist families to participate in their state or employment healthcare plan.

Evaluate risk factors for threats to oral health such as tobacco use, particularly chewing tobacco (see quote from Jeremy in the chapter-opening scenario). A risk for oral injury exists with engagement in certain sports. Ask about physical activity and recommend that a mouth guard be worn if the youth engages in hockey, football, or some other sports. Some teens may wish to whiten the teeth or obtain orthodontia to improve appearance. The nurse can help the youth and parents to find resources for needed care.

Expected outcomes for oral health include dental visits twice annually; daily positive oral health habits; absence of risk factors for poor oral health, injury, or tobacco use; and obtaining recommended follow-up care for problems.

Mental and Spiritual Health

Adolescents have many challenges to their mental health and need support to emerge from adolescence with mental and spiritual strengths. Mental health topics must be addressed at each health supervision opportunity to promote mental health among teens. Mental health is closely linked to developmental tasks such as growing independence, formation of close relationships with peers, becoming confident in accomplishments, and setting goals for the future. Some chronic mental health disorders such as schizophrenia can emerge during adolescence, so mental health screening is important to perform with this age group.

As during other developmental stages, the self-concept continues to evolve, influencing how the adolescent reacts to the environment. Self-regulation—making decisions to govern oneself—becomes critically important. Self-esteem, or a positive feeling about the self, is key to meeting life's challenges. Ask what the teen is proud of and has accomplished and what disappointments have occurred as well. Provide resources to deal with disappointments and praise the teen's accomplishments.

The adolescent's self-esteem is connected to perception of body image. Factors such as early or late maturation,

overweight or underweight, or the role of the media can influence the teen's body image. A healthy image includes the realization that the body has positive and less positive attributes and that the individual can influence the body by healthy eating and physical activity. Be alert for the teen whose wish for a different body leads to eating disorders and excessive exercise or intake of nutritional supplements.

Sexuality involves both body changes that signal mature sexual development, and the mental concept of oneself as a sexual being. Body changes and mental concepts do not necessarily mature at the same time, and adolescents may not be ready for sexual maturity; decisions about sexual behavior are not necessarily equivalent to achieving sexual maturation. Most young adolescent girls have begun menstruating, and by early to middle adolescence, boys are having nocturnal emissions and ejaculations. Ask teens if they have received information about puberty, body changes, and sexuality. Tell young adolescents that most teens have questions and that they may ask about any areas of interest, including contraception and sexually transmitted infections. Ask older adolescents directly if they have had sexual intercourse and if so, what they are doing to protect against pregnancy and sexually transmitted infections. Provide support for adolescents who have decided not to have sexual intercourse, encouraging them to continue this plan, telling them that sexual feelings are normal, but that decisions about sexual intercourse are their right and privilege. Ask if the adolescent has ever experienced unwanted pressure for intercourse and if there has been help and support to deal with the situation. Intimate partner violence, date rape, and other trauma signal a need for referral to a mental health specialist. See Chapter 42 for further information.

Ask if teens have confusion about their sexuality. If teens have self-identified as being gay, let them know they are welcome and ask about decisions regarding sexual practices, reinforcing the need for protection against sexually transmitted infections. Provide community resources to support gay or lesbian teens so that they can develop a social group in which they feel comfortable. Some adolescents are seen for health care at the time they become sexually active. Use this opportunity to reinforce and correct prior knowledge about the body and protection against pregnancy and sexually transmitted infections.

Clinical Tip

The nurse who works with adolescents dealing with sexuality issues may find that the values of some teens are very different from one's personal values. How do you react when a teen decides to have sexual intercourse or has become pregnant? Can you help teens to make wise decisions without telling them what they should do?

It is important for adolescents to learn the significance of sexual intercourse and the meaning of close relationships. Teaching them early about this will enable them to respect others at the time they do have intimate relations. Respect is also the key to working with teens. Nurses should treat them with respect, expecting them to consider options and make wise decisions. Nurses who cannot work with certain groups of teens because of moral values differing from their own have the obligation to refer the teens for care to resources where they can receive the information and services they are requesting.

Most adolescents still need discipline or guidance from parents at certain times. Rather than a constant battle over daily events, it is best if there are just a few important rules that parents have to enforce only rarely. When working with parents, nurses can assist them to set useful boundaries for teens and offer resources such as parenting groups and websites for assistance.

Sleep is necessary for anyone to function safely and at a level of one's potential. Unfortunately, many youth do not get the sleep needed for healthy functioning. Teens have an increased need for sleep due to their growth rates and activity levels. At the same time, their internal clocks change, making it more difficult to get to sleep at the usual time. It is thought that a decrease in secretion of melatonin occurs, so the teen does not feel tired in the late evening. However, they often do not have the number of hours of sleep needed by the time they wake up for school or work. The problem may be worsened if the student participates in sports or other activities. They may need to get to school before normal starting hours for music, sports, or other activities, or perhaps stay late into the evening for practices. Some adolescents work weekends or evenings as well. And of course social activities usually fill much of their time. Although about 9 hours of sleep is needed, most adolescents get about 6 hours (Mayo Clinic, 2013). The effects of sleep deprivation can be serious. Teens cannot perform to their potential in school or at work. Many parents state that adolescents are moody and difficult to communicate with when they are tired. There may be a connection between lack of sleep and substance abuse, and teens commonly use caffeinated beverages to stay awake. Some people tend to eat more when they are tired, and get less physical activity. Perhaps one of the most serious consequences deals with the danger of driving while sleepy; this is a common cause of accidents. Ask adolescents about what time they go to bed, when they awaken, and whether they are frequently tired. Provide suggestions for regular sleep schedules, avoiding caffeine products in the evening, making screen technology unavailable during sleep time, and planning a day of relaxation into every week.

Healthy People 2020

(SH-3) Increase the proportion of students in grades 9 through 12 who get sufficient sleep on school nights

- Less than 31% of adolescents have 8 hours of sleep on school nights. *Healthy People 2020* has set a modest goal to increase this percentage to 33% who achieve at least 8 hours of sleep on school nights.

School plays an increasingly important role in adolescent mental health. School provides peer support, meaningful activities, and a forum for learning time management and other skills. At the same time, some youth stress because of inability to fit in, worry about grades and their futures, and violent or unsupportive school situations. Discuss the elements of school that adolescents like and those they do not like. Determine what support is available in the schools. Ask the adolescent about future plans and how those are influencing choices for courses and friends in school.

Temperament or personality type characteristics continue into adolescence and generally do not change from earlier years. For example, the active infant and young child is usually an active teenager. The slow-to-warm-up baby may be the adolescent who needs more time to adjust to a new school or teachers. If the adolescent or parent has trouble with personality characteristics, it may be helpful to talk about these traits, help them to establish a positive sense about the attributes, and discuss ways to adapt the environment as needed. For example, parents should not expect a slow-to-warm-up teen to be interested in running for a class office. Someone with irregular sleep

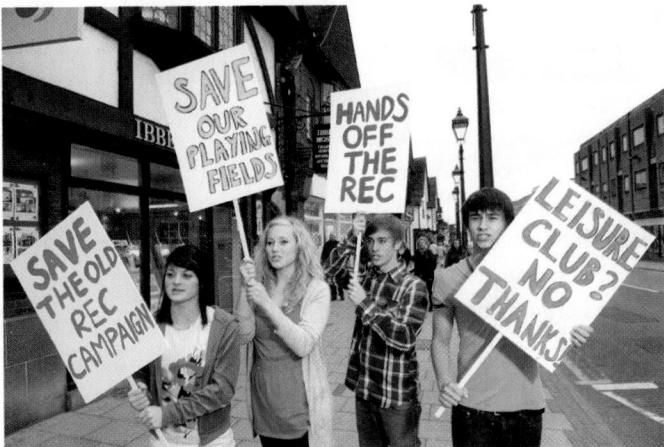

Figure 36–8 Spiritual health for teens. Teens often become associated with causes. This helps them to feel part of a social group and also provides opportunities for examining belief systems and making decisions about meaningful activities.

and eating habits will find it difficult to have a job at a set time and will need to set alarms and other reminders.

Spirituality offers comfort and support for the adolescent. Being a member of a teen group in a faith-based home can offer a peer group with similar values and bring meaning to life. Some adolescents reject the faith of their parents and seek a different group; others seek to leave religious practices totally, while others become more committed to them. Ask them if they have the resources they need to bring meaning to their lives; provide them if needed. Realize that participation in community food kitchens, raising money for causes, and other activities also provide meaning for many adolescents (Figure 36–8).

The nurse actively promotes the mental health of youth by understanding their developmental needs and providing information and resources. Gentle guidance and active partnership with youth help to provide the resources to ensure healthy self-concept, sexuality, and personality development. While most teenagers have many protective factors that can be identified and fostered, a few have risks that can harm mental health. It is important to identify the risks, and to use health maintenance techniques to lessen the risk factors. Depression and substance use are two common risks to mental health. Depression is discussed in Chapter 55, and substance abuse is discussed in Chapter 42. See the quick checklists in Table 36–5 to help in identifying these problems during health supervision visits.

Although health promotion and health maintenance activities commonly occur in office or clinic settings, there are many other settings where nurses work with adolescents, and mental health activities are often integrated into these settings. Consider offering health promotion/maintenance wherever students might be found. Some nontraditional settings include correctional facilities, school-based health centers, and programs for pregnant teens. Adolescents in these facilities can benefit from services to improve diet, physical activity, and lifestyle behaviors that influence mental health.

The desired outcomes for mental and spiritual health promotion and maintenance include meaningful activities in the adolescent's life, emerging independence, good choices about lifestyle behaviors, and development of successful coping skills.

TABLE 36–5 Signs of Depression and Substance Abuse

DEPRESSION	SUBSTANCE ABUSE
Changes in appetite and weight	Changes in school performance, sleep, and appetite
Changes in sleep schedules and patterns	Unusual behavior, such as getting into trouble at school
Changes in school performance	Accidents and other unexplained events
Physical complaints	Lack of responsibility for actions
Loss of interest and pleasure in usual activities and friends	Increased mood changes
Depression, irritability, poor concentration	Inability to set goals
Feelings of worthlessness, helplessness	A variety of physical changes depending on the substance used
Thoughts of death or suicide	

Source: Adapted from Tanski, S., Garfunkel, L. C., Duncan, P. M., & Weitzman, M. (2011). *Performing preventive services*. Elk Grove Village, Il: American Academy of Pediatrics.

Relationships

Adolescents form stronger bonds with friends than at any time earlier in development; at the same time, they need their parents for guidance and reassurance as they become more independent. As teenagers strive for independence, they frequently strike out at parents, test limits, and have conflicts with parents. Interactions in the family provide consistent and important ties at the same time that social interactions become a central part of life. Health promotion helps teens to form strong friendships with peers and to continue to value and participate in the family. It helps parents to understand the developmental needs and their role in establishing a new type of relationship with the emerging young adult in the family. Partnerships with healthcare providers are important to help families work together to achieve these outcomes.

When adolescents are seen for healthcare visits, assess relationships with others. Provide time alone with both the adolescent and the parents (if they are present) so that everyone has time to talk freely and to ask questions. Some areas already discussed, such as school performance and activities, provide information about the adolescent's friends and how time is spent. Ask teens to describe their best friends and what they do together. Ask parents their opinions of the youth's friends. Inquire about the youth's roles in the family. Does the teen have jobs and responsibilities? What freedom is allowed? What are relationships like with siblings and extended family members such as grandparents and cousins? What activities are done together as a family? Are there differences in the teen's and the parents' answers to these questions? What are the teen's and parents' desires for how the family unit functions?

Provide an opportunity to talk with the teen alone about issues such as domestic violence. Is the youth abused or is there violence between adults in the family? Are there stressors such as lack of sufficient finances, an ill parent, or a lost job? How have these occurrences affected the adolescent? Minor adjustments can be helped by discussion, whereas some major problems will need referral to mental health specialists.

In their relationships with peers, adolescents often have many of the same issues that emerge with parents. They may have disagreements with friends or feel hurt by things that are said or done. Ask teens about how things are going with friends and what problems they have. Talk about negotiating, joining groups to form new friendships, and the importance of respecting and not making fun of others. Give them strategies for living up to their own standards even when friends are enticing them to do other things. Suggest that having friends one can trust and who have the same ideals can be very supportive and fun in adolescent years. Expected outcomes are the formation of strong relationships both within and outside of the family, along with independence in decision making.

Disease Prevention Strategies

Teenagers typically do not have many diseases and most are minor illnesses like respiratory and gastrointestinal illness. However, there are some diseases that occur and nurses must always be aware of signs of potential disease. Some common health issues that are described throughout this book include the following:

- Acne and skin infections (see Chapter 57)
- Body piercing and tattooing (see Chapter 42)
- Sports overuse injuries (see Chapter 56)
- Constipation and diarrhea (see Chapter 51)

Other observations may signal more serious health concerns and need to be referred for further evaluation. Examples include the following:

- Scoliosis (see Chapter 56)
- Anemia (see Chapter 49)
- Excessive tiredness (see Chapter 50)
- Bruising (see Chapter 49)
- Depression, suicidal thoughts, other mental health issues (see Chapter 55)
- Sexually transmitted infections (see Chapter 52)
- Eating disorders (see Chapter 42)
- Abuse or severe bullying (see Chapter 42)

Several screening tests should be performed during health supervision visits with adolescents, including vision, hearing, smoking, depression, stress, alcohol or other substance use, blood pressure, urinalysis, sexually transmitted infection risk, and, in some cases, Pap smears and breast examinations. Screening tests with abnormal results require follow-up and intervention. For example, if the adolescent is anemic, iron tablets may be needed and teaching about high-iron foods should be done. Vision impairment requires referral to an eye specialist. Presence of sexually transmitted infections requires teaching and medication treatment. History of sexual activity will guide the nurse to tests that should be included in the examination (see *Clinical Tip*).

The adolescent should receive extensive information about ways to protect health and prevent disease. The hazardous outcomes of smoking are discussed, and smoking cessation programs are encouraged for smokers. Unprotected sexual activity is presented as a serious health threat. Use of sunscreens to prevent burns and future skin cancer is encouraged. Females are taught breast self-examination, and males are taught testicular examination. For youth who are overweight and sedentary, the possible outcomes such as type 2 diabetes and cardiovascular disease are mentioned. While it would not be advisable to threaten or frighten an adolescent with descriptions of diseases, an understanding of the potential serious outcomes can be motivators for behavior change.

In addition to teaching to prevent disease, the nurse also administers any needed immunizations. Many adolescents have not had immunizations since about school entry time, so their record should be carefully reviewed (see Chapter 43). When checking the adolescent's record, consider the following questions about some common immunizations that are needed:

- *When was the last tetanus-diphtheria (Td) booster?* It is recommended every 10 years if no wounds have required an update in the interim. If the child received it at age 5 years, a booster is needed at 15 years. A Tdap (tetanus-diphtheria-acellular pertussis) booster is given, with the preferred age of 11 to 12 years.
- *Was a second measles-mumps-rubella administered?* A second dose may not have been routine when teens were younger so they may need it now.
- *Is hepatitis A common in your state?* If so, the teen needs to get that vaccine.

- *Has the youth had hepatitis B vaccine?* This is important for all youth, and some may not have received it as infants.
- *Did the youth have a documented history of varicella disease?* If not, two doses of the vaccine are needed.
- *Has the youth received meningococcal vaccine?* Meningococcal vaccine is now recommended for all youth.
- *Have the adolescent female and male received the human papillomavirus vaccine?* Human papillomavirus vaccine (three-dose series) is recommended for females and males from 11 to 12 years, or for those 13 to 26 years not previously immunized. The vaccine can be given as early as 9 years of age.
- *Has the youth received the annual influenza vaccine?* Annual influenza vaccine is now recommended for all children and adolescents.

The results of health screening are shared with the teen and with the parent as appropriate. Teaching and other interventions for disease prevention are examples of health maintenance activities. Expected outcomes are increasing knowledge of common diseases and methods of prevention among teen and parent, use of screening tests by the healthcare provider, and use of the healthcare home by the adolescent for treatment of diseases.

Injury Prevention Strategies

Injury is the greatest health hazard for adolescents, so injury prevention must be integrated into every health contact with youth. The major hazard is automobile crashes (see Chapter 1). Many teens learn to drive and have a license by 16 years of age. They often transport friends, get distracted by social interactions in the car, have little experience about what to do if a car slides or has mechanical problems, may drink and drive, talk or text on cell phones while driving, and are often tired when driving (Figure 36–9). Many states have instituted graduated driving

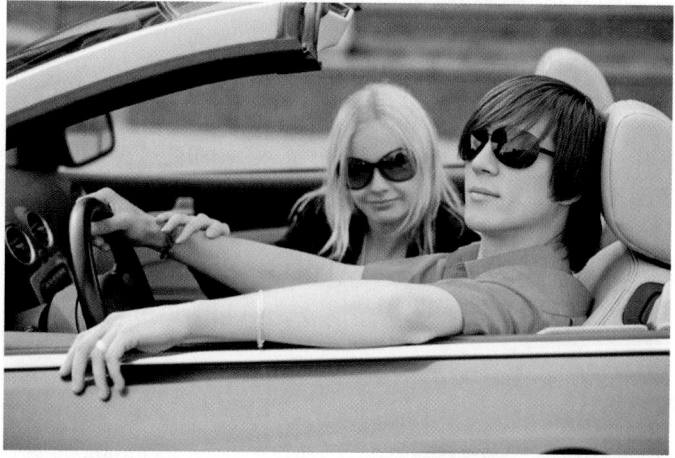

Figure 36–9 **Injury prevention for teens. Adolescents often drive motorized vehicles and may be at risk for injury if not properly prepared or protected. What teaching and experience do these youth need for safe enjoyment of the experience of driving and riding with friends? Do schools in your area offer driver education classes? What are the state requirements for youth driver licensure?**

SOURCE: wrangler/Shutterstock.

licensing to help decrease some risks. Know the graduated driver license laws in your state and reinforce them with youth and families. Driving should always be presented as a privilege and a responsibility. Suggest that parents consider enforcing serious consequences such as losing the ability to drive for a time after any infraction. Because of the great risk of injury and death from motor vehicle crashes, ask at each health visit if the teen drives, rides with other teens, what rules parents have established about driving, and whether the teen ever drinks and drives or rides with someone who does. Reinforce the need to wear a lap and shoulder belt at all times and to never drink and drive.

SAFETY ALERT!

Major risk factors for teen drivers include inexperience (especially vulnerable time is the first 6 months of driving), transporting other teens, night driving, non-use of seat belt, and distractions such as texting and playing music. Graduated driver licensing is an approach used to decrease motor vehicle crashes among novice teen drivers. The CDC recommends that no learners' permits be allowed before 16 years of age, that permits must be held for at least 6 months, that driving from 10 p.m. to 5 a.m. not be allowed except with adult chaperone, that other youth not be transported, and that regular licenses (without youth restrictions) not be allowed until 18 years of age. Zero-tolerance policies for drinking, texting or cell phone use, and non-use of seat belts should be enforced (CDC, 2011b). How can nurses be active in political discussions to promote graduated driver licensing and support parents of novice teen drivers?

Youth are at risk for injury with other motorized vehicles. Motorcycles, four-wheelers, boats, jet skis, farm machinery, and tools are other sources of injury. Ask about the youth's exposure to various machines and teach about avoiding alcohol and drug use and safety gear and precautions to be used. Every health visit should include other questions that help to identify a wide variety of injury hazards. Be sure to discuss and provide written material to perform injury prevention teaching. Such measures are important health maintenance activities (Tables 36–6 and 36–7). Desired outcomes for nursing care include absence of serious injury, the ability to state sources of risk for injury, and emergency plans for assistance when engaging in any risky activities.

Nursing Management

For the Health Promotion and Maintenance of the Adolescent

Nursing Assessment and Diagnosis

Nurses assess adolescents in a variety of settings, including offices, clinics, schools, homes, correctional facilities, extended care facilities, sports-related facilities, and family planning clinics. A wide array of health concerns should be included in these assessments:

- Measurement of growth
- Presence of any unusual findings on physical examination
- Lifestyle choices related to dietary intake, physical activity, and oral hygiene

- Assessment of mental status, family interactions, and social connections with peers
- Any risky behaviors the adolescent engages in such as smoking, unprotected sexual relations, alcohol or drug use, or unsafe driving practices

The people and organizations around the adolescent such as family, school, and neighborhood are all assessed. Remember to list both risks and protective factors. The protective factors can be used during implementation to enhance the youth's resilience.

Based on a thorough assessment, you will establish nursing diagnoses that are appropriate for the adolescent and family. Some possible nursing diagnoses might include the following (NANDA-I © 2014):

- *Rape-Trauma Syndrome* related to date rape
- *Dentition, Impaired,* related to ineffective oral hygiene
- *Obesity* related to lack of basic nutritional knowledge and obesity in both parents
- *Nutrition, Readiness for Enhanced,* related to increasing interest in nutritional knowledge
- *Sleep Pattern, Disturbed,* related to frequently changing sleep–wake schedule
- *Self-Esteem, Situational Low,* related to situational crisis of friends making fun of adolescent
- *Injury, Risk for,* related to psychomotor and cognitive factors

Planning and Implementation

Whatever the setting, the nurse partners with the adolescent, the parents, and other persons such as teachers or school counselors to plan appropriate goals and related interventions. Nurses work with individual adolescents in offices, schools, and other settings, and often work with groups of adolescents to perform teaching. Apply communication skills that are effective with teens, such as listening to concerns, allowing for discussion, and bringing in peers who have had experiences related to the topic being discussed.

Many nursing interventions involve teaching, so it is wise to develop a number of resources for working with teens. Consult the resources on this textbook's companion website, and visit agencies in your community to gather appropriate materials. Teaching topics should be directed both at health promotion (providing information to enhance the adolescent's state of health) and health maintenance (sharing tips about how to avoid disease and injury). A good starting point is to have the adolescent identify a personal health goal and begin teaching there. In addition to teaching, direct care is provided when administering immunizations, performing vision screening, and examining the spine and posture for scoliosis.

One of the challenges during health supervision for adolescents is including the right mix of teen and parent decision making and involvement. It is again important to apply communication skills by tactfully allowing time for both parent and adolescent to be seen alone. Realize that health supervision provides support and information for parents, such as useful discipline techniques, recognition of common parental feelings about teens, and the need for growing independence

TABLE 36–6 Injury Prevention in Adolescence

	HAZARD	DEVELOPMENTAL CHARACTERISTICS	PREVENTIVE MEASURES
	Motor vehicle crashes	Adolescents learn to drive, enjoy new independence, and often feel invulnerable.	Insist on driver's education classes. Enforce rules about safe driving. Seat belts should be used for every trip. Discourage drug and alcohol use. Get treatment for teenagers who are known substance abusers.
	Sporting injuries	Adolescents may participate in physically challenging sports such as soccer, gymnastics, or football. They may be allowed to drive motorboats.	Encourage use of protective sporting gear. Teach safe boating practices. Perform teaching related to hazards of drug and alcohol use, especially when using motorized equipment.
	Drowning	Adolescents overestimate endurance when swimming. They take risks diving.	Encourage swimming only with friends. Reinforce rules and teach them about risks.

by their youth. When providing teaching to groups of teens in schools, there may be policies about what needs to be sent home to parents. For topics such as sexually transmitted infections or substance use, some schools require that an outline be sent home for parents to read. Parents may call with questions about content and approach, or some may choose to attend the presentation. To create an effective presentation, the nurse must partner with the school administration, teachers, parents, and others. The ability to collaborate successfully with many individuals and agencies is an important skill for the nurse.

Wherever adolescents are seen, whether in offices or other private settings, schools, correction facilities, or other places with groups present, it is important to leave information about how to contact the nurse or another care provider. Provide brochures, referral numbers, names, and emails related to the topics discussed. Encourage annual visits for health supervision and suggest a variety of places to obtain this care. For example, if a youth will soon graduate from high school, find out if the youth will be working or attending college and provide links to health insurance or care providers in the new location.

Evaluation

Expected outcomes for care of adolescents and their families during health promotion and health maintenance include the following:

- Normal growth patterns and healthy weight are maintained.
- The adolescent is physically active for 60 minutes daily.
- Debris and plaque are absent on dental surfaces.
- The adolescent establishes a positive self-concept.
- The adolescent establishes positive relationships with peers, family members, teachers, and others.
- Healthy lifestyle habits are maintained that promote prevention of disease and injury.

TABLE 36–7 Injury Prevention Topics for Adolescents

TOPIC	INJURY PREVENTION TEACHING
Driving	Always wear seat and shoulder belts.
	Do not drink alcohol or take drugs and drive or ride with others who do.
	Do not talk or text on a cell phone as you drive.
	Do not drive when you are tired.
	Drive with parents or other adults for several months in winter driving conditions if you live where there is snow, ice, or heavy rains.
	Keep your car in good repair.
Sun	Wear sunscreen. Limit direct exposure to the sun, especially early in the summer when the skin is most sensitive to burns. This can be achieved by wearing sunscreen, hats, and clothing that prevent sunburns.
Machinery	Learn how to use power tools correctly.
	Always have someone near when you use tools or machinery.
	Follow guidelines for agricultural safety (CDC, 2011c).
Emergency care	Learn first aid, CPR, and airway obstruction removal.
Water safety	Learn to swim well.
	If you supervise younger children near water, never leave them alone, even for a minute.
Fires	Do not play with fire.
	Follow guidelines to avoid igniting gasoline.
	Test smoke alarms in your house every 6 months and change batteries annually.
Firearms	Know and follow rules to keep firearms locked, with ammunition locked in a separate place.
	Never take out a gun to show a friend unless your parent is also present.
	Take firearm safety classes if you hunt or target shoot.
Hearing	Avoid loud music especially for long periods and through ear phones.
Sports	Wear protective gear recommended for your sport.
Abuse	Report any abuse to an adult you trust.
	Date with other couples whenever possible and report date rape.
	Do not drink or take drugs.

Source: Data from Hagan, J. F., Shaw, J. S., & Duncan, P. M. (2008). *Bright futures: Guidelines for health supervision of infants, children, and adolescents* (3rd ed.). Elk Grove Village, IL: American Academy of Pediatrics.

Focus Your Study

- Health promotion visits are recommended annually and should take place in any setting where the child is seen, even for episodic or emergency care.

- Developmental surveillance, growth measurement, and physical examination provide the basis for establishing risk and protective factors for each child and adolescent.

- School-age children and adolescents are increasingly independent in making choices about nutrition and physical activity, while peer influence continues to grow.

- Establishment of affirmative self-esteem is important for school-age children and adolescents in order to develop positive mental health.

- Injury and disease prevention for school-age children and adolescents focuses on common causes of morbidity and mortality, such as firearms, abuse, motor vehicle crashes, alcohol and substance use, lack of immunizations, and sports-related injuries.

- The nurse integrates information from the health supervision visit to plan appropriate interventions for school-age children, adolescents, and their families.

Clinical Reasoning in Action

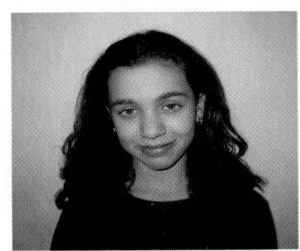

Tammy is a 13-year-old coming into the office for her yearly checkup and she has never been in the hospital or had surgery. She is a good student and is excited to start seventh grade next year. She has not had any immunizations since going into kindergarten. Tammy arrives with her mother, with whom she lives; she has no contact with her biologic father. Her mother decides to stay in the waiting room, but did note on the written history form that there is a family history of high cholesterol and heart disease in family members under 50 years old. Tammy's mother is a single parent working full time with two other children at home. Tammy's body mass index is in the 85th percentile and she passed her hearing and vision tests. Her blood pressure is 115/70 and her urinalysis shows blood, but Tammy has her menses today. Tammy has a period every month and menarche started at 10 years old. Her menses lasts 5 to 7 days and she denies experiencing cramping or excessively heavy menses. Tammy enjoys being a member of the volleyball team and is involved in a church youth group. She does not get to spend much time with her friends because she watches her two younger siblings in the afternoons while her mother is at work. When her mother is away, she admits to sitting and playing video games or watching TV most of the day. Tammy says she has had a boyfriend, but denies sexual activity. She also denies any experimentation with substance use.

1. What vaccines is Tammy due for at this age if she has not already had them?
2. A dietary assessment demonstrates that Tammy frequently skips meals and eats fast food almost daily. What are some of the suggestions you can give Tammy to improve her nutritional status?
3. What are some of the injury prevention topics you can discuss with Tammy?
4. Based on the additional information you collected about Tammy, what are some of the areas of recommended health teaching?
5. Develop a concept map for Tammy that includes all of the health promotion areas important to all youth, such as nutrition, oral health, physical activity, social interactions, family relationships, and disease/injury prevention. How can her development be enhanced to draw on strengths and improve areas of need? What part does the healthcare provider play in promoting her health?

References

American Academy of Pediatric Dentistry (AAPD). (2012). *Policy on third-party reimbursement of fees related to dental sealants.* Retrieved from http://www.aapd.org /media/Policies_Guidelines/P_3rdPartSealants .pdf#xml=http://pr-dtsearch001.americaneagle .com/service/search.asp?cmd=pdfhits&DocId= 330&Index=F%3a%5cdtSearch%5caapd%2eo rg&HitCount=16&hits=18+46+57+11f+149+ 155+162+18e+1b6+1d2+207+228+246+269+ 2a8+2ca+&hc=314&req=sealants

American Academy of Pediatrics (AAP). (2011a). *Discipline.* Retrieved from http://www.healthychildren.org

American Academy of Pediatrics (AAP). (2011b). *Car safety seats.* Retrieved from http://www .healthychildren.org

American Academy of Pediatrics (AAP). (2014). *Car seats: Information for families for 2014.* Retrieved from http://www.healthychildren.org/English/safety -prevention/on-the-go/Pages/Car-Safety-Seats -Information-for-Families.aspx

American Academy of Pediatrics Committee on Practice and Ambulatory Medicine, Bright Futures Periodicity Schedule Workgroup. (2014). 2014 Recommendations for pediatric preventive health care. *Pediatrics, 133,* 568–570.

Bandura, A. (1986). *Social foundations of thought and actions: A social cognitive theory.* Englewood Cliffs, NJ: Prentice Hall.

Bandura, A. (1997a). *Self-efficacy in changing societies.* New York, NY: Cambridge University.

Bandura, A. (1997b). *Self-efficacy: The exercise of control.* New York, NY: Freeman.

Ben-Arye, E., Traube, Z., Schachter, L., Jaimi, M., Levy, M., Schiff, E., & Lev, E. (2011). Integrative pediatric care: Parents/attitudes toward communication of physicians and CAM practitioners. *Pediatrics, 127*(1), 384–395.

Centers for Disease Control and Prevention (CDC). (2011a). *How much physical activity do children need?* Retrieved from http://www.cdc.gov /physicalactivity/everyone/guidelines/children/html

Centers for Disease Control and Prevention (CDC). (2011b). *Policy impact: Teen driver safety.* Retrieved from http://www.cdc.gov/Motorvehiclesafety /teenbrief/

Centers for Disease Control and Prevention (CDC). (2011c). *Agricultural safety.* Retrieved from http://www.cdc.gov/niosh/topics/aginjury

Centers for Disease Control and Prevention (CDC). (2013). *Bicycle-related injuries.* Retrieved from http://www .cdc.gov/HomeandRecreationalSafety/Bicycle/

Centers for Disease Control and Prevention (CDC). (2014). Youth risk behavior surveillance—United States, 2013. *Morbidity and Mortality Weekly Report, 63*(SS04), 1–172.

Child Trends. (2013). *Health care services.* Retrieved from http://www.childtrends.org/wp-content /uploads/2013/10/2013-10HealthCareServices.pdf

Connor, J. P., George, S. M., Gullo, M. J., Kelly, A. B., & Young, R. M. (2011). A prospective study of alcohol expectancies and self-efficacy as predictors of young adolescent alcohol misuse. *Alcohol and Alcoholism, 46*(2), 161–169.

Davies, M. A., Terhorst, L., Nakonechny, A. J., Skukla, N., & ElSaadawi, G. (2014). The development and effectiveness of a health information website designed to improve parents' self-efficacy in managing risk for obesity in preschoolers. *Journal for Specialists in Pediatric Nursing.* doi: 10.1111/jsph.12086

Devoe, J. E., Tillotson, C. J., Wallace, L. S., Lesko, S. E., & Pandhi, H. (2012). Is health insurance enough? A usual source of care may be more important to ensure a child receives preventive health counseling. *Maternal and Child Health Journal, 16,* 306–315.

Hagan, J. F., Shaw, J. S., & Duncan, P. M. (Eds.). (2008). *Bright futures: Guidelines for health supervision of infants, children, and adolescents* (3rd ed.). Elk Grove Village, IL: American Academy of Pediatrics.

KidsHealth. (2011). *Developing your child's self-esteem.* Retrieved from http://kidshealth.org/parent/emotions /feelings/self_esteem.html

Kuo, D. Z., Houtrow, A. J., Arango, P., Kuhlthau, K. A., Simmons, J. M., & Neff, J. M. (2011). Family-centered care: Current applications and future directions in pediatric health care. *Maternal Child Health Journal, 16*(2), 297–305.

Mayo Clinic. (2013). *Teen sleep: Why is your teen so tired?* Retrieved from http://www.mayoclinic.org /healthy-living/tween-and-teen-health/in-depth /teens-health/art-20046157

National Highway Traffic Safety Administration. (2012). *Car seats and booster basics.* Retrieved from http: //www.safercar.gov/parents/RightSeat.htm

Pender, N. J., Murdaugh, C. L., & Parsons, M. A. (2015). *Health promotion in nursing practice* (7th ed.). Upper Saddle River, NJ: Pearson Prentice Hall.

Santrock, J. W. (2012). *Child development* (12th ed.). Boston, MA: McGraw-Hill.

Tanski, S., Garfunkel, L. C., Duncan, P. M., & Weitzman, M. (2011). *Performing preventive services.* Elk Grove Village, IL: American Academy of Pediatrics.

Thai, K. T., McIntosh, A. S., & Pang, T. Y. (2014). Bicycle helmet size, adjustment and stability. *Traffic Injury Prevention,* June 20.

U.S. Department of Health and Human Services. (2011). *Strengthening families and communities.* Washington, DC: Author.

World Health Organization (WHO). (2014). *Adolescent responsive health systems.* Retrieved from http://www.who.int/maternal_child_adolescent /topics/adolescence/health_services/en/

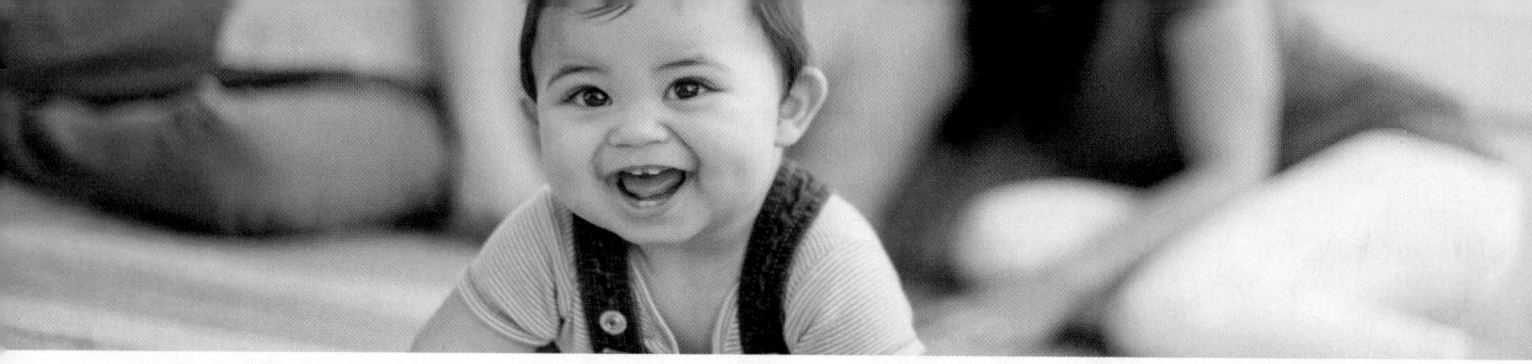

Chapter 37
Family Assessment and Concepts of Nursing Care in the Community

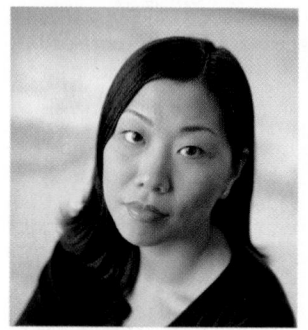

Sometimes Jessica's asthma attacks really frighten me because she struggles so hard to breathe. She has a lot of trouble with asthma in the summertime with all the heat. I'm afraid to let her play outside with her friends for fear that she will have another attack. I'd really like to know how to keep Jessica's asthma under control.

—Mother of Jessica, 8 years old

Ryan McVay/Getty Images

∨ Learning Outcomes

37.1 Contrast the categories of family strengths that help families cope with stressors.

37.2 Summarize the advantages of using a family assessment tool.

37.3 Assemble a list of family support services that might be available in a community.

37.4 Discuss the community healthcare settings where nurses provide health services to children.

37.5 Compare the roles of the nurse in each identified community healthcare setting.

37.6 Summarize the special developmental needs of children to consider in disaster preparedness planning.

Children receive most of their health care in community settings. Depending on the community, healthcare resources, and age of the child, nurses have an important role related to the care provided in each of these settings. When providing health care to the child and family, it is important for the nurse to assess the family's strengths, be aware of community resources, help families manage the complex health care that is often provided in the home, and prepare for emergencies and disasters.

Family Assessment

A **family** is defined as two or more individuals who are joined together by marriage, birth, or adoption and live together in the same household (U.S. Census Bureau, 2013). A family may also be a self-identified group of two or more persons joined together through the sharing of resources and emotional closeness. Families are guided by a common set of values or beliefs about the worth and importance of certain ideas and traditions. Each family and its members are unique in their strengths and their responses to complex and often conflicting demands for time and attention.

Children and families live within a variety of home environments, and interactions within those settings directly or indirectly influence behaviors and learning. Because of these environmental influences on the family, it is important to consider the relationship of the family with the social networks within the community.

Nurses must be able to assess family strengths and support mechanisms, to identify strategies for **coping** (the use of learned behavioral and cognitive strategies to manage or relieve perceived stress), and to determine when families have overextended their resources and need additional support. In some cases, nurses can provide the additional support needed, and at other times, referral to other healthcare professionals and community resources is appropriate to address the family's needs.

Family Stressors

Family stress theory focuses on the family's ability to cope and adjust to stressful events, such as having a child with a significant health condition (Ramisch, 2012). Most families know their resources and have developed coping strategies to deal with daily routine stressors (e.g., completion of household chores, homework). Family stressors may pile up from many sources, such as work demands, school issues, extended family demands, the desire to achieve quality family time, and community roles. Additional stressors may include inadequate finances, healthcare concerns, and relationship challenges.

Nonroutine stressors (such as surgery or the birth of a child) and unexpected events (a child's sudden illness or injury) are often more stressful because the family has not had time to review resources and prepare a response. A child's illness or injury affects every member of the family. Family members respond to this stress, sometimes in a way that changes interactions among family members and with the environment. The nurse should identify how families respond to the stress of a child's illness or injury so that nursing interventions include support that may reduce the impact on the entire family.

Family Strengths

Family strengths are the relationships, processes, and resources that families can use during times of adversity and change to manage stressors. Nurses can support families by helping them to identify and use these strengths to manage the stressors associated with family challenges or crises. Strengths that enable families to develop and adapt to stressors include (Lester et al., 2013):

- Resources such as education, prior experiences, and finances
- Effective communication and collaborative problem solving
- Being emotionally aware and working to maintain emotional stability
- Developing shared meaning about the experience

The nurse should identify a **family's resilience**—the family's capacity to develop strengths and abilities, to "bounce back" from stress and challenges. Resilience is often a dynamic interaction between protective processes (strengths and capacities) and vulnerabilities, such as life event stressors, health status, or environmental risks (Herrman et al., 2011). When a family can gain some control and deal with events satisfactorily, its members acquire a sense of competence, making them more resilient, in contrast to families who are overwhelmed by traumatic experiences. Resilience of children is discussed in Chapter 42.

Most families have the capacity to develop resilience. Nursing support may be needed to help family members learn new skills, make adaptations, and gain confidence in their abilities to manage the challenges of the child's health condition. Potential resources to foster resilience include the faith community, finances, social support, physical health, family flexibility, and family coping mechanisms. Families with fewer resources will be more susceptible to disruption when a healthcare crisis or event occurs.

Functional families use their strengths and a variety of coping strategies to successfully reduce stress. Coping strategies of dysfunctional families are defensive (e.g., denial of family problems, exploiting a family member, use of threats or withdrawal of affection and support, dominance and submissive patterns, and family substance abuse).

After developing a rapport and relationship with the family, the nurse can help families identify their strengths and areas for improvement that can lead to increased resiliency. Focus on family competence, and acknowledge and validate family members' emotions. Help families to recognize that strengths and strategies used in prior life experiences may transfer to the current healthcare experience. Once family members recognize the strengths they bring to the management of their child's healthcare problem, the family is more likely to become an effective partner in the process.

Clinical Tip

Family strengths helpful in managing stressors include the following:

- *Communication skills*—the ability of family members to listen, gather information, and to discuss their concerns in an honest and open manner
- *Shared family values and beliefs*—the family's common perceptions of reality and willingness to have hope and to appreciate that change is possible; family celebrations; family traditions
- *Intrafamily support*—the support and reinforcement provided by extended family members to promote family cohesion and a sense of belonging; family time and routines
- *Self-care abilities*—the family's ability to take responsibility for health problems and the demonstrated willingness of individual members to care for themselves
- *Problem-solving skills*—the family's use of collaboration and negotiation for problem solving, using daily and prior life experiences as resources, and focusing on the present rather than past events or disappointments; effective utilization of healthcare resources
- *Community linkages*—maintenance of active linkages with the community; reaching out to others in the social network including extended family and friends

Collecting Data for Family Assessment

Establish a trusting relationship with the child and family to obtain an accurate and concise family assessment. Identify the primary concerns of the parent(s) and child, noting that they may be different. Acknowledge these multiple concerns and demonstrate respect for the diversity of the family. The goal is to obtain family information to plan nursing interventions that help the family care for the child and improve the child's outcomes while valuing each family member.

Information about the family is collected continuously during the healthcare process, through interviews, observations of family interactions, reports from other healthcare providers or agencies working with the family, and with a family assessment tool.

Additional data for the family assessment include the psychosocial history and daily living patterns (see Chapter 33). Observation of the home and family members is recommended in some cases to obtain valuable information about family functioning.

Family Assessment Tools

Family assessment tools help in gathering information about the family's functioning. Some tools specifically focus on family strengths, coping strategies, and family stresses. Learning about how the family nurtures its members, solves problems, and communicates may help identify strategies that can be effective for managing the child's health care. The nurse may learn how to work more effectively with the family, such as by collaborating with the family in planning for health maintenance and health promotion strategies.

GENOGRAM

Information about family structure can be illustrated on a **genogram** (a pedigree that displays information about a family's health history over at least three generations). (See Chapter 3 for examples of pedigrees.) Additional identifying features such as social class, occupation, place of residence, faith, and ethnicity may be added for the family assessment process.

Clinical Tip

Family assessment data that may be helpful:

- Name, age, gender, and family relationship of all people residing in the household
- Family type, structure, roles, and values
- Cultural associations, including cultural norms and customs related to childrearing and infant feeding
- Faith-based group participation
- Support systems network, including extended family, friends, work associates, faith-based affiliations, and community associations
- Communication patterns, including language barriers
- Environmental data—place of residence, housing condition, number of persons living in the residence, sleeping arrangements, play areas, transportation, neighborhood characteristics

---

FAMILY ECOMAP

An **ecomap** is an illustration of a family's relationships and social networks that may be prepared by nurses in partnership with family members. The nurse may learn information about how the family perceives or receives social support, and the strength of family relationships with significant other persons and organizations. Community resources being used by the family and other potential community resources that may help promote the family's health may be identified. Figure 37–1 shows a sample ecomap.

CALGARY FAMILY ASSESSMENT MODEL

This tool, developed by Lorraine Wright and Maureen Leahey (2013), uses three categories of information (structural, developmental, and functional family data) to assess a family's strengths and problems. The complete model is available in their textbook *Nurses and Families: A Guide to Family Assessment and Intervention*. The model enables collection of extensive family information, and it can facilitate assessment of family challenges, such as problems integrating a treatment plan in family routines. A family genogram or ecomap may also be helpful in completing the assessment.

HOME OBSERVATION FOR MEASUREMENT OF THE ENVIRONMENT (HOME)

The HOME Inventory is an assessment tool developed to measure the quality and quantity of stimulation and support available to a child in the home environment (Caldwell & Bradley, 1984). The tool is used to identify relationships between the home environment, child care, and a child's development (Hackman et al., 2013; Sarsour et al., 2011).

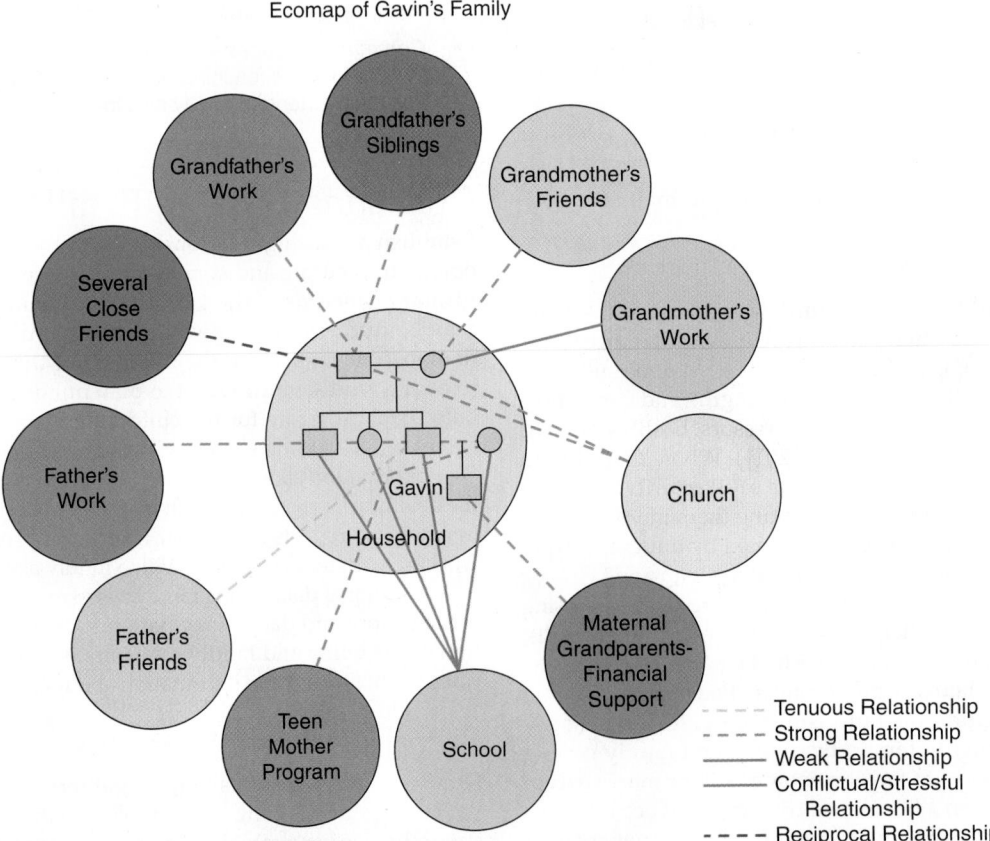

Ecomap of Gavin's Family

Tenuous Relationship
Strong Relationship
Weak Relationship
Conflictual/Stressful Relationship
Reciprocal Relationship

Figure 37–1   An ecomap illustrates the family's relationships and interactions with groups and individuals in the immediate external environment.

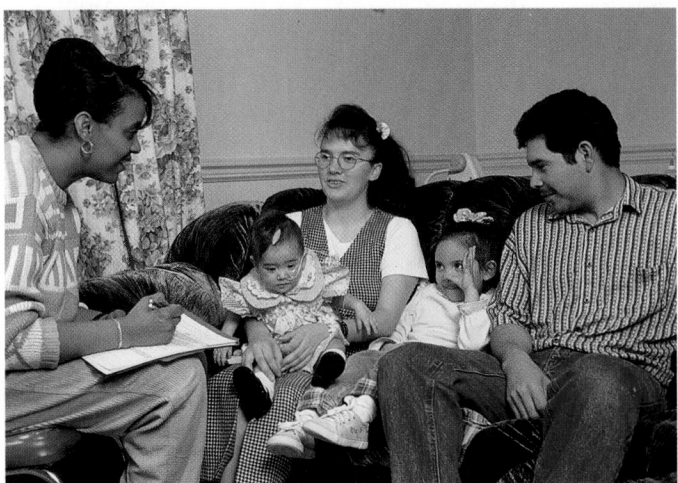

Figure 37-2 **A visit to the home when all family members are present provides the best information for completion of an assessment tool such as the Home Observation for Measurement of the Environment (HOME).**

Four age-specific scales are available (birth to 3 years, 3 to 6 years, 6 to 10 years, and 10 to 15 years). Examples of subscales contained in each age-specific HOME Inventory include parental responsivity, acceptance of child, the physical environment, learning materials, variety in experience, and parental involvement. Data are collected during an informal, low-stress interview and observation over 45 to 90 minutes in the home setting (Figure 37-2). The child's primary caregiver and the child must be present and awake so their interaction can be observed. Family members are encouraged to act normally. Assessment of the home environment may help to identify nursing interventions that promote the child's growth and development, such as items in the home that can be used for toys and strategies for parent interaction with the child to promote learning.

Family Support Services in the Community

Family support services exist in all communities to help families with the rearing of healthy children and managing family stressors. Community programs often exist to support the health and development of children, parental competencies, and positive family relationships. Most programs are designed with the premise that no family is entirely self-sufficient and most can benefit from some external support. Examples of these family support services include the following:

- Head Start and Early Head Start
- Before- and after-school programs for children of working parents
- School-based health and counseling services
- Play groups for preschool children
- Peer support groups
- Social service programs offered by the faith community
- Home visiting programs for high-risk children and parents
- Job skills training, adult education, and literacy programs
- Crisis care and respite care programs
- Funding for military family support programs

Compile a list of the formal and informal family support services in your community. Nurses play an important role in linking families to the types of community support services they need after performing a family assessment and collaborating with families to identify and seek assistance most beneficial to their needs.

Community-Based Health Care

Health plans and healthcare providers continue to explore options to provide safe, high-quality care in the community with fewer hospitalizations or shorter stays when hospitalization is needed. Patterns of healthcare delivery have changed due to technologic developments and efforts to reduce healthcare costs. For example:

- Surgery and invasive diagnostic procedures are performed in ambulatory settings.
- Short-stay or observation units in hospital settings reduce the number of hospital admissions.
- Long-term intravenous antibiotic therapy can be provided in the home.
- Pediatric hospice and palliative care services occur in the home setting.

The trend in out-of-hospital care continues to increase for children with chronic health conditions and advanced disease states. Families are often willing to care for their child who is **medically fragile** (having significant health conditions that require skilled nursing, with or without medical equipment, to support vital functions) in the home because of their desire to have the child integrated into the family and community (Miles, Holditch-Davis, Burchinal, et al., 2011). Technologic advances, such as portable medical equipment, enable families to provide complex healthcare services in the home and other community settings, and such care in the community is less costly. Home care services and other support services have been developed to support these families.

Pediatric health care in the community occurs along a continuum that covers the entire child healthcare system. This continuum is reflected in the Bindler-Ball Continuum of Pediatric Health, including health promotion and health maintenance services, care for chronic conditions, acute illnesses and injuries, and end-of-life care (see Chapter 1 for this model). Health care for individual children is improved when there is continuity of care and communication between healthcare settings.

The nurse working with families in a community setting uses knowledge of how the larger environment influences the child's health and development and the family's functioning, and integrates that information into the nursing care plan. To work effectively in the community, the nurse needs to gain experience and skills in:

- Conducting a child and family assessment and collaborating with the family to plan, implement, and evaluate healthcare strategies that fit the family's economic, cultural, and social situation
- Working with community agencies (schools, faith-based groups, military-based groups, and other community-based resources) to assess, plan strategies, and implement and evaluate approaches addressed to the healthcare needs of the community's children

Community Healthcare Settings

Children receive most of their health care (health promotion and episodic health care for acute illnesses and injuries) in community settings. Depending on the community, healthcare resources, and age of the child, care may be received in all or only a few of the following settings:

- A healthcare center or a physician's office is the usual site for health promotion, health maintenance, episodic acute care, and health management of children with chronic conditions.

- A public health clinic may provide health promotion and health maintenance services as well as treatment for specific health conditions. A homeless shelter may also have the capacity to offer such services.

- A hospital outpatient center may provide specialized services to children with chronic conditions or the full range of services offered in a healthcare center.

- Schools usually provide health promotion and health maintenance services, plus first aid and emergency care as needed. School-based healthcare centers exist in some schools to provide health care, counseling, health education, and care for acute conditions. Some school settings also offer preschool and after-school childcare services.

- Childcare centers provide first aid for emergencies and some health promotion services.

- The home is where the family provides care for minor illnesses and injuries and for chronic and complex health conditions, including end-of-life care when the child's family is supported by home health services.

A nurse may serve as a community health nurse, home health nurse, school nurse, pediatric nurse in an office setting, and nurse practitioner or advanced practice nurse in these settings. The nurse in any of the above settings has an important role in promoting the health and safety of the child, being a leader in setting policies in the healthcare center, and using the nursing process to help families meet the healthcare needs of their children. The nurse may assume the role of direct care provider, educator, advocate, or planner.

Nursing Roles in the Office or Healthcare Center Setting

The nursing process is used when providing care for children in the healthcare center. The range of assessment responsibilities may vary by setting as well as the nurse's preparation and experience (Figure 37–3). Specific functions of the pediatric nurse in this setting include the following:

- Identifying children in need of urgent care or isolation

- Performing nursing assessments, including the health history, vital signs, growth and development, nutritional status, immunization status, family strengths and challenges

- Conducting physical examinations

- Performing age-appropriate screening tests to detect health problems such as vision or hearing loss, anemia, and lead poisoning to ensure that the child has access to all needed health services

- Assisting with health examinations, diagnostic tests, and procedures

- Developing nursing diagnoses and implementing a plan of care

- Providing immunizations

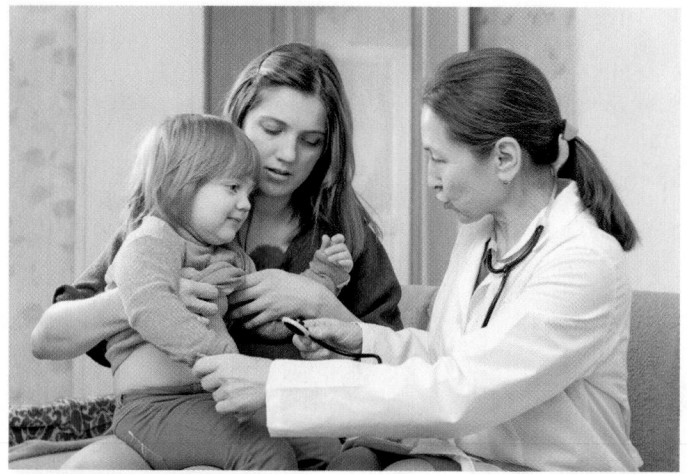

Figure 37–3 Nurses carefully assess children in the office setting who present with an acute care illness to identify how serious the child's illness is. Monitor the child for symptom changes during the visit. Gather information about the child's illness, and identify the education needed for the family to care for the child at home.

SOURCE: Iakov Filimonov/Shutterstock.

- Providing information about procedures and offering reassurance

- Providing family and client education for health promotion or management of the health condition

- Linking families with community resources

- Ensuring a safe healthcare setting and adherence to infection control guidelines (See the *Clinical Skills Manual* SKILLS for infection control methods.)

- Participating in the healthcare center's performance improvement program to identify ways to enhance services provided to children and their families

An important goal is to develop a positive relationship with the child and family so that optimal health care is provided. This relationship is strengthened during future healthcare visits.

IDENTIFYING SEVERELY ILL AND INJURED CHILDREN

Each child with an episodic illness or injury presenting to the healthcare center must be assessed on arrival to determine the urgency of care needed. Quickly assess for changes in mental status, airway patency, labored breathing, or poor circulation to identify a child who needs immediate medical attention. The child with an urgent condition must be monitored frequently to detect any worsening of condition and need for emergency care.

Clinical Tip

Developing a relationship with the child and family in a community setting is equally as important as it is in the hospital. The initial interaction often sets the stage for a long-term relationship with the family that returns to the same setting for health care over many years. Remember to put aside the stressors you may be feeling before you approach the child and family. Take a few moments to play with the infant or child and to comment on a positive attribute of the child to the parents. This should help reduce the parents', and perhaps the child's, stress level, which helps set the stage for a long-term partnership with the child and family.

EMERGENCY RESPONSE PLANNING

The nurse collaborates with all health professionals and the office manager to develop an emergency response plan for the healthcare center. The nurse teaches office staff to recognize a child needing immediate assessment by the nurse. The nurse is often responsible for ensuring that all emergency care equipment, supplies, and medications are organized and readily available in a central treatment room. The nurse may also coordinate mock drills so that all health professionals and support staff know and perform their designated role when a true emergency occurs.

SAFETY ALERT!

Required emergency equipment for managing a pediatric emergency in a healthcare center includes the following in various pediatric sizes (Wright & Krug, 2016):

- Oxygen delivery system (bag-valve masks in 450- and 1000-mL sizes, clear oxygen face masks with and without reservoir)
- Airway equipment (oral and nasopharyngeal airways, Magill forceps, suction devices, laryngoscope handle and blades, endotracheal tubes and stylet, end-tidal CO_2 detector, nasogastric tubes)
- Pulse oximeter, automated external defibrillator with pediatric capabilities
- Intravenous (IV) and intraosseous needles, IV tubing and microdrip, and 500-mL bags of normal saline, lactated Ringer, and 5% dextrose 0.45 normal saline IV solution
- A length-based resuscitation tape and preprinted drug dosage chart to quickly identify equipment sizes and drug dosages by the length or weight of the child
- Essential drugs, including oxygen, epinephrine 1:1000, and albuterol for inhalation; suggested drugs, including activated charcoal, naloxone, 25% dextrose, diphenhydramine, antibiotics, oral and parenteral corticosteroids, atropine, and sodium bicarbonate

Locate the emergency equipment in every clinical setting where you have assignments so that you can quickly take the child to it or bring the equipment to the child if an emergency occurs.

EDUCATING THE CHILD AND FAMILY

Family and client education regarding injury prevention, growth and development, nutrition, healthy lifestyles, and the home care of episodic illnesses and injuries are important nursing roles. The nurse may be responsible for selecting client education materials for the waiting area and those specifically used to teach families about various conditions. Knowledge of the community and population served by the healthcare center enables the nurse to select appropriate education materials for the culture and literacy level served.

Nurses teach families to provide the condition-specific care for the child at home. Examples of information provided include:

- Signs that the condition is not improving as expected and when to return to the healthcare provider
- How and when to administer prescribed medications and their potential side effects
- Recommended diet and activity
- Other supportive care for the child's condition
- Education to help the child and family recognize when to initiate care for a new episode of a chronic condition (e.g., asthma and sickle cell disease) to avoid a healthcare visit or reduce the episode severity

IDENTIFYING COMMUNITY RESOURCES

Nurses are often involved in identifying community resources needed by the child and family to help promote the child's health. Compiling a manual of community resources and regularly updating names, phone numbers, and websites of contacts will make it easier to provide information efficiently. Examples of community resources that might be included are early intervention programs, support groups, translation services, food banks, lead paint abatement services, social services, and mental health services.

ENSURING A SAFE ENVIRONMENT FOR CHILDREN

The healthcare center has many potential hazards such as equipment, cleaning supplies, sharps, medications, and laboratory chemicals and supplies from which the child needs to be protected. The child must be attended at all times when in the examination area. Develop and implement infection control guidelines to reduce the transmission of infectious diseases among child patients and among the healthcare providers and children.

Nursing Roles in the Specialty Healthcare Setting

Pediatric nurses also provide care for children with acute and chronic conditions within hospital outpatient or specialty care ambulatory settings. Children may be referred to physician specialists for diagnostic workups or for the long-term management of their chronic conditions. In some cases, health promotion, health maintenance, and episodic illness care are provided to children with chronic conditions in these settings. With experience, pediatric nurses working in a hospital ambulatory setting develop specialized knowledge and skill to meet the specific needs of the children cared for in that setting. The roles for nurses in these settings are similar to those described for the healthcare center.

Nursing Roles in the School Setting

School nursing is a specialized practice of professional nursing in the education setting that advances the well-being, academic success, and lifelong achievement of students. School nurses care for children and youth with a wide range of physical and mental health challenges. They advocate for the children as policies are developed for the school community, such as nutritious school breakfasts and lunches or recess and physical education classes for all students. Because of their role in the education system, they are able to educate teachers and administrators about how health conditions affect student functioning and ways to integrate children with special healthcare needs into the school setting (Taras, 2014).

Healthy People 2020

> (EMC-4) Increase the proportion of elementary, middle, and senior high schools that require school health education
>
> (NWS-2) Increase the percentage of schools with a school breakfast program and offer nutritious foods and beverages outside of school meals

---

In 2013, 61.7 million children and adolescents attended public and private elementary and secondary schools in the United States. An estimated 12.9% of the enrolled children had a known medical condition or disability for which they received Individuals with Disabilities Education Act services (U.S. Department of Education, National Center for Education Statistics, 2014). Approximately 11% to 13% of children and adolescents require daily medication administered at school for at least 3 months for conditions such as asthma, diabetes, and seizures. Additional children need medications for a shorter interval for an acute health problem (Center for Health and Healthcare in Schools, 2013). Children who have complex health conditions (e.g., dependent on medical technology, such as peritoneal dialysis, tracheostomies, and ventilators) need school nurses to develop and coordinate the plan for their care during school. These include children who are medically fragile. (See Chapter 38 for a discussion of children with chronic conditions and planning for their care in the school setting.)

The breadth of school health issues addressed by school nurses is illustrated in national health objectives published in *Healthy People 2020*. Additional examples of objectives addressing children and youth in the school setting include (U.S. Department of Health and Human Services, 2015):

- (ECBP-2) Increase the proportion of elementary, middle, and senior high schools that provide comprehensive school health education to prevent health problems in the following areas: unintentional injury, violence, suicide, tobacco use and addiction, alcohol or other drug use, unintended pregnancy, HIV/AIDS and sexually transmitted infections, unhealthy dietary patterns, and inadequate physical activity
- (PA-4) Increase the proportion of the nation's public and private schools that require daily physical education for all students
- (IVP-27) Increase the proportion of public and private schools that require students to wear appropriate protective gear when engaged in school-sponsored physical activities
- (DH-14) Increase the proportion of children and youth with disabilities who spend at least 80% of their time in regular education programs
- (ECBP-5) Increase the proportion of elementary, middle, and senior high schools that have a full-time registered school nurse-to-student ratio of at least 1:750

The school nurse plans, develops, manages, and evaluates healthcare services to all children in the educational setting. Other roles of the nurse in the school setting include the following: maintaining infection control, participating on teams to develop student individualized education plans (IEPs) and individualized health plans (IHPs), updating health records, collecting data on services provided to students, consulting with health teachers about educational topics, investigating environmental safety hazards, developing an emergency preparedness plan, and planning for crisis intervention and support services. The traditional tasks of screening, first aid, and monitoring immunization status are still performed (Figure 37–4). In many cases, the nurse works with families of the students to ensure that needed care is provided. See Chapter 38 for more information on IEPs and IHPs.

Collaboration with the other health professionals in the community is also important to promote health in the school setting, as the following examples illustrate:

- Partnering with the school physician consultant to discuss and update standing orders for the care of children. These standing orders usually address urgent and emergency care potentially needed by students and the variety of student healthcare problems that may occur.

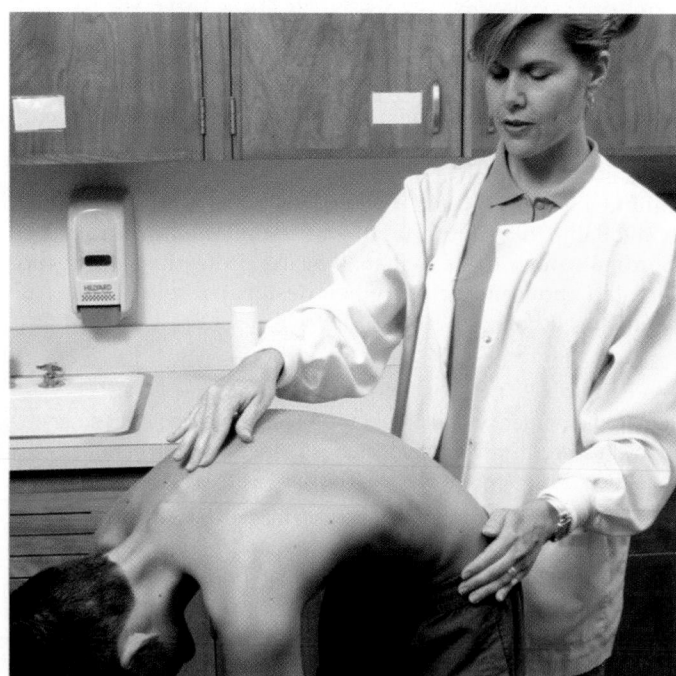

Figure 37–4 The school is often the setting for screening tests of large groups of students to identify those who may have a health problem that could interfere with learning. Screening tests are often organized so all children in a particular grade are assessed, such as scoliosis screening for children in fifth grade.

- Working with the parent–teacher association and other community organizations to organize health fairs and injury prevention programs for students.
- Communicating with the child's primary healthcare provider or pediatric specialist about a child's specific health condition that needs to be effectively managed in the school setting. Obtain the parent's permission to request confidential client information. The school nurse has regular opportunities to monitor the child's health status and to provide information that may help the primary healthcare providers with the child's ongoing management.

In some communities, school-based healthcare centers provide comprehensive physical, dental, reproductive, and mental health services plus health education to students. They provide service coordination and collaboration to address the health needs of youth with health problems or poor access to healthcare services, especially those not readily available in the community (American Academy of Pediatrics [AAP], 2012). A multidisciplinary team of nurse practitioners, physicians, physician assistants, mental health providers, and other supporting staff often provides care.

PREPARATION FOR EMERGENCIES

Because children spend so much of their day in school, this setting is a common location of injury and acute illnesses. The school nurse often works with school administrators, the physician consultant, and the local emergency medical services (EMS) agency to develop a response plan for true emergencies. School personnel (administrators, secretaries, and health aides) also need training to identify an emergency that requires activation of the local EMS system and to provide emergency care until the EMS providers arrive.

Other potential emergencies can occur during school hours, such as natural and man-made disasters, and behavioral crises (e.g., school shootings). Nurses may participate in planning committees to develop an **emergency preparedness plan**, a community-based coordinated response plan for the incident (see information later in the chapter). Children experiencing a traumatic event may need psychologic support (see Chapter 42).

Clinical Reasoning   Acute Asthma Episode at School

Jessica, 8 years old, is anxious because she is having more trouble breathing than usual. Her teacher notices her breathing difficulty and sends Jessica to the school nurse for treatment. Jessica has a rescue inhaler at school, and this treatment often relieves her symptoms and allows her to return to classes. In this case, Jessica's acute asthma episode does not respond to the treatment, so the school contacts her mother. Because it will take Jessica's mother at least 45 minutes to reach the school, the school nurse and mother decide that 9-1-1 should be called to get Jessica to the emergency department more quickly.

What special arrangements are needed to permit a child to receive care for asthma or another chronic condition while at school? See Chapter 46 and *Evidence-Based Practice: Improving Asthma Management at School* for more information about asthma management.

FACILITATING A CHILD'S RETURN TO SCHOOL

The school nurse also helps the child return to the classroom following an acute illness or injury. Examples include making environmental adaptations, creating an IHP when a new health condition is diagnosed, or revising the IHP when a significant change in the status of the child's chronic condition has occurred (see Chapter 38). The child's parents or the pediatric nurse in the hospital or community setting may initiate the request to coordinate the child's return to school. Educational materials about the child's condition can be recommended to educate students, faculty, and staff. The school nurse then begins to work with the family to prepare teachers and school administrators for the child's special needs, such as limited mobility or medications. The child's teacher and classmates can be prepared for the child's physical changes if appropriate. Sometimes the teacher's expectations of the child need to be modified, such as a child with a mild brain injury who may have decreased ability to concentrate for several weeks during recovery.

Nursing Roles in the Childcare Setting

An estimated 12.5 million children under 5 years of age receive care in out-of-home childcare settings while parents are at work (U.S. Census Bureau, 2011). Many types of childcare arrangements exist, such as in-home care by a family member or nanny, a babysitter cooperative, a licensed childcare family home setting for up to five children, or a licensed childcare center for six or more children.

EVIDENCE-BASED PRACTICE | Improving Asthma Management at School

Clinical Question

Because of the potential for frequent absences and the need to manage their condition at school, what are some strategies for helping children with asthma to improve their school performance?

The Evidence

A study recruited 530 children with persistent asthma, ages 3 to 10 years, from 67 schools for a randomized controlled trial with school daily-observed therapy compared to parent-administered therapy. Families of all children received a diary to track the child's symptoms, which were retrieved by a monthly telephone interview. Children in the school treatment group had more symptom-free days, significantly fewer nights with symptoms, fewer days with activity limitations, and fewer school absences than the children in the control group. Children in the school treatment group were also less likely to have an asthma episode requiring oral prednisone treatment (Halterman et al., 2011).

A subsequent study recruited 100 children with persistent asthma, ages 3 to 10 years, from 19 schools to participate in a pilot study to compare a web-based screening process and school daily-administered therapy to parent-administered therapy. Parents were expected to administer therapy on nonschool days for children in the intervention group. The web-based screening tool integrated national guidelines for assessment of asthma severity, selected prescribed medications for severity level, and sent information to the child's primary care provider. At the end of the school year, children in the school treatment group had fewer school absences related to asthma, fewer nighttime symptoms, and fewer days needing rescue medications compared to the comparison group. Primary care providers and school nurses reported support

for the school-observed therapy program after learning study outcomes (Halterman et al., 2012).

A questionnaire was used to investigate the knowledge of 38 elementary school teachers from two schools about the care of children with asthma. More than 50% of teachers missed questions about characteristics of children with severe asthma, signs that asthma is under good control, signs of a life-threatening asthma episode, proper technique for medication administration, and the common symptoms after rescue inhaler medication (Lucas, Anderson, & Hill, 2012).

Best Practice

Children with persistent asthma are often unable to perform their best in school. Teachers also need increased awareness of asthma symptoms to help identify children who need rescue medications during the school day. School health programs can offer effective strategies to help manage asthma, such as identifying children needing daily asthma medications, offering supervised medication administration, and educating children to manage their asthma. Prior research revealed a relationship between how well the children self-manage their asthma and the children's asthma symptoms and morbidity (Kaul, 2011).

Clinical Reasoning

During a school clinical experience, identify the number of children with asthma and how many children report to the school nurse with asthma episodes in a month. What strategies has the school nurse used to work with children who have persistent asthma (e.g., educating students about self-management, providing medication at school, or seeking an asthma action plan)? Have those strategies helped to reduce the number of asthma episodes?

States establish minimum licensure requirements and guidelines for the safe operation of childcare settings that address the staff qualifications, staff-to-child ratio, staff training requirements, safe food handling, safe health practices, and environmental safety. Guidelines for the safe operation of childcare centers are available through the National Resource Center for Health and Safety in Child Care.

Healthy People 2020

(NWS-1) Increase the number of States with nutrition standards for foods and beverages provided to preschool-aged children in child care

(PA-9) Increase the number of States with licensing regulations for physical activity provided in child care

---

Nurses can assume an important consultant role in the establishment of a childcare center's policies for healthcare practices, teaching staff about safe healthcare practices, and monitoring and promoting healthcare practices in the setting. The nurse consultant can also teach staff to identify children with illnesses and to provide first aid for injured children. Nurses may provide health screening and direct care in childcare centers that care for ill children.

REDUCING DISEASE TRANSMISSION

Children attending childcare centers are at increased risk for infectious diseases. Children are close together in large numbers, put things in their mouths, may be contagious before symptoms occur, and are susceptible to most infectious agents. The nurse can educate and work with the childcare center manager and staff to reduce disease transmission in the following ways (American Academy of Pediatrics, American Public Health Association, & National Resource Center for Health and Safety in Child Care, 2013):

- Teach staff when and how to perform hand hygiene, manage a child's secretions, sanitize toys and surfaces, and treat a child's cuts and scrapes.

- Develop guidelines for diapering infants and toddlers to reduce disease transmission.

- Check each child's health daily for signs of acute illness (e.g., behavior changes, rashes, fever, vomiting, diarrhea, or eye drainage). Isolate and care for ill children until they return home.

- Monitor the immunization status of children and plan for the exclusion of unimmunized children and children with immune deficiencies and disorders when a vaccine-preventable disease occurs in a child attending the facility (see Chapter 43).

- Develop and follow guidelines for safe food preparation and handling.

HEALTH PROMOTION AND HEALTH MAINTENANCE

Health promotion activities within a childcare center promote the child's highest level of functioning and development, such as activities to stimulate physical, cognitive, and emotional development, and nutritious food to foster growth. Health maintenance activities are those that prevent injury or disease, such as immunization monitoring, infection control, and practices like putting infants on their backs to sleep. See the *Sudden Infant Death Syndrome* section in Chapter 46 for additional information.

Health Promotion

Nurses working with a childcare center can design and offer health education programs for the children (such as toothbrushing, hand hygiene, blowing the nose into a tissue, and coughing or sneezing into the elbow or shirt sleeve if a tissue is not available) to promote healthy habits.

Growth and Development Childcare Outcomes

When children receive quality child care that addresses their health and developmental needs, there are numerous benefits in cognitive development, language, math proficiency, social skills, interpersonal relationships, and self-regulation of behavior. These benefits lead to improved school readiness (Hillemeier, Morgan, Farkas, et al., 2013).

ENVIRONMENTAL SAFETY

To prevent child abduction, ensure that the childcare center maintains a current list of family members who may take a child from the facility and has guidelines for verifying identity when necessary.

The nurse should inspect the childcare environment to identify hazards that could cause injury to the children. Cleaning supplies and other toxins must be stored in a locked cabinet to prevent exposure. Inspect toys used by children to ensure that there are no sharp edges or points, small parts, or pinching parts. Check the safety of playground equipment (Figure 37–5).

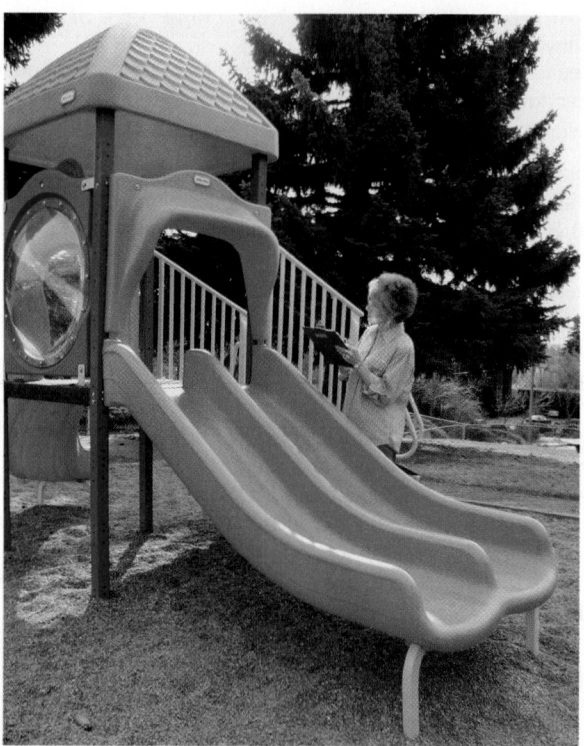

Figure 37–5 Assess the childcare center's environment for safety hazards. Check the area around playground equipment, making sure there are wood chips or cushioned tiles under the equipment. Inspect the playground equipment for protruding screws, loose nuts and bolts, and instability at least monthly.

EMERGENCY CARE PLANNING

As in the school setting, guidelines for assessing and identifying the child with an emergency health condition and the development of an emergency care plan for an acutely ill or injured child is essential. This plan should include giving first aid, calling EMS to transport the child to the emergency department, notifying the parent, and accompanying the child to the emergency department until the parent arrives.

Nursing Roles in the Home Healthcare Setting

Home health care is a component of the continuum of comprehensive health care provided to children and families. Children with episodic or long-term health conditions can benefit from home healthcare services to promote their optimal function and participation in the family. Home healthcare services may be provided to children with complex health conditions, short-term acute care conditions, and even for hospice care.

Pediatric in-home healthcare services for children with complex healthcare conditions or who are medically fragile have increased because of the increased survival of preterm infants, infants with complex congenital conditions, children with severe trauma, and children with life-limiting or life-threatening conditions (Mendes, 2013). Technologies now used in the home include ventilators, suction, peritoneal dialysis, enteral feeding tubes, pumps for feeding tubes, intravenous fluids, and medications.

The home environment is believed to improve the long-term care of these children by integrating them into the family, promoting their growth and development, and minimizing the number of hospitalizations. The family may feel as if some control over family life is achieved by having the child in the home. However, the health and well-being of parents is affected by limited sleep, chronic distress, and less time to engage in social and personal health-oriented activities (Murphy, Carbone, & the Council on Children with Disabilities, 2011). Many families feel like they were offered no choice about assuming responsibility for the nursing and technologic care of their child who is medically fragile (Mendes, 2013). This causes stress as the family attempts to balance the child's constant care requirements and needs of the entire family. Healthcare providers and insurers are challenged to simultaneously address the child's illness and developmental needs while supporting families when these children are transitioned to care at home.

Home health care is considered by health payers to be a cost-effective alternative to hospital inpatient care. Many different options for health insurance payment exist, such as family health insurance, the Child Health Insurance Program (CHIP), Social Security, and state Medicaid programs. The family also has a financial burden because of paying some costs out of pocket—for medications, supplies, and transportation. A parent may need to give up employment to care for the child and to qualify for Medicaid.

Nurses need a variety of skills, knowledge, and experience to work in the pediatric home care setting, such as:

- Knowledge and experience in pediatric assessment and acute care practice using various medical technologies. These skills enable nurses to provide direct care, teach the family and child self-care practices, and monitor the child's progress.
- The ability to adapt, be creative, and be prepared to deal with the unexpected, such as equipment malfunctions.

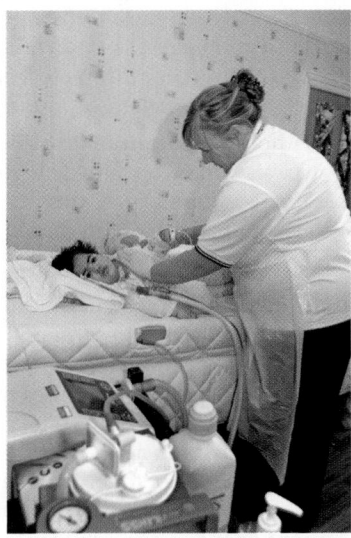

Figure 37–6 Nurses provide both short-term and long-term services to families in the home setting. In some cases, families need support for a short time after the child is discharged from the hospital following an acute illness. In other cases, families need assistance with complex nursing care for the child assisted by technology.

SOURCE: Paula Solloway/Alamy.

- An understanding of community resources, financing mechanisms, and multiagency collaboration; and good communication skills.
- Knowledge of the community's health resources to help families obtain services that match the child's and family's needs.
- An understanding of the community's cultural diversity and the cultural values of the families served.
- Skill in collaborating with other healthcare team members.

Home care nursing is focused on assisting a family to gain a greater ability to more independently manage the child's care related to a chronic condition or an acute condition following hospital discharge. Nurses also work with the family in the home care setting to promote or restore the child's health while attempting to minimize the effects of the disability and illness, including life-limiting illness (Figure 37–6).

Nursing Management

For the Child in the Home Healthcare Setting

Nursing Assessment and Diagnosis

Home health nurses assess the home, the child, and the family during intermittent skilled nursing visits. Assessment of the home is focused on environmental safety, adapting the environment for the child's care, and identifying needed resources. When working with the hospital discharge planner or case manager to initiate home health services, the following aspects of the home are assessed:

- Home readiness (safe sleeping arrangements, adequate supplies, ability to meet nutritional and fluid needs, telephone access, heat, electricity, refrigeration, lack of any communicable diseases in the home, and safe access into and out of the home)

- Potential hazards related to the child's age, condition, and requirements for technology-assisted care (e.g., extension cords used to plug equipment into electrical outlets and inadequate space for a wheelchair or walker)
- Features of the home environment that could cause an acute illness (e.g., use of a woodstove or fireplace for heating that could cause respiratory distress, active renovation of a house releasing lead dust, and family members who smoke)

Assessment of the child is focused on the current health status, growth, developmental progress, and social interaction with family members and healthcare providers. The potential for abuse and neglect is assessed in children with complex health conditions who are at higher risk.

Family strengths and coping abilities are evaluated along with parenting methods. Parents' skills in giving the child needed medications, performing care procedures, and detecting signs of an urgent change in the child's health status are assessed. The presence of siblings, their developmental and physical status, and their needs should also be assessed.

Developing Cultural Competence Assessment

When assessing the child and family in the home, recognize when any potential conflicts might exist between recommended medical care and the family's preferences. Identify which family member is most influential in decisions about the child's care. Use open-ended questions to talk with families and understand the issue from their point of view. Ask family members to identify the issue, why it is a concern, and the impact on their lives. Information gained can be used to educate the family, communicate with healthcare providers about potential alternate care options, and develop a nursing care plan that integrates the family's preferences.

Examples of nursing diagnoses that could apply to the family as the child transitions from the hospital to home setting include the following (NANDA-I © 2014):

- *Home Maintenance, Impaired,* related to insufficient family organization and planning
- *Coping: Family, Compromised,* related to multiple stressors in caring for a child with a complex health condition
- *Health Management, Family, Ineffective,* related to complexity of medical interventions
- *Social Interaction, Impaired,* related to therapeutic isolation

Planning and Implementation

Nursing care should focus on promoting an environment within the home for the child to develop, learn social skills, and gain a sense of identity based on family values. Nurses help families in the home setting in the following ways:

- Ensuring that the child will be safe at home
- Providing competent nursing care to the child
- Educating parents about the child's condition and signs that may indicate an urgent change in health status
- Educating family members to safely administer medications and feedings, and perform medical procedures

- Demonstrating methods to promote the child's development
- Linking families to community resources, including support groups, respite care, and therapeutic recreation
- Assisting families in time management skills
- Advocating for increased health insurance coverage or locating other sources of financial assistance

COLLABORATING WITH THE FAMILY

The nurse works in partnership with the family in the home to promote the health of the child and of the family unit. The nurse must develop a respectful and trusting relationship with the family, remembering that the family maintains control in the home care setting. Open communication is essential so the nurse can learn what is important to the child and family, and then modify the nursing care plan when appropriate.

Role expectations of the nurse, especially when in the home for extended hours, must be clearly understood to reduce stress in the family. House rules for such things as parking, private areas in the home, door to use, where to store belongings, and routines need to be negotiated, and then those rules need to be followed. The success of home care is also based on effective cultural communication. For example, some Jewish families follow strict dietary guidelines that do not permit dairy products and meat to be served together in the same dishes or during the same meal. The nurse needs to abide by the dietary guidelines and observe the family's food preparation practices.

The range of nursing care that may be included in a child's home care plan may include sensory stimulation, routines of daily living, positioning and skin care with gentle handling, respiratory care, nutrition and elimination, medications, and other supportive therapies. Other providers, such as physical therapists, speech-language therapists, occupational therapists, and social workers, may provide other healthcare services in collaboration with the home health nurse.

A parent or guardian should be present when nurses provide home care. Informed consent is needed for invasive treatments and decisions for provision of needed emergency care to prevent serious consequences. A plan for communication about key client-care information (e.g., daily notes written by both the family members and nurse) and scheduled meetings with family members are important to ensure that needed information is shared. This also helps the family members evaluate how well the nurse meets their expectations for care of the child.

SUPPORTING THE FAMILY

When home health nursing is episodic, parents of children with complex conditions often feel stressed by the constant care demands. They may be sleep deprived when caring for the child 24 hours a day and need some assistance in identifying alternative care options, such as **respite care**, short-term home care to relieve the primary caregiver and allow time away from home (see Chapter 38 for more information). Families often need support in identifying and advocating for potential services that may be of value to their child and financial resources for which they may be eligible.

EMERGENCY PREPAREDNESS

The nurse should help the family develop an emergency care plan for any child whose condition could worsen rapidly and become life threatening (e.g., severe congenital heart defect, tracheostomy, or apnea), or be more than the parents or home health nurse can provide with resources available. The plan should provide guidelines for when to call 9-1-1. The emergency care plan should include an essential medical history

---

TEACHING HIGHLIGHTS | Home Evacuation Plan

Developing a home evacuation plan is important when the family has one or more children with special healthcare needs. Important steps to have families take in developing the plan include:

- Have working smoke and carbon monoxide detectors in the home and teach children what the alarm means. Make sure batteries are changed twice a year.
- Draw a diagram of your house. Mark all windows and doors. Plan two routes out of every room. Think about an escape plan if the fire starts in the kitchen, bedroom, or basement.
- Figure out the best way to get infants and young children out of the house. Will you carry them? Is there more than one small child, and if so, how will you get all the small children out if you are the only adult?
- Teach preschool and school-age children to follow the escape plan by crawling, touching doors, and going to the window if the door is hot. Show children how to cover their nose and mouth to reduce smoke inhalation.
- Prepare an alternate fire escape plan in case you are alone with the child when the fire begins.
- Keep home exits clear of toys and debris.
- Select a safe meeting place outside the home. Teach children not to go back inside the burning home.

---

that provides the emergency care providers with enough information to understand the child's health condition, to prevent delays in disease-specific treatment, and to minimize unnecessary interventions until the child's personal physician can be consulted. Refer to the American Academy of Pediatrics website for an emergency information form.

Families should develop a plan for safe evacuation of the home in case of fire or other emergency. This is very challenging when the child cannot mobilize independently and requires equipment for continued survival or quality of life. See *Teaching Highlights: Home Evacuation Plan* for information to help families develop a plan for safe evacuation of the home.

When the child is dependent on technology, the family should notify the power company so that the home is on the high-priority list for service after power outages. Backup generators may be needed if electrical power for life-sustaining equipment is essential. The child should also be registered for a disaster shelter that can accommodate the healthcare needs of the child and at least one caregiver when major power outages occur.

Evaluation

Expected outcomes of nursing care include the following:

- Care of the child's medical needs is integrated into the family's routines when possible.
- The family has an emergency care plan for the child in the event of a disaster, a weather emergency, or if the child's condition suddenly worsens.
- The home health nurse and family work in partnership to promote the child's health and growth and development.

Preparation for Disasters

Disasters are serious and massive events that impact many people in a community and cause extensive damage, hardship, deaths, injuries, and psychologic trauma. Natural disasters include floods, ice storms, hurricanes, earthquakes, volcanic eruptions, tornados, and wild fires. Trains or trucks carrying toxic chemicals and nuclear waste that crash or explode may also cause a disaster. Terrorism is another potential cause of disasters and may involve the use of infectious organisms, bombs, toxic chemicals, or radioactive agents. (See Chapter 43 for information about infectious agents used for bioterrorism.)

Disasters may cause death, injury, physical damage, psychologic trauma, and economic disruption.

Children have special vulnerabilities during a disaster. Disasters are very traumatic for the children involved, and there may be immediate and delayed responses. Disbelief, fright, and grief reactions are among immediate responses (Jones & Schmidt, 2013). Children may lose their homes and personal possessions. They may be separated from their families. Friends, pets, and family members may be injured or dead. They may also have problems expressing their feelings about the disaster.

Growth and Development

Developmental considerations must be considered during disaster planning because young children may be unable to do the following (AAP, 2013a):

- Walk or mobilize to escape danger.
- Understand what is happening.
- Understand the need to flee or take evasive action.
- Follow the instructions regarding evacuation or safe actions.
- Tell others they need help.
- Distinguish between reality and fantasy.

Fear, anxiety, sadness, and confusion are some common initial responses to a disaster, whether it is natural or man-made. The responses of children may be even greater if parents are also anxious or overwhelmed. Developmental stage, prior life experience, and the ability of the primary caregiver to meet safety and security needs will determine a child's response to disaster. Support for early responses to the disaster include the following (Jones & Schmidt, 2013):

- *Infants*—disrupted routine such as changes in sleeping and eating patterns, crying, and irritability associated with family responses to the disaster. Support involves providing a consistent caregiver and maintaining normal routines as much as possible.
- *Toddlers*—disrupted sleep, nightmares, night terrors, regressive behaviors such as clinging behaviors, withdrawal, and temper tantrums. Support involves re-establishing routines for sleep, meals, and play as much as possible as well as a comfort item and storytelling.

- *Preschoolers*—similar to toddlers, regressive behaviors (bedwetting, thumb sucking, fear of the dark), disrupted sleep, anxiety, and complaints of stomachaches or headache. Support involves reestablishing routines, allowing regression during stress, and promoting play and storytelling to express feelings.

- *School-age children*—preoccupation with the disaster details and anxiety about consequences, fear of more harm for themselves and their family. Support involves restricting media exposure, explanations of the event in age-appropriate terms, opportunities to express their feelings, and play therapies.

- *Adolescents*—more awareness of the disaster's severity and its significance that may complicate responses, anxiety, unrealistic fears, anger, changes in mood, stomachaches, and headaches. Support involves engaging adolescents in disaster response efforts when it is safe, encouraging them to talk with peers and teachers about their feelings, relaxation techniques, exercise, and journal writing.

Nursing Management

DISASTER PREPARATION

Pediatric nurses in schools and other community settings like schools play an important role in preparing families for a disaster. They can guide families to developmentally appropriate resources for talking with their children about disaster planning and disasters that occur. Families who discuss disaster planning with health professionals are more likely to follow disaster preparedness recommendations, and children may cope better if involved in the family's disaster planning (Jones & Schmidt, 2013). Children need to know what to do in case of a disaster and that police officers, fire fighters, and emergency medical personnel are available to help them. They should be taught areas that are safest in the home, how to respond to smoke detector alarms and community alerts, when to call the emergency number, and how to contact the family members when separated (AAP, 2013b).

Help the family develop a disaster plan for staying at home or for evacuation. Families must prepare to manage for 72 hours within their own home following a major disaster or epidemic. The family needs a 3-day supply of nonperishable food and bottled water, flashlights and batteries, a battery-powered radio, over-the-counter medications, and many other resources. Remember to have formula, diapers, bottles, powdered milk, moist towelettes, and diaper rash ointment for infants and children if needed. A plan for family pets should also be made. Refer to the Federal Emergency Management Agency (FEMA) website for the most current recommendations for family supplies to have on hand.

Parents should also carry phone numbers of out-of-town contacts, schools, and neighbors at all times. Developing a list of each family member's medications, clothing, food, water, and other essentials is important so the family can quickly pack and respond to an evacuation order.

Advance planning is needed to ensure that children assisted by technology have the resources needed in the event of a disaster. Help the family register with the designated community shelter caring for individuals needing electrical power for their medical equipment. Batteries for medical equipment should be fully charged at all times. Additionally, parents need to arrange for a durable power of attorney so that consent for emergency medical care can be available should the child and parents become separated during a disaster.

EMERGENCY RESPONSE

Nurses are important first responders during disasters. They provide emergency health care for rescued victims and first aid for the walking wounded, work in disaster shelters, and perform general public health interventions (e.g., vaccines, sanitation, food and water). Nurses can provide a safe place for children, away from media and unfolding traumatic events, such as the rescue of dead and injured. Do not allow children to leave a scene unaccompanied by a parent or other responsible adult. Assess for panic reactions, unexpected behaviors, and changing conditions.

Clinical Tip

A 12-volt inverter is an inexpensive device that can be plugged into a car's cigarette lighter and delivers 110 to 120 volts of alternating-current power. This device can be powered with the car's battery or by turning on the engine and can be used to keep a patient's life-support device working.

PSYCHOLOGIC SUPPORT

Nurses with knowledge of child and adolescent development can meet the psychologic needs of youth after a disaster. Respond to families in a compassionate and supportive manner, comfort and console children, and provide information and some guidelines for positive coping.

Once the initial disaster is managed and children return to home or other settings, children may need extra time with their parents. Parents should attempt to reestablish daily routines for school, meals, play, and rest as soon as possible. Encourage parents to listen and answer the child's questions about the disaster honestly and in language the child can understand. If they cannot answer a question, it is better to be honest and say so. Reassure the child that they are trying to do everything to keep the child safe. Encourage older children and adolescents to discuss the disaster with family members and peers if desired.

Because disasters may cause disruption for extended periods, the child may have prolonged periods of emotional distress. Identify children and families who do not return to normal life patterns. Worrisome signs include persistently reliving the event in dreams or memories, hypervigilance, difficulty sleeping, irritability, difficulty concentrating, and avoiding stimuli associated with the event. Children who may be more vulnerable to posttraumatic stress reactions (PTSD) include those who change schools, witness destruction, lose a parent, lose a home, or remain in a shelter (Jones & Schmidt, 2013). (See Chapter 55 for a discussion of PTSD.) Use these signs to identify children for whom more psychologic help is needed and to promote access to those services.

Focus Your Study

- Categories of family strengths that help families cope with stressors include effective family communication, collaborative problem solving, family assets such as education and finances, being emotionally aware and working to maintain emotional stability, and developing shared meaning about the experience.

- Pediatric care in the community occurs in many settings such as physician offices, mobile vans, healthcare centers, hospital outpatient clinics, schools, childcare centers, the home, and disaster shelters.

- Working with the child and family in the community setting requires an understanding of how the larger environment influences the child's health and development.

- Nurses working in many community healthcare settings develop a long-term relationship with the child and family over time that helps to promote the provision of optimal health care.

- Examples of community family support services include Head Start education programs, before- and after-school programs, peer support groups, faith community social service programs, crisis care, and respite care programs

- Pediatric nurses in community settings assist with diagnostic workups and management of children with chronic health problems, including family and client assessment, health education, health promotion, and linking families with community resources.

- School nursing focuses on removing or minimizing health barriers to learning so children can perform academically. Services include prevention, health promotion, health education, emergency care, and managing chronic health problems.

- Nurse consultants to childcare settings assist the administrators in the establishment of the childcare center's policies for healthcare practices, teach staff about safe healthcare practices, and monitor healthcare practices.

- Home care nursing goals include promoting or restoring the health of the child while attempting to minimize the effects of the disability and illness.

- Pediatric nurses help families to prepare for a disaster by helping them to develop a disaster plan, use developmentally appropriate information to talk with children about what to do when disasters occur, provide direct care in a disaster shelter, and provide psychosocial support to families and children.

Clinical Reasoning in Action

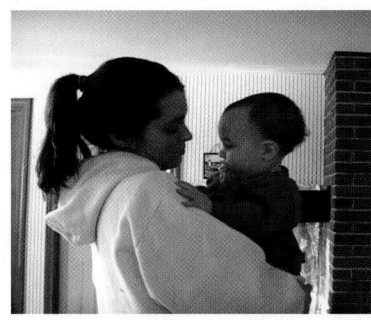

Gavin is a 1-year-old coming into the clinic for his well-child checkup. The clinic is set up to see teen mothers and their babies for well-child visits and immunizations. Tanika, his mother, has been bringing him there since he was born. Gavin qualifies for healthcare coverage through the Medicaid system in his state. He was born full term and has never been in the hospital or had surgery. Tanika is still attending high school and plans to graduate this year. She and Gavin are living with her boyfriend's (Gavin's father) parents until they can raise enough money to live on their own. Gavin's father does not come to the well-baby visits. Gavin attends child care while his mother is at school. He is up-to-date on immunizations so far and there is no significant family medical history, but there is smoking in the home. Gavin has been walking since he was 9 months old. He is able to point, wave, clap, and speak two words. He is able to drink from a cup and put objects into a cup. He has been growing and thriving at an appropriate pace. Tanika describes him as a good eater and tells you that he is currently on whole milk. He has soft stools daily and five to six wet diapers per day. He sleeps through the night and takes two naps per day. Tanika describes him as an extremely active child and has worked on childproofing everything in the house.

1. What is the role of the nurse in caring for Gavin and his parents in the clinic?

2. What data does the nurse collect to perform a family assessment?

3. What strengths and stressors are likely to be present in this family?

4. What information should the nurse provide to help Tanika prepare for evacuation with Gavin since springtime flooding is anticipated?

References

American Academy of Pediatrics (AAP). (2012). School-based health centers and pediatric practice. *Pediatrics, 129*(2), 387–393.

American Academy of Pediatrics (AAP). (2013a). *Pediatric preparedness resource kit*. Retrieved from http://www.aap.org/en-us/advocacy-and-policy/aap-health-initiatives/Children-and-Disasters/Documents/PedPreparednessKit.pdf

American Academy of Pediatrics (AAP). (2013b). *Safety and prevention: Getting your family prepared for disasters*. Retrieved from: http://www.healthychildren.org/English/safety-prevention/at-home/Pages/Getting-Your-Family-Prepared-for-a-Disaster.aspx

American Academy of Pediatrics, American Public Health Association, & National Resource Center for Health and Safety in Child Care. (2013). *Stepping stones to caring for our children: National health and safety performance standards; Guidelines for early care and education programs* (3rd ed.). Retrieved from http://www.cfoc.nrckids.org/

Caldwell, B. M., & Bradley, R. H. (1984). *The home observation for measurement of the environment*. Little Rock, AR: University of Arkansas.

Center for Health and Healthcare in Schools. (2013). *Medication management*. Retrieved from http://www.healthinschools.org/Health-in-Schools/Health-Services/School-Health-Services/School-Health-Issues/Medication-Management.aspx

Hackman, D. A., Betancourt, L. M., Brodsky, N. L., Kobrin, L., Hurt, H., & Farah, M. J. (2013). Selective impact of early parental responsivity on adolescent stress reactivity. *PLOS One, 8*(3), e58250.

Halterman, J. S., Szilagyi, P. G., Fisher, S. G., Fagnano, M., Tremblay, P., Conn, K. M., … Borrelli, B. (2011). Randomized controlled trial to improve care for urban children with asthma. *Archives of Pediatric and Adolescent Medicine, 165*(3), 262–268.

Halterman, J. S., Fagnano, M., Montes, G., Fisher, S., Tremblay, P., Tajan, R., … Butz, A. (2012). The school-based preventive asthma care trial: Results of a pilot study. *Journal of Pediatrics, 161*(6), 1109–1015.

Herrman, H., Stewart, D. E., Diaz-Granados, N., Berger, E. L., Jackson, B., & Yuen, T. (2011). What is resilience? *Canadian Journal of Psychiatry, 56*(5), 258–265.

Hillemeier, M. M., Morgan, P. L., Farkas, G., & Maczuga, S. A. (2013). Quality disparities in child care for at-risk children: Comparing Head Start and non-Head Start settings. *Maternal and Child Health Journal, 17*, 180–188.

Jones, S. L., & Schmidt, C. K. (2013). Psychosocial effects of disaster in children and adolescents: Significance and management. *Nursing Clinics of North America, 48*, 229–239.

Kaul, T. (2011). Helping African American children self-manage asthma: The importance of self-efficacy. *Journal of School Health, 81*(1), 29–33.

Lester, P., Stein, J. A., Saltzman, W., Woodward, K., McDermid, S. W., Milburn, N., … Beardslee, W. (2013). Psychological health of military children: Longitudinal evaluation of a family-centered prevention program to enhance family resilience. *Military Medicine, 178*(8), 838–845.

Lucas, T., Anderson, M. A., & Hill, P. D. (2012). What level of knowledge do elementary school teachers possess concerning the care of children with asthma? A pilot study. *Journal of Pediatric Nursing, 27*, 523–527.

Mendes, M. A. (2013). Parents' descriptions of ideal home nursing care for their technology-dependent children. *Pediatric Nursing, 39*(2), 91–96.

Miles, M. S., Holditch-Davis, D., Burchinal, M. R., & Brunssen, S. (2011). Maternal role attainment with medically fragile infants: Part 1. Measurement and correlates during the first year of life. *Research in Nursing and Health, 34*, 20–34.

Murphy, N. A., Carbone, P. S., & the Council on Children with Disabilities. (2011). Parent-provider-community partnerships: Optimizing outcomes for children with disabilities. *Pediatrics, 128*(4), 795–802.

Ramisch, J. (2012). Marriage and family therapists working with couples who have children with autism. *Journal of Marital and Family Therapy, 38*(2), 305–316.

Sarsour, K., Sheridan, M., Jutte, D., Nuru-Jeter, A., Hinshaw, S., & Boyce, W. T. (2011). Family socioeconomic status and child executive functions: The roles of language, home environment, and single parenthood. *Journal of the International Neuropsychological Society, 17*, 120–132.

Society of Pediatric Nurses. (2014). *Disaster management for children and families.* Retrieved from http://www.pedsnurses.org/p/cm/ld/fid=57&tid=28&sid=50

Taras, H. L. (2014). School nursing: Beyond medications and procedures. *JAMA Pediatrics, 168*(7), 604–606.

U.S. Census Bureau. (2011). *Child care: An important part of life.* Retrieved from https://www.census.gov/how/pdf/child_care.pdf

U.S. Census Bureau. (2013). *Current population survey (CPS)—Definitions and explanations.* Retrieved from http://www.census.gov/cps/about/cpsdef.html

U.S. Department of Education, National Center for Education Statistics. (2014). *Digest of education statistics, 2013 (NCES 2011-015).* Retrieved from http://nces.ed.gov/programs/digest

U.S. Department of Health and Human Services. (2015). *Healthy People 2020.* Retrieved from http://www.healthypeople.gov/2020/topicsobjectives2020/default.aspx

Wright, J. L., & Krug, S. E. (2016). Emergency medical services for children. In R. M. Kliegman, B. F. Stanton, J. W. St. Geme, & N. F. Schor (Eds.), *Nelson textbook of pediatrics* (20th ed., p. 478). Philadelphia, PA: Elsevier.

Wright, L., & Leahey, M. (2013). *Nurses and families: A guide to family assessment and intervention* (6th ed.). Philadelphia, PA: F. A. Davis.

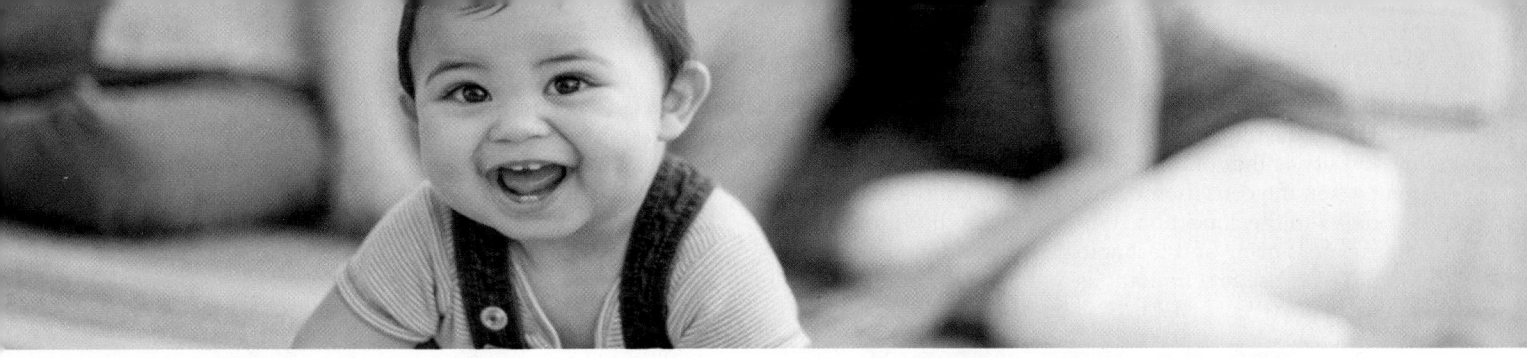

Chapter 38

Nursing Considerations for the Child and Family With a Chronic Condition

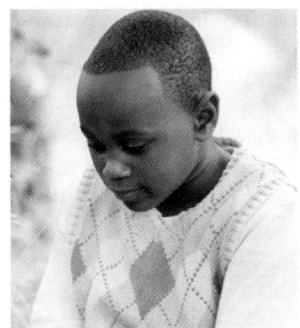

I'm nervous about going to school for the first time since my diabetes was diagnosed. I'm worried that my friends will make fun of me because I have to check my blood and give myself a shot at lunchtime. I wish this would just go away, but I know it's something I will have for the rest of my life. My mom and dad were really upset, but they are getting used to the idea now and will do anything to make sure I am doing okay.

—Mark, 10 years old

Ethno Images/Alamy

Learning Outcomes

38.1 Explain the causes of chronic conditions in children.

38.2 Identify the categories of chronic conditions in children.

38.3 Describe the nurse's role in caring for a child with a chronic condition.

38.4 Assess the family of a child with a chronic condition.

38.5 Prepare the family of a child with a chronic condition to effectively care for the child in the home.

38.6 Summarize nursing management for the child with a chronic condition to support transition to school and adult living.

38.7 Discuss the family's role in care coordination.

Overview of Chronic Conditions

A **chronic condition** is generally thought of as one that is expected to last at least 3 months (Kennedy, 2011). An estimated, 14.6 million children under the age of 18 in the United States have special healthcare needs related to some type of chronic condition (Data Resource Center for Child & Adolescent Health, 2012). Chronic conditions vary in etiology, manifestations, severity, and their effect on the child's physical, psychosocial, and cognitive development. Chronic conditions develop from multiple causes:

- Genetic or inheritable conditions may manifest as a chronic condition. Examples include muscular dystrophy, hemophilia, sickle cell disease, and cystic fibrosis.

- Conditions may result from a congenital defect or insult to the infant during fetal development, such as neural tube defect, maternal substance abuse, cleft palate, and cerebral palsy.

- Insult or injury may be associated with birth and care following birth (sepsis, prematurity, intraventricular hemorrhage) that lead to conditions such as bronchopulmonary dysplasia, attention deficit disorder, and vision or hearing impairment.

- Conditions can be acquired through injury or acute medical condition such as brain injury, cancer, HIV infection, drowning, and mental health problems.

These and additional chronic illnesses are discussed in the systems chapters later in this text.

In most cases, these chronic conditions become lifelong disorders, but the impact on the affected child varies according to the severity of the condition, the stage of growth and development when the condition occurs, and the child's and family's responses to the condition. Whereas some conditions require intense monitoring and technologic support for survival, other conditions cause few limitations and have a minimal effect on quality of life (Figure 38–1).

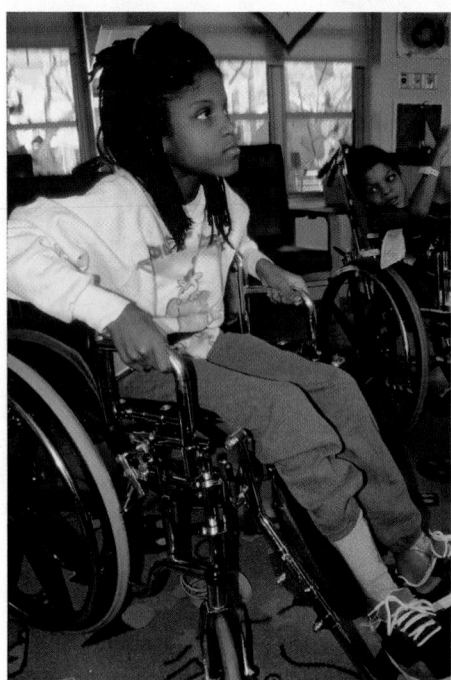

A

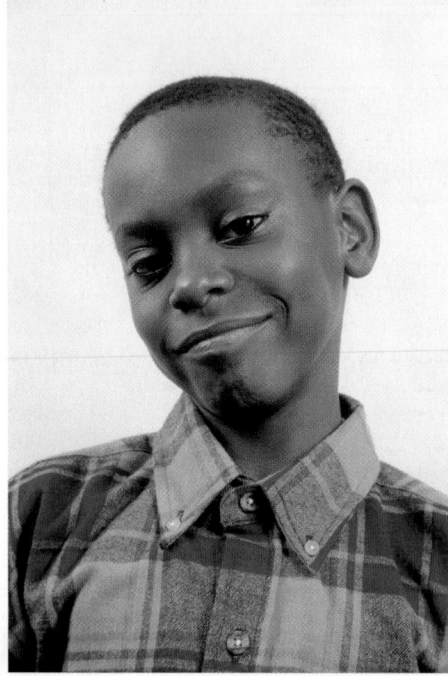

B

Figure 38–1 Children with chronic conditions may have a visible or nonvisible health condition, or nonvisible until an acute episode of their condition makes the condition visible. *A,* The child in a wheelchair has a visible disability. *B,* The child with a seizure disorder may have no visible signs of the condition unless a seizure is witnessed.

TABLE 38–1 Examples of Conditions by Special Healthcare Need Category

SPECIAL HEALTHCARE NEED CATEGORY	CHRONIC HEALTH CONDITION EXAMPLES
Dependent on medications or special diet	Diabetes mellitus, asthma, seizures, phenylketonuria, organ transplantation, cystic fibrosis, celiac disease
Dependent on medical technology	Renal failure, bronchopulmonary dysplasia
Increased use of healthcare services	Cancer, sickle cell disease, cystic fibrosis
Functional limitations	Down syndrome, brain injury, autism, myelodysplasia, cerebral palsy

Categories of chronic conditions may include functional limitations, developmental disorders, behavioral issues, anatomical problems, and limb dysfunction (Goodman, Posner, Huang, et al., 2013). The condition may also be further defined based on the amount of care that is needed, such as special medications, special diet, or medical technology. Children with chronic conditions require more care than healthy children require.

See Table 38–1 for examples of chronic conditions that may fall into a specific category. Many children with chronic conditions have special healthcare needs that fall into several of these areas. In the majority of cases, the more severe the chronic condition, the greater the number of categories of special healthcare needs. Many children with a chronic condition and children dependent on technology require specialized health care. The term **children with special healthcare needs (CSHCN)** is applied to "those who have one or more chronic physical, developmental, behavioral, or emotional conditions for which they require an above routine type or amount of health and related services" (U.S. Department of Health and Human Services, Health Resources and Services Administration [USDHHS/HRSA], 2011).

Many of these children have a **disability,** a limitation that interferes with a child's ability to fully participate in society, which can be related to medical impairment (chronic health condition), functional limitation (mobility, self-care, communication, or learning behavior impairment), or a mental condition that interferes with social interactions.

Data show that 19.8% of children in the United States have a special healthcare need (Data Resource Center for Child & Adolescent Health, 2012). Although these children represent a small percentage of the nation's children, they require significantly more healthcare resources than those without special healthcare needs, including more visits to clinics and emergency departments, dental visits, inpatient hospital days, and prescription medications. Efforts to reduce health costs have resulted in fewer hospitalizations and more care in the community for children with special healthcare needs.

The child with a life-threatening illness or a chronic condition as the result of a complex illness, prematurity, or a congenital defect may be considered **medically fragile** (Miles, Holditch-Davis, Burchinal, et al., 2011). Some of these children are **technology assisted,** dependent on a medical device that is required to sustain life or to maintain health status (mechanical ventilators, intravenous nutrition or drugs, tracheostomy,

Healthy People 2020

(DH-5) Increase the proportion of youth with special health-care needs whose healthcare provider has discussed transition planning from pediatric to adult health care

(MICH-30) Increase the proportion of children, including those with special healthcare needs, who have access to a medical home

(MICH-31) Increase the proportion of children with special healthcare needs who receive their care in family-centered, comprehensive, coordinated systems

suctioning, oxygen, or nutritional support with tube feedings) (Figure 38–2). Other children depend on medical devices that compensate for vital body functions and require nursing care management such as renal dialysis, urinary catheters, and colostomies.

Children assisted by technology can be cared for at home because compact portable equipment is available. Home-based equipment used for the child with a chronic condition may include ventilators, enteral feeding tubes, intravenous catheters, infusion pumps, dialysis equipment, and oxygen. With the support of home health services, parents can learn to manage the child's care. The benefit of home health services to the child is support of physical, emotional, and cognitive growth and development within the normal environment of the home.

All families with children experiencing a chronic condition need to make lifestyle adjustments, ensuring a baseline of care that helps maintain the child's health status and promotes growth and development. In many cases, the child has a baseline level of home management with episodic exacerbations that require the family to make sudden adjustments in family routines, such as may occur with the child who has seizures or an infection. These exacerbations often cause stress and disrupt family routines. In other cases, the chronic condition requires the family to learn and provide care that is complex and time intensive, such as cystic fibrosis, diabetes mellitus, bronchopulmonary dysplasia, and significant cognitive impairment. These more severe chronic conditions often impact the child's physical and psychologic development. Table 38–2 outlines healthcare

needs of these children and families and the nursing implications related to planning health services delivery to children and their families.

Role of the Nurse

The nurse's role in caring for the child with a chronic condition includes the following:

- Providing health supervision from infancy to transition into adulthood
- Collaborating with the multidisciplinary healthcare team
- Partnering with parents or caregivers to manage the child's care at home
- Referring the family to appropriate community services
- Assisting with planning for education services
- Promoting positive parenting behaviors and psychosocial adaptation and well-being of the child and family
- Promoting growth and development of siblings

Assess each family member's level of understanding of the condition, treatment, and anticipated outcome of the condition. Determine the family's stage of acceptance of the child's chronic illness, and how well the child's care is integrated into family routines. Evaluate the child's home care environment to determine the potential for abuse, lack of adequate care, or neglect, or for opportunities to enhance care provided. Assess the family's strengths, stressors, risk factors, and coping strategies. Provide information related to community resources. See *Nursing Care Plan: The Child With a Chronic Condition*. See Chapter 41 for stages that a family might progress through when faced with a diagnosis of a life-threatening illness or injury in a child.

The Child With a Newly Diagnosed Chronic Condition

Informing the child of a newly acquired chronic condition is individualized and is based on the child's developmental level and age. See *Growth and Development: Developmental Considerations for the Child With a Chronic Condition*. Questions the child may ask vary, but often focus on the cause of the condition, how to make it better, and how it will affect daily life. Provide information tailored to the child's level of understanding and answer questions honestly. The nurse should also address the fears and concerns of the family. Provide condition-specific education to help prepare the family for care at home and begin discharge planning. See *Teaching Highlights: Discussing a Child's Condition* and *Teaching Highlights: Informing Parents of Their Child's Chronic Illness or Disability*. The parents' heightened anxiety level may reduce the comprehension of information heard. See *Developing Cultural Competence: Cultural Sensitivity in Healthcare Providers for Children With Special Healthcare Needs*.

Most children with chronic conditions live at home, which causes other family members, including siblings, to be affected as well (Nielsen et al., 2012). Siblings of children with a chronic condition are affected in a variety of ways. These children experience some degree of disruption in their lives and demonstrate a variety of emotional responses (Fleary & Heffer, 2013). They may feel powerless and may receive less attention from their parents than the ill child. Siblings may have feelings of jealousy, anger, depression, guilt, resentment, worry, and anxiety (Fleary & Heffer, 2013; Vermaes, van Susante, & van Bakel, 2012). Siblings may fear that they themselves will have the same disease or condition as the affected child.

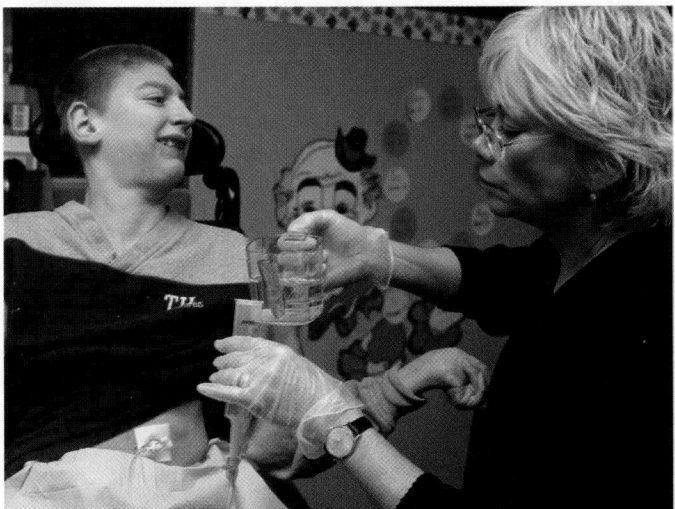

Figure 38–2 This child needs a gastrostomy tube to ensure adequate nutrition is obtained to support growth and promote resistance to infection.

TABLE 38–2 Healthcare Needs of Children With Chronic Conditions

HEALTHCARE NEED	DEFINITION	NURSING ACTIONS
Access to care	Care includes the availability and accessibility of providers with knowledge as well as ancillary services needed by children and their families.	Assist the family in obtaining transportation assistance if required. Assist the family in identifying healthcare providers who provide health promotion and other services to address the child's specific healthcare needs.
Appropriateness of care	Services and care are delivered by individuals with expertise and experience and are developmentally and culturally appropriate for the child and family.	Support the family by outlining educational and health services needed when developing an individualized education plan (IEP) and individualized health plan (IHP).
Comprehensiveness of care	Care includes coverage of the preventive, primary, and tertiary care needs of children, and linkages with other service systems, such as education, social services, and family support systems.	Provide the family with resource contacts such as social services, family support groups, and other systems to help the family manage the child's condition. Assist the family in identifying a care coordinator or developing the skills to take on the care coordination role themselves.
Coordination of care	Families are linked to medical care, financial health resources, and educational and community-based services; information is centralized.	Assist the family to identify a care coordinator or to develop the skills to become the care coordinator. See additional information in this chapter related to care coordination. Provide guidance and resources if the family decides to assume the role of care coordinator. Encourage the family to partner with the healthcare team to ensure continuity of care.
Continuity of care	Care is provided through a medical home or pediatric healthcare home; linkages between primary, specialty, therapeutic, and home care exist throughout childhood.	Facilitate communication between all the child's healthcare providers. Include the family and older child in all decision making.
Degree to which family-centered services are provided	The importance of the family is reflected in the way services are planned and delivered, building on individual and family strengths, and respecting the diversity of each family.	Determine the needs of the child and the family to ensure they are being addressed. Assist the family in identifying local and specialized healthcare providers. Recognize and respect the culture and cultural practices of the child and family.

Developing Cultural Competence Cultural Sensitivity in Healthcare Providers for Children With Special Healthcare Needs

The 2009/2010 National Survey of Children with Special Health Care Needs found that the majority of physicians and other healthcare providers were sensitive to family values and customs. Specific results indicated that 69.6% of physicians or other healthcare providers were always sensitive to family values and customs, 19.3% were usually sensitive, and 11.1% were sometimes or never sensitive (Child and Adolescent Health Measurement Initiative, 2012). It is essential for all healthcare providers to be sensitive to family values and customs of children with special healthcare needs.

Siblings may also have positive responses related to growing up with a chronically ill sibling, including an increased awareness of illness, maturity, family bonding and support, and an increased appreciation for life (Fleary & Heffer, 2013). See Chapter 39 for siblings' responses to the child experiencing an illness.

Discharge Planning and Home Care Teaching

As the child with a newly diagnosed chronic condition transitions to the home, parents often feel overwhelmed with preparations for home care, the anxiety of caring for a child with special healthcare needs, and supporting the child's growth and development needs. Work with the parents to ensure a smooth transition from hospital to the home environment. Assist the family in the initial discussions with the multidisciplinary team that participates in developing the child's care plan. Ensure that the family understands the role of each care provider. Provide contact numbers for parents to call should any issues arise at home.

Education to provide care of the child at home may be initiated by the hospital nursing staff, and then transitioned to special nurse educators or the home health nurses. Care is taken to ensure that all aspects of management are discussed with the family and that they demonstrate an understanding of and ability to perform the care required.

During discharge planning it may be helpful to identify a parent peer or peer support group to provide support to the

Nursing Care Plan: The Child With a Chronic Condition

1. Nursing Diagnosis: *Knowledge, Deficient (Child),* related to learning self-care skills (NANDA-I © 2014)

GOAL: The child will acquire self-care skills for lifetime management.

INTERVENTION	RATIONALE
• Assess the child's developmental level and select an educational approach and self-care activities to match.	• Learning goals for the child must match knowledge and skill expectations appropriate for developmental stage.
• Review with the child all steps involved in the self-care skill and how to perform the skill.	• The child may have watched the routine used by parents many times, and asking the child to list each step helps the nurse identify extra training needed.
• Use demonstration/return demonstration until the child is comfortable with procedures.	• Evaluation permits positive reinforcement and guidance for modification of techniques.
• Help parents develop a planned sequence of self-care skills to teach the child.	• Parents need guidance to identify appropriate self-care skills that the child is developmentally ready to learn.
• Discuss a plan for increased responsibility for self-care with the child and parents.	• Parents often need encouragement to transition responsibility to the child, becoming a supervisor rather than the person controlling care.

EXPECTED OUTCOME: Child will demonstrate the proper technique in the self-care skill and be able to assume responsibility for that skill with supervision by the parent. Responsibility for self-care increases as new skills are learned.

2. Nursing Diagnosis: *Family Processes, Interrupted,* related to management of chronic disease (NANDA-I © 2014)

GOAL: The child and family will manage the required treatments, monitoring, and medication regimen for the child's condition while maintaining family routines and functioning.

INTERVENTION	RATIONALE
• Assess the child's and family's lifestyle and attempt to fit the child's care needs into those schedules.	• Fitting the child's care to the child's and family's lifestyle promotes adherence to regimen and healthier family processes.
• Discuss the family's routines for special occasions and vacations and any activities important to the child. Identify ways to modify the child's management for these occasions and activities.	• It is important for the child to participate in special events with the family and peers as a normal child to promote psychologic development.

EXPECTED OUTCOME: Child and family will maintain important family routines and successfully manage the child's condition.

3. Nursing Diagnosis: *Coping: Readiness for Enhanced,* related to self-care management of chronic condition (NANDA-I © 2014)

GOAL: The child will develop a support system network.

INTERVENTION	RATIONALE
• Talk with the child about how to tell friends, teachers, and other important people about the chronic condition.	• These important people can assist the child in an emergency if they have enough information to assess the problem.
• Discuss ways to explain the condition to important people and how to answer questions.	• Having an opportunity to plan and role-play the conversation will reduce the child's anxiety about condition disclosure.
• Role-play ways to talk about the condition with friends and teachers.	• Sharing information about the condition helps others understand changes in lifestyle needed by the child.
• Encourage the child to attend peer support groups or camps specific to the child's condition.	• Learning and support networks developed at camp can promote development of problem-solving skills that increase coping abilities.

EXPECTED OUTCOME: Child will identify the friends, teachers, and other important persons informed about the chronic condition who can provide support when needed.

Growth and Development Developmental Considerations for the Child With a Chronic Condition

Newborns and Infants

- Newborns and infants who are medically fragile are at risk for chronic conditions related to brain injury, oxygen deprivation, and respiratory problems.
- Newborns cared for in the NICU are exposed to an environment of bright lights and high-pitched noises that can negatively affect their development (Aita, Johnston, Goulet, et al., 2013).
- Promote development and parent–infant bonding by encouraging the parents to spend time with the infant and engage in face-to-face interaction. When the newborn is stable, provide opportunities for parents to touch, soothe, and care for the infant.
- Provide sensory stimuli such as mobiles, soft music, and different textures for the infant to touch.

Toddlers

- Chronic illness can interfere with the achievement of autonomy and development of self-control. Some parents are overprotective and may do simple tasks they feel the child is incapable of accomplishing, rather than encouraging the child to try to do things independently. The child can lose independence and lack opportunities to meet developmental tasks.
- Nurses can promote the development of toddlers with chronic conditions by offering the child choices when possible, such as which color gown to wear or which food to eat first.
- Help parents recognize the toddler's capabilities, and allow the child to take the time to practice and learn a skill. Identify the next most appropriate developmental tasks for the child to learn and give the parents some strategies they can use to offer learning opportunities.

Preschoolers

- Preschool children recognize the association between body parts and problems associated with the chronic condition. The preschooler engages in magical thinking during this stage, and the child may believe that his or her thoughts or behaviors caused the condition. The child may also think the condition is a form of punishment.
- Hospitalization or implementation of a treatment plan, such as a new medication, may interfere with the preschool-age child's developing independence (University of Michigan Health System, 2014).
- Nurses can promote development by explaining the purpose of treatments and procedures in terms the preschooler can understand, and by emphasizing that treatments and procedures are not punishment for any wrongdoing.
- Look for ways to use play so the child can learn an aspect of self-care, perform an activity, and feel a sense of accomplishment. Encourage social interactions with other children when possible. Give positive feedback to the child for appropriate efforts and successes.

School-Age Children

- Early school-age children have an increased understanding of their condition and are capable of participating in certain aspects of monitoring and care. Older school-age children begin to understand about managing their condition and the long-term needs associated with their condition. They can assume more responsibility for their care such as serum glucose monitoring, intermittent self-catheterization, or monitoring the condition of skin under braces.

- Some children with chronic conditions have learning difficulties and other limitations that interfere with education and social competence. The child needs to gain social skills, interact with peers, master new information, learn to cope with stress, and acquire skills that lead to self-sufficiency in order to develop a sense of industry.
- The school-age child senses that he or she is different from peers and may feel left out, especially if functional limitations affect his or her ability to participate in extracurricular activities. It is important that children with chronic health conditions be allowed to participate in activities as much as their condition allows and their physician approves (University of Michigan Health System, 2014).
- Nurses can promote development of school-age children by encouraging their interaction with children in the same age group. When possible, this should occur with children who have the same type of chronic condition. Link the child to a peer support group to promote social interaction and to help the child recognize that others also have the same condition. When the child has an extended absence from school because of the chronic condition, encourage contact from school peers and friends through cards and computer messages, as well as the completion of school assignments.
- Begin to identify aspects of the child's care that the child can learn to assume under the parents' supervision. Inform families of the benefit of special camps for children with the chronic condition (when available) to promote recreation, social interaction, and learning skills of self-care.

Adolescents

- The adolescent with a chronic condition has numerous challenges with the rapid changes in growth and sexual maturation; ongoing development of identity, body image, and self-concept; and the need to plan for vocational and healthcare transitions. Cognitive development and abstract thinking skills are achieved during this stage, allowing the adolescent to develop an understanding of the short-term and long-term consequences related to the condition.
- The adolescent becomes more aware of differences between self and peers. Some adolescents are unable to cope with the recognizable differences between themselves and healthy peers, and they withdraw from social activities and relationships. Others may engage in risky behavior (e.g., alcohol, sexual activity, eating foods that interfere with therapy) that may be harmful to themselves or to management of their condition, just to be accepted by peers.
- Nursing actions to promote development of the adolescent include client education to help the adolescent learn about the chronic condition, care needed to manage or control the condition, and problem solving and specific skills for integrating self-care management into daily life. Parents need to be coached to transition care over to the adolescent and to support the adolescent to make healthy decisions regarding care.
- Encourage the adolescent to build a safety net of friends who know enough about the chronic condition to assist if a problem occurs, such as a seizure, asthma episode, or insulin reaction.
- Discuss sexual maturation and the importance of protected sexual activity, and discourage risky behaviors by the adolescent.
- Provide adolescents an opportunity to express concerns regarding self-management, vocational planning, and future independent living. Refer them to their local vocational rehabilitation services.

family. Parent peers who have had similar experiences may be very helpful in identifying strategies for the initial care transition in the home and additional issues that arise over time. If the family has a computer that family members frequently use, Internet resources for information and family support should be provided.

Collaborate with the family and healthcare team to ensure that the child has a medical or healthcare home in the local community to provide health promotion and maintenance and to assist with the coordination of local community resources. Promote communication and joint planning of care between the specialty care provider and local healthcare provider. Nurses working in hospital specialty clinics and other community settings can help ensure that children with chronic conditions receive multidisciplinary referrals and have appointments scheduled. Social services may be called to assist the family with identifying financial resources and other community resources for home management. Ongoing assistance may be required to help families deal with financial issues, time management, and other challenges.

Coordination of Care

Care coordination is the process of planning and integrating health care services among providers in an effort to achieve and promote good health in the child. Care coordination in a medical home facilitates transition from a pediatric healthcare provider to an adult healthcare provider (American Academy of Pediatrics, 2012). Care coordination also improves the quality and safety of client care (Taylor et al., 2012). See *Evidence-Based Practice: Care Coordination for Children With Special Healthcare Needs*. A **case manager**, often a nurse or social worker, may be given responsibility to help the family with care coordination. Case managers are often paid by a healthcare insurer to reduce

healthcare costs by coordinating the healthcare team, determining family needs, identifying financial and local support resources, and arranging for needed healthcare services.

Care coordination may help families who have children with special healthcare needs (Lawson, Bloom, Sadof, et al., 2011; Taylor et al., 2012). It may include helping the family modify the home to support required technology, such as mechanical ventilation or wheelchair use. Assistance may be required in purchasing or leasing ventilators, infusion pumps, or other specialized equipment. The coordination plan also includes determining the potential need for home health nursing, physical therapy, or other home health services. See *Developing Cultural Competence: Disparities in Care Coordination*.

Developing Cultural Competence Disparities in Care Coordination

Research by Toomey, Chien, Elliott, et al. (2013) found that children with special healthcare needs (CSHCN) were more likely to have inadequate care coordination than children without special healthcare needs. The study also found that Black and Latino children were more likely to have unmet care coordination needs than White children. Effective care coordination is essential for all CSHCN.

Families become very well educated about their child's condition and the services that would make managing the condition easier. Once management goals are established by the multidisciplinary team, the case manager partners with the family to help in the decision-making process regarding how goals will be met. An important role is helping the family to determine cost-effective strategies to meet healthcare goals

Clinical Question

How can care coordination enhance the care that children with special healthcare needs (CSHCN) and their families receive?

The Evidence

Taylor et al. (2012) evaluated the effectiveness of a care coordination program for CSHCN. The goal of the program was to assist families in achieving competency in care coordination and to support healthcare providers in the care coordination process. This study evaluated the effectiveness of a care coordination counselor implemented at a children's hospital with 430 beds and 50 outpatient care sites. The care coordination counselor was a BSN-prepared nurse who was made available to clients and families with complex needs. Additional tools provided to the families included a care binder, Care Coordination Network Committee, and the Community Resources for Families database. A survey was used to compare responses from families who received services from the care coordination counselor and those who only received a care binder. Twenty-five families who received services from the care coordination counselor and 50 families who received only the care binder completed the survey. Eighty-three percent of those receiving services responded positively overall to the survey, compared with 55% of those receiving only the binder. Additionally, 67% of those receiving services stated that care coordination for their child had improved over the past 6 months, compared to 47% of those who only received the care binder.

Looman et al. (2013) examined the importance of the role of the advanced practice nurse in relationship-based care coordination of children with complex special healthcare needs. Outcomes were measured using the Tele-Families study, a 4-year randomized controlled study whose goal is to evaluate the effectiveness of an enhanced interactive telehealth program and care coordination by the advanced practice nurse for children with complex special healthcare needs. Preliminary findings based on qualitative data from 94 families receiving telenursing interventions from an advanced practice nurse indicate increased parent satisfaction with having one person to coordinate care. Parents also expressed satisfaction with decreased time needed to have forms and prescriptions updated.

Petitgout, Pelzer, McConkey, et al. (2013) described the development of a hospital-based care coordination program for CSHCN. The program includes inpatients and outpatients and utilizes a family-centered approach to provide care coordination and a medical home. Over the past 10 years, improved client outcomes have been noted and include a decrease in length of stay, high family satisfaction, and decreased cost. In this program, the pediatric nurse practitioners collaborate with other healthcare providers and services to provide care coordination.

Best Practice

Care coordination is essential when working with CSHCN and their families. Care coordination in which nurses work with families to facilitate coordination of services is effective and leads to greater satisfaction with care and improved client outcomes. The nurse assists families to identify needed programs and services and is in an excellent position to serve as a liaison between these programs and the family to decrease the risk for fragmentation of care.

Clinical Reasoning

Why is care coordination a vital aspect of care for CSHCN? Provide an example of coordination of services for CSHCN. How do nurses play a role in care coordination for CSHCN?

---

and to delay the time when the child reaches the cap on health insurance benefits.

Some families assume the role of care coordinator for their child. It is essential for the family to understand that care coordination is time consuming and requires ongoing assessment and evaluation of the child's status and anticipated outcomes. Support family members in their decision to lead the care coordination process by helping the parents to become knowledgeable about the child's condition and treatment regimen. Encourage the parents to take an active role in the treatment planning and decision-making process so that they gain confidence in their abilities. Many hospitals have workshops for parents who are managing the complex care of their children. Parent-to-parent support groups can provide advice, support, and suggestions for referrals. Review the care coordination to ensure that the child has access to the most appropriate care and resources. Provide positive feedback to the parents as their advocacy skills increase.

Suggest that the family maintain a log of the healthcare team members, their roles, when the child was seen and any interventions, the results of interventions, and future planned interventions or treatments. The family can use this information when communicating with the healthcare providers, particularly in an emergency, and it may also help eliminate unnecessary duplication of procedures.

Community Sites of Care

Most children with chronic conditions are cared for in the home with or without home nursing or other health services. The healthcare provider for children with chronic conditions varies by the type of condition, type of health insurance coverage, preferences of the family, and availability of pediatric specialty resources.

Office or Health Center

Every child should have a "healthcare home" or "medical home," a consistent, continuous, comprehensive, family-centered, and compassionate source of primary health care. A healthcare home or medical home for these children is especially important because children with chronic conditions need regular preventive health care just as healthy children do. Health promotion, disease prevention, and anticipatory guidance have greater significance for the child with special healthcare needs. These children already have a condition that places them at higher risk for additional problems, such as infectious diseases, injury, or developmental delay. Information about community resources that may help the child and family is usually more extensive when the child's healthcare home is in the local community. The goal is for the child to have as normal a childhood as possible.

Ideally, this healthcare provider is located in the community where the family resides, making it more convenient for the family to obtain routine health care as well as care for episodic illnesses. Having a regular healthcare provider has many advantages for the family:

- Because the child and family are seen more frequently, a trusting, family-centered relationship can develop. The healthcare provider learns about the family's strengths and coping abilities.

- The healthcare provider sees the child and family when things are going well and during exacerbations. This may enable the healthcare provider to identify strategies that help the family to better coordinate the child's care.

- When the provider is based in the same community as the child, it is likely that information about community resources is known; this will reduce the efforts that families must make to identify appropriate services needed by the child.

Specialty Referral Centers

An optimal healthcare arrangement for the child with a chronic condition exists when the medical or healthcare home provider collaborates with a pediatric team or specialist that specializes in the care of children with a specific chronic condition. Pediatric specialists, advanced practice nurses, and other healthcare providers (e.g., physical therapists, social workers, and nutritionists) often function as a team providing coordinated care to the family and child with a chronic condition, such as spina bifida, cystic fibrosis, or diabetes. These specialty teams are often found in major medical centers, requiring travel to the facility. When communication flows from the team to the child's healthcare provider and back to the team, new treatments can be monitored by the child's physician, and consultation can be sought if the child's health status changes (Figure 38–3).

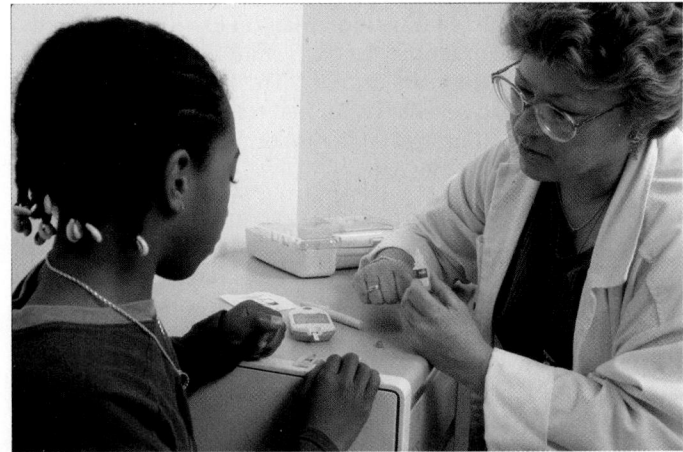

Figure 38–3 Nurses often assume a larger role in working with children and families with a chronic health condition in the ambulatory setting. Developing a care plan and educating the child and family to manage type 1 diabetes is an important role of this pediatric nurse, who is also a certified diabetes educator.

Nurses working in hospital specialty clinics and other community settings can help ensure that these children receive the appropriate health promotion services. The nurse in a tertiary care facility needs to identify appropriate resources and to help the family connect with local community resources. This is a greater challenge if the child and family have traveled a distance to obtain the specialty services, supporting the need for a primary care provider in the home community to provide regular care and to help coordinate local community resources.

Schools

All children, including those with chronic conditions and special healthcare needs, are entitled by federal law to a free education that is matched to their developmental and functional capabilities (Individuals with Disabilities Education Act [IDEA] and Section 504 of the Rehabilitation Act of 1973). **Early intervention** provides special services for infants and toddlers up to age 3 years who have a developmental delay or are at risk for a developmental delay. Early intervention programs are federal programs administered by the states. Children are evaluated at age 3 to determine continued eligibility in preschool (Caley, 2012; Pacer Center, 2012). IDEA has led to support of communities that are developing early childhood education programs and to schools with students who are blind, deaf, or have autism or traumatic brain injury. Provisions for adolescent transitional planning for adult living, including vocational training and independent living, are also included in the Individuals with Disabilities Education Act (U.S. Department of Education [USDOE], 2011).

Attending school is an important transition for children with chronic conditions and their families. Sending the child to school has several benefits for the child and family, including opportunities for socialization with children and adults outside of the family. School attendance promotes a feeling of normalcy in the family and provides a break for the primary care provider. Integration into the school system requires collaboration of family, school personnel, the nurse, and other members of the healthcare team.

EDUCATIONAL SYSTEM PLANNING

Careful planning is needed when a child with special needs attends school or receives other education services. Many children have chronic medical conditions that require management during the day in the school environment, such as asthma, diabetes, and attention deficit disorder. Some children simply need medications administered regularly or episodically. Other children require more extensive interventions integrated into the school day, such as blood glucose monitoring or intermittent self-catheterization. The education system is obligated to provide reasonable accommodations to ensure that the child's medical needs are met during the school day. The education system's obligation is negotiated with the family in formalized plans. The school nurse is an active participant on the team that collaborates with the family to develop these formalized plans.

- An **individualized family service plan (IFSP)** is developed for the early intervention process for infants with special healthcare needs and their families. The IFSP contains information about the services required to support a child's development and enhance the family's capacity to facilitate the child's development. The family and education service providers work as a team to plan, implement, and evaluate services specific to the family's unique concerns, priorities, and resources.

Clinical Tip

Federal laws for providing education services for children with special healthcare needs include:

- The Rehabilitation Act, PL 93-112, of 1973 prohibited discrimination against people with a disability. Section 504 specifies that each student who has a disability is entitled to **accommodations**—services or special assistance provided in the school setting to ensure that a student with a physical or mental impairment has access to an appropriate education and is able to participate as fully as possible in school activities. Examples of accommodations might include allowing additional time to take a test, using strategies that decrease exposure to peanuts in a child who has an allergy to peanuts, or allowing the child to test his or her blood glucose level. Students with disabilities must be provided with educational services to meet their needs just as services are provided to those without disabilities. See Chapter 37 for further discussion on the nurse's role in the school setting.

- The Education for All Handicapped Children Act, PL 94-142, of 1975 mandated that all children, even those with disabilities, be provided with free public education and related services. Safeguards were put into place to ensure that the rights of children with disabilities and their parents are protected. Additional purposes of this legislation were to assist states to provide education to children with disabilities and to evaluate the effectiveness of efforts to educate children with disabilities.

- The Education for All Handicapped Children Amendments, PL 99-457, of 1986 expanded the scope of PL 94-142 to include appropriate services for infants and toddlers with disabilities and their families.

- The Individuals with Disabilities Education Act (IDEA), PL 105-17, of 1997 and the Individuals with Disabilities Education Act of 2004, PL 108-446, with final regulations published in 2006 (reauthorization of the 1997 legislation), ensure that all children with disabilities have available to them a free and appropriate public education that emphasizes special education and related services designed to meet their unique needs and prepare them for employment and independent living. Every child with a disability must have a written individualized education plan (IEP), and parents have the right to question placement decisions and to due process when settling differences. In addition, the 2004 legislation focused more on state and local accountability to educate children with disabilities. This legislation also added a requirement that the child be invited to the IEP meeting.

Source: Data from Kim, D., & Samples, E. (2013). Comparing individual healthcare plans and Section 504 plans: School districts' obligation to determine eligibility for students with health related conditions. *Urban Lawyer, 45*(1), 263–279; Project Ideal. (2013). *Special education public policy.* Retrieved from http://www.projectidealonline.org/v/special-education-public-policy/; Yell, M. L., Conroy, T., Katsiyannis, A., & Conroy, T. (2013). Individualized education programs and special education programming for students with disabilities in urban schools. *Fordham Urban Law Journal, 41*(2), 669–714.

- An **individualized education plan (IEP)** is developed for a child with cognitive, motor, social, and communication impairments who needs special education services. The IEP is jointly planned with the school administrator, teacher, parents, and other special support professionals as appropriate for the child's condition. The child is also included in the process when possible. The plan is developed after an assessment of the child's abilities and specific functional limitations.

- An **individualized health plan (IHP)** is developed for the child with medical conditions that need to be managed

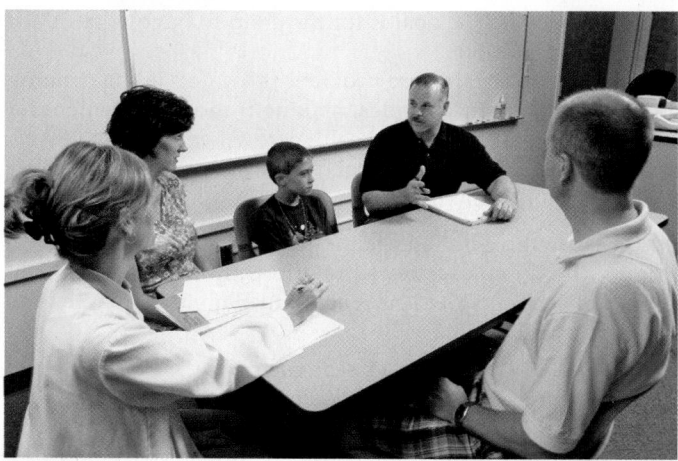

Figure 38–4 Because some children need medications or other therapies during school hours, the parents and child, school nurse, teacher, and school administrators develop a plan to manage the child's condition during school hours. The resulting document is the child's individualized health plan.

within the school setting. An IHP may be developed simultaneously with the IEP for the child with a health problem and a coexisting functional impairment. Some children only need an IHP for management of their chronic medical condition at school, such as daily medication administration or for glucose monitoring and insulin injection. An order from a licensed healthcare provider is required for medication administration and special treatments. Learning may be challenged when the child has frequent acute illness episodes that result in missed days of school, and the IHP often integrates methods to prevent the child from being penalized for those absences (Figure 38–4).

- An Individualized Section 504 Accommodation Plan may be used rather than an IHP for children with physical or mental impairments. The same process is used for development of the plan.

- An **individualized transition plan (ITP)** is included in the development of an IEP for each child with a chronic disability who is 14 years or older. The ITP focuses on helping individuals receive vocational training and in moving successfully from the home into other community living settings as they grow older.

Parents have an important role in advocating for their child to ensure that the child receives the most appropriate educational services. School systems must provide a full range of educational services for the children with special healthcare needs, including services that support cognitive development, self-care skills, mobility, improved communication, and social skills. Because each child's severity and combination of impairments is unique, identifying and matching the specific services for each child requires discussion and negotiation. Parents should make an effort to learn about the different types of educational services that address a child's specific disability in preparation for the IEP meeting. Parents often need a mentor or experienced parent to help with the development of the IEP the first few times. In this way, the parents are better prepared to participate in the educational planning and development of the child's IEP. School nurses are employees of the school system and may be limited in their

The elements of an IEP are as follows:

- Student's name
- Date of meeting to develop or review the IEP
- Statement of transition service needs of student beginning at age 14 years
- Present level of assessments and education performance, including how the child's disability affects the child's involvement and progress in a general curriculum or participation in appropriate activities
- Measurable annual goals that include short-term objectives in meeting the child's needs that enable the child to be involved in or progress in the general curriculum or participate in appropriate activities
- Special education and related services, supplementary aids and services, and program modifications or supports for school personnel needed to enable the child to make advancements toward attaining annual goals
- Explanation of the extent to which the child will or will not participate with nondisabled children
- Any specific modification in the administration of state or districtwide assessments of achievement that are needed for the child to participate in the assessment, or reasons for excluding the child from assessment
- How the child's progress toward annual goals will be measured
- How the child's parents will be regularly informed of the child's progress toward annual goals and the extent to which the child's progress is sufficient to meet goals by the end of the year

Source: Data from U.S. Department of Education (USDOE). (2000). *A guide to the individualized education program*. Retrieved from http://www.ed.gov/parents/needs/speced/iepguide/index.htm; U.S. Department of Education. (2006). *Individualized education programs*. Retrieved from http://idea.ed.gov/explore/view/p/%2Croot%2Cdynamic%2CTopicalBrief%2C10%2C; Yell, M. L., Conroy, T., Katsiyannis, A., & Conroy, T. (2013). Individualized education programs and special education programming for students with disabilities in urban schools. *Fordham Urban Law Journal, 41*(2), 669–714.

advocacy role on behalf of individual students. However, school nurses are in a good position to educate the IEP team about specific interventions needed by children with medical conditions and ways to integrate those interventions into the school day.

Teachers will need to learn to identify specific health problems, such as increased respiratory effort in a child with asthma or sweating, and pallor and loss of concentration in a child with diabetes. The child's teachers become part of the child's safety net for rapid access to needed healthcare intervention. With support from the school administration and school nurse, teachers can learn about the child's condition and special care that may be needed during the school day, such as a snack for the child with diabetes, management of the child who has a seizure, and ways to reduce the spread of infection within the classroom.

THE CHILD'S RESPONSE TO ENTERING SCHOOL

Children with chronic conditions—whether the conditions cause minimal interference in the child's daily life or significant interference, such as dependence on technology—face certain challenges in the school setting. They may for the first time recognize differences between themselves and other children, such as appearance, abilities, social skills, or special treatment needs. Limitations in abilities may cause the child to be shy or embarrassed. Affected children may also be teased or bullied by other children because of their disability (Vessey & O'Neill, 2011).

Some children, particularly adolescents, may attempt to hide their condition or fail to adhere to necessary recommendations, such as dietary restrictions, to appear like their peers.

EDUCATION FOR CHILDREN WHO ARE MEDICALLY FRAGILE

Children who are medically fragile or technology assisted are also entitled to education and education services in the school setting. The parents and the school system must carefully consider the child's need for skilled supportive nursing care. Parents are often anxious about how well the child will be cared for by others during the school day. Risks for the child in the school setting include safety issues related to ventilators, tracheostomy, and medication therapy, as well as exposure to infectious diseases. The school administration must provide the personnel resources and equipment needed to ensure that care and a care provider are consistently available. Modifications to the school setting for the child, such as wheelchair ramps or an elevator, may be needed. Sometimes the child is placed in a classroom with healthy children, and the teacher is expected to monitor the child with a chronic condition and provide care as needed. Health aides may be assigned to provide care for one or more children with school nurse supervision. Some children are placed in classes composed of children with special healthcare needs where health aides are more available to provide needed care.

Nurses play a key role in assisting the family to understand that a teacher's primary responsibility is to teach, not to provide health care. The teacher is responsible for the health and safety of all children in the classroom. Parents need to have realistic expectations about the level of skilled support services that can be provided to a child who is medically fragile in a classroom. The need to balance the obligations for a child's special education services with the needs of all other children in a classroom can be a challenge for teachers and education leaders.

HOME SCHOOLING

The family of a child who is medically fragile or technology dependent may choose the option of home schooling the child, with resources provided through the school system. Home schooling may be used for all of the child's education or for periods when the child is experiencing exacerbations or more complications from the condition. The benefits of home schooling include continuity of education when the child would otherwise be unable to attend school and reductions in the child's stress and fatigue levels. Potential negative effects of home schooling include lack of peer and social interaction and decreased opportunity to develop social skills. The family that chooses home schooling needs to establish a routine for the education process.

TRANSITION TO ADULTHOOD

The number of adolescents with special healthcare needs transitioning to adulthood has increased as medical advances have increased life expectancy for many people with disabilities and chronic healthcare conditions (Oswald et al., 2013). Effective transition from pediatric-focused to adult-focused healthcare systems is essential in adolescents with these chronic health conditions (Huang et al., 2014). When their chronic condition could affect their future ability to work and live independently, customized transition planning is needed in preparation for adulthood and self-determination. A transition plan is developed in collaboration with the family based on the needs that have been identified in relation to the adolescent's goals for health care, employment, and community living. The plan should be individualized with psychosocial support provided to the adolescent during the transition planning and process (Oswald et al., 2013). Healthy & Ready to Work services may be particularly helpful to adolescents and families in planning for transition to adulthood (HRTW National Resource Center, 2014).

Clinical Reasoning Transitioning to Adulthood

Martin is a 17-year-old with sickle cell anemia. As he reaches adulthood, the need to transition from a pediatrician to an adult healthcare provider will arise. What factors should be taken into consideration in deciding when this healthcare transition should occur?

Professionalism in Practice Health Insurance Coverage

Health insurance helps to ensure that young adults have access to comprehensive healthcare services. The Patient Protection and Affordable Care Act of 2010 (PPACA) includes legislation that prevents denial of healthcare benefits based on preexisting conditions (Sorrell, 2012). This legislation also allows young adults to stay on their parents' insurance policies up to age 26 (Slive & Cramer, 2012). Nurses who work with adolescents with special healthcare needs should collaborate with the care coordinator, advanced practice nurse, physician, social worker, and other members of the healthcare team to facilitate a successful transition to adulthood without interruption in quality health care and health insurance coverage.

Home Care

Many families become the primary caregiver for the child with a chronic condition, assuming responsibility for assessment and treatment despite the level of skill and complexity involved in that care. The numerous benefits of home care include the promotion of health, well-being, and development for the child, decreased financial costs to health insurance companies and the healthcare system, and a sense of satisfaction to families when they are able to care for their child at home. The family faces numerous challenges for home care, including modification of the home. Management of the condition involves technologic support, medications, and treatment regimens, all potential necessities to maintain the child in the home. Family members must decide who has responsibility for different aspects of the child's care. Many families must also decide whether both spouses will continue to work or if one parent will stay home to care for the child. Home health nursing care may be needed if both parents continue to work or to cover the night shift so parents can sleep.

Moving the child who is chronically ill, or a technology-assisted child, to the home setting is a life-changing decision for the family and it must be done with collaboration between the family and the healthcare team. Preparation for the child's transition to the home requires that the family receive extensive training and instructions on the child's care. Management of the condition involves technologic support, medications and treatment regimens, and all potential necessities to maintain the child in the home.

This transition is often challenging and intimidating for the family who now must assume the role of independent caregiver for a child who may have been hospitalized for several months. Family members often feel unprepared to handle the complex situation of the chronic condition and/or technologic supports. They are at risk to develop **caregiver burden**, the unrelenting

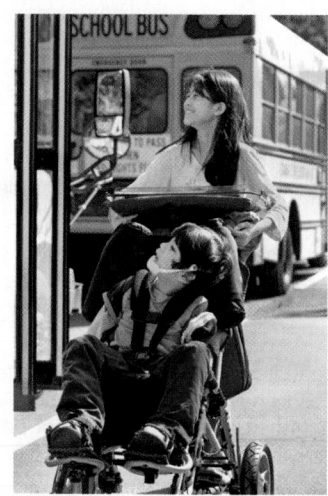

Figure 38–5 Daily caregiving demands of the child who is medically fragile continue 24 hours a day, 7 days a week. Parents need to identify ways to share the care of the child and other family care management. When the child lives with a single parent, additional healthcare resources are needed so the parent can sleep.

SOURCE: Jaren Jai Wicklund/Shutterstock.

pressure and anxiety related to providing daily care to a child with disabilities while meeting other family obligations. The family needs to be highly motivated and possess strength and resiliency factors to overcome the obstacles that will arise. These characteristics will help them be successful in assuming management responsibility for the child's care (Figure 38–5).

RESPITE CARE

Respite care is an important support service that involves caring for the child with a chronic condition while the parents take a short break away from the daily care. Whiting (2014) identified respite care as the greatest unmet need of parents of children with complex healthcare needs. Respite care may be provided by extended family, friends, or an agency, and may take place in the home or an area outside of the home. An example of respite might be skilled nursing care in a facility or the home so the family can have a weekend away. Assist the family in identifying respite care that meets the individual family's needs from the services available in the community. Many states have passed legislation for in-home family support services that include respite care. Because many respite services charge for their assistance, the family may require help in identifying respite waiver subsidies available to them. Reliable childcare and enrollment in school are other mechanisms for families to obtain respite care.

EMERGENCY PREPAREDNESS

Advance planning is needed to ensure that medically fragile children who require technology for survival or have the potential for life-threatening episodes have the necessary resources in the event of a disaster. The designated shelter for such children, with health professionals and electrical power for the needed equipment, should be identified and known to the family. In the meantime, battery packs for power backup should be available at all times. Additionally, parents need to arrange for durable power of attorney so that consent for emergency medical care can be available as needed. The child and parents may become separated during the disaster, or the parents may become injured and unable to care for the child. Refer to Chapter 37 for more information related to emergency preparedness.

Focus Your Study

- A chronic condition is a long-term, ongoing condition that is expected to last 3 months or more and may involve functional limitations, developmental disorders, behavioral issues, anatomic problems, and limb dysfunction or require special medications, a special diet, or more healthcare services than a healthy child would require.

- Approximately 14.6 million children in the United States have special healthcare needs related to a chronic condition.

- Chronic conditions can occur as a result of a genetic condition, congenital anomaly, injury during fetal development or at birth, complication of care after birth, serious infection, or significant injury.

- Children who are medically fragile are dependent on a medical device for survival or prevention of further disability.

- A developmental delay results when there is failure to achieve anticipated milestones during specific developmental stages.

- Families with children experiencing a chronic condition need to make lifestyle adjustments, ensuring a baseline of care that helps maintain the child's health status and promotes growth and development.

- Siblings of the child with a chronic illness may have feelings of jealousy, anger, depression, guilt, resentment, worry, and anxiety.

- The time of diagnosis is one of the most stressful times for families of children with chronic conditions as the parents wait anxiously for the outcome of diagnostic procedures. Other times associated with significant stressors for the family include developmental milestones, school entry, adolescence, and planning for the transition to adult health and vocational services.

- Moving the child with a chronic illness who is dependent on technology to the home setting is a life-changing decision for the family, and it must be done with collaboration between the family and the healthcare team.

- Caregiver burden is the unrelenting pressure and anxiety related to providing daily care to a child with disabilities while meeting other family obligations.

- The financial burden of caring for a child with special health-care needs is significant even when the family has health insurance.

- Sending the child to school has several benefits for the child and family, including socialization for the child beyond the immediate family and respite for parents.

- An individualized education plan (IEP) is developed for a child with cognitive, motor, social, or communication impairments who needs special education services in the school setting. An individualized health plan (IHP) is developed for the child with medical conditions that need to be managed within the school setting.

- All children, including those with chronic conditions and special healthcare needs, are entitled by federal law to a free education that is matched to their developmental and functional capabilities.

- An individualized transition plan (ITP) is developed for adolescents with a chronic condition in collaboration with the family to assist in identifying appropriate support programs, living arrangements, and employment for adult life.

- Children with chronic health conditions require regular health promotion, health screening, and health maintenance care, as well as specialized health services to assist the child and family in management of the condition.

- The role of the nurse in caring for the child with a chronic condition includes providing health supervision from infancy to transition into adulthood, collaborating with the multidisciplinary healthcare team, partnering with the family to manage the child's care at home, referring the family to appropriate community services, assisting with planning for education services, promoting positive parenting behaviors and psychosocial adaptation and well-being of the child and family, and promoting growth and development of siblings.

- Nurses who specialize in caring for children with complex chronic conditions may experience compassion fatigue as they continue their efforts to meet the ongoing needs of these families.

Clinical Reasoning in Action

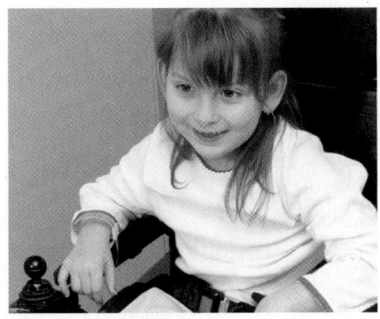

Haley is an 8-year-old child with cerebral palsy who will be attending school for the first time. Her mother had initially preferred home schooling for Haley and now wants to support her social development with other children. A case manager is asked to assist with facilitating Haley's entry into school. The case manager coordinates a multidisciplinary meeting of the clinic nurse, physical therapist, physician, and Haley's family to review her health status and to discuss the transition to school.

They also discuss potential accommodations needed for Haley's mobility limitations. The multidisciplinary team assists the parents in developing a plan for Haley's transition to school.

1. What role will the clinic nurse and case manager have in helping develop Haley's IEP and IHP?

2. What role will the school nurse have with the child, caregivers, teacher, and classmates during the facilitation of school entry?

3. What actions will the mother need to take in preparing the school personnel for Haley's health needs?

4. Haley's 10-year-old sister attends the same school. What effects of Haley's entry into school might the sibling experience?

References

Aita, M., Johnston, C., Goulet, C., Oberlander, T. F., & Snider, L. (2013). Intervention minimizing preterm infants' exposure to NICU light and noise. *Clinical Nursing Research, 22*(3), 337–358.

American Academy of Pediatrics. (2012). *Care delivery management.* Retrieved from http://www.medicalhomeinfo.org/how/care_delivery/

Caley, L. (2012). Risk and protective factors associated with stress in mothers whose children are enrolled in early intervention services. *Journal of Pediatric Health Care, 26*(5), 346–355.

Child and Adolescent Health Measurement Initiative. (2012). *National survey of children with special health care needs (NS-CSHCN 2009/10).* Retrieved from http://www.childhealthdata.org

Data Resource Center for Child & Adolescent Health. (2012). *Who are children with special health care needs?* Retrieved from http://childhealthdata.org/docs/nsch-docs/whoarecshcn_revised_07b-pdf.pdf

Fleary, S. A., & Heffer, R. W. (2013). Impact of growing up with a chronically ill sibling on well siblings' late adolescent functioning. *ISRN Family Medicine, 2013,* 1–8.

Goodman, R. A., Posner, S. F., Huang, E. S., Parekh, A. K., & Kokh, H. K. (2013). Defining and measuring chronic conditions: Imperatives for research, policy, program, and practice. *Preventing Chronic Disease, 10*(April 25). doi: http://dx.doi.org/10.5888/pcd10.120239

HRTW National Resource Center. (2014). *Systems and services.* Retrieved from http://www.syntiro.org/hrtw/systems/index.html

Huang, J. S., Terrones, L., Tompane, T., Dillon, G., Pian, M., Gottschalk, M., . . . Bartholomew, K. (2014). Preparing adolescents with chronic disease for transition to adult care: A technology program. *Pediatrics, 133*(6), e1639–e1646.

Kennedy, A. P. (2011) Systematic ethnography of school-age children with bleeding disorders and other chronic illnesses: Exploring children's perceptions of partnership roles in family-centred care of their chronic illness. *Child: Care, Health & Development, 38*(6), 863–869.

Kim, D., & Samples, E. (2013). Comparing individual healthcare plans and Section 504 plans: School districts' obligation to determine eligibility for students with health related conditions. *Urban Lawyer, 45*(1), 263–279.

Lawson, K. A., Bloom, S. R., Sadof, M., Stille, C., & Perrin, J. M. (2011). Care coordination for children with special health care needs: Evaluation of a state experiment. *Maternal Child Health Journal, 15,* 993–1000.

Looman, W. S., Presler, E., Erickson, M. M., Garwick, A. W, Cady, R. G., Kelly, A. M., & Finkelstein, S. M. (2013). Care coordination for children with complex special health care needs: The value of the advanced practice nurse's enhanced scope of knowledge and practice. *Journal of Pediatric Health Care, 27*(4), 293–303.

Miles, M. S., Holditch-Davis, D., Burchinal, M. R., & Brunssen, S. (2011). Maternal role attainment with medically fragile infants: Part 1. Measurement and correlates during the first year of life. *Research in Nursing and Health, 34,* 20–34.

Nielsen, K. M., Mandleco, B., Roper, S. O., Cox, A., Dyches, T., & Marshall, E. S. (2012). Parental perceptions of sibling relationships in families rearing a child with a chronic condition. *Journal of Pediatric Nursing, 27*(1), 34–43.

Oswald, D. P., Gilles, D. L., Cannady, M. S., Wenzel, D. B. Willis, J. H., & Bodurtha, J. N. (2013). Youth with special health care needs: Transition to adult health care services. *Maternal Child Health Journal, 17,* 1744–1752.

Pacer Center. (2012). *Preparing for transition from early intervention to an individualized education program.* Retrieved from http://www.pacer.org/parent/php/php-c158.pdf

Petitgout, J. M., Pelzer, D. E., McConkey, S. A., & Hanrahan, K. (2013). Development of a hospital-based care coordination program for children with special health care needs. *Journal of Pediatric Health Care, 27*(6), 419–425.

Project Ideal. (2013). *Special education public policy.* Retrieved from http://www.projectidealonline.org/v/special-education-public-policy/

Slive, L., & Cramer, R. (2012). Health reform and the preservation of confidential health care for young adults. *Journal of Law, Medicine & Ethics, 40*(2), 383–390.

Sorrell, J. (2012) Ethics: The Patient Protection and Affordable Care Act: Ethical perspectives in 21st century health care. *OJIN: The Online Journal of Issues in Nursing, 18*(1). Retrieved from http://www.nursingworld.org/MainMenuCategories/ANAMarketplace/ANAPeriodicals/OJIN/Columns/Ethics/Patient-Protection-and-Affordable-Care-Act-Ethical-Perspectives.html

Taylor, A., Lizzi, M., Marx, A., Chilkatowsky, M., Trachtenberg, S. W., & Ogle, S. (2012). Implementing a care coordination program for children with special health-care needs: Partnering with families and providers. *Journal for Healthcare Quality, 35*(5), 70–77.

Toomey, S. L., Chien, A. T., Elliott, M. N., Ratner, J., & Schuster, M. A. (2013). Disparities in unmet need for care coordination: The National Survey of Children's Health. *Pediatrics, 131*(2), 217–223.

U.S. Department of Education (USDOE). (2000). *A guide to the individualized education program.* Retrieved from http://www.ed.gov/parents/needs/speced/iepguide/index.htm

U.S. Department of Education (USDOE). (2006). *Individualized education programs.* Retrieved from http://idea.ed.gov/explore/view/p/%2Croot%2Cdynamic%2CTopicalBrief%2C10%2C.

U.S. Department of Education (USDOE). (2011). *Q and A: Questions and answers on secondary transition.* Retrieved from http://idea.ed.gov/explore/view/p/%2Croot%2Cdynamic%2CQaCorner%2C10%2C

U.S. Department of Health and Human Services (USD-HHS). (2015). *Healthy People 2020.* Retrieved http://www.healthypeople.gov/2020/topicsobjectives2020/default.aspx

U.S. Department of Health and Human Services, Health Resources and Services Administration (USDHHS/HRSA). (2011). *Children with special health care needs in context: A portrait of states and the nation 2007.* Rockville, MD: Author.

University of Michigan Health System. (2014). *Children with chronic conditions.* Retrieved from http://www.med.umich.edu/yourchild/topics/chronic.htm

Vermaes, P. R, van Susante, A. M. J., & van Bakel, H. J. A. (2012). Psychological functioning of siblings in families of children with chronic health conditions. *Journal of Pediatric Psychology, 37*(2), 166–184.

Vessey, J. A., & O'Neill, K. M. (2011). Helping students with disabilities better address teasing and bullying situations: A MASNRN study. *The Journal of School Nursing, 27*(2), 139–148.

Whiting, M. (2014). Support requirements of parents caring for a child with disability and complex health needs. *Nursing Children and Young People, 26*(4), 24–27.

Yell, M. L., Conroy, T., Katsiyannis, A., & Conroy, T. (2013). Individualized education programs and special education programming for students with disabilities in urban schools. *Fordham Urban Law Journal, 41*(2), 669–714.

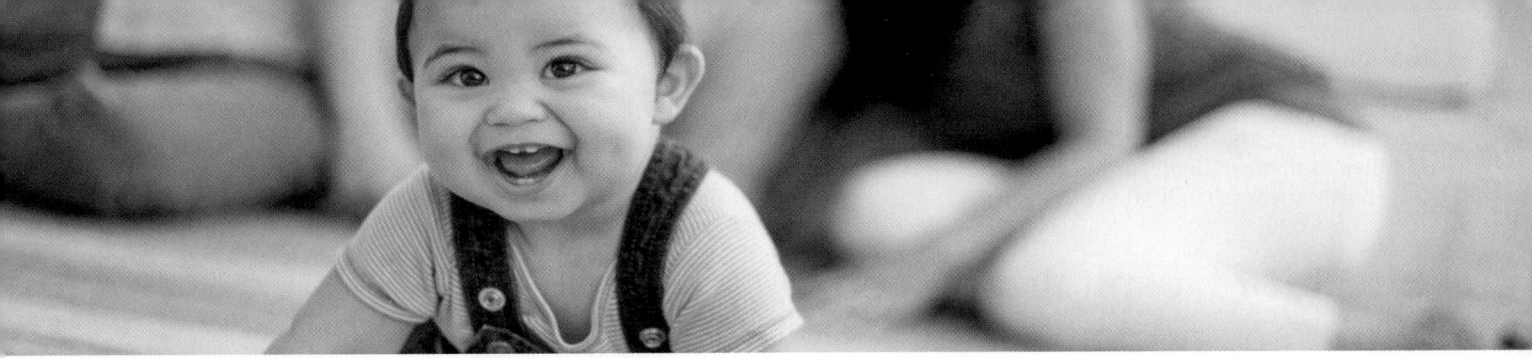

Chapter 39
Nursing Considerations for the Hospitalized Child

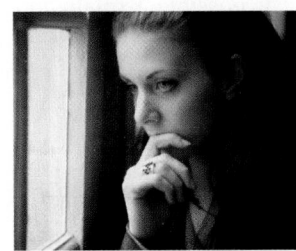

Mel Curtis/Getty Images

We live 50 miles from the hospital and have three other children. We were worried about how we were going to be able to stay with Sabrina. She's only 4, and it's her first time in the hospital. Fortunately, they have beds for parents, so one of us can always be by her side throughout her procedure and recuperation.

—Mother of Sabrina, 4 years old

⌄ Learning Outcomes

39.1 Compare and contrast the child's understanding of health and illness according to the child's developmental level.

39.2 Explain the effect of hospitalization on the child and family.

39.3 Describe the child's and family's adaption to hospitalization.

39.4 Apply family-centered care principles to the hospital setting.

39.5 Identify nursing strategies to minimize the stressors related to hospitalization.

39.6 Integrate the concept of family presence during procedures and nursing strategies used to prepare the family.

39.7 Summarize strategies for preparing children and families for discharge from the hospital setting.

Hospitalization, whether it is elective, planned in advance, or the result of an emergency or trauma, is stressful for children of all ages and their families. Because most pediatric conditions can be managed within the home and community, hospitalization is not always required to manage the child with an illness. Additionally, many pediatric surgical procedures are being performed on an outpatient basis. However, for children who are hospitalized, the illness acuity is frequently high. Because of advances in medical technology in recent years, children with complex medical conditions have improved survival rates, resulting in an increase in the rate of chronically ill children who require frequent and sometimes long-term hospitalization (LeGrow, Hodnett, Stremler, et al., 2014).

Hospitalized children experience a variety of emotions because they are in an unknown environment, surrounded by strangers, unfamiliar equipment, and frightening sights and sounds. These children are subjected to unfamiliar procedures, some of which are invasive or painful and may even require surgery. For both children and families, routines are disrupted and normal coping strategies are tested.

Nurses today are challenged to provide individualized care for the hospitalized child with complex medical conditions, acute illnesses, or injury. As a key aspect of that role, nurses must address the psychosocial and developmental concerns that accompany hospitalization. (Developmental theorists and stages are presented in Chapter 31.) To minimize the stress of hospitalization, nurses provide support and education to children and their families before, during, and after hospitalization.

During hospitalization, nurses use a family-centered approach and work collaboratively with parents to implement various strategies that promote coping and adaptation and to prepare children for necessary procedures. Nurses also collaborate with members of a multidisciplinary team and partner with families to prepare them for discharge home or transfer to a long-term care or rehabilitation facility.

Effects of Hospitalization on Children and Their Families

Children's Understanding of Health and Illness

Can you remember as a child thinking that yelling at your mother caused your strep throat? Young children have limited knowledge about the body and its relation to health and illness. They do not understand what causes them to get sick. Their understanding is based primarily on their cognitive ability at various developmental stages and on previous experiences with healthcare professionals. As children become older, they develop a more accurate understanding of illness. For example, perhaps as an adolescent you believed that you would never become ill or have an accident; or maybe you feared being in a car crash like that of a friend. Knowledge of a child's understanding of health and illness is essential in assisting a child to adapt to the hospital experience.

Hospitalization and the accompanying medical procedures are very stressful for children, especially very young children such as toddlers and preschoolers. The child's attempts to deal with these stressors impact both the psychologic and physiologic well-being of the child. Infants, toddlers, and preschoolers lack the cognitive skills to understand hospitalization and are the age groups most likely to exhibit regressive behaviors. Young children have fears and anxieties related to things such as the dark, strangers, and monsters. A hospital's unfamiliar environment can exacerbate those anxieties. Significant stressors for hospitalized children include:

- Separation from parents, the primary caretaker, or peers
- Loss of self-control, autonomy, and privacy
- Painful and/or invasive procedures
- Fear of bodily injury and disfigurement

Nursing care of the hospitalized child focuses on minimizing the child's fears, anxieties, and disruption of the child's usual routine, and supporting the family through the stressful experience. Strategies include minimizing separation anxiety, loss of control, pain related to procedures, and fear. Table 39–1 highlights key stressors of hospitalization for children at each developmental stage.

INFANT

By about 6 months of age, infants have developed an awareness of themselves as separate from their mothers or fathers. They are able to identify primary caretakers and to feel anxious when in contact with strangers. Hospitalization can be a traumatic time for an infant, particularly if the parents are not staying with the child. Infants can sense the anxiety their parents are experiencing during a hospitalization.

Common stressors to the infant include painful procedures, immobilization of extremities, and the sleep deprivation caused by the disruption of the infant's normal sleep patterns and routines. However, the most common stressor of hospitalization for the infant is separation from parents, which is manifested by **separation anxiety**. Characteristic behaviors of children in

the three phases of separation anxiety are listed in Table 39–2. Infants and toddlers between 6 and 19 months of age who are hospitalized often display some of these behaviors, particularly if parents are unable to remain with the child. In addition to separation anxiety, children between 6 and 18 months of age may display **stranger anxiety** (wariness of strangers) when confronted with unfamiliar healthcare professionals. See *Evidence-Based Practice: Anxiety and Fears in Children Related to Hospitalization and Surgery.*

Encourage family members to be active participants in the care of the hospitalized infant through touch, sight, and sound. Infants get satisfaction from meeting their oral needs, so parents and nurses should provide sources for oral stimulation, such as pacifiers and age-appropriate teething toys. The infant should be rocked and touched with light stroking to provide tactile stimulation for developmental growth. However, minimize excessive noise and prolonged stimuli to allow the infant periods of rest.

Encourage parents to stay with the hospitalized infant. If family members are unable to remain at the hospital, encourage them to visit their infant as often as possible. Explain and emphasize the importance of parent–newborn attachment and bonding to the parents.

Clinical Tip

Children encounter many members of the healthcare team, in addition to other hospital personnel, when hospitalized. Children ages 6 to 18 months perceive these people as strangers and may cry when someone new enters the room. As the child sees a person over and over again, the stranger anxiety for that person subsides. Providing consistent nursing staff as much as possible will limit the number of "strangers" that the child encounters while hospitalized.

TODDLER

Toddlers are the group most at risk for a stressful experience as a result of illness and hospitalization. This age group is old enough to understand that their routine has been disrupted, but they do not understand why. Separation from parents is the major stressor, and toddlers protest vigorously when their parents depart. When one or both parents cannot be present, they can leave mementos to comfort the child. These might include an object belonging to a parent, a picture, or an audiotape or videotape with messages from the parents.

Disruption of routine also causes stress for the toddler. The nurse encourages parents to remain present as much as possible for important rituals such as toileting, carrying out bedtime routines, and singing favorite nursery rhymes. Autonomy is the developmental task of the toddler (see Chapter 31). Having their activities limited and being confined especially threaten children in this age group. When possible, maintain the toddler's normal home routines for bathing and other activities. Offer the toddler choices when possible, such as choosing the color of Jell-O or which gown/pajamas to wear.

Clinical Tip

Toddlers may challenge a nurse by refusing to cooperate with treatments and procedures, including physical assessments. To diffuse such confrontations, encourage cooperation by offering the toddler some sense of control. For example, a nurse might let the child handle the stethoscope first before listening to the child's heart.

TABLE 39–1 Stressors of Hospitalization for Children at Various Developmental Stages

DEVELOPMENTAL STAGES AND STRESSORS	RESPONSES	NURSING MANAGEMENT
INFANT Separation anxiety Stranger anxiety Painful, invasive procedures Immobilization Sleep deprivation, sensory overload	Sleep–wake cycle disrupted. Feeding routines disrupted. Displays excessive irritability.	Encourage parental presence. Adhere to infant's home routine as much as possible. Utilize topical anesthetics or preprocedural sedation as prescribed (see Chapter 40). Promote a quiet environment and reduce excess stimuli.
TODDLER Separation anxiety Loss of self-control Immobilization Painful, invasive procedures Bodily injury or mutilation Fear of the dark	Cries if parents leave the bedside. Is frightened if forced to lie supine. Wonders why parents do not come to the rescue. Associates pain with punishment.	Encourage parental presence. Allow parents to hold child in their lap for examinations and procedures when possible. Allow choices when possible. Utilize topical anesthetics or preprocedural sedation as prescribed. Explain all procedures using simple developmentally appropriate language. Provide a night-light.
PRESCHOOLER Separation anxiety and fear of abandonment Loss of self-control Bodily injury or mutilation Painful, invasive procedures Fear of the dark and monsters	Displays difficulty separating reality from fantasy. Fears ghosts and monsters. Fears body parts will leak out when skin is not intact. Fears that tubes are permanent. Demonstrates withdrawal, projection, aggression, regression.	Encourage parental presence. Allow choices when possible. Utilize topical anesthetics or preprocedural sedation as prescribed. Explain all procedures. Provide a night-light or flashlight.
SCHOOL-AGE CHILD Loss of control Loss of privacy and control over bodily functions Bodily injury Separation from family and friends Painful, invasive procedures Fear of death	Displays increased sensitivity to the environment. Demonstrates detailed recall of events to self and other patients.	Encourage parental participation. Allow the child choices when possible. Explain all procedures and offer reassurance. Utilize topical anesthetics or preprocedural sedation as prescribed. Encourage peer interaction via Internet, phone calls, and other methods of communication.
ADOLESCENT Loss of control Fear of altered body image, disfigurement, disability, and death Separation from peer group Loss of privacy and identity	Displays denial, regression, withdrawal, intellectualization, projection, displacement.	Include the adolescent in the plan of care. Encourage discussion of fears and anxieties. Explain all procedures. Ask the adolescent about the desire for parental involvement. Encourage peer interaction.

TABLE 39–2 Stages of Separation Anxiety

PROTEST	DESPAIR	DENIAL (DETACHMENT)
Screaming, crying	Sadness	Lack of protest when parents leave
Clinging to parents	Quiet, appear to have "settled in"	Appearance of being happy and content with everyone
May resist attempts by other adults to comfort them	Withdrawal or compliant behavior	Show interest in surroundings
	Crying when parents return	Close relationships not established

Clinical Question

What fears do children experience related to hospitalization and surgery, and how do they best express them?

The Evidence

In the past several years, many research studies have focused on the child's response to procedures and hospitalization and how best to prepare children of different ages. Recent studies have focused specifically on the child's fears related to this experience, how they express those fears, and how nurses can provide support.

A study by Salmela, Aronen, and Salanterä (2011) examined how children experience fears related to the hospital in 90 children ages 4 to 6. The children were interviewed in either a kindergarten classroom or hospital setting. Interviews were semistructured and accompanied by pictures of a fairy-tale figure in a hospital setting. The main fears identified were those related to nursing interventions and pain, separation from parents and being alone, lack of information, and equipment and instruments. The children described their fears in a variety of ways, including verbally expressing the fear, shouting, crying, fooling around, downplaying the fear, or expressing the fear in a picture or in their surroundings. The meanings of the hospital-related fears were grouped into four categories: insecurity, being injured, helplessness, and rejection.

Wilson, Megel, Enenbach, et al. (2010) explored the views of 93 children ages 5 to 9 related to hospitalization. Both hospitalized and never-hospitalized children were included in the study. The Barton Hospital Picture Test, a tool consisting of eight drawings related to situations that occur in the hospital, was shown to the children. The children were asked to tell a story about the pictures. The main theme that emerged from the stories was fear of being alone. Other feelings included being scared, mad, sad, bored, and lonely. The stories also indicated that the children wanted to be protected from uncertainty and scary things, and they wanted companions because they were not at home.

Karlsson, Rydström, Enskär, et al. (2014) discussed fears of children related to needle-related medical procedures and described the experience of nurses providing support during these procedures. The study utilized video-recorded observations of 20 needle-related medical procedures with follow-up interviews with a nurse. Fourteen different nurses took part in the study, which was conducted in both inpatient and outpatient settings. The interviewers asked the nurses about their experiences supporting children during needle-related medical procedures. Findings of the study indicated that children experience needle-related medical procedures in a variety of ways, and that it is essential to assess each child and their ability to cope, taking into account their age, developmental level, and previous experiences.

Six components of supportive actions were identified in the study, including developing relationships through conversation with both the parent and the child and being sensitive to the body language expressed by the child and the parents.

Another component was identified as balancing between tact and use of restraint. This sometimes involved the use of preparation and play to distract the child, but at times, the child needed to be restrained in order to complete the procedure.

Being an advocate for the child was an additional supportive action identified. While parents are generally the primary advocate for children during procedures, the nurse may take on this primary role if the parent is unable to do so.

Adjusting time is a component that refers to the need for nurses to give the child the right amount of time for the procedure, including time for the child to become familiar with the environment.

The final component of support identified in the study was maintaining belief, which referred to giving hope and courage prior to the procedure and praising the child afterwards. This might entail the use of the words "brave" and "good" and the opportunity for the child to look in the gift box prior to the procedure.

Best Practice

Research demonstrates that children have fears related to health care and hospitalization. These fears vary among children of different ages and those in well settings versus the hospital setting. Children fear medical staff, equipment, instruments, pain, procedures, and needles, and they fear being left alone. Policies that provide open visitation for parents and include them in the care of the child will decrease fears related to being alone. Therapeutic nursing interventions that provide developmentally psychosocial care and education to hospitalized children is essential to decrease fear and anxiety related to staff and procedures.

Clinical Reasoning

How can children in school settings be prepared for future encounters with health care? Describe policies that promote parental presence for hospitalized children. How can fears related to medical staff, equipment, instruments, pain, procedures, and needles be reduced in hospitalized children?

PRESCHOOLER

The greatest stressors for preschoolers are their fears: fear of being alone, fear of being in the dark, fear of abandonment, fear of loss of self-control related to the body and emotions, and fear of bodily injury or mutilation. Preschoolers may also feel guilty about being sick, or they may view illness and hospitalization as punishment.

Similar to the toddler, preschoolers desire a normal routine, and the nurse can partner with the family to maintain routines as much as possible. Developmentally, preschoolers exhibit a sense of initiative (see Chapter 31) as they explore the world around them. To promote that initiative, the nurse can encourage the preschool child's independence by offering choices such as, "Do you want to take the red medicine or the purple medicine first?"

Parents should be encouraged to stay with the child if possible. For those who cannot stay, preschoolers need to know when to expect their parents to return to the hospital. Because most preschoolers lack a conception of time measurements like "2 hours," "half-past 4," or "3 o'clock," respond with simpler statements of time, such as "after supper" or "before breakfast." Encourage parents to make telephone calls to the preschooler if possible. Some parents are able to make calls from work.

Preschoolers get a sense of security from hearing their parent's voice confirming that the parent will return to the hospital.

Parents often believe it is better to leave the hospital room after their child has fallen asleep, as their departure will not stress the child. In fact, the opposite is true. If a child awakens to find the parent gone unexpectedly, the child may become anxious and may develop a lack of trust. Instead, encourage parents to tell their child when they need to leave and why (e.g., has to go to work or go home). By providing honest information to the child, parents or caregivers demonstrate that they can be trusted.

SCHOOL-AGE CHILD

The school-age child relies on parents and others for support and understanding during stressful events and procedures. Although school-age children attempt to maintain their composure during painful or invasive procedures, generally they still require a great deal of support. Major sources of stress for hospitalized school-age children include:

- Loss of control related to bodily functions
- Privacy issues
- Fear of bodily injury, pain, and concerns related to death
- Separation anxiety from family and friends

School-age children understand concepts, so parents who cannot remain at the bedside are encouraged to tell the child what time they will return and to let them know if the time changes. Parents are encouraged to be available for telephone calls to provide support and comfort to their child. Stressful procedures can lead to regression or other behavioral changes, although this is less likely than with younger patients. Inform the parents that this behavior is normal during stressful situations.

Developmentally, school-age children exhibit a sense of industry (see Chapter 31), taking pride in their achievements at home, at school, and in sports. To foster that sense of industry, allow children to participate in their care as much as possible. Encourage them to continue with schoolwork and engage in creative outlets such as art or crafts.

Growth and Development

School-age children between the ages of 5 and 8 years believe that the internal body consists mainly of a heart and bones. They view the digestive system as having two parts, the mouth and the stomach. Showing them how parts of the body are related can be helpful to enhance their understanding. However, young adolescents, ages 11 to 13 years, can describe the location and function of major body parts such as the brain, nose, eyes, heart, and stomach. However, they usually have gaps in understanding and may have misconceptions, so evaluating their knowledge is a part of the nursing plan in order to plan teaching to meet their knowledge needs.

ADOLESCENT

Preoccupation with appearance and body image are paramount in this age group. By offering education and explanations that focus on these issues, nurses can provide significant reassurance to the adolescent. Nevertheless, adolescents often try to maintain independence and rigid self-control when undergoing painful and invasive procedures. Because hospitalization may increase dependence on their parents, adolescents may respond with frustration and anger. The nurse who respects the adolescent's desire for privacy and independence is often successful in establishing a trusting relationship and assisting the adolescent to cope with the hospitalization and illness. Encourage the adolescent to discuss thoughts and feelings about experiences. Careful listening by the nurse is essential for establishing a positive rapport.

Major stressors for hospitalized adolescents include:

- Loss of independence, control, and privacy
- Fear of bodily injury or changes in body image
- Fear of disability, pain, and even death
- Separation from peers, home, and school

Adolescents are in the process of establishing their identity and becoming independent of their parents' influence, so control over aspects of their care is important. Partner with the family and multidisciplinary team to ensure that the adolescent is an active participant in decisions and the plan of care. Privacy and modesty are major concerns, as adolescents' physical characteristics are rapidly changing. To demonstrate respect for their feelings, knock on the door before entering and ask permission before conducting assessments or other procedures. By allowing choices in clothing, hair, and music, the nurse can acknowledge the importance of the adolescent's self-image.

The peer group is a major influence in adolescents' lives. Allowing flexible visiting hours for friends helps teens maintain their social network and provides needed support. When friends are not able to visit, providing teens with Internet access provides a means of accessing their friends for support. Encouraging participation in recreation and teen lounge facilities available during hospitalization provides the adolescent with additional peer group support opportunities.

Family Responses to Hospitalization

The illness and hospitalization of a child disrupt a family's usual routines. Parental roles change when the child is hospitalized and care is being provided by nursing staff. Roles may be altered as one parent stays at the hospital with the child while the other parent or siblings take on additional tasks at home. Family members may experience anxiety and fear, especially when the outcome is unknown or a potentially serious health condition prompted the hospitalization.

Family members' ability to cope can be challenged by a serious emergency, lengthy illness, chronic condition, poor prognosis, lack of family support, and lack of financial or community services. The stress on parents can be compounded by the burden of missed work, additional expenses, and concerns about feeding and caring for children at home. (See Chapter 41 for a description of nursing support for the child with life-threatening illness or injury.) Stress interferes with the parents' ability to provide support to the hospitalized child (Agazio & Buckley, 2012).

It is essential that nurses assess parental needs and attend to those needs in order to establish a trusting relationship. Parents who have support from nursing staff have less anxiety and more self-confidence, and are better equipped to make decisions and participate in their child's care.

Nurses also need to be alert to family members' cultural views about health, illness, and the causation of illness, which can influence their response to hospitalization and the family's management of the experience. Cultural influences may also determine which family member is the decision maker regarding healthcare practices, and provide guidelines for acceptable treatments.

The siblings of a hospitalized child may receive little attention from the parents who are overwhelmed and anxious about their hospitalized child's health. How siblings respond depends on their developmental level and ability to understand what is going on. Younger siblings who do not understand the causes of illness and hospitalization may feel guilty about fighting with or being mean to their brother or sister in the past. Some siblings may fear becoming ill themselves. Some may believe that they played a role in the child's illness or injury and need reassurance that they did not cause it. If the sibling did in some way contribute to the illness or injury, help that child to cope with the guilt by providing an opportunity to discuss these feelings. Siblings often have nightmares about the illness or injury their brother or sister has sustained and about the ill child dying (see Chapter 41).

As hospitalization causes family roles and routines to change, siblings may feel insecure and anxious. Education and support for siblings of hospitalized children promotes coping and adaptation to a sibling's illness.

As appropriate, encourage siblings to visit. Such a visit is especially encouraged if the child could potentially die, as it allows the sibling the opportunity to say good-bye. (See Chapter 41 for further discussion of the dying child.) These visits often help to improve the mood of the hospitalized child and assist the sibling to overcome misconceptions or negative emotions. Because children's fantasies are often worse than reality, unfounded fears may be relieved by a visit.

Before the visit, prepare the siblings by explaining what they will likely encounter. Describe the hospital environment, including equipment, sounds, and smells. Describe how the ill brother or sister will appear. If the hospitalized child acts, moves, talks, or appears differently than before the hospitalization, provide an explanation beforehand. A child-life specialist may be involved with this preparation (see specific information related to this role later in the chapter). Consider using a doll, drawing pictures, or showing an actual photograph of the hospitalized child to help prepare the siblings. (See *Teaching Highlights: Strategies for Working With the Sibling of a Hospitalized Child*.)

During the visit, demonstrate how to talk to and touch the ill child and encourage the siblings to do the same. After the visit, discuss with siblings what they saw and felt, and answer any questions they may have. When a sibling cannot visit, contact with the hospitalized child can be maintained by sending pictures, drawings, cards, and messages recorded on iPods or other electronic devices, and through email, instant messaging, or webcam. Partner with the family to determine the most appropriate and effective method of communicating if the sibling is unable to visit. If parents are staying at the hospital with the hospitalized child, partner with them to help establish communication routines for the well siblings. For example,

encourage the parents to call the siblings at home at a regular time each night. Allowing the siblings at home the opportunity to share their day, and to receive an update on the hospitalized child, provides a feeling of connectedness and may minimize feelings of worry and resentment. The phone call offers siblings a consistent link to the parent and the reassurance that they are important and loved.

Family Assessment

To support the hospitalized child and provide family-centered care, nurses develop an understanding of the family dynamics and individualize the nursing care according to the needs of the child and family. To develop a plan of care that involves all family members, the nurse assesses the impact of the child's illness or hospitalization on the family. Table 39–3 provides a list of questions to guide the nurse in determining the roles of family, knowledge of family, support systems, and effects on siblings. (See Chapter 37 for further discussion of family assessment.)

Collaborate with the family to determine their resources, such as:

- Coping strategies of family members
- Financial resources
- Access to health care
- Availability of community services

One family with limited financial support may manage quite well because they have effective coping strategies, whereas another family with greater financial resources may have difficulty if their coping strategies are ineffective. Staying with a hospitalized child can be a financial drain for parents if one or both must take a leave of absence from work, miss scheduled workdays, or travel to the hospital. Additional expenses may include hotel rooms, meals, parking fees, and child care for other children. Assess the family's ability to manage these additional expenses. To evaluate the burden of hospitalization, use a multidisciplinary approach, which may lead to increased access to community resources and support for families.

Assess the family dynamics by evaluating:

- The quality of communication
- Methods of coping with stress
- Risk factors
- Sources of strength

TEACHING HIGHLIGHTS | Strategies for Working With the Sibling of a Hospitalized Child

The nurse working with siblings of a hospitalized child can implement the following strategies to assist the siblings in understanding what is happening to their brother or sister:

- *Be truthful.* Explain why the child is hospitalized, what the treatment involves, and how long the hospitalization is expected to last.
- *Assure siblings that they did not cause the illness and that the hospitalized child did nothing wrong.* If a sibling had some involvement in or responsibility for the health crisis, referral for mental health counseling may be needed.
- *Allow siblings to ask questions and discuss fears and other feelings.*
- *Encourage siblings to visit if possible.* Cover tubes and wires with a sheet. Wash off blood or cover bloody bandages if possible. Prepare the siblings for any equipment, dressing, and procedures they might see and any sounds they might hear.
- *Warn siblings if the hospitalized child is not speaking.* Say something like, "John can't talk now. He seems to be sleeping deeply. He may be able to hear, though, so you can touch him and talk to him."
- *Encourage siblings to express their feelings related to the disruptive effect of the child's hospitalization on family life.*

TABLE 39–3 Family Assessment

FAMILY ROLES

- What changes will the child's illness create in the family?
- Will household tasks need to be reallocated?
- What specific burdens will be placed on family members?
- Will one parent stay with the child or spend a great deal of time in the hospital?
- Will one parent or guardian be primarily responsible for communicating with other family members?

KNOWLEDGE

- What knowledge does the family have about the child's condition and treatment? Does the family need further information?
- How quickly can discharge planning and teaching begin?

SUPPORT SYSTEMS

- Does the child or family have health insurance? What percentage of costs will it cover? Will other financial support be needed? Will costs continue for ongoing care after hospitalization? If so, will existing health insurance cover those costs?
- Are close friends or family available to provide care for other children, assist with family tasks, or help in other ways?
- Are there community services such as support groups, camps for children with disabilities, education sessions, or equipment and financial resources to which the nurses can refer the family?

SIBLINGS

- Have siblings been informed of the ill child's condition and the expected outcome?
- Have they been reassured that they did not cause the illness?
- Do they understand the change in roles and family routines?
- Are they able to visit the ill child?
- Have their teachers been informed of the family stress?
- If the hospitalized child's life is threatened, are the siblings involved in a plan to promote coping?

Common sources of strength and support include friends and relatives, religious leaders, hospital chaplains, and social workers.

Examine how the family has dealt with the health needs of the child if the child has been hospitalized or required home care in the past. (See *Developing Cultural Competence: Supporting Alternative Health Practices*.) Determine the family members' level of understanding related to the child's hospitalization and anticipated therapy. Collaborate with family members to determine their desired role in the child's care. Assess the family's needs for referral to family service agencies or other community organizations that may be required. Evaluate the need for support groups or agencies that provide medical equipment or other assistance.

Developing Cultural Competence Supporting
Alternative Health Practices

Many cultural groups, such as Asians, African Americans, Europeans, Hispanics, and American Indians, may continue to use their traditional healthcare practices (Spector, 2013). They may not share this information with nurses or healthcare providers, both out of respect and in fear that they will be told not to use these methods. Recognizing and supporting use of traditional practices along with Western medicine can promote health and provide comfort for children and families. Ask the families about the use of traditional, complementary, or alternative therapies. Examples include herbal remedies, healers, acupuncture, prayer, and hot and cold foods.

Teaching the child and family, providing support, and referring them to community resources are key elements in providing family-centered care. Additional resources available for the child and family include social workers, child and family mental health professionals, and advanced practice nurses. Additionally, hospital programs and parent support groups are available to assist families in coping with a child's illness.

Nurse's Role in the Child's Adaptation to Hospitalization

Hospitalization of the child may be planned or unexpected. A child may be hospitalized for any of the following reasons:

- The child develops an acute illness or exacerbation of chronic illness.
- The child requires diagnostic or treatment procedures or requires elective surgery.
- The child who was previously healthy suffers an injury, necessitating unexpected hospitalization.

Planned Hospitalization

When hospitalization is planned, both children and their parents have time to prepare for the experience. Assess the family's knowledge and expectations and then provide information about likely experiences. A variety of approaches can be used to provide information and allay fears:

- Tours of the hospital unit or surgical area are helpful. This activity assists the child and family to become familiar with the environment they will encounter. During tours,

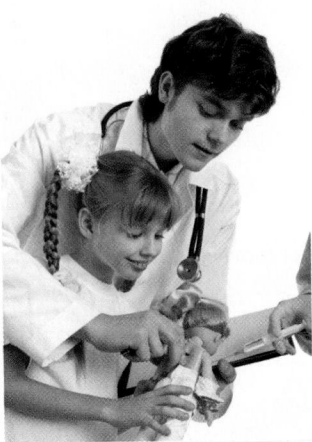

Figure 39–1 The child's anxiety and fear often will be reduced if the nurse explains what is going to happen and demonstrates how the procedure will be done by using a doll. Based on your experience, can you list five things you can do to prepare a school-age child for hospitalization?

SOURCE: Poznyakov/Shutterstock.

preschoolers and school-age children can see and handle items with which they will come in contact. If a tour is not possible, photographs or a DVD can be used to demonstrate the medical setting and procedures.

- The surgical team's attire is less frightening if the child has a chance to try it on and engage in play while wearing the attire.
- Medical equipment is not as frightening when the child learns what it does and observes how it is used, for example, through demonstration on a doll (Figure 39–1).
- Puppets and skits can be used to help explain procedures to children.
- Offer health fairs, as many hospitals do, to explain health procedures to children. During a tour, while hospitalized, or at home, the child can be exposed to books or media that explain in age-appropriate terms what to expect during various procedures.
- Reinforce teaching through coloring books or other educational materials.

Different approaches may be more effective in helping adolescents prepare for hospitalization. In addition to written materials, models, and DVDs, adolescents also learn from talking with peers who have had similar experiences. To demonstrate respect for their sense of independence and privacy, offer adolescents an opportunity to ask questions without their parents present.

Include the family in preparing the child of any age for hospitalization. Parents can be instrumental in preparing a child for hospitalization by reviewing material presented, being available to answer questions, and being truthful and supportive (Tables 39–4 and 39–5).

Unexpected Hospitalization

An unanticipated admission places the child at emotional risk for several reasons, including:

- Lack of preparation for the experience
- Uncertainty and unpredictability of events that follow

TABLE 39–4 Parental Preparation of Children for Hospitalization

The nurse can assist the parents in preparing the child for hospitalization by suggesting the following interventions:

- Read stories to the child about the experience. Numerous books and pamphlets are available (see Table 39–5).
- Talk about going to the hospital, what it will be like. Talk about coming home.
- Encourage the child to ask questions about the hospital and surgery.
- Encourage the child to draw pictures of what the hospital will be like.
- Visit the hospital unit before hospitalization if possible.
- Let the child touch or see equipment if possible.
- Provide a doctor or nurse kit for the child to play with.
- Provide clothing so the child can dress up like a nurse or healthcare provider if desired.
- Plan for support via parents' presence, telephone calls, special items belonging to the parents that child can keep during the stay.
- Be honest.

- Unfamiliarity of the environment
- Heightened anxiety of the child's parents

An admission for exacerbation of a disease, such as cystic fibrosis or leukemia, can provoke feelings of depression or hopelessness. See Chapter 38 for information related to coping with chronic illness.

Assist the child and family who are not prepared for hospital admission to adapt to the experience by orienting them to the environment, providing an opportunity for questions, offering truthful responses, and explaining all procedures and expectations. Discuss the anticipated plan of care for the child and involve the family in the child's care. Give the family an opportunity to express their fears and concerns. Refer to social services and/or parent support groups if additional support is needed.

TABLE 39–5 Examples of Children's Books Regarding Hospitalization

The Berenstain Bears Go to the Doctor, by S. Berenstain & B. Berenstain

Clifford Visits the Hospital, by N. Bridwell

Corduroy Goes to the Doctor, by D. Freeman & L. McCue

Curious George Goes to the Hospital, by M. Rey & H. A. Rey

Do I Have to Go to the Hospital? A First Look at Going to the Hospital, by P. Thomas

Franklin Goes to the Hospital, by P. Bourgeois & B. Clark

Going to the Hospital, First Experiences, by M. Bates

Lions Aren't Scared of Shots: A Story for Children About Visiting the Doctor, by H. J. Bennett & M. S. Weber

Nursing Care of the Hospitalized Child

Family-centered nursing care of the hospitalized child focuses on promoting the child's and family's coping strategies to deal with the stressors of hospitalization, promoting optimal development and safety and minimizing disruption of the child's usual routine as much as possible.

Special Units and Types of Care

Children admitted to a hospital may be cared for in one or more of the following units: general pediatric unit, short-stay unit, outpatient unit, ambulatory surgical unit, emergency department, or pediatric intensive care unit. Hospitalized children may require surgical treatment involving preoperative and postoperative care. Children with infectious diseases require isolation precautions. Other children may need rehabilitative care to achieve or restore maximum potential.

GENERAL PEDIATRIC CARE UNIT

Smaller facilities typically incorporate all pediatric care specialties in one unit or area, whereas larger medical centers and children's hospitals have separate medical units for different specialties. Specialized units may include medical and/ or surgical units, orthopedic units, oncology units, mental health units, and units specific to developmental levels (e.g., adolescent unit). Admission to a specialized unit may be the result of an acute condition, such as pneumonia or trauma, or the result of an exacerbation of a chronic condition, such as asthma. Other causes for admission include surgical procedures requiring longer than a 24-hour stay and the need for inpatient treatments and services. Nursing care for regular hospital admission includes orienting the child and family to the unit and procedures, adhering to the child's normal routine as much as possible, including both the child and the family in the decision-making process, providing direct care to the child, promoting a safe environment for the child, and promoting the child's growth and developmental needs.

SHORT-STAY, OUTPATIENT, AND AMBULATORY SURGICAL UNITS

Hospital stays for children have generally become short, with many procedures being performed in outpatient units such as minor surgery (in ambulatory surgical centers), diagnostic tests (such as cardiac catheterizations), radiology studies requiring sedation, and treatments (such as chemotherapy). The child may be admitted in the morning and discharged that afternoon. In addition, children who have potentially serious illnesses may be placed on a short-stay or observation unit for monitoring or limited treatment, after which medical staff decide either to hospitalize the child for additional treatment or, if improvement occurs, to discharge the child. These short stays are considered beneficial primarily because they cause minimal disruption of family patterns and are cost effective for the institution, health insurance company, and family. Nurses assist parents to prepare the child properly for planned admissions, monitor the child during the procedures, encourage family participation in care, and keep families well informed (Table 39–6).

Nursing care of the child in short-stay, outpatient, and ambulatory surgical units is the same as for regular hospital admission. However, time for teaching is compressed, requiring the nurse to implement teaching methods in a minimal amount of time to ensure the family understands discharge instructions.

TABLE 39–6 Nursing Considerations When Preparing Parents and Child for Planned Short-Stay Admission

- Are there special requirements prior to arrival, such as not being permitted food or drink or needing extra fluid intake?
- At what time and where must the child arrive?
- Are any special forms, insurance numbers, or previous records needed?
- How long will the child stay in the hospital?
- Can the child bring something familiar from home such as a blanket or stuffed animal?
- Are parents expected or encouraged to be with the child or stay in the health facility?
- Is there a chance the child may need to remain longer than expected?
- What will the child's condition be for discharge home?
- Will special equipment or care be needed?
- What symptoms can indicate problems?
- Where can the family go or whom can they call in case of problems or questions?

Effective teaching methods on this accelerated schedule include demonstration, videos, pamphlets with verbal review, and informal teaching sessions.

EMERGENCY CARE

When a child is brought to an emergency department, the parents are usually frightened and insecure and may even be in a state of shock. The fast pace and critical nature of the unit creates an atmosphere in which parents are hesitant to ask questions and are anxious about the outcome. Many factors can contribute to the parents' anxiety and stress (see Chapter 41), including the unexpected nature of the situation; uncertainties

---

Clinical Reasoning Preparing Children for Hospitalization or Short-Stay Surgery

Six-year-old Kate has had several nosebleeds and fainting spells recently. After examination by her healthcare provider and a number of diagnostic studies such as chest x-ray examination, echocardiography, and electrocardiography, coarctation of the aorta is diagnosed. Kate will come in this week for a cardiac catheterization. She is scheduled to have open heart surgery in 2 weeks.

Kate has had few health problems, and her experiences with healthcare professionals are limited. Her parents, who are anxious about the heart surgery, are concerned about how their daughter will adapt to hospitalization.

How should you prepare Kate for the cardiac catheterization and later for the surgery? Include knowledge of her developmental stages and cognitive understanding in your planned intervention approaches. How far in advance should teaching take place? What teaching aids are helpful? How can Kate's parents be involved in and reinforce the teaching? What kind of support do her parents, siblings, and friends need during hospitalization?

Professionalism in Practice Parental Presence During Procedures and Resuscitation

Emergency Nurses Association (ENA) (2012) recommends that family members be allowed to be at the bedside during invasive procedures and resuscitation following the written policy of the institution. The clinical practice guideline developed by the ENA recommends that a healthcare professional be designated for explanations and support for the family. During development of the guideline, research by the ENA concluded that family presence during invasive procedures and resuscitation is not detrimental to the patient, family, or healthcare professionals. The ENA also concluded that development of a written policy can provide some structure and support for the healthcare team.

Parents who wish to remain with a child even during invasive procedures or resuscitation efforts should be allowed to do so. The nurse collaborates with the family members to determine their desired presence in critical situations and keeps them informed about the health care provided.

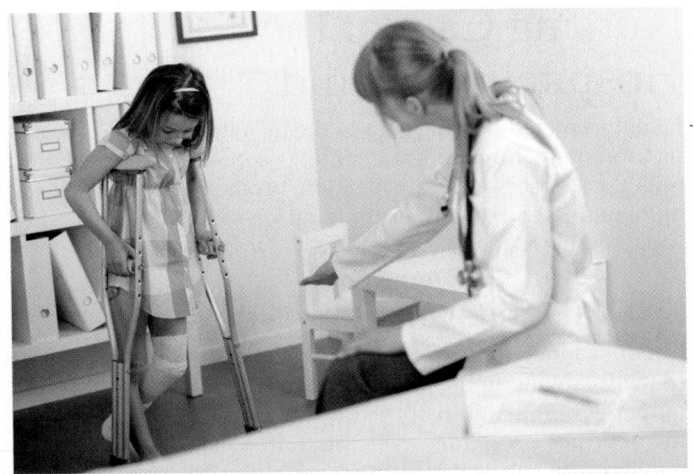

Figure 39–2 Rehabilitation units provide an opportunity for the child to relearn tasks like walking and climbing stairs. They provide an important transition from hospital to home community.

SOURCE: CandyBox Images/Shutterstock.

in the emergency environment; the necessity for quick decision making; the need for numerous procedures, tests, and treatments; and fear of pain. The nurse keeps both the child and the family informed about what is being done and when more news may be available. The parents and child are encouraged to remain together as much as possible (see Chapter 41).

INTENSIVE CARE UNIT

Intensive care units provide nursing care to infants and children, including children with life-threatening illnesses and injuries, acute exacerbations of chronic illness (such as severe or life-threatening asthma exacerbation), or any other condition requiring advanced support and continuous monitoring (see Chapter 41). Parents of a critically ill or injured child admitted to the pediatric intensive care unit (PICU) experience high levels of stress (Ames, Rennick, & Baillargeon, 2011). They are likely to be anxious, particularly since the child's condition may be severe and the prognosis may be guarded. The unfamiliar equipment may create an atmosphere of fear or anxiety. Numerous healthcare professionals work in the intensive care environment, and without effective and open communication, parents may not know whom to question or even what questions to ask. Partner with the family and encourage them to write down their questions and direct them to the appropriate source if you are unable to answer the question.

ISOLATION

Children who require isolation to prevent spread of infection may experience lack of stimulation due to limited contact with other children and visitors. Frequent family visits are important and should be encouraged. Family members may be reluctant to wear protective garments either out of fear of using them incorrectly or because they believe they are unnecessary. The nurse ensures that the family understands the reason for isolation and any special procedures. Having contact with and holding the child are encouraged when possible.

REHABILITATION

Rehabilitation is the process of assisting a child with physical or mental challenges to reach full potential through therapy

and education. Rehabilitation units provide children with ongoing care and support to continue recovery beyond the initial period of illness or injury (Figure 39–2). These may be separate units within a hospital or independent centers. The objective of rehabilitation is to assist children with physical, psychosocial, or educational challenges to reach their fullest potential and to promote achievement of developmentally appropriate skills. Collaboration with a multidisciplinary team including parental involvement is essential.

Parental Involvement and Parental Presence

Family members are essential to the child's care during illness. Integrity of the family unit is fostered through parental involvement during the child's hospital stay. Involvement provides parents with control and a feeling that they are active participants in their child's progress, and it also prepares the family for care that will be required when the child goes home. The child benefits greatly from parental presence and participation and experiences less emotional distress and anxiety if the parents are present (see *Developing Cultural Competence: Support Systems*). If the parent–child attachment remains uninterrupted, the child experiences fewer behavioral maladjustments.

A positive relationship between the parents and the healthcare team is an essential component of family-centered care. Parental satisfaction is enhanced when parents' questions about their child's care and condition are answered; when the healthcare team is kind, caring, and takes experiences of parents seriously; and when prompt and consistent care is provided (Fisher & Broome, 2011). Parents need to feel valued. Romaniuk, O'Mara, and Akhtar-Danesh (2014) found a significant difference in parents' desires to participate in their child's care and their actual level of participation. Parents indicated that they wanted to be more involved in the care of their child, especially in activities related to being an advocate for their child. The nurse should partner with the family to determine the extent to which parents desire to be involved in the child's care.

PREPARATION FOR PROCEDURES

Hospitalized children may experience numerous procedures during hospitalization, from collection of urine or blood specimens to lumbar punctures and surgery. Fear of the unknown increases the child's anxiety. Maintain a positive attitude when preparing the child and reassure the child that it is normal to be frightened of unknown experiences. Special techniques can help the child to understand and cope with feelings about these procedures. Techniques used to prepare the child depend on developmental age, coping abilities, and previous experience.

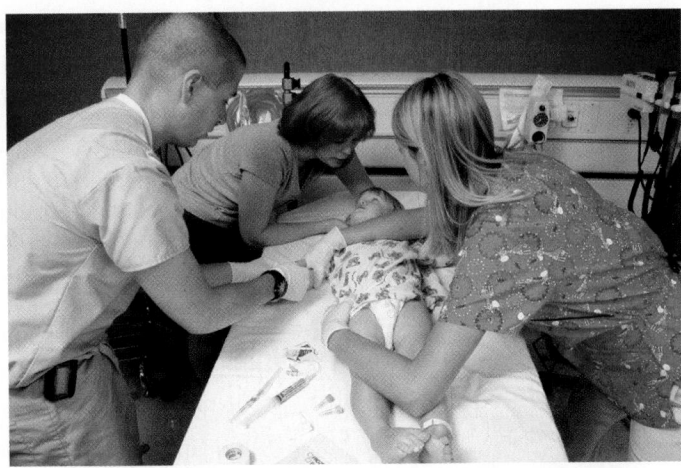

Figure 39–3 Health facility policies that permit parents to be present during a procedure performed on their child are an example of a family-centered care policy. The parent plays an important role in providing security and comfort to this child who is having blood drawn.

Developing Cultural Competence Support Systems

Culture can have a significant influence on health beliefs and practices. For example, Mexican Americans view family as a strong support. Extended family may want to be with a hospitalized child. The father of the child is often the spokesperson, and mothers commonly are influential in decisions regarding child health care. The nurse should incorporate all the people the family wishes to have present in the hospital and include them in explanations about health care.

PSYCHOLOGIC PREPARATION

Preparation may begin a few moments to several days before the procedure, depending on the child's age and developmental level. In providing sensitive care to the child, nurses assume that a procedure can potentially be traumatic for the child. Even providing urine in a specimen cup or undergoing radiologic examination can be frightening if the child does not understand the reason for the procedure or know what to expect. Administration of medication can also make the child frustrated or anxious. When preparing the child for medication administration using techniques appropriate to the developmental level of the child, the nurse ensures that the medication is safely given (see Table 39–7).

Use developmentally appropriate techniques to assess the child's knowledge and feelings about an upcoming procedure. For example, with a school-age child, the nurse might explain the procedure using drawings, stories, body outline dolls, anatomically correct dolls, and conversation. When assessing the child's perception about procedures, the nurse should consider the following:

- Does the child know the purpose of the procedure?
- Has the child experienced this procedure before? If so, was the experience painful, frightening, or reassuring?
- What does the child think will happen? Are the child's beliefs accurate?
- Is the procedure painful?
- What techniques does the child use to gain control in challenging situations?
- Will the parents or other caregiver be present to provide support?

When explaining a procedure and its purpose, use words that the child understands. Older children require explanations geared to their cognitive level and previous experiences. They will want to know what is happening, why, and what they can do to cope during the procedure (see Table 39–8).

For adolescents, provide written information, DVDs, and other available media. Schedule time for questions and discussions. Allow adolescents to make choices about their own health care when possible. For example, ask them to make those choices with questions such as, "Do you want your hand numbed for the IV start?" Maintain a positive attitude when preparing the adolescent and reassure them that it is normal to be frightened of unknown experiences.

Parental presence can provide comfort and support to the child during procedures. Parents should be allowed to choose whether they want to stay for the procedure (Figure 39–3). Some parents may feel that they will be too upset to support the child; many choose to stay. Some adolescents want their parents to be involved in their care; others prefer to minimize their parents' roles. Partner with the adolescents to ensure that their wishes are known regarding parental presence.

PHYSICAL PREPARATION

Physical preparation depends on the age of the child and the procedure. Preprocedural sedation may be required. If sedation is required, the child will not be able to have anything by mouth (NPO) for a period of time. Young infants might be provided sucrose for procedures (see Chapter 40 for pain management). Procedural checklists are often utilized.

Performing the Procedure

Procedures on young children are generally performed in a **treatment room** (a room designated for performing treatments such as intravenous starts, blood draws, and lumbar punctures) to promote the children's sense of security that their own room is a "safe" and relatively pain-free site unless this is contraindicated, such as in the presence of skeletal traction or isolation. Older children can be given the option of having a procedure performed in the treatment room or in their own hospital room. Older school-age children and adolescents may prefer to remain in their room for the procedure.

Perform the procedure as quickly and efficiently as possible. If the parents wish to participate, ask them to hold the

TABLE 39–7 Variations in Medication Administration to Children

ROUTE	DEVELOPMENTAL CONSIDERATIONS	TECHNIQUES
Oral	Children under 5 years cannot generally swallow pills and capsules. Children may not want to take medicine.	• Medications are usually given in liquid form (e.g., elixir, syrup, or suspension). • Sometimes tablets are crushed or capsules are opened and mixed with a small amount of food. Check with pharmacy to be sure this does not inactivate the drug. Never crush enteric-coated or timed-release medicine. • When choosing a vehicle for crushed tablets, use only 1 spoonful of applesauce, pudding, jelly, or similar food or 1–2 mL of liquid so that it is easier to ensure that the entire dose will be taken. • Use an oral syringe to increase accuracy when administering a liquid medication. • Position young children upright to avoid choking and aspiration. • Give liquid medicines slowly by oral syringe (for infants) aimed at the inside of the cheek or by medicine cup (for toddlers and preschoolers) for drinking. • Communicate with the child that you expect that the medicine will be taken. Let children choose the type of fluid to drink after, but do not ask if they will take their medicine now.
Rectal	Colon is small in size.	• Lubricate the tip of the suppository before placement. • Place the suppository at the rectal opening and advance past the sphincter. • For children younger than 3 years, the nurse's gloved fifth finger is used for insertion. After this age, the index finger can usually be used.
Ophthalmic and otic	Young children may be fearful of medicines placed in the eyes or ears.	• Adequate immobilization is needed to avoid injury. • The nurse's hand can be stabilized by resting the wrist on the child's head. • Explanations and therapeutic play can be used with children old enough to explain the process of administration. • Have medication at room temperature.
Topical	Skin of infants is thin and fragile.	• Only prescribed doses and medicines appropriate for young children should be used on the skin. • Covering the area or keeping the child's hands occupied may be necessary to ensure adequate contact of medication with the skin.
Intramuscular	Anatomy and physiology of children differ from those of adults.	• The gluteus maximus muscle (dorsal gluteal site) is not recommended in children because of danger of injury to the sciatic nerve (Tschudy & Arcara, 2011). • The vastus lateralis site is preferred for children. • The deltoid muscle is rarely used in young children except for the small amounts injected in some vaccines. • Amounts to be administered should be limited to no more than 1–2 mL for ventrogluteal and vastus lateralis sites and 0.5 mL for deltoid depending on muscle size. Refer to the *Clinical Skills Manual* SKILLS for illustrations. • Z-track technique (retracting tissue to the side and releasing it after injection to prevent seepage into tissue) is often used.
Intravenous	Veins are small and fragile. Fluid balance is critical.	• Careful maintenance of sites is needed. • Common infusion sites include hands and feet, although scalp veins are sometimes used in infants. • Infusion pumps require frequent monitoring. • Syringe pumps are often used to administer medications when minimal fluid is to be given. • Central lines are commonly used for long-term intravenous medication therapy.

Note: See *Clinical Skills Manual for Maternity and Pediatric Nursing, Fifth Edition,* for further medication administration techniques. See Appendix E for information related to how drug dosages are determined for children.

Source: Bindler, R. C., Ball, J. W., London, M. L., & Davidson, M. R. (2017). *Clinical skills manual for maternity and pediatric nursing* (5th ed.). Hoboken, NJ: Pearson.

child's hand or stand close by for comfort. Utilize nursing staff instead of parents to immobilize the child as needed. The parents, or another nurse, can be designated to support the child by means of a gentle touch, talking, singing, giving reassurance, or illustrating stress-reduction techniques.

After the procedure, no matter how the child responded, the child should be praised. A choice of reward often soothes the young child. If the procedure is performed in a treatment room, the child is returned to the room for comfort and reassurance.

TABLE 39–8 Assisting Children Through Procedures

DEVELOPMENTAL STAGE	BEFORE PROCEDURE	DURING PROCEDURE
Infant	None for infant. Explain to parents the procedure, the reason for it, and their role. Allow parents the option of being present for procedures. Parents may be able to touch a foot, rub a cheek, and talk soothingly to the infant.	• Nursing staff should immobilize the infant securely and gently. Parents should not be asked to hold the child down. • Perform procedure quickly. Use touch, voice, pacifier, and bottle as distractions. • Ask parent to hold, rock, and sing to infant after procedure.
Toddler	Give explanation just before procedure, since toddler's concept of time is limited. Explain that child did nothing wrong; the procedure is simply necessary.	• Perform in treatment room. • Nursing staff should immobilize the child securely. • Give short explanations and directions in a positive manner. • Avoid giving choices when none is available. For example, "We are going to do this now" is better than "Is it okay to do this now?" • Allow child to cry or scream. • Comfort child after procedure. Give child a choice of favorite drink, if allowed, or special sticker.
Preschool child	Give simple explanations of procedure. Basic drawings may be useful. While providing supervision, allow the child to touch and play with equipment to be used, if possible. Since any entry into the body is viewed as a threat, state that the child's body will remain the same, and use adhesive bandages to reassure the child that the body is intact and parts will not "fall out."	• Perform in treatment room. Nursing staff should immobilize the child securely. • Give short explanations and directions in a positive manner. Encourage control by having the child count to 10 or spell name. • Allow child to cry. Give positive feedback for cooperation and getting through procedure. • Encourage the child to draw afterward to explore the experience.
School-age child	Clear, thorough explanations are helpful. Use drawings, pictures, books, and contact with equipment. Teach stress-reduction techniques such as deep breathing and visualization. Offer a choice of reward after procedure is completed.	• Be ready to immobilize the child if needed. Allow child to remain in position by self if child is able to be still. • Explain throughout procedure what is happening. • Facilitate use of stress-control techniques. • Praise cooperative efforts.
Adolescent	Give clear explanations orally and in writing. Teach stress-reduction techniques. Explore fear of certain procedures, such as staple removal or venipuncture.	• Assist adolescent in self-control. Assist with use of stress-control techniques. • Explain expected outcome and tell when results of test will be completed.

Refer to Chapter 40 for discussion of pain management and sedation for procedures.

Preparation for Surgery

A child's surgical experience may be elective, planned in advance, or the result of an emergency or trauma. How a child responds to the experience is related to the psychologic and physical preparation the child receives. Preoperative preparation, including familiarization with the environment and equipment and explaining surgical procedure, can decrease anxiety in both the child and the parent (Healy, 2013). The accompanying *Nursing Care Plan* provides information related to care of the child undergoing surgery. Additional nursing diagnoses include (NANDA-I © 2014):

• *Infection, Risk for*, related to exposure to hospital-acquired infection
• *Injury, Risk for*, related to exposure to hospital-acquired infection and use of preoperative medication
• *Skin Integrity, Impaired*, related to disruption of skin surface and limited mobility after surgery
• *Constipation, Risk for*, related to surgical procedure and anesthetics
• *Fluid Volume: Imbalanced, Risk for*, related to intravenous infusion and NPO status
• *Gas Exchange, Impaired*, related to anesthetics and pain

Nursing Care Plan: The Child Undergoing Surgery

1. Nursing Diagnosis: *Knowledge, Deficient*, related to preoperative and postoperative events (NANDA-I © 2014)

GOAL: The child and family will acquire knowledge related to the operation.

INTERVENTION	RATIONALE
• Ask questions of the parent and child about surgery.	• Prior knowledge and understanding can be reinforced and used to guide your presentation.
• Teach about preoperative and postoperative events using appropriate developmental methods such as dolls, drawings, stories, and tours.	• Developmental level determines the cognitive approach that works best for teaching.
• Reinforce information the family has received about the purpose of surgery.	• The healthcare provider may have explained operation.
• Have the children demonstrate postoperative events that pertain to their care such as deep breathing, putting bandage on doll, taping intravenous line on doll, and pressing patient-controlled analgesia button.	• Concrete experience promotes learning.
• Allow the parents and child to ask questions.	• Learners must have opportunity to ask questions.

EXPECTED OUTCOME: Child and family will be able to verbalize details about expected preoperative and postoperative events. They will ask questions that demonstrate understanding. Child will demonstrate skills needed in the postoperative period.

2. Nursing Diagnosis: *Anxiety* related to planned surgery (NANDA-I © 2014)

GOAL: The child and family will show decreased behavior indicating anxiety.

INTERVENTION	RATIONALE
• Question the child about expectations of hospitalization and previous experiences.	• Previous experiences can influence present anxiety level.
• Orient the child to the hospital setting, routines, staff, and other patients.	• Familiarity with the setting and people can decrease anxiety by removing unknown factors.
• Institute age-appropriate play and interactions with the child.	• Play can increase trust level and decrease anxiety.
• Explain procedures and prepare for those that might cause trauma. Encourage parents to support the child.	• The child is more likely to trust healthcare providers if they are truthful and if parents are present.
• Allow the parents and child to ask questions.	• Questioning provides an opportunity to explain the unknown, which decreases anxiety.

EXPECTED OUTCOME: Child and family will demonstrate less anxiety. They will verbalize understanding and comfort in hospital routines. Parents will support the child during traumatic procedures.

3. Nursing Diagnosis: *Pain, Acute*, related to surgical procedure (NANDA-I © 2014)

GOAL: The child will maintain an adequate comfort level.

INTERVENTION	RATIONALE
• Assess behavioral cues (e.g., crying, movement, guarding ability to participate in activities of daily living).	• Behavior of preverbal children provides clues to pain experience.
• Use an appropriate pain assessment tool for verbal and nonverbal children.	• An age-appropriate pain assessment tool allows verbal children to quantify the amount of pain. Pain assessment tools designed for nonverbal children allow the nurse to quantify the amount of pain when the child cannot provide a self-report. (See Chapter 40 for descriptions of a variety of pain assessment tools.)
• Administer prescribed pain medications around the clock.	• Narcotics and nonnarcotic analgesics alter pain perception.
• Use age-appropriate nonpharmacologic methods of pain control (e.g., distraction, repositioning, massage).	• Nonpharmacologic interventions interfere with pain perception and may decrease the child's anxiety.

EXPECTED OUTCOME: Child's pain will be controlled as demonstrated by a low number on the pain assessment tool (behavioral or verbal).

4. Nursing Diagnosis: *Knowledge, Deficient*, related to care at home (NANDA-I © 2014)

GOAL: The child and family will verbalize self-care required at home.

INTERVENTION	RATIONALE
• Provide oral and written home care instructions regarding surgical wound care, medications, activities, and diet.	• Teaching regarding home care is necessary early in hospitalization.
• Provide a number to call for questions or concerns. Instruct on follow-up visits.	• Parents need to know emergency information and that follow-up care is required.

EXPECTED OUTCOME: Child and family will demonstrate skills needed for home care following discharge. They will verbalize plans for future care.

PREOPERATIVE CARE

Preoperative care of the child includes both psychosocial and physical preparation for surgery. The goal of preoperative teaching is to reduce the fear associated with the unknown and decrease stress and anxiety associated with surgery.

Psychosocial Preparation.   Preoperative teaching is geared to the child's developmental level. If child-life specialists are available, they can play an important role in preparing the child for surgery. When the child will be transferred to an intensive care unit or recovery room after surgery, a visit to the area before surgery can reduce the fear and anxiety associated with waking up in a strange environment filled with frightening sights, sounds, and smells. The use of DVDs, body outline dolls, anatomically correct puppets and dolls, drawings, and models is encouraged to teach the child about the surgical procedure (Figure 39–4). Playing with stethoscopes, gowns, masks, and syringes without needles also helps the child feel more in control (see discussion about dramatic play later in this chapter). Children are reassured that their parents can accompany them to the operating room floor and will be waiting when they awaken from surgery. Parents should be allowed to carry infants and young toddlers to the pediatric holding area or have them ride

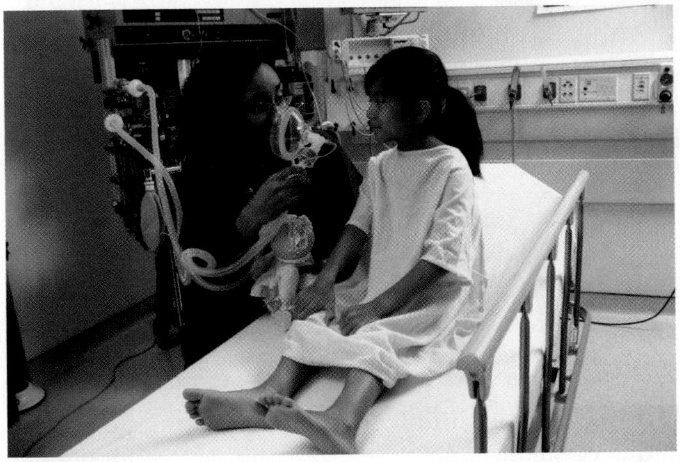

Figure 39–4 Showing young school-age children equipment that will be used in surgery will help to decrease anxiety related to the unknown. What are other methods the nurse can use to teach young school-age children about surgery?

in one parent's lap in a wheelchair. Older toddlers and preschoolers should be allowed to ride in a special wagon if possible. Special teddy bears and blankets are generally allowed in the preoperative holding area and provide comfort to the child. The nurse should make sure that the item is labeled with the child's name. Prepare family members for what to anticipate and what is expected of them. Explain the purpose of special equipment such as intravenous setups and monitoring devices. In some hospitals, only one or two immediate family members are allowed to visit the child at one time. Visitors may be required to wear special gowns, shoes, or hats, and they may be restricted to certain areas.

Parental Presence During Anesthesia Induction.   Many hospitals now allow parents to be present with their child during anesthesia induction and again in the postanesthesia recovery area. Parents often want to support their child before and immediately after a surgical procedure, and their presence offers reassurance and comfort to the child. The decision to allow parents to be present during anesthesia induction must be made on an individual basis. The nurse explains expectations, such as surgical gown, cap, shoe covers, and the parent's role during induction. The nurse offers the parents an opportunity to ask questions and voice concerns.

Physical Preparation.   Preparation for surgery may occur in designated preoperative areas. Procedures generally conducted in preoperative areas include premedication, intravenous start (if not performed following general anesthesia), and preparation of the surgical site. If urinary catheterization is necessary, it is usually not performed until the child has been anesthetized.

Preoperative procedures and guidelines vary among hospitals and outpatient surgical centers. Preoperative checklists, such as the sample shown in Table 39–9, are used in ambulatory and acute care settings to ensure proper physical preparation of patients for surgery. Weigh the preoperative child accurately, measure vital signs, and ask about last fluid intake amount and type. Monitor urinary output. NPO status in an infant and young child is distressing to both the child and the parents. Reinforce teaching regarding necessary NPO status and provide support to the family as needed.

Nursing management during the preoperative period includes establishing accurate baseline data, administering prescribed fluids, and performing assessments of fluid status. When an intravenous infusion is prescribed, start the infusion (see the *Clinical Skills Manual* SKILLS), ensuring that the type of fluid and flow rate match those that are ordered and that would be expected for the weight of the child.

TABLE 39–9 Preoperative Checklist

_____	Check that consent forms are witnessed and signed and in the patient's chart.
_____	Be sure the child's name band is in place.
_____	Be sure any allergies are prominently noted in the child's chart and on a special name band.
_____	Remove any prosthetic devices, including orthodontic appliances and body piercings.
_____	Check the child's mouth for loose teeth and tongue piercings.
_____	Remove eyeglasses, jewelry, and nail polish.
_____	Bathe and cleanse the operative site if ordered.
_____	Put the child in a hospital gown, allowing the child to wear underwear.
_____	Check that all special tests have been completed and the results are in the child's chart.
_____	Have the child void before surgery.
_____	Keep the child NPO before surgery.
_____	Give the child prescribed medications.
_____	Check vital signs and record on chart.
_____	Transport the child safely to the operating room.

Of necessity, the young child who undergoes surgery usually is restricted from consuming oral foods and fluids just before, during, and for a period after surgery, thus creating a risk of fluid imbalance. The length of time the child is kept without oral intake before surgery varies. Recommendations from the American Society of Anesthesiologists indicate that clear liquids may be given up until 2 hours before surgery, breast milk until 4 hours before surgery, and infant formula 6 hours before. Milk and a light meal may be consumed up until 6 hours before surgery (American Society of Anesthesiologists, Committee on Standards and Practice Parameters, 2011).

Infants will generally have very specific orders related to what time they should be made NPO for breast milk, formula, and clear liquids. This time will depend on what time the infant is scheduled for surgery. Because children beyond infancy do not usually eat or drink during the night, orders are usually written for NPO after midnight. However, if surgery is not scheduled for the morning, more specific orders should be written, especially for the toddler and preschool-age child, who will not be as tolerant of an extended NPO status. The ultimate decision on how long the child is NPO lies with the anesthesiologist. Sometimes, because of emergencies, planned surgeries for infants and young children may be postponed for several hours. These children are NPO and generally do not have IV access. What action should the nurse take in this case?

POSTOPERATIVE CARE

Postoperative care of the child includes both physical and psychologic care. In the immediate postoperative period, the nurse should perform baseline monitoring of vital signs according to hospital protocol, maintain effective airway clearance and monitor for evidence of respiratory depression or distress (see Chapter 46), evaluate the child's level of consciousness, evaluate the surgical site for evidence of drainage or bleeding, and record urine output and output from drainage tubes. The nurse should also examine the postoperative orders and ensure that the child receives the correct type and amount of intravenous fluid prescribed. In addition, the nurse should provide comfort and pain relief (see Chapter 40).

Resumption of oral intake depends on the surgical procedure, the child's condition, and surgeon protocol. Once oral fluids are resumed, the nurse should monitor for emesis. When the child is consuming adequate fluids, the rate of intravenous fluids should be decreased or discontinued according to healthcare provider orders.

Parents are encouraged to visit with the child as soon after surgery as possible (Figure 39–5). In some facilities, children are brought to postoperative anesthesia care units (PACUs) after surgery, where they recover from anesthesia. Depending on the child's condition, he or she may be discharged home directly from an outpatient surgical procedure or admitted to a short-stay, general pediatric, or intensive care unit.

POSTOPERATIVE HOME CARE INSTRUCTIONS

Routine postoperative instructions for the family of the child undergoing outpatient or 1-day-stay surgical procedures include monitoring for signs of infection such as drainage, redness, or swelling of the surgical incision, fever, and change in behavior. Instructions for follow-up visit, medications, other treatments, wound care, and signs and symptoms that require medical attention are also provided. Additional instructions are tailored according to the surgical procedure and the child's condition. The nurse ensures the family understands home care instructions through their return demonstration statement of understanding.

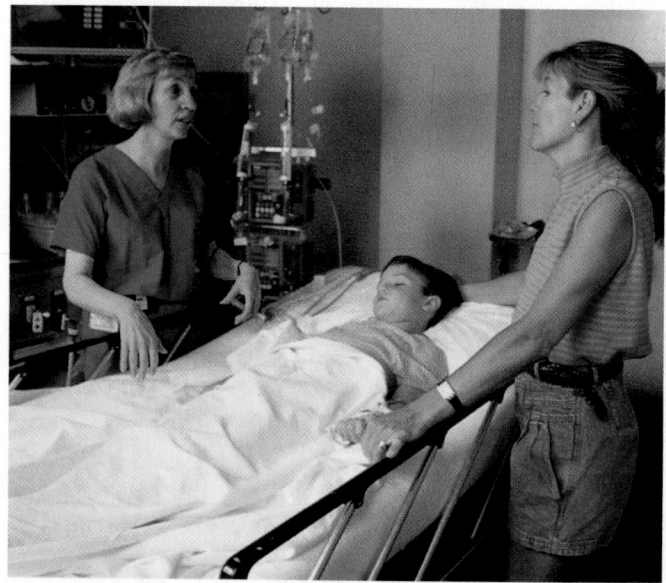

Figure 39–5 This child has just undergone surgery and is in the postanesthesia care unit. Although the child's physical care is immediate and important, remember that both the child and the family have strong psychosocial needs that must be addressed concurrently. It is important to reunite the family as soon as possible after surgery.

Strategies to Promote Coping and Normal Development of the Hospitalized Child

During hospitalization, care of the child focuses not only on meeting physiologic needs, but also on meeting psychosocial and developmental needs. Nurses can employ several strategies to help children adapt to the hospital environment, promote effective coping, and provide developmentally appropriate activities, such as child-life programs, rooming in, therapeutic play, and therapeutic recreation.

Rooming In

The practice of **rooming in** involves a parent staying in the child's hospital room during the course of the child's hospitalization. Some hospitals provide cots, others have special built-in beds on pediatric units, and, in some institutions, a parent is provided a separate room on the unit. Parents who stay at the bedside usually want to help care for their child to some degree. Most parents are comfortable providing basic care to their child, such as feeding and diapering, while parents of chronically ill children might be comfortable participating in more technical aspects of care (Romaniuk et al., 2014). Communication between the nurse and family is important so that the parents' desire for involvement is understood and supported.

Rooming in provides the child with the comfort and security of parental presence. Some parents may feel more comfortable staying with their child and participating in care, others may experience more stress if they are missing work and are away from home and other children. Partner with the parent to assist them in establishing a rooming-in plan that is beneficial to both the child and family. For example, in longer hospital stays, parents may alternate turns staying with the child. Grandparents, aunts and uncles, and grown siblings may be included in the plan.

Some facilities offer free or reduced-cost meals to the parent rooming in. The parent who does not receive these meals may often skip many meals because of the financial impact on an already overburdened budget related to illness and hospitalization. The nurse should be alert to the parent who never leaves the bedside and should make sure parents are eating. Emphasize the importance of the child's need for a healthy parent. Social services or other departments may be able to assist the family in obtaining meals while rooming in with the hospitalized child.

Parents rooming in with their child for an extended hospitalization can be encouraged to take advantage of facilities such as the Ronald McDonald House or other housing available for parents, at some point during the stay, as a respite for a few hours. This break will provide them with an opportunity for needed rest and privacy.

Child-Life Programs

Many hospitals have child-life programs that focus on the psychosocial needs of hospitalized children. Professional child-life specialists, paraprofessionals, and volunteers staff these departments (Figure 39–6). A **child-life specialist** plans activities to provide age-appropriate playtime for children either in the child's room or in a specialized playroom. Some of the planned activities are designed to assist children in working through feelings about illness. Examples include playing with medical equipment, acting out procedures or treatments on dolls, using games to act out feelings, or drawing pictures about hospital treatments.

Therapeutic Play

Play is a significant component of childhood, and the stress of illness and hospitalization increases the value of play. Yet, because of the need to contain costs, hospitals may minimize their play programs. Therefore, nurses should document the

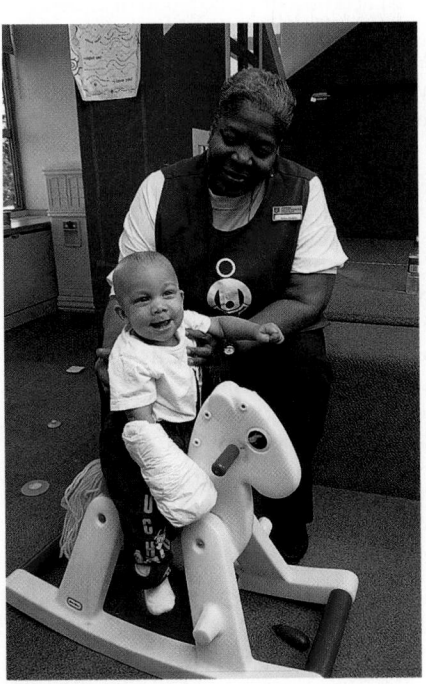

A

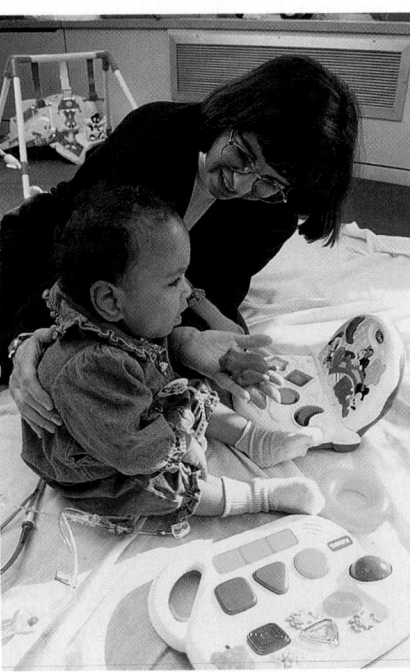

B

Figure 39–6 *A*, **Volunteers such as this grandmother can provide stimulation and nurturing to help young children adapt to lengthy hospitalizations.** *B*, **Child-life specialists plan activities for young children in the hospital to facilitate play and stress reduction.**

need for and benefits of play. Beyond facilitating normal development, play sessions can provide a means for the child to:

- Learn about health care
- Express anxieties
- Work through feelings
- Achieve a sense of mastery or control over frightening or little-understood situations

Play that presents an opportunity to deal with the fears, concerns, and stressors of health experiences is called **therapeutic play**. Therapeutic play has many benefits for both the child and the health professional. It allows the child an opportunity to relive, understand, and integrate fearful healthcare experiences. The child can achieve a sense of mastery by being in control of the occurrences during play. This helps to lower the child's stress and anxiety about the events. In addition, the healthcare professional can observe the child's play to learn more about the type of events that cause anxiety to the child. The child's coping methods can be observed and additional techniques offered to the child. *Play therapy* is a mental health technique used to treat children with mental health problems rather than normal life events that have caused anxiety. This technique is discussed in Chapter 55.

Through therapeutic play, children's knowledge of their illnesses or injuries can be assessed. A common technique involves using an outline drawing of the body (Figure 39–7) or having the child draw a picture about the hospitalization. Drawings can be used to determine what the child knows and understands about the hospitalization. In addition to assessment, drawing can be used as a nursing intervention. Demonstrate to the child on a drawing what will occur during surgery or a treatment. Children's drawings of healthcare experiences allow them to express fears and gain mastery over the situation.

Dramatic play, in which medical situations encountered are reenacted by the child, often helps the child cope with painful treatments and intrusive procedures. Play using safe medical equipment, such as bandages and syringes without needles, and providing scrubs and uniforms for dress-up are effective materials for encouraging dramatic play. Dramatic play offers an outlet for anxiety in children trying to deal with stressful and confusing situations. At the same time, these activities allow the nurse to observe and assess the child's perception of the illness and procedures. The nurse is then able to clarify any of the child's misconceptions.

A variety of techniques may be used to promote therapeutic and dramatic play (Table 39–10), depending on the child's developmental stage. The nurse can ensure that a selection of age-appropriate toys, distraction materials (stress balls, bubbles, music), and "prizes" are available.

Many hospitals, particularly children's hospitals, provide playrooms on each of the units to allow children a place to play and socialize with same-age peers. These rooms are generally brightly decorated in children's themes, and provide numerous opportunities for play, such as board games, video games, supplies for painting or drawing, and age-appropriate toys for each developmental level. For younger children, families may be encouraged to bring the child's favorite age-appropriate toys from home. For older children, there may be options for computer communication with children in other hospitals. Portable electronic gaming equipment may be available to children in isolation or those unable to come to the playroom or teen lounge. Specific interventions according to developmental level are discussed below.

INFANT

Infants require external stimuli for growth. The use of mobiles, music, mirrors, and other methods promotes stimulation and offers comfort to the newborn or infant. Parents and family are encouraged to cuddle or rock the infant and sing lullabies. Talking to the infant encourages interaction and play.

TODDLER

Approach toddlers slowly and make the initial approach in their parents' presence, if possible, to decrease feelings of stranger anxiety. Playing a variation of peek-a-boo or hide-and-seek using the curtain surrounding the toddler's crib or bed helps promote the realization that objects out of sight, such as parents, do return. Transitional objects, such as a familiar blanket or stuffed animal, can temporarily substitute for the security of parents. The toddler can be read familiar stories. Repetition of stories promotes a sense of stability in the unfamiliar hospital environment.

A doll is a familiar toy that can be used to re-create a stressful environment, thereby providing an opportunity for the child to express and work through feelings. Children's hospitals may have condition-specific and anatomically correct dolls for this purpose. Other developmentally appropriate toys for toddlers include familiar objects from home such as measuring cups or spoons, wooden puzzles, building blocks, and push-and-pull toys. Playing with safe hospital equipment helps toddlers overcome the anxiety associated with these items. Supervise these play sessions and remove hospital equipment when you leave.

PRESCHOOLER

The nurse can intervene to reduce the stress produced by preschoolers' fears through the use of some kinds of play. A simple outline of the body or a doll can be used to address the child's

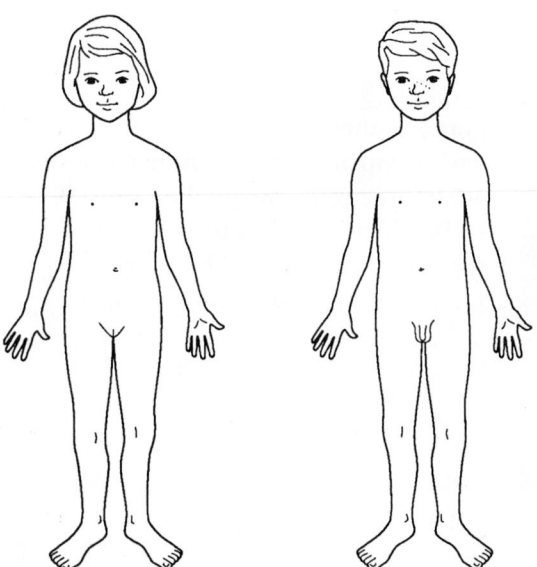

Figure 39–7 The nurse can use a simple gender-specific outline drawing of a child's body to encourage children to draw what they think about their medical problem. Such drawings reveal a child's interpretation, which the nurse can work with to provide appropriate care.

TABLE 39–10 Therapeutic Play Techniques

TECHNIQUE	ASSESSMENT	INTERVENTIONS
Stories	Have the child make up a story about a picture. Analyze content and emotional clues in the story. Have child tell a story about an important experience in a group of other children.	Read or make up stories to explain illness, hospitalization, or other specific aspects of health care. Emotions such as fear can be included.
Drawings	Ask the child to draw a picture about being in the hospital. Consider subject matter, size, and placement of items in drawings, colors used, presence or absence of physical barriers, and general emotional feeling.	Use the child's drawings or outlines of the body to explain care, procedures, or conditions. Provide an opportunity for children to draw pictures of their choices or directed topics such as a picture of the child's family or healthcare encounter. Ask the child: "Tell me about your picture." Be alert to the child's emotions: "This child must be frightened by the big x-ray machine."
Music	Observe types of music chosen and effects of played music on behavior.	Encourage parents and children to bring favorite tapes to the hospital for stress relief. Have tapes playing during tests and procedures. Parents can tape their voices to play for infants and young children during separations. During longer hospitalizations children can tape messages for siblings or classmates, who are then encouraged to retape their responses. Playtime can include the opportunity to play instruments and sing.
Puppets	The puppets can ask questions of young children, who are often more likely to answer the puppet than a person.	Perform short skits to teach children necessary healthcare information. Include emotional content when appropriate.
Dramatic play	Provide dolls and medical equipment, and analyze the roles assigned to dolls by the child, the behavior demonstrated by the dolls in the child's play, and the apparent emotions. Dolls with health problems like those of the child are especially helpful.	Provide dolls and equipment for play sessions. To ensure safety, supervise closely when actual equipment is used. Respond to emotions and behavior shown. Use dolls and equipment such as casts, nebulizer, intravenous apparatus, and stethoscope to explain care. Use dolls with problems or handicaps similar to those of the child when available. Provide toys that foster expression of emotion, such as a pounding board and indoor darts.
Pets	Provide animal-assisted therapy. Watch the interaction between child and animal.	Respond to emotions the child shows. Facilitate touch and stroking of animals.

Note: Additional techniques, such as sand or water play, may be appropriate in specific situations.

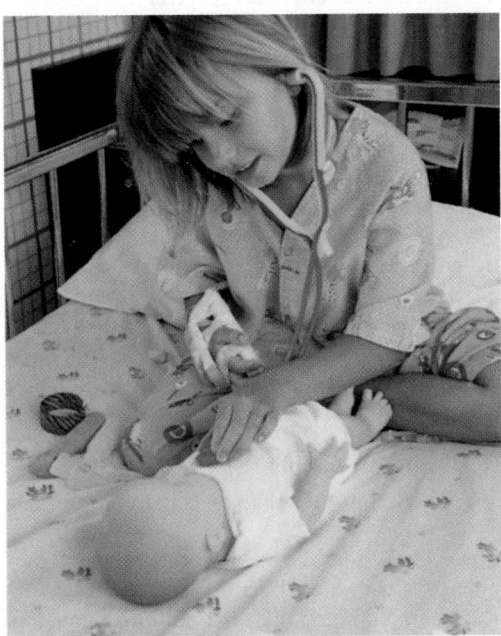

Figure 39–8 Age-appropriate play will help the child adjust to hospitalization and care.

fantasies and fears of bodily harm. Playing with safe hospital equipment may help preschoolers to work through feelings such as aggression (Figure 39–8).

Preschoolers prefer crayons and coloring books, puppets, felt and magnetic boards, play dough, books, and recorded stories. Preschoolers and older children often enjoy animal-assisted therapy. Some hospitals and units may have scheduled visits from pets, most commonly dogs. **Animal-assisted therapy (AAT)** is goal directed and individualized for each child while animal-assisted activity (AAA) may include visits to several children without specific goals. Both of these have positive benefits for hospitalized children (Goddard & Gilmer, 2015) (Figure 39–9).

SCHOOL-AGE CHILD

Although play begins to lose its importance in the school-age years, the nurse can still use some techniques of therapeutic play to help the hospitalized child deal with stress. School-age children often regress developmentally during hospitalization, demonstrating behaviors characteristic of an earlier state, such as separation anxiety and fear of body injury. Outlines of the body and anatomically correct dolls or condition-specific dolls can be used to illustrate the cause and treatment of the child's

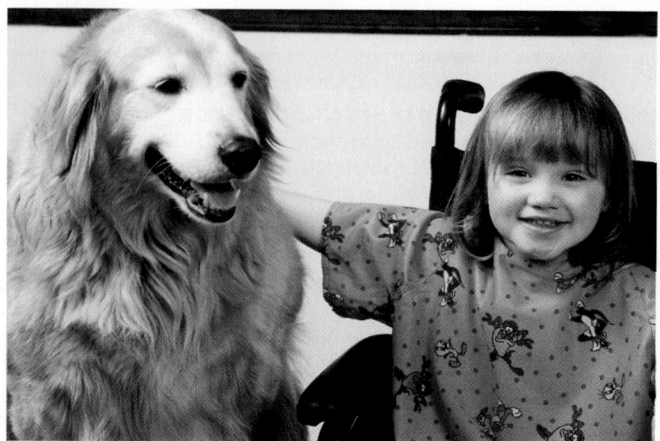

Figure 39-9 Hospitals may have animal-assisted therapy from specially trained animals to provide comfort and distraction during health care. Both the child and the dog seem to be smiling.

illness (Figure 39-10). Use terms for body parts that are suitable for older children. Drawings provide an outlet for expression of fears and anger.

School-age children enjoy collecting and organizing objects and often ask to keep disposable equipment that has been used in their care. They may use these items later to relive the experience with their friends. Games, books, puzzles, schoolwork, crafts, tape recordings, and computers provide an outlet for aggression and increase self-esteem in the school-age child. The type of play used should promote a sense of mastery and achievement.

Therapeutic Recreation

Many of the special play techniques used with younger children are not suitable for adolescents, but adolescents do need a planned recreation program to help them meet developmental needs during hospitalization. Peers are important, and the

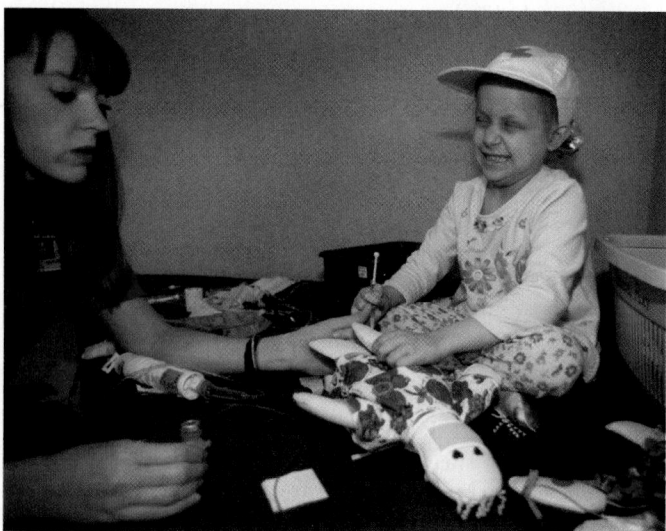

Figure 39-10 Having the child play with specialty dolls will help the child adjust. Such play helps the child realize what activities are possible.

SOURCE: John F. Rhodes/Newscom.

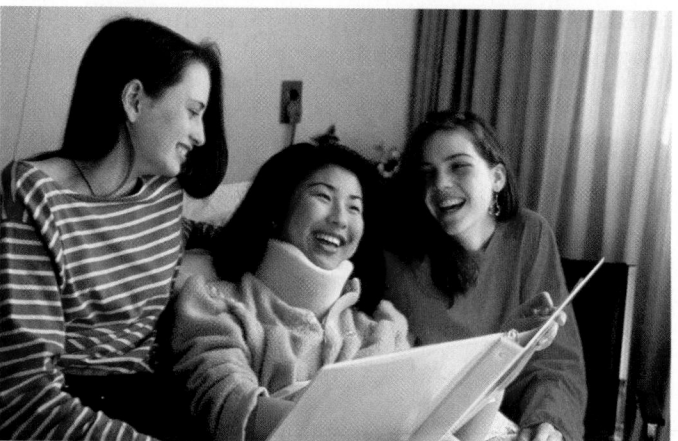

Figure 39-11 Having interaction with other hospitalized adolescents and maintaining contact with friends outside the hospital are very important so that the teenager does not feel isolated and alone.

SOURCE: Cusp/Superstock.

isolation of hospitalization can be difficult. Telephone contact with other teenagers and visits from friends should be encouraged. Interactions with other teenagers at a pizza party, video game, or movie night or during other activities can help adolescents feel normal (Figure 39-11). Physical activities that provide an outlet for stress are recommended. Even adolescents on bed rest or in wheelchairs can play a modified form of basketball. Some hospitals provide a teen room or teen lounge with age-appropriate activities such as a pool table, video games, and computers.

The independence of adolescence is interrupted by illness. Nurses can provide choices for teenagers to assist them in regaining control. Providing adolescents options and encouraging them to choose an evening recreational activity can promote their feelings of independence.

Strategies to Meet Educational Needs

Some hospitalizations are so short that the absence of the child or adolescent from school and peers is of minimal concern. However, if hospitalization is expected to last longer than a few days or if the child's condition changes so that the child needs special school arrangements, the nurse should assess the effects of hospitalization on the child's education.

When an elective procedure occurs, encourage families to assist in the arrangement of the extended school absence with teachers. The child can then be provided with schoolwork to complete in the hospital or at home when capable. This minimizes educational deficits and future problems for the child. Pencils, paper, comfortable work areas, computers, and quiet work times are provided to meet the child's educational needs. Telephone calls, Internet connections, and live video conferencing with teachers can be arranged as needed. The hospital teachers collaborate with the child's school teachers to ensure the child is meeting the educational objectives to avoid deficits upon return to school.

Nurses should also consider the social aspects of school and peers. Peers can be encouraged to visit a hospitalized classmate, send cards and letters, call on the phone, or communicate via the Internet. Classmates may even videotape a class session, allowing everyone the opportunity to send messages to the hospitalized child. When the child returns to school, information may be shared about the child's special needs. Maintain the child's and family's privacy by discussing with them the information needed by others, and obtaining written permission before disclosing any information. The hospital and school nurse often collaborate with each other, as well as the child and family, to plan for the child's needs. The child with chronic health problems or who requires long-term hospitalization has additional needs with regard to school. See Chapter 38 for information related to the child with a chronic condition in a school setting.

Hospitals or rehabilitation units may have classrooms, teachers, and facilities to promote learning. Many school districts provide tutors or computer connections for students who are hospitalized or receiving home care for extended periods. Teachers can visit children at the hospital or at home. Parents are often pivotal in making arrangements to meet the child's educational needs, since they interact with the child, the school, and the healthcare team.

Growth and Development

For children who are given the opportunity to hear, touch, see a model or equipment, read, look at pictures, or even smell things like alcohol swabs, learning is more complete. This is particularly important for the school-age child in the stage of concrete operational thought, who must be able to manipulate material in order to learn.

CHILD AND FAMILY TEACHING

Teaching is an essential part of the nurse's role in care of hospitalized children and their families and begins with the initial contact between the family and healthcare providers. Teaching may be informal, as when the nurse integrates an explanation during routine care, or structured, as when the nurse plans and implements a formal teaching program.

Nurses emphasize to the family that most teaching will occur in informal sessions rather than in formalized programs. The family should be aware of the teaching process to encourage active listening and participation. Actively involve the family in the learning process to ensure their understanding. The nurse and family partner together to identify the family's learning needs and appropriate teaching method to best convey the information. Recall that family members may be at various cognitive and anxiety levels and therefore have needs for different types of teaching. Develop a plan with both the family and other healthcare professionals to facilitate learning among the child and family members.

Prior to implementing teaching for the child, it is essential to assess the child's developmental level. Teaching directed at parents must also be geared to their level of understanding. If English is not spoken or is the parents' second language, an interpreter may be necessary. If interpreters are needed to facilitate understanding, be sure they are contacted and are available for teaching sessions.

Depending on the information to be presented, teaching may use the cognitive, psychomotor, or affective domains of learning. Teaching that includes all three domains is more effective. Explanations or reading materials, including pamphlets, booklets, DVDs, and models, are tailored to a level the parent can understand. The choice of tools used varies depending on the child's diagnosis and available materials.

Timing is a critical factor in teaching. Parents and children are less receptive to teaching when they are preoccupied with stress or activities. Collaborating with the parents in scheduling specific times for teaching sessions may be helpful.

TEACHING PLANS

A teaching plan is a written plan that includes goals and expected outcomes, interventions needed to achieve the specified goals, and a method and time for evaluation of the expected outcomes. The teaching plan may also specify teaching methods and types of materials to be used. By developing a teaching plan, a nurse helps to ensure that all the necessary information is included and taught efficiently. Additionally, this written documentation of teaching allows for continuity of care between nurses and other disciplines. Multidisciplinary teaching plans provide clear communication for all healthcare team members in the teaching process.

The child's primary caretaker should be an active participant in the development and implementation of the teaching plan. The primary caretaker is most often a parent but may be a close family member (uncle, aunt, or grandparent). Before establishing a teaching plan, the nurse should assess the child's or parent's knowledge, skills, and feelings by considering the following questions:

- What does the parent/caretaker or child know about the health issue?
- What are the expectations of the child and family?
- What is the cognitive level or ability to learn?
- Is there a desire to learn?
- What previous experiences affect the learning experience, either positively or negatively?
- What previous interventions have been the most useful for the child and family?
- What resources are available to the parents, child, and nurse that enhance understanding of the health condition?
- Are there feelings or beliefs that might interfere with the learning process?
- What complementary care does the family use, and how does this relate to the teaching plan?

The second step involves deciding what knowledge, skill, or change in attitude is desired. Outcome criteria or objectives are established with the parent and child. Possible teaching methods and a range of approaches are explored. A variety of resources, including written materials (books, pamphlets, handouts, and stories), computer software, audiovisual presentations, dolls, and body models are available to encourage interest from the child and family. Refer to Chapter 1 for information on reading level of patient education materials. In some settings, audiovisual and computer resources may be limited. Small group teaching sessions (e.g., for children with recently diagnosed diabetes) may be another option and provide the child with an opportunity to interact and learn from peers experiencing the same condition. Gathering two or three parents together on a unit to learn and share experiences may also be helpful. For some conditions, standardized teaching plans are available in books and from healthcare agencies. These plans can serve as a guide in developing an individualized teaching plan.

TEACHING FOR CHILDREN WITH SPECIAL HEALTHCARE NEEDS

Children who have disabilities may have special learning needs. If the child has a visual impairment or perceptual difficulty, material is presented in auditory and tactile ways. Children who have hearing deficits require visual and tactile presentations. Children who have learning disabilities may require more frequent reinforcement and shorter teaching sessions. These children are evaluated often for comprehension in order to adjust teaching as necessary.

Children who have chronic conditions or special healthcare needs may have been hospitalized numerous times and have received other health care at home and in the community. They usually have adapted coping mechanisms that help them deal with their illness. Nurses can talk with the child to determine what has helped in the past, provide information about what to expect during the current hospitalization, assign staff members who are familiar when possible, and follow each child's lead in assisting the child in coping. Do not assume that the child with a history of numerous hospitalizations understands all activities since each hospitalization is different. Even the most routine activities should be explained. Regularly review the updated plan of care with the parents and child. Provide the child with opportunities to ask questions and express concerns and fears. Assess the child's individual learning needs. Older children can be asked how they best like to learn. Determine the necessity for special equipment or teaching methods.

Preparation for Home Care

Nurses play an important role in preparing the child and family for discharge home; this preparation starts early during the hospitalization. The nurse works with the social service department, home care agencies, and the family to plan for equipment, procedures, and other home care needs. Home care nurses collaborate with the hospital nurse and assist families to meet the child's healthcare needs.

Assessing the Child and Family in Preparation for Discharge

Preparations for the discharge process are best started upon admission to the hospital. The healthcare team, including the primary healthcare provider, nurse, social worker, and discharge planner partner with the family to ensure a smooth transition. Assess the family's ability to manage the child's care and if any special adaptation to the home environment is necessary.

When a child who has been hospitalized for an extended time is to be discharged home, the school district is contacted by the hospital school teacher (if available) or social worker, and plans for education or reentry into school are made. This involves an assessment of the child by the school district and formulation of an individualized education plan (IEP). The IEP may include home tutors, specialized services from persons such as physical or speech therapists, or arrangements for transport of the child with a disability to the school and provisions for special medical care as needed. An individualized health plan (IHP) may also be required. See Chapter 38 for definitions and a detailed discussion on IEPs and IHPs. Some common problems that interfere with successful discharge planning include financial concerns, the family's unavailability for teaching and planning, lack of equipment, and lack of teamwork among involved healthcare disciplines. Nurses who assess for these potential problems from the initial contact with the child and family can intervene and assist the family to resolve them as soon as possible.

Preparing the Family for Home Care

The family may need to learn physical and rehabilitative procedures for the child's care. Short-term care may be necessary until the child regains full function. In other situations, care may be required throughout the child's life. This may involve measuring vital signs or assessing blood glucose levels.

For the child requiring complex long-term care, parents may need to learn about intravenous lines, medications, oxygen administration, or ventilators (Figure 39–12). See Chapter 38 for discussion of the child with a chronic condition.

Parents need to be taught how to use the equipment needed for the child's care and must show that they can use it correctly. They must be able to identify symptoms of distress and report them immediately to the healthcare provider. The education provided and the parents' ability to perform care are discussed with a visiting nurse or individual who manages the home care program. Parents should be encouraged to learn cardiopulmonary resuscitation (see the *Clinical Skills Manual* SKILLS). Help parents explore options for respite care. If they cannot provide daily care or need a break, they should be able to rely on others for a short period. Some agencies are available to provide respite care. Ongoing assistance may be needed to help families deal with finances, time, and other challenges. If parents must take a leave of absence from work to provide care for the child, inform them about the coverage provided by the Family Medical Leave Act (U.S. Department of Labor, 2012).

Preparing Parents to Act as Case Managers

The family is an integral part of the plan of care for an ill or hospitalized child. The child with a chronic illness or an injury requiring long-term care will probably require the services of numerous healthcare personnel or healthcare agencies. One person needs to be identified as a **case manager** to coordinate health care and to prevent gaps and overlaps. In some hospitals, nurses act as case managers. They may organize a patient care conference while the child with a chronic condition is hospitalized. Management goals are set and decisions are made about which healthcare provider or agency is responsible for helping the child meet each goal.

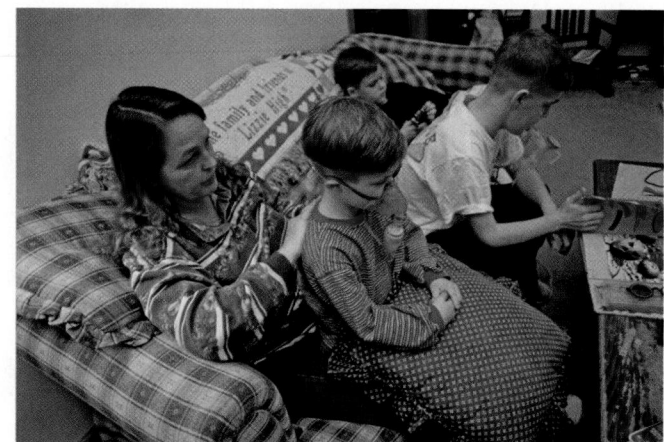

Figure 39–12 This child with chronic medical problems is being cared for at home. Are there any legal implications for the hospital and the nurse associated with the preparation of the child and family for home care?

SOURCE: Karen Kasmauski/Corbis.

Parents can also be case managers. The parent as case manager coordinates medical care, hospital stays, and visits to specialists; meets with school district representatives to plan the individualized education program for the child; finds equipment, personnel, and other services for home care; and manages the child's overall care.

Nurses should strongly encourage parents who want to take over case management to do so. Help them learn the management skills required. Many community agencies such as social service or home health agencies hold workshops for parents managing the complex care of their children.

Focus Your Study

- Hospitalization is a stressful event for all children and their families and affects families in a variety of ways, including disruption of usual routines, anxiety and fear related to the unknown, sibling concerns, financial difficulties, and parental anxiety over changing roles.

- The understanding of children about their illnesses and hospitalizations is based on cognitive and psychosocial stage/level and upon previous healthcare experiences.

- Nurses assess the impact of the child's illness or hospitalization on the family unit and provide individualized family-centered care. Supporting rooming in by parents or other family members, promoting development and safety, minimizing disruption of routines, and orientation to special units and expectations are specific strategies that can be implemented.

- Families are always disrupted by a child's hospitalization, and various approaches can help them to understand the process and cope more successfully. Specific examples include promoting parental involvement in care; orienting the child and family to the hospital setting, routines, and staff; age-appropriate explanations of procedures; and encouraging parents to support the child.

- When hospitalization is planned, both the child and family can prepare for the experience. Nurses assist this process by teaching them what to expect. Preparation may include tours, therapeutic play, books, and developmentally appropriate explanations.

- When hospitalization is unplanned, nurses can prepare the child and family by orienting them to the environment and use of developmentally appropriate explanations of procedures and equipment.

- A teaching plan includes goals and expected outcomes, interventions needed to achieve the specified goals, and a method and time for evaluation of the expected outcomes. How the teaching plan is implemented depends on the unique characteristics of the child/family to be taught.

- The child is prepared for procedures using a variety of techniques, taking into consideration the child's developmental age, coping abilities, and previous experience.

- Strategies such as child-life programs, therapeutic play, and therapeutic recreation help meet the psychosocial needs of the hospitalized child.

- The nurse assists the family to plan for the child's long-term healthcare needs and home care issues. Culturally competent care is integrated throughout all provisions of care.

Clinical Reasoning in Action

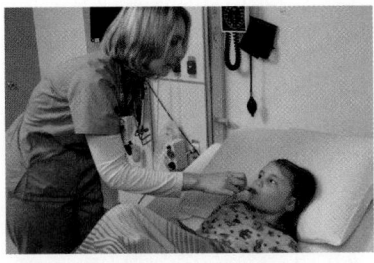

Five-year-old Tiona has a history of frequent tonsillitis and was scheduled for a tonsillectomy and adenoidectomy (T&A). Following the operation, Tiona refused to drink liquids because she was afraid it would hurt when she swallowed. After receiving intravenous pain medication, Tiona realized that she could swallow without too much pain and began to eat popsicles and drink liquids. She was then switched to oral pain medication. Later in the day, Tiona was drinking liquids well enough to be discharged home.

1. What information should the nurse include in the discharge teaching plan for Tiona's mother?

2. As Tiona and her mother are preparing to leave the hospital, Tiona states, "I am going to be good so I do not have to come to the hospital anymore!" How should the nurse respond?

3. Tiona's mother states that she is worried that her daughter will not drink enough at home. What can the nurse suggest to Tiona's mother to encourage her to drink fluids? What are the symptoms of dehydration that Tiona's mother should watch for over the next few days?

4. Children Tiona's age have many fears and stressors related to hospital and surgery. How can Tiona's mother assist her daughter to express her feelings about the hospital experience once she is home?

References

Agazio, J. G., & Buckley, K. M. (2012). Revision of a parental stress scale for use on a pediatric general care unit. *Pediatric Nursing, 38*(2), 82–87.

Ames, K. E., Rennick, J. E., & Baillargeon, S. (2011). A qualitative interpretive study exploring parents' perception of the parental role in the paediatric intensive care unit. *Intensive and Critical Care Nursing, 27*, 143–150.

American Society of Anesthesiologists, Committee on Standards and Practice Parameters. (2011). Practice guidelines for preoperative fasting and the use of pharmacologic agents to reduce the risk of pulmonary aspiration: Application to healthy patients undergoing elective procedures. *Anesthesiology, 114*(3), 495–511.

Bindler, R. C., Ball, J. W., London, M. L., & Davidson, M. R. (2017). *Clinical skills manual for maternity and pediatric nursing* (5th ed.). Hoboken, NJ: Pearson.

Emergency Nurses Association. (2012). *Emergency nursing resource: Family presence during invasive procedures and resuscitation in the emergency department.* Retrieved from http://www.ena.org /practice-research/research/CPG/Documents/ FamilyPresenceCPG.pdf

Fisher, M. J., & Broome, M. E. (2011). Parent–provider communication during hospitalization. *Journal of Pediatric Nursing, 26*(1), 58–69.

Goddard, A. T., & Gilmer, M. J. (2015). The role and impact of animals with pediatric patients. *Pediatric Nursing, 41*(2), 65–71.

Healy, K. (2013). A descriptive survey of the information needs of parents of children admitted for same day surgery. *Journal of Pediatric Nursing, 28*, 179–185.

Karlsson, K., Rydström, I., Enskär, K., & Englund, A. D. (2014). Nurses' perspectives on supporting children during needle-related medical procedures. *International Journal of Qualitative Studies on Health and Well-Being, 9.* Retrieved from http://dx.doi .org/10.3402/qhw.v9.23063

LeGrow, K., Hodnett, E., Stremler, R., & Cohen, E. (2014). Evaluating the feasibility of a parent-briefing intervention in a pediatric acute care setting. *Journal for Specialists in Pediatric Nursing, 19*, 219–228.

Romaniuk, D., O'Mara, L., & Akhtar-Danesh, N. (2014). Are parents doing what they want to do? Congruency between parents' actual and desired participation in the care of their hospitalized child. *Issues in Comprehensive Pediatric Nursing, 37*(2), 103–121.

Salmela, M., Aronen, E. T., & Salanterä, S. (2011). The experience of hospital-related fears of 4- to 6-year-old children. *Child: Care, Health and Development, 37*(5), 719–726.

Spector, R. E. (2013). *Cultural diversity in health and illness* (8th ed.). Upper Saddle River, NJ: Pearson.

Tschudy, M. M., & Arcara, K. M. (2011). *The Harriet Lane handbook* (19th ed.). St. Louis, MO: Elsevier Mosby.

U.S. Department of Labor. (2012). *Fact sheet #28: The Family and Medical Leave Act of 1993.* Retrieved from http://www.dol.gov/whd/regs/compliance /whdfs28.pdf

Wilson, M. E., Megel, M. E., Enebach, L., & Carlson, K. L. (2010). The voices of children: Stories about hospitalization. *Journal of Pediatric Health Care, 24*(2), 95–100.

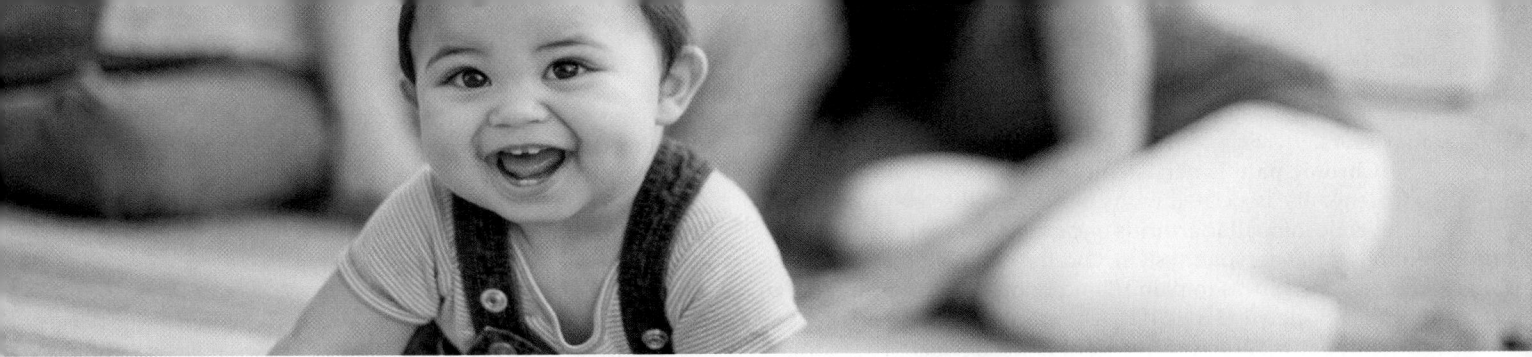

Chapter 40
Pain Assessment and Management in Children

Felicia must be in pain so soon after her surgery. I know I would have pain if it were me. Can she get pain medicine without getting another needle?

—Mother of Felicia, 5 years old

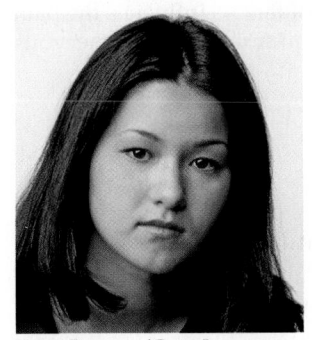

Kevin Peterson/Getty Images

Learning Outcomes

40.1 Summarize the physiologic and behavioral consequences of pain in infants and children.

40.2 Analyze the behaviors of an infant or a child to assess for pain.

40.3 Assess the developmental abilities of children to perform a self-assessment of pain intensity.

40.4 Plan the nursing care for a child receiving an opioid analgesic.

40.5 Examine the role of nonpharmacologic (complementary) interventions in effective pain management.

40.6 Plan nursing care for a child in acute pain that integrates pharmacologic interventions and developmentally appropriate nonpharmacologic (complementary) therapies.

40.7 Develop a nursing care plan for the child with a chronic painful condition.

40.8 Develop a nursing care plan for assessing and monitoring the child having sedation and analgesia for a medical procedure.

Every child has an individual perception of pain. A neurologic response to tissue injury, **pain** is an unpleasant sensory and emotional experience associated with actual or potential tissue damage. Much of the acute pain infants and children feel associated with medical conditions and procedures can be prevented or greatly relieved. Effective pain management is every child's right.

Pain

Pain may be either acute or chronic. **Acute pain** is sudden, of short duration, and may be associated with a single event, such as surgery, injury, or an acute exacerbation of a condition such as a sickle cell crisis. An immediate pain response occurs at the time of tissue damage, and the inflammatory response that follows causes a sustained pain response that decreases as healing occurs.

Chronic pain is persistent, lasting longer than 3 months, and generally associated with a prolonged disease process such as juvenile idiopathic arthritis or cancer. Chronic pain affects the entire central nervous system, and the child has increased neuron responsiveness to painful and nonpainful stimuli (American Pain Society [APS], 2012). Chronic pain may be nociceptive or neuropathic. **Nociceptive pain** is the normal processing of pain stimuli caused by tissue injury or damage. **Neuropathic pain** is an abnormal processing of pain stimuli by the peripheral or central nervous system. It may be initiated or caused by a primary lesion or dysfunction of the nervous system. Chronic pain is discussed more fully later in this chapter.

Pain transmission to the brain occurs through specialized nerve fibers (see *Pathophysiology Illustrated: Pain Perception*). The pain signal may be modified depending on the presence of other stimuli, either from the brain or from the periphery.

If pain is untreated or poorly treated, neurons become hyperexcited by the N-methyl-D-aspartic acid receptor system, which sensitizes the central nervous system. This leads to initiation of a pain memory and potentially to permanent alterations in pain pathways of young infants that may result in chronic pain syndromes (Rosen & Dower, 2011; Tobias, 2014a).

Misconceptions About Pain in Children

Healthcare professionals once believed that children feel less pain than adults. Undertreatment of pain was based on these attitudes about pain and the difficulty and complexity of pain assessment in children. Healthcare professionals now recognize that infants and children of all ages feel pain, just as adults do. For a review of past myths and the contrasting reality, see Table 40–1.

Developmental Aspects of Pain Perception, Memory, and Response

Although every infant and child perceives pain, their understanding, response to pain, and memory of painful events change as they develop. A number of factors influence the pain perceived by the child, including maturation of the nervous

Pathophysiology Illustrated: **Pain Perception**

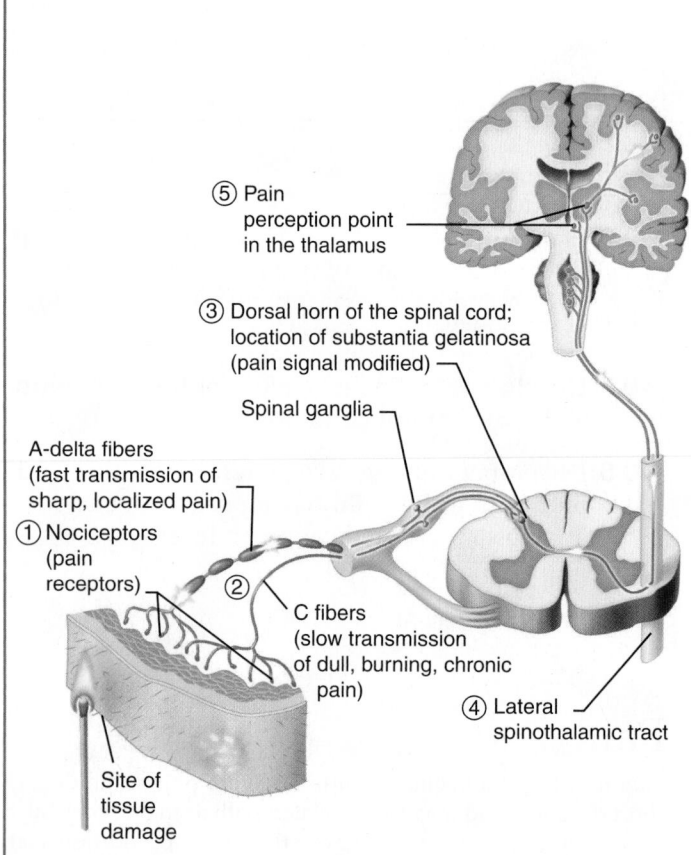

⑤ Pain perception point in the thalamus

③ Dorsal horn of the spinal cord; location of substantia gelatinosa (pain signal modified)

Spinal ganglia

A-delta fibers (fast transmission of sharp, localized pain)

① Nociceptors (pain receptors)

②

C fibers (slow transmission of dull, burning, chronic pain)

④ Lateral spinothalamic tract

Site of tissue damage

1. **Nociceptors (free nerve endings at the site of tissue damage that are able to detect and respond to chemical, mechanical, and thermal stimuli) transmit information via specialized nerve fibers to the spinal cord.**

2. **Unmyelinated C fibers slowly transmit dull, burning, diffuse pain as well as chronic pain. Large, myelinated A-delta fibers quickly transmit sharp, well-localized pain. Inflammatory mediators (e.g., bradykinin, prostaglandins, leukotrienes, serotonin, and substance P) are produced in response to tissue damage. These substances help move the pain impulse from the nerve endings to the spinal cord.**

3. **After the sensory information reaches the substantia gelatinosa in the dorsal horn of the spinal cord, the pain signal may be modified depending on the presence of other stimuli. Nonpainful touch, vibration, or pressure at the periphery and endogenous opioids from the brain can interfere with and reduce the transmission of pain to the brain.**

4. **The pain signal is then transmitted through the lateral spinothalamic tract, to the thalamus of the brain where perception occurs.**

5. **Once the sensation reaches the brain, interpretation of pain occurs, and emotional responses may increase or decrease the intensity of the pain perceived.**

TABLE 40–1 Misconceptions About Pain in Infants and Children

MYTH	REALITY
Newborns and infants are incapable of feeling pain. Children do not feel pain with the same intensity as adults because a child's nervous system is immature.	The anatomic, physiologic, and neurochemical structures for pain transmission are well developed at birth, even in preterm infants (Huether, 2014, p. 495). Children feel a similar amount of pain as adults postoperatively (Tobias, 2014a).
Infants are incapable of expressing pain.	Infants express pain with both behavioral and physiologic cues that can be assessed.
Infants and children have no memory of pain.	Children remember painful episodes, fear procedures that cause pain, and may have increased pain responses during future procedures (Fein, Zempsky, Cravero, et al., 2012).
Parents exaggerate or aggravate their child's pain.	Parents know their child and are able to identify behaviors associated with pain.
Children are not in pain if they can be distracted or if they are sleeping.	Children use distraction to cope with pain, but they soon become exhausted when coping with pain and fall asleep.
Repeated experience with pain teaches the child to be more tolerant of pain and cope with it better.	Children who have more experience with pain respond more vigorously to pain. Experience with pain teaches how severe the pain can become.
Children recover more quickly than adults from painful experiences such as surgery.	Children heal quickly from surgery, but they have the same amount of tissue injury and pain from surgery as an adult.
Children tell you if they are in pain. They do not need medication unless they appear to be in pain.	Children may be too young to express pain or afraid to tell anyone other than a parent about the pain. The child may fear treatment for pain will be worse than the pain itself.
Children without obvious physical reasons for pain are not likely to have pain.	The cause of pain cannot always be determined. The feeling of pain is subjective and should be accepted.
Children run the risk of becoming addicted to pain medication when used for pain management.	Children may develop physical dependence and tolerance after prolonged use of opioids for a serious injury, but addiction is uncommon (Galinkin, Koh, & Committee on Drugs and Section on Anesthesiology and Pain Management, 2014).

system, the child's developmental stage, and previous pain experiences. See Table 40–2 to learn more about the child's understanding of pain as well as the behavioral and verbal responses to pain at each age.

Children's responses to acute or chronic pain are influenced by factors such as memory of a past painful experience, their temperament, their ability to control what will happen, their use of a pain-coping mechanism, and emotions like fear or anxiety. Pain may be expressed as anger, anxiety, feeding problems, and sleep disturbances (Rosen & Dower, 2011).

Depending on their developmental stage, children use different coping strategies to deal with pain, such as escape, postponement or avoidance, diversion, and imagery. Children may not complain of pain for several reasons:

• Young children cannot give a description of their pain because of a limited vocabulary or few pain experiences.

• Some children believe they need to be brave and not worry their parents.

• Preschoolers and adolescents may assume the nurse knows they have pain.

• Some children are afraid it will hurt more to have the pain treated.

Cultural Influences on Pain

Pain sensitivity is believed to vary by race and ethnicity, with evidence that Blacks and Latinos perceive greater pain than Whites (Sadhasivam et al., 2012). In addition, culture and social learning greatly influence the child's expression of pain. Children observe family members in pain and try to imitate their responses. Through the process of parental approval and disapproval, they learn how to behave when in pain, how much pain should be tolerated, how much discomfort justifies a complaint, how to express a complaint of pain, and who to approach for pain relief. See *Developing Cultural Competence: Examine Your Own Experience.*

Developing Cultural Competence Examine Your Own Experience

Think about your childhood pain experiences and how your family encouraged you to be stoic or to express pain. Such childhood experiences often contribute to a health professional's attitudes about the pain experienced by children. For example, some healthcare providers may believe that being in pain for a little while is not so bad, that pain helps build character, or that using pain medication is a sign of a weak character. However, all nurses need to acknowledge the child's right to pain management because it is the standard of care.

Many ethnic groups, such as Irish, Japanese, Russian, Amish, and Appalachian, encourage a stoic response with a diminished expression of pain. Other ethnic groups, such as

TABLE 40–2 The Child's Understanding of Pain, Behavioral Responses, and Verbal Descriptions by Developmental Stage

AGE GROUP	UNDERSTANDING OF PAIN	BEHAVIORAL RESPONSE	VERBAL DESCRIPTION
INFANT			
0–6 months	Has no understanding of pain; is responsive to parental anxiety	Generalized body movements, chin quivering, facial grimacing, poor feeding	Cries
6–12 months	Has a pain memory; responsive to parental anxiety	Reflex withdrawal to stimulus, facial grimacing, disturbed sleep, irritability, restlessness	Cries
TODDLER			
1–3 years	Lacks understanding of what causes pain and why it might be experienced	Demonstrates fear of painful situations; may resist with entire body or localized withdrawal; aggressive behavior, disturbed sleep	Cries or wails, cannot describe intensity or type of pain Uses common words for pain such as *owie* and *boo-boo*
PRESCHOOLER			
3–6 years (preoperational)	Pain is a *hurt* Does not relate pain to illness; may relate pain to an injury Often believes pain is punishment or someone else is responsible for the pain Unable to understand why a painful procedure will help them feel better	Active physical resistance, directed aggressive behavior, strikes out physically and verbally when hurt, easily frustrated	Has the language skills to express pain on a sensory level Can identify location and intensity of pain, may deny pain, may believe their pain is obvious to others
SCHOOL-AGE CHILD			
7–9 years (concrete operations)	Understands simple relationships between pain and disease Understands the need for painful procedures to monitor or treat disease May associate pain with feeling bad or angry May recognize psychologic pain related to grief and hurt feelings	Passive resistance, clenches fists, holds body rigidly still, suffers emotional withdrawal, engages in plea bargaining	Can specify location and intensity of pain; can describe physical characteristics of pain in relation to body parts
10–12 years (transitional)	Better understanding of the relationship between an event and pain Has a more complex awareness of physical and psychologic pain, such as moral dilemmas and mental pain	May pretend comfort to project bravery, may regress with stress and anxiety	Able to describe intensity and location with more characteristics, able to describe psychologic pain
ADOLESCENT			
13–18 years (formal operations)	Has a capacity for sophisticated and complex understanding of the causes of physical and mental pain Recognizes that pain has both qualitative and quantitative characteristics Can relate to the pain experienced by others	Wants to behave in a socially acceptable manner, shows a controlled behavioral response May immerse self in an activity as a pain distraction May not complain about pain if given cues that nurses and other healthcare providers believe it should be tolerated	More sophisticated descriptions as experience is gained; may think nurses are in tune with their thoughts, so they do not need to tell the nurse about their pain

TABLE 40–3 Physiologic Consequences of Unrelieved Pain in Children

RESPONSES TO PAIN	POTENTIAL PHYSIOLOGIC CONSEQUENCES
RESPIRATORY CHANGES	
Rapid shallow breathing	Alkalosis
Inadequate lung expansion	Decreased oxygen saturation, atelectasis
Inadequate cough	Retention of secretions, pneumonia
NEUROLOGIC CHANGES	
Increased sympathetic nervous system activity and release of catecholamines	Tachycardia, elevated blood pressure, vasoconstriction, and decreased tissue oxygenation
	Increased intracranial pressure, change in sleep patterns, irritability
METABOLIC CHANGES	
Increased metabolic rate with stress response, increased release of hormones, suppressed release of insulin	Increased fluid and electrolyte losses
	Altered nutritional intake, hyperglycemia
IMMUNE SYSTEM CHANGES	
Depressed immune and inflammatory responses	Increased risk of infection, delayed wound healing
GASTROINTESTINAL CHANGES	
Decreased gastric acid secretions and intestinal motility	Impaired gastrointestinal functioning, nausea, poor nutritional intake, ileus
ALTERED PAIN RESPONSE	
Increased pain sensitivity	Hyperalgesia, decreased pain threshold, exaggerated memory of painful experiences

Source: Data from Greenwald, M. (2010). Analgesia for the pediatric trauma patient: Primum non nocere? *Clinical Pediatric Emergency Medicine*, *11*(1), 28–40; Huether, S. E. (2014). Pain, temperature regulation, sleep, and sensory function. In K. L. McCance, S. E. Huether, V. L. Brashers, & N. S. Rote (Eds.), *Pathophysiology: The biologic basis for disease in adults and children* (7th ed., pp. 481–524). St. Louis, MO: Mosby Elsevier; Clark, L. (2011). Pain management in the pediatric population. *Critical Care Nursing Clinics of North America*, 23, 291–301; Tobias, J. D. (2014a). Acute pain management in infants and children—Part 1: Pain pathways, pain assessment, and outpatient pain management. *Pediatric Annals*, *43*(7), e163–e168.

people of Puerto Rican, Jewish, and Arabic heritage, are more likely to use both verbal and nonverbal methods (moans and groans) to express pain freely (Purnell, 2014). However, not all members of a cultural group will demonstrate the same pain response. Children will have individualized responses to pain based on past experiences, and younger children have had less time to acquire culturally learned behaviors.

Consequences of Pain

Unrelieved pain is stressful and has many undesirable physiologic consequences (Table 40–3). For example, the child with acute postoperative pain takes shallow breaths and suppresses coughing to avoid more pain. These self-protective actions increase the potential for respiratory complications. Unrelieved pain may also delay the return of normal gastric and bowel functions and cause a stress ulcer. Anorexia associated with pain may delay the healing process. Pain drains the body of energy resources needed for healing and growth.

Pain Assessment

The goal of pain assessment is to provide accurate information about the location and intensity of pain and its effects on the child's functioning.

Pain History

Parents can provide a great deal of information about the child's response to pain, such as the following:

- How the child typically expresses pain. Children and parents use similar terms to describe pain. Knowing the appropriate word to use makes communicating with the child easier. See *Growth and Development*.

- The child's previous experiences with painful situations and reactions.

- How the child copes with and manages pain. The child with several past pain experiences may not exhibit the same types of stressful behaviors as the child with few pain experiences.

- What works best to reduce the child's pain?

- The parent's and child's preferences for analgesic use and other pain interventions.

Growth and Development

Children slowly acquire words for pain over the first 6 years of life. Toddlers and preschoolers use *ouch, pinch,* and *hurt* to describe pain. Other pain words include *owie, boo-boo, ache, stinging, cutting, burning, itching, hot,* and *tight*. Expressions of pain intensity by young children may include "hurts a lot" or "a really bad hurt" (Rashotte et al., 2013).

Ask older children to give a history of painful procedures. Keep in mind that children may modify their pain descriptions depending on the type of questions asked and what they expect will happen as a result of their response. Examples of questions to ask include the following:

- What kinds of things caused hurt in the past? What made it feel better?

- What do you tell your mother or caregiver when you hurt or are in pain? What do you, your caregiver, or your mother do for the pain?

- What would you like the nurse to do for the hurt? What should the nurse or other caregiver do for your pain?

- Where do you hurt? What does it feel like? What do you think is causing the pain?

Pain Assessment Tools

Various scales and tools are used to assess pain in children. After a pain assessment tool is designed, it is must be evaluated for **validity** (accurately measures the concept it was designed to measure) and **reliability** (consistent results are obtained when measured by the same rater or other raters). All of the following pain assessment tools have validity and reliability established.

PAIN BEHAVIOR SCALES FOR NONVERBAL CHILDREN

Physical and behavioral indicators are used to quantify pain in infants and nonverbal children. For example, the Neonatal Infant Pain Scale (NIPS) and the Faces, Legs, Activity, Cry, and Consolability (FLACC) Observational Tool rely on the nurse's observation of the child's behavior (expression, positioning, movement, and crying).

Neonatal Infant Pain Scale (NIPS). The NIPS is designed to measure procedural pain in preterm and full-term newborns up to 6 weeks after birth. The newborn facial expression, cry quality, breathing patterns, arm and leg position, and state of arousal are observed. See Table 40–4.

The Faces, Legs, Activity, Cry, and Consolability (FLACC) Observational Tool. The FLACC scale is designed to measure acute pain in infants and young children following surgery, and it can be used until the child is able to self-report pain with another pain scale. The tool has validity and reliability for evaluation of postoperative pain. See Table 40–5.

Pain Location. Young children (3 years and older) can localize pain if given an outline of the front and back of the body. The child can mark where the pain is located or color the area of pain with crayons. The child should use one color for the place where it hurts the most, and another color for areas with less pain.

ASSESSING CHILDREN WITH INTELLECTUAL DISABILITY

Assessing the pain of a child with severe intellectual disability is challenging. Many children with intellectual disability are able to use simple self-report pain tools. In other cases, behavioral pain assessment tools are appropriate.

The FLACC scale with some modifications can be successfully used by parents and nurses to assess postoperative pain in children with intellectual disability. Before surgery the parent identifies pain behaviors the child displays, such as a specific facial expression, body posture, leg position, and vocalizations to help guide the assessment. These behaviors are added to the descriptors for the scores in each of the FLACC scale categories. This tool has shown good validity and inter-rater reliability for use in this population (Ely et al., 2012).

SELF-REPORT PAIN SCALES

Self-report assessment tools of pain intensity are considered to be the best method of assessing pain in children and adolescents who can use such tools (see the *Clinical Skills Manual* SKILLS). Examples of self-report tools developed for children include the Faces Pain Rating Scale, the Oucher Scale, and the Poker Chip Tool.

TABLE 40–4 Neonatal Infant Pain Scale (NIPS)

CHARACTERISTIC	SCORING CRITERIA
FACIAL EXPRESSION	
0 = Relaxed muscles	• Restful face with neutral expression
1 = Grimace	• Tight facial muscles; furrowed brow, chin, and jaw (*Note*: At low gestational ages, infants may have no facial expression.)
CRY	
0 = No cry	• Quiet, not crying
1 = Whimper	• Mild moaning, intermittent cry
2 = Vigorous cry	• Loud screaming, rising, shrill, and continuous (*Note*: Silent cry may be scored if infant is intubated, as indicated by obvious facial movements.)
BREATHING PATTERNS	
0 = Relaxed	• Relaxed, usual breathing pattern maintained
1 = Change in breathing	• Change in drawing breath; irregular, faster than usual, gagging, or holding breath
ARM MOVEMENTS	
0 = Relaxed/restrained (with soft restraints)	• Relaxed, no muscle rigidity, random movements of arms
1 = Flexed/extended	• Tense, straight arms; rigid; or rapid extension and flexion
LEG MOVEMENTS	
0 = Relaxed/restrained (with soft restraints)	• Relaxed, no muscle rigidity, occasional random movements of legs
1 = Flexed/extended	• Tense, straight legs; rigid; or rapid extension and flexion
STATE OF AROUSAL	
0 = Sleeping/awake	• Quiet, peaceful, sleeping; or alert and settled
1 = Fussy	• Alert and restless or thrashing; fussy

Source: From Lawrence, J., Alcock, D., McGrath, D. P., Kay, J., MacMurray, S. B., & Dulberg, C. (1993). The development of a tool to assess neonatal pain. *Neonatal Network, 12*(6), 61; Taddio, A., Hogan, M. E., Moyer, P., Girgis, A., Gerges, S., Wang, L., & Ipp, M. (2011). Evaluation of the reliability, validity and practicality of 3 measures of acute pain in infants undergoing immunization injections. *Vaccine, 29*, 1390–1394.

TABLE 40–5 FLACC Behavioral Pain Assessment Scale

CATEGORIES	SCORING		
	0	**1**	**2**
Face	No particular expression or smile	Occasional grimace or frown; withdrawn, disinterested	Frequent to constant frown, clenched jaw, quivering chin
Legs	Normal position or relaxed	Uneasy, restless, tense	Kicking or legs drawn up
Activity	Lying quietly, normal position, moves easily	Squirming, shifting back and forth, tense	Arched, rigid, or jerking
Cry	No cry (awake or asleep)	Moans or whimpers, occasional complaint	Crying steadily, screams or sobs; frequent complaints
Consolability	Content, relaxed	Reassured by occasional touching, hugging, or being talked to; distractible	Difficult to console or comfort

Instructions: Observe the child for 5 minutes or longer. Observe the legs and body uncovered. Reposition the child or observe activity. Assess body for tenseness and tone. Initiate consoling interventions if needed. Each of the five categories is scored from 0 to 2, resulting in a total score between 0 and 10. A total score of 0 = relaxed and comfortable; 1–3 = mild discomfort; 4–6 = moderate pain; 7–10 = severe discomfort or pain.

Source: Used with permission from Merkel, S. I., Voepel-Lewis, T., Shayevitz, J. R., & Malviya, S. (1997). The FLACC: A behavioral scale for scoring post-operative pain in young children. *Pediatric Nursing*, 23(3), 293–297; Gomez, R. J., Barrowman, N., Elia, S., Manias, E., Royle, J., & Harrison, D. (2013). Establishing intra- and inter-relater agreement of the Faces, Legs, Activity, Cry, Consolability scale for evaluating pain in toddlers during immunization. *Pain Research & Management*, 18(6), e124–e128.

To use pain scales, the child must understand the concept of a little or a lot of pain well enough to tell the nurse and to follow simple directions. Children 2 to 3 years of age can usually understand the concept of "more or less." Only three choices should be offered these children when assessing pain (none, some, a lot). Most children at ages 4 to 5 years can distinguish a larger number from a smaller number or correctly put different sized blocks in largest to smallest order. These children can use a self-report pain rating tool.

Faces Pain Rating Scale.
This scale has a series of six or seven cartoon-like faces with expressions from smiling (or neutral) to tearful depending upon the model selected. The Wong-Baker scale is commonly used for children from 3 years through adolescence (Figure 40–1). After explanations about the meaning for each face, the child selects the face that is the closest match to the pain felt. The nurse should not use the tool to compare with the child's facial expression to determine pain level. Older children can use the words associated with the tool to provide a pain rating. The Faces Pain Rating Scale has good validity and reliability for measuring pain intensity (Wood et al., 2011).

Oucher Scale.
The Oucher Scale presents a series of six photographs of a child expressing increasing pain intensity in combination with a vertical Visual Analog Scale (Figure 40–2). The tool has been developed and tested in four cultural groups: White, African American, Hispanic, and Asian.

Poker Chip Tool.
This tool uses four checkers or poker chips to quantify acute procedural pain. The child is asked to pick the number of chips that best match the pain felt, with one chip being a little pain and four being the most pain one could have.

School-age children and adolescents have better number concepts and language skills, so additional tools can be used to assess their pain. The nurse should ask the child to describe the pain and give its location. Providing some words such as *sharp, dull, aching, pounding, cold, hot, burning, throbbing, stinging, tingling,* or *cutting* can help children describe their pain.

Numeric Pain Scale.
This tool, also called the Visual Analog Scale, is a single 10-cm horizontal or vertical line that has descriptors of pain at each end (no pain, worst possible pain). Marks and numbers are placed at each centimeter on the line. The child marks the amount of pain felt, and the numbers on the line are used to score the pain. Younger school-age children often have less understanding of numbers and directions to use this tool.

Word-Graphic Rating Scale.
This tool has words rather than numbers describing increasing pain intensity across a 10-cm Visual Analog Scale without numbers. The child marks the line

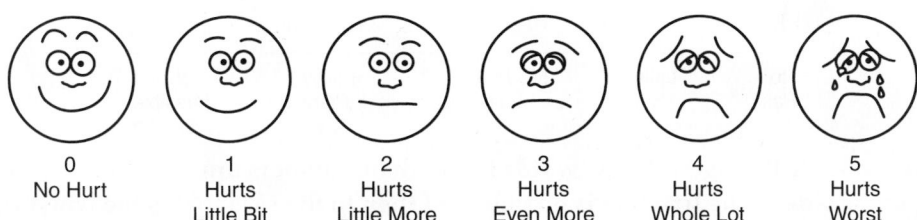

0	1	2	3	4	5
No Hurt	Hurts Little Bit	Hurts Little More	Hurts Even More	Hurts Whole Lot	Hurts Worst

Figure 40–1 Teach the child to use the Faces Pain Rating Scale by pointing to each face and using the words under the picture to describe the amount of pain felt. Then ask the child to select the face that comes closest to the amount of pain felt. Use the number under the selected face to score the pain.

SOURCE: Used with permission from Wong, D. L., & Baker, C. M. (1988). Pain in children: Comparison of assessment scales. *Pediatric Nursing, 14,* 9–16.

that is closest to the level of pain felt. A millimeter ruler can be used to quantify the pain and record the pain score (Figure 40–3).

Adolescent Pediatric Pain Tool. This tool includes a human figure drawing, the Word-Graphic Rating Scale, and a choice of descriptive words, for example, *burning, ache, sharp*, and *dull*. Adolescents indicate pain sites on the human figure outline, use the Word-Graphic Rating Scale as described, and use the word

choices to characterize the pain felt. This tool may be used to assess acute and chronic pain.

Acute Pain

Children experience acute pain related to a variety of illnesses and injuries, surgery, and invasive procedures. Just as with adults, children must have their pain assessed and managed.

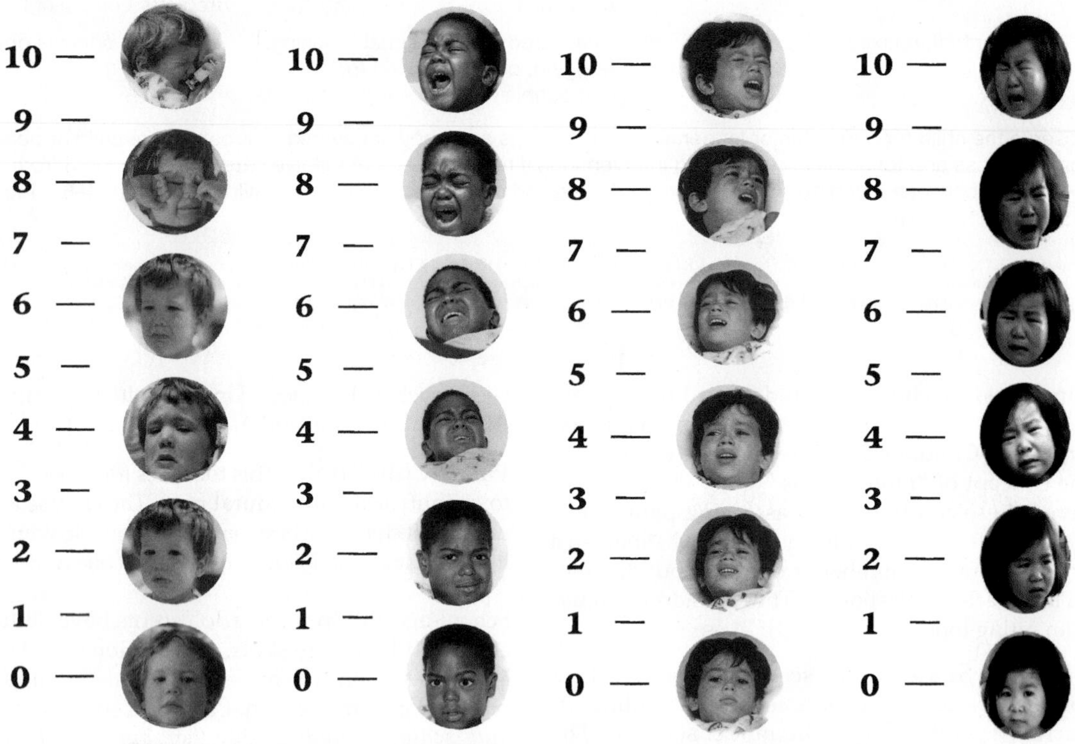

Figure 40–2 Use the Oucher Scale with the best match for the child's ethnicity. Teach the child to use the scale. Point to each photograph and explain that the bottom picture is "no hurt," the second picture is a "little hurt," the third picture is "a little more hurt," and so on until the sixth picture which is the "biggest or most hurt you could ever have." The young child selects a face that matches the level of pain. The numbers beside the photos are used to score the amount of pain the child reports. The older child can select a pain intensity number between 0 and 10. The nurse should not compare the photos with the child's expression to determine a pain level. See http://www.oucher.org for more information.

SOURCE: The White version of the Oucher Scale used with permission from Judith E. Beyer, RN, PhD, 1983. The African American version of the Oucher Scale used with permission from Mary J. Denyes, RN, PhD, and Antonia M. Villarruel, RN, PhD, 1990. The Hispanic version of the Oucher Scale used with permission from Antonia M. Villarruel, RN, PhD, 1990. The Asian version of the Oucher Scale used with permission from C. H. Yeh, RN, PhD, and C. H. Wang, BSN, 2003.

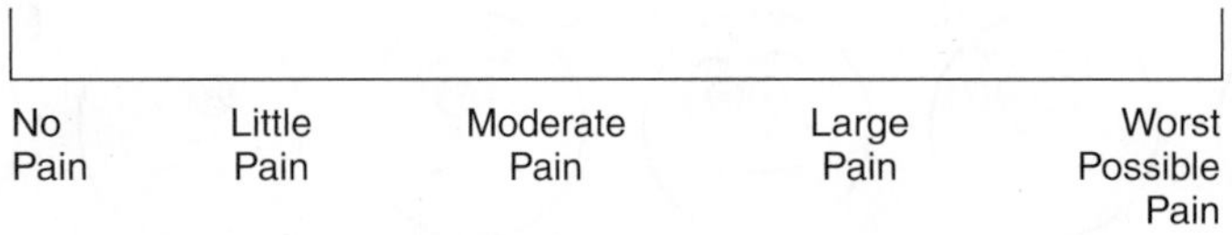

| No Pain | Little Pain | Moderate Pain | Large Pain | Worst Possible Pain |

Figure 40–3 The Word-Graphic Rating Scale has words rather than numbers under the line. Teach the child to use the tool by pointing to the side of the line that is no pain and then to the side that is the worst possible pain. Ask the child to make a mark along the line that matches the amount of pain felt. Use a millimeter ruler to measure from the "no pain" end of the line to the marked location to identify the pain score. Make sure the line is 10 cm each time pain is assessed so comparisons can be made.

SOURCE: Used with permission from Sinkin-Feldman, L., Tesler, M., & Savedra, M. (1997). Word placement on the Word-Graphic Rating Scale by pediatric patients. *Pediatric Nursing, 23,* 31–34.

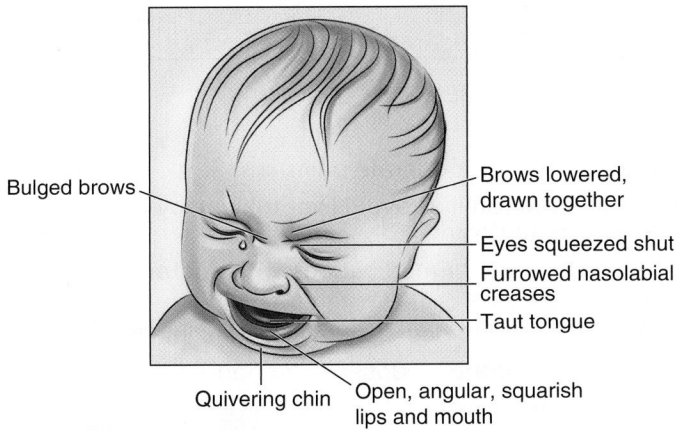

Bulged brows

Brows lowered, drawn together

Eyes squeezed shut

Furrowed nasolabial creases

Taut tongue

Quivering chin

Open, angular, squarish lips and mouth

Figure 40–4 Characteristic neonatal pain facial expressions include bulged brow, eyes squeezed shut, furrowed nasolabial creases, open lips, pursed lips, stretched mouth, taut tongue, and a quivering chin.

SOURCE: Adapted from Carlson, K. L., Clement, B. A., & Nash, P. (1996). Neonatal pain: From concept to research questions and the role of the advanced practice nurse. *Journal of Perinatal Neonatal Nursing, 10*(1), 64–71.

Clinical Manifestations

PHYSIOLOGIC INDICATORS

Acute pain stimulates the adrenergic nervous system and results in physiologic changes, including tachycardia, tachypnea, hypertension, pupil dilation, pallor, increased perspiration, and increased secretion of stress hormones such as the catecholamines and cortisol (Huether, 2014). These signs demonstrate a complex stress response. The body adapts physiologically to acute pain; after several minutes, the vital signs return to near normal and perspiration decreases, so these signs cannot be used for monitoring acute pain. Persistent or continuous chronic pain of long duration permits physiologic adaptation, so normal heart rate, respiratory rate, and blood pressure levels are often seen (Huether, 2014).

BEHAVIORAL INDICATORS

Newborns and infants demonstrate knitted brows, squinted eyes with cheeks raised, eyes closed, crying, jerky or flailing movements, and stiff posture in response to pain. See Figure 40–4. A preterm or sick newborn may have a weaker cry, a less expressive face, or not have the energy to make as many body movements as the well infant (Badr, 2013).

Children in acute pain are often distressed and anxious, especially if they have experienced pain previously. Behaviors that could indicate pain or anxiety in infants and toddlers include crying, restlessness or agitation, hyperalertness or vigilance, sleep disturbances, and irritability. Children and adolescents may demonstrate the following additional behaviors:

- Short attention span (child is easily distracted)
- Posturing (guarding a painful joint by avoiding movement), remaining immobile, or protecting the painful area
- Drawing up knees, flexing limbs, massaging affected area
- Lethargy, remaining quiet, or withdrawal
- Sleep disturbances
- Depression and/or aggressive behavior, especially for those who fear that the discomfort will worsen

Clinical Therapy

Acute pain management includes both drug and nondrug measures. Children need adequate pain medication, but complementary therapies can enhance pain management and ultimately reduce the amount of pain medication needed.

ACETAMINOPHEN AND NONSTEROIDAL ANTI-INFLAMMATORY DRUGS

Nonsteroidal anti-inflammatory drugs (NSAIDs) such as ibuprofen, primarily given orally, are effective for the relief of mild to moderate pain and chronic pain. Acetaminophen is a nonnarcotic analgesic and antipyretic that is used like an NSAID; however, it does not have a systemic anti-inflammatory action. NSAIDs are most commonly used for bone, inflammatory, and connective tissue conditions. An NSAID may be prescribed in combination with an opioid to increase the effectiveness of the opioid drug, and potentially reduce the amount of opioids needed. See *Medications Used to Treat: Pain.*

OPIOIDS

Opioids are analgesics commonly given for severe pain, such as after surgery or a severe injury. Opioids (e.g., morphine) are commonly administered by oral, subcutaneous, intramuscular (IM), and intravenous (IV) routes. Oral and IV routes are preferred for use in children because the intramuscular and subcutaneous routes cause pain and stress at the time of administration.

Oral administration of opioids is as effective as IM and IV routes when the drug is given in an **equianalgesic dose** (the amount of drug needed to produce the same analgesic effect regardless of the route used). The optimal analgesic dose is not specific for age or ethnicity of clients. See *Medications Used to Treat: Pain.* Meperidine is rarely prescribed for children because of adverse effects on the central nervous system, including seizures, agitation, and depressed mood (Tobias, 2014b). Codeine must also be used with caution in children.

SAFETY ALERT!

Codeine acquires its analgesic properties with its conversion to morphine by the liver, and it requires metabolism by the CYP2D6 enzyme. About 10% of White people and varying frequencies in other ethnic groups are poor metabolizers and therefore do not receive adequate pain relief from codeine (Pasero & McCaffery, 2011, p. 330). Children of North African, Ethiopian, and Saudi heritage are more likely to be ultrarapid metabolizers and risk a life-threatening overdose, even at recommended dosages (Watt & Arnstein, 2013). Genetic testing is not currently recommended.

After reports of several pediatric deaths and overdoses associated with codeine, the U.S. Food and Drug Administration issued a boxed warning that contraindicates the use of codeine after tonsillectomy or adenoidectomy (Aschenbrenner, 2013).

Clinical Tip

Analgesics were often withheld from children with acute abdominal pain until surgeons could complete an assessment, as it was believed that analgesia would interfere with diagnosis. Studies involving children with appendicitis revealed that giving morphine did not delay the diagnosis or cause complications associated with opioid use (Fein et al., 2012). Be an advocate for pain management in these children.

Medications Used to Treat: Pain

MEDICATION AND ACTION	NURSING MANAGEMENT
Nonopioid Analgesic	
Acetaminophen (Tylenol), *Oral, Rectal, IV* Inhibits prostaglandin synthesis in the central nervous system (CNS) and blocks pain impulse generation in the periphery	• Use for mild or moderate pain. • Ensure that families avoid liver toxicity by using appropriate dosing. • Avoid using other medications with acetaminophen as an ingredient. • Give with food to decrease gastrointestinal (GI) upset. • Give no more than 5 doses in 24 hours.
Nonsteroidal Anti-Inflammatory Drugs (NSAIDS)	
Acetylsalicylic Acid (Aspirin), *Oral, Rectal* Inhibits prostaglandin synthesis involved in pain synthesis in periphery Ibuprofen (Motrin), *Oral* Cyclooxygenases 1 and 2 (COX-1 and COX-2) NSAID inhibitors that block prostaglandin synthesis Naproxen (Naprosyn, Aleve), *Oral* Inhibits prostaglandin synthesis by inhibiting COX1 and COX2 isoenzymes Ketorolac (Toradol), *IV, IM* Inhibits prostaglandin synthesis by decreasing activity of the COX enzyme, which decreases prostaglandin precursors	• Use for short-term management of mild or moderate pain. • Do not use aspirin in children recovering from chickenpox or influenza because of concern about Reye syndrome. • Give with food to decrease GI upset. • Monitor for prolonged bleeding time with extended use. • Run periodic lab tests for blood counts with differential, serum electrolytes, liver function tests with extended use. • Monitor for hypersensitivity reaction, especially if child is allergic to aspirin. • Educate parents about signs of GI bleeding if prescribed for extended use.
Opioids	
Morphine Sulfate, *IV, IM, Subq, Oral* Agonist that binds with mu receptors in the brain and spinal cord to provide analgesia; gold standard for comparison of other analgesics Hydromorphone (Dilaudid) Opiate receptor agonist in central nervous system (CNS) leading to changes in pain perception Levorphanol (Levo-Dromoran) Synthetic morphine derivative with opiate receptor agonist activity, more potent and longer duration of action than morphine Methadone (Dolophine), *Oral, IV* Synthetic narcotic that has increased duration of action with repeated doses	• Use for moderate to severe pain. • Carefully calculate the dosage to be administered and verify with another nurse. • Obtain baseline vital signs before administration for future comparison. • Assess pain regularly for pain relief and duration. • Carefully monitor for signs of respiratory depression, especially during drug-specific peak action time. • Anticipate and provide preventive treatment for constipation. • Monitor for other adverse effects and notify healthcare provider. • For severe pain, administer every 4 hours or continuously to avoid pain breakthrough.
Fentanyl, *IV, Intranasal, Transmucosal, Transdermal* Synthetic and potent narcotic agonist that causes analgesia and sedation, short action time	• May be used for sedation and analgesia for painful procedures. • Monitor vital signs. • Observe the child for thoracic and skeletal muscle rigidity and weakness that may depress respirations. • Respiratory depression effect may last 4 hours longer than analgesic effect; be prepared to support ventilations and give naloxone.

Oxycodone (Roxicodone), *Oral*

Semisynthetic derivative of an opium agonist that binds with receptors in the CNS to alter the perception of pain and emotional response to pain

- Use for moderate pain.
- Monitor respiratory status for respiratory depression.
- Note adverse effects such as nausea, dizziness, and sedation.
- Determine child's continued need for medication, as the potential for drug abuse is high.

Codeine, *Oral*

Opiate receptor agonist in CNS leading to changes in pain perception

- Use for mild or moderate pain.
- Assess pain regularly for pain relief and duration.
- Observe for nausea, a common side effect.
- See *Safety Alert!*.

Source: Data from: Taketomo, C. K., Hodding, J. H., & Kraus, D. M. (2014). *Pediatric dosage handbook* (21st ed.). Hudson, OH: American Pharmacists Association; Barnes, S. (2014). Analgesia and sedation. In B. Engorn, & J. Flerlage (Eds.), *The Harriet Lane handbook* (20th ed.). Philadelphia, PA: Elsevier; Wilson, B. A., Shannon, M. T., & Shields, K. M. (2016). *Nurse's drug guide 2016*. Hoboken, NJ: Pearson Education.

Common opioid side effects include sedation, nausea, vomiting, constipation, urinary retention, and itching. These may be treated by rotating the opioids used or with specific therapies as follows:

- *Sedation*—supplement lower opioid dose with nonsedating analgesia or psychostimulant such as methylphenidate (Pasero & McCaffery, 2011, p. 512; Rosen & Dower, 2011)
- *Nausea and vomiting*—antiemetic medication, alternate opioid
- *Constipation*—prophylactic stool softener, a stimulating laxative, and increased fluids and dietary fiber
- *Urinary retention*—place child in bathtub, run water, intermittent catheterization
- *Pruritus*—antihistamine, alternate opioids, or naloxone 0.1 to 0.2 mcg/kg/hr continuous IV infusion (given simultaneously with opioid) (Pasero & McCaffery, 2011, p. 500)

The major life-threatening complication of opioid administration is **respiratory depression** (unresponsiveness and progressively decreasing respiratory rate that may progress to respiratory arrest). Clinical signs that indicate the development of respiratory depression include sleepiness, small pupils, and shallow breathing. Children at higher risk for opioid-induced respiratory depression have an altered level of consciousness, an unstable circulatory status, a history of apnea, a known airway problem such as obstructive sleep apnea, or are receiving another medication that potentiates the CNS effect of the opioid (e.g., benzodiazepines or barbiturates). Starting opioid dosages for these children may be 50% of the recommended dose (Tobias, 2014b).

Frequent visual assessments and cardiorespiratory monitoring or pulse oximetry are important safety guidelines when the infant or child is at increased risk for respiratory depression.

SAFETY ALERT!

Respiratory depression is most likely to occur when the child is sleeping and the tongue may obstruct the airway. Carefully monitor the child's vital signs during the drug-specific peak action time to detect respiratory depression. Monitor the respiratory rate because pulse oximetry does not measure ventilation.

If respiratory depression occurs, naloxone is administered at a rate of 1 to 2 mcg/kg every 1 to 2 minutes to gradually reduce the opioid effects without losing analgesia effects (Tobias, 2014b). Continue to monitor the child for respiratory depression because the half-life of naloxone is shorter than the opioid's half-life.

When given opioids over an extended period of time, children develop **physical dependence**, the physiologic adaptation to an analgesic or sedative drug by the peripheral and central nervous systems that may lead to **withdrawal**, the physical signs and symptoms that occur when a sedative or pain drug is stopped suddenly. Physical dependence is not addiction. **Tolerance** is an adaptation to an opioid dosage that results in a shorter duration of drug effectiveness over time. An increasing dosage is needed to produce the same level of pain relief. For example, a child might develop physical dependence or tolerance after being in an intensive care setting long term with pain management for life-threatening injuries, multiple surgeries, and invasive procedures. See Table 40–6 for signs and symptoms of withdrawal. The child is weaned off

TABLE 40–6 Clinical Manifestations of Opioid or Sedative Withdrawal

SYSTEM	SIGNS AND SYMPTOMS
Central nervous system	Anxiety, irritability, increased wakefulness, tremors, increased muscle tone, inability to concentrate, frequent yawning, sneezing, delirium, visual or auditory hallucinations
Gastrointestinal system	Decreased appetite, nausea, vomiting, diarrhea, uncoordinated suck and swallow
Sympathetic nervous system	Tachycardia, tachypnea, increased blood pressure, nasal stuffiness, lacrimation, sweating, fever, increased salivation

Source: Data from Pasero, C., & McCaffery, M. (2011). *Pain assessment and pharmacologic management*. St. Louis, MO: Mosby Elsevier; Suddaby, E. C., & Josephson, K. (2013). Satisfaction of nurses with the Withdrawal Assessment Tool-1 (WAT-1). *Pediatric Nursing, 39*(5), 238–242, 259; Galinkin, J., Koh, J. L., & Committee on Drugs and Section on Anesthesia and Pain Management. (2014). Recognition and management of iatrogenically induced opioid dependence and withdrawal in children. *Pediatrics, 133*(1), 152–155.

opioids over 2 to 4 weeks to prevent withdrawal symptoms. One plan is to switch the child to oral opioids and reduce the daily dose by 10% over several days. The longer the child has been taking the opioids, the longer the tapering should take.

DRUG ADMINISTRATION

Pain from surgery, major trauma, acute episodes such as vaso-occlusive crisis, or cancer is present for predictable periods because of the effects of tissue damage. Pain relief should be provided around the clock. Every effort should be made to give the child analgesics without causing more pain. The preferred routes of administration are intravenous, local nerve block, and oral.

Continuous infusion analgesia is recommended for children with persistent severe pain, as it keeps blood levels constant. Analgesics may also be given intravenously on a scheduled basis (e.g., every 3 to 4 hours). Delays in analgesia administration increase the chances of **breakthrough pain** (pain that emerges as the pain medication wears off, resulting in the loss of pain control) and the subsequent anticipation of pain. Giving analgesics on an as-needed (PRN) basis for acute pain results in the loss of pain control. More medication is often needed to restore pain control than would have been required with continuous infusion analgesia.

Patient-Controlled Analgesia. **Patient-controlled analgesia (PCA)** is a method of administering an intravenous analgesic, such as morphine, using a computerized pump programmed by the healthcare professional and controlled by the child (see the *Clinical Skills Manual* SKILLS). After pain control has been achieved with a continuous IV infusion of morphine (basal dose) by the nurse, the child presses a button to receive a smaller analgesic dose (bolus dose) for episodic pain relief. This method of pain management is especially useful for pain control in the first 48 hours after surgery or until oral pain management is possible. Safety features to prevent overdoses include the ability to set the maximum number of bolus infusions per hour and the maximum amount of drug received in a specific time period. Once oral analgesics can be taken, PCA is discontinued.

PCA is prescribed mostly for children ages 6 years and older, but may be offered to children as young as 5 years. The child should be able to self-report pain with a pain scale and understand that pushing the button will give them medication to relieve pain. See *Teaching Highlights: Patient-Controlled Analgesia (PCA)*. Nurse-controlled analgesia, with the nurse taking responsibility for bolus infusions, is sometimes provided for younger children or those with cognitive impairments. The nurse must assess pain before pushing the device button to reduce risks for adverse events.

SAFETY ALERT!

PCA by proxy, such as giving a parent permission to push the PCA button, has been used for some children with disabilities or too young to be responsible. Many facilities no longer permit parents to administer PCA to their child. If permitted, parents must be taught to follow guidelines for pain assessment and PCA use, and adherence to guidelines must be monitored to reduce the risk for an adverse event associated with too much medication.

REGIONAL PAIN MANAGEMENT

Epidural pain control provides selective analgesia for a body region, and it has become more common for postoperative pain management. A catheter is inserted into the epidural space during general anesthesia through which anesthetics and opioids may be administered in small doses. Analgesia may be administered by intermittent bolus, continuous infusion by a small pump, or PCA to maintain pain control for the first 24 to 48 hours after surgery. Urinary retention may be a complication and a urinary catheter may be required for the duration of epidural pain management. Monitor vital signs, pain level, and degree of motor and sensory block.

Regional nerve blocks, such as a popliteal or femoral for the lower extremity, or interscalene (in a muscle of the cervical vertebrae) for the upper extremity, are used for anesthesia and to control pain after surgery. A subcutaneous catheter is inserted into the local area for infusion of the medications. The single dose administered during surgery may last up to 15 hours postoperatively (Guarin, 2013). A continuous infusion may also be given using a pump.

Clinical Tip

Assess the extremity receiving the local nerve block for color, temperature, and capillary refill. Assess motor function by asking children if they can move their legs, wiggle their toes, and lift their buttocks off the bed. Ensure proper positioning of the extremity to prevent nerve damage. Protect the extremity from injury because the child has reduced feeling in the limb. Monitor the child every 2 hours for tingling felt in the fingers or toes of the affected extremity, the first sign that the nerve block is receding. Effective oral analgesia should be initiated to maintain pain control when the nerve block begins to recede.

TEACHING HIGHLIGHTS | Patient-Controlled Analgesia (PCA)

- What is PCA? *Analgesia* means pain relief: you get to control the amount of medicine you receive by using the PCA machine.
- The machine gives the medicine by passing it through the tube that is connected to your IV line. When you push the button, the machine pumps pain medicine into the IV line to make you feel better.
- The machine limits the amount of medicine you can get to what the healthcare provider prescribes. You can get any amount up to the maximum hourly limit by pushing the button at times during the hour. The push button will not let you make a mistake if you drop it or roll on it.
- Whenever you feel pain, hurt, or discomfort, push the button to get more medicine. You should be the only one to push the button. Do not let another family member push the button.
- No needles for pain shots are needed as long as the IV line is in place.
- The PCA may not relieve all of your pain, but it should make you feel comfortable. Let the nurse know if you think your PCA is not working.
- The PCA will be used until you can take pain medicine by mouth.

Nonpharmacologic Methods of Pain Management

Complementary therapies are nonpharmacologic methods used for pain management that can enhance the effect of analgesics and potentially reduce the amount of analgesics needed. One or more of these methods may provide adequate pain relief when the child has low levels of pain.

DISTRACTION

Distraction involves engaging a child in a pleasant activity to help focus attention on something other than pain and the anxiety. Teach the parent to be a distraction coach and suggest developmentally appropriate distraction activities to use. Examples of distraction activities are provided in *Growth and Development: Distraction Activities* later in the chapter. Note that children in severe pain cannot be distracted and do not assume that pain is gone if a child can be distracted.

GUIDED IMAGERY

Imagery is a cognitive behavioral process that encourages the child to relax (often with progressive muscle relaxation techniques) and focus on vivid mental images as if they were real, and to ignore things, such as a painful procedure. For example, help the child to visualize and explore a favorite place, do a fun activity, remember a funny story, or be a superhero. Ask the child to think about all the sights, sounds, smells, tastes, and feelings that will enhance the image and experience. Imagery has been used successfully by school-age children to reduce the pain associated with sickle cell disease (Dobson & Byrne, 2014).

RELAXATION TECHNIQUES

Progressive muscle relaxation is used to reduce muscle tension that may worsen pain. Teach children to tense and relax different muscle groups, starting with the hands and feet, and then moving to more central muscles. Ask the child to tense a muscle group for 10 seconds and notice how it feels, and then ask the child to relax the muscle group for 10 seconds and compare the feelings. With practice, the child should be able to detect the difference between tense and relaxed muscles and then to reduce the tension. Relaxation techniques may be combined with rhythmic breathing.

BREATHING TECHNIQUES

Rhythmic deep breaths can be used with distraction or muscle relaxation during a painful procedure or as a mechanism to reduce stress. Ask the child or adolescent to take a deep breath, hold it for 5 seconds, and blow out through the mouth, as if to push the tension out or the needle away. Another breathing technique is patterned, shallow breathing. The young child is encouraged to take shallow breaths in through the nose and blow out through the mouth while thinking of a particular image. For example, the short breaths could be the "toot, toot" of a train horn.

CUTANEOUS STIMULATION

Gently rub the painful area, massage the skin gently, and hold or rock the child. Touching competes with the pain stimuli that are transmitted from the peripheral nerves to the spinal cord and brain and may reduce the pain felt by the child. Swaddling and skin-to-skin contact are methods to reduce neonatal pain responses.

HYPNOSIS

Hypnosis is an altered state of awareness facilitating heightened concentration, decreased awareness of external stimuli, increased relaxation, and increased suggestibility. The hypnotic or positive therapeutic suggestion often uses muscle relaxation and guided imagery, and posthypnotic suggestions are given for the relief of anxiety, tension, and pain. Children more easily respond to hypnosis than adults because of their imaginative powers for fun and fantasy. Hypnosis has been successful in helping children and adolescents manage the stress and pain associated with invasive medical procedures and chronic pain such as daily headaches and surgery (Kohen, 2011; Martin, Smith, Newcomb, et al., 2014).

SUCROSE SOLUTION

A sucrose solution (2 mL of 24% solution) is effective for pain relief during painful procedures (venipuncture, heel sticks, cannulation) in preterm and term newborns up to 1 month of age (Cooper & Petty, 2012). The sweet taste is believed to activate the endogenous opioid pathways, leading to the release of endogenous opioids. The effectiveness of sucrose solution beyond 4 weeks of age for immunizations has not been consistently demonstrated in research (Wilson, Bremner, Mathews, et al., 2013). Give the solution 2 minutes before the procedure, and the analgesic effect of sucrose lasts approximately 3 to 5 minutes. Allow the infant to continue sucking on a pacifier or to breastfeed during the procedure to enhance the effect of sucrose.

APPLICATION OF HEAT AND COLD

Heat application promotes dilation of blood vessels. The increased blood circulation permits the removal of cell breakdown debris from the site. Heat also promotes muscle relaxation, breaking the pain–spasm–pain cycle. To reduce edema, do not apply heat in the first 24 hours after an injury.

The application of cold is believed to slow the ability of pain fibers to transmit pain impulses to help control pain. Apply ice for 20 to 30 minutes and then remove for about 10 minutes before continuing therapy. Assess the skin for redness or signs of irritation. Discontinue cold applications immediately if the skin alternately blanches and reddens afterwards.

ELECTROANALGESIA

Also known as transcutaneous electrical nerve stimulation (TENS), **electroanalgesia** delivers small amounts of electrical stimulation to the skin by electrodes. This electronic stimulation is stronger than the pain impulses and is thought to interfere with the transmission of pain impulses from the peripheral nerves to the spinal cord and brain. TENS may be used for both acute and chronic pain management. The only known side effect is skin irritation at the electrode site.

ACUPUNCTURE

A traditional Chinese treatment for pain relief, acupuncture has been gaining greater acceptance in Western medicine. Acupuncture is based on the theory that energy, or chi, flows along channels through the body (meridians) that are connected by acupuncture points. Placement of acupuncture needles at specific pain points interferes with the transmission of pain impulses to the brain, and it also stimulates the release of endogenous opioids (Chon & Lee, 2013). Limited research has been conducted about the use and effectiveness of acupuncture in children.

Nursing Management

For the Child With Acute Pain

Nursing Assessment and Diagnosis

Nurses have an ethical obligation to relieve a child's suffering. Unrelieved pain has consequences, and appropriate pain management may have benefits such as earlier mobilization, shortened hospital stays, and reduced costs. Anticipate the presence of pain and recognize the child's right to pain control.

Professionalism in Practice Pain Management

In 2001, the Joint Commission introduced standards for the assessment and management of pain in clients treated in healthcare facilities. Nurses have a responsibility to assess a child's pain during their initial assessment and as appropriate during subsequent care. Pain management should be provided, and children and parents should be educated about managing pain (Joint Commission, 2014).

When assessing pain in children, keep the following questions in mind:

- What is happening in tissues that might cause pain? Assume that children who have had surgery, injury, a vaso-occlusive episode, or illness are experiencing pain since these events also cause pain in adults.
- What external factors could be causing pain? For example, is the cast too tight or is the child poorly positioned in bed?
- Are there any indicators of pain, either physiologic or behavioral?
- How is the child responding emotionally?
- How does the child or parent rate the pain?

Physiologic symptoms such as nausea, fatigue, dyspnea, bladder and bowel distention, and fever may influence the intensity of pain felt by a child. The child's behavior or responses to pain stimuli may also be affected by fear, anxiety, separation from parents, anger, culture, age, or a previous pain experience.

When working with an infant or child, determine which pain scale is the most appropriate for the circumstance and developmental stage. When using a self-report pain assessment tool, *use the same tool each time* you assess for pain or for the evaluation of pain management. This makes comparison of assessment results possible. A chronologic record of the child's pain assessments must be documented along with actions taken to relieve pain in addition to the follow-up assessments to determine the effectiveness of those actions.

Remember that surgery and trauma can result in multiple sites of pain (incision or laceration, cut or bruised muscles, interrupted blood supply, nasogastric tube placement, insertion sites of IV lines). Attempt to evaluate the intensity of pain at each site.

Examples of nursing diagnoses for children in pain include the following (NANDA-I © 2014):

- *Pain, Acute*, related to injury and femur fracture
- *Anxiety* related to anticipation of pain from an invasive procedure
- *Mobility: Physical, Impaired*, related to pain
- *Nausea* related to opioids used for pain medication

Other nursing diagnoses are included in *Nursing Care Plan: The Child With Postoperative Pain.*

Planning and Implementation

Nursing management involves the following actions to increase and maintain client comfort: pharmacologic intervention; complementary therapy; monitoring, evaluating, and documenting

---

Nursing Care Plan: The Child With Postoperative Pain

1. Nursing Diagnosis: *Pain, Acute (severe abdominal)*, related to surgery and injury (NANDA-I © 2014)

GOAL: The child will report relief.

INTERVENTION	RATIONALE
• Have the child select a pain scale and rate the amount of pain perceived before and 30–60 minutes after analgesia is given to ensure pain relief.	• The child's pain rating is the best indicator of pain. Maintenance of pain control requires less analgesia than treating each acute pain episode.
• Assess pain control each hour to ensure that the child's pain is relieved.	• Frequent monitoring identifies inadequate pain control before it becomes significant.
• Reposition the child every 2 hours to maintain good body alignment.	• New positions decrease muscle cramping and skin pressure.
• Provide therapeutic touch or massage. Encourage the parents to read a story or play favorite music.	• Complementary therapy reduces stress and enhances the analgesic action.

EXPECTED OUTCOME: Child will report pain relief after administration of analgesia, respositioning, and complementary therapy, as indicated by a lower level on the pain scale.

2. Nursing Diagnosis: *Sleep Pattern, Disturbed*, related to inadequate pain control (NANDA-I © 2014)

GOAL: The child will experience fewer disruptions of sleep by pain.

INTERVENTION	RATIONALE
• Give analgesia by continuous infusion or every 3–4 hours around the clock.	• Pain breakthrough occurs even during sleep and disturbs its healing effects.

EXPECTED OUTCOME: Child will sleep for age-appropriate number of hours per day, undisturbed by pain.

3. Nursing Diagnosis: *Health Management, Readiness for Enhanced*, **related to self-management of pain control and use of nonpharmacologic pain-control measures (NANDA-I © 2014)**

GOAL: The child and family will effectively use patient-controlled analgesia (PCA) and complementary therapy pain-control measures.

INTERVENTION	RATIONALE
• Teach the child how the PCA works and when to push the button.	• The child must know that pain can be relieved by pushing the PCA button and how the button works.
• Teach the family and the child how to use age-appropriate complementary therapies for pain management.	• Complementary therapy pain-control measures may reduce the amount of analgesia needed.

EXPECTED OUTCOME: Child's pain rating will stay low. Child and family will independently use complementary therapies for pain control.

GOAL: The child and family will use appropriate analgesia after discharge.

INTERVENTION	RATIONALE
• Explain why managing pain is helpful for the child's healing.	• The family and child may not know the benefits of relieving pain.
• Discuss how to assess the child's pain and ways to manage it at home after discharge.	• The family and child may be anxious about pain management at home.

EXPECTED OUTCOME: Family will understand pain assessment and pain-relief measures and state appropriate dose and frequency for pain medication use at home.

4. Nursing Diagnosis: *Breathing Pattern, Ineffective*, **related to opioid overdose (NANDA-I © 2014)**

GOAL: The child will maintain adequate ventilations.

INTERVENTION	RATIONALE
• Verify that correct opioid dose is given for the child's weight.	• Respiratory depression is a significant complication when too much opioid medication is given.
• Monitor vital signs and depth of respirations before analgesic is administered and at time of peak drug action. Withhold opioid if vital signs fall within parameters set by the healthcare provider or policy.	• A respiratory depression episode must be identified before it progresses to respiratory arrest. All opioids act on brainstem center, which decreases responsiveness to CO_2 tension.
• Calculate agonist dose prescribed by healthcare provider to be sure it will reverse respiratory depression, but not counteract effect of analgesia.	• Valuable time will be saved if agonist is needed to treat respiratory depression. Complete reversal of analgesia will cause the child to have significant pain.

EXPECTED OUTCOME: Child will not have episodes of respiratory depression associated with analgesia.

5. Nursing Diagnosis: *Constipation, Risk for*, **related to opioid administration and decreased motility of gastrointestinal tract (NANDA-I © 2014)**

GOAL: The child will have minimal constipation.

INTERVENTION	RATIONALE
• Assess bowel sounds and abdominal distention, and palpate the abdomen.	• Signs of constipation must be anticipated and identified.
• Request healthcare provider order for stimulating laxative and stool softener.	• Opioids increase the transit time of feces and interfere with bile enzymes needed for evacuation.
• Provide fluids of choice to increase fluid intake when IV fluids are decreased.	• Extra fluids will counteract opioid action of increasing the absorption of water from the large intestine.
• Inform family and child that constipation is a side effect of pain medication.	• Parents can become partners in increasing fluid intake and monitoring bowel movements.

EXPECTED OUTCOME: Child will have bowel movements at least every 2 days while on opioid pain control.

EVIDENCE-BASED PRACTICE | Challenges to Adequate Pain Management

Clinical Question

Why does adequate management of children with acute pain continue to be a problem despite the increased knowledge about children's needs for pain relief?

The Evidence

A children's hospital committed to pain management conducted a survey of nurses (n = 272) to rate 18 potential barriers to optimal pain management. The five leading barriers identified were inadequate healthcare provider orders, insufficient premedication orders before procedures, insufficient time allowed to premedicate before procedures, low priority given to pain management by medical staff, and parents' reluctance to have children receive medication (Czarnecki et al., 2011).

After implementation of some quality improvement projects related to the identified barriers to optimal pain management, a follow-up survey using the same questions was conducted with nurses (n = 442) in the same hospital. Consistency in barriers perceived by nurses was found for four of the five leading barriers. Insufficient time allowed to premedicate before procedures was less of a barrier, perhaps due to development of a hospitalwide procedure guideline. A significant decrease in perceptions related to the barriers of inadequate healthcare provider orders and insufficient premedication orders before procedures was found, both also having been the focus of quality improvement efforts. A new barrier was identified related to the time taken to process and deliver pain medications from pharmacy (Czarnecki, Salamon, Thompson, et al., 2014). Findings revealed that more work is needed.

Thirty nurses working in a general hospital participated in focus groups to identify their perceptions about barriers and facilitators to pediatric pain management and the effectiveness of the facility's 3-year-old pediatric pain practice guideline. One nursing barrier related to knowledge deficiencies about pain management and analgesics and the potential of overdosing a child. The nurses expressed an expectation that parents and children inform them when in pain rather than being proactive in assessing for pain, and they were concerned about parents requesting pain medication when the child's behavior did not reflect pain. It was not evident that all nurses knew about or used the pain practice guideline since participating nurses requested pediatric pain assessment tools and a pain medication flow chart that was part of the practice guideline (Twycross & Collins, 2013).

Best Practice

Pain management is a complex process that requires the nurse to assess the child and make clinical judgments about treatment. The expectations that children must display pain behaviors to have their pain believed or that pain assessment and management is a low nursing priority are ongoing concerns. The facility's structure and culture also have an important influence on pain management. The Czarnecki studies focused on organizational contributors to pain management and efforts to change the system. Findings revealed some improvements but illustrate the challenges of making systemwide improvements, even in a pediatric hospital. System changes to improve pain management require collaboration among healthcare providers and the development of practice guidelines. Hospitals then need to educate healthcare providers about the care expectations in the practice guidelines and evaluate how well they are implemented. Nurses must take responsibility for learning and consistently using the guidelines.

Clinical Reasoning

In the clinical setting, identify the infrastructure supports to promote pain management of children, such as pain assessment tools, pain flow sheets, pain management policies and guidelines, education, and resources for complementary therapies. Identify additional supports that would help you as an inexperienced nurse to gain competence in pediatric pain management.

---

the effectiveness of pain-control measures to provide optimal comfort; and client education. See *Evidence-Based Practice: Challenges to Adequate Pain Management.*

PHARMACOLOGIC INTERVENTION

Give analgesics as ordered by the healthcare provider, ensuring that the dose is appropriate for the child's weight. When administering an opioid by intravenous infusion or PCA, monitor the flow rate and the site for infiltration. Follow facility guidelines for monitoring vital signs, and use a pulse oximeter or cardiorespiratory monitor with audible alarm for children at risk for respiratory depression. Vital signs (heart rate and blood pressure) may not change in response to effective analgesia when infection, trauma, or other stressors keep them elevated. Make sure that naloxone is available in case adverse effects develop. The dose should be precalculated and the medication immediately available when an opioid is used.

Check for the presence of other side effects of analgesics, such as sedation, nausea, vomiting, itching, urinary retention, and constipation. An alternative opioid or medications to treat the side effects may be prescribed when analgesia is needed long term.

Oral NSAIDs, sometimes in combination with an opioid, are generally ordered for less severe pain or chronic pain. These drugs may mask fever. Be alert to the potential complication of gastrointestinal hemorrhage in critically ill children who have increased gastric acids as a physiologic stress response to pain.

Assess the child for pain using a behavioral or self-report pain scale 15 to 30 minutes following intravenous pain medication and 1 hour after oral pain medication to determine if adequate pain control was achieved. Evaluate the child's level of pain frequently to identify any increase in pain intensity. Use information collected from the child and parent. Dramatic reductions in pain should occur, although not all pain may disappear. Be certain to record results of pain-control measures to guide future nursing actions. Use a flow sheet to document assessments, medication administration, complementary therapies, and other comfort measures during the postoperative period.

Many children sleep after receiving an analgesic. This sleep is not a side effect of the drug or a sign of an overdose, but the result of pain relief. Pain interrupts sleep, and once pain is relieved, the child can sleep comfortably. However, sleep does not always indicate pain control. A child in pain may fall asleep in exhaustion. Look for other symptoms of pain, such as excess movement or moaning.

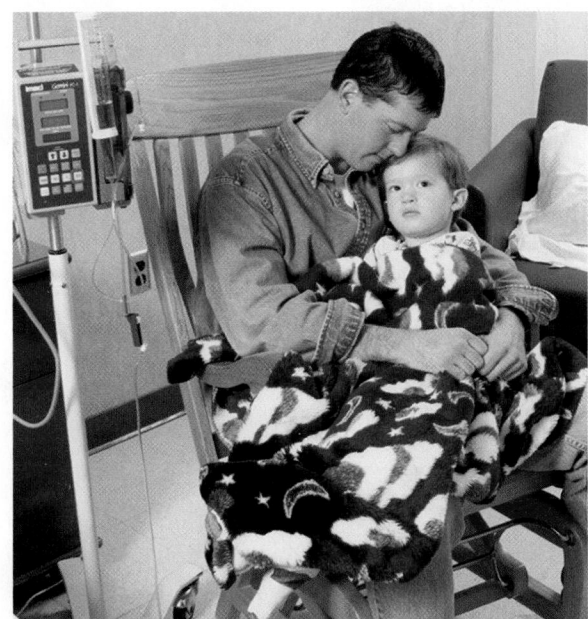

Figure 40–5 The presence of the parent is an important part of pain management. Children often feel more secure telling their parents about their pain and anxiety.

Become an advocate for the child when the dose or type of analgesic ordered is inadequate. When the child with severe pain has been taking opioids for several days, tolerance may occur and an increasing amount of the opioid may be needed to produce or maintain the same level of pain relief. The duration of effective analgesia becomes shorter than expected, and breakthrough pain occurs. Review the child's record to verify that the opioid was given at the appropriate dose and frequency before asking the healthcare provider to modify the child's pain medication.

COMPLEMENTARY THERAPY

Complementary therapies can be implemented for all children with discomfort and pain, with or without pain medication. Parents are one of the most powerful nonpharmacologic methods of pain relief available to children (Figure 40–5). When parents are actively participating in the child's care during hospitalization, provide suggestions for some age-appropriate interventions to improve comfort (see *Growth and Development: Distraction Activities*).

Growth and Development Distraction Activities

Children of all ages feel more secure and may have less pain and anxiety when parents are present. Parents can actively participate during their child's care with selection of age-appropriate distraction strategies, such as the following:

- *Infants:* holding, rocking, pacifier, mobiles, music, soft toys, massage
- *Toddlers:* massage, pinwheels, stories, bubbles, touch, holding, rocking, music
- *Preschoolers:* puzzles, action figures and other toys, being a superhero, kaleidoscopes, books, videos
- *School-age children:* rhythmic breathing, muscle relaxation, guided imagery, talking about pleasant experiences, playing games, watching a video, video games
- *Adolescents:* rhythmic breathing, muscle relaxation, guided imagery, having visitors, video games, watching videos, listening to CD player or iPod

Clinical Reasoning Determining When a Child Is in Pain

Felicia, who is 5 years old, was struck by a car. Six hours ago, she had surgery to repair a liver laceration, but she also has numerous bruises and abrasions on her body. After spending 3 hours in the postanesthesia unit, she was moved to the pediatric inpatient unit. She has an intravenous line in place, as well as a nasogastric tube attached to low suction. Her abdominal dressing is clean and dry. Felicia has orders for morphine IV every 3 hours around the clock for the first 24 hours.

Felicia's mother is rooming in with her during her hospital stay. Twelve hours after surgery, Felicia is dozing but is responsive to verbal stimuli. Her most recent IV morphine was given 2 hours ago. The nurse attempts to determine how well Felicia's pain is managed. Her facial expression indicates that she is not in pain. Felicia's mother feels that she is resting comfortably.

How do you know whether Felicia is in pain? Can you expect her to tell you if she feels pain? What other pain-relief measures could reduce or help to control her pain in the first 24 hours? What is the appropriate dose of IV morphine for Felicia, who weighs 25 kg? What is the timing of assessments of the response to pain medication and potential side effects? What signs of respiratory distress indicate a need for naloxone administration?

MEASURES TO INCREASE COMFORT DURING PAINFUL PROCEDURES

Make every effort to increase the child's comfort during painful procedures, including the use of complementary therapies. Topical anesthetics can be used to reduce the pain associated with an immunization, other injection, intravenous insertion, venipuncture, heel lance, or the first needlestick of another procedure. Give time for the medication to become effective. Mechanisms for administration of topical anesthetics include the following:

- Vapocoolant sprays can be used for injections. Spray the site or soak a cotton ball and apply to intact skin for about a minute.
- EMLA (eutectic mixture of local anesthetics) cream, an emulsion of 2.5% lidocaine and 2.5% prilocaine, is effective if applied 60 minutes before a needlestick, venipuncture, or circumcision procedure on intact skin in infants and children (Barnes, 2014). The depth of penetration deepens if left on longer.
- L-M-X4, 4%, liposomal lidocaine (formerly called ELA-MAX), is effective if applied 30 minutes before a needlestick. It is available without a prescription. See Figure 40–6.
- The Synera anesthetic patch, containing 70 mg of lidocaine and 70 mg of tetracaine, can be applied to intact skin for 20 to 30 minutes prior to a procedure. It becomes heated on application and results in more rapid anesthesia.
- Buzzy for Shots is a device that has a cold pad placed against the skin and a buzzing bee that vibrates. Buzzy is placed over the site of a needlestick for 30 seconds and then moved and placed proximally during the needlestick. The cold and vibration stimulation interferes with pain

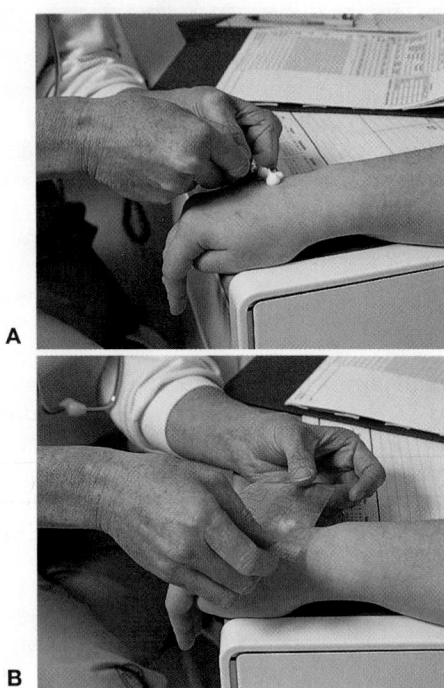

Figure 40–6 Anesthetizing cream (e.g., L-M-X4 or EMLA) may be prescribed for use prior to a painful needlestick. *A,* Apply a thin layer on selected sites and wait 30 seconds, and then apply a thick layer of cream over intact skin. *B,* Cover the cream with plastic wrap or a transparent adhesive dressing to keep the cream in place and to prevent ingestion. Depending upon the cream used, the dermal surface is anesthetized in 30 to 60 minutes.

transmission, and it also provides distraction for the child (Buzzy, 2014). See Figure 40–7.

- A needle-free powder lidocaine delivery system (J-Tip) produces rapid analgesia (within 1 to 3 minutes) for IV starts and venipuncture. The system has a sterile, single-use, prefilled, and disposable cartridge that is pressed against the skin. Pressurized carbon dioxide gas ruptures the cartridge and forces lidocaine particles to penetrate the skin. Prepare the child for the small pop sound when it is used.

- LET (lidocaine, epinephrine, and tetracaine) is a topical anesthetic for laceration repair. The LET liquid is applied to a cotton ball and the skin, or LET gel is applied to the skin and covered with an occlusive dressing. The anesthetic works in 30 minutes (Barnes, 2014).

A local anesthetic such as lidocaine buffered by sodium bicarbonate or bupivacaine is often injected subcutaneously to provide analgesia for emergent invasive procedures.

Assemble a pain management kit to promote distraction, imagery, and relaxation in children. Include items such as magic wands, pinwheels, bubble liquid, a Slinky spring toy, a foam ball, party noisemakers, and pop-up books. It may also be helpful to include items for therapeutic play such as syringes, adhesive bandages, alcohol swabs, and other supplies from a medical kit. The pain management kit may be especially helpful for distracting children who are being prepared for medical procedures.

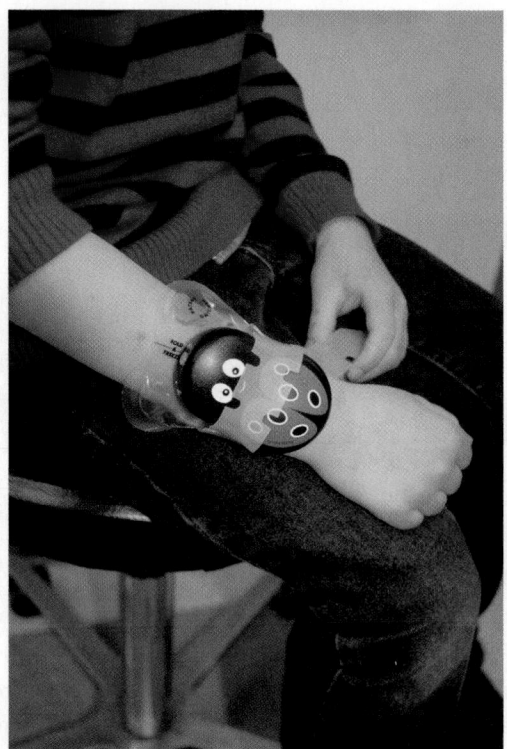

Figure 40–7 Buzzy for Shots is a device that uses cold and vibration stimulation to interrupt and reduce pain transmission due to immunization and venipuncture needlesticks. The vibration and colorful bee distract the child. Start by attaching the cold pack to Buzzy and placing this on the target area. Turn the buzzer on for 30 seconds. Then move Buzzy to an area proximal to the planned needle site, turn on the buzzer, and keep in place during the needlestick. This child is being prepared for an IV start on his arm.

SOURCE: Photo courtesy of Jane Ball, RN, DrPH.

Clinical Tip

Teach parents about the use of anesthetic cream (e.g., L-M-X4 or EMLA) or other pain management tool when the child is scheduled for an immunization or venipuncture. Anesthetic cream can be applied to the skin before departing for the healthcare visit. Provide directions regarding the correct placement of the cream on the arm or leg. Have the parents follow the directions from the package regarding the amount to use and how to cover the site with plastic wrap during the trip to the health center.

DISCHARGE PLANNING AND HOME CARE TEACHING

Children are frequently discharged from the hospital with oral analgesics following surgery, injury, or treatment of acute medical conditions. The child usually leaves the hospital or surgical center pain free, and the parents may not anticipate pain. Provide information about the child's need for pain medication around the clock for the first 1 to 2 days to prevent the child from feeling pain, and the benefits of pain management in promoting the child's healing.

Provide guidance to help parents assess their child's pain, and for school-age children and adolescents to assess their own pain. Teach parents and children about the dosage and frequency of administration and the side effects of the analgesic ordered. Consider providing a calendar or recommended schedule for daily pain medication and other medications for at least a week. Parents can post this on the refrigerator and check off doses as administered. This strategy may improve adherence with recommendations. Review complementary therapies and encourage children and parents to use the techniques that work best for them.

SAFETY ALERT!

Parents may make common dosing errors when using teaspoons or tablespoons to measure medications such as liquid acetaminophen or ibuprofen for their children, especially if abbreviations (tsp or tbs) are used on the label instructions. For example, use of a tablespoon rather than the recommended teaspoon dose leads to 3 times the appropriate dose. Additionally, the size of tableware spoons varies, which can also affect dose accuracy. Use of dosing devices measured in millimeters (mL) (e.g., oral syringe, dosing spoon, or measuring cup) is an effective way to reduce medication errors that can lead to adverse effects associated with medications prescribed for pain. Educate parents about the correct milliliter dose when labels specify medication volume by teaspoon or tablespoon. The American Academy of Pediatrics (AAP) now recommends that all oral liquid medications be prescribed using metric units or milliliters (AAP, 2015).

Remember that many common health problems (otitis media, pharyngitis, and urinary tract infection) have pain as one of the presenting symptoms. Often the only medication prescribed is an antibiotic to clear the infection. The child may be in pain for 48 to 72 hours until the antibiotic controls the infection. Give parents recommendations for pain control and comfort measures during this period. Review the dose, dosing device, and formulation of acetaminophen or ibuprofen used by parents to identify any risk for overdose. Avoid using any left-over pain medications prescribed for other conditions. See Chapter 43.

SAFETY ALERT!

Warn parents who are sent home with a prescription for an opioid for their child about the need to dispose of the remaining medication or to lock it up after it is no longer needed. Adolescents may share unprotected tablets with friends leading to and supporting substance abuse. The rate of poisoning death due to prescription drug misuse has increased dramatically in recent years (see the *Healthy People 2020* objective). Check with local law enforcement or the pharmacy about the availability of medication disposal sites or options.

Healthy People 2020

(SA-19) Reduce the past-year nonmedical use of prescription drugs

Evaluation

Expected outcomes of nursing care include the following:

- The child's pain level is assessed frequently and pain management is effective in improving the child's comfort.

- The child successfully uses a PCA pump to control acute pain.
- Age-appropriate complementary therapies enhance the comfort provided by medications.
- Parents maintain the child's pain management after discharge.

Chronic Pain

Some children have medical conditions that cause chronic pain or recurrent episodes of acute pain, sometimes in more than one body system. Medical conditions such as juvenile idiopathic arthritis, sickle cell disease, cancer, headaches, recurrent abdominal pain, and HIV infection all cause chronic and recurrent pain. Approximately 20% to 35% of children and adolescents are estimated to have chronic pain (APS, 2012). These children and adolescents often have functional limitations related to school, social activities and relationships, physical activity, and family responsibilities. Chronic pain has social and emotional consequences for the child and family.

Clinical Manifestations

Behavioral indicators of chronic pain may include fatigue, inactivity, posturing, difficulty concentrating and sleeping, withdrawal from activities, and mood disturbances. Persistent or continuous chronic pain permits physiologic adaptation so the elevated heart rate, respiratory rate, and blood pressure levels associated with the initial response to acute pain are rarely seen (Huether, 2014). However, the child with intermittent acute painful episodes may have initial vital sign changes. Varying levels of disability may also exist.

Clinical Therapy

An interdisciplinary team that collaborates on addressing the factors that stimulate and contribute to the child's pain in an individualized treatment plan should focus on improving function and comfort. Cognitive behavioral therapies are used to address the connection between thoughts, feelings, and behaviors; reduce stress; and promote coping. Physical and occupational therapy may help restore function. Treatment for sleep disturbances and strategies for school functioning are addressed. Complementary therapies such as relaxation strategies, ice, or heat should be used when appropriate (APS 2012). Analgesics rarely include opioids except for acute painful episodes. NSAIDs or acetaminophen may be prescribed. Complete pain relief may not be possible. A tricyclic antidepressant may be prescribed for its analgesic properties and because depression may be a coexisting condition.

Health Promotion

Children with chronic pain should learn a cognitive behavioral therapy (e.g., hypnosis, guided imagery) that helps the child to reduce stress, cope with pain, and enhance pain management. Use of relaxation techniques with guided imagery that includes positive suggestions for comfort has helped many children with a chronic painful condition reduce their pain. Improved quality of life scores have been noted (Gottsegen, 2011).

Nursing Management

When assessing chronic pain in the child, approach pain as if it were the primary problem for attention. Consider the physical, behavioral, and psychologic signs and symptoms together. Focus on the following topics to assess and evaluate chronic pain in children (APS, 2012):

- Obtain the history of pain onset, its development over time, intensity, duration, variability, location, and what worsens or relieves it. Ask what the family and child believe causes the pain. Identify past pain problems in the family.

- Learn about the impact of the pain on the child's daily life (sleep, appetite, school, activity, and social interactions). Identify how much distress the child and family experience with pain.

- Identify the child's methods for coping with pain. How does the pain impact the child's emotional function?

- Ask about the current treatment methods, including complementary therapies.

- Observe the child's appearance, posture, gait, and emotional and cognitive state. Perform a complete neurologic examination. Assess muscle spasms, trigger points, and areas sensitive to light touch.

Encourage older school-age children and adolescents with chronic pain or recurrent episodes of acute pain to keep a pain diary to describe the pain intensity, characteristics, timing, activities, and potential triggers of their pain, as well as their response to pain treatment measures. A pain assessment scale should be used to rate the pain intensity before and after medications and other pain-control measures are used. This record can help improve pain management when shared with healthcare providers.

Monitor pain intensity at each office visit and frequently during hospitalizations. Believe the child who reports chronic pain or recurrent episodes of pain, and use pharmacologic and nonpharmacologic methods to reduce or relieve the child's pain. Remember the child may have increased pain sensitivity in anticipation of and during needlesticks and other procedures.

Work with the pain management team to individualize the pain management plan to meet the child's needs, family's beliefs and values, and their cultural preferences for care. Develop a care plan for acute painful episodes associated with the condition. Assist the child and family to identify age-appropriate and acceptable complementary therapies to help cope with discomfort. Encourage daily exercise to promote function.

Sedation and Analgesia for Medical Procedures

Children undergo a wide variety of painful diagnostic and treatment procedures in the hospital and in outpatient settings. Procedures such as chest tube insertion, arterial puncture, lumbar puncture, bone marrow aspiration, fracture reduction, laceration repair, insertion of a central or peripheral intravenous line, and burn debridement cause significant pain in children. The anticipation of these procedures causes anxiety and emotional distress that can lead to greater pain intensity. For example, children with prior painful cancer treatment procedures may express greater pain during later procedures, even when provided with adequate analgesia (Rosen & Dower, 2011).

Sedation is a medically controlled state of depressed consciousness (light to deep) used for painful diagnostic and therapeutic procedures. **Moderate sedation** (formerly called conscious sedation) occurs with lower doses of sedatives and enables the child to maintain protective reflexes independently, continuously maintain a patent airway, and respond to tactile and verbal stimuli. **Deep sedation** is a controlled state of depressed consciousness or unconsciousness in which protective airway reflexes are lost. See Table 40–7 for characteristics of different sedation levels.

Drugs used for sedation include the following:

- Benzodiazepines: midazolam (Versed), diazepam (Valium), and lorazepam (Ativan); antagonist agent is flumazenil

- Hypnotics or barbiturates: methohexital

- Ketamine

- Propofol (Diprivan) or Etomidate

- Chloral hydrate

- Analgesics: fentanyl, alfentanil; antagonist agents are naloxone and nalmefene

Every healthcare facility should have guidelines for the use of sedation to ensure safe healthcare practices. Healthcare providers monitoring the child should have specific qualifications, such as training in pediatric advanced life support. Potential complications of sedation include respiratory depression, a compromised airway, delayed awakening, agitation, nausea and vomiting, and tachycardia or bradycardia (Krauss & Green, 2013).

TABLE 40–7 Clinical Manifestations of Light, Moderate, and Deep Sedation

ASSESSMENT FACTORS	LIGHT SEDATION	MODERATE SEDATION	DEEP SEDATION
Airway	Maintains airway independently and continuously	Maintains airway independently and continuously	Airway may not be maintained, may need ventilation assistance
Cough and gag reflexes	Reflexes intact	Reflexes intact	Partial or complete loss of reflexes
Level of consciousness	Responds normally to verbal stimuli	Purposeful response to verbal or gentle tactile stimuli	Difficult to arouse, purposeful response after repeated or painful stimuli

Source: Data from Jest, A. D., & Tonge, A. (2011). Using a learning needs assessment to identify knowledge deficits regarding procedural sedation for pediatric patients. *AORN Journal, 94*(6), 567–574; Barnes, S. (2014). Analgesia and sedation. In B. Engorn, & J. Flerlage (Eds.), *The Harriet Lane handbook* (20th ed.). Philadelphia, PA: Elsevier Mosby; Krauss, B., & Green, S. M. (2014). Systemic analgesia and sedation for procedures. In J. R. Roberts, & C. B. Custalow (Eds.), *Roberts and Hedges' clinical procedures in emergency medicine* (6th ed., pp. 586–610). Philadelphia, PA: Elsevier Saunders.

Sedation is a continuum, and the child may move from one level of sedation to another. The child must be carefully monitored for respiratory depression and signs of deep sedation, so the airway can be protected and ventilatory support can be provided if needed. A pediatric code cart, resuscitation bag-valve-mask and drugs, oxygen, and suction must be available, along with antagonist agents (naloxone and flumazenil) for opioids and benzodiazepines, when the effects of sedation and respiratory depression must be reversed.

Nursing Management

When the child receives sedation, continuously assess the child's status to include visual confirmation of respiratory effort, chest wall movement, color, vital signs, level of consciousness, and oxygen saturation. Document vital signs every 5 minutes (Jest & Tonge, 2011). A cardiorespiratory monitor, pulse oximeter, and expiratory CO_2 monitor should be used, but the equipment must not replace visual assessment. Be prepared to suction emesis or excessive salivation that could obstruct the airway. After the procedure, check vital signs every 15 minutes until the child regains full consciousness and level of functioning, usually within 30 minutes.

Criteria for discharging the child after sedation include the following (Krauss & Green, 2013):

- Stable vital signs, airway patency, and intact protective reflexes
- Child sits up without assistance, infant holds head up
- Discharge status is the same as admission status
- Fluid intake is not essential as some sedation medications stimulate vomiting in children.

Inform parents that the child may have mild adverse effects from sedation, such as crying, lethargy, and vomiting. Avoid food and fluids for 2 hours if the child has nausea. For the next 12 hours, do not permit activities such as bicycle riding or gymnastics that require coordination, and do not leave the child unattended in the bathtub or pool.

Focus Your Study

- Pain is an unpleasant sensation that is either acute or chronic. It is perceived in response to tissue damage that increases the stress in children of all ages. Neuropathic pain is one form of chronic pain.

- Unrelieved pain causes many undesirable physiologic consequences on body systems, such as inadequate lung expansion and coughing, increased metabolic rate, increased sympathetic nervous system activity, decreased gastric acids and intestinal motility, depressed inflammatory responses, and increased pain sensitivity.

- A child's responses to and understanding of pain depend on age, stage of development, culture, and prior painful experiences.

- Assessment of acute and chronic pain should include physical, behavioral, and emotional factors to obtain the most accurate information about the location and intensity of the child's pain and how the child responds to it.

- Pain assessment should include the use of a valid and reliable pain assessment tool that is appropriate for the child's age, cognitive development, and condition.

- Every infant, child, and adolescent has the right to adequate pain control.

- Pharmacologic interventions for pain control include opioids, nonsteroidal anti-inflammatory drugs (NSAIDs), and acetaminophen.

- Analgesia for continuous or severe pain should be given around the clock to maintain pain control.

- Complementary therapies for pain management include the following: parental presence, distraction, cutaneous stimulation, sucrose solution, electroanalgesia, guided imagery, breathing techniques, progressive muscle relaxation techniques, hypnosis, application of heat and cold, biofeedback, and acupuncture.

- Methods to reduce pain associated with needlesticks include vapocoolant spray, LMX-4 cream, Synera patch, Buzzy for Shots, and needle-free lidocaine delivery system.

- Epidural and regional nerve blocks are pain-control methods used more frequently for postsurgical pain management because they have fewer side effects than systemic medications.

- Parents need education and preparation to provide pain management for children who are discharged home following surgery and injuries.

- Children with recurrent and chronic painful conditions need an individualized pain management plan that includes cognitive behavioral therapies, physical and occupational therapy, and other measures to improve function, quality of life, and comfort.

- The child receiving sedation should be continuously and visually monitored for respiratory effort, vital signs, color, level of responsiveness, vomiting, and excessive salivation.

Clinical Reasoning in Action

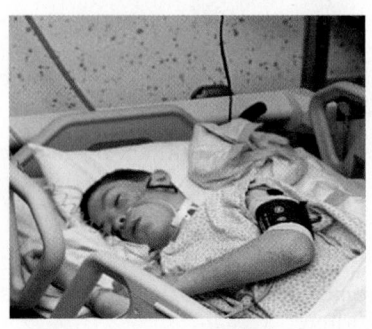

A 12-year-old boy, Kevin, is recovering at a local children's hospital from a four-wheeler ATV crash. He was riding the ATV unsupervised and without permission while his parents were at work. He suffered three broken bones, several lacerations, and an abdominal injury that required surgery. His parents are very worried about his injuries and at the same time angry with him for not following the rules. Kevin appears expressionless in his hospital bed, but cries and grimaces at any slight movement. When asked on a scale of 1 to 10 (10 being the most pain) how much pain he is feeling, he says a 10. His parents are reluctant to let him have any pain medications because they fear he may become dependent on the medication. His father states that Kevin should be a man and tolerate the pain, and he thinks enduring the pain will teach him a lesson about responsibility. The nurse explains that pain management is necessary to improve Kevin's healing, help him mobilize sooner, and potentially shorten his hospital stay. She explains the physiologic consequences of ineffective pain management and discusses how the medication will help him sleep and rest. She explains that some of the pain medications can be addicting, but the chances of Kevin becoming addicted to pain medications for this injury are extremely rare. She also reviews the nonpharmacologic methods of relieving pain. The parents are still reluctant to allow the medications, but agree to conform to the healthcare provider's orders.

1. What are some of the potential physiologic consequences of letting Kevin suffer pain?
2. What are some examples of opioid analgesics appropriate for Kevin?
3. What are some examples of NSAIDs available to Kevin?
4. What are the signs of tolerance to the prescribed opioid?

References

American Academy of Pediatrics Committee on Drugs (AAP). (2015). Metric units and the preferred dosing of orally administered medications. *Pediatrics, 135*(4), 784–787.

American Pain Society (APS). (2012). *Assessment and management of children with chronic pain.* Retrieved from http://www.americanpainsociety.org/uploads/pdfs/aps12-pcp.pdf

Aschenbrenner, D. S. (2013). Drug watch. *American Journal of Nursing, 113*(6), 23–24.

Badr, L. K. (2013). Pain in premature infants: What is conclusive evidence and what is not? *Newborn & Infant Nursing Reviews, 13,* 82–86.

Barnes, S. (2014). Analgesia and sedation. In B. Engorn & J. Flerlage (Eds.), *The Harriet Lane handbook* (20th ed., pp. 111–126). Philadelphia, PA: Elsevier Mosby.

Buzzy. (2014). *Buzzy drug free pain relief.* Retrieved from http://buzzy4shots.com/

Chon, T. Y., & Lee, M. C. (2013). Accupuncture. *Mayo Clinic Proceedings, 88*(10), 1141–1146.

Clark, L. (2011). Pain management in the pediatric population, *Critical Care Nursing Clinics of North America, 23,* 291–301.

Cooper, S., & Petty, J. (2012). Promoting the use of sucrose as analgesia for procedural pain management in neonates: A review of the current literature. *Journal of Neonatal Nursing, 18,* 121–128.

Czarnecki, M. L., Simon, K., Thompson, J. J., Armus, C. L., Hanson, T. C., Berg, K. A., . . . Malin, S. (2011). Barriers to pediatric pain management: A nursing perspective. *Pain Management Nursing, 12*(3), 154–162.

Czarnecki, M. L., Salamon, K., Thompson, J. J., & Hainsworth, K. R. (2014). Do barriers to pediatric pain management as perceived by nurses change over time? *Pain Management Nursing, 15*(1), 292–305.

Dobson, C. E., & Byrne, M. W. (2014). Using guided imagery to manage pain in young children with sickle cell disease. *American Journal of Nursing, 114*(4), 26–36.

Ely, E., Chen-Lim, M. L., Zarnowsy, C., Green, R., Shaffer, S., & Holtzer, B. (2012). Finding the evidence to change practice for assessing pain in children who are cognitively impaired. *Journal of Pediatric Nursing, 27,* 402–410.

Fein, J. A., Zempsky, W. T., Cravero, J. P., & The Committee on Pediatric Emergency Medicine and the Section on Anesthesiology and Pain. (2012). Relief of pain and anxiety in pediatric patients in emergency medical systems. *Pediatrics, 130*(5), e1391–e1405.

Galinkin, Koh, & Committee on Drugs and Section on Anesthesiology and Pain Management. (2014). Recognition and management of iatrogenically induced opioid dependence and withdrawal in children. *Pediatrics, 133*(1), 152–155.

Gomez, R. J., Barrowman, N., Elia, S., Manias, E., Royle, J., & Harrison, D. (2013). Establishing intra- and inter-relater agreement of the Faces, Legs, Activity, Cry, Consolability scale for evaluating pain in toddlers during immunization. *Pain Research & Management, 18*(6), e124–e128.

Gottsegen, D. (2011). Hypnosis for functional abdominal pain. *American Journal of Clinical Hypnosis, 54*(1), 56–69.

Greenwald, M. (2010). Analgesia for the pediatric trauma patient: Primum non nocere? *Clinical Pediatric Emergency Medicine, 11*(1), 28–40.

Guarin, P. L. B. (2013). How effective are nerve blocks after orthopedic surgery? A quality improvement study. *Nursing 2013, 43*(6), 63–66.

Huether, S. E. (2014). Pain, temperature regulation, sleep, and sensory function. In K. L. McCance, S. E. Huether, V. L. Brashers, & N. S. Rote (Eds.), *Pathophysiology: The biologic basis for disease in adults and children* (7th ed., pp. 481–524). St. Louis, MO: Mosby Elsevier.

Jest, A. D., & Tonge, A. (2011). Using a learning needs assessment to identify knowledge deficits regarding procedural sedation for pediatric patients. *AORN Journal, 94*(6), 567–574.

Joint Commission. (2014). *Facts about pain management.* Retrieved from http://www.jointcommission.org/pain_management

Kohen, D. P. (2011). Chronic daily headache: Helping adolescents help themselves with self-hypnosis. *American Journal of Clinical Hypnosis, 54,* 32–46.

Krauss, B., & Green, S. M. (2014). Systemic analgesia and sedation for procedures. In J. R. Roberts, & C. B. Custalow (Eds.), *Roberts and Hedges' clinical procedures in emergency medicine,* (6th ed., pp. 586–610). Philadelphia, PA: Elsevier Saunders.

Lawrence, J., Alcock, D., McGrath, D. P., Kay, J., MacMurray, S. B., & Dulberg, C. (1993). The development of a tool to assess neonatal pain. *Neonatal Network, 12*(6), 61.

Martin, S., Smith, A. B., Newcomb, P., & Miller, J. (2014). Effects of therapeutic suggestion under anesthesia on outcomes in children post tonsillectomy. *Journal of PeriAnesthesia Nursing, 29*(2), 94–106.

Merkel, S. I., Voepel-Lewis, T., Shayevitz, J. R., & Malviya, S. (1997). The FLACC: A behavioral scale for scoring post-operative pain in young children. *Pediatric Nursing, 23*(3), 293–297.

Pasero, C., & McCaffery, M. (2011). *Pain assessment and pharmacologic management.* St. Louis, MO: Elsevier Mosby.

Purnell, L. D. (2014). *Guide to culturally competent care* (3rd ed.). Philadelphia, PA: F. A. Davis.

Rashotte, J., Coburn, G., Harrison, D., Stevens, B. J., Yamada, J. Abbott, L. K., & CIHR Team on Children's Pain. (2013). Healthcare professionals' pain narratives in hospitalized children's medical records: Part 1, Pain descriptors. *Pain Research and Management, 18*(5), e75–e83.

Rosen, D. A., & Dower, J. (2011). Pediatric pain management. *Pediatric Annals, 40*(5), 243–252.

Sadhasivam, S., Chidambaran, V., Ngamprasertwong, P., Esslinger, H. R., Prows, C., Zhang, X., . . . McAuliffe, J. (2012). Race and unequal burden of perioperative pain and opioid related adverse effects in children. *Pediatrics, 129*(5), 832–838.

Suddaby, E. C., & Josephson, K. (2013). Satisfaction of nurses with the Withdrawal Assessment Tool-1 (WAT-1). *Pediatric Nursing, 39*(5), 238–242, 259.

Taddio, A., Hogan, M. E., Moyer, P., Girgis, A., Gerges, S., Wang, L., & Ipp, M. (2011). Evaluation of the reliability, validity and practicality of 3 measures of acute pain in infants undergoing immunization injections. *Vaccine, 29,* 1390–1394.

Taketomo, C. K., Hodding, J. H., & Kraus, D. M. (2014). *Pediatric dosage handbook* (21st ed.). Hudson, OH: American Pharmacists Association.

Tobias, J. D. (2014a). Acute pain management in infants and children—Part 1: Pain pathways, pain assessment, and outpatient pain management. *Pediatric Annals, 43*(7), e163–e168.

Tobias, J. D. (2014b). Acute pain management in infants and children—Part 2: Intravenous opioids, intravenous nonsteroidal anti-inflammatory drugs, and managing adverse events. *Pediatric Annals, 43*(7), e169–e175.

Twycross, A., & Collins, S. (2013). Nurses' views about the barriers and facilitators to effective management of pediatric pain. *Pain Management Nursing, 14*(4), e164–e172.

Watt, L. D., & Arnstein, P. (2013). Codeine for children: Weighing the risks. *Nursing 2013, 43*(11), 62–63.

Wilson, B. A., Shannon, M. T., & Shields, K. M. (2016). *Nurse's drug guide 2016.* Hoboken, NJ: Pearson Education.

Wilson, S., Bremmer, A. P., Mathews, J., & Pearson, D. (2013). The use of oral sucrose for procedural pain relief in infants up to six months of age: A randomized controlled trial. *Pain Management Nursing, 14*(4), e95–e105.

Wood, C., von Baeyer, C. L., Falinower, S., Moyse, D., Annequin, D., & Legout, V. (2011). Electronic and paper versions of a faces pain intensity scale: Concordance and preference in hospitalized children. *BMC Pediatrics, 11,* 87–95

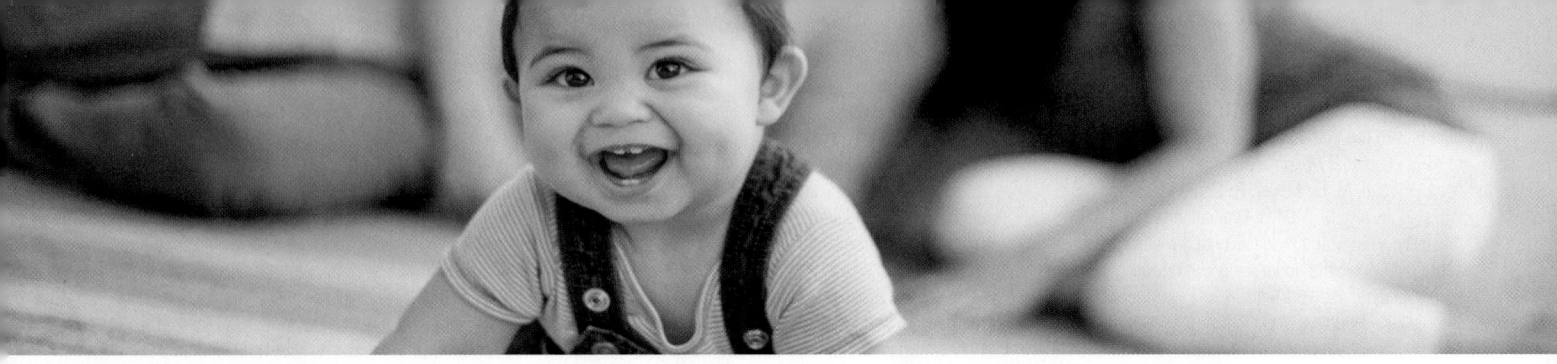

Chapter 41
The Child With a Life-Threatening Condition and End-of-Life Care

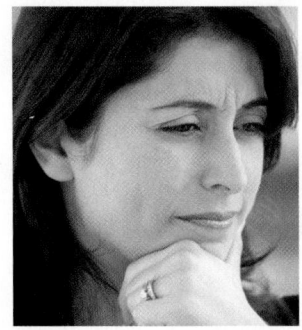

It all happened so fast. No one saw the car coming. Next thing I knew, we were in the emergency room talking about abdominal and head injuries. Now Alexa is in the intensive care unit, and I'm worried because she is still unconscious and on a ventilator. It was helpful for the nurse to tell me that even though Alexa couldn't respond, it was good to talk to her, because she will probably hear me and be comforted.

—Mother of Alexa, 6 years old

Michael Matisse/Getty Images

∨ Learning Outcomes

41.1 Summarize the effects of a life-threatening illness or injury on children.

41.2 Examine the family's experience and reactions to having a child with a life-threatening illness or injury.

41.3 Identify the coping mechanisms used by the child and family in response to stress.

41.4 Develop a nursing care plan for the child with a life-threatening illness or injury.

41.5 Apply assessment skills to identify the physiologic changes that occur in the dying child.

41.6 Develop a nursing care plan to provide family-centered care for the dying child and family.

41.7 Plan bereavement support for the parents and siblings after the death of a child.

41.8 Evaluate strategies to support nurses who care for children who die.

The intense emotional and physical demands placed on the critically ill or injured child present a challenge to nurses' attempts to provide developmentally appropriate care. The child's parents and siblings are confronted with a stressful situation. A family-centered model of nursing practice offers a framework for performing interventions that help to minimize stress and enhance coping by the ill or injured child, parents, and siblings.

Life-Threatening Illness or Injury

A **life-threatening condition** is one in which there is a likelihood that the child will die prematurely (Randall, Cervenka, Arday, et al., 2011). A threat to a child's life may be expected, as

in a chronic illness or progressive disabling disease. More often, the death is unexpected as a result of an unintentional injury, the leading cause of death in children, or an acute illness. How children, parents, and siblings cope with the threat will depend on the anticipated or unanticipated nature of the event and the conditions surrounding the child's admission to the hospital.

When death results from a chronic disease or terminal illness, the child and family have time to adjust to episodes of life-threatening crisis and impending death. Although the child could die unexpectedly during treatment, parents have some knowledge of the condition, the hospital setting, and the healthcare team and have had an opportunity to become involved in the child's therapy as integral members of this team. Emergency admission for an acute illness or unintentional injury, in contrast, brings with it sudden stressors as the child and family are thrust into an unfamiliar environment, confronted with frightening or invasive procedures, and faced with an uncertain outcome.

Nursing care of children and families coping with specific chronic diseases or terminal illnesses such as cancer, cystic fibrosis, or muscular dystrophy is discussed elsewhere in this text. The following discussion focuses on care of children with life-threatening illnesses or injuries and care of the dying child.

Child's Experience

Admission to the hospital, emergency department, or pediatric intensive care unit (PICU) is one of the most frightening experiences a child can have. Critically ill children may appear extremely anxious and fearful, or withdrawn, solemn, and preoccupied with their own physical condition. The illness or injury often brings pain, decreased energy, and changes to the affected child's level of consciousness.

Young children admitted to the PICU may be unable to understand what is happening to them. The PICU environment appears overwhelming, fast paced, and frightening, secondary to the numerous machines, noises, people, and procedures the child encounters. The child's normal sleep patterns can be disrupted because of the lack of day–night patterns in many intensive care units (Figure 41–1). Being cared for by strangers contributes to the child's anxiety. The child's limited ability to move intensifies feelings of powerlessness and vulnerability.

Children's responses to stress are influenced by their developmental levels, past experiences, types of illness, coping mechanisms, and available emotional support. Nurses must consider how their developmental level and coping skills will influence their ability to deal with the emergency department or PICU experience. Successful coping can provide these children with the skills to handle difficult situations in the future.

An unanticipated admission places the child at emotional risk because of the lack of preparation for the experience, the uncertainty and unpredictability of events that follow, the unfamiliarity of the environment, and the heightened anxiety of parents. An admission for an acute exacerbation of a disease such as cystic fibrosis or leukemia can provoke feelings of depression or hopelessness. Chapter 39 describes the stressors and responses to hospitalization of children by age group.

The child cared for in the PICU will experience the same stressors as any child who is hospitalized. However, the PICU environment is more intense and is very stressful for children. Treatment, disease, and/or environmental related stressors place these children at risk for posttraumatic stress disorder. They are exposed to strangers, unfamiliar equipment, other sick children, and noises from alarms, phones, and pagers (Dow, Kenardy, Long, et al., 2012).

Coping Mechanisms

Coping refers to the cognitive and behavioral responses that help a person manage specific internal and external demands that exceed personal resources, enabling the person to solve problems and to respond appropriately. The child may mirror the parents' behaviors and responses, which may help or hinder the child's response to stress. The child's temperament, previous coping experiences, and availability of **support systems** (extended network of family, friends, and religious and community contacts that provide nurturance, emotional support, and direct assistance to parents) all combine to influence the child's ability to cope with the current experience.

The nature and severity of the illness and an emergency admission to the hospital stress a child's coping capabilities. Defense mechanisms displayed by children in these situations include **regression**, or return to an earlier behavior (a common reaction to stress), denial, **repression** (involuntary forgetting), postponement, and bargaining.

Nursing Management

For the Child With a Life-Threatening Illness or Injury

Nursing care of the child with a life-threatening illness or injury and the child's family includes assessing the child's physical and psychosocial needs, assessing the family's psychosocial needs, providing physical and psychosocial care for the child, and providing support for parental physical and emotional needs.

Nursing Assessment and Diagnosis

Nursing assessment involves physiologic parameters, plus skilled observation of the child's psychosocial and emotional needs. An understanding of normal psychosocial and cognitive development is necessary to plan developmentally appropriate interventions. Assessment should include the child's response to illness, the environment, coping strategies, and the need for information and support.

The accompanying *Nursing Care Plan* includes common nursing diagnoses for the child with a life-threatening illness or injury. The following nursing diagnoses may also be appropriate (NANDA-I © 2014):

- *Communication: Verbal, Impaired,* related to the effects of endotracheal intubation and mechanical ventilation
- *Spiritual Distress* related to the crisis of illness or suffering
- *Sleep Pattern, Disturbed,* related to circadian asynchrony, excessive stimulation, pain, and anxiety caused by the critical care unit environment
- *Activity, Deficient Diversional,* related to forced inactivity

Planning and Implementation

Nursing care focuses on promoting a sense of trust, providing education about the illness or injury, preparing the child for

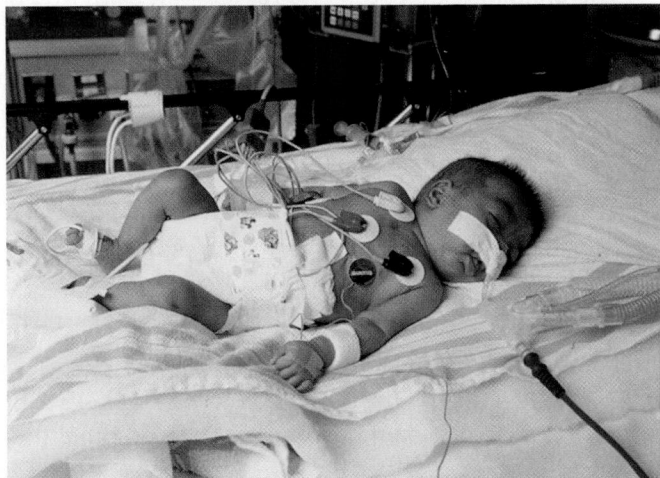

Figure 41–1 Jooti feels pain, hears noises, has her sleep disrupted, and has limited mobility because of all the equipment attached to her.

Clinical Reasoning PICU Stressors

The PICU receives a call from a community hospital requesting transport for an unstable 12-year-old boy, Gavin, who is in status epilepticus. Gavin has a seizure disorder controlled with medications, but several days ago he decided to stop taking his medications. After receiving several medications in the community hospital emergency department to stop the seizures, Gavin experienced some respiratory depression. He is currently intubated to maintain his airway until the medications wear off.

The transport team is in the air within minutes and arrives at the rural community hospital 25 minutes later. The team stabilizes Gavin, receives reports from the medical and nursing teams, meets briefly with his parents, answers a few questions, and is back in the air.

Gavin is admitted directly to the PICU and connected to cardiorespiratory and noninvasive blood pressure monitors. His existing intravenous lines and endotracheal tube are evaluated for patency as team members quickly complete a head-to-toe assessment. When Gavin's parents arrive, his nurse meets them and prepares them for what they will see.

What stressors do children like Gavin face after sudden admission to the PICU? What stressors will parents face during the initial period when you work with them?

procedures, facilitating the use of play, and promoting a sense of control. Physiologic care for the child in the PICU may include the following: frequent physiologic assessment, pain and sedation management, nutritional support, medication administration, management of multiple IV lines and pumps, maintenance of ventilatory and hemodynamic monitoring equipment, and wound care.

PROVIDE PSYCHOSOCIAL CARE FOR THE CHILD

Children admitted to a PICU need support for the stressful experience. Children often feel and hear even when unconscious, so touch and talking to the child are important. Nurses play a key role in providing developmentally appropriate support to the child. Nursing interventions are directed at building a trusting relationship, minimizing the stressors experienced by the child, and promoting coping. Ongoing reassessment of progress in meeting the child's needs is critical.

PROMOTE A SENSE OF SECURITY

For children of all ages, feeling secure depends on a sense of physical and psychologic safety. A sense of physical security is difficult to attain within the PICU because frequent procedures are part of the child's treatment plan. Parental presence at the bedside is one of the best ways to decrease anxiety and promote a sense of security. Including parents as partners in the child's care provides comfort and reassurance to the child. Children whose parents have high anxiety levels pick up their parents' emotional cues and become more anxious. Consistency of staff

---

Nursing Care Plan: The Child Coping With a Life-Threatening Illness or Injury

1. Nursing Diagnosis: *Anxiety (Child)* related to separation from parents, unfamiliar environment, strangers as caretakers, invasive procedures (NANDA-I © 2014)

GOAL: The child will exhibit or express an increased sense of security.

INTERVENTION	RATIONALE
• Encourage parents to remain at the bedside (open visitation) and to participate in the child's care by touching, talking to, reading to, and singing to the child.	• Presence of the parents is comforting to the child.
• Talk with the child. Avoid discussions at bedside that the child should not overhear.	• The child may overhear and remember, even if unconscious.
• Offer to arrange a visit from the chaplain or other spiritual support.	• Spiritual support often provides comfort and sustenance in a time of crisis.
• Provide the child with developmentally appropriate explanations when possible. Encourage the child to ask questions and express concerns.	• Information reduces anxiety and builds trust.
• Make the child's bedside more personal and familiar by encouraging parents to bring in security objects, family photos, and favorite toys from home.	• Security objects decrease foreignness of hospital environment. The child derives comfort from presence of personal items.
• Involve the child in play appropriate to developmental age (see Chapter 31).	• Play provides familiarity, decreases fantasy, and provides motor activity.
• Provide care using a primary nursing care model.	• Consistency in healthcare givers helps to build the child's trust. Healthcare giver learns child's cues.

EXPECTED OUTCOME: Child will appear more relaxed and acknowledge parents' presence. Behavioral manifestations of anxiety will be absent. Restful periods of sleep will be noted.

2. Nursing Diagnosis: *Powerlessness* related to inability to communicate and control relinquished to the healthcare team (NANDA-I © 2014)

GOAL: The child or adolescent will have an increased sense of control over the situation.

INTERVENTION	RATIONALE
• Provide opportunities for choices when possible. Encourage participation in self-care.	• Such opportunities provide sense of control and autonomy through decision making.
• Prepare the child or adolescent in advance (timing dependent on developmental level) for procedures. Describe the sensations that will be experienced. Allow some choice in timing or method of pain relief.	• Providing information to children or adolescents lets them know what to expect. Allowing choices gives them a sense of involvement and lets them know their input is important.
• Provide routines for the child both within a 24-hour period and for scheduled care. Tell the child before the procedure (timing dependent on developmental level), repeat explanation of why procedure is necessary, complete procedure in a consistent manner, and offer praise or a special story when completed. When possible, incorporate rituals from home.	• Routines and rituals provide a sense of continuity and comfort for the child.
• Provide other means of communication to the intubated child (e.g., a word board or finger board).	• Fostering communication by some means helps the child maintain some sense of control.
• For the child requiring restraints or immobilizers, use as seldom as possible, provide appropriate explanations, and release at regular intervals. Wrapping IV lines well can help maintain lines and avoid the need for restraints.	• Release from restraints or immobilizers helps diminish the sense of powerlessness that accompanies their use.

EXPECTED OUTCOME: Child or adolescent will express satisfaction over ability to control some elements of situation. Child or adolescent will participate in self-care and decision making.

3. Nursing Diagnosis: *Pain, Acute,* related to injuries, invasive procedures, surgery (NANDA-I © 2014)

GOAL: The child will experience reduced pain and improved comfort.

INTERVENTION	RATIONALE
• Assess the child's pain location, intensity, and what makes it better or worse.	• Assessment provides baseline information from which a plan of care can be developed.
• If appropriate, use a pain assessment scale (see Chapter 40).	• Use of a scale provides continuity and consistency in monitoring of the child's pain.
• Provide optimal pain relief with prescribed analgesics. Provide comfort measures such as position changes and back rubs. Provide diversional activities as appropriate or possible. Incorporate the family in pain-relief modality.	• Physiologic and psychologic methods of pain control can be used in combination to maximally improve outcomes.

EXPECTED OUTCOME: Child will experience a perceived or actual improvement in comfort level.

is invaluable in developing familiarity and a trusting relationship with the child.

Personalizing the child's bedside can promote comfort and a sense of security. Pictures from home, a favorite blanket or toy, music tapes, or posters can make the environment friendlier and more familiar to the child (Figure 41–2). Religious or spiritual symbols may also provide psychologic support.

PROVIDE EDUCATION AND PREPARE THE CHILD FOR PROCEDURES

The ability of children to understand the cause of their illness and its therapy depends on their cognitive abilities. Help younger children to understand that illness and hospitalization are not a punishment.

Preparation for procedures is important at all ages, even for the unconscious or sedated child. Toddlers will benefit from being talked to, soothed, and touched during and after the procedure. Provide preschoolers, school-age children, and adolescents with an explanation of the sensations they can expect to experience (temperature, vibrations, sounds, smells, tastes, sight). (See Chapter 39.)

FACILITATE THE USE OF PLAY

Play can be used to alleviate stress and to help prepare children for procedures. The nurse can also use play to assess the child's developmental level. Even within the PICU, therapeutic play diminishes negative fantasies, provides motor activity, and helps the child cope with stressors (see Chapter 39). Children with

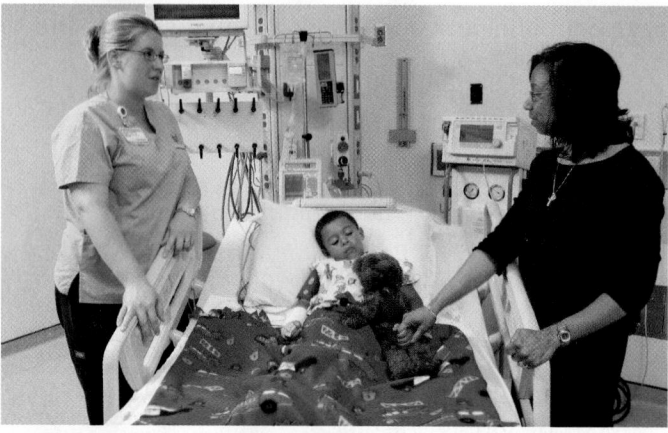

Figure 41–2 By their very nature, PICUs are ominous and sterile. To lessen this effect, it can help to personalize the child's space. Being there with the child and parent, answering questions, or just talking can be a comfort to both.

limited mobility due to tubes and immobilizers can still feel a sense of accomplishment, for example, by completing a puzzle, even if the nurse points and moves each piece as the child responds through nods and gestures to indicate where the puzzle piece should be placed. Play can help children work through a painful situation, making it more tolerable. The child-life specialist may also be able to facilitate coping by assisting in preparation for procedures and providing distraction during procedures. See a discussion of the role of the child-life specialist in Chapter 39.

PROMOTE A SENSE OF CONTROL
Children between toddlerhood and adolescence experience a loss of control during a life-threatening illness. This loss of control may be related to the body, emotions, normal routines, or privacy. Nursing interventions should promote a sense of control over these areas.

Children hospitalized in an intensive care unit experience a heightened sense of loss of control secondary to the many machines, noises, and limits on mobility. These children often self-remove or threaten to self-remove technologic equipment or devices employed in their care such as an endotracheal tube, peripheral IV line or central line, nasogastric tube, or arterial line. Physical immobilizers are sometimes used in children with altered levels of consciousness to prevent them from pulling out tubes and lines. Although immobilizers are sometimes necessary, they contribute to the child's sense of powerlessness. Nurses should position these devices in a way that maintains comfort as much as possible.

Enhance the child's coping skills by teaching the child and family a combination of relaxation, visual imagery, or distraction techniques, and comforting self-talk phrases, such as "This will be over soon," "If I stay calm, it will be all right," and "It will be over fast so I can do something fun." Help the parents become the child's coping coaches.

Evaluation

Expected outcomes of nursing care include the following:

- A trusting relationship is developed with the child and family.
- The child is given preparation and support for procedures.
- The child's coping is promoted by family presence and therapeutic play.

Clinical Tip
The Joint Commission requires that hospitals have policies and procedures for the use of restraints or immobilizers and a plan to release them for short periods. Documentation in the medical record according to hospital policy is also required. Restrain all children as little as possible, and explain the rationale for immobilizers, emphasizing that they are not a punishment (see the *Clinical Skills Manual* SKILLS).

Parents' Experience of a Child's Life-Threatening Illness or Injury

The uncertainty and unpredictability of a child's life-threatening illness or injury challenge a family's coping and stability. Admission of a child to the pediatric intensive care unit (PICU) is one of the most stressful events that a parent can experience (Jee et al., 2012). The sudden loss of the parenting role with the child's emergency admission causes stress. Families display many different responses and coping mechanisms such as crying, emotional outbursts, fear, and demanding information. Parents are at risk for long-term psychologic effects, including the development of posttraumatic stress disorder (PTSD), when the child is hospitalized in an intensive care unit (Jee et al., 2012). Parents may find it difficult to support the child if their own needs are not met. They may also transmit their anxiety to the child, who then becomes even more anxious. Family-centered care must be provided to meet the needs of parents with a variety of personalities, coping mechanisms, and responses to the crisis. Clear, concise communication is imperative.

The Family in Crisis

The critical care environment and the implications of a child's life-threatening illness or injury are far removed from the everyday experiences of most families. The unfamiliarity of the environment and the uncertainty and seriousness of the illness or injury create a **family crisis**, which occurs when the family encounters a problem that seems insurmountable and usual coping skills are not effective.

Since families have little time to prepare for the experience, a sudden admission threatens family integrity, causing enormous stress and separation from loved ones. The interruption of the unique parent–child relationship can be more stressful to parents than the physical PICU environment. Siblings are also affected. See the section on *The Siblings' Experience* later in this chapter. In addition, extended family members such as grandparents must be considered. Stresses are further intensified in the case of divorce, separation, and stepparenting. Financial problems, a long distance from home to hospital, or another ill or injured family member can compound the crisis.

Clinical Tip
In addition to dealing with the child's life-threatening condition, parents may need to quickly arrange for the care of other children. For example, the child's siblings may be at band practice or other activities and a ride home must be planned. Parents must decide if one of them will leave the hospital to pick up the siblings and inform them about their brother's or sister's illness/injury, or whether a family member or friend will do it for them. This decision may not be easy and will depend in part on the condition of the hospitalized child. The parents may need assistance to make these arrangements when they are in a state of crisis.

Parental Reactions to Life-Threatening Illness or Injury

When faced with a threat to their child's life, parents typically progress through stages that might include shock and disbelief, anger and guilt, deprivation and loss, anticipatory waiting, and readjustment or mourning. Some families progress through these stages in a linear fashion, while others go back and forth between stages, especially if the child's condition improves and then worsens.

SHOCK AND DISBELIEF

The universal reaction to a child's life-threatening condition is shock and disbelief. As the familiar is disrupted, parents experience a loss of control, an inability to regain their bearings, and feelings of immobility. The hospital environment, emergency department, or PICU may seem unreal. The emotions parents experience initially are intensified by the physical appearance of their child (particularly after a major injury); the presence of monitors, tubing, and equipment; and the actual injury or illness.

Shock and disbelief begin in the first few moments after hearing the "news" and can last for days. The shock helps postpone the full impact of the crisis. During this period, parents search for answers and explanations about the illness or injury. Information must be repeated many times to parents, since in this stage they are often unable to assimilate information easily.

ANGER AND GUILT

Anger and guilt surface as parents become more aware of their child's illness or injury. Their anger may be directed toward themselves or each other because they could not protect the child. Other individuals may be blamed such as the driver of a motor vehicle who injured the child. Parents may also be angry with their child. This anger may be a result of injuries the child sustained when breaking known rules such as drinking and driving, playing with matches, or riding a bike without a helmet. Lastly, the anger may not be directed at anyone specifically. Injuries caused by natural disasters such as an earthquake, flood, or hurricane provoke just as much anger as those that result from the actions of people, and they may pose a challenge to the parents' spiritual beliefs.

Parents typically react to their child's illness or injury with some degree of guilt. This reaction may be magnified in the PICU environment. The fact that the guilt usually has no basis in real events does not lessen the feeling. A question parents frequently ask at this stage is, "Why not me instead of my child?" Parents' feelings of guilt may be related to the following:

1. They may feel responsible for causing the illness or injury. Statements such as "If only I hadn't sent him to the store on his bike, this wouldn't have happened" reflect feelings of guilt for causing or failing to prevent the injury.

2. They may feel guilty about not noticing the onset of an illness or disregarding earlier illness symptoms. The mother of a 1-year-old with meningitis may repeatedly say, "I shouldn't have waited so long to take her to the doctor!"

DEPRIVATION AND LOSS

As the shock associated with the child's life-threatening condition slowly recedes, new stressors emerge. Within minutes or hours, parents are deprived of their familiar role as the parent of a healthy child and find themselves in an unexpected and unfamiliar role as the parent of a critically ill child.

The difficulty and ambivalence parents feel in releasing a part of their responsibility as the child's primary caretakers can threaten their self-esteem and self-control. If parents cannot participate in the child's care, they may feel helpless or worthless.

ANTICIPATORY WAITING

Once the child's condition is stabilized and survival seems likely, parents often move into a period of anticipatory waiting. This stage is characterized as "life suspended in time." Parents spend a great deal of time waiting: for test results, for explanations, for their child to become conscious, or for surgery to be over. Parents may fear leaving the area because they may miss an important procedure, healthcare provider visit, or decisions or changes in treatment. Lack of mobility decreases the parents' use of typical coping mechanisms, so anxiety and the sense of powerlessness may increase. If the parents have a cell phone, write down the number and ensure them that they will be called for any change in the child's condition. This allows parents to feel like they can leave at least for a few minutes. If the parents do not have a cell phone, provide a pager if available.

Parents may have a preoccupation with medical details. During this period, they may ask questions about the long-term effects of the illness or injury on the child, about the potential for brain damage, or about the need for additional surgeries. Parents may place demands on staff and be frustrated when the child's progress is slow.

READJUSTMENT OR MOURNING

The last stage that parents experience is readjustment or mourning. Readjustment is experienced as the child recovers, improves steadily, and prepares for transfer and discharge. In contrast, parents of the child who dies reenter the cycle of emotions characteristic of grief. Parents also mourn when the child remains seriously ill or unresponsive, when the outcome remains uncertain for an extended period, or when long-term care is required.

Table 41–1 lists the most important needs of parents when a child is hospitalized with a life-threatening illness or injury.

Nursing Management

For the Parents of a Child With a Life-Threatening Illness or Injury

Nursing care of the family includes assessing the family's psychosocial needs and providing support for parental physical and emotional needs.

Nursing Assessment and Diagnosis

Nurses who work with families of critically ill children have a unique opportunity to help them adapt and to promote family functioning. Begin by assessing the family's reaction to the illness, coping skills, stressors, and needs. (See Chapter 38.) This initial assessment provides a baseline of information for developing a care plan and strategies to meet the psychosocial as well as physiologic needs of families.

Several nursing diagnoses may apply to parents who are dealing with their child's life-threatening condition. Examples include the following (NANDA-I © 2014):

- *Family Processes, Interrupted,* related to the impact of a critically ill child on the family system
- *Spiritual Distress* related to the child's life-threatening condition, suffering, or death
- *Fatigue* related to extreme stress, sleep deprivation, and crisis

TABLE 41–1 Nursing Interventions to Meet Parental Needs When a Child Is Hospitalized With a Life-Threatening Illness or Injury

PARENTAL NEEDS	NURSING INTERVENTIONS
Information	• Provide information and frequent updates about the child's condition using terminology that parents can understand. • Repeat the information and provide other materials frequently because parents forget or cannot concentrate on details with all the stress they are under. • Explain the child's condition, equipment being used, and procedures of care. • Facilitate a discussion with the healthcare provider at least daily. • Provide general information about unit policies, team members, and phone numbers.
Proximity to their child	• Provide permission for the parents to remain at the bedside. • Encourage parents to touch and speak with the child and demonstrate ways if parents are hesitant. • Work within the unit to provide open, flexible visiting hours.
Reestablishment of their parental role and control	• Implement family-centered care so parents feel recognized as important to their child's recovery and as the decision maker for the child's treatment options.
Participation in their child's care	• Encourage parents to participate in care (e.g., bathing and hair care, diaper changes, feeding, range-of-motion exercises, massages). • Encourage parents to help with diversional activities (e.g., reading, singing, telling stories). • Encourage parents to explain equipment and procedures to the child to reduce the child's fears.
Confidence in the treatment plan and caregivers	• Try to maintain continuity in staffing and healthcare contacts. • Demonstrate caring for the child. • Provide assurance that the child is receiving appropriate treatment and pain management.
Psychologic support	• Acknowledge that the situation is difficult. • Help parents to focus on the positive or unchanged aspects of the child's appearance. • Encourage parents to get rest and nutrition to help them maintain physical resources necessary for coping. • Provide space and privacy as needed. • Give hope if realistic—an essential component of coping. • Offer the choice of other family members to be present. • Discuss the possible responses of siblings and the long-term emotional responses of the patient.

• *Hopelessness* in parents related to the child's deteriorating physical condition
• *Grieving* related to potential death of the child or loss of body functions
• *Coping: Family, Compromised,* related to the severity of the illness or injury in the child

Planning and Implementation

Nursing care focuses on providing family-centered care to help meet the needs of families, minimize stress, and enhance family coping (see Table 1–1). Nurses are challenged to blend and balance technology with caring.

PROVIDE INFORMATION AND BUILD TRUST

Orienting parents to the hospital, as well as to the unit routines, helps them to adapt to their surroundings. Parents will gain a sense of control and independence if they know where to get supplies and how to find the lounge, cafeteria, and restrooms.

Provide frequent and accurate information. Deliver information on the child's illness, condition, and plan of care in a manner and language readily understandable to parents. Upon admission, provide the parents with an idea of what to expect in the days ahead and to be prepared for special procedures or major changes in therapy. Parents also need to be prepared before they see the child the first time. Explain the tubes and monitors that are present and how the child will look and react.

Honesty in discussions is extremely important. If parents feel misled or that information is being withheld, a trusting relationship will be impossible. However, informed parents will feel that they are active participants in decision making and care planning for their child. Trust is facilitated when parents believe that the staff truly cares about the child and sees the child as a special individual. Trust is especially important when difficult decisions must be made, such as withdrawal of life support, or to reduce the risk for conflict.

Parents also need a sense of hope regarding their child's condition to help them cope. Focus on the positives as the child progresses through the different phases of the life-threatening condition.

FACILITATE POSITIVE STAFF–PARENT RELATIONSHIPS AND COMMUNICATION

Given the intensity of the parents' experience when their child is critically ill, it is easy to see how problems can arise between staff and parents. Each healthcare team member must be aware of the child's current status so that parents receive consistent information from all staff. A consistent message can instill confidence. Provide explanations geared to the parents' level of understanding, using language the parents can understand.

Introduce the parents to the nurse and healthcare provider with overall responsibility for the child's care. This is especially important in teaching hospitals that have rotating interns and residents. The attending healthcare provider with the overall responsibility should meet with parents as often as necessary to talk about changes in the child's condition or treatment plan and to allow time for parents to ask questions (Figure 41–3). Encourage parents to keep a daily log or notebook to record information on the child's care, progress, and needs, as well as questions they want to ask. Family care conferences can be helpful when a large number of team members provide care. Arrange for daily visits by an interpreter if the family does not speak or understand English. Have information about the child's condition and care summarized for communication at that time.

PROMOTE PARENTAL INVOLVEMENT

An important role of nurses is to encourage and support parents in their parenting role. The parents' place when possible is at the bedside. Parents can provide comfort to their child and

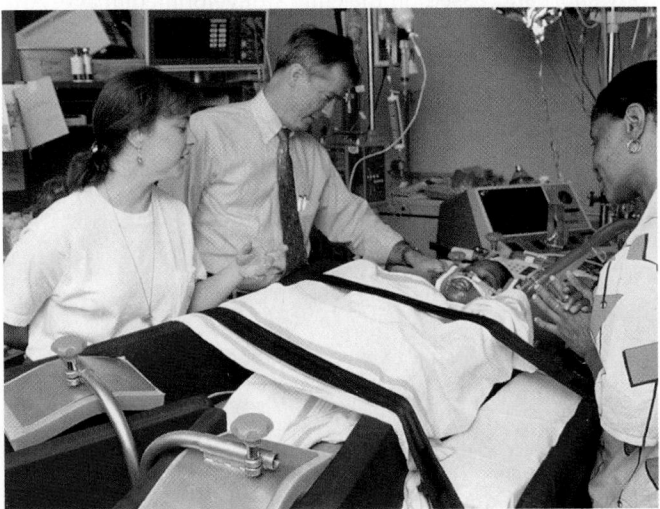

Figure 41–3 In times of crisis, everyone likes to know that someone is in charge and who that person is. The parents should meet and talk with the healthcare provider in charge and the nurses as often as possible. Parents need to know that someone is responsible, even if different people are providing care.

can assist in explanations that offer reassurance to their child. They may also be able to assist with basic care needs such as bathing and changing diapers (Ames, Rennick, & Baillargeon, 2011). Parents provide continuity and may notice subtle condition changes that an assigned nurse may miss. Throughout the child's hospitalization, parents will continue to need reassurance and encouragement.

Participation in care of the child is an integral aspect of family-centered care and enhances the family's ability to cope with the child's illness or injury. Open communication with the family about the child's treatments and plan of care is essential. Parents need to know how their child is doing, understand the care being provided to their child, and know what to expect next (Ames et al., 2011). Parents who do not remain at the child's bedside may feel that they are not an important team member. When parents are unable to remain at the bedside, they should be allowed to call the unit at any time to check on their child.

FAMILY PRESENCE DURING RESUSCITATION AND INVASIVE PROCEDURES

Many hospitals are implementing policies that permit families to be present during resuscitation and invasive procedures. Healthcare professionals have expressed concern that parents who are allowed to witness resuscitation efforts might lose control and interfere. Another concern is that medical staff, especially those in training, might feel uncomfortable, and that there is an increased risk for litigation. However, reports related to family presence during resuscitation have failed to demonstrate any increase in litigation (Jabre et al., 2013). Families have reported that they felt being present during resuscitation and invasive procedures helped their child and helped them (Meert, Clark, & Eggly, 2013). In addition, studies have failed to show that family presence interrupts care or interferes with the healthcare providers' ability to intervene in the care of the child (Emergency Nurses Association [ENA], 2012).

The Emergency Nurses Association supports the option of family presence during invasive procedures and resuscitation (ENA, 2012). Parents and other family members (e.g., grandparents) may wish to be present during invasive procedures (such as lumbar puncture) or resuscitation of the child. The nurse partners with the family to determine their needs at the time. To better facilitate the needs of the family, the following should be determined:

- Who desires to be present during resuscitation or invasive procedures?
- What role will they play during the procedure (e.g., snuggle child for comfort)?

Healthcare agencies should have an established policy for family presence during invasive procedures or resuscitation (ENA, 2012). Care must be family centered and individualized to each situation according to the child's and family's needs. A designated healthcare professional should be available to stay with family members during resuscitation and provide comfort and explanations as needed (ENA, 2012).

PROVIDE FOR PARENTAL PHYSICAL AND EMOTIONAL NEEDS

The experience of having a child with a life-threatening condition drains the parents' physical and emotional reserves. Parents often need encouragement to take care of themselves and to periodically take a break. A statement such as "It is important for you to eat and rest because Alexa is really going to need you when she wakes up" helps parents to realize that becoming exhausted benefits neither them nor the child.

Many communities have a residence for families of hospitalized children. This is often an inexpensive but warm and supportive environment for families. The Ronald McDonald Children's Charities supports many of these residences. A Ronald McDonald Family Room may be found in some hospitals and is provided as a comfortable setting where families of hospitalized children can get away from the high-tech hospital atmosphere while remaining close to the child. Computer resources in one of these locations or in a Family Resource Center may make it possible for parents to stay in contact with concerned family and friends. When financial burdens are a consideration, parents may need family support and social service referrals.

Parents are often at different levels of coping during a crisis. The severity of the child's illness or injury may foster cohesion between the parents and build a stronger relationship. Unfortunately, the reverse may also be true—differences in styles or levels of coping may foster a sense of isolation, placing a strain on the couple's relationship. Nurses should be alert to family dynamics and refer the family for counseling or therapy if indicated.

MAINTAIN OR STRENGTHEN FAMILY SUPPORT SYSTEMS

Support systems enable parents to cope with overwhelming problems and crises. Most parents indicate that having family or friends nearby is crucial as a support system. Some families seek support through prayer and support from religious or faith-based leaders.

Extended family, especially grandparents and friends, frequently offer the family assistance, but parents may need to be reassured that it is all right to ask for help as well. Some parents are uncomfortable asking for help, instead attempting to handle multiple responsibilities themselves, often to the point of exhaustion. Some parents are so overwhelmed that they are unable to respond to offers of help because it requires too great a mental effort on their part. The nurse should assist the parents in responding to these offers for assistance.

Nurses may need to intervene on parents' behalf when they have inadequate support. Parents may be frustrated by people who come to visit unannounced, stay too long, or visit too often. They may find it difficult to tell well-meaning but insensitive friends that they cannot deal with visitors right now. In these situations, it may be helpful for the nurse to offer to serve as a gatekeeper. Suggest that parents inform family and friends about specific times for visits or phone calls to allow for rest periods. An extended family member may be given the responsibility of relaying information to others.

Families of children with a life-threatening illness or injury often have emotional needs beyond the support capabilities of the nurse caring for the child. Referrals to family and support services or pastoral care may be beneficial in these instances.

Evaluation

Expected outcomes of nursing care include the following:

- The nurse establishes a trusting relationship and effective communication with the family.
- Parents participate in their child's care as much as desired.
- Parents and extended family members receive emotional support and nurturance needed to sustain them through the child's illness.

The Siblings' Experience

As the parents' focus shifts to the critically ill child, they may need support in dealing with the healthy siblings. Siblings of a critically ill child may experience stress related to parental absence, being cared for by others, changes in routine, and lack of information about their ill sibling (Meert et al., 2013). Nurses should recognize that siblings may fear becoming ill themselves or believe that they played a role in the child's illness. Siblings often have nightmares about the illness or injury their brother or sister has sustained and about the ill child dying. Inform siblings about their brother's or sister's condition using language and concepts appropriate to their ages and developmental levels. Being allowed to visit the sick child may help siblings to cope (Meert et al., 2013).

Before the visit, talk with the siblings about what to expect and describe how their brother or sister will look. If the ill child acts, moves, talks, or looks different than usual, provide an explanation beforehand. Describe the hospital environment, including equipment, sounds, and smells. Use a doll, draw pictures, or show an actual picture of the child to prepare the siblings. See *Teaching Highlights: Strategies for Working With the Sibling of a Hospitalized Child* in Chapter 39. The child life specialist may also be able to assist in preparing siblings for a visit to the intensive care unit (see Chapter 39).

During the visit the nurse should demonstrate how to talk to and touch the ill child and encourage the siblings to do the same (Figure 41–4). The length of the visit should be relatively short and based on the child's developmental age. After

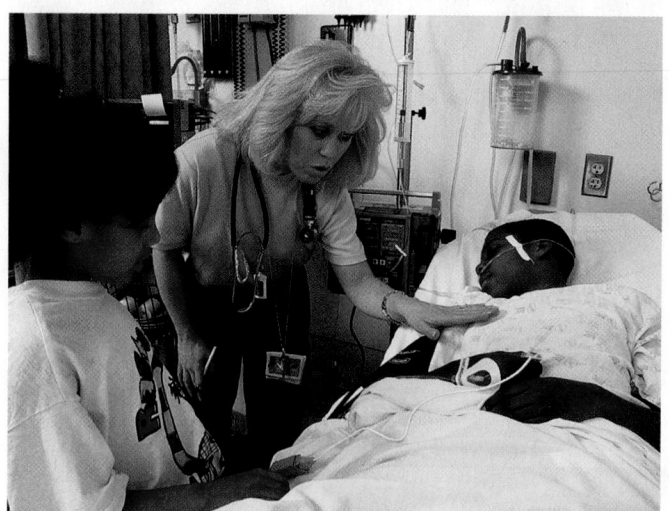

Figure 41–4 During the sibling's visit to the ill child, it is important to talk with the sibling and answer any questions in an honest manner at a level the child can understand.

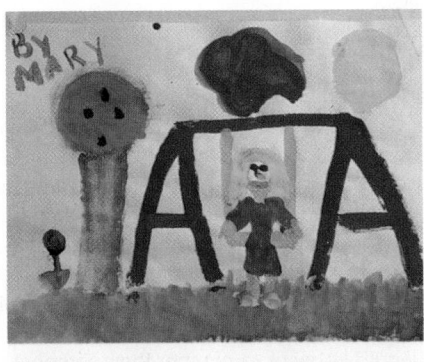

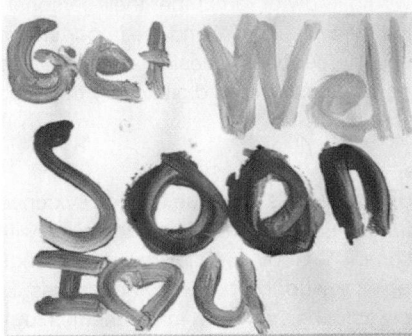

Figure 41–5 It is important that parents and siblings feel comfortable communicating with the seriously ill child. If siblings cannot visit, they should be encouraged to paint or record messages. They need to be able to express themselves and to feel that they are helping.

the visit, the nurse should talk with siblings about what they saw and felt, and answer their questions. When a sibling cannot visit, contact with the ill child can be maintained by sending pictures, drawings, cards, and messages recorded on audiotapes or cell phones if allowed (Figure 41–5).

If parents are staying at the hospital with the ill child, encourage them to call the siblings at home daily. This allows the siblings at home to feel connected by the opportunity to share their day and to receive an update on the ill child. The phone call offers siblings a consistent link to the parents and the reassurance that they are important and loved. Internet contact or text messaging may be another way to communicate with older siblings. Arrange for parents to access a computer, if possible, for families who might find this contact supportive.

Evaluation

Expected outcomes of nursing care include:

- Siblings are prepared for visits to the child with a life-threatening illness or injury.
- Siblings receive emotional support and assistance to cope with the unfamiliar environment.

End-of-Life Care

When the family is faced with end-of-life decision making and care because of a child's chronic condition or multiple acute care episodes, the family needs honest information about various treatment options and potential outcomes. Depending on cognitive abilities, developmental stage, physical and mental status, and prior experiences with health care, the child may also participate in the decision-making process. The family may need to consider issues such as palliative care, hospice care, do-not-resuscitate requests, continuation of schooling, organ/tissue donation, and autopsy.

Palliative and Hospice Care

Pediatric **palliative care** is a multidisciplinary care approach for children with life-shortening disorders and their families. It is intended to relieve suffering of all types (physical, psychologic, spiritual, and social); to enhance quality of life for patients and their families; to facilitate informed decision making by the patient, family, and health professionals; and to improve care coordination (American Academy of Pediatrics [AAP] Section on Hospice and Palliative Medicine and Committee on Hospital Care, 2013). Palliative care may be provided along with curative care, life-prolonging care, or as the main focus of care. Palliative care may be seen as the holistic care provided to a child until the family decides to view dying as a natural process and stops curative care (Trotzuk & Gray, 2012). Children may require these services for many years.

Hospice is a form of palliative care that is provided by licensed agencies and for children is most often provided in the home but may also be provided in special centers or the hospital. Federal regulations outline the required bundle of services that include nursing, healthcare provider, psychosocial, and spiritual services; medications; durable medical equipment; and a range of diagnostic tests and therapeutic interventions (AAP, 2013). Hospice care is provided to the child near the end of life, and it is focused on supporting the family and ensuring that the remaining time for the child is lived as comfortably and as fully as possible.

About 75% of all children who die each year in a hospital, often in an intensive care unit from a life-threatening condition, do not have palliative or hospice care management (Keim-Malpass, Hart, & Miller, 2013). It is estimated that 5000 children in the United States on any day are within the last 6 months of dying and could benefit from palliative or hospice services (Crozier & Hancock, 2012). These services are also an option for neonates on the edge of viability.

When a child receives hospice care, the family and healthcare providers collaborate to determine which treatments are appropriate to continue with the child's end-of-life care, such as IV fluids, gastrostomy feedings, and certain medications. The child is maintained as alert and comfortable as possible. Hospice also provides grief counseling and support to parents for 1 year following the death of the child. See *Evidence-Based Practice: Responding to the Needs of the Family.*

Ethical Issues Surrounding a Child's Death

Because the death of a child is so emotionally charged, potential misunderstandings and conflicts can develop between families and healthcare providers. The more common ethical issues that need to be addressed include withdrawing or withholding treatment, parental treatment refusal, and do-not-resuscitate orders.

Brain Death Criteria

A commonly accepted definition of death in the United States is **brain death**, the irreversible cessation of all functions of the brain. Specific medical protocols are used to declare

EVIDENCE-BASED PRACTICE | Responding to the Needs of the Family

Clinical Question

The families of children with life-limiting conditions often have difficulty expressing their needs for support. What are some of the most important focus areas for nursing support in palliative care programs for children and their families?

The Evidence

A survey of 50 parents whose child died as a result of advanced heart disease in the intensive care unit setting was conducted to gain information about the care provided at the child's end of life. The majority of parents (66%) believed they had little or no preparation for the way their child died or about the child's medical problems in the last month of life. Many (40%) reported receiving conflicting information from the child's healthcare team about expectations of the child's end of life. Parents (66%) reported that the child's quality of life was poor to fair during the final month, and half of children experienced suffering. Most did not realize their child would not survive until death was imminent, indicating a gap in understanding the child's prognosis (Blume et al., 2014).

A pilot study explored a method to promote advance care planning for 30 adolescents (with a mean age of 16 years) with cancer and a parent. Dyads were randomly assigned to the intervention group or control group. The control group received a brochure about advance care planning and no additional information. Six different end-of-life scenarios with possible care options for additional medical interventions or limiting treatment were provided by the research team during education and data collection sessions. Intervention adolescents were encouraged to write five wishes for their own care if a bad outcome were to occur in the future. Adolescents in the intervention group were significantly better informed about advance care planning, and adolescent–parent dyads were more likely to agree about when to limit treatment than control dyads. The

intervention adolescents (100%) wanted their parents to select the best option at the time compared to control adolescents (60%) (Lyon, Jacobs, Briggs, et al., 2013).

A focus group qualitative research process was used to help plan a legacy-making project. Eight children (7 to 12 years old) with cancer and their parents were asked to provide feedback to the legacy-making project and the questions that would guide children when they shared their story. Children wanted to participate, and said they wanted to leave a story in which others would know or remember their personal characteristics, things they like to do, and the important people in their lives. Based on feedback, questions were revised to help guide the script for a customized digital story that a child could develop (Akard et al., 2013).

Best Practice

Palliative care professionals continue to seek evidence-based care interventions to support children and families with life-limiting conditions. The above studies reveal challenges in care and strategies to support patients and families. Each of these topics was consistent with major themes found in systematic analysis of 21 qualitative and survey-based studies about patient and family needs, including accurate and clear information about the child's illness, treatments, and prognosis; spiritual needs and ways to remember the child after death; and decision making with regard to treatment decisions (Stevenson, Achille, & Lugasi, 2013).

Clinical Reasoning

When in a clinical setting where children with life-limiting conditions receive treatment, seek information about the resources and strategies used by the palliative care team to meet the needs of children and their families. What additional resources would be helpful for nursing support in this population?

---

brain death before withdrawal of life support or when organ transplantation is planned. To declare brain death, the child must be unresponsive in an irreversible coma from a known cause and have absence of brainstem reflexes, and apnea testing must reveal hypercarbia. Before an evaluation for brain death is performed, it is confirmed that the child does not have hypothermia, conditions, or medications that could contribute to brain death findings. The two required examinations by different healthcare providers for brain death to be declared are separated by 24 hours for newborns and 12 hours for infants and children (Nakagawa, Ashwal, Mathur, et al., 2011).

Withdrawal of or Withholding Treatment

The decision to withdraw or withhold life-sustaining treatments, such as mechanical ventilation or dialysis, from the dying child is very difficult and emotional for parents. Parents may feel that agreeing to withdraw treatment is a form of abandonment. When treatments are withdrawn, reassure parents the child will receive comfort measures, including pain medication. Reinforce the fact that the underlying disease process is

causing the child to die rather than withdrawing life-sustaining treatments.

Medically provided nutrition and hydration (through nasogastric or gastrostomy tubes and IV catheters) support a child's existence at the end of life, but research has not demonstrated an association with survival or improved quality of care (Rapoport, Shaheed, Newman, et al., 2013). Food and fluids may be withheld when they would be of no benefit to the child, but this is a difficult decision for parents because food and fluid are associated with nurturing and love.

Conflicted opinions often develop if parents and the healthcare provider are unable to discontinue aggressive therapies that may also cause discomfort. The nurse may experience moral distress, believing that the child's suffering is being extended without much hope for improvement. Consultation with a member of the hospital ethics committee can help clarify the issues involved and reduce the emotions of health professionals associated with the conflict. During the consultation an unbiased professional collects facts about the child's condition, clarifies the beliefs and values of parents and health professionals, and improves communication while investigating options for compromise. Families are often invited to a meeting in which the ethical dilemmas regarding their child's care are discussed so they are better informed to make decisions.

Developing Cultural Competence End-of-Life Care

Discussing the option with parents about withholding or withdrawing therapy is challenging as they are struggling to accept that no further curative care is possible for their child. The focus becomes what is best for the child within the context of the culture, faith, and values of the family. Latino families may believe that all care and every effort should be provided to their child. African American families with a strong Christian belief may want all efforts continued in the hope of divine intervention. Palliative care with a focus on reducing suffering, promoting comfort, and providing information about end-of-life care planning may not be viewed by these families as the best care (Wiener, McConnell, Latella, et al., 2013).

Professionalism in Practice DNAR Order in the School Setting

The National Association of School Nurses position statement on Do Not Attempt Resuscitation (DNAR) provides guidelines for the development of a plan for students who have such an order. The school nurse should work with the family, school administrators, the child's healthcare team, local emergency medical services providers, and others such as a local funeral director to develop plans for the supportive response when a child has an arrest. This plan is spelled out in the child's individualized health plan. The nurse must also educate school personnel about the planned response and their role, permitting discussion about their feelings concerning a child's death in the school setting. Keep in mind that a plan for bereavement support of faculty, staff, and students should also be developed for implementation when a child dies (National Association of School Nurses, 2014).

Do-Not-Resuscitate Orders

Parents faced with a child's end-stage, irreversible life-limiting condition may be asked to consider a do-not-resuscitate (DNR) order. Terms becoming more common are "**allow natural death" (AND)** and comfort care, which involve the continuation of ongoing care, managing pain, and choosing not to initiate cardiopulmonary resuscitation if the child stops breathing or the heart stops beating. Medical care is not discontinued; rather the DNR order is part of the child's management plan. Palliative care is provided, and, in some cases, curative care continues for these children.

A DNR order is part of advance care planning. A recent survey of healthcare providers and nurses revealed that advance care planning discussions often occur later in the child's care than they should, either during an acute illness or when death is imminent rather than during a period of stability (Sanderson, Zurakowski, & Wolfe, 2013). This planning process is becoming more important in pediatrics because of the increasing number of children with complex health conditions that have a variable but prolonged disease trajectory that leads to death. Honest and compassionate discussions between healthcare professionals and families, including adolescents, should occur. The family should be informed about significant condition changes and what to expect. Some time should be provided for the family and adolescent to consider what is important to them at the end of life. Families can participate in planning the child's end-of-life care with healthcare providers.

The Americans with Disabilities Act of 1990 and the Education for All Handicapped Children Act mandate that all children with disabilities—including those with complex chronic conditions and terminal illnesses—are entitled to the same education as other students. It is estimated that in the United States nearly 4000 children and adolescents attend school and may be within 6 months of dying from their chronic condition (National Association of School Nurses, 2014). These children may be at higher risk of dying while at school, and many school districts have established policies and protocols for dealing with a student's DNR order. Advance planning with an individualized health plan and emergency care plan are needed for the school setting.

Care of the Dying Child

Caring for a dying child is challenging and requires the utmost sensitivity and compassion. Children as young as 5 years of age can sense when they are seriously ill. Their awareness of death develops more rapidly when they are experiencing the progression of a disease and ongoing medical treatment. Children with life-limiting illnesses often learn about death and their own illness from exposure to other seriously ill and dying children during hospitalization or clinic visits.

Awareness of Dying by Developmental Age

Infants and toddlers are not actually aware of death, but they are aware of and react to changes in normal routines and the behavior of parents. Toddlers know they feel tired and sick, but they do not understand that their physical symptoms are associated with impending death (Figure 41–6).

Preschool children can see their bodies deteriorate and feel the effects of medications used during disease progression and treatment. Changes in self-concept occur as they perceive these body changes. They often describe their illness in terms of mutilation to their body. These physical changes may make them realize that they are dying.

School-age children also have subtle fears about body integrity and anxieties about the seriousness of their illness. This greater preoccupation with illness is considered by many professionals as the child's version of **death anxiety**, a feeling of apprehension or fear of death. Children may express death anxiety as a concern with treatments that invade the body or interfere with normal body functions.

Adolescents have a mature understanding of death, but the normal developmental milestones of adolescence add to their problems in facing a terminal illness. They are struggling to establish their own identity and plans for the future. At a time when body image is extremely important, they may be faced with the possibility of mutilation and disfigurement. Dying adolescents are often isolated from their peers during a period when peers are the most essential social group. Adolescents nearing the end of life may be angry because they recognize that

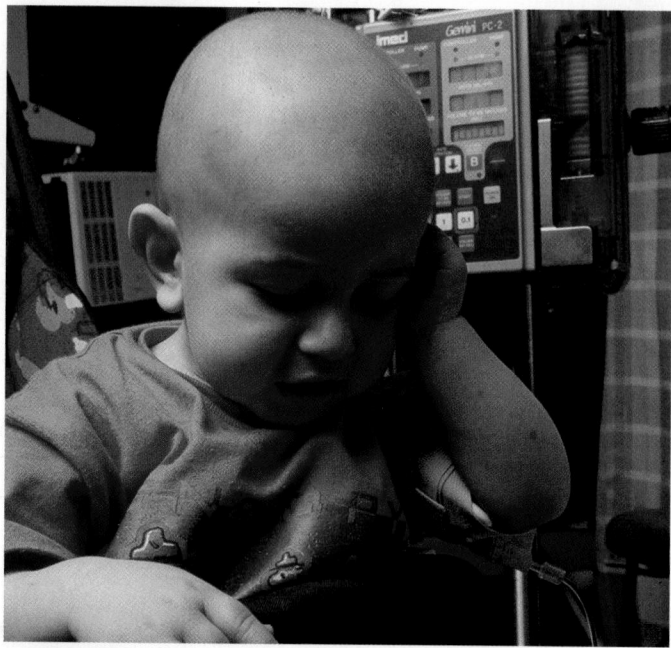

Figure 41–6 The toddler with a life-limiting condition recognizes that he feels sick and that routines are different. His anxiety may increase because of the concern and feelings of sadness exhibited by his parents.

their loss is occurring at a time when the whole world is opening up to them.

Do not expect adolescents to handle feelings in the same way that adults do. They often avoid expressing anger against the family, seeking to control and direct these feelings elsewhere. Adolescents may become angry at changes in treatment procedures, lack of explanations, and threats to their independence. As death nears, the adolescent may permit comforting and support and may accept care from warm and loving family members, as long as it is not given in a condescending manner.

Nursing Management
For the Dying Child

Nursing care of the dying child and family focuses on providing family-centered support for their physical and psychosocial needs.

Nursing Assessment and Diagnosis

Assess the child's physiologic status and comfort level. Physiologic changes in the dying child may be directly related to the child's disease process or injury. Signs and symptoms of approaching death are provided in Table 41–2.

Assess the child's awareness of impending death. Examples of questions the child may ask include: "What will death be like? Will it hurt? What happens to me when I die? Will I be

TABLE 41–2 Clinical Manifestations of the Dying Child

SYSTEM	CLINICAL MANIFESTATIONS
Cardiovascular system (decreased cardiac output and peripheral circulation)	• The heart rate may initially increase as hypoxia develops; then the heart rate and blood pressure decrease. • A change in pulse pressure and a decrease in the volume of Korotkoff sounds indicate imminent death. • Diaphoresis, clammy cool skin, and changes in skin coloring (mottled to cyanotic). Mottling is a sign of imminent death.
Respiratory system (pulmonary congestion due to impaired cardiac function)	• Tachypnea, diminished breath sounds, and hypoxia. • Dyspnea; **air hunger**, the most severe form of dyspnea, may cause the child to look panicked, gasp for breath, and sit upright; it may not be relieved by oxygen. • Cheyne-Stokes breathing (periods of shallow breathing alternating with apnea) is a sign of imminent death. • As muscles relax, secretions accumulate in the oropharynx and bronchi causing noisy breathing as air passes through the secretions. • Moaning or grunting with breathing is common.
Neurologic system (neurologic dysfunction due to decreased cerebral perfusion, metabolic acidosis, and accumulated toxins from renal and liver failure)	• Hypoxemia. • Agitation or restlessness, withdrawal, increasing drowsiness, confusion. • May be unconscious during final hours. • May speak of visions (persons or objects) not visible to others. • Deterioration of hearing and vision acuity. Remember that hearing is one of the last senses to diminish before death.
Musculoskeletal system	• Extreme muscle weakness and fatigue. • May be unable to reposition self or toilet self. • Difficulty swallowing; may be unable to cough effectively and clear secretions.
Renal system (decreased renal function)	• Decreased urine production. • Sphincters relax and incontinence can occur.
Gastrointestinal system	• Decreased oral fluid intake and anorexia are common. • Sphincters relax and bowel incontinence can occur.

with [a deceased person whom the child was close to] again? Will my parents be all right? Will you remember me?" Assess the ability of the parents to talk with the child about dying.

Assess the family for coping skills and need for social supports. Identify any cultural or spiritual traditions, rituals, and beliefs related to loss and grieving that may provide comfort to the family.

Examples of nursing diagnoses that apply to the dying child and family include the following (NANDA-I © 2014):

- *Fear (Child)* related to unanswered questions and concerns of abandonment
- *Anxiety, Death (Child),* related to own impending death
- *Grieving (Parents)* related to imminent death of child
- *Hopelessness (Parents)* related to failure of therapies to prolong life

Planning and Implementation

Nursing care for the dying child and the family includes providing comfort, assisting the child in a peaceful death, assisting the child and family with coping strategies, and facilitating grief.

PHYSIOLOGIC CARE

A major goal in care of the dying child is to promote comfort and keep the child pain free. Opioids may be prescribed to promote optimal pain relief. Oral, transdermal, or rectal analgesia is available for families who choose to withhold IV fluids. Complementary therapies for comfort and pain management can be used by the nurse and family members (see Chapter 40).

If dyspnea, or air hunger, occurs, position the child to maintain the airway and promote breathing. Open a window or use a circulating fan to ease the child's distress. An opioid may be prescribed for air hunger or tachypnea as its action dilates the pulmonary vessels, reduces oxygen consumption, and decreases pulmonary congestion.

Other physiologic care includes keeping the airway clear of secretions, bathing and keeping the skin dry and intact, changing the child's position frequently, and encouraging favorite foods and liquids as tolerated. Decrease excessive stimulation and reduce unnecessary activities. Involve the parents in physical care and encourage them to hold and comfort the child.

COMMUNICATING WITH THE CHILD ABOUT HIS OR HER IMPENDING DEATH

The dying child may be aware of impending death before being told, and parents may not understand this. When the child has no opportunity to talk about death, the child may feel isolated and distressed. The child may believe that initiating the conversation about an awareness of death and related fears will add to the family's emotional burden.

Some parents wish to protect the child from bad news and avoid talking to the child about the child's serious illness and potential death. Parents often do not know how to talk with their child about dying. Some parents feel emotionally unable to answer the child's questions about dying. They may fear that talking about the impending death will take away the child's hope. A professional who has special training in bereavement counseling can assist children and families with the discussion. When the family is ready to talk with the child about the child's death, suggest some developmentally appropriate words to use. Emphasize to the parents that the child may actually need to hear the word *dying* in order to understand. Strategies for talking with a dying child are described in Table 41–3. Families who have talked with their child about dying report they have rarely regretted having the discussion (Gaab, Owens, & MacLeod, 2013).

Provide the child with opportunities for fantasy play, drawing, and storytelling, without emphasizing or reinforcing death themes. Listen to what children tell you about themselves and their lives. **Death imagery**, references to death or death-related topics (going away, separation, funerals), may be a theme of their stories.

Some dying children want to leave a legacy so they will be remembered or to express their good-byes through photography, journals, poetry, writing letters, or music. Some children choose to make crafts or a memory box for others, or to give away special possessions.

When caring for adolescents, outbursts of frustration and anger are common, but these are not personally directed at the nurse. Provide activities to help adolescents channel their feelings. Continue providing support in spite of their behavior. This approach may encourage adolescents to accept comforting without losing face. Be available to listen when the adolescent wants to talk and express feelings and frustrations. Promote friendships with other adolescents who have similar interests or problems.

FAMILY SUPPORT

Parents need to be present when possible as the child is dying, a pivotal event in their parent–child relationship. Work closely with the family when the child's death is imminent; they will remember the experience and words spoken for the rest of their lives. Prepare the family for changes in the child's appearance and behavior. Providing the parents with a room to be alone with the child ensures privacy at this extremely personal time.

TABLE 41–3 Strategies for Communicating With Dying Children

- Be receptive when dying children initiate a conversation, or look for opportunities to talk with them, such as when their physical health or behavior is changing.
- Ask dying children what they know. Correct any misunderstood information with language appropriate for their age. Ask what they want to know. Be honest when answering questions, but do not provide more information than requested.
- Encourage dying children to talk about what worries them. Allow them to express their feelings and to be upset. Empathize with these children's feelings.
- Ask dying children what is most important to them with the time they have left.
- Offer opportunities for nonverbal expression of feelings, such as art, music, and writing. Ask what the art represents.
- Let dying children know they will not be abandoned and that any suffering they may have will be treated.
- Let dying children know they will always be loved and remembered.

Source: Data from Evan, E. E., & Cohen, H. J. (2011). Child relationships. In J. Wolfe, P. S. Hinds, & B. M. Sourkes (Eds.), *Textbook of interdisciplinary pediatric palliative care* (pp. 125–134). Philadelphia, PA: Elsevier Saunders; You, J. J., Fowler, R. A., & Heyland, D. K. (2014). Just ask: Discussing goals of care with patients in hospital with serious illness. *Canadian Medical Association Journal, 186*(6), 425–432; MacPherson, C. F. (2013). The final chapter. *Clinical Journal of Oncology Nursing, 16*(5), e190–e191.

Ask the family what is important to them in the final moments and hours of the child's life and what will be important to them in the grief process. Each culture has its own way of defining, addressing, and acknowledging death. Customs, ceremonies, religious laws, and beliefs are strongly connected with dying (see Table 41–4 for rituals regarding dying and after death). Accommodate desired spiritual or cultural practices when possible. Holding the child is a universal request and should be permitted, along with touching, stroking, kissing, and talking soothingly.

Many families find that saying good-bye as a group is helpful. Families need to cry together and to tell each other how much they will miss each other. Assure them that the vigil with the child prevents the child from feeling isolated or abandoned

TABLE 41–4 Spiritual Traditions Regarding Dying and After-Death Rites

RELIGIOUS GROUP	RITUALS YOU MIGHT OBSERVE
American Indians	• Beliefs and practices vary widely among tribes • Autopsy is generally acceptable
Buddhism	• Family presence is important • Last-rite chanting at bedside • Cremation is common
Catholicism	• Sacrament of the sick, baptism of newborn • Obligated to take ordinary but not extraordinary means to prolong life • Burial is common
Christian Science	• No medical help is sought to prolong life • No donation of body parts. Disposal of body and parts decided by family
Hinduism	• Family presence with chanting, prayers, and singing • Final rites by a religious leader; a thread tied around neck or wrist signifies a blessing; do not remove • Autopsy if required by law; organ donation may be acceptable • Cremation is common
Islam	• Deathbed should be turned to face Mecca, reading from the Qur'an stressing hope and acceptance • Body is washed 3 times, only by Muslim of the same gender • Autopsy only for medical or legal reasons; organ donation is acceptable • Burial as soon as possible
Jehovah's Witness	• Prayer and reading the Bible • Organ donation is forbidden • Autopsy acceptable for legal reasons • Burial determined by family preference
Judaism	• Autopsy if required by law and organ donation in some cases • Prefer natural death rather than technologic support • Body ritually washed, and a living person is always with the body after death • Burial occurs as soon as possible; all body parts buried together • Seven-day mourning period
Mormonism	• If death inevitable, promote a peaceful and dignified death; laying on of hands, anointing with oil • Organ donation is an individual choice • Burial in "temple clothes"
Protestantism	• Variable rituals, laying on of hands, anointing with oil, communion, final blessing • Organ donation, autopsy, and burial or cremation are individual decisions • Means to prolong life is individual decision
Seventh Day Adventist	• Prayer, anointing with oil • Prefer prolonging life • Organ donation and autopsy are individual decisions • Disposal of body and burial are individual decisions

Source: Adapted from Spector, R. E. (2013). *Cultural diversity in health and illness* (8th ed., pp. 151–152). Upper Saddle River, NJ: Prentice Hall Health; Purnell, L. D. (2014). *Guide to culturally competent health care* (3rd ed.). Philadelphia, PA: F. A. Davis; Wiener, L., McConnell, D. G., Latella, L., & Ludi, E. (2013). Cultural and religious considerations in pediatric palliative care. *Palliative and Supportive Care, 11*, 47–67.

as death approaches. The dying child should never be left alone when dying is imminent.

Developing Cultural Competence Diverse Perspectives on Death

Consider cultural differences when working with families who are dealing with the death of a loved one, for example (Evans & Ume, 2012; Purnell, 2014; Weiner et al., 2013):

- African Americans often place great importance on the presence and involvement of their families in their care. They embrace religion and spirituality. They may be less likely to request medications for pain and other symptoms because of an expectation to suffer. They may seek more aggressive care.

- Some Asian families desire to protect the terminally ill from knowledge of their condition, so their final days will be peaceful. Decision making is often collectively decided by the family, and a spokesperson for the family is often the oldest male or head of household. Some families may believe that making plans for the child's death could cause the child's premature death or having a visit by the chaplain may signify an impending death.

- Hispanics generally believe the entire family makes important decisions. They see death as a natural part of life, and they do not want to be a burden for their families. Cultural customs related to grief and loss vary. Crying openly is seen as appropriate. Faith is very important in times of death. The anniversary of a loved one's death is celebrated every year.

TISSUE AND ORGAN DONATION

Healthcare professionals are obligated to ask families about making an anatomic gift. Become familiar with national guidelines for organ collection and donation so you will be better prepared to serve the family of the dying child and potential organ recipients. An organ procurement coordinator collaborates with the healthcare team to help explain the organ donation process to the family, and to assure family members that the organ donation process is totally separate from decisions regarding their child's care. Organ donation costs are paid by the organ procurement organization, but recipients pay transplantation costs.

NEED FOR AUTOPSY

When the exact cause of death is unclear, an autopsy may be suggested. An autopsy may be required by state law for an unnatural or unexpected death, such as suicide, homicide, child abuse, or sudden infant death syndrome. When parents have a choice, they may be hesitant to consent to autopsy because it further invades the child's body. Support the family during the decision-making process by explaining that the autopsy will likely reveal the cause of death or inevitability of death.

POSTMORTEM CARE AND FAMILY SUPPORT

Offer ongoing support after the child dies. Questions like the following may help begin the conversation: "I am sorry for your loss. How can I help?" "What are your traditions when an infant or child dies?" "Is there someone I can call for you?" Nurses should feel free to express their sorrow and grief for the child and family. Crying with families is recognized as an expression of caring and empathy.

Identify the family's wishes for postmortem care before performing any care. Ask before removing any jewelry or other item from the child because cultural and spiritual practices may specify that the article remain on the child after death. Follow the healthcare facility's guidelines for postmortem care. Position the child according to guidelines or cultural/religious practices, clean the room, and remove medical equipment.

After the child's death, allow the family to spend as much time as they need with the child's body. Never rush family members who are saying good-bye to the child. Save all of the child's personal items—especially in the case of an infant. A lock of hair, hand- or footprints, the infant's identification band, the child's weight and height, or a picture of the infant can be sources of comfort and remembrance for families. Ask for permission before cutting a lock of hair as some cultural and religious groups prohibit it. Seal the last clothes or patient gown used by the child, or the infant's blanket, in a plastic bag to retain the child's scent. Use a special remembrance box or container for this purpose. If parents refuse to take the items, give them to another family member or retain them. Document the collection of the mementos and who received them in case parents ask for them at a later time.

Clinical Tip

When a sudden violence-related death of a child or adolescent occurs, steps to preserve forensic evidence are taken. Removal of medical equipment is not permitted. Follow facility guidelines for evidence collection (e.g., child's clothing, sheet used during resuscitation) and the chain of possession prior to giving evidence to law enforcement authorities. The child may be swaddled in a clean sheet for family member access. Depending on the injuries and circumstances, the family may not be permitted to have physical contact with the child's body (O'Malley et al., 2014).

When a newborn or young infant has died, wrap the baby in a blanket and offer the mother and other family members the opportunity to hold the baby. Parents may want to bathe and dress the infant. The family experiencing the death of a newborn may appreciate an offer to take pictures of the baby and family together, if picture taking is not prohibited by religious or cultural traditions. Some families may feel uncomfortable taking pictures and refuse the offer. The nurse should question the family about baptism or other ritual requests for the newborn, and facilitate arrangements for a religious or spiritual leader at the family's request. Ensure that the mother experiencing the death of a newborn receives information about lactation suppression or milk donation options if she has been breastfeeding.

A bereavement folder should be provided to parents with information that includes resources available to help with a memorial service or funeral and potential sibling responses. Include grief counseling resources and support groups and encourage the family to use these resources for the first year after the child's death. Inform parents that certain dates, such as the day of the week the child died, the child's birthday, or family holidays, will be difficult and may trigger intense sadness. Parents may benefit from keeping a journal of their thoughts and memories, or writing letters or poems to or about their child. Follow-up phone calls from healthcare providers are appreciated by families.

Evaluation

Expected outcomes of caring for the dying child and family may include the following:

- The child is pain free and comfortable, and the child's physiologic needs are met.
- The cultural and spiritual needs of the dying child and family are met.
- The dying child and family receive support during the dying process.
- The family receives continued support after the child's death.

Bereavement

Parents' Reactions

The death of one's child is likely the most traumatic event a parent will experience. Grief, an individual's feelings and behaviors in response to death or loss, is painful, individualized, and exhausting. Many factors influence the parents' grief responses, including their perception of whether the death could be prevented, the suddenness and other circumstances of the death, the nature of their attachment to the child, previous losses, spiritual or religious orientation, and culture.

Sudden Death of a Child

An estimated 25% of child and adolescent deaths each year are related to complex chronic conditions (Klein & Saroyan, 2011). The majority of child and adolescent deaths are sudden and unexpected, such as from sudden infant death syndrome, injury, illness, suicide, or violence. Parents need additional support to deal with the sudden and unexpected death of their child and with their surviving children.

Death of a Newborn or Young Infant

In 2013, in the United States, 29,138 infants died shortly after birth or during their first year of life (Centers for Disease Control, National Center for Health Statistics, 2015). The death of a newborn forces the parents to experience their child's entire life cycle in a short period of time, and they are faced with overwhelming grief at a time when they anticipated the experience of joy. Refer parents to a perinatal bereavement program or support group. See Chapter 21.

Grief and Bereavement

Although parents progress through distinct stages of grief, as described previously in this chapter, the timeline and nature of the grief process differ for each individual. The intense pain and shock initially felt by parents gradually give way to feelings of anger, guilt, depression, and loneliness. Very slowly, and with much support, energy returns and parents again begin to enjoy life experiences. Parents may experience friction due to differing intensities of grief and coping processes. Additional support may be needed to prevent a sense of loneliness and isolation.

Clinical Tip

The following strategies can assist the nurse in working with parents whose child dies suddenly and who are not present during the resuscitation:

- Identify a spokesperson for the medical team to keep the family informed during resuscitation efforts. Call support resources (e.g., chaplain service, social worker, or interpreter).
- Create time for families to assimilate the child's worsening status by providing two to three updates during the resuscitation. Prepare them for what is to come.
- Ensure that the right family members are present for discussions after the death, or have a family support member for a single parent. Provide a private space with telephone access.
- Turn off your phone and beeper, sit close, and make eye contact. If the family arrived after resuscitation ended, ask them what they know about what happened. Prepare them by saying you are sorry to give them this bad news. Verify that the child (use the child's name) has died. Let the family know that everything possible was done to save the child, but the injuries or illness complications were too severe to survive.
- Allow the family time to absorb the information. Accept whatever emotions family members express. Let the family be first to talk. Answer any questions asked. Be prepared to repeat information.
- Offer to telephone family or friends.
- After the death, prepare the body for viewing in a private place, covering disfiguring wounds. Escort the family to the body and explain any tubes or lines that must remain in place. Allow them time to say goodbye.
- Convey information to the family about the cause of death, autopsy, funeral preparations, and the normal grief process. Provide contact information for the family in case of questions.
- Arrange for family follow-up to see how they are responding to the child's loss and to review autopsy findings.

Source: Data from Shoenberger, J. M., Yeghiazarian, S., Rios, C., & Henderson, S. O. (2013). Death notification in the emergency department: Survivors and physicians. *Western Journal of Emergency Medicine, 14(2),* 181–185; O'Malley, P. J., Barata, I., Snow, S., American Academy of Pediatrics Committee on Pediatric Emergency Medicine, American College of Emergency Physicians Pediatric Emergency Medicine Committee, & Emergency Nurses Association Pediatric Committee. (2014). Death of a child in the emergency department. *Pediatrics, 134(1),* e313–e330; Old, J. L. (2011). Communicating bad news to your patient. *Family Practice Management.* Retrieved from http://www.aafp.org/fpm/2011/1100/p31.html

---

Let parents know that caring for themselves physically and mentally is important, even though the period surrounding their child's death is difficult. Refer parents to local support groups for bereaved parents and siblings (e.g., Compassionate Friends, First Candle, and SHARE Pregnancy and Infant Loss Support), and provide books and articles for later use. Some facilities and most palliative care programs have formal follow-up programs for bereaved parents to encourage a healthy progression through the grieving process.

Siblings' Reactions

Siblings experiencing the death of a brother or sister grieve and require supportive and compassionate care. Siblings anticipating the addition of a new baby to the family will also feel the loss. The siblings may have received less attention from parents during the child's illness. Depending on their development, they may fear that they caused their brother's or sister's illness or injury, or worry that their bad thoughts caused the illness. Table 41–5 highlights children's understanding of

TABLE 41–5 Children's Understanding of Death, Their Potential Behaviors, and Nursing Management

UNDERSTANDING OF DEATH	POTENTIAL BEHAVIORS	NURSING MANAGEMENT
INFANT *Cognitive stage: sensorimotor* Senses emotions of caregivers, and altered routines Senses separation	Resists cuddling and eats less May have feeding problems Cries excessively, clingy Sleeps more than usual	Provide a sense of security by holding and hugging and a soothing voice by a caring person if the parent is too distraught. Try to return to usual routines.
TODDLER *Cognitive stage: preoperational* No understanding of true concept of death Aware someone is missing—separation anxiety Unable to distinguish death from temporary separation or abandonment	Regresses to younger stage of development Clingy, does not want to let parent out of sight Whiney, irritable, may show distress by biting, hitting, tears Problems eating and sleeping Sleep disturbances Fearfulness	Encourage parents to hold and cuddle the toddler to help reduce the fear of separation. Follow familiar routines. Be tolerant of regressive behaviors. Use distraction (toys, games, videos) when the child is fussy or clingy.
PRESCHOOLER *Cognitive stage: preoperational* Believes death is temporary and the dead person will return Experiences magical thinking (believes own thoughts or actions potentially caused the death) Confuses death with being away or asleep Has beginning experience with death of animals and plants	Regression to earlier developmental stage, problems with bowel and bladder control, tantrums, may withdraw from activities, disobedience May fear going to sleep, has nightmares, afraid of the dark, separation anxiety Crying spells Seems morbidly fascinated with death Asks when deceased will return Asks many questions Complaints of abdominal pain	Provide honest and consistent responses to the child's questions; say the person is not coming back. Try to follow usual routines. Be tolerant of regressive behaviors; provide play activities. Keep memories alive with pictures and items that remind the child of the loved one. Participate in rituals, e.g., going to the cemetery, releasing helium balloons, and planting flowers.
SCHOOL-AGE CHILD *Cognitive stage: concrete operations* Understands difference between temporary separation and death By 6 years, knows death is permanent. By 9–10 years, understanding of death is same as adult May have guilt or assume blame for the death May not realize that death can occur at any age	Crying, moody, may become more withdrawn and distant, may have angry outbursts or disruptive behaviors, may dwell on absence of loved one Decreased concentration for school work, may refuse to go to school Psychosomatic complaints—stomachache or headache May try to comfort parents by taking over tasks May fear another loved person will die	Listen to the child and answer questions honestly. Return to usual routines and activities. Have the parent let the child know when parents will return and a how to contact them. Keep memories alive through activities such as art, music, creating a memory book, sewing a quilt, and planting a garden. Share Internet resources; suggest coping support groups. Encourage the family to seek faith-based support.
ADOLESCENT *Cognitive stage: formal operations* Intellectually capable of understanding death Recognizes all people and self will die Understands the association between illness and death Sense of invincibility conflicts with fear of death Able to recognize effect of death on others	May have severe depression, mood swings, withdrawal from friends, may feel angry or guilty Girls may seek comfort from friends Eating and sleeping problems May act-out or display risk-taking behaviors May assume responsibility for family well-being Uses abstract and philosophical reasoning to try to make sense of life	Be available and encourage open communication. Share your own grief and feelings with the adolescent. Keep memories alive with pictures and items that remind the teen of the loved one. Access counseling and support groups; share Internet resources. Encourage the child to seek support from the family's faith group.

Source: Data from Lancaster, J. (2011). Developmental stages, grief, and a child's response to death. *Pediatric Annals, 40*(5), 277–281; DeFrancis Sun, B., Richards J. T. (Eds.). (2011). *The grieving child: Helping children cope with grief when an infant dies* (2nd ed.). Retrieved from http://www.mchlibrary.info/suid-sids/documents/SIDRC/HelpingChildrenCope.pdf; Machajewski, V., & Kronk, R. (2013). Childhood grief related to death of a sibling. *Journal of Nurse Practitioners*, 9(7), 443–448.

death at different developmental stages, some of the possible behavioral responses, and nursing considerations for family education.

When possible, siblings should have the opportunity to visit when the child is dying so that they feel nothing was hidden from them. Memories about the death process are part of the grieving process (Lancaster, 2011). Nurses and other support personnel can assist the surviving children to adapt to their parents' distraction, grief, and increased protectiveness of them. The siblings need to hear that the parents' grief in no way diminishes the love felt for them.

When talking to the siblings of a child who has died, be honest and answer questions truthfully. Provide information about the child's death in a manner they can understand. Use developmentally appropriate terms, such as, "Adam's heart will never beat again," "He will never get cold or hungry," and "He will never come home again." Reassure siblings that they did not cause their brother or sister to die (unless they did contribute to the child's death) and that death was not a punishment for wrongdoing. Allow the siblings to ask questions and acknowledge the emotions they are feeling. Emphasize that it is okay for them to be sad, angry, frightened, or tearful. Use the same amount of energy and concern to acknowledge the sibling's and the adult's grief.

Encourage the parents, if appropriate, to allow siblings to participate in planning the child's memorial or funeral service. A funeral service director can be supportive to provide family time for the sibling to say good-bye. Attending the service assists the sibling to grieve, and being able to grieve as a family provides a sense of connectedness to parents and security at a vulnerable time. When siblings attend the funeral, they should be prepared for what to expect, such as an open casket and the behaviors of mourners. Suggest that parents designate a family member or close friend to monitor the siblings' needs while the parents attend to other matters. Keep the family together as much as possible.

As with parental bereavement, sibling bereavement is intense and a lifelong process. Sad feelings may return repeatedly as understanding about death increases. Be open and available when children wish to talk about a dead sibling to support their grieving. Encourage parents to make sure other caregivers and teachers know about the sibling's loss. Books for the family that might help children with grief include *Tell Me, Papa: Answers to Questions Children Ask About Death and Dying* by M. Johnson, J. Johnson, and A. C. Blake; *What Happens When Someone Dies: A Child's Guide to Death and Funerals* by M. Mundy and R. W. Alley; and *A Complete Book About Death for Kids* by E. Grollman and J. Johnson.

Staff Reactions to the Death of a Child

Caring for dying children is especially stressful and demanding for healthcare professionals. Some nurses cope by distancing themselves socially from the dying child and family to maintain composure and a professional demeanor. Nurses with young children may have more difficulty caring for the dying child. They tend to identify with the child, making it more difficult to recognize the dying child's anxiety and fears because of their own personal defenses against a sense of helplessness to alter the course of the child's disease.

When the child dies, the bond that was developed with the child and family is lost, and feelings of helplessness or powerlessness may be related to failed efforts to relieve suffering (Duvall, 2011). Nurses may feel extreme sadness and helplessness in association with a child patient's death and the grief observed among the child's family members. Nurses may alternate between dealing with their grief and suppressing it, which permits them to avoid becoming consumed by the loss.

Nurses who work with terminally ill children and their families need special preparation to care for children and families and to manage personal stress simultaneously. Mentoring by experienced hospice nurses, as well as additional educational experiences, may be helpful. Nurses must learn to cope effectively with grief and develop empathy, competence, and confidence in their ability to provide more humane and effective nursing care. Nurses should feel free to express their sorrow and grief for the child and family. Some nurses attend funeral and memorial services when invited by the patient's family.

Nurses working in emergency departments caring for children who die suddenly or in hospice settings and hospital units that care for terminally ill children need support systems to help balance the stresses of working with dying children. An important support system often gives an opportunity to discuss the experience with a supportive peer (Figure 41–7). Many facilities offer debriefing group sessions with mental health professionals to discuss feelings and concerns, as well as resources to help nurses learn about self-care activities, relaxation techniques, and how to maintain a balance between their work and personal lives.

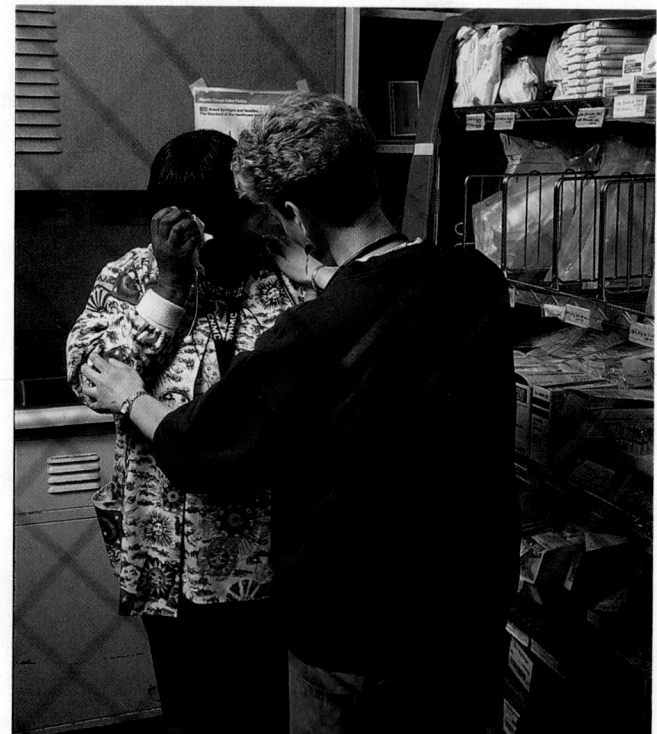

Figure 41–7 Nurses need to express grief in a supportive environment after a child's death. Sharing the sadness and grief or futility of resuscitation efforts with colleagues can often help nurses continue to provide supportive care to the next families who need compassionate care.

Focus Your Study

- A life-threatening illness or injury places intense emotional and physical demands on the child and family due to the unfamiliar environment of the emergency department or intensive care unit, frightening or invasive procedures, and an uncertain outcome.

- Defense mechanisms displayed by children in stressful situations such as a life-threatening illness or injury include regression (return to an earlier behavior), denial, repression (involuntary forgetting), postponement, and bargaining.

- Nursing interventions to promote a child's psychologic health include permitting parents to be present, preparing children for procedures, using play to help the child manage anxiety, and allowing the child some choices to gain a sense of control.

- Parents typically progress through the stages of shock and disbelief, anger and guilt, deprivation and loss, anticipatory waiting, and readjustment or mourning when their child has a life-threatening illness or injury.

- A family-centered approach will help meet the needs of families, minimize stress, and enhance family coping. Appropriate nursing care includes providing information and building trust, promoting family involvement (including presence during invasive procedures and resuscitation if desired), encouraging parents to meet physical and emotional needs, facilitating effective communication, and maintaining family support systems.

- The nurse should ensure siblings receive information about their critically ill or injured brother or sister in preparation for a visit, and they should support the parents to provide regular messages to help them control feelings of jealousy, guilt, fear, and insecurity. Allowing the siblings to visit the child may help them to cope.

- Palliative care is a service for persons with life-limiting conditions that provides therapies to reduce suffering, to improve the quality of remaining life, to facilitate decision making regarding end of life, and to coordinate care. Hospice is one category of palliative care.

- The families of dying children face many decision-making issues such as when to begin palliative and/or hospice care, advance care planning, the withholding or withdrawal of treatments, and DNR requests.

- One commonly accepted definition of death in the United States is brain death, or the irreversible cessation of all functions of the brain, including the cerebral cortex and brainstem.

- Children with life-threatening illnesses often learn about death and their own illness through exposure to other ill and dying children. Children recognize that their condition is worsening when receiving extra treatments, feeling ill, and noticing cues from their parents, even if they are not told they are dying.

- It is essential to work closely with the family when a child's death is imminent, helping to provide the support and services most important to them in the last moments or hours of their child's life.

- The nurse caring for the dying child and family offers physiologic and psychosocial support during end-of-life care.

- Bereavement support must be provided to the family, making sure that siblings are not overlooked. Allow siblings to participate in planning the memorial service. Encourage parents to allow siblings to express their emotions.

- Caring for a dying child is difficult, and nurses need special preparation to meet the needs of the child and family, and to manage their own responses when a child they care fore dies.

Clinical Reasoning in Action

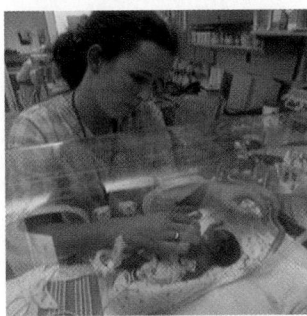

Kelly is a premature baby weighing 500 g (1.1 lb) when born at 24 weeks' gestation after her mother had premature rupture of membranes. Her parents, Shawn and Lori, are of Navajo Indian descent. Kelly's condition is extremely critical and she is on life support. You know that any amount of touch can be extremely stressful for newborns this small and in critical condition. The mother has been pumping and freezing breast milk for future use. The parents are encouraged to assist the nurse in any way they can, but they are not able to touch Kelly. While the parents know how critical Kelly's condition is and have learned about the machines and medications being used, they are still confused and uncertain about the situation. They have not left the hospital at all. The grandparents have been helping care for Roseanne, Kelly's 7-year-old sister, and she has visited her sister once. On her third day of life, Kelly gained weight and started to show an increase in activity. The parents thought this could be a positive sign, but the nurse explained that swelling caused the weight gain and the increased activity was from agitation as Kelly struggled to breathe. When the parents were at the bedside, Kelly started to become cyanotic and her oxygen saturation level dropped to the 60s. The healthcare team tried to save her but were unsuccessful. This was a devastating loss for the family and all the medical personnel involved.

1. What are some of the stressors Kelly experienced while in the hospital?

2. What are the stages of grief Kelly's family is likely to experience?

3. What are some strategies that can be used to help Roseanne deal with the loss of her sister?

4. What are some of the strategies for supporting Kelly's parents?

References

Akard, T. F., Gilmer, M. J., Friedman, D. L., Given, B., Hendricks-Ferguson, V. L., & Hinds, P. S. (2013). From qualitative work to intervention development in pediatric oncology palliative care research. *Journal of Pediatric Oncology Nursing, 30*(3), 153–160.

American Academy of Pediatrics (AAP) Section on Hospice and Palliative Medicine and Committee on Hospital Care. (2013). Pediatric palliative care and hospice care: Commitments, guidelines, and recommendations. *Pediatrics, 132*(5), 966–972.

Ames, K. E., Rennick, J. E., & Baillargeon, S. (2011). A qualitative interpretive study exploring parents' perception of the parental role in the paediatric intensive care unit. *Intensive and Critical Care Nursing, 27*, 143–150.

Blume, E. D., Balkin, E. M., Aiyagari, R., Ziniel, S., Beke, D. M., Thiagarajan, R., . . . Wolfe, J. (2014). Parental perspectives on suffering and quality of life at end-of-life in children with advanced heart disease: An exploratory study. *Pediatric Critical Care Medicine, 15*(4), 336–342.

Centers for Disease Control and Prevention, National Center for Health Statistics. (2015). *Underlying Cause of Death 1999–2013 on CDC WONDER Online Database*. Retrieved from http://wonder.cdc.gov/ucd-icd10.html

Crozier, F., & Hancock, L. E. (2012). Pediatric palliative care: Beyond the end of life. *Pediatric Nursing, 38*(4), 198–203, 227.

DeFrancis Sun, B., & Richards, J. T. (Eds). (2011). *The grieving child: Helping children cope with grief when an infant dies* (2nd ed.). Retrieved from http://www.mchlibrary.info/suid-sids/documents/SIDRC/HelpingChildrenCope.pdf

Dow, B., Kenardy, J., Long, D., & Le Brocque, R. (2012). Children's post-traumatic stress and the role of memory following admission to intensive care: A review. *Clinical Psychologist, 16*, 1–14.

Duvall, A. (2011). Care of the caretaker: Managing the grief process of health care professionals. *Pediatric Annals, 40*(5), 266–273.

Emergency Nurses Association (ENA). (2012). *Emergency nursing resource: Family presence during invasive procedures and resuscitation in the emergency department*. Retrieved from http://www.ena.org/practice-research/research/CPG/Documents/FamilyPresenceCPG.pdf

Evan, E. E., & Cohen, H. J. (2011). Child relationships. In J. Wolfe, P. S. Hinds, & B. M. Sourkes (Eds.), *Textbook of interdisciplinary pediatric palliative care* (pp. 125–134). Philadelphia, PA: Elsevier Saunders.

Evans, B., & Ume, E. (2012). Psychosocial, cultural, and spiritual health disparities in end-of-life and palliative care: Where we are and where we need to go. *Nursing Outlook, 60*, 370–375.

Gaab, E. M., Owens, G., & MacLeod, R. D. (2013). Primary caregivers' decisions around communicating about death with children involved in pediatric palliative care. *Journal of Hospice and Palliative Nursing, 15*(6), 322–329.

Jabre, P., Belpomme, V., Azoulay, E., Jacob, L., Bertrand, L., Lapostolle, F., . . . Adnet, F. (2013). Family presence during cardiopulmonary resuscitation. *The New England Journal of Medicine, 368*(11), 1008–1018.

Jee, R. A., Shepherd, J. R., Boyles, C. E., Marsh, M. J., Thomas, P. W., & Ross, O. C. (2012). Evaluation and comparison of parental needs, stressors, and coping strategies in a pediatric intensive care unit. *Pediatric Critical Care Medicine, 13*(3), e166–e172.

Keim-Malpass, J., Hart, T. G., & Miller, J. R. (2013). Coverage of palliative and hospice care for pediatric patients with a life-limiting illness: A policy brief. *Journal of Pediatric Health Care, 27*(6), 511–516.

Klein, S. M., & Saroyan, J. M. (2011). Treating a child with a life-threatening condition. *Pediatric Annals, 40*(5), 259–265.

Lancaster, J. (2011). Developmental stages, grief, and a child's response to death. *Pediatric Annals, 40*(5), 277–281.

Lyon, M. E., Jacobs, S., Briggs, B., Cheng, Y. I., & Wang, J. (2013). Family-centered advance care planning for teens with cancer. *JAMA Pediatrics, 167*(5), 460–467.

Machajewski, V., & Kronk, R. (2013). Childhood grief related to death of a sibling. *Journal of Nurse Practitioners, 9*(7), 443–448.

MacPherson, C. F. (2013). The final chapter. *Clinical Journal of Oncology Nursing, 16*(5), e190–e191.

Meert, K. L., Clark, J., & Eggly, S. (2013). Family-centered care in the pediatric intensive care unit. *Pediatric Clinics of North America, 60*(3), 761–772.

Nakagawa, T. A., Ashwal, S., Mathur, M., Mysore, M., & the Society of Critical Care Medicine, Section on Critical Care and Section on Neurology of the American Academy of Pediatrics, and the Child Neurology Society. (2011). Guidelines for the determination of brain death in infants and children: An update of the 1987 task force recommendations. *Pediatrics, 128*(3), e720–e740.

National Association of School Nurses. (2014). *Do not attempt resuscitation (DNAR)—The role of the school nurse*. Retrieved from http://www.nasn.org/Portals/0/positions/2014psdnr.pdf

Old, J. L. (2011). Communicating bad news to your patient. *Family Practice Management*. Retrieved from http://www.aafp.org/fpm/2011/1100/p31.html

O'Malley, P. J., Barata, I., Snow, S., American Academy of Pediatrics Committee on Pediatric Emergency Medicine, American College of Emergency Physicians Pediatric Emergency Medicine Committee, & Emergency Nurses Association Pediatric Committee. (2014). Death of a child in the emergency department. *Pediatrics, 134*(1), e313–e330.

Purnell, L. D. (2014). *Guide to culturally competent health care* (3rd ed.). Philadelphia, PA: F. A. Davis.

Randall, V., Cervenka, J., Arday, J., Hooper, T., & Hanson, J. (2011). Prevalence of life-threatening conditions in children. *American Journal of Hospice and Palliative Care, 28*, 310–315.

Rapoport, A., Shaheed, J., Newman, C., Rugg, M., & Steele, R. (2013). Parental perceptions of forgoing artificial nutrition and hydration during end of life care. *Pediatrics, 131*(5), 861–869.

Sanderson, A., Zurakowski, D., & Wolfe, J. (2013). Clinician perspectives regarding the do-not-resuscitate order. *JAMA Pediatrics, 167*(10), 954–958.

Shoenberger, J. M., Yeghiazarian, S., Rios, C., & Henderson, S. O. (2013). Death notification in the emergency department: Survivors and physicians. *Western Journal of Emergency Medicine, 14*(2), 181–185.

Spector, R. E. (2013). *Cultural diversity in health and illness* (8th ed., pp. 151–152). Upper Saddle River, NJ: Prentice Hall Health.

Stevenson, S., Achille, M., & Lugasi, T. (2013). Pediatric palliative care in Canada and the United States: A qualitative metasummary of the needs of patients and families. *Journal of Palliative Medicine, 16*(5), 566–577.

Trotzuk, C., & Gray, B. (2012). Parents' dilemma: Decisions concerning end-of-life care for their child. *Journal of Pediatric Health Care, 26*(1), 57–61.

Wiener, L., McConnell, D. G., Latella, L., & Ludi, E. (2013). Cultural and religious considerations in pediatric palliative care. *Palliative and Supportive Care, 11*, 47–67.

You, J. J., Fowler, R. A., & Heyland, D. K. (2014). Just ask: Discussing goals of care with patients in hospital with serious illness. *Canadian Medical Association Journal, 186*(6), 425–432.

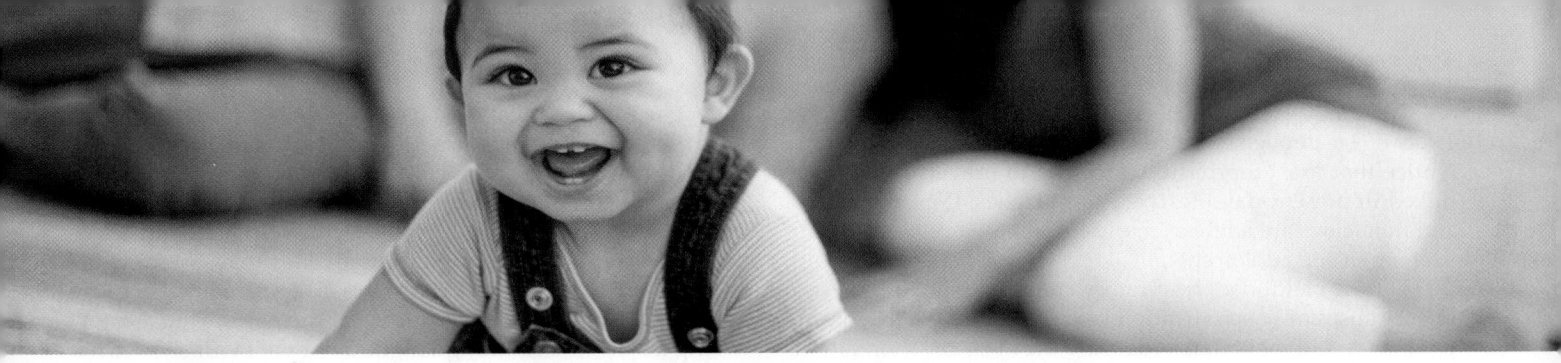

Chapter 42
Social and Environmental Influences on the Child

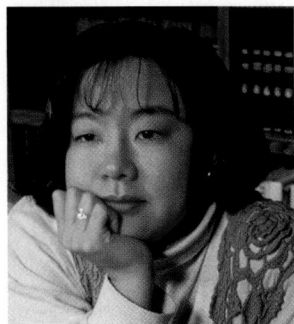

Amy has always been a challenge! She has already left home a couple of times and lived on the streets, which was very hard on us. Lately, she has been more interested in school and is living at home and trying to do well. We want her to succeed and learn the skills she needs in her life. I wish she would not have all of these body piercings, but we don't want to make too big an issue of it as long as she is doing well in school.

—Mother of Amy, 15 years old

Steve Skjold/Alamy

⌄ Learning Outcomes

42.1 Identify major social and environmental factors that influence the health of children and adolescents.

42.2 Apply the ecologic model and resiliency theory to assessment of the social and environmental factors in children's lives.

42.3 Examine the effects of substance use, physical activity, and other lifestyle patterns on health.

42.4 Plan nursing interventions for children who experience violence.

42.5 Evaluate the environment for hazards to children, such as exposure to harmful substances and potential for poisoning.

42.6 Explore the nursing role in prevention and treatment of child abuse and neglect and other forms of violence.

42.7 Plan nursing interventions for children related to social and environmental situations.

Many of the major causes of mortality and morbidity in children and adolescents are closely linked with social influences in the child's world. The social contexts for young children growing up today are different from those of even a decade ago. Examining the social contexts in which children live and grow can provide insights into behavior, and present opportunities for nursing interventions. All nurses must examine the social influences and apply the knowledge gained to plan health care that will benefit youth as they grow into adulthood.

Children and adolescents are also influenced by their environments. The physical setting, exposure to chemical agents, and other environmental factors are increasingly identified as being instrumental in determining health. Nurses assess the environment for its risk and protective factors, and then use this information to plan nursing care appropriate to enhance the health status of children and adolescents.

What are the settings where nurses might work with youth in the community? What are the challenges of today's society that children must often face at very young ages? How can nurses help children face these challenges and emerge as healthy and contributing members of society? What roles do nurses play in identifying and using the protective factors and in minimizing the risk factors of youth? This chapter will examine and apply these social and environmental concepts in a variety of nursing settings.

Examine again the major causes of death for children from 1 year of age through adolescence that are presented in Chapter 1. Notice that most morbidity is related to preventable causes linked to present-day lifestyles. Car crashes, fires, drowning, and homicides are a few examples of common causes of death in children and adolescents.

During childhood, respiratory conditions and injuries are major causes of hospitalization in children. By the teen years, pregnancy and mental disorders are the most common admitting diagnoses to hospitals (Agency for Healthcare Research and Quality, 2013). All of these conditions are related, at least in part, to the social and environmental settings in which children live. These settings and their influences must be examined to understand how best to intervene with children. Consult other chapters for additional information on related topics. For example, Chapter 31 fully discusses growth and development of children, Chapter 36 addresses health promotion topics of adolescents including homosexuality, Chapter 38 discusses chronic conditions, and Chapter 55 details cognitive variations and mental health issues such as suicide.

Basic Concepts

In this chapter, two main theories provide a framework for examining societal influences on children. The ecologic model and resiliency theory are discussed in Chapter 31, and should be reviewed now to assist in evaluating the environmental settings that influence children.

The ecologic theory views the child and the environment as interacting forces, with children influencing systems around them, even while they are influenced by these systems (Bronfenbrenner, 2005). The systems with which the child has daily contact are microsystems (e.g., family, child care, school), but other systems such as parental work and political or cultural environments are also important. Understanding these systems, or the forces in which children function, can provide information that guides healthcare providers. For example, if the parents' employers do not provide healthcare insurance, their children may not get needed health care such as immunizations, treatment for diseases, and growth monitoring.

Resiliency theory examines risk and protective factors in the child's environment and their influence on the child's ability to adapt to stressful events. Such factors can be modified to lead to more productive and healthy outcomes. Resilience is the ability to exhibit healthy responses even when faced with significant stress and adversity (see Chapter 31 for a further description of resiliency theory) (Benard, 2014; Henderson, Bernard, & Sharp-Light, 2007). Families may have protective factors that provide strength and assistance in dealing with crises and risk factors that contribute to healthcare challenges. For example, if a young child is hospitalized for treatment of an acute infectious illness, some **protective factors** might include the ability of one parent to stay with the child at all times, the ability of a grandmother to care for siblings at home during this time, and the child's ability to adapt to new situations and communicate readily with staff members. On the other hand, **risk factors** might include lack of comprehensive health insurance to pay for the hospitalization, lack of an identified healthcare "home" (consistent healthcare provider) for the child, and incomplete immunizations. The concepts of resiliency theory can be applied to Amy's family as described in the chapter-opening quotation. She experienced disruption in family stability. The risk and protective factors interacted with her own personality in ways that resulted in her desire to be an independent person, establishing her identity through body art, and, finally, a desire to return to school.

The National Longitudinal Study of Adolescent Health was conducted with over 100,000 adolescents in the United States, and found that parent–family connectedness, school connectedness, a belief in a higher being, and academic success were predictive of youth having lower health risks. Follow-up interviews are currently being carried out with the participants, who are now young adults; the resulting longitudinal data will show what characteristics and influences persist into adult life (Add Health Study, 2014). Nurses can assist adolescents and their families in establishing a sense of attachment to each other. Encourage families to include adolescents in activities, attend their sports and other school events, have meals together regularly, and attend faith-based activities or other community events as a family.

Theoretical frameworks are discussed in Chapter 31 and are useful when examining social and environmental influences on children because they guide us to examine certain factors that can be altered or understood. They suggest the assessment data to collect and pertinent nursing interventions to use. They also foster partnerships with other care providers who use these and similar theories to plan social, psychologic, and other types of care for children and their families.

Social Influences on Child Health

Poverty

An important risk factor that influences the health of children is poverty. Conversely, basic financial stability is a protective factor that contributes to the general health and well-being of children. Twenty percent (14.7 million) of U.S. children are poor and living in a family earning less than $23,624 annually for a family of four (Federal Interagency Forum on Child and Family Statistics, 2015).

Children who are poor are more likely to have unmet health needs, to have difficulty in school, to become teen parents, and to experience multiple health problems, including stunted growth and lead poisoning. Inadequate or unsafe housing, food insecurity, and poor dietary quality are more common (Federal Interagency Forum on Child and Family Statistics, 2015). What is the face of poverty? Some statistics that may prove surprising include the following:

- Children most likely to be living in poor households are those below 5 years of age.

- About 48% of children living in a single-headed household are poor, while only 11% in married-couple households are poor.

- Ethnic variations are startling: 13% of White children, 39% of African American children, and 34% of Hispanic children live in poverty.

- Poverty rates are higher in suburban and rural areas than in central cities.

- Nearly 70% of poor children have at least one parent working full time (Federal Interagency Forum on Child and Family Statistics, 2015).

Poverty leads to homelessness for some children. Families with children are the fastest growing group of homeless people; families experiencing homelessness comprise one third of the total homeless population. Each year, 1 in 30, or 2.5 million, children experience homelessness (National Center on Family Homelessness, 2015). The reasons for homelessness are also common risks for a number of the other challenges to health discussed in this chapter, including poor finances, abuse or other violence, and mental instability.

Children who experience homelessness often have multiple physical and mental health problems, and lack health insurance to provide care for these problems. Some of the common problems faced by homeless children and families include trauma, substance use, respiratory and skin infections, tuberculosis and HIV, and nutritional disorders. Children may have developmental delays, learning problems, or growth disruptions (American Academy of Pediatrics Council on Community Pediatrics, 2013; Kerker et al., 2011). Teens who have been homeless are more likely to engage in risky behavior such as unprotected sex, sex with multiple partners, and substance abuse. They are more likely than other teens to need emergency care, to be depressed or have some other mental illness, and to become pregnant (National Center on Family Homelessness, 2015).

Health problems related to homelessness, and other family characteristics, continue even after finding a place to live. Even after families leave homeless shelters, children frequently become separated from their mothers because of parent stress, lack of access to resources, and inability of parent(s) to provide adequate homes for the children. Complex, ongoing care is needed. This may begin in a shelter for the homeless, but should continue while the family obtains a place to live, accesses other community services, gets the children safely enrolled in school, and has financial and mental stability.

Nursing management for families with children that are poor or homeless focuses on identification of poverty, careful assessment of health risks, and linking the family to resources that can assist with stability and health. There is often no way to identify a poor child from appearance, and they may hide their status when they are in school or come to a healthcare facility. Addresses given may not be accurate, or the address of a shelter might be used. Children living at shelters or in cars and on the street usually do not take the school bus but prefer to walk to avoid stigma. Alternatively, they may be picked up by the bus first, and dropped off last, to reduce embarrassment. Be alert for children who have multiple health problems and repeated infectious diseases. They may be hungry and without adequate nutrition either at times or consistently. Degrees of personal hygiene may vary depending on access to laundry and bathing facilities. See Table 42–1 for examples of nursing care needs for homeless children and families. See *Evidence-Based Practice: Developmental and Health Implications of Homelessness*.

Stress

The adverse effect of stress on adults is well documented and the impact of stress on children has also been recognized. Stress can be acute, such as when a child has an argument with a friend, a test in school, or a family crisis. Stress can also become chronic when the family frequently does not have enough food, when fighting or abuse is frequent, or when the child is overscheduled and feels under constant pressure to perform (Elkind, 2007). Children manifest stress in a variety of ways, including regressive behavior, interrupted sleep, hyperactive behavior, gastrointestinal symptoms, crying, and withdrawal from normal events. Common stressful events for children include moving to a new home or school, marital difficulties in the family, abuse, one or both parents deployed in the military (Figure 42–1), and being expected to achieve at an extremely high level in school or sports. The busy pace of today's lifestyles and the media's encouragement of early development in children may put undue stress on some children and preteens (Elkind, 2007). Adolescents may be stressed by fulfilling many roles, such as student, part-time worker, and active member of a family. They may be in school all day, be in sport or music practice for 2 to 3 hours after school, and then have a job for several additional hours. Lack of adequate sleep is common and adds further to stress, in addition to putting the teen at risk for car crashes and poor school performance. For poor families, commonly reported stressors are related to food, shelter, transportation, medical care, and personal-time needs.

EVIDENCE-BASED PRACTICE | Developmental and Health Implications of Homelessness

Clinical Question
Children are the age group showing the fastest growth in homelessness. Because of their ages, children are vulnerable to developmental delays, mental health problems, poor school achievement, and effects of violence. Mothers are the main support for young children, but when they are homeless, they may not be able to provide the care children need for healthy growth and development. Most nurses have not been homeless and do not understand the experience of homelessness for children. What is the experience of homelessness like for children?

The Evidence
A 15-week nutrition education and physical activity program in a homeless shelter had 162 child participants. The researchers found that the children's past experiences of hunger and food insecurity influenced their present food choices. Their life experiences must be understood to influence changes in nutrition (Rodriguez, Appelbaum, Stephenson-Hunter, et al., 2013). Children from 11 to 14 years in a homeless shelter reported 13 times less suicide ideation following family strengthening approaches to care (Lynn et al., 2014). A report of an undergraduate nursing student experience in a service-learning research project in homeless shelters resulted in many changes in students. These included increased understanding of the needs of homeless people, recognition of mental health disorders, identification of vulnerable populations, and increased advocacy in social justice (August-Brady & Adamshick, 2013).

Best Practice
Youth and families in homeless shelters have multiple healthcare, educational, and social needs. Understanding the backgrounds and offering programs that are most needed can benefit families and children. Developmental screening, identification of health issues, and provision of educational programs are needed.

Clinical Reasoning
Find at least two agencies that provide health care for persons who are homeless in your community. What are some of the common health problems treated? How are youth engaged in care? What explanations are provided? Are mothers of young children offered parenting classes and stress-reduction interventions? What links are available to other community resources? What is the nursing role in the community agencies you located?

TABLE 42–1 Common Health Problems and Nursing Management of Children Who Are Poor and/or Homeless

COMMON HEALTH PROBLEMS	NURSING MANAGEMENT
Lack of immunizations	Check immunization records.
	Provide immunizations at schools and in homeless shelters.
Common infectious diseases	Facilitate free clinics in shelters, schools, community settings.
	Teach hygiene measures.
	Provide information about resources for bathing and hygiene.
	Provide resources for disease management.
	Arrange for medications when needed.
Sleep deficits	Inform parents about respite facilities.
	Arrange for children to have quiet sleep time in school if possible.
Vision and hearing deficits	Perform screening for deficits.
	Provide resources for eyeglasses, hearing aids, care for ear infections. (Service organizations such as the Lion's Club are good options.)
Nutritional deficits	Perform height and weight checks and a nutritional assessment.
	Evaluate the family for food security (see Chapter 32).
	Be sure the child is registered for school breakfast and lunch programs if available.
	Ensure that children are linked to summer food programs at the end of the academic year.
	Link to the Special Supplemental Nutrition Program for Women, Infants and Children (WIC).
	Inform about resources for meals and field gleaning (collecting unused farm produce) in the community.
Dental care problems	Teach oral hygiene.
	Provide toothbrushes and toothpaste.
	Provide bottled water if the child lives in a car or on the street.
	Perform oral assessment.
	Refer to dental programs for people with low incomes.
Injuries	Teach basic safety precautions.
	Visit the living situation if possible to assess for safety hazards.
	Provide helmets, car seats, or other gear as needed.
	Teach "street safe" skills.
	Provide resources for violence prevention and intervention.
Adolescent pregnancy and sexually transmitted infections	Provide sexuality teaching in accordance with state law.
	Inform about access to family planning services.
	Assess for child abuse and prostitution.
Mental illness	Assess for depression.
	Evaluate for suicide potential.
	Provide links to services.
	Plan programs to foster self-esteem.
	Arrange for a Big Brother or Big Sister.
	Refer to extracurricular activities in the school and community.
	Arrange for a school bus stop away from a shelter so other students do not stigmatize the homeless child.

The child experiencing stress has more frequent respiratory and gastrointestinal illnesses and is more likely to be the victim of an injury. The negative long-term effects of stress on body organs and systems suggest that children under stress are more likely to develop illnesses such as strokes, hypertension, and heart attacks later in life (Balodis, Wynne-Edwards, & Olmstead, 2010; Slopen, McLaughlin, & Shonkoff, 2014).

Nurses help children manage stress by encouraging good coping strategies (Sapienza & Masten, 2011). Emphasize healthy lifestyles with all children, including good nutrition, exercise, and plenty of sleep. Classes in yoga or martial arts may be stress-reducing for some children. Encourage parents to provide youth with activities that foster self-esteem, and to avoid unrealistic expectations about performance in sports and other activities. Provide resources to help with food acquisition, shelter, transportation, and medical care for families needing them. Adolescents may benefit from various approaches for stress management such as massage, rest, physical activity, and yoga.

Since military deployment can create family stress, partner with military families to assist them as one or both parents are

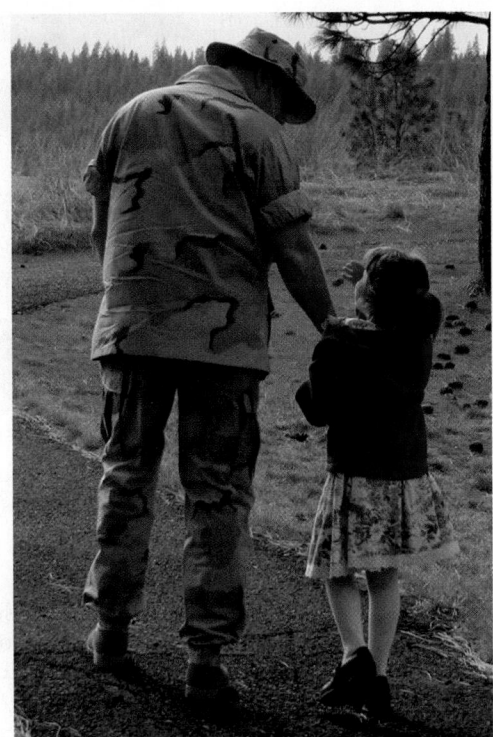

Figure 42–1 Stress from military deployment. The special relationship between a father about to be deployed in the military and his young daughter is clear. This father has two other children and is spending time with each of them, as well as with the family together, before leaving. The cycle of leaving and returning home can be stressful for families. Nurses can assist military families in making plans for health care, finances, and communication while gone and providing resources for emotional support for the entire family.

Clinical Reasoning Demographics and Nursing Care

Nurses should understand the demographics in the areas where they work. What is the poverty rate in your community? What ethnic groups are overrepresented among the poor? Locate needed resources such as food services, health care for the underserved, and enhanced school programs in order to refer poor families. Recognize that health promotion services may not be a high priority when a family does not have adequate housing or food. When children are seen in any setting, such as in school or in an emergency department or hospital for acute care, perform needed assessments and intervention. Measure growth, assess vision and hearing, evaluate dietary intake, and check immunization status. Find out the stresses the family experiences and what resources they need to meet basic necessities. Construct a nursing care plan for a family living in poverty with two young children.

---

deployed for duty in a remote location. Connect parents with resources for child care, mental health services, and arrangements that need to be made to prepare for the absence. If the family has had frequent moves, they may not be strongly connected to resources in the community. During deployment the remaining parent may return to the home of origin; some family support may then be present. Help families explain to children why and where the parents are going, and how they will keep in touch during their absence. Children need to know who they will stay with, whether they will attend the same school, and how food and other needs will be provided. Parents need family, mental health, and financial support whether they are being deployed or remaining at home (Allen, Rhoades, Stanley, et al., 2011; Aranda, Middleton, Flake, et al., 2011).

Families

The families into which children are born influence them greatly. Children are supported in different ways and acquire different worldviews depending on such factors as whether one or both parents work, how many siblings are present, and whether an extended family is close by. Examine the family structure such as two parents present, single parent, adolescent parent, same sex parents, extended family, grandparents raising grandchildren, and stepparents. Financial challenges influence work requirements and lifestyle stability. Resources in the community interact with family structures and can provide support and foster resilience in the face of challenges. All of these factors influence the physical and mental health of children, and can determine their needs for nursing interventions.

One common occurrence in the lives of many children is divorce of parents. The divorce rate in the United States is estimated to be around 50% of all marriages. Each year, an additional 1 million children are affected by divorce (Children and Divorce, 2013). Children are inevitably affected by the parents' divorce, even if the divorce was preceded by many periods of stress and tension in the home.

Many children believe they are at fault for the separation and divorce, that they said or did something to make the parent leave. When one parent leaves, the children may feel abandoned by that parent and may fear being abandoned by the remaining parent. Also, children may become engaged in the disputes of parents, and experience conflicts of loyalty when parents fight for their affection.

In divorces involving conflict and hostility, the children may have increased problems with adjustment. When children must make a series of changes in their lives in addition to the parents' separation (new home, different school), their adjustment is made more difficult as their sense of order is upset. Predictable routines have changed, and children may test limits to see if they still apply; academic and behavior problems may manifest.

The age of the child also influences understanding of and reactions to the divorce. For 3- to 5-year-olds, anxiety, temper tantrums, and other behavioral changes may occur; children ages 6 to 8 years are frequently worried and blame themselves for the divorce; 9- to 10-year-old children are predominantly angry; 11- to 13-year-olds feel lonely and deny the permanence of divorce; 14- to 17-year-olds are angry at parents and may act out frustration by abusing substances or challenging parents (Dunn & Craig, 2013).

A family's risk factors (e.g., recent separation, parental stress, and limited healthcare coverage) and its strengths (e.g., loving relationships, influential grandparents or other extended family members, and general good health) should be identified and used in planning care. Parents who are divorced can be assisted to plan strategies to ensure that the child does not feel responsible for the divorce and is able to form strong relationships with both parents. Encourage the family to ensure that the child has a relationship with both parents, using phone, Internet, and other methods to remain in close contact. See Chapter 2 for a thorough discussion of family factors as they relate to family-centered care and a description of strategies for assessment and intervention with families.

School and Child Care

Once a child is 5 or 6 years of age, several hours daily are spent in a school setting. Children develop physical skills through participation in education and sports. Psychosocial stages are met as the child interacts with children and adults and achieves social interaction patterns and pride in accomplishments. The presentation of concepts that challenge thought processes enhances cognitive development.

Although the primary role of schools is educational, they also perform several health-related functions. School health screening programs identify children with problems such as hearing loss, visual impairment, and scoliosis. Nurses provide assessment, teaching, and clinical management related to some health problems. Some schools have clinics that examine and provide even more complete health care for children. Many schools teach good nutrition, healthful living, safe sexual practices, and other health-related subjects. A school nurse may be present, at least part time, to plan these classes or to work with teachers. Nurses assist school districts in providing plans for emergency health care when needed. With the increase in mainstreaming, school staff now have the responsibility for administering medications, maintaining urinary catheters, and providing respiratory care and other treatments to ensure children's proper growth and development. See Chapter 37 for further discussion of school nurse activities.

Some children spend part or nearly all of their days in child care settings (Figure 42–2). Over 60% of children under 6 years receive some type of child care regularly. Children spend an average of 33 hours/week in childcare settings (Laughlin, 2013). The closeness of the parent–child relationship, the quality of care, and the length of the childcare day are important in determining childcare effects on children. The mother's sensitivity to her child is the best indicator of child behavior regardless of childcare arrangements (ChildStats, 2011).

Nursing management involves helping parents to explore types of daycare options available and to evaluate programs in their communities (Table 42–2). Care options for young school-age children, either before or after school, can also be shared with parents. When available, recommend early intervention programs with at-risk children, such as the Zero to Three Project and Head Start, which contribute to children's health and welfare. Nurses frequently manage the health programs in early intervention, providing screening, doing health evaluations, and

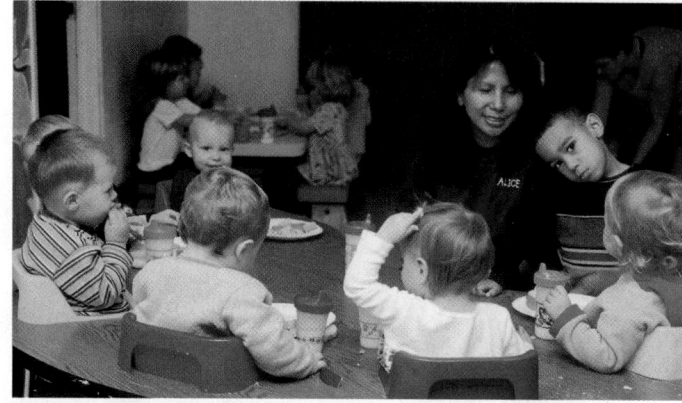

Figure 42–2 **Most children will spend time in childcare settings. It is important to explore options and find the best fit for the child's needs.**

establishing early intervention education plans. Nurses assist families in evaluation of childcare centers and share information about accreditation. The National Association for the Education of Young Children (2010) has established childcare criteria.

Community

The community in which a child lives may support the child's development or, conversely, expose the child to hazards. Social programs such as Head Start preschools, sports activities, after-school programs, and child abuse treatment centers offer valuable services that improve the experience of growing children. On the other hand, an economically depressed community with scant services and a high homicide rate is unsupportive and hazardous for growing children.

The physical environment is supportive when the child has sidewalks on which to walk to school, open spaces in which to learn and play, and clean air to breathe. Children who must walk to school on unsafe roads, have access to contaminated drinking supplies, or live near polluting manufacturing companies or in crowded housing or old structures are at risk for injuries and health problems such as lead poisoning (see discussion of poisoning later in this chapter).

TABLE 42–2 Types of Child Care

TYPE OF CARE/DESCRIPTION	ADVANTAGES	DISADVANTAGES
In home (caretaker comes to home of the child)	Child can remain at home Little exposure to infectious diseases No need for alternative care when child is ill	Limited contact with other children to encourage development Limited ability to rapidly locate alternate when provider is ill Most costly
Family child care (parent brings child to home of a caretaker)	Limited number of children Family-type atmosphere Some exposure to other children and encouragement of development	Little governmental regulation or examination Care provider may be distracted by activities in the home
Parent brings child to a center where many children receive care	A learning curriculum plan is in place Contact with other children can enhance development Subject to regulation and licensing Care providers are focused solely on the children	Exposure to multiple children increases infectious disease risk Demands of multiple children may distract or tire care providers

TEACHING HIGHLIGHTS | Evaluation of Child Care

The nurse can help parents to evaluate childcare options and make decisions about placement for their children. Parents should always be welcomed to visit an agency or home childcare site—this is essential so they can see the routines in action. Some questions they can ask are suggested as follows:

Administration

- Is the facility licensed?
- Who are the administrators? What is their training and experience?
- How many staff are employed? What is their training?
- Is there a parent board? What part does it play in administering the center?

Physical Environment, Health, and Safety

- What is the neighborhood like? Is transportation to the center convenient?
- What is the condition of the lighting, heat, cooling, and ventilation systems; play spaces (inside and out); and the building's general condition?
- Is playground equipment safe?
- Is there a soft material such as bark, sand, or rubber tiles under climbing equipment?
- Are the children always supervised?
- Are there emergency medical forms and signed forms for field trips?
- Who may pick up children? How are they signed in and out?
- What is the immunization policy and how are records examined and maintained?
- Are criminal background checks of staff done for potential child abuse and other problems?
- What is the policy for children with infectious diseases and other illness?
- How are foods prepared? Are staff licensed in food handling?
- What is the state of general cleanliness?
- Who changes diapers? Are recommendations for standard precautions to prevent pathogen transfer followed?
- What arrangements and routines are made for naps and quiet times?

Developmental Approaches

- Is the curriculum appropriate for different age groups?
- Are there materials and plans for gross motor, fine motor, language, and social development?
- How much time do children spend in structured time? Free time?
- How is discipline handled?
- Do the children appear occupied and happy?
- What reading materials are available?
- What type and quantity of field trips are planned?
- What is the educational level and longevity of the childcare workers?
- Is there a diversity among the children's backgrounds and experiences?

Source: Adapted from the National Association for the Education of Young Children. (2010). *Introduction to the NAEYC early childhood program standards and accreditation criteria: Program standards.* Retrieved from http://www.naeyc.org/accreditation.

Culture

The child's cultural group may influence the use of traditional and contemporary healthcare practices. If the parents or children are recent immigrants, they may still be learning the English language and finding out about healthcare resources. Children and adolescents of immigrants may feel stress as they combine their family's traditional culture with the new culture in which the family now lives. They may also have a great deal of responsibility to interpret for the family since they often can speak two languages and understand practices in the new culture.

Recent immigrants may experience culture shock, a state of crisis related to the difference in values and lifestyle between the two cultures they have experienced. This can lead to stress-related symptoms, and create a need for healthcare intervention. Children whose parents emigrated from another country may feel different from peers and develop conflict with their parents, particularly during adolescence.

All cultural groups have rules about patterns of social interaction. Schedules of language acquisition are determined by the number of languages spoken and the amount of speech in the home. The particular social roles assumed by men and women in the culture affect school activities and ultimately career choices. Attitudes toward touching and other methods of encouraging developmental skills vary among cultures.

Nurses must become aware of common characteristics of the cultural groups they serve so that they can provide culturally competent nursing care. Arrange for interpreters when needed. Be aware that families often accept and use both traditional and westernized health care, and remain nonjudgmental about traditional healing practices. Provide access to foods for a variety of ethnic backgrounds in healthcare facilities. Evaluate youth in immigrant families for conflict between family and societal expectations. Incorporate communication with the school nurse, who often has experience with a diversity of ethnic and racial groups and their cultural practices. See Chapter 2 for further exploration of cultural awareness.

Lifestyle Activities and Their Influence on Child Health

Many patterns of daily life play a part in determining the length and quality of one's life. A child's use of tobacco products and controlled substances influences both physical and mental health. Patterns of exercise and use of protective gear protect against early disabilities. The use of decorative patterns to tattoo or scar the skin and can introduce pathogens is an example of a lifestyle pattern that influences mental health, body image, and the body's physical health.

Tobacco Use

Tobacco use is the most preventable cause of adult death in the United States. It leads to 438,000 premature deaths annually, and will be responsible for the premature death of 5 million of today's youth as they reach adult years (U.S. Department of Health & Human Services [USDHHS], 2011). Major health problems linked to tobacco use include cardiovascular disease, cancer, chronic lung disease, increased prevalence of car crashes, low birth weight, and other maternal problems. Cigarette use is most common; however, chewing tobacco, snuff, cigars, hookahs (water pipe for smoking flavored tobacco), and bidis (small, brown, hand-rolled cigarettes) also pose significant health hazards. Even passive smoking (secondhand smoke) or environmental tobacco smoke (ETS) is linked to increased heart disease, blood pressure, respiratory problems, sudden infant death syndrome (SIDS), middle ear infections, and decreased youth academic performance (U.S. Environmental Protection Agency, 2014). "Third-hand" tobacco exposure refers to the smoking residues that remain on clothing and room/automobile surfaces.

Clinical Tip

Electronic cigarettes, known as e-cigarettes, provide an aerosol that contains nicotine and other substances. Flavorings such as spices or chocolate are frequently added. In just a 1-year period, from 2011 to 2012, e-cigarette use in 6th to 12th graders doubled, from 3.3% to 6.8%. The effects of e-cigarettes and the additives are unknown at this time, but concerns are warranted. Whether they lead to smoking of traditional cigarettes is a question yet unanswered (Centers for Disease Control and Prevention [CDC], 2013a, 2014a). When inquiring about tobacco use, specifically mention new and popular trends such as e-cigarettes and hookah pipes. Ask about frequency, type, and other details of use.

Many nurses view tobacco use as an adult issue, but each day 3200 youths try their first cigarette, and the usual age for trying tobacco is 9 to 14 years (Figure 42–3). Peer pressure is a powerful incentive for trying some form of tobacco. Nicotine is highly addictive, and most people become addicted to the substance in adolescent years. Early initiation of smoking is an extremely risky behavior because 90% of adult smokers began smoking before 18 years of age (CDC, 2011a, 2013b; 2014a). Although sale of tobacco products to children and advertisements aimed at this age group are forbidden by federal law,

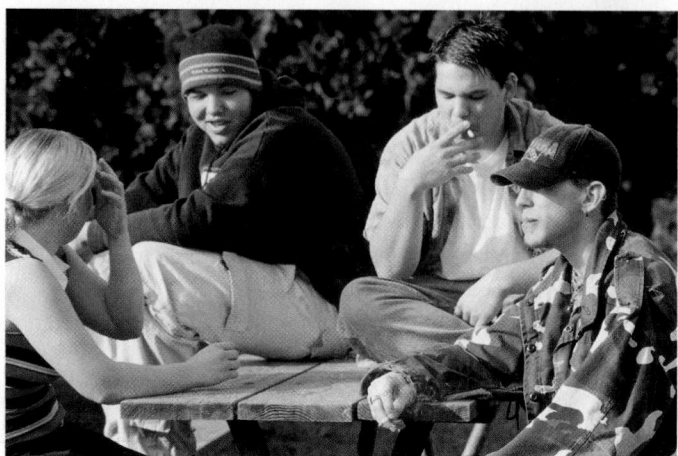

Figure 42–3 Approximately 70% of children have tried smoking by their high school years. Early intervention can begin with discussions about smoking starting at 9 or 10 years of age.

many youths obtain and use tobacco. About 16% of high school students in the United States have smoked within the past 30 days, and one half of all youth have tried tobacco, making this an important health risk (CDC, 2014a).

Developing Cultural Competence Smoking Rates Among Youth

Among youth in the United States, White youth are significantly more likely to smoke than either Hispanic or African American peers. About 19% of White students reported smoking in the previous month, while 14% of Hispanic and 8% of African American students reported this behavior (CDC, 2014a). American Indian and Alaska Natives also have high smoking rates, while Asian Americans have low rates. Youth smoking rates also vary by state, ranging from 4% to 20% among various states (CDC, 2014a; USDHHS, 2011).

Certain characteristics contribute to the likelihood of tobacco use. They include increasing age, male gender, ethnic group, ease of obtaining tobacco products, and smoking among family members. Low socioeconomic group membership, access to tobacco products, low price of products, advertising, and lack of parental involvement in the youths' lives are associated with tobacco use (USDHHS, 2011). Gender differences may exist for youth who are beginning or seeking to quit tobacco use. For example, girls may be more worried about the smell and effect of tobacco on clothing and appearance, while boys more commonly express concern about smoking's effects on sports or activities (Sullivan, Bottorff, & Reid, 2011).

Several programs have been developed to encourage youth to avoid tobacco use. In addition, smoking cessation programs are available to assist youth who are already regular smokers to successfully achieve the goals of cessation or decrease in tobacco use. Use of counseling, tobacco-free environments, and peer cessation programs have been useful. Aids such as patches, gum, lozenges, nasal spray, and medications have not been adequately tested for safety in adolescents (Broberg & Nield, 2013). Once a teen is identified as a tobacco user, a biologic marker such as urine cotinine (a by-product of tobacco) levels can help to identify the frequency of smoking. This information can be used to make suggestions to the teen about the potential outcomes of the behavior and the cessation program that is most likely to be helpful.

Nursing Management

Tobacco Use

Nursing Assessment and Diagnosis

Nurses are in a unique position to inquire about the incidence of smoking and other tobacco use among youth. Insert questions into all well-child visits, beginning at about 9 to 10 years of age. Inquire about whether family members (especially parents and siblings) smoke or chew, and ask if some of the child's friends have tried smoking. Try to find out the child's knowledge and beliefs about the benefits and risks of tobacco use. As the child gets older, ask more direct and detailed questions. A nonjudgmental and collegial approach will be best to obtain a truthful response. School nurses can make observations about numbers of teens smoking and general attitudes about tobacco use. When children come to hospitals and other health facilities for care, use of tobacco should be part of general admission questions. Include questions about chew and hookah or flavored tobacco exposure.

Some nursing diagnoses that may apply to youth who smoke or show potential for this behavior include the following (NANDA-I © 2014):

- *Activity Intolerance* related to lowered oxygen supply
- *Gas Exchange, Impaired,* related to ventilation-perfusion imbalance
- *Self-Esteem, Chronic Low,* related to negative self-appraisal
- *Knowledge, Deficient,* regarding dangers of tobacco use related to developmental focus on present
- *Nutrition, Imbalanced: Less than Body Requirements,* related to effects of chemical dependence

Planning and Implementation

The roles of nurses in preventing and intervening in youth smoking are to inform youth, identify smokers, and implement programs (Table 42–3). Provide developmentally appropriate information about the hazards of tobacco use in all settings where youth are present. Addicted teens who share their stories

of difficult withdrawal from tobacco and adults who have had cancer of the lungs or larynx may be effective speakers. Offer information on prevention and cessation programs to youths and families in clinics, outpatient surgery centers, community activities, and hospitals. Use opportunities such as adolescent pregnancy and illness to reinforce the hazardous effects of tobacco on the individual and on those around. Adolescent mothers should understand the risks for small-for-gestational age babies when they smoke in pregnancy and the increased risk of sudden infant death syndrome (SIDS) when infants are exposed to secondhand smoke (see Chapter 46). Speak to young athletes about the effects of tobacco on athletic performance. Show youth the ways this product can interfere with meeting life goals. Role play how to tell other youth "no" when tobacco is offered. Establish programs that increase the sense of self-esteem without tobacco use. Be sure to include parents in the programs so that they see and acknowledge their role in setting an example about tobacco use and in providing guidelines for the child. Provide information on the influence of environmental tobacco smoke (secondhand smoke).

Adopt a nonjudgmental attitude when asking questions about smoking so that youth using tobacco can be identified. Ask questions without parents present and assure youth that the information will not be shared. Encourage youth to cut back and to quit use of tobacco products. Offer assistance to them in these efforts. Encourage positive coping techniques for youth who are engaged in cessation. Such techniques include keeping busy, avoiding smoking situations, using oral stimulation such as a toothpick or gum, exercising, relaxing, and using nicotine replacement approaches (Audrain-McGovern et al., 2011).

Work with the schools and school districts to help establish preventive and cessation programs. There should be clear guidelines about school policies regarding tobacco use on school grounds. Keeping occasional youth tobacco users from becoming regular users should be a goal in order to avoid nicotine addiction. Find out what positive incentives can be offered to youth who are successful in quitting tobacco use. Contract with them to achieve their goals.

Evaluation

Expected outcomes of nursing interventions regarding tobacco use are lowered rates of regular use, delayed initiation of use, and success of cessation programs. *Healthy People 2020* objectives can be used to plan programs.

TABLE 42–3 Nursing Role in Youth Tobacco Use Prevention

INFORM

- Hang posters, provide brochures, and facilitate presentations about tobacco risks in all settings where youth are present. Include contemporary uses such as e-cigarettes and hookahs.
- Target tobacco users with special information about the effects of nicotine on their bodies.

IDENTIFY

- Ask questions about smoking and other tobacco use at every health encounter beginning at about 9 to 10 years of age. Ask if the child's parents, siblings, and/or friends use tobacco.
- For users, ask amount and type of tobacco and nicotine.
- Find resources where youth obtain tobacco in the community and become proactive in stopping sales.

IMPLEMENT

- Encourage youth tobacco users to quit.
- Facilitate referral to cessation programs.
- Arrange positive rewards for youth successful in cessation.

(TU-15.2 and 15.3) Increase smoke-free and tobacco-free environments in schools, including all school facilities, property, vehicles, and school events, to 100%

(TU-18.1–18.4) Reduce exposure to tobacco advertising and promotions that influence adolescents and young adults

(TU-7) Increase smoking cessation attempts by adolescent smokers to 64%

(TU-2.2) Reduce tobacco use by adolescents to 21%

(TU-2.3) Reduce smokeless tobacco use by adolescents to 6.9%

(TU-3.2) Reduce initiation of tobacco use among adolescents to 4.3%

Alcohol Use

Alcohol use by the young is common. An estimated 66.6% have tried alcohol, which is the drug of choice and convenience for youth. By 12th grade, 76.3% of females and 74.9% of males have had alcoholic drinks (CDC, 2014a). Current use is also common with 34% of high school students admitting to drinking within the last month, and 20.8% having engaged in binge drinking, or having five or more drinks within a 2-hour period. Even very young adolescents are affected since 40% of eighth graders have tried alcohol and 11% have had one or more episodes of binge drinking (National Institute on Alcohol Abuse and Alcoholism, n.d.). About 18.6% of high school students report that their first drink was before age 13 (CDC, 2014a).

Many factors influence the child and adolescent who drink alcohol. Patterns in the family, media advertisements, and social environments in high school and college that honor or expect drinking all contribute to the problem. Access to alcohol is easy for most youth because older siblings or classmates often obtain drinks for them. It is a "rite of passage" for many at teen birthday parties or college events. Alcohol is the most common and accepted drug in today's society and, as such, youth are exposed to it. They often experiment with alcohol and experience its effects without understanding or considering the implications of its use. A significant risk factor for initiation of alcohol use is a transition time, such as change from middle to high school, or a major family stress, such as parental separation or divorce.

Drug Use

Substance use occurs in children and adolescents of all socioeconomic levels and is a growing health problem. The use of any drug can pose a serious psychologic and physical risk to children and adolescents.

In addition to alcohol, a variety of other drugs are used by youth. Over 41% of U.S. high school students have used marijuana, and 23% have used it in the last month; 5.5% have used cocaine, with nearly 3% having used it in the last month; 6.6% have used ecstasy. Inhalant use of glue, paints, or other substances is more common, with nearly 9% reporting use. Approximately 3.2% report methamphetamine use (Figure 42–4), and 2.2% use heroin (CDC, 2014a). Synthetic drugs (commonly referred to as "designer" drugs), such as phencyclidine (PCP), mimic other narcotics, stimulants, and hallucinogens and are also dangerous. "Bath salts" are a contemporary drug that has effects similar to those of amphetamines. These drugs are synthetic versions of cathinone, which occurs naturally in the khat plant (Lehner & Baumann, 2013; McGraw & McGraw, 2012). Common contemporary drugs and street names are listed in

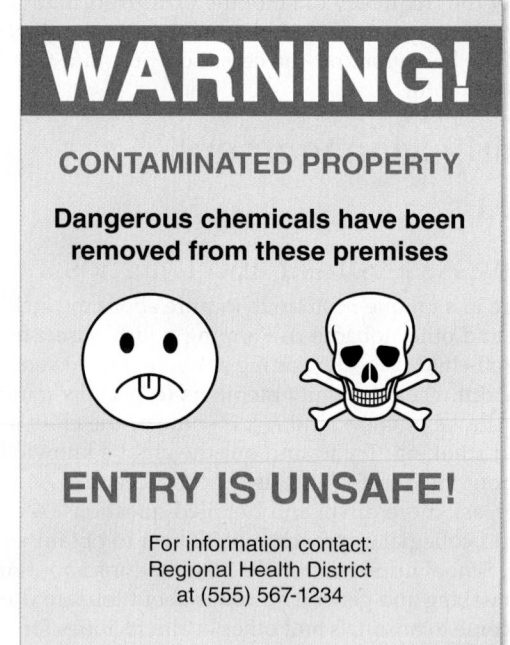

WARNING!

CONTAMINATED PROPERTY

Dangerous chemicals have been removed from these premises

ENTRY IS UNSAFE!

For information contact:
Regional Health District
at (555) 567-1234

Figure 42–4 Methamphetamine is a popular drug because it can be manufactured with items that are available to the lay public. Manufacture of the substance in homes has become a concern of health departments and communities at large. Children can be harmed by the chemicals produced and may experience neglect and abuse. They may suffer even after the home is found and adults are apprehended as they must be placed in foster homes.

Table 42–4. Some youth use these drugs with alcohol, which can lead to deadly consequences.

Prescription drugs are sometimes used for nonmedical purposes. For example, methylphenidate (Ritalin) is used for treatment of attention deficit hyperactivity disorder (ADHD) and generally acts as a stimulant. Its unprescribed use among youth has increased dramatically during the past few years. Prescription pain medications are another example of drugs that are easily abused by youth who are treated with them after surgery or other procedures.

Over-the-counter medications are legal, but frequently abused. Easily obtainable at grocery stores and drug stores, these drugs include antihistamines, atropine, bromides, caffeine, ephedrine, pseudoephedrine, phenylpropanolamine, and amphetamine-like substitutes. Volatile inhalants, such as glues, are dangerous substances of abuse, and their use appears to be rising among school-age children and adolescents. Anabolic steroids are the drugs of abuse most commonly used by athletes (see Chapter 32 for further information on enhancing substances).

ETIOLOGY AND PATHOPHYSIOLOGY

In most cases, substance use represents a maladaptive coping response to the stressors of childhood and adolescence. Individual, peer, family, and community risk factors all contribute to increased incidence of use (American Academy of Child and Adolescent Psychiatry [AACAP], 2013). A child may begin using drugs or alcohol to deal with stress because family members or peers do so. Children in families with a history of

TABLE 42–4 Common Contemporary Club Drugs, Street Names, and Drug Information

DRUG	ACTION	STREET NAMES	ROUTE	TIME OF ACTION
Methylenedioxymethamphetamine (MDMA)	Stimulant; appetite suppressant; increased pulse, BP, temperature; overhydration; hyponatremia; memory loss	Ecstasy, XTC, X, Adam, Clarity, Lover's speed, E	PO (tablets, capsules)	3–6 hr
Cathinone ("bath salts")	Similar to amphetamines: agitation, combative behavior, hallucinations, delusions, hyperthermia, tachycardia, hypertension	Many names such as Bliss, Blue Silk, Charge, Energy-1, Gold Rush, K2, Meph, Mephisto, Ocean Burst, Rave ON, Rush, Special Gold, Spice, Tranquillity, White Knight	PO (capsules), snorted, IV, IM, rectal	2–4 hr but up to 8 hr possible
Gamma-hydroxybutyrate (GHB) (Xyrem)	CNS depressant, euphoria, growth hormone release, hypersalivation, hypotonia	Grievous Bodily Harm, G., Liquid Ecstasy, Georgia Home Boy, date-rape drug	PO (liquid, powder, tablets, capsules)	4 hr
Ketamine	Anesthetic; decreased memory, attention, learning; increased BP; respiratory collapse	Special K, K, Vitamin K, Cat Valiums, Jet	IV, respiratory (injected, snorted, or smoked; liquid or powder)	1–2 hr
Rohypnol (benzodiazepine; flunitrazepam)	Amnesia, sedative; decreased BP, urinary retention; given prior to sexual assault	Roffies, Rophies, Roche, Forget-me Pill	PO, respiratory (snorted; tablets)	8–12 hr
Methamphetamine	Stimulant; highly addictive; memory loss; violence, psychosis; cardiac and neurologic damage	Speed, Ice, Chalk, Meth, Crystal, Crank, Fire, Glass, Tina, Tweak, Yaba (meth and caffeine)	PO, respiratory, IV (smoked, snorted, injected)	Several hours; long-term permanent effects
Lysergic acid diethylamide (LSD)	Hallucinogen; increased pulse, BP, temperature; psychosis, flashbacks	Acid, Boomers, Blotters, Dots, Yellow Sunshines	PO (liquid, tablets, capsules)	1–2 hr; trips last 12 hr; possible flashbacks later

Source: Data from National Institute on Drug Abuse. (2011). *NIDA InfoFacts: Club drugs*. Retrieved from http://www.nida.nih.gov/Infofacts/clubdrugs.html and http://www.drugabuse.gov/drugpages .clubdrugs.html

substance abuse are at higher risk of abusing drugs and alcohol. Other risk factors include rebelliousness, aggressiveness, low self-esteem, dysfunctional parental relationships, lack of adequate support systems, academic underachievement, poor judgment, and poor impulse control.

Initial experimentation with alcohol or drugs may be unpleasant. However, with continued use, the adolescent learns to "achieve the high," an illusion of power and well-being. The adolescent wants the high more frequently and actively seeks alcohol or drugs. Tolerance to the substance occurs with continued use, and ever-increasing amounts are required to achieve a pleasurable high. Physical and psychologic dependence ensues as the body's tissues require the substance to function properly. Withdrawal symptoms occur when the child or adolescent is deprived of the substance.

Clinical Tip

Following are common inhalant agents:

AEROSOLS
Cooking spray
Whipped cream
Spray paint
Cosmetic sprays

ADHESIVES
Model glues
Rubber cements

SOLVENTS
Nail polish remover
Paint thinner or cleaner
Lighter fluid
Degreaser

OTHER
Gasoline
Helium

CLINICAL MANIFESTATIONS

Substance abuse in children and adolescents is commonly overlooked and underdiagnosed by healthcare providers, in part because of the wide range of clinical presentations, which vary according to type of drug used, amount, frequency, time of last use, and severity of drug dependence (Table 42–5).

Common physical manifestations include alterations in vital signs, weight loss, chronic fatigue, chronic cough, respiratory congestion, red eyes, and general apathy and malaise. Withdrawal may be shown by anxiety, headache, tremors, nausea and vomiting, malaise, weakness, insomnia, depressed mood or irritability, and hallucinations. The mental status examination (refer to Chapter 33) may reveal alterations in level of consciousness, impaired attention and concentration, impaired thought processes, delusions, and hallucinations. Low self-esteem, feelings of guilt or worthlessness, and suicidal or homicidal thoughts are also common.

Poor school performance and changes in mood, sleep habits, appetite, dress, and social relationships are nonspecific characteristics of the child or adolescent who is using substances.

CLINICAL THERAPY

Multiple psychiatric diagnostic criteria exist for each drug class. Children and adolescents who have other psychosocial disorders commonly use or abuse drugs or alcohol. Treatment should therefore focus not only on the substance use or abuse, but also on the issues underlying the problem. Intervention includes the family as well as the substance-abusing child or adolescent.

TABLE 42–5 Clinical Manifestations of Commonly Abused Drugs

DRUG	POTENTIAL FOR DEPENDENCE	CLINICAL MANIFESTATIONS
DEPRESSANTS		
Alcohol, barbiturates (amobarbital, pentobarbital, secobarbital)	Physical and psychologic: high; varies somewhat among drugs	Physical: decreased muscle tone and coordination, tremors Psychologic: impaired speech, memory, and judgment, confusion; decreased attention span; emotional lability
STIMULANTS		
Amphetamines (e.g., Benzedrine), caffeine, cocaine, "bath salts"	Physical: low to moderate Psychologic: high; withdrawal from amphetamines and cocaine can lead to severe depression	Physical: dilated pupils, increased pulse and blood pressure, flushing, nausea, loss of appetite, tremors Psychologic: euphoria; increased alertness, agitation, or irritability; hallucinations; insomnia
OPIATES		
Codeine, heroin, meperidine (Demerol), methadone, morphine, opium, oxycodone (Percodan)	Physical and psychologic: high; varies somewhat among drugs; withdrawal effects are uncomfortable but rarely life threatening	Physical: analgesia, depressed respirations and muscle tone (may lead to coma or death), nausea, constricted pupils Psychologic: changes in mood (usually euphoria), drowsiness, impaired attention or memory, sense of tranquility
HALLUCINOGENS		
Lysergic acid diethylamide (LSD), mescaline, phencyclidine (PCP)	Physical: none Psychologic: unknown	Physical: lack of coordination, dilated pupils, hypertension, elevated temperature; severe PCP intoxication can result in seizures, respiratory depression, coma, and death Psychologic: visual illusions and hallucinations, altered perceptions of time and space, emotional lability, psychosis
VOLATILE INHALANTS		
Glues, typing correction fluid, acrylic paints, spot removers, lighter fluid, gasoline, butane	Physical and psychologic: varies with drug used	Physical: impaired coordination, liver damage (in some cases) Psychologic: impaired judgment, delirium
MARIJUANA		
	Physical: low Psychologic: usually low; occasionally moderate to high	Physical: tachycardia, reddened conjunctiva, dry mouth, increased appetite Psychologic: initial anxiety followed by euphoria; giddiness; impaired attention, judgment, and memory

---

TEACHING HIGHLIGHTS | Identifying the Youth Who Is Abusing Substances

Families are often confused about the behavior of adolescents and unsure whether it represents normal development or abuse of substances. Some characteristics of normal development that help to differentiate these occurrences are listed as follows. When concerned about possible substance use, the parent can confront the child or talk with school nurses or counselors.

- Many youth are periodically distant with parents but remain involved with peers in school sports and other activities. Withdrawal from all activities and friends may indicate substance abuse.
- Adolescents often complain about school, but when teachers report the student meets expectations and is consistently performing in the classroom, this is normal behavior.
- Teens may be weepy on occasion when having a difficult time with friends or not performing as desired. Continued, consistent weepiness is more likely to indicate depression or substance abuse.
- Teens like to stay up late and are frequently tired in the morning, whereas abusing teens may "nod off" frequently during the day.
- Many adolescents like to achieve a disheveled look in clothing, but the teen who frequently neglects basic hygiene or does not seem to have the energy to wash and dress may be depressed or be abusing substances.
- All teens get some infections, but teens who are abusing substances may have reddened eyes, oral sores, and constant respiratory discomfort from "snorting" substances.

The primary goal of treatment is to teach the child and other family members to develop and sustain positive coping patterns, and to support them during this process. Most treatment programs offer inpatient and outpatient services, as well as after-care programs. These programs usually consist of peer support that focuses on developing a drug- and alcohol-free lifestyle, healthy family relationships, and positive coping skills. Family involvement is strongly encouraged. Hospitalization is required if the physical dependence is significant and withdrawal places the child at risk for complications such as seizures, depression, or suicidal behavior.

Nursing Management

Alcohol and Drug Use

Nursing Assessment and Diagnosis

Mental health assessment of all older children and adolescents requires screening for alcohol and other substances, including screening for over-the-counter and prescription medication use (American Academy of Pediatrics Committee on Practice and Ambulatory Medicine, 2014; Havens, Young, & Havens, 2011). Maintaining a confidential approach will increase the ability to obtain truthful information about use of substances. Assessment tools provide useful information for the healthcare provider.

Nurses may encounter the substance-abusing child or adolescent in the emergency department or outpatient clinic, in schools and other community settings, or during hospitalization for an injury or other acute problem. Diagnosis includes assessment of both the family and the substance-abusing child or adolescent. Nursing assessment includes taking a thorough history from the parents and child, observing the child's behavior, and performing a physical examination. The history should include the age at which drug use began, pattern of use, length of time the drug has been used, amount of drug used, and psychologic state while on drugs. A history of parental drug use and noninvolvement in parenting the child puts the child at higher risk for substance abuse, reflecting the combined effects of genetic and environmental influences. Environmental factors such as access to the substance, use with other teens or adults, and resources for treatment are important to consider. Evaluate the home, education, alcohol, drugs, smoking, and sex practices of the teen.

PHYSIOLOGIC ASSESSMENT

Look for physical signs and symptoms of substance use, including bloodshot eyes, dilated pupils, slurred speech, and weight loss. Blood and urine levels of substances and metabolite are sometimes measured. The adolescent may appear sleepy or restless, or may show signs of clumsiness or inconsistent behavior. Consider all types of substances, including model glue, gasoline, and other sources. Consider signs of withdrawal as well as current intoxication.

PSYCHOLOGIC ASSESSMENT

Changes in social habits may indicate substance use. Parents may report a drop in the school-age child's or adolescent's grades or decreased interest in school activities. The adolescent does not introduce new friends to parents, and has less contact with parents, teachers, and other adults who were previously important. The youth may appear more energetic than usual, always "on a high," or exhibit weight loss. Note the child's current drug use, potential for violence, and motivation to make changes. Assess the degree of family support available.

FAMILY ASSESSMENT

In families with substance-using adults, children may experience neglect and abuse, as well as exposure to drugs. When family members are substance users, young children may experience periods when adults cannot provide supervision and do not encourage healthy activities, or they may be exposed to potentially unsafe or violent episodes. When parents are manufacturing products such as methamphetamine, young children are exposed to toxic chemicals and run the risk of suffering burns and other sequelae from home laboratory production and explosions. Be alert for unusual injuries, signs of inconsistent parenting, and delays in or disturbed growth and development. Be prepared to refer parents for care and for following protocols for child abuse prevention (see sections on abuse and neglect later in this chapter).

Nursing diagnoses for children and adolescents who abuse drugs or alcohol might include the following (NANDA-I © 2014):

- *Social Interaction, Impaired,* related to altered thought processes
- *Self-Esteem, Chronic Low,* related to dysfunctional family and social relationships
- *Injury, Risk for,* related to altered perceptions and sensorium
- *Violence: Self-Directed or Other-Directed, Risk for,* related to physiologic dependence on drugs, alcohol, and other substances

Planning and Implementation

Care of children and adolescents who abuse drugs, alcohol, and other substances is challenging and often frustrating. Long-term mental health counseling may be necessary to resolve underlying issues and foster lifestyle and behavioral changes.

Prevention is the most desirable intervention. The nurse can play a major role in teaching children and their families about substance abuse. Education should begin in primary school, and continue with intensification during middle school and high school. Nurses also can play a major role in community education. Various prevention programs have been developed by federal and private organizations. Referral to support organizations may be beneficial for the child, parents, and other family members. Self-help groups, available in most communities, include Alcoholics Anonymous, Narcotics Anonymous, Al-Anon, Nar-Anon, and Ala-Teen. Parents may receive support from a group such as Parents Anonymous.

The youth's protective factors can be identified and used in planning appropriate interventions. For example, a child with goals for a future career can be helped to see how substance use will interfere with goal attainment. Identifying a strong role model through a program like Big Brothers or Big Sisters can assist children who lack that strength in their families.

The child who has begun to use and abuse drugs needs an intensive intervention program. Referral to a psychiatric health specialist is needed for diagnosis and intervention. Group programs and those that integrate the family are most effective. Find out what resources are present in your community to treat youth who are using alcohol or other drugs. Nurses are active in treatment programs as well as sustaining treatment effects and avoiding relapse during visits to community agencies once the youth returns to family, school, and other surroundings.

Evaluation

Expected outcomes of nursing interventions include abstention from alcohol and street drugs, successful participation in substance abuse programs, and developmentally appropriate social and cognitive skills.

Physical Inactivity and Sedentary Behavior

In the past few decades, children have become increasingly sedentary. This change is a reflection of lifestyles in which car travel is valued, computers and televisions are part of daily life, neighborhoods are sometimes unsafe places for play, and schools do not routinely require daily physical education classes (Figure 42–5). Children and adolescents spend an astounding amount of time with media (television, computers, games, and phone applications)—an average of 2 hours of television daily for those under 6 years, and 4 hours of television and an additional 2 hours of other media use daily for older youth (KidsHealth, 2014). Excessive screen time influences behavior because there is physical inactivity during viewing, a lack of social interaction and cognition, and a tendency to eat high-fat snacks with high caloric content. While screen time increases, physical activity decreases, with only 25% of youth engaged in the recommended moderate to vigorous physical activity for 60 minutes daily (Fakhouri et al., 2014).

Physical inactivity leads to many health concerns. A primary outcome is overweight or obesity (see Chapter 32 for a definition and further information on obesity). Other outcomes can be an increased rate of type 2 diabetes (see Chapter 53), increased exposure to television/computer game violence and sexual activity at early ages, and early progression of cardiovascular disease (see Chapter 47).

However, patterns of physical activity established in childhood can lead to increased exercise behaviors in adulthood, contributing to lower rates of low back pain, overweight, osteoporosis, heart disease, diabetes, colon cancer, and high blood pressure, and also lead to a more positive self-image.

Although many children demonstrate low levels of physical activity, a profound decrease in vigorous activity is common in grades 9 through 12. Boys more commonly participate in team sports than girls. Although about 48% of students attend physical education (PE) classes at least once a week, only 29% have daily PE classes (CDC, 2014a).

Health providers can integrate assessment of physical activity into all health care, and make recommendations to children and families that will help to increase opportunities for physical activity. Nurses can assess height, weight, and body mass index (BMI) to look for signs of overweight (see Chapter 32). Children should be asked about how they like to spend free time. Community and school activities should be encouraged and rewarded. Examples include fun runs, walks for benefit causes, aerobics classes, team sports, roadside cleanups, fairs, and carnivals. Help parents and children learn what they can do for physical fitness. Work with school physical education personnel to plan activities both in and out of physical education class that promote lifelong exercise routines. Work toward the goal of 60 minutes of daily moderate intensity physical activity for all children (CDC, 2014a). During health promotion visits, help children identify ways to gradually increase physical activity and decrease sedentary time.

Injury and Protective Equipment

In the discussion of causes of childhood and adolescent morbidities and mortalities in Chapter 1, unintentional injuries are listed as a common problem. In fact, a majority of deaths from age 10 years onward result from four causes: motor vehicle crashes, other unintentional injury, homicide, and suicide (National Center for Health Statistics & National Vital Statistics System, 2012). Chapters 34, 35, and 36 discuss the frequent injuries seen in children at different developmental ages, and safety precautions to avoid injuries from car crashes, falls, poisonings, and other developmentally related injuries. Many common injuries are preventable with simple use of protective gear and following of safety guidelines (Figure 42–6). Some sports and activities that require safety gear include rollerblading,

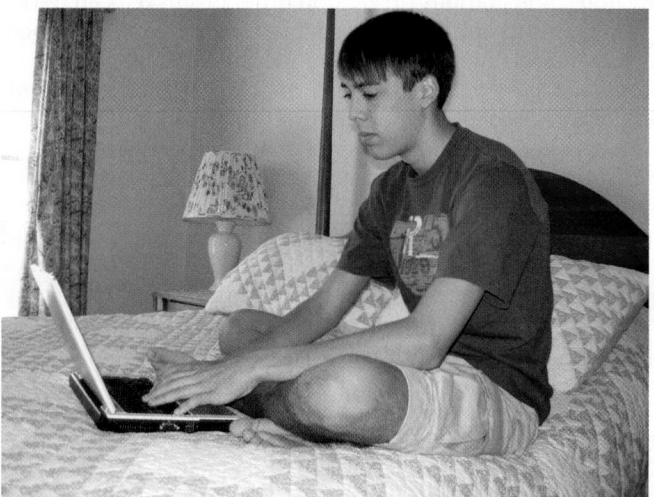
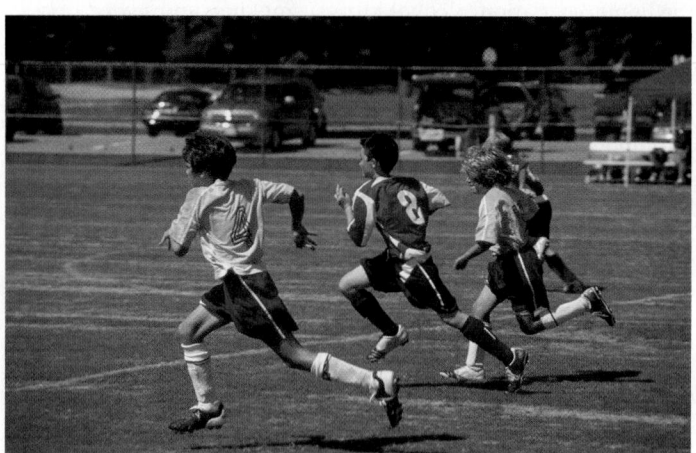

Figure 42–5 **Role of sports in development. Physical inactivity is a growing problem among children and can contribute to poor health. It is important to balance sedentary activities, such as playing computer games, with physical and social activities. Sports are an excellent way for children to develop their psychosocial, cognitive, and motor skills.**

SOURCE: Soccer photo courtesy of Robert Young/Fotolia.

TEACHING HIGHLIGHTS | Physical Activity Guidelines for Youth

- Engage in moderate to vigorous physical activity (such as bike riding, walking, baseball, and rollerblading) for at least 60 minutes daily.
- Engage in vigorous activity that causes sweating and hard breathing (such as soccer, running, and ice hockey) at least 3 times weekly.
- Engage in muscle strengthening activity at least 3 times weekly.
- Engage in bone strengthening activity at least 3 times weekly.
- Encourage schools to offer physical education to all students, and have students sign up when this is an elective.
- Encourage walking and bike riding to friends' homes and stores whenever safe.
- Plan physical activities together as a family.
- Get a pet and plan to walk the pet together daily.
- Limit television and other similar sedentary activities to no more than 2 hours daily.
- On days home, allow the child to watch television for up to 1 hour, and then insist on 1 hour of reading, 1 hour of physical activity, and 1 hour of socializing with others before returning to more television.

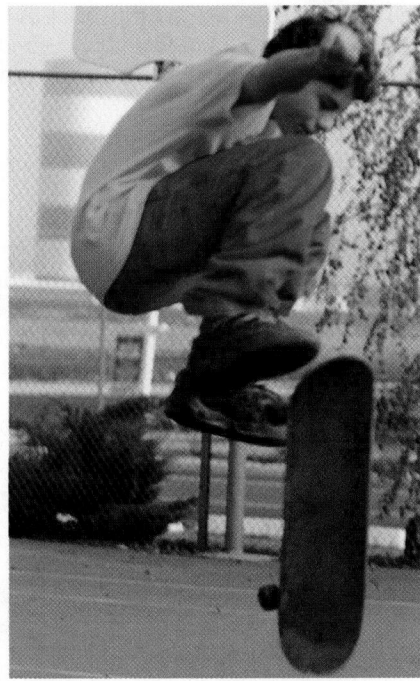

Figure 42–6 **Use of protective gear. What protective gear should children use for skateboarding? How would you convince them to use the protection?**

skateboarding, roller hockey, ice hockey, football, soccer, baseball, scooters, all-terrain vehicles, and skiing or snowboarding fast or using jumps.

Over 8% of youths rarely or never wear car safety belts in automobiles; 22% have recently ridden with someone who had been drinking alcohol (CDC, 2014a). Emphasize safe automobile and motorcycle behaviors in adolescence, with the recognition that risks increase if driving is combined with use of alcohol and controlled substances. Adolescents sometimes engage in practices that put them at particular risk, and nurses should be alert for such activities in their communities. Examples include car surfing (standing on the trunk, hood, or roof of a moving vehicle) or street racing (racing cars down a street at extremely high speed), or "extreme" sports.

About 44 million U.S. children ride bicycles, a beneficial physical activity. However, only about 12% are protected by helmet use, even though bicycling is the most common activity associated with injury (CDC, 2014a). Strategies to make helmet use more attractive to children and adolescents are needed. Nurses can play a major role in programs to educate and reward children for helmet use, and can assist families to find affordable helmets. Nurses can be active in identifying behaviors in youths in specific communities and working with schools and other community groups to support legislation for helmet use, evaluate proper fits of helmets, and work to locate sources for incentives and low-cost helmets. Efforts should also include adequate conditioning for sports, proper treatment of injuries, and prevention of overuse injuries.

A growing number of children engage in "extreme" sports, those that carry a high degree of risk and have not traditionally been common. Some examples are mountain biking, skateboarding with ramps, motocross racing, three-wheeling, ski racing, snowboarding through trees and on courses with pikes and other challenges, ice climbing, rock climbing, and wakeboarding. While the nurse is probably unable to dissuade youth from engaging in these activities, safety measures should be emphasized. Find out what protective gear the youth wears and what is recommended. Provide examples of stories of youth who have been saved by use of such gear. Encourage the youth to engage in sports activities only when others are present and to have a plan for emergencies, including a working cell phone, leaving information with an adult about plans and expected return, and planning for harsh weather with items such as emergency blankets, gear, and food. Encourage the youth to talk with parents and other adults about the risks and responsibilities of the activities.

Developing Cultural Competence Ethnic Disparity in Unintentional Childhood Injuries

Although the unintentional injury rate in children under 19 years declined 39% from 1987 to 2013, striking ethnic disparity rates exist in the rates of unintentional injury among children. These differences are mainly due to living in impoverished communities rather than any innate biologic variations. The rate of death from unintentional injury ranges from 23.8/100,000 in American Indian/Alaska Native, to 12.8 among African Americans, 11.5 among Whites, and 8.8/100,000 in Hispanics (CDC, 2012a). What are the major causes of unintentional injury in your community and state? What ethnic and age groups are at greatest risk? How can you integrate teaching in your practice that is specific to the findings in your community?

Body Art

Body art in the form of painting, tattooing, and piercing has been used by humans throughout history. In recent years, there has been a resurgence of interest in this decorative art among teens. Many adolescents have multiple body piercings and tattoos, and they may even resort to performing these decorations on themselves or friends.

Approximately 21% of adolescents and young adults have tattoos, and even more have at least one body piercing (Owen, Armstrong, Koch, et al., 2013). In some states, teens must be 18 years of age or have parental permission to obtain body art, but students often report that it is easy to have an adult present who signs and claims to be a parent. Amy, described at the opening of this chapter, had her piercing done by a friend. In some states, tattoo and body piercing businesses must be licensed and comply with certain regulations; other states have no regulations. Amy demonstrates some common characteristics of teens who choose to use body art. It may be seen as a way to establish individualism and independence, and it may help some teens to feel part of a peer group. Multiple tattoos and piercings are common, as is the case with Amy (Figure 42–7).

Body art is a common source of infections with skin pathogens. Infections can range from mild inflammatory reactions to bacterial and viral infections and serious long-term infections. Body piercing is a major method of transmission of hepatitis C, a disease that may not be manifested until years later (see Chapter 51). It can be a source of HIV if proper techniques are not followed. Serious systemic infections such as endocarditis have occurred after some piercings. Piercings in parts of the body such as the mouth or navel are most prone to bacterial infection and continued redness and irritation. The pierced site may not appear infected, but transfer of organisms can lead to serious infection and heart damage. Examples of serious infective agents include *Neisseria, Mycobacterium, Staphylococcus, Pseudomonas, Streptococcus, hepatitis B,* and *hepatitis C* (Juhas & English, 2013). A number of cases of *Mycobacterium chelone* skin infection from contaminated ink were identified across the country in 2012 (CDC, 2012b). When noting signs of systemic infection such as fever, weakness, malaise, and arthralgia (see Chapter 47 for full discussion of endocarditis), gather history about body piercings and refer for care to the primary healthcare provider. Pierced tongues can lead to chipped teeth or even be the cause of choking if the piercing is dislodged from the site.

Another issue that the teen should consider is the relationship of the tattoos to future lifestyle changes. Advise teens to avoid tattooing the name of a person or musical group since relationships change and tastes in music evolve. Be sure they know the meaning of phrases, foreign words, or Asian symbols. Consider the visibility of the tattoo and its effect on future employment. Tattoos on the face, neck, or other readily visible places may be a detriment during employment interviews. Tattoos should always be considered permanent. Methods for removal may be costly, painful, and unsuccessful.

Another form of body art that is regarded as disfigurement is *deliberate self-harm* or *nonsuicidal self-injury.* One example is *branding,* or scarification, whereby the skin is burned to result in a scar. Commonly a desired sign, symbol, or word is inscribed. Results are usually not precise and do not adhere to expected designs. This procedure is done on the self or friend, using common household metal implements heated in fires or stoves. Others cut themselves in the form of a desired design, a process called *cutting.* This type of self-harm or self-injury is performed with razor blades, knives, scissors, broken glass, needles, or sharp pencils. These practices can result in infection, often do not yield the desired result, and may indicate underlying problems. Adolescent screenings should ask about cutting or intentional injury to skin. Using a nonjudgmental attitude, the youth involved should be referred for further assessment by primary care providers or counselors (Catledge, Scharer, & Fuller, 2012; Smith, 2011).

Because teens may choose to obtain body art even if parents object and even when there are state laws to prohibit or make it difficult to do so, nursing care must focus on providing information for the teen, assessing sites, identifying infections, and referring if needed. Care is almost always provided in community settings such as clinics or schools. Consider asking teens if they are thinking about body art since they often do not seek advice before obtaining the body art and may not get adequate teaching.

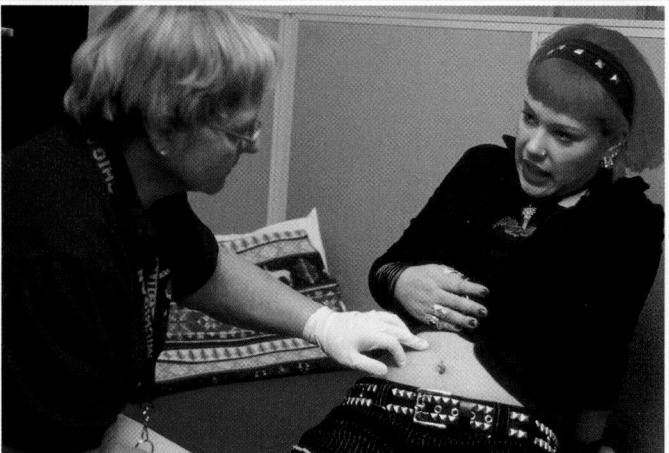

Figure 42–7 **Health risks to adolescents. Talk openly with adolescents about their health and teach them to avoid health risks connected with tattoos and piercing.**

Clinical Reasoning The Adolescent With Body Piercings

Amy is 15 years old and attends an alternative high school. She recently had an ear piercing and it is painful. She comes to the health room to ask the advice of the school nurse. The area around the piercing is inflamed and mildly edematous. After asking some questions, the nurse learns that Amy's ear was pierced by a friend, using a needle that had been "sterilized" by passing it through a match flame. She has had a slight fever, but otherwise feels fine.

In her home state, adolescents under 18 years of age must have the signature of a parent for body piercings and tattoos, so Amy chose to have the procedure done by a friend. She believes this is safe since her friend has done many piercings on others. She admits that her parents are not very pleased with her body art, but that they allow her to do it as long as she agrees to stay in high school. She had previously run away and spent several weeks living on the streets.

- What healthcare and social needs does Amy have?
- How can you support both Amy and her parents?
- What physical care does Amy need to treat potential infection at her piercing site?
- What systemic infectious diseases is Amy at risk of acquiring due to repeated body piercings using an unsterile technique?

TEACHING HIGHLIGHTS	Care for Tattoos and Body Piercings

Before the Procedure

- Does the studio look clean?
- Visit several studios to make comparisons of techniques, quality, and cleanliness.
- Ask to watch a tattoo or piercing done on someone else.
- What are the artist's sterilization and hygiene practices?
- Is the artist licensed? Trained?
- Look at pictures of completed art and talk with former clients.
- Insist that new, sterile equipment be opened in front of the person to be decorated.
- Consider if this permanent body decoration is desired for a lifetime.
- Consider what the tattoo or piercing will look like in several years.
- Consider the possible side effects such as infection, future dislike for the art, and allergy to dyes or metals.
- Be sure that hepatitis B vaccination is completed before the procedure.
- Be aware that no immunization is available to protect against the health risks of hepatitis C and HIV.

Care After the Procedure

- Touch the area only after carefully washing your hands.
- Keep the area elevated and use ice for the first 2 days to minimize swelling.
- Avoid contact with another person's body fluids until well healed.
- Turn the piercing jewelry gently several times daily using washed hands.
- Use antibacterial mouthwash or cleaner or ointment as recommended.
- Avoid pressure and rubbing on the site (such as belts on navel piercings).
- Watch carefully for signs of infection and report them to a healthcare provider:
  - Increased redness
  - Swelling
  - Pain
  - Hot feeling
  - Discharge
- Ask the artist how long healing will take. It varies from 2 months in the mouth or up to 6 or 8 months for a navel.
- Metal is dangerous during some medical procedures such as magnetic resonance imaging (MRI) or during surgery. Be sure to tell doctors and nurses about your piercings when you are hospitalized or receiving medical care, especially if they are in a part of the body not readily visible.
- If you decide to remove a piece of jewelry soon after it is placed, the skin may heal with only a slight scar.

Sexual Orientation

Adolescence is a time of identifying emerging sexuality. Most teens establish relationships with members of the opposite sex and learn how to interact in ways guided by their peer group, family, and culture. For some youth, the transition into adult sexuality can be more challenging if they feel an emotional and sexual attraction to people of the same sex (**homosexuality**). The term **gay** is often used for homosexual males and **lesbian** for homosexual females. Other youth are **bisexual**, or attracted to both men and women, and some are **transgendered**, or attracted to dress and act like members of the opposite sex. The abbreviation LGBT is sometimes used to refer to lesbian, gay, bisexual, or transgendered, and LGBT/Q indicates those who are questioning their sexual orientation. About 5% to 12% of persons report an experience with someone of the same sex, and about 3% identify as being LGBT/Q (Chandra, Mosher, Copen, et al., 2011). Data on youth are not often reported; however, the National Survey of Family Growth reports that about 90% of adolescents and young adults report that they are heterosexual, with the remainder reporting that they are homosexual,

bisexual, or not sure (Sexuality Information and Education Council of the United States, n.d.).

Sexual attractions and practices different than the mainstream are not deviant nor symptoms of a mental disorder but should be viewed as part of a continuum of sexual expression. No known gene, early life experience, or other event causes homosexuality (American Psychiatric Association, 2012).

LGBT/Q youth are at risk for a variety of problems related to emotional and physical health. These include rejection by family members and peers, verbal harassment, sexual abuse and physical assault, a high rate of suicide, substance abuse, a high rate of homelessness, and sexual risks of HIV and other sexually transmitted infections. Their health risks need to be identified and appropriate care provided in welcoming and nonjudgmental healthcare facilities.

Nurses can provide health care for LGBT/Q youth in a variety of settings. School nurses and clinics can display a sign to demonstrate that they are accepting of persons with minority sexual orientation. These signs are rainbows or triangles with several colors shown and can be obtained from local gay or lesbian community groups. Terminology in assessment should be gender free. Ask "Do you have one or more sexual partners?" rather than "Do you have a boyfriend?" When youth identify as LGBT/Q, provide usual care of all kinds. This includes preventive care such as immunizations, sports assessments, and injury prevention teaching. Be alert that the youth may have additional health challenges. Ask about peer and parental support; refer to support groups if needed. Provide resources for homelessness and when the teen is depressed or suicidal (see Chapter 55). Perform testing for sexually transmitted infections if the teen is having sexual contact, and teach preventive measures. Foster a positive sense of self-esteem through encouraging positive activities such as sports, music, and friendships with peers.

Effects of Violence

Violence is a threatened or actual use of physical force or power that leads to actual or potential physical or emotional trauma. Violence can be directed at oneself, another person, or against a group or community. Violence can result in injury, death, psychologic harm, disruption of development, or deprivation (Child Trends, 2015). In the past several years, adults and children alike have been shocked by violent episodes in schools. Although these incidents had much media coverage, they are just one type of violence to which children may be regularly exposed. Children can be the recipients of violence during child abuse and homicides, and they themselves can perform acts of violence on others. They may be touched by violence when parents, siblings, or other family members are killed in gang conflicts, in terrorist attacks, or in wars. The effects of violence are far reaching and ongoing; they permeate the victim's entire lifetime. This section explores some types of violence affecting children.

Schools and Communities

At a time when firearm deaths are decreasing overall, unintentional deaths and suicides have increased among children. Many of these deaths are committed with firearms found in the home. Over 4000 youth from 10 to 19 years old die from firearm homicides annually, and another approximately 15,000 die from firearm suicide. Firearm homicide is the second leading cause of injury death for youth, and firearm suicide is the fifth leading cause of injury death for youth (CDC, 2011b). Forty percent of households with children have guns (2 million children live in these homes), and in many of those homes, the firearms are stored loaded or are not secured under lock. Parents often report that children do not know firearm locations when 39% of the children are actually able to state the locations and 22% have handled the guns (Children's Defense Fund, 2014).

Homicide in children has gained attention in the past several years because of several shootings at schools, universities, and other community sites. While homicide is an extreme example, there are other types of violence. Children report being threatened verbally and with guns or knives at home, in schools, and in their neighborhoods. They may be beaten up or bullied or harassed. An estimated 3 to 10 million children are exposed to acts of domestic violence by adults in their homes. They may be subjected to dangerous situations in their neighborhoods or during times of homelessness. Date rape or other sexual violence is reported by up to 10% of teens (CDC, 2014a).

SAFETY ALERT!
When a group of children is attacked or killed in a school shooting, this tragic occurrence has the attention of the media. Little do many realize that this tragedy is part of daily life across the country. A firearm kills about seven children every day in the United States, or about 50 per week. An additional 200 to 300 children suffer from nonfatal firearm injuries (Children's Defense Fund, 2014). Nurses must intervene in this national tragedy. Become familiar with firearm injury statistics in your community. Teach families, children, and youth about the dangers of firearms. Urge safe storage. Help schools establish programs to ensure safety for students.

Internationally, millions of children experience violence annually, and decreasing violence against children has become a focus of the World Health Organization and the United Nations (World Health Organization, 2014). Common forms of violence worldwide are war and terrorism. War affects children in several ways: Parents leave home to fight in wars; children may be forced to take on adult roles in families when parents leave; children become orphans when parents are killed; children may be raped, sexually trafficked, or forced to be sex slaves; and some children are trained and forced to fight in battles, carry messages, or otherwise engage in combat themselves. Children who live through wars or have a parent or sibling die in war can be permanently affected by these events. Depression and other mental health problems are common in youth who have experienced war.

Natural disasters and terrorism also take a large toll on the mental health of children and adolescents. Most children and adolescents who live through terrorism experience profound sadness, cling to adults who provide security, and have a variety of somatic complaints. Interventions should be directed at different phases of violence, such as preevent preparation (emergency preparation and training) and postevent activity (offering special services and resources).

Several resources have been developed to help families and health professionals help children deal with war and violence. See the resources at the National Center for Children Exposed to Violence, Society of Pediatric Nurses, and American Academy of Child and Adolescent Psychiatry websites.

Bullying

One type of violence that frequently occurs in schools is **bullying**, or aggressive behavior that is intended to cause harm, exists in a relationship with imbalance of power, and occurs repeatedly. Bullies are aggressive, impulsive, and need to dominate others. Bullying behaviors include verbal abuse (taunting, teasing), name calling, threats, spreading rumors, social exclusion, and physical abuse (hitting, shoving, kicking, tripping). About 20% of children suffer bullying at school each year, and about 5% did not go to school at least 1 day in the previous month because of safety concerns due to bullying (CDC, 2014a). Although bullying is most commonly reported in schools, it can occur in neighborhoods as children go to and from school, on school buses, on sports teams, and in other settings.

Bullying can also occur through the Internet and is reported by 20% (with a range of 9% to 40% in various studies) of young people (Cyberbullying Research Center, 2011; Schneider, O'Donnell, Stueve, et al., 2012). **Cyberbullying** occurs when a child or adolescent is targeted by another via an Internet posting or other digital technology and threatened, tormented, harassed, humiliated, or embarrassed. Personal information may be disclosed or fabricated, persons are excluded, offensive messages are sent, or harmful messages are sent out under the target person's name. Such attacks are socially aggressive and often anonymous.

Bullies themselves are at risk and are more likely than other youth to abuse substances, be depressed, and carry weapons to school, putting other children at risk. Bullying is associated with future delinquent behavior, depression, low self-esteem, loneliness, suicidal ideation, and suicide attempts (Tsitsika et al., 2014).

Children who are bullied are more commonly socially isolated and anxious. Health problems such as migraines, stomach pains, suicidal thoughts, and other problems can result. Academic performance commonly deteriorates and rates of school absenteeism increase (American Academy of Pediatrics, 2011). Realizing the serious effects of such behaviors, a number of states have now passed legislation that reiterates the rights of all children to attend school in a safe and peaceful manner. Some state education departments mandate school district programs for students about bullying, and clear school policies about dealing with the behavior. See the Health Resources and Services Administration (HRSA) Maternal and Child Health Bureau website at www.stopbullyingnow.hrsa.gov.

Nurses can be active in setting up school policies about bullying and integrating assessment and interventions related to bullying into health promotion visits. School programs should:

- Inform all students that bullying is not tolerated.
- Train teachers and other personnel about signs of bullying.
- Ensure adult supervision in hallways and on playgrounds, sites where bullying is most common.
- Teach children to promptly report bullying that is experienced or observed.
- Set up peer support for those who are bullied.
- Arrange therapeutic treatment through school counselors and other resources for those who bully; involve parents in the treatment plan.
- Measure incidence of bullying, monitor outcomes of policies, and use data to evaluate policies in schools.

Nurses who are in clinics, offices, and other health promotion settings can:

- Be alert for children with behavior changes (irritability, anxiety, poor self-concept).
- Consider bullying as a potential cause when fear or refusal to attend school is reported by child or parents.
- Ask questions during visits, such as "Have you ever been afraid to go to school?," "What are the best and worst things about going to your school?," and "What are the other kids in your neighborhood like?"
- Ask parents what they have done about any situations identified. Partner with the parent to act as liaison to the school or other agency.
- Refer identified bullies and victims of bullying to mental health specialists.

Incarceration

A growing number of children are entering the judicial system, and many are admitted at young ages. About 3.4% of youth in the United States are incarcerated at any given time (Annie E. Casey Foundation, 2011). Children in detention,

courts, and other facilities have frequently been victims as well as perpetrators of violence. They often have multiple risks such as substance abuse, early sexual activity, multiple sexual partners, sexual abuse, lack of a healthcare home, and mental health problems. The incarceration facility itself may subject youth to additional violence, abuse, and other maltreatment (Annie E. Casey Foundation, 2011). Nurses work within the juvenile justice system to provide episodic care for children or to partner with others to establish health-related programs within facilities. Youth who are incarcerated need the following:

- Basic physical care such as immunizations, vision, and hearing screening
- Nutrition assessment and teaching
- Skin assessment and hygiene practice teaching
- Information about sexuality, sexual practices, and sexually transmitted infections
- Assessment for substance abuse
- Teaching about hazards of substance use and assistance with quitting
- Mental health services
- Developmental assessment
- Individualized education plans to meet cognitive needs

Hazing

Hazing is an activity that is forced on an individual, causes humiliation, and is required for membership in an organization or group. It can sometimes be harmful and even lead to death. Sports teams, music groups, and Greek sororities and fraternities are examples of groups commonly associated with hazing. Activities might include removing clothes, drinking large amounts of alcohol, using snuff or other substances, being locked in small places, being beaten, and many other behaviors. In spite of its common practice, many students do not know what to do about hazing practices; coaches or other adult leaders may or may not be aware of hazing practices. Youth often believe that they must experience and uphold the traditions of hazing to belong to their group (Allan & Madden, 2011). Ask during health visits if the student has ever had to do something to belong to a group or team. Ask about "scary" things others have had them do. Assist schools and colleges in setting up anti-hazing policies. Encourage students to report hazing. Be aware of the possibility of hazing when seeing children with traumatic injuries (Hazing Prevention, 2011).

Domestic Violence

Domestic violence occurs between members of a family. The specific type of violence known as *intimate partner abuse* occurs between adult partners in the family. It may involve the parents of a child, or one parent and a significant other. This type of abuse injures the child or adolescent because it is traumatic to witness a close family member or loved one become the recipient of violence. About 3.3 million children annually in the United States are exposed to violence against their mothers or other female care providers; children who live in homes where intimate partner abuse occurs are significantly more likely to be abused themselves (Cross, Matthews, Tonmyr, et al., 2012; Davidov, Nadorff, Jack, et al., 2012). Children may also be the direct victims of domestic violence in a family. See the section on child abuse later in this chapter.

Dating Violence

Dating violence is another type of intimate partner abuse; this type occurs in relationships among youth. Over 10% of adolescent males and females report being victims of dating violence (CDC, 2014a). Such behaviors include being hit, slammed into something, or intentionally injured with an object or weapon. Girls who reported dating violence were also more likely to report other risk behaviors, such as feeling sad, having attempted suicide, or having used substances such as tobacco and drugs. Early sexual activity, having a higher number of sex partners, and being less likely to use birth control are also associated with a higher incidence of dating violence. A risk profile with a cluster of potentially dangerous behaviors may therefore put adolescents more at risk for dating violence.

Date rape is a term used when dating violence takes the form of rape. This can be particularly harmful to females who often do not want to share the event or press charges against the attacker.

Nurses should screen for violence at each health promotion visit, including gynecologic visits and prenatal care. Ask what is going well and not going well in intimate relationships, and whether the person ever feels unsafe or is forced to do things she does not wish to do. Recognize that while not as common, males may even be victims of violence in close relationships. Recognize that alcohol and other drugs are often connected with violence in relationships so ask about their use. Organize peer discussion groups about intimacy in order to help youth develop a sense of self-confidence and self-efficacy that will empower them to refuse participation in activities in which they do not wish to engage.

Nursing Management

Violence

Nursing Assessment and Diagnosis

Nurses are in key positions to identify children at risk of being recipients and victims of violence. The ecologic framework can be used to assess children. Some questions that can be asked are listed in Table 42–6. It is important to detect both the risks that lead to vulnerability and the protective factors that can promote resilience and safety. (Refer to Chapter 31 for explanations of these factors and the systems that influence the child.) Adapt questions to each age group and insert them in every healthcare encounter.

Nursing care for violence is discussed in the *Nursing Care Plan*. The following nursing diagnoses may be appropriate (NANDA-I © 2014):

- *Violence: Self-Directed, Risk for,* related to history of violence
- *Self-Esteem, Chronic Low,* related to history of abuse
- *Family Processes, Dysfunctional,* related to situational crises
- *Development: Delayed, Risk for,* related to environmental deficiencies

Planning and Intervention

Prevention is an important role for the nurse. Interventions such as providing resources for family planning; teaching self-regulation/control techniques; and applying technology such as kiosks in health centers, virtual training for healthcare

TABLE 42–6 Assessment Questions to Identify Violence Risk and Protective Factors

MICROSYSTEM
- Have you been hurt by your parents or anyone else at home?
- When was the last time you were made fun of or bullied at school? What did you do?
- Have you ever brought a gun or knife or other weapon to school?
- Do you have access to guns and knives at home? At friends' houses?
- What stresses are there in your family now?
- Tell me about school—what you like and don't like.

MESOSYSTEM
- Do your parents attend school meetings? Talk with your teachers?
- Do you participate in any church, synagogue, or mosque services?
- Do you participate in any community activities?

EXOSYSTEM
- What stresses do your parents have at work, in their families, with their health or finances?
- Do you feel like your school helps to keep you safe?
- Are there plans for handling violent episodes at your school if they were to occur?
- Do you feel safe in your neighborhood?
- Where would you go or who would you call if you felt unsafe or were hurt and no one was at home?

providers, and positive media messages are all important measures in preventing violence (Child Trends 2015). Nurses intervene with individual children, with families, and in schools and communities to increase safety and decrease violence. Help children and families meet basic needs and access resources to assist with finances, respite care, domestic violence, and other issues. Education is a key element of intervention.

PROVIDING INFORMATION

Teach the family the dangers of firearms and the necessity for using gun locks and locked cabinets, storing guns unloaded, and storing guns and ammunition in separate places. Suggest alternative activities to minimize child exposure to violence in the media. Inform parents about rating systems for television and other media, and about lockout mechanisms for televisions and computers. Discuss the harmful effects of verbal and physical abuse to the child or other family members and explore alternatives.

Present the school-age child and adolescent with information about bullying and strategies for dealing with it. Provide school and community resources where the child can go if there are threats of any kind. Discuss date rape and violence with all teens and encourage them to report it.

COMMUNITY-BASED NURSING CARE

Both in schools and in community settings, nurses can plan peer mentoring to provide assistance to children at high risk of experiencing violence. Nurses can link and coordinate school and community programs for children to provide for parent involvement and child support. Discuss safety issues,

Nursing Care Plan: The Child and Violent Behavior

1. Nursing Diagnosis: *Violence: Other-Directed, Risk for*, related to history of family violence (NANDA-I © 2014)

GOAL: The child will demonstrate impulse control.

INTERVENTION	RATIONALE
• Identify violent behaviors in the child.	• Violence in the child usually develops over time.
• Provide a safe place for exploration of feelings by referral to school or other counseling, support groups, and other resources.	• The child needs an opportunity to explore feelings and vulnerability.
• Provide strategies for managing anger and alternative ways for coping with problems.	• Coping strategies can be learned from others and can help in dealing with a stressful home situation.

EXPECTED OUTCOME: Child will express the ability to manage problems in acceptable ways.

GOAL: The child will be secure in a safe environment.

INTERVENTION	RATIONALE
• Perform a thorough assessment of hazards to the physical and emotional state in the child's home, neighborhood, and school.	• Hazards to physical and emotional health promote violence to and from the child.
• Institute actions that will result in removal of child from unsafe situations.	• Removal from family, community, or school may be needed to ensure child safety.
• Use community resources to provide respite care, teaching for families, and safety instructions for the child.	• Stress reduction measures may help to decrease violent behaviors.

EXPECTED OUTCOME: Child will express a sense of physical and emotional safety in daily life.

2. Nursing Diagnosis: *Injury, Risk for,* related to physical or psychologic conditions in the environment (NANDA-I © 2014)

GOAL: Risk for physical and emotional injury to the child is decreased.

INTERVENTION	RATIONALE
• Identify physical and psychologic factors that affect the child's safety.	• Multiple factors in the family can contribute to risk of violence and lack of safety for the child.
• Assist family to deal with issues such as mental status challenges, fatigue, financial concern, substance abuse, and lack of adequate childcare resources.	
• Instruct family on methods of keeping the child safe.	• Families need information about the impact of unsafe settings on the child and methods that can decrease risk of injury.

EXPECTED OUTCOME: Child will not be injured in physical or emotional ways in the home or other immediate settings.

3. Nursing Diagnosis: *Post-Trauma Syndrome* related to physical or psychosocial abuse (NANDA-I © 2014)

GOAL: The child will demonstrate abuse or violence recovery.

INTERVENTION	RATIONALE
• Assess the child's affect and behaviors.	• Disturbed child behaviors can demonstrate a sense of mistrust and insecurity.
• Evaluate social interactions and sense of trust in others.	
• Assist the child in identifying feelings and coping strategies by providing counseling, art therapy, and other strategies.	• Establishment of close interactions with others demonstrates reestablishment of a sense of trust.

EXPECTED OUTCOME: Child will identify feelings related to violent episode(s) and express healing of the self.

both risk factors and protective actions, in schools and community groups. Report children who are at risk. Work to establish extended programs for children so that they are safe after school. Help children learn behaviors that will help them to be safe in their communities and at home. Teach positive problem-solving and conflict-management techniques to children and parents.

Youth with special needs are a special concern of nurses. Jails and detention centers often have a nurse who visits youth on a regular basis or when health problems occur. Health teaching may be provided in some facilities. Halfway houses and homeless shelters are examples of settings where violence prevention and intervention can occur with youth. Mental health centers and other programs have nurses that work with children who are victims of violence (for example, have witnessed domestic violence, have witnessed or had a family member murdered, have been abused at home or school) or perpetrators of violence. See Chapter 55 for a discussion of posttraumatic stress disorder and its effects on the child and adolescent.

Partner with families to assist them in talking to children about war and terrorism. Recognize that youth who have experienced such events themselves are more at risk for mental health disruptions with future events. Answer questions from children honestly but reassure them that many people are trying to make the situation safe. Other suggestions for parents include the following:

- Limit television viewing and other media exposure because of its constant replaying of the events of terrorism or war. Preschoolers may think the events continue to happen, rather than being a one-time occurrence. Watch with children and talk with them about what is happening.

- Continue with structured family events such as meals, recreation, and faith-based activities. Spend time with your child.

- Take cues from the child about how much to discuss. Use words the child or adolescent can understand.

- Partner with the school so teachers know what parents have discussed and parents are aware of how events are discussed at school.

- If youth decide to become active by writing letters or joining campaigns, allow them to participate in this way.

- Be alert for regression in behavior, sleep and eating problems, or other indications of stress. Consider talking with the healthcare provider or a counselor in such situations.

- Expect that even after the child has adjusted, there may be delayed reactions. Anniversaries of events, holidays, and birthdays often bring renewed pain and sadness.

- Realize that adults must care for themselves, obtain stress relief, and talk with others in order to have strength and resources available for children.

Evaluation

The expected outcomes of nursing care for violence prevention include a decrease in incidents of homicides, firearm injuries, abuse, date rape, and other violence among children. Additional outcomes are establishment of programs to decrease violence, and verbalization by all children of what to do if violence occurs and how to solve problems without becoming violent.

Child Abuse

One of the most common types of violence against children is child abuse. Children from all socioeconomic groups and both genders are victims of abuse. This type of violence can have implications for both the physical and mental health of children, and can influence their health status even long after the abuse has occurred. Awareness of the problem of child abuse is increasing. More cases are being reported; however, these are probably only a small percentage of the total.

There are 3.4 million reports of abuse and neglect annually, with 78% of them due to neglect, 18% related to physical abuse, 9% to sexual abuse, and 11% to other types of abuse; about 1640 children die annually (5 children daily) from abuse (CDC, 2014b; Childhelp, 2013). Infants have the highest rate of abuse (21.9 per 1000 children,) with decreasing rates as children get older. Twenty-seven percent of victims are under 3 years of age, and 20% are 3 to 5 years old (CDC, 2014b).

Physical abuse is only one part of a larger problem. The definition of child abuse has expanded during the past decades and includes physical neglect, emotional abuse and neglect, verbal abuse, and sexual abuse, as well as physical abuse. Abuse generally involves an act of commission, that is, actively doing something to a child physically, emotionally, or sexually, such as hitting, belittling, or molesting. Neglect more often involves an act of omission, such as not providing adequate nutrition, emotional contact, or necessary physical care, or abandoning a child. Because the evidence is often not visible, emotional abuse and neglect are more difficult to identify and prove than physical abuse or neglect. Risk factors for abuse and neglect are listed in Table 42–7.

Physical Abuse

Physical abuse is the deliberate maltreatment of another individual that inflicts pain or injury and may result in permanent or temporary disfigurement or even death. Common methods of physical abuse in children are listed in Table 42–8.

TABLE 42–7 Risk Factors for Child Abuse and Neglect

FACTORS INCREASING RISK FOR PHYSICAL ABUSE
Poverty
Violence in the family
Prematurity or low birth weight
Unrelated male primary caretaker
Parents who were abused as children
Age less than 3 years
Child disability or condition that requires a great deal of care (e.g., intellectual disability, attention deficit hyperactivity disorder)
Parental substance abuse or social isolation

FACTORS INCREASING RISK FOR SEXUAL ABUSE
Absence of natural father or having a stepfather
Being female
Mother's employment outside the home
Poor relationship with parent
Parental relationship characterized by conflict
Parental substance abuse or social isolation

TABLE 42–8 Methods of Physical Abuse in Children

Hitting, slapping, kicking, or punching	Throwing the child against a wall, down stairs, or against a window
Whipping with belts, shoes, or electrical cords (**A**)	Choking or gagging the child
Inflicting burns with a lit cigarette or lighter (**B**)	Fracturing the legs, arms, ribs, or skull
Immersing child or body part in scalding water (commonly legs, perineal area, hands, or feet; see Figure 57–16)	Deliberately administering excessive doses of prescribed or nonprescribed drugs
Shaking the child violently ("shaken child" syndrome)	Deliberately withholding prescribed medication
Tying the child to a fence, bed, tree, or other object	

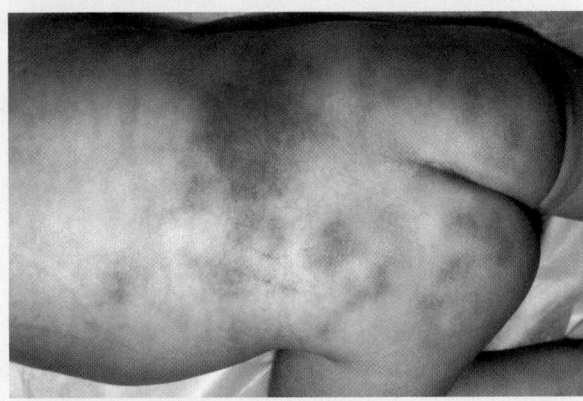

A

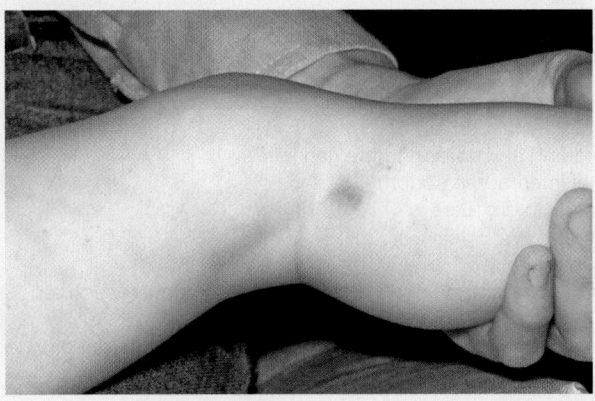

B

SOURCE: *A,* BioPhoto Associates/Science Source; *B,* Mediscan/Alamy.

Physical Neglect

Physical neglect is the deliberate withholding of or failure to provide the necessary and available resources to the child. Behaviors constituting physical neglect include failure to provide for the following basic needs: supervision appropriate for child's age, adequate nutrition and hydration, hygiene (e.g., clean diapers and clothes, bathing and toileting facilities), shelter (e.g., warmth in winter), and appropriate health care (e.g., immunizations, dental care, medications, eyeglasses).

Abandoned Babies

There are no accurate statistics on numbers of babies that are abandoned in dumpsters, on doorsteps, and in other locations. This tragedy has been addressed by Safe Haven laws in some states that allow women to drop unwanted babies at certain locations such as hospitals and fire stations without legal recrimination. In spite of these laws, babies continue to be abandoned, perhaps because mothers do not know about the laws or because they do not believe they will not be found guilty. Young teen mothers may not want others to know they had a baby. In addition, placement of these babies in adoptive homes is difficult because of paternity suits. Nurses should know their state's Safe Haven law details. Inform adolescents and young women about the law and post information in community sites frequented by women. Partner with young pregnant women to link them to resources such as adoption agencies when they might not want to keep a baby.

Emotional Abuse

Emotional abuse usually involves shaming, ridiculing, embarrassing, or insulting the child. It can also include the destruction of a child's personal property, such as tearing up the child's favorite family photographs or letters or harming, killing, or giving away the child's pet. These actions are frequently used as a means of frightening or controlling the child.

Verbal abuse is a common method of emotional abuse. Words can be a violent and volatile weapon against a child, eroding the child's fragile sense of self and destroying self-esteem. Common examples of verbal abuse include yelling obscenities at the child, calling the child names, threatening to "put the child away" or to give away or kill the child's pet, telling the child "I wish you were never born" or "You're worthless," and using words to humiliate, shame, or degrade the child.

Emotional Neglect

Emotional neglect is characterized by the caretaker's emotional unavailability to the child. The usual style of interaction is cold and lacking in sensitive personal attention. The child suffers from a lack of nurturance and failure of the parent or caretaker to meet basic dependency needs. An example of emotional neglect is the parent who is mentally ill, or abusing alcohol or other substances, and cannot respond adequately to the child's developmental needs.

Sexual Abuse

Child sexual abuse is the exploitation of a child for the sexual gratification of an adult. About 1.2 per 1000 children (almost 100,000) children in the United States are sexually abused each year. Approximately 10% of schoolchildren report that they have been sexually abused. Many children who are sexually abused are under the age of 5 years, some as young as 3 months. The perpetrator is often the parent, stepparent, or someone else known to the child such as a friend, neighbor, or babysitter. Methods of sexual abuse may be sexual acts, allowing others to commit sexual abuse, threats, exploitation via video or other means, and a variety of other actions (Childhelp, 2013; National Center for PTSD, 2011). Use of the word *child* in relation to sexual abuse and molestation refers to anyone who has not reached the age of consent, even if a teenager. **Incest** is sexual activity between close family members, so that marriage would be legally or culturally prohibited. Abusers often threaten to harm or kill the child or another family member if the child discloses the abuse. Some abusers are pedophiles, people who have sexual impulses toward preadolescent children. The pedophile is at least 16 years of age and is at least 5 years older than the victim, and the victim is 13 years of age or younger. Another form of sexual abuse is *exhibitionism*, or obtaining sexual arousal by exposing one's genitals to a stranger. Some children are victims of prostitution, forced to offer themselves for money or the pleasures of others, either in person or through videos and Internet sources.

Clinical Tip

Following are common forms of sexual abuse:
- Oral–genital contact
- Fondling and caressing the genitals
- Anal intercourse/sodomy
- Sexual intercourse
- Rape
- Prostitution
- Forced viewing of or participation in pornography such as sexually explicit or nude photographs
- Encouraging nude photos or sexual activity via Internet or video

---

ETIOLOGY AND PATHOPHYSIOLOGY

Regardless of the type of abuse, the most common abuser is the child's parent or guardian or a male friend of the child's mother. Substance abuse is a major contributor to the problem, with one half of cases related to parental alcohol or drug abuse (Childhelp, 2011). Risk factors associated with abusive behavior in adults include the following:

- Psychopathology, such as drug addiction or alcoholism, low self-esteem, poor impulse control, and other personality disorders

- Poor parenting experiences, such as abuse in the abuser's own childhood, rejection by the abuser's own parent(s), lack of knowledge of alternative methods of discipline, strong belief in or family tradition of harsh discipline, and lack of parental affection

- Marital stressors and problems with partners, such as hostile-dependent, abusive, or nonsupportive relationships, and one-sided decision making

- Environmental stressors, such as legal, financial, medical, or housing problems

- Social isolation, such as few friends and limited use of sitters, family, or other resources

- Inappropriate expectations for the developmental level of the child

CLINICAL MANIFESTATIONS

See Table 42–9 for clinical manifestations of physical abuse in children and adolescents. Behaviors inconsistent with developmental stage may be apparent. For example, the toddler or preschool child may be indiscriminately friendly with unfamiliar adults, including healthcare providers, rather than demonstrating shyness or anxiety. For the infant or young child with shaken baby syndrome or shaken child syndrome, the symptoms are those of central nervous system injury from repeated coup and contrecoup injury (see Chapter 54). These may include vomiting, irritability, fatigue, poor feeding, bradycardia, apnea, enlarged fontanelle, and seizures. Bruises are usually not present, but computerized tomography (CT) is often definitive for

---

TABLE 42–9 Clinical Manifestations of Physical Abuse in Children and Adolescents

- Multiple bruises in various stages of healing
- Scald burns with clear lines of demarcation and in a glove or stocking distribution (see Figure 57–16)
- Rope, belt, or cord marks, usually seen on the mouth, buttocks, back, legs, and arms (see Figure A in Table 42–8)
- Burn scars in various stages of healing
- Multiple fractures in various stages of healing, spiral fractures not explained by accident
- Shortness of breath and distress upon being moved, indicating chest contusions and possible rib fractures
- Sedation from overmedication
- Exacerbation of chronic illness (such as diabetes or asthma) because of withholding of medication
- Cranial and abdominal injuries
- Change in behavior or school performance
- Fear and avoidance of certain people or situations

---

the diagnosis with radiographs and MRI used to provide a thorough diagnostic profile (National Center for PTSD, 2011).

Manifestations of physical neglect include undernourishment (evidenced by constantly feeling hungry, hoarding or stealing food, and being underweight), unclean clothes and body, poor dental health (extensive cavities or generally poor condition of teeth), and inappropriate clothing for the season.

Manifestations of emotional abuse, verbal abuse, and emotional neglect include fear, poor physical growth, and failure to meet appropriate developmental milestones. The child may have difficulty relating to adults, impaired communication skills, and developmental delays. Behavioral manifestations include anxiety, fear, shame, aggression, delinquency, and depression.

Children who have been sexually abused may exhibit a variety of physical and behavioral signs and symptoms (Table 42–10). Bruising, bleeding, and laceration of the genital area are obvious signs of trauma (National Center for PTSD, 2011). However, sexual abuse does not always result in apparent injury. Among the many long-term consequences of child sexual abuse are ongoing feelings of shame, guilt, anger, and hostility; decreased self-esteem, which leads to increased self-destructive behavior, risk of suicide, and decreased ability to establish positive relationships in adulthood; recurrence of victimization experiences; substance abuse; and eating disorders. The results can be long lasting, with children experiencing posttraumatic stress disorder (PTSD) or substance abuse in adulthood. Factors associated with greater psychologic harm to the child include (1) a long period of abuse, (2) use of violent force or threat of violence, (3) abuse involving penetration (intercourse or oral–genital sex), and (4) abuse involving family members, especially the father or stepfather.

CLINICAL THERAPY

Diagnosis of abuse is made on the basis of a careful history and thorough physical examination. X-ray, CT, and MRI studies may be ordered to identify signs of recurrent abuse (e.g., healed fractures). Laboratory studies may involve urine culture for signs of infection or screening for sexually transmitted infections; they can also rule out other causes of bleeding such as hemophilia. Genitourinary

TABLE 42–10 Clinical Manifestations of Sexual Abuse in Children and Adolescents

- Vaginal discharge
- Blood-stained underpants or diaper
- Genital redness, pain, itching, or bruising
- Difficulty walking or sitting
- Urinary tract infection
- Sexually transmitted infection
- Somatic complaints, such as headaches or stomachaches
- Sleeping problems, such as nightmares or night terrors
- Bed-wetting
- Unwillingness to go to babysitter, family member, neighbor, or other person
- New or excessive sexual curiosity or play
- Fear of strangers
- Constant masturbation
- Curling into fetal position
- Phobias about particular places, people, or things
- Abrupt changes in school performance and attendance
- Changes in eating habits
- Abrupt changes in behavior (especially withdrawal)
- Child or adolescent female acts like a wife or mother
- Excessively seductive behavior

examination may be performed if sexual abuse is suspected. Some children are admitted directly to the hospital with the diagnosis of suspected abuse or neglect. Less obvious as a victim of abuse is the child admitted with a skull fracture who "fell off a chair."

Clinical Tip

About 8000 to 9000 U.S. children are hospitalized with fractures each year, and it is estimated that 20% to 25% of children under 1 year of age and 6% to 7% of older children experience abuse as the cause of fracture. Current guidelines of the American Academy of Pediatrics recommend skeletal survey in fractures known to be due to abuse, domestic violence, or being hit by a toy, or when there is no history of trauma that caused the fracture. From 12 to 23 months, all fractures must be evaluated by skeletal survey, and in children older than 24 months, the fracture type determines the need for skeletal survey (Wood et al., 2014).

Neglect, which is more difficult to define and identify, frequently requires hospitalization with a comprehensive medical, social, and psychiatric evaluation. Five basic categories must be considered when attempting to diagnose neglect: (1) medical care neglect (lack of necessary medical care), (2) gross safety neglect (lack of appropriate supervision), (3) physical neglect (lack of food and shelter), (4) emotional neglect, and (5) educational neglect.

All 50 states have extensive, complex statutes about reporting child abuse and neglect. A specialist must be consulted, especially if the child's testimony will be used in court.

Children do not routinely make false allegations of abuse. If indeed there is reason to believe the allegations are false, a child and adolescent therapist (psychiatrist, psychologist, psychiatric clinical nurse specialist, or social worker) with special expertise should be consulted to determine the truth. Keep in mind that children who withdraw their accusations may have been threatened or coerced into doing so. Because children who have been physically, emotionally, or sexually abused are at risk for major depression, they require skilled care by mental healthcare providers who are specially trained in this area. Initially, the treatment goals include prevention of self-destructive or other dangerous acts. Children must be encouraged to express their fears and feelings in a safe and supportive environment. Equally important is the child's need to build coping skills and self-esteem. These children must be reassured and convinced that they are in no way responsible or to blame for what happened.

Professionalism in Practice Laws Regarding Child Abuse Reporting

Every state has a child abuse law specifying the particular behaviors that define every type of abuse. Any professional who works with children and reasonably suspects that a child has been abused is required to report suspicions of abuse or neglect to the local agency for child protective services. Reports made in good faith are not liable to countersuits. However, professionals who suspect abuse and do not report it may be held responsible by the judicial system. In some states, all citizens are mandated to report suspected abuse. Check the law in your state to learn those particular details. See the U.S. Department of Health and Human Services website for state laws (www.childwelfare.gov/systemwide/laws_policies/state/can).

Individual treatment with art therapy is used initially because it is the least threatening method in the early stages of treatment, it can easily be tailored to meet the child's individual needs, and it prepares the child for other forms of treatment such as family and group therapy (Figure 42–8). Family or group therapy may be of benefit in exploring the child's concerns and feelings. Anger is common, especially in children who were abused by a trusted adult such as the father or stepfather.

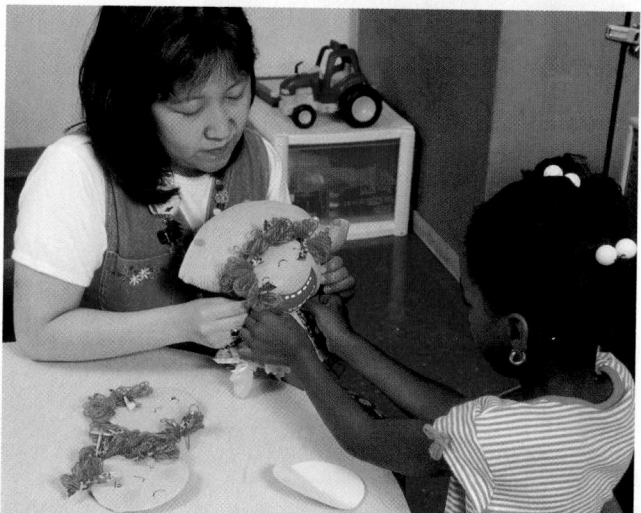

Figure 42–8 **Clinical interventions with children. Therapeutic strategies with young children involve various methods of communication, such as dramatic play and art.**

Nursing Management

Child Abuse and Neglect

Nursing Assessment and Diagnosis

Nursing assessment in instances of suspected child abuse or neglect requires a comprehensive history and physical examination, with documentation of findings. Consultation with social service agencies in the community is important if the family is receiving services.

Obtaining the history can be stressful for both the nurse and the parent. Use of therapeutic communication techniques and a quiet, unhurried environment are helpful. Be open, nonjudgmental, and calm. A statement such as "Hello, Mr. S. My name is Joan T. I'm Jonathan's nurse, and I will be asking you some questions about his overall health" may be a good start. It is important to differentiate true child abuse from cultural variations that might inaccurately be assumed to indicate abuse (Figure 42–9*A* and *B*). Obtaining information about abusive and neglectful behaviors requires a trusting relationship with parents, who are often afraid to trust any professional.

The health history sequence should include (1) parental concerns, (2) general family history, and (3) specific child history. This sequence begins with nonthreatening topics and allows the nurse to demonstrate concern before asking about abuse-related concerns. Obtain details about how injuries occurred. Document the parents' and child's own words verbatim using quotation marks. Compare reports obtained from each family member for lack of consistency and details that change over time.

It is desirable to interview the parent and child separately as well as together. Parent–child interaction during an intensive history-taking session provides an opportunity to observe the child's behavior and the parent's method of handling and responding to the child.

Data gathered during history taking are particularly important in light of physical findings. Are there discrepancies between the history and physical assessment data? Do the parents give a history of an uncontrollable, inattentive toddler when the nurse observes a child who is attentive throughout a 15-minute examination? Assess the child's general appearance, including dress and behavior during the assessment. How do the child's affect, behavior, and development compare with those of other children the same age? Document all lesions and bruising, including site, size, and color. Be aware of mongolian spots that can mistakenly be interpreted as a sign of child abuse (see Chapter 33). If there are fractures, follow the guidelines above regarding need for skeletal survey. Be alert for the signs of shaken child syndrome; this most often appears as a subtle neurologic condition. Measure head circumference and perform a neurologic examination (see Chapter 54).

Documentation of findings is important in all situations but is essential in cases of suspected child abuse and neglect. Each person who handles a laboratory specimen or other item (e.g., clothing soiled with semen) in cases of suspected child abuse must be identified in the client's record, and the specimen must never be left unattended. Record physical findings as observed. Use figure diagrams to document skin injuries. Take photographs as directed to document the location, nature, and extent of injuries.

Among the nursing diagnoses that might be appropriate for the physically abused or neglected child are the following (NANDA-I © 2014):

- *Pain, Acute,* related to inflicted injuries
- *Skin Integrity, Impaired,* related to inflicted injuries
- *Development: Delayed, Risk for,* related to lack of supportive parenting and environment
- *Nutrition, Imbalanced: Less than Body Requirements,* related to inadequate caloric intake

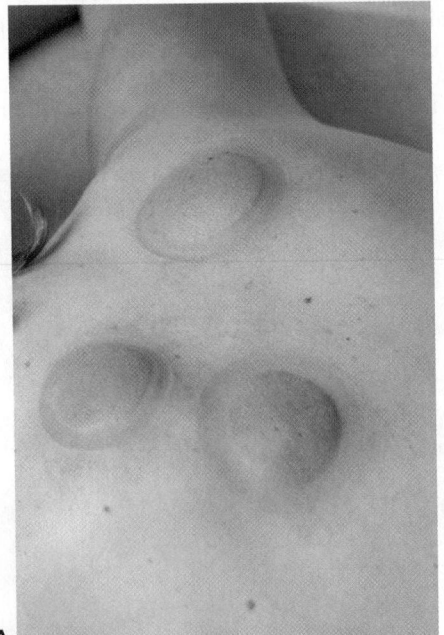

A

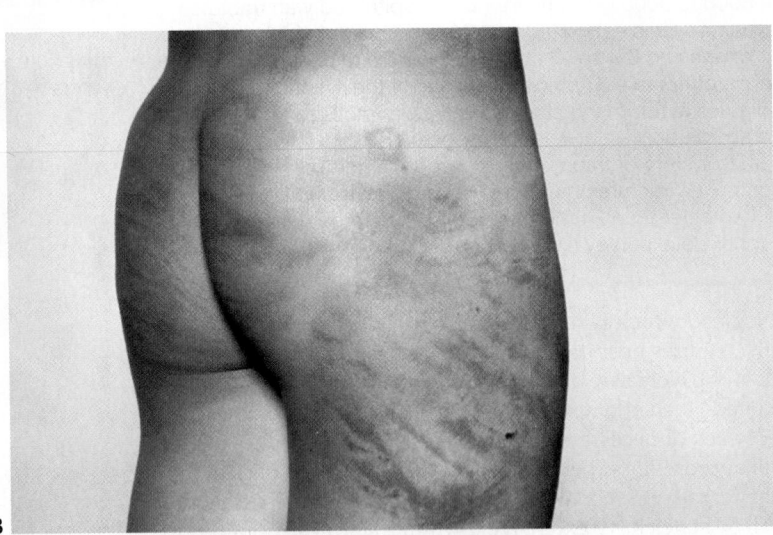

B

Figure 42–9 It is important to differentiate cultural practices, such as *A*, cupping, and *B*, coining, from signs of child abuse. Traditional treatment practices are sometimes mistaken for signs of physical abuse. Inquire about what treatments have been tried for the child at home. If unfamiliar with the treatment, ask the family members to explain what they have done. When there is lack of clarity, work with other professionals to decide if child abuse is a potential concern.

SOURCE: *A*, Doc-stock/Alamy; *B*, Biophoto Associates/Science Source.

- *Health Maintenance, Impaired,* related to lack of parental provision of child's essential needs
- *Fear* related to actual physical harm or repeated risk of injury
- *Injury, Risk for,* related to physical abuse
- *Violence: Other-Directed, Risk for (Parent),* related to inability to manage anger

Additional diagnoses that might apply to the emotionally abused or neglected child include the following (NANDA-I © 2014):

- *Coping, Defensive,* related to psychologic impairment
- *Self-Esteem, Chronic Low,* related to lack of appropriate emotional support from parents
- *Coping: Family, Disabled,* related to dysfunctional family dynamics and pattern of physical abuse

Diagnoses that might apply to the sexually abused child include the following (NANDA-I © 2014):

- *Anxiety* related to potential separation from parent
- *Rape-Trauma Syndrome* related to sexual exploitation
- *Role Performance, Ineffective,* related to domestic violence
- *Personal Identity: Disturbed,* related to disturbance of usual activities of childhood

Developing Cultural Competence Cupping and *Cao Gio*

Traditional treatment practices are sometimes mistaken for signs of physical abuse. The Chinese practice of cupping, which involves heating a bamboo cup and placing it on the skin, is a traditional treatment for headaches or abdominal pain. The Vietnamese practice of *cao gio* ("rubbing out the wind"), in which a coin or the fingers are forcefully rubbed on the chest, back, or neck, is used to treat minor ailments. Ask about marks on the skin, how they occurred, and what health practices the family uses.

Planning and Implementation

Nursing care focuses on helping to remove the child from an abusive environment, preventing further injury, providing supportive care, and reinforcing the importance of follow-up care and counseling.

PREVENT FURTHER INJURY

Work with social services and community agencies to assess the child's home environment, individuals living in the home, and the actions surrounding the abuse. Assist in removing the child from the home to temporary custody of the court or foster care of another relative if indicated. Counsel family members about abuse and refer them for appropriate therapy.

PROVIDE SUPPORTIVE CARE

Protect and treat the child's injuries (e.g., fractures, burns). Include parents in the child's treatment plan, and keep them informed about the child's progress. Even if suspected of inflicting injuries to the child, the parent is still the child's primary caretaker. Talk with the parent as you would with any parent. Be supportive of any guilt expressed. Encourage the parent to assist with the child's care. Observe parent–child interactions

and document supportive behaviors and the child's response to the parent versus other healthcare providers.

Interacting nonjudgmentally with a parent suspected of child abuse can be difficult. Nurses should talk with a colleague about any anger they feel toward such a parent or about the child's injuries or specific actions surrounding the abuse. Use team meetings to develop strategies that enable healthcare providers and other professionals to work with the parents and child.

Clinical Tip

When children have been abused, they are often frightened in new situations. Sexually abused children may resist removing clothes and may become very anxious during a physical examination or medical test. They may distrust members of the gender that abused them. When aware of a history of abuse, ask the parents or guardians how to best facilitate the child's health care. Be sensitive to fears and allow the child to wear clothing, have a support person present, or whatever may provide a sense of security. Consistency of nurses assigned to the child and the presence of a counselor may help to increase rapport and trust.

HOME CARE TEACHING

If there is any question about the child returning to a potentially dangerous situation, support the child's removal from the situation. The child may receive supervised care in the home by court order. Day care, home nursing, and social worker visits may be arranged. Parents should be referred to parent effectiveness classes, family therapy, and support groups as necessary. When a neighbor or friend is the abuser, the family may need support and legal advice when a term of incarceration is finished and the perpetrator returns to the community. Some states and communities have sexual offender laws that publicize the presence of an offender on parole within neighborhoods.

Encourage the family to inform other care providers when the child's abuse history may affect a response to care. They should be alert to signs of PTSD so they can seek assistance if the child has continuing problems (see Chapter 55).

Evaluation

Expected outcomes of nursing care for the child who has been abused or neglected include the following:

- The child maintains normal growth and development.
- A positive sense of self-esteem emerges in the child.
- Parents are provided with information and resources for stress relief.
- The child is provided with a nurturing environment.
- The child experiences no further episodes of abuse.

Münchausen Syndrome by Proxy (Factitious Disorder)

Münchausen syndrome by proxy is a potentially deadly form of child abuse that involves the fabrication of signs and symptoms of a health condition in a child. In most cases, the mother creates these fictitious signs in her child (the proxy). The victim is usually less than 6 years, and commonly less than 1 year of age. Frequently, the child's symptoms of illness are used to gain entry into the medical system to meet the abuser's own psychologic needs for attention. The perpetrator may induce illness by giving the child medications or perform other actions such as adding blood to the child's urine specimen (National Center for Biotechnology Information, 2011).

The issues of abuse are multidimensional. The child is a victim of the feigned illness, repeated hospitalizations, and invasive procedures. Equally disruptive is the deprivation of the child's daily routine caused by the periodic medical crises.

Münchausen syndrome by proxy should be suspected when unexplained, recurrent, or extremely rare conditions occur; illness is unresponsive to treatment; and the history and clinical findings are inconsistent. The most commonly reported signs and symptoms are central nervous system dysfunction, apnea, diarrhea, vomiting, fever, seizures, signs of bleeding (in urine or stool), and rashes. The parent may overdose the child on medications, such as nonprescription drugs and even syrup of ipecac, causing a variety of side effects. The symptoms occur in the presence of the same caretaker and disappear when the child is separated from that caretaker.

The child often appears uncooperative, extremely anxious, fearful, and negative. The caretaker, who in contrast appears very cooperative, competent, and loving, often expresses a desire for the child to recover. The caretaker may even suggest diagnostic procedures to try to determine "what's wrong." Characteristically, the caretaker thrives in the healthcare environment.

The cause of factitious disorder is often complex and rooted in the caretaker's own abusive or neglectful childhood. The disorder occurs in all socioeconomic classes. Often the perpetrator has some type of healthcare background, such as nursing or another allied health profession. The abuser is often young and married, and appears very involved with and interested in the child (National Institutes of Health, 2013).

A suspicion of Münchausen syndrome by proxy requires a coordinated evaluation by a collaborative care team. Members of the team must organize and communicate a strategic plan regarding collection of evidence, confrontation of the abuser, and management of the hospitalized child. The child's safety is the ultimate concern. The case must also be reported to the appropriate child protective services. Remember also that some health conditions are very hard to diagnose and that sometimes unexplained health problems are related to an underlying disease. As one possible example, see mitochondrial disease that is described in Chapter 53.

Nursing Management

Take special care to maintain a trusting relationship with the parent or guardian so that person does not become suspicious and leave the hospital. Often the best person on the team to function in the role of "trusted other" is a member of the psychiatric consultation team.

Careful documentation of parent–child interactions, presence or absence of symptoms, and other pertinent observations is essential. The child must be closely monitored. If blood is present in the child's urine, stool, or vomitus, carefully document whether the nurse was present or whether the sample was provided by the parent. Covert video surveillance may be ordered by the hospital when the syndrome is highly suspected in a particular situation. Expert consultants may be needed to ensure legal requirements for investigation are met. When enough evidence is collected to prove Münchausen syndrome by proxy, the caretaker is confronted by the healthcare provider or a member of the psychiatric team in planning with law enforcement officials.

Environmental Influences on Child Health

Environmental contaminants, poisoning, and accidental respiratory ingestion are discussed in this section. See Chapter 37 for a discussion of the effects of disasters on children and related nursing management.

Environmental Contaminants

Contaminants are **toxins**, harmful or poisonous chemicals produced by metabolism or an organism (e.g., ricin), or **toxicants**, harmful natural or synthetic chemicals not metabolically produced by an organism (Genius, Sears, Schwalfenberg, et al., 2013). These products are commonly produced during industrial manufacture, but could be released as a form of terrorism. Children are generally more vulnerable than adults to such exposures because of their developing bodies. They consume high amounts of food, water, and air per unit of body weight. Consequences to the neurologic system are particularly important to developmental and behavioral outcomes (Magzamen, Van Sickle, Rose, et al., 2011).

Knowledge of environmental contaminants and their effects on children is limited. Environmental contaminants may be found in the air, water, soil, food, complementary therapies, and various objects, such as jewelry. Ground and surface water can be contaminated by manufacturing processes, agricultural and urban runoff into streams, sewage treatment plants, landfills, and particulates in the air. Some toxicants associated with deleterious effects on the child's developing nervous system include phthalates, bisphenol A, brominated flame retardants, polycyclic aromatic hydrocarbons, and gas cooking (Jurewicz, Polanska, & Hanke, 2013).

Contaminants in the environment can influence children in complex ways. Prenatal exposure can affect the developing fetus. Exposure during lactation may bring contaminants to the breastfed baby. Environmental effects may occur as the child grows through skin contact, inhalation, or food and water ingestion. Because children are exposed to many chemicals on a daily basis, harmful exposures are often difficult to identify. One example of a known harmful agent is environmental tobacco smoke (ETS). The mother who smokes or is exposed to ETS runs an increased risk of having a baby that is small for gestational age or who dies of sudden infant death syndrome (SIDS) (see Chapter 46). The child exposed to ETS has an increased risk of occurrence and severity of asthma and other respiratory diseases. The homes of smokers have higher nicotine levels even if adults are not smoking in the house (Kassem et al., 2014).

One to 2 million migrant workers travel from their homes, often in Central or South America, to work in the U.S. farm industry each year (Schmalzried & Fallon, 2012). The children of migrant farm workers constitute a group that is at particular health risk. The farm industry presents many environmental health risks: exposure to pesticides, unsanitary drinking water, overcrowding, insect exposure, equipment hazards, poor transportation, social isolation, and poverty (Shelton et al., 2014). Children living in migrant farm worker families are more likely to have respiratory and ear infections, gastroenteritis, intestinal parasites, skin infections, unmet dental needs, poor nutrition and anemia, delayed development, and occupation injuries (Schmalzried & Fallon, 2012). Families travel frequently so provision of coordinated health care is difficult, leading to low immunization rates and academic challenges. Adolescents may even travel alone, lacking supervision by parents or other adults.

Some potentially harmful environmental exposures across various settings include the following (American Academy of Pediatrics Council on Environmental Health, 2011; Karr, 2012; Meadows-Oliver, 2012):

- Pesticides such as organophosphates, organochlorine, chlorpyrifos, dialkyl phosphates, carbamates, pyrethroids (Children may be exposed through home use, parents who work in pesticide manufacturing, garden/farm/agricultural use, and ingestion through food treated with pesticides.)
- Outdoor air pollution from automobiles, power plants, and other sources (Children spend time outside and therefore have increased exposure.)
- Indoor air pollution from dust mites, molds, lead particles from old housing, wood smoke, and other sources
- Heavy metal exposure, including lead, mercury, arsenic, and chlorine
- Substances such as polychlorinated biphenyls (PCBs) stored in fatty tissues of the mother and causing fetal exposure or in animal fats; also present in electrical wiring
- Phthalates used to make flexible plastic products, such as catheters, intravenous tubing and bags, food packaging, and toys
- Bisphenol A (BPA) used to make hard plastics, such as baby bottles, containers used for microwaving, toys, and linings of food cans (Recent legislation mandates that BPA can no longer be used in baby bottles.)

Nursing Management

Nurses are instrumental in identifying exposure to environmental toxic agents. Inquire about:

- Parental work with harmful substances such as dust and chemicals
- Age of home (homes built before 1978 or renovated in the last 6 months are at risk for contamination with chemicals)
- Safety items in home such as radon, carbon monoxide, and smoke alarms
- Child and family member with hobby requiring use of toxic materials, such as lead with stained glass work or glue with model building
- Child's consumption of nonfood products

Nurses in public health agencies often coordinate care for migrant farm workers. Evaluating living conditions and hazards through home visits is necessary. Provision of care and electronic and paper records can enhance care with distant sites where the family spends part of the year. Screening for health and developmental progression should be carried out whenever children are evaluated. In some northern U.S. communities, Head Start or other daycare centers open additional facilities during summer months when migrant families need such care while adults work in fields.

For children in all settings, consider the possibility of environmental exposure and refer for blood testing and further evaluation whenever delayed development or behavioral problems are evident. Test blood levels for contaminants such as lead (see later section). Hair, urine, and other testing may be possible as well. Identification of the toxic exposure and its removal from the environment are critical. Removal from the body by drug treatment is possible for some substances. Instruct the family in prevention of further exposure. Perform periodic growth and developmental measurements on the child and ensure return for further blood tests and other monitoring.

Poisoning

Young children are at risk for ingestion of foreign substances because of their characteristic behaviors, which involve exploration of the environment. Poisonings are the second leading cause of unintentional home-injury death and account for nearly one third of all unintentional home injuries. Annually, over 2 million calls are made for human ingestions to poison control centers, 80% for children under 6 years. About 130,000 visits to emergency departments occur, and over 800 children die from poisoning (Bronstein, Spyker, Cantilena, et al., 2012; CDC, 2013c).

Infants and toddlers commonly place objects in their mouths. Although most poisons are ingested, other routes of contamination include dermal, inhalation, and ocular. The Poison Prevention Packaging Act of 1970 mandates child protective devices for all potentially toxic substances, such as household cleansers and medications. However, many are still ingested by children.

The most dangerous toxic substances a small child may ingest include iron, antidepressants, hypoglycemic agents, cardiovascular drugs, salicylates, anticonvulsants, and illicit drugs. The five most common classifications of poisons ingested by children less than 5 years of age are cosmetics and personal care products, analgesics, household cleaning products, miscellaneous foreign bodies and toys, and topical preparations (Bronstein et al., 2012). Other common causes of poisoning include vitamins, cold and cough preparations, pesticides, and plants (e.g., Boston ivy, poinsettia, philodendron, lily-of-the-valley, daffodil bulbs, azalea, and rhododendron). Some household items are nontoxic and cause little harm; however, items that contain caustic agents or toxic chemicals can cause irreversible damage or death. Substances most often associated with a fatality in children less than 6 years of age include analgesics, plants, cold and cough preparations, and hydrocarbons (Bronstein et al., 2012).

SAFETY ALERT!

Most of the deaths resulting from poisoning occur in teens and are related to use or abuse of prescription pain medications. Pain relievers, tranquilizers, sedative, and stimulants are frequently available in homes and pose a risk for young children who take them out of curiosity and teens who may take them in an experimental manner (CDC, 2013c). When youth combine alcohol with prescription medications, the outcomes can be even more serious. Another contemporary exposure involves marijuana; states that have legal medical and personal-use marijuana practices create another potential exposure for children. The median age for children requiring care for marijuana exposure is 1.5 to 2 years (Wang et al., 2014). Nurses should inquire about toxic substances in the homes of all youth and provide safety teaching regarding ways to keep children of all ages from having access to these substances.

CLINICAL MANIFESTATIONS

The manifestations of poisoning depend on the toxin. Some common effects include altered mental status, respiratory or cardiac symptoms, seizures, vital sign changes, and gastrointestinal symptoms. See Table 42–11.

TABLE 42–11 Clinical Manifestations of Commonly Ingested Toxic Agents

TYPE	SOURCES	CLINICAL MANIFESTATIONS	CLINICAL THERAPY
Corrosives (strong acids and alkaline products that cause chemical burns of mucosal surfaces)	Batteries Oven and drain cleaners Clinitest tablets Denture cleaners Bleach Toilet bowl cleaners Hair relaxers	Severe burning pain in mouth, throat, or stomach Swelling of mucous membranes; edema of lips, tongue, and pharynx (respiratory obstruction) Violent vomiting; hemoptysis Drooling; inability to clear secretions Signs of shock Anxiety Agitation	• Do not induce vomiting! • Dilute toxin with water to prevent further damage.
Hydrocarbons (organic compounds that contain carbon and hydrogen; most are distillates of petroleum)	Gasoline Kerosene Furniture polish Lighter fluid Paint thinners	Gagging Choking Coughing Nausea Vomiting Alteration in sensorium (lethargy) Weakness Respiratory symptoms of pulmonary involvement, tachypnea, cyanosis, retractions, grunting	• Do not induce vomiting! (Aspiration of hydrocarbons places the child at high risk for pneumonia.) • Use gastric lavage for highly toxic hydrocarbons. • Provide supportive respiratory care. • Decontaminate skin by removing clothing and cleansing skin.
Acetaminophen	Many over-the-counter products	Nausea Vomiting Sweating Pallor Hepatic involvement (pain in upper right quadrant, jaundice, confusion, stupor, coagulation and bilirubin abnormalities)	• Administer the antidote *N*-acetylcysteine, which binds with the metabolite, preventing absorption and protecting the liver. • Activated charcoal may be used.
Salicylate	Products containing aspirin	Nausea Disorientation Vomiting Dehydration Diaphoresis Hyperpnea Hyperpyrexia Bleeding tendencies Oliguria Tinnitus Convulsions Coma	• Depends on amount ingested. • Induce vomiting. • Administer intravenous sodium bicarbonate, fluids, and vitamin K.
Mercury	Broken thermometers Chemicals Paints Pesticides Fungicides	Tremors Memory loss Insomnia Weight loss Diarrhea Anorexia Gingivitis	• Similar to that for lead poisoning (see text discussion).

Iron	Multiple vitamin supplements and therapeutic iron tablets	Vomiting Hematemesis Diarrhea Bloody stools Abdominal pain Metabolic acidosis Shock Seizures Coma	• Activated charcoal may be used. • Administer intravenous fluids and sodium bicarbonate. • Deferoxamine chelation therapy.

Cardiac medications	Calcium channel blockers
	Beta blockers
	Digoxin
		Bradycardia, arrhythmias, heart block
		Hypotension
		Dizziness, unsteady gait
		Altered mental status, seizures
		Nausea, vomiting
			• Administer IV fluids.
			• Administer prescribed medications:
			  • Vasopressor therapy
			  • Calcium chloride
			  • Glucagon, or high-dose regular insulin with supplemental glucose to achieve euglycemia
			  • Digoxin immune Fab

Hypoglycemic agent	Sulfonylurea	Hypoglycemia
		Tachycardia
		Diaphoresis, clammy skin
		Mental status changes, coma
			• Administer prescribed medications:
			  • Glucagon
			  • Octreotide

Source: Data from O'Donnell, K. A., & Ewald, M. B. (2011). Poisonings. In R. M. Kleigman, R. B. F. Stanton, J. St. Geme, N. F. Schor, & R. E. Behrman (Eds.), *Nelson textbook of pediatrics* (19th ed., pp. 250–270). Philadelphia, PA: Elsevier Saunders; McGregor, T., Parkar, M., & Rao, S. (2009). Evaluation and management of common childhood poisonings. *American Family Physician, 79*(5), 397–403; and Smollin, C. G. (2010). Toxicology: Pearls and pitfalls in the use of antidotes. *Emergency Medical Clinics of North America, 28,* 149–161.

CLINICAL THERAPY

Specific information about the poison is obtained from the parent to guide medical management. Blood and urine toxicology screens, as well as arterial blood gas and electrolyte testing, are performed. Testing of vomitus for the presence of medication or other poisonings may be helpful in determining the amount ingested. Other tests may include serum glucose, an electrocardiogram, serum electrolytes, and arterial blood gases. Testing of vomitus for the presence of medications or poisons may be helpful in determining the amount ingested.

In the emergency department the child's airway, breathing, circulation, and level of consciousness are assessed. The goal of treatment is to prevent further absorption of the poison and to reverse or eliminate its effects. The Poison Control Center is consulted to obtain guidance for treatment. An antidote is prescribed if one is available. Gastric lavage and activated charcoal are no longer routine therapy but may be used in some children if within 1 hour of ingestion. Cathartics or whole bowel irrigation with polyethylene glycol may be used for heavy metals or for long-acting or sustained-release medications. Syrup of ipecac is no longer recommended for treating suspected poisoning. Vomiting is rarely induced because too much of the poison may be absorbed before the agent used to cause vomiting is effective. In addition, vomiting is actually harmful when corrosives have been ingested and must absolutely be avoided in these situations.

Children with severe poisoning are admitted to the intensive care unit to carefully monitor the child and provide supportive care for the toxin's effects (e.g., arrhythmias, depressed respirations, seizures, hypotension, hypoglycemia, and electrolyte abnormalities). Potential complications of poisoning, depending on the type of poison, include respiratory and/or cardiac arrest, hypovolemic shock, liver failure, renal failure, seizures, and esophageal or tracheal burns.

Nursing Management

Poisoning

Nursing care focuses on initial emergent care and stabilization of the child with poisoning, followed by family education to reduce the risk of repeated poisoning.

Nursing Assessment and Diagnosis

Parents who suspect that their child has ingested a poison should immediately call the Poison Control Center (PCC). The PCC will advise parents about treatment to begin at home, and if the child needs treatment in the emergency department. If the child has vomited, the vomitus should be brought to the emergency department. With older children, the possibility of intentional ingestion needs to be considered.

Take a history from the family about the child's suspected ingestion substance, time, amount, and symptoms. Initial assessment focuses on airway, vital signs, and neurologic status. Assess drooling, diaphoresis, and increased or depressed respirations. Assess for wheezing, respiratory distress, or stridor. Assess for decreased responsiveness and seizure activity. Assess heart rate, skin color, capillary refill, peripheral and central pulses, and blood pressure. Assess pupils (abnormally large or pinpoint pupils may be observed). Assess mouth, lips, and tongue for corrosive burns or edema. Assess breath for unusual odor. Assess the child for vomiting and diarrhea. Assess vomitus for presence of medication or other ingested substances. Determine the child's height and weight or use a length-based tape to determine medication dosages and equipment sizes.

Nursing diagnoses for the child with ingestion of a toxic substance may include (NANDA-I © 2014):

- *Airway Clearance, Ineffective,* related to excessive secretion effect of toxic substance
- *Gas Exchange, Impaired,* related to depressed neurologic status
- *Aspiration, Risk for,* related to depressed neurologic status and vomiting
- *Cardiac Output, Decreased,* related to effects of toxic substance
- *Injury, Risk for,* related to repeated occurrence of poisoning
- *Family Processes, Interrupted,* related to poisoning of a family member

Planning and Implementation

Emergency care focuses on airway and hemodynamic stability, removal of toxic agents, and support of the family. The child is attached to pulse oximetry and cardiorespiratory monitors. An intravenous line is started for the administration of fluids and an antidote, if available. When activated charcoal is prescribed, it may be in a ready-to-drink solution in an opaque container, or it may need to be mixed with sorbitol or apple juice to encourage the child to drink it. Cover the cup so the child does not see the black liquid, and provide a straw to prevent spillage. Once immediate care has been provided, nursing care shifts to providing emotional support and preventing recurrence.

PROVIDE EMOTIONAL SUPPORT

Wait until the child is out of immediate danger before questioning parents in detail about the incident. Encourage parents to express feelings of anger, guilt, or fear about the incident.

PREVENT RECURRENCE

Discuss with parents the need to supervise infants and young children at all times. Ask parents how medicines and cleaning agents are stored and whether the house contains any plants. Teach parents proper methods of childproofing the home. Have the PCC number readily available. Suggest measures for preventing recurrence of poisoning. (See *Teaching Highlights: Avoiding Childhood Poisoning.*)

The toll-free number for the American Association of Poison Control Centers (AAPCC) is 1-800-222-1222. The number can be accessed from anywhere in the United States and Puerto Rico, and the caller will be connected to the nearest poison control center.

Evaluation

Expected outcomes for nursing care of the child with poisoning include:

- The child maintains an open airway, effective gas exchange, and ventilatory function.
- The child is free from wheezing, coughing, pneumonia, or other signs indicating aspiration.
- The child's heart rate and blood pressure remain stable and appropriate for age.
- Neurologic status is appropriate for age.
- The family and child (if older) verbalize understanding of preventive measures and demonstrate measures to improve home environment safety.

Ingestion of Foreign Objects

There are about 100,000 cases of ingestion of foreign objects by children under 5 years of age annually in the United States. Coins, parts of toys, buttons, batteries, and glass are common objects ingested by young children (Bronstein et al., 2012). Adults often witness infants and young children ingesting foreign bodies, and older children will usually report swallowing a foreign object. Most small, round, smooth objects may not cause any clinical distress. However, if the foreign body is lodged in the esophagus, children may present with substernal pain, drooling, and dysphagia. Some children may exhibit respiratory symptoms including wheezing or coughing.

Serious complications can occur following foreign body ingestion. These complications include perforation of the intestinal tract, the most serious sequela of foreign body ingestion. Sharp objects are associated with a higher perforation rate than dull objects; perforations commonly occur in the region of the ileocecal valve. Development of strictures at the site of a retained foreign body may also occur. Respiratory complications arise if the object becomes lodged in the trachea, bronchi, or lungs. See Chapter 46 for care of the child with a foreign body airway obstruction.

Many ingested foreign bodies in children are radiopaque, so radiographs of the neck, chest, esophagus, and abdomen are useful tools for verifying ingestion and identifying the location of the object. Most foreign bodies pass spontaneously through the gastrointestinal system and are eliminated through stool. However, foreign bodies may become lodged in the esophagus and pose a significant risk to the child. Endoscopic examination

---

TEACHING HIGHLIGHTS | Avoiding Childhood Poisoning

Families with children require instructions for avoiding childhood poisoning. Teach family members these interventions to help avoid childhood poisonings:
- Place household cleaners, medications, vitamins, and other potentially poisonous substances out of the reach of children or in locked cabinets.
- Keep alcohol, marijuana, and prescription medications out of access for all youth, including teens.
- Use warning stickers such as Mr. Yuk on all containers.
- Buy products with child-resistant caps.
- Store products in their original containers.
- Never place household cleansers or other products in food or beverage containers.
- Remove all houseplants from the child's play areas.
- Put the poison control center phone number by every phone in the house.
- Use caution when visiting other settings that are not childproofed (e.g., grandparents' homes). Remember that visitors may have pills in their purses or pockets that are easily reached by children.

and retrieval of the ingested foreign body may be necessary. Potentially harmful objects such as batteries, sharp objects, and magnets are removed surgically.

Nursing Management

Nursing care centers on supporting the child, providing collaborative assistance in the identification and removal of the foreign body, and teaching the child and family measures to reduce reoccurrence. Assess the child for drooling, wheezing, substernal pain, dysphagia, and coughing. Obtain a thorough history from the family. Determine, if possible, what was ingested, when the ingestion occurred, and any symptoms that the child experienced. Assess breath sounds.

Prepare the child for radiologic studies. Explain the procedures and reassure the child and family during the studies. Prepare for endoscopic examination and/or retrieval if necessary. If the foreign object is in the stomach and the child is to be observed for natural excretion of the object, explain monitoring of stools to parents. Suggest the use of tongue blades to examine stools for presence of the foreign body and to report if the object has not been passed within the expected time frame (generally 48 hours). Encourage the family to return for further radiologic examinations to determine the foreign object's progress of passage.

Partner with the family and assist them in establishing a safe home environment for the child. Encourage the family to keep all small items out of the child's reach and to ensure the child is monitored at all times. Expected outcomes for nursing care of the child who has ingested a foreign body include removal of the foreign body, reduction in risk, and family verbalization of preventive measures to reduce risk of ingestion of foreign bodies.

Lead Poisoning

Lead poisoning has been successfully prevented in many areas of the United States, with a substantial decline in lead levels from the mid-1970s. The average blood lead level for children is now 1.9 mcg/dL, down from 15 mcg/dL in 1976. Approximately 450,000 U.S. children (1%) from 1 to 5 years of age have blood lead levels above the recommended upper level of 5 mcg/dL. There is no safe level of lead exposure—even children with blood lead levels lower than 10 mcg/dL have been reported to have a decrease in cognition (CDC, 2012c).

Lead in paint is the most common source of lead exposure for preschool children. Children are also exposed to lead when they ingest contaminated food, water, and soil or when they inhale dust contaminated with lead. Paints on toys and crafts from some foreign countries may contain lead; unless such products are certified safe they should not be used by children.

Children are at greater risk for lead poisoning because they absorb and retain more lead in proportion to their weight than adults do. Lead is particularly harmful to children under the age of 7 years.

CLINICAL MANIFESTATIONS

Lead interferes with normal cell function, primarily of the nervous system, blood cells, and kidneys, and adversely affects the metabolism of vitamin D and calcium. Clinical manifestations depend on the degree of toxicity. Neurologic effects include decreased IQ scores, cognitive deficits, impaired hearing, and growth delays. Impaired mental function can occur with blood levels even lower than 5 mcg/dL. Lead ingestion by a woman during pregnancy can result in fetal malformations, reduced

TABLE 42–12 Clinical Manifestations of Lead Poisoning

LEVEL	CLINICAL MANIFESTATIONS
Less than 9 mcg/dL	Generally asymptomatic although subtle neurologic effects may be present with any exposure
10–19 mcg/dL	Mild impairment in growth, fine motor skills, and cognition Anemia
20–44 mcg/dL	General fatigue and motor impairment Difficulty concentrating Paresis or paralysis, tremor Headache Diffuse abdominal pain, vomiting, weight loss, constipation Anemia
45–69 mcg/dL	Colic (intermittent, severe abdominal cramps), anorexia, vomiting Hyperirritability Increased lethargy Lead line (blue-black) on gingival tissue
Over 70 mcg/dL	Encephalopathy, which may lead abruptly to seizures, changes in consciousness, coma, and death Ataxia

Source: Adapted from Agency for Toxic Substances & Disease Registry. (2011). *Lead toxicity clinical evaluation.* Atlanta, GA: Author.

birth weight, and premature birth. Severe lead poisoning, which can result in encephalopathy, coma, and death, is now rare in developed countries.

Once in the body, lead accumulates in the blood, soft tissues (kidney, bone marrow, liver, and brain), bones, and teeth. Lead that is absorbed by the bones and teeth is released slowly; thus exposure to even small doses, over time, can result in dangerously high levels of lead in the body. See Table 42–12.

CLINICAL THERAPY

An environmental history should be obtained for all children. For those with risk of elevated lead (Pb) levels (living in homes completed before 1978, receiving Medicaid, and/or living in poverty), blood screening should be considered (CDC, 2012c, 2014c). Follow-up testing is required in 2 to 3 months. Because most children are asymptomatic, careful history and identification of risk factors will guide healthcare providers in identifying children who need blood testing for lead. Children with elevated Pb levels require a full medical evaluation, including a detailed environmental and behavioral history, physical examination, and tests for iron deficiency. Interventions to remove sources of lead from the child's environment are necessary. Blood screening is performed at 12 and 24 months, as well as for children in these groups who are 36 to 72 months but not previously screened. A venous blood sample is preferred because it reduces the risk of specimen contamination from lead on the skin. Capillary specimens are used in some cases with careful skin preparation. Any elevation in a capillary specimen must be confirmed by a venous sample. A blood Pb level below 5 mcg/dL is considered acceptable, although it may still not screen out all children with impaired development due to lead. *Healthy People 2020* objectives aim at decreasing blood levels of children and the number of children with elevated levels (USDHHS, 2011).

Healthy People 2020

(EH-8.1) Eliminate elevated blood levels in children

(EH-8.2) Reduce the mean blood levels in children from 1 to 5 years to 1.4 mcg/mL

Children with very high blood Pb levels require medical treatment. For levels above 45 mcg/dL, chelation therapy is considered for administration. Children with blood Pb levels greater than 70 mcg/dL are critically ill from lead poisoning and require immediate chelation therapy and interventions to provide a lead-free environment.

Chelation is a reaction in which an organic compound, containing carbonyl (CO) and hydroxyl (OH) groups, coordinates with a metal to form a firmly bound ringlike structure. Chelation therapy for lead poisoning involves the administration of an agent that binds with lead, decreasing its effects and increasing its rate of excretion from the body. Calcium disodium ethylenediamine tetraacetate ($CaNa_2$ EDTA) IM or IV, dimercaprol (BAL) deep IM, penicillamine PO, or succimer (DMSA) PO may be used. Children with blood Pb levels between 25 and 69 mcg/dL receive $CaNa_2$ EDTA for 5 to 7 days, followed by a rest period and then a second chelation treatment. Children with Pb-B levels greater than 70 mcg/dL are given both BAL and $CaNa_2$ EDTA, followed by a rest period and a second chelation treatment using $CaNa_2$ EDTA alone. Chelation therapy has the potential for serious side effects. $CaNa_2$ EDTA can cause tubular necrosis and cardiac arrhythmia; IM administration is painful, so it is generally given IV. BAL can lead to hypertension, tachycardia, headache, fever, or nephrotoxicity. Penicillamine is used only when treatment with other drugs is not effective because of its multisystem side effects. Succimer is associated with GI side effects, rash, headache, and neurologic symptoms. Long-term follow-up of children receiving chelation therapy is essential. The child should never be discharged unless a lead-free home environment has been ensured.

Nursing Management

Nursing care centers on screening, education, and follow-up. Nurses often work with state and local health officials to plan screening for children at high risk of lead exposure. Ask parents about the child's development and eating habits and be alert for risk of lead exposure. Educate parents about sources of lead in the environment and techniques to reduce exposure. Make home visits to evaluate exposure to lead and to perform individualized teaching. Emphasize the importance of housekeeping interventions to reduce exposure to lead dust. These interventions include damp mopping of hard surfaces, floors, window sills, and baseboards; washing the child's hands and face before meals; and frequent washing of toys and pacifiers. Be alert that home renovation can significantly increase the levels of lead in dust.

Teach parents the importance of including foods high in iron and calcium in the child's diet to counteract losses of these minerals associated with lead exposure. The child should eat meals at regular intervals because lead is absorbed more readily on an empty stomach.

Be sure that parents understand the importance of follow-up testing of lead levels. If the child is developmentally delayed, refer the family to an infant stimulation or early intervention program. Referral to social services and either a visiting nurse or home healthcare nurse may also be appropriate.

Nurses who administer chelating drugs are challenged by the complexity of treatment and required care. Chelation should always be managed by experts in such care, and in consultation with the Lead Poisoning Prevention Branch of the National Center for Environmental Health of the CDC. Careful monitoring of liver and kidney function, cardiac, GI, and neurologic systems is needed for all chelating drugs. Administration for some drugs is via IM route and is painful; children will need skilled nursing and child life specialist care.

Expected outcomes of nursing care for the child with lead or other poisoning include the following:

- The child exhibits normal growth and development, including cognition.
- Adequate nutritional intake is ensured for the child.
- Lead or other poisons are removed from the child's environment.
- The family expresses understanding of measures to establish a safe environment for the child.

Focus Your Study

- Many of the major morbidities and mortalities of childhood and adolescence are related to social and environmental factors.
- The theories of ecologic development and resilience provide frameworks to assess interactions of children and their environments, and to mitigate risk factors.
- Poverty and homelessness are pervasive and influence many health outcomes.
- Substance use, particularly of alcohol and drugs, poses risks to youth and requires screening, prevention, and cessation programs appropriate for developmental age.
- Violence can be directed at children, and children can be the perpetrators of violence. The nurse plans interventions for an array of abusive situations such as child abuse, sexual abuse, and domestic violence.
- Environmental contaminants affect the health of children, from the prenatal period through childhood. Medicines, plants, pesticides, lead, and other household products pose risks at all ages, even though most poisonings occur in children under 5 years of age.

Clinical Reasoning in Action

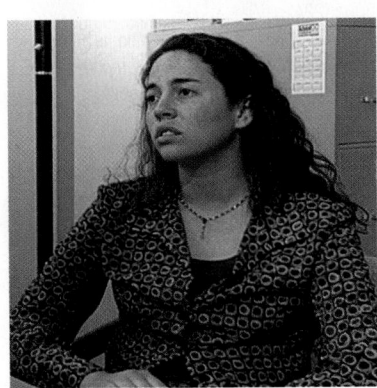

You are working at the inpatient adolescent psychiatric unit where there are approximately 20 teens between the ages of 12 and 17 years old. The teens are admitted for several different diagnoses, including depression, suicide attempts, bipolar disorders, and eating disorders. The nurses are in charge of medication administration, vital signs, unit safety issues, physical assessments, and basic therapeutic interventions. You are working with a client named Cindy, 15 years old, who was admitted because of a suicide attempt and has been given a dual diagnosis of bulimia nervosa and depression. She has had extreme weight loss and gain over the past year and is currently 67 inches tall and weighs 140 lb. She has stated she tried to commit suicide with a knife because she was upset over the loss of her boyfriend. She thought she was fat and was trying to

lose weight by using laxatives and vomiting after meals. There is a family history of depression and substance abuse, but Cindy denies any substance use. She lives with her mother and has no contact with her father. She does not feel she has anyone to discuss her feelings with, and states her mother is gone from the house frequently. Cindy admits to often eating fast food and snacking on other junk food and soda. She has been in the hospital for 2 weeks and was resistant to treatment at first, but seems to be improving with therapy and medication. She has lost 3 lb while she has been hospitalized, and her average vital signs are temperature 98.7°F, pulse 70, respirations 12, and blood pressure 110/70 mmHg. (Review the content on bulimia in Chapter 32 to answer the following questions.)

1. What are some of the signs of bulimia Cindy may exhibit?
2. What can you tell the mother about Cindy's vital signs and stability at this time? How can you explain the weight loss?
3. What behavioral signs of bulimia should be part of your nursing assessment of Cindy while she is hospitalized?
4. What are the treatment recommendations for Cindy?

References

Add Health Study. (2014). *Add Health: The National Longitudinal Study of Adolescent Health*. Retrieved from http://www.cpc.unc.edu/projects/addhealth

Agency for Healthcare Research and Quality (AHRQ). (2013). *Most frequent conditions in U.S. hospitals*. Rockville, MD: Author.

Agency for Toxic Substances & Disease Registry. (2011). *Lead toxicity clinical evaluation*. Atlanta, GA: Author.

Allan, E. J., & Madden, M. (2011). The nature and extent of college student hazing. *International Journal of Adolescent Medicine and Health, 24*(1), 83–90.

Allen, E. S., Rhoades, G. K., Stanley, S. M., & Markman, H. J. (2011). On the home front: Stress for recently deployed army couples. *Family Process, 50*, 235–247.

American Academy of Child and Adolescent Psychiatry (AACAP). (2013). *Substance use resource center*. Retrieved from http://www.aacap.org/AACAP/AACAP /Families_and_Youth/Resource_Centers/Substance _Use_Resource_Center/Home.aspx

American Academy of Pediatrics. (2011). *Bullies beat down self-esteem*. Retrieved from http://www .healthychildren.org

American Academy of Pediatrics Council on Community Pediatrics. (2013). Providing care for children and adolescents facing homelessness and housing insecurity. *Pediatrics, 131*, 1206–1210.

American Academy of Pediatrics Council on Environmental Health. (2011). Chemical-management policy: Prioritizing children's health. *Pediatrics, 127*(5), 983–990.

American Academy of Pediatrics Committee on Practice and Ambulatory Medicine, Bright Futures Periodicity Schedule Workgroup. (2014). 2014 recommendations for pediatric preventive health care. *Pediatrics, 133*, 568–570.

American Psychiatric Association. (2012). *LGBT—Sexual orientation*. Retrieved from http://www.psychiatry .org/mental-health/people/lgbt-sexual-orientation

Annie E. Casey Foundation. (2011). *No place for kids: The case for reducing juvenile incarceration*. Baltimore, MD: Author.

Aranda, M. C., Middleton, L. S., Flake, E., & Davis, B. E. (2011). Psychosocial screening in children with wartime-deployed parents. *Military Medicine, 176*, 402–407.

Audrain-McGovern, J., Stevens, S., Murray, P. J., Kinsman, S., Zuckoff, A., Pletcher, J., . . . Wileyto, E. P. (2011). The efficacy of motivational interviewing versus brief advice for adolescent smoking behavior change. *Pediatrics, 128*(1), e101–e111.

August-Brady, M., & Adamshick, P. (2013). Oh, the things you will learn: Taking undergraduate research to the homeless shelter. *Journal of Nursing Education, 52*, 342–345.

Balodis, I. M., Wynne-Edwards, K. E., & Olmstead, M. C. (2010). The other side of the curve: Examining the relationship between pre-stressor physiological responses and stress reactivity. *Psychoneuroendocrinology, 35*, 1363–1373.

Benard, B. (2014). *The foundations of the resiliency framework*. Retrieved from http://www.resiliency .com/free-articles-resources/the-foundations-of-the -resiliency-framework/

Broberg, M. C., & Nield, L. S. (2013). Helping adolescents kick the habit. *Consultant for Pediatrics, August 2013*, 375–377.

Bronfenbrenner, U. (2005). *Making human beings human: Bioecologic perspectives*. Thousand Oaks, CA: Sage.

Bronstein, A. C., Spyker, D. A., Cantilena, L. R., Rumack, B. H., & Dart, R. C. (2012). 2011 annual report of

the American Association of Poison Control Centers' National Poisoning Data System (NPDS): 29th annual report. *Clinical Toxicology, 50*, 911–1164.

Catledge, C. B., Scharer, K., & Fuller, S. (2012). Assessment and identification of deliberate self-harm in adolescents and young adults. *The Journal for Nurse Practitioners, 8*, 299–305.

Centers for Disease Control and Prevention (CDC). (2011a). *Youth and tobacco use*. Retrieved from http://www.cdc.gov/tobacco/data_statistics/fact _sheets/youth_data/tobacco_use/index.htm

Centers for Disease Control and Prevention (CDC). (2011b). Violence-related firearm deaths among residents of metropolitan areas and cities—United States, 2006–2007. *Morbidity and Mortality Weekly Report, 60*, 573–578.

Centers for Disease Control and Prevention (CDC). (2012a). Vital signs: Unintentional injury deaths in persons aged 0–19 years—United States, 2000–2009. *Morbidity and Mortality Weekly Report, 61*, 270–276.

Centers for Disease Control and Prevention (CDC). (2012b). Tattoo-associated nontuberculous mycobacterium skin infections, multiple states 2011–2012. *Morbidity and Mortality Weekly Report, 61*, 653–656.

Centers for Disease Control and Prevention (CDC). (2012c). *Low level lead exposure harms children: A renewed call for primary prevention*. Retrieved from http://www.cdc.gov/nceh/lead/acclpp/final _document_030712.pdf

Centers for Disease Control and Prevention (CDC). (2013a). Notes from the field: Electronic cigarette use among middle and high school students—United States, 2011–2012. *Morbidity and Mortality Weekly Report, 62*, 729–730.

Centers for Disease Control and Prevention (CDC). (2013b). *National youth tobacco survey*. Retrieved from http://www.cdc.gov/tobacco/data_statistics /surveys/nyts

Centers for Disease Control and Prevention (CDC). (2013c). *A national action plan for child injury prevention: reducing poisoning injuries in children*. Retrieved from http://www.cdc.gov/safechild/NAP /overviews/poison.html

Centers for Disease Control and Prevention (CDC). (2014a). Youth risk behavior surveillance—United States, 2013. *Morbidity and Mortality Weekly Report, 63*(SS04), 1–172.

Centers for Disease Control and Prevention (CDC). (2014b). *Child maltreatment*. Retrieved from http://www.cdc.gov/violenceprevention/pdf /childmaltreatment-facts-at-a-glance.pdf

Centers for Disease Control and Prevention (CDC). (2014c). Lead screening and prevalence of blood lead levels in children aged 1–2 years—Child blood lead surveillance system, United States, 2002–2010, and National Health and Nutrition Examination Survey, United States, 1999–2010. *Morbidity and Mortality Weekly Report, 63*(02), 36–42.

Chandra, A., Mosher, W. D., Copen, C., & Sionean, C. (2011). Sexual behavior, sexual attraction, and sexual identity in the United States: Data from the 2006–2008 National Survey of Family Growth. *National Health Statistics Report, 36*, 1–36.

Childhelp. (2013). *Child abuse statistics and facts*. Retrieved from https://www.childhelp.org/child-abuse-statistics/

Child Trends. (2015). *Preventing violence: Understanding and addressing determinants of youth violence in the United States*. Retrieved from http://www.childtrends .org/wp-content/uploads/2015/03/2015-10 PreventingViolence21.pdf

Children and Divorce. (2013). *Children divorce statistics*. Retrieved from http://www.children-and-divorce .com/children-divorce-statistics.html

Children's Defense Fund. (2014). *State of America's children 2014*. Retrieved from http://www .childrensdefense.org/child-research-data-publications /data/2014-soac.pdf?utm_source=2014-SOAC -PDF&utm_medium=link&utm_campaign=2014 -SOACChildStats. (2011). *Child care*. Retrieved from http://www .childstats.gov/americaschildren09 /famsoc3.asp

Cross, T. P., Matthews, B., Tonmyr, L., Scott, D., & Ouimet, C. (2012). Child welfare policy and practice on children's exposure to domestic violence. *Child Abuse and Neglect, 36*(3), 210–216.

Cyberbullying Research Center. (2011). *Research*. Retrieved from http://cyberbullying.us/research.php

Davidov, D. M., Nadorff, M. R., Jack, S. M., Coben, J. H., & NFP IPV Research Team. (2012). Nurse home visitors' perspective of mandatory reporting of children's exposure to intimate partner violence to child protection agencies. *Public Health Nursing, 29*(5), 412–423.

Dunn, W. L., & Craig, G. J. (2013). *Understanding human development* (3rd ed.). Upper Saddle River, NJ: Pearson Education.

Elkind, D. (2007). *The hurried child: 25th anniversary edition*. Cambridge, MA: Da Capo Lifelong Publishing.

Fakhouri, T. H. I., Hughes, J. P., Burt, V. L., Song, M., Fulton, J. E., & Ogden, C. L. (2014). *Physical activity in U.S. youth aged 12–15 years, 2012*. NCHS data brief, no 141. Hyattsville, MD: National Center for Health Statistics.

Federal Interagency Forum on Child and Family Statistics. (2015). *America's children: Key national indicators of well-being*. Washington, DC: U.S. Government Printing Office. Retrieved from http://www.childstats .gov/americaschildren/eco1.asp

Genius, S. J., Sears, M. E., Schwalfenberg, G., Hope, J., & Bernhoft, R. (2013). Clinical detoxification: Elimination of persistent toxicants from the human body. *Scientific World Journal, June 6*, 238–347. doi: 10.0055/2013/238347

Havens, J. R., Young, A. M., & Havens, C. E. (2011). Nonmedical prescription drug use in a nationally representative sample of adolescents: Evidence of greater use among rural adolescents. *Archives of Pediatrics and Adolescent Medicine, 165*, 250–255.

Hazing Prevention. (2011). *Hazing information*. Retrieved from http://www.hazingprevention.org/hazing -information.html

Henderson, N., Bernard, B., & Sharp-Light, N. (2007). *Resiliency in action*. Ojai, CA: Resiliency in Action.

Juhas, E., & English, J. C. (2013). Tattoo-associated complications. *Journal of Pediatric and Adolescent Gynecology, 26*, 125–129.

Jurewicz, J., Polanska, K., & Hanke, W. (2013). Exposure to widespread environmental toxicants and children's cognitive development and behavioral problems. *International Journal of Occupational Medicine and Environmental Health, 26*, 185–204.

Karr, C. (2012). Children's environmental health in agricultural settings. *Journal of Agromedicine, 17*(2), 127–139.

Kassem, N. O., Daffa, R. M., Liles, S., Jackson, S. R., Kassem, N. O., Younis, M. A., . . . Hovell, M. F. (2014). Children's exposure to secondhand and thirdhand smoke carcinogens and toxicants in homes of hookah smokers. *Nicotine and Tobacco Research, 16*, 961–75.

Kerker, B. D., Bainbridge, J., Kennedy, J., Bennani, Y., Agerton, T., Marder, D., . . . Thorpe, L. E. (2011). A population-based assessment of the health of homeless families in New York City, 2001–2003. *American Journal of Public Health, 101*, 546–553.

KidsHealth. (2014). *How TV affects your child*. Retrieved from http://kidshealth.org/parent/positive/family /tv_affects_child.html

Laughlin, L. (2013). *Who's minding the kids? Child care arrangements: Spring 2011*. Retrieved from http: //www.census.gov/prod/2013pubs/p70-135.pdf

Lehner, K. R., & Baumann, M. H. (2013). Psychoactive "bathsalts": Compounds, mechanisms, and toxicities. *Neuropsychopharmacology Reviews, 38*, 242–244.

Lynn, C. J., Acri, M. C., Goldstein, L., Bannon, W., Beharie, N., & McKay, M. M. (2014). Improving youth mental health through family-based prevention in family homeless shelters. *Child and Youth Service Review, 44*, 243–248.

Magzamen, S., Van Sickle, D., Rose, L. D., & Cronk, C. (2011). Environmental pediatrics. *Pediatric Annals, 40*(3), 144–151.

McGraw, M., & McGraw, L. (2012). Bath salts: Not as harmless as they sound. *Journal of Emergency Nursing, 38*(6), 582–588.

Meadows-Oliver, M., (2012). Environmental toxicants: Lead and mercury. *Journal of Pediatric Health Care, 26*, 213–215.

National Association for the Education of Young Children. (2010). *Introduction to the NAEYC early childhood program standards and accreditation criteria: Program standards*. Retrieved from http://www .naeyc.org/accreditation

National Center for Biotechnology Information. (2011). *Münchausen syndrome by proxy*. Retrieved from http://www.ncbi.nih.gov/pubmedhealth /PNH0002522/

National Center for Health Statistics & National Vital Statistics System. (2012). *Fatal injury reports, 2008*. Retrieved from http://webapppa.cdc.gov/cgi-bin /broker.exe

National Center for PTSD. (2011). *Child sexual abuse*. Retrieved from http://www.ptsd.va.gov/public/pages /child-sexual-abuse.asp

National Center on Family Homelessness. (2015). *The characteristics and needs of families experiencing homelessness*. Retrieved from http://www .familyhomelessness.org

National Institute on Alcohol Abuse and Alcoholism. (n.d.). *Snapshot of underage drinking*. Retrieved from http: //www.niaaa.nih.gov

National Institute on Drug Abuse. (2011). *NIDA InfoFacts: Club drugs*. Retrieved from http://www.nida/nih.gov /Infofacts/clubdrugs.html and http://www.drugabuse .gov/drugpages.clubdrugs.html

National Institutes of Health. (2013). *Münchausen syndrome by proxy*. Retrieved from http://www.nlm.nih .gov/medlineplus/ency/article/001555.htm

O'Donnell, K. A., & Ewald, M. B. (2011). Poisonings. In R. M. Kleigman, R. B. F. Stanton, J. St. Geme, N. F. Schor, & R. E. Behrman (Eds.), *Nelson textbook of pediatrics* (19th ed., pp. 250–270). Philadelphia, PA: Elsevier Saunders.

Owen, D. C., Armstrong, M. L., Koch, J. R., & Roberts, A. E. (2013). College students with body art: Well-being or high-risk behavior? *Journal of Psychosocial Nursing and Mental Health Services, 51*, 20–28.

Rodriguez, J., Applebaum, J., Stephenson-Hunter, C., Tinio, A., & Shapiro, A. (2013). Cooking, health eating, fitness and fun (CHEFFs): Qualitative evaluation of a nutrition education program for children living at urban family homeless shelters. *American Journal of Public Health, 103*(Suppl 2), S361–S367.

Sapienza, J. K., & Masten, A. S. (2011). Understanding and promoting resilience in children and youth. *Current Opinion in Psychiatry, 24*, 267–273.

Schmalzried, H. D., & Fallon, L. F. (2012). Reducing barriers associated with delivering health care services to migratory agricultural workers. *Rural and Remote Health, 12*(3), 2088.

Schneider, S. K., O'Donnell, L., Stueve, A., & Coulter, R. W. S. (2012). Cyberbullying, school bullying, and psychological distress: A regional census of high school students. *American Journal of Public Health, 102*, 171–177.

Sexuality Information and Education Council of the United States. (n.d.) *Questions and answers: LGBTQ youth*. Retrieved from http://www.siecus.org/index .cfm?fuseaction=page.viewpage&pageid=605& gran dparentID=477&parentID=591

Shelton, J. F., Geraghty, E. M., Tancredi, D. J., Delwiche, L. D., Schmidt, R. J., Ritz, B., . . . Herty-Picciotto, I. (2014) Neurodevelopmental disorders and prenatal residential proximity to agricultural pesticides: The CHARGE study. *Environmental Health Perspectives, 122*, 1103–1109.

Slopen, N., McLaughlin, K. A., & Shonkoff, J. P. (2014). Intervention to improve cortisol regulation in children: A systematic review. *Pediatrics, 133*, 312–326.

Smith, B. D. (2011). Adolescent self-injury: Evaluation, referral, and treatment. *Consultant for Pediatricians, June 2011*, 190–195.

Smollin, C. G. (2010). Toxicology: Pearls and pitfalls in the use of antidotes. *Emergency Medical Clinics of North America, 28*, 149–161.

Sullivan, K. M., Bottorff, J., & Reid, C. (2011). Does mother's smoking influence girls' smoking more than boys' smoking? A 20-year review of the literature using a sex- and gender-based analysis. *Substance Use and Misuse, 46*, 656–668.

Tsitsika, A. K., Barlou, E., Andrie, E., Dimitropoulou, C., Tzavela, E. C., Janidian, M., & Tsolia, M. (2014). Bullying behaviors in children and adolescents: "An ongoing story." *Frontiers in Public Health, 2.* doi: 10.3389/fpubh.2014.00007

U.S. Department of Health and Human Services (USDHHS). (2011). *Healthy People 2020.* Retrieved from http://www.healthypeople.gov/2020

U.S. Environmental Protection Agency. (2014). *Information for child care providers on environmental tobacco smoke.* Retrieved from http://www2.epa.gov/childcare /information-child-care-providers-about-environmental -tobacco-smoke

Wang, G. S., Roosevelt, G., Le Lait, M. C., Martinez, E. M., Bucher-Bartelson, B., Bronstein, A. C., & Heard, K. (2014). Association of unintentional pediatric exposure with decriminalization of marijuana in the United States. *Annals of Emergency Medicine, 63*, 684–689.

Wood, J. N., Fakeye, O., Feudtner, C., Mondestin, V., Localio, R., & Rubin, D. M. (2014). Development of guidelines for skeletal survey in young children with fractures. *Pediatrics, 134*, 45–53.

World Health Organization. (2014). *Global status report on violence prevention.* Geneva, Switzerland: World Health Organization.

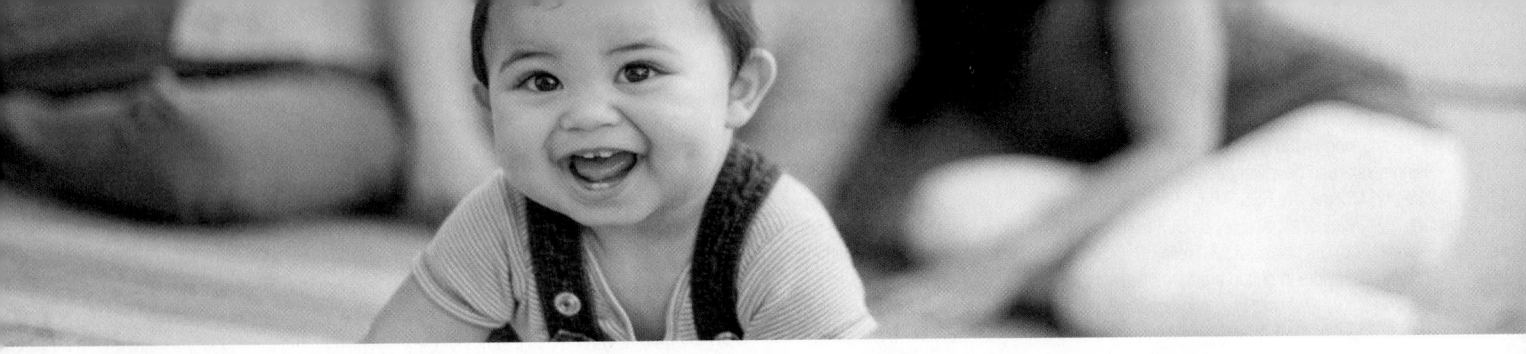

Chapter 43
Immunizations and Communicable Diseases

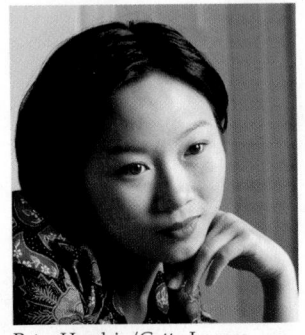

Peter Hendrie/Getty Images

We came in today because Chang has a fever. I know Lian and Chang need immunizations. Lian will be going to kindergarten in the fall, so it's very important for her to get all of the immunizations she needs now.

—Mother of Lian, 5 years old, and Chang, 2 years old

Learning Outcomes

43.1 Compare the vulnerability of young children and adults to communicable diseases.

43.2 Propose strategies to control the spread of infection in healthcare and community settings and the home.

43.3 Examine the role that vaccines play in reducing and eliminating communicable diseases.

43.4 Select the appropriate vaccines to administer to an infant, a toddler, a child entering kindergarten, an older school-age child, and an adolescent.

43.5 Plan the nursing care for children of all ages needing immunizations.

43.6 Outline a plan to maintain the potency of vaccines.

43.7 Create a parent education session that focuses on the care of infants and children with a fever.

43.8 Recognize common infectious and communicable diseases.

43.9 Develop a nursing care plan for the child with a common communicable disease.

A **communicable disease** is an infection often caused by **direct transmission** (from one person or animal to another by body fluid contact), via **indirect transmission** (to a person by contact with contaminated objects), or by *vectors* (ticks, mosquitoes, other insects). An **infectious disease** is any communicable disease caused by microorganisms transmitted from one person to another or from an animal to a person. Children can develop complications or secondary infections that require health care and can sometimes result in death.

For a communicable disease to occur three factors need to be in place:

1. An infectious agent or pathogen

2. An effective means of transmission

3. Presence of susceptible host (See *Pathophysiology Illustrated: The Chain of Infection Transmission.*)

Special Vulnerability of Infants and Children

Infants and young children are often susceptible hosts. Newborns are more susceptible because the immune system is not fully mature at birth and disease protection from vaccines is

1044

Pathophysiology Illustrated: **The Chain of Infection Transmission**

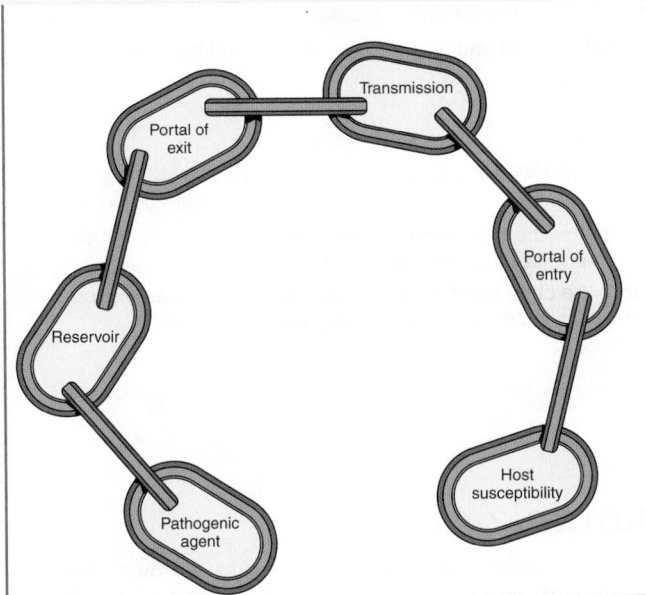

An effective chain of infection transmission requires a suitable habitat or reservoir for the pathogen. To prevent or control the spread of infection, one of the links in the chain must be broken, such as eliminating one or more of the habitats or reservoirs (e.g., insecticide spraying to kill mosquitoes that carry malaria). Isolating an infected individual interferes with disease transmission, and killing the pathogen eliminates the causal agent.

incomplete. Maternal **antibodies** (proteins capable of responding to specific infectious agents) transferred through the placenta and breast milk provide **passive immunity** to the newborn. Passive immunity may also be provided with immune globulin. These antibodies provide limited protection for some infections, and this protection decreases over several months after birth. Immunodeficiency and poor health may also increase a child's risk for a communicable disease.

Infants and children develop **active immunity**, antibody development for specific infections through immunization or exposure to the natural disease. Exposure to infectious agents leads children to naturally develop antibodies that prevent or reduce the response to future exposure to the same infectious agent (Figure 43–1). (Refer to Chapter 48, *Anatomy and Physiology of Pediatric Differences.*)

The poor hygiene behaviors of young children promote transmission of communicable diseases in environments where children are in close contact. The fecal–oral and respiratory routes are the most common sources of transmission in children. Children do not wash their hands after toileting unless closely supervised. They then put their hands in their mouth and rub their nose and eyes. Diapers may leak stool and provide the fecal exposure to organisms. In some cases, the child may be contagious before disease symptoms occur (e.g., varicella and parvovirus B-19) and before the child can be isolated. See Table 43–5 for more information about these and other communicable diseases.

Public Health and Communicable Diseases

Reducing the number of preventable childhood illnesses is a national goal of *Healthy People 2020*. Approximately 300 children in the United States die each year from vaccine-preventable diseases. Routine immunization, with all recommended vaccines administered to children beginning at birth, is estimated to save 33,000 lives, prevent 14 million cases of disease, and reduce direct healthcare costs by $9.9 billion (U.S. Department of Health and Human Services, 2015).

Healthy People 2020

> (IID-1) Reduce, eliminate, or maintain elimination of cases of vaccine-preventable diseases
>
> (IID-3) Reduce meningococcal disease
>
> (IID-4) Reduce invasive pneumococcal infections

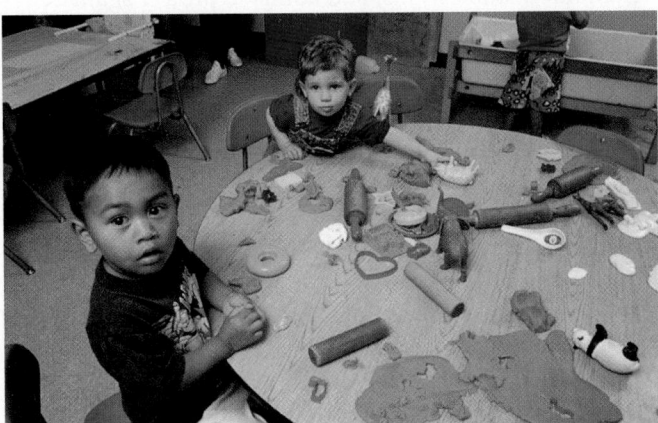

Figure 43–1 Infectious diseases are easily transmitted in settings such as childcare centers where multiple children handle common objects that have been sneezed, coughed, or drooled upon.

Nurses have an important health promotion role in reducing the transmission of infectious diseases by immunization and in educating families to interrupt the transmission of infection. Preventing the spread of infectious diseases involves several strategies that must be well coordinated. Nurses have

---

TEACHING HIGHLIGHTS | Reducing the Transmission of Infection

Teach families how to reduce the spread of infection among family members with the following practices:

- Wash hands thoroughly with soap and water or cleansing gels after all contact with the child's diaper, used tissues, runny nose, and mucous membranes.
- Use disposable tissues and discard immediately after use.
- Teach children to cough or sneeze into their elbow rather than their hands.
- Teach children to wash their hands with soap and water after toileting and before eating.
- Do not allow children to share dishes and utensils.
- Wash hands before preparing food and again several times during the food preparation process. Follow guidelines for safe food preparation and storage. Use warm soapy water to wash dishes and cutting boards.
- Wipe counters and surfaces that are used for diaper changes or that the child touches with a disinfectant such as bleach solution, Lysol, or isopropyl alcohol. Make sure the diaper-changing area is well away from food preparation areas.
- Dispose of diapers in closed containers.

---

a significant role in this process and are responsible for implementing several infection-control strategies:

- Use proper hand hygiene. Wash hands with soap and water when visibly dirty, when contaminated by blood or other body fluids, when in contact with a contaminated surface, and after using the toilet (Centers for Disease Control, 2014a). Use alcohol-based hand sanitizer to clean the hands in all other routine clinical situations.
- Use standard and transmission-based precautions (see the *Clinical Skills Manual* **SKILLS** for more information).
- Promote and provide immunizations.
- Separate and quarantine ill children from well children. Separate children at high risk for infection from those with infections in all clinical settings.
- Eliminate the habitat or reservoir of the host (e.g., eliminate standing water where mosquitoes breed).
- Kill the pathogen (e.g., sanitize toys and surfaces exposed to organisms).
- Educate parents and caregivers to reduce the transmission of infectious diseases. (See *Teaching Highlights: Reducing the Transmission of Infection*.)

Professionalism in Practice **Infection Control in Schools**

School nurses have an important leadership role in targeting communicable diseases because of their professional knowledge and public health perspective (National Association of School Nurses, 2011). School nurses document the student immunization records and encourage families to have their children fully immunized. Students with communicable diseases are identified so they can be sent home for care, reducing exposure to other students. It is important for school nurses to stay informed about communicable disease outbreaks in the community and then to be vigilant about monitoring illness patterns among students and faculty. When a communicable disease outbreak occurs in the school setting, the school nurses reports the outbreak to local health officials so that communitywide infection-control information can be shared. They also develop programs and teach students how to reduce the spread of infection.

Immunization

The development and wide use of vaccines is one of the great achievements of modern medicine. A vaccine introduces an **antigen** (a foreign substance that triggers an immune system response) into the body, and the vaccinated person produces antibodies that provide active immunity to a disease without having the clinical disease.

When a child needs antibodies faster than the body can develop them, passive immunity may be provided by giving the child antibodies produced by another human or animal host (e.g., immune globulin). This approach is used with children at risk for a disease to prevent the disease from occurring or to reduce its severity after an exposure. For example, if an unimmunized toddler receiving chemotherapy for cancer is exposed to chickenpox, the child needs immediate protection (passive immunity). Varicella immune globulin is given to reduce the child's risk for developing chickenpox, a potentially fatal infection for this child. Passive immunity does not last long, so the child needs to receive the varicella vaccine at a later time in order to develop active immunity.

Since the first vaccines were developed in the late 1800s, the incidence of many diseases has decreased dramatically. The average infant born in 2015 receives vaccines for 14 childhood diseases by age 6 years. Vaccines have also been developed for older children, adolescents, and adults to protect against pertussis, meningococcus, human papillomavirus, pneumococcus, and herpes zoster. Vaccines improve the health of children and reduce the parents' burden of caring for ill children.

The following lists the types of vaccines against childhood illnesses used in the United States:

- **Killed virus vaccine.** A microorganism has been killed but is still capable of causing the human body to produce antibodies. Example: inactivated poliovirus.
- **Toxoid.** A toxin has been treated (by heat or chemical) to weaken its toxic effects but retain effective antigens. Example: tetanus toxoid.
- **Live virus vaccine.** A microorganism is in a live but attenuated, or weakened, form. Example: measles and varicella vaccines.
- **Recombinant forms.** A genetically altered organism is used in vaccines. Examples: hepatitis B and **acellular pertussis vaccine** (a vaccine that uses pertussis proteins rather than the whole cell to stimulate active immunity).

- **Conjugated forms**. An altered organism is joined with another substance to increase the immune response. Examples: The *Haemophilus influenzae* type b (Hib) vaccine is conjugated with a protein-carrier like tetanus toxoid. No immunity to tetanus develops with this vaccine.

Today's vaccines are often produced synthetically with recombinant DNA technology or genetic engineering to improve vaccine safety and efficacy and to reduce their side effects. See Table 43–1 for recommended pediatric vaccines.

TABLE 43–1 Pediatric Vaccines

IMMUNIZATION TYPE	SIDE EFFECTS	CONTRAINDICATIONS	NURSING CONSIDERATIONS
Diphtheria, Pertussis (Whooping Cough), and Tetanus Toxoid (DTaP, Tdap)			
Type: Inactivated **Dosage:** 0.5 mL, IM **Age(s) given:** 2, 4, 6, 15–18 months; 4–6 years (5 doses); 11–12 years (Tdap) **Caution:** For a prior serious reaction to the pertussis component of DTaP vaccine, use DT (children less than 7 years) and Td (children 7 years and older) vaccines. **Storage:** Refrigerate, do not freeze. Tripedia and Infanrix vial stopper contains latex.	**Common:** Redness, pain, swelling, nodule at injection site; fever up to 38.3°C (101.0°F); drowsiness, irritability, fussiness; anorexia within 2 days of injection Increase in frequency and magnitude of local reactions with fourth and fifth doses (e.g., entire limb swelling) **Serious:** Allergic reaction, anaphylaxis; shock or collapse (an episode with sudden loss of muscle tone, pallor, fever, and unresponsiveness), fever above 40.5°C (104.8°F); febrile seizure; persistent inconsolable crying	Gelatin allergy (do not use Tripedia) Serious side effects after a prior dose: e.g., anaphylaxis, encephalopathy within 7 days of vaccine dosage ***Precautions and temporary deferral for DTaP and Tdap administration:*** • Infants under age 1 year with evolving neurologic disorder • Guillain-Barré syndrome less than 6 weeks after previous dose • Moderate to severe febrile illness • Older children with a progressive neurologic condition	• Use same brand for all doses if possible. • Ask about previous vaccine reactions. • Shake vaccine before withdrawing. Solution will be cloudy. Do not use if it contains clumps that do not resuspend. • If a child has a history of seizures with or without fever, give acetaminophen at the time of vaccine and then every 4 hr for 24 hr. • Inform parents about an increased potential reaction to the fourth and fifth doses. • A tetanus booster may be given for a contaminated wound or burn, if 5 or more years since the last dose (AAP, 2015, p. 775).
***Haemophilus influenzae* Type B (Hib)**			
Type: Inactivated **Dosage:** 0.5 mL, IM **Age(s) given:** 2, 4, 6, 12–15 months; (4 doses for PRP-T[a] [ActHIB]) *or* 2, 4, 12–15 months (3 doses for PRP-OMP[a] [PedvaxHIB]) **Storage:** Refrigerate, loss of potency if frozen. Vial stopper with Pentacel and MenHibRix contains no latex.	**Common:** Pain, redness, or swelling at site **Serious:** Anaphylaxis (extremely rare); fever	Prior anaphylactic reaction. Comvax is contraindicated if yeast allergy exists. **Precautions:** Moderate or severe acute illness with or without fever Ask if child is immunosuppressed. Some children benefit from additional doses (AAP, 2015, p. 373).	• Solution is clear and colorless. • Since different product preparations (e.g., single and combination vaccines) affect the immunization schedule, read package inserts carefully. • Follow directions for reconstituting, refrigerating, and discarding unused reconstituted vaccine.
Hepatitis A (HepA)			
Type: Inactivated **Dosage:** 0.5 mL (1.0 mL over age 19 years), IM **Age(s) given:** 12–23 months; second dose 6–12 months after first dose. **Storage:** Refrigerate, loss of potency if frozen.	**Common:** Pain and induration at injection site; fever **Serious:** Anaphylaxis reactions are rare	Known hypersensitivity to any component of vaccine, including neomycin Anaphylactic reaction to prior vaccine dose **Precautions:** Pregnancy	• Shake well, slightly opaque white suspension. No reconstitution is needed. • Some Havrix and all Vaqta vials have a latex stopper. • Can be given for postexposure prophylaxis against hepatitis A (AAP, 2015, p. 398). • Immune globulin and vaccine can be given at the same time in different sites.

(continued)

TABLE 43–1 Pediatric Vaccines (*continued*)

IMMUNIZATION TYPE	SIDE EFFECTS	CONTRAINDICATIONS	NURSING CONSIDERATIONS
Hepatitis B (HB)			
Type: Inactivated **Dosage:** 0.5 mL (1.0 mL at 20 years), IM **Age(s) given:** Birth, 1–2 months, 6–18 months; 3 doses; a 3-dose series can be started at any age. **Storage:** Refrigerate, do not freeze. Vaccine brands can be interchanged for 3-dose series. Use the monovalent (single vaccine) preparation for newborns up to 6 weeks of age.	**Common:** Pain or redness at injection site **Serious:** Anaphylaxis is uncommon	Anaphylaxis reaction to prior dose Serious hypersensitivity reaction to prior dose related to vaccine component (e.g., yeast) **Precautions:** Newborn weighing less than 2000 g (4.4 lb) may receive dose at birth, but receive 3 additional doses starting at 1 month of age Moderate or severe acute illness with or without fever	• Check status of mother's hepatitis B test. If mother has HBsAg+ or unknown status, give vaccine to newborn within 12 hr of birth along with hepatitis B immune globulin in another site. • Shake vaccine before withdrawing. Solution will appear cloudy. • Formulations (pediatric, adult, dialysis) and combination vaccines are available. Read package insert carefully and follow directions for the product used. • Check the anti-HB and HBsAg levels in infants of HBsAG+ mothers at age 9–18 months, after series completion (AAP, 2015, p. 421).
Human Papillomavirus (HPV4 or HPV2)			
Type: Recombinant **Dosage:** 0.5 mL, IM **Age(s) given:** 11–12 years, second dose 2 months later, third dose 6 months after the first dose. May be administered to males and females between 9 and 26 years of age. HPV2 is not licensed for males (Markowitz et al., 2014). **Storage:** Refrigerate, do not freeze. Light exposure reduces vaccine potency.	**Common:** Pain, swelling, erythema at the injection site, headache, nausea, pruritus, and fever **Potential serious reactions:** Guillain-Barré syndrome, blood clot, bronchospasm, asthma, arthritis	Severe allergic reaction to prior dose or hypersensitivity to a vaccine component (e.g., yeast) Pregnancy **Precautions and deferral:** Moderate to severe acute illness with or without fever. Can be given when mild acute illness is present.	• Use same brand for each dose if possible. • Shake well before use. Solution is a white cloudy liquid. No dilution or reconstitution. • Observe adolescent for 15 min when seated because of risk of fainting and syncope. • Administer vaccine before onset of sexual activity. • Educate adolescents that this vaccine prevents only one sexually transmitted infection.
Influenza (IIV4 or LAIV4)			
Type: Inactivated (IIV), or live attenuated (LAIV) for intranasal (IN) use **Route:** IM (all ages), IN (2 years and older) **Dosage:** 0.25 mL in infants 6–35 months, 0.5 mL starting at 3 years for IIV; 0.2 mL for LAIV **Age(s) given:** Annually in the fall, beginning at 6 months of age; then annually. Children under age 9 years receiving IIV or LAIV for the first time should receive a second dose 4 weeks later (AAP, 2015, p. 483). **Storage:** **IIV:** Refrigerate, do not use if frozen. **LAIV:** Keep frozen. May thaw and refrigerate for 24 hr before use.	**Common after IIV:** Soreness at injection site, fever, aches **Common after LAIV:** Runny nose or nasal congestion, decreased appetite, irritability, sore throat, fever	**IIV and LAIV:** Severe allergic reaction to eggs or prior vaccine dose, such as anaphylaxis **LAIV:** Contraindicated in children less than 2 years old with immunosuppression, asthma or wheezing episode in prior 12 months, or receiving an aspirin-containing product. **Precautions:** **LAIV:** Postpone vaccine when child has nasal congestion. **IIV:** May be given with minor illness, with or without fever. Give IIV if close contact with a severely immunocompromised person.	• Thawed LAIV is pale yellow, clear to slightly cloudy. • Split LAIV dose with a dose divider clip. Administer while child is sitting upright. Insert the tip of the sprayer inside each nostril and depress the plunger. • Reimmunize with 1 dose each year as immunity wanes, and vaccines are modified to include the new season's viruses. • If the child has received at least 2 doses of IIV since July 2010, only 1 annual dose is needed (Grohskopf et al., 2014).

IMMUNIZATION TYPE	SIDE EFFECTS	CONTRAINDICATIONS	NURSING CONSIDERATIONS
Measles, Mumps, Rubella (MMR)			
Type: Live attenuated *Dosage:* 0.5 mL, subcutaneously (SQ) *Age(s) given:* 12–15 months; 4–6 years (2 doses) Give MMR and varicella vaccines on the same day or at least 4 weeks apart. *Storage:* Freeze or refrigerate vaccine before reconstitution. When reconstituted, keep refrigerated and away from light; discard if unused within 8 hr. Diluent is stored at room temperature or in a refrigerator; do not freeze.	*Common:* Fever 6–12 days after immunization; redness or pain at injection site; noncontagious rash; joint pain *Serious:* Allergic reaction or anaphylaxis; febrile seizure; meningitis (usually mild); encephalopathy; thrombocytopenia purpura; and rare cases of coma and permanent brain damage Children, ages 12–23 months, receiving the combined MMR and varicella vaccine have an increased risk of febrile seizures compared to children receiving MMR as separate vaccines (CDC, 2014h).	Prior anaphylactic reaction to neomycin Severe allergic reaction to prior vaccine dose or vaccine component Pregnancy Severe immunodeficiency due to malignancy, congenital immunodeficiency disease, long-term immunosuppressive therapy, or child with HIV infection *Precautions and deferral:* Receipt of immune globulin or blood product in last 3–11 months. History of thrombocytopenia or thrombocytopenic purpura Moderate or severe acute illness with or without fever Personal or family history of seizures may increase risk of febrile seizures after immunization (McLean, Fiebelkorn, Temte, et al., 2013).	• Ask about immune suppression. • Reconstituted vaccine is a clear, yellow solution. • Give entire contents of reconstituted vial even if more than 0.5 mL. • May give to a child with an egg allergy (AAP, 2015, p. 541). • Give to children with HIV unless severely immunocompromised. • Give tuberculosis (TB) test at same time as MMR or 4–6 weeks later. • Educate adolescent girls to avoid pregnancy for 28 days after immunization.
Meningococcal Tetravalent Conjugate (MenACWY-D, MenACWY-CRM)			
Type: Conjugate *Dosage:* 0.5 mL, IM *Age(s) given:* 11–12 years, and booster dose 16–18 years MenACWY-CRM may be given to high-risk children (2 months and older). Infants under 7 months get 4 doses (2, 4, 6, and 12 months); older children get 2 doses, with second dose 3 months later or after 12 months of age (MacNeil et al., 2014). *Storage:* Refrigerate until used, do not freeze.	*Common:* Swelling and pain at injection site, irritability, headache, fatigue, anorexia, and diarrhea	Severe allergic reaction (e.g., anaphylaxis) after prior dose or to a vaccine component (e.g., diphtheria toxoid) *Precautions:* Previous history of Guillain-Barré syndrome, unless at high risk for meningococcal disease	• Protect vaccine from light. • Verify that correct vaccine licensed for used for infants and children less than 24 months of age. • Give a booster dose to children 2–6 years old with immunosuppression 3 years after first dose for children 2–6 years and then every 5 years. • Give a booster dose to children 7 years and older with immunosuppression 5 years after first dose and then every 5 years (AAP, 2015, p. 555).
Pneumococcal Conjugate (PCV13)			
Type: Conjugate *Dosage:* 0.5 mL, IM *Age(s) given:* 2, 4, 6, 12–15 months *Storage:* Refrigerate, do not freeze.	*Common:* Pain, redness, swelling, induration at injection site; fever; irritability, decreased appetite, increased or decreased sleep *Severe:* Allergic reaction or anaphylaxis	Severe allergic reaction (e.g., anaphylaxis) after a prior dose of PCV7, PCV13, or vaccine containing diphtheria toxoid, or a component of one of the listed vaccines *Precautions and deferral:* Moderate or severe acute illness with or without fever	• Clear, colorless, or slightly opalescent liquid. • Give a supplemental dose using PCV13 if a child 6–18 years is at risk for invasive pneumococcal disease who also received PPSV23 (AAP, 2015, p. 635).

(continued)

TABLE 43–1 Pediatric Vaccines (*continued*)

IMMUNIZATION TYPE	SIDE EFFECTS	CONTRAINDICATIONS	NURSING CONSIDERATIONS
Poliovirus Vaccine (IPV) **Type:** Inactivated **Dosage:** 0.5 mL, subcutaneously or IM, follow guidance for brand used **Age(s) given:** 2, 4, 12–18 months; 4–6 years (4 doses) **Storage:** Refrigerate, do not freeze.	**Common:** Swelling and tenderness, irritability, tiredness **Serious:** Allergic reaction or anaphylaxis	Severe allergic reaction, e.g., anaphylaxis, after prior dose or to vaccine components (neomycin, streptomycin, polymyxin B) ***Precautions and deferral:*** Pregnancy Moderate or severe acute illness with or without fever	• Ask about an allergy to the antibiotic contained in the specific IPV product available. • Clear, colorless suspension. Do not use if it contains particulate matter, becomes cloudy, or changes color.
Rotavirus Vaccine (RV1, RV5) **Type:** Live **Dosage:** 1 mL or 2 mL, oral **Age(s) given:** RV1 at 2 and 4 months (2 doses); RV5 at 2, 4, and 6 months (3 doses); all 3 doses of vaccine should be completed by 8 months of age. Complete the series with the same vaccine. **Storage:** Refrigerate, do not freeze.	**Common:** Irritability, cough, runny nose, loss of appetite, vomiting **Severe:** Potential increased risk for intussusception	Severe allergic reaction to a previous dose or to a vaccine component Severe combined immunodeficiency disease Uncorrected gastrointestinal malformation that puts infant at risk for intussusception History of intussusception ***Precautions and deferral:*** Altered immunosuppression Moderate or severe acute illness with or without fever, including diarrhea and vomiting Preexisting chronic gastrointestinal disease Spina bifida or bladder exstrophy	• Pale yellow clear liquid. Protect vaccine from light. • Ask about contacts that might have immunodeficiency; viral shedding is known to occur. • Squeeze the liquid into the infant's mouth toward the inner cheek until the dosing tube is empty. • RV1 applicator has latex; RV5 applicator is latex-free. • Do not repeat the dose if the infant spits out, vomits, or regurgitates during or after the dose. • There are no food or liquid restrictions before or after vaccine.
Varicella Virus Vaccine **Type:** Live attenuated **Dosage:** 0.5 mL, subcutaneously **Age(s) given:** 12–18 months, 4–6 years May be given in combined vaccine with MMR. **Storage:** Keep frozen at 5°F (−15°C) or colder. May be stored for up to 72 hr in refrigerator prior to reconstitution. Diluents kept at room temperature. Once reconstituted, use vaccine within 30 min or discard.	**Common:** Pain or redness at injection site; fever; a vaccine-related rash (2–5 maculopapular or vesicular lesions may occur 5–26 days after injection). **Severe:** Allergic reaction or anaphylaxis; rare cases of encephalitis, pneumonia, erythema multiforme, Stevens-Johnson syndrome, thrombocytopenia, seizure, and Guillain-Barré syndrome	Severe allergic reaction (e.g., anaphylaxis) after a prior dose or to a vaccine component (e.g., neomycin or gelatin). Known severe immunodeficiency due to malignancy, chemotherapy, congenital immunodeficiency disorder, long-term immunosuppressive therapy, or clients with HIV infection who are severely immunocompromised Pregnancy Active untreated tuberculosis ***Precautions and deferral:*** Receipt of blood products or immune globulin within past 3–11 months Moderate or severe acute illness with or without fever	• Ask if child is immunodeficient or has an allergy to a vaccine component. • Clear, colorless to pale yellow liquid when reconstituted. • Give the entire contents of the vial even if more than 0.5 mL. • Instruct adolescent girls of childbearing age to avoid pregnancy for 3 months after immunization. • Antiviral agents should not be used 1 day before or for 21 days after vaccine. • Avoid exposure to immunodeficient persons for 6 weeks after vaccinated.

Source: Data from American Academy of Pediatrics. (2015). *Red Book: Report of the Committee on Infectious Disease* (30th ed.). Elk Grove Village, IL; McLean, H. Q., Fiebelkorn, A. P., Temte, J. L., & Wallace, G. S. (2013). Prevention of measles, rubella, congenital rubella syndrome, and mumps, 2013: Summary recommendations of the Advisory Committee on Immunization Practices. *Morbidity and Mortality Weekly Report, 62*(4), 1–34; Markowitz, L. E., Dunne, E. F., Saraiya, M., Chesson, H. W., Curtis, C. R., Gee, J., . . . Unger, E. R. (2014). Human papillomavirus vaccination: Recommendations of the Advisory Committee on Immunization Practices. *Morbidity and Mortality Weekly Report, 63*(5), 1–30; Grohskopf, L. A., Olsen, S. J., Sokolow, L. Z., Bresee, J. S., Cox, N. J., Broder, K. R., . . . Walter, E. B. (2014). Prevention and control of seasonal influenza with vaccines: Recommendations of the Advisory Committee on Immunization Practices (ACIP)—United States, 2014–15 influenza season. *Morbidty and Mortality Weekly Report, 63*(32), 691–697; MacNeil, J. R., Rubin, L., McNamara, L., Briere, E. C., Clark, T. A., & Cohn, A. C. (2014). Use of MenACWY-CRM vaccine in children aged 2 through 23 months at increased risk for meningococcal disease: Recommendations of the Advisory Committee on Immunization Practices, 2013. *Morbidity and Mortality Weekly Report, 63*(24), 527–530.

Clinical Manifestations

Children have a variety of reactions to the antigens in different vaccines, and those reactions occur because of the child's immune system response. Common local reactions at the injection site include erythema, swelling, pain, and induration. Systemic reactions such as fever, fussiness or irritability, malaise, and anorexia may occur. A rash or arthralgia may occur with some vaccines. Highly anxious adolescents may have syncope or a vasovagal reaction within 15 minutes of immunization, leading to fall-related injuries (American Academy of Pediatrics [AAP] Committee on Infectious Disease, 2015, p. 26–27).

Allergic reactions to vaccines occur occasionally, such as a wheal and urticaria, within minutes to hours after the injection. A severe local allergic reaction is manifested by warmth, erythema, edema, petechiae, or ulceration occurring 2 to 8 hours after vaccination. A non-life-threatening systemic allergic reaction, such as generalized urticaria or transient petechiae, may occur within minutes. Anaphylaxis, a life-threatening reaction manifested by hypotension, generalized urticaria, angioedema, and laryngeal edema, rarely occurs with any vaccine. Allergic reactions are most often associated with vaccine components such as eggs, gelatin, yeast, and neomycin (AAP, 2015, pp. 54–56). See Table 43–1 for potential vaccine allergies.

Collaborative Care

Vaccines are recommended for administration at specific ages and intervals. Timing for first immunizations is determined by the age at which **transplacental immunity** (passive immunity transferred from mother to infant) decreases or disappears, and the infant or child develops the ability to make antibodies in response to the vaccine. Scientists continue to study the duration of protection from vaccines. Many vaccines are repeated at a later age to boost immunity.

Clinical Tip

Make every effort to stay current on immunization guidelines and information about vaccines, safe administration, adverse effects, and so on. Major resources provide more extensive information about immunization schedules and specific vaccines, as well as infectious and communicable diseases. The American Academy of Pediatrics' *Red Book: Report of the Committee on Infectious Diseases* is updated about every 3 years. Another resource is *Epidemiology and Prevention of Vaccine-Preventable Diseases*, commonly called the *Pink Book*, published by the Public Health Foundation, which has comprehensive information on communicable diseases and vaccines. The revised immunization schedule is published each January in several pediatric medical and nursing journals. The Centers for Disease Control and Prevention (CDC) maintains a website with detailed information about immunizations, the recommended vaccine schedule, and infectious and communicable diseases.

IMMUNIZATION SCHEDULES

The recommended immunization schedule is updated at least annually to reflect new vaccine information. The Advisory Committee on Immunization Practices (ACIP) of the Centers for Disease Control and Prevention (CDC), the American Academy of Pediatrics (AAP), and the American Academy of Family Practitioners (AAFP) collaborate to provide a uniform recommended schedule. See Figure 43–2 for the 2015 recommendations for vaccines that all children should receive. Schedules and recommendations vary for children who begin immunizations later in childhood or need catch-up doses.

Children with **asplenia** (loss of the spleen due to surgery or nonfunctioning due to sickle cell disease) are at higher risk for invasive pneumococcal and meningococcal infections. After completion of the PCV13 series, these children should receive pneumococcal polysaccharide vaccine (PPSV23) beginning at age 24 months. A second dose is given 5 years later. Some children who are American Indians or Alaska Natives living in areas of increased incidence of invasive pneumococcal disease may also be given PPSV23 (AAP, 2015, p. 92). See Table 43–1 for MCV4 guidelines.

IMPROVING IMMUNIZATION RATES

The effort to increase the numbers of children protected from vaccine-preventable diseases and to monitor immunization status is a national public health initiative.

Healthy People 2020

(IID-7) Achieve and maintain effective vaccination coverage levels for universally recommended vaccines among young children

(IID-10) Maintain vaccination coverage levels for children in kindergarten

(IID-11) Increase routine vaccination coverage levels for adolescents

---

For children between 19 and 35 months of age in 2013, the reported level of full immunization (four DTP/DT/DTaP, three IPV, one MMR, three Hib, three HB, one varicella, and four PCV13) was 70.4%. Rates were higher for individual vaccine series. Variations were found by racial and ethnic groups and family income level (Elam-Evans, Yankey, Singleton, et al., 2014). In 2012, adolescents between 13 and 17 years of age were found to have the following vaccination coverage: one Tdap since age 10 years (84.6%), one to two MCV4 (74%), second MMR (91.4%), three HB (92.8%), second varicella or disease (82.6%), and three HPV (in females, 33.4%, and in males, 6.8%) (Curtis et al., 2013). Increasing the immunization rate of adolescents has many challenges.

Lower immunization rates are often associated with economic factors, limited access to health care, lack of primary care at hours convenient for working parents, inadequate education about the importance of immunization, and cultural or religious prohibitions. The federal Vaccines for Children program provides free vaccines for qualified children and adolescents less than 19 years of age and has resolved some of the economic factors associated with vaccine coverage. However, the cost of vaccines, approximately $2091 for all approved vaccines for fully immunizing a child through the adolescent years in 2014, is a barrier for children with private health insurance (CDC, 2014b).

An increasing number of parents are choosing not to immunize their children for philosophic, religious, or other reasons, such as (Hendrix et al., 2014):

- Belief that vaccine-preventable diseases are not dangerous, and they occur rarely today
- Concerns that the frequency and number of vaccines to be administered cause pain and may overwhelm an infant's immune system
- A vaccine's potential harm to the child because of the amount of its chemical and biologic content and its side effects
- Concerns that vaccines are related to autism
- Mistrust in healthcare provider recommendations

Figure 1. Recommended immunization schedule for persons aged 0 through 18 years – United States, 2015.
(FOR THOSE WHO FALL BEHIND OR START LATE, SEE THE CATCH-UP SCHEDULE [FIGURE 2]).

These recommendations must be read with the footnotes that follow. For those who fall behind or start late, provide catch-up vaccination at the earliest opportunity as indicated by the green bars in Figure 1. To determine minimum intervals between doses, see the catch-up schedule (Figure 2). School entry and adolescent vaccine age groups are shaded.

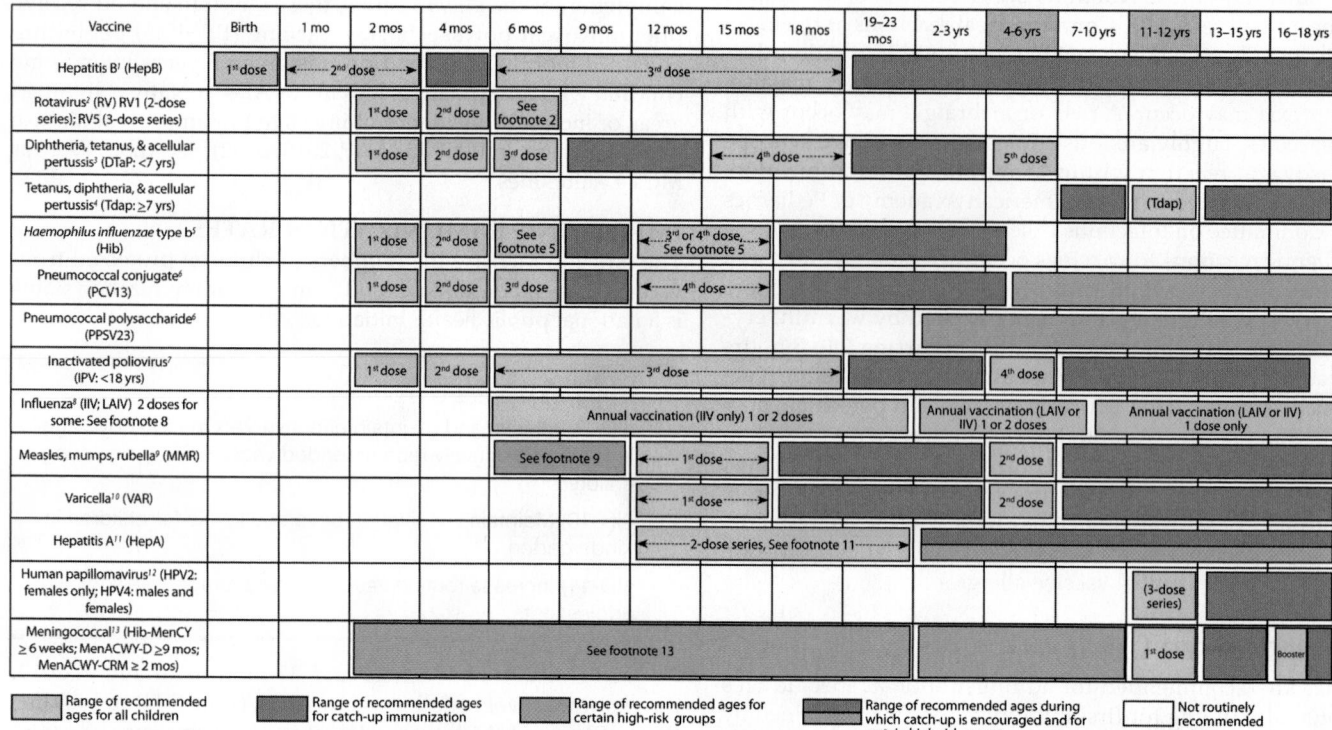

This schedule includes recommendations in effect as of January 1, 2015. Any dose not administered at the recommended age should be administered at a subsequent visit, when indicated and feasible. The use of a combination vaccine generally is preferred over separate injections of its equivalent component vaccines. Vaccination providers should consult the relevant Advisory Committee on Immunization Practices (ACIP) statement for detailed recommendations, available online at http://www.cdc.gov/vaccines/hcp/acip-recs/index.html. Clinically significant adverse events that follow vaccination should be reported to the Vaccine Adverse Event Reporting System (VAERS) online (http://www.vaers.hhs.gov) or by telephone (800-822-7967). Suspected cases of vaccine-preventable diseases should be reported to the state or local health department. Additional information, including precautions and contraindications for vaccination, is available from CDC online (http://www.cdc.gov/vaccines/recs/vac-admin/contraindications.htm) or by telephone (800-CDC-INFO [800-232-4636]).

This schedule is approved by the Advisory Committee on Immunization Practices (http://www.cdc.gov/vaccines/acip), the American Academy of Pediatrics (http://www.aap.org), the American Academy of Family Physicians (http://www.aafp.org), and the American College of Obstetricians and Gynecologists (http://www.acog.org).

NOTE: The above recommendations must be read along with the footnotes of this schedule.

Footnotes — Recommended immunization schedule for persons aged 0 through 18 years—United States, 2015

For further guidance on the use of the vaccines mentioned below, see: http://www.cdc.gov/vaccines/hcp/acip-recs/index.html

For vaccine recommendations for persons 19 years of age and older, see the Adult Immunization Schedule.

Additional information

- For contraindications and precautions to use of a vaccine and for additional information regarding that vaccine, vaccination providers should consult the relevant ACIP statement available online at http://www.cdc.gov/vaccines/hcp/acip-recs/index.html.
- For purposes of calculating intervals between doses, 4 weeks = 28 days. Intervals of 4 months or greater are determined by calendar months.
- Vaccine doses administered 4 days or less before the minimum interval are considered valid. Doses of any vaccine administered ≥5 days earlier than the minimum interval or minimum age should not be counted as valid doses and should be repeated as age-appropriate. The repeat dose should be spaced after the invalid dose by the recommended minimum interval. For further details, see *MMWR, General Recommendations on Immunization and Reports / Vol. 60 / No. 2; Table 1. Recommended and minimum ages and intervals between vaccine doses* available online at http://www.cdc.gov/mmwr/pdf/rr/rr6002.pdf.
- Information on travel vaccine requirements and recommendations is available at http://wwwnc.cdc.gov/travel/destinations/list.
- For vaccination of persons with primary and secondary immunodeficiencies, see Table 13, "*Vaccination of persons with primary and secondary immunodeficiencies,*" in *General Recommendations on Immunization* (ACIP), available at http://www.cdc.gov/mmwr/pdf/rr/rr6002.pdf.; and American Academy of Pediatrics. "Immunization in Special Clinical Circumstances," in Pickering LK, Baker CJ, Kimberlin DW, Long SS eds. *Red Book: 2012 report of the Committee on Infectious Diseases. 29th ed. Elk Grove Village, IL: American Academy of Pediatrics.*

1. **Hepatitis B (HepB) vaccine. (Minimum age: birth)**
   Routine vaccination:
   At birth:
   - Administer monovalent HepB vaccine to all newborns before hospital discharge.
   - For infants born to hepatitis B surface antigen (HBsAg)-positive mothers, administer HepB vaccine and 0.5 mL of hepatitis B immune globulin (HBIG) within 12 hours of birth. These infants should be tested for HBsAg and antibody to HBsAg (anti-HBs) 1 to 2 months after completion of the HepB series at age 9 through 18 months (preferably at the next well-child visit).
   - If mother's HBsAg status is unknown, within 12 hours of birth administer HepB vaccine regardless of birth weight. For infants weighing less than 2,000 grams, administer HBIG in addition to HepB vaccine within 12 hours of birth. Determine mother's HBsAg status as soon as possible and, if mother is HBsAg-positive, also administer HBIG for infants weighing 2,000 grams or more as soon as possible, but no later than age 7 days.
   Doses following the birth dose:
   - The second dose should be administered at age 1 or 2 months. Monovalent HepB vaccine should be used for doses administered before age 6 weeks.
   - Infants who did not receive a birth dose should receive 3 doses of a HepB-containing vaccine on a schedule of 0, 1 to 2 months, and 6 months starting as soon as feasible. See Figure 2.
   - Administer the second dose 1 to 2 months after the first dose (minimum interval of 4 weeks), administer the third dose at least 8 weeks after the second dose AND at least 16 weeks after the **first** dose. The final (third or fourth) dose in the HepB vaccine series should be administered **no earlier than age 24 weeks.**
   - Administration of a total of 4 doses of HepB vaccine is permitted when a combination vaccine containing HepB is administered after the birth dose.
   Catch-up vaccination:
   - Unvaccinated persons should complete a 3-dose series.
   - A 2-dose series (doses separated by at least 4 months) of adult formulation Recombivax HB is licensed for use in children aged 11 through 15 years.
   - For other catch-up guidance, see Figure 2.

2. **Rotavirus (RV) vaccines. (Minimum age: 6 weeks for both RV1 [Rotarix] and RV5 [RotaTeq])**
   Routine vaccination:
   Administer a series of RV vaccine to all infants as follows:
   1. If Rotarix is used, administer a 2-dose series at 2 and 4 months of age.
   2. If RotaTeq is used, administer a 3-dose series at ages 2, 4, and 6 months.
   3. If any dose in the series was RotaTeq or vaccine product is unknown for any dose in the series, a total of 3 doses of RV vaccine should be administered.
   Catch-up vaccination:
   - The maximum age for the first dose in the series is 14 weeks, 6 days; vaccination should not be initiated for infants aged 15 weeks, 0 days or older.

- The maximum age for the final dose in the series is 8 months, 0 days.
- For other catch-up guidance, see Figure 2.

3. **Diphtheria and tetanus toxoids and acellular pertussis (DTaP) vaccine. (Minimum age: 6 weeks. Exception: DTaP-IPV [Kinrix]: 4 years)**
   Routine vaccination:
   - Administer a 5-dose series of DTaP vaccine at ages 2, 4, 6, 15 through 18 months, and 4 through 6 years. The fourth dose may be administered as early as age 12 months, provided at least 6 months have elapsed since the third dose. However, the fourth dose of DTaP need not be repeated if it was administered at least 4 months after the third dose of DTaP.
   Catch-up vaccination:
   - The fifth dose of DTaP vaccine is not necessary if the fourth dose was administered at age 4 years or older.
   - For other catch-up guidance, see Figure 2.

4. **Tetanus and diphtheria toxoids and acellular pertussis (Tdap) vaccine. (Minimum age: 10 years for both Boostrix and Adacel)**
   Routine vaccination:
   - Administer 1 dose of Tdap vaccine to all adolescents aged 11 through 12 years.
   - Tdap may be administered regardless of the interval since the last tetanus and diphtheria toxoid-containing vaccine.
   - Administer 1 dose of Tdap vaccine to pregnant adolescents during each pregnancy (preferred during 27 through 36 weeks' gestation) regardless of time since prior Td or Tdap vaccination.
   Catch-up vaccination:
   - Persons aged 7 years and older who are not fully immunized with DTaP vaccine should receive Tdap vaccine as 1 dose (preferably the first) in the catch-up series; if additional doses are needed, use Td vaccine. For children 7 through 10 years who receive a dose of Tdap as part of the catch-up series, an adolescent Tdap vaccine dose at age 11 through 12 years should NOT be administered. Td should be administered instead 10 years after the Tdap dose.
   - Persons aged 11 through 18 years who have not received Tdap vaccine should receive a dose followed by tetanus and diphtheria toxoid (Td) booster doses every 10 years thereafter.
   - Inadvertent doses of DTaP vaccine:
     - If administered inadvertently to a child aged 7 through 10 years may count as part of the catch-up series. This dose may count as the adolescent Tdap dose, or the child can later receive a Tdap booster dose at age 11 through 12 years.
     - If administered inadvertently to an adolescent aged 11 through 18 years, the dose should be counted as the adolescent Tdap booster.
   - For other catch-up guidance, see Figure 2.

Figure 43–2 *A*, Recommended immunization schedule for children 0 to 18 years, United States, 2015. For further guidance on the vaccines listed see http://www.cdc.gov/vaccines/hcp/acip-recs/index.html

B. Catch-up immunization schedule for persons aged 4 months through 18 years who start late or who are more than 1 month behind —United States, 2015.

The figure below provides catch-up schedules and minimum intervals between doses for children whose vaccinations have been delayed. A vaccine series does not need to be restarted, regardless of the time that has elapsed between doses. Use the section appropriate for the child's age. Always use this table in conjunction with Figure 1 and the footnotes that follow.

Vaccine	Minimum Age for Dose 1	Minimum Interval Between Doses			
		Dose 1 to Dose 2	**Dose 2 to Dose 3**	**Dose 3 to Dose 4**	**Dose 4 to Dose 5**
Children age 4 months through 6 years					
Hepatitis B[1]	Birth	4 weeks	8 weeks *and* at least 16 weeks after first dose. Minimum age for the final dose is 24 weeks.		
Rotavirus[2]	6 weeks	4 weeks	4 weeks[2]		
Diphtheria, tetanus, and acellular pertussis[3]	6 weeks	4 weeks	4 weeks	6 months	6 months[3]
Haemophilus influenzae type b[5]	6 weeks	4 weeks if first dose was administered before the 1st birthday. 8 weeks (as final dose) if first dose was administered at age 12 through 14 months. No further doses needed if first dose was administered at age 15 months or older.	4 weeks[5] if current age is younger than 12 months **and** first dose was administered at younger than age 7 months, **and** at least 1 previous dose was PRP-T (ActHib, Pentacel) or unknown. 8 weeks *and* age 12 through 59 months (as final dose)[5] • if current age is younger than 12 months **and** first dose was administered at age 7 through 11 months; OR • if current age is 12 through 59 months **and** first dose was administered before the 1st birthday, **and** second dose administered at younger than 15 months; OR • if both doses were PRP-OMP (PedvaxHIB; Comvax) **and** were administered before the 1st birthday. No further doses needed if previous dose was administered at age 15 months or older.	8 weeks (as final dose) This dose only necessary for children age 12 through 59 months who received 3 doses before the 1st birthday.	
Pneumococcal[6]	6 weeks	4 weeks if first dose administered before the 1st birthday. 8 weeks (as final dose for healthy children) if first dose was administered at the 1st birthday or after. No further doses needed for healthy children if first dose administered at age 24 months or older.	4 weeks if current age is younger than 12 months and previous dose given at <7months old. 8 weeks (as final dose for healthy children) if previous dose given between 7-11 months (wait until at least 12 months old); OR if current age is 12 months or older and at least 1 dose was given before age 12 months. No further doses needed for healthy children if previous dose administered at age 24 months or older.	8 weeks (as final dose) This dose only necessary for children aged 12 through 59 months who received 3 doses before age 12 months or for children at high risk who received 3 doses at any age.	
Inactivated poliovirus[7]	6 weeks	4 weeks[7]	4 weeks[7]	6 months[7] (minimum age 4 years for final dose).	
Meningococcal[13]	6 weeks	8 weeks[13]	See footnote 13	See footnote 13	
Measles, mumps, rubella[9]	12 months	4 weeks			
Varicella[10]	12 months	3 months			
Hepatitis A[11]	12 months	6 months			
Children and adolescents age 7 through 18 years					
Tetanus, diphtheria; tetanus, diphtheria, and acellular pertussis[4]	7 years[4]	4 weeks	4 weeks if first dose of DTaP/DT was administered before the 1st birthday. 6 months (as final dose) if first dose of DTaP/DT was administered at or after the 1st birthday.	6 months if first dose of DTaP/DT was administered before the 1st birthday.	
Human papillomavirus[12]	9 years	Routine dosing intervals are recommended.[12]			
Hepatitis A[11]	Not applicable (N/A)	6 months			
Hepatitis B[1]	N/A	4 weeks	8 weeks **and** at least 16 weeks after first dose.		
Inactivated poliovirus[7]	N/A	4 weeks	4 weeks[7]	6 months[7]	
Meningococcal[13]	N/A	8 weeks[13]			
Measles, mumps, rubella[9]	N/A	4 weeks			
Varicella[10]	N/A	3 months if younger than age 13 years. 4 weeks if age 13 years or older.			

NOTE: The above recommendations must be read along with the footnotes of this schedule.

Figure 43–2 *(Continued) B*, Catch-up immunization schedule for children 4 months to 18 years, United States, 2015. For further guidance on the vaccines listed see http://www.cdc.gov/vaccines/hcp/acip-recs/index.html

SOURCE: Centers for Disease Control (CDC).

Other parents are selecting an alternate immunization schedule to delay or space out vaccines, such as the Sears Alternative Vaccine Schedule. However, this approach is not supported by evidence or public health officials.

See Table 43–2 for common misconceptions some parents have about vaccines and vaccine safety information. Increasing immunization rates of children whose parents are hesitant is a challenge. See *Evidence-Based Practice: Immunization Challenges.*

VACCINE INJURY COMPENSATION

Vaccines are tested for safety before being licensed by the U.S. Food and Drug Administration; however, serious vaccine reactions occur in rare instances. When a link between a child's immunization and a serious adverse reaction is identified, the National Vaccine Injury Compensation Program provides compensation for the family. The Vaccine Adverse Event Reporting System (VAERS) was established in 1988 to track serious vaccine reactions. See Table 43–3 for the serious reactions specific to each vaccine that are eligible for compensation.

Nursing Management
For the Child Receiving Immunizations

Nursing Assessment and Diagnosis

Nurses are responsible for reviewing a child's health record to determine whether the child needs vaccines. Identify any potential contraindications to vaccines by asking the following:

- Has the child had a serious reaction to any vaccine? Has the child had any vaccines in the last 4 weeks?
- Are there allergies to any vaccine components (e.g., eggs, neomycin, gelatin, or yeast) or latex?

Text continues on page 1056

TABLE 43–2 Common Misconceptions About Vaccines and Correct Information

COMMON MISCONCEPTIONS	CORRECT VACCINE INFORMATION
Vaccine-preventable diseases have been eliminated.	The incidence of vaccine-preventable diseases is low in the United States, but these diseases occur elsewhere in the world. Unvaccinated travelers have reintroduced diseases from a country or a U.S. community where the disease exists. Recent outbreaks of measles have been linked to unimmunized travelers who became infected in one of 18 countries (Gastañaduy et al., 2014). Children with lowered immune status (e.g., treatment for cancer) are at higher risk for exposure to infection because of lowered herd immunity. **Herd immunity** is the protection provided by a large group of persons who have immunity to a disease and indirectly protect others without immunity by reducing the risk for exposure and infection.
Immunization weakens the immune system. Multiple vaccines overload the immune system and cause harmful effects.	Vaccines use the body's immune system to prevent a future infection. Infants are capable of developing protective immune responses to multiple vaccines simultaneously. The number of antigens in these vaccines is substantially fewer than the immune challenges associated with daily environmental exposures (DeStefano, Price, & Weintraub, 2013).
Thimerosal use in vaccines may cause mercury poisoning.	Thimerosal, a bacteriostatic agent that contains ethyl mercury, previously was used to sterilize vaccines in multidose vials. Because of concerns about mercury poisoning and related nerve and brain damage, thimerosal has been eliminated from all but the influenza vaccine. A thimerosal-free influenza vaccine is available for children (AAP, 2015, p. 18).
It would be better to let the child get the disease than get immunized.	Most parents have never seen these diseases and do not understand how dangerous they may be, sometimes leading to hospitalization, disability, and even death. Infected children can spread the infection to pregnant women, exposing the fetus, and to infants and children with serious medical conditions.
Vaccines do not work; children still get the disease.	No vaccine is 100% effective, and immunity does wane over time, leading to the need for a booster dose.

EVIDENCE-BASED PRACTICE | Immunization Challenges

Clinical Question
What strategies are needed to increase acceptance of vaccines in hesitant parents?

The Evidence
A randomized trial study using web-based interactions with 1759 parents investigated the effectiveness of public health messages about the safety of the MMR vaccine or the danger of measles, mumps, and rubella diseases. The four messages integrated CDC vaccine language and included (1) corrected misinformation that vaccines cause autism, (2) presented information on disease risks, (3) a story about a child hospitalized with measles, and (4) photographs of infected children to emphasize the disease risks. The outcome measure was intent to give the MMR vaccine to a future child. None of the messages increased parents' intent to immunize a future child with the MMR vaccine. Provaccine messages were least effective in parents with negative attitudes about vaccines. In some cases, messages increased beliefs about MMR side effects (Nyhan, Reifler, Richey, et al., 2014).

A randomized trial survey of 802 parents of infants less than 12 months of age were presented four vaccine messages to identify which one increased a parent's intent to immunize their child with the MMR vaccine. The Vaccine Information Sheet (VIS) was the control message. The other three messages included the VIS plus (1) the benefits of the vaccine to the child, (2) the benefits of immunizing the child to society, and (3) the benefits of the vaccine to the child plus society. Parents had a significantly higher intent to immunize their infant when the benefits of the vaccine to the child or the benefits to the child plus society messages were used when compared to the control message (Hendrix et al., 2014).

A study using data from the National Immunization Survey for Teens focused on reasons parents gave for adolescents who were not up-to-date on Tdap/Td, MCV4, and HPV as not receiving the vaccines. The reasons given for Tdap/Td and MCV4 were the same: not recommended by a healthcare provider, not needed, lack of knowledge, or don't know. The HPV vaccine was not accepted more commonly for these reasons: not sexually active, not needed or not necessary, and vaccine safety concerns (Darden et al., 2013).

Best Practice
With the increased trend in undervaccination of children, efforts have shifted to finding messages that will increase a parent's acceptance of vaccines. One study identified a higher acceptance occurred when the discussion with the parent about a vaccine focused on the benefit for their child rather than societal benefits. Exposure to viruses and bacteria causing vaccine-preventable diseases is unpredictable, so vaccines are given before an exposure. For adolescents, it is important to emphasize the reduced risk of cervical cancer that may occur 20 to 40 years after exposure to HPV. Since the virus is acquired during sexual activity, it is important for adolescents to receive the vaccine before sexual activity begins.

Clinical Reasoning
Think about some specific benefits to a child for each of the vaccines administered (e.g., no discomfort due to the disease, fewer days of school missed, fewer days the parents have to miss work because of a sick child). When in a clinical setting, identify and include the specific benefits for the child for each vaccine in the education provided to parents when seeking consent for vaccine administration.

TABLE 43–3 National Vaccine Injury Act—Vaccine Injury Table

VACCINE	ILLNESS, DISABILITY, INJURY, OR CONDITION COVERED	TIME PERIOD FOR FIRST SYMPTOM OR MANIFESTATION OF ONSET OR OF SIGNIFICANT AGGRAVATION AFTER VACCINE ADMINISTRATION
Vaccines containing tetanus toxoid-containing vaccines (e.g., DTaP, Tdap, DTP-Hib, DT, Td, or TT)	Anaphylaxis or anaphylactic shock	4 hr
	Bacterial neuritis	2–28 days
	Any acute complication or sequela (including death) of above events occurring in the specified time period	Not applicable
Vaccines containing whole cell pertussis bacteria, extracted or partial cell pertussis antigen(s) (e.g., DTaP, Tdap, DTP, P, DTP-Hib)	Anaphylaxis or anaphylactic shock	4 hr
	Encephalopathy (or encephalitis)	72 hr
	Any acute complication or sequela (including death) of above events occurring within the specified time period	Not applicable
Measles, mumps, rubella virus–or any of its components (e.g., MMR, MR, M, R)	Anaphylaxis or anaphylactic shock	4 hr
	Encephalopathy (or encephalitis)	5–15 days
	Any acute complication or sequela (including death) of above events occurring within the specified time period	Not applicable
Vaccines containing rubella virus (e.g., MMR, MR, R)	Chronic arthritis	7–42 days
	Any acute complication or sequela (including death) of above events occurring within the specified time period	Not applicable
Vaccines containing measles virus (e.g., MMR, MR, M)	Thrombocytopenic purpura	7–30 days
	Vaccine strain measles viral infection in an immunodeficient recipient	6 months
	Any acute complication or sequela (including death) of above events occurring within the specified time period	Not applicable
Vaccines containing live polio (OPV)	Paralytic polio	
	• in a nonimmunodeficient recipient	30 days
	• in an immunodeficient recipient	6 months
	• in a vaccine-associated community case	Not applicable
	Vaccine-strain polio viral infection	
	• in a nonimmunodeficient recipient	30 days
	• in an immunodeficient recipient	6 months
	• in a vaccine-associated community case	Not applicable
	Any acute complication or sequela (including death) of above events	Not applicable
Vaccines containing polio inactivated virus (IPV)	Anaphylaxis or anaphylactic shock	4 hr
	Any acute complication or sequela (including death) of above events occurring within the specified time period	Not applicable
Hepatitis B vaccines	Anaphylaxis or anaphylactic shock	4 hr
	Any acute complication or sequela (including death) of above events occurring within the specified time period	No limit
Haemophilus influenzae type b polysaccharide conjugate vaccines	No condition specified	Not applicable
Hepatitis A vaccines	No condition specified	Not applicable
Varicella vaccine	No condition specified	Not applicable
Rotavirus vaccine	No condition specified	Not applicable
Pneumococcal conjugate vaccine	No condition specified	Not applicable
Meningococcal vaccines	No condition specified	Not applicable
Trivalent influenza vaccines	No condition specified	Not applicable
Human papillomavirus (HPV) vaccines	No condition specified	Not applicable
Any new vaccine recommended by the CDC for routine administration to children after publication by the Secretary of the Department of Health and Human Services of notice of coverage	No condition specified	Not applicable

Effective date: November 12, 2013. For guidance in further interpretation of this table, visit the website below.

Source: From Health Resources and Services Administration. (2013). *Vaccine injury table.* Retrieved from http://www.hrsa.gov/vaccinecompensation/vaccineinjurytable.pdf

- Does the child have a serious medical condition (seizures, cancer, HIV infection, immune diseases, blood disorder, asthma) or wheezing in the past 12 months?
- Has the child received any blood products, immune globulin, or any antiviral drugs in the past year?
- Has the child taken cortisone, prednisone, other steroids, or anticancer drugs or had radiation treatments in the past 3 months?
- If the client is a female, is pregnancy possible now or in the next month?

SAFETY ALERT!

Immune globulin, blood products, and immunosuppressive agents inhibit the child's response to live virus vaccines (MMR, varicella), so ask parents about any recent administration of these products. When possible, administer inactivated vaccines 2 or more weeks before and live virus vaccines 4 or more weeks before immunosuppressive therapy is begun (Rubin et al., 2013). Refer to the most current guidelines from the Centers for Disease Control and Prevention's Advisory Committee on Immunization Practices (ACIP) to identify the correct interval (3 to 11 months) between the administration of the blood product, immune globulin, or completion of immunosuppression therapy and administration of a live virus vaccine (Kroger, Sumaya, Pickering, et al., 2011).

If immune globulin or blood products were given 14 days before or up to several months following a vaccine, readminister the vaccine after the period specified by the CDC, unless serologic testing determines that the child developed adequate serum antibodies (AAP, 2015, pp. 38–39).

Healthcare providers miss many opportunities to immunize children. Assess the immunization status of children (and siblings present) during all healthcare visits and hospitalizations and in schools. Use the most current immunization schedule to identify needed vaccines. When a child needs immunizations, determine the best combination of vaccines to give at this visit to better protect the child. However, make sure the appropriate interval has occurred between vaccine dosages, using the catch-up vaccine schedule. Ways to reduce the number of missed opportunities for full immunization of children include the following:

- Place a reminder in the child's health record to alert health professionals about the child's need for immunizations. Establish a system to send parents a reminder when the child's immunizations are due or overdue.
- Give vaccines when the child has a minor illness, even with a low-grade fever and antibiotic treatment, or has a recent exposure to an infectious disease.
- Use combination vaccines (e.g., DTaP-HepB-IPV) to reduce the number of injections from 20 to 13 in the first 2 years (see Table 43–4).
- Give multiple vaccines at the same time using separate syringes and injecting in separate sites. If using the same extremity, separate injection sites by an inch (AAP, 2015, p. 36).
- Give medically stable low-birth-weight infants all vaccines appropriate for chronologic age as full-term infants. Use the full dose (AAP, 2015, pp. 68–69).
- Give the vaccine even when a prior dose caused a local reaction or a family member had an adverse response.

TABLE 43–4 Combination Vaccines

VACCINE NAME	VACCINE COMPONENTS	AGES USED
Comvax	Hib and HepB	2, 4, and 12–15 months of age, 3 doses
TriHIBit	DTaP and Hib	15–18 months, fourth dose of HIB and DTaP series
Twinrix	HepA and HepB	18 years and older
Pediarix	DTaP, HepB, and IPV	2, 4, and 6 months of age, 3 doses
ProQuad	MMR and Varicella	12–15 months of age, and 4–6 years of age
Kinrix	DTaP and IPV	4–6 years, fifth dose of DTaP and fourth dose of IPV
Pentacel	DTaP, IPV, and Hib	2, 4, 6, and 15–18 months of age, 4 doses
MenHibrix	Hib, Meningococcal CY serotypes	2, 4, 6, and 12–15 months of age

Source: Adapted from Kroger, A. T., Sumaya, C. V., Pickering, L. K., & Atkinson, W. L. (2011). General recommendations on immunization: Recommendations of the Advisory Committee on Immunization Practices (ACIP). *Morbidity and Mortality Weekly Report, 60*(2), 37; MacNeil, J. R., Rubin, L., McNamara, L., Briere, E. C., Clark, T. A., & Cohn, A. C. (2014). Use of MenACWY-CRM vaccine in children aged 2 through 23 months at increased risk for meningococcal disease: Recommendations of the Advisory Committee on Immunization Practices, 2013. *Morbidity and Mortality Weekly Report, 63*(24), 527–530.

The accompanying *Nursing Care Plan* explores two potential nursing diagnoses that apply to the child needing immunizations. Additional nursing diagnoses may include the following (NANDA-I © 2014):

- *Skin Integrity, Risk for Impaired,* related to vaccine response
- *Health Maintenance, Ineffective,* related to philosophical beliefs regarding routine immunization
- *Anxiety* related to fear of needles

Planning and Implementation

Nursing management focuses on protecting the potency of vaccines, being a strong advocate for immunization, educating parents about immunizations and possible side effects, addressing their fears about possible reactions, obtaining consent, and reporting adverse reactions.

PROTECT VACCINE POTENCY

Take special care to ensure vaccine potency, so all children develop adequate immune response (CDC, 2014c).

- Store vaccines properly in the refrigerator or freezer (i.e., separate doors for refrigerator and freezer, storage conditions should be adequate: Refrigeration: 35°F to 46°F [2°C to 8°C]; Freezer: 5°F [–15°C] or lower as stated in vaccine package inserts).
- Keep jugs of water in the refrigerator and trays of ice in the freezer to help maintain a consistent temperature.
- Store the vaccines on the middle shelves of the units, 2 to 3 in. away from the walls, with space for air to circulate between boxes; place older vaccines in the front.
- Check the refrigerator and freezer temperatures twice daily and record the temperatures on a log or use an automatic temperature measurement system.
- Make an emergency plan for safe storage of vaccines in case of a power outage or natural disaster.

Nursing Care Plan: The Child Needing Immunizations

1. Nursing Diagnosis: *Infection, Risk for*, related to incomplete immunizations for age (NANDA-I © 2014)

GOAL: The child will become adequately protected from disease-preventable illnesses.

INTERVENTION	RATIONALE
• Review the child's immunization record for needed vaccines at each healthcare visit.	• Children who need vaccines can be identified.
• Identify all due vaccines that can be provided simultaneously.	• Multiple vaccines given at the same visit more adequately protect the child.
• Identify potential contraindications to needed vaccines. Review past reactions to vaccines.	• Identifying contraindications and past reactions reduces the risk for adverse reactions to vaccines.

EXPECTED OUTCOME: Child will be adequately protected for age from vaccine-preventable illnesses.

2. Nursing Diagnosis: *Health Management, Family, Ineffective* (NANDA-I © 2014)

GOAL: Parents will sign consent for vaccines to be given.

INTERVENTION	RATIONALE
• Educate the parents and adolescents about the need for specific vaccines and the risk if not given. Obtain signed consent before giving vaccines.	• Informed consent is required for all treatments.

EXPECTED OUTCOME: Parent(s) will complete the consent forms, which are placed in the child's file.

GOAL: Parents and adolescents will state the side effects of vaccines given.

INTERVENTION	RATIONALE
• Review past reactions to vaccines and describe common potential reactions and why they occur.	• Parents should expect common reactions and know they indicate the child's body is building protection to the illness.
• Describe serious side effects that should be reported to the healthcare provider.	• Parents need to be prepared for potential serious side effects so they can obtain care if needed.

EXPECTED OUTCOME: Parents will report all serious side effects to the healthcare provider.

GOAL: Parents will manage common side effects of vaccines.

INTERVENTION	RATIONALE
• Teach parents general comfort measures for common side effects, for example: • Cool pack to tender leg • Acetaminophen or ibuprofen for fever and discomfort • Rocking and holding the infant • Gentle movement of affected extremity	• Parents will know how to make the child more comfortable during the 24–48 hr after the vaccine is given.

EXPECTED OUTCOME: Child will be given comfort measures after vaccine administration.

OBTAIN CONSENT

Federal legislation requires written consent before administering a vaccine. The nurse often has the responsibility to inform the child's parents or legal guardian, and supply the most current Vaccine Information Statement (VIS) for each vaccine to be given, a requirement of the National Vaccine Injury Act.

Explain the risks and benefits of each vaccine and common local reactions. Answer all of the parents' questions. Parents may have heard sensational stories about vaccines, and correct information is needed to help them make informed decisions.

Developing Cultural Competence Vaccine Information Statements (VIS)

Consider literacy and reading level when giving a VIS to a parent. The VIS is written at a sixth-grade level, but parents may have poor literacy. The VIS has been translated into 40 languages, and these are available through the CDC website. Ask rather than assume the parent can read the preferred spoken language. It is acceptable to read the VIS to parents and make sure that they understand the information.

TEACHING HIGHLIGHTS | Care of the Child After Immunizations

When a child receives an immunization, educate parents to observe for any reactions that might occur and call the child's healthcare provider if there is concern about any of the symptoms listed.

- Local pain, redness, and swelling are common. Use ice on the injection site to help reduce swelling and pain. Acetaminophen or ibuprofen may be given to reduce a fever and pain. The symptoms should disappear in a day or two.
- The child may have a fever, joint pain, muscle aches, or fatigue within hours to days after the vaccine is given. Give acetaminophen or ibuprofen for pain.
- With a mild allergic reaction to the vaccine, a few hives may be noted around the injection site.
- A severe allergic reaction is indicated by a flushed face; swelling of the face, mouth, or throat; wheezing or other difficulty breathing; shock (confusion, lack of movement or response, or unconsciousness); and abdominal cramping. Call 9-1-1 for emergency treatment. Have the child lie down with the legs raised higher than the level of the heart until the ambulance arrives to promote blood return to the vital organs.

When a parent refuses to accept a particular vaccine, have the parent sign an informed refusal document. If a disease outbreak occurs, the unimmunized child must be kept out of school or child care. See section on Fever, later in this chapter, for guidance on home care of the child with an infectious disease.

For each vaccine administered, the nurse is required to record the (1) month, day, and year of administration, (2) vaccine given, (3) manufacturer, (4) lot number and expiration date of the immunization given, (5) site and route of administration, and (6) name, title, and address of the person who administers the vaccine. Provide parents with a record of the child's immunizations, and enter the information on vaccines administered into the healthcare agency's official records.

Provide guidance for managing expected mild reactions at home (see *Teaching Highlights: Care of the Child After Immunizations*). Provide information about the proper dose of acetaminophen or ibuprofen to give the child.

ADMINISTER VACCINES

Check the expiration of vaccines before use. Follow the manufacturer's directions for reconstituting vaccines and use the solution provided. Write the date and time on the bottle if it is a multidose vial. Reconstitute vaccines immediately before use as some have a short shelf life.

Use 1-in. needles rather than 5/8 in. (25 mm rather than 16 mm) for infants for IM injections to give the vaccine deep in the muscle mass. Stretch the skin to decrease the amount of subcutaneous tissue the needle must go through. Follow facility needle length guidelines for children of other ages. For vaccines given subcutaneously, select a 5/8-in. 23- to 25-gauge needle. Use the upper thigh in infants less than 12 months of age, and the upper outer triceps region for older children (Kroger et al., 2011).

SAFETY ALERT!

Adolescents who are extremely fearful of getting an injection are at a greater risk for fainting, syncope, or vasovagal response after a vaccine injection. Provide the injection when the adolescent is sitting or lying down. Observe the adolescent while sitting or lying down for 15 minutes to prevent secondary injury in case of syncope.

REDUCE PAIN AND ANXIETY

Make an effort to reduce the pain associated with vaccine injections, especially since infants and children must return for more injections. Give the appropriate immunizations to the child as efficiently as possible, while providing support to the child

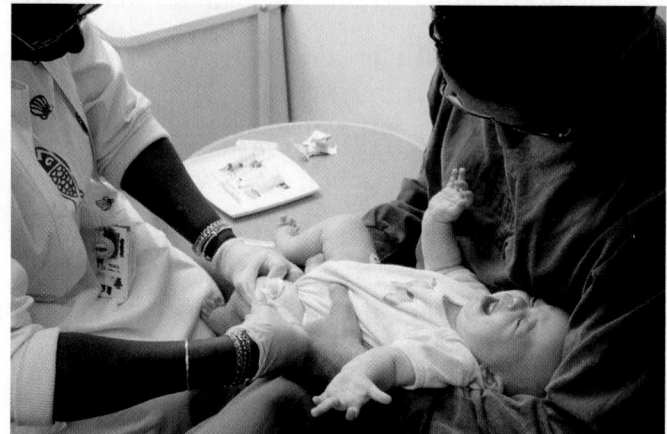

Figure 43–3 **Give immunizations quickly and efficiently. Do not prolong the wait and let fear grow. The child will be anxious, especially if more than one injection must be given.**

(Figure 43–3). Suggestions for pain management include the following techniques:

- Coach the parent to hold and talk with the child during the injections. Funny faces, a toy, or age-appropriate distraction might also help. Encourage parents to give comfort measures after the injection.
- Give infants up to 4 months of age 24% sucrose water to drink (e.g., Sweetease or mix 1 packet of table sugar with 10 mL of tap water) prior to the injection (see Chapter 40). Then allow the infant to suck on a pacifier or breastfeed during the injections.
- Apply pressure at the site for 10 seconds before the injection.
- Provide information about obtaining L-M-X4 (a topical anesthetic available without a prescription) prior to the next visit. Instruct parents how to apply L-M-X4 cream to one or more sites prior to the child's appointment. See Chapter 40 for information regarding use of L-M-X4.
- Spray the planned injection site with vapocoolant spray immediately before the injection, or spray it on a cotton ball and hold that against the skin.
- Have two providers each give an injection simultaneously in different extremities.

- Do not prolong the process of giving immunizations. Give the child honest answers that the needles will cause some pain.
- Let the child select the arm or leg for the injection and forms of distraction to promote coping.

PREPARE FOR EMERGENCIES

Be prepared for potential vaccine anaphylaxis even though it is a rare event. Keep epinephrine and resuscitation equipment immediately available. The dose for epinephrine (aqueous 1:1000) is 0.01 mL/kg per dose (maximum dose is 0.5 mL) intramuscularly. The dose can be repeated every 5 to 15 minutes in order to control symptoms and maintain blood pressure. When the child is stable, oral antihistamines and corticosteroids may be prescribed for an additional 24 to 48 hours (AAP, 2015, pp. 66–68).

Remember to report anaphylaxis and other severe reactions following immunization to the Vaccine Compensation Injury Program. See Table 43–3.

Evaluation

Expected outcomes of nursing care include the following:

- Parents are fully informed and give consent for immunizations.
- All vaccines appropriate for the child's age are given at each health visit.
- The parents are prepared to identify serious vaccine reactions and manage mild reactions at home.

Clinical Reasoning Immunizations

A 5-year-old girl, Lian, has accompanied her mother and 2-year-old brother Chang to the pediatric clinic. Lian's mother is concerned because Chang has had a fever of 38.3°C (101.0°F) for the past 3 days. Although Chang has visited this clinic several times in the past few months for health care, this is the first time Lian has come along.

When asked, Lian's mother says Lian had a healthcare visit about 2 years ago, but she does not know if she had all of her shots. In checking Lian's health records, the nurse notes that she needs DTaP, IPV, PCV13, MMR, varicella, and HepA vaccines. Chang needs MMR, varicella, HepA, and PCV13 vaccines.

Should Lian receive any of these vaccines today, even though her brother is ill? Which vaccines could be given during one visit? Should Chang receive any vaccines today?

Communicable Diseases in Children

Communicable diseases cause acute illnesses resulting from bacterial, viral, protozoan, or fungal organisms. Infants and children are more susceptible and develop communicable diseases more frequently than adults do. Active immunity to microorganisms does not occur until there is natural exposure or immunization that leads to antibody production.

The epidemiology, clinical manifestations, treatment, prevention, and nursing care of selected communicable diseases of childhood are described in Table 43–5. Infectious diseases transmitted by animal vectors are detailed in Table 43–6. See Chapter 6 for information on sexually transmitted infections, Chapter 45 for information about conjunctivitis, Chapter 46 for information on tuberculosis, and Chapter 51 for information on hepatitis and parasites.

Clinical Manifestations

The child with an infectious or communicable disease has a cluster of symptoms specific to the disease that appear at the end of the **incubation period**, the time interval between exposure and development of symptoms. Some diseases have a **prodrome**, the phase of early manifestations of the infection until the development of the overt clinical syndrome. Fever is the most common sign of communicable disease in infants and children. Other nonspecific signs are related to the specific disease and may include fatigue, malaise, weakness, decreased responsiveness or inability to concentrate, skin rash, poor appetite, vomiting, diarrhea, and body aches.

Developing Cultural Competence Disease Causation

In some cultures, infectious diseases are seen as punishment or the result of curses or evil spirits. For example, American Indians (e.g., Navajo) traditionally view illnesses as the result of disharmony or displeasing the spirits. They may not believe in the germ theory of disease causation (Purnell, 2014).

FEVER

Fever is an increased body temperature of 38.0°C (100.4°F) or higher taken by rectal or tympanic route, and 37.8°C (100.°F) or higher by the oral or temporal route. The hypothalamus is the body's thermostat or control center for the regulation of body temperature (see *Pathophysiology Illustrated: Fever*). As blood circulates through the hypothalamus, the body is directed to conserve or release heat, depending on the temperature of the blood.

FEVER MANAGEMENT

A fever can be a beneficial physiologic response to infection, helping to slow the growth and reproduction of organisms that thrive at lower body temperatures. A fever decreases the serum levels of zinc, iron, and copper needed by bacteria for reproduction. It also encourages the body to shift to a metabolism that burns fat and proteins rather than glucose, which deprives bacteria of a food source (Huether, 2014). Fever is not inherently harmful until it reaches 41.0°C (105.9°F). Medical management may include postponing treatment of low-grade fevers (under 38.9°C [102.0°F]) to promote the body's natural defenses against an infection.

Fevers are often treated if they cause discomfort with acetaminophen or ibuprofen. Aspirin is no longer recommended in children because of its association with Reye syndrome (see Chapter 54). Antipyretics inhibit prostaglandin synthesis, which results in lowering of the body's temperature set point and reducing the fever.

Developing Cultural Competence Hot and Cold Therapy

Many Latino and Asian cultures subscribe to the hot and cold theory of disease causation. Fever, a hot condition, is treated by giving the ill person cold substances (either foods or medicines). Cold foods include dairy products, fresh vegetables, fruits, chicken, goat meat, and fish. Cold medicines include orange flower water, linden, and sage (Purnell, 2013). See Table 2–2, *Hot and Cold Conditions and Foods*.

Text continues on page 1072

TABLE 43–5 Selected Infectious and Communicable Diseases in Children

DISEASE	CLINICAL MANIFESTATIONS	CLINICAL THERAPY	NURSING MANAGEMENT
CHICKENPOX (VARICELLA)[a, b]			
Causal agent: Varicella-zoster, human herpesvirus 3. **_Epidemiology:_** Humans are the source of infection. Peak occurrence is in the late fall, winter, and spring. Maternal antibodies disappear 2–3 months after birth. **_Transmission:_** Direct contact of the virus to the mucous membranes or conjunctiva primarily through airborne secretions and sometimes with lesion contact. **_Incubation period:_** 14–21 days. **_Period of communicability:_** Most contagious 1–2 days before the rash to shortly after onset of rash. Contagious until all lesions are crusted over. Contagious state may be prolonged after passive immunization or in immunodeficient children. 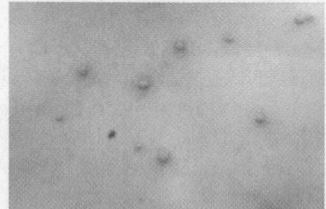 Kasiap/Shutterstock	Acute onset of mild fever, malaise, anorexia, headache, mild abdominal pain, and irritability occurs before and with eruption. Begins as a macular rash that progresses to a papule, then clear fluid-filled vesicle before crusting. Rash erupts for 1–5 days, and up to 250–500 lesions of all stages may be present at any one time. Crusts may remain for 1–3 weeks. Lesions begin on the trunk, scalp, and face, and spread to the rest of the body. Mucous membranes may have ulcerative lesions. Mouth lesions may lead to decreased fluid intake. **_Complications:_** Complications are rare but can include secondary infection (cellulitis, local abscesses, sepsis, meningitis, encephalitis, pneumonia), thrombocytopenia, and Reye syndrome. Chickenpox can be fatal in newborns of infected mothers and immunocompromised children. Carefully monitor children undergoing chemotherapy, steroid treatment, or transplant therapy after exposure to the disease.	**_Diagnostic testing:_** Polymerase chain reaction or direct fluorescent antibody testing of fluid from vesicle or scab. **_Medical management:_** Supportive care. IV acyclovir is used for immunocompromised clients and those on high-dose corticosteroids (AAP, 2015, p. 851). Give varicella-zoster immune globulin as soon as possible (within 10 days) to newborns of infected mothers, hospitalized premature neonates, and immunocompromised, unimmunized children (Marin, Bialek, & Seward, 2013). **_Prognosis:_** Most children recover fully. Children who are immunocompromised must be treated aggressively. **_Prevention:_** Varicella is vaccine preventable (see Table 43–1). The vaccine may be given within 72 hr after exposure to prevent or to significantly modify the disease. Wild virus (varicella strain not covered in the vaccine) cases occur in vaccinated children.	• Use airborne and contact precautions. • Isolate all hospitalized children with a recent exposure to varicella to protect newborns and immunocompromised clients. Nurses caring for the child should have documented immunity. • At home, isolate the child from susceptible individuals (medically fragile and immunocompromised children or adults, and women early in pregnancy). Notify the school or childcare facility of the child's illness. • Secondary cases are often more severe than the primary case. The child with atopic eczema or sunburn may have a more severe rash. • Give acetaminophen or ibuprofen to control fever. • Control itching with oral antihistamines, soothing oatmeal and Aveeno baths, or Caladryl lotion. • Keep the child's fingernails trimmed and clean. Place soft cotton mittens over the hands of young children when itching cannot be controlled. • Change bed linens frequently. • Reassure the child that the lesions are temporary and will go away. • Monitor for signs of complications (e.g., drowsiness, meningeal signs, respiratory distress, and dehydration). Disorientation and restlessness may indicate viral encephalitis. • Monitor for acyclovir side effects. Monitor renal function if the child has renal insufficiency.

DISEASE	CLINICAL MANIFESTATIONS	CLINICAL THERAPY	NURSING MANAGEMENT
DIPHTHERIA[a, b] ***Causal agent:*** *Corynebacterium diphtheriae.* ***Epidemiology:*** Occurs mostly in colder months in unimmunized and inadequately immunized children. Cases of cutaneous and wound diphtheria occur sporadically in the tropics. The disease is endemic in parts of Africa, Latin America, Asia, the Middle East, and states of the former Soviet Union. ***Transmission:*** Contact with respiratory droplets, nasal or eye discharge, or skin lesion; less commonly by indirect contact with contaminated items; or unpasteurized milk. ***Incubation period:*** 2–7 days or longer. ***Period of communicability:*** Usually 2–4 weeks or until 4 days after antibiotics are started.	The characteristic lesion is an adherent grayish pharyngeal membrane that in severe cases may extend into the trachea or cause airway obstruction. Attempts to remove the membrane result in bleeding. Symptoms can be mild or severe with a gradual onset over 1–2 days. A sore throat and enlarged tender cervical lymph nodes are present. The child may have a swollen neck. ***Complications:*** The organism produces an endotoxin that causes myocarditis and peripheral neuropathy (diplopia, slurred speech, difficulty swallowing, or paralysis of the palate) or ascending paralysis that may be confused with Guillain-Barré syndrome.	***Diagnostic testing:*** Culture from any mucosal or cutaneous lesion. ***Medical management:*** IV equine antitoxin (for respiratory diphtheria) is given after the child is tested for sensitivity. Antibiotic therapy is prescribed for 14 days with IV or IM penicillin G, changing to oral erythromycin when the child can swallow. ***Prognosis:*** Respiratory diphtheria may be complicated by life-threatening airway obstruction. ***Prevention:*** Diphtheria is a vaccine-preventable disease (see Table 43–1). This is a reportable disease.	• Use transmission-based precautions and isolate the child. • Monitor closely for signs of increasing respiratory distress, as well as cardiac and neurologic complications. • Have emergency airway equipment available. Provide humidified oxygen as necessary. • Administer antitoxin and antibiotics as prescribed. Give no medications containing caffeine or other stimulants. • Use oral suction gently as necessary. • Allow children to use mouthwash if desired. Gargling is not permitted because it can irritate the pharyngeal surfaces. • Encourage liquids as tolerated. Intravenous fluids may be necessary. • Provide emotional support to the family. • Initiate the search for client contacts to give antibiotics and immunization boosters.
ENTEROVIRUSES ***Causal agent:*** Group A and B coxsackieviruses, human enteroviruses. ***Epidemiology:*** Occurs worldwide, most commonly in summer and early fall. More common in settings with poor hygiene and overcrowding. Immunity to specific virus probably occurs after infection, but duration is unknown. ***Transmission:*** Fecal–oral and respiratory routes. ***Incubation period:*** 3–6 days. ***Period of communicability:*** Viral shedding may occur for weeks or months after infection.	Irritability, fever, anorexia, malaise, rash, and a sore throat. Each virus causes additional manifestations. ***Herpangina:*** Small, grayish papulovesicular ulcerative pharyngeal lesions that gradually increase in size. ***Hand, foot, and mouth disease:*** Diffuse lesions on the mucous membranes of the mouth; papulovesicular lesions on the hands and feet last for 7–10 days. ***Enterovirus D-68:*** Severe respiratory illness in children with history of asthma or wheezing (Midgley et al., 2014). ***Complications:*** Children with immune deficiency may have more severe manifestations.	***Diagnostic testing:*** Polymerase chain reaction or culture of stool, throat, or other primary site may be obtained. ***Medical management:*** Supportive care. IV immune globulin may be used in life-threatening neonatal infections and in immunodeficient children with chronic meningoencephalitis (AAP, 2015, p. 336). ***Prognosis:*** Recovery is generally good with supportive care. ***Prevention:*** Avoid contact with infected persons early in the disease.	• Use standard and contact precautions if the child is hospitalized. • Use good hand hygiene. • Apply topical lotions and give systemic medications as ordered to lessen the pain and relieve the irritation. • Offer cool drinks and soft, bland foods (no citrus, salty, or spicy foods). Swallowing may be painful. Observe for dehydration. • Offer warm saline mouth rinses. • Provide reassurance and support to parents. • Give acetaminophen or ibuprofen for fever. • Keep the child out of school or child care while febrile.

[a]Indicates that a vaccine or antitoxin is available for use in high-risk or as-needed situations.
[b]Indicates that the disease has a safe and effective vaccine.

(continued)

TABLE 43–5 Selected Infectious and Communicable Diseases in Children (*continued*)

DISEASE	CLINICAL MANIFESTATIONS	CLINICAL THERAPY	NURSING MANAGEMENT

ERYTHEMA INFECTIOSUM (FIFTH DISEASE)

Causal agent: Human parvovirus B19.

Epidemiology: Occurs worldwide, most often in winter and spring. Also occurs in epidemics, with peak activity every 3–4 years (CDC, 2012). The incidence is highest in children between the ages of 5 and 14 years.

Transmission: Respiratory secretions and blood.

Incubation period: 4–20 days.

Period of communicability: No longer contagious once rash appears.

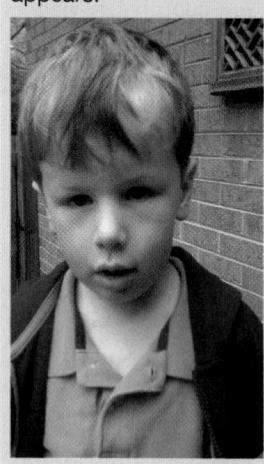

Erythema infectiosum

Stage 1: Begins as a mild illness (fever, headache, chills, malaise, nausea, body ache) lasting 2–3 days, followed by a symptom-free period of 1–7 days.

Stage 2: Fiery-red rash on the cheeks giving a "slapped face" appearance (see figure); circumoral pallor. In 1–4 days a lacelike symmetric, erythematous, maculopapular rash appears on the trunk and spreads to the extremities; spares the palms and soles. The rash may last 7–10 days or longer.

Stage 3: Over 1–3 weeks the rash fades, but can reappear if the skin is irritated or exposed to sunlight.

Complications: Children with hemolytic conditions may have transient aplastic crisis. Polyarthropathy is rare in children.

Diagnostic testing: Diagnosis by physical signs or positive serum immunoglobulin (Ig) M parvovirus B19-specific antibody (important when exposure to a pregnant woman is likely).

Medical management: Supportive care usually leads to spontaneous recovery. Children with hemolytic conditions may need blood transfusions if an aplastic crisis occurs. Administer IV immune globulin to immunodeficient clients who develop a chronic infection (AAP, 2015, p. 595).

Prognosis: Fetal infection may occur resulting in fetal hydrops, anemia, or spontaneous abortion.

Prevention: Avoid contact with infected persons. Exposed pregnant women should seek prompt medical attention.

- Use standard and droplet precautions. Isolation is needed only for children hospitalized with aplastic crisis or when immunosuppressed.
- Give acetaminophen or ibuprofen to control fever.
- Use soothing oatmeal or Aveeno baths if the rash is pruritic. Antipruritics may also help to relieve itching.
- Encourage rest and offer frequent fluids.
- Keep children out of direct sunlight if possible. Provide protective, light, loose clothing if exposure to sunlight cannot be avoided.
- Provide quiet diversionary activity.
- Allow the child to return to school or child care once the rash appears (AAP, 2015, p. 596).
- Explain the three stages of rash development to parents.

HAEMOPHILUS INFLUENZAE, TYPE B[b]

Causal agent: Coccobacilli *H. influenzae* bacteria (several serotypes, encapsulated or nonencapsulated).

Epidemiology: Occurs most often in the spring and summer. Unimmunized and inadequately immunized infants and young children are most commonly affected. Neonates may acquire the organism by aspirating amniotic fluid or contact with vaginal secretions.

Transmission: Direct contact or respiratory droplet inhalation. Asymptomatic colonization in the nose and throat is common.

Incubation period: Unknown, but may be a few days.

Period of communicability: 3 days from onset of symptoms.

Begins with a viral upper respiratory infection. The organism passes through the mucosal barrier to directly invade the bloodstream. It can cause severe invasive illnesses, including meningitis, epiglottitis, pneumonia, infectious arthritis, and cellulitis. It may cause sepsis in infants. Other illnesses caused by the organism include sinusitis, otitis media, bronchitis, and pericarditis. Each disease has specific clinical manifestations.

Invasive disease has decreased 99% since introduction of the vaccine (AAP, 2015, p. 369).

Complications: Responds to antibiotic therapy. If untreated, severe sequelae and death can occur from conditions such as meningitis, epiglottitis, sinusitis, pneumonitis, and cellulitis, especially in young infants.

Diagnostic testing: Culture of blood, cerebrospinal fluid, or middle ear aspirate may be obtained.

Medical management: Treatment for invasive disease is IV antibiotics for 10 days. Dexamethasone may be given to reduce the neurologic sequelae of meningitis. Infections such as otitis media can be managed with oral antibiotics.

Rifampin may be given to unprotected household contacts if another child 4 years or younger has not had the vaccine series.

Prognosis: With rapid diagnosis and treatment, recovery is good. When treatment is delayed, disability may occur.

Prevention: *H. influenzae* type b is a vaccine-preventable disease (see Table 43–1).

- Use droplet precautions until 24 hr after the initiation of antibiotics.
- Identify potential contacts and review their immunization status. Determine the need for rifampin. Inform parents to seek health care rapidly if the exposed child becomes ill.
- Administer acetaminophen or ibuprofen to increase the child's comfort.
- Closely monitor IV sites for patency and infiltration.
- Perform nursing care measures specific to the illness.
- Inform family members that rifampin turns urine and other body fluids orange, and it will cause stains.

DISEASE	CLINICAL MANIFESTATIONS	CLINICAL THERAPY	NURSING MANAGEMENT
INFLUENZA[b] *Causal agent:* Orthomyxoviruses, types A, B, and C. Type A can be subtyped based on surface proteins: hemagglutinin (H) and neuraminidase (N). *Epidemiology:* Prevalent in the United States from October to March, but the virus is active in other parts of the world year-round. The influenza A virus mutates each season. The number of infections peak in about 3 weeks from the initial case and continue for about 3 months. Incidence of infection is often greater in young children who have fewer prior influenza infections and antibodies. *Transmission:* Spreads by aerosolized particles and direct contact with respiratory secretions. *Incubation period:* 1–4 days. *Period of communicability:* 1 day before symptoms to 5–7 days after symptom onset.	Abrupt onset of fever 100.4–104.0°F (38–40°C), chills, cough, runny nose, sore throat, malaise, aches, headache, and anorexia. Children may have nausea and vomiting, diarrhea, and abdominal pain. Recovery usually occurs in 3–5 days. *Complications:* Pneumonia, otitis media, asthma exacerbations, tracheitis, myocarditis, myositis, febrile seizures, sinusitis, and neurologic conditions such as meningitis, encephalitis, encephalopathy, or Guillain-Barré syndrome. Children with chronic pulmonary, hematologic, metabolic, and cardiovascular conditions are at greater risk for severe infection. In the 2013–2014 influenza season, 924 children aged 0–17 years were hospitalized, and 50 children died due to influenza (Arriola et al., 2014).	*Diagnostic testing:* Rapid antigen testing from throat swabs, nasopharyngeal washings, and sputum detects antigens of influenza A and B. Viral cultures, direct fluorescent antibody, or indirect immunofluorescent antibody staining. *Medical management:* Treatment is supportive. Antiviral therapy may be used to treat symptomatic children or for prevention. Oseltamivir (Tamiflu), amantadine (Symmetrel), zanamivir (Relenza), and rimantadine (Flumadine) are approved for children with specific age guidelines. Antiviral therapy should be started within 48 hr of symptoms for best results. (AAP, 2015, pp. 481). *Prognosis:* Most children recover. *Prevention:* Annual influenza immunization beginning at age 6 months (see Table 43–1).	• Use droplet and contact precautions for hospitalized infants and children. • For home care, encourage parents to wash hands frequently and to isolate the child from other family members. • Provide fluids to keep nasal secretions moist and to prevent dehydration. • Provide acetaminophen or ibuprofen for fever management and mild pain. • If antiviral medications are given, be alert for nausea and vomiting. Zanamivir can exacerbate asthma. • Provide rest and quiet diversional activities. • Children should be kept home until 24 hr after fever is gone. • Teach parents to be alert to signs of complications from the viral infection. • Become familiar with community pandemic infection plans.
MEASLES (RUBEOLA)[a, b] *Causal agent:* Morbillivirus, a member of the paramyxovirus group. *Epidemiology:* Occurrence peaks in the late winter and early spring. In 2014, 592 cases and 18 outbreaks occurred in the United States, mostly in unimmunized children. Most outbreaks were linked to cases imported from other countries (CDC, 2014d). *Transmission:* Direct contact with respiratory droplets and airborne spread. *Incubation period:* About 8–12 days. *Period of communicability:* From 4 days before the rash until 4 days after its appearance. 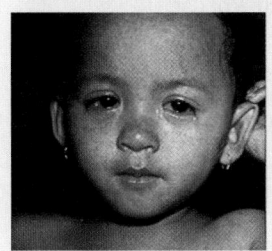 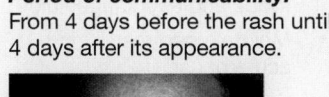Barbara Rice/Centers for Disease Control and Prevention	*Prodromal stage:* High fever (up to 105.0°F [40.5°C]), malaise, cough, coryza, conjunctivitis. Koplik spots (1–3 mm gray or blue-gray spots on an erythematous base) appear opposite the second molars on the buccal mucosa. They slough before or during the onset of the rash. This stage lasts 1–3 days. *Stage 2:* Maculopapular rash (dark red to purple), reaching a peak in 2–4 days when it becomes confluent. The mildly pruritic rash begins on the face and spreads to the trunk and extremities. Other symptoms include fatigue, photophobia, and generalized lymphadenopathy. *Complications:* About 30% of cases develop pneumonia, otitis media, diarrhea, or encephalitis (CDC, 2014d). Complications and death occur most often in children who are malnourished or immunocompromised.	*Diagnostic testing:* Serologic test for immunoglobulin (Ig) M measles antibody. *Medical management:* Supportive care. No antiviral therapy is available. Antibiotics are used for secondary bacterial infections. MMR vaccine within 72 hr of exposure or immune globulin within 6 days of exposure may help prevent or reduce disease severity. *Prognosis:* Increased risk of death in children under age 5 years and immunocompromised persons (AAP, 2015, p. 535). *Prevention:* Measles is a vaccine-preventable disease (see Table 43–1). This is a reportable disease.	• Maintain airborne precautions when the child is hospitalized. • Use a cool-mist vaporizer to help clear respiratory passages. Suction nose and oral cavity gently if needed. • Give nonaspirin antipyretics for fever and antipruritics for itching. Cough medication may be prescribed. • Teach parents to observe for complications and to seek care as needed. • Keep lights dim, and cover windows if the child has photophobia. • Keep skin clean and dry. Avoid using soap. • Offer cool liquids frequently in small amounts. Blended, pureed, and mashed foods are most easily tolerated. • Maintain bed rest. Visitors should be immune to measles. Provide diversional activities.

[a]Indicates that a vaccine or antitoxin is available for use in high-risk or as-needed situations.

[b]Indicates that the disease has a safe and effective vaccine.

(continued)

TABLE 43–5 Selected Infectious and Communicable Diseases in Children (*continued*)

DISEASE	CLINICAL MANIFESTATIONS	CLINICAL THERAPY	NURSING MANAGEMENT
MENINGOCOCCUS			

Causal agent: *Neisseria meningitidis,* a gram-negative diplococcus.

Epidemiology: Often occurs in winter or early spring. Serogroups B, C, and Y cause the most disease in the United States. Highest rates occur in infants under 1 year of age and adolescents 16–21 years. Outbreaks have occurred in childcare centers, college dormitories, and military recruit camps. There are fewer than 1000 cases annually in the United States (CDC, 2014e).

Transmission: Spread by direct contact with respiratory secretions from human carriers.

Incubation period: 3–7 days.

Period of communicability: Until 24 hr of treatment with an effective antibiotic.

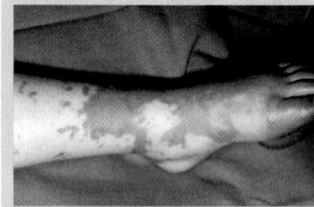

Medical-on-Line/Alamy

Meningitis: Most common invasive disease. Abrupt onset of flulike symptoms of fever, malaise, stiff neck, nausea, vomiting, decreased mental status, seizures, and coma.

Meningococcemia (sepsis caused by meningococcus): Fatigue; vomiting; cold hands and feet; chills; severe aches and pains in muscles, joints, chest, and abdomen; rapid breathing; diarrhea. An urticarial, maculopapular or petechial rash appears that may progress to purpura (see figure) and severe septic shock.

Complications: Approximately 11%–19% of survivors have serious sequelae (CDC, 2014e). Survivors of meningitis may develop hearing loss or neurologic disability. Survivors of meningococcemia may have permanent disabilities from digit or limb amputations, and scarring from skin grafts.

Diagnostic testing: Cultures of the blood and cerebrospinal fluid, and a Gram stain of petechial skin scrapings.

Medical management: IV antibiotics with penicillin G, cefotaxime, ceftriaxone, or ampicillin; chloramphenicol for children allergic to penicillin.

The child is treated in the ICU for shock with IV fluids and vasopressors, and with respiratory support. Blood products are used to treat disseminated intravascular coagulation.

Several surgeries may be needed for removal of necrotic tissue.

Prognosis: Even with antibiotic treatment about 10%–15% of clients die (CDC, 2013e).

Prevention: Several serotypes are vaccine preventable (see Table 43–1).

Close contacts receive an antibiotic. Community contacts should also receive the meningococcal vaccine to prevent an outbreak (AAP, 2015, p. 557). This is a reportable disease.

- Use standard and droplet precautions until an effective antibiotic has been administered for 24 hr.
- Be alert for development of shock and respiratory compromise as the disease progresses quickly. Have emergency equipment available.
- Avoid overloading the child with IV fluids and blood products. Administer medications as prescribed.
- Monitor the child with meningitis for signs of increased intracranial pressure.
- Help the family mobilize its support system, and keep the family informed of the child's status and treatment as the disease progresses.
- Help identify contacts who should receive prophylactic antibiotics. Educate them about the expected side effects (i.e., orange urine with rifampin).
- Teach contacts to be observant for signs of illness and to seek health care promptly if they occur.
- The surviving child will often need rehabilitation for limb amputations or hearing loss. Work with the social worker to transition the child to long-term care.

MONONUCLEOSIS			

Causal agent: Epstein-Barr virus (EBV), human herpesvirus type 4.

Epidemiology: The virus infects the oral mucosa and salivary glands. Occurs worldwide in no seasonal pattern. Infection is common in adolescents and young adults in the United States.

Transmission: Direct contact with saliva or exposure to body fluids (e.g., blood or semen).

Incubation period: Estimated to be 4–6 weeks.

Young children may have a mild infection with no distinguishing clinical signs.

Symptoms include fever, malaise, headache, anorexia, abdominal pain, a painful sore throat (exudative pharyngotonsillitis), and enlarged cervical lymph nodes. An enlarged spleen and liver may occur.

The syndrome typically lasts 2–4 weeks, but fatigue may continue for weeks.

Complications: Peritonsillar abscess, sinusitis, mastoiditis.

Diagnostic testing: A heterophil antibody response test. Greater than 10% atypical lymphocytes and a positive heterophil antibody response test are diagnostic (AAP, 2015, p. 337–338).

Medical management: Supportive care. Corticosteroids may be used for tonsillar swelling and impending airway obstruction, massive splenomegaly, myocarditis, or hemolytic anemia.

Antibiotics (ampicillin and amoxicillin) are not used because a nonallergic rash often develops (AAP, 2015, p. 339).

- Use standard precautions if the child is hospitalized.
- Give antipyretics and analgesics for fever and sore throat. Offer warm salt water for gargling. Offer soft foods and encourage fluids.
- Maintain bed rest during acute phase.
- Educate the teen to avoid intimate contact and not to share food and beverages until recovered.

DISEASE	CLINICAL MANIFESTATIONS	CLINICAL THERAPY	NURSING MANAGEMENT
Period of communicability: May be weeks before symptoms occur, and becomes latent after infection. Contagious if reactivation occurs (CDC, 2014f).	Rare conditions include neurologic disorders (e.g., meningitis, encephalitis, and Guillain-Barré syndrome), hematologic disorders (lymphocytosis), and immune disorders. Those with immune disorders have more severe disease.	**Prognosis:** Rarely fatal. After recovery, the virus becomes latent in the lymphoid system and can reactivate during periods of immunosuppression. **Prevention:** No known prevention.	• Return to contact sports and strenuous activity (e.g., weight lifting) is approved by the healthcare provider when the liver and spleen are normal size, usually in about 4 weeks. • If splenomegaly is present, alcohol should be avoided for 3 months after liver function test results return to normal.

MUMPS (PAROTITIS)[b]

| **Causal agent:** *Rubulavirus* in the Paramyxoviridae family.

Epidemiology: Occurs worldwide in unvaccinated children, most often in winter and spring. Infection and vaccination induce lifelong immunity.

Transmission: Inhalation of respiratory secretion droplets.

Incubation period: 12–25 days.

Period of communicability: Up to 5 days before and after parotid swelling onset.

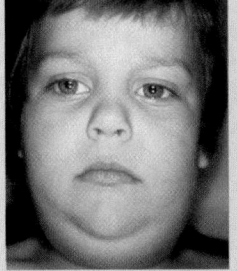 Centers for Disease Control and Prevention | Acute onset of malaise, fever, muscle aches, and swelling of one or more salivary glands (parotid, sublingual, or submaxillary) are the classic signs. Other signs include earache, headache, pain with chewing, and decreased appetite and activity. May be asymptomatic in some children.

Complications: Orchitis (inflammation of the testicles) that rarely leads to fertility problems, encephalitis, oophoritis (inflammation of ovaries), temporary or permanent deafness. Viral meningitis occurs in less than 10% of cases (AAP, 2015, p. 564). | **Diagnostic testing:** Viral culture from a throat washing, urine, or cerebrospinal fluid. A serologic test for mumps-specific IgM antibodies may be performed.

Medical management: Supportive care focused on symptom relief.

Prognosis: Mumps is usually self-limiting.

Prevention: Mumps is a vaccine-preventable disease.

This is a reportable disease. | • Use standard and droplet precautions for hospitalized children while contagious.

• Children are cared for at home. They may be uncomfortable but rarely very ill. Provide diversion.

• Avoid exposure to immunocompromised or susceptible individuals.

• Give acetaminophen or ibuprofen to control fever and pain.

• Encourage fluid intake. Offer soft and blended foods as chewing and swallowing may be painful. Avoid foods and beverages that increase salivary flow and cause pain (e.g., citrus, spices, and candies).

• Be alert for signs of complications.

• Keep children out of school or child care until 5 days after parotid swelling occurs. |

PERTUSSIS (WHOOPING COUGH)[b]

| **Causal agent:** *Bordetella pertussis*.

Epidemiology: Occurs worldwide and year-round. Rates have increased because of waning immunity with 28,639 cases in 2013 (CDC, 2013a). Children with waning immunity can spread the disease to unimmunized young infants at greatest risk for death from the infection.

Transmission: Inhalation or direct contact with respiratory droplets.

Incubation period: 5–10 days. | **Catarrhal stage:** The onset is insidious with cold symptoms, a runny nose, mild cough, and fever, lasting about 1–2 weeks.

Paroxysmal stage: A series of rapid coughs followed by a forceful inspiration through a narrowed glottis causes stridor, or the "whoop." The child has cyanosis, vomiting, and exhaustion associated with coughing paroxysms. Infants under 6 months of age may have gagging, gasping, or apnea rather than whooping. Sucking on a bottle may trigger coughing, leading to poor oral intake and dehydration. The "whoop" may be absent in immunized children. | **Diagnostic testing:** Nasopharyngeal culture, polymerase chain reaction (PCR) testing, and serology.

Medical management: Supportive care. Macrolide antibiotics (erythromycin, clarithromycin, azithromycin, and trimethroprim-sulfamethoxazole). Symptoms are reduced only if initiated in the catarrhal stage (CDC, 2013a).

Prognosis: The disease is most severe in infants younger than 6 months, of which 1.6% will die (CDC, 2013a). | • Use droplet precautions until 5 days after effective antibiotic is initiated.

• Monitor respirations and oxygen saturation with a cardiac monitor and pulse oximetry. The smaller the infant, the greater the risk for apnea.

• Meet infant needs promptly to reduce crying, which can precipitate coughing. Remain with the child during coughing spells, when hypoxic and apneic episodes are most likely. Give oxygen if ordered. Have emergency equipment available. |

[a]Indicates that a vaccine or antitoxin is available for use in high-risk or as-needed situations.
[b]Indicates that the disease has a safe and effective vaccine.

(continued)

TABLE 43–5 Selected Infectious and Communicable Diseases in Children (*continued*)

DISEASE	CLINICAL MANIFESTATIONS	CLINICAL THERAPY	NURSING MANAGEMENT
PERTUSSIS (WHOOPING COUGH) (*continued*)			
Period of communicability: Most contagious prior to the paroxysmal cough stage and for 2 weeks after cough onset if untreated. Communicable for 5 days after beginning effective antibiotic.	*Convalescent stage:* Up to 6–10 weeks later paroxysms gradually subside. *Complications:* Among infants: pneumonia, seizures, apnea, encephalopathy, and death. In adolescents: sleep disturbance, incontinence, syncope, rib fractures, and pneumonia (CDC, 2013a).	*Prevention:* Pertussis is a vaccine-preventable disease (see Table 43–1). The vaccine protection wanes over time. All adults should receive a Tdap booster every 10 years. Pregnant women should be immunized to protect their newborns from pertussis during the third trimester. The father and family members who will have close contact with the newborn should receive a Tdap booster prior to the newborn's birth (CDC, 2015). Close contacts should receive macrolide antibiotic prophylaxis.	• Provide humidification. Gentle suctioning may be necessary. • Give nonaspirin antipyretics as needed for fever. • Encourage frequent rest periods. • Provide small frequent feeding of desired foods. Encourage fluids. The child may need IV hydration if oral intake is not tolerated. • Provide emotional support to parents. • Teach parents to watch for signs of respiratory failure and dehydration if the child is managed at home.
PNEUMOCOCCAL INFECTION[b]			
Causative agent: Strepto-coccus pneumoniae, a gram-positive diplococcus, many serotypes. *Epidemiology:* Found in the pharynx of healthy people. Outbreaks occur in winter and spring in temperate climates, and only a few of the 90 serotypes account for most of the invasive pediatric infections. *Transmission:* Direct contact with respiratory secretions, and droplets and self-innoculation. *Incubation period:* 1–3 days. *Period of communicability:* Unknown. Probably within 24 hr after effective antibiotic therapy is initiated.	Causes invasive disease with signs and symptoms related to the focal area of infection. *Otitis media*—upper respiratory infection, fever, ear pain, and decreased appetite. *Bacteremia*—unexplained fever, reduced responsiveness, and no localized infection site. *Pneumonia*—fever, chills, chest pain, dyspnea, malaise, and a productive cough. *Meningitis*—inconsolable crying, increased irritability, lethargy, refusal to eat, nausea, vomiting, diarrhea, myalgia, photophobia, and seizures. The organism also causes sinusitis, pharyngitis, cellulitis, and laryngotracheobronchitis. Children under age 2 years, or having immunodeficiency (e.g., asplenia, malignancy, sickle cell disease, HIV infection, and nephrotic syndrome) and cochlear implants are at higher risk of invasive disease. *Complications:* Hearing loss or developmental delay from meningitis, empyema or pericarditis from pneumonia, and death.	*Diagnostic testing:* Bacterial culture from the site of infection. *Medical management:* Symptomatic care. Antibiotic selection is based upon culture sensitivity. Many pneumococcal strains are resistant to penicillin, cefotaxime, and ceftriaxone. Vancomycin may be required. Dexamethasone may be an adjunctive therapy for meningitis. *Prognosis:* An estimated 200 children die annually from pneumococcal disease (CDC, 2013b). Pneumococcal meningitis is associated with neurologic sequelae (e.g., hearing loss, motor deficits). *Prevention:* Many serotypes are vaccine preventable (see Table 43–1). Pneumococcal vaccine with 23 serotypes (PPSV23) is used for children at high risk of pneumococcal invasive disease.	• Maintain standard precautions. • Provide nonaspirin antipyretics for control of fever and comfort. • Encourage fluids, and monitor intake and output. • Monitor vital signs and level of consciousness to identify signs of worsening condition. • Educate parents about the need for the vaccine. The unimmunized child can become infected repeatedly with different serotypes. • Many children with mild disease will be treated at home. Educate parents about signs indicating a need to seek urgent medical care, medication administration, and comfort measures for the child.

DISEASE	CLINICAL MANIFESTATIONS	CLINICAL THERAPY	NURSING MANAGEMENT
POLIOMYELITIS[b]			
Causal agent: Poliovirus is an enterovirus with three serotypes. **Epidemiology:** Global eradication efforts have interrupted the transmission of polio in all but three countries—Afghanistan, Nigeria, and Pakistan (CDC, 2013c). Imported and wild polio is a threat to inadequately immunized children. **Transmission:** Direct contact with respiratory secretions and body fluids. **Incubation period:** Usually 7–10 days (range 3–36 days). **Period of communicability:** Greatest shortly before and with onset of clinical symptoms. The virus is excreted in the feces for 3–6 weeks.	More than 90% of infections are asymptomatic. **Mild illness:** A low-grade fever and sore throat. This minor illness may be followed by aseptic meningitis and paresthesias. **Serious illness:** Asymmetric flaccid paralysis may occur acutely in up to 1% of cases. Site of paralysis is commonly the legs, but it may affect the respiratory muscles. Residual paralysis may occur in more than half of those affected (AAP, 2015, p. 644). **Complications:** Permanent motor paralysis, respiratory arrest, postpolio syndrome, and death.	**Diagnostic testing:** Cell culture from stool or throat swabs. **Medical management:** Supportive therapy. No effective chemotherapeutic agents exist. **Prognosis:** Respiratory paralysis may lead to death. Motor paralysis may result in long-term disability. **Prevention:** Poliomyelitis is a vaccine-preventable disease (see Table 43–1). The vaccine is believed to confer lifelong immunity. This is a reportable disease.	• Use standard and droplet precautions. • Monitor for respiratory paralysis (ineffective cough, talking with frequent pauses, shallow and rapid respiratory rate). Have emergency equipment at bedside. Assist ventilations as needed until mechanical ventilation is set up. • Use moist hot packs, which may relieve discomfort. • Encourage fluids. • Keep the child on bed rest. Position the child to promote body alignment. • Perform range of motion exercises to prevent contractures after the acute phase. • Provide emotional support. Keep the child and family informed about the illness and therapies. • Help coordinate rehabilitation, such as long-term physical therapy when needed.
ROSEOLA (EXANTHEM SUBITUM, SIXTH DISEASE)			
Causal agent: Human herpesvirus type 6 (HHV-6). **Epidemiology:** Occurs worldwide year-round with no seasonal pattern. Occurs primarily in children 6–24 months of age (as maternal antibodies decline). Nearly all children are infected by 3 years of age. Congenital infection is also possible (AAP, 2015, p. 451). **Transmission:** Contact with saliva or respiratory secretions. **Incubation period:** Appears to be 9–10 days. **Period of communicability:** Healthy persons shed the virus (AAP, 2015, p. 450).	**Prodromal stage:** Sudden fever greater than 39.5°C (103.0°F) for 3–7 days, during which the child has a normal appetite and behavior, no rash or specific disease signs. **Rash stage:** A characteristic pale pink, discrete, maculopapular rash starts on the trunk and spreads to the face, neck, and extremities, lasting hours to days. The child may have characteristic postoccipital lymphadenopathy, tympanic membrane redness, and respiratory and gastrointestinal signs. **Complications:** Febrile seizures are common; encephalopathy or encephalitis may occur.	**Diagnostic testing:** Polymerase chain reaction (PCR) testing for HHV-6 in the blood or cerebrospinal fluid. **Medical management:** Supportive treatment for this self-limiting condition. **Prognosis:** Full recovery is usual. **Prevention:** No preventive measures.	• Use standard precautions if the child is hospitalized. • Give nonaspirin antipyretics to control fever. • Observe closely for any seizure activity, especially during the acute febrile periods. • Encourage fluids to maintain hydration. • Reassure parents that the rash will disappear in a few days.
ROTAVIRUS[b]			
Causal agent: RNA viruses of the Reoviridae family. Groups A, B, and C infect humans. **Epidemiology:** Occurs more often in cool periods, peaking in the spring in the United States. A common cause of severe diarrhea in children less than age 5 years.	Acute onset of fever and vomiting followed by watery diarrhea 1–2 days later. Up to 10–20 diarrheal stools a day. Symptoms lasting 3–8 days.	**Diagnostic testing:** Enzyme immunoassay or latex agglutination assay of a stool specimen. **Medical management:** Treatment involves adequate amounts of fluid and electrolyte replacement with oral rehydration solution. Antimotility drugs should not be used. If severely dehydrated, IV fluid resuscitation is performed. No antiviral therapy is available.	• Use standard and contact precautions. • Use good hand hygiene with soap and water or gel cleansers. • Clean and disinfect contaminated surfaces. • Assess hydration status frequently.

[a]Indicates that a vaccine or antitoxin is available for use in high-risk or as-needed situations.

[b]Indicates that the disease has a safe and effective vaccine.

(continued)

TABLE 43–5 Selected Infectious and Communicable Diseases in Children (*continued*)

DISEASE	CLINICAL MANIFESTATIONS	CLINICAL THERAPY	NURSING MANAGEMENT
ROTAVIRUS (*continued*)			
Transmission: Fecal-oral route, direct contact with contaminated objects. ***Incubation:*** 1–3 days. ***Period of communicability:*** Virus may persist in stool when child is immunocompromised.	***Complications:*** Dehydration and electrolyte disturbances. Immunocompromised children may develop persistent infection and diarrhea (AAP, 2015, p. 684).	***Prevention:*** Vaccine prevents several common viral groups (see Table 43–1).	• Breastfeeding is continued during oral rehydration therapy, but wait up to 24 hr before giving formula. • Feed older children complex carbohydrates and lean meats, yogurt, fruits, and vegetables 12–24 hr after starting oral rehydration therapy.
RUBELLA (GERMAN MEASLES)[b]			
Causal agent: An RNA virus, member of the family Togaviridae, genus *Rubivirus*. ***Epidemiology:*** Occurs worldwide. Most prevalent in winter and spring. No longer endemic in the United States (AAP, 2015, p. 689). Most U.S. cases occur among persons from other countries and those underimmunized. Congenital rubella syndrome occurs between 12 weeks of gestation to the end of the second trimester. ***Transmission:*** Droplet spread, direct contact with nasal secretions. ***Incubation period:*** 14–21 days. ***Period of communicability:*** 7 days before until 7 days after rash onset. Infants with congenital rubella may shed the virus for 1 year or longer after birth.	***Prodromal stage:*** Asymptomatic or low-grade fever, malaise, coryza, and sore throat, 1–5 days before the rash. Forschheimer spots (discrete, erythematous pinpoint or larger lesions on the soft palate) are seen. Posterior auricular and suboccipital lymphadenopathy may precede the rash. ***Rash stage:*** 1–5 days later a pink, maculopapular rash appears on the face and neck. The rash spreads to the trunk and legs, and fades in the same sequence. ***Complications:*** Transient arthralgia in adolescents; encephalitis. Pregnant females infected during the first trimester may have a fetus with congenital rubella syndrome birth defects (e.g., cataracts, heart defects, hearing impairment, thrombocytopenia, and purpuric skin lesions that give a "blueberry muffin" appearance) (see figure).	***Diagnostic testing:*** Cell culture from a nasal swab, and detection of IgM or IgG antibodies. ***Medical management:*** Supportive treatment. Rubella is a self-limiting in children. ***Prognosis:*** Full recovery is expected. Congenital rubella syndrome may result in death or congenital anomalies. ***Prevention:*** Rubella is a vaccine-preventable disease (see Table 43–1). 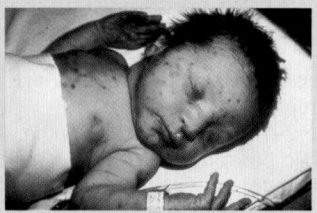 Centers for Disease Control and Prevention	• Maintain standard and droplet precautions. • Maintain contact precautions for infants with congenital rubella syndrome until 1 year of age unless nasopharyngeal and urine cultures are repeatedly negative after 3 months of age (AAP, 2015, p. 691). • Children are usually treated at home. Provide quiet activities. • Isolate the child from pregnant women. • Give nonaspirin analgesics and antipyretics for any pain and fever. • Encourage the child to consume preferred fluids and food. • Exclude children from child care or school for 7 days after onset of rash. Notify the school or childcare facilities of the child's illness.
STREPTOCOCCUS A			
Causal agent: Group A streptococci (GAS), numerous serotypes. ***Epidemiology:*** Pharyngeal infections tend to occur more in late fall, winter, and spring when closer person-to-person contact occurs. Pyodermal infections more often occur in warmer seasons with minor skin trauma and insect bites. Different serotypes are associated with pharyngeal and pyodermal infections, rheumatic fever, and acute glomerulonephritis (AAP, 2015, p. 733). ***Transmission:*** Contact with respiratory secretions for pharyngitis or skin lesions for pyoderma.	***Pharyngeal:*** Abrupt onset with a sore throat, dysphagia, tender cervical lymph nodes, malaise, high fever, chills, headache, abdominal pain, anorexia, and vomiting. The pharynx is beefy red with exudates, and palatal petechiae may be seen. ***GAS respiratory tract infection:*** Children younger than 3 years may have serous rhinitis, moderate fever, irritability, and anorexia rather than pharyngitis.	***Diagnostic testing:*** Rapid strep test or a culture of secretions from the pharynx and tonsils, blood culture for invasive disease. Cultures of skin lesions do not reveal primary organism (AAP, 2015, p. 737). ***Medical management:*** Prompt oral antibiotic therapy with penicillin V or amoxicillin or IM penicillin G benzathine. Clindamycin or oral macrolide may be used if the child is allergic to penicillin.	• Use standard and droplet precautions for pharyngeal infections and contact precautions for skin infections. • Promote bed rest during the febrile stage. • Give nonaspirin antipyretics to control fever. Teach parents important signs of a worsening condition. • For pharyngeal infections, offer warm salt water for gargling and nonacidic beverages. Encourage cool, clear liquids and a soft diet. Swallowing may be difficult.

DISEASE	CLINICAL MANIFESTATIONS	CLINICAL THERAPY	NURSING MANAGEMENT
Incubation period: Pharyngeal: usually 2–5 days. Pyodermal: usually 7–10 days. **Period of communicability:** For weeks in untreated pharyngeal infections; not contagious within 24 hr of starting antibiotics. 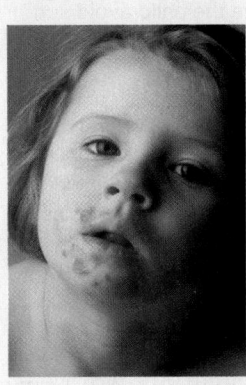 Bubbles Photolibrary/Alamy	**Scarlet fever:** A characteristic erythematous, confluent, sandpaper rash, starting on the neck and spreading to the trunk and extremities. The rash blanches with pressure, concentrates in flexor skin creases, and spares the circumoral area. In 3–4 days, the rash begins to fade and the tips of the toes and fingers peel. The classic strawberry tongue is seen on days 4–5. Most often occurs after pharyngeal symptoms. **Pyodermal:** Lesions (impetigo) are honey-colored crusts at the site of open lesions (see figure). **Complications:** If untreated, acute otitis media, sinusitis, peritonsillar or retropharyngeal abscess, cervical lymphadenitis, acute rheumatic fever, and acute glomerulonephritis. Invasive disease with toxic shock syndrome, bacteremia, necrotizing fasciitis, or myositis can be fatal.	Uncomplicated impetigo is treated with mupirocin or retapamulin ointment. See Chapter 57 for more information about bacterial skin infections and toxic shock syndrome. See Chapter 47 for treatment of acute rheumatic fever. **Prognosis:** Recovery is usually good with antibiotic therapy. Children can become long-term carriers of streptococcus A in their pharynx. **Prevention:** None.	• Explain to parents the importance of giving the full course of antibiotics. • Encourage other family members with sore throats to have throat cultures taken. • For impetigo, encourage good hand hygiene. Teach the parents to wash the skin, remove crusts, and apply antibiotic ointment. • Replace the child's toothbrush after treatment to prevent reinfection.
TETANUS[a, b] **Causal agent:** *Clostridium tetani,* an anaerobic gram-positive bacillus. **Epidemiology:** Bacillus is common and exists as a spore in soil, dust, and manure. The organism produces an endotoxin that affects the central nervous system. **Transmission:** Wounds (e.g., superficial, puncture, burns, crush injuries) exposed to contaminated soil or objects. **Incubation period:** 3–21 days (average 10 days). **Period of communicability:** No direct person-to-person contact.	Fever, diaphoresis, headache, and neck and jaw stiffness with painful facial spasms and difficulty chewing and swallowing, seizures, painful muscle stiffness, hypertension, tachycardia. Facial muscle spasms may produce a grinning expression (risus sardonicus). Eventual rigidity of the abdomen and trunk produce **opisthotonos** (rigid hyperextension of the entire body). Respiratory muscles may be affected and cause airway obstruction and suffocation. Newborns have increasing difficulty with sucking, irritability, and neck stiffness. **Complications:** Laryngospasm, respiratory distress, death.	**Diagnostic testing:** Based on clinical signs; cultures often ineffective. **Medical management:** IM human tetanus immune globulin with some injected into the wound site. The wound is cleaned and debrided. Antibiotics and medications to relieve muscle spasms are administered. Intensive care is provided with assisted ventilation, nutrition, and supportive care. Complete recovery may take weeks. **Prognosis:** Fatality rates are 10%–20%, depending on quality of supportive care (CDC, 2013d). **Prevention:** Tetanus is a vaccine-preventable disease (see Table 43–1). A tetanus booster is needed every 10 years, or, if a contaminated wound occurs, in 5 years.	• Use standard precautions. • Assist with wound debridement. • Monitor the child's condition. Handle as little as possible. Reduce stimulation by placing the child in a quiet, darkened room. • Offer skin and respiratory care. The child may need an endotracheal tube, suctioning, and supplemental oxygen for airway support. • Provide feedings via total parenteral nutrition or feeding tube. • Maintain hydration with IV fluids and electrolytes. • Try to reduce the child's anxiety, as mental status may be unaffected by disease process. • Prepare the family for a possible poor prognosis.

[a]Indicates that a vaccine or antitoxin is available for use in high-risk or as-needed situations.
[b]Indicates that the disease has a safe and effective vaccine.

TABLE 43–6 Selected Infectious Diseases Transmitted by Insect or Animal Hosts (Zoonosis)

DISEASE	CLINICAL MANIFESTATIONS	CLINICAL THERAPY	NURSING MANAGEMENT

LYME DISEASE

Causal agent: *Borrelia burgdorferi,* a spirochete transmitted by ixodid ticks.

Epidemiology: It occurs in most U.S. states, with greatest number of cases in the Northeastern, Mid-Atlantic, and North Central states. Exposure occurs in any outdoor setting where ticks are endemic. Most cases occur between May and November, with the highest rate in the summer.

Among children, the highest incidence in the United States is in 5- to 9-year-olds (AAP, 2015, p. 518).

Transmission: The tick is attached for 36–48 hr before the infection is transmitted (CDC, 2014g). Lyme disease is the most common vectorborne illness in North America.

Incubation period: 1–32 days after an infected tick bite.

Period of communicability: The infection is not communicable from person to person.

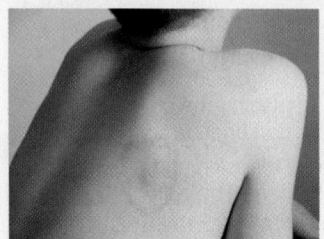

Kevin Shields/Alamy

Localized disease (LD): Erythema migrans, a painless annular red rash that expands over days or weeks to 5–30 cm (2–12 in.) in diameter. It may have partial central clearing (bull's eye) or look like a bruise in clients with dark skin. It occurs in about 70%–80% of cases, an average of 7 days after the tick bite (CDC, 2014g). The client may only have fever, chills, fatigue, body aches, malaise, and swollen lymph nodes. Some clients have both the rash and illness.

Early disseminated disease (EDD): In 3–10 weeks after the tick bite, multiple smaller erythema migrans lesions, generalized lymphadenopathy, and fatigue. Meningitis, facial nerve palsy, carditis, and migratory muscle and joint pain may occur.

Late disseminated disease (LDD): In 2–12 months, Lyme arthritis develops, commonly in the large joints such as the knee. Joint swelling, pain, and tenderness are seen.

Complications: Left untreated, Lyme disease progresses to LDD with cranial nerve palsies, carditis, encephalitis, or meningitis.

Diagnostic testing: Enzyme-linked immunosorbent assay (ELISA) plus the Western blot test.

Medical management: Oral amoxicillin, cefuroxime axetil, or doxycycline for 14–21 days for LD, 21–28 days for EDD, and up to 28 days for LDD. Intravenous antibiotics may be administered for up to 28 days for persistent arthritis, carditis, meningitis, or encephalitis.

Prognosis: Treatment during LD or EDD rarely progresses to LDD. May result in significant morbidity when chronic Lyme disease develops.

Prevention: No vaccine is available. There is no acquired immunity, so reinfection may occur.

Avoid areas that are heavily tick infested, and wear protective clothing. Check for ticks (especially hidden in hair) after every outing. Check pets that may carry home ticks that can transfer to the child. Remove ticks as soon as possible.

- Use standard precautions if the child is hospitalized.
- Educate parents about the importance of giving the full course of antibiotics.
- Have the child avoid sun exposure when taking doxycycline.
- Provide nonaspirin analgesics and antipyretics for relief of fever, headache, and muscle or joint aches.
- Children with Lyme disease may tire easily. Promote rest and avoid vigorous activities.
- Teach parents to safely remove ticks. Grasp the tick gently but firmly with fine-point tweezers where the mouthparts are attached. Pull gently until the tick releases. Clean the area with soap and water.

MALARIA

Causal agent: Plasmodium, four species (*P. falciparum, P. vivax, P. ovale, P. malariae*)

Epidemiology: Occurs in tropical and subtropical regions on four continents (Africa, Americas, Asia, and Oceana). Children have the highest mortality. The disease is acquired during travel to an endemic area, most often among immigrants visiting their home country who did not take preventive measures. *P. falciparum* causes the most serious disease. In 2011, 1947 cases were reported in the United States; 15% of all reported cases occurred in children 18 years old and younger (Cullen & Arguin, 2013).

Malaria begins with nonspecific signs such as high fever alternating with chills, profuse diaphoresis, and fatigue. Periods of symptomatic improvement may be seen between cycles lasting 48 or 72 hr depending upon type of infection.

Children may also have fever, anorexia, vomiting, jaundice, splenomegaly, and anemia. Additional symptoms include nausea, vomiting, diarrhea, cough, tachypnea, arthralgia, and body aches.

Diagnostic testing: Blood smears for parasites, or a PCR assay. A rapid malaria test is available. Blood tests may show anemia and thrombocytopenia.

Medical management: The child is hospitalized for fluid replacement, anemia management, and antipyretics. The blood is regularly monitored for parasite density.

IV or oral antimalarial medication (e.g., chloroquine, quinine sulfate, doxycycline, mefloquine, and atovaquone-proguanil) is selected based on region visited and resistance of species to the medication. Hypoglycemia may result from quinine treatment or because parasites consume large quantities of glucose.

- Use standard precautions.
- Maintain fluid intake. Monitor intake and output.
- Monitor the hematocrit and hemoglobin, as well as the blood glucose level.
- Observe for signs of increasing illness severity such as confusion, seizures, and shock. Be prepared to protect the child from injury and provide emergency support with airways and oxygen until the child can be transferred to the ICU.

DISEASE	CLINICAL MANIFESTATIONS	CLINICAL THERAPY	NURSING MANAGEMENT
Transmission: An infected female mosquito introduces the parasite through a bite. The parasite infects hepatic cells and reproduces leading to hepatic cell rupture. Parasites are released and infect the red blood cells. Transmission can occur by blood transfusion or transplacentally *Incubation period:* Varies by type, generally 8–25 days after a mosquito bite, but may be up to 1 year. *Period of communicability:* Communicable by blood, blood product transfusion, or organ transplant from an infected person.	Attacks may recur over the course of the year after infection, but the parasites die out gradually if no reinfection. Children who live in endemic areas and survive the first 5 years of life develop immunity to the severe effects of the disease as long as they have frequent reexposure to the infection. *Complications:* Severe anemia and cerebral malaria in young children. Pulmonary edema, respiratory failure, renal failure, spontaneous bleeding, and shock in older children and adolescents. Children with asplenia are at high risk for death.	Children may need blood transfusions. Primaquine may be prescribed to prevent relapse. *Prognosis:* Certain species have dormant liver-stage parasites, which can reactivate several months or years after initial infection. *Prevention:* While traveling in endemic areas, use DEET insect repellent, screened rooms, DEET-treated mosquito netting, and cover the body with light-colored clothing. Antimalarial chemoprophylaxis may be prescribed when traveling in an endemic region. A vaccine is being tested in children. This is a reportable disease.	• Administer antipyretics to control the fever and promote comfort. • Educate families traveling to endemic areas about the need for and correct administration of antimalarial drugs, despite the nausea and vomiting side effects. • Discuss protecting children during mosquitoes' nocturnal feeding times with protective clothing, mosquito repellent, and mosquito netting around the bed.

RABIES (HYDROPHOBIA)

Causal agent: *Lyssavirus* in the Rhabdoviridae family, two types (urban, in dogs; wild, in wildlife). *Epidemiology:* Occurs worldwide. Urban rabies is generally controlled by vaccination of dogs and cats. The most common carriers of rabies are raccoons, bats, skunks, and foxes (CDC, 2013e). *Transmission:* Infected saliva from the bite of a rabid animal introduces the virus into the wound. The virus travels along the nerves to the brain where it multiplies and migrates along the efferent nerves to the salivary glands. Rare cases of human-to-human transmission through exposure to mucous membranes, aerosol droplets, and organ transplant. *Incubation period:* Highly variable but usually 1–3 months.	No signs during the long incubation period. *Prodromal stage:* Over 2–10 days the child has fever, headache, malaise, apprehension, and paresthesia at the site of the bite. *Neurologic stage:* Cerebral signs of agitation, anxiety, confusion followed by abnormal behavior, delirium, hallucinations, and insomnia. The child progresses to coma and respiratory failure. *Complications:* Usually results in death.	*Diagnostic testing:* Confirmed by direct fluorescent antibody staining of the dead animal's brain tissue or detection of the virus in the client's saliva or cerebrospinal fluid. *Medical management:* Immediately wash animal bites thoroughly with soap and water and irrigate well with a virucidal agent such as povidone-iodine. Antibiotics and wound suturing are determined for individual cases. Postexposure prophylaxis— one dose of human rabies immune globulin (HRIG) and human diploid cell rabies vaccine (HDCV) is given IM the day of the bite when the animal may be rabid. HRIG is infiltrated locally around the bite with remaining volume given IM at a site distant from the vaccine. HDCV is repeated on days 3, 7, and 14 after the bite (4 doses) (CDC, 2013e). The vaccine is of no value once rabies symptoms are present. *Prognosis:* Usually fatal. *Prevention:* Immunize all domestic animals against rabies.	• Alert the local animal control to find and quarantine the unimmunized animal for observation. • Administer human rabies immunoglobulin (HRIG) and human diploid cell vaccine (HDCV) as ordered. Inject vaccine into the muscle to prevent vaccine failure. • Support the family while reinforcing the urgency for the vaccine and series of injections. • Educate parents about the vaccine side effects— irritation and itching at the injection site, headache, muscle aches, nausea, and dizziness. • If the child acquires rabies, the child will be hospitalized. Use standard and contact precautions. • Make the child as comfortable as possible. • Keep liquids out of sight of the hydrophobic child. • Provide emotional support to the family of the dying child. • Teach children to avoid contact with all unknown animals, dead or alive. • Participate in local education about rabies and safe interactions with dogs. See Chapter 57.

(continued)

TABLE 43–6 Selected Infectious Diseases Transmitted by Insect or Animal Hosts (Zoonosis) *(continued)*

DISEASE	CLINICAL MANIFESTATIONS	CLINICAL THERAPY	NURSING MANAGEMENT
ROCKY MOUNTAIN SPOTTED FEVER (TICKBORNE TYPHUS FEVER, SAO PAULO TYPHUS)			

ROCKY MOUNTAIN SPOTTED FEVER (TICKBORNE TYPHUS FEVER, SAO PAULO TYPHUS)

DISEASE	CLINICAL MANIFESTATIONS	CLINICAL THERAPY	NURSING MANAGEMENT
Causal agent: *Rickettsia rickettsii,* a gram-negative coccobacillus. **Epidemiology:** Occurs throughout the United States, southern Canada, and Central and South America. In the United States, 60% of cases occur in North Carolina, Oklahoma, Arkansas, Tennessee, and Missouri (CDC 2013f). Most infections generally occur between April and September. **Transmission:** Transmitted by bites of ticks, principally dog and wood ticks. **Incubation period:** 2–14 days (most commonly 7 days) after bite of an infected tick. **Period of communicability:** There is no evidence of person-to-person transmission. 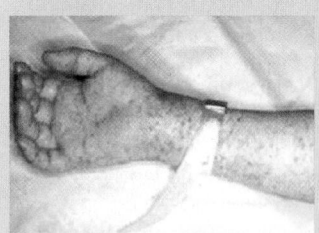 Science Source	Onset may be gradual or rapid with vague signs that mimic other diseases. Early symptoms are fever, malaise, headache, muscle aches, anorexia, nausea, vomiting, and diarrhea. The red maculopapular rash that blanches generally occurs 2–5 days after the fever. It appears first on the wrist, forearms, and ankles and then spreads to trunk and sometimes the palms and soles. The rash may be difficult to see on children with dark skin. A petechial rash appearing about day 6 is a sign of progression to severe disease. **Complications:** Vasculitis resulting in bleeding, disseminated intravascular coagulation (DIC), reduced circulation resulting in gangrene of digits or extremities, and neurologic deficits.	**Diagnostic testing:** Immunofluorescent antibody testing; direct immunofluorescence or immune-peroxidase tests may be performed on skin biopsies. Blood test may reveal thrombocytopenia. **Medical management:** Doxycycline regardless of client's age for 7–14 days (at least 3 days after fever subsides). The client with severe disease needs IV antibiotics. **Prognosis:** Delay in treatment can cause severe disease. A mortality rate of 1% is associated with delayed treatment (CDC 2013f). **Prevention:** Avoid areas that are heavily tick infested, and wear protective clothing. Check children for ticks and remove promptly if found.	• Use standard precautions. • The child may require care in the ICU. Have hemodynamic monitoring equipment and emergency supplies readily available. • Administer antibiotics as ordered. • Observe for any purpura development or abnormal bleeding. • Make the child as comfortable as possible. • Provide quiet diversion activities. • Provide emotional support, and keep parents informed about the child's condition. • Educate parents about prevention and the appropriate technique for tick removal.

ANTIBIOTIC USE

Antibiotics are often prescribed to treat bacterial infectious diseases; however, strains of bacteria have developed resistance to many antibiotics. Examples are community-acquired methicillin-resistant *Staphylococcus aureus* and drug-resistant strains of tuberculosis. Children with chronic conditions may be more susceptible to infection by drug-resistant pathogens. Many specialty organizations and medical centers have developed best practice guidelines for the use of antibiotics in treating common infections, such as acute otitis media.

Antiviral medications may be prescribed for viral infections, such as chickenpox and influenza. When the child is immunocompromised, antiviral medication should be started early to minimize the potential life-threatening consequences of the infection.

Cases of many communicable diseases must be reported to the state health department, using standardized state forms or on a designated website.

Nursing Management

For the Child With a Communicable Disease

Nursing Assessment and Diagnosis

Assess the child's hydration status and fluid intake, vital signs, comfort level, and appetite. Observe for seizures and for a **toxic appearance** (lethargy, poor perfusion, hypoventilation or hyperventilation, and cyanosis). The child with a fever may be irritable and restless, sleep fitfully, and have nonspecific muscular pain. Identify febrile children who may be at higher risk for a serious illness, in particular:

• Infants and children having a toxic appearance.

• Newborns less than 28 days of age with a temperature over 38.0°C (100.4°F).

• Children less than 4 years of age with a temperature over 41.0°C (105.8°F).

• Children with conditions such as a congenital heart disease, ventriculoperitoneal shunt, asplenia, and sickle cell disease.

Observe the child for other signs of infection, such as a rash, nausea and vomiting, or diarrhea, as well as generalized symptoms of a poor appetite, muscle aches, and malaise.

The following nursing diagnoses may be appropriate for children with communicable diseases (NANDA-I © 2014):

• ***Hyperthermia*** related to infectious disease process

• ***Skin Integrity, Impaired,*** related to skin lesions and scratching

• ***Mucous Membrane: Oral, Impaired,*** related to infectious disease process

• ***Fluid Volume: Deficient*** related to repeated episodes of vomiting and diarrhea

• ***Health Management, Family, Ineffective,*** related to complexity of care required by child

Pathophysiology Illustrated: **Fever**

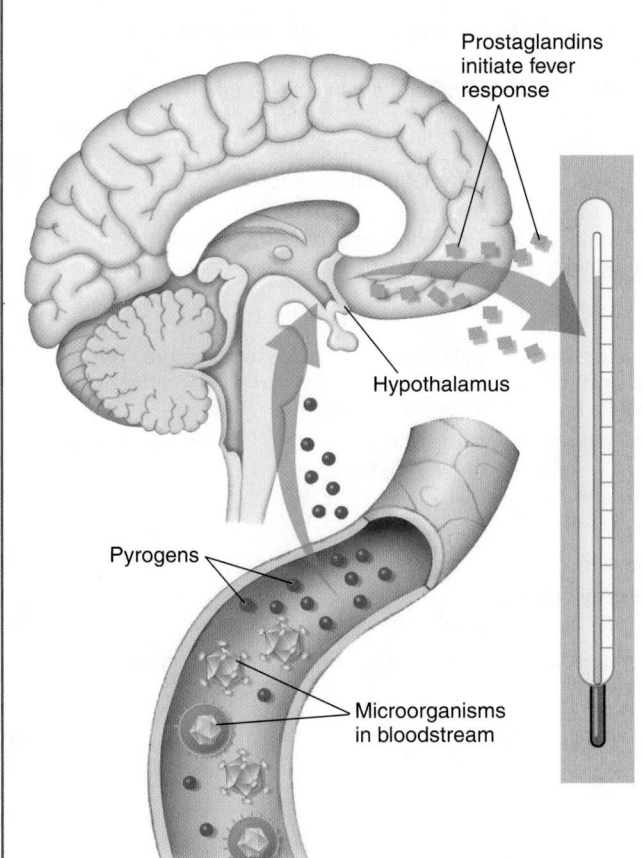

Prostaglandins initiate fever response

Hypothalamus

Pyrogens

Microorganisms in bloodstream

The hypothalamus functions as the body's thermostat, directing the body to conserve or dissipate heat. When microorganisms invade the body, **endogenous pyrogens** (interleukins, interferons, and tumor necrosis factor) are released by macrophages into the bloodstream. These substances travel to the hypothalamus where they trigger the production and release of prostaglandins, resulting in the fever response. A rise in the hypothalamus's set point leads to heat generation with shivering and chills, vasoconstriction, and decreased peripheral perfusion. Blood is diverted from the extremities to more central vessels to decrease heat loss. Shivering increases both metabolic action and heat production. The hypothalamus then maintains the temperature at the new set point. When the temperature is elevated, the heart rate, respiratory rate, and metabolic rate increase. Vasodilation occurs and the skin flushes, becoming warm to the touch.

Planning and Implementation

Most children with communicable diseases are cared for at home; however, infected children are seen in all healthcare settings. Nursing care includes collecting cultures, providing supportive care, administering antibiotics on schedule, monitoring antibiotic blood levels if indicated to ensure appropriate results, promoting the child's comfort, and educating parents.

PREVENT DISEASE TRANSMISSION

Nursing care of children with communicable diseases in healthcare settings focuses on preventing the spread of infection. Isolate children with suspicious rashes and respiratory infections. Cover draining wounds and dispose of dressings appropriately. All items with which the infected child comes into contact are considered contaminated (e.g., linens, toys, medical equipment). Use standard precautions and good hand hygiene. Recall that the fecal–oral and respiratory routes are the most common routes of transmission in children. Wipe down hard surfaces in the examining room with an antiseptic solution before another child uses the room. If possible, wipe down toys in the waiting room daily with a nontoxic antiseptic solution. Dispose of linens in appropriately marked linen bags. Ensure that all healthcare providers are fully immunized or that unimmunized or pregnant healthcare providers are not exposed to children with certain infections (e.g., pertussis, rubella, or varicella). See *Teaching Highlights: Reducing the Transmission of Infection* earlier in this chapter.

Children with severe infections are often admitted to the hospital for treatment. In addition, countless numbers of **nosocomial** (hospital-acquired) **infections** occur each year. Follow the facility's standard and transmission-based precautions to reduce the spread of infectious diseases to staff and other children. Discuss any concerns with the hospital's infection control nurse. (See the *Protective Methods* chapter in the *Clinical Skills Manual* SKILLS for more detailed information.)

FEVER MANAGEMENT

Nursing care for treatment of fever includes removing unnecessary clothing, encouraging increased fluid intake, and administering nonaspirin antipyretics. Identify clear fluids the child prefers to drink to encourage greater intake. Parents often fear a fever, believing it is a disease rather than a symptom of an illness. Provide information and reassurance. Help them to recognize signs that the child's condition is worsening. See *Teaching Highlights: Guidelines for Evaluating and Treating Fever in Children.*

EDUCATING THE FAMILY

Teach parents to care for their child at home. This includes how and when to give antipyretics and antibiotics if ordered, when over-the-counter medications may be used, appropriate fluids and foods to provide, and the care of rashes and other symptoms.

Teach parents to give all the antibiotic doses for the full number of days prescribed. Help develop a schedule that matches the family's routines. Make sure they know whether to give the antibiotic by mouth with or without food or apply topically. Inform them to discard the antibiotic when all doses have been given, and not to share the antibiotic with any other family member. These efforts will help fully treat the infection and reduce the chance that the infectious organism develops resistance to the antibiotic.

| TEACHING HIGHLIGHTS | Guidelines for Evaluating and Treating Fever in Children |

Facts about fevers:

- A fever is not a disease; it is the body's response to an infection. It means the child's body is using natural defenses to fight an infection.
- If the child has a fever and does not look sick, it may be better to let the child use natural defenses to fight off the virus or bacteria causing the fever.

Treating the fever:

- Use a thermometer to check the child's temperature every 4 to 6 hours, or more often if the fever returns.
- Use acetaminophen or ibuprofen (do not use aspirin) to lower the temperature. Use the correct dose and preparation for the child's weight, and mark down when the medication is given. Do not exceed the number of doses per day listed on the bottle to prevent an overdose. If the child is taking a cold medication with acetaminophen, call the healthcare provider for advice about acetaminophen dosage.
- Remove all but a light layer of the child's clothing.
- Monitor the child's behavior and response to fever medication. The medication will reduce the child's temperature. The temperature may rise again in 4 to 6 hours after the medicine has worn off. Check the temperature and give another dose of medication. The temperature will return to normal when the child is recovering from the illness.
- Sponging the child is not recommended. The lukewarm water may increase shivering and discomfort. Do not use alcohol for sponge baths.
- Give the child lots of fluids to drink and allow the child to rest.

Contact your healthcare provider immediately if:

- The infant is under 2 months old and has a fever over 38.0°C (100.4°F).
- The child has a fever over 40.1°C (104.2°F) and any of the following symptoms:
  - The child acts or looks very sick.
  - Inconsolable crying or whimpering. The child cries when moved or otherwise touched by the parent or other family members.
  - Difficult to awaken.
  - A stiff neck.
  - Purple spots on the skin.
  - Difficulty breathing that does not improve after the nose is cleared.
  - Unable to swallow and drooling saliva.
  - The child has a seizure.

Call your healthcare provider within 24 hours if:

- The child is 2 to 4 months old (unless fever occurs within 48 hours of a DTaP shot and the infant has no other serious symptoms).
- The child's fever is higher than 40.1°C (104.2°F), especially if the child is younger than age 3 years.
- The child complains of burning or pain with urination.
- The fever has been present more than 24 hours without an obvious cause or location of infection.
- The fever went away for more than 24 hours and then returned, or the fever has been present for more than 72 hours.

SAFETY ALERT!

Acetaminophen and ibuprofen preparations are available as infant drops, liquid syrup, chewable tablets, and adult-strength tablets or capsules. Identify the preparation used in the home to recommend the correct dosage for the child. The dose of acetaminophen is 10–15 mg/kg/dose and of ibuprofen is 4–10 mg/kg/dose. Alert parents that many over-the-counter medications also contain acetaminophen or ibuprofen; they should not be used at the same time as the antipyretic for fever to prevent an overdose.

ACETAMINOPHEN	IBUPROFEN
Infant drops—160 mg/5 mL using package dispenser	Infant drops—50 mg/1.25 mL using package dispenser
Children's liquid—160 mg/5 mL	Children's liquid—100 mg/5 mL
Chewable tablets—80 mg and 160 mg	Chewable and junior tablets—50 mg and 100 mg
Adult tablets or caplets—325 mg and 500 mg	Adult tablets or caplets—200 mg

Educate parents about methods to reduce disease transmission in the home. Encourage parents to limit the exposure of elderly family members, those with impaired immunity, infants, and visitors to the ill child. Make sure that the ill child's dishes and utensils are washed in hot soapy water or sanitized in a dishwasher. Place dressings with drainage in a plastic bag for disposal to prevent contact by other family members.

Encourage children to rest. Provide quiet diversional activities such as board games, computer games, DVDs, and music. Promote fluid intake and provide foods that the child prefers and do not cause discomfort. Reduce itching of rashes with lukewarm baths with Aveeno or oatmeal and topical lotions. Keep the child's hands clean and nails trimmed. Cover the hands with clean socks or mittens if scratching cannot be controlled.

Evaluation

Expected outcomes of nursing care include the following:

- Opportunities for spread of infection between clients and family members are minimized.
- The child's fever is effectively managed with antipyretics.
- The full treatment with antibiotics, if ordered, is completed.

Sepsis and Septic Shock

Sepsis or septicemia is a systemic inflammatory response syndrome (SIRS) in the presence of infection, such as bacteria invading the bloodstream. Infants and children who are at high risk include those with a chronic condition, burns, multiple invasive procedures, invasive catheters, a compromised immune system, or those on long-term antibiotics. Severe sepsis that progresses to septic shock is a significant health problem with an estimated in-hospital mortality rate of up to 10% (Hazinski, Mondozzi, & Baker, 2014).

Sepsis is caused by the effects of the infectious agent and its toxins. At least one of these significant events leads to the development of sepsis: an infectious agent causes severe tissue injuries that result in multiple system organ failure, the child's excessive inflammatory response triggers a secondary response, or counterregulatory mechanisms are ineffective (Roberts & Coffin, 2013). Septic shock results from a disrupted balance between proinflammatory mediators and anti-inflammatory mediators. The disrupted inflammatory mediators lead to greater tissue injury, abnormalities in coagulation and fibrinolysis, disseminated intravascular coagulation (DIC), vasodilation, major organ dysfunction, and increased susceptibility to other infections (see Chapter 49 for more information on DIC). Fibrin deposits in the microcirculation disrupt the blood flow and the delivery of oxygen and nutrients to the tissues. Cellular hypoxia and major multiple organ system dysfunction result.

Early signs of SIRS in children include fever or hypothermia, tachycardia, and tachypnea. Signs of septic shock include fever, tachycardia, tachypnea, and inadequate perfusion (altered responsiveness, prolonged capillary refill time, either diminished or bounding pulses, mottled cool extremities, and decreased urine output). Hypotension may be present despite adequate fluid resuscitation.

Diagnosis is often suspected from clinical signs and symptoms. Cultures of the blood, urine, cerebrospinal fluid, and skin lesions are obtained, as well as a complete blood count with differential. The white blood cell count may be elevated or low for age. Clinical therapy focuses on preserving vital organ function with oxygen, IV fluid resuscitation, vasopressor medications, and antibiotics. The treatment plan focuses on restoring the blood pressure, returning the heart rate and capillary refill rate to more normal levels, maintaining the cardiac output, and increasing oxygen delivery to the tissues and vital organs. Acid–base, glucose, and electrolyte level imbalances are managed. Enteral or parenteral nutritional support may be initiated early. Septic shock may progress to cardiac arrest if interventions are unsuccessful.

Nursing Management

Nursing care of the infant or child with sepsis occurs in the neonatal or pediatric intensive care unit. Nursing care of children with sepsis involves careful assessment and management of the child's vital signs, fluid and electrolyte balance, perfusion, hemodynamic stability, and response to clinical therapy. Families need extensive support for this life-threatening infection. Encourage the parents to participate in the child's care as much as possible. Observe for signs that the condition is worsening or resolving.

Emerging Infection Control Threats

Public health officials are conducting disease surveillance to identify emerging infections, such as **pandemic flu**, a worldwide influenza epidemic, or other epidemics such as Ebola. Some infectious agents have the potential to be weapons of terrorists (anthrax, smallpox, plague, botulism, hemorrhagic fever, or tularemia). Early recognition and reporting of clusters of patients with similar symptoms is essential to initiate public health measures that will reduce disease transmission. Additionally, confirmation of an epidemic triggers the mass casualty response needed to care for large numbers of ill adults and children. See Table 43–5 for influenza information.

Nursing Management

Maintain a high level of suspicion when greater than the expected number of individuals with similar signs and symptoms come to school or seek care in any healthcare facility. Initiating airborne and contact precautions and instituting isolation before a definitive diagnosis is appropriate when the level of suspicion is high. Assess children and provide supportive nursing care for the identified infection.

Focus Your Study

- Reducing the number of preventable childhood illnesses is a major national public health goal.

- A communicable disease is an illness caused by microorganisms that are commonly transmitted from one host (animal or human) to another.

- Newborns and infants are especially vulnerable to infectious diseases because their immune systems are immature, their passively acquired maternal antibodies provide limited protection, and disease protection through immunization is not yet complete.

- For a child to acquire a communicable disease, an infectious agent or pathogen, an effective means of transmission, and a susceptible host need to be present.

- Infection control measures caregivers can take include the following: good hand hygiene with soap and water or alcohol-based gels, disinfecting hard surfaces touched by the child or the child's body fluids, disinfecting toys, and making sure all children are fully immunized.

- The average infant born in 2015 will receive immunizations for 16 communicable diseases by 18 years of age.

- The Vaccines for Children program provides free immunizations for low-income children to ensure that finances are not a barrier to full immunization of those children.

- When parents resist immunizations for religious or philosophic reasons, the nurse should provide them with accurate information and help them understand how their child may benefit from immunization. If they still resist, inform them that their child may be at a significant risk for an infection and will need to be held out of school if an outbreak occurs.

- The potency of vaccines must be protected with storage in the refrigerator or freezer at the appropriate temperature.

- The National Vaccine Injury Acts of 1986 and 1993 provide compensation if a link between immunization and a serious adverse effect is found. The Vaccine Adverse Event Reporting System has been established to track serious vaccine reactions.

- Immunization information is updated frequently. It is the nurse's responsibility to regularly obtain current information about vaccines, immunization schedule, and important information to share with parents and adolescents.

- Infectious and communicable diseases are caused by bacterial, viral, protozoan, or fungal organisms.

- Fever is often a sign of infectious disease in children. When pathogens invade the body, endogenous pyrogens travel to the hypothalamus, where they trigger the production and release of prostaglandins, which initiate the fever response.

- The child with a toxic or septic appearance has the following signs: lethargy, poor perfusion, tachypnea or bradypnea, and pallor or cyanosis.

- The appropriate use and administration of antibiotics to help reduce the development of antibiotic-resistant bacteria includes the following: Give antibiotic dosages as prescribed for the full number of days ordered, do not share with other family members who might be ill, and discard when all doses have been given.

- Sepsis is a systemic response to infection that has a high mortality rate.

- The public health system conducts disease surveillance to detect the emergence of rare infections, an epidemic, or the presence of infectious disease potentially caused by terrorists.

Clinical Reasoning in Action

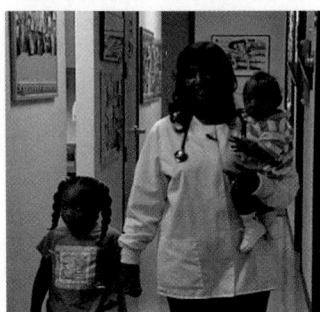

Keisha, 7 years old, and Brandon, 6 months old, are brought to the pediatric clinic, needing immunizations. Even though Brandon is sick today, their mother would still like Keisha to have her vaccines, and she would also like both children to have a complete checkup before their vaccines to make sure they are healthy.

You examine Keisha's vital signs as: 80th percentile in height, 40th percentile in weight, temperature 98.9°F, blood pressure 105/62 mmHg, urinalysis with a trace of leukocytes, and she passes her hearing and vision screening. She seems extremely anxious about having to get a needle. There is evidence of eczema and allergic rhinitis.

You examine Brandon as a sick visit while he clings to his mother. His vital signs are: temperature 102°F, respiratory rate of 30 breaths per minute, and heart rate of 90 beats per minute. In

Brandon's mouth, grayish, papulovesicular, ulcerative lesions are observed, evidence of an enterovirus. This type of illness does not respond to antibiotics. You advise the mother to avoid exposing Brandon to other persons because it is contagious and to offer cool drinks and bland foods. You also suggest that warm saline mouth rinses may be helpful. You advise the mother to observe for dehydration, and to give ibuprofen or acetaminophen as needed.

1. Since Brandon has been in to the office several times for various infections, what education can be given to his mother to reduce the chances of future infections?

2. Keisha has eczema and allergic rhinitis. Would this be a contraindication to giving vaccines?

3. What are questions the nurse should ask the mother before administering vaccines to Keisha to make sure there are no contraindications to giving them?

4. What should the mother be told about caring for Keisha after her vaccines?

5. How should the mother be told to manage Brandon's fever?

References

American Academy of Pediatrics of Pediatrics (AAP) Committee on Infectious Disease. (2015). *Red book: Report of the Committee on Infectious Disease* (30th ed.) Elk Grove Village, IL: Author.

Arriola, C. S., Brammer, L., Epperson, S., Blanton, L., Kniss, K., Mustaquim, D., . . . Jhung, M. (2014). Update: Influenza activity—United States, September 29, 2013–February 8, 2014. *Morbidity and Mortality Weekly Report, 63*(07), 148–154.

Centers for Disease Control and Prevention (CDC). (2012). *Fifth disease.* Retrieved from http://www.cdc.gov /parvovirusB19/fifth-disease.html

Centers for Disease Control and Prevention (CDC). (2013a). *Pertussis.* Retrieved from http://www.cdc .gov/pertussis/index.html

Centers for Disease Control and Prevention (CDC). (2013b). *Pneumoccocal disease.* Retrieved from http://www .cdc.gov/pneumococcal/about/index.html

Centers for Disease Control and Prevention (CDC). (2013c). *Polio.* Retrieved from http://www.cdc.gov/polio/about /index.htm

Centers for Disease Control and Prevention (CDC). (2013d). *Tetanus.* Retrieved from http://www.cdc.gov/tetanus /index.html

Centers for Disease Control and Prevention (CDC). (2013e). *Rabies.* Retrieved from http://www.cdc.govz/rabies/

Centers for Disease Control and Prevention (CDC). (2013f). *Rocky Mountain spotted fever.* Retrieved from http://www.cdc.gov/rmsf/index.html

Centers for Disease Control and Prevention (CDC). (2014a). *Hand hygiene basics.* Retrieved from http://www.cdc .gov/handhygiene/Basics.html

Centers for Disease Control and Prevention (CDC). (2014b). *CDC vaccine price list.* Retrieved from http://www .cdc.gov/vaccines/programs/vfc/awardees/vaccine -management/price-list/#pediatric

Centers for Disease Control and Prevention (CDC). (2014c). *Vaccine storage and handling.* Retrieved from http://www.cdc.gov/vaccines/recs/storage/default.htm

Centers for Disease Control and Prevention (CDC). (2014d.) *Measles.* Retrieved from http://www.cdc.gov/measles/index.html

Centers for Disease Control and Prevention (CDC). (2014e). *Meningococcal disease.* Retrieved from http://www.cdc.gov/meningococcal/index.html

Centers for Disease Control and Prevention (CDC). (2014f). *Epstein-Barr virus and infectious mononucleosis.* Retrieved from http://www.cdc.gov/epstein-barr/index.html

Centers for Disease Control and Prevention (CDC). (2014g). *Lyme disease.* Retrieved from http://www.cdc.gov/lyme/

Centers for Disease Control and Prevention (CDC). (2014h). *Vaccines and immunizations: Possible side effects from vaccines.* Retrieved from http://www.cdc.gov/vaccines/vac-gen/side-effects.htm

Centers for Disease Control and Prevention (CDC). (2015). *Pregnancy and whooping cough.* Retrieved from www.cdc.gov/pertussis/pregnant/index.html

Cullen, K. A., & Arguin, P. M. (2013). Malaria surveillance—United States, 2011. *Morbidity and Mortality Weekly Report, 62*(5), 1–18.

Curtis, C. R., Yankey, D., Jeyarajah, J., Dorell, C., Stokley, S., MacNeil, J., & Hariri, S. (2013). National and state vaccination coverage among adolescents aged 13–17 years—United States, 2012. *Morbidity and Mortality Weekly Report, 62*(34), 685–693.

Darden, P. M., Thompson, D. M., Roberts, J. R., Hale, J. J., Pope, C., Thompson, D. M., . . . Jacobson, R. M. (2013). Reasons for not vaccinating adolescents: National immunization survey of teens, 2008–2010. *Pediatrics, 131*(4), 645–651.

DeStefano, F., Price, C. S., & Weintraub, E. S. (2013). Increasing exposure to antibody-stimulating proteins and polysaccharides in vaccines is not associated with risk of autism. *Journal of Pediatrics, 163*(2), 561–567.

Elam-Evans, L. D., Yankey, D., Singleton, J. A., & Kolasa, M. (2014). National, state, and selected local area vaccination coverage among children aged 19–35 months—United States, 2013. *Morbidity and Mortality Weekly Report, 63*(34), 741–748.

Gastañaduy, P. A., Redd, S. B., Fiebelkorn, A. P., Rota, J. S., Rota, P. A., Bellini, W. J., . . . Wallace, G. S. (2014). Measles—United States, January 1–May 23, 2014. *Morbidity and Mortality Weekly Report, 63*, 1–4.

Grohskopf, L. A., Olsen, S. J., Sokolow, L. Z., Bresee, J. S., Cox, N. J., Broder, K. R., . . . Walter, E. B. (2014). Prevention and control of seasonal influenza with vaccines: Recommendations of the Advisory Committee on Immunization Practices (ACIP)—United States, 2014-15 influenza season. *Morbidty and Mortality Weekly Report, 63*(32), 691–697.

Hazinski, M. F., Mondozzi, M. A., & Baker, R. A. U. (2014). Shock, multiple organ dysfunction syndrome and burns in children. In K. L. McCance, S. E. Huether, V. L. Brashers, & N. S. Rote (Eds.), *Pathophysiology: The biologic basis for disease in adults and children* (7th ed., pp. 1699–1727). St. Louis, MO: Elsevier Mosby.

Health Resources and Services Administration. (2013). *Vaccine Injury Table.* Retrieved from http://www.hrsa.gov/vaccinecompensation/vaccineinjurytable.pdf

Hendrix, K. S., Finnell, M. E., Zimit, G. D., Sturm, L. A., Lane, K. A., & Downs, S. M. (2014). Vaccine message framing and parents' intent to immunize their infants for MMR. *Pediatrics, 134*(3), e675–2683.

Huether, S. E. (2014). Pain, temperature regulation, sleep, and sensory function. In K. L. McCance, S. E. Huether, V. L. Brashers, & N. S. Rote (Eds.), *Pathophysiology: The biologic basis for disease in adults and children* (6th ed., pp. 481–524). St. Louis, MO: Mosby Elsevier.

Kroger, A. T., Sumaya, C. V., Pickering, L. K., & Atkinson, W. L. (2011). General recommendations on immunization: Recommendations of the Advisory Committee on Immunization Practices (ACIP). *Morbidity and Mortality Weekly Report, 60*(2), 1–62.

MacNeil, J. R., Rubin, L., McNamara, L., Briere, E. C., Clark, T. A., & Cohn, A. C. (2014). Use of MenACWY-CRM vaccine in children aged 2 through 23 months at increased risk for meningococcal disease: Recommendations of the Advisory Committee on Immunization Practices, 2013. *Morbidity and Mortality Weekly Report, 63*(24), 527–530.

Marin, M., Bialek, S. R., & Seward, J. F. (2013). Updated recommendations for use of VariZIG—United States, 2013. *Morbidity and Mortality Weekly Report, 62*(28), 574–576.

Markowitz, L. E., Dunne, E. F., Saraiya, M., Chesson, H. W., Curtis, C. R., Gee, J., . . . Unger, E. R. (2014). Human papillomavirus vaccination: Recommendations of the Advisory Committee on Immunization Practices. *Morbidity and Mortality Weekly Report, 63*(5), 1–30.

McLean, H. Q., Fiebelkorn, A. P., Temte, J. L., & Wallace, G. S. (2013). Prevention of measles, rubella, congenital rubella syndrome, and mumps, 2013: Summary recommendations of the Advisory Committee on Immunization Practices. *Morbidity and Mortality Weekly Report, 62*(4), 1–34.

Midgley, C. M., Jackson, M. A., Selvarangan, R., Turabelitze, G., Obringer, E., Johnson, D., . . . Gerber, S. I. (2014). Severe respiratory illness associated with Enterovirus D68—Missouri and Illinois, 2014. *Morbidity and Mortality Weekly Report, 63*(36), 798–799.

National Association of School Nurses. (2011). *Infectious disease management in the school setting.* Retrieved from http://www.nasn.org/PolicyAdvocacy/PositionPapersandReports/NASNPositionStatementsFullView/tabid/462/ArticleId/34/Infectious-Disease-Management-in-the-School-Setting-Revised-2011

Nyhan, B., Reifler, R., Richey, S., & Freed, G. L. (2014). Effective messages in vaccine promotion: A randomized trial. *Pediatrics, 133*(4), e835–e842.

Purnell, L. D. (2013). *Transcultural health care: A culturally competent approach* (4th ed.). Philadelphia, PA: F. A. Davis.

Purnell, L. D. (2014). *Culturally competent health care* (3rd ed., pp. 48–75). Philadelphia, PA: F. A. Davis.

Roberts, K. E., & Coffin, S. E. (2013). Immunology and infectious disease, In M. F. Hazinski (Ed.), *Nursing care of the critically ill child* (3rd ed., pp. 851–867). St. Louis, MO: Elsevier.

Rubin, L. G., Levin, M. J., Ljungman, P., Davies, E. G., Avery, R., Tomblyn, M., . . . Kang, I. (2013). 2013 IDSA clinical practice guideline for vaccination of the immunocompromised host. *Clinical Infectious Diseases.* doi: 10.1093/cid/cit684

U.S. Department of Health and Human Services. (2014). *Healthy People 2020.* Retrieved from http://www.healthypeople.gov/2020/default.aspx

U.S. Department of Health and Human Services. (2015). *Immunizations and infectious diseases.* Retrieved from http://www.healthypeople.gov/2020/topics-objectives/topic/immunization-and-infectious-diseases

Chapter 44
The Child With Alterations in Fluid, Electrolyte, and Acid–Base Balance

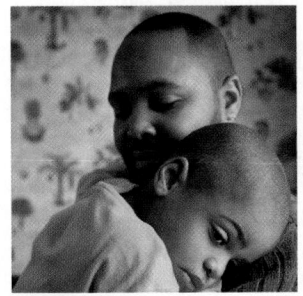

LeShan always likes to eat, so when he won't even drink I know he is sick. We just didn't know how sick he was or that he had gotten dehydrated. I wonder if we should have done something else for him at home.

—Father of LeShan, 18 months old

Iofoto/Shutterstock

Learning Outcomes

44.1 Describe normal fluid and electrolyte status for children at various ages.

44.2 Identify regulatory mechanisms for fluid and electrolyte balance.

44.3 Interpret threats to fluid and electrolyte balance in children.

44.4 Describe acid–base balance and recognize disruptions common in children.

44.5 Analyze assessment findings to recognize fluid-electrolyte problems and acid–base imbalance in children.

44.6 Plan appropriate nursing interventions for children experiencing fluid-electrolyte problems and acid–base imbalance.

A thorough understanding of fluid, electrolyte, and acid–base homeostasis and imbalances is essential when providing nursing care to children like LeShan described in the chapter opener. This chapter presents information about the processes that maintain fluid and electrolyte balance and describes the common imbalances that may occur in children. It also describes how the body regulates acid–base status and explains the management of acid–base imbalances.

Many health conditions cause changes in body fluids that must be regulated and managed. Sometimes management of fluid status in the home or in a short-term ambulatory facility can prevent more serious illness or hospitalization.

Anatomy and Physiology of Pediatric Differences

Infants and young children differ physiologically from adults in ways that make them vulnerable to fluid, electrolyte, and acid–base imbalances.

Fluid in the body is in a dynamic state. Much of the human body is composed of water. **Body fluid** is body water that has solutes dissolved in it. Some of the solutes are **electrolytes**, or charged particles (ions). Electrolytes such as sodium (Na^+), potassium (K^+), calcium (Ca^{2+}), magnesium (Mg^{2+}), chloride

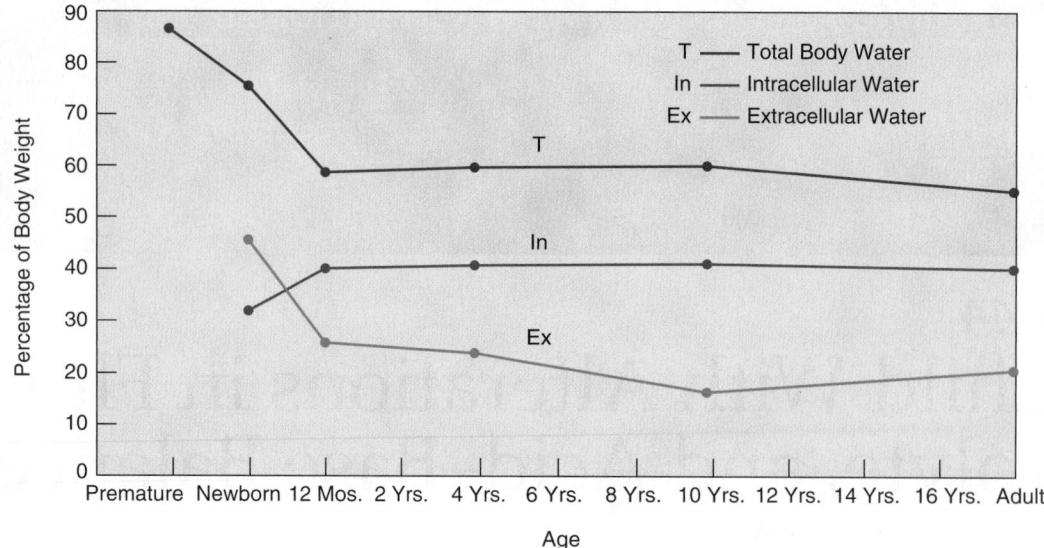

Figure 44–1   The major body fluid compartments. Extracellular fluid is composed mainly of intravascular fluid (fluid in blood vessels) and interstitial fluid (fluid between cells and outside the blood and lymphatic vessels). Intracellular fluid is that within cells.

(Cl^-), and inorganic phosphorus (P_i) ions must be present in the proper concentrations for cells to function effectively. In people of all ages, fluid continuously leaves the body through the skin, in feces and urine, and during respiration. **Sensible water loss** is that which is measurable and observable, such as urine. **Insensible water loss** cannot be directly measured or observed, such as that lost through the skin and respirations. For adults and children, intake of oral fluid is approximately equivalent to urinary output in normal circumstances. Likewise, water provided in food and by the body's metabolic processes is approximately the same as insensible loss from feces, skin, and respirations.

In people of all ages, body fluid is located in several compartments. The two major fluid compartments contain the **intracellular fluid** (fluid inside the cells) and the **extracellular fluid** (outside the cells). The extracellular fluid is made up of **intravascular fluid** (within the blood vessels) and **interstitial fluid** (between the cells and outside the blood and lymphatic vessels) (Figure 44–1). Extracellular fluid accounts for about one third of total body water, and intracellular fluid for about two thirds. The concentrations of electrolytes in the fluid differ depending on the fluid compartment. For example, extracellular fluid is rich in sodium ions; intracellular fluid, by contrast, is low in sodium ions but rich in potassium ions (Table 44–1).

TABLE 44–1 Electrolyte Concentrations in Body Fluid Compartments

	EXTRACELLULAR FLUID (ECF)		
COMPONENTS	**VASCULAR**	**INTERSTITIAL**	**INTRACEL- LULAR FLUID**
Na^+	High	High	Low
K^+	Low	Low	High
Ca^{2+}	Low	Low	Low (higher than ECF)
Mg^{2+}	Low	Low	High
P_i	Low	Low	High
Cl^-	High	High	Low
Proteins	High	Low	High

Fluid moves between the intravascular and interstitial compartments by a process called *filtration*. Water moves into and out of the cells by the process of *osmosis*. These processes are discussed later in the chapter. Electrolytes move across cell membranes both by **diffusion** of particles from a location of greater to less concentration and by active transport that is effective even against the concentration gradient.

The percentage of body weight composed of water varies with age. The percentage of total body water is highest at birth (and higher in premature than in full-term infants) and decreases with age (see *As Children Grow: Fluid and Electrolyte Differences*). Newborns and young infants also have a proportionately larger extracellular fluid volume than older children and adults because their brain and skin (both rich in interstitial fluid) occupy a greater proportion of their body weight. Much of the body's extracellular fluid is exchanged each day. Infants have a high daily fluid requirement with little fluid volume reserve; this makes the infant vulnerable to dehydration. As an infant grows, the proportion of water inside the cells increases.

Infants and children under 2 years of age lose a greater proportion of fluid each day than older children and adults and are thus more dependent on adequate intake. They have a greater amount of skin surface or body surface area (BSA) and thus have greater insensible water losses through the skin. Because of this relatively large BSA, they are also at greater risk when skin is affected, such as in burns. In addition, respiratory and metabolic rates are high during early childhood, so children have greater water loss from the lungs and greater water demand to fuel the body's metabolic processes (Figure 44–2). Because of these factors, the exercising child dehydrates easily and must consume more fluid during physical activity, particularly during hot weather (Mayo Clinic, 2011).

When fluid status is compromised, a number of body mechanisms are activated to help restore balance. Several of these mechanisms occur in the kidney. The kidneys conserve water and needed electrolytes while excreting waste products and drug metabolites. However, in children under 2 years of age, the glomeruli, tubules, and nephrons of the kidneys are immature. They are thus unable to conserve or excrete water and solutes effectively (see Chapter 52). Because more water

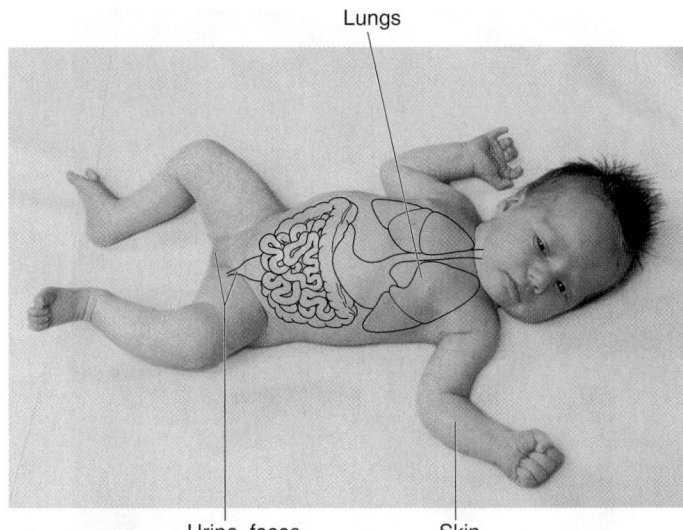

Figure 44–2 **Normal routes of fluid excretion from infants and children.**

is generally excreted, the infant and young child can become dehydrated quickly or develop electrolyte imbalances. In addition, infants have a weaker transport system for ions and bicarbonate, placing them at greater risk for acidosis and acid–base imbalances. Children under 2 years of age also have difficulty regulating electrolytes such as sodium and calcium. Renal response to high solute loads is slower and less developed, with function improving gradually during the first year of life.

Finally, in addition to the immaturity of physiologic processes, many health conditions make young children more vulnerable to fluid deficit. Examples include water loss due to phototherapy used to treat newborns with hyperbilirubinemia; water loss with increased respiratory rate during illness, fever, vomiting, and diarrhea; and drainage from blood loss or drainage tubes.

FLUID VOLUME IMBALANCES

When fluid excretion and losses are balanced by the proper volume and type of fluid intake, fluid balance will be maintained. However, if fluid output and intake are not matched, fluid imbalance may occur rapidly. The major types of fluid imbalances are:

- Extracellular fluid volume deficit (dehydration)
- Extracellular fluid volume excess
- Interstitial fluid volume excess (edema)

Extracellular Fluid Volume Imbalances

Extracellular Fluid Volume Deficit (Dehydration)

Extracellular fluid volume deficit occurs when there is not enough fluid in the extracellular compartment (vascular and interstitial). Depending on the cause of dehydration, sodium

As Children Grow: **Fluid and Electrolyte Differences**

Newborn

75% Total body water
- ECF 45%
- ICF 30%

Brain and skin occupy a greater proportion of body weight and are high in interstitial fluid

Infant

65% Total body water
- ECF 25%
- ICF 30–40%

High BSA promotes fluid loss

Little fluid reserve in intracellular fluid

5–6x greater fluid exchange daily

High metabolic rate requires generous fluid intake

Child/Adolescent

50% Total body water
- ECF 10–15%
- ICF 40%

Kidneys are immature until 2 years and unable to conserve water and electrolytes or fully assist in acid–base balance

The newborn and infant have a high percentage of body weight composed of water, especially extracellular fluid, which is lost from the body easily. Note the small stomach size, which limits a newborn's ability to rehydrate quickly.

may be at normal, low, or elevated levels. (Hyponatremia and hypernatremia are described later in the chapter.) The state of body water deficit is called **dehydration**. There are three major types of dehydration:

- **Isotonic dehydration** (or **isonatremic dehydration**) occurs when fluid loss is not balanced by intake, and the loss of water and sodium are in proportion. The serum sodium is therefore within normal limits or slightly low even though the circulating blood volume is lowered. Most of the fluid lost is from the extracellular component. This type of dehydration is commonly manifested in the illnesses of young children such as vomiting and diarrhea.

- **Hypotonic dehydration** (or **hyponatremic dehydration**) occurs when fluid loss is characterized by a proportionately greater loss of sodium than water. Serum sodium is below normal levels. Compensatory fluid shifts occur from the extracellular to intracellular components in an attempt to establish normal proportions, thus leading to even greater extracellular dehydration. Severe and prolonged vomiting and diarrhea, burns, and renal disease can lead to this condition, as well as administration of intravenous fluid without electrolytes in treatment of dehydration.

- **Hypertonic dehydration** (or **hypernatremic dehydration**) occurs when fluid loss is characterized by a proportionately greater loss of water than sodium. Serum sodium is above normal levels. Compensatory fluid shifts occur from the intracellular to extracellular components in an attempt to establish normal proportions. The extracellular component therefore remains fairly normal, delaying the onset of signs and symptoms of dehydration until the condition is quite serious. Neurologic symptoms reflecting intracellular imbalance may occur simultaneously with more common symptoms of dehydration. The condition may be caused by health problems such as diabetes insipidus (see Chapter 53) or administration of intravenous fluid or tube feedings with high electrolyte levels.

The body continuously attempts to compensate for fluid and electrolyte imbalance by shifting fluid and electrolytes from one component to another. Therefore, it is rare for only one type of dehydration to occur; the child's fluid and electrolyte status and symptoms are constantly changing. Ongoing assessment and management are needed.

ETIOLOGY AND PATHOPHYSIOLOGY

Extracellular fluid volume deficit is usually caused by the loss of sodium-containing fluid from the body. Vomiting, diarrhea, nasogastric suction, hemorrhage, and burns most often cause loss of fluid containing sodium. Vomiting and diarrhea are common manifestations of disease in children throughout the world, and each year up to 5 million children die from dehydration related to diarrhea. In the United States, about 300 to 500 die annually from this problem, about 220,000 are hospitalized, and 1.5 million receive outpatient care (Kinlin & Freedman, 2012).

Type 1 diabetes may become a cause of dehydration as the child exhibits polydipsia and polyuria (see Chapter 53 for a detailed description of diabetes). Another cause of extracellular fluid volume deficit in infants is increased water loss in low-birth-weight infants kept under radiant warmers to maintain heat (Figure 44–3). Less frequently, adrenal insufficiency, accumulation of extracellular fluid in a "third space" such as the peritoneal cavity, and overuse of diuretics may be the cause.

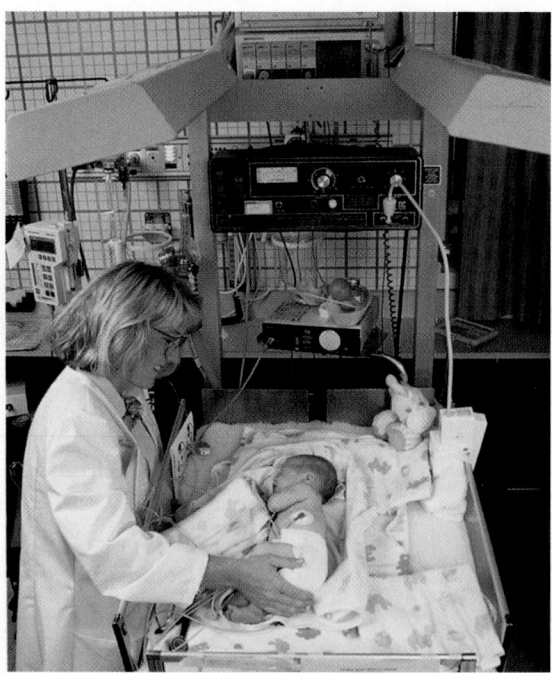

Figure 44–3 Fluid loss from overhead warming. Use of an overhead warmer or phototherapy increases insensible fluid excretion through the skin, thus increasing the fluid intake needed.

The latter etiology is most often seen in adolescents with bulimia (see Chapter 32).

Excessive exercise during very hot weather without sufficient fluid replacement can lead to fluid and electrolyte imbalance. Physiologic differences can place children at high risk, especially when they have vigorous outdoor activity in extreme heat with inadequate rest periods. Children may not feel thirsty and therefore may fail to drink adequately even when dehydrated. Additional risk factors include obesity and a combination of high temperature, high humidity, wind, and exposure to radiant heat (American Academy of Pediatrics [AAP] Council on Sports Medicine and Fitness & Council on School Health, 2011).

Burns and gastroenteritis are characterized by initial dehydration in the first 3 days due to a high loss of extracellular fluid. About 80% of the fluid loss is extracellular and only about 20% is intracellular. However, with time, the relationship begins to change, so that in illnesses over 3 days, about 60% of fluid loss is extracellular while 40% is intracellular (Engorn & Flerlage, 2015). Since the electrolyte composition of extracellular and intracellular fluids differs (see Table 44–1), electrolyte management will need to change for long-term conditions.

CLINICAL MANIFESTATIONS

The signs of dehydration relate to the severity or degree of the body water deficit (Table 44–2). They are a result of both the decreased fluid (e.g., diminished turgor and mucous membrane moisture) and the body's response to the fluid deficit (e.g., pulse and blood pressure changes).

Mild dehydration is hard to detect because children appear alert and have moist mucous membranes. Infants may be irritable and older children are thirsty. In moderate dehydration, the child is often lethargic and sleepy, but there may be periods of restlessness and irritability, especially in infants. Skin turgor is diminished, mucous membranes appear dry, and urine is dark in color and diminished in amount. Pulse rate is usually increased, and blood

TABLE 44–2 Severity of Clinical Dehydration

	MILD	MODERATE	SEVERE
Percentage of body weight lost	Up to 5% (40–50 mL/kg)	6–9% (60–90 mL/kg)	10% or more (100 mL/kg)
Level of consciousness	Alert, restless, thirsty	Irritable or lethargic (infants and very young children); alert, thirsty, restless (older children and adolescents)	Lethargic to comatose (infants and young children); often conscious, apprehensive (older children and adolescents)
Blood pressure	Normal for age	Normal or low; postural hypotension (older children and adolescents)	Low to undetectable
Pulse	Regular and strong	Rapid	Rapid, weak to nonpalpable
Skin turgor	Immediate	Poor	Very poor
Mucous membranes	Moist	Dry	Parched
Urine	Usual output	Decreased output (<1 mL/kg/hr); dark color; increased specific gravity	Very decreased or absent output
Thirst	Slightly increased	Moderately increased	Greatly increased unless lethargic
Fontanelle	Normal	Sunken	Sunken
Extremities	Warm; rapid capillary refill	Delayed capillary refill (>2 sec)	Cool, discolored; delayed capillary refill (>3–4 sec)
Respirations	Regular, usual rate	Usual or rapid rate	Changing rate and regularity
Eyes	Normal	Slightly sunken, decreased tears	Deeply sunken, absent tears

TABLE 44–3 Clinical Manifestations of Extracellular Fluid Volume Deficit

CLINICAL MANIFESTATIONS	ETIOLOGY
Weight loss	Decreased fluid volume; 1 L of fluid weighs 1 kg
Postural blood pressure drop (older children)	Inadequate circulating blood volume to offset the force of gravity when in upright position
Increased small vein filling time	Decreased vascular volume
Delayed capillary refill time	Decreased vascular volume
Flat neck veins when supine (older children)	Decreased vascular volume
Dizziness, syncope	Inadequate circulation to brain
Oliguria	Inadequate circulation to kidneys
Thready, rapid pulse	Cardiac reflex response to decreased vascular volume
Sunken fontanelle (infants)	Decreased fluid volume
Decreased skin turgor	Decreased interstitial fluid volume

pressure can be normal or low. Severe dehydration is manifested by increasing lethargy or nonresponsiveness, markedly decreased blood pressure, rapid pulse, nonelastic skin turgor, dry mucous membranes, sunken and dry eyes, and markedly decreased or absent urinary output (Feld & Kaskel, 2012). See Table 44–3.

CLINICAL THERAPY
Diagnosis of dehydration is best accomplished by clinical observations. Medical management depends on accurate identification of the degree of dehydration. In addition to physical signs and symptoms (see Table 44–2), elevated blood urea nitrogen (BUN) (over 17 mg/dL) and low serum bicarbonate (16–17 mEq/L or mmol/L) are useful to identify dehydration from moderate and severe diarrhea (Corbett & Banks, 2013; Dzierba & Abraham, 2011). The treatment of extracellular fluid volume deficit is administration of fluid containing sodium, by oral rehydration therapy or by intravenous fluids.

Oral rehydration is the treatment of choice to treat mild and moderate dehydration in children. The therapy successfully treats the dehydration caused by many gastrointestinal illnesses and prevents hospitalization for many infants and young children (Engorn & Flerlage, 2015; Freedman, Ali, Oleszczuk, et al., 2013; Jablonski, 2012). Commercially available solutions contain water, carbohydrate (sugar), sodium, potassium, chloride, and lactate. Examples include Pedialyte, Infalyte, Rehydralyte, Ricelyte, Resol, Nutrilyte, Hydralyte, and Lytren. Some clinicians allow lactose-free milk, breast milk, or half-strength milk to be given in addition to oral rehydration therapy solution. Oral rehydration may be accompanied by ondansetron to decrease vomiting in the child and its resultant continued dehydration (Freedman et al., 2013). In developing countries, an oral rehydration solution with zinc added has been effective in diarrhea treatment (Frohna, 2011). Prebiotics (oral supplements that stimulate growth of probiotic bacteria to positively alter intestinal flora) have also been found to be effective in decreasing the number of diarrheal stools in children with acute gastrointestinal disease (Frohna, 2011).

TABLE 44–4 Common Intravenous Solutions, Uses, and Components

IV SOLUTION	USES	CHO (g/100 mL)	PROTEIN (g/100 mL)	CAL/L	Na⁺ (mEq/L)	K⁺ (mEq/L)	Cl⁻ (mEq/L)	HCO₃⁻ (mEq/L)	Ca²⁺ (mEq/L)
					COMPONENTS				
D₅W	Restores water loss, plasma volume, and calories; lowers sodium levels	5	—	170	—	—	—	—	—
Normal saline (0.9% NaCl)	Restores water and sodium loss; maintains sodium and chloride at present levels	—	—	—	154	—	154	—	—
Ringer solution	Expands intracellular fluid; replaces extracellular losses	0–10	—	0–340	147	4	155.5	—	4
Lactated Ringer solution	Replaces fluid loss from burns, bleeding, and severe diarrhea	0–10	—	0–340	130	4	109	28	3
Albumin 25% (salt-poor albumin)	Restores major plasma protein in blood loss that has been treated with NS (plasma expander)	—	25	1000	100–160	—	<120	—	—

Note: A normal saline (NS) solution is a salt solution that has the same percentage of salt as the human body. This is a 0.9% solution of sodium chloride. The term *normal* indicates that there is the same weight, in grams, of sodium and chloride in the solution. Variations and combinations are available to tailor intake to needs of the child. For example, ½ NS (0.45% NaCl) or ¼ NS (0.225% NaCl) is often used in young children; the lower sodium content helps to avoid inadvertent hypernatremia. D₅½NS and D₅¼NS are combinations of D₅W and NS; they provide both carbohydrate and sodium.

Source: Adapted from Engorn, B. & Flerlage, J. (2014). *The Harriet Lane handbook* (20th ed.) St. Louis, MO: Elsevier Saunders; LeMone, P., Burke, K. M., Bauldoff, G., & Gubrud, P. (2015). *Medical surgical nursing* (6th ed.). Hoboken, NJ: Prentice Hall Health.

When the child is severely dehydrated, electrolytes are measured by laboratory analysis, and isotonic intravenous fluid is given, often accompanied by oral rehydration. The intravenous fluid is commonly Ringer lactate or dilute saline, such as one half or one quarter normal saline (see Table 44–4 for types of intravenous fluids and their uses). The fluid combination replenishes the extracellular fluid volume and adds solutes to return the body fluid back to normal. Note that only isotonic solutions are used for rapid infusion, and D₅W is avoided for this treatment (Carcillo, 2014; Engorn & Flerlage, 2015; Wang, Xu, & Xiao, 2014). The child may be hospitalized or treated with intravenous fluids in a short-stay unit until the dehydration is controlled. Once hydrated, the child resumes an age-appropriate diet.

Growth and Development

Urine specific gravity may increase in older children who are dehydrated, but children under 2 years of age are not able to concentrate urine effectively. A rising specific gravity may not be seen in the younger dehydrated child.

Nursing Management

For the Child With Extracellular Fluid Volume Deficit (Dehydration)

Nursing Assessment and Diagnosis

Weigh the child daily with the same scale and without clothing. Compare to past weights and calculate weight loss. Carefully measure intake and output, urine specific gravity, level of consciousness, pulse rate and quality, skin turgor, mucous membrane moisture, quality and rate of respirations, and blood pressure. For older children and adolescents, the nurse can compare the blood pressure when the child is supine with the pressure when the child is sitting with legs hanging down or standing. If the child is dehydrated, the sitting or standing blood pressure will be lower than the supine blood pressure

because blood accumulates in the dependent legs. Obtain samples of urine and blood as needed for dehydration evaluation. Urinalysis can usually be completed on a very small urine sample, such as 1 mL.

The nursing diagnosis *Fluid Volume: Deficient* applies to all children who have an extracellular fluid volume deficit. Other diagnoses depend on the severity of the condition and the age of the child. Several nursing diagnoses that might be appropriate for the mildly to severely dehydrated child are included in the accompanying *Nursing Care Plans*. Additional care of the child with dehydration from gastroenteritis can be found in Chapter 51. Nursing diagnoses might include the following (NANDA-I © 2014):

- *Fluid Volume: Deficient* related to active fluid volume loss or failure of regulatory mechanisms
- *Tissue Perfusion: Peripheral, Risk for Ineffective*, related to hypovolemia
- *Injury, Risk for*, related to postural hypotension

Clinical Reasoning The Dehydrated Child

LeShan is 18 months old. Several days ago he developed vomiting and diarrhea. His parents tried to get him to eat, but he had little appetite. He drank a little water and a few sips of juice, but the next morning he was listless and would not drink anything. The diarrhea continued.

His father has brought him to the urgent care center. LeShan is irritable on arrival, and his father reports that he has been alternately irritable and lethargic. His mucous membranes and tongue appear dry, and his skin turgor over the abdomen is slightly decreased. His father notes that LeShan has had only two wet diapers today and says the urine in his diaper was dark in color. He also reports that LeShan weighed 12 kg (26 lb) at the clinic last week. However, when the nurse weighs him, the scale reads only 11 kg (24.5 lb). What do LeShan's symptoms suggest about his degree of dehydration? What nursing interventions should be planned?

Nursing Care Plan: The Child With Mild or Moderate Dehydration

1. Nursing Diagnosis: *Health Management, Family, Ineffective*, **related to knowledge deficit about diarrhea and vomiting (NANDA-I © 2014)**

GOAL: The parents will describe appropriate home management of fluid replacement for diarrhea and vomiting.

INTERVENTION	RATIONALE
• Explain how to replace body fluid with an oral rehydration solution. Encourage parents to keep the solution at home and begin use with the first sign of diarrhea.	• Use of an oral rehydration solution can enable successful treatment of vomiting and diarrhea at home.
• Teach parents to continue the child's normal diet in addition to providing replacement fluids for diarrhea.	• Diet plus fluid supplementation leads to faster recovery.
• Provide verbal and written instructions to parents at each well-child visit. Teach hand hygiene for general use and during illness.	• Parents are provided with a reference for later use. Hand hygiene is the most effective measure to prevent illness that leads to dehydration.

EXPECTED OUTCOME: Parents will be able to successfully treat the child's diarrhea and vomiting at home.

2. Nursing Diagnosis: *Knowledge, Deficient (Parent)*, **related to causes of dehydration (NANDA-I © 2014)**

GOAL: The parents will state common causes of childhood dehydration.

INTERVENTION	RATIONALE
• Teach parents childhood conditions that commonly lead to dehydration.	• If parents recognize situations that can lead to dehydration, they will be more alert to its appearance.

EXPECTED OUTCOME: Parents will recognize conditions of risk for dehydration in children.

3. Nursing Diagnosis: *Fluid Volume: Deficient, Risk for*, **related to worsening of child's condition (NANDA-I © 2014)**

GOAL: The parents will seek health care for the child's worsening condition.

INTERVENTION	RATIONALE
• Teach parents to seek care when the child's vomiting or diarrhea worsens, when urine output via diaper or toilet decreases, or when the child's mental alertness changes.	• Severe dehydration may occur if milder forms are not successfully treated.

EXPECTED OUTCOME: Parents will seek prompt attention for the child's worsening condition, preventing the development of severe dehydration.

Planning and Implementation

Nursing care of the dehydrated child focuses first on prevention of the problem, and then on providing oral rehydration fluids, teaching parents oral rehydration methods, and, if necessary, administering intravenous fluids to restore fluid balance. The accompanying *Nursing Care Plans* summarize care of the child with mild to severe dehydration.

Clinical Tip

To obtain urine from an infant for testing specific gravity, place two cotton balls in the diaper. When they are wet, push them into a 10-mL syringe and squeeze out the urine with the plunger. Remember to use gloves for this procedure.

PREVENT DEHYDRATION

Nursing care can often prevent dehydration. Carefully monitor temperature probes in radiant warmers and isolettes for newborns to prevent overheating and resulting dehydration. Teach parents proper clothing for infants to prevent overheating. Nurses play an important role in educating parents, youth, school personnel, and coaches about the dangers of heat-related illness. Prevention is essential, so that children can exercise safely. Prior to a new exercise regimen, assessment for risk factors is performed. This includes medical conditions that put the child at high risk, such as cystic fibrosis, diabetes, obesity, or intellectual disability. Prior history of heat-related illness or recent change from a cooler to a hotter environment increases risk. Long exercise periods increase the stress on the body. The major nursing interventions are partnering with families and athletic coaches to prevent problems and to recognize and treat them promptly.

PROVIDE ORAL REHYDRATION FLUIDS

In mild or moderate dehydration, oral rehydration fluid is the first intervention. It is given in frequent small amounts; for example, 1 to 3 teaspoons of fluid every 10 to 15 minutes is a

Nursing Care Plan: The Child With Severe Dehydration

1. Nursing Diagnosis: *Fluid Volume: Deficient*, related to excess losses and inadequate intake (NANDA-I © 2014)

GOAL: The child will return to normal hydration status and will not develop hypovolemic shock.

INTERVENTION	RATIONALE
• Monitor weight daily. Assess intake and output every shift. Assess heart rate, postural blood pressure, skin turgor, small vein filling time, capillary refill time, fontanelle (infant), and urine specific gravity every 4 hours or more frequently as indicated.	• Frequent assessment of hydration status facilitates rapid intervention and evaluation of the effectiveness of fluid replacement.
• Administer intravenous fluid as ordered. Monitor for crackles in dependent portions of the lungs.	• Replace fluid lost from the body. Excessive replacement of sodium-containing fluids could cause extracellular fluid volume excess.
• Provide care hand hygiene and instruct family members to perform this also.	• Hand hygiene is the most important measure to prevent spread of microorganisms that can cause disease that leads to dehydration.

EXPECTED OUTCOME: The child will exhibit signs of normal hydration.

2. Nursing Diagnosis: *Injury, Risk for*, related to decreased level of consciousness (NANDA-I © 2014)

GOAL: The child will not experience injury.

INTERVENTION	RATIONALE
• Raise the side rails of the bed. Ensure that a small child does not become tangled in bed covers.	• Safety measures protect the child.
• Monitor level of consciousness every 2–4 hr or more often as indicated.	• Frequent assessment provides evidence of the need for safety interventions and of the effectiveness of therapy.
• Monitor serum sodium concentration daily or more often.	• Elevated serum sodium concentration causes brain cell shrinkage and decreased level of consciousness.
• Have the child sit before rising from bed and assist to stand slowly.	• Slow adjustment to upright posture reduces lightheadedness from decreased blood volume.

EXPECTED OUTCOME: Child will not fall or suffer other injuries.

3. Nursing Diagnosis: *Activity Intolerance* related to bed rest immobility (NANDA-I © 2014)

GOAL: The child will engage in normal activity for age.

INTERVENTION	RATIONALE
• Plan activities appropriate for the age of the child that can be done in bed.	• Activities will provide distraction and promote recovery.
• Group nursing interventions to provide time for the child to rest.	• The child will require more rest than usual.
• Provide assistance during meals and other activities as needed.	• Prevention of overexertion will conserve body fluid and promote healing.

EXPECTED OUTCOME: Child will engage in normal developmental activities and receive adequate rest.

---

useful guideline for starting oral rehydration. For the first 2 to 4 hours of treatment, 50 mL of fluid for each kilogram of the child's weight should be the target intake (Children's Mercy Hospital, 2011). Instruct parents to continue to administer 1 teaspoon every 2 to 3 minutes even if the child vomits, because small amounts of the fluid may still be absorbed. Table 44–5 outlines guidelines for oral rehydration therapy.

TEACH PARENTS ORAL REHYDRATION METHODS

Instruct parents about the types of fluids and amounts to be given. Begin teaching with parents of all newborns and reinforce teaching at each well-child visit. Advise parents to continue the child's normal diet in addition to providing the rehydration solution. Cereal, starches, soup, fruits, and vegetables are all

TABLE 44–5 Oral Rehydration Therapy Guidelines

CHILD'S CONDITION	RECOMMENDATION
No diarrhea, no dehydration	Continue on age-appropriate diet.
Minimal dehydration	If the child weighs less than 22 lb (10 kg), give 60–120 mL oral rehydration solution (ORS) for each diarrheal stool or vomiting episode; if over 22 lb (10 kg) in weight, give 120–240 mL ORS for each diarrheal stool or vomiting episode. Meanwhile, continue breastfeeding, or resume age-appropriate diet after initial hydration.
	Start slowly, administering 3–5 mL in a small cup or spoon every few minutes. Increase amounts gradually if no vomiting occurs.
	Recommend or provide samples of ORS; suggest ready-to-feed or powdered forms to use by parents.
Moderate dehydration	Give 50–100 mL/kg ORS in 3–4 hr in addition to replacing fluids lost as described above.
Severe dehydration	The child is hospitalized and treated with intravenous fluids. When hydrated adequately or concurrently with intravenous rehydration, begin oral rehydration therapy with 100 mL/kg of fluid in 4 hr and stool replacement as described above. Recalculate fluid needs after first 4 hr and adjust as needed.
Rehydration complete	Resume normal diet.

Source: Data from Children's Mercy Hospital. (2011). *Guidelines for oral rehydration*. Retrieved from http://www.childrensmercy.org/Content/view.aspx?id=8130.

allowed. Tell parents to avoid simple sugars, which can worsen diarrhea because of osmotic effects. This includes soft drinks (if used, they should be diluted with equal parts of water), undiluted juice, Jell-O, and sweetened cereal.

SAFETY ALERT!
Encourage parents to keep an oral rehydration solution in liquid or powder form on hand at all times and to use these solutions rather than juice, soda, or other drinks when the child first develops diarrhea or vomiting.

If an oral rehydration solution is too concentrated, it can make diarrhea worse. Juice, cola, and many sports drinks are very concentrated and should be diluted to half strength if they are the only fluids available to be given to a child who has diarrhea. Sugar facilitates the absorption of sodium in oral rehydration fluids. In addition, tell parents not to give diet beverages for oral rehydration because they contain no sugar and will not be effectively absorbed.

Repeated vomiting of large volumes of fluid, increasing diarrhea, or a worsening of the child's condition can indicate the need for intravenous therapy. Teach parents when to seek further medical care. If the child's condition worsens or does not improve after 4 hours of oral rehydration therapy, parents should contact a healthcare provider. Dizziness or lethargy are symptoms that can be manifestations of dehydration and indicate the need for further health care.

MONITOR INTRAVENOUS FLUID ADMINISTRATION

The hospitalized child usually requires intravenous fluids. Use volume control devices for measuring and monitoring intake. Be sure that the amount of fluid administered corresponds with the diagnosed dehydration state of the child (Table 44–6). Usually, about one half of the 24-hour total maintenance and replacement needs is given in the first 6 to 8 hours, with a slower rate infused for the remainder of the 24 hours. During the first 1 to 3 hours, the infusion rate may be highest to rapidly expand the vascular space. Electrolytes, such as potassium, are not added until the child has voided a sufficient quantity of urine for age in order to avoid hyperkalemia. Rapid infusion of a bolus of isotonic fluid (normal saline or lactated Ringer but *not* D_5W) in

the amount of 20 mL/kg over 20 minutes is sometimes used in outpatient settings, followed by oral fluids (Kliegman, Stanton, St. Geme, et al., 2011). Careful monitoring of intake and output is needed to ensure that the intravenous line remains in place until the child is tolerating oral fluids and taking in enough to maintain hydration. Verify that the type of fluid prescribed is being administered. When oral fluids are maintained, the child may be discharged and hospitalization avoided.

Maintain the intravenous line carefully so fluid infusion can be kept on schedule (refer to the *Clinical Skills Manual* SKILLS). Use a pump to prevent inadvertent, rapid infusion, which can lead to fluid overload and electrolyte imbalance (Figure 44–4). Play with the toddler and preschool child frequently and use diversionary methods as necessary to distract the child from the intravenous line. Monitor the child carefully and implement safety precautions as necessary. Once the child begins to tolerate some oral fluids, substitute oral rehydration therapy for intravenous fluids. Frequent administration of appropriate fluids is needed.

TABLE 44–6 Calculation of Intravenous Fluid Needs

STEP	CALCULATION	
Calculate the maintenance fluid needs of the child, using guidelines at right.	Usual Weight	Maintenance Amount
	Up to 10 kg	100 mL/kg/24 hr
	11–20 kg	1000 mL + (50 mL/kg for weight above 10 kg)/24 hr
	>20 kg	1500 mL + (20 mL/kg for weight above 20 kg)/24 hr
Calculate replacement fluid for that loss, using formula at right to obtain mL/kg/24 hr required.	Percentage of body weight loss × 10 × normal weight = mL/kg/24 hr required	
Calculate continued losses; add them to total of maintenance and replacement needs.		

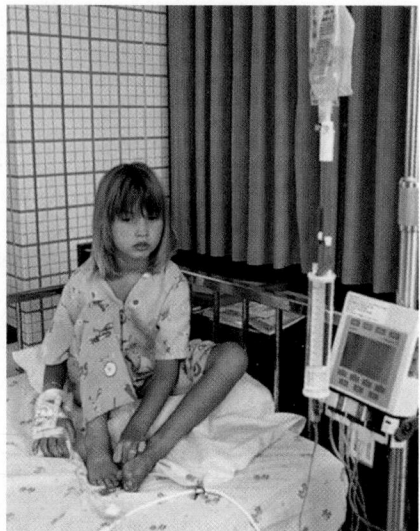

Figure 44–4 The use of a volume control device with an intravenous saline solution is important to prevent a sudden extracellular fluid volume overload.

DISCHARGE PLANNING AND HOME CARE TEACHING

Prior to discharge, parents need instructions about types of fluids and amounts to encourage. Teach the signs of dehydration (see Table 44–2) so that if the child does not take in adequate fluids, parents can seek help immediately. Instruct them to begin the child's normal diet once hydration is completed, determined by adequate urinary output and normal behaviors. Review methods of minimizing the child's chance of acquiring gastrointestinal infections (e.g., avoiding contact with other children who are infected; using careful handwashing and dishwashing procedures when another child in the home is sick). During well-child visits, encourage all parents to keep oral rehydration fluids at home in case they are needed; they are available in most grocery stores and pharmacies. Address the needs for increasing fluids in hot weather and when the child is exercising. See *Evidence-Based Practice: Treatment for Mild and Moderate Dehydration.*

Evaluation

Expected outcomes of nursing care include the following:

- Water and electrolytes in intracellular and extracellular compartments show adequate balance.
- The child has normal urinary output.
- The child maintains adequate fluid intake for maintenance needs.
- Vital signs remain within normal limits.

Extracellular Fluid Volume Excess

Extracellular fluid volume excess occurs when there is too much fluid in the vascular and interstitial compartment. This imbalance may also be called saline excess or extracellular volume overload. If this disorder occurs by itself (without saline disturbance), the serum sodium concentration is normal. There is simply too much extracellular fluid, even though it has a normal concentration.

Infants and children who develop an extracellular fluid volume excess have a condition that causes them to retain **saline** (sodium and water) or have been given an overload of sodium-containing isotonic intravenous fluid (Figure 44–5).

EVIDENCE-BASED PRACTICE | Treatment for Mild and Moderate Dehydration

Clinical Question

In spite of recommendations that children with mild or moderate dehydration be treated with oral rehydration therapy for gastroenteritis, many healthcare facilities and providers administer intravenous fluids to these children. How can nurses work to improve dehydration treatment to be consistent with current guidelines?

The Evidence

In the United States alone, gastroenteritis leads to 1.5 million healthcare visits annually and 200,000 hospitalizations. Most children can effectively be treated with a solution of glucose, electrolytes, and water. Such treatment is less invasive and painful than intravenous therapy for young children and is safe, effective, and easy to administer in the home setting. It is also recommended by the World Health Organization (WHO, 2014) and the American Academy of Pediatrics (AAP, 2013). However, many healthcare providers continue to use intravenous fluid treatment for mild to moderate rehydration (Jablonski, 2012). Even though nasogastric feeding is recommended when oral rehydration fails, all healthcare providers in a study of 113 emergency department personnel bypassed nasogastric feeding and began an intravenous line (Freedman, Keating, Rumatir, et al., 2012). A majority of 75 parents who visited an emergency department with a child who had gastroenteritis and dehydration expected the child to have an intravenous line, even when dehydration was mild or moderate (Nir, Nadir, Schechter, et al., 2013). A meta-analysis of 19 studies on use of oral rehydration solution found that social marketing, media education, and distribution of product increased parental acceptance and use of oral rehydration therapy (Lenters, Das, & Bhutta, 2013).

Best Practice

Nurses can partner with other healthcare providers to establish clinical pathways for dehydration treatment that follow recommendations for oral or nasogastric feedings. Implementing oral rehydration therapy immediately after assessment of the child assists in effective treatment. Appropriate oral rehydration solutions should be available on pediatric units, in emergency departments, and in all homes with children. Educate parents and healthcare providers about the benefits of oral rehydration for mild or moderate dehydration.

Clinical Reasoning

What questions can you ask a parent and what assessments can you perform to accurately evaluate if the child has mild or moderate dehydration? What oral rehydration solutions can the parent have available in the home setting? How will you inform colleagues of the current recommendations for the treatment of mild or moderate dehydration? How will you teach parents to administer oral rehydration in the home and what symptoms indicate that they need to seek additional care for the child?

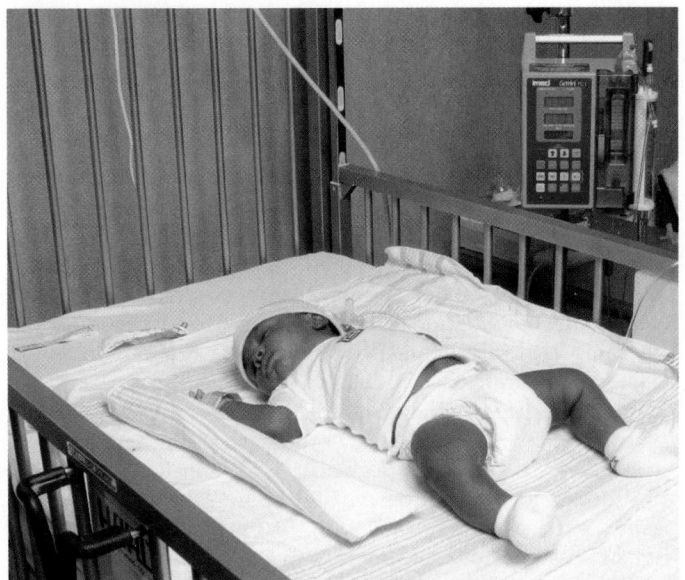

Figure 44–5 **Preventing extracellular fluid volume overload. If isotonic fluid containing sodium is given too rapidly or in too great an amount, an extracellular fluid volume excess will develop. Carefully monitor fluid intake, excretion, and retention in infants and children.**

What conditions cause retention of saline? The hormone aldosterone is secreted by the adrenal cortex. One of its normal functions is to cause the kidneys to retain saline in the body (see *Pathophysiology Illustrated: Aldosterone Effects*). Saline excess can be caused by any condition that results in excessive aldosterone secretion, such as adrenal tumors that secrete aldosterone, congestive heart failure, liver cirrhosis, and chronic renal failure. Most glucocorticoid medications (such as prednisone) have a mild saline-retaining effect when taken on a long-term basis. Intravenous fluid volume regulation is important, especially in young children. Either inaccurate calculation of needed fluid or inadvertent infusion of excess fluids can cause overload.

Extracellular fluid volume excess is characterized by sudden weight gain. A gain of 0.5 kg (1 lb) in a day is related to fluid, and represents 500 mL of saline. An overload of fluid in the blood vessels and interstitial spaces can cause clinical manifestations such as bounding pulse, distended neck veins in children (not usually evident in infants), periorbital edema, hepatomegaly, dyspnea, orthopnea, and lung crackles. Edema is the sign of overload of the interstitial fluid compartment. In an infant, edema is often generalized (Figure 44–6). Edema in children with extracellular fluid volume excess occurs in the dependent parts of the body, that is, in the parts closest to the ground. Thus, edema is evident in sacral areas in a child supine in bed. Scrotum or labia may be edematous. (Edema that develops from other causes is described in the next section of this chapter.)

The clinical therapy for extracellular fluid volume excess focuses on treating the underlying cause of the disorder. For example, a child who has congestive heart failure is given medications to strengthen the heart's ability to contract. Managing the cause also helps to reduce the extracellular fluid volume

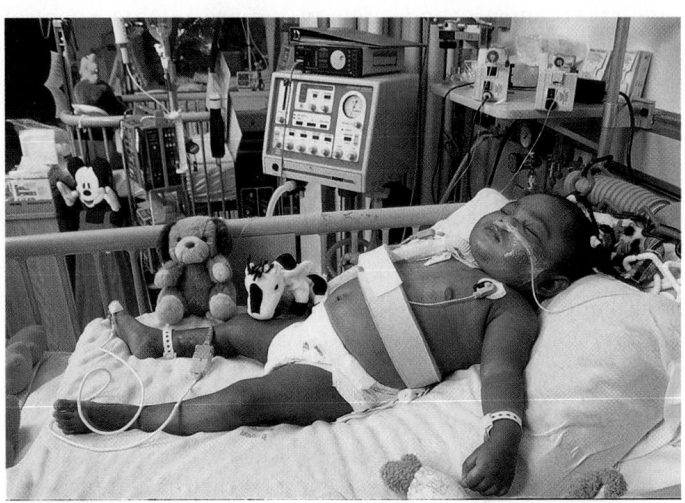

Figure 44–6 **This infant with congenital heart disease has signs of generalized edema. Note the fluid retention in the face and abdomen.**

Pathophysiology Illustrated: **Aldosterone Effects**

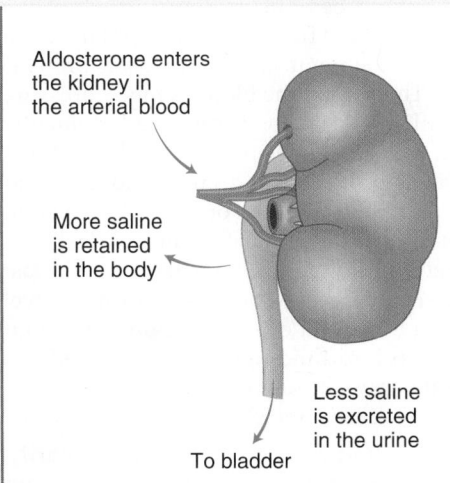

Aldosterone enters the kidney in the arterial blood

More saline is retained in the body

Less saline is excreted in the urine

To bladder

Aldosterone has a saline-retaining effect. Increased aldosterone secretion can be caused by adrenal tumors or congestive heart failure.

excess. Diuretics may be given to remove fluid from the body, thus reducing the extracellular fluid volume directly.

Nursing Management

Rapid weight gain is the most sensitive index of extracellular fluid volume excess. Therefore, daily weighing with the same scale and articles of clothing is an important nursing assessment. Measure the child's intake and output. For babies in diapers, a diaper is weighed dry and then wet, with grams of weight increase equal to urine volume in milliliters. When treatment is successful, output is greater than intake. Assess the character of the pulse and observe for neck vein distention when the child is sitting (usually visible only in older children). Monitor for signs of pulmonary edema (an indication of severe imbalance) by listening to lung sounds in the dependent lung fields (crackles) and assessing for respiratory distress (rapid respiratory rate, use of accessory muscles of respiration). Observe for edema.

A child may develop a fluid overload whenever an isotonic intravenous solution containing sodium, such as normal saline or Ringer solution, is administered. Therefore, monitor the infusion rate frequently and carefully and use a volume control device and pump whenever possible to aid in accurate administration. Use only small bags (e.g., 250 or 500 mL) for infants and young children, and check pumps frequently. If an excess of fluid has already developed, administer the medical therapy as prescribed and monitor for any complications of the medical therapy. For example, many diuretics increase potassium excretion in the urine, which may lead to an abnormally low plasma potassium concentration unless potassium intake is increased. (Refer to the discussion of hypokalemia later in this chapter.) It is also important to monitor for the development of extracellular fluid volume deficit as a result of diuretic therapy.

If edema is present, provide careful skin care and protection for edematous areas. Teach parents how to provide skin care and perform position changes at home. See the following section for additional interventions related to edema.

If a child has a long-term condition such as chronic renal failure that predisposes to extracellular fluid volume excess, a dietary fluid and sodium restriction may be prescribed (see Chapter 52 for further details). Teach parents how to manage sodium restriction. Plan low-sodium meals that fit the family's cultural practices. If the child is old enough to participate, incorporate games into the teaching. If a scale is available, teach parents to take and record an accurate daily weight.

Desired outcomes include electrolyte balance, maintenance of intact skin, and dietary intake as prescribed.

Interstitial Fluid Volume Excess (Edema)

Edema is an abnormal increase in the volume of the interstitial fluid. It may be caused by an extracellular fluid volume excess or it may result from other causes.

The causes of edema are best understood in the context of normal capillary dynamics. Fluid moves between the vascular and interstitial compartment by the process of **filtration**. Filtration is the net result of forces that tend to move fluid in opposing directions. The strongest forces determine the direction of fluid movement.

At the capillary level, two forces (blood hydrostatic pressure and interstitial osmotic pressure) tend to move fluid from the capillaries into the interstitial fluid, while two other forces (blood colloid osmotic pressure and interstitial fluid hydrostatic pressure) tend to move fluid in the opposite direction (from the interstitial fluid into the capillaries). The net result of these forces

---

Developing Cultural Competence Low-Sodium Diets

To adapt teaching about low-sodium diets to the cultural practices of a family, ask clients what types of food they usually eat. Help them to choose low-sodium foods from their diets and to avoid high-sodium foods. This approach is more effective than giving the same list of restricted foods to each family.

For example, some Asians may use monosodium glutamate to flavor foods and can be encouraged to add this at the table for family members who can have extra sodium rather than during cooking. Many Hispanic groups use large amounts of cheese, which can provide significant sodium. Encourage them to look for low-sodium cheese and substitute cottage cheese for other types since it is lower in sodium.

Canned foods tend to have high sodium, so teach all families to use fresh or frozen produce rather than canned when possible. Low-sodium milk is available and is a good option for young children. Teach families how to read and interpret food labels to identify salt (sodium) content

---

usually moves fluid from the capillaries into the interstitial compartment at the arterial end of the capillaries, and fluid from the interstitial compartment back into the capillaries at the venous end of the capillaries. This process brings oxygen and nutrients to the cells and removes carbon dioxide and other waste products.

Edema occurs if the balance of these four forces is altered so that excess fluid either enters or leaves the interstitial compartment (see *Pathophysiology Illustrated: Capillary Dynamics and Edema*). This may occur through:

1. Increased blood hydrostatic pressure
2. Decreased blood colloid osmotic pressure
3. Increased interstitial fluid osmotic pressure
4. Blocked lymphatic drainage

Many clinical conditions are associated with these altered forces (Table 44–7), as described in the following list:

1. Increased blood hydrostatic pressure. When extracellular fluid volume excess occurs, the increased fluid volume in the vascular compartment congests the veins. The pressure against the sides of the capillary is increased and more fluid then enters the interstitial compartment.

2. Decreased blood colloid osmotic pressure. Much of the osmotic pressure that pulls fluid into the capillaries is a result of the presence of albumin and other plasma proteins made by the liver. The part of the blood osmotic pressure that results from plasma proteins is often called **oncotic pressure**, or blood colloid osmotic pressure. Any condition that decreases plasma proteins will decrease blood colloid osmotic pressure and cause edema. For example, if a clinical condition causes large amounts of albumin to leak into the urine, the liver will not be able to make albumin fast enough to replace it. As a result the plasma protein level will fall, decreasing the blood osmotic pressure. Without this pulling force to return fluid to the capillaries, edema will occur. This is the cause of edema in children who have nephrotic syndrome (see Chapter 52).

3. Increased interstitial fluid osmotic pressure. Ordinarily, only a few small proteins enter the interstitial fluid, and the interstitial fluid osmotic pressure is small. However, if

bee sting or a sprained ankle. It occurs to a greater extent in burns, leading to swelling at the same time that there is a great loss of fluid volume through the burned skin (see Chapter 57).

4. Blocked lymphatic drainage. The lymph vessels normally drain small proteins and excess fluid from the interstitial compartment and return them to the blood vessels. If lymph vessels are blocked, fluid accumulates in the interstitial compartment. This may occur when a tumor blocks lymphatic drainage.

Edema causes localized or generalized swelling, which may cause pain and restrict motion. Edema due to extracellular fluid volume excess or right-sided heart failure usually occurs in the dependent portion of the body. In a child who is walking, dependent edema is observed in the ankles; in a bedfast, supine child, it is seen in the sacral area. The skin over an edematous area often appears thin and shiny.

The main focus of clinical therapy for edema is to treat the underlying condition that caused the edema. Such conditions are discussed throughout this book. The edema from inflammation of an injury is initially treated with cold to reduce capillary blood flow and thus reduce blood hydrostatic pressure.

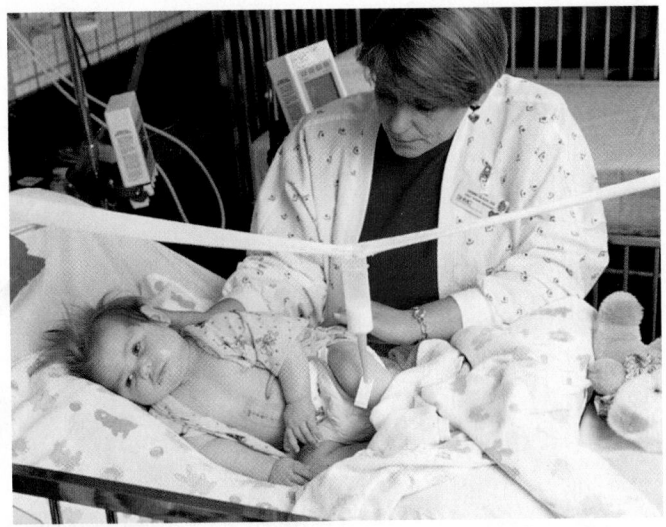

Figure 44–7 Care of edematous tissue. Edematous tissue is easily damaged. It must be kept clean and dry and free of pressure.

Nursing Management

A child or parent may make comments that alert the nurse to the development of edema. Shoes may become tight by the end of the day (dependent edema); the waistband of pants or a skirt may be "outgrown" suddenly (generalized edema or ascites [accumulation of fluid in the peritoneal cavity]); the eyes may be puffy (periorbital edema); a ring may be too tight; fingers may "feel like sausages." In many cases, visual inspection is sufficient to recognize edema. Observe for **pitting edema**, a "pit" or concave indentation that remains after an edematous area is pressed downward by the examiner's fingers. To detect changes in the amount of swelling, measure around the edematous part. If the edema is caused by extracellular fluid volume excess, daily measurements of weight and intake and output are a necessary part of the daily assessment. Nursing assessment should also focus on the integrity of the skin, presence of pain, restricted motion, and alterations in the child's body image.

Elevation of an area of localized edema helps to reduce the swelling. The skin over an edematous area needs extra care because it is fragile and prone to breakdown (Figure 44–7). Carefully position an infant or child on bed rest and turn frequently to prevent pressure sores. Perform turning carefully to avoid skin abrasion by rubbing against the sheets. Pat the skin dry after cleansing rather than rubbing it. Trim the child's fingernails smooth to prevent scratching. Teach parents skin care for the child at home. Teach older children to inspect their skin carefully to identify areas needing special care.

If restricted mobility is a problem, make specific plans to help the child manage activities. For example, if an edematous finger restricts the motion of a hand, food can be cut into bite-sized portions before the meal is served, so that the child can still eat independently.

Discomfort from edema may require creative nursing interventions. Distraction with toys or activities appropriate to the child's developmental level can be useful. Interventions to treat the underlying problem can also reduce the edema and its accompanying discomfort. Interventions for edema should be added to the nursing management of the underlying condition that causes the edema. Administration of the prescribed

medical therapy and observation for the complications of therapy are nursing responsibilities.

Discuss with school-age children and adolescents feelings of embarrassment about the edematous appearance. They need to understand the reason for edema and be able to explain it to peers. Arrange for the child to meet other children with similar concerns.

Desired outcomes of care include maintenance of intact skin, normal respiratory sounds and effort, and normal weight patterns.

ELECTROLYTE IMBALANCES

All body fluids contain electrolytes, although the concentration of those electrolytes varies depending on the type and location of the fluid. When a serum electrolyte value is reported from the laboratory, it provides information about the concentration of that electrolyte in the blood. It may not necessarily reflect the concentration of the electrolyte in other body compartments. Refer to Table 44–1 to see which electrolytes have the highest and lowest concentrations in the blood and other fluid compartments.

Electrolytes are normally gained and lost in relatively equal amounts so that the body remains in balance. However, when a child has an abnormal route of loss, such as vomiting, wound drainage, or nasogastric suction, electrolyte balance can be disturbed. In addition, supplementation with electrolytes via intravenous fluids in proportions different than body fluids can also cause electrolyte imbalance. Children with disease states that interfere with normal mechanisms of electrolyte regulation, such as renal disease, also have disturbance in electrolyte levels. Monitoring for signs of imbalance becomes important in all of these situations.

Sodium Imbalances

The serum sodium concentration reflects the **osmolality** of body fluids, that is, their degree of concentration or dilution. It refers to the number of moles of the substance per kilogram of water in the solution. Serum sodium concentration reflects the proportion

the capillary becomes abnormally permeable to proteins, the influx of large amounts of proteins into the interstitial fluid causes a dramatic increase in interstitial fluid osmotic pressure. The increased pulling force keeps an abnormal amount of fluid in the interstitial compartment. This mechanism plays an important part in the edema caused by a

Pathophysiology Illustrated: **Capillary Dynamics and Edema**

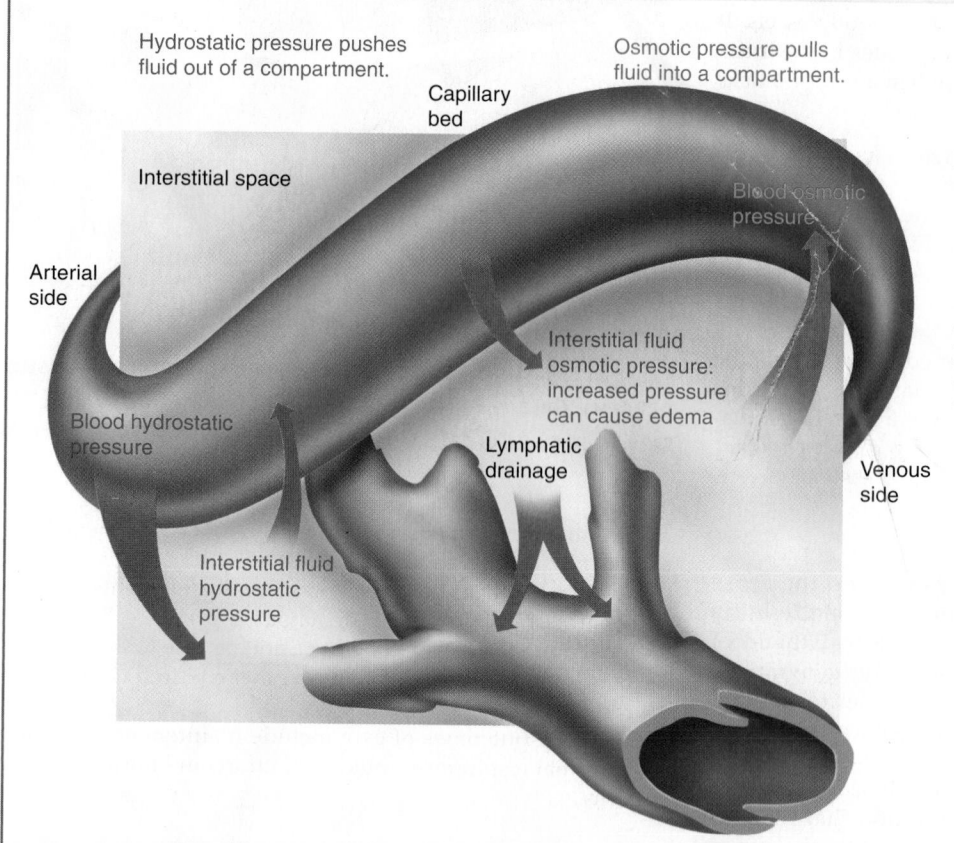

Hydrostatic pressure pushes fluid out of a compartment.

Osmotic pressure pulls fluid into a compartment.

Capillary bed

Interstitial space

Blood osmotic pressure

Arterial side

Blood hydrostatic pressure

Interstitial fluid osmotic pressure: increased pressure can cause edema

Lymphatic drainage

Venous side

Interstitial fluid hydrostatic pressure

With normal capillary dynamics, fluid moves out of the compartment by the force of hydrostatic pressure in the blood vessel and is pulled out by interstitial osmotic pressure. Fluid is forced into the compartment by interstitial hydrostatic pressure and pulled in by compartment osmotic pressure. Abnormal capillary dynamics can cause edema.

TABLE 44–7 Clinical Conditions That Cause Edema

CONDITION	RESULTING HEMODYNAMIC CHANGE	RESULT
Increased blood hydrostatic pressure	Increased capillary blood flow	Inflammation
		Local infection
	Venous congestion	Extracellular fluid volume excess
		Right heart failure
		Venous thrombosis
		External pressure on vein
		Muscle paralysis
Decreased blood osmotic pressure	Increased albumin excretion	Nephrotic syndrome (albumin leaks into urine)
		Protein-losing enteropathies (excess albumin in feces)
	Decreased albumin synthesis	Kwashiorkor (low-protein, high-carbohydrate starvation diet provides too few amino acids for liver to make albumin)
		Liver cirrhosis (diseased liver unable to make enough albumin)
Increased interstitial fluid osmotic pressure	Increased capillary permeability	Inflammation
		Toxins
		Hypersensitivity reactions
		Burns
Blocked lymphatic drainage	Venous congestion	Tumors
		Goiter
		Parasites that obstruct lymph nodes
		Surgery that removes lymph nodes

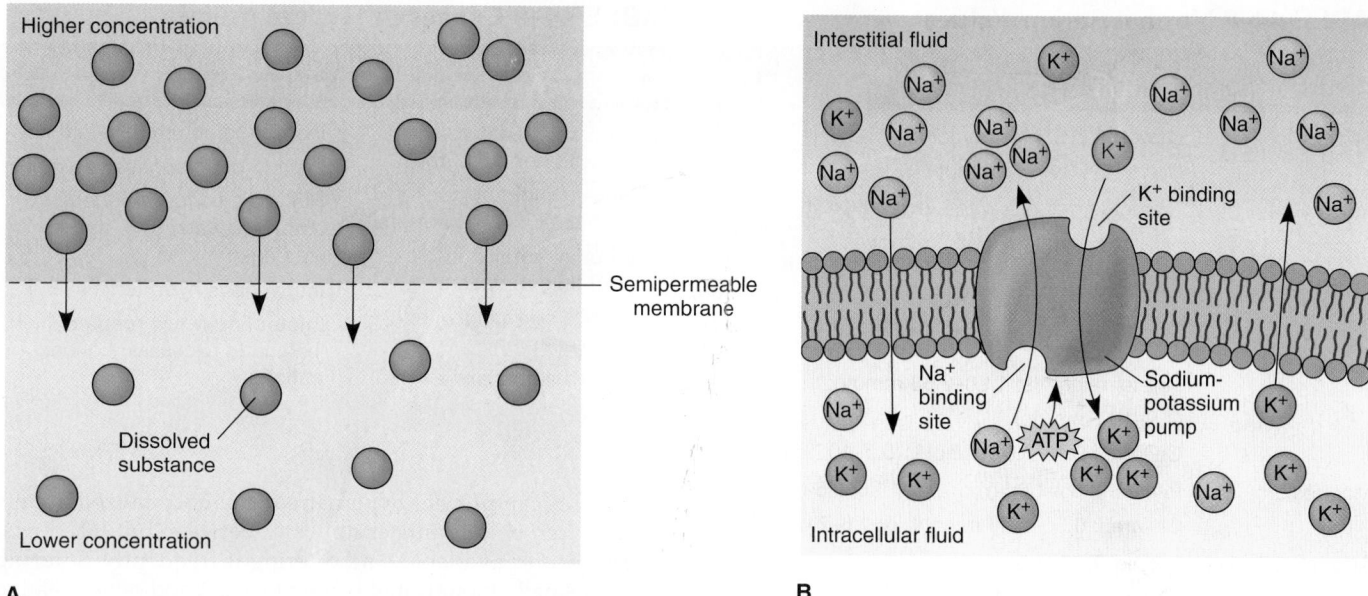

Figure 44–8 The sodium-potassium pump. *A*, Water balance is maintained by the simple passage of molecules from greater to lesser concentration across cell membranes. *B*, Sodium levels are maintained by an active transport system, the sodium-potassium pump, which moves these electrolytes across cell membranes in spite of their concentration.

of water and sodium in the extracellular compartment. When the osmolality of body fluids becomes abnormal, the cells swell or shrink. These cell size changes are due to **osmosis**, the movement of water across a semipermeable membrane into an area of higher particle concentration. Sodium levels are maintained at high extracellular and low intracellular levels by the sodium-potassium pump, which moves these electrolytes against their expected concentration gradients (Figure 44–8).

Hypernatremia

Hypernatremia is a condition of increased osmolality of the blood. The body fluids are too concentrated, containing excess sodium relative to water. Sodium level generally falls between 132 and 141 mmol/L, and a serum sodium level above 146 mmol/L in children (146 mmol/L in newborns) is diagnostic of hypernatremia (Engorn & Flerlage, 2015; Greenbaum, 2011) (Table 44–8).

Hypernatremia is caused by conditions that cause the body to lose relatively more water than sodium or to gain relatively more sodium than water (Table 44–9). Special circumstances in which a high solute intake may occur without adequate water include an infant formula that is too concentrated or one that is prepared with salt instead of sugar. A breastfed baby not receiving adequate breast milk who has normal water loss may develop hypernatremic dehydration. This is a risk at 2 to 3 days of age, when babies generally have a diuresis, if the baby does not feed well or the mother does not yet produce an adequate amount of breast milk (Bolat et al., 2013).

An infant or child who has hypernatremia is generally thirsty. The urine output is small unless the hypernatremia is caused by diabetes insipidus. A decreased level of consciousness manifested by confusion, lethargy, or coma results from shrinking of the brain cells. Seizures can occur when hypernatremia occurs rapidly or is severe. Severe hypernatremia can be fatal.

Serum sodium, specific gravity of urine, antidiuretic hormone (ADH), and 24-hour urine are common diagnostic tests. Hypernatremia is treated by intravenous administration of **hypotonic fluid**, or fluid that is more dilute than normal body fluid. This therapy dilutes the body fluids back to normal concentration. If a child is dehydrated, **isotonic fluids** (those with the osmolality of body fluids) may be administered first to replenish the volume, followed by hypotonic fluid to correct the osmolality. The underlying cause of the disorder is also treated.

Nursing Management

Monitor serum sodium level and measure intake and output and urine specific gravity. Normal specific gravity under 2 years is 1.001 to 1.018, while in children over 2 years 1.001 to 1.030 is the normal range (Corbett & Banks, 2013). Specific gravity changes toward normal levels as therapy progresses. Frequently assess responsiveness to monitor the effect of hypernatremia on brain cells. As the concentration of body fluids returns to normal, the child will become more alert and responsive. Watch for rebound hyponatremia while monitoring the fluid replacement. Implement safety interventions such as raised bed rails for protection. Ensure adequate rest and introduce developmentally appropriate activities when the child is alert.

Water deprivation is a form of child neglect or abuse. In neglect, the parents simply do not provide adequate water for the child. A form of child abuse that sometimes includes water deprivation is Munchausen syndrome by proxy (see Chapter 42). A small child who is hospitalized with hypernatremia that does not have a detectable cause may be subject to water deprivation. Assess the child's general condition, developmental tasks, the family dynamics, and the parents' understanding of formula preparation and the child's fluid intake needs.

Teaching can prevent many cases of hypernatremia. Be sure the breastfeeding mother has instruction and resources about lactation before discharge after birth. If the newborn is discharged

TABLE 44–8 Normal Serum Values

BLOOD COMPONENT	VALUES
Sodium	Newborn: 131–144 mmol/L
	Children: 134–143 mmol/L
Potassium	Premature infants: 4.5–7.2 mmol/L
	Full-term infants: 3.2–5.7 mmol/L
	Children: 3.7–5.0 mmol/L
Calcium (total)	Premature infants: 1.7–2.3 mmol/L (6.9–9.2 mg/dL)
	Full-term infants: 1.98–2.68 mmol/L (7.9–10.7 mg/dL)
	Children: 2.18-2.68 mmol/L (8.7–10.7 mg/dL)
Magnesium	Infants: 0.65–1.02 mmol/L or 1.6–2.5 mg/dL
	Children: 0.66–0.99 mmol/L or 1.6–2.4 mg/dL
Arterial pH	Infants: 7.18–7.5
	Children: 7.27–7.49
	Adolescents: 7.35–7.41
Arterial P_{O_2}	Infants: 60–70 mmHg (8–9.3 pKa)
	Children: 80–108 mmHg (10.7–14.4 pKa)
	Adolescents: 80–100 mmHg (4.3–6.4 pKa)
Arterial P_{CO_2}	Infants: 27–41 mmHg (3.6–5.5 pKa)
	Children and adolescents: 32–48 mmHg (4.3–6.4 pKa)
Arterial bicarbonate	Infants: 19–24 mmol/L
	Children: 18–25 mmol/L
	Adolescents: 20–29 mmol/L

Note: Laboratories may have slightly different levels for normal depending on assays performed. Always consult the normal values for your particular laboratory.

Source: From Greenbaum, L. A. (2011). Electrolyte and acid–base disorder. In R. M. Kliegman, B. F. Stanton, J. W. St. Geme, N. F. Schor, & R. E. Behrman (Eds.), *Nelson textbook of pediatrics* (19th ed., pp. 212–242). Philadelphia, PA: Saunders; Soldin, S. J., Wong, E. C., Brugnara, C., & Soldin, O. P. (2011). *Pediatric reference ranges* (7th ed.). Washington, DC: American Association for Clinical Chemistry.

soon after birth, be sure to schedule an appointment to check weight within the first few days, and alert the parents to expected output of at least six wet diapers daily. By about 10 days, newborns should have regained the birth weight.

When an infant is sick or developing slowly, parents sometimes want to feed the infant more concentrated formula to make the baby stronger. Parents and caregivers of bottlefed babies should be taught never to give undiluted formula concentrate or evaporated milk. Parents should be cautioned to keep salt out of reach, since eating handfuls of salt has caused hypernatremia. Teach parents to offer extra fluids during hot weather. Teach oral rehydration therapy for use at home during mild vomiting and diarrhea.

TABLE 44–9 Causes of Hypernatremia

LOSS OF RELATIVELY MORE WATER THAN SODIUM	GAIN OF RELATIVELY MORE SODIUM THAN WATER
Inadequate breastfeeding intake with normal output	Inability to communicate thirst
Diabetes insipidus (not enough antidiuretic hormone)	Limited or no access to water
Diarrhea or vomiting without fluid replacement	High solute intake without adequate water (e.g., tube feedings)
Excessive sweating without fluid replacement	Intravenous hypertonic saline
Increased aldosterone	Improper formula preparation leading to excessive concentration

Nurses can prevent hypernatremia in hospitalized infants and children by administering water between tube feedings, keeping water available, and offering it frequently. Offering frequent small amounts and using popsicles and other creative interventions can increase children's intake.

Desired outcomes of treatment for hypernatremia include balance of electrolytes and fluid in the intracellular and extracellular compartments and an alert level of consciousness.

Hyponatremia

In hyponatremia, the osmolality of the blood is decreased. The body fluids are too dilute, containing excess water relative to sodium. Hyponatremia is the most common sodium imbalance in children (Kliegman et al., 2011). A serum sodium level below 134 to 135 mmol/L in children (131 mmol/L in newborns) is diagnostic of hyponatremia (Greenbaum, 2011).

ETIOLOGY AND PATHOPHYSIOLOGY

Hyponatremia is caused by conditions that cause gain of relatively more water than sodium or loss of relatively more sodium than water (Table 44–10). Oral intake of water causes hyponatremia in unusual conditions such as forced fluid intake. More commonly, parents feed an infant only water or dilute formula to save money instead of using regular-strength formula or breast milk. Excessive swallowing of swimming pool water by an infant can have the same effect. Infants are vulnerable to the type of hyponatremia caused by water intoxication since they have a poorly developed thirst mechanism and may continue to drink, and then are unable to excrete excess water quickly because of immature kidney function. Forced water intake is another cause and form of child abuse. Exercise-induced hyponatremia can occur when people in prolonged physical activity such as marathon running consume

---

TEACHING HIGHLIGHTS | Preparing Infant Formula

Careful teaching about how to mix powdered formula is needed so that it is not too concentrated; this can help to prevent hypernatremia in the infant. Demonstrate the technique so that parents are well informed. Pictures are an important teaching tool if the parents are not able to read labels or instructions. When families use concentrated formula, equal amounts of concentrate and water should be mixed. Caution parents that even if an infant is premature or small, they should mix the formula as instructed. A useful strategy is to have the parents bring the formula being used to a healthcare visit and ask them to mix it as you watch. Any errors in technique can easily be corrected.

TABLE 44–10 Causes of Hyponatremia

GAIN OF RELATIVELY MORE WATER THAN SODIUM	LOSS OF RELATIVELY MORE SODIUM THAN WATER
Excessive intravenous D$_5$W (5% dextrose in water)	Diarrhea or vomiting with replacement by tap water only instead of fluid containing sodium
Excessive tap water enemas	
Irrigation of body cavities with distilled water	Excessive sweating
Excessive antidiuretic hormone	Diuretics, especially thiazides
Forced excessive oral intake of tap water	
Congestive heart failure	

hypotonic fluids in the form of water or sports drinks above the levels lost in respiratory, gastrointestinal, skin, and urinary routes (AAP Council on Sports Medicine and Fitness & Council on School Health, 2011).

CLINICAL MANIFESTATIONS

The child with hyponatremia has a decreased level of consciousness, which results from swelling of brain cells. This can manifest as anorexia, nausea, vomiting, headache, muscle weakness, decreased deep tendon reflexes, agitation, lethargy, or confusion. The condition can progress to respiratory arrest, dilated pupils, decorticate posturing, and coma. If hyponatremia arises rapidly or is extreme, seizures may occur. Hyponatremia is a frequent cause of seizures in infants under 6 months of age. Severe hyponatremia can be fatal.

CLINICAL THERAPY

Laboratory studies are the same as those used to diagnose hypernatremia. In most cases, hyponatremia is treated by restricting the intake of water. This therapy allows the kidneys to correct the imbalance by excreting excess water from the body. If a child is having seizures from hyponatremia, intravenous **hypertonic saline** (more concentrated than body fluid) may be administered. Use of this concentrated fluid rapidly increases body fluid concentration, but the process must be monitored carefully because it can easily cause rebound hypernatremia. For exercise-associated hyponatremia, intravenous access is established at the first-aid site, hypertonic saline is administered, and oxygen is delivered (AAP Council on Sports Medicine and Fitness & Council on School Health, 2011). In cases of diabetes insipidus, treatment for the condition is needed (see Chapter 53).

Nursing Management

For the Child With Hyponatremia

Nursing Assessment and Diagnosis

Hyponatremia should be prevented in hospitalized children receiving intravenous solutions (particularly postoperatively) by administering isotonic rather than hypotonic solutions. Monitor serum sodium level and measure intake and output. If an infant with hyponatremia has normal antidiuretic hormone (ADH) levels, and other causes have been ruled out, carefully question parents about proper preparation of formula and feeding practices. A toddler or school-age child may be subjected to

forced fluid intake as a form of child abuse. Sensitive interviewing and a caring manner can help identify such problems in a family.

Because hyponatremia is characterized by a decreased level of consciousness, frequently assess responsiveness to monitor the response to therapy. The child will become more alert and responsive as the concentration of body fluids returns to normal.

The highest priority nursing diagnosis for hyponatremia is *Injury, Risk for,* as it relates to the child's decreased level of consciousness. The following diagnoses might also apply (NANDA-I © 2014):

- *Self-care Deficit* related to weakness and tiredness
- *Health Maintenance, Impaired,* related to parental misinterpretation about infant formula preparation
- *Breastfeeding, Ineffective,* related to inadequate sucking by infant or inadequate milk production

Planning and Implementation

Nurses can prevent hyponatremia in hospitalized children by using normal saline instead of distilled water for irrigations and by avoiding tap water enemas. Verify intravenous fluid types and amounts and question use of hypotonic fluids in a child with no intake of sodium. Help the child comply with any prescribed fluid restrictions. Allow the child to choose favorite fluids to drink. Teach parents to replace body fluids lost through diarrhea or vomiting with oral electrolyte solutions.

Evaluation

Expected outcomes are maintenance of safety, balance of fluid and electrolytes, and establishment of adequate formula or breastfeeding intake.

Potassium Imbalances

Potassium, an essential electrolyte, performs many necessary functions in the body such as muscle contraction and enzymatic reactions. Potassium intake in healthy children comes from potassium-rich foods such as fruits and vegetables. Potassium is absorbed easily from the intestine. A normal potassium distribution is important for proper function.

A potassium imbalance arises when the serum potassium concentration rises or falls outside the normal range. Potassium imbalances are caused by alterations in potassium intake, distribution, or excretion; or by loss of potassium through an abnormal route such as burns, emesis, or renal failure.

Most potassium ions in the body are found inside the cells. The sodium-potassium pump in cell membranes moves potassium ions into cells to maintain the high intracellular potassium concentration. Potassium ions can be shifted into or out of cells by various physiologic factors (see *Pathophysiology Illustrated: Potassium Ions*). Potassium is excreted from the body through urine, feces, and sweat. The hormone aldosterone increases potassium excretion in the urine.

Hyperkalemia

Hyperkalemia is an excess of potassium in the blood. Potassium levels generally range from 3.2 to 5.7 mmol/L for newborns, and 3.7 to 5.0 mmol/L for infants and children. Hyperkalemia is reflected by a level above 5.7 mmol/L in newborns or above 5.5 mmol/L in children (see Table 44–8).

Pathophysiology Illustrated: **Potassium Ions**

Factors that shift potassium ions into or out of cells.

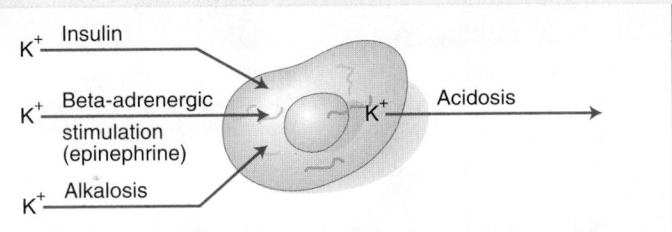

ETIOLOGY AND PATHOPHYSIOLOGY

Hyperkalemia is caused by conditions that include increased potassium intake, shift of potassium from cells into the extracellular fluid, and decreased potassium excretion. Renal insufficiency is a primary cause of hyperkalemia. Premature infants commonly have low systemic blood flow and resultant poor renal function, leading to hyperkalemia. Increased potassium intake is frequently due to intravenous potassium overload. Excessive or too rapid intravenous administration of potassium-containing solutions can occur if the potassium requirement is overestimated or if the intravenous infusion runs in too fast.

Blood transfusion is another source of potassium intake that may cause hyperkalemia. Potassium ions leak out of red blood cells that are stored in a blood bank. The longer the blood is stored, the more the potassium leaks out of cells and accumulates in the fluid portion of the transfusion. Hyperkalemia from administration of stored blood arises when multiple units are transfused, as when infants receive exchange transfusions or children receive multiple blood transfusions after a serious injury or during surgery.

Shift of potassium from cells into the extracellular fluid occurs when there is massive cell death, as with a crush injury, in sickle cell disease (hemolytic crisis), or when chemotherapy for a malignancy is rapidly effective (tumor lysis syndrome). In these situations, the dead cells release their high-potassium contents into the extracellular fluid. Potassium ions also shift out of cells in metabolic acidosis caused by diarrhea and in diabetes mellitus when insulin levels are low.

Decreased potassium excretion occurs with acute or chronic oliguria during renal failure, severe hypovolemia, and conditions that decrease the secretion of aldosterone by the adrenal cortex (lead poisoning, Addison disease, hypoaldosteronism). Several medications can cause hyperkalemia, including some cancer chemotherapies, potassium-sparing diuretics, angiotensin-converting enzyme inhibitors, and nonsteroidal anti-inflammatories.

CLINICAL MANIFESTATIONS

The clinical manifestations of hyperkalemia are all related to muscle dysfunction since potassium plays a vital role in muscle activity. Hyperactivity of gastrointestinal smooth muscle causes intestinal cramping and diarrhea in some children. The skeletal muscles become weak, typically beginning with leg weakness and ascending. Weakness can progress to flaccid paralysis. The child is often lethargic. Dysfunction of cardiac muscle causes cardiac arrhythmias such as tachycardia and may result in heart failure and cardiac arrest. Abnormalities in the electrocardiogram include a prolonged QRS complex, a peak in T waves, atrioventricular block, and ventricular dysrhythmia (Engorn & Flerlage, 2015).

CLINICAL THERAPY

The major diagnostic test is the serum potassium level. Hyperkalemia is treated by management of the underlying condition that caused the imbalance. If the serum potassium concentration is very high or is causing dangerous cardiac arrhythmias, treatment to decrease the serum potassium level may be ordered. These treatments may remove potassium from the body or drive it from the extracellular fluid into the cells. Potassium is removed from the body by peritoneal dialysis or hemodialysis, by potassium-wasting diuretics, or with a cation exchange resin (Kayexalate) administered orally or rectally. Medical treatments that drive potassium ions into cells are intravenous sodium bicarbonate, intravenous insulin, glucose, and calcium gluconate.

Nursing Management

For the Child With Hyperkalemia

Nursing Assessment and Diagnosis

Monitor serum potassium levels with prescribed laboratory analysis. Ongoing assessment of muscle strength is important because the muscle weakness may progress to flaccid paralysis. This paralysis is reversible on correction of the potassium imbalance. Diarrhea can occur in infants and children. An older child may complain of intestinal cramping. Monitor the pulse rate carefully.

Nursing diagnoses for a child who has hyperkalemia depend on the severity of the clinical manifestations. The cause of the imbalance may also lead to useful diagnoses that guide teaching for the child and the parents. The following nursing diagnoses may apply (NANDA-I © 2014):

- *Activity Intolerance* related to decreased cardiac output secondary to cardiac arrhythmias
- *Injury, Risk for,* related to muscle weakness
- *Self-care Deficit: Bathing and Dressing* related to neuromuscular impairment
- *Anxiety* related to change in health status
- *Health Maintenance, Ineffective,* related to parental lack of exposure about potassium intake in chronic renal failure
- *Health Management, Family, Ineffective,* related to complexity of therapy

Planning and Implementation

Nursing care includes measures to prevent hyperkalemia from developing in hospitalized children. If hyperkalemia does develop, care shifts to administering intravenous solutions, monitoring cardiopulmonary status, ensuring safety, promoting adequate nutrition, and preparing the child and family for discharge.

Growth and Development

The nursing diagnoses for hyperkalemic children will prompt a nurse to provide safety measures appropriate to the child's developmental level and to assist the child with activities that muscle weakness makes difficult. It is important to provide play and diversional activities that take into account the child's degree of muscle strength as well as the appropriate developmental level.

PREVENT HYPERKALEMIA

Any child receiving an intravenous infusion that contains potassium is at risk for hyperkalemia. Check that urine output is normal (1 to 2 mL/kg/hr) before administering intravenous potassium solutions. Turn over intravenous solutions to which potassium has been added several times to mix the contents thoroughly before connecting them to the infusion tubing. Double-check the potassium order and intravenous dosage with another nurse. Observe the child closely and perform cardiorespiratory monitoring.

Be sure blood or packed red blood cells are fresh, especially for the child receiving multiple transfusions and for all newborns. Use a cardiac monitor during infusion of these products to watch for arrhythmias.

ADMINISTER INTRAVENOUS SOLUTIONS

Once a child is diagnosed as being hyperkalemic, ensure that any infusions with added potassium are stopped. Several other infusions may need to be managed, including those containing glucose, sodium bicarbonate, and calcium gluconate. Maintain these infusions at the prescribed rates and monitor the child's condition frequently.

MONITOR CARDIOPULMONARY STATUS

Upon diagnosis of hyperkalemia, an electrocardiogram is performed and a cardiac monitor applied. Monitor for any changes in cardiac status and for cardiac arrhythmias. Report abnormal rate and character of pulse as well as shortness of breath.

ENSURE SAFETY

Since the child is weak, raise side rails. Position the child carefully. Assist the child with activities requiring leg muscle strength, such as climbing into bed or pushing up in bed. Encourage quiet activities with frequent rest periods. Document and report any change in muscle weakness.

PROMOTE ADEQUATE NUTRITIONAL INTAKE

Adequate caloric intake is necessary to prevent tissue breakdown and the resultant potassium release from cells. If the child's appetite is decreased, offer nourishing snacks. Restrict potassium-rich foods.

DISCHARGE PLANNING AND HOME CARE TEACHING

If the child has chronic renal failure or another condition that decreases aldosterone secretion, teach parents and children to restrict foods high in potassium. Most oral rehydration solutions, including Pedialyte, contain potassium and should not be used to provide fluid for the child. Instruct the family not to use salt substitutes, which commonly contain potassium. Parents should check with the healthcare provider and pharmacist before giving even over-the-counter products to the child because some of these medications contain potassium. Management of renal failure at home with frequent visits for dialysis and other treatments can be challenging. Refer to Chapter 52 for further suggestions to help parents handle this condition.

Evaluation

Expected outcomes for the child with hyperkalemia include the following:

- The child returns to a state of fluid and electrolyte balance.
- The child's safety is maintained.
- The child has adequate nutritional intake to provide essential potassium.
- The child maintains normal cardiac rate and rhythm.

Hypokalemia

Hypokalemia occurs when the serum potassium concentration is too low. Total body potassium may be decreased, normal, or even increased when the serum level is low, depending on the cause of the imbalance. Serum potassium levels below 3.7 mmol/L in children (3.2 mmol/L for newborns) are diagnostic of hypokalemia.

ETIOLOGY AND PATHOPHYSIOLOGY

Hypokalemia is caused by increased potassium excretion, decreased potassium intake, shift of potassium from the extracellular fluid into cells, and loss of potassium by an abnormal route.

Increased potassium excretion through the gastrointestinal tract is the major cause of hypokalemia in children. In addition to diuretics and other medications, causes of increased urinary potassium excretion are osmotic diuresis (glucose present in urine), hypomagnesemia, increased aldosterone (hyperaldosteronism, congestive heart failure, nephrotic syndrome, cirrhosis), and increased cortisol (Cushing disease and syndrome) (Engorn & Flerlage, 2015). Eating large amounts of black licorice increases renal excretion of potassium.

Decreased potassium intake will lead to hypokalemia slowly or more rapidly if combined with increased excretion or loss of potassium. Hospitalized children who are placed on NPO status and receive prolonged intravenous therapy should have added potassium. Adolescents concerned about weight loss or those with anorexia nervosa may embark on fad diets low in potassium.

A shift of potassium from the extracellular fluid into cells occurs in alkalosis and hypothermia (unintentional or induced for surgery). Hyperalimentation often causes hypersecretion of insulin, which also shifts potassium into cells.

Vomiting is a route for the loss of potassium; for example, self-induced vomiting in bulimia can cause hypokalemia. Nasogastric suctioning (Figure 44–9) and intestinal decompression

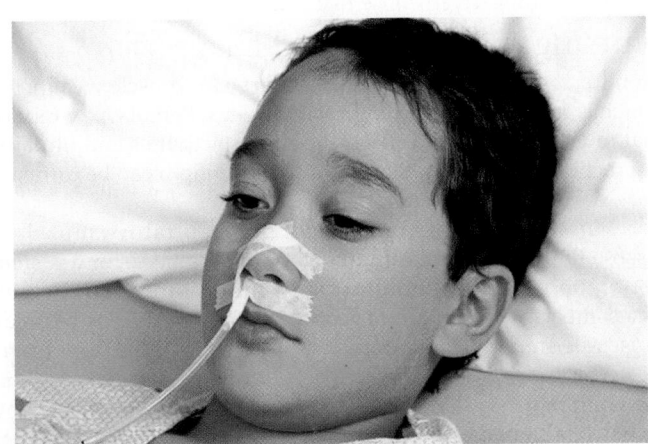

Figure 44–9 Nasogastric tubes and potassium levels. Because this child has a nasogastric tube in place, it is important to monitor his potassium levels.

TABLE 44–11 Drugs That May Cause Electrolyte Disturbance

HYPERKALEMIA	HYPOKALEMIA	HYPOCALCEMIA	HYPERMAGNESEMIA	HYPOMAGNESEMIA
Potassium-containing medications	Beta-adrenergic agonists	Antacids (if overused)	Magnesium antacids	Magnesium-wasting diuretics
Potassium-sparing diuretics	Insulin	Laxatives (if overused)	Magnesium-containing cathartics	Antineoplastics
Angiotensin-converting enzyme inhibitors	Potassium-wasting diuretics	Oil-based bowel lubricants		Systemic antifungals
Cytotoxic agents	Parenteral penicillins	Anticonvulsants		Aminoglycoside antimicrobials
	Glucocorticoids	Phosphate-containing preparations		Laxatives
	Aminoglycoside anti-microbials	Protein-type plasma expanders during rapid infusion		
	Systemic antifungals	Antineoplastics		
	Antineoplastics			
	Laxatives			

can cause potassium loss. Hypokalemia can also be caused by several medications (Crawford & Harris, 2011a) (Table 44–11).

CLINICAL MANIFESTATIONS

Since the ratio of intracellular to extracellular potassium determines the responsiveness of muscle cells to neural stimuli, it is not surprising that the clinical manifestations of hypokalemia involve muscle dysfunction. Gastrointestinal smooth muscle activity is slowed, leading to abdominal distention, constipation, or paralytic ileus. Skeletal muscles are weak and unresponsive to stimuli, and weakness may progress to flaccid paralysis. The respiratory muscles may be impaired. Cardiac arrhythmias can occur. Symptoms may range from mild fatigue to flat or absent T waves. Polyuria results from changes in the kidney caused by hypokalemia.

CLINICAL THERAPY

Serum measurement of potassium is the major diagnostic tool, and electrocardiograph may be used. Medical management of hypokalemia focuses on replacement of potassium while treating the cause of the imbalance. Potassium replacement may be given intravenously or orally.

Nursing Management

For the Child With Hypokalemia

Nursing Assessment and Diagnosis

Monitor serum potassium levels. Observe for muscle weakness, which is frequently detected first in the legs. Parents may report that muscle weakness restricts the child's activities and impairs interactions with peers. Skeletal muscle strength can be difficult to assess if the child is lethargic.

Muscle weakness may affect the respiratory muscles. Assess the child frequently to determine the need for assisted ventilation. Cardiac monitoring is important for continued assessment of hypokalemia-associated arrhythmias. Apical pulse rate should be monitored.

Assess for diminished bowel sounds. Ask the parents if the child has recently been awakening to use the toilet at night or has begun bed-wetting after previously being dry at night. These may be symptoms of polyuria associated with chronic hypokalemia.

The most important nursing diagnoses in the child with severe hypokalemia relate to cardiac arrhythmias and respiratory muscle weakness. The following nursing diagnoses may apply (NANDA-I © 2014):

- *Activity Intolerance, Risk for,* related to decreased cardiac output secondary to cardiac arrhythmia
- *Breathing Pattern, Ineffective,* related to respiratory musculoskeletal impairment
- *Injury, Risk for,* related to muscle weakness
- *Self-care Deficit: Bathing and Dressing* related to neuromuscular impairment
- *Constipation* related to decreased motility
- *Anxiety* related to change in health status
- *Health Maintenance, Ineffective,* related to management of potassium supplements or high-potassium diet
- *Health Management, Family, Ineffective,* related to complexity of potassium therapy
- *Nutrition, Imbalanced: Less than Body Requirements,* related to lack of basic nutritional knowledge regarding safe weight-loss diet

Planning and Implementation

Nursing care of the child with hypokalemia focuses on ensuring adequate potassium intake, monitoring cardiopulmonary status, promoting normal bowel function, ensuring safety, providing dietary counseling, and preparing the child and family for discharge.

Growth and Development

Bradycardia occurs at a different level for children of various ages. For infants, a pulse rate below 100 is considered bradycardia. For young children, 80 may be the identified number, whereas for adolescents, a pulse below 60 is bradycardia. Look at the child's age and normal pulse range to find changes that indicate bradycardia.

ENSURE ADEQUATE POTASSIUM INTAKE

Since potassium is excreted from the body every day, daily potassium intake is necessary to prevent hypokalemia. A hypokalemic child who is able to eat should be given a high-potassium diet. Teach parents (and the child if old enough) which foods are high in potassium and how to incorporate them into the daily diet (Table 44–12).

TABLE 44–12 Food Sources of Electrolytes

POTASSIUM-RICH FOODS		CALCIUM-RICH FOODS		MAGNESIUM-RICH FOODS
Apricots	Orange juice	Milk	Nuts	Whole-grain cereal
Bananas	Peaches	Cheese	Figs	Dark green vegetables
Cantaloupe	Potatoes	Yogurt	Chicken	Soy
Cherries	Prunes	Pudding	Salmon (canned with bones)	Almonds
Dates	Raisins	Egg yolks		Peanut butter
Figs	Strawberries	Grains (cream of wheat, farina, bran muffins)	Tofu	Bananas
Molasses	Tomato juice	Sardines (canned)	Fruit drinks with added calcium	Egg yolk
		Legumes		

Children who have no oral intake for a period of time should receive intravenous fluids that contain potassium. Calculate the dosage to be sure it is accurate. Ensure that the infusion runs on schedule. Sometimes the child will complain of burning along the vein when potassium is infused. The infusion may need to be slowed temporarily to allow it to continue. Check serum potassium to watch for high or low potassium levels. Monitor urine output. A child with oliguria can develop hyperkalemia when receiving supplements.

MONITOR CARDIOPULMONARY STATUS

Hypokalemia potentiates digitalis toxicity. A hypokalemic child receiving digitalis needs careful surveillance for digitalis toxicity, which is manifested as anorexia, nausea, vomiting, and bradycardia. Observe for these effects. Take the pulse rate and rhythm regularly. Monitor respirations and ease of breathing to watch for decreased respiratory muscle activity.

PROMOTE NORMAL BOWEL FUNCTION

Ensure adequate fluids and fiber in the diet. Monitor and record the number of stools and report inadequate stools.

ENSURE SAFETY

Keep bed side rails up. Assist the child as needed to move into and out of bed. Reposition the child frequently to preserve skin integrity of limbs that are not moved regularly. Perform passive range of motion if the child is not moving. Use supportive pillows to position the child properly.

PROVIDE DIETARY COUNSELING

The adolescent trying to lose weight and not consuming a nutritious diet needs dietary teaching. More intensive treatment will be needed for teens who are anorexic or bulimic (see Chapter 32 for interventions).

DISCHARGE PLANNING AND HOME CARE TEACHING

Teach parents how to give potassium supplements, if prescribed. Liquid or powdered potassium supplements can be mixed with juice or sherbet to improve the bitter taste. The parent should call the mixture "medicine" so that the child does not learn to dislike all juices. Teach the parents signs of hypokalemia and hyperkalemia and whom to call to report these symptoms. These signs must be reported promptly so medications can be adjusted.

Evaluation

Expected outcomes for the child with potassium imbalance include normal rate and rhythm of heart and respiratory system, regular bowel movements, maintenance of safety, and knowledge of child and family regarding food sources of potassium.

Calcium Imbalances

A normal serum calcium concentration is important for many physiologic functions, including muscle and nerve function, secretion of hormones, bone formation and strength, and clotting of the blood. Calcium is the most abundant mineral in the body, with about 98% of it being present in bones (AAP, 2013). There are three forms of calcium in plasma: calcium bound to protein, calcium bound to small organic ions (e.g., citrate), and free ionized calcium (Ca^{2+}), which is physiologically active. A discussion of dietary calcium intake and its importance in bone formation can be found in Chapter 32. (See *Developing Cultural Competence: Calcium Intake and Osteoporosis*.)

Parathyroid hormone is the major regulator of the plasma calcium concentration. It increases the plasma calcium concentration by increasing calcium absorption, increasing calcium withdrawal from bones, and decreasing calcium excretion in the urine. The plasma calcium concentration has an important influence on cell membrane permeability and influences the threshold potential of excitable cells. For this reason, calcium imbalances alter neuromuscular irritability.

Calcium imbalances are caused by alterations in calcium intake, absorption, distribution, or excretion. Calcium absorption requires vitamin D for maximum efficiency and is greatest

---

Developing Cultural Competence Calcium Intake and Osteoporosis

Ingestion and absorption of calcium are important for the growing child to ensure formation of strong bones. Adolescents who ingest more calcium have less risk of osteoporosis later in life. It has been noted that Black women have less bone loss and fewer fractures than White women. Studies with these two groups of women have demonstrated that Blacks absorb more calcium from the diet, and lose less in their urine, leading to increased bone density. However, this has led to an underidentification of osteoporosis in Black women who have relative risks of lactose intolerance and low dairy intake. Assess calcium intake for all and suggest appropriate interventions for your population group and individuals (NIH Osteoporosis and Related Bone Diseases National Resource Center, 2011).

Pathophysiology Illustrated: **Calcium Imbalances**

Some causes of excess calcium in the blood (hypercalcemia)

- Vitamin D overdose
- Hyperparathyroidism
- Bone tumors and other cancers
- Thiazide diuretics
- Familial hypercalcemia

Ca²⁺
Ca²⁺
Ca²⁺

Some causes of decreased calcium in the blood (hypocalcemia)

- Insufficient dietary calcium and vitamin D intake
- Chronic diarrhea
- Laxative abuse
- Malabsorption
- Chronic renal insufficiency
- Hypoparathyroidism
- Alkalosis
- Large transfusion of citrated blood
- Rapid infusion of plasma expanders

Ca²⁺
Ca²⁺
Ca²⁺

A variety of conditions can lead to hypercalcemia and hypocalcemia.

in the duodenum. Calcium distribution involves calcium entry into and exit from bones and the distribution of different forms of calcium in the plasma. Ionized calcium is the only physiologically active form; additional calcium is bound to protein or ions. Calcium is excreted in urine, feces, and sweat (see *Pathophysiology Illustrated: Calcium Imbalances*).

Hypercalcemia

Hypercalcemia refers to a plasma excess of total calcium (above 2.7 mmol/L in infants and children) (see Table 44–8). Because so much calcium is stored in the bones, however, the serum levels of calcium may not reflect body stores.

ETIOLOGY AND PATHOPHYSIOLOGY

Hypercalcemia is caused by conditions that include increased calcium intake or absorption, shift of calcium from bones into the extracellular fluid, and decreased calcium excretion. Hypercalcemia due to increased calcium intake or absorption may occur if an infant is fed large amounts of chicken liver (source of vitamin A) or is given megadoses of vitamin D or vitamin A, or if a child or adolescent consumes large amounts of calcium-rich foods concurrently with antacids (milk-alkali syndrome). Infants with very low birth weight can develop hypercalcemia if they have inadequate phosphorus intake because bone phosphorus and calcium will be resorbed. Hypercalcemia may also occur when children receiving total parenteral nutrition are given excessive doses of calcium.

Most cases of hypercalcemia in children are due to a shift of calcium from bones into the extracellular fluid. The excessive amounts of parathyroid hormone produced in hyperparathyroidism cause calcium withdrawal from bones. Prolonged immobilization also causes withdrawal of calcium from bones. Often, the excess calcium ions are excreted in the urine. However, if calcium is withdrawn from bones faster than the kidneys can excrete it, hypercalcemia results. Hypercalcemia also occurs

with many types of malignancies, such as leukemias. The malignant cells produce substances that circulate in the blood to the bones and cause bone resorption. The calcium from the bones then enters the extracellular fluid, causing hypercalcemia. Bone tumors destroy bone directly, leading to the release of calcium. Familial hypercalcemia and infantile hypercalcemia are rare congenital disorders.

Thiazide diuretics (e.g., thiazide and hydrochlorothiazide) decrease calcium excretion in the urine and may contribute to development of hypercalcemia. Lithium and theophylline can induce hypercalcemia (Ruppe, 2011).

CLINICAL MANIFESTATIONS

Hypercalcemia may have nonspecific symptoms, making diagnosis difficult. Many signs and symptoms of hypercalcemia are manifestations of decreased neuromuscular excitability. Constipation, anorexia, nausea, and vomiting can occur. Fatigue and skeletal muscle weakness dominate. Confusion, lethargy, and decreased attention span are common. Polyuria develops. Severe hypercalcemia may cause cardiac arrhythmias and arrest. Newborns with hypercalcemia have flaccid muscles and exhibit failure to thrive. Hypercalcemia increases sodium and potassium excretion by the kidneys and can lead to polyuria and polydipsia.

CLINICAL THERAPY

Serum calcium is tested although the blood level may not accurately reflect bone stores. Additional laboratory tests include serum albumin, phosphate, magnesium, alkaline phosphate, electrolytes, blood urea nitrogen, creatinine, and parathyroid hormone. Hypercalcemia is treated by increasing fluids and administering the diuretic furosemide (Lasix) to increase excretion of calcium in the urine. Treatment to decrease intestinal absorption of calcium involves effective use of glucocorticoids. Bone resorption can be decreased by administration of glucocorticoids and calcitonin. Phosphate is sometimes given to treat hypercalcemia, but it may cause dangerous precipitation of calcium phosphate salts in body tissues. Dialysis may be used, if necessary. The underlying condition causing the imbalance is treated.

Nursing Management
For the Child With Hypercalcemia

Nursing Assessment and Diagnosis

Nursing assessment of a child with hypercalcemia includes monitoring serum calcium levels, level of consciousness, gastrointestinal function, urine volume, specific gravity, cardiac rhythm, and pH. With chronic hypercalcemia, assessment of activity tolerance and developmental level becomes important.

Many nursing diagnoses are appropriate for children who have hypercalcemia. Diagnoses that address cardiac and neuromuscular manifestation are especially important. The following nursing diagnoses may apply (NANDA-I © 2014):

- *Activity Intolerance, Risk for,* related to decreased cardiac output secondary to cardiac arrhythmia
- *Injury, Risk for,* related to decreased level of consciousness
- *Injury, Risk for,* related to neuromuscular impairment
- *Injury, Risk for,* related to possibility of spontaneous fractures
- *Self-care Deficit: Bathing and Dressing* related to neuromuscular impairment
- *Anxiety* related to change in health status
- *Constipation* related to decreased motility
- *Nutrition, Imbalanced: Less than Body Requirements,* related to anorexia and nausea
- *Urinary Elimination, Impaired,* related to renal calculi

Planning and Intervention

Carefully calculate calcium in total parenteral nutrition and other solutions, administer these solutions with caution, and use cardiac monitoring to prevent hypercalcemia in hospitalized children.

Interventions to increase fluid intake are important for children with hypercalcemia or those who are immobilized. An increased fluid intake, appropriate to the child's age, is necessary to keep the urine dilute and to help reduce constipation (a common symptom of hypercalcemia). An acidic urine helps to keep calcium from forming stones. Because urinary tract infections may cause the urine to be alkaline, institute nursing interventions to prevent urinary tract infection. Thiazide diuretics, which decrease calcium excretion, should not be given to the hypercalcemic child. Provide a high-fiber diet to help reduce constipation.

Increasing mobility through assisted weight bearing helps decrease the withdrawal of calcium from bones that is caused by immobility. If the hypercalcemia is caused by withdrawal of calcium from bones, the child is at risk for fractures with minor trauma and must be handled with special care. See Chapter 56 for further discussion of care following fractures and prolonged casting.

Teach parents to avoid giving calcium-rich foods (such as dairy products) and calcium antacids (e.g., Tums) to children with hypercalcemia. Vitamin D supplements should be avoided as they increase calcium absorption from the gastrointestinal tract.

Evaluation

Expected outcomes include cardiac pump effectiveness, safety, normal bowel excretion, and adequate nutritional status.

Hypocalcemia

Hypocalcemia is a serum deficit of calcium (below 2.1 mmol/L in infants and children). Recall that serum calcium levels may not reflect body stores of this mineral, as most of the body's calcium is stored in bone.

ETIOLOGY AND PATHOPHYSIOLOGY

Hypocalcemia is caused by conditions that include decreased calcium intake or absorption, shift of calcium to a physiologically unavailable form, increased calcium excretion, and loss of calcium by an abnormal route.

Decreased calcium intake or absorption causes hypocalcemia in children with chronic generalized malnutrition or with a diet low in vitamin D and calcium. Adolescent girls trying to lose weight or maintain a low weight often decrease foods that contain calcium and may develop chronic hypocalcemia. They may have premature bone loss and inadequate bone. (See Chapter 32 for further discussion of calcium intake during adolescence.) This deficit cannot be made up later in life, increasing the risk of osteoporosis.

Even with a normal calcium intake, hypocalcemia occurs if the mineral is not absorbed. If a child does not have enough vitamin D, calcium is not absorbed efficiently from the duodenum. Sunlight speeds formation of vitamin D in the skin. Children institutionalized without access to sunlight (e.g., severely developmentally delayed children), those with very dark skin, or children kept well covered when outside may become hypocalcemic because of the lack of vitamin D (see Chapter 32). Uremic syndrome is another cause of vitamin D deficiency. It interferes with the kidney's ability to activate vitamin D. High phosphate intake can cause hypocalcemia. Chronic diarrhea and steatorrhea (fatty stools) also reduce calcium absorption from the gastrointestinal tract.

About 40% of calcium is bound to proteins and not available for interactions, 10% is bound to small organic ions such as citrate, and 50% is ionized and physiologically active. Calcium becomes physiologically unavailable when calcium shifts into bone or free ionized calcium in plasma binds to proteins or small organic ions in the plasma. Excessive calcium shifts into bones in various types of hypoparathyroidism, including DiGeorge syndrome (congenital absence of the parathyroid glands). Hypomagnesemia impairs parathyroid hormone function and may cause hypocalcemia. Some types of neonatal hypocalcemia are associated with delayed parathyroid hormone function or hypomagnesemia. Calcium shifts rapidly into bone when rickets is treated. A high plasma phosphate concentration causes plasma calcium to decrease. Ionized hypocalcemia, due to an increased binding of plasma ionized calcium, occurs very rapidly. The ionized hypocalcemia persists until the alkalosis resolves or the citrate is metabolized by the liver. Children who receive liver transplants are hypocalcemic for several days because of impaired citrate metabolism.

Increased calcium excretion occurs in steatorrhea, when calcium secreted into the gastrointestinal fluid binds to the fecal fat in addition to the dietary calcium that is bound in the feces. A similar situation occurs in acute pancreatitis.

Loss of calcium by an abnormal route may contribute to hypocalcemia; calcium is lost through burn or wound drainage or sequestered in acute pancreatitis. Many medications can cause hypocalcemia (see Table 44–11).

CLINICAL MANIFESTATIONS

The signs and symptoms of hypocalcemia are manifestations of increased muscular excitability (tetany). In children, they include twitching and cramping, tingling around the mouth or in the fingers, carpal spasm, and pedal spasm. Laryngospasm, seizures, and cardiac arrhythmias are more severe manifestations of hypocalcemia and may be fatal. Hypocalcemia may cause congestive heart failure, especially in newborns.

Although these symptoms are diagnostic of acute calcium deficiency, a more common state in children and adolescents is chronic low intake of calcium. This may be manifested by spontaneous fractures in infants and in adolescents who exercise excessively.

CLINICAL THERAPY

Laboratory measurement of serum calcium and cardiac monitoring are used for diagnosis. Hypocalcemia is treated by oral or intravenous administration of calcium. The original cause of the imbalance is also treated. If the hypocalcemia is due to hypomagnesemia, the magnesium must be replenished before the calcium replacement can be successful. When the cause is chronic low dietary intake, counseling is needed about high-calcium foods, and perhaps the necessity for vitamin D intake or supplements.

Nursing Management

For the Child With Hypocalcemia

Nursing Assessment and Diagnosis

Carefully assess growth in the young woman who is trying to diet. Whenever an adolescent girl is very thin, be sure to ask about excessive sports and other activities, and about regularity of menstrual periods. If periods are irregular or not occurring, collect additional dietary information to help determine whether the girl is lacking in intake of calcium, calories, and other nutrients. These assessments are needed even if serum calcium values are normal. Look for signs of inadequate nutrition such as fat and muscle wasting, dry hair, and cold hands and feet. Assess for muscle cramps, stiffness, and clumsiness; grimacing caused by spasms of facial muscles and twitching of arm muscles; and laryngospasm. Increased neuromuscular excitability may be detected by testing for Trousseau sign or Chvostek sign (see Chapter 33). Many healthy newborns have a positive Chvostek sign; however, this assessment should be reserved for children over several months of age. Monitor serum calcium levels and perform cardiac monitoring to observe for cardiac arrhythmias.

Growth and Development

Hypocalcemia in infants is more often seen as tremors, muscle twitches, and brief tonic–clonic seizures. Perform careful neurologic assessments on infants at risk of electrolyte imbalance.

The effects of increased neuromuscular excitability in the child with hypocalcemia are the basis for several nursing diagnoses. These include the following (NANDA-I © 2014):

- *Injury, Risk for,* related to potential for fractures
- *Injury, Risk for,* related to increased neuromuscular excitability
- *Breathing Pattern, Ineffective,* related to laryngospasm

- *Activity Intolerance* related to decreased cardiac output secondary to cardiac arrhythmias
- *Anxiety* related to change in health status
- *Nutrition, Imbalanced: Less than Body Requirements,* related to lack of basic nutritional knowledge of sources and recommended amounts of calcium intake

Planning and Implementation

To correct calcium deficiency in the hospitalized child, give oral or intravenous calcium as prescribed. Monitor for complications of calcium supplementation. Monitor for the side effect of constipation with oral supplements; or for tissue sloughing, elevated serum calcium, or decreased serum phosphate with intravenous supplementation. Verify dosage of calcium gluconate with another nurse, and monitor heart rate and rhythm. Calcium is never given subcutaneously or intramuscularly because it causes tissue necrosis. A 10% calcium gluconate intravenous solution should be readily available for emergency use in severe hypocalcemia.

Take measures to ensure safety for the child who is hospitalized with hypocalcemia. Seizure precautions may be necessary. Explain the cause of muscle cramps to parents and older children.

Counsel the family about dairy products and nondairy foods rich in calcium (see Table 44–12). For the adolescent girl whose weight and menstrual patterns show irregularities, total calories and calcium intake should be increased. Teaching may also be needed about proper calcium intake and its importance both to athletic performance and to the prevention of osteoporosis. Encourage three glasses of nonfat milk per day. Teach ways to use milk in the diet. For example, sprinkle nonfat dry milk on cereal and other foods. If the child is lactose intolerant, emphasize nondairy sources of calcium and advise parents to purchase special milk treated with lactase. However, be aware that this milk is more costly, and inadequate family finances may prevent its use. If a child has a health condition leading to chronic diarrhea, encourage increased intake of calcium-rich foods. Calcium supplements in the form of calcium carbonate tablets may be used.

Evaluation

Expected outcomes of nursing care include ingestion of recommended dietary allowances for calcium, absence of discomfort related to calcium imbalance, and freedom from injury.

Magnesium Imbalances

Magnesium is necessary for enzyme function in cells, acetylcholine release, glycolysis, stimulation of ATPases, and bone formation. Since magnesium is a component of chlorophyll, dark green leafy vegetables are a good dietary source of magnesium. Nuts and grains are also good sources of magnesium. Magnesium is absorbed primarily from the terminal ileum. It is distributed among the extracellular fluid (small amounts), the cells (larger amounts), and the bones (large amounts). Magnesium is excreted in urine, feces, and sweat.

Magnesium imbalances are caused by alterations in magnesium intake, distribution, or excretion; by loss of magnesium through an abnormal route; or by a combination of these factors. The plasma magnesium concentration influences the release of acetylcholine at neuromuscular junctions. Thus, magnesium imbalances are characterized by alterations in neuromuscular irritability.

Hypermagnesemia

Hypermagnesemia occurs when the plasma magnesium concentration is too high (above 2.4 mg/dL [0.99 mmol/L]) (see Table 44–8). Keep in mind that the serum levels measured in the laboratory may not reflect body magnesium stores because most magnesium in the body is located in the bones and inside the cells.

Hypermagnesemia is caused by conditions that involve increased magnesium intake and decreased magnesium excretion. Impaired renal function leading to decreased magnesium excretion is the most common cause of hypermagnesemia in children. In both oliguric renal failure and adrenal insufficiency, magnesium ions that cannot be excreted in the urine accumulate in the extracellular fluid.

Less frequently, increased magnesium intake may cause hypermagnesemia. Magnesium sulfate ($MgSO_4$) given to treat eclampsia in the mother before birth causes hypermagnesemia in the newborn. Abnormally high amounts may also be taken in magnesium-containing enemas, laxatives, antacids, and intravenous fluids. Epsom salt is a readily available product that is a nearly pure magnesium sulfate preparation; its use as an enema has caused death in children (see Table 44–11). Aspiration of seawater, as in near-drowning, is an uncommon but potentially serious source of excessive magnesium intake. Children with Addison disease can have abnormally high magnesium levels.

Clinical manifestations of hypermagnesemia include decreased muscle irritability, hypotension, bradycardia, drowsiness, lethargy, and weak or absent deep tendon reflexes. In severe hypermagnesemia, flaccid muscle paralysis, fatal respiratory depression, cardiac arrhythmias, heart block, and cardiac arrest can occur (Crawford & Harris, 2011b).

Hypermagnesemia is managed primarily by increasing the urinary excretion of magnesium. This is usually accomplished by increasing fluid intake (except in oliguric renal failure) and by the administration of diuretics. Dialysis may sometimes be necessary.

Nursing Management

Monitor serum magnesium levels. Take the child's blood pressure (to watch for hypotension), heart rate and rhythm (to monitor for bradycardia and cardiac arrhythmias), respiratory rate and depth (to observe for respiratory depression), and deep tendon reflexes (to assess muscle tone and paralysis or movement). Keep the side rails of the bed raised. Children with hypermagnesemia or oliguria should not be given magnesium-containing medications or sea salt.

Teach parents of children with chronic renal failure that these children should never be given milk of magnesia, antacids that contain magnesium, or other sources of magnesium. When hypermagnesemia is treated with diuretics, monitor potassium levels to watch for hypokalemia.

Expected outcomes of nursing care include maintenance of electrolyte balance, normal neuromuscular tone, safety, and regular heart rate and rhythm.

Hypomagnesemia

Hypomagnesemia refers to a plasma magnesium concentration that is too low (below 1.6 mg/dL [0.66 mmol/L]). Remember that the serum levels of magnesium may not reflect body stores, since most of the magnesium in the body is found in cells and bones.

Hypomagnesemia is caused by conditions that include decreased magnesium intake or absorption, shift of magnesium to a physiologically unavailable form, increased magnesium excretion, and loss of magnesium by an abnormal route.

Decreased magnesium intake or absorption can occur if a child who is not eating has prolonged intravenous therapy without magnesium. Chronic malnutrition is another cause of decreased magnesium intake. Magnesium absorption is decreased in chronic diarrhea, short bowel syndrome, malabsorption syndromes, and steatorrhea.

Magnesium may shift to a physiologically unavailable form after transfusion of many units of citrated blood products; magnesium bound to the citrate is not physiologically active. Such transfusions cause prolonged hypomagnesemia in liver transplant patients, who have impaired citrate metabolism. Magnesium shifts rapidly into bones that have been deprived of adequate stores.

Increased magnesium excretion in the urine occurs with diuretic therapy, the diuretic phase of acute renal failure, diabetic ketoacidosis, and hyperaldosteronism. Chronic alcoholism, occasionally seen in adolescents, increases urinary magnesium excretion. Magnesium contained in gastrointestinal secretions is bound to fat and excreted in the stool.

Clinical Tip

Instruct parents of a child with chronic renal failure to read labels to detect magnesium in antacids and cathartics. Encourage them to check with their pharmacist and other healthcare providers before administering any over-the-counter medication to the child.

Loss of magnesium by an abnormal route occurs with prolonged nasogastric suction and through sequestration of magnesium in acute pancreatitis. Several medications may cause hypomagnesemia (see Table 44–11).

Hypomagnesemia is characterized by increased neuromuscular excitability (tetany). The clinical manifestations are hyperactive reflexes, skeletal muscle cramps, twitching, tremors, and cardiac arrhythmias. Seizures can occur with severe hypomagnesemia.

Hypomagnesemia is managed by administering magnesium and treating the underlying cause of the imbalance.

Nursing Management

In addition to monitoring serum magnesium levels, nursing assessment of hypomagnesemia includes monitoring deep tendon reflexes, testing for Trousseau and Chvostek signs, monitoring cardiac function, and observing for muscle twitching. Children who are able to talk may report muscle cramping. Because magnesium levels are not routinely measured in many settings, request the test for any child who has risk factors and early manifestations of hypomagnesemia. When intramuscular or intravenous magnesium is ordered, administer carefully as directed and monitor vital signs. Electrocardiogram and renal studies may precede drug administration. Have resuscitative drugs and equipment readily available during drug administration.

Teach parents of a child with hypomagnesemia or continuing risk factors such as chronic diarrhea to include magnesium-rich foods in the diet (see Table 44–12). Before administering magnesium supplements, verify that the child's urine output is adequate. Monitor deep tendon reflexes if intravenous magnesium is given, and observe for complications of magnesium supplementation. Oral magnesium may lead to diarrhea, and intravenous magnesium can cause flushing, elevated serum magnesium, cardiac arrhythmias, or decreased deep tendon reflexes.

Expected outcomes of nursing care for the child with an imbalance in magnesium are restoration and maintenance of electrolyte balance.

CLINICAL ASSESSMENT OF FLUID AND ELECTROLYTE IMBALANCE

How can a nurse assess children appropriately for fluid and electrolyte imbalance without thinking through the clinical manifestations of every possible disorder one after the other? First, perform a rapid risk factor assessment on each child to see which factors are present (Tables 44–13 and 44–14).

A risk factor assessment may be performed mentally while providing care. Look for factors that alter the intake, retention, and loss of isotonic fluid and water. Use this information to evaluate which fluid imbalance is most likely to occur in a particular child. Next, look for factors that alter electrolyte intake and absorption, distribution between plasma and other electrolyte pools, excretion, and abnormal routes of electrolyte loss. Use this information to evaluate which electrolyte imbalances are most likely to occur in the child. A review of pathophysiology is important to understand the role of the other electrolytes and substances, such as phosphorus, in the body.

After evaluating possible imbalances for the child, perform a clinical assessment. Assess for fluid imbalances by assessing

TABLE 44–13 Risk Factor Assessment for Fluid Imbalances

TYPE OF FLUID	FACTORS TO ASSESS
Isotonic fluid (extracellular fluid volume imbalances)	Source of increased intake?
	Aldosterone secretion increased or decreased?
	Source of loss from the body?
Water	Source of increased intake?
	Antidiuretic hormone secretion increased or decreased?
	Source of unusual loss from the body?

TABLE 44–14 Risk Factor Assessment for Electrolyte Imbalances

POTENTIAL ELECTROLYTE IMBALANCE	ASSESSMENT FINDING
Electrolyte intake and absorption	Increased?
	Decreased?
Electrolyte shifts	From electrolyte pool to plasma?
	From plasma to electrolyte pool?
Electrolyte excretion	Increased?
	Decreased?
Electrolyte loss by abnormal route	Vomiting?
	Diarrhea?
	Nasogastric suction?
	Wound?
	Burn?
	Excessive sweating?

weight changes, vascular volume, interstitial volume, and cerebral function (Table 44–15). Assess for electrolyte imbalances by assessing serum electrolyte levels, skeletal muscle strength, neuromuscular excitability, gastrointestinal tract function, and cardiac rhythm (Table 44–16). Next, check for other manifestations specific to a particular high-risk imbalance (e.g., polyuria in hypokalemia). Evaluate any serum laboratory values available. This method of risk factor assessment followed by clinical assessment provides a rapid yet thorough approach to assessment for fluid and electrolyte imbalances.

Physiology of Acid–Base Balance

Normal acid–base balance is necessary for proper function of the cells and the body. The number of hydrogen ions (H^+) present in a fluid determines how acidic it is. Increasing the hydrogen ion concentration makes a solution more acidic. Because the hydrogen ion concentration in body fluids is very small, acidity is expressed as **pH** (the negative logarithm of the hydrogen ion concentration) rather than as the hydrogen ion concentration itself. The range of possible pH values is 1 to 14. A pH of 7 is neutral. The lower the pH, the more acidic the solution. A pH above 7 is basic. The higher the pH, the more basic the solution. Body fluids are normally slightly basic (see Table 44–8).

The pH of body fluids is regulated carefully to provide a suitable environment for cell function. The pH of the blood influences the pH inside the cells. **Acidemia** refers to a decreased blood pH below normal levels, while **alkalemia** is an increased blood pH. Normal arterial blood pH ranges are 7.36 to 7.42 for infants, 7.37 to 7.43 for children, and 7.35 to 7.41 for adolescents. For the enzymes outside the cells to function optimally, the pH must be in the normal range. If the pH inside the cells becomes too high or too low, then the speed of chemical reactions becomes inappropriate for proper cell function. Cell protein function relies on the correct level of hydrogen ions. Thus, acid–base imbalances result in clinical signs and symptoms, and, in severe cases, they may cause death.

In the course of their normal function, all cells in the body produce acids. Cells produce two kinds of acids: carbonic acid (H_2CO_3) and metabolic (noncarbonic) acids. Carbonic acid is formed from carbon dioxide and water, while common metabolic acids are pyruvic, sulfuric, lactic, and hydrochloric acids. These acids are released into the extracellular fluid and must be neutralized or excreted from the body to prevent dangerous accumulation. They can be neutralized to some degree by the buffers in body fluids. The lungs excrete carbonic acid in the form of carbon dioxide and water. Metabolic acids are excreted by the kidneys.

Buffers

The maintenance of hydrogen ions within normal range relies heavily on buffers. A **buffer** is a compound that binds hydrogen ions when their concentration rises and releases them when the concentration falls (see *Pathophysiology Illustrated: Buffer Responses to Excess Acid or Base*). Several kinds of buffers are present in the body, such as bicarbonate, protein, hemoglobin, and phosphate. Various body fluids have buffers to meet their special needs. The bicarbonate buffer system neutralizes metabolic acids (see *Pathophysiology Illustrated: The Bicarbonate Buffer System*); however, it cannot neutralize carbonic acid.

TABLE 44–15 Summary of Clinical Assessment of Fluid Imbalances

ASSESSMENT CATEGORY	SPECIFIC ASSESSMENTS	CHANGES WITH FLUID IMBALANCES
Rapid changes in weight	Daily weights	Weight gain—extracellular volume excess
		Weight loss—extracellular volume deficit; clinical dehydration
Vascular volume	Small vein filling time	Increased—extracellular volume deficit; clinical dehydration
	Capillary refill time	Increased—extracellular volume deficit; clinical dehydration
	Character of pulse	Bounding—extracellular volume excess
		Thready—extracellular volume deficit; clinical dehydration
	Postural blood pressure measurements	Postural drop—extracellular volume deficit; clinical dehydration
	Lung sounds in dependent portions	Crackles—extracellular volume excess
	Central venous pressure	Increased—extracellular volume excess
		Decreased—extracellular volume deficit; clinical dehydration
	Tenseness of fontanelle (infants)	Bulging—extracellular volume excess
		Sunken—extracellular volume deficit; clinical dehydration
	Neck vein filling (older children)	Full when upright—extracellular volume excess
		Flat when supine—extracellular volume deficit; clinical dehydration
Interstitial volume	Skin turgor	Skin tents—extracellular volume deficit; clinical dehydration
	Presence or absence of edema	Edema—extracellular volume excess
Cerebral function	Level of consciousness	Decreased—clinical dehydration

TABLE 44–16 Summary of Clinical Assessment of Electrolyte Imbalances

ASSESSMENT CATEGORY	SPECIFIC ASSESSMENTS	CHANGES WITH ELECTROLYTE IMBALANCES
Skeletal muscle function	Muscle strength	Weakness, flaccid paralysis—hyperkalemia; hypokalemia
Neuromuscular excitability	Deep tendon reflexes	Depressed—hypercalcemia; hypermagnesemia
		Hyperactive—hypocalcemia; hypomagnesemia
	Chvostek sign (not seen in infants)	Positive—hypocalcemia; hypomagnesemia
	Trousseau's sign	Positive—hypocalcemia; hypomagnesemia
	Paresthesias	Digital or perioral—hypocalcemia
	Muscle cramping or twitching	Present—hypocalcemia; hypomagnesemia
Gastrointestinal tract function	Bowel sounds	Decreased or absent—hypokalemia
	Elimination pattern	Constipation—hypokalemia; hypercalcemia
		Diarrhea—hyperkalemia
Cardiac rhythm	Arrhythmia	Irregular—hyperkalemia; hypokalemia; hypercalcemia; hypocalcemia; hypermagnesemia; hypomagnesemia
	Electrocardiogram	Abnormal—hyperkalemia; hypokalemia; hypercalcemia; hypocalcemia; hypermagnesemia; hypomagnesemia
Cerebral function	Level of consciousness	Decreased—hyponatremia; hypernatremia

Pathophysiology Illustrated: **The Bicarbonate Buffer System**

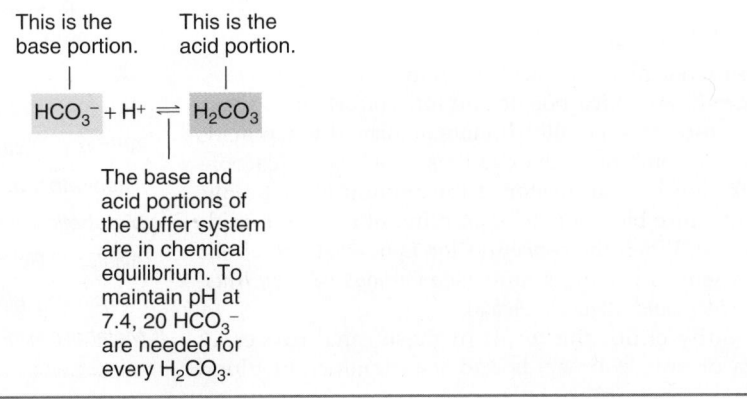

This is the base portion.

This is the acid portion.

$$HCO_3^- + H^+ \rightleftharpoons H_2CO_3$$

The base and acid portions of the buffer system are in chemical equilibrium. To maintain pH at 7.4, 20 HCO_3^- are needed for every H_2CO_3.

Pathophysiology Illustrated: **Buffer Responses to Excess Acid or Base**

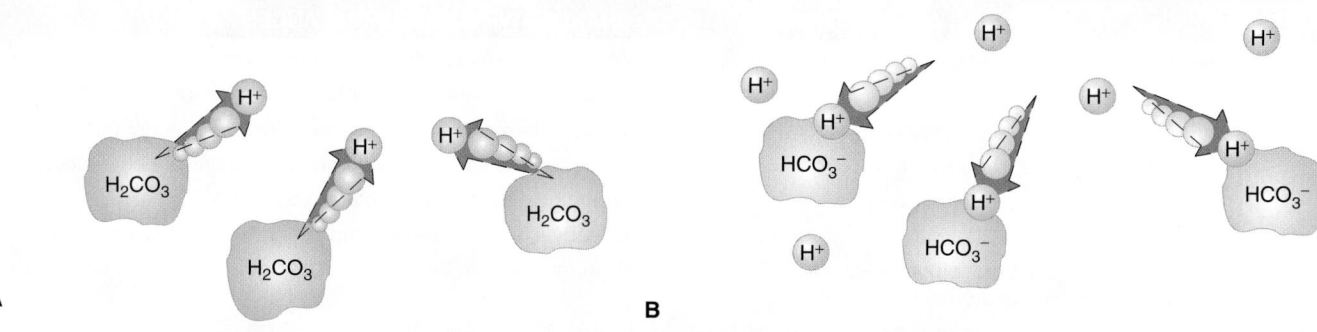

A, How buffers respond to an excess of base. If the blood has too much base, the acid portion of a buffer pair (e.g., H_2CO_3 of the bicarbonate buffer system) releases hydrogen ions (H^+) to help return the pH to normal.

B, How buffers respond to an excess of acid. If the blood has too much acid, the base portion of a buffer pair (e.g., HCO_3^- of the bicarbonate buffer system) takes up hydrogen ions (H^+) to help return the pH to normal.

All buffer systems have limits. For example, if there are too many metabolic acids, the bicarbonate buffers become depleted. The acids then accumulate in the body until they are excreted by the kidneys. Clinically, this is seen as a decreased serum bicarbonate concentration and decreased blood pH.

Role of the Lungs

The lungs are responsible for excreting excess carbonic acid from the body. A child breathes out carbon dioxide and water, the components of carbonic acid, with each breath. With faster and deeper breaths, more carbonic acid is excreted. Since carbonic acid is converted in the body to carbon dioxide and water by the enzyme carbonic anhydrase, an indirect laboratory measurement of carbonic acid is Pco_2 (see Table 44–8).

Although a child can voluntarily increase or decrease the rate and depth of respirations, they are usually involuntarily controlled. Chemoreceptors in the hypothalamus of the brain and in the aorta and carotid arteries monitor the Pco_2 and pH of the blood. These arteries also monitor the Po_2 of the blood. The input from the chemoreceptors is combined with other neural input to change breathing according to needs. Rate and depth increase or decrease according to the amount of carbonic acid that needs to be excreted.

If a child has a condition that decreases the excretion of carbonic acid or causes breathing to be too slow or shallow (such as overmedication following surgery), carbonic acid accumulates in the blood. Clinically, this is seen as an increased blood Pco_2. The reverse will also be true.

Role of the Kidneys

The kidneys excrete metabolic acids from the body in two ways. They reabsorb filtered bicarbonate and form bicarbonate when needed to restore balance. Bicarbonate is formed when acids and ammonium combine with extra ions. The blood bicarbonate concentration is an indicator of the amount of metabolic acids present, since bicarbonate is used in buffering the acids (see Table 44–8). When the concentration is normal, metabolic acids are present in usual amounts (see *Pathophysiology Illustrated: The Kidneys and Metabolic Acids*).

In a healthy child, the result of these renal processes is excretion of metabolic acids and maintenance of blood bicarbonate concentration within normal limits. However, a child whose kidneys are not producing enough urine may be unable to excrete metabolic acids effectively. Accumulation of these acids uses up many of the available bicarbonate buffers, resulting in a decreased serum bicarbonate concentration.

Role of the Liver

The liver also plays a role in maintaining acid–base balance by metabolizing protein, which produces hydrogen ions. It also synthesizes proteins needed to maintain osmotic pressures in the fluid compartments.

Acid–Base Imbalances

There are four acid–base imbalances. Two are the result of processes that cause too much acid in the body and are referred to as **acidosis**. The other two are the result of processes that cause too little acid in the body and are called **alkalosis**. An acid–base disorder caused by too much or too little carbonic acid is called a *respiratory acid–base imbalance*. A disorder caused by too much or too little metabolic acid is called a *metabolic acid–base imbalance*.

Arterial blood gas measurements (ABGs) provide a laboratory evaluation of a child's current acid–base status. In addition, oxygen saturation, or the percentage of hemoglobin saturated with arterial blood, is normally 95% to 100%. Table 44–17 provides a method that can help interpret the pH, Pco_2, and bicarbonate concentrations, the most important acid–base measures. End-tidal CO_2 can provide a continuous noninvasive measurement. (Remember that Pco_2 reflects carbonic acid status, and bicarbonate concentration reflects the metabolic acid status.)

Clinical Tip

Acidosis: Relatively too much acid in the body

Respiratory acidosis: Relatively too much carbonic acid

Metabolic acidosis: Relatively too much metabolic acid

Alkalosis: Relatively too little acid in the body

Respiratory alkalosis: Relatively too little carbonic acid

Metabolic alkalosis: Relatively too little metabolic acid

Pathophysiology Illustrated: **The Kidneys and Metabolic Acids**

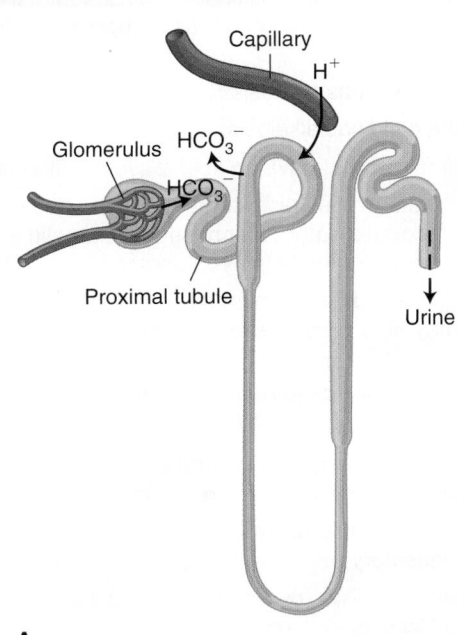

A

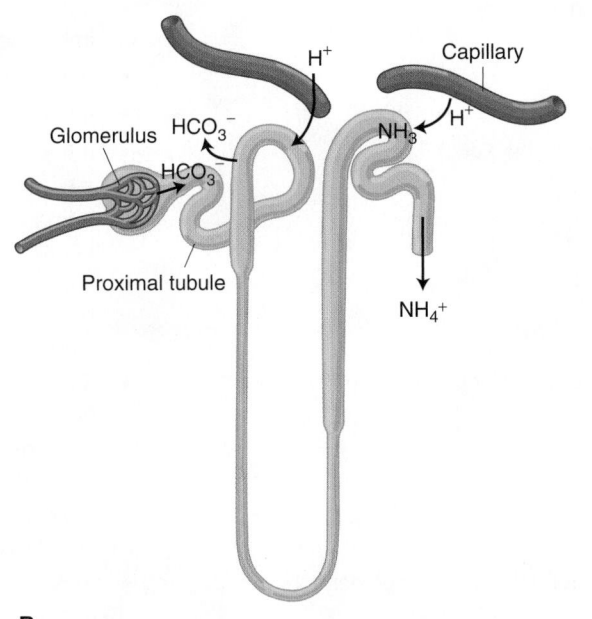

B

A, Recycling of bicarbonate by the kidneys. Bicarbonate ions that are in the blood are filtered into the renal tubules at the glomerulus. In the proximal tubules, bicarbonate ions are reabsorbed into the blood at the same time that hydrogen ions are transported from the blood into the renal tubular fluid.

B, Secretion and buffering of hydrogen ions in the kidneys. If the urine is too acidic, the cells that line the urinary tract could be damaged. To prevent this problem, hydrogen ions secreted into the distal tubules are neutralized by phosphate buffers or bound to ammonia and excreted in the form of ammonium ions.

Respiratory Acidosis

Respiratory acidosis is caused by an accumulation of carbon dioxide in the blood. Since carbon dioxide and water can be combined into carbonic acid, respiratory acidosis is sometimes called carbonic acid excess. The condition can be acute or chronic. It is controlled by the lungs.

ETIOLOGY AND PATHOPHYSIOLOGY

Any factor that interferes with the ability of the lungs to excrete carbon dioxide can cause respiratory acidosis. These factors may interfere with the gaseous exchange within the lungs, may impair the neuromuscular pump that moves air in and out of the lungs, or may depress the respiratory rate (Table 44–18 and Figure 44–10).

As the Pco_2 begins to increase, the pH of the blood begins to decrease. Compensatory mechanisms begin to act in the form of nonbicarbonate buffers, additional hydrogen ion excretion by the kidneys, and formation and decreased bicarbonate excretion by the kidneys. These compensatory mechanisms take several days to become active so the child manifests a changing clinical situation, depending on the underlying cause and the amount of compensation occurring (Table 44–19).

CLINICAL MANIFESTATIONS

Acidosis in the brain cells causes central nervous system depression, manifested by confusion, lethargy, headache, increased

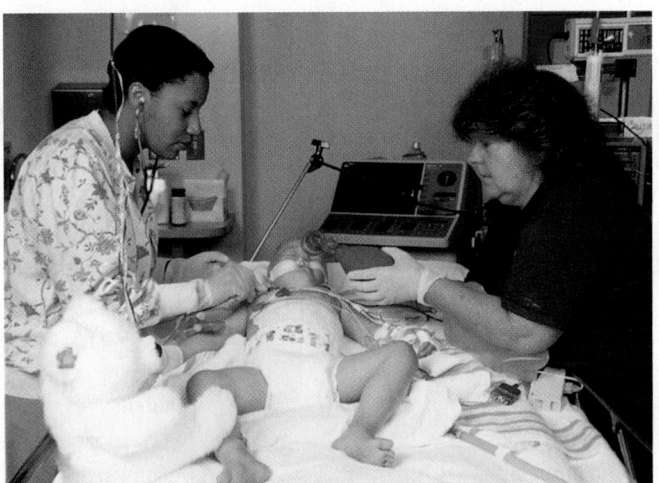

Figure 44–10 **Respiratory acidosis/alkalosis and mechanical ventilation. This child may develop respiratory acidosis or respiratory alkalosis. If the tidal volume is set too low during mechanical ventilation, carbon dioxide (carbonic acid) will accumulate in the body (respiratory acidosis) because it is not being excreted by the lungs. If the tidal volume is set too high, carbon dioxide will be depleted in the body (respiratory alkalosis) because it is being excreted in great quantities.**

TABLE 44–17 Questions to Ask to Interpret Arterial Blood Gas Measurements

QUESTION TO ASK	CONCLUSION
What is the pH?	• If the pH is normal, the child has no imbalance or has compensated for an imbalance. • If the pH is below normal, the child has acidosis. • If the pH is above normal, the child has alkalosis.
What is the P_{CO_2}?	• If the P_{CO_2} is normal, the child does not have an acid–base imbalance. • If the P_{CO_2} is above normal, the child has respiratory acidosis. This may be the primary disorder or may be a compensatory response to metabolic alkalosis. Looking at the bicarbonate concentration helps you decide. • If the P_{CO_2} is below normal, the child has respiratory alkalosis. Again, this can be the primary disorder or may be a compensatory response to metabolic acidosis.
What is the bicarbonate concentration?	• If the bicarbonate concentration is within normal range, the child does not have a metabolic acid–base imbalance. • If the bicarbonate is above normal, the child has metabolic alkalosis. This can be a primary disorder or can be compensatory in respiratory acidosis. • If bicarbonate is below normal, the child has metabolic acidosis, either as a direct disorder or as a compensatory response to respiratory alkalosis.
What do the results together tell you?	• If the pH is abnormal and either the P_{CO_2} or bicarbonate concentration is normal, there is an uncompensated acid–base disorder. • If all three values are abnormal, the child has a partially compensated disorder and the pH will provide the definitive answer. • If P_{CO_2}, pH, and bicarbonate are all decreased, then partially compensated metabolic acidosis is most likely. • If pH is normal and P_{CO_2} and bicarbonate are abnormal, there is a fully compensated acid–base disorder.
What are the child's history and clinical signs?	• Does your interpretation fit with what you know about the child's medical condition and with assessments you are making? • This last step helps you to integrate laboratory data with the clinical picture to strengthen your nursing care of the child with an acid–base imbalance.

TABLE 44–18 Causes of Respiratory Acidosis

FACTORS AFFECTING THE LUNGS	FACTORS AFFECTING THE NEUROMUSCULAR PUMP	FACTORS AFFECTING CENTRAL CONTROL OF RESPIRATION
Aspiration	Flail chest	Sedative overdose
Spasm of the airways	Pneumothorax or hemothorax	General anesthesia
Laryngeal edema	Mechanical underventilation	Head injury
Epiglottitis	Hypokalemic muscle weakness	Brain tumor
Croup	High cervical spinal cord injury	Central sleep apnea
Pulmonary edema	Botulism	
Atelectasis	Tetanus	
Severe pneumonia	Kyphoscoliosis	
Cystic fibrosis	Poliomyelitis	
Bronchopulmonary dysplasia	Muscular dystrophy	
Pulmonary embolism	Congenital diaphragmatic hernia	
	Guillain-Barré syndrome	

intracranial pressure, and even coma. Acute respiratory acidosis can lead to tachycardia and cardiac arrhythmias. The child's arterial blood gases always show an increased P_{CO_2}, the laboratory sign of increased carbonic acid. Serum pH can be decreased or normal.

CLINICAL THERAPY
Treatment of respiratory acidosis requires correction of the underlying cause. For example, treatment may include bronchodilators for bronchospasm, mechanical ventilation for neuromuscular defects, decreasing sedative use, or surgery for kyphoscoliosis.

TABLE 44–19 Laboratory Values in Uncompensated and Compensated Respiratory Acidosis

TYPE OF RESPIRATORY ACIDOSIS	HCO$_3^-$	pH	Pco$_2$
Uncompensated	Normal	Decreased	Increased
Partially compensated	Increasing	Decreasing but moving toward normal	Increased
Fully compensated	Increased	Normal	Increased

Nursing Management
For the Child With Respiratory Acidosis

Nursing Assessment and Diagnosis

Nursing assessment plays a pivotal role in decisions about interventions for respiratory acidosis. This is especially true in chronic conditions such as cystic fibrosis and kyphoscoliosis. Assess respiratory rate, rhythm, and depth carefully. Take the apical pulse and be alert for tachycardia or arrhythmia. A cardiac monitor may be used. Obtain serial arterial blood gas measurements in acute conditions to evaluate changing status. Assess the level of consciousness and energy. Observe for chronic fatigue, headache, or decreased level of consciousness.

Several nursing diagnoses may apply to the child with respiratory acidosis. The most important addresses the child's *Injury, Risk for*. Other nursing diagnoses depend on the specific clinical manifestation and the particular cause of the acidosis. Examples include the following (NANDA-I © 2014):

- *Injury, Risk for,* related to decreased level of consciousness
- *Activity Intolerance* related to decreased cardiac output secondary to cardiac dysrhythmias
- *Breathing Pattern, Ineffective (Hypoventilation),* related to neuromuscular impairment
- *Pain (Headache)* related to cerebral vasodilation
- *Health Management, Family, Ineffective,* related to complexity of bronchodilator therapy

Planning and Implementation

COMMUNITY-BASED NURSING CARE

Teach children at risk for respiratory acidosis and their parents preventive measures to use at home. For the child with a chronic condition such as cystic fibrosis, muscular dystrophy, or kyphoscoliosis, demonstrate deep breathing and encourage its use several times each day. Teach the family signs of infection—including fever, increased respiratory secretions, and discomfort with breathing—so that these problems can be treated promptly, preventing further respiratory involvement. Position the child to facilitate chest expansion. Teach parents about proper administration of any necessary medications. For example, the child with cystic fibrosis may receive antibiotics to prevent respiratory infections. Teach parents and older children about home respirator use (Figure 44–11).

HOSPITAL-BASED NURSING CARE

For the hospitalized child, the focus is on ensuring safety. Keep bed side rails raised, and turn and position the child frequently.

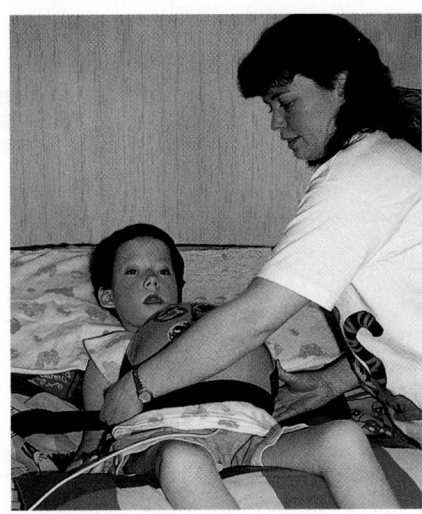

Figure 44–11 Home respirator use. This child, who has muscular dystrophy, uses a "turtle" respirator at home to assist with breathing. His parents required instructions from the nurse on use of the respirator. The family has a generator to provide electricity for the respirator during power outages.

Evaluate mental status and document and report any changes in alertness. When laboratory values of blood pH and Pco$_2$ are available, evaluate them promptly and report any changes or abnormalities. Administer medications as ordered. Carefully monitor the doses of sedatives to avoid further respiratory depression. Provide suctioning and encourage deep breathing.

Evaluation

Expected outcomes of nursing care for the child with respiratory acidosis include maintenance of safety, adequate rate and rhythm of respirations, and management of causative disorders.

Growth and Development

It is usually difficult to get a young child to do deep breathing or to use the "blow bottle" that is often given to older children and adults. To make deep breathing fun, use a pinwheel and have the child turn it during play. Alternatively, give a child a straw to blow bubbles in a glass of water or to blow scraps of paper across the bedside table.

Respiratory Alkalosis

Respiratory alkalosis occurs when the blood contains too little carbon dioxide. This condition is sometimes called *carbonic acid deficit*.

Excess carbon dioxide loss is caused by hyperventilation, in which more air than normal is moved into and out of the lungs. Some common causes of hyperventilation are hypoxia due to severe asthma, salicylate poisoning, and sepsis. Other causes are anxiety, fear, pain, meningitis, septicemia, and mechanical overventilation.

In many cases, respiratory alkalosis lasts for several hours only. Renal compensation does not occur because these compensatory mechanisms take several days to begin action. An example is the hyperventilation that occurs with acute anxiety. However, if the condition persists, the kidneys will begin to retain more acid and excrete more bicarbonate. Hydrogen ions will be released from body buffers to decrease plasma

TABLE 44–20 Laboratory Values in Uncompensated and Compensated Respiratory Alkalosis

TYPE OF RESPIRATORY ALKALOSIS	HCO$_3^-$	pH	Pco$_2$
Uncompensated	Normal	Increased	Decreased
Partially compensated	Decreasing	Increasing but moving toward normal	Decreased
Fully compensated	Decreased	Normal	Decreased

bicarbonate. While the imbalance continues, cellular function is thus protected by returning pH to normal levels (Table 44–20).

Arterial blood gas measurements show a decreased Pco$_2$ in respiratory alkalosis. Blood pH is generally elevated. The lack of carbon dioxide causes neuromuscular irritability and paresthesias in the extremities and around the mouth. Muscle cramping and carpal or pedal spasms can occur. The child may be dizzy or confused.

Medical management focuses on correcting the condition that caused the hyperventilation so that the body's compensatory mechanisms can return carbon dioxide levels to normal.

Nursing Management

For the Child With Respiratory Alkalosis

Nursing Assessment and Diagnosis

Assess the child's level of consciousness and ask if the child feels light-headed or has tingling sensations or numbness in the fingers or toes or around the mouth. Assess the rate and depth of respirations. Monitor the hospitalized child's Po$_2$ with serial arterial blood gas measurements to evaluate changes in status. Make a careful assessment about the cause of hyperventilation. Did an occurrence cause anxiety for the child? Is the child in pain? (See Chapter 40.) Has the child received salicylates in any form? Is the child mechanically ventilated? Is there a central nervous system infection such as meningitis?

Planning and Implementation

Nursing care for the child with respiratory alkalosis centers on teaching stress management techniques, maintaining pain control, promoting respiratory function, ensuring safety, regulating fluid status, and providing health supervision and home care.

SAFETY ALERT!

Check the Po$_2$ before any therapy for respiratory alkalosis is started because it is dangerous to stop hyperventilation if oxygenation is poor.

TEACH STRESS MANAGEMENT TECHNIQUES

When anxiety is the cause of respiratory alkalosis, instruct the child to breathe slowly; demonstrate the rhythm. Use a calm voice, stuffed toys, and supportive reassurance. Teach stress-control techniques such as relaxation and imagery for situations that cause anxiety.

MAINTAIN PAIN CONTROL

Use medications, imagery, distraction, positioning, massage, and other techniques to decrease pain and maintain pain

management. See Chapter 40 for a description of these and other measures to assist with pain control.

PROMOTE RESPIRATORY FUNCTION

Have the child cough, or apply suction as needed. Be certain that mechanical ventilation systems are working properly.

ENSURE SAFETY

Provide a safe environment for the child who has a decreased level of consciousness. Be sure the child is supervised when sitting or standing up. Keep bed rails up.

REGULATE FLUID STATUS

Renal compensation to manage ongoing respiratory alkalosis requires adequate urinary output. Regulate fluid intake to ensure urine output unless fluids are restricted because of a medical condition.

COMMUNITY-BASED NURSING CARE

Teach parents to keep aspirin and other salicylate products out of reach of children, preferably in a locked medicine box. Provide stickers with the number of the Poison Control Center.

Evaluation

Expected outcomes of nursing care for the child with respiratory alkalosis include normal respiratory rate and rhythm, maintenance of safety, and regulation of fluid status.

Metabolic Acidosis

Metabolic acidosis is a condition in which there is an excess of any acid other than carbonic acid. For this reason, it is sometimes *called noncarbonic acid excess.*

ETIOLOGY AND PATHOPHYSIOLOGY

Metabolic acidosis is caused by an imbalance in production and excretion of acid or by excess loss of bicarbonate. Excess accumulation occurs by one of two mechanisms. First, a child can eat or drink acids or substances that are converted to acid in the body. Examples include aspirin, boric acid, and antifreeze. Second, cells can make abnormally high amounts of acid that cannot be excreted. This is the case in ketoacidosis of untreated diabetes mellitus, untreated growth hormone deficiency, bladder construction that uses part of the bowel, or the starvation that can occur in anorexia or bulimia. A disorder of excretion occurs in conditions such as oliguric renal failure (Figure 44–12).

The body can lose bicarbonate through the urine or through excessive loss of intestinal fluid. Diarrhea, fistulas, and ileal drainage are all possible sources. Carbonic anhydrase inhibitors can cause loss of excess bicarbonate in the urine.

Below-normal pH of the blood stimulates the chemoreceptors in the brain and arteries and respiratory compensation begins. The child's rate and depth of breathing increase and carbonic acid is removed from the body. The blood pH shifts to a more normal range even though the cause is not corrected. The underlying condition and the degree of compensation alter the clinical laboratory values observed (Table 44–21).

TABLE 44–21 Laboratory Values in Uncompensated and Compensated Metabolic Acidosis

TYPE OF METABOLIC ACIDOSIS	HCO$_3^-$	pH	Pco$_2$
Uncompensated	Decreased	Decreased	Normal
Partially compensated	Decreased	Decreased	Decreasing but moving

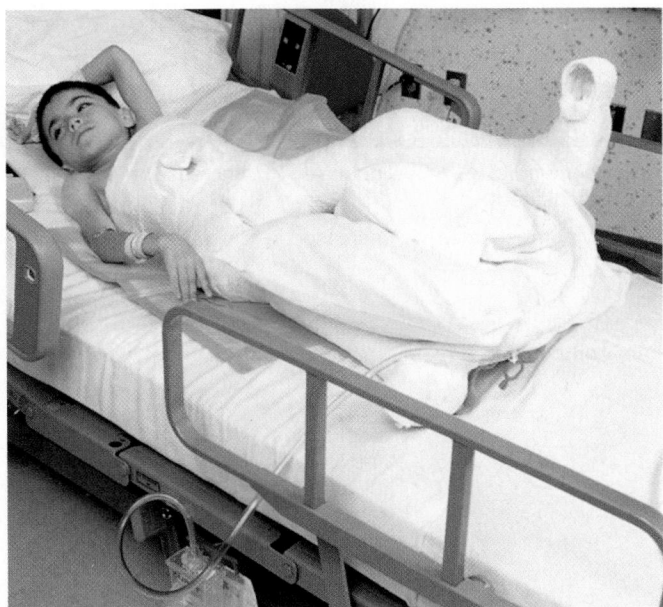

Figure 44–12 Disorders of excretion. With any postoperative or immobilized child, it is important to monitor urine output to detect oliguria. If the kidneys do not produce sufficient urine, the metabolic acids accumulate in the body and cause metabolic acidosis. Inadequate fluid intake in the postoperative or immobilized child can lead to oliguria and, potentially, metabolic acidosis.

CLINICAL MANIFESTATIONS

Laboratory values show decreased blood pH and decreased HCO_3^- and Pco_2. An attempt at respiratory compensation causes one of the most important signs of metabolic acidosis, increased rate and depth of respirations (hyperventilation) or **Kussmaul respirations**. Severe acidosis can cause decreased peripheral vascular resistance and resultant cardiac arrhythmias, hypotension, pulmonary edema, and tissue hypoxia. Confusion or drowsiness may result, as well as headache or abdominal pain.

CLINICAL THERAPY

Treatment of metabolic acidosis depends on identification and treatment of the underlying cause. In severe metabolic acidosis, intravenous sodium bicarbonate may be used to increase the pH and to prevent cardiac arrhythmias. This treatment is difficult to manage because renal excretion can cause excess retention of bicarbonate; therefore, intravenous sodium bicarbonate is used only in severe situations, such as prolonged cardiac arrest.

Nursing Management

For the Child With Metabolic Acidosis

Nursing Assessment and Diagnosis

Teach prevention of poisoning at each health promotion visit. For the child admitted with acidosis, assess the rate and depth of respirations. Evaluate the child's level of consciousness frequently. Be alert for signs or complaints of headache and abdominal pain. Serial arterial blood gas measurements will usually be obtained to evaluate changes in status.

Several nursing diagnoses can apply to the child with metabolic acidosis, including the following (NANDA-I © 2014):

- *Injury, Risk for,* related to confusion/drowsiness or decreased responsiveness
- *Cardiac Output, Decreased,* related to cardiac arrhythmias
- *Tissue Perfusion: Cerebral, Risk for Ineffective,* related to tissue hypoxia
- *Health Management, Family, Ineffective,* related to complexity of management of diabetes mellitus

Planning and Implementation

Ensure safety, taking into account the child's level of consciousness and alertness. Change the child's position to prevent pressure on the skin. Limit the child's activities to decrease cardiac workload.

Position the child to facilitate chest expansion. Provide oral care during rapid respirations since the mouth may become dry.

Monitor intravenous solutions and laboratory values indicating acid–base balance. Report changes promptly.

Once the child is stabilized, provide teaching to compensate for knowledge deficits. Teach parents of young children to keep medications and acids locked up and out of reach to prevent poisoning (Figure 44–13). This includes medicines with aspirin as well as substances commonly kept in the garage for car maintenance. Teach about home management of diabetes and about early identification and treatment to avoid diabetic ketoacidosis.

Evaluation

Expected outcomes of nursing care relate to prevention of acidosis and restoration of normal body balance during disease processes.

Metabolic Alkalosis

Metabolic alkalosis occurs when there are too few metabolic acids. It is sometimes called *noncarbonic acid deficit*.

A gain in bicarbonate or a loss of metabolic acid can cause metabolic alkalosis. Bicarbonate is gained through excessive intake of bicarbonate antacids or baking soda or through metabolism of bicarbonate precursors such as the citrate contained in blood transfusions. Increased renal absorption of bicarbonate can occur in profound hypokalemia, primary hyperaldosteronism, or extreme deficit in extracellular fluid volume. Use of

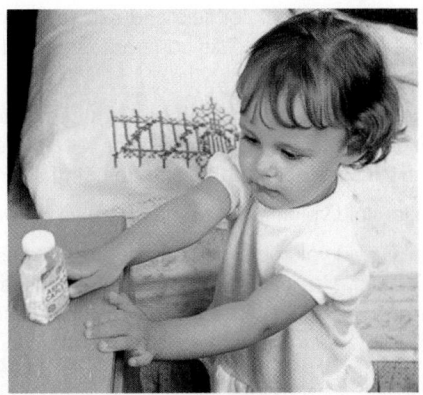

Figure 44–13 Prevent metabolic acidosis from poisoning. Teaching parents to use safety latches on cabinets to keep aspirin away from small children can help prevent one cause of metabolic acidosis.

enhanced water to constitute powdered formula can be a cause of metabolic alkalosis. Acid can be lost through severe vomiting, such as that seen in infants with pyloric stenosis, and through continued removal of gastric contents through suction.

When the chemoreceptors in the brain and arteries detect the rising pH of metabolic alkalosis and respirations decrease, the body retains carbonic acid. This carbonic acid can neutralize the bicarbonate and return pH toward normal.

Blood pH, bicarbonate, and Pco_2 are usually elevated in metabolic alkalosis (Table 44–22). Hypokalemia often occurs simultaneously. Respiratory rate and depth usually decrease. Increased neuromuscular irritability, cramping, paresthesia, tetany, seizures, and excitation can occur. Finally, this state can progress to weakness, confusion, lethargy, and coma.

Clinical therapy is directed at treating the underlying cause of the condition. Increasing the extracellular fluid volume with intravenous normal saline facilitates renal excretion of bicarbonate.

Nursing Management

Assess the child's level of consciousness frequently. Alertness may decrease after an initial period of excitement, so regular assessments are needed. Monitor neuromuscular irritability. Observe for nausea and vomiting. Assess the rate and depth of respirations carefully. Obtain serial arterial blood gas measurements as ordered.

Facilitate ease of respirations. Ensure safety by keeping bed rails elevated and by turning the child frequently. Position the child on the side to avoid aspiration of vomitus.

If antacids or improper formula constitution were the cause of the alkalosis, teach the child and parents about correct use of these medications.

Mixed Acid–Base Imbalances

It is possible for two acid–base imbalances to occur at the same time. For example, a child with cystic fibrosis can develop

TABLE 44–22 Laboratory Values in Uncompensated and Compensated Metabolic Alkalosis

TYPE OF METABOLIC ALKALOSIS	HCO₃⁻	pH	Pco₂
Acute condition; uncompensated	Increased	Increased	Normal
Partially compensated	Increased	Increased but moving toward normal	Increasing
Fully compensated	The need for oxygen drives respirations and limits full compensation for metabolic alkalosis.		

respiratory acidosis from lung problems and concurrent metabolic alkalosis from vomiting during an illness. Treatment with diuretics may cause concurrent metabolic alkalosis resulting from extracellular volume depletion and hypokalemia in a child with congestive heart failure and chronic respiratory acidosis. In these cases, all underlying causes must be identified and treated. Care of children with mixed acid–base imbalances is often complicated, requiring hospitalization and careful management. On discharge, the nurse can teach parents about signs of imbalance that need to be reported and treated to prevent further complications. Evaluation of care is based on outcomes of adequate respiratory ventilation and metabolic balance.

Focus Your Study

- Young children are at risk for fluid and electrolyte imbalance due to differences in body fluid compartments and regulation systems.

- Nurses institute health promotion and health maintenance measures to maintain normal body fluids for children who exercise in hot weather and those undergoing surgery.

- Extracellular fluid volume deficit manifests as dehydration.

- Extracellular fluid volume excess is due to an excess of saline in the body. Interstitial fluid volume excess manifests as edema and weight gain. Nurses carefully manage fluid status of young children and teach parents prevention and treatment

of fluid imbalances caused by gastroenteritis and other disease states.

- The most common electrolyte imbalances are hypernatremia and hypokalemia, and thus involve sodium and potassium.

- Normal acid–base balance is necessary for proper function of cells in the body.

- The lungs, kidneys, and liver play a role in maintaining acid–base balance.

- Acid–base imbalance can involve alkalosis or acidosis; either can have a respiratory or metabolic origin.

Clinical Reasoning in Action

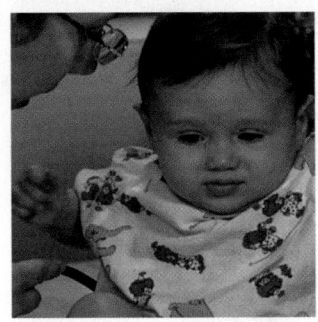

A 10-month-old named Devin comes to the emergency department by ambulance at 3:00 a.m. for respiratory distress. His parents state that he was experiencing a cough for the past week and developed a fever of over 103.0°F (39.4°C) tonight. He woke up crying with a frightening cough and could barely catch his breath; the parents called 9-1-1. Devin's respiratory rate is 50 times per minute with moderate retractions, his temperature is 104.2°F (40.1°C), his heart has a regular rhythm with a rate of 150 beats per minute, and he has stridor while breathing. At the hospital, after a breathing treatment with racemic epinephrine, his

respiratory rate decreases to 40 and retractions improve. The arterial blood gas measurements show an increased Pco_2, a decreased pH, and a normal HCO_3^-. A diagnosis of croup syndrome and resultant respiratory acidosis is made. Devin is admitted for monitoring.

1. What are some of the other possible causes of respiratory acidosis in children such as Devin?
2. What are some of the signs and symptoms of respiratory distress and the central nervous system problems associated with Devin's particular acid–base imbalance?
3. Devin's heart rate and rhythm are monitored closely in the hospital. What is the reason for these assessments?
4. What is the treatment for Devin's acid–base imbalance?
5. What are some of the measures taken in the hospital to ensure Devin's safety?

References

American Academy of Pediatrics (AAP). (2013). *Pediatric nutrition handbook* (7th ed.). Elk Grove Village, IL: Author: Author.

American Academy of Pediatrics (AAP) Council on Sports Medicine and Fitness & Council on School Health. (2011). Policy statement—Climatic heat stress and exercising children and adolescents. *Pediatrics, 128*, e741–e747. doi: 10.1542/peds.2011–1664

Bolat, F., Oflaz, M. B., Guven, A. S., Ozdemir, G., Alaygut, D., Dogan, M. T., . . . Fultekin, A. (2013). What is the safe approach for neonatal hypernatremic dehydration? A retrospective study from a neonatal intensive care unit. *Pediatric Emergency Care, 29*, 808–813.

Carcillo, J. A. (2014). Intravenous fluid choices in critically ill children. *Current Opinion in Critical Care, 20*, 396–401.

Children's Mercy Hospital. (2011). *Guidelines for oral rehydration.* Retrieved from http://www.childrensmercy .org/Content/view.aspx?id=8130

Corbett, J. V., & Banks, A. (2013). *Laboratory tests and diagnostic procedures* (8th ed.). Upper Saddle River, NJ: Pearson.

Crawford, A., & Harris, H. (2011a). Balancing act: Sodium and potassium. *Nursing 2011, 41*, 44–50.

Crawford, A., & Harris, H. (2011b). Balancing act: Hypo-magnesemia and hypermagnesemia. *Nursing 2011, 41*, 52–55.

Dzierba, A. L., & Abraham, P. (2011). A practical approach to understanding acid–base abnormalities in critical illness. *Journal of Pharmacy Practice, 24*, 17–26.

Engorn, B. & Flerlage, J. (2014). *The Harriet Lane handbook* (20th ed.) St. Louis, MO: Elsevier Saunders.

Feld, L. G., & Kaskel, F. J. (2012). *Fluid and electrolytes in pediatrics.* New York: Humana Press, Springer Publishers.

Freedman, S.B., Ali, S., Oleszczuk, M., Gouin, S., & Hartling, L. (2013). Treatment of acute gastroenteritis in children: An overview of systematic reviews of interventions commonly used in developed countries. *Evidence Based Child Health, 8*, 1123–1137.

Freedman, S. B., Keating, L. E., Rumatir, M., & Schuh, S. (2012). Health care provider and caregiver preferences regarding nasogastric and intravenous rehydration. *Pediatrics, 130*, e1504–e1511.

Frohna, J. G. (2011). Oral rehydration solution with zinc and prebiotics decreases duration of acute diarrhea in children. *Journal of Pediatrics, 158*, 288–292.

Greenbaum, L. A. (2011). *Electrolyte and acid–base disorder.* In R. M. Kliegman, B. F. Stanton, J. W. St. Geme, N. F. Schor, & R. E. Behrman (Eds.), *Nelson textbook of pediatrics* (19th ed., pp. 212–242). Philadelphia, PA: Saunders.

Jablonski, S. (2012). Oral rehydration of the pediatric patient with mild to moderate dehydration. *Journal of Emergency Nursing, 38*, 185–187.

Kinlin, L. M., & Freedman, S. B. (2012). Evaluation of a clinical dehydration scale in children requiring intravenous rehydration. *Pediatrics, 129*, e1211–e1219.

Kliegman, R. M., Stanton, B. F., St. Geme, J., Schor, N. F., & Behrman, R. E. (Eds.) (2011). *Nelson textbook of pediatrics* (19th ed.). Philadelphia, PA: Saunders.

LeMone, P., Burke, K. M., Bauldoff, G., & Gubrud, P. (2015). *Medical surgical nursing* (6th ed.). Hoboken, NJ: Prentice Hall Health.

Lenters, L. M., Das, J. K., & Bhutta, Z. A. (2013). Systematic review of strategies to increase use of oral rehydration solution at the household level. *BMC Public Health, 13* (Suppl 3), S3–S28.

Mayo Clinic. (2011). *Dehydration and youth sports: Curb the risk.* Retrieved from http://www.mayoclinic.com

NIH Osteoporosis and Related Bone Diseases National Resource Center. (2011). *Osteoporosis and African American women.* Retrieved from http://www.niams .nih.gov/Health_Info/Bone/Osteoporosis/Background /default.asp

Nir, V., Nadir, E., Schechter, Y., & Kline–Kremer, A. (2013). Parents' attitudes toward oral rehydration therapy in children with mild–to–moderate dehydration. *Scientific World Journal Nov 4*, doi: 10.1155/20

Ruppe, M. D. (2011). Medications that affect calcium. *Endocrine Practice, 17* (Suppl. 1), 26–30.

Soldin, S. J., Wong, E. C., Brugnara, C., & Soldin, O. P. (2011). *Pediatric reference ranges* (7th ed.). Washington, DC: American Association for Clinical Chemistry.

Wang, J., Xu, E., & Xiao, Y. (2013). Isotonic versus hypotonic maintenance IV fluid in hospitalized children: A meta-analysis. *Pediatrics, 133*, 105–113.

World Health Organization (2014). *Oral rehydration solutions.* Retrieved from http://rehydrate.org/solutions /homemade.htm

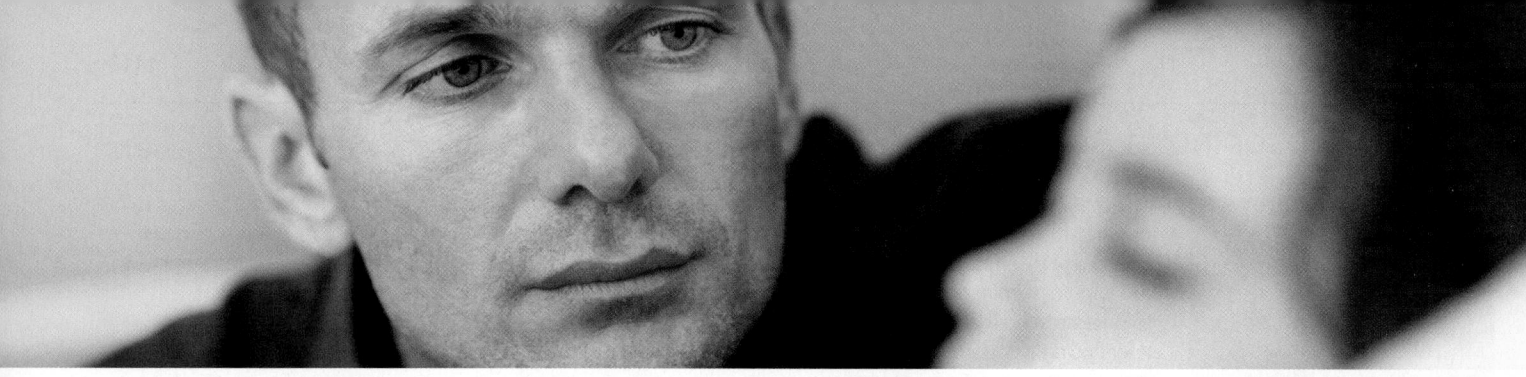

Chapter 45
The Child With Alterations in Eye, Ear, Nose, and Throat Function

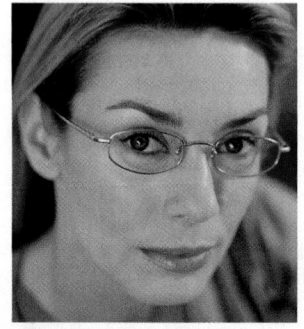

Digital Vision/Getty Images

The early intervention program that Raeanne attended to help her deal with her visual impairment prepared her well for preschool. We learned a lot too about how to help her. We are still really nervous about her starting at preschool and being with a lot of other children. We want it to go well for her.

—Mother of Raeanne, 3 years old

Learning Outcomes

45.1 Identify anatomy, physiology, and pediatric differences in the eye, ear, nose, and throat of children and adolescents.

45.2 Describe abnormalities of the eyes, ears, nose, throat, and mouth in children.

45.3 Carry out screening programs to identify children with vision and hearing abnormalities.

45.4 Plan nursing care for children with vision or hearing impairments.

45.5 Select and apply latest recommendations when implementing care and teaching for children with abnormalities of eyes, ears, nose, throat, and mouth.

45.6 Integrate preventive and treatment principles when implementing health promotion for children related to eyes, ears, nose, and throat.

The eye, ear, nose, and throat are connected, so a malformation, infection, or other condition in one of these structures may affect them all. Intact sensory structures enable children to reach developmental milestones; thus alterations, especially to the eye and ear, may delay a child's development. Most children with eye, ear, nose, and throat disorders are treated at home or in the community rather than in the hospital. How are conditions of the eye, ear, nose, and throat related? Which conditions have the potential to affect a child's growth, development, and behavior? In what settings do children with eye, ear, nose, and throat conditions receive care? How can parents be helped to foster development in their children when they have a visual or hearing disorder?

Anatomy and Physiology of Pediatric Differences

Eye

How are the eyes of children different from those of adults? Chapter 33 provides a detailed discussion of the assessment of the eyes and visual acuity, the ability to discriminate letters or other objects. The eyes of newborns differ from the eyes of adults in several ways. **Visual acuity** in newborns ranges between 20/100 and 20/400. The lens is more spherical and cannot accommodate to both near and far objects, which

TABLE 45–1 Visually Related Developmental Milestones

AGE	MILESTONE
Term neonate	Demonstrates alertness to light and visual stimulus presented 20–30 cm (8–12 in.) from eyes.
1 month	Follows an object 60 degrees horizontally and 30 degrees vertically; blinks at an approaching object.
2 months	Follows a person or moving object for 180 degrees from 2 m (6 ft) away; smiles in response to a face; raises head 30 degrees from prone.
3 months	Tracks an object through 180 degrees; regards own hand; begins visual–motor coordination.
4–5 months	Social smile; reaches for a cube 30 cm (12 in.) away; notices a raisin 30 cm (12 in.) away; stares at own hand.
7–8 months	Reaches and grasps an object, picks up a raisin by raking, transfers objects from hand to hand.
8–9 months	Pokes at holes in a peg board; well-developed pincer grasp; crawls; uncovers toy after seeing it hidden.
12–14 months	Stacks blocks; places a peg in a round hole; stands and walks.

Source: Data from Rudolph, C., Rudolph, A., Lister, G., First, L., & Gershon, A. (Eds.) (2011). *Rudolph's pediatrics* (22nd ed.). New York, NY: McGraw-Hill; Kliegman, R. M., Stanton, B. F., St. Geme, J., Schor, N. F., & Behrman, R. E. (Eds.) (2011). *Nelson textbook of pediatrics* (19th ed.). Philadelphia, PA: Saunders.

means that the newborn sees best at a distance of about 20 cm (8 in.). Since the optic nerve is not yet completely myelinated, the ability to distinguish color and other details is decreased. If the infant is preterm, especially less than 32 weeks' gestation, retinal vascularization, particularly in the periphery of the retina, may be incomplete (Hou et al., 2011; Wang, Spencer, Leffler, et al., 2012). The rectus muscles that control binocular vision may be somewhat uncoordinated at birth. The eyes should be aligned and movement coordinated by the age of 3 months.

The cornea of the infant and young child occupies a larger portion of the orbit than in the adult; the eyeball is about three quarters of its adult size. Since the eyeball is relatively unprotected laterally, it is more easily injured. The sclera of the newborn is thin and translucent with a bluish tinge, and the iris is blue or gray. Eye color changes during the first 6 months of life. Infants produce tears to nourish and oxygenate the outer layers of the cornea. Parents do not see tears when a young infant cries because the infant's lacrimal system drains them efficiently into the nasal cavity.

As infants grow, their eyes mature and their vision improves. By the age of 2 or 3 years, most children have a visual acuity of 20/50, and by the age of 6 or 7 years, it is 20/20. Visual acuity is measured using standardized letter or picture charts (see Chapter 33). **Vision** refers to the complex process of acquiring meaning from what is seen, involving the eye, brain, and related neurologic and physiologic structures. Development interacts with a child's maturing physiologic system to bring increasing meaning to objects in sight (Table 45–1).

Ear

Why do infants and young children have more ear problems than adults? The eustachian tube, which connects the nasopharynx to the middle ear, is proportionately shorter, wider, and more horizontal in infants than in older children or adults (see *As Children Grow: Eustachian Tube*). During sucking, yawning, and other movements, the tube opens for milliseconds, allowing free passage of air between the nasopharynx and the middle ear. This predisposes young children to development of otitis media, or middle ear infection.

The external ear canal is small at birth, although the internal ear and middle ear are relatively large. As a result, the tympanic membrane is close to the surface and can be easily injured. Babies can hear at about 20 weeks' gestation, and the auditory nerve function is mature at about 5 months of age in the infant.

As Children Grow: **Eustachian Tube**

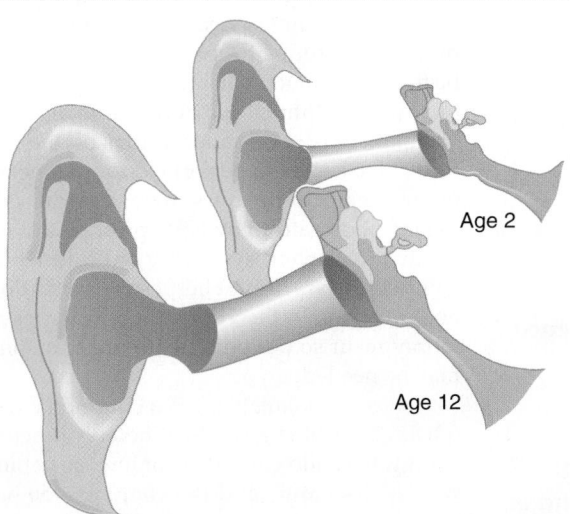

Age 2

Age 12

Position of eustachian tube is at less of an angle in the young child, resulting in decreased drainage (more horizontal).

End of eustachian tube in nasal pharynx opens during sucking.

Eustachian tube equalizes air pressure between the middle ear and the outside environment and allows for drainage of secretions from middle ear mucosa.

Of the three anatomic differences in the eustachian tube between adults and small children (shorter, wider, more horizontal), which do you think could cause more problems for the child and why?

Before 34 weeks' gestation, the exterior ear is soft with little cartilage apparent. When the ear of a preterm is folded forward and released, its recoil is slow, while with term newborns, the recoil is strong and fast.

Nose, Throat, and Mouth

Up to 6 months of age, infants breathe primarily through the nose and not through the mouth. Edema and nasal discharge may interfere with adequate air intake and feeding. Mucosal swelling and exudate may block the small nasal passages of young children.

The palatine tonsils, visible on oral examination, are located on each side of the oropharynx. The method for examining a child's throat is discussed in Chapter 33. Although tonsils vary in size considerably during childhood, they are normally large, especially in school-age children. Lymph tissue decreases in size by about 10 years, so its appearance after this age can indicate abnormality. The nasopharyngeal tonsils (adenoids) lie in the posterior wall of the nasopharynx, just above the oropharynx. In children the adenoids may become enlarged, harboring bacteria and interfering with breathing.

The mucosal membranes of the mouth are expected to be intact and without lesions at all ages. The first teeth commonly erupt at about 6 months of age, and the first loss of teeth begins at about 6 years. See Chapter 33 for thorough descriptions of assessment of the oral cavity in infants and children.

Disorders of the Eye

Infectious Conjunctivitis

Conjunctivitis is an inflammation of the conjunctiva, the clear membrane that lines the inside of the lid and sclera. Bacteria, viruses, allergies, trauma, or irritants cause the conjunctiva to become swollen and red with a yellow or white discharge (Figure 45–1). Parents commonly refer to all conjunctivitis as "pink eye."

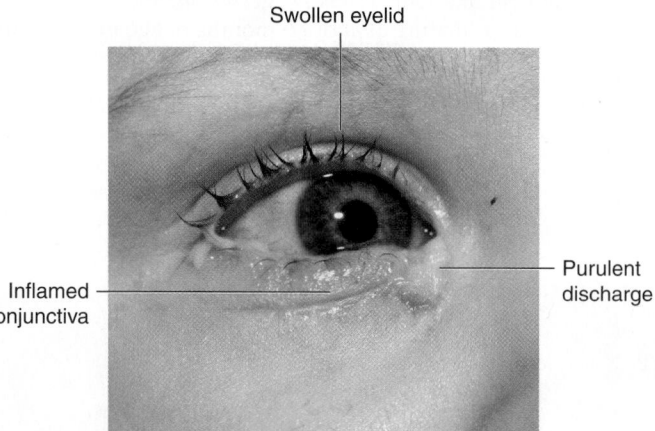

Swollen eyelid

Inflamed conjunctiva

Purulent discharge

Figure 45–1 **Acute conjunctivitis. The major difference between bacterial and viral conjunctivitis is that bacterial conjunctivitis has a purulent discharge that may result in crusting, whereas the discharge from viral conjunctivitis is serous (watery). Allergic conjunctivitis produces watery to thick drainage and is characterized by itching.**

SOURCE: Dr. P. Marazzi/Science Source.

Conjunctivitis in a newborn or infant under 30 days of age is called *ophthalmia neonatorum*. These infections are usually acquired from the mother during vaginal birth as a result of contact with infected vaginal discharge containing organisms such as *Chlamydia trachomatis* and *Neisseria gonorrhoeae*. See Chapter 25 for information on prophylactic eye treatment. Newborns occasionally get chemical conjunctivitis in response to prophylactic eye treatment. This may be a cause when the conjunctivitis develops within 24 to 48 hours after instillation of the medication.

Another cause of infection in infants is herpesvirus, which requires prompt and vigorous treatment to prevent eye injury or blindness. Infants with herpesvirus infections of the eye are treated with intravenous acyclovir as well as topical drops.

In infants who have frequent tearing and "mattering" (eyelid discharge that has formed a crust) on awakening, a plugged lacrimal duct may mimic conjunctivitis. Treatment involves massaging the tear duct every 4 hours when the infant is awake. Lacrimal ducts that remain plugged after the age of 1 year may have to be opened surgically.

Bacterial conjunctivitis can occur in children of any age. It is characterized by edema of the eyelid, red conjunctiva, and enlarged preauricular lymph glands. There is usually mucopurulent exudate that causes mattering, making the eyes difficult to open upon awakening. Older children with conjunctivitis complain of itching or burning, mild photophobia, and a feeling of scratching under the lids. Parents may notice increased tearing or a mucoid or mucopurulent discharge, redness and swelling of the conjunctiva, a pink sclera, and crusty eyelids, especially in the morning. There is no change in vision. Common infectious organisms include *Staphylococcus aureus*, *Haemophilus influenzae*, *Streptococcus pneumoniae*, and *Moraxella catarrhalis* (Gold, 2011). Most cases are caused by hand-to-eye contact, and the disease can rapidly spread whenever groups of youth spend time together, such as among young children and adolescents in schools and childcare centers, and even among college students in dormitories, sororities, fraternities, and on sports teams. Although bacterial conjunctivitis can be bilateral, it is more commonly unilateral.

Other infections in newborns and children can be caused by viruses. *Viral conjunctivitis* is more often bilateral than unilateral. Adenovirus is a common cause and spreads from respiratory adenovirus infection in hand-to-eye transmission. Signs and symptoms are similar to those of bacterial conjunctivitis, although they are sometimes milder in severity and slower in onset.

Herpes simplex virus (HSV) can also cause infection, either by transfer from a herpes-infected mother to her baby during birth or by contact with an infected person in infants or children of any age. Ophthalmic herpes infection is often accompanied by characteristic vesicular lesions on the skin of the face. A culture of the lesions is performed for diagnosis, and any accompanying conjunctivitis is assumed to be caused by herpesvirus. For the infection caused by HSV, prompt and vigorous treatment is needed to prevent eye injury or blindness, which can occur in children with recurrent herpesvirus infections as a result of antibody reaction to the viral antigen. Herpesvirus infections commonly recur so periodic treatment and sometimes prophylaxis may be needed.

Allergic conjunctivitis is a common cause of eye discomfort (Ortiz, 2013; Steele, 2012). When conjunctivitis is caused by an allergy, the child complains of intense itching. Eyes are red with watery discharge, and the conjunctivae have a "cobblestone" appearance.

In most cases, a diagnosis of the cause of conjunctivitis is made based on the history and symptoms. Cultures can be taken, especially in infants or in cases suspected of being an unusual bacterial illness or herpesvirus infection. A Gram stain of discharge and conjunctival scraping for potential chlamydial infection or herpesvirus infection are performed. Infants and children must be promptly referred to primary healthcare providers or eye specialists for treatment of possible eye infections. When diagnosed in the neonatal intensive care unit, the infant is isolated to prevent spread to other infants.

Antibiotic eye medication is prescribed in droplet or ointment form if a bacterial infection is suspected. Treatment may be started after a laboratory sample is obtained but before the results are known. Fluoroquinolones are now frequently used to treat bacterial conjunctivitis; drops or ointment can be used (O'Brien, 2012). Other drugs used to treat bacterial infections include bacotracom, erythromycin, azithromycin, and aminoglycosides (Granet, 2011; O'Brien, 2012). Newborn gonococcal conjunctivitis is treated with ceftriaxone. Chlamydial infections are treated with oral erythromycin. Careful total evaluation of the newborn with any conjunctivitis is also performed to watch for other signs of infection. Instructions for instilling eye medication are provided in the *Clinical Skills Manual* SKILLS .

Viral conjunctivitis may be treated with comfort measures such as cleaning drainage away with a warm clean cloth and avoiding bright lights and reading to the child. Ophthalmic antibiotics may sometimes be given to prevent bacterial invasion due to frequent rubbing of the eyes. Herpes simplex virus infections of the eye are treated promptly by an ophthalmologist, neonatologist, or others who are trained in this serious disease. Topical drugs are used, and often are combined with a systemic antiviral agent such as acyclovir. Neonatal herpes simplex virus infection is treated vigorously with parenteral acyclovir for 14 days (or longer if central nervous system involvement is found upon lumbar puncture) and with topical ophthalmic medication (trifluridine, iododeoxyuridine, or vidarabine). Recurrent lesions may necessitate suppressive or prophylactic treatment with oral acyclovir, the dosage of which must be adjusted according to the child's age and weight (Liu, Pavan-Langston, & Colby, 2012).

If an allergen is diagnosed as the cause of conjunctivitis, systemic or topical antihistamines may be prescribed. Topical steroids and vasoconstrictors may also be used. Decongestants can be combined with systemic antihistamines for short-term therapy. Mast-cell stabilizers may be used to decrease the activation of mast cells that accompanies allergic reactions; their use is safe in children 3 years of age and older.

Nursing Management

Nurses routinely instill antibiotics into the eyes of newborns after birth. Perform a careful examination so that any cases of ophthalmia neonatorum can be referred promptly to an ophthalmologist. Women infected with gonococcus or chlamydia should be identified so their babies can receive attention and medication at birth to prevent infection. Babies born at home should have ocular examinations soon after birth.

In suspected conjunctivitis, gentle pressure for several seconds with a gloved index finger placed next to the inner corner of the eye may cause a discharge of mucopurulent drainage. Refer for care and report the findings. Since infectious conjunctivitis is extremely contagious, tell parents that children should not return to child care or school until they have been taking an antibiotic for 24 hours. Teach parents the importance of careful hand hygiene and the avoidance of shared towels. Tell parents that children should not rub their eyes. Mittens may help prevent infants from rubbing their eyes. Toddlers may be distracted by activities that keep their hands busy. Teach parents the proper techniques for instilling eye medications. For children with allergies, alert parents to signs of infection so if the child gets an eye infection, they will seek prompt treatment.

Periorbital Cellulitis

Periorbital cellulitis is a bacterial infection of the eyelid and surrounding tissues that is usually caused by *Streptococcus* or *Staphylococcus*. Children present with swollen, tender, red or purple eyelids; restricted, painful movement of the area around the eye; and fever. Periorbital cellulitis should be treated promptly to prevent the spread of the infection to the posterior orbit. Orbital cellulitis is a serious outcome that can lead to bacterial meningitis. Management includes hospitalization for intravenous antibiotics and the application of hot packs. Children usually respond favorably within 48 to 72 hours (Cohen, 2011; Seltz, Smith, Durairaj, et al., 2011).

Visual Disorders

Vision, the complex process of acquiring meaning from what is seen, depends on many factors. The eyes must move quickly

---

TEACHING HIGHLIGHTS | Instilling Eye Medications in Children

It can be challenging to safely instill medication into young children's eyes. Give parents the following suggestions:

- Wash your hands well.
- Be sure the medicine is warmed at least to room temperature.
- Remove any drainage from the eye with a clean or sterile, moist, warm cloth or gauze.
- Wash your hands again.
- Have the child lying on the back with eyes closed.
- Gently pull the lower lid down to form a small pocket.
- Apply a thin string (for ointment) or drops of the medicine.
- Allow the eyelid to return to normal position.
- Have the child keep the eye closed for several seconds.
- Help prevent spread of the infection by keeping the child's hands clean.
- Enhance comfort by keeping the head elevated to decrease swelling and avoid exposure to bright light.

TABLE 45–2 Assessment Questions for Identifying Visual Disturbances in Children

YOUNG CHILD

Ask the parents:

Do your child's eyes follow you as you come into a room?

Are other objects followed with ease?

Do both eyes work together or does one seem to wander off?

At what age did your baby sit, stand, walk?

Does your child have any difficulty picking up objects?

SCHOOL-AGE CHILD

Ask the parents:

Does your child like to look at pictures and read?

Does your child hold toys or books close or sit very close to the television?

Does your child squint or rub the eyes?

Is your child at grade level in all subjects?

Has your child demonstrated any learning difficulties?

Does your child use a computer, watch television, or play computer games?

Does your child play sports and games at the same level of ability as peers?

and in a coordinated manner. (See Chapter 33 for discussion of eye movement assessment.) They must function together for clear, single vision to occur. If this ability, called **binocularity**, is not present (perhaps because of strabismus or amblyopia), the child may have double vision and the brain cannot make sense of the images it receives. Normally, perceptions of objects seen are integrated with other senses through eye–hand coordination, and with the brain through visual imagery and discrimination of objects seen. Although visual acuity is essential, the child's movements, mental processes, and other senses all interact to give meaning to objects that are viewed. Vision therefore influences learning and school performance (Davidson & Quinn, 2011).

Visual disturbances must be diagnosed and treated promptly to prevent impairment or loss of vision. Most children undergo a simple test for visual acuity during healthcare visits as soon as they can cooperate with the examiner. Once in school, children's visual acuity is screened every 2 to 3 years during the elementary years. Nurses often organize vision screening programs for children. Table 45–2 provides a series of questions that can be used to identify visual disturbances in children. A child who does not pass vision screening is referred to an ophthalmologist or optometrist for more detailed examination of near and far vision, eye structure and movement, and color discrimination.

Some of the common visual disorders in children are:

- *Hyperopia (farsightedness):* Light rays focus posterior to the retina, resulting in an inability to focus on nearby objects. All children have some degree of hyperopia until 9 to 10 years of age. However, their eyes can accommodate sufficiently to enable them to see near objects clearly. Blurring of vision occurs only in children with excessive hyperopia, or a difference in accommodation between the two eyes. *Amblyopia,* or a weakening of the poorer eye, can occur in these children if treatment is not obtained.

- *Myopia (nearsightedness):* Light rays focus anterior to the retina, resulting in an inability to see far-off objects.

Although children of any age can manifest myopia, it most commonly develops at about 8 years of age. The child may complain of headaches and often squints to improve distance vision.

- *Astigmatism:* Light rays are refracted differently depending on their place of entry to the eye. The curvature of the cornea or lens is not uniformly spherical, causing blurred images. The child with astigmatism often holds pages very close to the face to obtain the best visual image.

For the description and management of four disorders that can significantly affect vision—strabismus, amblyopia, cataracts, and glaucoma—see Table 45–3.

Compensatory lenses are prescribed for most visual disorders. A significant difference in visual acuity between the eyes is often a result of amblyopia or strabismus, and further treatment may be needed. The visual acuity of a child with compensatory lenses should be reevaluated every 1 to 2 years. More frequent visits to an eye specialist are needed when a child is being treated for amblyopia or strabismus.

Nursing Management

The nurse plays an important role in identifying visual disorders in children and performing careful eye examinations of newborns and children. Observe for symmetry of placement and movement, ability to follow objects with each eye, and any abnormalities in appearance. The light reflex, cover–uncover test, and visual acuity testing are essential tests for every child. See Chapter 33 for a description of eye examination and the *Clinical Skills Manual* for visual acuity tests SKILLS .

Nurses in preschools and schools plan and carry out visual acuity screening on children. Generally, certain grades (such as kindergarten, 2, 4, 6, and 8) are screened annually along with any children new to a district. The nurse performs and records the screening results and informs the school and families of any children with abnormal results, who are then referred to an eye specialist for care. An important part of the screening process is following up on referrals to be certain that children receive the diagnostic care they need.

Healthy People 2020

(V-1) Increase the proportion of preschool children aged 5 years and under who receive vision screening

- Currently, only 40% of preschool children receive vision screening, while the goal is for 44% to have such screening by 2020. Clearly, nurses can play a role in increasing the number of young children who have vision screening.

When abnormalities are found on screening, nurses refer families to the care of an eye specialist. When prescriptive lenses are used, the nurse instructs the parent and child on correct wear practices and care. If surgery is required, surgical and postoperative follow-up are needed. This will include pain control, observing for signs of infection (ophthalmic or systemic), and administering needed eye medications. Sterile technique is used postoperatively to provide eye care. Promptly report deviations from normal such as increased pain, redness, discharge, or edema of the eye; increased temperature or pulse, which may indicate infection; increased sensitivity to light; or other abnormalities. Children are usually discharged home with instructions to minimize certain vigorous activities for a certain period of time. Perform postoperative and discharge teaching and emphasize the importance of follow-up visits.

TABLE 45–3 Clinical Manifestations of Visual Disorders

ETIOLOGY	CLINICAL MANIFESTATIONS	CLINICAL THERAPY
STRABISMUS Can be congenital or acquired. Seen in up to 4% of all children; 30%–50% of children with strabismus develop amblyopia Most common types: **Esotropia:** inward deviation of eyes ("crossed eyes") **Exotropia:** outward deviation of eyes ("wall-eyes") 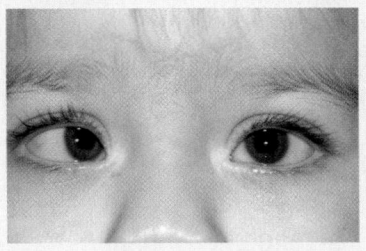 Strabismus. Biophoto Associates/Science Source.	Eyes appear misaligned to observer. May occur only when child is tired. Symptoms include squinting and frowning when reading; closing one eye to see; having trouble picking up objects; dizziness and headache. Corneal light reflex and cover–uncover tests confirm diagnosis. Child may have no other abnormalities but certain conditions such as cerebral palsy, hydrocephalus, Down syndrome, and seizure disorder are more commonly accompanied by strabismus.	Occlusion therapy (patching the fixating or good eye for 1–2 hr daily to force use of the weak eye) Compensatory lenses Surgery of the rectus muscles to correct muscle imbalance Eye drops to cause blurring of the good eye Prisms Vision therapy (eye exercises) If treatment is begun before 24 months of age, amblyopia (reduced vision in one or both eyes) may be prevented.
AMBLYOPIA (LAZY EYE) Reduced vision in one or both eyes; affects up to 4% of children and is the leading cause of vision loss in children. Amblyopia can result from anything that causes visual deprivation to one eye. The most common causes are untreated strabismus, with the child "tuning out" the image in deviating eye, congenital cataract, or uncorrected refractive errors causing visual differences between eyes.	Symptoms are the same as for strabismus. Vision testing can be used to diagnose condition.	Compensatory lenses Occlusion therapy for 2–6 hr daily through patching the eye or eye glass Occasionally, vision therapy (eye exercises) is used in an attempt to improve the weaker eye. Atropine 1% 1 drop/day in unaffected eye. Treatment is discontinued when visual acuity no longer improves; 20/20 acuity rarely attained. Treatment is most successful if received by 5–6 years of age.
CATARACTS Occurs when all or part of lens of eye becomes opaque, which prevents refraction of light rays onto retina Seen in 1–2/10,000 newborns 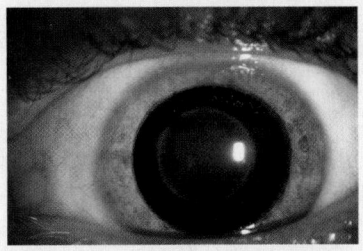 Congenital cataract. Sue Ford/Science Source.	Can affect one or both eyes and may be congenital or acquired. Examples include a variety of genetic syndromes and maternally transmitted intrauterine infections. Clouding of lens indicates presence of cataract; however, cataracts are not always visible to naked eye. Symptoms include distorted red reflex, symptoms of vision loss (see strabismus), white pupil. May be present alone but sometimes associated with other conditions such as fetal alcohol syndrome, Down syndrome, and Turner syndrome.	Must be diagnosed at a young age for successful treatment; many cases are missed. When diagnosed, a thorough examination is warranted because of genetic systemic disorders that are sometime associated with pediatric cataracts. Specific treatment depends on whether one or both eyes are affected, extent of clouding, and presence of other ocular abnormalities. Surgical removal of lens and corrective lenses; contact lenses frequently used; results of surgery are good; surgery before the age of 2 months is associated with the best results; visual acuity in 55% of children is 20/40 or better. Lens implant may be used. Eye protectors and restraints are used postoperatively to prevent injury; antibiotic or steroid drops may be used for several weeks; treatment for amblyopia may be necessary.

(continued)

TABLE 45–3 Clinical Manifestations of Visual Disorders (*continued*)

ETIOLOGY	CLINICAL MANIFESTATIONS	CLINICAL THERAPY
GLAUCOMA		

GLAUCOMA

Increased intraocular pressure damages eye and impairs visual function; ciliary body of eye produces aqueous fluid that flows between iris and lens into anterior chamber; if enough fluid accumulates, blindness results; about 1 in 10,000 newborns have glaucoma.

May be congenital (occurring in first 3 years of life) or juvenile (occurring from 3–30 years) and affect one or both eyes. Acquired cases can be related to conditions such as eye trauma or neoplasm.

Primary glaucoma (50% of cases) is an isolated anomaly of drainage; secondary glaucoma (50% of cases) is associated with other ocular or systemic abnormalities.

Symptoms of congenital glaucoma include tearing, blinking, corneal clouding, eyelid spasms, and progressive enlargement of eye; photophobia (extreme sensitivity to light).

Symptoms of juvenile glaucoma include constant bumping into objects in child's periphery (painless visual field loss); seeing halos around objects.

Diagnosis is made using a tonometer, which measures intraocular pressure.

Surgery to reduce intraocular pressure is treatment of choice, since medications used to combat glaucoma in adults are not as effective in children.

Compensatory lenses used following surgery.

Treatment is not always successful, especially if the child has congenital glaucoma, so parents' feelings regarding care of a child with a visual impairment should be explored.

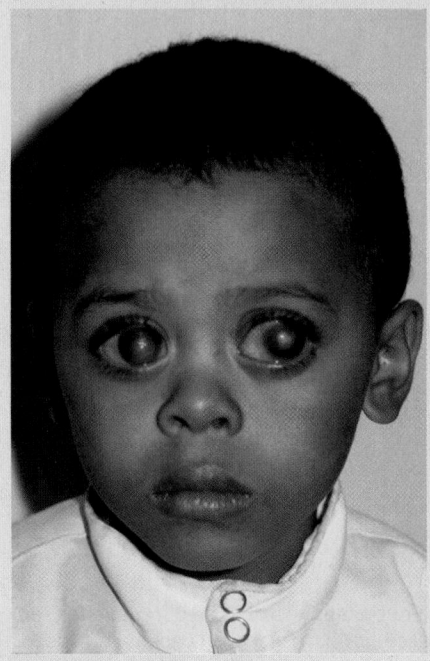

Congenital glaucoma.
Custom Medical Stock Photo/Newscom.

Source: Data from American Association for Pediatric Ophthalmology and Strabismus. (2014). *Strabismus*. Retrieved from http://www.aapos.org/terms/conditions/100; Bradfield, Y. S. (2013). Identification and treatment of amblyopia. *American Family Physician, 87,* 348–352; Yeung, H. H., & Walton, D. S. (2012). Recognizing childhood glaucoma in the primary pediatric setting. *Contemporary Pediatrics, 29*(5), 32–40; Trumler, A. A. (2011). Evaluation of pediatric cataracts and systemic disorders. *Current Opinion in Ophthalmology, 22,* 365–379; Kliegman, R. M., Stanton, B., St. Geme, J., Schor, N., & Behrman, R. E. (Eds.) (2011). *Nelson textbook of pediatrics* (19th ed., pp. 2569–2615). Philadelphia, PA: Saunders.

Color Blindness

Color blindness is an X-linked recessive disorder found in 10% of males and very rarely in females; it is more common in White than Black males. The most common form affects the ability to distinguish between the colors red and green; blue-yellow discrimination and other colors can also be involved. Preschool boys are tested for color blindness in some clinics to identify those with the disorder (Adams, Verdon, & Spivey, 2012). Color blindness is not treatable, and management focuses on issues of safety (e.g., problems in distinguishing between red and green traffic signals) and techniques to improve discrimination of colors in the affected color groups.

Retinopathy of Prematurity

Retinopathy of prematurity (ROP) occurs when immature blood vessels in the retina constrict and become necrotic. This condition, which may occur in infants of low birth weight or of short gestation, can heal completely or lead to mild myopia or retinal detachment and blindness.

ETIOLOGY AND PATHOPHYSIOLOGY

Retinopathy of prematurity results from injury to the developing capillaries of the retina. Oxygen therapy is associated with the development of ROP (Figure 45–2), but other factors such as respiratory distress, artificial ventilation, apnea, cerebral palsy,

Pathophysiology Illustrated: **Visual Abnormalities**

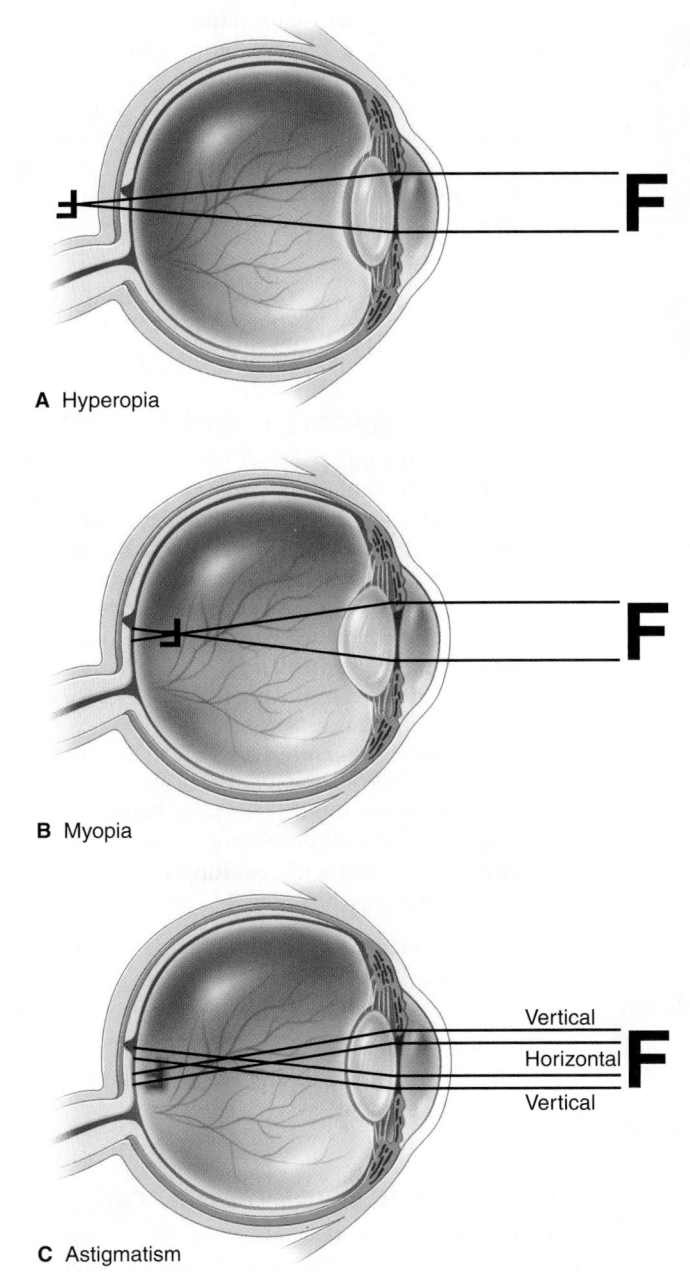

A Hyperopia

B Myopia

C Astigmatism

Vertical
Horizontal
Vertical

A, In hyperopia, light rays focus behind the retina, making it difficult to focus on objects at close range. *B*, In myopia, light rays focus in front of the retina, making it difficult to focus on objects that are far away. *C*, In astigmatism, light rays do not uniformly focus on the eye because of abnormal curvature of cornea or lens.

bradycardia, heart disease, multiple blood transfusions, infection, hypoxia, hypercarbia, acidosis, shock, and sepsis have also been linked with the disorder. It is most common in male infants born before 28 weeks of gestation and weighing under 1600 g (3 lb, 8 oz) at birth. A genetic link may be present because White infants are more commonly affected than those of African heritage, and Alaskan Natives have a high rate of the disorder. In developed countries, ROP is the second most common cause of blindness, with increasing prevalence in infants of lesser gestational age (Hartnett et al., 2014; National Eye Institute, 2014).

The retina is normally vascularized by about 8 months' gestation. However, for the premature infant, this process must continue after birth, and the environmental and other conditions listed in the preceding paragraph appear to affect its course. Arteriole constriction, followed by vascular proliferation of abnormal vessels, occurs. In most cases, the abnormal vessels gradually regress and normal vascularization occurs. Sometimes, however, the abnormal vascularization continues into the vitreous cavity, causing abnormalities of the retina, optic disc, and macula. It is not known why the disease progresses in some cases, but progression is directly linked to lower birth weight, greater prematurity, and duration (not necessarily concentration) of oxygen therapy. Raeanne, the child described in the scenario at the beginning of this chapter, developed retinopathy of prematurity after receiving oxygen therapy to aid her underdeveloped lungs.

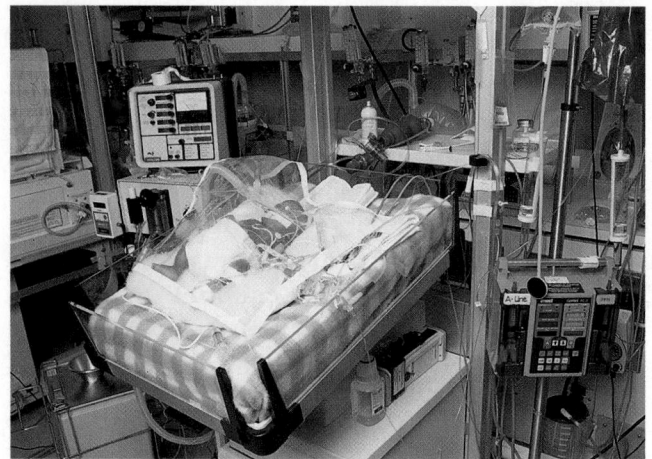

Figure 45–2 Artificial ventilation and risk for retinopathy of prematurity. This premature infant in the neonatal intensive care unit is receiving artificial ventilation—a risk factor for retinopathy of prematurity. The infant will need careful management of oxygen exposure and periodic eye examinations.

Although the developing capillaries are lost, in many cases, some degree of revascularization occurs later (National Eye Institute, 2014). The degree of visual loss, varying from slight to total, is determined by the degree of revascularization.

CLINICAL MANIFESTATIONS

Retinopathy of prematurity is characterized by progressive changes in the retinal blood vessels, and in severe disease, by retinal detachment. Premature and low-birth-weight infants at risk for the disease are given frequent ocular examinations to ensure early detection of these changes. For infants who do not receive ophthalmologic examinations, resulting visual impairment may be detected only later in infancy when the child progresses slowly in meeting developmental milestones, fails to reach for objects, and does not follow objects or faces with the eyes. When visual impairment is present, the child usually manifests myopia. Total loss of vision can occur in the child who suffers a retinal detachment.

CLINICAL THERAPY

Diagnosis is made by ophthalmologic examination. A classification system that includes zone (area of retina with abnormal vasculature), stage (severity of disease), and plus disease (vascular dilation and tortuosity in posterior pole near optic nerve) is used to describe the location, extent, and severity of the disease (International Committee for the Classification of Retinopathy of Prematurity, 2005; National Institutes of Health, 2013). All infants at risk, namely, those born before 32 weeks of gestation and under 1500 g (3 lb, 7 oz) or those born after 32 weeks gestation with birth weight from 1500 to 2000 g (3 lb, 7 oz to 4 lb, 3 oz), are assessed frequently, using binocular ophthalmoscopy, by an ophthalmologist experienced with the condition. The disease is not manifested before 4 to 6 weeks after birth, so it is important that the infant receive regular eye examinations until the risk is discounted. Eye examinations continue every 1 to 3 weeks, with the frequency being determined by the location of disease, progress of disease, and the infant's degree of immature vascularization. Involvement of blood vessels in the periphery of the retina rarely leads to visual impairment. With involvement in other areas of the retina, risk of visual problems is more common.

Treatment of infants with retinopathy of prematurity may include laser therapy or cryotherapy to stop progression of the disease process. New therapies such as injections are being explored in research protocols. Surgical procedures such as a scleral buckle procedure and vitrectomy have been used in retinal detachments. Prompt treatment of accompanying problems such as strabismus, amblyopia, and myopia can promote maximal development.

Nursing Management
For the Child With Retinopathy of Prematurity

Nursing Assessment and Diagnosis

Assessment of the infant at risk for retinopathy of prematurity begins at birth by identifying infants who may require oxygen therapy or assisted ventilation. Look for risk factors such as prematurity and low birth weight. Assess the infant's breathing efforts and report any changes. Be certain the ventilation equipment is properly set to deliver the correct ventilatory pressure and amount of oxygen, evaluated by pulse oximetry saturation (see the *Clinical Skills Manual* SKILLS). Note the cumulative risks in a particular case and suggest the need for a referral to an ophthalmologist, as necessary.

The following *Nursing Care Plan: The Child With a Visual Impairment Secondary to Retinopathy of Prematurity* outlines several nursing diagnoses. Other nursing diagnoses may be appropriate for an infant with the potential to develop retinopathy of prematurity or a child with resulting visual impairment. They include the following (NANDA-I © 2014):

- *Gas Exchange, Impaired*, related to ventilation-perfusion imbalance
- *Development: Delayed, Risk for*, related to effects of visual impairment
- *Family Processes, Interrupted*, related to a child with a visual impairment

Planning and Implementation

The nurse plays an important role in preventing retinopathy of prematurity. Encourage early and regular prenatal care to prevent unnecessary premature births. Administer oxygen only to newborns who need it, and in the amount specified by the physician to maintain prescribed oxygen saturation. Ensure that the proper ventilatory settings are used. Shield newborns from excessive exposure to light, since that may decrease susceptibility to retinopathy of prematurity. Be alert for infants with multiple risk factors and refer them, when appropriate, for ophthalmologic examination. Parents of infants at risk for retinopathy of prematurity require information about the disorder, as well as support, because the long-term effects on the child's vision are often identified only after subsequent examinations as the child grows.

The accompanying *Nursing Care Plan* summarizes care for the child with a visual impairment resulting from retinopathy of prematurity. The nurse is instrumental in case management for such children. Reinforce to parents the importance of follow-up eye examinations. Teach methods of stimulating development for a child with a visual impairment (refer to the next section).

Nursing Care Plan: The Child With a Visual Impairment Secondary to Retinopathy of Prematurity

1. Nursing Diagnosis: *Communication, Readiness for Enhanced*, related to altered reception, transmission, and integration resulting of visual images (NANDA-I © 2014)

GOAL: The child will receive adequate sensory input.

INTERVENTION	RATIONALE
• Provide kinesthetic, tactile, and auditory stimulation during play and in daily care (e.g., talking and playing). Provide music while bathing an infant, using bells and other noises on each side of infant. Verbally describe to a child all actions being carried out by adult.	• Because visual sensory input is not present, the child needs input from all other senses to compensate and provide adequate sensory stimulation.

EXPECTED OUTCOME: Child will demonstrate minimal signs of sensory deprivation.

2. Nursing Diagnosis: *Injury, Risk for*, related to impaired vision (NANDA-I © 2014)

GOAL: The child will be protected from safety hazards that can lead to injury.

INTERVENTION	RATIONALE
• Evaluate environment for potential safety hazards based on age of child and degree of impairment. Be particularly alert to objects that give visual cues to their dangers (e.g., stairs, stoves, fireplaces, candles). Eliminate safety hazards and protect the child from exposure. Take the child on a tour of new rooms, explaining safety hazards (e.g., schools, hotel room, hospital room).	• The child may be at risk for injury related both to developmental stage and to inability to visualize hazards.

EXPECTED OUTCOME: Child will experience no injuries.

3. Nursing Diagnosis: *Development: Delayed, Risk for*, related to impaired vision (NANDA-I © 2014)

GOAL: The child has experiences necessary to foster normal growth and development.

INTERVENTION	RATIONALE
• Help parents plan early, regular social activities with other children.	• The child with a visual impairment benefits developmentally from contact with other children.
• Provide opportunities and encourage self-feeding activities.	• To obtain adequate nutrients, the child needs to feel comfortable feeding self.
• Provide an environment rich in sensory input.	• Sensory input is needed for normal development to occur.
• Assess growth and development during regular examinations to identify the child's strengths and needs.	• Regular examinations aid in early identification of growth problems or developmental delays, so that appropriate interventions can be planned.

EXPECTED OUTCOME: Child will demonstrate normal growth and development milestones.

4. Nursing Diagnosis: *Family Processes, Interrupted*, related to child's prolonged disability from sensory impairment (NANDA-I © 2014)

GOAL: The family will identify methods for coping with their child with a visual impairment.

INTERVENTION	RATIONALE
• Provide explanation of visual impairment as appropriate.	• The parents may feel guilt about the child's visual impairment, which can be allayed by knowledge of the cause.
• Refer parents to organizations, early intervention programs, and other parents of children with visual impairments.	• The parents will receive needed information and support from others.
• Assist parents to plan for meeting the developmental, educational, and safety needs of their child with a visual impairment. Offer resources for changing home environment to assist child.	• The child may require an enhanced environment in order to foster developmental progress.

EXPECTED OUTCOME: Family will successfully cope with the experience of having a child with a visual impairment.

Clinical Reasoning The Child With ROP

Raeanne, 3 years old, has a severe visual impairment. Born prematurely at 25 weeks of gestation, she received oxygen therapy, which damaged her retinal blood vessels. As a result, Raeanne developed retinopathy of prematurity (ROP). While in the hospital, Raeanne was given frequent ophthalmoscopic examinations. She received cryotherapy to the retinal vessels—a treatment designed to prevent detached retinae and the resulting total vision loss. Although this treatment halted progression of the disorder, Raeanne was left severely myopic (nearsighted).

For the first 3 years of life, Raeanne and her mother attended an early-intervention program, which provided stimulation for Raeanne and helped teach her mother techniques for enhancing her developmental progress. Raeanne will soon begin attending preschool. Her speech is well developed for a 3-year-old; she is socially mature, converses readily, and shows no developmental delays. However, she has had little contact with other children.

As the nurse in the preschool Raeanne will be attending, how will you assist both her parents and the preschool staff in helping Raeanne adapt to the preschool experience?

Evaluation

Expected outcomes of nursing care for the child with retinopathy of prematurity include the following:

- Visual impairment is identified early in life.
- The child achieves normal developmental milestones.
- The family effectively manages the child's visual condition.

Visual Impairment

Visual impairment related to refractive errors, amblyopia, strabismus, and astigmatism occurs in 5% to 10% of young children (Granet & Khayali, 2011). About 500,000 children in the United States have visual impairment and about 60,000 are legally blind (vision 20/200 or worse) (American Foundation for the Blind, 2011).

Many conditions discussed earlier in this chapter lead to temporary or permanent visual impairment. Infants who are premature; whose mothers were infected prenatally with rubella, toxoplasmosis, or other viruses; and who have certain congenital and hereditary conditions have a high risk of visual problems (Table 45–4). Fetal alcohol syndrome (FAS) is a major cause of visual disturbance; 90% of children with FAS have eye abnormalities. See Chapter 55 for further description of FAS.

The signs of visual impairment depend on the cause and degree of the problem and the age of the child (Table 45–5). The child's eyes may appear crossed or watery, and the lids may be crusty. Verbal children may complain of itching, dizziness, headache, or blurred, double, or poor vision.

Diagnostic tests include vision screening, followed by referral to an eye specialist for full examination. Tests that are commonly performed include responses to visual stimuli, symmetry of eye movements, location of corneal light reflex, cover–uncover testing, visual field testing, and funduscopic examination of the retina. The U.S. Preventive Services Task Force (2011) recommends screening to detect amblyopia, strabismus, and defects in visual acuity in children at least once between 3 and 5 years of age. The American Academy of Pediatrics (2011) recommends age-appropriate eye evaluations at

TABLE 45–4 Common Causes of Visual Impairment in Children

CONGENITAL OR HEREDITARY	ACQUIRED
Cataracts	Injury to eye or head
Glaucoma	Infections
Tay-Sachs disease	Rubella
Marfan syndrome	Measles
Down syndrome	Chickenpox
Fetal alcohol syndrome	Brain tumor
Prenatal infections (maternal infection):	Retinopathy of prematurity
Rubella	Cerebral palsy
Toxoplasmosis	
Herpes simplex	
Retinoblastoma	

TABLE 45–5 Signs of Visual Impairment

INFANTS	TODDLERS AND OLDER CHILDREN
May be unable to follow lights or objects	May rub, shut, or cover eyes
Do not make eye contact	Tilt or thrust head forward
Have a dull, vacant stare	Blink frequently
Do not imitate facial expressions	Hold objects close
	Bump into objects
	Squint

health visits from birth through 4 years and age-appropriate visual acuity testing and ophthalmoscopy in children 5 years and older.

Clinical therapy depends on the child's condition and may include surgery, medication, and supportive aids. In the case of a disorder that results in permanent visual impairment, a collaborative care team of specialists works with the child and family. Nurses have an important role in this team to ensure developmental progression for the child and ongoing support for the family.

Growth and Development

Infants with visual impairment use kinesthesia, touch, and language to socialize. They appreciate and use touch more than other children and respond to verbal explanations when others use nonverbal communication. Vision affects both fine and gross motor skills, so skills such as hand-to-mouth coordination and walking may be delayed in children who have visual impairments.

Nursing Management

For the Child With Visual Impairment

Nursing Assessment and Diagnosis

Prevent visual deficits by teaching safety in activities that can injure the eye, engage in activities for early identification of the condition, and enhance the development of children with low vision. Vision screening facilitates early detection and treatment of conditions that can lead to vision loss. Visual testing can be

Clinical Question

Screening for visual ability is important to identify children with impairments. The American Academy of Pediatrics recommends that children be screened at every well-child visit, beginning in the newborn period. Screenings should include vision history, vision assessment, external inspection of the eyes and lids, eye movement assessment, pupil examination, and elicitation of red reflex. Once the child can cooperate, usually by about age 3 years, a vision test such as HOTV or tumbling E, along with ophthalmoscopic examination, should be added to the examination (Chou, Dana, & Bougatsos, 2011; U.S. Preventive Services Task Force, 2011). Worldwide, 13 million children are visually impaired because of uncorrected refractive errors, so vision screening is critical as the first step in providing corrective lenses (Sharma, Congdon, Patel, et al., 2012). How can nurses integrate into their practice the completion of vision examinations, provision of training for other screeners, evaluation of results, referral to specialists when abnormalities are found, and provision of follow-up care after diagnosis and treatment?

The Evidence

A study of the outcomes of school vision screening of 2726 children in North Carolina found that 3 children in 100 were identified upon follow-up with a vision problem, such as myopia, hyperopia, and astigmatism (Kemper, Helfrich, Talbot, et al., 2012). This study also found that no follow-up information was obtained on the outcome of referral for a full eye examination for 35% of the children with potential problems. School nurse staffing issues have made vision screening for children in schools a challenge, but innovative programs for training and supervising screeners such as volunteer parents, nursing students, and others have been successful. Key components of programs are to ensure that the nurse is present during screening for monitoring accuracy and consistency checks, performs the questionable results found by screeners, performs referrals, and conducts follow-up of vision referral results (National Association of School Nurses [NASN], 2012; Sides & Sigmon, 2013).

Best Practice

Nurses play a vital role in ensuring that children receive early, periodic, and regular visual and eye screening. Evidence that suggests the most accurate methods should be closely examined. While identification of problems is important, the nursing roles of training screeners, referral for care, identifying barriers to care, and ensuring that follow-up care has been received are also integral to vision care.

Clinical Reasoning

What vision screening methods are available in the offices, clinics, and schools in your community? How could you perform vision screening in the hospital setting if a child did not demonstrate expected visual ability for age? Design a program to train and supervise nursing students to perform vision screening. What are the essential components of a follow-up program for a school that screens all kindergartners and first graders for visual acuity? What questions will you ask parents during a well-child visit for a 2-year-old to determine if vision is normal? How will you combine your knowledge of developmental milestones with screening for vision?

---

done at any age, including immediately after birth. Developmental milestones that require vision, such as following bright lights, reaching for objects, or looking at pictures in a book, can be used to assess vision. For children over the age of 3 years, visual acuity is most frequently measured by means of an age-appropriate acuity test (see the *Clinical Skills Manual* SKILLS). Vision screening should begin at 3 years of age and take place during annual healthcare visits. See *Evidence-Based Practice: Nursing Role in Vision Screening and Follow-Up.* Most states mandate school screening of vision (see Chapter 33). The photo screener, a device that can be used to take a photo of the child's eyes, is useful for infants, toddlers, and preschoolers. The photo can be used to diagnose refraction errors, eye opacities, and misalignment. Visual fields and the ability to discriminate colors are tested at school age, when children can cooperate.

Children who have a visual impairment may lag in development of cognitive and other skills. Sighted children learn the word *cup* using four senses—sight, touch, hearing, and taste—to obtain the information necessary to connect words with the objects they represent. In contrast, children with visual impairments rely on only three senses—touch, hearing, and taste. They learn concepts through differences in sounds, textures, and shapes.

Many visual disorders are linked with conditions that influence development. Thus a child with cerebral palsy or fetal alcohol syndrome should be assessed frequently to identify a visual disorder, as well as to evaluate normal developmental milestones.

Nursing diagnoses for the child with impaired vision might include the following (NANDA-I © 2014):

- *Mobility: Physical, Impaired*, related to altered sensory perception
- *Injury, Risk for*, related to poor vision
- *Development: Delayed, Risk for*, related to visual impairment
- *Family Processes, Interrupted*, related to demands of a child with a sensory impairment

Planning and Implementation

Promote safety in sports and other activities to prevent visual impairment when possible. Nursing care for a child with a visual impairment focuses on encouraging the child's use of all senses, promoting socialization, helping parents to meet the child's developmental and educational needs, and providing emotional support to parents. Refer the parents to an early intervention program as soon as the diagnosis is made. Nearly all care occurs in community and home settings.

ENCOURAGE USE OF ALL SENSES

Children who are partially sighted or blind use other senses to a great extent. Encouraging the use of the eyes as much as possible is important even if a child has poor vision (Figure 45–3).

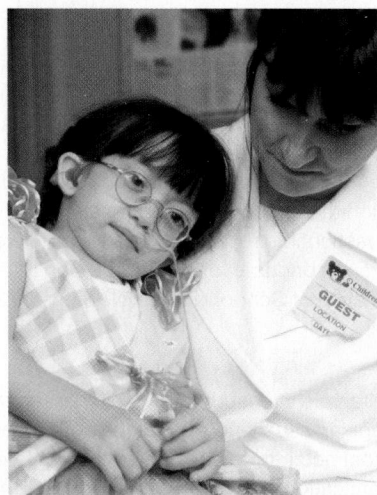

Figure 45–3 Encouraging use of the senses. This child needs ongoing developmental assessment and a comprehensive individualized education plan. Since she has impaired vision, the nurse uses touch and speaks with her throughout procedures to ensure sensory input.

PROMOTE SOCIALIZATION

The child's interactions and socializations should be as normal as possible (similar to those of sighted children of the same age and development).

- Stroke, rock, and hug infants and children who have a visual impairment. Sing and talk to them. These infants do not make eye contact and have rather blank expressions.
- Call the child's name and speak before touching the child. Tell the child when the nurse and others are leaving the room. Describe locations of foods on the plate and tray to orient the child.
- Teach parents to read body language and vocalization as expressions of emotion. Facial expressions give a great deal

of information, but infants and children with poor vision do not have the ability to learn by visual imitation. Show parents how to use tactile means to teach appropriate facial expressions. For example, a touch on the arm can be soft and stroking to indicate a smile, but firmer to indicate dismay or frown.

- Describe procedures such as blood pressure, ear examination, or cast application so the child knows what they will feel like. Let the child touch the equipment.
- Explain to parents that discipline and rewards for children with poor vision should be the same as those for other children in the family. The child should be given age-appropriate tasks.
- Encourage contact with peers as the child grows older. Teach children to look directly at persons who are talking to them. Play, sports, and other activities can be modified to give the child with a visual impairment the same social experiences as a sighted child.

COMMUNITY-BASED NURSING CARE

Public laws require that each state provide educational and related services for children with disabilities (see Chapter 1). Parents and healthcare providers should develop an individualized education plan (as discussed in Chapter 38) that maximizes the child's learning ability. If possible, the child with a vision problem should attend child care and preschool with children who have normal visual acuity. What nursing actions are needed to help a child with a visual impairment adjust to child care or school?

- Provide parents with information about educational options before their child reaches school age. Education should take place in a setting that allows the child to have contact with other children and to participate in social activities.
- The child may be mainstreamed with a tutor, be partially mainstreamed in a resource room, attend special classes, or be tutored at home. If the child is to attend public school, suggest to parents that they contact the school well before enrollment to ensure that school personnel understand the child's disability.
- Make sure that equipment such as large-print books, Braille materials, audio equipment, or an Optacon (described in

---

TEACHING HIGHLIGHTS | Enhancing Development of the Child With a Visual Impairment

- Encourage a toddler or preschooler who has a visual impairment to look at pictures in well-lit settings. Have a school-age child read large-print books. Computers designed for people with visual impairments are also available. The Optacon (a device that raises print so it can be felt by the child) and View Scan (which magnifies print) improve reading capability.
- Expose the infant and child to everyday sounds.
- Encourage the infant to use the sense of touch to explore people and objects. Have the parents purchase toys with sound and texture in mind. Directional concepts can be taught using games. Responding to the infant's and child's vocalizations encourages the use of speech.
- Teach specific techniques for toileting, dressing, bathing, eating, and safety.
- When the child becomes mobile, furniture and other objects in the environment should be kept in the same positions so the child can safely move around independently.

Extra care must be taken to prevent injuries when a child does not see.

- Emphasize the child's abilities. Adolescents can use seeing-eye dogs or a white cane to function independently.
- Encourage the child to function independently within normal developmental parameters.
- If the child goes to a hospital or another strange environment, orient the child to the placement of objects and do not rearrange them.
- Teach those around the child to:
  - Announce their presence to the child when approaching.
  - Walk slightly ahead of the child so the child can sense the movement of the accompanying person.
  - Let the child hold the seeing person's arm rather than the reverse.
  - Identify the contents of meals and encourage the child to feed self.

Teaching Highlights: Enhancing Development of the Child With a Visual Impairment) is available. Ensure that frequent eye examinations are performed and assist with proper use and care of prescribed glasses or contact lenses as necessary. Clean glasses daily with warm water and dry with a clean, soft cloth. Follow directions that the family provides, which describe the methods they use for cleaning contact lenses.

- Familiarize the child with the new environment.

Growth and Development

Children with visual impairment may take longer to master self-help skills such as feeding and dressing. Perform regular developmental assessments and suggest adaptive ways that parents can help the child learn these skills.

PROVIDE EMOTIONAL SUPPORT

The family often needs help to understand the child's abilities and disabilities. Support them as they learn about their child's visual problems, tell friends and family, and then adjust to supporting the child.

- Encourage habilitation as soon as realistically possible. Make the adjustment easier by providing information about the child's specific type of visual impairment, available community services, and groups or associations for children with similar vision conditions.

- Suggest resources to families of children with visual disorders.

- Be supportive and listen to the family's concerns about the child's visual deficit.

- Make sure the parents meet their own physical and emotional needs so they are better able to care for and provide support to their child.

Evaluation

Expected outcomes of nursing care for the child with a visual impairment include the following:

- The child is protected from injury.
- The child manifests growth and development to maximum potential.
- The child establishes a successful individualized education plan.

Injuries of the Eye

In the United States, eye injuries are common in children of all ages, especially from 11 to 14 years, and particularly in boys. Sports, darts, fireworks, air-powered BB guns, blunt and sharp objects, chemical and thermal burns, physical irritants, and abuse are causes of eye trauma. Sports injuries are most common, with 100,000 occurring annually; they are a common cause of blindness in children (National Eye Institute, n.d.).

Prevention is an important part of health promotion. Protective eyewear should be used by participants in all sports with a risk of eye injury, with extreme caution in those with diminished vision or only one functional eye. Common injuries occur in baseball, basketball, swimming, bicycling, and football so preventive measures should be taken such as proper training and use of protective gear. Chemicals and objects such as scissors and knives should be placed out of reach.

Some injuries can be treated at home but many require emergency care or hospitalization. The nurse will document the history of the injury, perform an assessment of the eye, and measure the visual acuity. If a tetanus booster has not been given in the last 5 years, the child is reimmunized. Table 45–6 summarizes emergency treatment of common eye injuries.

TABLE 45–6 Emergency Treatment of Eye Injuries

INJURY	TREATMENT
Subconjunctival hemorrhage (caused by coughing, mild trauma, or increased physical activity)	Usually heals spontaneously; child should see ophthalmologist if most of sclera is covered or if condition does not clear up in 1–2 weeks
Periorbital ecchymosis ("black eye")	Apply ice to eye area (both eyes) for 5–15 min every hour for the first 1–2 days after injury (even if only one eye is affected, both eyes may discolor); then apply warm compresses
Foreign body on conjunctiva	Do not let child rub eye; remove material on surface of eye by closing upper lid over lower lid, irrigating or everting upper lid, visualizing material, and removing it with slightly damp handkerchief; patch eye and transport child to emergency department if foreign body cannot be removed
Corneal abrasion	Superficial corneal abrasions are diagnosed by touching sterile fluorescein strip to lower conjunctiva; dye remains where corneal epithelial cells are disrupted; most corneal abrasions heal spontaneously although antibiotic ointment may be prescribed and eyes patched in some children
Burns (alkaline burns readily penetrate cornea and are more serious than acid burns)	For child with chemical burn, irrigate eye for 15–30 min; transport child to emergency department where irrigation should continue (see *Clinical Skills Manual* SKILLS); pupils are dilated to reduce pain and prevent adhesions; after irrigation is complete, eyes are patched and antibiotics are prescribed
Penetrating and perforating injuries	Obtain medical assistance immediately; never try to remove an object that has penetrated the child's eye; such objects should be removed by an ophthalmologist; prevent the child from rubbing injured eye; cover both eyes with shield before transportation to emergency department
Eye injuries caused by severe blows to head and eye (blunt trauma can seriously injure all eye structures, including orbit, which can be fractured)	Transport immediately to ophthalmologist's office or emergency department for evaluation and treatment; retinal hemorrhage is a common presentation of the type of child abuse called "shaken child syndrome"

Disorders of the Ear

Otitis Media

Otitis media, or inflammation of the middle ear, is sometimes accompanied by infection. This condition is one of the most common childhood illnesses, with a majority of infants having at least one case of acute otitis media by 3 years of age (Qureishi, Lee, Belfield, et al., 2014). Otitis media occurs more frequently among boys and in children who attend childcare centers, in those with allergies, in children exposed to tobacco smoke, and in those who use pacifiers several hours daily. It is most common during the winter months. Children with conditions such as cleft lip and palate or Down syndrome more often experience otitis media. Breastfeeding appears to be protective against otitis media. In the past decade, an increased number of cases have been observed, and recent changes have been made in recommendations for treatment.

Growth and Development

Fluid accumulation in the middle ear prevents the efficient transmission of sound and can result in hearing loss over time, potentially delaying speech and language development. These delays may manifest as cognitive deficits or behavior problems. Motor development has been found to be impaired in children with chronic ear infections.

ETIOLOGY AND PATHOPHYSIOLOGY

The specific cause of otitis media is unknown, but it appears to be related to eustachian tube dysfunction. Often, an upper respiratory infection precedes otitis media. This infection causes the mucous membranes of the eustachian tube to become edematous. As a result, air that normally flows to the middle ear is blocked, and the air in the middle ear is reabsorbed into the bloodstream. Fluid is pulled from the mucosal lining into the

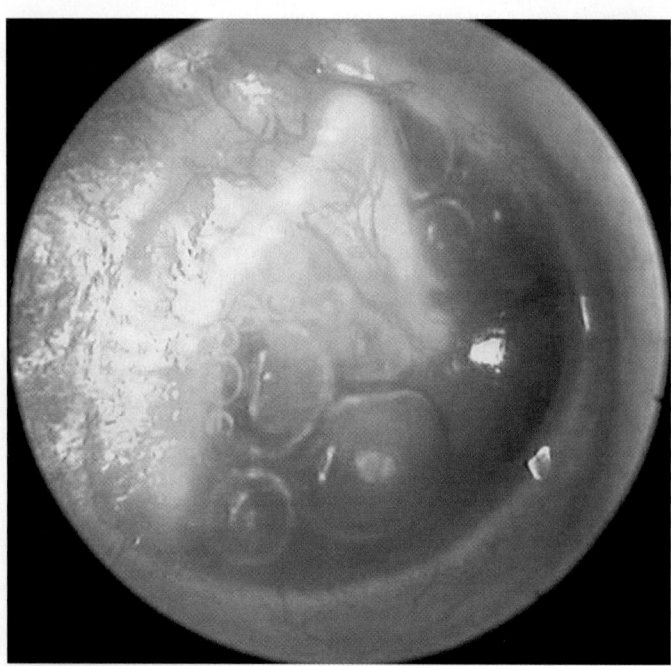

Figure 45–5 Otitis media with effusion is noted on otoscopy by fluid line or air bubbles.

SOURCE: Dr. Kevin T. Kavanagh, MD, FACS/Cumberland Otolaryngology Consultants.

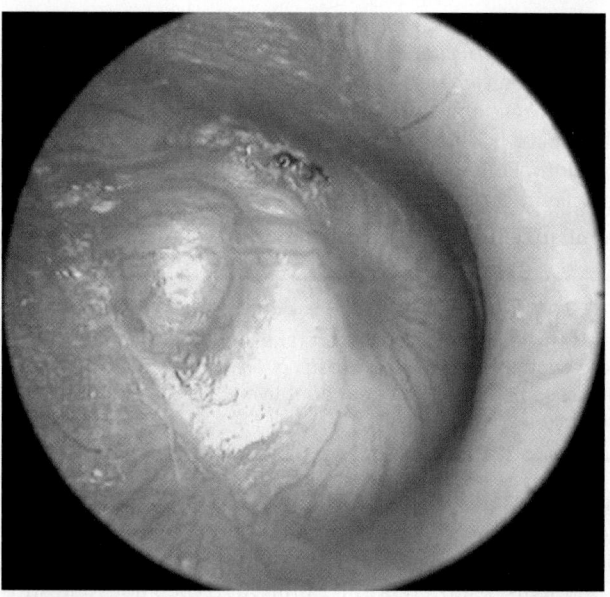

Figure 45–4 Acute otitis media is characterized by pain and a red, bulging, nonmobile tympanic membrane.

SOURCE: Dr. Kevin T. Kavanagh, MD, FACS/Cumberland Otolaryngology Consultants.

former air space, providing a medium for the rapid growth of pathogens. The tympanic membrane and fluid behind it become infected. The most common causative organisms are *Streptococcus pneumoniae, Haemophilus influenzae,* and *Moraxella catarrhalis* (Harmes et al., 2013).

Conditions such as enlarged adenoids or edema from allergic rhinitis can also obstruct the eustachian tube and lead to otitis media. Pacifier use raises the soft palate and may alter dynamics in the eustachian tube, providing for entry of microorganisms from the nasopharynx. Recurrent otitis media has an increased frequency in children of parents who smoke. Children with multiple siblings and those who attend childcare centers have increased rates of recurrent acute otitis media. Ethnicity appears to be a factor (see *Developing Cultural Competence: Otitis Media*).

CLINICAL MANIFESTATIONS

Otitis media is the general term for inflammation of the middle ear. *Acute otitis media (AOM)* is diagnosed when the child has acute onset of ear pain, bulging of the tympanic membrane upon otoscopy, and middle ear effusion (Figure 45–4). Recurrent acute otitis media is defined as three or more separate AOM episodes in 6 months, or four or more episodes in 12 months with at least one episode in the past 6 months (Lieberthal et al., 2013). *Otitis media with effusion (OME)* is evidence of fluid in the middle ear without inflammation (Figure 45–5). OME sometimes becomes chronic in nature (continuing more than 3 months) and is more commonly associated with hearing loss (Williamson, 2011).

Infants and young children have characteristic behaviors that indicate otitis media may be present. Pulling at the ear is a sign of ear pain (Figure 45–6). Diarrhea, vomiting, and fever are typical of otitis media. Irritability and "acting out" may be signs of a related hearing impairment. The child with otitis media often has night awakenings with crying due to increased pressure when prone or supine. Some children with otitis media are asymptomatic; therefore, an ear examination should be performed at every healthcare visit (see Chapter 33). See Table 45–7.

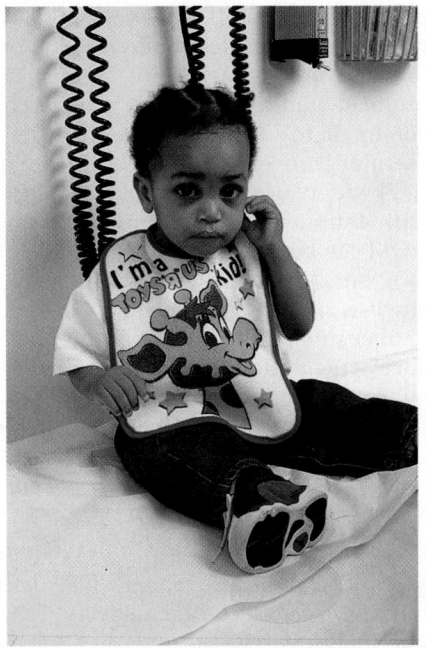

Figure 45–6 **This young child is pulling at the ear, an important sign of otitis media. Ask the parents about fussiness, presence of fever, and night awakenings; these are additional signs that are often observed in children with this condition.**

CLINICAL THERAPY

Otoscopic examination includes visualization and pneumatic otoscopy. The trained clinician can perform pneumatic otoscopy in which positive air pressure in the external canal is used to measure the movement of the tympanic membrane. Special gradient acoustic reflectometry (SGAR) measures the condition of the middle ear by introducing a sound and measuring the tympanic membrane response. A "flat" tympanogram is also suggestive of otitis media. (The tympanogram is described in a later section on hearing impairment.)

TABLE 45–7 Clinical Manifestations of Acute Otitis Media and Otitis Media With Effusion

ETIOLOGY	CLINICAL MANIFESTATIONS	CLINICAL THERAPY
Acute otitis media—bacterial infection in the middle ear from pathogens transferred from the nasopharynx; most common infectious agents are *S. pneumoniae, H. influenzae, M. catarrhalis*	*Behavioral*—ear pain, pulling at ear, rapid onset, irritability, malaise, poor feeding *Examination*—bulging tympanic membrane, air or fluid bubbles present behind tympanic membrane; immobile or poorly mobile tympanic membrane, red (or other color change such as white, gray, or yellow as long as bulging is present) tympanic membrane, reduced visibility of tympanic membrane landmarks with displaced light reflex	Treat ear pain with anesthetic ear drops, herbal pain products instilled into the auditory canal, or systemic acetaminophen or ibuprofen. Verify that the tympanic membrane is intact before inserting ear drops. In cases of nonsevere unilateral disease, consult with parents of children under 2 years to decide together on observation or antibiotic treatment. For child 2 years and above with nonsevere disease, observe the child's condition for 48–72 hr and, if not improved, treat with course of antibiotics. Severe and bilateral disease is always treated with antibiotic.
Otitis media with effusion—collection of fluid in the middle ear behind the tympanic membrane, which is not infected with bacteria	*Behavioral*—difficulty hearing or responding as expected to sounds *Examination*—signs of acute inflammation are NOT present; tympanic membrane is retracted or neutral; immobile or partly mobile tympanic membrane; yellow or gray tympanic membrane; opaque or thickened tympanic membrane with visibility of landmarks reduced	Symptomatic treatment and pain relief Careful assessment of hearing acuity over several months Speech assessment if loss of hearing acuity occurs Developmental assessment

Since otitis media with effusion may only involve fluid in the middle ear, it is best diagnosed by pneumatic otoscopy and tympanometry. Since this type of otitis media is most commonly associated with hearing loss, audiologic testing should be performed in the pediatric healthcare home (medical home) (see Chapter 34) if the effusion persists for 3 months or longer.

Concern has developed about the increasing appearance of drug-resistant microbials as causative agents in otitis media. These organisms may explain the increase in otitis media observed in the past decade. Based on current knowledge, the American Academy of Pediatrics (AAP) established recommendations for diagnosis and management of otitis media in 2004, which were updated in 2013 (Lieberthal et al., 2013). Consistent with current guidelines, for children from 6 months to 23 months with nonsevere unilateral disease, the healthcare provider and parent should consult about whether antibiotic use or observation for 48 to 72 hours is best. If nonsevere bilateral AOM is present or if severe AOM is present (temperature of 39.0°C [102.2°F] with pain for 48 hours) the young child should be treated with antibiotic. For children 24 months and older, nonsevere AOM can be treated with antibiotic or by observation for 48 to 72 ours (Lieberthal et al., 2013). In all cases where 48- to 72-hour observation is implemented, a method for follow-up is needed to ensure that the child has improved. When not improved during the period of watchful waiting, acute otitis media is treated with antibiotic therapy for 10 days in children under 6 years, and 5 to 7 days for children 6 years and over (Hoberman et al., 2011).

Professionalism in Practice Clinical Guidelines

In recent years, the American Academy of Pediatrics and other bodies have established new guidelines for treatment of conditions such as acute otitis media and sinusitis (described later in this chapter). Parents often expect antibiotics for any illness their child may have and do not understand the rationale for guidelines that recommend watchful waiting for a limited time to see if the child improves. Nurses should be familiar with recommendations and guidelines for preventive care (e.g., vision and hearing screening) and treatments (e.g., acute otitis media and sinusitis) so that they can explain the rationale for these approaches to parents. Such explanations can often allay concern and worry, and help build confidence in healthcare providers as partners with parents in care for their children.

When prescribed, the choice of antibiotic depends on the probable organism, ease of administration, cost, previous effectiveness, and any history of allergies. First-line therapy is amoxicillin, unless it has been given to the child in the previous 30 days. Amoxicillin with clavulanate and cefuroxime are second-line drugs. If an intramuscular drug is preferred, cefdinir at 14 mg/kg/day, cefpodoxime at 10 mg/kg/day, or cefuroxime at 30 mg/kg/day can be prescribed (Tschudy & Arcara, 2012).

OME is not treated with antibiotics but is evaluated periodically to be sure there is not an additional AOM that needs treatment. Children with OME generally improve within 3 months. Because this type of otitis is more commonly associated with hearing loss and cochlear damage, follow-up with audiology is essential. If hearing is abnormal, speech testing should be performed (Farboud, Skinner, & Pratap, 2011; Williamson, 2011).

Neither decongestants nor antihistamines have been shown to be effective in the treatment of otitis media with or without effusion. If infection recurs in spite of antibiotic treatment, **myringotomy** (surgical incision of the tympanic membrane) may be performed and **tympanostomy tubes** (pressure equalizing tubes) inserted to drain fluid from the middle ear. (See *Teaching Highlights: Care of the Child With Tympanostomy Tubes*.)

Nursing Management
For the Child With Otitis Media

Nursing Assessment and Diagnosis

Assess the tympanic membrane for color, transparency, mobility, presence of landmarks, and light reflex. Ask the parents whether the child has had a fever, been fussy, or been pulling at the ears. Observe for signs of impaired hearing.

Inquire about what the family has done at home to treat the ear infection and its associated pain. Some home remedies, such as rocking and singing to the child, are safe. Some other practices may be harmful.

Several nursing diagnoses that may apply are included in *Nursing Care Plan: The Child With Otitis Media*. Additional nursing diagnoses might include the following (NANDA-I © 2014):

- *Body Temperature: Imbalanced, Risk for*, related to infectious process
- *Fatigue (Child and Parent)* related to sleep deprivation
- *Health Maintenance, Ineffective*, related to chronic ear infections and altered sensory reception

Planning and Implementation

Most children with otitis media are not hospitalized; therefore, nursing management centers on care of the child in the home. The child having tympanostomy tubes inserted is generally treated in a day surgery setting. Occasionally, children admitted to the hospital for other problems have a concurrent ear infection. The accompanying *Nursing Care Plan* summarizes nursing care for the child with otitis media.

TEACHING HIGHLIGHTS | Care of the Child With Tympanostomy Tubes

After Surgery
- Encourage the child to drink generous amounts of fluids.
- Reestablish a regular diet as tolerated.
- Give pain medication (acetaminophen) as ordered for discomfort and at bedtime.
- Place drops in child's ears if prescribed.
- Restrict the child to quiet activities.

Following Postoperative Period
- Follow the care provider's instructions regarding swimming and water (some caution against swimming and other activities that might get water in ears; others do not).
- Ear plugs can be used to prevent water from getting into ears.
- Be alert for tubes becoming dislodged and falling out and alert healthcare provider (they usually fall out within 1 year).
- Report purulent discharge from the ear, which may indicate a new ear infection. Contact the healthcare provider.

Nursing Care Plan: The Child With Otitis Media

1. Nursing Diagnosis: *Pain, Acute*, related to inflammation and pressure on tympanic membrane (NANDA-I © 2014)

GOAL: The child or parent will indicate absence of pain.

INTERVENTION	RATIONALE
• Give analgesic such as acetaminophen. Use analgesic ear drops.	• Analgesics alter perception or response to pain.
• Have the child sit up, raise head on pillows, or lie on unaffected ear.	• Elevation decreases pressure from fluid.
• Apply warmth to the ear.	• Heat increases blood supply and reduces discomfort.
• Have the child blow a pinwheel to relieve pressure in ear.	• Attempts to open the eustachian tube may help aerate the middle ear.

EXPECTED OUTCOME: Verbal child will state that pain is relieved. Nonverbal child will exhibit improved disposition and comfort.

2. Nursing Diagnosis: *Infection, Risk for*, related to presence of pathogens (NANDA-I © 2014)

GOAL: The child will be free of infection.

INTERVENTION	RATIONALE
• Encourage breastfeeding of infants.	• Breastfeeding affords natural immunity to infectious agents.
• Instruct the parents to administer antibiotics exactly as directed and to complete prescribed course of medication.	• Taking antibiotics as prescribed minimizes chance for overgrowth of pathogens.
• Telephone the parents 2 or 3 days after initial examination.	• If symptoms have not improved in 36 hours, treatment should be evaluated.
• Examine ear 3 or 4 days after completion of antibiotic treatment, or if symptoms worsen in child on symptomatic treatment.	• Checkup determines whether treatment is effective.

EXPECTED OUTCOME: Child's temperature will be normal, symptoms will disappear, and tympanic membrane will show no signs of infection.

3. Nursing Diagnosis: *Development: Delayed, Risk for*, related to hearing loss (NANDA-I © 2014)

GOAL: The child will have normal hearing.

INTERVENTION	RATIONALE
• Assess hearing ability frequently.	• Monitoring detects hearing loss early.

EXPECTED OUTCOME: Child's general health and hearing will improve, and incidence of the condition will decrease.

GOAL: The child will have normal motor and language development.

INTERVENTION	RATIONALE
• Assess motor and language development at each healthcare visit.	• Early detection of developmental delays can lead to appropriate intervention.

EXPECTED OUTCOME: Child will have language and motor development within norms for age group.

Emphasize preventive measures. Exposure to secondhand smoke in the home increases the incidence of otitis media in children, so encourage parents who smoke to avoid smoking near the child or in the home. Wood-burning stoves should also be avoided when possible. If young children are in child care with fewer than 10 children, incidence decreases. Breastfeeding provides some protection from the disease. Placing infants or toddlers to sleep with a pacifier may increase incidence and should be avoided in the infant with prior infections. Many cases of otitis media are related to microbials such as *H. influenzae* and *Pneumococcus pneumoniae*, so immunization against these pathogens (see Chapter 43) can be effective preventive measures.

Help parents understand why there is a waiting period before prescriptions are given for antibiotics. When antibiotics are prescribed, review administration techniques, side effects, and the need for a repeat appointment when the medication is completed.

Chronic otitis media can create problems for the family. The child's waking at night with ear pain results in lack of sleep and parental fatigue. Since many children with otitis media experience ear pain that can disrupt their sleep and that of family members, anesthetic ear drops have been used for their analgesic effect on the tympanic membrane, and some families might prefer use of natural remedies for ear pain. Herbal extract ear drops (a naturopathic herbal extract of *Allium sativum, Verbascum thapsus, Calendula flores, Hypericum perforatum*, lavender, and vitamin E) with a local anesthetic of amethocaine and phenazone have been used. Parents often become frustrated and disillusioned by the healthcare system's inability to cure the child and may fear a permanent hearing impairment. Reassure parents that as the child grows older, the recurrent infections eventually cease. Teach them that asking for courses of antibiotics for every infection may not be the best treatment.

Provide pain relief techniques such as teaching correct administration of ear drops, oral administration of acetaminophen, and positioning the baby with the head slightly elevated.

Provide hearing and language examinations at regular intervals, inform parents of results, and refer to an audiology specialist if hearing problems are identified. Make sure parents of children with tympanostomy tubes know how to care for the child and what symptoms to report. For the child with some hearing loss due to otitis media with effusion, a home environment that fosters cognitive skills can overcome the effects of lowered hearing during the time of infection. Focus interventions on helping parents to read and talk with children frequently who have otitis media with effusion.

Evaluation

Expected outcomes of nursing care for the child with otitis media include the following:

- The child returns to normal sleep and feeding patterns.
- The child maintains normal hearing and speech development.
- Pain and temperature are effectively managed.
- Parents demonstrate understanding of the treatment regimen.

Otitis Externa

Otitis externa is an inflammation of the skin and surrounding soft tissue of the ear canal. It is sometimes called "swimmer's ear" because it is common in children who swim frequently, especially during hot and muggy weather. The ear canal can also be injured by use of cotton-tipped applicators, foreign objects, or sprays used near the face. If the tympanic membrane is not intact because of tympanostomy tubes or breakage of the membrane, drainage may be visible in the canal; this drainage may irritate the canal and lead to otitis externa. Any irritation of the canal can become infected with bacteria, virus, or fungi; sometimes it represents an allergic reaction. The child usually complains of pain and itching, and may have intense pain when the examiner presses on the tragus, or skin tab in front of the ear. Sometimes the ear appears swollen, and redness or drainage of the canal may be seen upon otoscopic examination.

Treatment of otitis externa requires removing the dried and flaking epithelium and cerumen. Burrow solutions or normal saline is used to irrigate and clean the canal if the tympanic membrane is intact. Steroid ear drops are used to decrease inflammation, and antibiotic drops are also used if a bacterial infection is suspected. If the child has tympanostomy tubes or a perforated tympanic membrane, nonototoxic ear antibiotic such as quinolone antibiotic ear drops are used. Ibuprofen or acetaminophen may be helpful for pain control. The ear canal should then be kept dry by using ear plugs or a swim cap for swimming and gently blow-drying the canal after bathing. The child should not return to swimming for about 5 days. Cotton-tipped applicators or other objects should not be placed in the ear canal so that the skin in the canal can heal. If hair sprays or other solutions are irritating, they should not be used by the child or adolescent.

Nurses should be aware of the signs of otitis externa such as a painful ear, drainage, and irritated canal. Verify that the tympanic membrane is intact during otoscopic examination. Teach families to avoid the irritants identified such as cotton-tipped applicators, sprays, and frequent swimming. Demonstrate proper instillation of drops (see the *Clinical Skills Manual* `SKILLS`) and give instructions for use of acetaminophen for pain relief in the acute period.

Hearing Impairment

About 1.6% of newborns do not pass the newborn hearing examination (Centers for Disease Control and Prevention [CDC], 2012). Additional children receive a diagnosis after the newborn period, and approximately 1 million children (2–3 of every 100 births) in the United States have some form of hearing impairment (National Institute of Deafness and Other Communication Disorders, [NIDCD], 2014). Hearing impairment is expressed in terms of **decibels (dB)**, which are units of loudness, and rated according to severity (Table 45–8). Children who have a mild hearing loss (35 to 40 dB) may miss 50% of everyday conversation and are considered at high risk for school failure. Children with a hearing loss of more than 80 dB are considered legally deaf.

Hearing disorders can be classified according to the location of the deficit. **Conductive hearing loss** occurs when conditions in the external auditory canal or tympanic membrane prevent sound from reaching the middle ear. **Sensorineural hearing loss** occurs when the hair cells in the cochlea or along the vestibulocochlear (acoustic) nerve (cranial nerve VIII) are damaged. This leads to permanent hearing loss. A **mixed hearing loss** indicates a hearing loss having a combination of conductive and sensorineural causes.

ETIOLOGY AND PATHOPHYSIOLOGY

About 50% of hearing loss is genetically caused, generally in a recessive inheritance pattern with *GJB2* gene abnormalities (American Speech-Language-Hearing Association [ASLHA], 2011). Another 25% is due to environmental causes around the time of birth. Acquired causes are due to injury or disease later in life such as frequent ear infections, infectious diseases, ototoxic drugs, head injury, and noise exposure (ASLHA, 2011). This type of loss is increasing; hearing loss among all populations has doubled in the past 30 years, and now approximately 14.9% of U.S. children have low-frequency or high-frequency hearing loss of at least 16-dB hearing level in one or both ears (ASLHA, 2014). Infants at risk for hearing loss include those with:

TABLE 45–8 Severity of Hearing Loss

TYPE OF LOSS	HEARING ABILITY
Slight/mild (20–40 dB)	Some speech sounds are difficult to perceive, particularly unvoiced consonant sounds.
Moderate (41–60 dB)	Most normal conversational speech sounds are missed.
Severe (61–80 dB)	Speech sounds cannot be heard at a normal conversational level.
Profound (81–90 dB)	No speech sounds can be heard; considered legally deaf.
Deaf (over 90 dB)	No sound at all can be heard.

Source: Data from American Speech-Language-Hearing Association. (2011). *Type, degree, and configuration of hearing loss.* Retrieved from http://www.asha.org/public/hearing/disorders/types .htm

- Family history of congenital hearing loss
- Positive titer for TORCH infections (toxoplasmosis, rubella, cytomegalovirus, syphilis, herpes)
- Craniofacial abnormalities
- Very low birth weight (less than 1500 g [3.3 lb])
- Stay in neonatal intensive care unit of over 5 days, or need for extracorporeal membrane oxygenation (ECMO), assisted ventilation, administration of ototoxic medications (e.g., gentamicin, tobramycin) or loop diuretics (e.g., furosemide), or hyperbilirubinemia that requires exchange transfusion
- Chemotherapy, particularly with aminoglycoside medications over 5 days
- Low Apgar score at 1 or 5 minutes
- Bacterial or viral meningitis
- Head trauma, especially basal skull/temporal bone fractures requiring hospitalization
- Mechanical ventilation for more than 5 days
- Caregiver concern regarding speech, language, hearing, developmental delay
- Presence of syndromes associated with hearing loss (Down syndrome, Pierre Robin syndrome, Arnold-Chiari malformation, neurofibromatosis, osteopetrosis, Hunter syndrome) (Joint Committee on Infant Hearing, 2007, 2008)

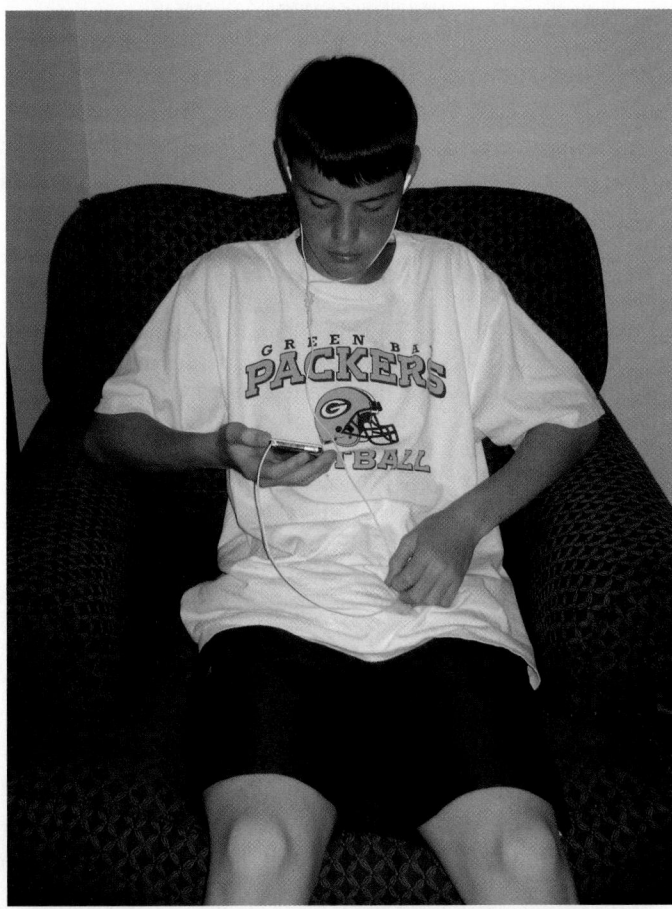

Figure 45–7   **Listening to loud music with headphones or at rock concerts is a frequent cause of hearing loss among teenagers and young adults. This adolescent needs to be informed about the possible outcomes of this activity.**

Common causes of conductive hearing loss include impacted cerumen, the most frequent reason for conductive loss; outer ear infection ("swimmer's ear"); trauma; or a foreign body. Conductive loss also occurs if the tympanic membrane does not fully vibrate, as in otitis media. In these cases, hearing loss may be restored after the infection clears. Chronic and untreated ear infections may lead to structural changes in the ear and permanent hearing impairment. The loss of acuity may be gradual or rapid and results in diminished hearing in all ranges.

Conditions leading to sensorineural hearing loss may be congenital (maternal rubella), genetic (Tay-Sachs disease), or acquired (such as from ototoxic drugs, bacterial meningitis, or loud noise). In sensorineural hearing loss, high-frequency sounds are most affected. Such hearing loss may be preceded by **tinnitus** or ringing in the ears. Teenagers who use earphones at high volumes or attend many rock concerts are at risk for hearing loss (Figure 45–7). Other noise hazards include firecrackers, guns, and power and farm equipment.

CLINICAL MANIFESTATIONS

Hearing is both an innate and a learned behavior. Infants and children who have hearing impairments exhibit a range of behaviors, depending on their age and the severity of the deficit. Infants who hear normally respond to sound in both obvious and subtle ways that do not occur in those who have hearing impairments (Table 45–9). As children mature, their hearing

TABLE 45–9 Behaviors Suggestive of Hearing Impairment

AGE	BEHAVIOR
Infant	Has a diminished or absent startle reflex to loud sound.
	Does not awaken when environment is very noisy.
	Awakens only to touch.
	Does not turn head to sound at 3–4 months.
	Does not localize sound at 6–10 months.
	Babbles little or not at all.
Toddler and preschooler	Speaks unintelligibly, in a monotone, or not at all.
	Communicates needs through gestures.
	Appears developmentally delayed.
	Appears emotionally immature, yells inappropriately.
	Does not respond to doorbell or telephone.
	Appears more interested in objects than people and prefers to play alone.
	Focuses on facial expressions rather than verbal communications.
School-age child and adolescent	Asks to have statements repeated.
	Answers questions inappropriately, except when able to view speaker's face.
	Daydreams and is inattentive.
	Performs poorly at school or is truant.
	Has speech abnormalities or speaks in a monotone.
	Sits close to or turns television or radio up loudly.
	Prefers to play alone.

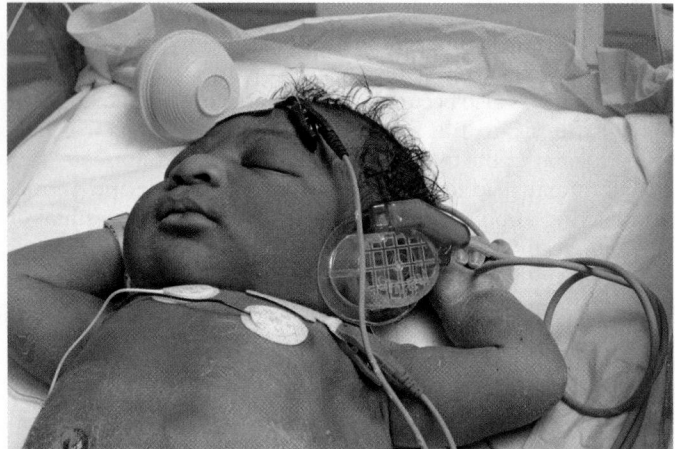

Figure 45–8 Newborn hearing screening is an effective tool in diagnosing some causes of hearing impairment very early in life.

impairments affect their language skills. Hearing loss is often manifested as a cognitive deficit, a behavioral problem, or both.

CLINICAL THERAPY

Early identification of hearing loss is a key element in successful treatment (see *Growth and Development*). Detection of hearing loss in infants is important to ensure optimal development. Universal screening of all infants is recommended before 1 month of age, with diagnostic audiologic evaluation before 3 months, and beginning of early intervention programs by 6 months of age for those with hearing impairment. State laws now mandate screening of newborns, and national data are maintained on outcomes. Observations of response to noise in all newborns should be accompanied by more sophisticated testing such as auditory brain stem response or transient evoked otoacoustic emissions, especially in those at high risk of deficits (Figure 45–8). All children should be evaluated for communication development beginning at 2 months of age during all well-child visits (American Academy of Pediatrics Committee on Practice and Ambulatory and Bright Futures Periodicity Schedule Work Group, 2014). See Table 45–10.

Growth and Development

Children with hearing loss can easily fall behind their peers in language milestones since they cannot hear and speak in the same manner as other children. Without interventions to enable them to learn language, they can also fail to develop reading and other literacy skills, related cognitive processes, and social-emotional development (Joint Committee on Infant Hearing, 2007). Carefully evaluate hearing and all developmental milestones during each regularly scheduled healthcare visit. Refer infants and children with abnormalities for further evaluation. When hearing loss is identified as a cause of delayed development, interventions guided by healthcare providers with expertise in hearing loss are needed.

An otoscopic examination with a tympanogram can be performed on an older infant to determine conductive hearing loss. The **tympanogram** is a test that provides a graph of the ability of the middle ear to transmit sound. An airtight probe is inserted into the external ear canal and a tone is emitted. The probe measures the pressure, which is plotted on a graph. A "flat" tympanogram suggests conductive hearing loss. **Audiography** can be used with cooperative children over 3 years of age. Sounds

TABLE 45–10 Screening Tests for Newborn Hearing

TEST	MECHANISM OF ACTION
Otoacoustic emission (OAE) (either transient-evoked [TEOAE] or distortion-product [DPOAE])	A measure of low-intensity sounds from the cochlear hair cells in response to clicks from a probe placed in the ear canal
	Sensitive in frequency range above 1500 Hz
	May show false negative for loss below 1000–1500 Hz
	Detects inner ear hearing loss by evaluating cochlear and hair cell function
	Does not detect neural damage to cranial nerve VIII
	Can be sensitive to outer ear canal obstruction or middle ear effusion, leading to false positive result
Auditory brainstem response (ABR)	Electrical response to auditory stimuli from three surface scalp electrodes
	Reflects activity of cochlea, cranial nerve VIII, and auditory brainstem pathways
	Detect hearing loss from 1000–8000 Hz
	May show false-negative results for losses in the 500- to 2000-Hz levels
	Will give a positive result if there is damage to cranial nerve VIII or brainstem pathways even if cochlear loss is not present

of various frequencies and intensities are presented to the child through earphones, and the child is instructed to raise a hand when the sound is heard. Audiography cannot detect hearing loss caused by middle ear effusion but can indicate sensorineural loss.

The hearing of preschool and school-age children is tested by asking them to repeat whispered words. Hearing of school-age children and adolescents also is assessed with the Weber and Rinne tests (see Chapter 33).

If a hearing loss is uncorrectable, a collaborative care team composed of pediatrician, audiologist, otolaryngologist, speech–language pathologist, nurse, teacher, and social worker should help the child and family adapt to the disability. If the deficit is due to recurrent ear infections, tympanostomy tube insertion may improve hearing.

A hearing aid may be prescribed for a conductive loss. A sensorineural loss is more difficult to treat, but cochlear implants and bone conduction hearing aids have been used in some children. A cochlear implant is a small electronic device that helps to provide sound for those who are deaf or profoundly hard of hearing. It consists of the following:

1. A microphone to pick up sound that is located outside of the body; worn as a headpiece behind the ear

2. A speech processor that organizes sound from the microphone; worn behind the ear or on a belt

3. A transmitter that transfers the sound into electrical impulses; part of the headpiece behind the ear

4. Electrodes that send the signals to the brain; this receiver is implanted in the skin behind the ear with a wire leading to the cochlear fluid in the middle ear

TABLE 45–11 Communication Techniques for Children Who Have a Hearing Impairment

TECHNIQUE	DESCRIPTION
Cued speech	Supplement to lipreading; eight hand shapes represent groups of consonant sounds and four positions about the face represent groups of vowel sounds; based on the sounds the letters make, not the letters themselves; child can "see-hear" every spoken syllable a hearing person hears
Oral approach	Uses only spoken language for face-to-face communication; avoids use of formal signs; uses hearing aids and residual hearing
Total communication	Uses speech and sign, fingerspelling, lipreading, and residual hearing simultaneously; child selects communication technique depending on the situation

For children with uncorrectable hearing loss, several approaches are used to enhance communication (Table 45–11). Children with hearing impairments may receive speech therapy and instructions in lipreading, sign language, cuing, and fingerspelling.

Growth and Development

Infants and young children respond automatically with a blink or the startle reflex to unexpected or loud noises. As they mature, they localize the sound source, then understand speech, and then communicate verbally.

Nursing Management

For the Child With a Hearing Impairment

Nursing Assessment and Diagnosis

Nurses conduct newborn hearing tests soon after birth and make observations of the infant's responses to sound. As the child grows, assess hearing at every well-child visit. The best judges of hearing are parents; ask them if they have any concerns about their child's hearing. An infant's reaction to rattles, bells, or handclapping (about 30 cm [12 in.] from the ear) is an important observation. Evaluate language milestones when examining the older infant and child. Language development is a major area of focus in deaf children. Deaf infants begin to babble at about 5 to 6 months of age, the same age as hearing infants. However, this babbling ceases several months later in the child who has a hearing impairment.

School nurses use audiometers to evaluate hearing during screening programs in schools, and refer children who do not pass the screening test (see the *Clinical Skills Manual* `SKILLS`). Measures to promote speech and communication development as well as safety are implemented.

Common nursing diagnoses for the child with impaired hearing include the following (NANDA-I © 2014):

- *Communication: Verbal, Impaired*, related to abnormal sound transmission
- *Development: Delayed, Risk for*, related to communication impairment
- *Coping: Family, Readiness for Enhanced*, related to caring for a child with a hearing impairment

Planning and Implementation

Nurses can encourage prevention of hearing loss from exposure to loud noises such as loud music and power and farm equipment. Music should be turned down and ear protection worn for other activities. School nurses should be active in hearing conservation education programs in school. Several programs are available to assist the school nurse in teaching children at targeted ages about noise-induced hearing loss. The nurse should develop and deliver hearing conservation curricula to children at elementary, middle, and high school levels; inform teachers and other healthcare professionals about noise-induced hearing loss; and train volunteers to assist with school programs.

Newborn screening, developmental assessment, and childhood hearing screening facilitate identification of hearing loss in newborns, infants, and children. Newborns and infants should be tested for hearing loss by 1 month of age. In cases of loss, intervention should begin before 6 months of age (Joint Committee on Infant Hearing, 2007).

Nursing care of the child with a hearing impairment focuses on facilitating the child's ability to receive spoken language and to send information, helping parents meet the child's schooling needs, and providing emotional support to parents. Refer the parents to an early intervention program as soon as the diagnosis of hearing impairment is made, in order to foster the child's development. If a cochlear implant is planned, the child needs surgical care and follow-up to monitor results and integrate sound gradually into the child's life. Pneumococcal and meningococcal vaccines and ongoing speech therapy are needed.

FACILITATE ABILITY TO RECEIVE SPOKEN LANGUAGE

Be aware of how the child compensates for hearing loss and use these strategies in communication:

- If hearing loss is mild or temporary or if the child reads lips, first obtain the child's visual attention by lightly touching the child or saying the child's name.
- Position your face 1 to 2 m (3 to 6 ft) from the child's face and make sure that the child's eyes are focused on your face and lips. Make sure the room is well lit, with no backlighting. Speak at a normal rate and tone, and use facial expressions that show caring or concern. If the child does not understand, rephrase the information in shorter, simpler sentences. Use specific, concrete explanations, and give the child time to comprehend. Watch for subtle signs of misinterpretations and give consistent and immediate feedback since only 30% of the English language is visible on the lips.
- Be familiar with the different types of hearing aids. Hearing aids, which are microphones that amplify all sounds, can be worn in or behind the ear, in the frame of glasses, or on the body with a wire attached to the ear. Place the hearing aid in the ear with the volume off, then slowly turn up to half volume. Adjust as needed. When talking to a child with a hearing aid, speak slowly within 15 to 45 cm (6 to 18 in.) of the microphone using a normal conversational tone. Talk to the child even if the child is not looking at you. Make sure the batteries are fresh for the best reception. Since all sound is amplified, reduce background noise as much as possible. Clean the hearing aid daily with a damp cloth. Change the batteries as needed, usually about once a week. The child's growth necessitates a new fitting, usually about once annually.

Health Promotion The Child With a Hearing Impairment

Growth and Developmental Surveillance

- Ensure that the child receives all immunizations at scheduled times. All children with cochlear implants should have pneumococcal vaccine (PCV7 for under 5 years of age or PPV23 for over 5 years). The immunization should be completed 2 weeks before surgery for cochlear implant. Children should be up-to-date on all immunizations, but rubella, mumps, and measles are especially important since infections with the diseases could cause further hearing loss.

- Complete developmental assessment, including receptive and expressive verbal skills at each visit.

- Teach about safety precautions for those with hearing impairment, such as inability to hear announcements at school, fire alarms at home, or sirens when traveling. Assist the family to install visual stimuli for fire alarms and other safety needs.

Communication

- Review the type of communication used by the child and the family's satisfaction.

- Ask about relationships with other children, both those with hearing impairments and those without.

- Review discipline techniques used by the parents and consistency of limit setting.

Nutrition and Physical Activity

- Complete 24-hour diet recall and be sure the child receives adequate nutrition appropriate in energy for activities.

- Review the child's exercise patterns since some children with hearing impairment may avoid interactions with other children in sports.

- Refer the family to community activity programs as needed.

Mental Health

- Determine stressors parents may feel.

- Locate community resources for early intervention and ongoing programs.

- Assist the youth and family to plan for moves to new schools and communities, and for plans related to transition to young adulthood, including college, trade schools, or work in the community.

Disease Prevention Strategies

- Be sure signs of ear infection such as fever, irritability, disturbed sleep, rubbing ear, or ear drainage are promptly evaluated in the pediatric healthcare home.

- Teach parents to administer antibiotics for ear infections exactly as prescribed.

- Encourage breastfeeding of infants and avoiding smoking to minimize incidence of ear infections.

- Be sure the child has all recommended immunizations.

Injury Prevention Strategies

- Encourage family to preserve any hearing the child may have by avoiding exposure to loud sounds; when children are old enough to understand, be sure they safeguard against exposure to loud music, guns, and other risks.

- Teach the child and family to plan for safety when crossing streets, driving cars, escaping house fires, and other situations that normally rely on hearing.

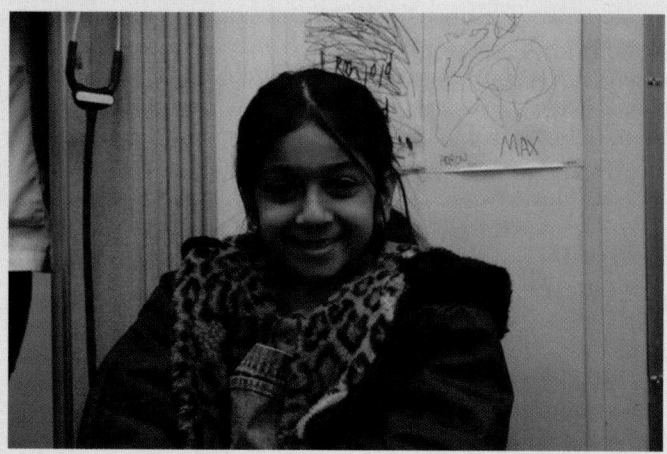

Acoustic feedback, an audible whistling sound that cannot always be heard by the child, is one of the most common problems with hearing aids. To eliminate this sound, readjust the hearing aid to make sure that it is inserted properly and that no hair or ear wax is caught between the ear mold and canal. Turning down the volume may also help. (See *Health Promotion: The Child With a Hearing Impairment*.)

A remote microphone system is another type of device designed to improve hearing. This is often used in the classroom situation because it eliminates background noise. The speaker wears a transmitter that picks up the voice and transmits it to a receiver worn by the child.

FACILITATE ABILITY TO SEND INFORMATION

Maintain the child's hearing aid in proper condition. Many children with impaired hearing communicate using speech, which is enhanced through speech therapy. In addition, they are taught to sign, fingerspell, or use cued speech (Figure 45–9). Articulation may be difficult, and understanding what the child is trying to say may be frustrating for both the nurse and the child. Taking time to listen carefully is important.

Take measures to promote speech and communication development as well as safety. Ask the parents to explain the child's communication techniques and to help interpret words. Have younger children point to pictures. Use assisted technologies such as a computer or picture board as well as drawings or gestures if necessary. This is especially helpful for communicating feelings of pain and hunger during hospitalization. If the child signs or fingerspells, make sure that you understand the signs for important functions. Give older children a pad of paper and pencil to write requests. People other than parents should be able to understand what the child is trying to communicate. Have an interpreter available if the child uses American Sign Language. Learn some common signs to communicate

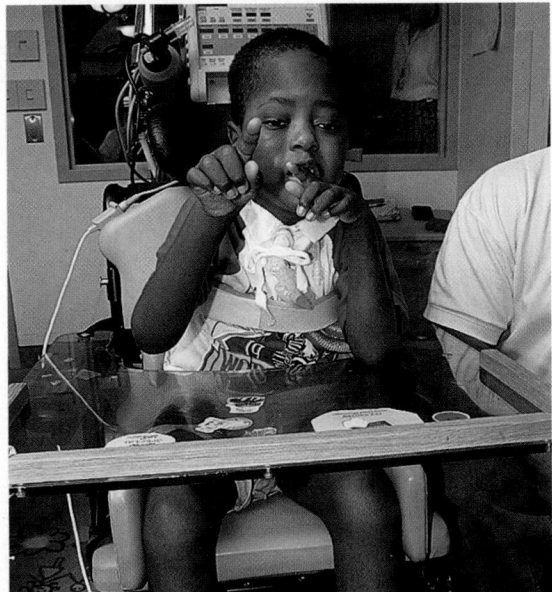

Figure 45–9 **This child with a hearing impairment and tracheostomy is communicating by means of American Sign Language (ASL).**

simple words or phrases. Orient the child carefully to new settings such as the hospital room or a new school.

HELP PARENTS TO MEET CHILD'S EDUCATIONAL NEEDS

Public laws apply to the education of children who have a hearing impairment (see Chapter 1). After diagnosis, the parents and professionals together agree on an individualized education plan (see discussion in Chapter 38). Day care and preschool are recommended for children with hearing problems.

- Give parents information about adjustments that may have to be made for a child with a hearing impairment who attends public school. By sitting at the front of the classroom, the child may be able to hear and see more clearly. The teacher should always face the child when speaking, and background noise should be reduced.

- Tell parents that children who have hearing impairments have the same intelligence quotient (IQ) distribution as children without a hearing impairment. However, communication and learning can be difficult, and extra support is needed.

- Children with a hearing impairment should reach their intellectual potential, although development in certain areas may take place more slowly than it does in children without a hearing impairment.

PROVIDE EMOTIONAL SUPPORT

By recognizing the effects of the diagnosis on the family, the nurse can help the family deal with their reaction to the child's hearing loss. Supporting healthy coping is an important intervention to help the parents carry on with their lives.

- Help the parents understand the child's disability and its effect on speech and language development. Provide accurate information about their concerns. Work jointly with other professionals and social service workers if necessary.

- Tell the family about the community services available for medical, nursing, psychologic, and financial assistance.

Evaluation

Expected outcomes of nursing care for a child with a hearing impairment include the following:

- The child is assisted in establishment of communication method.
- The child manifests growth and development to maximum potential.
- A successful individualized education plan is established.
- The family demonstrates positive coping and healthcare management.

Injuries of the Ear

Ear injuries of many types commonly occur in children. Lacerations, infections, and hematomas may occur in the external ear structures, especially the pinna. Children may place foreign objects in the ear, and insects may enter the ear canal. Rupture of the tympanic membrane may result from head injuries, blows to the ear, or insertion of objects into the ear canal. Caution children and parents not to place anything into the ear, including cotton swabs for cleaning.

See Table 45–12 for information on the emergency treatment of ear injuries. Any injury resulting in earache, decreased hearing, persistent bleeding, or other discharge should be seen by a healthcare provider.

Disorders of the Nose and Throat

Epistaxis

Epistaxis, or nosebleed, is common in school-age children, especially boys. The Kiesselbach plexus, an area of plentiful veins located in the anterior nares, is the most common source of bleeding. The most common cause is irritation from nosepicking, foreign bodies, or low humidity. Other causes include forceful coughing, allergies, or infections resulting in congestion of the nasal mucosa. Posterior nosebleeds have a variety of causes, some of which may indicate systemic disease (i.e., bleeding disorder) or injury. Bleeding from the posterior septum is more serious and may be life threatening. Hospitalization may be necessary.

Nursing Management

Children with nosebleeds are sometimes brought to the emergency department by a parent who has been unable to stop the flow of blood within a few minutes. Both parent and child may be frightened. Ask the parent briefly about any history of nosebleeds and other contributing factors, including medications. Take the child's pulse and blood pressure to assess for excessive blood loss. Carefully examine the nasal mucosa by asking the child to blow any clots out gently, if possible. Suctioning may be necessary.

Observing the flow may help determine whether the blood is coming from an anterior or a posterior location. A nosebleed confined to one side of the nose is almost always anterior, but posterior bleeding can flow on one or both sides. If blood cannot be seen, the child may be swallowing it and may become nauseated. Suspect posterior bleeding in children who have sustained blunt trauma to the head.

TABLE 45–12 Emergency Treatment of Ear Injuries

INJURY	TREATMENT
PINNA	
Minor cuts or abrasions	Wash thoroughly with soap and water and rinse well; leave exposed to air if possible or apply adhesive bandage; monitor for infection.
Hematomas	Needle aspiration should be performed and pressure dressing applied; undrained hematomas may become fibrotic; "cauliflower ear" deformity may develop.
Cellulitis or abscesses	Apply moist heat intermittently; make sure that prescribed antibiotic is taken; minor surgery may be performed for an abscess.
Deep lacerations	Apply pressure to stop bleeding; transport to healthcare provider's office or emergency department for suturing.
EAR CANAL	
Foreign bodies	Have child lie on back and turn head over edge of bed, with affected side down; wiggle earlobe and have child shake head; foreign object may fall out as result of gravity; if object remains in ear, call healthcare provider; do not try to remove foreign body with tweezers since this may push the object further into the ear.
Insects	Shine flashlights into ear to try to attract insect; instilling a few drops of mineral oil, olive oil, or alcohol kills insect, and irrigating ear canal gently may remove dead insect. See the *Clinical Skills Manual* `SKILLS`.
TYMPANIC MEMBRANE	
Ruptures	Call healthcare provider if child has persistent ear pain after blow, blast injury, or insertion of foreign object; cover external ear loosely with piece of sterile cotton or gauze; if tympanic membrane has been ruptured, systemic antibiotics are prescribed.

The child with anterior bleeding should sit upright quietly. The head should be tilted forward to prevent blood from trickling down the throat, which can lead to vomiting. The nares should be squeezed just below the nasal bone and held for 10 to 15 minutes while the child breathes through the mouth. If the bleeding does not stop, a cotton ball or swab soaked with Neo-Synephrine, epinephrine, thrombin, or lidocaine may be inserted into the affected nostril to promote topical vasoconstriction or anesthesia. Once the bleeding has stopped, the nostril may have to be cauterized with silver nitrate or electrocautery. If the bleeding cannot be stopped, absorbable packing may be used.

Posterior bleeding must also be stopped by packing, and the child must be monitored carefully. Arterial ligation is occasionally needed. Repeated or severe nosebleeds need further evaluation (Montague, Whymark, Howatson, et al., 2011).

Assess the child's hematocrit or hemoglobin if significant bleeding has occurred. Take a complete history and do a physical examination of children with frequent epistaxis to rule out systemic disease. (See *Teaching Highlights: Prevention and Home Management of Epistaxis*.)

After the nosebleed has stopped, the child is more vulnerable to recurrent bleeding and should avoid bending over, stooping, strenuous exercise, hot drinks, and hot baths or showers for the next 3 to 4 days. Sleeping with the head elevated on two or three pillows and humidifying the air with a vaporizer may also prevent a recurrence. Give parents suggestions for prevention and home management of epistaxis.

TEACHING HIGHLIGHTS | Prevention and Home Management of Epistaxis

Prevention

- Humidify the child's room, especially during the winter.
- Discourage the child from picking or rubbing the nose or inserting foreign objects in the nose.
- Instruct the child to blow the nose gently and release sneezes through the mouth.

Home Management

- Keep the child calm.
- Sit the child upright with head tilted slightly forward so blood does not run down the nasopharynx.

- Press a roll of cotton under the upper lip to compress the labial artery.
- Apply steady pressure to both nostrils just below the nasal bone with the thumb and forefinger for 15 to 20 minutes. Time by the clock.
- Apply an ice pack or cold compress to the bridge of the nose or the back of the neck.
- Call healthcare provider if the bleeding does not stop.
- Avoid vigorous exercise and aspirin or other noncoagulant drugs during the first few days after an episode of epistaxis.

Source: Adapted from Melia, L., & McGarry, G. W. (2011). Epistaxis: Update on management. *Current Opinion in Otolaryngology & Head and Neck Surgery, 19*, 30–35.

Nasopharyngitis

Nasopharyngitis, also known as upper respiratory infection (URI) or the "common cold," causes inflammation and infection of the nose and throat and is a common illness of infancy and childhood. More than 200 viruses and numerous bacteria can cause this condition. The most common viruses include rhinovirus and coronavirus, and the most frequently occurring bacterium is group A *Streptococcus*. See Chapter 46 for a discussion of respiratory syncytial virus (RSV), a common cause of both upper and lower respiratory illness. The organisms incubate in 1 to 3 days, and the infection is communicable several hours before symptoms develop and for 1 to 2 days after they begin. Symptoms may last 4 to 10 days or longer. The pathogens spread when the infected person touches the hand of an uninfected person, who then touches the mouth or nose, resulting in self-inoculation with infected droplets.

A red nasal mucosa with clear nasal discharge and an infected throat with enlarged tonsils may be apparent in children with nasopharyngitis. Vesicles may be present on the soft palate and in the pharynx. Accompanying symptoms may vary, depending on the child's age (Table 45–13).

Between episodes of nasopharyngitis, the child should be asymptomatic. If a child continues to have upper respiratory infections, an underlying condition such as allergy, asthma, or polyps should be ruled out.

Nursing Management

For infants who cannot breathe through the mouth, normal saline nose drops can be administered every 3 to 4 hours, especially before feeding, and followed by bulb suctioning if needed (see the *Clinical Skills Manual* SKILLS). For infants over 9 months of age, nasal stuffiness can be treated with normal saline. Children over 6 years of age can use nasal sprays.

TABLE 45–13 Manifestations of Nasopharyngitis

INFANTS YOUNGER THAN 3 MONTHS OF AGE

Lethargy	Feeding poorly
Irritability	Fever (may be absent)

INFANTS 3 MONTHS OF AGE OR OLDER

Fever	Anorexia
Vomiting	Irritability
Diarrhea	Restlessness
Sneezing	

OLDER CHILDREN

Dry, irritated nose and throat

Chills, fever

Generalized muscle aches

Headache

Malaise

Anorexia

Thin nasal discharge, which may later become thick and purulent

Sneezing

Decongestant nose drops and sprays should not be used for more than 4 or 5 days or more often than recommended. Antihistamines may be helpful for children with allergic rhinitis or profuse nasal drainage. Long-acting nasal sprays and medications with several ingredients are not recommended. (See *Teaching Highlights: Over-the-Counter Cough and Cold Medications*.)

Room humidification may help prevent drying of nasal secretions. Antipyretics such as acetaminophen reduce fever and make the child more comfortable. Aspirin is not recommended because of its association with Reye syndrome (refer to Chapter 54).

TEACHING HIGHLIGHTS | Over-the-Counter Cough and Cold Medications

Parents may try to treat children who have upper respiratory infections with the same medications they are accustomed to taking for a cold. Work with parents during a health promotion visit and help them plan for how to handle medications for the child. Guidelines are as follows:

- Do NOT use cough and cold products in children under 2 years of age unless given specific directions to do so by a healthcare provider.
- Read the label to be sure the medication is recommended for the child's age and condition. Give only the dose recommended for the age and weight of the child. Do NOT use products packaged for adults.
- Be sure you know how to measure the medication. Tablespoon and teaspoon are not the same, and using household spoons may lead to incorrect dosing. Use only the measuring device that is provided with liquid medications to ensure accuracy. If one is not provided, purchase one at the pharmacy that is precisely labeled. Use only a measuring device with the precise marking to match the dose you need to give.

- Consult the pharmacist, nurse, or other healthcare provider if you have questions, if the child is taking other medicines, if the medication is not recommended for the age of the child, if the child's condition does not improve, or if other symptoms appear.
- Use the child-resistant cap after each opening of the bottle. Store the medication out of reach of all children, preferably in a locked location.
- Inspect containers and do not buy those that may have tears, imperfections, or tampering. Review all of the information in the "Drug Facts" box on the package label.
- If you use home remedies or other herbal products to treat colds, be sure to check on their safety with your healthcare provider first.
- If the child becomes more ill or does not improve, stop the medicine and contact the healthcare provider. If you do not understand instructions on the package contact a healthcare provider before using it.

Source: Adapted from Budnitz, D. S., Lovegrove, M. C., & Rose, K. O. (2014). Adherence to label and device recommendations for over-the-counter pediatric liquid medications. *Pediatrics, 133,* e283–e290; U.S. Food and Drug Administration. (2011). *Public Health Advisory—FDA recommends that over-the-counter (OTC) cough and cold products not be used for infants and children under 2 years of age.* Retrieved from http://www.fda.gov/drugs/drugsafety; U.S. Food and Drug Administration. (2014). *OTC cough and cold products—Not for infants and children under 2 years of age.* Retrieved from http://www.fda.gov /ForConsumers/ConsumerUpdates/ucm048682.htm

Children should avoid strenuous physical activity and engage in quiet play such as reading, listening to music or stories, or watching television or videotapes. Children should not be forced to eat. Encourage the intake of favorite fluids to liquefy secrètions. Tell parents that no medicine or vaccine can prevent the common cold, but eliminating contact with infected persons can reduce the spread of infection. Proper hand hygiene and disposal of tissues helps to decrease the spread of the infection. Cleaning counters, toys, door knobs, and other surfaces on a daily basis can decrease the spread of infections. Discourage sharing of food, dishes, and utensils at meals.

Developing Cultural Competence Hot and Cold Disease Theory

Many Hispanic and Asian cultural groups believe in the "hot and cold theory" of disease, in which health problems are viewed as the result of imbalance. For example, some Mexican Americans traditionally treat a "cold disease" such as an earache or common cold with "hot" substances. Ask families if they prefer to eat certain foods or use complementary treatments during an illness. Incorporating such preferences may help the child and increase the confidence of the family in healthcare providers.

Sinusitis

Sinusitis is an inflammation of one or more of the paranasal sinuses. These sinuses, which have respiratory epithelium and are continuous with the respiratory tract, include the maxillary, ethmoid, frontal, and sphenoid sinuses. The sinuses may become infected with bacteria following a viral upper respiratory infection or allergic inflammation, and therefore sinusitis is a common occurrence in children (Wald et al., 2013).

Sinusitis can be viral or bacterial. Signs and symptoms of sinusitis in children are sometimes nonspecific. A history of recent upper respiratory infection is common, persistent cough from postnasal drip can occur, and nasal discharge or swelling can be apparent. Malodorous breath, fever, mouth breathing, hyponasal speech, and cervical lymphadenopathy may be present. Young children may be anorexic or have difficulty feeding, and older children may complain of headache.

Diagnosis of sinusitis is usually based on history and physical examination findings. Acute bacterial sinusitis is diagnosed when a child with upper respiratory infection (URI) presents persistently (10 days or more) with nasal discharge and or daytime cough, worsening course, or severe onset with temperature 39.0°C (102.2°F) or above and purulent nasal discharge for 3 days or more (Wald et al., 2013). Percussion and illumination of sinuses, computed tomography (CT), magnetic resonance imaging (MRI), and ultrasound are not generally useful in diagnosing sinusitis in children. CT or MRI may be used when orbital or central nervous system complications are suspected. For the child with repeated sinusitis or who appears toxic, aspiration of sinus aspirate may be performed for culture by an otolaryngologist.

Antibiotics are prescribed if there is severe onset or worsening course of illness, and often when there is persistent illness (Wald et al., 2013). Amoxicillin is the first choice for therapy; amoxicillin/clavulanate, cefuroxime, cefdinir, azithromycin, and clarithromycin are also sometimes used. Children with recurrent sinusitis should be referred for further care by an otolaryngologist and allergy specialist. Efficacy of decongestants, antihistamines, and nasal irrigation has not been demonstrated (Shaikh & Wald, 2014).

Parents whose child has persistent and purulent nasal drainage should be told to see a healthcare provider, particularly if the drainage is accompanied by facial pain, headache, and fever. Nurses should teach parents to correctly administer antibiotics (e.g., to take medications for the full course) if prescribed, and to use saline nose drops if needed for comfort. Infants may need their noses cleared with nose drops and a bulb syringe prior to feedings. (Refer to the *Clinical Skills Manual* SKILLS for correct use of a bulb syringe.) Antipyretics can be given for fever and to relieve pain.

Pharyngitis

Acute pharyngitis is an infection that primarily affects the pharynx, including the tonsils. It is seen most frequently in children 4 to 7 years of age and is rare in children less than 1 year of age. Approximately 80% of these infections are caused by viruses; the rest are caused by bacteria. Bacterial pharyngitis is commonly known as "strep throat," since in many cases it is caused by group A beta-hemolytic streptococcus (GABHS) (Ebell, 2014).

The major complaint is a sore throat. Children with symptoms of strep throat who have minimal throat redness and pain, exudate, mild lymphadenopathy, and a low-grade fever, and who have been exposed to someone who has strep pharyngitis should have a throat culture. The classic signs of purulent drainage and white patches are not present in all cases of strep throat.

A child who finds swallowing difficult or extremely painful, who drools, or who exhibits signs of dehydration or respiratory distress should be seen by a healthcare professional immediately. These signs could be indicators of serious conditions such as peritonsillar or retropharyngeal abscess, epiglottitis (Chapter 46), or diphtheria (Chapter 43).

Peritonsillar abscess (a tonsil infection that spreads into surrounding tissues and causes cellulitis) or retropharyngeal abscess (an infection of the lymph nodes that drain the adenoids, nasopharynx, and paranasal sinuses) are serious conditions. These conditions may have additional symptoms such as decreased neck movement, neck edema or pain, and respiratory distress. CT scan or MRI may be helpful in diagnosis of abscess. See Table 45–14 for manifestations of viral pharyngitis, strep throat, peritonsillar abscess, and retropharyngeal abscess.

The diagnosis of strep throat is made by throat culture, using the rapid or traditional strep tests (see the *Clinical Skills Manual* SKILLS). Results of the rapid strep test may be available within minutes; those for the traditional test are available in 24 to 48 hours. A negative rapid test is followed by a traditional test in order to verify results.

Streptococcal pharyngitis is treated with oral penicillin for 10 days or with long-acting penicillin given in one injection. If the child is allergic to penicillin, erythromycin, azithromycin, or clarithromycin is given. Acute symptoms should resolve within 24 hours of therapy, at which time, the child is no longer contagious. For viral pharyngitis, symptomatic treatment alone is used.

Clinical Tip

Throat cultures must be properly performed for accurate diagnosis. Swab a sterile cotton-tip applicator across the tonsils, posterior edge of the soft palate, and uvula. Ask cooperative children to put their hands under their buttocks, open their mouth, and laugh or pant like a dog. Quickly swab the throat. You can place uncooperative and young children on their backs with their hands next to their heads and have a parent or an assistant hold them. Depress the tongue gently with a tongue blade and swab the throat and both tonsils.

TABLE 45–14 Clinical Manifestations of Viral Pharyngitis, Strep Throat (Group A Beta-Hemolytic Streptococcus [GABHS]), Peritonsillar Abscess, and Retropharyngeal Abscess

VIRAL PHARYNGITIS	STREP THROAT	PERITONSILLAR ABSCESS	RETROPHARYNGEAL ABSCESS
Nasal congestion	Abrupt onset	Fever	Fever
Mild sore throat	Tonsillar exudate	Malaise	Sore throat
Conjunctivitis	Painful cervical lymphadenopathy	Sore throat, more severe on one side	Inability to eat
Cough	Anorexia, nausea, vomiting, abdominal pain	Marked erythema and edema, especially of one side of throat, tonsil, and soft palate, sometimes with deviated uvula	Neck pain and edema
Hoarseness			Pharyngitis
Mild pharyngeal redness	Severe sore throat		Respiratory distress and stridor
Minimal tonsillar exudate	Headache, malaise	Mouth odor	
Mildly tender anterior cervical lymphadenopathy	Fever > 38.3°C (101.0°F)	Difficulty speaking	
Fever < 38.3°C (101.0°F)	Petechial mottling of soft palate	Difficulty opening mouth wide	
		Cervical lymphadenitis	
		Ear pain	

Note: Children 6 months to 3 years of age may have streptococcal pharyngitis with symptoms that resemble those of viral pharyngitis. Children with scarlet fever have the symptoms of strep throat plus a sandpaper-textured erythematous generalized rash and pallor around the lips.

Source: Data from Hsiao, H. J., Huang, Y. C., Hsia, S. H., Wu, C. T., & Lin, J. J. (2012). Clinical features of peritonsillar abscess in children. *Pediatric Neonatology, 53*, 366–370; Hoffman, C., Pierrot, L., Contencin, P., Morisseau-Durand, M. P., Manach, Y., & Couloigner, V. (2011). Retropharyngeal infections in children: Treatment strategies and outcomes. *International Journal of Pediatric Otorhinolaryngology, 75*, 1099–1103.

Peritonsillar abscess is treated by draining the abscess, providing antibiotics effective in treating the fluid cultured from the abscess, and hydration. Commonly administered antibiotics include ampicillin/sulbactam, penicillin G, and clindamycin. Once treatment has resolved the infection, the child is evaluated for possible tonsillectomy (Hsaio, Huang, Hsia, et al., 2012). Retropharyngeal abscess is also frequently treated by drainage of the abscess, although intravenous antibiotics alone are effective in some cases. Ampicillin/sulbactam, clindamycin, cephalosporin, and penicillin are common antibiotics. Respiratory management may be needed.

Nursing Management

Nursing care focuses on symptomatic relief. Acetaminophen reduces throat pain and generalized fever. Cool, nonacidic fluids and soft foods, ice chips, or frozen juice pops given frequently in small amounts facilitate swallowing and prevent dehydration. Humidification and gargling with warm salt water (5 g [1 teaspoon] salt to 250 mL [8 oz] water) soothe an irritated throat. Alternatively, the salt water can be placed in a spray bottle and sprayed gently toward the throat. Commercial throat sprays or throat lozenges are not generally more effective than these home remedies. Encourage the child to rest to conserve energy and promote recovery.

Teach parents the importance of completing the 10-day course of antibiotics if prescribed for bacterial pharyngitis. Reinforce to parents the importance of treating streptococcal infections because untreated infections may lead to rheumatic fever, cervical adenitis, sinusitis, glomerulonephritis, or meningitis.

Tonsillitis and Adenoiditis

Tonsillitis is an infection or inflammation (hypertrophy) of the palatine tonsils. Although most children with pharyngitis may have infected tonsils, they do not necessarily have tonsillitis. The adenoids are lymphatic tissue located on the posterior pharyngeal wall and are sometimes called the pharyngeal tonsils; they can manifest with acute or chronic infection.

ETIOLOGY AND PATHOPHYSIOLOGY

Like pharyngitis, tonsillitis and adenoiditis may be caused by a virus or bacterium. The primary site of infection is the tonsils.

CLINICAL MANIFESTATIONS

Symptoms suggestive of tonsillitis include frequent throat infections with breathing and swallowing difficulties, persistent redness of the anterior pillars, and enlargement of the cervical lymph nodes. If children breathe through their mouths continuously, the mucous membranes may become dry and irritated. Adenoiditis is characterized by nasal stuffiness, discharge, and postnasal drip, which result in coughing or excessive clearing of the throat.

CLINICAL THERAPY

Diagnosis is made on the basis of visual inspection and clinical manifestations. Tonsils appear large and inflamed. Enlarged adenoids are diagnosed by radiologic studies.

Symptomatic treatment for tonsillitis is the same as for pharyngitis. Recent guidelines provide clear recommendations for surgery involving repeated infections and sleep-disordered breathing. Watchful waiting is recommended in most cases. Tonsillectomy can be considered when there are at least seven episodes of tonsillitis in the previous year, at least five episodes per year for 2 years, or at least three episodes annually for 3 years. In these cases, tonsillitis diagnosis requires a sore throat and at least one of the following symptoms: temperature above 38.3°C (101.0°F), cervical adenopathy, tonsillar exudate, and positive group A beta-hemolytic streptococcal infection (Giordano et al., 2011). Sleep-disordered breathing that exists with tonsillar hypertrophy and a condition such as growth abnormality, poor school performance, enuresis, or behavioral problem is also appropriate reason for surgical tonsillectomy (Mitka, 2011). One intraoperative dose of intravenous dexamethasone is recommended, but routine operative antibiotics are not needed.

Nursing Management
For the Child With Tonsillitis and Adenoiditis

Nursing Assessment and Diagnosis

Assess the throat carefully during each physical examination. Observe for tonsils that are simply large (a common finding in childhood) and those that are inflamed. Look for the degree of redness and presence of any exudate. Ask if the child has pain or difficulty swallowing. Ask about the history of past tonsillar infections and the length of time of the present discomfort.

If surgery is indicated, take a complete history of the child preoperatively. Monitor vital signs and observe for respiratory distress, hemorrhage, and dehydration postoperatively.

Several nursing diagnoses may apply to the child with tonsillitis. They include the following (NANDA-I © 2014):

- *Pain, Acute*, related to inflammation of the pharynx
- *Fluid Volume: Deficient, Risk for*, related to inadequate intake
- *Breathing Pattern, Ineffective*, related to obstruction by enlarged tonsils
- *Swallowing, Impaired*, related to inflammation and pain
- *Knowledge, Readiness for Enhanced*, related to home care following discharge

Planning and Implementation

The nurse provides general supportive care and, if medication is prescribed, encourages completion of the full course of treatment. The nursing management of children with tonsillitis is similar to that of children with pharyngitis (see earlier discussion).

If surgery is indicated, help the parents prepare their child for a short-term surgical procedure with a possible overnight stay in the hospital (see Chapter 39). Children should be free of sore throat, fever, or upper respiratory infection for at least 1 week before surgery. They should not be given aspirin or ibuprofen for 2 weeks before surgery since these medications can increase postoperative bleeding. Check if any herbal medications are taken and report them to the surgeon and anesthesiologist since some may interfere with anesthetic drugs used in surgery.

DISCHARGE PLANNING AND HOME CARE TEACHING

Discharge planning includes teaching parents about pain management, fluid and nutrition intake, activity restrictions, and possible complications in the postoperative period. Most children have a sore throat for 7 to 10 days after tonsillectomy. Advise parents how to relieve the child's throat pain. (See *Teaching Highlights: Care After Tonsillectomy*.)

Children may experience ear pain, especially when swallowing, between 4 and 8 days after tonsillectomy. Advise parents that this pain is referred from the tonsillar area and does not indicate an ear infection.

Emphasize to parents the importance of adequate fluid intake. Children should be given any liquid they prefer for the first week, except citrus juices, which may produce a burning sensation in the throat. Soft foods such as gelatin, applesauce, frozen juice pops, and mashed potatoes can be added as tolerated.

Children do not need to be confined to bed, but they should avoid vigorous exercise for the first week after surgery. Advise parents that the child may return to school approximately 10 days after tonsillectomy.

TEACHING HIGHLIGHTS | **Care After Tonsillectomy**

After tonsillectomy, the parent can take the following measures to increase the child's comfort:

- Have the child drink adequate cool fluids to reduce spasms in the muscles surrounding the throat.
- Ensure that the child drinks recommended amount of fluid to avoid dehydration.
- Apply an ice collar around the child's neck.

- Give acetaminophen elixir or other analgesic as prescribed.
- Have the child gargle with a solution of 2.5 g (1/2 teaspoon) each of baking soda and salt in a glass of water.
- If ordered by the healthcare provider, have the child rinse the mouth well with viscous lidocaine or other local anesthetic.

TEACHING HIGHLIGHTS | **Complications of Tonsillectomy and Adenoidectomy**

Bleeding

- To prevent bleeding, aspirin or ibuprofen should not be given for pain for the first postoperative week. Use acetaminophen instead.
- Bleeding is most likely to occur within the first 24 hours or 7 to 10 days after the tonsillectomy, when the scar is forming. Report any trickle of bright red blood or increased swallowing to the healthcare provider immediately.

Infection

- The back of the throat will look white and have an odor for the first 7 to 8 days after the surgery. The child may

also have a low-grade fever. These are not signs of infection.

- For temperatures over 38.3°C (101.0°F), acetaminophen may be used.
- Call the healthcare provider if the child develops a fever above 38.8°C (102.0°F).

Pain

- Administer acetaminophen as ordered.
- Offer frequent small amounts of cool liquids. Avoid citrus juice.
- Provide for rest and quiet activities for several days.

TEACHING HIGHLIGHTS	Care of a Tooth Avulsion

When a tooth is removed during an injury, prompt treatment may improve the chance that it can be reimplanted. If the child's condition is stable, try to reimplant the tooth and then transfer to an emergency dental facility.

- Handle the tooth only by the crown (its top) rather than the root to avoid further damage.
- Gently rinse the tooth with a stream of sterile saline. Do NOT place it under running water.
- Insert into the socket.

- Have the child provide gentle pressure by biting a piece of gauze or a moistened tea bag. If the child is unstable or has other injuries, enlist emergency medical transportation (call 9-1-1). In this case, the tooth is transported with the child.
- If a dental aid kit is available, it may contain a transport liquid such as ViaSpan or Hank's Balanced Salt Solution. If these are not available, alternatives include cold milk, saline, saliva, or water. Place the tooth in one of these transfer liquids to keep it moist and send it with the child to the healthcare facility.

Source: Adapted from American Association of Endodontists. (2013). *The treatment of traumatic dental injuries*. Retrieved from http://www.nxtbook.com/nxtbooks/aae/traumaguidelines/index.php#/0

Any surgery carries the risk of postoperative complications. Teach parents the normal signs of healing in the postoperative period, as well as signs of complications. (See *Teaching Highlights: Complications of Tonsillectomy and Adenoidectomy*.)

Evaluation

Expected outcomes of nursing care for the child with tonsillitis include the following:

- The child has adequate intake of food and fluids.
- Pain and fever are effectively managed.
- There is an absence of postoperative complications such as bleeding, hemorrhage, and dehydration.
- Healing occurs without impairment following tonsillectomy.

Disorders of the Mouth

The mouth is an important structure that is directly linked to both the gastrointestinal and respiratory systems. Structural problems can occur in the mouth, often in conjunction with other defects such as tracheoesophageal fistula or cleft lip and palate (see Chapter 51). A second type of mouth disorder in children is ulceration. Children sometimes have changes in the mucous membranes of the mouth, associated with illnesses, infections, or as a side effect of drug treatments. Trauma is a third cause for mouth disorders in children. Accidents can cause fractures of the jaw, dental emergencies, or other trauma.

Nursing Management

Most mouth ulcers are treated symptomatically. Since the oral mucosa is fast growing, the cells can rapidly heal. Keeping the mouth clean and administering systemic or topical analgesics can assist with comfort. Foods should be mild and nonirritating. Acyclovir may be administered for treatment of herpes infections. Antibiotics are needed for bacterial infection of oral lesions. Stevens-Johnson syndrome necessitates removing the drug that causes the reaction, and treating the child with oral antihistamines and supportive therapy.

Nurses inform parents of proper treatment for injuries and may provide emergency treatment in schools and other community settings. Injury prevention is encouraged through use of protective gear during sports. Mouth guards can be helpful to prevent dental damage. See Chapter 42 for a discussion of protective sporting gear and of body piercing that may involve the oral cavity. Because the mouth has a profuse blood supply, bleeding may be extensive for even minor injuries. It is best to use clean cloths to absorb the blood and prevent choking on it, and get the child to an emergency facility to have the lesion examined.

Dental injuries may involve fracture of a tooth, luxation (partial extrusion), or avulsion (complete removal). The periodontal ligament holds the tooth in the socket but its attachment is torn during a tooth avulsion. When avulsion has occurred, fast care improves the chance that a permanent tooth can be reimplanted and kept alive. When reimplanted within 30 minutes, the chances of survival of the tooth are best (American Association of Endodontists, 2013). The nurse or family provides immediate care and the child should be transported immediately to an emergency facility. (See *Teaching Highlights: Care of a Tooth Avulsion*.)

Focus Your Study

- Health conditions affecting the eyes and ears are common in childhood, partially because of anatomic differences in structure, and can lead to developmental and communication disorders.

- Conjunctivitis can occur in the newborn and throughout childhood.
- Children manifest a wide array of visual disorders, such as hyperopia, myopia, and astigmatism.

- Strabismus, amblyopia, cataracts, glaucoma, and retinopathy of prematurity are serious conditions that can affect vision.

- Nurses commonly screen vision of children in schools and healthcare facilities to identify those with visual impairment.

- Otitis media is a common childhood health condition, with monitoring and antibiotics as potential treatments.

- Newborns should be screened for response to sounds, and those at high risk of hearing impairment should be carefully monitored in early childhood.

- Hearing loss may be conductive, sensorineural, or mixed.

- Nursing interventions for the child with vision or auditory impairment should focus on maximizing development and communication.

- Common disorders of the nose, throat, and mouth include epistaxis, nasopharyngitis, pharyngitis, tonsillitis, and oral ulcers.

- Nurses are influential in providing preventive teaching and emergency care when trauma occurs to the eyes, ears, and mouth.

Clinical Reasoning in Action

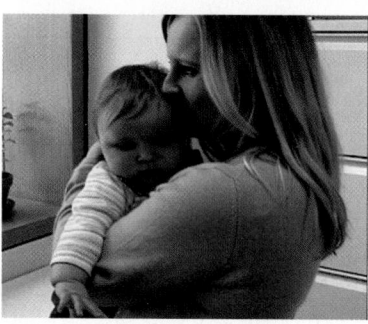

You are working at a local children's urgent care facility when a couple comes in carrying their screaming 9-month-old child, Becky. The parents are worried, as Becky has been crying steadily for the past 2 hours. You ask about recent illnesses or injuries and they tell you that she has had only two colds in her life and the most recent was about a week ago.

You assess Becky's vital signs as follows: weight 19 lb (8.6 kg), temperature 101°F, respirations 60 breaths per minute without retractions, and heart rate 120 beats per minute. She does not have any rashes or evidence of injuries, and upon examination, she appears well nourished but clearly in distress. Her heart rate is regular and rhythm and breath sounds are equal bilaterally and clear to auscultation. Both tympanic membranes are red and bulging. Her abdomen is soft and without organomegaly. The healthcare provider diagnoses bilateral acute otitis media and administers analgesic ear drops and ibuprofen in the office. Within 15 minutes, Becky has settled down, stopped crying, and is resting in her father's arms. The family is sent home with instructions to administer analgesics and return within 48 hours for further assessment.

1. What are the three main organisms that may have caused Becky's otitis media?

2. What are some of the guidelines you can give Becky's parents about otitis media treatment?

3. The mother says she has family members who have had tubes placed in their ears because of ear infections and wants to know if this is something that Becky will need to have done. How will you answer the mother's question?

4. What are some methods parents can use to prevent future otitis media episodes?

References

Adams A. J., Verdon W. A., & Spivey B. E. Color vision. In W. Tasman, & E. A. Jaeger (Eds.) *Duane's foundations of clinical ophthalmology* (2012). Philadelphia: Lippincott Williams & Wilkins.

American Academy of Pediatrics (AAP). (2011). *Vision screenings.* Retrieved from http://healthychildren.org

American Academy of Pediatrics (AAP) Committee on Practice and Ambulatory Medicine and Bright Futures Periodicity Schedule Work Group. (2014). Policy statement: 2014 recommendations for pediatric preventive health care. *Pediatrics, 133*(3), 568–570.

American Association for Pediatric Ophthalmology and Strabismus. (2014). *Strabismus.* Retrieved from http://www.aapos.org/terms/conditions/100

American Association of Endodontists. (2013). *The treatment of traumatic dental injuries.* Retrieved from http://www.nxtbook.com/nxtbooks/aae /traumaguidelines/index.php#/0

American Foundation for the Blind. (2011). *Children and youth with vision loss.* Retrieved from http://www.afb .org/Section/asp?SectionID=15&TopicID=411&Docu mentID=4896

American Speech-Language-Hearing Association (ASLHA). (2011). *Type, degree, and configuration of hearing loss.* Retrieved from http://www.asha.org /public/hearing/disorders/types.htm

American Speech-Language-Hearing Association (ASLHA). (2014). *The prevalence and incidence of hearing loss in children.* Retrieved from http://www .asha.org/public/hearing/disorders/children.htm

Bradfield, Y. S. (2013). Identification and treatment of amblyopia. *American Family Physician, 87,* 348–352.

Budnitz, D. S., Lovegrove, M. C., & Rose, K. O. (2014). Adherence to label and device recommendations for over-the-counter pediatric liquid medications. *Pediatrics, 133,* e283–e290.

Centers for Disease Control and Prevention (CDC). (2012). *Summary of 2009 national CDC EHDI data.* Retrieved from http://www.cdc.gov/ncbddd/hearingloss /2009-data/2009_ehdi_hsfs_summary_508_ok.pdf

Chou, R., Dana, T., & Bougatsos, C. (2011). *Screening for visual impairment in children ages 1–5 years: Systematic review to update the 2004 U.S. Preventive Services Task Force recommendation* (Report No. 11-05151-EF-1). Rockville, MD: Agency for Healthcare Research and Quality.

Cohen, S. M. (2011). Orbital cellulitis as a complication of sinusitis. *Journal for Nurse Practitioners, 7,* 38–44.

Davidson, S., & Quinn, G. E. (2011). The impact of pediatric vision disorders in adulthood. *Pediatrics, 127,* 334–339.

Ebell, M. H. (2014). Diagnosis of streptococcal pharyngitis. *American Family Physician, 89,* 976–977.

Farboud, A., Skinner, R., & Pratap, R. (2011). Otitis media with effusion ("glue ear"). *British Medical Journal, 343.* doi:10.1136/bmj.d3770

Giordano, T., Litman, R. S., Li, K. K., Mannix, M. E., Schwartz, R. H., Setzen, G., ... Patel, M. M. (2011). Clinical practice guideline: Tonsillectomy in children. *Otolaryngology—Head and Neck Surgery, 144.* doi:10.1177/0194599810389949

Gold, R. S. (2011). Treatment of bacterial conjunctivitis in children. *Pediatric Annals, 40,* 95–105.

Granet, D. B. (2011, May). Treating bacterial conjunctivitis. *Infectious Diseases in Children,* 10–15.

Granet, D. B., & Khayali, S. (2011, February). Amblyopia and strabismus. *Pediatric Annals,* 89–94.

Harmes, K. M., Blackwood, A., Burrows, H. L., Cooke, J. M., Van Harrison, R., & Passamani, P. P. (2013). Otitis media: Diagnosis and treatment. *American Family Physician, 88,* 435–440.

Hartnett, M. E., Morrison, M. A., Smith, S., Yanovitch, T. L., Young, T. L., Colaizy, T., ... Cotton, C. M. (2014). Genetic variants associated with severe retinopathy of prematurity in extremely low birth weight infants. *Investigative Ophthalmology and Visual Science, 55,* 6194–6203.

Hoberman, A., Paradise, J. L., Rockette, H. E., Shaikh, N., Wald, E. R., Kearney, D. H., ... Barbadora, K. A. (2011). Treatment of acute otitis media in children under 2 years of age. *New England Journal of Medicine, 364,* 105–115.

Hoffman, C., Pierrot, L., Contencin, P., Morisseau-Durand, M. P., Manach, Y., & Couloigner, V. (2011). Retropharyngeal infections in children: Treatment strategies and outcomes. *International Journal of Pediatric Otorhinolaryngology, 75*, 1099–1103.

Hou, C., Norcia, A. M., Madan, A., Tith, S., Agarwal, R., & Good, W. V. (2011). Visual cortical function in very low birth weight infants without retinal or cerebral pathology. *Investigative Ophthalmology and Visual Science, 25*, 9091–9098.

Hsiao, H. J., Huang, Y. C., Hsia, S. H., Wu, C. T., & Lin, J. J. (2012). Clinical features of peritonsillar abscess in children. *Pediatric Neonatology, 53*, 366–370.

International Committee for the Classification of Retinopathy of Prematurity. (2005). The international classification of retinopathy of prematurity revisited. *Archives of Ophthalmology, 123*, 991–999.

Joint Committee on Infant Hearing. (2007). Year 2007 position statement: Principles and guidelines for early hearing detection and intervention programs. *Pediatrics, 120*, 898–921.

Joint Committee on Infant Hearing. (2008). *Clarification for year 2007 JCIH position statement.* Retrieved from http://www.jcih.org/clarification%20year%20207%207%20statement.pdf

Kemper, A. R., Helfrich, A., Talbot, J., & Patel, N. (2012). Outcomes of an elementary school–based vision screening program in North Carolina. *Journal of School Nursing, 28*, 24–30.

Kliegman, R. M., Stanton, B., St. Geme, J., Schor, N., & Behrman, R. E. (Eds.) (2011). *Nelson textbook of pediatrics* (19th ed.). Philadelphia, PA: Saunders.

Lieberthal, A. S., Carroll, A. E., Chonmaitree, T., Ganiats, T. G., Hoberman, A., Jackson, M. A., ... Tunkel, D. E. (2013). The diagnosis and management of acute otitis media. *Pediatrics, 131*, e964–e999.

Liu, S., Pavan-Langston, D., & Colby, K. A. (2012). Pediatric herpes simplex of the anterior segment: Characteristics, treatment, and outcomes. *Ophthalmology, 119*, 2003–2008.

Melia, L., & McGarry, G. W. (2011). Epistaxis: Update on management. *Current Opinion in Otolaryngology & Head and Neck Surgery, 19*, 30–35.

Mitka, M. (2011). Guideline cites appropriateness criteria for performing tonsillectomy in children. *Journal of the American Medical Association, 305*, 661–662.

Montague, M. L., Whymark, A., Howatson, A., & Kubba, H. (2011). The pathology of visible blood vessels on the nasal septum in children with epistaxis. *International Journal of Otorhinolaryngology, 75*, 1032–1034.

National Association of School Nurses (NASN). (2012). *The use of volunteers in school health services.* Silver Spring, MD: Author.

National Eye Institute. (n.d.). *Sports-related eye injuries.* Retrieved from http://www.nidcd.nih.gov/health/hearing/coch.asp

National Eye Institute. (2014). *Facts about retinopathy of prematurity (ROP).* Retrieved form https://www.nei.nih.gov/health/rop/rop

National Institute of Deafness and Other Communication Disorders (NIDCD). (2014). *Quick statistics.* Retrieved from http://www.nidcd.nih.gov/health/statistics/Pages/quick.aspx

National Institutes of Health. (2013). *Retinopathy of prematurity.* Retrieved from http://www.nlm.nih.gov/medlineplus/ency/article/001618.htm

O'Brien, T. P. (2012). Comparative analysis of current antibiotics' potency, safety, and efficacy in treating bacterial conjunctivitis as well as potential impact on bacterial resistance. *Infectious Diseases in Children,* (Suppl), 9–14.

Ortiz, G. (2013). Vasomotor rhinitis and allergic conjunctivitis. *Clinical Advisor, January 2013*, 24–35.

Qureishi, A., Lee, Y., Belfield, K., Birchall, J. P., & Daniel, M. (2014). Update on otitis media—Prevention and treatment. *Infection and Drug Resistance, 7*, 15–24.

Rudolph, C., Rudolph, A., Lister, G., First, L., & Gershon, A. (Eds.) (2011). *Rudolph's pediatrics* (22nd ed.). New York, NY: McGraw-Hill.

Rye, M. S., Blackwell, J. M., & Jamieson, S. E. (2012). Genetic susceptibility to otitis media in childhood. *Laryngoscope, 122*, 665–675.

Seltz, L. B., Smith, J., Durairaj, V. D., Enzenauer, R., & Todd, J. (2011). Microbiology and antibiotic management of orbital cellulitis. *Pediatrics, 127*, e566–e572.

Shaikh, N., & Wald, E. R. (2014). Decongestants, antihistamines and nasal irrigation for acute sinusitis in children. *Cochrane Database Systematic Review, 9*, CD007909.

Sharma, A., Congdon, N., Patel, M., & Gilbert, C. (2012). School-based approaches to the correction of refractive error in children. *Survey of Ophthalmology, 57*, 272–283.

Sides, M., & Sigmon, P. (2013). Innovative solutions for mandated vision screenings. *NASN School Nurse, 28*, 185–186.

Steele, R. W. (2012). Differentiating pediatric acute bacterial conjunctivitis from other etiologies. *Infectious Diseases in Children,* (Suppl), 3–8.

Trumler, A. A. (2011). Evaluation of pediatric cataracts and systemic disorders. *Current Opinion in Ophthalmology, 22*, 365–379.

Tschudy, M. M., & Arcara, K. M. (2012). *The Harriet Lane handbook* (19th ed.). St. Louis, MO: Elsevier Mosby.

U.S. Food and Drug Administration. (2011). *Public health advisory—FDA recommends that over-the-counter (OTC) cough and cold products not be used for infants and children under 2 years of age.* Retrieved from http://www.fda.gov/drugs/drugsafety

U.S. Food and Drug Administration. (2014). *OTC cough and cold products—Not for infants and children under 2 years of age.* Retrieved from http://www.fda.gov/ForConsumers/ConsumerUpdates/ucm048682.htm

U.S. Preventive Services Task Force. (2011). *Vision screening.* Retrieved from http://www.ahrq.gov/news/visioneng.htm

Wald, E. R., Applegate, K. E., Bordley, C., Darrow, D. H., Glode, M. P., Marcy, M., ... Weinberg, S. T. (2013). Clinical practice guideline for the diagnosis and management of acute bacterial sinusitis in children ages 1 to 18 years. *Pediatrics, 132*, e262–e280.

Wang, J., Spencer, R., Leffler, J. N., & Birch, E. E. (2012). Characteristics of peripapillary retinal nerve fiber layer in preterm children. *American Journal of Ophthalmology, 153*, 850–855.

Williamson, I. (2011, January 12). Otitis media with effusion in children. *Clinical Evidence,* pii:0502.

Yeung, H. H., & Walton, D. S. (2012) Recognizing childhood glaucoma in the primary care setting. *Contemporary Pediatrics, 29*(5), 32–40.

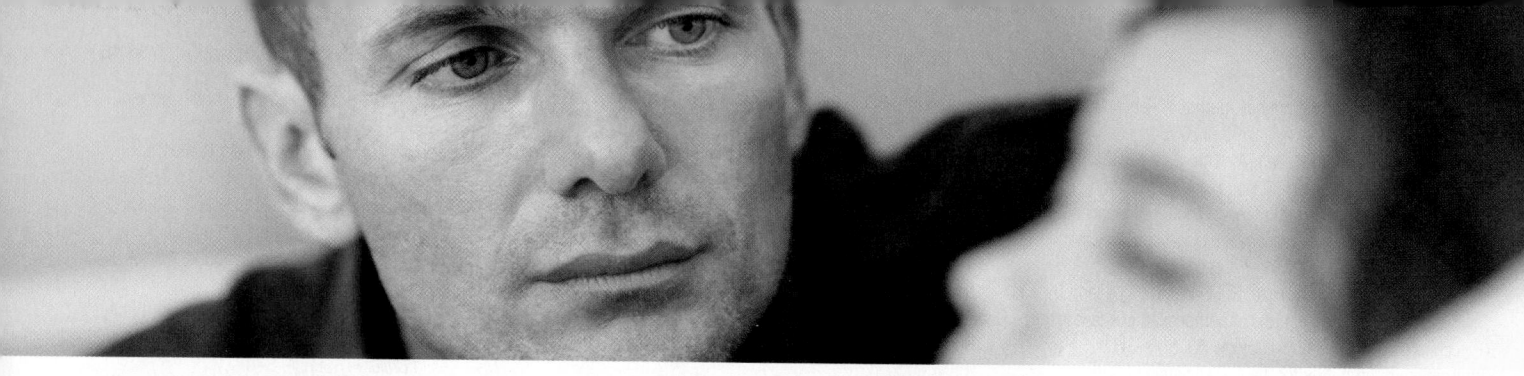

Chapter 46
The Child With Alterations in Respiratory Function

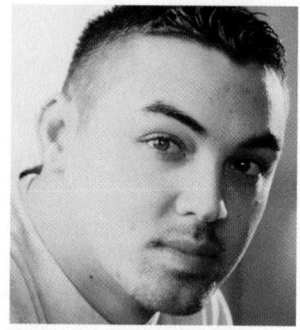

Ron Chapple/Getty Images

Emily gets sick so much faster than my other children. I guess the bronchopulmonary dysplasia and her tracheostomy make her more susceptible to infections. I really get concerned because she struggles so hard to breathe when she gets an infection. I have learned to suction and change her tracheostomy, but I'm afraid that one day her tracheostomy tube will get completely blocked. I just hope I remember all the things I've learned if that happens, and that the emergency medical personnel come quickly.

—Father of Emily, 8 months old

∨ Learning Outcomes

46.1 Describe unique characteristics of the pediatric respiratory system anatomy and physiology and apply that information to the care of children with respiratory conditions.

46.2 Contrast the different respiratory medical conditions that can cause respiratory distress in infants and children.

46.3 Explain the visual and auditory observations made to assess a child's respiratory effort or work of breathing.

46.4 Assess the child's respiratory status and analyze the need for oxygen supplementation.

46.5 Distinguish between conditions of the lower respiratory tract that cause illness in children.

46.6 Create a nursing care plan for a child with a common acute respiratory condition.

46.7 Develop a school-based nursing care plan for the child with asthma.

46.8 Develop a home nursing care plan for the child with cystic fibrosis.

46.9 Contrast the signs of different injuries to the respiratory system.

Respiratory problems may result from structural problems, functional problems, or a combination of both. Structural problems involve alterations in the size and shape of parts of the respiratory tract. Functional problems involve alterations in gas exchange and threats to this normal process from irritants (such as large particles and chemicals), infections, or injuries. Alterations in the immune and neurologic systems may also threaten respiratory function. (See Chapter 45

for upper respiratory conditions such as colds, otitis media, sinusitis, and pharyngitis.)

Most respiratory problems in children produce mild symptoms, last a short time, and can be managed at home. However, respiratory conditions are the most common cause of hospitalization in children between 1 and 17 years of age when numbers for pneumonia and asthma are combined (Pfuntner, Wier, & Stocks, 2013). Some respiratory conditions are chronic and have a significant impact on the child's growth and development.

Anatomy and Physiology of Pediatric Differences

The child's respiratory tract constantly grows and changes until about 12 years of age. The young child's neck is shorter than an adult's, resulting in airway structures that are closer together.

Upper Airway Differences

The child's airway is shorter and narrower than an adult's. These differences create a greater potential for obstruction (see *As Children Grow: Airway Development*). The infant's airway is approximately 4 mm (0.16 in.) in diameter, about the width of a drinking straw, in contrast to the adult's airway diameter of 20 mm (0.8 in.). The trachea primarily increases in length rather than diameter during the first 5 years of life. The child's little finger is a good estimate of the child's tracheal diameter. The child's trachea divides into two bronchi at a higher and different angle than an adult's (see *As Children Grow: Trachea Position*). The airway can be more easily compressed because the cartilage supporting the trachea is more flexible than an adult's. The child's narrower airway causes an increase in **airway resistance**, the effort or force needed to move oxygen through the trachea to the lungs, when airway inflammation is present (see *Pathophysiology Illustrated: Airway Diameter*).

Newborns are obligatory nose breathers. The only time newborns breathe through the mouth is when they are crying. The coordination of mouth breathing is controlled by maturing neurologic pathways; thus, infants up to 2 to 3 months of age do not automatically open the mouth to breathe when the nose is obstructed. Keep the newborn's nasal passages patent for such activities as breathing and eating.

Lower Airway Differences

The tracheobronchial tree is complete in the full-term newborn, but the child's lower airway is constantly growing. Beginning at 24 weeks' gestation, the lung sacs begin forming to support future gas exchange. The lung sacs begin differentiating into alveoli at 36 weeks' gestation (Rozance & Rosenberg, 2012). Alveoli continue developing and increasing in number for the first 5 to 8 years of age, followed by further development in size and complexity (Brashers & Huether, 2014).

The bronchi and bronchioles are lined with smooth muscle, but these are undeveloped in newborns. However, by 5 months of age an infant has enough muscle to react to irritants by bronchospasm and muscle contraction.

Children under age 6 years use the diaphragm to breathe because the intercostal muscles are immature. By 6 years of age, the child uses the intercostal muscles more effectively. The ribs are primarily cartilage and very flexible. In cases of respiratory distress, the negative pressure caused by the diaphragm movement causes the chest wall to be drawn inward, causing **retractions**, seen as sunken areas between the ribs during inspiration (see *Pathophysiology Illustrated: Retraction Sites*).

Children consume more oxygen than adults because of a higher metabolic rate. More oxygen is consumed when the child is in respiratory distress. The child also has fewer glycogen reserves, leading to more rapid muscle fatigue when accessory muscles must be used for breathing (Brashers & Huether, 2014).

Respiratory Distress and Respiratory Failure

Many respiratory conditions associated with breathing difficulty can progress to respiratory distress. If the condition is not managed effectively, it can progress to respiratory failure. Foreign-body aspiration is a common cause of airway obstruction and respiratory distress.

Foreign-Body Aspiration

Foreign-body aspiration is the inhalation of any object (solid or liquid, food or nonfood) into the respiratory tract. It is a major health threat for infants and young toddlers because of their increasing mobility and tendency to put objects into their mouths. Aspiration occurs most often during feeding and reaching activities, while crawling, or during playtime. However, aspiration may occur in children of any age. Approximately 100,000 cases occur each year, most often in children between 1 and 3 years old (Brashers & Huether, 2014). Some children die as a result of complete airway obstruction.

ETIOLOGY AND PATHOPHYSIOLOGY

In infants over 6 months of age and young children, any number of small objects that enter the child's mouth may cause aspiration. Foods such as nuts, popcorn, or small pieces of raw vegetables or hot dog and small objects such as toy parts, beads, safety pins, coins, buttons, or latex balloon pieces are frequent causes of airway obstruction. Partial and sometimes complete airway obstruction can occur.

The severity of the obstruction depends on the size and composition of the object or substance and its location within the respiratory tract. Most aspirated foreign bodies (AFBs) usually cause bronchial, not tracheal, obstruction. An object lodged high in the airway above the vocal cords is more easily removed by coughing or by back blows and chest thrusts.

The right lung is the most common site of the AFB because of the angle of its mainstem bronchus. Objects may migrate from higher to lower airway locations. An object may also move back up to the trachea, creating extreme respiratory difficulty. If the AFB is lodged in the trachea, it becomes life threatening.

CLINICAL MANIFESTATIONS

In many cases, the aspiration is unobserved. The child may have a sudden onset of choking, spasmodic coughing, shortness of breath, or **dysphonia** (muffled, hoarse, or absent voice sounds). These signs may be brief or may persist for several hours if the object drops below the trachea into a mainstem bronchus. Some children become asymptomatic after coughing for 15 to 30 minutes. The child may develop increased respiratory effort such as **dyspnea** (difficulty breathing), tachypnea, nasal flaring, and retractions. As respiratory distress progresses, the child may have a concentrated focus on breathing, an anxious expression, and an upright position with the neck extended. As **hypoxia** (lower than normal oxygen in the tissues) increases, behavior changes such as irritability and decreased responsiveness are seen.

If the AFB drops into the right bronchus and lower airway and is not removed, the child may present weeks later with a chronic cough, persistent or recurrent pneumonia, or a lung abscess.

CLINICAL THERAPY

Clinical therapy focuses on taking a careful history to determine whether aspiration could have occurred. Witnessed coughing, gagging, or choking associated with feeding or crawling on the

As Children Grow: **Airway Development**

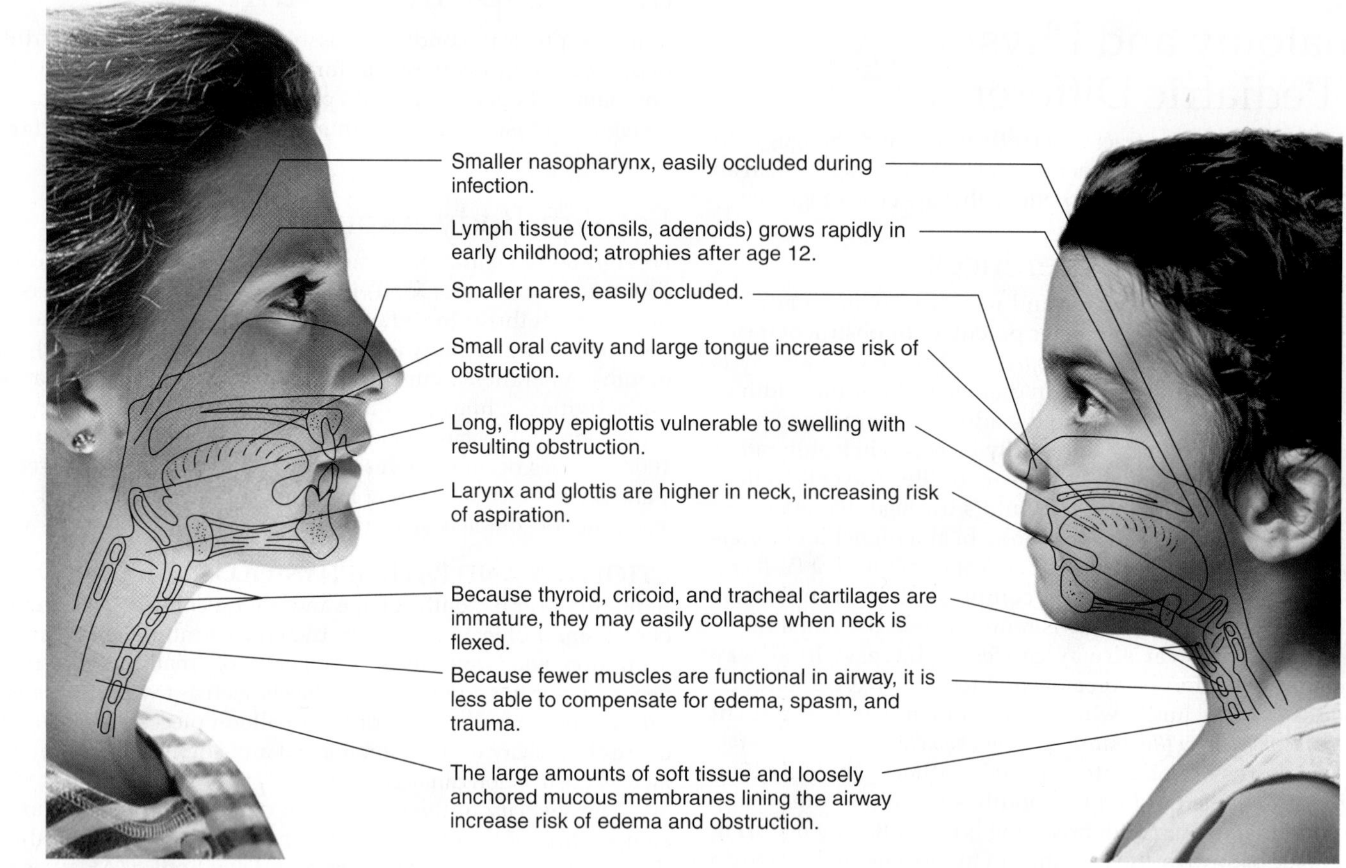

Smaller nasopharynx, easily occluded during infection.

Lymph tissue (tonsils, adenoids) grows rapidly in early childhood; atrophies after age 12.

Smaller nares, easily occluded.

Small oral cavity and large tongue increase risk of obstruction.

Long, floppy epiglottis vulnerable to swelling with resulting obstruction.

Larynx and glottis are higher in neck, increasing risk of aspiration.

Because thyroid, cricoid, and tracheal cartilages are immature, they may easily collapse when neck is flexed.

Because fewer muscles are functional in airway, it is less able to compensate for edema, spasm, and trauma.

The large amounts of soft tissue and loosely anchored mucous membranes lining the airway increase risk of edema and obstruction.

It is easy to see that a child's airway is smaller and less developed than an adult's airway, but why is this important? An upper respiratory tract infection, allergic reaction, positioning of the head and neck during sleep, and the small objects children play with can have serious consequences in the child.

As Children Grow: **Trachea Position**

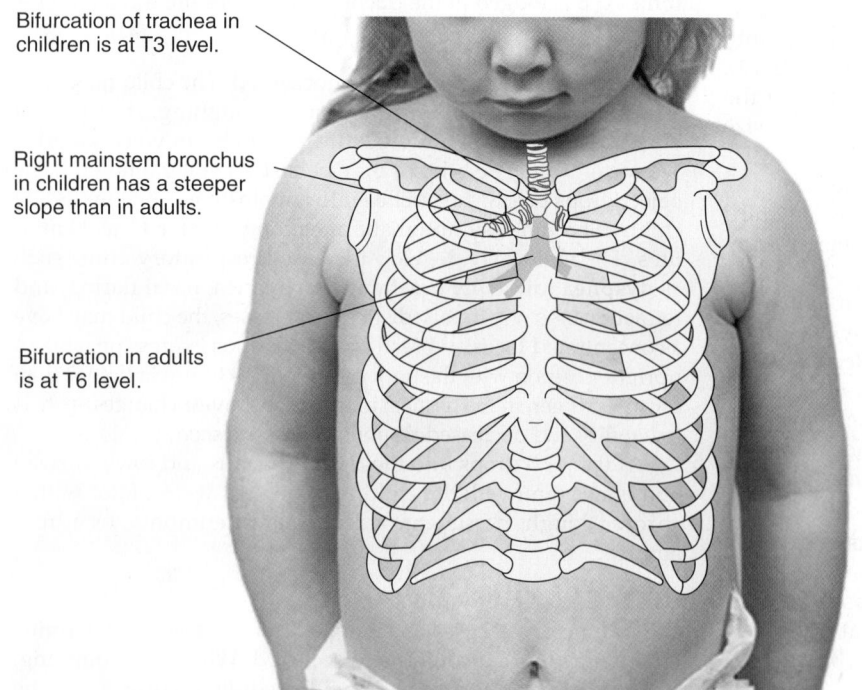

Bifurcation of trachea in children is at T3 level.

Right mainstem bronchus in children has a steeper slope than in adults.

Bifurcation in adults is at T6 level.

In children, the trachea is shorter and the angle of the right bronchus at bifurcation is more acute than in the adult. When you are resuscitating or suctioning, you must allow for these differences. Do you think that the angle of the right bronchus is significant in foreign-body aspiration? Why?

Pathophysiology Illustrated: **Airway Diameter**

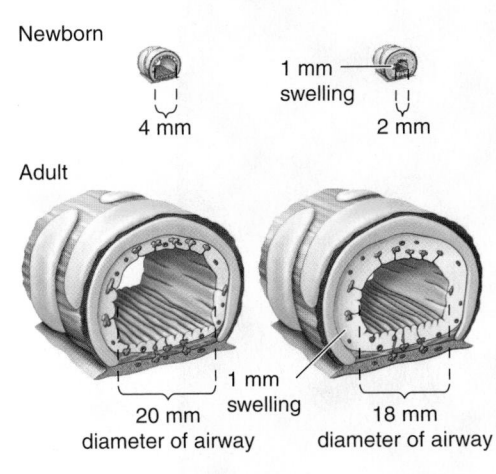

An infant's airway diameter is approximately 4 mm (0.16 in.), in contrast to the adult's 20-mm (0.8-in.) airway diameter. An inflammatory process in the airway causes swelling that narrows the airway, and airway resistance increases. Note that swelling of 1 mm (0.04 in.) reduces the infant's airway diameter to 2 mm (0.08 in.), but the adult's airway diameter is only narrowed to 18 mm (0.7 in.). Air must move more quickly in the infant's narrowed airway to get the needed amount of air into the lungs. The friction of the quickly moving air against the side of the airway increases airway resistance. The infant must use more effort to breathe and must breathe faster to get adequate oxygen.

floor may confirm the aspiration. Decreased breath sounds, stridor, and respiratory distress increase suspicion in the child without a witnessed aspiration. Many aspirated objects are organic, such as food, and cannot be seen on a radiograph. See Figure 46–1. A special radiograph, called a forced expiratory film, may show local hyperinflation (air trapping) and a mediastinal shift away from the affected side, abnormalities that an AFB may cause.

An object lodged in the trachea is life threatening. Back blows and chest thrusts or abdominal thrusts are used to remove an object from an obstructed airway. (See the *Clinical Skills Manual* **SKILLS** .) Fluoroscopy and fiberoptic bronchoscopy may be used to identify, locate, and extract the AFB. The child may develop pneumonia if an AFB is not recognized as a cause of respiratory distress. See the section on pneumonia later in the chapter.

Nursing Management

For the Child With Foreign-Body Aspiration

Nursing Assessment and Diagnosis

PHYSIOLOGIC ASSESSMENT

Perform the respiratory assessment following the guidelines given in *Assessment Guide: The Child in Respiratory Distress*. The child with an acute AFB will be in respiratory distress and must be constantly monitored. If the object remains lodged, observe the child for signs of increasing respiratory distress, especially vital signs, altered mental status, and audible wheezing on auscultation. Note changes in breath sounds, from noisy to decreasing to

Pathophysiology Illustrated: **Retraction Sites**

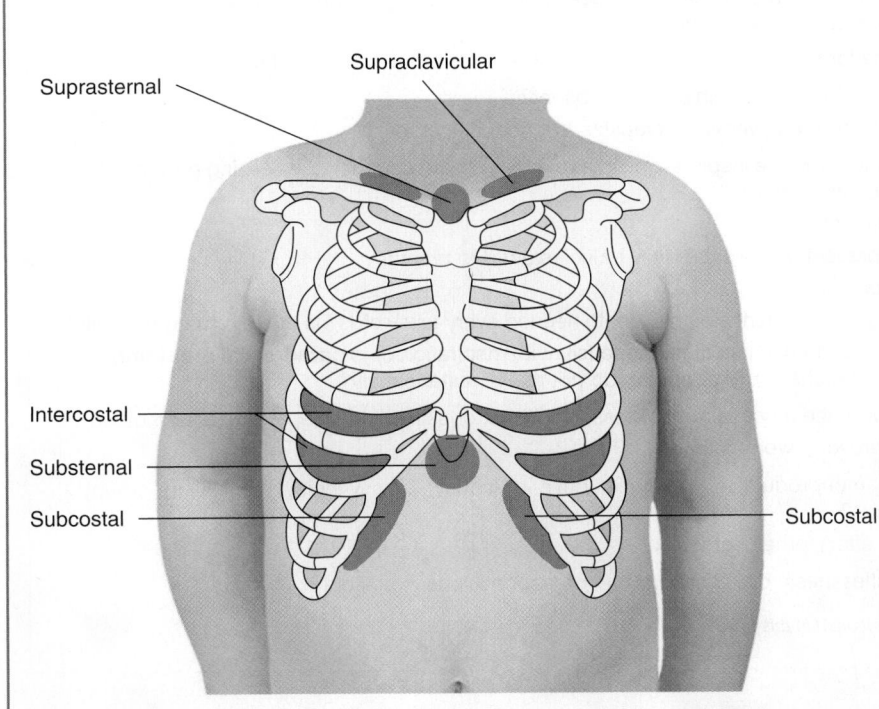

Infants and young children have immature chest muscles, and ribs of cartilage making the chest wall very flexible. The negative pressure created by the downward movement of the diaphragm is increased in cases of respiratory distress, and the chest wall is pulled inward, causing retractions. Intercostal retractions are seen in mild respiratory distress. As respiratory distress severity increases, substernal and subcostal retractions are seen. In cases of severe distress, supraclavicular and suprasternal retractions occur as the accessory muscles (sternocleidomastoid and trapezius muscles) are used.

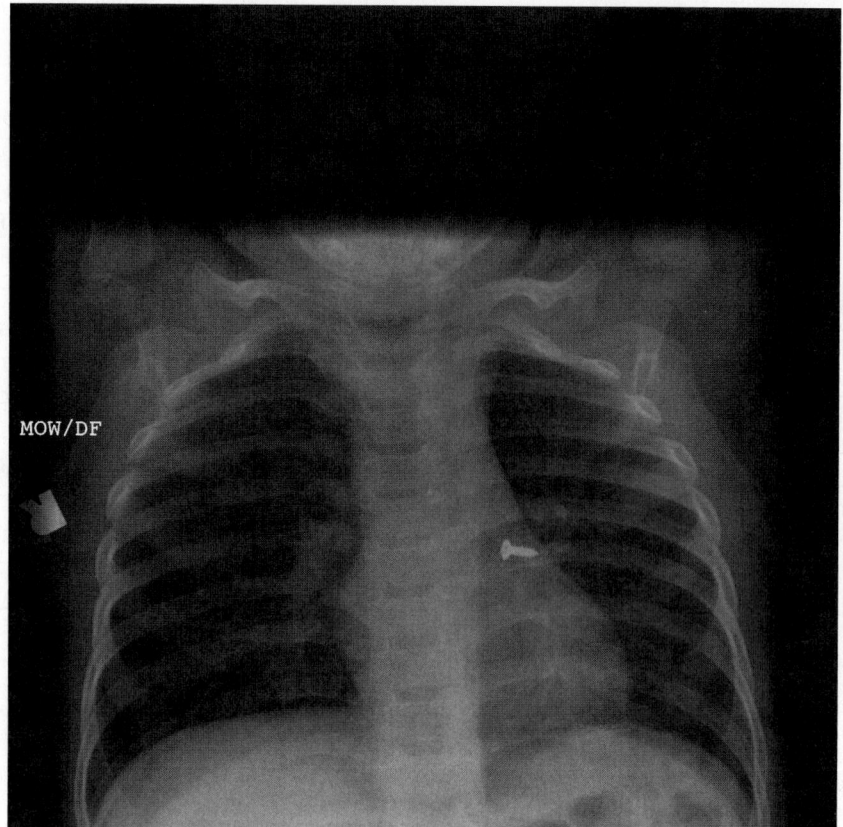

MOW/DF

Figure 46–1 An aspirated screw is clearly visible in the child's left mainstem bronchus on this chest radiograph.

SOURCE: Courtesy of Evelyn Anthony, MD, Department of Radiology, Brenner Children's Hospital, Wake Forest University Health System.

ASSESSMENT GUIDE | The Child in Respiratory Distress*

Assessment Focus	Assessment Guideline
Position of comfort	• Is the child comfortable lying down? • Does the child prefer to sit up or in the **tripod position** (sitting forward with arms on knees for support and extending the neck)?
Vital signs	• Assess the rate and depth of respirations. See Table 33–9 for age-related respiratory rates. Is **tachypnea** (abnormally rapid respiratory rate) present? • Assess the pulse for rate and rhythm. See Table 33–11 for age-related heart rates.
Lung auscultation	• Are breath sounds bilateral, diminished, or absent? • Are **adventitious sounds** (wheezes, crackles, or rhonchi) present?
Respiratory effort (work of breathing)	• Is **stridor** (audible crow-like inspiratory and expiratory breath sounds) or wheezing present? Is grunting heard on expiration? • Is breathing easy or labored? • Are retractions present or are accessory muscles used to breathe? • Is nasal flaring present? • Can the child say a full sentence or is a breath needed every few words? Is the cry strong or weak? • Do the chest and abdomen rise simultaneously with inspiration or is **paradoxical breathing** present in which the chest and abdomen do not rise simultaneously?
Color	• What is the color of the mucous membranes, nail beds, or skin (pink, pale, cyanotic, or mottled)? • Does crying improve or worsen the color?
Cough	• Is the cough dry (nonproductive), wet (productive, mucousy), brassy (noisy, musical), or croupy (barking, seal-like)? • Is the coughing effort forceful or weak?
Behavior change	• Is irritability, restlessness, or change in level of responsiveness present?

*Refer to Chapter 33 for the assessment techniques mentioned in this table.

absent, on the affected side. This can indicate that the object is moving and blocking a mainstem bronchus. Document any subtle changes in the child's respiratory status and report promptly.

Attach the child to a cardiorespiratory monitor and pulse oximeter (a transcutaneous assessment method to detect the amount of hemoglobin saturated with oxygen [SpO_2]) to assess the child for subtle signs of increasing hypoxia. A pulse oximetry reading (SpO_2) of less than 95% indicates **hypoxemia** (lower than normal oxygen level in the blood).

PSYCHOSOCIAL ASSESSMENT

The unexpected and acute nature of the event creates anxiety for both parents and child. The child will be fearful because of difficulty breathing. Assess the family's level of distress and coping ability.

DEVELOPMENTAL ASSESSMENT

As the child's condition stabilizes, observe how well the child's abilities match the parents' understanding of age-appropriate behaviors. See Chapter 31.

Common nursing diagnoses for a child with an AFB include the following (NANDA-I © 2014):

- *Airway Clearance, Ineffective*, related to obstruction by a foreign body
- *Ventilation: Spontaneous, Impaired*, related to respiratory muscle fatigue
- *Anxiety (Child)* related to difficulty breathing, unfamiliar surroundings, and procedures
- *Injury, Risk for*, related to small objects in environment

Planning and Implementation

Be prepared to perform back blows and chest thrusts for an infant or abdominal thrusts for the child with complete obstruction. (See the *Clinical Skills Manual* SKILLS .) When the child has a partial obstruction, remain with the child and have resuscitation equipment at the bedside. Permit the child to stay in a position of comfort. Avoid performing procedures that increase the child's anxiety because sudden movements and increased respiratory efforts may cause the obstruction to move and completely obstruct the airway.

After the AFB is removed, the child is stabilized and observed for a few hours in a short-stay unit to ensure that there are no respiratory complications.

Clinical Tip

Accuracy of pulse oximetry readings (SpO_2) can be improved by doing the following:

- Place the sensor over clean dry skin (e.g., finger, foot, ear lobe). Select a site or extremity that will not be moved extensively and where perfusion is adequate. Make the sensor secure to prevent movement of the sensor.
- Position the sensor for a reading at the level of the heart.
- Avoid placing the sensor probe over sites covered with dark nail polish or false nails.
- Cover the sensor with a light barrier when the child is in intense internal or external light to reduce interference.
- Confirm that the child's heart rate matches that detected by the pulse oximeter.
- Shivering, vasoconstriction, poor capillary refill, hypothermia, intravenous dyes, and electromagnetic interference may result in a false low reading (Fouzas, Priftis, & Anthracopoulos, 2011). Anemia may result in a false high reading.

DISCHARGE PLANNING AND HOME CARE TEACHING

Prevention of future aspirations is a major focus for nursing care. Educate the family on the child's developmental characteristics and how to identify potential safety hazards in the home. Food should be cut in small pieces. Check toys for small or broken parts and remove from young children. Store small objects (e.g., batteries, screws, buttons, earrings, and coins) out of a child's reach. Encourage the parents to learn rescue breathing, back blows, chest thrusts, or abdominal thrusts.

Evaluation

Expected outcomes of nursing care include the following:

- The child breathes spontaneously after removal of the foreign body.
- Parents complete a home safety check to prevent future aspiration incidents.

Respiratory Failure

Respiratory failure occurs when the body can no longer maintain effective gas exchange. Poor ventilation of the alveoli initiates the process that leads to respiratory failure. Hypoventilation occurs when oxygen need exceeds oxygen intake, the airway is partially occluded, or the exchange of oxygen and carbon dioxide in the alveoli is disrupted. This disruption may occur when a malfunction of respiratory center stimulation occurs (the alveoli do not receive the message to diffuse, e.g., a narcotic overdose), muscles of ventilation are fatigued and do not work effectively (e.g., status asthmaticus), or the relationship between ventilation and blood flow to the alveoli (perfusion) is impaired. Hypoxemia and **hypercapnia** (an excess of carbon dioxide in the blood) result from hypoventilation. When the blood levels of oxygen and carbon dioxide reach abnormal levels, hypoxia occurs and respiratory failure begins.

Signs of impending respiratory failure include worsening respiratory distress with increased respiratory effort (dyspnea, tachypnea, nasal flaring, and intercostal retractions), irritability, lethargy, and cyanosis. Grunting in infants is a sign of severe disease and the potential need for mechanical ventilation (Prodhan, Sharoor-Karni, Lin, et al., 2011). *Hypoxemia that persists when supplemental oxygen is given is a sign of respiratory failure.* See Table 46–1.

CLINICAL THERAPY

Arterial blood gas values help to identify hypoxemia and hypercapnia. Pulse oximetry helps determine when an arterial blood gas measurement is needed. When pulse oximetry (SpO_2) readings are between 76% and 90%, an arterial blood gas should be obtained as the SpO_2 reading may be falsely high (Ross, Newth, & Khemani, 2014) See Appendix B for expected arterial blood gas values and the *Clinical Skills Manual* SKILLS . Refer to Chapter 44 for interpretation of acidosis and alkalosis that must be considered simultaneously.

Medical management is focused on treating the cause of respiratory failure and reversing the severe hypoxemia with oxygen, mechanical ventilation, and positive end-expiratory pressure (PEEP) to increase functional residual capacity. These children are admitted to the pediatric intensive care unit (PICU).

The child's ability to maintain an open airway decreases as the level of responsiveness declines. Endotracheal (ET) intubation is a short-term, emergency measure to stabilize the airway by placing a tube in the trachea. The ET tube must be protected and stabilized to prevent its displacement. End-tidal

TABLE 46–1 Clinical Manifestations of Respiratory Failure and Imminent Respiratory Arrest

PHYSIOLOGIC CAUSE	CLINICAL MANIFESTATIONS
INITIAL SIGNS OF RESPIRATORY FAILURE The child is trying to compensate for oxygen deficit and airway blockage. Oxygen supply is inadequate; behavior and vital signs reflect compensation and beginning hypoxia.	Restlessness Tachypnea Tachycardia Diaphoresis
EARLY DECOMPENSATION The child tries to use accessory muscles to assist oxygen intake; hypoxia persists and efforts now waste more oxygen than is obtained.	Nasal flaring Retractions Grunting Wheezing Anxiety, irritability Mood changes Headache Hypertension Confusion
SEVERE HYPOXIA AND IMMINENT RESPIRATORY ARREST The oxygen deficit is overwhelming and beyond spontaneous recovery. Cerebral oxygenation is dramatically affected; central nervous system changes are ominous.	Dyspnea Bradycardia Cyanosis Stupor and coma

CO_2 monitoring is used to ensure that the tube is correctly positioned in the trachea (see the *Clinical Skills Manual* SKILLS). A **tracheostomy**, the creation of a surgical opening into the trachea through the anterior neck at the cricoid cartilage, is performed when long-term airway management is needed.

Assisted ventilation may be needed until mechanical ventilation is provided or the child breathes spontaneously. Children are often sedated to improve ventilation. Continuous positive airway pressure is one therapy used to improve oxygenation and lung compliance. Respiratory arrest results if respiratory failure cannot be managed.

Nursing Management

Early recognition of impending respiratory failure is the most important aspect of care for a child with any signs of respiratory compromise. Assess the child using guidelines found earlier in this chapter in the *Assessment Guide*. Monitor the child for changes in vital signs, respiratory status, SpO_2, and level of responsiveness. When the child has a chronic respiratory condition, development of respiratory failure may be gradual and signs will be subtle. Be particularly alert to behavior changes in addition to respiratory signs. Serial blood gases may be needed to monitor the child.

SAFETY ALERT!

As the child tires from the prolonged effort of breathing, the respiratory rate may begin to decrease. This is an ominous sign and may progress to respiratory arrest without intervention.

Place a child who has respiratory compromise in an upright position (elevate the head of the bed). Respiratory distress,

anxiety, excessive crying, and even fever can deplete metabolic reserves and increase the child's need for oxygen. Administer oxygen as ordered and keep emergency equipment at the child's bedside. Be prepared to provide assisted ventilation if the respiratory status deteriorates. (See the *Clinical Skills Manual* SKILLS .)

Clinical Reasoning Oxygen Delivery Devices

Oxygen delivery devices are selected to match the concentration of oxygen needed by the child. In respiratory failure, a higher concentration of oxygen is needed to reverse the hypoxemia. Which oxygen delivery device should be used? Are there any contraindications to oxygen use in a child who is hypoxic?

The child with an endotracheal or tracheostomy tube cannot talk or cry because vocal cord vibration is obstructed. Infants and young children often express initial frustration when they realize they cannot communicate verbally. When the child is alert, provide a bell or noisemaker as a way to gain attention. A communication board can be used with older children. Suction airway secretions as needed and provide tracheostomy care if present. See the *Clinical Skills Manual* SKILLS .

Many children are discharged from the hospital and cared for at home for an extended period with a tracheostomy tube in place. Parents must demonstrate competence in all aspects of tracheostomy care (how to maintain and suction the airway, clean the tracheostomy site, and change the tube), as well as emergency resuscitation skills adapted to the tracheostomy. A home healthcare nurse can provide follow-up care and support for the child and family. (See the *Clinical Skills Manual* SKILLS .)

Apnea

Infants commonly have **periodic breathing**, an irregular rhythm, and may have pauses of up to 20 seconds between breaths. This breathing pattern is not apnea. **Apnea** is the cessation of respiration lasting longer than 20 seconds, or any pause in respiration associated with cyanosis, marked pallor, hypotonia, or bradycardia. Apnea may be the first major sign of respiratory dysfunction in the newborn (see *Care of the Newborn With Respiratory Distress* in Chapter 27).

Apparent Life-Threatening Event (ALTE)

Apparent life-threatening event (ALTE) is defined as a frightening episode of apnea accompanied by a color change (e.g., cyanosis or pallor), limp muscle tone, choking, or gagging. Most affected infants are younger than 6 months of age (Chu & Hageman, 2013).

Potential causes of ALTE include gastroesophageal reflux, seizures, and lower respiratory disorders. Other causes may include ear, nose, and throat abnormalities; trauma; metabolic disorder; cardiac arrhythmias; sepsis; pertussis; and child abuse. ALTE and sudden infant death syndrome (SIDS) have different clinical and epidemiologic factors; however, some infants with ALTE are at increased risk for mortality (Chu & Hageman, 2013).

A detailed history helps identify the potential condition associated with ALTE. Diagnostic tests may include an electrocardiogram, complete blood count with differential, serum electrolytes, swallowing studies, gastrointestinal imaging, cultures, serum ammonia levels, and a chest radiograph. A medical cause is found for about 50% of ALTE cases (Chu & Hageman, 2013).

Physical stimulation or emergency resuscitation may be required to revive the infant. Treatment is targeted at the underlying condition.

Nursing Management

After ALTE, many infants are admitted to the hospital for evaluation and cardiorespiratory monitoring. Assess the infant's responsiveness and behavior (e.g., irritability or unexplained sleepiness). Monitor vital signs, and assess the child's growth. The focus of the physical examination is to detect signs of injury, infection, neurologic abnormalities, or features suggestive of a genetic or metabolic syndrome.

Attach a cardiorespiratory monitor and pulse oximeter to continuously assess the heart rate, respiratory rate, and oxygenation status while the infant is awake and asleep. Because the infant who has had ALTE may be at risk for cardiopulmonary arrest, keep emergency resuscitation equipment and drugs readily accessible at all times.

Provide emotional support. Establishing rapport and open communication with the parents is essential for creating a sense of trust. To obtain further information about the episode, use open-ended questions and active listening skills. Parents are fearful and anxious about the infant's prognosis. Explanations of tests and treatment help to decrease their anxiety and increase their understanding of the situation.

Encouraging parents' participation in the infant's care helps to promote the infant's sense of security, and it promotes family bonding. Teach parents how to hold the infant without disconnecting the monitoring cables. Wrapping the cable inside the infant's blanket helps secure the wires, increasing parents' feelings of confidence in handling the infant.

Support the mother to continue breastfeeding and maintaining a supply of breast milk by pumping, if necessary. Ensure that the mother gets adequate fluids and nutrition. Provide privacy for breast pumping, and store breast milk for future feedings.

DISCHARGE PLANNING AND HOME CARE TEACHING

Address home care needs in advance of the infant's discharge. Review guidelines for safe sleep positions. Some infants may be discharged with a cardiorespiratory monitor. Teach parents how to operate the monitor, what to do when the infant has an apnea episode, and how to perform cardiopulmonary resuscitation (CPR) and choking-intervention techniques (see the *Clinical Skills Manual* SKILLS). See *Teaching Highlights: Home Care Instructions for the Infant Requiring a Cardiorespiratory Monitor.*

Obstructive Sleep Apnea

Obstructive sleep apnea syndrome (OSAS) is a disorder of breathing during sleep that involves increased respiratory resistance leading to recurrent episodes of partial and complete upper airway obstruction that disrupt normal ventilation during sleep and sleep patterns (Marcus et al., 2012). This results in labored breathing and snoring when the child tries to move air past the obstruction. OSAS is believed to affect 1% to 5% of school-age children (Marcus et al., 2012).

The upper airway contains about 30 muscles that permit the pharynx to collapse, enabling the child to talk and swallow, but also maintain airway patency. When the child is awake, muscle tone is maintained and the airway remains patent even when potential obstructions are present. During sleep, the airway muscles relax, the pharynx becomes obstructed, and airway

---

TEACHING HIGHLIGHTS | Home Care Instructions for the Infant Requiring a Cardiorespiratory Monitor

Apnea Equipment
- Review how the monitor operates, the lead wires, placement of skin electrodes and pulse oximetry sensor, and how to set the event recorder. Keep the battery fully charged, and keep the manual for troubleshooting handy.

Emergency Preparation
- Have an emergency plan and complete an emergency information form about the infant's health problem. Notify the telephone company, electric company, local ambulance service, and the local emergency department (to get priority service status).
- Post the emergency response phone numbers by all phones and save in cell phones, along with the phone numbers for the healthcare provider, medical equipment company, power company, neighbor, and key family members.
- Take a cardiopulmonary resuscitation (CPR) course.

Safety Precautions
- Place monitor on firm surface; keep away from other appliances (television, microwave oven) and water.
- Ensure that alarms are audible from all locations.
- Double-check that the monitor and event recorder are on before putting the infant down for a nap or at bedtime.
- Thread cable and wires through lower end of infant's clothes.
- Ensure integrity of leads, monitor cable, and power cord (replace if frayed).

Routine Care
- Explain the reasons for the apnea monitor and frequency of use. Use it whenever the infant sleeps. Review the manual for troubleshooting.
- Show how to attach and detach infant chest leads and belt. Evaluate the skin for irritation or sores under the electrodes, and move the electrode if skin is irritated. Use no oils or lotions on the chest.

Responding to an Alarm
- Observe the infant for breathing first to determine if this is a real event or a loose lead.
- Stimulate the infant if respirations are absent or infant is lethargic. Start by calling the infant's name and gently touching, proceeding to vigorous touch if needed.
- If no response, proceed with CPR and call 9-1-1.
- If a loose lead is suspected, determine if electrode patches are loose. Check the wires from the electrode or monitor cable. Check the power supply. Is the monitor malfunctioning?

resistance increases, leading to snoring. Reduced upper airway tone and obstruction cause apnea episodes that lead to hypoxemia, hypercapnia, and an elevated blood pressure. Hypertrophy of the adenoids and tonsils is the most common cause of OSAS, followed by craniofacial abnormalities, obesity, and neuromuscular disorders (e.g., cerebral palsy, muscular dystrophy).

Children with OSAS snore and have labored breathing during sleep such as retractions and paradoxical breathing. After snoring or breathing pauses, the child may snort, gasp, choke, move, or arouse to take a breath. Sleep is restless and the child may sleep in unusual positions to hyperextend the neck and airway. Symptoms of sleep deprivation (daytime sleepiness, poor attention, aggression, acting-out behavior, and poor school performance) may be noted. The child may also have enuresis, a morning headache, obesity, hypertension, failure to thrive, and cardiac dysfunction.

Healthy People 2020

(SH-1) Increase the proportion of persons with symptoms of obstructive sleep apnea who seek medical evaluation

---

Initial diagnosis occurs with a detailed history about snoring. **Polysomnography**, a sleep study that simultaneously records the sleep state, gas exchange, breathing efforts, cardiac rhythm, and muscle activity and movement, is performed. Adenotonsillectomy (adenoidectomy and tonsillectomy) is the most common treatment for OSAS, and the condition resolves in the majority of children. Children are evaluated 6 to 8 weeks after adenotonsillectomy to determine if some degree of OSAS persists that needs other treatment. Continuous positive airway pressure (CPAP) is used for children with surgical contraindications or those with persistent OSAS (craniofacial anomalies or neuromuscular disorders) after adenotonsillectomy. Weight loss strategies may be implemented for children with obesity. Some children with mild OSAS may be treated with nasal steroids. Without treatment, complications can include failure to thrive, pulmonary hypertension, **cor pulmonale** (obstruction of pulmonary blood flow that leads to right ventricular hypertrophy and heart failure), systemic hypertension, and cognitive impairment.

Nursing Management

In the community setting, all children should be screened for snoring as part of their routine health care. Assess the child for signs of nasal obstruction, mouth breathing, and enlarged tonsils. Determine if the child has symptoms of sleep deprivation or if a condition is present that places the child at high risk for OSAS. When snoring is present, encourage the family to keep a sleep diary.

When a polysomnogram is ordered, talk with the parents about how to prepare the child for the strange setting and wires that will be attached during the sleep study. Most pediatric centers will allow the parent to stay with the child during the study.

Following adenotonsillectomy, the child with OSAS is commonly hospitalized overnight because respiratory complications may occur. The hospital nurse monitors the child for bleeding and respiratory distress, such as obstructive sleep apnea and pulmonary edema. Continuous pulse oximetry is used to detect oxygen desaturation. See Chapter 45 for care of the child having adenoidectomy and tonsillectomy.

Sleep center nurses provide education and support to families of children who need to use CPAP to treat OSAS. The nurse helps identify the best fitting mask or nasal prong system for CPAP delivery. Parents may need guidance about helping children go to sleep wearing the mask until they are accustomed to it.

Sudden Infant Death Syndrome

Sudden and unexpected infant death (SUID) is a leading cause of infant mortality. Sudden infant death syndrome (SIDS), a subset of SUID, is defined as the sudden death during sleep of an infant under 1 year of age that remains unexplained after a thorough investigation, including an autopsy, a review of the circumstances of death, and the clinical history. Some unexpected infant deaths may be classified as accidental suffocation or positional asphyxia (e.g., face against bedding or rolled from side to abdomen) depending upon the circumstances. SIDS is the third leading cause of infant mortality in the United States (Heron, 2013). Most SIDS deaths occur in infants between 2 and 4 months of age, and it accounts for 50% of SUID cases (Matthews & Moore, 2013). SIDS is currently unpredictable and, in some cases, unpreventable.

SIDS is called a "syndrome" because infants are believed to have a vulnerability that increases their risk for sudden death during the first 6 months of life, a critical period of developing homeostatic control. An environmental stressor (e.g., secondhand smoke, overheating, soft bedding, prone or side-lying position) compounds the vulnerability. Abnormalities associated with the neurotransmitter serotonin in the medulla oblongata may interfere with arousal responses during sleep in a critical development period (Matthews & Moore, 2013). See Table 46–2 for factors that place infants at risk for sudden infant death.

Typically, parents find the infant unresponsive in the crib in the morning or after a nap. They usually report hearing no cries or disturbances during the night. Clinical findings include evidence of a struggle or change in position during sleep and the presence of frothy, blood-tinged secretions from the mouth and nose.

TABLE 46–2 Risk Factors for Sudden Infant Death

INFANT RISK FACTORS

- Preterm or low birth weight, small for gestational age, multiple birth
- Native American and African American infants are at higher risk; Whites, Asians, and Hispanics are at lower risk
- Males are at higher risk
- Maternal smoking, alcohol use disorder, or substance abuse
- Socioeconomic disadvantages

ENVIRONMENTAL RISK FACTORS

- Sleeping prone or side-lying position
- Bed sharing—higher risk in infants 0–3 months old
- Soft bedding, pillows, blankets, and stuffed animals that infants roll into—higher risk in infants over 3 months old
- Overheating
- Secondhand tobacco smoke exposure

Source: Data from Gelfer, P., & Tatum, M. (2014). Sudden infant death syndrome. *Journal of Pediatric Health Care, 28*(5), 470–474; Colvin, J. D., Collie-Akers, V., Schunn, C., & Moon, R. Y. (2014). Sleep environment risks for younger and older infants. *Pediatrics, 134*(2), e406–e412; Van Nguyen J. M., & Abenhaim H. A. (2013). Sudden infant death syndrome: Review for the obstetric care provider. *American Journal of Perinatology, 30*(09), 703–714.

Nursing Management

The sudden, unexpected nature of the infant's death is often confirmed in the emergency department. The nurse's role is to be empathetic and provide support during one of the greatest crises a family must face. The focus is on supporting the family during the communication of bad news and the shock of the infant's death. See Chapter 41.

Reassure the parents that they are not responsible for the infant's death and help them contact other family members and mobilize support. Older children may need reassurance that SIDS will not happen to them. They may also believe that bad thoughts or wishes about their baby brother or sister caused the death. Support groups can help parents, siblings, and other family members express these fears and work through their feelings about the infant's death. The First Candle organization can help families locate a support group in their area.

Nurses play an important role in SUID and SIDS prevention. Educate the parents of all newborns and infants about the recommended infant sleep position—on the back on a firm surface. The Safe to Sleep Campaign, encouraging the placement of infants in the supine position for sleeping, was initiated in 1992 and has led to a 50% decrease in SIDS deaths (Flook & Vincze, 2012). However, no further reduction in deaths due to SUID or SIDS has been noted for the last decade. Ask parents to make sure the infant is placed to sleep on the back when cared for by another family member or childcare provider. Parents should also use a firm mattress and avoid the use of loose bedding, toys, and pillows. A sleeper suit rather than a blanket should be used to keep the infant warm while sleeping. See *Evidence-Based Practice: Infant Sleep Environment and Positioning*. A pacifier is also recommended for nap and bedtime (Task Force on Sudden Infant Death Syndrome, 2011). See Chapter 54 for issues related to infant skull flattening from sleeping on the back.

EVIDENCE-BASED PRACTICE | Infant Sleep Environment and Positioning

Clinical Question

In 2010, 13.5% of all infants were reported to be placed to sleep in the prone position (Matthews & Moore, 2013). An unknown number of infants are placed to sleep in a manner that increases their risk of suffocation. What strategies might help increase safe sleep environments and positioning for young infants?

The Evidence

A study used focus groups and interviews with 83 African American mothers from diverse socioeconomic groups to learn about surfaces and soft bedding used for their infants. Findings revealed that parents had different interpretations of firm bedding, and they believed that soft bedding (pillows, blankets, and crib bumper pads) increased the infant's comfort and, in some cases, safety. For example, parents believed that the surface was firm if a pillow or blanket was placed between the mattress and the sheet and the sheet was tucked tautly around the pillow or blanket. Misconceptions about firm and soft bedding increase the risk for suffocation and SIDS as the infant sleeps (Ajao, Oden, Joyner, et al., 2011).

A bed audit in a large neonatal intensive care unit (NICU) identified that only 39% of infants were sleeping in supine position, and 45% had no soft objects in their bed. A telephone survey to parents of infants discharged from the NICU identified only 23% of infants had safe sleep practices that met all criteria. A quality improvement initiative led to nursing guidelines and nursing education on safe sleep practices. An algorithm was developed to assess when an infant could be transitioned to supine sleep position. Cue cards were placed in an infant's crib when the infant met criteria to begin supine sleep positioning. The card reminded nurses to use and to begin educating parents about safe sleep practices. Parent education about safe sleep practices included a DVD and written discharge guidelines. A crib audit revealed an increase in supine sleep position use in eligible infants from 39% before interventions to 83% 3 months after the intervention. Rates also increased for firm bedding surface and no soft items in the bed. A follow-up survey of parents after discharge also reflected a significant increase in safe sleep practices (23%

before interventions and 82% after the intervention) (Gelfer, Cameron, Masters, et al., 2013).

A study investigated factors in the sleep environment by age of infants who died of SIDS or SUID. Data collected by state child death review teams for infants less than 12 months of age who died during sleep or in the sleep environment were analyzed for the following factors: infant and caregiver characteristics, object (e.g., clothing, blanket, bumper pads, stuffed toys) in the sleep environment, and sleep place and position. Bedsharing was associated with 69.2% of study infant deaths, and the rate was significantly higher in infants less than 3 months of age (73.8%) than in older infants (58.9%). Deaths in younger infants were less likely to be associated with an object in the sleep environment or a change in sleep position for supine or side-lying to prone. Older infants were more likely to die in the prone position and to have objects in the sleep environment (Colvin, Collie-Akers, Schunn, et al., 2014).

Best Practice

While the Safe to Sleep Campaign has successfully promoted supine sleep positions for infants, additional sleep environment factors can increase the risk for an infant's death during sleep. Parent education needs to focus on more than just supine positioning. Modeling the safe sleep environment and position for parents when infants are hospitalized is an effective message. As infants develop an ability to roll over and move in the bed, parents should be reminded to keep objects out of the bed, especially soft objects that can suffocate when the infant rolls from supine to prone. Nurses also need to understand a parent's perspective on issues such as bedding and bedsharing so that education can appropriately address beliefs and concerns.

Clinical Reasoning

Identify if policies exist for infant sleep position in the maternity and pediatric sections of your hospital. Conduct an audit of cribs and bassinets to determine what proportions of infants are sleeping in the supine position and if any objects are in the bed.

While African American infants are at higher risk for SIDS, many of these families do not follow guidelines for safe sleep practices, even when stating they have heard about recommendations to avoid bed sharing and to use supine sleep positioning for the infant. Reasons parents gave for not following medical advice included perceived safety (less risk of aspiration), convenience (do not have to walk to the crib), and better infant sleep quality when prone. Cultural and familial influences were a factor in not following medical advice (Gaydos et al., 2015). Nurses, when counseling about safe sleep, should more thoroughly explain the rationale for the safe sleep recommendations and address cultural and familial beliefs.

Clinical Tip

A review of several studies evaluated the relationship between breastfeeding and SIDS. Findings revealed that breastfeeding for any period of time is protective, and greater protection occurs if breastfeeding is exclusive (Hauck, Thompson, Tenabe, et al., 2011). Place hospitalized infants to sleep in supine position rather than side-lying or prone.

Croup Syndromes

Croup is a term applied to a broad classification of upper airway illnesses that result from inflammation and swelling of the epiglottis and larynx. The swelling usually extends into the trachea and bronchi. Viral croup syndromes include acute spasmodic laryngitis (spasmodic croup) and laryngotracheobronchitis (LTB). Bacterial croup syndromes include bacterial tracheitis and epiglottitis (see *Pathophysiology Illustrated: Airway Changes With Croup*).

Acute spasmodic laryngitis, LTB, and bacterial tracheitis affect a large number of children across all age groups in both sexes. Epiglottitis, previously a common serious respiratory illness, is rare in the United States because of the *Haemophilus influenzae* type B vaccine. The initial symptoms of all four conditions include inspiratory stridor (a high-pitched, musical sound that is created by narrowing of the airway), a "seal-like" barking cough, and hoarseness. Acute spasmodic croup and LTB are the most common disorders, but epiglottitis and bacterial tracheitis are more serious. See Table 46–3 for information on the etiology, clinical manifestations, and clinical therapy for these disorders.

SAFETY ALERT!

Throat cultures and visual inspection of the inner mouth and throat are contraindicated in children with LTB and epiglottitis. These procedures can cause **laryngospasms** (spasmodic vibrations that close the larynx) as a result of the child's anxiety or of probing this reactive and already compromised area. A complete airway obstruction may result.

Pathophysiology Illustrated: **Airway Changes With Croup**

Upper airway tissues respond to the invading virus with inflammation and edema. The epiglottis swells, occluding the airway, and the trachea swells against the cricoid cartilage, narrowing the airway. Copious secretions increase the respiratory distress and can obstruct the airway.

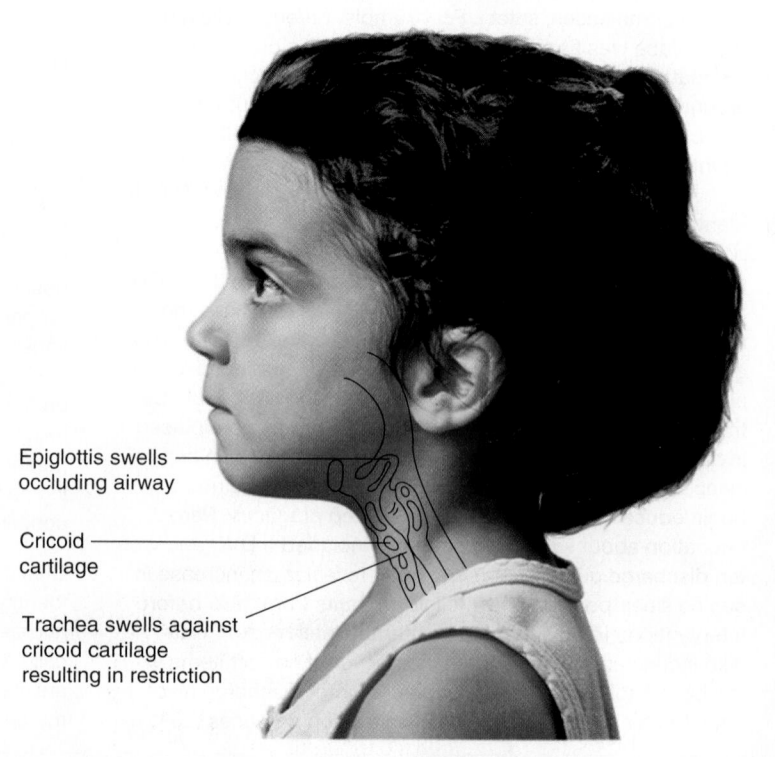

Epiglottis swells occluding airway

Cricoid cartilage

Trachea swells against cricoid cartilage resulting in restriction

TABLE 46–3 Summary of Croup Syndromes

| | VIRAL SYNDROMES | | BACTERIAL SYNDROMES | |
	ACUTE SPASMODIC LARYNGITIS (SPASMODIC CROUP)	LARYNGOTRACHEITIS/ LARYNGOTRACHEO-BRONCHITIS (LTB)	BACTERIAL TRACHEITIS	EPIGLOTTITIS (SUPRAGLOTTITIS)
Etiology	Recurrent; suspect allergies with sensitivity to viruses that cause LTB; also associated with gastroesophageal reflux	Parainfluenza, types I, II and III, RSV, influenza, enteroviruses, adenoviruses, or *Mycoplasma pneumoniae*	*Staphylococcus, Moraxella catarrhalis*, and nontypeable *H. influenzae*; may follow viral LTB as a secondary infection	*Haemophilus influenzae*, Group A beta-hemolytic streptococcus, staphylococcus
Severity	Least serious	Serious; progresses if untreated	Can be life threatening; requires close observation	Most life threatening (medical emergency)*
Age affected	3 months to 8 years	3 months to 3 years	1 month to 13 years*	2 years to 8 years
Onset	Abrupt nighttime onset; resolves over 24 to 48 hours; recurs*	Gradual onset as a URI, progressing to respiratory distress and potential airway obstruction over 24 to 48 hr	Progressive over 2 to 5 days, may present like LTB initially but condition worsens after LTB treatment	Progresses rapidly (hours)*; may progress to complete airway obstruction
Clinical manifestations	Afebrile; mild respiratory distress; barking-seal cough; signs of respiratory infection are not present*	*Early:* mild fever (less than 40.0°C [102.2°F]); barking-seal, brassy, croupy cough; rhinorrhea; sore throat; stridor (inspiratory); apprehension; restless or irritable May progress to retractions; increasing stridor; cyanosis	High fever (higher than 39.0°C [102.2°F]); URI appears as viral croupy cough and croup initially; stridor (tracheal); purulent secretions; child often prefers to lie flat; toxic appearance; dysphagia and drooling are rarely present	High fever (higher than 39.0°C [102.2°F]); URI; intense sore throat; dysphagia*; drooling*; increased pulse and respiratory rate; prefers upright position (tripod position with neck extended)*; cherry red epiglottis; barking cough is absent*
Clinical therapy	Oral dexamethasone; treatment for gastroesophageal reflux may reduce recurrences; other airway disorders may need to be considered such as aspirated foreign body	Oral dexamethasone; nebulized epinephrine for severe symptoms; supplemental oxygen if hypoxic; monitor for airway obstruction	May have initial treatment for LTB but condition worsens; blood cultures, endotracheal intubation to protect the airway, and intravenous antibiotics	Immediate endotracheal intubation to protect the airway, supplemental oxygen, blood cultures, culture of epiglottis, intravenous antibiotics for gram-positive organisms that are changed as needed to match culture sensitivities

*Classic signs that distinguish the condition.

Source: Data from Roosevelt, G. E. (2016). Acute inflammatory upper airway obstruction (croup, epiglottitis, laryngitis, and bacterial tracheitis). In R. M. Kliegman, B. F. Stanton, J. W. St. Geme, & N. F. Schor (Eds.), *Nelson textbook of pediatrics* (20th ed., pp. 2031–2036). Philadelphia, PA: Elsevier; Sharma, G. D., & Conrad, C. (2011). Croup, epiglottitis, and bacterial tracheitis. In American Academy of Pediatrics Section on Pediatric Pulmonology, *Pediatric pulmonology* (pp. 347–363). Elk Grove Village, IL: Author; Zoorob, R., Sidani, M., & Murray, J. (2011). Croup: An overview. *American Family Physician*, 83(9), 1067–1073.

Emergency management consists of maintaining and improving respiratory effort with medications, and, in some cases, supplemental oxygen. Children with acute spasmodic croup and LTB who respond well to oral medication are often sent home from the emergency department after an observation period. Children with moderate to severe symptoms may need additional nebulized epinephrine, and may be admitted for further treatment if the respiratory status does not improve. Most children who are admitted respond to medications and oxygen therapy and are discharged within 48 to 72 hours.

Clinical Tip

No studies of therapies for acute spasmodic croup or LTB support routine exposure of the child to cold air, decongestants, or cough medications (Zoorob, Sidani, & Murray, 2011). However, some children with mild recurrent acute spasmodic croup get relief from exposure to cold air or warm humidity in a closed bathroom with warm steam. Children who do not have relief from these complementary therapies should be seen by a healthcare provider for treatment.

Children with bacterial tracheitis and epiglottitis have a more severe airway obstruction. These children usually are intubated in the operating room because the obstruction can rapidly become life threatening. These children are then transferred to the PICU for care.

Nursing Management

For the Child With Croup Syndrome

Nursing Assessment and Diagnosis

The initial and ongoing physical assessment of the child with one of the croup syndrome disorders focuses on adequacy of respiratory functioning and severity of illness. Attach a cardio-respiratory monitor and pulse oximeter. Have the child in an area where continuous visual monitoring is possible to detect changes in severity of respiratory distress. Assess vital signs, including temperature.

Pay particular attention to any progressive changes in the child's respiratory effort that may signal the need for intubation. Regularly assess the respiratory rate, heart rate,

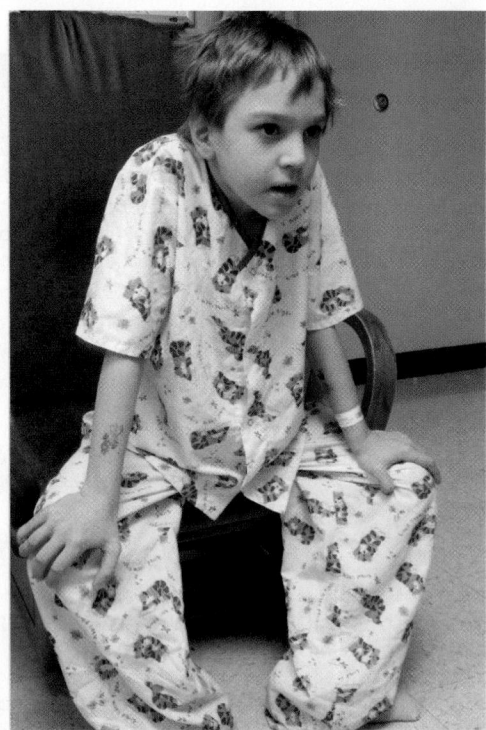

Figure 46–2 Children with severe respiratory distress and a narrowed airway often sit in a tripod position, leaning forward with arms on the legs. The head and neck are extended with the jaw thrust forward to help keep the airway open. This position may also be seen in a child with an acute asthma flare.

retractions, use of accessory muscles, stridor, breath sounds, preferred position, and responsiveness (Figure 46–2). Exhaustion can diminish the intensity of retractions and stridor. As the child uses remaining energy reserves to maintain ventilation, breath sounds may actually diminish. Noisy breathing (audible airway congestion, coarse breath sounds) in this situation verifies adequate energy stores. Responsiveness decreases as hypoxemia increases.

SAFETY ALERT!

If the child is suspected of having epiglottitis or a severe airway obstruction, do not leave the child's side until intubation occurs. Observe the child continuously for inability to swallow, absence of voice sounds, increasing degree of respiratory distress, and acute onset of drooling. A change in the child's level of consciousness—from anxiety to lethargy to stupor—occurs as hypoxia increases. If any of these signs occur, get medical assistance immediately. The quieter the child, the greater the cause for concern.

The following nursing diagnoses might be appropriate for the child with a croup syndrome disorder (NANDA-I © 2014):

• *Breathing Pattern, Ineffective*, related to airway narrowing, decreased energy, and fatigue

• *Fluid Volume: Deficient, Risk for*, related to fever and swallowing difficulty

• *Fear (Child)* related to dyspnea, unfamiliar surroundings, procedures, and separation from support system

Planning and Implementation

MAINTAIN AIRWAY PATENCY

Allow the child to assume a comfortable position. Be immediately available to attend to the child's respiratory needs, and keep resuscitation equipment and an intubation tray at the bedside. Supplemental oxygen with humidity may be needed for hypoxemia. Ensure that a means of communication (sign language or simple word cues) is established so the older child can alert nursing staff to respiratory difficulty.

Postpone anxiety-provoking procedures such as venipuncture until the airway is considered to be secure. Anxiety associated with procedures often causes increased respiratory distress. Crying stimulates the airway, increases oxygen consumption, and in some cases, such as epiglottitis, can precipitate laryngospasm that can obstruct the airway.

When the child is intubated, care is provided in the PICU to ensure continual observation (see the *Clinical Skills Manual* SKILLS). Provide humidified air or supplemental oxygen if prescribed. The child with bacterial tracheitis needs frequent suctioning because of thick tracheal secretions that pool in the upper airway.

MEET FLUID AND NUTRITIONAL NEEDS

The illness preceding the emergency department visit may have compromised the child's fluid status, or the child may have difficulty swallowing because of inflammation. Recognize the potential fluid deficit and monitor the child's hydration and nutritional status. Fluids help thin secretions and provide calories for energy and metabolism.

When the child can drink fluids provide cool, noncarbonated, nonacidic drinks such as oral rehydration fluids or fruit-flavored drinks, gelatin, and popsicles. Encourage the parents to gain the child's cooperation in taking oral fluids. When the child's airway is compromised an intravenous infusion is needed to rehydrate the child, maintain fluid balance, or provide emergency access.

ADMINISTER MEDICATIONS

Administer medications as prescribed. Children with acute spasmodic laryngitis and LTB are treated with oral dexamethasone, and some children need nebulized epinephrine. Children with bacterial tracheitis or epiglottitis are initially treated with IV antibiotics until inflammation is reduced and the airway becomes stable without an endotracheal tube. Antibiotics are then administered orally.

PROVIDE FAMILY SUPPORT

Support parents who may be very anxious about the abrupt onset of life-threatening respiratory distress. When the child is intubated, reassure the child and family that their inability to make sounds is temporary. Explain the need for various pieces of equipment to help reduce the child's stress.

DISCHARGE PLANNING AND HOME CARE TEACHING

During the child's observation period for acute spasmodic laryngitis and LTB, educate the parents about actions to take if symptoms recur. For example, the child should return to the healthcare provider if:

• Mild symptoms do not improve after 1 hour of exposure to cool outdoor air or air conditioning.

• The child's breathing is rapid and labored with nasal flaring and retractions.

• The child does not drink adequate fluids and the urine output is reduced.

Ensure that parents of children with bacterial tracheitis or epiglottitis understand the importance of completing the full course of antibiotics.

Evaluation

Expected outcomes of nursing care include the following:

- The child responds to medications with decreased respiratory distress.
- The child's fear and anxiety is managed with family support and explanations about care.

Lower Airway Disorders

Lower airway disorders occur because a structural or functional problem interferes with the lungs' ability to complete the respiratory cycle. Disorders of the lower airway include bronchitis, bronchiolitis, pneumonia, and tuberculosis.

Bronchitis

Acute bronchitis, inflammation of the trachea and bronchi, rarely occurs in childhood as an isolated problem. The bronchi can be affected simultaneously with adjacent respiratory structures during a respiratory illness. Bronchitis occurs most commonly in the winter months.

The classic symptom of bronchitis is a dry, hacking cough that increases in severity at night. The cough may or may not be productive. The child may swallow sputum and vomit as a result. The chest and ribs may be sore because of the deep and frequent coughing. Over several days breath sounds may become coarse with fine crackles, and some scattered high-pitched wheezing may be heard. Treatment is palliative unless a secondary bacterial infection occurs that needs antibiotic therapy.

Nursing Management

Nursing management includes supporting respiratory function through rest, humidification, hydration, and symptomatic treatment. Refer to the sections in this chapter on asthma and pneumonia for detailed information on treatment measures.

Home care should emphasize the self-limiting nature of the disorder. Advise parents who smoke that quitting or not smoking in the child's presence may benefit the child.

Bronchiolitis and Respiratory Syncytial Virus

Bronchiolitis is a lower respiratory tract illness that occurs when a viral or bacterial organism causes inflammation and obstruction of the bronchioles. It is a leading cause of hospitalization during the first year of life (Weinberger, 2011). Infants who develop bronchiolitis have an increased risk for recurrent wheezing during the first year of life (Blanken et al., 2013).

ETIOLOGY AND PATHOPHYSIOLOGY

Respiratory syncytial virus (RSV) is the most common cause of bronchiolitis, but adenovirus, parainfluenza virus, and human metapneumovirus may also be responsible. RSV occurs in annual epidemics from October to March. It is transmitted through direct contact with respiratory secretions or indirectly through contaminated surfaces. The infected child sheds the virus for 3 to 8 days, and the incubation period is 2 to 8 days. Nearly all children have been infected with RSV by 2 years of age, and reinfection throughout life is common (American Academy of Pediatrics [AAP], 2015, p. 667–668). Risk factors for severe RSV infection include immunosuppression, very low birth weight, lung disease, severe neuromuscular disease, or complicated congenital heart defects (Brashers & Huether, 2014).

Viruses, acting as parasites, are able to invade the mucosal cells that line the small bronchi and bronchioles. The invaded cells die when the virus bursts from inside the cell to invade adjacent cells. The membranes of the infected cells fuse with adjacent cells, creating large masses of cells or "syncytia." The resulting cell debris clogs and obstructs the bronchioles and irritates the airway. In response, the airway lining swells and produces excessive mucus. Despite this protective effort by the bronchioles, the actual effect is partial airway obstruction and bronchospasms.

The cycle is repeated throughout both lungs as the airway cells are invaded by the virus. The partially obstructed airways allow air in, but the mucus and airway swelling cause air trapping, and hyperinflation of the alveoli. Areas of atelectasis may occur. Normal gas exchange is affected, leading to hypoxemia. The child with severe RSV is at risk for apnea and respiratory failure as hypoxemia and hypercarbia develop.

CLINICAL MANIFESTATIONS

Some children have mild symptoms such as rhinitis, cough, low-grade fever, wheezing, tachypnea, poor feeding, vomiting, and diarrhea. Dehydration may be present if the child has been sick for several days. Parents report that the infant or child is acting more ill—appearing sicker, less playful, and less interested in eating. Infants, especially, may refuse to feed or may spit up what they eat along with thick, clear mucus.

The infant or child with a more severe infection has tachypnea greater than 70 breaths per minute, grunting, increased wheezing, crackles, retractions, nasal flaring, irritability, lethargy, poor fluid intake, and a distended abdomen from overexpanded lungs. As hypoxia develops the infant becomes cyanotic and has decreasing mental status. As the airflow continues to decrease, breath sounds diminish. Thus the noisier the lungs, the better, as this indicates that the child is still able to move air in and out of the lungs. While RSV bronchiolitis resolves in 5 to 7 days, increased airway resistance and airway hypersensitivity may persist for weeks or even months.

CLINICAL THERAPY

The history and physical examination provide the data needed to diagnose bronchiolitis. Chest radiographs show hyperinflation, patchy atelectasis, and other signs of inflammation. Enzyme-linked immunoabsorbent assay (ELISA) or immunofluorescent assay performed on a posterior nasopharyngeal wash or swab specimen are used to identify the virus causing bronchiolitis (see the *Clinical Skills Manual* SKILLS).

Treatment is supportive. Most children have mild disease and can be managed at home. See *Teaching Highlights: Home Care for the Infant With Mild Bronchiolitis.* The child is placed on respiratory and contact isolation when hospitalized to minimize the spread of the virus to other hospitalized children. Humidified oxygen is provided to infants with severe hypoxemia. Other supportive care includes hydration with oral or IV fluids and nasal suctioning before feeding. Continuous positive airway pressure (CPAP) may be used in the child with moderate to severe bronchiolitis. Chest physiotherapy does not affect severity or length of hospital stay and is not recommended (Zentz, 2011).

Few medications are prescribed for RSV and bronchiolitis. Antipyretics may be used. Nebulized hypertonic saline (3%) can

| TEACHING HIGHLIGHTS | Home Care for the Infant With Mild Bronchiolitis |

General care instructions:

- Use the bulb syringe to suction the nares of an infant under 1 year of age.
- Give fluids to help thin secretions and provide calories for energy.
- Encourage active toddlers to rest and take naps during recovery.

Advise parents to call the physician if:

- Respiratory symptoms interfere with sleeping or eating.
- Breathing is rapid or difficult.
- Symptoms persist in a child who is less than 1 year old, has heart or lung disease, or was premature and had lung disease after birth.
- The child acts sicker—appears tired, less playful, and less interested in food (parents just "feel" the child is not improving).

improve clinical severity score and reduce hospital length of stay. Bronchodilators and corticosteroids have not been demonstrated to be effective therapies. Antibiotics are used only when a bacterial infection is present.

Prevention of RSV is a focus for children at highest risk for severe bronchiolitis. Examples include infants born prematurely (less than 32 weeks' gestation) and those who required supplemental oxygen for several weeks after birth. Some children less than 2 years of age being treated for chronic lung disease of prematurity, congestive heart failure, or pulmonary hypertension are also at higher risk. The American Academy of Pediatrics has specific criteria for selecting infants and children up to age 2 years to receive passive immunity protection (AAP, 2015, pp. 673–675).

Intramuscular palivizumab (Synagis) provides passive immunity to help protect these high-risk infants. A dose of 15 mg/kg is given every 30 days for 5 months beginning in October or November at the onset of the RSV season. Palivizumab is expensive, but it is believed to offer benefits to the infants at high risk who might require hospitalization for RSV. Palivizumab does not interfere with administration of normal recommended childhood vaccines (AAP, 2015, p. 40).

Nursing Management

For the Child With Bronchiolitis and RSV

Nursing Assessment and Diagnosis

PHYSIOLOGIC ASSESSMENT

Assess airway and respiratory function carefully. Good observation skills are important to ensure timely interventions for worsening respiratory symptoms and prevention of respiratory failure (see the *Assessment Guide* and Table 46–1 earlier in this chapter). Assess the child's hydration status, weigh the child daily, and monitor the intake and output. Attach a cardiorespiratory monitor and pulse oximeter. An oxygen saturation level below 90% is the best indicator of the condition's severity.

SAFETY ALERT!

RSV bronchiolitis often increases in severity before beginning to resolve. Stay alert for signs of increasing respiratory distress and a greater need for oxygen. Signs of life-threatening illness include central cyanosis, respiratory rate greater than 70 breaths a minute, listlessness, diminished breath sounds, and apneic episodes. Inform the physician immediately of any significant changes in respiratory status.

PSYCHOSOCIAL ASSESSMENT

Observe children and their parents for signs of fear and anxiety. The unfamiliar hospital environment and procedures can increase stress. Parents' questions, as well as their nonverbal cues, help direct nursing interventions during admission and throughout hospitalization.

The accompanying *Nursing Care Plan: The Child With Bronchiolitis* lists common nursing diagnoses for the child with bronchiolitis. Others that might also be appropriate include (NANDA-I © 2014):

- *Airway Clearance, Ineffective*, related to increased airway secretions in bronchioles
- *Activity Intolerance* related to imbalance between oxygen supply and demand
- *Family Processes, Interrupted*, related to sudden acute illness of the infant

Planning and Implementation

Nursing management of the hospitalized child with bronchiolitis focuses on maintaining respiratory function, supporting overall physiologic function and hydration, reducing the child's and family's anxiety, and preparing the family for home care.

MAINTAIN RESPIRATORY FUNCTION

Close monitoring is essential to evaluate the child's improvement or to spot early signs of deterioration. Patent nares are important to promote oxygen intake. A bulb syringe and saline nose drops can be used to quickly clear the nasal passages. Elevate the head of the bed to ease the work of breathing and drain mucus from the upper airways. Supplemental oxygen with humidity may be provided via nasal cannula, mask, hood, or tent. When the child resists or is frightened by the oxygen apparatus, engage the parent to soothe the child and promote acceptance of the therapy.

SUPPORT PHYSIOLOGIC FUNCTION

Group nursing tasks to decrease stress and promote rest. Medications may be administered to control temperature and promote comfort as needed. Infants may have feeding difficulty and are at risk for aspiration. Suction the nasal passages before giving oral feedings. Feed smaller volumes more frequently to help conserve energy in infants who are formula-fed or breast-fed. When the risk of aspiration is high, nasogastric tube feedings may be used to provide nutrition. An IV infusion may be ordered to rehydrate the child and maintain fluid balance until oral fluid intake is adequate.

Nursing Care Plan: The Child With Bronchiolitis

1. Nursing Diagnosis: *Breathing Pattern, Ineffective,* **related to increased work of breathing (NANDA-I © 2014)**

GOAL: The child will return to respiratory baseline and will not experience respiratory failure.

INTERVENTION	RATIONALE
• Assess respiratory status (see *Assessment Guide*) when child is calm and not crying at least every 2–4 hr, or more often as indicated for an increasing or decreasing respiratory rate and episodes of apnea.	• Changes in breathing pattern may occur quickly as the child's energy reserves are depleted. Baseline and subsequent assessments help detect changes in the respiratory rate and respiratory effort.
• Attach a cardiorespiratory monitor and pulse oximeter with alarms set. Record and report changes promptly to physician.	• The alarm can alert the nurse to any sudden respiratory changes and lead to more rapid interventions.

EXPECTED OUTCOME: Child will return to respiratory baseline within 48–72 hr.

GOAL: The child's oxygenation status will return to baseline.

INTERVENTION	RATIONALE
• Administer humidified oxygen via mask, nasal cannula, hood, or tent.	• Humidified oxygen loosens secretions, helps maintain oxygenation status, and eases respiratory distress.
• Assess and compare the child's SpO_2 level on room air and when on supplemental oxygen.	• Comparison of SpO_2 levels provides information about improvement status.
• Note child's response to ordered medications.	• Medications act systemically to improve oxygenation and decrease inflammation.
• Position head of bed up or place child in position of comfort on parent's lap, if crying or struggling in crib or bed.	• Position facilitates improved aeration and promotes decrease in anxiety (especially in infants) and energy expenditure.
• Assess tolerance to feeding and activities.	• Provides an assessment of condition improvement.

EXPECTED OUTCOME: Child's respiratory effort will ease. The SpO_2 level will remain above 90% during treatment. Child will tolerate therapeutic measures with no adverse effects. Child will rest quietly in position of comfort.

2. Nursing Diagnosis: *Fluid Volume: Deficient, Risk for,* **related to inability to meet body requirements and increased metabolic demand (NANDA-I © 2014)**

GOAL: The child's immediate fluid deficit will be corrected.

INTERVENTION	RATIONALE
• Evaluate need for intravenous fluids. Maintain IV, if ordered.	• Previous fluid loss may require immediate replacement.

EXPECTED OUTCOME: Child's hydration status will be maintained during acute phase of illness as demonstrated by appropriate urine output and moist mucous membranes.

GOAL: The child will be adequately hydrated, be able to tolerate oral fluids, and progress to normal diet.

INTERVENTION	RATIONALE
• Calculate maintenance fluid requirements and give oral fluids, IV fluids, or both.	• Assessment of fluid requirements enables the child to maintain hydration while transitioning to oral fluids.
• Offer clear fluids and incorporate parent in care. Offer fluid choice when tolerated.	• Choice of fluid offered by parent gains the child's cooperation.
• Maintain strict intake and output monitoring and evaluate specific gravity at least every 8 hours.	• Monitoring provides objective evidence of fluid loss and ongoing hydration status.
• Perform daily weight measurement on the same scale at the same time of day. Evaluate skin turgor.	• Further evidence of improvement of hydration status.
• Assess mucous membranes and presence of tears.	• Moist mucous membranes and tears are signs of adequate hydration.

EXPECTED OUTCOME: Child will take adequate oral fluids after 24–48 hr to maintain hydration. Child will accept beverage of choice from parent or nursing staff. Child's weight will stabilize after 24–48 hr; skin turgor will be supple. Child will show evidence of improved hydration.

(continued)

Nursing Care Plan: The Child With Bronchiolitis (continued)

3. Nursing Diagnosis: *Anxiety (Child and Parent)* **related to acute illness, hospitalization, uncertain course of illness and treatment, and home care needs (NANDA-I © 2014)**

GOAL: The child and parents will demonstrate behaviors that indicate less anxiety.

INTERVENTION	RATIONALE
• Encourage parents to express fears and ask questions; provide direct answers and discuss care, procedures, and condition changes.	• Parents have the opportunity to vent feelings and receive timely, relevant information. This helps reduce parents' anxiety and increase trust in nursing staff.
• Incorporate parents in the child's care. Encourage parents to bring familiar objects from home. Ask about and incorporate in care plan the home routines for feeding and sleeping.	• Familiar people, routines, and objects decrease the child's anxiety and increase parents' sense of control over an unexpected, uncertain situation.

EXPECTED OUTCOME: Parents and child will show less anxiety as symptoms improve and as child and parents feel more secure in hospital environment. *Parents* will freely ask questions and participate in the child's care. *Children* will cry less and allow themselves to be touched or held by staff.

GOAL: Parents will verbalize knowledge of bronchiolitis symptoms and use of home care methods before the child's discharge from the hospital.

INTERVENTION	RATIONALE
• Explain symptoms, treatment, and home care of bronchiolitis.	• Anticipating the potential for recurrence assists the family to be prepared should respiratory symptoms recur after discharge.
• Provide written instructions for follow-up care arrangements, as needed.	• Written and verbal instructions reinforce knowledge. Parents may not "hear" and remember details if only given verbally.
• Make sure parents can read the instructions provided in family's primary language.	• Many families have reading difficulties or may read a language other than English.

EXPECTED OUTCOME: Parents will accurately describe respiratory symptoms and initial home care actions.

REDUCE ANXIETY

The need for hospitalization and assistive therapies creates anxiety and fear in the child and parents. The parents may be frightened by the child's continued respiratory difficulty. Infants may respond to their parents' anxiety and be more irritable. Provide parents with thorough explanations and daily updates, and encourage their participation in the child's care. Reassure them that holding or touching the child will not dislodge wires or tubing, and that their presence will calm and support the child.

If the child has been ill for a few days before admission, the parents are likely to be tired. Acknowledging parents' physical and emotional needs creates a spirit of caring and enhances communication between staff and family. Encourage the parents to take turns at the child's bedside and to take breaks for meals and rest.

DISCHARGE PLANNING AND HOME CARE TEACHING

The child is discharged once oxygenation is stable (pulse oximetry at least 90%) on room air and full oral feedings have been possible for at least 12 hours (Weinberger, 2011). In most children, respiratory efforts and decreased mucus production decrease within 24 to 72 hours, but all symptoms like coughing may take weeks to resolve.

Teach the parents proper administration of medications. Acetaminophen or ibuprofen may be prescribed for persistent low-grade fevers and general discomfort. Advise parents that RSV infection can recur. Educate them to recognize symptoms and when to call the healthcare provider.

Evaluation

Expected outcomes of nursing care for the child with bronchiolitis are provided in the *Nursing Care Plan*.

Pneumonia

Pneumonia, an inflammation or infection of the bronchioles and alveolar spaces of the lungs, occurs most often in infants and young children. More than 150,000 children are hospitalized for pneumonia annually in the United States (Queen et al., 2014). Pneumonia can be community acquired (CAP) or hospital acquired (e.g., associated with mechanical ventilation). The focus of this discussion is CAP.

Pneumonia may be viral, mycoplasmal, or bacterial in origin. Viral-bacterial coinfection also occurs. Children under 5 years of age most often have viral pneumonia caused by RSV, human metapneumovirus, influenza virus, parainfluenza virus, or adenovirus. Bacterial pneumonia occurs in all age groups. Mycoplasmal pneumonia is more common in children 5 years and older. Common bacterial organisms include *Streptococcus pneumoniae*, *Chlamydophila pneumoniae*, and *Staphylococcus aureus*. Group B streptococcus, enteric gram-negative bacilli, and

Chlamydia trachomatis are found in infants younger than 3 months of age. Children with cystic fibrosis or immunosuppression are susceptible to other bacterial, parasitic, or fungal infections.

Bacterial and viral invaders act differently within the lungs:

- Bacteria enter the lungs after aspiration of nasopharyngeal bacteria and colonize in the trachea and bronchi. Prior damage by a viral infection may damage the epithelium and reduce the child's ability to clear the organisms. Inflammation leads to edema and purulent exudates. Cellular debris and mucus cause airway obstruction. Bacteria tend to be distributed evenly throughout one or more lobes of a single lung, a pattern termed *unilateral lobar pneumonia*.

- Viruses enter through the upper respiratory tract, damaging the ciliated epithelium in the distal airway. Viruses invade and kill cells causing cell debris. The alveoli become infiltrated nearest the bronchi of one or both lungs. Adjacent areas become invaded in a scattered, patchy pattern referred to as bronchopneumonia.

- Aspiration of food, emesis, gastric reflux, or hydrocarbons causes a chemical injury and inflammatory response, which sets the stage for bacterial invasion.

CAP is often preceded by an upper respiratory tract infection including rhinitis and a cough. Other symptoms include fever, rhonchi, crackles, wheezes, dyspnea, tachypnea, chest pain, restlessness, and abdominal pain. Newborns and infants may have tachypnea, grunting, nasal flaring, retractions, irritability, lethargy, and a poor appetite. Diminished breath sounds may be noted.

Diagnosis is based on history and physical findings. Rapid influenza and other respiratory virus testing is recommended to help distinguish between viral and bacterial causes of CAP. Bacterial pneumonia is more often associated with a higher fever, absolute neutrophil count, and percentage of bands (Brashers & Heuther, 2014). A chest radiograph and blood cultures may be performed when the child requires hospitalization.

Clinical management for all types of pneumonia includes pain and fever control, and supportive care through airway management, fluids, and rest. Children with severe CAP are hospitalized, and may be treated with antibiotics, supplemental oxygen, and IV fluids. Current antibiotic guidelines are high-dose ampicillin or amoxicillin for 5 days in children with uncomplicated CAP (Greenberg, Givon-Lavi, Sadaka, et al., 2014). Antiviral therapy is prescribed for some children.

Nursing Management

If the child with CAP is hospitalized, assess the child, paying particular attention to respiratory rate, heart rate, and temperature, and observe color for pallor or cyanosis. Attach a pulse oximeter to monitor the SpO_2 level. Assess hydration status. Assess for the presence of pain with coughing.

Nursing measures used for the child with bronchiolitis are generally applicable (see earlier section in this chapter). Teach the child and parent how to splint the chest by hugging a small pillow or teddy bear to make coughing less painful. Acetaminophen or ibuprofen may be prescribed for pain management and temperature control. Administer antibiotics as prescribed. Promote hydration and nutrition by encouraging the intake of preferred clear liquids and small servings of soft foods.

For home management, teach parents about administering prescribed antibiotics, any potential side effects, and the need to give the full course. Educate parents about signs that the child's condition may be worsening (increased breathing difficulty or refusal to take fluids). Most children recover uneventfully, but some continue to have worsening reactive airway problems or abnormal results on pulmonary function tests.

Preventive measures are limited. The *Haemophilus influenzae* type B (Hib) and pneumococcal conjugate (PCV13) vaccines protect against some causes of pneumonia. The 23-valent pneumococcal vaccine is recommended for children over 2 years of age with immunosuppression or some chronic conditions (see Chapter 43).

Tuberculosis

Tuberculosis (TB) is an infection caused by *Mycobacterium tuberculosis*, which is transmitted through the air in infectious particles called *droplet nuclei*. About 1000 active TB cases occur in children each year, and rates are highest among children and adolescents with at least one foreign parent (Starke & Cruz, 2014). Children account for 7% of all cases reported in the United States each year (Winston & Menzies, 2012).

ETIOLOGY AND PATHOPHYSIOLOGY

Children usually acquire a TB infection from infected adults who cough, sneeze, speak, or sing, and send out tiny droplets containing the bacillus. When inhaled, the bacillus is small enough to travel directly to the alveoli and cause infection. When the organism reaches the alveoli, an immune response is initiated, and macrophages surround and wall off the bacillus in a small hard capsule, called a *tubercle*. The tubercle bacilli grow slowly, dividing every 25 to 32 hours. The bacilli grow for 2 to 12 weeks until they number 1000 to 10,000, at which point the cellular immune response to a TB skin test (TST) would occur if the test were administered.

In persons with intact cell-mediated immunity, activated T cells and macrophages form granulomas around the tubercles that limit multiplication. The proliferation of TB is arrested, but small numbers of viable bacilli remain in the tubercle. These individuals have latent tuberculosis infection (LTBI), a positive TST, and no clinical or radiographic signs of disease. They are not infectious and cannot transmit the disease.

Active TB can develop as the bacilli grow, divide within the tubercle, and break free. Progression to active TB generally occurs within 1 year of infection in infants and adolescents, who have the greatest risk of transitioning from LTBI to active TB (Perez-Velez & Marais, 2012). Factors further increasing that risk include immunosuppressive therapy, HIV coinfection, immunodeficiency, malnutrition, and chronic medical conditions (AAP, 2015, p. 808). Most children under age 10 years with active TB are not contagious because they have small pulmonary lesions and unproductive coughing during which few or no bacilli are expelled (AAP, 2015, pp. 827).

Disseminated, or extrapulmonary, TB occurs more commonly in infants and young children. Bacilli are released from the primary site into the bloodstream, spreading to the liver, spleen, kidney, bone marrow, or meninges (miliary TB).

CLINICAL MANIFESTATIONS

Children with LTBI are asymptomatic. Children with pulmonary TB may have a persistent cough, weight loss or failure to gain weight, fever, fatigue, wheezing, and decreased breath sounds. Adolescents may have fever, anorexia, weight loss or growth delay, productive cough, and night sweats. **Hemoptysis** (coughing up blood from the respiratory tract) is a late sign of advanced pulmonary TB. When TB spreads outside the pulmonary system, additional signs are specific to the system invaded:

- *Superficial lymphadenitis:* firm, nontender, matted lymph nodes
- *Miliary:* high fever, vomiting, lethargy, headache, seizures, nuchal rigidity, cranial nerve palsies, and irritability; also hepatosplenomegaly and generalized lymphadenopathy
- *Osteoarticular:* inflammation, pain, swelling, fever, and limited range of motion of the affected bone or joint

CLINICAL THERAPY

Screening to identify a child's risk for LTBI should occur during the first health visit, every 6 months until age 2 years, and then annually. Administer a tuberculin skin test (intradermal purified protein derivative [PPD]) or interferon-gamma release assay (IGRA) if one or more of these risk factors are present (AAP, 2015, p. 812; Desale, Bringardner, Fitzgerald, et al., 2013; Rose et al., 2014; Seddon, Hesseling, Godfrey-Faussett, et al., 2013):

- The child's parents or family members immigrated from a country or region where TB is an established health problem, such as Asia, India, the Middle East, Africa, or Latin America.
- The child was born in one of the countries or regions mentioned above.
- The child traveled to any of the countries or regions mentioned above and had close contact with residents, such as residing in the home of residents, for a week or longer.
- A family member has tested positive with a PPD or IGRA.
- The child has clinical signs or radiologic findings that could be associated with TB.
- The child infected with HIV should have annual tuberculin testing.

A positive PPD or IGRA indicates that the child has been exposed to and infected with TB, and antibodies have been produced against the bacillus.

An interferon-gamma release assay (IGRA; e.g., quantiFERON or T.Spot.TB) may help clarify PPD findings. For example, a child vaccinated with bacille Calmette-Guérin (BCG) may have a false-positive response to multiple PPDs, but IGRA does not cross-react with BCG and gives a more accurate result (Riazi et al., 2012). Like the PPD, the IGRA cannot distinguish between latent or active TB. Other diagnostic tests include acid-fast stains of blood, gastric aspirate, sputum cultures, and a chest radiograph.

Active and latent TB are treated with isoniazid, rifampicin, pyrazinamide, and ethambutol. Therapy for active TB usually involves a 6-month regimen consisting of isoniazid, rifampin, pyrazinamide, and ethambutol for the first 2 months and isoniazid and rifampin for the remaining 4 months. LTBI in children less than 12 years of age is treated with a single daily dose of isoniazid for 9 months (or rifampin for 6 months if TB is drug resistant to isoniazid). Direct-observed drug therapy administered by a healthcare provider 2 times a week for the duration of treatment is recommended for children with active TB and when daily therapy adherence is not assured for children with LTBI (AAP, 2015, pp. 816). Healthy youth with LTBI, ages 12 years and older, may receive once-weekly direct-observed drug therapy with isoniazid and rifampin for 12 weeks (Jereb, Goldberg, Powell, et al., 2011). Children with a positive PPD and negative IGRA who do not receive treatment for LTBI should be followed for 1 to 2 years to monitor for transition to active disease (Amanatidou, Syridou, Mavrikou, et al., 2012).

The local public health department is notified to search for disease contacts of the child with newly diagnosed LTBI or active TB. The child is considered a sentinel case and the adult contact with active TB must be identified.

Nursing Management

Assessment focuses on identifying children at high risk of TB exposure and performing a PPD as appropriate. Infant and young children with a positive PPD are at greater risk to develop active TB, so assess them carefully for weight loss, fever, fatigue, coughing, and respiratory status. Consider the child's immunosuppression status. If active TB is suspected, implement airborne isolation precautions until the infection status is known.

SAFETY ALERT!

Airborne isolation precautions are intended to protect the nurse as well as to reduce the risk for transmission of infection to other clients. Use all recommended personal protective equipment (PPE) correctly, perform hand hygiene, and appropriately dispose of linens, PPE, and trash to protect yourself and others from infection.

Nursing care of the child with LTBI focuses on administering medications and providing supportive care. Teach parents about the disease process, medications, possible side effects, and the importance of completing long-term therapy. Emphasize the importance of taking medications as prescribed on an empty stomach. Initiate direct-observed drug therapy twice a week if poor adherence is suspected.

Encourage proper nutrition and rest to promote normal growth and development. The child can return to school or child care when effective therapy has been instituted, adherence to therapy has been documented, and clinical symptoms have diminished substantially (AAP, 2015, p. 829). Children should receive all usual immunizations. Most children treated for TB can lead essentially normal lives. See the discussion of pneumonia earlier in this chapter and of tubercular meningitis in Chapter 54 for other nursing care measures.

Chronic Lung Diseases

Bronchopulmonary Dysplasia (Chronic Lung Disease)

Bronchopulmonary dysplasia (BPD), also called chronic lung disease of prematurity, is defined as the need for supplemental oxygen for at least 28 days after premature birth. BPD more commonly develops in infants born at less than 28 weeks' gestation when lungs are immature. BPD is estimated to occur in 35% to 50% of newborns born at less than 28 weeks' gestation (Strueby & Thébaud, 2014).

ETIOLOGY AND PATHOPHYSIOLOGY

Preterm infants less than 28 weeks' gestation are born before alveolar development occurs. BPD results from positive-pressure ventilation and oxygen needed to treat respiratory failure and respiratory distress syndrome. (See newborn respiratory distress information in Chapter 27.) The treatment injures the immature lungs leading to fewer and larger alveoli with less functional surface area and a smaller vascular bed in the lungs, which has greater tone and reactivity. These changes potentially lead to long-term chronic lung disease (Strueby & Thébaud, 2014). A patent ductus arteriosus may also contribute to BPD development. Antenatal corticosteroids and surfactant replacement therapy have reduced the incidence of BPD in more mature preterm infants.

Pathophysiology Illustrated: **Barrel Chest**

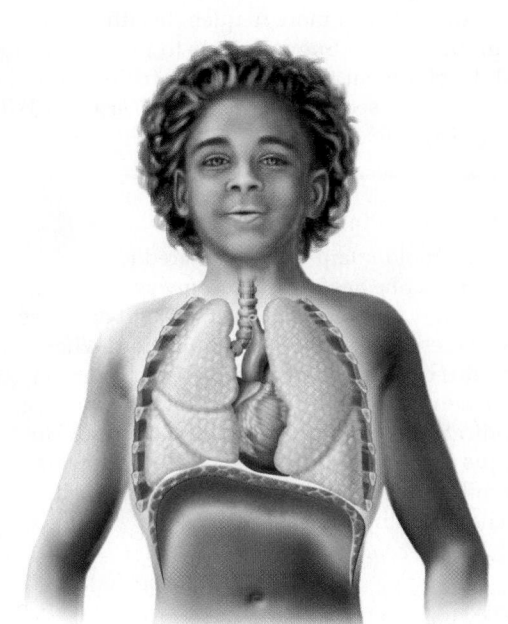

A barrel chest may result from chronic respiratory conditions such as asthma or bronchopulmonary dysplasia, in which air trapping or hyperinflation of the alveoli occurs. The chest's anterioposterior diameter increases to give a rounded chest shape.

CLINICAL MANIFESTATIONS

The infant with BPD has persistent signs of respiratory distress: tachypnea, nasal flaring, grunting, retractions, wheezing, crackles, and irritability. Normal activities like feeding create increased oxygen demands and fatigue that may lead to failure to thrive. The infant has intermittent bronchospasms, mucous plugging, and chronic air trapping, which may lead to a barrel-shaped chest (see *Pathophysiology Illustrated: Barrel Chest*). Cyanosis may be seen in severe cases.

CLINICAL THERAPY

See Chapter 27 for initial respiratory management of the low-birth-weight infant. Medical management for BPD involves therapies to support respiratory function and good nutrition, which helps to accelerate lung maturity. Medications are administered such as surfactant, corticosteroids, vitamin A, and caffeine (Strueby & Thébaud, 2014). Supplemental oxygen with humidity is used. Nasal continuous or intermittent positive pressure ventilation is often used. An endotracheal tube or tracheostomy may be needed for long-term airway management to prevent narrowing of the trachea in more severe cases. Infants with severe BPD are carefully weaned off of assisted ventilation. Increased calories are needed to support growth, but fluids are restricted to prevent pulmonary edema. Some infants need gastrostomy or nasogastric tube feeding to get adequate calories.

Severity of BPD is determined at 36 days' corrected gestational age by the ongoing need for supplemental oxygen or positive-pressure ventilation in an infant who required supplemental oxygen at 28 days of life. Pulmonary artery hypertension is a complication when severe lung disease exists (see Chapter 47). Surviving infants are at risk for cognitive delays, cerebral palsy, growth failure, and abnormal lung function. Infants with severe BPD often have chronic lung disease.

After discharge from the neonatal ICU (NICU), some infants require ongoing oxygen therapy and some may have a tracheostomy. Infants with severe BPD often require frequent hospitalization because of respiratory infections or pulmonary hypertension. Antibiotics are used to aggressively treat infections. An annual influenza vaccine is recommended, and palivizumab may be given monthly to prevent RSV (see section earlier in this chapter on bronchiolitis). Infants and children with continuing airway hyperactivity may have bronchodilator therapy and asthma controller medications prescribed (see section on asthma later in this chapter).

Nursing Management

For the Child With Bronchopulmonary Dysplasia

Nursing management focuses on assessing and managing the infant's acute episodes, ensuring adequate nutrition, and promoting growth and development.

Nursing Assessment and Diagnosis

At each healthcare visit, assess the infant's respiratory status and growth. The infant may have poor weight gain because the work of breathing requires extra calories. Assess how well the family is managing care for the child in the home and any stressors that might exist. Evaluate development regularly because the infant may have motor, language, and cognitive delays. Coordinate a periodic assessment of hearing and vision. Infants with BPD may become acutely ill at any time, so observe for signs of infection.

During hospitalization for acute infections, a cardiorespiratory monitor and pulse oximeter are used. Assess airway and respiratory function, vital signs, color, and behavior changes to identify signs of worsening respiratory symptoms even when oxygen is provided. Observe for airway obstruction when the infant has a tracheostomy and suction as needed. See the *Clinical Skills Manual* SKILLS for tracheostomy care.

Nursing diagnoses that may be appropriate include (NANDA-I © 2014):

- *Gas Exchange, Impaired*, related to ventilation-perfusion imbalance
- *Nutrition, Imbalanced: Less than Body Requirements*, related to high metabolic needs and fatigue associated with feeding
- *Caregiver Role Strain* related to 24-hour responsibility for infant with BPD
- *Development: Delayed, Risk for*, related to chronic condition and limited opportunities to practice motor skills

Planning and Implementation

Organize care for the hospitalized child to reduce unnecessary physical stimulation. Position the infant to facilitate breathing.

Administer medications as prescribed. Careful fluid management is essential to reduce the risk for pulmonary edema. Provide nutrition to meet energy needs. Support the mother who desires to breastfeed. A high-calorie formula (24 to 30 calories/oz) may be given to promote weight gain. Some children need nasogastric or enteral feedings to get adequate nutrition when cyanosis is noted with feeding.

Once home, many infants need oxygen, tracheostomy care, multiple medications, and high-calorie feedings (Figure 46–3). Make referrals for needed oxygen, respiratory supplies, medications, an early intervention program, and follow-up care well in advance of the infant's discharge. Some families need home health nursing assistance, especially during the initial transition

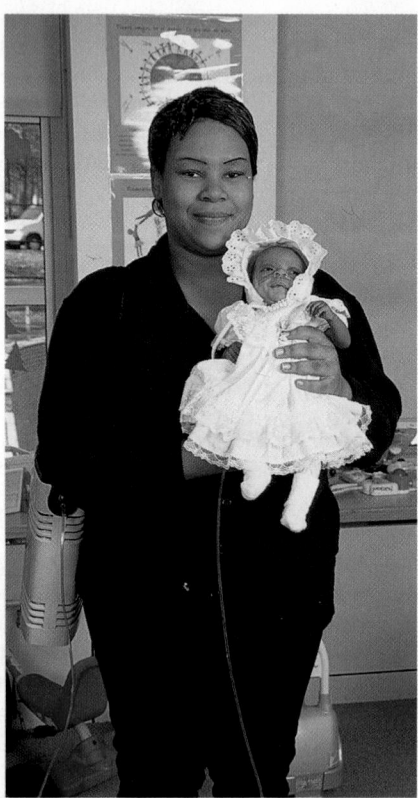

Figure 46–3 **Many children with BPD are cared for at home, with the support of a home care program to monitor the family's ability to provide airway management, oxygen, and ventilator support. This premature infant girl, who is now 4 months old but weighs only about 5 lb, still requires supplemental oxygen.**

period. Teach parents to provide the complex care needed by the infant and to identify the signs of respiratory compromise indicating a need for rapid intervention.

All infants with BPD need more frequent health promotion visits and all immunizations. Suggest ways to provide for the infant's normal development through rest, nutrition, stimulation, and family support (see *Health Promotion: The Child With Bronchopulmonary Dysplasia*).

Clinical Reasoning Infant With BPD

Emily is an 8-month-old infant with BPD cared for at home by her parents. She has a tracheostomy and receives humidification. Emily has periodic infections and episodes of respiratory distress that require hospitalization. When she develops a fever, more secretions than usual collect in the trachea. Suctioning is needed to ease Emily's breathing. What signs indicate that Emily needs to be suctioned? How do you select the correct size of suction catheter? How do you suction Emily without causing hypoxia? When is it necessary to change Emily's tracheostomy tube?

Evaluation

Expected outcomes of nursing care may include:

- The infant receives adequate calories to sustain growth.
- The family identifies acute illness episodes rapidly and seeks appropriate care.
- The infant's acute respiratory decompensation episodes are effectively managed.

Asthma

Asthma is a common chronic disorder in children characterized by bronchial constriction, hyperresponsive airways, and airway inflammation. An estimated 10.5 million (14%) of children in the United States have received an asthma diagnosis, and 7.1 million children continue to have asthma episodes. Children report that asthma episodes result in missing 1 or more days of school and some activity limitation (Centers for Disease Control and Prevention, 2013). Asthma results in an increased number of health center and emergency department visits for treatment; sometimes hospitalization is necessary. The rate of death due to asthma in children and youth in the United States is 2.6 per million (Centers for Disease Control and Prevention, 2013). See *Developing Cultural Competence: Asthma Prevalence*.

Healthy People 2020

(RD-1) Reduce asthma deaths

(RD-2) Reduce hospitalizations for asthma

(RD-3) Reduce emergency department (ED) visits for asthma

Developing Cultural Competence Asthma Prevalence

Current asthma prevalence in children was higher among males (10%) compared to females (7.1%). Among racial and ethnic groups, Black children (14.0%) and multirace children (13.2%) have a higher prevalence than White children (7.4%) (Centers for Disease Control and Prevention, 2013).

Health Promotion The Child With Bronchopulmonary Dysplasia

Health Supervision

- Assess blood pressure to detect abnormal findings associated with pulmonary hypertension.
- Coordinate vision screening by an ophthalmologist every 2 to 3 months during the first year of life. Myopia and strabismus are common in premature infants.
- Coordinate pulmonary function tests annually or as needed for clinical condition.
- Perform hearing and other screening tests as recommended for age.

Growth and Developmental Surveillance

- Assess growth and plot measurements on a growth chart corrected for gestational age. Even if length and weight are lower than normal, monitor for continued growth following the growth curves.
- Perform a developmental assessment, correcting for gestational age.

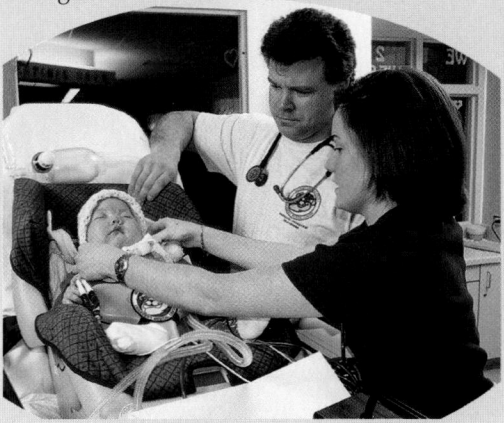

Nutrition

- Review caloric intake. Ensure that increased calories are provided to support growth. Assess feeding difficulties related to oral motor function associated with long-term enteral feeding. Refer to a nutritionist as necessary.

Physical Activity

- Organize care to provide rest periods during the day.
- Give parents ideas for promoting the infant's motor development, such as reaching for and moving toward toys and objects of interest.

Family Interactions

- Identify ways to coordinate nighttime care to reduce child and family sleep disturbances.
- Provide discipline appropriate for developmental age.

Disease Prevention Strategies

- Reduce exposure to infections. Encourage selection of a childcare provider who cares for a small number of children, if one is used. If possible, avoid the use of childcare centers during RSV season.
- Immunize the child with the routine vaccine schedule based on chronologic age.
- Administer the 23-valent pneumococcal vaccine at 2 years of age.
- Provide monthly injections of palivizumab throughout the RSV season.

Condition-Specific Guidance

- Develop an emergency care plan for times when the infant's condition rapidly worsens.

ETIOLOGY AND PATHOPHYSIOLOGY

Asthma is a chronic inflammatory disease caused by multiple factors (e.g., environmental exposures, viral illnesses, allergens, and a genetic predisposition) that occur at a crucial time in the immune system's development. Asthma is now considered to be a collection of several diseases that have similar characteristics and symptoms (Custovic, Lazic, & Simpson, 2013).

Many potential genes or regions of chromosomes are associated with asthma, such as those that are associated with increased immune and inflammatory response and airway remodeling. Approximately 70% of children have an allergic or atopic form of asthma, while other children have genetic factors that reduce their responsiveness to beta-adrenergic inhaled medications (Brashers & Huether, 2014; Chang, 2012). Environmental exposures also increase the risk for asthma, including passive tobacco smoke, indoor air contaminants (e.g., pet dander, cockroach feces), and outdoor air pollutants. Recurrent respiratory viral infections also increase risk. Protective factors are believed to include a large family size, later birth order, childcare attendance, and exposure to certain organisms. In theory, these factors increase exposure to infections early in life, enabling the child's immune system to develop along a nonallergic pathway (Brashers & Huether, 2014).

Persistent inflammation causes the normal protective mechanisms of the lungs (mucous formation, mucosal swelling, and airway muscle contraction) to overreact in response to a **trigger** (an inflammatory or noninflammatory stimulus that initiates an asthma episode). Triggers include exercise, infectious agents, allergens, fragrances, food additives, pollutants, weather changes, emotions, and stress. Inflammatory mechanisms enhance airway responsiveness, and triggers stimulate bronchospasms (smooth muscle contractions).

The trigger leads B cells to activate IgE and cytokines that then activate the migration and proliferation of eosinophils and the release of proinflammatory mediators. Direct tissue injury, increased bronchial hyperresponsiveness, fibroblast proliferation, and airway scarring result. An exaggerated inflammatory response leads to vasodilation, increased capillary permeability, mucosal edema, contraction of smooth bronchial muscle, and secretion of thick mucus, which narrow and obstruct the airways. Impaired expiration leads to air trapping, hyperinflation, and dyspnea, the physiologic sequence that results in an acute asthma episode (see *Pathophysiology Illustrated: Asthma*). Decreased perfusion of the alveolar capillaries results from hypoxic vasoconstriction and increased pressure due to hyperinflation of the alveoli. Hypoxemia leads to an increased respiratory rate, but because of airway resistance, less air is inspired per minute, worsening hypoxemia.

Pathophysiology Illustrated: **Asthma**

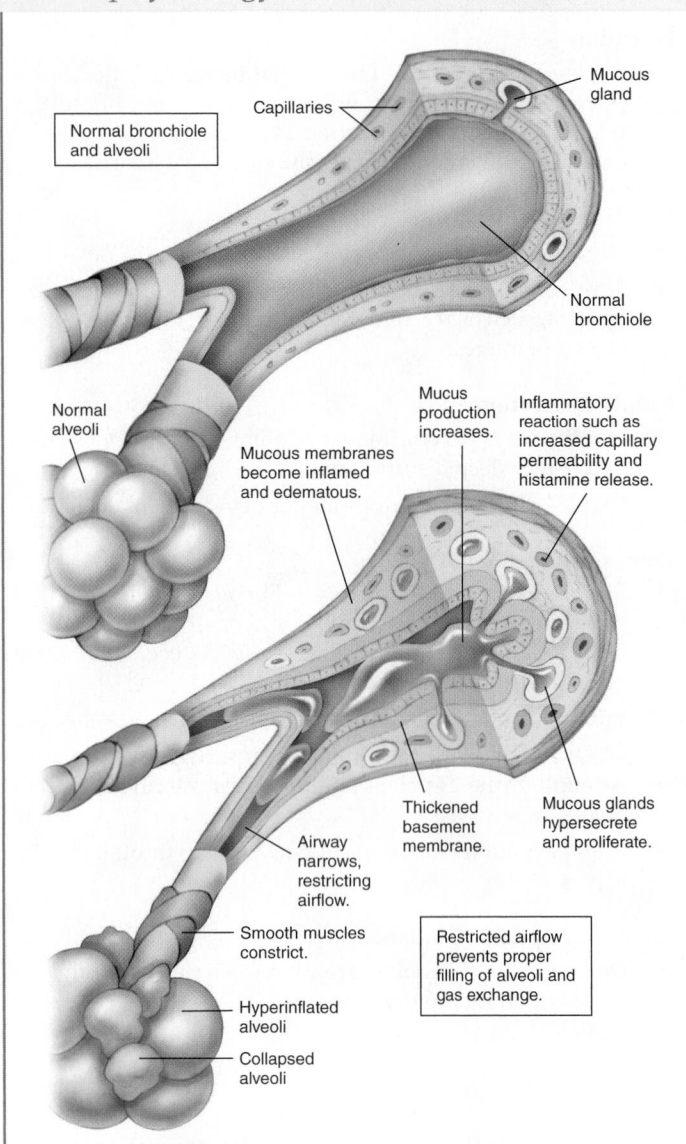

Normal bronchiole and alveoli

Capillaries

Mucous gland

Normal bronchiole

Normal alveoli

Mucous membranes become inflamed and edematous.

Mucus production increases.

Inflammatory reaction such as increased capillary permeability and histamine release.

Thickened basement membrane.

Mucous glands hypersecrete and proliferate.

Airway narrows, restricting airflow.

Smooth muscles constrict.

Hyperinflated alveoli

Collapsed alveoli

Restricted airflow prevents proper filling of alveoli and gas exchange.

Some asthma triggers are exercise, infection, and allergies. Airflow is obstructed through constriction and narrowing of the airway, along with increased production of mucus. Alveoli may become hyperinflated or collapse because of obstruction, leading to impaired gas exchange.

CLINICAL MANIFESTATIONS

The sudden onset of breathing difficulty (cough, wheeze, or shortness of breath) is an acute asthma episode or asthma attack. The infant or child who has had frequent episodes of coughing or respiratory infections should be evaluated for asthma. Frequent coughing, especially at night, is a signal that the child's airway is very sensitive to stimuli, and this could be a sign of "silent" asthma.

During an acute episode, respirations are rapid and labored and the child often appears tired because of the ongoing effort to breathe. Nasal flaring and intercostal retractions may be visible. The child exhibits a productive cough and expiratory wheezing, a prolonged expiratory phase, decreased air movement, accessory muscle use, and respiratory fatigue. The child may complain of chest tightness. Anxiety increases as the acute episode worsens, and the increasing anxiety intensifies the child's physical responses.

In a severe acute episode, wheezing may not be heard because of low airflow. Head bobbing may be seen in young children using the accessory muscles to breathe. Hypoxia and the cumulative effect of administered medications may cause behaviors ranging from wide-eyed agitation to lethargic irritability. In children who have repeated acute episodes, a barrel chest and accessory muscle use are common findings.

CLINICAL THERAPY

Diagnosis is made by history, physical examination and pulmonary function testing (spirometry) that shows evidence of episodic airflow obstruction (that is at least partially reversible) and airway hyperresponsiveness. Spirometry readings are most commonly measured as forced expiratory volume in 1 second (FEV_1) and expressed as a percentage of predicted FEV_1 for the child's height, age, gender, and race. A chest radiograph may help determine if a foreign body could account for symptoms. Skin testing may be used to identify allergens (asthma triggers).

Clinical Tip

Spirometry testing is performed when the child is able to cooperate, usually by 5 to 6 years of age. Coughing interferes with a good result, so perform testing when asthma is well controlled. Coach the child to give the best effort each time. Allow children to practice using the mouthpiece and nose clip. To perform the test, have the child exhale forcefully. With the mouth forming a tight seal around the mouthpiece, ask the child to take a rapid deep breath without breathing through the nose. Have the child to keep a tight seal around the mouthpiece and to exhale forcibly for at least 6 seconds. Three acceptable readings are obtained, but limit the child to eight efforts (Banasiak, 2014). Be sure to record the child's age, height, weight, gender, race, and time and dose of the last medications, which are used for interpretation of the test.

Several clinical patterns (phenotypes) of asthma have been noted and can sometimes be identified from the history. Asthma management that specifically addresses a child's clinical pattern is being investigated. Examples of clinical patterns include the following (Howrylak et al., 2014):

- Intermittent asthma that is triggered only by a viral respiratory infection. No allergic component exists, and lung function is not impaired. Symptoms are seasonal, matching the timing of increased viral infections. The most effective asthma maintenance treatments do not prevent the viral infection trigger.
- Persistent or chronic asthma daily and year-round symptoms. Most have an allergic component to their disease, such as atopic dermatitis. Viral infections may also trigger symptoms. Airway hyperresponsiveness is present and lung function is affected. Symptom-free days occur only with effective maintenance treatment.
- Seasonal allergic asthma is triggered by inhalant allergens (mold, grasses, other pollens) and cause daily symptoms during that allergy season. Seasonal asthma treatment versus continuous asthma treatment may be an effective strategy.

Asthma may go into remission or increase in severity over time. Asthma severity is categorized by how often the child has symptoms and nighttime awakening, how many days a week a short-acting beta$_2$-agonist (SABA) medication is needed, and how many times a year a child needs oral corticosteroid therapy. Spirometry measurement of lung function is an additional method used to determine asthma severity in children 5 years and older. See Table 46–4 for classification of asthma severity in children. See accompanying *Medications Used to Treat: Asthma*.

TABLE 46–4 Classification of Asthma Severity in Children

ASTHMA SEVERITY	CHARACTERISTICS
Intermittent	Symptoms 2 or fewer days a week
	No nighttime awakenings
	SABA use for symptom control 2 or fewer days a week
	No interference with activity
	Oral corticosteroid use no more than once a year
	Normal FEV$_1$ between exacerbations, FEV$_1$ greater than 80% predicted, FEV$_1$/FVC greater than 85% (5–11 years) or normal (12 years and older)
Mild persistent	Symptoms greater than 2 days a week, but not daily
	Nighttime awakenings 1 to 2 times a month (less than 5 years) or 3 to 4 times a month (5 years and older)
	SABA use for symptom control 2 or more days a week, but not daily
	Minor activity limitation
	Oral corticosteroid use 2 or more times a year
	FEV$_1$ greater than 80% predicted, FEV$_1$/FVC greater than 80% (5–11 years) or normal (12 years and older)
Moderate persistent	Daily symptoms
	Nighttime awakenings 3 to 4 times a month (less than 5 years) or more than once a week but not nightly (5 years and older)
	SABA use for symptom control daily
	Some activity limitation
	Oral corticosteroid use 2 or more times a year
	FEV$_1$ equals 60%–80% predicted, FEV$_1$/FVC equals 70%–80% (5–11 years) or FEV$_1$/FVC reduced more than 5% (12 years and older)
Severe persistent	Symptoms throughout the day
	Nighttime awakening greater than 1 time a week (less than 5 years) or every night (5 years and older)
	SABA use several times a day
	Extremely limited activity
	Oral corticosteroid use 2 or more times a year
	FEV$_1$ less than 60% predicted, FEV$_1$/FVC less than 75% (5–11 years) or FEV$_1$/FVC reduced more than 5% (12 years and older)

Note: SABA = short-acting beta$_2$-agonist; FEV$_1$ = forced expiratory volume in 1 second; FVC = forced vital capacity.

Source: Adapted from National Asthma Education and Prevention Program (NAEPP). (2007). *Expert panel report 3: Guidelines for the diagnosis and management of asthma* (pp. 307–309). Bethesda, MD: National Heart Lung and Blood Institute, National Institutes of Health. Retrieved from http://www.nhlbi.nih.gov/guidelines/asthma

Medications Used to Treat: Asthma

QUICK RELIEF MEDICATIONS, ROUTE, AND ACTION	NURSING MANAGEMENT
Short-acting beta$_2$-agonists (SABA) Albuterol, levalbuterol, pirbuterol *Metered-dose inhaler or nebulizer* Relaxes smooth muscle in airway leading to rapid bronchodilation (within 5–10 min) and mucus clearing. Drug of choice for acute therapy and prevention of exercise-induced bronchospasm.	• Use before inhaled steroid, wait 1–2 min between puffs, wait 15 min to give inhaled steroid. Child should hold breath 10 sec after inspiring. Then rinse mouth and avoid swallowing medication. Use a spacer. • Differences in potency exist, but all products are comparable on a per puff basis. • Dose-related side effects include tachycardia, nervousness, nausea and vomiting, headaches. • Regular use more than 2 days a week for symptom control indicates a loss of control and need for additional therapy.
Corticosteroids Methylprednisolone, prednisone, prednisolone *Oral* Diminishes airway inflammation, secretions, and obstruction, enhances bronchodilating effect of beta$_2$-agonists. Used for acute episodes not fully responsive to beta$_2$-agonists; reduces hospitalization rates.	• Short-term therapy should continue until child achieves 80% peak expiratory flow personal best, or until symptoms resolve. • Give with food to reduce gastric irritation. • Give oral dose in early morning to mimic normal peak corticosteroid blood level. • Assess for potential adverse effects of long-term therapy, such as decreased growth, unstable blood sugar, immunosuppression.
Anticholinergic Ipratropium *Metered-dose inhaler or nebulizer* Inhibits bronchoconstriction and decreases mucus production.	• Not for primary emergency treatment because of 30- to 90-min time of onset. • Rinse mouth afterward to get rid of bitter taste. • Side effects include increased wheezing, cough, nervousness, dry mouth, tachycardia, dizziness, headache, palpitations. • Prevent medication contact with eyes.
DAILY CONTROL MEDICATIONS, ROUTE, AND ACTION	NURSING MANAGEMENT
Long-acting beta$_2$-agonists (LABA) Salmeterol, formoterol *Dry powder inhaler* Relaxes smooth muscle in airway, increases ciliary motility. Used for nocturnal symptoms and prevention of exercise-induced bronchospasm. Used as an add-on therapy.	• Do not use for acute asthma episode. • Take preexercise dose 30–60 min before activity. Do not use additional dose before exercise if already using twice daily doses, which should be 12 hr apart. • Caution against overdosage because side effects such as tachycardia, tremor, irritability, insomnia will last 8–12 hr. • Report failure to respond to usual dose because this may indicate need for stepped-up therapy.
Inhaled corticosteroids (ICS) Beclomethasone, budesonide, flunisolide, fluticasone, mometasone, triamcinolone *Metered-dose inhaler or nebulizer* Anti-inflammatory, controls seasonal, allergic, and exercise-induced asthma; effectively reduces mucosal edema in airways.	• Administer with spacer or holding chamber. • Separate parts and clean inhaler daily. • Rinse mouth and gargle following treatment to remove drug from oropharynx to reduce chance of cough, thrush, and dysphonia. • Prevent eye exposure through proper metered-dose inhaler, nebulizer, or dry powder inhaler (DPI) administration. • Monitor for headache, gastrointestinal upset, dizziness, infection. • Use exactly as prescribed.

Methylxanthines

Theophylline

Oral

Relaxes muscle bundles that constrict airways; dilates airway; provides continuous airway relaxation.

Used for long-term control, may help reduce need for increased corticosteroid dosages. Less commonly used than inhaled medications because of side effects.

- Do not crush or chew tablet. Give at same time each day.
- Maintain therapeutic serum level of 10–20 mcg/L; requires serum level checks and dose adjustment.
- Limit caffeine intake.
- Side effects include tachycardia, dysrhythmias, restlessness, tremors, seizures, insomnia, hypotension, severe headaches, vomiting, and diarrhea.

Mast cell inhibitors

Cromolyn sodium, nedocromil

Metered-dose inhaler or nebulizer

Anti-inflammatory, inhibits activation and release of inflammatory mediators for early and late phase asthma response to allergens and exercise-induced bronchospasm.

May be used for unavoidable allergen exposure.

- Do not use at time of symptom development or acute episode.
- Must be used up to 4 times a day to be effective.
- Therapeutic response seen in 2 weeks, maximum benefit may not be seen for 4–6 weeks.
- Adverse reactions include wheezing, bronchospasm, throat irritation, nasal congestion, and anaphylaxis. Immediately report these symptoms to physician.

Leukotriene receptor antagonist (LTRA)

Montelukast, zafirlukast

Oral

Reduces inflammation cascade responsible for airway inflammation; improves lung function and diminishes symptoms and need for quick-relief medications.

- Available in granules for infants and chewable tablets for young children.
- Administer montelukast in the evening; may be given with food or without.
- Make sure child chews montelukast chewable tablet rather than swallowing whole. Granules may be mixed in applesauce or ice cream; do not mix in liquid.
- Administer zafirlukast 1 hour before or 2 hr after meal.
- Report fever, acute asthma episodes, flulike symptoms, severe headaches or lethargy.
- Take as prescribed; do not withdraw abruptly.

Immunotherapy

Omalizumab

Subcutaneous

A therapeutic antibody that blocks IgE from causing reactions leading to asthma symptoms.

- Approved for children 12 years and older with moderate or severe persistent asthma.
- Injections required every 2–4 weeks based on serum IgE levels.
- Be alert for anaphylaxis; it should be administered in a health center prepared to treat anaphylaxis.

Other

Hyposensitization (allergy shots)

Subcutaneous

Series of injections with gradual dose increase that can increase the child's tolerance of unavoidable allergens (e.g., mold, pollen)

- May be of value for child with persistent asthma having allergies that can be addressed by immune therapy.

Source: Data from Wilson, B. A., Shannon, M. T., & Shields, K. M. (2016). *Nurse's drug guide 2016*. Hoboken, NJ: Pearson; Taketomo, C. K., Hodding, J. H., & Kraus, D. M. (2014). *Pediatric and neonatal dosage handbook* (21st ed.). Hudson, OH: Lexicomp; Chang, C. (2012). Asthma in children and adolescents: A comprehensive approach to diagnosis and management. *Clinical Reviews in Allergy and Immunology, 43*(1–2), 98–137.

Recommended therapy is tied to asthma severity classification. Clinical therapy includes medications, hydration, education, and support of parents and child. Pharmacologic treatment is matched to the severity of asthma for daily control and for management of acute episodes. The goal is to maintain asthma control long term, using the least amount of medication and reducing the risk for adverse effects.

Clinical Tip

Signs of good control in children during a week include few or no episodes of dyspnea or wheezing during the day or waking the child at night, no interference with normal activity, school, or exercise, and few uses of a short-acting beta₂-agonist for symptom control (Nguyen et al., 2014). Various questionnaires to measure asthma control in children have been proposed and studies to validate them are in process.

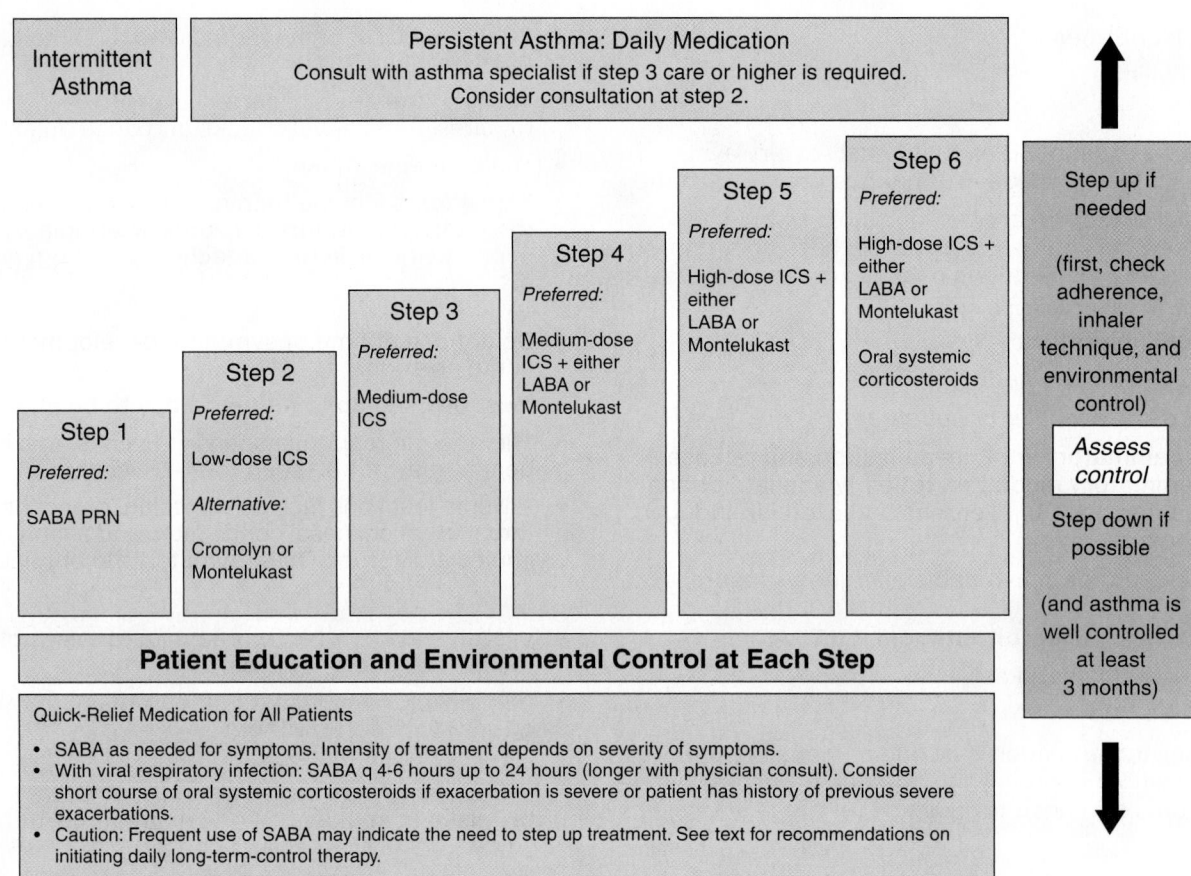

Key: **Alphabetical order is used when more than one treatment option is listed within either preferred or alternative therapy.** ICS, inhaled corticosteroid; LABA, inhaled long-acting beta₂-agonist; SABA, inhaled short-acting beta₂-agonist

Figure 46–4 Stepwise approach to managing asthma in children 0 to 4 years of age.

SOURCE: From National Asthma Education and Prevention Program. (2007). *Expert panel report 3: Guidelines for the diagnosis and management of asthma* (p. 305). Bethesda, MD: National Institutes of Health, National Heart Lung and Blood Institute. Retrieved from http://www.nhlbi.nih.gov/guidelines/asthma.

The main goal of asthma therapy is to manage symptoms and the disorder. Medication therapy and other therapies are divided into six progressive steps intended to match the child's asthma severity. Specific step guidelines are established for different age groups: 0 to 4 years, 5 to 11 years, and 12 years and older. The child's response to therapy is reviewed periodically to determine if medications should be stepped up or down to correspond to the child's symptoms. See Figure 46–4 for the nationally recommended stepwise approach for children aged 0 to 4 years. An asthma action plan is recommended to guide home management of asthma symptoms.

Recommendations for children with persistent asthma include the use of daily inhaled corticosteroids and additional long-term control medications as severity increases. A peak flow meter is often recommended in addition to an asthma management plan to guide the parents and child in treating asthma episodes (see *Teaching Highlights: Using a Peak Expiratory Flow Meter* later in this section). Children with intermittent asthma may only need short-acting beta₂-agonists. When asthma control is difficult to achieve, the child is referred to an asthma specialist.

Acute Asthma Episodes. Most children with acute exacerbations respond to aggressive management in the emergency department with continuous albuterol by nebulizer, oral systemic corticosteroids, and inhaled ipratropium. Children who do not respond or who are already being managed at home on corticosteroids have a greater chance of hospital admission.

Exercise-Induced Asthma. Up to 70% of children and youth report shortness of breath, wheezing, coughing, difficulty taking a deep breath, noisy breathing, or chest tightness to occur during and after exercise. Pretreatment with a short-acting beta₂-agonist 5 to 20 minutes before exercise often prevents exercise-induced asthma and provides relief for 2 to 4 hours (Parsons et al., 2013).

Severe Asthma Episodes. Some asthma episodes do not respond to repeated doses of albuterol and corticosteroids, and progress to potentially life-threatening episodes. The child has increased hypoxemia, decreased expiration due to air trapping, and ineffective ventilation. Respiratory acidosis develops. Children often require treatment in the intensive care unit. Intravenous magnesium sulfate may be added to other medications, such as theophylline and intravenous beta₂ agonists, for the acute episode. Heliox (70% helium:30% oxygen or 80% helium:20% oxygen) gas is less dense than supplemental oxygen and causes less airflow resistance in narrowed airways. Ketamine and inhaled anesthetics are used in some critical cases along with assisted ventilation (Wong, Lee, Turner, et al., 2014). A few children progress to respiratory failure and die.

Nursing Management

For the Child With Asthma

Nursing Assessment and Diagnosis

The nurse usually encounters the child and family in the emergency department, health center, or nursing unit. Often, acute care has become necessary because the child's level of respiratory compromise cannot be managed at home. In some cases, the child and family are seen following acute episodes to have education for asthma management at home or in school.

PHYSIOLOGIC ASSESSMENT

Identify the child's current respiratory status first by assessing the ABCs—airway, breathing, and circulation—to make sure the child's condition is not life threatening. If the child is moving air or talking, assess the quality of breathing. Observe the child's color, and assess the respiratory and heart rates. Auscultate the lungs for the quality of breath sounds and for the presence or absence of wheezing. Note whether a cough or stridor is present. Inspect the chest for retractions to assess the severity of respiratory distress. Move on to other aspects of assessment only after finding no life-threatening respiratory distress.

Attach a pulse oximeter; a SpO_2 reading of less than 92% indicates hypoxemia. Assess skin turgor, intake and output, and urine specific gravity. A spirometry reading may be attempted, but the child may be unable to use the spirometer because of respiratory distress. Because asthma symptoms can be associated with an infection or other condition, perform a head-to-toe assessment to identify other associated problems. See the *Assessment Guide* at the beginning of this chapter.

ASSESS ASTHMA MANAGEMENT

Key questions to consider asking parents and older children or adolescents include the following:

- How often in the past month has the child had shortness of breath, coughing, chest tightness, or chest pain during the day? During the night?
- How many times a week does the child need to use rescue medications?
- Have asthma symptoms limited the child's work or play at school or home?
- Which medicines is the child currently taking? How often?
- Have any medication dosages been missed in the last week? How many?
- What are your concerns about the medicines prescribed (e.g., not really needed, side effects, worried about "steroids")?
- Is there any issue with the cost or ability to obtain the medicines?
- Have you tried any other treatments for asthma (e.g., complementary therapies recommended by a healer)?
- Show me how you use your inhaler.

Additionally, several questionnaires have been developed to help health professionals assess an adolescent's asthma control, such as the Asthma Control Test.

PSYCHOSOCIAL ASSESSMENT

Assess the child's anxiety or fear related to the asthma episode or hospitalization. How are parents responding to the current acute episode? Are they anxious, concerned, or frustrated? Do they potentially have concerns about finances, missing work, or other family members at home? Assess whether the child thinks this episode could have been avoided if medications had been used.

Examples of nursing diagnoses for the child experiencing an acute asthma episode include the following (NANDA-I © 2014):

- ***Airway Clearance, Ineffective***, related to airway compromise, copious mucous secretions, and coughing
- ***Gas Exchange, Impaired***, related to airway obstruction
- ***Fluid Volume: Deficient, Risk for***, related to inability to drink adequate fluids when in respiratory distress
- ***Anxiety/Fear (Child and Parents)*** related to difficulty breathing
- ***Health Management, Family, Ineffective***, related to lack of understanding about the need for daily management of a chronic disease

Planning and Implementation

Pharmacologic and supportive therapies are used to reverse the airway obstruction and promote respiratory function. Nursing interventions focus on maintaining airway patency, meeting fluid needs, promoting rest and stress reduction for the child and parents, supporting the family's participation in care, and providing the family with information to enable them to manage the child's disease.

MAINTAIN AIRWAY PATENCY

If the child is exhibiting breathing difficulty, give supplemental humidified oxygen by nasal cannula or face mask. Humidity prevents drying and thickening of mucous secretions. Place the child in a sitting (semi-Fowler) or upright position to promote and ease respiratory effort. Evaluate the effectiveness of positioning and oxygen administration by pulse oximeter and by observing for improved respiratory status. (See the *Clinical Skills Manual* SKILLS .)

The respiratory distress and need for supplemental oxygen can be stressful for parents and child alike (Figure 46–5). Encouraging the parents' presence can be reassuring for the child. Keep the parents informed of procedures and results, and get their input when developing the treatment plan.

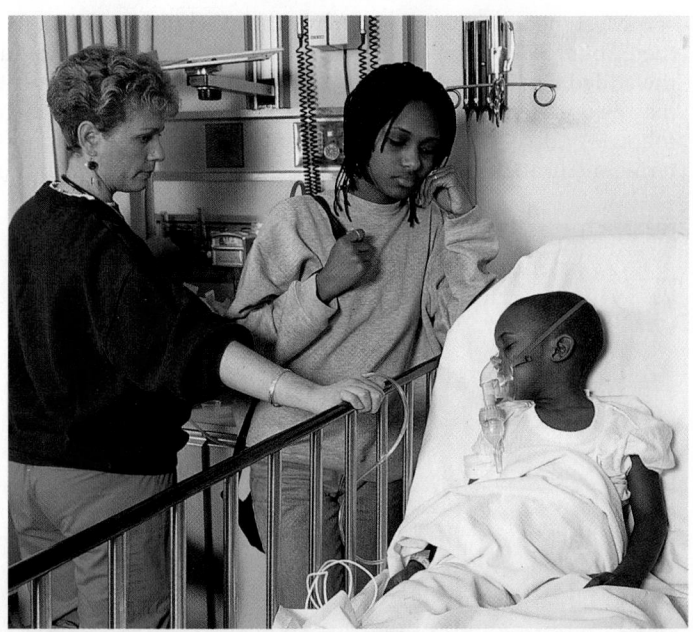

Figure 46–5 An acute asthma episode requires management in the emergency department. The child is placed in a semi-Fowler position to facilitate respiratory effort. Support both the child and parent during these acute episodes. This mother looks exhausted after a sleepless night of caring for her son.

Growth and Development

Metered-dose inhalers (MDIs), nebulizers, and dry powder inhalers (DPIs) are devices used for inhalation therapy. These devices cause special challenges for infants and young children because many devices require cooperation and coordination. The appropriate technique must be taught and reinforced frequently.

- Children over 5 years usually have the ability to use an MDI. Using the closed mouth technique, have the child insert the mouthpiece in the mouth between the teeth and seal the lips. Look straight ahead, and keep the tongue away from the mouthpiece opening. Just as the child starts to breathe, press down on the canister to release the medication. Continue to breathe in slowly through the mouth for at least 5 seconds, and then hold the breath for another 10 seconds. No mist should be seen coming from the mouth after the breath or from the top of the inhaler after actuation, both of which are signs the technique was not good. Teach the child to use an MDI without a spacer, by breathing slowly through a straw.

- Younger children need a spacer with a mask attachment, while other children prefer to use a spacer with the MDI. Select a spacer with a mask for infants and young children that fits from the top of the nose to just under the mouth. The seal should be flexible to prevent an air leak. Crying leads to prolonged exhalation and short inspiration, reducing lung deposition. Use play and distraction to improve cooperation for medication delivery. When use of a spacer or holding chamber is preferred, put the mask on firmly over the nose and mouth or the mouthpiece in the mouth with mouth closed around it. Release a puff of medication and have the child take 4 to 6 quiet deep breaths over 10 seconds. Move the spacer away from the face or mouth, and have the child hold a breath for 10 seconds. Follow this with the second puff. Wash the child's face after using a spacer with a mask. Wash the plastic spacer with household detergent and air dry it to reduce the static charge that can attract medication particles.

- A nebulizer changes liquid medication into aerosol particles. No coordination of breathing is required, making nebulizers easier for young children to use. Nebulizers are not more efficient than MDIs with a spacer, but the outcome may be better since the child can breathe normally. Make sure the nebulizer mouthpiece is sealed by the lips, and mouth breathing is used. If the child cannot coordinate mouth breathing, use a face mask. Nebulizers take 8 to 10 minutes per treatment, so distraction may be needed to improve the cooperation of infants and young children for that duration.

- DPIs are activated when the child takes a breath, so puffs do not need to be coordinated with inhalation. No spacer or propellant is used. Children starting at age 5 years may be able to take the rapid, deep, and sustained breath needed to effectively use the device. Children less than 6 years of age who are wheezing may not be able to inspire at a rate fast enough to obtain the optimal amount of medication. Steps for using DPI include the following: Remove the lid, load the dose (puncturing the blister or capsule), fully breathe out away from the device, put the mouthpiece between the lips and teeth, and breathe in deeply and forcefully. Hold the breath for 10 seconds and remove the mouthpiece from the mouth.

- Some MDIs or DPIs have a whistle. It may warn that the inhaled breath is too fast or too shallow, but in other devices, it indicates the breath was adequate. Be sure to inform the child and family about what the whistle on the child's inhaler indicates.

Source: Data from Dinakar, C., & Welch, M. J. (2014). Device how-tos. *Contemporary Pediatrics, 31*(May). Retrieved from http://contemporarypediatrics.modernmedicine.com/contemporary-pediatrics/content/tags/asthma/device-how-tos; Sleath, B., Ayala, G. X., Gillette, C., Williams, D., Davis, S., Tudor, G., Washington, D. (2011). Provider demonstration and assessment of child device technique during pediatric asthma visits. *Pediatrics, 127*(4), 642–648; Asthma Initiative of Michigan for Healthy Lungs. (2011). *How to use a metered-dose inhaler the right way.* Retrieved from http://www.getasthmahelp.org/inhalers_main.asp.

Most medications are given by inhalation (Figure 46–6). (See the *Clinical Skills Manual* SKILLS.) The aerosol droplets provide the added benefit of moisture. Continuous nebulizer treatments may be used for some children with severe acute episodes. See the following *Growth and Development* for considerations in administering medications with inhalation devices. Monitor the child for medication side effects. The frequency of vital sign assessment is determined by the severity of symptoms.

MEET FLUID NEEDS

Fluid therapy is often necessary to restore and maintain adequate fluid balance. Adequate hydration is essential to thin and break up trapped mucous plugs in the narrowed airways. An intravenous infusion may be needed if the child cannot meet fluid needs by mouth, and for administering certain medications and glucose. Monitor the child's intake, output, and specific gravity to avoid overhydration that could lead to pulmonary edema in severe asthma episodes.

As respiratory difficulty diminishes, offer oral fluids slowly. The child's fluid preferences should be determined and choices given where possible. Involve parents to help gain the child's cooperation in taking oral fluids.

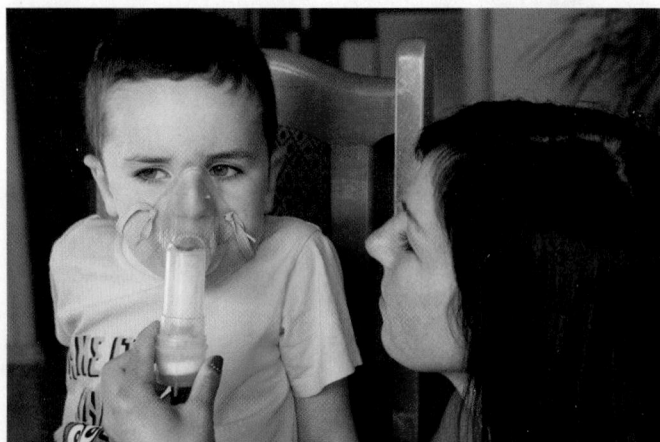

Figure 46–6 **Medications given by inhalation therapy reach the bloodstream rapidly while minimizing the systemic effects. A nebulizer works well for young children because it does not require coordination of breathing with medication inhalation.**

SOURCE: greenland/Shutterstock.

Clinical Tip

Iced beverages precipitate bronchospasms in some children with asthma. Offer room-temperature or slightly cooled fluids instead.

PROMOTE REST AND STRESS REDUCTION

The child having an acute asthma episode is usually very tired from prolonged labored breathing when admitted to the nursing unit. Put the child in a quiet room that is accessible for frequent monitoring to promote relaxation and rest. Group tasks to avoid repeatedly disturbing the child.

SUPPORT FAMILY PARTICIPATION

Recognize that parents may be exhausted after spending hours with their child in respiratory distress. Give parents the *option* of assisting with the child's treatments, rather than *expecting* them to help, in addition to comforting the child. Provide frequent updates about the child's condition and encourage the parents to take breaks as needed.

Length of hospitalization depends on the child's response to therapy. Any underlying or accompanying health problem, such as preexisting lung disease or pneumonia, can complicate and extend the child's hospital stay. Communicate with the family of the hospitalized child frequently about the child's condition.

DISCHARGE PLANNING AND HOME CARE TEACHING

Parents need a thorough understanding of asthma—how to prevent asthma episodes and how to follow the child's asthma action plan to manage symptoms. Support of parents and the child should focus on helping them to understand and cope with the diagnosis and the need for daily management to promote near-normal respiratory function while the child continues to grow and develop normally.

Discharge planning for the child with asthma focuses on increasing the family's knowledge about the disease, medication therapy, and the need for follow-up care. Make sure the child receives an appointment with an allergist or asthma specialist if moderate to severe persistent asthma exists. Refer the child and parents to a healthcare provider for more comprehensive education that considers cultural factors for asthma management. See *Developing Cultural Competence: Asthma Disparity Factors.*

COMMUNITY-BASED NURSING CARE

Nurses provide care to children with asthma in pediatricians' offices, specialty asthma clinics, schools, and summer camps. The child's asthma control and management should be assessed at each visit.

Promoting Asthma Management Skills

Review the family's daily plan for monitoring the child's respiratory status. Encourage the school-age child or the parents of younger children to keep a symptom diary that includes peak exploratory flow rate (PEFR) for 2 weeks prior to a health visit as well as all daytime and nighttime symptoms. The Asthma Tracker is one tool a family can use to monitor the young child's asthma symptoms (Nkoy et al., 2014). Evaluate the child's use of the MDI or DPI, and correct the child's technique as needed. Teach the family or review the child's technique about how to measure and interpret peak expiratory flow readings (see *Teaching Highlights: Using a Peak Expiratory Flow Meter*).

Clinical Tip

A study revealed that using a peak expiratory flow meter provided parents with an objective measure of the child's asthma symptoms and empowered them to initiate treatment earlier than without the meter. Communication with the child's healthcare provider was more effective when a peak expiratory flow meter was used (Burkhart, Rayens, & Oakley, 2012).

Assess the parent's ability to identify the timing and type of stepped-up care needed to manage worsening symptoms identified on the child's asthma action plan. The asthma action plan should include the daily control medications, quick-relief medications to take once symptoms of an asthma episode are identified, and when to call the healthcare provider. Identify routines that may improve adherence to daily medication use, such as keeping

Developing Cultural Competence Asthma Disparity Factors

African American and Hispanic children have a higher prevalence rate for asthma. A major factor may be lower access to high-quality ambulatory care that does not provide education within the cultural beliefs of the family. Other factors associated with the high prevalence rate may include (Kueny, Berg, Chowdhury, et al., 2013):

- Environmental housing conditions (indoor allergen exposure to rodents, molds, and cockroaches)
- Employment options that increase potential introduction of allergens into the home
- Air pollution in urban areas such as nitrogen dioxide from engine exhaust fumes
- Medication beliefs associated with concerns over safety of inhaled corticosteroids and development of tolerance with daily use, or following the advice of healers
- Emotional stress within the home

Identify potential factors contributing to child's asthma to provide effective education and support to the child and family.

medications where they will be seen at mealtime. The goal is to bring asthma episodes under control with stepped-up care before emergency care is needed. Reassure the family that most children with asthma can lead a normal life with some modifications.

Healthy People 2020

(RD-6) Increase the proportion of persons with current asthma who receive formal patient education

(RD-7.1) Increase the proportion of persons with current asthma who receive written asthma management plans from their healthcare provider according to National Asthma Education and Prevention Program (NAEPP) guidelines

Refer parents to a local support group to gain additional knowledge and confidence in asthma management. Many hospitals have family resource centers that can assist parents to find helpful information on the Internet.

Child-Focused Education

Engage the child in learning about how the lungs work and what happens when an acute asthma episode occurs. Teach the child how to begin steps toward self-management as appropriate. Encourage the child to ask questions. Provide an activity or coloring book for the child and printed educational materials for the parents. See *Teaching Highlights: Home Care for the Child With Asthma* to guide asthma education for the child and family.

Encourage school-age children to assume more responsibility for care, including avoidance of known triggers, early symptom recognition, relaxation breathing, and the proper use of inhaled medication. Help the child learn the early signs of an asthma episode (coughing, breathlessness, or peak expiratory flow meter reading) and to take quick-relief medication before signs become more serious.

TEACHING HIGHLIGHTS	Using a Peak Expiratory Flow Meter

A peak expiratory flow meter is a useful tool for asthma self-management. It measures the child's ability to push air forcefully out of the lungs. Changes in the peak expiratory flow rate (PEFR) signal worsening lung function and the beginning of an asthma episode. To use a peak expiratory flow meter:

- Set the device at zero or the base level.
- Stand up and take as deep a breath as possible.
- Put the mouthpiece of the meter in the mouth and firmly close the lips around it. Do not cough or let your tongue block the mouthpiece. Blow out as hard and fast as possible over 1 to 2 seconds. To help toddlers learn how to use a peak flow meter, have them practice by blowing into a noisemaker or party favor.
- Write down the reading.
- Repeat the process 2 times and record the highest of the 3 numbers on the chart.
- Measure and record the best PEFR reading twice a day for 2 weeks so the healthcare provider can determine the child's personal best reading. (Make sure the child is optimally treated with medications during the day to obtain the best reading.)
- The physician will use the child's personal best average readings to set the green, yellow, and red color zones to guide treatment in the child's asthma action plan. The child's personal best changes as the child grows taller, so the child's personal best should be measured every year.
- The physician provides guidelines for the child and family to use when monitoring the PEFR. If the child or parent suspects the child might have the onset of breathing difficulty, the peak flow meter can be used. Some children have problems identifying early symptoms of an acute asthma episode onset (increased cough, wheezing, or shortness of breath). The peak flow meter measures the change in how hard the child can blow out air. Using the zones established by the healthcare provider, the child and family can determine what action to take.
- **Green zone:** The PEFR reading is between 80% and 100% of the child's personal best. Air is moving well in the child's lungs. In this case, the child has good asthma control and can continue daily activities. No modification of the treatment plan is needed.
- **Yellow zone:** The PEFR reading is between 50% and 80% of the child's personal best. In this case, the child is developing breathing problems. The parents should follow directions in the child's asthma action plan, which usually involves quick-relief medications. The child should feel better and the PEFR should improve over the next hour. If symptoms and the PEFR do not improve, contact the child's healthcare provider for additional treatment guidance.
- **Red zone:** The PEFR is less than 50% of the child's personal best. In this case, the child has a severe asthma episode and needs urgent treatment with quick-relief medication. Call the child's healthcare provider for additional care guidelines or take the child to the emergency department.

Source: Data from American Academy of Allergy, Asthma, and Immunology (AAAAI). (2014). *Peak flow meter.* Retrieved from http://www.aaaai.org /conditions-and-treatments/library/at-a-glance/peak-flow-meter.aspx; Johns Hopkins Medicine. (2012). *Peak flow measurement.* Retrieved from http:// www.hopkinsmedicine.org/healthlibrary/test_procedures/pulmonary/peak_flow_measurement_92,P07755;WebMD. (2012). *Asthma and the peak flow meter.* Retrieved from http://www.webmd.com/asthma/guide/peak-flow-meter.

Health Maintenance

Provide routine health promotion and maintenance care, including immunizations. Live virus vaccines may need to be postponed if the child has used oral corticosteroids recently. Carefully monitor the child's growth, especially when the child uses inhaled corticosteroids and episodic oral corticosteroids, which can slow growth and result in reduced adult height by an average of 1.2 cm (0.47 in.) (Kelly et al., 2012).

Assess the child's activity and exercise level, and any symptoms experienced such as chest tightening, wheezing, or shortness of breath. Exercise-induced bronchospasm typically occurs 5 to 10 minutes after stopping the activity and resolves 20 to 30 minutes later. First, make sure the child gets some exercise to improve fitness, and then assess how frequently the child has exercise-induced symptoms. Compare that information to the classification of asthma severity in Table 46–4. Teach the child about the timing of rescue medications before exercise to prevent exercise-induced bronchospasm. Make sure the child uses the daily control and quick-relief medication asthma action plan.

Environmental Control

Reducing allergens in the environment is an important part of asthma management. Focus efforts on reducing molds in the home with lowered humidity and removal of houseplants. When possible, remove pets from the home (especially from the child's bedroom). Dust mites live in the carpets,

Professionalism in Practice Asthma Management by School Nurses

The National School Nurses Association joined eight organizations in a position statement to improve asthma management in school settings. School nurses are encouraged to implement a comprehensive asthma plan for the management of students with asthma in the school setting that includes identifying and monitoring all students with asthma and obtaining their asthma action plans. School nurses are additionally encouraged to collaborate with school officials to adopt and implement an environmental assessment and management plan that addresses environmental asthma triggers (American Lung Association, 2013). See Chapter 37 for more information on nursing care in the school setting.

mattresses, upholstered furniture, bedcovers, soft toys, and clothes. Vacuum carpets and upholstered furniture frequently using a high-efficiency vacuum filter. Buy soft toys that can be washed. Controlling dust mites in the child's bed and bedroom is a high priority. Encase the child's mattress and pillow in plastic covers. Bathe pets frequently to reduce pet dander. Initiate cockroach eradication. Smoke from cigarettes, wood stoves, and fireplaces should be eliminated when possible. See

TEACHING HIGHLIGHTS | Home Care for the Child With Asthma

Identify current knowledge about the condition and its impact on the child:

- What happens in the lungs during an asthma episode?
- What are the child's early warning signs of an asthma episode?
- What are the child's symptoms (wake up at night, cough a lot)? How does the child respond to them?
- Is the child involved in any exercise activity? If no, why not? Do asthma symptoms occur when the child is exercising?
- Does asthma interfere with social activities or activities with friends?
- What are the child's personal asthma triggers? (Suggest keeping a log of symptoms that occur during the day and night, including when and where, to help identify triggers [e.g., home, school, outdoors, with exercise].) The symptom diary is very helpful in determining the need for more education or for stepped-up or stepped-down medications.

Set up a schedule for parents to learn asthma management:

- Make sure the parents and child know that asthma is a chronic condition that needs daily management and environmental control to reduce or prevent acute asthma episodes.
- Review the asthma action plan for daily management, quick relief, and when to call the physician or to seek emergency care.
- Assess the child's technique with a peak expiratory flow meter, and correct technique as needed. Discuss when to use the meter and how to interpret and use the results for asthma control. Keep a record of peak flow readings for 2 weeks prior to each health visit.

Review parents' understanding of medication therapy:

- Provide information about medications: name, type of drug, dose, method of administration, expected effect, possible side effects. Make sure families understand that daily control medications help prevent acute asthma episodes; the child will not feel them work like the quick-relief medications. Discuss any concerns the family has about the use of "steroid" medication, and describe how they differ from the anabolic steroids abused by athletes.
- Assess the child's MDI or DPI technique and correct as needed.
- When a nebulizer is used to treat an infant or young child, suggest diversions to promote cooperation during the 8- to 10-minute treatment.

Address associated issues:

- What are the financial considerations of medication cost and lifestyle changes?
- Have arrangements been made for the child to use medications at childcare or school?
- Does the child have a medical identification bracelet or tag?
- Would a self-help group or camp experience be helpful for the child?

Chapter 48 for *Teaching Highlights: Removing Common Allergens From the Home.*

School Management

Provide a healthcare provider order so the child's asthma symptoms can be treated at school or at child care. The parents should work with school administrators to have an individualized health plan (that includes an asthma action plan) developed so the child can carry a rescue inhaler and medications can be administered, including pretreatment for exercise. Provide a supply of medications to the school or childcare organization. Make sure teachers of young children can help recognize signs of an acute asthma episode and reduce a child's anxiety about going to the nurse for quick-relief medications. Many schools are attempting to improve the environment and reduce asthma triggers.

Clinical Tip

All 50 states and the District of Columbia have legislation that entitles a child with asthma to carry and self-administer asthma medications at school (Allergy and Asthma Network, 2014). Families of children old enough to recognize worsening asthma symptoms and to self-administer rescue medications should make sure the school knows about the state law.

Evaluation

Expected outcomes of nursing care include the following:

- The child recognizes early asthma symptoms and promptly uses quick-relief medications, fluids, and

relaxation breathing before severe respiratory distress occurs.

- The child learns to identify and avoid asthma triggers.
- The child and family implement the prescribed daily treatment plan and asthma action plan to reduce the number of asthma episodes the child has.
- The child with a serious asthma episode responds to oxygen, fluids, and medication therapy, avoiding hospital admission.

Cystic Fibrosis

Cystic fibrosis (CF) is a common inherited autosomal recessive disorder of the exocrine glands, leading to physiologic alterations in the respiratory, gastrointestinal, and reproductive systems. The incidence of CF varies by race—1:2500–3500 in non-Hispanic Whites, 1:4000–10,000 in Hispanics, 1:15,000–20,000 in non-Hispanic Blacks, 1:32,000 in Asian Americans, and 1:1500–3970 in Native Americans (Nakano & Tluczek, 2014). Gender is not a factor in disease incidence. Approximately 30,000 children and adults have CF in the United States, and approximately 50% are older than age 18 years. The median life span for individuals with CF is mid-40s (Cystic Fibrosis Foundation [CFF], 2014) (Figure 46–7).

ETIOLOGY AND PATHOPHYSIOLOGY

A gene isolated on the long arm of chromosome 7 directs the function of the transmembrane conductance regulator (CFTR), which regulates the hydration of epithelial cells of many body

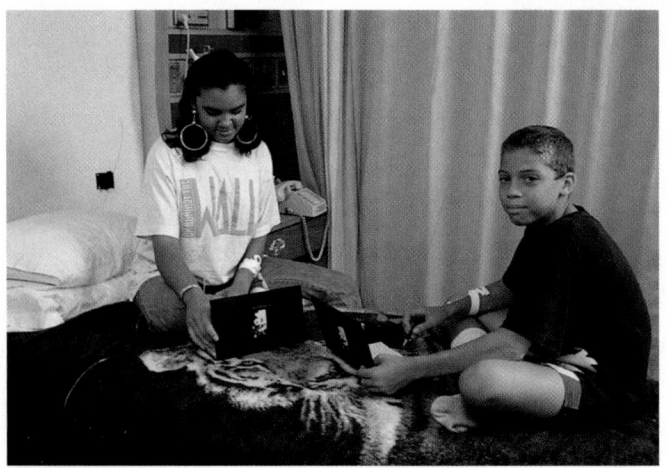

Figure 46–7 Cystic fibrosis is an inherited autosomal recessive disorder of the exocrine glands, so it is not uncommon to see siblings with it such as this brother and sister.

organs. More than 1900 mutations of the *CFTR* gene have been identified, but only 127 of these mutations produce CF symptoms (Nakano & Tluczek, 2014). An estimated 10 million persons in the United States are carriers of a defective *CFTR* gene,

and have no symptoms (Brashers & Huether, 2014). Disease severity varies by number of symptom-causing CFTR mutations. Children with more severe CF have 2 symptom-causing CFTR mutations (Nakano & Tluczek, 2014).

With a defective CFTR protein, chloride-ion transport across the exocrine and epithelial cells is impaired and increased sodium absorption reduces water movement across cell membranes. Secretions become thickened in the sweat ducts, the airways, pancreas, intestine, bile ducts, and vas deferens. The small airways in the lungs become clogged with thickened mucus that can harbor bacteria. The lubricating layer between the airway epithelium and mucus inhibits normal ciliary action and cough clearance.

Air becomes trapped in the small airways, leading to hyperinflation, atelectasis, and secondary respiratory infections. Even with antibiotics and a good response, over time the airways develop chronic bacterial and fungal colonization and **bronchiectasis** (a persistent abnormal dilation of the bronchi), and respiratory failure occurs. Pneumothorax and hemothorax may occur in older children. The rate of disease progression is related to disease severity.

Obstructions in the pancreatic ducts impede the natural enzyme flow that enables the body to digest fats, fat-soluble vitamins, and proteins. Nutritional deficits may cause failure to thrive. As the child ages, the pancreas may stop producing sufficient insulin, leading to glucose intolerance and the development of cystic fibrosis–related diabetes mellitus. See Table 46–5.

TABLE 46–5 Clinical Manifestations of Cystic Fibrosis

PATHOPHYSIOLOGY	CLINICAL MANIFESTATIONS
UPPER RESPIRATORY	
Clogged sinuses	Nasal polyps
	Chronic sinusitis, frontal headaches, purulent nasal discharge, postnasal discharge
LOWER RESPIRATORY	
Reduced ciliary clearance; obstructed airways; air trapping and hyperinflation; bacterial colonization	Chronic moist, productive cough; wheezing; coarse crackles
	Frequent infections
Chronic fibrotic lung changes	Shortness of breath, decreased exercise tolerance
	Barrel chest
	Clubbing of fingers and toes (Figure 46–8)
PANCREAS	
Damaged pancreatic ducts obstruct enzymes needed for digestion	Poorly digested food
	Vitamin A, D, E, and K deficiencies
Produced enzymes damage the pancreas, leading to inadequate insulin secretion	Poor weight gain or failure to thrive; delayed onset of puberty
	CF-related diabetes mellitus
GASTROINTESTINAL	
Thickened intestinal secretions and decreased gut mobility	Meconium ileus at birth
Obstructed bile ducts	Abdominal distention
	Greasy, bulky stools (steatorrhea) that are frothy, foul smelling, and floating
	Constipation or intestinal obstruction
	Rectal prolapse
	Liver cirrhosis
REPRODUCTIVE	
Males—absence of vas deferens, low sperm count	Males—infertility
Females—thick vaginal discharge and decreased cervical secretions	Females—may have difficulty conceiving
SWEAT GLANDS	
Excess chloride and sodium electrolyte loss in the sweat	Salty sweat
	Salt depletion, hyponatremia

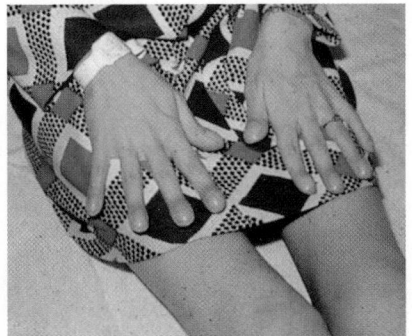

Figure 46–8 Digital clubbing, enlargement of the distal phalanges, occurs in children with cystic fibrosis because of chronic fibrotic changes within the lungs.

Failure to secrete enough chloride and fluid into intestines causes meconium ileus (a small bowel obstruction in newborns), affecting 15% of newborns with CF (Henderson et al., 2012). Older children may have intermittent and recurrent episodes of partial small bowel obstruction that can progress to total obstruction, abdominal distention, and vomiting. Chronic inflammation may occur in the intestines, leading to the development of Crohn disease. In rare cases, children with CF develop liver disease.

The imbalances created by excessive electrolyte loss through perspiration, saliva, and mucous secretion alter metabolic function. These children are at risk for hyponatremic dehydration secondary to electrolyte imbalance.

CLINICAL MANIFESTATIONS

One of the first signs of CF is that newborns fail to pass meconium in the first few days of life. Parents may notice a salty taste to the skin of their infant. Other primary symptoms are associated with thick, sticky mucus. See Table 46–5.

CLINICAL THERAPY

CF is usually diagnosed in infancy. Newborn screening is performed (in all 50 states and the District of Columbia) on dried blood samples to measure pancreatic enzyme immunoreactive trypsinogen (IRT) concentrations, which are high in newborns with CF. If the reading is high, a second IRT concentration test is performed in 2 to 3 weeks. Some states perform a DNA analysis for the most common *CFTR* mutations on the same blood sample if the second IRT concentration is high. Newborn screening is positive if the IRT is elevated and DNA analysis identifies one or more *CFTR* mutations (Nakano, & Tluczek, 2014).

A sweat chloride test by pilocarpine iontophoresis, the gold standard for diagnosis of CF, is performed if the newborn screening is positive (Figure 46–9). A chloride concentration of 60 mEq/L or higher is diagnostic for all age groups. A sweat chloride concentration of 30 to 59 mEq/L in infants less than 6 months old or a concentration between 40 to 59 mEq/L for children and adults is suspicious. If suspicious, a repeat sweat chloride test or DNA analysis for additional *CFTR* mutations maybe performed. Genetic testing is also available for adults with a positive family history, partners of individuals with CF, and couples seeking prenatal testing to identify carriers of CF gene mutations.

A spirometer is used to monitor pulmonary function in children 6 years and older (see clinical tip on spirometry testing in section on asthma). Forced vital capacity (FVC) and forced expiratory volume in 1 second (FEV_1) readings are taken. Sputum cultures are obtained to identify infectious organisms and antibiotic sensitivities.

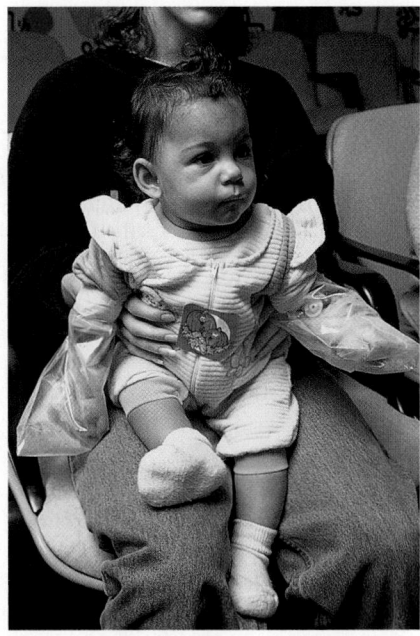

Figure 46–9 This 6-month-old girl is being evaluated for cystic fibrosis using the sweat chloride test.

Clinical therapy focuses on maintaining respiratory function, managing infections, promoting optimal nutrition and exercise, and preventing gastrointestinal blockage (Table 46–6). Newly diagnosed children without symptomatic lung disease are aggressively treated to slow the development of inflammation, chronic respiratory infections, reduction in pulmonary function, and to improve nutrition and support growth.

Treatment is focused on controlling inflammation of the airways, treating infection, and on reducing mucus accumulation. Various devices and airway clearance techniques are used regularly to reduce the accumulation of mucus in the lungs, such as chest physiotherapy, forced expiratory technique (huffing), oscillating positive expiratory pressure, and high-frequency chest wall oscillation. Chest physiotherapy is often performed on infants and young children, but older children can learn to use other airway techniques independently.

Frequent prolonged courses of antibiotics for infections may be prescribed to improve pulmonary function, exercise tolerance, and quality of life. Sputum culture results and sensitivities help guide the selection of the specific antibiotics. Children with *Pseudomonas aeruginosa* or *Burkholderia cepacia* infections have a poorer outcome. Medications are used to reduce sputum viscosity and to dilate the airways. Anti-inflammatory treatment is sometimes prescribed. Vitamins and pancreatic enzymes are also provided to improve the child's nutritional status. A new medication, ivacaftor (Kalydeco), has been approved only for children 6 years and older who have the G551D *CFTR* mutation. See the following *Medications Used to Treat: Cystic Fibrosis.*

Collaborative care by healthcare providers including physicians, nurses, respiratory therapists, and nutritionists has resulted in improved medical management and nutrition that prolongs the lives of children and adults with CF. However, new complications such as CF-related diabetes (often with insulin insufficiency and insulin resistance) that develops in 20% of adolescents must be carefully managed along with the progression of the disease (see Chapter 53) (Brunzell, Hardin, Moran, et al., 2011). CF-related diabetes is difficult to manage because the child needs a large caloric intake that must be balanced by insulin dosage.

End-stage lung disease from cystic fibrosis is the third most common reason for a lung transplant in the United States. About

Medications Used to Treat: Cystic Fibrosis

MEDICATIONS AND ACTIONS	NURSING MANAGEMENT
Beta₂-adrenergic receptor agonist bronchodilators *Aerosol* Used for airway hyperresponsiveness; may help prevent bronchospasm associated with inhaled therapies.	• Use before airway clearance procedure. Have the child hold the breath 10 sec after inhalation. • Avoid swallowing the medicine, and rinse the mouth afterward.
Dornase alpha (DNAse or Pulmozyme) *Aerosol* Loosens, liquefies, and thins pulmonary secretions to reduce exacerbations.	• Keep refrigerated until placed in the nebulizer. • Monitor for improvement in dyspnea and mucus clearance.
Hypertonic saline (7%) *Aerosol* Hydrates the airway mucus and stimulates coughing to improve lung function and reduce exacerbations.	• Use following a bronchodilator.
Ivacaftor (Kalydeco) *Oral* Promotes chloride ion transport and improves regulation of salt and water absorption and secretion in the tissues (Taketomo, Hodding, & Kraus, 2014). Only for children with G551D *CFTR* mutation.	• Monitor child's hepatic enzyme levels; hold medication if levels are significantly elevated. • Administer with high-fat foods. • Do not eat grapefruit or Seville oranges while taking medication.
Ibuprofen *Oral* Can slow the progression of lung pulmonary function decline (Mogayzel et al., 2013).	• Educate the child and parents to monitor for signs of gastrointestinal bleeding. • Ensure that the child does not take aspirin or other NSAIDs unless approved by healthcare provider.
Antibiotics (e.g., tobramycin, azithromycin, aztreonam, and others identified by culture sensitivity) *Aerosol, oral, or IV* Used to treat and suppress infections.	• Higher doses than normal and prolonged courses may be prescribed. • Teach the child and family to develop a schedule to give the correct dose at appropriate intervals.
Pancreatic enzyme supplements (Cotazym-S, Pancrease, Viokase) *Oral* Assists in digestion of nutrients decreasing fat and bulk.	• Given prior to food ingestion. • Ensure that enzymes are taken with meals and snacks.
Vitamins (A, D, E, and K) and antioxidants (selenium, zinc, and ascorbate) *Oral* Supplements vitamins not produced.	• Ensure that vitamins are prescribed in non–fat-soluble form to promote absorption. • Give twice a day.

67.8% of cases survive 1 year, 60% survive 5 years, and 43% survive 10 years (Dorgan & Hadjiliadis, 2014). Persons infected with *Burkholderia cepacia* have a lower rate of survival, making them ineligible for transplant at many centers. Respiratory failure from end-stage lung disease is the cause of death in most patients with CF.

Nursing Management

For the Child With Cystic Fibrosis

Care of the child with previously diagnosed CF is the focus of the following discussion.

Nursing Assessment and Diagnosis

PHYSIOLOGIC ASSESSMENT

Physical assessment of the child focuses on respiratory function. Inquire about the frequency and characteristics of the child's cough and sputum. Compare this information with the child's baseline. Changes in the cough may be more important than its presence or absence related to the development of a new infection. Auscultate the chest for breath sounds, crackles, and wheezes. Note any cyanosis or clubbing of the extremities. Obtain SpO₂ and spirometry readings if changes in respiratory status are suspected.

TABLE 46–6 Clinical Therapy for Cystic Fibrosis

CLINICAL THERAPY	RATIONALE
RESPIRATORY THERAPY	
Exercise and physical fitness	Promotes maintenance of lung function.
Airway clearance techniques—chest physiotherapy twice a day for all lung segments (percussion or vibration with the child positioned to promote sputum drainage), oscillating chest vests, or other expiratory techniques	Helps secretions move to bronchi from smaller airways. Coughing and breathing airway clearance techniques help expel secretions.
Immunizations	Prevents viral and some bacterial infections.
Chest tube drainage of air leaks	Resolves pneumothorax.
Thoracoscopy to sew over ruptured alveoli	Repairs area of recurrent pneumothorax and prevents future episode in same location.
Lung transplantation	Reverses respiratory failure.
GASTROINTESTINAL TRACT THERAPY	
Acid suppression therapy	Gastroesophageal reflux worsens lung function; enteric coating of enzyme supplements is affected by high acid content in duodenum.
Hyperosmolar enemas, isotonic fluid lavage of the intestines (oral or by nasogastric tube)	Enema relieves meconium ileus in most infants; fluid lavage reduces distal intestinal obstruction.
NUTRITION	
Well-balanced, high-calorie, high-fat diet	Promotes essential nutrient balance for health, growth, weight maintenance, and increased lung capacity and survival.
Pancreatic enzyme supplements	Promotes digestion of fats and proteins.

Determine if the child is maintaining an appropriate growth pattern by plotting the weight, height, and body mass index on a growth curve. Children with significantly lower percentiles for height and weight should be considered malnourished. Inquire about the child's appetite and dietary intake. Ask how nutritional supplements, pancreatic enzymes, and vitamins are used. Observe the adolescent for the appearance of secondary sex characteristics, which are often delayed because of nutritional status.

Assess the child's stooling pattern. Identify whether the child has problems with abdominal pain or bloating, and whether these problems can be related to eating, stooling, or other activities. Palpate the abdomen for liver size, fecal masses, and evidence of pain.

PSYCHOSOCIAL ASSESSMENT

The emotional stress of this chronic disease may not be readily apparent, particularly if the child's symptoms are mild and not imminently life threatening. Ongoing observation of child and parent behaviors helps direct nursing interventions. Parents may feel guilt as carriers of the disease. Siblings may also show signs of difficulty in dealing with the illness, particularly if not affected by the disease. Siblings with CF may be affected if the child is showing signs of significant deterioration, being forced to acknowledge their own future course with the disease.

Ask parents how the child's illness has affected day-to-day functioning, potential conflicts with family activities, and how they have adapted to the child's plan of care. Investigate the need for respite care. Ask what the parents have told the child and siblings about the disease. What questions have the child and siblings asked about CF, and how have parents answered them? Has the child ever asked about the life expectancy of someone with CF? If not, what would parents say if asked?

Common nursing diagnoses for the child with CF include the following (NANDA-I © 2014):

- *Airway Clearance, Ineffective*, related to thick mucus in lungs

- *Nutrition, Imbalanced: Less than Body Requirements*, related to need for increased calories to meet growth and metabolic needs
- *Infection, Risk for*, related to the presence of mucous secretions conducive to bacterial growth
- *Role Conflict, Parental*, related to interruptions in family life due to the home care regimen and child's frequent exacerbations

Planning and Implementation

Nursing management involves supporting the child and family initially, when the diagnosis is made, during subsequent hospitalizations, and during visits to specialty and primary healthcare providers. The nurse's role begins with implementing specific medical therapies and providing nursing care to meet the child's physiologic and psychosocial needs. Airway clearance techniques, medications, and nutrition must be coordinated to promote optimal body function. Psychosocial support and reinforcement of the child's daily care needs are important in preparation for home care.

Children with CF require periodic hospitalization when a severe infection occurs or for a pulmonary and nutritional assessment. The child is often placed in a private room with standard precautions to reduce the spread of infectious organisms. Children with CF are not roomed together to reduce the risk for transmission of *Pseudomonas aeruginosa* and *Burkholderia cepacia* between them.

Respect the parents' experiences as the child's primary care provider and include them in the child's routine care as much as possible. However, parents may view the hospital stay as a break from the rigorous daily pulmonary routine at home and need support to take advantage of the respite. While the family is often proficient at providing physical care to the child, the nurse should take the opportunity to review basic and new information about airway clearance techniques, medications,

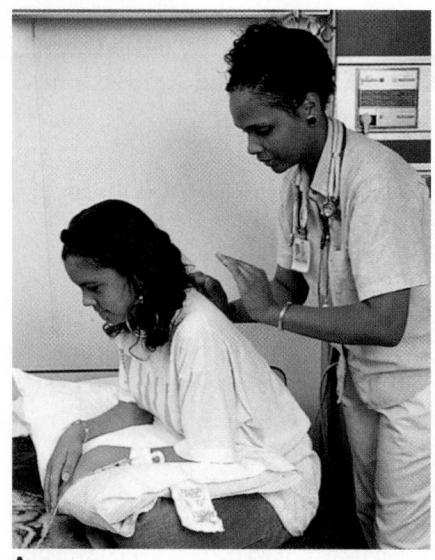
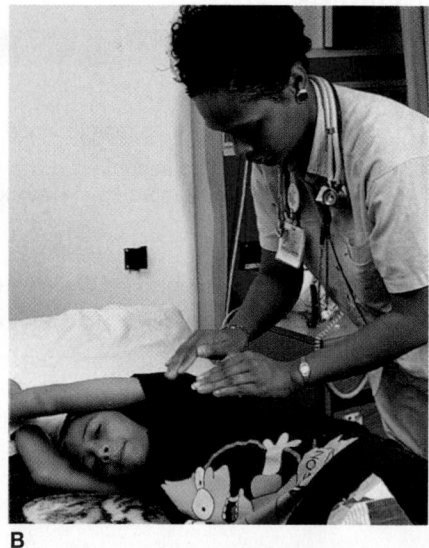
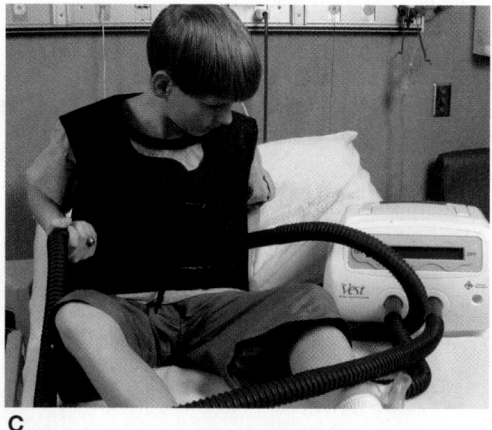

A B C

Figure 46–10 Chest physiotherapy with postural drainage can be achieved by clapping with a cupped hand on the chest wall over the segment to be drained to create vibrations that are transmitted to the bronchi to dislodge secretions. *A*, If the obstruction is in the posterior apical segment of the lung, the nurse can do this with the child sitting up. *B*, If the obstruction is in the left posterior segment, the child should be lying on the right side. Several other positions can be used depending on the location of the obstruction. *C*, A high-frequency chest wall oscillation vest is another option for airway clearance that the child can independently manage.

and nutrition. This is especially important as the child matures and begins to assume some self-care responsibilities.

PROVIDE RESPIRATORY THERAPY
Chest physiotherapy or an alternate airway clearance technique is usually performed 1 to 3 times per day to facilitate the removal of secretions from the lungs. (See the *Clinical Skills Manual* SKILLS .) Perform this before meals because coughing may stimulate vomiting. Aerosol treatments with a bronchodilator, as well as DNAse and hypertonic saline to help thin respiratory secretions, may precede the airway clearance procedure. Respiratory therapists and nurses often collaborate in teaching parents and other family members the skills for these necessary treatments. Some children use an oscillating vest for 30 minutes twice a day rather than chest physiotherapy (Figure 46–10).

ADMINISTER MEDICATIONS AND MEET NUTRITIONAL NEEDS
Antibiotics for acute exacerbation are provided by oral, inhalation, and intravenous routes. Because children with CF have an increased clearance of most antibiotics, they need higher doses and longer treatment courses, often for at least 14 days until the child achieves the best possible lung function. Serum antibiotic drug levels may be ordered to ensure therapeutic dosing; however, monitor renal function tests to detect problems related to higher antibiotic dosages. In some cases, a portacath or peripherally inserted central catheter (PICC) line is placed so that IV antibiotics can be given at home.

Digestive problems can be eased with pancreatic enzymes and dietary modification. Pancreatic enzyme supplements come in powder sprinkles and capsule form and are taken orally with all meals and large snacks. The amount needed is individualized based on the child's nutritional needs and digestive response to these supplements. Help families identify any foods that contribute to a child's gastrointestinal problems. The goal is to achieve near-normal, well-formed stools and adequate weight gain.

Fat-soluble vitamins (A, D, E, and K) are not completely absorbed from food; therefore, they must be taken in water-soluble form. Multivitamins taken twice daily usually are sufficient to prevent deficiency.

Respiratory complications and a higher metabolic rate make additional calories essential. Some children and youth need supplemental nasogastric or gastrostomy feedings to gain and maintain weight. The diet should be well balanced, with an emphasis on high caloric value and high-fat content. Salt is also needed in the diet.

PROVIDE PSYCHOSOCIAL SUPPORT
Help the parents and child learn what they must do to maintain health after discharge. Emotional support is essential because the diagnosis of CF creates anxiety and fear in both the parents and the child. They need assistance with emotional and psychosocial issues relating to discipline, body image (stooling odor, barrel chest), frequent rehospitalization, the potential terminal nature of the illness, the child's feeling of being different from friends, and overall financial, social, and family concerns. Because CF is inherited, families may have more than one child with CF. Refer families to genetic counseling and support groups.

DISCHARGE PLANNING AND HOME CARE TEACHING
The financial burden of medications, supplies, and medical follow-up may not be recognized immediately by a family overwhelmed by the diagnosis. Initially, parents need assistance in obtaining necessary equipment. If the parents require financial assistance, refer them to social services and the Cystic Fibrosis Foundation. Home care of the child with CF is expensive and can impact the family's finances.

COMMUNITY-BASED NURSING CARE
Nurses may encounter the child with CF in specialty clinics, health centers, and schools. Use the assessment guidelines found earlier

in this chapter to assess the child. Observe the child's physical appearance, noting overall body proportions and any changes characteristic of CF. Respiratory function tests are usually performed every 6 months during CF visits. Assess hearing acuity on a regular basis, especially if the antibiotic tobramycin is used.

A psychosocial assessment is especially important when the child is going through major developmental stages. School-age children and adolescents are often embarrassed at being viewed as different from peers. Ask how the child or adolescent feels about the need to consume such a large amount of food, to take medications, and to follow the daily respiratory care routine.

Review the child's airway clearance technique. If additional short-term therapies are prescribed to help improve pulmonary status, educate the child and family about the techniques to use and help them identify the best time to fit the additional treatment into the daily schedule. Having to do the chest physiotherapy regimen 3 or 4 times a day has a significant impact on family time. Alternate airway clearance therapy techniques, such as a vest, huffing, or oscillating positive expiratory pressures, may be more easily accepted by the family, especially since the parent does not have to physically perform the percussion and vibration. Daily aerobic exercise is recommended to promote airway clearance and overall health.

Managing the child's nutrition is important and takes time and energy. Refer the parents to a nutritionist to customize a meal plan for the child's caloric needs. Despite the child's voracious appetite, parents may have difficulty getting the child with CF to eat enough calories for optimal nutrition and growth. Parents need suggestions for preparing calorie-dense meals and snacks. A gastrostomy tube for nighttime feeding may be needed when the child's weight is 85% to 90% of ideal for height. Children with adequate nutrition have a longer life expectancy.

Clinical Tip

Use of cream or half and half added to soups, casseroles, and puddings; cream cheese spread on breads, muffins, and crackers; sour cream added to casseroles; and powdered milk added to regular milk, meatloaf, and custards are all ways to increase the calories in food eaten. Adolescents should have high-calorie snacks they can store in their school locker to eat before after-school activities.

Children with CF lose more than normal amounts of salt in their sweat, especially during hot weather, strenuous exercise, and fever. During periods of exercise and increased sweating, encourage the child to drink more fluids and increase salt intake. Allow the child to add extra salt to food and permit some salty snacks (pretzels with salt, pickles, carbonated soda). Teach parents to recognize early symptoms of salt depletion, including fatigue, weakness, abdominal pain, and vomiting, and to contact the child's healthcare provider if these symptoms occur.

Gradual assumption of responsibility for daily disease management is necessary and may be challenging if the child rebels or is defiant regarding therapy. Individualize the child's daily care regimen to facilitate time for interaction with peers and participation in school activities. Link adolescents to vocational service planning programs to help plan for their future. Initiate palliative care planning when the child's disease progresses toward respiratory failure.

Adolescents with CF need special assistance in coping with their disorder, especially since the median survival is now more than 40 years. Help them identify normal adolescent changes versus those related to CF. Discuss ways to cope with the difference they know exists between themselves and peers. They need to develop normal relationships and establish intimacy with a partner. Information about potential infertility must be provided along with the guidelines for safe sexual practices to reduce the risk for sexually transmitted infections. Females with CF may be able to conceive and should be offered contraception.

Evaluation

Expected outcomes of nursing care include the following:

- The child and family develop proficiency in providing the daily pulmonary care and reducing the incidence of respiratory infections.
- The child and family develop a schedule and routine for daily pulmonary care that fits into family and school activities.
- The child consumes adequate calories and pancreatic enzymes to support growth and to stay within desirable weight ranges.
- The child and family cope effectively with the child's disease.

Injuries of the Respiratory System

Airway compromise after an injury to the respiratory system can cause death if not managed quickly and effectively. Children are vulnerable to changes in respiratory function after injury because their airway is small and can become easily obstructed. Airway obstruction can be caused by the tongue, small amounts of blood, mucus, or foreign debris, and swelling in the respiratory tract or adjacent neck tissue, leading to hypoxia. If the child's neck is flexed or hyperextended, the soft laryngeal cartilage may also compress and obstruct the airway.

Smoke-Inhalation Injury

Exposure of the child's face and airway to smoke or extreme heat leads to dramatic responses in the child's respiratory tract. Smoke and heat increase the child's risk for airway obstruction, carbon monoxide poisoning, acute respiratory distress syndrome, late complications such as pneumonia, and death. The child's higher respiratory rate also increases exposure to noxious chemicals.

The severity of the smoke-inhalation injury is influenced by the type of material burned and is more severe if the child was found in a closed space. Smoke, a product of the burning process that is composed of gases and particles, such as cyanide from synthetic materials, is generated in varying volumes and density. The type and concentration of toxic gases, which are usually invisible, affect the severity of pulmonary damage. The duration of exposure to the smoke and toxic gases contributes significantly to the child's prognosis.

Exposure to extreme heat, common in house fires, leads to surface injury and upper airway damage. The upper airway normally removes heat from inhaled gases, sparing the lower airway from thermal damage. Airway edema develops rapidly over a few hours and potentially leads to acute respiratory distress syndrome.

Carbon monoxide (CO) is a clear, colorless, odorless, and tasteless gas that develops as a fire consumes oxygen or from poorly ventilated heating systems. The CO molecule binds more firmly to hemoglobin than does oxygen. As a result, reduced amounts of oxygen in the blood rapidly produce tissue hypoxia in the child. The brain receives inadequate oxygen, resulting in confusion and progressing to loss of consciousness. This is one reason fire victims have difficulty escaping. The process can be rapidly reversed by the timely administration of 100% oxygen, if provided before hypoxia becomes too severe (Hampson, Piantadosi, Thom, et al., 2012).

Damage to the lower airway often results from chemical or toxic gas inhalation. Soot carried deeply into the lungs combines with water to deposit acid-producing chemicals on the lung tissue. These acids burn the tissue and destroy the cilia and surfactant. Tissue destruction, pulmonary edema, and disrupted gas exchange are the initial insult to the lungs. Days later, the damaged tissue sloughs off, obstructing the airways. The lungs become a breeding ground for microorganisms, leading to pneumonia. Healing leaves scars in the damaged alveoli that can reduce future lung function.

Clinical manifestations of inhalation injury associated with fire include burns of the face and neck, singed nasal hairs, soot around the mouth or nose, and hoarseness with stridor or voice change, even when the child initially has no respiratory distress. Edema develops rapidly over a few hours and may lead to airway obstruction with signs such as tachypnea, stridor, coughing, and wheezing. Respiratory distress develops and can lead to respiratory failure. If carbon monoxide poisoning is present, the child may have headache, dizziness, confusion, shortness of breath, and loss of consciousness.

Diagnosis is based on history of smoke exposure in a closed area, and physical signs of soot around the nose and mouth. Arterial blood gases and a carboxyhemoglobin level are obtained. The child with minimal signs and symptoms when seen in the emergency department may be admitted to monitor for progression of respiratory distress. Initial treatment is 100% humidified oxygen. If respiratory distress develops, aggressive airway management with endotracheal tube insertion and monitoring are provided in the PICU. Mechanical ventilation and high concentration oxygen may be necessary. Chest physiotherapy and suctioning may be provided in an effort to keep the airway clear. All other injuries sustained in the fire are treated.

Nursing Management

Assess the child for the development of respiratory distress. Check vital signs frequently, and monitor the SpO₂. Auscultate the lungs for crackles, wheezes, and decreased breath sounds. Assess for level of consciousness and behavior changes that could indicate increasing hypoxia.

Provide oxygen as ordered. Position the child to promote respiratory function. If the child's condition deteriorates, assist with procedures to secure the child's airway and prepare the child for transfer to the ICU. Assess the family's response to the life-threatening crisis and offer support with information about the child's condition (see Chapter 41).

Blunt Chest Trauma

Blunt chest trauma in infants and toddlers is most often due to motor vehicle crashes and abuse. Bicycles, scooters, skateboards, and skates are more commonly associated with blunt chest trauma in school-age children. Injuries from high-energy motor vehicle crashes more commonly occur in adolescents. Chest injuries may not be obvious and can be extremely difficult to evaluate.

Most children who die after sustaining severe blunt chest trauma were hypoxic because of poor airway and ventilatory control. A child's elastic, pliable chest wall and thin abdominal muscles provide minimal protection to underlying organs. This elasticity of the ribs often prevents rib fractures in children less than 12 years of age, but the energy from blunt trauma is transferred directly to the internal organs. A pulmonary contusion or pneumothorax may result.

Pulmonary Contusion

A pulmonary contusion is defined as bruising damage to the tissues of the lung that often results from the transfer of energy from a strong blow to the chest. It often occurs without rib fracture. The lung tissue is indirectly injured, causing capillaries to bleed into the alveoli. Edema develops in the lower airways. The blood and fluid from damaged tissues accumulate over a couple of days and may interfere with gas exchange. Acute respiratory distress syndrome and long-term respiratory dysfunction may result.

The child may initially appear asymptomatic if it is an isolated injury. With a large pulmonary contusion the child may develop respiratory distress, along with fever, wheezing, hemoptysis, and crackles over several hours. Careful observation is required during the first 12 hours after the injury to detect decreased perfusion related to ventilatory impairment.

Chest radiographs or computed tomography may be diagnostic for a pulmonary contusion several hours after the injury. Therapy includes supplemental oxygen, pain control, incentive spirometry, and avoiding prolonged immobilization. Children with severe injury to the lungs will require mechanical ventilation with low airway pressures. Pneumonia is a potential complication.

Nursing Management

Nursing care centers on providing necessary physiologic support, such as oxygen therapy, positioning, incentive spirometry, fluid management, and comfort measures. Observe for hemoptysis, dyspnea, decreased breath sounds, wheezes, crackles, and a transient temperature elevation. Agitation and lethargy can signal increasing hypoxia. Inspect the thorax for symmetric chest wall movement, and auscultate for breath sounds in both lungs. The child may initially appear well but requires careful monitoring to detect signs of deterioration. Children with significant injuries are cared for in the ICU. Some children require ventilator support as the pulmonary tissues heal.

Pneumothorax

A pneumothorax occurs when air enters the pleural space because of a penetrating chest injury or tears in the tracheobronchial tree, the esophagus, or the chest wall. If blood collects in the pleural space, it is called a *hemothorax*, and if blood and air collect, it is called a *pneumohemothorax*. A pneumothorax is one of the more common thoracic injuries in pediatric trauma patients. The three types of pneumothorax are open, closed, and tension.

An *open pneumothorax* results from any penetrating injury that exposes the pleural space to atmospheric pressure, thereby collapsing the lung. A sucking sound may be heard as the air moves through the opening on the chest wall. The child may show signs of restlessness, cyanosis, and subcutaneous emphysema (air leakage in the tissue). Emergency treatment involves placing a water-tight bandage sealed on three sides over the opening to prevent more air from entering the chest during inspiration. The fourth side is left open so accumulated air can escape on expiration. A thoracostomy is performed, and a chest tube is inserted (see the *Clinical Skills Manual* SKILLS). A closed

Pathophysiology Illustrated: **Pneumothorax**

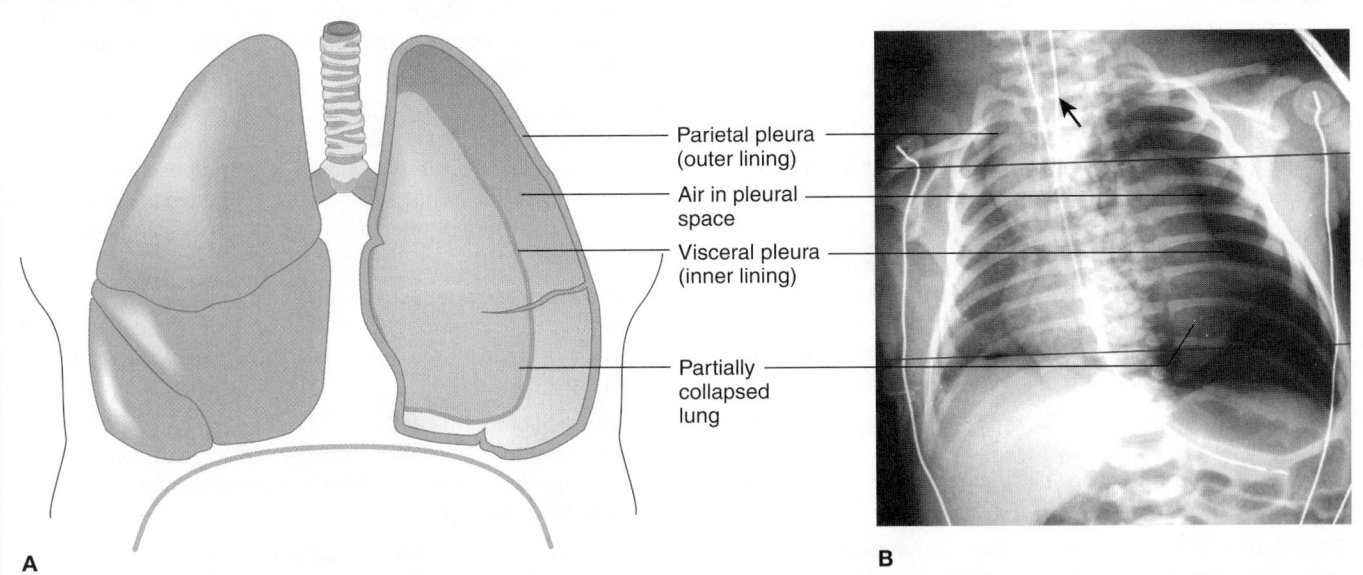

A   **B**

A, A pneumothorax is air in the pleural space that causes a lung to collapse. Whether the air results from an open injury or from bursting of alveoli due to a blunt injury, it is important to focus on airway management and maintain lung inflation. *B*, Tension pneumothorax. Note the collapsed lung on the child's left side and the deviation of the child's heart and trachea to the right side of the chest (see arrow).

SOURCE: Courtesy of Dorothy Bulas, MD, Professor of Radiology and Pediatrics, Children's National Medical Center, Washington, DC.

drainage system is attached to remove the air and reinflate the lung by reestablishing negative pressure.

A *closed pneumothorax* is sometimes caused by blunt chest trauma with no evidence of rib fracture (see *Pathophysiology Illustrated: Pneumothorax*). The chest may be compressed against a closed glottis (such as with breath holding), causing a sudden increase in pressure within the thoracic cavity. The pressure increase is transferred to the alveoli, causing them to burst. A single burst alveolus may be able to seal itself off, but the lung collapses when many alveoli are damaged. Breath sounds are decreased or absent on the injured side, and the child is in respiratory distress. A thoracostomy is performed and a chest tube inserted and attached to a closed drainage system.

A *tension pneumothorax* is a life-threatening emergency that results when the air leaks into the chest during inspiration but cannot escape during expiration. Internal pressure continues to build, compressing the chest contents and collapsing the lung. Venous return to the heart is impaired as the mediastinum shifts and the trachea, heart, vena cava, and esophagus are compressed

toward the unaffected lung, leading to decreased cardiac output. Signs of tension pneumothorax include increasing respiratory distress, decreased breath sounds, and paradoxical breathing. Immediate care for a tension pneumothorax is a needle thoracentesis to allow air to escape and relieve the tension. A chest tube is then inserted and attached to a closed drainage system.

Nursing Management

Nursing management focuses on airway management and maintaining lung inflation. The child arrives on the nursing unit with a chest tube and drainage system in place. Continued close observation for respiratory distress is essential. Carefully monitor vital signs. When the chest tube is removed, the site is covered with an occlusive dressing and the child's respiratory status is monitored for signs of respiratory distress. Complications include hemothorax (if the thoracostomy and chest tube are improperly placed), lung tissue injury, and scarring from poor tube placement (especially if the tube is placed too near the breast in girls).

Focus Your Study

- Respiratory conditions are a leading cause of hospitalization for all children between 1 and 19 years of age.

- The child's airway is shorter and narrower than an adult's, increasing the risk for obstruction. The lungs have no muscles; the diaphragm and intercostal muscles power ventilation.

- Foreign-body aspiration is a major health problem for infants and toddlers, often related to their increasing mobility and tendency to put small objects such as food and small toy parts in their mouths.

- Signs of impending respiratory failure in infants and children include worsening respiratory distress, irritability, lethargy, mottled color or cyanosis, diaphoresis, and increased respiratory effort such as dyspnea, tachypnea, nasal flaring, grunting, and retractions.

- An apparent life-threatening event (ALTE) is an episode of apnea accompanied by a color change (e.g., cyanosis or pallor), limp muscle tone, choking, or gagging in an infant less than 12 months of age.

- Obstructive sleep apnea syndrome (OSAS) in children is commonly caused by enlarged tonsils and adenoids. Children snore loudly and have labored breathing during sleep.

- Sudden infant death syndrome (SIDS) is a leading cause of death in infants. Onset of the fatal episode occurs during sleep and remains unexplained after a thorough investigation, including an autopsy, a review of the circumstances of death, and the clinical history.

- Laryngotracheobronchitis (LTB) is a viral croup syndrome with signs of an upper respiratory illness, hoarseness, tachypnea, inspiratory stridor, and a seal-like barking cough. Fever may or may not be present.

- Epiglottitis is a bacterial infection that can cause a life-threatening airway obstruction. It is commonly prevented by the pneumococcal vaccine. Classic signs include dysphonia, dysphagia, drooling, and distressed respiratory effort.

- Respiratory syncytial virus (RSV) is the most common cause of bronchiolitis, a lower respiratory tract infection that causes inflammation and obstruction of the bronchioles.

- Symptoms of pneumonia in infants and children include elevated temperature, rales, crackles, wheezes, cough, dyspnea, tachypnea, restlessness, and decreased breath sounds if consolidation occurs.

- Children under 2 years are at increased risk for developing active tuberculosis, including tubercular meningitis and disseminated TB.

- Chronic lung disease or bronchopulmonary dysplasia (BPD) usually develops in neonates with a birth weight of 1000 g (2.2 lb) or less. Treatment with oxygen and positive-pressure ventilation causes inflammation and damages the bronchioles, resulting in fibrosis, edema of the bronchioles, and smooth muscle hypertrophy.

- An asthma episode results from inflammation and a stimulus causing excessive mucus formation, mucosal swelling, and airway muscle contraction, leading to airway obstruction.

- In cystic fibrosis, defective chloride-ion transport across the exocrine and epithelial cell walls results in an abnormal accumulation of viscous, dehydrated mucus that affects the respiratory, gastrointestinal, and reproductive systems.

- Signs of smoke-inhalation injury in children include burns of the face and neck, singed nasal hairs, soot around the mouth or nose, and hoarseness with stridor or voice change.

- A pneumothorax may become life threatening when air leaking into the chest cavity during inspiration cannot escape during expiration, increasing compression. Venous blood return to the heart is impaired as the mediastinum shifts toward the unaffected lung.

Clinical Reasoning in Action

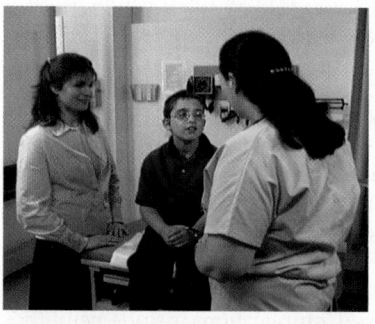

Adam and his mother have come to the health center to follow up on his hospitalization to get an asthma action plan and to discuss how to reduce his asthma episodes. Adam, who is 7 years old, has a history of episodic wheezing and nebulizer treatments, but he had never been hospitalized for asthma until last week. During his 2-day hospitalization, his parents were given initial education about how to manage his moderate persistent asthma.

His mother has brought along Adam's medications (inhaled corticosteroid and salmeterol MDI for daily control, and an albuterol MDI for quick relief), his peak flow meter, spacer, and his asthma action plan. She tells you that he is also completing a dose of oral corticosteroids. You discuss the peak flow meter, the guidelines, and what type of action to take as needed. Based on his height of 48 in., his peak flow meter green zone is 160–128, his yellow zone is 128–80, and his red zone is 80 or below. Adam is to use his daily control medications twice a day. If he has symptoms, he is to take his albuterol MDI with spacer, two puffs every 4–6 hours as needed.

1. What are some of the side effects associated with Adam's albuterol MDI?

2. What is the benefit to using a spacer on Adam's albuterol and inhaled corticosteroid MDI?

3. Address the concerns of Adam's mother about the daily use of inhaled corticosteroids.

4. What are the signs of respiratory distress to observe for with Adam?

5. What information should be shared with the school nurse for Adam's symptom management while at school?

References

Ajao, T. I., Oden, R. P., Joyner, B. I., & Moon, R. Y. (2011). Decisions of black parents about infant bedding and sleep surfaces. A qualitative study. *Pediatrics, 128*(3), 494–502.

Allergy and Asthma Network. (2014). *Medications at school.* Retrieved from http://www.aanma.org /advocacy/meds-at-school/

Amanatidou, V., Syridou, G., Mavrikou, M., & Tsolia, M. N. (2012). Latent tuberculosis infection in children: Diagnostic approaches. *European Journal of Clinical Microbiologic Infectious Disease, 31,* 1285–1294.

American Academy of Allergy, Asthma, and Immunology (AAAAI). (2014). *Peak flow meter.* Retrieved from http://www.aaaai.org/conditions-and-treatments /library/at-a-glance/peak-flow-meter.aspx

American Academy of Pediatrics (AAP). (2015). *Red book: 2015 report of the Committee on Infectious Diseases* (30th ed.). Elk Grove Village, IL: Author.

American Lung Association. (2013). *Joint statement on improving asthma management in schools.* Retrieved from http://www.lung.org/lung-disease/asthma /becoming-an-advocate/national-asthma-public -policy-agenda/joint-statement-improve-asthma -mgmt-schools.pdf

Asthma Initiative of Michigan for Healthy Lungs. (2011). *How to use a metered-dose inhaler the right way.* Retrieved from http://www.getasthmahelp.org /inhalers_main.asp

Banasiak, N. C. (2014). Spirometry in primary care for children with asthma. *Pediatric Nursing, 40*(4), 195–198.

Blanken, M. O., Rovers, M. M., Molenaar, J. M., Winkler-Seinstra, P. L., Meijer, A., Jan, L. L., ... Bont, L. (2013). Respiratory syncytial virus and recurrent wheeze in healthy preterm infants. *New England Journal of Medicine, 368*(19), 1791–1799.

Brashers, V. L., & Huether, S. E. (2014). Alterations in pulmonary function. In K. L. McCance, S. E. Huether, V. L. Brashers, & N. S. Rote (Eds.), *Pathophysiology: The biologic basis for disease in adults and children* (7th ed., pp. 1290–1318). St. Louis, MO: Elsevier Mosby.

Brunzell, C., Hardin, D. S., Moran, A., & Schindler, T. (2011). *Managing cystic fibrosis–related diabetes (CFRD): An instruction guide for patients and families* (5th ed., p. 7). Retrieved from http://www.cff.org /UploadedFiles/LivingWithCF/StayingHealthy/Diet /Diabetes/CFRD-Manual-5th%20Edition-05-2012.pdf

Burkhart, P. V., Rayens, M. K., & Oakley, M. G. (2012). Effect of peak flow monitoring on child asthma quality of life. *Journal of Pediatric Nursing, 27,* 18–25.

Centers for Disease Control and Prevention. (2013). *Asthma facts—CDC's national asthma control program grantees.* Retrieved from http://www.cdc.gov /asthma/pdfs/asthma_facts_program_grantees.pdf

Chang, C. (2012). Asthma in children and adolescents: A comprehensive approach to diagnosis and management. *Clinical Reviews in Allergy and Immunology, 43*(1–2), 98–137.

Chu, A., & Hageman, J. R. (2013). Apparent life-threatening events in infancy. *Pediatric Annals, 42*(2), 78–83.

Colvin, J. D., Collie-Akers, V., Schunn, C., & Moon, R. Y. (2014). Sleep environment risks for younger and older infants. *Pediatrics, 134*(2), e406–e412.

Custovic, A., Lazic, N., & Simpson, A. (2013). Pediatric asthma and development of atopy. *Current Opinion in Allergy and Clinical Immunology, 13*(2), 173–180.

Cystic Fibrosis Foundation (CFF). (2014). *About cystic fibrosis: What is cystic fibrosis?.* Retrieved from http://www.cff.org/AboutCF/

Desale, M., Bringardner, P., Fitzgerald, S., Page, K., & Shah, M. (2013). Intensified case-finding for latent tuberculosis infection among the Baltimore City Hispanic population. *Journal of Immigrant Minority Health, 15,* 680–685.

Dinakar, C., & Welch, M. J. (2014). Device how-tos. *Contemporary Pediatrics, 31*(May). Retrieved from http://contemporarypediatrics.modernmedicine.com /contemporary-pediatrics/content/tags/asthma /device-how-tos

Dorgan, D. J., & Hadjiliadis, D. (2014). Lung transplantation in patients with cystic fibrosis: Special focus to infection and comorbidities, *Expert Reviews in Respiratory Medicine, 8*(3), 315–326.

Flook, D. M., & Vincze, D. L. (2012). Infant safe sleep: Efforts to improve education and awareness. *Journal of Pediatric Nursing, 27*(2), 186–188.

Fouzas, S., Priftis, K. N., & Anthracopoulos, M. B. (2011). Pulse oximetry in pediatric practice. *Pediatrics, 128*(4), 740–751.

Gaydos, L. M., Blake, S. C., Gazmararian, J. A., Woodruff, W., Thompson, W. W., & Dalmida, S. G. (2015). Revisiting safe sleep recommendations for African-American infants: Why current counseling is insufficient, *Maternal Child Health Journal, 19,* 496–503.

Gelfer, P., Cameron, R., Masters, K., Six Sigma Black Belt, & Kennedy, K. (2013). Integrating "Back to Sleep" recommendations into neonatal ICU practice. *Pediatrics, 131*(4), e1264–e1270.

Gelfer, P., & Tatum, M. (2014). Sudden infant death syndrome. *Journal of Pediatric Health Care, 28*(5), 470–474.

Greenberg, D., Givon-Lavi, N., Sadaka, Y., Ben-Shimol, S., Bar-Ziv, J., & Dagan, R. (2014). Short-course antibiotic treatment for community-acquired alveolar pneumonia in ambulatory children: A double-blind, randomized, placebo-controlled trial. *Pediatric Infectious Disease Journal, 33*(2), 136–142.

Hampson, N. B., Piantadosi, C. A., Thom, S. R., & Weaver, L. K. (2012). Practice recommendations in the diagnosis, management, and prevention of carbon monoxide poisoning. *American Journal of Respiratory Critical Care Medicine, 186*(11), 1095–1101.

Hauck, F. R., Thompson, J. M. D., Tenabe, K. O., Moon, R. Y., & Vennemann, M. M. (2011). Breastfeeding and reduced risk of sudden infant death syndrome: A meta-analysis. *Pediatrics, 128*(1), 103–110.

Henderson, L. B., Doshi, V. K., Blackman, S. M., Naughton, K. M., Pace R. G., Moskovitz, J., ... Cutting, G. R. (2012). Variation in MSRA modifies risk of neonatal intestinal obstruction in cystic fibrosis. *PLoS Genetics, 8*(3), e1002580.

Heron, M. (2013). Deaths: Leading causes for 2010. *National Vital Statistics Reports, 62*(2), 1–96.

Howrylak, J. A., Fuhlbrigge, A. L., Strunk, R. C., Zeiger, R. S., Weiss, S. T., & Raby, B. A. (2014). Classification of childhood asthma phenotypes and long-term clinical responses to inhaled anti-inflammatory medications. *Journal of Allergy and Clinical Immunology, 133*(5), 1289–1300.

Jereb, J. A., Goldberg, S. V., Powell, K., Villarino, M. E., & LoBue, P. (2011). Recommendations for use of an isoniazid-rifapentine regimen with direct observation to treat latent *Mycobacterium tuberculosis* infection. *Morbidity and Mortality Weekly Report, 60*(48), 1650–1653.

Johns Hopkins Medicine. (2012). *Peak flow measurement.* Retrieved from http://www.hopkinsmedicine. org/healthlibrary/test_procedures/pulmonary /peak_flow_measurement_92,P07755

Kelly, H. W., Sternberg, A. L., Lescher, R., Fuhlbrigge, A. L., Williams, P., Zeiger, R. S., ... Strunk, R. C. (2012). Effect of inhaled glucocorticoids in childhood on adult height. *New England Journal of Medicine, 367*(10), 904–912.

Kueny, A., Berg, J., Chowdhury, Y., & Anderson, N. (2013). Poquito a poquito: How Latino families with children who have asthma make changes in their home. *Journal of Pediatric Health Care, 27*(1), e1–e11.

Marcus, C. L., Brooks, L. J., Draper, K. A., Gozal, D., Halbower, A. C., Jones, J., ... Shiffman, R. N. (2012). Clinical practice guideline: Diagnosis and management of childhood obstructive sleep apnea syndrome. *Pediatrics, 130*(3), 576–584.

Matthews, R., & Moore, A. (2013). Babies are still dying of SIDS. *American Journal of Nursing, 113*(2), 59–64.

Mogayzel, P. J., Naureckas, E. T., Robinson, K. A., Mueller, G., Hadjiliadis, D., Hoag, J. B., ... Pulmonary Clinical Practice Guidelines Committee. (2013). Cystic fibrosis pulmonary guidelines: Chronic medications for maintenance of lung health. *American Journal of Respiratory Critical Care Medicine, 187*(7), 680–689.

Nakano, S. J., & Tluczek, A. (2014). Genomic breakthroughs in the diagnosis and treatment of cystic fibrosis. *American Journal of Nursing, 114*(6), 36–43.

National Asthma Education and Prevention Program (NAEPP). (2007). *Expert panel report 3: Guidelines for the diagnosis and management of asthma.* Bethesda, MD: National Institutes of Health, National Heart Lung and Blood Institute. Retrieved from http://www.nhlbi .nih.gov/guidelines/asthma

Nguyen, J. M., Holbrook, J. A., Wei, C. Y., Gerald, L. B., Teague, W. G., & Wise, R. A. (2014). Validation and psychometric properties of the Asthma Control Questionnaire among children. *Journal of Allergy and Clinical Immunology, 133,* 91–97.

Nkoy, F. L., Stone, B. L., Fassl, B. A., Uchida, D. A., Koopmeiners, K., Sarah Halbern, S., ... Maloney, C. G. (2014). Longitudinal validation of a tool for asthma self-monitoring. *Pediatrics, 132*(6), e1554–e1561.

Parsons, J. P., Hallstrand, T. S., Mastronarde, J. G., Kaminsky, D. A., Rundell, K. W., Hull, J. H., ... Anderson, S. D. (2013). An official American Thoracic Society clinical practice guideline: Exercise-induced bronchoconstriction. *American Journal of Respiratory Critical Care Medicine, 187*(9), 1016–1027.

Perez-Velez, C. M., & Marais, B. J. (2012). Tuberculosis in children. *New England Journal of Medicine, 367*(4), 348–361.

Pfuntner, A., Wier, L. M., & Stocks, C. (2013). Most Frequent Conditions in U.S. Hospitals, 2011, *H-CUP Statistical Brief # 162.* Retrieved from http://www .hcup-us.ahrq.gov/reports/statbriefs/sb162.pdf

Prodhan, P., Sharoor-Karni, S., Lin, J., & Noviski, N. (2011). Predictors of respiratory failure among previously healthy children with respiratory syncytial virus infection. *American Journal of Emergency Medicine, 29,* 168–173.

Queen, M. A., Myers, A. L., Hall, M., Shah, S. S., Williams, D. J., Auger, K. A., ... Tieder, J. S. (2014).

Comparative effectiveness of empiric antibiotics for community-acquired pneumonia. *Pediatrics, 133*(1), e23–e29.

Riazi, S., Zeligs, B., Yeager, H., Peters, S. M., Benavides, G. A., Mita, O. D., & Bellanti, J. A. (2012). Rapid diagnosis of *Mycobacterium tuberculosis* infection in children using interferon-gamma release assays (IGRAs). *Allergy and Asthma Proceedings, 33*(3), 217–226.

Roosevelt, G. E. (2016). Acute inflammatory upper airway obstruction (croup, epiglottitis, laryngitis, and bacterial tracheitis). In R. M. Kliegman, B. F. Stanton, J. W. St. Geme, & N. F. Schor (Eds.), *Nelson textbook of pediatrics* (20th ed., pp. 2031–2036). Philadelphia, PA: Elsevier Saunders.

Rose, W., Kitai, I., Kakkar, F., Read, S. E., Behr, M. A., & Bitnun, A. (2014). Quantiferon gold-in-tube assay for TB screening in HIV infected children: Influence of quantitative values. *BMC Infectious Diseases, 14*, 516–521.

Ross, P. A., Newth, C. J. L., & Khemani, R. G. (2014). Accuracy of pulse oximetry in children. *Pediatrics, 133*(1), 22–29.

Rozance, P. J., & Rosenberg, A. A. (2012). The neonate. In S. G. Gabbe, J. R. Niebyl, H. L. Galen, E. Jauniaux, M. B. Landon, J. L. Simpson, D. A. Driscoll (Eds.), *Obstetrics: Normal and problem pregnancies* (6th ed., pp. 481–516). Philadelphia, PA: Elsevier Saunders.

Seddon, J. A., Hesseling, A. C., Godfrey-Faussett, P., Fielding, K., & Schaaf, H. S. (2013). Risk factors for infection and disease in child contacts of multidrug-resistant tuberculosis: A cross-sectional study. *BMC Infectious Diseases, 13*, 392–401.

Sharma, G. D., & Conrad, C. (2011). Croup, epiglottitis, and bacterial tracheitis. In American Academy of Pediatrics Section on Pediatric Pulmonology, *Pediatric Pulmonology* (pp. 347–363). Elk Grove Village, IL: Author.

Sleath, B., Ayala, G. X., Gillette, C., Williams, D., Davis, S., Tudor, G., … Washington, D. (2011). Provider demonstration and assessment of child device technique during pediatric asthma visits. *Pediatrics, 127*(4), 642–648.

Starke, J. R., & Cruz, A. T. (2014). The global nature of childhood tuberculosis. *Pediatrics, 133*(3), e725–e727.

Strueby, L., & Thébaud, B. (2014). Advances in broncho-pulmonary dysplasia. *Expert Reviews in Respiratory Medicine, 8*(3), 327–338.

Taketomo, C. K., Hodding, J. H., & Kraus, D. M. (2014). *Pediatric and neonatal dosage handbook* (21st ed.). Hudson, OH: Lexicomp.

Task Force on Sudden Infant Death Syndrome. (2011). SIDS and other sleep-related infant deaths: Expansion of recommendations for a safe infant sleeping environment. *Pediatrics, 128*(5), 1030–1039.

Van Nguyen J. M., & Abenhaim H. A. (2013). Sudden infant death syndrome: Review for the obstetric care provider. *American Journal of Perinatology, 30*(09), 703–714.

WebMD. (2012). *Asthma and the peak flow meter.* Retrieved from http://www.webmd.com/asthma/guide/peak-flow-meter

Weinberger, M. M. (2011). Bronchiolitis. In American Academy of Pediatrics Section on Pediatric Pulmonology, *Pediatric pulmonology* (pp. 377–390). Elk Grove Village, IL: Author.

Wilson, B. A., Shannon, M. T., & Shields, K. M. (2016). *Nurse's drug guide 2016.* Hoboken, NJ: Pearson.

Winston, C. A., & Menzies, H. J. (2012). Pediatric and adolescent tuberculosis in the United States, 2008–2010. *Pediatrics, 130*(6), e1425–e1432.

Wong, J. J. M., Lee, J. H., Turner, D. A., & Rehder, K. J. (2014). A review of the use of adjunctive therapies in severe acute asthma exacerbation in critically ill children. *Expert Reviews in Respiratory Medicine, 8*(4), 423–441.

Zentz, S. E. (2011). Care of infants and children with bronchiolitis: A systemic review. *Journal of Pediatric Nursing, 26*(6), 519–529.

Zoorob, R., Sidani, M., & Murray, J. (2011). Croup: An overview. *American Family Physician, 83*(9), 1067–1073.

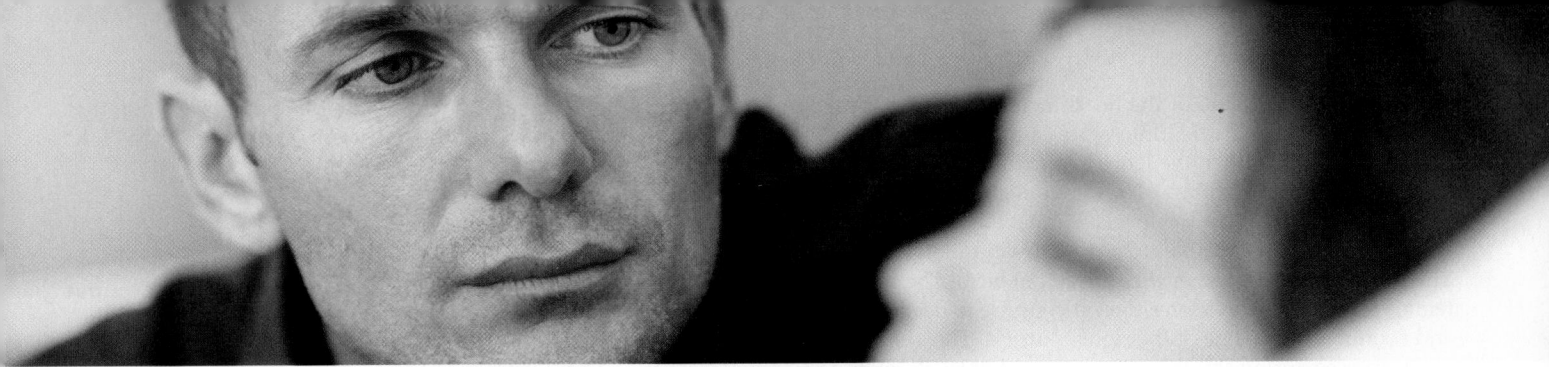

Chapter 47
The Child With Alterations in Cardiovascular Function

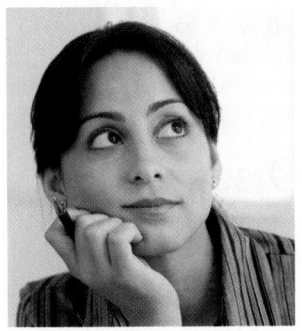

Brandy got sick so fast. Look how fast she is breathing. She gets tired before she can finish her formula. We didn't expect her to need heart surgery when she was still so small. We were told her chances for successful surgery would improve if she grew some more. I just want her to get stronger and have the chance to grow up to be like other kids.

—Mother of Brandy, 1 month old

Blend Images/Shutterstock

∨ Learning Outcomes

47.1 Describe the anatomy and physiology of the cardiovascular system, focusing on the flow of blood and the action of heart valves.

47.2 Describe the pathophysiology associated with congenital heart defects with increased pulmonary circulation, decreased pulmonary circulation, mixed defects, and obstructed systemic blood flow.

47.3 Develop a nursing care plan for the infant with a congenital heart defect cared for at home prior to corrective surgery.

47.4 Create a nursing care plan for the child undergoing open heart surgery.

47.5 Recognize the signs and symptoms of congestive heart failure in an infant and child.

47.6 Develop a nursing care plan for a child with congestive heart failure.

47.7 Differentiate among the heart diseases that are acquired or begin development during childhood.

47.8 Develop a nursing care plan for a child with Kawasaki syndrome.

47.9 List strategies to reduce a child's risk of adult-onset cardiovascular disease.

47.10 Plan the nursing management of hypovolemic shock.

Alterations in cardiovascular function may result from a congenital defect, acquired infection, or injury. Congenital heart defects are one of the most common birth defects, occurring in approximately 1% of all live births (Peterson et al., 2014). More than 35 types of heart defects have been documented. Examples of acquired cardiovascular conditions include rheumatic fever, Kawasaki disease, and hypertension.

Anatomy and Physiology of Pediatric Differences

The transition from fetal to pulmonary circulation that occurs at birth is described in Chapter 24. Systemic vascular resistance increases after the umbilical cord is cut. Blood flow to the lungs and then to the left side of the heart increases, stimulating closure of the foramen ovale, unless pressures on the right side of the heart are higher than the left. The ductus arteriosus normally constricts and closes within 10 to 15 hours after birth in response to higher oxygen saturation levels. Permanent closure occurs by 10 to 21 days after birth unless the oxygen saturation remains low. The right ventricle is larger than the left at birth. The higher systemic vascular pressures force the left ventricle to develop quickly and soon match the size of the right ventricle. The systolic blood pressure rises during childhood, reaching adult levels by puberty.

The heart is divided into four chambers: two atria and two ventricles. A septum, or wall, separates the left and right sides of the heart. The tricuspid and mitral valves open and close to control the flow of blood between the atria and the ventricles. The pulmonary and aortic valves open when the ventricles pump blood and close to prevent the backflow of blood to the ventricles. The great arteries (aorta and pulmonary artery) carry blood away from the heart to either the body or the lungs. Pulmonary veins and the superior and inferior venae cavae return blood to the heart. See Table 47–1 for **hemodynamics** (passage of blood through the heart and pulmonary system of the normal heart).

Oxygenation

Oxygen bound to hemoglobin is transported to the tissues by the systemic circulation. Hematocrit and hemoglobin concentrations appropriate for the child's age are necessary for adequate oxygen transport (see Chapter 49). The oxygen arterial saturation is the amount of oxygen that can potentially be delivered to the tissues. **Desaturated blood** results when oxygenated and unoxygenated blood mix because of a congenital heart defect. Cyanosis, which indicates **hypoxemia** (lower than normal amounts of oxygen in the blood), results from a decreased concentration of oxygenated hemoglobin.

Clinical Tip

A pulse oximeter provides a noninvasive measurement of the percutaneous arterial oxygen saturation level (SpO_2) and may provide an early clue that hypoxemia is developing before cyanosis is visualized. A reading of 95% to 98% is normal in children. See Chapter 46 for a review of pulse oximetry use.

The child's bone marrow responds to chronic hypoxemia by producing an excess number of red blood cells (**polycythemia**) to increase the amount of hemoglobin available for oxygenation. A hematocrit value of 50% or higher is common in children who have heart defects causing cyanosis. A hemoglobin concentration greater than 20 g/dL is considered extreme polycythemia.

Polycythemia is also associated with a platelet dysfunction that increases the risk for thromboembolism, especially if the child becomes dehydrated (see Chapter 49).

Cardiac Functioning

The infant's metabolic rate and oxygen requirements double at birth, so the heart rate is high to maintain a high **cardiac output** (volume of blood ejected from the left ventricle each minute) and adequate oxygen transport. Stress, exercise, fever, or respiratory distress cause tachycardia, which increases cardiac output and oxygen transport.

Infants have a greater risk of heart failure than older children because the immature heart is more sensitive to volume or pressure overload. The cardiac output in newborns and young children depends primarily on heart rate until the heart muscle is fully developed at 5 years of age. During infancy the heart's muscle fibers are less developed and less organized, resulting in limited increase in functional capacity. Infants have less **compliance** (amount of expansion the ventricles can achieve to increase stroke volume) of the heart muscle, so the **stroke volume** (the amount of blood ejected with each contraction) cannot increase substantially. The newborn has little cardiac reserve capacity until oxygen requirements begin to decrease at about 2 months of age (McDaniel, 2014).

Congenital Heart Disease

Congenital heart disease refers either to a defect in the heart or great vessels or to persistence of a fetal structure (e.g., patent foramen ovale or patent ductus arteriosus) after birth. The incidence is about 8 to 12 per 1000 live births (Park, 2014, p. 7). A critical congenital heart defect is life threatening and requires emergency care, surgery, or catheter intervention within the first days or weeks of life. These defects account for 25% of infant deaths related to a birth defect during the first year of life (Peterson et al., 2014).

Etiology and Pathophysiology

Most congenital heart defects develop during the first 8 weeks of gestation. They can develop as the result of a combined or interactive effect of genetic and environmental factors, such as:

- Fetal exposure to drugs (e.g., phenytoin, angiotensin-converting enzyme [ACE] inhibitors, lithium, warfarin, valproic acid, retinoic acid) and alcohol
- Maternal viral infections such as rubella or coxsackievirus B5
- Maternal metabolic disorders such as phenylketonuria, diabetes mellitus, and hypercalcemia
- Increased maternal age

TABLE 47–1 Hemodynamics of the Normal Heart

ACTION	RIGHT SIDE OF HEART	LEFT SIDE OF HEART
Blood return to heart	From systemic circulation by way of the superior and inferior venae cavae.	From the lungs by way of the left and right pulmonary veins.
Diastolic phase	Pulmonary valve closes and tricuspid valve opens.	Aortic valve closes and mitral valve opens.
	Blood flows from the venae cavae through the right atrium and tricuspid valve into the right ventricle.	Blood flows from the pulmonary veins through the left atrium and mitral valve into the left ventricle.
Systolic phase	Tricuspid valve closes and pulmonary valve opens.	Mitral valve closes and aortic valve opens.
	Blood is pumped into the pulmonary artery and passes into the right and left pulmonary arteries and lungs.	Blood is pumped into the aorta where it enters the systemic circulation.

- Multifactorial genetic patterns
- Chromosomal abnormalities (e.g., Turner, Noonan, Marfan, DiGeorge, and trisomy [13, 18, 21] syndromes)

Because of the genetic component, the incidence of congenital heart defects (CHDs) is expected to slowly rise; for example, a mother with a CHD has an increased risk of having an affected child.

Congenital heart defects are categorized by pathophysiology and hemodynamics rather than by the presence of cyanosis. These categories are described in more detail later in this chapter and include the following:

- Increased pulmonary blood flow
- Decreased pulmonary blood flow
- Obstructed systemic blood flow

Mixed defects fall into one of these three classifications, but the infant's survival depends on mixing systemic and pulmonary blood. Children with mixed defects and decreased pulmonary blood flow have similar clinical therapy and nursing management, so these categories will be discussed together.

Clinical Manifestations

The presence of a heart murmur is often the first indication of a congenital heart defect. A murmur indicates blood is flowing with higher pressure than normal to get through a narrowed valve or vessel or through a **shunt** (an abnormal anatomic opening in the septum between the systemic and pulmonary circulation). Other clinical manifestations and the timing of their appearance vary by the pathophysiology and severity of the defect. See Table 47–2. Newborns may become symptomatic as soon as the umbilical cord is cut or within the first few days of life. Some children may be asymptomatic except for a heart murmur. Signs and symptoms in older children may include exercise intolerance, chest pain, arrhythmias, syncope, and sudden death.

Clinical Therapy

Multiple tests are used to diagnose cardiac defects (Table 47–3). Blood tests such as a hematocrit and hemoglobin are taken to assess for anemia or polycythemia. Arterial blood gases may be obtained, especially when cyanosis or a complex heart defect is suspected. Newborn screening with pulse oximetry is used to identify critical congenital heart disease (Association of Maternal and Child Health Programs, 2013).

Treatment for congenital heart defects depends on the severity of symptoms and whether the condition is imminently life threatening. Interventional cardiac catheterization or surgical correction with restoration of normal hemodynamics and physiology is the treatment of choice for many defects. A

TABLE 47–2 Clinical Manifestations of Heart Defects by Pathophysiology

PATHOPHYSIOLOGY AND TYPE OF DEFECT	CLINICAL MANIFESTATIONS
Increased pulmonary blood flow (PDA, ASD, VSD, AV canal)	Tachypnea, tachycardia, murmur, congestive heart failure (CHF), poor weight gain, diaphoresis, periorbital edema, frequent respiratory infections
Decreased pulmonary blood flow (PS, TOF, pulmonary or tricuspid atresia, TGA)	Cyanosis, hypercyanotic spells, poor weight gain, polycythemia
Obstruction to systemic blood flow (COA, AS, HLHS, MS, interrupted aortic arch)	Diminished pulses, poor color, delayed capillary refill time, decreased urine output, CHF with pulmonary edema
Mixed defects—postnatal survival is dependent on mixing of systemic and pulmonary blood (TGA, TAPVR, truncus arteriosus, double outlet right ventricle)	Cyanosis, poor weight gain, pulmonary congestion, CHF may occur with increased shunting

Key: AS, aortic stenosis; ASD, atrial septal defect; AV, atrioventricular; COA, coarctation of aorta; HLHS, hypoplastic left heart syndrome; MS, mitral stenosis; PDA, patent ductus arteriosus; PS, pulmonic stenosis; TAPVR, total anomalous pulmonary venous return; TOF, tetralogy of Fallot; TGA, transposition of great arteries; VSD, ventricular septal defect

TABLE 47–3 Diagnostic Tests Used in Children With Congenital Heart Disease

DIAGNOSTIC TEST	PURPOSE
Radiographic studies (chest radiograph, computed tomography, magnetic resonance imaging)	Reveals size and contour of the heart and characteristics of pulmonary vascular markings, anatomic characteristics of the heart
Electrocardiogram (ECG)	Records quality of major electrical activity in the heart, identifies arrhythmias. A Holter monitor allows for continuous 24- to 48-hr ECG recordings
Echocardiogram (two-dimensional and transesophageal)	Identifies heart's structures, the pattern of movement, hemodynamics, pressures, and the presence of anatomic defects
Magnetic resonance imaging	Identifies the precise location, anatomy, and severity of heart defects and assesses the function of the ventricles
Cardiac catheterization	Invasive procedure to obtain a precise measurement of oxygen saturation, cardiac output, and pressures in each heart chamber and blood vessel; used when anatomic alternations are not well defined by echocardiogram or specific pressures in heart chambers are needed prior to surgery (Ofori-Amanfo & Cheifetz, 2013)
Exercise testing	Enables ECG recording with controlled increase in activity to identify significant cardiac compensation or inadequate cardiac output
Hyperoxia test	Measures differences in arterial blood gas level when child is on room air and on 100% oxygen

palliative procedure (a surgical procedure that does not create normal anatomic or hemodynamic results) may be performed in children with a potentially fatal or lethal condition. It may also be performed as an initial procedure, allowing an infant to grow before definitive corrective surgery. Table 47–4 lists the types of interventions during cardiac catheterization and surgical procedures performed on children with congenital heart defects.

Nursing Management
For the Child Having Cardiac Catheterization

Cardiac catheterization performed for examination or for therapeutic intervention is often an outpatient procedure. The child is NPO for several hours, except for medications, and arrives at the catheterization laboratory 1 to 2 hours before the procedure.

TABLE 47–4 Clinical Interventions for Congenital Heart Defects

CARDIAC CATHETERIZATION INTERVENTIONS AND THERAPEUTIC USE	PURPOSE
Balloon atrial septostomy—Rashkind, or with transatrial needle puncture and balloon dilation Palliative for TGA	Creates a larger defect (at the foramen ovale) between atria to increase blood mixing.
Balloon dilation procedure Corrective for PS and MS; palliative for AS, COA	A deflated balloon is inserted and inflated to open a narrowed valve or blood vessel. A stent may be inserted to keep the vessel (e.g., ductus arteriosus) open.
Device closure Corrective for PDA, ASD, VSD	Closure of ductus arteriosus by an umbrella or coil device, and closure of a septal defect by a septal occluder.

SURGICAL PROCEDURES AND THERAPEUTIC USE	PURPOSE
Aorta end-to-end anastomosis Corrective for COA	Resection of the narrowed section of the aorta and connection of the proximal and distal sections.
Blalock-Taussig shunt, modified Palliative for TOF, single ventricle lesions with pulmonary outflow obstruction	Creation of aortopulmonary conduit (from the brachiocephalic artery to pulmonary artery) to increase pulmonary blood flow.
Brock Corrective for PS	Blind incision of pulmonary valve.
Damus-Kaye-Stansel—pulmonary artery-to-aortic anastomosis Corrective for TGA, complex single ventricle defects	Pulmonary artery is cut in two with the proximal section attached to the ascending aorta; the distal section is sewn over, and a shunt is created between the systemic circulation and the pulmonary artery to send blood to the lungs.
Fontan Palliative for HLHS, single ventricle defects	Creation of a conduit between inferior vena cava and pulmonary artery to increase pulmonary blood flow—total right heart bypass. The single ventricle assumes responsibility for the systemic circulation and ejects blood into the aorta.
Glenn or Bidirectional Glenn Palliative for HLHS, single ventricle defects	Superior vena cava connected to right pulmonary artery along with closure of aortopulmonary shunt. Systemic venous blood from the head is sent to the lungs directly without ventricular pumping.
Jatene—arterial switch Corrective for TGA	Aorta and pulmonary arteries are transected and reattached to the opposite stumps; coronary arteries are moved to new aorta area.
Norwood Palliative for aortic hypoplasia, single ventricle defects (e.g., HLHS)	Atrial septectomy, anastomosis of the main pulmonary artery to the aorta, and an arterial-pulmonary shunt (e.g., modified Blalock-Taussig shunt).
Norwood with Sano modification Palliative for HLHS	Creation of a right ventricle to pulmonary artery conduit so that both the direct pulmonary and aorta blood flow originate in the right ventricle.
Nikaidoh Corrective for TGA when a VSD and severe PS are present	The aortic route is translocated from the right ventricle, with attached coronary vessels to the left ventricle after reconstructing the left and right outflow tracts and patching the VSD.
Patch aortoplasty Corrective for COA	Insertion of a Dacron patch or opened left subclavian vein to expand the lumen of the aorta.

SURGICAL PROCEDURES AND THERAPEUTIC USE	PURPOSE
Pulmonary artery banding	
Palliative for VSD, AV canal, single ventricle defects	Placement of constricting band around pulmonary artery to reduce pulmonary blood flow and pressure.
Rastelli	
Corrective for TGA with pulmonic stenosis, TOF, tricuspid atresia, truncus arteriosus, and some cases of double outlet right ventricle	Creation of a conduit between the right ventricle to pulmonary artery with closure of the ventricular septal defect. In the case of truncus arteriosus, the pulmonary arteries are removed from the truncus.
Ross	
Corrective for AS	The diseased aortic valve is replaced with the patient's pulmonic valve (pulmonary autograft), and a homograft (valve from a human donor) replaces the pulmonic valve.
Subclavian flap aortoplasty	
Corrective for COA	Division of the distal subclavian artery and insertion of a flap into the aorta through the coarcted segment.
Transplant	
Corrective for HLHS, complex defects, cardiomyopathies	Replacement of diseased heart with donor heart.

Key: AS, aortic stenosis; ASD, atrial septal defect; AV, atrioventricular; COA, coarctation of aorta; HLHS, hypoplastic left heart syndrome; MS, mitral stenosis; PDA, patent ductus arteriosus; PS, pulmonic stenosis; TOF, tetralogy of Fallot; TGA, transposition of great arteries; VSD, ventricular septal defect

In preparation for the procedure, the child is asked to void and is given an oral sedative. Infants and young children often need sedation to keep them still during the procedure.

Nursing Assessment and Diagnosis

Before the procedure, assess the child using the assessment guidelines found in the accompanying *Assessment Guide: The Child With a Cardiac Condition*. Collect baseline data on skin temperature, color, strength of pedal and popliteal pulses, and hematocrit and hemoglobin levels for comparison with postcatheterization assessments.

After the procedure, monitor the child for potential complications such as arrhythmia, bleeding, hematoma development, thrombus formation, and infection for several hours. No bleeding should occur at the catheterization site. Assess vital signs and perfusion of the lower extremities (pulses, temperature, color, capillary refill, and sensation) and compare to precatheterization status. The child's temperature and vital signs should remain stable. Monitor intake and output because the contrast medium may cause diuresis.

The following nursing diagnoses may apply to the child who undergoes cardiac catheterization (NANDA-I © 2014):

- *Fear* related to separation from support system in a stressful situation
- *Fluid Volume: Imbalanced, Risk for*, related to inadequate fluid intake due to NPO status and diuretic effect of contrast medium
- *Tissue Perfusion: Peripheral, Risk for Ineffective*, related to mechanical reduction of arterial and venous blood flow to lower extremity

Planning and Implementation

Prepare the child for cardiac catheterization with age-appropriate information. Because the child will be sedated but arousable for the procedure, explain the sensations that will be experienced (e.g., restraints on arms, equipment noises, cold liquid cleanser for catheter site, and warm feeling of contrast injection).

Nursing care during a cardiac catheterization focuses on monitoring the child's vital signs, reassuring the child, and providing emergency care if necessary. After the catheters and guidewires are removed at the end of the procedure, direct pressure must be applied for 15 minutes. A pressure dressing is then placed over the site for several hours.

SAFETY ALERT!

Assess the pressure dressing over the catheterization site every 5 minutes for 15 minutes, every 15 minutes for 1 hour, and hourly, or as directed by the healthcare provider. Do not remove or loosen the dressing to observe the site until the ordered time for the pressure dressing has elapsed. Check under the buttocks to make sure blood does not ooze out and run under the child. Seek immediate medical intervention if the leg has reduced warmth and decreased perfusion, or bleeding is noted.

The child is kept on bed rest for 4 to 6 hours with an effort to keep the leg straight for several hours. Avoid elevating the head of the bed as flexion of the hips is not permitted during this period. Activity is limited for 24 hours, and in some cases, the child is hospitalized. Provide quiet diversional activities.

Encourage the child to drink small amounts of clear liquids initially, and then progress to other fluids and food as the child tolerates them. Provide adequate fluids to maintain hydration status, especially if the child takes diuretics. The child's intake and output should be balanced.

DISCHARGE PLANNING AND HOME CARE TEACHING

Children are routinely discharged several hours after the cardiac catheterization. Teach the parents to watch the child for signs of complications and make sure they know when to notify the healthcare provider. See *Teaching Highlights: Home Care After Cardiac Catheterization*.

Evaluation

Expected outcomes of nursing care include the following:

- Any potential complications (thrombosis or hemorrhage) following cardiac catheterization are rapidly identified and cared for.
- The child maintains fluid balance.

ASSESSMENT GUIDE | The Child With a Cardiac Condition*

Assessment Focus	Assessment Guidelines
Respirations	• What is the respiratory rate and depth?
	• Are signs of increased respiratory effort present (e.g., tachypnea, dyspnea, retractions, nasal flaring, expiratory grunting)?
	• Is a cough present?
	• Auscultate breath sounds. Are any adventitious sounds present (e.g., wheezes, crackles)?
Pulse characteristics	• Assess the pulse rate, rhythm, and quality.
	• Compare pulse sites for strength and rate (apical to brachial, radial, femoral, pedal).
Blood pressure	• Compare the blood pressure to expected value for age, gender, and height percentile. (See Appendix D.)
	• Compare blood pressure values between upper and lower extremities.
Color	• Observe overall color. Note pallor, dusky color, or cyanosis.
	• Compare the color in peripheral and central locations (e.g., nail beds to mucous membranes). Does crying improve or worsen the color?
	• Assess pulse oximetry.
Chest	• Inspect the anterior chest for bulging or **heaving** (lifting of the chest wall during contraction).
	• Palpate the chest wall over the heart for pulsations, heaves, or vibrations.
	• Locate the point of maximum intensity.
Heart auscultation	• Auscultate the heart for the heart sounds and their quality (loud versus weak, distinct versus muffled).
	• Are any extra heart sounds or murmurs present? Describe murmurs by their intensity, location, radiation, timing, and quality.
	• Auscultate the heart with the child sitting and reclining to detect differences in heart sounds.
Fluid status	• Observe for signs of periorbital, facial, or peripheral edema, or for dehydration.
	• Observe for abdominal distention.
	• Palpate the liver to detect hepatomegaly.
	• Assess capillary refill.
Activity and behavior	• Is exercise tolerance present? Does the child tire with feeding?
	• Note presence of diaphoresis and when it occurs.
	• Identify changes in activity level or behavior (lethargy, restlessness, irritability, and decreased responsiveness).
General	• Assess pattern of growth.

*See Chapter 33 for assessment.

TEACHING HIGHLIGHTS | Home Care After Cardiac Catheterization

- Check for signs of complications several times in the first 24 hours after catheterization and notify the healthcare provider immediately if any of these signs are noted:
  - Bleeding or a bruise increasing in size at the catheterization site
  - Foot on side of catheterization site is cooler than other foot
  - Loss of feeling in foot on side of catheterization
  - Fever
- If the child is treated with diuretics, observe for signs of dehydration (dry mucous membranes, absence of tears, and strong urine).
- Encourage fluids to help flush the dye out of the body and to prevent dehydration.
- Permit quiet play such as computer games, puzzles, and videos for the first 24 hours after the procedure.

Congenital Heart Defects That Increase Pulmonary Blood Flow

The most common congenital heart defects result from a connection between the left and right side of the heart (septal defect) or between the great arteries (patent ductus arteriosus) that allows blood to flow between the left and right side of the heart.

Etiology and Pathophysiology

The pressures on the left side of the heart are higher. When a connection occurs between the left and right side of the heart, blood shunts from the left to the right side of the heart and increases the amount of blood pumped to the lungs. The size of the connection and how much blood passes through it determine how quickly the child develops signs of congestive heart failure (CHF) (see section on CHF later in this chapter). The increased blood flow to the lungs causes increased pulmonary vascular resistance (constriction of the pulmonary vascular bed) in an effort to reduce the blood flow, and pulmonary artery hypertension (see section later in this chapter). Right ventricular hypertrophy (RVH) develops to overcome the increasing pulmonary vascular resistance and to deliver the blood to the lungs.

Clinical Manifestations

The infant's heart rate, respiratory rate, and metabolic rate are increased because of the high pulmonary blood flow. Sucking to feed takes energy and diaphoresis often occurs. If the infant is unable to take in enough calories to support the metabolic rate and growth, poor weight gain is noted. If CHF develops, signs include dyspnea, tachypnea, intercostal retractions, and periorbital edema. Frequent respiratory infections occur as the wet environment in the lungs caused by CHF supports bacterial growth. See Table 47–5 for the pathophysiology, clinical manifestations, diagnostic tests, clinical therapy, and prognosis for the specific congenital heart defects that increase pulmonary blood flow.

TABLE 47–5 Pathophysiology, Clinical Manifestations, Diagnostic Tests, Clinical Therapy, and Prognosis for Defects That Increase Pulmonary Blood Flow

ANATOMY

PATENT DUCTUS ARTERIOSUS (PDA)

Pathophysiology

A common congenital defect caused by persistent fetal circulation that accounts for 5% to 10% of all infants with congenital heart disease (Park, 2014). When pulmonary circulation is established and systemic vascular resistance increases at birth, pressures in the aorta become greater than in the pulmonary arteries. Blood is then shunted from the aorta to the pulmonary arteries, increasing circulation to the pulmonary system. It is a common problem of preterm infants who have respiratory distress syndrome or hypoxemia that work to keep the ductus arteriosus open (Park, 2014).

Clinical Manifestations

Dyspnea; tachypnea; tachycardia; full, bounding pulses; widened pulse pressure; hypotension may be noted when cardiac output is low. May be asymptomatic.

CHF, intercostal retractions, hepatomegaly, and poor growth when a large PDA exists.

A continuous "machinery" murmur during systole and diastole, and a thrill in the pulmonic area.

High risk for frequent respiratory infections and pneumonia.

Diagnostic Tests

The chest radiograph and ECG show left ventricular hypertrophy.

The PDA can be visualized, and PDA blood flow can be measured on echocardiogram.

Clinical Therapy

Transcatheter closure by obstructive device is the standard therapy in most centers. Video-assisted thoracoscopic surgery with clip ligation of the PDA may be performed.

Intravenous ibuprofen or indomethacin often stimulates closure of the ductus arteriosus in preterm infants, but cannot be used if CHF is present; it is not used in term infants.

Prognosis

No long-term sequelae occur if treated before pulmonary vascular disease (pulmonary hypertension or pulmonary vascular obstructive disease) develops.

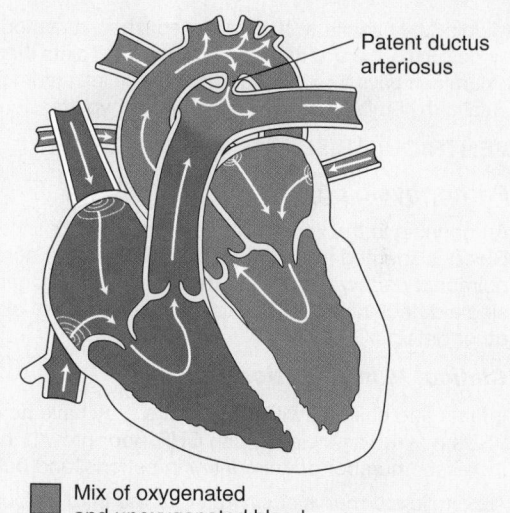

Patent ductus arteriosus

Mix of oxygenated and unoxygenated blood

ATRIAL SEPTAL DEFECT (ASD)

Pathophysiology

The opening in the atrial septum permits left-to-right shunting of blood. The opening may be small, as when the foramen ovale fails to close, or large (the septum may be completely absent). Of children with congenital heart disease, 30% to 50% have an ASD in combination with other defects, but it may occur as an isolated defect in 5% to 10% of children (Park, 2014).

Clinical Manifestations

Infants and young children with small or moderate-size ASDs usually have no symptoms. Large ASDs may cause CHF, easy tiring, and poor growth.

A soft systolic ejection murmur occurs in the pulmonic area with fixed, wide splitting of S_2 through all phases of respiration.

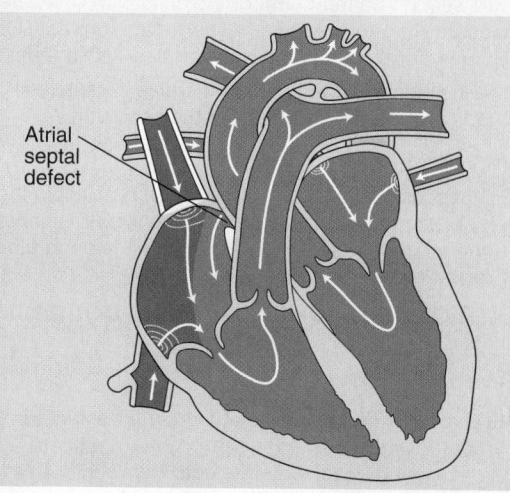

Atrial septal defect

(continued)

TABLE 47–5 Pathophysiology, Clinical Manifestations, Diagnostic Tests, Clinical Therapy, and Prognosis for Defects That Increase Pulmonary Blood Flow (*continued*)

ANATOMY

Diagnostic Tests

Echocardiogram identifies a dilated right ventricle due to blood overload and the shunt size.

The chest radiograph and ECG reveal little information unless the ASD is large, has excessive shunting, and right ventricular hypertrophy is present.

Clinical Therapy

Spontaneous closure of some small ASDs occurs within the first 4 years of life. No activity limitations are needed.

Secundum ASDs are usually closed by a septal occluder during cardiac catheterization. Aspirin at 81 mg per day is prescribed for 6 months after the procedure.

Surgery to close or patch the ASD is performed when significant increased pulmonary blood flow causes CHF. Arrhythmias may develop in postoperative period.

Prognosis

Middle-aged adults with uncorrected small- and moderate-size ASDs may have no symptoms but are at risk for a stroke. Small clots that commonly develop in the right atrium can pass through the ASD into the left atrium and systemic circulation. CHF, atrial arrhythmias, and pulmonary artery hypertension may develop in untreated adults.

VENTRICULAR SEPTAL DEFECT (VSD)

Pathophysiology

An opening in the ventricular septum results in increased pulmonary blood flow. Blood is shunted from the left ventricle directly across the open septum into the pulmonary artery. This is the most common congenital heart defect. It occurs as a single defect in about 15% to 20% of cases but also is found in combination with other defects (Park, 2014).

Clinical Manifestations

Infants and children with small VSDs may have no symptoms. Moderate or large VSDs may be associated with CHF, poor growth, decreased exercise tolerance, an increased number of pulmonary infections, and pulmonary hypertension.

A systolic murmur is auscultated at the third or fourth left intercostal space at the sternal border. A thrill may be present.

Diagnostic Tests

A chest radiograph and ECG reveal little when VSDs are small. An enlarged heart and pulmonary vascular markings on chest radiograph occur in cases of large VSDs with shunting. Right and left ventricular hypertrophy may be seen on ECG.

Echocardiogram identifies the size and location of the defect.

Clinical Therapy

Most small VSDs close spontaneously within the first 6 months of life. Treatment is conservative when no signs of CHF or pulmonary artery hypertension are present.

See section on treatment of the child with CHF later in this chapter. VSD surgical closure is performed after 1 year of age unless CHF cannot be managed medically. Surgery for these infants is performed within the first 6 months of life.

Device closure of VSD during cardiac catheterization may be attempted for some VSDs that are not too close to the heart valves.

Prognosis

Highest risk associated with surgical repair is in the first 2 months of life. Children respond well to surgery and experience substantial catch-up growth. Arrhythmias, right bundle branch block, and complete heart block are possible complications. Some children need a pacemaker.

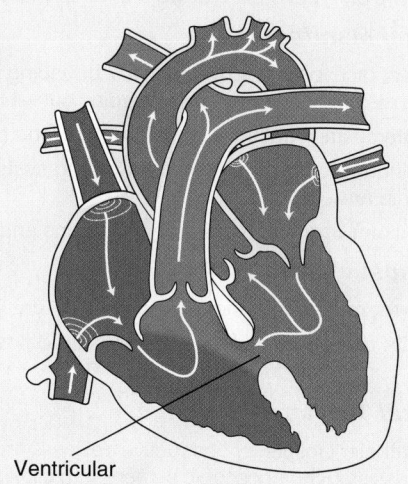

Ventricular septal defect

ATRIOVENTRICULAR CANAL (ENDOCARDIAL CUSHION) DEFECT (AV CANAL)

Pathophysiology

Endocardial cushions are fetal growth centers for the mitral and tricuspid valves and atrioventricular (AV) septum. The most complex AV canal defect results in one AV valve and large septal defects between both atria and ventricles. An AV canal defect occurs in about 2% of congenital heart defect cases, and 70% of these children have Down syndrome (Park, 2014).

Clinical Manifestations

Infants often develop CHF, tachypnea, tachycardia, avoidant/restrictive food intake disorder (failure to thrive), recurrent respiratory infections, and repeated respiratory failure.

S_1 is accentuated and S_2 is split. A holosystolic murmur is loudest at the left lower sternal border, and a thrill may be palpated. The murmur may be transmitted to the left axilla when mitral regurgitation is present (see Chapter 33 for a description of heart sounds).

Diagnostic Tests

On chest radiograph, cardiomegaly and pulmonary vascular markings are present. On ECG, a prolonged PR interval and enlarged ventricles are noted.

Echocardiogram reveals dilation of the ventricles, septal defects, and details of valve malformation.

Clinical Therapy

CHF is treated as described later in this chapter.

Surgery is performed between 2 and 4 months of age to prevent pulmonary vascular disease. Patches are placed over septal defects, and valve tissue is used to form functioning valves. The mitral valve may be replaced.

Infective endocarditis prophylaxis is required until 6 months after corrective surgery.

Prognosis

Arrhythmias and mitral valve regurgitation, a residual septal defect, and subaortic stenosis may occur postoperatively. Short-term survival rates among infants with and without Down syndrome are similar.

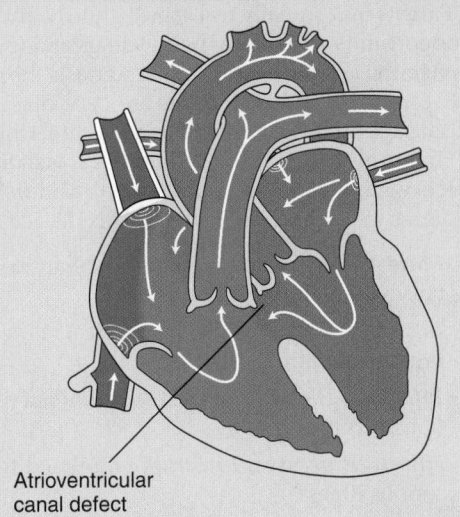

Atrioventricular canal defect

Clinical Therapy

See Table 47–3 for tests used to diagnose the condition. In addition to a chest radiograph, complete blood count, and urinalysis, coagulation studies, platelet counts, and serum electrolytes are often obtained for children having open heart surgery.

Surgery is often performed early in infancy to prevent irreversible pulmonary vascular disease. Unless complications develop before surgery, infants and children usually make a complete recovery without limitations. The major complication of these defects is pulmonary artery hypertension, which is described later in this chapter.

Conservative treatment, such as waiting until the child is symptomatic or older, may be selected for some children with these defects. See Figure 47–1. For example, a small ventricular septal defect may close spontaneously, or closure of an atrial septal defect may be postponed until preschool or early school-age years. Ibuprofen or indomethacin may be given to preterm infants with a patent ductus arteriosus when immediate closure of the ductus is needed. Interventional cardiac catheterization with a septal closing device is performed in an increasing number of cases.

Postpericardiotomy syndrome occurs as a complication in 25% to 30% of children when surgery involves an incision through the pericardium, leading to pericardial and pleural inflammation (Park, 2014, p. 364). It may result from an autoimmune response to damaged myocardium or pericardium or blood in the pericardial sac. The syndrome generally develops within a few weeks to a few months after surgery, more often in children over 2 years of age. It is characterized by a high fever up to 40°C (104°F) and sometimes severe chest pain that worsens with deep inspiration. The median duration of the condition is 2 to 3 weeks. Mild cases are treated with bed rest and NSAIDs or indomethacin. Severe cases may need corticosteroids, diuretics, or emergency pericardiocentesis.

Nursing Management

For the Child Prior to Surgery

Nursing Assessment and Diagnosis

PHYSIOLOGIC ASSESSMENT

Prior to surgery, the infant or child is seen regularly to assess growth and for signs of worsening CHF. See *Assessment Guide: The Child With a Cardiac Condition* for assessment guidelines. Failure to gain weight is an indication of an increased metabolic rate and inability to consume adequate calories for both metabolic function and growth. Assessment of length and head circumference helps to determine the full impact of the condition on growth.

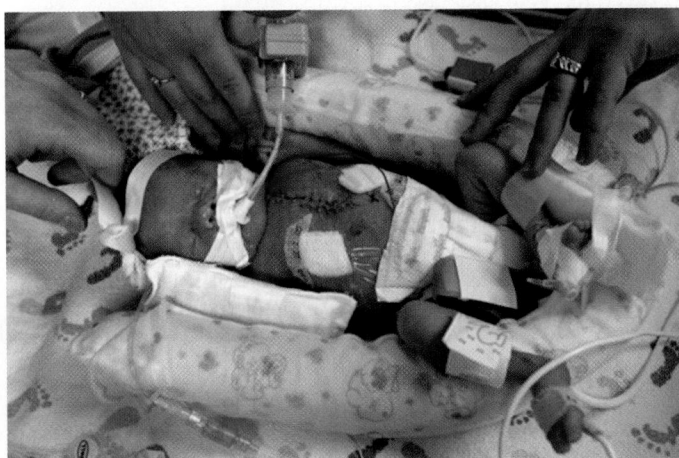

Figure 47–1 **An infant with a ventricular septal defect repair. Surgery is performed with this type of defect to prevent pulmonary vascular disease and pulmonary artery hypertension.**

SOURCE: Barbara Davidson/Dallas Morning News/KRT/Newscom.

PSYCHOSOCIAL ASSESSMENT

Assess the ability of the parents to cope with the infant's diagnosis. Parents may initially feel shock, guilt, or anxiety. Parents need an opportunity to express their feelings and to begin learning to manage the child's illness. The diagnosis, hospitalization, and early care of the infant at home are very stressful. Parents need special support if their infant has a life-threatening heart defect.

Examples of nursing diagnoses associated with heart defects having increased pulmonary blood flow and their complications include the following (NANDA-I © 2014):

- *Fluid Volume: Excess* related to heart failure and pulmonary vasculature overload
- *Infant Feeding Pattern, Ineffective*, related to shortness of breath and fatigue
- *Infection, Risk for*, related to pulmonary vascular congestion and chronic illness
- *Family Processes, Interrupted*, related to crisis of child's serious illness

Planning and Implementation

When the child has a large defect, CHF may be present. See section on CHF later in this chapter for care guidelines.

FAMILY EDUCATION

Participate with members of the cardiology team to provide information and educate the family about the child's condition. Information may include the following:

- General information about the congenital heart disease, including a description of the heart's anatomy and physiology and the defect
- Information about genetic and environmental influences associated with congenital heart disease
- Signs of CHF and treatment if it develops
- Overview of the child's prognosis and timing of medical and surgical interventions, including some sample cases with good and poor outcomes

PSYCHOSOCIAL SUPPORT

Parents are often anxious about an uncertain surgical outcome. Determine if parents have a support system as they learn about the infant's diagnosis and make difficult decisions about the child's surgery. Some parents may be concerned that signing consent for surgery places the child in even more danger of illness or even death. Identify some resources for support, such as social services, pastoral services, or a parent of a child with a similar heart defect.

Parents should be offered genetic counseling if planning a future pregnancy.

Clinical Tip

Some valuable resources for parents of a child with a congenital heart defect are as follows:

- *It's My Heart* by the Children's Heart Foundation
- *Hope for Families of Children with Congenital Heart Defects* by Lynda T. Young
- *The Heart of a Child: What Families Need to Know About Heart Disorders in Children* by C. A. Neill, E. A. Clark, and C. Clark, Johns Hopkins Press
- *Heart Warriors: A Family Faces Congenital Heart Disease* by Amanda Rose Adams, Behler Publications

---

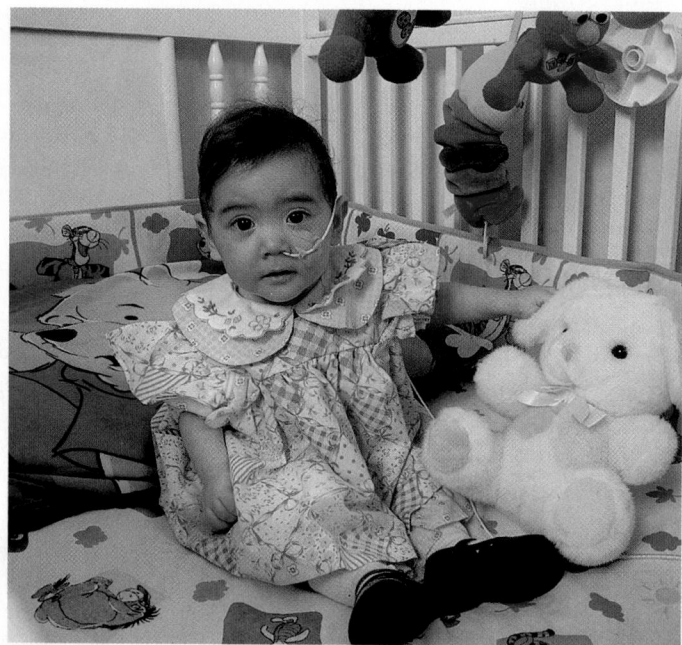

Figure 47–2 **Infants with cardiac conditions often require supplemental feedings to provide sufficient nutrients for growth and development. The parents of this infant girl have been taught how to give her nasogastric feedings at home.**

HOME CARE

Children are managed at home until surgery. Parents should encourage feeding to promote growth, but allow the infant to feed only for 30 minutes or as directed by healthcare providers for infants with complex heart defects or CHF. Breastfeeding or breast milk is encouraged because of its beneficial effects for the infant. Infants should be held at a 45-degree angle to reduce tachypnea. If the infant has difficulty gaining weight, formula or breast milk can be pumped and fortified with products that increase calorie density. Transpyloric, nasogastric, or gastrostomy tube feedings may also be given at night or 24 hours a day to ensure that adequate calories are ingested. See Figure 47–2. Salt intake is rarely limited in infants. When tube feedings are used, encourage the infant to take some formula orally to provide positive oral stimulation. See feeding suggestions for the infant with CHF later in this chapter.

Reduce the infant's exposure to infectious diseases, and encourage frequent hand hygiene. Respiratory infections increase hypoxemia in children with cyanosis. Fever increases the metabolic rates and oxygen demands. Vomiting and diarrhea may cause an electrolyte disturbance. Notify the healthcare provider about fever, poor feeding, vomiting, and diarrhea.

Health promotion visits are important and all immunizations are provided according to the recommended schedule. Provide monthly prophylaxis for respiratory syncytial virus (RSV) with palivizumab to infants who have complex heart defects during the peak season. See Chapter 46.

PREPARATION FOR SURGERY

When the child is preschool age or older, prepare the child for the settings, equipment, and experiences to expect before and after surgery. Follow guidelines for preoperative treatment described in Chapter 39. If an infant or toddler is having surgery, inform the parents about how the child will look, equipment that will be used, and what care will be provided in the immediate postoperative period.

Evaluation

- Nutritional intake is adequate with oral and supplemental tube feeding as necessary.
- The child maintains a growth pattern that follows the established growth curve percentile.
- The child receives all immunizations and RSV prophylaxis to reduce the potential for acute illnesses.

Nursing Management

For the Child Having Surgery for Increased Pulmonary Blood Flow

The goal of nursing management is to perform assessments, provide supportive care to the family, and meet the child's nursing care needs before and after surgery.

Nursing Assessment and Diagnosis

At the time of surgery, the child needs a careful history and physical examination to detect any acute illnesses as well as the child's physiologic status. Assess the child's behavioral patterns, cardiac function, respiratory function, weight, and fluid status. See the *Assessment Guide* earlier in this chapter.

In the immediate postoperative period, the child will be cared for in the intensive care unit. When the child returns to the general nursing unit, assessment focuses on signs of surgical complications such as infection, arrhythmias, and impaired tissue perfusion. Monitor the child's temperature and inspect the surgical incision site. Fever, excessive incisional pain, spreading erythema around the incision, and wound drainage beginning 3 to 4 days postoperatively may be early signs of infection. Assess the chest and lungs for breath sounds, respiratory effort, and signs of distress that may indicate pneumonia or fluid in the pleural space.

Monitor the vital signs, including blood pressure and SpO_2. Auscultate the apical pulse to detect an irregular heart rate or bradycardia because either finding is a sign of reduced cardiac output that requires immediate intervention. Check capillary refill, extremity warmth, pedal pulses, level of consciousness, and urine output to assess tissue perfusion. Reduced urine output is a sign of decreased cardiac output. Continue to assess the child's pain.

Examples of nursing diagnoses following cardiac surgery include the following (NANDA-I © 2014):

- *Breathing Pattern, Ineffective*, related to respiratory muscle fatigue
- *Pain, Acute*, related to surgical incision and expansion of chest with coughing and deep breathing exercises
- *Fluid Volume: Imbalanced, Risk for*, related to impact of surgery on heart's pumping action
- *Infection, Risk for*, related to surgery and chronic disease status

Planning and Implementation

PAIN MANAGEMENT

Pain management with 24-hour intravenous opioids is provided for 1 to 2 days postoperatively or until the child is taking fluids. Then give oral analgesics around the clock. Follow the guidelines for pain management provided in Chapter 40. Teach parents and caregivers to move the child without lifting under the arms to reduce stress on the incision and pain.

PROMOTE RESPIRATORY FUNCTION

Encourage the child to take deep breaths and cough or to perform spirometry exercises regularly to promote full lung expansion (see the *Clinical Skills Manual* SKILLS). Bubbles or pinwheels may help young children to take deep breaths. Splint the chest with a pillow or stuffed animal to reduce pain from coughing and deep breathing. Chest physiotherapy may be performed in children under 3 years of age.

NUTRITION AND GENERAL CARE

Encourage the infant or child to begin oral fluids and nutrition when permitted. Oral fluids are rarely limited following surgery for defects with increased pulmonary blood flow, but assess intake and output carefully. Allow parents to bring in the child's favorite foods to encourage eating when they can be tolerated. Promote bowel elimination following surgery and when opioids are used.

Administer antibiotics as prescribed. If intravenous antibiotics are continued after the child's oral intake is established, the IV line can be converted to a heparin or saline lock.

Encourage the child to increase activity gradually with longer periods out of bed every day, but ensure adequate rest periods to promote healing. Provide diversional activities and opportunities for therapeutic play so the child can better manage the stresses associated with pain and frightening procedures.

DISCHARGE PLANNING AND HOME CARE TEACHING

Infants and children may be discharged from the hospital within a few days of surgery. Parents need information spread over several days to prepare for care of the child at home. See *Teaching Highlights: Care of the Child After Cardiac Surgery.*

Prepare parents for potential behavior problems of young children that may result from the stress of hospitalization, such as nightmares, separation anxiety, and overdependence on parents. Encourage parents to reassure children about their security, and to promote play and other means to deal with their feelings. If the child's behavioral symptoms continue for several weeks, referral for psychologic assessment and support may be needed for posttraumatic stress disorder. See Chapter 55.

Reassure parents of children with a complete correction of the cardiac defect that no further cardiovascular problems should occur. Provide parents with full information about the child's defect and the surgery performed to share with the child's healthcare providers. Encourage parents to allow the child to live a normal and active life.

Evaluation

Examples of expected outcomes of nursing care include the following:

- Full lung expansion is achieved with spirometry exercises or chest physiotherapy.
- The child's pain is effectively managed.
- The child's incision heals without infection.
- Catch-up growth occurs over the next few months to years.

Defects Causing Decreased Pulmonary Blood Flow and Mixed Defects

Information about these defect categories is combined in this section because the clinical therapy and nursing interventions are similar.

Etiology and Pathophysiology

DEFECTS CAUSING DECREASED PULMONARY BLOOD FLOW

Defects that obstruct the flow of blood from the right side of the heart to the lungs decrease the amount of blood that gets oxygenated by the lungs. If an atrial or ventricular septal opening exists, the obstructed pulmonary blood raises pressures on the heart's right side higher than the left, leading to right-to-left shunting. Hypoxemia and cyanosis result because of the increased amount of unoxygenated blood in the systemic circulation.

The bone marrow is stimulated to produce more red blood cells so more hemoglobin is available to carry oxygen. **Polycythemia**, an above-normal increase in the number of red blood cells, may result and place the child at risk for thromboembolism. Over time, platelet survival is reduced and clotting factors are impaired, increasing the infant's risk of bleeding with surgery. Bacteria in the unoxygenated blood (which is usually filtered out by the lung's capillaries) may cross into the systemic circulation through the septal defect, leading to a brain abscess (Park, 2014, p. 141).

When infants and children with cyanosis rise in the morning, they may experience an abrupt decrease in systemic vascular resistance. This increases the blood shunted from right to left across the VSD, and less blood flows to the lungs, leading to increased hypoxemia. Crying, feeding, increased activity, a warm bath, and straining with defecation are all events that can suddenly lower the systemic vascular resistance and trigger a hypoxic episode or spell. Hypovolemia may also trigger a hypoxic episode. The partial pressure of oxygen (PO_2) is lowered, and the partial pressure of carbon dioxide (PCO_2) rises. Hypoxemia becomes progressively worse as the respiratory center in the brain overreacts, increasing the respiratory effort. The extra respiratory effort further worsens the hypoxic episode that can become life-threatening unless rapid intervention is successful.

MIXED DEFECTS

Many complex congenital heart defects involve a combination of defects that increase and decrease pulmonary blood flow, making the newborn dependent on mixing of the pulmonary and systemic circulations for survival during the postnatal period. The mixed oxygen-saturated and oxygen-desaturated blood results in a general desaturated systemic blood flow and cyanosis. Pulmonary congestion occurs because of increased pulmonary blood flow and obstruction of systemic flow.

Clinical Manifestations

DEFECTS CAUSING DECREASED PULMONARY BLOOD FLOW

Clinical manifestations in infants initially include cyanosis shortly after birth, dyspnea, and a loud murmur. The skin may initially be ruddy or mottled before cyanosis is observed. Cyanosis that does not respond as expected to supplemental oxygen is a classic sign of decreased pulmonary blood flow. Signs and symptoms of chronic hypoxemia include fatigue, clubbing of the fingers and toes, exertional dyspnea, and delayed developmental milestones (Figure 47–3). Infants may need to stop sucking periodically during feedings to breathe, and diaphoresis may be seen with the increased work of feeding. These infants have a higher metabolic rate, and inadequate calories may be

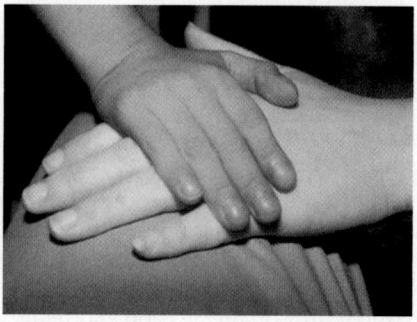

Figure 47–3 Clubbing of the fingers in an older child is one manifestation of a heart defect that reduces pulmonary blood flow.

consumed, resulting in poor weight gain. See Table 47–6 for the pathophysiology, clinical manifestations, diagnostics tests, clinical therapy, and prognosis for these defects.

Toddlers with uncorrected cyanotic heart disease often squat in the knee–chest position to relieve dyspnea (Figure 47–4). This position reduces the cardiac output by decreasing the blood return from the lower extremities and by increasing the systemic vascular resistance. Blood flow to the lungs is increased. Hypoxic episodes can occur suddenly between 2 months and 2 years of age. Signs include increased cyanosis, increased rate and depth of respirations, tachycardia, poor tissue perfusion, diaphoresis, and seizures and loss of consciousness.

TABLE 47–6 Pathophysiology, Clinical Manifestations, Diagnostic Tests, Clinical Therapy, and Prognosis for Defects That Decrease Pulmonary Blood Flow

ANATOMY

PULMONIC STENOSIS (PS)

Pathophysiology

Stenosis (narrowing of a valve or valve area) can be above, below, or at a valve. Stenosis obstructs blood flow into the pulmonary artery, increases preload, and results in right ventricular hypertrophy. PS as a single defect accounts for 8% to 12% of all congenital heart defects, but it also occurs with other defects (Park, 2014). Stenosis in the subvalvular area may develop as the heart muscle grows.

Clinical Manifestations

Children with mild stenosis may have no symptoms and grow normally.

In moderate to severe stenosis, dyspnea and fatigue occur on exertion. Signs of CHF, heart failure, and chest pain on exertion occur in severe cases.

A loud systolic ejection murmur with a widely split S_2 and thrill may be found in the pulmonic listening area. A murmur heard louder and longer indicates increased severity.

Diagnostic Tests

The chest radiograph may show an enlarged pulmonary artery with normal heart size and normal pulmonary vascularity.

The ECG may show right atrial enlargement and right ventricular hypertrophy.

An echocardiogram provides information about the thickness of the valve, the pressure gradient across the valve, and size of the valve ring.

Cardiac catheterization findings include increased right ventricular pressure and a normal or slightly lowered pulmonary artery pressure.

Clinical Therapy

Balloon dilation of the valve, performed during cardiac catheterization, is the preferred treatment. Pulmonary regurgitation may result but is not a significant problem.

Surgical valvotomy is performed when balloon dilation is not indicated or unsuccessful. On occasion the pulmonary valve is replaced.

Prognosis

Newborns with critical PS have a mortality rate of 10%. PS does not typically increase in severity. Lifelong infective endocarditis prophylaxis may be needed.

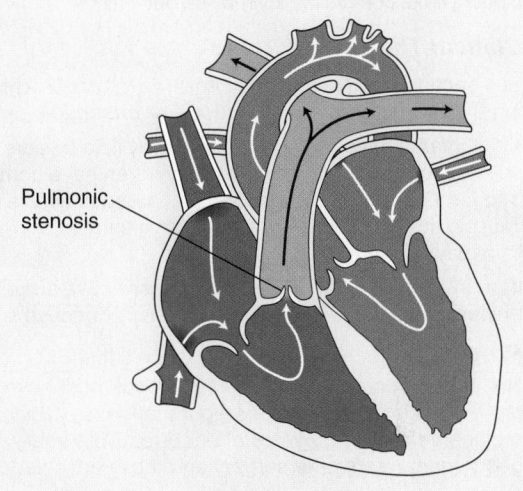

Pulmonic stenosis

☐ Decreased unoxygenated blood flow

TETRALOGY OF FALLOT (TOF)

Pathophysiology

Four defects are involved: stenosis of the pulmonary outflow tract or valve, right ventricular hypertrophy, ventricular septal defect (VSD), and overriding of aorta. The overriding aorta and VSD allow unoxygenated blood to pass into the systemic circulation. TOF accounts for about 5% to 10% of all cases of congenital heart disease (Park, 2014).

Clinical Manifestations

The newborn becomes hypoxic and cyanotic as the ductus arteriosus closes. The degree of pulmonary stenosis determines severity of symptoms. Older infants and children have tachypnea and cyanosis.

Polycythemia, hypercyanotic spells, metabolic acidosis, poor growth, clubbing, and exercise intolerance may develop.

Toddlers with uncorrected defects instinctively squat (assume a knee–chest position) to decrease the return of systemic venous blood to the heart. See Figure 47–4.

A systolic murmur is heard in the pulmonic area and transmitted to the suprasternal notch. A thrill may be palpated in the pulmonic area.

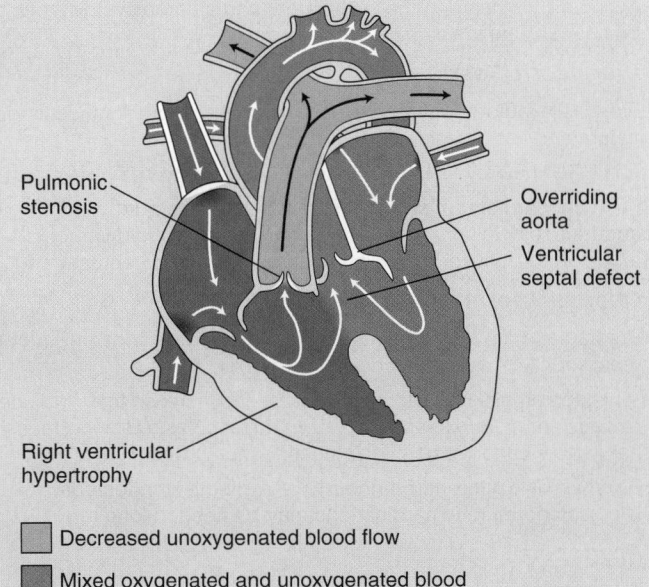

Pulmonic stenosis

Overriding aorta

Ventricular septal defect

Right ventricular hypertrophy

☐ Decreased unoxygenated blood flow

☐ Mixed oxygenated and unoxygenated blood

(continued)

TABLE 47–6 Pathophysiology, Clinical Manifestations, Diagnostic Tests, Clinical Therapy, and Prognosis for Defects That Decrease Pulmonary Blood Flow (*continued*)

ANATOMY

Diagnostic Tests

A chest radiograph shows the boot-shaped heart due to the large right ventricle, decreased pulmonary vascular markings, and a prominent aorta. The ECG shows right ventricular hypertrophy.

The echocardiogram shows the VSD, obstruction of pulmonary outflow, an overriding aorta, and the size of the pulmonary arteries. The condition may be detected by fetal echocardiography.

Blood tests reveal an elevated hematocrit and hemoglobin and an increased clotting time. Iron deficiency may be detected.

Clinical Therapy

See section on hypercyanotic episode management later in this chapter. Monitoring the child for metabolic acidosis or prolonged unconsciousness is critical.

Most infants have corrective surgery by 1 to 2 years of age unless a hypercyanotic spell occurs earlier. Symptomatic children have corrective surgery any time after 3 to 4 months of age. Some children need palliative surgery (modified Blalock-Taussig shunt) to delay total corrective surgery. A right bundle branch rhythm pattern may result from surgery.

If prosthetic material is used for the corrective surgery, infective endocarditis prophylaxis is required until 6 months after corrective surgery.

Prognosis

Not all children are cured by surgery, but most have improved quality of life and improved longevity. Pulmonary regurgitation may become severe and require a valve replacement 10 to 20 years after corrective surgery. Ventricular arrhythmias may occur many years after surgery and may cause sudden death (Park, 2014, p. 231).

PULMONARY OR TRICUSPID ATRESIA

In pulmonary atresia (a severe form of PS), no valve or opening exists to allow blood to flow between the right atrium and right ventricle. In tricuspid atresia, no valve or opening exists to allow blood to flow between the right atrium and ventricle. The right ventricle is **hypoplastic** (small and nonfunctional). Blood flows to the left side of the heart through the foramen ovale. The ductus arteriosus provides the only flow of blood to the pulmonary arteries and lungs. Tricuspid atresia accounts for 1% to 3% of congenital heart defects, while pulmonary atresia accounts for less than 1% (Park, 2014).

Clinical Manifestations

Cyanosis is present and severe at birth.

Tachypnea, poor feeding, CHF, pulmonary edema, hepatomegaly, acidosis, hypoxic spells, clubbing, polycythemia, and growth delays occur.

A continuous murmur from the PDA is heard in the pulmonic area. A single S_2 is heard in the aortic area, and a harsh systolic murmur may be heard at the lower left sternal border.

Diagnostic Tests

The chest radiograph may reveal a normal size or slightly enlarged right atrium and left ventricle.

The ECG may reveal left ventricular hypertrophy.

The echocardiogram shows a small hypoplastic right ventricular cavity and tricuspid valve, an absent right ventricular outflow tract, a dilated right atrium, and right-to-left shunting across the atrial septum.

Clinical Therapy

Prostaglandin E_1 is given immediately to maintain a patent ductus arteriosus. Treatment for CHF may be needed.

A balloon atrial septostomy is performed to increase the atrial opening size. Other palliative procedures may be performed, such as a Blalock-Taussig shunt or pulmonary artery banding, before a staged Fontan procedure for the single ventricle defect.

Prophylaxis for thromboembolism and infective endocarditis is recommended. Digoxin and diuretic medications may be needed long term.

Prognosis

The child has an increased risk for arrhythmia and right ventricular dysfunction. Survival after a successful Fontan procedure is greater than 95% (Park, 2014).

Labels: Patent ductus arteriosus; Pulmonary atresia; Atrial septal defect; Underdeveloped right ventricle

■ Decreased unoxygenated blood flow
■ Mixed oxygenated and unoxygenated blood

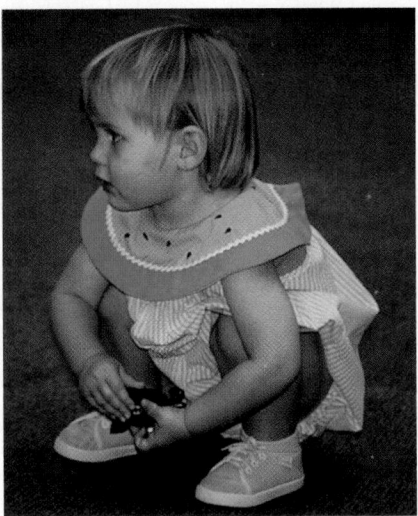

Figure 47–4 Children compensate for inadequate blood flow. A young child with an uncorrected or partially corrected defect that reduces pulmonary blood flow may squat (assume a knee–chest position) to reduce systemic blood flow return to the heart.

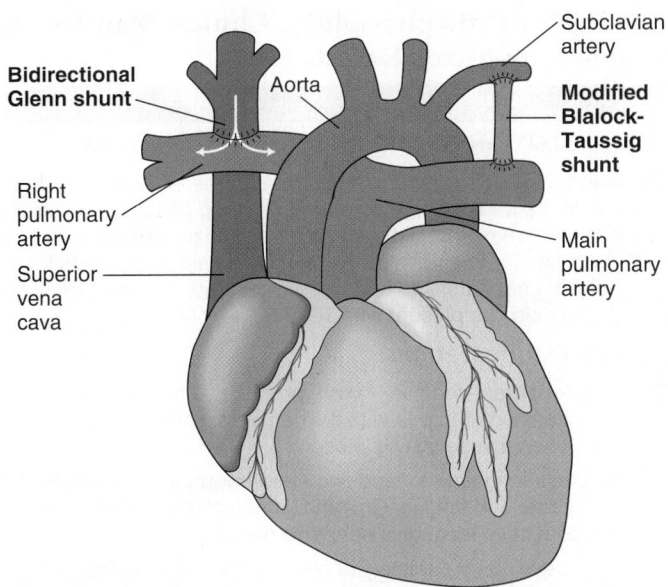

Figure 47–5 Anatomic location of the modified Blalock-Taussig and Glenn shunts for palliative procedures.

SAFETY ALERT!

Infants and young children respond to severe hypoxemia with bradycardia. Cardiac arrest in children often results from prolonged hypoxemia related to respiratory failure or shock rather than from a primary cardiac arrhythmia as in adults (Perkin, deCaen, Berg, et al., 2013). Bradycardia is a significant warning sign that cardiac arrest is imminent. Treating hypoxemia often reverses bradycardia and prevents cardiac arrest.

Older children may have additional symptoms such as exercise-induced dizziness and **syncope** (transient loss of consciousness and muscle tone), which are both serious signs indicating a need for medical evaluation.

MIXED DEFECTS

These complex congenital heart defects cause varying degrees of cyanosis and CHF. See Table 47–7 for the pathophysiology, clinical manifestations, diagnostic tests, clinical therapy, and prognosis for these complex mixed defects.

Clinical Therapy

Early management of these defects is important to prevent secondary damage to the heart, lungs, and brain, including the adverse effects of hypoxemia on the child's cognitive and psychomotor development. Corrective surgery is usually performed on newborns and young infants. A palliative procedure may be performed first for some potentially lethal conditions. See Figure 47–5 for various palliative shunts (surgically created channels for blood flow) that may be performed. In other cases, corrective surgery is preferred to give the newborn a better outcome. CHF is treated aggressively as described later in this chapter. See Tables 47–6 and Table 47–7 for clinical therapy for specific congenital heart defects.

If closure of the ductus arteriosus causes life-threatening cyanosis in newborns, prostaglandin E_1 (PGE_1) is given to reopen the ductus arteriosus and improve pulmonary or systemic blood flow. Treatment with PGE_1 provides time to transfer the newborn to a cardiac center for diagnostic evaluation and surgical intervention. Adverse effects include respiratory depression and apnea, so the infant must be closely monitored and sometimes ventilation must be assisted.

The child's hemoglobin and hematocrit values are monitored for polycythemia or anemia. If the blood viscosity becomes too high, red cell apheresis may be performed. Anemia is not well tolerated because the infant has less oxygen-carrying hemoglobin.

HYPOXIC EPISODES

Hypoxic (hypercyanotic) episodes are treated aggressively. Place the child in the knee–chest position to reduce blood return to the legs, increasing systemic vascular resistance. Reduce any irritating or painful stimuli, and try to calm the child. Provide supplemental oxygen. If these measures do not relieve the hypercyanotic spell, more aggressive treatment may include IV morphine, sedation (ketamine), sodium bicarbonate to treat acidosis, or a vasoconstrictor medication such as phenylephrine. Metabolic acidosis is treated if present. Postpone all unpleasant procedures. Immediate palliative or corrective surgery is often scheduled. Propanolol may be prescribed to prevent hypoxic episodes.

INFECTIVE ENDOCARDITIS

Prophylactic antibiotics for infective endocarditis are required for most children with complex cardiac defects prior to surgery and for 6 months after surgery. See *Medications Used for: Infective Endocarditis Prophylaxis for Dental and Invasive Respiratory Procedures* later in this chapter. Children whose surgery involved prosthetic valves or patches and those who have unrepaired cyanotic congenital heart disease, including palliative shunts and conduits, need lifelong infective endocarditis prophylaxis (Kharouf & Torchen, 2011).

OUTCOMES AND PROGNOSIS

Most children with congenital heart disease have normal IQ scores, and children with corrected simple defects can lead normal lives; however, neurologic insults can occur for many

TABLE 47–7 Pathophysiology, Clinical Manifestations, Diagnostic Tests, Clinical Therapy, and Prognosis for Mixed Defects

ANATOMY

TRANSPOSITION OF THE GREAT ARTERIES (TGA)

The pulmonary artery is the outflow tract for the left ventricle, and the aorta is the outflow tract for the right ventricle, creating parallel circulations. The condition is life threatening at birth, and survival initially depends on an open ductus arteriosus and foramen ovale. This common defect accounts for 5% to 7% of all congenital heart defects and is more common in males (Park, 2014). An ASD or VSD may also be present with TGA.

Clinical Manifestations

Cyanosis, apparent soon after birth, progresses to hypoxemia and acidosis. Cyanosis does not improve with oxygen administration. Cyanosis may be less apparent when a large VSD is present.

Infants take a long time to feed and need frequent rest periods because of rapid respiratory rate and fatigue. Growth failure may be evident as early as 2 weeks of age if corrective surgery is not performed.

CHF may develop immediately or over days or weeks. Tachypnea (60 breaths/min) is often present without retractions or dyspnea unless CHF is present.

A systolic murmur is present if a VSD is present; no other murmur is generally heard. S_2 is loud and heard as a single sound.

Diagnostic Tests

A chest radiograph may reveal a classic egg-shaped heart on a string with enlarged ventricles and increased pulmonary vascular markings.

The ECG reveals right ventricular hypertrophy.

The echocardiogram often shows the abnormal position of the great arteries rising from the ventricles and any associated defects.

Blood tests reveal an increased hematocrit and hemoglobin or polycythemia and acidosis.

Clinical Therapy

Prostaglandin E_1 is ordered to maintain a patent ductus arteriosus until a palliative procedure (balloon atrial septostomy) is performed during cardiac catheterization to permit oxygenated and unoxygenated blood to mix.

CHF is treated with diuretics and digoxin.

Corrective surgery (arterial switch) is usually performed in the neonatal period.

Prognosis

Survival without surgery is impossible. Complications may occur such as stenosis of the pulmonary artery or aorta in the vessels beyond the valves or coronary artery obstruction. Arrhythmias (sick sinus syndrome, atrial flutter, and atrial fibrillation), tricuspid valve insufficiency, right ventricular dysfunction or failure, and sudden death may be long-term complications associated with formerly used surgical procedures (e.g., Mustard and Senning) (Park, 2014, p. 213).

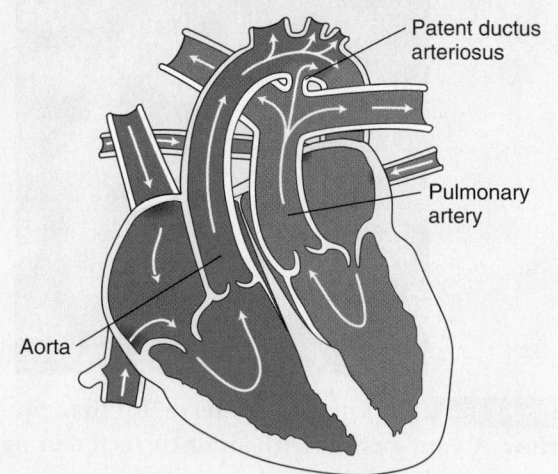

Patent ductus arteriosus

Pulmonary artery

Aorta

TRUNCUS ARTERIOSUS

A single large vessel empties both ventricles and provides circulation for the pulmonary, systemic, and coronary circulations. A VSD is usually present. This occurs in about 1% of congenital heart defects (Park, 2014).

Clinical Manifestations

Cyanosis develops soon after birth; however, this is also a condition of increased pulmonary blood flow. CHF develops within 2 weeks after birth with tachypnea, dyspnea, retractions, poor feeding, poor growth, clubbing, increased pulse pressure, bounding peripheral pulses, a widened pulse pressure, and frequent respiratory infections.

A systolic click may be heard in the apex and pulmonic area. The VSD produces a harsh systolic murmur in the lower sternal border.

Diagnostic Tests

The chest radiograph shows cardiomegaly, increased pulmonary vascular markings, and sometimes a right aortic arch.

The ECG reveals bilateral ventricular hypertrophy.

The echocardiogram shows a VSD, a large single great artery, and one semilunar valve.

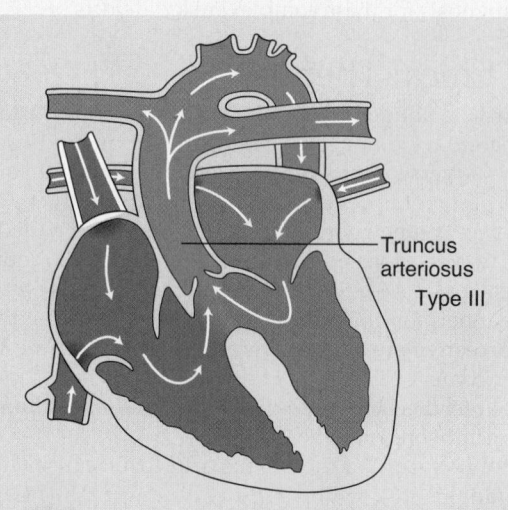

Truncus arteriosus

Type III

■ Mixed oxygenated and unoxygenated blood

Clinical Therapy

CHF is treated with diuretics and digoxin.

A Rastelli procedure is performed within a week of birth to close the VSD, enabling the left ventricle to empty into the single large great artery. A conduit is created to the pulmonary arteries. Repeated surgery is necessary to enlarge the pulmonary artery conduit or to repair the truncal valve.

Prophylaxis for infective endocarditis is needed for life.

Prognosis

Surgical mortality varies from 10% to 30% (Park, 2014). Ventricular arrhythmias may develop. The child should not participate in competitive or strenuous sports.

TOTAL ANOMALOUS PULMONARY VENOUS RETURN

The pulmonary veins empty into the right atrium or veins leading to the right atrium rather than into the left atrium. Mixed blood must pass through the foramen ovale or an ASD to provide the systemic circulation. Any obstruction of the pulmonary veins increases the condition's severity. This accounts for 1% of congenital heart defects (Park, 2014).

Clinical Manifestations

The newborn may have mild cyanosis and tachypnea. Signs of CHF (tachypnea, dyspnea, tachycardia, and enlarged liver) and pulmonary edema develop along with poor growth and frequent respiratory infections.

A precordial bulge may be palpated. The S_2 has a wide, fixed split when there is no pulmonary vein obstruction. A systolic murmur is heard in the pulmonic area.

Diagnostic Tests

The chest radiograph shows enlargement of the right atrium and ventricle and increased pulmonary blood flow.

The ECG reveals right ventricular hypertrophy.

The echocardiogram shows a dilated right atrium and ventricle, smaller left-sided chambers, dilated pulmonary arteries, and a patent foramen ovale. It can determine the type of pulmonary drainage and if the pulmonary venous return is obstructed.

Clinical Therapy

Prostaglandin E_1 is given to maintain the patent ductus arteriosus for some newborns.

Diuretics are given to treat CHF.

Surgery is performed to move or create a conduit to connect the pulmonary veins to the left atrium.

Prognosis

Surgery is required for survival. Postoperative mortality ranges from 5% to 10% (Park, 2014). Children may develop pulmonary hypertension, pulmonary vein obstruction, or atrial arrhythmias.

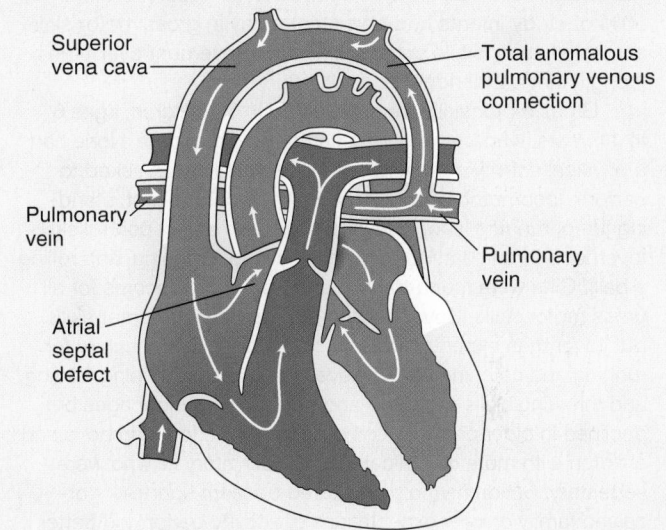

reasons. Conditions such as congestive heart failure and cyanosis can affect gross motor development. Infants with complex congenital heart defects are at risk for preoperative neurologic insult. Inadequate nutrition during the first year of life, when rapid brain development occurs, places the infant at greater risk. Some infants have structural brain abnormalities, abnormal cerebral blood flow, chromosomal abnormalities, cerebral ischemia, and other chromosomal disorders documented prior to surgery. Infants with cyanosis who also have iron deficiency anemia may develop a stroke. See *Evidence-Based Practice: Neurodevelopmental Outcomes in Children With Complex Congenital Heart Disease.*

Children with complex congenital heart defects need multiple stages of surgery, revisions of previous surgeries, valve replacements, or interventional catheterization to reopen valves or vessels that have become obstructed. However, rates of survival to adulthood have been improving for children with complex CHD. A pacemaker may be needed for children with potential life-threatening AV block or ventricular dysfunction (Park, 2014, pp. 442).

| Neurodevelopmental Outcomes in Children With
Complex Congenital Heart Disease

Clinical Question

What information do parents and school officials need to plan for educational supports for children who have had surgery for complex congenital heart defects?

The Evidence

Fifty infants who had cardiac surgery at less than 8 weeks of age were assessed for gross motor performance at 4, 8, 12, and 16 months of age using the Alberta Infant Motor Scale. Infants with chromosomal abnormalities were excluded. Gross motor skill development was delayed at all ages. More than 50% of study infants had persistent delay in gross motor skills across all ages, while some showed improvement over time (Long, Harris, Elderidge, et al., 2012).

Gross motor skills were evaluated in 55 children, ages 6 to 11 years, who previously had a Fontan procedure. None had a physical activity contraindication. Each child was asked to perform locomotor skills (run, gallop, hop on one foot, standing jump, running leap, sideways slide) and object control skills (overhand throw, batting, kicking, dribbling, catching, and rolling a ball). Girls were found to have age-appropriate scores for all gross motor skills. Boys had age-appropriate locomotor skills but lower than expected object control skills. Skill mastery for running and catching were delayed at all ages. Jumping, sliding, and throwing skills were age-appropriate at younger ages but declined in older children. Lower scores were found in boys and children with more complicated medical history or who were sedentary. Children who participated on team sports or perceived family or peer expectations of activity performed better than expected for age (Longmuir, Banks, & McCrindle, 2012).

Forty children who had had corrective or palliative surgery for a significant congenital heart defect (CHD) were evaluated

for behavior and competencies at school age. Children with diagnosed chromosomal abnormalities were excluded from the study. Healthy siblings closest in age to study children served as a comparison group. Parents completed the Child Behavior Checklist, while teachers completed the teacher version of the same test. Results indicated that in comparison with siblings, parents perceived that children with CHD had more behavior problems. Both teachers and parents identified reduced school competencies. Children with CHD missed more days of school, participated less in physical education, needed more remedial help, and had lower attainment than siblings (McCusker, Armstrong, Mullen, et al., 2013).

Best Practice

Children with complex CHDs and subsequent surgery often have motor and cognitive problems, such as difficulties with executive functioning skills, problem solving, and memory. These cognitive deficits may lead to learning disabilities, and poorly developed motor skills may interfere with social interactions with peers. Regular developmental screening is needed to identify the specific neurodevelopmental problems that a child could have prior to school entry. Educating families to encourage the child's participation in physical activities may help improve motor skills. Children with complex CHD may need an individualized education plan when disabilities affect learning.

Clinical Reasoning

Develop an outline of important information for a parent of a child with a complex congenital heart defect to discuss with the child's teacher and school officials when the child enters school, including physical and education issues.

Nursing Management

For the Child With Decreased Pulmonary Blood Flow

Nursing management of the hospitalized child focuses on monitoring PGE₁ therapy for newborns, treating hypercyanotic episodes, supporting families to care for the child at home, and providing postsurgical care.

Nursing Assessment and Diagnosis

PHYSIOLOGIC ASSESSMENT BEFORE SURGERY

Infants receiving PGE₁ therapy are cared for in an intensive care nursery where their cardiovascular status can be closely monitored until palliative procedures or corrective surgery is performed.

Prior to or between stages of surgery, the infant or child is seen regularly to assess growth and monitor for signs of CHF (tachycardia, tachypnea, crackles, frothy secretions, low urine output, and pulmonary edema) or worsening condition. The child's poor growth may affect weight, height, and head circumference, so plot serial measurements on the same growth curve to monitor the significance of the growth problems. Monitor physiologic status using the guidelines given in the *Assessment Guide* at the beginning of this chapter.

The child needs careful observation for signs of increased cyanosis in the morning or at other high-risk times. Observe for neurologic signs of thromboembolism due to polycythemia such as headache, dizziness, excessive irritability, and paralysis. Older children with cyanotic defects may have clubbing of the fingers and toes.

ASSESSMENT FOLLOWING SURGERY

Children are admitted to the ICU following surgery. Children undergoing video-assisted thoracostomy surgery may go to the postanesthesia unit and a short-stay unit for discharge the same day. See the nursing care guidelines in the section on nursing assessment of the child following cardiac surgery for increased pulmonary blood flow earlier in this chapter. Once the child returns to the general nursing unit, monitor the child's heart functioning. Assess vital signs, pulse oximetry, skin color, and perfusion of the skin by capillary refill and distal pulses. Monitor fluid intake and output. A sudden sustained increase in pulse and respirations and a decrease in peripheral perfusion may be early signs of hemorrhage. Signs of respiratory distress may indicate the development of a pneumothorax or CHF.

PSYCHOSOCIAL ASSESSMENT

Assess the parents' need for information and emotional support. In some cases, the infant's condition is first identified at birth; however, defects are often identified by fetal sonography.

The parents will be grieving the loss of a perfect newborn and be extremely anxious about the infant's condition and prognosis.

Examples of nursing diagnoses that may apply to a child with decreased pulmonary blood flow include the following (NANDA-I © 2014):

- *Cardiac Output, Decreased*, related to ventricular restriction and an obstructed outflow tract
- *Infection, Risk for*, related to unfiltered bacteria in the blood and sites of blood shunting that promote bacterial growth
- *Health Management, Family, Ineffective*, related to complexity of therapeutic regimen: assessment and management of hypoxic spells, which are unpredictable events
- *Activity Intolerance* related to cyanosis and dyspnea on exertion
- *Development: Delayed, Risk for*, related to profound hypoxemia

Planning and Implementation

HOME CARE OF THE CHILD BEFORE SURGERY

Some infants with tetralogy of Fallot and other serious defects are managed at home to grow and potentially improve surgical outcome. Parents are usually anxious during the wait for surgery. They may fear that the infant will not survive until surgery or that they will be unable to manage any problems the infant may have. Provide information and teach parents how to care for the infant at home. Arrange for home health nursing and other community services if required. Many of these children require supplemental nutrition and oxygen for emergencies. Because unoxygenated and oxygenated blood mix, supplemental oxygen does not improve the child's usual oxygen saturation (SpO$_2$) level.

Cyanosis with or without CHF often results in delayed gross motor skills. Make referrals to community-based early intervention programs to help parents learn about realistic developmental goals and to promote the infant's development. Encourage parents to treat the infant as normally as possible.

SAFETY ALERT!
The infant with moderate to severe disease should be able to tolerate crying for a few minutes. Do not permit prolonged crying because it worsens cyanosis and causes more hypoxemia.

Hypoxic episodes become life threatening if not treated immediately. The child becomes progressively more hypoxic and limp, loses consciousness, is likely to have a seizure or stroke, and may die. Teach parents to observe for signs of worsening cyanosis, particularly in the morning, that could signal the beginning of a hypercyanotic episode. Some families use a pulse oximeter daily to monitor the infant's SpO$_2$ and identify a change that may indicate an emergency.

Provide guidelines for the initial care of a hypoxic episode. The parents should call for an ambulance and try to calm and reassure the infant. The infant should be placed in a knee–chest position by holding the infant facing the parent's chest, placing one arm under the knees, and folding the legs upward toward the infant's chest. Use the other arm to support the infant's head and back. Alternatively, the infant can be placed supine with knees bent up to the chest. If oxygen is available, provide it in a manner that does not further upset the infant. If none is available in the home, it will be administered in the ambulance during transport to the emergency department.

Teach parents to report signs of illness to the healthcare provider. Vomiting and diarrhea may cause dehydration, a particular risk in children with polycythemia (the blood becomes more viscous and may form thrombi). Fever increases the metabolic rate and further stresses the heart. Aggressive management with antipyretic medication and fluid volume replacement is necessary.

Signs of infective endocarditis (low-grade fever, fatigue, and malaise) occurring within 2 months of surgery or a high-risk procedure should be reported. Teach parents to request antibiotic prophylaxis for the child when appropriate.

Although parents may travel with cyanotic children, they should talk with the healthcare provider before taking them to areas of high altitude or on an airplane. Supplemental oxygen when traveling may be necessary.

Clinical Tip
Develop an emergency plan for the infant in anticipation of acute problems such as a hypoxic episode or respiratory distress. The parents should learn cardiopulmonary resuscitation. Provide the parents with a card or form that has information about the child's condition, medications, necessary emergency care, and the healthcare provider's name so emergency care providers have vital information for initial medical care.

HOSPITAL-BASED CARE OF THE INFANT AND CHILD

The newborn receiving continuous infusion of PGE$_1$ is cared for in the NICU. Side effects of prostaglandin E$_1$ treatment such as cutaneous vasodilation, bradycardia, tachycardia, hypotension, seizure activity, fever, and apnea are monitored and managed.

Avoid any unpleasant or anxiety-provoking procedures in an effort to prevent a hypoxic episode. If a hypoxic episode occurs, follow guidelines for treatment.

Following surgery, the child is initially cared for in the ICU until heart function has stabilized. Once the child returns to the general nursing unit, nursing care is the same as described for the child having surgery for increased pulmonary blood flow earlier in this chapter.

COMMUNITY-BASED NURSING CARE AFTER SURGERY

Support adolescents to transition to self-care, especially those with a complex congenital heart defect. Coordination between a primary healthcare provider and cardiologist with expertise in adults with CHD is recommended when adolescents transition to adult healthcare providers. See *Health Promotion: The Adolescent With Congenital Heart Disease.*

Evaluation

Examples of expected nursing care outcomes include the following:

- The parents recognize a hypoxic episode and initiate appropriate emergency treatment.
- The parents manage fever and medical illnesses to prevent dehydration and thromboembolism.
- The family copes with the stress of the child's condition and other family demands.
- The child demonstrates progressive development in gross motor, fine motor, and language skills following surgical repair.

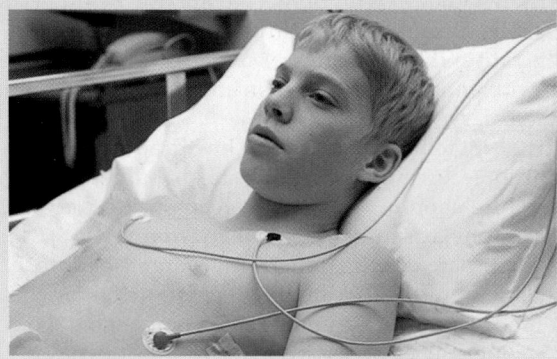

Preventive Care

- Ensure that the adolescent has a healthcare home for general health and illness care. Perform health screening according to recommended schedules (see Chapter 36). Give all recommended immunizations, including the influenza vaccine.
- Encourage routine dental visits twice a year. Make sure the adolescent knows that regular dental care can help reduce endocarditis risk and to seek antibiotic prophylaxis if needed.
- Encourage female adolescents to initiate gynecologic care to ensure that appropriate care is provided for sexual health and contraception. For example, contraceptives containing estrogen are not recommended for individuals with cyanosis, mechanical prosthetic heart valves, or Fontan circulation because of the risk of venous thrombosis (Warnes, 2014). Educate the adolescent about the potential need for special care during pregnancy.
- Provide counseling about health risks associated with tobacco use, alcohol and drug use, and unprotected sex.

Physical Activity

- Ensure that the adolescent with complex CHD has graded exercise testing on a treadmill or bicycle to determine the sports, exercises, and physical activity recommended.
- Clearly explain the importance of physical activity for long-term health. Inquire about the adolescent's beliefs about allowable exercise and activity level, and provide education if differences in recommended and perceived activity levels are found. Explain any activity limitations, such as avoidance of body blocking if a pacemaker is used.

Nutrition

- Encourage the adolescent to eat nutritious meals and snacks, and to avoid excess weight gain that could stress the heart function.
- Educate adolescents with polycythemia to maintain hydration.

Mental and Spiritual Health

- Talk with adolescents about their self-identify, as they have scars, may be smaller than their peers, may be less physically active, and have more frequent healthcare visits.
- Discuss the adolescent's concerns for the future because there may be significant uncertainty about the disease course and outcome.
- Identify and refer adolescents as needed for counseling or to a support group of adolescents of similar age with congenital heart disease.

Education for Self-Care

Begin the process of transitioning the adolescent to adult health care. Provide education about the congenital heart defect, surgeries that have been performed, and the types of symptoms resulting. Provide information about specific signs that require healthcare provider notification. Remember that previous education has been targeted to the parents. Correct any misperceptions that prior surgery resulted in a normal heart if that is not the case.

- Provide a written succinct summary of the adolescent's condition and medical management that can be shared with other healthcare providers.
- Provide education about infective endocarditis prophylaxis if needed. Describe situations that may increase risk, such as tattooing, acupuncture, dental care, electrolysis, and various diagnostic and surgical procedures.
- Discuss the medications needed and why. Develop plans for the adolescent to assume responsibility for self-administration. Educate the adolescent to seek guidance before using over-the-counter medications and herbal medications because of the potential for medication interaction.
- Discuss the genetic aspects of the condition and provide resources for genetic counseling if desired.
- Discuss the danger signs of the condition (such as arrhythmias, or the potential of dehydration in an adolescent with cyanosis) and how to seek urgent or emergency care.

Vocational Education

- Reassure adolescents who have had complete repairs of the congenital heart defect and have no disabilities that they have no limitations in their career or vocational selection.
- Provide career and vocational counseling to adolescents with cardiac disabilities that matches their interests, academic abilities, and clinical limitations. Encourage preparation for employment that can be maintained throughout the working career. Inform adolescents about their rights under the Americans with Disabilities Act of 1990.
- Encourage families and adolescents to identify health insurance options and policies that are a better match for the level of healthcare interventions needed.

Defects Obstructing Systemic Blood Flow

Etiology and Pathophysiology

An anatomic stenosis (narrowing of a valve, of the area around a valve, or in the great artery above a valve) causes obstruction to blood flow and results in a pressure load on the left ventricle and decreased cardiac output. The greater the narrowing, the more obstructed the blood flow is to the circulation. This results in higher pressure in the ventricle and decreased cardiac output. Newborns with severe left outflow obstruction or left ventricular dysfunction may develop decreased cardiac output and shock.

Clinical Manifestations

Low cardiac output is responsible for the following clinical manifestations: diminished pulses, poor color, delayed capillary refill time, and decreased urinary output. The blood cannot move past the obstruction, so it backs up into the left atrium and then the lungs, causing CHF and pulmonary edema. The child with mild obstructions may have leg cramps, cooler feet than hands, and stronger pulses in the arms than the legs.

Decreased blood supply to the gastrointestinal tract may lead to necrotizing enterocolitis. See Chapter 51. See Table 47–8 for the pathophysiology, clinical manifestations, diagnostic tests, clinical therapy, and prognosis for congenital heart defects that obstruct systemic blood flow.

TABLE 47–8 Pathophysiology, Clinical Manifestations, Diagnostic Tests, Clinical Therapy, and Prognosis for Defects That Obstruct the Systemic Blood Flow

ANATOMY

AORTIC STENOSIS (AS)

Narrowing of the aortic valve obstructs blood flow to the systemic circulation. The valve often has two valve leaflets (bicuspid), rather than three, that may be partially fused. The left ventricle must work harder to force blood past the narrowed valve opening. Aortic stenosis accounts for up to 10% of congenital heart defects (Park, 2014, p. 188).

Clinical Manifestations

Most infants and children with mild AS are asymptomatic. Life-threatening AS occurs in some newborns. CHF develops in infants with significant stenosis. Peripheral pulses may be weak and thready. The child may complain of chest pain after exercise, and exercise intolerance may be noted. Fainting and dizziness (syncope) are serious signs that require intervention.

The systolic blood pressure may be higher in the right arm than the left.

A systolic heart murmur and thrill may be detected in the aortic area with transmission to the neck. An ejection click may be heard. Splitting of the S$_2$ may be noted. Interventions may result in aortic insufficiency causing a high-pitched diastolic decrescendo murmur along the left sternal border near the mitral area.

Diagnostic Tests

The chest radiograph may reveal a normal-sized heart, but a dilated ascending aorta may be seen.

The ECG may show mild left ventricular hypertrophy in severe AS.

An echocardiogram reveals the number of valve leaflets, pressure gradient across the valve, and size of the aorta.

Exercise testing may be used in asymptomatic children to determine the amount of obstruction present.

Clinical Therapy

Newborns with life-threatening AS need PGE$_1$ to maintain a patent ductus arteriosus as well as dopamine and diuretics to treat CHF until the aortic valve can be dilated.

Treatment involves balloon dilation during cardiac catheterization or surgical valvotomy. Surgical treatment is palliative rather than curative.

Aortic valve replacement is performed when stenosis is severe or if significant regurgitation results from other interventions.

Prognosis

Chest pain, syncope, and sudden death can occur in symptomatic children, particularly during vigorous exercise. Untreated mild AS may progress after several decades as the valve calcifies. Stenosis may also reoccur after intervention. Valve replacement may become necessary, requiring lifelong anticoagulant therapy.

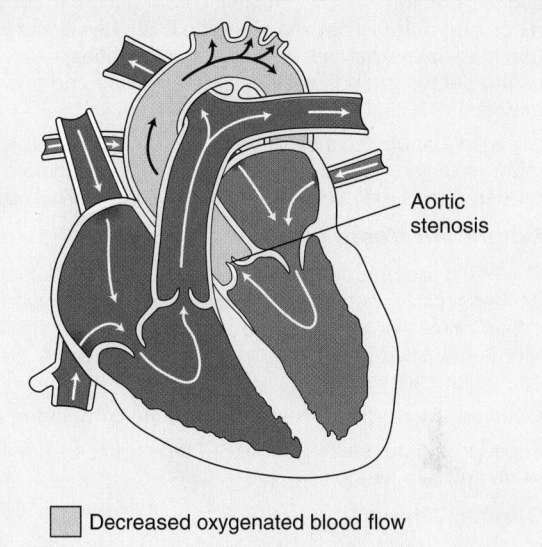

Aortic stenosis

☐ Decreased oxygenated blood flow

COARCTATION OF THE AORTA (COA)

Narrowing or constriction in the descending aorta, often near the ductus arteriosus or left subclavian artery, obstructs the systemic blood outflow. This defect occurs in 8% to 10% of congenital heart defects and is found in 30% of children with Turner syndrome (Park, 2014, p. 195).

(continued)

TABLE 47–8 Pathophysiology, Clinical Manifestations, Diagnostic Tests, Clinical Therapy, and Prognosis for Defects That Obstruct the Systemic Blood Flow (*continued*)

ANATOMY

Clinical Manifestations

Many children are asymptomatic and grow normally. Reduced blood flow through the descending aorta causes lower blood pressure in legs and higher blood pressure in arms, neck, and head. Brachial and radial pulses are typically bounding, but femoral and leg pulses are weak or absent. Older children may complain of weakness and pain in the legs after exercise.

Infants with moderate constriction are pale; may have poor feeding, avoidant/restrictive food intake disorder (failure to thrive), and increased respiratory effort. They may develop CHF. Newborns with severe constriction may have cyanosis in the lower extremities, heart failure, and shock as the ductus arteriosus closes. Renal failure and necrotizing enterocolitis may develop.

On auscultation, S_2 is heard as a loud single sound. A systolic ejection murmur may be heard at the upper right and middle or lower left sternal border. A thrill may be palpated in the suprasternal notch.

Diagnostic Tests

The chest radiograph may reveal cardiomegaly, pulmonary venous congestion, and indentation of the descending aorta. Dilation of the ascending aorta may be seen. Rib notching is rarely seen before 5 years of age. MRI is preferred for imaging to see the aortic arch, site of coarctation, and collateral circulation.

ECG may be normal or show left ventricular hypertrophy.

Echocardiogram shows the size of the aorta and functioning of the aortic valve and left ventricle.

Clinical Therapy

In symptomatic newborns, PGE_1 is given to reopen the ductus arteriosus and promote blood flow to the kidneys and lower extremities. Treatment to prevent CHF may be initiated with inotropic medications, diuretics, and oxygen (Park, 2014, p. 198).

Surgical resection is often preferred to balloon dilation during cardiac catheterization to reduce the risk for recoarctation. Balloon dilation with stent placement may be performed for sick newborns who will eventually need surgical repair and stent removal (Park, 2014, p. 199). Balloon angioplasty may be performed if coarctation recurs.

Prognosis

Balloon dilation and surgical resection are palliative because coarctation may recur with either procedure. Lifelong follow-up is necessary. Persistent hypertension occurs in some children.

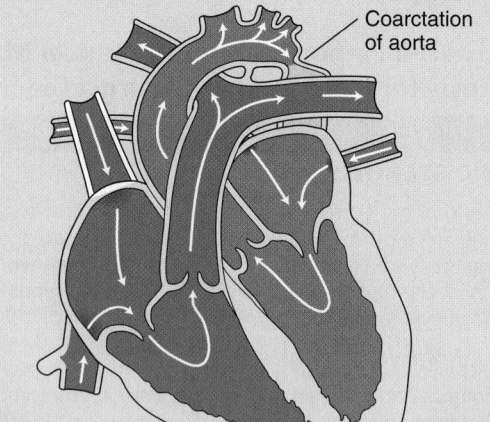

Coarctation of aorta

HYPOPLASTIC LEFT HEART SYNDROME (HLHS)

The mitral and aortic valves are absent or stenosed along with an abnormally small left ventricle and small aorta. HLHS accounts for about 1.5% of congenital heart defects (Awad & Busse, 2011). About 10% of cases are associated with Turner syndrome, trisomy 18, and other genetic disorders (Park, 2014, p. 258).

Clinical Manifestations

Within hours after birth, the newborn has progressive cyanosis and signs of CHF (tachycardia, tachypnea, dyspnea, retractions, and decreased peripheral pulses) as the ductus arteriosus closes.

Poor peripheral perfusion, pulmonary edema, and CHF lead to shock, acidosis, and death, without intervention.

On auscultation, S_2 is single and loud. No heart murmur is present.

Diagnostic Procedures

The chest radiograph shows cardiomegaly and increased pulmonary venous congestion.

The ECG shows right ventricular hypertrophy.

The echocardiogram shows the small left ventricle and enlarged right ventricle. This condition is often diagnosed prenatally.

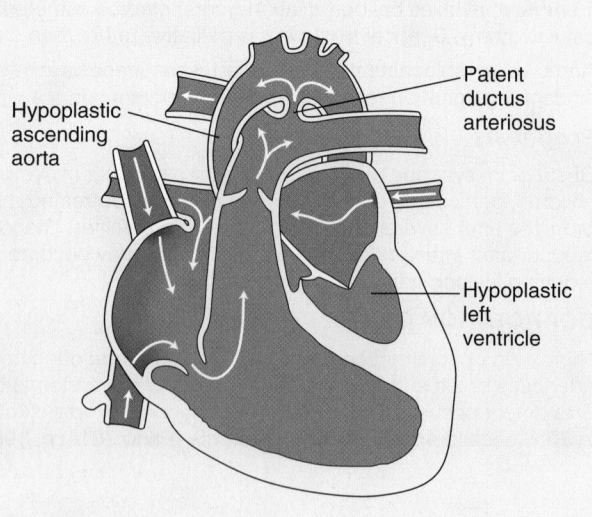

Hypoplastic ascending aorta

Patent ductus arteriosus

Hypoplastic left ventricle

■ Mixed oxygenated and unoxygenated blood

Clinical Therapy

Prostaglandin E$_1$ is given immediately to maintain a patent ductus arteriosus.

Intubation and ventilation are performed, and supplemental oxygen is provided. Metabolic acidosis is treated.

Genetic, ophthalmologic, and neurologic evaluations are often performed before surgery.

Treatment options include surgery or a heart transplant (see heart transplantation section later in chapter). Comfort or palliative care is chosen less often with advances in surgery.

Norwood surgery is performed in three stages. Stage 1 procedure is performed by 1 week of age. The aorta is reconstructed and the right ventricle is committed to pumping blood through the pulmonary valve to the aorta. The atrial septum is removed so blood can mix. A shunt is created to send adequate blood to the lungs. Stage 2, performed at 3 to 6 months of age, connects the superior vena cava directly to the pulmonary artery (Glenn shunt). Stage 3 Fontan procedure, performed at 1 to 2 years of age, connects the inferior vena cava to the pulmonary circulation, ending the mixing of oxygenated and unoxygenated blood.

Few infant hearts are available for transplantation.

Prognosis

Surgery is essential for survival, and the survival rate after stage 3 Fontan is 95% after 4 years (Park, 2014, p. 261). However, some infants die during intervals between surgical stages. Heart failure, arrhythmias, and sudden cardiac death may occur in children and adolescents several years after stage 3 Fontan surgery. The child will have physical activity limitations because of a single ventricle. Approximately 50% of surviving children have significant cognitive and neurologic impairment (Paris, Moore, & Schreiber, 2012) (see the *Evidence-Based Practice* feature earlier in this chapter).

Clinical Tip

The systolic blood pressure is usually 10 to 15 mmHg higher in the legs than the arms in healthy children. In children with coarctation of the aorta, the systolic blood pressure in the legs may be equal to or lower than in the arms, as the defect obstructs systemic blood flow to the abdomen and lower extremities.

Clinical Therapy

Neonates with severe systemic outflow obstruction or left ventricular dysfunction may develop decreased cardiac output and shock. PGE$_1$ and inotrope medications may be required to support the systemic circulation until the obstruction is relieved or ventricular function improves.

Some children (e.g., after Fontan procedure or aortic valve replacement) need long-term treatment with aspirin or warfarin to prevent the development of thrombi. Caution parents of children who take warfarin (Coumadin) to avoid using herbal products because of interactions. For example, children will have an increased warfarin effect with ginkgo biloba or a decreased effect with St. John's wort (Yu, Bostwick, & Hallman, 2011).

Nursing Management

See the sections on *Congenital Heart Defects That Increase Pulmonary Blood Flow* for nursing care management of children with aortic stenosis and coarctation of the aorta earlier in this chapter and on *Defects Causing Decreased Pulmonary Blood Flow and Mixed Defects* for nursing care management of infants with hypoplastic left heart syndrome (HLHS) earlier in this chapter.

Parents of children with life-threatening defects such as HLHS are under intense pressure to make a decision about the best treatment for their newborns (palliative care, Norwood procedure, or heart transplant). Nurses have an important role in providing parent support during the decision making process as they may get conflicting recommendations by neonatologists and surgeons (Toebbe, Yehle, Kirkpatrick, et al., 2013). Share information with the parents so they are fully informed about treatment options and their associated mortality, the intense care needed by the surviving child, the potential for disabilities, and the unknown long-term survival. Identify family members, clergy, or social workers who can support the parents through this period. If parents choose comfort or palliative care, interventions such as PGE$_1$ are discontinued, and the infant is given appropriate pain medication and comfort (see Chapter 41). Reassure parents that they are good parents, no matter what decision they make.

Congestive Heart Failure

Congestive heart failure (CHF) occurs when heart function is impaired and cardiac output is inadequate to support the body's circulatory and metabolic needs. It may result from a congenital heart defect that either increases pulmonary blood flow or obstructs the systemic blood outflow tract. Other causes include arrhythmias, pathologic conditions that require high cardiac output (e.g., severe anemia, acidosis, or bronchopulmonary dysplasia), and acquired heart disease (e.g., cardiomyopathy or Kawasaki disease).

Etiology and Pathophysiology

Pulmonary blood volume overload associated with congenital heart defects is a common cause of CHF in infants. Many infants with this pathophysiology develop CHF within the first 6 months of life (McDaniel, 2014). Defects that allow blood to shunt from the left side of the heart to the right increase the amount of blood pumped to the lungs. The pulmonary system is overloaded, and if prolonged can lead to pulmonary artery hypertension (see the section later in this chapter). Obstructive congenital defects restrict the flow of blood, so the heart muscle hypertrophies to work harder to force blood through these structures. Eventually the heart muscle cannot keep up with the demand.

When cardiac output remains insufficient, blood pressure is decreased and hypoxia occurs in the organs and tissues. The sympathetic nervous system is activated and catecholamines are released, leading to tachycardia, improved heart muscle contraction, and improved smooth muscle tone that returns blood to the heart. The sympathetic nervous system also reduces blood flow to the kidneys, which in turn stimulates the release of rennin, angiotensin, and aldosterone. Sodium and fluid are retained to increase circulatory volume. The myocardium stretches temporarily to manage the increased blood flow and force of contraction. These physiologic responses are unable to maintain the cardiac output and maintain blood pressure as CHF progresses and the maximum myocardial stretch is reached. Progressive systemic edema and pulmonary congestion leads to right- or left-sided heart failure that may become bilateral.

Clinical Manifestations

Initial signs of CHF may be subtle and not immediately recognized. The infant tires easily, especially during feeding. Weight loss or lack of normal weight gain, diaphoresis, irritability, and frequent respiratory infections may be evident. Pallor or mottling of the skin may be present. Older children may have exercise intolerance, dyspnea, abdominal pain or distention, and peripheral edema.

As the disease progresses, tachypnea, tachycardia, pallor or cyanosis, nasal flaring, grunting, retractions, cough, or crackles may develop. A third heart sound may be auscultated. Generalized fluid volume overload is seen more commonly in toddlers and older children. Periorbital and facial edema and hepatomegaly are signs of fluid volume excess. Peripheral edema is less common in infants and young children. Jugular vein distention is seen in older children. See Table 47–9 for more detailed clinical manifestations.

Cardiomegaly, enlargement (hypertrophy) of the heart muscle, occurs in an effort to maintain cardiac output. Cyanosis, weak peripheral pulses, cool extremities, hypotension, and heart murmur are precursors of cardiogenic shock, which can occur if CHF is not adequately treated (see the section on cardiogenic shock later in this chapter).

Clinical Therapy

Diagnosis is based primarily on physical findings. A chest radiograph reveals cardiac enlargement and venous congestion or signs of pulmonary edema. Echocardiography confirms the diagnosis and severity of CHF. An electrocardiogram may identify an arrhythmia cause of CHF. Electrolytes, lactic acid, arterial blood gases, and a complete blood count are obtained. Renal function is evaluated with creatinine and blood urea nitrogen (BUN) levels. Liver function tests may be elevated.

TABLE 47–9 Clinical Manifestations of Congestive Heart Failure

PATHOPHYSIOLOGY	CLINICAL MANIFESTATIONS
Pulmonary venous congestion	Mild resting tachypnea, wheezing, crackles, retractions, cough, grunting, nasal flaring, recent onset of poor feeding, increased tachypnea and diaphoresis with feeding
	Tiring with play and orthopnea may be seen in older children
Systemic venous congestion	Hepatomegaly, ascites, periorbital edema, fluid retention weight gain
	Jugular venous distention and dependent edema in older children
Impaired cardiac output	Tachycardia, weak pulses, hypotension, capillary refill time greater than 2 sec, pallor, cool extremities, oliguria, restlessness, irritability
High metabolic rate	Avoidant/restrictive food intake disorder (failure to thrive) or slow weight gain, diaphoresis

The initial goal is identify and treat the cause of CHF, such as an arrhythmia or surgical correction of a heart defect. Then efforts are made to decrease the work of the heart and improve systemic circulation. Diuretics, such as furosemide, thiazides, and spironolactone, are given to promote fluid excretion. Afterload-reducing agents (angiotensin-converting enzyme [ACE] inhibitors) are often prescribed to lessen the workload on the heart. Digoxin is less commonly prescribed with availability of ACE inhibitors. Inotropic medicines such as dopamine, dobutamine, isoproterenol, and epinephrine are used for critical care management. See *Medications Used to Treat: Congestive Heart Failure.*

Surgery or interventional cardiac catheterization for a congenital heart defect may become the treatment of choice. Cardiac transplantation may be performed for children with end-stage cardiomyopathy or complex congenital heart defects such as hypoplastic left heart syndrome.

Supportive medical therapies (supplemental oxygen, positioning to reduce respiratory distress, rest, and fluid and nutrition management) are part of the treatment plan. Most children improve rapidly after medication is administered.

Nursing Management
For the Child With Congestive Heart Failure

Nursing Assessment and Diagnosis

PHYSIOLOGIC ASSESSMENT
The diagnosis of CHF depends primarily on physical symptoms. Assess the child's vital signs, behavioral patterns, cardiac function, respiratory function, and fluid status using guidelines in the *Assessment Guide* earlier in this chapter. Use the age-specific heart and respiratory rates in Chapter 33 to identify tachycardia

Medications Used to Treat: Congestive Heart Failure

MEDICATIONS AND ACTIONS	NURSING MANAGEMENT
Digoxin (Lanoxin) Slows the heart rate, increases cardiac filling time, and increases cardiac output; used with increased pulmonary blood flow.	• Assess the heart rate for bradycardia for 1 min prior to giving a dose or for changes in heart rhythm or quality. • Monitor the child for digoxin toxicity. • See the CHF nursing management section for more information.
Furosemide (Lasix) Rapid diuresis; blocks reabsorption of sodium and water in renal tubules.	• Monitor patients during rapid diuresis for vital signs, intake and output, and fluid and electrolyte imbalances (e.g., hypokalemia and hypochloremia). • Assess for digoxin toxicity if hypokalemia is present.
Thiazides (Diuril) Chlorothiazide (suspension); hydrochlorothiazide (tablets) Maintains diuresis, decreases absorption of sodium, water, potassium, chloride, and bicarbonate in renal tubules.	• Monitor blood pressure and intake and output rates and patterns. • Monitor lab values for hypokalemia. Assess for digoxin toxicity if present.
Spironolactone (Aldactone) Maintains diuresis (potassium sparing).	• Assess for signs of fluid and electrolyte imbalance and digitoxicity.
ACEi (angiotensin-converting enzyme inhibitor) (e.g., Captopril, Enalapril) Promotes vascular relaxation and reduced peripheral vascular resistance, reduces afterload.	• Monitor for hypotension with initiation of therapy and dosage changes. • Assess for common side effects such as cough, hyperkalemia, and worsening renal function.
Carvedilol (Coreg) Improves left ventricular function, promotes vasodilation of systemic circulation; used for chronic heart failure and dilated cardiomyopathy.	• Give with food. • Assess the heart rate for bradycardia when the dose is increased. • Assess cardiac output by monitoring tissue perfusion, peripheral pulses, blood pressure, and urine output. • Monitor for dizziness and hypotension. • Monitor digoxin levels because drug may increase plasma digoxin concentration. • Monitor liver function periodically.

Source: Data from Wilson, B. A., Shannon, M. T., & Shields, K. M. (2016). *Pearson nurses' drug guide 2016.* Hoboken, NJ: Pearson Education; Park, M. K. (2014). *Pediatric cardiology for practitioners* (6th ed., pp. 457–464). Philadelphia: Elsevier Saunders; Satou, G. M., & Halnon, N. J. (2013). *Pediatric congestive heart failure.* Retrieved from http://emedicine.medscape.com/article/2069746-medication#1

and tachypnea. Obtain a detailed history of the onset of symptoms from the parents because CHF often develops slowly.

Measure intake and output carefully. Weigh the infant's diapers before use and after changing (each 1-g difference in weight equals 1 mL of urine). Weigh the child at the same time each day. Observe for periorbital or peripheral edema and circulatory changes. If ascites is present, take serial abdominal measurements to monitor changes. (See the *Clinical Skills Manual* SKILLS for guidelines.) Turn the child frequently and assess the skin for redness and breakdown.

FAMILY ASSESSMENT

Review the child's previous hospitalizations and assess the family's knowledge about the child's condition. Families of children with CHF are anxious about the potential deterioration of the child's condition and their ability to provide ongoing care.

Assess the family's anxiety level and coping strategies. Evaluate the family's economic status. Medication is crucial to treatment, and a family's inability to obtain the necessary medications jeopardizes the child's outcome. Identify the parent's ability to recognize changes in the child's condition and to provide needed care. Determine if another family member is available who could assist young parents or provide respite care.

DEVELOPMENTAL ASSESSMENT

Because fatigue limits the activities of the infant and young child with CHF, the opportunity to practice the skills needed to attain normal developmental milestones is more limited. Use a developmental assessment tool to document current status (see Chapter 34). Ask parents when the child attained expected developmental milestones such as sitting, manipulating objects, standing, or walking. Ask parents about contact and play with other children and a typical day's activity schedule. Parents may limit the child's contact with other children because of frequent infections and exercise intolerance. When CHF is well controlled, the child's energy level increases and developmental skills often improve. Repeating assessments every 2 to 3 months in infants and toddlers provides useful information about development and disease management.

Several nursing diagnoses that may apply to the child with CHF can be found in the accompanying *Nursing Care Plans*. The primary nursing diagnosis is **Cardiac Output, Decreased**, related to cardiac anomaly (NANDA-I © 2014).

Planning and Implementation

Nursing care for the child with CHF focuses on administering and monitoring effects of medications, maintaining adequate oxygenation and myocardial function, promoting rest, fostering development, providing adequate nutrition, and providing emotional support to the child and family (Figure 47–6). (See *Nursing Care Plan: The Child Hospitalized With Congestive Heart Failure*.)

ADMINISTER AND MONITOR PRESCRIBED MEDICATIONS

Children with CHF usually receive furosemide and an ACE inhibitor, and they may receive intravenous inotropic medications while in the PICU. In some cases, digoxin is prescribed. These medications are potent and must be administered correctly.

SAFETY ALERT!

Before giving the digitalizing dose of digoxin (a higher dose to establish a blood level more rapidly), assess baseline vital signs, the quality of peripheral pulses, and clinical symptoms, and also obtain an electrocardiogram (ECG). Check the levels of serum electrolytes, and check hepatic and renal functions. Assess hydration status, and hydrate if hypovolemic. The risk for digoxin toxicity is increased when hypokalemia is present. Repeated ECGs are used for early detection of toxicity for several days after digitalization (Park, 2014, p. 461).

Before giving any dose of digoxin, take the apical pulse for 1 minute. Call for a healthcare provider's advice before administering the digoxin in the following conditions:

- The heart rate is less than 60 to 100 beats/min, depending upon the age, or is higher or lower than the guideline noted in the healthcare provider's order.
- Changes in heart rhythm or quality are noted.

MAINTAIN OXYGENATION AND MYOCARDIAL FUNCTION

Oxygen therapy may be ordered. Make sure that tubing is patent, the oxygen flow rate is correct, the oxygen delivery device is working properly, and humidification is provided. Keep the child calm and quiet. Position the child in semi-Fowler or a 45-degree angle position to promote maximum oxygenation. An infant car safety seat is an option.

PROMOTE REST

Group assessments and interventions together to ensure that the child has some uninterrupted rest each hour. Rocking is restful for infants. Encourage older children to engage in quiet activities such as computer games and videos.

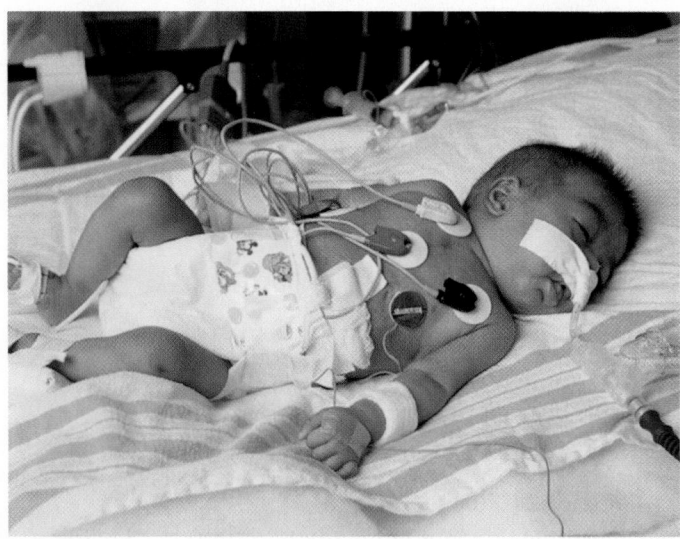

Figure 47–6 Jooti is receiving intravenous fluids and oxygen. Her condition is being continuously monitored for congestive heart failure.

FOSTER DEVELOPMENT

Encourage parents to play with the child, using toys to stimulate eye–hand coordination and fine motor movements. Such toys include rattles, blocks, and stuffed animals for infants and books, paper and crayons, and dolls for older children. Encourage sitting, standing, or walking for short periods with adequate rest afterward to promote the development of large muscles. Singing, talking, and playing music facilitate cognitive and language skills.

PROVIDE ADEQUATE NUTRITION

Teach parents about feeding techniques. Encourage the mother who chooses to breastfeed the infant. The antibodies in breast milk reduce infections, and the milk is naturally low in sodium. However, the sucking involved in breastfeeding or bottle feeding may cause dyspnea that forces the infant to rest frequently during feeding. Feedings should last no more than 30 to 40 minutes, but some infants should feed no longer than 20 minutes. Frequent small feedings generally work best, with burping after every half ounce of intake to minimize vomiting. Holding the infant at a 45-degree angle or positioned in an infant seat decreases venous return to the heart and decreases its metabolic demand. Make sure parents understand that changes in feeding habits (decreased intake, vomiting, sleeping through feedings, and increased perspiration with feedings) may indicate deteriorating cardiac status.

Infants with CHF need adequate nutrition to support growth because their metabolic rate is elevated. Some infants need a higher caloric formula (24 to 30 calories per ounce) to obtain adequate nutrition. For example, regular powdered formula can be prepared with less water or a human milk fortifier can be added to breast milk. In some cases, low-osmolarity glucose polymers or medium-chain triglyceride (MCT) oil is recommended for addition to standard formula (Park, 2014, p. 457). Nutritional supplementation by nasogastric, transpyloric, or gastrostomy tube may be prescribed. Parents are often advised to have the infant feed normally for a specific period to promote oral stimulation and bonding. The remainder of the formula is then given by tube feeding. (See the *Clinical Skills Manual* SKILLS .)

Nursing Care Plan: The Child Hospitalized With Congestive Heart Failure

1. Nursing Diagnosis: *Cardiac Output, Decreased*, related to cardiac anomaly (VSD) (NANDA-I © 2014)

GOAL: The child's cardiac output will be sufficient to meet the body's metabolic demands.

INTERVENTION	RATIONALE
• Administer digoxin as ordered.	• Digoxin increases contractility of the heart and force of contraction.
• Regularly count the apical pulse and listen to heart sounds, especially before each dose of digoxin. Record the apical pulse rate with each dose of digoxin.	• Digoxin may cause bradycardia. Pulse and heart sounds provide information about heart functioning.
• Use cardiac monitor if prescribed.	• Monitor notes bradycardia and arrhythmias.
• Monitor serum potassium level and for digitoxicity.	• Hypokalemia increases risk of digoxin toxicity.
• Provide for rest periods each hour.	• Rest decreases need for high cardiac output.

EXPECTED OUTCOME: Child's cardiac output will be sufficient as indicated by increased energy, adequate feeding intake, and decreased edema. Child will maintain normal serum potassium levels and therapeutic levels of digoxin. Child will rest hourly and have adequate energy to eat and play.

GOAL: The child will manifest adequate oxygenation.

INTERVENTION	RATIONALE
• Evaluate respiratory rate and breath sounds. Observe for diaphoresis, a sign of increased respiratory effort. Use pulse oximetry to determine oxygen saturation readings.	• Provides information about oxygenation and ease of respiration.
• Provide oxygen and humidification if prescribed.	• Supplemental oxygen decreases tachypnea, and humidification moistens secretions to keep airway clear.
• Place child in semi-Fowler position.	• This position facilitates lung expansion.

EXPECTED OUTCOME: Child will maintain a normal SpO_2 level and respiratory rate for age without evidence of adventitious sounds or diaphoresis.

2. Nursing Diagnosis: *Fluid Volume: Excess*, related to heart failure (NANDA-I © 2014)

GOAL: Intake and output will be balanced once excess fluid is excreted.

INTERVENTION	RATIONALE
• Administer diuretics as ordered.	• Diuretics mobilize fluids and facilitate excretion.
• Measure intake and output carefully. Weigh diapers to assess output of infants. Weigh daily. Measure abdominal girth daily. Observe for peripheral edema.	• Adequate output is a good indicator of renal perfusion. Assessments demonstrate effectiveness of treatment.
• Monitor electrolytes.	• Electrolyte imbalance is common when diuretics are given.
• Maintain fluid restrictions if prescribed.	• Fluid restriction may help decrease the cardiac load.

EXPECTED OUTCOME: Child's intake and output will be proportional, and electrolyte levels will remain within normal ranges.

3. Nursing Diagnosis: *Skin Integrity, Risk for Impaired*, related to altered fluid status (NANDA-I © 2014)

GOAL: The child's peripheral and central edema will decrease.

INTERVENTION	RATIONALE
• Change child's position frequently.	• Position changes promote circulation to skin over pressure points.
• Inspect skin frequently for redness and skin breakdown over pressure points.	• Inspection identifies earliest stages of skin breakdown.

EXPECTED OUTCOME: Child will have no skin breakdown after edema resolves.

(continued)

Nursing Care Plan: The Child Hospitalized With Congestive Heart Failure (continued)

4. Nursing Diagnosis: *Nutrition, Imbalanced: Less than Body Requirements*, related to high metabolic needs and rapid tiring while feeding (NANDA-I © 2014)

GOAL: The child will receive adequate nutrition to meet metabolic needs.

INTERVENTION	RATIONALE
• Hold infant at 45-degree angle for feeding.	• Position facilitates breathing while eating.
• Record intake carefully.	• Evaluation of intake indicates whether caloric and other nutritional needs are met.
• Weigh child daily.	• Weight gain indicates growth (in absence of fluid retention).
• Give frequent small meals with rest periods in between.	• Digesting small meals requires less energy.
• Use high-calorie formula or give high-calorie snacks.	• High-calorie formulas and snacks provide calories efficiently.
• Use soothing approaches such as holding infants for feeding and having parents eat with older child.	• Restful approach facilitates intake with minimum cardiac work.
• Transition to supplemental tube feedings if the infant is not able to gain weight.	• Tube feedings provide added calories without taxing the infant's energy.

EXPECTED OUTCOME: Infant or child will gain recommended weight according to growth grids. All dietary requirements will be met, and mealtimes will be pleasant.

PROVIDE EMOTIONAL SUPPORT

The family is often anxious about the condition of the child hospitalized with CHF. Give parents a chance to express concerns about their child's condition. Explain the child's treatment regimen, and make sure family members understand the child's need for nutrition and rest. Refer parents to the appropriate support groups; talking with parents of children with cardiac conditions may be a source of emotional support.

DISCHARGE PLANNING AND HOME CARE TEACHING

Identify and address home care needs well in advance of discharge. Show parents how to prepare formula or supplement breast milk, and then offer guidance to help maximize the child's nutritional intake. While the child is hospitalized, teach the family about medication administration and signs of a worsening condition (e.g., increased feeding difficulty, irritability, lethargy, breathing difficulty, and puffiness around the eyes or extremities). Arrange for home care nursing visits to reinforce the education provided, to monitor the child's condition, and to assess the family's ability to manage the child's care. Ensure that the family has a phone contact for questions and emergency assistance. (See *Nursing Care Plan: The Child With Congestive Heart Failure Being Cared for at Home.*)

Demonstrate administration of drugs, and then supervise while the parents measure and administer medications. If digoxin is prescribed, teach parents about the signs of digoxin's toxic effects. Parents are frequently taught to take the child's pulse and to report any significant change to the healthcare provider and any signs of medication side effects. Teach parents about the potential interaction between digoxin and macrolide antibiotics so they can remind the primary care provider to prescribe safe antibiotics when they are needed.

Teach parents to take special care with an acute illness that involves a fever and diarrhea or vomiting. An acute illness could lead to dehydration more quickly when the child takes diuretics, and urgent care will be needed.

These children are evaluated frequently by healthcare providers for progression in signs and symptoms, appropriate weight gain, and developmental progress. Families are evaluated for their ongoing ability to manage the child's condition and cope with the stress of caring for a sick child.

Evaluation

Expected outcomes of nursing care can be found in the *Nursing Care Plans.*

Clinical Reasoning The Infant With Ventricular Septal Defect

Brandy, who is 1 month old, was diagnosed with a ventricular septal defect (VSD) at birth and started developing signs of respiratory distress and difficulty with feeding.

Brandy's mother had been alerted to watch for these signs as a possible indication of CHF. Brandy was quickly hospitalized so her CHF could be treated with intravenous furosemide, dopamine, and potassium. Over the next 2 days, she lost the weight she had gained as a result of fluid retention.

Corrective surgery was performed to place a patch over the septal opening. Brandy was cared for in the intensive care unit before being transferred to another unit.

- Why did Brandy develop CHF? Why was corrective surgery performed when she is so young?
- What teaching and support do Brandy's parents need to care for her at home after the heart surgery?

Acquired Heart Diseases

Cardiomyopathy

Cardiomyopathy is a serious disorder of the heart's muscle that affects chamber size, wall thickness, or contraction and leads to problems with ventricular systolic or diastolic function.

Nursing Care Plan: The Child With Congestive Heart Failure Being Cared for at Home

1. Nursing Diagnosis: *Development: Delayed, Risk for*, related to effects of physical disability (NANDA-I © 2014)

GOAL: The child will meet developmental milestones for age group.

INTERVENTION	RATIONALE
• Perform baseline developmental assessment.	• Assessment provides comparison for later assessments and basis for planning specific games, toys, and activities.
• Plan for short play periods after rest.	• Short play periods maintain energy and facilitate play.
• Introduce age-appropriate toys and activities such as rattles and blocks for infants and art projects for older children.	• Play activities facilitate learning and mastery of developmental tasks.
• Plan for interactions with healthy children.	• Social skills are learned through contact with others.

EXPECTED OUTCOME: Child will display normal language, fine motor, and gross motor activity.

2. Nursing Diagnosis: *Health Management, Family, Ineffective*, related to complexity of therapeutic regimen (NANDA-I © 2014)

GOAL: Parents will demonstrate correct administration of medications.

INTERVENTION	RATIONALE
• Have parents prepare the medication dosages and administer the digoxin, diuretics, and other medications to the child while observed by the nurse.	• Demonstrating techniques used to administer medications provides opportunities to identify dosage errors and to suggest methods to help ensure the child gets all needed medications.

EXPECTED OUTCOME: Parents will demonstrate ability to prepare correct medication dosage and administer it to the child.

GOAL: Parents will state side effects of medications and symptoms of congestive heart failure.

INTERVENTION	RATIONALE
• Describe side effects of medications. Give parents handouts with telephone number to call to ask questions or report side effects.	• If side effects are understood, serious complications can be avoided.
• Describe subtle onset of CHF symptoms (increasing weakness, exhaustion, irritability, difficulty feeding, cough or difficult respirations, edema).	• Parents can evaluate child regularly and note subtle changes requiring medical management.

EXPECTED OUTCOME: Parents will report that child continues to demonstrate improvement and adequate cardiac output without signs of congestive heart failure.

3. Nursing Diagnosis: *Nutrition, Imbalanced: Less than Body Requirements*, related to chronic illness and tiring while feeding (NANDA-I © 2014)

GOAL: The infant or child will demonstrate normal weight gain for age.

INTERVENTION	RATIONALE
• Teach parents methods to promote food intake related to positioning, size of feedings, and food choices.	• Positioning, frequency of feedings, size of feedings, and use of high-caloric foods can enhance nutritional intake.
• Observe feeding during home visit.	• Feedback can assist parents in integrating positive feeding techniques.

EXPECTED OUTCOME: Infant or child will show normal weight gain. Parents will report and demonstrate successful feedings of child.

4. Nursing Diagnosis: *Activity Intolerance* related to poor cardiac output (NANDA-I © 2014)

GOAL: The child will perform all necessary activities of daily living without undue tiring.

INTERVENTION	RATIONALE
• Suggest activities parents can alternate with rest throughout the child's day.	• Activities to promote development must be alternated with rest because of decreased cardiac output.
• Have parents limit child's exposure to persons with contagious disease.	• When the child is ill and tired, the immune system can be compromised.
• Help family plan quiet surroundings to provide for child's rest.	• Home setting may need to be altered to promote rest.

(continued)

Nursing Care Plan: The Child With Congestive Heart Failure Being Cared for at Home
(*continued*)

EXPECTED OUTCOME: Child will perform necessary activities and rest frequently each day.

5. Nursing Diagnosis: *Caregiver Role Strain* related to 24-hour responsibility for child's care (NANDA-I © 2014)

GOAL: Parents will express ability to meet own needs.

INTERVENTION	RATIONALE
• Assess family and community supports. Provide information related to respite care.	• Variable family and community supports are available.
• Encourage parents to seek activities to meet personal needs.	• Parents need time for own personal needs to successfully care for child.

EXPECTED OUTCOME: Parents will report some time away from the child and report renewal in caring for the child.

Dilated cardiomyopathy is the most common form, in which the four chambers dilate and systolic contraction is weakened. Clots may form as blood pools in the heart, increasing the child's risk for pulmonary or brain embolism. An estimated 20% to 35% have an inherited form with autosomal dominant, autosomal recessive, X-linked, or mitochondrial inheritance pattern (Park, 2014, p. 330). Other common causes are myocarditis, neuromuscular disease, such as muscular dystrophy, or other infections. The child usually presents with fatigue, weakness, and exertional dyspnea. Arrhythmias may develop that can cause cardiac arrest. The child is treated for CHF (diuretics, digoxin, and ACE inhibitors), including aspirin to reduce thromboembolisms, antiarrhythmic medications, and beta-adrenergic medications (e.g., carvedilol). Ultimately a heart transplant may be considered. Activity is restricted.

In hypertrophic cardiomyopathy, enlargement or hypertrophy of the left ventricle and the ventricular septum occurs, making the ventricular walls rigid. About 50% of hypertrophic cardiomyopathy cases are genetically transmitted as an autosomal dominant trait involving mutations on 1 of 10 genes (Park, 2014, p. 321). Myocardial cells become enlarged with some scarring, and coronary arteries may be affected. The outflow tract may become obstructed. Because the left ventricle is stiff, diastolic filling is affected, potentially causing enlargement of the left atrium and pulmonary venous congestion. Symptoms include exertional dyspnea, fatigue, dizziness, fainting, and angina-like chest pain. Palpitations may occur because of atrial or ventricular arrhythmia. It is the most common cause of sudden unexpected cardiac death in adolescents and young adult athletes (Park, 2014, p. 321). Treatment involves beta-adrenergic blockers (e.g., propranolol or metoprolol) or calcium channel blockers (e.g., verapamil). An implantable cardioverter/defibrillator or surgical myomectomy to relieve the obstruction may be considered. Strenuous exercise and competitive sports are prohibited.

Nursing Management

Nursing management for dilated cardiomyopathy is similar to that for children with CHF unless or until a heart transplant is performed. Nursing management for cardiomyopathy involves frequent visits to assess the child's condition and to review treatments.

Heart Transplantation

Approximately 450 heart transplants are performed on children and adolescents each year in the United States (Meaux et al., 2014). The number of donor hearts available for transplantation in children is limited. Ventricular assist devices are used in some pediatric centers to maintain function in other vital organs until a heart is available for transplant. In 2010, the median survival of infants receiving heart transplants was 18.3 years and for adolescents 11.3 years (Meaux et al., 2014). The primary reasons for heart transplantation in infants and children are cardiomyopathy and congenital heart disease. The number of adults with complex congenital heart defects who seek heart transplantation is increasing as survival through childhood has increased.

Acute rejection is a leading cause of early mortality after transplantation. Signs in infants and children are often nonspecific, including low-grade fever, increasing resting heart rate, fatigue, abdominal pain, nausea, vomiting, decreasing exercise tolerance, and irregular rhythm. Endomyocardial biopsy performed during cardiac catheterization is used to diagnose rejection and may be performed frequently. Research continues for identify biomarkers that can be used to diagnose and monitor rejection in children. The immunosuppression regimen usually includes calcineurin inhibitors (cyclosporin or tacrolimus), azathioprine or mycophenolate mofetil, and corticosteroids. Selecting the correct dosage for children is essential as too much increases the risks for infection, malignancy, and toxic effects, while too little increases the risk for rejection (Andrikopoulou & Mather, 2014).

Early deaths are due to graft failure or infection. Hyperlipidemia and blood vessel thickening in the transplanted heart are leading causes of death for long-term survivors. Statin medications are prescribed to control hyperlipidemia, and hypertension is treated with calcium channel blockers.

While bacterial, fungal, and viral (i.e., cytomegalovirus) infections are a cause of mortality, more common childhood illnesses (acute otitis, colds) may be well tolerated. Antibiotics and other new medications prescribed must be carefully considered because of potential interactions with immunosuppression medications.

Nursing Management

Depending on the age at time of transplant, the child may not have had all immunizations (see Chapter 43). Live virus vaccines should be given at least 1 month prior to the heart transplant, and are usually contraindicated following the transplant (AAP, 2015, pp. 84–86). Help parents arrange for schools and childcare centers to provide early notification of cases of measles, mumps, rubella, and chickenpox. Provide preventive treatment for the child as needed. Encourage good hand hygiene to reduce the spread of infection at home and at school.

After recovery from surgery, children may have near-normal exercise capabilities, normal heart function, and be able to return to school and other activities. Immunosuppressive medications will be continued long term and can cause a variety of physical side effects such as hirsutism, gum hyperplasia, weight gain, moon face, acne, rashes, and osteoporosis. Children and adolescents may need support to develop positive self-esteem.

Organ rejection is a major concern of families. Provide education for the parents and child about the need to adhere to the immunosuppression protocol and to keep appointments for evaluation. Adolescents need special attention to promote adherence to the immunosuppression protocol.

Pulmonary Artery Hypertension

Pulmonary artery hypertension (PAH) is a sustained increased pressure in the pulmonary artery. It is a complication of congenital heart defects that increases pulmonary blood flow, pulmonary conditions (e.g., meconium aspiration and acute respiratory distress syndrome in the newborn), and congenital diaphragmatic hernia.

Local mediators help the pulmonary vascular smooth muscles stay relaxed to allow blood to flow easily to the lungs. Excessive pulmonary blood flow, such as from a patent ductus arteriosus or ventricular septal defect, causes blood to backup in the lungs and pulmonary vascular constriction to decrease blood flow to the lungs. If excess pulmonary blood flow is not controlled, pulmonary vasoconstriction is maintained. Right ventricular hypertrophy develops to increase the pulmonary artery pressure and push blood across the constricted pulmonary vascular bed. Inflammation, hypertrophy of small pulmonary arteries, and fibrosis develop. The increased pressure leads to a right-to-left shunt, and right heart failure may occur. PAH may become progressive and irreversible.

The child has dyspnea with activity, retractions, fatigue, tachypnea, cyanosis with or without clubbing, diaphoresis, feeding difficulty, and avoidant/restrictive food intake disorder (failure to thrive). Cough with wheezing may occur. As right-sided heart failure occurs, signs of CHF develop. Older children also have distended neck veins, palpitations, chest pain, and syncope.

Cardiac catheterization is used to diagnose the severity of the condition. Therapy for pulmonary hypertension involves supplemental oxygen as needed. Surgery is used to treat the condition in cases of CHD that increases pulmonary blood flow. Treatments for other pulmonary conditions causing PAH, such as meconium aspiration and acute respiratory distress disorder, are initiated. Medications used to treat chronic PAH include calcium channel blockers, diuretics, and anticoagulants. Other medications used but still being tested for use in children include bosentan, ambrisentan, and sildenafil (Buck, 2013). No cure is available, but life can be prolonged with these measures.

Nursing Management

Nursing care in the community focuses on promoting rest for oxygen conservation, monitoring fluid intake and output carefully, and administering medications and oxygen. Airplane travel may be possible with supplemental oxygen. Exercise should be tailored to avoid dyspnea. Give parents needed support and information about their child.

Infective Endocarditis

Infective endocarditis is a potentially life-threatening but uncommon infection in an individual with endocardial cell damage. While it is a rare condition in children, it may be associated with a congenital heart defect (CHD), rheumatic heart disease, a central venous catheter, heart surgery, or intravenous drug abuse. Among children with a CHD, those with a bicuspid aortic valve, cyanotic lesion, or cardiac surgery within the prior 6 months are at greater risk for endocarditis (Leggiadro, 2014; Park, 2014, p. 343). The rate of endocarditis has increased, potentially because of the use of medical devices and hospital-acquired infections (Bor, Woolhandler, Nardin, et al., 2013).

The endocardium may be injured by a high-velocity or turbulent blood flow due to a heart defect or an indwelling catheter in the right side of the heart. Implanted vascular grafts, patches, prosthetic valves used during cardiac surgery, or implanted devices (e.g., for dialysis) may be a site of infection. Staphylococcal and streptococcal organisms are the most commonly reported bacteria causing endocarditis (Williams & Fagan, 2014). Infectious organisms introduced into the bloodstream by dental or medical procedures adhere to the injury site and colonize (See *Pathophysiology Illustrated: Infective Endocarditis*).

The onset is often slow with symptoms such as recurrent low-grade fever, fatigue, weakness, joint and muscle aches, loss of appetite, weight loss, and diaphoresis. Other signs may include a new heart murmur, or a change in intensity of an existing murmur, and splenomegaly. Petechiae, splinter

---

Pathophysiology Illustrated: **Infective Endocarditis**

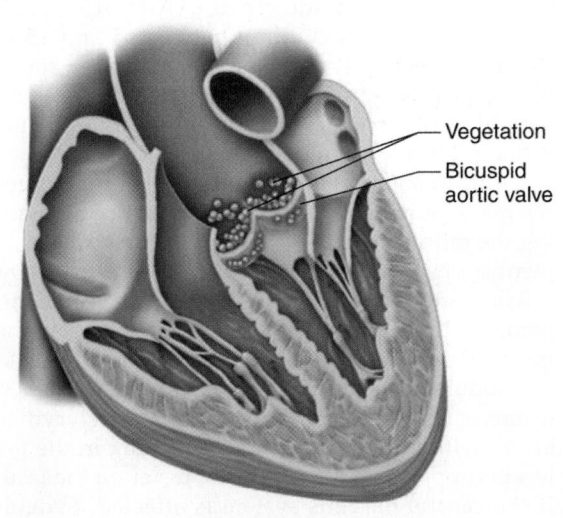

Vegetation

Bicuspid aortic valve

The endocardium is injured by high velocity blood flow through a stenotic valve, by turbulent blood flow across a septal defect, or by the positioning of a central venous catheter. Fibrin and platelets migrate to the site of the endothelial damage, becoming the foundation for nonbacterial thrombotic emboli where the infective organisms settle. In some cases, a vegetation forms near the site of the injury, as in this illustration around the aortic valve.

Medications Used for: Infective Endocarditis Prophylaxis for Dental and Invasive Respiratory Procedures

ANTIBIOTIC RECOMMENDATIONS	NURSING MANAGEMENT
Amoxicillin for oral use	• Give 1 large dose 30–60 min before procedures, or up to 2 hr after the procedure if preprocedure dose is missed.
Ampicillin for IM or IV use	• Teach parents and the child to keep at least 1 dose in the home for dental visits or emergencies.
If allergic to penicillin:	• Have parents inform each healthcare provider of the child's need for prophylaxis.
Cephalexin	
Clindamycin	
Azithromycin	
Clarithromycin	

Source: Data from American Academy of Pediatrics (AAP). (2015). *Red book: 2015 report of the Committee on Infectious Diseases* (30th ed., p. 971). Elk Grove Village, IL: Author; Sabe, M. A., Shrestha, N. K., & Menon, V. (2013). Contemporary drug treatment of infective endocarditis. *American Journal of Cardiovascular Drugs, 13,* 251–258; Park, M. K. (2014). *Pediatric cardiology for practitioners* (6th ed., p. 349). Philadelphia: Elsevier Saunders.

hemorrhages under nails, Roth spots (exudative lesions of the retina), Osler nodes (red, painful nonhemorrhagic nodules on the pads of the fingers and toes), and Janeway lesions (nontender, blanching macular lesions on the palms and soles) may be seen in adolescents (Park, 2014, pp. 343–344). Signs of CHF may be seen in some children. Those with indwelling catheters may initially have pulmonary signs related to septic pulmonary embolism.

The Duke criteria, a positive blood culture, echocardiographic findings, and clinical signs provide guidelines for diagnosis and management of infective endocarditis. The condition is most often diagnosed by transthoracic and transesophageal echocardiography, which reveals the site of infection, valve damage, and heart function. Blood culture identifies the infective organism.

Clinical therapy consists of intravenous antibiotics such as nafcillin, oxacillin, or methacillin and gentamycin initially until blood cultures reveal the specific organism. Vancomycin is used in some cases. Once the organism is identified, the antibiotics are changed and administered for a minimum of 4 to 6 weeks depending upon the infective organism. Surgery to replace an affected valve is performed in some children. The majority of children recover.

Prevention of infective endocarditis is preferred. Antibiotic prophylaxis is recommended for dental procedures and invasive respiratory procedures for selected individuals at highest risk for adverse outcomes from infective endocarditis (see the section on defects causing decreased pulmonary blood flow earlier in this chapter). See the accompanying *Medications Used for: Infective Endocarditis Prophylaxis for Dental and Invasive Respiratory Procedures*.

Nursing Management

Nursing care focuses on assessing the child's respiratory and cardiovascular status, administering medications, and teaching the parents about the child's care. Assess the child's vital signs, SpO_2, and level of consciousness because CHF and embolism may occur. The parents will be anxious about the child's condition, especially if this occurs following surgery for a congenital heart defect or in a critically ill child or newborn. Monitor the parents' coping skills and need for information.

Administer medications as prescribed and monitor serum antibiotic levels. Monitor for side effects of antibiotics and for infiltration at the infusion site. Keep invasive procedures to a

minimum. Use careful aseptic technique when managing central lines and venous access devices.

The child is often lethargic and on bed rest. Encourage parents to participate in the child's care and plan quiet age-appropriate activities. Home infusion therapy is often ordered so care can continue on an outpatient basis. Instruct parents about care procedures and reinforce the importance of follow-up visits. Home schooling may be needed during the recovery period.

Nursing care also focuses on prevention of endocarditis. Good oral hygiene and regular dental care are important preventive measures. Stress the importance of telling future healthcare providers, including dentists and surgeons, about the child's infective endocarditis history so prophylactic antibiotics can be given for invasive dental and respiratory procedures.

Acute Rheumatic Fever

Acute rheumatic fever (ARF) is an inflammatory disorder of connective tissue that results from an autoimmune response to some strains of group A beta-hemolytic streptococci (GAS). This disorder may cause long-term damage to heart valves, and affects the joints, brain, and skin tissues. While ARF is a significant health problem in developing countries, the incidence is very low in the United States and developed countries because GAS infections are treated earlier.

Only a small number of individuals infected with the strain of GAS that causes pharyngitis develop ARF, but specific serotypes have not been identified (AAP, 2015, p. 733). It occurs most commonly in children between 5 and 15 years old. A genetic susceptibility to the disease may exist, such as in Pacific Islanders, predisposing children to the disorder. An estimated 60% of patients with ARF develop rheumatic heart disease (Chang, 2012).

One to 3 weeks after an untreated streptococcal infection, the major or hallmark signs of ARF may occur. Carditis involving the mitral or aortic valve may be detected by the development of a new murmur. Chest pain may be caused by pericardial inflammation. Two or more large joints become inflamed with pain, swelling, tenderness, erythema, and heat. The signs may migrate from joint to joint (migratory polyarthritis). Subcutaneous nodules may be palpated over bony prominences and along extensor tendons. A nonpruritic skin rash (erythema marginatum) with pink macules and blanching in the middle of the lesions appears on the trunk, but never on the face and hands. If the central nervous system is affected, Sydenham chorea

(St. Vitus dance), characterized by aimless movements of the extremities and facial grimacing, is present.

Diagnosis is based on the Jones criteria, the presence of two or more of the major signs noted above and evidence of a recent streptococcal infection (e.g., a positive throat culture or an elevated or rising antistreptolysin-O titer of 333 Todd units). ARF is suspected when one major sign, evidence of a recent streptococcal infection and one or more minor signs (arthralgia, fever, elevated erythrocyte sedimentation rate or C-reactive protein, or a prolonged PR interval on electrocardiogram) are present (Park, 2014, p. 368). Echocardiography is used to diagnose subclinical signs of carditis that are not evident by auscultation (Gerwitz, Baltimore, Tani, et al., 2015).

Clinical therapy includes antibiotics (penicillin or erythromycin) to eradicate the streptococcal infection. Aspirin is used for fever, arthritis, and arthralgias. Corticosteroids are recommended in cases of severe carditis. Most children recover fully, but they are at risk for subsequent episodes of rheumatic fever. Children should be monitored carefully by echocardiogram for potential cardiac complications. Antibiotic prophylaxis (oral penicillin V or amoxicillin, or intramuscular benzathine penicillin G) is prescribed to children with ARF to reduce the risk for recurrent episodes until at least 21 years of age or 10 years after ARF (Park, 2014, p. 373). Persons allergic to penicillin are often prescribed azithromycin or clindamycin (Chang, 2012).

Nursing Management

An important role of the nurse is prevention of ARF. Nurses in clinics, offices, and schools need to ensure that all children with possible streptococcal infections obtain a rapid strep test or throat culture. Even if the sore throat is mild, testing is needed if family members or other contacts have had a streptococcal infection. Emphasize to the family the importance of giving all doses of the antibiotic prescribed when the test result is positive.

The child with ARF is hospitalized for a period of time. During the acute inflammatory phase, monitor temperature and vital signs at least every 4 hours. Auscultate the child's heart and note any unusual sounds. Observe the child for changes in skin, joints, or behavior. The child is on bed rest for several weeks if carditis is present, or only a week if arthritis is the major manifestation. Be sure family members obtain throat cultures to identify possible asymptomatic streptococcal carriers.

Administer antibiotics and aspirin as prescribed. The child is usually lethargic and often has joint pain. Aspirin often relieves pain dramatically after a few doses. Position and handle the child's joints carefully. Provide quiet activities, and encourage visits or telephone calls from family members and friends. Provide emotional support for the child with chorea; the purposeless involuntary movements are disturbing and can last for 5 to 15 weeks.

The child is generally cared for at home during the recovery phase. Activities may be limited, especially if heart damage is suspected. Help parents plan quiet activities, such as playing board games or computer games, watching videos, or reading. Arrange rest periods after the child returns to school. Reassure the child and parents that the effects of chorea will eventually subside.

After discharge, long-term antibiotic prophylaxis is initiated. Make sure the child and parents understand the importance of taking prescribed medication until adulthood to prevent recurrent rheumatic fever. Make sure the parents understand that the child's future sore throats may be streptococcal and a rapid strep test or throat culture should be obtained even when the child is taking daily antibiotics. The child may need a different antibiotic for the infection. Emphasize the importance of follow-up care to prevent new infections and to monitor heart function.

Kawasaki Disease

Kawasaki disease is an acute febrile, systemic vascular inflammatory disorder that affects small and midsize arteries, including the coronary arteries. It is the leading cause of acquired heart disease in children in the United States and leads to more than 5000 hospitalizations per year (O'Connell & Sloand, 2013). Children under 5 years of age account for 80% of cases, and 50% of cases occur in children under 2 years (AAP, 2015, p. 497). In the United States, Kawasaki disease has a higher incidence in children of Asian and Pacific Island origin (Park, 2014, p. 354).

ETIOLOGY AND PATHOPHYSIOLOGY

The etiology of Kawasaki disease is unknown. It is thought to be caused by or related to an infectious agent that has not yet been identified. The disorder appears to result in an exaggerated immune response to the infection in a genetically susceptible child. The inflammatory disease involves the small and midsize arteries and sometimes causes coronary artery aneurysms. Coronary artery abnormalities may occur within a week of fever onset (Rowley, 2012). Without treatment, up to 25% of children develop coronary artery aneurysms that can lead to a myocardial infarction (Park, 2014, p. 360).

CLINICAL MANIFESTATIONS

The three stages of the disease are acute, subacute, and convalescent:

- The acute stage of Kawasaki disease, lasting 1 to 2 weeks, is characterized by irritability, high fever that persists for more than 5 days, hyperemic conjunctivae, red throat, swollen hands and feet, maculopapular or erythema multiforme–like rash on the trunk and perineal area, unilateral enlargement of the cervical lymph nodes, diarrhea, and hepatic dysfunction.

- The subacute stage, lasting 2 or more weeks, is characterized by no fever, cracking lips and fissures, desquamation of the skin on the tips of the fingers and toes, joint pain, cardiac disease, and thrombocytosis (Figure 47–7).

- In the convalescent stage, 6 to 8 weeks after disease onset, the child appears normal but lingering signs of inflammation may be present. Deep transverse grooves (Beau lines) may appear across nails on the hands and feet.

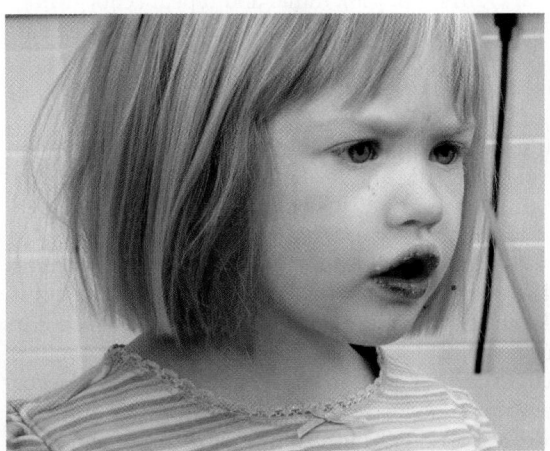

Figure 47–7 This child shows many of the signs of the subacute stage of Kawasaki disease: strawberry tongue, dry cracking lips, and buccal mucosa erythema.

TABLE 47–10 Diagnostic Criteria for Kawasaki Disease

Kawasaki disease is diagnosed when a high spiking fever over 39.0°C (102.2°F) for 5 days or longer is accompanied by four of the five principal features not explained by another disease process. When fewer than four criteria are present, but echocardiography or angiography reveals coronary artery abnormalities, Kawasaki disease is also diagnosed.

BODY PART AFFECTED	PRINCIPAL FEATURES
Eyes	Bilateral bulbar conjunctivitis without exudate
Skin	Intense erythema of the buccal and pharyngeal surfaces with dry, swollen, cracked, and fissuring lips and a strawberry tongue
	Erythema of the palms and soles, edema of the hands and feet, and then desquamation after 2 or more weeks of symptoms
	Dermatitis of the trunk with an erythematous maculopapular rash
Lymph nodes	Cervical lymphadenopathy, frequently unilateral, with a lymph node over 1.5 cm (0.60 in.) in diameter found early in the disease

Source: Data from McLellan, M. C., & Baker, A. L. (2011). At the heart of the fever: Kawasaki disease. *American Journal of Nursing, 111*(6), 57–63; Rowley, A. H. (2012). Kawasaki disease genetics, pathology, and need for earlier diagnosis and treatment. *Contemporary Pediatrics, 29*(12), 18–24; Park, M. K. (2014). *Pediatric cardiology for practitioners* (6th ed., pp 355–357). Philadelphia: Elsevier Saunders.

Other clinical manifestations may occur during the acute phase, such as arthralgias, abdominal pain with diarrhea, liver dysfunction, gallbladder hydrops, and aseptic meningitis. During the acute phase of Kawasaki disease, its signs and symptoms are commonly confused with other diseases.

CLINICAL THERAPY

Diagnosis is based on clinical signs using the criteria given in Table 47–10 because there is no specific diagnostic laboratory test. Blood studies may reveal elevations of the erythrocyte sedimentation rate, white blood cell count, C-reactive protein, platelet counts, bilirubin, alanine aminotransferase levels, and lipid levels (Park, 2014, pp. 356). Initial and repeat echocardiography is used to identify specific vascular changes in the heart and coronary arteries.

Kawasaki disease is treated with a single high dose (2 g/kg) IV infusion of immune globulin (IVIG) over 10 to 12 hours. Administering IVIG within 7 to 10 days of onset reduces the risk for coronary artery aneurysm. Some children receive IV diphenhydramine before IVIG to reduce the risk of allergic response. High doses of aspirin (80 to 100 mg/kg/day in 4 divided doses) are given for the high fever and to promote comfort. A lower aspirin dose (2 to 5 mg/kg once daily) is given once the child is afebrile for 2 to 3 days. Low-dose aspirin is continued to reduce clot formation until the platelet count is normal or longer term if coronary artery abnormalities occur. When the fever persists or returns within 36 hours after the first IVIG dose, a second IVIG infusion of 2 g/kg is given. If the second IVIG dose is not effective, corticosteroid therapy may be used. Infliximab, a monoclonal antibody, has been used in some U.S. children, but studies of its effectiveness have not yet been completed (Park, 2014, p. 360).

The duration of hospitalization depends on the presence of cardiac lesions and how long the fever persists. Most children recover fully, but they are monitored for cardiac disease for several months. Coronary aneurysms develop in 5% and giant aneurysms occur in 1% of children treated with IVIG, but about 50% to 67% of coronary artery aneurysms resolve within 2 years (Park, 2014, pp. 360–361). Some children with coronary artery involvement have a myocardial infarction, often within the first year after disease onset.

Nursing Management

Nursing care focuses on promoting comfort, monitoring for early signs of complications or disease progression, and supporting the family.

When the child is hospitalized, take the temperature every 4 hours and before each aspirin dose. Assess the extremities for edema, redness, and desquamation every 8 hours. Examine the eyes and the mucous membranes for inflammation. Monitor the child's dietary and fluid intake, and weigh the child daily. Carefully assess heart sounds and rhythm.

Administer aspirin and monitor for side effects such as bleeding and gastrointestinal upset. Administer IVIG as a blood product. Start the infusion rate at a rate of 0.5 mL/kg/hr for 30 minutes and gradually increase the rate to 2 mL/kg/hr. Carefully monitor the child and stop the infusion immediately if a reaction occurs (see Chapter 48).

Promote the child's comfort. Assess pain and provide analgesics and complementary therapies to manage pain. Keep the child's skin clean and dry, and lubricate the lips. Use cool compresses and tepid sponges to make the feverish child more comfortable. Change the child's clothes and bed linens frequently. Give the child frequent small feedings of soft foods and liquids that are neither too hot nor too cold.

Use passive range-of-motion exercises to facilitate joint movement. Because the child with Kawasaki disease is often lethargic and irritable, plan rest periods and quiet age-appropriate activities. Encourage the parents to participate in their child's care to promote comfort and reassure the child. Give the parents information about the disease and the child's treatment.

Before the child is discharged, teach the parents to administer aspirin as ordered and to watch for side effects. Have them measure the child's temperature daily for the first 2 weeks and record it on a log. Any fever above 38.3°C (101.0°F) should be reported to the healthcare provider. Advise the parents that the child needs to avoid contact sports or other activities that could cause bleeding when aspirin or warfarin is prescribed long term. The child who recovers without cardiovascular complications is encouraged to live an active lifestyle without exercise limitations. Limitation of strenuous activity is recommended for all children with coronary aneurysms or stenoses.

Emphasize the need for follow-up care to monitor for cardiac complications, hypertension, and hyperlipidemia. Postpone needed live virus vaccines (measles and varicella) for 11 months after IVIG administration, but other immunizations may be given on schedule.

Cardiac Arrhythmias

Cardiac **arrhythmias** (abnormal heart rhythms or dysrhythmias) occur frequently in children, but less often than in adults. Three categories of arrhythmias are tachyarrhythmias (sinus tachycardia), bradyarrhythmias (sinus bradycardia), and no pulse (ventricular tachycardia, ventricular fibrillation, pulseless electrical activity, or asystole). Less common arrhythmias are often associated with postoperative complications of congenital heart disease, Kawasaki disease with coronary artery involvement, rheumatic heart disease, cardiomyopathy, and electrolyte abnormalities. Arrhythmias may cause decreased cardiac output and CHF. More serious arrhythmias may result in syncope or sudden death.

BRADYCARDIA

Bradycardia is a heart rate less than the lower limit of normal for the child's age (usually a heart rate less than 80 in infants and less than 60 in children and adolescents). Some athletes may normally have a heart rate of 60. It is associated with beta-adrenergic medications and conditions such as hypothermia, hypoxia, hyperkalemia, and increased intracranial pressure. See Chapter 33 for normal heart rate ranges by age.

General symptoms of bradycardia include fatigue, exercise intolerance, dizziness, and syncope. The underlying cause is treated. Other treatment may include supplemental oxygen and medications (epinephrine, atropine, isoproterenol, glucagon). Chronic bradycardia may require a pacemaker.

SUPRAVENTRICULAR TACHYCARDIA

Supraventricular tachycardia (SVT), the most common pathologic tachycardia, is the abrupt onset of a rapid, regular heart rate, often too fast to count. The presenting heart rate with SVT will be greater than 220 beats/min in infants and greater than 180 beats/min in children. Potential causes include Wolff–Parkinson–White syndrome, congenital heart defects (e.g., single ventricle and corrected transposition of the great arteries), and postoperative cardiac surgery. Often no heart disease is present. Cardiac output is affected because diastolic filling cannot occur with such a rapid heart rate. Prolonged episodes of continuous SVT (more than 6 to 12 hours) can progress to CHF or cardiogenic shock if untreated.

Early signs in infants include poor feeding, irritability, and pallor. Older children may have palpitations, chest pain, dizziness, shortness of breath, decreased exercise tolerance, and syncope. Palpitations felt in the neck may be present. Recurrent attacks are common.

Treatments focus on reducing the heart rate. Initial steps involve vagal stimulation (applying ice-water bag to the face for 10 seconds or rectal stimulation with a thermometer) or having the child perform a Valsalva maneuver (e.g., holding the breath and straining, or blowing forcefully on the thumb to increase intrathoracic and venous pressures). Amiodarone by IV bolus is the preferred medication to lower the heart rate. Synchronized cardioversion is used for life-threatening episodes unresponsive to medications. Recurrent episodes of SVT are common, and propranolol, verapamil, or atenolol may be prescribed long term to reduce the frequency of episodes. **Radio-frequency ablation**, the use of radio energy (heat) to destroy a very small section of the myocardium through which an accessory conduction pathway passes, may be performed during cardiac catheterization.

LONG QT SYNDROME

Long QT syndrome (LQTS) is an inherited rhythm disturbance of ventricular tachycardia with a prolonged QT interval and abnormal T waves that puts children at risk for ventricular fibrillation and sudden death. Electrolyte disorders and certain drugs may trigger long QT arrhythmia in some children genetically predisposed to the disorder. In some children, arrhythmia is triggered by demanding physical exercise (e.g., swimming), a strong emotional reaction, or an abrupt loud noise (e.g., doorbell or alarm clock). In some genetic forms, the arrhythmia

more often occurs during rest or sleep. Arrhythmia may occur without warning and result in sudden death. Presenting signs include episodic dizziness, palpitations, syncope, seizure, or cardiac arrest.

Professionalism in Practice Sports Preparticipation Screening

The American Academy of Pediatrics recommends sports preparticipation screening to identify children and youth at risk for sudden cardiac death (American Academy of Pediatrics Section on Cardiology and Cardiac Surgery, 2012). Nurses can play an important role in identifying children and youth at risk by asking questions during the history for any child symptomatic of an arrhythmia or presenting for a physical assessment to play sports. Important questions include the following:

- Has the child passed out or had a seizure suddenly and without warning, either during exercise or in response to a loud noise (e.g., doorbell, alarm clock)?
- Has the child ever experienced chest pain or shortness of breath when exercising?
- Has any family member died suddenly and unexpectedly before age 50 years?
- Has any family member been diagnosed with an enlarged heart (cardiomyopathy) or rhythm disorder like long QT syndrome?

If the child is resuscitated or evaluated because of presenting signs or family history, the arrhythmia is commonly detected by electrocardiogram. The disorder is treated by beta-blockers (e.g., propranolol). A cardioverter/defibrillator (ICD) may be implanted in children and adolescents considered at high risk for sudden death. Do not permit the child to participate in competitive sports and supervise the child when swimming. Other triggers and medications that prolong the QT interval are avoided.

Nursing Management

Children with severe arrhythmias are treated in the emergency department or intensive care unit. The child is placed on a cardiac monitor and pulse oximeter. Frequently assess the vital signs and keep the healthcare provider informed about continuing abnormal rates or rhythms. Observe and record changes in level of consciousness, color, weakness, irritability, and feeding patterns. Administer medications as ordered. Have emergency drugs and resuscitation equipment available at the bedside. When sedation is ordered for invasive procedures such as synchronized cardioversion, follow the institution's guidelines for frequent assessment and intervention.

Episodes of arrhythmia and the potential for future episodes are frightening for both the child and parents. Provide written information about the danger signs indicating an arrhythmic episode and how to obtain emergency care. Educate the child and parents about the home treatment plan, including the importance of medication adherence that may prevent or reduce the frequency of episodes. Encourage parents to obtain cardiopulmonary resuscitation training. Help the child and family to avoid medications that can trigger another episode: for SVT, cardiac stimulant drugs such as decongestants; and for

LQTS, medications that prolong the QT interval (e.g., antihistamines, antidepressants, and macrolide antibiotics). An updated list of these medications can be found online. If the child has an ICD, parents need education about signs of defibrillation discharges (crying, grabbing chest, chest pain) and when to notify the healthcare provider.

Dyslipidemia

Dyslipidemia is an abnormal concentration of one or more lipids (total cholesterol, low-density lipoproteins [LDL], triglycerides, high-density lipoproteins [HDL]) in the blood. Children who have a genetic history or lifestyle that makes them more susceptible to future coronary heart disease (atherosclerosis) should be identified so preventive health measures can be implemented. A high LDL level, reduced HDL level, elevated blood pressure, type 1 or 2 diabetes mellitus, cigarette smoking, and obesity are major risk factors (National Heart Lung and Blood Institute [NHLBI], 2012).

Abnormalities in the lipid levels may be the result of excessive production, lack of clearance of the lipoprotein particles, a genetic defect in lipid metabolism, or other defects such as enzyme deficiencies. Some children have dyslipidemia due to genetic factors that cause abnormalities in lipid-metabolizing enzymes or abnormal cellular lipid receptors. Obesity is another leading cause of dyslipidemia. Examples of other causes include hypothyroidism, diabetes, nephritic syndrome, and certain drugs such as corticosteroids, beta-blockers, and isotretinoin (Brashers, 2014). More commonly, children have mild lipid abnormalities due to a combination of heredity and lifestyle factors. The child with dyslipidemia has no clinical manifestations of the condition.

A blood test for total cholesterol, HDL, and triglycerides identifies the condition. The LDL level is calculated from the triglyceride, HDL, and total cholesterol levels. See Table 47–11. Children between 2 and 8 years of age with the following risk factors should be screened for hyperlipidemia with a fasting lipid panel: a positive family history of dyslipidemia or cardiovascular disease (e.g., myocardial infarction, angina, stroke, coronary bypass surgery, or angioplasty) before 55 years in men or 65 years in women, parent with total cholesterol of 240 mg/dL or higher, or the child has cardiovascular risk factors (body mass index greater than 95th percentile, hypertension, cigarette smoking, diabetes mellitus, or a condition that causes secondary dyslipidemia). All children should have lipid screening once between 9 and 11 years of age and again between 17 and 21 years of age (NHLBI, 2012).

The primary management of dyslipidemia in most children includes dietary modifications, exercise, and other changes in lifestyle. The child's diet is carefully analyzed and changes are made to satisfy the dietary guidelines so that saturated fats are less than 7% and monosaturated fats are 20% of total caloric intake, cholesterol intake is less than 200 mg/day for treatment of elevated LDL levels, and trans fats are avoided (NHLBI, 2012). A healthy total fat intake is 20% to 35% of daily calories. High dietary fiber is encouraged. If the child is obese, weight loss is encouraged.

If a child age 10 years or older continues to have high serum lipid levels after dietary changes and increased physical activity, medications may be prescribed. Cholestyramine or colestipol, which bind bile acid in the intestine, niacin, statins, and fish oil may be prescribed. The goal is to lower LDL concentration to less than 130 mg/dL or a 50% level reduction (Giddings, 2012). Children and adolescents taking statins should have periodic creatine kinase and liver transaminase monitoring.

TABLE 47–11 Laboratory Values for Assessment of Dyslipidemia in Children Between 2 and 19 Years Old

TEST	RECOMMENDED LEVEL	LEVELS OF HIGHER RISK
Total cholesterol	Under 170 mg/dL	Borderline: 170–199 mg/dL
		Abnormal: 200 mg/dL or higher
LDL-C	Under 110 mg/dL	Borderline: 110–129 mg/dL
		Abnormal: 130 mg/dL or higher
Triglyceride 0–9 years	Under 75 mg/dL	Borderline: 75–99 mg/dL
		Abnormal: 100 mg/dL or higher
10–19 years	Under 90 mg/dL	Borderline: 90–129 mg/dL
		Abnormal: 130 mg/dL or higher
HDL-C	45 mg/dL or higher	Borderline: 40–45 mg/dL
		Abnormal: Under 40 mg/dL

Source: Adapted from National Heart Lung and Blood Institute (NHLBI). (2012). *Expert panel on integrated guidelines for cardiovascular health and risk reduction in children and adolescents*. Retrieved from http://www.nhlbi.nih.gov/guidelines/cvd_ped/index.htm

Nursing Management

Nursing care focuses on identifying children at risk for dyslipidemia, providing education about diet and exercise, and monitoring eating patterns. Identification and management of dyslipidemia takes place in many community settings. Office and clinic nurses identify children who need to have serum lipid measured. Nurses in schools provide education on ways to reduce risk factors. The child's history of exercise patterns, weight percentile, and dietary intake provides important information. Obtain information on familial heart disease, hypertension, diabetes, and smoking to determine risk factors.

Work with nutritionists to provide dietary teaching and monitor family eating patterns. The food plan for the child and entire family should consist primarily of fruit, vegetables, whole grain breads and cereals, low-fat and nonfat dairy products, lean meat and fish, legumes, and nuts. Processed foods, juices, sugar-sweetened drinks, and simple carbohydrates (foods with sugar and white flour) should be limited. Help parents understand that modeling food choices helps children learn to select and eat better food choices and reduce lipid levels. For children with familial hypercholesterolemia, lifelong dietary management is essential.

Healthy People 2020

(NWS-18) Reduce consumption of saturated fat in the population aged 2 years and older

Help the child select an enjoyable moderate to intense activity for daily participation, and then perform 30 minutes of aerobic exercise (e.g., jogging, swimming, biking, roller blading, soccer) at least 3 to 4 times a week to promote cardiovascular fitness. Discourage smoking by the child or the parents to reduce the risk for cardiovascular disease.

Educate children and adolescents taking statin medications to report any adverse effects to their healthcare provider: myalgia, muscle soreness, weakness, tenderness, or dark-colored urine. Include the entire family in the treatment plan; it is difficult for a single family member to change eating and exercise patterns.

Hypertension

Hypertension in children and adolescents is defined as a systolic or diastolic blood pressure reading that is equal to or greater than 95th percentile for age, gender, and height percentile. Normal blood pressure is defined as a systolic or diastolic reading that falls below the 90th percentile for age, gender, and height percentile. An estimated 3% to 5% of children and adolescents have hypertension (Hylick, Grubbs, Johnson, et al., 2014). Detection during childhood is important as it is a major risk factor for heart disease and stroke during adulthood.

Healthy People 2020

(HDS-5) Reduce the proportion of persons in the population with hypertension

---

Primary hypertension occurs in about 5% of the pediatric population and is related to the increasing rate of obesity in children (Dennison, 2012). The most common causes of secondary hypertension in children include coarctation of the aorta, renal disorders, neurofibromatosis, obstructive sleep apnea, and endocrine disorders (Daniels, 2013).

Because children rarely have symptoms of hypertension, the condition is detected during a health examination. Symptoms of severe hypertension may include headaches, epistaxis, dizziness, and visual changes.

CLINICAL THERAPY

Hypertension is diagnosed after three or more separate blood pressure readings a week apart or ambulatory blood pressure monitoring shows systolic or diastolic readings at the 95th percentile or higher for gender, age, and height. Initial evaluation includes a urinalysis, serum creatinine, electrolyte levels, blood urea nitrogen, and a complete blood count. A urine culture and renal ultrasound are performed if an initial test is positive. Serum lipid studies, fasting glucose, and serum insulin are obtained to identify dyslipidemia or diabetes. Other potential testing may include thyroid and adrenal hormone levels to identify hyperthyroidism and an echocardiogram to assess for coarctation of the aorta or left ventricular hypertrophy. Polysomnography may be performed to identify a sleep disorder.

Developing Cultural Competence **Blood Pressure**

A recent study investigated the blood pressure readings of 199,513 children between 3 and 17 years of age along with height, weight, and body mass index (BMI). The sample was well represented by the following racial and ethnic groups: White, Black, Asian, and Hispanic. The rate of prehypertension (90th to less than 95th percentile) was 12.7%, while 5.4% were in the hypertension range (95th percentile or greater). The highest prevalence of hypertension was found among the Black and Asian children in the study (Lo et al., 2013).

Nonpharmacologic measures for reduction of blood pressure include weight reduction and increased exercise (30 to 60 minutes a day). The Dietary Approaches to Stop Hypertension (DASH) diet is recommended for children and adolescents with elevated blood pressure. It is low in sodium and encourages fruits, vegetables, low-fat or fat-free dairy products, whole grains, fish, poultry, beans, seeds, and nuts (NHLBI, 2012). Discourage the child from smoking and the use of alcohol or drugs.

Medications are used for children with persistent, severe hypertension that is not resolved with dietary changes and exercise. Medications prescribed may include diuretics, beta-blocking agents, angiotensin-converting enzyme (ACE) inhibitors, angiotensin receptor blockers (ARB), and calcium channel blockers (Daniels, 2013).

Nursing Management

Children should have their blood pressure measured annually beginning at 3 years of age. Take a complete history for the child with persistent high blood pressure to identify potential risk factors such as family history for hypertension, smoking, or a systemic disease. Is the child obese? Assess the diet for salt intake and servings of fruits and dairy products eaten daily. What are the child's daily exercise routines? Review any medications or other potential agents used by the child or adolescent.

Assess the child's blood pressure and consistently use the right arm and an appropriately sized cuff (see the *Clinical Skills Manual* SKILLS). Compare the leg blood pressure to that in the arm. Compare readings to the blood pressure values for gender, age, and height percentile (see Appendix D). Monitor the child with borderline hypertension every 3 to 6 months. Take at least two readings during the visit and average them if they differ.

Teach both the child and the parents how to improve the diet and develop exercise routines. Provide suggestions about seasoning substitutes for salt and a list of salty foods to avoid. Increasing intake of low-fat dairy products and fruits can contribute to blood pressure control.

Discuss ways to increase activity and reduce time watching television or playing computer games. Provide suggestions for the management of stress and stressful situations. Emphasize the need to avoiding smoking, alcohol, and drugs. Teaching that involves the entire family is usually the most effective. Instruct the family on correct administration of prescribed medications when used.

Injuries of the Cardiovascular System

Shock

Shock is an acute, complex state of circulatory dysfunction resulting in failure to deliver sufficient oxygen and other nutrients to cells and tissues. It can be caused by a variety of conditions such as hemorrhage, dehydration, sepsis, obstruction of blood flow, and cardiac pump failure.

Hypovolemic Shock

Hypovolemic shock is a clinical state of inadequate tissue and organ perfusion resulting from inadequate blood or plasma volume in the vascular space (see *Pathophysiology Illustrated: Hypovolemic Shock*). The blood or plasma in the vascular space may be decreased because of hemorrhage or fluid movement into the interstitial spaces.

Pathophysiology Illustrated: **Hypovolemic Shock**

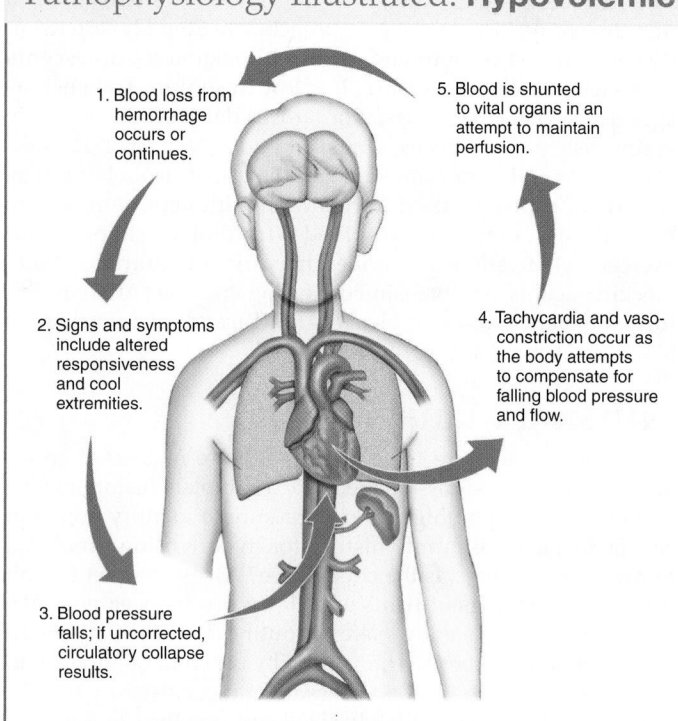

1. Blood loss from hemorrhage occurs or continues.

2. Signs and symptoms include altered responsiveness and cool extremities.

3. Blood pressure falls; if uncorrected, circulatory collapse results.

4. Tachycardia and vaso-constriction occur as the body attempts to compensate for falling blood pressure and flow.

5. Blood is shunted to vital organs in an attempt to maintain perfusion.

If hemorrhage reduces the circulating blood volume, the body compensates by increasing the heart rate and constricting the peripheral blood vessels. This allows the remaining blood to be circulated to the vital organs. When blood loss exceeds 20% to 25%, the child's body can no longer compensate; blood pressure falls, and circulatory collapse is imminent.

ETIOLOGY AND PATHOPHYSIOLOGY

Major causes of decreased intravascular blood volume include the following:

- Hemorrhage from significant injury
- Plasma loss from burns, nephrotic syndrome, and sepsis
- Fluid and electrolyte loss associated with dehydration, diabetic ketoacidosis, and diabetes insipidus

Decreased blood volume results in inadequate delivery of oxygen and nutrients to cells and accumulation of toxic wastes in the capillaries. Less blood returns to the heart to fill the ventricles, resulting in a lower stroke volume. Decreased cardiac output and mean arterial pressure then occur. The kidneys receive less blood, leading to decreased ability to filter toxins. Cellular hypoxia (reduced oxygenation of the tissues) and acidosis develop simultaneously. The accumulation of toxins and inadequate tissue oxygenation cause cellular damage.

When the child's brain senses inadequate oxygen, adrenergic and renal mechanisms help compensate:

- Catecholamine and cortisol levels rise to increase the heart rate, blood pressure, and heart muscle contractions to improve cardiac output.
- The renin–angiotensin–aldosterone system works to retain sodium and fluid in the vascular space when kidney perfusion is decreased.
- Antidiuretic hormone is secreted when the atria have reduced blood volume leading to water retention.
- Glucagon is released to provide energy for life-preserving functions.
- An increased respiratory rate improves oxygenation and decreases waste accumulation in the cells.
- The hydrostatic pressure falls, permitting fluid to shift into the vascular space and increase circulating blood volume.

- Peripheral vessels constrict to maintain systemic vascular resistance and increase perfusion to vital organs as long as possible.

When the child can no longer compensate (20% to 25% of volume loss), hypotension results. Life-threatening end-organ failure occurs without immediate therapy.

CLINICAL MANIFESTATIONS

Signs of early hypovolemic shock in children are nonspecific as the child is compensating for decreased blood volume. The blood pressure may be normal for age. The child has sustained tachycardia (usually higher than 130 beats per minute), increased respiratory effort, delayed capillary refill (greater than 2 seconds), weak peripheral pulses, pallor, and cold extremities (signs of decreased perfusion). Urine output decreases (to less than 0.5 to 1 mL/kg/hr in infants and young children) when renal blood flow drops. In cases of dehydration, dry mucous membranes and poor skin turgor are also present. See Table 47–12.

CLINICAL THERAPY

Clinical signs are used to diagnose the condition as no laboratory tests detect the blood volume deficit quickly enough. After hypovolemic shock is diagnosed or suspected, treatment is initiated. The hematocrit and hemoglobin, arterial blood gases, serum electrolytes, glucose, osmolality, blood urea nitrogen, and urinalysis are obtained during initial care.

Emergency care focuses on improving tissue perfusion. An open airway is established, oxygen is administered, and ventilation is assisted if necessary. Bleeding is controlled, and an IV or intraosseous line is inserted to provide large volumes of crystalloid fluids (normal saline or lactated Ringer). A fluid bolus of 20 mL/kg is administered rapidly over 5 minutes. The same amount of fluid is given in 5 minutes if the child's physiologic condition does not improve after the first fluid bolus. When the child is injured and no improvement is seen after the second

TABLE 47–12 Clinical Manifestations of Hypovolemic Shock

SYSTEM	EARLY COMPENSATED SHOCK	MODERATE UNCOMPENSATED SHOCK	SEVERE UNCOMPENSATED SHOCK
Cardiac	Mild tachycardia, weak distal pulses, strong central pulses, normal blood pressure	Moderate tachycardia, thready distal pulses, weak central pulses, decreasing systolic blood pressure	Extreme tachycardia, hypotension, narrow pulse pressure, absent distal pulses, thready central pulses
Respiratory	Mild tachypnea	Moderate tachypnea	Severe tachypnea
Neurologic	Normal, anxious, irritable, or combative behavior	Confusion, agitation, combativeness, lethargy, decreased pain response	Comatose state
Skin	Mottled appearance; capillary refill time greater than 2 sec; cool, clammy extremities	Pallor; capillary refill time greater than 3 sec; cold, dry extremities; sunken eyes	Pale, cold skin; cyanosis; capillary refill greater than 5 sec
Renal	Decreased urine output; increased specific gravity in older infants and children (newborns cannot concentrate urine)	Oliguria; increased specific gravity	No urine output

Source: Data from Chamiedes, L., Samson, R. A., Schexnadyer, S. M., & Hazinski, M. F. (Eds.). (2011). *Pediatric advanced life support* (p. 97). Dallas, TX: American Heart Association; Hazinski, M. F., Mondozzi, M. A., & Baker, R. A. U. (2014). Shock, multiple organ dysfunction syndrome, and burns in children. In K. L. McCance, S. E. Huether, V. L. Brashers, & N. R. Rote (Eds.), *Pathophysiology: The biologic basis for disease in adults and children* (7th ed., pp. 1699–1727). St. Louis, MO: Mosby Elsevier; Steffen, K. M. (2011). Trauma, burns, and common critical care emergencies. In M. M. Tschudy & K. M. Arcara (Eds.), *The Harriet Lane handbook* (19th ed., p. 109), Philadelphia, PA: Elsevier Mosby.

fluid bolus, blood is often administered. Once the child's physiologic condition is stabilized, the cause of the hypovolemic shock becomes the focus of examination and treatment.

Nursing Management

For the Child With Hypovolemic Shock

Nursing Assessment and Diagnosis

Ask the parent (or child, if appropriate) about possible injuries or the duration and severity of acute illnesses. If no external bleeding is evident, determine whether an injury may be causing internal bleeding. For example, the liver and spleen are highly vascular organs and if injured could bleed enough to cause hypovolemic shock without evidence of bleeding. An acute illness such as gastroenteritis with prolonged vomiting and diarrhea can also result in dehydration and hypovolemic shock.

If external bleeding is apparent, determine the amount of blood lost. Although children lose the same amount of blood from a laceration as adults, the total volume of blood lost is proportional to their weight.

Growth and Development

The child's total blood volume varies by weight. The child has approximately 80 mL of blood for every kilogram of body weight.

- Newborn: 3 kg × 80 mL = 240 mL (1 cup)
- 5-year-old child: 25 kg × 80 mL = 2000 mL (2 quarts)
- 13-year-old child: 50 kg × 80 mL = 4000 mL (1 gallon)

Frequently assess the child's heart rate, respiratory rate, blood pressure, capillary refill time, level of consciousness with the Glasgow Coma Scale (see Chapter 54), color, and skin temperature to identify any changes that indicate improvement or deterioration in the child's condition. Monitor urine output and specific gravity hourly. Signs of the child's improved status include:

- A decrease in heart rate, respiratory rate, and capillary refill time
- An increase in systolic blood pressure and urine output

- Improved color, level of consciousness, and skin temperature
- Regaining of lost weight

Assess the parents' response and coping mechanisms to the child's potentially life-threatening injury. Families are unprepared for the abrupt change in the child's condition because of the unpredictability of the injury. See Chapter 41.

Examples of nursing diagnoses that may apply to the child with hypovolemic shock include (NANDA-I © 2014):

- *Cardiac Output, Decreased*, related to hypovolemia
- *Fluid Volume: Deficient* related to active fluid volume loss
- *Tissue Perfusion: Peripheral, Ineffective*, related to impaired transport of oxygen across alveolar and capillary membrane
- *Coping: Family, Compromised*, related to life-threatening condition of the child

Planning and Implementation

Nurses in the emergency department, operating room, and intensive care unit more commonly participate in the resuscitation of the child in hypovolemic shock, often using guidelines or protocols for nursing actions. Assist with the child's assessment and establish IV access. Calculate and prepare the amount of IV fluid needed for the child's weight (20 mL/kg). The IV fluid is often warmed because hypothermia interferes with the child's response to treatment. Ensure rapid fluid administration by IV push or pressure bag. Monitor the child's physiologic response to the fluid bolus within 5 minutes. Prepare a second and third fluid bolus. Keep the child covered or use heat lamps to reduce body-heat loss.

When packed red blood cells are administered, verify that the correct blood has been obtained for the child. Ensure that the IV fluid is normal saline to prevent clotting during blood administration (see the *Clinical Skills Manual* SKILLS). Assess the child carefully for a transfusion reaction (see Chapter 49). Monitor the child's physiologic circulatory responses for improvement or deterioration in status. Notify the healthcare provider of any deterioration.

Parents and children with hypovolemic shock resulting from injury are usually apprehensive. The child may be fearful because of the sudden hospitalization or agitated because of

Pathophysiology Illustrated: **Obstructive Shock Due to Mediastinal Shift**

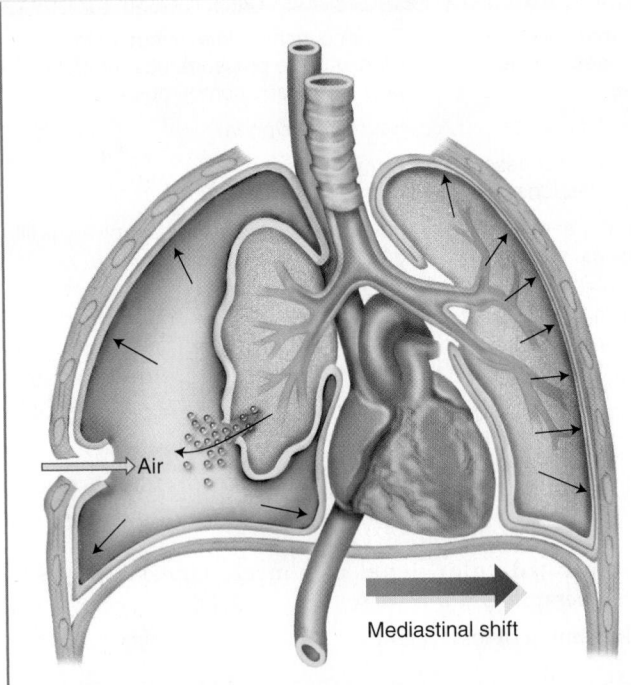

Mediastinal shift

Obstructive shock can occur when a tension pneumothorax obstructs blood flow to and from the heart (see Chapter 46). Here, the great vessels are compressed during the mediastinal shift, obstructing blood return to the heart.

an altered level of consciousness. Because parents often fear for the child's life in cases of severe injury, update them about the child's condition frequently. Provide support and explain the care being provided and how it helps the child. Listen to their concerns and correct any misconceptions.

Evaluation

Examples of expected nursing care outcomes include the following:

- The child receives adequate fluid resuscitation or blood to prevent progression to severe uncompensated shock.
- The family copes with the stress of the child's injury.

Distributive Shock

Distributive shock is an abnormal distribution of blood volume, usually resulting from a decrease in systemic vascular resistance. The blood accumulates in the extremities because of vasodilation and capillary permeability. Less blood is returned to the heart, so **preload** (amount of blood in the ventricle at the end of diastole that stretches the heart muscle before contraction) drops and cardiac output falls. Blood flow is inadequate to all tissue beds. Causes of distributive shock include anaphylaxis, sepsis, and spinal cord injury. See Chapter 43 for a discussion of sepsis and septic shock.

Nursing Management

The child with distributive shock is cared for in the intensive care unit. Nursing care focuses on detecting and managing subtle changes in the child's physiologic status to improve the child's condition. Parents are supported as described in Chapter 41.

Obstructive Shock

Obstructive shock occurs from a mechanical blockage of blood flow into and through the heart and great vessels (see *Pathophysiology Illustrated: Obstructive Shock Due to Mediastinal Shift*). Causes in children include compression of the vena cava, pericardial tamponade, pulmonary embolism, tension pneumothorax, pleural effusion, and congenital heart defects with outflow obstruction (e.g., severe aortic stenosis, coarctation of the aorta). Management is focused on treatment of the underlying condition to relieve the obstruction.

Nursing Management

The child is usually cared for in the intensive care unit with nursing care focused on supporting the child's respiratory and cardiovascular functioning. See Chapter 46 for care of the child with a tension pneumothorax.

Cardiogenic Shock

Cardiogenic shock is an impairment of myocardial function that causes low cardiac output and poor tissue perfusion even though blood volume is adequate. Causes of cardiogenic shock in children may include pump failure, severe obstructive congenital heart disease such as hypoplastic left heart syndrome, cardiomyopathy, myocarditis, severe electrolyte or acid–base imbalance, a complication of shock, and early septic shock (Hazinski, Mondozzi, & Baker, 2014).

Compensatory responses divert blood to the heart and brain; however, reduced blood flow to the kidneys, liver, and intestines can lead to ischemia and end-organ failure. Increased systemic vascular resistance puts more stress on the failing heart. Each contraction causes more blood to accumulate in the heart and pulmonary vessels, eventually leading to CHF, metabolic acidosis, and circulatory collapse.

Clinically, cardiogenic shock resembles hypovolemic shock with low cardiac output. Tachycardia, tachypnea, decreased oxygen saturation, hypotension, diminished peripheral pulses, and cool, mottled extremities are common signs. Disorientation and restlessness occur as the compensatory mechanisms fail. Signs of respiratory distress associated with CHF and pulmonary edema are often present.

An enlarged heart and pulmonary congestion may be seen on a chest radiograph. The goals of medical treatment are rapid restoration of myocardial function. Diuretics and vasodilators are given along with adequate ventilatory support, sedatives, analgesics, and antipyretics. Inotropic agents may be used in some cases.

Nursing Management

The child will be cared for in the intensive care unit. Nursing care focuses on monitoring and supporting the respiratory and cardiovascular status, fluid management, and medication administration. See Chapter 41 for care of the child with a life-threatening condition.

Myocardial Contusion

Myocardial contusion, a rare injury in children, results from a strong, blunt force against the chest wall that injures the heart muscle in the right ventricle. Blood flow to areas of the heart muscle is disrupted, or myocardial cells are directly destroyed. This potentially life-threatening condition most often occurs with striking the steering wheel of a motor vehicle during a crash, a crush injury, or a fall.

A myocardial contusion should be suspected in cases of injury to the anterior chest. The child has chest wall tenderness or pain because of fractured ribs or chest wall contusion. An electrocardiogram reveals arrhythmias or signs of myocardial infarct. A two-dimensional echocardiogram may show an abnormality in heart wall movement. Cardiac troponin I levels may be elevated.

Because of the risk of sudden arrhythmias, the child is admitted to the intensive care unit for cardiac monitoring.

Commotio Cordis

Commotio cordis, also known as a cardiac concussion, is a blunt, nonpenetrating blow to the precordium that causes ventricular fibrillation and sudden death. The majority of victims are healthy children and youth without an underlying cardiovascular disease participating in sports such as baseball, softball, ice hockey, and lacrosse. In some cases, the event is triggered by physical contact with another person, such as a fist, elbow, knee, or head. The impact timing on the precordium is believed to coincide with the period of vulnerable cardiac repolarization.

The most common arrhythmias recorded after the victim's collapse include ventricular fibrillation and ventricular tachycardia. Survival improves if prompt cardiopulmonary resuscitation or defibrillation is provided.

Nursing Management

The role of the nurse is to implement rapid cardiopulmonary resuscitation and to facilitate defibrillation. Nursing care is then focused on monitoring for cardiac arrhythmias, often in the intensive care unit.

Focus Your Study

- Congenital heart defects occur in approximately 1% of all live births, making them the most common birth defect.

- Infants and children under 5 years of age increase their cardiac output by increasing the heart rate. After that age, the muscle fibers in the myocardium are developed enough to stretch and increase stroke volume.

- Most congenital heart defects develop during the first 8 weeks of gestation, often the result of genetic and environmental factors.

- Congenital heart defects are categorized by pathophysiology and hemodynamics:

  - Defects that increase pulmonary blood flow include the following: patent ductus arteriosus, atrial septal defect, ventricular septal defect, and atrioventricular canal.

  - Defects that decrease pulmonary blood flow include the following: pulmonic stenosis, tetraology of Fallot, pulmonary atresia, and tricuspid atresia.

  - Defects that decrease systemic blood flow include the following: aortic stenosis, coarctation of the aorta, and hypoplastic left heart syndrome.

- Transposition of the great arteries and truncus arteriosus are examples of mixed defects that require mixing of the pulmonary and systemic circulations for survival during the neonatal period.

- Cardiac catheterization is more commonly used in children to intervene or repair some heart defects rather than to evaluate the hemodynamics and pressure gradients within the heart.

- Infants with congenital heart defects that increase pulmonary blood flow are at high risk for development of congestive heart failure.

- The child with a congenital heart defect that decreases pulmonary blood flow may have life-threatening hypoxic episodes requiring emergency treatment.

- Congenital heart defects that obstruct systemic blood flow cause signs and symptoms associated with low cardiac output: diminished pulses, poor color, prolonged capillary refill time, and decreased urinary output.

- Infants are at risk of heart failure as they are more sensitive to volume or pressure overload.

- Signs of congestive heart failure may include tachypnea, tachycardia, pallor or cyanosis, nasal flaring, grunting, retractions, cough, crackles, periorbital and facial edema, jugular vein distention, and hepatomegaly.

- Cardiomyopathy during childhood occurs most often in infancy and adolescence.

- Heart transplantation is performed in infants and children for complex heart defects or cardiomyopathy. Rejection and infection are the major causes of mortality and morbidity during the first year following the transplant.

- Pulmonary artery hypertension is a life-threatening complication of congenital heart disease with excessive pulmonary blood flow. Irreversible pulmonary vascular changes include inflammation, hypertrophy of pulmonary vessels, and fibrosis.

- Infective endocarditis is a risk for children who have some congenital heart defects, following heart surgery with patching or artificial valves, rheumatic heart disease, or a central venous catheter. Not all cases of infective endocarditis are preventable.

- Rheumatic fever is an inflammatory connective tissue disease following a streptococcal infection that may affect the heart, joints, skin, or central nervous system.

- Kawasaki disease is an acute febrile, systemic inflammatory illness with an unknown etiology. Coronary artery inflammation or aneurysms may be a significant complication.

- Two potentially life-threatening cardiac arrhythmias are supraventricular tachycardia and long QT syndrome.

- Some children have familial or lifestyle-related dyslipidemia that causes undesirable levels of cholesterol or triglycerides. These children need dietary intervention and exercise regimens as initial therapies.

- All children with systolic or diastolic blood pressure at the 95th percentile for age, gender, and height percentile have hypertension.

- Hypovolemic shock is an acute, complex state of circulatory dysfunction resulting in failure to deliver sufficient oxygen and other nutrients to meet cell and tissue demands.

- Signs that a child is in compensated hypovolemic shock include tachycardia, increased respiratory effort, prolonged capillary refill time, weak peripheral pulses, pallor, and cold extremities.

- Distributive shock is an abnormal distribution of the blood volume that results from a decrease in vascular resistance. It may be caused by anaphylaxis, sepsis, or spinal cord injury.

- Obstructive shock occurs when circulation is impeded by conditions such as compression on the vena cava due to tension pneumothorax, aortic stenosis, or coarctation of the aorta.

- Myocardial contusion results from a strong, blunt force against the chest wall that injures the heart muscle and causes an arrhythmia.

Clinical Reasoning in Action

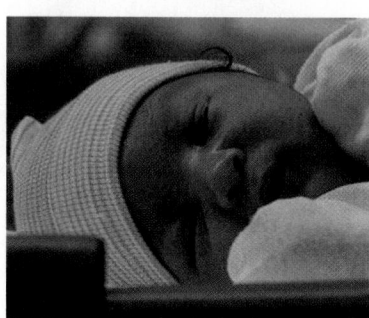

You are working in the hospital when Samantha, a 2-day-old newborn, is diagnosed with a continuous, systolic, grade 3 heart murmur in the pulmonic area of the chest. This is the parents' first child and they are extremely worried about their 6-week-premature baby. Samantha has full, bounding pulses and weighed 5 lb 6 oz at birth, but has lost 3 oz in the past 2 days. The mother's pregnancy was healthy until her water broke suddenly. The day after Samantha was born, the parents were told about the heart murmur. After an echocardiogram and chest radiograph are performed, Samantha is diagnosed with a patent ductus arteriosus (PDA). The healthcare provider prescribes 3 doses of a medication to aid in the closure of the duct.

You explain that her vital signs and urine output will need to be monitored closely for decreases while she is on this medicine.

Several days later, the heart murmur is still heard; the medicine did not work. The parents want to avoid surgery if possible and the doctor explains that if the ductus closes by the time she is 9 to 12 months old, and she is without symptoms, surgery could be avoided. If the PDA is not corrected, her life span will be shortened. She is discharged from the hospital, thriving and breastfeeding well. The parents are educated to observe for poor weight gain, swelling, intercostal retractions, and breathing more than 60 times per minute. A follow-up appointment is made for 1 week later.

1. How would you explain a PDA to the parents?
2. What was the most likely cause of Samantha's initial weight loss? Is it the PDA that caused the weight loss?
3. What is the physiologic reason Samantha's life span would be shortened if the PDA does not close or get surgical correction?
4. How would you describe congestive heart failure to the parents?

References

American Academy of Pediatrics (AAP). (2015). *Red book: 2015 report of the Committee on Infectious Disease* (30th ed.). Elk Grove Village, IL: Author.

American Academy of Pediatrics Section on Cardiology and Cardiac Surgery. (2012). Pediatric sudden cardiac arrest. *Pediatrics, 129*(4), e1094–e1102.

Andrikopoulou, E., & Mather, P. J. (2014). Current insights: use of Immuknow in heart transplant recipients. *Progress in Transplantation, 24*(1), 44–50.

Association of Maternal and Child Health Programs. (2013). *Issue brief: State newborn screening and birth defects program role in screening for critical congenital heart defects (CCHD).* Retrieved from http://www.amchp.org/programsandtopics/CHILD-HEALTH/projects/newborn-screening/Documents/AMCHP_Screening_for_CCHD_Issue_Brief_FINAL-Oct2013.pdf

Awad, S. M. M., & Busse, J. (2011). Hypoplastic left heart syndrome. In R. Abdulla (Ed.), *Heart disease*

in children (pp. 273–282). New York, NY: Springer.

Bor, D. H., Woolhandler, S., Nardin, R., Brusch, J., & Himmelstein, D. U. (2013). Infective endocarditis in the U.S., 1998–2009: A nationwide study. *PLOS One, 8*(3), e60033.

Brashers, V. L. (2014). Alterations in cardiovascular function. In K. L. McCance, S. E. Huether, V. L. Brashers, & N. R. Rote (Eds.), *Pathophysiology: The biologic basis for disease in adults and children* (7th ed., pp. 1129–1193). St. Louis, MO: Elsevier Mosby.

Buck, M. (2013). Update on therapies for pulmonary arterial hypertension in children. *Pediatric Pharmacotherapy, 19*(6), 1–4.

Chamiedes, L., Samson, R. A., Schexnadyer, S. M., & Hazinski, M. F. (Eds.). (2011). *Pediatric advanced life support* (p. 97). Dallas, TX: American Heart Association.

Chang, C. (2012). Cutting edge issues in rheumatic fever. *Clinical Reviews in Allergy and Immunology, 42*(2), 213–237.

Daniels, S. R. (2012). Diagnosis and management of hypertension in children and adolescents. *Pediatric Annals, 41*(7), e144–e153.

Dennison, B. A. (2012). Bright futures and NHLBI integrated pediatric cardiovascular health guidelines. *Pediatric Annals, 41*(1), 31–35.

Gerwitz, M. H., Baltimore, J. S., Tani, L. Y., Sable, C. A., Shulman, S. T., Carapetis, J., . . . Kaplan, E. L. (2015). Revision of the Jones Criteria for the diagnosis of acute rheumatic fever in the era of doppler echocardiography: A scientific statement from the American Heart Association. *Circulation, 131,* 1806–1818.

Giddings, S. S. (2012). An emerging dyslipidemia: New NHLBI and NLA treatment guidelines. *Contemporary Pediatrics, 29*(7), 24–33.

Hazinski, M. F., Mondozzi, M. A., & Baker, R. A. U. (2014). Shock, multiple organ dysfunction syndrome, and burns in children. In K. L. McCance, S. E. Huether, V. L. Brashers, & N. R. Rote (Eds.), *Pathophysiology: The biologic basis for disease in adults and children* (7th ed., pp. 1699–1727). St. Louis, MO: Mosby Elsevier.

Hylick, E. V., Grubbs, C. R., Johnson, J., & Oliver, B. (2014). Pediatric hypertension. *US Pharmacist. 39*(2), 57–60.

Kharouf, R., & Torchen, L. (2011). Infective endocarditis. In R. Abdulla (Ed.), *Heart disease in children* (pp. 333–342). New York, NY: Springer.

Leggiadro, R. J. (2014). Infective endocarditis in children with congenital heart disease. *Pediatric Infectious Disease Journal, 33*(2), 173.

Lo, J. C., Sinaiko, A., Chandra, M., Daley, M. F., Greenspan, L. C., Parker, E. D., . . . O'Connor, P. J. (2013). Prehypertension and hypertension in community-based pediatric practice. *Pediatrics, 131*(2), e415–e424.

Long, S. H., Harris, S. R., Eldridge, B. J., & Galea, M. P. (2012). Gross motor development is delayed following early cardiac surgery. *Cardiology in the Young, 22,* 574–582.

Longmuir, P. E., Banks, L., & McCrindle, B. W. (2012). Cross-sectional study of motor development among children after the Fontan procedure. *Cardiology in the Young, 22,* 443–450.

McCusker, C. G., Armstrong, M. P., Mullen, M., Doherty, N. N., & Casey, F. A. (2013). A sibling-controlled, prospective study of outcomes at home and school in children with severe congenital heart disease. *Cardiology in the Young, 23,* 507–516

McDaniel, N. L. (2014). Alterations in cardiovascular function in children. In K. L. McCance, S. E. Huether, V. L. Brashers, & N. R. Rote (Eds.), *Pathophysiology: The biologic basis for disease in adults and children* (7th ed., pp. 1194–1224). St. Louis, MO: Elsevier Mosby.

McLellan, M. C., & Baker, A. L. (2011). At the heart of the fever: Kawasaki disease. *American Journal of Nursing, 111*(6), 57–63.

Meaux, J. B., Green, A., Nelson, M. K., Huett, A., Boateng, B., Pye, S., . . . Riley, L. (2014). Transition to self-management after pediatric heart transplant. *Progress in Transplantation, 24,* 226–233.

National Heart Lung and Blood Institute (NHLBI). (2012). *Expert panel on integrated guidelines for cardiovascular health and risk reduction in children and adolescents.* Retrieved from http://www.nhlbi.nih.gov/guidelines/cvd_ped/index.htm

O'Connell, J., & Sloand, E. (2013). Kawasaki syndrome and streptococcal scarlet fever: A clinical review. *The Journal for Nurse Practitioners, 9*(5), 259–264.

Ofori-Amanfo, G., & Cheifetz, I. M. (2013). Pediatric postoperative cardiac care. *Critical Care Clinics of North America, 29,* 185–202.

Paris, J. J., Moore, M. P., & Schreiber, M. D. (2012). Physician counseling, informed consent and parental decision making for infants with hypoplastic left-heart syndrome. *Journal of Perinatology, 32,* 748–751.

Park, M. K. (2014). *Pediatric cardiology for practitioners* (6th ed.). Philadelphia: Elsevier Saunders.

Perkin, R. M., deCaen, A. R., Berg, M. D., Schexnayder, S. M., & Hazinski, M. F. (2013). Shock, cardiac arrest, and resuscitation. In M. F. Hazinski (Ed.), *Nursing care of the critically ill child* (3rd ed., pp. 101–154). St. Louis, MO: Elsevier.

Peterson, C., Ailes, E., Riehle-Colarusso, T., Oster, M. E., Olney, R. S., Cassell, C. H., . . . Gilboa, S. M. (2014). Late detection of critical congenital heart disease among US infants: Estimation of the potential impact of proposed universal screening using pulse oximetry. *JAMA Pediatrics.* doi:10.1001/jamapediatrics .2013.4779.

Rowley, A. H. (2012). Kawasaki disease genetics, pathology, and need for earlier diagnosis and treatment. *Contemporary Pediatrics, 29*(12), 18–24.

Sabe, M. A., Shrestha, N. K., & Menon, V. (2013). Contemporary drug treatment of infective endocarditis. *American Journal of Cardiovascular Drugs, 13,* 251–258.

Satou, G. M., & Halnon, N. J. (2013). *Pediatric congestive heart failure.* Retrieved from http://emedicine .medscape.com/article/2069746-medication#1

Steffen, K. M. (2011). Trauma, burns, and common critical care emergencies. In M. M. Tschudy, & K. M. Arcara (Eds.), *The Harriet Lane handbook* (19th ed., p. 109). Philadelphia, PA: Elsevier Mosby.

Toebbe, S., Yehle, K., Kirkpatrick, J., & Coddington, J. (2013). Hypoplastic left heart syndrome: Parent support for early decision making. *Journal of Pediatric Nursing, 28,* 383–392.

Warnes, C. A. (2014). Pregnancy and heart disease. In D. L. Mann, D. P. Zipes, P. Libby, R. O. Bonow, & E. Braunwald (Eds.), *Braunwald's heart disease: A textbook of cardiovascular medicine* (10th ed., pp. 1755–1770). Philadelphia, PA: Elsevier Saunders.

Williams, J. T. B., & Fagan, H. A. (2014). A 15-year-old boy with congenital heart disease, fevers, and acute onset of dysarthria. *Pediatric Annals, 43*(2), 64–67.

Wilson, B. A., Shannon, M. T., & Shields, K. M. (2016). *Pearson nurses' drug guide 2016.* Hoboken, NJ: Pearson Education.

Yu, M. A., Bostwick, J. R., & Hallman, I. S. (2011). Warfarin drug interactions: Strategies to minimize adverse drug events. *Journal for Nurse Practitioners, 7*(6), 506–512.

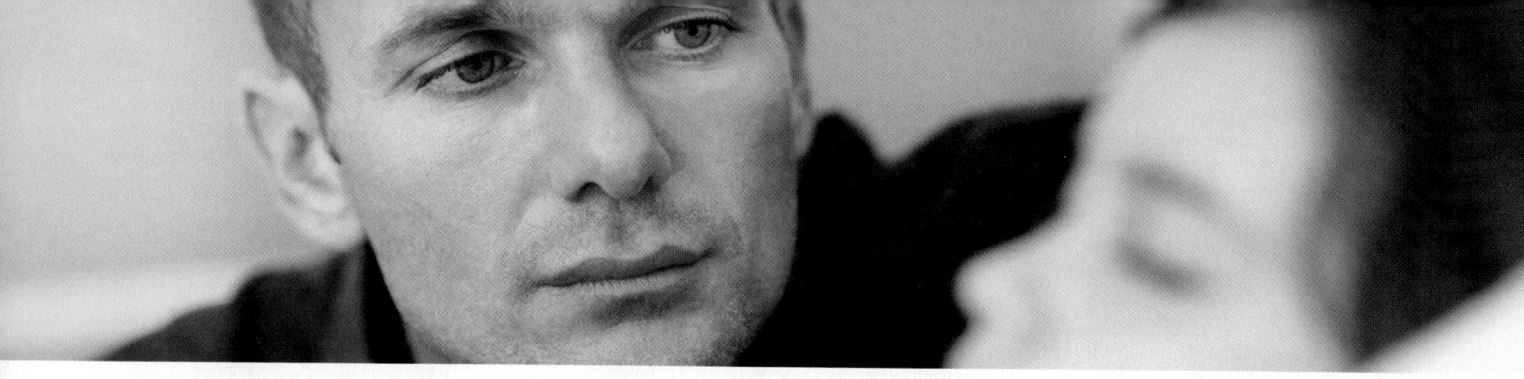

Chapter 48

The Child With Alterations in Immune Function

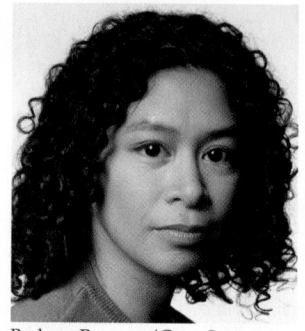

We knew that Raymond might have AIDS—my sister was HIV positive. But we have taken him in as our own child and cared for him. Somehow we thought he would be fine. Now, to find out that he does have AIDS is devastating, especially since my sister is also very ill. We need to learn a lot about how to help him. Can we send him to a preschool next year as we had planned? How will we get money to pay for his medicines? What do we tell other people? How do we get him to eat better? We just don't know where to turn right now.

—Aunt of Raymond, 2 years old

Barbara Penoyar/Getty Images

⌄ Learning Outcomes

48.1 Describe the structure and function of the immune system and apply that knowledge to the care of children with immunologic disorders.

48.2 Summarize infection control measures needed for children with an immunodeficiency.

48.3 Develop a nursing care plan in partnership with the family for a child with human immunodeficiency virus (HIV infection).

48.4 Plan nursing care for the child with an autoimmune condition such as systemic lupus erythematosus or juvenile arthritis.

48.5 Identify exposure prevention measures for the child with latex allergy.

48.6 Determine nursing interventions and prevention measures for the child experiencing hypersensitivity reactions.

Signs and symptoms of immunologic disorders in children are often nonspecific. The immune system is one of the few body systems that regulate, either directly or indirectly, all other body functions. Thus a problem with the immune system can result in multisystem consequences and may be life threatening. The child with recurring infections may have an undiagnosed immunologic disorder. Congenital abnormalities sometimes signal a defect in cellular immunity. This chapter will examine some of the more common disorders of immune function and discuss nursing care of children and families who have these diseases.

Anatomy and Physiology of Pediatric Differences

The function of the immune system is to recognize any foreign substances within the body—in simple terms, to distinguish "nonself" from "self"—and to eliminate foreign substances as efficiently as possible. Whenever the body recognizes the presence of a substance that it cannot identify as part of itself, the body protects itself through the immune response. Normally, the immune system responds to an invasion of foreign substances, or antigens, in numerous ways. It produces **antibodies**, or proteins that work against **antigens**, the foreign substances that trigger the immune response. There are many types of antibodies, described later in this section. The immune system also produces other types of cells, such as T lymphocytes and natural killer (NK) cells.

Immunity is either natural or acquired. **Natural immunity** comprises the defenses present at birth, such as intact skin, body pH, natural antibodies from the mother, and inflammatory and phagocytic properties. **Acquired immunity** consists of humoral (antibody-mediated) and cell-mediated immunity and is not fully developed until a child is about 6 years of age.

Humoral immunity is responsible for destroying bacterial antigens. B lymphocytes, produced in the bone marrow, gut, and other lymphoid tissue, are the central factors in humoral immunity and develop into plasma cells that produce antibodies. Antibodies are a type of protein called **immunoglobulins** of which there are five types: IgM, IgG, IgA, IgD, and IgE (Table 48–1). IgM, IgG, and IgA act to control a number of body infections, whereas IgE is useful in combating parasitic infections and is part of the allergic response. The role of IgD is not clear (Orduño, Grimaldi, & Diamond, 2013).

Antibodies are found in serum, body fluids, and certain tissues. When a child is first exposed to an antigen, the B lymphocyte system begins to produce antibodies that react specifically to that antigen (see *Pathophysiology Illustrated: Primary Immune*

TABLE 48–1 Classes of Immunoglobulins

IMMUNO-GLOBULIN	LOCATION	ACTION
IgM	Present in intravascular spaces (blood and lymph)	Mediates cytotoxic response and activates complement
		First antibody produced with primary immune response
IgG	Present in all body fluids	Active against bacteria, bacterial toxins, and viruses
		Activates complement
		Only immunoglobulin to cross the placenta
IgA	Present in secretions of gastrointestinal, respiratory, and genitourinary tracts	Prevents binding of viruses to cells of the respiratory and gastrointestinal tracts
IgD	Present in blood, lymph, and surfaces of B cells	Function not fully understood
IgE	Present in internal and external body fluids	Releases chemical mediators responsible for immediate hypersensitivity response

Pathophysiology Illustrated: **Primary Immune Response**

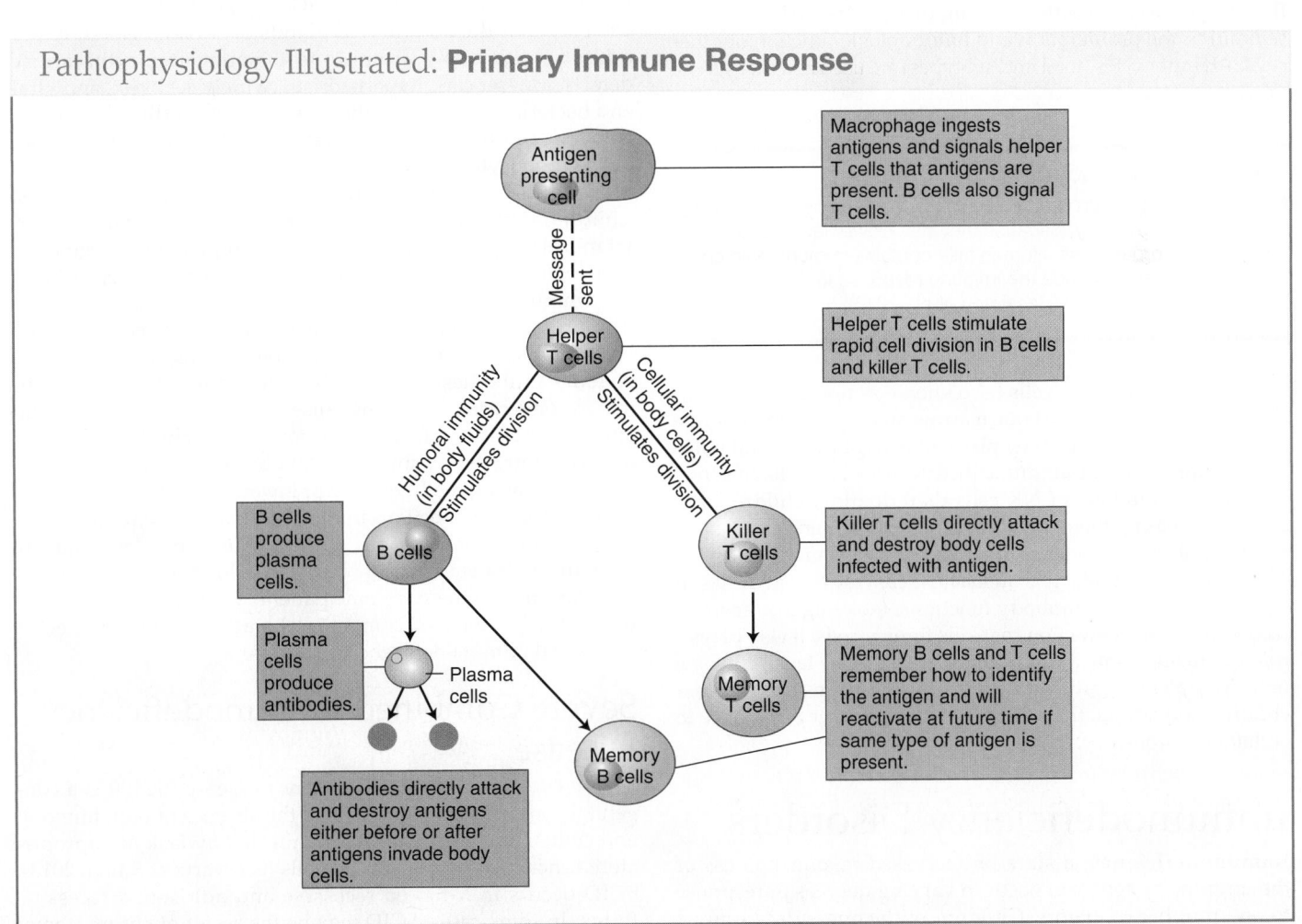

Macrophage ingests antigens and signals helper T cells that antigens are present. B cells also signal T cells.

Helper T cells stimulate rapid cell division in B cells and killer T cells.

Killer T cells directly attack and destroy body cells infected with antigen.

Memory B cells and T cells remember how to identify the antigen and will reactivate at future time if same type of antigen is present.

Antibodies directly attack and destroy antigens either before or after antigens invade body cells.

B cells produce plasma cells.

Plasma cells produce antibodies.

Response). It takes approximately 3 days for this process, known as a **primary immune response**, to occur. Subsequent encounters with the antigen trigger memory cells, resulting in a **secondary immune response** within 24 hours.

Infants and children have differing amounts of some immunoglobulins. IgG is the only immunoglobulin that crosses the placenta; as a result, a newborn's levels are similar to those of the mother (Buckley, 2016a). This maternal IgG disappears by 6 to 8 months of age. The infant's IgG then increases gradually until mature levels are reached at 7 to 8 years of age. IgM levels are low at birth, rise markedly at 1 week of age, and continue to increase until adult levels are reached at about 1 year. IgA and IgE are not present at birth. The manufacture of these immunoglobulins begins by 2 weeks of age; however, normal values are not achieved until 6 to 7 years of age. Thus it is easy to see why children under 6 years of age become ill so often—they do not have a full complement of immunoglobulins.

In contrast, cell-mediated immunity achieves full function early in life. The thymus begins producing T lymphocytes in the fetus and by birth many of these cells are present. The thymus is large at birth, grows during childhood and adolescence, and decreases in size in adulthood (Buckley, 2016a). Other lymphoid tissues such as the spleen and tonsils are also comparatively large in young children. Because of this well-developed cellular immunity, any blood infused into newborns is generally irradiated to prevent **graft-versus-host disease** (a series of immunologic reactions in response to transplanted cells) from transfused lymphocytes.

Specialized types of T lymphocytes include killer T cells, suppressor T cells, and helper T cells. Suppressor T cells inhibit B lymphocytes from differentiating into plasma cells. Helper T cells aid in the proliferation and immunologic function of other cells. T lymphocytes (total and subtypes) are used as a measure of immune response.

Growth and Development

Newborns are most prone to development of infection, particularly when born prematurely, because they have lower levels of their own immune protections. Human milk contains immunologic components that can influence the immune response in the infant and protect against infection (Hassiotou et al., 2013).

Natural killer (NK) cells (also known as non-B/non-T lymphocytes) originate in the bone marrow and thymus and migrate to the blood and spleen. They play a role in control of viral infection, tumors, and autoimmune disease. Newborns have somewhat lower numbers of NK cells than do older children and adults, decreasing their ability to respond to certain antigens.

Complement is a component of blood serum consisting of 11 protein compounds. It is an inactive enzyme that activates in response to antigen–antibody functions, resulting in a generalized inflammatory reaction that kills foreign cells. It also plays a role in causing some autoimmune diseases. The levels of some of the complement proteins are lower in newborns than in older children and adults, thus delaying and hampering response to certain infections.

Immunodeficiency Disorders

Immunodeficiency, a state of decreased responsiveness of the immune system, can occur to varying degrees in response to any number of events. Children with congenital immune deficiency, or **primary immune deficiency**, are born with a failure of humoral antibody formation (B-cell disorder), a deficient cellular immune system (T-cell disorder), or a combination of both defects. In congenital disorders, the immune deficiency is not caused by another condition. However, immunodeficiency may also be acquired, as in human immunodeficiency virus (HIV) infection. Acquired immune deficiency is also called **secondary immune deficiency**.

B-Cell and T-Cell Disorders

In B-cell disorders, immunoglobulins may be present in inadequate numbers or nearly absent. X-linked agammaglobulinemia, selective IgA deficiency, and common variable immunodeficiency are examples of such disorders (Michaels & Green, 2016). Because newborns are protected from infection by maternal antibodies in the first months after birth, symptoms of B-cell disorders usually become apparent after 3 months of age once the infant loses maternal antibodies. Infants with these disorders have frequent recurrent bacterial infections and failure to thrive. With treatment, consisting of intravenous immunoglobulins and antibiotics, most children survive into adulthood. Prognosis depends on the degree of antibody deficiency.

T-cell disorders are characterized by inadequate numbers of T lymphocytes or absence of T-cell functions. Isolated T-cell disorders are rare, are usually accompanied by a B-cell disorder, and may be associated with congenital abnormalities (as in DiGeorge syndrome) or of unknown cause. DiGeorge syndrome, a T-cell disorder caused by chromosome deletion at 22q11.2, is usually diagnosed soon after birth. The syndrome is characterized by the absence (complete DiGeorge) or hypoplasia (partial DiGeorge) of the parathyroid glands or thymus gland, hypocalcemia with tetany within 24 to 48 hours after birth, cardiac defects, low-set ears, hypertelorism (widely set eyes), and viral and bacterial infections in the neonatal period (Buckley, 2016b; Fernandez, 2013). There is generally a mild to moderate decrease in T-lymphocyte counts (McDonald-McGinn & Sullivan, 2011). Prophylactic antibiotics are used to prevent bacterial infections. Children with partial DiGeorge are treated with calcium and vitamin D supplements. Those with complete DiGeorge need thymus transplantation in order to survive (Fernandez, 2013).

Immunodeficiency with hyper-IgM is a T-cell disorder that primarily affects males and causes decreased T-cell function, variable abnormal levels of immunoglobulins, and high titers of some antibodies. It is usually X linked but may be autosomal in some cases. Infections caused by viruses, bacteria, fungi, and opportunistic infections are common in children with this disorder. Intravenous immune globulin (IVIG) therapy is helpful in decreasing the frequency of lower respiratory tract infections and severe infections but does not affect the frequency of upper respiratory infections or other infections. Bone marrow or stem cell transplantation with cord blood has been used as an aspect of treatment in some patients with varying outcomes (Park, 2012). Table 48–2 compares laboratory values for selected congenital immunodeficiency disorders.

Severe Combined Immunodeficiency Disease

Severe combined immunodeficiency disease (SCID) is a congenital condition characterized by the absence of both humoral and cellular immunity that is manifested by lack of appropriately functioning T cells and B cells (Schwartz & Sinha, 2013). SCID occurs in X-linked recessive and autosomal recessive forms. In some cases, SCID may be the result of chromosomal

TABLE 48–2 Laboratory Findings for Selected Congenital Immunodeficiency Disorders

DISORDERS	LABORATORY FINDINGS
B CELL	
X-linked hypogammaglobulinemia	Reduced IgA, IgM, IgE, IgG (<100 mg/dL), absence of B cells in peripheral blood, normal T cells
Selective IgA deficiency	IgA less than 10 mg/dL
Common variable immunodeficiency	Reduced IgG, IgA, and IgM
T CELL	
DiGeorge syndrome	Lymphopenia; absent T-cell functions, decreased T cells, normal B cells
X-linked immunodeficiency with hyper-IgM	Reduced IgG, IgA; elevated IgM; mutations in T-cell surface proteins
COMBINED	
Severe combined immunodeficiency syndrome (SCID)	Complete absence of T- and B-cell and NK immunity
Wiskott-Aldrich syndrome	Thrombocytopenia, low platelet volume, nonfunctional B-cells, normal IgG, decreased IgM, increased IgA, increased IgE; inability to respond to polysaccharide antigens

abnormalities. The disorder is estimated to occur in 1 per 50,000–100,000 live births (Pai & Notarangelo, 2013). Without appropriate treatment, children born with SCID usually do not survive more than 1 year (Buckley, 2016c)

ETIOLOGY AND PATHOPHYSIOLOGY

Severe combined immunodeficiency disease is caused by genetic mutations that lead to absence of immune function and, in some cases, absence of natural killer (NK) cells (Buckley, 2016c). The B lymphocytes are also generally defective, but even

if they are normal, their function is compromised because of the severe T-cell deficiency (Kwan et al., 2014).

CLINICAL MANIFESTATIONS

Symptoms of SCID develop early in life. The infant often demonstrates a susceptibility to infection, presenting during the first few months of life with persistent respiratory infections and diarrhea (Buckley, 2016c). Recurrent oral candidiasis, failure to thrive, and skin infections are also frequently seen in affected children. Additionally, failure to recover completely from infection, frequent reinfection, and infection with viruses such as cytomegalovirus and the bacterium *Pneumocystis jiroveci* (formerly called *P. carinii*) are common in the child with SCID (Buckley, 2016c). Children are also highly susceptible to serious infections such as meningitis, skin or organ infection, osteomyelitis, or sepsis.

CLINICAL THERAPY

Refer to Table 48–2 for laboratory findings in SCID. Diagnosis is usually made only after extensive laboratory testing. In addition to a complete blood count, erythrocyte sedimentation rate, and B- and T-cell lymphocyte counts, other studies including IgA, IgG, and IgM antibody titers to immunizations received, and neutrophil count, may be performed (Table 48–3). A chest radiograph is conducted to assess thymus size.

The standard therapy for severe combined immunodeficiency disease is the administration of intravenous immune globulin (IVIG), which is administered to provide protection until humoral immunity is established. Hematopoietic stem cell transplantation (see Chapter 49) offers the best hope for children with SCID. T-cell function is restored with the transplantation, and new cells appear 3 to 4 months after infusion of the donor stem cell. Gene therapy may also be used to treat SCID. Prognosis for the child is poor without aggressive therapy and transplant.

Prevention and prompt treatment of infection are essential. Antibiotic therapy is targeted at infectious agents. Antibiotic prophylaxis and special immunization recommendations are needed. Children with T-cell deficiencies should receive lymphocyte-depleted and irradiated blood products because of the risk of infection and graft-versus-host disease from lymphocytes in the donor blood (Schwartz & Sinha, 2013).

TABLE 48–3 Cells Evaluated in Laboratory Studies for Immune Conditions

TEST AND TYPE OF CELL EVALUATED	ACTION	IMPLICATION OF INCREASED OR DECREASED LEVELS
WHITE BLOOD CELL (WBC) COUNT		
Neutrophil (54%–62%)	Phagocytic cell that defends against bacteria	Increased in bacterial infection, inflammatory processes, and some malignancies
Eosinophil (1%–3%)	Associated with antigen–antibody reaction	Increased in allergic reaction; decreased in children receiving corticosteroids
Basophils (0%–3%)	Phagocytic cell; involved in immediate hypersensitivity reaction; stores histamine and has receptor sites for IgE	Increased in leukemia; decreased in allergy, acute infection, collagen, and chronic diseases
Monocytes (4%–9%)	Phagocytic cell active in chronic infection	Increased in tuberculosis, protozoan infection, monocytic leukemia
Lymphocytes (T, B, non-B/non-T [NK]) (25%–33%)	Major components of immune system	Increased in many infections; decreased in children with immune deficiency
IMMUNOGLOBULINS		
(IgM, IgG, IgA, IgD, IgE) (See Appendix B for age-specific values.)	Many roles in a number of immunologic reactions	Increased in presence of infection or allergic response; decreased in children with immune deficiency

Nursing Management
For the Child With SCID

Nursing Assessment and Diagnosis

Obtain a thorough history of infections, including age of onset, type of causal organism, frequency, and severity. Assess family history, and determine if the child has had any unusual reactions to vaccines, medications, or foods. Measure the child's height and weight and plot on a growth chart to identify failure to thrive. Assess the child's nutritional intake and fluid and electrolyte balance. Assess for evidence of infections involving the skin, subcutaneous tissues, respiratory system, and mucous membranes. Palpate the abdomen for hepatomegaly and the lymph nodes for lymphadenopathy. Perform a developmental assessment and assess for delays in achievement of developmental milestones. Assess family support systems and coping mechanisms when a child is diagnosed with the disorder.

The primary nursing diagnosis for a child with SCID is *Infection, Risk for*, related to immunodeficiency. Other nursing diagnoses may include the following (NANDA-I © 2014):

- *Nutrition, Imbalanced: Less than Body Requirements*, related to illness
- *Skin Integrity, Risk for Impaired*, related to immunologic deficit
- *Caregiver Role Strain, Risk for*, related to a child with a chronic, life-threatening illness
- *Development: Delayed, Risk for*, related to physical disability and chronic illness

Planning and Implementation

Nursing care of the immunodeficient child focuses on preventing infection (see *Teaching Highlights: Reducing Risk of Infection in the Child With Immunodeficiency Disease*). However, even with the use of environmental controls, such as keeping children inside special units (positive-pressure rooms) to maintain a sterile environment, these children are prone to **opportunistic infections** (those caused by normally nonpathogenic organisms in persons who lack normal immunity).

PREVENT SYSTEMIC INFECTION

Frequent and thorough handwashing is important. Standard precautions are always used and transmission-based precautions are established when indicated. Implement sterile aseptic technique when caring for all sites where needles, catheters, central lines, endotracheal tubes, pressure-monitoring lines, and peripheral intravenous lines, or other invasive equipment enter the child's body (see the *Clinical Skills Manual* SKILLS). The

child should be placed in a positive-pressure isolation room, and contact with infectious individuals should be avoided. Inform parents that because of the risk of infection to the child, live vaccines are avoided for the child as well as siblings, parents, and other household members. Refer to the current recommendations for immunizations for the immunocompromised child. (See Chapter 43.)

PROMOTE SKIN INTEGRITY

The skin is the only intact defense that many immunodeficient children have. Provide thorough and frequent skin care, and observe all possible pressure areas closely for signs of breakdown or infection. Reposition the child frequently and encourage range-of-motion exercises.

PROMOTE NUTRITIONAL BALANCE

Encourage adequate fluid and nutritional intake. Provide foods that the child prefers and those with high nutritional value. Offer small frequent feedings of high-calorie, protein-rich foods. Refer to a dietitian as needed to plan with parents for the best individualized diet for the child.

MANAGE MEDICATION THERAPY

Many medications used long term in the treatment of children with SCID have numerous side effects. Monitor closely for side effects of antibiotics, such as overgrowth of resistant organisms (e.g., thrush infections in the mouth, *Clostridium difficile* infections of the gastrointestinal tract) and administer IVIG safely.

PROVIDE EMOTIONAL SUPPORT AND REFERRALS

SCID is a life-threatening and devastating disease. Even with aggressive therapy, the prognosis is poor for children who do not receive a hematopoietic stem cell transplant. Evaluate the family's knowledge about the disease and provide education about infection control measures and signs of infection. The parents may experience guilt because of the genetic nature of the disease and the difficulties of treatment. Listen closely to their concerns and encourage them to discuss their fears. Refer them to an appropriate support group or counselor if needed. Encourage genetic counseling if the parents plan to have more children. Evaluate the family's ability to care for the child at home. Offer financial resource information and other referrals as needed.

The family of a child who undergoes hematopoietic stem cell transplantation requires additional support and referrals. The transplantation procedure involves surgery for both the ill child and the donor, often another child in the family. After the transplant the ill child will be hospitalized for several months until T-lymphocyte levels are sufficient to provide resistance to infection. During this period, parents may need to rely on social services to help manage the family situation, particularly if the child is hospitalized at a medical center far from the family's home. Assess the family's situation and make appropriate

---

TEACHING HIGHLIGHTS | Reducing Risk of Infection in the Child With Immunodeficiency Disease

Teach family members the following practices to reduce the risk of transmission of infection:

- Wash all bottles, nipples, and pacifiers with hot water and soap, or in the dishwasher.
- Do not allow child to share utensils, cups, bottles, or pacifiers.
- Use safe food preparation practices such as peeling fruit and vegetables and using different surfaces and utensils for preparing meats versus other foods.
- Change diapers frequently and cleanse skin with mild soap and dry thoroughly.
- Wash hands before handling child, after changing diapers, and before feeding child.
- Maintain clean pets and keep the pet's environment clean.
- Avoid exposing the child to other family members' illnesses, such as colds.

referrals to social services and support groups. Introduce parents to other families undergoing hematopoietic stem cell transplantation. (See Chapter 49 for discussion of hematopoietic stem cell transplantation.)

Evaluation

The success of nursing care for the child with SCID is measured by outcomes such as the following:

- The child is free of infection.
- The child has adequate nutritional status as determined by normal growth patterns.
- The child's skin remains intact.
- The family adapts to and copes with the demands of a chronic illness.
- The child performs developmentally within normal level for age.

Wiskott-Aldrich Syndrome

A combined congenital immunodeficiency syndrome, Wiskott-Aldrich syndrome (WAS) is an X-linked disorder that causes mutation in the *WAS* gene and changes in the WAS protein. The gene resides on Xp11.22–11.23 (Buckley, 2016c). The incidence is 1 in 250,000 live male births (Schwartz & Siperstein, 2013). The IgM levels are low, IgG levels are normal or slightly low, and IgA and IgE levels are elevated (Buckley, 2016c).

The diagnosis is made in the early neonatal period on the basis of the thrombocytopenia, which leads to bleeding as evidenced by petechiae, hematuria, bloody diarrhea, and hematemesis. In addition to thrombocytopenia and related symptoms, Wiskott-Aldrich syndrome is characterized by eczema and recurrent infections in infancy and childhood. Infections including otitis media, bacterial pneumonia, and skin infections are common (Albert, Notarangelo, & Ochs, 2011; Schwartz & Siperstein, 2013).

Treatment is supportive and includes antibiotic prophylaxis, platelet transfusions, and intravenous gamma globulin (IVIG). Splenectomy may reduce the risk of bleeding; however, this is done sparingly because of the risk of life-threatening infection following the procedure. The treatment of choice and the only cure for Wiskott-Aldrich syndrome is hematopoietic stem cell transplantation (HSCT). Following HSCT, the child is at risk for both rejection and graft-versus-host disease (Albert et al., 2011; Schwartz & Siperstein, 2013).

Nursing Management

Nursing care is similar to that for the child with SCID. Refer the parents for genetic counseling to help them understand the disease transmission and the probability of having another child with the same disorder. Arrange for psychologic support for parents overwhelmed with guilt from learning that the illness is inherited.

Help the parents and family cope with the knowledge that the child has a chronic and potentially fatal illness (see Chapters 38 and 41). Referral to family counseling may be appropriate. Expected outcomes are the child's return to normal immunologic function, absence of hemorrhage, and successful coping with a life-threatening illness.

Human Immunodeficiency Virus and Acquired Immune Deficiency Syndrome

Acquired immune deficiency syndrome (AIDS) is caused by the human immunodeficiency virus (HIV-1 primarily; HIV-2 less commonly) (American Academy of Pediatrics [AAP], 2015, p. 453).

Because HIV destroys the body's ability to fight infection, opportunistic infections that would normally not affect healthy people destroy the immune system. AIDS is the advanced stages of HIV infection.

Most cases of HIV in children are the result of perinatal transmission. The Centers for Disease Control and Prevention (CDC) (2014a) estimates that 162 infants were born with HIV infection in the United States in 2010. The incidence of perinatally acquired HIV infection in the United States has declined by an estimated 90% since the early 1990s. This improvement is primarily due to more effective identification and treatment of mothers who are infected with HIV (CDC, 2014a). The leading cause of newly acquired HIV infection in teens is unprotected sexual intercourse, while intravenous substance use is responsible for most other cases. In many cases, both of these factors are involved.

ETIOLOGY AND PATHOPHYSIOLOGY

Children can acquire HIV in a form of **vertical transmission** from their mothers transplacentally or during delivery. Transmission can occur during birth from blood, amniotic fluid, and exposure to genital tract secretions, and after birth through breast milk from HIV-infected mothers. However, risk for perinatal transmission has been significantly reduced since mothers identified as being infected receive antiretroviral therapy (ART) during pregnancy, undergo a cesarean section, and are advised not to breastfeed (CDC, 2014a). If the mother is not treated during pregnancy, labor, or delivery, there is a 25% chance that the newborn will be infected (U.S. Department of Health and Human Services [USDHHS], 2012) Prenatal testing is essential for identifying mothers who are HIV positive so that treatment can be started and decrease the infant's chances of acquiring the infection to less than 1% (CDC, 2014a).

The virus affects multiple systems and eventually destroys the ability of the child's immune system to respond to infection. An understanding of the natural history of HIV disease is still evolving, and there are several important differences in the disease progression and clinical manifestations of pediatric and adult HIV infections.

HIV selectively targets and destroys T cells, thereby decreasing and eventually eliminating cellular immunity. HIV destroys CD4 T cells (helper cells), which are crucial to normal function of the immune system. HIV selectively targets T cells, decreasing cellular immunity, and affecting humoral immunity as well. Thus the untreated child is left unprotected against a myriad of bacterial, viral, fungal, and opportunistic infections, which are ultimately fatal. Every organ system can be affected. (See *Pathophysiology Illustrated: Human Immunodeficiency Virus.*)

CLINICAL MANIFESTATIONS

The neonate is asymptomatic at birth. The time period for the development of opportunistic infections varies; however, the interval from HIV infection to the onset of overt AIDS is shorter in children than in adults. See Table 48–4.

Early clinical signs for children with HIV infection are nonspecific findings, including lymphadenopathy, hepatosplenomegaly, oral candidiasis, failure to thrive and weight loss, delayed development, swelling of the parotid gland, and chronic diarrhea (AAP, 2015, p. 457; Kronman & Smith, 2015). Recurrent bacterial infections, lymphoid interstitial pneumonitis (LIP), and progressive neurologic deterioration are more common in children than adults. *Pneumocystis jiroveci* (formerly known as *P. carinii*) pneumonia is also common and may present early in infancy (Kronman & Smith, 2015).

CLINICAL THERAPY

There is no cure for HIV or AIDS. Care focuses on the prevention of HIV transmission, the detection of the presence of HIV, aggressive therapy to reduce progression to AIDS, and promotion of the infant's or child's growth and development and survival.

Most children with HIV infection are diagnosed early in life. Virologic tests for detection of the virus are monitored in infants born to mothers infected with HIV. Testing is recommended at 14 to 21 days, 1 to 2 months, and 4 to 6 months. The preferred tests are the HIV DNA polymerase chain reaction (PCR) or the HIV RNA assay (viral load). Any positive result is confirmed by retesting. In addition, CD4 cell counts and percentages should

be performed at least every 3 to 4 months to evaluate the child's immune status. This monitoring may change to every 6 to 12 months in children and adolescents who are compliant with therapy and have stable CD4 values and clinical status for over 2 to 3 years (Panel on Antiretroviral Therapy and Medical Management of HIV-Infected Children, 2014).

Antibody tests are performed in children with no clinical signs or virologic evidence of HIV infection to see if the maternal HIV antibodies have disappeared. A diagnosis of HIV infection is definitively excluded in children with two negative antibody tests at age 6 months or older. Repeat testing is recommended between 12 and 18 months of age in children who have not yet had two negative antibody tests (Panel on Antiretroviral

Pathophysiology Illustrated: **Human Immunodeficiency Virus**

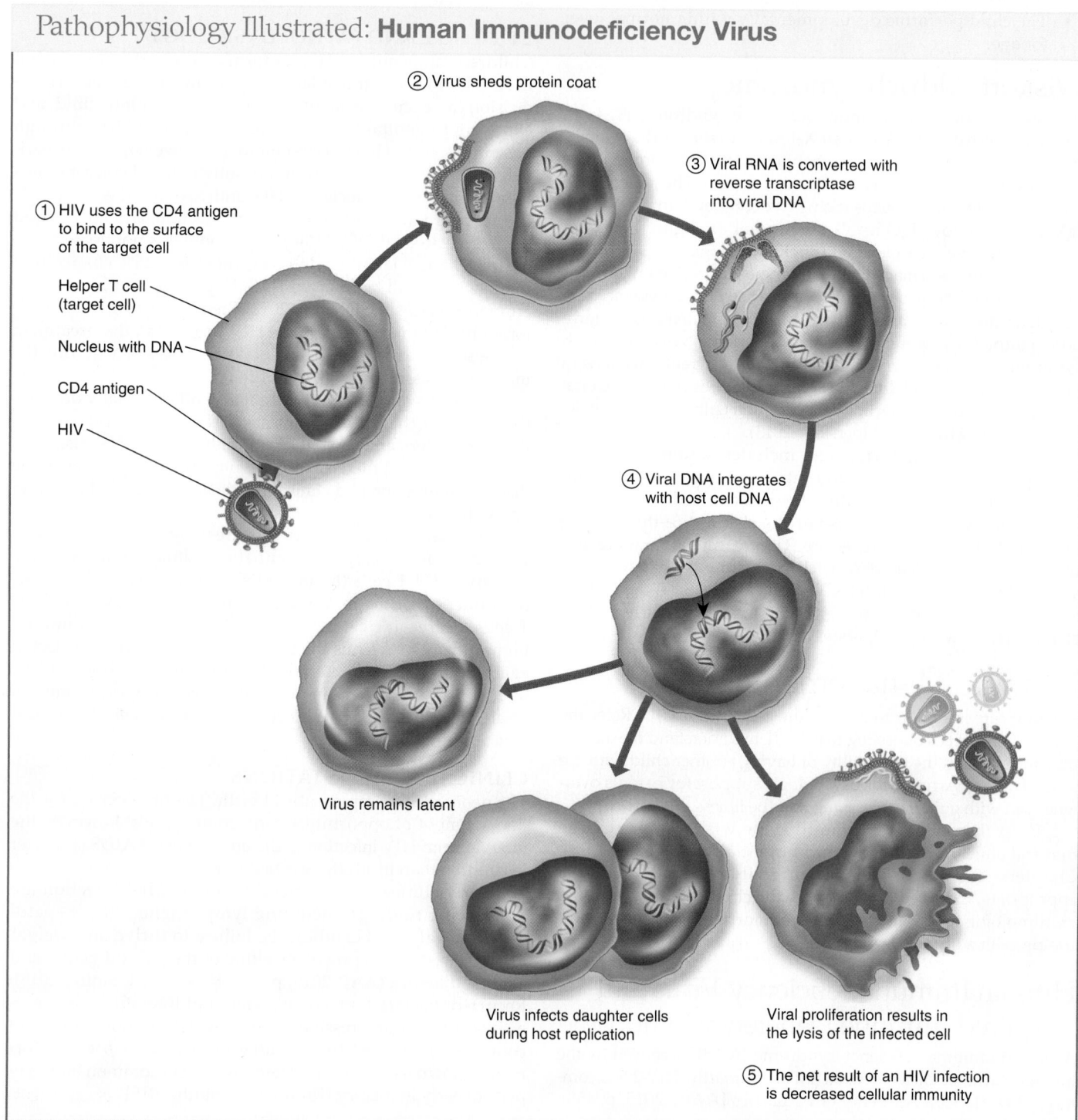

① HIV uses the CD4 antigen to bind to the surface of the target cell

Helper T cell (target cell)

Nucleus with DNA

CD4 antigen

HIV

② Virus sheds protein coat

③ Viral RNA is converted with reverse transcriptase into viral DNA

④ Viral DNA integrates with host cell DNA

Virus remains latent

Virus infects daughter cells during host replication

Viral proliferation results in the lysis of the infected cell

⑤ The net result of an HIV infection is decreased cellular immunity

TABLE 48–4 Clinical Manifestations of Human Immunodeficiency Virus in Children

ETIOLOGY	CLINICAL MANIFESTATIONS	CLINICAL THERAPY
Frequent, chronic, or unusual infections due to poor immune response	Chronic bilateral otitis media Oral candidiasis *Pneumocystis jiroveci* pneumonia Skin disorders Fever Parotitis	Antimicrobial therapy for treatment of infections Recommended immunizations Limit exposure to groups of people or to individuals with known infections of any kind
Poor nutritional intake due to lack of appetite caused by disease and medications	Failure to thrive (eating disorder of childhood) Weight and body mass index below 10th percentile Chronic diarrhea Skin irritation	Monitor growth Supplemental intake such as enteral feedings at night, and total parenteral nutrition (TPN) if needed Meticulous skin care to prevent breakdown
Immune system overgrowth to compensate for lack of proper immune response	Hepatosplenomegaly and lymphadenopathy	Assess abdomen frequently Teach about safe transport to avoid injury to liver and spleen

Note: Be alert for the possibility of HIV infection in infants with combinations of listed clinical manifestations, especially in infants known to be at risk.

Source: Data from American Academy of Pediatrics (AAP). (2015). *Red book: 2015 report of the Committee on Infectious Diseases* (30th ed.). Elk Grove Village, IL: Author; Kronman, M. P., & Smith, S. (2015). Infectious diseases. In K. J. Marcdante & R. M. Kliegman, *Nelson essentials of pediatrics* (7th ed., pp. 315–416). Philadelphia, PA: Elsevier Saunders.

Therapy and Medical Management of HIV-Infected Children, 2014). See Table 48–5.

Medical management begins with prevention of the spread of HIV from mother to newborn. Because of the rapidity of disease progression in perinatally transmitted HIV infection, early identification of infected infants is important to ensure the most effective treatment. Mothers infected with HIV should be identified during pregnancy, and their infants should undergo periodic laboratory testing, as described earlier. All infected mothers should receive zidovudine antiretroviral therapy after the 14th week of pregnancy (AAP, 2015, p. 472). Early identification of mothers infected with HIV and implementation of antiretroviral therapy will lead to a decrease in the numbers of infants and children with HIV infection.

Clinical Tip

Many people who are at risk of HIV infection may not have HIV testing readily available. To reduce barriers to early detection of the virus, rapid HIV tests have been made available. Specimens are obtained from saliva or fingerstick for blood sample. Oral fluids are obtained by gently swabbing both the upper and lower outer gums of the mouth. Results are available in 20 minutes. Follow-up testing is performed to confirm positive rapid HIV tests (CDC, 2014b). Health professionals must be prepared to offer counseling during the same visit as when the test is administered.

All infants of infected mothers with indeterminate HIV infection status should start prophylaxis against *P. jiroveci* pneumonia by the age of 4 to 6 weeks and continue to 1 year of age unless the

TABLE 48–5 HIV Pediatric Classification System: Clinical Categories

WHEN INFECTED, THE CHILD WITH HIV IS CLASSIFIED AS:

- Category N (not symptomatic)
- Category A (mildly symptomatic)
- Category B (moderately symptomatic)
- Category C (severely symptomatic; multiple, recurrent serious bacterial infections)

Source: Adapted from Panel on Antiretroviral Therapy and Medical Management of HIV-Infected Children. (2014). *Guidelines for the use of antiretroviral agents in pediatric HIV infection.* Retrieved from http://aidsinfo.nih.gov/contentfiles/lvguidelines/pediatricguidelines.pdf

diagnosis of HIV infection is excluded. Prompt therapy with anti-infectives is used for bacterial and viral opportunistic infections. The need for prophylaxis after 1 year of age is dependent on the child's degree of immunosuppression (AAP, 2015, p. 641).

Treatment for the child diagnosed with HIV involves combination antiretroviral therapy (cART). Initial medication therapy should include a combination of several antiretroviral (AVR) drugs. At least three drugs from a minimum of two different categories should be used. See *Medications Used to Treat: Human Immunodeficiency Virus in Children* for information related to antiretroviral drugs that may be used in children. Families should be advised that these drugs neither cure HIV nor prevent transfer from the person infected to others.

Children on antiretroviral therapy should be monitored closely for side effects and toxicity related to the medications. A complete blood count and blood chemistry along with a clinical history should be evaluated prior to beginning treatment, 4 to 8 weeks later, and then every 3 to 4 months. In addition, CD4 cell counts and HIV RNA levels are recommended at the same time intervals to evaluate compliance with the medication regimen and effectiveness of the treatment. A lipid panel is also recommended prior to initiating treatment and every 6 to 12 months to monitor for signs of elevated cholesterol and triglyceride levels. Additional testing may be recommended depending on the particular drug regimen (Panel on Antiretroviral Therapy and Medical Management of HIV-Infected Children, 2014). With rapid advances in the treatment of HIV infection, HIV is thought of more as a chronic illness as opposed to a terminal disease (Mawn, 2012).

Nursing Management

For the Child With HIV Infection

Nursing Assessment and Diagnosis

For infants at risk of HIV infection, obtain the HIV test results of the mother if available. When the mother's results are positive, the infant will need to be screened for HIV infection according to CDC guidelines as described in the previous section. Facilitate the screening and explain its necessity to the family.

Medications Used to Treat: Human Immunodeficiency Virus in Children

MEDICATION AND ACTION/INDICATION	NURSING IMPLICATIONS
Nucleoside and nucleotide analog reverse transcriptase inhibitors	
Inhibits action of viral reverse transcriptase, an enzyme in the conversion of RNA to DNA. Abacavir Didanosine Emtricitabine Lamivudine Stavudine Tenofovir Zidovudine (AZT)	Common side effects include fever, headache, insomnia, myalgia, nausea, vomiting, diarrhea, anorexia, bone marrow suppression with resulting granulocytopenia and anemia, dyspnea, cough, skin rash. Teach signs and symptoms of infection.
Protease inhibitors	
Blocks the function of the enzyme protease needed for viral formation and growth. Atazanavir Darunavir Fosamprenavir Lopinavir/Ritonavir Nelfinavir Ritonavir Tipranavir	Side effects include CNS, CV changes, life-threatening hematologic changes, respiratory distress, and allergy; monitor for specific side effects of the particular drug administered. Oral forms taken within 2 hr of a full meal.
Nonnucleoside reverse transcriptase inhibitors (NNRTIS)	
Binds to viral reverse transcriptase and disrupts the conversion of RNA to DNA. Efavirenz Etravirine Nevirapine	Side effects include fever, headache, nausea, diarrhea, hepatitis, altered liver function, anemia, neutropenia, drowsiness and fatigue, altered mental status, rash, Stevens–Johnson syndrome. Teach the family to notify healthcare provider immediately if rash appears.
Fusion inhibitors	
Prevents viral entry. Enfuvirtide	Requires subcutaneous injection twice a day. There is a high incidence of local reaction at the injection site, limiting the use of this medication in children.
Integrase inhibitors	
Blocks the action of the viral enzyme integrase. Raltegravir	Side effects include rash, nausea, diarrhea, headache, insomnia, fever, and muscle weakness. Give orally without regard to food intake.

Source: Data from Panel on Antiretroviral Therapy and Medical Management of HIV-Infected Children. (2014). *Guidelines for the use of antiretroviral agents in pediatric HIV infection.* Retrieved from http://aidsinfo.nih.gov/contentfiles/lvguidelines/pediatricguidelines.pdf; Rivera, D. M., & Frye, R. E. (2014). *Pediatric HIV infection treatment & management.* Retrieved from http://emedicine.medscape.com/article/965086-treatment#aw2aab6b6b2

PHYSIOLOGIC ASSESSMENT

Assessment centers on observation and evaluation of potential sites of infection. Assess breath sounds, respiratory status, arterial blood gases, level of consciousness, and mental status, and report any abnormal findings. Assess the child's height and weight frequently. Observe for signs of failure to thrive and assess for anemia. Assess for *Candida* infections in the mouth and the diaper area. Note any developmental delays in motor skills or intellectual functioning, which could result from encephalopathy and poor nutrition, and can signal an increasing severity in symptom level. These findings should be reported immediately so that further medical evaluation can be implemented.

PSYCHOSOCIAL ASSESSMENT

Assess family support systems and coping mechanisms because the stress of caring for a child with HIV infection may overwhelm the parents. Assess the family's ability to care for the child. Inquire about the extended family's ability to provide daily care as well as emotional support. Support the family when they decide to inform a school-age child or adolescent of the diagnosis. When assessing an adolescent with HIV infection, evaluate the teen's understanding of how HIV is transmitted and the response to the diagnosis.

The accompanying *Nursing Care Plan* includes common nursing diagnoses that may apply to a child hospitalized with HIV infection. Other nursing diagnoses may include the following (NANDA-I © 2014):

- *Diarrhea* related to gastrointestinal infection, malignancy, or drug reactions
- *Mucous Membrane: Oral, Impaired*, related to infection
- *Development: Delayed, Risk for*, related to chronic infection and poor nutrition
- *Coping: Family, Compromised*, related to life-threatening illness
- *Caregiver Role Strain* related to anxiety about child's condition and demands of providing care

Planning and Implementation

The first step in managing HIV infection is prevention. Nurses must be active in instituting measures to prevent vertical transmission of HIV to the infants of infected mothers. Measures advised include adequate testing, prophylaxis for HIV-exposed infants and opportunistic infections, and follow-up visits for evaluation of general health and development for all infants at risk of the disease.

Education related to HIV infection, transmission of the disease, and testing should be a routine part of anticipatory guidance provided to adolescents. Adolescents who are sexually active should be offered HIV testing. Nurses can be instrumental in developing educational programs related to HIV prevention in school settings.

If the child is diagnosed with HIV, close health supervision is needed to ensure that medications are taken and examinations are carried out. When HIV progresses to clinical AIDS, nursing care is similar to that of a child with any serious, chronic, life-threatening disease. Nursing care centers on preventing infection, managing pain, promoting respiratory and other organ function, promoting adequate nutritional intake, and providing emotional support to the parents and child, while promoting the child's growth and development. The accompanying *Nursing Care Plan* summarizes nursing care for the child hospitalized with AIDS.

PREVENT INFECTION

Immunosuppressed children become infected with bacteria as well as other organisms that are common in the environment. Protect the neonate from HIV-infected maternal secretions. Bathe the newborn as soon as possible after delivery and wash the eyes and face before administering prophylactic eye drops or ointment. Avoid invasive procedures in the newborn and encourage the mother to formula-feed the baby rather than breastfeed.

Proper disposal of needles and contaminated materials or equipment is essential to reduce the transmission of HIV (Figure 48–1). Standard precautions (see the *Clinical Skills Manual* SKILLS) are implemented to prevent exposure to HIV.

Frequent hand hygiene and limiting exposure of the child to individuals with upper respiratory or other infections are the best interventions to protect the child with HIV from acquiring other infections. Vaccines are administered to children with HIV infection following guidelines that have been established (see Chapter 43). Benefits and risks of vaccines are weighed and the child should receive the immunization if appropriate. The live measles-mumps-rubella and the varicella vaccine can

be administered to children and adolescents with HIV infection who are asymptomatic and have adequate T-lymphocyte and CD4 values (AAP, 2015, p. 469). See Chapter 43 for further immunization recommendations for the child who is immunocompromised. Educate sexually active adolescents on the importance of practicing safe sex and the ramifications of high-risk sexual behaviors and intravenous drug abuse.

Clinical Tip

Older school-age children and adolescents with HIV should be informed of their diagnosis and counseled appropriately regarding sexual transmission. Telling the child is difficult for parents and they often avoid doing so. Because parents usually want to be the ones to tell the child, they need help to plan how to discuss the issue and ongoing support in the process of communication. Nurses can assist in the following ways:

- Help parents understand the need to discuss the diagnosis with the child.
- Provide information about how to tell the child. Role play with the parents how to tell the child and use information at the child's developmental understanding to assist parents to be honest.
- Provide sources of hope—the success of treatment, children living with HIV, and maintaining an active life.
- Assist the family to join support groups or web-based groups.
- Help the family plan for respite care as needed.
- Provide emotional support for this difficult task and allow for ongoing opportunities to express concerns, fears, and anxieties.

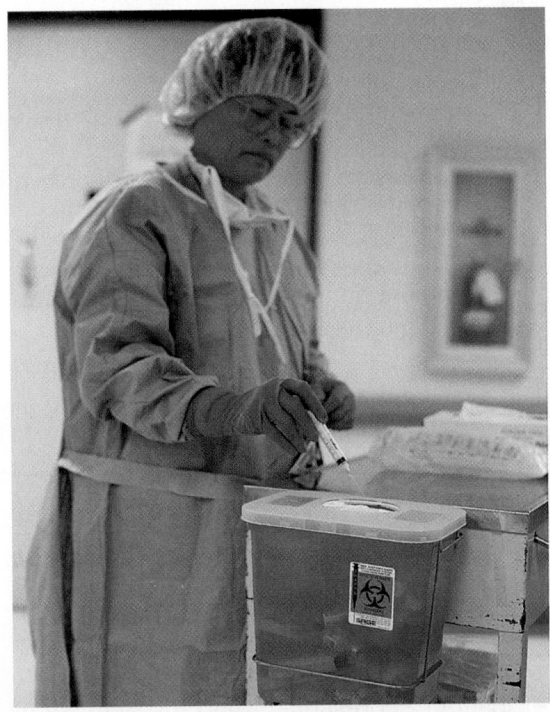

Figure 48–1 **Biohazard disposal. This nurse is disposing of a needle and syringe in a biohazard container, a necessary practice to avoid the transmission of HIV through needlesticks with contaminated needles. Standard precautions provide protection even when the immune status of the patient is not known.**

Nursing Care Plan: The Child With Acquired Immunodeficiency Syndrome

1. Nursing Diagnosis: *Infection, Risk for,* **related to immunosuppression (NANDA-I © 2014)**

GOAL: Risk factors for infection will be reduced as evidenced by absence of signs of infection.

INTERVENTION	RATIONALE
• Assess the child every 2–4 hr for fever; lesions in the mouth; and redness, inflammation, soreness, and lesions on the skin or around intravenous lines.	• Fever is one of the few signs of infection in the immunosuppressed child who does not have a sufficient number of white blood cells.
• Auscultate for changes in breath sounds every 2 hr. Perform pulmonary toilet (coughing, deep breathing, incentive spirometry) every 2–4 hr.	• Pneumonia is a likely infection in the child HIV infection.
• Enforce good hand hygiene. Allow no fresh flowers, fruits, or vegetables in child's room. Screen visitors for colds or recent exposure to varicella. Use blood and body fluid precautions (refer to the *Clinical Skills Manual* SKILLS). Practice strict asepsis for dressing changes and suctioning.	• Control of environmental factors helps prevent infection.
• Coordinate patient care assignments to avoid exposing the child to individuals with recent infections or immunizations.	• Planning minimizes chances for infection.
• Organize patient care activities to allow for adequate periods of rest.	• Rest periods allow the child to regain energy.
• Follow recommendations of CDC and AAP for immunizing immunosuppressed children. Avoid varicella vaccine. Perform annual TB testing.	• Special recommendations consider the child's decreased immune response and the danger of acquiring disease from certain live virus vaccines.

EXPECTED OUTCOME: Child will have no fever and show no other signs of infection.

2. Nursing Diagnosis: *Nutrition, Imbalanced: Less than Body Requirements,* **related to loss of appetite and decreased absorption of nutrients (NANDA-I © 2014)**

GOAL: The child will demonstrate adequate nutritional status to meet metabolic needs as evidenced by adequate weight gain for age.

INTERVENTION	RATIONALE
• Encourage frequent small meals to promote nutritional and fluid intake.	• Additional nutrition is required to rebuild the immune system.
• Maintain nasogastric tube feeding, if ordered. Total parenteral nutrition may be necessary to ensure adequate nutrition.	• Supplementation may be needed to ensure adequate calories.
• Eliminate unpleasant stimuli and odors from the environment during meals.	• Unpleasant stimuli decrease the desire for food.
• Monitor skin turgor every shift.	• Skin turgor reflects hydration status.
• Weigh daily.	• It is important to monitor weight status.
• Involve a nutritionist in planning a diet for the child that includes favorite foods.	• Including favorite food encourages intake.

EXPECTED OUTCOME: Child will eat frequent meals of adequate nutritional content. Child's weight will stay within normal limits.

3. Nursing Diagnosis: *Skin Integrity, Risk for Impaired,* **related to skin infection, immobility, or diarrhea (NANDA-I © 2014)**

GOAL: The child will have intact skin.

INTERVENTION	RATIONALE
• Observe all pressure areas closely for signs of infection or breakdown.	• Skin care is important in the immunocompromised child. The skin may be the only intact defense the child has.
• Keep skin clean and dry. Provide perineal care to minimize irritation from diarrhea.	• Prevents breaking or cracking of skin.

EXPECTED OUTCOME: Child will be free of preventable skin breakdown.

4. Nursing Diagnosis: *Knowledge, Deficient (Parent)*, **related to home care of child with AIDS** (NANDA-I © 2014)

GOAL: The parent(s) will demonstrate knowledge about home care including medication regimen, measures to prevent infection, and signs and symptoms to report to healthcare providers.

INTERVENTION	RATIONALE
• Explain the importance of optimizing the child's health status and reducing risk of complications through diet, rest, and meticulous personal hygiene. Be sure that parents and other family members understand how HIV infection is spread and take appropriate precautions.	• Knowledge about the disorder and preventive measures is necessary to provide safe and effective home care for the child.
• Be sure that parents understand the need for adherence to the medication regimen and understand how to administer medications.	• Knowledge of rationale increases compliance.
• Inform the family about signs and symptoms of infection that should be reported promptly to the healthcare provider or nurse (fever, chills, cough, mild erythema).	• Prompt treatment increases outcome.

EXPECTED OUTCOME: Parent will describe appropriate home care and preventive measures for a child with AIDS.

Clinical Tip

Work with the family of the child with HIV infection to establish a plan for medication administration. Assist them to establish a time schedule that limits the administration of several large amounts of medication at the same time. Stress the importance of disguising the taste of bitter medications to increase the child's willingness to take the medication.

PROMOTE MEDICATION REGIMEN ADHERENCE

The treatment regimen with the use of antiretroviral therapies for the child with HIV infection may be complex, time consuming, and costly, presenting an overwhelming challenge to the child and the family. Adherence to the prescribed antiretroviral regimen is imperative as nonadherence will likely result in disease progression (Buchanan et al., 2012). Some common reasons for nonadherence include frequent dosing, restrictions on daily schedules, pill taste, side effects, and dietary restrictions (Malee et al., 2011). Strategies for achieving optimal management of the treatment regimen include educating the parent or childcare provider, and the affected child when doing so is developmentally appropriate, about the purpose of the medication, the benefits of adhering to the regimen, and the potential consequences of failure to adhere to the regimen. Behavior modification techniques, using positive reinforcement, can be very effective in promoting the child's adherence. Provide support to the family, and tailor the medication regimen to the family's routine when possible. Offer praise to the child and parent for adhering to the regimen. If problems exist in managing the treatment regimen, carefully listen to the family to help determine the cause. Collaborate with the family in establishing goals to help meet the prescribed treatment regimen. If further intervention is required, options include direct observational therapy or home visits. Consider the effect of cultural beliefs on medication adherence (see *Developing Cultural Competence: HIV/AIDS and African Americans* and *Evidence-Based Practice: Adolescents With HIV Infection and Medication Regimen Adherence*).

Developing Cultural Competence HIV/AIDS and African Americans

HIV affects African Americans more than any other racial/ethnic group. The incidence of HIV in African Americans is 8 times greater than that of Whites. According to 2010 data, African Americans accounted for approximately 44% of new HIV infections in adults and children over 13 years of age. The CDC has implemented programs focusing on maximizing the effectiveness of HIV prevention methods (CDC, 2015). It is essential that efforts are focused on high-risk populations so that they receive education regarding prevention, testing, and resources.

PROMOTE RESPIRATORY FUNCTION

Because many children with HIV infection develop pneumonia, encourage the child to cough and deep breathe every 2 to 4 hours. In the community, regular physical activity encourages lung aeration. When in the hospital, blowing cotton balls with a straw, blowing bubbles, or other games may engage the interest of a younger child. Reposition infants frequently so all areas of the lungs can aerate. The plan of care should include rest periods to conserve energy and lower the body's demand for oxygen.

PROMOTE ADEQUATE NUTRITIONAL INTAKE

Because many children with HIV infection fail to thrive, nutrition is an important part of their care. (See Chapter 32 for information to include in a detailed nutritional assessment.) A nutritionist should be involved in planning an appropriate diet for the child that provides necessary calories, protein, and other nutrients. Vitamins may be especially lacking in the diets of infected children. Antioxidants (vitamin A, vitamin E, zinc, and selenium) are known to enhance general immune system function; children should consume these nutrients at recommended levels. It is important, however, to verify that there are no interactions between specific vitamins and the child's prescribed antiretroviral medications. Periodic dietary analysis and teaching are needed. Adequate nutrition is sometimes provided through total parenteral nutrition or through nasogastric or gavage feeding.

Diarrhea resulting from gastrointestinal infection and lactose intolerance is a common finding in children with HIV infection, and it complicates other nutritional disturbances. Alternative formulas may be recommended. Although antidiarrheal medications are not generally used in infants, they may be prescribed for older children. Carefully monitor hydration status, skin turgor, and urine output. Provide careful perineal skin care to prevent infection.

The frequency of *Candida* infections leads to blisters, cracking, and discharge involving the oral mucous membranes. To keep the child's lips and mouth moist, mouth care should be performed every 2 to 4 hours with a non–alcohol-based solution such as normal saline. The child may need a prescription mouthwash.

PROVIDE EMOTIONAL SUPPORT

The family of the child with HIV infection is under emotional stress, and this is compounded if others in the family are infected. The infected teen may see progression of disease in the parent and lose hope. Integrate social services and support groups into the care of the child as soon as the diagnosis is made. Spend time talking with the family to provide them with an opportunity to discuss their fears and feelings. In many parts of the United States, HIV infection still carries a tremendous stigma, and the family may not be able to discuss their feelings outside the healthcare environment. Safeguard the family's wishes about the privacy of the diagnosis.

Clarify any misconceptions the older child with HIV infection may have about transmission of the disease. Routes of transmission and the need for safe sexual practices must be discussed openly and clearly with adolescents. Providing support for adolescents is particularly important because the dependence on family or other caregivers that this chronic and terminal disease brings can make it difficult to meet the

---

EVIDENCE-BASED PRACTICE | Adolescents With HIV Infection and Medication Regimen Adherence

Clinical Question
What factors are associated with medication adherence in the adolescent with HIV infection?

The Evidence
MacDonell, Naar-King, Huszti, et al. (2013) utilized a cross-sectional multisite sample to examine barriers to antiretroviral medication adherence in behaviorally and perinatally HIV-infected youth. The subjects for the study were 484 youth, ages 12 to 24, who were prescribed medication for HIV. The most common barriers reported were forgetting to take the medication, not feeling like taking the medication, and not wanting to be reminded of their disease. While the top barriers were similar for behaviorally and perinatally infected participants, those infected perinatally reported significantly more barriers. There was a significant correlation in those with perinatally acquired infection between the number of barriers and percentage of doses missed, psychologic distress, and viral load. For those with behaviorally acquired infection, there was a significant correlation between number of barriers and number of doses missed, psychologic distress, and substance use. Forgetting to take the medication was the top barrier listed for the full study sample. Other top barriers included not feeling like it/needing a break, medicine reminded them of the disease, medication made them sick to their stomach/tasted bad, and running out of the prescription.

A qualitative study by Udomkhamsuk, Fongkaew, Grimes, et al. (2014) examined the concerns and needs related to adherence to treatment for HIV infection. Data were collected using participatory activities and interviews with 25 youth ages 14 to 21. Five themes emerged from the interviews: Lack of drug knowledge; boredom, discouragement, and denial; fear of disclosure; not managing medication; and risk taking. Some of the subthemes included not knowing about side effects of antiretroviral therapy (ART), being bored with repeatedly taking medications, feeling discouraged by having an incurable disease, denial, fear of losing friendships, disclosure of their infection, forgetting to carry the medicine with them, not taking medicine on time, lack of negotiation skills, curiosity, and poor safe sex planning skills. The study concluded that lack of full adherence to the ART regimen was related to cognitive and psychosocial factors and that youth with HIV infection lack knowledge related to ART.

Navarra, Neu, Toussi, and colleagues (2014) used a cross-sectional descriptive survey design to evaluate the relationship between functional literacy (the ability to read and write), health literacy (the skill to access and understand health information), beliefs about antiretroviral therapy (ART), media use, and adherence to ART. Fifty youth ages 13 to 24 participated in the study. The instruments used in the study included The Test of Functional Health Literacy in Adults (TOFHLA), the Rapid Estimate of Adult Literacy in Medicine-teen (REALM-teen), the Media Use Questionnaire, and the Beliefs About Medication Scale (BAMS). The BAMS assessed intent regarding oral medication adherence, perceived threat of illness, negative outcome expectancy, and positive outcome expectancy. Data from these instruments were collected during a clinic visit using face-to-face interviews after the investigator asked the youth to recall how many doses of their antiretroviral medication had been missed in the past 3 days. While health literacy was not a predictor of adherence in these subjects, higher positive outcome expectancy scores were associated with increased adherence. Subjects with below-grade level reading were associated with a lower level of adherence. This study indicated the importance of a comprehensive care model that includes assessing both health beliefs and reading skills in HIV-infected youth.

Best Practice
Adherence to antiretroviral therapy is a concern in the adolescent population. Concerns and knowledge related to the disease and the treatment plan should be assessed. It is essential that adolescents have adequate medical care and receive comprehensive education related to the importance of adherence to their medication regimen and the positive effects of adhering to antiretroviral therapy. Regimens that are simple, palatable, and with the fewest side effects possible are important in order to increase adherence (MacDonnell et al., 2013). Measures that increase adolescents' confidence in their ability to comply with the treatment plan should be implemented. Discuss strategies with adolescents that will assist them in remembering to take their medication.

Clinical Reasoning
What barriers does your health center address in its care of children with HIV that may lead to medication nonadherence in the HIV-infected adolescent? What support does the adolescent need to improve medication adherence? What measures can the nurse take to improve medication adherence in the adolescent?

developmental task of independence. Adolescents may benefit from contact with other infected peers.

DISCHARGE PLANNING

The diagnosis of HIV infection is surrounded by strong emotions and fears. Be honest and direct. Education is essential. Explain that there is no evidence that casual contact among family members can spread the infection. For the child who has been hospitalized, home care needs should be identified in advance of discharge.

Discuss the family's finances as well as health insurance coverage for the child's care. Assess the family's ability to provide nutritious food, pay for required medications, and to provide a supportive environment. Refer to services as needed to ensure provision of quality care after discharge.

Support groups, home healthcare nursing services, financial assistance, and psychologic counseling are usually needed at some point during the child's illness, and the family should be aware that such services are available. Assist the family with coping mechanisms to deal with feelings of guilt and/or fear about the child's condition.

Clinical Reasoning The Toddler With HIV Infection

Raymond, a 2-year-old child, has had recurrent infections since he was born. After a recent illness with fever, vomiting, and diarrhea, blood tests were done to evaluate his immune function. He was diagnosed with HIV infection and admitted to the hospital for children.

- What physical needs does Raymond have at this time?
- What information does Raymond's family need?
- What can you do to provide emotional support to Raymond's family?

COMMUNITY-BASED NURSING CARE

Much of the care of the child with HIV infection takes place in the community. With the continued success of aggressive therapy, the majority of children infected with HIV can be expected to attend child care and school. Additionally, a substantial number of these children will reach adolescence, and some will reach adulthood. Assess the family and community support systems and provide resources and referrals as needed to help parents provide adequate care for their child and to assist adolescents as they transition to adulthood. Many children with HIV infection are placed in foster homes, and these families need careful instruction to manage this multifaceted illness.

School attendance guidelines recommend unrestricted school attendance and/or childcare center attendance for children with HIV infection. In addition, children should be allowed to participate in all activities to the extent that their health and other recommendations for management of infectious diseases permit (AAP, 2015, pp. 158–159). Contraindications to school attendance include lack of control of body secretions, biting, and open wounds that cannot be covered. CDC guidelines for standard precautions should always be followed in the school,

child care, and home settings. The nurse or assigned school personnel may be responsible for providing medicines or other care at school for children infected with HIV.

Assist the family in altering the home environment to provide standard precautions during care. To reduce the likelihood of transmission of HIV, make sure the child and family understand that the virus is transmitted through blood, urine, stool, and other body fluids. Instruct parents to use recommended precautions when handling body fluids. Explain that they should wear gloves when changing diapers; disposing of urine, stool, and emesis; or treating the child's cuts and scrapes. In addition, teach them to wash their hands immediately after contact with blood or other body fluids. To reduce the risk of spread of infectious organisms to the child with HIV, educate family members about the importance of proper hand hygiene. Instruct parents to use a bleach solution for disinfection of objects when necessary and to avoid contact with people with infectious illnesses.

Precautions to guard against foodborne illness are particularly important for the child with HIV infection. Parents also need instruction on correct administration and side effects of any medications the child is taking. Giving a child a complicated combination of drugs can be challenging for all families; therefore, teaching should be tailored to the particular family and should be followed by repeated evaluation of the family's success with medication administration.

Emphasize the importance of promoting the child's development. Perform frequent developmental screenings. Teach the parents how to support the child in achieving developmental milestones. Encourage contact with other children and adults, provide for appropriate toys, teach parents how to encourage the child's communication, and praise the family for what the child has already accomplished. Children who manifest decreasing achievement of developmental milestones or other neurologic symptoms should be assessed by the primary healthcare provider for HIV-induced encephalopathy. The nurse's record of development will be of great importance in this situation. The child needs regular health maintenance care, such as child health supervision visits, immunizations, and care for any other health conditions.

Evaluation

There are many desired outcomes of care for the child with HIV infection or AIDS. Expected outcomes of nursing care include the following:

- The numbers of cases of pediatric HIV due to vertical transmission from known infected mothers decrease.
- Infectious diseases in children with HIV infection are prevented.
- The child has adequate respiratory function and perfusion.
- The child has adequate nutritional intake to support normal growth patterns and prevent malnutrition.

TEACHING HIGHLIGHTS | Food Safety

The child with HIV infection is more prone to foodborne disease. Instruct parents to practice the following:

1. Use a separate cutting board for meats, and wash it with hot soapy water after use.
2. Wash all utensils with hot soapy water between any uses.
3. Wash and peel fresh fruits and vegetables. Consider use of canned varieties to limit exposure to microorganisms.
4. Use a disposable cloth or cloth that is washed after each meal to clean dishes. A sponge can harbor microorganisms and should not be used.
5. If well water is the source of drinking water, have it checked for contaminants regularly.
6. Do not allow the child to eat raw or undercooked meats, fish, eggs, or cookie dough. Avoid natural honey.
7. Bleach solution (2 tablespoons liquid chlorine bleach added to 1 quart cold water) is a good low-cost sanitizer for cleaning surfaces in the kitchen.

- The family adequately copes with the stress of a chronic disease.
- The child attends school and is supported in the educational process.

Autoimmune Disorders

In an immune system damaged by pathologic changes, an immune response may occur to some of the body's own proteins, resulting in the production of autoantibodies. These pathologic conditions in which the body directs the immune response against itself—identifying "self" as "nonself"—are called *autoimmune disorders*.

The primary feature of autoimmune disorders is tissue injury caused by a probable immunologic reaction of the host with its own tissues. Structural or functional changes occur as immune cells attack other cells in the body. Autoimmune disorders are grouped into systemic and organ-specific diseases. Systemic diseases, which generally involve more than one organ, include systemic lupus erythematosus and juvenile arthritis, which are discussed in this chapter. Organ-specific diseases, which primarily affect a single organ, include type 1 diabetes (see Chapter 53) and thyroiditis. Immune thrombocytic purpura is an immune disease affecting blood platelets and clotting and is discussed in Chapter 49. Psoriasis is a T-cell–mediated autoimmune disease of the skin and is discussed in Chapter 57.

Systemic Lupus Erythematosus

Systemic lupus erythematosus (SLE) is a chronic inflammatory, autoimmune disease of unknown origin that involves many organ systems (Silverman & Eddy, 2011). Although it is primarily diagnosed in adulthood, approximately 15% to 20% of cases are diagnosed in childhood (Fortuna & Brennan, 2013). SLE affects 1.5 million people in the United States. It is more common among African Americans, Native Americans, Hispanics, and Asians than Whites. More severe disease and higher morbidity and mortality are seen in African Americans with SLE (Mattingly, 2011). SLE is 9 times more common in females than males (Ferenkeh-Koroma, 2012).

ETIOLOGY AND PATHOPHYSIOLOGY

The exact etiology of SLE is unknown. A genetic component is suspected because the disease is often more prevalent in members of the same family. It is believed that in those genetically predisposed, an outside environmental agent causes the body to initiate an abnormal immune system response to its own tissues (Lupus Foundation of America, 2014; Silverman & Eddy, 2011).

The body produces autoantibodies and combines with antigens to form immune complexes. These antigen–antibody complexes are deposited in the connective tissue, triggering an inflammatory response. The chronic inflammation then destroys connective tissue. The tissue damage varies according to the organ involvement, although the tissues most likely to be affected are the small blood vessels, glomeruli, joints, spleen, and heart valves. Because many systems can be affected simultaneously, organ damage with subsequent multisystem failure may occur.

CLINICAL MANIFESTATIONS

Manifestations of SLE may be acute, with onset of nephritis, arthritis, or vasculitis, or may be noted as a gradual onset with nonspecific symptoms. Symptoms depend on the organ involved and the amount of tissue damage that has occurred and include fever, fatigue, malaise, and weight loss. Other clinical manifestations include rash, arthritis, and nephritis (Defendi, 2011; Mattingly, 2011). A butterfly rash on the face, consisting of a pink or red rash over the bridge of the nose extending to the cheeks, is a characteristic finding (Ferenkeh-Koroma, 2012) (Figure 48–2). Children with SLE may have anemia, leukopenia, and thrombocytopenia (Mattingly, 2011). Renal disease, the leading cause of morbidity and mortality in children with SLE, is evident at diagnosis in 50% of these children and in 80% to 90% within the first year of diagnosis.

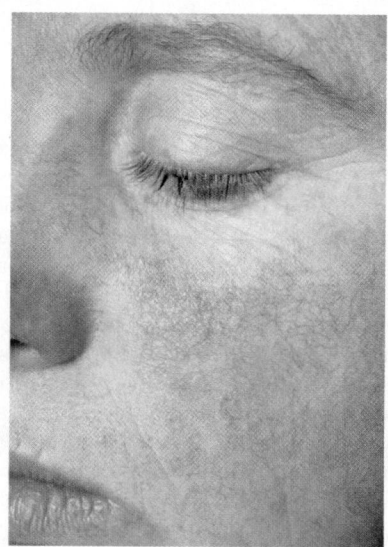

Figure 48–2 This child displays a "butterfly" rash across the cheeks and bridge of the nose. It is often seen in the child with SLE.

SOURCE: BSIP/Science Source.

Central nervous system disorders may occur in children with SLE and include headaches, mood disorders, seizure disorders, and cerebrovascular disease (Silverman & Eddy, 2011). See Table 48–6.

TABLE 48–6 Clinical Manifestations of Systemic Lupus Erythematosus

SYSTEM	CLINICAL MANIFESTATIONS
Integumentary	A butterfly rash on the face, consisting of a pink or red rash over the bridge of the nose extending to the cheeks, is a characteristic finding Photosensitivity Alopecia Mouth or nose ulcers
Hematologic	Fatigue Fever Easy bruising Nosebleeds
Musculoskeletal	Joint pain Swollen inflamed joints Myalgias Muscle weakness
Neurologic	Headache Peripheral neuropathy Psychosis Seizures Mood disorder Cognitive disorder Stroke
Pulmonary	Chest Pain Dyspnea Pulmonary hypertension Pulmonary embolism
Cardiac	Arrhythmias Chest pain Friction rub Raynaud phenomenon (fingers turning white and/or blue in the cold)
Renal	Hematuria Hypertension Proteinuria Edema
Gastrointestinal	Abdominal pain (may radiate to the shoulder) Diarrhea

Source: Adapted from Mattingly, E. (2011). Lupus in adolescents. *Advance for NPs & PAs*, 2(4), 27–32; Klein-Gitelman, M. S. (2013). *Pediatric systemic lupus erythematosus.* Retrieved from http://emedicine.medscape.com/article/1008066-overview; Silverman, E., & Eddy, A. (2011). Systemic lupus erythematosus. In J. T. Cassidy, R. E. Petty, R. M. Laxer, & C. B. Lindsley (Eds.), *Textbook of pediatric rheumatology* (6th ed., pp. 315–343). Philadelphia, PA: Elsevier Saunders.

Systemic lupus erythematosus is characterized by periods of remission and exacerbation (flares). Flares are triggered by a variety of causes, including sun exposure, an upper respiratory infection or other infection, and stress. The child or family may be able to identify other triggers to flares, such as particular events, activities, or situations.

CLINICAL THERAPY
Blood tests reveal anemia, an elevated blood urea nitrogen (BUN), abnormal plasma proteins, abnormal erythrocyte sedimentation rate (ESR), presence of antinuclear antibodies, and a positive LE (lupus erythematosus) cell reaction, which indicates nonspecific inflammation. The Coombs test is positive. Radiologic examinations include chest radiographs and computed tomography (CT) scans, as well as magnetic resonance imaging (MRI) of affected joints. A 24-hour urine collection and imaging studies, as well as renal biopsies, may be performed to evaluate lupus nephritis. Urinalysis may reveal proteinuria.

The goals of medical management are to create a remission of symptoms and to prevent complications. Corticosteroids, such as prednisone or methylprednisolone, are prescribed to control inflammation. Antimalarial preparations, such as hydroxychloroquine, are used to treat symptoms associated with skin lesions and renal and arthritic problems. Although the exact action of these drugs on SLE is not known, they often permit continued remission with a lowered dose of steroids. Nonsteroidal antiinflammatory drugs (ibuprofen, naproxen) are used to relieve muscle and joint pain. Immunosuppressant drugs, such as cyclophosphamide, azathioprine, mycophenolate mofetil, cyclosporine, and methotrexate, have been used to help control SLE. (Klein-Gitelman, 2013; Mattingly, 2011; Silverman & Eddy, 2011). Patients with SLE who are on corticosteroids or those who have arthritis are at increased risk for osteopenia. Vitamin D_3 and calcium carbonate improve bone health in these patients (Klein-Gitelman, 2013). Diet may be restricted if the child has excessive weight gain or fluid retention from steroids and renal damage. Prognosis depends on the severity of the internal organ involvement. Whereas SLE was once considered a fatal disease, 5-year survival rates for SLE are 92% or as high as 100%, and 10-year survival rates of 85% have been cited (Defendi, 2011). Survival rates decrease to 80% at 15 years after diagnosis (Mattingly, 2011). Kidney failure is managed by hemodialysis or peritoneal dialysis. Renal transplantation has been very successful for treatment of renal failure secondary to lupus nephritis.

Growth and Development
The side effects of the corticosteroids, immunosuppressants, and antimalarial drugs used in the treatment of children with SLE include hair loss, susceptibility to infection, "moon face," retinal damage, and bone loss. These are significant side effects for the adolescent, who is commonly concerned about appearance. Teens with SLE may need special teaching, guidance, and support. Support groups or Internet chat rooms may be helpful.

Nursing Management
For the Child With SLE
Nursing Assessment and Diagnosis

PHYSIOLOGIC ASSESSMENT
Assess the child's nutritional status, including comparison of prior and current weight for evidence of recent weight loss or weight gain. Assess the skin for rashes, ulcers, photosensitivity, ecchymosis, petechiae, cyanosis, and hair loss. Respiratory assessment includes breath sounds, respiratory rate, and assessing for extra sounds associated with pleural effusion or pleuritis. Cardiovascular assessment includes vital signs as well as assessing heart sounds and for signs of pericarditis or friction rub. Musculoskeletal assessment includes joint pain, joint swelling, joint deformity, pain, weakness, and ability to perform activities of daily living. Assess the neurologic system for changes in affect or cognitive abilities and seizure activity. Palpate the spleen to detect splenomegaly.

PSYCHOSOCIAL ASSESSMENT

Because SLE is a chronic disease that primarily affects adolescents, psychosocial assessment is indicated. Assess family interactions, exploring stressful situations such as divorce or trauma. Treatment-related restrictions associated with medications and changes in appearance such as weight gain, cushingoid appearance, and skin rashes can lead to withdrawal, depression, and risk for suicide. Perform psychosocial assessments periodically as the child grows and adapts to the disorder or faces new developmental challenges with a chronic disease.

Several nursing diagnoses may apply to the child with SLE. These include the following (NANDA-I © 2014):

- *Skin Integrity, Risk for Impaired*, related to photosensitivity
- *Activity Intolerance, Risk for*, related to joint pain and fatigue
- *Body Image, Disturbed*, related to side effects of medications and skin alterations
- *Infection, Risk for*, related to immunosuppressive medications
- *Pain, Acute*, related to joint inflammation and injury
- *Health Management, Family, Ineffective*, related to complexity of therapeutic regimen

Planning and Implementation

The goals of nursing care are to assist the child to manage and cope with a chronic disease, prevent infection, maintain fluid balance, promote adequate nutrition, promote skin integrity, promote rest and comfort, manage side effects of medication, avoid triggers for disease flares, and provide emotional support.

PREVENT INFECTION

Infections are a leading cause of death for those with SLE. Prophylactic antibiotics may be required for dental work and surgical procedures. Instruct the patient and family to inform all healthcare providers of the disease to plan for prophylactic measures. Emphasize the importance of receiving recommended immunizations including pneumococcal, meningococcal, and influenza. Instruct the family on hand hygiene and infection control measures in the home. Warn adolescents about the dangers of tattooing and body piercing because of the risk of infection.

MAINTAIN FLUID BALANCE

Because most children with SLE have renal involvement, nursing care includes maintaining accurate intake and output measurements and frequent evaluation of the child's fluid and electrolyte status and weight.

PROMOTE ADEQUATE NUTRITION

Currently, there are no specific dietary plans for the child with SLE; however, the diet may be restricted according to renal involvement, weight gain, weight loss, or other complications. The child is at risk for weight gain associated with treatment with steroids and a decreased activity level during exacerbations of this disease. A well-balanced, nutritious diet with calcium and vitamin D supplements to support bone density as well as appropriate fluid intake for age should be encouraged.

PROMOTE SKIN INTEGRITY

The presence of ulcers on mucous membranes can cause weakening of the tissues, placing the child at increased risk for infection. Provide instructions on oral care to maintain intact oral mucosa. Encourage the use of good hygienic measures and a mild soap for the skin. Recommend that adolescents limit their use of cosmetics, especially oil-based ones. Reinforce the importance of avoiding sunlight as much as possible and the use of sun protection factor (SPF) of 30 or higher at all times when in the sun. Encourage the child to wear protective clothing to limit exposure to sunlight (see Chapter 57 for discussion of sun exposure). Additionally, avoidance of unprotected fluorescent lighting is recommended since exacerbations of systemic lupus erythematosus have been reported following this type of exposure. Advise adolescents with lupus to avoid the use of tanning beds since these devices produce ultraviolet light and can cause or worsen lupus skin lesions (Lupus Foundation of America, 2014). Provide instructions on oral care to maintain intact oral mucosa. Provide instructions on the care of the head if alopecia occurs.

PROMOTE REST AND COMFORT

The child with SLE experiences fatigue and joint pain, leaving little energy reserve during acute episodes of the disease. Encourage frequent rest periods and a nutritious diet to maximize energy stores. A physical therapist can plan a program to encourage mobility and increase muscle strength. Implement measures such as application of heat to painful areas.

MANAGE SIDE EFFECTS OF MEDICATIONS

Observe for side effects of medications used for treatment, and teach the child and family about these effects. For example, immunosuppressant drugs can reduce the body's resistance to infection, and nonsteroidal anti-inflammatory drugs commonly cause gastric distress and bleeding of the gastrointestinal tract. The antimalarial drug hydroxychloroquine increases the risk of retinopathy and blindness; therefore, eye examinations should be performed every 6 months (Ilowite & Laxer, 2011). Corticosteroid side effects include cushingoid effects, weight gain, and hypertension. Sulfa drugs should be avoided because they increase photosensitivity.

AVOID TRIGGERS FOR DISEASE FLARES

Many children and their parents can recognize the signs of an impending flare and the triggers that precede them. Some of the triggers that might cause a flare include sunlight, stress, illness, and medications. Partner with the parents and child to implement measures to avoid these triggers. Discuss preventive behaviors such as avoiding sun exposure and avoiding stressors. Stress-reducing techniques such as guided imagery, reading, yoga, and quiet games can benefit the child or adolescent and reduce exacerbations of SLE. It may be necessary to discontinue a sport, music lesson, or other activity temporarily to provide a chance for the child to relax each day. Adolescents should be warned that alcohol, smoking, and drugs also pose an increased risk due to the potential to stimulate flares. Female adolescents who are sexually active should avoid birth control pills that contain the hormone estrogen, since the extra estrogen may exacerbate symptoms. Alternative birth control methods should be discussed with the adolescent.

PROVIDE EMOTIONAL SUPPORT

Adolescents may have an altered body image as a result of rash, alopecia, arthritic changes in the joints, and chronic disease. Referral to a lupus support group, social services, or counseling may be helpful. The Lupus Foundation of America can provide information to help parents and children adjust to the disease. Internet support groups are also available for those with SLE.

Evaluation

Successful outcomes of nursing care involve management of this chronic disease. Expected outcomes of nursing care include the following:

- The child has absence of pain.
- The child has absence of infection.
- The child has adequate intake and output levels, with demonstrated fluid and electrolyte balance and renal function.
- The child maintains intact skin.
- The child has a positive body image.

Juvenile Idiopathic Arthritis

Arthritis in children has long been referred to as *juvenile rheumatoid arthritis (JRA)* in the United States. The International League of Associations for Rheumatology now uses the term *juvenile idiopathic arthritis (JIA)* to describe arthritis with an unknown cause in children (Wedderburn & Nistala, 2013).

Juvenile idiopathic arthritis refers to inflammation involving one or more joints, lasting more than 6 weeks, and diagnosed prior to 16 years of age (Wedderburn & Nistala, 2013). This disease results in decreased mobility, swelling, and pain. The peak age of onset for JIA is between 1 and 3 years of age, with the illness occurring twice as often in females as in males (Petty & Cassidy, 2011). Approximately 1 of every 1000 children in the United States has JIA (Stanley & Ward-Smith, 2011).

Juvenile arthritis affects joints and surrounding tissues in addition to potential effects on other organs such as the heart, lungs, liver, and eyes. During the disease's course, the child may experience pain, impaired mobility, and interference with normal growth and development. Children may enter remission or manifest continued symptoms of a chronic disease. Remission may last for months, years, or a lifetime. Rarely, the disease is unresponsive to treatment or the child may suffer lasting impairment such as bone and joint changes. Children with early onset have a better prognosis for complete recovery.

ETIOLOGY AND PATHOPHYSIOLOGY

The cause of JIA is unknown, but it is thought to have an autoimmune basis. Inflammation begins in the joint and leads to pain and swelling (Figure 48–3). Scar tissue eventually develops,

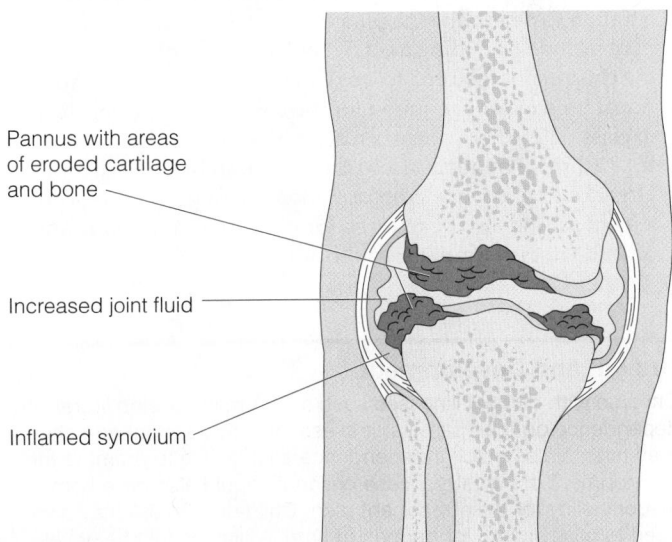

Pannus with areas of eroded cartilage and bone

Increased joint fluid

Inflamed synovium

Figure 48–3 **Joint inflammation and destruction in juvenile arthritis.**

resulting in limited range of motion. Altered growth related to early closure of epiphyseal plates, small joint contractures, and synovitis may occur. Although terminology varies among the different classifications, the three major types of juvenile arthritis under the most current classification of JIA are oligoarthritis, polyarthritis, and systemic arthritis (Petty & Cassidy, 2011):

- *Oligoarthritis* involves one to four joints and is the most common type of JIA. Approximately 30% to 60% of children with JIA have oligoarthritis. **Uveitis** (inflammation of the middle layer of the eye) occurs in approximately 17% to 26% of children with oligoarthritis (Hsu, Lee, & Sandborg, 2013).
- *Polyarthritis* involves five or more joints. Rheumatoid factor–negative polyarthritis affects 10% to 30% of children with JIA, while rheumatoid factor–positive polyarthritis affects 5% to 10% of children with JIA. Uveitis occurs in approximately 4% to 25% of children with rheumatoid factor–negative JIA and 0% to 2% of those with rheumatoid factor–positive JIA (Hsu et al., 2013).
- *Systemic arthritis* is characterized by high fever; swollen, painful joints; and rash. Systemic arthritis affects internal organs and joints. Approximately 10% of children with JIA have systemic arthritis (Hsu et al., 2013; Nierengarten & Oski, 2014).

CLINICAL MANIFESTATIONS

JIA may be restricted to a few joints or be systemic with involvement of multiple joints. Symptoms can include fever, rash, lymphadenopathy, splenomegaly, and hepatomegaly. The child with JIA may develop a limp or obviously favor one extremity over the other. A slow rate of growth or uneven growth of extremities may also be noted. Pain, stiffness, loss of motion, and swelling occur in the large joints such as the knees. Older children may develop symmetric involvement of the small joints of the hand. The disease is frequently chronic, extending over several years after an initial manifestation with pain and other symptoms. Remissions and exacerbations are characteristic.

CLINICAL THERAPY

No specific laboratory tests confirm the diagnosis; however, there are some tests to help support the diagnosis. The child may present with anemia and leukocytosis. Erythrocyte sedimentation rate (ESR) and C-reactive protein (CRP) tests may be helpful in determining the amount of inflammation. Rheumatoid factor and antinuclear antibody (ANA) tests may be positive (Petty & Cassidy, 2011). Radiographs are generally performed to exclude other causes, such as fractures, rather than as a definitive diagnosis, although radiographs are useful in monitoring for joint damage and bone development.

The goals of treatment are to relieve pain, control inflammation, preserve joint function, prevent deformities, achieve remission of the disease, minimize side effects of the disease and treatment, and promote normal growth and development (Petty & Cassidy, 2011). Nonsteroidal anti-inflammatory drugs (NSAIDs) such as ibuprofen, naproxen, indomethacin, diclofenac, and meloxicam are used to reduce inflammation and pain. Children who do not respond to NSAIDs may be treated with disease-modifying antirheumatic drugs such as methotrexate. Steroids such as prednisone and methylprednisolone may be used with children with more severe forms of juvenile arthritis. Biologic response modifiers such as etanercept, infliximab, and adalimumab have also been used to treat JIA (Petty & Cassidy, 2011; Stanley & Ward-Smith, 2011).

Complications such as chronic uveitis, which results from chronic inflammation, may occur in children with juvenile arthritis. Children with oligoarthritis and polyarthritis will need eye examinations either every 3 to 4 months or 4 to 6 months depending on their age and the presence or absence of ANA. Because uveitis is rare in children with systemic arthritis, the recommended frequency for eye examinations is every 12 months (Petty & Rosenbaum, 2011).

Growth interference for the child with JIA is a potential complication. The specific disorder may result in bone growth disturbance such as contractures or effusions. The administration of corticosteroids can also inhibit growth.

Nursing Management
For the Child With JIA

Nursing Assessment and Diagnosis

A careful history is important, as it is sometimes the primary mode of diagnosis. Assess for joint swelling and deformities, pain, decreased mobility, morning stiffness, fever, nodules under the skin, growth delays, and enlarged lymph nodes. The following nursing diagnoses may apply to the child with juvenile arthritis (NANDA-I © 2014):

- *Activity Intolerance* related to chronic pain
- *Mobility: Physical, Impaired*, related to joint stiffness and inflammation
- *Pain, Chronic*, related to joint inflammation
- *Body Image, Disturbed*, related to condition and physical appearance

Planning and Implementation

Nursing care focuses on promoting mobility, encouraging adequate nutrition, and teaching the parents and child about the disease and its management. Most care will occur in the community, including physical therapy, with only occasional hospitalizations at the time of an exacerbation of the disease.

PROMOTE IMPROVED MOBILITY

The goals of physical therapy are to maintain joint function, strengthen muscles, increase tone, maintain body alignment, and prevent permanent deformities such as contractures. Range-of-motion exercises, stretching, hydrotherapy, and swimming exercises help to prevent deformities (Figure 48–4). Encourage the child to perform activities of daily living. Exercise may be painful or even difficult for the child, but it is important because

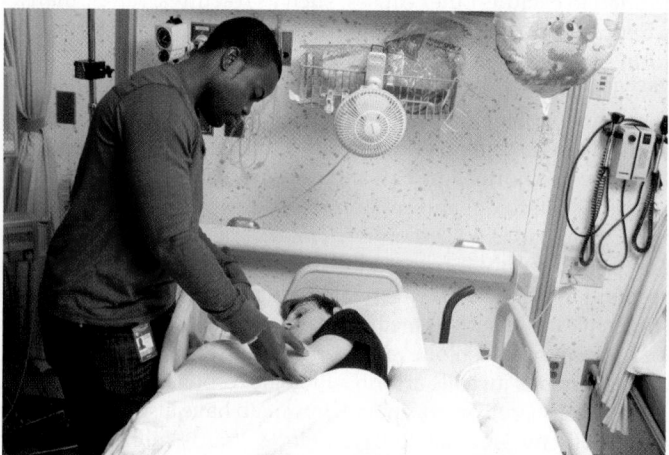

Figure 48–4 Passive range-of-motion exercises are an important aspect of physical therapy for a child or adolescent with juvenile idiopathic arthritis.

it strengthens and stretches the muscles and prevents potential contractures. Emphasize the importance of establishing a regular exercise and activity routine. Encourage periods of rest during exacerbations, as the child fatigues more easily. Medications may be given to reduce joint swelling and inflammation. In addition, warm compresses to the involved joints are soothing.

PROMOTE ADEQUATE NUTRITION

Promote general health by encouraging a well-balanced diet. Children with decreased mobility may have reduced metabolic needs, and excess weight causes additional muscle strain. Periodically perform diet recalls and nutritional assessments. Plot growth carefully and watch for changes in growth percentiles. (See Chapter 32 for additional information regarding nutrition assessment.)

COMMUNITY-BASED NURSING CARE

The child with JIA may never, or rarely, be hospitalized. Most care takes place during visits to healthcare offices, clinics, and physical therapy. Educate parents on the child's condition and prognosis, and answer their questions about the child's treatment. The child may need support to adjust to the diagnosis of a chronic illness. Allow the child to express anger and frustration about the diagnosis of arthritis. Allow the opportunity for the child and parents to express feelings regarding the crippling effects of the disease. Social services, a child-life specialist, or a psychologist may be consulted as needed.

Encourage the child to maintain contact with peers and to attend school whenever possible. Explain to the child and parents that overexertion may exacerbate the disease. Inform parents about possible complications of JIA, such as altered growth related to early closure of epiphyseal plates, small joint contractures, and synovitis. Partner with the family and school officials to meet the child's needs.

Professionalism in Practice **Accommodations for Children With JIA**

Section 504 of the Rehabilitation Act of 1973 and the Individuals with Disabilities Education Act (IDEA) protect children with disabilities from discrimination. A formal plan such as an individualized education plan (IEP) should be developed for the child with arthritis that outlines accommodations and modifications that are needed at school (Solomon, 2014). The school nurse can work with the family and school administration to determine the plan. Accommodations at school may include providing a set of books for the home so that the child is not required to carry the books home daily. Additional time may be required for the child to move from class to class. The school nurse can refer parents and children to the Arthritis Foundation and the American Juvenile Arthritis Organization for further information and support. The adolescent should also be referred for vocational counseling and offered support for transition to adult services.

Growth and Development

Children with chronic illnesses such as JIA may develop increased dependence on their parents. It is essential that school-age children maintain as much independence as possible to promote their development of industry. These children should also have some responsibility for their treatment plan. Children with JIA may also need to miss school for periods of time. A plan should be developed so that the child is able to keep up with school assignments. In addition, ongoing contact with peers should be maintained to promote the child's social development.

TABLE 48–7 Characteristic Findings in Children With Allergies

SYSTEM/ORGAN	FINDINGS
Respiratory system	Wheezing, rhinitis (seasonal and perennial), cough, adventitious breath sounds, inspiratory stridor, edema of glottis, nasal congestion or discharge
Gastrointestinal system	Abdominal pain and colic, mouth sores, constipation, diarrhea, bloody stools, geographic tongue, vomiting
Skin	Angioedema, urticaria, eczema, atopic dermatitis, erythema multiforme, purpura, drug and food rashes, contact dermatitis
Nervous system	Headache, tension, fatigue, seizures, tremors, irritability, sleep disorders, decreased concentration
Eye	Conjunctivitis, ciliary spasm, iritis, itching of eyes, tearing
Blood	Thrombocytopenic purpura, hemolytic anemia, leukopenia, agranulocytosis
Musculoskeletal system	Arthralgia, myalgia, torticollis
Genitourinary system	Dysuria, vulvovaginitis, enuresis
Miscellaneous	Anaphylactic shock, serum sickness

Evaluation

Expected outcomes of nursing care for the child with juvenile arthritis include the following:

- The child maintains joint mobility and has absence of joint deformity.
- The child has absence of pain.
- The child has a positive body image.
- The child has absence of infection.
- The parents understand and support the therapeutic process.

Allergic Reactions

For unclear reasons, an increasing number of children are diagnosed with some types of allergy, such as allergic rhinitis and asthma. Why are some children allergic to cats, for instance, while no one else in the family has allergies? To answer this question, the nurse needs a basic understanding of the mechanisms of allergy.

An **allergy** is an abnormal or altered reaction to an antigen. Antigens responsible for clinical manifestations of allergy are called **allergens**. Allergens can be ingested in food or drugs,

injected or absorbed through contact with unbroken skin, and inhaled. Food allergies are discussed in Chapter 32. Common allergens in children include:

- Medications (such as penicillin)
- Animal dander
- Dust, mites, and mold
- Plant pollens
- Foods (such as nuts, seafood, or egg white)

An allergic reaction is an antigen–antibody reaction and can manifest itself as anaphylaxis, atopic disease, serum sickness, or contact dermatitis. Therefore, the symptoms can be mild to severe or life threatening, and they can be localized or systemic. Characteristic findings in children with allergies are summarized in Table 48–7.

The **hypersensitivity response**, an overreaction of the immune system, is responsible for allergic reactions. Hypersensitivity reactions have been classified into four types (Table 48–8). Type I hypersensitivity reactions, the most common allergic reactions, occur within seconds or minutes of exposure to the antigen and may progress to anaphylaxis. The release of chemical substances such as histamine is responsible for the signs and symptoms exhibited. The first time a child is exposed to the

TABLE 48–8 Clinical Manifestations of Types of Hypersensitivity Reactions

TYPE	ETIOLOGY	CLINICAL MANIFESTATIONS	EXAMPLES
Type I: localized or systemic reactions (anaphylaxis)	Antibodies bind to certain cells, causing release of chemical substances such as histamine that produce an inflammatory reaction.	Hypotension, wheezing, spasm of smooth muscle; stridor, wheal, urticaria edema, vomiting, diarrhea	Anaphylaxis Extrinsic asthma
Type II: tissue-specific reactions	Antibodies cause activation of complement system, which leads to tissue damage.	Variable; may include dyspnea or fever	Transfusion reaction ABO incompatibility Hemolytic anemia
Type III: immune-complex reactions	Immune complexes are deposited in tissues, where they activate complement, which results in a generalized inflammatory reaction.	Urticaria, fever, joint pain	Acute glomerulonephritis Serum sickness
Type IV: delayed reactions	Antigens stimulate T cells that release lymphokines, which cause inflammation and tissue damage.	Variable; may include fever, erythema, pruritus, contact dermatitis, blistering	Contact dermatitis Tuberculin skin test Graft-versus-host disease Stevens–Johnson syndrome Allograft rejection

allergen, there is no reaction. With every exposure thereafter, however, the allergic child may have a reaction to the allergen.

Type II sensitivity reactions occur within 15 to 30 minutes after exposure to the antigen. Type III hypersensitivity reactions may be difficult to distinguish from type II reactions. Hypersensitivity reactions generally peak within 6 hours.

Type IV reactions are delayed responses that do not appear until several hours after exposure and require 24 to 72 hours to fully develop. A type IV reaction, which is not confined to any specific tissue, is elicited by relatively complex antigens such as those of bacteria and viruses and by simple antigens such as drugs and metals.

Assessment of the child with an allergy includes a complete physical examination; laboratory, radiography, and pulmonary function studies; tests of nasal function; and serum and/or skin testing. Treatment generally involves avoidance of the allergen, such as substitution of a different drug when the child has a drug allergy. Desensitization may sometimes be used with increasing doses of the allergen administered subcutaneously in an office where resuscitation is readily available. This treatment is useful for allergy to bees or some pollens. For skin allergies, the allergen is avoided, skin is kept well lubricated, and topical steroids may be used. Oral antihistamines are sometimes used to treat allergy. Emergency medical care may be required to treat anaphylaxis.

Nursing Management

The child with allergies requires a thorough assessment, including a complete past medical history, family history, personal and social history, and review of symptoms. The history focuses on the following areas:

- What symptoms does the child experience? Children should be encouraged to describe the difficulty in their own words.

- Are the symptoms continuous or intermittent? What are the frequency and duration of episodes?

- When did the child first begin to experience symptoms? Did the child have eczema/atopic dermatitis or a feeding problem in infancy or childhood? Did the infant have frequent bouts of colic or skin problems when new foods were introduced? Was there a change in symptoms at puberty? Are the symptoms becoming worse or spontaneously improving?

- What known agents in the environment cause difficulties?

- Are there seasonal variations in symptoms? At what time of the day or night do symptoms usually occur?

The nurse may be responsible for performing intradermal skin tests for allergies (Figure 48–5). Nursing care focuses on treating the symptoms, alleviating the anxiety of the child and parents, and identifying the allergens. Educating the child and family on methods to minimize or avoid exposure to allergens

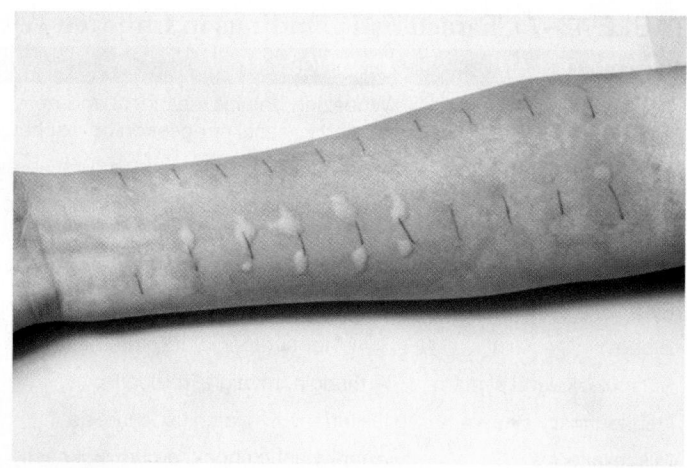

Figure 48–5 **Results of intradermal skin testing on the forearm. Injections are given on each side of the markings. Note the positive results marked by induration and erythema in response to certain antigens.**

SOURCE: Southern Illinois University/Science Source.

is important. Teach parents of children who have had severe reactions to bee or wasp stings how to take precautions and how to provide emergency treatment if the child is stung. An EpiPen may be prescribed, and the parents and child will require instructions on its proper use.

Families may need instructions on allergy-proofing the home. Pets, dust, carpets, fabrics, feather pillows and bedding, and cigarette smoke can all cause allergic reactions. If families are reluctant to give up pets, frequent baths can reduce dander, which is the usual allergen. Instruct the family on proper use of epinephrine.

When the child has type I reactions to an environmental substance, avoidance of the allergen is most critical. In addition, childcare providers, families, and school personnel must be able to treat anaphylaxis if exposure to the allergen occurs. When the child is hospitalized, be sure to label the child's chart and bed and apply a red armband to alert others to allergies. School nurses keep records about children's allergies and inform school personnel about the allergies and cautions that need to be followed. See Chapter 32 for more information about serious reactions to food, such as peanut allergy. Nurses must be aware of the resuscitation procedures and equipment in all facilities such as hospital units, offices, childcare centers, and schools. See Chapter 45 for airway maintenance.

Latex Allergy

Latex is a sap from the rubber tree. It is prevalent in the environment and is a component of many commercial products (Asthma and Allergy Foundation of America, 2014). Latex allergy is caused by an IgE-mediated response that develops after repeated exposure to latex. A reaction to latex products can be manifested as an irritant reaction of the skin; as a type IV delayed hypersensitivity reaction with contact dermatitis; or as a type I hypersensitivity, which is immediate and often has systemic manifestations (itchy eyes, asthma, or anaphylaxis) (Katrancha & Harshberger, 2012; Wade, 2012).

Latex allergy is present in approximately 1% of the general population (Katrancha & Harshberger, 2012). It is more common among certain occupations, including healthcare workers, and in specific types of clients. An estimated 8% to 17% of healthcare workers and up to 68% of children with spina bifida are allergic to latex (American Latex Allergy Association, 2014). In addition, children who have frequent medical procedures or multiple surgeries involving latex are at increased risk of developing allergy to latex (Asthma and Allergy Foundation of America, 2014).

Clinical Tip

In 1998, the U.S. Food and Drug Administration ordered that warning labels be placed on any medical products that contain latex, advising that use of the product might cause an allergic reaction (U.S. Food and Drug Administration, 2014). Check product labels in your healthcare facility for this warning. What products should have a label?

Children and adolescents at high risk should receive allergy testing for latex. When a positive skin test has occurred or when the person has had a reaction to latex, all latex products must be removed from the allergic individual's environment. Alternative products, such as nonlatex gloves and catheters, must be used when providing health care. People allergic to latex should also wear a medical identification bracelet at all times and should have an epinephrine kit readily available at home and school. Nurses should be alert for any signs of hypersensitivity when the child is receiving health care, and be prepared with drugs and equipment to treat anaphylaxis. This is especially important in operative settings when acute anaphylaxis is often life threatening. Nurses should emphasize to parents and children that many everyday products contain latex, including latex balloons and condoms (Table 48–9).

TABLE 48–9 Latex Sources in the Home and Community

• Art supplies	• Diapers
• Balloons	• Feeding nipples
• Koosh balls	• Handles on racquets, tools, and bikes
• Tennis balls	• Kitchen cleaning gloves
• Gym mats	• Pacifiers
• Chewing gum	• Paints and sealants
• Sneakers	• Condoms
• Sandals	• Rubber bands
• Toothbrushes	• Water toys and equipment

Source: Data from Spina Bifida Association. (2012). *Latex in the home and community.* Retrieved from http://www.spinabifidaassociation.org/atf/cf/%7B85f88192-26e1-421e-9e30-4c0ea744a7f0%7D/SBA-LATEXLIST-2012-ENGLISH.PDF

Clinical Tip

Healthcare personnel are at high risk of developing latex allergy because of intense exposure to products containing latex. Nurses can protect themselves by using the following measures:

- Decrease exposure by using alternative products whenever available (use synthetic rubbers, polyethylene, nitrile, neoprene, vinyl gloves).
- Use powder-free gloves if using latex gloves (the powder has high amounts of latex, which are inhaled).
- Avoid oil-based hand creams and lotions before putting on latex gloves, as these preparations break down the latex.
- When symptoms of sensitivity to latex occur on exposure (rash, hives, nasal congestion, conjunctivitis, cough, or wheeze), contact the employee health department of your facility.
- If diagnosed as latex allergic, avoid all contact and wear a medical identification bracelet.

Graft-Versus-Host Disease

Graft-versus-host disease can occur when organs are transplanted or when bone marrow or stem cells are transfused into a recipient, typically as treatment for leukemia or severe combined immunodeficiency disease. The donated cells attach to the recipient child's bone marrow and begin production. The child's lymphocyte production increases and an immune response

---

TEACHING HIGHLIGHTS | Removing Common Allergens From the Home

Preventing exposure to the known allergens in the home setting is important. Families can take several measures to minimize contact with allergens. These include:

- Keep pets out of the child's bedroom.
- Clean frequently with moist cloths and mops to remove dust.
- Use plastic covers on mattresses and pillows.
- Avoid using carpeting whenever possible; hard-surface floors are preferable.
- Avoid toys that collect dust (plastic and wood toys are better alternatives than stuffed fabric toys).
- Use high-efficiency air filters.
- Repair homes to prevent entry of water and subsequent molds.
- Consider dehumidification in moist climates, especially in the child's bedroom.

develops. However, despite blood and tissue typing, sometimes the donor cells are incompatible with the recipient cells and the new cells begin to mount an immunologic response in the child who has received the transplant. The incidence of the disease is lower in matched siblings than in matched nonsibling transplants (Velardi & Locatelli, 2016).

Graft-versus-host disease may be either acute or chronic. Acute disease has generally been thought of as occurring during the first 100 days after transplant, while chronic disease has been labeled as occurring 100 days posttransplant. In acute disease, the skin, liver, and upper and lower gastrointestinal tract are affected. Symptoms include a pruritic or painful rash, diarrhea, and abdominal pain. The diarrhea may be voluminous and lead to fluid and electrolyte imbalance. Liver enzymes and bilirubin are also elevated (Mandanas, 2014).

Chronic graft-versus-host disease is similar to an autoimmune reaction in the recipient's body and affects multiple systems, including skin, oral cavity, eyes, gastrointestinal tract, liver, lungs, and joints. Specific symptoms may include but are not limited to a rash, mouth sores, diarrhea, anorexia, nausea, vomiting, shortness of breath, chronic cough, itching, muscle weakness, and photophobia (Liu & Hockenberry, 2011).

Careful physical examination and laboratory tests assist in determining the presence of the disease and stage of reaction. Early identification is key to beginning therapy and stopping

progression of this life-threatening condition. Several drugs have been used in treatment of graft-versus-host disease and include cyclosporine, tacrolimus, and prednisone or methylprednisolone. Topical corticosteroids such as triamcinolone 0.1% may be used for skin involvement (Mandanas, 2014).

Nursing care focuses on careful physical assessment of all children who have received transplants to assist in early identification of the disease process. All body systems can be involved, especially in chronic disease, so frequent and thorough assessments are needed. Place particular emphasis on skin examination and report rashes that occur. Monitor gastrointestinal functioning by asking about nausea, vomiting, diarrhea, abdominal pain, bloody stools, and dietary intake. Weigh and measure the child and compare to earlier findings. Auscultate the lungs and be alert for signs of infection. Inquire about pain in joints or other body parts. Perform regular eye examinations and ask about burning or itching of eyes. Perform prescribed blood tests to monitor for liver and bone marrow function.

Nursing care for the child who has had a bone marrow or stem cell transplant is complex. Emphasize the need for regular examinations to identify any signs of disease. Children and their families need information and support about this immune system complication of transplantation of bone marrow or stem cells.

Focus Your Study

- The immune system recognizes any foreign substances within the body and eliminates them as efficiently as possible.

- The immune system is composed of antibodies, leukocytes (white blood cells), and lymphoid tissue.

- The infant is born with natural immunity from the mother and develops acquired immunity gradually in the first 6 years of life.

- Acquired immunity is humoral (antibody mediated) and cell mediated.

- B cells, T cells, natural killer (NK) cells, and complement proteins are the major components of a healthy immune system.

- Disorders of the immune system can have genetic causes (primary immunodeficiency) or they can be acquired (secondary immunodeficiency).

- Severe combined immunodeficiency disease (SCID) is life threatening and requires careful medical and nursing management.

- Human immunodeficiency virus (HIV) can lead to acquired immune deficiency syndrome (AIDS); care focuses on prevention of this viral infection.

- When the child is infected with HIV/AIDS, nursing care centers on preventing infection, promoting adherence to the medication regimen, managing pain, promoting respiratory and other organ function, promoting adequate nutritional intake, and providing emotional support to the

parents and child while promoting the child's growth and development.

- Autoimmune disorders such as juvenile idiopathic arthritis and systemic lupus erythematosus occur when the body perceives its own tissue as being foreign and mounts a defense against it.

- Systemic lupus erythematosus (SLE), a generalized disorder mainly occurring in females, is a chronic inflammatory, autoimmune disease of unknown origin that involves many organ systems.

- Juvenile idiopathic arthritis (JIA) is a chronic autoimmune inflammatory disease characterized by joint inflammation resulting in decreased mobility, swelling, and pain. JIA occurs twice as often in females as in males.

- There continues to be a rise in the number of children diagnosed with some types of allergy. A thorough assessment and careful teaching can help the child with allergies to successfully manage reactions.

- Allergy to latex products is commonly seen in children, healthcare workers, and the general population. Children most at risk for latex allergy include those with spina bifida and those undergoing frequent medical procedures or multiple surgeries involving latex.

- Graft-versus-host disease can occur when organs are transplanted or when bone marrow or stem cells are transfused into a recipient.

Clinical Reasoning in Action

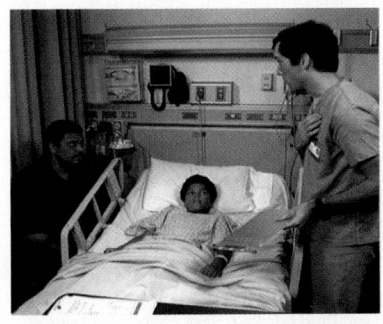

You are working at a pediatrician's office when 11-year-old Nirah and his parents come in. The husband, wife, and Nirah have all been infected with the human immunodeficiency virus (HIV). Nirah does not know he is HIV infected, but he has been very compliant with taking his antiretroviral medications. However, he has recently developed a cough and his parents decided to visit the pediatrician's office.

The pediatrician finds that Nirah has a fever of 102.0°F (38.8°C), respiratory rate of 60 breaths per minute, no visible retractions during respiration, and a pulse of 120 beats per minute. The healthcare provider decides to admit him to the hospital.

After the laboratory tests and radiographs are completed in the hospital, the healthcare provider tells the family that Nirah has pneumonia and strep throat. Nirah is started on IV antibiotics and shows improvement after 3 days of treatment. You monitor Nirah frequently and have him deep breathe. You also teach the parents how to encourage deep-breathing exercises.

1. How does HIV interfere with normal function of the child's immune system?
2. What are some of the measures of infection control for Nirah while he is hospitalized with HIV?
3. How can you promote Nirah's respiratory function?
4. When children, especially those with an immune system problem, are on antibiotics, they can develop thrush (*Candida* in the mouth). What is the treatment to prevent this side effect?

References

Albert, M. H., Notarangelo, L. D., & Ochs, H. D. (2011). Clinical spectrum, pathophysiology, and treatment of the Wiskott-Aldrich syndrome. *Current Opinion in Hematology, 18,* 42–48.

American Academy of Pediatrics (AAP). (2015). *Red book: 2015 report of the Committee on Infectious Diseases* (30th ed.). Elk Grove Village, IL: Author.

American Latex Allergy Association. (2014). *About latex allergy.* Retrieved from http://latexallergyresources.org/about-latex-allergy

Asthma and Allergy Foundation of America. (2014). *Latex allergy.* Retrieved from http://www.aafa.org/display.cfm?id=9&sub=21&cont=383

Buchanan, A. L., Montepiedra, G., Sirois, P. A., Kammerer, B., Garvie, P. A., Storm, D. S., & Nichols, S. L. (2012). Barriers to medication adherence in HIV-infected children and youth based on self- and caregiver report. *Pediatrics, 129*(5), e1244–1251.

Buckley, R. H. (2016a). T lymphocytes, B lymphocytes, and natural killer cells. In R. M. Kliegman, B. F. Stanton, J. W. St. Geme, & N. F. Schor (Eds.), *Nelson textbook of pediatrics* (20th ed., pp. 1006–1012). Philadelphia, PA: Elsevier.

Buckley, R. H. (2016b). Primary defects of cellular immunity. In R. M. Kliegman, B. F. Stanton, J. W. St. Geme, & N. F. Schor (Eds.), *Nelson textbook of pediatrics* (20th ed., pp. 1019–1022). Philadelphia, PA: Elsevier.

Buckley, R. H. (2016c). Primary combined antibody and cellular immunodeficiencies. In R. M. Kliegman, B. F. Stanton, J. W. St. Geme, & N. F. Schor (Eds.), *Nelson textbook of pediatrics* (20th ed., pp. 1022–1032). Philadelphia, PA: Elsevier.

Centers for Disease Control and Prevention (CDC). (2014a). *HIV among pregnant women, infants, and children.* Retrieved from http://www.cdc.gov/hiv/risk/gender/pregnantwomen/facts/

Centers for Disease Control and Prevention (CDC). (2014b). *HIV/AIDS.* Retrieved from http://www.cdc.gov/hiv/default.html

Centers for Disease Control and Prevention (CDC). (2015). *HIV among African Americans.* Retrieved from http://www.cdc.gov/hiv/risk/racialethnic/aa/facts/index.html

Defendi, G. L. (2011). Systemic lupus erythematosus. *Consultant for Pediatricians, 10* (1), 26–27.

Ferenkeh-Koroma, A. (2012). Systemic lupus erythematosus: nurse and patient education. *Nursing Standard, 26*(39), 49–57.

Fernandez, J. (2013). DiGeorge. *Merck Manual Online.* Whitehouse Station, NJ: Merck Research Laboratories. Retrieved from http://www.merckmanuals.com/professional/immunology_allergic_disorders/immunodeficiency_disorders/digeorge_syndrome.html

Fortuna, G., & Brennan, M. T. (2013). Systemic lupus erythematosus: Epidemiology, pathophysiology, manifestations, and management. *Dental Clinics of North America, 57*(4), 631–655.

Hassiotou, F., Hepworth, A. R., Metzger, P., Lai, C. T., Trengove, N., Hartmann, P. E. & Filgueira, L. (2013). Maternal and infant infections stimulate a rapid leukocyte response in breastmilk. *Clinical and Translational Immunology, 2*(e3), 1–10.

Hsu, J. J., Lee, T. C., & Sandborg, C. I. (2013). Treatment of juvenile idiopathic arthritis. In G. S. Firestein, R. C. Budd, R. C. Gabriel, I. B. McInnes, & J. R. O'Dell (Eds.), *Kelley's textbook of rheumatology* (9th ed., pp. 1752–1770). Philadelphia, PA: Elsevier Saunders.

Ilowite, N., & Laxer, R. M. (2011). Pharmacology and drug therapy. In J. T. Cassidy, R. E. Petty, R. M. Laxer, & C. B. Lindsley (Eds.), *Textbook of pediatric rheumatology* (6th ed., pp. 71–126). Philadelphia, PA: Elsevier Saunders.

Katrancha, E. D., & Harshberger, L. A. (2012). Nursing students with latex allergy. *Nurse Education in Practice, 12,* 328–332.

Klein-Gitelman, M. S. (2013). *Pediatric systemic lupus erythematosus.* Retrieved from http://emedicine.medscape.com/article/1008066-overview

Kronman, M.P., & Smith, S. (2015). Infectious diseases. In K. J. Marcdante & R. M. Kliegman (Eds.), *Nelson essentials of pediatrics* (7th ed., pp. 315–416). Philadelphia, PA: Elsevier Saunders.

Kwan, A., Abraham, R. S., Currier, R., Brower, A., Andruszewski, K., Abbott, J. K., ... Puck, J. M. (2014). Newborn screening for severe combined immunodeficiency in 11 screening programs in the United States. *JAMA, 312*(7), 729–738.

Liu, Y-M., & Hockenberry, M. (2011). Review of chronic graft-versus-host disease in children after allogeneic stem cell transplantation: Nursing perspective. *Journal of Pediatric Oncology Nursing, 28*(1), 6–15.

Lupus Foundation of America. (2014). *Living well with lupus.* Retrieved from http://www.lupus.org/answers/topic/living-well-with-lupus

MacDonell, K., Naar-King, S., Huszti, H., & Belzer, M. (2013). Barriers to medication adherence in behaviorally and perinatally infected youth living with HIV. *AIDS and Behavior, 17*(1), 86–93.

Malee, K., Williams, P., Montepiedra, G., McCabe, M., Nichols, S., Sirois, P. A., ... Kammerer, B. (2011). Medication adherence in children and adolescents with HIV infection: Associations with behavioral impairment. *AIDS Patient Care and STDs, 25*(3), 191–200.

Mandanas, R. A. (2014). *Graft versus host disease.* Retrieved from http://emedicine.medscape.com/article/429037-overview

Mattingly, E. (2011). Lupus in adolescents. *Advance for NPs & PAs, 2*(4), 27–32.

Mawn, B. E. (2012). The changing horizons of U.S. families living with pediatric HIV. *Western Journal of Nursing Research, 34*(2), 213–229.

McDonald-McGinn, D. M., & Sullivan K. E., (2011). Chromosome 22q11.2 deletion syndrome (DiGeorge syndrome/velocardiofacial syndrome). *Medicine, 90*(1), 1–18.

Michaels, M. G., & Green, M. (2016). Infections in immunocompromised persons. In R. M. Kliegman, B. F. Stanton, J. W. St. Geme, & N. F. Schor (Eds.), *Nelson textbook of pediatrics* (20th ed., pp. 1287–1295) Philadelphia, PA: Elsevier.

Navarra, A-M, Neu, N., Toussi, S., Nelson, J., & Larson, E. L. (2014). Health literacy and adherence to antiretroviral therapy among HIV-infected youth. *Journal of the Association of Nurses in AIDS Care, 25*(3), 203–213.

Nierengarten, M. B., & Oski, J. A. (2014). Juvenile idiopathic arthritis: Rethinking remission. *Contemporary Pediatrics, 31*(7), 14–19.

Orduño, N. M., Grimaldi, C., & Diamond, B. (2013). B cells. In G. S. Firestein, R. C. Budd, R. C. Gabriel, I. B. McInnes, & J. R. O'Dell (Eds.), *Kelley's textbook of rheumatology* (9th ed., pp. 191–214). Philadelphia, PA: Elsevier Saunders.

Pai, S-Y, & Notarangelo, L. D. (2013). Congenital disorders of lymphocyte function. In R. Hoffman, E. J. Benz, L. E. Silberstein, H. Heslop, J. I. Weitz, & Anastasi, J. (Eds.), *Hematology: Basic principles and practice* (6th ed., pp. 674–685). Philadelphia, PA: Elsevier Saunders.

Panel on Antiretroviral Therapy and Medical Management of HIV-Infected Children. (2014). *Guidelines for the use of antiretroviral agents in pediatric HIV infection.* Retrieved from http://aidsinfo.nih.gov/contentfiles /lvguidelines/pediatricguidelines.pdf

Park, C. L. (2012). *X-linked immunodeficiency with hyper IgM.* Retrieved from http://emedicine.medscape.com /article/889104-overview

Petty, R. E., & Cassidy, J. T. (2011). Chronic arthritis in childhood. In J. T. Cassidy, R. E. Petty, R. M. Laxer, & C. B. Lindsley (Eds.), *Textbook of pediatric rheumatology* (6th ed., pp. 211–235). Philadelphia: Elsevier Saunders.

Petty, R. E., & Rosenbaum, J. T. (2011). Uveitis in juvenile idiopathic arthritis. In J. T. Cassidy, R. E. Petty, R. M. Laxer, & C. B. Lindsley (Eds.), *Textbook of pediatric rheumatology* (6th ed., pp. 305–314). Philadelphia: Elsevier Saunders.

Rivera, D. M., & Frye, R. E. (2014). *Pediatric HIV infection treatment & management.* Retrieved from http://emedicine.medscape.com/article/965086-treatment#aw2aab6b6b2

Sampson, H. A., Wang, J., & Sicherer, S. H. (2016). Anaphylaxis. In R. M. Kliegman, B. F. Stanton, J. W. St. Geme, & N. F. Schor (Eds.), *Nelson textbook of pediatrics* (20th ed., pp. 1131–1136). Philadelphia, PA: Elsevier.

Schwartz, R. A., & Sinha, S. (2013). *Pediatric severe combined immunodeficiency.* Retrieved from http://emedicine.medscape.com/article/888072-overview

Schwartz, R. A., & Siperstein, R. (2013). *Pediatric Wiskott-Aldrich syndrome.* Retrieved from http://emedicine.medscape.com/article/888939-overview

Silverman, E., & Eddy, A. (2011). Systemic lupus erythematosus. In J. T. Cassidy, R. E. Petty, R. M. Laxer, & C. B. Lindsley (Eds.), *Textbook of pediatric rheumatology* (6th ed., pp. 315–343). Philadelphia, PA: Elsevier Saunders.

Solomon, L. (2014). *Educational rights for your child with juvenile arthritis: Understanding the educational rights of your child with arthritis is the key to school success.* Retrieved from http://www.arthritistoday .org/about-arthritis/types-of-arthritis/juvenile-arthritis/daily-life/educational-rights-and-resources /individual-education-plan.php

Spina Bifida Association. (2012). *Latex in the home and community.* Retrieved from http://www. spinabifidaassociation.org/atf/cf/%7B85f88192

-26e1-421e-9e30-4c0ea744a7f0%7D/SBA -LATEXLIST-2012-ENGLISH.PDF

Stanley, L. C., & Ward-Smith, P. (2011). The diagnosis and management of juvenile idiopathic arthritis. *Journal of Pediatric Health Care, 25*(3), 191–194.

Udomkhamsuk, W., Fongkaew, W., Grimes, D. E., Viseskul, N., & Kasatpibal, N. (2014). Barriers to HIV treatment adherence among Thai youth living with HIV/AIDS: A qualitative study. *Pacific Rim International Journal of Nursing Research, 18*(3), 203–215.

U.S. Department of Health and Human Services (USDHHS). (2012). *Can I transmit HIV to my baby?* Retrieved from http://aids.gov/hiv-aids-basics /prevention/reduce-your-risk/pregnancy-and-childbirth/

U.S. Food and Drug Administration. (2014). *New type of latex glove cleared.* Retrieved from http://www.fda .gov/forconsumers/consumerupdates/ucm048052 .htm

Velardi, A., & Locatelli, F. (2016). Graft versus host disease, rejection, and venoocclusive disease. In R. M. Kliegman, B. F. Stanton, J. W. St. Geme, & N. F. Schor (Eds.), *Nelson textbook of pediatrics* (20th ed., pp. 1069–1071). Philadelphia, PA: Elsevier.

Wade, J. (2012). Care of the type 1 latex allergy patient. *Australian Nursing Journal, 12*(19), 30–33.

Wedderburn, L. R., & Nistala, K. (2013). Etiology and pathogenesis of juvenile idiopathic arthritis. In G. S. Firestein, R. C. Budd, R. C. Gabriel, I. B. McInnes, & J. R. O'Dell (Eds.), *Kelley's textbook of rheumatology* (9th ed., pp. 1741–1751). Philadelphia, PA: Elsevier Saunders.

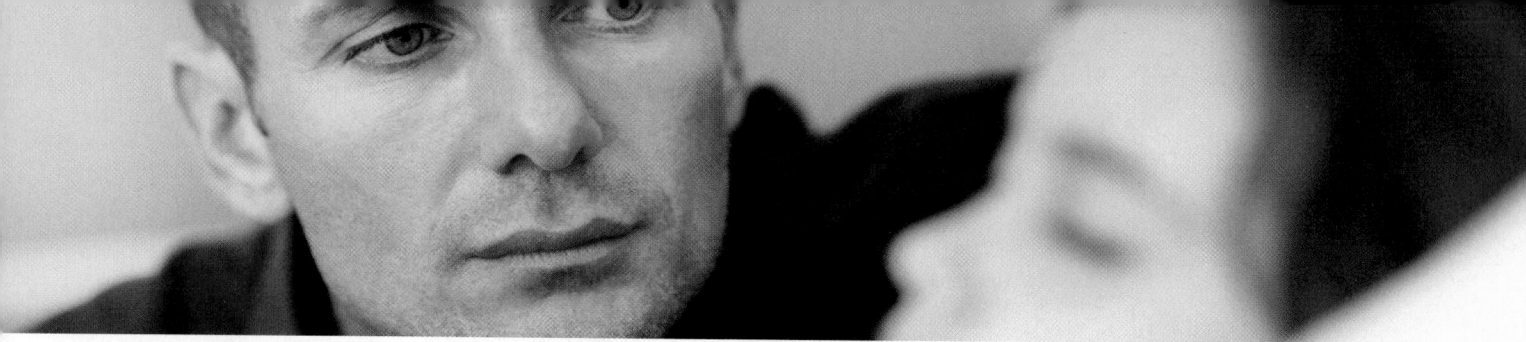

Chapter 49
The Child With Alterations in Hematologic Function

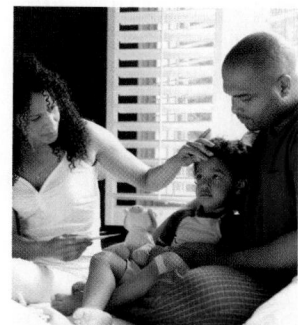

Having a child with sickle cell disease is very difficult for us. We know this is a genetic disease, and we feel responsible for Michael's pain. We also never seem to expect the bad times when they come. He'll be doing well and we almost forget . . . then he gets sick or doesn't drink enough and we're in the hospital again. His older sister has started talking about how she worries that sometime she'll have a child with sickle cell disease and we don't know what to tell her.

—Father of Michael, 3 years old

Blend Images/Alamy

⌄ Learning Outcomes

49.1 Describe the function of red blood cells, white blood cells, and platelets.

49.2 Discuss the pathophysiology and clinical manifestations of the major disorders of red blood cells affecting the pediatric population.

49.3 Discuss the pathophysiology and clinical manifestations of the selected disorders of white blood cells affecting the pediatric population.

49.4 Discuss the pathophysiology and clinical manifestations of the major bleeding disorders affecting the pediatric population.

49.5 Plan the nursing management and collaborative care of a child with a hematologic disorder.

49.6 Prioritize nursing interventions for a child receiving hematopoietic stem cell transplantation (HSCT).

The hematologic system is one of a few body systems that regulate, directly or indirectly, all other body functions. Because blood is involved in the function of all tissues and organs, changes in the blood may result in altered functioning of many body organs and structures. This chapter discusses the most common disorders of the blood and blood-forming organs in children. (See Chapter 50 for a discussion of leukemia.)

Anatomy and Physiology of Pediatric Differences

Blood has two components: a fluid portion called *plasma* and a cellular portion known as the *formed elements* of the blood. The cellular portion consists of red blood cells (erythrocytes),

white blood cells (leukocytes), and platelets (thrombocytes) (Figure 49–1). Table 49–1 gives normal values for these blood components in children.

Production of *red blood cells (RBCs)* begins in the embryo by the second week of gestation. White blood cell and platelet production begins at 8 weeks. Most of this early production occurs first in the embryonic yolk sac and then in the liver; however, by 20 to 24 weeks' gestation, liver production decreases as bone marrow production begins to dominate (Christensen & Ohls, 2016). At birth, **hematopoiesis**, or blood cell production, occurs in the marrow of almost every bone. The flat bones, such as the sternum, ribs, pelvic and shoulder girdles, vertebrae, and hips, retain most of their hematopoietic activity throughout life.

At birth, the newborn has a naturally occurring elevation in RBCs due to a high level of erythropoietin, which stimulates red cell production. Once the newborn begins breathing air and

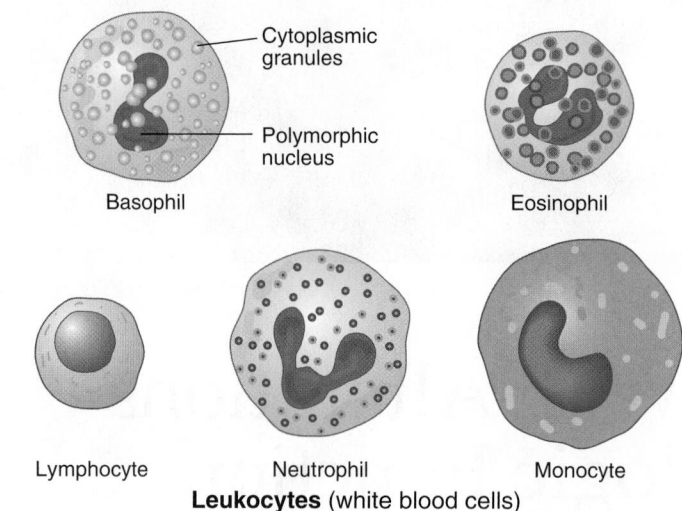

Basophil

Eosinophil

Lymphocyte · Neutrophil · Monocyte

Leukocytes (white blood cells)

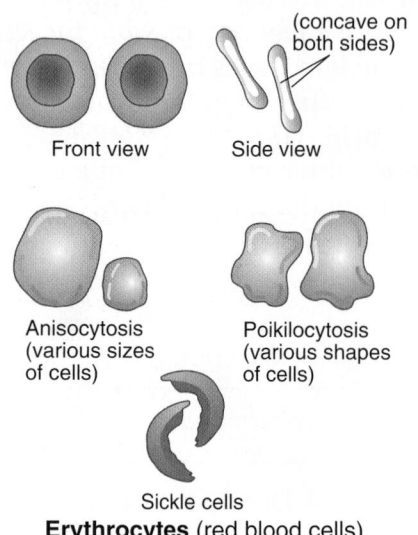

Front view · Side view · (concave on both sides)

Anisocytosis (various sizes of cells) · Poikilocytosis (various shapes of cells)

Sickle cells

Erythrocytes (red blood cells)

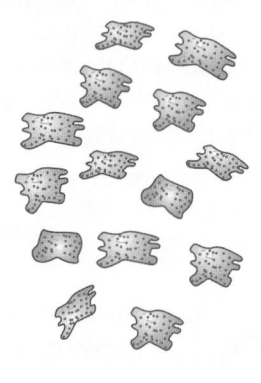

Thrombocytes (platelets)

Figure 49–1 **Types of blood cells.**

the oxygen level in the blood increases, this production slows. Levels of RBCs fall until about 2 to 3 months of age (to about 9 to 11 g/dL) and then begin increasing. Adult levels are reached during adolescence. Teenage boys have RBC levels slightly higher than those of teenage girls (see Appendix B).

TABLE 49–1 Mean Values for Common Hematology Tests in Children

TEST*	MEAN VALUE
Red blood cell (RBC)	$3.8–5.03 \times 10^{12}$/L
Hemoglobin (Hb)	10.2–13.4 g/dL
Hematocrit (Hct)	31.7%–39.8%
White blood cell (WBC)	$4.86–11.4 \times 10^9$/L
Platelets	$203–367 \times 10^9$/L

*See additional blood values in Appendix B.

Source: Adapted from Soldin, S. J., Wong, E. C., Brugnara, C., & Soldin, O. P. (2011). *Pediatric reference ranges* (7th ed.). Washington, DC: AACC Press; data from Lo, S. F. (2016). Reference intervals for laboratory tests and procedures. In R. M. Kleigman, B. F. Stanton, J. W. St. Geme, & N. F. Schor (Eds.), *Nelson textbook of pediatrics* (20th ed., pp. 3464–3473). Philadelphia, PA: Elsevier.

The white blood cell count is highest at birth, although levels vary greatly among newborns. Values begin to decline after 12 hours of life and continue to do so during the first week. By 1 week of age, white blood cell values stabilize and remain stable until 1 year of age. After that, the white blood cell count slowly decreases until the adult value is reached in adolescence (Walovich & Newberger, 2016).

Platelet levels in newborns are lower than in older children and adults. Levels of many clotting factors are also lower in newborns (Scott & Raffini, 2016). Vitamin K is required for the synthesis of clotting factors II, VII, IX, and X. For this reason, all newborns receive a prophylactic injection of vitamin K at birth (Greenbaum, 2016).

Red Blood Cells

Red blood cells, or erythrocytes, are the most abundant of the cellular elements of blood. They are formed through a process called **erythropoiesis**. The primary function of red blood cells is to transport oxygen from the lungs to the tissues. These cells also help to carry carbon dioxide from the tissues back to the lungs. Hemoglobin, a red pigment composed of protein and iron, is essential to this function.

TABLE 49–2 White Blood Cells and Their Functions

TYPE	FUNCTION
Neutrophils	Phagocytosis
Eosinophils	Allergic reactions
Basophils	Inflammatory reactions
Monocytes (macrophages)	Phagocytosis, antigen processing
Lymphocytes	Humoral immunity (B cell), cellular immunity (T cell)

Polycythemia is an above-average increase in the number of red cells in the blood. **Anemia** is a reduction in the number of red blood cells; the various types of anemia are discussed in the following main section.

White Blood Cells

White blood cells, or leukocytes, are the mobile units of the body's protective system. They are formed in bone marrow and lymph tissue. There are five types of white blood cells, each with a distinct function (Table 49–2).

A differential blood count indicates the percentages of the different types of white cells in the blood and is sometimes useful in identifying the cause of an illness. For example, infections cause an increase in neutrophils; and allergies are related to an increase in eosinophils. The role of lymphocytes is discussed with acquired immunodeficiency syndrome in Chapter 48. A decrease in the number of white blood cells is called **leukopenia**, and can be caused by immune or bone marrow disorders.

Platelets

Platelets, or thrombocytes, are cell fragments that can form hemostatic plugs to stop bleeding. They are synthesized from components in the red bone marrow and are stored in the spleen. A deficiency of platelets can lead to bleeding disorders and is termed **thrombocytopenia**. See the accompanying *Assessment Guide* for assessment guidelines for a child with a hematologic condition.

Anemias

Anemia is defined as a reduction in the number of RBCs, the quantity of hemoglobin, and the volume of packed red cells to below-normal levels. This condition can be caused by loss or destruction of existing RBCs or by an impaired or decreased rate of red cell production. Anemia also can be a clinical manifestation of an underlying disorder, such as lead poisoning or **hypersplenism** (a syndrome characterized by splenomegaly and blood cell deficiencies). Common childhood anemias are discussed in this section.

Iron Deficiency Anemia

Iron deficiency anemia is the most common type of anemia and the most common nutritional deficiency in children. Iron deficiency anemia can occur secondary to blood loss, malabsorption, or poor nutritional intake. See Chapter 32 for a discussion of iron deficiency anemia due to deficits in nutritional intake. Increased physiologic demands (such as rapid growth periods) for blood production can also lead to anemia.

Rapidly growing adolescents whose diets are high in fat and low in vitamins and minerals are particularly susceptible to iron deficiency anemia. Infants who do not consume adequate solid foods after 6 months of age and are fed only breast milk or formula that is not fortified with iron are also at risk for iron deficiency because neonatal iron stores have been depleted by this time and their iron needs are not being met. In addition, if the mother's nutritional status during pregnancy was inadequate, or the infant was born prematurely or as part of a multiple birth, insufficient iron may have been stored in the latter part of pregnancy, placing the infant at higher risk for anemia in the first months of life.

Chronic blood loss is always a potential cause of iron deficiency anemia. Those at risk of anemia include the infant who has had bleeding in the neonatal period; the child who loses blood as a result of conditions such as Crohn disease, celiac disease, or parasitic gastrointestinal illness; and the adolescent girl who has **menorrhagia** (heavy menstrual bleeding).

Clinical manifestations and severity of symptoms are directly related to the amount of iron deficiency or degree of iron deficiency anemia. Infants with mild to moderate anemia may be asymptomatic, while those with severe anemia may present with pallor, fatigue, irritability, poor feeding, tachypnea, and cardiomegaly (Mahoney, 2014). *Pica*, or consumption of nonfood items, is also a symptom of iron deficiency anemia (Harper & Conrad, 2014).

Diagnosis is made on the basis of clinical presentation and laboratory studies. The hemoglobin, hematocrit, mean corpuscular volume, mean corpuscular hemoglobin, red blood cell count, and reticulocyte count are evaluated to confirm the diagnosis (Harper & Conrad, 2014). A hemoglobin value less than 11 g/dL

ASSESSMENT GUIDE | The Child With a Hematologic Condition

Assessment Focus	Assessment Guidelines
Family history	• Does a family member have sickle cell disease/trait or other blood disorder? • Does a family member have hemophilia or other inherited clotting alteration?
Growth and development	• Measure height and weight on a regular basis and plot on standardized growth charts. • Perform nutritional assessment to see if child is getting enough calories. • Assess child for attainment of developmental milestones.
Skin	• Assess for pallor, flushing, rashes, and ecchymosis. • Observe for prolonged bleeding/clotting time and easy bruising.
Joints	• Observe for edema, pain, inflammation, and range-of-motion.
Additional assessments	• Assess pain in various body parts. • Identify frequency of infections. • Assess for history of fatigue and lethargy.

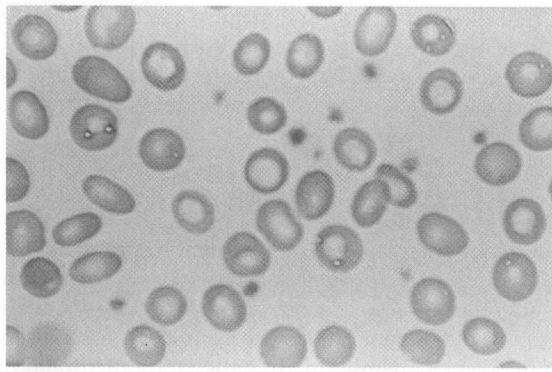

Figure 49–2 In iron deficiency anemia, red blood cells appear hypochromic as a result of decreased hemoglobin synthesis.

SOURCE: Biophoto Associates/Science Source.

is indicative of anemia. For children with severe anemia, additional recommended testing includes serum iron, serum ferritin, total iron-binding capacity, transferrin saturation levels, and stool testing for occult blood. Microscopic analysis reveals RBCs to be microcytic (small) in size and hypochromic (pale) in appearance (Mahoney, 2014) (Figure 49–2). A diet history and analysis can provide information about food intake; see Chapter 32 for guidelines about diet history.

Treatment involves correction of the iron deficiency with oral elemental iron preparations. Ferrous sulfate at a dose of 3 to 6 mg/kg/day is a common treatment, followed by evaluation for its effectiveness (Mahoney, 2014; Powers & Buchanan, 2014). Oral iron preparations cause several side effects such as constipation and gastrointestinal discomfort; therefore, the child may receive iron medications (to restore blood levels of iron) while the iron content of the diet is increased above the recommended dietary allowances (RDAs). Oral iron medications can then be tapered off once the child's food intake can supply the needed iron; the child is evaluated in about 6 months for recurring anemia.

Nursing Management

Children with iron deficiency anemia are usually identified and treated in the community unless they have another serious illness. Nursing care focuses on screening for the disorder and educating the parents and child about the causes of iron deficiency anemia, dietary management, and the importance of complying with the medication regimen.

Screening for iron deficiency is recommended for all children at approximately 12 months of age (Mahoney, 2014; Powers & Buchanan, 2014). Rescreening is needed in children if risk factors are identified (Mahoney, 2014). Frequency of screening for anemia during adolescence should be determined on an individual basis. Boys should be screened at least once during peak growth spurts. Girls should be screened at least every 5 years beginning at 13 years of age. Risk assessment for anemia should be performed annually in adolescents. If risk factors are identified, the adolescent is screened more frequently (Abrams, 2014) (see Chapters 34 and 36). A hematocrit or hemoglobin level is obtained for screening. More detailed tests are performed if the blood test is abnormal. Children at high risk for nutritional deficiencies, such as those in low-income groups and WIC programs (Special Supplemental Nutrition Program for Women, Infants, and Children), may require tests earlier. Most

children in Head Start are screened annually by nurses. In addition, children showing signs of anemia such as low energy and pallor should be screened. Height and weight measurements are obtained at each healthcare visit, plotted on growth charts, and compared with percentiles obtained at previous visits. Slow downward trends in percentiles are of concern and require further nutritional analysis (see Chapter 32). Perform developmental screening tests to assess for developmental delays (see Chapter 31).

Dietary management is the preferred long-term treatment for iron deficiency anemia. Teach the child and family to plan for foods that are rich in iron. Include teaching about foods with vitamin C since this vitamin may increase the absorption of iron (Powers & Buchanan, 2014). The infant over 6 months of age should have a diet that includes breast milk or iron-fortified formula and baby cereals with iron fortification. Avoid cow's milk in the first year of life because it can cause bleeding from the gastrointestinal tract, contributing to anemia. If the older infant or toddler consumes large quantities of milk and refuses to eat solid food, restrictions on milk intake may be required. Older infants and toddlers can eat finger foods such as thinly sliced meats. Adolescents can be encouraged to eat foods with high iron content and vitamin C such as hamburgers with a slice of tomato.

Oral iron preparations are given to correct anemia. Instruct the family about side effects such as black stools, constipation, and a foul aftertaste. Emphasize the importance of drinking fluids and eating foods high in dietary fiber to minimize constipation. The medicine should be stored safely to avoid accidental poisoning. Expected outcomes of care are intake of recommended levels of iron and return to normal hematocrit level.

Normocytic Anemia

In normocytic anemia, there is an increase in the destruction of red blood cells or decreased production of red blood cells. This type of anemia may be related to parvovirus B19, Epstein-Barr virus or other infections; bone marrow disorders such as leukemia; renal disease, G6PD (glucose-6-phosphate dehydrogenase) deficiency; inflammatory disorders or several other conditions (Lerner, 2016; Panepinto, Punzalan, & Scott, 2015). Clinical manifestations of normocytic anemia are similar to those seen in iron deficiency anemia, with the possible occurrence of hepatomegaly and splenomegaly as well.

Treatment of normocytic anemia depends on the underlying cause. When the anemia is associated with inflammation or infection, the underlying condition is treated. When hemorrhage is the underlying cause, the source of the bleeding is identified and treated. In acute emergencies, blood products are infused to make up for some of the losses.

Nursing Management

Nursing management of normocytic anemia depends on the cause of the decreased RBCs. Children with inflammatory or infectious diseases require careful assessment and management of medication and other treatment regimens. Administer blood products and other intravenous fluids as ordered to restore blood volume. Use follow-up or home visits to assess hematocrit, hemoglobin, and dietary intake. (Refer to the discussion later in this chapter for management of disseminated intravascular coagulation, to Chapter 51 for management of intestinal infections, and to Chapter 52 for management of hemolytic uremic syndrome.)

TABLE 49–3 Types of Sickle Cell Disease

DISORDER	CHARACTERISTICS
Sickle cell anemia (HbSS)	Most common type of sickle cell disease
	RBCs are crescent shaped
	Homozygous condition (child has two sickle hemoglobin genes)
	Child is subject to sickle cell crises
	Average life span is 45 years of age
Sickle C disease (HbSC)	Child inherits one HbS gene and one HbC gene
	RBCs are C shaped
	Anemia is generally milder than in Hb SS disease
	Painful crises occur about 50% as often as in Hb SS disease
	Average life span is 64 years of age
Sickle beta + thalassemia disease (Hb + Sβ) and sickle beta 0 thalassemia disease (Hb0 Sβ)	Combination of sickle cell trait and thalassemia trait. In sickle cell beta+, there is a reduced amount of hemoglobin A, and the life span is near normal. In sickle cell beta 0, there is no hemoglobin A and the life span is mid-50s.

Source: Data from DeBaun, M. R., Frei-Jones, M., & Vichinsky, E. (2016). Hemoglobinopathies. In R. M. Kliegman, B. F. Stanton, J. W. St. Geme III, N. F. Schor, & (Eds.), *Nelson textbook of pediatrics* (20th ed., pp. 2336–2353). Philadelphia, PA: Elsevier Saunders; Saunthararajah, Y., & Vichinsky, E. P. (2013). Sickle cell disease: Clinical features and management. In R. Hoffman, E. J. Benz, L. E. Silberstein, H. Heslop, J. I. Weitz, & J. Anastasi (Eds.), *Hematology: Basic principles and practice* (6th ed., pp. 548–572). Philadelphia, PA: Elsevier Saunders; Vichinsky, E. P. (2014). *Variant sickle cell syndromes*. Retrieved from uptodate.com.

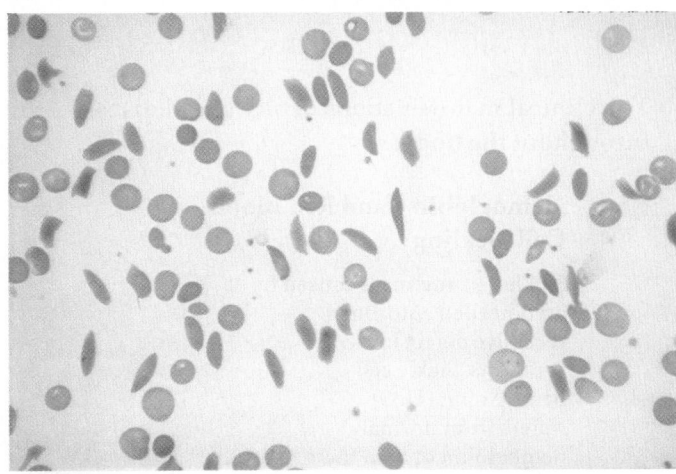

Figure 49–3 **Many of these red blood cells show the elongated crescent shape characteristic of sickle cell disease.**

SOURCE: BRUCE COLEMAN INC./Alamy.

Sickle Cell Disease

Sickle cell disease (SCD) is a hereditary **hemoglobinopathy** characterized by the partial or complete replacement of normal hemoglobin with abnormal hemoglobin S (Hgb S) in red blood cells (Table 49–3). This causes occlusion of small blood vessels, ischemia, and damage to affected organs. Sickle cell trait (carrying one gene for the disease) affects approximately 2 million Americans. Approximately 1 in 12 African Americans are carriers of the disease (Maakaron & Taher, 2014). Individuals with sickle cell trait have one sickle cell hemoglobin gene and one normal hemoglobin gene. They are carriers of the disease and generally do not have symptoms, although symptoms have been known to occur when the body is under extreme conditions (Centers for Disease Control and Prevention, 2014)

ETIOLOGY AND PATHOPHYSIOLOGY

Sickle cell disease is an autosomal recessive disorder. If both parents have the trait, with each pregnancy the risk of having a child with the disease is 25%. (See Chapter 3 for a discussion of recessive gene transmission.)

In the most common type of sickle cell disease (HbSS, also referred to as sickle cell anemia), the hemoglobin in the RBC acquires an elongated crescent or sickle shape (Figure 49–3). The sickled cells are rigid and obstruct capillary blood flow. Microscopic obstructions lead to engorgement and tissue ischemia. This local tissue hypoxia causes further sickling and ultimately large infarctions. Organ tissues become damaged by infarctions, leading to scarring and impaired function by 2 to 3 months of age. Levels of fetal hemoglobin decline, leading to splenic impairment (Yawn et al., 2014). Most children with HbSS disease will have functional asplenia by 5 years of

age (DeBaun, Frei-Jones, & Vichinsky, 2016). Children with sickle cell disease may suffer from splenic sequestration when blood is trapped in the spleen, a life-threatening complication. Many children must undergo splenectomy in early childhood, leading to severely compromised immunity. Infection rate is high because of impaired immunity. Bacterial infections are the leading cause of death in young children with sickle cell disease.

A stroke occurs in some children with sickle cell disease. Eleven percent of children experience this complication by 20 years of age (Lovett, Sule, & Lopez, 2014). Other complications of sickle cell disease may include acute chest syndrome with pulmonary infiltrate and infection, priapism (sustained and painful penile erection), retinopathy, kidney damage, and gallstone formation (de Montalembert, Ferster, Colombatti, et al., 2011; Meier & Miller, 2012; Tanabe, Dias, & Gorman, 2013).

Sickling may be triggered by fever, hypoxia, emotional stress, or physical stress. Precipitating factors for sickle cell crisis include increased blood viscosity (such as from a low fluid intake or fever) and hypoxia or low oxygen tension. Potential causes of hypoxia or low oxygen tension include high altitudes, poorly pressurized airplanes, hypoventilation, vasoconstriction when cold, or an emotionally stressful event. Any condition that increases the body's need for oxygen or alters the transport of oxygen (such as infection, trauma, or dehydration) may result in sickle cell crisis.

Sickled cells can resume a normal shape when rehydrated and reoxygenated. However, the membranes of these cells become more fragile, and cell life is shortened to about 10 to 20 days rather than the usual 120 days. Chronic hemolytic anemia develops because of the continued destruction of RBCs (Maakaron & Taher, 2014; Myers & Eckes, 2012 (See *Pathophysiology Illustrated: Sickle Cell Disease*.)

CLINICAL MANIFESTATIONS

Affected children are usually asymptomatic until 4 to 6 months of age because sickling is inhibited by high levels of fetal hemoglobin. Clinical manifestations are directly related to the shortened life span of blood cells (hemolytic anemia) and tissue destruction resulting from **vaso-occlusion** (blockage of a blood vessel). Illness results from recurrent vaso-occlusive events that involve painful crises and chronic organ damage. Pathologic

Pathophysiology Illustrated: **Sickle Cell Disease**

The clinical manifestations of sickle cell disease result from pathologic changes to structures and systems throughout the body.

Hemoglobin S and Red Blood Cell Sickling

Sickle cell anemia is caused by an inherited autosomal recessive defect in Hb synthesis. Sickle cell hemoglobin (HbS) differs from normal hemoglobin only in the substitution of the amino acid valine for glutamine in both beta chains of the hemoglobin molecule.

When HbS is oxygenated, it has the same globular shape as normal hemoglobin. However, when HbS loses its oxygen, it becomes insoluble in intra-cellular fluid and crystallizes into rodlike structures. Clusters of rods form polymers (long chains) that bend the erythrocyte into the characteristic crescent shape of the sickle cell.

Incorrect amino acids

β chains

Hemoglobin S molecule

α chains

Polymerized deoxyhemo-globin S

Oxyhemoglobin S

Oxygenated erythrocyte

O₂

Deoxyhemoglobin S

Deoxygenated erythrocyte

Sickled erythrocyte

The Sickle Cell Disease Process

Sickle cell disease is characterized by episodes of acute painful crises. Sickling crises are triggered by conditions causing high tissue oxygen demands or that affect cellular pH. As the crisis begins, sickled erythrocytes adhere to capillary walls and to each other, obstructing blood flow and causing cellular hypoxia. The crisis accelerates as tissue hypoxia and acidic metabolic waste products cause further sickling and cell damage.

Sickle cell crises cause microinfarcts in joints and organs, and repeated crises slowly destroy organs and tissues. The spleen and kidneys are especially prone to sickling damage.

Microinfarct

Necrotic tissue

Damaged tissue

Inflamed tissue

Hypoxic cells

Mass of sickled cells obstructing capillary lumen

Capillary

changes happen in most body systems, resulting in multiple signs and symptoms. Examples of common organs affected include the following:

- Brain—stroke, often manifested by headache, aphasia, convulsions, visual changes
- Eyes—retinopathy, retinal detachment, diminished vision
- Bones—chronic ischemia of bones with susceptibility to infection and bone degeneration, manifested by osteoporosis, osteomyelitis, spinal deformities, or aseptic necrosis of the femoral head
- Liver—impaired blood flow from capillary obstruction leads to enlargement and scarring of the liver, manifested by hepatomegaly or cirrhosis
- Spleen—splenic infarct leads to fibrosis and increased rates of infection
- Kidneys—ischemia of kidneys causes enuresis, hematuria, inability to concentrate urine
- Penis—microcirculatory obstruction and engorgement (priapism)
- Extremities—vaso-occlusion and chronic ischemia manifests as peripheral neuropathy, weakness, or arthralgia
- Skin—decreased peripheral circulation causes ulcerations

Sickle cell crises are acute exacerbations of the disease that vary markedly in severity and frequency. Table 49–4 outlines the most common types of crises affecting children with sickle cell disease. The most common reason for a visit to the emergency department for the child with sickle cell disease is acute pain crisis (Shihabuddin & Scarfi, 2014). Additionally, 60% to 80% of hospitalizations for children with SCD are related to pain (Meier & Miller, 2012). The sickled RBCs cannot move through the blood vessels and capillaries. Blood vessel occlusion occurs, leading to restricted blood flow and subsequent tissue ischemia. This is referred to as vaso-occlusive crisis (Myers & Eckes, 2012). Pain results from tissue ischemia. Pain is typically experienced in the back or extremities but can occur in other areas (Lovett et al., 2014). Children with sickle cell disease can also develop acute chest syndrome (ACS), a life-threatening complication of sickle cell disease in which a new pulmonary infiltrate is present on chest radiograph. Symptoms of ACS include fever, chest pain, tachypnea, coughing, and wheezing (Meier & Miller, 2012).

CLINICAL THERAPY

Newborns are screened for sickle cell disease. If the test is positive, hemoglobin electrophoresis should be repeated to confirm the diagnosis (Maakaron & Taher, 2014). (See *Developing Cultural Competence: Sickle Cell Disease*.)

Developing Cultural Competence Sickle Cell Disease

Historically, sickle cell disease has been thought of as occurring only in the African American population. In recent years, the disease has been diagnosed in those of Mediterranean, South American, Arabian, and East Indian descent. All newborns in the United States are screened for sickle cell disease as part of the newborn screening panel (March of Dimes, 2014). While African American families may be familiar with the need for screening, parents of children from other cultures may question this practice. Explain the importance of early diagnosis of sickle cell disease and reinforce the fact that heritage cannot be predicted from appearance or name alone.

Management focuses on pain control, hydration, oxygenation, prevention of infection, and prevention of associated complications. Treatment of crises involves aggressive hydration, oxygen administration, pain management, and bed rest to reduce energy expenditure. Parenteral analgesics, such as morphine and hydromorphone (Dilaudid), are generally administered around the clock or via patient-controlled analgesia. In addition to parenteral narcotics, the child may also receive intravenous ketorolac (Toradol) or oral ibuprofen (Motrin) every 6 hours around the clock as adjunctive therapy. Oral and

TABLE 49–4 Types of Sickle Cell Crises

TYPE	CAUSE/PRECIPITATING EVENTS	CLINICAL MANIFESTATIONS	SEVERITY
Vaso-occlusive crisis (pain crisis); most common type of crisis	Stasis of blood with clumping of cells in the microcirculation, ischemia, and infarction Precipitated by: • Dehydration • Temperature extremes • Infection • Localized hypoxemia • Physical or emotional stress	Extremely painful Symptoms include: • Fever • Tissue engorgement • Painful swelling of joints in hands and feet • Priapism • Severe abdominal pain	Thrombosis and infarction of local tissue may occur if the crisis is not reversed. Cerebral occlusion can result in stroke, manifested by paralysis and/or other central nervous system complications.
Splenic sequestration	Pooling of blood in the spleen	Profound anemia, hypovolemia, and shock	Life-threatening crisis—death can occur within hours.
Aplastic crisis	Triggered by infection with parvovirus B19 or depletion of folic acid	Diminished production and increased destruction of red blood cells Signs include profound anemia, pallor	Is life threatening.

Source: Data from Lovett, P. B., Sule, H. P., & Lopez, B. L. (2014). Sickle cell disease in the emergency department. *Emergency Medicine Clinics of North America, 32*(3), 629–647; Maakaron, J. E., & Taher, A. T. (2014). *Sickle cell anemia*. Retrieved from http://emedicine.medscape.com/article/205926-overview; Meier, E. R., & Miller, J. L. (2012). Sickle cell disease in children. *Drugs, 72*(7), 895–906; Myers, M., & Eckes, E. J. (2012). A novel approach to pain management in persons with sickle cell disease. *MEDSURG Nursing, 21*(5), 293–298.

intravenous fluid replacement also promotes pain relief since dehydration is often a cause of crisis. Fluids also reduce the viscosity of the blood, so adequate hydration is essential. Oxygen is usually administered to provide comfort and decrease the incidence of pulmonary complications.

Infection in a child with sickle cell disease is a serious condition requiring immediate attention. When an infection is suspected, cultures (blood, urine, and throat) are obtained to identify the source of infection and the offending organism. Aggressive antibiotic therapy is implemented immediately.

Penicillin prophylaxis should be started in the newborn period or as soon as the child is diagnosed and continued until 5 years of age to prevent a potentially life-threatening bacterial infection with the *Streptococcus pneumoniae*. Newborn screening has led to earlier diagnosis and, therefore, earlier initiation of prophylaxis (Yawn et al., 2014). The medication may be continued past 5 years of age if the child has a history of severe pneumococcal sepsis, or if the healthcare provider feels the child is still at high risk for infection caused by *S. pneumoniae* (Saunthararajah & Vichinsky, 2013).

To prevent life-threatening infection in the child with sickle cell disease, it is essential for the child to receive recommended immunizations including the pneumococcal conjugate vaccine, HIB vaccine, hepatitis B vaccine, and influenza vaccine (see Chapter 43). In addition, children with SCD should receive the 23-valent pneumococcal vaccine (Pneumovax) at age 2 and age 5 and every 5 years as an adult (Saunthararajah & Vichinsky, 2013). Children with anatomic or functional asplenia should also receive the meningococcal vaccine beginning at 2 months of age. Specific guidelines are provided by the CDC (Centers for Disease Control and Prevention, 2015). Blood transfusions improve tissue oxygenation, reduce sickling, correct anemia, and temporarily reduce the percentage of HbS (Inati, Khoriaty, & Musallam, 2011).

Annual transcranial Doppler testing is recommended for children with SCD between the ages of 2 and 16 (Maakaron & Taher, 2014). Prophylactic transfusions are recommended for children with abnormal transcranial Doppler testing to prevent or decrease the risk of stroke (Lovett et al., 2014; Maakaron & Taher, 2014). However, frequent transfusions may result in an overload of iron in the body. The iron is stored in tissues and organs (**hemosiderosis**) because the body has no way of excreting it (Lovett et al., 2014). An iron-chelating drug such as deferoxamine (Desferal), which binds excess iron so it can be excreted by the kidneys, is administered. An oral chelator, deferasirox (Exjade), has been used in some patients since approval by the U.S. Food and Drug Administration (FDA) in 2005 and has demonstrated similar efficacy to deferoxamine infusion (Meier & Miller, 2012). Deferasirox could potentially simplify treatment and improve compliance by use of oral administration for patients requiring chelation therapy.

Treatment with hydroxyurea has been helpful in adults, and is being used frequently in children. This medication improves fetal hemoglobin levels and increases total hemoglobin concentration (Strouse & Heeney, 2012). The presence of fetal hemoglobin reduces sickling and subsequently the frequency of painful crisis secondary to vaso-occlusion. Although studies have demonstrated the effectiveness of hydroxyurea in children, the FDA labeling related to indications for the use of this drug refers only to adults, necessitating off-label usage in the pediatric population (Strouse & Heeney, 2012).

Hematopoietic stem cell transplantation (HSCT) is the only known cure for sickle cell disease and has been used in children with severe complications related to SCD. Only a few hundred people with sickle cell disease worldwide have received a stem cell transplant as a cure for sickle cell disease because its use is limited to those children who have a human leukocyte antigen (HLA)–compatible sibling. It is estimated that less than 20% of children with SCD have a sibling who is a match. The survival rate for children with sickle cell disease who have been able to receive a stem cell transplant is 93% to 97% (Meier & Miller, 2012). (See discussion regarding HSCT later in this chapter.)

SAFETY ALERT!

It is important for all health facilities to have current guidelines for transfusion protocols. Become familiar with the policies and procedures where you work. For example, the child's blood type and patient identification need to be checked by two registered nurses before starting the infusion. See the *Clinical Skills Manual* `SKILLS` for further information on blood transfusions.

Prognosis depends on the severity of the child's disease; children with more frequent exacerbations and hospitalizations have poorer prognosis. Newborn screening has led to early intervention in babies who have SCD (Maakaron & Taher, 2014). Early diagnosis, prophylactic antibiotics, and monthly transfusions for those at risk for stroke have extended life spans in individuals with sickle cell disease, with a median life span of 42 years of age for males and 48 for females (Tanabe et al., 2013). The life span of individuals with sickle cell trait is normal (Sickle Cell Information Center, 2012).

Nursing Management

For the Child With Sickle Cell Disease

Nursing Assessment and Diagnosis

The nurse may be involved in sickle cell gene testing to identify carriers and children who have the disease. Once a child is diagnosed with the disease, a comprehensive physical assessment is essential because sickle cell disease can affect any body system.

Professionalism in Practice Newborn Screening for SCD

Newborn screening for sickle cell disease is mandatory in all 50 states (National Newborn Screening and Genetics Resource Center, 2014). Nurses play an important role in educating parents about the importance of newborn screening and about the diagnosis and treatment plan once a diagnosis of sickle cell disease is made.

PHYSIOLOGIC ASSESSMENT

In children who are known to have sickle cell disease, obtain a detailed history from the parents or child about past crises, precipitating events, medical treatment, and home management. Measure the child's height and weight accurately and compare to past measurements since failure to thrive is common. Ask about chronic or acute pain that the child is experiencing. Pain may occur in nearly any body part, but most commonly manifests as headache, extremity pain, or abdominal discomfort. The ill child with sickle cell disease should receive a careful multisystem assessment. Fever, neurologic changes such as decreased alertness or behavioral changes, and respiratory symptoms are emergency conditions that necessitate prompt treatment. When

TABLE 49–5 Clinical Manifestations of Blood Transfusion Reactions

TYPE OF REACTION AND ETIOLOGY	CLINICAL MANIFESTATIONS
Allergic reaction related to immune response to protein in the blood	Urticaria, itching, respiratory distress
Hemolytic reaction related to mismatched blood, history of multiple transfusions, or infusion with a solution containing dextrose or other additives	Fever, chills, hematuria, headache, chest pain; can progress to shock
Febrile or septic related to contamination of blood; may also be caused by idiopathic conditions	Chills, fever, headache, decreased blood pressure, nausea or vomiting, and leg and back pain
Circulatory overload related to infusions of excessive amounts of fluid or too rapid administration	Labored breathing, chest or low back pain, productive cough, rales upon auscultation, distended neck veins, increased central venous pressure

the child is in crisis, assess pain and note the presence of any signs of inflammation or infection. Carefully monitor the child for signs of shock (see Chapter 47).

Clinical Reasoning Sickle Cell Disease

Michael is a 3-year-old African American child with sickle cell disease who is admitted to the hospital with severe abdominal pain. What are the most important nursing assessments and interventions to integrate within Michael's care?

PSYCHOSOCIAL ASSESSMENT

The family of a child with sickle cell disease requires a thorough psychosocial assessment. Ask if other family members have the diagnosis. If the child is newly diagnosed with the disorder, the family needs assistance to deal with feelings related to the serious, life-threatening nature of the disease. Assess parents' understanding of the disease transmission and ask whether genetic counseling has been obtained. Determine whether the family has adequate healthcare coverage to pay for the child's medical expenses and whether the child qualifies for assistance because of the disability associated with the disease. Ask older children about their knowledge of the disease, and explore their feelings related to the management of a chronic condition. When siblings or other family members are carriers, periodic counseling is needed so they can understand implications for dating, marriage, and having children.

Several nursing diagnoses that might apply to the child with sickle cell disease are presented in the accompanying *Nursing Care Plan*. Other nursing diagnoses might include the following (NANDA-I © 2014):

- *Caregiver Role Strain* related to illness chronicity
- *Parenting, Risk for Impaired*, related to having a child with a physical illness
- *Development: Delayed, Risk for*, related to effects of physical disability
- *Mobility: Physical, Impaired*, related to pain
- *Knowledge, Deficient (Child or Parents)*, related to lack of exposure about cause and treatment of sickle cell disease

Planning and Implementation

The accompanying *Nursing Care Plan* summarizes nursing care for the child with sickle cell disease. Nursing management for the child in crisis focuses on increasing tissue perfusion, promoting hydration, controlling pain, preventing infection, ensuring adequate nutrition, preventing complications, and providing emotional support to the child and family.

INCREASE TISSUE PERFUSION

Administer blood transfusions and oxygen as ordered. To prevent hemolysis, the intravenous fluid used before and after a blood transfusion must be saline rather than D_5W. Monitor for transfusion reactions (Table 49–5). Encourage the child to rest. Work with the child and family to avoid emotional stress. Any activities that increase cellular metabolism also result in tissue hypoxia. Schedule caregiving activities and play to allow for optimal rest.

PROMOTE HYDRATION

The child with sickle cell disease is adversely affected by dehydration. Calculate the child's fluid maintenance requirements (minimum daily fluid intake) (see Chapter 44) and monitor the child's oral fluid intake. Administer intravenous fluids as ordered. Adjust oral intake as necessary to keep the child well hydrated.

CONTROL PAIN

Administer prescribed analgesics around the clock during crises. If patient-controlled analgesia is used, be sure that the constant infusions run as ordered and that the parent or child understands the use of the button for dosing when needed (see Chapter 40). Help the child assume a comfortable position. Avoid putting stress on painful joints. See *Evidence-Based Practice: Sickle Cell Disease and Pain Management.*

SAFETY ALERT!

Blood reactions can occur as soon as a blood transfusion begins. Administer the first 20 mL of blood slowly and observe the child carefully for a reaction. Assess the child according to agency policy and promptly report changes in condition. If a reaction occurs, stop the transfusion immediately, call the healthcare provider, monitor vital signs, keep the intravenous line open with normal saline, check for hematuria, and administer medications as ordered.

PREVENT INFECTION

Infection makes the child more susceptible to a crisis, and the crisis, in turn, increases susceptibility to infection. Teach the parents how to administer antibiotics for prophylaxis or treatment of infection. Because infections are particularly virulent in these children, tell parents to get immediate care when the child is ill. Emphasize the importance of immunizations. See the discussion earlier in this chapter and Chapter 43 for further information about recommended and supplemental immunizations.

Nursing Care Plan: The Child With Sickle Cell Disease

1. Nursing Diagnosis: *Tissue Perfusion: Peripheral, Ineffective,* **related to affinity of hemoglobin for oxygen (NANDA-I © 2014)**

GOAL: The child will show few signs and symptoms of tissue hypoxia.

INTERVENTION	RATIONALE
• Instruct child to avoid physical exertion, emotional stress, low-oxygen environments (e.g., airplanes, high altitudes), and known sources of infection.	• Decreased activity and exposure reduce the body's need for oxygen.

EXPECTED OUTCOME: Child will have no shortness of breath and shows no signs of hypoxia.

GOAL: Repeated stroke will be avoided.

INTERVENTION	RATIONALE
• Administer blood transfusions as ordered.	• Packed cells increase number of red blood cells available to carry oxygen to tissue cells. Transfusions promote circulation.
• Perform several caregiving activities together whenever possible.	• Grouping activities allows for optimum rest.
• Give oxygen as ordered.	• A high concentration of oxygen in alveoli increases diffusion of gas across membranes.
• Administer and teach the family about prophylactic transfusions for the child who has had a stroke.	• Lowers potential for a future stroke.

EXPECTED OUTCOME: Child does not suffer a stroke.

2. Nursing Diagnosis: *Fluid Volume: Deficient, Risk for*, **related to inadequate fluid intake and dehydration (NANDA-I © 2014)**

GOAL: The child will maintain or be restored to adequate hydration.

INTERVENTION	RATIONALE
• Calculate the child's daily fluid requirements. Monitor the child's usual fluid consumption and make necessary adjustments. Encourage the child to take fluids. Observe for signs of dehydration.	• Optimizing fluid intake ensures that the child gets needed fluid. Dehydration exacerbates crises.
• Record intake and output.	• Early intervention can be effective in minimizing complications from dehydration. Child may need oral or intravenous rehydration therapy.

EXPECTED OUTCOME: Child will show signs of adequate hydration.

3. Nursing Diagnosis: *Pain, Chronic*, **related to physical disability and clustering of sickled cells (NANDA-I © 2014)**

GOAL: The child will verbalize that pain is controlled.

INTERVENTION	RATIONALE
• Administer analgesics, such as morphine or hydromorphone (Dilaudid), as ordered. Continuous intravenous infusion is used for the duration of a painful crisis.	• Pain of sickle cell crises is excruciating.
• Position carefully.	• Joints and extremities can be extremely painful.

EXPECTED OUTCOME: Child will be pain free or pain control will be significantly improved.

4. Nursing Diagnosis: *Infection, Risk for*, related to chronic disease and splenic malfunction (NANDA-I © 2014)

GOAL: The child will not develop infection.

INTERVENTION	RATIONALE
• Ensure adequate nutrition by providing high-calorie, high-protein diet. Ensure that the child's immunizations are up-to-date and that children less than age 5 years are receiving prophylactic antibiotics. Make sure that parents have a thermometer in the home and know how to use it. Report any signs of infection to a healthcare provider immediately.	• Children with a chronic illness are at greater risk of infection.
• Isolate the child from possible sources of infection. Instruct parents about signs of infection and encourage them to seek prompt health care.	• Restriction of persons with infection decreases the child's contact with infectious agents. Prompt care for infection reduces the chance of sickle cell crisis.

EXPECTED OUTCOME: Child will be free of infection.

EVIDENCE-BASED PRACTICE | Sickle Cell Disease and Pain Management

Clinical Question

What are effective pain management strategies for children with sickle cell disease? How well is pain assessed and managed in children with sickle cell disease?

The Evidence

Severe episodes of sickle cell crisis require visits to the emergency department (ED) and/or hospitalization for pain management. Relief of pain is the primary goal for healthcare providers and is most significant to the child experiencing pain.

Zempsky, Corsi, and McKay (2011) performed a retrospective chart review of 77 patients with sickle cell disease (SCD), ages 3 to 21 years, to evaluate the relationship between pain scores and time to administration of pain medication. Triage pain scores using the visual analog scale (VAS) in the ED for patients with sickle cell disease averaged 7.7, whereas those for patients with long bone fractures averaged 6.7. For every point increase on the VAS for patients with fractures, the time to administration of pain medication decreased by 5.6 minutes. There was no relationship between the pain score for patients with SCD and time to administration of pain medication. This suggests that pain scores are not used initially when making decisions in the ED regarding pain management for individuals with sickle cell disease but are used for patients with other painful conditions.

Ender et al. (2014) evaluated the use of a clinical pathway in the acute management of pain in children with sickle cell disease. Data were collected from 35 patients before the pathway was introduced and from 33 patients after the pathway was introduced. All patients with sickle cell disease older than 6 months of age who presented to the pediatric ED with sickle cell pain were eligible to be included in the study. Patients with SCD with pain from another cause or those in whom a stroke was suspected were excluded from the study. Data collected at triage included time of patient registration and first set of vital signs, patient weight, time of first pain medication administration, type of medication and dosage administered, pain score, and whether or not the child was admitted to

the hospital. The pathway included a checklist that provided instructions for triage, monitoring, timing of assessments and interventions, and medication administration. Results of the study showed that after the clinical pathway was introduced, the mean time interval for administration of the first analgesic was reduced from 74 minutes to 42 minutes. The mean time interval for administration of the first opioid was reduced from 94 minutes to 46 minutes. This represented significant improvement in administration of the first analgesic and first opioid and was statistically significant. The mean time interval for pain reassessment showed improvement, with the time reduced from 110 minutes to 72 minutes, but was not statistically significant. The study concluded that use of a clinical pathway can lead to improvement in pain management of patients with SCD.

Dobson and Byrne (2014) evaluated the effects of guided imagery training on school-age children ages 6 to 11 years with a diagnosis of sickle cell disease. Changes in pain perception, use of analgesia, self-efficacy, and imaging ability were described. Twenty children who had been treated in the clinic for at least a year served as the sample for the study. The children completed pain diaries every day for 2 months. Baseline and end-of-treatment imaging ability and self-efficacy was measured. The results of the study showed that training in the use of guided imagery led to reductions in pain intensity, decreased use of analgesics, and a significant increase in self-efficacy. The study concluded that guided imagery is effective in the management of pain related to sickle cell disease.

Best Practice

Children and adolescents with sickle cell disease who present to the ED with a painful episode have high levels of pain. These patients may have been in pain for several days prior to coming to the hospital. They may wait for a period of time before receiving opioid pain medication.

Protocols or clinical pathways should be established to ensure that children and adolescents who present to the ED with a painful episode receive pain medication in a timely

(continued)

manner. While in the ED and if hospitalized, pain intensity should be evaluated on a regular basis using an appropriate pain scale and the pain regimen adjusted as needed.

Clinical Reasoning
How will you determine which pain assessment tool is most appropriate to assess pain in children of different ages? How will you determine if the child in sickle cell crisis is obtaining adequate pain relief? (Consult Chapter 40 for ideas.) In addition to analgesics, what are appropriate nonpharmacologic methods that you can use to decrease pain in children with SCD?

ENSURE ADEQUATE NUTRITION

Emphasize the importance of adequate nutrition to promote growth. Encourage the child to eat a high-protein, high-calorie diet. Stress the importance of folic acid and vitamin C as supplements as prescribed. Perform regular growth measurements, and if slow growth is apparent, perform 24-hour recalls and other nutritional assessments.

Growth and Development

To encourage fluid intake in a small child:

- Use a favorite cup or glass.
- Use straws.
- Take advantage of times the child is thirsty, such as on awakening or after play.
- Leave a cup within easy reach of the child.
- Offer frozen juice pops and crushed ice drinks.

PREVENT COMPLICATIONS OF CRISES

Observe the child for signs of increasing anemia, infection, shock, and acute chest syndrome. Assess vital signs frequently and note changes that might be indicative of complications. Maintain ongoing monitoring of the child's neurologic status for evidence of altered cerebral function. Monitor the child's respiratory status for signs of acute chest syndrome. Assess for an enlarged spleen by gentle palpation. Administer blood transfusions and observe the child for any adverse reaction. Assess growth and developmental milestones.

PROVIDE EMOTIONAL SUPPORT

Sickle cell disease is a chronic disease accompanied by life-threatening episodic crises. Family members often need help to deal with their feelings about the diagnosis and its implications. Explore resources in the home and community to see if parents will be able to administer medications and fluids and to provide adequate nutrition. Assess parents' knowledge of signs of infection and of sickle cell crisis and when to seek medical care for the child. Refer the parents for genetic counseling, particularly if they plan to have more children. Encourage adolescents and young adults in the family to receive genetic counseling and testing as well. Referrals to support groups and contact with others with the disease can be helpful.

DISCHARGE PLANNING AND HOME CARE TEACHING

Identify and address home care needs well in advance of discharge. Give parents information about sickle cell disease and the child's treatment. Even parents of a child previously diagnosed with the disorder may benefit from information about the disease process and its management. Explain the basic effect of tissue hypoxia and the effects of sickling on circulation. Assist the family to explore resources in the home and community and determine if parents will be able to administer medications and fluids and to provide adequate nutrition.

Teach parents to look for signs of dehydration, such as dry mucous membranes, weight loss, and a sunken fontanelle in infants. Give specific instructions about how many ounces of liquid the child needs to drink each day. Emphasize that increased fluid intake is needed to replace the fluids lost from overheating or exposure to hot weather. Make sure both the child and family understand the triggers and precipitating factors for sickle cell crises. Encourage them to avoid situations that cause crises. Instruct the child and parents about signs and symptoms of crises that should be reported to their healthcare provider.

When regular blood infusions are used, the resulting iron overload is damaging to body organs. Provide the family with instructions about the treatment for iron overload.

Tell parents that it is important to inform all treating healthcare providers and dentists of the child's medical condition. The child should also wear medical identification (e.g., a medical identification bracelet). Special precautions are necessary when the child undergoes surgery of any kind because hypoxia resulting from anesthesia is a major surgical risk.

Family members need ongoing support to deal with the stress of having a child with a chronic condition. Provide resources, respite care for parents, and information as needed for siblings.

Encourage older children with sickle cell disease to participate in activities with other children between crises but to avoid strenuous physical exertion and contact sports. Play and social interactions that promote learning and development are important.

Evaluation

Expected outcomes of nursing care for the child with sickle cell disease include the following:

- Pain is managed to facilitate comfort level.
- The child maintains an adequate hydration state to prevent cell sickling.
- Side effects of the disease are absent in the respiratory system, central nervous system, and body organs.
- The child maintains a normal immune status and prevents infection.
- The family or child promptly recognizes and treats the complications of the disease.
- The child maintains normal growth and development.
- The nurse provides necessary services and resources for the parents and other family members.
- The family has knowledge of disease and its treatment.

TEACHING HIGHLIGHTS | Home Care Considerations for the Child With Sickle Cell Disease

- Follow recommended schedules for health promotion visits.
- Keep scheduled appointments with the child's hematologist.
- Be sure the child's immunizations are up-to-date.
- Special testing, such as heart and eye examinations, may be needed periodically to check for sequelae of the disease.
- Follow instructions for antibiotic administration.
- Assess the child's pain and give pain medication as prescribed for acute and chronic pain.
- Ensure that the child gets extra fluids in hot weather, when ill, during physical activity, and during travel. Dehydration can lead to crisis.
- As the child develops, provide information about the disease and encourage self-care.
- Be sure the school personnel understand the child's diagnosis and any care required during school hours.
- Contact your healthcare provider if the child has a high fever, a common illness that lasts more than 1 day, seizures, change in behavior, severe pain, abnormal skin color or breathing pattern, or any other symptoms that concern you.
- Inform all care providers of the child's condition and need for special planning prior to surgery.

Thalassemias

The thalassemias are a group of inherited blood disorders of hemoglobin synthesis characterized by anemia that can be mild or severe. There are three types of beta-thalassemias (β-thalassemias): thalassemia minor, or thalassemia trait (produces mild anemia); thalassemia intermedia (produces moderate anemia and may require transfusions); and thalassemia major, also known as Cooley's anemia (produces anemia requiring transfusion). Clinical manifestations of β-thalassemia are caused by the defective synthesis of hemoglobin, structurally impaired RBCs, and the shortened life span of the RBCs. Symptoms of thalassemia major generally develop during the second 6 months of age and include pallor, jaundice, growth retardation, irritability, hepatomegaly, and splenomegaly (Giardina & Rivella, 2013). In alpha-thalassemia (α-thalassemia), the child may have a one-gene defect (α-thalassemia silent carrier) and generally be symptom free; have a two-gene defect (α-thalassemia trait) and have mild anemia; or have α-thalassemia major, which results in hydrops fetalis. Intrauterine transfusion can increase the survival rate in the fetus with α-thalassemia major. Those who survive will be transfusion dependent. Hematopoietic stem cell transplant is the only cure (DeBaun et al., 2016).

Diagnosis is made by hemoglobin electrophoresis, which reveals a decreased production of one of the globin chains in hemoglobin and an elevated F and A hemoglobin. A complete blood count shows a decreased hemoglobin, hematocrit, and reticulocyte count (DeBaun et al., 2016). Prenatal testing using chorionic villi sampling or amniocentesis can detect the disease in the fetus. Treatment is supportive. The goal of medical management is to maintain normal hemoglobin levels. A chronic transfusion program, in which blood transfusions are administered every 2 to 4 weeks, is the conventional therapy used to treat children with severe disease. Since iron overload is a side effect of this treatment, children may need to receive an iron-chelating drug such as deferoxamine or deferasirox (Exjade). (See previous discussion.) A splenectomy may be required for the child with splenomegaly. Hematopoietic stem cell transplantation (HSCT) may be offered as an alternative therapy for children newly diagnosed with the disorder.

Nursing Management

Nursing care focuses on observing for complications of transfusion therapy, supporting the child and family in dealing with a chronic life-threatening illness, and referring the family for genetic counseling. Encourage parents to take an active role in the child's treatment regimen. Teach parents the technique for subcutaneous infusion of deferoxamine if that route is to be used for therapy at home.

Compliance with transfusion therapy often becomes an issue as children reach adolescence. Offering the adolescent treatment options, such as when to undergo transfusion, can help improve compliance. Adolescents with β-thalassemia and parents of newly diagnosed children can be referred to the Thalassemia Action Group, a national organization for those with this disease, or to the Cooley's Anemia Foundation. Expected outcomes of nursing care include maintenance of normal hemoglobin and hematocrit, safe transfusion of blood products, maintenance of recommended body iron levels, and family understanding about the genetic transmission of the disease.

Hereditary Spherocytosis

Hereditary spherocytosis (HS) is a hemolytic disorder occurring in 1 in 5000 people of Northern European descent. The inheritance pattern of hereditary spherocytosis is most commonly autosomal dominant, but in some cases is autosomal recessive. Additionally, up to 25% of cases have no family history (Segel & Casey, 2016). Erthrocytes assume a spherical shape due to an intrinsic membrane defect. Spectrin deficiency is most common (Gonzalez & Eichner, 2014). The erythrocytes are retained and removed by the spleen, leading to splenomegaly in the child (Hsiao et al., 2013).

Clinical manifestations appear in the neonatal period or during early infancy. Severity of the anemia varies, but mild jaundice is usually evident. Aplastic crisis (discussed in Table 49–4) is the most serious complication the child experiences. Gallstones are a complication associated with hereditary spherocytosis. Complete blood count reveals anemia, and microscopic examination reveals the abnormally shaped cells (Gonzalez & Eichner, 2014).

Treatment of children with hereditary spherocytosis includes daily folic acid and red blood cell transfusions when indicated. Children with mild, uncomplicated disease may be managed without surgery (Gonzalez & Eichner, 2014). Splenectomy is indicated in children with severe disease and in those with moderate disease who show signs of growth failure or significant signs and symptoms of anemia. Removal of the spleen increases the risk of infection and sepsis (Das et al., 2014; Gonzalez & Eichner, 2014). Infants and young children are especially at risk. Delaying the surgery until after age 6 reduces the risk of bacterial infection and sepsis (Gonzalez & Eichner, 2014). Nursing care for the child with hereditary spherocytosis is the same as care for the child with anemia.

Aplastic Anemia

Aplastic anemia is a deficiency in the number of blood cells that results from failure of the bone marrow to produce adequate numbers of all types of circulating blood cells. The condition may be congenital or acquired. Eighty percent of cases of aplastic anemia are acquired, and it is thought to be an autoimmune disease (Bakhshi, 2014).

Acquired aplastic anemia in children can develop after treatment with radiation or after ingestion of drugs such as chloramphenicol, NSAIDS, or anticonvulsants. This type of anemia can also be a result of an infectious process such as viral hepatitis, mononucleosis, or cytomegalovirus; related to nutritional deficiencies in vitamin B_{12} or folic acid; or related to exposure to chemicals such as insecticides and pesticides (Hartung, Olson, & Bessler, 2013).

Symptoms are related to the degree of bone marrow failure and include **petechiae** (small pinpoint red or purple spots on the mucous membranes or skin), **purpura** (irregular bluish purple areas of bleeding into the tissues), menorrhagia in postmenarchal girls, and epistaxis. Symptoms associated with anemia include pallor, fatigue, and exercise intolerance. Symptoms related to neutropenia include fever and bacterial infections (Hartung et al., 2013). Death can result from complications associated with hemorrhage and sepsis.

Diagnosis is made by complete blood count studies, which reveal leukopenia with marked neutropenia, thrombocytopenia, and **pancytopenia** (decreased number of blood cell components), and by bone marrow aspiration, which reveals yellow, fatty bone marrow instead of red bone marrow.

Supportive treatment includes transfusions of packed cells, platelets, or both. Immunosuppressive drug therapy is effective for many children because it is believed the child's immune system is attacking the bone marrow. Immunosuppressive agents generally include antithymocyte globulin (ATG) and cyclosporine. The treatment of choice for children with severe aplastic anemia is hematopoietic stem cell transplantation (HSCT) from an HLA-matched sibling donor (Bakhshi, 2014).

Nursing Management

Nursing interventions focus on preventing bleeding, administering and monitoring blood transfusions, preventing infection, encouraging mobility as tolerated, educating the parents and child about the disorder, and providing emotional support. Families need support in dealing with a child who has a life-threatening disease. Refer them to support groups for counseling, if indicated, and to social services. Expected outcomes of nursing care include absence of infection, no bleeding, and parental education related to the disease and treatment.

Bleeding Disorders

Hemophilia

Hemophilia refers to a group of hereditary bleeding disorders that result from a deficiency in specific clotting factors. Hemophilia A, or classic hemophilia, is caused by a deficiency of factor VIII in the blood and occurs in 1 in 5000 male births (Özgönenel et al., 2013). Hemophilia B, also known as Christmas disease, is caused by a deficiency of factor IX and occurs in 1 in 25,000–30,000 male births (Zaiden, 2014). Hemophilia A accounts for 85% of persons with hemophilia, and 10% to 15% have hemophilia B (Scott, 2016).

ETIOLOGY AND PATHOPHYSIOLOGY

Hemophilias A and B are X-linked recessive disorders, which manifest almost exclusively as affected males and carrier females. Genes for clotting factors VIII and IX are located near the terminal long arm of the X chromosome (Scott, 2016). A daughter will inherit the gene from her father with hemophilia and may transmit it to her sons. (See Chapter 3 for a description of genetic transmission.) Some children affected by hemophilia do not have a family member with a history of a clotting disorder. In these cases, the disorder is caused by a new mutation. (Scott, 2016). The degree of bleeding is related to the amount of clotting factor and the severity of the injury.

CLINICAL MANIFESTATIONS

Hemophilia is manifested in different children by bleeding tendencies that range from mild to moderate or severe. Children with hemophilia often do not demonstrate symptoms until after 6 months of age as they become more mobile and incur injuries and bleeding from falls.

Spontaneous bleeding, **hemarthrosis** (bleeding into a joint space), and deep tissue hemorrhage occur. Affected children frequently experience bleeding into the joint spaces of the knees, ankles, and elbows. Bleeding into joint spaces causes the child to have limited motion because of pain and swelling. Bone changes and flexion deformities can result from the effects of blood in the joint structures (Rodriguez-Merchan, 2012).

Males may have bleeding after circumcision. Other symptoms include easy bruising (**ecchymosis**), hematuria, and bleeding after tooth extraction, minor trauma, or minor surgical procedures. Subcutaneous, intramuscular hemorrhages and gastrointestinal bleeding can occur. Intracranial bleeding occurs in 10% of patients with severe hemophilia and has a mortality rate of 30%. Females who carry the trait for hemophilia do not usually manifest symptoms of the disease (Zaiden, Furlong, Crouch, et al., 2014).

CLINICAL THERAPY

Diagnosis of affected children and carriers can be done before birth through chorionic villus sampling or amniocentesis. Genetic testing of family members is increasingly being used to identify carriers. Diagnosis can also be made on the basis of the history, physical examination, and laboratory data. Laboratory tests show low levels of factor VIII or IX, and prolonged activated partial thromboplastin time (aPPT). Prothrombin time (PT), thrombin time (TT), fibrinogen, and platelet count are normal.

The goal of medical management is to control bleeding by replacing the missing clotting factor. Desmopressin (DDAVP), an analog of vasopressin, stimulates the release of factor VIII stored in the blood vessels, thereby increasing the percentage of available factor by approximately threefold. DDAVP is effective in some patients with mild and moderate hemophilia A (Roman, Larson, & Manno, 2013).

Many recombinant factor VIII concentrates are available as replacement therapy for hemophilia A (Zaiden et al., 2014). Factor IX concentrates are also available to treat hemophilia B (Zaiden, 2014). The child with severe hemophilia may be on a prophylactic regimen of replacement therapy, whereas the child with mild to moderate hemophilia may only receive episodic therapy. Prophylaxis decreases bleeding episodes and joint damage that may result from repeated episodes of hemarthrosis (Koerper, 2012). Prompt and adequate treatment is needed to prevent serious bleeding episodes and their sequelae. Gene therapy is being explored for treatment of hemophilia in hopes that an eventual cure will be found (Chuah, Evens, & Vandendriessche, 2013).

Nursing Management
For the Child With Hemophilia

Nursing Assessment and Diagnosis

PHYSIOLOGIC ASSESSMENT
Obtain a complete medical history from the parents or child. In particular, ask about previous episodes of bleeding and the occurrence of hemophilia or any other bleeding disorders in family members. The history of bleeding will vary, depending on the severity of the disease.

Assess the child for any joint pain, swelling, or permanent deformity, particularly around the knees, elbows, ankles, and shoulders. Observe for prolonged bleeding or oozing of blood. Note the presence of hematuria and mild flank pain. Conduct a neurologic assessment because the risk for intracranial hemorrhage and bleeding can lead to peripheral neuropathies.

PSYCHOSOCIAL ASSESSMENT
It is difficult for families to manage care of the child with hemophilia, especially if the disease is severe. Assess the family's coping mechanisms and support systems. Determine the family's ability to manage procedures and treatments; the factor concentrates and infusion equipment are costly. Assess older children's understanding of the disease, limitations, and their adaptation to the disease.

DEVELOPMENTAL ASSESSMENT
Because the child with hemophilia may have physical activity restrictions, physical skills may be delayed. Perform frequent developmental assessments, being particularly attentive to fine and gross motor skills.

The most important nursing diagnosis for the child with hemophilia is *Injury, Risk for,* related to bleeding disorder. Some of the other nursing diagnoses that might apply include the following (NANDA-I © 2014):

- *Pain* related to bleeding episodes
- *Mobility: Physical, Impaired,* related to joint stiffness or contractures
- *Home Maintenance, Impaired,* related to challenges of hemophilia
- *Family Processes, Interrupted,* related to family role shift required to care for a child with a chronic illness
- *Development: Delayed, Risk for,* related to effects of physical disability

Planning and Implementation
Nursing care focuses on preventing and controlling bleeding episodes, limiting joint involvement and managing pain, and providing emotional support. Both short-term interventions and long-term management are necessary.

PREVENT AND CONTROL BLEEDING EPISODES
Bleeding problems are rare in infants with hemophilia. However, as children learn to walk and develop other motor skills they often fall and suffer cuts and bruises. The risk of injury can be reduced by emphasizing to parents the need for close supervision and a safe environment. Parents should encourage children to play with safe, age-appropriate toys.

When the child is hospitalized, use nursing approaches to minimize the possibility of bleeding. Ensure that the hospital environment is safe by orienting the child to the room and keeping the floor and room clear of hazards as much as possible. If significant bleeding does occur, offer supportive measures and assist with factor replacement therapy. Carefully monitor the child's condition for any side effects when factor replacement therapy is administered. Control any superficial bleeding by applying pressure to the area for at least 15 minutes. Immobilize and elevate the affected area, and apply ice packs to promote vasoconstriction.

LIMIT JOINT INVOLVEMENT AND MANAGE PAIN
During bleeding episodes, hemarthrosis is managed by the administration of factor replacement as quickly as possible, elevating and immobilizing the joint and applying ice packs, and administering analgesics for pain. Once bleeding has been controlled, range-of-motion exercises strengthen muscles and joints and prevent flexion contractures. Physical therapy may be needed. Because excessive weight can place added stress on joints, encourage the child to maintain an appropriate weight.

PROVIDE EMOTIONAL SUPPORT
The needs of families with children who have hemophilia are best met through a comprehensive team approach. Refer the parents for genetic counseling as soon as possible after diagnosis. It is important to identify family members who carry the trait because they may suffer excessive bleeding during surgery.

Encourage the parents to verbalize their feelings. Be understanding and sensitive to their needs. Teach the parents about hemophilia and explain how the disorder affects both the child and other family members. Refer the parents and child to organizations such as the National Hemophilia Foundation for further information.

DISCHARGE PLANNING AND HOME CARE TEACHING
The child may be hospitalized briefly during the first manifestation of bleeding for diagnosis and management. Most care will subsequently take place in the home. Home care needs should be identified and addressed well in advance of discharge. Advise parents to have the child wear a medical identification bracelet. Dentists and all other healthcare providers should be aware of the diagnosis.

Explain the cause of bleeding so both the child and parents understand the disease process. Teach the child and family how to identify internal bleeding. Signs and symptoms such as joint pain, abdominal pain, and obvious bleeding are indicators for immediate factor infusion. Make sure the child and parents know what situations could cause bleeding to occur. Teach parents to give acetaminophen instead of aspirin and aspirin-containing products.

Instruct the parents and the child, when appropriate, to prepare and administer factor concentrate. If infusion of the missing factor is scheduled regularly, bleeding episodes can be controlled or avoided. Have the parents demonstrate the procedure and make sure they can administer the product correctly. Ensure that parents know where they can get the factor concentrate.

The child will need an individualized school health plan (see Chapter 38). Members of the school staff should be instructed in management of emergencies. The nurse can identify key staff members in the school and teach them the actions that need to be taken.

Help the family and school plan an appropriate schedule of activities for the child. Explain how the parents can coordinate their child's care with a number of health professionals. Provide ongoing case management, assisting the family to take on this task if able.

Hemophilia is a debilitating disorder for the child, and it also can be financially draining for the family. Frequent outpatient visits, emergency department visits, hospital admissions, and the cost of factor replacement can exhaust a family's resources. If indicated, refer families to appropriate social services (e.g., the state's maternal and child health program for children with special healthcare needs) and organizations such as the National Hemophilia Foundation. Sharing experiences with other families of children with hemophilia can provide support.

Evaluation

Expected outcomes of nursing care include the following:

- Injury to the child is prevented.
- Pain is managed to promote comfort level.
- The nurse and family promote normal growth and development for the child.
- The child and family have adequate knowledge of disease management, including recognition of bleeding and prompt initiation of infusions.

Clinical Tip

Use the acronym RICE (**r**est, **i**ce, **c**ompression, **e**levation) to help you remember important measures to control a bleeding episode.

Clinical Tip

Take the following precautions when caring for children with bleeding disorders:

- Avoid taking temperatures rectally or giving suppositories.
- Avoid intramuscular injections unless absolutely necessary and only after factor replacement has been given. Children should receive recommended immunizations subcutaneously with firm pressure to the injection site for 5 minutes following the injection.
- Apply firm, continuous pressure to venipuncture sites 5 minutes after any venipuncture procedure.
- Do not give aspirin or aspirin-containing products.

Von Willebrand Disease

Von Willebrand disease is the most common hereditary bleeding disorder. The various subtypes of this disorder are classified based on the amount and functionality of the von Willebrand factor (vWF), a plasma protein and the carrier for clotting factor VIII. The most common form of the disorder is transmitted as an autosomal dominant trait, and can occur in both males and females (Acharya, 2014).

The characteristic manifestations are prolonged and excessive mucocutaneous bleeding. In children, this is generally exhibited through easy bruising and recurrent epistaxis. Increased bleeding also occurs during surgery and dental extractions. Affected teenage girls may have menorrhagia (increased menstrual bleeding) (Acharya, 2014; Weickert, Miesbach, Alesci, et al., 2014).

Growth and Development

Encourage children with hemophilia to participate in leisure activities such as computer games, reading clubs, and crafts as well as social clubs such as Boy Scouts. Swimming, bicycle riding, hiking, and other noncontact sports are excellent options for the child. Protective equipment appropriate to the sport or recreational activity the child is participating in should be worn. Activities important to development can be encouraged when coaches, teachers, and others know how to treat bleeding episodes.

Diagnosis of von Willebrand disease is made after laboratory studies reveal decreased von Willebrand factor levels, von Willebrand factor antigen levels, and factor VIII activity; reduced platelet agglutination; and prolonged or normal activated partial thromboplastin time (aPPT).

Treatment is similar to that for the child with hemophilia and involves infusion of von Willebrand protein concentrate. Desmopressin (DDAVP) is administered to promote release of stored vWF and to prevent bleeding associated with dental or surgical procedures (Thiagarajan, 2014).

Nursing Management

Teach parents about the disorder and instruct them not to give the child any aspirin or other drugs that can cause bleeding or inhibit platelet function. Teach management of bleeding episodes and intravenous infusion techniques, as for hemophilia. The prognosis is good, and children with von Willebrand disease usually have a normal life expectancy. Expected outcomes of nursing care include prompt management of bleeding and prevention of disease complications.

Disseminated Intravascular Coagulation

Disseminated intravascular coagulation (DIC) is a life-threatening, acquired pathologic process in which the clotting system is abnormally activated, resulting in widespread clot formation in the small vessels throughout the body. Excess thrombin is generated, followed by deposition of fibrin strands in body tissues. The circulating fibrin fragments later begin to interfere with platelet aggregation and other aspects of the clotting mechanism, resulting in bleeding or hemorrhage (LeMone, Burke, Bauldoff, et al., 2015).

The most common cause of DIC is sepsis. Infections caused by gram-negative and gram-positive bacteria, fungi, viruses, and protozoa may lead to DIC (LeMone et al., 2015). Symptoms can include gingival bleeding, mucosal bleeding, hemoptysis, petechiae, purpura, bruising, oozing of blood after an injection, hematuria, frank bleeding from incisions, tachycardia, and hypotension (LeMone et al., 2015; Levi & Schmaier, 2014).

Medical management includes platelet and factor replacement so that platelets and clotting factors are restored. Although controversial, heparin may be administered to treat uncontrolled thrombosis (LeMone et al., 2015; Levi & Schmaier, 2014).

Nursing Management

DIC is a complex disorder managed by a critical care team. Nursing care focuses on assessing the bleeding, preventing further injury, and administering prescribed therapies. Observe for petechiae, ecchymoses, and all body orifices and skin breaks for oozing every 1 to 2 hours. Careful monitoring of dependent areas is essential because blood will pool in these locations. Intravenous sites are particularly prone to oozing and should be assessed every 15 minutes. Examine stool for the presence of blood, and measure blood loss as accurately as possible. Measure intake and output.

Because all body systems can be involved, careful, continuous assessment of all systems is needed. Institute bleeding control precautions, monitor prescribed therapy (transfusion, anticoagulant therapy), and report any signs of complications. Desired outcomes of nursing care are management of bleeding and adequate function of all body systems. Adequate family support in this life-threatening situation is a focus of nursing care.

Immune Thrombocytopenic Purpura

Immune thrombocytopenic purpura (ITP) also known as *idiopathic thrombocytopenic purpura,* is a bleeding disorder characterized by increased destruction of platelets in the spleen. Platelets are destroyed as a result of the binding of autoantibodies to platelet antigens (Kessler & Sandler, 2014). When the rate of platelet destruction exceeds the rate of platelet production, the number of circulating platelets decreases and blood clotting slows. The cause of ITP is unknown, but it usually follows an infectious illness.

Symptoms include multiple ecchymoses and petechiae and mucosal bleeding in the mouth or nose. Diagnosis is made by history and through physical and laboratory findings, which show a decreased platelet count (generally less than 20,000 mm^3/dL) (Kessler & Sandler, 2014; Warrier & Chauhan, 2012). The child has normal hemoglobin and white blood cell counts. A bone marrow aspiration may be performed to rule out other diagnoses (Warrier & Chauhan, 2012).

Patients with a platelet count greater than 10,000 and little bleeding may be carefully observed without the need for additional treatment. Modalities of treatment vary among healthcare providers and may include corticosteroids, intravenous immune globulin (IVIG), and intravenous anti-D immunoglobulin. Platelet administration is not generally an aspect of treatment, except in cases of severe hemorrhage (Heiner & Morgan, 2014). With ITP, platelet administration will control bleeding temporarily since the administered platelets will be destroyed.

It is estimated that 20% of children with ITP will develop chronic disease (Warrier & Chauhan, 2012). Children who fail to respond to treatment for acute ITP and persist with thrombocytopenia for longer than 12 months are considered to have chronic ITP (Generali & Cada, 2013). Splenectomy may be an option for children with persistent or chronic disease, significant bleeding, lack of response to drug therapy, or altered quality of life (Neunert, 2011).

Nursing Management

Nursing care focuses on controlling and reducing the number of bleeding episodes. Preventive measures are similar to those for the child with hemophilia. Teach parents to use acetaminophen, rather than aspirin, to control pain. Provide emotional support to the family. Have the child avoid contact sports. Perform careful assessments of bleeding and take vital signs. Expected outcomes of care are prevention of bleeding and restoration of normal coagulation patterns.

Hematopoietic Stem Cell Transplantation

Hematopoietic stem cell transplantation (HSCT) is a treatment used for diseases such as severe combined immunodeficiency disease, severe and unresponsive aplastic anemia, and leukemia (refer to Chapters 48 and 50). Hematopoietic stem cells exist primarily in the bone marrow but also circulate in the peripheral blood. These cells can grow into new body cells, and have become useful in treatment of immune and hematologic diseases when restoration of normal cells is needed. Stem cells can be obtained from bone marrow, cord blood, or peripheral blood (Kolins, Zbylut, McCollom, et al., 2011; Moore & Ikeda, 2014).

Hematopoietic stem cell transplants are either autologous or allogeneic. In **autologous transplantation**, the child's own marrow is taken, treated, stored, and reinfused after the child has received chemotherapy. **Allogeneic transplantation** may be syngeneic (from an identical twin), related, or unrelated. In allogeneic transplantation, the donor, often a sibling (related), has a compatible human leukocyte antigen (HLA). HLAs are proteins found on the surface of nearly all nucleated cells within the body, and they are responsible for regulating the immune response. When no relative is found to match the child, a histocompatible donor (unrelated) may be sought from the National Marrow Donor Program or a cord blood bank (Kolins et al., 2011; Moore & Ikeda, 2014). With the development of this registry, bone marrow transplantation from HLA-matched unrelated donors has become possible for some children.

The transplantation procedure begins with chemotherapy and, sometimes, total body irradiation directed at destroying circulating blood cells and the diseased bone marrow in the ill child. The chemotherapy program for destruction of bone marrow ranges from 7 to 10 days (Moore & Ikeda, 2014). During this time, the child is cared for in strict isolation in a special unit that provides a germ-free environment (Figure 49–4). Following

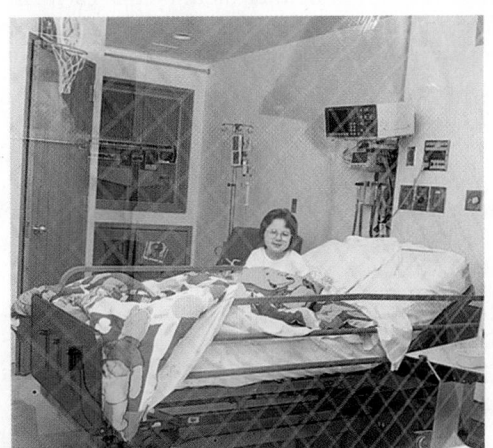

Figure 49–4 The child undergoing bone marrow transplantation is hospitalized in a special sterile unit while receiving chemotherapy before the transfusion. The child remains in the unit for several weeks afterward until the new marrow produces enough cells to maintain health.

the immunosuppression procedure, the child receives an intravenous transfusion with the donor stem cells. This procedure is similar to administration of a blood product. The healthy stem cells migrate to the bone marrow. Healthy bone marrow, capable of making blood cells, is the anticipated result. If the transplantation is successful, the cells implant in the child's marrow and begin to produce blood cells within approximately 2 to 4 weeks.

Pancytopenia (marked decrease in RBCs, WBCs, and platelets) lasts for several weeks following the transplant. Major risks during this period are anemia, infections, and bleeding. Once the bone marrow begins to produce new cells, graft-versus-host disease (rejection) is the major threat. Refer to Chapter 48 for a discussion of graft-versus-host disease.

Monitor the child undergoing HSCT by assessing the skin, mucous membranes, gastrointestinal function, respiratory function, cardiac function, and hydration status. Because graft-versus-host disease may occur at any time, even after the child returns home, frequent thorough assessments are necessary after discharge.

Supportive care after the transplantation procedure focuses on preventing infection, controlling bleeding, maintaining a nutritious diet and hydration, monitoring for signs of rejection, and providing psychosocial support. The treatment is lengthy, the child is often critically ill, and parents may have traveled to a medical center many miles from home for the procedure. Ask parents about other family members and how they are managing. Provide information about inexpensive housing available near the medical center. Encourage parents to discuss their feelings with other parents of children receiving bone marrow transplantation. Organizations such as the Bone Marrow Transplant Family Support Network can serve as resources for families.

When the child is ready for discharge, be sure the family is prepared to administer medications, recognize signs of graft-versus-host disease, provide adequate nutrition for the child, and perform other necessary care. Arrange for follow-up visits and provide the names of local healthcare contact people who can offer support and provide information. The child may need tutors or other educational assistance to promote integration back into the school setting. The major expected outcome of nursing care is the proper activity of bone marrow in the child with resulting normal levels and function of blood cells. Other outcomes are provision of family support, ongoing care and education for the child, adequate nutrition, and prevention of infection. See *Health Promotion: The Child With Hematopoietic Stem Cell Transplantation [HSCT]*.

Health Promotion   The Child With Hematopoietic Stem Cell Transplantation (HSCT)

Growth and Development

- Measure and plot height and weight at each visit using standard growth curve charts.

- Measure onset and progression of puberty using Tanner staging.

- An individualized education plan (IEP) should be performed yearly to identify learning problems.

- Routine hearing screening is advised since hearing loss may occur as a result of ototoxic drug therapy.

- Vision should be screened at each primary care visit since corticosteroid use can cause cataracts, graft-versus-host disease (GVHD) can result in keratoconjunctivitis, and cytomegalovirus (CMV) can cause retinitis.

- Blood pressure should be monitored at each visit because children are commonly placed on medication for hypertension after HSCT because of nephrotoxic medications.

- Instruct parents to measure and record blood pressure at home if necessary.

Nutrition

- Teach family to avoid foods with potential vectors for infection, such as unpasteurized products and undercooked meats.

- A low-sodium diet may be required if the child has hypertension.

- Calcium supplements may be administered to reduce the risk of osteopenia.

Physical Activity

- If the child has thrombocytopenia, physical activity may be restricted.

- The child may experience fatigue. Ask about activity tolerance.

Oral Health

- Dental screening and any required restorative care should be done before transplant to reduce potential sources of infection.

- Routine dental care is resumed once the child's immune system is restored. Ask the family about the child's routine dental care.

Mental and Spiritual Health

- Apply developmental approaches to assess the child's feelings after a HSCT.

- Ask the child about coping with being in the hospital and at home rather than attending school.

- Many physical changes occur with treatment that may interfere with body image. Assess the child's or adolescent's body image in a manner appropriate to age.

Relationships

- In-hospital or in-home schooling is required after HSCT for 6 to 12 months until immune function has been obtained to reduce the risk of infection.

- Encourage peer contact, telephone calls, e-mail, and letters to reduce the child's feelings of isolation.

- On returning to school, the child is encouraged to participate fully in school activities.

- For the adolescent, sex education is important, especially to avoid sexually transmitted infections.

Disease Prevention Strategies

- Teach the family that hand hygiene is essential to prevent the spread of infection.

- Dishes should be washed in a dishwasher. Teach safe food preparation techniques.

- In-home child care is recommended because of the risk of infection in other childcare settings.
- Teach the family that the child should have minimal direct contact with animals to avoid infections.

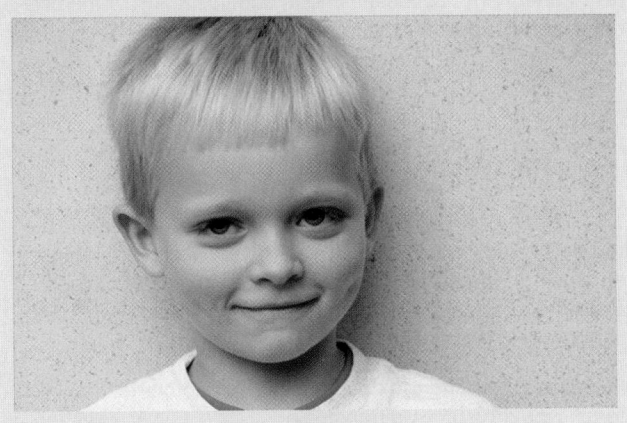

- Determine the child's need for an altered immunization schedule after HSTC.
- Instruct parents to monitor the child for infection and report any temperature elevation to the healthcare provider.
- Encourage the family to obtain an influenza vaccine annually for the child and all household or close contacts.
- Teach signs and symptoms of infection and stress the importance of prompt reporting.

Injury Prevention Strategies

- Review safe medication storage with the family.
- Help the family develop a plan for the safe disposal of used needles and syringes.

Focus Your Study

- Erythrocytes (red blood cells) are a major component of the blood and transport oxygen from the lungs to body tissues.
- Polycythemia is an increase in the number of red blood cells. Anemia is characterized by a decrease in red blood cell number.
- Leukocytes (white blood cells) are important in the cell's defenses against disease.
- Thrombocytes (platelets) are necessary for normal clotting of blood.
- The major anemias of childhood include iron deficiency anemia, normocytic anemia, sickle cell disease, thalassemia, hereditary spherocytosis, and aplastic anemia.
- Sickle cell disease is a genetic disease in which an abnormal shape, or sickling, of red blood cells prevents the normal flow of blood.
- Children with sickle cell disease are at risk for vaso-occlusive (pain) crisis, splenic sequestration, and aplastic crisis.
- Complications of sickle cell disease include stroke, acute chest syndrome with pulmonary infiltrate and infection, priapism, retinopathy, kidney damage, and gallstone formation.
- Nurses assist families in dealing with chronic diseases such as sickle cell disease by providing information about the disorder and resources that can provide assistance, monitoring child growth and development, instituting preventive care, and managing exacerbations of the disease.
- The thalassemias are a group of genetic diseases of red blood cells, which cause defective synthesis of hemoglobin.

- Children who receive chronic blood transfusions for sickle cell disease or thalassemia are at risk to develop iron overload and may need to receive an iron-chelating drug such as deferoxamine or deferasirox (Exjade).
- Hereditary spherocytosis (HS) is a hemolytic disorder in which the erythrocytes assume a spherical shape due to an intrinsic membrane defect. The erythrocytes are retained and removed by the spleen, leading to splenomegaly in the child.
- Aplastic anemia is a deficiency of all blood cells related to poor bone marrow function; it can be congenital or acquired after exposure to certain drugs or harmful environmental toxins.
- Hemophilia is a bleeding disorder transmitted by genes; hemophilia A is most common and results in a decrease in clotting factor VIII.
- The goal of treatment for hemophilia is to control bleeding by preventive care and replacement of the missing factor.
- Major nursing concerns for the child with hemophilia include managing bleeding episodes, controlling pain during bleeds, minimizing physical immobility, supporting the family in learning management of this chronic disease, and explaining genetic implications of the disease.
- Von Willebrand disease is a hereditary bleeding disorder characterized by a deficiency of von Willebrand factor, a plasma protein that is a carrier for clotting factor VIII.
- Disseminated intravascular coagulation is a serious condition in which clotting mechanisms are disturbed, leading to extensive clotting and tissue damage.

- Immune thrombocytopenic purpura causes destruction of platelets and most frequently follows a childhood viral disease.

- Management of immune thrombocytopenic purpura includes corticosteroids, intravenous immune globulin (IVIG), and intravenous anti-D immunoglobulin. The disease is considered to be autoimmune in nature.

- Hematopoietic stem cell transplant (HSCT) is a useful treatment in some diseases of the hematologic system and some

cancers; it involves infusion of bone marrow, peripheral stem cells, or neonatal stem cells from a donor into the blood of the recipient where it circulates, implants into the bone marrow, and begins making new blood cells.

- Nursing care before and after HSCT includes infection prevention, careful physical assessment, administration of medications, and support for the family.

Clinical Reasoning in Action

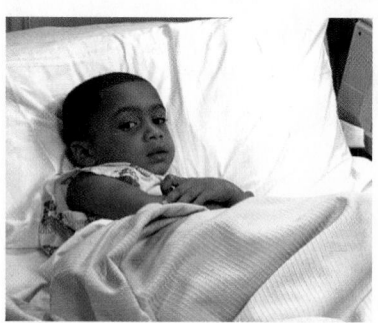

Frederick is admitted to the hospital with severe abdominal pain. He has been hospitalized for his sickle cell disease several times in the past and now, as an 8-year-old, he and his mother are very familiar with the routine. The disease is stable most of the time, but about twice annually he is admitted to the hospital for complications of the disorder. His mother expresses how upsetting it is to watch her son suffer pain from this disease.

In the hospital, a priority nursing intervention is to control Frederick's pain. The doctor diagnoses that the abdominal pain is

caused by sickled cells in his spleen. Frederick's hemoglobin is 6 g/dL, and a blood transfusion is ordered. Fluids and oxygen are also administered. Frequent vital signs and other monitoring are performed to identify any infections.

1. Besides correcting the anemia, what is another reason Frederick would be given a transfusion?
2. What is happening to Frederick's spleen such that it is causing his abdominal pain?
3. In what way does sickle cell disease affect the various systems of the body?
4. When giving a blood transfusion to Frederick, should warm or cold blood be given? What is the reason for your answer?

References

Abrams, S. A. (2014). *Iron requirements and iron deficiency in adolescents.* Retrieved from www.uptodate.com

Acharya, S. S. (2014). *Pediatric Von Willebrand disease.* Retrieved from http://emedicine.medscape.com/article/959825-overview

Bakhshi, S. (2014). *Aplastic anemia.* Retrieved from http://emedicine.medscape.com/article/198759-overview

Centers for Disease Control and Prevention. (2014) *What you should know about sickle cell trait.* Retrieved from http://www.cdc.gov/ncbddd/sicklecell/documents/SCD%20factsheet_Sickle%20Cell%20Trait.pdf

Centers for Disease Control and Prevention. (2015). *Summary of recommendations for child/teen immunization.* Retrieved from http://www.immunize.org/catg.d/p2010.pdf

Christensen, R. D., & Ohls, R. K. (2016). Development of the hematopoietic system. In R. M. Kliegman, B. F. Stanton, J. W. St. Geme III, N. F. Schor (Eds.), *Nelson textbook of pediatrics* (20th ed., p. 2304–2309). Philadelphia, PA: Elsevier Saunders.

Chuah, M. K., Evens, H., & Vandendriessche, T. (2013). Gene therapy for hemophilia. *Journal of Thrombosis and Haemostasis, 11*(Suppl 1), 99–110.

Das, A., Bansal, D., Ahluwalia, J., Das, R., Rohit, M. K., Attri, S. V., . . . Marwaha, R. K. (2014). Risk factors for thromboembolism and pulmonary artery hypertension following splenectomy in children with hereditary spherocytosis. *Pediatric Blood and Cancer, 61*(1), 29–33.

DeBaun, M. R., Frei-Jones, M., & Vichinsky, E. (2016). Hemoglobinopathies. In R. M. Kliegman, B. F.

Stanton, J. W. St. Geme III, N. F. Schor (Eds.), *Nelson textbook of pediatrics* (20th ed., pp. 2336–2353). Philadelphia, PA: Elsevier Saunders.

de Montalembert, M., Ferster, A., Colombatti, R., Rees, D. C., & Gulbis, B. (2011). ENERCA clinical recommendations for disease management and prevention of complications of sickle cell disease in children. *American Journal of Hematology, 86*(1), 72–75.

Dobson, C. E., & Byrne, M. W. (2014). Using guided imagery to manage pain in young children with sickle cell disease. *American Journal of Nursing, 114* (4), 26–36.

Ender, K. L., Krajewski, J. A., Babineau, J., Tresgallo, M., Schechter, W., Saroyan, J. M., & Kharbanda, A. (2014). Use of a clinical pathway to improve the acute management of vaso-occlusive crisis pain in pediatric sickle cell disease. *Pediatric Blood & Cancer, 61*(4), 693–696.

Generali, J. A., & Cada, D. J. (2013). Dexamethasone: Idiopathic thrombocytopenic purpura in children and adolescents. *Hospital Pharmacy, 48*(2), 108–110.

Giardina, P. J., & Rivella, S. (2013). Thalassemia syndromes. In R. Hoffman, E. J. Benz, L. E. Silberstein, H. Heslop, J. I. Weitz, & J. Anastasi (Eds.), *Hematology: Basic principles and practice* (6th ed., pp. 505–535). Philadelphia, PA: Elsevier Saunders.

Gonzalez, G., & Eichner, E. R. (2014). *Hereditary spherocytosis.* Retrieved from http://emedicine.medscape.com/article/206107-overview

Greenbaum, L. A. (2016). Vitamin K deficiency. In R. M. Kliegman, B. F. Stanton, J. W. St. Geme III, N. F.

Schor (Eds.), *Nelson textbook of pediatrics* (20th ed., pp. 342–343). Philadelphia, PA: Elsevier Saunders.

Harper, J. L., & Conrad, M. E. (2014). *Iron deficiency anemia.* Retrieved from http://emedicine.medscape.com/article/202333-overview

Hartung, H. D., Olson, T. S., & Bessler, M. (2013). Acquired aplastic anemia in children. *Pediatric Clinics of North America, 60*(6), 1311–1336.

Heiner, J. D., & Morgan, T. L. (2014). Progressive bruising in an otherwise healthy child: Immune thrombocytopenia purpura. *Canadian Journal of Emergency Medicine, 16*(2), 158–159.

Hsiao, M., Sathya, C., Nathens, A. B., de Mestral, C., Hill, A. D., & Langer, J. C. (2013). Is activity restriction appropriate for patients with hereditary spherocytosis? A population-based analysis. *Annals of Hematology, 92*(4), 523–525.

Inati, A., Khoriaty, E., & Musallam, K. M. (2011). Iron in sickle-cell disease: What have we learned over the years? *Pediatric Blood and Cancer, 56,* 182–190.

Kessler, C. M., & Sandler, S. G. (2014). *Immune thrombocytopenic purpura.* Retrieved from http://emedicine.medscape.com/article/202158-overview

Koerper, M. (2011). *Keeping up to date on prophylaxis and treatment strategies in patients with hemophilia.* Retrieved from http://www.medscape.org/viewarticle/750012

Kolins, J. A., Zbylut, C., McCollom, S., & Aquino, V. M. (2011). Hematopoietic stem cell transplantation in children. *Critical Care Nursing Clinics of North America, 23,* 349–376.

LeMone, P., Burke, K. M., Bauldoff, G., & Gubrud, P. (2015). Nursing care of patients with hematologic disorders. In P. LeMone, K. M. Burke, G. Bauldoff, & P. Gubrud (Eds.), *Medical surgical nursing: Clinical Reasoning in Patient Care* (6th ed., pp. 1014–1061). Hoboken, NJ: Pearson.

Lerner, N. B. (2016). The anemias. In R. M. Kliegman, B. F. Stanton, J. W. St. Geme III, N. F. Schor (Eds.), *Nelson textbook of pediatrics* (20th ed., pp. 2309–2312). Philadelphia, PA: Elsevier Saunders.

Levi, M. M., & Schmaier, A. H. (2014). *Disseminated intravascular coagulation.* Retrieved from http://emedicine.medscape.com/article/199627-overview

Lo, S. F. (2016). Reference intervals for laboratory tests and procedures. In R. M. Kliegman, B. F. Stanton, J. W. St. Geme, & N. F. Schor (Eds.), *Nelson textbook of pediatrics* (20th ed., pp. 3464–3473). Philadelphia, PA: Elsevier.

Lovett, P. B., Sule, H. P., & Lopez, B. L. (2014). Sickle cell disease in the emergency department. *Emergency Medicine Clinics of North America, 32*(3), 629–647.

Maakaron, J. E., & Taher, A. T. (2014). *Sickle cell anemia.* Retrieved from http://emedicine.medscape.com/article/205926-overview

Mahoney, D. H. (2014). *Iron deficiency in infants and young children: Screening, prevention, clinical manifestations, and diagnosis.* Retrieved from www.uptodate.com

March of Dimes. (2014). *Sickle cell disease and your baby.* Retrieved from http://www.marchofdimes.org/baby/sickle-cell-disease-and-your-baby.aspx

Meier, E. R., & Miller, J. L. (2012). Sickle cell disease in children. *Drugs, 72*(7), 895–906.

Moore, T., & Ikeda, A. K. (2014). *Bone marrow transplantation.* Retrieved from http://emedicine.medscape.com/article/1014514-overview

Myers, M., & Eckes, E. J. (2012). A novel approach to pain management in persons with sickle cell disease. *MEDSURG Nursing, 21*(5), 293–298.

National Newborn Screening and Genetics Resource Center. (2014). *National Newborn Screening Status Report.* Retrieved from http://genes-r-us.uthscsa.edu/sites/genes-r-us/files/nbsdisorders.pdf

Neunert, C. (2011). Idiopathic thrombocytopenic purpura: Advances in management. *Clinical Advances in Hematology & Oncology, 9*(5), 404–406.

Özgönenel, B., Zia, A., Callaghan, M. U., Chitlur, M., Rajpurkar, M., & Lusher, J. M. (2013). Emergency department visits in children with hemophilia. *Pediatric Blood and Cancer, 60*(7), 1188–1191.

Panepinto, J. A., Punzalan, R. C., & Scott, J. P. (2015). Hematology. In K. J. Marcdante & R. M. Kliegman (Eds.), *Nelson essentials of pediatrics* (7th ed., pp. 506–533). Philadelphia, PA: Elsevier Saunders.

Powers, J. M., & Buchanan, G. R. (2014). Iron deficiency anemia in toddlers to teens: How to manage when prevention fails. *Contemporary Pediatrics, 31*(5), 12–17.

Rodriguez-Merchan, E. C. (2012). Prevention of the musculoskeletal complications of hemophilia. *Advances in Preventive Medicine, 2012,* 1–8.

Roman, E., Larson, P. J., & Manno, C. S. (2013). Transfusion therapy for coagulation factor deficiencies. In R. Hoffman, E. J. Benz, L. E. Silberstein, H. Heslop, J. I. Weitz, & J. Anastasi (Eds.), *Hematology: Basic principles and practice* (6th ed., pp. 1705–1715). Philadelphia, PA: Elsevier Saunders.

Saunthararajah, Y., & Vichinsky, E. P. (2013). Sickle cell disease: Clinical features and management. In R. Hoffman, E. J. Benz, L. E. Silberstein, H. Heslop, J. I. Weitz, & J. Anastasi (Eds.), *Hematology: Basic principles and practice* (6th ed., pp. 548–572). Philadelphia, PA: Elsevier Saunders.

Scott, J. P., (2016). Factor VIII or factor IX deficiency (hemophilia A or B). In R. M. Kliegman, B. F. Stanton, J. W. St. Geme III, N. F. Schor (Eds.), *Nelson textbook of pediatrics* (20th ed., pp. 2384–2388). Philadelphia, PA: Elsevier Saunders.

Scott, J. P., & Raffini, L. J. (2016). Hemostasis. In R. M. Kliegman, B. F. Stanton, J. W. St. Geme III, N. F. Schor (Eds.), *Nelson textbook of pediatrics* (20th ed., pp. 2379–2381). Philadelphia, PA: Elsevier Saunders.

Segel, G. B., & Casey, D. (2016). Hereditary spherocytosis. In R. M. Kliegman, B. F. Stanton, J. W. St. Geme III, N. F. Schor (Eds.), *Nelson textbook of pediatrics* (20th ed., pp 2330–2333). Philadelphia, PA: Elsevier Saunders.

Shihabuddin, B. S., & Scarfi, C. A. (2014). Fever in children with sickle cell disease: Are all fevers equal? *The Journal of Emergency Medicine, 47*(4), 395–400.

Sickle Cell Information Center. (2012). *FAQ: Sickle cell disease.* Retrieved from https://scinfo.org/faq/faq-sickle-cell-disease

Soldin, S. J., Wong, E. C., Brugnara, C., & Soldin, O. P. (2011). *Pediatric reference ranges* (7th ed.). Washington, DC: AACC Press.

Strouse, J. J., & Heeney, M. M. (2012). Hydroxyurea for the treatment of sickle cell disease: Efficacy, barriers, toxicity, and management in children. *Pediatric Blood & Cancer, 59,* 365–371.

Tanabe, P., Dias, N., & Gorman, L. (2013). Care of children with sickle cell disease in the emergency department: Parent and provider perspectives inform quality improvement efforts. *Journal of Pediatric Oncology Nursing, 30*(4), 205–217

Thiagarajan, P. (2014). *Platelet disorders.* Retrieved from http://emedicine.medscape.com/article/201722-overview#aw2aab6c21

Vichinsky, E. P. (2014). *Variant sickle cell syndromes.* Retrieved from uptodate.com

Walovich, K. J., & Newberger, P. E. (2016). Leukopenia. In R. M. Kliegman, B. F. Stanton, J. W. St. Geme III, N. F. Schor (Eds.), *Nelson textbook of pediatrics* (20th ed., pp. 1047–1053). Philadelphia, PA: Elsevier Saunders.

Warrier, R., & Chauhan, A. (2012). Management of immune thrombocytopenic purpura. *The Ochsner Journal, 12*(3), 221–227.

Weickert, L., Miesbach, W., Alesci, S. J., Eickholz, P., & Nickles, K. (2014). Is gingival bleeding a symptom of type 1 von Willebrand disease? A case-control study. *Journal of Clinical Peridontology, 41,* 766–771.

Yawn, B. P., Buchanan, G. R., Afenyi-Annan, A. N., Ballas, S. K., Hassell, K. L., James, A. H., . . . John-Sowah, J. (2014). Management of sickle cell disease: Summary of the 2014 evidence-based report by expert panel members. *JAMA, 312*(10), 1033–1048.

Zaiden, R. A. (2014). *Hemophilia B.* Retrieved from http://emedicine.medscape.com/article/779434-overview

Zaiden, R. A., Furlong, M. A., Crouch, G. D., & Besa, E. C. (2014). *Hemophilia A.* Retrieved from http://emedicine.medscape.com/article/779322-overview

Zempsky, W. T., Corsi, J. M., & McKay, K. (2011). Pain scores: Are they used in sickle cell pain? *Pediatric Emergency Care, 27*(1), 27–28.

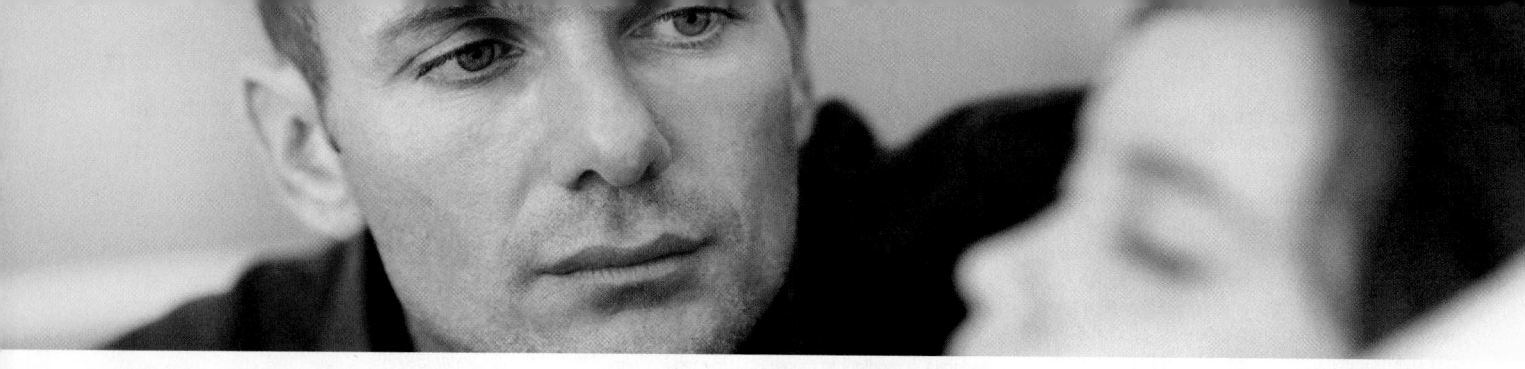

Chapter 50
The Child With Cancer

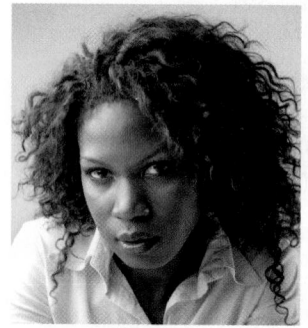

Rasheed was just diagnosed with leukemia seven months ago, but already he has been in the hospital five times. This time he had enterocolitis, an infection of the intestines. But he has now improved and is determined to fight the disease. It's his will and strength that help us all to be strong and to know that he will do well after his treatment is finished.

—Mother of Rasheed, 12 years old

Ollyy/Shutterstock

⌄ Learning Outcomes

50.1 Describe the incidence, known etiologies, and common clinical manifestations of cancer.

50.2 Synthesize information about diagnostic tests and clinical therapy for cancer to plan comprehensive care for children undergoing these procedures.

50.3 Integrate information about oncologic emergencies into plans for monitoring all children with cancer.

50.4 Recognize the most common solid tumors in children, describe their treatment, and plan comprehensive nursing care.

50.5 Plan care for children and adolescents of all ages who have a diagnosis of leukemia.

50.6 Prioritize elements of comprehensive care planning for children with soft-tissue tumors.

50.7 Analyze the impact of cancer survival on children and use this information to plan for ongoing physiologic and psychosocial care in the children's futures.

Cancer is a daunting diagnosis at any age, but in children, it seems even more profound. The diagnosis and treatment are met with shock and disbelief, they require a change in the roles of everyone in the family, and challenge all children and families involved in many ways. Nurses who work in pediatric oncology have unique opportunities to assist children and families in mobilizing resources and learning about maximizing physical, emotional, and developmental health while dealing with the challenges of the illness and treatment.

Why do children develop different types of cancers than adults? Cancers in children often have a different etiology than those in adults. Most adult cancers are epithelial in origin, whereas in children, nonepithelial or embryonal cell types are predominant. Whereas many adult cancers are slow growing

and result from exposure to carcinogens over time, most childhood cancers are fast growing, and a child who appears healthy may suddenly appear ill over a period of days or weeks. Cancer in adults is often the result of dietary practices or habits such as smoking. Some adult-onset cancers are the result of oncogenic responses to stimuli—that is, responses that stimulate cancerous changes in cells. Other cancers that occur in adults result from prolonged exposure to toxins such as coal dust and asbestos. Some cancers are known to be related to genetic causes. In adults, prevention through general lifestyle changes is a major focus of interventions. However, in children, cancer is usually embryonic (occurring during development of the fetus) or oncogenic in origin. Thus, lifestyle changes that begin in childhood have little effect on the incidence of childhood cancer, although they may help reduce the incidence of later cancer or other diseases. Occasionally, an environmental exposure is linked to the incidence of cancer in children.

Abnormal cellular growth can occur in any area of the body. Why are some growths called cancer and others not? Changes in cellular growth within the body are called **neoplasms** (meaning "new growth"). A neoplasm is further classified as benign or malignant. **Benign** means that a growth does not endanger life or health; it tends not to recur after treatment. **Malignant** means that if not treated, a tumor will continue to grow, and will spread to other sites in the body (**metastasis**), ending in death. The common term for this type of cellular growth is *cancer*.

Anatomy and Physiology of Pediatric Differences

The major physiologic difference between adults and children that affects cellular growth involves the immune system and how well it defends the body. The rate of cell growth in children also can play a role in the rapid progression of some childhood cancers. The continuing presence of fetal cells in small children is related to some cancers.

The immune system defends the body against foreign organisms and substances through two responses: nonspecific and specific. In a nonspecific response, the components of the immune system attack a variety of targets. Nonspecific components include phagocytic (cell-destroying) cells such as mononuclear leukocytes, polymorphonuclear (PMN) leukocytes, natural killer (NK) cells, and complements (noncellular proteins) that work together to destroy invading cells and substances. During the first month of a child's life, the nonspecific response is immature, so phagocytic cells have little ability to move toward cancer cells and fulfill their function. The nonspecific response is also impaired in premature and small-for-gestational-age (SGA) infants.

In a specific response, T lymphocytes and various proteins called immunoglobulins (Igs) attack only one type of invader. The specific response capability also is immature in infants. B-cell production of immunoglobulins (IgM, IgG, and IgA) is below adult levels, so that the infant is vulnerable to bacterial and viral infections. (For a discussion of immune function, see Chapter 48.)

In children, many cells grow quickly. This fast growth can lead to the proliferation of cancerous as well as normal cells. Cell division that is out of control may normally trigger a mechanism called **apoptosis**, whereby the cell "realizes" something is wrong and destroys itself. The process of apoptosis, or physiologic cell death, may not be well developed in young children.

Childhood Cancer

The care of children who have cancer is a challenging specialty in pediatric nursing. In some cases, the child undergoes treatments that may continue for years and result in a variety of side effects. Today, treatments for cancer have improved prognoses in many cases, but in some, the prognosis still requires that the family deal with a life-threatening illness (see Chapter 41). The child is often cared for at home with outpatient visits for treatment and occasional hospitalization when needed. The periods of hospitalization are times of intense physical vulnerability for the child and intense emotional vulnerability for both the child and the family. To monitor the child closely, nurses need a sound knowledge of physiologic and psychologic responses,

medical interventions, and nursing care. Integration of developmental knowledge into assessment and intervention is essential. Effective communication skills are necessary to support the child and family and promote realistic hope. See the *Nursing Management* sections and the *Nursing Care Plans* later in this chapter for specific interventions required.

Incidence

In the United States, cancer is diagnosed annually in approximately 11,000 children under 15 years of age, and about 1500 die from cancer annually (American Cancer Society [ACS], 2011). In children under 15 years of age, cancer is the leading cause of disease-related death, and it is the second leading cause of overall death after unintentional injury (ACS, 2011). However, mortality rates have declined by about 47% since 1975. The overall survival rate is 80% for childhood cancer. Survival rates vary related to the stage of disease at time of diagnosis and differ for specific types of cancer, ranging from 66% for neuroblastoma to 95% for Hodgkin disease (ACS, 2011; Arndt, 2011a). Figure 50–1 shows the most common forms of childhood cancers among children in different age groups.

Etiology and Pathophysiology

Alterations in cellular growth occur in response to external and internal stimuli. Neoplasms are caused by one or any combination of three factors: (1) external stimuli that cause genetic mutations, (2) immune system and gene abnormalities, and (3) chromosomal abnormalities.

EXTERNAL STIMULI

External stimuli may affect the child's general health and cause mutations in body cells. **Carcinogens** are chemicals or industrial processes that, when combined with genetic traits and in interaction with one another, result in cancer. Several carcinogens cause cancers that are diagnosed during childhood. Others cause cancers that begin in childhood but are not identified until adulthood. Some chemicals suspected of causing childhood cancer include diethylstilbestrol (maternal use of therapeutic estrogen hormones), anabolic androgenic steroids, alkylating chemotherapeutic agents, and immunosuppressants used for organ transplantation. Radiation exposure has been known to cause cancers such as leukemia and thyroid tumors in children exposed to nuclear fallout from atomic bombs, other nuclear accidents, and other excessive radiation sources.

External stimuli may also lead to secondary cancers in children, or those occurring after treatment for a primary cancer and of a different cellular type than the primary cancer. Secondary cancers can result when the child is treated for a primary cancer with high doses of radiation. Excessive exposure to ultraviolet radiation from the sun predisposes children to development of skin cancer in adolescence and adulthood (see Chapter 57).

IMMUNE SYSTEM AND GENE ABNORMALITIES

One critical function of a normal immune system is immune surveillance, in which phagocytic cells circulate throughout the body, detecting and destroying abnormal and cancerous cells. Children with congenital immune deficiencies, such as Wiskott-Aldrich syndrome, in which immune surveillance may fail, are at high risk for cancer. A form of non-Hodgkin lymphoma develops in some children treated with immune system–suppressing drugs. Children with acquired immunodeficiency syndrome (AIDS) may also be at higher risk of certain types

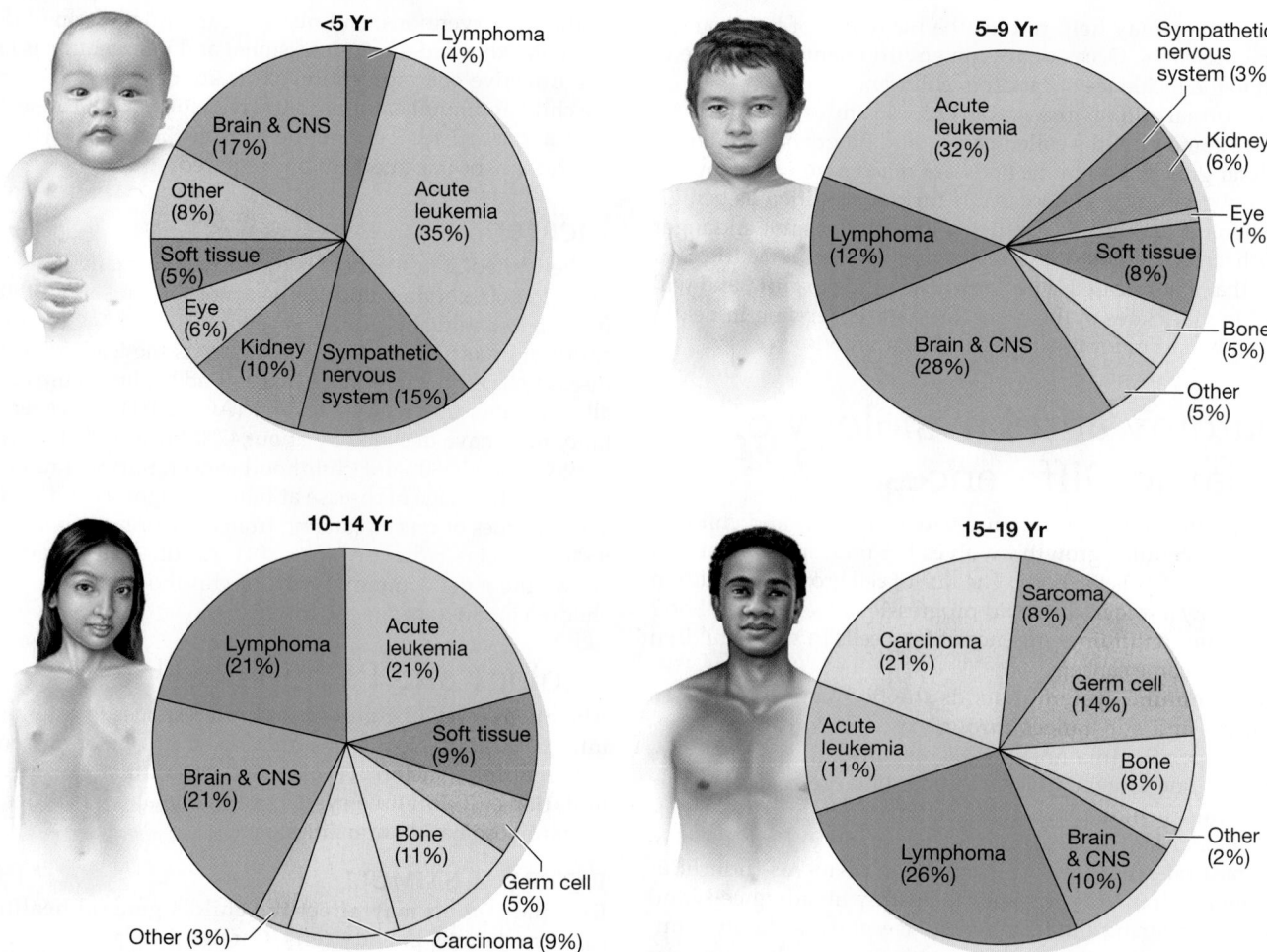

Figure 50–1 Percentage of primary tumors by site of origin for different age groups.

SOURCE: Data from Asselin, B. (2011). Epidemiology of childhood and adolescent cancer. In R. M. Kliegman, B. F. Stanton, J. W. St. Geme, N. F. Schor, & R. E. Behrman (Eds.), *Nelson textbook of pediatrics* (19th ed., pp. 1725–1727). Philadelphia, PA: Elsevier Saunders.

of cancer, such as Hodgkin disease, non-Hodgkin lymphoma, Kaposi sarcoma, and leiomyosarcoma (Sigel et al., 2011).

Viruses and other substances may alter the immune system, thereby allowing cancer to occur (see *Pathophysiology Illustrated: Proto-Oncogene Alteration*). Their action is based on changing certain genes that normally regulate cellular growth and development (called **proto-oncogenes**) into related genes that allow unregulated cell division and cancerous growth (called **oncogenes**). Among the cancers thought to be linked to viral action and the change of proto-oncogenes to oncogenes are certain leukemias, rhabdomyosarcoma, Burkitt lymphoma, and some forms of Hodgkin disease.

Genetic changes can include autosomal dominant, autosomal recessive, and X-linked transfer. In these cases, the resulting cancers often occur relatively early in life. Cancers of these types are typically aggressive since the child has inherited the abnormal gene and it is within each cell, rather than a single mutation of one gene in a specific cell. Because of the progress made in the Human Genome Project, there is increasing ability to perform genetic testing for certain familial cancers. Examples of cancers that are sometimes caused by genetic abnormalities within families include retinoblastoma and Wilms tumor (described later in this chapter), multiple endocrine neoplasia, type 2 (thyroid cancer), and familial adenomatous polyposis (invasive colon cancer). Not all cases of these cancers are familial, but their incidence suggests the need for careful history

taking to identify any other cases in the family. Providing recommendations for referral to genetic counseling services and following up with further education and psychologic support are important nursing roles.

Professionalism in Practice Nursing Genomics Competencies

Cancer's relationship with genetic characteristics is increasingly recognized, and treatments may target certain genes. For these reasons, it is important that nurses who work in oncology nursing achieve genomic competency. The Genomic Nursing Concept Inventory (GCNI) has been developed and evaluated to measure genomic literacy and advance evidence-based nursing education (Ward, Haberman, & Barbosa-Leiker, 2014). Nurses believe that genomic competency is important, but it has been found that a deficit in this knowledge affects nurses regardless of academic preparation (Calzone, Jenkins, Culp, et al., 2014). Genetic and genomic competencies have been developed to encompass risk assessment and interpretation; genetic education, counseling, testing, and results interpretation; clinical management; ethical, legal, and social implications; professional role; leadership; and research (Greco, Tinley, & Seibert, 2011). See Chapter 3 for further information about genetics and genomics.

Pathophysiology Illustrated: **Proto-Oncogene Alteration**

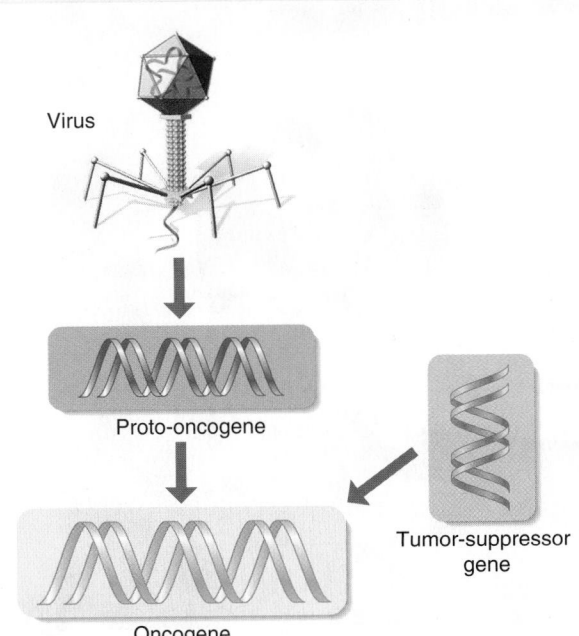

Virus

Proto-oncogene

Tumor-suppressor gene

Oncogene

A proto-oncogene normally regulates cellular growth and development. When altered by a virus or other external cause, it can change to an oncogene, which allows unregulated genetic activity and tumor growth. Tumor suppressor genes regulate the effects of oncogenes to decrease wildly proliferating cellular growth.

Tumor suppressor genes counteract the effect of oncogenes, keeping cellular growth within normal limits. When tumor suppressor genes are missing, unstemmed cellular growth can occur. These genes are commonly missing in children with retinoblastoma and Wilms tumor.

CHROMOSOMAL ABNORMALITIES

Normal chromosomes undergo change as a part of the genetic process. Most changes are not harmful. However, some result in chromosomal abnormalities such as hyperploidy (more than the normal number of chromosomes), deletion, translocation, and breakage.

Some chromosomal abnormalities have been linked to an increased incidence of cancer. Children with Down syndrome have a much higher incidence of leukemia than nonaffected children; the risk varies greatly according to the type of leukemia (Roberts & Izraieli, 2014). Children missing a band of genetic material on chromosome 13 often have retinoblastoma. Similarly, a Wilms tumor often develops in children missing part of the genetic material from chromosome 11.

Regardless of the location and cause of abnormal cellular growth, the pathophysiologic process of cancer is similar. The altered cell begins to multiply as directed by the altered genetic structure of its DNA and the absence or inactivation of tumor suppressor genes. Each new cell transmits the new or altered pattern to the next generation. As the abnormal cells replicate, they form a growing neoplastic mass. Normal cells usually die as the increased metabolic rate of the neoplastic cells depletes available nutrition. The altered DNA in the tumor cells may also

TEACHING HIGHLIGHTS | Ways to Decrease the Incidence of Cancer in Children

Many parents ask what they can do to decrease the incidence of cancer in children as they grow into adulthood. Three major teaching areas should be addressed:

1. Have children increase intake of fruits and vegetables. Most children do not eat enough of these foods, and increased intake is associated with lower rates of many cancers. Aim for a minimum of five servings daily.
2. Protect skin with sunscreen. Early excessive exposure to sun, and having had one or repeated severe sunburns during childhood, increases chances of skin cancers developing in adulthood. Tanning bed exposure is a prime risk factor for skin cancer; all children and adolescents, and particularly those with cancer, should strictly avoid tanning beds (Greinert & Boniol, 2011).
3. Discourage smoking among children and be sure children are not exposed to environmental tobacco smoke. This will decrease the future chance of developing lung cancer.

When there is a history of cancer in the family, particularly of a type associated with familial incidence such as some breast or ovarian cancers, encourage the family to learn more about the cancer and teach their children to receive regular surveillance as they enter young adulthood.

Inform youth in all families about screening, such as the Papanicolaou test, breast self-examination, and testicular examination, that can lead to early detection. Encourage youth to receive the human papillomavirus quadrivalent vaccine recombinant (Gardasil) to prevent cervical cancers and other health problems caused by human papillomavirus (HPV). (See Chapter 43 for further information.)

cause the abnormal cells to invade adjoining tissue. Through continued growth the mass expands until it enters and disrupts a major vessel or a vital organ.

Clinical Manifestations

Each type of childhood cancer signals its presence differently. Because many of the presenting signs and symptoms of cancer are typical of common childhood illnesses, diagnosis may be delayed. In some cases, no symptoms are noted until the cancer is advanced. Some of the common presenting symptoms of cancer follow:

- *Pain* may be the result of a neoplasm either directly or indirectly affecting nerve receptors through obstruction, inflammation, tissue damage, stretching of visceral tissue, or invasion of susceptible tissue.

- *Cachexia* is a syndrome characterized by anorexia, weight loss, anemia, asthenia (weakness), and early satiety (feeling of being full).

- *Anemia* may be experienced during times of chronic bleeding or iron deficiency. In chronic illness, the body uses iron poorly. Anemia is also present in cancers of the bone marrow when the number of red blood cells (RBCs) is reduced, in part because of the presence of large numbers of other bone marrow products. Treatment of cancer often promotes further anemia.

- *Infection* is usually a result of an altered or immature immune system. In addition, infection occurs when bone marrow cancers inhibit maturation of normal immune system cells. Infection may also occur in children treated with corticosteroids. Because their immune response is altered, the normal signs of infection may not appear.

- *Bruising* and *petechiae* can occur if the bone marrow cannot produce enough platelets; bleeding after even minor trauma can lead to ecchymosis.

- *Neurologic symptoms* may result from impingement on the brain or nervous system. Signs of increased intracranial pressure, decreased or altered consciousness, eye abnormalities, or other neurologic or behavioral changes may be evident.

- *Palpable mass* may be present for certain cancers. This is most commonly abdominal but may be mediastinal, in the neck, or at other sites.

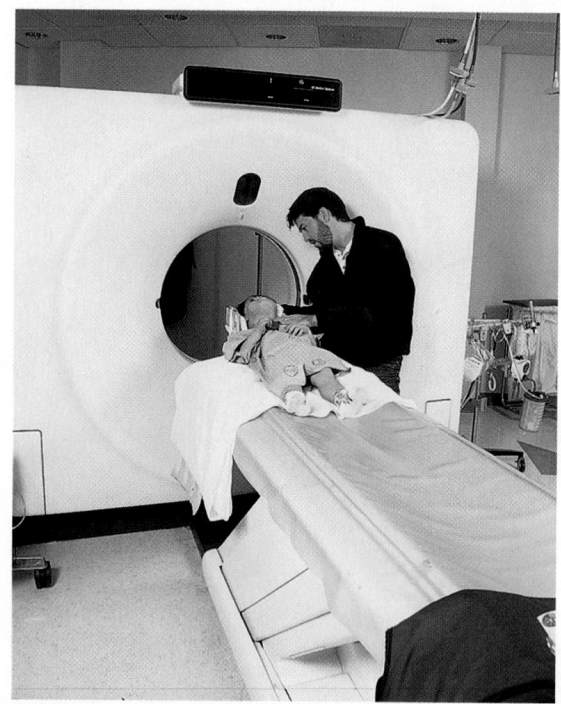

Figure 50–2 Computed tomography can be a frightening procedure for children. This 2-year-old boy is comforted by his father before the procedure.

A variety of other symptoms can occur depending on the location of the cancer. Subcutaneous nodules may appear if leukocytosis is present. Superior vena cava syndrome or respiratory difficulty can occur with mediastinal tumors (such as neuroblastoma), and enlarged lymph nodes are common with lymphomas.

DIAGNOSTIC TESTS

The most common diagnostic tests performed on children with cancer are a complete blood count (CBC) with differential, bone marrow aspiration (BMA), bone marrow biopsy (BMBX), lumbar puncture (LP), peripheral blood studies, radiographic examination, magnetic resonance imaging (MRI), computed tomography (CT; Figure 50–2), ultrasound, and biopsy of tumor. See Table 50–1.

TABLE 50–1 Selected Diagnostic Tests for Childhood Cancer

TEST	PURPOSE	NORMAL LABORATORY VALUES	DIAGNOSTIC VALUES
Bone marrow aspiration	Examines bone marrow.	Less than 5% blast cells (immature)	Greater than 25% blast cells in acute lymphoblastic leukemia, most with hypercellular marrow
Lumbar puncture	Examines cerebrospinal fluid.	Cell count (microliters) Polymorphonuclear leukocytes 0 Monocytes 0–5 RBCs 0–5	Presence of malignant cells indicates central nervous system involvement
Complete blood count and differential	Examines cellular components of blood.	WBC less than 10,000/mcL Platelets 150,000–400,000/mcL Hemoglobin 12–16 g/dL	WBC greater than 10,000/mcL OR depressed levels of WBCs Platelets 20,000–100,000/mL Hemoglobin 7–10 g/dL
Absolute neutrophil count (ANC)	Examines blood component ratio: (% of segmental neutrophils plus % of bands [immature neutrophils]) times WBC count; this number is then divided by 100.	ANC greater than 1000	ANC less than 1000 = risk of infection

Additional studies helpful for certain cancers are nuclear medicine scans with radioactive isotopes such as gallium or iodine, bone scan with technetium 99m, or positron emission tomography (PET) and single-photon emission computed tomography (SPECT), which combine nuclear medicine with CT. Specific tests such as pulmonary function tests and echocardiograms may be used in certain situations. Urine analysis is also performed.

The blood work is very detailed and includes RBC, WBC, platelets, hematocrit and hemoglobin, serum electrolytes, liver studies, and markers that are elevated in specific types of tumors. Absolute neutrophil count (ANC) is important; it uses both the segmented (mature) and bands (immature neutrophils) as a measure of the body's infection-fighting capability. ANC is calculated by adding the percentage of segmented neutrophils to the percentage of bands, and then multiplying this percentage by the WBC count.

The tests are aimed at identifying the source of the cancer and any metastases to additional sites. This enables the oncology specialist to stage the cancer. *Staging* refers to the process of labeling the type of cancer cells, severity, and spread, which will determine the recommended treatment and assist in teaching the family about treatment and prognosis. Stage 1 indicates less severe cancer without spread to other parts of the body; higher numbers indicate both greater severity and spread to other sites.

CLINICAL THERAPY

Clinical therapy for cancer is extremely complex and is managed by a specialist in pediatric oncology. The cancer itself is treated, its effects on the body are addressed, and the side effects of treatment are managed. Examples of the effects of cancer on the body include altered nutritional status from anorexia due to the cancer diverting nutrients to itself, decreased immune response from impaired manufacture of white blood cells and other immune components, and a variety of symptoms as a tumor presses on vital organs. In addition, cancer treatment itself has many potential side effects that require constant monitoring and adjustments in treatment.

Cancer is treated with one or a combination of therapies: surgery, chemotherapy, radiation, **biotherapy** (treatment that uses and/or enhances the body's abilities to fight disease, particularly by using biologic agents to promote immune response), and bone marrow transplantation. The choice of treatment is determined by the type of cancer, its location, and staging. Treatments all have side effects and these will also require clinical management. Many families also choose to use some type of complementary therapy in addition to traditional medical approaches.

The goal of treatment may be curative, supportive, or provision of end-of-life care. Curative treatment rids the child's body of the cancer. Supportive treatment includes transfusions, pain management, antibiotics, and other interventions to assist the body's defenses and increase the child's comfort. End-of-life treatment is designed to make the child as comfortable as possible when no curative treatment is possible. (See Chapter 41 for a detailed discussion of end-of-life care for children.) Whatever combination of treatment is used, families have many questions and need resources for information.

Surgery.   Surgery is used to remove or debulk (reduce the size of) a solid tumor. An example of a cancer that is commonly treated with surgery is a Wilms tumor. Surgery may also determine the stage and type of cancer.

Chemotherapy.   **Chemotherapy** is the administration of specific drugs that kill both normal and cancerous cells. The administration of various chemotherapeutic drugs is timed to achieve the greatest cellular destruction. The cell's cycle of replication determines the schedule (see *Pathophysiology Illustrated: Chemotherapeutic Drug Action*). Several chemotherapeutic drugs are administered simultaneously to maximize their lethal impact on cells at all stages of activity (see *Medications Used for: Cancer Chemotherapy*). Medications are most commonly oral, intravenous, or **intrathecal** (into spinal canal). Whereas DNA in a normal cell can repair itself after chemotherapy, the DNA in a neoplastic cell cannot. The particular chemotherapeutic treatment protocol used is based on research into different types of cancer cells. A **protocol** is a plan of action for chemotherapy based on the type of cancer, its stage, and the particular cell type (Figure 50–3).

Other drugs used in the treatment of children with cancer include colony-stimulating factors, antiemetics, and nutritional supplements. Colony-stimulating factors are hormone-like glycoproteins that enhance blood cell production and counteract the myelosuppressive effects of chemotherapeutic drugs. For example, erythropoietin is produced in the kidney, and a recombinant form (epoetin) is available that can be used to treat anemia of cancer, thereby decreasing the number of transfusions needed. Filgrastim (Neupogen) increases production of

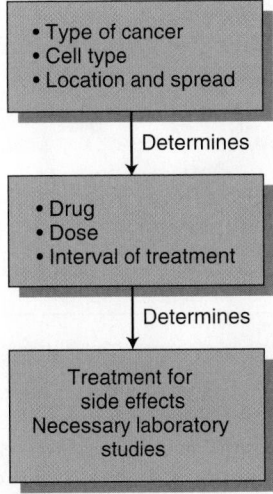

Protocol = Map or plan of action

- Type of cancer
- Cell type
- Location and spread

Determines

- Drug
- Dose
- Interval of treatment

Determines

Treatment for side effects Necessary laboratory studies

Figure 50–3   Chemotherapy protocol. A protocol is a map or plan of action that directs therapy by identifying the drug and its accompanying treatment.

Pathophysiology Illustrated: **Chemotherapeutic Drug Action**

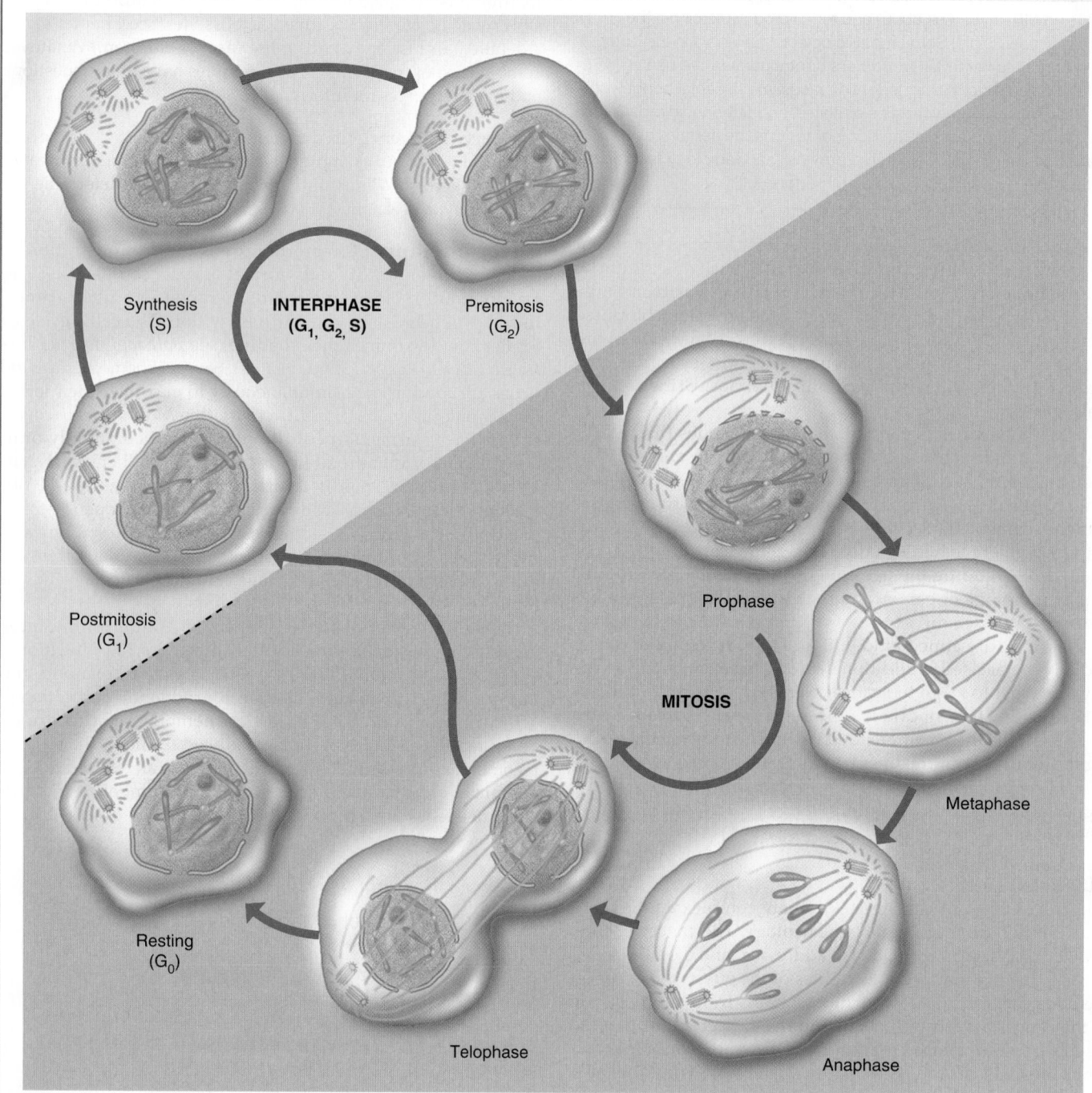

Synthesis
(S)

**INTERPHASE
(G$_1$, G$_2$, S)**

Premitosis
(G$_2$)

Prophase

Postmitosis
(G$_1$)

MITOSIS

Metaphase

Resting
(G$_0$)

Telophase

Anaphase

Chemotherapeutic drugs either act at specific parts of the cell cycle or are nonspecific for action (act throughout all cell phases). See *Medications Used for: Cancer Chemotherapy* for further information about specific drugs and their site of action in the cell cycle.

neutrophils by the bone marrow (see *Medications Used During Cancer Treatment: Colony-Stimulating Factors*). Antiemetics, such as ondansetron (Zofran), can be used to treat the nausea and vomiting that are common side effects of therapy. Nutritional supplements help maintain nutritional status.

Radiation. **Radiation** therapy involves unstable isotopes that release varying levels of energy to cause breaks in the DNA molecule and thereby destroy cells. Radiation has been used as a treatment method since the early 1900s, shortly after its discovery. It is often used for the local and regional control of cancer, and in combination with surgery and chemotherapy; it may be curative or palliative.

The area to be irradiated (treatment field) includes the tumor site and sometimes other involved areas, such as lymph glands. The goal is to irradiate the tumor but not healthy

Medications Used for: Cancer Chemotherapy

MEDICATION AND ACTION/INDICATION	NURSING IMPLICATIONS
Cell Cycle–Specific Agents	
Antimetabolites • 5-Azacytidine • 5-Fluorouracil • 6-Mercaptopurine • 6-Thioguanine • Cytosine arabinoside (cytarabine) • Hydroxyurea • Methotrexate The antimetabolites work at the synthesis phase of cell division; interfere with function of nucleic acid; inhibit DNA or RNA synthesis.	Various routes are used for individual agents, such as oral, intravenous, and intrathecal. Most common side effects are nausea and vomiting, myelosuppression, stomatitis. Specific agents such as methotrexate and cytarabine can cause neurologic toxicity with high doses. Consult drug books and package inserts for a detailed list of side effects. Obtain baseline CBC, liver function, renal function. Monitor intake and output and body weight. Ensure hydration and output levels ordered by oncologist. Monitor vital signs and cardiovascular and respiratory function. Watch for bleeding and signs of infection. Monitor carefully during administration for signs of anaphylaxis.
Vinca alkaloids • Etoposide • Teniposide • Irinotecan • Paclitaxel • Vinblastine • Vincristine Act during mitosis; bind with cell proteins to inhibit nucleic acid and protein synthesis.	Most are given intravenously with some drugs also available for oral route. Common side effects include nausea and vomiting, abdominal cramping and diarrhea, constipation, paralytic ileus, hair loss, hypotension or hypertension, peripheral neuropathy and neurologic toxicity (latter especially with vinblastine and vincristine). Obtain baseline blood work. Consult specific drug information for period of maximum myelosuppressive effect. Be alert for bruising, infection, and other signs of myelosuppression. Monitor carefully during administration for signs of anaphylaxis, particularly with etoposide and paclitaxel.
Miscellaneous—G_1 phase activity • L-asparaginase Causes depletion of asparagine, needed by cancer cells; makes cell in G_1 phase vulnerable to other agents; interferes with synthesis. Used in combination with other agents in leukemia and other cancers.	Administered intravenously or intramuscularly. Major side effects are severe nausea and vomiting, hypersensitivity, renal failure, myelosuppression, acid–base imbalance. Because of the risk of life-threatening hypersensitivity reactions, emergency medications and care must be immediately available. Perform CBC, serum amylase, glucose, coagulation factors, bone marrow function, liver function tests before therapy and twice weekly. Monitor intake and output, neurologic status, gastrointestinal symptoms, abdominal pain.
Miscellaneous—G_2 phase activity • Etoposide Works at G_2 phase; binds cellular proteins to cause metaphase arrest; also acts on S phase of DNA synthesis. Used with other agents, particularly in recurrent disease.	Administered orally and intravenously. Common side effects are nausea and vomiting, myelosuppression, hair loss, diarrhea. Can cause anaphylaxis; hypotension and IV site pain with rapid infusion. Perform baseline CBC, liver, and renal function tests. Check IV site frequently since extravasation can cause necrosis. Monitor vital signs during infusion and stop drug if hypotension occurs. Keep emergency drugs and equipment readily available.

(continued)

Medications Used for: Cancer Chemotherapy (*continued*)

Cell Cycle–Nonspecific Agents

Alkylating agents

- Cyclophosphamide
- Carboplatin
- Cisplatin
- Busulfan
- Chlorambucil
- Ifosfamide
- Thiotepa
- Mechlorethamine
- Melphalan
- Procarbazine
- Dacarbazine

Substitute an alkyl group for a hydrogen atom, leading to blockage of DNA replication. Used for treatment of many cancers, either alone or in conjunction with other agents.

Most are administered orally and/or intravenously. Array of side effects depending on specific drug. Some common side effects are nausea and vomiting, diarrhea, myelosuppression, hair loss, neuropathies, pulmonary toxicity, renal damage; secondary tumors later in life associated with some agents.

Obtain CBC and full blood work before and during treatment. Mesna may be administered with some alkylating agents to lower the risk of hemorrhagic cystitis. Monitor for side effects of the specific agents administered.

Ensure generous hydration and monitor intake and output.

Teach family the importance of long-term monitoring for secondary tumors.

Antibiotics

- Doxorubicin
- Mitomycin-C
- Dactinomycin
- Bleomycin
- Daunorubicin
- Idarubicin
- Mitoxantrone

Interfere with nucleic acid, inhibiting DNA or RNA synthesis. Used in combination with other agents to treat leukemia and other childhood cancers.

Most are administered intravenously.

Common side effects include nausea and vomiting, myelosuppression, oral ulcers, skin and pulmonary toxicity. Several have cumulative dose toxicity, such as cardiac abnormalities (doxorubicin) and skin/pulmonary (bleomycin); total dose the child has received must be monitored.

Obtain baseline CBC and other blood studies and monitor throughout therapy.

Monitor vital signs, lung function, cardiac function, and neurologic status throughout and following therapy. Be alert for signs of myelosuppression and mucosal ulcers.

Nitrosoureas

- Carmustine
- Lomustine

Cross-breakage in DNA strands so that DNA and RNA replication cannot occur. Used in lymphomas and other childhood cancers. Can cross blood–brain barrier.

Administered orally (lomustine) or intravenously (carmustine). Major side effect is myelosuppression.

Others include pulmonary fibrosis, eye infarction, skin changes, hair loss, nausea, and vomiting.

Obtain baseline and periodic CBC and other studies.

Monitor pulmonary function, skin, and signs of infection or bleeding such as ecchymosis or petechiae.

Hormones

- Prednisone
- Prednisolone
- Dexamethasone

Analog of hydrocortisone; anti-inflammatory; delayed and depressed immune response. Used in conjunction with other agents for many types of childhood cancer.

Often administered orally.

Numerous side effects including edema, moon face, mood lability, increased appetite, disturbed sleep, immunosuppression, disturbed glucose control, osteoporosis.

Teach child and family the effects of the drug. Minimize exposure to persons with infection. Monitor for infections in all systems.

Monitor weight regularly. Take vital signs. Teach to take as directed. Drug must be tapered slowly at end of therapy.

Topoisomerase I inhibitor

- Irinotecan
- Mitoxantrone
- Topotecan

Inhibit the enzyme topoisomerase I in the cell nucleus, relaxing DNA and preventing its duplication.

Used in conjunction with other agents to treat acute lymphocytic leukemia and other childhood cancers.

Administered intravenously: topotecan can be given intrathecally. Common side effects include nausea and vomiting, diarrhea, fever, dehydration, myelosuppression. Can alter liver function and cause skin changes.

Obtain baseline and periodic CBC and other studies, including liver function.

Monitor for signs of myelosuppression, gastrointestinal distress, change in liver function.

adjacent tissue. The total dose of radiation is divided (or fractionated) and given over several weeks. A common course of radiation treatment might be once daily 4 or 5 days per week for a period of 2 to 7 weeks.

SAFETY ALERT!

Nurses who care for a child receiving implant radiation or who work in a radiation department need to wear a dosimeter film badge at all times to measure their radiation exposure.

Examples of cancers treated with radiation include Hodgkin disease, Wilms tumor, retinoblastoma, rhabdomyosarcoma, and central nervous system disease in leukemia. Tumors that have a low sensitivity to radiation, such as osteosarcoma and soft-tissue sarcomas, require higher doses of radiation, or other treatments may be preferred.

Biotherapy. Biotherapy is the use of biologic retooling and molecular intervention to produce targeted cancer therapy. Biologic retooling uses parts of the human body that are programmed to destroy cells, and applies them to the cancer cells. An example of this technique includes development of antibodies that are tumor specific to certain cancers, and produced by the body in response to antigens of cancer cells (Smith & Reaman, 2015). These antibodies promote apoptosis or death of the cancerous cells. Another example is the group of drugs that stimulate the body's own immune response. Cancer vaccines are under development that may work to help the body fight cancers; already developed is human papillomavirus vaccine (see Chapter 43). The actions of many of these agents are not completely understood and may have different effects in children versus adults, and some agents have more than one effect. For example, interferon has both antiviral and antiproliferative effects on some malignant cells. Interferon and tumor necrosis factor (TNF) are undergoing clinical trials to study their effectiveness and to develop protocols for their safe use against selected cancers.

Molecular targeting involves interference with metabolic pathways (e.g., through enzyme disruption) in the tumor cells. It may therefore disturb the cell's growth and development and thereby depress proliferation.

TEACHING HIGHLIGHTS | Cancer Therapy

Most parents are not aware of the effects of cancer treatment and how they can help children through this experience. Depending on the stage and type of treatment, there are several ways to help:

- Children in radiation therapy and chemotherapy become fatigued because of cancer and treatment effects. Provide extra rest periods with shorter activity periods between them.
- Have a suitcase ready in case the child develops a complication and needs to be taken to stay in the hospital for a few days. Several hospital stays of a few days are normal during treatment.
- Parents are often key in identifying problems early. They should be encouraged to share their observations and concerns about symptoms the child is experiencing.
- Parents are usually concerned about providing central line care but feel more comfortable after a few days of caring for the line.
- Children may not feel hungry because of anorexia from the disease and as a side effect of treatment. When they are ready to eat, intake should be nutritious.
- Remember that children with cancer are still at their normal developmental age. Treat them appropriately for their age, not as if they are older or younger. Utilize the child-life specialist in the hospital to assist with planning activities appropriate to the child's developmental age.
- Try to maintain contact with the child's peer group and family members. When school attendance or direct contact is not possible because of immune suppression, arrange for phone calls, videocam exchanges, and other methods of communication.
- Seek information from other parents, the Internet, and other resources on cancer care.
- Many families use complementary approaches to deal with the child's cancer. Most of these approaches are not contraindicated. However, be sure to tell the oncologist about what treatments you are choosing to use to be sure none of them will injure your child.
- Take time to get away and relax so that you have enough energy and are better able to deal with your child's therapy.

Medications Used During Cancer Treatment: Colony-Stimulating Factors

MEDICATION AND ACTION/INDICATION	NURSING IMPLICATIONS
Epoetin alfa (human recombinant erythropoietin) This glycoprotein stimulates the bone marrow in RBC formation; useful when numbers of RBCs are low because of chemotherapeutic effects.	Give subcutaneously or intravenously. Do not shake and do not use if discolored or particles are present. Single-dose vials only, so discard any solution that is not used. Obtain red blood cell tests before therapy and periodically after; improvement in hematocrit should be seen in 7–14 days. Monitor blood pressure before and during therapy because hypertension can result. Monitor for change in neurologic response and headache; both seizures and strokes are possible side effects.
Filgrastim (Neupogen) and pegfilgrastim (Neulasta) These human granulocyte colony-stimulating factor preparations (G-CSF) increase the bone marrow's production of neutrophils.	Administered subcutaneously and intravenously; prepare as directed for IV infusion to prevent its absorption by IV tubing. Single-dose vials only so discard any solution that is not used. Incompatible with many medications; check package insert; do not give within 24 hr before or after chemotherapeutic drugs or their effect may be decreased. Obtain baseline and twice weekly CBC. Monitor for side effects such as bone pain and heart arrhythmias; report fevers and be alert for other signs of infection when neutrophil count is low.
Oprelvekin (Neumega) A hematopoietic growth factor, interleukin-11, that increases platelet count; useful in low platelet count due to chemotherapeutic effects on bone marrow.	Administered subcutaneously. Single-dose vials only, so discard any solution that is not used. Obtain baseline CBC and platelet count; monitor platelets throughout treatment. Monitor for side effects such as edema, fever, CNS changes, tachycardia, respiratory problems, and skin rash. Take daily weights and monitor for fluid retention.

An additional type of biologic therapy is gene therapy, or attempting to replace a faulty gene with one that is normal. Genetic technology is growing rapidly and shows promise for future treatment of cancer and other childhood diseases. This complex field includes research to identify genes that lead to disease, recombinant techniques to enable genetic engineering, and studies of enzymes active in DNA and RNA formation. Nurses need to have enhanced knowledge of this important work as technologies are increasingly applied in cancer treatment (Calzone et al., 2014; Greco et al., 2011).

Bone Marrow and Hematopoietic Stem Cell Transplantation. Bone marrow and hematopoietic stem cell transplantation (HSCT) are used to treat leukemia, neuroblastoma, and some noncancerous conditions such as aplastic anemia. The goal of therapy is to administer a lethal dose of chemotherapy and radiation that will kill the cancer, and then to resupply the body with stem cells either from the child's own bone marrow that was previously removed (autologous transplant) and stored or from a compatible donor (allogeneic transplant). Umbilical cord blood is a potential source of stem cells used for transplant, as are peripheral blood stem cells (obtained from the donor's circulating blood rather than from bone marrow). The donor, whether autologous or allogeneic, can be given growth factors prior to donation to stimulate production of stem cells. An advantage of peripheral stem cells is that they can be easily collected somewhat less painfully and invasively than by the procedure of a bone marrow aspiration.

Transplantation has become the treatment of choice for some cancers when a relapse occurs while the child is receiving another form of cancer therapy and for primary treatment of certain cancers. First, a histocompatible donor must be located. The child then receives intensive chemotherapy, often followed by total body irradiation. Beginning 7 to 10 days before the transplant, this treatment kills all circulating blood cells and bone marrow contents. Following this treatment, the child is intravenously transfused with the donor bone marrow or other source of stem cells. New blood cells usually form within 2 to 8 weeks. (See Chapter 49 for a description of care for the child undergoing transplantation.)

Stem cells that become established in the host child's bone marrow can also be obtained from newborn umbilical cord blood. For some children this has become a better option than waiting for a matching bone marrow donor. Cord blood can be easily collected at birth from a sibling of the ill child because histocompatible matches often occur in siblings, or cord blood banks may offer a match. The umbilical cord blood is then infused into the child undergoing treatment, and the same mechanism occurs as in transplantation of bone marrow—implantation of the stem cells into the child's bone marrow and production of normal blood cells over about 2 to 6 weeks. Advantages of umbilical cord blood are that, unlike bone marrow collection, it is not painful for the donor and does not require anesthesia, there is an opportunity to easily collect samples from many ethnic groups that are underrepresented in bone marrow donor registries, graft-versus-host disease after treatment is less prevalent, and storage of umbilical cord blood for use later in life is possible. A variety of federally funded and private blood banks are available to store and provide umbilical blood.

Complementary Therapies. Many families use **complementary therapies** in treatment of a child's cancer. These approaches to care are also referred to as alternative or unconventional, and may involve nutritional supplements, oral herbal supplements, touch therapy, and mind/body interventions. Little research has been done on complementary therapies, although up to 80% of children with cancer have used at least one such therapeutic approach (Paisley, Kang, Insogna, et al., 2011). Healthcare providers should be aware of these practices, inquire in a nonjudgmental manner about the therapies, and attempt to learn about specific therapies and practices. Although some herbs and nutritional products such as St. John's wort may decrease serum concentration of chemotherapeutic agents, or some may act as hormones in the body, most are not known to negatively affect contemporary medical treatment. The families should be assisted in seeking information and supported in use of their chosen therapies. Eating fruits and vegetables is associated with lower cancer incidence in adults, and some foods such as garlic and oranges may slow cancer growth or enhance medical chemotherapy. Some individuals use herbal supplements to treat cancer; these include cat's claw (bark of a tree root), mistletoe, and shark cartilage. The U.S. Food and Drug Administration has allowed testing of the efficacy of some herbal treatments for cancer. Some herbs can decrease nausea and vomiting, and others can boost the immune system's function. Several cancer drugs such as vincristine and paclitaxel are obtained from plant products.

End-of-Life Care. In spite of modern medical practices and complementary therapies, some children do not survive childhood cancer. In these cases, the focus of health care is to provide comfort and emotional support for the child and family. Too often, healthcare providers feel uncomfortable when a child is expected to die and may withdraw from close contact with the child or family, fail to provide adequate comfort measures, and leave the family without access to needed resources. When recognition of prognosis is delayed, children suffer more and end-of-life care is less integrated. Some symptoms for which children are commonly undertreated include pain, dyspnea, nutrition, elimination, and fatigue. Additionally, care may be required from a wide array of specialists, which can lead to fragmentation of care and lack of integrated palliative approaches.

Care for the dying child can be enhanced by an end-of-life or palliative care team; an integrated plan of care; collaboration among families and healthcare providers; and a focus on the child's developmental level and family needs. Parents state that an advanced care directive that outlines the medical care plans for the child is helpful in preserving the child's quality of life and increases the child's comfort. See Chapter 41 for a detailed description of terminal care for children with terminal disease.

SPECIAL ISSUES IN CHILDHOOD CANCER

Oncologic Emergencies. Oncologic emergencies can be organized into three groups: metabolic, hematologic, and those involving space-occupying lesions. The most common metabolic emergencies include tumor lysis syndrome and septic shock, while common hematologic emergencies include bone marrow suppression, gastrointestinal and central nervous system bleeding, and disseminated intravascular coagulation. The most common emergencies involving space-occupying lesions include brain herniation, spinal cord compression, and superior vena cava compression from a superior mediastinal mass. The next sections describe these and other oncologic emergencies in more detail.

Metabolic Emergencies. Metabolic emergencies result from the lysis (dissolving or decomposing) of tumor cells, a process called *tumor lysis syndrome*. This cell destruction results in hypocalcemia, hyperkalemia, hyperphosphatemia, and hyperuricemia. It is seen most commonly in children with non-Hodgkin lymphoma (especially the subtype Burkitt lymphoma), acute lymphocytic leukemia, and acute myeloid leukemia (Burns, Topoz, & Reynolds, 2014; Kishimoto et al., 2014). (See Table 50–2.) The nurse collects laboratory studies, including CBC, absolute neutrophil count (ANF), serum electrolytes, bicarbonate, uric

TABLE 50–2 Clinical Manifestations and Management of Tumor Lysis Syndrome

ETIOLOGY	CLINICAL MANIFESTATIONS	CLINICAL THERAPY	NURSING IMPLICATIONS
Breakdown of malignant cells releases intracellular components into blood.	Hyperuricemia Hyperkalemia Hyperphosphatemia Hypocalcemia	• Vigorous hydration with 2–4 times maintenance fluid • Correction of electrolyte imbalances • Administration of allopurinol or urate oxidase (Rasburicase) to reduce conversion of metabolic by-products to uric acid?	• Administer fluids, beginning before therapy. • Carefully measure intake and output. • Record daily weight. • Monitor urine specific gravity; it should remain less than 1.010. • Monitor for desired and side effects of drug therapy.
Electrolyte imbalance causes metabolic acidosis and serious abnormalities.	Cardiac arrhythmias Impaired renal function Tetany, neurologic and mental status changes	• ECG monitoring • Medications such as furosemide to facilitate potassium excretion • Dialysis may be needed	• Administer electrolytes and medications. • Urine pH should remain 7.0–7.5. • Perform Trousseau and Chvostek signs for tetany monitoring and assess neurologic function. • Perform mental status examination. • Obtain laboratory specimens as needed.

acid, blood urea nitrogen (BUN) and creatinine, and urinalysis. The emergency can be life threatening, and the family will need ongoing support and explanations about care.

A second type of metabolic emergency is septic shock. During periods of immune suppression, the child is vulnerable to overwhelming infection, resulting in circulatory failure, inadequate tissue perfusion, and hypotension. Septic shock can be fatal (see Chapter 47 for a description of septic shock), so early and aggressive treatment improves outcome. Factors contributing to massive infection include inadequate neutrophil production, abnormal granulocytes (not able to be actively phagocytic), erosions through normal barriers such as blood vessels and mucous membranes, and altered bone marrow production caused by chemotherapy and some forms of radiation. Such infections may manifest with hyperthermia or hypothermia, tachycardia, tachypnea, hypotension, mental changes, and peripheral cyanosis and coolness, and must be vigorously treated with antimicrobial therapy and hydration management.

A third type of metabolic emergency occurs when treatment destroys large amounts of bone, resulting in hypercalcemia (elevated calcium in the serum). Hypercalcemia is most common in children with acute lymphocytic leukemia and rhabdomyosarcoma. Treatment includes hydration and adequate oral phosphate supplement (Demirkaya, Sevinir, Yalcinkaya, et al., 2012; Kolyva, Efthymiadou, Gkentizi, et al., 2014).

Some children develop syndrome of inappropriate antidiuretic hormone (SIADH) and have excessive release of ADH. The resulting decreased urinary output leads to water intoxication. See Chapter 53 for a detailed description of SIADH.

Hematologic Emergencies. Hematologic emergencies result from bone marrow suppression or infiltration of brain and respiratory tissue with high numbers of leukemic blast cells (hyperleukocytosis). Bone marrow suppression results in anemia and thrombocytopenia with resultant hemorrhage. Gastrointestinal and central nervous system bleeding (strokes) are common. Disseminated intravascular coagulation (DIC) occurs in some children and is a life-threatening complication. See Chapter 49 for a thorough description of this condition. Disruption of normal WBC production and resulting hyperleukocytosis can lead to obstruction of small blood vessels throughout the body.

Treatment involves infusion of packed red blood cells for anemia; and platelet transfusion, vitamin K, and fresh frozen plasma for thrombocytopenia and hemorrhage. Hyperviscosity is treated by plasmapheresis, hydroxyurea, and close management of chemotherapy. Respiratory and other vital support is needed (Henry & Sung, 2015; Lewis, Hendrickson, & Moynihan, 2011).

Space-Occupying Lesion. Extensive tumor growth may result in spinal cord compression, increased intracranial pressure, brain herniation, seizures, massive hepatomegaly, and superior vena cava syndrome (obstruction of the superior vena cava by tumor). These emergencies are often caused by neuroblastoma, medulloblastoma, astrocytoma, Hodgkin disease, or lymphoma. After biopsy of the mass, treatment involves radiation therapy, chemotherapy, and corticosteroids.

Psychosocial Needs. The diagnosis of cancer is devastating for families. They cannot believe that their vibrant, young child or adolescent has a potentially life-threatening disease. Families are in a state of crisis when the diagnosis is made, with the first response being one of shock. At the same time that they are in a state of shock about the diagnosis, parents must gather resources to support the child, make treatment decisions, and adjust family life to integrate the needs of the child with cancer. Some families

need to travel a great distance for the child's treatments, and others may have financial constraints that make healthcare costs a major concern. For nearly everyone, parental work schedules as well as arrangements for other children must be adjusted. Most cancer treatment will last for a minimum of several months up to several years, necessitating nearly constant adaptation. Parents, siblings, and extended families should all be included in plans of care.

The child reacts to the diagnosis based on age. Infants and toddlers are unaware of the severity of the disease, but react to a change in routine and to the anxiety of the care providers. Preschoolers are beginning to understand illness; however, they may think they caused their illness and are confused about why the parent cannot make the illness go away. School-age children can understand a diagnosis of cancer and benefit from opportunities to talk about the experience. Adolescents find contact with others who have gone through their experience reassuring and supportive. Nearly all children are hospitalized after diagnosis, and care should include proximity to parents, involvement in self-care appropriate for age, positive relationships with staff, and emotional care. Programs such as group therapy sessions, computer programs about cancer and treatment, and school reintegration all show potential for assisting youth who are adjusting to cancer. Children with cancer are commonly anxious about the treatments and disturbed schedules and routines (National Cancer Institute, 2011d).

Nursing Management
For the Child With Cancer

Nursing Assessment and Diagnosis

HISTORY
During health promotion visits of all children, nurses take into account the importance of a history of cancer in the family. Particularly when more than one person has had cancer, and when young children in the extended family have been affected, complete a family history, or genogram, to isolate cases in the family (see Chapter 3 for examples of genograms). A history of exposure to known carcinogens is also important. Does a parent work in an industry with substances like chemicals or asbestos that might remain on clothing worn home? Was the child treated with radiation or chemotherapy for a previous cancer? Does the child have an identified condition with a high incidence of some type of cancer, such as Down syndrome? Does the child have any recognized congenital anomalies? A number of conditions are more commonly associated with certain types of cancer.

PHYSIOLOGIC ASSESSMENT
When performing any physiologic assessment on children, consider the possible signs and symptoms of cancer. These include anemia, frequent infections, bleeding disorders, loss of weight, fatigue, pain, and changes in mental health and neurologic status. Assessment of children with the most significant types of childhood cancers is presented later in the chapter.

Once cancer has been diagnosed, a thorough physical assessment of all systems is needed to help identify the presence and extent of cancer (see Chapter 33). Systems needing particularly thorough assessments are neurologic, respiratory, cardiac, and gastrointestinal. Assess hydration status and the tumor site if it is visible. Carefully measure height and weight, and compare with prior findings for the child. Observe gait and coordination, as well as any changes in mental status. Evaluate immunization status, pain, nutritional intake, fatigue, infections,

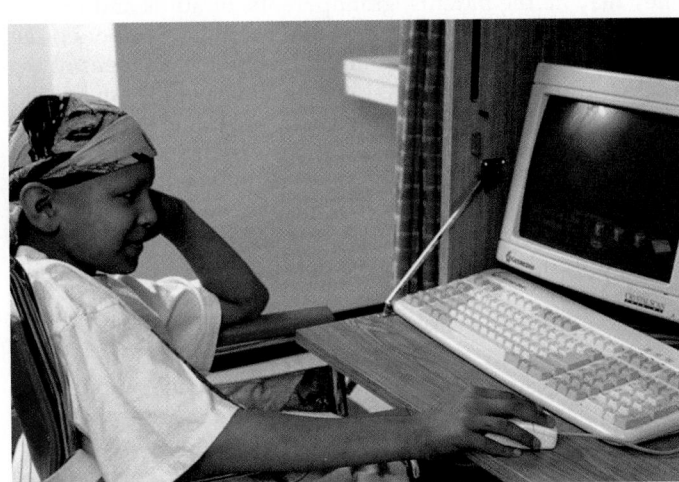

Figure 50–4 One of the most common threats to a child's body image at any age is hair loss induced by chemotherapy. Use of hats can improve self-concept.

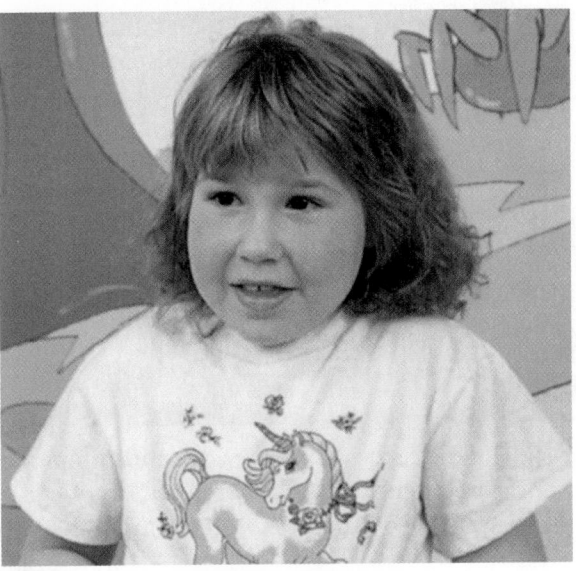

Figure 50–5 The child with cushingoid changes frequently has a rounded face and prominent cheeks.

bruising, shortness of breath, and elimination problems. Periodic laboratory studies will be performed. Tailor assessments to the side effects of particular treatments. For example, the child on chemotherapy is likely to experience a **nadir** (lowest point) of WBC count about 10 days after drug administration so blood counts are needed then.

PSYCHOSOCIAL ASSESSMENT

Assessment of body image, stress and coping abilities, knowledge of the condition and cognitive level, support systems, and developmental level provides data that help determine the appropriate nursing interventions for the child with cancer and the family.

Body Image

Hair loss, surgical scars, and cushingoid changes are three common treatment-induced threats to body image. Most children being treated for cancer experience hair loss (Figure 50–4). Children who have cranial surgery lose hair as part of the surgical preparation. Chemotherapy frequently results in some degree of hair loss. The speed of hair loss is unique to the child and can

be as rapid as overnight or slower, with hair left on the pillow and in the hairbrush.

A second challenge to the child's body image is surgery. The scars of cranial and neck surgery are obvious, as are amputation and limb salvaging. Abdominal surgery for lymphoma is more easily concealed but is still a threat to the child's body image.

A third source of altered body image is the cushingoid features, such as round and flushed face, prominent cheeks, double chin, and generalized obesity (Figure 50–5), that result from the use of corticosteroids. As the child's weight increases, stretch marks similar to those of pregnancy may occur. These stretch marks often remain after the corticosteroids are decreased.

Body image disturbances occur when a child cannot integrate changes and continues to cling to old images despite their inconsistency with reality. Common means for assessing body image are drawings, colored pictures cut out by the child to form a collage, discussion, and observation. See Chapter 39 for further discussion of these and other assessment techniques that can be used with children.

As Children Grow: **Children Need Help in Coping With the Physical Effects of Cancer Treatment**

Children of different ages experience differing threats to body image as a result of cancer treatment. A preschool girl may be most upset at hair loss because she now looks like a boy. For many parents, especially of daughters, the loss of the child's hair can be devastating. Ask the parents and the child what the loss is like for them. Prepare them for the fact that hair loss can be rapid or slow. Find out how they will plan to cope. Some children want the hair cut very short so its loss will not be as traumatic. Offer resources for wigs, hats, or other ideas. Put them in touch with children who have lost hair and with those who have now regrown it.

A school-age child has the most difficult time with changes that interfere with the developmental task of industry. Amputation, which decreases the child's ability to participate in activities such as sports, dancing, and schoolwork, can be a major challenge during the school-age years. Assist children to adapt to new sports when they are able to do so. Partner with schools, coaches, and families to facilitate children's participation in activities they choose.

Teenagers are often most worried about changes like hair loss and cushingoid features, which cause them to look different from peers. Introducing adolescents to others of their own age who are coping with similar conditions can assist them in their developmental tasks.

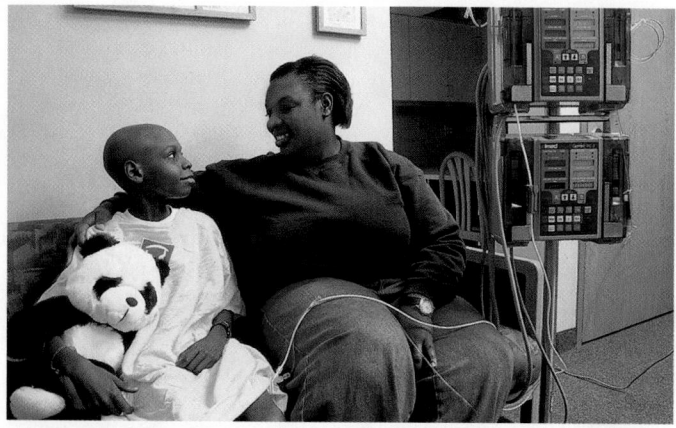

Figure 50–6 The child with cancer depends on parents and family members to provide support. Nurses can assist families and draw on their strengths to help the child.

Stress and Coping

The diagnosis of cancer is a major stressor for both the child and the family. Although each child's prognosis and each family's coping mechanisms are unique, most families deal with the diagnosis in a manner similar to that of other families who have a child with a life-threatening illness (see Chapter 41). Assess the family (and child if old enough) for their understanding and acceptance of the diagnosis. Find out if the family has told the child and siblings about the diagnosis and if they need assistance in deciding how to do this. Assess the level of anxiety during healthcare visits and scheduled treatments (Figure 50–6). Evaluate the family's methods of coping, such as the ability to integrate relaxing and meaningful activities into family life, the use of support systems in the extended family and community, and the ability to alter expectations to take into account the child's health status. Some families demonstrate resilience and the ability to assist the child and all of their members. Other families, however, may be experiencing multiple stresses, making adaptation to the new diagnosis particularly difficult. Concurrent stressors increase the difficulty of coping with childhood cancer. Evaluate the family for stressors such as illness or death of another family member, occupational changes, financial problems, relocation, and change in vacation plans. Evaluate the family's knowledge of the U.S. Family and Medical Leave Act benefits, which enable parents to use sick time, vacation, and leave without pay to care for an ill family member while safeguarding employment.

Knowledge

Anxious people tend to narrow their scope of attention and may read unintended messages into the behaviors of healthcare personnel. Anxiety also limits a person's ability to retain information.

Assess the child's knowledge of cancer and its treatment throughout the treatment period. As the child matures cognitively, reevaluate knowledge. Cancer and its treatment are complex topics. Parents are exposed to information in various forms, including written material, news reports, and Internet websites and resources. Evaluate their knowledge and information sources and provide them with opportunities to ask questions. Evaluate the learning style of the child and family in order to adapt approaches to meet their needs.

Support Systems

Cancer treatment generally occurs over a long time. The extended family is crucial in providing necessary support to the child, parents, and siblings. Identify key people in the family. They may be the parents, grandparents, or aunts and uncles. Support groups for children or other family members often help individuals and the family to meet the challenges of the disease. Thoroughly assess the coping strategies the family uses to meet the various challenges posed by the child's illness. This information helps to predict the success of interventions, such as home care with intravenous medications, and to decide when referrals for other supportive therapies are needed.

The return to school may pose difficulties for the child with cancer or it may be a source of support to be connected again to peers. The child is encouraged to go to school, even if only for half a day per week, to stay connected to peers. Evaluate the school's ability to accept a child who is medically vulnerable into the classroom. Assess whether the other children and teachers have been prepared for the appearance and needs of the child with cancer. Nurses who work in the oncology department of the hospital or clinic can ask if the family would give consent to visit the school, meet with the school nurse, and plan together to meet the child's educational needs. Help the teacher devise a plan to prepare the children, and offer to visit the classroom to explain what the child with cancer is experiencing. Arrangements can be made for tutors to help children keep up with schoolwork if they cannot attend school. An individualized education plan is needed. Parents need information about the legal right to home schooling and a specialized plan since the child is newly ill and they will likely not have been exposed to this in the past.

Assess family resources to identify support systems available to help the family during crises and if a child is expected to die. Extended supports include friends, jobs, insurance coverage, religious affiliations, cultural support systems, and the school system. Parents commonly lose contact with close friends after the diagnosis of cancer in a child. This is an additional stressor for the family. Jobs are often a source of support because coworkers may have gone through the same experience. It may also be comforting for parents to return to their jobs where they can feel a sense of security in tangible accomplishments. However, jobs can also be a source of stress if employers are unsympathetic to the demands of the child's hospitalization and clinic or office visits.

The nurse caring for a child and family in the end-of-life care phase can best support family members by helping them to view the child's unique characteristics, conveying care and concern for the family, and continuing to have close contact with the dying child. Faith-based affiliations can be an important source of support. Evaluate whether such affiliations are meaningful for the family and, if so, plan for visits from the appropriate clergy. In some cultures, spiritual leaders are an important part of the family's support system. Enable a healer to visit the child and conduct a healing ceremony if that will be supportive to the family and child.

DEVELOPMENTAL ASSESSMENT

Developmental assessment of children should be performed regularly during treatment for cancer at times when the child is feeling well so that results are accurate. Assessment of the child's physical and neurologic development helps determine the progress made during treatment and provides a baseline for evaluating the long-term effects of treatment. Children under 6 years of age who have cancer should receive regular developmental assessment with a standardized screening tool (see Chapter 34). A home healthcare nurse can perform such testing, or it can be done by a nurse in the pediatric healthcare home (medical home) who sees the child for a general health supervision visit. Recommend referral to a neuropsychologist for testing early in treatment and if changes in developmental performance are noted. Children who have received cranial radiation and intrathecal chemotherapy need regular scholastic evaluations. Impaired neurocognitive performance may be a long-term effect of treatment. Observe developmental milestones at each contact with the child and refer for further assessment if regression has occurred. Performance in school and engagement in social activities with friends provide important information about expected developmental milestones in older children. If the parents have signed up for a clinical trial (research) treatment for the child, children should also give verbal or written assent when they have the cognitive maturity to do so.

ASSESSMENT FOR IMPACT OF CANCER SURVIVAL

Children with cancer have a variety of common psychologic and physiologic problems regardless of their specific type of cancer. They and their families are dealing with a complex illness that will influence their lives for years. The impact of this experience extends into all areas of function. During the past 20 to 30 years, treatment for childhood cancers has been increasingly successful, and 80% of children with cancer are now expected to have long-term survival. However, the success of new modalities and treatment combinations has created special healthcare needs for many survivors (Landier, Armenian, & Bhatia, 2015; Rueegg et al., 2013) (Figure 50–7).

Healthy People 2020

(C-14) Increase the mental and physical health-related quality of life of cancer survivors

---

Surgery can have many results. Body organs may be removed and manipulated, leading to adhesions, intestinal obstruction, visual impairment, neurologic disruption, and sterility. Removal of the spleen can lead to serious infections. Amputation necessitates the need for prosthetic devices and physical rehabilitation.

Radiation has several long-term effects. It can impair the growth of bones and teeth, leading to conditions such as scoliosis, leg length discrepancy, or poor dental health. Chronic pain can result from skeletal toxicity. Hypothyroidism can be observed in those who have had head and neck radiation. Cardiotoxicity and pulmonary toxicity can result from mediastinal radiation. Delayed puberty and sterility can result from radiation effects to the cranium and spinal regions. Impaired neurocognitive performance may occur as long-term effects of treatment, especially with higher doses of radiation.

Secondary cancers, most commonly solid tumors, occur in some survivors. **Secondary cancers** are also called *second malignant neoplasms (SMNs)*. They occur subsequent to the primary cancer and treatment but are of a different histologic type. Cancers of the central nervous system, skin, breast, bone, and thyroid are examples of secondary neoplasms (Reulen et al., 2011). Most of these cancers can be effectively treated, emphasizing the need for thorough and frequent monitoring of the treated patient with cancer. Other chronic conditions, such as heart failure, congestive heart failure, cognitive dysfunction, and reproductive problems are more common in cancer survivors who are adults than in the general population, whereas cardiovascular risk and insulin resistance may even be more prevalent in child cancer survivors (Steinberger et al., 2012).

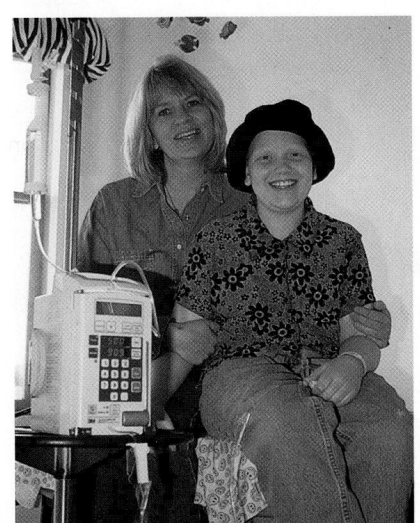
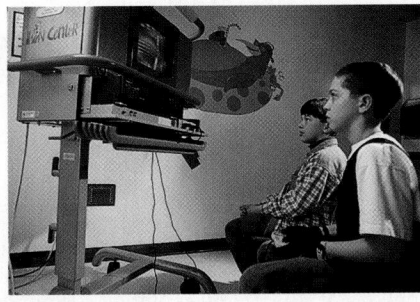
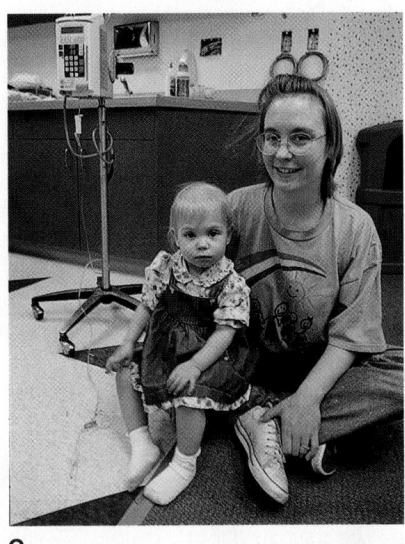

A **B** **C**

Figure 50–7 Survivors of childhood cancer. *A*, Nicole, 11 years old, is undergoing chemotherapy for Ewing sarcoma. Her mother emphasizes, "It's our faith that has gotten us through this. The hardest part is how busy you are coming to treatments all the time. Nicole's younger brother sometimes feels neglected." *B*, According to Jesse, who is 10 years old and waiting for a bone marrow transplant, "The thing that has helped me the most [in dealing with acute lymphoblastic leukemia] is all the mail I got from my friends." His mother adds, "We're just really positive and think that everything will turn out all right." *C*, Cassie, 19 months old, has been diagnosed with neuroblastoma. At this age, it is hard for her to understand what is happening to her. Her mother has stayed with her each time she has come to the hospital, which has helped Cassie adjust to therapy. Her caregivers are confident that she will respond well to her treatment.

Chemotherapy can cause a wide variety of effects, both during its administration and for years afterward (Table 50–3). Cardiomyopathy can occur with some drugs, especially the anthracyclines. Temporary or permanent pulmonary toxicity and renal complications can develop. Neurologic effects of some drugs can lead to hearing loss (e.g., cisplatin and ifosfamide), cataracts, and paraplegia (e.g., intrathecal methotrexate for leukemia). Learning disabilities or change in intelligence quotient (IQ) occurs in some children; infertility may result (Kirchhoff et al., 2011).

TABLE 50–3 Common Side Effects of Chemotherapy

SIDE EFFECT	CLINICAL MANIFESTATIONS	CLINICAL THERAPY
Bone marrow suppression	Evidence of suppression usually appears 7–10 days after administration of chemotherapy; recovery is usually complete within 3–4 weeks.	Blood transfusions are administered when anemia is severe (Hgb less than 7–8 g/dL) or platelets are very low and clinical examination reveals signs and symptoms of anemia or bleeding. Some institutions use a low-microbial diet to decrease the possibility that infectious organisms will colonize the intestine. Septra is used for *Pneumocystis jiroveci* pneumonia (formerly known as *P. carinii*) prophylaxis; additional drugs for antifungal and antibacterial prophylaxis are under investigation. Instruct the family and child about the importance of protecting the body from bruising during periods of mild to moderate thrombocytopenia (platelet count: 5000–20,000/mm^3). Careful hand hygiene is essential. Encourage use of masks if family or staff have nasopharyngeal infections.
Nausea and vomiting	Symptoms may occur immediately or 5–6 hr after administration of chemotherapy and may last 48 hr.	Antiemetics, such as ondansetron (Zofran), granisetron (Kytril), metoclopramide (Reglan), and diphenhydramine (Benadryl), are used to treat this side effect. Teach relaxation techniques, hypnosis, and systematic desensitization (a hypnotic process that progressively reduces reactions to objects that cause strong emotional or physical responses) to help decrease the child's symptoms. Encourage mild exercise and change of diet (eating only easily digestible foods) 12 hr before chemotherapy.
Anorexia and weight loss	May occur at any time.	Hyperalimentation is necessary if dietary changes are unsuccessful in halting the child's weight loss. Pay careful attention to changes in taste that affect food preferences. Referral to a dietitian may be helpful to achieve successful modification of the child's diet.
Oral ulcers	The oral mucositis resulting from chemotherapy usually occurs within 3–4 days and is often a contributing factor in anorexia.	Antifungal agents, such as nystatin or clotrimazole, lessen the possibility of candidal infection. Promote good oral hygiene, use soft foam wand or water irrigation to clean teeth; commercial mouthwashes are not recommended because they contain alcohol and increase drying of the oral cavity; specially formulated pharmacologic mouthwash may promote comfort.
Constipation	Can occur at any time in treatment but becomes more common as therapy progresses and dietary intake and physical activity decrease.	Stool softeners and laxatives are used to treat this side effect (e.g., MiraLAX). Advise parents to increase fluids and fibrous foods in the child's diet.
Pain	Pain can occur at any time and is best understood by subjective explanations of the child.	Acetaminophen, morphine, steroids, and antidepressants may be used to manage pain; nonsteroidal anti-inflammatory drugs are often avoided because of their promotion of bleeding. Careful pain assessment is important; the location of the pain may provide a clue to its cause, for example, metastasis to the skull, infiltration of joints, or damage to soft tissue; pain associated with chemotherapy may also be related to oral mucositis, myalgia, or tumor embolization; painful polyneuropathy can follow treatment with vincristine or cisplatin. Acetaminophen for pain can mask the presence of fever, which signals infection; careful and complete physical assessment is needed to identify infection. Pharmacologic, nonhypnotic (deep breathing, self-control), and hypnotic methods of pain control may be used; the nonpharmacologic methods often prove helpful to children with pain from multiple etiologies.

The diagnosis and stress of treatment, along with the risk of recurrence, are significant stressors for the child with cancer. Families may find it difficult to obtain full insurance coverage for the child who has had a prior cancer. Employment can be a potential problem for cancer survivors if employers have concerns about the earlier cancer diagnosis. Most people with cancer report fear of recurrence of the disease, which is a stressor. Some children report decreased quality of life (QOL) and emotional distress (Rueegg et al., 2013; Winick, 2011). Conversely, hopefulness and the sense of having an added purpose in life can be positive outcomes for many cancer survivors. Some meet with others who have a recent diagnosis, or work on fund-raising events that financially support cancer research. Survivorship services and care plans promote positive health outcomes (Eshelman-Kent et al., 2011).

Nurses are involved with families when a diagnosis of cancer is made, during the therapy process, and in the years that follow. For a child who survives cancer, ongoing care is essential. Evaluate the child regularly with thorough physical, psychosocial, developmental, and cognitive assessments. Carefully monitor all body systems (e.g., cardiovascular; respiratory; musculoskeletal; eye, ear, nose, and throat; genitourinary). Record height and weight, growth patterns, and nutritional patterns. Ask about the child's interactions with peers and performance at school. Children who have received cranial radiation and intrathecal chemotherapy need regular scholastic evaluations. Be alert for signs and symptoms that could indicate a secondary tumor. Periodic laboratory studies will be performed. Ask the parents about insurance coverage and other financial difficulties during ongoing care.

Plan care to assist the family to manage any long-term effects of cancer treatment. This may involve physical rehabilitation, support related to visual impairment, or treatment for cardiac or musculoskeletal abnormalities. Provide resources for information and support. Facilitate periodic evaluations in a healthcare agency so that serious outcomes of treatment can be identified early.

The accompanying *Nursing Care Plans* include several diagnoses that may be appropriate for the child with cancer who is receiving care in the hospital or at home. Among the many other diagnoses that may be appropriate for a child with cancer are the following (NANDA-I © 2014):

- *Diarrhea* related to radiation therapy and toxins
- *Urinary Elimination, Impaired*, related to chemotherapy
- *Tissue Integrity, Impaired*, related to effects of chemotherapy and radiation therapy on oral mucosa
- *Skin Integrity, Impaired*, related to altered nutritional state, effects of medication, radiation, and immobilization
- *Coping, Ineffective*, related to situational crisis of chronic and acute illness
- *Caregiver Role Strain* related to anxiety and disruption in family roles and patterns
- *Sleep Pattern, Disturbed*, related to biochemical agents, anxiety, and unfamiliar surroundings
- *Body Image, Disturbed*, related to chronic illness and treatments
- *Knowledge, Deficient (Child or Parents)*, related to lack of exposure to disease or treatments
- *Grieving* related to actual or potential loss

Nursing Care Plan: Hospital Care of the Child With Cancer

1. Nursing Diagnosis: *Pain, Acute*, **related to tissue injury (NANDA-I © 2014)**

GOAL: The child will report reduced pain that is manageable.

INTERVENTION	RATIONALE
• Give analgesics as ordered.	• Adequate medications can reduce pain.
• Teach relaxation techniques, deep breathing, and distraction.	• Nonpharmacologic methods work with the medication to reduce pain.
• Insert pain management techniques appropriate for developmental age (see Chapter 40).	• Developmental level determines the pain assessment method that should be used, as well as the most appropriate intervention methods, from rocking, to distraction, to providing information.

EXPECTED OUTCOME: Child will experience pain reduced to the level that allows the child to interact appropriately and gain rest.

2. Nursing Diagnosis: *Nutrition, Imbalanced: Less than Body Requirements*, **related to inability to ingest or digest food or absorb nutrients (NANDA-I © 2014)**

GOAL: The child will maintain adequate nutritional intake. The child will experience reduced effects of chemotherapy (i.e., nausea and vomiting).

INTERVENTION	RATIONALE
• Offer small feedings. Encourage favorite foods. Refer to dietitian for special meals. Weigh daily.	• Measures can increase caloric intake. Taste changes and mouth sores alter desire for food.
• Teach the child distraction and relaxation techniques. Give antiemetics according to orders.	• Pharmacologic and nonpharmacologic methods are effective in helping to reduce nausea.

EXPECTED OUTCOME: Child will maintain admission weight or preillness weight. The child will have minimal side effects of nausea and vomiting.

(continued)

Nursing Care Plan: Hospital Care of the Child With Cancer (*continued*)

3. Nursing Diagnosis: *Fluid Volume: Excess or Deficient*, related to medications (NANDA-I © 2014)

GOAL: The child will be adequately hydrated.

INTERVENTION	RATIONALE
• Record all intake and output. Monitor intravenous rate and solution as appropriate. Monitor output from urine and other output routes such as vomiting or diarrhea.	• Some drugs (e.g., cyclophosphamide) necessitate a high level of fluid intake to prevent complications. Careful balance of intake and monitoring of output are required.
• Test specific gravity of urine daily.	• Renal function may be affected by chemotherapy.

EXPECTED OUTCOME: Child will demonstrate adequate hydration. Mucous membranes will be hydrated. Specific gravity will remain within normal range.

4. Nursing Diagnosis: *Infection, Risk for,* related to immunosuppression, invasive procedures, malnutrition, or pharmaceutical agents (NANDA-I © 2014)

GOAL: The child will remain free of infection.

INTERVENTION	RATIONALE
• Wash hands often. Maintain in isolation if needed.	• Hand hygiene is effective to reduce organisms. Transmission-based precautions may be needed to safeguard child.
• Monitor temperature. Use a noninvasive method such as tympanic; report method used when recording temperature. Report elevation to healthcare provider.	• Elevated temperature is a sign of infection. Children with oral or intestinal mucositis should not have temperature taken in these mucous cavities since it may cause increased irritation.

EXPECTED OUTCOME: Child will remain infection-free.

GOAL: The child will return to normal, uninfected state.

INTERVENTION	RATIONALE
• Administer intravenous antibiotics as ordered. Monitor temperature. Use cooling mattress as ordered. Report elevations over 38°C (101°F) to healthcare provider.	• Multiple antibiotics are needed to deal with bacterial and fungal infections during neutropenia. Blood cultures may be taken to identify organism.

EXPECTED OUTCOME: The child with an infection will be effectively treated.

5. Nursing Diagnosis: *Coping, Ineffective,* related to situational crisis (NANDA-I © 2014)

GOAL: The child will demonstrate normal adaptive coping methods.

INTERVENTION	RATIONALE
• Encourage drawings and other therapeutic play for expression of feelings. Allow for expression of angry feelings, such as hitting dolls and throwing sponge balls. Discuss how to behave during treatments.	• Expression of feelings helps identify avoidance coping for further intervention. Play is a normal way for the child to express self and ideas. Misinterpretations can be corrected. Knowledge of appropriate and helpful behaviors supports self-esteem.

EXPECTED OUTCOME: Child will continue to use usual coping strategies expected for developmental stage.

Planning and Implementation

Nurses have many resources to assist in planning and implementing nursing care for the child with cancer. Oncology Nursing Society and the Association of Pediatric Hematology and Oncology Nurses are examples of organizations helpful to nurses. The nursing care of children newly diagnosed with cancer and their families includes immediate physiologic and psychologic support, along with anticipatory guidance about imminent and future medical interventions. Assist and support the family as they make decisions about types of treatment that are appropriate for the child.

Nursing care of the hospitalized child with cancer and the child receiving ongoing therapy at home is summarized in the accompanying *Nursing Care Plans*. These care plans are designed for the child who has progressed beyond cancer diagnosis and is receiving chemotherapy.

Physiologic care of the hospitalized child focuses on providing support during treatment. This includes ensuring optimal nutritional intake, administering medications, managing the multiple side effects of chemotherapy and radiation, ensuring adequate hydration, preventing infection, and managing pain during diagnostic procedures and treatment.

Nursing Care Plan: Home Care of the Child With Cancer

1. Nursing Diagnosis: *Health Management, Family, Ineffective,* related to complex chemotherapeutic therapy (NANDA-I © 2014)

GOAL: The child will comply with oral medication regimen.

INTERVENTION	RATIONALE
• Educate parents and child about the importance of taking medication as prescribed.	• Understanding can assist parents and child in placing importance on medication intake.
• Set up calendar with dates, times, and medications clearly labeled.	• Visual reminders can help them recall instructions.
• Reward the child for taking medications.	• Reinforcing desired behaviors through rewards is effective with children.

EXPECTED OUTCOME: Child will take all medications according to prescription.

2. Nursing Diagnosis: *Development: Delayed, Risk for,* related to serious illness (NANDA-I © 2014)

GOAL: The child will demonstrate normal physical, emotional, and cognitive development.

INTERVENTION	RATIONALE
• Encourage play appropriate to age.	• Normal activities support self-esteem and self-knowledge.
• Encourage the child to attend school when able to do so. Arrange for tutors at home when unable to attend.	• School is the work of the child and promotes cognitive and social growth.
• Encourage seeing peers when unable to attend school.	• Peer contacts help the child in normal developmental tasks.
• Work with teachers to support reentry to school. Use puppets, videotape, and discussion with classmates.	• Classmates need to understand what has happened to their friend without asking the child directly.

EXPECTED OUTCOME: Child will continue to develop physically, emotionally, and cognitively at a normal pace.

3. Nursing Diagnosis: *Fatigue* related to disease state (NANDA-I © 2014)

GOAL: The child will maintain energy levels necessary for normal activities.

INTERVENTION	RATIONALE
• Problem solve ways to save energy for play and school.	• The child and parents are assisted to see school and play as important.
• Plan with child for quiet activities during low-energy times.	• The child is empowered to select and plan own activities.

EXPECTED OUTCOME: Child will plan use of time effectively to maintain energy for school and play. The child conserves energy during times of increased fatigue.

ENSURE OPTIMAL NUTRITIONAL INTAKE

The high metabolic rate of cancer growth depletes the child's nutritional stores. In addition, the catabolic effect of chemotherapy and radiation on normal cells necessitates additional cellular replacement. The child needs increased nutritional intake at a time when nausea and vomiting are occurring as drug side effects, and when decreased activity, treatment protocols, and general health status result in diminished appetite. This often leads to extreme concern on the part of parents, and they may focus excessive attention on the child's intake.

Administer antiemetic drugs to lessen nausea from chemotherapy. Integrate feeding methods and foods that the family and the child find most helpful for ensuring adequate intake. Allow the family to bring the child's favorite foods to the hospital. Ask the family what treatments they use to decrease the child's nausea and vomiting. Perform 24-hour dietary recalls to assess the child's intake, and evaluate height and weight regularly. Special nutritional products may be given orally, nasogastric or nasoduodenal tube feedings may be given, or total parenteral nutrition may be necessary.

ADMINISTER MEDICATIONS

An important intervention of the oncology nurse is administering medications safely. Most chemotherapeutic drugs are prescribed and calculated as dose per meter squared (dose/m²), with m² being calculated from the child's height and weight. (See the *Clinical Skills Manual* SKILLS .)

A number of chemotherapeutic drugs are commonly used in combinations. These drugs are prepared with special techniques under laminar flow devices to minimize potential toxic effects on healthcare providers. Gloves and other hazardous drug protocols are used. The Occupational Safety and Health Administration (OSHA) publishes an instruction manual entitled *Controlling Occupational Exposure to Hazardous Drugs* that outlines general guidelines, protective equipment, and procedures. Care must be taken to protect the patient as well; the

TEACHING HIGHLIGHTS	Nutrition and the Child With Cancer

Because of the effects of cancer and chemotherapy or other treatment, the child often has a poor appetite. Mucosal sores lead to difficulty chewing and swallowing. Parents can enhance the nutritional intake of the child in a variety of ways:

- Provide frequent small feedings rather than three meals daily.
- Integrate the child's favorite foods and the cultural foods common to the family into daily menus.
- Have nutritious snacks available for times when the child feels like eating.
- Sprinkle dried milk on top of cereals and other foods.
- Smooth, soft foods are usually preferred. Avoid acidic or spicy foods. Milkshakes with added peanut butter, puddings, and soft casseroles may be well tolerated. Try a variety of liquid protein-calorie supplements to find those the child likes.
- Avoid making food an area for disagreement. Do not force foods but rather make them readily available.
- If therapy is causing the child to vomit, do not encourage food at that time. The child may develop food aversions to foods that are vomited.
- Administer antiemetics as ordered during therapy since they can prevent nausea and vomiting.
- Report weight loss and increased fatigue.
- Bring the child in for scheduled health visits so growth, development, and effects of therapy can be monitored.
- Some children need a temporary feeding tube to ensure adequate nutrition. Feedings at night can often increase intake and promote health. Occasionally, a central line is inserted to provide total parenteral nutrition.
- Supplements and tube feedings will usually be covered by insurance if the healthcare provider writes an order for them.

nurse should avoid **extravasation** of intravenous drugs (leakage into the soft tissue around the infusion site) because permanent tissue damage can result.

In addition to chemotherapeutic drugs, the nurse administers other medications, such as antiemetics to control nausea, vitamin supplements, and antibiotics. Antiemetics such as ondansetron are given prophylactically when a cancer agent is administered that has known emetic effects. Ask parents about complementary therapy and medications they are obtaining from other sources and using at home. All medications must be safely administered and the child should be monitored for side effects. **Polypharmacy** (the use of several drugs at one time to treat multiple health conditions) can lead to multiple side effects and can challenge the body's ability to metabolize and excrete drugs.

Some children receive fluids and medications at home via central lines or by intramuscular or subcutaneous injection. Consider referral to home healthcare infusion agencies for monitoring of these treatments and provision of supplies for home use.

MANAGE TREATMENT OF SIDE EFFECTS

All cancer treatments affect some normal body cells as well as cancer cells, causing a wide variety of side effects. Know all side effects of specific drugs administered and monitor for them. A frequent occurrence is **myelosuppression**, or suppression of blood cell production in the bone marrow. Be alert for signs of a decreased white blood cell count, such as infections. **Neutropenia** is present when the absolute neutrophil count is less than 500 cells/mm³ or if between 500 and 1000 cells/mm³ when chemotherapy is being given and falling levels are anticipated. At these levels, children will be given a broad-spectrum antibiotic; granulocyte colony-stimulating factor (G-CSF) may be given (see *Medications Used During Cancer Treatment: Colony-Stimulating Factors*). Take the child's temperature, isolate the child from others with infections, and perform serum laboratory studies as ordered. Although an elevated temperature generally indicates infection, in a child with immunosuppression, the temperature may be low even in overwhelming infection. A colony-stimulating factor for white cell production may be administered if necessary. A treatment known as *leucovorin rescue* is used in conjunction with high-dose methotrexate chemotherapy. Leucovorin (citrovorum factor) is a form of folic acid that helps to protect normal cells from

the destructive action of methotrexate. It is started within 36 hours of methotrexate administration and is given along with hydration therapy (Cohen & Wolff, 2013).

Protect the child from bruises and be alert for hemorrhage or signs of bleeding such as petechiae or the presence of blood in vomit and urine. These are all effects of **thrombocytopenia**, or decreased platelets. When thrombocytopenia occurs, minimize needlesticks and other intrusive procedures. Be ready to deal with nosebleeds and watch for bleeding gums. Report any bleeding episodes to the oncology specialist. Be sure parents know that the child should avoid contact sports or other rough activities and that any healthcare provider, such as a dentist, should be informed of the child's treatment and condition. Infusions to increase platelets are sometimes administered.

Inadequate red blood cell production can result in anemia. Encourage the child to eat iron-rich foods, and administer nutritional supplements as needed. Blood transfusions are sometimes needed to treat severe anemia.

Chemotherapy affects all rapidly growing cells in the body, but especially those of the mucous membranes. Provide good oral hygiene with a soft toothbrush, foam wand, or water irrigation device. Report oral breakdown promptly. See *Teaching Highlights: Oral Care* for common techniques to manage oral hygiene. Be alert for blood in vomit and stool or dark-colored stools, all of which can indicate bleeding in the gastrointestinal tract. Blood in the urine may also occur. Know all side effects of specific drugs administered and monitor for them. Some side effects are late and may be seen after therapy is completed. Emphasize importance of all follow-up visits scheduled in the future for monitoring of late effects.

Radiation can cause burns to the skin. Examine the skin daily during hospitalization or weekly when making home visits. Leave the marks on the skin that outline the radiation target area. Avoid use of lotions, powders, and soaps on the target skin area. Some children may need to be anesthetized to ensure correct positioning for radiation; postanesthesia care will then be needed.

ENSURE ADEQUATE HYDRATION

Hydration management can be a challenge because the child may not be thirsty but is excreting large numbers of cell fragments and other substances as a result of treatment. Offer frequent

Since cancer treatment and poor nutritional status can adversely affect the oral status of children, families need help to plan and carry out prophylactic and treatment measures. Children continue to lose teeth, have new teeth erupt, and require nutrients to help in building teeth not yet erupted even during cancer treatment. Some suggestions are:

- Provide a visit to the dentist early in treatment for assessment, treatment of dental disease, and establishment of a prevention plan.
- Brush teeth twice daily with a soft bristle brush and rinse with water.
- When granulocyte counts fall below 500/mm^3 or platelets fall below 40,000/mm^3, toothettes or gauze can be used to clean the teeth. Avoiding brushes will help to prevent bleeding and infection.
- Toothpaste can be used unless it causes discomfort.
- Medications may be used to prevent infection. They may include antibacterial mouthwash, nystatin, or fluconazole. Continue oral fluoride if it is not present in the drinking water.
- If bleeding, infection, or other oral care needs emerge, consult with the dentist and pediatric oncologist to develop a treatment plan.

small amounts of fluid. Include frozen ice pops or other fluid-containing foods such as Jell-O. Measure intake and output. To ensure adequate excretion, a number of chemotherapeutic drugs are given with intravenous fluids. It is important to administer fluids as ordered and ensure that the recommended urinary output excretion rate is maintained after drug administration.

PREVENT AND TREAT INFECTION

Children with cancer have an altered immune system, both from the disease and from the effects of immunosuppressant drugs, and must be kept away from persons with known infections. Teach parents to avoid taking the child to places that attract large gatherings of people, such as department stores, once the child returns home. Teach administration of any drugs being used to prevent infection such as pentamidine or sulfa preparations for *Pneumocystis* pneumonia prophylaxis. Emphasize the need to report any exposure to contagious diseases, especially chickenpox. Some drugs may mask signs of infection, so be alert for any signs of mild infection. Fever, malaise, and mild respiratory infection must all be reported promptly (see *Teaching Highlights: Reportable Events for Children Receiving Chemotherapy*). Keep the child's immunization record so immunizations that have not been given yet can be administered in regular clinic visits after therapy is complete,

using Centers for Disease Control and Prevention (CDC) recommendations for timing after treatment. Follow recommendations for the immunization of children with cancer as published by the CDC and the American Academy of Pediatrics (AAP). Usually, no immunizations are given to the child until 6 months after completing chemotherapy.

Management of infections is critical. Children are often hospitalized and central lines are used for antibiotic administration. Blood cultures and cultures of infected body parts help to establish the causative organisms. Because of lowered immune status, unusual agents are sometimes identified. Administer medication treatment on time and as ordered. Ensure standard precautions and transmission-based precautions are followed. Temperature and vital signs are taken and all body systems are assessed at admission and at least every 4 hours.

MANAGE PAIN

The child with cancer may experience pain from the disease itself and from the medical interventions, such as lumbar puncture, bone marrow aspiration, and frequent intravenous infusions and blood draws. Use all possible pain management techniques to keep the child comfortable because this encourages cooperation throughout the long treatment period.

Parents require verbal and written instructions about signs and symptoms to report to the child's oncologist while the child is receiving chemotherapy. Have parents report the following events to the child's oncologist if they occur while the child is receiving chemotherapy:

- Temperature above 38°C (101°F)
- Any bleeding, such as nosebleeds, blood in stool or urine, petechiae, bruising
- Pain or discomfort with urination or defecation
- Sores in the mouth
- Vomiting or diarrhea
- Persistent pain anywhere, including headache
- Signs of infection, such as cough, fever, runny nose, tugging at ears
- Signs of infection in central lines, such as redness, drainage, or tenderness
- Exposure to communicable diseases, especially varicella (chickenpox)

Parents should also inform dentists and other healthcare providers that the child is receiving chemotherapy prior to procedures. Prophylactic antibiotics should be given before and after dental care.

Source: Adapted from Bindler, R. M., & Howry, L. B. (2005). *Pediatric drug guide*. Upper Saddle River, NJ: Prentice Hall.

Whenever possible, include the parents in comforting the child after painful procedures. (See Chapter 40 for suggestions on methods of pain management.) Nurses must examine research on effective pain management for children and integrate findings into practice (Fielding, Sanford, & Davis, 2013).

Sedation for diagnostic and therapeutic procedures (see Chapter 40) may be used for pain management. Administer sedation as ordered for young children who are undergoing lumbar punctures, radiation, and other procedures, and monitor them after the procedure. Coordinate other painful or intrusive tests so they can be done while the child is sedated for radiation.

Topical anesthetics such as eutectic mixture of local anesthetic (EMLA) cream may be used to numb the skin before an intravenous start, lumbar puncture, or bone marrow aspiration. Do not use EMLA on infants who are a gestational age of less than 37 weeks. Doses are individualized for infants and young children; follow guidelines for drug administration. For all infants, be certain that parents realize the importance of limiting the area and duration as ordered and to keep the cream in a safe place to avoid ingestion by any children. Other pain-prevention measures include fast-acting sprays, intradermal injection of anesthesia with lidocaine, iontophoresis (local anesthetic and electrical current), and sedation. Follow sedation monitoring protocols. (See the *Clinical Skills Manual* SKILLS.) Additional pain management techniques such as relaxation training and hypnosis may be beneficial. Having parents or other support persons present is helpful to most children.

PROVIDE PSYCHOSOCIAL SUPPORT

A diagnosis of cancer brings with it many emotions for the family. Initially, parents experience shock and anger. They need basic information about the disease and the purpose of the tests that will be performed. Instructions often need to be repeated as parents may not process information the first time it is presented because of their increased stress levels. Help the parents plan how and when to tell the child the diagnosis. What the child needs to know is based on the child's developmental level and understanding.

Once family members have progressed from their initial state of shock about the diagnosis, they need to learn more about the disease. They may be interested in the pathophysiology, treatment, and expected outcome or the prognosis. Clarify their understanding of these areas and ask what questions they have. Provide verbal explanations and written material. Parents may talk with friends, purchase books, or search the Internet for information. Find out where they are getting information and provide additional resources when appropriate. Correct misconceptions and misinformation.

The family needs many strategies to deal with the challenge of long-term treatment for cancer. As the child experiences remissions and exacerbations or complications, the family feels alternately hopeful and discouraged. Identify the family's support systems and intervene as needed to enhance these systems. Facilitate contact with extended family members who might be of help, religious or spiritual connections, social service agencies, and other resources such as Internet and parent support groups. For parents who are concerned about job obligations and financial concerns, help them identify sources of financial assistance, respite from child care, and ways to take time for themselves.

Consider the impact on siblings when a child is being treated for cancer. They may alternately resent and feel guilty for the sibling's illness. They may not understand the treatments or disease. School progress may be slowed and teachers may not be aware of the sibling's stress. (See *Evidence-Based Practice: Cancer, Sleep, and Fatigue*.)

Children undergoing treatment for cancer need support appropriate to their developmental stage and cognitive level. (See Chapters 31 and 39 for developmental levels and effective support strategies for children of different ages.) Younger children primarily need support during painful procedures

---

EVIDENCED-BASED PRACTICE | Cancer, Sleep, and Fatigue

Clinical Question

Inadequate amounts and quality of sleep are common problems among youth. Busy schedules and use of screen technologies contribute to poor sleep habits. Daytime sleepiness and other outcomes can result (Bartel, Gradisar, & Williamson, 2014). The child or adolescent with cancer is even more likely to have disturbed sleep, due to the cancer itself, the treatment protocols, and associated symptoms. What assessments and interventions should the nurse implement to understand sleep needs in the child with cancer?

The Evidence

A systematic review by nurses examined the measurement of sleep in adolescents with cancer by measures such as questionnaires, sleep diaries, and actigraphy (a watchlike device that measures movement and accurately displays sleep time). Primary reasons for disturbed sleep in cancer treatment included pain, frequent awakenings or fragmented sleep, and symptoms such as nausea (Erickson et al., 2011). Both mothers and children with acute lymphoblastic leukemia had disturbed sleep patterns, difficulty falling asleep, and fatigue (Matthews, Neu, Cook, et al., 2014).

Sleep disturbance may even continue after cancer treatment is completed because of brain changes that resulted from a tumor, or from treatment such as radiation or chemotherapy. In over 1400 survivors of childhood cancer, fatigue and poor sleep quality were identified (Clanton et al., 2011).

Best Practice

Cancer interfaces with normal developmental progression in several ways, one of which is sleep. Question sleep patterns at each oncology visit, provide suggestions for sleep hygiene, and refer the child and parents for sleep intervention as needed. Inquire about daytime sleepiness and fatigue. Have the family remove televisions and cell phones from the youth's bedroom, arrange for rest periods each day, and maintain routines that enable sleep.

Clinical Reasoning

Plan a series of questions to ask children and teens with cancer about the amount of sleep obtained on weekdays and weekends, patterns of sleep, and any changes in sleep since the cancer was diagnosed. Inquire about how the disease and its treatment have influenced sleep in the parents. What sleep hygiene measures can assist in acquiring needed sleep time and quality?

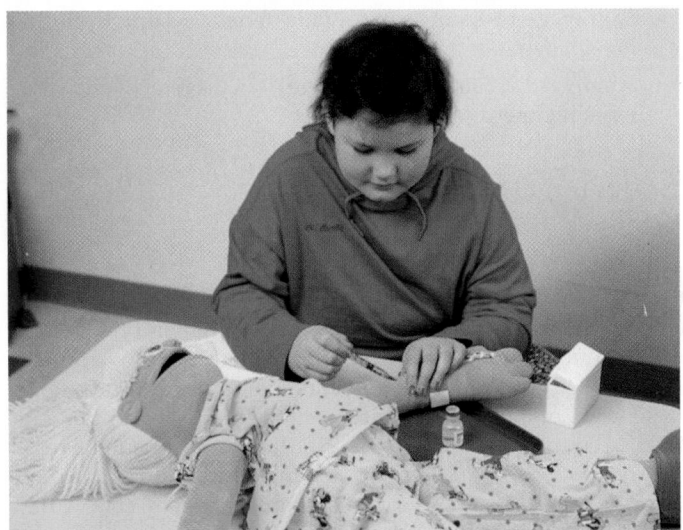

Figure 50–8 **A child in a pediatric oncology clinic giving injections to a doll. This type of play therapy helps the child deal with fear, thus lowering her stress level.**

and separation from parents. Older children need intervention strategies to help work through feelings about treatments (Figure 50–8). A major developmental task of adolescence is to attain independence and control, but cancer often interferes with adolescents' ability to achieve this task. Therefore, plan nursing strategies that empower adolescents as much as possible. Introduce them to other teens with similar diagnoses and allow them to make decisions and choices independent of parents when possible. An adolescent can decide which type of medication port would be best (e.g., an implantable port under the skin or a venous access device with tubing outside the body). Making this choice enables the teen to feel more in control of the disease and treatment.

Talk with the child's teachers before the return to school after treatment to explain the child's condition. Ask them to notify the family immediately of diseases or infections in other children so the child with cancer treatment who is immunocompromised can be kept home. Arrange for tutors if necessary to assist the child with schoolwork during hospitalization and home care. Explore the option of summer camp for children with cancer. The Make-A-Wish Foundation strives to make dreams come true for ill children by sponsoring them for a desired activity or outing. Refer the child to this foundation if appropriate.

The siblings of a child who has cancer may grieve over the ill brother or sister and may feel sad and depressed. Inquire about what they know about the child's condition and their reactions or behavior changes. Ask the parents if the siblings are demonstrating symptoms such as depression, behavioral changes, or decrease in school performance and suggest interventions as appropriate. Find out who is caring for siblings and whether their teachers have been informed about the family situation. Invite them to play therapy sessions and recreational activities with the ill child. They may benefit from speaking with a school counselor or can be referred to a support group for siblings of children with cancer. Some cancer summer camps welcome siblings as well as children with cancer.

Chapter 41 offers strategies to help the family of a child with cancer cope with the stressor of a life-threatening illness. For some types of cancer, the child may experience a remission with treatment, but a recurrence of disease later as cancer cells

grow again. The family may become angry or depressed about the relapse. Repeated treatments challenge the family's support systems. Waiting for the outcome of diagnostic tests can be an especially challenging time. Provide information as soon as possible. If the child's illness progresses, refer the family to hospice to help them care for the terminally ill child and work through the grieving process. Explore cancer support groups and share this information with families.

DISCHARGE PLANNING AND HOME CARE TEACHING

Preparation for home care centers on creating a normal environment while supporting the child's physiologic and psychosocial responses to the cancer and treatments. Education is the primary focus of discharge planning. Teach the parents how to ensure adequate nutritional intake, to be alert for signs of infection, to protect the child from exposure to communicable diseases during times of neutropenia, to administer medications at home, and to handle vomiting and pain. Help the parents and child deal with any obstacles to normal development and functioning. Teach the parents and family about symptoms that need to be treated immediately.

Home management of a vascular access device or central line, such as a Broviac catheter, initially challenges parents (Figure 50–9). An implanted port, which allows the child freedom to swim and engage in other activities, may be used. Parents will need information about whatever device the child has received. Demonstrate details about cleaning the site, instilling heparin in the line or reservoir, and other needed care. After teaching the parents, observe them performing the procedure before the child is discharged.

Emphasize the need for the child and family to have fun and be as normal as possible. Play distracts the child and is essential in reducing fears. Children, parents, and siblings often benefit from participation in cancer support groups and cancer

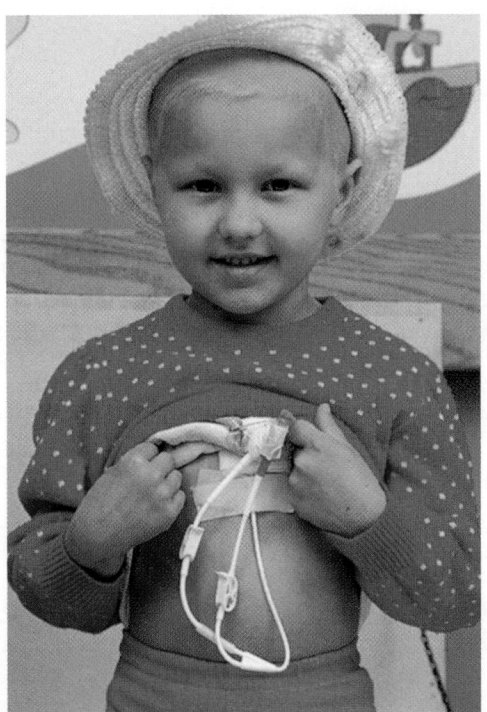

Figure 50–9 **Comfort and convenience. A vascular access device allows chemotherapeutic agents to be administered without the need for repeated "sticks" to the child.**

summer camps. These activities create additional support systems, build the child's self-esteem, and enhance coping skills through role modeling. (See *Teaching Highlights: Cancer Therapy* earlier in this chapter.)

Make home visits to evaluate the family's strengths and needs in the home setting. Be sure that the family has adequate support from hospice and other end-of-life services when a child's condition is terminal.

Most children are treated for cancer over a period of 2 to 3 years. Since normal developmental stages progress during this time, health promotion and health maintenance visits should still occur. Some usual care may have to be altered, but many of the same developmental concerns of all children should be addressed. Help parents to view the child as a "normal" child who is ill for a period of time, but still needs to have limits set on behavior, to develop healthy lifestyles, and to have environmental stimulation to learn to talk, read, or perform motor and cognitive tasks.

Evaluation

Expected outcomes of nursing care for the child with cancer relate to the specific disease, treatments, and responses. Some examples of outcomes include the following:

- The child demonstrates adequate intake to promote normal growth.
- Hydration is adequate to support body processes and ensure drug and cancer cell product elimination.
- Treatment side effects are promptly identified.
- Pain is managed to a level of comfort satisfactory to child and family.

- Family uses resources to provide necessary support during hospitalizations and treatments.
- Family demonstrates knowledge of management and treatment regimens.

Solid Tumors

Brain Tumors

Central nervous system (CNS) or brain tumors are the most commonly occurring solid tumors in children and the second most common malignancy, after leukemia. Each year approximately 1300 children under 5 years of age and 2200 youth up to 20 years of age are diagnosed with tumors of the brain and CNS, accounting for one in five childhood cancers; the overall survival rate is 70% ("Brain Tumor Incidence," 2011; Kuttesch, Rush, & Ater, 2011; McLendon, Adekunle, Rajaram, et al., 2011).

ETIOLOGY AND PATHOPHYSIOLOGY

The cause of most brain tumors is unknown. About 5% to 10% of brain tumors are genetic in origin. Exposure to radiation is a known risk factor, such as CNS radiation used for treatment of some other cancers. There is a higher incidence in children than adults with certain other cancers or diseases such as retinoblastoma, renal tumors, neurofibromatosis, tuberous sclerosis, or endocrine syndromes (Faria, Rutka, Smith, et al., 2011; Pollack & Jakacki, 2011).

Brain tumors in children usually occur below the roof of the cerebellum and involve the cerebellum, midbrain, and brainstem (see *Pathophysiology Illustrated: Brain Tumors*). In contrast, brain tumors in adults are usually located above the areas between the cerebrum and cerebellum.

Pathophysiology Illustrated: **Brain Tumors**

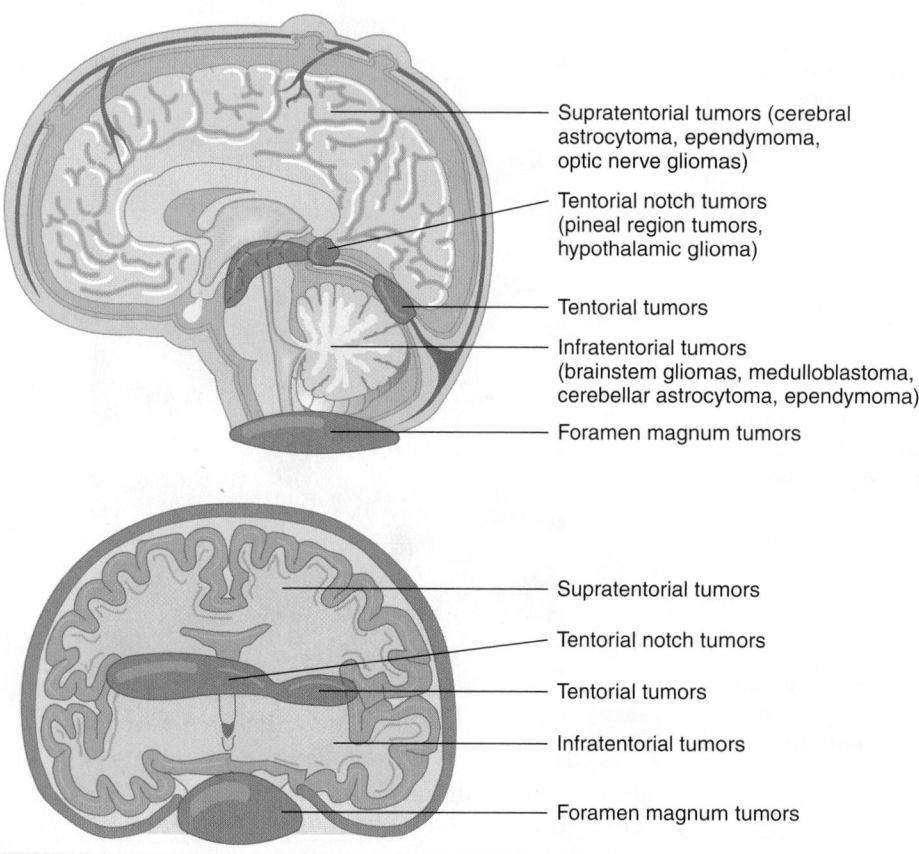

Supratentorial tumors (cerebral astrocytoma, ependymoma, optic nerve gliomas)

Tentorial notch tumors (pineal region tumors, hypothalamic glioma)

Tentorial tumors

Infratentorial tumors (brainstem gliomas, medulloblastoma, cerebellar astrocytoma, ependymoma)

Foramen magnum tumors

Supratentorial tumors

Tentorial notch tumors

Tentorial tumors

Infratentorial tumors

Foramen magnum tumors

Approximately 1700 children under the age of 14 years are diagnosed annually as having tumors of the brain and CNS. The four most common brain tumors in children are medulloblastoma, cerebral astrocytoma, ependymoma, and brainstem glioma ("Brain Tumor Incidence," 2011; Kuttesch et al., 2011; McLendon et al., 2011).

Health Promotion The Child Receiving Cancer Treatment

Cancer treatment often extends for several years, so the child needs to continue health promotion and health maintenance visits.

Growth and Development Surveillance

- The child is assessed for height, weight, and body mass index. This provides information about growth patterns, which may be altered by cancer treatment. If indicated, 24-hour diet recalls and other nutritional assessments are performed.

- Teaching is provided about age-appropriate foods. Since appetite may be impaired during periods of treatment, the child may be lacking fruits, vegetables, or other foods, as well as the nutrients they include. Encourage parents to be sure the child has a well-balanced diet during periods of remission.

- Perform developmental screening of young children. Provide suggestions for parents about the stimulation that is appropriate for the child's age. Include quiet activities that can be used when the child is fatigued or receiving therapy. These might include reading books, listening to tapes and music, and working on a computer. Have the parent plan for these activities on days that the child goes for chemotherapy or other treatment.

- Ask about the school-age child's progress in school. Performance may be altered because of neurologic effects of treatment as well as missing school. Plan for the family to partner with the school personnel for provision of tutors, computer programs, or other needed assistance.

- Encourage continued social contact with peers when blood counts are adequate to prevent infection.

Physical Assessment and Screening

- Careful physical assessments are performed to identify any abnormalities that may result from cancer or its treatment. Cardiopulmonary and neuromuscular assessments are particularly important. Vision and hearing should be assessed prior to treatment and periodically throughout. Include measurements of fine and gross motor activity.

Elimination

- Toddlers may have an interruption in toilet training during periods when they do not feel well. Help parents to understand this regression and encourage them to start again when the child is feeling better.

- Some medications cause diarrhea or constipation so evaluate bowel patterns and provide guidance as needed. Skin care instruction may be needed if the child has diarrhea and is relatively immobile. Increasing fluids and fiber foods may be needed for constipation.

- Evaluate urinary output since many medications have effects on kidney function. Encourage adequate fluids for age to ensure elimination of medications.

Sleep and Fatigue

- Children undergoing treatment often have disturbed sleep patterns. Parents of young children may become exhausted working all day, getting the child to treatments, and having disturbed sleep at night. Assess both the child's sleep patterns and the family's experiences. Encourage plans for respite care to enable rest periods.

- Provide cots, rocking chairs, and other comfortable settings for child and family members during treatments.

- Both child and parents may not expect or understand the profound fatigue that occurs during cancer treatment. They can be helped to plan for providing quiet times, and replenishing energy through naps, massage, relaxing baths, and spending time with family.

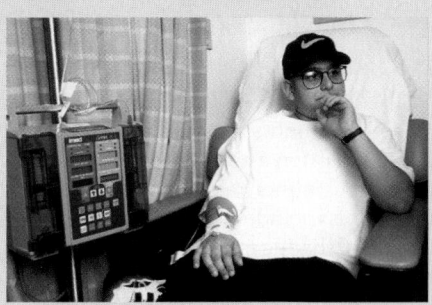

Physical Activity

- Since the child has periods of fatigue, patterns of physical activity may decrease. Emphasize the importance of integrating physical activity when the child feels well, since it is needed for learning gross motor skills, facilitating blood flow, improving mental status, and setting patterns for the future.

Disease and Injury Prevention Strategies

- The child with cancer has the same safety hazards as other children of the same age, and such topics as car safety seats, fire prevention, water safety, and violence prevention should be addressed.

- An important hazard for children with cancer is infection due to decreased immune response. Keep records of immunization status. Follow the recommendations of the CDC and AAP for other immunizations. Teach the hazards of large groups when the child's immune system is compromised. Teach care of central lines and other potential sources of infection. Have families report signs of infection and exposure to known illnesses promptly.

Mental and Spiritual Health

- Evaluate the child and family for signs of anxiety and depression. Ask how they are managing the cancer treatment and what poses the greatest challenges. Refer to other families with similar circumstances for support.

- Ensure that the child has contact with friends through child care, school, or via phone, letters, and a computer.

- Find out the impact of the child's cancer on the parent's jobs. Ask how the siblings have been coping, what changes there are in school performance, and whether teachers and others are aware of the stress the sibling may be experiencing.

Transitional Care

- As the child's treatment ends, instruct the child's parents about needed periodic follow-up with the oncologist. Continue to perform neurologic examinations and ascertain school performance. Be alert for signs of secondary tumors.

- Ask about worries regarding the future. As teens grow older, have them take over more responsibility for informing healthcare providers of their cancer history and assist them to transition to adult healthcare providers.

TABLE 50–4 Clinical Manifestations of Brain Tumors

TUMOR	ETIOLOGY	CLINICAL MANIFESTATIONS	CLINICAL THERAPY
Medulloblastoma	External layer of cerebellum	Headache, vomiting, ataxia	Surgery; chemotherapy with lomustine, vincristine, cisplatin; radiation
Astrocytomas	Glial cells, supratentorial or infratentorial	Seizures, visual disturbances, increased intracranial pressure, vomiting	Surgery; chemotherapy with vincristine, dactinomycin; radiation
Ependymoma	Fourth ventricle, posterior fossa	Hydrocephalus	Surgery, radiation
Brainstem gliomas	Pons	Cranial nerve (VI + VII) tract signs, nystagmus, ataxia, motor symptoms	Surgery, radiation

CLINICAL MANIFESTATIONS

Children with brain tumors can manifest behavioral and nervous changes. These are often a result of increased intracranial pressure and may occur either rapidly or slowly and subtly. Some common symptoms include headache, nausea, vomiting, abnormal gait, dizziness, change in vision or hearing, fatigue, and mental status changes such as educational or behavioral problems.

Brainstem tumors can present with weight deficits and may be mistakenly diagnosed as an eating disorder of infancy and childhood (failure to thrive). This may delay proper treatment. See Table 50–4 for common manifestations of certain types of brain tumors.

Medulloblastomas are brain tumors in the external layer of the cerebellum. They account for 35% to 40% of childhood brain tumors, and commonly occur in children 5 to 6 years of age. *Astrocytomas* arise from glial cells and can be either above or below the area between the cerebrum and cerebellum. They account for 35% to 40% of childhood brain tumors. The presenting symptoms vary depending on the location of the tumor. Endocrine, vision, and behavioral changes are all possible, as well as increased intracranial pressure and seizures. *Ependymomas* commonly occur in the fourth ventricle of the posterior fossa and comprise 10% to 15% of childhood brain tumors. Impaired growth, hydrocephalus, seizures, and cranial nerve impairments are the most common manifestations. *Brainstem gliomas* are located in the pons and typically spread into the surrounding tissue. They account for 10% to 15% of childhood brain tumors (Kuttesch et al., 2011).

CLINICAL THERAPY

Brain tumors are diagnosed with computed tomography (CT), magnetic resonance imaging (MRI), positron emission tomography (PET), single-photon emission computed tomography (SPECT), myelography, and angiography. New technologies combine imaging with angiography to more specifically image the lesion. Examples include magnetic resonance angiography (MRA), magnetic resonance spectroscopy (MRS), perfusion and diffusion imaging, digital subtraction angiography (DSA), and CT angiography (CTA) (Paldino, Faerber, & Poussaint, 2011). Neurophysiologic tests (electroencephalography and brainstem evoked potentials) are used to assess sensory pathway integrity and disease-related or drug-related sensory dysfunction. Other tests that may be performed are tumor markers and cerebrospinal fluid cytology. Lumbar puncture identifies abnormal cells in the cerebrospinal fluid. Bone marrow aspiration and bone scans identify extracranial primary neoplastic growth since cancers in other sites can metastasize to the brain.

Treatment depends on the type of brain tumor. Surgery is common. It may be performed to obtain a biopsy specimen, to debulk (reduce the tumor by partial removal) or excise the tumor, or to treat any hydrocephalus that may be present. During surgery, radiologic images allow the neurosurgeon to see computerized images of the brain while stimulating nerves to determine their functioning. These techniques provide rapid feedback to the neurosurgeon. Laser surgery, which has delicate precise control and accuracy, is used when tumors are close to sensitive neural or vascular structures.

Use of radiation after surgery and chemotherapy has improved the survival of children with medulloblastoma and ependymoma. High-dose chemotherapy is often used, and this modality has improved the survival of children with CNS tumors. Low-dose chemotherapy can shrink and help manage some tumors. Intrathecal administration of chemotherapy is useful in some cases. An Ommaya reservoir, a dome-shaped device with a catheter, may be surgically placed under the scalp to administer chemotherapy directly to the central nervous system.

However, the blood–brain barrier reduces the effectiveness of chemotherapy for children with brain tumors. For example, when methotrexate is administered intrathecally (in the spinal canal), only a small amount crosses normal brain capillaries. Radiation is not used in children under 3 years old because of resultant damage to brain cells. Hematopoietic stem cell transplantation is increasingly used. Numerous new approaches are being investigated and will be used increasingly in the years ahead. New combinations of chemotherapeutic agents, precision-guided delivery of medications and radiotherapy, gene therapy, cytokine-producing therapy to activate the immune system, molecular analysis and epigenetic markers to guide treatment, and blood–brain barrier disruption are examples of emerging treatments (Faria et al., 2011; Pollack, 2011).

Clinical Tip

The following are examples of drugs that may be used to treat brain tumors (Kuttesch et al., 2011):

- Cyclophosphamide
- Ifosfamide
- Lomustine
- Methotrexate
- Vincristine
- VP-16
- Cisplatin
- Carboplatin
- Nitrosourea
- Temozolomide

Complications of treatment for children with brain tumors are significant. They include severe infections (associated with high-dose chemotherapy), seizure activity, sensorimotor defects, hydrocephalus, and growth problems. Care is taken to treat infections early and aggressively. If a cerebrospinal shunt is used, infection or blockage can occur. (See Chapter 54 for further discussion of cerebrospinal shunts in children.) Anticonvulsants are commonly given prophylactically after surgery. Endocrine problems, such as growth hormone changes, hypothyroidism, and panhypopituitarism, may occur when the tumor is in the hypothalamic–pituitary area. Treatment may also lead to impaired cognitive function and emotional or behavioral problems in some children. Memory deficits and selective attention deficits are the most common problems.

Diabetes insipidus is a special consideration in children with midline brain tumors, such as those that compress the hypothalamus, pituitary stalk, or posterior pituitary gland. Manifestations of diabetes insipidus include voiding of large amounts of dilute urine with a specific gravity of less than 1.005 to 1.010 (see Chapter 53).

Nursing Management

For the Child With a Brain Tumor

Nursing Assessment and Diagnosis

The focus of physiologic assessment of the child with a brain tumor is determined by its presentation (Table 50–5). Presenting signs can be categorized as follows:

- Nonspecific signs related to increasing intracranial pressure
- Secondary signs related to displacement of intracranial structures
- Focal signs suggesting direct involvement of the brain and cranial nerves

Thorough neurologic examination before surgery is essential to provide a record of baseline functioning. The neurologic examination also allows the evaluation of the child's changing physiologic status before surgery. Ask if the child has manifested slow changes over time or has had quickly developing symptoms. Measurement of head circumference and assessment of the anterior fontanelle are necessary in children under the age of 18 months.

Perform developmental screening on young children using the Denver II or other developmental test (see Chapter 34). Ask about the child's social interactions, school performance, and any behavior changes that have occurred.

Several nursing diagnoses can be identified for the child with a brain tumor depending on the type and location of the tumor. Some common examples follow (NANDA-I © 2014):

- *Nutrition, Imbalanced: Less than Body Requirements*, related to loss of appetite
- *Mobility: Physical, Impaired*, related to tumor pressure on coordination centers

TABLE 50–5 Physiologic Assessment of Brain Tumors

CLINICAL MANIFESTATIONS	ASSESSMENT
Nonspecific signs: headache, morning vomiting, somnolence, irritability	Level of consciousness, pupil response, pupil shape and size
Secondary signs: disturbances of cranial nerves; other signs depend on site of tumor	All cranial nerves
Focal signs: truncal ataxia (midline brain tumors), general nystagmus, head tilting	Motor ability, head positions when watching television or looking at people (double vision, sixth cranial nerve involvement)

- *Development: Delayed, Risk for*, related to effects of disability
- *Memory, Impaired*, related to neurologic disturbance
- *Pain, Acute*, related to compression of brain tissue

Planning and Implementation

The child with a brain tumor requires multidisciplinary care by, among others, a neurologist, neurosurgeon, pediatrician, dietitian, and social worker. Other specialists are also often needed. The nurse can act as a case manager to coordinate the complex care needed by the child.

For the nursing care of children immediately following surgery, refer to Chapter 39. In addition, close monitoring of neurologic status is needed postoperatively (refer to Chapter 54). Be especially alert for signs of increased intracranial pressure and infection. Observe for seizure activity. Administer drugs such as antibiotics and anticonvulsants as ordered.

Signs and symptoms of diabetes insipidus may occur following brain surgery (see Chapter 53 for a description of diabetes insipidus). Nursing care includes hourly measurement of intake and output, measurement of serum sodium levels every 4 to 6 hours, accurate fluid replacement, and frequent assessment of neurologic status. An indwelling urinary catheter is useful for accurate measurement of urinary output.

DISCHARGE PLANNING AND HOME CARE TEACHING

Teach the parents to watch for an increase in voiding of dilute urine. Be sure they can recognize the signs of infection and changes in the child's neurologic status. Once the child is ready for discharge, chemotherapy or radiation may begin; tell parents the reason and potential side effects of these treatments. Help the family get any special equipment they may need to care for the child at home, such as a wheelchair, bed rails, or dressings. The American Cancer Society is a potential resource for assistance with these needs.

Children with brain tumors, especially those who have received radiation, often have some permanent sequelae. They may have slowed development, incoordination, learning disabilities, or other effects. These sequelae are most common in children who are 3 years of age or younger at the time of radiation therapy. Perform accurate height and weight measures at each healthcare visit. Assess developmental milestones. Ask about progress in school and any special services that might be needed. Perform thorough neurologic assessments. Support the family as they learn to deal with unknown or changed expectations for the child's performance.

Evaluation

Expected outcomes of nursing care for the child with a brain tumor depend on the site of tumor, clinical therapy, and medical outcome. Some outcomes might include the following:

- Nutritional intake is adequate to support growth and prevent malnutrition.
- A safe environment is maintained for the child.
- Physical mobility is maintained to the limits of developmental level and alterations of disease.
- An environment that supports normal developmental milestones within the capability of the child is maintained.
- Pain is managed to a level of comfort.
- Parents understand the diagnosis and treatment plan.

TABLE 50–6 International Neuroblastoma Staging System

STAGE	DESCRIPTION
1	Localized tumor confined to the area of origin; complete gross excision, with or without microscopic residual disease; identifiable ipsilateral and contralateral lymph nodes negative microscopically
2A	Unilateral tumor with incomplete gross excision; identifiable ipsilateral and contralateral lymph nodes negative microscopically
2B	Unilateral tumor with complete or incomplete gross excision; with positive ipsilateral regional lymph nodes; identifiable contralateral lymph nodes negative microscopically
3	Tumor infiltrating across the midline with or without regional lymph node involvement; or unilateral tumor with contralateral regional lymph node involvement; or midline tumor with bilateral regional lymph node involvement
4	Dissemination of tumor to distant lymph nodes, bone, bone marrow, liver, and/or other organs (except as defined in stage 4S)
4S	Localized primary tumor as defined for stage 1 or 2 with dissemination limited to liver, skin, and/or bone marrow; bone marrow involvement should be minimal (less than 10% of cells); if greater it is stage 4 disease

Source: Data from National Cancer Institute. (2011e). *Stages of neuroblastoma*. Retrieved from http://www.cancer.gov/cancertopics/pdq/treatment/neuroblastoma/HealthProfessional/page2.

Neuroblastoma

Neuroblastoma is the solid tumor most commonly occurring outside the cranium of children. It is responsible for 8% to 10% of childhood cancers and 15% of cancer deaths in children. The average age at diagnosis is 17 to 22 months; it is the most common tumor in infants during the first year of life. Nearly all cases (90%) are diagnosed before 5 years of age (Zage & Ater, 2011). Prognosis varies, depending on the staging of the tumor (Table 50–6) and the age of the child, with more favorable outcomes in infants under 1 year of age and in presenting sites in the pelvis or thorax. Less favorable outcomes are associated with the presence of N-*myc* oncogen amplification. Survival rates are 90% for stages 1 and 2, but drop to 25% to 35% for stage 4 (Zage & Ater, 2011). As compared to White, Hispanic, and Asian children, more African American and Native American children have advanced disease upon diagnosis and therefore lower survival rates (Henderson et al., 2011). It is unknown if genetic differences or lack of consistent primary care contributes to this disparity.

Neuroblastoma is commonly a smooth, hard, nontender mass that can occur anywhere along the sympathetic nervous system chain. A frequent location is the abdomen, although other sites are the adrenal, thoracic, and cervical areas.

ETIOLOGY AND PATHOPHYSIOLOGY

Neuroblastoma originates in primitive neurocrest cells that form the adrenal medulla, paraganglia, and sympathetic nervous system of the cervical sympathetic chain and the thoracic chain. Approximately 50% of neuroblastomas develop in the adrenal medulla; 30% develop in the cervical, thoracic, or pelvic ganglia; and the remaining are elsewhere along the sympathetic chain (Zage & Ater, 2011). Lymph node metastasis is common because of the proximity of the tumor origin to the lymph system drainage.

The cause of neuroblastoma is unknown. A genetic defect found in many cases of neuroblastoma is a deletion of the short arm of chromosome 1 (1p del); other abnormalities include 11q, 14q, and 17q. Amplification of the proto-oncogene N-*myc* or mutation of *Phox2B* and *ALK* genes may be seen (Shuangshoti et al., 2011; Zage & Ater, 2011).

CLINICAL MANIFESTATIONS

The location of the mass determines the symptoms. A retroperitoneal mass causes altered bowel and bladder function; characteristic signs are weight loss, abdominal distention, enlarged liver, irritability, fatigue, and fever. Dyspnea or infection may occur when the tumor is mediastinal. Neck and facial edema may result from vena cava syndrome if the tumor is mediastinal and large. Intracranial lesions may be present with periorbital ecchymosis. Malaise, fever, and a limp can occur if there has been metastasis to the bone. Bone marrow disease can manifest as **pancytopenia** (abnormal depression of all cellular blood components) with neutropenia (causing infections) and anemia (causing fatigue). Metastatic spread can result in an array of symptoms affecting multiple organs.

CLINICAL THERAPY

The International Neuroblastoma Staging System (INSS) recommends different diagnostic and laboratory evaluations for diagnosis of the primary disease and of metastases (see Table 50–6). Biopsy of the tumor is used for initial diagnosis, and metastases are diagnosed by bone marrow biopsy, radiolabeled scanning, x-ray, CT, and MRI. Tumor markers include vanillylmandelic acid (VMA), homovanillic acid (HVA), dopamine, ferritin, NSE (an enzyme in neural tissue), lactic dehydrogenase (LDH), and a ganglioside GD2 (a sugar and lipid molecule on the surface of neural cells). VMA and HVA are by-products of adrenal hormones, and their levels are usually elevated in the urine and blood (see Appendix B for normal values). Areas of necrosis and calcification are readily identifiable with radiologic tests. These tests also help in the staging of the disease by identifying metastases. Urinary catecholamines are often increased.

Routine blood cell counts are needed, including CBC with differential. The test may reveal anemia and thrombocytopenia. There is no classic WBC response, although thrombocytopenia may occur in association with disseminated intravascular coagulation. **Leukocytosis** (higher than normal leukocyte count) and **leukopenia** (lower than normal leukocyte count) have been observed with bone marrow involvement. Serum electrolytes, liver function studies, LDH, coagulation studies, and urinalysis are performed. Elevations in dopamine, ferritin, NSE, LDH, and GD2 are seen. All of these laboratory findings are used initially to diagnose the disease and later to follow its progress. A biopsy or surgical removal of the tumor will be followed by analysis of its type and genetic abnormalities. Areas of necrosis and calcification in major organs are readily identifiable with radiologic tests and MRIs. These tests also help in the staging of the disease by identifying metastases.

The stage of the tumor determines the treatment protocol. Surgical excision of the mass is performed and may be the only treatment in low-risk stages. With higher risk, surgery is followed by chemotherapy with a combination of drugs. Radiation is often used, especially in disseminated disease or when tumors are not receptive to chemotherapy. Autologous stem cell transplantation may be performed for advanced disease, sometimes followed by the biologic modifier *cis*-retinoic acid and fenretinide (to promote apoptosis) (Zage & Ater, 2011).

Nursing Management

For the Child With Neuroblastoma

Nursing Assessment and Diagnosis

Assess the presenting site of the tumor, such as the neck or abdomen, by observation and inspection. Palpation is contraindicated to avoid seeding tumor cells. Carefully document related functioning, such as bowel and bladder function. Take vital signs to watch for elevated temperature and vital sign changes caused by a thoracic mass. Observe gait and coordination. Take weight and height and compare to earlier percentiles for the child. Specific assessments during treatment will depend on the treatment methods used (refer to the earlier discussions of chemotherapy and radiation treatment). Psychosocial assessment and emotional assessment of the family are needed.

A variety of nursing diagnoses may be appropriate for the child with neuroblastoma, depending on the location and extent of the presenting disease. Some common diagnoses might include the following (NANDA-I © 2014):

- *Gas Exchange, Impaired*, related to ventilation-perfusion imbalance
- *Mobility: Physical, Impaired*, related to neuromuscular impairment
- *Pain* related to tumor pressure and injury
- *Grieving (Family)* related to potential loss of significant person

Planning and Implementation

The nursing management of the child with neuroblastoma can encompass the three phases of medical treatment: chemotherapy, surgery, and radiation. Specific postsurgical care depends on the size and site of the tumor. Normal postoperative care includes providing fluid support and respiratory care and preventing infection.

Nursing care during the chemotherapy phase includes minimizing side effects, preventing infection, teaching parents about the medications their child is receiving, and monitoring physical and emotional growth and development of the young child. When radiation is part of the treatment, use common nursing measures described earlier in the chapter.

Topics for parent and family teaching and discharge planning are presented in *Teaching Highlights: The Child With a Neuroblastoma*. Ongoing support and connection to resources to assist in management of the child's treatment at home will be needed. When the prognosis is poor, parents may appreciate referrals to hospice, to other parents who have experienced similar child illnesses, and to other community resources. See Chapter 41 for additional nursing care for the end of life.

Evaluation

Expected outcomes of nursing care for the child with neuroblastoma include the following:

- Ventilatory exchange is adequate to support daily activities.
- Physical mobility is maintained to the level possible considering developmental age.
- Sensory/perceptual alterations are managed to provide for safety and sensory input.
- Pain is managed to a level of comfort.
- Family members accept and integrate the diagnosis.

Wilms Tumor (Nephroblastoma)

Nephroblastoma, an intrarenal tumor of which the most common type is Wilms tumor, is a common abdominal tumor of childhood and accounts for 6% of all childhood tumors. The incidence is approximately 7.6 cases per million children

---

TEACHING HIGHLIGHTS | The Child With a Neuroblastoma

Surgery Phase

- Teach the parents to observe for signs of infection at the wound site and to take the child's temperature, if necessary.
- Assist the family to provide pain management including medication administration and various comfort measures.
- Teach the parents the importance of keeping accurate records of urine output and bowel movements and to notify the healthcare provider if the child does not have a bowel movement at least every 3 days.
- Continue with progression to a regular diet.

Chemotherapy Phase

The child frequently has a central line placed early in the chemotherapy phase. The central line greatly reduces the emotional trauma associated with chemotherapy and blood tests.

- Teach the child how to help the parents with cleaning of the central line.
- Teach the child how to protect the central line.
- Teach the parents how to clean and dress the site of the central line.
- Have the parents practice central line care with a model and then on the child before discharge to increase the parents' confidence.
- Give the parents written and illustrated information about care of a central line.
- Arrange for home care dressing supplies before discharge.
- Give the parents detailed chemotherapy information.
- Teach administration of any medications that the parent will administer via central line or other routes.
- Refer the family to the American Cancer Society for coloring books for children receiving chemotherapy.

annually. Wilms tumor occurs most frequently between 2 and 3 years of age, with young ages being more commonly associated with bilateral disease (Buckley, 2011).

ETIOLOGY AND PATHOPHYSIOLOGY

Wilms tumor is associated with several congenital anomalies: aniridia (absence of the iris), hemihypertrophy (abnormal growth of one half of the body or a body structure), genitourinary anomalies, nevi, and hamartomas (benign, nodule-like growths). These connections suggest a genetic link; chromosomal deletions at 11p13 and 11p15 (locations for *WT1* and *WT2* genes) have been associated with Wilms tumor. It has a high incidence in Beckwith-Wiedemann syndrome, which is characterized by macroglossia and hypoglycemia. However, most children with Wilms tumor have no other abnormalities. Wilms tumor grows very quickly, doubling its size in 11 to 13 days. Such fast growth generally contributes to a large tumor by the time of diagnosis. However, chemotherapeutic drugs have significantly increased survival rates for children with Wilms tumor, with 90% survival rates (Anderson, Dhamne, & Huff, 2011; Buckley, 2011; Huff, 2011).

CLINICAL MANIFESTATIONS

Wilms tumor is usually an asymptomatic, firm, lobulated mass located to one side of the midline in the abdomen. Often a parent discovers the mass during the child's bath. Hypertension caused by increased renin activity related to renal damage is reported in 25% of cases. Hematuria or abdominal pain is sometimes present.

CLINICAL THERAPY

The diagnosis of Wilms tumor is based on an ultrasound study of the abdomen and an intravenous pyelogram. CT scanning or MRI of the lungs, liver, spleen, and brain may be performed to identify any metastasis. This information is used in staging the tumor (Table 50–7). A complete blood count is obtained, as well as BUN and creatinine levels. Liver function tests are performed.

Treatment is multifaceted and increasingly successful; about 90% of early stages and 70% of metastatic cases have long-term survival (Anderson et al., 2011). Surgery is performed to remove the affected kidney, to examine the opposite kidney, and to look for other sites of metastasis. Chemotherapy or radiation therapy, alone or in combination, is sometimes used before surgery to reduce the size of the tumor. Radiation, chemotherapy, or both may also follow surgery. Children whose tumors are almost completely excised and who have a favorable prognosis do not require irradiation of the tumor bed and may receive limited chemotherapy.

Long-term complications of treatment include liver damage, portal hypertension, and mild cirrhosis, which may occur in children treated for right-sided Wilms tumor. Radiation damage (such as thinning or weakening) of the skeleton, pelvis, and thorax has been reported. Kyphosis and scoliosis may occur from irradiation of vertebral bodies and the pelvis. Glomerular damage to the remaining kidney may also occur. Second malignancies in the original radiation field have occurred with orthovoltage radiation, but recent changes in radiation therapy have reduced this risk.

Clinical Tip

The following are examples of drugs that may be used to treat Wilms tumor:

- Vincristine
- Actinomycin D
- Doxorubicin
- Cyclophosphamide

TABLE 50–7 National Wilms Tumor Study Staging System

STAGE	DESCRIPTION
I	The tumor is limited to the kidney and completely excised. The surface of the renal capsule is intact. The tumor is not ruptured before or during removal. No residual tumor is apparent beyond the margins of the excision.
II	The tumor extends beyond the kidney but is completely excised. Regional extension of the tumor is present (i.e., penetration through the outer surface of the renal capsule into the perirenal soft tissues). Vessels outside the kidney substance are infiltrated or contain tumor thrombus. Biopsy may have been performed on the tumor, or local spillage of tumor confined to the flank has occurred. No residual tumor is apparent at or beyond the margin of excision.
III	Residual nonhematogenous tumor is confined to the abdomen. Any of the following may occur: • Lymph nodes on biopsy are found to be involved in the hilus, the periaortic chains, or beyond. • Diffuse peritoneal contamination by the tumor has occurred, such as by spillage of tumor beyond the flank before or during surgery, or by tumor growth that has penetrated through the peritoneal surface. • Implants are found on peritoneal surfaces. • The tumor extends beyond the surgical margins either microscopically or grossly. • The tumor is not completely resectable because of local infiltration into vital structures.
IV	Hematogenous metastasis: deposits are present beyond stage III (e.g., lung, liver, bone, and/or brain).
V	Bilateral renal involvement is present at diagnosis. An attempt should be made to stage each side according to the above criteria on the basis of extent of disease before biopsy.

Source: Data from National Cancer Institute. (2011f). *Wilms tumor and other childhood kidney tumors treatment: Stage information.* Retrieved from http://www.cancer.gov/cancertopics/pdq/treatment/wilms/HealthProfessional/page3.

Nursing Management

For the Child With Wilms Tumor (Nephroblastoma)

Nursing Assessment and Diagnosis

Perform a thorough baseline assessment of the child. Do not palpate the abdomen because of the potential for spreading the cancerous cells. Monitor the child's blood pressure carefully because hypertension is a common finding that may require treatment.

Nursing diagnoses for a child with Wilms tumor will differ depending on the phase of treatment. Some common nursing diagnoses might include the following (NANDA-I © 2014):

- *Infection, Risk for*, related to inadequate defenses
- *Urinary Elimination, Impaired*, related to anatomic obstruction
- *Tissue Perfusion: Cardiac, Risk for Decreased*, related to hypertension caused by mechanical reduction of blood flow
- *Caregiver Role Strain, Risk for*, related to child's illness severity
- *Home Maintenance, Impaired*, related to child's disease

Planning and Implementation

Nursing management can be divided into two phases: the postrenal surgery phase and the chemotherapy phase. (See Chapter 39 for general care of the child after surgery.) Drawings and special teaching dolls with removable kidneys can be used to teach young children about the surgery. Although chemotherapy may occur at two different times, before and after surgery, nursing management considerations remain the same.

Nursing care during the postrenal surgery phase focuses on pain management and close monitoring of fluid levels. A large incision is necessary to remove the kidney, and the resultant postoperative shift of organs and fluid in the abdominal cavity may create discomfort for the child. Frequently reposition the child and use noninvasive and pharmacologic pain interventions to improve the child's comfort. Gentle handling is important. Monitor fluids closely following surgery to prevent hypovolemia and to assess the shift of fluids out of the third space and out of the body. Assess daily weight, intake and output (I&O), and urine specific gravity. Monitor the function of the remaining kidney. Take blood pressure frequently to watch for signs of shock and to assess the functioning of the remaining kidney.

SAFETY ALERT!

If you feel a mass during palpation of a child's abdomen, stop palpating immediately and report the finding to the child's primary healthcare provider. Never palpate the liver or abdomen of a child with Wilms tumor as this could cause a piece of the tumor to dislodge. Place a sign on the child's bed and in the chart alerting healthcare providers not to palpate the abdomen.

During the chemotherapy phase, monitor the child for side effects of drugs, the potential for infection from the central line site, and the function of the remaining kidney. Advise parents about home care needs, administration of medications, and monitoring for drug side effects and ongoing needs for healthcare monitoring. A long-term complication in children who receive doxorubicin treatment is congestive heart failure, so ongoing periodic healthcare evaluations are needed. Be sure care is well coordinated among all healthcare providers.

Evaluation

Desired outcomes for nursing care of the child with nephroblastoma include balanced intake and output, normal vital signs, recovery from surgery, and successful family management of postsurgical care and ongoing treatments.

Bone Tumors

Osteosarcoma

Osteosarcoma is the most common tumor affecting the skeleton of children, with an incidence of seven cases per million children. Its peak incidence is during the rapid growth years, at age 13 years for girls and age 14 years for boys (Arndt, 2011b). The tumor is usually located at the metaphysis of the distal femur, proximal tibia, or proximal humerus.

ETIOLOGY AND PATHOPHYSIOLOGY

Bone tissue produced by osteosarcoma never matures into compact bone. Although the cause of osteosarcoma is unknown, radiation exposure (either environmental or treatment related) is associated with its development. Survivors of retinoblastoma have a greatly increased incidence of osteosarcoma. An abnormality of gene *p53* has been noted in some cases of this cancer, leading to oncogene malformations and possibly to an absence of tumor suppressor genes (Chen et al., 2014).

CLINICAL MANIFESTATIONS

The common initial symptoms are pain, swelling, and a limp. The pain can be referred to the hip or back, which can delay diagnosis. Deep bone pain causing night awakenings should be investigated (Arndt, 2011b). Pulmonary metastasis occurs in 20% of cases. Other metastatic sites include kidney, adrenals, brain, and pericardium. When lung metastasis is the only site, lung resection may be successful for treatment. Disseminated metastases and bone lesions have poorer prognoses.

CLINICAL THERAPY

Diagnosis is made through radiographic studies of the affected area, bone scan, CT or MRI scans of involved bone, blood test for serum alkaline phosphatase and lactic dehydrogenase (levels may be elevated), and tumor biopsy (to confirm the diagnosis). Arteriography may be performed if limb-sparing surgery is contemplated. Complete blood count, liver studies, and renal studies are performed for information about possible metastases.

Clinical Tip

The following are examples of drugs that may be used to treat osteosarcoma:

- Methotrexate with leucovorin rescue
- Doxorubicin
- Cisplatin
- Ifosfamide with mesna

Treatment involves both surgery and chemotherapy. The surgery is either a limb-salvage procedure or limb amputation. In limb-salvage procedures, the tumor is removed and a bone graft or internal prosthesis is inserted. A limb-salvage procedure is often possible if bone growth has taken place and a neurobundle (area where several nerves converge) is not involved in the tumor (Manfrini, Tiwari, Ham, et al., 2011). Other criteria such as joint involvement and possibility of prosthetic use in the future are weighed in the decision about a salvage procedure or amputation. Physical rehabilitation will be needed after either amputation or limb-salvage procedure. Aggressive chemotherapy following surgery has improved the survival rate. At the time of diagnosis, most children have metastases (even though they may not be identifiable), so chemotherapy is needed. Chemotherapy is started before surgery to shrink the tumor, especially when limb-salvage surgery is planned. It is also given postoperatively to treat and prevent metastasis.

Ewing Sarcoma

Ewing sarcoma is a malignant, small, round cell tumor usually involving the diaphyseal (shaft) portion of the long bones. The most common sites are the femur, pelvis, tibia, fibula, ribs, humerus, scapula, and clavicle, but any bone may be involved. Ewing sarcoma occurs in two children per million, is most common in White and Hispanic children, and is rare in African American and Asian American children. The incidence is highest in children between the ages of 5 and 20 years (HaDuong, Martin, Skapek, et al., 2015; Moore & Haydon, 2014).

Translocations on chromosomes 11 and 22 have been identified in children with Ewing sarcoma; these are t(11;22)(q24;q12). In addition, these tumors express a proto-oncogene, c-*myc*.

The symptoms are similar to those of osteosarcoma and may include pain, swelling, fever, an elevated WBC count, an elevated erythrocyte sedimentation rate, and elevated C-reactive protein. Some children present with a fracture of the affected bone. A tumor biopsy is necessary for diagnosis. Diagnostic tests are the same as those for osteosarcoma.

Initial treatment for Ewing sarcoma is chemotherapy to reduce the tumor, followed by radiation and surgical removal of the tumor and/or bone. Limb-salvage procedures are now commonly performed rather than amputation. Chemotherapy is always used after initial treatment because undetectable metastases are nearly always present.

Clinical Tip

The following are examples of drugs that may be used to treat Ewing sarcoma (Meyer & Grier, 2014):

- Vincristine
- Cyclophosphamide
- Dactinomycin
- Doxorubicin
- Ifosfamide
- Irinotecan
- Etoposide
- Temozolomide
- Topotecan

Nursing Management

For the Child With a Bone Tumor

Nursing Assessment and Diagnosis

Carefully evaluate any child or adolescent who has a limp or complains of pain in an extremity. Confirm the onset and whether the symptoms were associated with injury. Refer for further evaluation if the discomfort persists or is not associated with injury. Physiologic assessment of the child with a bone tumor includes assessment of the site before surgery. Assess the child's pain or discomfort, mobility, and gait. Take careful vital signs, especially noting temperature and respirations. Psychologic assessments of the child and family are needed, especially if amputation is planned. Loss of a limb causes body image disturbances, particularly with school-age children and adolescents. Assess the child's understanding of the treatment and of care after surgery. Find out what support systems are available to the family.

Observe the wound postoperatively for infection and hemorrhage. Assess circulation above and below the operative site. If edema is found, elevate the limb. If a limb-salvage procedure is performed, the child's extremity will remain, but it will not function as before because muscle insertion sites and mass have been removed with the tumor during surgery. Detailed charting of the condition of the surgical site and limb function is important.

If the limb has been amputated, assess the child for the following signs indicating a disturbed body image:

- Refusal to look at or touch the altered or missing body part
- Preoccupation with loss or change
- Feelings of shame or embarrassment, either verbalized or demonstrated
- Distorted perception of normal body (easily seen in the child's drawings of the body)

- Fears of rejection or unwanted attention from others
- Overexposure or hiding of the affected body part
- Actual or perceived change in the structure and function of the body or body parts

Psychosocial assessment of the child and family is discussed in more detail earlier in the general section titled *Childhood Cancer*.

Nursing diagnoses for the child with a bone tumor are based on the treatment and needs of each child. The nursing diagnoses that might be appropriate include the following (NANDA-I © 2014):

- ***Infection, Risk for***, related to amputation or limb-salvage procedure
- ***Skin Integrity, Impaired***, related to mechanical forces of prosthesis
- ***Mobility: Physical, Impaired***, related to musculoskeletal impairment
- ***Body Image, Disturbed***, related to treatment and injury
- ***Pain, Acute***, related to physical injury of tissues

Planning and Implementation

Care of the child after surgery involves general postoperative care (see Chapter 39). The child who has had an amputation has special needs regarding skin care and rehabilitation. Inspect the tissue at the surgical site, using sterile technique, and turn the child at least every 2 hours. The site needs to heal completely before chemotherapy can begin and a prosthesis can be made. Pain management is a major nursing care need. When amputation has occurred, the adolescent will often experience phantom pain. This is pain that feels as if it were occurring in the amputated extremity and is caused by trauma to the nerves in the area of the amputation. Acknowledge that the pain is real since the nerve endings are intact and the patient is perceiving real discomfort. Medicate adequately and use additional pain control measures such as repositioning the limb using gentle movement, supporting the limb, and using distraction or deep breathing.

Discuss insurance and other financial arrangements with the parents, as prosthetics can be costly. Physical therapy will be needed as well. Referral to a Shriners Hospital is an option for some families.

Implement plans to help the child deal with body image disturbance. Plan for a visit from another child who is well adjusted to a prosthesis. Help the child gradually learn how to care for the stump. Slow progress may be made as the child first looks briefly, then for longer periods, and finally is willing to touch the stump. Show the child how it is possible to continue with sports such as baseball, skiing, or biking with a prosthesis. A discussion group with others can be very useful for adolescents. Plan with the child how to tell friends about the surgery and what issues the child may face upon return to school. Make plans for elevator access if needed and emergency evacuation procedures. Some children or adolescents may need referral for counseling to assist in dealing with body image disturbance.

The child will receive physical rehabilitation while hospitalized and after discharge. When the child is discharged, explain to the family the importance of bringing the child for outpatient chemotherapy and physical rehabilitation visits. Special arrangements may be needed at the child's school to accommodate a wheelchair, crutches, or ambulation with a new prosthesis. Call or visit the school to see whether there are buttons to open doors, wide doorways to facilitate passage, and any limitations of the building. Contact school personnel to plan the child's return.

Follow-up care is needed to monitor for progress and to be alert for signs of metastases. Fracture may be a sign of recurrent tumor. All body systems such as lungs, heart, kidneys, and liver are monitored for signs of recurrence.

Evaluation

Expected outcomes of nursing care for the child with a bone tumor focus on the treatments required and adaptation to changes in lifestyle. Examples include the following:

- The surgical site heals with no signs of infection.
- The child adapts to changes in mobility status.
- The child successfully adjusts to changes required in school settings.
- Skin remains intact.
- Positive body image is achieved.
- Pain is managed to a level of comfort.

Leukemia

Leukemia is the most commonly diagnosed pediatric malignancy in children under 14 years of age. A cancer of the blood-forming organs, leukemia is characterized by a proliferation of abnormal white blood cells in the body. Several types of leukemia are differentiated depending on the blood cells affected. The main types are acute lymphoblastic leukemia (ALL), acute myelogenous leukemia (AML), and the rare chronic leukemias of childhood. Because chronic leukemias such as chronic myelocytic, chronic myelomonocytic, and chronic lymphocytic leukemia are rare in children, the following discussion will focus on ALL and AML.

The most common type of childhood leukemia is acute lymphoblastic leukemia, which accounts for 25% of all childhood cancer and 78% of leukemias in children. The peak age at onset is 2 to 3 years. ALL is more common in White children and in boys (Tubergen, Bleyer, & Ritchey, 2011). Subtypes of ALL are based on the French-American-British (FAB) system of classification. There are three types of ALL in the FAB system: L1, L2, and L3. Rasheed, the 12-year-old boy who is described in the chapter-opening scenario, has ALL.

AML refers to all leukemias from myeloid cells. About 17% of childhood leukemias are AML. AML is most common in children younger than 2 years of age and in adolescents. It is more common in boys than girls and in Asians/Pacific Islanders, Hispanics, and Whites than in African Americans. There are several subtypes of AML in the FAB classification:

M0 = acute nonlymphocytic leukemia without maturation

M1 = acute nonlymphocytic leukemia with poor maturation

M2 = acute nonlymphocytic leukemia with maturation

M3 = acute promyelocytic leukemia

M4 = acute myelomonocytic leukemia

M5 = acute monocytic leukemia

M6 = erythroleukemia

M7 = acute megakaryocytic leukemia

Etiology and Pathophysiology

The causes of leukemia are not well understood. Some investigators theorize that exposure to infectious agents can predispose

> ### Developing Cultural Competence Prevalence of Leukemia
>
> African American, Hispanic, and Native American children have statistically poorer outcomes from leukemia treatment than do White and Asian children. Analysis of 5-year survival rates demonstrated poorer outcomes for African American children than White children with AML (Bhatia, 2011). It is unclear whether racial and ethnic groups with poorer outcomes have particular genetic characteristics placing them at risk, do not obtain treatment as soon, have more complications from the disease, enroll less often in clinical trials, or have less access to care at oncology centers. Clearly, more research is needed to describe and then eliminate the racial and ethnic disparity in leukemia treatment outcomes.

children to leukemia. Genetic factors are believed to play a role in some types of the disease. For instance, children with chromosomal defects such as Down syndrome, neurofibromatosis type I, Bloom syndrome, and Shwachman syndrome have an increased incidence of ALL (Messinger et al., 2012). Children with immune deficiency states, such as ataxia-telangiectasia, congenital hypogammaglobulinemia, and Wiskott-Aldrich syndrome, have an increased risk of ALL.

Ionizing radiation exposure when in utero and chemical agents such as treatment with chemotherapy for other cancers are thought to play some role in the development of AML. Several chromosomal and genetic abnormalities are associated with AML.

Leukemia occurs when the stem cells in the bone marrow produce immature WBCs that cannot function normally. These cells proliferate rapidly by cloning instead of normal mitosis, causing the bone marrow to fill with abnormal WBCs. The abnormal cells then spill out into the circulatory system where they steadily replace the normally functioning WBCs. As this occurs, the protective lymphocytic functions such as cellular and humoral immunity are reduced, leaving the body vulnerable to infections.

The malignant WBCs rapidly fill the bone marrow, replacing stem cells that produce erythrocytes (red blood cells) and other blood products such as platelets, thereby decreasing the amount of these products in circulation. The stem cells are replaced by leukemic clones, eventually resulting in anemia. Children with leukemia commonly experience abnormal bleeding, ecchymosis, or petechiae because of the reduced amounts of platelets.

Clinical Manifestations

Children with ALL and AML usually have fever, pallor, overt signs of bleeding, lethargy, malaise, anorexia, and large joint or bone pain. Petechiae, frank bleeding, and joint pain are cardinal signs of bone marrow failure. Enlargement of the liver and spleen (hepatosplenomegaly) and changes in the lymph nodes (lymphadenopathy) are common. If the leukemia has infiltrated the central nervous system (entered it by means of the circulatory or lymphoid system), the child may have signs such as headache, vomiting, papilledema, and sixth cranial nerve palsy (inability to move the eye laterally). These findings are caused by the leukemic cells massing and putting pressure on nerves. The testicles, spinal cord, and bone marrow are common sites for infiltration. The leukemic cells in the testicle become a mass that causes the testicle to enlarge, often painlessly.

Clinical Therapy

Diagnosis is based initially on blood counts and bone marrow aspiration. Blood counts commonly reveal a combination of abnormalities such as anemia, thrombocytopenia, and/or neutropenia. Bone marrow aspiration reveals immature and abnormal lymphoblasts and hypercellular marrow and is the differential test. The percentage of blast cells in marrow is measured. Other abnormal laboratory findings include elevated serum uric acid and hypocalcemia, as well as elevated potassium and phosphorus levels. Laboratory studies such as rapid flow cytometric assay are making the measurement of even very small numbers of leukemic cells possible, so that treatment can improve prognosis in children with minimal residual disease. Leukemic cells are examined and classified by FAB type, and DNA analysis may provide clues about genetic changes; all of these considerations are used to establish the protocol for treatment. Blood cells of children with ALL are B cell or T cell; these classifications are also used to establish treatment protocols.

Both ALL and AML are now approached by analysis of molecular targeting for the origin and type of disease identified (Masetti, Kleinschmidt, Biagi, et al., 2011; Pui, Carroll, Meshinchi, et al., 2011). Treatment of ALL involves radiation and chemotherapy (Rabin & Poplack, 2011). Radiation is used for central nervous system (CNS) disease, in T-cell leukemia, and for testicular involvement. Chemotherapy is commonly organized into four phases: (1) induction, (2) consolidation, (3) delayed intensification, and (4) maintenance of remission. Additional drugs may be used for treatment of CNS involvement. Maintenance therapy may continue for 2 to 3 years, causing decreased resistance to infection for this prolonged period. Treatment of AML involves use of a wide variety of drugs during the induction and consolidation phases.

Maximum cell death occurs during the *induction phase*. The cells that remain after this period are more resistant to treatment. After 3 to 4 weeks, bone marrow aspiration is reevaluated. Drugs are used in combination with CNS prophylaxis; cranial irradiation is used in some cases. During the *consolidation phase*, chemotherapy with L-asparaginase is administered. *Delayed intensification* uses additional drugs to target the leukemic cells that have survived. Treatment during the *maintenance phase* is aimed at destroying the remaining leukemic cells. Combinations of active drugs are used to prevent resistance. Occasionally, other drugs are added to the regimen, such as vincristine, prednisone, cyclophosphamide, intravenous methotrexate, cytosine arabinoside, doxorubicin, or anthracyclines.

The prognosis for children with leukemia is much improved with current therapy. An important factor is the initial leukocyte count; the higher the leukocyte count (over 50,000/mm^3) at diagnosis, the worse the prognosis. For children in the low-risk group, the probability of prolonged survival is as high as 90%; even higher risk ALL has a 75% to 80% cure rate with current treatments (Tubergen et al., 2011). Treatment methods and duration are adjusted for each child depending on that child's metabolic analysis and other risk factors (Rabin & Poplack, 2011).

Approximately 15% to 20% of children have a relapse within a year after completing treatment (Tubergen et al., 2011). Treatment for relapse consists of additional chemotherapeutic drugs. The prognosis is best if the relapse occurs late after the initial diagnosis and after the initial treatment is completed. Hematopoietic stem cell transplant (HSCT) is a treatment option for the child who has a relapse with ALL and who then achieves a second remission; the transplant is given when the

---

Clinical Tip

Following are the laboratory values in leukemia:

	Normal	Common Values in Leukemia
Leukocytes	Less than 10,000/mcL	Greater than 10,000/mcL
Platelets	150,000–400,000/mcL	20,000–100,000/mcL
Hemoglobin	12–16 g/dL	7–11 g/dL

Clinical Tip

The following are examples of drugs that may be used to treat ALL:

Induction Phase
- Prednisone
- Vincristine
- L-asparaginase
- Daunorubicin
- Intrathecal methotrexate (central nervous system prophylaxis)

Consolidation Phase
- L-asparaginase
- Doxorubicin

Delayed Intensification Phase
- Vincristine
- Ara-C
- Cyclophosphamide
- L-asparaginase

Maintenance Phase
- 6-Mercaptopurine or 6-thioguanine
- Methotrexate

---

child is in remission. Transplant is also used for children with AML; they do not need to be in remission for the transplant to be performed.

Overall, 80% of children with leukemia are cured. Chemotherapy itself can create numerous complications, affecting all body organs. Secondary malignancies sometimes occur later in life. See the section on cancer survival earlier in this chapter.

Clinical Tip

The following are examples of drugs that may be used to treat AML:

Induction Phase
- Daunorubicin
- Doxorubicin
- Mitoxantrone
- Cytarabine

Consolidation Phase
- Etoposide
- Teniposide

Nursing Management
For the Child With Leukemia

Nursing Assessment and Diagnosis

Thorough physical assessment is important to ensure prompt identification of problems without injuring the child who has deficient coagulation and immune function. Perform assessments every 8 hours or more often depending on the chemotherapeutic regimen. Observe carefully for bruising, petechiae, and other signs of bleeding; assess for fever or other signs of infection. Once chemotherapy has begun, closely monitor renal functioning through specific gravity, intake and output, and daily weight measurements. Monitor dietary intake, nausea, vomiting, and constipation. Observe for mucosal ulcers in the mouth. A central line is usually in place for intravenous infusion of medications, so carefully assess the line for proper functioning and for signs of infection. Ask the parents about any behavioral changes. CNS infiltration can affect the child's level of consciousness, causing irritability, vomiting, and lethargy. However, chemotherapeutic drugs and antiemetics can also induce these nonspecific signs. Frequent venipunctures, bone marrow aspirations, and lumbar punctures require pain assessment and an evaluation of the level of knowledge and coping skills of child and family.

Leukemia causes many changes in the body, and confirmation of the disease is difficult for families to face. Among the many nursing diagnoses that might be appropriate for the child with leukemia are the following (NANDA-I © 2014):

- *Nutrition, Imbalanced: Less than Body Requirements*, related to inability to ingest food
- *Infection, Risk for*, related to altered immune system functioning
- *Injury, Risk for*, related to bleeding
- *Activity Intolerance* related to generalized weakness
- *Pain* related to chemotherapy and disease process
- *Sleep Pattern, Disturbed*, related to chemotherapeutic drugs and disease process
- *Anxiety (Child and Parent)* related to change in health status

Planning and Implementation

Bone marrow suppression may necessitate transmission-based precautions. Instruct parents in the prevention of infection and use nursing care measures to prevent infection also. Perform careful hand hygiene; take temperature frequently; give mouth care with antibacterial mouthwashes; and inspect skin, mouth, rectal area, and central line site for any signs of infection. Care of mouth sores and other side effects of chemotherapy is presented in *Nursing Care Plan: Hospital Care of the Child With Cancer* earlier in this chapter.

Special attention to renal function is needed when the child receives cyclophosphamide. Gross hematuria is a side effect of this drug. Hydration with intravenous fluids to attain a specific gravity of less than 1.010 prevents or reduces the severity of hematuria. It also prepares the kidneys to manage products of tumor cell breakdown. To achieve the desired specific gravity, the child receives intravenous fluids at 1.5 times maintenance volume for at least 6 to 8 hours before and at least 1.5 hours after administration of the drug. Other chemotherapy drugs have different infusion times, while some do not require hydration prior to infusion. Check drug references carefully for recommendations with each drug. Evaluate the infusion site before and frequently during infusion. Although extravasation is not as common with central lines used in cancer treatment as in peripheral lines, it still can occur. Many chemotherapeutic agents are extremely toxic to tissues. In addition, lysis of the cancer cells can produce toxic side effects (see the *Oncologic Emergencies* section earlier in the chapter). Careful monitoring of intake and output is required to record the intravenous fluids, assess kidney functioning, and monitor excretion of byproducts from destroyed tumor cells. Monitor specific gravity every 8 hours, as well as before and during administration of the drug, and when the intravenous fluids are reduced to maintenance volume levels. Daily weight measurements are important to assist in planning adequate hydration during chemotherapy, as well as to measure nutritional status.

Drug side effects may necessitate infusion of platelets or packed red blood cells. See the *Clinical Skills Manual* SKILLS for techniques to be used in these situations.

Many children are treated in an oncology clinic, staying in the hospital only on the day of intravenous drug administration and receiving oral medications at home. The time at the hospital is used to assess how the family is managing issues such as nutrition, sleep, medication administration, and obtaining psychosocial support. Careful teaching for the family is needed to ensure safe drug administration and identification of issues requiring further care.

Nurses play a key role in the long-term multidisciplinary treatment of children with leukemia. The impact of a diagnosis of leukemia and the long-term nature of treatment can severely stress the coping abilities of both the child and the family. Ongoing psychosocial assessment and emotional support are essential (see the general discussion of psychosocial assessment in the *Childhood Cancer* section earlier in this chapter). Referral to support groups

---

TEACHING HIGHLIGHTS | Chemotherapy for Childhood Leukemia

Physical Care
- Have rest periods each day.
- Avoid exposure to people with illnesses.
- Drink generous amounts of water.
- Eat a healthy diet, using frequent, small, and nutritious meals to obtain enough nutrients.
- Take medicines prescribed to decrease nausea.
- Maintain good oral hygiene with a soft toothbrush and water irrigation device.
- Avoid sun exposure and check skin each day for any signs of bruises, pressure areas, cuts, or scratches.
- Allow time for and eat foods to promote bowel elimination.
- Promote bowel elimination through regular dietary and toileting practices.
- Report any signs of infection, changes in condition, or other concerns.

Emotional Care
- Be prepared for loss of hair with plans for hats, wigs, or other alternatives.
- Continue contact with friends via phone, Internet, and in person when possible.
- Try relaxation techniques to aid in sleep and management of treatments.
- Talk with clergy, teachers, parents, counselors, friends, or other supportive people about the experience of having leukemia.
- Keep a journal to record feelings and experiences.

and social services may be beneficial. Help the family explore alternative therapies such as relaxation, imagery, and nutritional support that may aid the child. Be alert for any interactions that could occur between complementary therapies and the medical regimen.

Evaluation

Expected outcomes for nursing care of the child with leukemia include the following:

- Infection and other secondary complications of chemotherapy are prevented.
- Adequate hydration is maintained.
- Normal urinary output is maintained.
- Blood values are within normal limits.
- The family adapts successfully to parenting a child with chronic illness.
- Parents demonstrate adequate knowledge related to the disease process.

Soft-Tissue Tumors

Hodgkin Disease

Hodgkin disease, a disorder of the lymphoid system, usually arises in a single lymph node or an anatomic group of lymph nodes (see *Pathophysiology Illustrated: Hodgkin Disease*). Hodgkin disease rarely occurs before 10 years of age. It accounts for just 5% of cancers in children under 14 years, but 15% of cancer in youth from 15 to 19 years. The disease has a bimodal peak with higher incidence in the early 20s and after 50 years (Waxman, Hochberg, & Cairo, 2011). Three forms of the disease exist: the young person form in those under 14 years, the young adult form in persons from 15 to 34 years, and the older adult form in those over 50 years. There is a slightly increased incidence in males, which is more pronounced in the disease manifested in younger children (Carbone, Spina, Gloghini, et al., 2011).

ETIOLOGY AND PATHOPHYSIOLOGY

Hodgkin disease occurs in clusters and has been reported in families. This suggests a possible genetic link as well as an infectious agent (such as Epstein-Barr virus) or environmental hazard (Waxman et al., 2011).

CLINICAL MANIFESTATIONS

The main symptom of Hodgkin disease is nontender, firm lymphadenopathy, usually in the supraclavicular and cervical nodes but occasionally in the mediastinal area. A mediastinal growth can cause respiratory difficulty because of pressure on the trachea or bronchi. A characteristic large cell with multiple nuclei, called the Reed-Sternberg cell, is characteristic of Hodgkin disease, although

Pathophysiology Illustrated: **Hodgkin Disease**

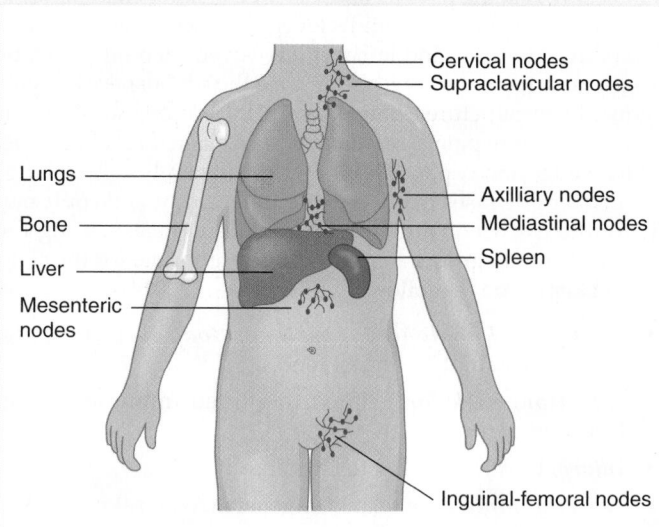

Lymph nodes and organs affected in Hodgkin disease in children.

the cell is found also in infectious mononucleosis and some other lymphomas. Fever, night sweats, and weight loss occur in one third of children with Hodgkin disease and are associated with a more aggressive form of the disease. The leukocyte count and erythrocyte sedimentation rate (ESR) may be elevated.

CLINICAL THERAPY

Diagnosis is based on the presence of Reed-Sternberg cells in a lymph node biopsy. A staging classification is used to determine disease severity (Table 50–8). The basis for staging is data obtained from the history, physical examination, chest x-ray study (for metastasis), chest CT scan, CT or MRI scans of the retroperitoneal nodes, lymphangiogram if there is retroperitoneal involvement, laboratory studies (complete blood count, ESR, serum copper level, C-reactive protein, liver and renal function tests), and a radionuclide scan with gallium. Bone marrow biopsy, bone scan, or a staging laparotomy may be performed if advanced disease is suspected. Minimally invasive surgery can be used to biopsy or remove the spleen for diagnosis, avoiding the potential complications of major surgery (Waxman et al., 2011).

Clinical Tip

The following are examples of drugs that may be used to treat Hodgkin disease:

- Doxorubicin
- Bleomycin
- Vinblastine
- Dacarbazine
- Etoposide
- Prednisone
- Cyclophosphamide
- Procarbazine
- Methotrexate
- Mechlorethamine

TABLE 50–8 Staging System for Hodgkin Disease

STAGE	DESCRIPTION
I	Disease within a single lymph node region
IE	Disease within a single extralymphatic organ or site outside of lymphatic system (extralymphatic organ)
II	Disease within two or more lymph node regions on same side of diaphragm
IIE	Disease within extralymphatic organ, and of one or more lymph node regions on same side of diaphragm
III	Disease of lymph node regions on both sides of diaphragm; stage III(1) indicates involvement of upper abdomen above the renal vein, whereas stage III(2) indicates involvement of pelvic or other lower abdomen nodes
IIIE	Disease of lymph node regions on both sides of the diaphragm with involvement of extralymphatic organ
IIIS	As in III, plus disease within spleen
IIISE	As in III, plus disease in extralymphatic organs and spleen
IV	Disseminated disease within one or more lymphatic organs with or without lymph node involvement

Source: Data from National Cancer Institute. (2011a). *Childhood Hodgkin lymphoma treatment: Staging and diagnostic evaluation.* Retrieved from http://www.cancer.gov/cancertopics/pdq/treatment/childhodgkins/HealthProfessional/page4.

Chemotherapy using a four-drug combination has been found to be the most effective drug treatment. Radiation is commonly added, with low doses for children who are still growing, and larger doses for those who are physically mature or those whose disease is more advanced at diagnosis. The 5-year survival rate is approximately 85% to 90%, depending on the stage of the disease at diagnosis.

Autologous stem cell or allogeneic stem cell transplant is a treatment option in children with advanced disease or relapse.

Non-Hodgkin Lymphoma

The four types of pediatric non-Hodgkin lymphoma (NHL) are (1) lymphoblastic lymphoma, (2) small noncleaved cell (Burkitt) lymphoma, (3) diffuse large B-cell lymphoma, and (4) anaplastic large cell lymphoma (Waxman et al., 2011). Lymphomas of all types are the third most common group of malignancies in children, following leukemia and brain tumors. Non-Hodgkin lymphomas are malignant tumors of lymphoreticular (internal framework of the lymph system) origin. The peak incidence for lymphomas occurs between the ages of 7 and 11 years, and they are three times more common in boys than in girls. The cure rate is 85% to 90% (Waxman et al., 2011).

Lymphoblastic non-Hodgkin lymphomas are caused by T-cell abnormalities. These abnormal T cells are diffuse, highly malignant, and very aggressive and do not mature. T-cell lymphomas produced by these cells often occur in children with congenital or acquired immunodeficiency states, chronic immune stimulation, or autoimmune disease. Some lymphomas have B-cell abnormalities, most specifically Burkitt lymphoma; 8q24 chromosomal translocation may be found in these cases (Waxman et al., 2011).

The incidence of lymphomas shows geographic variability. For example, a high incidence of Burkitt lymphoma is found in equatorial Africa, where it causes 50% of childhood cancers. Incidence in Hispanic children is higher than in White children, and African Americans have the lowest incidence. Boys are affected more than girls, and children with immune system compromise are most commonly affected. Epstein-Barr virus has been associated with Burkitt lymphoma, but in most cases of NHL, there are no known causes (Waxman et al., 2011).

Children with non-Hodgkin lymphoma frequently present with fever and weight loss. The lymph glands are usually enlarged or nodular, with the most frequent sites being the cervical, axillary, inguinal, and femoral nodes. However, the disease may be diffuse, without nodular glands. The anterior mediastinum is the primary site for T-cell lymphomas. Tumors that occur in this area may compress the airway (causing breathing difficulty) or superior vena cava (leading to swelling of the face, neck, or arms), and can cause pain. Jaw involvement is common in Burkitt lymphoma.

CBC is performed; additional blood tests include renal and liver function, electrolytes, uric acid, and LDH. Bone marrow aspiration and lumbar puncture are performed. Chest x-ray, bone scan, gallium scan, CT, and MRI can help to isolate affected body organs. Tissue biopsy confirms the diagnosis.

A staging system is used to describe the tumor mass and extension to other body areas (Table 50–9). Treatment is tailored to the type of cancer and its stage. Stages I and II may be treated with drugs such as vincristine, cyclophosphamide, prednisone, and methotrexate for several months. Intrathecal medication is added if head and neck cancers are present. Stages III and IV are treated with additional drugs (up to nine total) for longer periods (1 to 2 years). Radiation is uncommonly used and may be helpful to treat a tumor that is impinging on a body part. Surgery is used to biopsy the tumor mass and treat any complications caused by the cancer. HSCT is used for children with recurrent disease.

Rhabdomyosarcoma

Rhabdomyosarcoma is the most common soft-tissue tumor diagnosed in children, and is especially common in children under 5 years of age. The 5-year survival rate is 70% (Egas-Bejar & Huh, 2014). It occurs most often in the muscles around the eyes (extraorbital), in the neck, and less commonly in the abdomen, genitourinary tract, and extremities (Figure 50–10).

The cause of rhabdomyosarcoma is unknown. However, it is more common in children with neurofibromatosis and Li-Fraumeni syndrome. Mutations in tumor suppressor gene *p53* are sometimes seen. The abnormal cells arise from mesenchyme that normally grows into muscle, fat, and bone.

Tumors close to the eye produce swelling, ptosis, visual disturbances, and eye movement abnormalities. When the tumor occurs in the genitourinary tract, the result can be urinary obstruction, hematuria, dysuria, vaginal discharge, and a

TABLE 50–9 St. Jude Children's Research Hospital Staging Classification for Non-Hodgkin Lymphoma

STAGE	DESCRIPTION
I	Single tumor or node area involved; no tumor in abdomen or mediastinum
II	Single tumor with lymph node involvement; or two node areas or tumor on same side of diaphragm; or GI tumor in one site
III	Two tumors or node areas on different sides of diaphragm; or a primary mediastinal, intra-abdominal, or epidural tumor
IV	Any involvement with CNS or bone marrow metastases

Source: Adapted from National Cancer Institute. (2011b). *Childhood non-Hodgkin lymphoma treatment: Stage information.* Retrieved from http://www.cancer.gov/cancertopics/pdq/treatment/child-non-hodgkins/HealthProfessional.

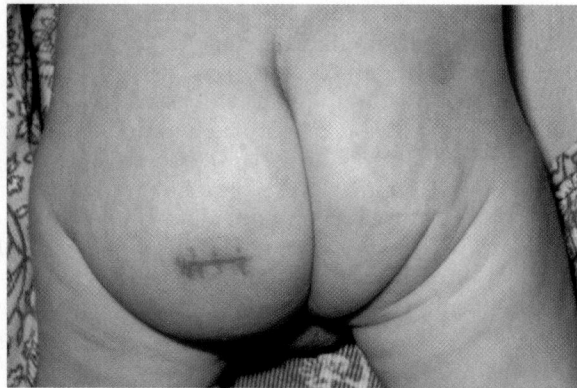

Figure 50–10 Rhabdomyosarcoma can occur in soft tissue throughout the body. Although the areas around eyes and neck are common sites, soft tissue around genitalia, in extremities, and in other sites can also be affected. A biopsy was performed on the buttock of this infant, who will now undergo chemotherapy and surgical removal of the rhabdomyosarcoma tumor, followed by further chemotherapy.
SOURCE: Dr. P. Marazzi/Science Source.

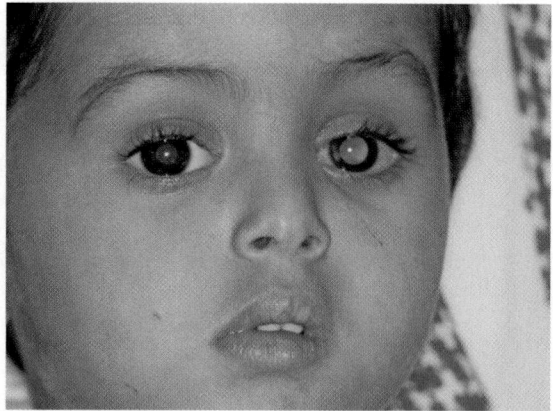

Figure 50–11 Retinoblastoma is characterized by leukokoria, a white reflection in the pupil.
SOURCE: Custom Medical Stock Photo/Newscom.

protruding vaginal mass. Rhabdomyosarcoma occurring in the abdomen may be asymptomatic. There is rapid metastasis to the lungs, bones, bone marrow, and distant lymph nodes.

Diagnosis is confirmed by CT, MRI, PET, bone marrow aspiration, and biopsy. CBC, renal and liver studies, and urinalysis are performed. Lumbar puncture may be used in head and neck tumors. A useful biologic marker, desmin, allows differentiation of rhabdomyosarcoma from other round cell tumors. A significant number of children have metastatic disease at the time of diagnosis, so chest and lung CT scans, as well as regional lymph node biopsies are performed (Arndt, 2011b).

Treatment includes surgical removal of the tumor when possible. However, if the tumor involves other structures, removal may not be possible. Many children have metastasis at the time of diagnosis, so the primary tumor may not be removed. Surgery is followed by wide-field radiation and chemotherapy with a combination of drugs. Some commonly used drugs include the following:

- Vincristine
- Actinomycin
- Cyclophosphamide (VAC therapy)

Prognosis depends on the site, staging (Table 50–10), and histologic findings.

Retinoblastoma

Retinoblastoma is an intraocular malignancy of the retina. It may be bilateral (20% to 30%) or unilateral. In 40% of children, the disease is inherited by an autosomal dominant gene. Family

TABLE 50–10 Classification of Rhabdomyosarcoma

STAGE	DESCRIPTION
I	Localized tumor, completely resected disease
II	Total gross resection with regional microscopic spread
III	Locally extensive tumor with residual microscopic spread
IV	Any size primary tumor with distant metastatic disease present

Source: Data from National Cancer Institute. (2011c). *Childhood rhabdomyosarcoma treatment: Stage information*. Retrieved from http://www.cancer.gov/cancertopics/pdq/treatment/childrhabdomyosarcoma/HealthProfessional.

history is therefore important to collect, although many cases occur with no family history of the cancer (Zage & Herzog, 2011). The tumor arises from embryonic retinal cells. It may be a new mutation or may be passed on to offspring of affected individuals in an autosomal dominant manner. The retinoblastoma gene, *RB1*, is on chromosome 13q14.

The first sign of retinoblastoma is a white pupil, termed *leukokoria* or *cat's-eye reflex* (Figure 50–11). The red reflex is absent, asymmetric, or of a differing color in the affected eye. Other symptoms may include a fixed strabismus (a constant deviation of one eye from the other), orbital inflammation, glaucoma, and heterochromia (irises of different colors).

Retinoblastoma is usually diagnosed when the child is between 1 and 2 years of age. A family history should alert healthcare providers so that regular ophthalmologic examinations can be performed frequently on infants and young children in the family. The appearance of a unilateral tumor demands regular examinations of the healthy eye since bilateral disease can develop. In some children, a pineal gland tumor can also develop, causing CNS symptoms. The overall tumor-free survival rate is 95% (Zage & Herzog, 2011).

Diagnostic tests for the cancer include full ocular examination and CT or MRI scans of the eye orbit. All children with a history of retinoblastoma in the family should be examined by an ophthalmologist after birth, at 6 weeks, every 2 to 3 months until 2 years, every 4 months until 3 years, and then annually to aid in early diagnosis. Tumors are classified according to a staging system, from a very small localized tumor (group I) to tumors involving more than half the retina and with seeding into the vitreous (group V).

Treatment for retinoblastoma may include removal of the eye (enucleation) when there is permanent retinal damage or failure to respond to other treatment. Other surgical treatments involve cryotherapy or photocoagulation (argon laser therapy). Radiation is nearly always used, either as the sole treatment or before surgery to shrink the tumor. Chemotherapy is sometimes used but is frequently ineffective because the drugs often fail to penetrate sufficiently into the eye. Chemotherapeutic drugs include carboplatin, etoposide, vincristine, and cyclosporine. Multiple therapies are more commonly used in children with bilateral retinoblastoma. Children with retinoblastoma are at increased risk of developing a secondary tumor, including another retinoblastoma or a sarcoma, most commonly osteogenic sarcoma. However, most young children who have been treated for the disease have good health and normal mental abilities several years after treatment. The most common sequela of retinoblastoma is decrease in visual acuity.

Nursing Management

For the Child With a Soft-Tissue Tumor

Nursing Assessment and Diagnosis

PHYSIOLOGIC ASSESSMENT

Physiologic assessment of the child with a soft-tissue tumor, such as Hodgkin disease, non-Hodgkin lymphoma, rhabdomyosarcoma, and other lymphomas, focuses on the child's general condition. Accurate height and weight measurements are essential to provide a baseline against which to measure the child's growth during treatment, as well as for calculation of chemotherapeutic drug dosages.

Observe the area of the tumor, such as the face, neck, and abdomen, and describe any changes. Monitor respiratory status if the tumor is in the face or neck. Report any changes in respiratory pattern to the oncology specialist. Avoid palpation of any tumor site or enlarged area; injudicious palpation and manipulation of a tumor site can influence metastasis. Notify the primary healthcare provider of a change in any lymph node or any other area of the body.

Gastrointestinal and genitourinary functions can be altered by the presence of a tumor and by treatment such as chemotherapy and radiation. Careful measurement of the child's intake and output is essential. Abdominal tumors may affect defecation, so charting of all bowel movements is important. Explain to the family and child why keeping accurate records is necessary.

Observe wounds closely for lack of healing as a result of chemotherapy or radiation. Examine the mouth and extremities for wounds or ulcers. Nutritional changes caused by treatment will affect the body's ability to support healthy cells and heal wounds.

A thorough eye examination is warranted for any child who has a family history of retinoblastoma or has undergone treatment for a prior tumor. Assess color and position of the iris and eye movements and perform the cover–uncover test and other eye tests described in Chapter 33. Ask whether the child has been evaluated by an ophthalmologist.

PSYCHOSOCIAL ASSESSMENT

Refer to the general discussion of psychosocial assessment in the *Childhood Cancer* section earlier in this chapter. Assessment of body image is needed when the child has a soft-tissue tumor affecting appearance of the head and neck.

The location and type of a soft-tissue tumor determine the specific nursing diagnoses for a particular child. Common nursing diagnoses might include the following (NANDA-I © 2014):

- *Tissue Perfusion: Peripheral, Risk for Ineffective*, related to interruption of blood flow
- *Breathing Pattern, Ineffective*, related to effect of tumor deformity on neck or chest wall
- *Swallowing, Impaired*, related to tumor or treatment
- *Development: Delayed, Risk for*, related to effects of treatment
- *Body Image, Disturbed*, related to illness and treatment

Planning and Implementation

Nursing management of children with soft-tissue tumors varies depending on the specific tumor. Children with lymphoma affecting the mediastinum may need respiratory support. Position the child so that the head is elevated. Administer chemotherapeutic drugs as ordered, maintaining adequate fluids to facilitate excretion of the resultant breakdown products. Monitor the central line used for chemotherapy administration, and teach parents care of the central line when the child is at home.

For the child with a rhabdomyosarcoma involving the bladder, monitor urinary output carefully. Report hematuria and painful urination. Monitor the changes that occur during therapy. For example, in children with eye tumors, observe for a decrease in ptosis, which may indicate successful treatment. Administer pain medications as needed and use distraction and other techniques to decrease the child's discomfort. Emphasize to parents the need for follow-up CT and MRI scans after completion of treatment.

When the child with retinoblastoma undergoes removal of the eye, the parents and child will need detailed instructions on postsurgical care. Demonstrate to the parents care of the socket and use of a conformer to maintain the eye socket shape. When healing is complete and the child receives a prosthetic eye, instruct parents about its insertion and care. The child can gradually be taught to take over this care when old enough. Encourage periodic healthcare visits to monitor for signs of a tumor in the other eye. Interventions to encourage normal developmental milestones are adapted if sensory alteration has resulted.

Pay attention to the body changes associated with the cancer and its treatment. Children and adolescents may need suggestions to deal with hair loss, disfigurement, and living with serious illness. Referral to other children and teens with similar concerns may be helpful. Parents of all children need help to encourage normal development in the child with cancer.

The child with a soft-tissue tumor often receives chemotherapy or radiation, or sometimes both modalities. Nursing management during chemotherapy and radiation is discussed earlier in this chapter in the general sections on these treatment measures and in *Nursing Care Plan: Hospital Care of the Child With Cancer*. Generally, the family needs help to adjust to the diagnosis of a life-threatening disease and to the care of the ill child. Refer to Chapter 39 for a description of postsurgical care. Consult Chapter 45 for strategies to assist the child and family if the child has a visual impairment resulting from a retinoblastoma. Topics for parent and family teaching and discharge planning are similar to those previously presented.

COMMUNITY-BASED NURSING CARE

Reinforce with families the importance of long-term follow-up after treatment for a soft-tissue tumor. Increased risk for secondary cancers for 2 to 3 decades is possible, and early identification can help with prompt diagnosis. Partner with other healthcare providers to provide instructions to families as the child transitions from oncology treatment back to the pediatrician so they understand the importance of telling all healthcare providers about the cancer and treatment. Establish oncology clinics to track and examine survivors. As children grow into teen and young adult years, help them to take over this important task in their care.

Some recommended annual examinations include the following:

- CBC
- Physical examination with special attention to skin, abdomen, and thyroid
- Monitoring for signs of hypothyroidism and hyperthyroidism
- Neurologic and developmental examinations; monitoring of school performance
- First mammogram at 25 years in those with chest radiation
- Pap and pelvic examinations for teen and young adult women
- Mental status assessment

TEACHING HIGHLIGHTS | Care of the Child With a Soft-Tissue Tumor

- Teach the family about the chemotherapeutic drugs and their side effects.
- Teach about the care of surgically placed venous access devices.
- Provide written and illustrated information about the chemotherapy protocol(s).
- Provide the family with radiation and surgery education specific to the tumor treatment.
- Refer the family to nutrition resources such as dietitians for ways to promote the child's adequate intake of food and fluid.

Evaluation

The following expected outcomes of nursing care for the child with a soft-tissue tumor are examples that illustrate the varied tumor presentations:

- Side effects of treatment are successfully managed.
- The surgical site heals with no signs of infection.
- The child adapts successfully to sensory loss resulting from cancer or treatment.
- The child adapts to an altered self-image.
- The child achieves growth and development to maximum potential.
- In cases of terminal disease, parents receive adequate support for the process of anticipatory grieving.

Focus Your Study

- Cancer is a leading cause of illness and death among children.
- Cancer may be influenced by chromosomal or genetic messages, environmental carcinogens, or infectious process; often a combination of factors is present.
- Cancer treatments include surgery, chemotherapy, radiation, biotherapy, and alternative therapies. Palliative care is needed when disease has relapsed and cure is no longer possible.
- Oncologic emergencies are life-threatening conditions caused by cancer or its treatment; the main types of emergencies are metabolic, hematologic, or space occupying.
- Key signs of childhood cancer are pain, cachexia, anemia, infection, bruising, petechiae, and neurologic symptoms.
- A protocol is a plan of action for chemotherapy that is based on the type of cancer, its stage, and the particular cell type,
- Nursing assessment for children with cancer involves detailed physical data, as well as psychologic factors, developmental achievements, and family social status.
- Common physical nursing interventions for children with cancer involve nutrition, medication administration, hydration, infection prevention, pain management, and measures to decrease side effects of treatment. Families require ongoing psychosocial support, information, and referral to diverse resources when caring for the child with cancer.
- While the numbers of children who are long-term survivors continue to grow, some of these children experience lasting effects such as cognitive or behavioral problems, recurrent or secondary cancers, or discrimination.

- Nursing care after cancer treatment is completed includes monitoring for any long-term physiologic or psychosocial sequelae.
- Common brain tumors in children include medulloblastoma, astrocytoma, ependyoma, and glioma; neuroblastoma is a tumor that is located along the sympathetic nervous system chain.
- Headache, vomiting, ataxia, seizures, increased intracranial pressure, hydrocephalus, and sensory disturbances are the major clinical manifestations of brain tumors.
- Nephroblastoma (Wilms tumor) is an intrarenal tumor; when suspected, the abdomen should not be palpated.
- Common bone tumors in childhood are osteosarcoma and Ewing sarcoma; both are most common among adolescents.
- Leukemia is a common childhood malignancy, with the major types being acute lymphoblastic leukemia (ALL) and acute myelogenous leukemia (AML).
- A variety of soft tissue tumors are seen in children and adolescents; they include Hodgkin disease, non-Hodgkin lymphoma, rhabdomyosarcoma, and retinoblastoma.
- Nurses are in a key position to assist families during the cancer diagnosis, treatment during adjustment to school and other life tasks, and in providing palliative care for children who do not survive.

Clinical Reasoning in Action

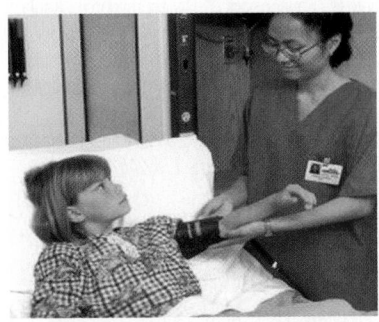

Seven-year-old Christina is brought to the hospital with an unusual rash, lethargy, and fever. Blood work is drawn, and the results are abnormal. The hematologist confirms that Christina has acute lymphoblastic leukemia (ALL), the most common childhood cancer. Her parents are in shock and disbelief about the news; she seems too young. Christina is immediately admitted to the hospital and put on an IV with orders for more blood work.

Christina's blood work demonstrates the following: hemoglobin 9 g/dL, leukocytes 20,000/mm^3, and platelets 90,000/mm^3.

Chemotherapy was initiated and precautions were taken to avoid infections. Recommendations for Christina include rest times daily, generous amounts of water, intake of healthy foods, and avoidance of sun exposure. The parents are happy when Christina comes home during the chemotherapy. The hematologist advises them it is not uncommon to return to the hospital because of a chemotherapeutic complication. The parents are encouraged to remember to take care of themselves. This will help them deal with Christina's therapy more effectively.

1. What are some of the common side effects of chemotherapy?
2. Why is it important to check Christina's daily weights?
3. What symptoms should Christina's parents report to the doctor while she is on chemotherapy?
4. What are some developmentally appropriate techniques you can encourage that will assist Christina to deal with her illness?

References

American Cancer Society (ACS). (2011). *Cancer in children.* Retrieved from http://www.cancer.org

Anderson, P. M., Dhamne, C. A., & Huff, V. (2011). Wilms tumor. In R. M. Kliegman, B. F. Stanton, J. W. St. Geme, N. F. Schor, & R. E. Behrman (Eds.), *Nelson textbook of pediatrics* (19th ed., pp. 1760–1762). Philadelphia, PA: Elsevier Saunders.

Arndt, C. A. S. (2011a). Neuroblastoma. In R. M. Kliegman, B. F. Stanton, J. W. St. Geme, N. F. Schor, & R. E. Behrman (Eds.), *Nelson textbook of pediatrics* (19th ed., pp. 1763–1768). Philadelphia, PA: Elsevier Saunders.

Arndt, C. A. S. (2011b). Soft tissue sarcomas. In R. M. Kliegman, B. F. Stanton, J. W. St. Geme, N. F. Schor, & R. E. Behrman (Eds.), *Nelson textbook of pediatrics* (19th ed., pp. 1760–1762). Philadelphia, PA: Elsevier Saunders.

Bartel, K. A., Gradisar, M., & Williamson, P. (2014). Protective and risk factors for adolescent sleep: A meta-analytic review. *Sleep Medicine Review, (Sept),* S1087–S0792.

Bhatia, S. (2011). Disparities in cancer outcomes: Lessons learned from children with cancer. *Pediatric Blood & Cancer, 56,* 994–1002.

Bindler, R. M., & Howry, L. B. (2005). *Pediatric drug guide.* Upper Saddle River, NJ: Prentice Hall.

Brain tumor incidence in the U.S. (2011). *Journal of the National Cancer Institute, 103*(9), 707.

Buckley, K. S. (2011). Pediatric genitourinary tumors. *Current Opinion in Oncology, 23,* 297–302.

Burns, R. A., Topoz, I., & Reynolds, S. L. (2014). Tumor lysis syndrome: Risk factors, diagnosis, and management. *Pediatric Emergency Care, 30,* 571–576.

Calzone, K. A., Jenkins, J., Culp, S, Caskey, S., & Badzek, L. (2014). Introducing a new competency into nursing practice. *Journal of Nursing Regulation, 5,* 40–47.

Carbone, A., Spina, M., Gloghini, A., & Tirelli, U. (2011). Classical Hodgkin's lymphoma arising in different host's conditions: Pathobiology parameters, therapeutic options, and outcome. *America Journal of Hematology, 86,* 170–179.

Chen, X., Bahrami, A., Pappo, A., Easton, J., Dalton, J., Hedlund, J., ... Dyer, M. A. (2014). Recurrent somatic structural variations contribute to tumorigenesis in pediatric osteosarcoma. *Cell Reports, 7,* 104–112.

Clanton, N. R., Klosky, J. L., Jain, N., Srivastava, D. K., Mulrooney, D., Zeltzer, L., ... Krull, K. R. (2011). Fatigue, vitality, sleep, and neurocognitive functioning in adult survivors of childhood cancer: A report from the childhood cancer survivor study. *Cancer.* doi:10.1002/cncr.25797

Cohen, I. J., & Wolff, J. E. (2013). How long can folinic acid rescue be delayed after high-dose methotrexate without toxicity? *Pediatric Blood & Cancer, 61,* 7–10.

Demirkaya, M., Sevinir, B., Yalcinkaya, U., & Yazici, Z. (2012). Disseminated rhabdomyosarcoma presenting as hypercalcemia. *Indian Pediatrics, 49,* 66–67.

Egas-Bejar, D., & Huh, W. W. (2014). Rhabdomyosarcoma in adolescent and young adult patients: Current perspectives. *Adolescent Health, Medicine and Therapeutics, 5,* 115–125.

Erickson, J. M., Beck, S. L., Christian, B., Dudley, W. N., Hollen, P. J., Albritton, K., ... Godder, K. (2011). Fatigue, sleep–wake disturbances, and quality of life in adolescents receiving chemotherapy. *Journal of Pediatric Hematology and Oncology, 33,* e17–e25.

Eshelman-Kent, D., Kinahan, K. E., Hobbie, W., Landier, W., Teal, S., Friedman, D., ... Freyer, D. R. (2011). Cancer survivorship practices, services, and delivery: A report from the Children's Oncology Group (COG) nursing discipline, adolescent/young adult, and late effects committees. *Journal of Cancer Survivorship, 5*(4), 345–357.

Faria, C. M., Rutka, J. T., Smith, C., & Kongkham, P. (2011). Epigenetic mechanisms regulating neural development and pediatric brain tumor formation. *Journal of Neurosurgery: Pediatrics, 8,* 119–132.

Fielding, F., Sanford, T. M., & Davis, M. P. (2013). Achieving effective control in cancer pain: A review of current guidelines. *International Journal of Palliative Nursing, 19,* 584–591.

Greco, K. E., Tinley, S., & Seibert, D. (2011). Development of the essential genetic and genomic competencies for nurses with graduate degrees. *Annual Review of Nursing Research, 29,* 173–190.

Greinert, R., & Boniol, M. (2011). Skin cancer—Primary and secondary prevention (information campaigns and screening)—With a focus on children and sunbeds. *Progress in Biophysics and Molecular Biology, 107*(3), 473–476.

HaDuong, J. H., Martin, A. A., Skapek, S. X., & Mascarenhas, L. (2015). Sarcomas. *Pediatric Clinics of North America, 62,* 179–200.

Henderson, T. O., Bhatia, S., Pinto, N., London, W. B., McGrady, P., Crotty, C., ... Cohn, S. L. (2011). Racial and ethnic disparities in risk and survival in children with neuroblastoma: A Children's Oncology Group study. *Journal of Clinical Oncology, 29,* 76–82.

Henry, M., & Sung, L. (2015). Supportive care in pediatric oncology: Oncologic emergencies and management of fever and neutropenia. *Pediatric Clinics of North America, 62,* 27–46.

Huff, V. (2011). Wilms tumours: About tumour suppressor genes, an oncogene and a chameleon gene. *Nature Reviews Cancer, 11,* 111–121.

Kirchhoff, A. C., Krull, K. R., Ness, K. K., Armstrong, G. T., Park, E. R., Stovall, M., ... Leisenring, W. (2011). Physical, mental, and neurocognitive status and employment outcomes in the childhood cancer survivor study cohort. *Cancer Epidemiology and Biomarkers Prevention, 20,* 1838–1849.

Kishimoto, K., Kobayashi, R., Ichikawa, M., Sano, H., Suzuki, D., Yasuda, K., ... Kobayashi, K. (2014). Risk factors for tumor lysis syndrome in childhood acute myeloid leukemia treated with a uniform protocol without rasburicase prophylaxis. *Leukemia and Lymphoma, 26,* 1–11.

Kolyva, S., Efthymiadou, A., Gkentizi, D., Karana-Ginopoulou, A., & Varvarigou, A. (2014). Hypercalcemia and osteolytic lesions as presenting symptoms of acute lymphoblastic leukemia in childhood. *Journal of Pediatric Endocrinology and Metabolism, 27,* 349–354.

Kuttesch J. F., Rush, S. Z., & Ater, J. L. (2011). Brain tumors in children. In R. M. Kliegman, B. F. Stanton, J. W. St. Geme, N. F. Schor, & R. E. Behrman (Eds.), *Nelson textbook of pediatrics* (19th ed., pp. 1746–1753). Philadelphia, PA: Elsevier Saunders.

Landier, W., Armenian, S., & Bhatia, S. (2015). Late effects of childhood cancer and its treatment. *Pediatric Clinics of North America, 62*, 275–300.

Lewis, M. A., Hendrickson, A. W., & Moynihan, T. J. (2011). Oncologic emergencies: Pathophysiology, presentations, diagnosis, and treatment. *Cancer Journal for Clinicians, 61*, 287–314.

Manfrini, M., Tiwari, A., Ham, J., Colangeli, M., & Mercuri, M. (2011). Evolution of surgical treatment for sarcomas of proximal humerus in children: Retrospective review of a single institute over 30 years. *Journal of Pediatric Orthopedics, 31*, 56–64.

Masetti, R., Kleinschmidt, K., Biagi, C., & Pession, A. (2011). Emerging targeted therapies for pediatric myeloid leukemia. *Recent Patents on Anticancer Drug Discovery, 6*, 354–366.

Matthews, E. E., Neu, M., Cook, P. F., & King, N. (2014). Sleep in mother and child dyads during treatment for pediatric acute lymphoblastic leukemia. *Oncology Nursing Forum, 41*, 599–610.

McLendon, R. E., Adekunle, A., Rajaram, V., Kocak, M., & Blaney, S. M. (2011). Embryonal central nervous system neoplasms arising in infants and young children. *Archives of Pathology and Laboratory Medicine, 135*, 984–993.

Messinger, Y. H., Higgins, R. R., Devidas, M., Hunger, S. P., Carroll, A. J., & Heerema, N. A. (2012). Pediatric acute lymphoblastic leukemia with a t(8;14) (q11.2;q32): B-cell disease with a high proportion of Down syndrome: A Children's Oncology Group study. *Cancer Genetics, 205*, 453–458.

Meyer, W. H., & Grier, H. E. (2014). Comparing oxozophosphorines for treating Ewing sarcoma. *Journal of Clinical Oncology, 32*, 2401–2402.

Moore, D. D., & Haydon, R. C. (2014). Ewing's sarcoma of bone. *Cancer Treatment Research, 162*, 93–115.

National Cancer Institute. (2011a). *Childhood Hodgkin lymphoma treatment: Staging and diagnostic evaluation.* Retrieved from http://www.cancer.gov.cancertopics /pdq/treatment/childhodgkins/HealthProfessional /page4

National Cancer Institute. (2011b). *Childhood non-Hodgkin lymphoma treatment: Stage information.* Retrieved from http://www.cancer.gov.cancertopics /pdq/treatment/child-non-hodgkins/HealthProfessional

National Cancer Institute. (2011c). *Childhood rhabdomyosarcoma treatment: Stage information.* Retrieved from http://www.cancer.gov/cancertopics/pdq/treatment /childrhabdomyosarcoma/HealthProfessional

National Cancer Institute. (2011d). *Pediatric considerations for depression.* Retrieved from http://www.cancer.gov .cancertopics

National Cancer Institute. (2011e). *Stages of neuroblastoma.* Retrieved from http://www.cancer.gov.cancertopics /pdq/treatment/neuroblastoma/HealthProfessional/page2

National Cancer Institute. (2011f). *Wilms tumor and other childhood kidney tumors treatment: Stage information.* Retrieved from http://www.cancer.gov .cancertopics/pdq/treatment/wilms/HealthProfessional /page3

Paisley, M. A., Kang, T. I., Insogna, I. G., & Rheingold, S. R. (2011). Complementary and alternative therapy use in pediatric oncology patients with failure of frontline chemotherapy. *Pediatrics & Blood Cancer, 56*, 1088–1091.

Paldino, M. J., Faerber, E. N., & Poussaint, T. Y. (2011). Imaging tumors of the pediatric central nervous system. *Radiology Clinics of North America, 49*, 589–616.

Pollack, I. F. (2011). Multidisciplinary management of childhood brain tumors: A review of outcomes, recent advances, and challenges. *Journal of Neurosurgery: Pediatrics, 8*, 133–148.

Pollack, I. F., & Jakacki, R. I. (2011). Childhood brain tumors: Epidemiology, current management and future directions. *Nature Reviews Neurology, 7*, 495–506.

Pui, C. H., Carroll, W. L., Meshinchi, S., & Arceci, R. J. (2011). Biology, risk stratification, and therapy of pediatric acute leukemias: An update. *Journal of Clinical Oncology, 29*, 551–565.

Rabin, K. R., & Poplack, D. G. (2011). Management strategies in acute lymphoblastic leukemia. *Oncology, 25*, 328–335.

Reulen, R. C., Frobisher, C., Winter, D. L., Kelly, J., Lancashire, E. R., Stiller, C. A., … Hawkins, M. M. (2011). Long-term risks of subsequent primary neoplasms among survivors of childhood cancer. *Journal of the American Medical Association, 305*, 2311–2319.

Roberts, I., & Izraeli, S. (2014). Haemotopoietic development and leukemia in Down syndrome. *British Journal of Haemotology, 167*, 587–599.

Rueegg, C. S., Gianinazzi, M. E., Rischewski, J., Beck Popovic, M., von der Weid, N. X., Michel, G., & Kuehni, C. E. (2013). Health-related quality of life in survivors of childhood cancer: The role of chronic health problems. *Journal of Cancer Survivorship: Research and Practice, 7*, 511–522.

Shuangshoti, S., Shuangshoti, S., Nuchprayoon, I., Kanjanapongkul, S., Marrano, P., Irwin, M. S., & Thorner, P. S. (2011). Natural course of low risk neuroblastoma. *Pediatrics & Blood Cancer.* doi:10.1002/pbc.23325

Sigel, K., Dubrow, R., Silverberg, M., Crothers, K., Braithwaite, S., & Justice, A. (2011). Cancer screening in patients with HIV. *Current HIV/AIDS Report, 8*, 142–152.

Smith, M. A., & Reaman, G. H. (2015). Remaining challenges in childhood cancer and newer targeted therapeutics. *Pediatric Clinics of North America, 62*, 301–312.

Steinberger, J., Sinaiko, A. R., Kelly, A. S., Leisenring, W. M., Steffen, L. M., Goodman, P., … Baker, K. S. (2012). Cardiovascular risk and insulin resistance in childhood cancer survivors. *Journal of Pediatrics, 160*(3), 494–499.

Tubergen, D. G., Bleyer, A., & Ritchey, A. K. (2011). The leukemias. In R. M. Kliegman, B. F. Stanton, J. W. St. Geme, N. F. Schor, & R. E. Behrman (Eds.), *Nelson textbook of pediatrics* (19th ed., pp. 1732–1739). Philadelphia, PA: Elsevier Saunders.

Ward, L. D., Haberman, M., & Barbosa-Leiker, C. (2014). Development and psychometric evaluation of the genomic nursing concept inventory. *Journal of Nursing Education, 53*, 511–518.

Waxman, I. M., Hochberg, J., & Cairo, M. S. (2011). Lymphoma. In R. M. Kliegman, B. F. Stanton, J. W. St. Geme, N. F. Schor, & R. E. Behrman (Eds.), *Nelson textbook of pediatrics* (19th ed., pp. 1739–1753). Philadelphia, PA: Elsevier Saunders.

Winick, N. (2011). Neurocognitive outcome in survivors of pediatric cancer. *Current Opinion in Pediatrics, 23*, 27–33.

Zage, P. E., & Ater, J. L. (2011). Neuroblastoma. In R. M. Kliegman, B. F. Stanton, J. W. St. Geme, N. F. Schor, & R. E. Behrman (Eds.), *Nelson textbook of pediatrics* (19th ed., pp. 1753–1757). Philadelphia, PA: Elsevier Saunders.

Zage, P. E., & Herzog, C. E. (2011). Retinoblastoma. In R. M. Kliegman, B. F. Stanton, J. W. St Geme, N. F. Schor, & R. E. Behrman (Eds.), *Nelson textbook of pediatrics* (19th ed., pp. 1768–1769). Philadelphia, PA: Elsevier Saunders.

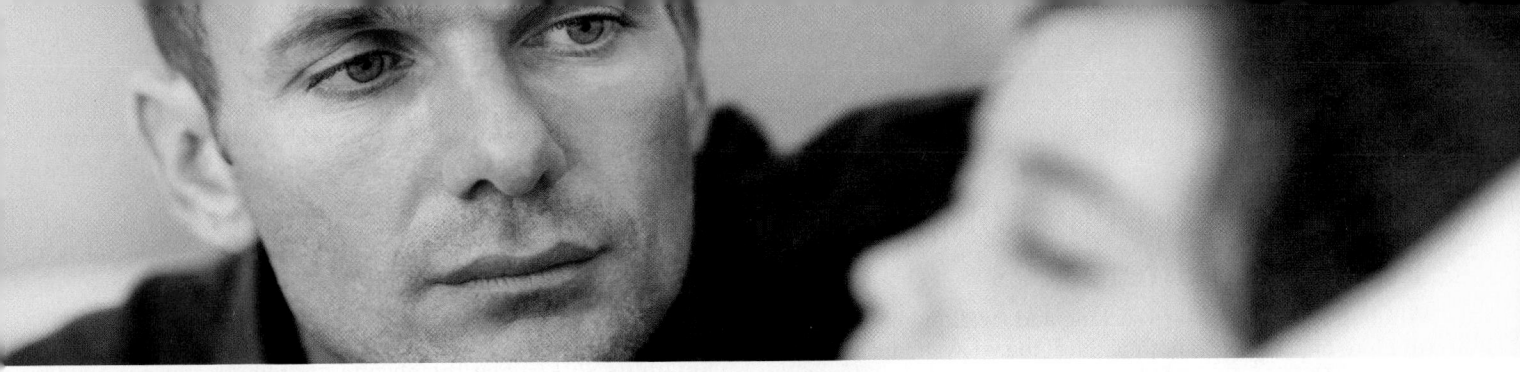

Chapter 51
The Child With Alterations in Gastrointestinal Function

I was so worried when Jerome was born. He had no anal opening and his esophagus did not lead to his stomach. Now that he's had several surgeries, he is growing and doing pretty well, and I'm so happy to see him starting to smile. I can't wait until his final surgery is completed and he no longer has the colostomy.

—Mother of Jerome, 6 months old

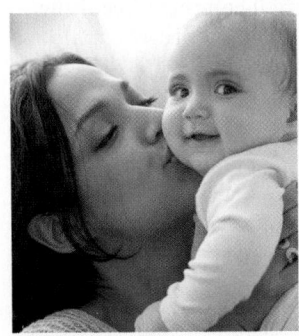

Monkey 3000/Fotolia

⌄ Learning Outcomes

51.1 Describe the general function of the gastrointestinal system.

51.2 Discuss the pathophysiologic processes associated with specific gastrointestinal disorders in the pediatric population.

51.3 Identify signs and symptoms that may indicate a disorder of the gastrointestinal system.

51.4 Contrast nursing management and plan care for disorders of the gastrointestinal system

for the child needing abdominal surgery versus the child needing nonoperative management.

51.5 Analyze developmentally appropriate approaches for nursing management of gastrointestinal disorders in the pediatric population.

51.6 Plan nursing care for the child with an injury to the gastrointestinal system.

What causes structural defects of the gastrointestinal tract such as the esophageal atresia and imperforate anus experienced by Jerome? What special care do children with gastrointestinal abnormalities need to promote growth and development during treatment for those anomalies? This chapter discusses the care of infants who have structural defects and those with other common disorders of gastrointestinal functioning.

Through the gastrointestinal (GI) tract, a child ingests and absorbs the foods and fluids necessary to sustain life and promote growth. Most GI disturbances produce short-term symptoms that interfere with nutrition and fluid balance only briefly. Some disorders or severe defects lead to complications that prevent optimal nutrition and adequate growth. This

chapter explores some common GI disorders in children. (See Chapter 44 for a discussion of specific fluid imbalances that may accompany GI disorders.)

GI disorders can result from a congenital defect, acquired disease, infection, or injury. Structural problems may occur when development is altered or ceases in the first trimester of gestation. Because various parts of the GI system are developing at this point in gestation, it is not unusual for infants to have more than one structural defect of the GI system. This was the case with Jerome, the child mentioned in the chapter-opening quotation. Infections can cause an increase or decrease in motility and prevent proper absorption of nutrients. Interruption or destruction of the GI system can also result from trauma. While reading this chapter, remember that any interruption or alteration in the GI system decreases the body's ability to obtain nutrients, thus impairing growth.

Anatomy and Physiology of Pediatric Differences

Although the fetus makes sucking and swallowing movements in utero and ingests amniotic fluid, the GI system is immature at birth. The processes of absorption and excretion do not begin until after birth because the placenta provides nutrients and removes waste. Sucking is a primitive reflex that occurs whenever the lips or cheeks are stroked. The infant does not have voluntary control over swallowing until about 6 weeks of age.

The stomach capacity of the newborn is quite small, and intestinal motility (**peristalsis**) is greater than in older children (see *As Children Grow: Stomach Capacity*). These characteristics explain the newborn's need for small, frequent feedings and the increased frequency and liquid consistency of bowel movements. Because of the relaxed lower esophageal sphincter, infants frequently regurgitate small amounts of feedings.

Digestion takes place in the duodenum. Infants have a deficiency of several enzymes: amylase (which digests carbohydrates), lipase (which enhances fat absorption), and trypsin (which catabolizes protein into polypeptides and some amino acids). Enzymes are usually not present in sufficient quantities to aid digestion until 4 to 6 months of age. Thus abdominal distention from gas is common.

Liver function is also immature. After the first few weeks of life, the liver is able to conjugate bilirubin and excrete bile. The processes of **gluconeogenesis** (formation of glycogen from non-carbohydrates), plasma protein and ketone formation, vitamin storage, and **deamination** (removal of amino group from amino compound) remain immature during the first year of life.

By the second year of life, digestive processes are fairly complete. Stomach capacity increases to accommodate a three-meals-per-day feeding schedule. Around 18 months of age, the child becomes aware of a full rectum and is physically able to have some control over excretory functions (Goldson & Reynolds, 2012). See the accompanying *Assessment Guide: The Child With a Gastrointestinal Condition* for guidelines for assessing the gastrointestinal system.

Structural Defects

Structural defects can involve one or more areas of the gastrointestinal tract. These defects occur when growth and development of fetal structures are interrupted during the first trimester. This can leave the structure incomplete, resulting in *atresia* (absence or closure of a normal body orifice), malposition, nonclosure, or other abnormalities.

Cleft Lip and Cleft Palate

Cleft lip and cleft palate are two distinct facial defects that can occur singly or in combination (Figure 51–1). Cleft lip with or without cleft palate occurs in 1 out of every 750 to 1000 live births. The incidence is higher in Asian (1 in 500) than in White children (1 in 750). The defect is less common in African Americans, with an incidence of 1 of every 2000 live births. Cleft lip

---

As Children Grow: **Stomach Capacity**

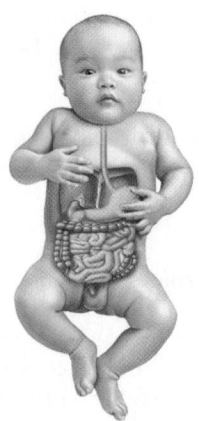

The young infant has a smaller stomach capacity than that of an older child or adolescent. A newborn has a stomach capacity of approximately 20 mL (Bergman, 2013). As infants grow, their stomach capacity increases, decreasing the frequency with which they need to be fed (American Academy of Pediatrics [AAP], 2014). Stomach capacity increases to approximately 90 mL in a 30-day-old term infant and to 360 mL around 1 year of age. An adult stomach holds 2 to 3 L (Collopy & Friese, 2010).

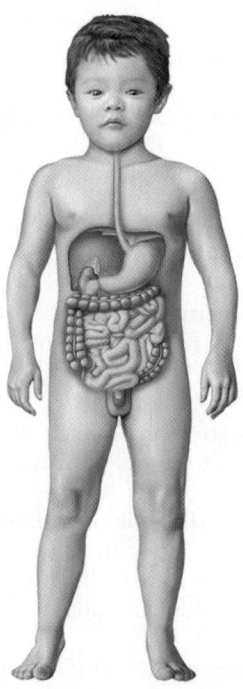

Source: Data from American Academy of Pediatrics. (2014). *Amount and schedule of formula feedings*. Retrieved from healthychildren.org/English/ages-stages/baby/feeding-nutrition/Pages/Amount-and-Schedule-of-Formula-Feedings.aspx; Bergman, N. J. (2013). Neonatal stomach volume and physiology suggest feeding at 1-h intervals. *Acta Paediatrica, 102*, 773–777; Collopy, K., & Friese, G. (2010). Pediatric drug administration. *Emergency Medical Services Magazine, 39*(6), 52–57.

ASSESSMENT GUIDE | The Child With a Gastrointestinal Condition

Assessment Focus	Assessment Guidelines
Abdomen—inspection	• Observe the shape of the abdomen. • Note any abdominal distention. Measure abdominal girth. • Observe the umbilicus for protrusion. • Observe for peristaltic waves (visible rhythmic contractions of the intestinal wall smooth muscle). • Observe for jaundice, bruising, and increased bleeding.
Abdomen—auscultation	• Auscultate for bowel sounds in all four quadrants prior to palpation.
Abdomen—palpation	• Palpate the abdomen and note if it is soft or firm. • Palpate the size of the umbilical ring. • Does the child complain of pain or tenderness during palpation? Does the infant cry? • Describe any masses palpated by location, shape, size, and consistency. • Palpate the liver for size and tenderness. • Palpate the spleen for size and tenderness.
Mouth and esophagus	• Note the presence of increased oral secretions. • Note the presence of cleft lip or palate.
Nutrition	• Note tolerance of feedings, spitting up, emesis, and recurrent respiratory infections. • Observe amount, color, and frequency of emesis. • Note if emesis is associated with feeding and whether or not it is projectile. • Note amount of intake, frequency of feedings, and growth.
Stool	• Observe color, consistency, and size of stool. Note any changes in stool patterns.
Family history	• Ask about history of gastrointestinal illness with genetic influences such as celiac disease and inflammatory bowel disease.

and palate occur together in approximately 45% of cases, while cleft palate occurs alone approximately 35% of the time, and cleft lip occurs alone approximately 20% of the time (Patel, Cohen, Ramaswamy, et al., 2014).

ETIOLOGY AND PATHOPHYSIOLOGY

Cleft lip with or without cleft palate results when the maxillary processes fail to fuse with the elevations on the frontal prominence during the sixth week of gestation. Normally, union of the upper lip is complete by the seventh week. Fusion of the secondary palate occurs between 5 and 12 weeks of gestation.

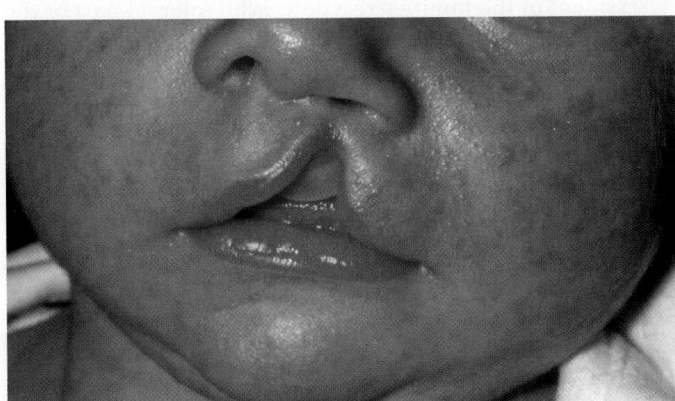

Figure 51–1 **Unilateral cleft lip.**

SOURCE: Dr. P. Marazzi/Science Source.

Failure of the tongue to move downward at the correct time prevents the palatine processes from fusing.

The intrauterine development of the hard and soft palates is completed in the first trimester. It is during this time that other major organ systems develop. Approximately 30% of children with cleft and/or palate will have another congenital anomaly (Setó-Salvia & Stanier, 2013). There is an increased incidence in families with a prior history of cleft lip or palate. The cause is believed to be multifactorial, involving a combination of environmental and genetic influences. Etiologic factors include smoking during pregnancy, maternal use of alcohol, and use of medications such as anticonvulsants and steroids during pregnancy (Setó-Salvia & Stanier, 2013). Additional studies have suggested that folate intake during pregnancy may reduce the incidence of cleft lip and palate (Blanton et al., 2011; Kelly, O'Dowd, & Reulbach, 2012).

CLINICAL MANIFESTATIONS

A cleft that involves the lip is readily apparent at birth. It may be a simple dimple in the vermilion border of the lip or a complete separation extending to the floor of the nose. The defect may be unilateral or bilateral and may occur alone or in combination with a cleft palate defect. Varying degrees of nasal deformity may also be present.

Cleft palate defects are less obvious when they occur without a cleft lip and may not be detected at birth. Clefts of the hard palate form a continuous opening between the mouth and nasal cavity and may be unilateral or bilateral, involving just the soft palate or both the soft and hard palates.

CLINICAL THERAPY

A multidisciplinary team is involved in cleft lip and palate management since these children have an increased risk for impairment in speech, hearing, and dentition. The team should include the pediatric primary healthcare provider and specialists in plastic and oral surgery, audiology, speech/language pathology, otolaryngology, dentistry, genetics, social work, and psychology (Crockett & Goudy, 2014).

Cleft lip and palate are usually diagnosed at birth or during the newborn assessment, but may be diagnosed in utero. Successful imaging of the face via transabdominal ultrasound can be performed as early as 13 to 14 weeks' gestation. Use of three-dimensional ultrasound or magnetic resonance imaging, if available, allows for a clearer picture of the defect and enhances the ability to detect isolated cleft palate prenatally (Wilkins-Haug, 2014). After the child is born, cleft lip and cleft palate are diagnosed by characteristic physical findings. The upper lip, alveolar arches, nostrils, and primary and secondary palates should be inspected and palpated (Crockett & Goudy, 2014).

The timing of cleft lip repair varies among surgeons. Repair generally occurs between 3 and 5 months of age, but may occur earlier or later depending on surgeon preference (Figure 51–2). If the defect is severe, the child may need more than one operation to achieve total repair. After surgery, soft elbow immobilizers (also known as restraints) are used for 2 weeks to protect the incision. (See the *Clinical Skills Manual* SKILLS.) The child should receive distraction and pain medication as needed because prolonged crying may disrupt the suture line. Antibiotics may also be prescribed (Crockett & Goudy, 2014).

Early closure of the lip enables the infant to form a better seal around the nipple for feeding. The sucking motion strengthens the muscles necessary for speech. Special feeding devices such as longer nipples with enlarged holes are available to help meet the infant's nutritional needs before surgical correction. A lactation consultant can assist with breastfeeding techniques.

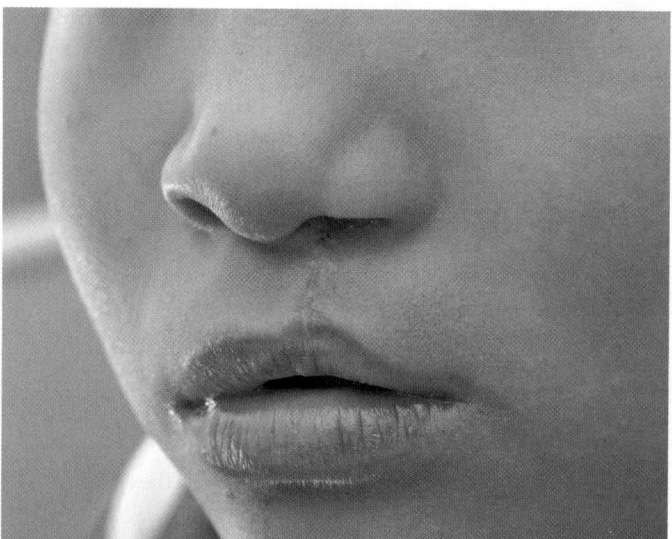

Figure 51–2 Repaired unilateral cleft lip.

SOURCE: jorgecachoh/Fotolia.

Timing of the cleft palate repair varies among surgeons and depends on the size and severity of the cleft. The palate should be closed by 12 months of age (Wiet, Biavati, & Rocha-Worley, 2013). This protects the formation of tooth buds and allows the infant to develop more normal speech patterns.

Infants with cleft lip and cleft palate are prone to recurrent otitis media, which can lead to hearing problems. (Refer to Chapter 45 for care of the child with chronic otitis media.) The child who has had a cleft palate repair requires orthodontic care. Early visits permit assessment of tooth eruption and the need for future orthodontic work.

Nursing Management

For the Child With Cleft Lip and Cleft Palate

Nursing Assessment and Diagnosis

PHYSIOLOGIC ASSESSMENT

A cleft lip defect is observable at birth. A cleft palate defect is usually noted during the newborn assessment by palpation of the primary and secondary palate (Crockett & Goudy, 2014). A description of the location and extent of the defect helps the nurse determine the correct method of feeding. Thorough and complete physical assessment is required since additional defects are sometimes present.

> ### Developing Cultural Competence Corrective Surgery for Cleft Lip and Palate
>
> In many developing countries, infants do not have access to surgery for correction of cleft lip and palate. They may grow into childhood and adulthood with these abnormalities. Medical teams from the United States, Canada, and other countries sometimes travel to developing nations for short medical missions, performing surgery on the children and teaching local doctors surgical techniques. Are there medical missions teams from your area that perform these surgeries? What planning is required for such trips to perform surgery safely and care for the children? What is the impact on the communities served?

PSYCHOSOCIAL ASSESSMENT

Assessment of the family's reactions is an integral part of the overall nursing assessment. Physical deformities, especially of the face, can be devastating to parents. A poorly corrected defect can lead to the development of low self-esteem in the older child. Assess the child's developmental level and social interactions with peers.

The accompanying *Nursing Care Plan* lists common nursing diagnoses for the infant with a cleft lip and/or palate. Other diagnoses that might be appropriate include the following (NANDA-I © 2014):

- *Anxiety (Parent)* related to situational crisis and threat to self-concept
- *Attachment, Risk for Impaired (Parent and Infant),* related to newborn's structural defect
- *Pain, Acute,* related to surgical repair of defect
- *Development: Delayed, Risk for,* related to structural defect and altered nutritional intake

Planning and Implementation

Nursing care involves providing emotional support, performing postsurgical care, educating parents on feeding techniques, helping parents coordinate care and maintain a healthy home environment, and making appropriate referrals. See *Nursing Care Plan: The Infant With a Cleft Lip or Palate* for a summary of nursing care.

PROVIDE EMOTIONAL SUPPORT

When a child is born with a cleft lip/cleft palate, parents may grieve the loss of the ideal child that they expected. Parents may need assistance to view their infant as a whole person, rather than focusing solely on the physical defect. Promote parent–infant bonding by explaining the nature of the structural defect and the procedure for correction. Interact and speak to the

---

Nursing Care Plan: The Infant With a Cleft Lip or Palate

Preoperative Care

1. Nursing Diagnosis: *Aspiration, Risk for*, related to anatomic defect (NANDA-I © 2014)

GOAL: The infant will have no episodes of gagging or aspiration.

INTERVENTION	RATIONALE
• Assess respiratory status and monitor vital signs at least every 2 hr.	• Allows for early identification of problems.
• Keep suction equipment and bulb syringe at bedside.	• Suctioning may be necessary to remove milk or mucus.
• Position upright for feedings.	• Minimizes passage of feedings through cleft.
• Feed slowly and use adaptive equipment as needed.	• Facilitates intake while minimizing risk of aspiration.
• Hold upright for 30 minutes after feeding.	• Prevents aspiration of feedings.
• Burp frequently (after every 15–30 mL of fluid).	• Helps to prevent regurgitation and aspiration.

EXPECTED OUTCOME: Infant will exhibit no signs of respiratory distress.

---

2. Nursing Diagnosis: *Coping: Family, Compromised*, related to birth of a child with a defect (NANDA-I © 2014)

GOAL: Parents will begin bonding process with the infant. The family's coping ability will be maximized. Parents will verbalize the nature and sequelae of the defect.

INTERVENTION	RATIONALE
• Help parents to hold the infant and facilitate feeding process.	• Contact is essential for bonding.
• Point out positive attributes of infant (e.g., hair, eyes, alertness.).	• Helps parents see the child as a whole, rather than concentrating on the defect.
• Explain surgical procedure and expected outcome. Show pictures of other children's cleft lip repair.	• Eliminating unknown factors helps to decrease anxiety.
• Assess parents' knowledge of the defect, their degree of anxiety and level of discomfort, and the interpersonal relationships among family members.	• Helps to determine the appropriate timing and amount of information to be given regarding the child's defect.
• Provide information about the etiology of cleft lip and palate defects and the special needs of these infants. Encourage questions.	• Concrete information allows parents time to understand the defect and reduces guilt.
• Explore the reactions of extended family members.	• Extended family is an important source of support for most parents of a newborn. Family members can often help promote acceptance and compliance with the treatment plan.
• Support rooming in.	• Rooming in allows parents to continue the bonding process.
• Encourage parents to participate in caretaking activities (holding, diapering, feeding).	• Participation in infant care decreases anxiety and provides parents with a sense of purpose.
• Refer to parent support groups.	• Support groups allow parents to express their feelings and concerns, to find people with concerns similar to their own, and to seek additional information.

(continued)

Nursing Care Plan: The Infant With a Cleft Lip or Palate (*continued*)

EXPECTED OUTCOME: Parents will hold, comfort, and show concern for the infant. Family will demonstrate ability to cope with and manage the infant's care. Parents receive necessary support to care for their infant.

3. Nursing Diagnosis: *Nutrition, Imbalanced: Less than Body Requirements,* **related to the infant's inability to ingest nutrients (NANDA-I © 2014)**

GOAL: The infant will gain weight steadily.

INTERVENTION	RATIONALE
• Assess fluid and calorie intake daily. Assess weight daily (same scale, same time, with infant completely undressed). Teach parents signs of adequate fluid intake such as frequency of wet diapers.	• Provides an objective measurement of whether the infant is receiving sufficient caloric intake to promote growth. Using the same scale and procedure when weighing the infant provides for comparability between daily weights.
• Observe for any respiratory impairment.	• Any symptoms of respiratory compromise will interfere with the infant's ability to suck. Feedings should be initiated only if there are no signs of respiratory distress.
• Provide weight-appropriate calories and fluid amounts. If the infant needs an increased number of calories to grow, referral to a nutritionist should be made. Higher calorie concentration formulas are available.	• Provides optimal calories and fluids for growth and hydration.
• Facilitate breastfeeding.	• Breast milk is recommended as the best food for an infant. The process of breastfeeding helps to promote bonding between mother and infant.
• Hold the infant in an upright position.	• Facilitates swallowing and minimizes the amount of fluid return from the nose.
• Give the mother information on breastfeeding the infant with a cleft lip or palate such as plugging the cleft lip and eliciting a letdown reflex before nursing.	• Information and specific suggestions may encourage the mother to persist with breastfeeding.
• Contact the La Leche League for the name of a support person.	• The La Leche League promotes breastfeeding for all infants. It can provide support people with experience who will aid the mother.
• If the mother is unable to breastfeed (or prefers not to), initiate bottle-feeding:	• Facilitates swallowing and minimizes the amount of fluid return from the nose.
• Place nipple against the inside cheek toward the back of the tongue. If needed, use a premature nipple (slightly longer and softer than regular nipple with a larger opening) or special cleft feeder.	• Use of longer, softer nipples makes it easier for the infant to suck. Special cleft feeders decrease the amount of pressure in the bottle and make the formula flow more easily.
• Initiate nasogastric feedings if the infant is unable to ingest sufficient calories by mouth.	• Adequate nutrition must be maintained. Use of a feeding tube allows the infant who has difficulty with oral feeding to receive adequate nutrition for growth.

EXPECTED OUTCOME: Infant will maintain adequate nutritional intake and gain weight appropriately. Successful breastfeeding will be achieved if desired. Feeding will provide necessary nutrients and will be a positive experience for parents and infant.

Postoperative Care

1. Nursing Diagnosis: *Breathing Pattern, Ineffective,* **related to surgical correction of defect (NANDA-I © 2014)**

GOAL: The infant will maintain an effective breathing pattern.

INTERVENTION	RATIONALE
• Assess respiratory status and monitor vital signs at least every 2 hr.	• Frequent assessment allows for early identification of problems.
• Apply a cardiorespiratory monitor.	• The monitor enables early detection of abnormal respirations, facilitating prompt intervention.
• Keep suction equipment and bulb syringe at the bedside. Gently suction oropharynx and nasopharynx as needed; avoid suture areas.	• Gentle suctioning will keep the airway clear. Suctioning that is too vigorous can irritate the mucosa.
• Provide cool mist for first 24 hr postoperatively if ordered.	• A mist moisturizes secretions to reduce pooling in the lungs. It also moisturizes the oral cavity.
• Reposition every 2 hr.	• Repositioning ensures expansion of all lung fields.

EXPECTED OUTCOME: Infant will show no signs of respiratory infection or compromise.

---

2. Nursing Diagnosis: *Tissue Integrity, Impaired,* **related to mechanical factors (NANDA-I © 2014)**

GOAL: The infant's lip and/or palate will heal with minimal scarring or disruption.

INTERVENTION	RATIONALE
• Position the infant with cleft lip repair on back.	• Prone positioning would allow the infant to rub the suture line.
• Use soft elbow immobilizers. Remove every 2 hr and replace. Do not leave the infant unattended when restraints are removed.	• Immobilizers prevent the infant's hands from rubbing surgical site. Regular removal allows for skin and neurovascular checks.
• Maintain suture line or Steri-Strips placed over cleft lip repair.	• Maintaining suture line will minimize scarring.
• Avoid metal utensils or straws after cleft palate repair.	• These devices may disrupt suture line.
• Do not allow pacifiers.	• Sucking can disrupt suture line.
• Keep the infant well medicated for pain in initial postoperative period. Have parents hold and comfort the infant.	• Good pain management minimizes crying, which can cause stress on the suture line. Increases bonding and soothes the child to decrease crying.
• Provide developmentally appropriate activities (i.e., mobiles, music).	• Appropriate activities soothe and keep the infant calm.

EXPECTED OUTCOME: Lip/palate will heal without complications.

---

3. Nursing Diagnosis: *Nutrition, Imbalanced: Less than Body Requirements,* **related to inability to ingest nutrients (NANDA-I © 2014)**

GOAL: The infant will receive adequate nutritional intake.

INTERVENTION	RATIONALE
• Maintain intravenous infusion as ordered.	• The IV provides fluid when the child is NPO (nothing by mouth).
• Begin with clear liquids, then give half-strength formula or breast milk as ordered.	• Ensures adequate fluids and nutrients.
• Use syringe or dropper inside of mouth.	• Avoids suture line and resultant accumulation of formula in that area.
• Give high-calorie soft foods after cleft palate repair.	• Rough foods, utensils, and straws could disrupt the surgical site.

EXPECTED OUTCOME: Infant will receive adequate nutritional intake. The infant resumes usual feeding patterns and gains weight appropriately.

infant in the parents' presence and point out positive attributes such as alertness, soft skin, or active movements. Self-blame is common among parents. Parents can also be referred to the American Cleft Palate Association for information about the disorder. Pictures of children who have had repair are available at this website. Seeing pictures of children who have had a successful repair offers reassurance to parents.

Parental anxiety is a typical response when children undergo surgery, and it is heightened when the surgery involves an infant. To minimize anxiety, give clear, concise explanations to parents. Allow sufficient time for parents to ask questions. Encourage parents to hold and cuddle the infant before surgery (see Chapter 39).

PROVIDE POSTOPERATIVE CARE

Provide general postoperative care for the infant. (See *Nursing Care Plan: The Infant With a Cleft Lip or Palate* in this chapter and *Nursing Care Plan: The Child Undergoing Surgery* in Chapter 39.) Additional postoperative nursing diagnoses may include (NANDA-I © 2014):

- *Infection, Risk for,* related to location of surgical procedure
- *Knowledge, Deficient (Parent),* related to lack of exposure and unfamiliarity with resources

Assess vital signs frequently and maintain the infant's airway. Measure intake and output. When oral fluids with clear liquids are started, they are usually given through a dropper, syringe, or special feeder. Position the infant in a sitting position for the feedings to avoid aspiration. Frequently burp the infant during feedings. The infant then progresses to half-strength formula or breast milk. After each feeding, cleanse the suture line with water or normal saline to avoid accumulation of feedings. In addition, the following specific interventions are necessary to ensure healing of the suture line:

- Prevent the infant from rubbing the suture line on the bedding by positioning the infant in a supine position.
- Maintain soft elbow immobilizers.
- Maintain the suture line or Steri-Strips placed over the incision. Place antibiotic body ointment on the incision site as ordered.
- Medicate the infant as prescribed to control pain and to minimize crying and stress on the suture line.
- After cleft palate surgery, avoid the use of metal utensils or straws, which may disrupt the surgical site.

COMMUNITY-BASED NURSING CARE

Identify and address home care needs well in advance of discharge. Discuss all aspects of the infant's care with the parents throughout hospitalization and after surgery. Involve parents in the infant's care to increase their comfort level before discharge and to promote bonding. Teach feeding techniques, how to recognize signs of infection, how to position the infant, and how to care for the suture line. Breastfeeding is usually possible with some assistance from a lactation specialist, even if the mother pumps her breasts and milk is fed by a special nurser. For infants requiring assistance to feed, several wide-based nipples, squeezable bottles, and other special bottles are available. Management involves many different healthcare professionals. In addition to hospital, clinic, and home health nurses, members of the healthcare team often include specialists such as a plastic surgeon, orthodontist, dentist, social worker, audiologist, speech pathologist, and pediatrician. The parents are the best coordinators of the child's care. Encourage them to keep a diary listing the professionals with whom they talk and the content of the discussions.

Teach parents how to care for the child after discharge. Teach them how to feed the infant, identify signs of complications (fever, vomiting, respiratory distress), administer any medications as prescribed, and care for the surgical site. Emphasize the importance of soft elbow immobilizers as prescribed.

Discuss with the parents the financial implications of long-term care. Private insurance does not always cover all the costs of care necessary for the child. Refer parents to programs and financial aid for which the parents and child may be eligible. Relief from financial worries enables parents to concentrate on

---

Growth and Development

An infant who has had a cleft lip repair needs stimulation to provide distraction. This approach will minimize crying, which can damage the suture line. Soft, colorful toys, mobiles, and other visual objects are helpful. Music also can be used to soothe the infant. Parental presence is comforting and reassuring.

---

caring for the child. Determine whether additional family supports are necessary.

Referral to a home healthcare agency for support may be helpful. Encourage follow-up visits with healthcare professionals (see *Health Promotion: The Child With Cleft Lip or Cleft Palate*). The child may need further evaluation of speech development, ear infections, or a recommendation for plastic surgery.

Evaluation

Expected outcomes of nursing care are provided in the accompanying *Nursing Care Plan*.

Esophageal Atresia and Tracheoesophageal Fistula

Esophageal atresia is a malformation that results from failure of the esophagus to develop as a continuous tube during the fourth and fifth weeks of gestation. The defect affects occurs in approximately 1 in 4500 neonates (Liszewski, Bairdain, Buonomo, et al., 2014). At least 90% of those affected also have a tracheoesophageal fistula (Khan & Orenstein, 2016a).

ETIOLOGY AND PATHOPHYSIOLOGY

In esophageal atresia, the foregut fails to lengthen, separate, and fuse into two parallel tubes (the esophagus and trachea) during fetal development. Instead the esophagus may end in a blind pouch or develop as a pouch connected to the trachea by a fistula (tracheoesophageal fistula) (see *Pathophysiology Illustrated: Esophageal Atresia and Tracheoesophageal Fistula*). Esophageal atresia is often associated with a maternal history of polyhydramnios (Khan & Orenstein, 2016a; Saxena, Blair, & Konkin, 2014). Other congenital anomalies occur in greater than 50% of children with esophageal atresia (Barman, Mandal, Shukla, et al., 2014). Jerome, the child described in the quotation at the beginning of the chapter, had esophageal atresia as well as an imperforate anus.

Health Promotion The Child With Cleft Lip or Cleft Palate

The child with cleft lip or cleft palate requires close monitoring and intervention to foster growth and development. The nurse can assist the child and family to achieve healthy outcomes.

Growth and Development Surveillance

- Monitor the child's growth and developmental patterns.
- Monitor for developmental delays.
- Explain to parents that regression following surgery in the toddler or older child is normal.

Nutrition

- Refer family to sources for nipples, nursers, and other special feeding devices.
- Assist mother with learning how to express breast milk and facilitate breastfeeding.
- Teach parents to avoid foods that can pose a choking hazard to the child.
- Teach parents to feed the infant in an upright position and to burp the child frequently during feedings.

Physical Activity

- Activity for the child having surgical procedures to correct cleft palate is generally restricted for approximately 2 to 3 weeks postsurgery to allow for healing.
- After healing has occurred, encourage the parents to promote the child's activities as they would any child without cleft lip or cleft palate.

Oral Health

- The child should be routinely screened for dental caries. Ask family about dental visits.
- Teach the parents to provide good dental hygiene to the child.
- Routine dental/orthodontic evaluation is necessary for the child with cleft palate.

Mental and Spiritual Health

- For uncorrected or poorly corrected cleft lip or palate, the child may experience poor self-esteem related to body image.

- Encourage family to adhere to treatment and surgical correction plan, including staged surgical corrections, dental care, and speech pathology assistance.
- Ask the family about financial ability regarding speech therapy, dental care, and other services that may be required. Financial constraints can impede compliance with recommended therapies.
- Be alert for the child who has had experiences with teasing associated with articulation or physical appearance.
- Refer parents to websites such as Project Smile and other resources.
- Refer the child for counseling if indicated.

Relationships

- Evaluate the parents for parent–infant bonding.
- Promote bonding by encouraging the parents to participate in the infant's care, to hold the infant, and to recognize the infant's positive attributes.

Disease Prevention Strategies

- Teach family to recognize signs and symptoms of ear or other infections and to seek immediate evaluation. Treatment of acute otitis media is necessary to prevent long-term effects of repeated infections.
- Emphasize to the parents the importance of audiology screening for children with cleft lip and palate to evaluate conductive hearing loss.

Injury Prevention Strategies (Safety)

- Assist parents to properly apply elbow restraints or to wrap child in mummy blanket to protect suture line in the postoperative period.
- Ask the parents about eating utensils the child uses.
- Teach parents to avoid straws, metal spoons, and other sharp utensils that may damage the palate.

Pathophysiology Illustrated: **Esophageal Atresia and Tracheoesophageal Fistula**

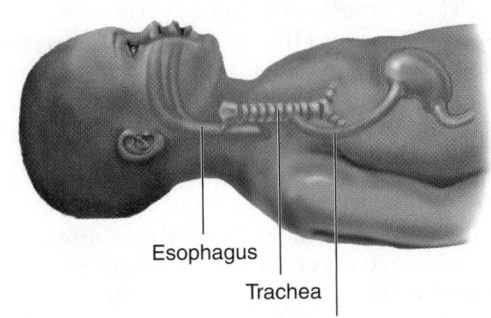

Esophagus

Trachea

Bottom portion of esophagus

In the most common type of esophageal atresia and tracheoesophageal fistula, the upper segment of the esophagus ends in a blind pouch connected to the trachea; a fistula connects the lower segment to the trachea.

CLINICAL MANIFESTATIONS

Symptoms in the newborn include excessive salivation and drooling, often accompanied by three classic signs for this defect: cyanosis, choking, and coughing. Sneezing may also be noted. During feeding, fluid returns through the infant's nose and mouth. Aspiration places the infant at risk for pneumonia. Depending on the type of defect, the infant's abdomen may be distended because of air trapping.

CLINICAL THERAPY

Esophageal atresia is suspected based on the presence of polyhydramnios and a small or absent fetal gastric bubble noted on prenatal ultrasound (Garabedian et al., 2014; Nowicki, 2013). After the child is born, passage of a radiopaque tube through the esophagus may be attempted. If the tube meets resistance, a chest and abdominal radiograph can confirm the presence of esophageal atresia. Radiologic examination may also reveal associated anomalies (Nowicki, 2013). Early diagnosis is essential to prevent aspiration of secretions, which can lead to pneumonia (Khan & Orenstein, 2016a).

Primary repair is preferred when possible and involves connecting the two ends of the esophagus and ligating the fistula if present (Nowicki, 2013). If primary repair of the esophageal atresia is not possible in the neonatal period, a gastrostomy tube is placed for feedings and the fistula is ligated (Nowicki, 2013; Saxena et al., 2014). Several procedures have been developed that allow for stretching of the esophagus over a period of time. Once the length of the esophagus is adequate, the two ends are reconnected in a delayed primary repair. The child will generally remain in the hospital setting until the repair. Potential postoperative complications include gastroesophageal reflux, aspiration, stricture formation, leak at the area of anatamosis, and tracheomalacia (Nowicki, 2013). The prognosis is usually good with surgery; however, some conditions are complicated, requiring repeated surgeries and long-term management. In the event that the two ends of the esophagus cannot be reconnected, colonic, jejunal, or gastric segments may be used to lengthen the esophagus (Khan & Orenstein, 2016a).

Nursing Management

The nurse may recognize the signs and symptoms in the immediate newborn period. Assess the infant for difficulty feeding and excessive drooling and the classic signs of choking, coughing, and cyanosis. Assess for respiratory distress and assess the lung sounds carefully.

Esophageal atresia is a surgical emergency. Preoperatively the infant requires close observation and intervention to maintain a patent airway. Specific interventions include:

- Have suction readily available to remove any secretions that accumulate in the nasopharyngeal airway.

- Place the infant with the head of the bed slightly elevated to minimize aspiration of secretions into the trachea.

- Use continuous or low intermittent suction to remove secretions from the blind pouch.

- Withhold oral fluids, and provide maintenance intravenous fluids.

- Constantly monitor the infant's vital signs and overall condition.

After surgery administer intravenous fluids and antibiotics. Monitor strict intake and output. Total parenteral nutrition may be needed until gastrostomy or oral feedings are tolerated. Monitoring and assessment of feeding tolerance are ongoing. Feedings are introduced slowly and in small amounts. Assess for respiratory difficulty during reintroduction of feedings. Monitor weight, growth, and developmental achievements.

The parents require emotional support throughout the infant's hospitalization. Clearly explain all procedures. Encourage parents to bond with the infant by stroking and talking to the infant. Eliciting questions and allowing parents to participate in the infant's care, especially feeding (when permitted), can facilitate bonding and help to prepare parents for care of the infant after discharge.

The specific details of discharge teaching depend on the types of procedures the child has had. Teach the parents about gastrostomy tube care and feedings if applicable, signs of infection, and how to prevent postoperative complications.

The outcomes of nursing care will depend on the extent of the defect and correction. Examples include the following:

- The child does not experience respiratory distress and maintains normal respirations.

- The child achieves and maintains a normal weight.

- Positive parent–infant bonding is established.

- The parent has knowledge of the defect, its corrections, and the child's needs.

Pyloric Stenosis

Pyloric stenosis is a hypertrophic obstruction of the circular muscle of the pyloric canal. Pyloric stenosis occurs in approximately 2 of every 1000 births (Lin et al., 2014). There is an increased incidence in firstborn males (Hunter & Liacouras, 2016; Taylor, Cass, & Holland, 2013). Pyloric stenosis is more common in the White population (Hunter & Liacouras, 2016; McAteer, Ledbetter, & Goldin, 2013)

ETIOLOGY AND PATHOPHYSIOLOGY

The exact cause of pyloric stenosis is unknown, although frequently there is a family history of the disorder. *Hypergastrinemia* (too much gastrin in the blood) is thought to play a role in the development of pyloric stenosis. Studies have indicated a higher incidence of the disorder in infants who received oral erythromycin before 2 weeks of age (Lozada, Royall, Nylund, et al., 2013).

Hypertrophy of the circular pylorus muscle results in stenosis of the passage between the stomach and the duodenum, partially obstructing the lumen of the stomach (see *Pathophysiology Illustrated: Pyloric Stenosis*). The lumen becomes inflamed and edematous, which narrows the opening until the obstruction becomes complete. At this time, vomiting becomes more forceful. As the obstruction progresses, the infant becomes dehydrated and electrolytes are depleted, resulting in metabolic imbalances.

CLINICAL MANIFESTATIONS

Symptoms usually become evident 2 to 8 weeks after birth, although onset may vary (Taylor et al., 2013). Initially, the infant appears well or regurgitates slightly after feedings. The parents may describe the infant as a "good eater" who vomits occasionally. As the obstruction progresses, the vomiting becomes projectile. In **projectile vomiting**, the contents of the stomach may be ejected up to 3 feet from the infant. The vomitus is nonbilious and may become blood tinged

TEACHING HIGHLIGHTS | Teaching the Family About Gastrostomy Tube Feedings

The infant or child who has difficulty swallowing, consuming oral feedings, or gaining weight may be a candidate for a gastrostomy tube. Indications for gastrostomy tube placement may include neurologic deficit; avoidant/restrictive food intake disorder (failure to thrive); severe gastroesophageal reflux; feeding aversions; short bowel syndrome; defects of the mouth, esophagus, or stomach; and cerebral palsy (Hannah & John, 2013). Depending on the condition, the child may need the gastrostomy tube for all feedings or supplementary feedings. Research indicates that the use of a standardized education protocol is beneficial. Patient outcomes were improved and caregiver confidence and knowledge increased (Schweitzer et al., 2014). See Chapter 39 for general guidelines related to teaching plans. See also the accompanying *Clinical Skills Manual* SKILLS .

General Principles

Preoperatively

- Assess what the family knows about a gastrostomy tube and gastrostomy tube placement.
- Assess what methods will be most effective in teaching care of the gastrostomy tube and enteral feedings.
- Show the family pictures or dolls with gastrostomy tubes and explain what the child's abdomen will look like in the immediate postoperative period.
- Provide the family with a booklet about gastrostomy tubes and enteral feedings.

Postoperatively

- Show the family the child's gastrostomy tube and reassess their understanding of the tube.
- When feedings are ordered, demonstrate the first feeding to the parents while explaining each step.
- Actively involve a family member in the second feeding. With subsequent feedings, have a family member feed the child with the nurse watching.
- Teach the family about:
  - Feeding administration
  - Medication administration
  - Daily care of the tube and the site surrounding the tube
  - How to handle common complications such as blockage, leaking, dislodgement, presence of hypergranulation tissue, and site irritation or infection
  - Phone numbers to call if needed
  - When to seek medical care related to the gastrostomy tube
- All family members who are involved in care of the child should practice feeding the child and administering medications to the child prior to discharge. This allows the nurse to assess for understanding of the procedure and gives the family confidence in their ability to care for the child. Some children will need bolus feedings, others may have continuous feedings via a feeding pump, and yet others may have bolus feedings during the day and continuous feedings at night.

Source: Data from Correa, J. A, Fallon, S. C., Murphy, K. M., Victorian, V. A., Bisset, G. S., Vasudevan, S. A., ... Lee, T. C. (2014). Resource utilization after gastrostomy tube placement: Defining areas of improvement for future quality improvement projects. *Journal of Pediatric Surgery, 49*, 1598–1601; Hannah, E., & John, R. M. (2013). Everything the nurse practitioner should know about pediatric feeding tubes. *Journal of the American Association of Nurse Practitioners, 25*, 567–577; Schweitzer, M., Aucoin, J., Docherty, S. L., Rice, H. E., Thompson, J., & Sullivan, D. T. (2014). Evaluation of a discharge education protocol for pediatric patients with gastrostomy tubes. *Journal of Pediatric Health Care, 28*(5), 420–428.

---

because of repeated irritation to the esophagus. The infant generally appears hungry, especially after emesis; irritable; fails to gain weight; and has fewer and smaller stools. The child may present with dehydration and metabolic alkalosis depending on how long the child has been vomiting (Tigges & Bigham, 2012). On physical examination, peristaltic waves may be observed across the abdomen as the stomach attempts to move contents past the narrowed pyloric canal (Lin et al., 2014). An olive-sized mass in the right upper quadrant may be evident (Lisonkova & Joseph, 2013; Markowitz, 2014).

CLINICAL THERAPY

An abdominal ultrasound to determine the diameter and length of the pyloric muscle is the preferred method performed to confirm the diagnosis (Castellani, Peschaut, Schippinger, et al., 2014; Markowitz, 2014). Blood tests will determine if the child is dehydrated or has an electrolyte or acid–base imbalance (see Chapter 44). Infants with pyloric stenosis are at risk for hypochloremia, hypokalemia, and metabolic alkalosis; however, recent studies show that normal laboratory values are found most often. This could be attributed to earlier diagnosis and the increased use of ultrasound to confirm the diagnosis (Taylor et al., 2013; Tutay, Capraro, Spirko, et al., 2013).

Surgery is performed as soon as possible after the infant's fluid and electrolyte balance is restored. Laparoscopic pyloromyotomy is the preferred surgical method to correct pyloric stenosis (Castellani et al., 2014). In a pyloromyotomy, the pyloric muscle is split to allow the passage of food and fluid. The prognosis is good. The infant is usually taking fluids within a few hours following surgery and discharged on full-strength formula within 24 hours after surgery.

Pathophysiology Illustrated: **Pyloric Stenosis**

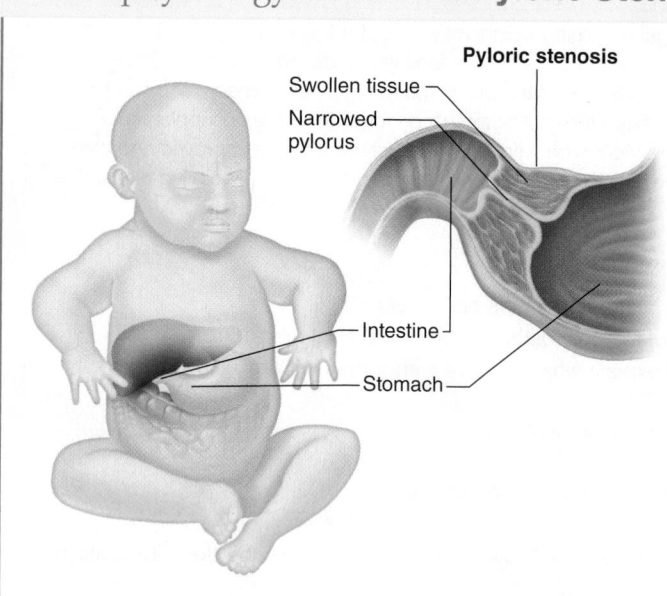

Pyloric stenosis

Swollen tissue

Narrowed pylorus

Intestine

Stomach

In pyloric stenosis, the hypertrophied pyloric muscle causes symptoms of projectile vomiting and visible peristalsis.

Nursing Management

For the Child With Pyloric Stenosis

Nursing Assessment and Diagnosis

Observe the infant's abdomen for the presence of peristaltic waves. Bowel sounds are hyperactive on auscultation. Auscultate before palpating the abdomen since palpation can cause a change in bowel patterns (see Chapter 33). Palpation reveals an olive-shaped mass in the right upper quadrant of the abdomen.

Assess the infant's history of vomiting, vital signs, weight, and nutritional status. Assess skin turgor, anterior fontanelle, urinary output (weigh diapers), urine specific gravity, and mucous membranes for signs of dehydration. Describe vomiting episodes and estimate emesis amount. Be alert for signs of an electrolyte and/or acid–base imbalance (See Chapter 44 for a discussion of electrolyte and acid–base imbalances.) Assess parental anxiety related to the child's condition. The child usually appears hungry. Crying and general discomfort are frequently observed.

Nursing diagnoses that might be appropriate for the child with pyloric stenosis include (NANDA-I © 2014):

- *Fluid Volume: Deficient,* related to vomiting
- *Nutrition, Imbalanced: Less than Body Requirements,* related to vomiting and inability to ingest nutrients
- *Sleep Pattern, Disturbed,* related to discomfort and hunger
- *Anxiety (Parents)* related to surgery
- *Pain, Acute,* related to surgical incision

Planning and Implementation

Nursing care focuses on meeting the infant's fluid and electrolyte needs, minimizing weight loss, promoting rest and comfort, preventing infection, and providing supportive care for parents.

MEET FLUID AND ELECTROLYTE NEEDS

Withhold oral feedings preoperatively because projectile vomiting will continue until the obstruction is relieved. Emphasize to the parents the importance of maintaining an NPO status preoperatively. Intravenous therapy is administered to correct fluid and electrolyte imbalances as needed and to maintain adequate hydration. Maintain nasogastric tube to suction if one is present and measure output from the tube. Inform parents that all diapers will be weighed to measure the infant's output of urine and stool.

MINIMIZE WEIGHT LOSS

The infant loses weight because of frequent vomiting. Monitor weight daily both preoperatively and postoperatively. Begin feedings postoperatively according to the healthcare provider's orders. Some surgeons prefer an NPO period following pyloromyotomy, with slow, incremental increases in volume and strength of feedings once feeding has resumed. Others will implement an earlier postoperative feeding approach.

PROMOTE REST AND COMFORT

During the preoperative period, the infant is hungry and cries often. The infant is swaddled to maintain warmth and provide comfort. Encourage the parents to hold and cuddle the infant. Provide a pacifier to meet the infant's need to suck.

Postoperatively, the infant is uncomfortable because of the surgical incision. Analgesics can be administered to relieve discomfort as ordered. (See Chapter 40 for a discussion of pain management.) Instruct parents to avoid pressure on the incision. When diapering the infant, slide the diaper gently under the buttocks rather than lifting the legs. Swaddling, rocking, and use of a pacifier provide comfort to the infant.

PREVENT INFECTION

Postoperatively, the incision is covered with collodion or Steri-Strips and should be kept clean and dry. Inspect the incision site for redness, swelling, or discharge. Monitor the infant's temperature every 4 hours. Auscultate the lungs to assess for any adventitious sounds.

PROVIDE SUPPORTIVE CARE

The need for hospitalization and surgery creates anxiety for parents. Encourage them to participate in the infant's care and to discuss their fears and concerns. Provide simple and clear explanations about the infant's condition and care. Advise parents that occasional vomiting after surgery may occur.

DISCHARGE PLANNING AND HOME CARE TEACHING

Instruct parents to observe the incision for redness, swelling, or discharge and to notify the healthcare provider immediately if these occur or if the infant develops a fever. To reduce the possibility of infection, advise parents to fold the infant's diaper so that it does not touch the incision. Provide instructions about feeding to ensure the infant's intake.

Evaluation

Expected outcomes of care include pain control, intake of recommended fluid and food with absence of vomiting, and manifestation of normal growth patterns.

Gastroesophageal Reflux

Gastroesophageal reflux (GER), the return of gastric contents into the esophagus, is the result of relaxation of the lower esophageal sphincter (Khan & Orenstein, 2016b; Marcdante & Kliegman, 2015). GER is the most common esophageal disorder in children (Khan & Orenstein, 2016b). Approximately 50% of infants have some degree of reflux (Lightdale & Gremse, 2013). Factors that increase the incidence of GER in the pediatric population include a short narrow esophagus, small stomach, large volume feedings, an immature lower esophageal sphincter, a liquid diet, and frequent horizontal position (Marcdante & Kliegman, 2015). Additional factors that increase the incidence of GER include prematurity, neurologic impairment, obesity, chronic respiratory disorders, and a history of repaired esophageal atresia (Lightdale & Gremse, 2013).

The primary symptoms of GER are regurgitation, spitting up, or vomiting (Lightdale & Gremse, 2013). Children with GER are frequently hungry and irritable. They eat often but still lose weight. Infants with reflux are at risk for aspiration and apnea.

Gastroesophageal reflux disease (GERD) is a more serious manifestation of GER. Symptoms of GERD in infants include vomiting or regurgitation associated with irritability, refusal of feedings, poor weight gain, sleep disturbance, respiratory symptoms including coughing, choking and wheezing and arching of the back during feedings (Lightdale & Gremse, 2013; Randel, 2014). Symptoms of GERD in older children include dysphagia, heartburn, and chest pain (Lightdale & Gremse, 2013).

Diagnosis is confirmed by a thorough history of the child's feeding patterns and by diagnostic evaluation. An upper GI series is helpful in assessing anatomy and possibly detecting an alteration in motility. Esophageal pH monitoring and intraluminal esophageal impedance are the preferred diagnostic tools for GER. Upper endoscopy with esophageal biopsy is the method used to determine the amount of damage to the esophagus in the presence of GERD and to rule out other conditions (Lightdale & Gremse, 2013; Randel, 2014).

Treatment depends on the severity of the condition. Generally, feeding modification, thickened feeds, and positioning are effective management for milder cases. A smaller feeding volume and increased frequency of feedings is recommended (Lightdale & Gremse, 2013). The healthcare provider may decide that rice cereal needs to be added to the infant's bottle to thicken feedings (Schwarz & Hebra, 2014). A special nipple may need to be used. Prethickened formulas are commercially available. For example, Enfamil AR contains added rice, is nutritionally balanced, and may be beneficial to young infants who are formula-fed (Schwarz & Hebra, 2014). Children may benefit from smaller, more frequent meals. Greasy and spicy foods, chocolate, peppermint, citrus, and caffeine should be avoided (Schwarz & Hebra, 2014). See *Professionalism in Practice: Guidelines for Management of Gastroesophageal Reflux.*

Professionalism in Practice Guidelines for Management of Gastroesophageal Reflux

The American Academy of Pediatrics has established guidelines related to the management of complicated GER and GERD. Included in these guidelines are recommendations related to infant feeding and positioning. Formula-fed infants may need a different formula and maternal diet may need to be modified in breastfed infants. Smaller, more frequent feedings and thickened feedings may decrease symptoms. Upright positioning is recommended. Semisupine positioning in a car seat or infant carrier should be avoided after feedings, as this may exacerbate symptoms (Lightdale & Gremse, 2013). Pediatric nurses care for infants with GER and GERD in both inpatient and outpatient settings. They have the opportunity to help families reduce the symptoms of reflux in the infant by educating parents about strategies related to feeding and positioning.

Use of medications to treat GERD in children varies among healthcare providers. See *Medications Used to Treat: Gastroesophageal Reflux Disease* for examples of medications that may be used.

Treatment for severe cases of GERD may include surgery that involves wrapping the greater curvature of the stomach (fundus) around the distal esophagus (fundoplication) (Khan & Orenstein, 2016b; Lightdale & Gremse, 2013; Randel, 2014). A gastrostomy tube may be inserted during surgery to serve as an access for venting and as a means for feeding if needed (Khan & Orenstein, 2016b).

Nursing Management

Nursing management focuses on supporting the infant's or child's nutritional intake, promoting interventions to reduce associated complications, and supporting the family.

Monitor the infant's weight daily and plot on a growth chart to note progress. Observe for any signs of respiratory distress, and keep the infant's nose and mouth clear of emesis.

Adequate nutrition must be maintained for the child to achieve normal growth and development. Infants receiving oral feedings should be given small, frequent feedings. Elevate the head of the bed to prevent aspiration if vomiting should occur. If the child has a gastrostomy tube, it is important to maintain skin integrity around the stoma site.

Medications Used to Treat: Gastroesophageal Reflux Disease

MEDICATION AND ACTION	NURSING IMPLICATIONS
Histamine H₂ Receptor Antagonists Zantac (ranitidine) Pepcid (famotidine) Inhibit the histamine H₂ receptor on the gastric parietal cell, thus blocking gastric acid secretion.	May be administered with or without food. Teach parents to avoid OTC medications without checking with healthcare provider. Monitor for side effects: Bradycardia Fatigue Rash Constipation Headache Confusion Nausea Irritability Thrombocytopenia Dizziness Diarrhea
Proton Pump Inhibitors Prevacid (lansoprazole) Prilosec (omeprazole) These powerful inhibitors of gastric acid secretion alleviate symptoms and help to heal esophagitis. Block the final common pathway of acid production by inhibiting activated proton pumps in the gastric parietal cell canaliculus.	Administer in the morning on an empty stomach. Monitor for side effects: Abdominal pain Fatigue Nausea Diarrhea Headache Proteinuria Dizziness Hematuria Rash Constipation Anorexia Teach family to inform primary healthcare provider if severe diarrhea occurs. Teach family to inform primary healthcare provider if changes in urinary elimination, such as pain or discomfort associated with urination, occur.

Source: Data from Blanco, F. C., Davenport, K. P., & Kane, T. D. (2012). Pediatric gastroesophageal disease. *Surgical Clinics of North America*, 92(3), 541–558; Lightdale, J. R., & Gremse, D. A. (2013). Gastroesophageal reflux: Management guidance for the pediatrician. *Pediatrics*, 131(5), e1684–e1695; Wilson, B. A., Shannon, M. T., & Shields, K. M. (2015). *Pearson nurse's drug guide 2015*. Hoboken, NJ: Pearson Education.

Clinical Tip

Parents are encouraged to hold their infant in an upright position for 20 to 30 minutes following feedings. Minimize seated positioning such as in an infant car seat because this increases intra-abdominal pressure and promotes reflux.

Clinical Tip

In older children, a pattern of chronic vomiting (low-grade, nearly daily emesis) or cyclic vomiting (repeated severe vomiting of an episodic nature) can occur. These patterns differ from vomiting seen in colic or gastroesophageal reflux. **Chronic vomiting** is often associated with upper gastrointestinal tract diseases such as gastritis and esophagitis, whereas **cyclic vomiting** (also called *cyclic vomiting syndrome*) is a functional disorder characterized by recurrent episodes of severe nausea and vomiting that last several hours to days. The affected children have symptom-free periods between episodes, in which they are able to participate in normal activities (Tarbell & Li, 2013). Continuous vomiting of any nature should be evaluated.

Discharge planning focuses on instructing parents in how to feed and position the infant, as well as providing comfort and emotional support. Encourage parents to hold and cuddle the infant during all feedings. Providing the infant with a pacifier helps to meet nonnutritive sucking needs. Teach parents how to suction the nose and mouth if vomiting occurs.

Omphalocele and Gastroschisis

Omphaloceles are congenital malformations in which intra-abdominal contents herniate through the umbilical cord (Figure 51–3). An omphalocele results when the intestines fail to return to the abdominal cavity during the 10th to 12th week of gestation (Ledbetter, 2012). The size of the sac varies depending on the extent of the protrusion. Large defects may contain intestines, stomach, liver, and the spleen (Hood & Zimmerman, 2013). The abdominal contents are contained in a sac that is composed of peritoneum, Wharton jelly, and amniotic membrane (Glasser, 2014). Rupture of the sac results in evisceration of the abdominal contents. Omphalocele with herniation of intestines into the umbilical cord occurs in 1 in 5000 births, while omphalocele with herniation of liver and intestines occurs in 1 in 10,000 births (Carlo & *Ambalavanan*, 2016). Fifty to seventy percent of infants with omphalocele will have an associated anomaly such as bladder exstrophy, cardiac defects, and Meckel diverticulum (Razmus, 2011).

Gastroschisis is a congenital defect of the abdominal wall, characterized by protrusion of bowel through a defect in the abdominal wall to the side (most often to the right) of the umbilicus. Unlike the omphalocele, no membrane covers the organs

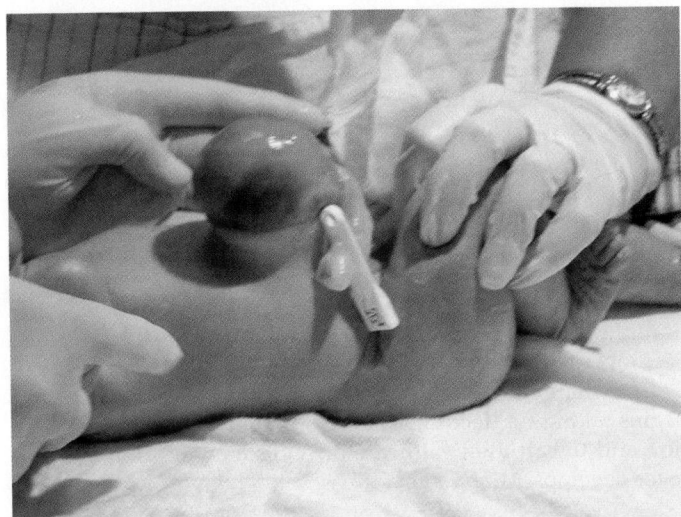

Figure 51–3 In omphalocele, the size of the sack depends on the extent of the protrusion of abdominal contents through the umbilical cord.

SOURCE: Courtesy of Carol Harrigan, RNC, MSN, NNP.

(Corey et al., 2013; Hood & Zimmerman, 2013; Ruano et al., 2011) (Figure 51–4). Gastroschisis occurs in 4 to 5 per 10,000 births (Benjamin & Wilson, 2014). Approximately 20% of infants with gastroschisis have an associated anomaly, most often atresia or intestinal stenosis (Razmus, 2011).

Care of the child with gastroschisis or omphalocele centers on protecting the protruding abdominal organs, correcting the defect, and preventing complications such as hypothermia, infection, and injury to involved organs.

Both gastroschisis and omphalocele are associated with elevation of maternal serum alpha-fetoprotein (MSAFP) (Glasser, 2014). Routine prenatal ultrasonography and determination of MSAFP levels lead to early diagnosis, education

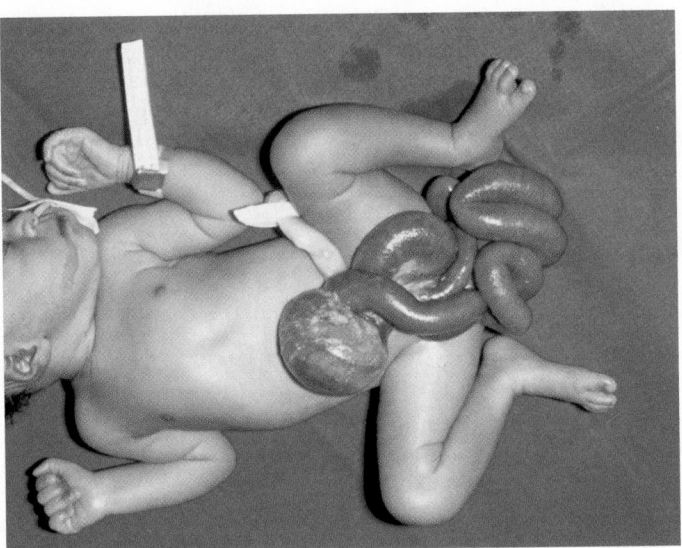

Figure 51–4 The newborn with gastroschisis has abdominal contents located outside the abdominal wall.

SOURCE: Ansary/Custom Medical Stock Photo/Newscom.

of the family, and coordination of the team of specialists needed to manage these congenital anomalies (Razmus, 2011).

The immediate action upon birth is to protect the sac (in omphalocele) or exposed abdominal contents (in gastroschisis) from injury by placing the infant feet first into a bowel bag (large sterile clear bag) that extends to the nipple line and is secured with ties. The bag is filled with warm saline to decrease heat loss, to keep organs moist, and to allow for visualization of the defect (Razmus, 2011). The child will often be transferred to a neonatal intensive care unit (NICU) with surgical capability for this defect.

One surgery may be all that is needed to repair a small defect. For larger defects, the first stage of repair may involve nonoperative placement of the abdominal contents or sac into a Silastic silo. Once the abdominal cavity can accommodate the intestinal contents, the child will have surgery to close the abdominal wall (Razmus, 2011).

Nursing Management

Be alert for signs of associated congenital anomalies. (Refer to the discussion of tracheoesophageal fistula earlier in this chapter, of genitourinary anomalies in Chapter 52, and of congenital heart defects in Chapter 47.)

Immediately after birth, follow healthcare provider protocol for maintaining the omphalocele sac or for the exposed abdominal contents in gastroschisis as discussed previously. Monitor vital signs at least hourly, paying close attention to temperature, as the infant can lose heat through the sac. The child should be in a warmer or isolette for maintenance of temperature control. Inspect the area for signs of infection.

Because the infant is NPO preoperatively, maintain fluid and electrolyte balance with intravenous fluids. Postoperative care includes measures to control pain, prevent infection, maintain fluid and electrolyte balance, and ensure adequate nutritional intake. Attainment of bowel motility and function varies and is often delayed for weeks after surgery. Total parenteral nutrition for the infant is used until full bowel function has returned (Hood & Zimmerman, 2013).

Throughout the infant's hospitalization, parents need clear, accurate explanations about the infant's condition. To help the parents deal with the crisis of an acutely ill newborn, provide emotional support and encourage parents to express their feelings. When the child has multiple anomalies, parents need ongoing support for the lengthy treatment, numerous hospitalizations, and management of nutritional intake.

Expected outcomes of nursing care depend on the severity of the defect and its correction, but may include:

- Fluid volume balance is maintained.
- The incision heals without signs of infection.
- Stable thermoregulatory function is maintained.
- Effective pain management is achieved.
- Parent–infant bonding and attachment are demonstrated.

Intussusception

Intussusception occurs when one portion of the intestine prolapses and then invaginates or telescopes into another. It is one of the most frequent causes of intestinal obstruction during infancy and occurs at a rate of 1 in 2000 infants and children.

Intussusception is more common in male babies. An estimated 65% of cases occur in children prior to 1 year of age (Deloach & Farber, 2013).

ETIOLOGY AND PATHOPHYSIOLOGY

Ninety percent of intussusception cases in children are idiopathic because a direct cause is not generally identified. Although the exact cause is unknown, there is frequently a current or recent enteritis or upper respiratory infection (Pepper, Stanfill, & Pearl, 2012).

The most common site of intussusception is the ileocecal valve (Cochran, Higgins, & Strout, 2011). Telescoping of the intestine obstructs the passage of stool. The walls of the intestine rub together, causing inflammation, edema, and decreased blood flow. This can lead to bowel wall edema, necrosis, and perforation (Territo, Wrotniak, Qiao, et al., 2014) (Figure 51–5).

CLINICAL MANIFESTATIONS

The onset of intussusception is usually abrupt. A previously healthy infant or child suddenly experiences acute abdominal pain with vomiting and passage of brown stool. There may be periods of comfort between acute episodes of pain. As the condition worsens, painful episodes increase. The child may have bilious emesis and a palpable abdominal mass. The stools become red and resemble currant jelly because of the mix of blood and mucus (Cochran et al., 2011; Deloach & Farber, 2013).

CLINICAL THERAPY

Diagnosis is made on the basis of the history and confirmed by radiographs and ultrasound of the abdomen. A contrast enema using air or barium can be both diagnostic and therapeutic. An air (or pneumatic) enema reduces the intussusception in approximately 90% of cases and is considered safer than a barium enema because of the decreased risk of perforation (Pepper et al., 2012).

A nasogastric tube is inserted for gastric decompression. If reduction of the intussusception does not occur during the contrast enema, surgical intervention to reduce the invaginated bowel and remove any necrotic tissue is necessary. Surgery is generally successful in correcting the problem; however, intussusception can recur after hydrostatic reduction or surgical correction.

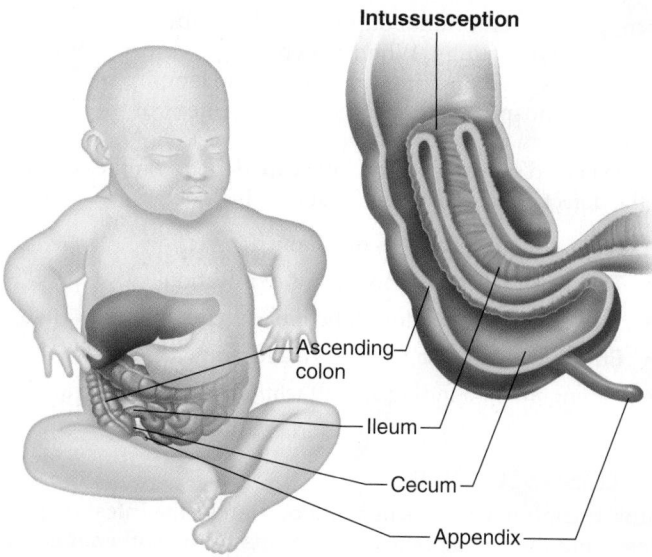

Intussusception

Ascending colon

Ileum

Cecum

Appendix

Figure 51–5 In infants, intussusception is commonly associated with viral illnesses and gastroenteritis.

Nursing Management

Nursing management focuses on maintaining or restoring fluid and electrolyte balance. Intravenous fluids are started immediately. Serum electrolyte monitoring is essential to correct imbalances.

Postoperative care focuses on monitoring for early signs of infection, managing the child's pain, and maintaining nasogastric tube patency. Assess vital signs, check for abdominal distention, and assess for return of bowel function. Feeding protocols vary among practitioners. Generally, after normal bowel function returns, clear liquid feeding or breastfeeding can resume. Feedings are then advanced as the infant or child tolerates them.

Discharge usually occurs shortly after the infant or child begins taking full feedings. Instruct parents to watch for infection and to call the healthcare provider if symptoms recur, a fever develops, or appetite decreases.

Clinical Tip

The passage of a normal brown stool may indicate that an intussusception has been reduced. Report this finding to the primary healthcare provider immediately, as the course of treatment may be altered, especially in the case of a planned surgical reduction.

Volvulus

During the 7th to 12th week of gestation the small intestine undergoes rapid growth. In normal development, the intestine rotates counterclockwise as it settles into its permanent position inside the abdominal cavity. Malrotation of the intestine occurs in approximately 1 of every 500 live births (Shalaby, Kuti, & Walker, 2013). When malrotation of the intestine occurs, the child is at risk for *volvulus*, a twisting of the intestine. Volvulus disrupts blood flow in the intestines and can lead to necrosis of the bowel, short bowel syndrome, and death. Volvulus is considered a surgical emergency. Early diagnosis and treatment is necessary to preserve the bowel and to save the child's life (Hebra & Cuffari, 2012; Shalaby et al., 2013).

Symptoms of volvulus in the infant include bilious vomiting, firm abdomen with distention, irritability secondary to pain, and passage of bloody stools. The diagnosis is confirmed through radiologic studies. Intravenous fluids are given to rehydrate the infant and to correct any electrolyte imbalance. Emergency exploratory surgery to untwist the bowel is essential (Zerpa & Shapiro, 2013). If a portion of the bowel is necrotic, that portion of the bowel is removed. An ostomy may need to be created, depending on the amount of bowel removed. See the section on ostomies later in this chapter. The child is at risk for developing short bowel syndrome if a significant amount of bowel is removed (see discussion later in this chapter).

Nursing Management

The infant or child who presents to the emergency department with bilious vomiting and a firm and distended abdomen should be assessed quickly to determine the cause of the symptoms. Once volvulus has been diagnosed, nursing management focuses on keeping the child NPO, administering intravenous fluids, assessing vital signs, and reporting symptoms of a worsening condition. The child who has had surgery to correct uncomplicated volvulus will need care similar to that described for the child with intussusception. If necrotic bowel was removed, the child may have an ostomy for a period of time.

Hirschsprung Disease

Hirschsprung disease, also known as *congenital aganglionic megacolon*, is a congenital anomaly in which inadequate motility causes mechanical obstruction of the intestine. The disease occurs in approximately 1 in 5000 live births, and is more common in males than females (Burkhardt, Graham, Short, et al., 2014). Hirschsprung disease can occur as a single anomaly or in combination with other anomalies such as congenital heart defects, Down syndrome, and urinary tract anomalies (Burkhardt et al., 2014; Langer, 2013).

ETIOLOGY AND PATHOPHYSIOLOGY

Hirschsprung disease is the congenital absence of ganglion cells (nerve cells) in the wall of a variable segment of rectum and colon. The absence of autonomic parasympathetic ganglion cells in the colon prevents peristalsis at that portion of the intestine, resulting in the accumulation of intestinal contents and abdominal distention. In most cases, the area lacking ganglion cells is limited to the rectosigmoid region of the colon (Fiorino & Liacouras, 2016).

CLINICAL MANIFESTATIONS

Clinical manifestations of Hirschsprung disease vary depending on the child's age at onset. Symptoms in newborns generally include abdominal distention, feeding intolerance, bilious vomiting, and failure to pass meconium within the first 24 to 48 hours after birth (Holder & Jackson, 2013; Langer, 2013; Nelville, 2014). *Enterocolitis* (inflammation of the intestines) is a complication of Hirschsprung disease that can be fatal if not recognized and treated early. Symptoms of enterocolitis include fever, foul smelling and/or bloody **diarrhea** (frequent, watery stools), abdominal pain, and vomiting (Nelville, 2014).

The older infant or child may have a history of failure to gain weight, malnutrition, and chronic severe **constipation** (difficult and infrequent defecation with passage of hard, dry stool), (Langer, 2013; Nelville, 2014).

CLINICAL THERAPY

Diagnosis is made on the basis of the history, bowel patterns, radiographic contrast studies, and rectal biopsy for presence or absence of ganglion cells. The rectum is small in size on palpation and does not contain stool. Abdominal radiographs generally show a distended bowel with dilated bowel loops throughout the abdomen. Water-soluble contrast studies reveal a transition zone between the normal and aganglionic bowel (Burkhardt et al., 2013; Langer, 2013). Rectal biopsy revealing the absence of ganglionic cells and the presence of hypertrophic nerve bundles has proven to be the most reliable test for confirmation of the diagnosis (Burkhardt et al., 2013; Fiorino & Liacouras, 2016; Langer, 2013).

Primary repair of Hirschsprung disease to remove the aganglionic portion of the bowel using a pull-through procedure. A primary repair may not be possible in the presence of extensive dilated proximal bowel, enterocolitis, or bowel perforation. In that case, a temporary colostomy is created and is closed when the definitive surgery takes place (Langer, 2013).

The return of normal bowel function depends on the amount of bowel involved. Some fecal incontinence and constipation may persist following surgery. Enterocolitis is a serious complication that can occur before or after surgery, resulting in ischemia and ulceration of the bowel wall. Treatment for enterocolitis associated with Hirschsprung disease includes rectal irrigations and antibiotics (Holder & Jackson, 2013).

Nursing Management

Nursing assessment in the newborn period includes careful observation for the passage of meconium. Because newborns are often discharged within 24 hours of birth, tell parents to notify the healthcare provider if no stool is passed or the abdomen becomes distended. When the disease is diagnosed later in infancy or in childhood, obtain a thorough history of weight gain, nutritional intake, and bowel elimination habits.

When Hirschsprung disease is diagnosed, nursing care includes monitoring for infection, managing pain, maintaining hydration, measuring abdominal circumference to detect any distention, and providing support to the child and family. Preoperative oral intake varies depending on the surgeon; however, intake is generally restricted to clear fluids the day before surgery. Rectal irrigations may be performed to evacuate the bowel prior to surgery.

Initial postoperative nursing care is the same as for any other infant or child having abdominal surgery: Maintain intravenous fluids and nasogastric tube. Monitor intake and output. Administer pain medications as prescribed and assess at least every hour for evidence of pain utilizing a pain scale and documenting assessment. If a colostomy was performed, the stoma should be assessed frequently as well as the return of bowel function. See the section on ostomies later in this chapter.

Children occasionally develop constipation and parents may need guidance to adapt the diet and fluid intake to manage this complication. Because some children develop malabsorption, be alert for signs of poor growth or malnutrition.

Expected outcomes of nursing care include:

- Fluid and electrolyte balance is maintained.
- Adequate nutritional intake to promote growth and development is evident.
- Adequate bowel function is demonstrated.
- The child's pain is managed effectively.
- The parents demonstrate effective coping with stress of the child's condition.

Anorectal Malformations

Anorectal malformations refer to anomalies of the rectum and distal anus, the urinary tract, and the genital tract. They have an incidence of approximately 1 in 5000 live births worldwide (Guardino & Pieper, 2013). Anorectal malformations are frequently associated with other anomalies. Some babies have VACTERL conditions. VACTERL refers to the presence of three or more of the following anomalies: **v**ertebral anomalies, **a**nal atresia, **c**ongenital heart disease, **t**racheoesophageal fistula, **r**enal anomalies, and **l**imb defects (Akay & Klein, 2016).

ETIOLOGY AND PATHOPHYSIOLOGY

The term *imperforate anus* (absence of the anal opening) is frequently used to refer to anorectal malformations and is classified according to the specific defect. Boys with imperforate anus frequently have a rectourethral fistula and girls generally have a rectovestibular fistula (Orr, 2011). Anal stenosis (narrowing of the anus) is a mild form of imperforate anus (Guardino & Pieper, 2013; Akay & Klein, 2016).

CLINICAL MANIFESTATIONS

Imperforate anus affects boys and girls equally. Perineal inspection at birth reveals the absent anal opening. Failure to pass meconium within the first 24 hours of birth may be indicative of imperforate anus. Stool in the urine usually indicates the presence of a fistula between the colon and urinary tract. Cloacal malformations in girls, in which the urinary tract, vagina, and rectum fuse together, forming a common channel, may occur. The child with a cloacal malformation has one opening in the perineum (Guardino & Pieper, 2013).

Diagnosis of anorectal malformation is usually made at birth or during the newborn assessment of anorectal structures and rectal patency. Ultrasound and lower gastrointestinal radiographic studies are used to confirm the diagnosis and demonstrate the extent of the anomaly.

CLINICAL THERAPY

Management depends on the extent of the malformation and presence of associated conditions. Anal stenosis may be treated with dilation alone. A single operation, anoplasty, may be used to repair rectoperineal defects (previously known as low defects). Higher defects require a three-stage procedure. A temporary colostomy in the newborn period provides for bowel decompression and for protection of the surgical site when the anomaly is repaired. Reconstructive surgery is accomplished via a posterior sagittal anorectoplasty (PSARP). This surgery generally occurs between 3 to 6 months of age, although timing varies among surgeons. When the operative site has healed, approximately 2 weeks after surgery, anal dilations are begun. When the desired size of the anal opening has been achieved, the colostomy is closed (Orr, 2011).

Nursing Management

During the initial newborn assessment, the perineal area is inspected for a poorly developed anal dimple or sacral anomalies. Observe and record passage of meconium.

Once the diagnosis has been made, intravenous fluids are initiated and a nasogastric tube is inserted to decompress the stomach. Monitor the child's intake and output (I&O) and cardiorespiratory functioning. Provide emotional support to the parents and give them information about the upcoming surgery.

Postoperative care specific to the child who has had a PSARP procedure centers on protection of the surgical site. A Foley catheter will be in place for 5 days to protect the new anal opening from urine. The colostomy that is still in place protects the surgical site from stool. The child should have nothing placed in the rectum. Provide adequate pain management for the child. Maintain intravenous fluids until the child is able to take liquids by mouth.

Nursing care for the child who has had colostomy closure is more complex because the bowel has been manipulated during surgery. It is essential to maintain the nasogastric tube to low wall suction until bowel function returns. Provide intravenous fluids or total parenteral nutrition through peripheral or central venous access until the child can tolerate fluids by mouth. Monitor intake and output. The child will frequently have a Foley catheter in place for accurate measurement of urine output.

Care of the operative site may include dressing changes in addition to assessment for signs of infection. As the child begins to pass stool through the anal opening for the first time, skin breakdown is likely. Protect the perineal area with a barrier cream or paste.

Provide intravenous pain medication on a regular basis. The nurse is also responsible for administering prescribed antibiotics that protect the child from infection.

The child with associated abnormalities may need several surgeries and interventions to treat all of the conditions

present. Partnering with families and a group of healthcare providers will assist in case management that facilitates the child's health and development. Health promotion and health maintenance that include support of family members, ensuring immunizations, and monitoring developmental status are important.

DISCHARGE PLANNING AND HOME CARE TEACHING

Infants are increasingly discharged shortly after birth, so parents need clear instructions about normal newborn stools and what abnormalities to report. The nurse should:

- Teach parents how to care for the ostomy site if a colostomy is performed in the newborn period (see discussion of ostomies later in this chapter).
- Reassure parents that the colostomy will be closed in the future, and help them plan for that hospitalization.
- Refer parents to ostomy support groups in the community or online.
- Discuss follow-up care and long-term management.
- Arrange follow-up visits and home care visits to evaluate the child's ostomy site and monitor growth.

Clinical Tip

Following colostomy closure in the child who has had a colostomy for several months, the perineal area is not accustomed to contact with stool. Without meticulous skin care, breakdown is very likely. Teach parents to change diapers frequently, clean the perineal area carefully, and apply a protective barrier ointment or cream at each diaper change.

After surgery to create the anal opening, teach parents how to take the infant's temperature using the axillary route (see the *Clinical Skills Manual* SKILLS). Once anal dilations have begun, the family will be taught how to perform them at home. After the final surgical procedure, discuss feeding regimens and bowel habits necessary to maintain adequate nutrition for growth and development. Advise parents that children with anorectal malformations may have difficulty achieving bowel control. Patience in toilet training is important. When the child reaches an age appropriate for toilet training, encourage the family to speak with a healthcare provider to discuss the child's progress.

Clinical Reasoning Imperforate Anus and Esophageal Atresia

Six-month-old Jerome was born with both imperforate anus and esophageal atresia. He had a colostomy created shortly after birth. His esophageal atresia has been repaired. He has just had surgery to create a new anal opening and will have the colostomy closed in approximately 6 weeks. What are the priorities of nursing care after an anorectoplasty? How can the surgical site be protected to ensure healing? What are essential components or preoperative and postoperative teaching related to the colostomy closure? What information related to toilet training should be given to Jerome's parents in the future?

Expected outcomes of nursing care include:

- The child's pain is effectively managed.
- Incisions heal without signs of infection.
- Fluid and electrolyte balance is maintained.
- Adequate bowel function is demonstrated.
- The parents demonstrate an understanding of ostomy care and other treatment protocols.

Hernias

A **hernia** is the protrusion or projection of an organ or a part of an organ through the muscle wall of the cavity that normally contains it. This protrusion may result from the failure of normal openings to close during fetal development or from weakness in the supporting musculature. When intra-abdominal pressure increases (as when the infant cries or strains to pass stool), the weakened area separates, causing a protrusion of underlying organs. Inguinal hernias are the most common type of hernia occurring in children (see Chapter 52). Other hernias that occur frequently in children are diaphragmatic and umbilical.

CONGENITAL DIAPHRAGMATIC HERNIA

In a diaphragmatic hernia, abdominal contents protrude into the thoracic cavity through an opening in the diaphragm. Sites of herniation include the substernal space, the posterolateral region, and the esophageal hiatus. The cause is a delay or failure in closure of the pleuroperitoneal musculature, which forms the diaphragm (Lee, Jun, & Lee, 2014). Intestines and other abdominal structures enter the thoracic cavity through the opening in the diaphragm. The overall incidence of diaphragmatic hernia is 1 in 2200 births (Rollins, 2012). Associated anomalies are present in 40% to 60% of infants born live with diaphragmatic hernia (Sfakianaki, 2012).

A diaphragmatic hernia is a life-threatening condition with an overall mortality rate of 20% to 35% in infants born alive with this condition (Rollins, 2012). Severe respiratory distress secondary to pulmonary hypoplasia occurs shortly after birth. As the infant cries, abdominal organs extend into the thorax, decreasing the size of the thoracic cavity. The infant becomes dyspneic and cyanotic. Characteristic findings include a barrel-shaped chest and sunken abdomen.

Congenital diaphragmatic hernia is diagnosed in utero by ultrasound in approximately two thirds of patients. Prenatal diagnosis improves survival rates, as it allows for early identification of infants who will require complex care after birth (Rollins, 2012).

Immediate respiratory support is essential in a neonatal intensive care unit (NICU). Ventilator support is necessary to manage respiratory compromise. Conventional mechanical ventilation, high-frequency oxygen ventilation, nitric oxide, and extracorporeal membrane oxygenation (ECMO) are the main methods used to treat respiratory failure in these children (Rollins, 2012; Sfakianaki, 2012; Sluiter, van de Ven, Wijnen, et al., 2011).

The infant is positioned with the head and thorax higher than the abdomen to facilitate downward movement of abdominal organs. A nasogastric tube is inserted to decompress the stomach. Intravenous fluids are administered through an umbilical artery catheter.

Once the infant's condition is stabilized, the defect is corrected surgically. The chance for a successful repair and survival is affected by the size of the defect. Children who survive will generally continue to have health concerns and should have continued evaluation of pulmonary, gastrointestinal, nutritional, and neurodevelopmental related problems (Rollins, 2012).

Nursing Management

The infant with a diaphragmatic hernia is admitted to the NICU and requires continuous monitoring. Preoperative management centers on providing supportive care to the infant and parents and includes the following:

- Note the infant's vital signs every 30 minutes on the cardio-respiratory monitor.
- Observe for worsening of respiratory compromise.
- Maintain intravenous fluid administration.
- Promote decreased stimulation to keep the infant calm and thus maintain low abdominal pressure.
- Keep parents informed about the infant's condition, and provide emotional support both before and after surgery.

Postoperative care includes:

- Positioning the infant on the affected side to facilitate expansion of the lung on the unaffected side
- Observing closely for signs of infection
- Maintaining respiratory support
- Managing pain
- Carefully monitoring fluid and electrolyte balance

Before discharge, instruct parents in wound care, prevention of infection, and feeding techniques.

UMBILICAL HERNIA

An umbilical hernia results from a weak or imperfectly closed umbilical ring. Umbilical hernia is a common condition in childhood and occurs more frequently in Black children and low-birth-weight infants (Carlo & *Ambalavanan*, 2016).

An umbilical hernia appears as a soft swelling covered by skin. Omentum and small intestine herniate or protrude through the opening with coughing, crying, or straining during a bowel movement. It is easily reduced by pushing the bowel back through the fibrous ring. Most defects that appear prior to 6 months of age will resolve spontaneously by 1 year of age. Surgery is indicated in cases of *strangulation* (closure of the muscular ring around a portion of the bowel, preventing it from moving back into the abdomen). Surgery is also recommended if the defect does not resolve by 4 to 5 years of age or if the defect becomes larger after 1 to 2 years of age (Carlo & *Ambalavanan*, 2016).

Nursing Management

Nursing management is generally supportive. Instruct parents not to apply tape, straps, or coins to reduce the hernia as these methods have not been proven to be effective. If surgery is required, it is usually performed in a short-stay unit. Postoperatively, teach parents how to care for the surgical site, to watch for bleeding, and to recognize signs of infection. Reinforce the importance of returning for follow-up evaluation.

Ostomies

An intestinal **ostomy** is an opening, or **stoma**, into the small or large intestine that diverts fecal matter, providing an outlet when a distal surgical anastomosis, obstruction, or nonfunctioning structure prevents normal elimination (Figure 51–6).

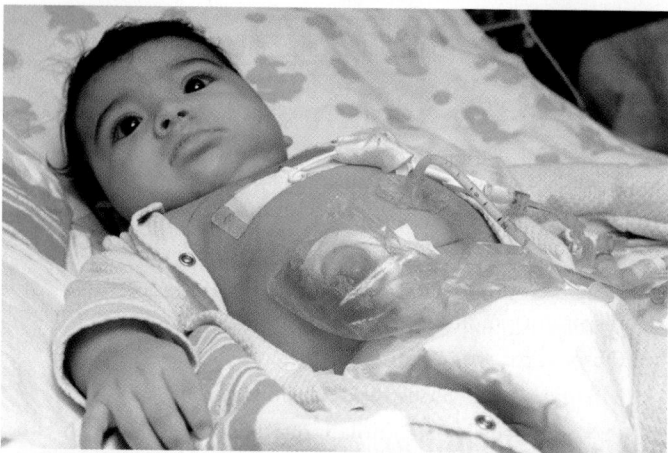

Figure 51–6 This infant has several gastrointestinal problems and requires ostomies for gastric feedings and for drainage of fecal material. Note the appearance of the healthy stoma.

Depending on the integrity and function of anatomic structures, the ostomy may be temporary or permanent. Infants and small children with imperforate anus, necrotizing enterocolitis, Hirschsprung disease, or volvulus may require a temporary or permanent colostomy or ileostomy. Ostomies may also be indicated for children with inflammatory bowel disease, intestinal tumors, or abdominal trauma.

An ostomy may be elective or considered a surgical emergency. In all cases, it affects a child's lifestyle, alters body image, causes anxiety, and increases the risk for alterations in physiologic processes (electrolyte imbalance, increased nutritional requirements). For adolescents, it may also result in dependence at a time when autonomy is a major developmental need.

When assessing the family and child approaching ostomy surgery, it is important to determine their ability to understand and accept the physical changes that will occur. Parents may feel guilt and anger about the need for an ostomy when the child has a genetically transmitted disease, is injured, or has developed an obstruction from necrosis of the bowel. Encourage the parents and child to express their feelings, and correct any misunderstandings. Parents and older children may be referred for counseling and to support groups to help them deal with their feelings. Adolescents often benefit from a visit with an adolescent ostomate (someone who has an ostomy) who can answer questions about living with an ostomy.

PREOPERATIVE CARE
Preoperative education focuses on educating the child and family and preparing them for postoperative management.

Growth and Development
The preschooler has some manual dexterity and can help with some parts of the procedure for changing an ostomy appliance and cleaning the stoma. Teach the child using a doll or stuffed animal. Many school-age children are able to care for their ostomy independently. Teach them how to avoid leakage around the bag, which could be embarrassing. Adolescents are generally totally independent in their self-care of ostomies. However, they may need support to deal with the fact that they are different from their peers.

Discuss how the appliance or ostomy pouch will look, and explain the purpose of the appliance in developmentally appropriate terms. Encourage the parents and child to touch and manipulate all equipment. Show a younger child how to place a pouch on a doll. Older children can practice placing a pouch on their skin. These measures help relieve anxiety by providing information and increasing familiarity with the appliance.

In addition to discussion of the appliance, preoperative education should include discussion of pain control and measures that will be used to prevent postoperative complications (turning, coughing, and breathing deeply). Gear the instructions to the child's developmental level. Encourage parental participation to promote compliance.

POSTOPERATIVE CARE
Postoperative care of a child with an ostomy is similar to that of any child who undergoes abdominal surgery. (See the discussion of nursing management for appendicitis later in this chapter and *Nursing Care Plan: The Child Undergoing Surgery* in Chapter 39.) Management of the stoma may be done by an "ostomy nurse" or other nurses. Major interventions involve ensuring proper function of the stoma, identifying complications, and instituting daily stoma care. Complications include skin breakdown, mucotaneous separation, necrosis, stenosis, prolapse, hernia, retraction, laceration, and leakage (Coha, 2013; Lindholm et al., 2013). Assess the stoma, quality and amount of fecal matter, skin condition, and adherence of the pouch. Evaluate the understanding and ability of the family to care for the ostomy.

Identify and address home care needs well in advance of discharge. Instructions include skin care, care of the stoma, appliance removal and application, and frequency of appliance changes (see the *Clinical Skills Manual* **SKILLS**). Begin teaching immediately after surgery with responsibility for care transferred gradually to the parents and child as they are ready. Discuss diet, activity level, hygiene, clothing, equipment, and financial considerations. Arrange for home visits to check periodically on the home management program.

Parents and children can be referred to the United Ostomy Association or a local ostomy group for information and support. Make referrals to social service, counseling, and a home health agency, if appropriate.

Expected outcomes of nursing care include successful adjustment to the ostomy, thorough evacuation of the bowel, absence of infection and other complications, intact skin, and formation of a positive self-image in the child.

Clinical Tip
Avoid adhesive enhancers on the skin of newborns and premature infants. Their skin layers are so thin that removal of the appliance can strip off the skin. Remember also that adhesive contains latex and its frequent use is not advised because of the risk of latex allergy development (see Chapter 48).

Inflammatory Disorders

Inflammatory disorders are reactions of specific tissues of the GI tract to trauma caused by injuries, foreign bodies, chemicals, microorganisms, or surgery. These disorders may be acute or chronic and may involve various segments of the GI tract.

Appendicitis

Appendicitis is an inflammation of the vermiform appendix, the small sac near the end of the cecum, and is the most common cause of emergency surgery in children (Hung, Lin, & Chen, 2012; Singh, Kadian, Rattan, et al., 2014). The condition occurs most often in children and adolescents ages 10 to 19 years. While the overall rate of perforated appendix is 20% to 35%, the rate in children less than 3 years of age is 80% to 100% as compared to 10% to 20% in children 10 to 17 years of age (Minkes & Alder, 2014). Other factors may affect the rate of appendiceal perforation. See *Evidence-Based Practice: Perforated Appendix*.

EVIDENCE-BASED PRACTICE | Perforated Appendix

Clinical Question

Early diagnosis and treatment is essential for positive outcomes for the child with appendicitis. Increased morbidity and mortality is associated with a perforated appendix. Young children have a higher rate of perforated appendix than older children. What are other factors that increase the rate of perforated appendix in children?

The Evidence

Ladd et al. (2013) conducted a retrospective study of 667 children who underwent appendectomy to determine if racial and socioeconomic factors were associated with an increased risk of perforated appendix. They also examined whether these factors were associated with symptom duration of greater than 48 hours. Results revealed that symptom duration and age had the strongest effect on the risk of perforated appendix, regardless of the race or ethnicity of the child. Children ages 0 to 4 and those presenting after 2 days of symptoms had significantly higher rates of perforation. Black and Hispanic children had significantly higher rates of perforated appendix than White children. Black children were more likely to have symptom duration of greater than 48 hours, leading the investigators to conclude that the increased incidence of perforated appendix in this population is related to delay in presentation to the hospital for treatment; however, they were not able to conclude that it was related to socioeconomic factors. The investigators found that the incidence of perforated appendix is higher in Hispanics regardless of other factors, leading them to conclude that being of Hispanic origin was a risk factor alone, and that perhaps there might be other cultural or economic factors not examined in this study that might contribute to the higher incidence in this group.

Levas et al. (2014) conducted a multicenter study to determine if there was an association between Hispanic ethnicity and limited English proficiency (LEP) and the rate of perforated appendix and the use of computed tomography (CT) and ultrasound in children presenting with abdominal pain. The sample comprised 2590 children ages 3 to 18 presenting with abdominal pain that was concerning for a diagnosis of appendicitis. A diagnosis of appendicitis was made in 1001 of these children. Perforated appendix was diagnosed in 25% of English-speaking non-Hispanics, 31% of English-speaking Hispanics, and 34% of Hispanics with LEP ($p < .01$). English-speaking non-Hispanics had a trend toward a higher incidence of perforated appendix, but it was not statistically significant. Twenty percent of Hispanics with LEP presented with a duration of pain greater than 72 hours, compared with 9.8% of English-speaking non-Hispanics. Hispanics with LEP were less likely to undergo CT or ultrasound. Those with mid-range Pediatric Appendicitis Scores (PAS) were significantly less likely to have these imaging studies, compared with English-speaking non-Hispanics. There was no significant difference in the timing between imaging studies and surgery based on English proficiency or ethnicity.

Lee, Yaghoubian, Stark, et al. (2012) examined whether being treated at a county hospital versus a private hospital affected the rate of perforated appendix, rate of laparoscopic appendectomy, and outcomes in children with appendicitis. For the study, 7902 cases of children treated for appendicitis between 1998 and 2007 were reviewed. Of these, 682 were treated at the county hospital and 7220 were treated at 1 of 11 private medical centers that are part of a larger system. The county hospital in this study was also referred to as a Safety Net hospital, which treats the highest number of uninsured patients and provides care to anyone regardless of financial, immigration, or insurance status. Results of the study showed that patients treated at the county hospital had a lower income, a higher rate of perforated appendix, and longer hospital stays. These patients also had a higher rate of laparoscopic appendectomy and a lower postoperative abscess drainage rate. The study showed that patients treated at the county hospital did not have poorer outcomes than those treated at private hospitals. They did have higher rates of perforated appendix, which the investigators attributed to delayed access to care. These patients had longer hospital stays, even though there was a higher rate of laparoscopic appendectomy, and a lower rate of postoperative abscess drainage. The delay in discharge could be related to fewer resources available, including transportation for discharge or insufficient care available at home for these children because parents are at work. Outcomes within the county hospital were similar regardless of income level or ethnic group. The investigators concluded that the differences in patients at the two hospitals might be related to differences in access to health care and other underlying ethnic and socioeconomic disparities as opposed to hospital type.

Best Practice

Young children have a higher incidence of perforated appendix. This is related to their inability to understand the concept of pain and verbalize this to their parents. Parents must be educated about the importance of recognizing cues in their children that could be indicative of pain. A longer duration of symptoms or delay in seeking health care was also identified as a risk factor for perforated appendix. This could be related to lack of knowledge related to symptoms requiring medical attention or lack of access to health care. Ongoing education for parents related to signs of illness in children is essential. Nurses play a key role in this education, especially in the outpatient clinic setting. Access to health care and resources continues to be a concern and demonstrates the need for improvement in access to all patients regardless of ethnic background, language proficiency, or socioeconomic status. Nurses play an important role in advocating for these patients.

Clinical Reasoning

Give specific examples of how nurses can work with children and families to decrease the incidence of perforated appendix. What are some factors that might attribute to the higher incidence of perforated appendix in Hispanics?

ETIOLOGY AND PATHOPHYSIOLOGY

Appendicitis almost always results from an obstruction in the appendiceal lumen. It can be caused by a fecalith (hard fecal mass), parasitic infestations, stenosis, hyperplasia of lymphoid tissue, or a tumor.

Continued secretion of mucus following acute obstruction of the lumen increases pressure, causing ischemia, cellular death, and ulceration. The appendix may perforate or rupture, resulting in fecal and bacterial contamination of the peritoneum. Peritonitis spreads quickly and if untreated can result in small bowel obstruction, electrolyte imbalances, septicemia, and hypovolemic shock.

CLINICAL MANIFESTATIONS

At onset, symptoms include periumbilical cramps, abdominal tenderness, anorexia, nausea, and fever. In adolescent and young adult females, symptoms must be differentiated from those associated with ruptured ectopic pregnancy, endometriosis, ovarian cysts, and pelvic inflammatory disease (Minkes & Alder, 2014).

As the inflammation progresses, pain in the right lower abdomen becomes constant. Pain is often most intense at the McBurney point, halfway between the anterior superior iliac crest and the umbilicus (see *Pathophysiology Illustrated: Appendicitis*). Symptoms progress to include guarding, rigidity, nausea, vomiting, onset of pain before vomiting, anorexia, and rebound tenderness following palpation over the right lower quadrant (Bishop & Carter, 2013; Minkes & Alder, 2014).

As appendicitis progresses, the child remains motionless, usually in a side-lying position with knees flexed. Sudden relief of pain usually means that the appendix has perforated.

CLINICAL THERAPY

Diagnosis of appendicitis in young children can be difficult because their pain may be less localized and their symptoms more diffuse than in the older child. Continuing evaluations over several hours are often needed to establish the diagnosis. The presence of an elevated white blood cell count (above $10,000/mm^3$), increased neutrophil ratio, and an elevated C-reactive protein combined with the symptoms supports a diagnosis of appendicitis (Bishop & Carter, 2013). A white blood cell count greater than $15,000/mm^3$ in a patient with appendicitis is a strong indicator that the appendix has perforated (Minkes & Alder, 2014). Abdominal ultrasound is preferred by some healthcare providers as the initial screening tool in the diagnosis of appendicitis; however, CT scans are more sensitive and may be used, especially when the appendix cannot be seen well on ultrasound or the results are inconclusive (Bishop & Carter, 2013; Minkes & Alder, 2014).

Treatment of uncomplicated appendicitis involves immediate surgical removal (appendectomy), generally through a laparoscopic appendectomy (Groves et al., 2013). Preoperatively, the child is kept NPO. Intravenous fluids and electrolytes, and antibiotics are administered (Minkes & Alder, 2014). Postoperatively, the child has an abdominal incision with a dressing covering the incision. Antibiotics may be administered. The child is generally discharged within 24 to 36 hours as long as they have adequate oral intake, are afebrile, and receive effective pain relief with oral pain medication (Bishop & Carter, 2013).

With perforated appendix, laparoscopic appendectomy is generally performed. While open appendectomy has been the treatment of choice in the past, recent studies have indicated that laparoscopic appendectomy is an effective approach for the treatment of perforated appendix as well. With laparoscopic appendectomy the abdominal cavity can be explored and lavaged (Groves et al., 2013). Postoperatively, the child with a perforated appendix may have a nasogastric tube to decompress the abdomen and will remain NPO until signs of bowel function return. Bowel function is best indicated by the passage

Pathophysiology Illustrated: **Appendicitis**

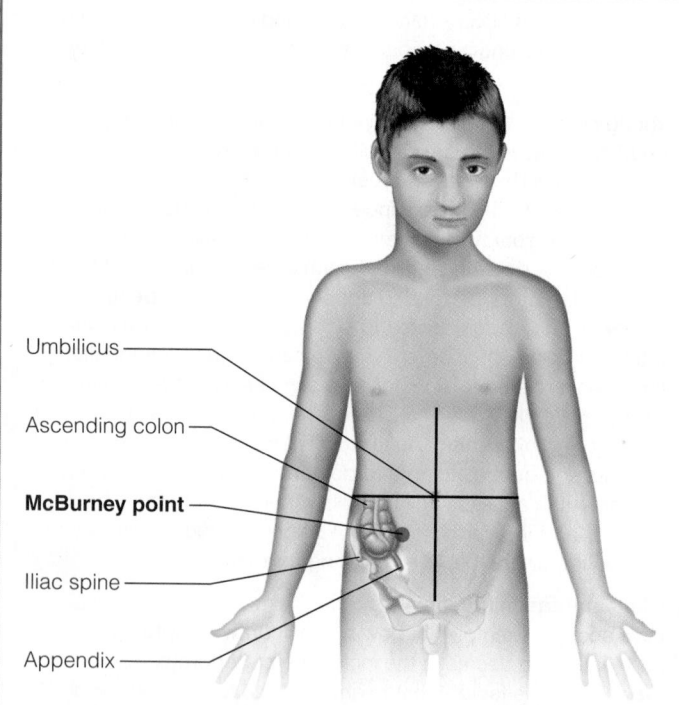

The McBurney point is the common location of pain in children and adolescents with appendicitis.

Umbilicus

Ascending colon

McBurney point

Iliac spine

Appendix

of flatus or stool. The child will also have a peripheral or temporary central line for administration of intravenous fluids and medications. After surgery for a perforated appendix, the child will receive antibiotics for several days. Morphine is generally given for pain.

In some cases, where an abscess is formed secondary to rupture of the appendix, the surgeon may choose to place a percutaneous drain, begin broad-spectrum antibiotics, and remove the appendix at a later time. This process is referred to as an interval appendectomy (Santacroce & Ochoa, 2013).

Nursing Management
For the Child With Appendicitis

Nursing Assessment and Diagnosis

PHYSIOLOGIC ASSESSMENT

A detailed assessment of the child's pain is necessary to differentiate appendicitis from other illnesses (see Chapter 40). Ask the child to point to the painful area and describe the pain. Recognize that localizing the pain may be difficult for young children. Note onset, location, and intensity of pain; precipitating factors; and relief measures tried. Remember to inspect, auscultate, and then palpate gently to identify distention and areas of pain. Rebound tenderness can also be assessed. Deep palpation of the left side of the abdomen followed by removing the hand quickly can lead to pain in the area of the appendix (rebound tenderness). However, once appendicitis is suspected or verified, avoid abdominal palpation in order to minimize pain to the child. Assess vital signs to determine baseline values, and monitor every 4 hours thereafter.

PHYSIOLOGIC ASSESSMENT

Because appendicitis usually occurs in school-age children and adolescents, assessment of the child's coping skills is important. Adolescents, because of their preoccupation with body image, may be concerned about the surgical scar. Assess the parents' and child's anxiety about the sudden hospitalization and need for emergency surgery.

Among the nursing diagnoses that might be appropriate for the child with appendicitis are the following (NANDA-I © 2014):

- *Pain, Acute,* related to inflammation and surgery
- *Fluid Volume: Deficient, Risk for,* related to fluid volume loss and inadequate fluid volume intake
- *Anxiety* related to physical condition
- *Infection, Risk for,* related to bowel trauma
- *Airway Clearance, Ineffective,* related to retained secretions

Planning and Implementation

Nursing management focuses on promoting comfort, maintaining hydration, providing emotional support, supporting respiratory function, providing care of the surgical site, and monitoring for symptoms of infection.

PROMOTE COMFORT

Preoperatively, a right side-lying position with knees bent is usually the most comfortable. If the appendix has perforated, lying on the right side helps the peritoneal cavity drain. Administer analgesics as ordered, and note relief from pain. Postoperatively, the child should be placed in a semi-Fowler or side-lying position on the right side. The child with a perforated appendix will require intravenous pain medication on a regular basis. The child who has an appendectomy for uncomplicated appendicitis will need oral or intravenous pain management for postoperative pain control.

MAINTAIN HYDRATION

An intravenous infusion is initiated preoperatively and continued until bowel function returns after surgery. Once bowel function returns and after the nasogastric tube has been removed, offer water in small amounts and then other clear fluids. The child should be monitored closely for nausea after beginning to take oral fluids.

PROVIDE EMOTIONAL SUPPORT

For many children, appendicitis may be their first hospitalization and their first experience with healthcare personnel other than their primary healthcare provider. The nurse must elicit a history, perform a physical examination, coordinate diagnostic tests, and prepare the child for surgery in a short period of time. Emotional support is essential for both child and parents. Good preoperative education can reduce anxiety. Answer any questions the child or parents may have.

SUPPORT RESPIRATORY FUNCTION

General anesthesia during surgery compromises respiratory function. It is important for the child to turn, cough, and breathe deeply to prevent atelectasis. Provide adequate analgesia and encourage the child to splint the incision area with a pillow during coughing to decrease pain. Incentive spirometry is frequently ordered for the child. Young children may be resistant to this procedure or may be too young to understand the procedure. An effective alternative approach is to give the child bubbles or a pinwheel to blow.

RECOGNIZE SYMPTOMS OF INFECTION

Assess vital signs and observe the abdominal incision every 4 hours for redness, edema, or drainage. If a drain is present, assess drainage for color, consistency, and amount. The amount of drainage from the wound should decrease gradually as the wound heals. If the appendix perforated, the child is hospitalized for several days of intravenous antibiotics.

DISCHARGE PLANNING AND HOME CARE TEACHING

Children with uncomplicated appendicitis are discharged once bowel function returns and they have a bowel movement. Children with perforated appendix will have a longer hospitalization since they require several days of intravenous antibiotics. When the child is ready for discharge, give parents instructions for home care. Teach parents to recognize the signs and symptoms of infection and to seek early treatment.

Normal activities can be resumed fairly quickly, but the child should avoid strenuous activities and contact sports in the immediate postoperative period. Parents should check with the child's healthcare provider before allowing the child to resume sports activities. Home tutoring may be needed for a short time so the child can keep up with schoolwork.

Evaluation

Expected outcomes of nursing care include the following:

- The child's pain is effectively managed.
- The child demonstrates effective airway clearance.
- The wound heals without the development of a secondary infection.
- Adequate hydration is achieved and maintained.

Necrotizing Enterocolitis

Necrotizing enterocolitis (NEC) is a potentially life-threatening inflammatory disease of the intestinal tract that occurs primarily in premature infants. While the overall incidence is 1 in 1000 live births. NEC affects up to 7% of infants of very-low-birthweight infants (weighing less than 1500 g). NEC is associated with a mortality rate of 5% to 24% (Huda, Chaudhery, Ibrahim, et al., 2013). The disease occurs most often in the ileum (Berman & Moss, 2011; Huda et al., 2013).

The etiology of NEC is multifactorial. Intestinal ischemia and inflammation, bacterial or viral infection (a result of the premature infant's decreased immune response and greater risk for infection), enteral feeding, and immaturity of the gastrointestinal mucosa may all be contributing factors (Gregory, DeForge, Natale, et al., 2011; Morgan, Young, & McGuire, 2011).

Manifestations generally occur during the second week of life after enteral feedings are started; however, NEC can develop before feedings are started, after several weeks of life, and long after feedings are started. The infant may initially show signs of feeding intolerance (increased gastric residuals, vomiting, irritability, and abdominal distention). Bloody diarrhea may be present because of the hemorrhagic bowel. The condition progresses to lethargy, periods of apnea and bradycardia, and temperature instability (Berman & Moss, 2011).

Diagnosis is made on the basis of characteristic clinical findings and the presence of free peritoneal gas, dilated bowel loops, bowel distention, and bowel wall thickening on abdominal radiographs. Stools and emesis are monitored for occult blood. Laboratory data reveal anemia, leukopenia, leukocytosis, thrombocytopenia, electrolyte imbalance, and metabolic or respiratory acidosis. Blood cultures are positive for the organism present.

Necrotizing enterocolitis requires prompt intervention to decrease the morbidity and mortality associated with this illness. Treatment includes bowel rest (NPO status), gastric decompression with nasogastric suction, and antibiotic therapy (Gregory et al., 2011; Rapoport & Nishii, 2013; Wright & Miller, 2012). The infant will need central venous access to provide nutrition (Rapoport & Nishii, 2013). Serial radiographs of the abdomen should be performed to detect worsening or resolution of the disease process (Wright & Miller, 2012). Perforation or necrosis of the bowel necessitates surgical resection of the bowel. An ileostomy or colostomy may be performed.

All cases of necrotizing enterocolitis are treated with strict enteric precautions to prevent the spread of infection to other premature infants on the unit.

Long-term complications of necrotizing enterocolitis include short bowel syndrome, strictures, cholestasis, impaired nutrition and growth, and delayed developmental performance.

Nursing Management

Nursing care centers on prevention and early detection of necrotizing enterocolitis to minimize bowel loss, and providing postoperative care. Observe for feeding intolerance by aspirating gastric residual (if the infant is receiving enteral feedings). Measure abdominal circumference and assess bowel sounds in the premature or high-risk infant every 4 to 8 hours. Even minimal changes in circumference can indicate necrotizing enterocolitis and should be reported to the primary care provider.

SAFETY ALERT!

The infant with NEC is at risk to develop sepsis. Signs of sepsis in the newborn or premature infant include:

- Hypothermia or hyperthermia
- Jaundice
- Respiratory distress
- Hepatomegaly
- Abdominal distention
- Poor feeding
- Vomiting
- Lethargy

Report these symptoms to the primary healthcare provider immediately.

Maintaining fluid and electrolyte balance is essential. Provide comfort by holding and cuddling an infant who is NPO, and offer a pacifier to meet nonnutritive sucking needs. Careful assessment for infection and maintenance of skin integrity are essential. Feedings are gradually reestablished once bowel function returns. Because the symptoms of necrotizing enterocolitis may not appear until several days after feedings begin, parents may not be prepared for the infant's decline. Recovery is slow and can be complicated. Give clear explanations and encourage parents to ask questions and express their fears and concerns. If the infant's condition worsens, offer the parents support (see Chapter 41).

Once the child is discharged, frequent follow-up is needed. Parents need specific education related to feedings, medications, and any other treatments prescribed. The infant requires regular and thorough physical assessments to check weight gain, assess development, and identify signs of complications. If the child had to have an ostomy created, the family must be taught ostomy care.

The infant requires regular and thorough physical assessments to identify any complications. Growth of the child is monitored and compared with previous findings. Developmental progress is assessed by regular administration of a developmental test such as the Denver II.

Clinical Tip

Cholestasis is a disruption of bile flow and the most common problem in survivors of necrotizing enterocolitis. It is a complication of total parenteral nutrition (TPN) and commonly occurs 2 weeks after TPN therapy has been initiated. It is characterized by hyperbilirubinemia, hepatomegaly, and elevated serum aminotransferase levels (Vitola & Balistreri, 2016).

Expected outcomes of nursing care for the child with necrotizing enterocolitis include:

- The child is free of signs and symptoms of infection.
- Fluid and electrolyte balance is achieved and maintained.
- Tissue perfusion is maintained following surgical removal of necrotic bowel.
- The child consumes adequate nutrition to support growth and development needs.

If surgery is performed, complete healing without infection or other complication is desired. If the infant is not successfully treated, support and comfort for the parents are necessary. When the child survives, desired long-term outcomes include normal developmental progression and nutrition to support growth.

Meckel Diverticulum

Meckel diverticulum results when the omphalomesenteric duct, which connects the midgut to the yolk sac during embryonic development, fails to atrophy. Instead, an outpouching of the ileum remains, usually located near the ileocecal valve. The pouch contains gastric or pancreatic tissue, which secretes acid, causing irritation and ulceration. Meckel diverticulum is the most common GI malformation and occurs in 1% to 4% of the population (Pepper et al., 2012).

Clinical manifestations usually appear by age 2. Meckel diverticulum most commonly presents as GI bleeding or obstruction. The child generally presents with bloody stool, irritability, fatigue, abdominal pain and distention, nausea, and vomiting (Pepper et al., 2012).

Diagnostic testing for Meckel diverticulum depends on the presentation and includes laboratory analysis to evaluate for the presence of anemia and dehydration (Pepper et al., 2012). Imaging studies are also used to assist in the diagnosis and include radiographs, ultrasound, CT scan, and radionuclide scanning (Kotecha, Bellah, Pena, et al., 2012). Technetium-99*m* pertechnetate nuclear medicine (also called a *Meckel scan*) is the current imaging test of choice for a bleeding diverticulum (Pepper et al., 2012).

Treatment is surgical excision of the diverticulum and removal of any involved bowel. The prognosis is good following surgical excision.

Nursing Management

Preoperatively, an intravenous infusion is initiated to correct fluid and electrolyte imbalances. Monitor intake and output. Observe for rectal bleeding, and test stools for **occult blood** (blood that is present in small quantities and is measurable only by laboratory testing). Keep the child on bed rest. Assess vital signs every 2 hours, and monitor for signs of shock. Postoperative care is similar to that for an infant or child undergoing abdominal surgery. (See the earlier discussion of postsurgical nursing management of appendicitis and *Nursing Care Plan: The Child Undergoing Surgery* in Chapter 39.)

At discharge, parents need instructions on caring for the surgical site, preventing infection, providing an adequate diet, and administering prescribed medications.

Inflammatory Bowel Disease

CROHN DISEASE AND ULCERATIVE COLITIS

Inflammatory bowel disease encompasses two distinct chronic disorders, Crohn disease and ulcerative colitis, that have similar symptoms and treatment. Inflammatory bowel disease differs from irritable bowel syndrome.

Crohn disease is a chronic, inflammatory process. The disorder can occur randomly throughout the GI tract with the ileum, colon, and rectum as the most common sites. A distinct feature of Crohn disease is the development of enteric fistulas between loops of bowel or nearby organs. Mucosal ulcers begin in small locations, and then grow in size and depth into the mucosal wall. Submucosal inflammation can be severe. The etiology is unknown. There is strong evidence to support a genetic association. Crohn disease is more common in

Whites than African Americans. It is rare in Asian and Hispanic populations (Grossman & Mamula, 2014). It most often develops in adolescents and young adults. Crohn disease has an incidence of approximately 4.56 per 100,000 (Grossman & Baldassano, 2016). The onset of Crohn disease is subtle. Crampy abdominal pain is usually reported first, followed by diarrhea. Other symptoms include fever, anorexia, growth failure or weight loss, general malaise, and joint pain. Diagnosis is based on laboratory evaluation, diffuse abdominal tenderness, and radiologic and biopsy examinations. Anemia, an elevated erythrocyte sedimentation rate, hypoalbuminemia, and thrombocytosis are other possible findings. Stools are positive for occult blood (Glick & Carvalho, 2011).

Clinical Tip

Irritable bowel syndrome (IBS) refers to a functional disorder of the gastrointestinal tract that is characterized as chronic and episodic. There is no structural cause, but it seems to be triggered by events such as gastroenteritis, major life events or stressors, or dietary intolerance. Other causative factors may include stress, diet, drugs, and alcohol. IBS is characterized by episodes of abdominal cramping and pain, diarrhea or constipation, and bloating (Mason, 2014). Management generally focuses on the symptoms. A change in lifestyle and diet might be effective in decreasing the frequency of symptoms. Medications such as antispasmodics, antimotility agents, and laxatives may also be used (Mason, 2014).

Ulcerative colitis is a chronic recurrent disease of the large intestine and rectal mucosa of unknown etiology. Inflammation is limited to the mucosa, as opposed to Crohn disease, which extends deep into the bowel wall. Ulcerative colitis can involve the entire length of the bowel with varying degrees of inflammation, ulceration, hemorrhage, and edema. Emotional and other psychosocial factors may influence the presentation and course of the disease. It is more prevalent among persons of Jewish heritage. The disease develops before 20 years of age with peak onset at about 12 years. The incidence of pediatric ulcerative colitis in North America is approximately 2 per 100,000 (Grossman & Baldassano, 2016). See Table 51–1 for a comparison of the two diseases.

The first symptom of ulcerative colitis is usually diarrhea. Lower abdominal pain and cramping are present before and during a bowel movement and are relieved by the passage of stool and flatus. The stool is often mixed with blood and mucus. Weight loss or delayed growth, nutritional deficiencies, and arthralgias often occur as effects of the disease.

Diagnosis centers on evaluating the cause and identifying the extent of involved bowel and differentiating an infectious process from ulcerative colitis. Upper endoscopy and colonoscopy are helpful to determine the extent and severity of the inflammatory process. Laboratory studies generally indicate an elevated erythrocyte sedimentation rate, elevated C-reactive protein, hypoalbuminemia, antineutrophil cytoplasmic antibodies (ANCA), and anti–*Saccharomyces cerevisiae* antibodies (ASCA) (Kelsen & Mamula, 2013).

Crohn disease and ulcerative colitis have periods of remission and exacerbation. Treatment for both diseases includes pharmacologic interventions, nutrition therapy, and, in severe cases, surgery. First-line pharmacologic treatment of Crohn disease involves aminosalicylates. Sulfasalazine inhibits prostaglandin synthesis, thereby decreasing inflammation. Corticosteroids and immunosuppressants are used in children with

TABLE 51–1 Clinical Manifestations of Ulcerative Colitis and Crohn Disease

	ULCERATIVE COLITIS	CROHN DISEASE
Type of lesions	Continuous, superficial involvement	Segmental, transmural (through the wall) involvement
Clinical manifestations		
Anal or perianal lesions	Rare	Common
Anorexia	Mild to moderate	Can be severe
Diarrhea	Often severe	Moderate
Growth retardation	Mild	Significant
Pain	Present	Common
Rectal bleeding	Present	Absent
Weight loss	Moderate	Severe
Risk of cancer	Slightly increased	Greatly increased

more severe disease. Biologic therapies such as infliximab (Remicade) have been effective in patients with Crohn disease and ulcerative colitis who fail to respond to other therapies (Glick & Carvalho, 2011).

A nutritionist is part of the team treating the child. The goal of nutrition therapy is to provide adequate caloric intake and nutrients necessary for growth. Vitamin, iron, zinc, and folic acid supplementation is frequently required. Total parenteral nutrition (TPN) is often given to treat nutritional deficiencies and malnutrition, which accompany inflammatory bowel disease (see the *Clinical Skills Manual* SKILLS). A high-protein, high-carbohydrate, low-fiber diet with normal amounts of fat is recommended.

Clinical Tip

The following drugs are used in the treatment of inflammatory bowel disease:

Aminosalicylates

Sulfasalazine

Mesalamine

Corticosteroids

Prednisone

Prednisolone

Hydrocortisone

Budesonide

Biologic Therapies

Infliximab (Remicade)

Adalimumab (Humira)

Certolizumab (Cimzia)

Immunosuppressants

6-Mercaptopurine (6-MP)

Azathioprine

Cyclosporine

Methotrexate

Antibiotics

Metronidazole

Ciprofloxacin

Source: Data from Glick, S. R., & Carvalho, R. S. (2011). Inflammatory bowel disease. *Pediatrics in Review, 32*(1), 14–25; Peyrin-Biroulet, L. (2011). Why should we define and target early Crohn's disease? *Gastroenterology & Hepatology, 7*(5), 324–326; Triantafillidis, J. K., Merikas, E., & Georgopoulos, F. (2011). Current and emerging drugs for the treatment. *Drug Design, Development and Therapy, 5*, 185–210.

If other treatment measures fail to reduce inflammation, surgery is generally indicated. A temporary colostomy or ileostomy is performed to allow the bowel to rest. However, in Crohn disease, ulcerations tend to recur elsewhere in the GI tract. In ulcerative colitis, removal of the diseased bowel provides a permanent cure.

Nursing Management

Nursing management occurs mainly in the community and home and focuses on helping the child and family adjust to the emotional impact of a chronic disease, administering medications and diet therapy, monitoring nutritional status, and providing appropriate referrals. Provide emotional support and counseling to help the child adjust to feeling "different" from peers. Inability to compete with peers and frequent absences from school can affect the child's self-esteem. Have the parents contact the school district to arrange for tutoring in case extended absences from school become necessary. Encourage the child who is not attending school regularly to maintain contact with friends through telephone calls, cards, and visits.

Body image is a major concern for children and adolescents with inflammatory bowel disease. Corticosteroid therapy causes growth retardation and delayed sexual maturation. Encourage the child to discuss feelings about these side effects. If a permanent colostomy or ileostomy is required, help the child and family understand the need for surgical treatment. (See the discussion of ostomies earlier in this chapter.) Introduce the child and family to other children who have stomas.

If the child is unable to eat or the intake of calories is insufficient to meet basic nutritional and metabolic needs, TPN is ordered (see the *Clinical Skills Manual* SKILLS). If the child is able to eat, parents need instructions about dietary needs. Frequently measure growth and assess nutrition.

Teach parents about medication administration and diet therapy. Reinforce to both the parents and child the importance of adhering to a strict medication regimen. Emphasize that medications should be continued even when the child is asymptomatic. Discuss side effects of the drugs and what to do if any of these symptoms occur. Since immune status may be altered by steroid use, have families avoid contact with infectious diseases when the child is taking steroids. Immunization schedules may need to be altered.

Growth and Development

Providing adequate stress reduction may be helpful in control of inflammatory bowel disease. Teach young children relaxation techniques, such as deep breathing, progressive tensing and relaxing of muscles, and visualization of favorite places. Encourage busy school-age children and teens to have quiet and restful times each day in addition to physical activity periods. Meditation might be effective in older children and teens.

TEACHING HIGHLIGHTS | Diet Instructions for Inflammatory Bowel Disease

- Several small feedings are usually better tolerated than three meals daily.
- Limiting fiber intake can help to decrease intestine motility and inflammation. Peel fruits and avoid large quantities of whole grains and nuts.
- If the child is not eating well, offer high-calorie meals. If lactose intolerance is not a problem for the particular child, cream soups, milkshakes, puddings, and custards can be offered.
- Liquid dietary supplements may be helpful to ensure protein and caloric requirements are met.
- Watch for foods that cause intestinal problems for the individual child, and avoid them in the future.
- Avoid having mealtime become a reason for family strife. Seek help of nurses and dietitians if needed.

Parents need instructions for TPN if this therapy is used, as well as information about care of a central venous catheter, including dressing changes, sterile and nonsterile techniques, signs of infection, how to handle infusion pumps and tubing, and how to measure the child's intake and output. Assist parents in obtaining equipment and supplies necessary for the child's care. Have parents demonstrate their mastery of care for the central venous catheter and their understanding of TPN techniques during home visits and appointments for health care.

Refer parents to social services, the visiting nurse association, and home healthcare agencies, if they are not receiving any of these services. For information about inflammatory bowel disease, refer families to the Crohn's and Colitis Foundation.

Expected outcomes of nursing care for the child with inflammatory bowel disease include the following:

- Normal growth and development are achieved.
- The child demonstrates the ability to cope with episodes of GI distress.
- The child adheres to the medication regimen.
- There is no evidence of central line infection.
- The child has a positive body image.
- The child is able to integrate stress-lowering practices into daily life.

Peptic Ulcer

A peptic ulcer is an erosion of the mucosal tissue in the lower end of the esophagus, in the stomach (usually along the lesser curvature), or in the duodenum. Peptic ulcers occur primarily in individuals receiving nonsteroidal anti-inflammatory drugs and those with *Helicobacter pylori* infection (Chason, Reisch, & Rockey, 2013).

Clinical manifestations vary according to the age of the child and location of the ulcer. The most common symptom is abdominal pain (burning) associated with an empty stomach, which may awaken the child at night. Vomiting and pain after meals, anemia, occult blood in stools, and abdominal distention may also be present.

Diagnosis is based on the history and radiologic studies. Bleeding from peptic ulcer disease is treated with acid-suppressant medications. These medications include histamine-2 receptor antagonists (H2RAs) such as rantidine and famotidine and proton pump inhibitors such as omeprazole, pantoprazole, and lansoprazole. *H. pylori* infection is generally treated with a proton pump inhibitor, amoxicillin, and clarithromycin for 7 to 14 days (Anand, 2015). Follow-up is important to ensure that the organism has been eradicated. The prognosis is usually good with early intervention.

Nursing Management

Assess the child for abdominal pain, vomiting, and abdominal distention. Assess for family history of *H. pylori* infection. Nursing care centers on interventions to promote adequate nutritional intake, promote healing, and prevent recurrences. Provide a nutritionally sound, age-appropriate diet. Omit foods only if they exacerbate the disorder.

Medications must be given as scheduled. Emphasize the importance of continuing medication therapy as prescribed. The family needs encouragement to continue the medications as ordered and to return for follow-up visits. Children who attend school may prefer to take medications in the form of tablets, which are easier to carry than liquid preparations. The appropriate form must be completed in order for the child to receive medication at school.

Parents should discuss any additional medications with the primary healthcare provider before administering to the child. Caution parents to avoid ibuprofen, which irritates the gastric mucosa. If an antipyretic or pain medication is needed, acetaminophen should be given. Advise parents to read medication labels if they are unsure of product contents.

Because psychologic stress can contribute to peptic ulcer disease, the parents and child should be assisted to identify sources of stress in the child's life. Assess coping mechanisms and provide referral for psychologic counseling, if appropriate. Teach relaxation techniques and recommend community classes on yoga or other stress reduction.

Disorders of Motility

Fluids are an important part of normal GI functioning. As food passes through the intestines, fluids are reabsorbed and moderately soft stool is formed and evacuated. In disorders such as diarrhea and constipation, fluid balance is altered, causing either more or less fluid to be reabsorbed. This can severely alter the characteristics of the stool. Reabsorption of too little water produces diarrhea and can lead to fluid and electrolyte alterations. Reabsorption of too much fluid can cause constipation, which if untreated can lead to bowel obstruction.

Gastroenteritis (Acute Diarrhea)

Gastroenteritis is an inflammation of the stomach and intestines that may be accompanied by vomiting and diarrhea.

Gastroenteritis can affect any part of the GI tract. It may be an acute problem, caused by viral, bacterial, or parasitic infections, or a chronic problem. Rotavirus is a leading cause of severe gastroenteritis in children less than 5 years of age worldwide. The rotavirus vaccine is recommended for infants in order to decrease the morbidity and mortality related to this organism (Agócs et al., 2014). Infants and small children with gastroenteritis or diarrhea can quickly become dehydrated and are at risk for hypovolemic shock if fluid and electrolyte losses are not replaced (see Chapter 44). A significant number of infants and young children are hospitalized each year for dehydration secondary to gastroenteritis.

ETIOLOGY AND PATHOPHYSIOLOGY

Diarrhea in children is related to many different causes (Table 51–2). The specific etiology is not always identified. The common mechanism is a decrease in the absorptive capacity of the bowel through inflammation, decrease in surface area for absorption, or alteration of parasympathetic innervation. Children in childcare centers and those living in substandard housing with improper sanitation are at increased risk.

TABLE 51–2 Causes of Diarrhea in Children

ETIOLOGY	BOWEL MANIFESTATIONS
Emotional stress (anxiety, fatigue)	Increased motility
Intestinal infection (bacteria [Escherichia coli, Salmonella, Shigella], viral [human rotavirus, enteric adenovirus], fungal overgrowth)	Inflammation of mucosa; increased mucus secretion in colon
Food sensitivity (gluten, cow's milk)	Decreased digestion of food
Food intolerance (lactose, introduction of new foods, overfeeding)	Increased motility; increased mucus secretion in colon
Medications (iron, antibiotics)	Irritation and suprainfection
Colon disease (colitis, necrotizing enterocolitis, enterocolitis)	Inflammation and ulceration of intestinal walls; reduced absorption of fluid; increased intestinal motility
Surgical alterations (short bowel syndrome)	Reduced size of colon; decreased absorption surface

Clinical Tip

Carbonated beverages and those containing high amounts of sugar should not be given when a child has diarrhea. Fermentation of sugar in the gastrointestinal tract causes increased gas, abdominal distention, and an increased frequency of diarrhea.

CLINICAL MANIFESTATIONS

Diarrhea may be mild, moderate, or severe. In mild diarrhea, stools are slightly increased in number and have a more liquid consistency. In moderate diarrhea, the child has several loose or watery stools. Other symptoms include irritability, anorexia, nausea, and vomiting. Moderate diarrhea is usually self-limiting, resolving without treatment within 1 or 2 days. In severe diarrhea, watery stools are continuous. The

child exhibits symptoms of fluid and electrolyte imbalance (see Chapter 44), has cramping, and is extremely irritable and difficult to console.

CLINICAL THERAPY

Diagnosis is based on the history, physical examination, and laboratory findings. Physical examination provides a guide to the severity of dehydration (see Chapter 44). The stool can be examined for the presence of ova, parasites, infectious organisms, viruses, fat, and undigested sugars. Laboratory evaluation of serum and urine helps identify electrolyte imbalances and other deficiencies.

Medical management depends on the severity of the diarrhea and fluid and electrolyte imbalances. The goal of treatment is to correct the fluid and electrolyte imbalances. For mild and moderate dehydration, oral rehydration therapy is the first intervention (see Chapter 44). This may be accomplished at home or in the short-stay observation unit in a hospital.

For severe dehydration, rehydration is accomplished by intravenous infusion with a solution chosen to correct the specific electrolyte imbalances. (See Chapter 44 for further information about solutions to correct dehydration.) As soon as possible, introduce clear liquids or breast milk and then encourage the child to progress to a regular diet. Foods generally are not withheld for more than 1 to 2 days.

If the diarrhea is caused by bacteria or parasites, antimicrobial therapy may be prescribed. Antiemetics and antidiarrheals are generally not used in young children since they can mask the signs and symptoms of more serious illness.

Nursing Management

For the Child With Gastroenteritis

Nursing Assessment and Diagnosis

The nurse may encounter the child and family in the emergency department, urgent care center, clinic, or office. The child may be cared for over several hours at a clinic or urgent care center so that dehydration is treated with intravenous infusion and/or oral rehydration, and then sent home with instructions for parents to care for the child. A thorough history may help in identifying the cause.

If the child is hospitalized, it is important to assess onset, frequency, color, amount, and consistency of stools. If the child is also vomiting, monitor the amount and type of vomitus. Initial and ongoing physical assessment of the child focuses on observing for signs and symptoms of dehydration, which reflect underlying fluid and electrolyte status. Evaluate urinary output and specific gravity. An accurate weight must be obtained on admission and daily thereafter. Monitor vital signs every 2 to 4 hours. A febrile child has increased water loss, contributing to the dehydration. Assess skin integrity, especially in the perineal and rectal areas, and note any breakdown or rashes.

The accompanying *Nursing Care Plan* lists common nursing diagnoses for a child with gastroenteritis. The following diagnoses may also be appropriate (NANDA-I © 2014):

- *Anxiety (Child and Parent)* related to change in health status
- *Sleep Pattern, Disturbed,* related to pain
- *Nutrition, Imbalanced: Less than Body Requirements,* related to inability to ingest sufficient nutrients

Nursing Care Plan: The Child Hospitalized With Gastroenteritis

1. Nursing Diagnosis: *Diarrhea* related to infectious process (NANDA-I © 2014)

GOAL: The child's bowel function will be restored to normal.

INTERVENTION	RATIONALE
• Obtain baseline vital signs and monitor every 2–4 hr.	• Fluid and electrolyte imbalances can alter vital body functions.
• Observe stools for amount, color, consistency, odor, and frequency.	• Aids in the diagnosis and in monitoring the child's status.
• Test stools for occult blood.	• Frequent defecation and some infectious organisms can cause bleeding.
• Monitor results of stool culture and sample for ova and parasites.	• Rapid notification of the healthcare provider will facilitate treatment.
• Wash hands well before and after contact with the child.	• Helps prevent transmission of microorganisms.
• Isolate the child until the cause of the diarrhea is determined.	• Prevents exposure of other patients and staff.
• Assist the child with toileting and hygiene.	• The child may be weak, incontinent, physically impaired, or anxious and require assistance to use the bathroom.
• Administer prescribed oral rehydration and intravenous solutions.	• Provides necessary fluids and nutrients.
• Notify the healthcare provider if diarrhea persists, stool characteristics change, or other symptoms of dehydration electrolyte imbalance occur.	• Ensures early intervention.

EXPECTED OUTCOME: Child's bowel function will return to normal.

2. Nursing Diagnosis: *Fluid Volume: Deficient*, related to active fluid volume loss (NANDA-I © 2014)

GOAL: The child will remain hydrated and will begin to drink fluids within 24 hours of admission.

INTERVENTION	RATIONALE
• Monitor intake and output. Document time of each voiding. Weigh all diapers.	• Will determine if output exceeds input. Long periods of time without urine output can be an early indicator of poor renal function. A child should produce 1–2 mL of urine/kg/hr.
• Compare admission weight to preadmission weight. Assess weight daily.	• The degree of dehydration can be determined by the percentage of weight loss. Daily weights aid in determining progress toward rehydration.
• Assess level of consciousness, skin turgor, mucous membranes, skin color and temperature, capillary refill, eyes, and fontanelles every 4 hours.	• Will determine degree of hydration and adequacy of interventions.
• Assess for vomiting.	• Vomiting frequently accompanies diarrhea and contributes to the child's fluid loss.
• Provide oral fluid and electrolyte replacement solution if able to tolerate.	• Less invasive than IV fluids. Provides for replacement of essential fluids and electrolytes.
• Provide and maintain IV replacement therapy, as ordered.	• Use of IV replacement is based on the degree of dehydration, ongoing losses, insensible water losses, and electrolyte results.

EXPECTED OUTCOME: Child will have normal fluid and electrolyte balance as indicated by laboratory evaluation and physical examination.

(continued)

Nursing Care Plan: The Child Hospitalized With Gastroenteritis (continued)

3. Nursing Diagnosis: *Skin Integrity, Risk for Impaired*, related to altered fluid status (NANDA-I © 2014)

GOAL: The child will remain free of skin breakdown and rashes.

INTERVENTION	RATIONALE
• Assess skin of perineum and rectum for signs of skin breakdown or irritation.	• Early assessment and intervention can prevent worsening of the condition.
• Provide prevention or restorative care for infants as follows:	
Preventive Care:	
• Change diapers every 2 hr or as needed.	• Minimizes skin contact with chemical irritants from stool and urine.
• Wash diaper area after each soiling.	• Removes traces of stool if present.
• Apply A&D ointment, Aquaphor, or another barrier ointment with each diaper change.	• Provides a barrier and protects intact or reddened skin from becoming excoriated.
Restorative Care:	
• Leave the buttocks open to air for a few minutes several times daily, placing absorbent pads under the infant.	• Promotes air circulation to the area.
• Notify the healthcare provider if the skin is severely broken or peeling or if a rash is present.	• Additional measures such as the use of a barrier cream or paste may be needed to ensure skin healing.
• *For toddlers and older children:* Tub bathe at least daily (if condition allows) in tepid water. Pat the area dry.	• Helps loosen any fecal matter without scrubbing, which can cause additional irritation to the skin.
• Discourage the wearing of underwear if possible.	• Allows air to circulate and prevents accumulation of moisture.
• Apply barrier ointment with each diaper change or as instructed.	• Provides a barrier and protects intact or reddened skin from becoming excoriated.

EXPECTED OUTCOME: Child's perianal and rectal tissue will remain pink and intact.

Planning and Implementation

Nursing care focuses on providing emotional support, promoting rest and comfort, and ensuring adequate nutrition.

PROVIDE EMOTIONAL SUPPORT

The child may have been ill for several days or become suddenly ill a short time before seeking health care. The child and parents are usually anxious, so it is important to allow them to talk and ask questions. The child may require blood tests to help direct rehydration therapy. Most children are cared for at home, although care in a 24-hour monitoring unit may occur. Using therapeutic play techniques, such as allowing the child to manipulate equipment, can reduce anxiety (see Chapter 39).

PROMOTE REST AND COMFORT

Children with gastroenteritis may awaken frequently with periods of vomiting and diarrhea. Provide a quiet, restful environment and cluster nursing care to allow for periods of uninterrupted rest. To reduce the child's anxiety, encourage parents to room-in. Place the child's favorite toys and comfort objects within reach. Keep the child's mouth moistened with a wet washcloth, or an occasional ice chip. Provide skin care after each diarrheal episode to maintain skin integrity. Avoid using commercial baby wipes that contain alcohol as these irritate the skin and cause discomfort for the child.

ENSURE ADEQUATE NUTRITION

Liquids are offered throughout the illness, even if an intravenous infusion is in place. Follow guidelines for oral rehydration therapy in Chapter 44. Small amounts of normal diet for age are provided. Infants are breastfed or given formula. The child's diet progresses according to protocol or the child's tolerance for feedings.

Clinical Tip

Instruct parents in the importance of and techniques for hand hygiene, especially when caring for the child with gastroenteritis. Teach children in childcare centers and school how to wash their hands effectively to prevent spread of infectious diseases.

DISCHARGE PLANNING AND HOME CARE TEACHING

Discharge teaching begins on arrival at the healthcare facility. Teach the parents about the symptoms of dehydration and what actions to take if diarrhea recurs. Be sure that parents understand the recommended diet progression. Emphasize the necessity of good hygiene practices to prevent the spread of microorganisms that can cause gastroenteritis. If the child attends child care, have the parent inform the care center about the infection so the staff can be alerted to watch for other cases and can take steps to prevent the spread of infection.

Evaluation

Expected outcomes of nursing care are provided on the accompanying *Nursing Care Plan.*

Constipation

Constipation is a common complaint in the pediatric population and accounts for 3% of all visits to the pediatric primary care provider (Nurko & Zimmerman, 2014). Up to 30% of the pediatric population experience constipation (Watson, 2014). Most children experience functional constipation. This refers to constipation that cannot be attributed to an underlying physiological or anatomic abnormality (Rogers, 2012).

Because stool patterns vary among children, identification of an abnormal pattern is sometimes difficult. Infants usually have several bowel movements a day. For a young child, one bowel movement a day may be normal. As the child grows, however, three to four bowel movements in a week may be a normal pattern. The diagnosis of constipation must take into account the child's normal stool patterns.

Constipation may be caused by an underlying disease, diet, or psychologic factor. It may result from defects in filling, or more commonly emptying, of the rectum. Pathologic causes of defective filling include ineffective colonic propulsive activity, caused by hypothyroidism or use of medication, and obstruction, caused by a structural anomaly (stricture or stenosis) or by an aganglionic segment (Hirschsprung disease). If the rectum fails to fill, stasis leads to increased water reabsorption and hard, dry stools. Emptying of the rectum depends on the defecation reflex. Lesions of the spinal cord, weakness of the abdominal muscles, and local lesions blocking sphincter relaxation all may impede attempts to defecate.

Constipation during infancy is rare and is most often caused by mismanagement of diet. The transition from formula to cow's milk may cause a transient constipation since the bowel must adjust to the increased protein content of cow's milk.

Constipation occurs most frequently in the toddler and preschool age groups. This increased incidence is often associated with learning to control body functions. Many children do not like the sensations of a bowel movement and may begin withholding stool, which accumulates in and dilates the rectum until the next urge to defecate. The increasingly hard and painful bowel movement reinforces the child's behavior, and a cycle begins (Rogers, 2012).

Constipation in the school-age child, older child, and adolescent is generally related to activity, diet, and toileting habits. The child may not be eating enough fiber and could be eating starchy foods that contribute to constipation. Constipation may occur because of limited time for toileting. The child may not take time during the day to have a bowel movement or may be hesitant to use an unfamiliar bathroom.

Diagnosis is based on a thorough history and physical examination. When constipation occurs along with growth failure, vomiting, or abdominal pain, further investigation is necessary to rule out other disorders. Tests may include thyroid function tests; measurements of calcium, glucose, and electrolytes; a complete blood count; and urinalysis.

CLINICAL THERAPY

Dietary management is the treatment of choice for constipation that has no underlying pathologic cause. Constipation in young infants can usually be corrected by increasing the amount of fluids or adding 2 oz of pear or apple juice to daily intake. Increasing physical activity and fluid intake may be effective for some children.

Removing constipating foods (e.g., bananas, rice, and cheese) from the child's diet often decreases constipation. Increasing the child's intake of high-fiber foods (e.g., whole-grain breads, raw fruits, and vegetables) and fluids also promotes bowel elimination. In older infants, increasing the intake of fluids, cereals, fruits, and vegetables in the diet should correct the problem. A single glycerin suppository or enema may be required to remove hard stool.

Encouragement from parents and relaxation of bathroom privileges at school promote regularity and return of usual bowel patterns within a short time for school-age children. Children may need to get up earlier to have breakfast to allow time for toileting before going to school.

Constipation may follow surgery, especially in children who are immobilized. Stool softeners and a diet high in fiber and fluids prevent and treat constipation. Pharmacologic management of severe constipation usually occurs in two stages. The first stage involves disimpaction, followed by maintenance therapy (Rogers, 2011).

Disimpaction is difficult for the child and those who are managing the child's constipation. Consider the most effective means to evacuate the stool while causing the least amount of stress and anxiety to the child. The oral route is less invasive, but if the child experiences nausea and vomiting, the rectal route might be used. Polyethylene glycol solution with electrolyte solution is recommended for disimpaction (Paul, Dewdney, & Lamb, 2012; Rogers, 2011, 2012). Once the stool has been evacuated, maintenance therapy that may include polyethylene glycol powder, docusate, lactulose, or other products is continued for several weeks after a regular bowel patterns are established (Rogers, 2012).

Behavior modification may prove beneficial to managing constipation and may include having the child sit on the toilet after meals. Providing rewards for toileting at routinely scheduled times is effective (Rogers, 2012).

Nursing Management

Nursing care focuses on teaching parents what constitutes normal bowel patterns in children and the importance of diet in maintaining normal bowel patterns. Assess the child's diet history and obtain a description of bowel patterns from parents. Ask what the family does to treat constipation. Assessment of the child's food likes and dislikes may provide a clue as to the cause of constipation. Regular bowel habits are encouraged by placing the child on the toilet 30 minutes after a meal or around the time defecation usually occurs. Providing positive reinforcement during toilet training helps prevent a withholding pattern.

Teach parents dietary measures to promote regularity of bowel movements. Children can be given a high-fiber diet that includes fruits and vegetables. Cut-up fresh fruits, dried fruits, and fruit juice can be offered as snacks. A glycerin suppository can be used periodically. This is a natural stimulant and lubricant of the bowel. Caution parents to avoid frequent use of laxatives, stool softeners, and enemas since overuse can cause bowel dependency. Herbal stimulant laxatives are discouraged for children younger than 12 years, whereas other intestinal motility aids are not generally harmful. Find out more about any herbs the family commonly uses.

Encopresis

Encopresis is an abnormal elimination pattern characterized by the recurrent soiling or passage of stool at inappropriate times by a child who should have achieved bowel continence. Encopresis is reported to occur in approximately 3% of children ages 3 to 12. Children with primary encopresis have never achieved bowel control. Children with secondary encopresis have been continent of stool for more than 6 months before developing encopresis (Coehlo, 2011).

Encopresis is usually associated with voluntary or involuntary retention of stool in the lower bowel and rectum, leading to constipation, dilation of the lower bowel, and incompetence of the inner sphincter. The retention of stool is usually a result of being "too busy"; the child puts off going to the bathroom because of the inconvenience of leaving an activity. The retention of stool leads to constipation that is untreated and chronic. Loose stool leaks around the hard feces, and the child becomes unaware of a need to eliminate. Soiling may occur during the day or night. Bowel movements are irregular, painful, small, and hard. The child may be ridiculed by peers because of offensive body odor. This rejection leads to withdrawal and behavioral problems, often resulting in altered school performance and attendance. The child continues to hold stool because the passage has become painful. Parents commonly seek health care, believing that the child has diarrhea or constipation.

The underlying constipation that leads to encopresis may be caused by the stress of environmental changes (e.g., birth of a sibling, moving to a new house, attending a new school), issues of anger and control related to bowel training, diet, a full schedule of activities, or a genetic predisposition.

A thorough history, physical examination, and diagnostic studies (possibly including barium or contrast enema) are necessary to rule out organic causes and anatomic abnormalities. Information about the child's toilet training habits and parents' attitudes concerning those habits is obtained. A dietary history, including eating habits and types of foods eaten, is often helpful. Physical examination sometimes reveals a nontender mass in the lower abdomen.

In addition to dietary management and treatment to evacuate the bowel if needed as discussed in the preceding section, bowel training, behavior management, and family support are important components in the management of encopresis. Bowel training involves having the child sit on the toilet for a specific amount of time after breakfast and after dinner. This allows the child to gain or regain control of their bowel and an awareness of a full rectum. Behavior management includes involving the child in their care and provides reward and positive reinforcement for successes. Treatment for encopresis may take 6 to 12 months. The family needs education and support during this process. Long-term management may include oral stool softeners (Coehlo, 2011).

Nursing Management

Prevention of encopresis is the nursing goal. Partner with parents to teach toilet training techniques, emphasizing the child's developmental readiness. Parents are encouraged to praise the child for successes and to avoid punishment and power struggles. Encourage high-fiber diets and regular times for elimination.

Nursing care centers on educating the child and parents about the disorder and its treatment and on providing emotional support. Explain the treatment plan, including dietary changes and use of laxatives or stool softeners. Reassure the child that he or she has a healthy body and, with treatment, will achieve normal functioning. The child is monitored during clinic visits for at least 6 months to be certain new patterns have been established.

Intestinal Parasitic Disorders

Intestinal parasitic disorders occur most frequently in tropical regions. Outbreaks take place where water is not treated, food is incorrectly prepared, or people live in crowded conditions with poor sanitation. In the United States, outbreaks of diseases caused by protozoa or helminths (worms) are increasing. Young children, especially those in day care, are most at risk of infection. Young children often lack good hygiene practices and are likely to put objects and their hands into their mouths. See Table 51–3 for common intestinal parasitic disorders.

Another common cause of young child infection is exposure to pets and wildlife. Pets should be checked regularly for parasites and treated for worms as needed. Sandboxes should be kept covered when not in use, and children should be taught good handwashing techniques after exposure to their pets (CDC, 2014b). Laboratory examination of stool specimens identifies the causative organism (protozoa, worms, larvae, or ova). Treatment usually involves an anthelmintic.

Nursing care centers on preventive teaching. Emphasize the importance of good hygiene practices, especially careful handwashing, after toileting and when handling food. Ensure the family understands proper medication administration. Instruct parents to administer prescribed medications as directed even if the child's condition seems to be improved.

Disorders of Malabsorption

Malabsorption occurs when a child cannot digest or absorb nutrients in the diet. Disorders of malabsorption include celiac disease, lactose intolerance, and short bowel syndrome. Celiac disease and lactose intolerance are discussed in Chapter 32. Cystic fibrosis, a common cause of malabsorption, is discussed in Chapter 46.

Short Bowel Syndrome

Short bowel syndrome is a decreased ability to absorb and digest a regular diet due to a shortened intestine. Loss of intestine may result from extensive bowel resection for treatment of necrotizing enterocolitis or inflammatory disorders or from a congenital bowel anomaly such as intestinal malrotation, gastroschisis, or atresia.

The extent and location of the involved bowel determine the severity of the disorder. Because specific types of absorption occur primarily in certain parts of the bowel, the section lost determines the particular vitamins and other nutrients that are inadequate.

During the first 3 months after bowel resection, watery diarrhea is common. In the transition period, the remaining bowel usually increases its absorptive surface area and partially compensates for the absent intestine. At first, the infant or young child requires nutritional support to provide sufficient nutrients for adequate growth and development. In the initial period, the child only receives total parenteral nutrition (TPN). Once the bowel begins to recover, in addition to TPN, start continuous enteral feedings. Continuous exposure to nutrients

TABLE 51–3 Common Intestinal Parasitic Disorders

PARASITIC INFECTION	TRANSMISSION, LIFE CYCLE, PATHOGENESIS	CLINICAL MANIFESTATIONS	CLINICAL THERAPY	COMMENTS
GIARDIASIS				
Organism: protozoan *Giardia lamblia* Centers for Disease Control (CDC)	Transmission is through person-to-person contact, unfiltered water, improperly prepared infected food, and contact with animals. Cysts are ingested and passed into the duodenum and proximal jejunum, where they begin actively feeding. They are excreted in the stool.	May be asymptomatic. *Infants:* diarrhea, vomiting, anorexia, avoidant/restrictive food intake disorder (failure to thrive) *Older children:* abdominal cramps; intermittent loose, foul-smelling, watery, pale, and greasy stools	Medications used to treat giardiasis include metronidazole, tinidazole, and nitazoxanide (drugs of choice). Quinacrine, furazolidone, and paromomycin may be used.	Most common intestinal parasitic organism in the United States. Symptoms last 2–6 weeks. Medication may decrease this time frame. Parents or caregivers should wear gloves when handling diapers or stool of an infant or child infected with parasites.
ENTEROBIASIS (PINWORM)				
Organism: nematode *Enterobius vermicularis* B.G. Partin; Dr. Moore/CDC	Transmission is from discharged eggs inhaled or carried from hand to mouth. Eggs hatch in the upper intestine and mature in 1–2 months. Larvae then migrate to the colon and lay eggs. Movement of worms causes intense itching. Scratching deposits eggs on the hands and under the nails.	Intense perianal itching, irritability, restlessness, and short attention span; in females, can migrate to the vagina and urethra to cause infection. Itching intensifies at night when the female comes to the anal opening to lay eggs.	Medications used to treat enterobiasis include mebendazole, pyrantel pamoate, and albendazole. The child and all household members should be treated at the same time. Treatment may be repeated in 2 weeks.	Most common worm infection in the United States. Transmission is increased in crowded conditions such as housing developments, schools, and childcare centers.
ASCARIASIS (TYPE OF ROUNDWORM)				
Organism: nematode *Ascaris lumbricoides* James Cavallini/BSIP SA/Alamy	Transmission is from discharged eggs carried from hand to mouth. The adult lays eggs in the small intestine. Eggs are excreted in stool. Swallowed eggs hatch in the small intestine. Larvae may penetrate intestinal villi, entering the portal vein and liver, then moving to the lung. Larvae that ascend to the upper respiratory tract are swallowed and proceed to the small intestine, where they repeat the cycle.	Mild infection may be asymptomatic. Severe infection may result in intestinal obstruction and impaired growth.	Medications used to treat ascariasis include ivermectin, mebendazole, and albendazole.	Most common in warm, moist climates. Associated with poor personal hygiene and poor sanitation.
HOOKWORM DISEASE				
Organism: nematode *Necator americanus* Centers for Disease Control (CDC)	Transmission is through direct contact with infected soil containing larvae. Worms live in the small intestine and feed on villi, causing bleeding. Eggs are deposited in the bowel and excreted in feces. Eggs hatch in damp, shaded soil. Larvae attach to and penetrate the skin, then enter the bloodstream, migrating to the lungs. Larvae then migrate to the upper respiratory passages and are swallowed.	In healthy individuals, mild infection seldom causes problems. Presence of larvae on the skin may cause itching and a rash. More severe infection may result in diarrhea, abdominal pain, anemia, weight loss, and fatigue.	Medications used to treat hookworm disease include mebendazole, albendazole, and pyrantel pamoate. Iron supplements may also be given.	Children should wear shoes when outdoors. Note, however, that other unprotected areas of the skin may still come in contact with larvae.

(continued)

TABLE 51–3 Common Intestinal Parasitic Disorders (*continued*)

PARASITIC INFECTION	TRANSMISSION, LIFE CYCLE, PATHOGENESIS	CLINICAL MANIFESTATIONS	CLINICAL THERAPY	COMMENTS
STRONGYLOIDIASIS (TYPE OF ROUNDWORM)				
Organism: nematode *Strongyloides stercoralis* 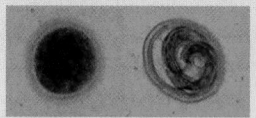 Centers for Disease Control (CDC)	Transmission is from the ingestion of discharged larvae in the soil. Life cycle is similar to that of the hookworm, except this roundworm does not attach to the intestinal mucosa, and feeding larvae (rather than eggs) may be deposited in the soil.	Mild infection may be asymptomatic. Severe infection may result in abdominal pain and distention, nausea, vomiting, diarrhea, dry cough, throat irritation, and itchy rash.	Medications used to treat strongyloidiasis include ivermectin and albendazole. Treatment may need to be repeated if symptoms recur after treatment.	Most common in older children and adolescents.
TOXOCARIASIS (TYPE OF ROUNDWORM)				
Organism: nematode *Toxocara canis* or *T. cati*, commonly found in dogs and cats Centers for Disease Control (CDC)	Transmission is through the ingestion of eggs in the soil. Ingested eggs hatch in the intestine. Mobile larvae then migrate to the liver and eventually to all major organs (including the brain). Once migration is complete, they encapsulate in dense fibrous tissue.	Most cases are asymptomatic. Severe symptoms include fever, coughing, pneumonia, and enlarged liver.	Medications used to treat toxocariasis include albendazole and mebendazole. Steroids may also be used.	Deworm household pets on a regular basis. Keep children away from areas contaminated with animal droppings.

Note: Some of the medications listed may not be available in the United States, and some of them may not be approved for use in all age groups.

Source: Data from American Academy of Pediatrics (AAP). (2015). Parasitic diseases. *Red book: 2015 report of the Committee on Infectious Diseases* (30th ed. pp. 588–591). Elk Grove Village, IL: Author; Centers for Disease Control and Prevention (CDC). (2014a). *Parasites*. Retrieved from http://www.cdc.gov/parasites; Gershon, A. A., & Hotez, P. J. (2011). Infectious diseases. In C. D. Rudolph, A. M. Rudolph, G. E. Lister, L. R. First, & A. A. Gershon (Eds.), *Rudolph's pediatrics* (22nd ed., pp. 878–1247). New York, NY: McGraw-Hill. Photos of *Giardia lamblia*, strongyloidiasis, hookworm, and toxocariasis are courtesy of the Centers for Disease Control and Prevention, Atlanta, GA.

allows the bowel to adapt (Cuffari, 2014). It is essential that the child receive the appropriate nutritional components regardless of the method in which nutrition is delivered.

SAFETY ALERT!

The child with short bowel syndrome will receive TPN via a central line. Aseptic technique in the care of the central line is essential to prevent a catheter-associated bloodstream infection and potential sepsis (Gutierrez, Kang, & Jaksic, 2011). Maintaining patency of the central line is also essential because this may be the child's only route for receiving nutrition. It is not uncommon for children with short bowel syndrome to require insertion of multiple central lines over time because of either infection or occlusion of the line, especially if they require long-term TPN. This not only places a stress on the child who must undergo yet another surgical procedure, but is a stressor for the family as well.

Nursing Management

Nursing care focuses on meeting the child's nutritional and fluid needs and teaching parents how to care for the child at home. Establishing an adequate nutritional intake and bowel pattern is a lengthy process. TPN is provided initially until a feeding regimen can be established. Oral and enteral feedings are instituted gradually to allow the bowel time to compensate. Provide support to the family and child throughout this period. Teach parents how to prepare and administer total parenteral feedings and care for the central line (see the *Clinical Skills Manual* SKILLS). Once enteral or tube feedings have started, teach management of the feeding pump and care of the feeding tube. Ensure regular bowel function and maintain skin integrity. Arrange home visits to monitor the child's growth and development, care of the central line and tube-feeding site, and any side effects such as fluid and electrolyte imbalance and diarrhea.

Hepatic Disorders

The liver is one of the most vital organs in the body. Its primary functions include production of blood clotting factors, fibrinogen, and prothrombin; secretion of bile and *bilirubin* (yellow pigment produced from the breakdown of red blood cells); metabolism of fat, protein, and carbohydrates; detoxification of hormones, drugs, and other substances; and storage of vitamins A, D, E, and K and glycogen. Thus any inflammatory, obstructive, or degenerative disorder that affects liver function can be life threatening. The following discussion focuses on three common liver disorders in children: biliary atresia, viral hepatitis, and cirrhosis. A discussion of hyperbilirubinemia can be found in Chapter 27.

Biliary Atresia

Biliary atresia results when the extrahepatic bile ducts fail to develop or are closed. The disorder leads to cholestasis, cirrhosis, portal hypertension, end-stage liver disease, and death by 2 years of age if left untreated (Flanigan, 2013; Moreira, Cabral, Cowles, et al., 2012; Sira, Taha, & Sira, 2014). Biliary atresia is the leading indication for pediatric liver transplantation (Moreira et al., 2012).

CLINICAL MANIFESTATIONS

Initially, the newborn is asymptomatic. Jaundice may not be detected until 2 to 3 weeks after birth. At that point, bilirubin levels increase, accompanied by abdominal distention and hepatomegaly (see Appendix B for bilirubin levels and other liver function tests). As the disease progresses, splenomegaly occurs. The infant experiences easy bruising, prolonged bleeding time, and intense itching. Stools have putty-like consistency and are white or clay colored because of the absence of bile pigments. Excretion of bilirubin and bile salts results in tea-colored urine. Avoidant/restrictive food intake disorder (failure to thrive) and malnutrition occur as the destructive changes of the disease progress.

The cause of biliary atresia is unknown. Absence or blockage of the extrahepatic bile ducts results in blocked bile flow from the liver to the duodenum. This altered bile flow soon causes inflammation and fibrotic changes in the liver. In addition to blockage, the disease can also be caused by hepatocellular dysfunction. Lack of bile acids also interferes with digestion of fat and absorption of fat-soluble vitamins A, D, E, and K, resulting in steatorrhea and nutritional deficiencies. Without treatment the disease is fatal.

CLINICAL THERAPY

Diagnosis is based on the history, physical examination, and laboratory evaluation. Laboratory findings reveal elevated bilirubin and serum aminotransferase and alkaline phosphatase levels, prolonged prothrombin time, and increased ammonia levels (Schwarz, 2014). Percutaneous liver biopsy suggests biliary atresia, and an exploratory laparotomy and intraoperative cholangiography confirms the diagnosis (Robie, Overfelt, & Xie, 2014).

Treatment involves surgery to attempt correction of the obstruction (hepatoportoenterostomy) and supportive care. In a hepatoportoenterostomy (Kasai procedure), a segment of the intestine is anastomosed to the porta hepatis. The primary purpose of this procedure is to promote bile flow from the liver. Intravenous antibiotics are administered in the postoperative period to prevent cholangitis. Prophylaxis with oral antibiotics is continued for 1 to 2 years after surgery (Flanigan, 2013).

Additional treatment includes administration of intramuscular vitamin K prior to invasive procedures and surgery to decrease the risk of bleeding afterwards and vitamins A, D, E, and K to provide supplementation since absorption of these vitamins is impaired. The infant is breastfed or is given Pregestimil or Nutramigen, formulas that contain medium-chain triglycerides. As the liver disease worsens, the child may need cholestyramine and antihistamines to help decrease itching. Enteral feedings may be needed as well (Flanigan, 2013).

Ursodeoxycholic acid (Actigall) may be given to the child to promote bile flow (Schwarz, 2014).

While bile flow is achieved with the Kasai procedure in many children with biliary atresia, approximately 70% to 80% of children having this surgery will eventually need a liver transplant (Mieli-Vergani & Tizzard, 2012). Advances in transplantation surgery now make it possible to perform partial liver transplants from living donor resections. This enables transplantation to be performed before the child develops end-stage liver disease (Flanigan, 2013).

Nursing Management

Nursing care in the initial stages of biliary atresia is the same as that for any healthy newborn. As symptoms develop, the focus of nursing care becomes long-term management and support.

Diagnosis of this potentially fatal disorder can be devastating to parents. Provide emotional support and offer frequent explanations of tests during the initial diagnostic evaluation. As the disease progresses, the infant becomes irritable because of intense itching and the accumulation of toxins. Tepid baths may help to relieve itching and provide comfort. Dry skin by patting rather than rubbing to avoid further skin irritation. Promote rest by grouping nursing activities while the infant is awake. Weigh the infant daily. Administer TPN, lipids, and fat-soluble vitamins A, D, E, and K as prescribed.

Care following a hepatoportoenterostomy is similar to that for a child undergoing abdominal surgery. (See the earlier discussion of postsurgical nursing management for appendicitis and *Nursing Care Plan: The Child Undergoing Surgery* in Chapter 39.) Posttransplant care includes immunosuppressant drugs and close monitoring for vascular complications. Discharge planning focuses on teaching parents how to care for the child's skin, provide for nutritional needs, administer medications, and monitor for increasing symptoms of liver disease. When the child has received a transplant, teach parents how to identify signs of rejection (nausea, vomiting, fever, and jaundice), as well as the administration and side effects of immunosuppressant medications. Refer parents to support groups, clergy, or social services if indicated. They will need ongoing visits from a home healthcare nurse to help them manage the child's complex care. Palliative care may need to be discussed with the family if it becomes evident the child will not survive (see Chapter 41). Expected outcomes for nursing care of the child with biliary atresia are as follows:

- The child consumes adequate nutrition in order to support growth and development.
- Parents cope effectively with stress of the child's condition.
- The child achieves growth and developmental milestones expected for age.

Viral Hepatitis

Hepatitis is an inflammation of the liver caused by a viral infection. Hepatitis may be an acute or chronic disease. Acute hepatitis is rapid in onset and, if untreated, may develop into chronic hepatitis. The most frequently diagnosed causative organisms are hepatitis A virus (HAV), hepatitis B virus (HBV), and hepatitis C virus (HCV). A lesser known type is hepatitis D virus (HDV). Hepatitis E (HEV) occurs primarily in developing countries and is rarely seen in the United States (CDC, 2012a). In 2012, the incidence of hepatitis A declined to 10.5 cases per

TABLE 51–4 Comparison of Hepatitis Types

TYPE	IMMUNIZATION AVAILABLE	PROPHYLAXIS	PRIMARY TRANSMISSION	INCUBATION PERIOD
Hepatitis A	Yes	Immune globulin Hepatitis A vaccine	Fecal–oral	15–19 days
Hepatitis B	Yes	Hepatitis B immune globulin Hepatitis B vaccine	Needlesticks or sharps exposure Intravenous drug use During birth Sexual activity	60–180 days
Hepatitis C	No	None	Needlesticks or sharps exposure Intravenous drug use During birth	14–160 days
Hepatitis D	No	Hepatitis B vaccine	Needlesticks or sharps exposure Intravenous drug use During birth Sexual activity	21–42 days
Hepatitis E	No	None	Fecal–oral	21–63 days

Source: Data from Centers for Disease Control and Prevention (CDC). (2012a). *Hepatitis E information for health professionals.* Retrieved from http://www.cdc.gov/hepatitis/HEV/index.htm; CDC. (2012b). *Hepatitis B information for health professionals.* Retrieved from http://www.cdc.gov/hepatitis/HBV/index.htm; CDC. (2014d). *Hepatitis A information for health professionals.* Retrieved from http://www.cdc.gov/hepatitis/HAV/index.htm; CDC. (2014e). *Hepatitis C information for health professionals.* Retrieved from http://www.cdc.gov/hepatitis/HCV/index.htm; CDC. (2014f). *Hepatitis D information for health professionals.* Retrieved from http://www.cdc.gov/hepatitis/HDV/index.htm; Jensen, M. K., & Balistreri, W. F. (2016). Viral hepatitis. In R. M. Kliegman, B. F. Stanton, J. W. St. Geme III, & N. F. Schor (Eds.), *Nelson textbook of pediatrics* (20th ed., pp. 1942–1953). Philadelphia, PA: Elsevier Saunders.

100,000 in the United States. The incidence of hepatitis B has also decreased remarkably during the past several years with an incidence of 0.9 cases per 100,000 in 2012 (CDC, 2014c). The decline in both of these illnesses is related to routine vaccine administration, especially in children.

ETIOLOGY AND PATHOPHYSIOLOGY

Hepatitis A is highly contagious and traditionally has been called *infectious hepatitis*. Infection occurs primarily through the fecal–oral route. Transmission is by direct person-to-person spread or through ingestion of contaminated water or food. Hepatitis A frequently occurs in children in childcare settings where hygiene practices are poor. Food handlers can spread hepatitis A if not aware of their infection; it is a common cause of foodborne illness. Because the virus is transmitted in the early stages of the disease when individuals are often asymptomatic or only mildly ill, large numbers of people may be exposed before the diagnosis is confirmed (Table 51–4). Most children recover from hepatitis A; however, in rare instances, acute liver failure may occur (Jensen & Balistreri, 2016).

Hepatitis B can result in acute or chronic infection and is transmitted by the parenteral route through the exchange of blood or any body secretion or fluids, sexual activity, and transmission from mother to fetus in utero (Peate & Jones, 2014). Adolescents who use intravenous drugs and have unprotected sexual intercourse are at risk for contracting hepatitis B. Major sources for the spread of HBV are healthy chronic carriers.

Hepatitis C is the most common chronic bloodborne infection in the United States. The hepatitis C virus is transmitted primarily through intravenous drug use, needlestick injury, and birth to a mother infected with hepatitis C. The virus can also be spread through blood transfusions, but the incidence of this route of transmission in the United States is rare because blood is screened for this infection. Chronic infection occurs in 75% to 85% of those individuals infected with hepatitis C (CDC, 2014e).

Hepatitis D (delta virus) is a defective virus that can gain entry to a human only in connection with hepatitis B (CDC, 2014f). It can occur as a coinfection along with hepatitis B or as a superinfection in someone already infected with hepatitis B.

Hepatitis E infection is primarily transmitted through contaminated water and is most common in developing countries (Jensen & Balistreri, 2016).

The liver's response to injury by the viruses that cause hepatitis is similar (see *Pathophysiology Illustrated: Viral Hepatitis*). Initially, invasion of the parenchymal cells by the virus results in local degeneration and necrosis. Subsequent infiltration of the parenchyma by lymphocytes, macrophages, plasma cells, eosinophils, and neutrophils causes inflammation that blocks biliary drainage into the intestine. Impaired bile excretion causes a buildup of bile in the blood, urine, and skin (jaundice). Structural changes in the parenchymal cells account for other altered liver functions.

CLINICAL MANIFESTATIONS

Symptoms of acute viral hepatitis infection include nausea, vomiting, fatigue, abdominal pain, joint pain, pruritus, and urticaria in the prodromal phase. In the icteric phase, the child develops jaundice, gray- or pale-colored bowel movements, gastrointestinal symptoms, right upper quadrant pain, and malaise. In the convalescent phase the jaundice resolves and laboratory values return to normal (Buggs, 2014; CDC, 2012c).

CLINICAL THERAPY

Diagnosis is often made on the basis of a thorough history and physical examination. A history of exposure to persons with the disease is significant. Physical examination reveals a tender, enlarged liver. Laboratory evaluation includes serologic testing (to detect the presence of antigens and antibodies to HAV, HBV, HCV, or HDV) liver function studies, serum bilirubin, and prothrombin time (Harris & Crawford, 2013; Jensen & Balistreri, 2016).

Early diagnosis is essential to follow the course of the illness and identify potential complications. Management includes bed rest, hydration, and adequate nutrition.

The spread of viral infections can be interrupted by elimination of the virus from the infected population, institution of proper hygiene, and passive or active immunization. To date, no antiviral agent has been developed to combat the hepatitis viruses. Prevention depends on breaking the cycle of infection.

Pathophysiology Illustrated: **Viral Hepatitis**

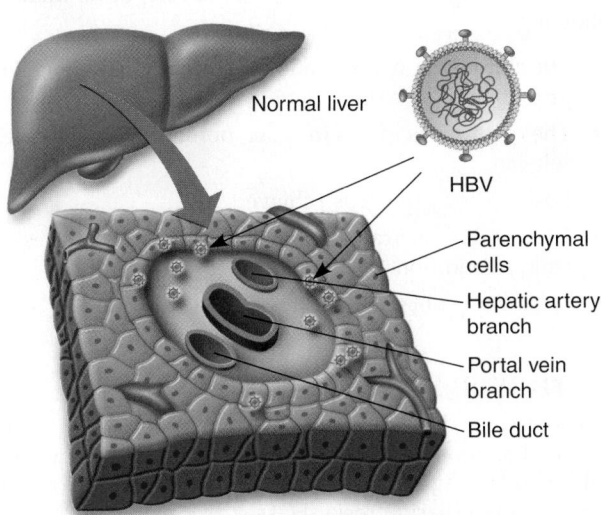

Normal liver

HBV

Parenchymal cells

Hepatic artery branch

Portal vein branch

Bile duct

① Virus invades parenchymal cells, causing local degeneration and necrosis

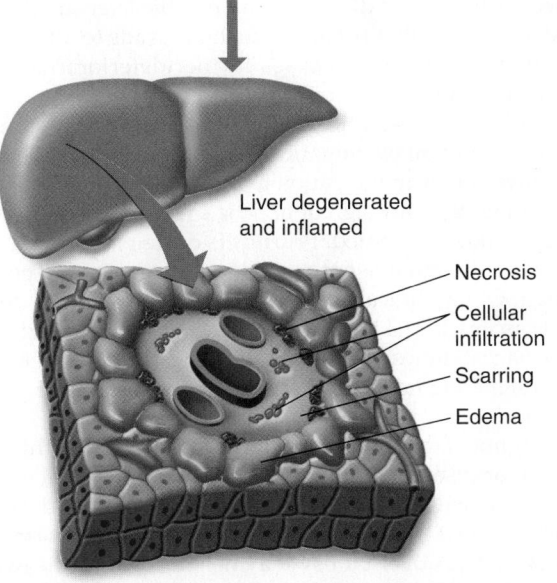

Liver degenerated and inflamed

Necrosis

Cellular infiltration

Scarring

Edema

② Infiltration by lymphocytes, macrophages, and other white blood cells causes inflammation that blocks drainage

③ Structural changes occur in parenchymal cells, resulting in altered liver function:

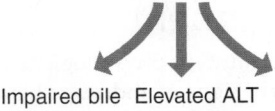

| Impaired bile excretion | Elevated ALT and alkaline phosphatase levels | Decreased albumin synthesis |

The hepatitis virus causes degeneration and necrosis of the liver, which results in abnormal liver function and illness.

Active immunization for hepatitis A, a two-dose series, is recommended for all people at increased risk of acquiring infection, for children, and for those who wish to acquire immunity to the illness. The CDC (2012c) recommends that all children receive the first hepatitis A vaccine at 1 year of age.

Hepatitis B immune globulin (HBIG) and the hepatitis B vaccine must be given to infants born to infected mothers within 12 hours of birth to provide protection against the virus. Administration of the first dose of the three-dose series of the hepatitis B vaccine shortly after birth to all infants further reduces the risk of perinatal infection in cases where the mother's status may be unknown or incorrectly documented (CDC, 2012b). (Chapter 43 provides specific information on immunization schedules.)

Individuals who have been exposed to hepatitis A and have not been previously immunized should receive immune globulin or the hepatitis A vaccine within 2 weeks of exposure. Healthy individuals, ages 12 months to 40 years of age, not previously immunized may receive the hepatitis A vaccine instead of immune globulin within 2 weeks of exposure (CDC, 2014d). Passive immunity to HBV can be achieved with hepatitis B immune globulin (HBIG). Used for one-time exposure and for infants of infected mothers, it is given within 12 hours after birth (CDC, 2012b).

Nursing Management
For the Child With Viral Hepatitis

Nursing Assessment and Diagnosis

The nurse usually encounters the child and family in an outpatient setting. In addition to observing the child for characteristic signs of hepatitis (jaundiced skin and sclera), assess for abdominal pain, anorexia, nausea and vomiting, malaise, and arthralgia. A history of the child's contacts in the past several weeks is also obtained. For an infant, the hepatitis history of the mother and other family members is important.

Common nursing diagnoses for the child with acute hepatitis might include the following (NANDA-I © 2014):

- *Nutrition, Imbalanced: Less than Body Requirements*, related to chronic illness
- *Fatigue* related to disease state
- *Body Image, Disturbed (Older Child)*, related to jaundice
- *Anxiety (Parent and Child)* related to threat to health status

Planning and Implementation

Nursing care involves home and community considerations because children with hepatitis are seldom admitted to the hospital. The hospitalized child is placed in isolation. Prevention of the disease is integrated into all health care by discussion of immunization and standard precautions. Parents need additional detailed information about health precautions and infection control measures if hepatitis cases have occurred in the family or community. Teach parents the importance of checking with health professionals before administering any medications (even nonprescription medicines). Also teach them to maintain adequate nutrition, promote rest and comfort, and provide diversional activities.

PREVENT SPREAD OF INFECTION

Teach the parents and the child infection control measures to help prevent transmission of the virus. For parents, reinforce good hygiene practices, such as washing hands before and after toileting and proper disposal of soiled diapers. Vaccination for those exposed to hepatitis A or B should occur as discussed above. All healthcare providers should receive the hepatitis B immunization series and use standard precautions at all times (see the *Clinical Skills Manual* SKILLS).

Clinical Tip

Nurses in childcare centers can provide assessment of the center's procedures and teaching to prevent hepatitis A transmission. Help the center to set standards about:

- Handwashing after each diaper change
- Proper disposal of diapers
- Cleaning diaper-changing surfaces after each diaper change
- Enforcing policy that food handlers never perform diaper changes
- Instructing parents to keep children at home for at least 2 weeks after a diagnosis of hepatitis A
- Informing parents of other children attending the childcare center when there is a case of hepatitis A and teaching them the symptoms of the condition

---

MAINTAIN ADEQUATE NUTRITION

Initially, the child is encouraged to eat favorite foods. Once the anorexia and nausea have resolved, a high-protein, high-carbohydrate, low-fat diet is recommended. Increased protein helps maintain protein stores and prevent muscle wasting. Increased carbohydrates ensure adequate caloric intake and prevent protein depletion. The use of low-fat foods lessens stomach distention. Offer the child small, frequent feedings.

PROMOTE REST AND COMFORT

Bed rest is necessary only if the child has severe fatigue and malaise. However, most children voluntarily limit their activities during the initial phase of the disease. Keep the child quiet and comfortable. Offer comfort items such as favorite toys, blankets, and pillows.

ADMINISTER MEDICATIONS

Drug metabolism is altered during hepatitis since the liver cannot detoxify medications readily. As with all liver disorders, medications need to be administered carefully, and the child's condition must be monitored for possible drug side effects, especially since so many drugs are metabolized by the liver. Caution parents to check with healthcare providers before giving any nonprescription medication. For example, acetaminophen is metabolized in the liver, and liver disease can interfere with its breakdown.

PROVIDE DIVERSIONAL ACTIVITIES

Hospitalized children with hepatitis are kept in isolation. Nonhospitalized children with hepatitis do not need to be isolated, but they should be kept at home for 2 weeks following the onset of symptoms. Parents who cannot take time off from work may need to arrange home sitters to stay with the child. Offer suggestions for diversional activities during this period. Young children can be given a new toy or favorite activities. Older children and adolescents can be given board games, puzzles, books or magazines, movies, or video games. Phone calls and short visits from friends help school-age children and adolescents maintain contact with peers.

Evaluation

Expected outcomes of nursing care for hepatitis include the following:

- The child demonstrates adequate nutritional intake to meet growth and development needs.
- The child participates in quiet, nonfatiguing activities and self-care.
- Positive body image is achieved.
- Parents demonstrate effective coping with the stress of the child's condition.
- Hepatitis is not spread to the child's contacts.

Cirrhosis

Cirrhosis is a degenerative disease process that results in fibrotic changes and fatty infiltration in the liver. It can occur in children of any age as the end stage of several disorders such as hepatitis and biliary atresia (Hassan & Balistreri, 2016; Squires & Balistreri, 2016). The diffuse destruction and regeneration of the hepatic parenchymal cells result in an increase in fibrous connective tissue and disorganization of the liver structure. Progressive scarring that occurs in cirrhosis leads to altered blood flow to the liver, which causes further deterioration of liver function (Squires & Balistreri, 2016).

Clinical manifestations of cirrhosis vary. Hepatomegaly may be evident on examination. Jaundice occurs as the disease progresses and is an indication of hyperbilirubinemia. Jaundice is sometimes the only sign of hepatic dysfunction, so its appearance must be investigated. Pruritus is common in children with cirrhosis, although it is not related to the degree of hyperbilirubinemia. Other clinical manifestations of cirrhosis in children include ascites, portal hypertension, encephalopathy, and variceal hemorrhage (Squires & Balistreri, 2016). Severe end-stage complications signaling hepatic failure can occur at any time and with little warning.

Diagnostic evaluation is based on the child's history of infection or disease with liver involvement. Physical examination may reveal jaundice, skin changes, ascites, and hemodynamic changes. Laboratory evaluation reveals abnormal liver function tests. A liver biopsy may help determine the extent of the parenchymal damage.

Medical management focuses on treating the child's symptoms and achieving optimal nutritional status and growth. Liver transplantation is the most common treatment for biliary atresia and metabolic disorders and is the only treatment for end-stage liver disease.

Nursing Management

Nursing care focuses on monitoring physiologic and psychosocial changes to identify early signs of end-stage hepatic failure. Monitor vital signs every 2 to 4 hours. Measure weight daily to assess for fluid retention. Close monitoring of electrolytes and liver function test results helps determine the need for fluid replacement therapy.

Careful administration of medications and monitoring for side effects are necessary because drug metabolism is altered in liver disorders. If ascites is present, provide a low-sodium, low-protein diet and restrict fluids. Remove all water pitchers, glasses, and straws to minimize the child's desire to drink.

Parents of a child with cirrhosis are coping with a life-threatening disorder, and their anxiety and stress are high. The child may be awaiting a liver transplantation that represents the only hope for recovery. Support parents and encourage them to talk about their fears and concerns (see Chapter 41). Encourage parents to participate in the child's care. Referral to a support group or counseling may be beneficial.

Injuries to the Gastrointestinal System

Refer to Chapter 42 for information related to injury to the GI system due to poisoning and ingestion of foreign objects.

Abdominal Trauma

Motor vehicle crashes, falls, and auto–pedestrian injury are the leading causes of blunt abdominal injury in children. Other causes include child abuse, all-terrain vehicle accidents, and bicycle accidents (Mendez, 2014). While blunt trauma is most common, penetrating injury accounts for 10% to 20% of pediatric trauma admissions. Gunshot wounds are the most common cause of penetrating injury. Other causes include stabbing or impalement on an object (Daley, Raju, & Lee, 2013). Children are more likely than adults to sustain abdominal injuries because of their small pliable rib cage and less developed abdominal muscles, which provide little protection for major solid organs such as the spleen, liver, and kidneys. In addition, the solid organs in children are larger in proportion to their body size compared to adults, so less surface area of the organs is protected by the ribs, making them more exposed and vulnerable to injury (Daley et al., 2013; Mendez, 2014; Saxena, 2013).

The kind of injury determines the extent of organ damage. High-velocity blunt trauma, which may occur in motor vehicle crashes, usually involves multiple organs. Solid organs such as the liver and spleen can be bruised or lacerated. The sudden increase in abdominal pressure that occurs with a lap belt injury causes hollow organs such as the stomach, intestines, and bladder to burst. Sports-related abdominal trauma is often associated with a direct blow to the abdomen, and a single organ is usually injured. Bicycle accidents account for 5% to 14% of blunt abdominal trauma in children. Serious abdominal injury can result if the handlebars hit the child in the abdomen (Alkan et al., 2012; Cevek, Boleken, Sogut, et al., 2013).

Penetrating trauma is generally apparent upon inspection. Blunt trauma may not be as obvious. The abdomen should be inspected for abrasions, bruising, or markings (e.g., tire tracks or lap belt marks) that provide a clue to injury beneath the skin surface (Mendez, 2014). Abrasions, erythema, and ecchymosis in the lower abdominal area are classic visible signs of seat belt trauma (Borgialli et al., 2014). See Chapter 33 for abdominal assessment techniques. Additional clinical manifestations of abdominal injury include pain and tenderness, abdominal distention, and signs of hypovolemic shock such as pallor, altered mental status, hypotension, and tachycardia (Wesson, 2013).

Suspected abdominal trauma in a child necessitates a thorough history and physical examination. The description of the event should be compared with the child's signs and symptoms. Plain abdominal radiographs may reveal air in the abdomen. A focused abdominal ultrasound can reveal free fluid in the abdomen. An abdominal CT scan identifies a solid organ injury. Urinalysis that shows blood in the urine may be indicative of damage to the urinary tract or kidneys (McKenna & Pieper, 2013). Serial hemoglobin and hematocrit evaluation is essential to determine hemodynamic stability. Type and cross-match of blood is also necessary in case the child needs a blood transfusion. In addition, liver function tests and pancreatic enzymes are monitored in the case of injury to the liver and pancreas (Saxena, 2013).

SAFETY ALERT!

The child who is restrained in a motor vehicle with only a lap belt is at high risk for abdominal injury in a crash. As the car stops rapidly, the child's body is restrained and flexes around the lap belt. The sudden increase in abdominal pressure causes injury to hollow organs, and sometimes solid organs. Children no longer using car safety seats should sit in a booster seat so that a shoulder restraint is used in addition to the lap belt. A booster seat should be used until the child is 8 years of age or weighs at least 80 lb.

The spleen and the liver are the organs most commonly injured in blunt abdominal trauma. Nonsurgical management is preferred. The spleen plays a major role in immune function; therefore, the organ is salvaged whenever possible to decrease the risk of infection (Saxena, 2013). Liver lacerations are treated much like spleen lacerations as long as major vessels have not been injured. Exploratory laparotomy is performed to resect hollow organ injuries or to repair liver or spleen lacerations when bleeding is not controlled.

Treatment of an abdominal, liver, or spleen injury takes place in the pediatric intensive care unit (PICU) and focuses on preventing or managing hemorrhage and monitoring for signs of shock. An intravenous infusion is initiated for fluid maintenance and to provide access for blood products. The child is kept NPO. A nasogastric tube is inserted. Blood transfusions and pharmacologic management are used to treat blood loss.

The child is maintained on strict bed rest until bleeding is controlled and the hemoglobin and hematocrit are stable. The length of time the child is hospitalized ranges from 2 to 5 days depending on the severity of the injury. The length of time for activity restrictions after discharge ranges from 3 to 6 weeks and also depends on the severity of the injury (McKenna & Pieper, 2013).

Nursing Management

Nursing care includes initial and ongoing assessments of the child's condition. Assess the abdomen for bruising, pain, guarding, rebound tenderness, distention, and obvious signs of injury such as bruising. Monitor hematocrit and vital signs every hour as warranted to detect hypovolemia (see Chapter 47). Tachycardia and hypotension may indicate hypovolemia or internal bleeding. Strict monitoring of intake and output will provide information about the child's fluid status. Monitor the respiratory status because abdominal injuries may also have thoracic involvement. The child with associated thoracic injuries may not take deep breaths if it is painful.

The child and parents are usually fearful and anxious when the child is admitted to the hospital. If the injury was preventable, parents may have feelings of guilt or anger. Provide emotional support and avoid judgmental comments or statements that assign blame. Additional nursing care includes maintenance of the nasogastric tube, intravenous fluids, and blood, and monitoring of lab studies as appropriate. Any concerns should be reported to the healthcare provider immediately.

Once the child's condition is stabilized, the focus of nursing care shifts to preventive teaching. Parents should be taught safety measures to prevent future injuries. Discuss the use of car safety restraint devices for riding in an automobile (see Chapters 34, 35, and 36). If the child's injury was the result of a bicycle fall or crash, discuss the importance of the proper bicycle size and safety measures such as use of a helmet and proper use of hand signals.

Focus Your Study

- A variety of structural defects caused by fetal development alterations can affect the gastrointestinal system of infants.

- Cleft lip and palate are structural defects that often involve care by a team of healthcare providers such as a plastic surgeon, pediatrician, nurse, audiologist, speech therapist, and orthodontist.

- A variety of defects of the esophagus and trachea can manifest as mild to life-threatening problems in the newborn period.

- Pyloric stenosis is a common cause of projectile vomiting in the newborn period.

- Gastroesophageal reflux is one of the most common gastrointestinal problems in infants and children.

- Abdominal wall defects and anorectal malformations are serious structural defects of infancy.

- Intussusception is one of the most common causes of intestinal obstruction in the pediatric population and primarily occurs in children less than 1 year of age.

- Hirschsprung disease, or aganglionic megacolon, leads to failure to pass normal stools and distention of the abdomen.

- Several of the intestinal problems of childhood necessitate temporary or permanent ostomy placement.

- Hernias can be present in the diaphragmatic area, umbilicus, or inguinal canal.

- The most common inflammatory disorder of the gastrointestinal tract is appendicitis.

- Necrotizing enterocolitis is a potentially life-threatening inflammatory disease of the intestines seen primarily in premature infants after enteral feedings are begun.

- Common inflammatory bowel diseases affecting primarily adolescent and young adult age groups are Crohn disease and ulcerative colitis.

- Peptic ulcers occur primarily in individuals receiving nonsteroidal anti-inflammatory drugs and those with *Helicobacter pylori* infection.

- Common disorders of motility include diarrhea, constipation, and encopresis.

- Gastroenteritis and parasitic disorders are common causes of gastrointestinal disturbance and distress in children, and may lead to fluid and electrolyte imbalance.

- Short bowel syndrome occurs when surgery is used to treat an intestinal disease and significant sections of the bowel are removed.

- Biliary atresia and hepatitis are the most common liver diseases in young children.

- Abdominal trauma most often occurs to children involved in motor vehicle crashes.

Clinical Reasoning in Action

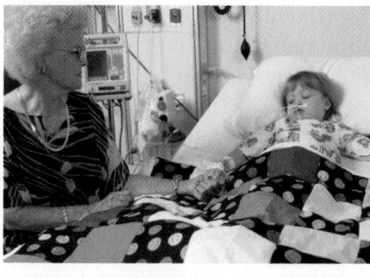

Four-year-old Jenna has just been admitted to the pediatric unit following surgery for a perforated appendix. She complained of her stomach hurting last night, but this morning her condition was worse and she had a temperature of 102°F. Worried that this was not just a virus, Jenna's mother took her to the pediatrician. On the way to the doctor's office Jenna told her mother that her pain "just went away." While at the pediatrician's office she complained of feeling bad all over. On examination, her abdomen was rigid and no bowel sounds were heard. A complete blood count revealed a white blood count (WBC) of 22,000/mm³. The pediatrician diagnosed that Jenna had appendicitis and most likely had a perforated appendix. He referred Jenna to the emergency department for assessment and surgical consultation. A CT scan confirmed a diagnosis of appendicitis. During surgery the appendix was found to have perforated.

Jenna had a laproscopic appendectomy. A dry dressing is in place. Jenna has a peripherally inserted central catheter (PICC) line for fluids, pain medication, and intravenous antibiotics. She also has a nasogastric tube to suction and a Foley catheter.

Jenna's parents are anxious about the surgery. They feel guilty that Jenna became ill so quickly and wonder if they could have done something to prevent it. This is Jenna's first hospitalization.

They are worried that she will have a lot of pain and wonder how she will cope with the hospitalization.

1. What is the priority of nursing care for Jenna in the immediate postoperative period?

2. What should the nurse include when teaching Jenna's parents about the postoperative course?

3. Jenna's parents ask why she needs all of the tubes. What information should the nurse include related to the purpose

of the nasogastric tube, the Foley catheter, and the central line?

4. Create a concept map for Jenna based on postoperative management of a 4-year-old with a perforated appendix. Include nursing interventions related to fluid and electrolyte balance, pain management, prevention of pulmonary complications, treatment of infection, and developmental and psychosocial care.

References

Agócs, M. M., Serhan, F., Yen, C., Mwenda, J. M., de Oliveira, L. H., Teleb, N., ... Kang, G. (2014). WHO Global Rotavirus Surveillance Network: A strategic review of the first 5 years, 2008–2012. *Morbidity and Mortality Weekly Report, 63*(29), 634–637.

Akay, B., & Klein, M. D. (2016). Anorectal malformations. In R. M. Kliegman, B. F. Stanton, J. W. St. Geme III, & N. F. Schor (Eds.), *Nelson textbook of pediatrics* (20th ed., pp. 1894–1897). Philadelphia, PA: Elsevier Saunders.

Alkan, M., Iskitt, S. H., Soyupak, S., Tuncer, R., Okur, H., Keskin, E., & Zorludemir, U. (2012). Severe abdominal trauma involving bicycle handlebars in children. *Pediatric Emergency Care, 28*(4), 357–360.

American Academy of Pediatrics (AAP). (2015). Parasitic diseases. *Red book: 2015 report of the Committee on Infectious Diseases* (30th ed. pp 588–591). Elk Grove Village, IL: Author.

American Academy of Pediatrics (AAP). (2014). *Amount and schedule of formula feedings*. Retrieved from healthychildren.org/English/ages-stages/baby/feeding-nutrition/Pages/Amount-and-Schedule-of-Formula-Feedings.aspx

Anand, B. S. (2015). *Peptic ulcer disease treatment & management*. Retrieved from http://emedicine.medscape.com/article/181753-overview

Barman, S., Mandal, K. C., Shukla, R. M., & Mukhopadhyay, B. (2014). Esophageal atresia with tracheoesophageal fistula associated with situs inversus totalis. *Indian Journal of Surgery, 76*(3), 239–240.

Benjamin, B., & Wilson, G. N. (2014). Anomalies associated with gastroschisis and omphalocele: Analysis of 2825 cases from the Texas Birth Defects Registry. *Journal of Pediatric Surgery, 49*, 514–519.

Bergman, N. J. (2013). Neonatal stomach volume and physiology suggest feeding at 1-h intervals. *Acta Paediatrica, 102*, 773–777.

Berman, L., & Moss, R. L. (2011). Necrotizing enterocolitis: An update. *Seminars in Fetal and Neonatal Medicine, 16*, 145–150.

Bishop, C. A., & Carter, M. E. (2013). Appendicitis. In N. T. Browne, L. M. Flanigan, C. A. McComiskey, & P. Pieper (Eds.), *Nursing care of the pediatric surgical patient* (3rd ed., pp. 407–416). Burlington, MA: Jones & Bartlett.

Blanco, F. C., Davenport, K. P., & Kane, T. D. (2012). Pediatric gastroesophageal disease. *Surgical Clinics of North America, 92*(3), 541–558.

Blanton, S. H., Henry, R. R., Yuan, Q., Mulliken, J. B., Stal, S., Finnell, R. H., & Hecht, J. T. (2011). Folate pathway and nonsyndromic cleft lip and palate. *Birth Defects Research (Part A): Clinical and Molecular Teratology, 91*, 50–60.

Borgialli, D. A., Ellison, A. M., Ehrlich, P., Bonsu, B., Menaker, J., Wisner, D. H., ... Holmes, J. F. (2014). Association between the seat belt sign and intra-abdominal injuries in children with blunt torso trauma in motor vehicle collisions. *Academic Emergency Medicine, 21*(11), 1240–1248.

Buggs, A. M. (2014). *Viral hepatitis*. Retrieved from http://emedicine.medscape.com/article/775507-overview

Burkhardt, D. D., Graham, J. M., Short, S. S., & Frykman, P. K. (2014). Advances in Hirschsprung disease genetics and treatment strategies: An update for the primary care pediatrician. *Clinical Pediatrics, 53*(1), 71–81.

Carlo, W. A. & Ambalavanan, N. (2016). The umbilicus. In R. M. Kliegman, B. F. Stanton, J. W. St. Geme III, & N. F. Schor (Eds.), *Nelson textbook of pediatrics* (20th ed., pp. 890–891). Philadelphia, PA: Elsevier Saunders.

Castellani, C., Peschaut, T., Schippinger, M., & Saxena, A. K. (2014). Postoperative emesis after laparoscopic pyloromyotomy in infantile hypertrophic pyloric stenosis. *Acta Paediatrica, 103*(2), e84–87.

Centers for Disease Control and Prevention (CDC). (2012a). *Hepatitis E information for health professionals*. Retrieved from http://www.cdc.gov/hepatitis/HEV/index.htm

Centers for Disease Control and Prevention (CDC). (2012b). *Hepatitis B information for health professionals*. Retrieved from http://www.cdc.gov/hepatitis/HBV/index.htm

Centers for Disease Control and Prevention (CDC). (2012c). *The ABCs of hepatitis*. Retrieved from http://www.cdc.gov/hepatitis/Resources/Professionals/PDFs/ABCTable.pdf

Centers for Disease Control and Prevention (CDC). (2014a). *Parasites*. Retrieved from http://www.cdc.gov/parasites

Centers for Disease Control and Prevention (CDC). (2014b). *Healthy pets, healthy people*. Retrieved from http://www.cdc.gov/Features/HealthyPets

Centers for Disease Control and Prevention (CDC). (2014c). *Viral hepatitis surveillance—United States, 2012*. Retrieved from http://www.cdc.gov/hepatitis/Statistics/2012Surveillance/PDFs/2012HepSurveillanceRpt.pdf

Centers for Disease Control and Prevention (CDC). (2014d). *Hepatitis A information for health professionals*. Retrieved from http://www.cdc.gov/hepatitis/HAV/index.htm

Centers for Disease Control and Prevention (CDC). (2014e). *Hepatitis C information for health professionals*. Retrieved from http://www.cdc.gov/hepatitis/HCV/index.htm

Centers for Disease Control and Prevention (CDC). (2014f). *Hepatitis D information for health professionals*.

Retrieved from http://www.cdc.gov/hepatitis/HDV/index.htm

Cevek, M., Boleken, M. E., Sogut, O., Gokdemir, M. T., & Karakas, E. (2013). Abdominal injuries related to bicycle accidents in children. *Pediatric Surgery International, 29*(5), 459–463.

Chason, R. D., Reisch, J. S., & Rockey, D. C. (2013). More favorable outcomes with peptic ulcer bleeding due to Helicobacter pylori. *The American Journal of Medicine, 126*(9), 811–818.

Cochran, A. A., Higgins, G. L., & Strout, T. D. (2011). Intussusception in traditional pediatric, nontraditional pediatric, and adult patients. *American Journnal of Emergency Medicine, 29*, 523–527.

Coehlo, D. P. (2011). Encopresis: A medical and family approach. *Pediatric Nursing, 37*(3), 107–112.

Coha, T. (2013). Care of the child with an ostomy. In N. T. Browne, L. M. Flanigan, C. A. McComiskey, & P. Pieper (Eds.), *Nursing care of the pediatric surgical patient* (3rd ed., pp. 121–148). Burlington, MA: Jones & Bartlett.

Collopy, K., & Friese, G. (2010). Pediatric drug administration. *Emergency Medical Services Magazine, 39*(6), 52–57.

Corey, K. M., Hornik, C. P., Laughon, M. M., McHutchison, K., Clark, R. H., & Smith, P. B. (2014). Frequency of anomalies and hospital outcomes in infants with gastroschisis and omphalocele. *Early Human Development, 90*, 421–424.

Correa, J. A, Fallon, S. C., Murphy, K. M., Victorian, V. A., Bisset, G. S., Vasudevan, S. A., ... Lee, T. C. (2014). Resource utilization after gastrostomy tube placement: Defining areas of improvement for future quality improvement projects. *Journal of Pediatric Surgery, 49*, 1598–1601.

Crockett, D. J., & Goudy, S. L. (2014). Cleft lip and palate. *Facial Plastic Surgery Clinics of North America, 22*(4), 573–586.

Cuffari, C. (2014). *Pediatric short bowel syndrome*. Retrieved from http://emedicine.medscape.com/article/931855-overview

Daley, B. J., Raju, R., & Lee, S. (2013). *Considerations in pediatric trauma*. Retrieved from http://emedicine.medscape.com/article/435031-overview

Deloach, R., & Farber, L. D. (2013). Intussusception. In N. T. Browne, L. M. Flanigan, C. A. McComiskey, & P. Pieper (Eds.), *Nursing care of the pediatric surgical patient* (3rd ed., pp. 399–406). Burlington, MA: Jones & Bartlett.

Fiorino, K., & Liacouras, C. A. (2016). Congenital aganglionic megacolon (Hirschsprung disease). In R. M. Kliegman, B. F. Stanton, J. W. St. Geme III, & N. F. Schor (Eds.), *Nelson textbook of pediatrics* (20th ed., pp. 1809–1811). Philadelphia, PA: Elsevier Saunders.

Flanigan, L. M. (2013). Biliary atresia and choledochal cyst. In N. T. Browne, L. M. Flanigan, C. A. McComiskey, & P. Pieper (Eds.), *Nursing care of the pediatric surgical patient* (3rd ed., pp. 435–446). Burlington, MA: Jones & Bartlett.

Garabedian, C., Verpillat, P. Czerkiewicz, I., Langlois, C., Muller, F., Avni, F., … Houfflin-Debarge, V. (2014). Does a combination of ultrasound, MRI, and biochemical amniotic fluid analysis improve prenatal diagnosis of esophageal atresia? *Prenatal Diagnosis, 34*, 839–842.

Gershon, A. A., & Hotez, P. J. (2011). Infectious diseases. In C. D. Rudolph, A. M. Rudolph, G. E. Lister, L. R. First, & A. A. Gershon (Eds.), *Rudolph's pediatrics* (22nd ed., pp. 878–1247). New York, NY: McGraw-Hill.

Glasser, J. G. (2014). *Pediatric omphalocele and gastroschisis.* Retrieved from http://emedicine.medscape.com/article/975583-overview

Glick, S. R., & Carvalho, R. S. (2011). Inflammatory bowel disease. *Pediatrics in Review, 32*(1), 14–25.

Goldson E., & Reynolds, A. (2012). Child development & behavior. In W. W. Hay, Jr., M. J. Levin, R. R. Deterding, M. J. Abzug, & J. M. Sondheimer (Eds.), *CURRENT diagnosis & treatment: Pediatrics* (21st ed.). New York, NY: McGraw-Hill. Retrieved from http://www.accessmedicine.com

Gregory, K. E., DeForge, C. E., Natale, K. M., Phillips, M., & VanMarter, L. J. (2011). Necrotizing enterocolitis in the premature infant: Neonatal nursing assessment, disease pathogenesis, and clinical presentation. *Advances in Neonatal Care, 11*(3), 155–164.

Grossman, A. B., & Baldassano, R. N. (2016). Inflammatory bowel disease. In R. M. Kliegman, B. F. Stanton, J. W. St. Geme III, & N. F. Schor (Eds.), *Nelson textbook of pediatrics* (20th ed., p. 1819–1831). Philadelphia, PA: Elsevier Saunders.

Grossman, A. B., & Mamula, P. (2014). *Pediatric Crohn disease.* Retrieved from http://emedicine.medscape.com/article/928288-overview

Groves, L. B., Ladd, M. R., Gallaher, J. R., Swanson, J., Becher, R. D., Pranikoff, T., & Neff, L. P. (2013). Comparing the cost and outcomes of laparoscopic versus open appendectomy for perforated appendicitis in children. *The American Surgeon, 79*(9), 861–864.

Guardino, K. O., & Pieper. (2013). Anorectal malformations in children. In N. T. Browne, L. M. Flanigan, C. A. McComiskey, & P. Pieper (Eds.), *Nursing care of the pediatric surgical patient* (3rd ed., pp. 359–372). Burlington, MA: Jones & Bartlett.

Gutierrez, I. M., Kang, K. H., & Jaksic, T. (2011). Neonatal short bowel syndrome. *Seminars in Fetal & Neonatal Medicine, 16*, 157–163.

Hannah, E., & John, R. M. (2013). Everything the nurse practitioner should know about pediatric feeding tubes. *Journal of the American Association of Nurse Practitioners, 25*, 567–577.

Harris, H., & Crawford, A. (2013). Hepatitis goes viral. *Nursing 2013, 43*(11), 38–43.

Hassan, H. H. A-K., & Balistreri, W. F. (2016). Neonatal cholestasis. In R. M. Kliegman, B. F. Stanton, J. W. St. Geme III, & N. F. Schor (Eds.), *Nelson textbook of pediatrics* (20th ed., pp. 1928–1932). Philadelphia, PA: Elsevier Saunders.

Hebra, A., & Cuffari, C. (2012). *Intestinal volvulus.* Retrieved from http://emedicine.medscape.com/article/930576-overview

Holder, M., & Jackson, L. (2013). Hirschsprung's disease. In N. T. Browne, L. M. Flanigan, C. A. McComiskey, & P. Pieper (Eds.), *Nursing care of the pediatric surgical*

patient (3rd ed., pp. 347–358). Burlington, MA: Jones & Bartlett.

Hood, E., & Zimmerman, B. T. (2013). Abdominal wall defects. In N. T. Browne, L. M. Flanigan, C. A. McComiskey, & P. Pieper (Eds.), *Nursing care of the pediatric surgical patient* (3rd ed., pp. 277–294). Burlington, MA: Jones & Bartlett.

Huda, S., Chaudhery, S., Ibrahim, H., & Pramanik, A. (2014). Neonatal necrotizing enterocolitis: Clinical challenges, pathophysiology and management. *Pathophysiology, 21*, 3–12.

Hung, M.-H., Lin, L.-H., & Chen, D. F. (2012). Clinical manifestations in children with ruptured appendicitis. *Pediatric Emergency Care, 28*(5), 433–435.

Hunter, A. K., & Liacouras, C. A. (2016). Hypertrophic pyloric stenosis. In R. M. Kliegman, B. F. Stanton, J. W. St. Geme III, & N. F. Schor (Eds.), *Nelson textbook of pediatrics* (20th ed., pp. 1797–1799). Philadelphia, PA: Elsevier Saunders.

Jensen, M. K., & Balistreri, W. F. (2016). Viral hepatitis. In R. M. Kliegman, B. F. Stanton, J. W. St. Geme III, & N. F. Schor (Eds.), *Nelson textbook of pediatrics* (20th ed., pp. 1942–1953). Philadelphia, PA: Elsevier Saunders.

Kelly, D., O'Dowd, T., & Reulbach, U. (2012). Use of folic acid supplements and risk of cleft lip and palate in infants: A population-based cohort study. *British Journal of General Practice, 62*(600), e466–e472.

Kelsen, J. R., & Mamula, P. (2013). *Ulcerative colitis in children.* Retrieved from http://emedicine.medscape.com/article/930146-overview

Khan, S., & Orenstein, S. R. (2016a). Esophageal atresia and tracheoesophageal fistula. In R. M. Kliegman, B. F. Stanton, J. W. St. Geme III, & N. F. Schor (Eds.), *Nelson textbook of pediatrics* (20th ed., pp. 1783–1784). Philadelphia, PA: Elsevier Saunders.

Khan, S., & Orenstein, S. R. (2016b). Gastroesophageal reflux disease. In R. M. Kliegman, B. F. Stanton, J. W. St. Geme III, & N. F. Schor (Eds.), *Nelson textbook of pediatrics* (20th ed., pp. 1787–1791). Philadelphia, PA: Elsevier Saunders.

Kotecha, M., Bellah, R., Pena, A. H., Jaimes, C., & Mattei, P. (2012). Multimodality imaging manifestations of the Meckel diverticulum in children. *Pediatric Radiology, 42*, 95–103.

Ladd, M. R., Pajewski, N. M., Becher, R. D., Swanson, J. M., Gallaher, J. R., Pranikoff, T., & Neff, L. P. (2013). Delays in treatment of pediatric appendicitis: a more accurate variable for measuring pediatric healthcare inequalities? *The American Surgeon, 79*(9), 875–881.

Langer, J. C. (2013). Hirschsprung disease. *Current Opinion in Pediatrics, 25*(3), 368–374.

Ledbetter, D. J. (2012). Congenital abdominal wall defects and reconstruction in pediatric surgery: Gastroschisis and omphalocele. *Surgical Clinics of North America, 92*, 713–727.

Lee, J. Y., Jun, J. K., & Lee, J. (2014). Prenatal prediction of neonatal survival in cases diagnosed with congenital diaphragmatic hernia using abdomen-to-thorax ratio determined by ultrasonography. *Journal of Obstetrics and Gynaecology Research, 40*(9), 2037–2043.

Lee, S. L., Yaghoubian, A., Stark, R., Sydorak, R. M., & Kaji, A. (2012). Are there differences in access to care, treatment, and outcomes for children with appendicitis treated at county versus private hospitals? *The Permanente Journal, 16*(1), 4–6.

Levas, M. N., Dayan, P. S., Mittal, M. K., Stevenson, M. D., Bachur, R. G., Dudley, N. C., … Kharbanda, A. B.

(2014). Effect of Hispanic ethnicity and language barriers on appendiceal perforation rates and imaging in children. *The Journal of Pediatrics, 164*(6),1286–1291.

Lightdale, J. R., & Gremse, D. A. (2013). Gastroesophageal reflux: Management guidance for the pediatrician. *Pediatrics, 131*(5), e1684–e1695.

Lin, C-Y, Chi, H., Hsu, C-H, Huang, F-Y, Lee, H-C, & Chiu, N-C. (2014). Peristaltic waves in infantile hypertrophic pyloric stenosis. *The Journal of Pediatrics, .164*(2), 423.

Lindholm, E., Persson, E., Carlsson, E., Hallén, A-M., Fingren, J., & Berndtsson, I. (2013), Ostomy-related complications after emergent abdominal surgery: A 2-year follow-up study. *Journal of Wound Ostomy & Continence Nursing, 40*(6), 603–610.

Lisonkova, S., & Joseph, K. S. (2013). Similarities and differences in the epidemiology of pyloric stenosis and SIDS. *Maternal Child Health Journal, 18*(7), 1721–1727.

Liszewski, M. C., Bairdain, S., Buonomo, C., Jennings, R. W. & Taylor, G. A. (2014). Imaging of long gap esophageal atresia and the Foker process: Expected findings and complications. *Pediatric Radiology, 44*(4), 467–475.

Lozada, L. E., Royall, M. J., Nylund, C. M., & Eberly, M. D. (2013). Development of pyloric stenosis after a 4-day course of oral Erythromycin. *Pediatric Emergency Care, 29*(4), 498–499.

Marcdante, K. J., & Kliegman, R. M. (2015). Esophagus and stomach. In K. J. Marcdante & R. M. Kliegman (Eds.), *Nelson essentials of pediatrics* (7th ed., pp. 430–437). Philadelphia, PA: Elsevier Saunders.

Markowitz, R. I. (2014). Olive without a cause: the story of infantile hypertrophic pyloric stenosis. *Pediatric Radiology, 44*(2), 202–211.

Mason, I. (2014). Supporting community patients with irritable bowel syndrome (IBS). *Journal of Community Nursing. 28*(1), 28–33.

McAteer, J. P., Ledbetter, D. J., & Goldin, A. B. (2013). Role of bottle feeding in the etiology of hypertrophic pyloric stenosis. *JAMA Pediatrics, 167*(12), 1143–1149.

McKenna, C., & Pieper, P. (2013). Pediatric trauma. In N. T. Browne, L. M. Flanigan, C. A. McComiskey, & P. Pieper (Eds.), *Nursing care of the pediatric surgical patient* (3rd ed., pp. 513–535). Burlington, MA: Jones & Bartlett.

Mendez, D. R. (2014). *Overview of blunt abdominal trauma in children.* Retrieved from uptodate.com

Mieli-Vergani, G., & Tizzard, S. A. (2012). Biliary atresia and Kasai's surgery—When is it too late? *Pediatric OnCall Journal, 9*(9). Retrieved from http://www.pediatriconcall.com/Journal/Article/FullText.aspx?artid=511&type=J&tid=&imgid=&reportid=358&tbltype=

Minkes, R. K., & Alder, A. C. (2014). *Pediatric appendicitis.* Retrieved from http://emedicine.medscape.com/article/926795-overview

Moreira, R. K., Cabral, R., Cowles, R. A., & Lobritto, S. J. (2012). Biliary atresia: A multidisciplinary approach to diagnosis and management. *Archives of Pathology and Laboratory Medicine, 136*(7), 746–760.

Morgan, J. A., Young, L., & McGuire, W. (2011). Pathogenesis and prevention of necrotizing enterocolitis. *Current Opinion in Infectious Disease, 24*, 183–189.

Nelville, H. L. (2014). *Pediatric Hirschsprung disease.* Retrieved from http://emedicine.medscape.com/article/929733-overview

Nowicki, D. E. (2013). Esophageal defects. In N. T. Browne, L. M. Flanigan, C. A. McComiskey, & P. Pieper (Eds.), *Nursing care of the pediatric surgical patient* (3rd ed., pp. 219–245). Burlington, MA: Jones & Bartlett.

Nurko, S., & Zimmerman, L. A. (2014). Evaluation and treatment of constipation in children and adolescents. *American Family Physician, 90*(2), 82–90.

Orr, S. (2011). Anal dilatation in children with anorectal malformations. *Gastrointestinal Nursing, 9*(8), 37–40.

Patel, P. K., Cohen, S., Ramaswamy, R., Grasseschi, M. F., & Morris, D. E. (2014). *Unilateral cleft lip repair.* Retrieved from http://emedicine.medscape.com /article/1279641-overview

Paul, S. P., Dewdney, C., & Lam, C. (2012) Managing children with constipation in the community. *Nurse Prescribing, 10*(6), 274–284.

Peate, I., & Jones, N. (2014). Caring for hepatitis B. *British Journal of Healthcare Assistants, 8*(8), 384–389.

Pepper, V. K., Stanfill, A. B., & Pearl, R. H. (2012). Diagnosis and management of pediatric appendicitis, intussusception, and Meckel diverticulum. *Surgical Clinics of North America, 92*, 505–526.

Peyrin-Biroulet, L. (2011). Why should we define and target early Crohn's disease? *Gastroenterology & Hepatology, 7*(5), 324–326.

Randel, A. (2014). AAP releases guideline for the management of gastroesophageal reflux in children. *American Family Physician, 89*(5), 395–397.

Rapoport, K., & Nishii, E. K. (2013). Necrotizing enterocolitis. In N. T. Browne, L. M. Flanigan, C. A. McComiskey, & P. Pieper (Eds.), *Nursing care of the pediatric surgical patient* (3rd ed., pp. 295–311). Burlington, MA: Jones & Bartlett.

Razmus, I. S. (2011). Assessment and management of children with abdominal wall defects. *Journal of Wound, Ostomy, Continence Nursing, 38*(1), 22–26.

Robie, D. K., Overfelt, S. R., & Xie, L. (2014). Differentiating biliary atresia from other causes of cholestatic jaundice. *American Surgeon, 80*(9), 827–831.

Rogers, J. (2011). Functional constipation in childhood. *Nurse Prescribing, 9*(7), 326–331.

Rogers, J. (2012). Assessment, prevention and treatment of constipation in children. *Nursing Standard, 26*(29), 46–52.

Rollins, M. D. (2012). Recent advances in the management of congenital diaphragmatic hernia. *Current Opinion in Pediatrics, 24*(3), 379–385.

Ruano, R., Picone, O., Bernardes, L., Martinovic, J., Dumez, Y., & Benachi, A. (2011). The association of gastroschisis with other congenital anomalies: How important is it? *Prenatal Diagnosis, 31*, 347–350.

Santacroce, L., & Ochoa, J. B. (2013). *Appendectomy.* Retrieved from http://emedicine.medscape.com /article/195778-overview

Saxena, A. K., (2013). *Pediatric abdominal trauma.* Retrieved from http://emedicine.medscape.com /article/1984811-overview

Saxena, A. K., Blair, G., & Konkin, D. E. (2014). *Esophageal atresia with or without tracheoesophageal fistula.* Retrieved from http://emedicine.medscape .com/article/935858-overview

Schwarz, S. M. (2014). *Pediatric biliary atresia.* Retrieved from http://emedicine.medscape.com/article /927029-overview

Schwarz, S. M., & Hebra, A. (2014). *Pediatric gastroesophageal reflux.* Retrieved from http://emedicine. medscape.com/article/930029-overview

Schweitzer, M., Aucoin, J., Docherty, S. L., Rice, H. E., Thompson, J., & Sullivan, D. T. (2014). Evaluation of a discharge education protocol for pediatric patients with gastrostomy tubes. *Journal of Pediatric Health Care, 28*(5), 420–428.

Sfakianaki. A. K., (2012). Congenital diaphragmatic hernia. *Contemporary OB/GYN, 57*(9), 26–36.

Shalaby, M. S., Kuti, K., & Walker, G. (2013). Intestinal malrotation and volvulus in infants and children. *British Medical Journal, 347*(7936), 33–35.

Singh, M., Kadian, Y. S., Rattan, K. N., & Jangra, B. (2014). Complicated appendicitis: Analysis of risk factors in children. *African Journal of Paediatric Surgery, 11*(2), 109–113.

Sira, M. M., Taha, M., & Sira, A. M. (2014). Common misdiagnoses of biliary atresia. *European Journal of Gastroenterology & Hepatology, 26*(11), 1300–1305.

Sluiter, I., van de Ven, C. P., Wijnen, R. M. H., & Tibboel, D. (2011). Congenital diaphragmatic hernia: Still a moving target. *Seminars in Fetal & Neonatal Medicine, 16*, 139–144.

Squires, J. E., & Balistreri, W. F. (2016). Manifestations of liver disease. In R. M. Kliegman, B. F. Stanton, J. W. St. Geme III, & N. F. Schor (Eds.), *Nelson textbook of pediatrics* (20th ed., pp. 1922–1928). Philadelphia, PA: Elsevier Saunders.

Tarbell, S. E., & Li, B. U. K. (2013). Health-related quality of life in children and adolescents with cyclic vomiting syndrome: A comparison with published data on youth with irritable bowel syndrome and organic gastrointestinal disorders. *Journal of Pediatrics, 163*(2), 493–497.

Taylor, N. D., Cass, D. T., & Holland, A. J. A. (2013). Infantile hypertrophic pyloric stenosis: Has anything changed? *Journal of Paediatrics and Child Health, 49*(1), 33–37.

Territo, H. M., Wrotniak, B. H., Qiao, H., & Lillis, K. (2014). Clinical signs and symptoms associated with intussusception in young children undergoing ultrasound in the emergency room. *Pediatric Emergency Care, 30*(10), 718–722.

Tigges, C. R., & Bigham, M. T. (2012). Hypertrophic pyloric stenosis: It can take your breath away. *Air Medical Journal, 31*(1), 45–48.

Triantafillidis, J. K., Merikas, E., & Georgopoulos, F. (2011). Current and emerging drugs for the treatment. *Drug Design, Development and Therapy, 5*, 185–210.

Tutay, G. J., Capraro, G., Spirko, B., Garb, J., & Smithline, H. (2013). Electrolyte profile of pediatric patients with hypertrophic pyloric stenosis. *Pediatric Emergency Care, 29*(4), 465–468.

Vitola, B. E., & Balistreri, W. F. (2016). Liver disease associated with systemic disorders. In R. M. Kliegman, B. F. Stanton, J. W. St. Geme III, & N. F. Schor (Eds.), *Nelson textbook of pediatrics* (20th ed., pp. 1954– 1957). Philadelphia, PA: Elsevier Saunders.

Watson, L. (2014). Constipation in children. *Nursing Standard, 28*(41), 18.

Wesson, D. E. (2013). *Liver, spleen, and pancreas injury in children with blunt abdominal trauma.* Retrieved from uptodate.com.

Wiet, G. J., Biavati, M. J., & Rocha-Worley, G. (2013). *Reconstructive surgery for cleft palate.* Retrieved from http://emedicine.medscape.com/article/878062- overview

Wilkins-Haug, L. (2014). *Etiology, prenatal diagnosis, obstetrical management, and recurrence of orofacial clefts.* Retrieved from uptodate.com. http:// emedicine.medscape.com/article/878062-overview

Wilson, B. A., Shannon, M. T., & Shields, K. M. (2015). *Pearson nurse's drug guide 2015.* Hoboken, NJ: Pearson Education.

Wright, K., & Miller, H. D. (2012). Evidence-based findings of necrotizing enterocolitis. *Newborn and Infant Nursing Reviews, 12*(1), 17–20.

Zerpa, J. A., & Shapiro, T. J. (2013). Malrotation and volvulus. In N. T. Browne, L. M. Flanigan, C. A. McComiskey, & P. Pieper (Eds.), *Nursing care of the pediatric surgical patient* (3rd ed., pp. 333–346). Burlington, MA: Jones & Bartlett.

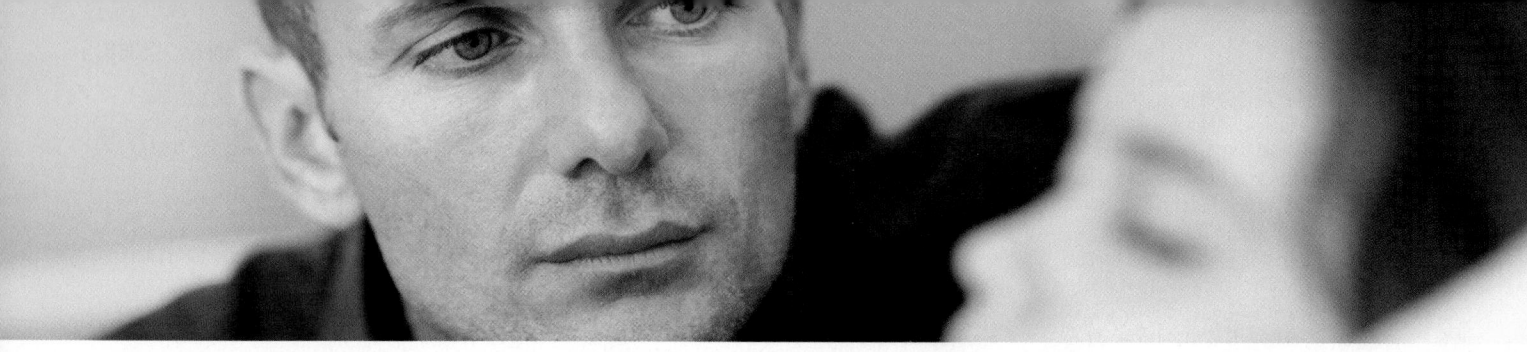

Chapter 52

The Child With Alterations in Genitourinary Function

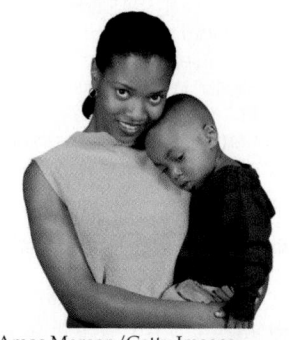

Planning Terrell's day can be a challenge, because his treatment often interferes with his activities. We all hope that Terrell receives a kidney transplant soon so his growth will improve and he will not have to miss school during treatment.

—Aunt of Terrell, 5 years old

Amos Morgan/Getty Images

∨ Learning Outcomes

52.1 Describe the pathophysiologic processes associated with genitourinary disorders in the pediatric population.

52.2 Develop a nursing care plan for the child with a urinary tract infection.

52.3 Discuss the nursing management of a child with a structural defect of the genitourinary system.

52.4 Outline a plan to meet the fluid and dietary restrictions for the child with a renal disorder.

52.5 Identify growth and developmental issues for the child with chronic renal failure.

52.6 Plan nursing care for the child with acute and chronic renal failure.

52.7 Summarize psychosocial issues for the child requiring surgery on the genitourinary system.

Many infections, structural disorders, and disease processes alter genitourinary function. Because the kidneys and other urinary system organs perform several essential body functions, including removal of waste products and maintenance of fluid and electrolyte balance, disorders that affect these organs pose a significant threat to the health of children.

Although the reproductive system is functionally immature until puberty, uncorrected structural defects can have both psychologic and physiologic implications for the developing child.

Anatomy and Physiology of Pediatric Differences

The genitourinary system is made up of the urinary and reproductive organs. The urinary system—kidneys, ureters, bladder, and urethra (Figure 52–1)—excretes wastes and maintains acid–base and fluid and electrolyte balance. The reproductive system consists of internal and external organs that at maturity promote the conception and healthy development of a fetus.

changes of puberty accelerate anatomic and functional development (see Chapter 33 for figures illustrating pubertal development). In girls, the mons pubis becomes more prominent and hair begins to grow. The vagina lengthens, and the epithelial layers thicken. The uterus and ovaries enlarge, and the musculature and vascularization of the uterus also increase. In boys, downy hair begins to appear at the base of the penis, and the scrotum becomes increasingly pendulous as the testes enlarge. The penis increases in length and width.

Urinary Tract Infection

An infection of the urinary tract may be of bacterial, viral, or fungal origin, and can occur in the lower or upper urinary tract. Cystitis is a lower urinary tract infection (UTI) that involves the urethra or bladder. Pyelonephritis is an upper UTI that involves the ureters, pelvis, and renal parenchyma. UTIs can be acute or chronic (the latter being either recurrent or persistent).

UTIs are very common in children, with 8% of girls and 2% of boys having at least one UTI by 7 years of age (White, 2011). It is further estimated that 1% of boys and 3% to 5% of girls will have a UTI during childhood and 30% to 50% of them will have at least more than one UTI (Paintsil, 2013).

Etiology and Pathophysiology

Most UTIs in children are caused by *Escherichia coli*, a common gram-negative enteric bacterium (White, 2011). Urinary stasis enhances the risk of UTI. Stasis may be caused by abnormal anatomic structures or abnormal function (e.g., **neurogenic bladder** in which an interrupted nerve supply from myelomeningocele or spinal cord trauma impairs the bladder's voiding function and leads to incomplete bladder emptying). Children normally void 5 to 6 times a day. Infrequent voiding, common in school-age children, results in incomplete emptying of the bladder and urinary stasis. Other factors associated with increased risk of UTI include poor hygiene, inadequate cleansing after bowel movements, and an irritated perineum. Uncircumcised males have a higher incidence of UTIs than circumcised males (Dubrovsky, Foster, Jednak, et al., 2012). This increased incidence is highest in the first year of life (Morris & Wiswell, 2013). Constipation in children and sexual activity in adolescent females also contribute to the incidence of UTI in the pediatric population (Fisher et al., 2014). **Vesicoureteral reflux**, the backflow of urine from the bladder into the ureters during voiding, is another cause of UTI and is discussed later in this chapter.

Growth and Development

Urinary tract infections are more common in males than females in the first few months of life. It is estimated that the incidence of UTI in uncircumcised males during the first year of life is 7 to 14 of 1000 as compared to 1 to 2 of 1000 circumcised infants (American Academy of Pediatrics Task Force on Circumcision, 2012). By 1 year of age, the incidence of UTI is much higher in females than males (Fisher et al., 2014). This is related to the shorter female urethra (2 cm [1 in.] in young girls) being closer to the anus and vagina, which increases the risk of contamination by fecal bacteria. See Chapter 25 for discussion of recommendations for circumcision in newborns.

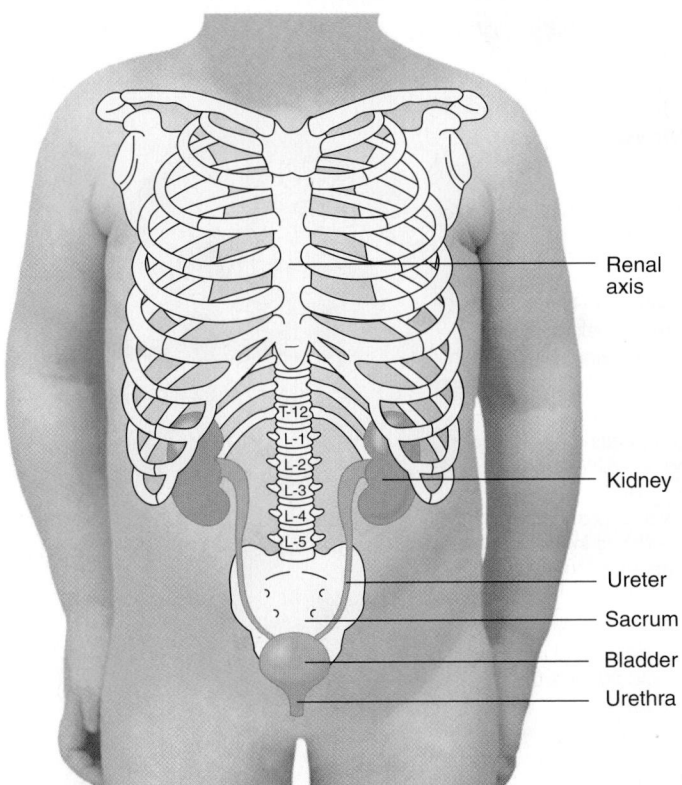

Figure 52–1 The urinary system is composed of the kidneys, ureters, bladder, and urethra. The kidneys are located between the twelfth thoracic (T12) and third lumbar (L3) vertebrae.

Labels: Renal axis, Kidney, Ureter, Sacrum, Bladder, Urethra; T-12, L-1, L-2, L-3, L-4, L-5

Urinary System

All of the nephrons that will make up the mature kidney are present at birth. The kidneys grow and the tubular system matures gradually during childhood, reaching full size by adolescence. Most renal growth occurs during the first 5 years of life. This increase in size is primarily a result of enlargement of the nephrons. The kidney's efficiency also increases with age. During the first 2 years of life, the kidneys are less efficient at regulating electrolyte and acid–base balance (see Chapter 44) and eliminating some drugs from the body. After age 2 years, the kidneys' efficiency increases markedly.

Bladder capacity increases with age. A child's bladder capacity (in ounces) can be estimated by adding 2 to the child's age (e.g., a 4-year-old has a bladder capacity of 6 ounces) (see *As Children Grow: Development of the Genitourinary System*). Stimulation of "stretch receptors" within the bladder wall initiates urination. Simultaneous contraction of the detrusor muscle of the bladder and relaxation of the internal and external sphincters result in emptying of the bladder. Children less than 2 years of age cannot maintain bladder control because of insufficient nerve development.

Normal renal function requires the following: unimpaired renal blood flow, adequate glomerular ultrafiltration, normal tubular function, and unobstructed urine flow.

Reproductive System

The reproductive system in children is functionally immature until puberty. Throughout childhood the genitalia (with the exception of the clitoris in girls) enlarge gradually. The hormonal

Renal scarring can result from pyelonephritis because of the ischemic effects of infection. Renal scarring has been associated with hypertension and chronic renal failure (White, 2011). The risk of renal damage increases in the following instances:

As Children Grow: **Development of the Genitourinary System**

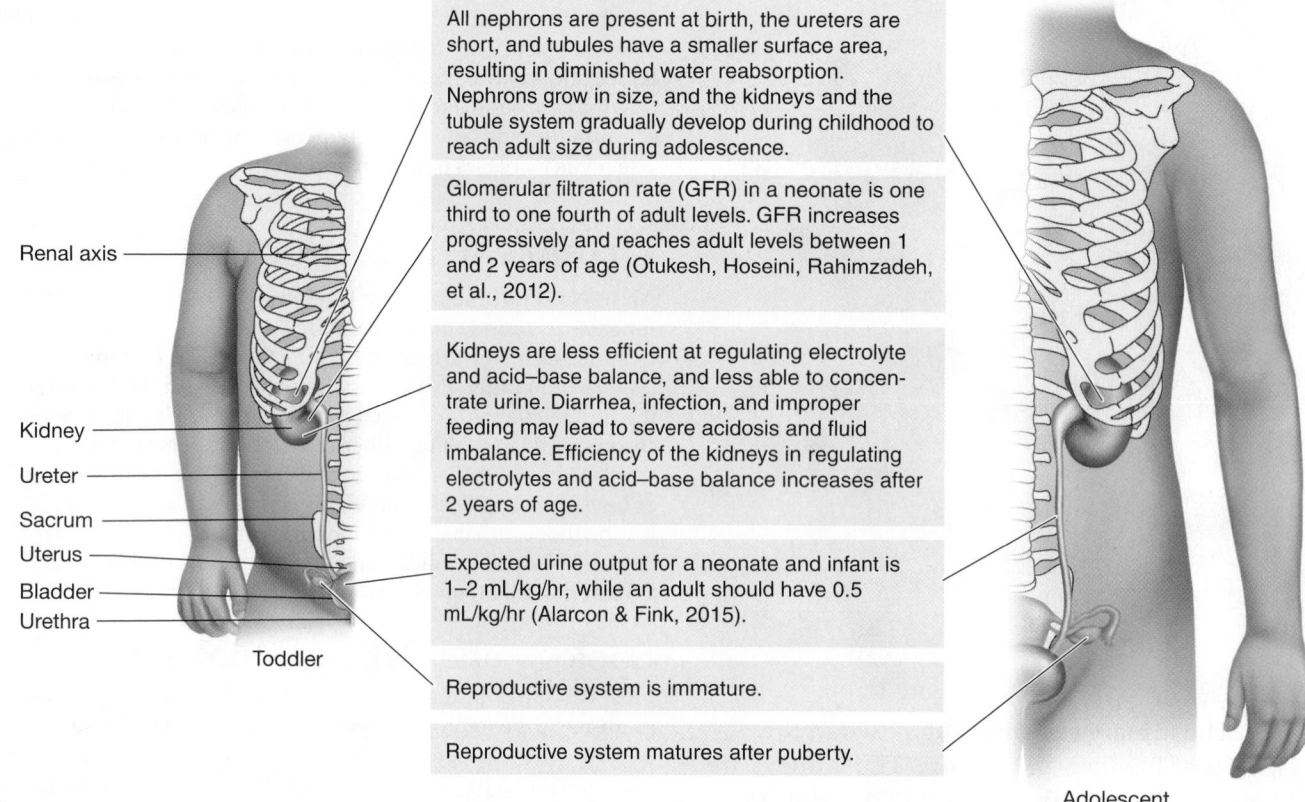

All nephrons are present at birth, the ureters are short, and tubules have a smaller surface area, resulting in diminished water reabsorption. Nephrons grow in size, and the kidneys and the tubule system gradually develop during childhood to reach adult size during adolescence.

Glomerular filtration rate (GFR) in a neonate is one third to one fourth of adult levels. GFR increases progressively and reaches adult levels between 1 and 2 years of age (Otukesh, Hoseini, Rahimzadeh, et al., 2012).

Kidneys are less efficient at regulating electrolyte and acid–base balance, and less able to concentrate urine. Diarrhea, infection, and improper feeding may lead to severe acidosis and fluid imbalance. Efficiency of the kidneys in regulating electrolytes and acid–base balance increases after 2 years of age.

Expected urine output for a neonate and infant is 1–2 mL/kg/hr, while an adult should have 0.5 mL/kg/hr (Alarcon & Fink, 2015).

Reproductive system is immature.

Reproductive system matures after puberty.

Renal axis
Kidney
Ureter
Sacrum
Uterus
Bladder
Urethra

Toddler

Adolescent

Source: Data from Otukesh, H., Hoseini, R., Rahimzadeh, N., & Hosseini, S. (2012). Glomerular function in neonates. *Iranian Journal of Kidney Diseases*, 6(3), 166–172; Alarcon, L. H., & Fink, M. P. (2015). Physiologic monitoring of the surgical patient. In F. C. Brunicardi, D. K. Andersen, T. R. Billiar, D. L. Dunn, J. G. Hunter, J. B. Matthews, & R. E. Pollock (Eds.), *Schwartz's principles of surgery* (10th ed.). Retrieved from http://www.accessmedicine.com

- UTI in infant less than 1 year of age
- Delay in diagnosis and effective antibacterial treatment for an upper UTI
- Anatomic obstruction or nerve supply interruption
- Recurrent episodes of upper UTIs

Clinical Manifestations

Symptoms depend on the location of the infection and the age of the child. Symptoms in the newborn period tend to be nonspecific (e.g., unexplained fever, hypothermia, failure to thrive, poor feeding, vomiting and diarrhea, strong-smelling urine,

and irritability). Any child under 2 years of age with a fever of unknown origin should be tested for a UTI. The more "classic" symptoms of lower UTI are not seen until the preschool years, as listed in Table 52–1. Many UTIs are asymptomatic and are discovered incidentally on routine examination.

Clinical Therapy

A urine specimen is examined for the presence of bacteria. Dipsticks can be used to screen for urinary tract infection. A dipstick-positive leukocyte esterase test identifies white blood cells and pyuria, and a positive nitrite dipstick detects gram-negative bacteria. The UTI is diagnosed when a midstream

TABLE 52–1 Clinical Manifestations of Urinary Tract Infection

TYPE OF UTI	CLINICAL MANIFESTATIONS
Lower UTI—cystitis	
Infants	Fever, diarrhea, vomiting, irritability, lethargy, foul-smelling diapers, poor feeding, failure to gain weight
Preschooler	Fever, hematuria, urgency, dysuria, frequency, cloudy urine, foul-smelling urine, dehydration, abdominal pain, enuresis
School-age	Fever, hematuria, urgency, dysuria, frequency, cloudy urine, foul-smelling urine, dehydration, abdominal pain, suprapubic or flank pain, enuresis
Upper UTI—pyelonephritis	High fever, chills, abdominal pain, nausea, vomiting, flank pain, costovertebral angle tenderness, moderate to severe dehydration

clean-catch urine culture yields greater than 100,000 colony-forming units (cfu) of a single bacteria, or when greater than 10,000 cfu of a single bacterium are cultured from a sterile catheterized specimen (Ammenti et al., 2012). See the *Clinical Skills Manual* for urine collection methods SKILLS. Once the presence of bacteria is confirmed, antibiotic sensitivity for the specific organisms cultured is then determined. Urinalysis reveals white blood cells (WBCs) in the urine. A complete blood count reveals an elevated WBC count. A renal ultrasound is recommended after the first urinary tract infection with fever to rule out structural abnormalities (Newman, 2011). A voiding cystourethrogram (VCUG) may be obtained to test for vesicoureteral reflux if the ultrasound results are abnormal or the child has recurrence of a urinary tract infection with fever (Fisher et al., 2014).

Antibiotic therapy is begun as soon as urine samples have been collected. Antibiotics are selected based on the age of the child, sensitivity of the cultured organism, and the child's signs and symptoms. The antibiotic is changed, if necessary, after culture sensitivity is determined. Routine antibiotic prophylaxis is no longer recommended after the first urinary tract infection in infants and children (Paintsil, 2013).

Table 52–2 lists diagnostic tests commonly used to identify urinary tract conditions.

Clinical Tip

Several procedures are available for evaluation of kidney and bladder function. It is important for the patient and family to understand the procedure. Examples of these procedures and their purpose include:

- *Renal ultrasound*—Noninvasive procedure that uses sound waves to visualize the kidneys, ureters, and bladder. Renal ultrasound is useful in determining the size and shape of the kidneys, blood flow to the kidneys, signs of injury or damage, blockage, tumors, or kidney stones.
- *Voiding cystourethrogram*—Determines if there is reflux of urine into the ureters (see the discussion of vesicoureteral reflux later in this chapter). A catheter is placed prior to the procedure so that the bladder may be filled with dye. Radiographs are used to visualize the bladder during the procedure and see if dye moves into the ureters.

TABLE 52–2 Diagnostic Tests and Laboratory Procedures for the Genitourinary System

DIAGNOSTIC PROCEDURES	LABORATORY TESTS
Computed tomography (CT)	Blood urea nitrogen (BUN)
Cystoscopy	Creatinine clearance
Diuretic renogram (a type of nuclear scan)	Urinalysis (UA) (see the *Clinical Skills Manual* SKILLS)
Intravenous pyelogram	
Magnetic resonance imaging (MRI)	Urine culture (see the *Clinical Skills Manual* SKILLS)
Radionucleotide renal scan with dimercaptosuccinic acid (DMSA)	Urine protein-to-creatinine ratio
Renal biopsy	
Renal or bladder ultrasound	
Voiding cystourethrogram (VCUG) or radionuclide cystography	

Children who appear ill and cannot tolerate oral antibiotics are often hospitalized because they need rehydration and initiation of parenteral antibiotic treatment until afebrile for 24 hours. Infants may develop permanent kidney damage or generalized sepsis if a UTI is not treated aggressively. If a structural defect is identified, surgical correction may be necessary to prevent recurrent infections that could lead to renal damage.

Children treated on an outpatient basis should receive follow-up by phone (or in person if needed) within 24 to 48 hours to validate the child's response to treatment and to make changes to the treatment plan, if needed, based on urine culture sensitivities. A follow-up visit 7 to 10 days after the initiation of treatment is important to see how the patient responded to treatment (Fisher et al., 2014).

Nursing Management

For the Child With Urinary Tract Infection

Nursing Assessment and Diagnosis

PHYSIOLOGIC ASSESSMENT

Obtain a history of urinary symptoms. Assess the infant for toxic (very ill) appearance, fever, and poor feeding. Evaluate the child's oral fluid intake. Assess for quality, quantity, and frequency of voiding. Assess the infant's or child's vital signs, including blood pressure. Palpate the abdomen and suprapubic and costovertebral areas for masses, tenderness, and distention. Assess for abdominal or flank pain, frequency, urgency, and dysuria. Observe the urinary stream, if possible, and perform a urinalysis, including specific gravity. Proper collection of the urine specimen is essential. Obtain a clean-catch urine specimen if the child is old enough to do this. If not, get a catheterized sample (see the *Clinical Skills Manual* SKILLS). An early morning urine specimen is preferred because the urine is more concentrated.

PSYCHOSOCIAL ASSESSMENT

Sexually active adolescents may deny having symptoms of a UTI because they fear disclosing their sexual activity to their parents. Careful questioning and a visit alone with the adolescent may be necessary to elicit these concerns. Be open and approachable and give the patient and family the chance to address their concerns.

Common nursing diagnoses for the child with a UTI include the following (NANDA-I © 2014):

- *Urinary Elimination, Impaired*, related to recurrent urinary tract infections
- *Urinary Retention* related to infrequent voiding habits or vesicoureteral reflux
- *Health Management, Family, Ineffective*, related to lack of knowledge of preventive UTI measures
- *Fluid Volume: Deficient, Risk for*, related to fever and inadequate intake

Planning and Implementation

Nursing care for the hospitalized child with a complicated UTI centers on administering prescribed medications, promoting rehydration, assessing renal function, and teaching parents and older children how to minimize the risk of future infection.

Administer antibiotics and antipyretics as prescribed to maintain therapeutic drug levels and reduce fever. Encourage fluid intake to dilute the urine and flush the bladder. Frequent voiding minimizes urinary stasis. Document intake and output.

Assess renal function by comparing the child's output to the expected urine output and weigh the child daily.

Because bladder training is such an important milestone for young children, any disorder that affects voiding may have developmental implications. A toddler who has been toilet trained may regress and require diapers temporarily as a result of UTI-related incontinence. An older child may develop enuresis after a prolonged period of being dry at night. Reassure parents that this is normal and emphasize that the child needs support. A preschooler may perceive the infection and any parental disapproval as punishment for an imagined wrong.

DISCHARGE PLANNING AND HOME CARE TEACHING

Children with UTIs are usually cared for at home. Teach parents that all doses of the antibiotic must be taken as prescribed and that they may be continued even after the infection has cleared to prevent a recurrence. Teach prevention through proper hygiene and avoidance of risk behaviors.

Give parents specific guidelines for oral fluid intake. Make sure the amount of fluids recommended for a 24-hour period equals the maintenance fluids needed plus additional fluids required because of fever and diuresis to flush out pathogens (see Chapter 44). Suggest that the parents avoid giving the child caffeinated and carbonated beverages because these have the potential to irritate the bladder mucosa. Teach parents the signs and symptoms of recurrent infection and to seek care promptly.

The child with a neurogenic bladder requires a clean intermittent catheterization to be performed several times a day to reduce urinary stasis and the potential for UTI. Although the procedure for inserting the catheter is the same as that for catheterization using sterile technique, children and families are generally taught to use clean technique. See *Teaching Highlights: Prevention of Urinary Tract Infections.*

Evaluation

Expected outcomes of nursing care include:

- The child increases fluid intake and number of times voiding each day.
- Future UTIs are prevented.

Structural Defects of the Urinary System

Bladder Exstrophy

Bladder exstrophy is a rare congenital defect in which the posterior bladder wall extrudes through the lower abdominal wall (Figure 52–2). Failure of the abdominal wall to close during fetal development results in eversion and protuberance of the bladder wall along with a wide separation of the rectus muscles and the symphysis pubis. The upper urinary tract is usually normal. The bladder mucosa appears as a mass of bright-red tissue, and urine continually leaks from the ureters onto the skin (Ring & Huether, 2014). Females have a bifid (split) clitoris. Males have a short, stubby penis, and the glans is flattened with dorsal chordee and a ventral prepuce. Undescended testicles and inguinal hernias are common in children with bladder exstrophy (Elder, 2016a).

The exposed bladder tissue is covered with plastic wrap to keep the bladder mucosa moist until surgery is performed (Elder, 2016a). The goal of primary closure of the bladder and anterior abdominal wall is an acceptable urinary reservoir (Bhatnagar, 2011). Primary closure is generally performed soon after birth but may be delayed if the bladder template is too small or other contraindications are identified (Inouye, Tourchi, DiCarlo, et al., 2014). The wound and pelvis are immobilized to promote healing. An osteotomy (see Chapter 56) to rotate the innominate bones of the pelvis to approximate the symphysis pubis reduces tension on the closed bladder and abdominal wall to promote healing. Epispadias repair is often performed between 1 and 2 years of age or at the same times as a surgical procedure to improve continence. Surgery to reconstruct the bladder neck and reimplant the ureters is performed when the bladder has achieved capacity of 80 to 90 mL (Elder, 2016a). The goals of surgical reconstruction include:

- Closure of the bladder and abdominal wall
- Urinary continence, with preservation of renal function

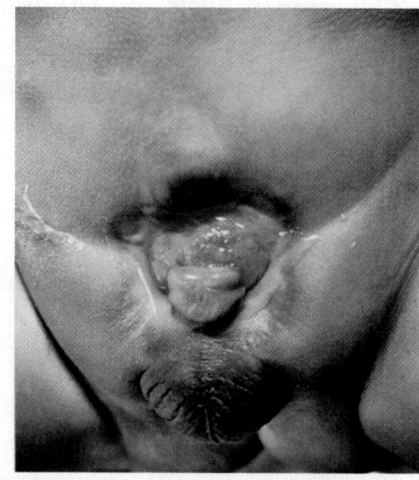

Figure 52–2 This child has bladder exstrophy, noted by extrusion of the posterior bladder wall through the lower abdominal wall.

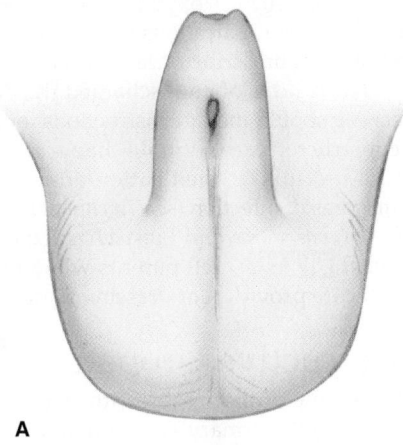
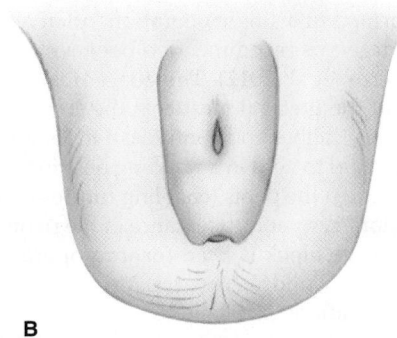

A   B

Figure 52–3 *A*, In hypospadias, the urethral canal is open on the ventral surface of the penis. *B*, In epispadias, the canal is open on the dorsal surface.

- Creation of functional and normal-appearing genitalia
- Correction to promote later sexual functioning

Some children require permanent urinary diversion because a functional bladder cannot be reconstructed.

Nursing Management

Preoperative nursing care centers on preventing infection and trauma to the exposed bladder. The bladder mucosa is protected with plastic wrap to keep the bladder mucosa moist (Elder, 2016a). The surrounding area is cleaned daily and protected from leaking urine with a skin sealant.

Postoperatively, the wound and pelvis are immobilized to facilitate healing. Internal and external immobilization techniques are used for pelvic closure (see Chapter 56). In addition to pain assessment and management, nursing care includes maintaining proper alignment, avoiding abduction of the infant's legs, monitoring peripheral circulation, and providing meticulous wound and skin care. Maintain aseptic technique for wound care and monitor for signs of infection including redness, drainage, and edema.

Monitor renal function by assessing the adequacy of urine output and blood and urine chemistries to detect signs of renal damage. Observe for any signs of obstruction in the drainage tubes such as increased intensity of bladder spasms, decreased urine output, or urine or blood draining from the urethral meatus. Promote comfort and give antibiotics as ordered.

Parents need emotional support to help them cope with the disfiguring nature of the infant's defect and the uncertainty of complete repair. To promote parent–infant bonding, encourage parents to participate in all aspects of the infant's care, including bathing, feeding, and wound care. Discharge teaching should include instructions about dressing changes and diapering and the need to immediately report any signs of infection or change in renal function. Emphasize the need for routine follow-up visits after surgery to assess urinary function and to ensure that the next stages of surgery for continence control are performed at the appropriate time in the child's development. The family should be aware that achievement of continence is more difficult in children with bladder exstrophy, and urinary diversion to achieve continence may be necessary if surgical procedures are not successful. Parents may require guidance to promote the child's self-esteem and self-confidence with sexual identity and

function. Psychologic counseling may be beneficial to the child during adolescence.

Hypospadias and Epispadias

Hypospadias and epispadias are congenital anomalies involving the abnormal location of the urethral meatus (Figure 52–3). The reported incidence of hypospadias is 1 in 300 male births (Snodgrass & Bush, 2014). The incidence of epispadias is 1 in 40,000 to 118,000 births. Epispadias occurs twice as often in males as females (Ring & Huether, 2014). See section on bladder exstrophy earlier in this chapter.

In hypospadias, the urethral meatus can be located anywhere along the course of the urethra on the ventral surface of the penile shaft, from the perineum to the tip of the glans. Most cases are mild, with the meatus slightly off center from the tip of the penis; in severe cases, the meatus is located on the scrotum. Hypospadias often occurs in conjunction with congenital *chordee*, a fibrous line of tissue that results in ventral curvature of the penile shaft. Associated defects may include inguinal hernia, cryptorchidism (undescended testes), and partial absence of the foreskin (Ring & Huether, 2014).

Clinical Tip

When children are not able to achieve continence, some type of urinary diversion may be created. A *vesicostomy* is a procedure in which an opening is created from the bladder to the skin. The urine drains from the opening (stoma) to the child's diaper or a drainage bag. In the *Mitrofanoff procedure*, a reservoir for urine and a stoma are created so that children can catheterize themselves through the umbilicus (see Chapter 54).

Epispadias and bladder exstrophy are the same condition, but epispadias is the milder expression of the condition. The opening may be small or a fissure may extend the entire length of the penis. Females with epispadias have a cleft of the ventral urethra that generally extends to the bladder neck (Ring & Huether, 2014). The remainder of this discussion will focus on hypospadias and males with distal epispadias because the treatment for severe epispadias in males and epispadias in females is similar to the final stage of repair of bladder exstrophy (Elder, 2016a).

The diagnosis of hypospadias is generally made at birth. If the parents would like to have their son to be circumcised, the procedure should be delayed until surgery to repair the hypospadias is performed (Chalmers, Wiedel, Siparsky, et al., 2014). Hypospadias is corrected surgically, usually during the first year of life, to minimize psychologic effects when the child is older. Surgery is usually performed in a single operation, often as an outpatient procedure. Surgery is recommended between 6 and 12 months of age (Kocherov et al, 2012). The goals of surgical repair are (1) placement of the urethral meatus at the end of the glans penis with satisfactory caliber and configuration for a urinary stream (enabling the child to void in a standing position), (2) release of chordee to straighten the penis (enabling future sexual function), and (3) satisfactory cosmetic appearance of the penis.

A caudal or penile nerve block is used for intraoperative and postoperative analgesia (Kundra, Yuvaraj, Agrawal, et al., 2011). Anticholinergic medications may be prescribed to relieve bladder spasms. A urethral **stent** (a device used to maintain patency of the urethral canal) or catheter is placed to maintain patency of the new urethral canal opening. The stent or catheter may drain directly into the diaper, using a double-diapering technique, or into a closed drainage collection bag.

Nursing Management

It is important to address parents' concerns at the time of birth. Preoperative teaching can relieve some of their anxiety about the future appearance and functioning of the penis.

Postoperative care focuses on protecting the surgical site from injury. The infant or child returns from surgery with the penis wrapped in a simple dressing, and a urethral stent or catheter for urinary drainage. Plan care to ensure that the stent does not get removed. Refer to the hospital's policy for the appropriate use of immobilizers in this situation.

Encourage fluid intake to maintain adequate urinary output and patency of the stent. Strict documentation of intake and output is essential to detect postoperative complications. Notify the healthcare provider if there is no urine drainage for 1 hour because this may indicate kinks in the system or obstruction. Pain may be associated with bladder spasms. Anticholinergic

medications such as oxybutynin may be prescribed. Acetaminophen or other medications may also be given for pain. Antibiotics are often prescribed until the stent is out.

The child is often discharged the day of surgery. Discharge teaching should include instructions for parents about care of the reconstructed area, double-diapering to protect the operative site, fluid intake, medication administration, and signs and symptoms of infection (see *Teaching Highlights: Caring for the Child After Hypospadias and Epispadias Repair* and the *Clinical Skills Manual* SKILLS). Tell parents when the child needs to see the healthcare provider for dressing removal.

Obstructive Uropathy

Obstructive uropathy refers to structural or functional abnormalities of the urinary system that interfere with urine flow and result in urine backflow into the kidneys. The pressure caused by urine backup compromises kidney function and often causes **hydronephrosis** (accumulation of urine in the renal pelvis as a result of obstructed outflow). Physiologic changes that may occur as a result of hydronephrosis include the following:

- Cessation of glomerular filtration occurs when the pressure in the kidney pelvis equals the filtration pressure in the glomerular capillaries. To compensate, the blood pressure increases to increase the glomerular filtration pressure; however, increasing pressure on the glomeruli leads to cell death.
- Metabolic acidosis results when the distal nephrons' ability to secrete hydrogen ions is impaired.
- Impairment of the kidney's ability to concentrate urine results in polydipsia and polyuria.
- Obstruction results in urinary stasis, promoting bacterial growth.
- Restriction of urinary outflow causes progressive renal damage and chronic renal failure if untreated.

Obstructive uropathy may be caused by several congenital lesions such as ureteropelvic junction (UPJ) obstruction,

---

TEACHING HIGHLIGHTS | Caring for the Child After Hypospadias and Epispadias Repair

- Use double-diapering to protect the operative site. See the *Clinical Skills Manual* SKILLS .
- Do not bathe the child in a tub until the stent (the small tube that drains the urine) or catheter is removed.
- Restrict the infant or toddler from activities (e.g., playing on riding toys) that put pressure on the surgical site. Avoid holding the infant or child straddled on the hip. Limit the child's activity for 2 weeks.
- Encourage the infant or toddler to drink fluids to ensure adequate hydration. Provide fluids in a pleasant environment or using a special cup. Offer fruit juice, fruit-flavored ice pops, fruit-flavored juices, flavored ice cubes, and gelatin.
- Administer the complete course of prescribed antibiotics to avoid infection.
- Observe for signs of infection: fever, swelling, redness, pain, strong-smelling urine, or change in flow of the urinary stream.
- The urine will be blood tinged for several days. Call the healthcare provider if urine is seen leaking from any area other than the penis.

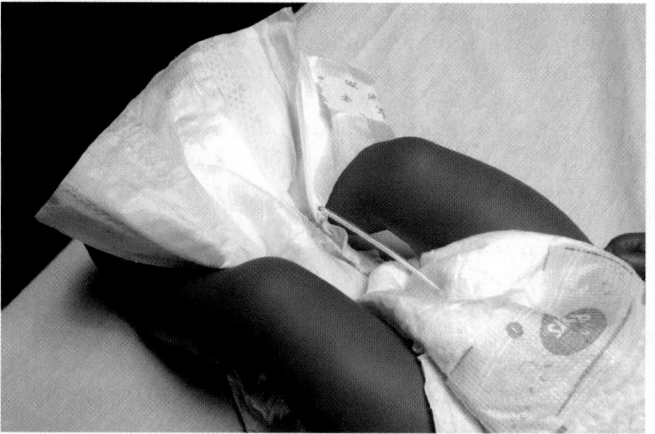

A double-diapering technique protects the operative site after surgery for hypospadias repair. The inner diaper collects stool; the outer diaper, urine.

Pathophysiology Illustrated: **Obstruction Sites in the Urinary System**

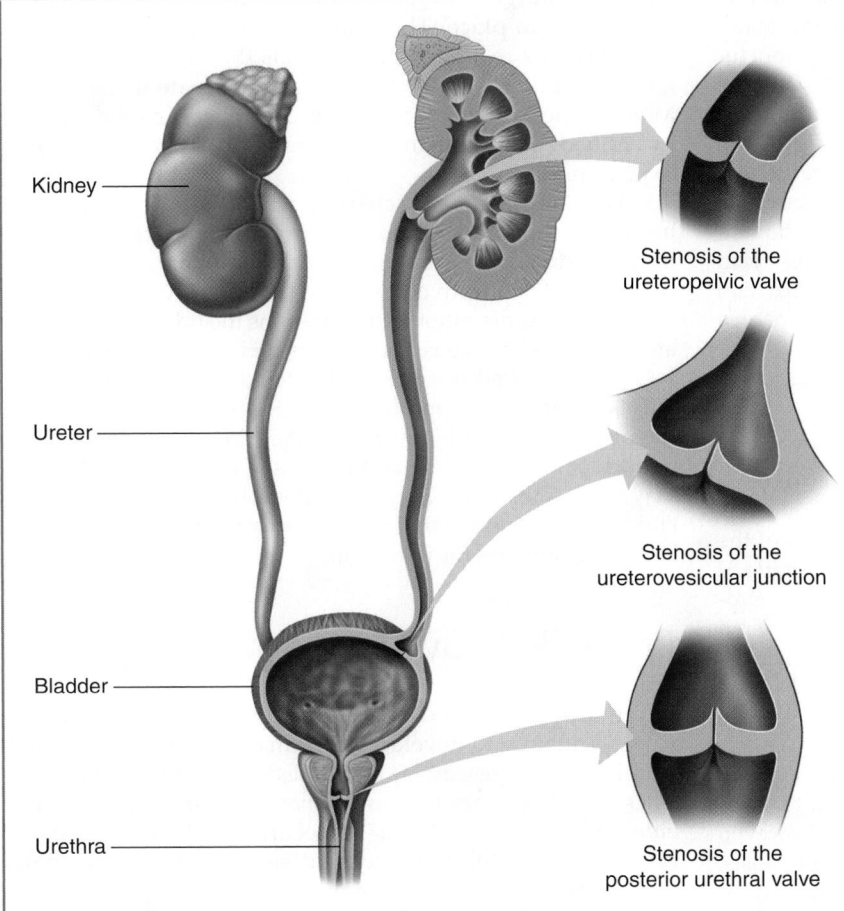

Kidney

Ureter

Bladder

Urethra

Stenosis of the
ureteropelvic valve

Stenosis of the
ureterovesicular junction

Stenosis of the
posterior urethral valve

Obstruction may occur in either the upper or lower urinary tract. Common sites of obstruction occur at the ureteropelvic valve, the ureterovesicular junction, or the posterior urethral valve. Renal failure is most likely to occur when both kidneys are affected by hydronephrosis.

posterior urethral valves (PUVs), and stenosis or hypoplasia of the ureterovesicular junction (see *Pathophysiology Illustrated: Obstruction Sites in the Urinary System*). The UPJ is the most common site of obstruction of the upper urinary tract in infants and children. UPJ obstruction occurs in 1 of every 1000 to 2000 newborns, making it the most common cause of hydronephrosis in newborns (Lee, Han, & Rah, 2014). PUVs (abnormal folds of mucosa in the male urethra) occur in 1 of every 5000 children and are a significant cause of end-stage renal disease in children (Kari et al., 2013). Stenosis of the distal ureter at the ureterovesicular junction leads to dilation of the entire ureter, renal pelvis, and kidney (Ring & Huether, 2014).

Clinical manifestations vary depending on the cause and location of the obstruction (Table 52–3). Early diagnosis and

treatment prevents kidney damage and deterioration of renal function. Prenatal ultrasound may detect hydronephrosis and PUV. A diuretic-enhanced radionuclide scan and voiding cystourethrogram are performed when UPJ or ureterovesicular obstruction is suspected.

The goals of surgical correction or diversion are to lower the pressure within the collecting system, which reduces renal damage, and to prevent stasis, which decreases the risk of infection. Surgical correction may necessitate **pyeloplasty** (removal of an obstructed segment of the ureter and reimplantation into the renal pelvis) or valve repair or reconstruction depending on the cause of the obstruction. Urinary incontinence resulting from sphincter weakness is a common problem after surgery.

TABLE 52–3 Clinical Manifestations of Obstructive Lesions of the Urinary System

OBSTRUCTIVE LESION	CLINICAL MANIFESTATIONS
Ureteropelvic junction obstruction	In infants: abdominal mass (enlarged kidney), hypertension, urinary tract infection
	In children: hematuria, pain, intermittent nausea and vomiting
Posterior urethral valves	In infants: abdominal mass (enlarged kidney), distended bladder, poor urinary stream, urinary tract infection, sepsis, low specific gravity, polyuria, increased creatinine level, failure to thrive
	In children: urinary frequency and incontinence
Ureterovesicular junction obstruction	Urinary tract infection (recurrent or chronic), hematuria, pain, abdominal mass (enlarged kidney), enuresis

Nursing Management

Preoperative nursing care focuses on preparing the parents and child for the procedure and addressing parents' concerns about the postsurgical outcome. Provide parents with an opportunity to discuss concerns about how the disorder will affect the child's long-term renal functioning.

Postoperative care involves monitoring vital signs and intake and output and observing for signs of urine retention, such as decreased output and bladder distention. Many children are discharged with stents or catheters. Teach parents how to change dressings, double-diaper, care for catheters, assess pain and give analgesics, and recognize signs of possible obstruction or infection. Parents should encourage the child to participate in age-appropriate activities. However, children should avoid contact sports because of their potential to injure the bladder.

Vesicoureteral Reflux

In vesicoureteral reflux (VUR), there is a retrograde flow of urine from the bladder into the ureters. Severity ranges from reflux of urine into the ureter only (grade 1) to severe dilation of the ureter and renal pelvis with severely blunted calyces (grade 5) (Estrada & Cendron, 2013). The reflux prevents complete emptying of the bladder, and because urine returns to the bladder, it creates a reservoir for bacterial growth (Ring & Huether, 2014). Bacteria in the urine may be swept up to the kidneys, leading to pyelonephritis, which is the most common cause of kidney damage in children (Wadie & Moriarty, 2012).

A renal ultrasound, voiding cystourethrogram (VCUG), and/or dimercaptosuccinic acid (DMSA) scan is used to diagnose, grade, and follow the progression of VUR. Note, however, that VCUG is the only test that provides a definitive diagnosis. The use of prophylactic antibiotics is controversial but may be prescribed to prevent UTIs. Surgical management with ureteral reimplantation may be needed depending on the grade of reflux (Passamaneck, 2011). Endoscopic management with the submucosal injection of Deflux has proven to be a successful alternative for some patients and may be considered as an alternative to surgery (Wadie & Moriarty, 2012).

Professionalism in Practice Screening Siblings for Vesicoureteral Reflux

Vesicoureteral reflux (VUR) occurs in 1% to 2% of the pediatric population and is present in 30% to 40% of children with a urinary tract infection (UTI). Research has shown that siblings of children with VUR have a much higher risk of having VUR than children without a family history, with a reported incidence of 26% to 50%. The American Urological Association Pediatric Vesicoureteral Reflux Guidelines have been revised to include recommendations related to screening siblings of children with VUR. It is especially important that siblings who present with a UTI be evaluated for VUR with a voiding cystourethrogram (Hunziker, Colhoun, & Puri, 2014). Nurses have opportunities to work with families of children being treated for urinary tract infections and/or VUR. Parents should be made aware of the increased incidence of VUR in siblings and the need for prompt attention to any signs of UTI. It is important that they include in the education of these families the relationship of recurrent UTI and subsequent kidney damage in children.

Nursing Management

Following surgery to reimplant the ureters, a urinary catheter will be in place. The urine will be bloody initially and clear within 2 to 3 days. Intravenous fluids will be administered at a rate sufficient to maintain adequate urine output. Monitor the catheter for patency. Administer medications as prescribed, including antibiotics and antispasmodics such as oxybutynin.

The child can be discharged when the urinary catheter has been removed and the child can void spontaneously. An ultrasound or cystogram may be performed prior to discharge to evaluate the effectiveness of the surgery. Educate the family about the administration of medications including prophylactic antibiotics and antispasmodics if needed. Inform parents of the need for increased fiber in the diet to address the constipating effects of the antispasmodic medication. Guidelines for calling the physician include fever over 38.5°C (101.5°F), abdominal or back pain, or swelling and redness of the incision. The child may take a short shower or tub bath when returning home. The child should avoid active play for 3 weeks following surgery. Provide guidelines for follow-up.

Prune Belly Syndrome

Prune belly syndrome, also known as *Eagle-Barrett syndrome*, is a congenital defect characterized by failure of the abdominal musculature to develop. The skin covering the abdominal wall is thin and resembles a wrinkled prune. Other characteristics include urinary tract anomalies, poor ureteral peristalsis, enlarged bladder, high risk for recurrent UTI, vesicoureteral reflux, and bilateral cryptorchidism in males. Prune belly syndrome occurs predominantly in males (95%), with an incidence of 1 in 29,000 to 40,000 live births (Caldamone & Woodard, 2012).

The etiology of prune belly syndrome is unknown; however, it is thought to be related to a fetal urinary tract obstruction or a specific injury to the mesoderm during the first trimester. In addition to urinary tract anomalies, cardiac, pulmonary, gastrointestinal, and musculoskeletal anomalies also occur (Hassett, Smith, & Holland, 2012).

Prune belly syndrome is frequently diagnosed prenatally by ultrasound. Mortality in the neonatal period is related to pulmonary hypoplasia and severe renal dysfunction (Hassett et al., 2012). Abdominal wall reconstruction and correction of genitourinary defects, including orchiopexy (or orchidopexy), are performed to repair defects. The mortality rate in infants has improved significantly in the past 3 decades with advances in surgical techniques. Approximately 30% of children with prune belly syndrome will develop end-stage renal disease in childhood or adolescence because of inadequate renal function (Elder, 2016b).

Nursing Management

Nursing management for the infant with prune belly syndrome is the same as for other defects of the genitourinary system, including preoperative and postoperative management. Additional management includes psychosocial support for the child and family related to the numerous congenital anomalies, body image concerns, and long-term consequences of the defect.

A discussion of Wilms tumor can be found in Chapter 50.

TABLE 52–4 Milestones in the Development of Bladder Control

AGE	DEVELOPMENTAL MILESTONE
1.5 years	Child passes urine at regular intervals.
2 years	Child announces when voiding is taking place.
2.5 years	Child makes known the need to void; can hold urine.
3 years	Child goes to the bathroom alone; holds urge if preoccupied with play.
2.5–3.5 years	Child achieves nighttime control.
4 years	Child shows great interest in going to bathrooms when away from home (shopping centers, movies).
5 years	Child voids approximately 5 to 6 times a day; prefers privacy; is able to initiate emptying of bladder at any degree of fullness.

Enuresis

Enuresis is repeated involuntary voiding by a child old enough that bladder control is expected, usually about 5 to 6 years of age. (See Table 52–4 for bladder control milestones.) Enuresis can occur either at night (nocturnal), during the day (diurnal), or both night and day.

Enuresis is further categorized as primary or secondary:

- *Primary enuresis*—Child has never had a dry night; attributed to maturational delay and small functional bladder; not associated with stress or psychiatric cause.

- *Secondary enuresis*—Child who has been reliably dry for at least 6 months begins bed-wetting; associated with stress, infections, and sleep disorders.

Growth and Development

Nighttime wetting episodes usually decrease as the child ages. An estimated 21% of children ages 4.5 years and 8% of children 9.5 years of age average less than two episodes of nighttime wetting per week. Wetting episodes occur more than 2 times per week in 8% of children ages 4.5 years and 1.5% of children 9.5 years of age (Jacques, 2013).

Primary nocturnal enuresis is the most common type of enuresis and occurs more frequently in males than females (Elder, 2016c). It occurs more often in children who have a positive family history and generally involves more than one causative factor. Factors may include maturational delay, sleep disorders, and reduced or small functional bladder capacity (Ray, 2011). Nocturnal enuresis is also more prevalent in children with obstructive sleep apnea syndrome (Bascom et al., 2011). Additionally, enuresis frequently occurs in children with constipation. The constipation should be treated prior to the implementation of any treatment for enuresis (Walle et al., 2012).

A thorough history can help identify potential causes of secondary enuresis. The child's lower spine is examined for fistulas, sacral dimples, or tufts of hair that could be signs of spina bifida occulta (see Chapter 54). Diabetes, urinary tract infection, and other conditions should also be ruled out. Prolonged hospitalization, family stressors, and preoccupation with school concerns also have been associated with secondary enuresis.

Clinical Tip

Questions to ask when taking an enuresis history include the following:

Family History

Is there a family history of renal or urinary structural abnormalities?

Is there a family history of bed-wetting? At what age did bed-wetting stop?

Family Management of Enuresis

How serious is the problem for the family?

What happens when the child wets? (Who gets up and changes sheets?)

How is the child treated? Is the child punished or blamed for wetting?

What remedies have been tried?

Toilet Training

When was it initiated and what method was used?

Has the child ever been dry during the day or night for an extended period?

How long was the child's longest dry period?

How often does the child void? Have a bowel movement?

Does the child have a history of constipation or encopresis?

Stressors

How is the child doing in school?

Are any new or chronic stressors present in the child's life?

How does the problem interfere with play and other activities?

Risk Factors

Diabetes—Are there any signs of polyuria or polydipsia?

Urinary tract infection—Does the child have frequency, urgency, burning on urination?

A multitreatment approach is usually most effective. Limiting excessive fluids at night, bladder training, enuresis alarms, and positive reinforcement are common approaches (Table 52–5). Alarms have about a 70% success rate but take 3 to 5 months to be effective (Ray, 2011).

Medications used in the treatment of primary nocturnal enuresis include desmopressin, imipramine, and oxybutynin:

- Desmopressin is the most common medication used for nocturnal enuresis and has an antidiuretic effect. Desmopressin is given at nighttime at the beginning of treatment. Once its effectiveness has been established, it may be used every night or as needed for times when the child is away from home for a short period (e.g., sleepovers or camp) (Nevéus, 2011).

- Oxybutynin, an anticholinergic medication, has an antispasmodic effect, improves storage function of the bladder, and decreases the overactivity of the detrusor muscle. Oxybutynin may also be used in combination with desmopressin in children who have not responded to desmopressin alone or in combination with an alarm (Norfolk & Wootton, 2012).

- Imipramine, a tricyclic antidepressant, has anticholinergic and antispasmodic effects and may be used in children who do not respond to other methods. This medication requires close monitoring because of its effects on mood and the associated danger of overdoses (Nevéus, 2011).

TABLE 52–5 Treatment Approaches for Enuresis

APPROACH	DESCRIPTION
Limiting fluids	Fluid intake is limited in the evening and before the child goes to bed. Fluids with caffeine should be avoided.
Bladder exercises	The child drinks a large amount and then holds urine as long as possible. The child practices stopping voiding midstream. Exercises should continue for at least 6 months.
Timed voiding	The child with diurnal enuresis is instructed to void every 2 hr and to use a double voiding pattern; this trains the bladder to empty completely and avoid overdistention.
Enuresis alarms	A detector strip is attached to the child's pants. The alarm sounds a buzzer that alerts the child when wetting occurs, so the child can get up and finish voiding in the bathroom. This works best for children over 7 years old, and takes 3 to 5 months for success.
Reward system	Set realistic goals for the child and reinforce dry days or nights with stars and stickers on a chart.
Medications	Desmopressin, oxybutynin, and imipramine are used as discussed in the text.

Nursing Management

Teach the child and parents about the physiologic development of bladder control and causes and treatment of enuresis. Explore feelings of guilt or blame. Make sure the parents are aware that the child cannot control the wetting. Psychosocial support is an essential part of care since stress is an important cause of secondary enuresis. Provide emotional support to the parents and child, and encourage the child's participation in the treatment plan. Refer the child for counseling or therapy if appropriate.

Assess the parents' and child's motivation and readiness for interventions. The child needs to be an active participant in the treatment plan for daytime and nighttime wetting. Before parents buy an enuresis alarm, suggest they use an alarm clock in the child's room for several nights to see if the child will arouse. Find out whether the child shares a room with others who will be disturbed by the alarm. Ask if the child and parents are willing to persist with an enuresis alarm because it may take months to work. Discuss potential strategies with the family to reduce stressors on the child or to help the child cope with the stressors. Expected outcomes of nursing care include:

- The child has an increased number of dry nights.
- The child and family choose one or more interventions that they prefer and persist in using them.

Renal Disorders

Nephrotic Syndrome

Nephrotic syndrome is an alteration in kidney function secondary to increased glomerular basement membrane permeability to plasma protein (see *Pathophysiology Illustrated: Nephrotic Syndrome*). Nephrotic syndrome does not refer to a specific disease, but rather to a clinical state characterized by edema, massive proteinuria, hypoalbuminemia, hypoproteinemia, hyperlipidemia, and altered immunity. Congenital nephrotic syndrome is generally related to a genetic defect (Holmberg & Jalanko, 2014). The term *primary nephrotic syndrome* is used when there is no identifiable cause. *Secondary nephrotic syndrome* results from a systemic disease, drugs, or toxins (Ring & Huether, 2014).

Approximately 85% of children with nephrotic syndrome have a type of primary disease called *minimal change nephrotic syndrome* (MCNS). It is estimated that more than 95% of these children respond to steroid therapy (Pais & Avner, 2016). MCNS derives its name from the normal or only minimally changed appearance of the glomeruli on light microscopic evaluation. MCNS is the focus of the following discussion.

ETIOLOGY AND PATHOPHYSIOLOGY
The cause of primary MCNS is not clearly understood but an immune system role is suspected (Pais & Avner, 2016). The mechanism of increased glomerular permeability is unknown because the glomeruli appear normal (Ring & Huether, 2014). In MCNS, increased permeability of the glomerular membrane permits large, negatively charged molecules such as albumin to pass through the membrane and be excreted in the urine. Proteinuria results in decreased oncotic pressure and edema because fluid remains in the interstitial spaces instead of being pulled back into the vascular compartment (Pais & Avner, 2016). Immunoglobulins are lost, resulting in altered immunity. Loss of protein in the urine, insufficient albumin production by the liver, and a decreased albumin concentration as a result of salt and water retention by the kidney contribute to hypoalbuminemia. Hypercoagulability occurs because of alterations in coagulation factors. The liver responds by increasing synthesis of lipoprotein, resulting in hyperlipidemia (Ring & Huether, 2014). Children who develop steroid-resistant nephrotic syndrome are at risk for end-stage renal disease (Lombel, Hodson, & Gipson, 2013).

CLINICAL MANIFESTATIONS
In most children, edema develops gradually over several weeks. Children may have a history of periorbital edema on waking that resolves during the day as fluid shifts to the abdomen and lower extremities. Other signs include snug fit of clothing and shoes, pallor, hypertension, irritability, anorexia, hematuria, decreased urine output, and nonspecific malaise. The child's urine may be frothy or foamy. Parents often do not seek medical treatment until generalized edema develops on the child's extremities, abdomen, or genitals (Figure 52–4). Respiratory distress from pleural effusion may occur in some cases.

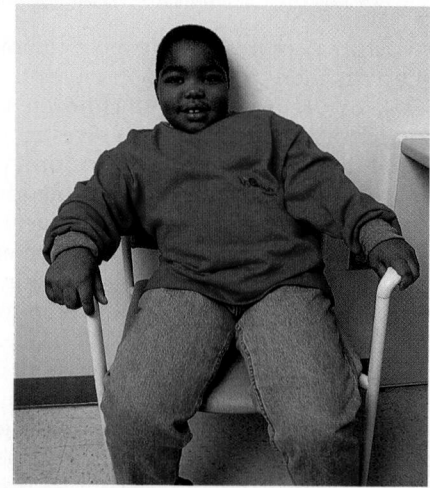

Figure 52–4 This boy has generalized edema, a characteristic finding in nephrotic syndrome.

Pathophysiology Illustrated: Nephrotic Syndrome

Note the contrast between the normal glomerular anatomy and the changes that exist in nephrotic syndrome, which permit protein to be excreted in the urine. The lower albumin blood level stimulates the liver to generate lipids and excessive clotting factors. Edema results from decreased oncotic plasma pressure, renin-angiotensin-aldosterone activation, and antidiuretic hormone secretion.

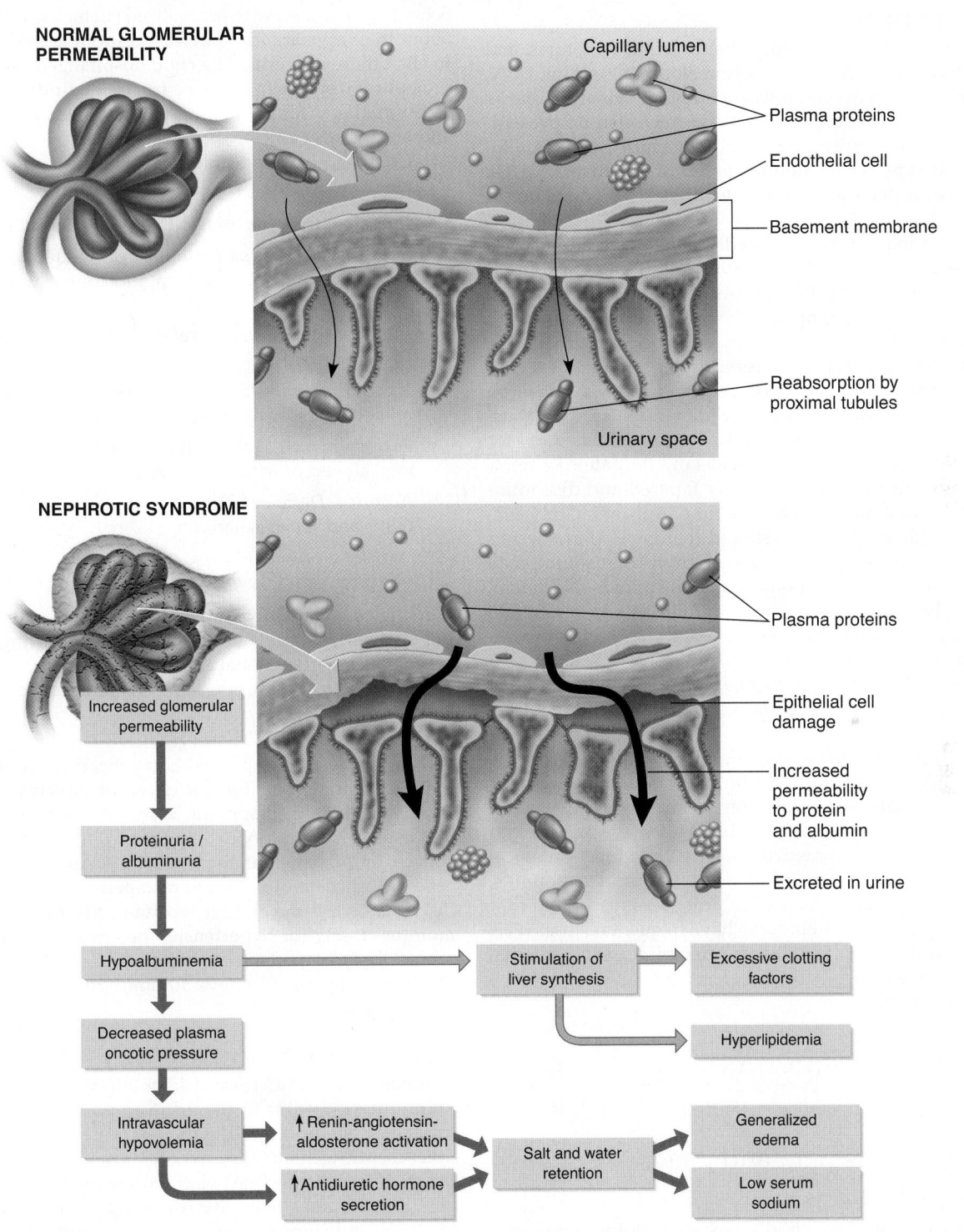

Massive edema resulting in a dramatic weight gain and abdominal pain, with or without vomiting, may occur depending on the amount of albumin lost and the amount of sodium ingested. The child becomes malnourished as a result of protein loss in the urine. The skin is pale and shiny with prominent veins, and the hair becomes more brittle. An increased risk of thrombosis is present.

CLINICAL THERAPY

Diagnosis is based on the history, characteristic symptoms, and laboratory findings. Urinalysis, serum albumin, sodium, BUN, cholesterol, and electrolytes tests are ordered. Urinalysis shows large protein. Microscopic hematuria may also be present. Other values that confirm the diagnosis include hypoalbuminemia indicated by serum albumin levels of less than 2.5 g/dL and urinary protein excretion of greater than 3.5 grams per 24 hours (Pais & Avner, 2016).

Children may be hospitalized when severe edema or a major infection is present, but are usually treated as outpatients. Clinical therapy focuses on decreasing proteinuria, relieving edema, managing associated symptoms, improving nutrition, and preventing infection. A corticosteroid (such as prednisone) is prescribed to decrease proteinuria. In most children, urine protein levels fall to trace or negative values within 2 to 3 weeks of the start of therapy. Children who respond successfully to therapy continue to take corticosteroids daily for 6 weeks, followed by at least 4 weeks of alternate-day treatment. The medication is then slowly tapered and discontinued over a 1- to 2-month period of time. Approximately 80% to 90% of children respond to steroid therapy within 4 weeks (Pais & Avner, 2016). Intravenous methylprednisolone may be used in children not responsive to oral steroids (Nachman, Jennette, & Falk, 2012). Intravenous administration of albumin followed by furosemide may be ordered in the child with massive edema who is unresponsive to fluid restriction and parenteral diuretics (Pais & Avner, 2016). Analgesics may be ordered for pain related to edema or flank pain from a urinary tract infection.

Relapses occur in many children with nephrotic syndrome (Pais & Avner, 2016). Children who have a relapse after drug therapy is discontinued receive repeat therapy. Other medications used include diuretics, antihypertensive agents, and antibiotics. Immunosuppressive or immunomodulator medications, including cyclophosphamide, cyclosporine, tacrolimus, and mycophenolate, may be used to prolong remissions in children with nephrotic syndrome who have frequent relapses (Pais & Avner, 2016). Since diuretics can precipitate hypovolemia, hyponatremia, and hypokalemia, electrolyte levels should be carefully monitored.

Nursing Management

For the Child With Nephrotic Syndrome

Nursing Assessment and Diagnosis

PHYSIOLOGIC ASSESSMENT

Careful assessment of the child's hydration status and edema is essential. Carefully monitor intake and output. Weigh the child daily using the same scale, and measure abdominal girth to monitor changes in edema and ascites (see the *Clinical Skills Manual* SKILLS). Monitor vital signs at least every 4 hours to watch for signs of respiratory distress, hypertension, or circulatory overload. Test urine for proteinuria and specific gravity

at least once each shift. In addition, assess for skin breakdown from edema, for hypovolemia during periods of diuresis, and for indications of infection.

PSYCHOSOCIAL ASSESSMENT

Children and parents are often fearful or anxious on admission. Because edema often develops gradually, parents may feel guilty if they did not seek medical attention immediately. School-age children with generalized edema are often concerned about their appearance. Careful questioning may be necessary to elicit these concerns. The child hospitalized for a recurrence of nephrotic syndrome may be frustrated or depressed. Assess individual and family coping mechanisms, support systems, and level of stress.

Common nursing diagnoses for the child with MCNS include the following (NANDA-I © 2014):

- *Infection, Risk for,* related to immunosuppressive therapy
- *Skin Integrity, Risk for Impaired,* related to edema, lowered resistance to infection and injury, immobility, and malnutrition
- *Fluid Volume: Excess,* related to renal dysfunction and sodium retention
- *Nutrition, Imbalanced: Less than Body Requirements,* related to loss of appetite and protein loss in urine
- *Fatigue* related to fluid and electrolyte imbalance, albumin loss, altered nutrition, and renal failure
- *Activity, Deficient Diversional,* related to fatigue, immobility, and social isolation

Planning and Implementation

Nursing care is mainly supportive and focuses on administering medications, preventing infection, preventing skin breakdown, meeting nutritional and fluid needs, promoting rest, and providing emotional support to the parents and child.

ADMINISTER MEDICATIONS

It is important to give prescribed medications at the scheduled times. Monitor closely for side effects of corticosteroids such as moon face, increased appetite, increased hair growth, abdominal distention, and mood swings, as well as adverse effects of corticosteroids such as hypertension, nausea, and hyperglycemia. Corticosteroids should be tapered rather than abruptly discontinued. If the child is receiving albumin intravenously, monitor closely for hypertension or signs of volume overload caused by fluid shifts. If diuretics are used, observe for shock. The child may need to have albumin infused simultaneously with diuretics.

PREVENT INFECTION

Children with MCNS are at risk for infection because of the loss of immunoglobulins in the urine and corticosteroid therapy. Implement careful hand hygiene and standard precautions. Strict aseptic technique is essential during invasive procedures. Monitor the child's white blood cell count when cytotoxic drugs are given because bone marrow suppression is a side effect. Monitor vital signs carefully to detect early signs of infection that may be masked by corticosteroid therapy. Decrease the child's social contacts during immunosuppressive treatment, and caution parents and children to avoid exposure to people with respiratory infections and communicable diseases. Emphasize the importance of avoiding shopping malls, sporting arenas, grocery stores, game stores, and other public areas where the risk of exposure to such infections is increased. Provide instructions to the parents on signs of infection, including fever and changes in behavior. Discuss with parents the need for maintenance of annual recommended influenza immunizations and avoiding those who have recently been vaccinated with live viruses.

PREVENT SKIN BREAKDOWN

Meticulous skin care is essential to prevent skin breakdown and potential infection. Assess the skin repeatedly, turn the child frequently, and use therapeutic mattresses (e.g., egg crate, airflow) to help prevent skin breakdown. Keep the skin clean and dry.

MEET NUTRITIONAL AND FLUID NEEDS

Keep the child's food preferences in mind when planning menus. Encourage the child to eat by presenting attractive meals in small portions. Socialization during meals may improve the child's appetite. Fluids are not usually restricted except during severe edema.

PROMOTE REST

Provide opportunities for quiet play as tolerated, such as drawing, playing board games, listening to CDs, and watching movies. Adjust the child's daily schedule to allow rest periods after activities. Signs of fatigue may include irritability, mood swings, or withdrawal. Tell the parents and child about the importance of rest. Limiting visitors during the acute phase of the illness may be necessary. Telephone and computer contacts may be encouraged as an alternative to visitors. To provide a sense of control, encourage these children to set their own limits on activity.

PROVIDE EMOTIONAL SUPPORT

Parents and children often need support to cope with this chronic disease. Thoroughly explain the child's disease and treatment regimen to parents. Parental anxiety in combination with the hospitalization may interfere with the child's independence. Help parents promote the child's independence by allowing the child to choose from the menu or to select the daily activity schedule. This gives the child some sense of control.

Children with MCNS may have a distorted body image because of sudden weight gain and edema. They may refuse to look in the mirror, refuse to participate in care, and take less interest in their appearance. Encourage children to express their feelings. Help them maintain a normal appearance by promoting normal grooming routines. Encourage children to wear their own pajamas rather than hospital gowns. Scarves or hats may be used to lessen the child's edematous appearance. Adolescents can be encouraged to write their feelings in a journal as a coping mechanism. These children may have a long-term psychosocial adjustment because of having a chronic condition with concerns about potential relapse.

DISCHARGE PLANNING AND HOME CARE TEACHING

Explain the disease process, prognosis, and treatment plan to parents and school-age children. Make sure parents know how to administer medications and can identify potential side effects. Inform parents about restricting fluid intake until the edema resolves. Instruct parents about the need to monitor urine daily for protein, and have them keep a diary to record results. Monitoring the child's weight each week may help parents identify early stages of fluid retention and signs of relapse before edema occurs.

Tutoring may be required for a short period after discharge. Encourage parents to allow the child to return to normal activities once the acute episode has resolved. Emphasize the importance of avoiding contact with people with infectious diseases because of the child's reduced immunity. Reinforce to parents that as long as the child is receiving corticosteroid therapy or shows signs of MCNS, a no-added-salt diet should be followed.

Most children do well with corticosteroid therapy; however, relapses are common. These relapses decrease as the child gets older. Children should have periodic bone density evaluations because of the repeated steroid therapy, which can weaken bones and lead to osteoporosis.

Evaluation

Expected outcomes of nursing care may include:

- The child responds to corticosteroid therapy.
- The child does not acquire an infection.
- Fluid, electrolyte, and acid–base balance is restored and maintained.
- Skin integrity is maintained.
- The child meets nutritional requirements and follows dietary guidelines.

Acute Postinfectious Glomerulonephritis

Glomerulonephritis is the most common inflammation of the glomeruli of the kidneys. In children, it is most often a response to a group A beta-hemolytic streptococcal infection of the skin or pharynx. It is also caused by other organisms, including *Staphylococcus* and *Pneumococcus* bacteria and coxsackieviruses. The incidence of acute postinfectious glomerulonephritis (APIGN) is highest in children between 2 and 6 years of age, and the disorder is more common in boys than in girls (Nachman et al., 2012).

ETIOLOGY AND PATHOPHYSIOLOGY

The child with APIGN usually becomes ill after contracting a nephrogenetic strain of group A beta-hemolytic streptococcal infection of the upper respiratory tract or the skin. Often the child contracts a streptococcal infection (e.g., strep throat), recovers, and then develops signs of APIGN after an interval of 10 to 21 days.

Glomerular damage occurs as a result of an immune complex reaction that localizes on the glomerular capillary wall. See *Pathophysiology Illustrated: Acute Postinfectious Glomerulonephritis*. Antibody–antigen complexes become lodged in the glomeruli, leading to inflammation and obstruction. The glomerular membranes thicken, and capillaries in the glomeruli become obstructed by damaged tissue cells, leading to a decreased glomerular filtration rate. Vascular permeability increases, allowing red blood cells and red cell casts to be excreted. Sodium and water are retained, expanding the intravascular and interstitial compartments and resulting in the characteristic finding of edema.

CLINICAL MANIFESTATIONS

Many children are asymptomatic. In other children, the onset is usually abrupt with flank or midabdominal pain, irritability, malaise, and fever. Microscopic hematuria is present in nearly all cases, and gross hematuria, resulting in tea-colored urine, is found in up to 50% of cases. Mild periorbital edema occurs early, along with dependent edema of the feet and ankles. Edema may progress in severity to cause pulmonary congestion

Pathophysiology Illustrated: **Acute Postinfectious Glomerulonephritis**

Infection from group A beta-hemolytic streptococci causes an immune response that leads to inflammation and damage to the glomeruli. Protein and red blood cells are allowed to pass through the glomeruli. Blood flow to the glomeruli is reduced because of obstruction with damaged cells. Renal insufficiency results, leading to the retention of sodium, water, and waste.

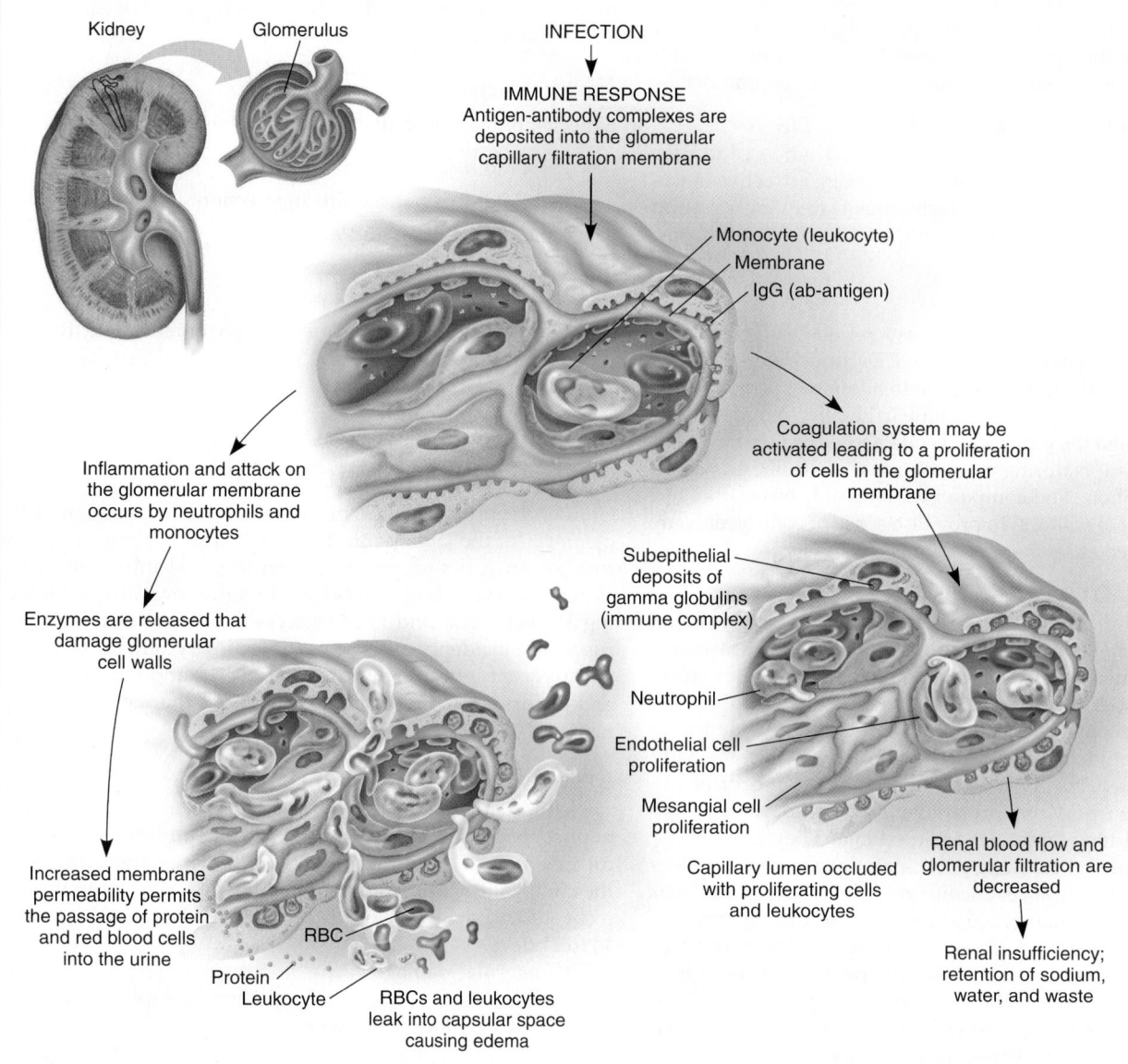

or ascites (Nachman et al., 2012). Acute hypertension may lead to headache, nausea, vomiting, lethargy, seizures, and other CNS symptoms. Oliguria may or may not be present (Ring & Huether, 2014).

CLINICAL THERAPY

The serum BUN and creatinine concentrations are elevated. Serum protein is decreased as a result of mild or moderate proteinuria. The white blood cell count and erythrocyte sedimentation rate may be elevated. An elevated antistreptolysin O (ASO) titer reflects the presence of antibodies from a recent streptococcal respiratory infection, but the ASO level associated with a recent skin infection is low. The anti-DNAse B titer is helpful

for detecting antibodies associated with recent skin infections. Most children have a reduced serum complement (C3) level due to the initial infection (Nachman et al., 2012). Urinalysis reveals hematuria, proteinuria, and red blood cell casts. Anemia is common in the acute phase, usually because extracellular fluid dilutes the serum. Hemoglobin and hematocrit levels reveal anemia, which is common in the acute phase and is generally caused by dilution of the serum by the extracellular fluid (Bhimma, 2014).

Treatment focuses on relief of symptoms and supportive therapy. Bed rest is a key component of the treatment plan during the acute phase. Edema and mild to moderate hypertension should be treated with sodium restriction and a diuretic such as furosemide (Nachman et al., 2012; Ring & Huether, 2014). A course of antibiotics may be given to ensure eradication of the original infectious agent. Immediate emergency care is needed for severe hypertension with cerebral dysfunction.

The prognosis for most children with APIGN is good. Clinical signs, proteinuria, and hematuria resolve within several weeks. Over 95% of children recover completely (Ring & Huether, 2014).

Nursing Management

For the Child With Acute Postinfectious Glomerulonephritis

Nursing Assessment and Diagnosis

As with other renal disorders, care of the child with APIGN requires careful monitoring of vital signs and fluid–electrolyte balance to evaluate renal functioning and identify complications. Frequent blood pressure monitoring is required since it can rise as high as 200/120 mmHg. With severe hypertension, assess for signs of central nervous system problems (headache, blurred vision, vomiting, decreased level of consciousness, confusion, and convulsions). Monitor urine for proteinuria and hematuria. Record output. Assess edema, which may be periorbital or dependent and may shift as the child's position is changed. Assess for a pulmonary effusion (crackles, dyspnea, and cough).

Nursing diagnoses may include the following (NANDA-I © 2014):

- *Fluid Volume: Excess,* related to decreased glomerular filtration and increased sodium
- *Infection, Risk for,* related to renal impairment and corticosteroid therapy
- *Skin Integrity, Risk for Impaired,* related to tissue edema
- *Nutrition, Imbalanced: Less than Body Requirements,* related to loss of appetite and proteinuria
- *Activity Intolerance* related to fluid and electrolyte imbalance, infectious process, and altered nutrition
- *Health Management, Family, Ineffective,* related to child's medication schedule and treatment regimen after discharge

Clinical Tip

Antibiotics are *not* a treatment for APIGN. Instead, antibiotics are prescribed to treat the original infection (such as strep throat) if the infection is still present.

Planning and Implementation

MONITOR FLUID STATUS

Monitor vital signs, fluid and electrolyte status, and intake and output. Hypovolemia can occur as a result of fluid shifting from vascular to interstitial spaces despite the outward clinical signs of excess fluid retention. Monitor the degree of ascites by measuring abdominal girth. Document urine specific gravity. Make sure parents and visitors understand the need to limit fluids to prevent excessive intake.

PREVENT INFECTION

Impaired renal function puts the child at risk for infection. Monitor for signs of infection, including fever, increased malaise, and an elevated white blood cell count. Screen family members for the presence of streptococcal infection and refer for treatment if necessary. Instruct the family in good hand hygiene technique. Limit visitors, and screen for upper respiratory infections.

PREVENT SKIN BREAKDOWN

Bed rest is required during the acute phase. Dependent areas and other pressure areas are vulnerable to skin breakdown. Turn the child frequently. Pad bony prominences or susceptible areas with sheepskin, or protect skin with a transparent dressing. Elevate lower extremities on pillows when in the dependent position or when the child is lying in bed. Make sure the child's bed is free of crumbs or sharp toys. Keep sheets tight and free of wrinkles. Maintain proper hygiene and dry skin.

MEET NUTRITIONAL NEEDS

A team approach (including the nurse, renal dietitian, parents, and child) is often needed to meet the child's nutritional needs. In most cases, the child follows a no-added-salt and low-protein diet. This diet may be challenging since the child may refuse to eat foods that taste different. Anorexia presents the greatest challenge to meeting daily nutritional requirements during the acute phase of the disease. To increase the child's appetite, encourage parents to bring the child's favorite foods from home, serve foods in age-appropriate quantities, and allow the child to eat with other children or with family members.

PROVIDE EMOTIONAL SUPPORT

Parents of a child with APIGN commonly feel guilty. Parents may blame themselves for not responding more quickly to the child's initial symptoms or may believe they could have prevented the development of glomerular damage. Discuss the etiology of the disease and the child's treatment, and correct any misconceptions. Emphasize that it is not possible to predict which of the few children with streptococcal infections will develop APIGN.

DISCHARGE PLANNING AND HOME CARE TEACHING

Children are hospitalized for a few days, although it may require 3 weeks for hypertension and gross hematuria to resolve and longer for the disorder to resolve completely. Discharge planning focuses on teaching parents about the child's medication regimen, potential side effects of medications, dietary restrictions, and signs and symptoms of complications. Teach parents how to take the child's blood pressure and how to test urine for blood or protein. Emphasize that it is important to avoid exposing the child to people with upper respiratory tract infections. The child should be allowed to return to the normal routine and activities after discharge, with periods being allowed for rest.

Evaluation

Expected outcomes of nursing care are the following:

- The child receives appropriate fluid volume each day and maintains normal urine output.
- The child develops no areas of redness, abrasions, or skin breakdown over pressure points.
- The child's temperature remains within normal limits and the child is free of secondary infection.

- The child maintains preillness weight and tolerates daily intake that meets nutritional requirements.
- The parents administer medications as prescribed. The child's sodium and potassium levels reflect adherence to dietary restrictions.

Renal Failure

Renal failure, which may be acute or chronic, occurs when the kidney is unable to excrete wastes and concentrate urine. Acute renal failure occurs suddenly (over days or weeks) and may be reversible, whereas in chronic renal failure, kidney function diminishes gradually and permanently over months or years.

Both types of renal failure are characterized by **azotemia** (accumulation of nitrogenous wastes in the blood) and sometimes **oliguria** (reduced urine volume for age), indicating the kidney's inability to excrete metabolic waste products. Chronic renal failure eventually results in **anuria** (absence of urine output).

Acute Renal Failure

Acute renal failure (ARF), also called *acute kidney injury*, is a sudden loss of adequate renal function in which the kidneys are unable to clear metabolic wastes and to regulate extracellular fluid volume, sodium balance, and acid–base homeostasis. Potential causes include hemolytic-uremic syndrome, acute glomerulonephritis, sepsis, poisoning, nephrotoxic medications, hypovolemia, obstructive uropathy, and complication of cardiac surgery.

ETIOLOGY AND PATHOPHYSIOLOGY

ARF may be caused by prerenal or postrenal factors as well as actual kidney damage. Prerenal ARF is a result of decreased perfusion to an otherwise normal kidney in association with a systemic condition. Hypovolemia secondary to dehydration is generally the cause; however, alterations in renal vasculature or cardiac function may also precipitate prerenal ARF. This is the most common type of ARF in infants and young children (Lum, 2014).

TABLE 52–6 Clinical Manifestations of Acute Versus Chronic Renal Failure

TYPE OF RENAL FAILURE	CLINICAL MANIFESTATIONS
Acute renal failure	Dark urine or gross hematuria, headache, edema, fatigue, crackles, gallop heart rhythm, hypertension, hematuria, lethargy, nausea and vomiting, oliguria
	Mass in flank area if a cyst, tumor, or obstructive lesion is present
Chronic renal failure	Fatigue, malaise, poor appetite, nausea and vomiting, failure to thrive or short stature
	May have oliguria or polyuria
	Headache, decreased mental alertness or ability to concentrate
	Chronic anemia, hypertension, edema
	Fractures with minimal trauma, rickets, valgus deformity

Primary kidney damage (intrinsic factors) may result from infection, diseases such as hemolytic-uremic syndrome, acute glomerulonephritis, and acute tubular necrosis, and nephrotoxic injury (Lum, 2014).

Postrenal ARF is generally found in newborns with urologic anatomic anomalies (Lum, 2014). Children may have oliguria or normal or increased urine output. Renal failure without oliguria usually indicates a less severe renal injury. Children who recover from ARF may have residual kidney damage and compromised renal function.

CLINICAL MANIFESTATIONS

Characteristically, a healthy child suddenly becomes ill with nonspecific symptoms that indicate a significant illness or injury (e.g., nausea, vomiting, lethargy, edema, gross hematuria, oliguria, and hypertension). These symptoms are a result of electrolyte imbalances, uremia, and fluid overload. The child appears pale and lethargic. See Tables 52–6 and 52–7 for more information.

Hyperkalemia is the most life-threatening electrolyte disorder associated with ARF. Hyponatremia affects central nervous system function, resulting in symptoms that range from fatigue to seizures. Edema occurs as a result of sodium and water retention. (Refer to Chapter 44 for a discussion of these fluid and electrolyte alterations.) Children with ARF are also more susceptible to infection because of depressed immune functioning. **Uremia** occurs when there is an excess of urea and other nitrogenous waste products in the blood. Neurologic symptoms from accumulating wastes may include headache, seizures, lethargy, and confusion.

CLINICAL THERAPY

Diagnosis of renal failure is based primarily on urinalysis and blood chemistry results, including BUN, serum creatinine, sodium, potassium, and calcium levels (Table 52–8). The kidneys are normal in size, and no signs of renal **osteodystrophy** (a complex bone disease process of chronic kidney disease in which there is increased resorption of bone caused by chronic hyperparathyroidism) are found on radiography. Various imaging studies to assess kidney structures, renal blood flow, and renal perfusion and function may be performed to determine whether the child has ARF or chronic renal failure. A renal biopsy may be required.

Treatment depends on the underlying cause of the renal failure. The goal is to minimize or prevent permanent renal damage while maintaining fluid and electrolyte balance and managing complications. Initial emergency treatment of children with fluid depletion focuses on rapid fluid replacement of saline or lactated Ringer solution at 20 mL/kg given rapidly over 5 to 10 minutes and repeated as needed to ensure renal perfusion and stabilize blood pressure. Albumin may also be administered when blood loss is the cause of circulatory depletion. If oliguria persists after restoration of adequate fluid volume, intrinsic renal damage is suspected.

Children with fluid overload, such as those with pulmonary edema, require diuretic therapy, and dialysis if they respond poorly to diuretics. Once the child is stabilized, fluid requirements are calculated to maintain zero water balance (intake should equal urine output and insensible fluid loss). All potential sources of potassium should be eliminated until hyperkalemia is controlled. Other electrolyte imbalances are treated. Nutrition must be maintained with extra carbohydrate intake during the catabolic state. Antibiotics are prescribed for infection if applicable. Nephrotoxic antibiotics such as aminoglycosides (e.g., gentamicin, vancomycin) should be avoided.

TABLE 52–7 Clinical Manifestations of Electrolyte Imbalances in Acute and Chronic Renal Failure

ELECTROLYTE IMBALANCE AND CAUSE	CLINICAL MANIFESTATIONS
HYPERKALEMIA Results from inability to adequately excrete potassium derived from diet and catabolized cells. In metabolic acidosis, there is also movement of potassium from intracellular fluid to extracellular fluid.	• Peaked T waves, widening of QRS waves on ECG • Dysrhythmias • Muscle weakness
HYPONATREMIA In the acute oliguric phase, hyponatremia is related to the accumulation of fluid in excess of solute.	• Change in level of consciousness • Muscle cramps • Anorexia • Abdominal reflexes, depressed deep tendon reflexes • Cheyne-Stokes respirations • Seizures
HYPOCALCEMIA Phosphate retention (hyperphosphatemia) depresses the serum calcium ion concentration. Calcium is deposited in injured cells. Hyperkalemia and metabolic acidosis may mask the common clinical manifestations of severe hypocalcemia.	• Muscle tingling • Changes in muscle tone • Seizures • Muscle cramps and twitching • Positive **Chvostek sign** (contraction of facial muscles after tapping facial nerve just anterior to parotid gland)

Note: See Chapter 44 for more information related to these alterations in electrolytes.

Source: Data from Hines, E. Q. (2012). Fluid and electrolytes. In *The Harriet Lane handbook* (19th ed., pp. 271–292). Philadelphia, PA: Elsevier Saunders; Sreedharan, R., & Avner, E. D. (2016). Renal failure. In R. M. Kliegman, B. F. Stanton, J. W. St. Geme, & N. F. Schor (Eds.), *Nelson textbook of pediatrics* (20th ed., pp. 2539–2547). Philadelphia, PA: Elsevier; Verive, M. J. (2013). *Pediatric hyperkalemia*. Retrieved from http://emedicine.medscape.com/article/907543-overview.

Some children whose ARF is unresponsive to management require dialysis to correct severe electrolyte imbalances, manage fluid overload, and cleanse the blood of waste products. The clinical situation and age of the child determine whether hemodialysis or peritoneal dialysis is used. Refer to the *Renal Replacement Therapy* section later in this chapter.

Prognosis depends on the cause of ARF. When renal failure results from drug toxicity or dehydration, the prognosis is generally good. However, ARF that results from diseases such as hemolytic-uremic syndrome or acute glomerulonephritis may be associated with residual kidney damage.

TABLE 52–8 Diagnostic Tests for Renal Failure

DIAGNOSTIC TESTS	FINDINGS IN RENAL FAILURE
URINALYSIS	
pH	Acidic urine
Osmolarity	Greater than 500: prerenal ARF
	Less than 350: intrinsic ARF
Specific gravity	Greater than 1.020: prerenal ARF
	Less than 1.010: intrinsic ARF
Protein	Positive
Blood	Positive
SERUM CHEMISTRY*	
Potassium	Elevated
Sodium	Normal, low, or high; depends solely on the amount of water in the body
Calcium	Low
Phosphorus	High
Urea nitrogen	Increased
Creatinine	Increased
pH	Low acidic

Note: *Please refer to Appendix B for normal values for various ages.
ARF = acute renal failure.

Source: Data from Sreedharan, R., & Avner, E. D. (2016). Renal failure. In R. M. Kliegman, B. F. Stanton, J. W. St. Geme, & N. F. Schor (Eds.), *Nelson textbook of pediatrics* (20th ed., pp. 2539–2547). Philadelphia, PA: Elsevier; Workeneh, B.T., Agraharkar, M., & Gupta, R. (2014). *Acute kidney injury*. Retrieved from http://emedicine.medscape.com/article/243492-overview

---

SAFETY ALERT!

Nephrotoxic drugs include the following:

• Antimicrobials: aminoglycosides, cephalosporins, tetracycline, sulfonamides
• Radiographic contrast media with iodine (typically used for CT scans)
• Heavy metals: lead, barium, iron
• Nonsteroidal anti-inflammatory drugs: indomethacin, aspirin, ibuprofen

---

Nursing Management

For the Child With Acute Renal Failure

Nursing Assessment and Diagnosis

A complete history and physical examination are necessary to identify progression of symptoms and possible causes of renal failure.

PHYSIOLOGIC ASSESSMENT

Assess vital signs, level of consciousness, and other neurologic indicators to help identify clinical signs of electrolyte imbalance (see Table 52–7). Measure the child's weight on admission

Pathophysiology Illustrated: Acute Renal Failure

The initial kidney injury is usually associated with an acute condition such as sepsis, trauma, or hypotension or is the result of treatment for an acute condition with a nephrotoxic medication. Injury to the kidney can occur because of glomerular injury, vasoconstriction of capillaries, or tubular injury. All consequences of injury lead to decreased glomerular filtration and oliguria.

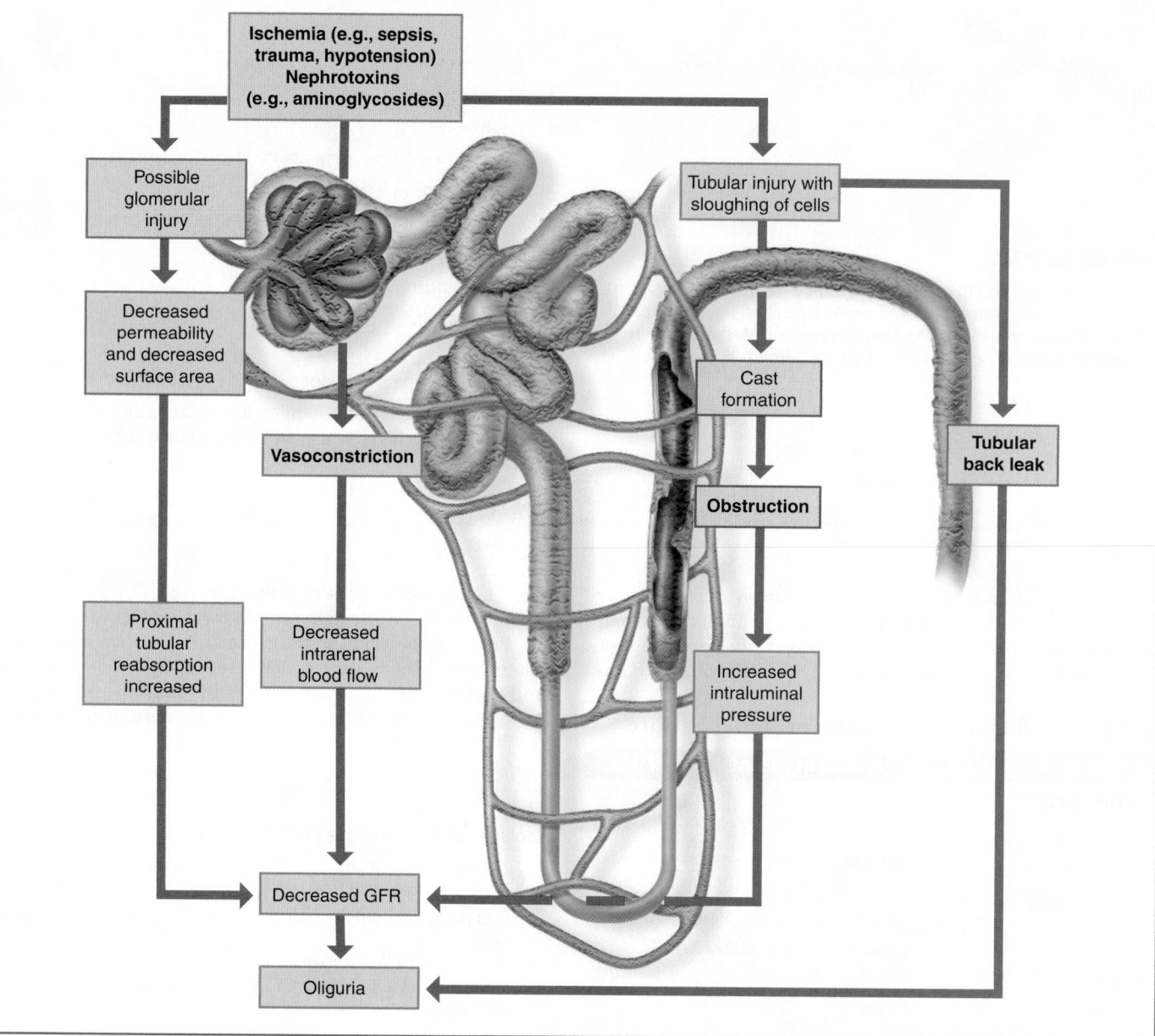

to provide a baseline for evaluating changes in fluid status. Monitor urinalysis, urine culture, and blood chemistry studies. Inspect urine for color, specific gravity, amount, and odor. Cloudy urine may indicate infection; tea-colored urine suggests hematuria. Assess urine specific gravity and intake and output.

PSYCHOSOCIAL ASSESSMENT

The unexpected and acute nature of the child's hospitalization creates anxiety for both parents and child. Assess for feelings of anger, guilt, or fear associated with the hospitalization. Such feelings are likely if ARF developed as a result of dehydration,

a preventable injury, or poisoning. Assess coping mechanisms, family support systems, and level of stress.

Several nursing diagnoses may apply to the child with ARF, including the following (NANDA-I © 2014):

- *Perfusion: Renal, Risk for Ineffective,* related to hypovolemia, sepsis, or drug
- *Fluid Volume: Excess,* related to renal dysfunction and sodium retention
- *Nutrition, Imbalanced: Less than Body Requirements,* related to anorexia, nausea, vomiting, and catabolic state

- *Infection, Risk for,* related to invasive procedures and monitoring equipment, and diminished immune functioning
- *Coping: Family, Compromised,* related to sudden hospitalization and uncertain prognosis of child

Planning and Implementation

Nursing care focuses on preventing complications, maintaining fluid balance, administering medications, meeting nutritional needs, preventing infection, and providing emotional support to the child and parents.

PREVENT COMPLICATIONS

Complications are best prevented by ensuring compliance with the treatment plan. Careful monitoring of vital signs, intake and output, serum electrolytes, and level of consciousness can alert the nurse to changes that indicate potential complications.

MAINTAIN FLUID BALANCE

Estimate the child's fluid status by monitoring of intake and output and blood pressure 2 or 3 times daily. Also obtain a weight at least daily on the same scale at the same time of day. Monitor serum chemistry values, especially for sodium and potassium.

If the child has oliguria, limit fluid intake (including parenteral nutrition) to replacement of insensible fluid loss (what is excreted by the lungs, skin, and gastrointestinal tract), which is about one third the daily maintenance requirements in afebrile children. If the child is febrile, fluid requirements are increased. See Chapter 44.

Clinical Tip

The child with **renal insufficiency** is at greater risk for fluid loss with illness. In cases of acute gastrointestinal illness, children are at greater risk for dehydration.

ADMINISTER MEDICATIONS

Because the kidney's ability to excrete drugs is impaired in ARF, dosages of all medications should be adjusted. The actual dosage of the drug can be reduced or the time interval between doses may be increased. Check drug levels to monitor for drug toxicity and know the signs of drug toxicity for each medication the child is receiving.

MEET NUTRITIONAL NEEDS

Children are at risk for malnutrition because of their high metabolic rate during ARF. Parenteral or enteral feeding may be used initially to minimize protein catabolism. The diet is tailored to the individual child's need for calories, carbohydrates, fats, and amino acids or protein hydrolysates. Depending on the degree of renal failure, sodium, potassium, and phosphorus may be restricted. Initiate oral feeding as soon as tolerated.

PREVENT INFECTION

The child with ARF is extremely susceptible to hospital-acquired infections because of altered nutritional status, compromised immunity, and numerous invasive procedures. Thorough hand hygiene and standard precautions are imperative to decrease the risk of infection. Use sterile technique for all invasive procedures and when caring for lines. Drainage from catheter sites should be cultured to check for the presence of infectious organisms. Assess vital signs and lung sounds frequently.

PROVIDE EMOTIONAL SUPPORT

The sudden onset of ARF presents parents with an unexpected threat to their child's life. Both the child and the parents experience anxiety because of the unexpected hospitalization and the uncertainty of the prognosis. Parents often feel guilty, regardless of the cause of renal failure. Guilt is intensified if the parents feel there is something they could have done to prevent the condition. Encourage parents to verbalize their fears and help them work through feelings of guilt. Explain procedures and treatment measures to decrease anxiety. Encouraging parents and older siblings to participate in the child's care can increase their sense of control.

Developing Cultural Competence Reducing Sodium in the Child's Diet

Special effort is often needed to reduce the sodium in the diet of an Asian child. Sauces and seasonings for foods (soy sauce, mustards, monosodium glutamate, and garlic salt) are sodium rich even though the foods seasoned (rice, vegetables, shrimp, and chicken) are low in sodium. A child eating a diet of predominantly Mexican cuisine may also require significant modification because many of the foods are high in sodium and potassium. Individualized counseling and motivation are needed to encourage families to reduce the child's sodium intake and to use spices low in sodium when preparing meals.

DISCHARGE PLANNING AND HOME CARE TEACHING

Encourage parental involvement early in the child's hospitalization. Be sure parents understand the importance of administering medications correctly. Teach family members proper technique for measuring blood pressure so they can monitor the child's hypertension, if ordered. Make sure the parents can identify signs of progressive renal failure (see the following chronic renal failure discussion).

Diet counseling is a key component of discharge planning and is usually performed by a renal nutritionist. Depending on the degree of renal failure, the child's diet may include restrictions on protein, water, sodium, potassium, and phosphorus.

The parents should be given written guidelines listing appropriate food choices to assist in menu planning. Ethnic and cultural preferences should be considered when listing menu options.

Continued monitoring of renal function during follow-up examinations is critical as deterioration may occur over time. Referral to support groups can be helpful for both parents and children. The National Kidney Foundation is a source of numerous publications that are helpful to the child and family.

Evaluation

Expected outcomes of nursing care include:

- Kidney function is restored.
- Fluid, electrolyte, and acid–base balance is restored and maintained.
- Nutritional needs are met.
- The child does not acquire a secondary infection.

Chronic Renal Failure

Chronic renal failure (CRF) (also called chronic kidney disease) is a progressive, irreversible reduction in kidney function. The prevalence of CRF in children is approximately 18 per 1 million (Sreedharan & Avner, 2016).

ETIOLOGY AND PATHOPHYSIOLOGY

In children, CRF usually results from developmental abnormalities of the kidney or urinary tract, obstructed urine flow and reflux, hereditary diseases such as polycystic kidney disease, infections such as hemolytic-uremic syndrome, and glomerulonephritis (Lum, 2014).

The gradual, progressive loss of functioning nephrons ultimately results in **end-stage renal disease (ESRD)**. In ESRD, the kidneys can no longer maintain homeostasis and the child requires dialysis (Sreedharan & Avner, 2016).

The kidneys excrete excess acid in the body and regulate the body's fluid and electrolyte balance. Renal failure disrupts this fluid and electrolyte balance. As renal failure progresses, metabolic acidosis occurs because the kidneys cannot excrete the acids that build up in the body. Renal osteodystrophy occurs because the kidneys are unable to produce activated vitamin D or to excrete phosphorus, causing phosphorus levels to rise and serum calcium levels to fall. The parathyroid gland responds by drawing calcium and phosphorus from the bones to maintain the adequate serum calcium and phosphorus levels. Hypocalcemia may occur as the parathyroid glands become less responsive to vitamin D and lower serum calcium levels. Osteodystrophy increases the child's risk for spontaneous fractures (Sreedharan & Avner, 2016).

Growth retardation is caused by disturbances in the metabolism of calcium, phosphorus, and vitamin D; decreased caloric intake; and metabolic acidosis. Healthy kidneys also produce erythropoietin (the growth factor responsible for the production and maturation of red cells); lack of erythropoietin and progressive renal disease are the underlying causes of the anemia of CRF.

CLINICAL MANIFESTATIONS

Children with CRF frequently have no symptoms initially. As progression continues, renal insufficiency occurs with polyuria as the kidneys become unable to concentrate the urine. Symptoms such as pallor, headache, nausea, and fatigue become more common. Decreased mental alertness and ability to concentrate may be seen. The child may have anemia leading to tachycardia, tachypnea, and dyspnea on exertion. As the disease progresses, the child experiences a loss of appetite and has complications of renal impairment, including hypertension, pulmonary edema, growth retardation, osteodystrophy, delayed fine and gross motor development, and delayed sexual maturation. Refer to Table 52–6 to see how these signs contrast with signs of acute renal failure.

In ESRD, renal failure adversely affects all body systems. As the severity of the clinical and biochemical disturbances resulting from progressive renal deterioration increases, uremic symptoms develop. Signs and symptoms of uremic syndrome include nausea and vomiting, progressive anemia, anorexia, dyspnea, malaise, *uremic frost* (urea crystals deposited on the skin), unpleasant (uremic) breath odor, headache, progressive confusion, tremors, pulmonary edema, and congestive heart failure.

CLINICAL THERAPY

Laboratory evaluation, including serum electrolytes, phosphate, BUN, creatinine levels, and pH, is used to confirm the diagnosis of CRF. An early morning urine sample is collected for culture and to calculate the protein-to-creatinine ratio. The child's glomerular filtration rate is calculated from prediction equations using the serum creatinine level and the patient's height and gender. Imaging studies are performed to identify renal diseases that could be causing the renal failure. A renal biopsy may sometimes be performed.

CRF is irreversible; however, the course of the disease is variable. Some children progress quickly to renal failure, necessitating dialysis. Other children are managed with a combination of medication and diet therapy for some time before significant renal impairment occurs. Frequent modifications in the treatment plan are often necessary to address the child's changing status.

Dietary management focuses on maximizing caloric intake for growth while limiting phosphorus, potassium, and sodium intake as needed to maintain electrolytes in balance (Sreedharan & Avner, 2016). Adequate calcium needs to be part of the meal plan. Enteral or parenteral feedings may be required to achieve optimal protein intake, especially in children under 1 year of age. Complex carbohydrates should be chosen along with vegetables and fruits that are lower in potassium. Vegetable oils, hard candy, sugar, honey, and jelly may be recommended to add calories to the child's diet. Medications used to treat children with CRF are discussed in the table on the top of the next page.

Children who progress to ESRD require renal replacement therapy. The timetable for dialysis or renal transplantation is different from that of adults; transplantation is the goal so the child has an optimal chance for a more normal childhood. Earlier initiation can prevent some complications of ESRD. In addition to the GFR, nonspecific signs such as uremic syndrome, poorly controlled hypertension, renal osteodystrophy, failure of head circumference measurement to increase normally, developmental delay, and poor growth are used in determining when to initiate renal replacement therapy. (Refer to the *Renal Replacement Therapy* section later in this chapter.)

Nursing Management

For the Child With Chronic Renal Failure

Nursing Assessment and Diagnosis

Nursing assessment focuses on identifying signs and symptoms of renal failure and associated complications as well as assessing the psychosocial effects of renal failure on the child and family.

PHYSIOLOGIC ASSESSMENT

The initial and ongoing assessment of the child focuses on identifying complications of renal failure. Observe for signs of hypertension, edema, poor growth and development, osteodystrophy, and anemia. Assess vital signs, particularly the blood pressure. Observe for signs of alterations in electrolyte balance.

PSYCHOSOCIAL ASSESSMENT

As renal disease progresses, the number of stressors on the child and family increases. Denial and disbelief are commonly the first reactions. A thorough family assessment can help to identify particular needs of the child and family. The development of ESRD is particularly challenging during childhood and adolescence because of differences in appearance and social, psychologic, and physical issues. Nonadherence to treatments can endanger the adolescent's life.

Nursing diagnoses for the child with CRF are similar to those previously listed for ARF. Additional diagnoses might include the following (NANDA-I © 2014):

- *Social Interaction, Impaired,* related to impaired immunity and hemodialysis schedule during school hours
- *Activity Intolerance* related to anemia and fatigue

Medications Used to Treat: Chronic Renal Failure

MEDICATION AND ACTION/INDICATION	NURSING IMPLICATIONS
Vitamin and mineral supplement (Nephrocaps) Adds vitamins and minerals missing from heavily restricted diet.	Only prescribed vitamins should be used; over-the-counter brands may contain elements that are harmful.
Phosphate binding agents: calcium carbonate (Tums), calcium acetate (PhosLo), or sevelamer hydrochloride (Renagel) Reduces absorption of phosphorus from the intestines.	Ensure that phosphate binding agent is aluminum-free.
Calcitriol (Rocaltrol) Replaces the calcitriol that kidneys are no longer producing to keep calcium balance normal.	Monitor serum calcium level. Ensure that calcium supplement is provided.
Epoetin alfa (Epogen, Procrit) Stimulates bone marrow to produce red blood cells, treats anemia due to CRF.	Given by IV or subcutaneous injection. Monitor blood pressure because hypertension is an adverse effect. Monitor hematocrit and serum ferritin levels according to facility guidelines.
Iron supplementation Treats iron deficiency when epoetin alfa is prescribed.	Give without food or other medications to maximize absorption.
Growth hormone (rhGH) Used to stimulate growth in children with CRF.	Record accurate height measurements at regular intervals.
Antihypertensive agents: angiotensin-converting enzyme (ACE) inhibitor (Enalapril, Lisinopril) Used with proteinuric kidney disease because it slows the progression to ESRD.	Monitor blood pressure.
Loop diuretics (Furosemide) Used when volume overload is present.	Monitor urine output and electrolyte balance.

Source: Data from Gulati, S. (2012). *Chronic kidney disease in children.* Retrieved from http://emedicine.medscape.com/article/984358-overview; Lum, G. M. (2014). Kidney & urinary tract. In W. W. Hay, M. J. Levin, R. R. Deterding, & M. J. Abzug, *CURRENT diagnosis and treatment: Pediatrics* (22nd ed.). New York, NY: McGraw-Hill. Retrieved from http://accessmedicine.com; Sreedharan, R., & Avner, E. D. (2016). Renal failure. In R. M. Kliegman, B. F. Stanton, J. W. St. Geme, & N. F. Schor (Eds.), *Nelson textbook of pediatrics* (20th ed., pp. 2539–2547). Philadelphia, PA: Elsevier; Wilson, B. A., Shannon, M. T., & Shields, K. M. (2015). *Pearson nurse's drug guide 2015*. Hoboken, NJ: Pearson Education.

- *Health Management, Family, Ineffective,* related to complexity of care plan and economic difficulties
- *Body Image, Disturbed,* related to short stature and visible external catheter for dialysis

Planning and Implementation

Children with CRF are usually hospitalized for one or more of the following reasons: initial diagnostic evaluation, dialysis treatment initiation, problems with the treatment plan or infection. Nursing care for the hospitalized child with CRF focuses on monitoring for side effects of medications, preventing infection, meeting nutritional needs, and providing emotional support and anticipatory teaching.

MONITOR FOR SIDE EFFECTS OF MEDICATIONS

Assess for signs of electrolyte imbalance such as weakness, muscle cramps, dizziness, headache, and nausea and vomiting in children who are taking diuretics. Supervise the child's activities closely to prevent falls resulting from dizziness, especially at the beginning of diuretic therapy. If antihypertensive medications such as hydralazine are being administered, monitor the child's weight to detect excessive gain resulting from water and sodium retention.

PREVENT INFECTION

The child with CRF is susceptible to infections. Be alert for signs of infection, such as elevated temperature; cloudy, strong-smelling urine; dysuria; changes in respiratory pattern; or productive cough. Emphasize to the child and family the importance of good hand hygiene practices. Make sure the child receives the 23-valent pneumococcal vaccine and meningococcal vaccines in addition to usual childhood immunizations.

TABLE 52–9 Nutritional Information for the Child With Kidney Disease

Children with kidney disease have restricted diets, generally low in sodium, potassium, and phosphorus. A renal dietitian works with families of children with chronic renal failure to develop meal plans that fit a restricted diet. The nurse can help families remember that certain foods must be avoided or eaten in very small quantities by reviewing this table.

HIGH-SODIUM CONTENT FOODS	HIGH-POTASSIUM CONTENT FOODS	HIGH-PHOSPHORUS CONTENT FOODS
Soups and sauces: e.g., gravy, spaghetti and tomato sauce, barbeque sauce, steak sauce	*Fruit:* apricots, avocados, bananas, citrus fruits, fresh pears, nectarines, dates, figs, cantaloupe and other melons, prunes, and raisins	*Dairy products:* milk, cheese, yogurt, custard, pudding, ice cream
Processed lunch meats: e.g., bologna, ham, salami, hot dogs	*Vegetables:* celery, dried beans, lima beans, potatoes, leafy greens, spinach, tomatoes, winter squash	Dried beans, peas
Smoked meat and fish: bacon, chipped beef, corned beef, ham, lox	*Whole grains:* especially those containing bran	Nuts, peanut butter
Sauerkraut, pickles, and other pickled foods	Sardines, clams	Chocolate
Seasonings: horseradish, soy sauce, Worcestershire sauce, meat tenderizer, and monosodium glutamate (MSG)	Peanuts	Dark cola
	Dairy products: milk, ice cream, pudding, yogurt	Sausage, hot dogs
	Potassium-containing salt substitutes	

MEET NUTRITIONAL NEEDS

Maintaining adequate nutritional intake in a child with CRF who has dietary restrictions is challenging. Provide small, frequent feedings and present meals attractively to encourage the child to eat. A nutritionist works with the child and family to develop meal plans that meet the nutritional requirements and acknowledge the child's preferences. See Table 52–9 for foods that children with CRF should avoid.

MAINTAIN FLUID RESTRICTIONS

Plan the child's oral intake through the entire 24 hours to ensure that the child has some fluids with meals, when taking medications, and when thirsty. Keep in mind that many foods have a high fluid content (gelatin, fruit-flavored ice pops) and must be counted toward the daily fluid allowance. Use medicine cups or small cups for fluids given. Encourage parents and visitors to avoid drinking in the child's presence. Ensure that all visitors know and understand the importance of maintaining the child's fluid restriction.

PROVIDE EMOTIONAL SUPPORT

Progressive CRF requires a total lifestyle change for the child and family. The parents and child need opportunities to express and work through their feelings related to the disease, prognosis, and treatment restrictions. Help children express their feelings through drawings or therapeutic play.

The need for ongoing dialysis treatments and the wait for a suitable donor kidney are stressful for both parents and children. Identify effective coping methods and family support systems to promote treatment compliance. The National Kidney Foundation and local support groups for kidney disease can give the family information or additional support.

DISCHARGE PLANNING AND HOME CARE TEACHING

Parents need to understand the necessity of long-term treatments and follow-up care. Help the family develop a schedule for medication administration that fits with their routine. Emphasize the importance of consistency in administration times. Teach parents how to recognize medication side effects and complications.

Appropriate referrals are made to home care nursing agencies as indicated. Parents of children receiving peritoneal dialysis at home are taught how to perform the treatment and how to identify complications. Strict aseptic technique is necessary to prevent infection at the catheter site and peritonitis.

COMMUNITY-BASED NURSING CARE

Children with CRF require frequent outpatient visits to monitor the progression of signs and symptoms, and to evaluate the effectiveness of current treatments. The blood pressure is monitored. Blood and urine tests are performed to monitor renal function. Radiographs of the bones are often taken at 6-month intervals to assess changes caused by osteodystrophy. See *Health Promotion: The Child With Chronic Renal Failure*.

Encourage parents to register the young child for an early intervention program to promote development and interaction with other children. The dialysis schedule for school-age children should enable the child to participate in school, or home tutoring should be provided.

School-age children and adolescents are often embarrassed about being seen as different from peers. Ask them how they feel about the need to follow a special diet, take medications, and undergo dialysis treatments. To minimize the psychologic consequences of coping with a chronic disease, encourage parents to promote the child's participation in age-appropriate activities. Attendance at school and contacts with peers promote normal growth and development. Work to promote the child's self-worth and a healthy self-esteem. Encourage adolescents to participate in a program that helps them transition to adult health services and job skill training. Begin teaching the child during early adolescence about the health condition, medications taken and their actions, how to access emergency help, and problems caused by nonadherence to treatment. As the adolescent ages, have the family begin giving more responsibility for self-care, such as making appointments for health care, obtaining prescription refills, and seeking out healthcare providers for adult patients and a dialysis program. (See *Evidence-Based Practice: Living With Chronic Kidney Disease*.) As the child's renal impairment progresses, give the parents timely information about the disease process, dialysis treatments, and issues related to renal transplantation.

Health Promotion The Child With Chronic Renal Failure

Growth and Development Surveillance

- Compare the child's height, weight, and head circumference to age-specific norms to identify growth retardation and to plot progress.
- Assess developmental progress using the Denver II or another screening tool (refer to Chapter 34).
- Educate parents on normal developmental milestones and measures to promote achieving those milestones.
- Assess the adolescent for signs of delayed sexual maturation and, in girls, amenorrhea.

Nutrition

- Review the dietary restrictions with the child and parents.
- Partner with the family to assist the child to make good food selections and to restrict fluids and sodium as necessary, taking into account the child's likes and dislikes and cultural background. Encourage the child and family to take a list of a few favorite foods to the dietitian to see if they can be integrated into the child's meal plan.
- Make mealtime pleasant and make foods taste more appealing with permitted spices.
- Discuss possible behavioral responses by older children and adolescents to dietary restrictions and limitations imposed by the treatment plan. Involve the child and adolescent in discussions about dietary restrictions, and when possible integrate their recommendations for dietary restrictions and fluid management throughout the day.
- Emphasize to the school-age child that dietary and other restrictions are not punishment.
- Use enteral feeding at night to provide the needed calories for growth.

Physical Activity

- Encourage child to participate in developmentally appropriate activities as tolerated.
- Partner with the child to establish a routine plan for physical activity as tolerated that will help promote strong bones.

Oral Health

- Promote good dentition and oral hygiene.
- Schedule regular dental visits for examination and cleaning to reduce infections.
- Partner with the family to ensure they understand the need for antibiotic prophylaxis before certain invasive procedures, including dental care.

Mental and Spiritual Health

- Ask children how they feel about the need to follow a special diet, take medications, and undergo dialysis treatments. Ask what might make it easier for them to cope with the treatments, and integrate at least one idea into the care plan.

- Encourage parents to promote their child's participation in age-appropriate activities to minimize the psychologic consequences of coping with a chronic disease.
- Adolescents often resent the dietary restrictions and ongoing dialysis treatments, which pose a threat to their independence, evolving sense of self, and their need for independence. Noncooperation, depression, and hostility are common responses.
- Assist adolescents to begin the transition to adult health services.

Relationships

- Attendance at school and contacts with peers promote normal growth and development.
- Work to promote the child's self-worth and a healthy self-esteem.
- Prepare the child for peer conflict.
- Ensure that parents understand the importance of encouraging normal socialization of their child.

Disease Prevention Strategies

- Partner with the child and family to establish plans to avoid large crowds, people with infections, or other risks that expose the child to infection.
- If possible, all immunizations should be provided before renal transplantation, as long-term immunosuppressive therapy will then be prescribed.
- Live vaccines should not be given to the child taking immunosuppressive agents.
- Encourage the family to maintain scheduled appointments for routine serum and urine diagnostic tests performed to monitor renal function.

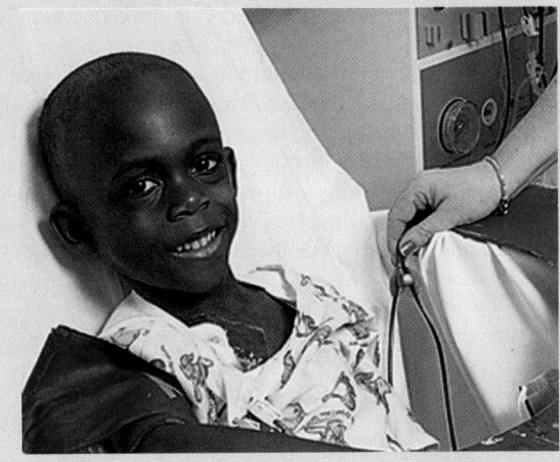

Evaluation

Expected outcomes of nursing care include:

- The child's fluid status is maintained.
- The child eats foods that meet nutritional needs while adhering to dietary restrictions.
- Growth and developmental milestones are achieved.

Renal Replacement Therapy

Renal replacement therapy is the treatment for renal failure and includes both dialysis and renal transplantation. The preferred method of dialysis is generally dependent on the age of the child. Currently, 88% of children 5 years of age and younger are treated with peritoneal dialysis, while 54% of children older than 12 years of age are treated with hemodialysis (Sreedharan & Avner, 2016).

EVIDENCE-BASED PRACTICE | Living With Chronic Kidney Disease

Clinical Question

Chronic kidney disease is a serious chronic condition that requires significant adaptations in lifestyle and complex medical treatments that take a toll on the child and family. What is the impact of this condition on children?

The Evidence

Heath et al. (2011) used the Generic Children's Quality of Life Measure to explore the impact of chronic kidney disease (CKD) on 225 pediatric patients ranging in age from 6 to 18 years. Of these patients, 49 had advanced CKD, 128 were posttransplant, and 47 were on dialysis. Results of the study showed that there was no difference between the mean quality-of-life scores in children who were in different treatment modalities. Age and gender did not affect the mean score. The study also showed that children ages 6 to 14 with CKD had significantly higher quality-of-life scores than children of the same age in the general population. While this was a surprising finding, it emphasized the fact that children with chronic conditions can perceive their quality of life as good despite having challenges with their health. These results could also be related to the psychosocial care provided by the renal team.

Al-Uzri et al. (2013) evaluated the effect of short stature on the health-related quality of life (HRQoL) in children with CKD. Short stature is common in children with CKD. Data collected as part of a larger multicenter Chronic Kidney Disease in Children study was used for the focus of this study. The participants were 483 children and/or parents who were enrolled in the larger study and had completed at least 2 evaluations of their HRQoL. The Pediatric Qualilty of Life Inventory (pedsQL) was used to assess physical, emotional, social, and school functioning. Parents completed the parent proxy version of the form. Results of the study demonstrated that parent-reported physical HRQoL was lower in the short stature group than the normal height group, although this was not statistically significant. Assessment of catch-up growth and its impact on HRQoL revealed that an increase in the height z score was related to a 7-point increase in the parents' perception of the child's physical and social functioning; however, there was no association between catch-up growth and the child's pedsQL score. Analysis of pedsQL scores in the 58 children who were taking growth hormone versus those who were not did not reveal a relationship; however, there was a significant impact of improved height z scores with growth hormone use on parents' perceptions of physical and social functioning. Additionally, children ages 15 to 17 with CKD had significantly higher rates

on the pedsQL inventory than their parents in all areas except for school functioning. There was a high level of agreement between children ages 8 to 14 and their parents on all aspects of the inventory except emotional functioning, with the child having lower scores than their parents' perception. The results of this study support the need for interventions that improve height in children with CKD. It also demonstrates the importance of evaluating both the perception of the child and the parents.

Research by Kilis-Pstrunsinska et al. (2013) evaluated the HRQoL in Polish children with CKD using the Pediatric Quality of Life Inventory. Participants in the study were 203 children with CKD and 388 parent/proxies. This study found that children with CKD had significantly lower HRQoL scores compared to international population norms for healthy children. Results also showed that children on dialysis had lower scores in physical and social functioning than those treated conservatively. Additionally, patients on hemodialysis had significantly lower overall scores than children treated conservatively or with peritoneal dialysis. In children who were treated conservatively, stage of disease did not affect scores. Differences were also noted between parent/proxy scores and the child. The differences varied depending on the severity of the disease and the intensity of the treatment plan.

Best Practice

Effects of chronic illness in children and adolescents can be both physically and psychosocially overwhelming. It is important to evaluate quality of life in children with chronic illness in order to better understand their responses to the illness and treatment (Heath et al., 2011). Children of different ages may view their quality of life differently. Their view may also be different depending on the severity of their disease, their current treatment plan, and the amount of support they have received. Parents' views of their child's quality of life may vary from that of the child. It is essential that nurses assess each child and family member individually to determine their view of the illness and its impact on their life. This will assist the nurse to develop an effective care plan for the child and family and coordinate additional support for them as needed.

Clinical Reasoning

Initiate a discussion with an older school-age child or adolescent with CKD. Listen to their description of living with the condition. Develop a nursing care plan to help the child take the next steps in self-management.

PERITONEAL DIALYSIS

In peritoneal dialysis, the peritoneum of the abdomen is the membrane through which the body's waste products pass from the blood to the abdominal cavity. A catheter is inserted through the abdominal wall into the peritoneal cavity. In children receiving peritoneal dialysis for ARF, a percutaneously placed catheter can be used for a few weeks. In children with CRF, a catheter is placed surgically for long-term use. The dialysis solution (**dialysate**) that enters the abdomen typically contains dextrose that pulls body wastes and extra fluid into

the abdominal cavity. These wastes and extra fluid leave the body with the drained dialysate. This method of dialysis is beneficial to small children since it allows continuous removal of fluids and waste products, decreasing the toxic effects of waste products on the child's developing body. The child can ambulate and interact with the environment. The timing of the treatment can be set to minimize the interruption of school, play, or other social events.

Two types of peritoneal dialysis are commonly used: continuous ambulatory peritoneal dialysis (CAPD) and automated

TABLE 52–10 Complications of Peritoneal Dialysis

COMPLICATIONS AND MANIFESTATIONS	CAUSE
PERITONITIS	
Cloudy dialysate, abdominal pain, tenderness, leukocytosis, fever (neonatal hypothermia), constipation	*Staphylococcus aureus, S. epidermidis*, fungal infections, gram-negative rods (risk is proportional to duration of dialysis and inversely proportional to age)
PAIN	
During inflow	Too rapid a rate of infusion, too large a volume of dialysate, encasement of catheter in a false passage, extremes in temperature of dialysate
During outflow at end of emptying	Omentum entering catheter at end of outflow
LEAKAGE	
Fluid around catheter, edema of penis or scrotum secondary to leakage into abdominal subcutaneous tissue, fluid leakage to pleural spaces through diaphragm	Overfilling of abdomen, catheter that has migrated from peritoneal cavity
RESPIRATORY SYMPTOMS	
Shortness of breath, decreased breath sounds in lower lobes, inadequate chest expansion	Abdominal fullness that compromises diaphragm movement, hole in diaphragm allowing dialysate into chest cavity

peritoneal dialysis (APD). Graduated cylinders are used to monitor the volume of fluid exchanged.

- CAPD uses gravity to instill prefilled bags of dialysate into the peritoneal cavity 4 or 5 times a day. The fluid remains in the cavity for 4 to 8 hours. The attached bag is folded under the child's clothes, permitting normal activity. After the allotted time, the dialysate is drained by hanging the bag lower than the pelvis. The repeated connections and disconnections with this method are time consuming for the child and family and increase the risk of infection.

- APD uses an automatic cycler to instill and drain the dialysate about 5 times over a 10-hour period, usually overnight. One additional exchange may be needed during the day. With this method, the number of connections and disconnections is minimized, which reduces demands on the family as well as the risk of infection. Infants and young children on peritoneal dialysis generally receive APD while they sleep (Zaritsky & Warady, 2011).

Peritonitis is a common complication of peritoneal dialysis. See Table 52–10. Peritonitis is treated with antibiotics infused in the dialysate (Mehrazma, Amini-Alavijeh, & Hooman, 2012).

Teach the family to perform peritoneal dialysis and to use sterile technique when performing dialysis and when doing catheter care. Peritoneal dialysis is time consuming, and family members must be committed to managing this procedure daily. Help the family develop home routines that minimize disruptions to daily family life. For additional information, refer to *Nursing Care Plan: The Child Receiving Home Peritoneal Dialysis.*

HEMODIALYSIS

Hemodialysis is a process in which the blood flows from the patient through a machine with a special filter that removes body wastes and extra fluids. Blood is pumped out of the body and through a dialyzer, where waste products and extra fluids diffuse out across a semipermeable membrane, before the blood is returned to the body. Dialysate is pumped in the direction opposite blood flow to promote waste extraction. Differences in osmolarity and concentration between the child's blood and the dialysate alter the intravascular electrolyte concentration and reduce the intravascular volume.

Clinical Tip

The dominant sign of peritonitis associated with peritoneal dialysis is cloudy dialysate. Other signs and symptoms may include fever, vomiting, diarrhea, abdominal pain, and tenderness. The nurse monitors for these symptoms and ensures that the child and family can recognize the symptoms and report them immediately.

Hemodialysis is used in the critical care setting and for those children with CRF when peritoneal dialysis is not possible for technical reasons, after repeated peritonitis, or when the family is unable to provide peritoneal dialysis safely. Hemodialysis for children is offered in a special dialysis center on an outpatient basis, or it can be performed at bedside during hospitalization. Treatment is usually performed 3 times a week, with each session lasting approximately 3 to 4 hours.

Children over 20 kg (44 lb) often have an arteriovenous (AV) fistula (connection between an artery and a vein) created for long-term vascular access. Alternatively, a synthetic tube can be implanted under the skin, creating a graft between the arterial and venous circulation to provide vascular access. Two needles are inserted into the arteriovenous fistula or the graft: one to carry blood to the dialyzer and one to return cleaned blood to the body. In emergencies and for infants, a double-lumen cannula is inserted into a large vein (e.g., the femoral, jugular, or subclavian vein) for hemodialysis.

Hemodialysis is more efficient than peritoneal dialysis but requires close monitoring for symptoms related to hypotension or rapid changes in fluid and electrolyte balance. Uncommonly, a **disequilibrium syndrome** (rapid changes in the body's water and electrolyte balance during treatment) may occur during or soon after the dialysis procedure is first initiated. Other complications include access thrombosis and infection. Heparin is used to reduce the risk of thrombosis.

Nursing management focuses on care of the child during dialysis and teaching the child and family about the administration of heparin and the control of bleeding from minor trauma. Carefully monitor fluid balance in the child undergoing hemodialysis. Check vital signs and blood pressure every half hour. Monitor oral intake and urinary output every half hour when the child is on the dialysis equipment. Weigh the child before

Nursing Care Plan: The Child Receiving Home Peritoneal Dialysis

1. Nursing Diagnosis: *Nutrition, Imbalanced: Less than Body Requirements*, **related to poor appetite, feeling of fullness after a small amount, and loss of protein in dialysate (NANDA-I © 2014)**

GOAL: The child will obtain adequate nutrients each day.

INTERVENTION	RATIONALE
• Develop a meal plan in collaboration with a nutritionist to identify the amounts of essential nutrients needed.	• Parents need concrete guidelines for food preparation.
• Provide small, frequent meals of needed nutrients.	• The child will feel full with smaller amounts of food because of the dialysate.
• Make mealtimes pleasant and avoid battles over the child's intake.	• The child will be more inclined to eat if there is less stress.
• Provide supplements by tube feeding if adequate oral intake is not possible.	• Adequate nutrition is important for growth and development, and must be supported if oral intake is inadequate.

EXPECTED OUTCOME: Child's intake will be adequate to maintain an expected growth pattern.

2. Nursing Diagnosis: *Infection, Risk for*, **related to daily invasive procedure (NANDA-I © 2014)**

GOAL: The child will not develop peritonitis.

INTERVENTION	RATIONALE
• Wash hands, use sterile gloves and aseptic technique for connection and disconnection of catheters.	• Aseptic technique reduces chance of introducing bacteria into the abdomen.
• Perform daily catheter site care.	• Skin around the catheter site will have fewer organisms that could potentially cause infection.

EXPECTED OUTCOME: Child will not develop peritonitis.

GOAL: If peritonitis occurs, it will be treated appropriately.

INTERVENTION	RATIONALE
• Observe for signs of infection (fever, abdominal pain, cloudy dialysate).	• Early identification of infection will reduce complications.
• Report signs of infection to healthcare provider immediately.	• Rapid intervention may reduce need for hospitalization.

EXPECTED OUTCOME: Hospitalization will not be needed for peritonitis because of early identification and prompt treatment.

3. Nursing Diagnosis: *Caregiver Role Strain* **related to daily dialysis treatments (NANDA-I © 2014)**

GOAL: The family will cope with daily demands for the child's dialysis treatments.

INTERVENTION	RATIONALE
• Discuss the importance of daily, consistent dialysis treatments for the child's overall health status.	• If parents understand the need for consistent dialysis treatments, they are more likely to adhere to guidelines.
• Collaborate with the family to identify strategies that could reduce the impact of dialysis on the family's life.	• When the family participates in planning care, adherence is more likely.
• Refer the family to local support groups for emotional support, treatment strategies, and respite care.	• Support groups may help the family develop effective coping strategies.

EXPECTED OUTCOME: Family will adhere to daily dialysis treatment guidelines.

and after the dialysis to determine any fluid imbalances that require adjustment during the next hemodialysis session.

SAFETY ALERT!
Monitor the child receiving hemodialysis for complications such as these that can occur suddenly:

- Hypotension—sudden nausea and vomiting, abdominal cramping, tachycardia, and dizziness
- Rapid fluid and electrolyte exchange—muscle cramping, nausea and vomiting, and dizziness
- Disequilibrium syndrome—restlessness, headache, nausea and vomiting, blurred vision, muscle twitching, and altered level of consciousness

Because fluid and dietary limitations (reduced intake of foods containing potassium, sodium, and phosphorus) are needed more often with hemodialysis than with peritoneal dialysis, make sure the family knows how to plan and provide for the child's daily nutritional needs. Review ways to reduce the risk of infection, including the daily care of the catheter site. Encourage showering rather than tub baths. Activities such as swimming may be discouraged.

KIDNEY TRANSPLANTATION

Kidney transplantation provides the only alternative to long-term dialysis for children with ESRD and generally yields good outcomes. The transplanted kidney can normalize physiology and provide a potential for normal growth. Because of the adverse effects on growth and development resulting from the delay of transplantation, children are given some priority over adults awaiting transplantation. Blood type compatibility between the donor and recipient is essential for a transplant to be successful. A human leukocyte antigen (HLA) system match also improves survival of the graft. A living relative donor kidney has a higher survival rate than a cadaver kidney (Scheinman, 2012). Children and their families are carefully screened prior to transplantation in an effort to identify problems that could lead to rejection of the kidney or infection that could be life threatening if the immune system is suppressed (Figure 52–5).

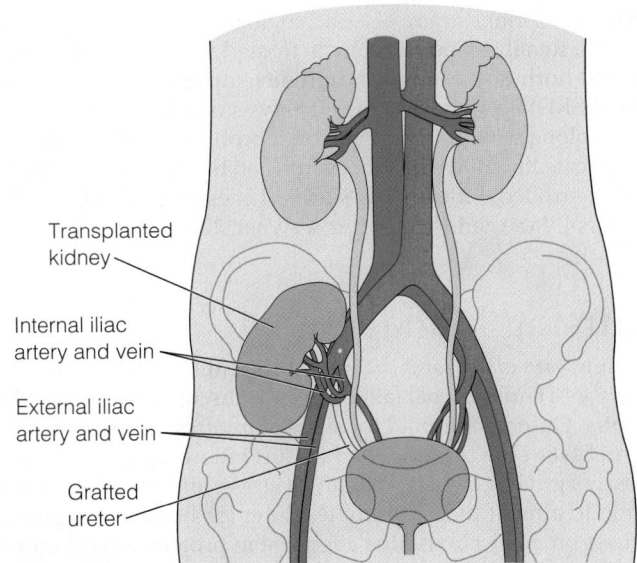

Figure 52–5 **The transplanted kidney is placed in the iliac fossa with anastomosis to the hypogastric artery, iliac vein, and bladder.**

Labels in figure:
- Transplanted kidney
- Internal iliac artery and vein
- External iliac artery and vein
- Grafted ureter

Clinical Reasoning The Child on Hemodialysis

Terrell, who is now 5 years old, was born with posterior urethral valves, which caused damage to his kidneys. Despite undergoing surgery to correct the defect during infancy, his kidney function continued to deteriorate. End-stage renal disease was diagnosed 2 years ago, and dialysis treatment was initiated. Terrell requires a kidney transplant, but in the meantime he is being treated with hemodialysis. He visits the dialysis center 3 afternoons a week for treatments lasting approximately 3 to 4 hours. This schedule permits him to attend kindergarten classes in the morning.

At his scheduled visit to the nephrologist, Terrell has gained weight and is edematous. In talking with him, the nurse discovers that Terrell has been drinking sodas and eating "junk food" at school. Terrell asks the nurse not to tell his mother because she will be mad, but that he just can't help eating and drinking what he isn't supposed to.

How does Terrell's growth and development level affect his adherence to the treatment regimen? What immediate intervention should the nurse take with Terrell? What approach should the nurse take when discussing this nutritional issue with the family?

After transplantation, the child must take immunosuppressive medications such as corticosteroids, azathioprine, cyclosporine, tacrolimus, and monoclonal antibodies to suppress rejection. Immunosuppression regimens use various combinations and sequences of these drugs to reduce the incidence of acute and chronic rejection.

Complications of immunosuppressive therapy include opportunistic infection, lymphomas and skin cancer, and hypertension. Adherence with therapy is essential for survival of the graft and for optimal medical outcomes after transplant. Nonadherence to the medication regimen in pediatric transplant patients ranges; it may be as high as 70% (Guilfoyle, Goebel, & Pai, 2011; Ingerski, Perrazo, Goebel, et al., 2011). Nonadherence is related to several factors, including forgetting to take medication and refusal to take medication because of expected side effects. Family dynamics, functioning, and flexibility also affect adherence (Guilfoyle et al., 2011). Adherence is higher in adolescents when their parents are knowledgeable and supportive, and when they promote the adolescent to become competent in self-care. Some primary kidney diseases, such as glomerulonephritis and hemolytic-uremic syndrome, can also recur in the transplanted kidney.

Nursing management includes teaching parents about the transplantation process before it occurs to help prepare them for the experience. Discuss all aspects of the child's care that will have an impact on the family's life, including follow-up appointments, medications, and general health promotion. Monitor adherence to immunosuppression treatment at each visit in an effort to identify issues early. Teach parents about the signs of acute rejection and infection, including when and how to notify the child's healthcare provider if immediate care is required.

Hemolytic-Uremic Syndrome

Hemolytic-uremic syndrome (HUS) is the most common cause of acute renal failure in young children, occurring primarily in those under 4 years of age (Ring & Huether, 2014). HUS has a classic triad of signs: (1) hemolytic anemia, (2) thrombocytopenia, and (3) acute renal failure (Tan & Silverberg, 2014).

HUS is most often caused by *Escherichia coli* strain O157:H7, which is found in undercooked meat and unpasteurized milk and juices (Tan & Silverberg, 2014). The bacteria has also been linked to petting zoos and other animal exhibits (Anderson & Weese, 2012).

E. coli strain O157:H7 produces a toxin that attaches to the glomeruli, collecting ducts, and distal tubules. The toxin damages the lining of the glomerular arterioles, causing the endothelial cells to swell and become occluded with platelets and fibrin clots. This partial occlusion damages the red blood cells, resulting in hemolytic anemia. Platelets cluster in areas of vascular endothelial damage, causing thrombocytopenia. Glomerular filtration is decreased, resulting in hematuria and proteinuria. Oliguria and ARF develop in nearly 50% of children with HUS (Ring & Huether, 2014).

An episode of severe gastroenteritis with diarrhea precedes the development of typical HUS by 1 to 2 weeks followed by 1 to 5 days without symptoms. Signs and symptoms of the onset of HUS include purpura, pallor, bruising, oliguria, and irritability. The child may have fever, anorexia, abdominal pain, vomiting, watery blood-stained diarrhea, mild jaundice, and circulatory overload. Signs of central nervous involvement include seizures and lethargy (Ring & Huether, 2014).

Treatment focuses on the complications of ARF and includes fluid restrictions and a high-calorie, high-carbohydrate diet that is low in protein, sodium, potassium, and phosphorus. Enteral nutrition is sometimes needed. Medications may include calcium gluconate or calcium chloride, aluminum hydroxide gel to bind to phosphorus, Kayexalate (sodium polystyrene) to remove excess potassium, and antihypertensive agents. Transfusions of fresh-packed red blood cells may be ordered to treat severe anemia. Platelets are given if the child is bleeding or if surgery is needed.

Transfusions are carefully administered to prevent hypertension caused by hypervolemia. Approximately 50% of children with typical HUS will need dialysis in the acute phase (Balestracci, Martin, Toledo, et al., 2012). Peritoneal dialysis is preferred unless the child has severe colitis and abdominal tenderness. Some children may develop chronic renal failure; however, most regain normal renal function (Ring & Huether, 2014).

Nursing Management

Monitor vital signs, neurologic signs, and laboratory values including electrolytes and blood counts. Monitor daily weights and assess intake and output. Observe the child carefully for signs of progressive renal impairment such as oliguria, elevated serum potassium, and elevated creatinine. Monitor for signs of bleeding related to thrombocytopenia, including petechiae and ecchymosis. Monitor the child for abdominal discomfort from diarrhea or other gastrointestinal disturbances.

Discharge planning focuses on teaching parents about medications and dietary and fluid restrictions. Follow-up visits are necessary to evaluate the effectiveness of the treatment plan. Make sure that parents understand that ground beef should be cooked to an internal temperature of 160°F (71°C) (U.S. Department of Agriculture, 2013). Teach the family to wash hands carefully when handling raw ground meats, and to make sure utensils touching raw meat do not come into contact with cooked meats. Encourage the use of a meat thermometer since the absence of pink in the center of the meat does not ensure that the appropriate temperature has been achieved.

Polycystic Kidney Disease

Polycystic kidney disease (PKD) is a genetic disorder that has autosomal recessive and dominant forms. Liver abnormalities are associated with both forms of the disease. The incidence of the autosomal recessive form is 1 per 20,000 live births (Zhou & Pollak, 2015). The autosomal dominant form is one of the most frequently inherited diseases with a prevalence of 1 in 800 live births in the United States (Watnick & Dirkx, 2015).

In PKD, cellular hyperplasia of the collecting ducts causes dilation of the ducts. Fluid secreted into these ducts enables cyst sacs to form. Initially, cysts are usually less than 2 mm in size and do not obstruct urinary flow. However, as the child grows, the cysts become larger and fibrosis occurs. The cysts slowly replace much of the kidney's mass and reduce kidney function. Tubular atrophy may occur in some children, whereas others have minimal changes in renal function. PKD is associated with liver abnormalities that progress in severity with age to fibrosis, portal hypertension, and biliary infection.

Newborns with autosomal recessive PKD may have enlarged kidneys, which are detected at birth. Approximately 60% of neonates with this disorder die within the first month from pulmonary hypoplasia. This complication is a result of deficient amniotic fluid (*oligohydramnios*) in utero secondary to severe intrauterine kidney disease (Zhou & Pollak, 2015).

Clinical manifestations in infants with autosomal recessive PKD include low-set ears, small jaw, and a flattened nose. Hypertension develops in early infancy and is often severe. Infants may have expected urine output or oliguria. Respiratory distress and feeding intolerance may develop from the enlarged kidneys (Porter & Avner, 2016). As uremia develops, infants and children develop renal osteodystrophy and progressive developmental delay and growth failure.

Sonography or renal biopsy confirms the diagnosis. The disease is often diagnosed on prenatal ultrasound. Liver function tests are usually normal initially. A liver biopsy may also be performed. Other family members should be screened for subclinical cases of PKD.

Treatment is supportive. Medications such as diuretics are prescribed for hypertension. Fluid and electrolyte abnormalities are managed. Antibiotics treat urinary tract infection. Growth hormones may be used in some children to promote growth. Renal osteodystrophy is treated to suppress the parathyroid hormone. Many children develop end-stage renal disease (ESRD) by 10 years of age. Dialysis or a kidney transplant will prolong survival; however, liver problems may continue to complicate the child's health, even when the kidney condition is well controlled. Fifteen-year survival is estimated to be at 70% to 80% of these children (Porter & Avner, 2016).

Nursing Management

Nursing care is the same as that for the child with renal insufficiency and chronic renal failure. See the discussion earlier in this chapter. Observe the child for signs of progressive renal impairment. Make sure the family schedules follow-up appointments to assess growth, developmental progress, and the effectiveness of the treatment plan. Family teaching for home management focuses on medications, diet adequate in protein and calories to support growth, management of acute gastrointestinal illnesses, and care for the child with progressive renal insufficiency and a liver disorder. Since the disease is inherited, the family should be referred for genetic counseling.

Structural Defects of the Reproductive System

Phimosis

In **phimosis**, the foreskin over the glans penis cannot be retracted. As a result of natural adhesion, phimosis is a normal finding in uncircumcised infants and young males. Circumcision, surgical removal of the foreskin, has long been a common practice performed in some countries and cultures during the newborn period. It is performed to prevent phimosis, for ease of proper male hygiene, and to prevent urinary tract infections and penile cancer. The procedure removes the skin covering the end of the penis. Circumcision is considered comparatively safe; however, complications such as damage to the urethra and disfigurement to the penis may occur. Nonsurgical treatment of phimosis involves the topical application of steroid cream and is an effective alternative to surgery (Shahid, 2012).

Cryptorchidism

Cryptorchidism (undescended testes) occurs when one or both testes fail to descend through the inguinal canal into the scrotum. Normally, the testes descend during the seventh to ninth month of gestation.

Cryptorchidism may be the result of a congenital defect of the gonads, a narrow inguinal canal, short spermatic cord, adhesions, insensitivity to gonadotropins, or lack of maternal gonadotropins. This disorder occurs in approximately 3% of term male infants and has a higher incidence in premature males (Rodway & McCance, 2014).

The higher temperature in the abdomen than in the scrotum results in morphologic changes to the testis. Complications of cryptorchidism include infertility and malignancy (Connolly & McComiskey, 2013; Lee & Houk, 2013).

Cryptorchidism is usually detected during the newborn examination when palpation of the scrotum fails to reveal one or both testes. It is not unusual for boys with cryptorchidism to have an inguinal hernia as well. In a majority of cases, the testes descend spontaneously by 3 months of age.

Although diagnosis is made on physical examination, diagnostic studies, including ultrasound, CT scan, and MRI, are utilized to determine the location of the testes. A diagnostic laparoscope may also be needed to locate the testis. When neither testis can be palpated, hormonal and chromosomal evaluation may be performed to detect an intersex disorder.

If the testes do not descend spontaneously, an orchiopexy should be performed. Timing of surgery may vary among healthcare providers. The current recommendation is that this procedure be performed at 6 months of age in full-term infants. Surgery may be delayed until 12 months of age in premature infants (Barthoid, 2012).

With an orchiopexy, an incision is made at the location of the testis, either in the abdomen or in the inguinal area. Blood vessels are disentangled to allow the testis to reach into the lower scrotum. A second incision is made in the scrotum at the point where the testis is stitched to the inside wall to keep it in place. A protective sealant is often put over the incision that peels off in 3 to 5 days. If the testis is defective or undeveloped, it may be removed surgically to decrease the risk of later malignancies and a prosthesis may be placed in the scrotum.

The goals of surgery are to repair any existing hernia, improve fertility, decrease the risk of malignancy, prevent testicular torsion, and provide the psychologic benefit of a normal appearing scrotum (Connolly & McComiskey, 2013). The risk of testicular cancer is 35 to 50 times greater in men with a history of cryptorchidism (Rodway & McCance, 2014).

Nursing Management

Preoperative nursing care includes preparing the parents and child for the procedure and addressing parents' concerns about the postsurgical outcome. Orchiopexy is often performed as an outpatient procedure. If the child is hospitalized, postoperative nursing care focuses on maintaining comfort and preventing infection. Encourage bed rest, and monitor voiding. Apply ice to the surgical area, and administer prescribed analgesics to relieve pain.

Discharge instructions should include demonstration of proper incision care. The diaper area should be cleaned well with each diaper change to decrease chances of infection. Sponge bathe the child for 2 days after surgery, and then a tub bath may be given. No medicine or ointment should be placed over the incision. Teach parents to identify signs of infection such as redness, warmth, swelling, and discharge and to notify the healthcare provider if present. Ibuprofen or acetaminophen may be given for pain. Inform parents to avoid straddling the infant across the hip and to permit no strenuous activity or straddle toy riding for 2 weeks after surgery to promote healing and to prevent injury.

Inguinal Hernia and Hydrocele

An **inguinal hernia** is a painless inguinal or scrotal swelling of variable size that occurs when abdominal tissue, such as bowel, extends into the inguinal canal. An inguinal hernia is found in 3.5% to 5.0% of full-term infants and 9% to 11% of preterm infants and occurs more often in boys than girls by a 8:1 ratio (Aiken & Oldham, 2016).

A hydrocele is a fluid-filled mass in the scrotum. The condition is found in 1% to 2% of male neonates. Most hydroceles resolve spontaneously by reabsorption by 1 year of age (Elder, 2016d).

During fetal development a peritoneal sac precedes the testicle's descent to the scrotum. The lower sac enfolds the testis to become the tunica vaginalis, and the upper sac atrophies before birth. Fluid may become trapped in the tunica vaginalis and cause the hydrocele. When the tunica vaginalis does not atrophy, an abdominal structure may move into it. Inguinal hernias are often associated with abdominal wall defects such as bladder exstrophy and prune belly syndrome, and are a common occurrence with undescended testes.

Diagnosis is made by physical examination at birth or in early infancy. Palpation of the scrotum reveals a round, smooth, nontender mass, which is noted with either a hernia or hydrocele. Parents may report an intermittent bulge in the groin or swelling in the scrotum. Swelling associated with a hernia may become more apparent with straining and reduced in size when quiet or asleep.

Outpatient surgery is performed as an elective procedure at an early age (usually after 3 months of age to reduce anesthesia risks) to avoid **incarceration** (hernia cannot be reduced and circulation is impaired), which is a medical emergency. A nerve block may be given in the operating room to reduce postoperative pain. The prognosis is generally excellent.

Nursing care for hydroceles and inguinal hernias includes assessment, explaining the disorder and its treatment, and providing preoperative and postoperative teaching, care, and support.

The incision is covered with a protective sealant rather than a dressing. Provide pain medication as ordered. Inform parents that the scrotum may be edematous and may appear bruised after surgery. Incision care involves careful cleaning of the diaper area.

Inguinal hernias can become incarcerated when a bit of bowel becomes trapped in the inguinal opening and the blood supply is constricted. Symptoms in the infant include irritability, poor feeding, and abdominal distention. An older child may complain of pain. Additional symptoms in infants and children may include an edematous, erythematous scrotum accompanied by fever, vomiting, and bloody stools (Aiken & Oldham, 2016). Efforts are made to reduce the hernia before surgery by applying pressure on the affected side, followed by semiurgent surgery. If the hernia cannot be reduced, emergency surgery is performed (Mishra et al., 2014).

Testicular Torsion

Testicular torsion is an emergency condition in which the testis suddenly rotates on its spermatic cord, cutting off its blood supply. The arteries and veins in the spermatic cord become twisted and interrupt the blood supply, leading to vascular engorgement and ischemia. Testicular torsion occurs in 3.8 per 100,000 males under 18 years of age each year (Sharp, Kieran, & Arlen, 2013). Often the testicles are positioned transversely in the scrotum, secondary to a congenital anomaly known as a *bell clapper deformity*. In this deformity, the tunica vaginalis has an inappropriately high attachment to the testes, allowing them to rotate freely and twist spontaneously on the spermatic cord. Approximately 12% of males have this deformity (Datta, Dhillon, & Voci, 2011; Govindarajan & Nelson, 2013).

Manifestations include severe pain and erythema in the scrotum, nausea and vomiting, abdominal pain, and scrotal swelling that is not relieved by rest or scrotal support. The testes are tender on palpation and become edematous. The cremasteric reflex is absent. Symptoms generally start when the child is sleeping or inactive, but they can occur after trauma, sexual activity, or exercise. Color Doppler ultrasonography is frequently used to confirm the diagnosis (Sharp et al., 2013).

Testicular torsion is a surgical emergency. When surgical treatment is implemented within 6 hours of the onset of symptoms, there is a 90% to 100% chance that the testicle can be saved. During surgery (orchiopexy), the testis is untwisted and stitched to the side of the scrotum in the correct position. The procedure is usually performed bilaterally to prevent future torsion in the other testis. If the testicle does not regain blood flow or is already necrotic, it is removed via orchiectomy (Sharp et al., 2013).

Nursing management involves psychologic support for the child and family related to the need for emergency surgery and concern about the child's future fertility. Reassure parents that because only one testis is usually involved, fertility should not be affected. The child often goes home within a few hours of surgery; thus the child and family need to be taught about proper care of the incision and pain management. Explain to parents that the child should not lift heavy objects for 4 weeks or participate in strenuous activity for 2 weeks after surgery to promote healing. Teach the adolescent testicular self-examination.

See Chapter 6 for information on sexually transmitted infections.

Focus Your Study

- Functions of the urinary system include excretion of wastes, maintenance of acid–base and fluid and electrolyte balance, regulation of blood pressure, production of erythropoietin, and regulation of calcium metabolism.

- Expected urine output for a neonate and infant is 1 to 2 mL/kg per hour while an adult should have 0.5 mL/kg per hour.

- Urinary tract infections are common infections in children. Factors placing the child at risk for a UTI include urinary stasis, infrequent voiding, irritated perineum, constipation, sexual abuse, and sexual activity in adolescent females.

- Structural defects of the urinary system—including bladder exstrophy, hypospadias and epispadias, obstructive uropathy, vesicoureteral reflux, and posterior ureteral valves—generally require surgical treatment.

- Bladder exstrophy is a congenital defect in which the abdominal wall does not fuse during fetal development, leading to exposure of the bladder wall, a separation of the rectus muscles, and widening of the symphysis pubis.

- Surgical correction of hypospadias and epispadias generally occurs during the first year of life to minimize psychologic effects on the child.

- Obstruction of the urinary tract interferes with urine flow and results in hydronephrosis or urine backflow into the kidneys.

This results in significant damage to the kidney and is a common cause of renal failure in children.

- Vesicoureteral reflux may result from a structural anomaly in which the ureters insert in an abnormal position into the bladder. Urinary tract infections are often a complication of this disorder.

- Prune belly (Eagle-Barrett) syndrome is a rare congenital disorder in which the skin covering the abdominal wall is thin and resembles a wrinkled prune. Anomalies associated with this syndrome include urinary tract anomalies, poor ureteral peristalsis, enlarged bladder, high risk for recurrent UTI, vesicoureteral reflux, and bilateral cryptorchidism in males.

- Nocturnal enuresis often occurs in children whose parents have a history of enuresis. Very few children have a structural or neurologic cause. Higher rates of enuresis have been noted in children with obstructive sleep apnea and constipation.

- Minimal change nephrotic syndrome is characterized by edema that develops over several weeks, weight gain, hypertension, irritability, hematuria, malaise, anorexia, and foamy or frothy urine.

- Acute postinfectious glomerulonephritis results most often from a beta-hemolytic group A streptococcal infection of the skin or pharynx. It is also caused by other organisms, including *Staphylococcus* and *Pneumococcus* bacteria and coxsackieviruses. Most children have a complete recovery of kidney function.

- Hemolytic-uremic syndrome is often associated with ingestion of *E. coli* strain 0157:H7, which produces a toxin that attacks the kidneys. The child develops hemolytic anemia, thrombocytopenia, and acute renal failure that can progress to chronic renal failure.

- Polycystic kidney disease is a genetic disorder with both autosomal recessive and autosomal dominant forms that lead to chronic renal failure. It may be detected prenatally or in young children by ultrasound.

- Acute renal failure occurs when kidney function diminishes abruptly and is often reversible. It may occur as a complication of trauma, sepsis, cardiac surgery, or drug toxicity. It is also seen in critically ill neonates with asphyxia, sepsis, or shock.

- Chronic renal failure is progressive and irreversible reduced function of the kidneys, eventually resulting in end-stage renal disease. It often results from developmental abnormalities of the kidneys or urinary tract.

- Children with end-stage renal disease are treated with renal replacement therapy, including hemodialysis, peritoneal dialysis, or kidney transplant.

- Structural defects of the male reproductive system include phimosis, cryptorchidism, inguinal hernia, hydrocele, and testicular torsion.

Clinical Reasoning in Action

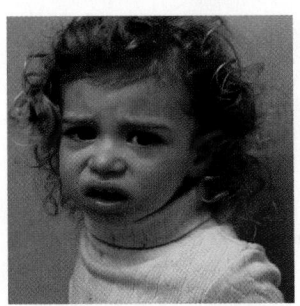

Kendra, a 2-year-old who appears ill, is brought into the urgent care center for a skin rash, fever, irritability, and edema. Her father is concerned she might also be dehydrated because her urine output is decreased. The healthcare provider determines her skin rash does not blanch when pressure is applied and notes a purplish color. Last week, Kendra was treated for an episode of abdominal pain, diarrhea, and vomiting. The healthcare provider immediately admits her to the hospital and orders a urine culture, blood work, and stool tests. The stool comes back positive for the strain of *E. coli* usually found in contaminated hamburger meat. Kendra has hemolytic-uremic syndrome (HUS) and is in acute renal failure (ARF). She also has low hemoglobin, elevated BUN and creatinine, hematuria, and electrolyte imbalances.

Kendra is given medication for her electrolyte imbalances, antihypertensive medications, and is placed on a high-calorie, high-carbohydrate diet with restrictions on protein, sodium, potassium, and phosphorus. You explain to her parents the extreme importance of adhering to her dietary and fluid restrictions to help keep her electrolytes and fluid level balanced. You educate them that in some cases children with HUS need dialysis and some children have long-term kidney damage. You teach them how to take her blood pressure, and how to observe for edema so that Kendra can be monitored after she goes home.

1. How is drug administration adjusted for Kendra since she has ARF? What is an important nursing role when administering various medications to her?

2. What is the reason ARF develops in HUS?

3. What is one way Kendra's condition could have been prevented?

4. Renal failure is characterized by azotemia and oliguria. Describe what these are.

References

Aiken, J. J., & Oldham, K. T. (2016). Inguinal hernias. In R. M. Kliegman, B. F. Stanton, J. W. St. Geme, & N. F. Schor, (Eds.), *Nelson textbook of pediatrics* (20th ed., pp. 1903–1909). Philadelphia, PA: Elsevier.

Alarcon, L. H., & Fink, M. P. (2015). Physiologic monitoring of the surgical patient. In F. C. Brunicardi, D. K. Andersen, T. R. Billiar, D. L. Dunn, J. G. Hunter, J. B. Matthews, & R. E. Pollock (Eds.), *Schwartz's principles of surgery* (10th ed.). Retrieved from http://www.accessmedicine.com

Al-Uzri, A., Matheson, M., Gipson, D. S., Mendley, S. R., Hooper, S. R., Yadin, O., ... Gerson, R. C. (2013). The impact of short stature on health-related quality of life in children with chronic kidney disease. *The Journal of Pediatrics, 163,* 736–741.

American Academy of Pediatrics Task Force on Circumcision. (2012). Male circumcision. *Pediatrics, 130*(3), e756–e785.

Ammenti, A., Cataldi, L., Chimenz, R., Fanos, V., LaManna, A., Marra, G., ... Montini, G. (2012). Febrile urinary tract infections in young children: Recommendations for the diagnosis, treatment and follow-up. *Acta Pædiatrica, 101,* 451–457.

Anderson, M. E., & Weese, J. S. (2012). Video observation of hand hygiene practices at a petting zoo and the impact of hand hygiene interventions. *Epidemiology & Infection, 140,* 182–190.

Balestracci, A., Martin., S. M., Toledo, I., Alvarado, C., & Wainsztein, R. E. (2012). Dehydration at admission increased the need for dialysis in hemolytic uremic syndrome children. *Pediatric Nephrology, 27,* 1407–1410.

Barthoid, J. S. (2012). Abnormalities of the testis and scrotum and their surgical management. In A. J. Wein, L. R. Kavoussi, A. C. Novick, A. W. Partin, & C. A. Peters (Eds.), *Campbell-Walsh urology* (10th ed., pp. 3557–3596). Philadelphia, PA: Elsevier Saunders.

Bascom, A., Penney, T., Metcalfe, M., Knox, A., Witmans, M., Uweira, T., & Metcalfe, P. D. (2011). High risk of sleep disordered breathing in the enuresis population. *Journal of Urology, 184*(4), 1710–1714.

Bhatnagar, V. (2011). Bladder exstrophy: An overview of the surgical management. *Journal of Indian Association of Pediatric Surgeons, 16*(3), 81–87.

Bhimma, R. (2014). *Acute poststreptococcal glomerulonephritis.* Retrieved from http://emedicine.medscape.com/article/980685-overview

Caldamone, A. A., & Woodard, J. R. (2012). Prune-belly syndrome. In A. J. Wein, L. R. Kavoussi, A. C. Novick, A. W. Partin, & C. A. Peters (Eds.), *Campbell-Walsh urology* (10th ed., pp. 3310–3324). Philadelphia, PA: Elsevier Saunders.

Chalmers, D., Wiedel, C. A., Siparsky, G. L. Campbell, J. B., & Wilcox, D. T. (2014). Discovery of hypospadias during newborn circumcision should not preclude completion of the procedure. *Journal of Pediatrics, 164,* 1171–1174.

Connolly, M. E., & McComiskey, C. A. (2013). Common outpatient pediatric surgical procedures: Inguinal and umbilical hernias, hydroceles, undescended testes, and circumcision. In N. T. Browne, L. M. Flanigan, C. A. McComiskey, & P. Pieper (Eds.), *Nursing care of the pediatric surgical patient* (3rd ed., pp. 383–390). Burlington, MA: Jones & Bartlett.

Datta, V., Dhillon, G., & Voci, S. (2011). Testicular torsion/detorsion. *Ultrasound Quarterly, 27*(2), 127–128.

Dubrovsky, A. S., Foster, B. J., Jednak, R., Mok, E., & McGillivray, D. (2012). Visibility of the urethral meatus and risk of urinary tract infections in uncircumcised boys. *Canadian Medical Association Journal, 184*(15), E796–E803.

Elder, J. S. (2016a). Anomalies of the bladder. In R. M. Kliegman, B. F. Stanton, J. W. St. Geme, & N. F. Schor (Eds.), *Nelson textbook of pediatrics* (20th ed., pp. 2575–2578). Philadelphia, PA: Elsevier.

Elder, J. S. (2016b). Obstruction of the urinary tract. In R. M. Kliegman, B. F. Stanton, J. W. St. Geme, & N. F. Schor (Eds.), *Nelson textbook of pediatrics* (20th ed., pp. 2567–2575). Philadelphia, PA: Elsevier.

Elder, J. S. (2016c). Enuresis and voiding dysfunction. In R. M. Kliegman, B. F. Stanton, J. W. St. Geme, & N. F. Schor (Eds.), *Nelson textbook of pediatrics* (20th ed., pp. 2581–2586). Philadelphia, PA: Elsevier.

Elder, J. S. (2016d). Disorders and anomalies of the scrotal contents. In R. M. Kliegman, B. F. Stanton, J. W. St. Geme, & N. F. Schor (Eds.), *Nelson textbook of pediatrics* (20th ed., pp. 2592–2598). Philadelphia, PA: Elsevier.

Estrada, C. R., & Cendron, M. (2013). *Vesicoureteral reflux.* Retrieved from http://emedicine.medscape .com/article/439403-overview

Fisher, D. J., Barton, L. L., Egland, A. G., Egland, T. K., Hellerstein, S., Howes, D. S., … Young, G. M. (2014). *Pediatric urinary tract infection.* Retrieved from http://emedicine.medscape.com/article/969643 -overview

Govindarajan, K. K., & Nelson C. P. (2013). *Pediatric testicular torsion.* Retrieved from http://emedicine .medscape.com/article/2035074-overview

Guilfoyle, S. M., Goebel, J. W., & Pai, A. L. (2011). Efficacy and flexibility impact perceived adherence barriers in pediatric kidney post-transplantation. *Families, Systems, & Health, 29*(1), 44–54.

Gulati, S. (2012). *Chronic kidney disease in children.* Retrieved from http://emedicine.medscape.com /article/984358-overview

Hassett, S., Smith, G. H. H., & Holland, A. J. A. (2012). Prune belly syndrome. *Pediatric Surgery International, 28,* 219–228.

Heath, J., MacKinlay, D., Watson, A. R., Hames, A., Wirz, L., Scott, S., … McHugh, K. (2011). Self-reported quality of life in children and young people with chronic kidney disease. *Pediatric Nephrology, 26,* 767–773.

Hines, E. Q. (2012). Fluid and electrolytes. In *The Harriet Lane handbook* (19th ed., pp. 271–292). Philadelphia, PA: Elsevier.

Holmberg, C., & Jalanko, H. (2014). Congenital nephrotic syndrome and recurrence of proteinuria after renal transplantation. *Pediatric Nephrology, 29,* 2309–2317.

Hunziker, M., Colhoun, E., & Puri, P. (2014). Renal cortical abnormalities in siblings of index patients with vesicoureteral reflux. *Pediatrics, 133*(4) e933–e937.

Ingerski, L., Perrazo, L., Goebel, J., & Pai, A. L. H. (2011). Family strategies for achieving medication adherence in pediatric kidney transplantation. *Nursing Research, 60*(3), 190–196.

Inouye, B. M., Tourchi, A., DiCarlo, H. M., Young, E. E., & Gearhart, J. P. (2014). Modern management of the exstrophy-epispadias complex. *Surgery Research and Practice, 2014.* Retrieved from http://dx.doi .org/10.1155/2014/587064

Jacques, E. (2013). Treating nocturnal enuresis in children and young people. *British Journal of School Nursing, 8*(6) 275–278.

Kari, J. A., El-Desoky, S., Farag, Y., Mosli, H., Altyieb, A. M., Al-Sayad, H., … Farsi, H. (2013). Renal impairment in children with posterior urethral valves. *Pediatric Nephrology, 28,* 927–931.

Kilis-Pstrusinska, K., Medynska, A., Chmielewska, I. B., Grenda, R., Kluska-Jozwiak, A., Leszczynska, B., … Zwolinska, D. (2013). Perception of health-related quality of life in children with chronic kidney disease by the patients and their caregivers: Multicentre national study results. *Quality of Life Research, 22,* 2889–2897.

Kocherov, S., Prat, D., Koulikov, D., Ioscovich, A., Shenfeld, O. Z., Farkas, A., & Chertin, B. (2012). Outcome of hypospadias repair in toilet-trained children and adolescents. *Pediatric Surgery International, 28,* 429–433.

Kundra, P., Yuvaraj, K., Agrawal, K., Krishnappa, C., & Kumar, L. T. (2011). Surgical outcome in children undergoing hypospadias repair under caudal epidural vs penile block. *Pediatric Anesthesia, 22,* 707–712.

Lee, H., Han, S. W., & Rah, K. H. (2014). *Pediatric ureteropelvic junction obstruction.* Retrieved from http://emedicine.medscape.com/article/1016988- overview

Lee, P. A., & Houk, C. P. (2013). Cryptorchidism. *Current Opinion in Endocrinology, Diabetes & Obesity, 20*(3), 210–216.

Lombel, R. M., Hodson, E. M., & Gipson, D. S. (2013). Treatment of steroid-resistant nephrotic syndrome in children: New guidelines from KDIGO. *Pediataric Nephrology, 28,* 409–414

Lum, G. M. (2014). Kidney & urinary tract. In W. W. Hay, M. J. Levin, R. R. Deterding, & M. J. Abzug (Eds.), *CURRENT diagnosis and treatment: Pediatrics* (22nd ed.). New York, NY: McGraw-Hill. Retrieved from http://accessmedicine.com

Mehrazma, M., Amini-Alavijeh, Z., & Hooman, N., (2012). Prognostic value of dialysis effluent leukocyte count in children on peritoneal dialysis with peritonitis. *Iranian Journal of Kidney Diseases, 6*(2), 114–118.

Mishra, P. K., Burnand, K., Minocha, A., Mathur, A. B., Kulkarni, M. S., & Tsang, T. (2014). Incarcerated inguinal hernia management in children: A comparison of the open and laparoscopic approach. *Pediatric Surgery International, 30,* 621–624.

Morris, B. J., & Wiswell, T. E. (2013). Circumcision and lifetime risk of urinary tract infection: A systematic review and meta-analysis. *The Journal of Urology, 189*(6), 2118–2124.

Nachman, P. H., Jennette, J. C., & Falk, R. J. (2012). Primary glomerular disease. In M. W. Taal, G. M. Chertow, P. A. Marsden, K. Skorecki, A. S. L. Yu, & B. M. Brenner (Eds.), *Brenner and Rector's the kidney* (9th ed., pp. 1100–1191). Philadelphia, PA: Elsevier Saunders.

Nevéus, T. (2011). Nocturnal enuresis-theoretic background and practical guidelines. *Pediatric Nephrology, 26,* 1207–1214.

Newman, T. B. (2011). The new American Academy of Pediatrics urinary tract infection guidelines. *Pediatrics, 128*(3), 572–575.

Norfolk, S., & Wootton, J. (2012). Nocturnal enuresis in children. *Nursing Standard, 27*(10), 49–56.

Otukesh, H., Hoseini, R., Rahimzadeh, N., & Hosseini, S. (2012). Glomerular function in neonates. *Iranian Journal of Kidney Diseases, 6*(3), 166–172.

Paintsil, E. (2013). Update on recent guidelines for the management of urinary tract infections in children: The shifting paradigm. *Current Opinion in Pediatrics, 25*(1), 88–94.

Pais, P., & Avner, E. D. (2016). Nephrotic syndrome. In R. M. Kliegman, B. F. Stanton, J. W. St. Geme, & N. F. Schor (Eds.), *Nelson textbook of pediatrics* (20th ed., pp. 2521–2528). Philadelphia, PA: Elsevier.

Passamaneck, M. (2011). The changing paradigm for the management of pediatric vesicoureteral reflux. *Urologic Nursing, 31*(6), 363–366.

Porter, C. C., & Avner, E. D. (2016). Autosomal recessive polycystic kidney disease. In R. M. Kliegman, B. F. Stanton, J. W. St. Geme, & N. F. Schor (Eds.), *Nelson textbook of pediatrics* (20th ed., p. 2513). Philadelphia, PA: Elsevier.

Ray, J. (2011). Enuresis. *Al Ameen Journal of Medical Sciences, 4*(2), 104–112.

Ring, R., & Huether, S. E. (2014). Alterations of renal and urinary tract function in children. In K. L. McCance & S. E. Huether (Eds.), *Pathophysiology: The biologic basis for disease in children and adults* (7th ed., pp. 1376–1392). St. Louis, MO: Elsevier Mosby.

Rodway, G., & McCance, K. L. (2014). Alterations of the male reproductive systems. In K. L. McCance & S. E. Huether (Eds.), *Pathophysiology: The biologic basis for disease in children and adults* (7th ed., pp. 885–917). St. Louis, MO: Elsevier Mosby.

Scheinman, J. I. (2012). Pediatric Transplantation. In M. W. Taal, G. M. Chertow, P. A. Marsden, K. Skorecki, A. S. L. Yu, & B. M. Brenner (Eds.), *Brenner and Rector's the kidney* (9th ed., pp. 2694–2718). Philadelphia, PA: Elsevier Saunders.

Shahid, S. K. (2012). Phimosis in children. *ISRN Urology, 2012,* 1–6.

Sharp, V. J., Kieran, K., & Arlen, A. M. (2013). Testicular torsion: Diagnosis, evaluation, and management. *American Family Physician, 88*(12), 835–840.

Snodgrass, W., & Bush, N. (2014). Recent advances in understanding/management of hypospadias. *F1000PrimeReports.* Retrieved from http://f1000 .com/prime/reports/m/6/101

Sreedharan, R., & Avner, E. D. (2016). Renal failure. In R. M. Kliegman, B. F. Stanton, J. W. St. Geme, & N. F. Schor (Eds.), *Nelson textbook of pediatrics* (20th ed., pp. 2539–2547). Philadelphia, PA: Elsevier.

Tan, A. J., & Silverberg, M. A. (2014). *Hemolytic uremic syndrome in emergency medicine.* Retrieved from http://emedicine.medscape.com/article/779218 -overview

U.S. Department of Agriculture. (2013). *Color of cooked ground beef as it relates to doneness.* Retrieved from http://www.fsis.usda.gov/wps/portal/fsis/topics /food-safety-education/get-answers/food-safety-fact -sheets/meat-preparation/color-of-cooked-ground -beef-as-it-relates-to-doneness/ct_index

Verive, M. J. (2013). *Pediatric hyperkalemia.* Retrieved from http://emedicine.medscape.com /article/907543-overview

Wadie, G. M., & Moriarty, K. P. (2012). The impact of vesicoureteral reflux treatment on the incidence of urinary tract infection. *Pediatric Nephrology, 27,* 529–538.

Walle, J., Rittig, S., Bauer, S., Eggert, P., Marschall-Kehrel, D., & Tekgul, S. (2012). Practical consensus guidelines for the management of enuresis. *European Journal of Pediatrics, 171,* 971–983.

Watnick, S., & Dirkx, T. (2015). Kidney disease. In S. J. McPhee, M. A. Papadakis, & M. W. Rabow (Eds.), *Current medical diagnosis and treatment 2015.* New York, NY: McGraw-Hill.

White, B. (2011). Diagnosis and treatment of urinary tract infections in children. *American Family Physician, 83*(4), 409–415.

Wilson, B. A., Shannon, M. T., & Shields, K. M. (2015). *Pearson nurse's drug guide 2015.* Hoboken, NJ: Pearson Education.

Workeneh, B. T., Agraharkar, M., & Gupta, R. (2014). *Acute kidney injury.* Retrieved from http://emedicine .medscape.com/article/243492-overview

Zaritsky, J., & Warady, B. A. (2011). Peritoneal dialysis in infants and young children. *Seminars in Nephrology, 31*(2), 213–224.

Zhou, J., & Pollak, M. R. (2015). Polycystic kidney disease and other inherited tubular disorders. In D. Kasper, A. Fauci, S. Hauser, D. Longo, J. L. Jameson, & J. Loscalzo (Eds.), *Harrison's principles of internal medicine* (19th ed.). New York, NY: McGraw-Hill. Retrieved from http://www.accessmedicine.com

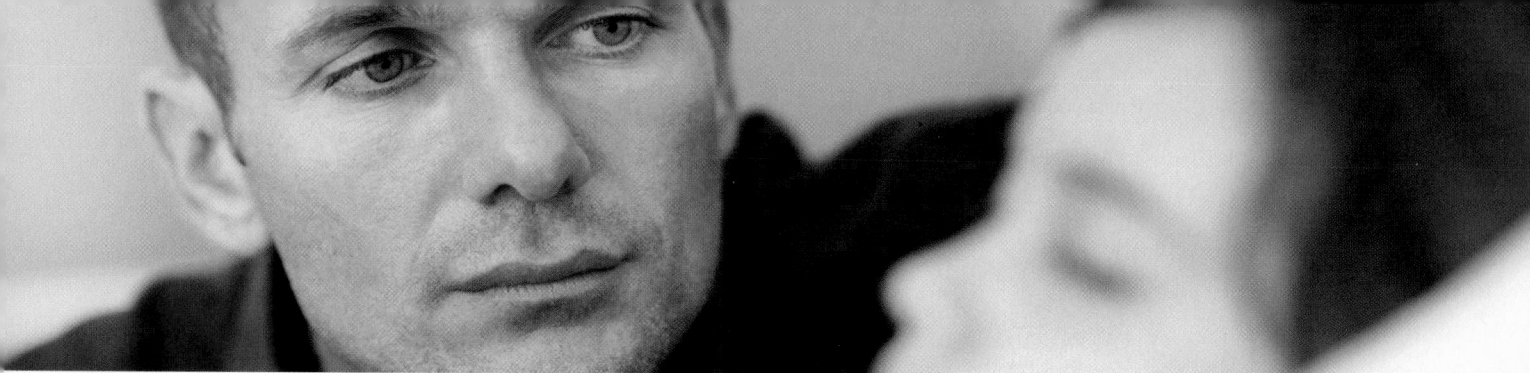

Chapter 53
The Child With Alterations in Endocrine Function

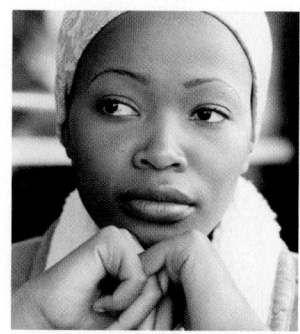

I am really worried about how Anthony is going to learn to manage all these aspects of diabetes care. Learning to check his blood sugar is pretty easy compared to counting calories and figuring out how much insulin to take and when to take it. I hope we have some time to get into a routine with his diabetes management before he gets sick. We have to work hard to keep the diabetes under control.

—Mother of Anthony, 12 years old

Stockbyte/Getty Images

⌄ Learning Outcomes

53.1 Identify the function of important hormones of the endocrine system.

53.2 Summarize signs and symptoms that may indicate a disorder of the endocrine system.

53.3 Identify all conditions for which short stature is a sign.

53.4 Prioritize nursing care for each type of acquired metabolic disorder.

53.5 Develop a family education plan for the child who needs lifelong cortisol replacement.

53.6 Distinguish between the nursing care of the child with type 1 and type 2 diabetes.

53.7 Plan care for the child with an inherited metabolic disorder.

The endocrine system controls the cellular activity that regulates growth and body metabolism through the release of hormones. Hormones are chemical messengers secreted by various glands that exert controlling effects on the cells of the body. Overlapping with all body systems, the general functions of the endocrine system include the following:

- Differentiation of the reproductive and central nervous systems in the fetus

- Regulation of the pace of growth and development in concert with the central nervous system throughout childhood and adolescence

- Coordination of the male and female reproductive systems, enabling sexual reproduction

- Maintenance of an optimal level of hormones for body functioning

- Maintenance of homeostasis, a healthy internal environment, in the presence of a constantly changing external environment

The endocrine and nervous systems interact to regulate responses within the body and with the external environment.

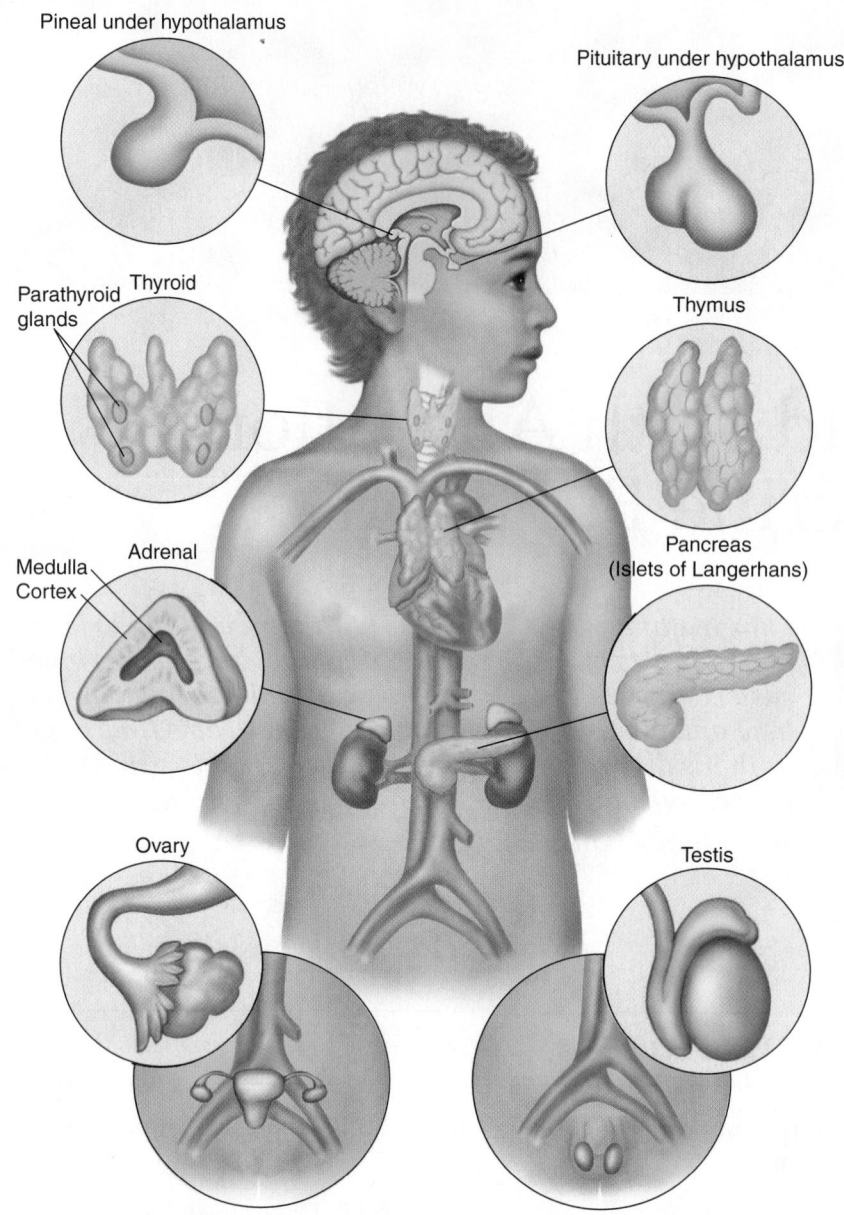

Pineal under hypothalamus

Pituitary under hypothalamus

Parathyroid glands

Thyroid

Thymus

Medulla
Cortex

Adrenal

Pancreas
(Islets of Langerhans)

Ovary

Testis

Figure 53–1 Major organs and glands of the endocrine system.

Anatomy and Physiology of Pediatric Differences

The hypothalamic-pituitary axis produces several releasing and inhibiting hormones that regulate the function of many endocrine glands, including the thyroid, adrenal, and male and female reproductive glands. The hypothalamus synthesizes many hormones and the pituitary gland works by stimulating or inhibiting the release of these hormones. The pituitary gland also secretes certain hormones. Hormones originating from this axis regulate growth. Other endocrine glands include the parathyroid glands and the islets of Langerhans in the pancreas (Figure 53–1). All of these glands secrete hormones into the bloodstream, which carries them to target organs or tissues. Most hormones exert their influence through interaction with receptors in the target cells of specific tissues (Table 53–1).

Hormone secretion regulation occurs through a *negative feedback* mechanism that functions to maintain an optimal internal environment in the body. Negative feedback occurs when an endocrine gland or secretory tissue receives a message that the target cells have received an adequate amount of hormone. In response, further secretion is inhibited. Secretion is resumed only when the secretory tissue receives another message indicating that levels of the hormone are low.

The endocrine system is responsible for sexual differentiation during fetal development and for stimulating growth and development during childhood and adolescence. This includes stimulating development of the reproductive system in both sexes.

Puberty (sexual maturation, lasting an average of 4.5 years) occurs when the gonads secrete increased amounts of the sex hormones estrogen and testosterone. At the average age of 9 years in girls and 11 years in boys, the hypothalamus produces increased amounts of gonadotropin-releasing hormone

TABLE 53–1 Endocrine Glands and Their Functions

GLAND/HORMONE	FUNCTION
ANTERIOR PITUITARY	
Growth hormone (somatotropin)	Regulates metabolic process related to growth.
Thyroid-stimulating hormone (TSH)	Stimulates thyroid hormone secretion.
Adrenocorticotropic hormone (ACTH) (corticotropin)	Stimulates secretion of glucocorticoids and androgens.
Follicle-stimulating hormone (FSH) (a gonadotropin)	Stimulates secretion of estrogen; stimulates follicle maturation in ovaries. Also critical for sperm production in males.
Luteinizing hormone (LH) and interstitial cell-stimulating hormone (ICSH) (male analog) (a gonadotropin)	Stimulates secretion of androgens in males and progesterone in females.
Prolactin-releasing hormone	Stimulates secretion of prolactin, which stimulates the secretion of milk during lactation.
Melanocyte-stimulating hormone (MSH)	Stimulates skin pigmentation.
Beta endorphins	Involved with pleasure during exercise and the alleviation of pain.
POSTERIOR PITUITARY	
Antidiuretic hormone (ADH)	Promotes water reabsorption back into blood, decreasing urine output.
Oxytocin	Stimulates uterine contractions and breast milk let-down reflex.
THYROID	
Thyroxine (T_4) and triiodothyronine (T_3)	Regulate metabolic rate of all cells, body heat production; protein, fat, and carbohydrate catabolism in all cells.
Thyrocalcitonin	Stimulates bone ossification and development.
PARATHYROID	
Parathyroid hormone	Regulates serum calcium levels and excretion of phosphorus.
ADRENAL	
Aldosterone	Increases sodium ion reabsorption, and increases potassium and hydrogen ion excretion in the kidneys.
Androgens	Stimulate bone development and secondary sexual characteristics.
Cortisol	Stimulates anti-inflammatory reactions.
	Protects from harmful stress responses.
Epinephrine	Activates sympathetic nervous system; stimulates increase in blood pressure and blood glucose levels.
PANCREAS (ISLETS OF LANGERHANS)	
Insulin	Facilitates cellular glucose utilization.
Glucagon	Increases blood glucose when low by stimulating glycogenolysis.
Somatostatin	Inhibits insulin and glucagon secretion; may prevent excess insulin secretion.
OVARIES	
Estrogen	Stimulates development of breasts and ova.
Progesterone	Stimulates breast glandular development; acts to maintain pregnancy.
TESTES	
Testosterone	Stimulates production of sperm, development of secondary sexual characteristics, and closure of epiphysis.

(GnRH). This hormone stimulates the anterior pituitary gland to secrete luteinizing hormone (LH) and follicle-stimulating hormone (FSH). In boys, LH stimulates testosterone production and FSH stimulates sperm production. In girls, LH and FSH stimulate development and maturation of the ova and ovulation. These hormones, in turn, stimulate the gonads to secrete more sex hormones, resulting in the development of primary and secondary sex characteristics (Figure 53–2).

Use the accompanying *Assessment Guide: The Child With an Endocrine Condition* to perform a nursing assessment of the endocrine system.

Disorders of Pituitary Function

Pituitary disorders such as growth hormone deficiency, hyperpituitarism, and precocious puberty directly affect a child's growth, while diabetes insipidus and the syndrome of inappropriate antidiuretic hormone are disorders affecting fluid balance. These disorders are discussed in the following subsections.

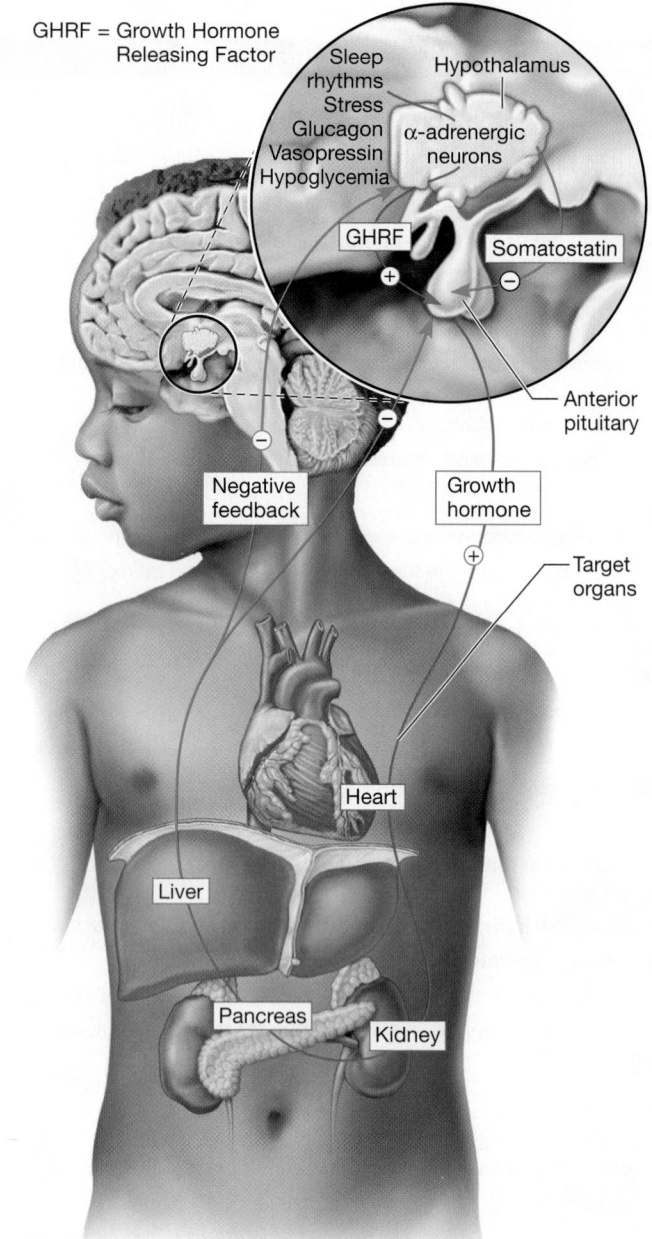

GHRF = Growth Hormone
Releasing Factor

Figure 53–2 **Feedback mechanism in hormonal stimulation of the gonads during puberty.**

Growth Hormone Deficiency (Hypopituitarism)

Growth hormone deficiency (GHD) is a disorder caused by decreased activity of the pituitary gland. Because most children with this disorder secrete inadequate amounts of growth hormone, the term *growth hormone deficiency* is often preferred to *hypopituitarism*. The disorder is estimated to occur in 1 of 4000 to 1 of 10,000 people (Stanley, 2012).

ETIOLOGY AND PATHOPHYSIOLOGY

The release of growth hormone from the anterior pituitary gland is controlled by the hypothalamus, which secretes releasing and inhibitory factors (somatostatin). Growth hormone (GH) (somatotropin) stimulates linear growth and bone mineral density, as well as the growth of all body tissues. Growth hormone

also stimulates the synthesis of proteins in the liver, among them the somatomedins, or insulin-like growth factors (IGFs), which promote glucose utilization by the cells and cell proliferation.

Infarction of the pituitary gland (related to sickle cell disease), central nervous system disease, tumors of the pituitary gland or hypothalamus (primarily craniopharyngiomas and gliomas), other brain tumors, cranial irradiation, brain trauma, chemotherapy, and psychosocial deprivation may cause GHD by interfering with the production or release of growth hormone. Other major causes of short stature include familial short stature, hypothyroidism, Turner syndrome, *constitutional growth delay* (delayed pubertal hormone secretion causes a late pubertal growth spurt), chronic renal failure, malnutrition, Cushing syndrome, Down syndrome, inborn error of metabolism, and severe cardiac, pulmonary, immunologic, or gastrointestinal disease. Psychosocial dwarfism is a syndrome of emotional deprivation that causes transient growth hormone deficiency; it is reversed by placing the child in a nurturing environment (Sirotnak, 2013). Refer to Chapter 56 for information about achondroplastic dwarfism.

CLINICAL MANIFESTATIONS

Children with GHD have normal birth weights and length. However, by the age of 1 year, they are below the 3rd percentile on the growth chart. The child characteristically grows at a rate of less than 5 cm (2 in.) per year. Other characteristic findings in infants include hypoglycemic seizures, hyponatremia, neonatal jaundice, pale optic discs, micropenis, and undescended testicles. Children with GHD tend to appear "cherubic" and exhibit youthful facial features, higher pitched voices, delayed dentition, "ripply" abdominal fat, decreased muscle mass, delayed skeletal maturation, and delayed sexual maturation. Slipped capital femoral epiphysis (see Chapter 56) has been associated with growth hormone therapy. Any child receiving growth hormone treatment who complains of hip pain or knee pain, or who manifests a limp, must be evaluated for this disorder (Cooke, Divall, & Radovick, 2011).

Any child whose height is 2 to 3 standard deviations below the mean height for age or whose measurement is falling off the normal growth chart should be evaluated for short stature (Table 53–2). A child whose screening tests reveal low levels of insulin-like growth factor (IGF-1) requires further evaluation by a pediatric endocrinologist. A careful history, physical examination, assessment of pubertal development and unusual facies, and radiologic studies are necessary to rule out familial short stature and constitutional growth delay, which are normal variants; skeletal dysplasias; or psychosocial short stature, which requires further evaluation.

CLINICAL THERAPY

Radiographic imaging of the hand or wrist bone is used to evaluate the stage of bone ossification and thus the **bone age** of the child. Using standardized norms for bone ossification, it can be determined if the child's chronologic and bone ages match. Significantly delayed (less than the child's age) or advanced (greater than the child's age) bone age may be indicative of the possibility of a systemic chronic disease or hormone abnormality requiring investigation (see *As Children Grow: Bone Age*). Provocative growth hormone testing, in which various medications (arginine, clonidine, glucagon, insulin, L-dopa) are administered to stimulate release of growth hormone, is a diagnostic test that may be used to confirm growth hormone deficiency (Guo, 2013).

For growth hormone deficiency, replacement therapy with growth hormone (GH) is administered to promote growth and development. Growth hormone replacement requires subcutaneous injections 6 to 7 times per week and generally continues

ASSESSMENT GUIDE | The Child With an Endocrine Condition

Assessment Focus	Assessment Guideline
Growth	• Carefully measure weight, length, or height and plot on a growth curve.
	• Compare measurements at different ages to assess the growth pattern over time and to assess the growth velocity.
Blood pressure	• Assess blood pressure and compare to expected norms for age. See Appendix D.
Facial characteristics	• Inspect the face for unusual features such as a protuberant tongue, protuberant eyes, or moon face.
Neck	• Palpate the neck for an enlarged thyroid or goiter.
Muscles	• Assess strength and muscle tone.
Genitalia and secondary sexual characteristics	• Assess external genitalia for signs of ambiguous genitalia or inappropriate development for age.
	• Determine the child's stage of development for each characteristic (breast and pubic hair for girls, genital and pubic hair for boys) by comparing to the images in Chapter 33 (Figures 33–28, 33–29, and 33–30).
	• Assess the sexual maturity rating with information given in Chapter 33 (Table 33–13). Compare the stage of development to the age of the boy or girl to determine early or delayed onset of puberty.
Body odor	• Assess body odor for unusual smell (e.g., sweet, musty, cheesy, sweaty feet).
Skin	• Assess skin color, noting areas of unusual pigmentation.
Family history	• Assess for family history of metabolic or endocrine disorders.

TABLE 53–2 Diagnostic Tests for Short Stature

TEST	PURPOSE RELATED TO SHORT STATURE
IGF-1 (insulin-like growth factor) and IGFBP-3 (insulin-like growth factor-binding protein 3)	Screens for growth hormone deficiency
MRI of the pituitary gland	Detects pituitary malformation or tumor
Provocative growth hormone testing	Tests for growth hormone deficiency
Bone age	Identifies skeletal maturation compared to chronologic age
Karyotype (girls)	Detects Turner syndrome
Thyroid function studies	Detects hypothyroidism
ACTH and cortisol levels	Detects other pituitary hormonal deficiencies
Urine creatinine, pH, specific gravity, urea nitrogen, electrolytes	Detects chronic renal failure (see Chapter 52)
Complete blood count and erythrocyte sedimentation rate	Screens for inflammatory bowel disease with anemia
Antigliadin antibodies	Screens for celiac disease

Source: Data from Parks, J. S., & Felner, E. I. (2016). Hypopituitarism. In R. M. Kliegman, B. F. Stanton, J. W. St. Geme, & N. F. Schor (Eds.), *Nelson textbook of pediatrics* (20th ed., pp. 2637–2644). Philadelphia, PA: Elsevier; Cooke, D. W., Divall, S. A., & Radovick, S. (2011). Normal and aberrant growth. In S. Melmed, K. S. Polonsky, P. R. Larsen, & H. M. Kronenberg (Eds.), *Williams textbook of endocrinology* (12th ed., pp. 935–1053). Philadelphia, PA: Elsevier Saunders.

for several years until growth is complete. The pediatric endocrinologist adjusts the dosage based on response to treatment (Ferguson, 2011).

The child usually experiences increased growth velocity for the first year of treatment, followed by a gradual decrease in growth for subsequent months or years. Growth should progress at least at the normal rate for age while the child continues on growth hormone treatment. If growth is slower than anticipated, compliance with therapy must be considered before the dosage is increased. Replacement therapy is continued until either the child achieves an acceptable height or growth velocity drops to less than 2 cm (1 in.) per year. Additionally, a bone age of greater than 14 years in girls and 16 years in boys is the criterion to stop treatment. In some cases, the onset of puberty is delayed with GnRH analogs to provide more time for growth hormone therapy to stimulate growth (Parks & Felner, 2016).

Nursing Management

Nursing care consists of monitoring growth, teaching the child and family about the disorder and its treatment, and providing emotional support. Collect blood samples in the manner and time ordered. Carefully measure the child's height and weight and plot them on a growth chart (see Appendix C and the *Clinical Skills Manual* SKILLS).

Teach the parents and child about the GH replacement therapy, preparation and administration of subcutaneous injections,

As Children Grow: **Bone Age**

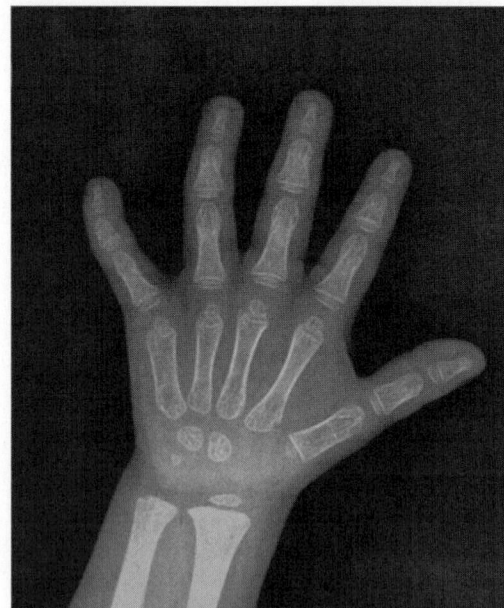

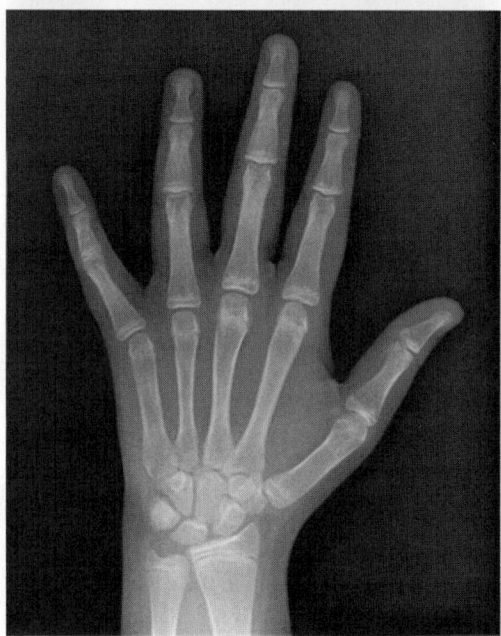

The radiographs of the hand and wrist of a 3-year-old girl and a 14-year-old girl reveal significant differences in skeletal maturation that are closely tied to physiologic maturation. The 3-year-old has many bones in the hand and wrist that have not fully developed. The secretion of estrogen during puberty has resulted in the development and calcification of secondary ossification centers of most of the bones in the hand and wrist of the 14-year-old.

SOURCE: Courtesy of Evelyn Anthony, MD, Department of Radiology, Brenner Children's Hospital, Wake Forest University Health System.

rotating injection sites, potential side effects, and actions to take if any side effects are noticed. Provide the parents with ideas about how to minimize the child's stress associated with daily injections. Give parents educational resources, such as information from the Magic Foundation and the Human Growth Foundation.

Replacement therapy is expensive and may not be covered by insurance (Ferguson, 2011).

Children with GHD, especially those whose deficiency is caused by tumors and trauma from radiation or surgery, may have academic problems because of acquired learning disabilities. Before the child enters or returns to school, a comprehensive evaluation should be performed to identify potential problems.

Encourage parents and teachers to treat the child in an age-appropriate manner. The child should dress in clothing that reflects chronologic age. Emphasize the child's strengths, support independence, and encourage participation in age-appropriate activities to aid in the development of a positive self-image. Suggest that the child take part in sports in which ability does not depend on size (e.g., swimming, gymnastics, wrestling, ice skating, and martial arts). Identifying positive role models, short people who accomplish their goals, also promotes a positive image. Refer the child for counseling if appropriate.

The best results occur when treatment begins at an early age, before the psychologic effects of short stature become apparent and when attainment of near-normal height is reached. People often treat short children on the basis of their size rather than their age, and such children experience social prejudice about height. Teasing is a common problem. The teenage years may be particularly stressful because of adolescents' characteristic preoccupation with body image.

Growth Hormone Excess (Hyperpituitarism)

Hyperpituitarism, a disorder in which excessive secretion of growth hormone increases the growth rate, is rare in children. If combined with precocious puberty, a tumor of the hypothalamus may be present. Affected children can grow to 7 or 8 feet in height when oversecretion occurs before closure of the epiphyseal plates. If the disorder occurs after closure of the epiphyseal plates, acromegaly occurs.

Because tall stature is valued in our society, assessment of children (particularly males) with accelerated linear growth is often delayed. Any child whose predicted height exceeds that consistent with parental height should be evaluated for possible growth problems and underlying pathologic conditions.

A complete history is obtained, and physical examination and laboratory testing are performed. Increased levels of insulin-like growth factor (IGF-1) establish the diagnosis of hyperpituitarism. Radiologic examination for bone age is obtained to determine if the epiphyseal plates have begun to fuse. Radiologic studies are used to detect a tumor. Thorough evaluation is required to differentiate hyperpituitarism from familial tall stature.

Treatment depends on the cause of the excessive growth and may involve surgical removal of a tumor or pituitary gland (hypophysectomy), radiation therapy, or radioactive implants. High doses of sex steroids are given to close the epiphyseal plates. The child may need lifelong pituitary hormone replacement following surgery.

Nursing Management

Tall stature, like short stature, can be stressful for children. Tall children are often treated as if they are older than their chronologic age. Tall adolescents may have problems with self-image, and girls in particular may worry about their appearance.

Nursing care focuses on teaching the parents and child about the disorder and its treatment, providing emotional support, and, if surgery is required, providing preoperative and postoperative teaching and care (see Chapter 39).

Diabetes Insipidus

Diabetes insipidus is a disorder of the posterior pituitary gland and is defined as an inability of the kidneys to concentrate urine. Two forms of diabetes insipidus occur: central (neurogenic) and nephrogenic diabetes insipidus. Central diabetes insipidus results from inadequate production of vasopressin (antidiuretic hormone), and nephrogenic diabetes insipidus results from ineffective action of vasopressin in the kidneys (Di Iorgi et al., 2012; McHugo & Harden, 2011).

ADH facilitates concentration of the urine by stimulating reabsorption of water from the distal tubule of the kidney. When ADH is inadequate, the tubules do not resorb, leading to **polyuria** (passage of a large volume of urine in a given period). Therefore, the body is unable to conserve water, resulting in severe dehydration.

The cause of 20% to 50% of cases of central diabetes insipidus is unknown and is classified as being idiopathic (Di Iorgi et al., 2012). Known causes of central diabetes insipidus include brain tumors, brain trauma, central nervous system infection, and neurosurgery (McHugo & Harden, 2011). Genetic nephrogenic diabetes insipidus is not as common as the acquired type, but its presentation is more severe. Acquired nephrogenic diabetes insipidus may be caused by drug toxicity, an adverse drug reaction, or illnesses that impair the ability of the kidneys to concentrate urine (Breault & Majzoub, 2016).

Polyuria and **polydipsia** (excessive thirst) are the cardinal signs of diabetes insipidus. Enuresis is common in children. Polydipsia is the body's attempt to preserve fluid balance. Additional manifestations observed in children with diabetes insipidus include hypernatremia, dilute urine, and dehydration (Table 53–3).

Clinical Tip

During the fluid deprivation test, advise parents that the child will be frustrated and irritable from thirst. No one should drink in front of the child during the testing period. Monitor the child's vital signs, intake, output, and weight carefully (McHugo & Harden, 2011).

Although the onset of symptoms is usually sudden, diagnosis is often delayed. Children who can quench their thirst may not complain to parents about symptoms. In infants, symptoms may include irritability, lethargy, vomiting, poor feeding, failure to thrive, and constipation (McHugo & Harden, 2011; Walsh & March, 2013).

In all forms of diabetes insipidus, the urine cannot be concentrated no matter how dehydrated the child becomes. A dehydration episode usually leads to the diagnosis. Serum sodium concentration and osmolality increase rapidly to pathologic levels. Often an unconscious child is admitted to the emergency department with dehydration and hypernatremia.

Initial testing involves serum electrolyte concentrations and a urinalysis including specific gravity and osmolality. Serum osmolality is increased (greater than 300 mOsm/kg), and urine osmolality is decreased (less than 300 mOsm/kg). Urine specific gravity is decreased (less than 1.005), and serum sodium is elevated (greater than 145 mEq/L). A CT scan or MRI may be ordered to visualize the pituitary gland to detect a tumor. A fluid-deprivation test evaluates the level of ADH and helps to confirm the diagnosis (Walsh & March, 2013).

Central ADH deficiency is treated by intranasal or oral desmopressin acetate (DDAVP). The medication reduces urinary output, enabling the child to live a more normal life with a decrease in thirst, urinary output, and nocturia. The dose of DDAVP is based on route of administration, age, and response to therapy (McHugo & Harden, 2011). Nephrogenic diabetes insipidus is treated with thiazide diuretics, which promote sodium excretion and stimulate the proximal tubule to reabsorb water. Indomethacin and amiloride may also be prescribed to have an additive effect on decreased water excretion (Breault & Majzoub, 2016). The child's sodium and potassium levels must be carefully monitored to prevent hypernatremia and hypokalemia (McHugo & Harden, 2011) (see Chapter 44).

Nursing Management

Educate parents about making fluids available to the child as needed, administering DDAVP, obtaining and recording daily weights, measuring intake and output, and recognizing signs of dehydration. Parents may need to weigh diapers to monitor urine output in infants. Cold fluids are often preferred and help relieve thirst. The child's fluid intake will need to be adjusted to prevent dehydration during an illness. Children often wake to drink fluids at night, but infants will need to have fluids provided. Many infants have coexisting brain damage and need nasogastric or gastrostomy feeding to maintain adequate hydration and nutrition. However, care should be taken to avoid the intake of excessive fluid as the child

TABLE 53–3 Clinical Manifestations of Diabetes Insipidus

CAUSE	CLINICAL MANIFESTATIONS	CLINICAL THERAPY
CENTRAL DIABETES INSIPIDUS		
ADH (vasopressin) deficiency	Polyuria, polydipsia	Desmopressin acetate
Familial or idiopathic	Nocturia, enuresis	
	Thirsty at night	
	Irritable if fluids withheld	
	Constipation, fever, dehydration	
NEPHROGENIC DIABETES INSIPIDUS		
Inherited or acquired	Polyuria, polydipsia	Diuretics
Decreased responsiveness of kidneys to ADH (vasopressin)	Hypernatremia in neonatal period	High fluid intake
	Dehydration, fever, vomiting	Salt- and protein-restricted diet
	Mental status changes	

will not be able to excrete the excess water load with DDAVP treatment.

The child with chronic diabetes insipidus should always wear a medical alert identification (tag, bracelet, or necklace) to indicate the presence of the disorder. Partner with the parents and school officials to make arrangements to provide the child unrestricted access to toilet facilities and water.

Syndrome of Inappropriate Antidiuretic Hormone (SIADH)

Syndrome of inappropriate antidiuretic hormone (SIADH) results from an excessive amount of serum ADH. It is seen in children with central nervous system infections, brain tumors, and brain trauma; in children with pulmonary disorders such as pneumonia, asthma, or cystic fibrosis; and in children receiving positive-pressure ventilation. Some medications, including diuretics and chemotherapy, have been associated with SIADH.

Failure of normal feedback mechanisms from the hypothalamus, pituitary gland, and kidney results in excessive secretion of ADH, leading to water reabsorption despite the presence of low serum osmolality. ADH secretion causes increased permeability of the distal renal tubules and collecting ducts and resulting in water reabsorption (Thomas & Fraer, 2014). Elevated ADH also causes suppression of the renin-angiotensin mechanism and sodium excretion. The outcome is **water intoxication** (an abnormal proportion of water to sodium in the extracellular fluid) and hyponatremia.

Signs of SIADH are related to water intoxication and hyponatremia, and include elevated blood pressure, distended jugular veins, crackles in lung fields, weight gain without edema, fluid and electrolyte imbalance, and concentrated urine with decreased urine output. As serum sodium levels continue to fall, lethargy, confusion, headache, altered level of consciousness, seizures, and coma occur because of cerebral edema.

Laboratory findings include a high urine osmolality, low serum osmolality, low serum sodium, high urine sodium, and decreased blood urea nitrogen (Pillai, Unnikrishnan, & Pavithran, 2011; Shoback & Funk, 2011).

Fluids are restricted to prevent further dilution of the blood. Medications include diuretics, demeclocycline to block action of ADH at the renal collecting tubules, and hypertonic saline IV fluids (Robinson & Verbalis, 2011; Shoback & Funk, 2011).

Nursing Management

Nursing care focuses on preventing injury, monitoring fluid balance, administering medications, and managing nutritional intake. Monitor intake and output, serum sodium, urine osmolality, and specific gravity. Educate the parents about the child's fluid restrictions and the hidden sources of water and fluids in foods to help avoid excessive fluid intake.

Teach the importance of checking weight daily and reporting weight gain, which may indicate fluid retention. Refer the family to a registered dietician to assist in identifying hidden sources of water and fluids, such as fruit-flavored ice pops, gelatin, watermelon, and citrus fruit, to prevent excessive fluid intake.

Depending on the cause of the disorder, lifelong medication may be required. If the child is prescribed demeclocycline, emphasize to the family the importance of follow-up care since the drug has nephrotoxic side effects. The child should wear a medical identification alert tag, bracelet, or necklace identifying the disorder and treatment.

Precocious Puberty

Precocious puberty is defined as the appearance of any secondary sexual characteristics before 8 years of age in girls (breast development or pubic hair) and 9 years of age in boys (pubic hair or genital development) (Bordini & Rosenfield, 2011).

Earlier than expected secretion of the normal hormones responsible for pubertal changes is not usually associated with an endocrine system abnormality (an idiopathic problem). External sources of hormones such as anabolic steroids or estrogen may be identified. Central precocious puberty or true precocious puberty occurs when the hypothalamus is activated to secrete gonadotropin-releasing hormone. Other potential causes of precocious puberty include tumors of the ovary or adrenal gland and a rare genetic condition known as McCune-Albright syndrome (Fuqua, 2013).

Isolated signs of premature sexual development such as **thelarche** (breast development), menarche (vaginal bleeding without other signs of sexual development), and **adrenarche** (development of pubic and axillary sexual hair) before 8 years of age in girls and 9 years in boys often needs no treatment.

Children with precocious puberty have an advanced bone age (premature skeletal maturation) and may appear unusually tall for their age. However, their growth ceases prematurely as the hormones stimulate closure of the epiphyseal plates, resulting in short stature. Behavioral changes may include mood swings and emotional lability.

Serum diagnostic studies include LH, FSH, testosterone, or estradiol. Provocative testing includes gonadotropin-releasing hormone (GnRH) stimulation to confirm the diagnosis. Radiologic imaging of the brain, as well as bone age tests, may be performed.

Treatment for central precocious puberty includes a GnRH analog to maintain a constant serum level of GnRH (Fuqua, 2013). Treatment often continues until a more normal age for puberty is reached (e.g., 11 years in girls and 12 years in boys). Simple monitoring of growth patterns may be the only intervention for children closer to the lower than expected age for puberty to begin. Tumors require surgery, radiation, and/or chemotherapy.

Nursing Management

Nursing care should focus on teaching the child and parents about the condition and its treatment, promoting growth, and providing emotional support. Inform the child in age-appropriate terms that the physiologic changes are normal but are occurring at an earlier than usual age. Reassure the child that friends will experience the same stages of development eventually. Emphasize to the family that the child's social, cognitive, and emotional development matches the child's age even though physical development is advanced.

Developing Cultural Competence Onset of Puberty

Differences exist by race in the onset of thelarche in girls of normal weight. Non-Hispanic African American girls and Mexican American girls normally undergo breast development during the seventh year, about 1 year earlier than non-Hispanic White girls (Bordini & Rosenfield, 2011).

Children with precocious puberty become self-conscious as body changes occur. Provide the child opportunities to express concerns and discuss issues related to body changes. The child may need to practice role-playing as a coping mechanism to manage teasing by other children. Partner with the family to encourage dressing the child in a manner appropriate to the child's chronologic age even though the child may look older. Provide privacy during physical examinations. Advise parents that they may need to discuss issues of sexuality with the child at an earlier age than normal. Refer the child and family for counseling if appropriate.

Teach the family proper medication administration and adherence to the treatment regimen. Determine the family's ability to financially manage the cost of treatment. Assistance in covering the cost of therapy may be available through pharmaceutical companies and third-party payers.

Disorders of Thyroid Function
Hypothyroidism

Hypothyroidism is a disorder in which levels of active thyroid hormones are decreased. It may be congenital or acquired. Congenital hypothyroidism occurs in approximately 1 in 3000 to 1 in 4000 live births worldwide (Seth & Maheshwari, 2013). It is twice as common in females as it is in males. In comparison to White infants, congenital hypothyroidism is less prevalent among Black infants but more prevalent in Hispanic, Asian American, Pacific Islander, and Native American infants (LaFranchi & Huang, 2016).

ETIOLOGY AND PATHOPHYSIOLOGY

Thyroid hormones are important for growth and development and for metabolizing nutrients and energy. When these hormones are not available to stimulate other hormones or specific target cells, growth is delayed and intellectual disability develops.

Congenital hypothyroidism is usually caused by a spontaneous gene mutation, an autosomal recessive genetic transmission of an enzyme deficiency, hypoplasia or aplasia of the thyroid gland, failure of the CNS–thyroid feedback mechanism to develop, or iodine deficiency. Intellectual disability is irreversible if the disorder is not treated.

Acquired hypothyroidism can be idiopathic or result from autoimmune thyroiditis (Hashimoto thyroiditis), late-onset thyroid dysfunction, isolated thyroid-stimulating hormone (TSH) deficiency caused by pituitary or hypothalamic dysfunction, or exposure to drugs or substances such as lithium that interfere with thyroid hormone synthesis. In the case of Hashimoto thyroiditis, the thyroid is infiltrated by lymphocytes that cause an autoimmune reaction and an enlarged thyroid. A genetic predisposition to autoimmune thyroiditis and an autosomal dominant inheritance of thyroid antibodies has been identified (LaFranchi & Huang, 2016).

CLINICAL MANIFESTATIONS

Infants with congenital hypothyroidism have few clinical signs of the disorder in the first weeks of life. Symptoms may include jaundice, thick tongue, hypotonia, umbilical hernia, hoarse cry, dry skin, constipation, and large fontanelles (Zeitler et al., 2014) (Figure 53–3).

Children with acquired hypothyroidism have many of the same signs as adults: decreased appetite; dry, cool skin; thinning hair or hair loss; depressed deep tendon reflexes; bradycardia; constipation; sensitivity to cold temperatures; abnormal menses; and a **goiter** (a nontender enlarged thyroid gland). Manifestations unique to children include change in past normal growth patterns with a weight increase, decreased height velocity, delayed bone and dental age, hypotonia with poor muscle tone, and delayed or precocious puberty.

CLINICAL THERAPY

Congenital hypothyroidism is usually detected during newborn screening, which is mandatory in all 50 states (National Newborn Screening and Genetics Resource Center, 2014). Newborn screening has greatly reduced the incidence of intellectual disability associated with this disorder (Shanholtz, 2013). A decreased T_4, normal T_3, and elevated thyroid-stimulating hormone level indicate hypothyroidism. An elevated TSH level indicates that the disease originated in the thyroid, not the pituitary. The two tests used to identify the disorder should occur: (1) before the newborn leaves the hospital, and (2) at the first healthcare visit at 1 to 2 weeks of age. Rapid response from the laboratory testing the samples is important to reduce the time to diagnosis and the effects of hypothyroidism on the infant's development.

Levothyroxine is the drug of choice for newborns with congenital hypothyroidism. The recommended starting dose is 10 to 15 mcg/kg per day (Zeitler et al., 2014). The dose is increased gradually as the child grows to ensure a **euthyroid** (thyroid hormones in appropriate balance) state. A pediatric endocrinologist monitors treatment. To ensure an adequate growth rate and prevent intellectual disability, the hormone must be taken throughout life. Periodic evaluation of T_4 and TSH serum levels, bone age, and growth parameters is necessary to assess for signs of excess or inadequate thyroid hormone.

Antithyroid antibodies are measured in children with a goiter and suspected Hashimoto thyroiditis because increased titers of antithyroglobulin and antimicrosomal antibodies are often found.

Children with congenital hypothyroidism that are diagnosed before 3 months of age have the best prognosis for optimal mental development. Children with acquired hypothyroidism usually have normal growth following a period of catch-up growth. Many adolescents with Hashimoto thyroiditis have a spontaneous remission.

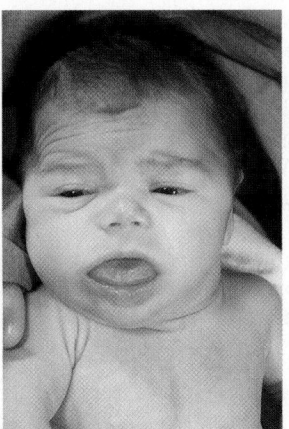

Figure 53–3 **Child with congenital hypothyroidism.**
SOURCE: Mediscan/Alamy.

Nursing Management

For the Child With Hypothyroidism

Nursing Assessment and Diagnosis

Routine neonatal screening is performed before discharge from the hospital and is often repeated at the infant's first health visit to evaluate levels of circulating thyroid hormones (see the *Clinical Skills Manual* SKILLS).

Record the length or height and weight at each follow-up visit and plot on a growth curve. The child is assessed for signs of inadequate growth to determine if the dose of thyroid hormone needs to be adjusted and to monitor compliance with medication. Conduct developmental screening to detect delays in developmental milestones.

Among the nursing diagnoses that might be appropriate for the child with hypothyroidism are the following (NANDA-I © 2014):

- *Development: Delayed, Risk for,* related to delayed initiation of thyroid replacement therapy
- *Growth: Disproportionate, Risk for,* related to poor adherence to thyroid hormone therapy
- *Body Image, Disturbed,* related to physical changes associated with condition
- *Fatigue* related to inadequate dose of thyroid medication

Planning and Implementation

Nursing care focuses on teaching the parents and child about the disorder and its treatment and monitoring the child's growth rate. Explain how to administer thyroid hormone (e.g., tablets can be crushed and mixed in a small amount of formula or applesauce as long as the child gets all of the medication). Advise parents that the child may experience temporary sleep disturbances or behavioral changes in response to therapy. Teach the parents how to assess for an increased pulse rate, which could indicate the presence of too much thyroid hormone, and advise them to report problems such as fatigue, which could indicate an improper drug dose that needs to be adjusted.

Caution parents to dress the child appropriately for the season to prevent hypothermia. Modify the child's diet by increasing the amount of fruits and bulk if constipation is a problem.

Reassure the family that the child has the best chance of normal development when the hormone replacement therapy is given as prescribed. Reinforce the importance of follow-up visits to assess growth rate and response to therapy and to regulate drug dosages as the child grows. Periodic assessments of educational achievement are needed. Even with good control, adolescents have persistent visual-spatial deficits and memory and attention problems. Parents should be informed that therapy will be lifelong and is needed to promote the child's mental development. When the cause is genetic, make a referral for genetic counseling.

Evaluation

Expected outcomes of nursing care of the child with hypothyroidism include the following:

- The child maintains adequate growth of height and weight, following a percentile curve throughout childhood.
- The child's diet contains adequate fruits and bulk to prevent constipation.
- The child's cognitive development is appropriate for age.

Hyperthyroidism

Hyperthyroidism occurs when thyroid hormone levels are increased, resulting in excessive levels of circulating thyroid hormones. Graves disease is the most common cause of hyperthyroidism in children, occurring more often in females and in children ages 11 to 15 years (Gastaldi et al., 2014).

ETIOLOGY AND PATHOPHYSIOLOGY

Graves disease is an autoimmune disorder. Immunoglobulins produced by the B lymphocytes stimulate oversecretion of thyroid hormones, resulting in the clinical symptoms. It has a high familial incidence.

Other less common causes of hyperthyroidism result from thyroiditis and thyroid hormone–producing tumors, including thyroid adenomas and carcinomas, and pituitary adenomas. Congenital hyperthyroidism can occur in infants of mothers with Graves disease as a result of transplacental transfer of immunoglobulins. This condition generally resolves by 6 to 12 weeks of age but can last longer (Huang & LaFranchi, 2016).

CLINICAL MANIFESTATIONS

Signs and symptoms are caused by hyperactivity of the sympathetic nervous system and may include an enlarged, nontender thyroid gland (goiter), prominent or bulging eyes (**exophthalmos**) (Figure 53–4), eyelid lag, tachycardia, nervousness, increased appetite with weight loss, emotional lability, moodiness, heat intolerance, hypertension, hyperactivity, irregular menses, insomnia, tremor, and muscle weakness (Bauer, 2011; Gastaldi et al., 2014). The thyroid gland may be slightly enlarged or grow to 3 to 4 times its normal size; feel warm, soft, and fleshy; and have an auditory bruit on auscultation. Onset is subtle, and the condition often goes unrecognized for 1 to 2 years.

Children with Graves disease usually have difficulty concentrating, behavioral problems, and declining performance in school. They become easily frustrated in the classroom and overheated and fatigued during physical education class. Children with this disorder find it difficult to relax or sleep. These symptoms usually prompt parents to seek medical treatment for the child.

The most serious complication of hyperthyroidism is severe **thyrotoxicosis**, also called *thyroid crisis* or *thyroid storm*. It is a life-threatening emergency resulting from extreme hyperthyroidism, in which elevated circulating levels of TH result in

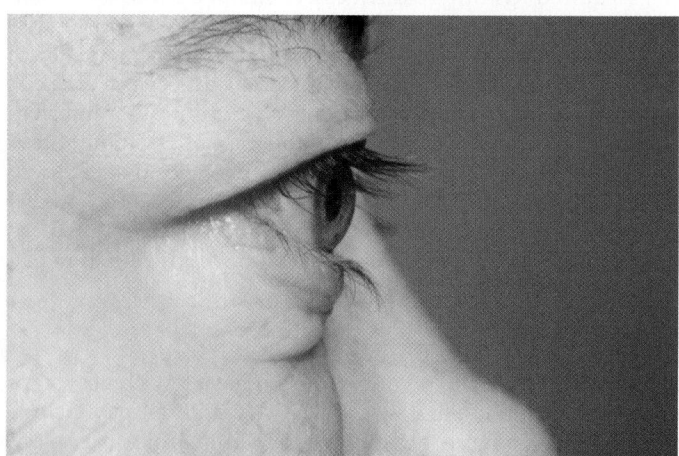

Figure 53–4 **Exophthalmos and an enlarged thyroid in an adolescent with Graves disease.**

SOURCE: Biophoto Associates/Science Source.

a hypermetabolic state. Symptoms include muscle weakness, diaphoresis, tachycardia, tremor, palpitations, diarrhea, irritability, nervousness, and anxiety (Bahn et al., 2011; Bauer, 2011; Fitzgerald, 2015).

CLINICAL THERAPY

Diagnostic studies include laboratory evaluation of serum TSH, T_3, and T_4 levels and a thyroid scan. T_3 and T_4 levels are markedly elevated, whereas the TSH level is decreased. Serum studies are also performed to detect thyroid autoantibodies anti-TG (anti-thyroglobulin) and anti-TPO (antiperoxidase), usually present in Graves disease and Hashimoto thyroiditis. A thyroid scan is performed to identify nodules or to confirm the high uptake of radioactive iodine associated with Graves disease.

The goal of clinical therapy is to inhibit excessive secretion of thyroid hormones. Treatment may include medication therapy, radiation therapy, or surgery. Medication therapy is most often the initial treatment, but compliance is often a problem because of side effects. Methimazole (Tapazole) and propylthiouracil (PTU) are antithyroid drugs that are used in children with hyperthyroidism. Because of the concern for severe liver disease with the administration of PTU, current recommendations are that children with hyperthyroidism receive methimazole instead (Bauer, 2011; Huang & LaFranchi, 2016; Rivkees, 2014).

Symptoms usually improve within weeks of starting treatment. Adjunct therapy with beta-adrenergic blocking agents such as propranolol or atenolol may be administered to relieve symptoms of tremors, tachycardia, lid lag, and excessive sweating (Bahn et al., 2011; Huang & LaFranchi, 2016).

Less than 30% of children achieve remission after a 2-year course of treatment with medication. Radiation therapy or thyroidectomy are other options if medication therapy is not effective (Leger et al., 2012). Thyroidectomy (removal of most of the thyroid) provides an immediate cure and avoids radiation and possible long-term complications of radioactive iodine. Removal of the thyroid gland results in hypothyroidism. Complications of thyroidectomy include hemorrhage, hypocalcemia, and damage to the laryngeal nerve paresis (Rivkees, 2014).

Nursing Management

For the Child With Hyperthyroidism

Nursing Assessment and Diagnosis

Assess the child's vital signs, as blood pressure and pulse may be elevated. Keep a record of food intake. Accurate measurement and recording of height and weight are important to establish baselines and identify patterns of growth. Observe the child's behavior, activity, and level of fatigue.

Common nursing diagnoses for the child with hyperthyroidism include the following (NANDA-I © 2014):

- *Thermoregulation, Ineffective,* related to illness and excessive activity of the sympathetic nervous system
- *Nutrition, Imbalanced: Less than Body Requirements,* related to high metabolic needs
- *Body Image, Disturbed,* related to physical changes caused by illness (prominent eyes, excessive perspiration, and tremors)
- *Fatigue* related to hypermetabolic state and sleep deprivation

Planning and Implementation

Nursing care focuses on teaching the child and parents about the disorder and its treatment, promoting rest, providing emotional support, and, if the child needs surgery, providing preoperative and postoperative teaching and care. Promote increased caloric intake by providing five or six moderate meals per day. Encourage the child and family to express their feelings and concerns about the disorder. Pointing out even slight improvements in the child's condition increases adherence with therapy.

Children with hyperthyroidism are easily fatigued. Rest periods should be scheduled at school and home and physical activities kept to a minimum until symptoms resolve. Encourage parents to provide a cool environment and allow the child to wear fewer clothes until symptoms subside.

Children who have partial or total removal of the thyroid gland receive antithyroid drugs, such as iodine, for approximately 2 weeks before surgery to reduce the vascularity and size of the thyroid gland and to decrease the risk of thyroid storm.

Teach the child and parents about drug therapy and instruct parents to watch for side effects of antithyroid drugs, including fever, urticaria, and lymphadenopathy. Provide preoperative teaching (see Chapter 39). Young children in particular may be fearful about having their throat "cut."

Postoperatively, elevate the head of bed to 30 degrees to promote patent airway. A tracheostomy kit, suction supplies, and IV calcium gluconate should be immediately available for emergency treatment of hypocalcemia and respiratory distress. If thyroidectomy is performed, thyrotoxicosis develops, and it does not immediately resolve because the half-life of T_4 is 7 to 8 days. Antithyroid medications should be slowly tapered (Sharma, 2014).

Teach the family about the need for lifelong thyroid hormone replacement if radiation or surgery is performed. The child should wear a medical alert identification bracelet, tag, or necklace. Make sure the child is monitored regularly to ensure that the T_4 level is adequate to sustain growth.

Evaluation

Expected outcomes of nursing care for the child with hyperthyroidism include the following:

- The child achieves balanced thermoregulation.
- The child participates in daily activities without experiencing fatigue.
- The child demonstrates a positive body image.

Disorders of the Parathyroid

Children usually have four parathyroid glands located posterior to the thyroid gland. Their primary function is to work in conjunction with vitamin D to regulate total body calcium.

Hyperparathyroidism

Primary hyperparathyroidism, rare during childhood, may result from a tumor (adenoma) or hyperplasia (Doyle, 2016a). Secondary hyperparathyroidism is due to disease outside of the parathyroid gland, leading to excessive secretion of parathyroid hormone. This is commonly seen in chronic renal failure when the kidneys are unable to reabsorb calcium, causing low serum calcium levels and stimulating continual secretion of parathyroid hormone (Kemper & van Husen, 2014). See Chapter 52.

At any age, symptoms of primary hyperparathyroidism may include bone pain, nephrolithiasis (kidney stones), and pathologic bone fractures. For primary hyperparathyroidism, unilateral surgical parathyroid exploration is recommended to remove the affected gland and biopsy the other gland on the same side. If bilateral disease is suspected, both sides are explored surgically (Belcher, Metrailer, Bodenner, et al., 2013). Treatment of secondary hyperparathyroidism focuses on prevention of hypercalcemia using vitamin D replacement and phosphorus binders (Kemper & van Husen, 2014).

Nursing Management

Nursing care centers on fluid management and electrolyte monitoring. In children who require surgery, assess for respiratory distress and a potential airway obstruction due to edema and a potential hematoma around the tracheal space. Monitor for signs of infection.

Following surgery, educate the child and parents to recognize signs of hypocalcemia and to provide appropriate amounts of calcium supplementation. After diagnosis or after surgical intervention, follow-up is important to monitor serum calcium and phosphorus levels to detect persistence of hyperparathyroidism.

Hypoparathyroidism

Primary hypoparathyroidism is rare, but it may result from congenital disorders (parathyroid aplasia, DiGeorge syndrome), surgical removal of the parathyroid glands (e.g., parathyroid adenoma, thyroidectomy), disease processes that destroy the parathyroid glands (Wilson disease, hemochromatosis), or medications (e.g., aluminum, asparagine, doxorubicin, cytosine, and arabinoside). Hypoparathyroidism can also be idiopathic. The primary result is hypocalcemia and hyperphosphatemia.

Infants may display hyperirritability, muscle rigidity, seizures, vomiting, abdominal distention, apneic episodes, intermittent cyanosis, or twitching. Muscle pain and cramps may progress to numbness, stiffness, and tingling of the hands and feet. A positive **Chvostek sign** (spasm of facial muscles after tapping facial nerve) may be present. Tetany and convulsions may occur with hypocalcemia (Doyle, 2016b).

Serum calcium and PTH levels are low and serum phosphorus is elevated. Radiographs often demonstrate increased bone density. Oral calcitriol and calcium are prescribed. Foods with high phosphorus content (dairy products and eggs) are limited (Doyle, 2016b).

Nursing Management

Assess and stabilize the airway, breathing, and circulation. In the acute care setting, children should be placed on a cardiorespiratory monitor. Maintain seizure precautions until normal serum calcium levels are attained. Obtain intravenous access and administer calcium supplementation as ordered.

SAFETY ALERT!
Dilute intravenous calcium per hospital protocol. Infiltration of IV calcium can cause extravasation and tissue sloughing. Always check the patency of the IV prior to administration. Monitor ECG during administration. Evaluate for hypocalcemia and hypercalcemia after administration.

Partner with the family to ensure their understanding of the need for calcium supplementation and reduced intake of phosphorus. Teach the family that periodic monitoring of calcium levels is important. Inform the family that hypoparathyroidism may require lifelong therapy.

Disorders of Adrenal Function
Cushing Syndrome and Cushing Disease

Cushing syndrome, also called *adrenocortical hyperfunction*, is characterized by a group of symptoms resulting from excess blood levels of glucocorticoids (especially cortisol). The most common cause of Cushing syndrome is the prolonged administration of glucocorticoid hormones (White, 2016a). Cushing disease is a type of Cushing syndrome and is caused by a pituitary tumor (Shah & Lila, 2011). During infancy most cases of endogenous Cushing disease are caused by a functioning adrenocortical tumor. The most common cause of endogenous Cushing syndrome in children older than 7 years of age is Cushing disease in which a pituitary tumor (adenoma) secretes excessive ACTH. This leads to bilateral adrenal hyperplasia (White, 2016a). The remainder of this discussion will focus on the child with Cushing syndrome caused by a pituitary tumor (Cushing disease). See *Clinical Tip* and *Safety Alert!* for discussions of Cushing syndrome caused by corticosteroid administration.

Clinical Tip

Cushingoid features occur most often in children receiving high doses of corticosteroids or corticosteroids over a prolonged period of time. Cushingoid features may develop in a shorter time than occurs with Cushing disease. Corticosteroids suppress adrenal function when administered long term. These children have exogenous Cushing syndrome and are at increased risk of hypertension, hyperglycemia, weight gain, linear growth retardation, and fractures (White, 2016a). These children may also exhibit mood swings and are at increased risk for infection (Wilson, Shannon, & Shields, 2016).

SAFETY ALERT!
Caution should be exercised with the use of topical steroid creams in children. Cases of exogenous Cushing syndrome have been reported with the prolonged use of these agents in the treatment of diaper dermatitis in infants and young children (Ho, Loke, Lim, et al., 2014).

Obesity is common in children with Cushing syndrome. Excessive weight gain is followed by slowed linear growth. The child develops the characteristic cushingoid features, which include a rounded (moon) face with prominent cheeks. Additional manifestations include hirsutism, acne, deepening of the voice, and hypertension (White, 2016a). Older children may also experience delayed puberty, irregular menstrual periods, headaches, weakness, pathologic fractures, emotional problems, and hyperglycemia (Pluta, Burke, & Golub, 2011; White, 2016a).

Diagnosis is based on characteristic physical findings and laboratory values, including increased 24-hour urinary levels of free cortisol and elevated nighttime salivary cortisol level. The child will also have an abnormal glucose tolerance test (White, 2016a). See Appendix B for laboratory values.

The adrenal-suppression test using an 11 p.m. dose of dexamethasone reveals that adrenal cortisol output is not suppressed overnight as would occur normally in children. Computed tomography (CT) and magnetic resonance imaging (MRI) are used to detect the specific location of tumors in the adrenal and pituitary glands.

Surgical removal of the pituitary adenoma is the current treatment of choice when this is the cause of Cushing syndrome. Irradiation of the pituitary is performed when surgical removal of the adenoma does not substantially reduce cortisol levels. Bilateral removal of the adrenal glands may be necessary in some cases to stop the excessive secretion of cortisol. Lifelong hormone replacement is required when both adrenal glands are removed (Pluta et al., 2011; White, 2016a).

Nursing Management

Nursing assessment includes monitoring the child's vital signs, fluid status, nutritional status, and weight. Additional assessment includes monitoring muscle strength and endurance during hospital play activities.

Teach the child and family about the disorder and its treatment. For children undergoing surgery, provide preoperative and postoperative teaching and care. Answer any questions the child and family may have and explain all laboratory and diagnostic tests. Explain to parents that the child's cushingoid appearance is reversible with treatment. Refer to Chapter 50 for general nursing care of the child with cancer. Provide nutritional guidance or refer the child and parents to a registered dietician to promote maintenance of an appropriate weight. Encourage the child to discuss feelings regarding changes in physical appearance. Assist the child and family to identify effective coping strategies.

For children who need cortisol replacement therapy following the surgical removal of both adrenal glands, administering the medication early in the morning or every other day causes fewer symptoms and mimics the normal diurnal pattern of cortisol secretion. Cortisol replacement in the postoperative period must be explained carefully to the parents. Hydrocortisone (Cortef, Solu-Cortef, cortisone acetate) is available in liquid, tablet, or injectable form. Parents may need to crush the tablet and mix with a small amount of applesauce, but the entire dose of medication must be taken. The oral preparations of cortisone have a bitter taste and can cause gastric irritation. Giving the dose at mealtimes and using antacids between meals help reduce these side effects. Teach parents how and when to administer the injectable form—usually when the child is vomiting, has diarrhea, or cannot take the oral medication. Failure to give medication when the child is ill may lead to severe illness and cardiovascular collapse.

Congenital Adrenal Hyperplasia

Congenital adrenal hyperplasia (CAH) is an autosomal recessive disorder occurring in 1 in 10,000 to 1 in 20,000 births (Boyse, Gardner, Marvicsin, et al., 2014). CAH is considered to be an inborn error of metabolism.

ETIOLOGY AND PATHOPHYSIOLOGY

Approximately 90% to 95% of children with congenital adrenal hyperplasia have a deficiency in 21-hydroxylase (Hird, Tetlow, Tobi, et al., 2015). Children with CAH have insufficient production of aldosterone and cortisol and an overproduction of androgen (Boyse et al., 2014; Hird et al., 2015).

Of the two classic forms of the disorder, 75% are salt-losing, caused by aldosterone deficiency and overproduction of androgen, and 25% are non–salt-losing with **virilization** (the production of masculine secondary sexual characteristics in females). In all forms, increased secretion of ACTH occurs in response to diminished cortisol levels (Nimkarn, Lin-Su, & New, 2011).

During fetal development the lack of cortisol triggers the pituitary to continue secretion of ACTH. This in turn stimulates overproduction of the adrenal androgens. Virilization of the female external genitalia begins in week 10 of gestation. If untreated, the overproduction of androgens results in accelerated height, early closure of the epiphyseal plates, and premature sexual development with both pubic and axillary hair.

CLINICAL MANIFESTATIONS

Congenital adrenal hyperplasia is the most common cause of **pseudohermaphroditism** (ambiguous genitalia) in newborn girls (see Figure 53–5). The female baby is born with an enlarged clitoris and partial or complete labial fusion. Females who are severely virilized may be mistaken for males with cryptorchidism, hypospadias, or micropenis (see Chapter 52). The uterus, ovaries, and fallopian tubes are normal. The male newborn may look normal at birth or may have a slightly enlarged penis and hyperpigmented scrotum. The boy may have tall stature and an adult-sized penis by school age, but the testes are appropriately sized for age. Partial enzyme deficiency produces less obvious symptoms. Precocious puberty, tall stature for age, acne, and excessive muscle development may be noted in both males and females as the child grows. As a result of early epiphyseal fusion, adult stature is shorter.

Signs of adrenal insufficiency may be the first indication of the disorder. Recurrent vomiting, dehydration, weakness, metabolic acidosis, hypotension, hypoglycemia, hyponatremia, and

---

TEACHING HIGHLIGHTS | Hydrocortisone Administration

Teach the family the following tips regarding hydrocortisone administration:

- Always give the medication at the times prescribed since the schedule follows the body's normal cortisol release pattern.
- Never abruptly discontinue the medication.
- Have the child wear a medical alert ID.
- If the child has vomiting or diarrhea and is unable to take the medication by mouth, administer the injections to replace oral doses as instructed and notify the healthcare provider immediately. Higher doses of hydrocortisone are needed when the child is ill.
- Always have injectable hydrocortisone available at home, at school, and everywhere the child travels. An emergency kit should be available at all times to supply cortisol to the child during acute illnesses and stressful situations. Check expiration dates frequently and maintain current medications in the emergency kit.

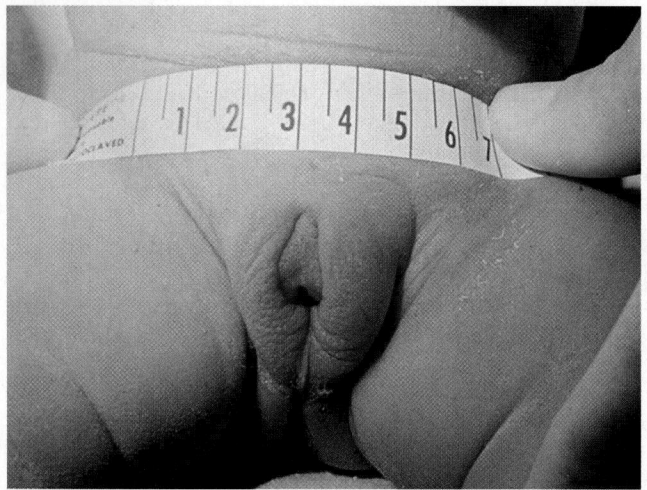

Figure 53–5 Newborn girl with ambiguous genitalia.

SOURCE: Courtesy of Patrick C. Walsh, MD.

hyperkalemia are characteristic signs of the salt-wasting form of the disorder (White, 2016b).

CLINICAL THERAPY

Diagnosis in infants and children is usually confirmed by laboratory evaluation of the serum 17-hydroxyprogesterone (17-OHP) level (Hird et al., 2015). Routine newborn screening for congenital adrenal hyperplasia is performed in all 50 states (National Newborn Screening and Genetics Resource Center, 2014). Prenatal diagnosis is available. In instances of ambiguous genitalia, a karyotype determines the infant's gender (see Chapter 3). Ultrasonography may be used to visualize pelvic structures.

In the salt-wasting form of the disorder, the child may have hyponatremia, hyperkalemia, acidosis, hypoglycemia, a high urine sodium level, and low serum and urinary aldosterone levels. Serum concentrations of testosterone in girls and androstenedione in boys and girls are elevated in affected infants. Measurement of ACTH and 17-hydroxyprogesterone levels reveals high readings, while the serum cortisol level is inappropriately low in comparison to ACTH (White, 2016b).

The goal of treatment is to suppress adrenal secretion of androgens by replacing deficient hormones. This is accomplished by the lifelong use of oral glucocorticoids (dexamethasone, prednisone, or hydrocortisone). The glucocorticoid replacement reduces secretion of ACTH, which had overstimulated the adrenal cortex. As a result, excessive adrenal androgen production is suppressed. The dose is individualized by monitoring growth parameters, bone age, and hormone levels. If the infant has the salt-wasting form of the disorder, salt is added to the infant's formula, and a mineralocorticoid is given to replace the missing hormone. Hormone dosage must be doubled or tripled during acute illnesses or injury and for surgery. Injectable hydrocortisone is used for severe stress. Generally, there are no side effects to the hormone; however, elevated doses can result in hypertension and growth impairment. Adrenalectomy is recommended only in cases when medical therapy is ineffective (Sharma & Seth, 2014; White, 2016b).

Reconstructive surgery of the enlarged clitoris is often performed on girls during the first year of life; however, some centers support waiting until adolescence, allowing the girl to participate in the decision for surgery.

Nursing Management
For the Child With Congenital Adrenal Hyperplasia

Nursing Assessment and Diagnosis

Assess the infant and child for signs of dehydration, electrolyte imbalance, and hypovolemic shock in the salt-wasting form of the disease (see the *Clinical Skills Manual* SKILLS). Monitor the airway, breathing, circulation, and responsiveness. Assess vital signs and peripheral perfusion (capillary refill, distal pulses, color and temperature of the extremities) frequently to detect early changes in condition such as hypovolemia.

Assess the parents' emotional response to a child with ambiguous genitalia and a chronic condition. Explore their values and beliefs regarding gender roles and sexuality while awaiting results of the karyotype.

Nursing diagnoses for the child with congenital adrenal hyperplasia might include the following (NANDA-I © 2014):

- *Parenting, Impaired,* related to a child with undetermined gender identity
- *Caregiver Role Strain* related to care of a child with a chronic, potentially life-threatening condition
- *Fluid Volume: Deficient, Risk for,* related to failure of regulatory mechanisms and excess excretion of salt by the kidneys
- *Growth: Disproportionate, Risk for,* related to accelerated growth and premature closure of epiphyseal plates

Planning and Implementation

Nursing care of the newborn with CAH focuses on teaching parents about the disorder and its treatment, offering emotional support, and providing preoperative and postoperative teaching for parents of infants undergoing reconstructive surgery. The administration of glucocorticoids and mineralocorticoids must be carefully controlled.

It is often difficult for parents to accept that their infant, whose genitalia look male, is really female. Reassure parents that with medication and surgery, the genitalia assume a female appearance and all organs necessary for future childbearing are usually functional. Several surgeries may be performed before 2 years of age and then during adolescence to dilate the vagina. Because of the risk for adrenal insufficiency, the child will most likely be hospitalized for surgery rather than having outpatient surgery.

Nurses can assist parents in educating the child's siblings, grandparents, other family members, and childcare workers about the condition. In the newborn nursery, the infant should be referred to as "your beautiful infant," not "your son" or "your daughter," until gender identity is confirmed.

Inform parents that genetic counseling should be provided for the child during adolescence. Inform parents considering a future pregnancy that prenatal testing may detect congenital adrenal hyperplasia in the fetus. Refer the family for counseling if indicated.

COMMUNITY-BASED NURSING CARE

Teach parents about the special problems that develop in the salt-wasting form of the disease during acute illness. Explain the medication regimen and help the family develop an emergency care plan. The child should wear a medical alert identification. Teach parents how to administer intramuscular injections of hydrocortisone. If injectable hydrocortisone is not available, the child needs urgent treatment in an emergency department. The child may become dehydrated quickly and need intravenous fluid and electrolyte replacement in addition to higher doses of hydrocortisone.

Evaluation

Expected outcomes of nursing care for congenital adrenal hyperplasia include the following:

- Parent–newborn attachment is achieved.
- The child maintains fluid volume balance.
- The child achieves age-appropriate growth and developmental milestones.
- The parents demonstrate understanding of treatment and respond appropriately when injectable medication is needed.

Adrenal Insufficiency (Addison Disease)

Adrenal insufficiency, also known as *Addison disease*, is a rare disorder in childhood characterized by a deficiency of glucocorticoids (cortisone) and mineralocorticoids (aldosterone). The lack of glucocorticoids affects the body's ability to handle stress. The majority of cases of Addison disease are caused by an autoimmune process. Other causes include infection, hemorrhage, medication use, and metastatic cancer (Michels & Michels, 2014).

Adrenal insufficiency usually develops slowly as the adrenal glands deteriorate. Symptoms generally worsen over a period of years. The early signs may not be noticed initially but include weakness, fatigue, weight loss, and gastrointestinal symptoms such as nausea, vomiting, diarrhea, constipation, and abdominal pain. Other symptoms include hyperpigmentation, hypotension, dizziness, joint pain, salt cravings, and hypoglycemia (Michels & Michels, 2014; National Endocrine and Metabolic Diseases Information Service, 2014).

CLINICAL THERAPY

The ACTH stimulation test is used to determine if the levels of cortisol are adequate. Serum cortisol is measured in the early morning. Low levels of serum cortisol are associated with adrenal insufficiency. The diagnostic workup also includes a complete blood count, serum electrolytes, and thyroid function tests. Hyponatremia and hyperkalemia are common in Addison disease. A CT scan may be used to visualize the adrenal glands (Ficorelli, 2013).

Treatment involves replacement of the deficient hormones with an oral glucocorticoid such as hydrocortisone, prednisone, or dexamethasone. Fludrocortisone acetate (Florinef), a mineralocorticoid, is given for aldosterone deficiency (Ficorelli, 2013).

Adrenal crisis (also called *Addisonian crisis* and *acute adrenal insufficiency*) may be caused by stressors such as infection, surgery, trauma, vomiting, and diarrhea. Noncompliance with the treatment plan may also be a precipitating factor (Ficorelli, 2013). The crisis is treated with aggressive fluid resuscitation, intravenous glucose, and intravenous glucocorticoids such as hydrocortisone. Children will also need increased doses of steroids during periods of increased physiologic stress, such as surgery, stressful procedures, and febrile illnesses. In these cases, the dose of hydrocortisone should be tripled and given every 6 to 8 hours while the stressor is present. Injectable hydrocortisone should always be available in case the child is vomiting or unable to take oral fluids (Speiser & Wilson, 2015).

Nursing Management

Nursing management focuses on restoring hemodynamic homeostasis in the child with Addison disease who is acutely ill. Educating the child and parents about the disorder, providing emotional support, and caring for the child during acute episodes are other aspects of nursing management. See the earlier discussion of congenital adrenal hyperplasia for further detail.

Pheochromocytoma

Pheochromocytoma is a tumor that arises from the adrenal gland. Tumors that are extra-adrenal with no anatomic connection are called *paragangliomas* (Mishra, Mehrotra, Agarwal, et al., 2014). In most cases, these tumors are benign and curable. They can occur in a familial pattern (autosomal dominant trait) with a male-to-female ratio of 3:2. Most tumors diagnosed in children are identified between the ages of 6 and 14 years; however, this only accounts for 10% of these tumors as most are identified during adult years (White, 2016c). Pheochromocytomas may also be associated with neurofibromatosis (see Chapter 54).

The tumor causes an excessive release of catecholamines. Clinical manifestations include hypertension, palpitations, sweating, anxiety, tremors, and headache for those with symptomatic pheochromocytoma. Twenty to 30% of these tumors are detected incidentally without a history of symptoms (Shuch, Ricketts, Metwalli, et al., 2014)

CLINICAL THERAPY

Diagnosis is based on biochemical studies measuring catecholamines in the blood and urine. Radiologic imaging with CT or MRI is used to provide the location of the tumor.

The treatment of choice is curative surgical removal of all identified tumors; however, the procedure is dangerous and may result in pheochromocytoma crisis. Removal of the tumor during surgery may cause a release of stored epinephrine and norepinephrine, leading to elevated blood pressure and changes in heart rate (pheochromocytoma crisis). If this occurs, alpha-adrenergic blocking agents are administered.

Medications to control hypertension, tachycardia, and catecholamine release are given for 7 to 21 days before surgery (Tsirlin, Oo, Sharma, et al., 2014). Plasma catecholamines are used to measure the effectiveness of the preoperative adrenergic blockade. Postoperatively, for several days, a 24-hour urine collection is measured for catecholamines to determine if all tumor sites were removed. With successful removal of all tumor sites, the prognosis is generally good. Follow-up is important to assess for recurrence.

Nursing Management

Nursing care is mainly supportive. Provide preoperative and postoperative teaching and care (see Chapter 39). Preoperatively, monitor vital signs and observe for signs of complications associated with pheochromocytoma crisis. Administer antihypertensives and watch for any signs of hyperglycemia, as discussed later in this chapter. Postoperatively, the child may be managed initially in an intensive care unit. Monitor blood pressure and glucose levels. Hypoglycemia and hypotension may occur following the withdrawal of excessive amounts of catecholamines. Observe for changes in neurologic status, respiratory distress, and signs of shock. Lifelong follow-up care with screening for hypertension and increased urinary catecholamine levels is required as symptoms recur if the child has other tumors not yet detected that activate at a later age (Tsirlin et al., 2014; White, 2016c).

Disorders of Pancreatic Function

Diabetes Mellitus

Diabetes mellitus, the most common metabolic disease in children, is a disorder of hyperglycemia resulting from defects in insulin secretion, insulin action, or both, leading to abnormalities in carbohydrate, protein, and fat metabolism (American Diabetes Association [ADA], 2014a). There are two main types of diabetes. Most children have immune-mediated type 1 diabetes, formerly called *insulin-dependent diabetes* mellitus or *juvenile diabetes*.

Type 1 Diabetes

In the United States, approximately 1 in every 400 to 600 children and adolescents have type 1 diabetes (Monaghan, Hoffman, & Cogen, 2013). According to the SEARCH for Diabetes in Youth Study, an estimated 18,436 people less than 20 years of age were diagnosed during 2008 to 2009. Non-Hispanic White children and adolescents had a higher incidence of new-onset type 1 diabetes than other groups (Centers for Disease Control and Prevention [CDC], 2014).

ETIOLOGY AND PATHOPHYSIOLOGY

Type 1 diabetes results from destruction of pancreatic islet beta cells, which fail to secrete insulin. The body becomes dependent on exogenous sources of insulin. Type 1 diabetes is a multifactorial disease caused by autoimmune destruction of insulin-producing pancreatic beta cells in individuals who are genetically predisposed (ADA, 2014a).

Type 1 diabetes has familial tendencies but does not show any specific pattern of inheritance. The number of autoantibodies helps predict the risk of developing type 1 diabetes. For children with one antibody, the risk is only 10% to 15%, while those with three or more antibodies have a risk of 55% to 90% (Marcdante & Kliegman, 2015). The child inherits a susceptibility to the disease rather than the disease itself. It is believed that an event such as a virus or other environmental factors trigger the inflammatory process, resulting in development of islet cell serum antibodies. These antibodies can be detected in the blood months to years before the onset of beta cell destruction (Marcdante & Kliegman, 2015).

Insulin helps transport glucose into the cells so that the body can use it as an energy source. It also prevents the outflow of glucose from the liver to the general circulation. Environmental factors such as enteroviruses or toxins are believed to lead to an autoimmune destruction of the beta cells in the islets of Langerhans (see *Pathophysiology Illustrated: Mechanism of Diabetes Mellitus*). Antigens are generated, leading to production of antibodies that indicate ongoing destruction of the islet cells. Chronic immune-mediated destruction of the beta cells continues over a period of time. Symptoms of type 1 diabetes are evident when approximately 90% of the beta cells have been destroyed (Craig et al., 2014)

As the secretion of insulin decreases, the blood glucose level rises and the glucose level inside the cells decreases. When the renal threshold for glucose (180 mg/dL) is exceeded, **glycosuria** (abnormal amount of glucose in the urine) occurs as a result of osmotic diuresis (Svoren & Jospe, 2016). Fluids follow the highly osmotic glucose and water is excreted in large volumes of urine (polyuria).

When glucose is unavailable to the cells for metabolism, free fatty acids provide an alternate source of energy. The liver metabolizes fatty acids at an increased rate, producing acetyl coenzyme A (CoA). The by-products of acetyl CoA metabolism (ketone bodies) accumulate in the body, resulting in a state of metabolic acidosis, or ketoacidosis. (Refer to Chapter 44 for a discussion of metabolic acidosis.)

CLINICAL MANIFESTATIONS

Children with type 1 diabetes generally present with polyuria, polydipsia, and weight loss. **Polyphagia** (excessive appetite) may be present. Enuresis may also occur in a previously toilet-trained child (Craig et al., 2014). The child may also present with a history of fatigue (Table 53–4). Children with new-onset diabetes may present with diabetic ketoacidosis (DKA). The prevalence varies but is higher in children less than 5 years of age with a reported incidence of 17.3% to 54.5% in that age group (Larsson et al., 2011). Other investigators report an overall incidence of DKA in youth at the time of diagnosis as being 15% to 67% (Szypowska & Skora, 2011). See the following *Clinical Tip* for information about cystic fibrosis–related diabetes.

Clinical Tip

Cystic fibrosis–related diabetes (CFRD) has similar features of types 1 and 2 diabetes; however, it is considered to be a separate condition. In cystic fibrosis, the pancreas is scarred and does not produce sufficient insulin (as in type 1 diabetes), which is referred to as **insulin deficiency**. Another mechanism of CFRD is **insulin resistance**, an impairment in insulin receptors on cell membranes, leading to inability to transfer sufficient amounts of glucose into cells, requiring higher levels of insulin for metabolism. Insulin deficiency and insulin resistance combined can lead to the development of diabetes more frequently in these patients than in the general population (Cystic Fibrosis Foundation, 2012).

CLINICAL THERAPY

Diagnosis is based on the presence of classic symptoms and one of the following plasma glucose levels (ADA, 2014a, p. S88; 2014b, p. S15):

- A_{1c} greater than or equal to 6.5%
- Fasting plasma glucose greater than or equal to 126 mg/dL (7 mmol/L), no caloric intake for at least 8 hours
- Two-hour plasma glucose greater than or equal to 200 mg/dL (11.1 mmol/L) during an oral glucose tolerance test
- Random plasma glucose concentration greater than or equal to 200 mg/dL (11.1 mmol/L) in a patient with classic symptoms of hyperglycemia

When an asymptomatic child's screening test reveals an elevated glucose level, confirmation of a second fasting plasma glucose level should be performed. An oral glucose tolerance test is rarely required. Other laboratory tests for known autoantibodies can indicate an autoimmune attack against the insulin-producing beta cells of the pancreas, and may be helpful in some cases to distinguish between types 1 and 2 diabetes. Plasma C-peptide levels are low or undetectable in type 1 diabetes, indicating little or no insulin secretion (ADA, 2014a). A careful history is necessary to rule out a stress-related illness,

Pathophysiology Illustrated: **Mechanism of Diabetes Mellitus**

Destruction of the alpha and beta cells in the islets of Langerhans produces multiple metabolic changes. Acute signs and symptoms are followed by short-term and long-term complications if the disease is not well managed.

corticosteroid use, fracture, acute infection, cystic fibrosis, pancreatitis, or liver disease.

Clinical therapy for type 1 diabetes combines insulin, nutrition management to support growth and maintain blood glucose at near-normal levels, an exercise regimen, and psychosocial support.

Insulin Therapy.   Multiple approaches to insulin therapy for children and adolescents are available, and an approach that works for the child and family should be selected. Children often need several daily injections of insulin before meals and at bedtime to maintain an optimal blood glucose level.

TABLE 53–4 Clinical Manifestations of Diabetes by Type

CAUSE	CLINICAL MANIFESTATIONS	CLINICAL THERAPY
Type 1—immune mediated, insulin deficiency due to pancreatic beta-cell destruction	Polyuria, polydipsia May have polyphagia Weight loss Ketoacidosis may be present at diagnosis, at continued risk for ketoacidosis Short duration of symptoms Initial period of decreased insulin requirement, then need insulin for survival	Blood glucose monitoring Insulin Dietary management, balancing carbohydrate intake to insulin Exercise
Type 2—insulin resistance with relative insulin secretory defect	Obese, little or no weight loss, or may have significant weight loss Acanthosis nigricans Long duration of symptoms Polyuria, polydipsia, may be mild or absent Glycosuria with or without ketonuria Ketoacidosis may be present Lipid disorders Hypertension Androgen-mediated problems such as acne, hirsutism, menstrual disturbances, polycystic ovary disease Excessive weight gain and fatigue due to insulin resistance	Diet with decreased calories and low-fat foods Decrease sedentary activity time or increase routine physical activity Blood glucose monitoring Oral medication (metformin) to improve insulin sensitivity May need insulin

Clinical Tip

The American Diabetes Association (2014b) considers a fasting glucose level of 100 to 125 mg/dL (5.6 to 6.9 mmol/L) to be an *impaired fasting glucose (IFG)*, and a 2-hour postload glucose level of 140 to 199 mg/dL (7.8 to 11.0 mmol/L) to be an *impaired glucose tolerance (IGT)*. Individuals with IFG or IGT are considered at increased risk for developing diabetes. A hemoglobin A$_{1c}$ value of 5.7% to 6.4% is an additional risk factor for the development of diabetes.

A basal-bolus insulin regimen has resulted in improved glycemic control in the pediatric population (ADA, 2014b). When multiple injections are used, basal insulin is administered once a day using a very long-acting insulin (Glargine or Detemir). A bolus of rapid-acting insulin (insulin lispro, insulin glulisine, or insulin aspart) is administered with each meal and snack based on the carbohydrate grams consumed and the blood glucose level. This means that a child may get six to seven injections a day. Stress, infection, and illness may either increase or decrease insulin needs. If basal-bolus therapy for type 1 diabetes is to be effective, the child and family need to do each of the following:

- Monitor the blood glucose appropriately to establish insulin requirements. For example, test glucose before and 2 hours after meals, as well as once a week at midnight and 3 a.m.
- Count carbohydrates consumed.
- Incorporate exercise into the daily routine.

Clinical Tip

Insulin is usually provided in prepackaged doses of 100 units/mL. Diluted insulin prepared by a pharmacist may be used for infants and toddlers who require a small insulin dosage. Insulin cartridges, disposable pens, and other devices are available, making insulin easy to carry by older children and adolescents who need frequent insulin injections during the day.

Clinical Tip

Very long-acting insulins (Glargine and Detemir) cannot be mixed with other insulins.

Continuous subcutaneous insulin infusion (CSII) pump therapy is being increasingly used by children and adolescents as the technology makes it possible to more closely match the plasma insulin levels found in children who do not have diabetes. CSII pump therapy has been used successfully in children of all ages and has been found to improve glycemic control with less hypoglycemia. Pump therapy requires the willingness of the patient or parent (with young children) to monitor blood glucose frequently, practice advanced insulin management skills, learn how to troubleshoot the pump, and be technology capable (Carchidi, Holland, Minnock, et al., 2011). Advantages and disadvantages of an insulin pump are outlined in Table 53–5.

Tight blood glucose control has long-term benefits and is becoming a standard of care for children of all ages. Maintaining tight control for young children is challenging because of the erratic eating patterns and difficulty in recognizing symptoms of hypoglycemia (Blackman et al., 2014). In the past, target blood glucose levels were higher in younger children because of these challenges and concerns over complications of hypoglycemia. While there are still concerns, better tools are available now to detect hypoglycemia. Additionally, there is now evidence that prolonged hyperglycemia in children can lead to early development of complications such as cardiovascular and renal disease. Based on this evidence, the American Diabetes Association (2014c) now recommends a target HbA$_{1c}$ goal of 7.5% across all pediatric age groups. It is important however that targets for blood glucose and HbA$_{1c}$ be individualized to achieve the best control and minimize the risk of both hypoglycemia and hyperglycemia (Chiang, Kirkman, Laffel, et al., 2014). The HbA$_{1c}$ is a

TABLE 53–5 Advantages and Disadvantages of an External Insulin Infusion Pump

ADVANTAGES	DISADVANTAGES
• Delivers a continuous infusion of insulin to match the basal rate needed plus an insulin bolus at mealtime to more closely simulate normal pancreatic function.	• Requires constant vigilance and adherence, including frequent blood sugar testing, carbohydrate counting, and dose calculations.
• Helps maintain blood glucose control between meals.	• Requires willingness to live connected to a device (can be disconnected for short periods by removing or clamping the catheter; however, DKA can occur within hours of interruption of insulin flow).
• Decreases HbA$_{1c}$ level.	
• Improves glycemic control.	
• Improves growth in children.	• Pump visibility and size.
• Reduces number of injections.	• Requires site to be changed every 2 to 3 days.
• New pumps calculate bolus insulin dose to number of carbohydrates consumed.	• Can increase risk of infection at the injection site.
	• Overuse of catheter-site locations may occur.
• Allows child to eat with less adherence to a schedule and have a more flexible lifestyle.	• Possible weight gain can occur when blood glucose control improves.
• Reduces number of injection sites, so variation in absorption decreases.	• Costs more than other insulin therapies.
• Results in fewer incidences of diabetic ketoacidosis.	• Can increase risk of DKA and ketonuria secondary to pump failure.
• Improves quality of life and psychosocial functioning.	

Source: Data from Alsaleh, F. M., Smith, F. J., & Taylor, K. M. (2012). Experiences of children/young people and their parents, using insulin pump therapy for the management of type 1 diabetes: Qualitative review. *Journal of Clinical Pharmacy and Therapeutics, 37*, 140–147; Blackman, S. M., Raghinaru, D., Adi, S., Simmons, J. H., Ebner-Lyon, L., Chase, H.P., . . . DiMeglio, L. A. (2014). Insulin pump use in young children in the T1D Exchange clinic registry is associated with lower hemoglobin A1c levels than injection therapy. *Pediatric Diabetes, 15*, 564–572; Carchidi, C., Holland, C., Minnock, P., & Boyle, D. (2011). New technologies in pediatric diabetes care. *MCN, 36*(1), 32–39; Woerner, S. (2014). The benefits of insulin pump therapy in children and adolescents with type 1 diabetes. *Journal of Pediatric Nursing, 29*(6), 712–713.

predictor of the average blood glucose over the past 3 months (National Diabetes Information Clearinghouse, 2014).

Complications of type 1 diabetes (retinopathy, heart disease, renal failure, and peripheral vascular disease) result from long-term hyperglycemic effects on the blood vessels. Without careful management, children with diabetes may develop renal failure and loss of vision in adulthood. Intensive therapy is expected to reduce the risk for or delay the development of these complications. Risk may be further reduced if the adolescent does not begin smoking and if the blood pressure is controlled.

Nutrition Therapy.   The goal of nutrition therapy is to provide adequate calories for the child's normal growth and development. An evaluation of the child's food intake, metabolic status, and lifestyle is necessary before establishing a nutrition plan. Daily caloric requirements are individualized for each child according to need. To facilitate adherence to the nutritional plan, an individualized approach with consideration of the child's and family's culture, lifestyle, and financial means should be incorporated. Careful instruction by a registered dietician or certified diabetes educator is essential in the management of diabetes.

Carbohydrate counting provides flexibility in meal planning and is simple for children and adolescents to use. One carbohydrate choice equals 15 g of carbohydrates. The number of carbohydrate choices needed at meals and snacks varies depending on the child's individualized nutrition plan. Generally, 1 unit of insulin covers 15 g of carbohydrates, making insulin dosage calculation for meal coverage relatively easy; however, a different ratio of insulin to carbohydrates may be calculated for individual children. If additional carbohydrates are eaten at a meal or snack, the number of insulin units can also be adjusted, providing further flexibility. A high-fiber diet is also recommended for improved control of blood glucose.

Exercise Program.   Physical activity is associated with increased insulin sensitivity. Regular exercise and fitness improve

glucose control, reduce cardiovascular risk factors, contribute to weight loss, and improve overall well-being. Blood lipid levels are also positively affected. However, the child must have an adequate caloric intake to prevent hypoglycemia. Excessive exercise associated with sports requires careful planning and management.

Nursing Management
For the Child With Type 1 Diabetes

Nursing Assessment and Diagnosis

PHYSIOLOGIC ASSESSMENT
Children with type 1 diabetes are frequently admitted to the hospital at the time of diagnosis. Assess the child's physiologic status, focusing on vital signs and level of consciousness. Assess hydration by checking mucous membranes, skin turgor, and urine output. Blood initially is collected to monitor blood gases, glucose, and electrolytes. The frequency of blood collection will depend on whether the child is in diabetic ketoacidosis. Once the child is stable, assess dietary and caloric intake and the ability of the child or family to manage care.

PSYCHOSOCIAL ASSESSMENT
Parents may feel guilty at the time of diagnosis if they waited to seek care until the child began to experience symptoms of diabetic ketoacidosis. Assess coping mechanisms, family strengths and resources, ability to manage the disease, and educational needs of both the child and parents. Examples of questions to ask in assessing the family's strengths and limitations in the child's disease management include:

• Do both parents or the single parent work? What hours?

• Who else is involved in the child's care?

• What is the child's usual daily schedule? Does the schedule vary on the weekend or any other days of the week?

- Does the child have health insurance? What coverage exists for diabetes education, treatment, and home management?
- Does the child have any cognitive, behavioral, motor, or visual problems coexisting with this condition?
- What other family stressors coexist with the diagnosis?

Clinical Reasoning Managing Adolescent Diabetes

Anthony, 12 years old, has just been diagnosed with diabetes mellitus. His parents took him to their family healthcare provider after Anthony complained of being constantly thirsty and hungry for over a week. Despite this, he has lost 5 lb. They note that he had a viral illness about 1 month ago but seemed to recover from it. His mother says that Anthony seemed lethargic for several days.

Anthony and his family must now learn to manage his diabetes using the combination of diet, exercise, and insulin therapy. Monitoring his blood glucose level is important in determining how much insulin he will need every day. Anthony's meals and activity will need to be coordinated with the insulin doses. Anthony and his parents will need to watch closely for signs of hypoglycemia. Develop a teaching plan that includes the following information:

- What causes diabetes?
- What potential problems need prompt treatment?
- What does Anthony need to monitor for when he gets sick?
- Intensive therapy will be a goal of Anthony's treatment. How can you help Anthony and his family decide if this should be accomplished with insulin injections or an insulin pump?
- What are some strategies to help an adolescent actively participate in his disease management and maintain optimal diabetic control?

DEVELOPMENTAL ASSESSMENT

Assess the child's developmental level, particularly fine motor skills and cognitive level. The child will need to learn how to obtain and read a blood glucose sample and how to inject insulin (see the *Clinical Skills Manual* SKILLS). Children can usually perform some of these tasks with supervision by 6 to 8 years of age.

Adolescents often perceive type 1 diabetes as a disability and may deny having the disease so they can be like their peers when eating and exercising. Talk with the adolescent and assess problem-solving skills associated with daily condition management, and the ability to manage special circumstances such as illness or changes in exercise. Self-management is the eventual goal, and the child's responsibilities are gradually increased.

Several diagnoses that may apply to the child newly diagnosed with type 1 diabetes are provided in the accompanying *Nursing Care Plans*. Additional diagnoses that may be appropriate include the following (NANDA-I © 2014):

- *Fluid Volume: Deficient, Risk for,* related to active fluid loss associated with hyperglycemia
- *Breathing Pattern, Ineffective,* related to metabolic acidosis
- *Coping, Ineffective,* related to inability to admit impact of disease on lifestyle

Planning and Implementation

Nursing care focuses on teaching the child and parents about the disease and its management, planning dietary intake, providing emotional support, and planning strategies for daily management in the community. Refer to the accompanying *Nursing Care Plans*, which summarize nursing care for the child who is hospitalized with newly diagnosed type 1 diabetes and the child who is receiving care in the community.

Nursing Care Plan: The Child Hospitalized With Newly Diagnosed Type 1 Diabetes Mellitus

1. Nursing Diagnosis: *Knowledge, Deficient (Survival Skills),* **related to lack of exposure to diabetic management in the newly diagnosed child (NANDA-I © 2014)**

GOAL: The child and parents will acquire survival skills for home management.

INTERVENTION	RATIONALE
• Assess the child's developmental level and select an educational approach and self-care activities to match.	• Learning goals for the child must match knowledge and skill expectations appropriate for developmental stage.
• Teach blood glucose monitoring, drawing up and injecting insulin, urine testing for ketones, record keeping, survival food guidelines, and when to call the healthcare provider.	• Diabetic management survival skills are needed for initial home management until more extensive education can be completed that permits more independent management.
• Use demonstration/return demonstration until the child and family are comfortable with procedures.	• Return demonstration permits evaluation, positive reinforcement and guidance for modification of techniques.

EXPECTED OUTCOME: Child and parents will demonstrate proper technique for blood glucose monitoring, urine testing for ketones, drawing up and injecting insulin doses, survival food guidelines, and record keeping.

GOAL: The child and parents will recognize signs and symptoms of hypoglycemia and hyperglycemia.

INTERVENTION	RATIONALE
• Teach signs and symptoms of hypoglycemic and hyperglycemic reactions.	• Recognition of and treatment of poor glucose control will prevent progression of symptoms.
• Teach the child to test blood glucose when feeling different than usual, and record the reading and symptoms felt.	• Permits child to learn his/her specific symptoms of hyperglycemia and hypoglycemia.

EXPECTED OUTCOME: Child and family will be able to describe symptoms of hypoglycemia and hyperglycemia.

---

2. **Nursing Diagnosis:** *Injury, Risk for (Complication)*, related to potential episodes of hypoglycemia and diabetic ketoacidosis (NANDA-I © 2014)

GOAL: The child will experience few episodes of hypoglycemia during hospitalization.

INTERVENTION	RATIONALE
• Assess the child at least every 2 hr for signs of hypoglycemia. If signs are present, check blood glucose to verify and administer source of quick sugar.	• Hypoglycemia commonly occurs during hospitalization because of change in diet, lack of food intake, or illness.
• When the child is NPO for a special procedure, verify with healthcare provider when food, fluids, and insulin are to be given, or if an intravenous infusion with dextrose is to be given.	• Giving insulin without food intake can lead to hypoglycemia. Intravenous dextrose and insulin can be used when the child must be NPO.
• Have glucose paste or 50% dextrose solution readily available.	• Glucose paste is used for oral treatment. Dextrose is used for emergency intravenous treatment of severe hypoglycemia.

EXPECTED OUTCOME: Child and staff will manage episodes of hypoglycemia without a crisis developing.

GOAL: The child's condition will be treated slowly to gradually reverse hyperglycemia and ketoacidosis and to prevent cerebral edema.

INTERVENTION	RATIONALE
• Assess the child's mental status for improvement or deterioration.	• Improvement in mental status may indicate successful treatment. Deterioration may indicate onset of cerebral edema.
• Check blood glucose and urine ketones frequently to confirm reduction in blood glucose level and ketosis, and to identify the insulin dose for administration.	• Frequent blood glucose and ketone level determination helps assess progress in treating ketoacidosis.
• Monitor and control IV fluid intake. Measure output.	• The child with ketoacidosis will be dehydrated. IV fluid intake needs to be carefully controlled to prevent cerebral edema.
• Have insulin doses checked by a second nurse.	• Doses are frequently small, and the possibility of error is great.

EXPECTED OUTCOME: Child's hyperglycemia and ketoacidosis will resolve without additional complications.

GOAL: The child and parents will demonstrate emergency management of hypoglycemia.

INTERVENTION	RATIONALE
• Identify sources of glucose to give in case of hypoglycemic reaction. Tell the child and parent to carry glucose tablets or paste with them at all times.	• Access to sources of glucose and its rapid administration are important for emergency care.

EXPECTED OUTCOME: Child and family will be able to identify several glucose sources for emergencies. The child and family have a source of glucose with them at each visit.

GOAL: The child and parents will demonstrate management of sick days.

INTERVENTION	RATIONALE
• Teach the child and family to test blood glucose and urine for ketones with acute symptoms and notify the healthcare provider.	• When the child is ill, hyperglycemia needs special management to prevent progression to ketoacidosis.

EXPECTED OUTCOME: Child's hyperglycemic episodes will not progress to ketoacidosis.

(continued)

Nursing Care Plan: The Child Hospitalized With Newly Diagnosed Type 1 Diabetes Mellitus (continued)

3. Nursing Diagnosis: *Nutrition, Imbalanced: Less than Body Requirements,* related to disorder of glucose and insulin (NANDA-I © 2014)

GOAL: The child will eat a well-balanced diet and maintain normal height and weight proportions.

INTERVENTION	RATIONALE
• Encourage and serve meals and snacks with consistent carbohydrates at the same time each day. • Provide a calorie nonrestricted diet.	• Keeps blood glucose levels stable during initial disease management stages. • Enables weight lost during onset of diabetes to be regained.

EXPECTED OUTCOME: Child will regain weight lost and demonstrate normal growth and stable blood glucose levels.

GOAL: The child and parents will state understanding of dietary management of diabetes mellitus.

INTERVENTION	RATIONALE
• Make an appointment with a registered dietician or certified diabetes educator who can assess the child's favorite foods and promote their integration into the child's diet. Reinforce the dietary information taught. • Provide sample menus and teach the use of carbohydrate counting.	• The registered dietician or certified diabetes educator can develop dietary recommendations that fit the specific needs of the child and include favorite foods, thereby increasing compliance with the diet. • Assists the family and adolescent with diet planning.

EXPECTED OUTCOME: Child and parents will describe nutritional needs of the child and select the dietary management best suited to the family's and child's eating habits.

Nursing Care Plan: The Child With Previously Diagnosed Type 1 Diabetes Being Cared for at Home

1. Nursing Diagnosis: *Nutrition, Imbalanced: Less than Body Requirements,* related to chronic illness (type 1 diabetes) (NANDA-I © 2014)

GOAL: The child will eat a well-balanced diet that maintains weight proportional to height.

INTERVENTION	RATIONALE
• Assess height and weight regularly and plot on growth chart. • Make an appointment with a registered dietician or certified diabetes educator who can assess the child's favorite foods and integrate them into a food plan that controls caloric intake. Encourage the child to keep a food diary.	• Assesses change in body mass index to identify potential weight problem early. • Inclusion of child's favorite foods helps child adapt to changes in the food plan.

EXPECTED OUTCOME: Diet records will indicate meals and snacks have the appropriate distribution of carbohydrates, protein, and fats, and daily caloric intake goals will be met.

2. Nursing Diagnosis: *Family Processes, Readiness for Enhanced,* related to management of a chronic disease (NANDA-I © 2014)

GOAL: The child and family will manage the food plan, exercise, blood glucose monitoring, and medication regimen.

INTERVENTION	RATIONALE
• Assess the family's lifestyle and attempt to fit the child's care needs into the family's schedule. • Discuss the family's routines for special occasions and vacations. Identify ways to modify the child's management for these occasions.	• Fitting the care to the family's lifestyle promotes adherence with the regimen. • It is important for the child to participate in special events with the family and peers as a normal child to promote psychologic development.

EXPECTED OUTCOME: Child and family will make minimal changes in usual lifestyle while managing the type 1 diabetes.

3. Nursing Diagnosis: *Coping, Ineffective (Individual)*, related to inadequate level of confidence in ability to cope (NANDA-I © 2014)

GOAL: The child will demonstrate enhanced coping skills.

INTERVENTION	RATIONALE
• Ask how the child has solved problems in the past. Review possible problems the child may encounter. Together evaluate the effectiveness of solutions. Suggest other solutions to consider.	• Children's success in mastering maturational conflicts and daily psychosocial problems will influence their pattern of coping.

EXPECTED OUTCOME: Child will demonstrate enhanced coping skills and express positive attitude toward self. Child will display warmth and affection toward family.

GOAL: The child will develop positive self-esteem.

INTERVENTION	RATIONALE
• Role-play ways to talk about diabetes with friends and teachers. Encourage the child to express feelings about diabetes to those the child trusts.	• Sharing information about the condition helps others understand changes in lifestyle needed by the child. Expressing feelings decreases anxiety.
• Encourage the child to attend diabetes camp.	• Learning and support networks developed at camp can promote self-esteem.
• Encourage the child to continue previous social activities and hobbies.	• Increased social interaction, especially in group sessions, improves self-esteem.

EXPECTED OUTCOME: Child will demonstrate confidence in interactions with peers and maintain social network.

PROVIDE EDUCATION

The nurse is an important member of the management team (physician, nurse, registered dietician, certified nurse educator, and social worker) and is usually responsible for educating the child and family. The majority of teaching may be performed by an advanced practice nurse or a certified diabetes nurse educator in the clinic setting, since children may be hospitalized only briefly following diagnosis.

The timing and amount of information provided are especially important in the first days following diagnosis. Both the child and parents are very tired, and they are often in a state of shock and disbelief. Information presented during this period needs to be repeated. This time should be used to assess learning needs and to answer the family's questions. Initial teaching focuses on the survival skills necessary for home management, including insulin administration, blood glucose testing, meal planning, and the recognition and treatment of both hypoglycemia and hyperglycemia (Figure 53–6). Partner with the child and family to identify barriers to management.

Explain the goals of insulin therapy. Teach the parents and child (if appropriate) how to draw up and administer insulin or how to use an insulin pen. Insulin pens might be accepted more readily than the traditional syringe and vial method; they are easier to transport, they provide more accurate dosing, and they decrease anxiety associated with needles and insulin administration in public (Hanas, de Beaufort, Hoey, et al., 2011). Rotating the injection sites is important to decrease the chances of *lipoatrophy*, loss of subcutaneous tissue, or hypertrophy

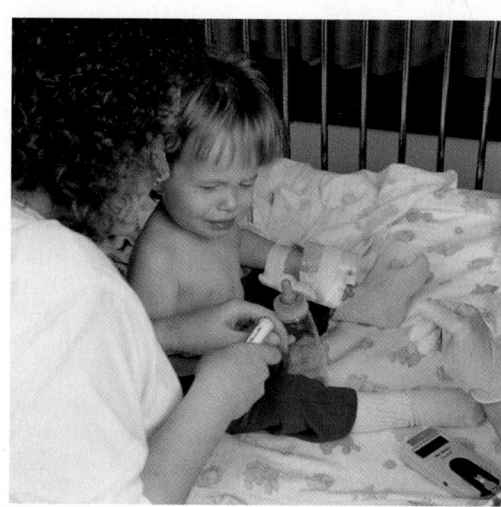

Figure 53–6 This mother is learning how to test her child's blood glucose level.

in which collagen is replaced by fat cells (Figure 53–7). The absorption rate of insulin varies by the site used. Insulin is usually absorbed most rapidly from the abdomen; however, insulin absorption is increased in the extremities with exercise. An understanding of the different types of insulin and their actions is essential.

TEACHING HIGHLIGHTS | Checking Blood Glucose Levels

Caution parents to check the blood glucose level of a toddler who is extremely sleepy or irritable, as these can be signs of either hypoglycemia or hyperglycemia.

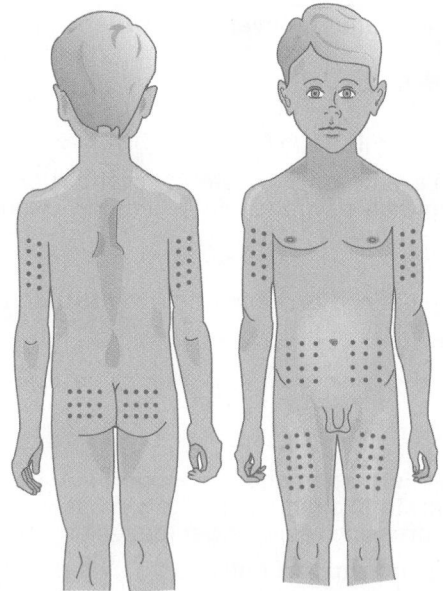

Figure 53–7 Insulin injection sites. Give all morning insulin in one site (e.g., arms) and all evening insulin in another (e.g., legs) because of different rates of absorption from these sites. Space injections about 1.25 cm (0.5 in.) apart.

Once the child and parents demonstrate understanding of this information, teach guidelines for managing episodes of hyperglycemia during acute illness and using an insulin correction scale. A correction scale indicates specific insulin dosages appropriate for a particular blood glucose level. The family also needs to learn "sick day" care guidelines to prevent diabetic ketoacidosis.

Initial teaching related to dietary management may be taught by the registered dietician. The nurse needs to assess understanding and reinforce principles taught. Assist the parent and child (if appropriate) to learn carbohydrate counting and how to plan nutritious meals for the child. See the accompanying *Nursing Care Plans* for additional guidelines.

Eating at consistent intervals is important for glycemic control, whether counting carbohydrates or following a conventional meal plan (three meals a day and three snacks a day). Although the child with diabetes is not restricted from eating any food, the child and parents need to learn about the relationship between foods eaten and insulin needed. Meal plans also need to be adjusted for exercise. Nonnutritive sweeteners such as aspartame and saccharin may be used in moderation. The child and family should learn how to read food labels. The meal plan should be customized, with the assistance of a registered dietician, to the child's age, cultural and family food preferences, and activity level.

PROVIDE EMOTIONAL SUPPORT

The diagnosis of type 1 diabetes often comes as a shock to the family. If there is a familial history, parents may feel guilty about having caused the disease. The diagnosis of a chronic disease that requires daily management can be difficult to accept. Provide the family with information about diabetes education programs, refer them to support groups with other parents of children with diabetes, and assist them in learning the role of disease management. Support for the child depends on age and developmental stage. Encourage the child to express feelings about the disease and its management. The adolescent may benefit from contact with other adolescents who have diabetes.

DISCHARGE PLANNING AND HOME CARE TEACHING

Home care needs should be identified and addressed before discharge. Initial survival skills described earlier are taught with the plans for ongoing outpatient education.

Make every effort to incorporate the diabetic regimen (insulin administration, food plan, blood glucose monitoring, and exercise) into the family's present lifestyle. The fewer changes the family has to make, the greater the chance of adherence.

The family and child newly diagnosed with diabetes should be made aware of the "honeymoon phase." This is a period during new-onset diabetes when the child has some residual beta-cell function, which reduces exogenous insulin requirements. The child and family may assume this is an indication that the diabetes "is better." However, the insulin requirement does eventually return. The duration of this phase varies among individuals.

Provide written materials and refer parents to books and other materials they can use in teaching the child about diabetes. The Juvenile Diabetes Research Foundation and the American Diabetes Association are excellent sources of information.

COMMUNITY-BASED NURSING CARE

During follow-up visits, ask the child or parents about signs indicating problems with diabetic control. Questions to ask that could help identify such problems include:

- Is the child hungry at meals? Between meals?
- How much fluid is the child drinking?
- Has the child been going to the bathroom frequently or had episodes of bed-wetting?
- Does the child have dry skin?

TEACHING HIGHLIGHTS | Sick Day Guidelines

Parents should receive written guidelines specific to their child related to sick-day management. Some general guidelines include the following (American Diabetes Association, 2013; Brink et al., 2014):

- Monitor the blood glucose levels every 2 to 3 hours or as instructed.
- Test urine ketones every 4 hours or as instructed by the healthcare provider.
- The usual dose of insulin may be increased for high blood glucose levels.
- Notify the healthcare provider if the child has fever or other signs of infection, is unable to tolerate fluids, has ketones in the urine, has blood glucose levels that are out of target range, or has signs of dehydration.

- Are there sores on the feet? Do scratches or scrapes take a long time to heal?

- Has the child had any skin infections?

- Does the child have changes in mood (depression, unexplained sadness, irritability) or energy level from day to day or throughout the day?

- Have there been any changes in vision?

Maintain a record of the child's growth measurements and vital signs. Review the child's typical dietary intake and exercise regimens. Assess the child's sexual development using Tanner staging guidelines (see Chapter 33). Puberty may be delayed if diabetic control is inadequate. Evaluation for the potential complications of diabetes should be performed annually, including blood for lipid levels, blood pressure, liver and renal function, urine for albumin, an ophthalmologic examination for retinopathy, and a neurologic examination of the extremities for neuropathies.

Education is ongoing, especially for children who develop diabetes at a young age. As they grow and assume more responsibility for their care, they need to learn more about the pathophysiology of the disease and the rationale for its management.

The child with diabetes should be treated as any other child without a chronic condition, including limit setting and consistent discipline for unacceptable behavior. Children with type 1 diabetes may learn maladaptive behaviors, using their disease to obtain something they want. Teach parents to be alert to signs of maladaption, such as helpless, demanding, or whining behaviors, and any evidence of poor coping. Additional behaviors may include skipping blood glucose testing and losing or damaging equipment. Food may become a battleground for toddlers who are picky eaters, but must eat enough for the insulin dose. Referral for counseling may be appropriate for some families.

Continually work with the child to encourage responsibility for self-care and with parents to promote the child's self-care (Figure 53–8). The child's developmental stage and cognitive level influence readiness to take on responsibility for self-care. Summer camps and other programs for children with diabetes are often helpful in providing education and support.

The preschool child's need for autonomy and control can be met by allowing the child to choose snacks or to pick which finger to stick for glucose testing and by helping parents to gather necessary supplies. School-age children can learn to test blood glucose, administer insulin, and keep records. They should be taught how to select foods and portion sizes appropriate for dietary management and how to plan food intake for an exercise program. School-age children need to learn to recognize the signs of hypoglycemia and hyperglycemia, and understand the importance of carrying a rapidly absorbed sugar product.

Although adolescents understand explanations about the potential complications of diabetes, they are present-time oriented and may rebel against the daily regimen of insulin injections, the food plan, and the exercise plan. Successful self-care depends in part on the adolescent's adjustment to the chronic nature of the disease and feelings of being different from peers. Although adolescents are able to manage self-care, the desire to be like peers may interfere with treatment adherence. Talk with adolescents to assess their mood and to evaluate their motivation to manage the meal plan, exercise regimen, blood glucose monitoring, and insulin therapy. Discuss how carbohydrate counting and insulin dose adjustment may provide the flexibility to participate in activities with peers. Collaborate with the adolescent in preparation to assume care, and assist parents in accepting the growing independence from adult supervision. A

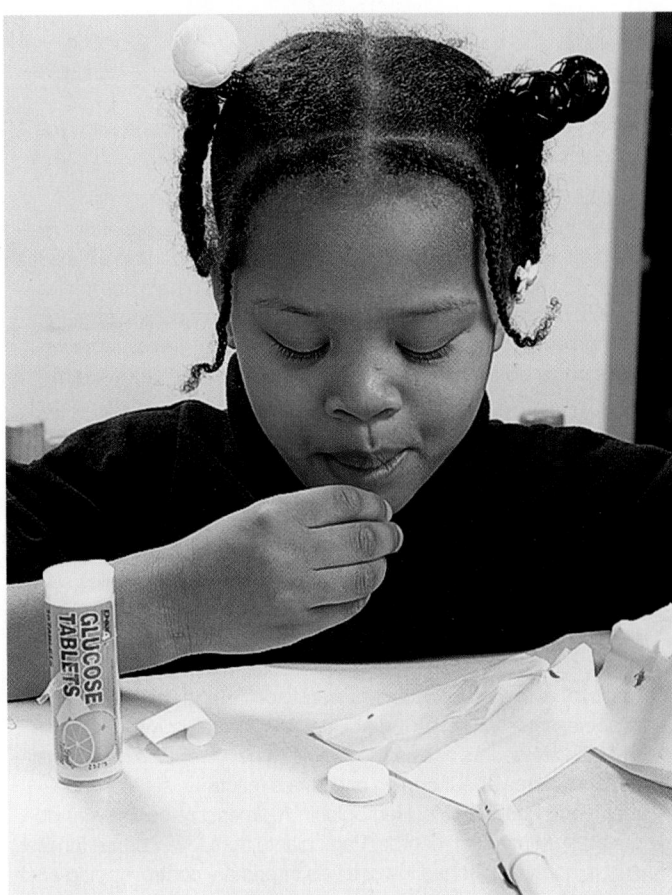

Figure 53–8 This girl is old enough to understand the need to take glucose tablets or another form of a rapidly absorbed sugar when her blood glucose level is low.

discussion of the hazards associated with having diabetes and the use of alcohol, drugs, and tobacco should occur. At every subsequent healthcare visit, the adolescent should be asked about alcohol intake. See *Evidence-Based Practice: Coping With Type 1 Diabetes in Adolescents*.

The child with type 1 diabetes may develop circulatory and neurologic changes over time. Emphasize the importance of good foot care from an early age, for example, wearing clean cotton socks, changing socks and shoes when they are damp, washing and drying feet, and keeping toenails short. Adolescents getting pedicures should inform the person performing them that they have diabetes.

Explain to parents that the child should wear some type of medical alert identification. Help them have an individualized school health plan developed (see Chapter 38) to ensure that school administrators and teachers can identify the signs of hypoglycemia or hyperglycemia and provide emergency management.

Evaluation

Expected outcomes of nursing care for children with type 1 diabetes can be found in the *Nursing Care Plans*.

Diabetic Ketoacidosis

Diabetic ketoacidosis (DKA) is a common and potentially life-threatening condition that occurs primarily in children with type 1 diabetes. Potential causes of DKA include incorrect or

---

EVIDENCE-BASED PRACTICE | Coping With Type 1 Diabetes in Adolescents

Clinical Question

What factors are associated with how adolescents cope with type 1 diabetes?

The Evidence

Jaser and White (2011) explored how coping strategies affect resilience in adolescents with type 1 diabetes. Thirty participant's ages 10 to 16 years with type 1 diabetes and their mothers completed questionnaires that focused on the teen's use of coping strategies, competence, and quality of life. Hemoglobin A_{1c} measurements were obtained from the teen's medical record. The study examined how adolescents use primary control and secondary control engagement strategies and/or disengagement strategies to cope with stress related to diabetes. Primary control coping strategies such as problem solving and emotional expression and secondary control coping strategies such as acceptance and distraction were associated with better metabolic control, better quality of life, and higher social competence. Use of disengagement strategies such as withdrawal or denial were associated with poorer metabolic control and lower social competence.

Jaser et al. (2012) studied the relationship of coping and stress reactivity with metabolic control, quality of life, and self-management in adolescents with type 1 diabetes. An ethnically diverse sample of 327 adolescents ages 11 to 14 with type 1 diabetes completed questionnaires about coping and stress reactivity, self-management, and quality of life. Hemoglobin A_{1c} measurements were obtained from medical records. Participants from low-income families and minority status had lower levels of primary control coping such as problem solving and secondary control coping such as acceptance. This group also had higher levels of disengagement coping such as avoidance. Results of the study also revealed that the use of primary and secondary control strategies to cope with stress related to diabetes was correlated with better self-management and better adaptation. The investigators concluded that there are differences in coping related to income and ethnicity and that coping strategies impacts self-management and metabolic control in adolescents with diabetes.

Iafusco et al. (2011) evaluated the effectiveness of a chat line for adolescents with type 1 diabetes on quality of life and metabolic control. The participants were 193 children and adolescents 10 to 18 years of age. Computer-based chats, moderated by a physician, took place once a week and covered topics such as diabetes management, fears related to hypoglycemia, anxiety related to the future, and relationships. At routine office visits, a research assistant gathered demographic data and assessed management of diabetes. Questionnaires, including the Diabetes Quality of Life for Youth Inventory (DQOLY), were completed at baseline, 1, and 2 years. A control group consisted of 203 adolescents who did not participate in the chat line. Results of the study found that participation at least once a month in the chat group improved well-being and metabolic control.

Best Practice

Adolescents with type 1 diabetes must cope with the increasing responsibility for complex self-management, including insulin administration, blood glucose testing, exercise, and nutrition. The types of coping strategies that are used affect the adolescent's quality of life and metabolic control. It is important that these adolescents learn effective coping strategies such as problem solving and distraction. Interventions that involve group discussions about concerns related to diabetes and routine follow-up to assess coping strategies, quality of life, and metabolic control are essential in maximizing outcomes for these adolescents with diabetes.

Clinical Reasoning

How can you address coping strategies and quality of life issues in adolescents with diabetes? What interventions can you think of that may improve quality of life and metabolic control in these adolescents?

Professionalism in Practice **Management of Diabetes in the School Setting**

Section 504 of the Rehabilitation Act of 1973 and the Americans with Disabilities Act of 1990 are federal laws that require that students with disabilities, including those with diabetes, be given an equal opportunity to participate in school activities. The position statement of the National Association of School Nurses states that a school nurse is required to develop an individualized health plan from the child's diabetes medical management plan. The school nurse oversees the implementation and evaluation of the plan (Butler, Fekaris, Pontius, et al., 2012). It is essential for the school nurse to work with parents to ensure that equipment and medications needed at school are provided so that children with disabilities are able to receive the care they need.

missed insulin doses, incorrect administration of insulin, or an illness, trauma, or surgery. DKA may be present in children with new-onset diabetes.

Insulin deficiency is accompanied by a compensatory increase in hormones (epinephrine, norepinephrine, cortisol, growth hormone, and glucagon) that are released when inadequate glucose is delivered to the cells. The muscle cells break down protein into amino acids that are then converted to glucose by the liver, leading to hyperglycemia. The adipose tissue releases fatty acids that are transformed by the liver into ketone bodies. Their accumulation leads to ketoacidosis. The hyperglycemia causes an osmotic diuresis resulting in dehydration, acidosis, and hyperosmolality. The rising ketones lead to metabolic acidosis. DKA is associated with severe metabolic, electrolyte, and fluid imbalances.

Characteristic signs of DKA include polyuria, polydipsia, weight loss, abdominal pain, nausea and vomiting, tachycardia, signs of dehydration, flushed ears and cheeks, Kussmaul respirations, acetone breath (fruity smell), altered level of consciousness, and hypotension. Hyperglycemia, glycosuria, and ketonuria are also present. In response to metabolic acidosis, children complain of abdominal or chest pain, nausea, and vomiting. The disorder may progress to electrolyte disturbances, arrhythmias, altered consciousness, pupillary changes, irregular respirations, inappropriate slowing of the heart rate, and widening pulse pressure. See Table 53–6 for clinical manifestations of hypoglycemia and hyperglycemia.

DKA is present with the following findings: blood glucose level greater than 250 mg/dL, serum ketones, acidosis (pH less than 7.3 and bicarbonate less than 15 mEq/L), and ketonuria.

Alteration in electrolytes occur. The blood urea nitrogen (BUN) and creatinine are elevated (Masharani, 2015).

The child with ketoacidosis is hospitalized. Medical management includes isotonic intravenous fluids and electrolytes for dehydration and acidosis. Intravenous insulin (0.1 unit/kg per hour) is administered by continuous infusion pump to decrease the serum glucose level at a rate not to exceed 100 mg/dL/hr. Faster reduction of hyperglycemia and serum osmolality increases the risk for cerebral edema. When glucose is lowered too rapidly, water is freed and attracted to the glucose, which has accumulated in large quantities in the brain. Cerebral edema is the most common complication of DKA and the most common cause of death in children with diabetes (Bialo, Agrawal, Boney, et al., 2015). As insulin and fluids are administered, potassium shifts to the cells, resulting in hypokalemia. Potassium replacement is needed as hypokalemia can lead to cardiac arrhythmia (McFarlane, 2011). See Chapter 54 for information about cerebral edema.

Nursing Management

Continuously monitor the child's vital signs, respiratory status, perfusion, and mental status. Assess for changes in neurologic status, respiratory pattern, blood pressure, and heart rate.

Monitor for cardiac arrhythmias associated with hypokalemia. Assess for signs of dehydration, including dry skin and mucous membranes and depressed fontanelles in infants. Monitor blood glucose levels hourly or as indicated. Frequently monitor the electrolytes and acid–base status, as well as urine glucose and ketone levels as indicated. Intake and output are monitored hourly. Assess for signs of hypoglycemia that may occur during insulin infusion.

Intravenous fluids are given in boluses of 10 to 20 mL/kg rapidly over 5 minutes if the child is in hypovolemic shock. Adequate fluids are given to reverse the fluid deficit. The insulin infusion must be carefully titrated to control the gradual reduction in hyperglycemia. The child is tapered off intravenous insulin and transitioned to subcutaneous insulin when clinically stable. Oral feedings are reintroduced when the child is alert and the glucose level is stabilized.

The prevention of future episodes of DKA is important. The parents and child need to learn strategies to keep hyperglycemic episodes from progressing to DKA. Parents should have specific instructions on how often to check the blood glucose and when to check the urine for ketones when the child is sick. If the child has an elevated blood glucose and moderate or large amounts of ketones, treatment with extra insulin and fluids can be initiated. Increased attention to blood glucose and urine ketone monitoring

---

Health Promotion **Child With Diabetes Mellitus**

Growth and Development Surveillance

- Compare the child's height, weight, and head circumfernce to age-specific norms to determine if growth is meeting expectations for age. Monitor body mass index (BMI) percentile at each healthcare visit.

- Assess developmental progress using the Denver II or another screening tool (refer to Chapter 34). Assess school performance.

- Assess for delays in development of secondary sexual characteristics and pubertal changes.

Nutrition

- Promote adherence to nutrition guidelines by including the child's personal preferences in the food plan.

Physical Activity

- Encourage regular physical activity and educate the child to modify insulin dosage or food intake for extra physical activity periods.

- Encourage the child to participate in sports when interested and work to balance exercise, food intake, and insulin dosage.

Oral Health

- Promote good dentition and oral hygiene.

- Regular dental visits are important to reduce risk of infections.

- The child with poorly controlled diabetes is at risk of gingivitis and cavities.

Mental and Spiritual Health

- Provide the child and adolescent an opportunity to discuss feelings regarding diabetes.

- Assess the adolescent for evidence of depression.

Relationships

- The child should attend school or child care as any other child. Parents may need support to find facilities able to monitor the child as needed and to provide the teaching required for facility employees.

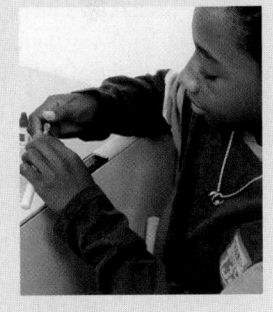

- Encourage the development of special friends who can be informed about the child's disorder and seek help when the child has signs of hypoglycemia or hyperglycemia.

Disease Prevention Strategies

- Encourage the family to ensure that the child receives all recommended immunizations, including an annual influenza vaccine.

- Refer the child for an annual ophthalmologic examination.

- Maintain appointments for regular evaluation of HbA$_{1c}$ to monitor glycemic control.

Injury Prevention Strategies

- Encourage the child to wear a medical alert identification.

- Encourage daily inspection of feet and foot care.

- Provide the family with strategies for safe disposal of needles and syringes.

is especially important when the child has significant stressors such as an illness. It is important for the child and family to understand that insulin is required even when the child is not eating to counter the hormones secreted in response to the stressor.

Hypoglycemia in the Child With Diabetes

Hypoglycemia can develop within minutes in children with type 1 diabetes mellitus. The symptoms outlined in Table 53–6 may occur when blood glucose levels suddenly drop or fall below 70 mg/dL. Children are at risk of hypoglycemia because of their rapid growth rates and unpredictable eating habits and physical activity. Severe hypoglycemic episodes may occur at night in children who are treated with two to three injections per day. Other common causes include an error in insulin dosage, errors in injection technique, inadequate calories because of missed meals, or exercise without a corresponding increase in caloric intake. Severe hypoglycemia can cause seizures.

Hypoglycemia can be diagnosed on the basis of the sudden onset of signs and symptoms. A blood glucose reading should be taken to confirm a low blood sugar is possible if equipment is readily available. Give a glucose source immediately by mouth. If the child becomes unconscious, administer an injection of glucagon, or, if unavailable, administer sugar gel or glucose paste squeezed onto the gums. In the hospital setting, administer an intravenous infusion of dextrose to prevent progression of symptoms. Since the effects of dextrose and glucagon are temporary, additional snacks or a meal is provided. The child should be continually observed for several hours after treatment.

Nursing Management

Teach parents and children to recognize the signs of hypoglycemia and take appropriate action. Parents are taught to give **glucagon** (a hormone produced by the pancreas that helps release stored glucose from the liver) by injection for cases of

---

TEACHING HIGHLIGHTS | Preventing DKA

When to Monitor for DKA

- Abdominal pain
- Nausea, vomiting, and anorexia
- 1- or 2-day history of polyuria and polydipsia
- Has illness (e.g., viral or other) and is unable to eat

Recognizing Signs of DKA

- Change in mental status
- Blood glucose greater than 250 mg/dL
- Moderate to large ketones present in urine
- Fruity breath odor
- Rapid, deep respirations
- Decreased urine output

Source: Data from Masharani, U. (2015). Diabetes mellitus & hypoglycemia. In M. A. Papadakis, S. J. McPhee, & M. W. Rabow (Eds.), *CURRENT medical diagnosis & treatment 2015*. New York, NY: McGraw-Hill; McFarlane, K. (2011). An overview of diabetic ketoacidosis in children. *Paediatric Nursing, 23*(1), 14–19.

TEACHING HIGHLIGHTS | Treating Hypoglycemic Episodes

- If the child shows signs of hypoglycemia (pallor, sweating, tremors, dizziness, numb lips or mouth, confusion, irritability, altered mental status), test the blood glucose level.
- Assist the child to perform the test. Skills needed to get an accurate reading deteriorate with altered mental status.
- If the blood glucose reading is less than or equal to 70 mg/dL, give glucose rapidly. Use one of the following to give 15 g of rapid-acting glucose to raise the blood sugar level:
  - ½ cup fruit juice
  - ½ cup of regular cola or soda
  - 1 small box raisins
  - 3 to 4 glucose tablets
- Wait 15 minutes and recheck the blood glucose level. Repeat the 15 g of rapid-acting glucose if it is still less than or equal to 70 mg/dL. Recheck the blood glucose level in another 15 minutes.
- Once blood sugar has returned to at least 80 mg/dL, give a more substantial snack such as cheese and crackers if the next meal will be more than 30 minutes later or an activity or exercise is planned.
- If the child is unconscious, administer glucagon by injection or spread glucose paste on the gums.

TABLE 53–6 Clinical Manifestations of Hypoglycemia and Hyperglycemia

CAUSE	CLINICAL MANIFESTATIONS	CLINICAL THERAPY
HYPOGLYCEMIA		
• Insulin dose too high for food eaten • Insulin injection into muscle • Too much exercise for insulin dose • Too long between meals/snacks • Too few carbohydrates eaten • Illness, stress	Rapid onset Irritability, nervousness, tremors, shaky feeling, difficulty concentrating or speaking, behavior change, confusion, repeating something over and over Unconsciousness, seizure, shallow breathing, tachycardia Pallor, sweating Moist mucous membranes, hunger Headache, dizziness, blurred vision, double vision, photophobia Numb lips or mouth	If conscious, give 15 g of carbohydrate. Wait 15 minutes and recheck blood glucose level. Give another 15 g of carbohydrate if 70 mg/dL or below. Recheck the blood glucose level in 15 minutes. If unconscious, give glucagon by injection.
HYPERGLYCEMIA		
• Insulin dose too low for food eaten • Illness or injury, stress • Too many carbohydrates eaten • Meals/snacks too close together • Insulin injected just under skin or injected into hypertrophied areas • Decreased activity	Gradual onset Lethargy, sleepiness, slowed responses, or confusion Deep, rapid breathing Flushed skin, dry skin Dry mucous membranes, thirst, hunger, dehydration Weakness, fatigue Headache, abdominal pain, nausea, vomiting Blurred vision Shock	Give additional insulin at usual injection time. Give correction scale insulin doses for specific blood glucose levels when ill or injured. Give extra injections if hyperglycemia and moderate to large ketones. Increase fluids.

severe hypoglycemia and to activate the emergency medical system (9-1-1). Reinforce the importance of balancing dietary intake, insulin, and exercise every day.

Type 2 Diabetes

Type 2 diabetes is a disease associated with insulin resistance (an alteration of the insulin receptor that signals the presence of insulin in the interior of cells). Significant risk factors for type 2 diabetes includes obesity, low levels of physical activity, intake of high-energy foods, low socioeconomic status, ethnicity, and family history of diabetes (Bacon, 2013; Dea, 2011; Svoren & Jospe, 2016). Over 75% of children with type 2 diabetes have a first- or second-degree relative with diabetes (Dea, 2011).

The increasing number of children being diagnosed with type 2 diabetes has caused significant concern in the healthcare community. According to the SEARCH for Diabetes in Youth Study, an estimated 5089 people younger than 20 years were newly diagnosed with type 2 diabetes annually during 2008 to 2009. The incidence was highest in children ages 10 to 19 and in U.S. minority populations (CDC, 2014). The true incidence is unknown because many children are undiagnosed.

Developing Cultural Competence Type 2 Diabetes Risk

Children of African American, Native American, Hispanic/ Latino, and Asian/Pacific Islander origins are at greater risk for developing type 2 diabetes (American Diabetes Association, 2015).

ETIOLOGY AND PATHOPHYSIOLOGY

Children who are obese are at risk to develop type 2 diabetes because the excess body fat decreases the body's ability to use insulin (Bacon, 2013). The onset of puberty and increased secretion of growth hormone are believed to be contributing factors in the development of insulin resistance (Dea, 2011). The pancreatic cells produce more insulin in an attempt to overcome the insulin resistance and maintain a normal glucose tolerance. When the beta cells are not able to produce enough insulin, blood glucose levels increase (Khan, Cooper, & Del Prato, 2014).

CLINICAL MANIFESTATIONS

Signs and symptoms of type 2 diabetes vary. The child may not have any symptoms or may present with polydipsia, polyuria, blurred vision, and fatigue (American Diabetes Association, 2015). **Acanthosis nigricans** is described as a hyperpigmentation and thickening of the skin with velvety irregularities in the skin folds of the back of the neck, axillae, and flexor skin surfaces. It has been established as a risk factor for the development of type 2 diabetes and is associated with insulin resistance (Abraham & Rozmus, 2012) (see Figure 53–9). The child with type 2 diabetes is usually obese with a high waist circumference. Approximately 5% to 25% of children with type 2 diabetes present with ketoacidosis at the time of diagnosis (Dea, 2011).

CLINICAL THERAPY

Blood glucose levels of 200 mg/dL or greater without fasting or a fasting glucose of 126 mg/dL or greater, are diagnostic of diabetes (ADA, 2014b). HbA$_{1c}$ predicts the average blood

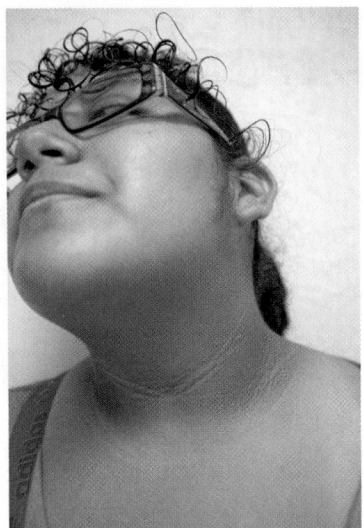

Figure 53–9 Acanthosis nigricans.

glucose over the past 3 months (National Diabetes Information Clearinghouse, 2014). Islet cell autoantibodies, fasting insulin levels, and C-peptide levels are used to help differentiate between type 1 and type 2 diabetes but are not definitive. Islet cell autoantibodies (GAD-65, islet cell antibodies, insulin) are suggestive for type 1 diabetes; however, autoantibodies specific to a certain antigen are not present in approximately 15% of children with type 1 diabetes. Additionally, some children with type 2 diabetes will have detectable autoantibodies. While insulin and C-peptide levels are usually low in children with type 1 diabetes, there is some overlap with type 2, so these values are not helpful with the initial classification (Cohee, 2012). A fasting lipid profile is obtained since dyslipidemia (primarily elevated triglycerides and LDL cholesterol) is usually present (Svoren & Jospe, 2016). High blood pressure for age, gender, and height percentile is also seen (see Appendix D).

The multiple goals for managing the child with type 2 diabetes include the following: normalizing the blood glucose and HbA$_{1c}$ levels, decreasing weight, increasing exercise, normalizing lipid profile and blood pressure, and preventing complications. Nutrition education and weight loss make up the major therapy. The child needs to have gradual, sustained weight loss, metabolic control of blood glucose levels, exercise, and emotional support.

If the child or adolescent presents with severe hyperglycemia or diabetic ketoacidosis, insulin will be required to gain initial glycemic control. Once metabolic control is achieved, oral medication (metformin) is initiated as the child is weaned off of insulin. Metformin is used when diet and exercise efforts are inadequate to control hyperglycemia. Metformin improves the sensitivity of target cells to insulin, slows the gastrointestinal absorption of glucose, and reduces hepatic and renal glucose production. It can be used when there is normal liver and kidney function and no ketosis. The dosage may be gradually increased to improve metabolic control. If additional medication is needed, sulfonylureas may be used if metformin alone is not adequate or is contraindicated, but their use in pediatrics is limited. Thiazolidinediones are not approved for use in children but may be used if metformin is contraindicated. Some children ultimately require insulin for glycemic control (Svoren & Jospe, 2016).

Nursing Management

For the Child With Type 2 Diabetes

Nursing Assessment and Diagnosis

Because the child with type 2 diabetes does not often have an acute onset, assess any child with a body mass index (BMI) greater than 85th percentile for age and gender for signs of insulin resistance (acanthosis nigricans, hypertension, and dyslipidemia). Family history of diabetes in an overweight child is a reason to begin screening for the condition. Once the child has been diagnosed, monitor the child's blood glucose levels and blood pressure. Assess the child's diet and activity patterns to determine appropriate changes for disease management. Consider evaluating the siblings for diabetes.

Nursing diagnoses that may apply to the child with type 2 diabetes include the following (NANDA-I © 2014):

- *Activity Intolerance* related to sedentary lifestyle and disease state (insulin resistance)
- *Health Management, Family, Ineffective*, related to family conflict over changing eating patterns
- *Self-Esteem, Situational Low,* related to situational crisis associated with diagnosis of new-onset chronic illness

Planning and Implementation

The child with type 2 diabetes may be hospitalized at the time of diagnosis because of ketoacidosis. However, the nurse in an inpatient setting is more likely to encounter this child when hospitalized for another condition or during visits for health care in clinics or schools. Nursing care focuses on managing the child's blood glucose levels and hypertension during the hospitalization, assessing growth and dietary intake, evaluating goals for weight loss and exercise programs, and reviewing the child's knowledge about diabetes and strategies for management at home.

COMMUNITY-BASED NURSING CARE

Since the child is initially diagnosed with type 2 diabetes and managed on an outpatient basis, nursing care focuses on teaching the child and parents about the disease and its management, managing dietary intake, providing emotional support, and planning strategies for daily management in the community.

Educate the child and family about the disease and lifestyle changes required for effective management of the condition. Focus on the need to increase activity with routine exercise of at least 30 to 60 minutes daily and to decrease sedentary activity time, such as computer and television viewing time to no more than 2 hours daily. Customize the activity strategy for each child with motivation to develop a regular routine.

Work with the family to substitute high-calorie and high-fat foods with a meal plan sensitive to the family's resources and ethnic preferences. Suggestions include limiting fast food and snacking on fruits and vegetables rather than foods high in fat and sugar. Assess the child's height, weight, and BMI on each visit, and plot on the appropriate growth curve for age and gender. A gradual sustained weight loss or decrease in BMI is the goal. If the child is experiencing a height growth spurt, maintenance of weight rather than weight loss is the goal. Encourage the entire family to make dietary changes, especially since other family members are also at risk for the condition.

Teach the child and family to perform home blood glucose testing to monitor glycemic control. This will let the child and family know that efforts to manage the disease are successful.

Take HbA$_{1c}$ levels at each visit to determine the average blood glucose level for the past 3 months. When dietary control and exercise are not successful in reducing blood glucose levels, teach the child and family about the prescribed oral medication.

Give the child and family opportunities to talk about the impact of the disease on their lives. Identify resources for information about strategies that have worked for other families. Identify local support groups and peer groups for the family and child. Suggest weekly activities, summer camps, and other ongoing programs to provide necessary support and motivation.

Make sure the child gets annual evaluations for potential complications of diabetes. The tests to be performed include blood for lipid levels, blood pressure, liver and renal function, urine for albumin, an eye examination for retinopathy, and a neurologic examination of the extremities for neuropathies. The child with type 2 diabetes has the same risk for developing long-term vascular complications as the child with type 1 diabetes when hyperglycemia is poorly controlled.

Evaluation

Examples of expected outcomes of nursing care include the following:

- The child decreases sedentary activity time to less than 2 hours a day.
- The child's daily intake of fruits and vegetables increases to five to eight servings daily, and total fat intake decreases to less than 30% of total calories.
- The child's BMI slowly and consistently decreases.

Disorders of Gonadal Function

Gynecomastia

Gynecomastia is a proliferation of glandular breast tissue in males that occurs in approximately 40% to 65% of adolescent boys. Gynecomastia results from an imbalance in estrogens and androgens in the breast tissue. Gynecomastia is generally idiopathic, although it can be associated with a chronic disorders, tumors, or drug use (Saito et al., 2014). The condition disappears in 75% of cases. If gynecomastia is causing pain or psychologic distress to the adolescent, treatment with a medication such as tamoxifen or surgical intervention with a minimally invasive approach may be indicated (Fischer et al., 2014).

Nursing care focuses on reassuring the child and his parents that gynecomastia is common and transient. Because of the body image concerns common during adolescence, embarrassment is a frequent problem. Recommend clothing styles and other methods to camouflage the enlarged breasts. If treatment is indicated, education regarding medication use or surgery is needed.

See Chapter 5 for a discussion of amenorrhea and dysmenorrhea.

Growth and Development

Girls competing in sports such as long-distance running and track and field may be at increased risk for musculoskeletal injury. The female athlete triad places the runner at increased risk for injury such as stress fractures and comprises these three components: low energy availability (with or without disordered eating), low bone mineral density, and menstrual dysfunction. Research indicates that oligomenorrhea (infrequent menstruation) or amenorrhea (lack of menstruation) and low bone mineral density are associated with injury in the lower extremities (Rauh, Barrack, & Nichols, 2014) (see Chapter 56).

Disorders Related to Sex Chromosome Abnormalities

Turner Syndrome

In Turner syndrome, girls have a missing or partial absence of one X chromosome. This condition occurs in approximately 1 in 2000 to 1 in 5000 live female births (Oliveira, Ribeiro, Lago, et al., 2013). An estimated 90% of fetuses with Turner syndrome are spontaneously aborted during the first trimester. Turner syndrome is primarily associated with short stature and infertility (Martin & Smyth, 2012).

Characteristic clinical findings in the newborn include edema of the hands and feet, a webbed neck, a low hairline, a high-arched palate, a small jaw, low-set ears, droopy eyelids, a short fourth toe, short fingers, a broad chest, and widely separated nipples (Figure 53–10). Some children may have only one or two mild symptoms, and the diagnosis may not be made until adolescence when pubertal delay and lack of the onset of menstruation are apparent (Martin & Smyth, 2012).

Growth usually proceeds at a normal rate until around 3 years of life and then slows, ceasing after puberty (Walker, 2014). Congenital heart defects frequently associated with Turner syndrome include coarctation of the aorta and bicuspid aortic valve (Levitsky, Luria, Hayes, et al., 2015). Other associated conditions include hearing loss, structural abnormalities of the kidney, and ophthalmic abnormalities (Martin & Smyth, 2012). Musculoskeletal disorders may include scoliosis and osteoporosis (Walker, 2014).

Diagnosis of Turner syndrome may be determined prenatally by amniocentesis or chorionic villi sampling (Martin & Smyth, 2012). The condition is diagnosed definitively by a karyotype. The most common and most severe phenotype is 45,X, indicating an absent X chromosome, which occurs in 40% to 60% of girls with Turner syndrome (Oliveira et al., 2013). Other types of Turner syndrome occur when the X chromosome is partially missing or rearranged, or when there are chromosomal changes in some of the cells (mosaicism) (Genetics Home Reference, 2012).

Treatment involves careful monitoring of the child's growth. A growth chart made especially for girls with Turner syndrome is available from the Turner Syndrome Society. Growth hormone therapy may be prescribed to promote growth during childhood. With treatment, final height generally reaches approximately 5 feet 2 inches; without treatment, the

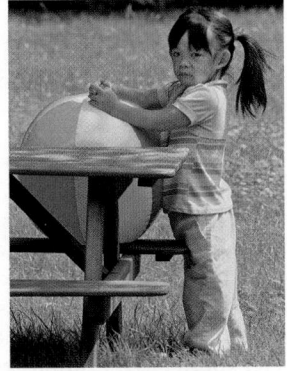

Figure 53–10 What characteristic physical manifestations of Turner syndrome can you identify in this girl?

SOURCE: Ed Suba Jr./Akron Beacon Journal/AP Photo.

final height is approximately 4 feet 8 inches (Martin & Smyth, 2012). Estrogen and progesterone therapy are generally prescribed to promote breast development and decrease the risk of osteoporosis (Walker, 2014).

Nursing Management

Nursing assessment is focused on monitoring growth rates and observing for signs of cardiac, renal, gastrointestinal, vision, hearing, musculoskeletal, or thyroid dysfunction. Carefully measure the child's height and plot on the growth curve. Teach the family the correct administration of growth hormone and potential side effects.

The lack of growth and sexual development associated with Turner syndrome presents problems not only for physical growth but also for psychosocial development. The girl's perception of her body and how she differs from peers affects self-image, self-consciousness, and self-esteem. In the United States, cultural values place importance on attaining normal to tall stature. Short children tend to be treated according to their size rather than their age. Emphasis is also placed on sexual maturity. Encourage parents to treat the child by her chronologic age rather than size. Even though the child's intelligence is generally normal, learning disabilities are common (Saenz, Tsai, Manchester, et. al., 2014).

Klinefelter Syndrome

Klinefelter syndrome is a genetic condition that occurs in boys who have an extra X chromosome (usually 47,XXY). It occurs in approximately 1 in 450 males. Klinefelter syndrome is associated with androgen deficiency, infertility in males, and tall stature (Bourke, Herlihy, Snow, et al., 2014).

Klinefelter syndrome may be diagnosed when the onset of puberty is delayed or an abnormal progression is evident. Testes are small and firm. Less facial and body hair may develop. Gynecomastia is a characteristic finding (Bourke et al., 2014).

Klinefelter syndrome may also be diagnosed during the school-age years when the child is having difficulty at school. The child may have delayed developmental milestones and a low verbal IQ. Language and learning problems including difficulty reading may be present. The child may have difficulty socializing with others and body image issues (Bourke et al., 2014).

Chromosomal analysis revealing one or more extra X chromosomes confirms the diagnosis. The goal of treatment is to stimulate masculinization and the development of secondary sex characteristics when adolescence is delayed. Testosterone replacement is begun at puberty when the male is 11 or 12 years of age. A testosterone preparation is given by intramuscular injection every 3 to 4 weeks to maintain serum testosterone levels within the normal range. The dose is increased gradually every 6 to 9 months until a maintenance dose is achieved in adults (Ali & Donohoue, 2016).

Nursing Management

Nursing care consists of educating the parents and child about the syndrome, evaluating the child's and family's coping mechanisms, assisting with school problems, and reinforcing the child's strengths. Encourage parents to channel their son's energy into areas that will provide opportunities for success and productive experiences. Emphasize the importance of rewarding the boy's successes in school, sports, or hobbies. Make genetic counseling available to adolescents, if indicated, because sexual functioning and fertility may be impaired.

Inborn Errors of Metabolism

Inborn errors of metabolism are inherited biochemical abnormalities of the urea cycle, amino acid, or organic acid metabolism. Therefore, protein, carbohydrate, fat, electrolyte, blood, and respiratory metabolism can be affected. Individually they are rare disorders; however, as a group they are a significant health problem in infancy.

The biochemical defect usually causes an abnormal chemical by-product to accumulate in the blood, urine, or tissues or results in a decreased amount of normal enzymes. Most disorders are associated with protein intolerance with symptoms developing shortly after formula or breast milk feedings begin.

Clinical manifestations usually occur within days or weeks of birth. Signs and symptoms may include lethargy and poor feeding, persistent vomiting, abnormal muscle tone and seizures, apnea and tachycardia, and an unusual urine or body odor (musty, sweet odor of maple syrup or burnt sugar, or cheesy or sweaty feet).

Newborn screening has been demonstrated to save lives and to prevent serious disability. The March of Dimes (2012) recommends newborn screening tests for 31 health conditions. In most states, newborn screening programs lead to the detection of several conditions before symptoms develop.

In some cases, disorders associated with inborn errors of metabolism are not detected until signs and symptoms are present. Initial laboratory tests include measurement of serum glucose, electrolytes, blood gases, and serum ammonia. Tests results make it possible to classify the disorder by the presence of hypoglycemia, metabolic acidosis, hyperammonemia, or liver dysfunction. Further diagnostic laboratory tests are then performed on newborns with positive results.

Treatment, when available, focuses on replacing or reducing the amount of the substance causing the biochemical abnormality.

Four of the more common inborn errors of metabolism—phenylketonuria, galactosemia, mitochondrial diseases, and maple syrup urine disease—are presented in this section. Congenital hypothyroidism and congenital adrenal hyperplasia, which are also considered inborn errors of metabolism, were discussed earlier in this chapter.

Phenylketonuria

Phenylketonuria (PKU) is an autosomal recessive inherited disorder of amino acid metabolism that affects the body's use of protein. It is caused by a mutation of the phenylalanine hydroxylase gene. The incidence is approximately 1 in 15,000 newborns in the United States (Araujo et al., 2013; Brosco & Paul, 2013). Approximately 275 children are born with PKU each year in the United States (Brosco & Paul, 2013). The defect results in an accumulation of phenylalanine in the blood or phenylalanine metabolites in the urine. If untreated, this disease leads to irreversible brain damage and severe intellectual disability. Phenylalanine levels above 20 mg/dL are indicative of classic PKU (Rezvani & Ficicioglu, 2016).

Children with PKU have a deficiency of the liver enzyme phenylalanine hydroxylase that normally breaks down the essential amino acid phenylalanine into tyrosine. As a result, phenylalanine accumulates in the blood, causing a musty or mousey body and urine odor, irritability, vomiting, hyperactivity, hypertonia, hyperreflexive deep tendon reflexes, seizures, and an eczema-like rash (Rezvani & Ficicioglu, 2016). Persistence of elevated phenylalanine leads to disruption of cellular processes of myelination and protein synthesis, and results in a seizure disorder and untreatable intellectual disability.

Babies appear normal at birth except for lighter skin complexion than their nonaffected siblings. If diagnosis is delayed, a mousy or musty body odor is noticed and intellectual disability may be severe. Other common findings in untreated children include microcephaly, growth retardation, enamel hypoplasia, prominent maxilla, and widely spaced teeth (Rezvani & Ficicioglu, 2016).

Screening for PKU is required by state law in all 50 states. For best results, the newborn should have begun formula or breast milk feeding before specimen collection. Early hospital discharge places newborns at risk for false-negative screening tests if screened within 24 hours of birth. Screening needs to occur no sooner than 48 hours after birth, or the test should be repeated at 1 to 2 weeks of age. If the test shows elevated levels of plasma phenylalanine, a repeat quantitative test is performed. If the second test is positive, the family is referred to an outpatient treatment center. Serum levels of phenylalanine should be measured periodically throughout life.

PKU is treated using special formulas and a diet low in phenylalanine to keep plasma phenylalanine levels between 2 and 6 mg/dL. The diet must also meet the child's needs for optimal growth. High-protein foods (meats and dairy products) are avoided because they contain large amounts of phenylalanine. Elemental medical foods (modified protein hydrolysates in which the phenylalanine has been removed) are used instead. The low-phenylalanine diet should be maintained throughout life for the best outcomes (Marcason, 2013).

Nursing Management

Nursing care is mainly supportive and focuses on teaching parents about the disorder and its management. The low-phenylalanine diet is a rigid, strict diet that excludes many foods. Educate the family about sources of phenylalanine, and refer the family to a registered dietician to establish an appropriate meal plan. Parents and children need a great deal of support to promote compliance. The formula and elemental medical food costs are relatively expensive. The formula is usually reimbursed by insurance, but negotiations with health plans may help parents obtain some support for medical foods. Parents of an affected child who are considering a future pregnancy and adolescents with the disorder should be referred for genetic counseling.

Galactosemia

Galactosemia, a disorder of carbohydrate metabolism, has an autosomal recessive inheritance pattern. It occurs in approximately 1 in 30,000 to 60,000 births in the United States (Screening, Technology, and Research in Genetics [STRG], 2012).

Galactosemia results from a deficiency of the liver enzyme galactose 1-phosphate uridyltransferase (GALT), one of three enzymes needed to convert galactose to glucose. The lack of enzyme leads to an accumulation of galactose metabolites in the eyes, liver, kidney, and brain, rapidly damaging the organs and causing life-threatening problems. Affected children become susceptible to gram-negative sepsis.

Early signs include poor sucking, failure to gain weight due to vomiting followed by diarrhea, hypoglycemia, and an enlarged liver. Later signs include intellectual disability, jaundice, ascites, sepsis, lethargy, seizures, hypotonia, cataracts, and coma. Babies may die within 1 month of birth without treatment, usually because of sepsis. When diagnosis is not made at birth, cirrhosis of the liver and intellectual disability progresses and becomes irreversible (Kishnani & Chen, 2016).

Routine newborn screening for galactosemia is performed in all 50 states (National Newborn Screening and Genetics Resource Center, 2014). (See the *Clinical Skills Manual* SKILLS.) Infants who are not screened at birth are identified once they become symptomatic. The diagnosis is based on history, physical examination, and laboratory tests (galactose, aspartate aminotransferase [AST], and alanine aminotransferase [ALT] levels are abnormally high). Urine specimens are checked for reducing substances (the Clinitest is positive and the Clinistix is negative) in several specimens while the infant is receiving human milk or formula with lactose.

Treatment involves placing infants on a lactose- or galactose-free formula. A lactose- and galactose-free diet must be followed for life. Calcium, vitamin D, and vitamin K supplements may be prescribed as well (STRG, 2012).

Despite compliance with the diet, complications (learning disabilities, speech defects, ovarian failure, and neurologic syndromes) develop in many children (Kishnani & Chen, 2016).

Nursing Management

Nursing management focuses on educating the parents and child about the disorder and required diet, assessing coping abilities, and providing emotional support. Refer the family to a registered dietician for diet counseling. Families must learn to screen foods for added milk solids and to avoid medications, such as antibiotics, that have lactose fillers. Calcium supplementation may be needed. Advise parents that several galactose-free cheeses are sold commercially. Because the disorder is inherited, refer the family for genetic counseling.

Mitochondrial Diseases

Mitochondrial diseases are a heterogeneous group of genetic disorders that result from a mutation in the nuclear or mitochondrial genes (Codier & Codier, 2014). It is estimated that 1 in 300 people have a genetic mutation that could affect mitochondrial function, but only a small fraction (1:5000) will develop mitochondrial disease (Codier & Codier, 2014).

Mitochondria are the cell's energy "powerhouses," producing energy through a process called *oxidative phosphorylation*, which uses glucose and oxygen to produce adenosine triphosphate (ATP) through the respiratory electron transport chain complexes I to V of the Krebs cycle (Codier & Codier, 2014). Point mutations, deletions, or duplications in mitochondrial DNA (mtDNA) can cause mitochondrial disorders that are transmitted from mothers to their children. Mitochondrial disorders can also result from mutations in the nuclear DNA (nDNA) of either parent and follow an autosomal recessive Mendelian pattern of inheritance (United Mitochondrial Disease Foundation [UMDF], 2011) (see Chapter 3 for further information about inheritance). Malfunction of the mitochondria results in the inability of the cell to produce sufficient energy and maintain metabolic regulation. Numerous mutations are known to cause mitochondrial disease. Some of the more common disorders are Leigh syndrome, Barth syndrome, Kearns-Sayers syndrome, fatty acid oxidation disease, mitochondrial encephalopathy with lactic acidosis and strokelike episodes (MELAS), neurogenic weakness with ataxia and retinitis pigmentosa (NAEP), and Pearson syndrome (Dassler & Allen, 2014).

Mitochondrial disease may present at any age, ranging from the newborn period into childhood and adulthood, with

TABLE 53–7 Affected Systems and Associated Symptoms of Mitochondrial Disease

SYSTEM	SYMPTOMS
Cardiovascular	Cardiomyopathy, heart block, arrhythmias, tachycardia, bradycardia
Endocrine	Short stature, diabetes mellitus, exocrine pancreatic failure, thyroid dysfunction, hypoglycemia
Eyes and ears	Vision loss and blindness, droopy eyelids, paralysis or weakness of the eye muscles, optic atrophy, degenerative eye disease, acquired strabismus, hearing loss, deafness
Gastrointestinal	Anorexia, vomiting, diarrhea, constipation, pseudo-obstruction, irritable bowel syndrome, dysphagia, dysmotility, gastroesophageal reflux, delayed gastric emptying
Genitourinary/renal	Glomerular disease, renal tubular acidosis, frequency, urgency, urinary retention
Hematologic	Bruising, bleeding, anemia, pancytopenia
Musculoskeletal	Exercise intolerance, low muscle tone, weakness, muscle pain,
Neurologic	Developmental delay, cognitive disabilities, seizures, migraines, strokes, ataxia, spasticity, temperature instability, fainting, absent reflexes
Respiratory	Obstructive sleep apnea, tachypnea, dyspnea
Systemic	Fatigue, failure to gain weight

Source: Data from Dassler A., & Allen, P. (2014). Mitochondrial disease in children and adolescents. *Pediatric Nursing, 40*(3), 150–154; Klehm, M., & Korson, M. (2014). *A clinician's guide to the management of mitochondrial disease*. Retrieved from http://www.mitoaction.org/guide/table-contents; United Mitochondrial Disease Foundation (UMDF). (2011). *MitoFIRST handbook: An introductory guide*. Retrieved from http://www.kintera.org/atf/cf/%7B858ACD34-ECC3-472A-8794-39B92E103561%7D/mito_first.pdf

a spectrum of possible signs and symptoms (see Table 53–7). Clinical presentation is very diverse but affects "high energy demand" organs (Codier & Codier, 2014). Hallmarks of mitochondrial disease include (1) more than one organ system involved, (2) atypical features of another type of known disease, and (3) recurrent setbacks or flare-ups during an infection or stress. Mitochondrial disease should be considered in any patient with unexplained multisystem involvement and progressive deterioration (UMDF, 2011). A single organ may be predominately affected, but a combination of dysfunction in unrelated organs, unexplained multisystem symptoms, or involvement of three or more organ systems without a unifying diagnosis should raise concern for mitochondrial disease (Codier & Codier, 2014).

Diagnosis is elusive, time consuming, laborious, and expensive, with limited evidence-based guidelines or biomarkers (Dassler & Allen, 2014). Clinical symptoms, family history, age of symptom onset, muscle biopsy, imaging, and genetic testing are considered in making a diagnosis (Dassler & Allen, 2014). Genetic testing is still in its infancy, remains expensive, and may not be covered by insurance. Many patients have delayed diagnoses or diagnoses of probable or possible mitochondrial disease.

There is no cure or well-studied pharmacologic treatment for mitochondrial disease. Treatment focuses on conserving energy; frequent intake of nutrients; regular sleep; maintaining health; maximizing mitochondrial function; symptom management; nutrition therapy; physical therapy; reducing physiologic stressors such as extremes in cold or heat; avoiding known mitochondrial toxins such as alcohol, cigarette smoke, and monosodium glutamate (MSG); and providing emotional care and family support (Codier & Codier, 2014; Dassler & Allen, 2014; UMDF, 2011). Nutritious foods and frequent hydration provide cells with nutrients to support mitochondrial function, while prolonged periods of fasting produce mitochondrial stress and should be avoided (Dassler & Allen, 2014). The only current pharmacologic treatments available consist of vitamin and dietary supplementation, known as a "mitochondrial cocktail" (Dassler & Allen, 2014). This cocktail often contains antioxidants such as thiamine, vitamin C, vitamin E, and alphalipoic acid, along with coenzyme Q10 (CoQ10) and levo-carnitine (Carnitor) as essential components of mitochondrial electron transport (UMDF, 2011).

Nursing Management

Nursing management for mitochondrial disease is multifaceted and includes physiologic, emotional, and spiritual care while educating parents about energy and fatigue management, nutritional support, physical therapy, acute and long-term symptom management, physiologic stress reduction, and immunizations (Codier & Codier, 2014). Multisystem care must be individualized to meet the needs of the patient. During an acute phase, nursing care involves extensive neurologic support, seizure management, cardiac respiratory support, tube feedings, nutritional supplementation, and frequent hydration. Children with the disease should usually go no longer than 8 to 12 hours without food. Infants should be fed around the clock every 2 to 4 hours. Small frequent meals are a better choice than three full meals a day. Consumption of a complex carbohydrate or protein before bed will help prevent overnight hypoglycemia. Children who are unable to sustain oral intake during an acute illness must be referred to the hospital for intravenous dextrose supplementation. Specialists should manage care during hospitalizations or surgery, especially the administration of anesthesia. Even simple infections such as otitis media or influenza can become life threatening. Long-term management includes assessment for mobility aids, home environment adaptations, educational care plans, vision and hearing aids, assessment of family functioning, stress and coping, genetic counseling, and end-of-life care. Nursing care also involves assisting parents to navigate the complex healthcare system and coordinate visits involving multiple specialists. Nurses should inquire about specific stressors related to travel, frequent hospitalizations, medical visits, school accommodations, care for siblings, and parental guilt, and suggest effective coping strategies to manage the many aspects of mitochondrial disease (Senger, 2013). If one child in the family is diagnosed with the disorder, the siblings should also be monitored or tested even if they are asymptomatic.

Maple Syrup Urine Disease

Maple syrup urine disease (MSUD) is a disorder of amino acid metabolism that has an autosomal recessive inheritance pattern (Cole, 2014). It is rare, occurring in approximately 1 in 150,000 to

1 in 185,000 of the general population, but it occurs as often as 1 in 760 in Mennonites (Burfield, Hussa, & Randall, 2012).

In MSUD leucine, isoleucine, and valine cannot be metabolized because of an enzyme defect in the branched chain of these three essential amino acids. All three amino acids are essential to form normal structures such as the hair, skin, and muscle. Accumulation of these three amino acids leads to encephalopathy and progressive neurologic impairment if left untreated (Bodamer & Lee, 2014).

Within 5 to 7 days of life, the newborn develops symptoms of poor sucking, irregular respirations, and rigidity with alternating flaccidity (Burfield et al, 2012). Ketosis and a sweet odor of maple syrup in urine are generally present when symptoms develop (Bodamer & Lee, 2014). If the child is not treated, symptoms progress to seizures, apnea, and death (Burfield et al., 2012).

All states require newborn screening for this condition (National Newborn Screening and Genetics Resource Center, 2014). Diagnosis is made with laboratory tests of the urine for positive ketones and blood tests for elevated levels of leucine, isoleucine, alloisoleucine, and valine.

Treatment during the acute stage involves removal of the branched-chain amino acids and their metabolites from the tissues and body fluids. Some critically ill infants may require dialysis to remove these compounds because their renal clearance is poor.

Lifelong treatment includes specially designed medical formulas and foods rich in amino acids, calories, vitamins, minerals, and other nutrients as prescribed. These special medical foods have the three amino acids removed. The child needs special low-protein foods that are adequate for growth with enough calories to support twice the child's basal metabolic rate. Daily urine testing is required to determine if ketones are being excreted, an indication that the body is in a catabolic state. Liver transplants have been performed in a few affected children who were subsequently able to tolerate a normal diet. The long-term prognosis of children with MSUD is guarded (Rezvani & Rosenblatt, 2016).

Nursing Management

Nursing care includes educating the family about the disorder and special dietary requirements. The parents need to learn how to mix the child's special formula with a natural protein source, amino acid supplements, and water. The child needs formula even when ill. Parents should have a sick day plan to prevent ketoacidosis. The child should be permitted moderate exercise only to prevent increases in leucine levels. Help families identify sources of information or support groups who can share recipes and tips for managing the child's condition.

Focus Your Study

- The hypothalamic-pituitary axis produces several releasing and inhibiting hormones that regulate the function of many endocrine glands.

- Puberty is the process of sexual maturation that occurs when the gonads secrete increased amounts of the sex hormones estrogen and testosterone, resulting in the development of primary and secondary sexual characteristics.

- Children with hypopituitarism have short stature as a result of growth hormone deficiency. Treatment with growth hormone early in life enables these children to potentially attain genetically appropriate heights.

- An excessive secretion of growth hormone or hyperpituitarism may cause children to have tall stature, growing up to 7 or 8 feet in height if no intervention is provided before the epiphyseal plates close.

- Diabetes insipidus is a disorder of the posterior pituitary gland and is defined as an inability of the kidneys to concentrate urine.

- Syndrome of inappropriate antidiuretic hormone (SIADH) results from an excessive amount of serum antidiuretic hormone (ADH), leading to water intoxication and hyponatremia.

- Precocious puberty is defined as the appearance of any secondary sexual characteristics before 8 years in girls and 9 years in boys. If no treatment is provided, the hormones will stimulate closure of the epiphyseal plates and the child will have short stature as an adult.

- Untreated or ineffectively treated congenital hypothyroidism results in impaired growth and intellectual disability.

- Signs of hyperthyroidism include an enlarged, nontender thyroid gland (goiter), prominent or bulging eyes, eyelid lag, tachycardia, nervousness, increased appetite with weight loss, emotional lability, moodiness, heat intolerance, hypertension, hyperactivity, irregular menses, insomnia, tremor, and muscle weakness.

- During infancy, most cases of endogenous Cushing disease are due to a functioning adrenocortical tumor. The most common cause of endogenous Cushing syndrome in children older than 7 years of age is Cushing disease, in which a pituitary tumor (adenoma) secretes excess ACTH.

- Congenital adrenal hyperplasia has two forms, salt-losing or non–salt-losing with virilization. The salt-losing form accounts for 75% of cases and is caused by aldosterone deficiency and overproduction of androgen. The non–salt-losing form accounts for the other 25% of cases.

- Congenital adrenal hyperplasia is the most common cause of pseudohermaphroditism (ambiguous genitalia) in newborn girls.

- Adrenal insufficiency, also known as *Addison disease*, is a rare disorder in childhood characterized by a deficiency of glucocorticoids (cortisone) and mineralocorticoids (aldosterone). Symptoms include weakness, fatigue, weight loss, and gastrointestinal symptoms such as nausea, vomiting, diarrhea, constipation, and abdominal pain. Other symptoms include hyperpigmentation, hypotension, dizziness, joint pain, salt cravings, and hypoglycemia.

- Pheochromocytoma is a tumor that arises from the adrenal gland and causes an excessive release of catecholamines. Clinical manifestations include hypertension, palpitations sweating, anxiety, tremors, and headache.

- Diabetes mellitus type 1 is the most common metabolic disease in children and one of the most common chronic diseases in school-age children. It is a disorder of carbohydrate, protein, and fat metabolism.

- Treatment of the child with diabetic ketoacidosis includes intravenous fluids and electrolytes for dehydration and acidosis. Insulin is given by continuous infusion pump to decrease the serum glucose level at a slow but steady rate to prevent the development of cerebral edema.

- Common causes of hypoglycemia in children with type 1 diabetes include an error in insulin dosage, inadequate calories because of missed meals, or exercise without a corresponding increase in caloric intake.

- Type 2 diabetes mellitus is a condition that results from insulin resistance. Children most commonly affected are obese, and many have family members with the same type of diabetes.

- Turner syndrome is diagnosed definitively by a karyotype. The most common and most severe phenotype is 45,X indicating an absent X chromosome.

- Signs of Klinefelter syndrome include gynecomastia, delayed onset of puberty with an abnormal progression, decreased testicular size, and less facial and body hair than normal.

- Inborn errors of metabolism—inherited biochemical abnormalities of the urea cycle and amino acid and organic acid metabolism—often have a significant impact on the endocrine system's ability to support growth and development. These disorders include phenylketonuria, galactosemia, defects in mitochondrial diseases, and maple syrup urine disease.

- Children with phenylketonuria (PKU) have a deficiency of the liver enzyme phenylalanine hydroxylase that normally breaks down the essential amino acid phenylalanine into tyrosine.

- Galactosemia results from a deficiency of a liver enzyme needed to convert galactose to glucose. This leads to an accumulation of galactose metabolites in the eyes, liver, kidney, and brain, rapidly damaging the organs and causing life-threatening problems.

- Mitochondrial diseases are a group of genetic disorders resulting from a mutation in the nuclear or mitochondrial genes.

- Maple syrup urine disease is a rare disorder in which leucine, isoleucine, and valine cannot be metabolized because of an enzyme defect in the branched chain of these three essential amino acids.

Clinical Reasoning in Action

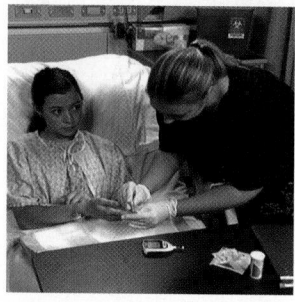

Fourteen-year-old Amanda is admitted to the hospital with newly diagnosed type 1 diabetes mellitus. She had initially been taken to her healthcare providers's office for enuresis, polyphagia, polydipsia, and lethargy, but when assessed, her urinalysis had glucose and ketones, and she had a weight loss of 15 lb.

Upon admission to the hospital, a full assessment is performed and the following vital signs are documented: weight 115 lb, temperature 98.8°F, respiratory rate 40 breaths per minute, heart rate 90 beats per minute, and blood pressure 106/63 mmHg. She has dry mucous membranes, but skin turgor is brisk. Blood is drawn immediately and will continue to be drawn every hour until she is stable.

After Amanda's condition stabilizes, education related to management of type 1 diabetes is initiated for Amanda and her parents. Amanda understands the nutritional guidelines associated with type 1 diabetes and how to, under adult supervision, perform blood glucose monitoring as well as how to draw up and administer insulin. Amanda and her parents spend most of the time in the hospital learning survival skills for managing her diabetes. Daily education and monitoring will occur in the diabetes clinic until the family is confident about taking care of Amanda. Regular follow-up visits will be scheduled with the diabetes nurse educator and endocrinologist.

1. What is the blood work most likely to be done on Amanda when admitted to the hospital for type 1 diabetes?

2. How should the family be told to manage hypoglycemic episodes?

3. What should the parents be told about preventing diabetic keto-acidosis in Amanda?

4. How often should blood glucose monitoring be performed once the condition is stabilized?

References

Abraham, C., & Rozmus, C. L. (2012). Is acanthosis nigricans a reliable indicator for risk of type 2 diabetes in obese children and adolescents? A systematic review. *The Journal of School Nursing, 28*(3), 195–205.

Alsaleh, F. M., Smith, F. J., & Taylor, K. M. (2012). Experiences of children/young people and their parents, using insulin pump therapy for the management of type 1 diabetes: Qualitative review.

Journal of Clinical Pharmacy and Therapeutics, 37, 140–147.

Ali, O., & Donohoue, P. A. (2016). Hypofunction of the testes. In R. M. Kliegman, B. F. Stanton, J. W. St. Geme, & N. F. Schor (Eds.), *Nelson textbook of pediatrics* (20th ed., pp. 2735–2741). Philadelphia, PA: Elsevier.

American Diabetes Association (ADA). (2013). *Sick days.* Retrieved from http://www.diabetes.org/living-with-diabetes/parents-and-kids/everyday-life/sick-days.html

American Diabetes Association (ADA). (2014a). Diagnosis and classification of diabetes mellitus. *Diabetes Care, 37*(Suppl. 1), S81–S90.

American Diabetes Association (ADA). (2014b). Standards of medical care in diabetes—2014. *Diabetes Care, 37*(Suppl. 1), S14–S80.

American Diabetes Association (ADA). (2014c). *Diabetes association sets new A1C target for children with type 1 diabetes.* Retrieved from http://www.diabetes

.org/newsroom/press-releases/2014/diabetes-association-sets-new-a1c-target-for-children-with-type-1-diabetes.html

American Diabetes Association (ADA). (2015). *Preventing type 2 in children*. Retrieved from http://www.diabetes.org/living-with-diabetes/parents-and-kids/children-and-type-2/preventing-type-2-in-children.html

Araujo, G. C., Christ, S. E., Grange, D. K., Steiner, R. D., Coleman, C., Timmerman, E., & White, D. A. (2013). Executive response monitoring and inhibitory control in children with phenylketonuria: Effects of expectancy. *Developmental Neuropsychology, 38*(3), 139–152.

Bacon, C. (2013). Supporting children and young people diagnosed with type 2 diabetes in school. *British Journal of School Nursing, 8*(5), 222–226.

Bahn, R. S., Burch, H. B., Cooper, D. S., Garber, J. R., Greenlee, C., Klein, I., ... Stan, M. N. (2011). Hyperthyroidism and other causes of thyrotoxicosis: Management guidelines of the American Thyroid Association and American Association of Clinical Endocrinologists. *Thyroid, 21*(6), 593–646.

Bauer, A. J. (2011). Approach to the pediatric patient with Graves' disease: When is definitive therapy warranted? *Journal of Clinical Endocrinology and Metabolism, 96*(3), 580–588.

Belcher, R., Metrailer, A. M., Bodenner, D. L., & Stack, B. C. (2013). Characterization of hyperparathyroidism in youth and adolescents: A literature review. *International Journal of Pediatric Otorhinolaryngology, 77*, 318–322.

Bialo, S. R., Agrawal, S., Boney, C. M., & Qunitos, J. B. (2015). Rare complications of pediatric diabetic ketoacidosis. *World Journal of Diabetes, 6*(1), 167–174.

Blackman, S. M., Raghinaru, D., Adi, S., Simmons, J. H., Ebner-Lyon, L., Chase, H. P., ... DiMeglio, L. A. (2014). Insulin pump use in young children in the T1D Exchange clinic registry is associated with lower hemoglobin A1c levels than injection therapy. *Pediatric Diabetes, 15*, 564–572.

Bodamer, O. A., & Lee, B. (2014). *Maple syrup urine disease*. Retrieved from http://emedicine.medscape.com/article/946234-overview

Bordini, B., & Rosenfield, R. L. (2011). Normal pubertal development: Part II: Clinical aspects of puberty. *Pediatrics in Review, 32*(7), 281–292.

Bourke, E., Herlihy, A., Snow, P., Metcalfe, S., & Amor, D. (2014). Klinefelter syndrome: A general practice perspective. *Australian Family Physician, 43*(1), 38–41.

Boyse, K. L., Garnder, M., Marvicsin, D. J., & Sandberg, D. E. (2014). "It was an overwhelming thing": Parents' needs after infant diagnosis with congenital adrenal hyperplasia. *Journal of Pediatric Nursing, 29*, 436–441.

Breault, D. T., & Majzoub, J. A. (2016). Diabetes insipidus. In R. M. Kliegman, B. F. Stanton, J. W. St. Geme, & N. F. Schor (Eds.), *Nelson textbook of pediatrics* (20th ed., pp. 2644–2646). Philadelphia, PA: Elsevier.

Brink, S., Joel, D., Laffel, L., Lee, W. W. R., Olsen, B., Phelan, H., & Hanas, R. (2014). Sick day management in children and adolescents with diabetes. *Pediatric Diabetes, 15*(Suppl. 20), 193–202.

Brosco, J. P., & Paul, D. B. (2013). The political history of PKU: Reflections on 50 years of newborn screening. *Pediatrics, 132*(6), 987–989.

Burfield, J., Hussa, C., & Randall, R. (2012). Hot topics in metabolism: A focus on phenylketonuria, liver transplantation, and galactosemia. *Topics in Clinical Nutrition, 27*(3), 181–195.

Butler, S., Fekaris, N., Pontius, D., & Zacharski, S. (2012). *Diabetes management in the school setting*. Retrieved from http://www.nasn.org/PolicyAdvocacy/PositionPapersandReports/NASNPositionStatementsArticleView/tabid/462/ArticleId/22/Diabetes-in-the-School-Setting-School-Nurse-Role-in-Care-and-Management-of-the-Child-with-Revised-20

Carchidi, C., Holland, C., Minnock, P., & Boyle, D. (2011). New technologies in pediatric diabetes care. *MCN, 36*(1), 32–39.

Centers for Disease Control and Prevention (CDC). (2014). *National diabetes statistics report, 2014*. Retrieved from http://www.cdc.gov/diabetes/pubs/statsreport14/national-diabetes-report-web.pdf

Chiang, J. L., Kirkman, M. S., Laffel, L. M. B., & Peters, A. L. (2014). Type 1 diabetes through the life span: A position statement of the American Diabetes Association. *Diabetes Care, 37*, 2034–2054.

Codier, E., & Codier, D. (2014). Understanding mitochondrial disease and goals for its treatment. *British Journal of Nursing, 23*(5), 254–258.

Cohee, L. (2012). Endocrinology. In *The Harriet Lane handbook* (19th ed., pp. 243–270). Philadelphia, PA: Elsevier.

Cole, C. (2014). Successful pregnancy and delivery with maple syrup urine disease. *Journal of Obstetric, Gynecologic & Neonatal Nursing, 43*(Suppl. 1), S95–S96.

Cooke, D. W., Divall, S. A., & Radovick, S. (2011). Normal and aberrant growth. In S. Melmed, K. S. Polonsky, P. R. Larsen, & H. M. Kronenberg (Eds.), *Williams textbook of endocrinology* (12th ed., pp. 935–1053). Philadelphia, PA: Elsevier Saunders.

Craig, M. E., Jefferies, C., Dabelea, D., Balde, N., Seth, A., & Donaghue, K. C. (2014). Definition, epidemiology, and classification of diabetes in children and adolescents. *Pediatric Diabetes, 15*(Suppl. 20), 4–17.

Cystic Fibrosis Foundation. (2012). *Cystic fibrosis-related diabetes*. Retrieved from http://www.cff.org/LivingWithCF/StayingHealthy/Diet/Diabetes/

Dassler, A., & Allen, P. (2014). Mitochondrial disease in children and adolescents. *Pediatric Nursing, 40*(3), 150–154.

Dea, T. L. (2011). Pediatric obesity & type 2 diabetes. *MCN, 36*(1), 42–48.

Di Iorgi, N., Napoli, F., Allegri, A. E. M., Olivieri, I., Bertelli, E., Gallazia, A., ... Maghnie, M. (2012). Diabetes insipidus—Diagnosis and management. *Hormone Research in Paediatrics, 77*, 69–84.

Doyle, D. A. (2016a). Hyperparathyroidism. In R. M. Kliegman, B. F. Stanton, J. W. St. Geme, & N. F. Schor (Eds.), *Nelson textbook of pediatrics* (20th ed., pp. 2694–2697). Philadelphia, PA: Elsevier.

Doyle, D. A. (2016b). Hypoparathyroidism. In R. M. Kliegman, B. F. Stanton, J. W. St. Geme, & N. F. Schor (Eds.), *Nelson textbook of pediatrics* (20th ed., pp. 2690–2693). Philadelphia, PA: Elsevier.

Ferguson, L. A. (2011). Growth hormone use in children: Necessary or designer therapy? *Journal of Pediatric Health Care, 25*(1), 24–30.

Ficorelli, C. T. (2013). Addison disease: The importance of early diagnosis. *Nursing Made Incredibly Easy!, 11*(2), 11–15.

Fischer, S., Hirsch, T., Hirche, C., Kiefer, J., Kueckelhaus, M., Germann, G., & Reichenberger, M. A. (2014).

Surgical treatment of primary gynecomastia in children and adolescents. *Pediatric Surgery International, 20*, 641–647.

Fitzgerald, P. A. (2015). Endocrine disorders. In M. A. Papadakis, S. J. McPhee, & M. W. Rabow (Eds.), *CURRENT Medical Diagnosis & Treatment 2015*. New York, NY: McGraw-Hill.

Fuqua, J. S. (2013). Treatment and outcomes of precocious puberty: An update. *Journal of Clinical Endocrinology & Metabolism, 98*(6), 2198–2207.

Gastaldi, R., Poggi, E., Mussa, A., Webber, G., Vigone, M. C., Salerno, M., ... Corrias, A. (2014). Graves disease in children: Thyroid-stimulating hormone receptor antibodies as remission markers. *The Journal of Pediatrics, 164*(5) 1189–1194.

Genetics Home Reference. (2012). *Turner syndrome*. Retrieved from http://ghr.nlm.nih.gov/condition/turner-syndrome

Guo, C. (2013). Diagnostic value of provocative test by insulin combined with clonidine for growth hormone deficiency in children. *Iranian Journal of Pediatrics, 23*(3), 315–320.

Hanas, R., de Beaufort, C., Hoey, H., & Anderson, B. (2011). Insulin delivery by injection in children and adolescents. *Pediatric Diabetes, 12*, 518–526.

Hird, B. E., Tetlow, L., Tobi, S., Patel, L., & Clayton, P. E. (2015). No evidence of an increase in early infant mortality from congenital adrenal hyperplasia in the absence of screening. *Archives of Disease in Childhood, 99*, 158–164.

Ho, C. W., Loke, K. Y., Lim, Y. L., & Lee, Y. S. (2014). Exogenous Cushing syndrome: A lesson of diaper rash cream. *Hormone Research in Paediatrics, 82*, 415–418.

Huang, S. A., & LaFranchi, S. (2016). Hyperthyroidism. In R. M. Kliegman, B. F. Stanton, J. W. St. Geme, & N. F. Schor (Eds.), *Nelson textbook of pediatrics* (20th ed., pp. 2680–2685). Philadelphia, PA: Elsevier.

Iafusco, D., Galderisi, A., Nocerino, I., Cocca, A., Zuccotti, G., Prisco, F., & Scaramuzza, A. (2011). Chat line for adolescents with type 1 diabetes: A useful tool to improve coping with diabetes: A 2-year follow-up study. *Diabetes Technology & Therapeutics, 13*(5), 551–555.

Jaser, S. S., Faulkner, M. S., Whittemore, R., Jeon, S., Delamater, A., & Grey, M. (2012). Coping, self-management, and adaptation in adolescents with type 1 diabetes. *Annals of Behavioral Medicine, 43*, 311–319.

Jaser, S. S., & White, L. E. (2011). Coping and resilience in adolescents with type 1 diabetes. *Child: Care Health and Development, 37*(3), 335–342.

Kemper, M. J., & van Husen, M. (2014). Renal osteodystrophy in children: Pathogenesis, diagnosis and treatment. *Current Opinion in Pediatrics, 26*(2), 180–186.

Khan, S. E., Cooper, M. E., & Del Prato, S. (2014). Pathophysiology and treatment of type 2 diabetes: Perspectives on the past, present, and future. *Lancet, 383*, 1068–1083.

Kishnani, P. S., & Chen, Y. (2016). Defects in metabolism of carbohydrates. In R. M. Kliegman, B. F. Stanton, J. W. St. Geme, & N. F. Schor (Eds.), *Nelson textbook of pediatrics* (20th ed., pp. 715–737). Philadelphia, PA: Elsevier.

Klehm, M., & Korson, M. (2014). *A clinician's guide to the management of mitochondrial disease*. Retrieved from http://www.mitoaction.org/guide/table-contents

LaFranchi, S. & Huang, S. A. (2016). Hypothyroidism. In R. M. Kliegman, B. F. Stanton, J. W. St. Geme, & N. F. Schor (Eds.), *Nelson textbook of pediatrics* (20th ed., pp. 2665–2675). Philadelphia, PA: Elsevier.

Larsson, H. E., Vehik, K., Bell, R., Dabelea, D., Dolan, L., Pihoker, C., ... Haller, M. J. (2011). Reduced prevalence of diabetic ketoacidosis at diagnosis of type 1 diabetes in young children participating in longitudinal follow-up. *Diabetes Care, 34,* 2347–2352.

Leger, J., Gelwane, G., Kaguelidou, F., Benmerad, M., Alberti, C., & French Childhood Graves' Disease Study Group. (2012). Positive impact of long-term antithyroid drug treatment on the outcome of children with Graves' disease: National long-term cohort study. *Journal of Clinical Endocrinology and Metabolism. 97*(1), 1–10.

Levitsky, L. L., Luria, A. H. O., Hayes, F. J., & Lin, A. E. (2015). Turner syndrome: Update on biology and management across the life span. *Current Opinion in Endocrinology, Diabetes, & Obesity, 22*(1), 65–72.

Marcason, W. (2013). Is there a standard meal plan for phenylketonuria (PKU)? *Journal of the Academy Of Nutrition And Dietetics, 113*(8), 1124.

Marcdante, K. J., & Kliegman, R. M (2015). Diabetes mellitus. In K. J. Marcdante & R. M. Kliegman (Eds.), *Nelson essentials of pediatrics* (7th ed., pp. 572–579). Philadelphia, PA: Elsevier Saunders.

March of Dimes. (2012). *Newborn screening.* Retrieved from http://www.marchofdimes.org/baby/newborn-screening-tests-for-your-baby.aspx

Martin, C. J. H., & Smyth, A. (2012). A midwives' guide to Turner syndrome. *British Journal of Midwifery, 20*(9), 628–631.

Masharani, U. (2015). Diabetes mellitus & hypoglycemia. In M. A. Papadakis, S. J. McPhee, & M. W. Rabow (Eds.), *CURRENT medical diagnosis & treatment 2015.* New York, NY: McGraw-Hill.

McFarlane, K. (2011). An overview of diabetic ketoacidosis in children. *Paediatric Nursing, 23*(1), 14–19.

McHugo, J., & Harden, A. (2011). Diabetes insipidus: Navigating troubled waters. *Advance for NPs and PAs, 2*(4), 20–24.

Michels, A., & Michels, N. (2014). Addison disease: Early detection and treatment principles. *American Family Physician, 89*(7), 563–568.

Mishra, A., Mehrotra, P. K., Agarwal, G., Agarwal, A., & Mishra, S. K. (2014). Pediatric and adolescent pheochromocytoma: Clinical presentation and outcome of surgery. *Indian Pediatrics, 51,* 299–302.

Monaghan, M., Hoffman, K. M., & Cogen, F. R. (2013). License to drive: Type 1 diabetes management and obtaining a learner's permit in Maryland and Virginia. *Diabetes Spectrum, 26*(3), 194–199.

National Diabetes Information Clearinghouse. (2014). *The A1C test and diabetes.* Retrieved from http://diabetes.niddk.nih.gov/dm/pubs/A1CTest/#1

National Endocrine and Metabolic Diseases Information Service (NEMDIS). (2014). *Adrenal insufficiency and Addison's disease.* Retrieved from http://endocrine.niddk.nih.gov/pubs/addison/addison.aspx

National Newborn Screening and Genetics Resource Center. (2014). *National newborn screening status report.* Retrieved from https://genes-r-us.uthscsa.edu/sites/genes-r-us/files/nbsdisorders.pdf

Nimkarn, S., Lin-Su, K., & New, M. I. (2011). Steroid 21 hydroxylase deficiency congenital adrenal hyperplasia. *Pediatric Clinics of North America, 58,* 1281–1300.

Oliveira, C. S., Ribeiro, F. M., Lago, R., & Alves, C. (2013). Audiological abnormalities in patients with Turner syndrome. *American Journal of Audiology, 22,* 226–232.

Parks, J. S., & Felner, E. I. (2016). Hypopituitarism. In R. M. Kliegman, B. F. Stanton, J. W. St. Geme, & N. F. Schor (Eds.), *Nelson textbook of pediatrics* (20th ed., pp. 2637–2644). Philadelphia, PA: Elsevier.

Pillai, B. P., Unnikrishnan, A. G., & Pavithran, P. V. (2011). Syndrome of inappropriate antidiuretic hormone secretion: Revisiting a classical endocrine disorder. *Indian Journal of Endocrinology and Metabolism, 15*(Suppl. 3), S208–S215.

Pluta, R. M., Burke, A. E., & Golub, R. M. (2011). Cushing syndrome and Cushing disease. *Journal of the American Medical Association, 306*(24), 2742.

Rauh, M. J., Barrack, M., & Nichols, J. F. (2014). Associations between the female athlete triad and injury among high school runners. *The International Journal of Sports Physical Therapy, 9*(7), 948–958.

Rezvani, I., & Ficicioglu, C. (2016). Phenylalanine. In R. M. Kliegman, B. F. Stanton, J. W. St. Geme, & N. F. Schor (Eds.), *Nelson textbook of pediatrics* (20th ed., pp. 636–640). Philadelphia, PA: Elsevier.

Rezvani, I., & Rosenblatt, D. S. (2016). Valine, leucine, isoleucine and related organic acidemias. In R. M. Kliegman, B. F. Stanton, J. W. St. Geme, & N. F. Schor (Eds.), *Nelson textbook of pediatrics* (20th ed., p. 649). Philadelphia, PA: Elsevier.

Rivkees, S. A. (2014). Pediatric Graves' disease: Management in the post–propylthiouracil era. *International Journal of Pediatric Endocrinology. 2014*(1), 1–23.

Robinson, A. G., & Verbalis, J. G. (2011). Posterior pituitary. In S. Melmed, K. S. Polonsky, P. R. Larsen, & H. M. Kronenberg (Eds.), *Williams textbook of endocrinology* (12th ed., pp. 292–323). Philadelphia, PA: Elsevier Saunders.

Saenz, M., Tsai, A. C., Manchester, D. K., & Elias, E. R. (2014). Genetics & dysmorphology. In W. W. Hay, M. J. Levin, R. R. Deterding, & M.J. Abzug (Eds.), *CURRENT diagnosis and treatment: Pediatrics* (22th ed.). New York, NY: McGraw-Hill. Retrieved from http://accessmedicine.com

Saito, R., Yamamoto, Y., Goto, M., Araki, Sh., Kubo, K., Kawagoe, R., ... Fukami, M. (2014). Tamoxifen treatment for pubertal gynecomastia in two siblings with partial androgen insensitivity syndrome. *Hormone Research in Paediatrics, 81,* 211–216.

Screening, Technology, and Research in Genetics (STRG). (2012). *Galactosemia.* Retrieved from http://www.newbornscreening.info/Parents/otherdisorders/Galactosemia.html

Senger, B. (2013). *Identifying disease characteristics, parent experience, and coping strategies when predicting pediatric illness-related stress in parents of children with mitochondrial disease* (doctoral dissertation). Retrieved from Washington State University Research Exchange, http://hdl.handle.net/2376/5035

Seth, A., & Maheshwari, A. (2013). Common endocrine problems in children (hypothyroidism and type 1 diabetes mellitus). *Indian Journal of Pediatrics, 80*(8), 681–687.

Shah, N. S., & Lila, A. (2011). Childhood Cushing disease: A challenge in diagnosis and management. *Hormone Research in Paediatrics. 76*(Suppl 1), 65–70.

Shanholtz, H. J. (2013). Congenital hypothyroidism. *Journal of Pediatric Nursing, 28*(2), 200–202.

Sharma, P. K. (2014). *Complications of thyroid surgery.* Retrieved from http://emedicine.medscape.com/article/852184-overview

Sharma, R., & Seth. A. (2014). Congenital adrenal hyperplasia: issues in diagnosis and treatment

in children. *Indian Journal of Pediatrics, 81*(2), 178–185.

Shoback, D., & Funk J. L., (2011). Humoral manifestations of malignancy. In D.G. Gardner & D. Shoback (Eds.), *Greenspan's basic & clinical endocrinology* (9th ed.). Retrieved from http://www.accessmedicine.com

Shuch, B., Ricketts, C. J., Metwalli, A. R., Pacak, K., & Linehan, W. M. (2014). The genetic basis of pheochromocytoma and paraganglioma: Implications for management. *Urology, 83,* 1225–1232.

Sirotnak, A. P. (2013). *Psychosocial dwarfism.* Retrieved from http://emedicine.medscape.com/article/913843-overview

Speiser, P. W., & Wilson, T. A. (2015). *Pediatric adrenal insufficiency (Addison disease).* Retrieved from http://emedicine.medscape.com/article/919077-overview

Stanley, T. (2012). Diagnosis of growth hormone deficiency in childhood. *Current Opinion in Endocrinology, Diabetes and Obesity, 19*(1), 47–52.

Svoren, B. M., & Jospe, N. (2016). Diabetes mellitus. In R. M. Kliegman, B. F. Stanton, J. W. St. Geme, & N. F. Schor (Eds.), *Nelson textbook of pediatrics* (20th ed., pp. 2760–2790). Philadelphia, PA: Elsevier.

Szypowska, A., & Skora, A. (2011). The risk factors of ketoacidosis in children with newly diagnosed type 1 diabetes mellitus. *Pediatric Diabetes, 12,* 302–306.

Thomas, C. P., & Fraer, M. (2014). *Syndrome of inappropriate antidiuretic hormone secretion.* Retrieved from http://emedicine.medscape.com/article/246650-overview

Tsirlin, A., Oo, Y., Sharma, R., Kansara, A., Gliwa, A., & Banerji, M. A. (2014). Pheochromocytoma: A review. *Maturitas, 77,* 229–238.

United Mitochondrial Disease Foundation (UMDF). (2011). *MitoFIRST handbook: An introductory guide* (web pamphlet). Retrieved from http://www.kintera.org/atf/cf/%7B858ACD34-ECC3-472A-8794-39B92E103561%7D/mito_first.pdf

Walker, K. A. B. (2014). Oral manifestations of Turner syndrome. *Access, 28*(5), 32–34.

Walsh, K., & March, P. (2013, August). Diabetes insipidus. *CINAHL Information Systems.*

White, P. C. (2016a). Cushing syndrome. In R. M. Kliegman, B. F. Stanton, J. W. St. Geme, & N. F. Schor (Eds.), *Nelson textbook of pediatrics* (20th ed., pp. 2723–2725). Philadelphia, PA: Elsevier.

White, P. C. (2016b). Congenital adrenal hyperplasia and related disorders. In R. M. Kliegman, B. F. Stanton, J. W. St. Geme, & N. F. Schor (Eds.), *Nelson textbook of pediatrics* (20th ed., pp. 2714–2723). Philadelphia, PA: Elsevier.

White, P. C. (2016c). Pheochromocytoma. In R. M. Kliegman, B. F. Stanton, J. W. St. Geme, & N. F. Schor (Eds.), *Nelson textbook of pediatrics* (20th ed., pp. 2727–2729). Philadelphia, PA: Elsevier.

Wilson, B. A., Shannon, M. T., & Shields, K. M. (2016). *Pearson nurse's drug guide 2016.* Hoboken, NJ: Pearson Education.

Woerner, S. (2014). The benefits of insulin pump therapy in children and adolescents with type 1 diabetes. *Journal of Pediatric Nursing, 29*(6), 712–713.

Zeitler, P. S., Travers, S. H., Nadeau, K., Barker, J. M., Kelsey, M. M., & Kappy, M. S. (2014). Endocrine disorders. In W. W. Hay, M. J. Levin, R. R. Deterding, & M.J. Abzug (Eds.), *CURRENT diagnosis and treatment: Pediatrics* (22th ed.). New York, NY: McGraw-Hill. Retrieved from http://accessmedicine.com

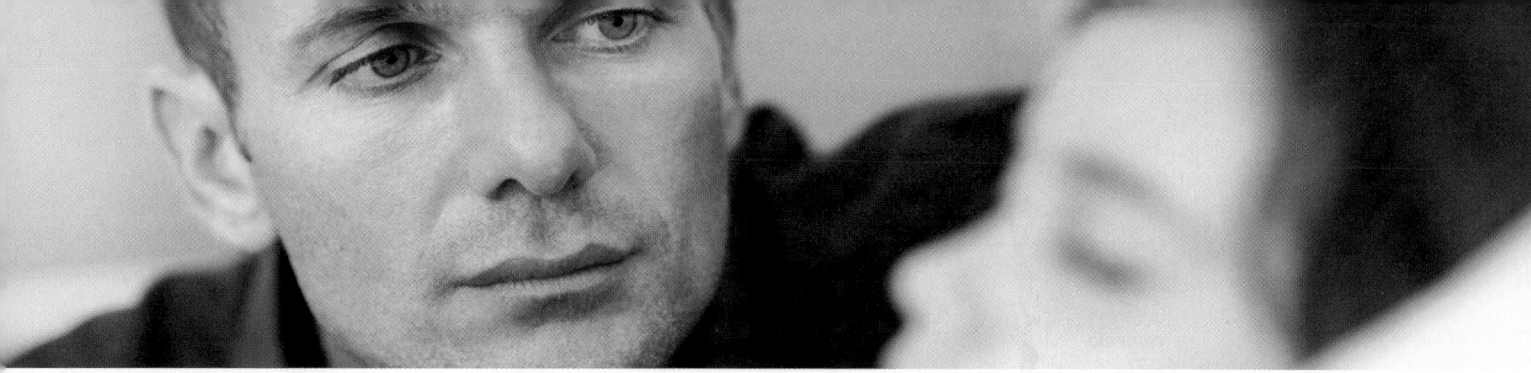

Chapter 54
The Child With Alterations in Neurologic Function

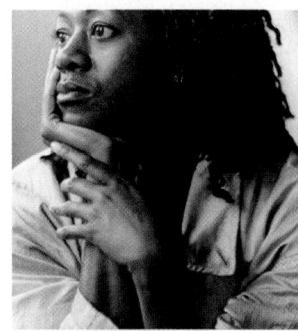

Mel Curtis/Getty Images

It's so hard to watch your child experience a brain injury and lie in a coma. All we can do is be here every day for Kirani. We keep talking to him and trying to get him to respond to us. We hope he will wake up soon.

—Mother of Kirani, 7 years old

⌄ Learning Outcomes

54.1 Describe the pediatric differences associated with the anatomy and physiology of the neurologic system.

54.2 Choose the appropriate assessment guidelines and tools to examine infants and children with altered levels of consciousness and other neurologic conditions.

54.3 Differentiate between the signs of a seizure and status epilepticus in infants and children, and describe appropriate nursing management for each condition.

54.4 Differentiate between signs of bacterial meningitis, viral meningitis, encephalitis, and Guillain-Barré syndrome in infants and children.

54.5 Develop a plan of nursing care for the child hospitalized with an acute neurologic condition.

54.6 Develop a nursing care plan for the infant with hydrocephalus and spina bifida.

54.7 Plan family-centered nursing care for the child with cerebral palsy in a community setting.

54.8 Contrast the appropriate initial nursing management for mild versus severe traumatic brain injury.

54.9 Discuss initiatives to prevent drowning in children.

Anatomy and Physiology of Pediatric Differences

Knowledge of the anatomy of the nervous system makes neurologic symptoms easier to understand. The brain, spinal cord, and nerves are the major structures of the nervous system

(Figure 54–1). The brain controls, regulates, or coordinates many body functions, including cognition, behaviors, the senses, and motor skills. The spinal cord transmits impulses to and from the brain, conveying sensory information and relaying impulses that stimulate motor responses. Alterations in neurologic function can have widespread effects on the body's metabolism.

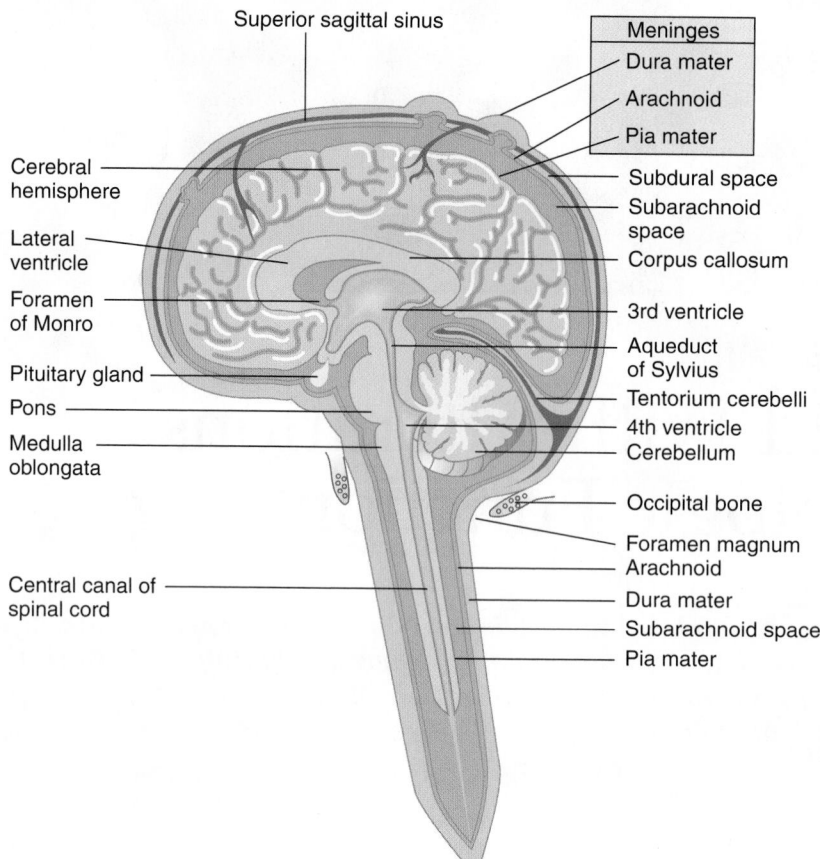

Figure 54-1 Transverse section of the brain and spinal cord. The brain is protected by the skull and covered by three layers of tissue called the *meninges*. Cerebral spinal fluid circulates within the ventricles of the brain and around the brain and spinal cord.

The neural tube from which the brain and spinal cord form develops early in gestation. The full-term newborn has a complete but immature central nervous system at birth. All the nerve cells the child will have throughout life are present at birth, but their maturation continues after birth. The number of glial cells (which build a structure around nerve cells) and dendrites (which carry nerve impulses from other nerve cells to the nerve cell body) continues to increase until about 4 years of age. Myelination, which increases the speed and accuracy of nerve impulses, continues after birth in a cephalocaudal direction. Myelination accounts for the progressive acquisition of fine and gross motor skills and coordination during early childhood.

The brain depends on a continuous blood flow to meet its high demands for oxygen. Through an autoregulatory process, the cerebral blood vessels dilate to maintain the cerebral blood flow in response to physiologic changes such as decreased cardiac output, increased intracranial pressure, or constriction of the neck's blood vessels due to positioning. Brain cells become damaged very quickly when blood flow and oxygenation are not maintained. Because the nervous system helps to control and coordinate many body functions, alterations in neurologic function can have widespread effects on the body's metabolism.

The anatomic and physiologic differences between children and adults help explain why children and adults have different neurologic problems. See *As Children Grow: Anatomic Differences Between Children's and Adults' Nervous System Structures.*

Altered States of Consciousness

Level of consciousness (LOC) is perhaps the most important indicator of neurologic dysfunction. *Consciousness,* the responsiveness to or awareness of sensory stimuli, has two components: *alertness,* or the ability to react to stimuli, and *cognitive power,* or the ability to process the data and respond either verbally or physically. *Unconsciousness* is depressed cerebral function, or the inability of the brain to respond to stimuli. Altered levels of consciousness can be further categorized as:

- *Confusion:* disorientation to time, place, or person; loss of clear thinking. Answers to simple questions may be correct, but responses to complex ones may be inaccurate.

- *Delirium:* state characterized by disorientation, fear, irritability or agitation, and mental or motor excitement.

- *Lethargy:* profound slumber in which speech and movement are limited. The child is aroused with moderate stimulation, but falls asleep easily once stimulation is removed.

- *Stupor:* deep sleep or unresponsiveness; the child is aroused only with repeated vigorous stimulation, but returns to the unresponsive state when the stimulus is removed.

- **Coma:** unconsciousness; cannot be aroused even by painful stimuli.

As Children Grow: **Anatomic Differences Between Children's and Adults' Nervous System Structures**

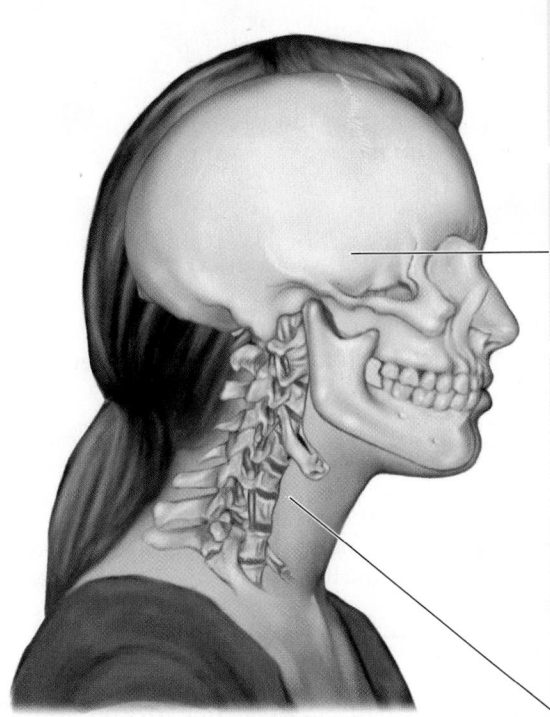

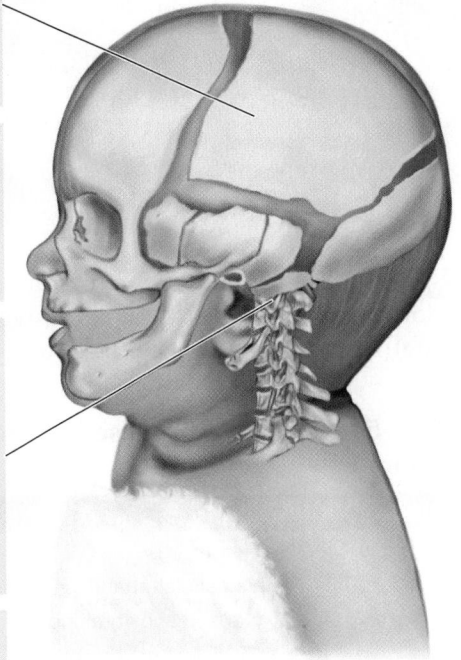

Top heavy, head is large in proportion to body; neck muscles poorly developed; thin cranial bones not well developed; unfused sutures; skull expands until age 2 years. *Prone to brain injury and skull fracture with falls.*

Head size proportional to body; neck muscles well developed, can reduce risk for brain injuries; sutures are ossified by age 12 years; no expansion of skull after 5 years.

Excessive spinal mobility; immature muscles, joint capsule, and ligaments of cervical spine; wedge-shaped, cartilaginous vertebral bodies; incomplete ossification of vertebral bodies. *Greater risk for high cervical spine injury at C1-C2 level or vertebral compression fractures with falls.*

Well-developed muscles and ligaments reduce spinal mobility; vertebral bodies completely formed and ossified.

The skull and brain grow and develop rapidly during early childhood. Infants and young children are at higher risk for injury to the brain and spinal cord because of developing anatomic structures.

Etiology and Pathophysiology

Infection of the brain and meninges is a common cause of an altered level of consciousness in children. Other causes include trauma, hypoxia, poisoning, seizures, alcohol or substance abuse, endocrine or metabolic disturbances (e.g., diabetic ketoacidosis), electrolyte or acid–base imbalance, brain tumor, stroke, or a congenital structural defect. Any of these pathologic processes can cause increased **intracranial pressure (ICP)** (force exerted by brain tissue, cerebrospinal fluid, and blood within the cranium). Decreased **cerebral perfusion pressure**, the amount of pressure needed to ensure that adequate oxygen and nutrients are delivered by the blood to the brain, often results when the increased ICP reduces brain arterial blood flow. Rapid diagnosis of the cause of altered consciousness and immediate treatment are essential to prevent poor outcomes.

Clinical Manifestations

Decline in a child's level of consciousness often follows a sequential pattern of deterioration. Initial changes may be subtle: a slight disorientation to time, place, and person. The child may become restless or fussy, and actions that normally calm or soothe only increase irritability. As responsiveness decreases, the child may become drowsy but still respond to loud verbal commands and withdraw from painful stimuli. Keeping the child awake is sometimes difficult. Then response to pain progresses from purposeful to nonpurposeful. The child may exhibit flexor or extensor **posturing**, the abnormal positions sometimes seen after serious injury to the brain (Figure 54–2). Clinical manifestations of increased ICP are provided in Table 54–1.

Clinical Therapy

Clinical therapy focuses on early diagnosis of the cause of altered consciousness and intervention to prevent further insult to the central nervous system (CNS). The Glasgow Coma Scale (GCS) is used to quantify the level of consciousness, most often for acute injury, and pediatric criteria for preverbal children are also available. See Table 54–2.

Laboratory tests may include a complete blood cell count, blood chemistry, clotting factors, and blood culture; toxicology assessments of blood and urine; and urinalysis with culture. A lumbar puncture may be performed if infection is suspected. An electroencephalogram (EEG) identifies damaged or nonfunctioning areas of the brain. Computed tomography (CT)

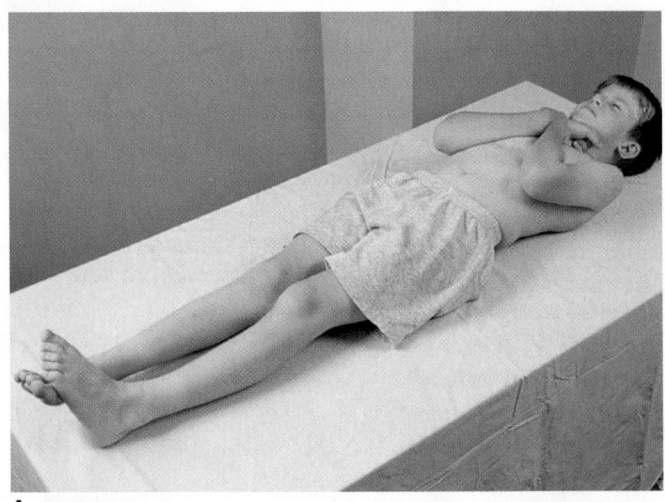
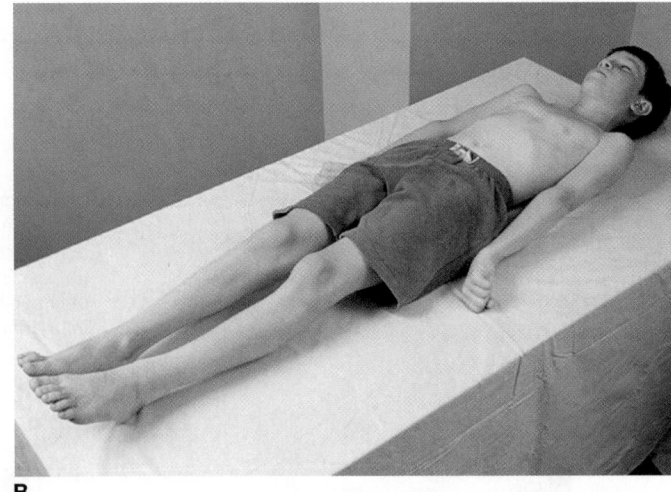

A

B

Figure 54–2 **Posturing associated with severe brain injury.** *A,* Flexor posturing (decorticate), characterized by rigid flexion, is associated with lesions above the brainstem in the corticospinal tracts. *B,* Extensor posturing (decerebrate), distinguished by rigid extension, is associated with lesions of the brainstem.

TABLE 54–1 Signs of Increased Intracranial Pressure

TIMING OF SIGNS	SIGNS
Early signs	Headache
	Visual disturbances, diplopia
	Nausea and vomiting
	Dizziness or vertigo
	Slight change in vital signs
	Pupils not as reactive or equal
	Sunsetting eyes (cranial nerve IV palsy; the iris of eye appears to be setting into the lower eyelid leaving sclera visible above the iris)
	Slight change in level of consciousness, restlessness
Infant has above signs plus:	Irritability
	Bulging fontanelle
	Wide sutures, increased head circumference
	Dilated scalp veins
	High-pitched, catlike cry
Late signs	Significant decrease in level of consciousness
	Seizures
	Cushing triad:
	• Increased systolic blood pressure and widened pulse pressure (systolic pressure increases as the diastolic pressure stays the same or decreases)
	• Bradycardia
	• Irregular respirations
	Fixed and dilated pupils, papilledema

or magnetic resonance imaging (MRI) is used to detect any lesions, structural abnormalities, vascular malformations, or edema. Skull radiographic studies may detect fractures or bony malformations.

SAFETY ALERT!
The lumbar puncture should be postponed if any signs of increased ICP (e.g., papilledema) are present, which could place the child at risk for brain **herniation** (protrusion of brain contents into the brainstem area).

The child is treated with oxygen, and assisted ventilation is provided when gas exchange is inadequate. Any metabolic, acid–base, or electrolyte imbalances are corrected. Antibiotics are initiated for suspected infection.

Maintenance of the cerebral perfusion pressure is important so that adequate oxygen and nutrients are supplied to the brain. Intravenous (IV) fluids or blood products are given if the child is hypovolemic. When poor perfusion and fluid overload exist, a vasopressor medication such as dopamine is administered to increase cardiac output and perfusion of the brain. If the ICP is markedly increased and is a result of obstruction of cerebrospinal fluid (CSF), a ventricular catheter may be inserted to drain CSF to decrease the ICP, temporarily relieving a life-threatening condition. See the *Clinical Skills Manual* SKILLS . See care specific to increased ICP and traumatic brain injury later in this chapter.

Nursing Management

For the Child With Altered Consciousness

Nursing Assessment and Diagnosis

General guidelines for assessing the child with a neurologic condition are provided in the accompanying *Assessment Guide: The Child With a Neurologic Condition.*

When consciousness is altered, initially assess the child's physiologic status, focusing on the child's responsiveness to the environment or stimuli, ability to maintain the airway, vital signs, and breathing patterns. When a cough or gag reflex is present, the child can protect the airway from aspiration. Assess the vital signs, respiratory effort, and color. Monitor pulse oximetry and arterial blood gas measurements. Adequate air exchange to keep oxygen and carbon dioxide levels within

TABLE 54–2 Glasgow Coma Scale for Assessment of Coma in Infants and Children

CATEGORY	SCORE*	PREVERBAL CHILD CRITERIA	OLDER CHILD AND ADULT CRITERIA
Eye opening	4	Spontaneous opening	Spontaneous
	3	To voice or sound	To sound
	2	To pain	To pressure
	1	No response to painful stimuli	No response
Verbal response	5	Smiles, coos, cries to appropriate stimuli	Oriented; uses appropriate words and phrases
	4	Irritable; spontaneous crying	Confused
	3	Cries to pain	Words
	2	Moans to pain	Sounds
	1	No response	No response
Motor response	6	Spontaneous movement	Obeys commands
	5	Purposeful, localizes pain	Localizes pain
	4	Withdraws to pain	Normal flexion
	3	Flexion to pain	Abnormal flexion; flexor posturing
	2	Extension to pain	Extension; extensor posturing
	1	No response; flaccid	No response; flaccid

*Add the score from each category to get the total. The maximum score is 15, indicating the best level of neurologic functioning. The minimum is 3, indicating total neurologic unresponsiveness

Source: From Teasdale, G., & Jennett, B. (1974). Assessment of coma and impaired consciousness. *Lancet*, 2, 81–84; James, H. E. (1986). Neurologic evaluation and support in the child with acute brain insult. *Pediatric Annals*, 15(1), 16–22; Bethel, J. (2012). Emergency care of children and adults with head injury. *Nursing Standard*, 26(43), 49–56; Teasdale, G., Allan, D., Brennan, P., McElhinney, E., & Mackinnon, L. (2014). Forty years on: Updating the Glasgow Coma Scale. *Nursing Times*, 110(42), 12–16; Teasdale, G., Maas, A., Lecky, F., Manley, G., Stocchetti, N., & Murray, G. (2014). The Glasgow Coma Scale at 40 years: Standing the test of time. *Lancet Neurology*, 13(8), 844–854; Worrall, K. (2004). Use of the Glasgow Coma Scale in infants. *Paediatric Nursing*, 16(4), 45–47.

ASSESSMENT GUIDE | The Child With a Neurologic Condition

Assessment Focus	Assessment Guidelines
Level of consciousness	• Is the infant or child lethargic or hard to arouse? • Is the infant or child irritable or difficult to console? • Use the Glasgow Coma Scale when a numeric score is important for future comparison. See Table 54–2.
Cognitive function	• Are the child's verbal skills appropriate for age? Can the child tell you his or her name and age? • Does the child follow directions appropriately?
Cranial nerves	• Assess the cranial nerves. See Table 33–19. See also Table 54–3 for methods to assess cranial nerves in the unconscious child.
Skull	• Palpate the fontanelles for bulging and suture lines for separation.
Pupils	• Check the pupils for size, reaction to light, and accommodation.
Vital signs	• Assess the heart rate, respiratory rate, and blood pressure. • Monitor for late signs of increased ICP (increased systolic blood pressure, a widened pulse pressure, bradycardia, and irregular respirations).
Posture and movement	• Assess the common newborn reflexes in the infant less than 4 months of age to evaluate posture and movement. See Chapter 24. • Observe the child's play or other spontaneous activity to assess strength, coordination, symmetry, and smoothness of movements. Are muscle tone and strength equal bilaterally? Is any weakness present? • Are the child's motor skills developmentally appropriate and acquired at the appropriate age? Has the child lost a previously acquired skill? • Assess the plantar reflex and deep tendon reflexes. See Table 33–20.
Neck stiffness	• Assess for neck stiffness (nuchal rigidity). See Figure 54–6.
Pain	• Assess level of pain when present.
Family history	• Is there a family history of headaches, seizures, neurofibromatosis, or other neurologic conditions?

normal ranges and maintenance of acid–base balance are critical to reduce the risk of hypoxemia and increased ICP.

A baseline neurologic assessment should be performed, including pupils, eye movements, and motor function (Figure 54–3). Assess the cranial nerves; however, be aware that assessment and interpretation may be more challenging in the unconscious child (Table 54–3). Observe for other physiologic signs of increased ICP (Table 54–1). See Table 54–4 for a method to rapidly assess an infant's responsiveness, referred to by the acronym AVPU (alert, verbal, pain response, unresponsive).

A cry with a loud, energetic quality, a strong suck and suck–swallowing coordination, and appropriate common newborn reflex responses for age are other signs of an infant's intact mental status.

TABLE 54–3 Assessment of Cranial Nerves in the Unconscious Child

CRANIAL NERVES	REFLEX	ASSESSMENT PROCEDURE AND NORMAL FINDINGS*
II, III	Pupillary	Shine a light source in eye. *Rapid, concentrically constricting pupils indicate intact cranial nerves II, III.*
II, IV, VI	Oculocephalic	Perform with eyes held open (doll's eyes) and head turned from side to side. *Eyes gazing straight up or lagging slightly behind head motion indicate intact cranial nerves II, IV, VI.* Precaution: Cervical spine injury must be ruled out before this assessment is performed.
III, VIII	Oculovestibular	Place the head in a midline and slightly elevated position. A physician injects ice water into ear canal. *Eyes deviating toward the irrigated ear indicate intact cranial nerves III, VIII.* Precaution: Ensure that the cervical spine is not injured and that the tympanic membranes are intact before this assessment.
V, VII	Corneal	Cornea is gently swabbed with sterile cotton swab. *A blink indicates intact cranial nerves V, VII.*
IX, X	Gag	Pharynx is irritated with tongue depressor or cotton swab. *Gagging response indicates intact cranial nerves IX, X.*

* Italics indicate normal findings.

TABLE 54–4 AVPU—Infant Responsiveness Assessment*

CRITERION	DESCRIPTION
Alert	Responsive to parents; cuddles, coos, or babbles; smiles
Verbal	Responsive to verbal stimulation
Pain response	Responsive to painful stimulation only
Unresponsive	No response to painful stimulation

*AVPU is the acronym formed from the first letter of each criterion.

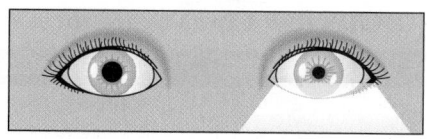

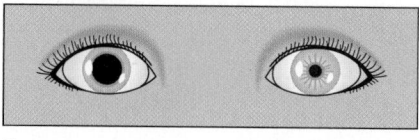

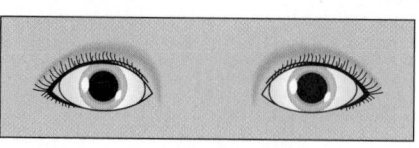

Figure 54–3 Pupil findings in various neurologic conditions with altered consciousness. *A,* A unilateral dilated and reactive pupil is associated with an intracranial mass. *B,* A fixed and dilated pupil may be a sign of impending brainstem herniation. *C,* Bilateral fixed and dilated pupils are associated with brainstem herniation from increased intracranial pressure.

Among the nursing diagnoses that might be appropriate for the child with an altered level of consciousness are the following (NANDA-I © 2014):

- *Breathing Pattern, Ineffective,* related to neuromuscular dysfunction associated with increased intracranial pressure
- *Aspiration, Risk for,* related to poor control of secretions with decreased level of consciousness
- *Skin Integrity, Risk for Impaired,* related to agitation and skin rubbing against bedding
- *Family Processes, Interrupted,* related to care of a child with an acquired disability

Planning and Implementation

HOSPITAL-BASED NURSING CARE

Nursing care of the child with altered consciousness or increased ICP focuses on maintaining airway patency, monitoring neurologic status, performing routine care, providing adequate nutrition, providing sensory stimulation, and providing emotional support to parents. Nursing care for the child with increased ICP is described later in this chapter.

Make sure the child's airway is patent at all times. If the child has difficulty managing secretions or has no gag reflex, endotracheal intubation or a tracheostomy is performed. Frequent suctioning may be required (see the *Clinical Skills Manual* SKILLS). Keep suction apparatus with catheters, oxygen, resuscitation bag and mask, and extra endotracheal or tracheostomy tubes at the bedside. Pulse oximetry or arterial blood gas measurement is performed at regular intervals to ensure that gas exchange is adequate.

Assisted ventilation may be required (see the *Clinical Skills Manual* SKILLS).

Anticipate that seizures may occur. Raise and pad the side rails to protect the child from injury.

Perform routine nursing care. If the corneal reflex is absent, place artificial tears in the eyes and keep them closed with gauze and tape. Perform routine mouth care by brushing the teeth and using swabs with water. Prevent complications associated with immobility (muscle atrophy, contractures, and skin breakdown). See Box 54–1.

Box 54–1 Care for the Child Who Is Immobile

- Massage child's skin gently using lotion.
- Change the child's position every 2 hours. Use splints or rolls made of towels or blankets to keep the body in proper alignment.
- Place child on a special mattress designed to relieve pressure points (airflow or foam), or use a sheepskin covering when a special mattress is not available.
- Place transparent dressing over skin surfaces exposed to rubbing or friction.
- Support physical therapy efforts with extra passive or gentle range-of-motion (ROM) exercises.
- Use sequential compression devices to prevent deep vein thrombosis.

Provide adequate nutrition. A nasogastric or transpyloric tube may be inserted if the child remains unconscious or is not alert enough to take food by mouth (see the *Clinical Skills Manual* SKILLS). A gastrostomy tube may be inserted for long-term enteral feeding.

Provide sensory stimulation. Because children with a severely altered level of consciousness may still be able to hear, talk to them. Listening to music or tapes of family members talking or reading can soothe the child when family members cannot be present. Encourage parents to stroke and touch the child in a soothing manner.

As the child becomes more alert, repeatedly orient the child to time, place, and person, depending on the child's age and level of understanding. Encourage parents to bring objects or toys from home to make the environment more familiar and promote a feeling of security.

Provide emotional support to the child and family. Explain the child's condition in simple terms. Encourage parents to take part in the child's care and therapy as much as possible. Give family members the opportunity to express their feelings. If the child's functioning has been permanently impaired, refer the family to the appropriate psychologic and social services. (See Chapter 41 for information about supporting families during a child's life-threatening illness.)

DISCHARGE PLANNING AND HOME CARE TEACHING

The child's transition from the hospital to home, a long-term care facility, or inpatient rehabilitation center must be planned well in advance of discharge. Identify a case manager or social worker to help plan the child's long-term care needs, including home health nursing and rehabilitation services, modifying the home, and purchasing special equipment.

COMMUNITY-BASED NURSING CARE

Home health nurses play a vital role in the care of the child with acquired neurologic dysfunction and prolonged altered consciousness. Teach the family how to care for the child with severe neurologic dysfunction and to perform routine procedures such as suctioning, maintaining the airway, skin care, feeding, positioning, ROM exercises, and stimulation. Regular follow-up visits are needed to assess the child's progress and to modify the treatment plan.

Link the child and family with community rehabilitation services through an early intervention program or school-based program. The home health nurse or case manager should help the family have an individual education plan (IEP) developed for the child (see Chapter 38).

Evaluation

Expected outcomes of nursing care include the following:

- The child's airway is maintained and the brain is adequately oxygenated.
- Complications of immobility are prevented.
- The family provides appropriate care to the child with prolonged altered consciousness to promote minimal long-term disabilities.

Seizure Disorders

Seizures are periods of abnormal electrical discharges in the brain that cause involuntary movement and behavior and sensory alterations. Epilepsy is a chronic disorder characterized by recurrent, unprovoked seizures, secondary to an underlying brain abnormality. Approximately 326,000 children under the age of 15 years live with epilepsy (Epilepsy Foundation, 2014a). The highest rate of onset occurs during the first 12 months of life (Kerr & Huether, 2014). See *Developing Cultural Competence: Seizures*.

Developing Cultural Competence Seizures

Some cultural groups have misperceptions of the cause of seizures, such punishment for sins, a lack of spiritual faith, or possession by spirits (Institute of Medicine, 2012, p. 32). For example, the Hmong people of Asia believe the child is experiencing *quag dab peg*, or "the spirit catches you and you fall down." Traditional Hmong view the condition as serious but take pride in the child who has the condition, as they have a link to the spirit world. In 1997, Anne Fadiman wrote a compelling story about the cultural conflict between a Hmong family and healthcare providers over the treatment of their daughter's seizures, *The Spirit Catches You and You Fall Down*.

Etiology and Pathophysiology

When an excessive number of neurons in the brain become overexcited, they discharge abnormally, leading to seizures. An imbalance of exciting and inhibiting mechanisms caused by poor regulation of the gamma-aminobutyric acid ionotropic receptor family A (GABA$_A$) neurotransmitters may be a cause of early childhood seizures (Kerr & Huether, 2014). Rather than being one distinct disorder, epilepsy and seizures are associated with CNS structural defects, or from disorders that affect CNS functioning, such as brain injury, infection, electrolyte disturbance, toxins, and brain tumor. Genetic factors or familial predisposition may lead to seizures. Some seizures have no known cause.

Partial, or **focal**, seizures are caused by abnormal electrical activity in one brain hemisphere or a specific area of the cerebral cortex, most often the temporal, frontal, or parietal lobes. The symptoms depend on the region of the cortex affected.

Generalized seizures are the result of diffuse electrical activity that begins in both brain hemispheres simultaneously, spreading throughout the cortex into the brainstem. The child's movements and spasms are bilateral and symmetric, and consciousness is impaired.

Febrile seizures occur in susceptible infants and children in connection with a rise in temperature to 39.0°C (102.2°F) or higher during the first 24 hours of an associated acute illness. They occur in 3% to 5% of children (Ismail et al., 2012). No evidence of intracranial infection or systemic metabolic disorder is present. A genetic predisposition may be present. These seizures are usually seen in children between 9 months and 5 years of age (Kerr & Huether, 2014). Simple febrile seizures last less than 15 minutes and do not recur during the same illness. Some children have complex febrile seizures that last 15 minutes or longer and recur within 24 hours, and they may be at greater risk for developing epilepsy.

Status epilepticus is a prolonged continuous seizure of 15 minutes or evidence of intermittent seizures noted from clinical signs or EEG tracings lasting more than 15 minutes without full recovery of consciousness between seizures (Wilkes & Tasker, 2013). Low levels of antiepileptic medications, fever, infection, and a recent medical condition change are risk factors in children. Among children, the highest incidence is in the first 12 months of life (Varelas, Spanaki, & Mirski, 2013). The basal metabolic rate rises during peak seizure activity and increases the demand for oxygen and glucose.

Clinical Manifestations

The symptoms of a seizure depend on the type and duration of the seizure. The characteristics of the various partial and generalized seizures are presented in Table 54–5.

Partial seizures often start with an aura or an abrupt, unprovoked alteration in behavior. The child may have time to get to the floor and avoid injury once the aura pattern is recognized.

Generalized seizures often begin with the **tonic** phase, characterized by unconsciousness, continuous muscular contraction, and sustained stiffness. The **clonic** phase that follows is characterized by alternating muscular contraction and relaxation or repeated rhythmic jerking. During the **postictal period** following seizure activity, the level of consciousness is decreased. The length of the postictal period varies. Children may have a partial seizure that progresses to a generalized seizure.

Growth and Development

Neonatal seizures may be subtle with roving eye movements, repetitive blinking, sucking, lip smacking, tongue thrusting, swimming movements of the arms, leg pedaling movements, and apnea or tachycardia (Beaulieu, 2013).

Simple febrile seizures are generalized seizures with tonic-clonic movements and eye rolling, followed by a brief postictal period. Complex febrile seizures have additional focal signs.

TABLE 54–5 Clinical Manifestations of Seizures

TYPE OF SEIZURE AND CAUSE	CLINICAL MANIFESTATIONS
PARTIAL SEIZURES	
Simple Partial Seizures **(focal seizures)**	
Focal damage (e.g., with cerebral palsy)	Onset: any age
Tumors or lesions	No loss of consciousness; lasts less than 30 sec; no postseizure confusion
Arteriovenous malformation	No **aura** (a visual, auditory, taste, or motor sensation preceding a seizure or migraine headache)
Brain abscesses	Signs depend on section of brain affected: motor activities such as twitching or lost muscle tone (may involve one extremity, part of an extremity, or ipsilateral extremities) or sensory sensations such as tingling, numbness, or a sensation involving sound, smell, or sight
	May progress to a generalized seizure
Complex Partial Seizures **(psychomotor seizures)**	
Lesions, cysts, or tumors	Onset: 3 years of age to adolescence
Perinatal trauma	Consciousness is impaired immediately; lasts 30 sec to 5 min; postseizure amnesia or confusion
Focal sclerosis (e.g., scarring of the medio-temporal lobe from prolonged febrile seizures)	Aura frequently present
Vascular anomalies (e.g., arteriovenous malformations)	May have abnormal motor activity, twitching, loss of tone, or posturing; **automatisms** (unusual body movements without purpose, e.g., lip smacking, lip chewing, sucking)
Brain trauma	May have sensory changes such as tingling or numbness, feeling of anxiety, fear, or déjà vu (sensation that event occurred before)
	May progress to a generalized seizure
	Abdominal pain

TYPE OF SEIZURE AND CAUSE	CLINICAL MANIFESTATIONS
GENERALIZED SEIZURES	
Tonic-Clonic Seizures **(grand mal seizures)**	
Cerebral damage from perinatal trauma, brain trauma, tumors, structural lesions, metabolic and neuromuscular degenerative disorders Genetic, strong familial incidence Many are idiopathic	Onset: any age, rare before 6 months of age Abrupt onset seizure, 1- to 2-min loss of consciousness, postseizure confusion (few minutes to hours) May or may not have aura Body becomes stiff and rigid when all muscles contract (tonic phase), followed by rhythmic jerking motions (clonic phase) Drooling as secretions are not swallowed Pupils dilated; eyes roll upward or deviate to one side Abdominal or chest wall rigidity with leg, head, and neck extended, and arms flexed or contracted Cry or grunt as air is forced out when diaphragm and chest muscles contract Urinary or bowel incontinence as muscles become flaccid during clonic phase Sleepiness, difficulty in arousal; hypertension; diaphoresis; headache, nausea, vomiting; poor coordination, decreased muscle tone; confusion, amnesia; slurred speech; visual disturbances; combativeness
Childhood Absence Epilepsy **(petit mal seizures)**	
Hyperventilation for 3 minutes Genetic (multifactorial) predisposition or mutations	Onset: ages 4–10 years with remission in adolescence More prevalent in females May develop other generalized seizures No aura; brief loss of consciousness, usually lasts 5–10 sec, rarely exceeds 30 sec, no postseizure confusion, lethargy, or sleepiness; amnesia regarding the seizure Frequent attacks (50–100 or more per day), may cluster, interfere with learning Eye blinking, eyelid fluttering, staring, glazed eye appearance, myoclonic jerks; interrupts voluntary activity, slight decrease or loss of muscle tone (head may droop, may drop objects) Verbal or touch stimulation does not interrupt seizure
Juvenile Myoclonic Epilepsy	
Genetic disorder	Onset often during puberty No loss of consciousness, child recovers in seconds, no postictal period Most often occur upon falling asleep or awakening Quick involuntary muscle jerks of the neck, shoulders, and arms Child usually has normal intelligence
Infantile Spasms **(West syndrome, salaam seizures)**	
Tuberous sclerosis (genetic syndrome) Mutation of several genes Intrauterine stroke Inborn errors of metabolism CNS malformations	Onset: age 4 and 18 months with peak onset at 3–7 months; more common in males Severe form of epilepsy; may occur with altered consciousness as part of a complex partial seizure; seizures occur in clusters, 5–150 per day Spasms with abrupt flexion and extension of muscle groups in the neck, trunk, and extremities, involving head nods or jackknife body contractions; occur as infant awakens or falls asleep. Spasms stop by 5 years of age when other seizure types occur. Developmental delays occur
Lennox-Gastaut Syndrome **(akinetic or atonic seizure)**	
Gray matter degenerative diseases and sub-acute seizures Sclerosing panencephalitis Many are idiopathic	Onset: first seen between 1 and 8 years, predominantly in boys Combination of generalized seizures including tonic-clonic, absence, and myoclonic activity; drop attack (falls to ground with sudden loss of postural tone, inability to break fall, is limp for period of time) Associated intellectual disability, delayed psychomotor development, and severe behavior problems

Clinical Therapy

After the child's first seizure, a thorough history is taken from the parent, primary caretaker, or witnesses to the event. The description and length of the seizure, presence or absence of an aura, and whether the child lost consciousness are noted. This information helps to identify the type of seizure according to the International Classification of Epileptic Seizures in Table 54–5.

Based on the physical findings and history, diagnostic tests ordered may include a complete blood cell count, blood chemistry, and urine toxicology. A urine culture, blood culture, and lumbar puncture are performed if meningitis is suspected. A lead level and tests for inborn errors of metabolism may be considered. Radiologic tests such as CT scanning or MRI and angiography may be performed to identify a cerebral lesion or metabolic disorder in the brain. An EEG is often performed at a follow-up visit between seizures. If the child is taking any anticonvulsants, a serum drug level is obtained.

Many seizures are self-limiting and require no emergency intervention. When the seizure is prolonged, emergency therapy includes airway management, supplemental oxygen, intravenous benzodiazepines, and careful monitoring of vital signs. Serum electrolytes, glucose, and blood gases may be monitored. The postictal period ranges from 30 minutes to 2 hours. When the child's seizure does not stop as expected with emergency intervention, treatment for status epilepticus is initiated (Table 54–6).

Children with simple febrile seizures are often not treated with an anticonvulsant at the time of the seizure because the seizure has stopped before arrival at the emergency department. Acetaminophen is given to lower the temperature. Long-term antiepileptic medications are not recommended for simple febrile seizures because of their adverse effects.

Most seizure disorders are treated with antiepileptic drugs (AEDs). A single (monotherapy) AED is preferred for seizure control to minimize the side effects such as sleepiness, decreased attention and memory, difficulty with speech, ataxia, and diplopia. A low dose is used initially and gradually increased until seizures are controlled. An alternate AED may be tried if seizure control is not achieved with a high therapeutic dose of the first medication or when unacceptable side effects occur. Some children have refractory or **intractable seizures**, requiring two or more AEDs. See *Medications Used to Treat: Seizures*. Medication dosage adjustments are often needed as the child grows. Blood tests to monitor for liver and hematologic problems and therapeutic drug levels are often performed.

SAFETY ALERT!

Because of the potential adverse effects of medications used to treat seizures, children are monitored for depression, suicidal thinking, and effects on learning. Medications should not be stopped abruptly, and dose is tapered when discontinuation is planned. When starting a new medication, adolescents should not engage in hazardous activities or drive a motorized vehicle until effects of the medication are known. Alcohol intake is contraindicated.

Surgery may be performed to remove a tumor, lesion, or portion of the brain that has been identified as causing the seizures, particularly when seizures do not respond to multiple AEDs. A vagal nerve stimulator with leads wrapped around the left vagus nerve may be implanted in children who are not candidates for surgery and are unable to tolerate multiple medications. The child activates the vagal nerve stimulator after experiencing an aura to reduce the spread of the seizure.

A ketogenic diet may be used for children with seizures that do not respond to AEDs. The diet is customized for the child to have high fat (80% of calories), adequate protein for growth, and very low carbohydrates that will maintain an ideal body weight, maximize ketosis, and achieve optimal seizure control. Each meal typically has about 3 to 4 g of fat for every 1 g of protein and carbohydrate (Epilepsy Foundation, 2014b). Ketosis is believed to produce anticonvulsant effects. Family motivation must be high to maintain the rigid diet for 1 or more years because improved seizure control is directly related to diet compliance. Diet side

TABLE 54–6 Status Epilepticus Clinical Therapy and Nursing Management

TYPE OF CARE	CLINICAL THERAPY AND NURSING MANAGEMENT
Emergency assessment and management	• Maintain a patent airway. Muscle rigidity may compromise the airway. Keep suction equipment at the bedside in case secretions are excessive. • Give supplemental oxygen because increased metabolic demands deplete oxygen stores. • Monitor vital signs and circulation with pulse oximeter and cardiorespiratory monitor. • Perform neurologic assessments every 5–10 min.
Ongoing urgent management	• Establish an IV line for fluid or medication administration. • Assess blood glucose level; administer glucose if the child is hypoglycemic; the physical stress of the seizure may result in declining glucose levels. • Insert a nasogastric tube to reduce the risk for aspiration due to vomiting. • Protect the child from injury. • Manage thermoregulation.
Medications	• Administer benzodiazepines such as diazepam, lorazepam, or midazolam. If there is no response, the dose may be repeated. Fosphenytoin or phenobarbital may be necessary if seizure activity continues. Cumulative doses of drugs may produce apnea, so be prepared to assist with endotracheal intubation and ventilations.

Source: Data from Shearer, P., & Riviello, J. (2011). Generalized convulsive status epilepticus in adults and children: Treatment guidelines and protocols. *Emergency Care Clinics of North America, 29,* 51–64; Varelas, P. N., Spanaki M.V., & Mirski, M. A. (2013). Status epilepticus: An update. *Current Neurology and Neuroscience Reports, 13*(7), 357–365; McLauchlan, D. J., & Robertson, N. P. (2012). Management of status epilepticus. *Journal of Neurology, 259,* 2261–2263.

Medications Used to Treat: Seizures

MEDICATION AND ACTION	NURSING MANAGEMENT
Benzodiazepines (diazepam, lorazepam) CNS depressant, anticonvulsant properties, used for status epilepticus	• Administer IV push medication very slowly into the IV entry site closest to the child's body. • Monitor for hypotension, tachycardia, and respiratory depression. • The rectal or nasal preparation may be prescribed for home administration to treat prolonged seizures.
Phenobarbital Enhances gamma-aminobutyric acid (GABA) neurotransmitter inhibition by prolonging the time that chloride channels are open in response to GABA.	• Administer IV push medication very slowly into the IV entry site closest to the child's body. • Monitor child's vital signs frequently when given IV. Monitor for excess sedation. • May crush tablets and mix with food or fluid. • Provide vitamin D and folic acid supplements when drug is used long term.
Phenytoin (Dilantin) **Fosphenytoin (Cerebyx)** Reduces voltage, frequency, and spread of electrical discharges within motor cortex to inhibit seizure activity.	• Monitor the child's vital signs frequently after IV dosage for respiratory depression. • Educate family to provide an adequate intake of vitamin D, folic acid, and calcium. • Promote frequent dental care for gingival hyperplasia. • Educate parents that urine may be pink, red, or brown color.
Carbamazepine (Tegretol) Inhibits sustained repetitive impulses and reduces synaptic transmission to the spinal cord, limiting the spread of seizure activity.	• Give with food to enhance absorption. Be aware that grapefruit may increase drug levels. • Educate parents about which tablets can be chewed and not chewed (sustained release). • Do not combine suspension with another liquid medication to prevent precipitation. • Causes photosensitivity reactions when skin is exposed to sunlight.
Valproic acid (Depacon, Depakote) Anticonvulsant; inhibits abnormal neuron discharges in the brain and decreases seizure activity.	• Do not use carbonated beverage to dilute syrup. Educate the child and parents that all tablets and capsules should be swallowed whole, not chewed. • Give with food to decrease gastrointestinal irritation. • Monitor platelet count and bleeding times. • Educate adolescent females about teratogenic effects of the medication, and the importance of contraception and planning pregnancy.
Ethosuximide (Zarontin) Suppresses spike and wave pattern in absence seizures; raises brain's seizure threshold.	• Monitor for weight loss or anorexia. • Give with food if gastrointestinal upset occurs. • Do not expose medication to light. Do not freeze.
Primidone (Mysoline) Raises the seizure threshold and changes seizure patterns.	• Give with food if gastrointestinal upset occurs. • Store medication away from light and moisture.
Felbamate (Felbatol) Blocks repetitive firing of neurons and increases seizure threshold.	• Monitor for weight gain or loss. • Monitor regularly for hematologic and liver problems as well as bruising or bleeding.
Gabapentin (Neurontin) Gamma-aminobutyric acid (GABA) neurotransmitter analog	• Monitor vision, concentration, and coordination as medication may cause impairments. • Do not take medication within 2 hr of an antacid.
Lamotrigine (Lamictal) Inhibits release of glutamate and aspartate in sodium channels to decrease seizure activity.	• Educate family about photosensitivity side effect. • Monitor for dizziness, lack of coordination, drowsiness, or depression if used with valproic acid. • Educate parents to notify healthcare provider if skin rash develops because of risk for Stevens–Johnson syndrome.

(continued)

Medications Used to Treat: Seizures (continued)

Medication	Nursing Considerations
Tiagabine (Gabitril filmtabs) Enhances activity of GABA, making it more available for postsynaptic neurons.	• Give with food. Avoid using with over-the-counter medications that cause drowsiness. • Monitor for signs of dizziness, tremor, and sleepiness.
Topiramate (Topamax) Sodium channel blocker and enhances ability of GABA to move chloride ions into the neurons.	• Monitor for weight loss. • Increase fluid intake to reduce risk of kidney stones. • Monitor mental status and for impaired cognitive function. • Inform parents to report speech and language problems.
Levetiracetam (Keppra) Unknown mechanism of action; inhibits seizure activity.	• Ensure that parents know whether tablet must be swallowed whole or can be chewed or crushed. • Monitor for gait and coordination problems.
Oxcarbazepine (Trileptal) Similar mechanism of action to carbamazepine.	• Monitor for hyponatremia and CNS impairment. • Educate adolescent females that oral contraceptives may be ineffective.
Zonisamide Facilitates dopaminergic and serotonergic transmission between neurons.	• Increase fluid intake to reduce risk of kidney stones. • Capsules should not be broken or crushed.
Rufinamide (Banzel) Modulation of sodium channels inhibits firing of sodium-dependent neuron transmission.	• Tablet may be crushed or swallowed whole. • Give medication with a meal because food increases drug absorption.
Clobazam (Onfi) Binds at GABA$_A$ receptor site to inhibit seizures; used for Lennox-Gastaut syndrome.	• Tablet may be crushed or swallowed whole. • Inform adolescent females that oral contraceptives may be ineffective.

Source: Data from Wilson, B. A., Shannon, M. T., & Shield, K. M. (2015). *Nurse's drug guide 2015*. Hoboken, NJ: Pearson; Taketomo, C. K., Hodding, J. H., & Crause, D. M. (2014). *Pediatric and neonatal dosage handbook* (21st ed.). Hudson, OH: Lexicomp; Zelleke, T. G., Depositario-Cabacar, D. F. T., & Gaillard, W. D. (2013). Epilepsy. In M. L. Batshaw, N. J. Roizen, & G. R. Lotrecchiano (Eds.), *Children with disabilities* (7th ed., pp. 487–506). Baltimore, MD: Paul H. Brooks Publishing Co.

effects include constipation, kidney stones, and slowed growth. Constipation is treated with medium-chain triglyceride (MCT) oil and increased fluids. Kidney stones are treated by increasing fluids and alkalinizing the urine. Approximately 10% to 15% of children become seizure-free, and nearly half of children have a 50% reduction in number of seizures (Epilepsy Foundation, 2014b).

A trial of medication withdrawal (slowly tapered over a few months) is often attempted for children who have been seizure-free for 2 years or longer. Approximately 25% to 36% of children have seizures recur after discontinuing medications (Zelleke, Depositario-Cabacar, & Gaillard, 2013). Children with epilepsy are more likely to have anxiety, depression, behavior problems, and disabilities (e.g., attention deficit hyperactivity disorder, developmental delay, or autism) than children who do not have epilepsy (Russ, Larson, & Halfon, 2012).

Nursing Management

For the Child With a Seizure Disorder

Nursing Assessment and Diagnosis

Assess and monitor the child's physiologic status. Observe the specific seizure activity, level of consciousness, vital signs, and signs of hypoxia. During the postictal period, monitor the child's vital signs, perform neurologic checks, and keep the environment safe. Once the child is stable, a more definitive assessment can be made. Level of consciousness is one of the most important indicators of neurologic function. Remember that the child's lack of response may be the result of the postictal state. Continuing motor activity, which may be less intense after benzodiazepines are given, is a potential sign of status epilepticus.

Collect and analyze historical information about the seizure activity. See Table 54–7.

Assess the family's adaptation to the seizure disorder, including how well the family is coping with the uncertainty of when the next seizure will occur.

Common nursing diagnoses for the child with a seizure disorder include the following (NANDA-I © 2014):

• **Breathing Pattern, Ineffective,** related to neuromuscular dysfunction during the tonic phase of a seizure

• **Airway Clearance, Ineffective,** related to inability to control secretions during seizure

• **Trauma, Risk for,** related to falls with seizures

• **Self-Esteem, Chronic Low,** related to refractory seizures and loss of bowel and bladder control during seizure activity

TABLE 54–7 Questions to Ask About Seizures

TIME PERIOD	QUESTIONS TO ASK
Just before the seizure	• What was the child doing? • Did the child complain of feeling unwell (headache, nausea, vomiting, muscle pain, fever) or feeling "funny"? • Did the child suffer any trauma? Did the child get into any medications or poisons?
During the seizure	• What movements of the arms and legs were seen? On one or both sides of the body or in one extremity only? • Did the child exhibit any chewing or other automatism? • Were the pupils dilated or the eyes deviated to one side? • Did the child's color change (pale, red, blue)? • Was the child incontinent of urine or stool? • Was the child aware of surroundings or able to respond to questions?
After the seizure	• How long did the episode last? • Was the child lethargic, weak, or uncoordinated when waking up? • Did the child have memory loss or confusion?

• *Anxiety* related to unpredictable nature of seizure disorder

• *Health Management, Family, Ineffective,* related to poor adherence with medications

Planning and Implementation

Children with a seizure disorder may be hospitalized for another condition. Nursing care focuses on preventing and managing a potential seizure by maintaining airway patency, ensuring safety, administering medications, and providing emotional support. Both acute care and long-term management are involved.

MAINTAIN AIRWAY PATENCY

Place nothing in the child's mouth during a seizure; loose teeth may be knocked out and aspirated. The child is put in side-lying position for secretions to drain. Monitor the child to ensure adequate oxygenation: The child's color should be pink, the heart rate at a normal or slightly above normal rate for age, and the SpO_2 greater than 95%. Oxygen is usually given at SpO_2 levels below 95% (see the *Clinical Skills Manual* SKILLS).

ENSURE SAFETY

Protect the child from self-harm during seizures (Figure 54–4). If the child is in bed, pad the side rails to prevent injury. Children who have frequent, recurrent seizures should wear helmets to protect their heads in case they fall. All children with seizure disorders should wear some form of medical alert identification.

ADMINISTER MEDICATIONS

Take special precautions when administering IV medications (benzodiazepines) for urgent seizure management. Give these medications very slowly over several minutes to minimize the risk of respiratory or circulatory collapse, and carefully monitor the child's vital signs.

Medications for the daily management of seizures are given orally. Ensure that extended-release medications are not crushed or chewed. When a child is NPO because of illness or on the day of surgery, seizure medications are usually given with a swallow of water. Obtain medication orders in these cases.

PROVIDE EMOTIONAL SUPPORT

Seizures are frightening to the child and family because control of body movements and consciousness are often lost. Parents often feel guilty about the child's seizure disorder and need guidance to treat the child as normally as possible. They may perceive that the child is treated differently by family, friends, and peers because of lack of understanding about seizures. Parents need additional support when seizures do not respond to one or more antiepileptic drugs and alternative therapies must be considered. Refer the child and family to support groups and counseling services if indicated. See *Evidence-Based Practice: Supporting Children With Epilepsy and Their Parents.*

Clinical Tip

When the child on a ketogenic diet is hospitalized, limit glucose and dextrose from all sources including IV fluids, elixirs, suspensions, and syrups. Use normal saline IV fluid. Obtain medications in pill form, crush them, and mix with an allowable food approved by the pharmacy.

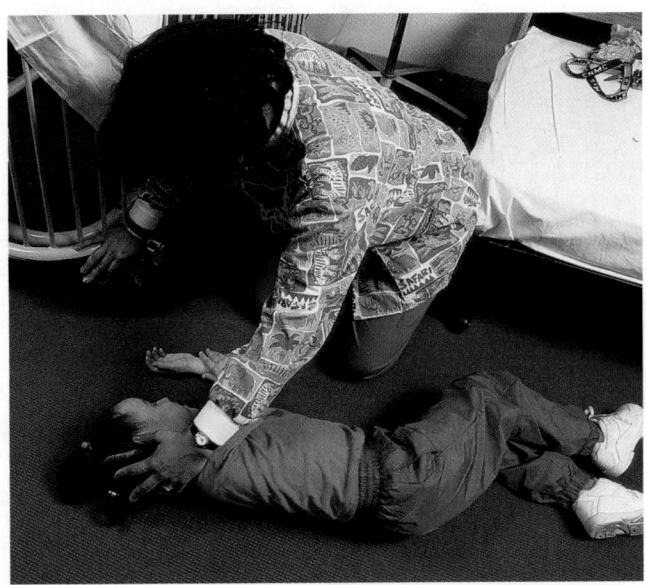

Figure 54–4 **Protect the child from injury during a seizure. The child who is standing should be gently assisted to the floor and placed in a side-lying position. Clear the area of any objects that might cause harm to the child.**

EVIDENCE-BASED PRACTICE | Supporting Children With Epilepsy and Their Parents

Clinical Question

What factors are related to stress and health quality of life for children with epilepsy and their families?

The Evidence

Twenty children, aged 9 to 15 years, and their parents completed a voluntary survey while attending a summer camp for children with epilepsy. The survey asked about seizure control and management, age at diagnosis, the worst thing about having epilepsy, and one thing they could change about having epilepsy. Feeling different or being teased was the most frequent response campers (50%) and parents (27%) gave to the worst thing about epilepsy, followed by the physical act of the seizure (campers, 38%; parents, 40%). Reducing the number or having no seizures was desired by 63% of campers and parents as the one change about having epilepsy. An additional 13% of campers wanted no seizures in public (VanStraten & Ng, 2012). While responses were not statistically significant, they do reveal important information about the impact of the condition on quality of life.

The risk for development of clinical depression among mothers of children with epilepsy participating in a multisite Health-related Quality of Life in Children with Epilepsy Study was identified at time of diagnosis and every 6 months for 24 months. Data were collected using the 20-item Center for Epidemiologic Depression Scale to assess mood, somatic complaints, interactions with others, and motor functioning. Data from several other research instruments helped identify factors such as family functioning, family resources, and epilepsy severity. Of the 338 mothers who agreed to participate in the project, 128 (38%) had a risk for clinical depression at the time of the child's diagnosis and were excluded from further evaluation. Of the remaining 210 mothers, a total of 58 (28%) mothers developed depressive symptoms at some point during the subsequent 24 months. Statistically significant factors associated with risk for clinical depression included a younger mother, the child's prescribed number of antiepileptic drugs,

worse family functioning, fewer family resources, and more family demands (Ferro & Speechley, 2011).

The same multisite Health-related Quality of Life in Children with Epilepsy Study also reported information on child health, well-being, and the impact of illness on life functions during the past 4 weeks for 374 children with a mean age of 7.4 years. The parent form of the Child Health Questionnaire was used at diagnosis and 24 months later for the study. Data from other research instruments helped identify factors such as parent depression, family functioning, family resources, and epilepsy severity. After controlling for physical and psychologic health at diagnosis, multiple regression analysis identified predictors at 24 months of better physical health (less severe cognitive problems and less parental depression) and better psychosocial health (less severe behavior problems, an older parent, better family functioning, and fewer demands) in participating children (Ferro, Landgraf, & Speechley, 2013). These studies further support the important role of the family environment on child health-related quality of life.

Best Practice

Epilepsy is a common neurologic condition that causes families and affected children to have social, psychologic, and physical challenges. Stressors can be related to the stigma associated with epilepsy, the unpredictable nature of when and where seizures may occur, loss of control, and even some of the disabilities associated with epilepsy. Research suggests that intervention programs to improve the family environment and to offer treatment for depression and anxiety may improve the family's healthy adaptation to epilepsy.

Clinical Reasoning

When caring for a child with epilepsy, what questions may help reveal the stressors that the parents and child are experiencing? Once stressors are identified, investigate resources with regard to parent mental health, improved epilepsy management, and support groups for children and their parents.

DISCHARGE PLANNING AND HOME CARE TEACHING

Encourage parents to express their fears and anxieties. Answer their questions honestly, and refer them to organizations such as the Epilepsy Foundation, where they can get more information about the child's disorder. Be sure parents know how to administer medications and keep the child safe. Provide information about whom to call with questions and when to return for follow-up.

COMMUNITY-BASED NURSING CARE

Educate the child and parents about medication regimens. Explain the purpose of each antiepileptic drug (AED), its administration schedule, and the importance of giving all doses. Provide information about the medication side effects, and alert parents to the signs of toxic reactions. Ensure that information is shared directly with older children so that they can begin taking more responsibility for self-care and gain a sense of self-control. A study explored nonadherence to AEDs in 124 newly diagnosed children ages 2 to 12 years. Researchers discovered that 58% of children had persistent nonadherence

and 42% had near perfect adherence during the first 6 months of therapy. The pattern of adherence was established within the first month of therapy. Socioeconomic status was the only factor associated with adherence, and lower socioeconomic status was associated with higher nonadherence (Modi, Rausch, & Glauser, 2011).

Ensure that adolescents understand that alcohol intake is contraindicated and may result in medication toxicity. Ask questions at each visit that may reveal actual medication adherence, such as inquiring about the number of pills remaining or difficulties paying for medications. Monitor the child's growth because a weight change may require dosage adjustment to maintain seizure control. Encourage the family to obtain regular dental care for the child treated with phenytoin and similar AEDs because of their effects on the gingivae.

The parents of children with recurrent febrile seizures should be taught to give the proper dose of acetaminophen or ibuprofen with fever onset. Parents need to know that fever management may not prevent a febrile seizure. Reassure parents that complications from febrile seizures are rare.

TEACHING HIGHLIGHTS | Safety for the Child With a Seizure Disorder

Children with epilepsy have more injuries of all sorts, including burns and falls. Children are at increased risk for death due to drowning. Planning for safety includes the following:
- Do not leave the child alone in the bathtub.
- Children who bathe alone should use the shower.
- A buddy and lifeguard should always be present when the child swims.
- A life vest should always be worn when boating.
- A child with frequent seizures should wear a helmet to protect the head in case of a fall.
- The child should not play or stand around open flames or outdoor grills.
- The child should avoid areas where fall risks are increased.
- A form of medical identification should be worn, such as a medical alert bracelet.

Educate adolescent females about the potential teratogenicity of some antiepileptic drugs (AEDs). Valproic acid and carbamazepine are associated with neural tube defects. Contraception should be used when the adolescent is sexually active, but ensure that barrier methods are used correctly when AEDs interact with oral contraceptives. When pregnancy is desired, an alternate AED may be prescribed with a lower risk for birth defects.

Teach families about safety guidelines for the child. See *Teaching Highlights: Safety for the Child With a Seizure Disorder.* Physical activity and exercise are important for all children. Encourage participation in sports when adequate supervision is provided. Children with well-controlled seizures may participate in most team sports, and activities such as bicycle riding. Activities such as rope climbing, rock or mountain climbing, tree climbing, snow skiing, scuba diving, and sky diving are more dangerous if seizures are not well controlled. Swimming and water sports require one-to-one supervision.

Assist the family to develop an individual health plan so the child can receive medications during school hours, if necessary. Provide information to teachers and school administrators about care of the child during a seizure and what information to report to the parents. Parents may want to provide a towel and clothing change for the child who has incontinence with a seizure.

The child may be afraid of having a seizure in front of friends. Reassure the child and family that taking medications regularly often controls seizures. Children need to be able to explain to peers what a seizure is and what to do if they are present when one occurs. Summer camps for children with seizures can be a safe and comfortable place for the child to enjoy outdoor activities. Teach parents to boost the child's self-image by emphasizing what the child can do, rather than focusing on contraindicated activities. Depending on state laws, most adolescents can drive after they have been seizure-free for at least 2 years.

Evaluation

Expected outcomes of nursing management include the following:
- The child achieves good seizure control with medication, ketogenic diet, or surgical intervention.
- The use of effective safety measures prevents injuries during seizures.

- The child gains enhanced self-esteem through participation in well-supervised sports and activities.

Infectious Diseases

Infections of the central nervous system need to be identified and treated rapidly because they can cause significant consequences in the developing child.

Bacterial Meningitis

Meningitis, an inflammation of the meninges, can be caused by either bacterial or viral agents. Bacterial meningitis is more serious than viral meningitis and is sometimes fatal. Meningitis may also be caused by tuberculosis. Newborns and infants are at greatest risk for bacterial meningitis. Infants and children who develop meningitis may have acute complications and long-term morbidity.

ETIOLOGY AND PATHOPHYSIOLOGY

Meningitis may occur secondary to other infections such as otitis media, sinusitis, pharyngitis, cellulitis, pneumonia, or septic arthritis; brain trauma; or a neurosurgical procedure. *Streptococcus pneumonia, Neisseria meningitides,* and staphylococcal and gram-negative microorganisms cause most cases of meningitis in children in the United States. Group B streptococcus causes some cases of meningitis in newborns. Rates of meningitis have fallen for children because of increased protection from several vaccines (Castelblanco, Lee, & Hasbun, 2014). Risk factors for meningitis include immunosuppression, a ventriculoperitoneal shunt, cochlear implant, skull fracture, neurosurgery, or a recent sinus or ear infection (Kerr & Huether, 2014).

In many cases, the infectious organism spreads to the CNS from the bloodstream (see *Pathophysiology Illustrated: Central Nervous System Infection*), triggering an inflammatory response. The brain becomes inflamed and edematous, leading to **cerebral edema** (an increase in intracellular and extracellular fluid in the brain that results from anoxia, vasodilation, or vascular stasis) and increased ICP. If the infection spreads to the ventricles, they can become obstructed and impede the flow of cerebrospinal fluid (CSF), causing cerebral edema and hydrocephalus as acute complications. The infection may trigger the syndrome of inappropriate antidiuretic hormone (SIADH).

Pathophysiology Illustrated: **Central Nervous System Infection**

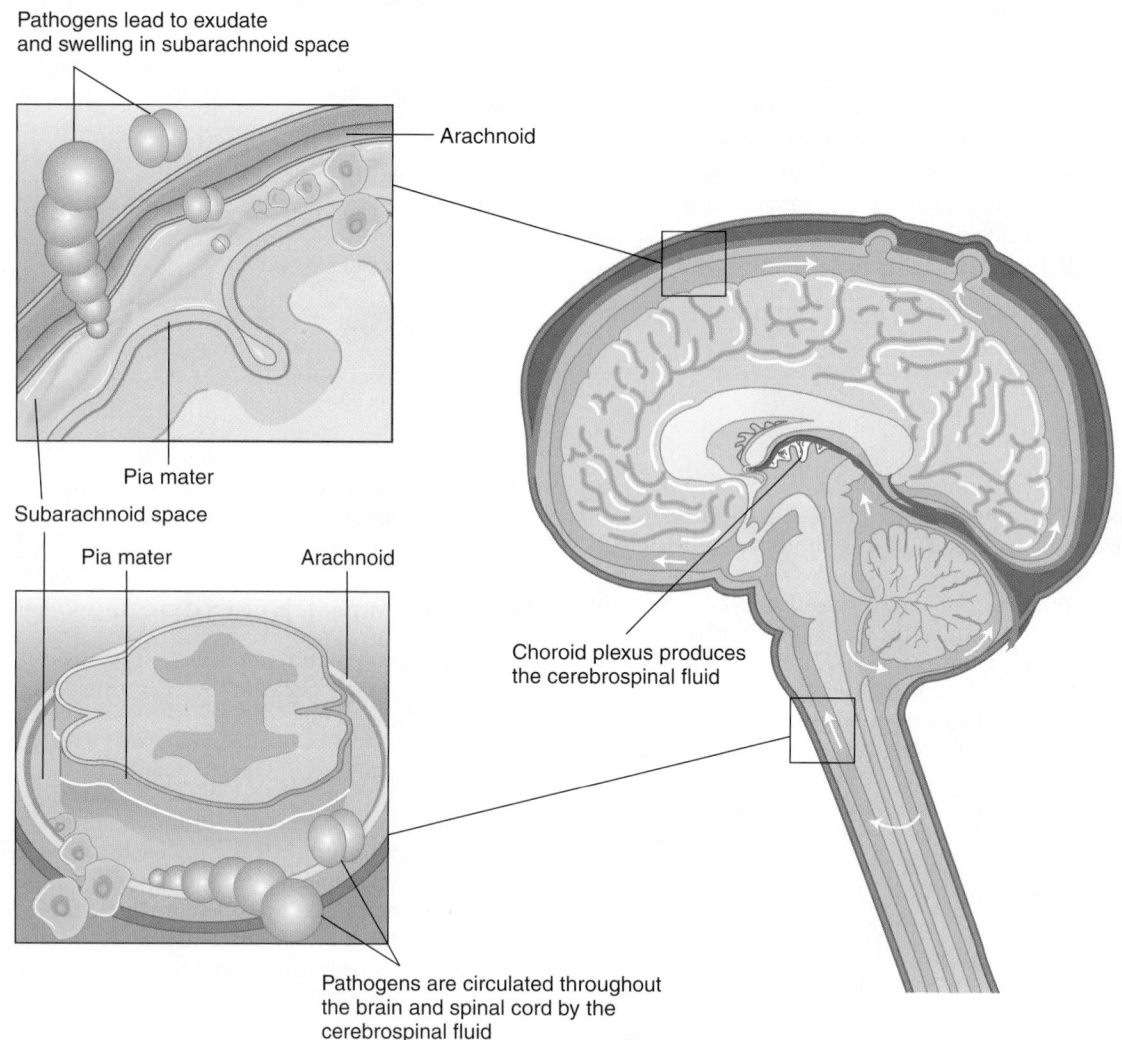

Pathogens lead to exudate and swelling in subarachnoid space

Arachnoid

Pia mater

Subarachnoid space

Pia mater

Arachnoid

Choroid plexus produces the cerebrospinal fluid

Pathogens are circulated throughout the brain and spinal cord by the cerebrospinal fluid

After bacteria reach the central nervous system, the pia mater, the arachnoid, and the cerebrospinal fluid–filled subarachnoid space become infected. The cerebrospinal fluid then circulates the pathogens throughout the brain and spinal cord.

CLINICAL MANIFESTATIONS

Symptoms vary by the child's age, the pathogen, and the length of the illness before diagnosis. Onset may be sudden or develop over 1 to 2 days. Symptoms in the young infant may include fever or hypothermia, change in feeding pattern, vomiting, or diarrhea. The anterior fontanelle may be bulging or flat. The infant may be alert, restless, lethargic, or irritable. Rocking or cuddling, which normally calms a fussy infant, irritates the infant with meningitis.

Older children are usually febrile, have altered consciousness (e.g., confusion, delirium, lethargy, irritability), and may have vomiting and complaints of muscle or joint pain. A hemorrhagic rash of petechiae that changes to purpura or large necrotic patches may be seen in meningococcal meningitis (see Chapter 43). Other symptoms consistent with meningeal irritation may include headache (most often frontal), photophobia, esotropia (inward eye deviation), and **nuchal rigidity** (resistance to neck flexion). The child is often comfortable only in an **opisthotonic position** (hyperextension of the head and neck) (Figure 54–5). The child may have a positive Kernig or Brudzinski sign, or both, on examination (Figure 54–6).

CLINICAL THERAPY

Diagnosis is based on the history, clinical presentation, and laboratory findings. Laboratory tests include a complete blood count, blood cultures, serum electrolytes, blood urea nitrogen, osmolality, and clotting factors. A lumbar puncture is performed to culture the CSF and evaluate it for white blood cells, protein, and glucose levels and also to determine CSF pressure. Real time polymerase chain reaction (PCR) assays of the CSF are also used for diagnosis. CT scanning may be performed when increased ICP or a brain abscess is suspected.

Antibiotics commonly used to treat bacterial meningitis include ampicillin, aminoglycosides, cefotaxime, ceftriaxone, penicillin G, and vancomycin. They are administered as soon as

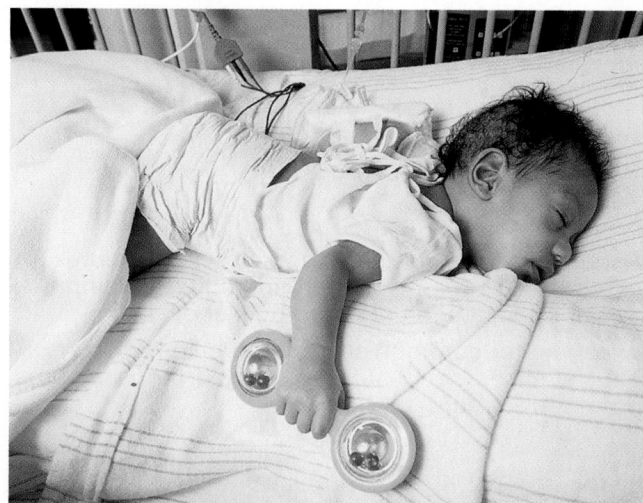

Figure 54–5 The child with bacterial meningitis may assume an opisthotonic position, with the neck and the head hyperextended, to relieve discomfort.

diagnostic tests are obtained and often changed once culture and sensitivity results are known since many organisms have antibiotic resistance. IV antibiotics are administered for 7 to 21 days, depending on the organism and the child's clinical response. Dexamethasone is given to children in cases of suspected *Haemophilus influenzae* type b infection to reduce the severity of potential sensorineural hearing loss (Le Saux & Canadian Paediatric Society Infectious Diseases and Immunization Committee, 2014). Other treatments include fever and seizure control, increased ICP management, and fluids and electrolytes.

Infants and children receive nothing by mouth and are started on IV fluids to manage cerebral perfusion pressure. The child is carefully monitored for increased ICP and SIADH (see Chapter 53). IV fluid volume is carefully managed to treat cerebral edema.

Approximately 20% of child survivors have significant disabilities (Martin, Sadarangani, Pollard, et al., 2014). Examples of disabilities include hearing impairment, gross neurologic deficits, and behavioral and intellectual disorders.

Nursing Management
For the Child With Bacterial Meningitis

Nursing Assessment and Diagnosis

Assess the child's physiologic status, including vital signs and level of consciousness. Measure head circumference often in hospitalized infants because of the potential for hydrocephalus. Be alert for signs of a change in the child's condition and response to treatment. Monitor the child's ability to control secretions and to drink sufficient fluids. Monitor intake and output. Assess for any sensory deficits. Identify parents' concerns about this potentially life-threatening condition.

Several nursing diagnoses that may apply to the child with bacterial meningitis appear in the accompanying *Nursing Care Plan*. Additional nursing diagnoses might include the following (NANDA-I © 2014):

- *Aspiration, Risk for,* related to altered level of consciousness and poor secretion control
- *Fluid Volume: Deficient, Risk for,* related to poor oral fluid intake
- *Spiritual Distress (Parent)* related to the child's life-threatening condition
- *Caregiver Role Strain* related to a hospitalized child and other family responsibilities

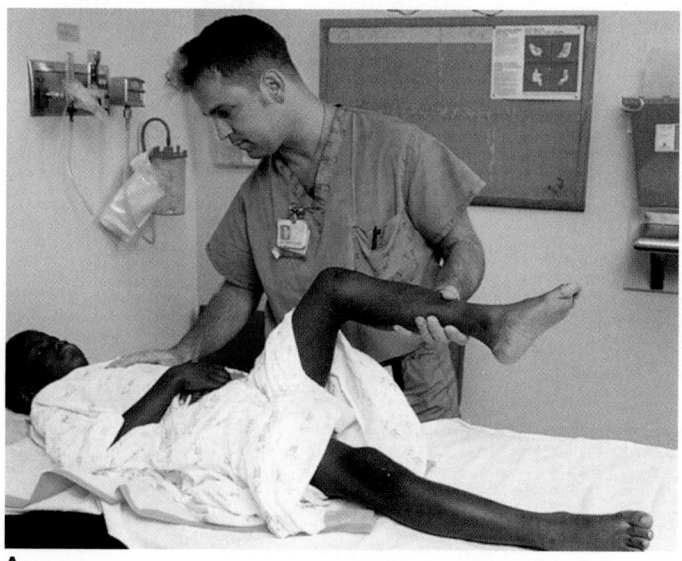

A

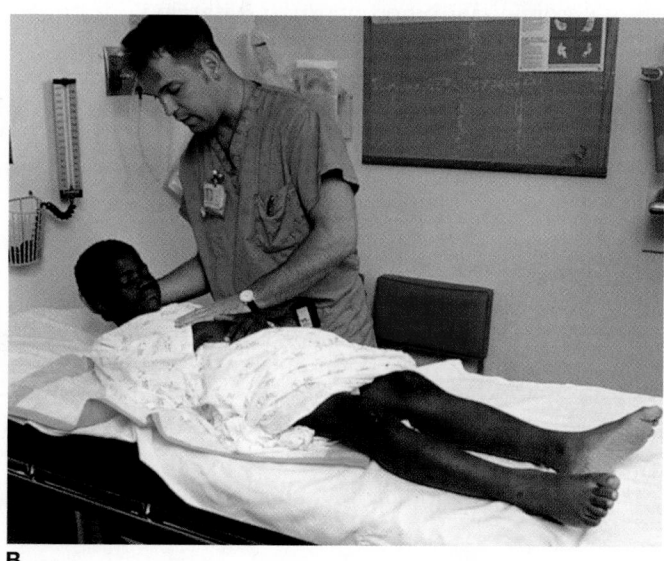

B

Figure 54–6 Testing for Kernig and Brudzinski signs, both common findings with meningitis. *A,* To test for Kernig sign, raise the child's leg with the knee flexed. Then extend the child's leg at the knee. If any resistance is noted or pain is felt, the result is a positive Kernig sign. *B,* To test for Brudzinski sign, flex the child's head while in a supine position. If this action makes the knees or hips flex involuntarily, a positive Brudzinski sign is present.

Nursing Care Plan: The Child With Bacterial Meningitis

1. Nursing Diagnosis: *Injury, Risk for,* related to infection of cerebrospinal fluid and potential sequelae (NANDA-I © 2014)

GOAL: The child will suffer minimal CNS injury secondary to infection.

INTERVENTION	RATIONALE
• Administer antibiotics and corticosteroids as prescribed.	• Antibiotics help eradicate the pathogen and prevent cerebral edema. Corticosteroids reduce inflammation and the chance of neurologic sequelae.
• Note return of fever, nuchal rigidity, or irritability. Monitor vital signs, assess for signs of increased ICP. Measure head circumference once or twice daily. Note changes in responsiveness. Notify the healthcare provider immediately if any signs are detected.	• Watching for common sequelae such as subdural effusions, hydrocephalus, or septic arthritis ensures prompt treatment.

EXPECTED OUTCOME: Child's condition will improve significantly within 48–72 hr (fever will decrease and no signs of neurologic sequelae will be detected).

GOAL: The child will not develop cerebral edema as a result of water retention.

INTERVENTION	RATIONALE
• Monitor for signs of increased ICP and SIADH.	• Early recognition is essential for management to be initiated quickly.
• Perform strict intake and output measurements. Determine urine specific gravity. Check electrolytes and osmolality of both serum and urine. Weigh the child daily. Restrict fluids and give sodium chloride as prescribed.	• Low urine output with a high specific gravity is a sign of fluid retention and SIADH. The child is maintained with lower fluids and is provided sodium supplements to reduce the possibility for cerebral edema.

EXPECTED OUTCOME: Cerebral edema will not develop. If SIADH or increased ICP occurs, the condition will be treated promptly so effects are minimized.

GOAL: The child will be free of injury resulting from disseminated intravascular coagulation (DIC).

INTERVENTION	RATIONALE
• Be aware of needlesticks and lesions that continue to bleed. Monitor clotting times.	• Prompt recognition leads to management of the coagulopathy.
• Administer blood products, vitamin K, or heparin as ordered.	• Prompt recognition allows for early initial treatment of DIC. The child may bleed to death if treatment is delayed.

EXPECTED OUTCOME: Child will not sustain injury from DIC.

GOAL: The child with any degree of hearing loss will be identified.

INTERVENTION	RATIONALE
• Arrange for hearing assessment prior to discharge.	• Hearing loss is a common complication. Early intervention is needed to promote growth and development.

EXPECTED OUTCOME: Child with identified hearing loss will be referred to an appropriate specialist or program for intervention.

2. Nursing Diagnosis: *Pain, Acute*, related to meningeal irritation (NANDA-I © 2014)

GOAL: The child will be as comfortable as possible.

INTERVENTION	RATIONALE
• Assess pain with age-appropriate pain scale.	• Pain scales provide ability to quantify pain for future comparison.
• Minimize tactile stimulation.	• Sensory stimulation increases discomfort.
• Allow the child to assume a comfortable position.	• The child determines the most comfortable position. The opisthotonic position may be the most comfortable.
• Keep the lights dim and maintain a quiet environment.	• Dim lights reduce the discomfort from photophobia. Noise can disturb the child.
• Provide pain medication as prescribed.	• Pain medication is appropriate for acute discomfort associated with illness.

EXPECTED OUTCOME: Child will be calm, and behaviors will indicate increased comfort.

3. **Nursing Diagnosis:** *Infection, Risk for (Family and Close Contacts)*, **related to exposure to child with meningitis** (NANDA-I © 2014)

GOAL: Caretakers or family members will have no apparent evidence of infection.

INTERVENTION	RATIONALE
• Explain rationale and dose schedule for taking rifampin or ciprofloxacin.	• Rifampin and ciprofloxacin provide prophylaxis for many bacterial pathogens responsible for meningitis.

EXPECTED OUTCOME: Family members and other close contacts will verbalize the schedule for rifampin or ciprofloxacin therapy.

Planning and Implementation

The accompanying *Nursing Care Plan* summarizes care for the child with bacterial meningitis. Nursing care begins with emergency treatment and continues as the child's condition stabilizes. Monitor respiratory and neurologic status, maintain hydration, administer medications, and prevent complications. Promote the child's comfort with reduced stimulation (dim lights, quiet room) and by placing in a side-lying position. Isolate the child according to hospital protocol until the causative organism is identified and effective treatment has been administered for 24 hours.

SAFETY ALERT!

Monitor the serum sodium concentration and urine specific gravity since the child is at risk for SIADH (see Chapter 53). Maintenance and replacement fluids are usually given to children with bacterial meningitis. If SIADH occurs, moderate fluid restriction with an isotonic solution is ordered until serum sodium levels return to normal.

Monitor the child's response to antibiotic therapy. Observe for signs of gastrointestinal bleeding, which is a potential complication of corticosteroid use.

Respond to parents' concerns about their child's condition, explaining all measures to reduce the child's discomfort and treat the illness. Identify ways parents can help meet the child's comfort needs.

Prevention is a major role for nurses. Encourage parents to get their infants and children fully immunized with the *Haemophilus influenzae*, pneumococcal, and meningococcal vaccines (see Chapter 43).

DISCHARGE PLANNING AND HOME CARE TEACHING

Identify and address home care needs well in advance of discharge. Follow-up visits are important to monitor for complications and sequelae. Help parents deal with any physical requirements resulting from the child's illness and any emotional, social, and financial repercussions of the child's condition. Teach parents what to do if the child has a seizure.

Infants and toddlers with neurologic sequelae should be referred to an early intervention program. Refer the child with a hearing loss to an otolaryngologist and speech and language specialist. Encourage early identification of other neurologic sequelae, such as learning problems. Children with neurologic sequelae need to have an individual education plan (IEP) developed (see Chapter 38), and parents may need help planning for the child's special educational needs. Refer parents to the appropriate social service agencies for support and assistance.

Evaluation

Expected outcomes of nursing care are provided in the accompanying *Nursing Care Plan*.

Viral (Aseptic) Meningitis

Viral meningitis is an inflammatory response of the meninges characterized by an increased number of blood cells and protein in the CSF. In the United States, an enterovirus is the most common cause of viral meningitis in children (Kelesidis, Mastoris, Metsini, et al., 2014).

Generally, the child with aseptic meningitis does not appear as ill as the child with bacterial meningitis. The child may have an abrupt onset of fever of 38.0°C to 40.0°C (100.4°F to 104°F) and have meningeal signs (headache, photophobia, stiff neck, and back pain), myalgia, irritability, and lethargy. Other symptoms include malaise, vomiting and diarrhea, upper respiratory symptoms, and a maculopapular rash. The infant may have a tense anterior fontanelle. Seizures are rare. Symptoms usually resolve spontaneously within 3 to 10 days.

The child with fever and meningeal signs is hospitalized. Blood, urine, and CSF analyses are performed. PCR and DNA testing of the CSF help detect viral meningitis, often within 24 hours. Until the diagnosis of aseptic meningitis is confirmed, the child is treated aggressively for bacterial meningitis. Other treatment is supportive of symptoms. Children usually make a full recovery.

Nursing Management

Initial nursing care focuses on providing supportive care as described for the child with bacterial meningitis. Give acetaminophen or ibuprofen as ordered to reduce fever, headache, and muscle or joint pain. Keep the room dark and quiet (to decrease stimuli and meningeal irritation), give IV or oral fluids, and promote comfort with proper positioning.

The child and family need information about the disease. Explain medical and nursing procedures in terms that the child and family can understand. Keep parents informed about the child's progress. Once the diagnosis of viral meningitis is made, immediately begin discharge planning and teaching for home care. Explain that recovery may take several weeks but that complete recovery is expected.

Encephalitis

Encephalitis is an acute inflammation of the brain often caused by an arbovirus that is transmitted by a mosquito, such as the West Nile, Eastern equine, Western equine, St. Louis, and La Crosse viruses. Other causes of encephalitis include Colorado tick fever, enteroviruses, and Epstein-Barr virus. Inflammation of the meninges is also common. Epidemics occur most often in warm weather seasons.

Encephalitis may occur as a direct or primary infection by an organism (virus, bacteria, fungi, or parasite) that successfully passes through the blood–brain barrier. Some children only have symptoms of a flulike illness after being infected and never develop encephalitis. Signs and symptoms include fever, irritability, severe headache, and bulging fontanelle, followed by altered mental status. The child may have flaccid or spastic paralysis. Meningeal irritation signs such as nuchal rigidity, photophobia, and positive Kernig or Brudzinski signs are common. Focal or generalized seizures may occur. Altered mental status may progress to coma over hours or days.

Diagnosis is based on history and laboratory findings. Information about recent immunizations, insect bites, or residence in or travel to areas where cases of encephalitis are present should be obtained (e.g., West Nile virus or Eastern equine encephalitis). CSF culture and analysis, blood serologic tests, and nasopharyngeal and stool specimens are evaluated to identify viral pathogens. Testing for virus-specific immunoglobulin M antibodies using the enzyme-linked immunosorbent assay (ELISA) test is performed after 5 days of acute illness. The PCR test is used to assay for herpes DNA in the CSF. A CT scan, MRI, and EEG may also be performed. An EEG may help assess seizure activity and help localize the area of the brain affected.

The child with encephalitis is at risk for seizures, respiratory failure, and increased ICP and receives supportive treatment in the intensive care unit (ICU). Physical therapy, occupational therapy, and speech therapy may be prescribed for these children. Children admitted to the ICU with serious symptoms are more likely to have persistent symptoms that last up to 6 months. Some fatalities occur, and significant neurologic sequelae may result.

Nursing Management

Nursing care focuses on monitoring cardiorespiratory function, preventing complications resulting from immobility, reorienting the child, and teaching the parents about the child's condition.

Monitor the child's cardiorespiratory function. Check the child's airway and ability to handle secretions. Assess the child's color, respiratory rate and effort, SpO$_2$, and arterial blood gases. Monitor the heart rate, blood pressure, capillary refill time, and urine output.

Provide seizure precautions. Prevent complications resulting from immobility (see Box 54–1). Maintain skin integrity. Proper positioning with frequent turning is important. When prescribed by the healthcare provider, perform chest physiotherapy to prevent pneumonia.

Give the parents information about their child's condition and prognosis. Provide support to parents as they cope with the serious nature of this condition.

As the level of consciousness begins to improve, the child may at first be confused and disoriented and may have residual effects of the disease. Orient the child to the hospital environment. Have the family take an active role in the child's physical and emotional recovery, such as by bringing favorite stuffed animals or music from home. Engage in therapeutic play (refer to Chapter 39 for techniques). Give the child age-appropriate toys to encourage a return to normal behavior.

Provide parents with instructions for home care. Plan follow-up visits so the child can be evaluated for neurologic sequelae. Ensure that children are referred for physical or speech therapy as needed. Refer parents to home care, social services, family counseling, and support groups as needed.

Reye Syndrome

Reye syndrome is an acute **encephalopathy**, which is a cerebral dysfunction caused by a toxic, inflammatory, or anoxic insult or injury that may result in permanent tissue damage, although the dysfunction may improve over time. In 1980, an association was identified between the use of aspirin for influenza or varicella and Reye syndrome. The condition is now rare in the United States (approximately 35 cases a year) since most parents give children acetaminophen or ibuprofen rather than aspirin for flulike symptoms and varicella (Ibrahim & Balistreri, 2016). The mortality rate associated with Reye syndrome is high.

Reye syndrome is classified as a secondary mitochondrial hepatopathy. It is caused by a drug toxic to the liver or other toxin, metal, or metabolite and results in a poorly functioning organ. In the case of Reye syndrome, an interaction between a viral illness and aspirin occurs in a susceptible individual (Ibrahim & Balistreri, 2016). The disorder is characterized by cerebral edema, hypoglycemia, and an enlarged, fatty, poorly functioning liver (due to an elevation of short-chain fatty acid levels and hyperammonemia).

Reye syndrome begins with a preceding viral illness that seems to be resolving, followed by an acute onset of vomiting, mental status changes, seizures, and progressive unresponsiveness. The condition progresses to cerebral edema and neurologic dysfunction, leading to a final stage with coma, seizures, flaccidity, loss of deep tendon reflexes, and respiratory arrest.

The diagnosis of Reye syndrome is based on an abrupt change in the child's level of consciousness and diagnostic laboratory tests that reveal liver dysfunction and no other identifiable cause. CSF analysis usually reveals white blood cells. Radiographic imaging reveals cerebral edema. Liver enzyme and ammonia levels are elevated, blood glucose levels are below normal, and prothrombin time is prolonged. Serum bilirubin levels are normal. A liver biopsy is sometimes performed to confirm the diagnosis.

The child with Reye syndrome receives supportive care in a pediatric ICU. Efforts are made to prevent the secondary effects of cerebral edema and metabolic injury associated with the elevated short-chain fatty acid and ammonia levels. Mechanical ventilation is often needed once the child is comatose. Arterial and venous blood pressure monitoring is performed. The child is monitored for signs of increased ICP secondary to cerebral edema (see the *Clinical Skills Manual*). Hypoglycemia is treated with IV glucose. Electrolytes, blood chemistry, and blood pH are monitored.

Clinical Tip

Make sure all parents know that they should use acetaminophen or ibuprofen rather than aspirin when the child has a viral illness such as influenza to prevent the development of Reye syndrome. Most over-the-counter medications for children are now made with acetaminophen or ibuprofen, but parents should be encouraged to verify this.

Nursing Management

Nursing care focuses on monitoring the child's physical status, providing emotional support, and teaching parents about disease prevention.

Check the child's respiratory and neurologic status frequently, and note any signs of improvement or deterioration. Refer to the discussion of nursing management of altered states of consciousness earlier in this chapter for specific nursing interventions.

Monitor laboratory tests for acidosis, elevation of ammonia levels, or hypoglycemia. Monitor the child's intake and output. Correct imbalances by administering fluids, electrolytes, or medications as ordered. Prevent complications associated with immobility. Support the family faced with the child's life-threatening illness (see Chapter 41).

The child who survives and is discharged is monitored for sequelae. Developmental and neurologic deficits may occur and are more severe in children under 2 years of age. Arrange for home nursing or frequent clinic visits during the recovery period for monitoring. Inform the parents about community resources that can assist them in promoting the child's recovery.

Guillain-Barré Syndrome (Postinfectious Polyneuritis)

Guillain-Barré syndrome is an acute inflammatory peripheral neuropathy with an acute onset of rapidly developing symmetric motor weakness that progresses in an ascending pattern. It is rare in children compared to adults.

Guillain-Barré syndrome is thought to be a postinfectious disorder that affects motor neurons, but may also affect sensory and autonomic neurons. The damaged neurons experience demyelination. Onset occurs within 6 weeks after an influenza-like or gastrointestinal illness (*Campylobacter jejuni* was the most common organism) in 60% of cases (Shui et al., 2012). An association between immunizations such as for influenza and the disorder has not been confirmed.

Infants have an onset of rapidly progressive severe hypotonia, possible respiratory distress, irritability, and feeding difficulties. Older children initially have pain, numbness, paresthesia, or weakness in all limbs. Weakness progresses bilaterally over days for up to 4 weeks. Maximum weakness is often reached in 2 to 4 weeks. Deep tendon reflexes may be diminished or absent. The child may develop acute ataxia or an inability to walk. Respiratory muscles and cranial nerves may not be affected, but difficulty swallowing and bilateral facial nerve weakness are signs of impending respiratory failure. If the autonomic nervous system is affected, blood pressure fluctuations and episodes of bradycardia and asystole may occur.

Diagnostic criteria of Guillain-Barré syndrome include varying degrees of progressive motor weakness (up to total paralysis of all extremities) and **areflexia** (no reflex response to stimulation). CSF protein levels rise to twice the upper limit of normal, and a few white blood cells are seen in the CSF. Bacterial and viral cultures are usually negative. Electroconduction tests such as electromyography show acute muscle denervation. An MRI of the spinal cord may be requested.

Clinical therapy for Guillain-Barré syndrome is intravenous immune globulin (IVIG) at a dose of 0.4 g/kg/day for 2 to 5 days when ascending paralysis is progressing rapidly. Guidelines for administration of IVIG can be found in Chapter 48. Responses to IVIG are dramatic, often within days. Plasma exchange to remove autoantibodies or immunosuppressive medications are alternate therapies. Corticosteroids are not effective. Pain management is important. Physical therapy and supportive care are initiated early to promote ambulation. The condition is rarely fatal; however, some disability may result.

Nursing Management

Nursing care focuses on monitoring respiratory status, meeting nutritional needs, managing autonomic nervous system dysfunction, preventing complications associated with weakness and immobility, providing emotional support, and teaching the parents how to care for the child after discharge.

Place the child on a cardiorespiratory monitor for continuous assessment in the early phase of the illness. Monitor the child for dyspnea, inability to handle secretions, inadequate respiratory effort, and mucous membrane color changes that may indicate the need for endotracheal intubation and mechanical ventilation.

Monitor the child's vital signs closely for episodes of tachycardia, bradycardia, blood pressure fluctuations, sweating, and bowel and bladder dysfunction. Observe frequently for decreased responsiveness. Promptly report the occurrence of these signs to the child's healthcare provider.

Assess the child's ability to swallow. If the child has no gag reflex, nutrition is provided with IV supplements or nasogastric tube feedings.

Prevent complications associated with immobility (see Box 54–1). Ensure good postural alignment, and turn the child every 2 hours. Maintaining skin integrity is also important.

Evaluate the child's muscle tone, strength, and symmetry. When the child's condition begins to improve, recovery of lost strength is the priority. Active exercise is emphasized in physical therapy. Encourage family members to participate in the child's care, especially during the recovery phase. They can help with the activities of daily living and reinforce what the child has learned in physical therapy.

Explain the progression of Guillain-Barré syndrome to the parents during the initial stages. Witnessing a rapid deterioration in their child's physical status can be frightening; therefore, inform parents that deterioration may continue until the treatment becomes effective. Be honest when discussing recovery and prognosis for the child. Have parents bring in favorite toys, dolls, or books to make the child feel more secure. Playing with or reading to the child can be comforting.

DISCHARGE PLANNING

Identify and address home care needs well in advance of discharge. Support the parents as they prepare for the child's return home, especially when return to full strength is expected to be slow. Outpatient physical therapy sessions may be needed several times a week in the early recovery stages. Frequent follow-up visits to the health center are essential to monitor the child's recovery. Refer the parents to home health services that can provide guidance for financial assistance.

COMMUNITY-BASED NURSING CARE

Help the child to adjust to any residual effects of Guillain-Barré syndrome. Help the child practice exercises learned in physical therapy sessions, and encourage the child to perform activities of daily living, such as brushing the teeth or combing the hair.

To promote a positive self-image, praise any effort the child makes to be self-sufficient. The child may be frustrated and angry. Allow the child to express these feelings in an appropriate way, either during play or in conversation. Home schooling may be needed until the child has strength to walk and participate in a full school day.

Headaches

An estimated 75% of children experience a headache by age 15 years, and headaches are a major reason for school absence (Antonaci et al., 2014). Up to 20% of children and adolescents experience migraine headaches (Sun et al., 2013). The incidence of headaches increases as children age. Headaches interfere with physical, social, and mental health aspects of daily life.

Etiology and Pathophysiology

Headaches have both benign (migraine, inflammatory, and tension) and structural causes, such as a tumor. See Table 54–8 for headache classifications and clinical manifestations.

- Migraine headaches may be triggered by stress; foods containing nitrates, glutamate, caffeine, tyramine, and salt; menses; fatigue; and hunger. Genetic predisposition may be a factor. Some children may also have abdominal migraine episodes (Catala-Beauchamp & Gleason, 2012).

- Tension headaches may be associated with stress related to school, anxiety, demanding schedules, fasting, and inadequate sleep.

- Medication overuse (rebound) headaches are associated with the frequent use (2 to 3 times a week) of medications for headaches (e.g., acetaminophen, nonsteroidal anti-inflammatory drugs [NSAIDs], decongestants, triptans, opioids, benzodiazepines, and ergotamines).

Clinical Manifestations

See Table 54–8 for the signs and symptoms associated with specific types of headaches.

Clinical Therapy

Diagnosis involves a detailed history of the headache characteristics (onset, duration, pain severity, quality, and location; aura; treatment or medications used) and associated symptoms (abdominal pain, nausea, vomiting). Assessment for neurologic signs such as altered consciousness, abnormal cranial nerves, papilledema, and motor or sensory deficits is performed. Radiologic studies (CT scan or MRI) are used only in cases of abnormal neurologic signs or a suspected structural problem. A lumbar puncture is performed if an infection or inflammatory process is suspected.

Treatment includes relaxation techniques, analgesics, and anti-inflammatory medications. A behavior management program may help reduce common headache triggers (inadequate sleep, stress, missed meals, caffeine, chocolate, or excessive extracurricular activities). Medications to abort migraines (e.g., almotriptan malate and rizatriptan benzoate by mouth) are approved by the U.S. Food and Drug Administration (FDA) for adolescents who can identify an aura or signs of an impending headache. Topiramate was recently approved by the FDA as a prophylactic medication for migraine headaches in adolescents. Medication overuse headaches are treated by withdrawal of all medications used for headaches for a 2- to 4-week period. Limited use of medications may be permitted after that period.

Nursing Management

Assess the child for potential neurologic signs associated with headaches. Encourage the child to keep a headache diary, either written or electronic, that tracks the events and stresses at the time of a headache to help identify patterns and potential triggers. Assist the child and family to see patterns in the headache diary and discuss potential strategies for relieving the headaches. Behavior changes that may reduce headaches include a consistent bedtime and wake-up time 7 days a week, a regular eating schedule, avoiding hunger, regular physical activity for 30 to 45 minutes at least 5 days a week, avoidance of identified food triggers, and avoidance of smoke and other strong odors.

Teach the child to take the prescribed medications at the first sign of a headache, but no more often than 2 to 3 days a week. See Chapter 50 for care of the child with a brain tumor.

Structural Defects

Common structural defects include microcephaly, hydrocephalus, neural tube defects, craniosynostosis, positional plagiocephaly, and neurofibromatosis.

Microcephaly

Microcephaly is a small brain with a head circumference below the third percentile on growth curves. Causes may include a genetic disorder or destructive insult during infancy, such as an infection, metabolic disorder, or hypoxia-ischemia. Intellectual disability is common (see Chapter 55 for more information).

Hydrocephalus

Hydrocephalus is the body's response to an imbalance between the volume of cerebrospinal fluid (CSF) produced and absorbed. The condition may be congenital or acquired as a result of intraventricular hemorrhage, meningitis, traumatic brain injury, or brain tumor. An estimated 1 to 2 infants per 1000 are born with hydrocephalus (National Institute of Neurological Disorders and Stroke [NINDS], 2014). It is commonly associated with myelomeningocele (described later in this chapter).

TABLE 54–8 Clinical Manifestations of Headaches by Classification

CLASSIFICATION OF HEADACHES	CLINICAL MANIFESTATIONS
MIGRAINE Vascular, acute recurrent	• Unilateral or bilateral pulsatile throbbing pain lasting for hours or days, moderate to severe pain intensity, aggravated by routine activity • Lasts 2–3 hr; may be relieved by sleep, but may last 48–72 hr if untreated • Nausea and vomiting • Photophobia and phonophobia • Visual or motor aura several minutes before headache starts; if no aura may have mood changes, food cravings, or anorexia hours before the attack • Preschool-age children may have irritability, restlessness, malaise, head banging, head holding, and sensitivity to light and sound • Recurrent abdominal pain
TENSION Muscular contraction Acute recurrent (less than 15 days a month)	• Intermittent or constant pain of mild to moderate intensity (may fluctuate), pressure or tightening (nonpulsatile) sensation • May last 30 min to 7 days • Unlikely to have nausea, vomiting, abdominal pain, or visual disturbances • Sensitive to light or sound
REBOUND OR MEDICATION OVERUSE Chronic nonprogressive (more than 15 days a month)	• Pain many be bandlike, over entire head, or crushing; may be bad enough to interfere with academic performance • Occurs at least 2–4 times a week or daily • Usually increases in frequency and severity over time, paralleling the increase in medication use • Recurs when medication wears off
INFLAMMATORY Sinusitis or dental abscess Acute localized	• Facial pain or tenderness over affected sinus, gum, or periorbital area; may be associated with nasal congestion • Dull, constant pressure; severity varies with head position • Fever may be present • No nausea, visual changes, light or sound sensitivity
STRUCTURAL Space-occupying lesion, hemorrhage, increased ICP Chronic progressive	• Severe pain, increases in frequency and severity, often in occipital or frontal location • Pain awakens child or is present in the morning; increases with coughing, sneezing, or straining • Vomiting that is persistent or preceded by recurrent headache • Abnormal neurologic signs (e.g., double vision, papilledema, strabismus, weakness, ataxia)

Source: Data from Blosser, C. G., Albers, A. C., & Reider-Demer, M. (2012). Headache. In C. Burns, A. M. Dunn, M. A. Brady, N. B. Starr, & C. G. Blosser (Eds.), *Pediatric primary care* (5th ed., pp. 606–614). Philadelphia, PA: Elsevier Saunders; Hershey, A. D., Kabbouche, M. A., & O'Brien H. L. (2016). Headaches. In R. M. Kliegman, B. F. Stanton, J. W. St. Geme, & N. F. Schor (Eds.), *Nelson textbook of pediatrics* (20th ed., pp. 2863–2874). Philadelphia: Elsevier; Paul, S. P., Debono, R., Walker, D. (2013). Clinical update: Recognising brain tumours early in children. *Community Practitioner, 86*(4), 42–45.

ETIOLOGY AND PATHOPHYSIOLOGY

Hydrocephalus may be either communicating or noncommunicating. In communicating hydrocephalus, the CSF flows freely among normal channels and pathways, but CSF absorption in the subarachnoid space and the arachnoid villi is impaired. It may be acquired or caused by a congenital malformation in the subarachnoid spaces.

Noncommunicating hydrocephalus accounts for most cases in children. It results from a blockage in the ventricular system

that prevents CSF from entering the subarachnoid space, resulting in enlargement of one or more ventricles (see *Pathophysiology Illustrated: Hydrocephalus*). This obstruction can be caused by infection, hemorrhage, tumor, surgery, or structural deformity. Congenital structural defects include the Chiari type II malformation (found in children with myelomeningocele), aqueduct of Sylvius stenosis, and the Dandy-Walker syndrome (includes hydrocephalus, a posterior fossa cyst, and hypoplasia of the cerebellum).

Pathophysiology Illustrated: **Hydrocephalus**

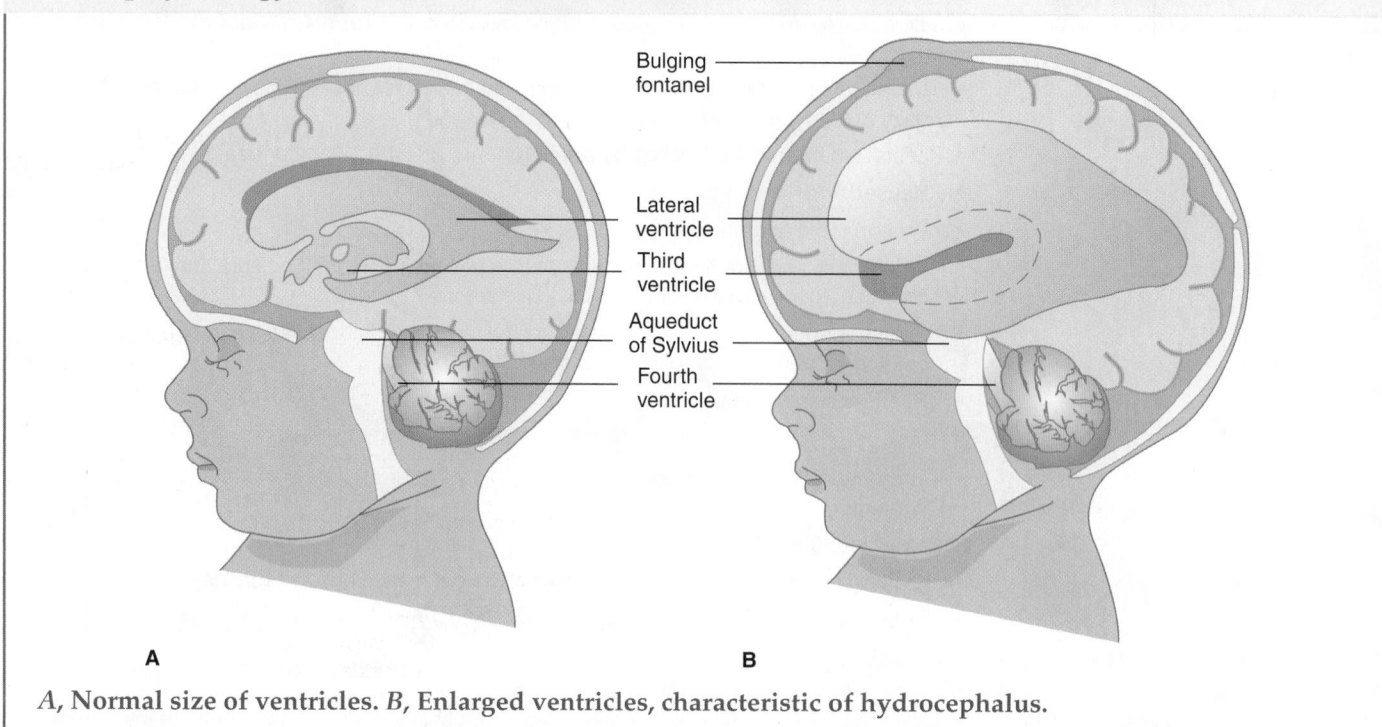

A, Normal size of ventricles. *B*, Enlarged ventricles, characteristic of hydrocephalus.

The Arnold-Chiari malformation (Chiari type II) involves a downward placement of the medulla and lower cerebellum through the foramen magnum of the skull into the cervical vertebrae. This displacement can cause sudden death, respiratory difficulty, swallowing difficulties, and the need for assisted ventilation. Symptoms during infancy may include stridor, a weak cry, and apnea. An older child may have an extremity weakness, difficulty swallowing, choking, hoarseness, vocal cord paralysis, and breath-holding episodes. This defect is also associated with intellectual disability and epilepsy.

CLINICAL MANIFESTATIONS
The signs and symptoms of hydrocephalus vary with the age of the child (Table 54–9). Infants have a rapidly increasing head circumference (Figure 54–7). Older children show signs of increased ICP. Signs of shunt malfunction in infants are nonspecific and include irritability, vomiting, poor appetite, disordered sleep, and fever. Older children with shunt malformation may have a headache, nausea, vomiting, and decreased level of consciousness.

CLINICAL THERAPY
The diagnosis of hydrocephalus may be made prenatally by ultrasound or based on physical findings and neuroimaging studies after birth. Daily head circumference measurements are essential for any infant at risk of developing hydrocephalus. CT and MRI imaging diagnose hydrocephalus, and in some cases reveal the anatomic cause. When the infant's fontanelle is still open, ultrasonography or echoencephalography may be used to confirm the diagnosis. CT and MRI imaging are also used to evaluate shunt failure.

Clinical therapy for hydrocephalus involves surgery to remove the obstruction (e.g., surgical removal of a tumor or endoscopic third ventriculostomy) or to create a pathway to divert excess CSF. A catheter or shunt is placed in the ventricle and passes the CSF to the peritoneal cavity, right atrium of the heart, the pleural spaces of the lungs, or the subgaleal space (space

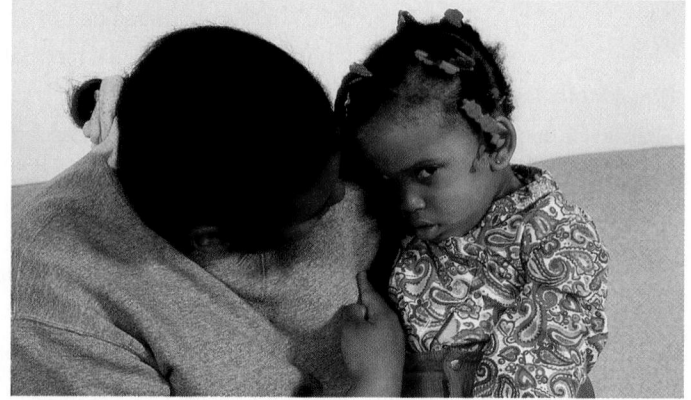

Figure 54–7 In communicating hydrocephalus, an excessive amount of cerebrospinal fluid accumulates in the subarachnoid space, producing the characteristic head enlargement seen here. Note the large forehead and facial features that seem small for the size of the head. When observing the child with hydrocephalus, look for a downward deviation of the eyes in which the lower half of the iris is hidden by the lower eyelid (sunsetting eyes). This finding occurs in severe hydrocephalus, but is not present in this child.

between the skull and scalp used for preterm infants with intraventricular hemorrhage) (Figure 54–8). Initial shunt placement is usually performed early in infancy with adequate tubing length for the child's future growth. Shunt revisions are often needed during childhood. Children with ventriculoatrial shunts receive perioperative IV antibiotics to reduce the risk for reinfection.

TABLE 54–9 Clinical Manifestations of Hydrocephalus

CAUSE	CLINICAL MANIFESTATIONS
CONGENITAL STRUCTURAL DEFECT	
Dandy-Walker syndrome	*Early signs*
Arnold-Chiari type II malformation	Rapidly increasing head circumference; tense, bulging fontanelle, split sutures
ACQUIRED DEFECT IN INFANCY	*Bossing* (protrusion) of frontal area, face is disproportionate for skull size
Intraventricular hemorrhage	Difficulty holding head up
	Macewen's or "cracked-pot" sign with percussion
	Prominent, distended scalp veins, translucent scalp skin
	Increased tone or hyperreflexia, Babinski sign
	Irritability or lethargy, poor feeding
	Decline in level of consciousness
	Late signs
	Sunsetting eyes (sclera visible above iris), sixth cranial nerve palsy
	Apnea spells
	Shrill, high-pitched cry
	Difficulty swallowing or feeding; vomiting
	Cardiopulmonary depression (severe cases)
ACQUIRED HYDROCEPHALUS IN OLDER CHILD AFTER CLOSURE OF SUTURES	
Postinfectious	Signs of increased ICP, no head enlargement
Tumor	Headache upon arising with vomiting
Hemorrhage	Irritability, sleepiness, confusion, lethargy, apathy, altered consciousness
	Personality change, loss of interest in daily activities
	Poor judgment or verbal incoherence, worsening school performance, memory loss
	Ataxia, spasticity, or other motor problems
	Visual defects secondary to pressure on second, third, and sixth cranial nerves

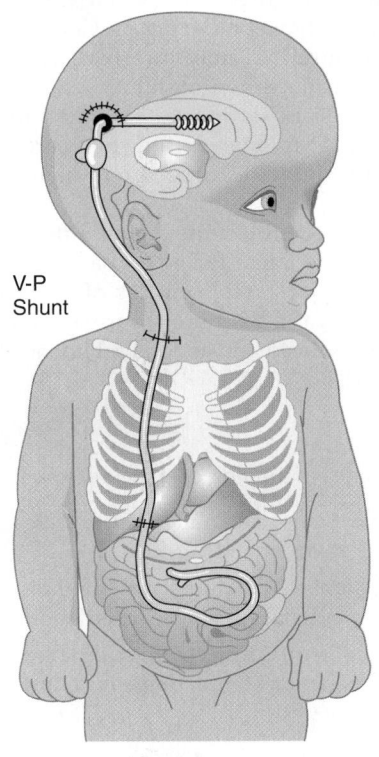

V-P Shunt

Figure 54–8 A ventriculoperitoneal shunt system consists of four parts: a ventricular catheter, a pumping chamber or reservoir, a one-way pressure valve, and a distal catheter. A shunt, commonly used to treat children with hydrocephalus, is often placed at 3 to 4 months of age.

SAFETY ALERT!

Technologic advances have led to the development of shunts with adjustable pressure valves that can be programmed with magnets. If the child receives an MRI, schedule time for the child to have the shunt pressure checked and adjusted as needed because the magnet from the MRI could affect the pressure setting.

Shunt mechanical complications may include a blocked catheter, kinked tube, or valve breakdown. Shunt materials and systems continue to be refined in an attempt to reduce mechanical problems.

Shunt infection is the most serious complication. To confirm the infection, a CSF culture is obtained from the shunt reservoir located in a burr hole placed in the skull. The shunt is surgically removed, and an external drainage device is placed. IV antibiotics are usually prescribed. A new shunt is inserted when the CSF cultures are sterile.

An upper cervical laminectomy may be performed in infants and children with the Arnold-Chiari malformation to prevent an emergency. Alternative treatment includes symptomatic care while maintaining the airway and preventing aspiration. Rapid surgical decompression may be needed to reduce brainstem compression and to prevent death.

Nursing Management

For the Child With Hydrocephalus

Nursing Assessment and Diagnosis

Nurses should assess all infants to promptly identify children with hydrocephalus. Measure the head circumference of all infants at each well-child visit and compare to prior measurements plotted on the growth curve (see the *Clinical Skills Manual* SKILLS). Note any signs of increased ICP, such as irritability, poor appetite, sunsetting eyes, or a shrill cry.

Monitor the child following placement of a ventriculoperitoneal shunt for signs of shunt failure and infection. Signs of infection in infants may include changes in responsiveness, unusual irritability, low-grade fever, diminished appetite, and sleep pattern disturbance. Measure the infant's head circumference daily and compare to prior measurements when shunt failure is suspected. Report any abnormalities to the healthcare provider immediately. Older children will have signs of increased ICP (Table 54–1).

Nursing diagnoses that might be appropriate for the child with hydrocephalus include the following (NANDA-I © 2014):

- *Infection, Risk for,* related to surgical procedure
- *Mobility: Physical, Impaired,* related to insufficient muscle strength to lift the increased weight of head
- *Caregiver Role Strain, Risk for,* related to care of a child with a chronic condition or life-threatening illness
- *Development: Delayed, Risk for,* related to repeated shunt infections and hospitalizations
- *Injury, Risk for,* related to potential shunt failure

Planning and Implementation

HOSPITAL-BASED NURSING CARE

Nursing care focuses on providing preoperative and postoperative care and providing emotional support.

Before surgery position the infant carefully; do not stretch or strain the neck muscles since they must support the large head. Holding the infant may be difficult because of the additional weight of the head. Reduce the risk for skin breakdown with an airflow mattress or by placing sheepskin under the head. Prevent any other complications associated with immobility (see Box 54–1). Attend to the child's special nutritional needs. Because the infant is prone to vomiting, frequent small feedings and frequent burping are beneficial.

After surgery the child is usually placed in a flat position to prevent rapid CSF drainage as the shunt begins working. The head of the bed is elevated gradually over a day or 2. Take vital signs, including the assessment of neurologic signs (such as pupil size and response to light, extraocular movements, and change in muscle tone) every 2 to 4 hours. Care for the child's surgical site as directed by healthcare provider order or agency guidelines. Monitor the child carefully for any signs of shunt malfunction, increased ICP, or infection. See Chapter 39 for other postoperative nursing care.

Support the parents and explain the child's condition and all procedures to be performed. Encourage parents and family to help with the child's care in the hospital when appropriate. Be sympathetic and understanding, and allow parents to express their concerns. If hydrocephalus occurs during early infancy, the parents will be anxious about the impact of the chronic condition and subsequent surgical procedures. If hydrocephalus is secondary to neoplasm or other acquired condition, however, the parents' anxieties are compounded by their child's life-threatening illness. Assure parents that most children with shunts lead normal lives, attending school and interacting with others no differently from their peers.

DISCHARGE PLANNING AND HOME CARE TEACHING

Identify and address home care needs well in advance of discharge. Parents must learn how to care for the surgical site until healed. Educate parents and other family members about important signs and symptoms of shunt failure (signs of increased ICP) and infection (changes in responsiveness, irritability, malaise, headache, nausea, and low-grade fever). Provide the telephone numbers of healthcare providers, and reinforce the need to contact a healthcare provider immediately if a problem with the shunt is suspected. Some children experience a seizure after shunt placement. Teach parents how to care for the child if a seizure occurs. Refer families to the appropriate home care, social services, and support groups such as the Hydrocephalus Association.

COMMUNITY-BASED NURSING CARE

Infants and children need frequent monitoring to ensure proper shunt functioning. Head circumference is measured at each visit to monitor growth. After shunt placement in an infant, head circumference may decrease 1 to 2 cm (0.39 to 0.79 in.) as the pressure is relieved. Head growth as a result of brain development may then be noted in 2 to 4 months. Alert the healthcare provider if head growth resumes sooner than 2 to 4 months, as the shunt may have malfunctioned or need a pressure setting change. Assess the child for visual problems and cognitive, speech, and motor developmental delays. Refer the child and family to an early intervention program to promote developmental progress. School-age children may need an IEP (see Chapter 38).

Encourage parents to provide good nutrition and reduce exposure to infections. Teach parents alternate positions for burping infants with an enlarged head and to use an infant seat after feeding to reduce regurgitation. Provide foods with fiber to promote regular bowel movements. Constipation increases abdominal pressure that may interfere with CSF drainage through the ventriculoperitoneal shunt.

Using a childcare setting with a small number of children, such as family or home-based child care, helps decrease exposure to infection. Encourage good hand hygiene by all caregivers.

Teach parents to protect the infant with an enlarged head from injury by using a rear-facing car safety seat regardless of age. This position decreases their risk of cervical spine injury and death in a car crash. Discourage participation in sports with a high potential for head and abdominal impact, but encourage other sports.

Evaluation

Expected outcomes of nursing care include the following:

- The infant develops adequate neck muscle control to interact with the environment.
- Shunt infections and malfunctions are rapidly identified by the parents, and medical attention is sought quickly.
- The child's potential for growth and development is maximized by care and a stimulating environment.

Neural Tube Defects

The neural tube is the tissue that ultimately develops into the CNS, including the brain and spinal cord. **Neural tube defects** occur in about 3000 pregnancies each year in the United States (Kerr & Huether, 2014). Neural tube defects include the following:

- *Anencephaly*—no development of the brain above the brain-stem, which is ultimately fatal
- *Encephalocele*—protrusion of meningeal tissue or meninges-covered brain through a defect in the skull
- *Spina bifida occulta*—a vertebral defect in which the posterior vertebral arches fail to fuse (usually the fifth lumbar or first sacral vertebrae), but the spinal cord and meninges are contained in the vertebral canal
- *Spina bifida cystica*—a posterior vertebral arch defect with protrusion of meninges through the bony spine
- *Meningocele*—protrusion of a meningeal sac filled with CSF through a vertebral defect, associated with no abnormalities of the spinal cord
- *Myelodysplasia (spina bifida or meningomyelocele)*—protrusion of a meningeal sac that contains CSF, a portion of the spinal cord, and nerves through a vertebral defect

MYELODYSPLASIA OR SPINA BIFIDA

Myelodysplasia (sometimes called *meningomyelocele*) refers to a malformation of the spinal cord and spinal canal. Spina bifida refers to a defect in one or more vertebrae that allows spinal cord contents to protrude. The malformation can occur anywhere along the vertebral column, but is most common at the lumbar or sacral portion of the spine. Each year in the United States, approximately 1500 infants are born with spina bifida (Centers for Disease Control and Prevention [CDC], 2014b). The incidence is higher among newborns of Hispanic women and lowest among non-Hispanic Black women (CDC, 2015).

Developing Cultural Competence Folate Deficiency

Mandatory fortification of all enriched grain products with folate was initiated in 1998. This public health initiative has prevented an estimated 1326 cases of spina bifida and anencephaly annually, a 28% reduction. Hispanic women have a lower intake of folic acid and a higher rate of folate deficiency, potentially because of a genetic susceptibility to folate deficiency or to the greater use of corn masa flour, which is not fortified like other cereal grains (CDC, 2015).

Etiology and Pathophysiology. The cause of spina bifida is unknown, although environmental factors have been implicated, such as chemicals (excessive use of alcohol), medications (e.g., valproic acid and carbamazepine used for seizures, isotretinoin for acne), genetic factors, and maternal health conditions (diabetes mellitus, gestational diabetes, folic acid deficiency, and maternal obesity). The increased incidence of the condition in families points to a possible genetic influence.

Healthy People 2020

(MICH-28) Reduce occurrence of neural tube defects

Clinical Manifestations. A saclike protrusion on the infant's back indicates meningocele or myelodysplasia (Figure 54–9). The clinical manifestations (paralysis, weakness, and sensory loss) depend on the location of the defect. The higher the defect on the spinal cord, the greater the neurologic dysfunction:

- *Thoracic level*—paralysis of the legs, weakness and sensory loss in the trunk and lower body region
- *Lumbar 1–2 level*—some hip flexion and adduction, cannot extend knees
- *Lumbar 3 level*—can flex hips and extend the knees; paralyzed ankles and toes
- *Lumbar 4–5 level*—can flex hips and extend the knees; weak or absent ankle extension, toe flexion, and hip extension
- *Sacral level*—mild weakness in ankles and toes

Sensory loss is more pronounced on the back of the legs, and the loss of lower extremity motor and sensory functioning may not be symmetric.

Bowel and bladder incontinence occurs with all but the sacral level lesions, but bowel and bladder function may still be affected at the sacral level. Renal damage may result from neurologic impairment and urinary retention (neurogenic bladder). Hydrocephalus is usually present in children with a myelomeningocele defect above the sacral level, along with the Arnold-Chiari type II malformation (see hydrocephalus earlier in this chapter). The range of problems associated with spina bifida is listed in Table 54–10.

Children with myelodysplasia have mobility problems, intellectual disability, and visual impairment. Additional complications include spinal curvatures, musculoskeletal and joint abnormalities, skin sores, precocious puberty, and sexual dysfunction.

Clinical Therapy. A high-resolution fetal ultrasound leads to the diagnosis, and an elevated maternal serum alpha-fetoprotein level is present. Fetal surgery prior to 26 weeks' gestation improved cognitive and motor function of infants at 30 months of age. It also reduces the need for a shunt for hydrocephalus; however, the surgery increases the risk for preterm birth (Adzick et al., 2011).

If fetal surgery is not performed, the lesion is examined after birth and the neurologic status is evaluated. Radiologic imaging by ultrasonography, CT scan, MRI, and flat films of the spinal column can pinpoint the bony defect and nerve

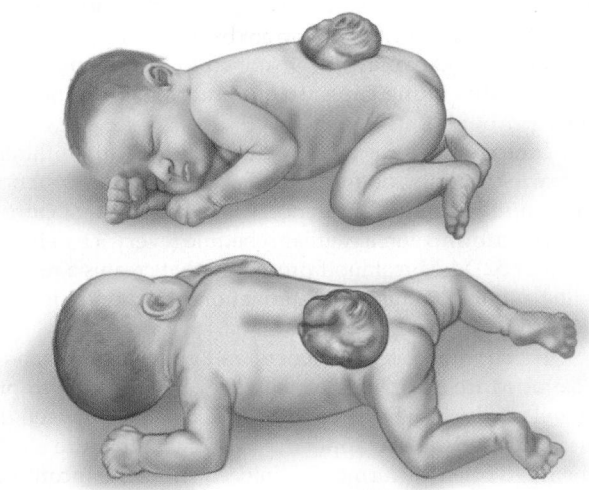

Figure 54–9 Lumbosacral myelomeningocele is caused by a neural tube defect in which the vertebral column is incompletely closed. The meninges (and sometimes the spinal cord) protrude as a saclike structure. Observe for leakage of cerebrospinal fluid.

TABLE 54–10 Clinical Manifestations of Myelodysplasia

CAUSE	CLINICAL MANIFESTATIONS
Interruption of the spinal cord at site of the spinal defect	Loss of motor and sensory function of the abdomen and lower extremities, dependent on defect level
	Scoliosis or kyphosis
	Incontinence of urine or urinary retention
	Incontinence of feces or constipation
	Sensory loss around genitalia
Muscle imbalance	Hip abnormalities, hip dysplasia
	Foot deformities (e.g., clubfoot)
Tethered spinal cord (the cord is abnormally attached to tissues around the spine that keeps it from moving freely within the spinal column)	Walking ability deteriorates
	Back pain, increasing scoliosis
	Leg pain, spasticity, progressive foot deformity
	Bladder and bowel function deteriorates
Brain abnormalities	Hydrocephalus, generalized seizures
	Learning problems, attention deficit disorder
	Problems with perceptual motor skills
	Memory and organization problems
	Problems with numeric reasoning

involvement. Subsequent testing is performed to evaluate bowel and bladder function, neurologic and motor function, and cognitive function.

Surgery to close and repair the lesion usually occurs within 24 to 48 hours of the infant's birth to reduce infection risk. As the child grows, braces are used to support joint position and mobility. Assistive devices such as walkers, crutches, and wheelchairs are used to enhance mobility. To minimize the risk for osteoporosis, the diet should ensure adequate calcium and vitamin D, and weight-bearing activities should be encouraged. Surgery to release a tethered spinal cord may be needed. An orthotic jacket may be prescribed to correct spinal deformities that affect lung capacity and interfere with mobility and sitting.

Interventions for a neurogenic bladder are initiated early to prevent kidney damage, to maintain bladder function, and to promote urinary continence. Clean intermittent catheterization is performed on a regular schedule (every 3 to 4 hours) (see Chapter 52). A Mitrofanoff procedure that creates a reservoir for urine and a stoma for catheterization in the umbilicus may be performed.

Dietary fiber, stool softeners, and glycerin or bisacodyl suppositories are prescribed for bowel evacuation and to promote bowel continence. Surgery to create a channel between the skin and bowel using the appendix (Malone antegrade continence enema) is often performed in children with fecal incontinence or severe constipation at the same time as the Mitranoff procedure. This procedure enables a child or adolescent to infuse an enema into the ascending and transverse colon to promote bowel evacuation to eliminate fecal soiling and incontinence.

Prognosis depends on the type of defect, the level of the lesion, and other complicating factors, such as renal dysfunction. In the United States, 90% survive to adulthood, and about 80% have normal intelligence (Spina Bifida Association, 2014). Children need multiple surgeries and invasive procedures. A team of healthcare providers, nurses, and therapists from the neurosurgery, orthopedic, urology, and physical medicine departments works with the child and family to form a comprehensive care plan.

Nursing Management

For the Child With Myelodysplasia or Spina Bifida

HOSPITAL-BASED NURSING CARE

The newborn is often transferred to a specialty center or neonatal intensive care unit until surgery is performed. Place the newborn in a prone position with hips slightly flexed and legs abducted to minimize tension on the sac. Monitor the sac for leakage of cerebrospinal fluid (CSF). Assess the extremities for deformities. Frequently assess the vital signs and stay alert for signs of infection, especially meningitis. Encourage the parents to interact with and soothe the newborn while waiting for surgery. Depending on when surgery will be performed, the newborn may be given small frequent feedings in the prone position.

Following surgery, inspect the surgical site for signs of infection and CSF leakage. Manage the infant's postoperative pain. Assess intake and output. Measure the head circumference daily to detect hydrocephalus. If a shunt was placed, provide care as described in the section on hydrocephalus.

Place the infant in a prone or side-lying position for sleep until healing has occurred, after which the supine sleep position may be used. Keep the diaper away from the incision site. Provide incision care according to agency guidelines. Assess the neonate regularly for signs of infection, motor deficits, and bladder and bowel involvement. Perform urinary catheterization on a regular schedule if needed.

Begin gentle range-of-motion (ROM) exercises as soon as possible to prevent muscle contractures and atrophy. Use caution because these children have brittle bones that fracture easily. Splints may be used to maintain extremity alignment.

Support the parents by keeping them informed about their child's status. Allow them to express their frustrations and anger. As soon as parents are able to cope with the child's condition, encourage them to become involved in the infant's care in the hospital.

The child with myelodysplasia may be hospitalized for surgery numerous times to correct deformities. Assess the child's vital signs, responsiveness, and level of pain. Because the child may have decreased pain sensation in the lower extremities, careful assessment is needed. Assess dressing sites for bleeding and drainage. Monitor the distal extremities for swelling and circulation.

SAFETY ALERT!

Children and adolescents with spina bifida are at high risk for latex allergy, thought to be related to frequent and cumulative numbers of exposure over time. See Table 48–9 for a list of products containing latex commonly found in the home.

DISCHARGE PLANNING AND HOME CARE TEACHING

Address home care needs well in advance of discharge. Help parents obtain special devices such as splints, wedges, and rolls, if needed, to prevent complications. Instruct parents how to position, handle, and feed the infant, and to perform ROM exercises. Teach parents to perform intermittent clean catheterization and establish a schedule for catheterization every 3 to 4 hours. See the *Clinical Skills Manual* SKILLS .

Teach parents the symptoms of increased ICP, hydrocephalus, shunt infection or malfunction, and urinary tract infection. Arrange for home care nursing to reinforce skills learned in the hospital as needed. Refer parents to resource groups such as the Spina Bifida Association.

COMMUNITY-BASED NURSING CARE

Because of multiple system involvement and to promote optimal development, children with myelodysplasia need comprehensive care planned and coordinated by a knowledgeable team of healthcare providers (e.g., orthopedics, neurosurgery, urology, developmental pediatrics, rehabilitation medicine, nursing, physical therapy, nutrition, and family support services). This care may be provided in partnership with the primary care healthcare provider. A case manager may be helpful to coordinate the health plan coverage and the child's care with numerous healthcare providers. Parents have many financial issues related to the child's need for medical supplies and new adaptive equipment to match growth.

At an appropriate age, teach the child to perform intermittent self-catheterization. When the child begins school, an individualized health plan should be developed so the child has access to the restroom, assistance as needed for toileting, and accommodations for mobility challenges.

Clinical Tip
The child who has clean intermittent catheterization performed usually has some bacteria in the urine. Symptoms indicating a urinary tract infection that should be treated include fever, dysuria, or new-onset incontinence.

Good nutrition planning is important to prevent obesity and to reduce constipation and fecal impaction. Bowel training is initiated to control bowel evacuation. A diet high in fiber helps ensure adequate stool. The child should have a bowel movement at least every 1 to 2 days to avoid impaction. Consistency in time of day for bowel evacuation is important to promote continence. A glycerin or bisacodyl suppository can be given to promote bowel evacuation at the appropriate time.

Promote safety and independent mobility with proper use of braces, walkers, crutches, canes, and in some cases custom-designed wheelchairs and car safety seats (Figure 54–10). For other safety guidelines, see *Teaching Highlights: Safety for the Child With Spina Bifida.*

Treat older children according to their intellectual level, not their motor development. Encourage them to take responsibility for self-care, and recognize their need to control their body functions. Monitor adolescents for mental health problems, especially as differences from peers and challenges in lifestyle become of greater concern. Refer for counseling as needed. See *Health Promotion: The Child With Myelodysplasia.*

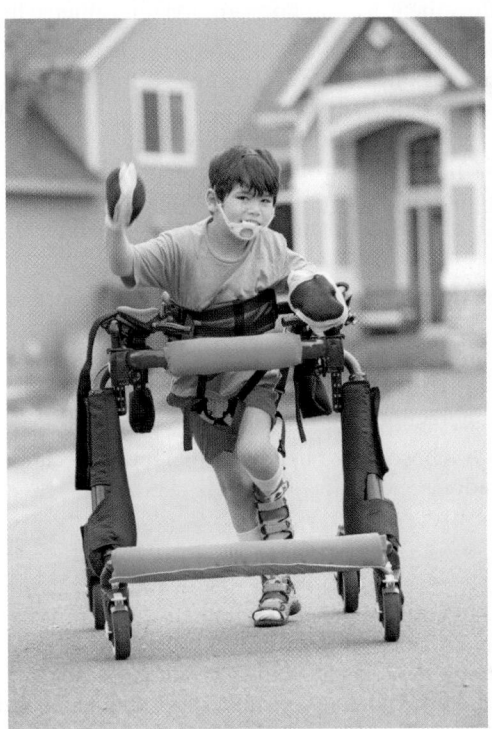
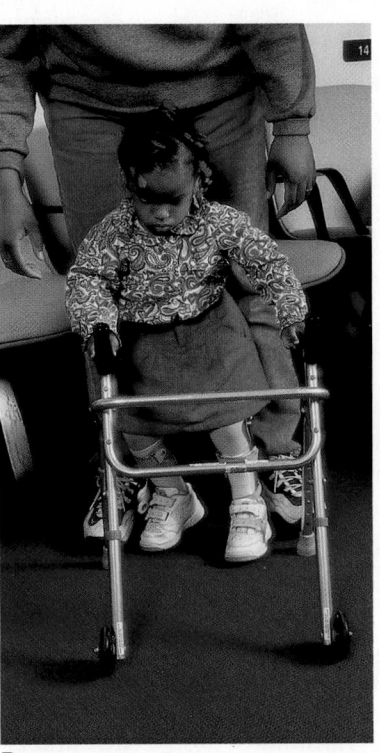
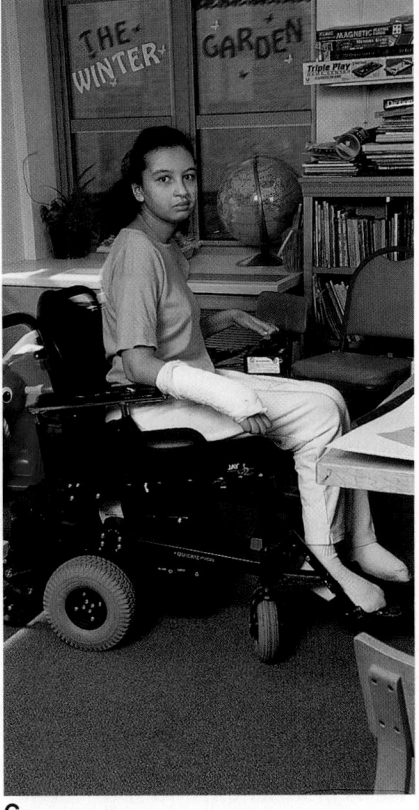

A **B** **C**

Figure 54–10 Help determine the best assistive device for the child to gain the most mobility independence and to promote development. The child may vary the devices used in different settings to promote optimal independence. *A* and *B,* Braces and walkers may be best for young children to promote an upright posture that encourages a normal interaction with the environment. *C,* A motorized wheelchair can assist the child with a significant neurologic impairment to achieve independence and mobility.

SOURCE: *A,* Jaren Wicklund / Fotolia.

| TEACHING HIGHLIGHTS | Safety for the Child With Spina Bifida |

Because of the loss of sensation in the lower extremities, injuries to the skin may not be immediately noticed by the child. Several routine actions will help reduce the risk for injury:

- Perform a daily check of all skin surfaces and pressure points associated with sitting, braces, and shoes to identify abrasions, scrapes, reddened areas, and other lesions. Stop using the braces or shoes until the skin heals or redness disappears.
- Keep all skin surfaces clean and dry. Wear socks under braces.
- Use a gel-filled cushion in the wheelchair, and teach the child to shift positions hourly to prevent pressure sores.
- Avoid burns to the lower extremities by checking the temperature of bath water and car safety seats in a hot car.
- Teach parents how to avoid the use of latex products and to inform all healthcare providers about the child's latex allergy or risk.
- Use safe ambulation techniques with walkers, canes, and crutches.

Health Promotion The Child With Myelodysplasia

Preventive Health Care

- Provide all recommended immunizations. If the child has a seizure disorder, alert parents that seizures may occur following immunizations.
- Perform all recommended routine screening procedures (vision, hearing, hematocrit, blood pressure).
- Obtain a urinalysis with culture in the newborn period and when signs of infection are noted.
- Screen for scoliosis annually beginning at birth.

Growth and Development Surveillance

- Monitor the growth of the child (length or height, weight, head circumference) and plot on growth curves. Monitor head circumference growth carefully because of hydrocephalus risk.
- Assess developmental status regularly. Motor skills are often delayed.
- Enroll the infant in an early intervention program to assist the parents to promote the child's development.
- Promote gradual independence in mobility and self-care.

Nutrition

- Teach families appropriate caloric intake and portion control for the child at each age to reduce the risk for obesity.

- Provide guidance about increased fluids and fiber in the diet to reduce the risk for constipation and urinary tract infections.
- Alert parents that allergies to foods like bananas, avocados, papaya, kiwi, and other foods may occur because of the risk of latex allergy.

Elimination

- Teach families the importance of performing intermittent catheterization on a regular schedule. Teach the child to perform self-catheterization and care for the catheter in preparation for school entry.
- Teach families to initiate bowel training so that a bowel regimen is established.

Sleep and Rest

- Position the child to prevent contractures. Change the child's position during the night to reduce pressure over skin surfaces.
- Teach parents to be alert for apnea spells or snoring that could be related to a Chiari type II malformation.

Relationships

- Encourage interaction with peers.
- Be alert for psychosocial adjustment problems, especially during the adolescent years.

Craniosynostosis

Craniosynostosis is the premature closure of cranial sutures in utero or during the first 18 months of life. This condition occurs in 1 per 1800 to 2200 live births, and boys are affected twice as often as girls (Kerr & Huether, 2014). Craniosynostosis may occur in association with chromosomal abnormality syndromes such as Apert and Crouzon syndromes, but most cases are not related to a syndrome (McCarthy et al., 2012).

When one or more sutures closes too early, bone growth continues in a direction parallel to the suture line. This leads to overgrowth at normal suture lines and classic skull deformities (Figure 54–11). Sagittal synostosis (scaphocephaly) occurs more

commonly in males and is the most common form of craniosynostosis (Brown & Proctor, 2011). Bicoronal synostosis is associated with Alpert or Crouzon syndromes.

Diagnosis of craniosynostosis is made by clinical appearance and palpation of a bony ridge along a skull suture line. Detection may occur during fetal ultrasound. Skull measurements, radiographs, and CT imaging confirm the diagnosis. Surgery is performed for cosmetic reasons and when increased ICP occurs. A custom orthotic helmet may be used for several months to promote optimal skull reshaping. Follow-up care is coordinated to manage potential associated problems, such as hypoplasia of the midface, orthodontic or ophthalmologic issues, and obstructive sleep apnea.

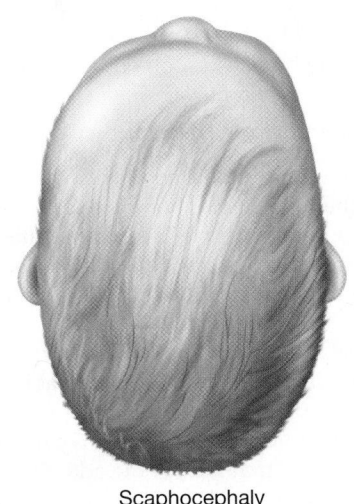
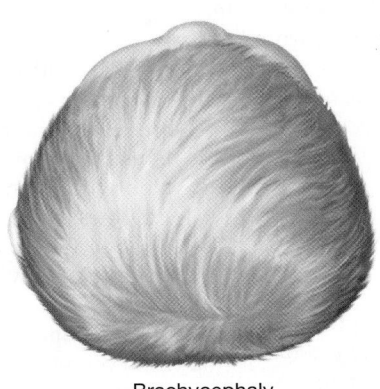
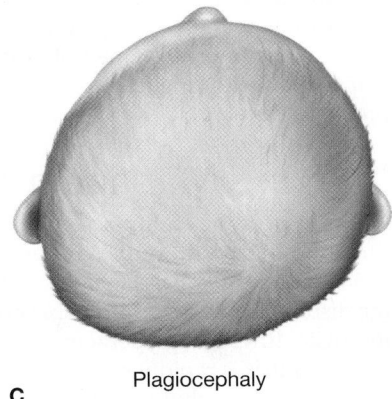

| A | Scaphocephaly | B | Brachycephaly | C | Plagiocephaly |

Figure 54–11 In craniosynostosis, the head shape is dependent on which sutures are involved. *A*, Scaphocephaly, premature closure of the sagittal suture causes a long, narrow skull, flattened parietal bones with a prominent occiput, a broad forehead, and a small or absent anterior fontanelle. *B*, Brachycephaly, premature closure of the bicoronal suture causes a head shape shortened anterior to posterior, and the occiput is flattened. *C*, Positional plagiocephaly is often asymmetric flattening of the occiput due to preferred sleep position when supine or due to torticollis.

After surgery, nursing care involves keeping the incision dry and intact. Observe the child for symptoms of increased ICP (see Table 54–1). The nurse should monitor intake and output, manage patient positioning, protect skin integrity, and monitor for infection. Explain to parents that surgery will improve the child's appearance. Assure them that most children with craniosynostosis are healthy, and that their brains develop normally.

Positional Plagiocephaly

Positional plagiocephaly (an asymmetric flattening of the skull) is associated with sleep position to prevent sudden infant death syndrome or in infants with neck problems such as congenital torticollis. Some infants have variable tone and developmental delay that reduces development of neck muscles strength (Looman & Flannery, 2012). The sutures do not close prematurely. If the infant's sleep position does not change, the weight of the head flattens the skull (see Figure 54–11C).

If torticollis is a factor in plagiocephaly, a physical therapy referral is important. In cases of severe positional plagiocephaly, a helmet device to correct the condition, especially when facial asymmetry is present. The helmet is most effective when treatment is initiated at 6 months of age when the skull bones are most malleable. The helmet is worn for 23 hours a day for 2 to 4 months. Remolding of the head shape continues naturally after that treatment period because the infant spends more time awake and upright.

Clinical Tip

To help prevent positional plagiocephaly, encourage parents to try to reduce the infant's preference for lying supine in one position. Rotate the side of the crib where an interesting toy is placed each day. Alternate the infant between the top and bottom of the crib each day, so the infant must turn the head in a different direction to look at who comes into the room. Put the infant in a bouncy seat while awake. Rotate the arm used for formula feeding the infant. When the child is alert and continuously supervised, place the infant in prone position on the floor for short periods (tummy time) to promote neck muscle strength and interaction with nearby objects.

Neurofibromatosis

Neurofibromatosis 1 (NF1), or von Recklinghausen disease, is an autosomal dominant genetic disorder in which tumors grow along nerves. One in 3500 individuals develops the disorder, and 50% of new cases result from a mutation (Julian, Edwards, DeCrane, et al., 2014).

The *NF1* gene is located on chromosome 17. Individuals with NF1 do not have adequate neurofibromin to control cell growth, and neurofibromas form from nerve sheath cells along peripheral nerves or at nerve endings. The neurofibroma may be an isolated growth, or extend along the length of a nerve and include nerve branches (plexiform neurofibroma). Dermal neurofibromas, which usually begin to appear around the time of puberty, may reside in the skin or project above the skin surface. Up to 5% of tumors become malignant in the brain or along nerves, and children may be at risk for leukemia, rhabdomyosarcoma, and pheochromocytoma (Julian et al., 2014). A higher prevalence of autism spectrum disorder may also occur in children with NF1 (Garg et al., 2013).

The disorder is characterized by six or more café au lait spots (darker than surrounding skin) 5 mm (0.20 in.) in diameter or larger seen at birth or by 2 years of age. The spots grow to 15 mm (0.6 in.) or larger by adulthood. Freckling in the axillary and inguinal areas is common. Multiple neurofibromas or benign tumors grow on or under the skin beginning during puberty. Pain may occur when a tumor compresses a nerve or grows in the spinal cord. Lisch nodules, tan or brown benign tumors on the iris of the eye, are characteristic. Vision deficits or blindness is found in some children because of a tumor along the optic pathway. Precocious puberty or delayed puberty and menarche may occur when the optic tumor invades the hypothalamus. The child often has a larger than expected head circumference. Other manifestations include thinning or bowing of the tibia, fractures that do not heal properly, and scoliosis.

Diagnosis is made in early childhood by the presence of two or more characteristic physical findings listed in the previous paragraph and a positive family history. Radiologic imaging (MRI of brain and radiographs of the spine and other bones) is performed when problems are detected. Ophthalmologic examinations are performed at least annually. Clinical therapy focuses on monitoring the child for signs of problems associated with the condition. The severity of the condition ranges from mild to severe with disabilities. Surgery may be performed to remove the tumor when neurofibromas become malignant, are painful or disfiguring, cause paralysis, or when life-threatening problems develop.

Nursing Management

Nurses assess the child for signs of neurofibromatosis. Assess the child's growth, pubertal development, vital signs, and vision on a regular basis to detect any problems associated with the disorder. School performance should be monitored as learning disabilities and hyperactivity may occur. Pay attention to any mass that is rapidly enlarging or causing new pain.

Provide psychologic support to the child and family. As tumor development increases during adolescence, problems with self-image and self-esteem are common. Adolescents may fear the response of peers to the tumors and isolate themselves. Identify potential peers or refer the adolescent to a support group.

Cerebral Palsy

Cerebral palsy (CP), a common syndrome of movement and posture development disorders, is caused by a nonprogressive lesion abnormality in the fetal or infant brain that results in activity limitations. The condition may also have associated hearing, vision, communication, perceptual, cognitive, and behavioral problems. An estimated prevalence of CP is 3.9 children per 1000 (Burkhard, 2013). Four types of motor dysfunction seen—spastic, dyskinetic, ataxic, and mixed—are related to the location of brain insult. Dystonia and athetosis are sometimes categorized together as dyskinesia.

Etiology and Pathophysiology

The majority of cases occur during the prenatal and perinatal periods. Risk factors include low birth weight, placental abnormalities, birth defects, meconium aspiration, birth asphyxia, neonatal seizures, respiratory distress syndrome, hypoglycaemia, and neonatal infections. Postnatal cases are related to meningitis, encephalitis, and traumatic brain injury (Colver, Fairhurst, & Pharoah, 2014).

Healthy People 2020

(MICH-27) Reduce the proportion of children with cerebral palsy born as low-birth-weight infants (less than 2500 grams)

Muscle growth is usually coordinated with bone growth, but muscle spasticity interferes. Contractures can develop that limit joint movement or cause deformities such as scoliosis. Because of more limited weight-bearing activity and potential nutritional problems with swallowing and independent feeding, children with CP are at greater risk for osteoporosis and fractures (Aronson & Stevenson, 2012).

Clinical Manifestations

Cerebral palsy is characterized by abnormal muscle tone and lack of coordination. Children have a variety of symptoms depending on their ages, and the pattern or extremities involved may vary:

- *Diplegia*—both legs are affected
- *Hemiplegia*—one side of the body is involved, the arm is usually more severely affected than the leg
- *Quadriplegia*—all four extremities are affected

All children with CP have motor impairment, with spasticity present more commonly than ataxia or athetosis and dystonia. Even if both sides of the body are affected, the impairment is usually more severe on one side. Spasticity is also associated with muscle weakness that interferes with gross motor activities.

See Table 54–11 for clinical manifestations of CP by type of brain injury. Symptoms are variable for this lifelong disability and depend on the area of the brain involved and the extent of brain injury. Behavioral and emotional problems may result from disruption of nerve pathways that reduce the adaptation of the brain.

Children with CP usually have delayed developmental milestones. The functional consequences of motor deficits become more obvious as the child grows even though the brain injury is nonprogressive. Other complications include intellectual disabilities, vision impairments, hearing loss, speech and language impairments, and seizures. Feeding may be difficult because of oral motor involvement, including hypotonia, with poor sucking and swallowing coordination that may result in aspiration or poor nutrition.

Clinical Therapy

Diagnosis is usually based on clinical findings of delayed development and increased or decreased muscle tone. CP is difficult to diagnose in the early months of life because it must be distinguished from other neurologic conditions and signs may be subtle. Suspicious historical findings include risk factors described in the *Etiology and Pathophysiology* section.

Ultrasonography can be used to detect fetal and neonatal abnormalities of the brain, such as intraventricular hemorrhage. Neuromotor tests are used to evaluate the presence of normal movement patterns, absence of common newborn reflexes, and abnormal tone. Once CP is suspected, CT and MRI imaging provide information about anatomic structures and help identify the cause of CP. Genetic and metabolic tests are performed if congenital anomalies are present. Hearing and vision should be evaluated. Standardized tools, such as the Functional Mobility Scale and Manual Ability Classification System, are used to describe the child's capabilities.

Clinical therapy focuses on helping the child develop to a maximum level of independence and to perform activities of daily living. This involves promoting mobility, an optimal range of motion, muscle control, balance, and communication with braces and splints, serial casting, and positioning devices (prone wedges, standers, and side-lyers). Referrals are made for physical, occupational, and speech therapy, as well as special education to improve motor function and ability.

Orthopedic surgery may be required to improve function by balancing muscle power and stabilizing uncontrollable joints. Surgical interventions may include Achilles tendon lengthening to increase the ankle range of motion, hamstring release to correct knee flexion contractures, procedures to improve hip adduction or correct spinal deformities, or dorsal rhizotomy (cutting the afferent fibers that contribute to spasticity).

Medications are given to control seizures, to control spasms (skeletal muscle relaxants, baclofen, and benzodiazepines), and to minimize gastrointestinal side effects (cimetidine or

TABLE 54–11 Clinical Manifestations of Cerebral Palsy by Type of Insult

CLASSIFICATION AND TYPE OF INSULT	CLINICAL MANIFESTATIONS
SPASTIC Cerebral cortex or pyramidal tract injury 75% of cases	Increased muscle tone through a joint's range of motion Leads to contractures and abnormal curvature of the spine Exaggerated deep tendon reflexes, clonus Persistent common newborn reflexes, positive Babinski sign
DYSKINETIC—ATHETOSIS Extrapyramidal, basal ganglia injury 10%–15% of cases	Muscle tone abnormalities affecting the entire body Difficulty with fine and purposeful movements or coordinating the timing of movement; tremors Slow involuntary writhing motions that interfere with ability to maintain a stable posture
DYSKINETIC—DYSTONIA Basal ganglia, extrapyramidal injury	Involuntary sustained muscle contractions that lead to sustained or intermittent exaggerated and distorted posturing, twisting, or repetitive movements Rigid muscles when awake; normal or decreased muscle tone when asleep
ATAXIC Cerebellar (extrapyramidal) injury 5%–10% of cases	Abnormalities of voluntary movement (muscle instability) involving balance and position of the trunk and limbs, difficulty maintaining posture, wide-based unsteady gait Difficulty controlling hand and arm movements during reaching Increased or decreased muscle tone, hypotonia in first couple of years
MIXED Multiple areas of brain are injured	No dominant motor pattern; may have mild spasticity, dystonia, and/or athetoid movement

ranitidine). Benzodiazepines affect brain control of muscle tone to help control spasticity. Dantrolene is a calcium channel blocker that is a muscle relaxant. Baclofen is administered orally or by intrathecal pump to decrease spasticity. See Figure 54–12. Botulinum toxin injection into specific muscles is a therapy that helps to temporarily control spasticity.

The prognosis for infants and children with CP depends on the level of motor disability and on the presence of intellectual, visual, or hearing deficits. Early intervention programs can help improve performance. Many children with hemiplegia or ataxia show some improvement with maturation and are able to ambulate. Others need assistance with mobility and

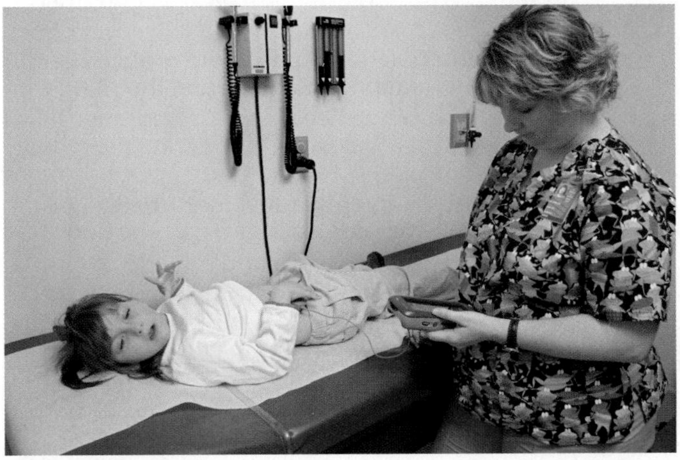

Figure 54–12 **Baclofen may be administered by an intrathecal pump. This child is having the reservoir of the baclofen pump filled.**

activities of daily living. Many of these children have difficulty with swallowing and aspiration, making feeding a challenge for families. A gastrostomy tube may ultimately be needed to ensure that the child has adequate nutrition and to prevent aspiration.

Nursing Management
For the Child With Cerebral Palsy

Nursing Assessment and Diagnosis

Be alert for children whose histories indicate an increased risk for CP. Assess all children at each healthcare visit for developmental delays. Note any orthopedic, visual, auditory, or intellectual deficits. When the common newborn reflexes persist beyond the normal age, refer for further evaluation (see Chapter 24). Identify infants who appear to have an abnormal muscle tone or abnormal posture (head lag beyond 6 months of age, arched back, poor trunk control and balance, toe walking or scissoring). Asymmetric or abnormal crawling by using two or three extremities and hand dominance prior to 18 months of age indicates a motor problem. Perform a simple screening test by placing a clean cloth on the infant's face. Infants normally use two hands to remove it. Be concerned if the infant over 6 months of age uses one hand or does not remove the cloth at all. Record dietary intake as well as height and weight percentiles for children suspected to have or diagnosed with the condition.

The child has many potential sources of pain. Pain could be associated with constipation, muscle spasms, physical therapy, bladder spasms, decubitus ulcers, headaches, and dental caries. Anticipate and take a careful history to identify potential causes of pain and pain patterns.

Nursing diagnoses for the child with CP often vary by the type of CP, the child's symptoms and age, and the family situation. *Nursing Care Plan: The Child With Cerebral Palsy* includes several nursing diagnoses. Additional nursing diagnoses might include the following (NANDA-I © 2014):

- *Constipation, Risk for,* related to low intake of fiber and fluids and insufficient physical activity
- *Tissue Integrity, Impaired,* related to decreased physical mobility and limited self-care ability
- *Communication: Verbal, Impaired,* related to hearing and/or motor speech impairment
- *Pain, Chronic,* related to spasticity and stretching exercises to prevent contractures
- *Development: Delayed, Risk for,* related to lack of muscle strength or limited social interaction

Planning and Implementation

The accompanying *Nursing Care Plan* summarizes care for the child with CP. Since the condition varies in severity and manifestations, interventions need to be customized to the child and family. Nursing care focuses on providing adequate nutrition, maintaining skin integrity, promoting physical mobility, promoting safety, promoting growth and development, teaching parents how to care for the child, and providing emotional support.

PROVIDE ADEQUATE NUTRITION

Children with CP require high-calorie diets because of feeding difficulties associated with spasticity or hypotonia. Many children have difficulty chewing and swallowing, and therefore are at risk for aspiration. Give the child small amounts of soft foods at a time. Utensils with large, padded handles may be easier for the child to hold. Make sure the child gets adequate fluids as the child may not be able to communicate thirst. Children with severe CP may need a gastrostomy tube to obtain adequate nutrition and fluids. Adequate fiber is needed to prevent constipation, and some children need a bowel management program to treat chronic constipation.

MAINTAIN SKIN INTEGRITY

Protect bony prominences from skin breakdown. Monitor splints and braces for proper fit and the skin under them for redness. If the skin is red or broken, the braces or splints should be removed and not worn until the skin is healed.

PROMOTE PHYSICAL MOBILITY

Proper body alignment should be maintained at all times. Support the child with pillows, towels, and bolsters whether the child is in bed or in a chair. Use splints and braces to help support joints in extension or a functional position and to reduce the risk for contractures. Support the head and body of a floppy infant. A spastic child with scissored, extended legs or a child with athetosis who writhes constantly is difficult to carry and transport.

Range-of-motion exercises are essential to maintain joint flexibility and to prevent contractures. Consult with the physical therapists who work with the child and assist with recommended exercises. Massage may be helpful when performing stretching exercises. Horseback riding is a therapeutic activity

---

Nursing Care Plan: The Child With Cerebral Palsy

1. Nursing Diagnosis: *Mobility: Physical, Impaired,* related to decreased muscle strength and control (NANDA-I © 2014)

GOAL: The child will attain the maximum physical abilities possible.

INTERVENTION	RATIONALE
• Perform development assessment and record age at which milestones are achieved (e.g., reaching for objects, sitting).	• Delayed development milestones are common with CP. As one milestone is achieved, interventions are revised to focus on the next skill.
• Plan activities to use gross and fine motor skills (e.g., holding eating utensils, toys positioned to encourage reaching). Allow time for the child to complete activities.	• Many activities of daily living and play activities promote physical development. The child may perform tasks more slowly than most children.
• Perform range-of-motion exercises every 4 hours for the child unable to move body parts. Position the child to promote tendon stretching (e.g., foot plantar flexion, legs extended at the knees and hips).	• Exercises and positioning promote mobility and increased circulation, and decrease the risk of contractures.
• Arrange for and encourage parents to keep appointments with a rehabilitation therapist.	• A regular and frequently reevaluated rehabilitation program assists in promoting development.
• Teach the family to use braces and other positioning devices.	• Adaptive devices are often necessary to maximize physical mobility.

EXPECTED OUTCOME: Child will reach maximum physical mobility and achieve developmental milestones.

2. Nursing Diagnosis: *Nutrition, Imbalanced: Less than Body Requirements,* related to difficulty chewing and swallowing and high metabolic needs (NANDA-I © 2014)

GOAL: The child will receive nutrients needed for normal growth.

INTERVENTION	RATIONALE
• Monitor height and weight and plot on a growth grid. Perform hydration status assessment.	• Insufficient intake can lead to impaired growth and dehydration.

• Teach the family techniques to promote caloric and nutrient intake:
  • Position the child upright for feedings.
  • Place foods far back in the mouth to overcome tongue thrust.
  • Use soft and blended foods. Allow extra time for chewing and swallowing.
  • Obtain adaptive handles for utensils and encourage self-feeding skills.
	• Special techniques can facilitate food intake. Adaptive handles may help the child better manage feeding self.

• Perform frequent respiratory assessment. Teach the family the preceding techniques to prevent aspiration. Teach care of the gastrostomy and tube-feeding technique as appropriate.	• Aspiration pneumonia is a risk for the child with poor swallowing coordination. Special feeding techniques or tube feeding may be needed.

EXPECTED OUTCOME: Child will show normal growth patterns for height, weight, and other physical parameters.

---

3. **Nursing Diagnosis:** *Health Management, Family, Ineffective,* related to excessive demands made on the family for the child's complex care needs (NANDA-I © 2014)

GOAL: The family will adapt to the growth and development needs of the child with CP.

INTERVENTION	RATIONALE
• Allow chances for parents to verbalize the impact of CP on the family. Provide referral to other parents and support groups.	• The family needs to explore the emotional and social impact of the child's care so they can integrate and grow from the experience.
• Explore community services for rehabilitation, respite care, child care, early intervention program, and refer family as appropriate.	• Diverse services are available and will be needed because of the multiple impacts of CP on the child.
• During home and office visits, review the child's achievements and praise the family for care provided.	• The child's achievements are positive reinforcement of the family's efforts.
• Teach the family skills needed to manage the child's care (e.g., medication administration, muscle stretching, seizure management).	• Complex skills must be learned before they can be performed efficiently.
• Teach case management techniques.	• The child requires care by many specialists, and many parents become case managers to coordinate care.
• Involve siblings in the care of the child with CP. Review with parents the needs of all children in the family.	• Siblings of the child with CP may feel left out because of the care provided. Special efforts help to meet the developmental needs of all family members.

EXPECTED OUTCOME: Child will demonstrate appropriate growth and developmental progress. Family will successfully support all of its members.

---

4. **Nursing Diagnosis:** *Activity, Deficient Diversional (Child),* related to poor social skills (NANDA-I © 2014)

GOAL: The child will engage in activities that maximize growth and development.

INTERVENTION	RATIONALE
• Refer the family to an early intervention program. Encourage contact with other children.	• The child needs a variety of activities and contact with other children and adults to maximize development.
• Work with the school to develop an individualized education plan that encourages interaction with peers and a variety of activities that support development.	• The education system is obligated to work with families to provide methods to enhance learning, including social interactions.
• Investigate recreational programs for children with disabilities and share information with the parents.	• Recreational programs for children with disabilities may promote social experiences and physical activity.

EXPECTED OUTCOME: Child will engage in activities to maximize development.

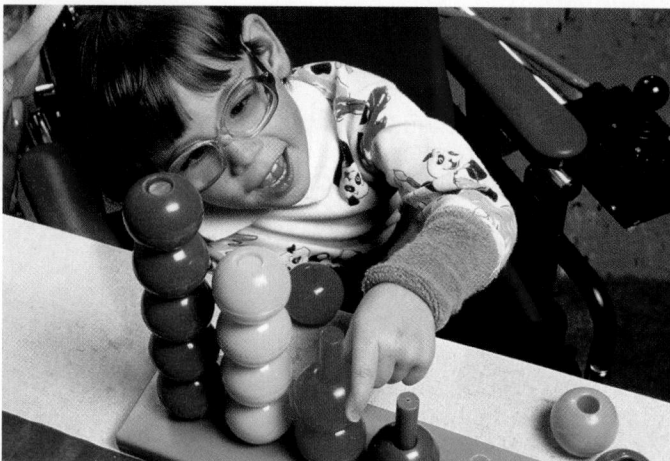

Figure 54–13 This child has cerebral palsy and wears glasses because of vision impairment. She uses a wheelchair for transport to the health center. Notice the planned placement and level of toys to promote her interaction.

SOURCE: Will & Deni McIntyre/Science Source.

as adjustment to the horse's gait helps improve balance and posture control.

Refer parents to the appropriate resources for help getting adaptive devices (Figure 54–13). To enhance interaction with the environment, teach the parents to position the child to foster flexion rather than extension (e.g., the child can bring objects closer to the face). Encourage parents to bring in the child's *adaptive appliances* (braces, positioning devices) for use during a hospitalization; however, secure them as the family may have difficulty replacing them if lost.

PROMOTE SAFETY

Safety belts should be used for children in strollers and wheelchairs (see the *Clinical Skills Manual* SKILLS). Determine if an adaptive car safety seat is needed so the child can be safely transported. A child with chronic seizures should wear a helmet to protect against further injury.

PROMOTE GROWTH AND DEVELOPMENT

Remember that many children with CP are physically but not intellectually disabled. Use terminology appropriate for the child's developmental level. Help the child develop a positive self-image to ensure emotional health and social growth. Children with a hearing impairment may need referral to learn American Sign Language or other communication methods. Provide audio and visual activities for the child who is quadriplegic.

Adaptive and assistive technology may be needed to promote mobility and communication. **Assistive technology** is any item, equipment, or product customized for use to promote the functional capabilities and independence of an individual with disabilities. Examples include computers, communication devices, adaptive utensils, and customized wheelchairs.

FOSTER PARENTAL KNOWLEDGE

Teach parents about the disorder and arrange sessions to teach them about all of the child's special needs. Teach administration, desired effects, and side effects of medications prescribed for seizures. Make sure parents are aware of the need for dental care for children because of the enamel defects and malocclusion that commonly occur in children with CP, and the gingival hyperplasia that occurs when taking some antiepileptic medications.

PROVIDE EMOTIONAL SUPPORT

Listen to the parents' concerns and encourage them to express their feelings and ask questions. Explain what they can expect from future treatment. Work with other healthcare providers to help families adjust to this chronic disease. Refer parents to individual and family counseling if appropriate.

COMMUNITY-BASED NURSING CARE

Children with CP need continuous support in the community. A case manager such as the parent or nurse is often needed to coordinate care. Parents may need financial assistance to provide the care that the child needs and to obtain appliances such as braces, wheelchairs, or adaptive utensils. Children need new adaptive devices, ongoing developmental assessment and care planning, and possibly surgery as they grow. Although the brain lesion does not change, it manifests differently as the child grows. For example, once the child begins to walk, the extensor tone may cause Achilles cord tightening. Braces may decrease deformities, but surgery may eventually be needed. Technology offers many new strategies to promote communication and self-care by these children.

Monitor the child's growth. If the child is unable to ambulate, use a scale that accommodates a wheelchair when weighing. Standing height measurements may be inaccurate. Other possible measures for stature include recumbent length, arm span, tibia length, and knee height. Schedule regular vision and hearing screening during health promotion visits. Give immunizations according to the recommended schedule, even though the pertussis, measles, mumps, and rubella vaccines may increase the risk of seizures in children with a seizure disorder. Educate parents about the possible risk for a seizure associated with the vaccines.

Early intervention programs can help parents learn to meet their child's special needs and obtain physical, occupational, and speech therapy. The child often needs an IEP to maximize learning potential (see Chapter 38). The nurse can help parents meet the needs of the child with CP in preschool, school, and healthcare settings. The nurse also makes referrals as appropriate to support groups and organizations such as the United Cerebral Palsy Association and Shriners Hospitals. Recreational activities may be identified through the National Association of Sports for Cerebral Palsy.

An individualized transition plan should be developed during adolescence to assist the family and adolescent with CP with plans for adult living. Vocational training options can be explored. Both the special mobility needs and educational support needed by the child must be addressed. See Chapter 38.

Evaluation

Expected outcomes of nursing care for the child with CP are provided in the *Nursing Care Plan.*

Injuries of the Neurologic System

Injuries to the brain and spinal cord are major causes of disability in previously healthy children. Drowning is another cause of brain injury in children.

Traumatic Brain Injury

A traumatic brain injury (TBI) is a blunt force or penetrating injury to the head that disrupts normal brain functioning, such as a loss of consciousness. More than 2600 children, ages 0 to 14 years, are estimated to die each year as a result of TBI (Brain Injury Association of America, 2014). Adolescents, 15 to 19 years, have the highest rate of death, followed by children less than age 5 years. The highest rate of hospitalization occurs in adolescents 15 to 19 years old, followed by children less than 5 years old (CDC, 2014a). TBI is a leading cause of death and disability in children and adolescents (Geyer, Meller, Kulpan, et al., 2013).

Growth and Development

Leading TBI mechanisms of injury resulting in emergency department visits or hospitalization vary by age (Quayle, Holmes, & Kuppermann, 2014):

- *Children 0 to 2 years old*—falls, usually from elevation or down stairs
- *Children 2 to 12 years old*—falls from elevation or associated with standing, running, or walking at ground level, or struck by or against an object
- *Adolescents 13 to 17 years old*—assault, sports, and motor vehicle related

ETIOLOGY AND PATHOPHYSIOLOGY

With a blunt injury the impact transfers energy through the skull and meninges to the brain. Primary injury occurs at the time of the impact when the initial cellular damage takes place, such as skull fracture, bruising, or hemorrhage. See *Pathophysiology Illustrated: Brain Injury* for an explanation of the primary injury. With a penetrating injury, additional brain damage occurs along the track of penetration. The secondary injury for both blunt and penetrating TBI is a biochemical and cellular response to the primary injury. Brain swelling begins immediately, leading to cerebral edema, inflammation, ischemia, and increased ICP. Decreased cerebral perfusion pressure limits the circulation, oxygen and nutrient delivery, and removal of toxins resulting from cell death. Brain cells are further damaged by the release of amino acids and an inflammatory response that increase the permeability of the blood–brain barrier.

CLINICAL MANIFESTATIONS

TBI signs and symptoms in children depend on the pathologic features and severity of the injury. The child with a mild TBI (concussion) may remain conscious or have brief loss of consciousness (seconds to a few minutes). The child with a moderate TBI loses consciousness for 5 to 10 minutes. Following mild or moderate TBI, children may have amnesia about the event, headache, nausea, and vomiting. See Table 54–12 for clinical manifestations of TBI by severity.

Unconsciousness may result from increased ICP, cerebral edema, intracranial hemorrhage, or extensive damage to the cerebral cortex or brainstem. Posttraumatic seizures are common. The presence of retinal hemorrhages, frenulum injuries, and fractures in an infant should raise the suspicion of child abuse (Fingarson & Pierce, 2012).

SAFETY ALERT!

Any infant who arrives in the emergency department with seizures, failure to thrive, respiratory irregularities, or coma should be evaluated for child abuse (shaken child syndrome). An infant has a large head and relatively weak neck muscles. Shaking an infant causes inertial injuries (acceleration and deceleration) that tear nerve fibers as the brain moves back and forth in the skull. Throwing the infant down onto a mattress further increases the forces with which the brain hits the back of the skull (Dubowitz & Lane, 2016).

Pathophysiology Illustrated: **Brain Injury**

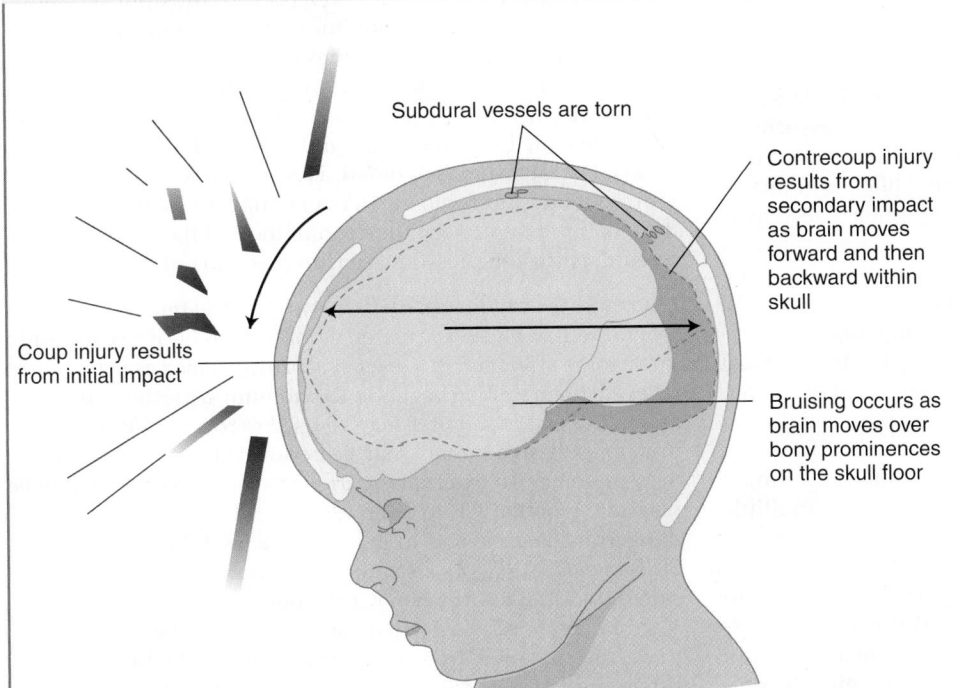

Subdural vessels are torn

Contrecoup injury results from secondary impact as brain moves forward and then backward within skull

Coup injury results from initial impact

Bruising occurs as brain moves over bony prominences on the skull floor

Brain injury can result from a direct blow to the head (coup injury) or the acceleration–deceleration movement of the brain (contrecoup injury) such as occurs from a motor vehicle crash. Movement of the brain in the skull tears nerves, fibers, and blood vessels, causing altered level of consciousness (LOC). Scalp injuries, skull fractures, contusions, and hematomas of brain tissue may also occur if the head experiences a direct blow.

TABLE 54–12 Clinical Manifestations of Traumatic Brain Injury by Severity

TYPE OF BRAIN INJURY	CLINICAL MANIFESTATIONS
Concussion or mild brain injury	Low-grade headache that will not go away
	Slowness in thinking, acting, speaking, reading
	Memory problems
	Loss of balance, unsteady walking
	Poor concentration, change in performance at school, lack of motivation or interest in favorite toys
	Feeling tired all the time, change in sleeping pattern
	Change in eating patterns
	Increased sensitivity to lights, sounds, distractions; easily irritated
Moderate brain injury	Glasgow Coma Scale score of 9–12
	Posttraumatic amnesia for 1–24 hr
	Loss of consciousness
Severe brain injury	Glasgow Coma Scale score of 8 or less
	Posttraumatic amnesia lasting longer than 24 hr
	Coma or unconsciousness
	Increased intracranial pressure
	Posttraumatic seizures

Changes in respiratory effort or periods of apnea can occur secondary to shock, injury to the spinal cord above C4, or damage to or pressure on the medulla. Heart rate and blood pressure provide information about brainstem function. Tachycardia can be a sign of blood loss, shock, hypoxia, anxiety, or pain. The Cushing triad (increased systolic blood pressure with a wide pulse pressure, bradycardia, and irregular respirations) is associated with significantly increased ICP, impending herniation, or compromised blood flow to the brainstem. Reflexes may be hyporesponsive, hyperresponsive, or nonexistent. The child may assume a flexor, extensor, areflexic, or flaccid posture (see Figure 54–2). Refer to Table 54–1 for signs of increased ICP. See Table 54–13 for clinical manifestations of specific brain injuries.

CLINICAL THERAPY

The severity of a brain injury is diagnosed from the history, physical examination, Glasgow Coma Scale (see Table 54–2), and diagnostic tests. Information about the events associated with and mechanism of injury, the child's initial and current responses, any loss of consciousness, and the child's memory of the event are obtained. The cranial nerves, pupillary response, palpation of the skull for depressions, deep tendon reflexes, and muscle strength are all evaluated.

Laboratory tests include a complete blood cell count, blood chemistry, coagulation tests, toxicology screening, and urinalysis. Radiographs detect fractures of the skull and cervical vertebrae. A CT scan detects fractures, intracranial bleeding, swelling, and diffuse axonal injury. An MRI scan is used during recovery to determine the extent of brain damage. PET scans measure the blood flow in the brain. A fracture indicates a more serious injury. Many children with brain injuries have multiple other injuries. Children with a moderate to severe TBI should be evaluated for a potential cervical spine injury.

The initial management of a child with a severe brain injury is based on the child's physiologic status (see *Concussion* section later in this chapter for management of a mild TBI). The airway must be clear and stable, and hypoxia must be prevented. The child is continuously monitored for hypercapnia, which causes vasodilation and increased ICP. The child may

be intubated and mechanically ventilated with 100% oxygen at a slightly increased respiratory rate in the first 24 hours after injury to maintain oxygenation levels and reduce ischemia (see the *Clinical Skills Manual* SKILLS).

Clinical Tip

In the child with moderate head injury, the oxygen saturation should remain over 95%. For the severely injured child who is intubated, monitor arterial blood gas results. A PaO_2 greater than 60 mmHg and a $PaCO_2$ between 35 to 38 mmHg are recommended (Geyer et al., 2013).

An intraventricular catheter (ventriculostomy) may be inserted and attached to a monitor to measure intracranial pressure. Efforts are made to maintain the cerebral perfusion pressure (difference between the mean arterial pressure minus the ICP or central venous pressure) so that the brain circulation is adequate to deliver oxygen and nutrients and to remove neurotoxins. Hypotension is avoided. Hypovolemic shock is treated if present and inotropic medications may be used to maintain the blood pressure. Keep the head of the bed flat until adequate cerebral perfusion pressure is ensured and maintained.

Increased Intracranial Pressure. Treatment is required when the ICP value is greater than 20 mmHg; it becomes life threatening at 40 mmHg (Geyer et al., 2013). If increased ICP is not relieved, brain shifting begins in the cranium, a precursor of herniation. Invasive procedures may be used to reduce ICP. Burr holes or more extensive surgery may be performed to evacuate a lesion or hematoma. An external ventricular drainage system may be placed to monitor ICP, to drain CSF when brain swelling reaches dangerous heights, and to help maintain CPP (see the *Clinical Skills Manual* SKILLS). Decompressive craniectomy may be considered as a last resort when ICP cannot be otherwise controlled.

Mannitol or IV hypertonic saline (3%) may be administered to decrease the ICP by shifting water out of the brain tissues. When prescribed, serum osmolality and electrolytes should be monitored. Sedation, analgesia, and paralytic agents may be administered to eliminate the child's resistance to mechanical

TABLE 54–13 Clinical Manifestations of Intracranial Hematomas

TYPE OF HEMATOMA	CLINICAL MANIFESTATIONS
SUBDURAL HEMATOMA Results from severe brain trauma, including shaken child syndrome. Is more common in infants less than age 1 year. Inertial forces tear veins bridging the subdural space; a venous hematoma forms beneath the dura and presses directly on the brain.	Symptoms that may occur 48–72 hr after the injury: • Gradual change in LOC (confusion, agitation, or lethargy) • Hemiparesis or eye deviation • Nausea or vomiting • Headache • Retinal hemorrhages in both eyes • Pupil on side of injury may be fixed and dilated • Seizures
EPIDURAL HEMATOMA Is rare in children, especially those less than 4 years of age. Results from blunt trauma such as falls, assaults, or baseball to temporal area. Arterial or venous bleeding occurs between the skull and the dura; associated with skull fracture.	• Minimal or absent symptoms at time of injury, followed by rapid deterioration in mental status and signs of increased ICP • Headache or full fontanelle • Paresis of cranial nerves III and VI • Papilledema • Fixed and dilated pupil
CEREBRAL CONTUSION Bruising on surface of brain is associated with coup and contrecoup injuries, including the base of the brain as it moves across the bony prominences in the base of the skull. Commonly occurs on frontal and temporal lobes. Is the most common TBI.	• Altered levels of consciousness ranging from confusion and disorientation to being obtunded • Focal symptoms depending on the area of injury
DIFFUSE AXONAL INJURY Results from rapid acceleration-deceleration injuries, such as with motor vehicle crash or shaken child syndrome. Nerve fibers are torn in both cerebral hemispheres and other brain areas. Other organ systems may also be injured.	• Immediate loss of consciousness • Unconsciousness lasting longer than 6 hr • Abnormal movements or posturing • Seizures • Increased ICP • Difficulty regulating blood pressure and breathing
SUBARACHNOID HEMORRHAGE Associated with severe head injuries such as intracranial hematomas or contusions; results from tearing of arteries or veins in the subarachnoid space.	• Progressive decrease in LOC • Severe headache, nausea, and vomiting • Ipsilateral pupil dilation • Diplopia • Hemiparesis • Nuchal rigidity
INTRACEREBRAL HEMATOMA Often results from acceleration-deceleration injury or penetrating injury; hemorrhage to frontal or temporal lobe.	• Focal symptoms depend on size and location of hematoma, such as epilepsy

ventilation, relieve pain, and lower the ICP. Medications to prevent seizures may be prescribed. Therapeutic hypothermia may be used. Sometimes despite all efforts, the child dies as a result of the consequences of the TBI.

If there is no cervical spine injury, the head of the bed is elevated up to 30 degrees. The child's head is kept in the midline to promote venous (jugular) drainage. Hip flexion is avoided. Normothermia is maintained. The environment is kept as quiet as possible. A urinary catheter is inserted to monitor output. Enteral nutrition support is started, using a postpyloric feeding tube to reduce the risk for aspiration.

Rehabilitation.   Initial stages of rehabilitation are made during the acute phase of management to prevent complications from immobilization, disuse, and neurologic dysfunction. Physical therapists, occupational therapists, speech-language specialists, and social workers all play vital roles. Moderate and severe TBI may result in a permanent disability, such as epilepsy, motor and cognitive impairments, learning problems, hearing and vision impairment, communication problems, and behavioral or emotional problems. Difficulties with learning skills are common. Reliable predictions of outcome in the child who has experienced a severe brain injury cannot be made until 6 to 12 months postinjury. One study reported that 61.6% of children with moderate and severe injuries were reported to receive services such as special education, 504 accommodations (see Chapter 38), tutoring, and occupational, physical, and speech therapy for disabilities 12 months after injury (Rivara et al., 2012).

Nursing Management
For the Child With Traumatic Brain Injury

Nursing Assessment and Diagnosis

Frequently assess the child's neurologic status using guidelines in *Assessment Guide: The Child With a Neurologic Condition* at the beginning of this chapter and the Glasgow Coma Scale (see Table 54–2). Compare findings to prior evaluations, and note improvement, stability, or deterioration. Assess the cranial nerves and pupils for size and reactivity. Monitor vital signs, responsiveness, and behavior carefully. Note any irritability or signs that might indicate increased ICP (see Table 54–1). Changes in these signs may indicate hypoxia, decreased perfusion, shock, or increased ICP. When the child has a decreased level of consciousness shortly after a brain injury, consider if a posttraumatic seizure occurred and if the child could still be in the postictal state. The cause of any deterioration must be quickly determined and appropriate interventions taken.

Observe for physiologic and behavioral signs of pain. Assume that the child with increased ICP is in pain, even when unresponsive. Assess the family's coping with the child's life-threatening injury and any support systems available to them (see Chapter 41).

Examples of nursing diagnoses appropriate for the child with TBI include the following (NANDA-I © 2014):

- *Tissue Perfusion: Cerebral, Risk for Ineffective,* related to hypoventilation, hypovolemia, and/or reduction of arterial blood flow to the brain due to increased ICP
- *Aspiration, Risk for,* related to decreased LOC and loss of protective reflexes
- *Fluid Volume: Imbalanced, Risk for,* related to therapies for reducing ICP
- *Coping: Family, Compromised,* related to life-threatening injury to child

Planning and Implementation

HOSPITAL-BASED NURSING CARE
The child with a severe TBI is initially cared for in the pediatric ICU. Nursing care focuses on maintaining cerebral perfusion pressure, minimizing increased ICP, reducing stimulation, preventing complications, and providing emotional support.

Once the child is on the general pediatric unit, maintain cardiopulmonary function. In the moderately injured child, observe breathing patterns and check color, neurologic signs, and LOC. The oxygen saturation should remain over 95%. Report any sign of decreased oxygenation or signs and symptoms of increased ICP to the healthcare provider immediately (see Table 54–1). Keep suction equipment at the bedside in case aspiration occurs.

Reduce physiologic stresses on the body that could increase ICP. Minimize unpleasant stimuli when possible, keep the environment quiet, and avoid jarring the bed. Pain management and temperature control are important. Position the child with the bed flat or elevated 15 to 30 degrees to avoid excessive flexion of the hips, and maintain the head and neck in neutral alignment to encourage venous return to the heart. The child may also be placed in a side-lying position with the head neither flexed nor extended. Monitor the effect of nursing procedures on ICP. Determine if clustering procedures is better than spreading procedures over time. Encourage parents to talk to the child and provide comforting touch.

Administer medications as prescribed. When the child is unresponsive, provide oral care to keep mucous membranes moist and intact and to reduce the risk for infection, especially if the child is being ventilated (see the *Clinical Skills Manual* SKILLS). Pad and cushion bony prominences, provide skin care, and change the child's position frequently. Protect the eyes from corneal irritation with ophthalmic ointment and patching.

Enteral feeding may be used initially, slowly progressing to oral foods as tolerated. Fluids are given to meet daily fluid requirements, or to maintain the child's blood pressure within normal ranges for age. Stool softeners and suppositories should be used as needed to prevent constipation. The side rails of the bed should be padded to protect the child if a seizure occurs.

Promote recovery and prevent physical deformities. Perform passive range-of-motion (ROM) exercises to prevent contractures. Splints may be used to position extremities in functional positions. Work with physical, occupational, and speech therapists to reinforce exercises and help teach parents the techniques so they can work with the child in the hospital and at home.

Provide stimulation and promote general awareness when the child is ready, based on the child's age and ability, by using toys, books, music, or games. Assist the family to provide stimulation but also to provide quiet time when the child displays agitation.

Provide emotional support to the family in collaboration with the social workers, healthcare providers, psychologists, rehabilitation therapists, and members of the clergy caring for the child and family. All can help the family adjust to having a child with a new disability.

Sometimes despite all efforts, the child dies as a result of the consequences of the brain injury. Provide support for the family while brain death testing is performed. See Chapter 41 for brain death criteria and methods for supporting the family when termination of life support and organ donation are discussed.

DISCHARGE PLANNING AND HOME CARE TEACHING
Children with serious TBIs may be transferred to an inpatient rehabilitation center to promote optimal achievement of function. Other children may have outpatient rehabilitation prescribed, and thus home care needs should be identified and addressed well in advance of discharge. A case manager is often needed to coordinate services and resources during rehabilitation. Social services intervention may be needed when brain injury results from child abuse.

Give parents information about caring for children with mild or moderate TBIs at home and possible behaviors to expect from the child. For children with disabilities, determine what adaptations and assistive technology are needed in the home to care for the child, such as a wheelchair, a walker, braces, or a special bed.

COMMUNITY-BASED NURSING CARE
Home care nursing may be important for the child with an acquired neurologic dysfunction and prolonged altered consciousness. The nurse can teach the family to meet the child's needs, monitor the intake of fluids and foods, position the child,

Marcus, 7 years old, was struck by a car and thrown several feet. He was unconscious on admission to the emergency department and showed some signs of increased ICP (dilated and fixed pupils). He was treated for shock, and his neurologic status and vital signs were frequently assessed. Marcus was found to have sustained several contusions of the brain, but no skull fracture. He was intubated and medicated to manage the increased ICP.

Marcus's ICP has now stabilized, but he has not totally regained consciousness. He is restless and agitated, and unable to follow directions. His parents stay at his bedside and provide auditory and tactile stimulation, hoping he will eventually respond. He receives physical therapy to prevent contractures and to maintain function. Marcus will need long-term rehabilitation to achieve the best outcome possible after this injury.

What is the role of the nurse in acute care of the child with a severe brain injury? What support does the family need to contribute to the child's care? How would you work with other healthcare providers to coordinate care during the acute care phase? How would you help plan the long-term care for a child such as Marcus?

and provide skin care. In-home physical therapists may teach parents to perform ROM exercises and other strategies to prevent contractures. Regular follow-up visits are needed to assess the child's recovery and to modify the treatment plan.

Children with moderate brain injuries often have long-term problems with attention, problem solving, speed of information processing, and behavior problems (e.g., impulsivity, irritability, apathy, aggression, and social withdrawal). Neuropsychologic testing is needed to identify subtle learning disabilities that are not usually revealed on standardized school achievement tests. Educational accommodations needed are usually different from those made for children with other learning disabilities.

The child or adolescent facing long-term rehabilitation needs support to adjust to the disability and to find the strength to maximize his or her abilities. Identify recreational opportunities for the child with disabilities to promote exercise and self-esteem. The adolescent may need to gain vocational skills and learn to live independently. Refer parents to the Brain Injury Association for further information.

Prevention of brain injury is another important role of the nurse. Encourage parents to obtain protective helmets and require children to use them for bicycling and skateboarding. Parents should be encouraged to wear a helmet themselves as role models. Encourage parents to monitor playgrounds for appropriate use of wood chips or cushioning tiles to reduce the severity of injuries associated with falls.

Evaluation

Examples of expected outcomes of nursing care for the family and child with TBI include the following:

- Cerebral perfusion pressure is maintained at an adequate rate to sustain oxygenation of the brain.
- Muscle function is maintained and physical deformities are prevented with ROM exercises and splinting during the recovery stages of the brain injury.

- Parents are supported through the child's acute recovery phase and learn to provide care the child will need at home.
- The child's school performance is monitored and appropriate educational resources are provided to support the child's learning.

Concussion

A concussion is a mild TBI that usually results from a direct blow to the head, face, neck, or other part of the body. Nearly a half million emergency department visits per year are associated with a concussion in children under age 15 years (Mason, 2013). Organized sports (football, hockey, rugby, soccer, and basketball) and other activities (snow skiing, skateboarding, falls from bicycles, and horseback riding) are associated with concussion.

The blow causes stretching and bruising of brain tissue that disrupts nerve transmission and metabolic function, but no structural abnormality is seen with radiographic imaging. While most children have concussion symptoms for up to 7 to 10 days, their cognitive recovery often takes longer.

The child with a concussion has a rapid onset of short-term functional impairment that may or may not involve loss of consciousness and cognitive, physical, emotional, and sleep symptoms that may persist for minutes to months (Meckler, 2014).

- *Physical*—headache, sensitivity to light or noise, dazed, visual problems, balance problems, fatigue, and nausea and vomiting
- *Cognitive*—feeling foggy or sluggish, difficulty concentrating and remembering, confused about recent events, answers slowly
- *Emotional*—irritable, sad, nervous, more emotional than usual
- *Sleep*—drowsy, sleeps more or less than normal, difficulty falling asleep

Pediatric concussive syndrome is thought to be caused by an injury to the brainstem and occurs in children younger than age 3 years. Toddlers seem stunned at the time of injury, but have no loss of consciousness. Later, these children become pale, clammy, and lethargic, and they may vomit.

Initial sideline evaluation of the child injured in an organized sport involves removing the child from play, and using a checklist to assess orientation, recent and remote memory, new learning, concentration, and balance (Harmon et al., 2013). Questions are asked about events before and after the injury to help identify amnesia, an important sign of a more serious injury. A history is taken and physical examination performed in the health center or emergency department. Because no findings are typically found on CT and MRI, radiologic imaging is not performed unless an intracranial structural injury is suspected. Computerized neuropsychologic tests are available to test a high school athlete's baseline performance for comparison after concussion to monitor recovery.

Treatment is supportive. Children are observed in the emergency department for several hours before being sent home with instructions to the parents to watch them closely for decreased responsiveness. The child who is unconscious for more than 5 minutes or has amnesia of the event may be admitted to the hospital or be observed in a short-stay unit to rule out other injury. All cognitive activities are limited in the first few days after injury, including time out of school, video games, watching television, and using a computer (Meckler,

2014). Before returning to organized sports, the child should be symptom-free and using no analgesia for headache. Symptoms usually disappear within several weeks but may last up to 6 months. Physical activities are gradually increased, and if symptoms recur, return to play is further delayed.

Even though the child looks normal following a brain injury, ensure that parents and teachers know that brain healing takes up to 6 weeks. Typical behaviors during this healing period may include tiring easily, memory loss or forgetfulness, easy distractibility, difficulty concentrating, difficulty following directions, irritability or short temper, and needing help starting and finishing tasks. Return the child to a full school schedule gradually to prevent fatigue and frustration. Educational assessment should be initiated if recovery takes longer than 6 weeks.

Young athletes who return to play too soon may have a delayed reaction time and be at greater risk for a second concussion. Long-term neurologic problems may result from recurrent concussions.

Professionalism in Practice Concussion
Management in the School Setting

The American Academy of Neurology recently updated guidelines for evaluation and management of concussions (Giza et al., 2013). Many activities in the school setting (e.g., sports, physical education, and playtime) can place the child at risk for a concussion. School nurses collaborate with school staff members, athletic trainers, and parents to prevent concussions and to assess the child with a potential concussion. Nurses may also coordinate the development of an individualized health plan to accommodate the child's graduated return to school and sports. They also help the teachers understand the emotional and behavioral responses of the child returning to the classroom (National Association of School Nurses [NASN], 2012).

Scalp Injuries

Injuries to the scalp, which can be caused by falls, blunt trauma, or penetration of a foreign body, are usually benign. Bleeding may be extensive, but hypovolemia or shock is uncommon unless the patient is an infant.

Lacerations should be irrigated with copious amounts of sterile normal saline solution and inspected for bony fragments or depressions, CSF leakage with a dural tear, or debris. If the injury is simple, the laceration can be sutured and the child discharged from the emergency department. If more severe, a neurosurgeon should be consulted.

Skull Fractures

A fracture to any of the eight cranial bones requires considerable force:

- *Linear fracture*—most common type of fracture, can potentially be caused by child abuse. May have overlying hematoma or soft tissue swelling; usually no symptoms.

- *Depressed skull fracture*—break in skull itself or an area shattered into many fragments. Pieces of bone may be depressed into brain tissue with hematoma forming on top.

- *Basilar fracture*—fracture at the base of the skull; may involve the frontal, ethmoid, sphenoid, temporal, or occipital bones; a dural tear may be present; increases risk for

meningitis. The child may have blood behind the tympanic membranes, CSF leakage (yellow to amber fluid) from the nose or ears, periorbital ecchymosis (raccoon eyes), or bruising of the mastoid (Battle sign).

Any area of the skull with swelling or a hematoma should be evaluated for possible fracture. Diagnosis is made by visual inspection, palpation, skull radiograph, or CT scan.

Treatment includes neurosurgical consultation. Surgery may be required for debridement or to elevate bone fragments of a depressed skull fracture. Tetanus prophylaxis and antibiotic therapy may be prescribed in some cases. Some skull fractures may be associated with intracranial bleeding, cranial nerve injuries, and posttraumatic epilepsy.

Penetrating Injuries

Gunshot wounds to the head can damage brain tissue, bone, and blood vessels. The child's level of consciousness quickly deteriorates because of the edema surrounding the penetration tract.

CT scans evaluate gunshot trauma and pinpoint the location of bullet and bone fragments as well as damaged brain tissue. Surgery is performed to debride the tract, evacuate any hematomas, and remove accessible bone or bullet particles. A high percentage of these children die. Those who survive may suffer multiple focal deficits and seizures.

Impalement injuries may occur in children in association with projectiles, dog bites, or other sharp objects. All objects must be left in place and removed in the operating room by a neurosurgeon. The child is at high risk for focal injury and infection. After surgery, children are managed in the same manner as other postoperative brain injuries, with attention focused on level of consciousness, management of increased ICP, and infection control.

Spinal Cord Injury

Injury to the spinal cord is a rare condition that causes major lifelong disabilities and a shortened life. Only 2% to 5% of spinal cord injuries occur in the pediatric population, and more commonly involve cervical spine injury (Pettiford et al., 2012). Mechanisms of injury in children and adolescents include motor vehicle crashes (passenger and pedestrian), recreational activities, and violence (child abuse, stabbing, and gunshot wounds).

The mechanism of injury and direction of forces determine the type of lesion that occurs (Figure 54–14). Hyperflexion injuries (e.g., bending around a car safety seat belt) produce tears or avulsions and fractures of vertebral bodies, as well as subluxation and dislocation. Rotation may cause joint dislocations or unstable spinal fractures. Hyperextension may result in the so-called hangman's fracture, ligament tears, avulsion fractures of vertebral bodies, and central or posterior spinal cord syndrome. Compression injuries may occur when a child falls from a height. Young children are prone to specific kinds of spinal cord injuries because of the mobility and flexibility of their spinal column.

Spinal cord injuries are classified as complete or incomplete. Complete lesions are irreversible and involve a loss of sensory, motor, and autonomic function below the level of the injury. Incomplete lesions involve varying degrees of sensory, motor, and autonomic function below the level of injury. Autonomic dysfunction is associated with hypotension, loss of bladder and bowel control, and loss of environmental thermoregulatory function. The higher the level of spinal cord injury, the more severe the neurologic damage. Table 54–14 describes the spinal cord injuries that occur in children.

At the time of injury due to compression, shear injuries, or other injury, the child is flaccid and loses reflexes below the

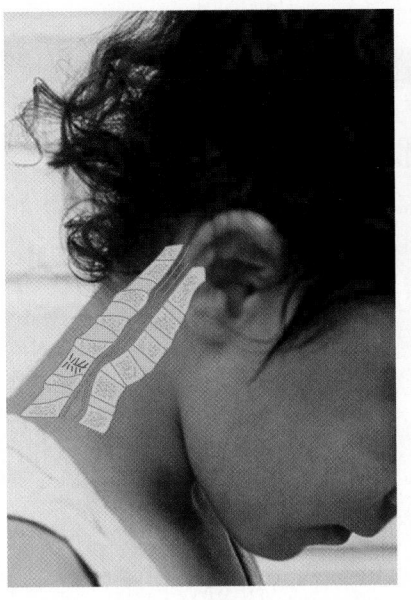
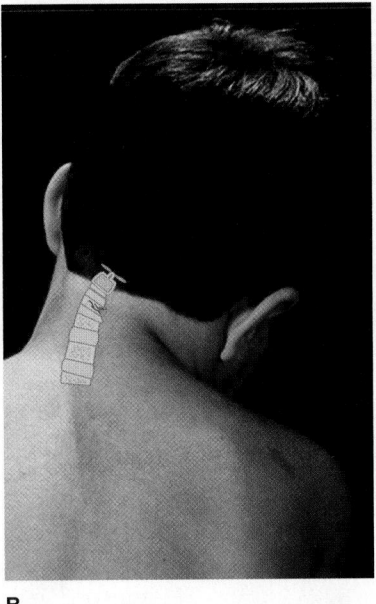
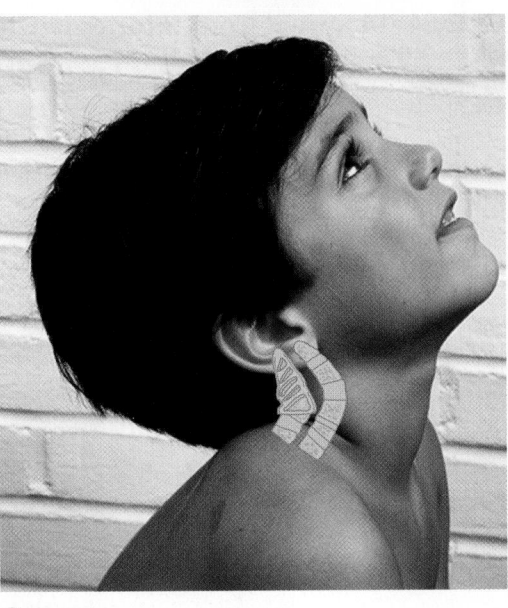

A   B   C

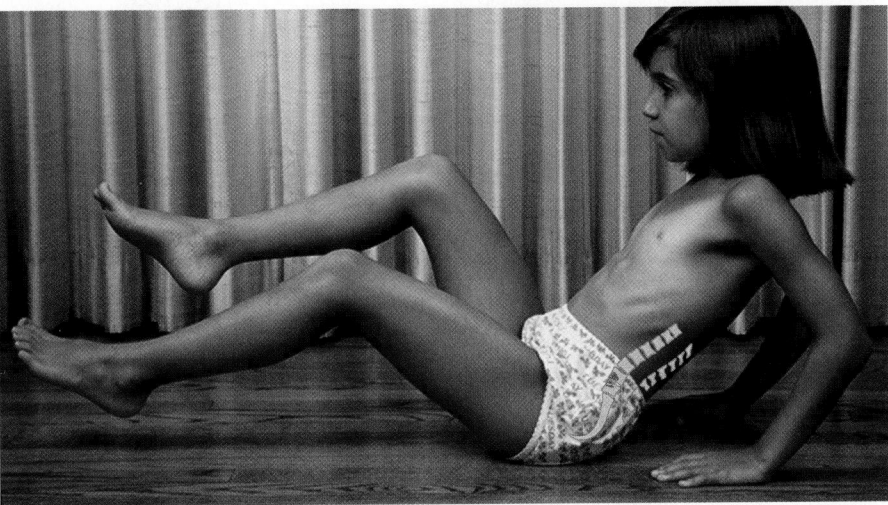
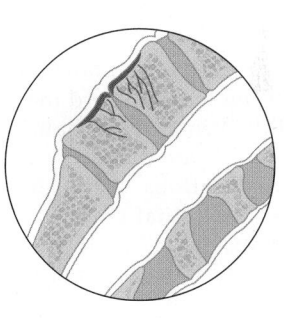

D

Figure 54–14 Mechanics of injury to the spinal cord. *A*, Hyperflexion. *B*, Lateral flexion. *C*, Hyperextension. *D*, Compression.

level of the lesion. Inflammation causes a secondary injury, resulting in ischemia and necrosis. **Spinal shock**, spinal cord concussion resulting in a transient suppression of nerve function below the level of the acute injury, occurs. Some return of function may occur within the first 72 hours of injury in an incomplete lesion. As neurologic recovery begins, spinal reflex activity returns and increasing spasticity is seen below the level of the injury.

The child can experience neurogenic shock in which there is loss of vasomotor tone and sympathetic innervations of the heart, resulting in hypotension, bradycardia, and peripheral vasodilation (a form of distributive shock). See Chapter 47. Priapism may be seen. Respiratory compromise may be present because of paralysis of the diaphragm.

Diagnosis is made by observation, neurologic examination, and radiologic studies of the cervical, thoracic, and lumbosacral spine to determine if a vertebral fracture or compression on the spinal cord is present. When a child with a suspected spinal cord injury was immobilized by prehospital providers,

cautious physical and radiologic evaluations are needed before the child is unrestrained. In addition, CT scanning, MRI, fluoroscopy, or myelography may be performed. Some young children have spinal cord injury without radiographic abnormality (SCIWORA) on a plain radiograph, but an MRI can detect the injury to ligaments and soft tissues.

Growth and Development

The vertebrae are not fully ossified in children younger than 9 years. The facet joints are more shallow and horizontal, allowing them to slide over each other more easily as the ligaments stretch. The young child's head is relatively large compared to the strength of the neck muscles. When the neck muscle strength is exceeded, the ligaments supporting the vertebrae can stretch much more than the spinal cord, leading to spinal cord tearing. Injuries to children under age 9 are more likely to occur at the C1 to C3 level, and at the C4 to C6 level in children ages 9 to 15.

TABLE 54–14 Spinal Cord Injuries in Children

SPINE REGION	INJURY CHARACTERISTICS
Cervical	• Site of the majority of spinal injuries in children under 10 years • Injury above C3 segment causes respiratory arrest and death without ventilatory support; many of these injuries are fatal • Diaphragm function is present when injury is at C5 level • **Tetraplegia,** can have loss of sensation and function of the head and neck and upper and lower extremities • Loss of sphincter function • Sensory level lost below the sternum
Thoracic	• More commonly, the site of spinal injuries in children between 8 and 14 years • Full control of upper extremities including hands • Poor trunk balance
Thoracolumbar	• Full control of muscles in abdomen and upper back • Good trunk balance
Lumbar	• Injuries at the L1–L3 level may occur in children 4–8 years using a car lap belt rather than a car safety seat • Below L3 may have functioning of muscles in upper leg • Loss of ankle and foot control

Spinal injuries are managed aggressively. The child with a confirmed spinal cord injury may be placed in external immobilization with a halo device. Surgery to reduce and internally fixate the fracture is performed for unstable fractures, dislocations, and progressive deformity. Decompression of the spinal cord and nerve roots may be performed if transection is not complete or if compression by a clot, herniated disk, or other lesion is present and can be relieved.

To decrease neurologic sequelae in children with motor deficits, a high-dose methylprednisolone is often administered intravenously if started within 8 hours of injury. Evidence does not clearly indicate a benefit to this treatment, and adverse effects include increased risk of infection, hyperglycemia, and gastrointestinal bleeding (Pettiford et al., 2012). Gastrointestinal prophylaxis is started to reduce the risk for an ulcer. Atropine and norepinephrine may be given to manage spinal shock. IV fluid resuscitation is also performed if the child could have hypovolemic shock from other injuries. Complications of spinal cord injury include:

- Impaired respiratory function due to a paralyzed diaphragm or diminished vital capacity
- Scoliosis if injury occurs before the skeleton is mature
- Hip instability due to poor acetabular development
- Pathologic fractures of the long bones due to immobilization hypercalcemia
- Pressure sores
- Deep vein thrombosis
- Autonomic dysreflexia

Spasticity, muscle atrophy, increased risk of respiratory problems, weight gain, osteoporosis, and other skeletal problems are long-term issues for many children. The goal of rehabilitation is to promote independence in daily activities, as well as mobility, strength, power, and endurance.

SAFETY ALERT!

Autonomic dysreflexia is a condition associated with injuries above the T6 level. It becomes a medical emergency when overactivity of the autonomic nervous system causes an abrupt onset of hypertension, cardiac arrhythmia, pupillary constriction, severe headaches, flushing above the level of the spinal cord lesion, and sweating. Below the level of the lesion, the skin is pale and cool with piloerection. Common triggers are constipation, a full bladder, or a pressure ulcer. Treatment involves positioning the patient upright, loosening tight clothing, emptying the bladder, eliminating any precipitating stimulus, and administering antihypertensive medication. Prevention of autonomic dysreflexia involves an effective bowel and bladder program and prevention of pressure ulcers (Stephenson & Berliner, 2014).

Nursing Management
For the Child With Spinal Cord Injury

HOSPITAL-BASED NURSING CARE

Nursing care focuses on monitoring vital signs, meeting nutritional needs, maintaining skin integrity, promoting independent functioning, providing emotional support, and promoting rehabilitation.

Be alert for any changes in vital signs, especially those that may signify increased respiratory difficulty, neurogenic shock (hypotension, bradycardia, and peripheral vasodilation), increased ICP (see Table 54–1), or autonomic dysreflexia. Monitor intake and output. Monitor bladder and bowel function. Assess the skin for integrity.

With higher cervical injuries, assess the cranial nerves as they may be affected by swelling around the spinal cord. Note the return of reflexes and change from flaccid tone to spasticity. Identify any changes in level of sensation or motor function. Carefully check the immobilizing device to ensure that the spine stays stable.

Some children with cervical lesions have tracheostomies performed to help maintain airway patency; others with high cervical lesions are dependent on ventilators. Keep suctioning equipment and other emergency equipment at the bedside at all times.

Ensure adequate nutrition. A child with complete paralysis may require a gastrostomy tube. When the child begins to eat, feed soft foods slowly as the child may have some swallowing difficulties.

Prevent skin breakdown (see Chapter 57). Observe surgical sites for signs of infection or inflammation. Provide regular traction pin site care according to hospital guidelines. Establish a schedule for patient repositioning.

Promote independent functioning by reinforcing the exercises and skills learned in physical and occupational therapy. Use supports, boots, footboards, splints, and braces as recommended by the therapists to prevent contractures. If hand mobility is limited, explore options for independence. Encourage the child to be as independent as possible in a wheelchair. An important mobility goal is to achieve wheelchair transfer and to perform self-care. Identify adaptive equipment that makes these goals possible.

Achieving bowel and bladder control may be difficult. Regular intermittent catheterizations may be necessary if urinary retention occurs (see the *Clinical Skills Manual* SKILLS). Anticipate that constipation will occur and initiate bowel training with a diet high in fiber and the use of stool softeners.

Therapeutic play appropriate for the child's developmental level is an important part of the healing process. Provide as many normal activities for the child as possible, but do not give the child tasks that will be difficult to complete. Child-life teachers or tutors can help the child keep up with schoolwork.

Television, DVDs, computer games, Internet connections, and music can offer diversion for prolonged hospitalization. Children with paraplegia can learn to use their arms and hands to play interactive games. Devices can also be adapted so that the child can play computer games or manipulate the television or radio. Identify assistive technology that may help the child with tetraplegia gain some level of independence.

Support the child emotionally. Encourage the child to meet small, short-term goals, including those that involve self-care. Encourage the child to express fears and frustrations.

Be compassionate and understanding. Encourage siblings to visit, answer their questions honestly, and help them to discuss their feelings. Involve the parents and siblings in the child's care as much as possible. When appropriate, encourage them to help with activities of daily living.

DISCHARGE PLANNING AND HOME CARE TEACHING

Many children are discharged to inpatient rehabilitation facilities. Assist with arrangements for the transfer. Work closely with the child, parents, and other members of the healthcare team concerning placement. Home care needs, reintegration into educational programs, and safety issues should be identified and addressed well in advance of discharge from the rehabilitation facility. Refer families to social services, family counseling, and support groups if indicated.

Hypoxic-Ischemic Brain Injury (Drowning)

Drowning is defined as the process resulting in primary respiratory impairment from submersion/immersion in a liquid medium. *Submersion injury* is the term used when the child survives. Drowning, a leading cause of unintentional injury death for children of all ages between birth and 19 years,

caused 866 deaths in the United States in 2013. Children 1 to 4 years and 15 to 19 years old had the highest rate of drowning deaths in 2013 (National Center for Injury Prevention and Control, 2015). Boys are affected more frequently than girls. For every death, an additional two children are hospitalized for nonfatal drowning events (Bowman, Aiken, Robbins, et al., 2012).

In young children, drowning is associated with bathing and falling in water (e.g., pools or large buckets). Older children are more likely to drown in open water, potentially associated with risk-taking behaviors, seizures, or alcohol use (Bowman et al., 2012).

It takes only enough water to cover the nose and mouth for a child to drown. The child trapped in water panics, struggles, tries to move using swimming motions, and holds the breath. The child aspirates a small amount of water from the oropharynx, causing a laryngospasm that lasts no more than 2 minutes and hypoxia. Because of increasing panic and hypoxia, the child swallows more liquid. As the laryngospasm passes, the child breathes water into the lungs. The child may also vomit and aspirate stomach contents. Aspirated water damages the lung surfactant and impairs alveolar gas exchange. Hypothermia may result because the child's body cools faster in water than in air, and systemic perfusion decreases as a result (see Chapter 57). With increasing hypoxia, the cardiac muscle becomes impaired and ultimately the heart stops.

Anoxia associated with drowning leads to cerebral edema and increased ICP and secondary cerebral injuries. With aggressive cardiopulmonary resuscitation the child may survive, but usually with neurologic impairment.

The signs and symptoms of submersion vary by the length of time underwater, temperature of the water, response to the episode, and the initial scene treatment. The child who has been submerged may be apneic and pulseless. When submerged for short periods (less than 5 to 10 minutes and resuscitated at the scene), children may have few symptoms and fully recover without neurologic impairment. Signs and symptoms in the rescued child may be decreased level of consciousness ranging from stupor to total unresponsiveness, apnea or irregular respirations, gastric distention, and seizures. The child submerged for longer than 10 minutes or who has delayed cardiopulmonary resuscitation is more likely to have neurologic impairment or to die.

Immediate cardiopulmonary resuscitation (CPR) performed at the scene is associated with the best outcomes. Emergency personnel with a defibrillator should assess the heart rhythm and defibrillate if ventricular fibrillation is present. The child should be transported to the hospital even if the child begins breathing spontaneously. Initial emergency treatment is 100% oxygen and rewarming. The airway may be secured with an endotracheal tube.

SAFETY ALERT!

All submersion victims should be observed in the hospital for 6 to 8 hours, even when initially asymptomatic. Signs of respiratory distress and cerebral edema develop within this timeline, and immediate care can be provided as needed.

The child who has a serious anoxic injury is cared for in the ICU. Mechanical ventilation may be used to keep the alveoli open, to promote adequate oxygenation, and to prevent respiratory acidosis. Treatment for cerebral edema is initiated (see earlier section on care of the child with a traumatic brain injury).

Nursing Management

Nursing care of the child who survives a submersion incident focuses on monitoring the child's neurologic and cardiopulmonary status and providing emotional support to the family.

Assess the child's responsiveness, spontaneous respiratory efforts, oxygenation, and vital signs. Perform frequent neurologic status assessments. Attach a cardiorespiratory monitor and pulse oximeter for continuous patient assessment information.

Implement the nursing interventions for a child with altered states of consciousness as described earlier in this chapter. If cerebral edema develops, implement nursing interventions as described in the earlier section on care of the child with a traumatic brain injury.

Provide emotional support to the family. Be nonjudgmental and provide a forum for parents to express their feelings. Reassure parents who exhibit guilt reactions that their child is receiving all possible medical treatment. Parents may be faced with an unknown prognosis. Encourage them to seek assistance from social workers, members of the clergy, close friends, and relatives. Arrange for appropriate referrals. If the child's prognosis is poor, an ethics consultation may be offered to educate the family about options for decision making regarding sustaining or terminating life support (see Chapter 41).

Identify and address rehabilitation or home care needs well in advance of discharge. Assist with arrangements for the child with minor deficits. Assign a case manager to the child with significant neurologic impairments so that long-term care options can be explored. Inpatient or outpatient rehabilitation options should be matched to the child's needs and family resources.

Drowning can be prevented by education, legislation, and changes in the environment. Pool owners should erect climb-proof 5-foot fences around all four sides of the pool. If fencing is on three sides, with the house serving as the fourth side, the house door to the pool area should be kept locked and have an alarm. Local ordinances may require such fences. Ensure that hot tubs and pools have drain covers or other safety devices that prevent a child from getting a limb or hair entrapped in a drain. Adolescents should learn the dangers of mixing alcohol or drugs and swimming. Keep 5- and 10-gallon buckets empty when not in use. Emphasize the importance of closely supervising children when near or in the water, whether at pools, at the beach, or in the bathtub. Children with seizure disorders should always have a buddy when swimming.

Focus Your Study

- The nervous system is complete with all nerve cells at birth. Myelination continues throughout childhood.

- Altered level of consciousness is caused by infection, trauma, hypoxia, poisoning, seizures, alcohol or substance abuse, endocrine or metabolic disturbances (e.g. diabetic ketoacidosis), electrolyte or acid–base imbalance, intracranial space-occupying lesion, stroke, and a congenital structural defect.

- Emergency care for the child or adolescent with a prolonged generalized seizure includes airway management, supplemental oxygen, intravenous benzodiazepines, and careful monitoring of vital signs and motor activity. Carefully document the duration of the seizure or series of seizures to detect status epilepticus.

- Neurologic damage from bacterial meningitis often occurs in infants and young children despite early, aggressive management. Complications may include hearing impairment, gross neurologic deficits, and behavioral and intellectual disorders.

- Encephalitis is an acute inflammation of the brain often caused by a virus that is transmitted by a mosquito, such as West Nile virus and Western Equine virus. Presenting signs include a severe headache, fever, irritability, and altered mental status.

- Reye syndrome is an encephalopathy with a high mortality rate that is associated with aspirin use for a mild viral illness. Because most parents give children acetaminophen or ibuprofen rather than aspirin for flulike symptoms and varicella, Reye syndrome has become rare.

- Guillain-Barré syndrome is a disorder of deteriorating motor function and paralysis that progress in an ascending pattern, paresthesia, and areflexia. It may be caused by an autoimmune response to an infectious organism, usually within 1 to 3 weeks of a gastrointestinal or respiratory illness.

- More than 75% of children experience a headache by age 15 years. Types of benign headaches include migraines, inflammatory (sinusitis), and tension.

- Microcephaly is a small brain that may be caused by genetic transmission, fetal or postnatal insult, or intrauterine infection.

- Hydrocephalus is caused by the blockage of cerebrospinal fluid flow through normal channels and pathways or the impaired absorption of cerebrospinal fluid in the subarachnoid space and the arachnoid villi. It can be associated with a congenital condition or acquired from meningitis or intraventricular hemorrhage, tumor, or structural deformity.

- The more common types of neural tube defects include anencephaly (no development of the brain above the brainstem), encephalocele (protrusion of meningeal or skin-covered brain through the skull), and myelomeningocele or spina bifida.

- Myelomeningocele or spina bifida is a malformation of the vertebrae and spinal canal with a protrusion of a meningeal sac filled with a portion of the spinal cord. It is the most common developmental disorder of the CNS.

- Positional plagiocephaly, an asymmetric flattening of the occiput, is associated with sleep position to prevent sudden infant death syndrome or with neck problems such as congenital torticollis. The weight of the infant head sometimes flattens the skull. Strategies to encourage the child to change the position of the head may help reduce its occurrence.

- Neurofibromatosis 1 is characterized by multiple café au lait spots, darker than the surrounding skin, that are 5 mm (0.2 in.) or larger in infants but grow to 15 mm (0.6 in.) in diameter during adolescence. Multiple benign tumors grow on or under the skin beginning during puberty.

- Most cases of cerebral palsy are characterized by spasticity and a lack of coordination. The risk for cerebral palsy is increased with prematurity, intraventricular hemorrhage, intrauterine infection, neonatal sepsis, and hyperbilirubinemia.

- Traumatic brain injury is a leading cause of death and disability during childhood. It results from falls, motor vehicle crashes, sports injuries, and child abuse.

- Concussions result from the stretching, compression, and shearing of nerve fibers after an impact injury to the head that causes signs such as transient altered mental status, amnesia, dizziness, and impairment of memory, orientation, and balance.

- Spinal cord injuries, although relatively rare in children, often result from significant forces such as from motor vehicle crashes. Because of the child's larger and heavier head and weaker neck muscles, cervical spine injuries are more common.

- Children who have the best outcomes following drowning include those submerged less than 5 minutes who receive immediate cardiopulmonary resuscitation.

Clinical Reasoning in Action

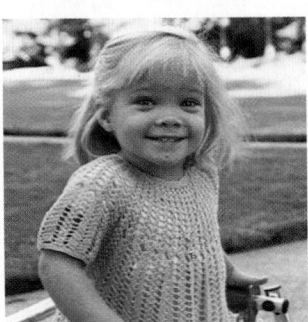

Abigail, a 3-year-old with myelodysplasia, is seen every few months with her parents in the multidisciplinary spina bifida clinic where you work. Her lesion is at the L3 level, so she can flex her hips and extend her knees, but her ankles and toes are paralyzed. She also has a ventriculoperitoneal shunt for hydrocephalus. She uses lower leg braces and a walker to mobilize and has minimal sensation in her lower legs and feet. Her bladder and bowel sphincters are also affected, so Abigail and her parents have worked hard to establish bowel control with a high-fiber diet and by establishing specific times for bowel evacuation. Abigail's parents learned to perform intermittent catheterization for bladder control to reduce the risk for kidney damage.

Her health history reveals she has experienced a case of otitis media since her last visit and responded well to antibiotics. Her legs are well protected by stockings to reduce rubbing by her braces. Her gait is becoming steadier with the walker, and her parents are encouraging exercise of her arms and upper trunk with swimming. You encourage Abigail's parents to promote her cognitive development with age-appropriate games and interaction with siblings. Her parents plan to enroll her in preschool in the fall.

1. What are the safety issues to discuss with Abigail's parents about spina bifida?

2. Describe spina bifida and its relationship with hydrocephalus.

3. Identify important health promotion issues to discuss with Abigail's parents.

4. Describe the issues that need to be addressed in planning for an IEP and individual health plan when Abigail enters preschool.

References

Adzick, N. S., Thom, E. A., Spong, C. Y., Brock, J. W., Burrows, P. K., Johnson, M. P., ... Farmer, D. L. (2011). A randomized trial of prenatal versus postnatal repair of myelomeningocele. *New England Journal of Medicine, 364*(11), 993–1004.

Antonaci, F., Voiticovschi-Iosob, C., Di Stefano, A. L., Galli, F., Ozge, A., & Balottin, U. (2014). The evolution of headache from childhood to adulthood: A review of the literature. *Journal of Headache and Pain, 15,* 15. Retrieved from http://www.thejournalofheadacheandpain.com/content/15/1/15

Aronson, E., & Stevenson, S. B. (2012). Bone health in children with cerebral palsy. *Journal of Pediatric Health Care, 26*(3), 193–199.

Beaulieu, M. J. (2013). Leviteracetam. *Neonatal Network, 32*(4), 285–288.

Bethel, J. (2012). Emergency care of children and adults with head injury. *Nursing Standard, 26*(43), 49–56.

Blosser, C. G., Albers, A. C., & Reider-Demer, M. (2012). Headache. In C. Burns, A. M. Dunn, M. A. Brady, N. B. Starr, & C. G. Blosser (Eds.), *Pediatric primary care* (5th ed., pp. 606–614). Philadelphia, PA: Elsevier Saunders.

Bowman, S. M., Aitken, M. E., Robbins, J. M., & Baker, S. P. (2012). Trends in US pediatric drowning hospitalizations, 1993–2008. *Pediatrics, 129*(2), 275–281.

Brain Injury Association of America. (2014). *Brain injury in children.* Retrieved from http://www.biausa.org/brain-injury-children.htm

Brown, L., & Proctor, M. R. (2011). Endoscopically assisted correction of sagittal craniosynostosis. *AORN Journal, 93*(5), 566–579.

Burkhard, A. (2013). A different life: Caring for an adolescent or young adult with severe cerebral palsy. *Journal of Pediatric Nursing, 28,* 357–363.

Castelblanco, R. L., Lee, M., & Hasbun, R. (2014). Epidemiology of bacterial meningitis in the USA from 1997 to 2010: A population-based observational study. *The Lancet Infectious Diseases, 14*(9), 813–819.

Catala-Beauchamp, A., & Gleason, R. P. (2012). Abdominal migraine in children: Is it all in their heads? *Journal of Nurse Practitioners, 8*(1), 19–26.

Centers for Disease Control and Prevention (CDC). (2014a). *TBI data and statistics.* Retrieved from http://www.cdc.gov/traumaticbraininjury/data/index.html

Centers for Disease Control and Prevention (CDC). (2014b). *Spina bifida.* Retrieved from http://www.cdc.gov/ncbddd/spinabifida/facts.html

Centers for Disease Control and Prevention (CDC). (2015). Updated estimates of neural tube defects prevented by mandatory folic acid fortification—United States, 1995–2011. *Morbidity and Mortality Weekly Report, 64*(1), 1–5.

Colver, A., Fairhurst, C., & Pharoah, P. O. D. (2014). Cerebral palsy. *Lancet, 383,* 1240–1249.

Dubowitz, H., & Lane, W. G. (2016). Abused and neglected children. In R. M. Kliegman, B. F. Stanton, J. W. St. Geme, & N. F. Schor (Eds.) *Nelson textbook of pediatrics* (20th ed., pp. 236–248). Philadelphia: Elsevier Saunders.

Epilepsy Foundation. (2014a). *Seizures in youth.* Retrieved from http://www.epilepsy.com/learn/seizures-youth

Epilepsy Foundation. (2014b). *Ketogenic diet.* Retrieved from http://www.epilepsy.com/learn/seizures-youth/about-kids/dietary-therapy

Fadiman, A. (1997). *The spirit catches you and you fall down.* New York, NY: Farrar, Strauss, Giroux.

Ferro, M. A., Landgraf, J. M., & Speechley, K. N. (2013). Factor structure of the Child Health Questionnaire Parent Form-50 and predictors of health-related quality of life in children with epilepsy. *Quality of Life Research, 22,* 2201–2211.

Ferro, M. A., & Speechley, K. N. (2011). Examining clinically relevant levels of depressive symptoms in mothers following a diagnosis of epilepsy in their children: A prospective analysis. *Social Psychiatry and Psychiatric Epidemiology, 47,* 1419–1428.

Fingarson, A. K., & Pierce, M. C. (2012). Identifying abusive head trauma. *Contemporary Pediatrics, 29*(2), 16–24.

Garg, S., Green, J., Leadbitter, K., Emsley, R., Lehtonen, A., Evans, G., & Huson, S. M. (2013). Neurofibromatosis type 1 and autism spectrum disorder. *Pediatrics, 132*(6), e1642–e1648.

Geyer, K., Meller, K., Kulpan, C., & Mowery, B. D. (2013). Traumatic brain injury in children: Acute care management. *Pediatric Nursing, 39*(6), 283–289.

Giza, C. C., Kutcher, J. S., Ashwall, S., Barth, J., Thomas, S. D., Getchius, T. S. D., Gioia, G. A., ... Ross Zafonte, R. (2013). Summary of evidence-based guideline update: Evaluation and management of concussion in sports: Report of the Guideline Development Subcommittee of the American Academy of Neurology. *Neurology, 80*(24), 2250–2257.

Harmon, K. G., Drezner, J., Gammons, M., Guskiewicz, K., Halstead, M. Herring, S., ... Roberts, W. (2013). American Medical Society for Sports Medicine position statement: Concussion in sport. *Clinical Journal of Sport Medicine, 23*(1), 1–18.

Hershey, A. D., Kabbouche, M. A., & O'Brien H. L. (2016). Headaches. In R. M. Kliegman, B. F. Stanton, J. W. St. Geme, & N. F. Schor (Eds.), *Nelson textbook of pediatrics* (20th ed., pp. 2863–2874). Philadelphia: Elsevier.

Ibrahim, S. H., & Balistreri, W. F. (2016). Mitochondrial hepatopathies. In R. M. Kliegman, B. F. Stanton, J. W. St. Geme, & N. F. Schor (Eds.), *Nelson textbook of pediatrics* (20th ed., pp. 1958–1961). Philadelphia: Elsevier Saunders.

Institute of Medicine. (2012). *Epilepsy across the spectrum: Promoting health and understanding.* Washington, DC: The National Academies Press.

Ismail, S., Lévy, A., Tikkanen, H., Sévère, M., Wolters, F. J., & Carmant, L. (2012). Lack of efficacy of phenytoin in children presenting with febrile status epilepticus. *American Journal of Emergency Medicine, 30*, 2000–2004.

James, H. E. (1986). Neurologic evaluation and support in the child with acute brain insult. *Pediatric Annals, 15*(1), 16–22.

Julian, N., Edwards, N. E., DeCrane, S., & Hingtgen, C. M. (2014). Neurofibromatosis 1: Diagnosis and management. *Journal for Nurse Practitioners, 10*(1), 30–35.

Kelesidis, T., Mastoris, I., Metsini, A., & Tsiodras, S. (2014). How to approach and treat viral infections in ICU patients. *BMC Infectious Diseases, 14*, 32.

Kerr, L. M., & Huether, S. M. (2014). Alterations in neurologic function in children. In K. L. McCance, S. E. Huether, V. L. Brashers, & N. S. Rote (Eds.), *Pathophysiology: The biologic basis for disease in adults and children* (7th ed., pp. 660–688). St. Louis, MO: Elsevier.

Le Saux, N., & Canadian Paediatric Society Infectious Diseases and Immunization Committee. (2014). Guidelines for the management of suspected and confirmed bacterial meningitis in Canadian children older than one month of age. *Paediatric Child Health, 19*(3), 141–146.

Looman, W. S., & Flannery, A. B. K. (2012). Evidence-based care of the child with deformational plagiocephaly: Part 1: Assessment and diagnosis. *Journal of Pediatric Health Care, 26*(4), 242–250.

Martin, N. G., Sadarangani, M., Pollard, A. J., & Goldacre, M. J. (2014). Hospital admission rates for meningitis and septicaemia caused by *Haemophilus influenzae, Neisseria meningitidis,* and *Streptococcus pneumoniae* in children in England over five decades: A population-based observational study. *The Lancet Infectious Diseases, 14*(5), 397–405.

Mason, C. N. (2013). Mild traumatic brain injury in children. *Pediatric Nursing, 39*(6), 267–272.

McCarthy, J. G., Warren, S. M., Bernstein, J., Burnett, W., Cunningham, M. L., Edmond, J. C., ... Yemen, T. A. (2012). Parameters of care for craniosynostosis. *Cleft Palate–Craniofacial Journal, 49*(1), 1S–24S.

Meckler, S. E. (2014). Clinical management of sports-related pediatric concussions. *Clinician Reviews, 24*(9), 24–32.

Modi, A. C., Rausch, J. R., & Glauser, T. A. (2011). Patterns of nonadherence to antiepileptic drug therapy in children with newly diagnosed epilepsy. *Journal of the American Medical Association, 305*(16), 1669–1679.

National Association of School Nurses (NASN). (2012). *Concussions—The role of the school nurse: Position statement.* Retrieved from http://www.nasn.org/portals/0/binder_papers_reports.pdf

National Center for Injury Prevention and Control. (2015). *10 leading causes of unintentional injury deaths, United States 2013, all races, both sexes.* Retrieved from http://webappa.cdc.gov/sasweb/ncipc/leadcaus10_us.html

National Institute of Neurological Disorders and Stroke (NINDS). (2014). *Hydrocephalus fact sheet.* Retrieved from http://www.ninds.nih.gov/disorders/hydrocephalus/detail_hydrocephalus.htm

Paul, S. P., Debono, R., & Walker, D. (2013). Clinical update: Recognising brain tumours early in children. *Community Practitioner, 86*(4), 42–45.

Pettiford, J. N., Bikhchandani, J., Ostlie, D. J., St. Peter, S. D., Sharp, R. J., & Juang, D. (2012). A review: The role of high dose methylprednisolone in spinal cord trauma in children. *Pediatric Surgery International, 28*, 287–294.

Quayle, K. S., Holmes, J. F., & Kuppermann, N. (2014). Epidemiology of blunt head trauma in children in U.S. emergency departments. *New England Journal of Medicine, 371*, 1945–1947.

Rivara, F. P., Koepsell, T. D., Wang, J., Temkin, N., Dorsch, A., Vavilala, M.S., ... Jaffe, K. M. (2012). Incidence of disability among children 12 months after traumatic brain injury. *American Journal of Public Health, 102*(11), 2074–2079.

Russ, S. A., Larson, K., & Halfon, N. (2012). A national profile of childhood epilepsy and seizure disorder. *Pediatrics, 129*(2), 256–264.

Shearer, P., & Riviello, J. (2011). Generalized convulsive status epilepticus in adults and children: Treatment guidelines and protocols. *Emergency Medical Clinics of North America, 29*, 51–64.

Shui, I. M., Rett, M. D., Weintraub, E., Marcy, M., Amato, A. A., Sheikh, S. I., ... Yih, W. K. (2012). Guillain-Barré syndrome incidence in a large United States cohort (2000–2009). *Neuroepidemiology, 39*, 109–115.

Spina Bifida Association. (2014). *What is spina bifida?* Retrieved from http://www.spinabifidaassociation.org/site/c.evKRI7OXIoJ8H/b.8277225/k.5A79/What_is_Spina_Bifida.htm

Stephenson, R. O., & Berliner, J. (2014). *Autonomic dysreflexia in spinal cord injury.* Retrieved from http://emedicine.medscape.com/article/322809-overview#a30

Sun, H., Bastings, E., Temeck, J., Smith, P. B., Men, A., Tandon, V., ... Rodriguez, W. (2013). Migraine therapeutics in adolescents: A systematic analysis and historic perspectives of triptan trials in adolescents. *JAMA Pediatrics, 167*(3), 243–249.

Taketomo, C. K., Hodding, J. H., & Crause, D. M. (2014). *Pediatric and neonatal dosage handbook* (21st ed.). Hudson, OH: Lexicomp.

Teasdale, G., & Jennett, B. (1974). Assessment of coma and impaired consciousness. *Lancet, 2*, 81–84.

Teasdale, G., Allan, D., Brennan, P., McElhinney, E., & Mackinnon, L. (2014). Forty years on: Updating the Glasgow Coma Scale. *Nursing Times, 110*(42), 12–16.

Teasdale, G., Maas, A., Lecky, F., Manley, G., Stocchetti, N., & Murray, G. (2014). The Glasgow Coma Scale at 40 years: Standing the test of time. *Lancet Neurology, 13*(8), 844–854.

VanStraten, A. F., & Ng, Y. (2012). What is the worst part about having epilepsy? A children's and parents' perspective. *Pediatric Neurology, 47*, 431–435.

Varelas, P. N., Spanaki, M. V., & Mirski, M. A. (2013). Status epilepticus: An update. *Current Neurology and Neuroscience Reports, 13*(7), 357–365.

Wilkes, R., & Tasker, R. C. (2013). Pediatric intensive care treatment of uncontrolled status epilepticus. *Critical Care Clinics, 29*, 239–257

Wilson, B. A., Shannon, M. T., & Shield, K. M. (2015). *Nurse's drug guide 2015.* Hoboken, NJ: Pearson.

Worrall, K. (2004). Use of the Glasgow Coma Scale in infants. *Paediatric Nursing, 16*(4), 45–47.

Zelleke, T. G., Depositario-Cabacar, D. F. T., & Gaillard, W. D. (2013). Epilepsy. In M. L. Batshaw, N. J. Roizen, & G. R. Lotrecchiano (Eds.), *Children with disabilities* (7th ed., pp. 487–506). Baltimore, MD: Paul H. Brooks Publishing Co.

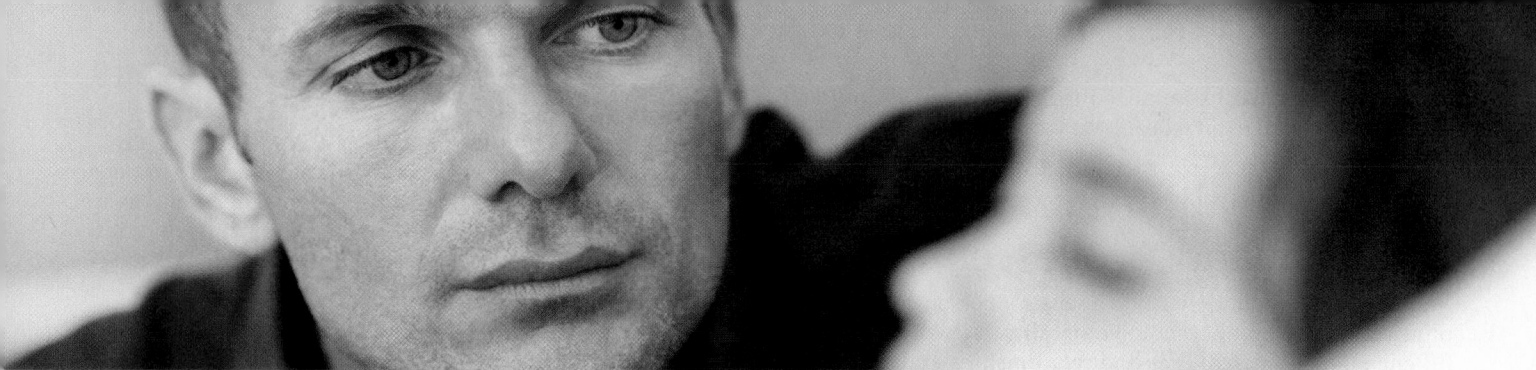

Chapter 55
The Child With Alterations in Mental Health and Cognitive Function

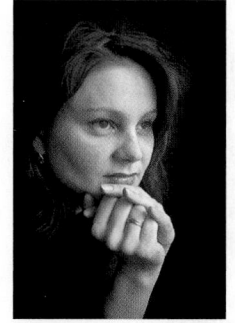

We've been so worried about Cassandra. After being in the car crash, she has become so frightened of everything. She wakes up at night screaming and has lost interest in school and friends. We hope that her work with the therapist will help to decrease her fears and get her involved in all of her activities again.

—Mother of Cassandra, 9 years old

Oleg Golovnev/Shutterstock

⌄ Learning Outcomes

55.1 Define mental health and describe major mental health alterations in childhood.

55.2 Discuss the clinical manifestations of the major mental health alterations of childhood and adolescence.

55.3 Plan for the nursing management of children and adolescents with mental health alterations in the hospital and community settings.

55.4 Describe characteristics of common cognitive alterations of childhood.

55.5 Use evidence-based practice to plan nursing management for children with cognitive alterations.

55.6 Establish and evaluate expected outcomes of care for the child with a cognitive alteration.

This chapter will provide the knowledge and tools needed to provide appropriate care for children with alterations in mental health and cognition. Mental health care is provided by psychiatric-mental health specialists, so the nurse's role often centers on identification, support of the therapy, teaching, and referral. Cognitive conditions are commonly managed by the family and the school personnel. The nurse also forms partnerships with families and school personnel to plan and evaluate care for the child with cognitive conditions such as intellectual disability (formerly called *mental retardation*). A thorough knowledge of development is a prerequisite to understanding both mental health alterations and cognitive conditions since developmental status is often altered in both mental health and cognitive conditions. Review Chapter 31 as

needed to understand the relationships of development to the conditions described in this chapter.

Some cognitive/mental health conditions in children originate from a genetic or physiologic cause. Examples include intellectual disability and childhood schizophrenia. The environments in which children live also influence their characteristics and contribute to dysfunctions such as anxiety, depression, and posttraumatic stress disorder.

Most mental health and cognitive conditions are treated in community settings, and nurses in these settings play an active role in the treatment and support of the child and family. Nurses may function as case managers, assisting a family to deal with all areas of the child's care. Occasionally, a child is hospitalized for treatment of a significant mental health alteration, or a child hospitalized for another health problem requires continued mental health services.

Mental Health Alterations of Children and Adolescents

Mental health is foundational to a sense of personal well-being, physical health, and psychologic stability. It involves successful engagement in activities and relationships and the ability to adapt and cope with change. **Cognition** refers to the change in thought, intelligence, and language that occurs over time as brain maturation and life experiences interact to mutually influence child performance (Santrock, 2011).

Approximately 15 million children in the United States suffer from mental illness that is severe enough to impair functioning at home or school. Overall, about 1 in 5 children and adolescents has a mental health disorder, and 1 in 10 has a disorder that profoundly interferes with daily functioning. Up to 75% to 80% of children with mental health disorders do not receive adequate comprehensive or multidisciplinary treatment, leading to unmet mental health needs. (National Center for Children in Poverty, 2014).

Etiology and Pathophysiology

From the ages of 10 to 21 years, mental health issues are among the top two leading causes of hospitalization (see Chapter 1). This high rate of hospitalization suggests that children are not receiving clinical therapy early, when outpatient care is appropriate and prognosis is best.

Certain population groups are at increased risk for mental disorders. Children from homes with low income are twice as likely to have mental health disruptions. Approximately 50% of children in the child welfare system and 70% of youth in the juvenile justice system have mental disorders (National Center for Children in Poverty, 2014). Children with special healthcare needs and those living in military families have particular barriers to accessing mental health services. More information about military family stress is found in Chapter 42.

Some mental health and cognitive alterations in children originate from a genetic or physiologic cause. Examples include intellectual disability and childhood schizophrenia. Often the family and surrounding environments in which children live influence their characteristics and contribute to dysfunctions such as anxiety, depression, and posttraumatic stress disorder. A unique and challenging interplay of genetics and the environment influences mental health and cognitive conditions, making prevention, diagnosis, and treatment challenging.

During all healthcare visits, mental health screening should be integrated into care so that alterations can be identified. See Chapters 34, 35, and 36 for specific questions to ask during health promotion and health maintenance visits.

Clinical Manifestations

The manifestations of mental health alterations in children are varied, but most can be identified through careful developmental and behavioral screening. Children with mental health conditions often do not display the usual developmental milestones at the times predicted. They may have social interaction problems with family members or other people, or they may have demonstrated a change in performance from former developmental achievement. Functional patterns of living such as the ability to feed and care for self, regulation of sleep and nutritional intake, and the ability to self-regulate during activities may be lacking. Repetitive actions, behavioral instability and outbursts, and withdrawal are other important signs of mental health disruption.

Clinical Therapy

Diagnosis of mental health conditions involves careful physical and psychologic assessment. Studies such as magnetic resonance imaging (MRI), radiographs, electroencephalograms, and toxicology screening may be useful. Mental health is linked to development so developmental screening tests are administered (see Chapter 34). Mental health status can influence activity level, physiologic parameters, and risk for certain conditions. Therefore, nurses should gather height and weight, review of systems, vital signs, and medication/substance use information. Family interactions, stressors, and methods of coping are assessed. When a potential mental health condition exists, the child receives further assessment from a mental health specialist. A resource commonly used is the *Diagnostic and Statistical Manual of Mental Disorders*, which lists diagnostic criteria for known mental health conditions. The current edition is the DSM-5 (American Psychiatric Association, 2013).

Professionalism in Practice *Diagnostic and Statistical Manual of Mental Disorders* **(DSM)**

The DSM-5 is the current compendium of psychiatric conditions, symptoms, and treatment. It includes screening tools and detailed information about pediatric mental health conditions such as attention deficit disorder, intellectual disability, and autism spectrum disorder. The pediatric nurse should access this information for screening tools and current evidence-based practice symptoms, and recognize the importance of acting as a person who identifies mental health disorders and refers children for appropriate care (American Psychiatric Association, 2013; Selekman & Diefenbeck, 2014).

The primary treatment goal for children and adolescents with psychosocial disorders is to assist the child and family to achieve and maintain an optimal level of functioning through interventions designed to reduce the impact of stressors. Therapeutic interventions and communication are based on the principle that feelings motivate behaviors. Parents and others close to the child often fall into the habit of reacting to the child's behaviors rather than trying to find out what feelings may be precipitating the undesirable actions. While behaviors may be considered in treatment, feelings and life experiences are often explored to provide insight and lead to behavior change. Medication may be used to enhance and support other therapy, or it may be the major therapeutic measure.

TREATMENT MODES

Three basic treatment modes are used: individual, family, and group therapy. The choice of treatment mode must take into account the child's age and developmental stage. Most therapists use several intervention strategies simultaneously. Different strategies are more or less effective and appropriate for children and adolescents in various stages of development. A thorough understanding of developmental needs, expectations, and abilities is therefore essential for mental healthcare providers.

Individual Therapy. Individual therapy involves only the child and the therapist. Treatment of specific emotional problems or disorders may involve various techniques such as play therapy, **psychodrama** (being assigned and playing out roles spontaneously in a therapeutic setting to assist in better understanding of the dynamics of a situation), art therapy, and cognitive therapy (a technique used to help a person recognize automatic negative thinking). Individual therapy may be short term (four to six sessions) or long term (lasting for several years).

Family Therapy.   Family therapy involves the exploration of a particular emotional problem and its manifestations among the family members. Family therapy is based on the idea that the emotional symptoms or problems of an individual are an expression of emotional symptoms or problems in the family. The focus is on the relationships among the family members, not the psychologic conflict within each individual member.

Group Therapy.   Group therapy involves an ongoing or limited number of sessions in which several individuals participate. The emphasis is on the interpersonal styles of relating to one another in the group. Group therapy is particularly effective with adolescents because of the importance of the peer group at this age. An advantage of group therapy is that stimuli and feedback come from multiple sources (the group members) instead of just one person (the therapist).

THERAPEUTIC STRATEGIES

Play Therapy.   Play is often called the language or work of the child. From a developmental perspective, children progressively learn to express feelings and needs through action, fantasy, and finally language. The special quality of play buffers children against the pressures and demands of daily life. Play helps children master developmental stages by strengthening physical and neurologic processes. Play also assists in cognitive learning, setting the stage for problem solving and creativity.

Play therapy is a technique that reveals problems on a fantasy level through the use of toys, dolls, clay, art, and other creative objects. It is often used with preschool and school-age children who are experiencing anxiety, stress, and other specific nonpsychotic mental disorders. Play therapy encourages children to act out feelings such as anger, hostility, sadness, and fear. It also gives the therapist a chance to help children understand, on a conscious or unconscious level, their own responses and behavior in a safe, supportive environment. This type of therapy was used for Cassandra, described in the chapter-opening quotation, who needed to gain some control over a frightening environment by acting out fears and trying solutions during play with a therapist. Play therapy is different from therapeutic play, which may be used with hospitalized children (see Chapter 39). Only a specialist is qualified to provide play therapy for mental health disorders.

Art Therapy.   Children who may be apprehensive about playing can sometimes be encouraged to participate in art therapy, using brief drawing exercises. This technique is appropriate for children of all ages, including adolescents. The drawings can help the therapist gain information about the child, the family, and the interactions between the child and family. However, children's drawings should never be the only basis for a definitive diagnosis.

When used in conjunction with a thorough history and appropriate psychologic testing information, art therapy can guide the child's treatment. These drawing exercises provide an opportunity to help in the healing process. The therapist can assist the child to release feelings of anger, pain, or fear onto paper, where they can be examined objectively. (Figures 55–1 to 55–4 present several examples of this technique.)

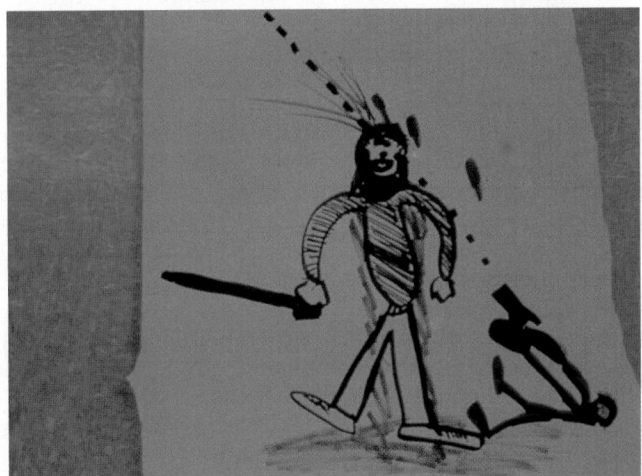

Figure 55–2   "Self-Portrait." Drawn by a 15-year-old boy who was admitted through the emergency department after a failed suicide attempt by hanging. He had a psychiatric diagnosis of depression and polysubstance abuse (including inhalants and alcohol), and he insisted that he was a member of a satanic cult in his hometown. Most of his drawings depicted a preoccupation with violence and suicide. The boy said that he always felt a "darkness" like a shadow that followed him around and wanted him dead. His family history was significant for depression and suicide on both his mother's and his father's side. His father also had a lengthy history of polysubstance abuse and alcoholism. The boy was discharged to a long-term residential treatment facility for adolescents.

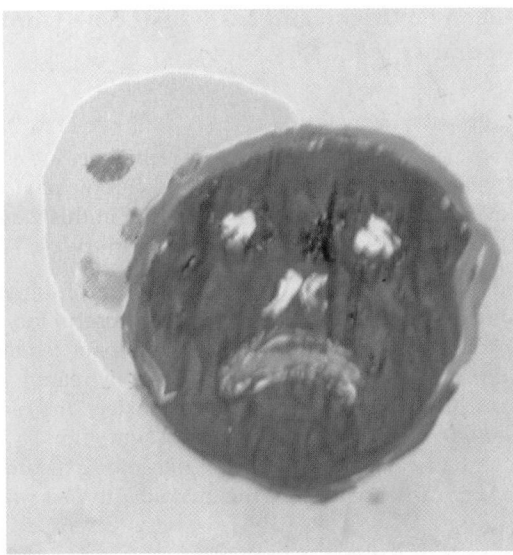

Figure 55–1   "Me." Drawn by a 14-year-old girl with major depression, anxiety, and school phobia who had experienced multiple losses over several years. Her mother had severe chronic lung problems and diabetes, and the girl had stopped attending school for fear that something would happen to her mother. This drawing represents the girl's obvious feelings of sadness and depression but also indicates a glimmer of hope (represented by the yellow mask coming from behind the dark mask of depression).

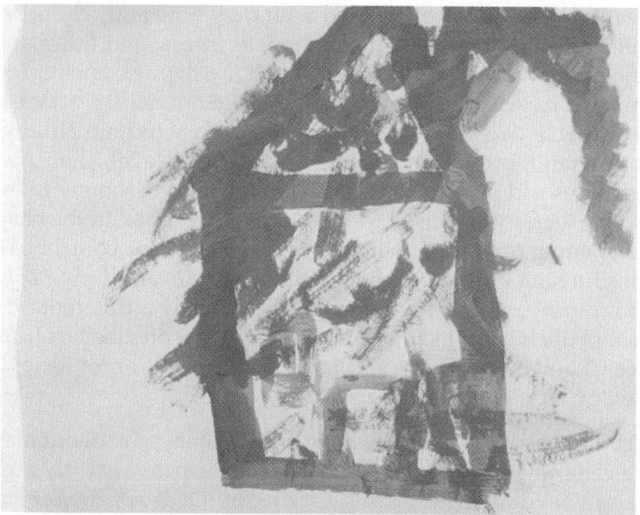

Figure 55–3 "An Activity." Drawn by an 8-year-old boy who was initially admitted to the medical–surgical floor of a pediatric hospital for dehydration resulting from vomiting and diarrhea. Psychiatric evaluation was ordered for extreme anxiety. These drawings, completed during the initial interview, led to further investigation, which revealed that the child had started a house fire in which his grandmother (his primary caretaker at the time) was killed. The family's home and all their belongings were lost. No one had known that the child had set the fire. Further sessions indicated that he had been setting neighborhood garage fires and watching them burn from a distance.

Cognitive and Behavioral Therapy (CBT). A combination of cognitive and behavioral therapy is useful in treating many mental health conditions in children. Cognitive therapy teaches thinking patterns to change reactions to situations that cause anxiety or other undesirable conditions. Children are taught how their brain and body are working; this understanding assists them in having control over the experience and responding with appropriate behaviors (Mayo Clinic, 2013a).

Behavior modification is a therapeutic technique that uses stimulus and response conditioning to alter inappropriate behaviors. It reinforces desirable behaviors, helping the child to replace maladaptive behaviors with more appropriate ones. This technique is based on the assumption that any learned behavior can be unlearned. Thus, if parents, nurses, teachers, and other adults consistently reinforce desirable behaviors, the child will eventually alter or discontinue undesirable behaviors.

Behavior modification may include (1) removing the child from the home to a more structured environment, such as a hospital, for a brief time, and (2) teaching the parents, teachers, and other appropriate adults to be agents of behavioral change. Several ongoing sessions may be required with the adults involved, using role playing and other techniques. Consistency is the most important principle in the success of behavior modification.

Visualization and Guided Imagery. The techniques of visualization and guided imagery begin with specific directions for progressive relaxation according to the child's ability. This form of therapy uses the child's own imagination and positive thinking to reduce stress and anxiety, decrease the experience of pain

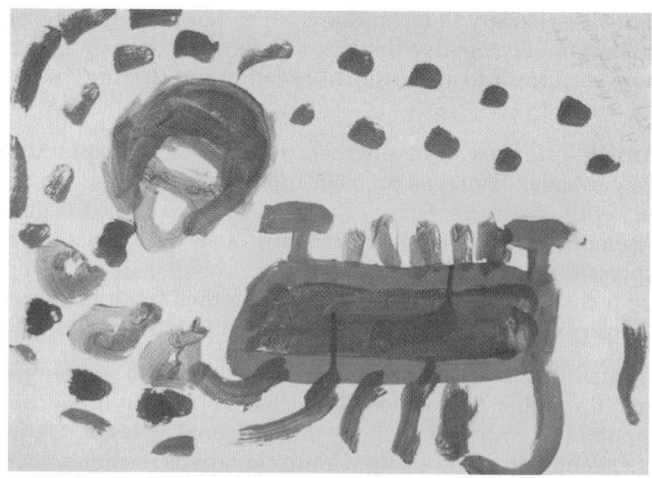

Figure 55–4 "A Family Activity." By the same boy who drew Figure 55–3. This drawing depicts a recurring incident of physical and emotional abuse by his mother's live-in boyfriend. It shows the family bathtub with feces and blood smeared on the floors and walls. The boy reported that when either he or his 3-year-old brother had a toileting accident the boyfriend would make them go into the bathroom and stand in the bathtub while he smeared the feces on the walls. He would then hit the children and make them clean up the mess. The boy had previously been removed from the mother's custody for neglect. He was transferred from the medical–surgical area to the inpatient children's psychiatric unit, where he received a diagnosis of depression, overanxious disorder, and child abuse (physical and emotional). Charges were filed against the mother's boyfriend and custody of both children was temporarily revoked.

or discomfort, and promote healing. The techniques are especially useful for managing anxiety disorders and chronic pain. It is not easy for all children to use their imagination in this way, so the technique may not work or be appropriate for everyone.

Hypnosis. Hypnosis involves varying degrees of suggestibility and deep relaxation effects. This technique is useful for children and adolescents because they can usually be hypnotized more easily than adults. Hypnosis is especially helpful in treating physical symptoms with a psychologic component, anxiety, and phobias. It is also useful in managing severe physical symptoms or discomfort (pain or nausea) associated with a physiologic disorder or its treatment (e.g., cancer or juvenile rheumatoid arthritis).

Nursing Management

Ongoing assessment of all children and their families for mental health risk should be performed from the beginning of life and throughout childhood and adolescence. When a potential mental health condition exists, the child should receive further assessment from a mental health specialist. Nursing assessment focuses on child behaviors, family interactions, lifestyle routines, developmental progression, and treatment for mental health or cognitive conditions (see accompanying *Assessment Guide: The Child With an Alteration in Mental Health or Cognition*).

ASSESSMENT GUIDE | The Child With an Alteration in Mental Health or Cognition

Assessment Focus	Assessment Guidelines
History	• Describe prenatal care and problems. Was there any trauma at birth?
	• Is there a diagnosed mental health disorder in the child or other family members?
	• Is there a history of any neurologic injuries or diseases such as cancer?
	• What medications is the child taking? What medications have been taken in the past?
	• Has there been exposure to environmental pesticides or other chemicals?
Growth	• Is growth progressing at a uniform rate so that the child maintains a similar growth percentile?
	• Is head circumference within normal limits?
Development	• Perform regular developmental screening to identify any variations from expected developmental milestones. Further testing is required if screening suggests any abnormalities.
	• What is the progression of skills reported by the family?
	• Are there any unusual capabilities or deficits?
	• Inquire about progression in school and extracurricular activities.
Social skills	• Describe the relationship between the child and significant adults. Is close attachment evident? Are there signs of attachment disorders such as lack of eye contact, smiles, or response to others in the environment?
	• Describe the school-age child's daily schedule, including family and peer activities. Does the child have friends and engage in several activities with them on a regular basis? Does the child generally interact well with others? Has the child recently had a change in school performance?
	• Ask the teen to describe daily activities and friends. Is there a combination of peer and family influence on personal decision making?
Affect	• Describe facial expression and response to nurse.
	• Observe body size, position, and posture.
	• Are interaction behaviors typical for the setting and age of the child?
	• Does the child display interest in surroundings?
	• Is the child dressed in an appropriate manner? Does the child establish eye contact?
Appearance	• Is the child's clothing appropriate for age, setting, and developmental level?
Behaviors	• Describe level of consciousness and interaction with surroundings.
	• Inquire about recent reported changes in behavior (e.g., sleep, eating patterns, communication with others, school performance, friendships, risky activities).
	• Has the child or parent identified any problem behaviors?
	• Are any particular events associated with the problem behaviors?
Life events	• Has the child or family experienced recent stress or trauma?
	• Have there been any changes in family structure?
	• Evaluate chronic health conditions in family members.

Many mental health disorders are managed effectively with therapy, medication, or both on an outpatient basis, while some necessitate admission to an inpatient psychiatric setting. Therefore, the nurse may encounter the child with a mental health disorder in a variety of community settings or during hospitalization for a concurrent psychiatric or physiologic problem.

In the hospital, nursing care includes carrying out the prescribed treatment plan and administering psychotropic medications. Evaluate the child's medication regimen for administration schedule, dosage, side effects, and effectiveness. See accompanying *Evidence-Based Practice: Pharmacogenetics and the Nursing Role.*

An important nursing intervention is to ensure safety of the child. Actions begin in the emergency department if a child is admitted for a mental health crisis. Remove or lock up potentially dangerous material such as medications, tubing, and sharps containers that may be in the child's room. A parent, guardian, or healthcare provider should remain with the child at all times. Inform the family member of the need to stay with the child and how to immediately notify the nurse if the adult needs to leave or if the child's condition changes. Part of the initial care is to evaluate risk by asking if the child has tried to hurt himself/herself or has been thinking about that. Ask about recent stresses, thoughts of hurting someone else, and why the

EVIDENCE-BASED PRACTICE | Pharmacogenetics and the Nursing Role

Clinical Question

Great variability is seen in the response to psychotropic medicines used to treat mental health disorders such as depression. Children and adolescents show even more variability than adults, related to developmental variation in absorption, distribution, metabolism, and elimination; therefore, close monitoring is essential (Madadi, 2015). How can the nurse apply new technologies about individualized treatments to medications when providing mental health care for youth?

The Evidence

The fields of genetics and genomics are growing rapidly (see Chapter 3). Currently, pharmacogenetic testing is being used so that clinicians can select the best psychotropic medications for particular clients. For example, a genetic test for a gene that codes for high manufacture of a body enzyme that metabolizes a particular medication predicts that the client will not respond well to that medication. Another psychotropic can be chosen to enhance response. On the other hand, if the client is a slow metabolizer of the medication, an increased risk of toxicity results. A tailored approach to treatment of attention deficit hyperactivity disorder (ADHD) has the potential to target specific gene patterns rather than using a trial-and-error approach to types of medications tried (Bruxel et al., 2014). Community treatment of mental health disorders has the potential to be enhanced by identification of the best drug to treat a given person. Nurses are called on to collect genetic samples (often from inside the mouth) and explain the procedure and results to families (Bartlett, 2011; Haga, O'Daniel, Tindall, et al., 2012). These roles demand that nurses understand genomics and pharmacogenetics in order to translate concepts to families (Knisely, Carpenter, & Von Ah, 2014).

Best Practice

The nurse in a setting where children and adolescents are treated for psychiatric disorders has an important role in applying new knowledge related to pharmacogenetics. First, the nurse needs to take a careful history of medications, over-the-counter products, and herbal remedies because many of these substances compete with psychotropic medications for metabolism in the body. When a DNA test is recommended prior to beginning medication, families need to understand the reason for the test. They will also need explanations about the test results and how they relate to the specific medication that has been prescribed. It is important that all children and adolescents receiving psychotropic medications be closely monitored for responses and side effects. The nurse is integral to the ongoing evaluation of the prescribed therapy (Kniseley et al., 2014).

Clinical Reasoning

What is the nursing role in history taking and in monitoring for the child or adolescent on psychotropic medication? What questions do you think a family is likely to ask when they learn that a genetic test is recommended before prescribing medication to an adolescent experiencing a mental health disruption such as severe depression? Where will you find the information about pharmacogenetics and pharmacogenomics that will provide necessary background for you and the family? How can pharmacogenetic testing enhance the treatment of individuals by both leading to a therapeutic response in a short time and avoiding serious side effects?

---

child thinks she/he has been brought to the emergency department. If the child is admitted to the psychiatric unit, follow unit policies for ensuring safety for children who are at risk of hurting themselves or others.

Developing Cultural Competence Spiritual **Beliefs and Mental Health**

In many cultures, care of the "spirit" is believed necessary to promote mental health. An identity with one's community and spiritual wholeness is promoted by storytelling, singing, rites of passage, and use of certain objects such as bags of herbs. Use of healers, family and community support, relaxation or meditation, exorcism, or other procedures may be used by families. Ask what the family believes about mental health, and integrate safe and culturally acceptable practices into the plan of care to enhance the child's mental health.

Psychiatric hospitalization is a stressful event for all families, and both the family and child need supportive care. Continuation of family involvement is critical. The nurse frequently is the liaison between the family and the therapist in making follow-up arrangements at the time of discharge. Be aware of the meaning of mental illness in various cultural groups and the treatments that may be commonly used. Integrate these complementary therapies into the care plan whenever safe. Families must feel that their responses and approaches to the child with a mental disorder are not judged by healthcare providers.

The nurse in the community assesses how a child with a mental health disorder is functioning in each microsystem, such as home, day care, school, and with friends. Assess risk and protective factors of the child and family (see Chapter 31). Evaluate involvement in therapy sessions and ability to manage prescribed pharmacologic interventions.

Developmental and Behavioral Disorders

Autism Spectrum Disorder (Neurodevelopmental Disorder)

Twelve to 16% of children are estimated to have a developmental or behavioral disorder. The most common group of disorders is called autism spectrum disorder (ASD), which affects about 14.7/1000 children (Centers for Disease Control and Prevention [CDC], 2012a, 2014a). ASD is a neurodevelopmental disorder that begins in early childhood and is characterized by impaired social interactions and communication, with restricted interests, activities, and behaviors, and repetitive patterns of behavior (American Psychiatric Association, 2013). ASD may be accompanied by other neurodevelopmental, mental, or behavioral conditions, so the manifestations can differ significantly among individuals. ASD is comprised of autism, Asperger syndrome, pervasive developmental disorder not otherwise specified, Rett syndrome, and childhood disintegrative disorder. The present incidence of ASD represents an increase from formerly described levels; before 1985, less than 1 child in 1000 was diagnosed with an autistic disorder. It is unclear whether there is a true increase in cases or simply improved techniques in making the diagnosis, as well as an enlarged diagnostic category that includes more children. The disorder is more common in males than females; peak age at diagnosis is 8 years, but symptoms often begin by 12 to 24 months of age (CDC, 2012a, 2014a).

ETIOLOGY AND PATHOPHYSIOLOGY

The etiology of autism spectrum disorder is unknown. Genes are clearly involved, although a complex array of genes appears to be responsible (Frye, 2014). Immune responses, environmental exposures, certain drugs during pregnancy, and neuroanatomy are being investigated as influences that interact with genetics to cause ASDs (CDC, 2014a; Won, Mah, & Kim, 2013). Neurotransmitters such as dopamine, serotonin, and opioids are abnormal in some children and are a focus of research. Fetal alcohol syndrome, fragile X syndrome, phenylketonuria, Down syndrome, and tuberous sclerosis are all associated with a higher than normal incidence of autism (Won et al., 2013). Despite concern expressed in earlier medical and lay press, no demonstrated relationship has been demonstrated between the measles-mumps-rubella vaccine or thimerosal (mercury-based preservative in some vaccines) and the incidence of ASDs (see Chapter 43 for further information on immunizations) (Maglione et al., 2014).

CLINICAL MANIFESTATIONS

The essential features of the disorder typically become apparent by the time a child is 3 years of age. They involve impairments in socialization, communication, and behavior (Harrington, 2013; Webb, 2011). Children with ASD are unable to relate to people in a manner that is common for young children, or to respond to social and emotional cues. In addition, they may engage in **stereotypy**, or rigid, repetitive, and machine-like movement with obsessive behavior (Figure 55–5). Characteristically, these repetitive behaviors in affected children include head banging, twirling in circles, biting themselves, and flapping their hands or arms. Frequently, a child's behavior is self-stimulating or self-destructive. Responses to sensory stimuli are frequently abnormal and include an extreme aversion to touch, loud noises, and bright lights. Emotional lability is common.

Communication difficulties or delays in speech and language are common, and are often the first symptoms that lead to diagnosis. Abnormal communication patterns include both verbal and nonverbal communication. Absence of babbling and other communication by 1 year, absence of two-word phrases by 2 years, and deterioration of previous language skills are characteristic. Children with ASD may eventually learn to talk, in some cases well, but their speech is likely to show certain abnormalities: use of *you* in place of *I*; **echolalia** (a compulsive parroting of what is heard); repeating questions rather than answering them; and fascination with rhythmic, repetitive songs and verses.

Behaviors of children with ASD show several differences from other children. They do not commonly explore objects but display stereotypy. They may line up objects, play with the same objects over and over, and have certain rituals that must be performed. They often become upset if these normal routines are disrupted. Rituals may involve eating only certain types or colors of foods or eating in specific patterns. Children may manifest disturbances in the rate or sequence of development. They frequently have cognitive impairment but can demonstrate a wide range of intellectual ability and functioning. Cognitive impairment may manifest early in life as slow developmental progression, particularly in social skills. Some children are impaired in particular areas of development, whereas others are above normal.

The clinical manifestations common in autistic spectrum disorder are listed in Table 55–1.

CLINICAL THERAPY

The first step in identifying children at risk of ASD is surveillance at each healthcare visit. Since diagnosis and treatment have often been delayed, the American Academy of Pediatrics has now identified a multistage process for surveillance and screening:

1. Perform surveillance at early healthcare visits to identify if a sibling has ASD, parents or other caregivers are concerned about the developmental progression of the child, or the healthcare provider notes abnormalities in child behavior.

2. The healthcare provider determines if the child appears to be at risk for ASD.

3. The healthcare provider evaluates the risks. If risk exists, the provider administers an age-appropriate and ASD-specific screening tool (e.g., Ages and Stages Questionnaire and Modified Checklist for Autism in Toddlers [M-CHAT]).

4. If no risk exists, an ASD-specific tool is administered at the 18- and 24-month visits.

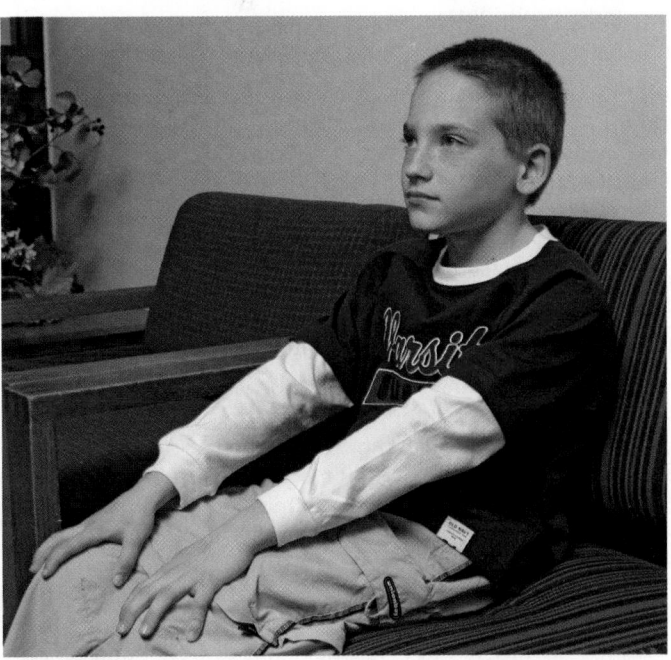

Figure 55–5 Stereotypy. **This child with ASD sits stiffly in the chair and engages in rhythmic rocking behavior. He has a disengaged look and does not readily interact with other children or adults who are in his environment.**

TABLE 55–1 Clinical Manifestations of Autistic Spectrum Disorder (Pervasive Developmental Disorder)

CLINICAL MANIFESTATIONS	CLINICAL THERAPY
Impaired social, communicative, and behavioral development, usually noted in first year of life.	Early intervention is key to maximal performance. Interventions focus on improving behaviors and communication skills, providing physical and occupational therapy, structuring play interactions with other children, and educating parents about the child's needs.
Impaired social interactions with normal language development for age; pitch, tone, and other speech characteristics may be abnormal. Verbal skills involving spelling and vocabulary are high but concept formation, language flexibility, and comprehension are low. Intellectual functioning may be at a high level, particularly in certain areas, while social skills are limited.	Social interactions are focus of therapy.
Early development often appears normal, but symptoms emerge at 6–18 months. Ataxia, handwringing, intermittent hyperventilation, dementia, and growth retardation show progressive increase. Appears only in females as an X-linked dominant disorder; mutations occur in the *MeCP2* gene, affecting methyl-CpG–binding protein 2, which is important in brain development.	Early intervention in areas of abnormal behaviors.
First 2–5 years of development appear normal followed by deterioration in many areas of functioning. Behaviors finally stabilize at some point without further deterioration.	Focus on areas of developmental function that show abnormality. Individualized education plans are needed in school to deal with communication, play, physical therapy, and teaching management skills to parents. Regression in toileting and other skills may occur.
Severe social impairment without meeting DSM criteria for other types of autistic spectrum disorder.	Behavioral therapy focuses on building social skills.

5. Select appropriate screening tool for age and risk profile of the child.

6. If screening is negative for a child with some risk, provide information to parents and evaluate again in 1 month. If screening is positive, refer for comprehensive ASD evaluation, including audiology, and begin early intervention programs (Harrington, 2013; Johnson et al., 2007, reaffirmed, 2010; Webb, 2011).

Several screening tests are available for use in health maintenance visits if autistic disorder is suspected. Additional testing is performed to rule out other causes of the child's behavior. Tests may include neuroimaging (CT scan or MRI), lead screening, metabolic studies, DNA analysis, and electroencephalogram. See Chapters 33 and 54 for further descriptions related to neurologic system assessment. Diagnosis is based on the presence of specific criteria, as described in the American Psychiatric Association's DSM-5 (see Table 55–2).

Early intervention helps maximize the child's potential by improving developmental skills and behaviors, as well as establishing helpful support for parents. Treatment focuses on behavior management to reward appropriate behaviors (called *applied behavior analysis [ABA]*), foster positive or adaptive coping skills, and facilitate effective communication. The goals of treatment are to reduce rigidity or stereotypy and other maladaptive behaviors. Some children must be physically restrained from aggressive or self-destructive behaviors. Speech therapy is an essential part of treatment. Instruction in social skills and occupational therapy to improve fine motor dexterity and sensory integration are provided. Some parents choose to use complementary therapies.

The overall prognosis for children with ASD to become functioning members of society varies. Successful adjustment is more likely for children with higher IQs, adequate speech, and access to specialized programs.

Nursing Management

For the Child With ASD or Neurodevelopmental Disorder

Nursing Assessment and Diagnosis

The nurse may encounter the child with ASD during routine well-child visits, or when parents seek care for a suspected hearing impairment, speech difficulty, or developmental delay. Early and frequent developmental screening of all children can help in referral for thorough assessment and identification of cases. Be alert to parental observations that the baby or young child does not look at them or provides other developmental or behavioral cues. Parents may report abnormal interaction such as lack of eye contact, disinterest in cuddling, minimal facial responsiveness, and failure to talk. Be alert for the "red flags": no babbling or communication gestures by 12 months, no single word by 16 months, no spontaneous two-word phrases by 24 months, or loss of language or social skills previously achieved (Johnson et al., 2007, reaffirmed 2010).

Assessment at every healthcare visit focuses on language development, response to others, and hearing acuity (see Chapters 31 and 33). Specialized screening tests for ASD may be administered. Pediatric nurses in outpatient settings should ensure that a variety of autism screening tools for different ages of children are available and used in healthcare settings (Webb, 2011).

When a child with a diagnosis of autistic disorder is hospitalized for a concurrent problem, obtain a history from the parents about the child's routines, rituals, and likes and dislikes, as well as ways to promote interaction and cooperation. Children with ASD may carry a special toy or object that they play with during times of stress. Ask parents about these objects and their use. Document this information in the clinical record.

TABLE 55–2 DSM-5 Diagnostic Criteria for Autistic Spectrum Disorder

1. Persistent deficits in social communication and social interaction across multiple contexts, as manifested by the following, currently or by history (examples are illustrative, not exhaustive):

   - Deficits in social-emotional reciprocity, ranging, for example, from abnormal social approach and failure of normal back-and-forth conversation; to reduced sharing of interests, emotions, or affect; to failure to initiate or respond to social interactions.
   - Deficits in nonverbal communicative behaviors used for social interaction, ranging, for example, from poorly integrated verbal and nonverbal communication; to abnormalities in eye contact and body language or deficits in understanding and use of gestures; to a total lack of facial expressions and nonverbal communication.
   - Deficits in developing, maintaining, and understanding relationships, ranging, for example, from difficulties adjusting behavior to suit various social contexts; to difficulties in sharing imaginative play or in making friends; to absence of interest in peers.

   Specify current severity:

   - Severity is based on social communication impairments and restricted, repetitive patterns of behavior.

2. Restricted, repetitive patterns of behavior, interests, or activities, as manifested by at least two of the following, currently or by history (examples are illustrative, not exhaustive; see text):

   - Stereotyped or repetitive motor movements, use of objects, or speech (e.g., simple motor stereotypies, lining up toys or flipping objects, echolalia, idiosyncratic phrases).
   - Insistence on sameness, inflexible adherence to routines, or ritualized patterns of verbal or nonverbal behavior (e.g., extreme distress at small changes, difficulties with transitions, rigid thinking patterns, greeting rituals, need to take same route or eat same food every day).
   - Highly restricted, fixated interests that are abnormal in intensity or focus (e.g., strong attachment to or preoccupation with unusual objects, excessively circumscribed or perseverative interests).
   - Hyper- or hyporeactivity to sensory input or unusual interest in sensory aspects of the environment (e.g., apparent indifference to pain/temperature, adverse response to specific sounds or textures, excessive smelling or touching of objects, visual fascination with lights or movement).

   Specify current severity:

   - Severity is based on social communication impairments and restricted, repetitive patterns of behavior.

3. Symptoms must be present in the early developmental period (but may not become fully manifest until social demands exceed limited capacities, or may be masked by learned strategies in later life).

4. Symptoms cause clinically significant impairment in social, occupational, or other important areas of current functioning.

5. These disturbances are not better explained by intellectual disability (intellectual developmental disorder) or global developmental delay. Intellectual disability and autism spectrum disorder frequently co-occur; to make comorbid diagnoses of autism spectrum disorder and intellectual disability, social communication should be below that expected for general developmental level.

Note: Individuals with a well-established DSM-IV diagnosis of autistic disorder, Asperger's disorder, or pervasive developmental disorder not otherwise specified should be given the diagnosis of autism spectrum disorder. Individuals who have marked deficits in social communication, but whose symptoms do not otherwise meet criteria for autism spectrum disorder, should be evaluated for social (pragmatic) communication disorder.

Specify if:
- With or without accompanying intellectual impairment
- With or without accompanying language impairment
- Associated with a known medical or genetic condition or environmental factor
- Associated with another neurodevelopmental, mental, or behavioral disorder

Source: Used with permission from American Psychiatric Association. (2013). *Diagnostic and statistical manual of mental disorders* (5th ed.). Washington, DC: Author. Copyright © 2013 American Psychiatric Association.

Ask about the child's behaviors and observe them on admission. Obtain a history of acute and chronic illnesses and injuries. Ask about eating patterns and food restrictions. Inquire about complementary and alternative medicine treatments in a nonjudgmental and supportive manner.

Nursing diagnoses must be tailored to fit the individual needs of the child. Examples of nursing diagnoses that might be appropriate for children with ASD include the following (NANDA-I © 2014):

- *Communication: Verbal, Impaired,* related to psychologic condition
- *Social Interaction, Impaired,* related to developmental disability
- *Injury, Risk for,* related to cognitive impairment
- *Caregiver Role Strain, Risk for,* related to chronicity and demands of child's condition

- *Coping: Family, Compromised,* related to having a child with prolonged disability

Planning and Implementation

Nursing care focuses on stabilizing environmental stimuli, providing supportive care, enhancing communication, maintaining a safe environment, giving the parents anticipatory guidance, and providing community-based care.

STABILIZE ENVIRONMENTAL STIMULI

Children with ASD interpret and respond to the environment differently from other individuals. Sounds that are not distressing to the average person may be interpreted by children with ASD as louder, more frightening, and overwhelming. The child needs to be oriented to new settings such as a classroom or the hospital room, and may adjust best to a small classroom or to a hospital room with only one other child. Encourage parents to bring the child's favorite objects from home, and try to keep these objects in the same places because the child does not cope well with changes in the environment.

PROVIDE SUPPORTIVE CARE

Developing a trusting relationship with the child with ASD is often difficult. Adjust communication techniques and teaching to the child's developmental level. Ask parents about the child's usual home routines, and maintain these routines as much as possible when the child is out of the home. Because self-care abilities are often limited, the child may need help meeting basic needs. School programs and individualized education plans (IEPs) (see Chapter 38) can help the child learn self-care skills. When possible, schedule daily care and routine procedures at consistent times to maintain predictability. Encourage parents to remain with the hospitalized child and to participate in daily care planning. Parents are integral parts of the treatment team when the child's learning goals are established in early intervention or school programs. Identify rituals for naptime and bedtime, and maintain them to promote rest and sleep. Establish patterns that help the child eat nutritious foods at mealtimes.

Use of complementary medicine for children with autistic spectrum disorder is common. Parents choose modalities such as special diets, use of supplements and vitamins, herbs, auditory training, hyperbaric treatment, chiropractic manipulation, and nonprescription medications such as melatonin (Valicenti-McDermott et al., 2014). Nurses should inquire about use of complementary therapies and provide information for the family to ensure safe practices.

ENHANCE COMMUNICATION

Since children with ASD have impaired communication, nursing care focuses on using and improving communication with the child. Speech is used when possible; short, direct sentences are usually most effective. When the child responds well to visual cues, pictures, computers, and other visual aids may form an important part of interactions. Some children use sign language.

MAINTAIN A SAFE ENVIRONMENT

Monitor children with ASD at all times, including bath time and bedtime. Close supervision is needed to ensure that the child does not obtain any harmful objects or engage in dangerous behaviors. Bicycle helmets and mittens are sometimes used to protect children with ASD so that they can safely participate in activities.

PROVIDE ANTICIPATORY GUIDANCE

Approximately half of all children with autistic disorder require lifelong supervision and support. This is especially true if the disorder is accompanied by intellectual disability (mental retardation). Some children may grow up to lead independent lives, although they will have social limitations with impaired interpersonal relationships. Encourage parents to promote the child's development through behavior modification and specialized educational programs. The overall goal is to provide the child with the guidance, education, and the support necessary for optimal functioning.

COMMUNITY-BASED NURSING CARE

Families need a great deal of support to cope with the challenges of caring for the child with ASD. The diagnosis may trigger feelings of grief and shock. Help the family identify resources for child care, such as special toddler programs, preschools, and parent support groups. The child will need an individualized education and health plan; the school nurse is instrumental in establishing these plans. The parent or primary caretaker often has a hard time getting respite care and may need assistance to find suitable resources. Siblings of the child with ASD may need help explaining the disorder to their friends or teachers. Family support programs are available in some states to provide assistance to parents.

Offer the family resources for genetic counseling. Parents need information about the need for immunizations since they may have heard erroneous information about a connection between immunization and the disorder. Encourage parents to have the child immunized on the recommended schedule. Parents may have questions about where to find information on complementary and alternative therapies.

Local support groups for parents of children with ASD exist in most areas. Parents can also be referred to the Autism Society of America, the American Academy of Pediatrics, and the Centers for Disease Control and Prevention for information.

Evaluation

Expected outcomes of nursing care for the child with ASD include the following:

- Behavioral symptoms are effectively managed.
- The child performs elements of self-care.
- The child remains free from injury.
- Consistent developmental progression is observed.
- The child develops successful communication strategies.

Attention Deficit Disorder and Attention Deficit Hyperactivity Disorder

Attention deficit disorder (ADD) is a variation in central nervous system processing characterized by developmentally inappropriate behaviors involving inattention. When hyperactivity and impulsivity accompany inattention, the disorder is called *attention deficit hyperactivity disorder (ADHD)*. The latter is the more common condition and affects about 11% of school-age children; boys (13.2%) are affected more often than girls (5.6%) (CDC, 2014b). It is also known to affect adolescents and adults, and those with the disorder often continue to manifest at least some of the symptoms as they grow into adulthood. Hyperactivity and impulsivity may improve as the child nears adulthood, with inattentiveness being the most persistent characteristic.

ETIOLOGY AND PATHOPHYSIOLOGY

Although a variety of physical and neurologic disorders are associated with ADHD, children with identifiable causes represent a small proportion of this population. Examples of known associations include exposure to high levels of lead or mercury in childhood and prenatal exposure to alcohol or tobacco smoke. Other prenatal factors associated with a higher incidence of ADHD include preterm labor, impaired placenta functioning, and impaired oxygenation. Seizures and serious head injury are other potential associations. Genetic factors may be important, as well as family dynamics and environmental characteristics. Although ADHD occurs more commonly within families (25% have a first-degree relative with the disorder), a single gene has not been located and a specific mechanism of genetic transmission is not known. It is believed that a genetic predisposition interacts with the child's environment, so that both factors contribute to the appearance of the condition. Family stress, poverty, and poor nutrition may also be contributing factors. Although daily television exposure at ages 1 to 3 years has been associated with attention symptoms of the condition later in childhood, not all studies verify this finding (Ferguson, 2011; van Egmond-Frohlich, Weghuber, & de Zwaan, 2012). It is likely that there are many types of attention deficit, resulting from several different mechanisms that involve interaction of genetic, biologic, and environmental risk factors.

The pathophysiology of ADD/ADHD is not totally known. However, some children exhibit a deficit in the catecholamines dopamine and norepinephrine, lowering the threshold for stimuli input. The disorder is marked by brain maturation delay in the area of self-regulation. Increased input from stimuli and decreased self-regulation cause the hallmark inability to inhibit stimuli and motor activity. Slow brain maturity, in the first 3 years of life, has now been demonstrated on imaging studies. The cortex is particularly affected and may explain the school and concentration difficulty associated with the disorder (National Institutes of Health [NIH], 2012).

CLINICAL MANIFESTATIONS

Children with ADD and ADHD have problems related to decreased attention span, impulsiveness, or increased motor activity. Symptoms can range from mild to severe. The disorders often coexist with various developmental learning disabilities. The child has difficulty completing tasks, fidgets constantly, is frequently loud, and interrupts others. Sleep disturbances are common. Because of these behaviors, the child often has difficulty developing and maintaining social relationships and may be shunned or teased by other children. This only increases the anxiety of the already compromised child, whose behavior is set on a downward-spiraling course.

Typically, girls with ADHD show less aggression and impulsiveness than boys, but far more anxiety, mood swings, social withdrawal, rejection, and cognitive and language problems. Girls tend to be older at the time of diagnosis. Children are frequently diagnosed with the disorder soon after beginning school, with its demands for attentive behavior.

CLINICAL THERAPY

Children are usually brought for evaluation when behaviors escalate to the point of interfering with the daily functioning of teachers or parents. Any child from ages 4 through 18 years who has academic problems, behavior difficulties, inattention, hyperactivity, or impulsivity should be evaluated for ADHD (Subcommittee on Attention-Deficit/Hyperactivity Disorder [Subcommittee on ADHD], 2011). When children have learning disabilities or anxiety disorders, the problem is commonly misdiagnosed as ADHD if full and accurate evaluation of the child's symptoms is not performed. Obtaining an accurate diagnosis after comprehensive testing by a pediatric mental health specialist is vital (NIH, 2012). Specific diagnostic criteria must be applied to all children with the potential diagnosis (see DSM-5 criteria in Table 55–3). The diagnosis of ADD is often difficult because of the absence of hyperactivity behaviors. Behaviors at home, school, or childcare centers must be evaluated because abnormal patterns in two settings are needed for diagnosis. A variety of tests are available for use by the trained professional in establishing the diagnosis.

Diagnosis begins with a careful history of the child, including family history, birth history, growth and developmental milestones, behaviors such as sleeping and eating patterns, progression and patterns in school, social and environmental conditions, reports from parents and teachers, and any other emotional or behavioral condition (Subcommittee on ADHD, 2011). A physical examination should be performed to rule out neurologic diseases and other health problems. The mental health specialist then performs testing of the child and administers questionnaires to the parent and teacher. It is important to identify other conditions that may either mimic ADD/ADHD or exist in conjunction with the disorders. These might include depression, anxiety, learning disorder, conduct disorder, or oppositional defiant disorder.

Treatment is established to meet the desired behavioral outcomes, and includes a combination of approaches, such as environmental changes, behavior therapy, and pharmacotherapy. The condition is chronic, so assessment should be ongoing for follow-up and evaluation of other mental health conditions (Brown, 2012).

Children often benefit from environmental changes. Decreasing stimulation—for example, by turning off television, keeping the environment quiet, and maintaining an orderly and clutter-free desk or study area without distraction—may help the child to stay focused on the task at hand. Another relatively simple change is appropriate classroom placement, preferably in a small class with a teacher who can provide close supervision and a structured daily routine. Consistent limits and expectations should be set for the child. Children living in chaotic homes and communities may function better if the environment can be simplified. When aggressive behaviors occur, therapeutic approaches such as play and group therapy may be useful.

Behavior therapy involves rewarding the child for desired behaviors and applying consequences for undesirable behaviors. Children may be rewarded by praise or earn points toward a movie or other desired outing for staying seated during meals or quietly listening in a classroom. All adults who are in close contact with the child, such as parents and teachers, must be educated to carry out the behavioral program (Subcommittee on ADHD, 2011).

Children with moderate to severe ADHD are treated with pharmacotherapy. Methylphenidate (Ritalin, Concerta) is most often prescribed, with alternatives of dextroamphetamine (Dexedrine or Adderall) and the nonstimulant medication atomoxetine. A skin patch that releases medication transdermally over a 9-hour period is available, facilitating ease of administration; a long-acting liquid medication formulation is also available (Findling & Dinh, 2014). Usually, a favorable response (a decrease in impulsive behaviors and an increase in the ability to sit still and attend to an activity for at least 15 minutes) is seen in the first 10 days of treatment and frequently with the first few doses. Guidelines recommend thorough evaluation of children before stimulant or other medication is prescribed in order to rule out any cardiac condition that could be affected by medication use.

A variety of complementary approaches, in addition to or instead of traditional behavioral therapy and medication, have been tried in children with ADD or ADHD. Chiropractic manipulation, biofeedback, yoga, massage, visual or auditory therapy, and dietary interventions have been used. Dietary therapies include elimination of dietary components such as highly processed foods, sugar, aspartame, or yeast and use of supplements such as omega-3 fatty acids, iron, magnesium, zinc, vitamin B_6, and herbs such as Pycnogenol (pine bark extract), melatonin, *Echinacea*, St. John's wort, and ginkgo biloba. Ask parents about alternative therapies used and investigate what is known about them in order to share this information with parents (Arnold, Hurt, & Lofthouse, 2013; Faraone & Antshel, 2014; Kemper, Gardiner, & Birdee, 2013).

TABLE 55–3 DSM-5 Diagnostic Criteria for Attention Deficit Hyperactivity Disorder

A. A persistent pattern of inattention and/or hyperactivity-impulsivity that interferes with functioning or development, as characterized by 1 and/or 2:

  1. *Inattention:* Six (or more) of the following symptoms have persisted for at least 6 months to a degree that is inconsistent with developmental level and that negatively impacts directly on social and academic/occupational activities:

    a. **Note:** The symptoms are not solely a manifestation of oppositional behavior, defiance, hostility, or failure to understand tasks or instructions. For older adolescents and adults (age 17 and older), at least five symptoms are required.

    b. Often fails to give close attention to details or makes careless mistakes in schoolwork, at work, or during other activities (e.g., overlooks or misses details, work is inaccurate).

    c. Often has difficulty sustaining attention in tasks or play activities (e.g., has difficulty remaining focused during lectures, conversations, or lengthy reading).

    d. Often does not seem to listen when spoken to directly (e.g., mind seems elsewhere, even in the absence of any obvious distraction).

    e. Often does not follow through on instructions and fails to finish schoolwork, chores, or duties in the workplace (e.g., starts tasks but quickly loses focus and is easily sidetracked).

    f. Often has difficulty organizing tasks and activities (e.g., difficulty managing sequential tasks; difficulty keeping materials and belongings in order; messy, disorganized work; has poor time management; fails to meet deadlines).

    g. Often avoids, dislikes, or is reluctant to engage in tasks that require sustained mental effort (e.g., schoolwork or homework; for older adolescents and adults, preparing reports, completing forms, reviewing lengthy papers).

    h. Often loses things necessary for tasks or activities (e.g., school materials, pencils, books, tools, wallets, keys, paperwork, eyeglasses, mobile telephones).

    i. Is often easily distracted by extraneous stimuli (for older adolescents and adults, may include unrelated thoughts).

    j. Is often forgetful in daily activities (e.g., doing chores, running errands; for older adolescents and adults, returning calls, paying bills, keeping appointments).

  2. *Hyperactivity and impulsivity:* Six (or more) of the following symptoms have persisted for at least 6 months to a degree that is inconsistent with developmental level and that negatively impacts directly on social and academic/occupational activities:

    a. **Note:** The symptoms are not solely a manifestation of oppositional behavior, defiance, hostility, or a failure to understand tasks or instructions. For older adolescents and adults (age 17 and older), at least five symptoms are required.

    b. Often fidgets with or taps hands or feet or squirms in seat.

    c. Often leaves seat in situations when remaining seated is expected (e.g., leaves his or her place in the classroom, in the office or other workplace, or in other situations that require remaining in place).

    d. Often runs about or climbs in situations where it is inappropriate. (**Note:** In adolescents or adults, may be limited to feeling restless.)

    e. Often unable to play or engage in leisure activities quietly.

    f. Is often "on the go," acting as if "driven by a motor" (e.g., is unable to be or uncomfortable being still for extended time, as in restaurants, meetings; may be experienced by others as being restless or difficult to keep up with).

    g. Often talks excessively.

    h. Often blurts out an answer before a question has been completed (e.g., completes people's sentences; cannot wait for turn in conversation).

    i. Often has difficulty waiting his or her turn (e.g., while waiting in line).

    j. Often interrupts or intrudes on others (e.g., butts into conversations, games, or activities; may start using other people's things without asking or receiving permission; for adolescents and adults, may intrude into or take over what others are doing).

B. Several inattentive or hyperactive-impulsive symptoms were present prior to age 12 years.

C. Several inattentive or hyperactive-impulsive symptoms are present in two or more settings (e.g., at home, school, or work; with friends or relatives; in other activities).

D. There is clear evidence that the symptoms interfere with, or reduce the quality of, social, academic, or occupational functioning.

E. The symptoms do not occur exclusively during the course of schizophrenia or another psychotic disorder and are not better explained by another mental disorder (e.g., mood disorder, anxiety disorder, dissociative disorder, personality disorder, substance intoxication or withdrawal).

  Specify whether:

  • **Combined presentation:** If both Criterion A1 (inattention) and Criterion A2 (hyperactivity-impulsivity) are met for the past 6 months.

  • **Predominantly inattentive presentation:** If Criterion A1 (inattention) is met but Criterion A2 (hyperactivity-impulsivity) is not met for the past 6 months.

  • **Predominantly hyperactive/impulsive presentation:** If Criterion A2 (hyperactivity-impulsivity) is met and Criterion A1 (inattention) is not met for the past 6 months.

  Specify if:

  • **In partial remission:** When full criteria were previously met, fewer than the full criteria have been met for the past 6 months, and the symptoms still result in impairment in social, academic, or occupational functioning.

  Specify current severity:

  • **Mild:** Few, if any, symptoms in excess of those required to make the diagnosis are present, and symptoms result in no more than minor impairments in social or occupational functioning.

  • **Moderate:** Symptoms or functional impairment between "mild" and "severe" are present.

  • **Severe:** Many symptoms in excess of those required to make the diagnosis, or several symptoms that are particularly severe, are present, or the symptoms result in marked impairment in social or occupational functioning.

Although ADHD was once thought to be a disorder of childhood that gradually improved with age, it is now known that ADHD is a chronic condition requiring ongoing management; for many individuals, symptoms continue into adulthood (American Psychiatric Association, 2013).

Nursing Management

For the Child With ADD or ADHD

Nursing Assessment and Diagnosis

The nurse often encounters the family who is concerned about the child's behavior before a diagnosis has been made. Ask about family and birth history and have the parents describe the child's behaviors. Perform developmental testing and look specifically for attention span and physical activity. Refer the family to their pediatric healthcare home for further assessment, and then to a mental healthcare specialist who is experienced in diagnosing ADHD. Schedule a visit for complete client and family history, physical examination, and electrocardiogram before medication is begun.

Nurses may encounter the child with ADHD in the hospital when parents bring the child for treatment of an injury (e.g., fracture) or other problem. Explore the parents' report of the child's attention span in detail. Usually within a few minutes in an unstructured setting or waiting area, the child with ADHD becomes restless and searches for distraction. Gather information about the child's activity level and impulsiveness. Be alert for information that reveals a serious problem, such as hurting animals or other children. Find out about distractibility, attention deficit in activities of daily living, characteristic ways of reacting, and the extent of impulsiveness when the child is receiving medication. Find out how the family manages at home. Ask about a family history of the disorder, because that is a common finding among children with ADHD.

Examples of nursing diagnoses that might be appropriate for a child with ADHD include the following (NANDA-I © 2014):

- *Communication: Verbal, Impaired,* related to altered perceptions
- *Social Interaction, Impaired,* related to chronic episodes of impulsive behavior
- *Self-Esteem, Chronic Low,* related to behaviors associated with ADD/ADHD
- *Injury, Risk for,* related to high level of impulsiveness and excitability
- *Caregiver Role Strain, Risk for,* related to management of child with unpredictable moods and high energy

Planning and Implementation

Prevention can focus on discouraging regular television exposure for young children from 1 to 3 years and encouraging daily vigorous physical activity for all children. Nursing care of the hospitalized child with ADD/ADHD focuses on administering medications, minimizing environmental distractions, implementing behavioral management plans, providing emotional support to the child and family, promoting self-esteem, and ensuring ongoing care.

ADMINISTER MEDICATIONS

Stimulant and nonstimulant medications increase the child's attention span and decrease distractibility. Be alert for the common side effects of these medications, including anorexia, insomnia, and tachycardia. Administering medication early in the day helps to alleviate insomnia. Anorexia can be managed by giving medication at mealtimes. Baseline cardiac examinations are needed, as well as periodic reevaluation. Careful monitoring of weight, height, and blood pressure is necessary. Instruct families about the abuse potential of stimulant drugs and teach them to keep the medications locked and to administer them only as directed.

MINIMIZE ENVIRONMENTAL DISTRACTIONS

The child may need an environment with minimal distractions. When hospitalized, this may mean a room with only one other child. Keep potentially harmful equipment out of reach. Monitor and limit television and video game time. Use shades to darken the room at nap- or bedtime, and minimize noise. Teach parents to minimize distractions at home during periods when the child needs to concentrate, for example, when doing schoolwork. Visits to areas such as shopping malls and playgrounds may need to be limited. Plenty of daily exercise and minimal use of television and video games may help the child concentrate when needed for school and other tasks.

IMPLEMENT BEHAVIORAL MANAGEMENT PLANS

Behavioral modification programs can help reduce specific impulsive behaviors. An example is setting up a reward program for the child who has taken medication as ordered or completed a homework assignment. The rewards may be daily as well as weekly or monthly, depending on the child's age. For example, one completed homework assignment might be rewarded with 30 minutes of basketball or a bike ride; assignments completed for a week might be rewarded with an activity of the child's choice on the weekend.

If punishment is necessary, the behavior should be corrected while simultaneously supporting the child as a person. Punishment is generally withdrawal of a privilege, and should follow the offense quickly, as the child may not otherwise connect the punishment with the behavior.

PROVIDE EMOTIONAL SUPPORT

Children with ADD or ADHD offer a special challenge to parents, teachers, and healthcare providers. Parents must cope simultaneously with managing the difficult needs and demands of a hard-to-handle child, obtaining appropriate evaluation and treatment, and understanding and accepting the diagnosis, even when the child exhibits different behaviors with different people. Family support is essential. Educate both the parents and the child about the importance of appropriate expectations and consequences of behaviors. Teach skills that will help as the child grows older: making lists of tasks to accomplish; having routines for eating, sleeping, recreation, and schoolwork; minimizing stimuli in the environment when completing work; and asking teachers and friends to identify when behavior is inappropriate.

PROMOTE SELF-ESTEEM

As the child grows, ask about school and friends in order to assess self-concept and self-esteem. Help the child understand the disorder at an appropriate developmental level, and facilitate a trusting relationship with healthcare providers. Assist the child with social skills through role-play, playing in small groups, and modeling. Promote the child's self-esteem by pointing out the positive aspects of behavior and treating instances of negative behavior as learning opportunities. Help the child to develop ego strengths (the consciousness to be able to screen outside stimuli and control internal demands), which will result in better impulse control and thus increase self-esteem over time (Houck, Kendall, Miller, et al., 2011).

COMMUNITY-BASED NURSING CARE

Most children with ADD or ADHD are hospitalized only when needing care for another condition. Parents need support to understand the diagnosis and to learn how to manage the child. Emphasize the importance of a stable environment, at home as well as at school. At home the child may have difficulty staying on task. Parents need to consider age and developmental appropriateness of tasks, give clear and simple instructions, and provide frequent reminders to ensure completion. Routines in the evening can promote good sleep patterns.

The nurse can serve as a liaison to teachers and school personnel, or as the case manager for the child. An individualized education plan may be needed (see Chapter 38), with clear expected outcomes stated for the child's behaviors. Special classrooms or periods of instruction free from the distractions of the entire class may enable the child to improve school performance. Parents may have difficulty understanding the need for these approaches because the child often tests with above-average intelligence. Reinforce the importance of providing a structured environment free from unnecessary external stimuli. Be sure that parents understand behavioral approaches that will help the child, how to administer prescribed medications, and the importance of returning for healthcare visits to monitor for side effects. Medication should be locked safely away at home to keep it away from other children and prevent illegal use of this controlled substance. An individual school health plan may be needed for medication management.

Parents may have heard about ADHD in the media and often have many questions about its cause and management. Providing information about complementary and alternative treatments is a nursing role.

As the child grows older, explain the disorder and teach about techniques that will assist in dealing with problems. Assist in planning for a quiet environment during work. Encourage children with attention deficits to write down instructions from teachers and to use checklists to help them accomplish specific tasks.

Evaluation

Expected outcomes of nursing care for the child with ADD or ADHD include the following:

- Parents and child demonstrate understanding of the condition.
- Medications are administered and managed safely and as prescribed.
- The child demonstrates increased attentiveness and decreased hyperactivity, impulsivity, and sleep disturbance.
- The child demonstrates formation of a positive self-image.
- Educational performance is achieved to maximum potential.

Mood Disorders

Depression

Depression is psychologic distress that can range from mild to severe. Only in recent years has depression in children been recognized as a clinical condition. Many children referred to child guidance centers and mental healthcare providers because of behavioral difficulties or poor achievement actually suffer from depression. The incidence of major depression is estimated to be about 2% in childhood and up to 8% in adolescence; by age 18 years approximately 11% have had a depressive episode (Chung & Soares, 2012; National Institute of Mental Health [NIMH], n.d.a). A history of substance abuse and anxiety disorder increases risk, and cultural variations in rates exist.

ETIOLOGY AND PATHOPHYSIOLOGY

Theories have been proposed to explain the cause of depression in children and adolescents. Depression may be biologic in origin or a result of learned helplessness, cognitive distortion, social skills deficit, or family dysfunction. The physiologic theory focuses on monoamine neurotransmission. These amines include indolamine, serotonin, norepinephrine, and dopamine, and decreases are sometimes found in depression. Magnetic resonance imaging has identified brain changes in individuals who are depressed, suggesting a biologic basis (NIMH, n.d.a).

Developing Cultural Competence Depression Rates

Ethnic/racial differences in depression rates exist. The highest rates of depression are observed with Hispanic and Native American youth. Although there are scant data with Asian American youth, their rates of depression appear to be low. Data do not provide a clear picture of depression in African American youth as compared to White youth; in some studies, rates are higher and in others they are lower. In general, more female youth than male youth report depression (Lee & Liechty, 2014). It is probable that genetics, environment, and culture interact to influence the differences in prevalence of depression.

Parental depression and stress are predictive of childhood depression. Abuse and neglect, family conflict, parental death, and low socioeconomic status predispose children to depression. Other psychiatric diagnoses are common in children with depression; these include conditions such as ADHD, anxiety disorder, bipolar disease, or substance abuse (Emslie, Kennard, & Mayes, 2011).

CLINICAL MANIFESTATIONS

Characteristic findings of major depression in children and adolescents include declining school performance; withdrawal from social activities; sleep disturbance (either too much or too little); appetite disturbance (too much or too little); multiple somatic complaints, especially headaches and stomachaches; decreased energy; difficulty concentrating and making decisions; low self-esteem; and feelings of hopelessness. There is much variation among children in the symptoms displayed, and they often have some, but not all, of the major criteria. Symptoms vary according to children's developmental levels.

CLINICAL THERAPY

Youth should be screened for depression during well-child examinations or when indicated at other healthcare encounters (Agency for Healthcare Research and Quality [AHRQ], 2014). Once depression or major depressive disorder is diagnosed, comprehensive assessment of the child should occur in order to rule out physical illness that can be linked to depressive symptoms, such as diabetes, cancer, and obesity. The child is tested for various mental health problems since comorbidities (combination with other disorders) are common. A history of bullying and substance abuse are examples of these comorbidities.

Initial assessment is performed by a child psychologist or child psychiatrist. A variety of scales and techniques are used; examples of useful tools are the Children's Depression Inventory (CDI), the Revised Children's Manifest Anxiety Scale, the Beck Depression Inventory (BDI-PC), the Guideline for Adolescent Preventative Services Questionnaire, the Patient Health Questionnaire for Adolescents (PHQ-A), the Reynolds Adolescent Depression Scale (RADS), and the Center for Epidemiological Studies Depression Scale for Children (CES-DC) (Stockings et al., 2014).

Treatment may include psychotherapy in combination with psychotropic medication. Often a combination of individual, family, and group therapy provides the greatest benefits for young children and adolescents. Involving parents, other family members, school personnel, and friends in the treatment plan is essential (Hughes & Asarnow, 2011). Group therapy is often effective for adolescents. Cognitive behavioral therapy (CBT) may be used with adolescents, and play therapy with younger children (see discussion of play therapy earlier in this chapter). CBT focuses on identification and restructuring of thoughts, feelings, and behaviors, leading to understanding of negative thoughts and increasing activities that provide pleasure (Mahoney, Kennard, & Mayes, 2011). Supportive interactions with healthcare providers and active problem solving are approaches that improve outcomes in adolescents. Healthcare providers should educate families about depression and counsel as needed. Confidentiality should be ensured. Refer to community resources as needed. Ensure a plan for safety of the adolescent.

Growth and Development

Symptoms of depression in children vary according to their developmental levels. Infants may fail to eat and grow. Toddlers can show regressive behaviors in toileting and other activities. Preschoolers have less symbolic and other play activities, may be irritable, and lack confidence. School-age children may show a decrease in academic performance, increased or decreased activity, somatic complaints, and loss of friends. Adolescents can have a wide array of symptoms such as anxiety, decreased social contact, poor school performance, lack of prior involvement in activities, poor self-care, difficulty with parents and teachers, or focus on violence (NIMH, n.d.a).

Antidepressant medications, most commonly the selective serotonin reuptake inhibitors (SSRIs), imipramine (Tofranil),

desipramine (Norpramin), and amitriptyline (Elavil), may be prescribed. The only antidepressant approved to treat major depressive disorders in children and adolescents is fluoxetine HCl (Prozac), but clinicians sometimes use others when the youth does not respond to Prozac.

SAFETY ALERT!

The SSRIs act to block reuptake of serotonin in the synapse, so that serotonin levels (which influence mood) increase. Although the SSRIs are generally considered safer than some other types of antidepressants, their use in children has been limited, so side effects must be monitored. Generally, the child is started with a low dose, which is increased slowly to minimize the chance of side effects. Because of some reports of increased suicidal ideation and the lack of efficacy evidence, a psychiatric-mental health specialist must closely monitor children and adolescents taking SSRIs (AHRQ, 2014; NIMH, 2012a). A patient medication guide with the risks and precautions, as well as drug label information, must be provided for every client and family.

The major serious and life-threatening side effect of SSRIs is serotonin syndrome, a condition characterized by agitation, muscle twitching, gastric upset, chills, fever, confusion, and dizziness. It is more likely to develop when the child or adolescent is also taking St. John's wort, other antidepressants, alcohol, diet pills, or drugs such as ecstasy and LSD (Mayo Clinic, 2013b; Morrison & Schwartz, 2014). Be certain to ask questions in a nonjudgmental way about intake of any alternative therapies, other medications, or substance use to identify those most at risk.

Sudden cardiac death has occurred in several children on tricyclic antidepressants (TCAs). Because of this risk, serum levels should be monitored and electrocardiograms (ECGs) performed. Specific ECG changes along with a resting heart rate above 100, systolic blood pressure above 130 mmHg, and diastolic blood pressure above 85 mmHg necessitate immediate reporting to the prescriber. A narrow margin exists between the therapeutic and lethal doses in children (Weeke et al., 2012).

Nursing Management
For the Child With Depression

Nursing Assessment and Diagnosis

Take a thorough history and physical examination, including observation of behavior, at the time of admission. Assess the child for common risk factors for depression (Table 55–4).

TABLE 55–4 Risk Factors for Child and Adolescent Depression

CHILD	FAMILY	SCHOOL AND SOCIAL SITUATIONS
• Frequent feelings of sadness, sleep problems, loss of interest in activities	• Parental neglect, abuse, or loss	• Academic pressures and underachievement
• Increase in risk taking and impulsivity	• Dysfunctional family relationships	• Stressful social relationships
• Previous suicide attempt	• Family history of depression, suicide, substance abuse, alcoholism, other psychopathology	• Declining participation in social events
• Alcohol or substance abuse		
• Diagnosed psychotic disorder		
• Chronic illness and frequent hospitalization		

Several nursing diagnoses that might be appropriate for the child or adolescent hospitalized with depression are included in the accompanying *Nursing Care Plan*. Other diagnoses might include the following (NANDA-I © 2014):

- *Self Neglect* related to lack of energy and inability to perform daily hygiene
- *Powerlessness* related to sense of helplessness
- *Self-Esteem, Chronic Low,* related to negative self-evaluation

Planning and Implementation

Nursing care of the child or adolescent hospitalized for depression includes administering medications and other therapy and providing supportive care. Monitor vital signs of youth receiving antidepressant medications. Watch for common side effects of the agent(s) used. Carefully monitor for serious side effects of TCAs or SSRIs and be aware that lower doses are used at initiation, with doses increasing slowly to the desired level. Frequent face-to-face follow-up visits are needed. When dosages are altered, behavior and ideation changes must be closely monitored. Monitor cardiovascular status, including hypertension and tachycardia, observe motor movement, and record dietary intake. Help parents to evaluate inpatient settings to be certain the care provided will best meet the needs of the child or adolescent. Refer to accompanying *Nursing Care Plan: The Child or Adolescent Hospitalized With Depression* for specific nursing interventions.

DISCHARGE PLANNING AND HOME CARE TEACHING

When the child has been hospitalized and is returning home, teach parents to recognize signs and symptoms of worsening depression. Also teach them dosages and side effects of any prescribed medications. Refer the family to appropriate healthcare providers and to support groups for family members dealing with depression.

COMMUNITY-BASED NURSING CARE

Most children with depression are cared for in the community. Maintain regular contact with the family through their healthcare visits to outpatient agencies and by making home visits. Monitor the child's affect, activity, and food intake. School teachers and counselors often are aware of the child's ability to perform in the school setting. Have the family schedule after-school care so young children are not left at home alone for extended periods. Assist the family in finding support for financial and emotional needs related to managing the child's depression. Major expected outcomes for nursing care of the child with depression are found on the accompanying *Nursing Care Plan*.

Bipolar Disorder (Manic Depression)

Bipolar disorder is a mental illness in which extreme changes in affect and energy are manifested. Moods most often alter between mania (high energy and euphoria) and depression.

Nursing Care Plan: The Child or Adolescent Hospitalized With Depression

1. Nursing Diagnosis: *Hopelessness* **related to long-term stress (NANDA-I © 2014)**

GOAL: The child or adolescent will discuss feelings of hopelessness.

INTERVENTION	RATIONALE
• Encourage open expression of feelings. Explore hopeless, sad, or lonely feelings. Point out the connection between feelings and behavior. Assess the child or adolescent to identify the precipitating event when feelings of sadness arose. Maintain an accepting and nonjudgmental attitude regarding any feelings expressed by the child.	• Expressing feelings may help to relieve sadness, loneliness, despair, and hopelessness.
• Encourage the child or adolescent to take part in self-care and unit activities. Use routines to establish feelings of control.	• An active role in self-care and treatment helps the child or adolescent to feel more in control.
• Medicate as ordered and document results.	• Antidepressants modify mood to a more hopeful outlook.

EXPECTED OUTCOME: By discharge, child or adolescent will express an interest in the future.

2. Nursing Diagnosis: *Coping, Ineffective,* **related to inadequate social support or disturbance in pattern of appraisal of threat (NANDA-I © 2014)**

GOAL: The child or adolescent will use effective coping skills.

INTERVENTION	RATIONALE
• Teach positive, effective coping strategies such as guided imagery and relaxation. Assist the child or adolescent to focus on strengths rather than weaknesses.	• Therapeutic techniques can help the child or adolescent to replace negative thoughts and images with more positive and effective beliefs and images. These interventions foster resilience.
• Assist the child or adolescent to identify friends, family members, and others who are positive and supportive.	• Helps the child or adolescent to become aware that people can be caring and supportive (thus validating self-esteem).

EXPECTED OUTCOME: Child or adolescent will verbalize and demonstrate ability to cope appropriately for his or her age.

3. Nursing Diagnosis: *Social Interaction, Impaired,* **related to self-concept disturbance (NANDA-I © 2014)**

GOAL: The child or adolescent will participate in and initiate activities and conversation.

INTERVENTION	RATIONALE
• Assist the child or adolescent to identify topics and activities of interest.	• The more the child or adolescent focuses on areas of interest, the less he or she will focus on internal anxiety and depression.
• Encourage interaction with peers and staff.	• Each positive interaction reinforces feelings of success. Each success reinforces the desire for future social interaction.
• Facilitate visits from family and friends.	• Reinforces positive and rewarding relationships.
• Provide guidance to family regarding interaction that promotes self-esteem.	• The family's existing interaction style is often negative.

EXPECTED OUTCOME: By discharge, child or adolescent will initiate conversation and activities with staff and peers.

4. Nursing Diagnosis: *Nutrition, Imbalanced: Less than Body Requirements,* **related to loss of appetite secondary to depression (NANDA-I © 2014)**

GOAL: The child's or adolescent's daily intake will be adequate to maintain optimal nutritional status.

INTERVENTION	RATIONALE
• Offer nutritious finger foods, sandwiches, and high-calorie liquid supplements frequently throughout the day.	• Convenient easy-to-eat foods encourage the child or adolescent to eat and maintain nutritional status.
• Offer easy-to-carry drinks that are high in vitamins, minerals, and calories.	• These are a convenient method for meeting hydration and electrolyte needs.
• Encourage daily vigorous physical activity of at least 30 min.	• Physical activity stimulates appetite.

EXPECTED OUTCOME: Child or adolescent's daily intake will be adequate to maintain optimal nutritional status by discharge.

Children often present with irritability or hyperactivity. About 1% of children and adults have bipolar illness, with a high rate of onset from 15 to 19 years, although onset as young as preschool age can occur. There is a high rate of attempted suicide in those with bipolar disease, as well as co-occurrence with other disorders such as ADHD, anxiety, and substance abuse, all of which complicate diagnosis (NIMH, n.d.b).

Bipolar disorder is classified into four types:

- *Bipolar I*—includes a severe manic episode that requires hospitalization or causes functional impairment in life
- *Bipolar II*—at least one episode of mild to moderate mania (hypomania) and one of depression
- *Cyclothymic disorder*—manifests as multiple mild manic and depressive episodes

TEACHING HIGHLIGHTS | Selecting Residential and Inpatient Care for the Child With Mental Illness

Families need guidelines to help them evaluate inpatient facilities when a child with a mental disorder must be placed in an institution. You can refer them to the National Alliance for the Mentally Ill website. Provide questions for the families to ask:
- What is the staff-to-youth ratio?
- What are the guidelines for chemical and physical restraint?
- Are children isolated when behaviors are inappropriate?
- Are children constantly monitored visually when in restraint or when potentially dangerous to self or others?
- Does the child have a full physical and psychologic evaluation by a specialist within 24 hours of entry to the facility?
- What professionals review the plan of care and how often?
- Who can the family speak to for regular updates on the child?
- How often can the family visit?
- What services will be covered by insurance?
- What subjective feelings do the family members have as they visit the unit and facility?
- What services will be offered on an ongoing basis on discharge?

- *Bipolar not otherwise specified*—rapid mood fluctuations, mania without depressive episodes, or chronic depression with hypomania episodes (NIMH, n.d.b).

When parents or close relatives are affected, the child is more likely to have the disorder. Thus a genetic etiology is probable. It is believed that genetics and environment interact to create the condition in youth. Brain imaging shows abnormalities of the frontal and prefrontal cortex, the hippocampus, the basal ganglia, and the left amygdala, which is the center for experiencing fear (NIMH, n.d.b).

The manic phase of bipolar illness is characterized by hyperactivity and high energy, irritability, aggression, and sometimes hallucinations. In the depressive phase, the child is sad, has alterations in sleep and eating patterns, and is socially withdrawn, similar to any depressive illness. Mania may be the persistent symptom in children, or rapid cycles of mania and depression can occur throughout the day (Dineen, 2014; Kloos & Robb, 2011; Scrandis, 2014).

Diagnosis and treatment of bipolar disorder should be performed by mental health specialists. Use of alcohol or illegal drugs should be ruled out as a cause of symptoms, even in children. Since the manic phase is often manifested by hyperactivity, the child may incorrectly be treated with stimulants (see treatment of ADHD earlier in this chapter), and the disease can be worsened. Irritability, elation, labile moods, and sleep disturbance are commonly seen in children (Dineen, 2014; Kloos & Robb, 2011; Scrandis, 2014).

The treatment of bipolar disease involves a variety of drugs used to stabilize mood. Lithium, valproate, divalproex, carbamazepine, olanzapine, oxcarbazepine, lamotrigine, quetiapine, and risperidone are examples of drugs used; antidepressants may be prescribed (Blake, 2012; NIMH, 2012a). Only lithium has been approved by the FDA for use in those ages 12 to 18 years. However, clinicians prescribe other drugs with careful monitoring being performed. Early treatment is key to preventing chronic, serious mental illness. Individual and family education and therapy can be helpful.

Nurses are instrumental in identifying children with the disorder, providing information to families, and monitoring the drugs and psychotherapy for the child. Nurses should observe for side effects to the specific drug regimen used and assist parents to find resources for health care since medications and other treatments may be costly. Parents and children need information about the disorder since it may recur several times during the child's life. Nurses can assist the child to find social events and groups that build a sense of self-esteem.

Anxiety and Related Disorders

A large group of anxiety disorders can affect youth as well as adults. Some of the more common types seen in children and adolescents are described in the following sections, with detailed nursing management described for posttraumatic stress disorder.

Generalized Anxiety Disorder

Anxiety is a subjective feeling of uncertainty and helplessness, usually accompanied by central nervous system (CNS) signs, including restlessness, trembling, perspiration, and rapid pulse. Anxiety is second only to substance abuse (see Chapter 42) in incidence for mental disorders and is a common mental disorder among children. From 4% to 20% of youth experience some type of anxiety disorder (Boydston, Hsiao, & Varley, 2012a; Sarvet & Brewer, 2011).

Anxiety disorders are strongly linked to familial and genetic factors. Diagnosis is performed by a mental health specialist, and treatment is usually cognitive behavioral therapy (CBT) and may involve medication. CBT can include child or family interventions that focus on relaxation, recognition of feelings, and self-talking (learned words or phrases said to oneself to aid in management of distress). Medications that have been reported to be successful in children include SSRIs and benzodiazepines (Boydston et al., 2012b).

Separation Anxiety Disorder

Separation anxiety disorder is characterized by an extreme state of uneasiness when in unfamiliar surroundings and often by refusal to visit friends' homes or attend school for at least 2 weeks. It is a common type of anxiety disorder manifested by children (Boydston et al., 2012a). Many children with separation anxiety disorder refuse to attend school at some point (see *School Phobia [Social Phobia]* section later in this chapter). This phobia may be recurrent and become worse at certain times. The condition may be acute in onset (preceded by a traumatic event) or slow in developing over time.

Children with separation anxiety disorder tend to be perfectionistic, overly compliant, and eager to please. They appear to cling to the parent or caretaker. They may use physical complaints such as headaches, abdominal pain, nausea, and vomiting in an attempt to avoid being away from the parent. Depression frequently accompanies separation anxiety disorder. The resulting avoidant behaviors can interfere with personal growth and development, academic achievement, and social functioning.

Diagnosis is made by a mental health specialist. Treatment includes CBT with both child and parents. Parents learn about the disorder and how to structure the setting so that the child is expected to attend school. Consistency in expectations is needed since if the child is permitted to stay home some days or has missed school and other activities for longer periods, treatment is more difficult. The child learns what situations cause anxiety and how to manage the situations and feelings elicited. Both parents and child work out the expectations for behavior for the child with the mental health therapist; school personnel are included in the treatment plan. Medication can be used if CBT is not helpful.

Growth and Development

The separation anxiety commonly experienced by a 2-year-old differs from the psychiatric disorder in age appropriateness, duration, and severity. Separation anxiety disorder affects children of preschool age or older, lasts for at least 2 weeks, and is characterized by excessive anxiety. In contrast, the separation anxiety experienced by the 2-year-old involves a single episode of separation from a familiar caretaker and is a characteristic response in toddlers.

Panic Disorder

Panic disorder is the presence of recurrent, unexpected panic attacks. Panic attacks are periods of intense fear and discomfort in the absence of real danger. The lifetime risk of panic disorder is 2% (Boydston et al., 2012a). Predictive factors for panic attacks in adolescence include a history of separation anxiety or other anxiety disorder in life and a history of parental panic attacks.

Examples of the physical symptoms experienced are palpitations, sweating, chills, hot flashes, shaking, shortness of breath, choking, chest pain, nausea, and dizziness. The person describes feelings of danger or doom. Some people may have accompanying agoraphobia. **Agoraphobia** is anxiety about being in places or situations from which escape may be difficult or embarrassing, or in which help may not be available. The attacks may be continuous or episodic, but generally are chronic.

Diagnosis is made by a mental health specialist. Similar to anxiety, treatment may involve individual and family therapy, with use of medication in some cases. Nurses can help identify the disorder, refer for evaluation, and provide care in the community so that the child attends therapy sessions and takes medication as ordered.

Obsessive-Compulsive Disorder

People with obsessive-compulsive disorder (OCD) may be mildly or severely affected. Up to 2% of children are affected, and about 80% of adults with OCD had the condition in childhood (Boydston et al., 2012a). Affected children have recurrent obsessive thoughts, commonly about contamination, harm, sex, or moral concerns. These obsessions are handled through a series of compulsive behaviors that interfere with daily life. Examples of behaviors are excessive handwashing, counting objects, and hoarding substances. These practices may take 1 hour or more of time each day. Children with OCD differ from adults in several ways. They have more aggressive obsessions, such as fears of catastrophe, more commonly hoard objects, and are more likely to have religious obsessions. The presence of comorbidity with other mental health disorders is common.

The basal ganglia of the brain are affected and a genetic link is observed. A neurochemical cause may be related to abnormal serotonin metabolism. MRI changes in the globus pallidus and anterior cingulated gyrus of the brain have been noted. Post-streptococcal autoimmune disorder may be a cause in some cases (NIMH, 2012b).

Clinical Tip

Pediatric autoimmune neuropsychiatric disorders (PANDAS) are characterized by obsessive-compulsive and/or tic disorder, childhood onset, association with group A beta-hemolytic streptococcal infection, and neurologic abnormalities. It is believed that in certain children, the strep infection leads to a neural autoimmune response, resulting in the psychiatric disorder. Research continues to identify possible mechanisms, results, and treatments for this cause of OCD (NIMH, 2012b). *Pediatric acute-onset neuropsychiatric syndrome (PANS)* is the term used to refer to all cases of abrupt-onset OCD, not only those following streptococcal infection.

Diagnosis is made by a mental health specialist. Treatment may involve CBT, where the feared occurrence is presented and the person learns that no harm will occur. Involvement of the family in treatment is important so that members learn how to handle the child's ritualistic behaviors. Medications, such as clomipramine and the SSRIs, are effective in most children and adolescents. Nurses can identify cases and refer for mental health evaluation and provide teaching and support for families.

School Phobia (Social Phobia)

School phobia (also called *social phobia, school avoidance,* or *school refusal*) is a persistent, irrational, or excessive fear of negative evaluation or embarrassment in social situations and therefore of attending school. The child may fear being harmed or losing control. Social and school phobias occur in children as young as 5 years of age, often being present at 11 or 12 years, but can occur in children up to 16 years (Boydston et al., 2012a).

Children with social phobia may fear asking for directions, ordering food at a restaurant, and speaking in the classroom. They commonly report that teachers and peers "pick on" them. Somatic complaints are similar to those in children with separation anxiety disorder. Characteristically, symptoms are present only on school days and not on weekends or holidays. The social withdrawal that occurs in this disorder further impairs the child since social interactions are needed for normal developmental progression.

Diagnosis is made by a mental health specialist. Treatment includes the family and child, and establishes firm limits for behavioral expectations and consequences. CBT is used, including education of the youth about the condition, body awareness of symptoms, and methods of changing feelings. SSRI medications may sometimes be needed to lessen anxiety in social situations.

Conversion Reaction

Conversion reaction is a disorder in which a disturbance or loss of sensory, motor, or other physical functions suggests neurologic or other somatic disease. The disturbance or loss cannot be explained by any known pathophysiologic mechanism. Instead, psychologic factors are involved. About 3% of the population experiences conversion reactions at some time. Adolescence and early adulthood are common times for the onset to occur, with onset being rare before 10 years or after 35 years of age (Kozlowska, Scher, & Williams, 2011).

Conversion reactions develop in response to a catastrophic event such as threat, loss, or harm. Clinical manifestations include altered sensations such as blindness or deafness; paralysis or ataxia, including inability to stand or walk and loss of ability to speak (aphonia); involuntary movements, such as pseudoepileptic convulsions; and constant complaints of pain with no physical basis (psychogenic pain). Children under 10 years old usually present with gait abnormalities or seizures. The onset of conversion symptoms is usually dramatic and sudden. Symptoms often appear to be neurologic, but on careful examination, obvious discrepancies are found. The person is usually calm about the symptoms even though they are serious. Often the child or family members appear indifferent or unconcerned over what healthcare providers consider an overwhelming physical disability.

Children suspected of having a conversion reaction require a complete physical and neurologic evaluation to rule out any possible physiologic basis for the symptoms. Individual and family therapy is usually necessary to identify the source of the psychologic conflict, pain, or need resulting in the conversion symptoms. Pharmacologic approaches may also be used.

Posttraumatic Stress Disorder

Acute stress disorder can occur after any life-threatening event and is manifested in the first month after exposure to the event. Symptoms include repeatedly reliving the traumatic experience, anxiety, and increased arousal. Similarly, people with *posttraumatic stress disorder* (PTSD) have experienced or witnessed a life-threatening event; however, the symptoms of distress continue for more than 1 month and cause impairment in functioning. Estimates of the incidence of PTSD are hard to obtain. It is assumed that about 40% of youth have an episode of trauma that could lead to PTSD, and there is a lifetime risk of 8.7% for the disorder. While 20% of children may experience PTSD after traumatic events, the prevalence rises to 90% when the trauma is severe (Boydston et al., 2012a).

Examples of events associated with posttraumatic stress include sexual or other child abuse, rape, car crash, fire, witnessing violence, and war experiences. Cassandra, described in the chapter-opening quote, was experiencing PTSD resulting from a frightening car crash as she was driven to school. She was too young to describe her feelings verbally to her mother or school personnel; however, she manifested the sleep abnormalities and other complaints common in the disorder.

The disorder involves both a traumatic event and the child's reaction to this event. It is believed that brain changes occur in trauma, leading to neurobiologic alterations that cause dysfunction of memory. Overreactivity of the amygdala, underreactivity of the prefrontal cortex, and increased dopamine in the medial prefrontal cortex are observed. Female gender, having other psychiatric disorders, a family history of psychiatric illness, and severe or lengthy trauma are all risk factors.

Common reactions in persons with PTSD are intrusive symptoms such as negative thoughts and feelings, avoidance of reminders of the event, and arousal or hyperreactivity to events (American Psychiatric Association, 2013). The child with PTSD has feelings of fear, terror, and helplessness, and may relive the event frequently in thought and nightmares. The child may become emotionally numb in a subconscious attempt to protect the self, but may have a persistently increased state of arousal. The child exhibits a state of hypervigilance and an exaggerated startle response, such as to touch or loud noises. The child with PTSD is often irritable, and has sleep problems and inattentiveness. The child feels detached from others and alone. Immediately after the event, the child may appear to have adapted and functions normally. However, after several weeks or even months, the symptoms of the disorder begin to appear.

The diagnosis is made by a mental health specialist; a variety of instruments assist in screening for the disorder. Counseling by a mental health specialist is the main therapy for PTSD. Cassandra saw a clinical psychologist who used play therapy to help her communicate her fears related to a car crash (Figure 55–6). CBT is the treatment of choice, with both the child and family members included. Young children show significant improvement in symptoms after a course of

CBT (Center for Injury Research and Prevention, 2011). A variety of antidepressants and SSRIs are used for pharmacologic treatment.

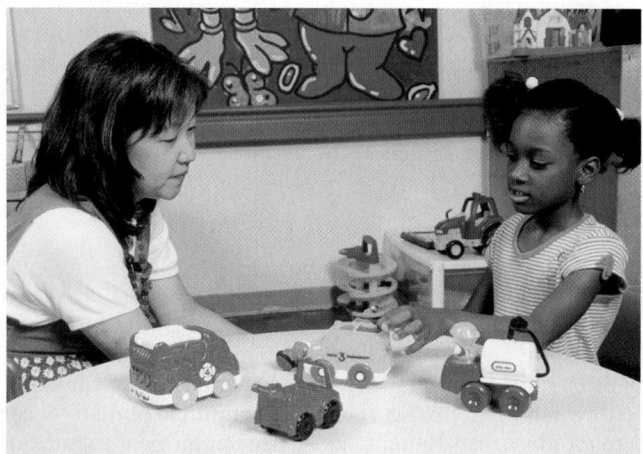

Figure 55–6 The psychologist uses play therapy to help Cassandra reenact her car crash. This helps her gain some control over the event so that it is not so frightening.

Clinical Reasoning Posttraumatic Stress Disorder

Cassandra is a 9-year-old girl who has recently become fearful about attending school and has awakened crying at night. She is in the third grade at a school she has attended for 2 years. A few weeks ago, she was in a car crash as her mother drove her to school. She received only minor injuries and returned to school the next day. However, her mother believes that Cassandra's behavior has been worsening since the car crash. She spoke with the school nurse, who is aware of no trauma at school, but did learn from the teacher that Cassandra has not been paying attention in class recently. Cassandra cannot explain why she does not want to go to school, only that her stomach aches or some other part of her body hurts.

Cassandra visited her pediatrician, who ruled out any physical cause for her complaints, and referred her to a child psychologist. The psychologist has scheduled several sessions with Cassandra to help her learn to verbalize her fears and learn strategies to deal with them. She uses dolls in an attempt to help Cassandra act out her fears and gain some understanding. The psychologist communicates Cassandra's progress to you, the school nurse.

- How can you ensure Cassandra's attendance at school?
- What does the teacher need to know to support Cassandra in the classroom?
- What is your role as liaison between the psychologist, family, and school personnel?
- Parents often feel guilty when a child experiences a mental health disorder. What type of information and support do Cassandra's parents need?

Nursing Management

Nurses often help identify PTSD victims so that care can be obtained. Ask about traumatic events in the past and how the child reacted. Inquire about recent changes in the child's behavior. Include school attendance, complaints of physical illness, sleep patterns, and rituals in behavior. A family history of mental disorders may be useful. Youth who run away from home and present at homeless shelters are often suffering from PTSD. Assessment for the condition should be part of the initial history.

Nursing care for anxiety disorders focuses on behavioral and cognitive therapies to enhance coping skills. Mental health nurses may conduct group therapy sessions (Figure 55–7). Group sessions for children often provide a forum for discussion of fears, an opportunity to enhance skills of working together, and an opportunity to learn coping skills. Being a member of a group with other children experiencing anxiety or trauma can remove the stigma and allow the child the freedom to explore the behavior and its causes. Several of the techniques described in the chapter, such as drawing pictures and discussing them or telling stories, are used by mental health nurses in child therapy groups (Boydston et al., 2012b).

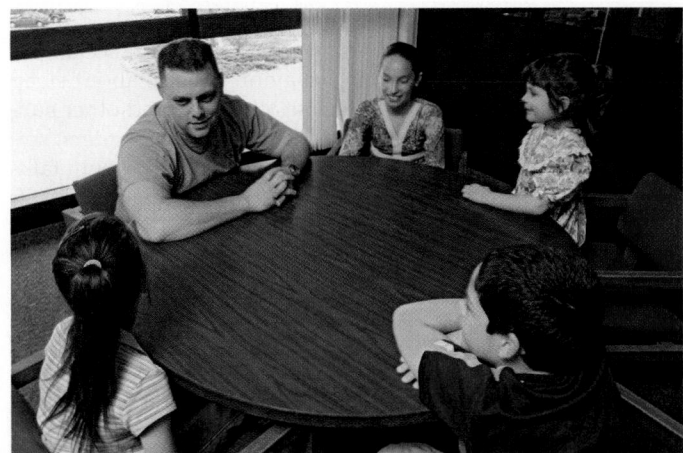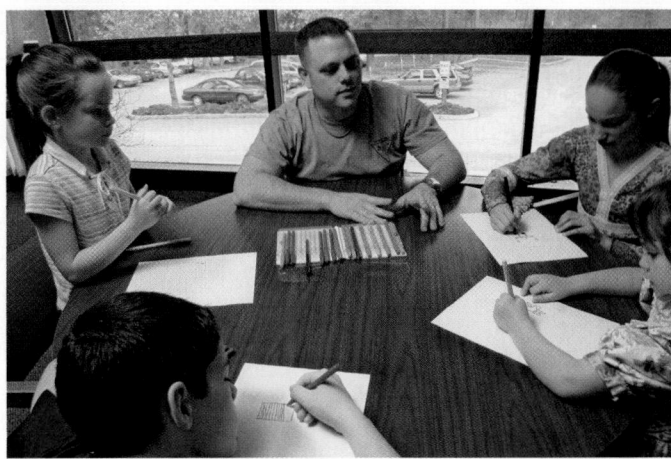

Figure 55–7 This nurse conducts a group therapy session for children who have experienced traumatic events and have resulting anxiety disorders. He is clearly engaged, has a positive rapport, and fosters exchanges among the children. Playing games and drawing are frequent techniques used in the group.

Children need to learn relaxation techniques and nurses may teach such techniques or recommend that the child consider participation in yoga or guided imagery classes. Inquire about alternative therapies that the child and family are using or have an interest in beginning, and refer as needed. Parents or other significant people should be included in the treatment program. Nurses often teach them basic information about the child's diagnosis and therapy. They should be in at least some therapy sessions with the child. Provide the family with resources that will assist with relief from worry about the child, guilt about causing an accident that triggered the child's symptoms, or other feelings related to the diagnosis.

Insurance companies may provide limited payment for mental health services. Help the family to see the importance of recommended therapy and assist them to find resources for care if needed. School personnel may need to know about the child's treatment. Partner with the families to provide needed information. Some schools have counselors that can be instrumental in carrying out treatment plans at school and acting as a resource in that setting. School personnel may be asked to provide feedback about the child's attendance, performance, and social skills as a measure of the success of therapy, and the community or school nurse can relay this information.

Nurses often administer medications to children being treated for PTSD and other mental health concerns. Be alert for side effects and ensure the family knows how to safely administer the drugs. These drugs should be kept locked securely. Have the child return for follow-up as needed since some medications may take several weeks to achieve effects, and close monitoring is essential. The child should wear a medication alert identification for drugs being taken.

Other Disorders

Suicide

Suicide is the third leading cause of death in adolescents between 15 and 19 years of age. About 4400 youth commit suicide annually, and an additional 149,000 receive care after attempted suicide. In any 1 year, over 15% of youth admit to contemplating suicide (CDC, 2012b). The prevalence of suicide is about 7.32 per 100,000, with 86% of the deaths among male adolescents. Firearms, suffocation, and poisoning are the most common means of suicide (CDC, 2012b).

TEACHING HIGHLIGHTS | Talking With Children About Traumatic Events

Whether a child or adolescent experiences trauma from a car crash, abuse, or environmental event, parents can help to decrease the effects of the stress and prevent the appearance of PTSD. Some suggestions for parents include:

- Be sure children feel free to ask parents, teachers, or others about the events and their feelings.
- Assure children that their feelings are common and the stress may return now and then over time.
- Be honest and open in responses, without overloading children with more details than they need.
- Be prepared to repeat answers and discuss the same topics many times.
- Get help from counselors who can suggest how to talk with the child.
- Use communication methods appropriate at various ages, such as reading books, doing art projects, or drawing.
- Show children that they are loved by spending time and planning activities with them.
- Limit the television and other media time where the child is exposed to violence and traumatic events.
- Restore a sense of normal routines into the child's life.
- Be alert for increasing signs of distress and seek care from a professional if they occur.

Developing Cultural Competence Suicide, Gender, and Ethnicity

Some ethnic groups have a high rate of suicide. For example, Native Americans and Alaskan Natives have a rate of suicide of 31/100,000, while for all youth the rate is 12.2/100,000. The historic pain experienced by this ethnic group and lack of opportunities for many youth may be some of the reasons for a high suicide rate. Hispanic female adolescents have a high rate of suicide attempts. Males have a high rate of suicide at 4 times that of females; males more often use firearms, while females more commonly use poisoning (CDC, 2012b).

Healthy People 2020 goals focus on eliminating such health disparities by finding the causes, decreasing rates of suicide, educating about risk factors, and establishing prevention programs (U.S. Department of Health and Human Services [USDHHS], 2015).

Healthy People 2020

(MHMD-2) Reduce suicide attempts by adolescents from the present 1.9/100 to 1.7/100 (a 10% improvement)

It is not unusual for healthcare providers and parents to label suicide attempts by children and adolescents "accidents." Up to one half of childhood suicides may be recorded as accidents; suicide data for children under age 10 years are not maintained. Adults may have difficulty believing that young children, in particular, would have any reason to want to end their lives. Because of this, many children brought to the emergency department with indications of a suicide attempt are often classified as unintentional injury victims and released without arrangements for appropriate follow-up care. Accurate identification and treatment are needed for youth at risk of suicide.

Many risk factors for suicide exist in children and adolescents, while some protective factors are influential as well (Table 55–5). The most common precursor to adolescent suicide is depression (see earlier discussion in this chapter). Common signs or symptoms of an underlying depression that could lead to suicide include boredom, restlessness, problems with concentration, irritability, lethargy, intentional misbehavior, preoccupation with one's own body or health, and excessive dependence on or isolation from others (especially adults or caregivers).

The child or adolescent at high risk for suicide may be admitted to a mental health unit for care or cared for in a community mental health facility. Treatment may include individual, group, or family therapy. Negotiating a "no suicide" contract is one method that may be used with a suicidal youth. In the contract, the child agrees not to attempt suicide during a specified time period. When a suicide attempt is made, the child or adolescent may be hospitalized for 24 hours, kept in a short-term monitoring unit, or sent home under close observation to ensure adequate assessment and monitoring. It is important to provide crisis intervention at the time of the suicide attempt to minimize the opportunity for repeat attempts and to begin a therapeutic treatment plan.

Nursing Management

The major nursing role is in prevention of suicide. All children and adolescents in health promotion visits and emergency departments should be evaluated for risk. Health promotion visits are an opportunity to be alert for children with depression (see previous discussion in this chapter), substance abuse, recent stresses, and changes in behavior. Inquire about sleep patterns, feelings of sadness, and use of alcohol and other substances. Gather a family history of mental health disorders, suicide attempts, and stresses. Ask about how often the youth talks with or has meals with the family. Be aware of the risk of self-inflicted strangulation.

Recall that all youth who receive medications for treatment of depression should be carefully monitored, especially in the first several weeks in order to identify those who may develop suicide ideation and risk. Although antidepressants have demonstrated efficacy for treating depression in youth, there is an increased risk of suicidal ideation or behaviors in children and adolescents treated with these drugs.

Most suicides are committed with firearms that are usually obtained from the home. Determine at each healthcare visit if the family has firearms. Teach them to keep the guns unloaded, with ammunition and firearms locked in separate locations. Be sure that children and adolescents do not have access to the keys for the locked firearms. Never underestimate the resourcefulness or abilities of a suicidal child or adolescent, regardless of age, IQ, or physical abilities.

Education in all school settings is appropriate to teach children about resources that can help them if they need it and to identify peers at risk. Mental health services of all types should be available and embedded in schools since that is the setting where

TABLE 55–5 Risk and Protective Factors for Suicide in Children and Adolescents

RISK FACTORS	PROTECTIVE FACTORS
History of previous attempted suicide	Emotional well-being
Friend committed or attempted suicide	Satisfactory school performance
School problems or changes in grades	Participation in sports or other group events
Pregnancy	Weight satisfaction
Drug use or abuse	Parent/family connectedness
Problems with a romantic relationship	Frequent discussions of important issues with family
Minority sexual practice	School connectedness
Loneliness, withdrawal	Safe school
Feelings of anxiety	Safe neighborhood
History of chronic family problems	Caring adult presence at school or elsewhere
Chronic illness	Availability of school counseling
Physical, emotional, or sexual abuse	School policies to limit and cope with fighting, bullying
History of suicide in a family member	
History of depression	
Chronic low self-esteem	
Change in behavior	
Change in weight	
Giving away special possessions	
Access to firearms and ammunition	

A tragic cause of unintentional suicide in children is the choking "game." About 25 children die each year in the United States from this practice with a mean age of 13 years. When the blood supply to the brain is interrupted and then rushes back, some people report a feeling of euphoria or a "high." Children and adolescents may seek the experience for the feelings it creates and may even become addicted to it. Unfortunately, some children become unintentionally strangled and die from the experience. Methods that children use to cut off oxygen include using their hands to apply pressure to the carotids in the neck, or tying belts, cords, towels, and other items to the neck and then around doorknobs or other solid objects. Some children perform these rituals with others who then rescue them so that they begin breathing; many of the injuries occur when children are alone since there is no one to perform a rescue. Teachers, parents, and other adults typically have not heard of or are unaware that children are performing these rituals. Adults can watch for signs such as conjunctival hemorrhage, headaches, bruising in the neck area, periods of disorientation, hoarseness, and finding items tied to doors and other solid objects. Parents can also be alert if the history of a family computer has shown the child's entry to a website that describes the practice. Nurses in schools and other settings should educate children about the dangers of strangulation and should provide materials for parents to inform them of the risk (CDC, 2008, 2010; Mechling, Ahern, & McGuinness, 2013).

youth spend much of their time (USDHHS, 2015). Be alert for children and adolescents at risk for suicide in any setting. Assess children and adolescents in schools, outpatient settings, and emergency departments for the possibility of suicidal behavior. Report threats of suicide and depressive behavior. When a child or adolescent persists in threatening suicide after establishment of a "no suicide" contract, hospitalization is necessary to ensure safety. Recognize that when a child or adolescent has committed suicide, friends of the victim may be at increased risk. Teach students to report to teachers, nurses, or counselors about friends who have threatened suicide or seem depressed or display behaviors different from usual. Nurses often plan with mental health specialists to implement suicide prevention programs in schools and communities. Provide supportive services to family and friends whenever suicide occurs. Consult websites and refer parents as appropriate. The Suicide Prevention Resource Center has helpful regional offices to facilitate networks at national, state, territorial, community, and tribal levels (Maheshwari & Joshi, 2012).

Professionalism in Practice Suicide Prevention

The U.S. Surgeon General and the National Action Alliance for Suicide Prevention presented the 2012 National Strategy for Suicide Preventions: Goals and Objectives for Action. Major strategies were focused around empowering individuals, families, and communities by increased knowledge; providing comprehensive clinical and community preventive services; providing treatment and support for individuals and families when needed; and conducting surveillance, research, and evaluation (USDHHS, 2012). Nurses have a role in each of these strategies by identifying risk and providing connections to services, integrating suicide prevention in all healthcare settings, and collecting evaluative data from their communities.

Nursing care during hospitalization for suicide centers on taking appropriate precautions to ensure the child's safety. Be alert for children and adolescents in the emergency department who may have attempted suicide (Schmid, Truong, & Damian, 2011). Monitor both the child and the hospital environment for any object that could be used for self-harm. Remove all potentially harmful objects, such as shoestrings, belts, pantyhose, and hair ribbons. Keep all personal care items (including toothbrush and shampoo) locked at the nursing station and monitor them constantly when used by the child.

Children or adolescents considered at high risk for suicidal behaviors are attended to by a nursing staff member at all times, including while using the bathroom and sleeping. It may be necessary for the child to dress in a plain hospital gown, be kept in a visually monitored seclusion room, or (if seriously impaired and self-abusive) be medicated for restraint for a period of time. Restraints are used only when ordered by the youth's physician and collaborative care team. Physical restraint is only a short-term approach to provide immediate safety if necessary. Chemical (medication) restraint may be needed to prevent self-injury by the suicidal person. See *Teaching Highlights: Selecting Residential and Inpatient Care for the Child With Mental Illness* earlier in this chapter for information to help families consider when choosing care for their suicidal child.

Hospitalization continues as long as the child's behavior is self-destructive. Children are referred for intensive individual and family therapy. Encourage parents to keep follow-up clinic appointments, to watch for self-destructive behaviors, and to administer any prescribed medications according to the treatment schedule. Arrange home visits and other community resources for families. Desired outcomes include an increase in coping skills for the child, no further suicide attempts, and an improved sense of well-being.

Tic Disorders and Tourette Syndrome

Tics are sudden, rapid, recurrent, nonrhythmic, and brief motor movements or vocalizations. They may involve movement of the head or upper body, blinking of eyes, or a variety of verbal noises. They may be worse during periods of stress or tiredness. Many children have mild motor tics at some time that gradually disappear with no intervention. When the tics are severe or last more than 1 year, they are considered chronic and may require attention from a mental healthcare provider.

Severe motor tics accompanied by verbal utterances are known as *Tourette syndrome*. The syndrome is often accompanied by other diagnoses such as attention deficit and learning disabilities. Children with Tourette syndrome may exhibit coprolalia, the involuntary utterance of obscenities, profanities, and racial slurs, or copropraxia, the involuntary use of obscene gestures. Tic disorders are characterized by disruptions in the levels of dopamine, serotonin, and other neurotransmitter and neuropeptide levels (National Institute of Neurological Disorders and Stroke, 2014).

Nursing care involves supporting parents and encouraging normal developmental progression for the child. Nurses should carefully monitor symptoms after medication is begun, minimize stress, and teach relaxation techniques.

Schizophrenia

Schizophrenia is a psychotic disorder that is relatively rare in young children and adolescents, occurring in 1 in 10,000 children. The condition can manifest in childhood but is more common in adolescence (Lachman, 2014; Mayo Clinic, 2014).

The cause of schizophrenia is unknown, but genetic predisposition or neurointegration deficits are suspected causes (Mayo Clinic, 2014). The brain is altered in the disease, with progressively enlarged ventricles and nervous system arousal. Impaired glucose metabolism is often present. Onset is usually slow with increasing intensity. Most often the child demonstrates restlessness, poor appetite, and social withdrawal over several weeks to months. Behavioral problems, slowed development, and minor neurologic symptoms may occur.

The clinical manifestations of schizophrenia are the same in children as in adults. Characteristic behaviors include social withdrawal, impaired social relationships, flat **affect** (outward appearance of feeling or emotion), regression, loose associations (thought characterized by speech in which ideas shift from one subject to another that is unrelated), poor judgment and problem solving, anxiety, delusions, and hallucinations. Motor abnormalities may include rocking and arm flapping.

During adolescence, acute schizophrenia can occur suddenly while the teenager is making plans to leave home and family to attend college, marry, or work in another area. Onset of symptoms may be triggered by an important loss (death of a significant other, parent, child, or friend).

Prompt diagnosis can lead to early treatment and more positive outcomes. Clinical therapy for childhood schizophrenia is multifaceted, including individual psychotherapy, family therapy, and various psychotropic medications (antipsychotics such as haloperidol [Haldol], clozapine, olanzapine, risperidone, antianxiety agents such as lorazepam [Ativan], and antidepressants such as imipramine [Tofranil]) (Lachman, 2014; Mayo Clinic, 2014). Drugs are only moderately effective at controlling hallucinations and delusions. Responses vary considerably, and children may have different responses than adults. Side effects determine what drugs are used and for how long. Antipsychotic medication is continued for at least 4 to 6 weeks before effectiveness can be determined. Medications often must be continued for several months or years after recovery from an acute schizophrenic episode, although medication-free trials may be tried in children who have not shown symptoms for 6 to 12 months.

Episodes of acute schizophrenia may require inpatient hospitalization on a psychiatric unit for thorough diagnosis and beginning management. Treatment may include an intensive school-based program in a structured, supervised setting with specially trained professionals. The goal of initial treatment is to reduce or control schizophrenic episodes and provide a safe, structured environment for the child or adolescent, enabling the child to live each day at an optimal level of functioning. Outpatient care is provided in the community following initial diagnosis and establishment of a treatment regimen.

Most children require long-term treatment, including intermittent periods of hospitalization. Children or adolescents whose symptoms are difficult to control and who present a safety risk to themselves or others may require long-term residential treatment. Earlier age at diagnosis and delay in treatment lead to poorer prognosis.

Nursing Management

The nurse may encounter the child or adolescent with schizophrenia during hospitalization for an acute episode, for treatment of another problem, or while working with the individual in the community. Nursing care centers on providing for physical safety and psychologic care, and normal growth and development for the child.

Family education and involvement in the treatment plan are essential. Teach the family to monitor the child's symptoms and progression. Educating the child and parents about the risk of recurrence and methods to alleviate side effects of prescribed medications may increase compliance with the treatment plan. Assess the child for common medication side effects. For example, when excess weight is a potential side effect, frequent growth measurements are made. Neurologic assessment and laboratory studies may be needed with some medications. Help the family establish educational plans and integration within the school system. Communicate with school personnel to ensure understanding of the child's condition and ongoing management of the individualized education plan.

Cognitive Alterations

A wide array of cognitive conditions occur in childhood. Some are mild and not diagnosed until a child has difficulty in school, while others may be associated with physical signs that are visible at birth. Two common conditions, learning disabilities and intellectual disabilities (mental retardation), are discussed in this section.

Learning Disabilities

Learning disabilities are a common problem of young children, affecting about 5% to 10% of school children (Boyle et al., 2011; CDC, 2013). They involve neurologic conditions in which the brain cannot receive or process information in the normal manner. Often the impairment is only in one or two types of learning, making diagnosis difficult. Common types of learning disorders are listed in Table 55–6.

Children may have difficulty processing visual information, which may be manifested in reading, writing, and mathematics performance. Others may have difficulty with oral information, leading to problems in language development and reading.

The causes of learning disorders are complex. Sometimes they are related to low birth weight or problems during the perinatal period. There may be a genetic component since their occurrence is more common when other family members are affected.

Learning disabilities should be diagnosed by a learning specialist such as a psychologist with special training. A series of cognitive and developmental tests are commonly used; magnetic resonance imaging (MRI) is sometimes used. Treatments involve learning how to compensate for the difficulties by using capabilities that are intact. Some children need to have all material written for them, and others need to have verbal presentations. Specific learning goals are established with the assistance of learning specialists. Children with learning disabilities should have individualized education plans (IEPs) established with realistic goals for school performance. (See Chapter 38 for further information about IEPs.)

TABLE 55–6 Examples of Learning Disabilities

DISORDER	CLINICAL MANIFESTATIONS
Dyslexia	Difficulty with writing, reading, spelling
Dyscalculia	Mathematics and computation problems
Dysgraphia	Difficulty with writing, spelling, and composition
Dyspraxia	Problems with manual dexterity and coordination

Nurses play a major role in identifying children with learning disabilities. The nurse may be in contact with families during health promotion visits or in other settings when parents relay concern about the child's performance or difficulty in some aspect of school. Nurses should assess the child for the following developmental milestones, which can indicate learning disability (National Joint Committee on Learning Disabilities, 2015):

- Tasks such as tying shoes, buttoning, or hopping
- Expressive and receptive speech
- Naming objects or reading
- Fine and gross motor milestones
- Following simple instructions

When a child may have a learning disability, the nurse should refer the family to the school or other testing resource. The nurse should partner with the family to plan for the child's learning needs, help the family to work closely with the child, suggest providing a setting at home to maximize potential for learning, and offer suggestions for building healthy self-esteem in the child. The nurse should assist the family to work with the school to establish annual goals for the child. Most children with learning disabilities can learn to perform well in their areas of strength and compensate for areas of difficulty. Early intervention is key to success and building a positive self-image regarding abilities.

Intellectual Disability (Formerly Called Mental Retardation)

Intellectual disability is now the preferred term for what was previously called *mental retardation*. **Intellectual disability** is defined as significant limitation in intellectual functioning and adaptive behavior. It is manifested as differences in conceptual, social, and practical adaptive skills, beginning before the age of 18 years (American Association on Intellectual and Developmental Disabilities, 2013). Later events that lead to limitations in function are commonly referred to as *brain injury*. Intellectual functioning is generally characterized by an intelligence quotient (IQ) below 70 to 75, accompanied by significant impairments in **adaptive functioning** (the ability to meet the standards expected for a cultural group). The child with intellectual disability has adaptive deficits in at least two areas such as communication, self-care, home living, social/interpersonal skills, use of community resources, self-direction, functional academic skills, work, leisure, health, or safety. A low IQ score by itself does not necessarily correlate with an impaired ability to carry out adaptive skills. The child should be evaluated within the contexts of the individual cultural and community environment. The IQ score and the level of adaptive skills together determine the degree of severity of intellectual disability.

Intellectual disability is one type of **developmental disability**, any of a variety of chronic conditions that are characterized by mental or physical impairments. Other examples include pervasive developmental disorder, cerebral palsy, and sensory loss. A developmental disability begins by age 21 years and lasts throughout life.

ETIOLOGY AND PATHOPHYSIOLOGY

Intellectual disability occurs in 12 per 1000 children, a decrease from 15.5 per 1000 1 decade ago (CDC, n.d.). Its causes can be grouped into three general categories: prenatal errors in the development of the central nervous system, prenatal or postnatal changes in the person's biologic environment, and external forces leading to central nervous system damage. In each instance, the precipitating factor changes the form, function, and adaptation of the central nervous system. Table 55–7 provides examples of common conditions associated with intellectual disability.

Three conditions from prenatal life that are associated with intellectual disability are Down syndrome, fragile X syndrome, and fetal alcohol syndrome. In the United States, about 1 in 700 infants, or 5500 infants each year, are born with Down syndrome (CDC, 2014c). The syndrome is caused by an extra chromosome; the child has 47 rather than 46 chromosomes. (See discussion of genetic transmission in Chapter 3.) The most common chromosome affected is 21 so that the child often has "trisomy 21," or three instead of two copies of number 21 chromosome. In addition to intellectual disability and physical signs, the child with Down syndrome is at higher risk of developing other conditions such as cardiac defects, hearing loss, gastrointestinal problems, orthodontic conditions, thyroid disease, dermatologic conditions, and leukemia (CDC, 2014c).

Fragile X syndrome is caused by a single recessive gene abnormality on the X chromosome. A permutation to the X chromosome may occur in males or females. When a father or mother passes the faulty X chromosome to a daughter, it may remain as a permutation or may change into a true mutation. The daughter has two X chromosomes and therefore does not manifest this recessive disorder. However, she can pass the mutated X chromosome to her son who becomes affected with fragile X. The mutation of fragile X is on gene *FMRP-1*, which instructs cells to make a protein necessary for normal brain development. The faulty gene creates a deficiency in the FMRI protein that leads to brain changes. The condition is often associated with other conditions such as sudden death heart disease (SDHD), anxiety, and autism (CDC, 2014d).

Fetal alcohol spectrum disorder (FASD) describes the wide range of effects of ethyl alcohol on the developing fetus. The condition ranges from alcohol-related birth defects (ARBDs), such as disorders of the heart, kidneys, bones, or hearing; to alcohol-related neurodevelopment disorder (ARND), such as intellectual disability; to fetal alcohol syndrome, which is the most severe end of the spectrum, leading to a combination of mental health and intellectual and physical problems (CDC, 2014e). Alcohol ingestion by the pregnant woman can influence development of many body organs, and effects can range from mild to severe. Despite many years of public health education, alcohol use remains a leading cause of intellectual disability. From 0.3 to 1.5 per 1000 births are affected by fetal alcohol syndrome (CDC, 2014e).

TABLE 55–7 Common Conditions Associated With Intellectual Disability

PRENATAL CONDITIONS	BIOLOGIC ENVIRONMENT	EXTERNAL FORCES
Down syndrome	Inborn errors of metabolism (e.g., phenylketonuria, hypothyroidism)	Traumatic brain injury (e.g., accident)
Fragile X syndrome		Poison ingestion (acute or chronic)
Fetal alcohol syndrome		Hypoxia/anoxic insult
Maternal infection (e.g., rubella, cytomegalovirus)		Infection (e.g., meningitis)
		Environmental deprivation

For a discussion of phenylketonuria and hypothyroidism, two common biochemical causes of intellectual disability, see Chapter 53. Other causes involve traumatic brain injury and infections of the central nervous system (see Chapter 54). Intellectual disability is more common in children born prematurely.

CLINICAL MANIFESTATIONS

Mild intellectual disability was originally described as an IQ between 50 and 70, moderate disability with IQ of 35 to 50, severe disability with IQ 20 to 35, and profound disability below 20. Although an IQ below 70 is generally considered indicative of intellectual disability, the functional assessment of the child is now considered a more accurate identification of children's performance and needs. Children who have intellectual disabilities manifest delays in all areas of development, including motor movement, language, and adaptive behavior. They usually achieve developmental milestones more slowly than the average child. These developmental delays may be the first indication to parents, teachers, and healthcare providers of the child's condition.

Intellectual disability is sometimes accompanied by sensory impairment, speech problems, motor and orthopedic disabilities, and seizure disorders. Of children with the disability, 10% to 30% manifest one of these other disorders. Table 55–8 lists several physical characteristics associated with Down syndrome, fragile X syndrome, and fetal alcohol syndrome.

Developing Cultural Competence Fetal Alcohol Syndrome

Fetal alcohol syndrome is more common in groups with higher intake of alcohol. Because some Native American tribes have a high rate of alcoholism, the federal government and some tribes have joined together to lower that risk among this ethnic group. Some reservations, such as the Yakama Nation in Washington State, do not sell alcoholic beverages and have put educational programs in place.

CLINICAL THERAPY

Intellectual disability is diagnosed and initial treatment is planned in a multistep process, and by involving a collaborative care team. Team members may include a developmental specialist, physician, geneticist, nurse, teacher, language therapist, occupational therapist, and physical rehabilitation specialist. See Table 55–9 for a description of the DSM-5 diagnostic criteria for intellectual disability. Diagnosis begins with a comprehensive history and evaluation of the child's physical characteristics, developmental level, and intellectual and adaptive functioning. Laboratory tests such as chromosome analysis, blood enzyme levels, lead levels, or cranial imaging provide valuable information in some circumstances. A three-generation family history is performed.

Developmental screening (see Chapter 34) can help identify children at risk. Tests of intellectual and adaptive functioning are performed when disability is suspected. A neurologic examination may indicate asymmetry of movement or strength, irritability or lethargy, or abnormal pitch to an infant's cry. Because intellectual disability may be accompanied by physical abnormalities, it is important to observe the child for facial symmetry, distance between the eyes, level of the ears, hair growth, and palmar creases. These abnormalities may be clues to other health problems.

TABLE 55–8 Characteristics Associated With Three Common Types of Intellectual Disability

SYNDROME	CHARACTERISTICS
Down syndrome (see Figures 33–8 and 33–33)	Small head (microcephaly)
	Flattened forehead
	Wide, short neck
	Epicanthal eye folds
	White spots on eye iris (Brushfield spots)
	Congenital cataracts
	Flat nose
	Small, low-set ears
	Protruding tongue
	Short broad hands
	Simian line on palm
	Wide space between first and second toes
	Hearing loss
	Increased incidence of diabetes, congenital heart defect, and leukemia
	Hypotonia
Fragile X syndrome	Long face
	Prominent jaw
	Large ears
	Frequent otitis media
	Large testicles
	Epicanthal eye folds
	Strabismus
	High arched palate
	Scoliosis
Fetal alcohol syndrome (see Figure 31–4)	Flat midface
	Low nasal bridge
	Long philtrum with narrow upper lip
	Short upturned nose
	Poor coordination
	Failure to thrive
	Skeletal and joint abnormalities
	Hearing loss

Based on the results of the evaluation, a multidisciplinary team plans the support needed to maximize the child's potential for development. Management focuses on early intervention to improve the degree of adaptive functioning. Associated physical, emotional, and behavioral problems are treated simultaneously. Depending on the child's condition, special education programs and physical or occupational therapy may be necessary (Figure 55–8). The Education for All Handicapped Children Act (PL 94-142) provides free appropriate education to all handicapped children between 2 and 21 years of age. Amendments to this act in 1986 (PL 99-457) encouraged states to provide early intervention services for infants and toddlers with developmental delay conditions through federal funding.

The child may require supportive care and assistance with activities of daily living. The plans for intervention need to change as the child grows and the family situation alters. Classes and special services are needed for youth and families when the adolescent with intellectual disability transitions into young adulthood.

TABLE 55-9 DSM-5 Diagnostic Criteria for Intellectual Disability

Intellectual disability (intellectual developmental disorder) is a disorder with onset during the developmental period that includes both intellectual and adaptive functioning deficits in conceptual, social, and practical domains. The following three criteria must be met:

1. Deficits in intellectual functions, such as reasoning, problem solving, planning, abstract thinking, judgment, academic learning, and learning from experience, confirmed by both clinical assessment and individualized, standardized intelligence testing.

2. Deficits in adaptive functioning that result in failure to meet developmental and sociocultural standards for personal independence and social responsibility. Without ongoing support, the adaptive deficits limit functioning in one or more activities of daily life, such as communication, social participation, and independent living, across multiple environments, such as home, school, work, and community.

3. Onset of intellectual and adaptive deficits during the developmental period.

Note: The diagnostic term *intellectual disability* is the equivalent term for the diagnosis of *intellectual developmental disorders*. Moreover, a federal statute in the United States (Public Law 111-256, Rosa's Law) replaces the term *mental retardation* with *intellectual disability*, and research journals use the term *intellectual disability*. Thus, *intellectual disability* is the term in common use by medical, educational, and other professions and by the lay public and advocacy groups.

Specify current severity as:
- **Mild**
- **Moderate**
- **Severe**
- **Profound**

Source: Used with permission from American Psychiatric Association. (2013). *Diagnostic and statistical manual of mental disorders* (5th ed.). Washington, DC: Author. Copyright © 2013 American Psychiatric Association.

Nursing Management
For the Child With Intellectual Disability

Nursing Assessment and Diagnosis

Nurses can help to identify children with intellectual disability through history taking, observation, and developmental screening during early childhood. The history should provide information about the mental and adaptive functioning of birth parents and other family members, as intellectual disability may cluster in some families, and conditions such as fragile X syndrome are genetic in origin. The pregnancy and birth history can provide important information about the mother's alcohol and drug use during pregnancy. Be alert for a history of difficult pregnancy and problems during birth. Prematurity places the child at risk of below-normal cognitive development. Frequent developmental testing during early childhood is needed for infants born prematurely. When genetic conditions in the family predispose family members to intellectual disability, assess the child carefully. Children from deprived environments or those at risk because of environmental factors such as lead poisoning (see Chapter 42) are more likely to manifest intellectual disability.

Many children with intellectual disability are not diagnosed until they reach school age, particularly if the condition is mild. Early intervention, however, can help to enhance the child's functioning later. During home visits, during clinic appointments, in childcare centers, and during hospitalization, be alert for signs such as developmental delays, multiple (more than three) physical anomalies associated with a specific condition (see Table 55-8), or neurologic alterations. Developmental assessment should be part of each healthcare visit; see Chapters 34, 35, and 36 for developmental surveillance recommended at each age.

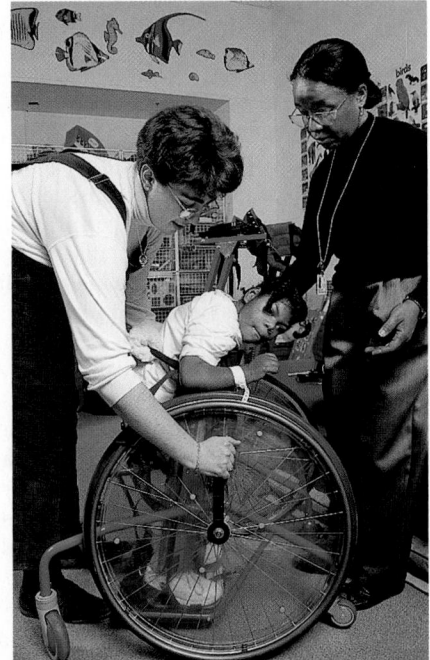

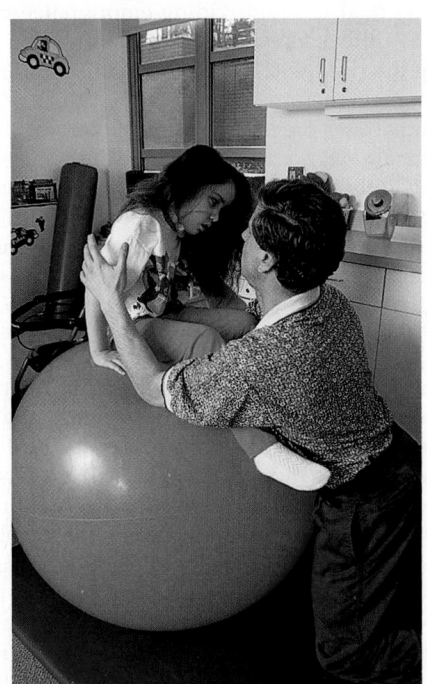

A   **B**

Figure 55-8 **Physical therapy is an important component of medical management for many children who have intellectual disabilities. *A,* This girl, who is severely intellectually disabled and uses a wheelchair, is being positioned in a mobile prone stander, which enables her to interact in a different manner with her therapists and the environment. *B,* Physical therapists also provide outpatient care in the community to children with varying degrees of disability.**

Once the diagnosis of intellectual disability has been made, assess the adaptive functioning of the child and family. Perform a functional assessment of the child, including toileting, dressing, and feeding skills. Assess the child's language, sensory, and psychomotor functioning. Assess the home and community for safety hazards. Observe how the family is managing with the child. Ask about family activities that include the child, community and school attitudes and support, and care management as well as planning for the future. Assess the availability of services such as groups for parents and special education opportunities for children. Evaluate the coping skills of family members.

Several nursing diagnoses may be appropriate for the child with intellectual disability, depending on the degree, cause, and outcome of the child's condition. Some of these diagnoses relate to impairments in adaptive functioning; others relate to the impact on the family. Examples include the following (NANDA-I © 2014):

- *Development: Delayed, Risk for,* related to neonatal disease or condition
- *Nutrition, Imbalanced: Less than Body Requirements,* related to inability to ingest sufficient food
- *Self-care Deficit: Dressing, Toileting, Bathing,* related to developmental disability
- *Communication: Verbal, Impaired,* related to developmental disability
- *Injury, Risk for,* related to lack of understanding of environmental hazards
- *Coping: Family, Compromised,* related to the child's developmental variations

Planning and Implementation

Nearly all children with intellectual disability are cared for in the community. However, they may have conditions that require periodic hospitalization or frequent healthcare visits. Nursing care focuses on providing emotional support and information to family members, maintaining a safe environment, assisting the child with adaptive functioning, and fostering parental management of the child's activities. Whenever possible, the nurse uses preventive teaching to lower the risk of disability. For example, nurses can integrate teaching into care for all women about the importance of avoiding all alcohol during any times when they might become pregnant. This helps prevent fetal alcohol syndrome, especially in early pregnancy when women may not know they are pregnant.

PROVIDE EMOTIONAL SUPPORT AND INFORMATION

Family members need empathy and support both at the time of diagnosis and in the ensuing years. Parents may be in an acute or chronic state of grief over the loss of the healthy child. Encourage them to verbalize their feelings. Introducing them to parents of other children who have intellectual disabilities may help and support them as they learn how to manage the child's needs. Discuss the availability of respite care to provide parents with a break from caretaking. Other family members such as grandparents and siblings may also feel grief or guilt and should be given an opportunity to talk about their feelings.

Parents need honest information and answers to their questions about the child's condition. Reinforce information provided by genetic counselors and other healthcare professionals. Parents need to know about community resources designed to assist children with intellectual disability. As mentioned earlier, the Education for All Handicapped Children Act (PL 94-142) provides free appropriate education to all handicapped children between 2 and 21 years of age. States and local communities may provide early intervention services for infants and toddlers with disabilities. Examples of programs include the Zero to Three early intervention programs, special education preschools and schools, county health services, and respite care. Ask parents if they have questions about IEPs and refer them to Internet sources if that is helpful. Review federal and state laws and services that might be helpful to the family, and help them interpret information they find to analyze its strengths and limitations.

MAINTAIN A SAFE ENVIRONMENT

Children with intellectual disabilities require close supervision because they may not understand common hazards. Ensure safety in the hospital. Assist parents to provide safety at home and school, and teach the child necessary skills such as pedestrian safety. Consider both physical and emotional safety. The child may be indiscriminately trusting and sometimes is at risk for physical or sexual abuse.

PROVIDE ASSISTANCE WITH ADAPTIVE FUNCTIONING

Encourage parents' efforts to maximize the child's areas of strength and identify needs related to adaptive behaviors. Refer them to resources to help with the child's impaired areas of adaptive functioning, such as communication, self-care, or social skills. During hospitalization, support parents' efforts to maintain the child's skills in toileting, dressing, and self-care by planning interventions to use the skills being taught at home.

COMMUNITY-BASED NURSING CARE

The child with intellectual disability needs ongoing care throughout childhood; interventions must be adapted as the child develops and the family's needs evolve. Parents often act as case managers for the child's care. Assist parents as necessary to acquire the skills required to coordinate the child's plan of care. Evaluate the child's needs regularly and help parents with the treatment plan as necessary. Provision of education including services such as physical or speech therapy is a primary goal. Most children with intellectual disability have an IEP designed to meet their specific learning needs. Parents, nurses, and others such as teachers and language therapists are part of the team that establishes the child's IEP. Promote optimal development and socialization. As the child reaches adolescence, education is directed toward a vocation, issues of sexuality, and the goal of independent living, when appropriate. Transition classes for adolescents with intellectual disability can teach self-care skills that may enable some to live in group homes or other community settings. Parents need help planning for the child's future and their own retirement.

Specific guidelines for care are available for the child with Down syndrome (Bull & Committee on Genetics, 2011). These guidelines suggest times for evaluation of hearing, growth, cardiac function, and other areas designed for early identification and treatment of associated disorders. There are growth grids for children with Down syndrome, and specific topics to suggest for anticipatory guidance during healthcare visits.

Evaluation

The expected outcomes of nursing care depend on the child's needs and developmental level. Early in the diagnostic phase, desired outcomes may involve the family's understanding of the diagnosis and the child's special needs. Later outcomes may focus on the child's communication of self-help skills. Outcomes related to cognitive performance and adaptive skills may be developed during childhood. Successful transition into adulthood at the maximal level of function is the ultimate desired outcome.

Focus Your Study

- Major treatment modes for children with mental health disorders include individual therapy, family therapy, and group therapy.

- Therapeutic strategies for treatment of children and adolescents with mental health disorders include play therapy, art therapy, cognitive behavioral therapy (CBT), visualization, and hypnosis.

- Nurses conduct mental health assessments, prevent disorders when possible, participate in intervention to treat disorders, and evaluate outcomes of treatment.

- Autism spectrum disorder is the major type of pervasive developmental disorder and is manifested by abnormal behavior, social interaction, and communication.

- Attention deficit hyperactivity disorder is characterized by developmentally altered behaviors involving inattention and hyperactivity.

- Mood disorders in childhood and adolescence are commonly manifested as depression or bipolar disorder.

- Several anxiety disorders occur in children and adolescents, most notably generalized anxiety, separation anxiety, panic, obsessive-compulsive disorder, social phobia, conversion reaction, and posttraumatic stress disorder (PTSD).

- Behavioral therapy and selective serotonin reuptake inhibitors (SSRIs) are used in treatment of anxiety; prescription drug use in children must be closely monitored.

- Suicide is a significant cause of death among youth; nurses play a key role in identifying youth at risk, instituting prevention programs, and counseling families and friends of suicide victims.

- Nurses play a role in identifying children with potential learning disabilities, referring for diagnosis, and partnering with the family to provide a positive learning experience for the child.

- Intellectual disability is subaverage intellectual and adaptive functioning, and may be caused by chromosomal, genetic, or environmental factors.

- A multidisciplinary team plans the care for children with intellectual disability and periodically evaluates the child's progress and the family's needs.

Clinical Reasoning in Action

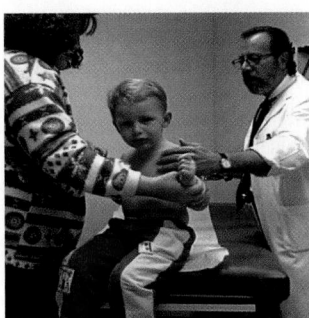

Cooper, a 5-year-old child with autism spectrum disorder, comes into the office for his annual checkup and school immunizations of diphtheria tetanus acellular pertussis (DTaP), inactivated polio vaccine (IPV), and measles-mumps-rubella (MMR). He is very combative and it takes four people to help hold him and administer the vaccines. He will be attending a special school for children with autism spectrum and related disorders. Diagnosed at 3 years old, he has never been in the hospital or had surgery. It is extremely difficult to examine him as he does not like to be touched. During prior visits in the office, Cooper has stood facing the wall and twisting his hands. He continues to be combative for most of the examination, even with the use of decreased stimuli, communication, and slow movements, but you are able to assess that his blood pressure is 95/53 mmHg. He is in the 50th percentile for both height and weight and his temperature is 99°F.

You give Cooper's mother information about local support groups for children with autism spectrum disorder and about local psychiatrists who can treat the condition with medication that helps control aggressive behavior. You also supply her with contact information for counselors in the area to help her deal with her own stress. She is appreciative of your help and support and looks forward to being able to send Cooper to school.

1. The mother has questions about the MMR vaccine and whether it causes autism. What can you tell her about that? Would you administer the vaccine today?

2. What can you tell the mother about safety issues with Cooper?

3. How can you enhance communication with Cooper when he comes into the office?

References

Agency for Healthcare Research and Quality (AHRQ). (2014). *Recommendations for children and adolescents: Guide to clinical preventive services.* Retrieved from http://www.ahrq.gov/professionals /clinicians-providers/guidelines-recommendations /guide/section3.html

American Association on Intellectual and Developmental Disabilities. (2013). *Definition of intellectual disability.* Retrieved from http://www.aaidd.org/content_100.cfm

American Psychiatric Association. (2013). *Diagnostic and statistical manual of mental disorders* (DSM-5) (5th ed.). Washington, DC: Author.

Arnold, L. E., Hurt, E., & Lofthouse, N. (2013). Attention-deficit/hyperactivity disorder: Dietary and nutritional treatments. *Child and Adolescent Psychiatric Clinics of North America, 22,* 381–402.

Bartlett, D. (2011). Drug therapy gets personal with genetic profiling. *American Nurse Today, 6*(5). Retrieved from http://www.americannursetoday.com /article.aspx?id=7814&fid=7770

Blake, T. (2012). Three medication pathways for bipolar disorder. *Nursing 2012, 42*(5), 28–35.

Boydston, L, Hsiao, R. C., & Varley, C. K. (2012a). Identifying anxiety disorders in the primary care setting. *Contemporary Pediatrics, 29*(6), 28–34.

Boydston, L, Hsiao, R. C., & Varley, C. K. (2012b). Anxiety disorders in adolescents: Assessment and treatment. *Contemporary Pediatrics, 29*(7), 36–42.

Boyle, C. A., Boulet, S., Schieve, L. A., Cohen, R. A., Blumberg, S. J., Yeargin-Allsop, M., . . . Kogan, M. D. (2011), Trends in the prevalence of developmental disabilities in U.S. children, 1997–2008. *Pediatrics.* doi: 10.1542/peds.2010-2989

Brown, P. (2012). ADHD guidelines: An update for your practice. *Consultant for Pediatricians, October Supplement,* S3–S7.

Bruxel, E. M., Akutagava-Martins, G. C., Salatno-Oliveira, A., Contini, V., Kieling, C., Hutz, M. H., & Rohde, L. A. (2014). ADHD pharmacogenetics across the life cycle: New findings and perspectives. *American Journal of Medical Genetics, 165B,* 263–282.

Bull, M. J., & Committee on Genetics. (2011). Clinical report—Health supervision for children with Down syndrome. *Pediatrics, 128,* 393–406.

Center for Injury Research and Prevention. (2011). *PTSD in children and parents.* Retrieved from http://injury .research.chop.edu/our_research/carit_research.php

Centers for Disease Control and Prevention (CDC). (n.d.). *Intellectual disabilities among children.* Retrieved from http://www.cdc.gov

Centers for Disease Control and Prevention (CDC). (2008). Unintentional strangulation deaths from the "choking game" among youths ages 6–19 years— United States 1995–2007. *Morbidity and Mortality Weekly Report, 57,* 141–146.

Centers for Disease Control and Prevention (CDC). (2010). *The choking game: Risky youth behavior.* Retrieved from http://www.cdc.gov

Centers for Disease Control and Prevention (CDC). (2012a). Prevalence of autism spectrum disorder among children aged 8 years—Autism and developmental disabilities monitoring network, 14 sites, United States, 2008. *Morbidity and Mortality Weekly Report (MMWR) Surveillance Summary, 61(SS03),* 1–19.

Centers for Disease Control and Prevention (CDC). (2012b). *Suicide.* Retrieved from http://www.cdc .gov/violenceprevention/pdf/Suicide-DataSheet-a.pdf

Centers for Disease Control and Prevention (CDC). (2013). *Developmental disabilities.* Retrieved from http://www.cdc.gov/ncbddd/developmentaldisabilities /index.html

Centers for Disease Control and Prevention (CDC). (2014a). Prevalence of autism spectrum disorder among children aged 8 years—Autism and developmental disabilities monitoring network, 11 sites, United States, 2010. *Morbidity and Mortality Weekly Report (MMWR) Surveillance Summary, 63(2),* 1–21.

Centers for Disease Control and Prevention (CDC). (2014b). *Attention-deficit/hyperactivity disorder.* Retrieved from http://www.cdc.gov/ncbddd/adhd /data.html

Centers for Disease Control and Prevention (CDC). (2014c). *Occurrence of Down syndrome.* Retrieved from http://www.cdc.gov/ncbddd/birthdefects /downsyndrome/data.html

Centers for Disease Control and Prevention (CDC). (2014d). *Facts about fragile X syndrome.* Retrieved from http://www.cdc.gov/ncbddd/fxs/facts.html

Centers for Disease Control and Prevention (CDC). (2014e). *Facts about FASDs.* Retrieved from http://www.cdc.gov/ncbddd/fasd/facts.html

Chung, P. J., & Soares, N. S. (2012). Childhood depression: Recognition and management. *Consultant for Pediatricians, September,* 259–267.

Dineen, W. K. (2014). Timely topics in pediatric psychiatry. *Journal of Clinical Psychiatry, 75,* 1224–1225.

Emslie, G. J., Kennard, B. D., & Mayes, T. L. (2011). Predictors of treatment response in adolescent depression. *Pediatric Annals, 40,* 300–306.

Faraone, S. V., & Antshel, K. M. (2014). Towards an evidence-based taxonomy of nonpharmacologic treatments for ADHD. *Child and Adolescent Psychiatric Clinics of North America, 23,* 965–972.

Ferguson, C. J. (2011). The influence of television and video game use on attention and school problems: A multivariate analysis with other risk factors controlled. *Journal of Psychiatric Research, 45,* 808–813.

Findling, R. L., & Dinh, S. (2014). Transdermal therapy for attention-deficit hyperactivity disorder with the methylphenidate patch (MTS). *CNS Drugs, 28,* 217–228.

Frye, R. E. (2014). Metabolic and mitochondrial disorders associated with epilepsy in children with autism spectrum disorder. *Epilepsy Behavior.* doi: 10.1016/j.yebeh.2014.08.134

Haga, S. B., O'Daniel, J. M., Tindall, G. M., Lipkus, I. R., & Agans, R. (2012). Survey of US public attitudes toward pharmacogenetic testing. *Pharmacogenomics Journal, 12,* 197–204.

Harrington, J. W. (2013). Autism in the school-aged child: Diagnostic dilemma, comorbid condition—or both? *Consultant for Pediatricians, Jan 2013,* 13–17.

Houck, G., Kendall, J., Miller, A., Mirrell, P., & Wiebe, G. (2011). Self-concept in children and adolescents with attention deficit hyperactivity disorder. *Journal of Pediatric Nursing, 26,* 239–247.

Hughes, J. L., & Asarnow, J. R. (2011). Family intervention strategies for adolescent depression. *Pediatric Annals, 40,* 314–318.

Johnson, C. P., Myers, S. M., & Council on Children with Disabilities. (2007, reaffirmed 2010). Identification and evaluation of children with autism spectrum disorders. *Pediatrics, 120,* 1183–1215.

Kemper, K. J., Gardiner, P., & Birdee, G. S. (2013). Use of complementary and alternative medical therapies among youth with mental health concerns. *Academic Pediatrics, 13,* 540–545.

Kloos, A. L., & Robb, A. S. (2011). Bipolar disorder in children and adolescents. *Pediatric Annals, 40,* 481–487.

Knisely, M. R., Carpenter, J. S., & Von Ah, D. (2014). Pharmacogenomics in the nursing literature: An integrative review. *Nursing Outlook, 62,* 285–296.

Kozlowska, K., Scher, S., & Williams, L. M. (2011). Patterns of emotional-cognitive functioning in pediatric conversion patients: Implications for the conceptualization of conversion disorders. *Psychosomatic Medicine, 73(9),* 775–788.

Lachman, A. (2014). New developments in diagnosis and treatment update: Schizophrenia/first episode psychosis in children and adolescents. *Journal of Child and Adolescent Mental Health, 26,* 109–124.

Lee, M. J., & Liechty, J. M. (2014). Longitudinal associations between immigrant ethnic density, neighborhood processes, and Latino immigrant youth depression. *Journal of Immigrant and Minority Health, May 7.* doi 10.1007/s10903-014-0029-4

Madadi, P. (2015). Ethical perspectives on translational pharmacogenetic research involving children. *Paediatric Drugs, 17(1),* 91–95. doi: 10.1007 /s40272-014-0111-3

Maglione, M. S., Das, Raaen, L., Smith, A., Chari, R., Newberry, S., . . . Gidengil, C. (2014). Safety of vaccines used for routine immunization of U.S. children: A systematic review. *Pediatrics, 134,* 325–337.

Maheshwari, R., & Joshi, P. (2012). Assessment, referral, and treatment of suicidal adolescents. *Pediatric Annals, 41,* 516–521.

Mahoney, J. R., Kennard, B. D., & Mayes, T. L. (2011). Cognitive behavioral treatment of depression in youth. *Pediatric Annals, 40,* 307–313.

Mayo Clinic. (2013a). *Cognitive behavioral therapy.* Retrieved from http://www.mayoclinic.org/tests-procedures/cognitive-behavioral-therapy/basics /definition/prc-20013594

Mayo Clinic. (2013b). *Depression (major depressive disorder).* Retrieved from http://www.mayoclinic .org/diseases-conditions/depression/in-depth/ssris /ART-20044825?pg=2

Mayo Clinic. (2014). *Childhood schizophrenia.* Retrieved from http://www.mayoclinic.org/diseases-conditions/childhood-schizophrenia/basics/causes /con-20029260

Mechling, G., Ahern, N. R., & McGuinness, T. M. (2013). The choking game: A risky behavior for youth. *Journal of Psychosocial Nursing and Mental Health Services, 51(12),* 15–20.

Morrison, J., & Schwartz, T. L. (2014). Adolescent angst or true intent: Suicidal behavior, risk and neurological mechanisms in depressed children and teenagers taking antidepressants. *International Journal of Emergency Mental Health, 16,* 247–250.

National Center for Children in Poverty. (2014). *Children's mental health.* Retrieved from http://www .nccp.org/topics/mentalhealth.html

National Institute of Mental Health (NIMH). (n.d.a). *Depression in children and adolescents.* Retrieved from http://www.nimh.nih.gov/health/publications /depression-in-children-and-adolescents/index.shtml

National Institute of Mental Health (NIMH). (n.d.b). *Bipolar disorder.* Retrieved from http://www.nimh.nih. gov/health/topics/bipolar-disorder/index.shtml

National Institute of Mental Health (NIMH). (2012a). *Mental health medications.* Retrieved from http://www.nimh.nih.gov/health/publications /mental-health-medications/what-medications-are-used-to-treat-bipolar-disorder.shtml

National Institute of Mental Health (NIMH). (2012b). *Information about PANDAS.* Retrieved from http://www.nimh.nih.gov/labs-at-nimh/research-areas/clinics-and-labs/pdnb/web.shtml

National Institute of Neurological Disorders and Stroke. (2014). *Tourette syndrome fact sheet.* Retrieved from http://www.ninds.nih.gov/disorders/tourette /detail_tourette.htm

National Institutes of Health (NIH). (2012). *Attention deficit hyperactivity disorder (ADHD).* Retrieved from http://www.nimh.nih.gov/health/publications /attention-deficit-hyperactivity-disorder /index.shtml

National Joint Committee on Learning Disabilities. (2015). *What is a learning disability?* Retrieved from http://www.ldonline.org/ldbasics/whatisld

Santrock, J. W. (2011). *Child development* (13th ed.). Boston, MA: McGraw-Hill.

Sarvet, B., & Brewer, S. (2011). Anxiety disorders in pediatric primary care. *Pediatric Annals, 40,* 499–505.

Schmid, A. M., Truong, A. W., & Damian, F. J. (2011). Care of the suicidal pediatric patient in the ED: A case study. *American Journal of Nursing, 111(9),* 34–43.

Scrandis, D. A. (2014). Identification and management of bipolar disorder. *Nurse Practitioner, 39(10).* 30–37.

Selekman, J., & Diefenbeck, C. (2014). The new DSM-5 and its impact on the mental health care of children. *Journal of Pediatric Nursing, 29,* 442–450.

Stockings, E., Degenhardt, L., Lee, Y. Y., Mihalopoulos, C., Liu, A., Hobbs, M., & Patton, G. (2014). Symptom screening scales for detecting major depressive disorder in children and adolescents: A systematic review and meta-analysis of reliability, validity and diagnostic utility. *Journal of Affective Disorders, 174C,* 447–463.

Subcommittee on Attention-Deficit/Hyperactivity Disorder, Steering Committee on Quality

Improvement and Management. (2011). ADHD: Clinical practice guideline for the diagnosis, evaluation, and treatment of attention-deficit/hyperactivity disorder in children and adolescents. *Pediatrics*. doi: 10.1542/peds.2011-2654

U.S. Department of Health and Human Services (USDHHS). (2012). *2012 national strategy for suicide prevention: Goals and objectives for action*. Washington, D.C.: Author

U.S. Department of Health and Human Services (USD-HHS). (2015). *Healthy People 2020*. Retrieved from http://www.healthypeople.gov

Valicenti-McDermott, M., Burrows, B., Bernstein, L., Hottinger, K., Lawson, K., Seijo, R., . . . Shinnar, S. (2014). Use of complementary and alternative medicine in children with autism and other developmental disabilities: Associations with ethnicity, child comorbid symptoms, and parental stress. *Journal of Child Neurology, 29*, 360–367.

Van Egmond-Frohlich, A. W., Weghuber, D., & de Zwaan, M. (2012). Association of symptoms of attention-deficit/hyperactivity disorder and childhood overweight adjusted for confounding parental variables. *International Journal of Obesity, 36*, 963–968.

Webb, P. L. (2011). Screening for autism spectrum disorders during well-child visits in a primary care setting. *Journal for Nurse Practitioners, 7*, 229–237.

Weeke, P., Jensen, A., Folke, F., Gislason, G. H., Olesen, J. B., Andersson, C., . . . Torp-Pedersen, C. (2012). Antidepressant use and risk of out-of-hospital cardiac arrest: A nationwide case-time-control study. *Clinical Pharmacology and Therapeutics, 92*, 72–79.

Won, H., Mah, W., & Kim, E. (2013). Autism spectrum disorder causes, mechanisms and treatments: Focus on neuronal synapses. *Frontiers in Molecular Neuroscience*. doi: 10.3389/fnmol.2013.00019

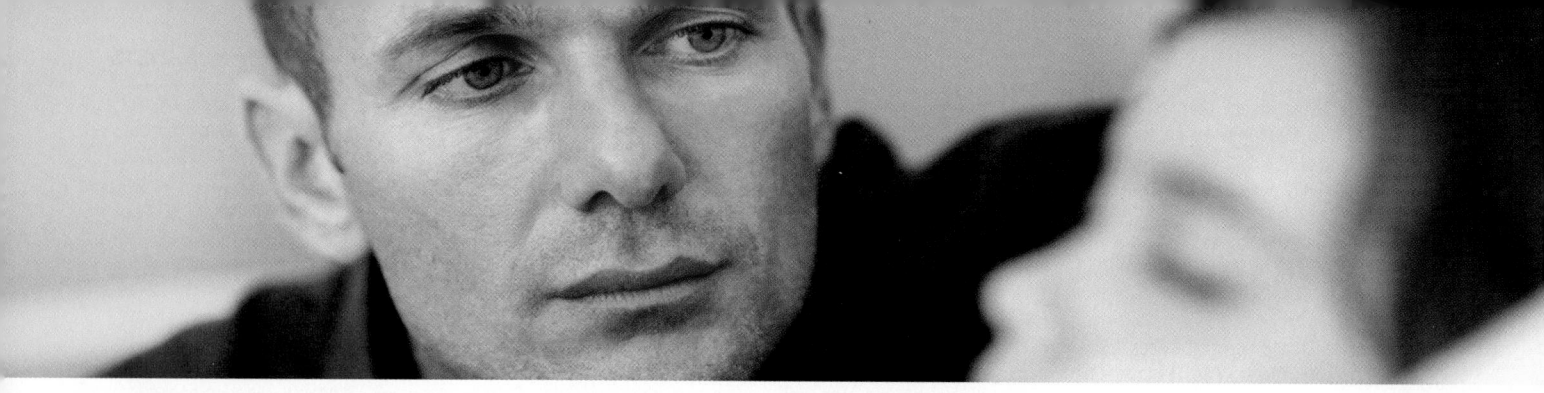

Chapter 56
The Child With Alterations in Musculoskeletal Function

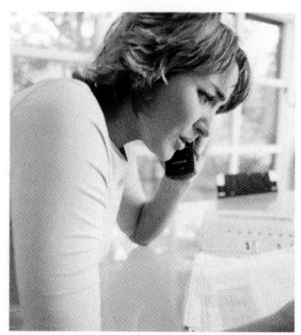

OMG/The Image Bank/Getty Images

When I got the call that Douglass was in the emergency room I was so scared. I guess we're lucky it was just a broken leg. I've never had a cast. What do you need to do with it? I also wonder if it's safe for him go back to his friend's house where he broke his leg on a trampoline. Should I tell him not to use the trampoline once he heals? It's hard to decide.

—Mother of Douglass, 12 years old

⌄ Learning Outcomes

56.1 Describe pediatric variations in the musculoskeletal system.

56.2 Plan nursing care for children with structural deformities of the foot, leg, hip, and spine.

56.3 Recognize signs and symptoms of infectious musculoskeletal disorders and refer for appropriate care.

56.4 Partner with families to plan care for children with musculoskeletal conditions that are chronic or require long-term care.

56.5 Prioritize nursing interventions to promote safety and developmental progression in children who require braces, casts, traction, and surgery.

56.6 Develop a nursing care plan for fractures, including teaching for injury prevention and nursing implementations for the child who has sustained a fracture.

The musculoskeletal system helps the body protect its vital organs, support weight, control motion, store minerals, and supply red blood cells. Bones provide a rigid framework for the body, muscles provide for active movement, and tendons and ligaments hold the bones and muscles together. Therefore, alterations in musculoskeletal functioning can have a significant impact on a child's growth and development.

What concerns do parents and children have when a child has musculoskeletal conditions? Will the child need any special adaptations in the home and school? Can musculoskeletal injuries be prevented? The information in this chapter will answer these questions, and enable nurses to provide effective care for children who have musculoskeletal disorders.

Musculoskeletal disorders may be congenital, such as clubfoot, or acquired, such as osteomyelitis. They may require short- or long-term management, and may be treated on an outpatient basis or require hospitalization. Some

Varus
An abnormal position of a limb that involves bending inward toward the midline of the body

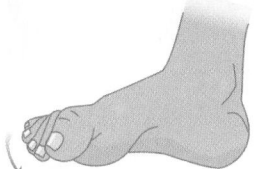

Valgus
An abnormal position of a limb that involves bending outward away from the midline of the body

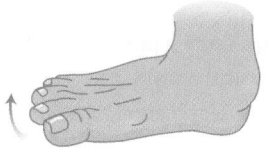

Supination
Lying on the back or placing the hand so that palm faces upward

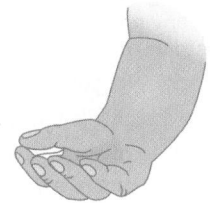

Pronation
Lying on the stomach or placing the hand so the palm faces downward

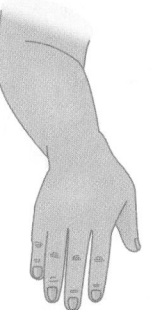

Adduction
Lateral movement of limbs toward the midline of the body

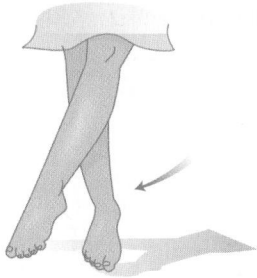

Abduction
Lateral movement of limbs away from the midline of the body

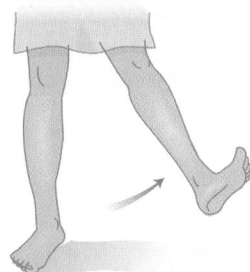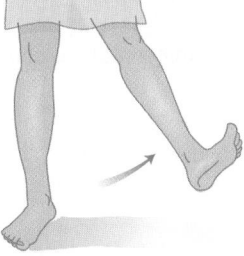

Flexion
A decrease in angle between bones forming a joint

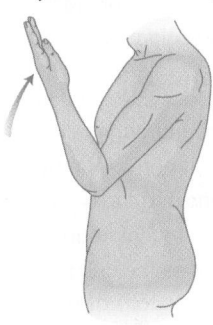

Extension
A movement that brings a limb into a straight position

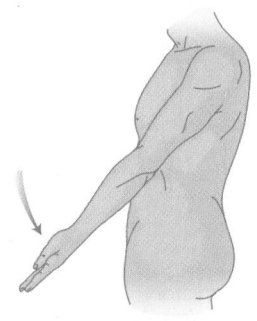

Inversion
Turning inward, usually more than normal

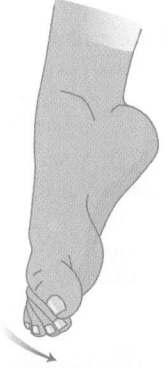

Eversion
Turning outward

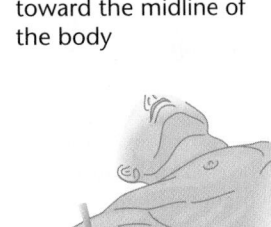

Internal rotation
Rotation of a body part toward the midline of the body

External rotation
Rotation of a body segment away from the midline of the body

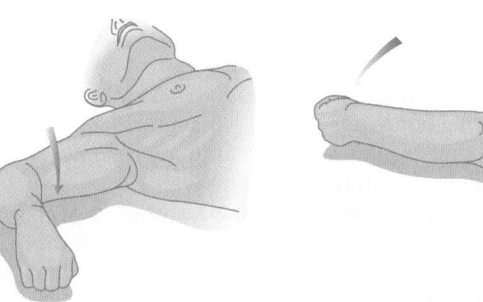

Figure 56–1   **Musculoskeletal positions and joint motions.**

disorders affect other body systems as well; for example, see cerebral palsy in Chapter 54. Many musculoskeletal disorders require surgical correction, casting, or braces.

Figure 56–1 reviews several terms that will be used throughout this chapter in describing the positioning of a child's limbs. See the accompanying *Assessment Guide* for assessment guidelines for the child with alterations in musculoskeletal function.

Anatomy and Physiology of Pediatric Differences

Bones

The bones of children and those of adults differ in several ways. Although primary centers of **ossification** (bone formation) are nearly complete at birth, a fibrous membrane still exists

ASSESSMENT GUIDE | The Child With a Musculoskeletal System Alteration

Assessment Focus	Assessment Guidelines
Muscles	• Is muscle mass symmetric?
	• Do fine and gross motor movements correspond to developmental expectations?
	• Can you identify any abnormal signs such as asymmetry of movement, tenderness, masses, weakness, hypotonia, hypertonia?
	• Can the school-age child get up from a lying or sitting position in the usual manner?
	• Can you describe the child's usual daily physical activity?
	• Has there been a loss of ability to perform developmental milestones?
Joints	• Are movements smooth and symmetric?
	• Are there any signs of tenderness, decreased range of motion, inflammation, crepitus/grinding, or masses?
	• Do the hips of newborns and infants manifest symmetric full range of motion?
	• Were there recent events of trauma such as in sports or a fall?
Bones	• Are any masses noted?
	• Are arms and legs the same length?
	• Is there a recent decrease or change in mobility, such as limping?
	• Are bones in alignment, or are abnormalities noted such as bowlegs or knock-knees?
	• Upon spinal screening, is the spine properly aligned (see screening procedure within this chapter)?
	• In what sports does the child participate? Is recommended protective gear worn?
Tendons and ligaments	• Do all joints move through full range of motion?
	• Is there any pain upon joint motion or palpation?
	• Are there feelings of grinding or crepitus as the joint moves?
	• Has there been a recent sports or other injury?
	• In what sports does the child participate?
Family history	• Is there a family history of disorders of the muscular or skeletal systems?

between the cranial bones (fontanelles). (See *As Children Grow: Sutures* in Chapter 33.) The posterior fontanelle closes between 2 and 3 months of age. The anterior fontanelle does not close until approximately 7 to 19 months of age, allowing for growth of the brain and skull (National Institutes of Health, 2012a). In addition, the ends of the long bones (epiphyses) remain cartilaginous (Figure 56–2). Long-bone growth continues until approximately age 20 years, when skeletal maturation is complete.

Secondary ossification occurs as the long bones grow. Cartilage cells at the epiphyses are replaced by osteoblasts (immature bone cells), resulting in the deposition of calcium. Calcium intake during childhood and adolescence is essential to provide adequate bone density that will prevent osteoporosis and fractures in adulthood. See Chapter 32 for a discussion of inadequate calcium intake during school age and adolescence.

The long bones of children are porous and less dense than those of adults. For this reason, children's bones can bend, buckle, or break as a result of a simple fall. Children and adolescents may suffer injuries to the musculoskeletal system from falls, car crashes, and sports. Fractures are one type of common injury. Because growth takes place at the epiphyseal plates, injuries to this portion of a long bone are of particular concern in young children.

In addition to the structural differences between the bones of children and adults, there are also functional differences in the skeletal system of children. (See *As Children Grow: Children Are Not Just Small Adults* in Chapter 33.) Before birth the thoracic and sacral regions of the spine are convex curves. As the infant

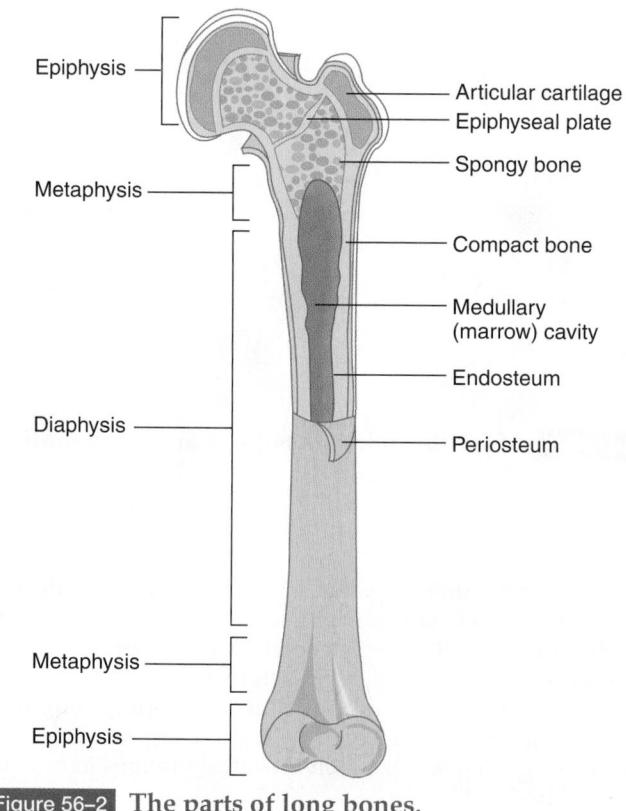

Figure 56–2 The parts of long bones.

learns to hold up the head, the cervical region becomes concave. When the child learns to stand, the lumbar region also becomes concave. Failure of the spine to assume these final curves results in an abnormal curvature of the spine (kyphosis or lordosis). The rapid bone growth of childhood facilitates healing after fractures, but may also lead to "growing pains," as muscles are pulled when bones grow quickly.

Muscles, Tendons, and Ligaments

The muscular system, unlike the skeletal system, is almost completely formed at birth. As a child grows, muscles do not increase in number, but rather in length and circumference. Until puberty, both ligaments and tendons are stronger than bone. When these structural differences are not recognized, a childhood fracture is sometimes mistaken for a **sprain**. A sprain is a tearing of ligaments, the structural support connecting bones, usually caused when a joint is twisted or otherwise traumatized. Tendons, which connect bones to muscles, grow in length and fibrous tissue as mechanical pressure is placed on them.

Disorders of the Feet and Legs

Metatarsus Adductus

Metatarsus adductus, the most common congenital foot deformity, is characterized by an inward turning of the forefoot at the tarsometatarsal joints (Figure 56–3). Often referred to as "intoeing," metatarsus adductus affects male and female infants equally and occurs in approximately 1 in 1000 births, with more common incidence being in first births and in families with prior cases of the disorder. It is sometimes accompanied by other problems such as developmental dysplasia of the hip (described later in this chapter) (Gilmore & Thompson, 2013; National Institutes of Health, 2012b). This condition is most likely caused by both intrauterine positioning and genetic factors. Metatarsus adductus is differentiated from other causes of intoeing, such as internal tibial torsion (more common in children ages 12 to 18 months who are learning to walk) and femoral anteversion (seen more often in preschool-age children).

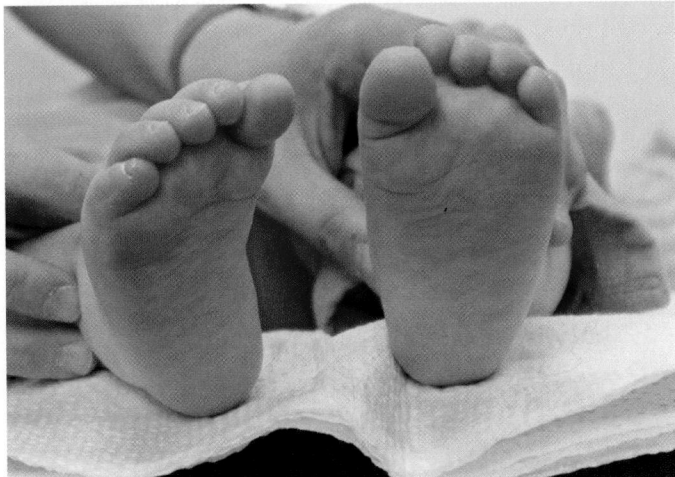

Figure 56–3 **Metatarsus adductus. This disorder is characterized by convexity (curvature) of the lateral border of the foot. The child's right foot demonstrates the disorder. Note that the forefoot turns inward and appears out of alignment with the remainder of the foot.**

Treatment depends on the degree of foot flexibility. If the foot can be readily maneuvered past the neutral position, simple exercises may correct the problem. Most cases resolve spontaneously by the time the infant is about 3 months of age. Serial casting is the treatment of choice for curvature angles greater than 15 degrees, or in cases that do not improve. The infant's feet are placed in a position as close to neutral as possible and are held secure with casts. Casts are changed weekly until the desired correction is achieved. Braces and orthopedic shoes may also be used to maintain correction after casting.

Nursing Management

Reassure parents that the child's condition can be corrected. If the child's deformity is mild, teach parents simple stretching exercises to perform at each diaper change. The foot is held securely by the heel, and the forefoot is moved outward from the body with the other hand. The position is maintained for 5 seconds, and repeated 5 times at each diaper change. If casting is necessary, provide cast care as outlined in Table 56–1 and teach parents how to care for the child in a cast at home. If metatarsus adductus persists into childhood without correction, the challenge is to find shoes that accommodate the unusual shape of the foot.

Clinical Tip

Casts are made out of plaster or fiberglass material. The former is durable and may be chosen for applications that will last for a long time. Plaster casts must be kept dry or they will deteriorate. Fiberglass casts are lighter and available in various colors and are therefore popular with children. While the outside of the cast can become moist without breakdown, the lining underside is not waterproof, so caution is still followed to preserve the cast integrity.

Clubfoot

Clubfoot is a congenital abnormality in which the foot is twisted out of its normal position. It occurs in approximately 1 to 2 in 1000 births, affects boys nearly twice as often as girls, and is bilateral in about half of affected infants (Gilmore & Thompson, 2013).

ETIOLOGY AND PATHOPHYSIOLOGY

The exact cause of clubfoot is unknown; however, several possible etiologies have been proposed. Some authorities believe abnormal intrauterine positioning causes the deformity. Others suspect neuromuscular or vascular problems as causes. There is a genetic component in some cases because the risk of having a second child with clubfoot when an earlier child is affected is 25% (Gilmore & Thompson, 2013).

CLINICAL MANIFESTATIONS

A clubfoot (talipes equinovarus) involves three areas of deformity: The midfoot is directed downward (**equinus**), the hindfoot turns inward (**varus**), and the forefoot curls toward the heel (adduction) and turns upward in partial supination. Muscles, tendons, and bones are all involved in the abnormality, and it cannot be corrected by exercise. Most children have this combination of findings. The foot is small with a shortened Achilles tendon. Muscles in the lower leg are atrophied, but leg lengths are generally normal (see *Pathophysiology Illustrated: Clubfoot*).

CLINICAL THERAPY

Diagnosis is made at birth on the basis of visual inspection. Radiographs are used to confirm the severity of the condition.

Early treatment is essential to achieve successful correction and reduce the chance of complications. Serial casting is the

TABLE 56–1 Nursing Care of the Child in a Cast

- A plaster cast takes anywhere from 24–48 hr to dry. When handling the wet cast, be gentle and use the palms of your hands, as fingertips can indent plaster and create pressure areas.
- After the cast is applied, elevate the extremity on a pillow above the level of the heart. Elevation helps reduce swelling and increases venous return.
- If the cast is applied after surgery, there may be drainage or bleeding through the cast material. Circle the stain and note the date and time on the cast to provide a way to assess the amount of fluid lost.
- Assess the distal pulses, and check the fingers and toes for color, warmth, capillary refill, and edema. Assess sensation as well as movement. Any deviation from normal may indicate nerve damage or decreased blood supply.
- During the first 24 hr, check the casted extremity every 15–30 min for 2 hr, then every 1–2 hr thereafter. The skin should be warm. It should blanch when slight pressure is applied and then return to its normal color within 3 sec (**A**). For the next 2 days, assess the casted extremity at least every 4 hr.

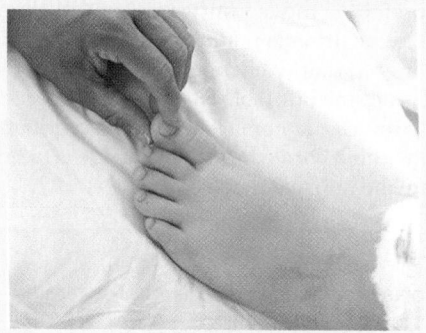

- Check the edges of the cast for roughness or crumbling. If necessary, pull the inner stockinette over the edge of the cast and tape in place.
- The rough edges of the cast may also be alleviated by "petaling." This is done by securing tape or padding to the inside of the cast and pulling it over the edge, covering the jagged or broken pieces of plaster, and securing it to the outer surface of the cast (**B, C, D**). Moleskin may be used on the cast as well.
- Keep the cast as clean and dry as possible. Cover the cast with plastic when the child bathes. Never leave the child alone to bathe, and discard the plastic safely so that the child cannot reach it because of suffocation hazard.
- The skin under the cast may itch; however, do not use powders or lotions near the edges or under the cast as they can cause skin irritation.
- Be sure that children do not put small objects between the casts and their extremities; that can cause skin irritation as well as neurovascular compromise.

A

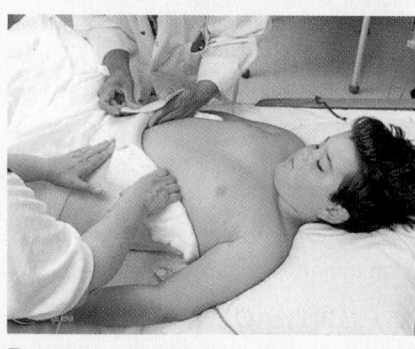

B

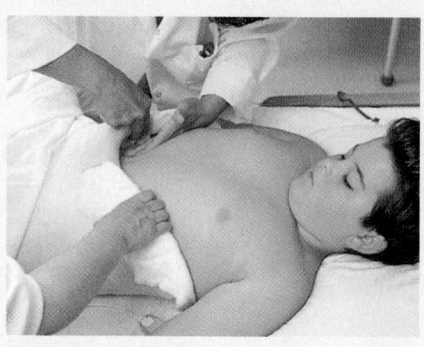

C

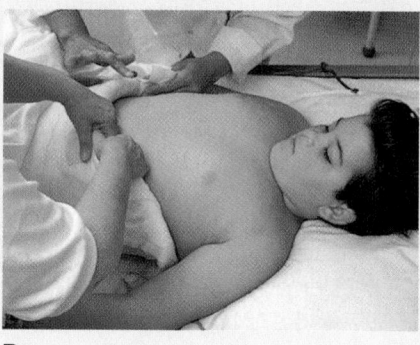

D

treatment of choice. Casting should begin as soon as possible after birth. Timing is critical because the short bones of the foot, which are primarily cartilaginous at birth, begin to ossify shortly thereafter. The foot is manipulated to achieve maximum correction first of the varus deformity and then of the equinus deformity. A long leg cast holds the foot in the desired position (Figure 56–4). The cast is changed every 1 to 2 weeks. This regimen of manipulation and casting continues for approximately 8 to 12 weeks until maximum correction is achieved. If the deformity has been corrected, the child may begin wearing a splint or reverse cast (shaped so that the foot turns outward away from the body instead of the normal inward turn) corrective shoes to maintain the correction. If the deformity has not been corrected, surgery is required. Casting holds the foot in position until surgery is performed.

The age at which a child undergoes clubfoot surgery varies among surgeons. However, most children have surgery between 3 and 12 months of age. The one-stage posteromedial release procedure, which involves realignment of the bones of the foot and release of the constricting soft tissue, is most common. The foot is held in the proper position by one or more stainless steel pins. A

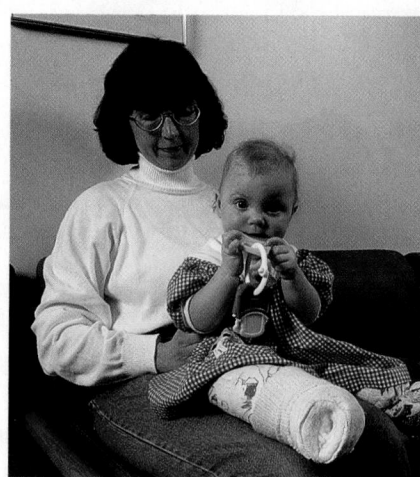

Figure 56–4 This girl has a long leg cast, which was applied after surgery to correct her clubfoot deformity.

Pathophysiology Illustrated: **Clubfoot**

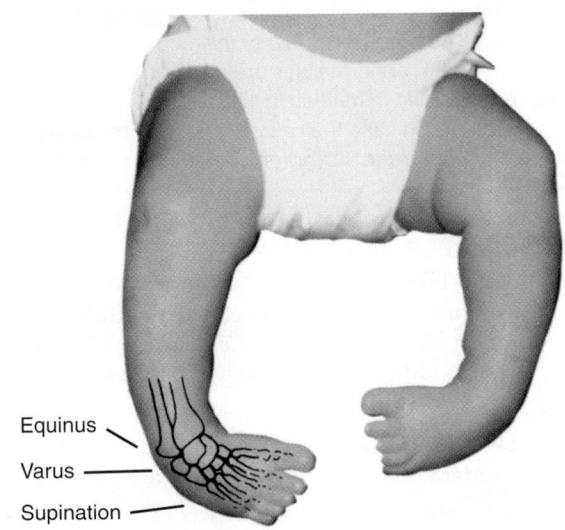

Equinus
Varus
Supination

Bilateral clubfoot deformity. Parents of a child with clubfoot will have many questions. Can the condition be treated? Will the child be able to walk normally after surgery? Will they need help caring for the infant? How much will surgery and other care cost? Will any subsequent children have a clubfoot?

cast is then applied with the knee flexed to prevent damage to the pin and to discourage weight bearing. Casting continues for 6 to 12 weeks. The child may then need to wear a brace or corrective shoes, depending on the severity of the deformity and the surgeon's preference (Gilmore & Thompson, 2013).

More severe cases or those not corrected in infancy may require more than one surgery to correct the foot.

Nursing Management

For the Child With Clubfoot

Nursing Assessment and Diagnosis

Nursing assessment, which begins at birth and continues throughout the child's subsequent outpatient casting visits and hospitalization for surgery, includes taking a genetic and birth history, performing a physical examination (including position and appearance of the foot), and assessing the child's motor development and family's coping mechanisms. Because parents will need to bring the child for frequent cast changes, assess access to transportation and other arrangements needed for these visits.

Among the nursing diagnoses that might apply to the child with a clubfoot deformity are the following (NANDA-I © 2014):

- *Mobility: Physical, Impaired*, related to prescribed movement restriction of cast
- *Skin Integrity, Risk for Impaired*, related to cast
- *Parenting, Impaired*, related to birth of a child with a physical defect
- *Health Maintenance, Ineffective*, related to lack of information about deformity, treatment, and home care

TEACHING HIGHLIGHTS | Care of the Child With a Cast

Skin Care
- Check the skin around the cast edges for irritation, rubbing, or blistering. The skin should be clean and dry.
- Cleanse the skin just under the cast edges and between the toes or fingers with a cotton-tipped applicator and rubbing alcohol. Avoid using lotions, oils, and powders near the cast as they may cause caking.
- Avoid poking sharp objects down inside the cast as this may result in sores.

Cast Care
- Keep the cast dry. Protect plaster with a cast shoe, thick sock, or sling.
- Allow a new, wet cast to air-dry for 24 hours. Raise it on pillows just above heart level to prevent swelling.
- Begin walking on a leg cast only when the physician gives permission.

Be Alert for Possible Complications
- Toes or fingers should be pink, not blue or white.
- Skin should be warm and the tips of the toes should blanch when pinched.

Notify Your Healthcare Provider if Any of the Following Occurs
- Unusual odor beneath the cast
- Burning, tingling, or numbness in the casted arm or leg
- Drainage through the cast
- Swelling or inability to move the fingers or toes
- Slippage of the cast
- Cast cracked, soft, or loose
- Sudden unexplained fever
- Unusual fussiness or irritability in an infant or child
- Fingers or toes that are blue or white
- Pain that is not relieved by any comfort measures (e.g., repositioning or pain medication)

Source: Courtesy of Shriners Hospital for Children, Spokane, WA.

Planning and Implementation

Nursing management involves providing emotional support, educating the family about home care of the child in a cast and the importance of keeping appointments at the outpatient facility for cast changes, preparing the family for the child's hospitalization if surgery is to occur, and providing postsurgical care.

PROVIDE EMOTIONAL SUPPORT

Clubfoot affects both the child and the family. The child's foot deformity is upsetting to parents, and they need emotional support to allay their fears. Helping parents understand the condition and its treatment is essential.

Promote bonding by encouraging parents to hold and cuddle the child and to take an active role in the child's care. Explain that, with treatment, the child is expected to grow and develop normally.

PROVIDE CAST AND BRACE CARE

Routine cast care is outlined in Table 56–1 and is important to ensure skin and neurovascular integrity. After serial casting is complete, or after surgery, the child may progress to wearing a brace or special shoe for 6 to 12 months. Braces should fit snugly but should not interfere with neurovascular function. Before the child begins to wear a brace, check the skin for any areas of redness or breakdown. Give parents guidelines for brace wear. Emphasize that proper skin care is essential. If skin redness develops, arrange to have the fit of the brace evaluated and modified if necessary.

PROVIDE POSTSURGICAL CARE

Routine postoperative care after surgical correction includes neurovascular status checks every 2 hours for the first 24 hours and observing for any swelling around the cast edges (see Table 56–1). Apply ice bags to the foot, and keep the ankle and foot elevated on a pillow for 24 hours. This promotes healing and helps with venous return. Check for drainage or bleeding. Administer pain medication routinely for 24 to 48 hours. Popliteal or epidural blocks may be placed during surgery and used in the immediate postsurgical period for pain control. Monitor these blocks for effectiveness and any undesired effects. (See Chapter 40 for detailed instructions on pain management.)

SAFETY ALERT!

The most serious complication of a cast is the obstruction to normal blood flow and nerve innervation. Monitoring of the child's distal extremity is important to identify this complication. If color, temperature, or other abnormalities are present, inform the nursing supervisor or physician immediately. Have a cast cutter readily available on the unit in case the cast needs to be removed. See the section on compartment syndrome later in this chapter.

DISCHARGE PLANNING AND HOME CARE TEACHING

Give parents written instructions for care of the child with a cast (see *Teaching Highlights: Care of the Child With a Cast* earlier in this chapter). In addition, assist them in the following ways:

- Demonstrate the use of a sponge bath to protect the cast from water breakdown. Have parents contact the healthcare provider if the cast gets wet with water or urine.
- Discuss options for clothing that accommodate a cast, for example, one-piece snap suits or sweatpants.
- Discuss potential safety hazards that may result from awkward positioning. Be sure the child is properly situated in a car safety seat for the trip home.
- Provide resources for strollers and other equipment that will support the cast so it does not hang down during the baby's activities.
- Suggest that parents try to place toys within the child's reach, since the movements of a child in a cast may be slowed.

Evaluation

Expected outcomes of nursing care include maintenance of skin integrity, recovery without complications after surgery, normal developmental progression of the child, and demonstrated parental knowledge of care of braces or casts, as needed.

Genu Varum and Genu Valgum

Genu varum (bowlegs) is a deformity in which the knees are widely separated while the ankles are close together and the lower legs are turned inward (varus). In genu valgum (knock-knees), the knees are close together and the lower legs are

---

TEACHING HIGHLIGHTS | Guidelines for Brace Wear

- Braces should be as comfortable as possible and the child should have adequate mobility while wearing the brace.
- Begin wearing the brace for periods of 1 to 2 hours and then progress to 2 to 4 hours.
- Check the skin at 1- to 2-hour intervals initially, then every 4 hours once skin has been clear for several days. If redness is apparent, leave the brace off and allow the skin to clear. If breakdown has occurred, the brace cannot be replaced until healing is complete. (See Chapter 57 for a discussion of pressure ulcers.)
- Always have the child wear a clean white sock, T-shirt, or other thin white liner beneath the brace. Be sure the liner is wrinkle-free under the brace. Avoid using powders or lotions that can cause skin to break down. Toughen any sensitive areas using alcohol wipes 3 to 4 times daily.
- Reapply the brace when the skin returns to its normal color.
- Return to the orthotic specialist or other specified healthcare provider if discomfort or red areas persist or if the brace needs adjustment or repair or is outgrown.
- Check the brace daily for rough edges.

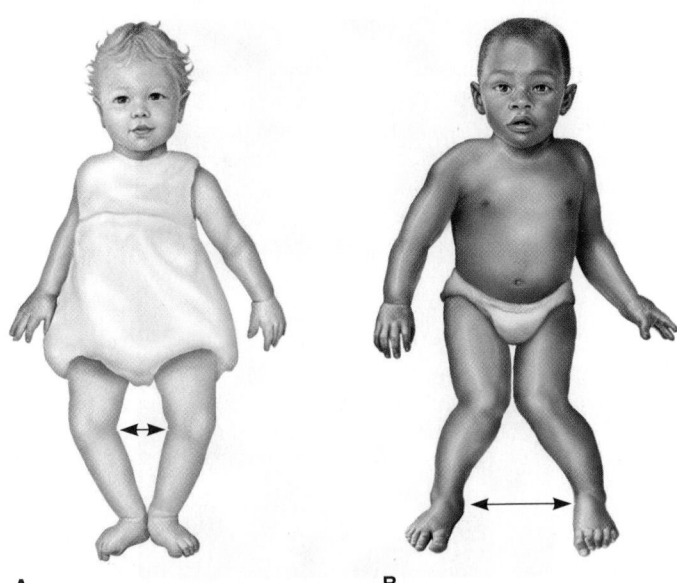

Figure 56–5 Genu varum and genu valgum. *A*, Genu varum, or bowlegs. The legs are bowed so that the knees are far apart as the child stands. *B*, Genu valgum, or knock-knees. Note that the ankles are far apart when the knees are together.

directed outward (valgus) (Figure 56–5). Chapter 33 discusses the assessment of bowlegs and knock-knees in children.

At certain stages of a child's development, the appearance of bowlegs or knock-knees is normal. Until 2 to 3 years of age, the knees are normally bowed, showing varus alignment, and by 4 to 5 years, some knock-knee or valgus alignment is common. However, the persistence of knock-knees beyond the age of 4 to 5 years necessitates further evaluation. The most common pathologic causes of bowed legs are Blount disease and rickets (see Chapter 32). Blount disease is characterized by abnormal growth on the medial side of the proximal tibia, which causes an increasing varus deformity. It is believed to be due to increasing compression forces across the medial knee and is more common in overweight, Black, and female children, and has been associated with low serum vitamin D levels (Sabharwal, 2015). Rickets is a result of inadequate bone mineralization, usually caused by a deficiency of calcium, vitamin D, or both. Since the bones are decalcified or softened, long bones such as those in the legs may bend into a bowed position. Occasionally, rickets is congenital and is caused by an X-linked autosomal dominant or recessive gene with the chromosomal location Xp22.31-p21.3. It results in an enzyme deficiency of alkaline phosphatase, which in turn leads to excessive inhibitors of bone mineralization. This type of rickets is rare and is called *familial hypophosphatemic rickets* (FHR).

Measurements, radiographs, arthrography (joint radiograph), magnetic resonance imaging (MRI), and computed tomography (CT) imaging may be used for accurate diagnosis. Braces are often used to correct mild deformities that could worsen as the child grows. Braces for bowlegs are worn at night; those for knock-knees both day and night. Duration of brace wear is determined by the severity of the deformity, which is usually evaluated by radiographs. If the deformity continues to worsen, surgery is necessary. Surgery is common in treatment of Blount disease. An **osteotomy** (cutting of the bone) is performed and the tibiofemoral angle surgically corrected. The

child is then placed in a cast for approximately 6 to 10 weeks, or until completely healed (Birch, 2013). When dietary rickets is the cause of varus deformity, supplementation with calcium and vitamin D is needed. FHR is treated with calcium and phosphorus in 5 to 6 daily doses.

Nursing Management

Reassure parents that bowlegs and knock-knees are usually a normal part of a child's growth and development. These conditions often resolve spontaneously and need no treatment other than continued observation.

Nursing care focuses on educating the parents and child about the condition and its treatment. Give the child and family guidelines for brace wear and maintenance (see *Teaching Highlights: Guidelines for Brace Wear* earlier in this chapter).

Disorders of the Hip

Developmental Dysplasia of the Hip

Developmental dysplasia of the hip (DDH) refers to a variety of conditions in which the femoral head and the acetabulum are improperly aligned. These conditions include hip instability, **dislocation** (displacement of the bone from its normal articulation with the joint), **subluxation** (in this instance, a partial dislocation), and acetabular **dysplasia** (abnormal cellular or structural development leading to instability) (Schwend, Shaw, & Segal, 2014). In the past, DDH was referred to as *congenital dislocated hip (CDH)*. The revised name of the disorder emphasizes that many cases of dislocation, subluxation, and dysplasia occur well after the neonatal period and involve more than a simple dislocation.

One in 100 newborns has hip instability, while dislocation occurs in 1.5 to 20 in 1000 births, depending on the studies examined. The condition affects girls four times as often as boys. It is unilateral in 80% of affected children, and the left hip is affected three times as often as the right (Roof, Jinguji, & White, 2013).

ETIOLOGY AND PATHOPHYSIOLOGY

Although the exact cause of DDH is unknown, genetic factors appear to play a role. DDH is 20 to 50 times more common in first-degree relatives of an infant with the condition than in the general population. If one child of a set of identical twins has DDH, the other twin is affected 30% to 40% of the time. Some types of DDH are linked to early gestational events at 12 and 18 weeks' gestation, as the lower limbs rotate and surrounding muscles develop. On the other hand, milder cases may be influenced by mechanical forces in the last month of pregnancy such as breech position, oligohydramnios, or fetal size, and can occur after birth as the hip assumes an extended rather than flexed posture (National Institutes of Health, 2013). The left hip is involved more often than the right hip as a result of intrauterine positioning of the left side of the fetus against the mother's sacrum. Maternal estrogen may cause laxity of the hip joint and capsule, leading to joint instability, especially in female infants who respond to these estrogen levels. Carrying infants with legs predominantly in extended position rather than with hips flexed may also be associated with DDH.

CLINICAL MANIFESTATIONS

Common signs and symptoms of DDH include limited abduction of the affected hip, asymmetry of the gluteal and thigh skinfolds, and telescoping or pistoning of the thigh

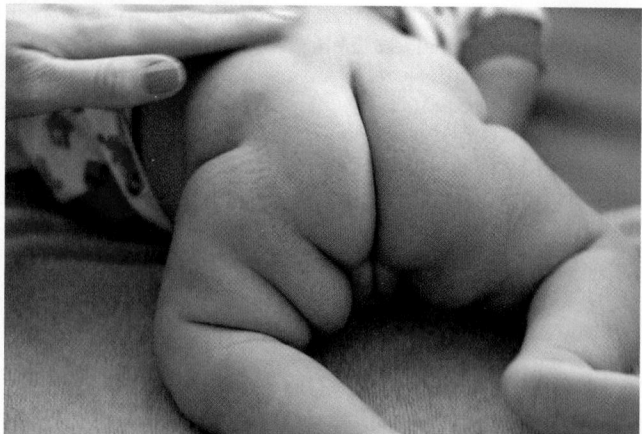

Figure 56–6 Common signs of developmental dysplasia of the hip (DDH). The asymmetry of the gluteal and thigh skinfolds is easy to see in this child with DDH.

(Figure 56–6). The older child with untreated DDH walks with a significant limp, which results from telescoping of the femoral head into the pelvis. The longer the disorder goes untreated and the more pronounced the clinical manifestations become, the more difficult the treatment.

CLINICAL THERAPY

Sixty to 80% of hip abnormalities noted in infants resolve by 2 months of age, so practitioners use care and caution in diagnosing DDH. However, only 15% to 25% of infants have known risk factors for the disorder. Therefore, the Pediatric Orthopaedic Society of North America recommends that all infants and young children should be screened for DDH until walking is well established at about 1 to 2 years of age (American Academy of Orthopaedic Surgeons [AAOS], 2014a; Roof et al., 2013). Physical examination reveals an Allis sign (one knee lower than the other when the knees are flexed) and positive Ortolani and Barlow maneuvers in babies under 8 to 12 weeks of age. Refer to Chapter 24 for a discussion of the assessment of hip dysplasia in newborns and infants. Radiographs are generally not reliable until approximately 4 months of age because the pelvis in a newborn is still primarily cartilaginous. Before 4 months of age, ultrasonography may be useful for diagnosis. Family history of DDH and a female baby in the breech position necessitate careful evaluation (AAOS, 2014a).

Treatment plans vary according to the child's age. For infants younger than 3 months, the Pavlik harness is the most commonly used method for hip reduction (Figure 56–7). The Pavlik harness is a dynamic splint—a splint that allows movement. It ensures hip flexion and abduction and does not allow hip extension or adduction. For infants older than 6 months of age, surgery with closed reduction is generally performed (positioning of the head of the femur into the acetabulum without an incision of the skin) followed by the application of a spica cast (Figure 56–8). Surgery may be preceded by a course of Bryant traction to facilitate stretching of the tissues that will promote positive surgical outcomes. In children over 18 months of age, open or closed reduction surgery and casting are usually necessary and bracing may also be required.

Early screening, detection, and treatment enable most affected children to attain normal hip function. A late diagnosis results in a lowered prognosis for full function.

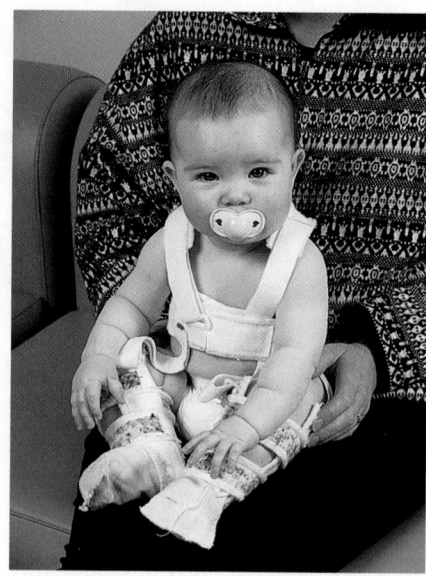

Figure 56–7 The most common treatment for DDH in a child under 3 months is a Pavlik harness. A shirt should be worn under the harness to prevent skin irritation. (It was omitted for clarity in this photograph.)

Nursing Management
For the Child With Developmental Dysplasia of the Hip

Nursing Assessment and Diagnosis

Assessment for DDH begins at birth and continues through all health promotion visits during the first 2 years of life. The family history or birth data may indicate a high-risk infant. Instructions for performing the physical examination to assess

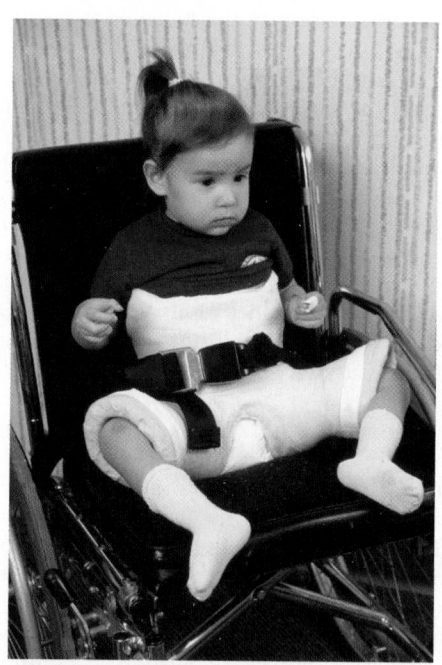

Figure 56–8 Surgery followed by spica cast application is commonly used in treatment of DDH.

the infant for DDH are provided in Chapter 33. Once treatment begins, assessments are performed based on risks of the treatment. Assess the skin of the child in traction or a cast every few minutes in the immediate postoperative period, progressing to once or twice daily at home. Include respiratory and circulatory assessments when the child is immobilized. Ongoing assessment of the child's growth and development is needed. Weigh the child in a cast once the cast is dry so a baseline casted weight can be used for comparison while the cast remains in place.

Several nursing diagnoses that may apply to the child with DDH include the following (NANDA-I © 2014):

- *Mobility: Physical, Impaired,* related to prescribed movement restriction (Pavlik harness, traction, spica cast, brace)
- *Skin Integrity, Risk for Impaired,* related to irritation from harness straps or skin traction
- *Urinary Elimination, Impaired or Constipation,* related to immobility caused by treatment
- *Nutrition, Imbalanced: Less than Body Requirements,* related to decreased appetite
- *Development: Delayed, Risk for,* related to limited mobility and potential decreased exposure to stimulation
- *Knowledge, Readiness for Enhanced (Parental),* related to lack of information about disease process and treatment

Planning and Implementation

The infant with DDH is often cared for at home and in outpatient facilities. If surgery is performed, the child is hospitalized for surgery and the immediate postoperative period. Nursing care varies according to the medical treatment and the child's age. Management includes maintaining traction, if ordered; providing cast care; preventing complications resulting from immobility; promoting normal growth and development; and teaching parents about the condition and care (e.g., management of a cast or a Pavlik harness). Because treatment may interfere with the child's normal movement, the treatment plan should take into consideration the age and developmental stage of the child in order to substitute activities to stimulate development.

PROVIDE CAST CARE AND CORRECT HARNESS ALIGNMENT

The principles of routine cast care presented in Table 56–1 apply to the care of spica casts. Special techniques should be used to help keep the cast clean and dry in children who are not toilet trained. Female and male urinals can be used for older children. Use a plastic lining to protect the cast edges during elimination for older children and use a small disposable diaper to cover the perineum in babies, tucking edges beneath the cast. Be sure to change the diaper frequently to prevent soiling of the cast.

The child in a Pavlik harness will have the harness applied in the healthcare facility. Parents need instructions on maintaining the child in the harness at all times. Return visits will be scheduled to ensure proper fit, maintenance of hip position, and skin condition.

PREVENT COMPLICATIONS RESULTING FROM IMMOBILITY

Immobilization from traction or a cast can cause alterations in physiologic functioning. To prevent complications:

- Assess breathing patterns and lung sounds frequently for congestion or respiratory compromise.
- Perform skin and neurovascular assessments approximately every 2 hours.

- Use adequate padding and skin wrapping to avoid placing pressure on the popliteal space. Such pressure could lead to nerve damage.
- For the child in a cast, change the child's position every 2 to 3 hours while awake to help avoid areas of pressure and promote increased circulation. The child can be placed either prone or supine or positioned on the floor and supported with pillows.
- Help prevent skin irritation and breakdown in the child with a cast. Use moleskin to protect from rough edges. Place tape around the perineal opening of the cast to prevent soiling.
- Increase fluids and fiber in the child's diet, as a change in bowel or bladder status is commonly associated with immobility.
- If permitted by physician orders, release the child from traction for meals and daily care. The time out of traction should not exceed 1 hour per day. Encourage parents to hold and cuddle the child at this time to promote comfort and bonding.

PROMOTE NORMAL GROWTH AND DEVELOPMENT

Engage the child in activities that stimulate the upper extremities and all five senses. Provide stimulating toys such as stacking blocks, brightly colored mobiles, soft balls, or musical toys. Position toys within the child's reach and interact with the child as much as possible. See Chapter 39 for specific recommendations for stimulating activities.

DISCHARGE PLANNING AND HOME CARE TEACHING

Teach parents how to care for a child in traction or a spica cast at home. Family members' active participation in the child's daily care during hospitalization gradually increases their confidence in their ability to provide care once home. Identify and address home care needs well in advance of discharge. Before discharge, be sure the parents have:

- Information about general cast care (see Table 56–1), positioning, bathing, toileting, and age-appropriate diversional activities. Include body mechanics for the adults moving the child.
- Knowledge of the importance of performing neurovascular checks and reporting any abnormalities immediately. Teach them circulation, motion, and sensitivity checks.
- The parents should understand that the bar between the legs on the cast is not to be used for holding or turning the child. The bar is used to position the legs at the proper distance; using it to lift can cause the cast to fracture, weaken, or disintegrate.
- Information on feeding the child.
- Safety teaching to minimize chance of injury to a casted child.
- Instruction about types of toys that are age appropriate and measures to prevent them from being placed into the cast (a T-shirt should be placed over the cast, covering its edges).
- Appropriate referrals for periodic assessment by a visiting nurse or home health nurse.
- Family resources to care for the child.

Before discharge, have parents demonstrate how to dress and feed a child in a spica cast. Ensure that safe travel arrangements have been made for the day of discharge. Help parents get an appropriate car safety seat in advance of discharge. Encourage parents to let the child interact with other children at home, and to provide the child in a cast with similar opportunities for play and social activities.

COMMUNITY-BASED NURSING CARE

Have parents of an infant in a Pavlik harness demonstrate care of the infant while in the harness. Teach family members about daily care (bathing, dressing, and feeding) of the infant. The harness is worn full time; instructions generally include sponge bathing while it is in place, although some physicians may allow it to be removed briefly each day for bathing. One shoulder strap is removed at a time to change a T-shirt while the legs are held in proper position. The hips and buttocks should be supported carefully in the abducted position at all times. Demonstrate how to feed the infant in an upright position to maintain abduction and how to change a diaper without removing the harness.

Instruct the parents of an infant with a harness or a child in a cast to look for any reddened or irritated areas near the harness or cast edges and to check toes frequently for proper circulation. Frequent repositioning reduces the risk of pressure sores or circulatory compromise. The infant should wear an undershirt and socks under the harness to prevent rubbing of the skin.

Safety precautions are important as the child will not have normal mobility. Parents will need to use a specially designed car seat that accommodates the child with abducted hips. Strollers and cribs should provide sufficient room to protect the legs from injury and to prevent hip adduction.

Evaluation

Expected outcomes for nursing care of the child with developmental dysplasia of the hip include the following:

- The skin remains intact.
- The child has no complications due to immobility.
- Parents demonstrate adequate knowledge regarding the condition, treatment, and necessary home care.
- A safe environment is maintained for the child.
- The child regains normal mobility.

Legg-Calvé-Perthes Disease

Legg-Calvé-Perthes disease (or simply Perthes disease) is a self-limiting condition in which there is avascular necrosis of the femoral head. The disease occurs in approximately 1 in 12,000

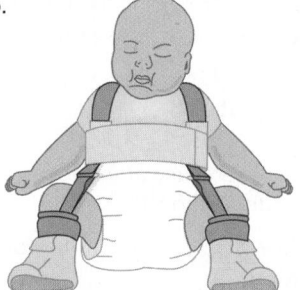
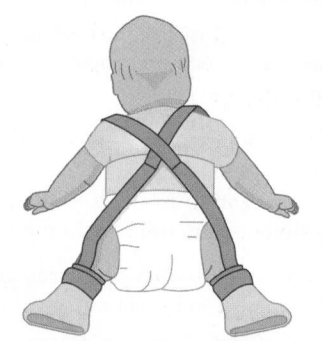

children and affects boys 4 times more often than girls. It usually occurs between the ages of 2 and 12 years, with an average age of 7 years at onset. The disease can be unilateral or bilateral (Kannu & Howard, 2014; Perry & Hall, 2011).

ETIOLOGY AND PATHOPHYSIOLOGY

The necrosis associated with Legg-Calvé-Perthes disease results from an interruption of the blood supply to the femoral epiphysis. How and why this occurs is not completely understood, but several predisposing factors have been identified. A coagulation system disorder causes repeated vascular interruptions to the proximal femur. Disturbed blood supply to the epiphyseal plate of the femoral bone is noted, leading to necrosis of the femoral head. The incidence of the condition is increased in families with a history of the disease, which suggests that genetic factors may play a role. In 17% of cases, onset of the disease is preceded by a mild traumatic injury, and 10% of children affected have a history of breech birth (Mazloumi, Ebrahimzadeh, & Kachooei, 2014). Trauma may cause a subchondral fracture and resultant synovitis, which in turn causes pressure that occludes the blood supply. Children with Legg-Calvé-Perthes disease often have delayed skeletal maturation, increased thyroid levels, and low somatomedin C (insulin-like growth factor). It is more common in those with low birth weight, increased parental age, and exposure to environmental tobacco smoke (Mazloumi et al., 2014).

CLINICAL MANIFESTATIONS

Legg-Calvé-Perthes disease progresses through four distinct stages, over a period of 1 to 4 years, after the original insult (usually unidentified) occurs (Table 56–2). Early symptoms of Perthes disease include a mild pain in the hip or anterior thigh and a limp, which are aggravated by increased activity and relieved by rest. The child favors the affected hip and limits hip movement to avoid discomfort.

As the disease progresses, range of motion becomes limited and weakness and muscle wasting develop. The affected thigh is 2 to 3 cm (0.8 to 1.2 in.) smaller than the unaffected thigh. Prolonged hip irritability may produce muscle spasms and increased pain. This period of the disease varies from 1 to 4 years. Gradually, revascularization begins and pain decreases.

CLINICAL THERAPY

Because the child's initial symptoms are mild, parents often do not seek medical attention until symptoms have been present for several months. Diagnosis is made using standard anteroposterior and frog-leg radiographs. However, radiographs taken early in the course of the disease may be normal or show vague widening of the cartilage space. Bone scans, MRI, and arthrography may be used in diagnosis. Laboratory studies of the blood, such as white blood cell count, help to rule out

TABLE 56–2 Clinical Manifestations of Legg-Calvé-Perthes Disease

STAGE	CLINICAL MANIFESTATIONS
Prenecrosis	An insult causes loss of blood supply to the femoral head.
I—Necrosis	Avascular stage (3–6 months); the child is asymptomatic, bone radiographs are normal, and the head of the femur is structurally intact but avascular.
II—Revascularization	Period of 1–4 years characterized by pain and limitation of movement. Bone radiographs show new bone deposition and dead bone resorption. Fracture and deformity of the head of the femur can occur.
III—Bone healing	Reossification takes place; pain decreases.
IV—Remodeling	The disease process is over, pain is absent, and improvement in joint function occurs.

inflammatory synovitis of the hip. Protein C, protein S, and APC-R (resistance to activated protein C) may sometimes be performed to evaluate if a coagulation abnormality is present (de Sanctis, 2011; Milani & Dobashi, 2011).

Medical management and prognosis depend on the degree of femoral involvement. Early detection is important. The desired outcome is a pain-free hip that functions properly. To promote healing and prevent deformity, the femoral head must be contained within the hip socket until ossification is complete. This can happen only if the hips remain in an abducted position. At the beginning of treatment, traction can be used to maintain the hips in an abducted and internally rotated position. Once abduction is accomplished, treatment consists of Petrie (leg abduction) casting, or surgical soft-tissue releases such as adductor tenotomy, followed by bracing. Toronto (Figure 56–9) and Scottish Rite braces are most commonly used. Prognosis

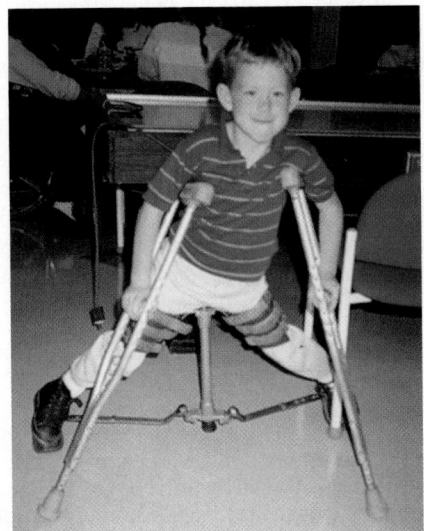

Figure 56–9 Although the Toronto brace may seem formidable for a child to wear, you can see by this photograph that, as usual, children adapt quite well to it.

is good if the femoral head can be contained long enough for proper healing to occur. Severe disease may be treated by surgery to release adductor muscles, treat the acetabulum or femur, and restore range of motion. Children with untreated disease or those diagnosed late in the disease process occasionally develop osteoarthritis, leg length discrepancy, or hip dysfunction later in life (Nakamura et al., 2014).

Nursing Management

For the Child With Legg-Calvé-Perthes Disease

Nursing Assessment and Diagnosis

Suspect Legg-Calvé-Perthes disease in any child, especially a boy 2 to 12 years of age, who complains of hip discomfort accompanied by a limp. The school nurse may be the first person to observe the child with symptoms of Legg-Calvé-Perthes disease. The child may complain of pain and have to rest during physical education classes. Refer the child to the healthcare provider immediately. Question the child who has an apparent limp about pain, and assess the child's range of motion. Ask if the child injured the hip at some time in the past.

Nursing diagnoses, which center on altered activities and compliance, might include the following (NANDA-I © 2014):

- *Mobility: Physical, Impaired,* related to restriction of brace or cast
- *Injury, Risk for,* related to potential complications resulting from noncompliance with the treatment regimen
- *Activity, Deficient Diversional,* related to forced inactivity
- *Body Image, Disturbed,* related to brace

Planning and Implementation

Children with Legg-Calvé-Perthes disease often receive all of their treatment at home. Helping the child and family comply with the prescribed treatment plan may be challenging because children develop the disease at an age when they are usually very active. The child, who may have little pain, often finds immobilization difficult.

PROMOTE NORMAL GROWTH AND DEVELOPMENT

Give parents suggestions to help redirect the child's energy within the limitations in mobility imposed by treatment. A return to school promotes a feeling of normality. Coordinate the return to school by facilitating the child's use of an elevator or ramp as needed in that setting. Partner with the family to provide instruction for school personnel and other children to foster understanding of the child's condition and treatment. Activities that involve peers also help the child achieve developmental milestones. Help the child adjust to wearing a brace.

Growth and Development

Legg-Calvé-Perthes disease primarily affects boys with an average age of 7 years. These school-age children are industrious and independent. Suggest activities that redirect energy and promote normal development. These may include horseback riding, which promotes hip abduction; swimming to increase mobility; handcrafts to promote fine motor skills; and computer activities to stimulate cognitive development.

COMMUNITY-BASED NURSING CARE

Both the child and the family should be aware that treatment generally takes more than 2 years. Emphasize the importance of following the treatment plan to ensure adequate hip containment and proper healing. Teach the family how to care for a child in traction and how to check the child's skin for breakdown (see Table 56–10 later in this chapter). Follow-up visits should be arranged at regular intervals in addition to home care visits during the period of traction.

Evaluation

Expected outcomes of nursing care are elimination of hip pain and discomfort, normal development during the period of immobilization, absence of complications, and parent and child knowledge of the treatment regimen.

Slipped Capital Femoral Epiphysis

Slipped capital femoral epiphysis (SCFE) occurs when the femoral head is displaced from the femoral neck. This condition is seen in 10 of 100,000 adolescents, commonly in the prepubertal growth spurt, between the ages of 12 to 15 years in boys and 10 to 13 years in girls. Boys are more often affected than girls. Black children and those with predisposing factors are affected more often than other children (Georgiadis & Zaltz, 2014).

ETIOLOGY AND PATHOPHYSIOLOGY

The cause of SCFE is unknown. Predisposing factors include obesity, a recent growth spurt, and endocrine disorders such as hypothyroidism and hypogonadism.

Slippage of the femoral head occurs at the proximal epiphyseal plate, and the femur displaces from the epiphysis (see *Pathophysiology Illustrated: Slipped Epiphysis*). Slippage is usually gradual (chronic), but may also result from acute trauma. The synovial membrane becomes inflamed, edematous, and painful. If untreated, callous formation occurs, resulting in a deformed hip with limited range of motion.

Growth and Development

Obesity is a known risk factor for SCFE. Increasing rates of obesity among children contribute to an increasing risk for the disorder. Research continues to demonstrate a relationship between body mass index (BMI) and SCFE. High rates of elevated BMI likely play a role in both bilateral SCFE occurrences and increasing incidence of the condition (Compton, 2014; Witbreuk et al., 2013). Nurses are well positioned to work with children and families to teach weight reduction strategies and to share information about the numerous health risks associated with elevated BMI.

CLINICAL MANIFESTATIONS

Symptoms include limp; knee, thigh, groin, or hip pain and loss of hip motion. Out-toeing, decreased internal rotation, and external rotation with flexion of the leg are symptomatic (Georgiadis & Zaltz, 2014). The condition is categorized as *acute* (sudden onset with less than 3 weeks' duration), *chronic* (longer than 3 weeks' duration), or *acute-on-chronic* (an additional slippage in a child with a chronic condition), depending on the onset and severity of symptoms. The child with an acute slip has sudden, severe pain and cannot bear weight. An acute slip may be associated with traumatic injury. The youth may be able to walk (stable) or unable to bear weight (unstable).

Pathophysiology Illustrated: **Slipped Epiphysis**

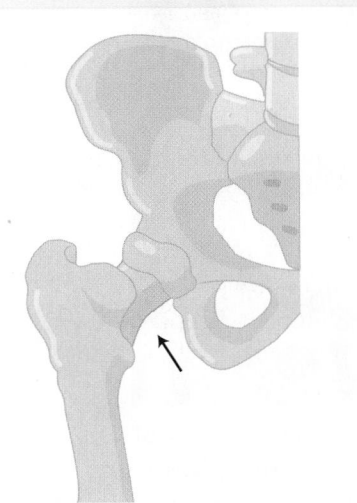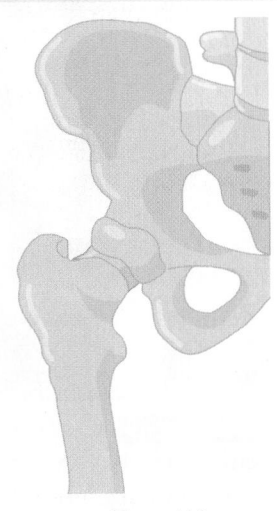

In slipped capital femoral epiphysis, the femoral head is displaced from the femoral neck at the proximal epiphyseal plate.

Slipped epiphysis

Normal hip

CLINICAL THERAPY

A complete history provides information about risk factors and the development of the condition. Radiographs confirm the diagnosis. A bone scan, ultrasound, CT, and MRI may also be performed.

The goal of medical management is to stabilize the femoral head while keeping displacement to a minimum and retaining as much hip function as possible. Surgical treatment is usually necessary; this involves fixation of the epiphysis with screws or pins. If the condition is stable, a single screw into the hip in an outpatient procedure is sufficient for stabilization; if unstable, surgical treatment may include traction and surgery.

Prognosis is related to the severity of the deformity and the occurrence of complications, such as avascular necrosis of the femoral head or **chondrolysis** (the breaking down and absorption of cartilage).

Nursing Management

For the Child With Slipped Capital Femoral Epiphysis

Nursing Assessment and Diagnosis

The child usually presents with hip pain or referred pain to the groin, thigh, or knee and limited mobility. A thorough history is needed to assess for injury as a cause. Assess the child's range of motion, pain, and limp, if apparent. Refer the child for treatment immediately if SCFE is suspected. This condition is considered to be an emergency, and it is essential that the child be treated immediately to keep weight off the affected joint (Georgiadis & Zaltz, 2014).

Among the nursing diagnoses that may apply to the child with SCFE are the following (NANDA-I © 2014):

- *Mobility: Physical, Impaired,* related to treatment
- *Pain* related to hip injury
- *Body Image, Disturbed,* related to treatment
- *Development: Delayed, Risk for,* related to mobility restrictions

- *Obesity* related to immobility
- *Tissue Perfusion: Peripheral, Ineffective,* related to traction, casting, and other treatments
- *Knowledge, Readiness for Enhanced (Child and Parent),* related to disease process and treatment

Planning and Implementation

Nursing management involves caring for the child in traction or after surgery, administering medications and other pain-control interventions, maintaining mobility within the limits imposed by treatment, providing adequate nutrition, educating the child and family about the disorder, providing emotional support, and promoting compliance with the treatment plan.

ENCOURAGE APPROPRIATE NUTRITIONAL INTAKE AND PHYSICAL ACTIVITY

A growing adolescent needs increased amounts of proteins, carbohydrates, and calcium to promote skeletal healing. Provide written instructions about nutritional requirements to promote bone healing and maintain an ideal body weight. If a child is overweight, encourage weight loss by decreasing the percentage of fat and sugar in the diet and by increasing physical activity that is safe to do. Weight loss decreases pressure on the femoral epiphysis and can also lead to a more positive self-image. Incorporate upper body exercises into treatment, both to assist in weight control and to build muscle. A few visits to physical therapy may facilitate a program of upper body exercise and teach safe ways of increasing the total amount of physical activity.

PROVIDE EMOTIONAL SUPPORT

Because the onset of SCFE is usually unexpected, the child and family may find themselves facing surgery with little warning. Explain the treatment plan simply and thoroughly. Reassure the child and family that with proper compliance, treatment should be successful.

DISCHARGE PLANNING AND HOME CARE TEACHING

Help the family plan for the child's return to school. If attendance is not possible for a time because of traction or surgery, arrange for tutors and computer communication with school as needed. Follow-up visits are necessary until the child's epiphyseal plates close. It is not uncommon for SCFE to occur in the other hip. Make sure the child and family are aware of symptoms such as decreased range of motion or pain that could indicate onset of the disorder in the other hip. Tell parents to contact their healthcare provider immediately if these symptoms occur.

Evaluation

Expected outcomes of nursing care for the child with slipped capital femoral epiphysis include maintenance of normal weight and recommended nutritional intake, absence of complications of immobility, successful adaptation to school following treatment, and family recognition of the need for ongoing monitoring for complications.

Disorders of the Spine

Scoliosis

Scoliosis is a lateral S- or C-shaped curvature of the spine that is often associated with a rotational deformity of the spine and ribs. Many people exhibit some degree of spinal curvature; curvatures of more than 10 degrees are considered abnormal. Curves are either idiopathic or compensatory, the latter occurring as the spine curves to compensate for a structural deformity such as leg length discrepancy. Idiopathic scoliosis occurs most often in girls, especially during the growth spurt between the ages of 10 and 13 years. From 1% to 3% of adolescents manifest with idiopathic scoliosis of greater than 10 degrees. A smaller number of children manifest infantile scoliosis before 3 years of age or juvenile scoliosis from 3 to 10 years (Lombardi, Akoume, Colombini, et al., 2011).

ETIOLOGY AND PATHOPHYSIOLOGY

The cause of scoliosis is complex. Structural scoliosis may be congenital, idiopathic, or acquired (associated with neuromuscular disorders such as muscular dystrophy or myelodysplasia, or secondary to spinal cord injuries).

In idiopathic structural scoliosis (the most common type), the spine for unknown reasons begins to curve laterally, with vertebral rotation. The most common curve is a right thoracic and left lumbar deformity. As the curve progresses, structural changes occur. The ribs on the concave side (inside of the curve) are forced closer together, while the ribs on the convex side separate widely, causing narrowing of the thoracic cage and formation of the rib hump. The lateral curvature affects the vertebral structure. Disc spaces are narrowed on the concave side and spread wider on the convex side, resulting in an asymmetric vertebral canal (Figure 56–10).

Scoliosis can also occur in congenital diseases involving the spinal structure and in the musculoskeletal changes seen in conditions such as myelomeningocele, cerebral palsy (see Chapter 54), or muscular dystrophy. Disturbances in platelet function, melatonin levels, and bone-related trace substances are sometimes evident (Lombardi et al., 2011). Scoliosis can also be acquired after injury to the spinal cord.

CLINICAL MANIFESTATIONS

The classic signs of scoliosis include truncal asymmetry, uneven shoulder and hip height, a one-sided rib hump, and a prominent scapula. The child does not usually complain of pain or discomfort.

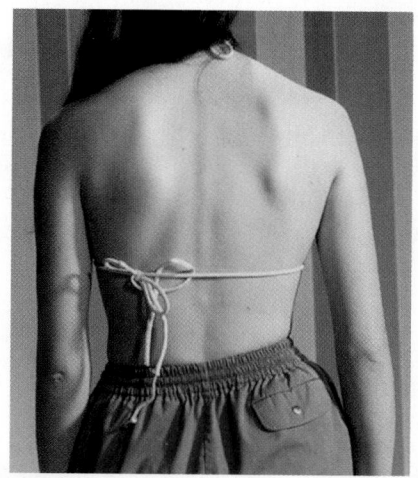

Figure 56–10 Clues for early detection of scoliosis. A child may have varying degrees of scoliosis. For mild forms, treatment will focus on strengthening and stretching. Moderate forms will require bracing. Severe forms may necessitate surgery and fusion. Clothes that fit at an angle, such as this teenage girl's shorts, and anatomic asymmetry of the back provide clues for early detection.

CLINICAL THERAPY

Generally, observation and radiographic examination are used to diagnose scoliosis. Additional diagnostic studies include MRI, CT, and bone scanning, which are used occasionally to assess the degree of curvature. The goal of medical management is to limit or stop progression of the curvature.

Early detection is essential to successful treatment. Adequate treatment and follow-up maximize the child's chances for proper spinal alignment. The treatment regimen chosen depends on the degree and progression of the curvature and the reaction of the child and family to medical management.

Treatment of children with mild scoliosis (curvatures of 10 to 20 degrees) consists of exercises to improve posture and muscle tone and to maintain, or possibly increase, flexibility of the spine. Emphasis is placed on building strength toward the outside of the curve while stretching the inside of the curve. However, these exercises are not a cure, and the child should be evaluated by a physician at 3-month intervals, with radiographic evaluation every 6 months.

Medical management of moderate scoliosis (curvatures of 20 to 40 degrees) includes bracing with a Boston brace. The goal of wearing a brace is to maintain the existing spinal curvature with no increase. Brace wear begins immediately after diagnosis. To achieve maximum effectiveness, the brace should be worn 23 hours per day. Brace treatment is lengthy, favorite sports may not be allowed, it can affect body image, and it requires a high degree of compliance, all of which can be difficult for adolescents.

Children with severe scoliosis (curvatures of 40 to 50 degrees or more) generally require surgery, which involves spinal fusion. The majority of spinal fusions are performed using segmental instrumentation of the spinal cord with hooks, wires, rods, and screws (Lubicky, Hanson, Riley, et al., 2011; Scottish Rite Hospital, 2011). Examples of surgical approaches include Luque wires, Cotrel-Dubousset (CD) instrumentation, Texas Scottish Rite Hospital system, and Moss-Miami system.

These treatments stabilize the spine well during surgery, may be accompanied by bone grafting to the spine, and require no long-term therapy or postoperative casting; instrumentation remains permanently in the back. Following surgery with wires or instrumentation, the child is on bed rest during a recovery period and then is generally fitted with anteroposterior plastic shells (also called thoracolumbar sacral orthotics) that are worn for several months to provide stability for the spine.

Nursing Management
For the Child With Scoliosis

Nursing Assessment and Diagnosis

School nurses often screen children for scoliosis, generally in the fifth and seventh grades. Several states mandate this screening, but it is not universal in all states, nor is it now recommended for all children (U.S. Preventive Services Task Force, 2014). When abnormalities are noted, refer the child to an orthopedic center for further evaluation. Children should be examined every 6 to 9 months thereafter. If scoliosis is detected, the child's brothers and sisters should be examined and observed closely. Scoliosis screening involves visual observations of the following.

From the front:

- Is the head midline?
- Are the shoulders at the same height?
- Is there the same amount of space between the arms and body on each side?

From the back:

- Is the head midline?
- Are the shoulders at the same height?
- Are the scapulae equally prominent and at the same height?
- Is the spine straight?
- Is there the same amount of space between the arms and body on each side?
- Are the hips at the same height?

With the adolescent holding hands together and bent over slightly:

- Are the scapula humps even?

With the adolescent holding hands together and bent over toward the floor:

- Are the flank humps even?
- Is the spine straight?
- Is there a marked roundness when viewed from the side? (evidence of kyphosis)

Once scoliosis has been identified, the focus becomes education and follow-up. Any child with scoliosis should have a comprehensive neurologic, cardiac, and respiratory examination, since the rib cage deformity can influence the functioning of these systems.

The following nursing diagnoses may apply to the child with scoliosis (NANDA-I © 2014):

- ***Health Behavior, Risk-Prone,*** related to duration and intensity of exercise prescription

- ***Mobility: Physical, Impaired,*** related to brace or movement restrictions and pain following surgery
- ***Skin Integrity, Risk for Impaired,*** related to brace
- ***Knowledge, Deficient,*** related to unfamiliarity with disease process and home care
- ***Body Image, Disturbed,*** related to deformity and brace wear

Common nursing diagnoses for the child having surgery can be found in the accompanying *Nursing Care Plan.*

Planning and Implementation

An important aspect of nursing care is client education. Client adherence to prescribed measures is critical to the success of treatment. Children and their families need to understand the condition and the stages of treatment; this is particularly true for adolescents undergoing treatment for scoliosis.

Children or adolescents facing surgery require education, reassurance, and support. Teach about pain control and the patient-controlled analgesia (PCA) pump. Often children donate some of their own blood prior to surgery, and the family may also donate so blood transfused in surgery is the children's or a family member's. Teach the child the safety that this ensures. The adolescent will benefit from learning about deep breathing, positioning, surgical incision, and all other aspects of postoperative care. The *Nursing Care Plan* summarizes nursing care for the child undergoing surgery for scoliosis.

PROMOTE ACCEPTANCE OF THE TREATMENT PLAN

Provide instructions about exercises that will help to decrease the severity of the spinal curvature, and obtain baseline exercise levels. Demonstrate the exercises, and explain their purpose (i.e., to strengthen back muscles). Help the child adjust to wearing a brace. Adolescents, in particular, may be reluctant to wear an external device such as a brace. To promote a sense of control, allow the adolescent to choose when to exercise and when to be out of the brace, within the treatment guidelines. Provide reassurance and encouragement and promote interaction with peers. Suggest that the adolescent work with a peer support person who is being treated for scoliosis or has had the condition in the past. Provide information about fashionable clothing that can be worn with the brace and facilitate visits to department stores that will help the teen shop for clothing.

Nursing Care Plan: The Child Undergoing Surgery for Scoliosis

1. Nursing Diagnosis: *Knowledge, Deficient (Child and Parents)*, related to lack of information about surgery (NANDA-I © 2014)

GOAL: The child and parents will verbalize understanding of the disease, its treatment, and the surgical procedure.

INTERVENTION	RATIONALE
• Teach the child and family about the course of the disease, its signs and symptoms, and treatment. Provide appropriate handouts. Encourage the child and parents to ask questions.	• Understanding and involvement increase motivation and compliance while reducing fear.
• Begin preoperative teaching at the time of admission. Orient the child to hospital and postoperative procedures. Before surgery, have the child demonstrate log-rolling, range-of-motion (ROM) exercises, and the use of an incentive spirometer. Discuss pain management.	• Preoperative teaching and familiarity with hospital procedures reduce the stress related to surgery and postoperative complications.

EXPECTED OUTCOME: Child and family will accurately verbalize knowledge about the disease and its treatment. Child and family will ask appropriate questions about postoperative care.

2. Nursing Diagnosis: *Breathing Pattern, Ineffective*, related to hypoventilation syndrome (NANDA-I © 2014)

GOAL: The child will show no signs of respiratory compromise.

INTERVENTION	RATIONALE
• Monitor respiratory status, especially after the administration of analgesics. Apply pulse oximeter.	• Evaluation of the child's respiratory condition anticipates and avoids complications. Analgesics such as morphine may increase or potentiate respiratory compromise.
• Administer oxygen if ordered.	• Oxygen increases peripheral oxygen saturation to 95%–100%.
• Have the child use an incentive spirometer.	• Spirometry increases lung expansion and aeration of the alveoli.
• Monitor intake and output.	• Adequate hydration promotes loose secretions and helps prevent infection.
• Reposition the child at least every 2 hr.	• Repositioning ensures inflation of the lung fields.

EXPECTED OUTCOME: Child will have normal respiratory patterns.

3. Nursing Diagnosis: *Injury, Risk for*, related to neurovascular deficit secondary to instrumentation (NANDA-I © 2014)

GOAL: The child's neurovascular system will remain intact as evidenced by circulation, sensation, and motor assessments. The child will feel no numbness or tingling.

INTERVENTION	RATIONALE
• Monitor the child's color, circulation, capillary refill, warmth, sensation, and motion in all extremities. Perform neurovascular assessments every 2 hr for the first 24 hr and then every 4 hr for the next 48 hr. Record presence of pedal and distal tibial pulses every hour for 48 hr. Report changes and abnormal findings immediately.	• When the spinal column is manipulated during surgery, altered neurovascular status, thrombosis formation, and paralysis are possible complications. Postoperative risks include loss of bowel or bladder control, weakness or paralysis, and impaired vision or sensation.
• Have the child wear antiembolism stockings until ambulatory. The stockings may be removed for 1 h 2–3 times daily.	• Antiembolism stockings prevent blood clots and promote venous return. Thrombus formation is a postoperative risk.
• Check for any pain, swelling, or a positive Homans sign (pain in the calf of the leg when the toes are dorsiflexed). Record any evidence of edema.	• Swelling may indicate a tight dressing and tissue damage. A positive Homans sign and pain may indicate thrombus formation.
• Monitor input and output.	• Abnormalities may indicate a fluid shift problem.
• Log roll while on bed rest. Encourage and assist the child with ROM exercises, both passive and active as prescribed.	• Log rolling maintains a straight spine. Exercises promote mobility and reduce risk of thrombus formation.

EXPECTED OUTCOME: Child will exhibit only temporary alteration (pale skin, faint pulse, and edema occur but they resolve within the initial postoperative phase). Child will return to the preoperative baseline state by discharge.

4. Nursing Diagnosis: *Pain* related to spinal fusion with instrumentation (NANDA-I © 2014)

GOAL: The child will verbalize an adequate level of comfort or show absence of pain behavior within 1 hour of a specific nursing intervention.

INTERVENTION	RATIONALE
• Assess the level of pain and initiate pain management strategies as soon as possible. Use patient-controlled analgesia if ordered.	• Adequate pain management allows for faster healing and a more cooperative patient. Patient-controlled analgesics may be effective.
• Administer pain medication around-the-clock to help ensure pain relief, especially during the first 48 hours. Monitor epidural blocks and patient-controlled analgesia or other methods used for pain control.	• Medicating around-the-clock helps to maintain comfort. Monitoring ensures patient safety.
• Use nonpharmacologic pain management techniques, such as imagery, relaxation, touch, music, application of heat and cold, and reduced environmental stimulation to supplement medications (see Chapter 40).	• Alternative treatments also interrupt the pain stimulus and provide relief. Nonpharmacologic methods can be an effective adjunct to pain management.
• Document pain assessment interventions and the child's response.	• Proper documentation guides the selection of the most effective means of pain control.
• Reassure the child that some discomfort is expected and that a variety of measures can be tried to reduce discomfort.	• Realistic expectations decrease anxiety and give the child a sense of control.

EXPECTED OUTCOME: Child will experience pain relief early in the postoperative period.

DISCHARGE PLANNING AND HOME CARE TEACHING

Identify and address home care needs well in advance of discharge after spinal surgery. The child will need to adapt to a new set of body mechanics. Show the child how to do simple tasks without bending or twisting the torso. Have the child demonstrate the ability to perform activities of daily living before discharge from the hospital. Partner with physical therapy/rehabilitation personnel to plan for the youth's needs related to safe and effective movement with the brace.

Activities for the child who has had spinal surgery are commonly limited for a period of time. The child can usually walk and perform physical activity such as gentle swimming, but lifting heavy loads, bending or twisting at the waist, or engaging in activities such as skiing, rollerblading, bicycle riding, and many other sports may not be allowed. Restrictions usually should be followed for 6 to 8 months, depending on the type of surgery and the surgeon. Emphasize to both the child and the family the importance of compliance. Give written discharge instructions to the child and family. Follow-up visits are important. The child should be examined 4 to 6 weeks after discharge, then every 3 to 4 months for 1 year, and every 1 to 2 years thereafter. The metal hardware in the back necessitates that after surgery the teen must carry a written physician explanation since the hardware will set off metal detectors at airports. Alternative screening methods are generally now available at most airports once the teen tells screeners about the metal implants.

Several organizations provide information and assistance to families of children with scoliosis. Make referrals as appropriate.

Evaluation

Expected outcomes of nursing care for the child with scoliosis treated by brace are maintenance of intact skin and compliance with prescribed therapy. Expected outcomes after surgical correction are given in the accompanying *Nursing Care Plan*.

Clinical Reasoning Adolescent Braces for Scoliosis

We know that adolescents are concerned about body image and that wearing a brace can be challenging. While there has been controversy about the efficacy of braces for scoliosis treatment, studies have found that bracing significantly decreases the progression of high-risk curves to the need for surgery (Brox, Lange, Gunderson, et al., 2012; Weinstein, Dolan, Wright, et al., 2013). Healthcare providers may need to address psychosocial coping issues in order to ensure compliance with brace therapy for scoliosis. What assessments can assist you in learning about the activity level, social interactions, and well-being of adolescents beginning scoliosis treatment?

Torticollis, Kyphosis, and Lordosis

Torticollis is tilt of the head caused by rotation of the cervical spine. The cause is generally an injury sustained to the sternocleidomastoid muscle at the time of birth or to a cervical spine abnormality. Stretching exercises or surgical lengthening of the sternocleidomastoid muscle are usual treatments. Occasionally, the cause of torticollis is visual impairment, leading to constant turning in one direction to see with the better eye.

Kyphosis (hunchback) and lordosis (swayback) are two other types of spinal curvature that may occur in children. Clinical therapy depends on the cause and degree of the curvature, and the age of the child at onset. Nurses can perform thorough musculoskeletal assessments of children (see Chapter 33) and refer any children with abnormalities for further evaluation. (See Table 56–3.)

Growth and Development

Postural lordosis is a characteristic finding in toddlers but should disappear by the school-age years.

TABLE 56–3 Clinical Manifestations of Kyphosis and Lordosis

CONDITION	CLINICAL MANIFESTATIONS	DIAGNOSTIC TESTS AND CLINICAL THERAPY	NURSING MANAGEMENT
KYPHOSIS			
Excessive convex curvature of the cervical thoracic spine	Visible hunchback or rounded shoulders; shortness of breath or fatigue; abdominal creases and tight hamstrings in severe cases	*Diagnostic tests:* Spinal curvature is assessed by having the child bend 90 degrees at the waist and looking at the scapular area from the side. Diagnosis is confirmed by radiograph. *Clinical therapy:* Exercises are prescribed for mild condition; bracing is commonly used; surgery is performed in severe cases.	Provide support. Encourage exercises and diligent brace wear. Help the child to deal with the psychologic stress of altered body image.
LORDOSIS			
Excessive concave curvature of the lumbar spine with an angle of more than 60 degrees; most common in prepubescent girls and African Americans	Presence of swayback; prominent buttocks; hip flexion contractures; tight hamstrings	*Diagnostic tests:* Spinal curvature is assessed by looking at the standing child from the side. Lumbar lordosis is confirmed by visualizing the spine on standing, lateral radiograph. *Clinical therapy:* Treatment focuses on exercises and postural awareness. Bracing and surgery are rarely prescribed.	Provide support. Reassure the child and family that the condition is often outgrown as the child matures. Encourage physical conditioning exercises and follow-up examinations on a yearly basis.

Additional Disorders of the Bones and Joints

Osteoporosis and Osteopenia

Osteoporosis, a condition in which there is decreased density and mass of bone, promotes the risk of fractures and is commonly associated with aging. However, children can have osteoporosis (also known as *metabolic bone disease* or a bone mineral density more than 2.5 standard deviations below the norm) related to imbalanced nutrition or other pathologic conditions. Osteoporosis is preceded by osteopenia or low bone mass, which is between 1.0 and 2.5 standard deviations below the norm (Szadek & Scharer, 2014).

ETIOLOGY AND PATHOPHYSIOLOGY

Very-low-birth-weight infants who are premature often have osteopenia of prematurity because much of the bone mass is usually acquired in the latter weeks of pregnancy. In addition, they may have other health problems after birth and be unable to ingest enough nutrients to meet metabolic needs for bone growth. Premature infants are often less active than others, which decreases the amount of mechanical loading on their bones, a factor known to increase bone resorption and decrease bone mass (Rack et al., 2011).

A group of children who may show signs of osteoporosis are those who have decreased mechanical loading. Children with spina bifida or cerebral palsy, conditions that interfere with ambulation, have limited pressure on bones and resultant lowered bone mass in affected extremities and spine. Some other conditions are associated with lower bone mass, including Turner syndrome, growth hormone deficiency, osteogenesis imperfecta, juvenile rheumatoid arthritis, and diabetes.

Children who are treated for disorders or injuries with casting and bracing are also at high risk of osteoporosis due to immobilization.

Finally, adolescence is a period when adequate intakes of calcium and vitamin D are needed to maximize bone formation and prevent osteoporosis later in life. Adolescents, particularly females, often do not meet the recommended daily allowance (RDA) for these nutrients and are at risk for osteoporosis even though it may not be manifested for years. Other lifestyle patterns of youth that decrease bone formation are smoking, alcohol use, excessive soda intake, and keeping weight at a very low level. Those with anorexia nervosa are at risk for osteoporosis and increased risk of fractures (Mehler, Cleary, & Guadiani, 2011).

CLINICAL MANIFESTATIONS

Osteoporosis is a silent disease, as is its precursor osteopenia; those who have the disorders are often without signs or symptoms for years. It may become apparent when a baby or child has a fracture and radiologic studies make the problem evident.

CLINICAL THERAPY

Bone mineral content and density are measured by single-photon absorptiometry (SPA), dual-photon absorptiometry (DPA), and dual-energy x-ray absorptiometry (DEXA); ultrasound may be used to assess preterm infants (Rack et al., 2011). Serum studies such as thyroid, bone-specific alkaline phosphatase, phosphorus, and type I collagen studies can be used to measure osteoblastic and osteoclastic activity. Vitamin D and calcium are measured, but since over 90% of the body's calcium is stored in bone, serum calcium is not accurately reflective of bone density.

Premature newborns at risk of osteopenia of prematurity need collaborative management by neonatologists, neonatal nutritionists, and neonatal nurses. Breast milk is enhanced by

Pathophysiology Illustrated: **Effects of Immobility**

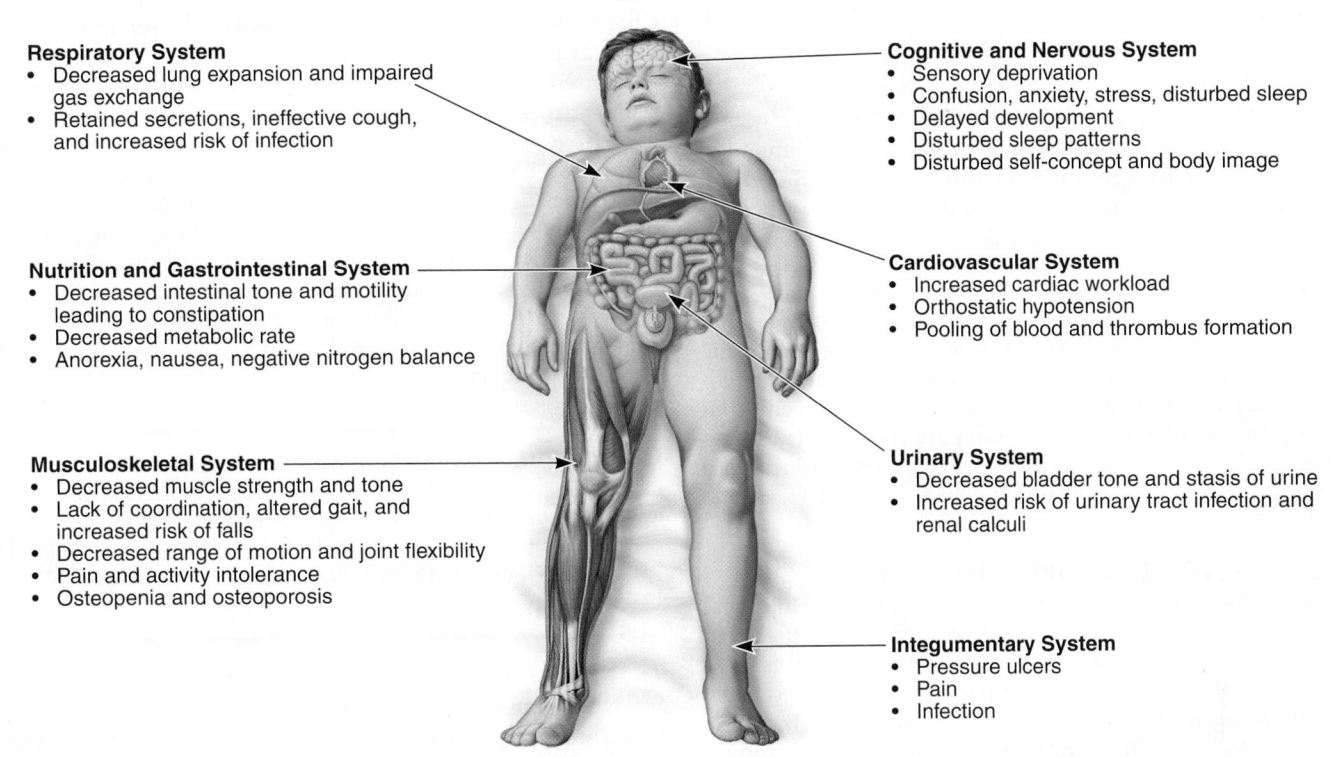

Respiratory System
- Decreased lung expansion and impaired gas exchange
- Retained secretions, ineffective cough, and increased risk of infection

Nutrition and Gastrointestinal System
- Decreased intestinal tone and motility leading to constipation
- Decreased metabolic rate
- Anorexia, nausea, negative nitrogen balance

Musculoskeletal System
- Decreased muscle strength and tone
- Lack of coordination, altered gait, and increased risk of falls
- Decreased range of motion and joint flexibility
- Pain and activity intolerance
- Osteopenia and osteoporosis

Cognitive and Nervous System
- Sensory deprivation
- Confusion, anxiety, stress, disturbed sleep
- Delayed development
- Disturbed sleep patterns
- Disturbed self-concept and body image

Cardiovascular System
- Increased cardiac workload
- Orthostatic hypotension
- Pooling of blood and thrombus formation

Urinary System
- Decreased bladder tone and stasis of urine
- Increased risk of urinary tract infection and renal calculi

Integumentary System
- Pressure ulcers
- Pain
- Infection

For older children at risk of developing osteoporosis, calcium and vitamin D intake is encouraged and oral supplements may be given. Standing therapy for those who are nonambulatory can provide mechanical weight and enhance bone density. Bisphosphonates, calcitonin, fluoride, and parathyroid hormone may be used to treat children and adolescents with osteoporosis (Szadek & Scharer, 2014). When a cast or other immobilizing device is removed from a child, a program of gradually increasing exercise in collaboration with physical rehabilitation professionals promotes bone strengthening and lowered risk for fractures or related sequelae.

adding special fortifiers; premature formula should be used rather than regular baby formula. When infants need enteral or parenteral feedings, calcium-to-phosphorus ratios are carefully balanced to enhance osteoblastic activity. There is evidence to suggest that assisted range-of-motion exercise can promote weight gain and bone mineralization in premature infants (Schulzke, Kaempfen, Trachsel, et al., 2014).

Nursing Management
For the Child With Osteoporosis or Osteopenia

Nursing Assessment and Diagnosis

Nurses identify newborns, children, and adolescents at risk of developing low bone mass and density. This is accomplished by identifying diseases and medications putting the child at risk, as well as history of fractures or malabsorption disorder. Ask about exercise and activity patterns, and physical therapy for children who are nonambulatory. Dietary intake is measured periodically for all youth at health promotion visits, and RDAs for calcium, phosphorus, and vitamin D are compared to intake.

Nursing diagnoses that may apply to the child with osteoporosis include the following (NANDA-I © 2014):

- *Nutrition, Imbalanced: Less than Body Requirements*, related to inability to consume essential nutrients
- *Injury, Risk for*, to bones related to decreased bone mass and density
- *Health Maintenance, Ineffective*, related to inadequate dietary intake

Planning and Implementation

Perform a dietary analysis of children at risk. (See Chapter 32 for detailed methods for diet assessment.) Refer children at risk to nutritionists and a physician for further education and diagnosis. Suggest referrals to physical rehabilitation to recommend weight-bearing exercise. Administer nutritional supplements when prescribed, and teach families how to give these medications. Partner with families to provide therapy that stimulates weight bearing for nonambulatory children. Teach parents how to recognize fractures in children who may not have normal sensation and are unable to report them. Edema, unusual shape of a limb, fussiness of the child, and falls should be reported promptly.

When osteoporosis is caused by immobility, many other symptoms occur as well. Be alert for these problems and integrate physical activity into care as much as possible to minimize their effects.

Evaluation

Expected outcomes of nursing care for the child with a potential for osteoporosis include adequate intake of recommended amounts of nutrients, absence of fractures, and normal findings on studies of bone mineral content and density.

Osteomyelitis

Osteomyelitis is an infection of the bone, most often one of the long bones of the lower extremity. It may be acute or chronic and may spread into surrounding tissues. Although osteomyelitis may occur at any age, it is most common in children between the ages of 1 and 12 years. Boys are affected 2 to 3 times as often as girls, primarily because they have a greater incidence of trauma. Overall incidence is 5 in 10,000 youth (Thomsen & Creech, 2011).

ETIOLOGY AND PATHOPHYSIOLOGY

Osteomyelitis is caused by a microorganism, usually bacterial but possibly viral or fungal. *Staphylococcus aureus* is the most common causative pathogen; others include *Escherichia coli*, *Neisseria meningitidis*, *Streptococcus pneumoniae*, *Mycobacterium tuberculosis*, *Borrelia burgdorferi*, and *Kingella kingae* (Bautista, Gholve, & Dormans, 2011; Thomsen & Creech, 2011). Common sources of infection are upper respiratory infection, trauma to the bone, and surgery.

The infecting organism spreads through the bloodstream or through a penetrating injury to the bone, where it becomes established. Infections in children often begin in the metaphysis (see Figure 56–2), which has a sluggish blood supply (Bautista et al., 2011). Eventually the infection may penetrate the bone cortex and periosteum. Inflammation and abscess formation can interrupt the blood supply to the underlying bone, affect the surrounding soft tissue, and, if the infection is left untreated, lead to necrosis.

CLINICAL MANIFESTATIONS

Symptoms include pain and tenderness with swelling, decreased mobility of the infected joint, and fever. Redness over the area may occur. The child may refuse to walk or may limp. The onset of acute osteomyelitis is generally rapid and is therefore sometimes misdiagnosed as a sports injury.

CLINICAL THERAPY

A history suggestive of osteomyelitis includes an upper respiratory infection or blunt trauma followed by pain at the area of a growth plate. Laboratory evaluation shows leukocytosis and an elevated erythrocyte sedimentation rate (ESR) and C-reactive protein. Radiographs and bone scans may identify the area of involvement. A needle aspiration of the site or a blood culture can confirm the diagnosis and provide a culture of the causative organism. Other studies may include enzyme-linked immunosorbent assay (ELISA) for Lyme antibody titer, antistreptolysin-O for recent streptococcal infections, or purified protein derivative (PPD) for exposure to tuberculosis (Thomsen & Creech, 2011).

Medical management begins with the intravenous administration of a broad-spectrum antibiotic, even before culture results are available. Since *S. aureus* is a common cause of infection, the antibiotic should be effective against this organism.

Treatment is influenced by the possibility of methicillin-resistant *S. aureus* (MRSA), so intravenous antibiotics are usually vancomycin or clindamycin, drugs effective against MRSA (see Chapter 43). Once the culture results are obtained, the antibiotic may be altered. Oral antibiotics are given once an adequate response has occurred. However, extended intravenous home therapy may be used. Antibiotic therapy continues for about 3 to 6 weeks. The cause of infection is not always identified from culture, so ESR and C-protein levels are followed carefully in these cases to identify if treatment is successful. When an adequate response is not obtained within 2 to 3 days, the area may be aspirated again or surgically drained. Intravenous fluids may be administered to ensure adequate hydration. In children with extensive orthopedic surgery or in those with immunosuppression, a short course of prophylactic antibiotic may be administered after surgery.

Growth and Development

Osteomyelitis in a newborn is of great concern because before 18 months of age the blood vessels cross the growth plates. This creates a higher risk of epiphyseal involvement with resultant limb length discrepancy. Poor feeding, crying when moved, and refusal to move a limb may indicate osteomyelitis.

Prompt diagnosis and treatment usually completely resolve the infection. The prognosis is related to the initiation of therapy—the earlier treatment begins, the better the outcome. Long-term unfavorable outcomes include disruption of the growth plate, which can interrupt growth, and damage to the joints from septic arthritis.

Nursing Management
For the Child With Osteomyelitis

Nursing Assessment and Diagnosis

A thorough history, including information about the onset of symptoms and a history of recent infections or puncture wounds, is essential. Ask about immunization status, especially tetanus vaccine. Assess the affected area for signs of redness, swelling, pain, and decreased range of motion. Measure vital signs; increased temperature and pulse in particular may provide clues about worsening infection. When osteomyelitis is possible, all cultures of blood or wound must be taken before antibiotic therapy is started.

Among the nursing diagnoses that may apply to the child with osteomyelitis are the following (NANDA-I © 2014):

- *Pain, Acute,* related to biologic injury
- *Mobility: Physical, Impaired,* related to discomfort
- *Infection, Risk for (Sepsis),* related to spread of infection
- *Imbalanced Nutrition: Less than Body Requirements,* related to loss of appetite
- *Knowledge, Readiness for Enhanced (Child and Parent),* related to lack of information about disease process

Planning and Implementation

Nursing management focuses on administering antibiotics, protecting the child from spread of the infection, and encouraging a well-balanced diet. Use standard precautions, with transmission-based precautions for any drainage from the site of infection.

OBTAIN CULTURES AND BLOOD WORK

Blood cultures and cultures of any open wound must be performed before the first dose of antibiotic when osteomyelitis is suspected. Obtain continuing blood samples as needed to monitor ESR and C-reactive protein levels. See the *Clinical Skills Manual* SKILLS.

ADMINISTER FLUIDS AND MEDICATIONS

Administer intravenous fluids as ordered to maintain the child's hydration status. Antibiotics are administered intravenously, at first, then orally. Monitor the intravenous site and provide care for the central line, if one is used. See the *Clinical Skills Manual* SKILLS.

In the early stages of the infection, analgesics are prescribed to relieve the associated pain and joint tenderness.

PROTECT FROM THE SPREAD OF INFECTION

Strict aseptic technique and transmission-based precautions should be used during all dressing changes. Children and family members should avoid direct contact with any dressings or drainage. Teach good hygiene practices, including hand hygiene, to maintain infection control. Take vital signs and evaluate the child frequently for symptoms indicating the spread of infection (e.g., increasing pain, difficulty breathing, increased pulse rate, fever).

ENCOURAGE A WELL-BALANCED DIET

Educate both the child and the parents about healthy dietary choices that promote healing. A high-protein diet and extra vitamin C will contribute to this process. Encourage increased fluid intake to provide adequate hydration and circulation.

DISCHARGE PLANNING AND HOME CARE TEACHING

Emphasize the importance of completing the full course of antibiotic therapy, especially for children who have had an abscess or lesion surgically drained. Some children may be discharged on intravenous antibiotics if the family is willing to learn the procedure for medication administration and care of the central line. Several sessions of demonstration and return demonstration are needed to ensure safe administration. If the family is unable to perform antibiotic therapy, a home infusion company may be available to come to the home and administer the medication. Explain that failure to follow the prescribed antibiotic therapy may result in chronic infection. Emphasize the importance of returning for blood analysis to monitor progression of healing.

Consider the child's age and developmental level and partner with the family to plan quiet activities and access to schoolwork. Provide suggestions for the family if the child will be immobilized at home.

Clinical Tip

If the child needs to remain home for a period of time during treatment for osteomyelitis, help the family plan for completion of school tasks. The nurse can partner with other health disciplines that are available to plan for the following:

- Contact the school and ask that work be sent home.
- Arrange for a tutor if needed.
- Facilitate computer communication between child, teacher, and other students.
- Help the family plan for help at home to monitor the child when the family needs to be at work or performing other tasks.
- Refer families to financial resources as appropriate for the services the child needs.
- Suggest activities that the child can do at home that foster developmental progress.

Evaluation

Expected outcomes of nursing care for the child with osteomyelitis include the following:

- The child has no signs of infection or sepsis.
- The child completes the prescribed course of antibiotics.
- Intake of fluids and nutrients is adequate for good health.
- The child's pain is effectively managed.
- The child is able to return to normal activities of daily living.

Skeletal Tuberculosis and Septic Arthritis

Skeletal tuberculosis (Figure 56–11) and septic arthritis are two infections that, although infrequent, may affect children and adolescents. See Table 56–4 for diagnostic tests and medical and nursing management for these infections.

Achondroplasia

Dwarfism is a genetic condition usually resulting in an adult height of 58 inches or less. The most common cause of dwarfism is achondroplasia, which causes short arms and legs. The torso and head are approximately normal size, but decreased growth of long bones causes short stature. This is known as *disproportionate short stature*. Achondroplasia is caused by an abnormal gene of chromosome 4 and occurs in 1 in 15,000 to 40,000 births (March of Dimes, 2012). The gene is coded to produce proteins

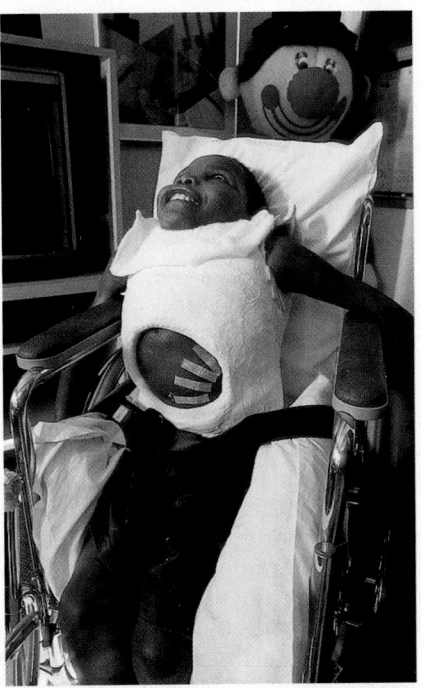

Figure 56–11 This boy from Kenya had surgery to correct severe kyphosis and scoliosis caused by tuberculosis of the spine. A Risser cast has been applied to maintain stability of the spine and thoracic cage during healing. Notice the area cut out of the cast to allow for auscultation of the abdomen, as well as to facilitate the child's comfort and adequate intake of food.

TABLE 56–4 Clinical Manifestations of Skeletal Tuberculosis and Septic Arthritis

CONDITION	CLINICAL MANIFESTATIONS	DIAGNOSTIC TESTS AND CLINICAL THERAPY	NURSING MANAGEMENT
SKELETAL TUBERCULOSIS			
Rare microbacterial infection that can be very destructive. The spine is the most frequent site of infection (Pott disease), with joints and other sites sometimes affected.	Depending on the site, pain, limp, severe muscle spasms, kyphosis, muscle atrophy, "doughy" swelling of joints, decreased joint motion, changes in reflexes, low-grade fever	*Diagnostic tests:* Diagnostic studies include tuberculosis skin test, complete blood count, synovial fluid analysis, and radiographs of affected limb or joint. *Clinical therapy:* Antibiotic therapy (using a combination of drugs) for 6–9 months is the treatment of choice. The affected site is immobilized. Disease may become resistant to these drugs, and additional drug therapy may be necessary.	Educate the child and family about the disorder and stress the importance of complying with long-term antibiotic therapy. Test all members of the family for tuberculosis. Report the disease to the local health department. Facilitate the immobilization and physical therapy of the child at home.
SEPTIC ARTHRITIS			
Joint infection of the synovial space most often caused by *Haemophilus influenzae, Staphylococcus,* and *Streptococcus.* The most common site of infection is the knee, followed by the hip, ankle, and elbow.	Fever, pain and local inflammation, joint tenderness, swelling, loss of spontaneous movement	*Diagnostic tests:* CBC with differential, ESR, blood cultures. Diagnosis is made based on joint aspiration findings. Results are commonly 100,000 WBCs and 75% neutrophils, ESR greater than 44 mm/hr. Radiographic changes may not be evident until later in the disease process. *Clinical therapy:* This is a medical emergency requiring prompt treatment to avoid permanent disability. Treatment involves joint aspiration, open drainage, and irrigation, followed by intravenous antibiotic therapy for 3–4 weeks and then oral antibiotics. If the full course of antibiotic treatment is not completed, the child risks recurrent infection and further degeneration of the infected joint.	Educate the child and family about the disorder and emphasize the importance of proper antibiotic therapy. Carefully position the painful joint. Administer antibiotics as prescribed. Use transmission-based precautions. Encourage fluids to ensure adequate hydration. Support and rest the joint; provide activities that do not require joint movement.

called *fibroblast growth factor receptors.* When fewer receptors are produced, the cells cannot respond normally to signals from growth factors. Achondroplasia may occur as a new genetic mutation with no previous family history or can occur when one or both parents are also dwarfs. There are other less common forms of dwarfism with about 200 identified types. (Refer to Chapter 3 for further information about genetic disease transmission.)

Children with achondroplasia have short legs and arms, short fingers with a separation between middle and ring fingers, and a large, prominent forehead. Hydrocephalus sometimes occurs in children with achondroplasia. (See Chapter 54 for a description of hydrocephalus.) Most children with the disorder inherit the gene from one parent. Since only one faulty gene must be present for manifestation of the disorder, it is a dominant characteristic. When a child inherits two copies of the gene from two affected parents, a fatal form of achondroplasia occurs, which is characterized by a small thorax, respiratory failure, and death in infancy.

Children with the disorder are diagnosed prenatally, at birth, or shortly after. When there is a family history, genetic testing before or after birth identifies the presence of the fibroplast growth factor receptor 3 (*FGFR3*) gene on chromosome 4. Characteristics common in the growth disorder include frequent otitis media, dental malocclusion, short fingers, bowing of legs, marked lordosis, and sleep apnea. The child may be slow at meeting gross motor developmental milestones (Ireland et al., 2012).

There is no treatment for the disorder at this time. Gene therapy and growth plate targeting are being explored as possible future treatments (Laederich & Horton, 2012). Some children and adults with dwarfism have undergone limb-lengthening procedures such as that described later in this chapter. Other orthopedic intervention may be needed to treat back pain or bone problems. For those children who develop hydrocephalus, insertion of a shunt to divert excess fluid may be needed. Treatment of conditions such as otitis media and malocclusion of teeth is provided.

Nursing Management

Nurses play an important role in helping families when a child is diagnosed with achondroplasia. If a parent is a dwarf or there is a positive family history of dwarfism, genetic counseling should be offered prenatally. Explain findings of testing and provide assistance with decision making about pregnancy if needed. Nurses assist parents who have a child with achondroplasia to adjust to the diagnosis, particularly if the parents have had no previous experience with the condition. They may feel guilt and anxiety; contact with other families who have children with achondroplasia can be a supportive intervention.

Nurses help the child with achondroplasia to develop a positive self-concept during childhood. Many resources, such as the Little People of America website, provide suggestions about how to foster a positive self-concept, adjust the home to facilitate the dwarf, and assist the child with adjustments in school settings. Partner with school nurses or counselors to ensure the child's successful inclusion in all school facilities and an individualized education plan. While some families decide to explore limb-lengthening procedures, most organizations state that focus should be placed on development of a healthy self-image rather than encouraging limb lengthening.

Nurses provide careful assessments of children throughout childhood. Head circumference is especially important in early childhood to identify hydrocephalus if it should occur. Carefully evaluate growth with specialized growth grids for achondroplasia, evaluate dental health at each visit, and perform developmental assessment with special emphasis on gross motor skills. Suggest activities such as swimming and biking that provide activity with little stress on bones. Assist the family by providing resources that assist with planning for car safety seats, methods of adjusting the home, and partnering with the school to provide a supportive atmosphere for the child. Some helpful organizations include Little People of America, Dwarf Athletic Association of America, Human Growth Foundation, Magic Foundation for Children's Growth and Related Adult Disorders, and March of Dimes. Refer for care for otitis media and provide postoperative care if tympanostomy tubes are inserted (see Chapter 45). Refer to dentists and orthodontists and encourage regular dental care.

Marfan Syndrome

Marfan syndrome is another example of a condition inherited in an autosomal dominant manner. About 1 in 5000 to 10,000 children are affected with the syndrome, which manifests with several conditions of connective tissue (Kumar & Agarwal, 2014; Rosenbush & Parker, 2014). The most common problems are cardiac (mitral valve prolapse, aortic regurgitation, abnormal aortic root dimensions), skeletal (pectus excavatum, long arms and digits, scoliosis, elongated head, high arched palate), ocular (lens subluxation), and respiratory (pneumothorax). The woman with Marfan syndrome has an increased risk of complications during pregnancy, primarily related to the extra requirements placed on the heart. The average age for diagnosis is 3 years, with a heart murmur as the usual finding. Careful assessment identifies additional characteristics of the condition along with a positive family history.

Diagnosis is made after a complete family history, a detailed physical examination, an eye examination, a thorough heart examination, radiographs of the chest, and MRI or CT.

There is no treatment for the syndrome, which causes abnormal formation of fibrillin matrix in connective tissue. However, early diagnosis can be successful in treating the cardiac abnormalities with medication or surgery to prevent dissection of the aorta, the major cause of death. Diagnosis in children is often difficult because many features of Marfan syndrome are not apparent until adolescence. Surgery may be needed to correct scoliosis, pectus excavatum, or pneumothorax. Careful monitoring throughout life is needed to prevent and treat abnormalities associated with the disorder.

Nursing Management

Nursing management of Marfan syndrome begins with identification of infants and children with symptoms of the disorder. Once diagnosed, collaboration with a cardiologist, ophthalmologist, and orthopedist is needed throughout the child's life. The child may require surgery for one or more conditions, can require antibiotics during elective procedures or dental care if the mitral valve is affected, and needs echocardiogram and other cardiac studies regularly. The nurse may need to explain the disorder to the family and provide referrals for genetic counseling. Case management for the numerous medical specialists will be advantageous. The child needs support during childhood to learn about the disorder and to manage the medication and monitoring required.

Osteogenesis Imperfecta

Osteogenesis imperfecta (OI), also known as *brittle bone disease*, is a connective tissue disorder that primarily affects the bones. Children with this condition have fragile bones that are more likely to fracture. Osteogenesis imperfecta occurs in 1 in 10,000 to 15,000 live births and affects boys and girls equally (van Dijk et al., 2011).

The underlying disorder is a biochemical defect in the production of collagen. The disease is genetically transmitted, generally in an autosomal dominant inheritance pattern, although some types are transmitted in a recessive pattern. The most common types are caused by mutations on the *COL1A 1* or *COL1A 2* genes on chromosomes 17 and 7, respectively (van Dijk et al., 2011).

Clinical manifestations include multiple and frequent fractures; blue sclerae; thin, soft skin; altered joint flexibility; short stature; enlargement of the anterior fontanelle; weak muscles; soft, pliable, brittle bones; and short stature. Conductive hearing loss can occur by adolescence or young adulthood.

The disease is classified into four main types. In type I disease, the most common form, children have fragile bones, blue sclerae, weakened tooth dentin, and possible hearing loss that manifests in adolescence. In type II disease, the ribs and skeleton are extensively involved; most children with this form of the disease die in utero or shortly after birth. Type III disease is identified in the newborn period or in infancy when the child sustains numerous fractures and manifests blue sclerae. Severe

---

Clinical Reasoning **Autosomal Dominant Disorders**

Both achondroplasia and Marfan syndrome are autosomal dominant disorders. Does this mean that the child needs one or two genes to manifest the disorders? If one parent has the disorder, what is the chance that a pregnancy will result in an affected child? Will there ever be a carrier who does not manifest the disease? See Chapter 3 for further information about autosomal dominant inheritance.

bone fragility and kyphoscoliosis are observed. Type IV disease is characterized by fractures without other symptoms of the disease. Bowing of the legs and other structural deformities can occur; however, the incidence of fractures decreases beginning in puberty. Recent genetic research has identified up to 11 different genetic mutations leading to various types of OI (Ben Amor, Rauch, Monti, et al., 2013; Womack, 2014).

Improved knowledge about the genetic transmission of this disease means that some cases of OI can be identified before birth using ultrasound or collagen analysis of chorionic villus cells or genetic testing. In many cases, however, diagnosis of OI is made only when the child has a delay in walking or sustains a fracture. Radiographic evaluation may detect old as well as new fractures. This may lead to an erroneous diagnosis of child abuse. Tests such as DEXA can be used to measure bone density. Serum alkaline phosphatase may be elevated; other measures of bone metabolism such as serum osteocalcin, procollagen 1 C-terminal peptide, collagen 1 teleopeptide, and urine deoxypyridinoline studies may be performed occasionally to measure effects of medication.

There is no cure for OI. Medical management consists primarily of fracture care and prevention of deformities. The goal is to maximize the child's independence and mobility while minimizing the risk of fractures. Treatment includes physical therapy; casting, bracing, or splinting; surgical stabilization; nutritional management with high vitamin D and calcium; and bisphosphonate medication such as pamidronate. Health supervision that includes dental examinations and hearing screening is important. Hematologic stem cell transplant has been used successfully in some children with severe OI and is under further research.

Nursing Management

Nursing care is primarily supportive and focuses on educating the parents and child about the disease and its treatment. The family may have been suspected of child abuse before the disease was diagnosed; explain the similar presenting symptoms of these cases. Ask about favorite activities of the child since these will need to be integrated into plans for physical activity and developmental progression. Perform careful growth measurements and developmental screening; ensure health promotion visits include dental and hearing screening.

To prevent fractures, children with osteogenesis imperfecta must be handled gently. Support the trunk and extremities using a blanket whenever moving the child. Tasks such as bathing and diapering may cause fractures and should be performed carefully. Never pull the legs upward during diaper changes, but slip a hand gently under the hips to raise them.

Children commonly have several fractures during childhood. The period of immobility and casting causes further bone breakdown due to decreased weight bearing, further increasing the chance of fracture. Children should have a well-balanced diet with additional vitamin C, vitamin D, and calcium to encourage healing and bone growth. Calories should be limited to maintain weight at recommended levels since immobility can lead to overweight and these children are generally short for their age. Partner with parents if the child is receiving experimental bisphosphonate medication so that doses are properly administered and serum/urine samples are obtained for monitoring.

When the child needs a fracture stabilized in surgery, or is having rods inserted to strengthen bones, surgical care management is important. Assess the child's vital signs and growth measurements. Obtain accurate weight before surgery and again after with the cast in place. Administer fluids and use pain-control techniques such as medication and other comfort measures. Be alert for signs of infection such as osteomyelitis, or respiratory or urinary tract infection. Begin fluids and perform dietary teaching before discharge to promote intake that fosters healing. Follow activity orders precisely to minimize safety hazards for the child. Partner with physical and occupational therapists to plan for the child's return to home and school, and to ensure the family can perform ROM exercises and other therapies. Ensure that the family has an approved car safety seat to transport the child.

Emphasize the importance of maintaining normal patterns of growth and development. Help toddlers explore and interact safely in their environment. Socialization is essential during the school-age and adolescent years. Encourage exercise, such as swimming, to improve muscle tone and prevent obesity. Adaptive equipment and motorized wheelchairs promote independent functioning. Maintenance of function can depend on proper rehabilitation services. Arrange and manage such services for the family.

The Osteogenesis Imperfecta Foundation provides information about the disease and can put families in touch with others who have the disease. Parents should receive genetic counseling. For parents who have a child with type II or III osteogenesis imperfecta, the terminal nature of the condition necessitates psychologic support, links to potential resources, and assistance with managing other tasks of family life. (See Chapter 41 for management of end-of-life care.) The siblings and extended family will need support to understand the disease and deal with their feelings and the affected child.

Expected outcomes include minimal fractures with optimal healing, normal range of motion, maintenance of a healthy diet and recommended weight, achievement of developmental milestones, family support, and adequate resources to provide necessary treatments for the child.

Muscular Dystrophies

The muscular dystrophies are a group of inherited diseases characterized by muscle fiber degeneration and muscle wasting. These disorders can begin early or late in life, and onset can be at birth or gradual. They are all terminal disorders, but the progression can vary from a few to many years.

Many types of muscular dystrophies affect children and adults. The most common form of childhood muscular dystrophy is Duchenne muscular dystrophy (pseudohypertrophic), which occurs in 1 per 3500 live male births (Theadom et al., 2014). **Pseudohypertrophy** refers to enlargement of the muscles as a result of their infiltration with fatty tissue. The gene for Duchenne muscular dystrophy was identified in 1987; it is carried in the Xp21.2 region of the chromosome and is either absent or deleted in affected children. This area codes for a protein called *dystrophin*, which is needed as a muscle membrane stabilizer. In the absence of dystrophin, a cascade of cellular events occurs, leading to necrosis in the fibers and their replacement by connective tissue. Since this is an X-linked disorder, it is seen only in males. There is similar incidence in various ethnic groups.

Becker muscular dystrophy is also X-linked and affects 1 in 30,000 boys (Becker Muscular Dystrophy, n.d.). Although the gene mutation is similar to Duchenne, it is milder in form. Other rare muscular dystrophies manifest in infancy, later childhood, or adolescence. There are a variety of genetic mutations ranging from X linked to autosomal.

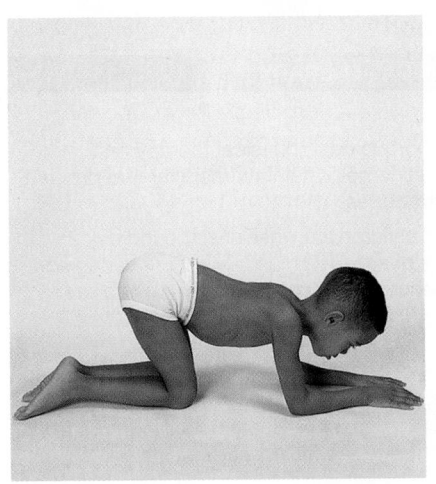

A

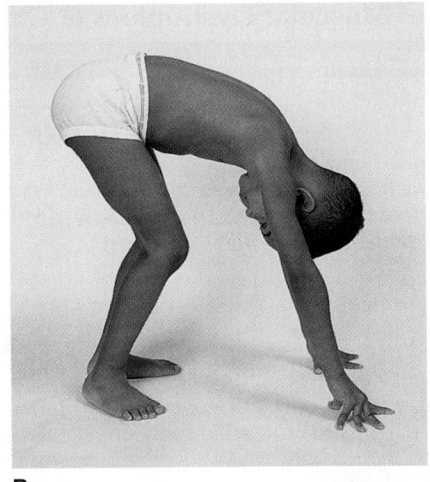

B

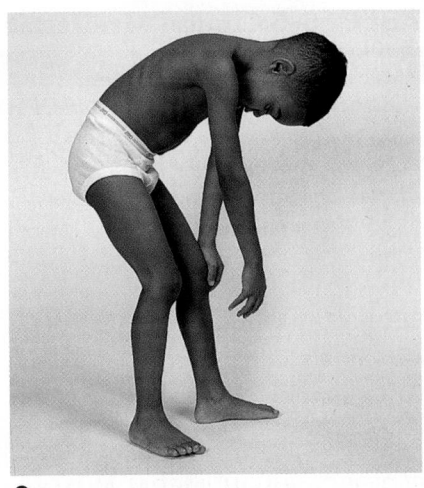

C

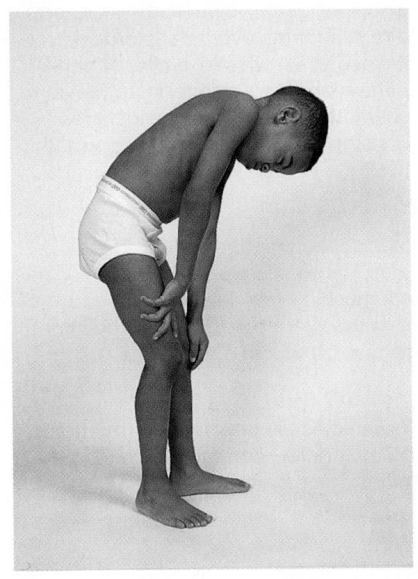

D

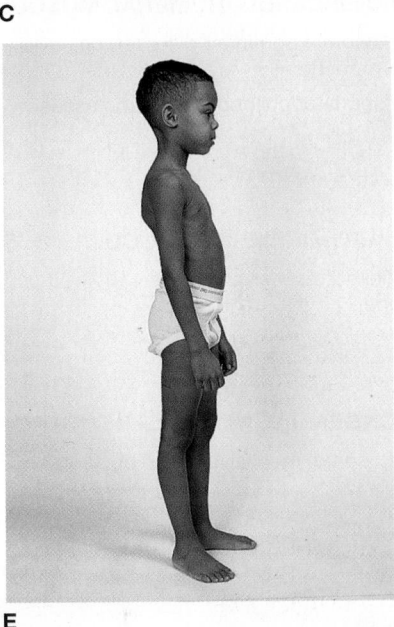

E

Figure 56–12 Gowers maneuver. Since the leg muscles of children with muscular dystrophy are weak, these children must perform the Gowers maneuver to raise themselves to a standing position. *A* and *B*, The child first maneuvers to a position supported by arms and legs. *C*, The child next pushes off the floor and rests one hand on the knee. *D* and *E*, The child then pushes himself upright.

Children with muscular dystrophy have generalized muscle weakness. They compensate for weak lower extremities by using the upper extremity muscles to raise themselves to a standing position (Gowers maneuver) (Figure 56–12). (See Table 56–5.)

Diagnosis and classification are most often based on clinical signs and the pattern of muscle involvement. Biochemical examinations such as serum enzyme assay, muscle biopsy, and electromyography confirm the diagnosis. Serum creatine kinase (CK) is elevated early in the disease. Muscle biopsy can measure dystrophin, the muscle protein that is deficient in muscular dystrophy. Genetic testing establishes the specific abnormality and type of disease present. Testing of newborns may be offered to families who have one child with the disease since this helps some families to adapt and prepare for the care the child will need. Respiratory function is measured periodically with pulmonary function tests and overnight pulse oximetry.

There is no effective treatment for childhood muscular dystrophy. Research is being directed at several techniques to repair mutations by gene therapy, override the genetic error in order to produce dystrophin, and apply stem cell therapy (Goyenvaile, Seto, Davies, et al., 2011). The steroids prednisone and deflazacort may preserve muscle function, preserving walking for a longer period. Rehabilitative therapy is needed to maximize independence and physical activity and to decrease hazards of immobility. Children and families can benefit from mental health support to help them in adapting to the progressive and terminal nature of the disease. A common complementary care used for muscular dystrophy is dietary enhancement. This enhancement includes giving vitamins A, C, E, D, and B-complex; minerals such as calcium, magnesium, zinc, and selenium; probiotic supplement; omega-3 fatty acids; herbal remedies such as green and rhodiola rosea teas; muscular and immunologic enzymes such as coenzyme Q10, N-acetyl cysteine, acetyl-L-carnitine, creatine, L-theanine; and melatonin to promote sleep. Massage is often used to assist with reduction of muscle spasms (University of Maryland Medical Center, 2011).

Progressive weakness and muscle deformity result in chronic disability (Figure 56–13). Respiratory infections are vigorously treated with deep breathing, coughing, nebulizer treatments, and antibiotics. Comprehensive and regular cardiac evaluations are recommended. The team approach to managing the child with muscular dystrophy ensures a comprehensive management plan. Team members should include physicians (pediatrician, orthopedic surgeon, neurologist), nurses, physical and occupational therapists, a nutritionist, psychologist or mental health therapist, and a social worker.

TABLE 56–5 Clinical Manifestations of Muscular Dystrophies of Childhood

TYPE OF DYSTROPHY	CLINICAL MANIFESTATIONS	CLINICAL THERAPY
DUCHENNE MUSCULAR DYSTROPHY		
X-linked recessive disorder seen in boys (on *Xp21* gene); however, 30%–50% of affected children have no family history *Onset:* within the first 3–4 years of life	Delayed walking; frequent falls; easily tired when walking, running, or climbing stairs; toe walking, hypertrophied calves; waddling gait; lordosis; positive Gowers maneuver; intellectual disability frequently seen	Supportive care; physical therapy and braces to help maintain mobility and prevent contractures Most children are wheelchair bound by 12 years of age; death usually occurs during adolescence from respiratory or cardiac failure
BECKER MUSCULAR DYSTROPHY		
X-linked recessive disorder *Onset:* usually after 5 years	Symptoms are similar to those of Duchenne muscular dystrophy, but milder and delayed; child is mobile until late teens; normal intelligence; congestive heart failure; contractures	Supportive care, same as for Duchenne muscular dystrophy Slow progression; death usually occurs from the third to the fifth decade of life
FACIOSCAPULOHUMERAL MUSCULAR DYSTROPHY		
Autosomal dominant disorder (on 4q35 chromosome) *Onset:* later childhood and adolescence	Face, shoulder girdle, lower limbs affected; unable to raise arms over head; lordosis; cannot close eyes, whistle, smile, or drink from a straw because of inability to move face; characteristic appearance includes facial weakness, winging of the scapula, thin arms, well-developed forearms	Physical therapy Slow progression; confined to wheelchair as older adult, but usually attains normal life span
EMERY-DREIFUSS MUSCULAR DYSTROPHY		
X-linked recessive disorder (on *Xq28* gene) *Onset:* childhood	Early onset of contractures followed by weakness; Achilles tendon, elbow, and spine affected; muscle weakness in upper body follows, with lower body weakness occurring later; cardiac conduction defect may occur	Physical therapy Surgery Pacemaker insertion
CONGENITAL MUSCULAR DYSTROPHIES		
Autosomal recessive group of disorders *Onset:* present at birth	Muscle weaknesses present at birth; motor development delay; contractures and joint deformities; hypotonia	Correction of skeletal deformity (orthosis or surgery) Usually nonprogressive

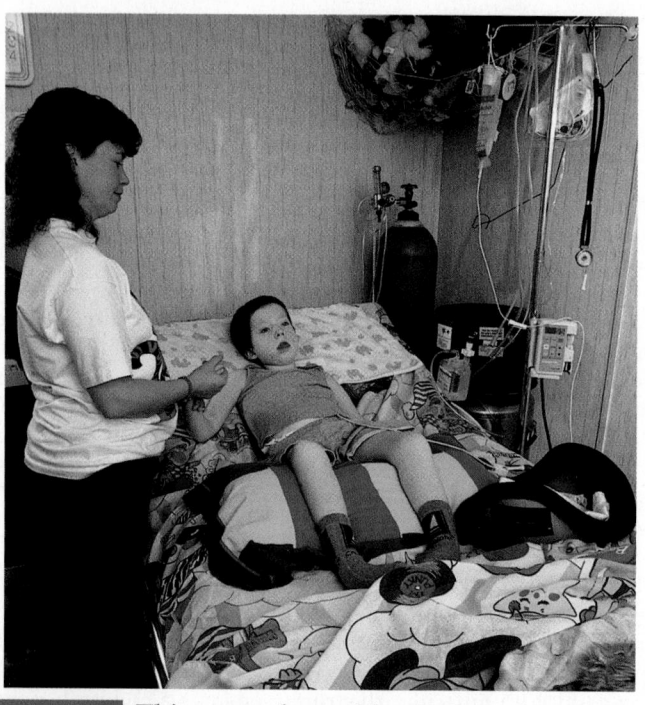

Figure 56–13 This young boy with muscular dystrophy needs to receive tube feedings and home nursing care. He attends school when possible and is able to use an adapted computer.

Nursing Management

Nursing care focuses on promoting independence and mobility and providing psychosocial support that helps the child and family deal with this progressive, incapacitating disease. Nearly all body systems become involved in the disease, and emotional care is important as well for child and family.

Monitor cardiac and respiratory functioning frequently. Assess urinary function and frequency of bowel movements. Periodically measure strength and range of motion. Assess mobility via ambulation or assisted device. Perform periodic developmental and nutritional assessments. Meet with teachers to evaluate the child's learning needs and functional level in the classroom. Evaluate the family's risk and protective factors for managing this chronic and fatal disorder.

Administer oxygen or respiratory therapy as ordered. Encourage the child to be independent for as long as possible. Concentrate on what the child can accomplish, and do not ask the child to complete tasks that may prove frustrating. Encourage parents to establish an individualized education plan with the school system. Reading books to the child, listening to tapes, and watching television offer the child stimulation during hospitalization. Exercise as tolerated contributes to muscle strength. Physical therapy helps the child ambulate and prevents joint contractures. It is important to provide back support and recommended posture by keeping the child's body in alignment when confined to a wheelchair. Provide information about complementary care that the family chooses to use.

Health Promotion The Child With Muscular Dystrophy

The child with muscular dystrophy needs close monitoring and intervention to foster growth and development in spite of a chronic and terminal disease. The nurse in health promotion can assist the child and family in many ways.

Growth and Development Surveillance

- Perform developmental screening of the young child.
- Refer to early intervention programs that establish educational plans to foster development.
- Provide resources and ideas for the parents based on the child's status rather than expected age norms. Plan interventions to maximize the highest level of function possible.
- Measure growth at each healthcare visit and plot on growth grids. Be alert for the child who is gaining weight related to decreased activity.
- Ensure visits with specialists in respiratory medicine and cardiology as recommended.

Nutrition

- Perform 24-hour analysis and evaluate for all essential nutrients. Base the analysis on the child's height and weight rather than chronologic age.
- Ask about appetite and food likes and dislikes.
- Encourage adequate fluid, whole grains, fruits, and vegetables to maintain bowel function.
- For the infant with muscular dystrophy, evaluate intake carefully; gavage feeding or nutritional supplementation such as with high-calorie formula may be needed.

Physical Activity

- Carefully monitor physical ability at each visit. Observe for decreases in movement, difficulty ambulating, or a history of falls.
- Partner with physical therapists to ensure range of motion and proper positioning of extremities.
- Explore activities that the child can do as mobility decreases. Swimming and upper body exercise may be good options.
- If the child is using a wheelchair, evaluate fit, safety, and ability to move the chair by arm controls.
- Physical activity should be regular and daily. Ensure that the family has resources to accomplish this need.

Activities of Daily Living

- Partner with occupational therapy to evaluate the child's ability to feed, bathe, dress, and provide own oral care. Provide adaptive devices as needed.
- Encourage the family to provide time for the child to perform own self-care as much as possible.
- Make a home visit or discuss with the family adaptations that could make it easier for the child to be independent in activities of daily living. Low drawers for clothing or open shelves that do not require pulling out to get items are examples of important adaptations.

Mental and Spiritual Health

- Inquire about the child's general mood.

- Ask the parents what is best and worst about their lives at this time. Use the information to establish a list of their meaningful activities and to identify the areas most in need of support.
- Ask about sources of support such as a group for parents of a child with muscular dystrophy, family participation in faith-based activity, and extended family or neighbors.

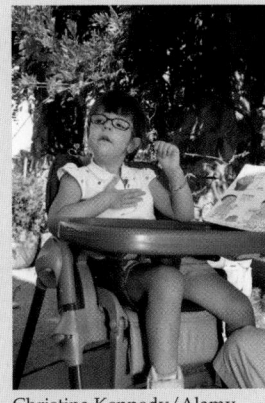
Christina Kennedy/Alamy

- Be alert for signs of depression in child or family (see Chapter 55).
- Assist the family to establish activities to increase self-esteem in the youth. The youth should be able to make choices appropriate for developmental age.
- If the child was diagnosed at a younger age, ask what the parents have now told the child about the disease. Provide support and role-playing opportunities for parents who wish to tell the child about the terminal nature of the disorder.
- Refer for services such as genetic counseling, grief counseling, or other supportive interventions.

Relationships

- Ask about siblings and their relationship with the child with muscular dystrophy.
- Inquire about the child's participation in early intervention or school programs, and community groups. Refer the family to resources that encourage the child's interactions with peers. This is particularly important for teens.
- Ask the parents if and how often they are able to spend time with other adults.

Disease Prevention Strategies

- Immunize the child at recommended times. If the child is ill and immunization is delayed, be sure to call the family back promptly to reschedule administration of vaccines so that infectious diseases can be avoided. Annual influenza vaccine is needed. If the child is treated with steroids for the disease, follow recommendations for immunization of children on steroids.
- Teach the family to avoid crowds and known infectious persons. The child may need to be out of school for a few days or weeks if there is an influenza or other disease outbreak in the school population.
- Teach the family signs of infection, especially of the respiratory tract. Have them report these symptoms promptly.
- Monitor effects of antibiotics when administered for infection.
- Encourage daily activities that encourage deep breathing. Swimming, blowing into an incentive spirometer, or playing with a pinwheel are examples.

(continued)

Injury Prevention Strategies

- Inquire about whether the family has an emergency evacuation plan for the child in case of house fire or other emergency. Assist them to develop a plan.

- If the child is using oxygen, teach about fire safety.

- When mechanical ventilation is used at home, help the family establish emergency backup systems for power outage, such as portable generators.

- Assist the family to learn proper body mechanics to safely transfer and provide care for the child.

Parents may feel guilty and hopeless. Encourage parents to express their feelings. Genetic counseling is recommended for the entire family, and it is especially important to identify female relatives who are carriers of one of the X-linked disorders. Siblings may feel neglected because their brother or sister is receiving so much attention. They may be concerned that they will develop the disease, and in some families, this indeed occurs. Encourage the parents to spend individual time with each child and to involve siblings in the child's care.

Refer family members to resource and support groups such as the Muscular Dystrophy Association. Provide ongoing support during hospitalizations, management of home care, and the child's changes in condition.

Injuries to the Musculoskeletal System

Musculoskeletal injuries are classified according to the mechanism, the location, and the force of the injury. Strains, sprains, dislocations, and fractures are the most common

musculoskeletal injuries in children; athletic participation and injuries from car crashes are frequent causes. Distinguishing among these injuries is often difficult. See Table 56–6. See accompanying *Evidence-Based Practice* for a discussion of backpack use by children. A detailed discussion of fractures follows.

Fractures

A fracture is a break in a bone that occurs when more stress is placed on the bone than the bone can withstand. Fractures may occur at any age; they are frequent in children because their bones are less dense and more porous than those of adults (see *Pathophysiology Illustrated: Classification and Types of Fractures*).

ETIOLOGY AND PATHOPHYSIOLOGY

Fractures in children may result from direct trauma to a bone (falls, sports injuries, abuse, motor vehicle crashes) or bone diseases that result in weakening of the bone (osteogenesis imperfecta). Children with osteoporosis or osteopenia are more prone to fractures (see description of these conditions earlier in the chapter). Trauma may be caused by an acute injury, by direct

TABLE 56–6 Clinical Manifestations of Strains, Sprains, and Dislocations

CONDITION	CLINICAL MANIFESTATIONS	CLINICAL THERAPY
STRAIN		
• Stretching or tearing of either a muscle or a tendon, usually from overuse (example: back strain resulting from improper or overly heavy lifting).	• Vary according to the type and severity of the strain. Pain can be acute or chronic.	• Rest and support of the injured part until the muscle or tendon heals and normal activity can occur.
SPRAIN		
• Stretching or tearing of a ligament, usually caused by falls, sports injuries, or motor vehicle crashes. For example, an anterior cruciate ligament (ACL) tear is a severe sprain requiring reconstruction.	• Edema, joint immobility, and pain.	• For the first 24–36 hr: Rest Ice Compression Elevation • After the first 24–36 hr, mobility is gradually increased.
DISLOCATION		
• Complete displacement of an articular joint surface, usually associated with falls, sports injuries, or motor vehicle crashes. Although almost any joint may be dislocated, most dislocations occur in the shoulder, knee, and hip.	• Pain and tenderness, swelling and obvious deformity, and instability of the joint.	• Varies according to the site and severity of the injury, and consists of: Shoulder: open or closed reduction followed by the application of a sling Knee: closed reduction with gentle traction, then immobilization with a splint Hip (posterior): immediate closed reduction or possibly open reduction, traction, or hip spica cast Hip (anterior): immediate closed reduction, extension traction, and hip spica cast

EVIDENCE-BASED PRACTICE | Do Heavy Backpacks Cause Back Pain?

Clinical Question
Many children wear backpacks that are heavy and are carried for large parts of the day. Low back, neck, and shoulder pain are prevalent in children, and a possible connection with backpacks has been suggested (Dockrell, Simms, & Blake, 2013). What can nurses do to reduce risk of back pain related to backpacks in children?

The Evidence
Several studies have investigated the relationships between backpack use and complaints of pain. Carrying a backpack over one shoulder, having heavier backpacks, and carrying the pack lower rather than higher were associated with greater back and shoulder pressure. Postural angle and lumbar curvature are altered by heavy backpacks. Children carrying backpacks that exceeded 10% of their body weight had a 50% increased chance of back pain, and girls more commonly experienced back pain (Rodriguez-Oviedo et al., 2012). Design, fit, and weight all may play a part in discomfort related to backpacks (Amiri, Dezfooli, & Mortezaei, 2012).

Best Practice
An association between backpack use and weight and complaints of pain appears to be evident, especially among girls.

Therefore, nurses should ask about backpack use at health promotion visits and advise on how to wear them. Encourage children to store backpacks in lockers when available throughout the day in order to decrease wearing time. The American Academy of Pediatrics and North American Spine Society list recommendations for backpack use:

- Have wide, padded shoulder straps and wear the pack on both shoulders, close to the body.
- Use a padded back and waist strap.
- Be sure the backpack is lightweight (no more than 10% to 15% of the youth's weight) or consider a rolling pack if it is heavy.
- Practice back strengthening exercises and learn to bend at the knees when lifting objects.

Clinical Reasoning
How will you partner with youth who are in sports after school to plan how to carry school items and sports gear safely? What exercises can you plan to help strengthen the back and thighs for carrying a pack? Which children are most at risk for back pain from heavy backpacks (consider gender and weight)?

Pathophysiology Illustrated: **Classification and Types of Fractures**

Classification

Complete (transverse) fracture

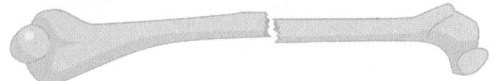

Break across entire section of a bone at a right angle to the bone shaft resulting in two or more fragments

Open fracture

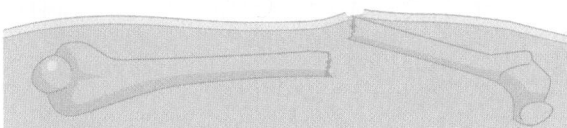

Broken bone protrudes through the skin leaving a path to the fracture site; high risk of infection exists

Greenstick fracture

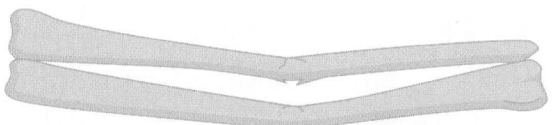

Caused by compression force; often seen in young children

Type

Spiral fracture

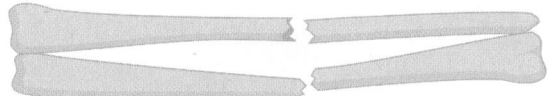

Associated with twisting force; fracture coils around the bone

Closed fracture

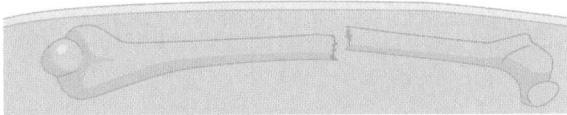

Broken bone does not protrude through the skin

Comminuted fracture

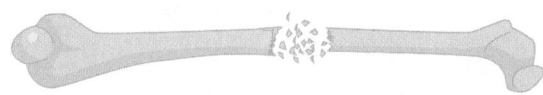

Associated with high-impact forces; bone breaks into three or more segments

Additional types of fractures include incomplete, in which the break occurs in only one side of the cortex; oblique, in which the fracture slants across the long axis of the bone; compression, in which two bones are jammed together (usually occurs in spinal area); and compacted, in which one bone fragment is wedged into another.

and forceful impact, or by overuse such as in chronic and repetitive activities. Child abuse is a cause of fracture and should be suspected when the type of fracture is uncommon for a given age (see Chapter 42).

CLINICAL MANIFESTATIONS

Signs and symptoms of fractures vary depending on the location, type, and nature of the causative injury. Fractures are generally characterized by pain, abnormal positioning, edema, immobility or decreased range of motion, ecchymosis, guarding, and crepitus. Childhood fractures most often involve the clavicle, tibia, ulna, and femur, with distal forearm fractures the most common type. Stress fractures are most common in the tibia, fibula, metatarsals, and calcaneus, while regular exercise can encourage bone development and be protective against fractures (Farr, Laddu, & Going, 2014; Harrington, Sochett, & Howard, 2014). Douglass, described in the chapter-opening vignette, had a fracture of his tibia. Fractures to the pelvis are often associated with motor vehicle crashes. Epiphyseal injuries are dangerous in children as they can interfere with bone growth at the site. These injuries are described using the Salter-Harris classification system (Figure 56–14).

CLINICAL THERAPY

Emergency care focuses on accurate diagnosis, pain management, and establishment of a treatment plan. Radiographs are useful for determining the exact location and type of the fracture. Medical management consists of two basic steps: (1) reduction to realign displaced or fragmented bones, and (2) immobilization so that healing can take place.

A closed reduction aligns the bone by manual manipulation or traction. Sedation and additional pain management techniques will be used during closed reduction. An open reduction requires surgical alignment of the bone, often using pins, plates, wires, or screws. For open fractures, surgery must also be performed for debridement, to remove dead tissue and clean the wound. Casting is the most common external method of immobilization. Casts may be placed on extremities (short or long leg or arm cast), the upper body to immobilize the spine, or from chest to legs to stabilize pelvis or hips (spica cast). Leg casts may be walking or nonwalking casts. Cast material is either plaster or a synthetic fabric. Other external methods of stabilization include traction and splinting (see Table 56–9 for types of traction). Pins may be inserted to stabilize the fracture, and can be used with or without casts or traction. A child with multiple fractures following a car crash or other trauma may need a combination of treatments.

Growth and Development

Stress fractures are becoming more common in adolescents and are most common in those who limit their intake of calories and calcium in an attempt to remain lean for sports such as distance running, cheerleading, or gymnastics (Field, Gordon, Pierce, et al., 2011). These fractures may present with chronic pain that changes in intensity. Be alert to this possibility when teenagers' diets and athletic activities place them at risk. The risk of bone fractures is increased with high cola consumption and television viewing time and with lower levels of physical activity and lower milk intake. Teach healthy diet and activity patterns to youth and their families to decrease these health risks.

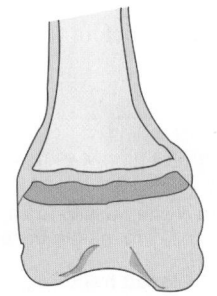

Type I
Common
Growth plate undisturbed
Growth disturbances rare

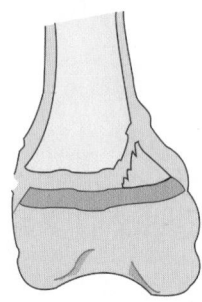

Type II
Most common
Growth disturbances rare

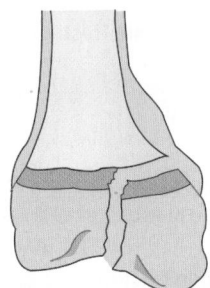

Type III
Less common
Serious threat to growth
    and joint

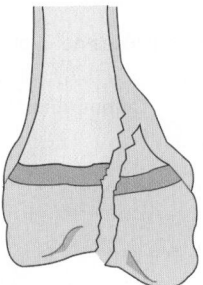

Type IV
Serious threat to growth

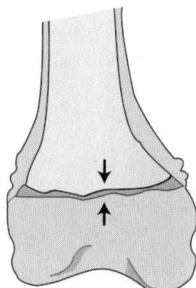

Type V
Rare
Crush injury causes cell death in growth plate,
    resulting in arrested growth and limited
    bone length
If growth plate is partially destroyed, angular
    deformities may result

Figure 56–14 The Salter-Harris classification system is based on the angle of the fracture in relation to the epiphysis.

TABLE 56–7 Complications of Fracture Reduction

COMPLICATION	CLINICAL THERAPY
Infection Acute (may occur with open fractures) Chronic (osteomyelitis)	Debridement, drainage, culture, and treatment with antibiotics
Neurovascular injury resulting from physical nerve damage	Nerve repair
Vascular injury	Vascular repair, amputation, tendon lengthening
Malunion (undesired healed alignment of bone) or delayed union	Corrective osteotomy; prolonged immobilization
Nonunion	Surgical intervention; internal fixation
Leg length discrepancy	Shoe lift

Immobilization is essential for the bone-healing process. Healing of fractures is influenced by factors including age, size of the involved bone, and fracture site. Fractures heal more quickly in children than in adults because the periosteum or vascular outer layer of bone is thicker and remains intact even during a fracture (AAOS, 2014b). If a fracture is properly reduced, complications should be minimal (Table 56–7). Fractures involving the epiphyseal growth plate must be treated properly to minimize the chance for limb length discrepancy, joint incongruity, and angular deformities.

Nursing Management

For the Child With a Fracture

Nursing Assessment and Diagnosis

When assessing an injured child, be alert to the signs and symptoms of fractures before moving the child. When in doubt about the type of injury, apply a splint to immobilize the joints above and below the injury. Try to identify the cause of the injury by asking the child, parents, or other family members what happened. Evaluate pain, edema, and any abnormal positioning of the injured area. When a child is admitted to the emergency department or hospital, nursing assessment includes the extent of the injury, the degree of pain, and the child's vital signs (respiratory status, pulse, and blood pressure). Monitor all systems since infection, fat emboli, and other problems can emerge during the treatment period.

Several nursing diagnoses may apply to the child with a fracture. They include the following (NANDA-I © 2014):

- *Pain* related to injury
- *Skin Integrity, Risk for Impaired,* related to treatment
- *Infection, Risk for,* related to open fracture or trauma
- *Mobility: Physical, Impaired,* related to treatment
- *Health Behavior, Risk-Prone,* related to peer group influence and chosen activities

Planning and Implementation

Nurses may be in community settings when children experience a fracture and may need to provide emergency care and arrange for transport. Inform emergency personnel of the assessment data to provide for safe care. In addition, be aware that repeated fractures in the same child can be a sign of other healthcare conditions. Young children may have osteogenesis imperfecta, an older child may be experimenting with risky behavior, and child abuse may have occurred if there are several fractures in various states of healing or if the parental explanation does not match the clinical presentation. Nursing care focuses on care of the child before and after fracture reduction, encouraging mobility as ordered, maintaining skin integrity, preventing infection, and teaching the parents and child how to care for the fracture. If sedation or pain blocks are used, nursing care for these procedures is needed. See the *Clinical Skills Manual* SKILLS.

When caring for a child who has undergone fracture reduction, it is important to know the signs of complications and follow protocols for assessment. Notify the physician immediately if these signs occur. The major serious complication is **compartment syndrome**, or a condition of increased pressure in a limited space such as the soft tissue of an extremity, which compromises circulation and nervous innervation (Schaffzin et al., 2013). (See Table 56–8.)

MAINTAIN PROPER ALIGNMENT

Immobilization maintains proper alignment of the fracture. Casts and traction are methods used for immobilizing an injured child. Cast care guidelines are included in Table 56–1, earlier in this chapter.

Different types of traction are used, depending on the location and type of fracture (Table 56–9). Nursing care for the child in traction is described in Table 56–10.

MONITOR NEUROVASCULAR STATUS

Neurovascular assessment is used for early detection of compartment syndrome. Compartment syndrome may occur with a crush injury or when a fracture is reduced. The swelling of inflammation reduces blood flow to the affected area, and

TABLE 56–8 Clinical Manifestations of Compartment Syndrome

Clinical manifestations begin about 30 min after tissue ischemia starts. Major manifestations include the following:

- Paresthesia (tingling, burning, loss of 2-point discrimination)
- Pain (unrelieved by medication, characterized by crying in the young child)
- Pressure (skin is tense, cast appears tight)
- Pallor (pale, gray or white skin tone)
- Paralysis (weakness or inability to move extremity)
- Pulselessness (weak or absent pulse)
- Poikilothermia (skin temperature assumes that of the environment)

Check extremities for:

• Color	• Edema
• Temperature	• Sensation
• Capillary refill	• Motor ability
• Peripheral pulses	• Pain

Document results and report changes or abnormal results immediately. Changes are a medical emergency.

Source: Data from Tschudy, M. M., & Arcara, K. M. (Eds.). (2012). *The Harriet Lane handbook.* Philadelphia: Mosby Elsevier; Schaffzin, J. K., Prichard, H., Bisig, J., Gainor, P., Wolfe, K., Solan, L. G., ... McCarthy, J. J. (2013). A collaborative system to improve compartment syndrome recognition. *Pediatrics, 132,* e1672–e1679; Wright, E. (2009). Neurovascular impairment and compartment syndrome. *Paediatric Nursing, 21*(3), 26–29.

TABLE 56–9 Types of Traction

SKIN TRACTION

Pull is applied to the skin surface, which puts traction directly on the bones and muscles. Traction is attached to the skin with adhesive materials or straps, or foam boots, belts, or halters.

DUNLOP TRACTION (CAN BE EITHER SKELETAL OR SKIN)

Used for fracture of the humerus. The flexed arm is suspended horizontally with straps placed on both the upper and lower portions for pull from both sides.

SKELETAL TRACTION

Pull is directly applied to the bone by pins, wires, tongs, or other apparatus that have been surgically placed through the distal end of the bone.

SKELETAL CERVICAL TRACTION

Used for cervical spine injuries to reduce fractures and dislocations. Crutchfield, Gardner-Wells, or Vinke tongs are placed in the skull with bur holes. Weights are attached to the apparatus with a rope and pulley system to the hyperextended head.

HALO TRACTION

Used to immobilize the head and neck after cervical injury or dislocation. Also used for positioning and immobilization after cervical injury.

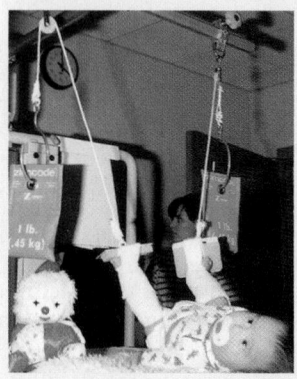

A

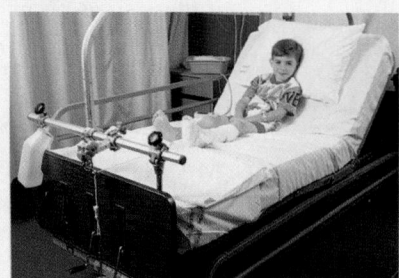

B

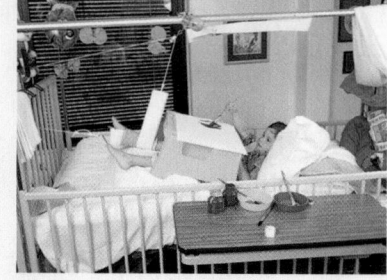

C

BRYANT TRACTION (A)

Used specifically for the child under 3 years of age and weighing less than 35.0 lb (17.5 kg) who has developmental dysplasia of the hip or a fractured femur. This bilateral traction is applied to the child's legs and kept in place by wrapping the legs from foot to thigh with elastic bandages. The hips are flexed at a 90-degree angle, with knees extended. This position is maintained by attaching the traction appliance to weights and pulleys suspended above the crib. The buttocks do not rest on the mattress, but are slightly elevated off the bed.

BUCK TRACTION (B)

Used for knee immobilization; to correct contractures or deformities; or for short-term immobilization of a fracture. It keeps the leg in an extended position, without hip flexion. Traction is applied to the extremity in one direction (straight line) with a single pulley system.

RUSSELL TRACTION (C)

Used for fractures of the femur and lower leg. Traction is placed on the lower leg while the knee is suspended in a padded sling. The slightly flexed hips and knees are immobilized. One force is applied by a double pulley to the foot and another force is applied upward using a sling under the knee and an overhead pulley.

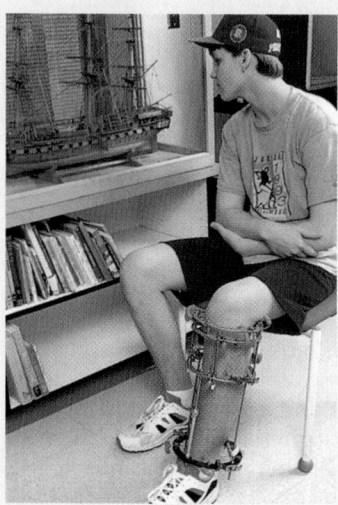

E

EXTERNAL FIXATORS (E)

These devices can be used in the treatment of simple fractures, both open and closed; complex fractures with extensive soft tissue involvement; correction of bony or soft-tissue deformities; pseudoarthroses; and limb length discrepancies. They are attached to the extremity by percutaneous transfixing of pins or wires to the bone. When used to lengthen an extremity, the device can be "distracted" or turned as ordered by the surgeon for a very small amount several times daily. This separates the bone and allows new growth, gradually lengthening the extremity.

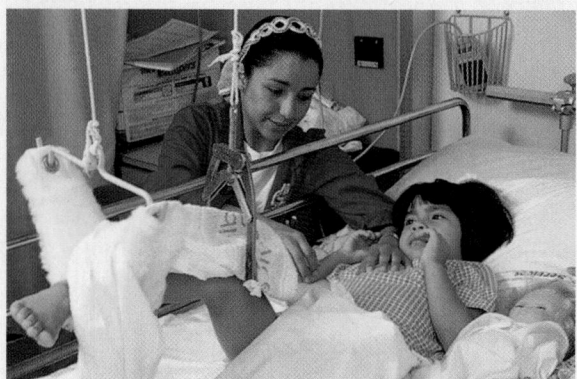

D

90–90 TRACTION (D)

Used for fractures of the femur or tibia. A skeletal pin or wire is surgically placed through the distal part of the femur, while the lower part of the extremity is in a boot cast. Traction ropes and pulleys are applied at the pin site and on the boot cast to maintain the flexion of both the hip and knee at 90 degrees. This traction can also be used for treatment of an upper extremity fracture.

TABLE 56–10 Care of the Child With Traction or External Fixator

1. Assess the child in traction by first checking the equipment. Make sure that the equipment is in the proper position. Observe both the body appliance and the attached weights and pulleys. Make certain that the child's body is in proper alignment.

2. Assess the skin under the straps and pin insertion sites for any signs of redness, edema, or skin breakdown.

3. Assess the extremity by checking neurovascular status frequently (check warmth, color, distal pulses, capillary refill time, movement, sensation).

4. Provide pin care when ordered using sterile technique. Clean the area surrounding the pin with cotton-tipped applicators saturated with normal saline or half-strength hydrogen peroxide. Clean the area again with sterile water or more saline. Apply an antibacterial ointment, if ordered, using another cotton-tipped applicator.

5. When external skin traction is used, perform skin care every 4 hr when the traction device is removed.

6. Place a sheepskin pad under the child's extremity if prescriptions permit.

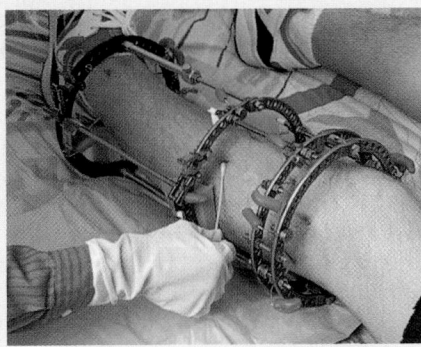

casting causes further constriction of blood flow. Douglass, who was described in the chapter-opening quotation, had a splint applied for several days, with casting later, to allow swelling to decrease and to minimize risk for compartment syndrome. Monitor the child's sensation to touch, temperature, movement, strength of the pulse, and capillary refill time in the extremity distal to the injury. Monitor every 15 minutes after the cast is applied for at least 2 hours and then every 1 to 2 hours, depending on the facility's policy and the child's condition. Keep the cast elevated above heart level to minimize edema. Report symptoms of compartment syndrome immediately as permanent damage to nerves and circulatory system can occur.

PROMOTE MOBILITY

The amount of mobility the child is allowed is ordered by the physician; restrictions depend on the extent and site of the fracture. Fractures of the hip or pelvis may involve body casts; wheeled carts make mobility possible. Children with leg fractures can sometimes bear weight on the cast, but if they cannot, they move around with crutches, walkers, or wheelchairs. See the *Clinical Skills Manual* SKILLS.

DISCHARGE PLANNING AND HOME CARE TEACHING

Most fractures can be easily managed at home. Activities are generally limited for approximately 8 weeks. Teach the parents and child cast care, activity restrictions, and how to identify problems that should be reported (see Table 56–1). Help parents to identify any modifications that may be needed at home and school. The child who has to manage steps at home or school may need special training with crutches or a temporary ramp. Refer parents to home health nurses or home teaching services if indicated. Provide pertinent teaching to prevent future injuries. Reinforce the need for protective gear for many sports (see Chapter 42).

Evaluation

Desired outcomes for treatment of injuries is proper healing of the body parts affected, return to usual strength and range of motion, and no impairment of musculoskeletal development.

Sports Injuries

Sports injuries are the most common type of injury in youth from 13 to 19 years of age. Football, soccer, cycling, and basketball are sports commonly associated with injury, and foot–ankle injuries are most common (Atay, 2014). Fractures, described earlier, are common sports injuries of young athletes, and may be treated on an outpatient basis or may require surgery and hospitalization. Douglass, in the opening scenario, is a good example of a youth with this type of injury. However, a variety of other injuries that affect the musculoskeletal system are common in sports; strains and sprains are examples. Overuse injuries can occur when tendons, muscles, or bones are stressed excessively without adequate rest periods (Luke et al., 2011). Children and adolescents have characteristics that put them at risk for injury. These include:

- Vulnerability of growth plates to injury, especially the distal tibia and fibula
- Increased joint mobility from lax tendons and ligaments, leading to injury of the knee, ankle, and hip
- More porous bones, leading to fractures and to more common injury to underlying organs
- Lack of experience in the sport and inadequate training
- Lack of acceptance of protective gear
- Impatience with taking the time to heal after injury
- Vulnerability to spinal injury related to high-impact sports and recreation such as diving in unsupervised locations

Common sports injuries are listed in Table 56–11. Treatments for sprains, strains, dislocations, and fractures are described in the preceding sections. Head and neck injuries are discussed in Chapter 54 and dental emergencies in Chapter 45. Clear guidelines for concussion injuries have been established (Harmon et al., 2013) and are discussed in Chapter 54. General approaches to minimize and treat injuries for youth athletes follow.

Athletes can benefit from teaching that enhances performance of their sports and also minimizes chance of injury. They should receive instruction in correct techniques from a person qualified to coach and supervise children. Nurses should encourage youths to gradually increase time and intensity at a sport, rather than immediately playing a new sport for long periods of time. Parents should be encouraged to inquire about the coach's experience and also verify that the coaching staff is prepared in emergency care.

The nurse should be alert for sports injuries during contacts with children and adolescents in health promotion visits. The nurse should ask about sports participation for all youths, but especially when there are complaints of sore muscles, edema of body parts, and bruises. Neurovascular assessment

TABLE 56-11 Common Sports Injuries

SPORT	TYPE OF INJURIES
Baseball/basketball	• Hand and finger fractures and sprains • Contusions and sprains of upper or lower extremities; wrists, elbows, knees, and ankles are common sites • Injury to body parts when hit by a ball (e.g., broken teeth, face, head, eye, and chest injuries)
Football	• Head and neck injuries such as skull or cervical vertebrae fracture • Pulled muscles or dislocations in shoulders and legs
Gymnastics	• Wrist and elbow fractures and strains • Tendonitis in elbows and ankles/legs
Hockey (ice and inline)	• Dental injury • Leg fractures • Head and neck injuries
Soccer	• Head and neck injury • Strains and fractures of legs
Wrestling	• Fractures and dislocations of upper and lower extremities

---

Clinical Reasoning The Child Wearing a Cast

Douglass was admitted to the clinic today for application of a short leg cast. He fractured his tibia nearly a week ago when he was on a trampoline with three friends, trying to see who could jump the highest. Douglass slipped and his leg hit the frame on the side. His friends helped him off the trampoline and found someone to transport Douglass to the emergency department. They then reached his mother by phone, who rushed to the hospital when she heard the news.

His mother states that he is now 12 years old and in middle school. He has been going to a friend's house nearly every day after school and spending time on activities such as the trampoline and rollerblading, as well as watching television and playing video games. She felt this was safer than him being at home alone during her work hours, but is now starting to wonder about whether to allow Douglass to engage in activities with his friend.

A splint has provided support for several days and has allowed the swelling to decrease before today's cast application. Douglass has been non–weight bearing on his leg and has been using crutches. He returned to school yesterday for part of the day and found it was hard to get to all of his classes.

• What teaching should you provide to help him keep the cast intact to ensure his safety and to alert him to signs of compartment syndrome?

---

of extremities, including color, temperature, capillary refill time, edema, pulses, sensation, and pain, should be performed. Questions should be phrased so that sports such as skateboarding or snowboarding, which might not be performed under supervision or in organized sports programs, can be identified. Youths might not consider these "sports."

Teach the importance of warming up for 10 to 15 minutes before participation and cooling down for a corresponding period at the end of activity. Encourage wearing recommended safety gear for the sport, including equipment such as a well-fitted protective helmet, face masks, eye protection, mouth guards, elbow and wrist guards, gloves, knee pads, and shin pads. Parents may need assistance to learn about the recommended equipment and resources for purchase. Frequent updates are needed as the child grows. The child should be taught not to ignore pain.

Injuries such as muscle strains should be treated promptly. They involve several steps:

• Resting the injury for 24 to 48 hours, applying ice for 20 minutes 4 times daily, compression with an elastic wrap to provide comfort and decrease edema, and elevating the affected part above heart level

• Gradually increasing motion to the part

• Adding flexibility and resistance or strengthening exercises

• Returning gradually to the sport, usually in 2 to 3 weeks after injury

The nurse should partner with the child, family, and other health professionals to plan for activity whenever an injury has occurred. Praise the family and youth for physical activity, an important part of a healthy lifestyle. Provide community resources to foster sports participation.

Amputations

Amputation—the complete absence of a body extremity—can be either congenital or acquired. Approximately two thirds of amputations in children are congenital and one third are acquired. Congenital amputations can be caused by constrictive amniotic bands, drugs, or irradiation. Acquired amputations are generally associated with trauma or the result of a disease or disorder. Children are prone to such injuries because of their small extremities and limited skeletal mass. Lawn mower injury, exercise equipment, and motor vehicle crashes are common causes. Most common traumatic amputations involve fingers or toes but hands and limbs are also at risk.

The child with an absent limb should be fitted with a prosthesis as soon as feasible and encouraged to use it several hours daily. This fosters a positive body image, independence, and self-confidence, and also ensures that motor skills develop as normally as possible (Ulger & Sener, 2011). The prosthetic device should be reevaluated as the child progresses physically and developmentally. Children with traumatic amputations may need frequent stump reconstructions because as children grow, so do their bones, and the skin tends to adhere to the bone. Bone may need to be cut and soft tissue added to keep the stump rounded. Joint fusions or stump lengthenings may also be needed to allow the effective use of a prosthesis. Several prosthetic revisions will be needed as the child grows and develops.

Nursing Management

Nursing care focuses on providing emotional support regarding altered body image, managing pain, maintaining skin integrity, and encouraging maximal independent functioning.

Recovering from the loss of a limb is one of the most difficult challenges facing children. Emphasize what children can do rather than what they cannot do. Good listening skills are important.

The child who has had surgery or a traumatic injury experiences pain. Many techniques discussed in Chapter 40 are useful interventions. After surgery, an epidural may be the treatment of choice. Oral analgesics are used during the period of adaptation to a prosthesis if the stump is tender. Children may have "phantom" limb pain in the lost extremity, although this phenomenon decreases significantly in the first year after amputation (Burgoyne et al., 2012; Wolff et al., 2011). The child usually begins wearing the prosthetic device for 1- to 2-hour intervals. Check the skin for any redness or breakdown. If redness or breakdown develops, leave the prosthesis off and allow the skin to clear before reapplying. Have the prosthesis adjusted if necessary, and increase wearing time as tolerated by the child.

Children with amputated limbs quickly learn how to accommodate to the prosthetic device. Use physical therapy programs specifically designed to help the child perform activities of daily living.

DISCHARGE PLANNING AND HOME CARE TEACHING

Answer any questions the family has about how to care for the prosthetic device and how to perform skin checks. Encourage parents to allow the child to participate in physically and emotionally challenging peer activities. Sporting activities that enable the child to participate using modified equipment are a good way to build self-confidence and motivation. For example, ski centers may offer programs that teach children with physical disabilities how to ski, or the Paralympics may be motivating for some children. Assess the need for counseling and offer referrals as appropriate.

Focus Your Study

- Children may develop musculoskeletal conditions as a result of congenital conditions, developmental variations, or trauma.

- Talipes equinovarus (clubfoot) is a common unilateral or bilateral variation in newborns that is treated by casting, traction, and/or surgery.

- Genu varum and genu valgum are normal variations at certain times in development that may need treatment if they persist.

- The nurse may identify developmental dysplasia of the hip (DDH) during newborn assessments and must refer the child for care to a specialist.

- Mild DDH is treated by a harness, but more severe cases may require surgery for the child to walk normally.

- Legg-Calvé-Perthes is a reversible disease most commonly seen in school-age boys, and causes necrosis of the femoral head.

- Slipped capital femoral epiphysis is treated by casting, tractions, or more commonly surgery with pinning, to stabilize the epiphysis.

- Scoliosis is a lateral curvature of the spine, and nurses commonly screen adolescents to identify the disorder.

- Scoliosis may require exercises, bracing, or surgery with instrumentation and spinal fusion.

- Osteoporosis can occur in premature infants, in children with conditions that lead to immobility and decreased weight bearing, and in youth with inadequate calcium or vitamin D intake.

- Osteomyelitis most commonly follows another infection and requires prompt treatment to prevent sepsis and serious injury to the bone.

- The child with osteogenesis imperfecta (brittle bone disease) requires careful handling by the nurse and parents to prevent fractures while fostering developmental progression.

- Muscular dystrophies are inherited diseases characterized by muscle wasting and degeneration.

- Children can experience a variety of fractures due to sports, car crashes, and other injuries.

- Many sports injuries experienced by youth can be avoided with proper equipment.

- Casts, braces, and traction are common interventions for musculoskeletal disorders; nursing interventions minimize development of complications related to these treatments.

Clinical Reasoning in Action

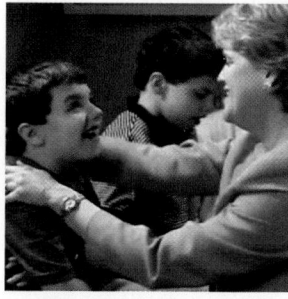

Peter, now 7 years old, was diagnosed at 5 years old with Duchenne muscular dystrophy. His parents are well informed about the disease since they had an older son who died of the disorder at 19 years. At the present time, he walks on his toes but is able to ambulate well with leg braces. Today, Peter is visiting the specialty clinic for children with muscular dystrophies. His braces will be checked for fit and performance, physical therapy will be performed, and he will attend a group session with other school-age children. During these visits, the parents also meet in a support group with other families and receive instruction and resources to help them with Peter's health management. As a nurse in the clinic you perform a physical and mental assessment on Peter. All findings are within normal limits, although he has had some constipation and several upper respiratory infections. You learn that he has an individualized education plan (IEP) in place at school that allows for periods of rest and physical therapy; the parents report that he is at grade level and excels at computer skills.

1. What are the main roles of the nurse working with Peter in the specialty clinic?

2. Children with muscular dystrophy often get to a standing position by mainly using arm muscles. What is the name of the maneuver?

3. What are some of the tests performed to see if a child has muscular dystrophy, and what are the expected results?

4. Who can Peter expect to meet with on the days he goes to the specialty clinic for muscular dystrophy?

5. Construct a concept map for Peter that demonstrates the multisystem involvement of his disease and how his developmental needs can be met in spite of his disability.

References

American Academy of Orthopaedic Surgeons (AAOS). (2014a). *Detection and management of pediatric developmental dysplasia of the hip in infants up to six months of age: Evidence-based clinical practice guideline.* Retrieved from http://www.aaos.org /research/guidelines/DDHGuidelineFINAL.pdf

American Academy of Orthopaedic Surgeons (AAOS). (2014b). *Forearm fractures in children.* Retrieved from http://orthoinfo.aaos.org/topic .cfm?topic=A00039

American Academy of Pediatrics. (1999, reaffirmed 2013). Transporting children with special health care needs. *Pediatrics, 104,* 988–992 (original policy); *Pediatrics, 132,* e281–e282 (reaffirmation).

Amiri, M., Dezfooli, M. S., & Mortezaei, S. R. (2012). Designing and ergonomics backpack for student aged 7–9 with user centred design approach. *Work, 41*(Suppl 1), 1193–1201.

Atay, E. (2014). Prevalence of sport injuries among middle school children and suggestions for their prevention. *Journal of Physical Therapy Science, 26,* 1455–1457.

Bautista, S. R., Gholve, P., & Dormans, J. P. (2011). Pediatric musculoskeletal infections: Managing the significant organisms. *Consultant for Pediatricians, 10*(2), 41–45.

Becker Muscular Dystrophy. (n.d.). *Becker muscular dystrophy.* Retrieved from http://www .beckermusculardystrophy.org

Ben Amor, M., Rauch, F., Monti, E., & Antoniazzi, F. (2013). Osteogenesis imperfecta. *Pediatric Endocrinology Reviews, 10*(Suppl 2), 397–405.

Birch, J. G. (2013). Blount disease. *Journal of American Academy of Orthopaedic Surgery, 21,* 408–418.

Brox, J. I., Lange, J. E., Gunderson, R. B., & Steen, H. (2012). Good brace compliance reduced curve progression and surgical rates in patients with idiopathic scoliosis. *European Spine Journal, 21,* 1957–1963.

Burgoyne, L. L., Billups, C. A., Jiron, J. L., Kaddoum, R. N., Wright, B. B., Bikhazi, G. B., ... Pereiras, L. A. (2012). Phantom limb pain in young cancer-related amputees: Recent experience at St. Jude Children's Research Hospital. *Clinical Journal of Pain, 28*(3), 222–225.

Compton, S. (2014). Childhood obesity and slipped capital femoral epiphysis. *Radiologic Technology, 85,* 321–324.

de Sanctis, N. (2011). Magnetic resonance imaging in Legg-Calvé-Perthes disease: Review of literature. *Journal of Pediatric Orthopaedics, 31*(2 Suppl.), S163–S167.

Dockrell, S., Simms, C., & Blake, C. (2013). Schoolbag weight limit: Can it be defined? *Journal of School Health, 83,* 368–377.

Farr, J. N., Laddu, D. R., & Going, S. B. (2014). Exercise, hormones and skeletal adaptation during childhood

and adolescence. *Pediatric Exercise Science, 26,* 384–391.

Field, A. E., Gordon, C. M., Pierce, L. M., Ramappa, A., & Kocher, M. S. (2011). Prospective study of physical activity and risk of developing a stress fracture among preadolescent and adolescent girls. *Archives of Pediatrics and Adolescent Medicine, 165,* 723–728.

Georgiadis, A. G., & Zaltz, I. (2014). Slipped capital femoral epiphysis: How to evaluate with a review and update of treatment. *Pediatric Clinics of North America, 61,* 1119–1135.

Gilmore, A., & Thompson, G. H. (2013). Common childhood foot deformities. *Consultant for Pediatricians,* (January), 28–34.

Goyenvaile, A., Seto, J. T., Davies, K. E., & Chamberlain, J. (2011). Therapeutic approaches to muscular dystrophy. *Human Molecular Genetics, 20*(Review Issue I), R69–R78.

Harmon, K. G., Drezner, J. A., Gammons, M., Guskiewicz, K. M., Halstead, M., Herring, S. A., ... Roberts, W. O. (2013). American Medical Society for Sports Medicine position statement: Concussion in sport. *British Journal of Sports Medicine, 47,* 15–26.

Harrington, J., Sochett, E., & Howard, A. (2014). Update on the evaluation and treatment of osteogenesis imperfecta. *Pediatric Clinics of North America, 61,* 1243–1247.

Ireland, P. J., Donaghey, S., McGill, J., Zankl, A., Ware, R. S., Pacey, V., ... Johnston, L. M. (2012). Development in children with achondroplasia: A prospective clinical cohort study. *Developmental Medicine Child Neurology, 54,* 532–537.

Kannu, P., & Howard, P. (2014). Perthes disease. *British Medical Journal.* doi: http://dx.doi.Org/10.1136/bmj .g5584

Kumar, A., & Agarwal, S. (2014). Marfan syndrome: An eyesight of syndrome. *Meta Gene, 2,* 96–105.

Laederich, M. B., & Horton, W. A. (2012). FGFR3 targeting strategies for achondroplasia. *Expert Reviews in Molecular Science, 19,* e11.

Lombardi, G., Akoume, M. Y., Colombini, A., Moreau, A., & Banfi, G. (2011). Biochemistry of adolescent idiopathic scoliosis. *Advances in Clinical Chemistry, 54,* 165–182.

Lubicky, J. P., Hanson, J. E., Riley, E., & Spinal Deformity Study Group. (2011). Instrumentation constructs in pediatric patients undergoing deformity correction correlated with Scoliosis Research Society scores. *Spine, 36,* 1692–1700.

Luke, A., Lazaro, R. M., Bergeron, M. F., Keyser, L., Benjamin, H., Brenner, J., ... Smith, A. (2011). Sports-related injuries in youth athletes: Is overscheduling a risk factor? *Clinical Journal of Sports Medicine, 21,* 307–314.

March of Dimes. (2012). *Achondroplasia.* Retrieved from http://www.marchofdimes.com/search.html

Mazloumi, S. M., Ebrahimzadeh, M. H., & Kachooei, A. R. (2014). Evolution in diagnosis and treatment of Legg-Calve-Perthes disease. *Archives of Bone and Joint Surgery, 2,* 86–92.

Mehler, P. S., Cleary, B. S., & Guadiani, J. L. (2011). Osteoporosis in anorexia nervosa. *Eating Disorders, 19,* 194–202.

Milani, C., & Dobashi, E. T. (2011). Arthrogram in Legg-Calve-Perthes disease. *Journal of Pediatric Orthopaedics, 31*(2 Suppl.), S156–S162.

Nakamura, J., Kamegaya, M., Saisu, T., Kakizaki, J., Hagiwara, S., Ohtori, S., ... Takahashik, K. (2015). Outcome of patients with Legg-Calve-Perthes onset before 6 years of age. *Journal of Pediatric Orthopedics, 35,* 144–150. doi: 10.1097 /BPO.0000000000000246

National Institutes of Health. (2012a). *Fontanelles.* Retrieved from http://www.nlm.nih.gov/medlineplus /ency/article/003310.htm

National Institutes of Health. (2012b). *Metatarsus adductus.* Retrieved from http://www.nlm.nih.gov /medlineplus/ency/article/001601.htm

National Institutes of Health. (2013). *Developmental dysplasia of the hip.* Retrieved from http://www.ncbi .nlm.nih.gov/pubmedhealth/PMH0001966/

Perry, D. C., & Hall, A. J. (2011). The epidemiology and etiology of Perthes disease. *Orthopedic Clinics of North America, 42,* 279–283.

Rack, B., Lochmuller, E. M., Janni, W., Lipowsky, G., Engelsberger, I., Friese, K., & Kuster, H. (2011). Ultrasound for the assessment of bone quality in preterm and term infants. *Journal of Perinatology.* doi:10.1038/jp.2011.82

Rodriguez-Oviedo, P., Ruano-Ravina, A., Perez-Rios, M., Garcia, F.B., Gomez-Fernandez, D., Fernandez-Alonso, A., ... Turiso. J. (2012). School children's backpacks, back pain and back pathologies. *Archives of Disease in Childhood, 97,* 730–732.

Roof, A. C., Jinguji, T. M., & White, K. K. (2013). Musculoskeletal screening: Developmental dysplasia a of the hip. *Pediatric Annals, 42,* 229–235.

Rosenbush, S. W., & Parker, J. M. (2014). Height and heart disease. *Reviews in Cardiovascular Medicine, 15,* 102–108.

Sabharwal, S. (2015). Blount disease: An update. *Orthopedic Clinics of North America, 46,* 37–47.

Schaffzin, J. K., Prichard, H., Bisig, J., Gainor, P., Wolfe, K., Solan, L. G., ... McCarthy, J. J. (2013). A collaborative system to improve compartment syndrome recognition. *Pediatrics, 132,* e1672–e1679.

Schulzke, S. M., Kaempfen, S., Trachsel, D., & Patole, S. K. (2014). Physical activity programs for promoting bone mineralization and growth in preterm infants. *Cochrane Database Systematic Reviews, 22,* 4:CD005387.

Schwend, R. M., Shaw, B. A., & Segal, L. S. (2014). Evaluation and treatment of developmental hip dysplasia in the newborn and infant. *Pediatric Clinics of North America, 61*, 1095–1107.

Scottish Rite Hospital. (2011). *Scoliosis and spine.* Retrieved from http://www.tsrhc.org/scoliosis -scoliometer.htm

Szadek, L. L., & Scharer, K. (2014). Identification, prevention, and treatment of children with decreased bone mineral density. *Journal of Pediatric Nursing, 29*, e3–e14.

Theadom, A., Rodrigues, M., Roxburgh, R., Balalla, S., Higgins, C., Bhattacharjee, R., ... Feigin, V. (2014). Prevalence of muscular dystrophies: A systematic literature review. *Neuroepidemiology, 43*, 259–268.

Thomsen, K., & Creech, C. B. (2011). Advances in the diagnosis and management of pediatric osteomyelitis. *Current Infectious Disease Reports, 13*, 451–460.

Tschudy, M. M., & Arcara, K. M., (Eds.). (2012). *The Harriet Lane handbook* (19th ed.). St. Louis, MO: Elsevier Mosby.

Ulger, O., & Sener, G. (2011). Functional outcome after prosthetic rehabilitation of children with acquired and congenital lower limb loss. *Journal of Pediatric Orthopaedics, 20*, 178–183.

University of Maryland Medical Center. (2011). *Muscular dystrophy.* Retrieved from http://www.wmm.edu /altmed/articles/musculardystrophy-000113.htm

U.S. Preventive Services Task Force. (2014). *Idiopathic scoliosis in adolescents: Screening.* Retrieved from http://www.uspreventiveservicestaskforce.org /Page/Document/RecommendationStatementFinal /idiopathic-scoliosis-in-adolescents-screening

van Dijk, F. S., Cobben, J. M., Kariminijad, A., Maugeri, A., Nikkels, P. G., van Rijn, R. R., & Pals, G. (2011). Osteogenesis imperfect: A review with clinical examples. *Molecular Syndromology, 2*, 1–20.

Weinstein, S. L., Dolan, L. A., Wright, J. G., & Dobbs, M. B. (2013). Effects of bracing in adolescents with idiopathic scoliosis. *New England Journal of Medicine, 369*, 1512–1521.

Witbreuk, M., van Kemenade, F. J., van der Sluijs, J. A., Jansma, E. P., Rottefeel, J., & van Royen, B. J. (2013). Slipped capital femoral epiphysis and its association with endocrine, metabolic and chronic diseases: A systematic review of the literature. *Journal of Children's Orthopaedics, 7*, 213–223.

Wolff, A., Vanduynhover, E., van Kleef, M., Huygen, F., Pope, J. E., & Mehhail, N. (2011). Phantom pain. *Pain Practice, 11*, 403–413.

Womack, J. (2014). Osteogenesis imperfect types I–XI: Implications for the neonatal nurse. *Advances in Neonatal Care, 14*, 309–315.

Wright, E. (2009). Neurovascular impairment and compartment syndrome. *Paediatric Nursing, 21*(3), 26–29.

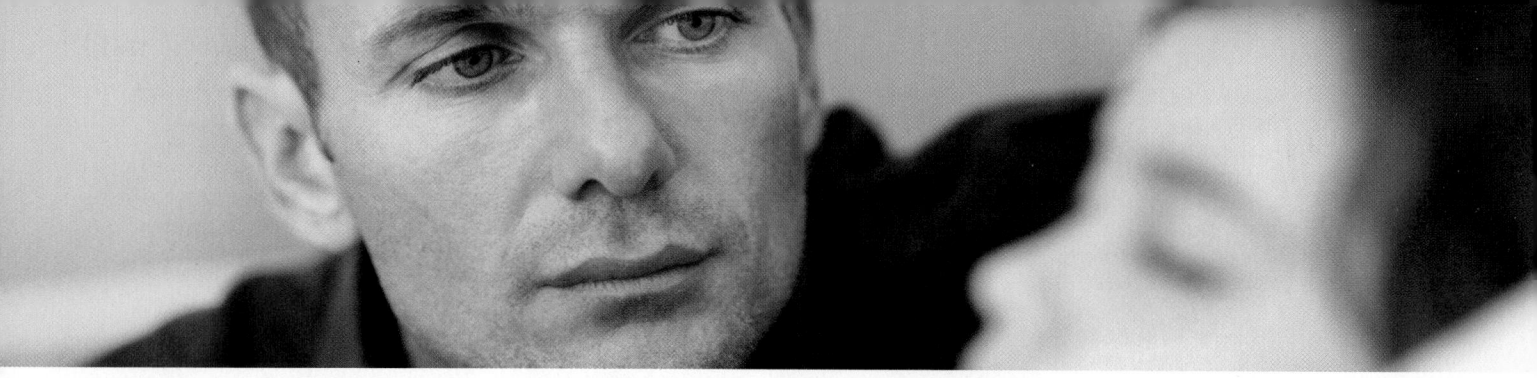

Chapter 57
The Child With Alterations in Skin Integrity

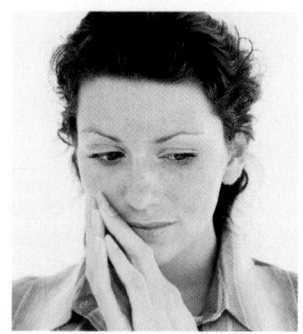

George Doyle/Getty Images

I didn't know that hot coffee could cause such a bad injury. I am worried about the scars Shanelle might have over her chest from this scald burn.

—Mother of Shanelle, 1 year old

Learning Outcomes

57.1 Classify the characteristics of skin lesions caused by irritants, drug reactions, mites, infection, and injury.

57.2 Differentiate among the stages of wound healing.

57.3 Compare skin conditions that have a hereditary cause or predisposition.

57.4 Plan the nursing care for the child with alterations in skin integrity, including dermatitis, infectious disorders, and infestations.

57.5 Prepare an education plan for adolescents with acne to promote self-care.

57.6 Summarize the process to measure the extent of burns and burn severity in children.

57.7 Develop a nursing care plan for the child with a full-thickness burn injury.

57.8 Contrast preventive strategies to reduce the risk of injury from burns, hypothermia, bites, and stings.

The skin has three distinct layers: the epidermis, the dermis, and the subcutaneous fatty layer that separates the skin from the underlying tissue (Figure 57–1). The epidermis is the thin, outermost layer of skin that grows rapidly and contains the melanocytes that synthesize and secrete melanin when the skin is exposed to ultraviolet light. Within the dermis are nerves, muscles, connective tissue, hair follicles, sebaceous and sweat glands, lymph channels, and blood vessels. The subcutaneous layer contains the sebaceous glands,

eccrine and apocrine sweat glands, and a layer of fat to help insulate the body from cold temperatures.

The infant's skin is thin with little underlying subcutaneous fat. Because of this, the infant loses heat more rapidly, has greater difficulty regulating body temperature, and becomes more easily chilled than an older child or an adult. The thinner skin also leads to increased absorption of harmful chemical substances and topical medications. The infant's skin contains more water than an adult's and has loosely attached cells. As

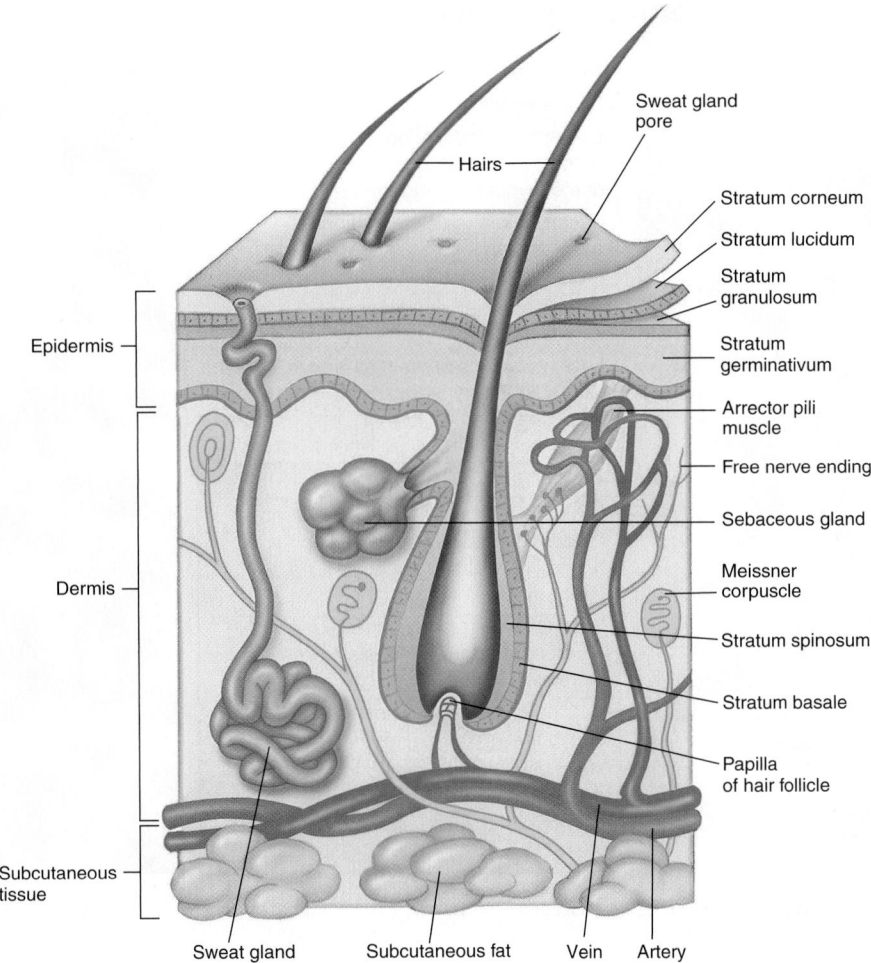

Hairs

Sweat gland pore

Stratum corneum

Stratum lucidum

Stratum granulosum

Stratum germinativum

Arrector pili muscle

Free nerve ending

Sebaceous gland

Meissner corpuscle

Stratum spinosum

Stratum basale

Papilla of hair follicle

Epidermis

Dermis

Subcutaneous tissue

Sweat gland

Subcutaneous fat

Vein

Artery

Figure 57–1 **Layers of the skin with accessory structures.**

the infant grows, the skin toughens and becomes less hydrated, making it less susceptible to bacteria. See changes in skin characteristics in *As Children Grow: Integumentary System Changes*.

Sebaceous glands function at birth, although somewhat immaturely. They vary in size and appear all over the body except on the hands and soles of the feet. Sebum, a lipid substance produced and secreted into the hair follicle or directly onto the skin, lubricates the skin and hair.

Eccrine glands, located in the dermis, open onto the skin surface. They secrete sweat, an odorless, watery fluid, primarily in response to emotional stress. These glands also respond to elevated body temperature by increasing production of sweat. Its evaporation cools the body. All eccrine sweat glands are present and functional at birth.

Apocrine glands, located mainly in the axillary and genital areas, secrete sweat with more lipids and protein. Body odor occurs when this sweat decomposes. Apocrine glands do not function until puberty.

Skin Lesions

Skin lesions vary in size, shape, color, and texture. The two major types of skin lesions are primary lesions and secondary lesions. Primary lesions arise from previously healthy skin and include macules, patches, papules, nodules, tumors, vesicles, pustules, bullae, and wheals. (See *Pathophysiology Illustrated: Common Primary Skin Lesions and Associated Conditions* in

Chapter 33.) Secondary lesions result from changes in primary lesions. They include crusts, scales, **lichenification** (thickening of the skin with more visible skin furrows), scars, keloids, excoriation, fissures, erosion, and ulcers (Table 57–1). It is important for the nurse to be able to identify and describe the primary and secondary skin lesions and understand their underlying cause and treatment.

Wound Healing

Wound healing occurs in three overlapping phases: hemostasis and inflammation, tissue formation, and maturation (see *Pathophysiology Illustrated: Phases of Wound Healing*).

Nursing responsibilities include wound cleansing and dressing changes. Wound cleansing is important because it removes loose material and bacteria from the site. Common cleansers are sterile water, normal saline, and commercial products that help loosen and suspend contaminants in water. Wound dressings have various properties that promote wound healing. See Table 57–2 for examples of primary dressings. Most primary dressings need a cover or secondary dressing. As the wound heals, the scar eventually achieves about 80% of the tissue's preinjury strength (Rote & Huether, 2014). A keloid results from an imbalance between collagen synthesis and collagen breakdown. The cause is unknown, but there is a familial tendency. A hypertrophic scar is raised but stays within the original wound boundaries.

As Children Grow: **Integumentary System Changes**

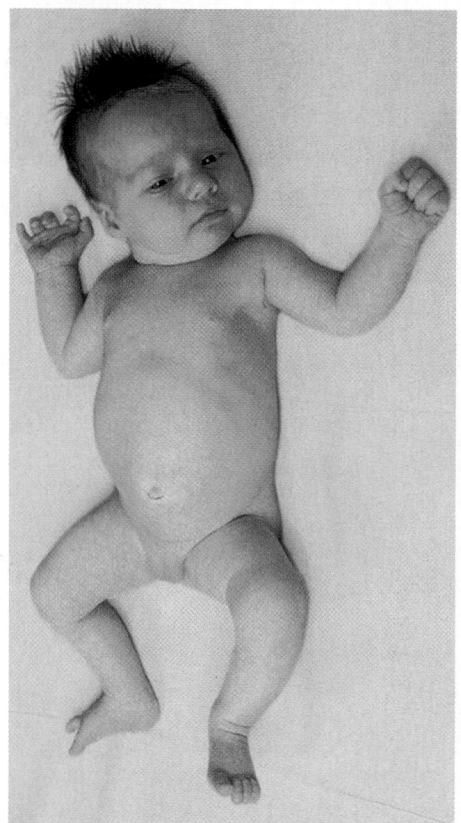

Newborns
Skin is very thin
Epidermis is loosely bound to the dermis, friction can cause separation of the layers with blistering
Eccrine sweat glands function, produce sweat in response to heat and emotional stimuli
Apocrine sweat glands are small and nonfunctional
Less melanin is present at birth so skin is lighter colored

Adolescents
Skin thickens
Epidermis and dermis are tightly bound, increasing resistance to infection and irritation
Eccrine sweat glands achieve full function, after puberty males sweat more than females
Apocrine sweat glands mature during puberty
Melanin is at adult levels, determining skin color and serving as a shield against ultraviolet radiation

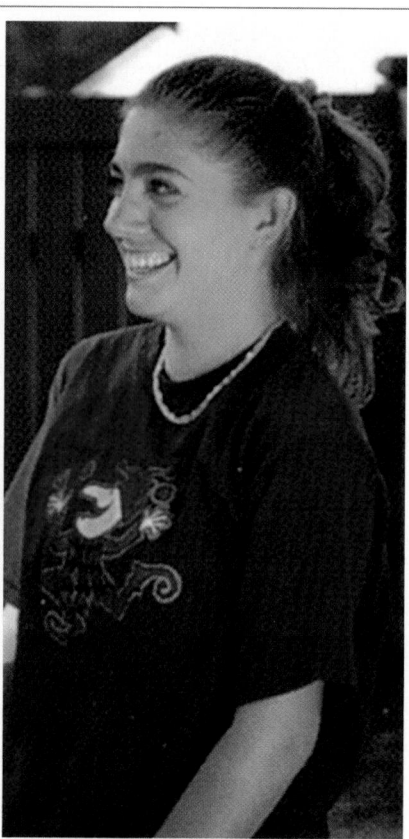

The structures of the skin mature during childhood, reaching adult function at puberty.

TABLE 57–1 Common Secondary Skin Lesions and Associated Conditions

LESION NAME	DESCRIPTION	EXAMPLE
Burrow	A narrow, raised irregular channel caused by a parasite	Scabies
Comedone	A plug of sebaceous and keratin material in a hair follicle	Acne
Crust	Dried residue of serum, pus, or blood	Impetigo
Erosion	Loss of superficial epidermis; moist but does not bleed	Ruptured chickenpox vesicle
Excoriation	Abrasion or scratch mark	Scratched insect bite
Fissure	Linear crack in skin	Tinea pedis (athlete's foot)
Keloid	Overdevelopment or hypertrophy of scar that extends beyond wound edges and above skin line because of excess collagen	Healed skin area following traumatic injury
Lichenification	Thickening of skin with increased visibility of normal skin furrows	Atopic dermatitis (eczema)
Scale	Thin flake of exfoliated epidermis	Dandruff, psoriasis
Scar	Replacement of destroyed tissue with fibrous tissue	Healed surgical incision
Telangiectasia	Dilated, superficial blood vessels	Birthmark
Ulcer	Deeper loss of skin surface; bleeding or scarring may ensue	Pressure ulcer

Dermatitis

Many skin inflammations occur in early childhood. Most are easily treated and have no long-term consequences. Dermatitis is a condition in which skin changes occur in response to external stimuli. The three most common types of acute dermatitis in infants, children, and adolescents are contact dermatitis, diaper dermatitis, and seborrheic dermatitis. See information on atopic dermatitis later in this chapter. These skin disorders may cause an emotional response in the child and family. Be supportive and reassure the family that the child is not infectious.

Contact Dermatitis

Contact dermatitis is an inflammation of the skin that occurs in response to direct contact with an allergen or irritant.

Pathophysiology Illustrated: **Phases of Wound Healing**

Wound healing occurs in three overlapping phases.

Hemostasis and Inflammation (3–5 days)

Platelets flow to site and form a clot to stop bleeding, sealing the wound with fibrin, trapped cells, and platelets.

Platelets release inflammatory mediators (cytokines, chemokines, and growth factors).

Increased blood flow to area delivers leukocytes, phagocytes, and lymphocytes.

Increased capillary permeability causes swelling and erythema.

Bacteria are destroyed and cellular debris and foreign particles are removed.

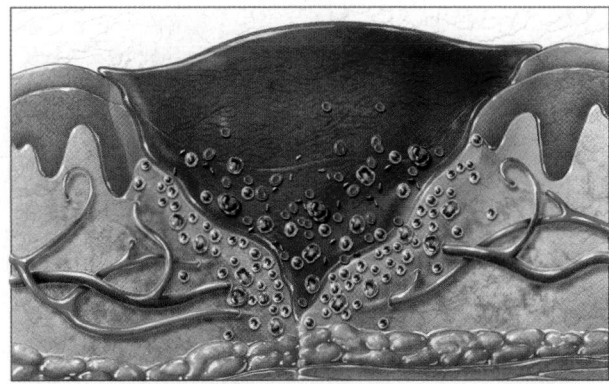

Tissue Formation (4 days to 2 weeks)

Natural debridement with fibrinolytic enzymes dissolves the fibrin clots.

Fibroblasts and endothelial cells in surrounding tissue direct the migration of cells to the newly developed fibrin matrix (replacing the clot), so remodeling can begin.

Granulation tissue forms and the wound is closed.

Capillary budding occurs for development of new blood vessels.

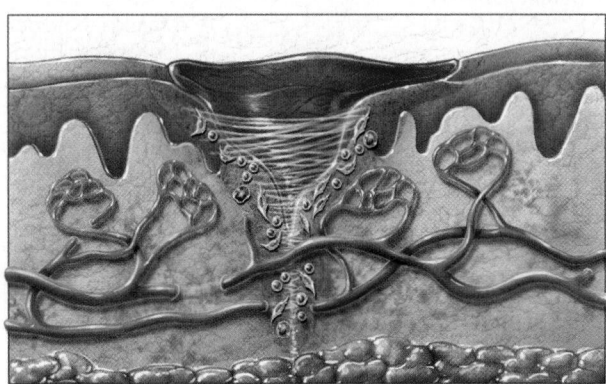

Maturation (months to 2 years)

Wound contraction occurs.

Epithelial cells migrate from the peripheral areas.

Collagen development leads to scar formation and strengthening.

Capillaries disappear from the scar tissue, returning the tissue to its original blood supply.

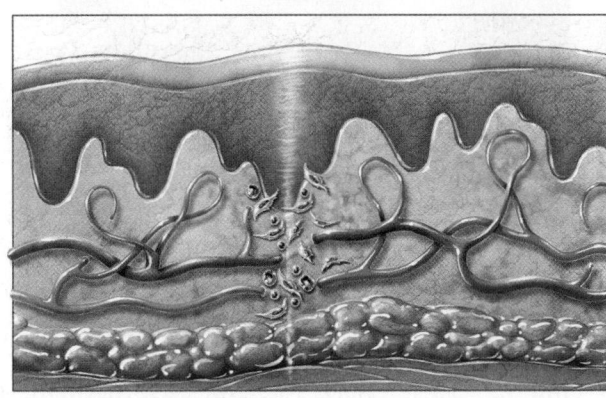

Source: Data from Reinke, J. M., & Sorg, H. (2012). Wound repair and regeneration. *European Surgical Research, 49*, 35–43; Yao, K., Bae, L., & Yew, W. P. (2013). Post-operative wound management. *Australian Family Physician, 42*(12), 867–870; Rote, N. S., Huether, S. E., & McCance, K. L. (2014). Innate immunity: Inflammation. In K. L. McCance, S. E. Huether, V. L Brashers, & N. S. Rote (Eds.), *Pathophysiology: The biologic basis for disease in adults and children* (7th ed., pp. 191–223). St. Louis, MO: Elsevier.

When contact dermatitis is caused by an external irritant, an inflammatory response occurs without an immune response. Common irritants include soaps, detergents, fabric softeners, bleaches, lotions, urine, and stool. An irritant can affect the skin any time there is adequate concentration and contact duration. Sweating and friction enhance the exposure to an irritant. Children with atopic dermatitis may be at risk for irritant contact dermatitis because of decreased skin barrier function.

Phytophotodermatitis can result when the child has skin contact with certain citrus fruits, celery, parsley, fennel, fig leaves, or ragweed. These plants have a chemical (furocoumarin) that sensitizes the skin to sunlight. Following sun exposure the child develops erythema and blistering at the site of the contact, and the skin then becomes hyperpigmented 1 to 2 weeks later. The hyperpigmentation fades over several months (Shulstad, 2012).

Allergic contact dermatitis is a delayed T-cell–mediated hypersensitivity reaction. An antigen is absorbed from the skin surface during the initial sensitization phase, and an immune memory is created. A repeated exposure or a long-term exposure is required to cause the immune response and the dermatitis. See Chapter 48 to review the immune response to allergens.

TABLE 57–2 Primary Wound Dressings

DRESSING TYPE	PROPERTIES	NURSING MANAGEMENT
Hydrocolloid—semiocclusive	Uses wound exudates to form a gel-like cover that adheres and protects wound bed from contaminants Maintains moist environment Promotes autolytic debridement	Use for granulating and epithelializing wounds with low or moderate amount of exudates. Use with caution in infected wounds. Cover at least 1 in. of intact skin around the wound.
Hydrogel—semiocclusive	Increases and maintains moisture content Promotes autolytic debridement Does not adhere, reducing pain with removal	Use with minimal or moderate exudate as limited exudates absorption. Cover at least 1 in. of intact skin around the wound.
Foam—semiocclusive	Absorbent—used for moderate to heavy exudate Nonadherent	Use for packing deep wounds. Use for heavy exudate when drainage is at peak.
Alginates—semiocclusive	Absorbs exudate and converts it to a gel Provides a moist environment	Use for moderate to heavy exudate. Use to pack wounds.
Transparent film—occlusive	Permeable to oxygen and water vapor Maintains moist environment Nonabsorbent Protects wound from contamination	Its use provides visible wound evaluation. Use on superficial wounds with little or no drainage or on areas of friction. Use care when removing film to prevent skin tearing.

Source: Data from Rolstad, B. S., Bryant, R. A., & Nix, D. P. (2012). Topical management. In R. A. Bryant & D. P. Nix (Eds.), *Acute & chronic wounds: Current management concepts* (4th ed., pp. 289–295). St. Louis, MO: Elsevier Mosby; Wound Care Information Network. (2013). *Wound care product and category index.* Retrieved from http://www.medicaledu.com/prodindx.htm; Wound Educators. (2015). *Wound dressings.* Retrieved from http://woundeducators.com/resources/wound-dressings/

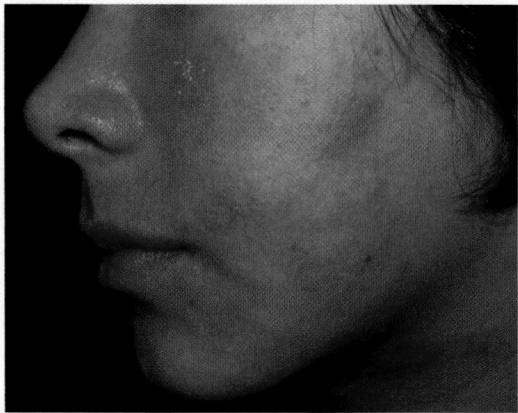

Figure 57–2 Contact dermatitis caused by poison ivy. Note the clustered tiny erythematous papules involving the face and neck. In some areas (particularly the neck), lesions are distributed in a linear fashion.

SOURCE: Courtesy of Daniel P. Krowchuk, MD, Professor of Pediatrics and Dermatology, Wake Forest School of Medicine, Winston-Salem, NC.

Common allergens include poison ivy, poison oak, lanolin, neomycin, rubber, chemicals in shoe leather, nickel, fragrances, and latex (Figure 57–2). Children may have both irritant and allergic reactions to latex, which is found in many types of hospital equipment and supplies and products in the home.

With irritant contact dermatitis, a discrete area of redness is seen that corresponds to the exposure location, and severity is related to duration of exposure. The rash usually develops within a few hours of contact, peaks within 24 hours, and quickly resolves with removal of the irritant. With longer exposure, reactions may include painful erythema, edema, vesicles, and exudate.

Allergic contact dermatitis is characterized by erythema, edema, pruritus, vesicles, or bullae that rupture, ooze, and crust. The rash is usually limited to the area of contact (Table 57–3). Symptoms of allergic contact dermatitis can develop several hours following exposure, after the immune response has been activated. Symptoms can last 3 to 4 weeks without treatment.

The history of potential exposures and distribution of lesions provide clues about the source and identity of the allergen or irritant. Secondary infection may occur. For irritant contact dermatitis, treatment involves removing the offending agent (e.g., clothes, plant, soap). Use emollients to restore the skin barrier. Decrease inflammation with hydrocortisone cream or ointment. Antihistamines may help relieve itching or be given for their sedative effect.

SAFETY ALERT!

Some children have allergic contact dermatitis associated with spices such as vanilla, clove, and cinnamon, as well as citrus peels. These children may develop systemic contact dermatitis through oral ingestion of these products that are in the Balsam of Peru family of flavorings in chewing gum, toothpaste, baked goods, and food condiments. These children may need special dietary guidelines to reduce exposure to Balsam of Peru products (Fonacier et al., 2012).

Acute allergic contact dermatitis is managed with medium-potency topical corticosteroids when less than 10% of the body surface area is affected. The topical corticosteroids are applied to the affected area twice a day for 2 to 3 weeks. Do not apply the medication to open lesions. Rebound dermatitis may occur if treatment is stopped early. Reactions to poison ivy or other allergens covering more than 10% of the body surface area require oral corticosteroid treatment for 7 to 14 days and a tapered dose for 7 to 10 additional days.

TABLE 57–3 Distribution of Lesions by Type of Allergen

DISTRIBUTION OF LESION	ALLERGEN
Face, eyelids, neck	Cosmetics, hair and skin care products, nail polish and cosmetics, fragrances, eyeglasses with nickel
Earlobes, area with body piercing	Jewelry with nickel, cell phone
Lips, mouth	Oral hygiene products, bubblegum, lipstick
Hands	Rubber or neoprene gloves, mouse pad
Dorsal aspects of toes and feet	Rubber or leather chemical in shoes, metal buckles on sandals
Trunk	Snaps or other metal fasteners on clothing, belt buckles, moisturizers, cleansers, sunscreen products

Source: Data from Kwan, J. M., & Jacob, S. E. (2012). Contact dermatitis in the atopic child. *Pediatric Annals, 41*(10), 422–428; Fonacier, L. S., Aquino, M. R., & Mucci, T. (2012). Current strategies in treating severe contact dermatitis in pediatric patients. *Current Allergy and Asthma Reports, 12*, 599–606; Krowchuk, D. P., & Mancini, A. J. (2012). *Pediatric dermatology: A quick reference guide* (2nd ed., pp. 43–53). American Academy of Pediatrics; Halloran, L. (2014). Developing dermatology detective powers: Allergic contact dermatitis. *Journal for Nurse Practitioners, 10*(4), 284–285.

Nursing Management

Assess the child's skin using guidelines found in accompanying *Assessment Guide: The Child With a Skin Condition*. Client education for home care management focuses on care of the skin and prevention of future exposures. Teach parents how to apply topical corticosteroids and to keep using the medication for 2 to 3 weeks even when the skin shows signs of healing. Wet dressings may be soothing and help loosen crusts. Burow solution used as a soak helps dry lesions. Familiarize parents with the symptoms of infection in the affected area (i.e., increased redness, oozing, fever) and tell them when to return for follow-up care.

Teach parents to avoid exposure to allergens or irritants. Advise parents to wash all clothes before the first wearing and to rinse clothes an extra time to remove all the soap. Mild soap should be used to clean the skin. An emollient may be used for dry skin. Place a barrier between the irritant (e.g., metal, shoe leather) and the skin. If a nickel allergy exists, avoid use of nickel jewelry and belt buckles.

Diaper Dermatitis

Diaper dermatitis, a common cause of irritant contact dermatitis, occurs in approximately one third of young children, usually in a mild form. It is more common in infants from 9 to 12 months and toddlers.

ASSESSMENT GUIDE | The Child With a Skin Condition

Assessment Focus

Skin characteristics

Hair

Lesions

Assessment Guidelines

- Inspect the skin for color, elevations, and imperfections.
- Palpate the skin for texture, moisture, temperature, turgor, and edema.
- Inspect the scalp hair for color, distribution, and cleanliness. Inspect for nits (lice eggs) that adhere to the hair.
- Inspect for areas of hair loss, bald spots, or broken hairs.
- Describe skin lesions according to characteristics listed in *Pathophysiology Illustrated: Common Primary Skin Lesions and Associated Conditions* in Chapter 33 and Table 57–1.
- Identify the location and distribution of lesions on the body.
- Palpate lesions for induration and temperature.
- Measure the size of lesions (length, width, and height).

TEACHING HIGHLIGHTS | Exposure to Poison Ivy or Poison Oak

- The rash is caused by contact with urushiol, a resin of the plants, either directly or indirectly, such as transfer from an animal or clothing. Avoid hugging a pet exposed to poison ivy until after the pet has been bathed. Once the rash develops, it is not contagious.
- Wash exposed skin with soap and water, and scrub under the nails as soon as possible after contact. Zanfel and Ivy X are products available over-the-counter that remove urushiol after poison ivy exposure to reduce itching and severity of rash if used promptly.
- Do not rub fingers exposed to poison ivy against broken skin or the eyes.
- Launder clothing worn during exposure, and wash hands after handling exposed clothing.
- Wear vinyl gloves to handle plants (cloth and rubber gloves allow sap to penetrate).
- Search the yard and remove all plants. Do not burn plants removed. A person with a sensitivity may inhale the smoke and develop severe airway inflammation.
- For children with sensitivity to poison ivy, an over-the-counter barrier cream such as Ivy X preexposure solution can be applied to help prevent skin penetration of plant oil.

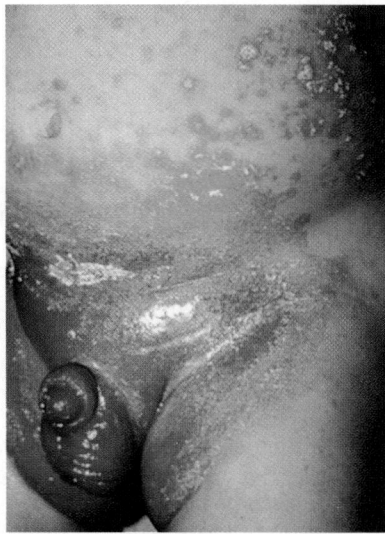

Figure 57–3 Diaper dermatitis. Note the skinfold that is free of inflammation.

SOURCE: Centers for Disease Control and Prevention.

Diaper dermatitis is a primary reaction to urine, feces, moisture, or friction. Urine and feces interact with the skin to cause dermatitis. The urine increases the wetness and pH of the skin, increasing abrasion and its permeability to irritants and microbes. Urine also metabolizes to ammonia, producing another irritant. Fecal organisms provide more irritants.

Infection with *Candida albicans* is a common complication of diaper dermatitis or antibiotic therapy for another condition. It is frequently the underlying cause of severe diaper rash. Diaper candidiasis often occurs simultaneously with oral candidiasis.

The rash is characterized by raw, moist, or weeping macules and papules of the skin in direct contact with the diaper. The skinfolds are usually spared. In severe cases, the infant develops a rash that is fiery red, raised, and confluent (Figure 57–3). Pustules with tenderness can also be present. When a *C. albicans* infection occurs, the rash has bright-red beefy plaques with sharp margins that may rupture and leave scales. Small papules and pustules may be seen, along with satellite lesions. Skinfolds may be affected.

Mild diaper dermatitis is treated with a water-impermeable barrier or protective sealant such as zinc oxide, Aquaphor, Desitin, or Balmex after every diaper change. In some cases, a diaper ointment combined with a protective powder (e.g., karaya powder) may be effective. An antifungal topical medication (e.g., nystatin) is applied to the skin before the barrier product when *C. albicans* is present, and is continued for 3 days after the rash clears. Topical corticosteroids are often avoided for diaper dermatitis because occlusion in the diaper area increases corticosteroid systemic absorption. If topical corticosteroids are necessary, a low-potency product is used.

Nursing Management

Diaper dermatitis can be a major source of stress for parents when the child is in constant discomfort. Instruct parents to change the diaper as soon as the infant is wet, or at least every 2 hours during the day and once during the night to minimize contact with urine and fecal irritants. Teach parents to apply barrier products and to remove them once or twice a day so fresh medication can be applied. Mineral oil and a soft cloth are effective for removing pastes. Encourage the parents to return for further care if the infant's skin is not greatly improved within a week.

Encourage parents to use superabsorbent disposable diapers, which tend to reduce the frequency and severity of diaper dermatitis. When wet, these diapers form a gel that keeps the skin drier than cloth diapers; however, diapers should still be changed every 2 to 3 hours. Exposing the diaper area to air aids healing. For example, allow the infant to go without a diaper while lying on an absorbent pad or cloth.

Advise parents to wash the perianal area with warm water or a waterless cleanser (Aquanil HC lotion or Cetaphil) after a bowel movement. Advise parents to use soft cloths or paper towels with warm tap water or to use baby wipes without alcohol if baby wipes are preferred. Pat the skin dry to reduce friction and skin injury. Avoid using powder or corn starch because they may increase friction.

Seborrheic Dermatitis

Seborrheic dermatitis is a recurrent inflammatory skin condition thought to be caused by an overgrowth of a yeast, *Malassezia furfur* (formerly *Pityrosporum ovale*). The condition is thought to be influenced by hormones. The rash is found over the areas of the body where the sebaceous glands are most plentiful: scalp (cradle cap), face, and postauricular and periorbital areas. The condition is frequently seen in infants up to 3 months of age and in adolescents.

Common symptoms are pruritus and a mildly erythematous, adherent, waxy scaling of the scalp (or "dandruff"). Yellow-red patches with greasy scaling may be present, typically on the scalp and nasolabial folds on the face, behind the ears, on the upper chest, and sometimes on the **intertriginous** (skinfolds of the neck, axillae, antecubital fossa) areas (Figure 57–4). Itching is less intense than with atopic eczema.

Treatment for young infants consists of daily shampooing with baby shampoo. An **emollient**, a topical product that soothes and softens the skin, such as warm mineral or olive oil, is left on the scalp for about 20 minutes to soften the crusts after shampooing. The scales are removed by brushing with the fingertips or a soft toothbrush. The hair is then shampooed again and rinsed

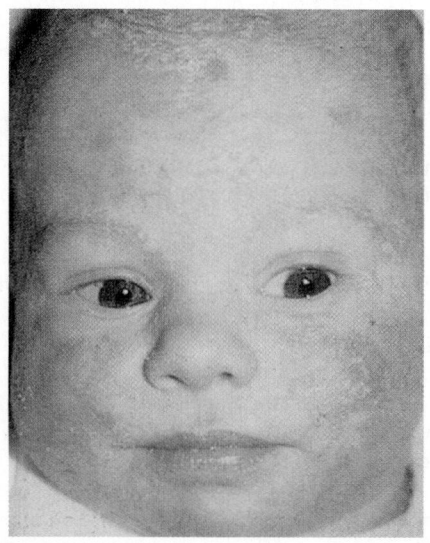

Figure 57–4 Seborrheic dermatitis.

thoroughly. A shampoo with 2% ketoconazole may be used in infants if baby shampoo is not effective (Ooi & Tidman, 2014).

Lesions on the body of adolescents can be treated with shampoos containing selenium sulfide or salicylic acid. Use baby shampoo to wash lesions on the eyelids and eyelashes. Treatments are continued for several days after the lesions disappear and may be repeated weekly to prevent recurrence. Topical corticosteroids are used to treat seborrhea that is not on the scalp, but avoid its use around the eyes.

Nursing Management

Teach new parents to wash the infant's hair daily with each bath. Reassure parents that gentle cleansing will not harm the infant's "soft spot." Demonstrate bathing to show them the proper technique, if necessary. Follow-up is seldom necessary, as the condition resolves with treatment. Advise adolescents that emotional distress may trigger future flare-ups and to initiate treatment promptly when symptoms begin.

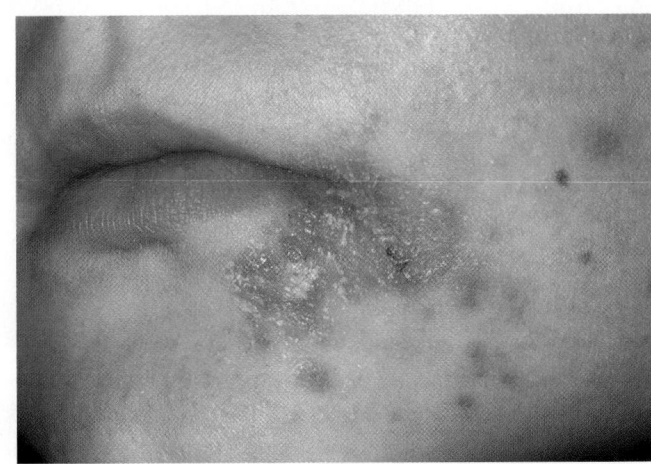

Figure 57–5 Impetigo. Note the honey-colored crusts over the lesion.

SOURCE: Dr. P. Marazzi/Science Source.

Bacterial Infections

Impetigo

Impetigo, the most common bacterial skin condition, is a highly contagious, superficial (epidermal) infection. The most common sites are the face, around the mouth, the hands, the neck, and the extremities. Minor skin injuries, insect bites, and dermatitis provide the portal for the infectious agent. Impetigo occurs more commonly in children who are in close physical contact with others, such as in childcare settings, or in those who have poor hygiene.

Either group A beta-hemolytic streptococcus, *Staphylococcus aureus*, or both together are usually responsible. *S. aureus*, the more common organism, colonizes on the skin and in the nose and throat. Children may pick their nose and infect themselves. Bullous impetigo results from a strain of *S. aureus* that produces an exfoliative toxin that blisters the epidermis.

The impetigo lesion begins as a papule that turns into a vesicle at the injury site. The vesicle ruptures and forms an erosion, and serous fluid forms the characteristic honey-colored crusts. Pruritus and regional lymphadenopathy may be present. The rash may spread to the face and extremities by self-inoculation (Figure 57–5). In bullous impetigo, vesicles stimulated by a toxin enlarge and coalesce to form bullae with sharp margins and no surrounding erythema. A thin honey-colored crust forms when the bullae rupture. When the crust is removed, a moist, erythematous lesion with a collar of skin around the erosion is seen. These lesions occur more commonly in moist skinfold areas. Impetigo is diagnosed by appearance or lesions or by bacterial culture.

Local treatment of nonbullous impetigo involves removal of the crusts and application of a topical antibiotic. A topical bactericidal ointment such as mupirocin or retapamulin is applied 3 times a day for 5 days (Stevens et al., 2014). Oral antibiotics are prescribed for bullous impetigo. Skin generally heals without scars. The infection is communicable for 24 hours after antibiotic ointment treatment is begun.

Potential complications are postinfectious streptococcal glomerulonephritis (see Chapter 52) and cellulitis.

Nursing Management

Teach parents to soak crusts in warm water and gently scrub them off with a gauze pad and antiseptic soap prior to using topical ointment. Teach parents to dispose of the gauze pad in a plastic bag to avoid spreading the infection to other family members. Advise parents to continue using the topical or oral medication for the full number of days prescribed. Inform the parents to observe all close contacts and family members for lesions. The infected child should not share towels or toiletries with others, and all linens and clothing used by the child should be washed separately with detergent and hot water. Keep fingernails short and clean to prevent spreading infection by scratching. Inform the childcare center about the infection, so staff can sanitize toys and surfaces.

Community-Acquired Methicillin-Resistant *Staphylococcus aureus*

Community-acquired methicillin-resistant *Staphylococcus aureus* (CA-MRSA) may cause a severe and aggressive skin and soft-tissue infection in healthy children. CA-MRSA is colonized on the skin, the mucous membranes, and nares of healthy individual carriers. Direct contact transmission and respiratory droplet transmission occur. Athletes are at high risk because of their potential for frequent skin-to-skin contact, cuts or abrasions, wound contact, and shared items.

Clinical manifestations include furuncles or abscesses that may invade deeper tissues. Localized swelling, redness, warmth, purulent drainage, fever, and pain may be present.

Incised abscesses are cultured to diagnose CA-MRSA. Simple abscesses are treated with incision, drainage, wound care, and systemic antibiotics. Children with repeated CA-MRSA infections may be encouraged to bathe in a tub with a diluted bleach solution (one half cup to a tub one quarter full) (Neville-Swensen & Clayton, 2011).

Clinical Tip

When the child has recurrent CA-MRSA infections, the child or family member may be a nasal carrier of *S. aureus*. All household members may be treated with nasal application of mupiricin 2 times a day for 5 days and bathe with diluted bleach solution (one half cup to a tub one quarter full) or chlorhexidine scrub for 5 days. Surfaces frequently touched and bed linens must be decontaminated. A second round of household treatment may be needed (Fritz et al., 2012).

Nursing Management

Ensure that parents and adolescents understand the importance of taking the full course of the prescribed antibiotic. Educate parents about meticulous wound care to prevent the spread of CA-MRSA:

- Keep the wound and drainage completely covered at all times.
- Change the dressing twice a day using vinyl gloves. Use good hand hygiene before and after dressing changes.
- Dispose of used dressings in a tightly closed plastic bag.
- Disinfect surfaces that come into contact with the wound or wound drainage using a bleach solution.
- Use hot water to wash linens and clothing used by the child, and dry clothes in a hot dryer.

Nurses have a major role in prevention of CA-MRSA infections. Nurses in contact with the wound should remove gloves before touching and contaminating surfaces in the examining room. Ensure that any equipment and linen used by the child are appropriately managed and the examining room is cleaned with an effective agent.

Educate parents, adolescents, coaches, and teachers about the importance of a regular schedule for cleaning equipment and having athletes take showers with soap and water after all practice sessions. Discourage athletes from sharing towels and clothing. Cover minor wounds to reduce exposure to other athletes. Skin infections that worsen rather than heal with regular topical antibiotics should be seen by a healthcare provider.

Folliculitis

Folliculitis is a superficial inflammation of the pilosebaceous follicle caused by infection, trauma, or irritation. The causative organism is usually *Staphylococcus aureus*. The condition is common in children and teenagers because of increased sweat production. Folliculitis may be associated with *Pseudomonas aeruginosa* exposure in a poorly chlorinated pool or hot tub.

Symptoms include pain or pruritus, localized swelling, and the formation of tiny dome-shaped, yellowish pustules and red papules at follicular openings with surrounding erythema. Individual lesions may become deeper and form an abscess (furuncle). Lesions are usually seen in clusters on the face, scalp, trunk, and extremities. Some children have fever, aching, and flulike symptoms. If associated with *Pseudomonas* exposure in a pool or hot tub, lesions may develop on areas covered by bathing suits.

Folliculitis is treated by washing the affected area with a topical antibacterial cleanser (e.g., chlorhexidine) and water. A benzoyl peroxide gel or wash or another drying agent will also help clear the infection. Ruptured lesions heal with hyperpigmentation and no scarring. Complications are rare. If the child or adolescent has systemic symptoms, oral antibiotics (e.g., clindamycin or doxycycline) may be prescribed. If a furuncle develops, incision and drainage may be needed. Children who are immunocompromised should not use hot tubs because of the potential for complications from *Pseudomonas*.

Nursing Management

Nursing management focuses on educating the parents and child about prevention. Advise children to shower daily and shortly after exercise, to cleanse with an antibacterial soap, and to wear loose cotton clothing. Talk with parents about the importance of maintaining the correct pH level and chlorine concentration in swimming pools and hot tubs. Bathing suits of affected children should be laundered and dried well before the next use.

Cellulitis

Cellulitis is an acute inflammation of the loose connective and subcutaneous tissues and the dermis. The condition usually occurs on the face and extremities as a result of trauma or a compromised skin barrier.

ETIOLOGY AND PATHOPHYSIOLOGY

The child may have a history of trauma, surgery, or skin lesions. Common causative organisms are *Staphylococcus aureus* and *Streptococcus pyogenes*. The condition may also result from a nearby abscess or sinusitis. Onset is usually rapid.

CLINICAL MANIFESTATIONS

Children with cellulitis have a rapid onset and they appear ill. Classic signs and symptoms include red or lilac, tender, warm, edematous skin around the infected site (Figure 57–6). The border is often indistinct because the infection is deep in the tissue. Other symptoms include fever, chills, malaise, and enlargement and tenderness of regional lymph nodes. **Lymphangitis**, inflammation of the lymphatic system draining the site of infection (seen as tender, erythematous streaks extending in a proximal direction), may be present.

CLINICAL THERAPY

Blood studies may show an increase in white blood cells. Cultures are taken by needle aspiration to identify the causative organisms. Blood cultures and a lumbar puncture are performed if the child has a toxic (very ill) appearance (see the *Clinical Skills Manual* SKILLS).

Children with severe cases or involvement of the face or a large affected surface area are hospitalized and treated aggressively with IV antibiotics and analgesics to avoid serious complications, such as sepsis, necrotizing fasciitis, or osteomyelitis. Children with less severe cellulitis on the trunk, limbs, or perianal area may be treated on an outpatient basis with

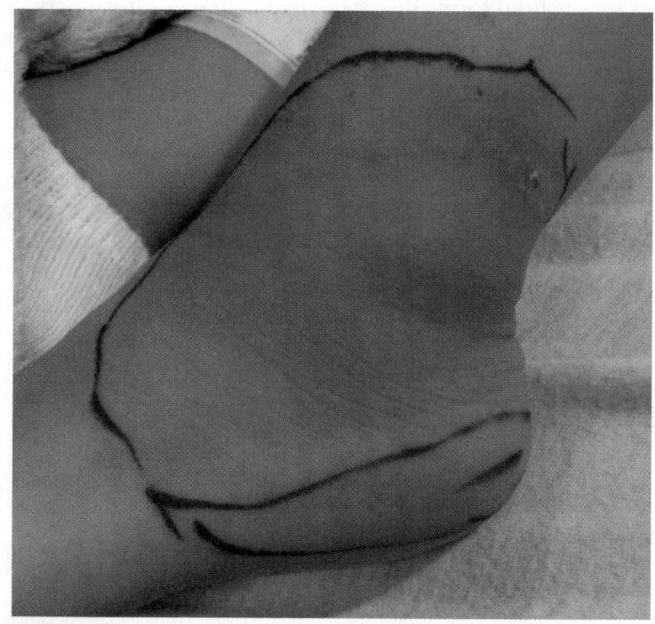

Figure 57–6 Characteristic appearance of cellulitis.

SOURCE: Courtesy of Daniel P. Krowchuk, MD, Professor of Pediatrics and Dermatology, Wake Forest School of Medicine, Winston-Salem, NC.

oral antibiotics. Recovery begins within 48 hours, but therapy should continue for at least 10 days (Juern & Drolet, 2016). See Chapter 45 for treatment of periorbital cellulitis.

Nursing Management

Assessment centers on recognition of the severity of infection, documentation of location and related symptoms, and monitoring of vital signs. Administer prescribed oral or IV antibiotics as scheduled. Supportive care includes warm compresses to the affected area 4 times daily, elevation of the affected limb, and bed rest. Outpatient follow-up is crucial to ensure response to therapy.

Advise parents about possible complications, such as abscess formation. Instruct parents of children treated at home to contact their healthcare provider if the child has any of the following signs:

- Spread of the infected area in the 24- to 48-hour period after the start of treatment
- Temperature over 38.3°C (101.0°F)
- Increased lethargy

Reinforce to parents the importance of compliance with the treatment regimen and the seriousness of the possible complications.

Viral Infections
Molluscum Contagiosum

Molluscum contagiosum is a skin infection caused by a poxvirus. It is transmitted by direct contact, contact with contaminated objects, or sexual contact. Spread occurs by autoinoculation. The incubation period is 2 to 7 weeks (American Academy of Pediatrics [AAP], 2015, p. 561). Children 2 to 11 years of age are most commonly affected, but increased risk is believed to be associated with atopic eczema and immunodeficiency.

Multiple pearl-like flesh-colored smooth papules (usually less than 30) are about 2 to 5 mm (0.08 to 0.2 in.) in size. The lesion has a central depression, and a plug of cheesy material can be expressed when punctured. Lesions may appear anywhere on the body, but are more often found on the face, trunk, and extremities. Adolescents may have lesions on the genital mucous membranes. If children have genital lesions, consider possible sexual abuse.

Supportive care is often preferred because aggressive treatments frequently cause scars or hyperpigmentation in children with darker skin. A single lesion may be present for 2 months, but the usual duration of the condition is 8 to 12 months, resolving spontaneously. Emollients, topical corticosteroids, or oral antihistamines are used for pruritus. When treatment is provided, options to destroy lesions include curettage, **cryotherapy** (freezing each lesion with liquid nitrogen), or pulsed-dye laser. Topical anesthesia is needed for curettage. Other treatment options include chemical treatment (e.g., salicylic acid or cantharidin), an immune modulator (e.g., imiquimod), or antiviral medication. No one treatment has demonstrated better effectiveness (Chen, Anstey, & Bugert, 2013). Secondary infections are a potential complication.

Nursing Management

Nursing education focuses on reducing disease transmission. Infected children should not use public swimming pools, hot tubs, or bathe with other children because the virus is more easily transmitted when the skin is wet. Transmission of the virus among household members is high. Towels, sponges, and clothing should not be shared. Wash the skin daily with gentle fragrance-free cleansers. Apply a hypoallergenic moisturizer or emollient to the entire skin surface. Teach parents to recognize potential secondary infections.

When intervention such as curettage or cryotherapy is performed, ensure that adequate topical anesthetic is used to minimize pain. Inform the child about what will happen, and provide distraction during the procedure to reduce anxiety.

Warts (Papillomavirus)

Warts commonly are found in children between 1 and 17 years, with a prevalence of 3.3% in the United States. The peak age is 9 to 10 years when 8.6% of children are affected (Silverberg & Silverberg, 2013). Several types of human papillomavirus infect epithelial cells and cause warts. Common warts appear on any skin surface, and plantar warts are found on the feet. The virus is commonly transmitted by direct skin-to-skin contact or mucous membrane contact. It also survives on various surfaces, and transmission can occur with contact, such as plantar warts from locker room floors. The incubation period may be 2 to 6 months; however, a latency period may exist in some cases. Children with immune compromise are more susceptible and often have numerous warts.

Common warts appear as skin-colored, rough, scaly papules and nodules on exposed skin surfaces. Individual and multiple warts may be seen, or large plaques may form if autoinoculation occurs. Warts usually cause no pain or itching unless on skin surface areas that becomes irritated. Plantar warts appear as papules and plaques on the bottom of feet that grow inward and cause pain. Small black dots result from thrombosed vessels on the surface of the warts caused by weight bearing.

No intervention may be recommended as warts often resolve spontaneously over a couple of years. Warts do not produce scarring unless treated surgically or in an aggressive manner. If warts cause pain or a social stigma, clinical therapy may be initiated. Treatment usually involves destruction by daily home application of salicylic acid plasters, and occlusion with tape is sometimes recommended. Other treatments include liquid nitrogen or pulsed-dye laser. No one treatment is fully effective. A keratolytic agent (imiquimod) may be used to treat external anogenital warts. Immunotherapy may also be used.

Nursing Management

Educate the parents and child about how warts are spread by picking at it or chewing on it. If the child will not stop sucking or chewing on the wart, bitter apple or a pepper solution may discourage the child. Teach parents about the application of peeling agents when prescribed for home use. If the reaction to the treatment is painful, encourage the parents to reduce the frequency of the treatment until the pain subsides and then to resume the original treatment schedule. Successful treatment may take several months, and parents may need encouragement to continue the therapy and remain optimistic.

Other viral skin conditions are described in Chapter 43.

Fungal Infections
Oral Candidal Infection (Thrush)

Thrush is a fungal infection, usually caused by *Candida albicans*. An acute infection may occur in newborns or in children who regularly use a corticosteroid inhaler or have received

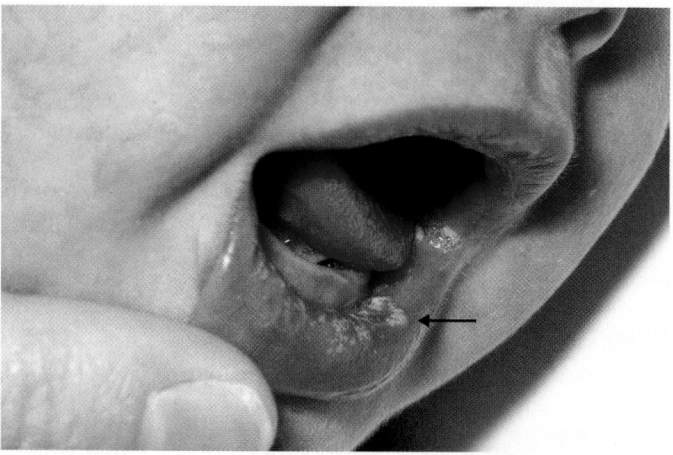

Figure 57–7 Oral thrush is an acute pseudomembranous form of candidiasis. It is a common fungal infection in infants and children.

SOURCE: Alamy.

antibiotics that disturb normal flora. An invasive *Candida* infection may occur in children with either an impaired immune status (immunodeficiency) or a central venous catheter receiving long-term parenteral alimentation therapy (AAP, 2015, p. 275). See Chapter 27 for newborn oral candidal infection.

Oral thrush is characterized by white patches that look like coagulated milk on the oral mucosa and may bleed when removed (Figure 57–7). Gentle attempts to remove patches are unsuccessful, while actual milk residue can be removed with gentle swabbing. The infant may refuse to nurse or feed because of discomfort and pain. The infant may also have diaper dermatitis. Fever is usually not present.

Diagnosis is made by clinical appearance, microscopic examination of a skin scraping suspended in potassium hydroxide, or fungal culture. Treatment involves oral nystatin suspension or clotrimazole applied to the mouth and tongue after feedings. Fluconazole or itraconazole may be used for immunocompromised patients with oropharyngeal candidiasis. Intravenous amphotericin B may be used for invasive and systemic *Candida* infections.

Nursing Management

Teach parents to give the medication by swabbing the suspension on the buccal mucosa and tongue surfaces, allowing the infant to swallow the remaining suspension. Teach older children to swish the solution around in the mouth before swallowing it.

To help prevent a reinfection, educate parents to use good hand hygiene and to sterilize bottle nipples and pacifiers. Teach parents and older children with asthma to rinse the mouth well with water after using a corticosteroid inhaler. If a spacer is used, it should also be rinsed with water after use. A commercial antiseptic spray may be used on toys put in the mouth that cannot be autoclaved, but follow directions carefully so the child does not ingest any harmful residue.

Dermatophytoses (Ringworm)

Dermatophytoses are fungal infections that commonly affect the skin, hair, or nails. Children of all ages may be affected. Dermatophytoses may be spread from another person or animal or by contact with a contaminated object. See Table 57–4 for the clinical manifestations of tinea infections.

Diagnosis is confirmed through microscopic examination of the hair and scalp scrapings using a potassium hydroxide (KOH) wet mount to reveal rows and chains of spores within the hair shaft. A fungal culture can also be taken from a scalp lesion by rubbing a cotton-tipped applicator across the scalp or body lesion. Shining a Wood lamp on the lesion helps identify some forms of tinea (e.g., microsporum fluoresces a brilliant green). The most common cause of tinea, *Trichophyton tonsurans*, does not fluoresce (AAP, 2015, p. 780). See Table 57–4 for clinical therapy.

Clinical Tip

Some children treated for tinea capitis develop an "id" reaction, an extensive, itchy papulovesicular rash on the trunk, extremities, and face similar to atopic dermatitis. This is a hypersensitivity reaction to the fungal antigen, not an allergic reaction to the oral medication (AAP, 2015, p. 779). Antifungal therapy must be continued to resolve the infection.

Nursing Management

Assess all members of the family and household pets for fungal lesions. Since person-to-person transmission is common, family members should not share hair accessories, brushes, and hats. Because a family member may be an asymptomatic carrier, all family members should be treated with selenium shampoo. Teach parents and older children or teenagers that fungi are found in soil and animals and are transmitted through direct contact.

Advise parents to give oral griseofulvin with fatty foods such as whole milk or peanut butter to enhance absorption. To prevent recurrence of the infection, the medications must be used for the entire prescribed period, even if the lesions are gone. Advise parents about the possibility of the "id" reaction so they will continue to give the medication.

Parents of children with tinea capitis should be told that hair regrowth is slow and may take 6 to 12 months. In rare cases, hair loss is permanent, which can be particularly stressful for older children or adolescents. Provide emotional support. Encourage children to wear shower shoes in public showers and locker rooms to prevent tinea pedis.

Drug Reactions

Adverse reactions to over-the-counter or prescription medications are relatively common. Children with drug allergies usually have reactions after ingestion (e.g., aspirin, antibiotics, sedatives), injection (e.g., penicillin), or direct skin contact with medications. Drug sensitivities may result from variations in an individual's ability to tolerate a particular drug or concentration of a drug or from allergic responses. (See Chapter 48 for a description of allergic reactions.)

Sensitivity reactions may occur after 1 or 2 doses when the child has previously taken the drug, but it may take up to 7 days for sensitivity to occur to a drug not previously administered. The most common reactions in children are erythematous macules and papules or urticaria, which may be pruritic. Drugs that may cause a sensitivity reaction include the following: sulfonamides, anticonvulsants, antibiotics, and nonsteroidal anti-inflammatory drugs (NSAIDs). Be alert to the possibility of serious drug reactions that may become a medical emergency. See Table 57–5 for clinical manifestations of drug reactions.

TABLE 57–4 Clinical Manifestations of Tinea Infections

INFECTION SITE AND CLINICAL MANIFESTATIONS	CLINICAL THERAPY
TINEA CAPITIS (SCALP) Scaly pustular bald areas with indistinct margins; may appear as seborrhea, with yellow, greasy scales; erythema or lesion lighter than skin color Broken hairs; black dotted stubbed appearance where weakened hair has broken off Mild itching **Kerion**—large purulent tender boggy mass on scalp with drainage 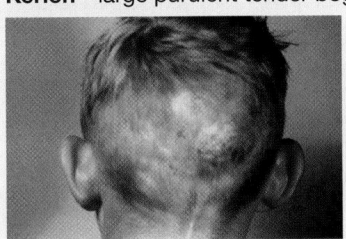 Tinea capitis. Centers for Disease Control and Prevention.	Oral griseofulvin for 8–12 weeks, OR oral terbinafine for 6 weeks in children over age 4 years. Fluconazole and itraconazole are not U.S. Food and Drug Administration (FDA) approved in children less than 12 years of age. Selenium sulfide or ketoconazole shampoo 2–3 times weekly, leaving the shampoo on the scalp for 10 min before rinsing. Encourage family members to use the shampoo 2–3 times a week to reduce the number of fungal spores in the household. For kerions with evidence of secondary bacterial infection, antibiotics are added to oral antifungal agents (AAP, 2015, p. 781).
TINEA CORPORIS (TRUNK) Pink, scaly circular patch with an expanding border, may be scaly or erythematous throughout; slightly raised borders with a clearing center Usually acquired from contact with infected human, animal, or contaminated object (e.g., hat) 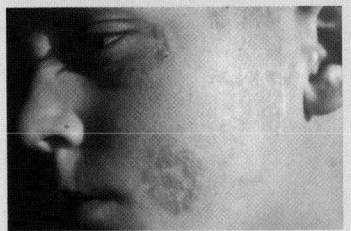 Tinea corporis. Centers for Disease Control and Prevention.	Topical cream (e.g., clotrimazole, miconazole, ketoconazole, terbinafine if 12 years and older or tolnaftate, naftifine, or ciclopirox if 10 years and older) twice a day for 4–6 weeks. Do not use a topical corticosteroid to prevent a persistent or recurrent infection. Selenium sulfide shampoo 2 times a week on the child's body to help reduce the number of spores. Family members may also use the shampoo. An oral antifungal agent when no response to topical therapy.
TINEA CRURIS ("JOCK ITCH") Scaly, erythematous annular lesions on groin and upper thighs, may spread to the abdomen and buttocks; usually spares the penis and scrotum May have elevated lesions, papules, or vesicles	Topical antifungal agent (e.g., clotrimazole, miconazole, and terbinafine for ages 12 years and older, tolnaftate or ciclopirox for 10 years and older) for 4–6 weeks. Topical corticosteroids are not used. Wash body area with selenium sulfide shampoo. Wear loose clothing to promote dryness in the groin area.
TINEA PEDIS ("ATHLETE'S FOOT") Vesicles or erosions on instep or between toes (fissures, red scaly); dry scaly patches or plaques with erythema on plantar and lateral surfaces of foot Peeling maceration and fissures in lateral toe web spaces indicate secondary bacterial involvement Pruritus	Broad-spectrum topical antifungal agent with antibacterial properties (e.g., econazole or ciclopirox) Allow feet to air dry. Use 100% cotton socks, change twice daily; put socks on before other clothing to reduce transmission of fungus to groin.

Source: Data from American Academy of Pediatrics, Committee on Infectious Disease. (2015). *Red book: Report of the Committee on Infectious Diseases* (30th ed., pp. 778–786). Elk Grove Village, IL: Author; Krowchuk, D. P., & Mancini, A. J. (2012). *Pediatric dermatology: A quick reference guide* (2nd ed., pp. 233–245). American Academy of Pediatrics; and Wyatt, H. (2013). Common skin infections in children. *Nursing Standard, 27*(46), 43–48.

The treatment of choice for most drug sensitivity reactions is discontinuation of the causative drug. In rare cases, a drug may be continued with careful monitoring when the child has a less severe sensitivity reaction because it is the best treatment choice. Supportive measures should be taken to decrease the intensity of the reaction. An antihistamine may be used to block the release of histamine, which causes the rash. Topical corticosteroids, cool compresses, and baths may also be prescribed for pruritus. For some severe drug reactions, the child must be hospitalized and treated on a burn unit.

TABLE 57–5 Clinical Manifestations of Drug Reactions

TYPE OF REACTION	CLINICAL MANIFESTATIONS
ALLERGIC DRUG REACTION	
Most commonly caused by sulfonamides, tetracyclines, NSAIDs, oral contraceptives, barbiturates, phenytoin, carbamazepine, benzodiazepines, and morphine	Erythematous, pruritic macules and papules; urticaria (hives) begins on the trunk and extends in a symmetric fashion, often sparing mucous membranes. Affected area darkens over 1–2 weeks, and skin peeling may occur. May heal with pigment changes.
ERYTHEMA MULTIFORME MINOR	
Hypersensitivity reaction to anticonvulsants, penicillins, salicylates, sulfa antibiotics, barbiturates, and phenytoin; infectious agents (e.g., herpes simplex virus)	Skin lesions may be preceded by fever, malaise, and upper respiratory symptoms. Widespread erythematous macules progress to target lesions (papules, vesicles, or bullae in a pale ring with an erythematous border). May progress to blisters and bullous lesions. Lesions may itch or burn. Lesions common on palms and soles, elbows, extensor surface of forearms and legs.
STEVENS–JOHNSON SYNDROME (SJS) AND TOXIC EPIDERMAL NECROLYSIS (TEN)	
Potentially life-threatening hypersensitivity reaction to penicillins, sulfonamides, cephalosporins, fluoroquinolones, antiepileptic medications, NSAIDs, acetaminophen, or reaction to infectious disease such as *Mycoplasma pneumoniae* Believed to be forms of the same disease and the most severe form of erythema multiforme.	Prodromal infection for 1–7 days with low-grade fever, sore throat, or malaise. Headache, muscle aches, joint pain, and vomiting and diarrhea may be seen. Erythematous skin is tender, progressing to blisters and bullae, and then to necrotic epidermis that sheds and weeps. Mucous membranes have blisters, erosions, ulcerations, and hemorrhagic crusting. Painful crusting and sloughing of the lips and oral membranes occur. Respiratory and gastrointestinal mucosa may also be affected. Erosions (similar to partial-thickness burns) may spread to cover up to 10% of the skin surface in SJS, 10%–30% in overlapping SJS and TEN, and more than 30% in TEN. Corneal blistering can lead to scarring and blindness.

Source: Data from Nicol, N. H., & Huether, S. E. (2014). Alterations in the integument in children. In K. L. McCance, S. E. Huether, V. L. Brashers, & N. S. Rote (Eds.), *Pathophysiology: The biologic basis for disease in adults and children* (7th ed., pp. 1653–1667), St. Louis, MO: Elsevier; Joyce, J. C. (2016). Vesiculobullous disorders. In R. M. Kliegman, B. F. Stanton, J. W. St. Geme, & N. F. Schor (Eds.), *Nelson textbook of pediatrics* (20th ed., pp. 3140–3150). St. Louis, MO: Elsevier; Feinberg, A. N., Shwayder, T. A., Ruqiya, T., & Therdpong, T. (2014). Pediatric dermatologic disorders. *Journal of Alternative Medicine Research, 6*(2), 95–137; Yang, M., Kang, M., Jung, J., Song, W., Kang, H.,Cho, S., & Min, K. (2013). Clinical features and prognostic factors in severe cutaneous drug reactions. *International Archives of Allergy and Immunology, 162*(4) 346–354.

Nursing Management

Teach parents to be alert for the signs of drug sensitivity reactions. Obtain a careful history of the child's past reactions to medications before starting new therapies. If a reaction occurs, discontinue the medication until the healthcare provider is notified. See the section on burns later in this chapter for nursing care the child with a severe drug reactions.

SAFETY ALERT!

Children with a true drug allergy (having a past serious systemic reaction) should never be treated with that drug again. Prominently mark the child's records so that all allergies are easily identified. The child should wear some type of medical alert identification.

Chronic Skin Conditions

Atopic Dermatitis

Atopic dermatitis (eczema) is a chronic, relapsing, superficial inflammatory skin disorder characterized by intense pruritus (Figure 57–8). The condition affects approximately 20% of infants, children, and adolescents (Nicol & Huether, 2014). Up to 60% of children who develop the condition do so during the first year of life (Roduit et al., 2012). Most children have or develop allergic conditions such as asthma or food allergy.

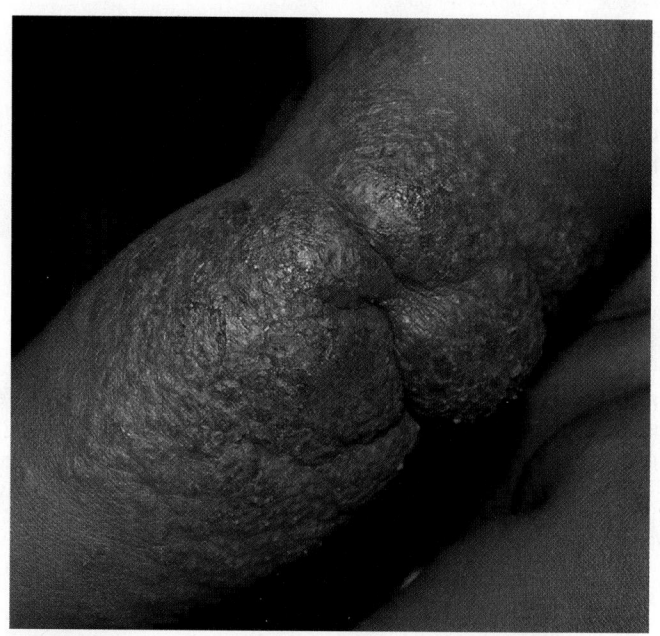

Figure 57–8 Severe atopic dermatitis in an infant. Note the thick (i.e., lichenified), hyperpigmented plaque on the extensor surface of the elbow.

SOURCE: Courtesy of Daniel P. Krowchuk, MD, Professor of Pediatrics and Dermatology, Wake Forest School of Medicine, Winston-Salem, NC.

ETIOLOGY AND PATHOPHYSIOLOGY

It is believed that mutations in the *filaggrin* gene are associated with a defective skin barrier that allows epidermal water loss that leads to **xerosis**, generally dry skin that is likely to crack and fissure. This also permits the penetration of allergens, irritants, and organisms. Both an IgE-mediated immediate immune response and T-cell–mediated delayed immune response are involved. The inflammatory response with cytokines, T-lymphocytes, and other cells plus scratching further damages the skin barrier (Tom, 2012). While food allergies often occur in children with atopic dermatitis, food allergies do not cause the condition (Tollefson, Bruckner, & Section on Dermatology, 2014).

Decreased recognition of pathogens by immune receptors and decreased response by neutrophils and natural killer cells after an infectious agent enters the skin leads to more skin infections, such as *Staphylococcus aureus*, which is colonized on the skin of 90% of affected children (Tollefson et al., 2014; Tom, 2012).

CLINICAL MANIFESTATIONS

Acute atopic dermatitis is characterized by patches with papules, vesicles, exudate, crusts, and excoriation. Some patches may weep. Chronic atopic dermatitis characteristics include darkened, thickened skin with prominent skin lines (lichenification), excoriation, dryness, and scaling. Inflammation usually occurs on the face, neck, and extensor surfaces in infants. The diaper area is usually spared in infants because the skin is damp and protected from scratching. The antecubital and popliteal skinfolds are often affected after age 2 years. Adolescents may additionally have these areas affected: the eyelids, where the earlobe touches the face, fingertips, toes, nipples, and the vulva.

The itching interferes with sleep and causes irritability. The child moves so much because of the itching discomfort that a perception of hyperactivity may occur. Erythema and warmth may indicate a secondary bacterial infection. Some children have repeated flares or chronic atopic dermatitis that persists into adulthood. Other children may have skin resolution when respiratory symptoms such as asthma develop.

CLINICAL THERAPY

Atopic dermatitis is distinguished by its history and clinical manifestations. Diagnostic features of atopic dermatitis include an early age of onset, parent or sibling with history of atopy, pruritus, dry skin, and the typical distribution of lesions for age, such as the cheeks, scalp, trunk, and extremities during infancy, the flexural areas during childhood, and the hands and feet during adolescence (Tollefson et al., 2014). No laboratory tests are diagnostic; however, children have an elevated IgE level. A skin culture may be obtained when secondary infection occurs.

Because there is no cure, the goals of treatment are to hydrate and lubricate the skin, reduce pruritus, minimize inflammatory responses, manage infectious triggers, and treat skin infections. The skin is hydrated by bathing, and then the entire body is lubricated by applying occlusive topical emollients within 3 minutes of leaving the water. This traps moisture in the skin and promotes flexibility of the skin without cracking. Moisturizing ointments and creams are applied 3 to 4 times a day, or when the skin feels dry.

Clinical Tip

Select fragrance-free emollients with a cream or ointment base that have the fewest preservatives. Lotions contain alcohol that will further dry the skin. Examples of emollients include Eucerin cream, Aveeno cream, Vanicream, Cetaphil cream, SBR-Lipocream, and petroleum jelly. Petroleum jelly (e.g., Vaseline) has the benefit of lower cost, especially since so much of the emollient must be used to cover the entire body each day.

Topical corticosteroids reduce inflammation and achieve quick control. Ointments are preferred over creams because of their occlusive effect, which ensures a stronger barrier and absorption into the skin. Many different preparations and seven categories of corticosteroid strength exist. Moderate-strength corticosteroids are used twice daily for 2 weeks under the emollient. Low-strength corticosteroids are used for thinner skin areas, such as the face, diaper area, and skinfolds. When the inflammation resolves, topical corticosteroids are tapered in frequency of application and potency and then discontinued. To reduce the risk for steroid side effects, topical steroids are not used on healthy skin. Oral corticosteroids are not commonly used because of a rebound effect may occur in which a more severe rash returns after the medication is discontinued (Tollefson et al., 2014).

SAFETY ALERT!

The potency or strength of a topical corticosteroid is based on whether it is fluorinated and contains other ingredients. Refer to a drug manual to identify the corticosteroid potency, not the percentage listed on the medication label. Avoid the use of higher potency corticosteroids on the face, genitalia, and skinfolds where absorption of the medication is increased because of the thinness of the skin. Intraocular hypertension, cataracts, skin atrophy, and adrenal suppression are potential adverse effects of higher potency topical corticosteroids.

Immunomodulator ointments such as tacrolimus (Protopic) and pimecrolimus (Elidel) are increasingly used as a second-line treatment for some children. Disadvantages include the cost of these medications and burning with application as perceived by some children. The medications are approved by the U.S. Food and Drug Administration (FDA) for children over 2 years of age, for short-term or intermittent treatment, who are not responsive to conventional therapy. The FDA has placed a black box warning on both drugs because of rare cases of malignancy (Tom, 2012).

The *Staphylococcus aureus* colonization on the child's skin may trigger an immune cascade that increases pruritus. Topical, oral, or IV antibiotics may be selected depending on severity of infection. Cephalexin is a common oral antibiotic used to treat *S. aureus* when CA-MRSA is not involved. When the child's skin condition does not respond, a skin culture may be needed to identify the correct antibiotic. Superinfections with herpes simplex may be treated with oral or intravenous acyclovir, depending on the severity of the infection. Children may be encouraged to soak in a tub with dilute chlorine bleach (one half cup to a tub one quarter full) once or twice a week to help reduce the number of *S. aureus* infections (Tollefson et al., 2014).

Pruritus is a significant problem, and treatment of flare-ups is the best way to reduce itching. Oral antihistamines have a limited effect on itching, but the sedative effect may help promote sleep. Tolerance to the sedating effects of these medications occurs, so their use is limited to 2 to 7 nights during a flare-up, when scratching interferes with sleep. Topical antihistamines are not recommended because of the potential for hypersensitivity reactions and contact dermatitis. Environmental control may be helpful. A humidifier in the winter counteracts dryness of the surrounding air, minimizing loss of skin moisture. Air conditioning in the summer limits unnecessary sweating that can exacerbate inflamed areas.

Food allergies causing urticaria and pruritus may aggravate atopic dermatitis. When the child younger than age 5 years has atopic dermatitis that does not respond to optimal management, efforts may be made to identify specific allergies to foods such as eggs, cow's milk, wheat, soy, and peanuts (Tollefson et al., 2014). See Chapter 32 for more information on food allergies and food elimination trials to identify food allergies.

Nursing Management

For the Child With Atopic Dermatitis

Nursing Assessment and Diagnosis

Take a thorough history, including any family history of allergy, environmental or dietary factors, past exacerbations, and what triggers a flare. For example, common triggers include harsh soaps and detergents, fragrances, rough nonbreathable clothing, sweat, and psychosocial stress. Note distribution and type of lesions, presence of weeping, or signs of infection.

Identify the impact that the skin disorder is having on the child and family. How much is the sleep of the child, siblings, or other family members disturbed? Is the child's self-esteem disturbed? What other stresses has the child's skin disorder placed on the family? Does the family have concerns about topical steroid medication use?

Common nursing diagnoses that may be appropriate for the child with atopic dermatitis include the following (NANDA-I © 2014):

- *Tissue Integrity, Impaired,* related to chemical irritants and mechanical factors (abrasive clothing)

- *Insomnia* related to prolonged physical discomfort (itching)

- *Infection, Risk for,* related to breaks in skin barrier

- *Self-Esteem, Chronic Low,* related to peer reaction to visible skin lesions

- *Health Management, Family, Ineffective,* related to excessive demands made on the family to keep the condition under control

Planning and Implementation

Nursing management focuses on education and emotional support. Atopic dermatitis can be controlled, but there is no cure. Advise parents that the lesions are not contagious and usually do not scar. Daily optimal management often reduces flares, but the time it takes is a family stressor. Emphasize the importance of following the daily treatment plan to promote healing of existing lesions and to reduce the risk of secondary infections. See *Teaching Highlights: Atopic Dermatitis Daily Skin Care.* Help parents and adolescents deal with the frustration of the acute flare-ups of the condition by reinforcing that remissions do occur with good home care.

Clinical Tip

Application of emollients daily to the entire body of newborns with a parent or sibling with atopic dermatitis or atopic condition has been suggested as a strategy to postpone the onset of atopic dermatitis. A pilot study involving 124 families demonstrated reduced incidence in newborns with daily emollient treatment compared to to babies with routine newborn skin care (Simpson et al., 2014). This may be a potential future strategy for newborns at high risk of atopic dermatitis.

The child, parents, and siblings are often tired because of lost sleep when the child scratches at night during an acute flare-up. School performance may be affected if the child has sleep deprivation or if the child is experiencing physical discomfort that interferes with learning. The itching and scratching may cause constant movement similar to attention-deficit hyperactivity. If an oral antihistamine has been ordered, make sure the parents understand when to give the medication to maximize its effectiveness for better sleep.

Atopic dermatitis produces visible changes that can affect a child's self-confidence and self-esteem. Identify activities that the child can participate in to improve self-esteem. Even though humidity and sweating can make eczema worse, encourage the child to participate in sports. The child should shower as soon as possible after strenuous activity and then apply needed medications and emollients.

Provide encouragement and positive reinforcement for improvements in the child's skin during healthcare visits. Ensure that a focus is on the child's health promotion during visits. See *Health Promotion: The Child With Atopic Dermatitis.* Encourage the parents to support the child's self-esteem. Atopic dermatitis is difficult to manage and may have a more profound effect on the child's and family's quality of life.

When atopic dermatitis is under control, educate parents that increased itching within hours of eating a food may be associated with a food allergy that aggravates atopic dermatitis. If a specific food allergy, such as eggs, has been identified, educate the parents about strategies for avoidance of food products that contain the allergen. Nutritional counseling may be needed to make sure the child has food options that meet daily nutritional requirements.

Evaluation

Expected outcomes of nursing care include the following:

- The child's atopic dermatitis is controlled and no infection occurs.

TEACHING HIGHLIGHTS | Atopic Dermatitis Daily Skin Care

- Have the child soak in the bathtub 10–15 minutes or shower once a day. Use mild, unscented soap only on dirty areas. Salt or baking soda added to the bath water may help if water stings the child's open lesions. Rinse and pat excess water from the skin and apply adequate emollient to the entire body within 3 minutes to trap moisture in the skin.
- Help the parents select an unscented emollient ointment or cream (Eucerin, Aveeno, Vanicream, Cetaphil, SBR Lipocream, or petroleum jelly) that fits into the family's budget. Large quantities are needed to cover the entire body twice a day. Petroleum jelly is inexpensive, safe, and easily applied.
- In regions with low humidity, apply emollients to the skin more frequently.
- Help ensure that parents receive adequate amounts of topical corticosteroids for effective treatment of a flare-up. When the child has a flare-up, bathe the child twice a day and apply the topical medications on inflamed areas, spreading thinly and rubbing in. Emollients are applied on top of medications as well as over the rest of the body.
- If immunomodulators are prescribed rather than topical corticosteroids, spread a pea-size amount to cover a 2-in. (5-cm) circle over the inflamed area. Apply emollients as for topical corticosteroids.
- Encourage the child to wear loose cotton clothing rather than wool or other irritating fabrics.
- Keep the child's fingernails trimmed and use clean cotton gloves or socks over the infant's or child's hands to decrease scratching and reduce the chance of secondary infection.
- Contact the child's healthcare provider if signs of infection are noted so that antibiotic treatment can be started.

Health Promotion The Child With Atopic Dermatitis

Growth and Development Surveillance

- Assess growth measurements and plot on a growth chart. Identify any changes that could be related to an altered meal plan due to food allergies.
- Assess developmental progress for age.

Nutrition

- Postpone adding eggs to the infant's diet if atopic dermatitis develops early in infancy. Provide nutritional counseling to ensure the child gets all essential nutrients when foods must be avoided.

Physical Activity

- Encourage physical activity, but have the child bathe and apply emollients soon afterwards.
- After swimming have the child immediately rinse off chlorine after leaving the pool and apply emollients.

Family Interactions

- Identify how frequently the sleep of the child and other family members is disturbed by scratching. Encourage the use of an antihistamine to promote sleep when a skin flare-up occurs.
- Discuss strategies to effectively use time for daily skin care.

Mental and Spiritual Health

- Assess the child's self-esteem and impact of skin lesions on relationships with peers.
- Identify how disturbed sleep affects behavior and learning.

Disease Prevention Strategies

- Provide all immunizations on schedule.
- Encourage good hand hygiene to reduce the risk of infection.
- Educate the child and parents to provide skin care as described in *Teaching Highlights: Atopic Dermatitis Daily Skin Care* to reduce skin inflammation and the risk for secondary infection.

- Parents identify triggers of the child's atopic dermatitis and avoid or eliminate them.
- The child's sleep is minimally disturbed by itching.

Acne

Acne is a chronic inflammatory disorder of the pilosebaceous hair follicles on the face and trunk. It is the most common skin disorder in the pediatric population, affecting 85% of the population ages 12 to 25 years (Nicol & Huether, 2014). Acne is found in all ethnic groups, and occurs equally in male and female adolescents. Severe acne is more common in male adolescents. Adolescents with severe acne often have a genetic predisposition.

ETIOLOGY AND PATHOPHYSIOLOGY

Keratin and sebum usually flow to the skin surface through the hair follicles. Androgens, released as puberty begins, trigger the sebaceous glands to increase the production of sebum. When the extra sebum mixes with the keratinocytes and causes them to clump together, the hair follicle canal becomes obstructed by **comedones** (whiteheads and blackheads). The sebum behind the comedone is an ideal environment for the anaerobic bacterium *Propionibacterium acnes*, which metabolizes the sebum, leading to an increased response by inflammatory mediators (Kim & Mancini, 2013). When the inflammatory reaction is close to the surface, a papule or pustule develops. If the inflammatory reaction is deeper, a larger papule or nodule develops. When the follicles rupture, bacteria spreads and the resulting inflammation in the deeper tissues leads to nodules and cysts that can result in scars.

Acne may occur in neonates in response to maternal androgen hormones and androgens produced by the fetal adrenal glands. Neonatal acne usually resolves spontaneously in a few months. When acne occurs in children between 1 and 7 years, it may be associated with true precocious puberty or an androgen-secreting tumor (Kim & Mancini, 2013).

CLINICAL MANIFESTATIONS

Lesions occur most often on the face, upper chest, shoulders, and back. Comedones are initial skin lesions. Closed comedones are whiteheads or flesh-colored papules with tiny follicular openings. Open comedones are blackheads in which the follicular plug has enlarged and dilated the follicular opening. As inflammation occurs, papules and pustules develop (Figure 57–9). Nodules are larger areas of inflammation that may involve more than one hair follicle. Cysts are compressible nodules without overlying inflammation. Scars form when the surrounding dermis is damaged and may be pitted, atrophic, or hypertrophic (keloid).

CLINICAL THERAPY

Diagnosis is based on the examination of the skin. Treatment is customized to the predominant type of lesion present and severity of the lesions. The goal of treatment is to suppress lesions until the condition is outgrown, thus preventing infection and scarring, and minimizing psychologic distress. A variety of topical and oral medications are prescribed (see *Medications Used to Treat: Acne*). Acne will recur gradually if the treatment is stopped, so maintenance therapy with topical retinoids is recommended once acne is controlled.

Skin irritation related to topical preparations may occur in adolescents with sensitive skin. Using a lower-concentration

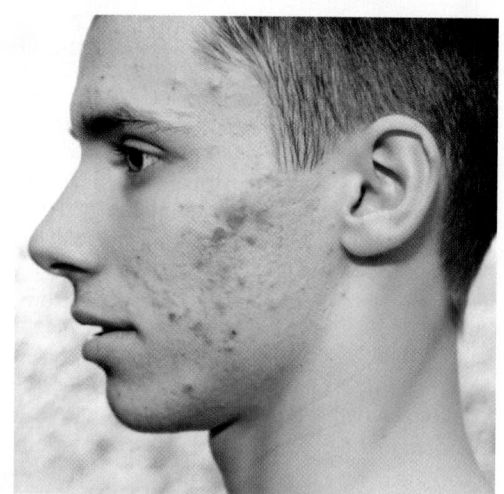

Figure 57–9 Note the comedones, papules, pustules, and healing lesions. Acne can have a significant effect on an adolescent's self-esteem.

SOURCE: bluecinema/Getty Images.

product and removing it after a few hours may reduce the initial irritation. With continued use the skin adapts, permitting the product concentration to be changed. Creams are used when skin is more sensitive, and gels are used when skin is oilier. (See *Developing Cultural Competence: Acne Lesions in Individuals With Dark Skin*.)

Isotretinoin (Accutane) is reserved for severe acne that is not responsive to other therapies. The daily 16- to 20-week course of treatment results in a dramatic improvement for up to 90% of patients (Studor-Heikenfeld & Colella, 2014). An intermittent lower-dose schedule over 6 to 18 months is also effective

Medications Used to Treat: Acne

MEDICATION AND ACTION	NURSING MANAGEMENT
Topical retinoids (tretinoin [Retin-A], adapalene, tazarotene) For mild or moderate papulopustular acne Regulates follicular keratinocyte shedding, has anti-inflammatory properties, helps to prevent new lesions, enhances penetration of topical antibiotics.	• Use lower concentrations initially as skin irritation is common. • Divide and spread a pea-sized amount over the entire face. Do not use as spot therapy. • Apply at night to reduce photosensitivity effect. • Use long term between flares for maintenance.
Benzoyl peroxide For mild or moderate papulopustular acne Topical antimicrobial with bacteriocidal action	• A lower strength may be used initially if skin irritation occurs. • Apply in the morning. • Inform clients that the product can bleach fabric.
Antibiotics (tetracycline, minocycline, erythromycin, doxycycline) Topical for mild inflammatory acne; oral for moderate to severe inflammatory acne Antimicrobial action reduces resident skin bacterial colonization.	• Combined with topical retinoid and benzoyl peroxide to reduce antibiotic resistance. • Takes 6–8 weeks to see improvement; antibiotic is changed if no response. Use is evaluated after 3 months to determine need for longer treatment. Avoid long-term use to reduce risk for antibiotic resistance.
Azelaic acid For mild or moderate papulopustular acne Keratolytic and anti-inflammatory properties	• Used in patients who cannot tolerate topical retinoids. • Apply twice daily.

MEDICATION AND ACTION	NURSING MANAGEMENT
Isotretinoin (Accutane) For severe nodular acne, especially when resistant to other treatment Causes sebaceous gland atrophy and decreases sebum production; reduces excess desquamation, bacteriocidal action, reduces inflammatory response, reverses effect of androgens on sebaceous glands.	• Requires informed consent. • Females need a monthly pregnancy test before each prescription refill as well as monthly tests for blood counts, lipid levels, and liver enzymes. • Females must use 2 forms of contraception, beginning 1 month prior to treatment, during treatment, and for 1 month after completing treatment to prevent pregnancy that would expose the fetus to teratogenic effects of the drug. • Take medication with food to increase oral absorption. • Encourage the use of sunscreen and protective clothing to prevent sunburn.
Oral contraceptives For persistent inflammatory papules and nodules Suppresses gonadotropin secretion and reduces ovarian androgen production.	• Use as an adjunct to other acne treatments. • May cause red, dry, and itching skin that can be treated with emollients. • Inform adolescent that acne may worsen during the first 3–6 weeks of treatment.
Spironolactone For severe acne Blocks the androgen receptor on the sebaceous gland.	• Prescribed for 1–3 months along with an antibiotic. • Not FDA approved for acne treatment, but commonly prescribed for that purpose.

Source: Data from Kim, W., & Mancini, A. J. (2013). Acne in childhood: An update. *Pediatric Annals, 42*(10), 418–427; Weinstein, M. (2013). Acne and the adolescent: A practical approach to management. *Contemporary Pediatrics, 30*(5), 30–36; Studor-Heikenfeld, J., & Colella, C. (2014). Isotretinoin: Reconsidering management of acne vulgaris in primary care. *Journal for Nurse Practitioners, 10*(9), 714–720.

Developing Cultural Competence Acne Lesions in Individuals With Dark Skin

Inflammatory acne in adolescents with darker skin color is associated with a dark discoloration as extra pigment gets deposited in the areas of inflammation. If protected from sun exposure, this darker coloration fades over 3 to 18 months. Encourage adolescents with dark skin to use noncomedonic sunscreen (SPF 30 or higher) whenever sun exposure is likely.

and has fewer side effects. Because isotretinoin is a teratogen, the FDA established the iPLEDGE program, a mandatory Internet-based registry for prescribers, patients, and pharmacies. See *Medications Used to Treat: Acne* for important guidelines. Inquire about prior episodes of depression and suicide attempts because of isotretinoin's potential association with both problems.

Nursing Management

For the Child With Acne

Nursing Assessment and Diagnosis

Physical assessment should include documentation regarding distribution, type, and severity of acne lesions. Assess the adolescent's and parents' knowledge about the cause and treatment of acne. Also explore the extent of emotional distress and low self-esteem that acne may be causing.

The accompanying *Nursing Care Plan: The Adolescent With Acne* lists common nursing diagnoses and summarizes nursing care.

Planning and Implementation

Nursing management focuses on educating the adolescent and parents about acne and its treatment. Encourage good hand hygiene before touching affected areas. Educate adolescents that picking and squeezing lesions may increase the inflammation when lesions rupture below the skin surface and may cause scarring. Excoriated acne lesions do not respond as well to the treatment used for the primary acne lesions. Inform the adolescent to avoid cleansing products with a greasy base, to shampoo the hair regularly, and to treat seborrheic dermatitis that can accompany acne. Correct misconceptions about dietary causes. Although no food is known to cause acne or increase the severity of lesions, good nutrition is important.

Topical medications should be spread in a thin film over the skin, according to directions. Inform the adolescent that treatment may seem to worsen acne as the comedones are being pushed out, and this is a sign that the medication is working. Emphasize that treatment is often long term. It may take at least 6 to 12 weeks for significant improvement to be seen after beginning treatment. Educate adolescents that healing lesions initially look like fading red areas, and, in some cases, hyperpigmented areas. Flare-ups are expected despite treatment, potentially caused by increased sweating, heat, humidity, and emotional stress.

Tretinoin is **phototoxic** (a rapid nonimmunologic reaction of the skin when exposed to sunlight), causing sunburn with even minimal exposure. Encourage adolescents to limit sun

Nursing Care Plan: The Adolescent With Acne

1. Nursing Diagnosis: *Health Maintenance, Ineffective,* related to daily hygiene and skin care (NANDA-I © 2014)

GOAL: The adolescent will verbalize proper hygiene, nutrition, and treatment of acne.

INTERVENTION	RATIONALE
• Teach good skin care:	• Good hygiene and appropriate skin care reduces irritation, surface oils, and bacteria, which intensify inflammatory reactions. Astringents and aftershave may contain alcohol and further dry the skin.
• Wash skin with mild soap and water twice a day.	
• Do not use astringents or abrasive cleansers.	
• Wash hands frequently, especially after eating greasy foods.	
• Apply topical retinoid 20 min after washing and drying face.	
• Praise good habits.	• Positive reinforcement encourages continued effort.
• Advise the adolescent to wash hair with antiseborrheic shampoo and to avoid oil-based cosmetics, pomades, or petroleum-based hair products.	• Seborrhea frequently accompanies acne. Oil-based products can obstruct sebaceous glands, exacerbating acne.
• Encourage the adolescent to keep a diary of skin care, menses, and diet habits.	• A record may help identify associations with flares that can be managed in the future.

EXPECTED OUTCOME: Adolescent will exhibit good hygiene habits and nutrition.

GOAL: The adolescent will verbalize understanding of treatment regimen.

INTERVENTION	RATIONALE
• Educate the adolescent about medications (action, side effects, dosage, method of application).	• Proper application of medication enhances healing of lesions.
• Encourage application of tretinoin at night. Encourage use of noncomedonic sunscreens of at least SPF 30 during the day.	• Nighttime application helps reduce sensitivity to sun and sunscreen helps to avoid sunburn.
• Educate the adolescent about time needed for a therapeutic response and importance of adhering to daily regimen.	• Up to 3 months may be needed for significant improvement. The adolescent needs a reason to continue with the care plan.
• Encourage continuation of daily therapies even when acne has improved significantly.	• Acne will return if treatment stops.

EXPECTED OUTCOME: Adolescent will implement the treatment regimen as outlined, resulting in a noticeable reduction in lesions.

2. Nursing Diagnosis: *Body Image, Disturbed,* related to biophysical factors (visible facial lesions) (NANDA-I © 2014)

GOAL: The adolescent will demonstrate increased self-confidence and self-esteem.

INTERVENTION	RATIONALE
• Establish a rapport with the adolescent.	• A trusting relationship promotes verbalization of concerns and fears.
• Provide education about the condition and therapy modalities.	• Providing information better enables the adolescent to take control of the condition.
• Encourage the adolescent to be responsible for treatment and follow-up, and give positive reinforcement.	• Responsibility reinforces sense of self-esteem.
• Encourage the adolescent to become involved with school activities and peers.	• Involvement in activities helps enhance self-esteem and allows the adolescent to explore new experiences and friendships.

EXPECTED OUTCOME: Adolescent will freely discuss concerns and fears. Adolescent will demonstrate active involvement in own care. Adolescent will show increased confidence, as demonstrated by involvement in extracurricular activities.

exposure and to use noncomedonic sunscreen products. Review instructions for taking other prescribed drugs, such as tetracycline and isotretinoin (Accutane), and discuss possible side effects. Emphasize the importance of return visits to the adolescent's healthcare provider to monitor medication side effects.

Psychologic support is an important aspect of care. Because adolescents are preoccupied with their body image and peer relationships, they often find having acne embarrassing. Monitor for signs of anxiety or depression. Encourage them to express their feelings and refer for counseling, if necessary.

Evaluation

Expected outcomes of nursing care can be found in *Nursing Care Plan: The Adolescent With Acne.*

Psoriasis

Psoriasis is a chronic, relapsing, pruritic, papulosquamous condition that affects the skin, scalp, and nails. It begins during childhood or adolescence in a third of cases (Bhutani, Kamangar, & Cordoro, 2012). A family history of psoriasis is often present, but a multifactorial inheritance is suspected.

Psoriasis is a T-helper cell–mediated autoimmune disease. Inflammatory cytokines from activated T cells cause chronic inflammation and are responsible for the skin changes (McCann & Huether, 2014). Cells proliferate so rapidly they do not mature and fully keratinize, leading to thickened epidermis and plaque formation. The onset of psoriasis may be triggered in children, particularly guttate-type psoriasis, by a streptococcal infection. Other triggers may include trauma, stress, and recent withdrawal from oral corticosteroids (Bhutani et al., 2012).

The typical psoriatic lesion is a thick, silvery, scaly erythematous plaque with an irregular border, surrounded by normal skin. Pruritus is often present. These lesions commonly are found on the scalp, elbows, knees, umbilicus, and genitals, or at the site of trauma. Nails may also be involved. Small points of bleeding may be noted when a scale is removed. Guttate psoriasis is characterized by an eruption of small round or oval papules on the trunk, face, and extremities. Some children also develop psoriatic arthritis.

Diagnosis is based on skin lesion characteristics or microscopic examination. Treatment includes topical steroids twice a day. Care must be taken to use lower-potency steroids in the diaper area and the face, and to switch from higher-potency to lower-potency steroids when lesions thin. Other topical medications include vitamin D, a retinoid, and tacrolimus or pimecrolimus. A tar shampoo may be used to clear scales in the scalp prior to topical steroid application. Salicylic acid may be used to remove some layers of plaques. Ultraviolet B phototherapy is used for children who do not respond to topical therapy. Systemic therapy with drugs such as methotrexate, oral retinoids, and cyclosporine is reserved for children with severe psoriasis. No cure exists, and lifelong relapses and remissions occur.

Nursing Management

Assess the child's skin for extent of the lesions and response to therapy. Spend time talking with the child and family to learn how the condition affects them. Educate them about the condition and reasonable expectations related to treatment. Families need to understand that lesions are not contagious, and periods of remissions and flare-ups are common. Actively involve the family and child in decision making regarding the treatment plan, such as the type of topical products (e.g., lotion, cream, ointment) they prefer to use. Teach them how to apply topical medications. Encourage the child to avoid situations in which chemical and physical trauma to the skin could occur.

Children and adolescents may have feelings of embarrassment, anger, and frustration related to their visible skin lesions. Psoriasis may impact their daily lives causing problems at school, with personal relationships, and with social acceptance. Children may anticipate rejection and withdraw from physical activities that require them to expose affected skin areas, such as swimming. The mental health of adolescents should be monitored to identify psychologic distress, depression, or substance abuse.

Epidermolysis Bullosa

Epidermolysis bullosa (EB) is a rare and severe chronic blistering skin disorder that occurs with minor trauma. EB is most often inherited in an autosomal dominant pattern (see Chapter 3). The incidence of the most common and least severe form, EB simplex (EBS), is estimated to be 1 per 25,000 live births (Coulombe & Lee, 2012).

Genetic changes in the intracellular proteins compromise their ability to provide structural support in keratinocytes of the epidermis. The basal keratinocytes are fragile and rupture easily with any mechanical injury trauma. One variant of EBS is localized to blistering of the hands, and another variant leads to more generalized blistering. It is often diagnosed when the child begins to walk or during puberty. With severe forms of EB, blistering and skin erosions are seen at birth and occur on all parts of the body, including the respiratory, gastrointestinal, and urologic systems. These children lose protein and have electrolyte and fluid imbalances, malnutrition, and anemia. Severe EB has a high mortality rate due to secondary infection.

Children with EB have extremely fragile skin, and blisters form with minor trauma, friction, or heat applied to the skin. In severe forms, the blistering can be extensive and damage to the skin is apparent. Fingers and toes may fuse with healing, leading to malformations. Children experience pain with blisters and may have difficulty walking when feet are affected. In the more common form of EB, blisters generally heal without scarring.

Diagnosis can be made prenatally by amniocentesis or chorionic villus sampling or by skin biopsy. The condition is managed by prevention of new blisters, wound care, good nutrition, and minimizing the risk for infection. Wound care is important to reduce the risk of infection. Blisters are pricked on two sides with a sterile needle each day and drained so that they do not extend. The blister roof is kept intact to act as a natural biologic dressing. Antibiotic ointments are applied to wounds, and changed monthly to reduce the risk for bacterial resistance. Wounds are covered, and care is taken to avoid placing adhesives directly on the skin. Biologic dressings may be used to cover larger wounds in some cases. Infants and children need additional protein and calories to support chronic wound healing. Pain management is customized to the severity of the child's condition and wound care provided.

Nursing Management

Teach the family to provide daily wound care at home. Wound care can be quite time consuming, so help the parents select the best time to do routine dressing changes. Perform dressing changes in a location without air currents to reduce pain from exposed wounds. Determine if financial support is needed to ensure that parents have the dressing supplies needed to effectively manage the child's wounds. Provide parents with guidance on all aspects of dressing changes.

- Precut dressings to reduce the wound exposure time.
- Gather all supplies and have an assistant present. Ask the assistant to gently hold the child's extremities to prevent movement of the extremity during blister lancing and dressing changes. Holding or grabbing the extremity too tightly can cause friction injury.
- Use soft music and distraction to help calm the infant.
- Soak off dressings that are stuck to the skin. Remove dressings from one area at a time as air exposure may cause pain.
- Inspect the skin each day for signs of infection.
- Use nonadherent dressings that can absorb the blister fluid to help prevent dressings from sticking to the skin. Place a bulky cover over the dressing to protect the skin and promote healing. Wrap fingers and toes separately so they do not fuse together with healing.

Help the parents to identify ways to protect the skin but still permit the child to interact with other children and have opportunities for development. Dress the child in soft cotton clothing that covers the skin, placing rough seams that can irritate the skin on the outside. Foam padding can be sewn into clothing over the knees and elbows for the infant who is crawling or walking. Shoes without seams on the inside should be worn with seamless cotton socks. Cotton socks can be used to mitten the infant's hands during sleep. The child should also avoid sun exposure and stay where temperatures are cool.

Protein is lost with blisters and chronic wound healing requires extra calories. Promote good nutrition with adequate calories and high protein to meet the child's growth and healing requirements. In infants, blistering in the mouth may interfere with feeding. A soft nipple with a larger hole may be easier for the infant to use. Vaseline on the lips may help reduce trauma to the mouth. Food temperature should be cool or room temperature and nonacidic to prevent injury to the gastrointestinal tract. In some cases, a gastrostomy tube is inserted for nutritional supplementation. Regularly measure height and weight and plot measurements on a growth curve to monitor growth and to identify growth deficiencies early.

Help parents and the child manage the psychologic impact of this disfiguring disorder and the inability to fully participate in all activities. An individualized health plan with educational accommodations will be necessary. Because the hands and feet are often involved, writing and test taking may be challenging. Mobility and walking throughout the school may also be a problem. Information needs to be provided to classroom teachers and classmates to help minimize injury.

Infestations

Pediculosis Capitis (Lice)

Pediculosis capitis is a lice infestation of the hair and scalp. Infestation occurs among children from all socioeconomic levels, and it is most common in children ages 3 to 11 years (Eisenhower & Farrington, 2012). Parents or teachers may be the first to notice lice, or healthcare providers may spot them during routine examination (see Chapter 33). Outbreaks occur periodically among children in child care and elementary school.

Head lice live and reproduce only on humans and are transmitted by direct hair-to-hair contact or indirect contact

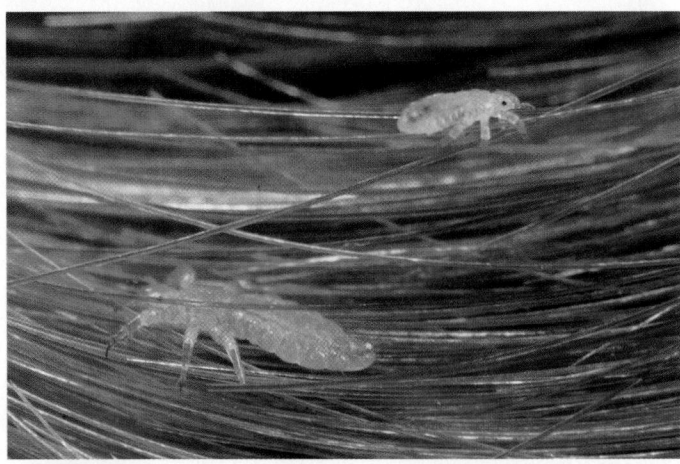

Figure 57–10 Note the presence of lice (highly magnified) crawling through the hair.

SOURCE: Darlyne A. Marawski/National Geographic Image Collection.

such as sharing of hair accessories, hats, towels, and bedding. Lice do not fly or jump, but they can crawl quickly. The female louse can lay up to 10 eggs (nits) a day on the hair shaft, close to the scalp. The incubation period for eggs to hatch is 7 to 10 days. Lice feed on human blood, sensitizing the child with their saliva to cause pruritus.

The child has intense pruritus and complaints of "dandruff" that sticks to the hair (actually the nits) and "bugs" in the hair. Nits look like silvery white, yellow, or darker 1-mm teardrops adhering to one side of the hair shaft, often near the scalp. Lice are wingless insects (2 to 3 mm long) that move away from light and are not easily seen (Figure 57–10). Scratching may lead to inflammation, pustules, and bacterial infection. Occipital and posterior cervical nodes are frequently palpable.

Treatment involves a pediculicide shampoo, such as pyrethrin within an enzymatic lice egg remover, or an ovicidal rinse, such as permethrin (Nix); however, resistance to these products has increased. Permethrin cream rinse is applied to dry hair and left in place for 10 minutes, before rinsing. The hair is towel-dried, and the nits are removed with a fine-toothed comb. A second treatment is needed in 7 to 10 days because the neurotoxin is not effective on nits. If live lice still persist after two treatments, a prescription ovicide such as malathion may be ordered. Some newer agents are available. See *Medications Used to Treat: Head Lice.*

SAFETY ALERT!

Lindane is a second-line treatment for head lice, and it must be used with caution in any child weighing less than 50 kg (110 lb) because of neurotoxicity and potential to cause seizures. High levels of resistance by lice have been documented. Lindane is no longer recommended for treatment of head lice (AAP, 2015, p. 600).

Nursing Management

Carefully assess children exposed to head lice using a bright light and magnifying glass to look for lice and nits along the hair shaft close to the scalp. To avoid potential infestation, change gloves with each child when assessing several children in a classroom setting.

Infestation with lice can be upsetting for both the child and family. Emphasize to the family that anyone can get lice. All

Medications Used to Treat: Head Lice

NAME OF MEDICATION/PREPARATION	NURSING MANAGEMENT
First-line pesticide treatment	
Permethrin 1% Crème Rinse—Nix	• Apply to the hair after shampooing and towel drying the hair. Leave on 10 min and rinse. Repeat in 7–10 days.
Pyrethrin shampoo (0.33%) or piperonyl butoxide (Rid, A-200, Bayer, and generic brands)	• Apply to *dry hair and scalp.* Lather, leave on 10 min, and rinse with cool water. Wet hair dilutes the product and may contribute to treatment failure. • Permethrin is approved for children 2 months of age and older.
Benzyl alcohol 5% (Ulesfia)—FDA-approved nonneurotoxic treatment for children ages 6 months and older; lice die by suffocation	• Apply to *dry hair,* saturating the hair and scalp. Rinse after 10 min. Repeat in 7 days. Protect eyes during use. Available by prescription.
Spinosad (Natroba)—FDA-approved for children 4 years and older; lice become paralyzed and die, ovicidal	• Apply topical suspension to *dry hair,* saturating the scalp and all hair. Rinse off after 10 min. May repeat in 7 days. Available by prescription and is expensive.
Sklice—FDA-approved 0.5% ivermectin lotion for children ages 6 months and older	• Apply to *dry hair,* completely covering the scalp and all hair. Leave on 10 min and rinse only with water; *do not* shampoo. No retreatment needed in most cases.
Second-line pesticide treatment	
Malathion 0.5%—Ovide lotion	• Apply to *dry hair.* Leave on 4 minutes and rinse. No retreatment is needed. May cause stinging sensation. Has potential to cause chemical burns. • Treatment is flammable; do not expose the child to electric heat sources.

Source: Data from Eisenhower, C., & Farrington, E. A., (2012). Advances in the treatment of head lice in pediatrics. *Journal of Pediatric Health Care, 26*(6), 451–461; Pariser, D. M., Meinking, T. L., Bell, M., & Ryan, W. G. (2012). Topical 0.5% Ivermectin lotion for treatment of head lice. *New England Journal of Medicine, 367*(18), 1687–1693; Bowden, V. R. (2012). Losing the louse: How to manage this common infestation in children. *Pediatric Nursing, 38*(5), 253–254, 277.

family members and contacts of the child should be examined for infestation and treated as necessary. Teach the child not to share clothing, headwear, or combs.

Explain to parents that the shampoo and rinses prescribed are pesticides and must be used for the time specified and as directed. An extra bottle of the product may be needed if the child has extra long hair. Inform parents that in order to avoid treatment failure no other shampoo or conditioner should be used before the lice shampoo or lotion. Do not wash the hair for 1 to 2 days after the pediculicide treatment. Keep these products out of the eyes and mouth of the child because they will irritate mucous membranes.

To remove nits, use a fine-toothed comb, tweezers, and a basin filled with water or isopropyl alcohol to dip and clean the comb and tweezers. Comb 1-inch sections from the scalp outward and pin these out of the way when done. Nits adhere to the hair shaft and must be manually pulled down the shaft with the comb, tweezers, or fingernails. All nits should be removed. Have blunt-nosed scissors available to cut a hair below the level of the nit when the nit cannot be removed. Put the child under a bright light and use distractions such as a video to keep the child entertained during the procedure. Check the hair every 2 to 3 days and remove any lice or nits seen. Giving boys a buzz haircut is one alternative. A shorter hair cut for girls may help with nit removal. Both the American Academy of Pediatrics and the National Association of School Nurses have policies that allow the child to stay in school even if all nits have not been removed.

Lice survive only about 3 days away from a human host, but nits may hatch after 8 to 10 days. For this reason, the child's bedding, towels, and clothing should be changed daily, laundered in hot water with detergent, and dried in a hot dryer for 20 minutes. Store nonessential bedding and clothing in a tightly sealed bag for 2 to 3 weeks and then wash. Discard hair accessories, brushes, and combs or soak them in hot soapy water (54.4°C [130.0°F]) for 10 minutes. Vacuum furniture and carpets and treat them with a hot iron when possible. Use of an insecticide in the home to kill the lice on carpets, furniture, and other items is not recommended when young children and pets may be exposed. Seal toys and other personal items that cannot be washed or dry-cleaned in a plastic bag for 2 weeks.

Scabies

Scabies is a highly contagious infestation caused by the mite *Sarcoptes scabiei.* It is spread by skin-to-skin and sexual contact. Transmission within a household is common. Children of all ages and both sexes can be affected. Because the mite usually takes at least 45 minutes to burrow into the skin, transient contact is unlikely to cause infestation.

The female mite burrows into the outer layer of the epidermis (stratum corneum) to lay her eggs, leaving a trail of debris and feces under the skin. The larvae hatch in approximately 3 to 4 days and proceed toward the surface of the skin. The cycle is repeated 14 to 17 days later. A delayed type IV hypersensitivity reaction to the mites, debris, and feces occurs within 4 weeks of infestation, causing irritation and intense pruritus (Cohen, 2014). Hypersensitivity response to reinfestation can occur within 24 hours.

Symptoms include a rash with papules and pustules, restlessness, and severe pruritus that worsens at night. Lesions may appear as linear, threadlike, grayish burrows 1 to 10 cm (0.4 to 4.0 in.) in length, which may end in a pinpoint vesicle. Lesions are usually located in the webs of the fingers, in the intergluteal folds, around the axillae, or on the palms, wrists, head, neck, legs, buttocks, chest, abdomen, and waist. In children under age 2 years, the head, neck, face, palms, and feet can be affected. The child's scratching and secondary infection often obliterate the linear burrow lesions. Nodules 2 to 20 mm (0.08 to 0.6 in.) in size occasionally develop as a granulomatous response to the dead mite antigens and feces and can persist for weeks after effective treatment.

Diagnosis is confirmed by microscopic examination of scrapings from a burrow, which reveals actively moving mites, fecal pellets, eggs, or nits. Treatment involves application of a scabicide, such as 5% permethrin lotion, over the entire body except the face, with special attention to the hands, fingers, feet, toes, and skin under the nails. Application of 5% permethrin lotion or malathion is preceded by a warm soap-and-water bath. When the skin is cool and dry, apply the lotion. The lotion is left in place for 8 to 48 hours before washing off. A second treatment is used 1 week later. Treat all members of the household and childcare contacts at the same time, even if they have no symptoms.

An oral antihistamine (e.g., Benadryl, Atarax) may be prescribed to help relieve itching. Antibiotics may be needed when a secondary infection occurs. Oral ivermectin, a new antiparasitic product with FDA approval for children weighing more than 15 kg, may be prescribed when treatment failure occurs.

Nursing Management

Advise parents that scabies is transmitted by close contact and is very contagious. All clothing, bedding, and pillowcases used by the child should be changed daily, washed with hot water, and ironed before reuse. Nonwashable toys and other items should be sealed in plastic bags for 5 to 7 days.

Educate the parents about the proper application of the scabicide. The child should have the scabicide reapplied to the hands if hands are washed or the child sucks the fingers or thumb. Socks over the young child's hands may reduce ingestion of the scabicide.

Treat all household members simultaneously. Uninfested individuals should avoid touching the affected child until after treatment is completed. If contact is made, they should wash their hands well. Inform the parents about signs of secondary infections and that itching and nodules may persist for weeks after effective treatment. Encourage the use of emollients because the treatment dries the skin.

Scabies, like pediculosis, can be embarrassing or upsetting for the child and family. Educate the child and parents about the condition, its spread, and treatment measures to prevent recurrence.

Vascular Tumors (Hemangiomas)

Vascular tumors, or hemangiomas, occur in 4% to 5% of infants (Lauren & Garzon, 2012). An increased incidence has been noted in women and infants who are non-Hispanic, White, low birth weight, and of multiple births (Chung & Cohen, 2014). An increased incidence is found in infants exposed to chorionic villus sampling, placental complications, or preeclampsia (Uihlein, Liang, & Mulliken, 2012).

Hemangiomas are vascular tumors believed to result from the proliferation of endothelium-like cells that could be caused by a mutation and some type of environmental exposure. These tumors undergo rapid growth and attain 80% of full size by age 3 months, and most growth will be completed by age 5 months (Chung & Cohen, 2014). This phase is followed by a slow **involution** (process of decreasing in size) phase that may take years. Hemangiomas may be superficial (in the epidermis), deep (in the dermis or subcutaneous tissue), or mixed superficial and deep. When multiple hemangiomas are found, some may be in major organs, such as the liver. Complications caused by the rapid growth pressure against or obstruction of vital structures (e.g., airway, eye, or ear canal) may occur.

Infantile hemangiomas begin as barely visible **telangiectasias** (dilated superficial blood vessels) or red macules that begin to grow rapidly and become bright red and compressible. Some lesions ulcerate with rapid growth. Superficial hemangiomas are bright-red vascular cutaneous plaques that resemble strawberries. Deep hemangiomas appear as bluish tumors covered with normal-appearing epidermis. Mixed hemangiomas have features of both superficial and deep tumors. The lesions, appearing any place on the body, are minimally compressible and have no bruit or thrill. As the vascular tumor involutes, signs of tissue atrophy, wrinkles, telangiectasias, and hypopigmentation may be noted.

Initial diagnosis is by physical examination and monitoring the growth of the vascular tumor. When a vital organ could become obstructed or a large facial hemangioma is present, ultrasound, computed tomography, or magnetic resonance imaging may be performed.

Simple hemangiomas are monitored and receive no treatment. Hemangiomas in problem areas may be treated with oral propranolol at 1 mg/kg twice daily. Vital signs are checked prior to first dose and at 1 and 2 hours after the first dose. The child is checked again at 1 week and then monthly with vital signs being checked each visit. If the child has cardiovascular, respiratory, or endocrine conditions, or hemangioma in a vital organ, the child may be admitted for initial propranolol dosing because of potential adverse effects. The medication may be stopped temporarily if the infant has wheezing or severe cough because it may worsen wheezing associated with asthma (Block & Blackmon, 2013). Photos are taken of lesions at each visit to document changes in the lesion.

Pulsed-dye laser treatment may be used after involution for residual telangiectasia. Light energy pulses target the lesion's oxyhemoglobin, which is heated after absorbing the wavelength of light. This ruptures the lesion's blood vessels. Provide topical anesthesia and eye protection. The lesion may darken for 1 to 2 weeks, as red blood cells are released from ruptured blood vessels. The treated skin surface eventually lightens. Surgical removal of ulcerated hemangiomatous tissue may be considered if a poor cosmetic outcome is expected.

Nursing Management

Assess the distribution of the hemangioma and consider the potential for complications as it goes through a rapid growth stage, such as potential compression of the airway for a hemangioma in the neck area. Monitor the child for signs of any complications, such as ulceration. Assess the parents' response to the infant's appearance and how they are managing interactions with friends and family about the infant's changing appearance.

Take photos of the infant at each visit so that parents have a record of improvements once therapy is initiated.

Educate the parents about the type of vascular lesion and the time when growth is most rapid. Inform parents about the possible ulceration, if a hemangioma is rapidly growing, and what signs to expect. Parents should return for care when concerned about the lesion, if watchful waiting has been selected.

When propranolol medication is administered in the outpatient setting, monitor the pulse and blood pressure as directed for the first dose to detect adverse effects such as hypotension, bradycardia, or arrhythmia. Vital signs are taken on each subsequent visit. Educate the parents that propranolol should be given with or after meals to prevent hypoglycemia. Inform parents about the need to wake the infant to feed once or twice during the night to prevent hypoglycemia. Educate them about the signs of hypoglycemia to watch for and if seen to feed the infant before the blood sugar drops lower. Other adverse effects include restless sleep, cold extremities, and delayed capillary refill time.

Talk with parents about comments people make about the infant's appearance and provide some possible responses that parents can make. To promote attachment, help the parents see the infant's positive characteristics, such as responsiveness and smiling. Show photos of other children with similar lesions who have completed therapy to show that improvements in appearance are gradual, but possible.

Prepare parents for the changes in the child's appearance with pulsed-dye laser therapy. Some swelling may occur after the treatment, so the application of ice packs for 10 minutes every hour during the first day may help. Teach parents to protect the skin surface from trauma after pulsed-dye laser treatments and to keep the infant's nails short to prevent scratching. Cleanse the area treated with water and pat it dry. Inform parents to avoid sun exposure for several weeks after the treatments, and to use sunscreen in the future.

Injuries to the Skin

Pressure Ulcers

Many children with disabilities are cared for in hospital, community, and home care settings, and they are at risk for skin breakdown and pressure ulcers. Children at greatest risk are those with limited mobility, the inability to change positions, sensory deficits, or incontinence. Infants and children at higher risk in hospital settings are those cared for in neonatal and pediatric intensive care units, sometimes associated with mechanical devices.

Soft tissues and capillary beds can be compressed between a bony prominence and an external surface. Tissue ischemia occurs when compression slows blood flow to the skin and deeper tissues. The cells are deprived of oxygen and nutrients, and metabolic waste products accumulate, resulting in hypoxia and soft-tissue injury. If compression is not relieved, the injury progresses rapidly and a pressure ulcer forms.

Stages 1 and 2 are the most common stages of pressure ulcers in children (Figure 57–11). In stage 3, an ulcer forms as the subcutaneous tissue is exposed, causing a full-thickness injury. In stage 4, the ulcer deepens and extends to muscle, bone, or supporting tissues. See Table 57–6 for common sites and potential causes of pressure ulcers in children.

Clinical Tip

The site of greatest pressure in infants and young children is the occiput. Older children have increased pressure on the sacral and occipital areas.

Initial treatment for early stages of skin damage is removing pressure from the affected site until the skin has healed. Children who use leg braces for alignment and mobility are

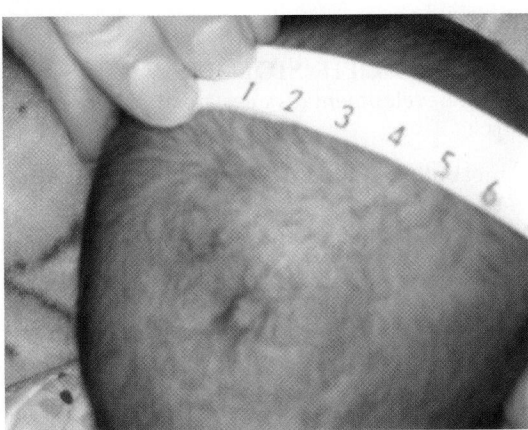

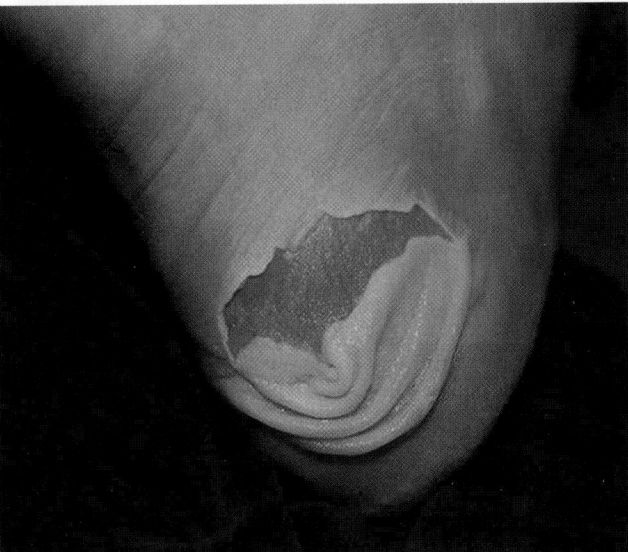

A   **B**

Figure 57–11 The initial stages of pressure ulcer formation. *A,* Stage 1, an area of redness does not go away within 30 minutes of removing the pressure or skin irritant. Children with dark skin may have persistent red, blue, or purple discoloration. *B,* Stage 2, the skin looks rubbed or raw like a blister or abrasion, a partial-thickness injury with damage through epidermis, dermis, or both.

SOURCE: Courtesy of Sandra Quigley, Children's Hospital, Boston, MA.

TABLE 57–6 Sites and Potential Causes of Skin Breakdown

SITES	POTENTIAL CAUSES
Occipital region of scalp	Inability to lift head
Sacrum and buttocks	Confinement to bed or wheelchair
Legs and feet	Orthotics, leg braces, casts
Spine and neck	Scoliosis brace
Knees, elbows, heels of feet	Rubbing against bed sheet
Sternum, iliac crest	Prone positioning for mechanical ventilation

often put in wheelchairs. Children who use wheelchairs may be put on bed rest with a pressure-reducing surface. Frequent repositioning is needed. A transparent film may be applied to affected red skin to minimize friction. Pressure ulcers are treated with dressings, such as hydrocolloids, gels or hydrogels, and calcium alginates that do not adhere to the wound.

Nursing Management

The Braden Q Scale (for children under age 5 years) or the Braden Scale are tools to assess the child's risk for pressure ulcers when hospitalized and when the child has a chronic condition with limited mobility. The nurse should assess the child for each of the following risk factors:

- Ability to change and control body position
- Amount of physical activity
- Ability to respond to the discomfort associated with pressure
- Degree to which the skin is exposed to moisture
- Movement of the skin against surfaces
- Food intake pattern
- Tissue perfusion and oxygenation

Carefully inspect the dependent skin surfaces of all infants and children confined to bed at least 3 times in each 24-hour period. Identify the size (length, width, and depth) and character of any skin lesion. Note any signs of infection, the appearance of wound edges, type of tissue at the wound base, and drainage. Describe any drainage amount, color, and type.

Develop protocols for pressure ulcer prevention so that children at high risk are identified and have appropriate interventions initiated (e.g., increased ambulation, frequent position changes, pressure-reducing surfaces, and moisture barriers). If the child is incontinent, change the diaper frequently to keep the skin clean and dry. Ensure an adequate intake of fluids, proteins, and vitamins to keep the skin healthy.

Moist wounds heal more rapidly than dry wounds because cell migration across the moist wound bed more effectively fights infection and removes cellular debris. Provide wound care and dressing changes according to agency guidelines. These guidelines may include saline irrigation, debridement, and a dressing appropriate for the wound condition. See Table 57–2 for types of wound dressings (see the *Clinical Skills Manual* SKILLS). Gauze wraps to hold the dressing in place help prevent skin damage caused by adhesives.

Teach parents of children with braces to inspect the skin under the braces every day for irritation (redness or blisters).

Help the child to use a mirror with a long handle to inspect skin on the bottom and sides of the feet, behind the knees, and on the lower legs. Check all edges of the braces for roughness or breakage that can pinch or scrape the skin. If any skin irritation is seen and redness does not go away within 30 minutes, do not put the brace back on until the skin heals. Inform the child's healthcare provider so that treatment can be started immediately. To reduce irritation, have the child wear cotton socks under the braces and make sure the shoes are large enough to accommodate the brace, socks, and the foot. Advise parents to return to a prosthetist regularly for brace refitting as the child grows.

Children who use a wheelchair are at risk for skin breakdown on the buttocks and lower back from the pressure of sitting for hours. A wheelchair cushion can distribute and shift the child's weight when sitting in the chair. Teach the child to change position frequently by doing wheelchair push-ups or by shifting the weight (leaning to the side or forward) for several minutes every 10 to 15 minutes. Make sure the child wears a safety belt when sitting in the wheelchair. Teach school personnel about the child's recommended protocol so they can provide opportunities in school to change positions and reinforce the routine.

Burns

Burns are among the top five leading causes of injury and death in children between 1 and 14 years of age (National Center for Health Statistics, National Vital Statistics System, 2015). In the United States, 128,765 children and adolescents under age 19 years were treated for burns in 2013 (Centers for Disease Control and Prevention [CDC], 2015). Of these children, the majority were less than age 5 years (Vloemans, Hermans, van der Wal, et al., 2014).

The four main types of burns are thermal, chemical, electrical, and radioactive. Thermal burns, the most common in children, result from flames, scalds (such as coffee or grease), or contact with hot objects (such as a wood stove or curling iron). Chemical burns occur when children touch or ingest caustic agents. Electrical burns are caused by direct or alternating current in electrical wires, appliances, or high-voltage wires. Radiation burns result from exposure to radioactive substances or sunlight. Burns are also found in 10% of cases of child abuse (Hazinski, Mondozzi, & Baker, 2014). See Chapter 42 for more information about child abuse.

ETIOLOGY AND PATHOPHYSIOLOGY

Children at different developmental stages are at risk for different types of burns:

- Infants are most often injured by thermal burns (scalding liquids, house fires).
- Toddlers are at risk for thermal burns (pulling hot liquids or grease onto themselves), electrical burns (biting electrical cords), contact burns, and chemical burns (ingesting cleaning agents, button batteries, and other substances) associated with exploring the environment (Figure 57–12).
- Preschool-age children are most often injured by scalding or contact with hot appliances (curling irons, ovens).
- School-age children are at risk for thermal burns (playing with matches, fireworks), electrical burns (climbing high-voltage towers, climbing trees, and contact with electrical wires), and chemical burns (combustion experiments).
- Adolescents also experience thermal, chemical, and electrical burns, as well as radiation burns associated with sunbathing.

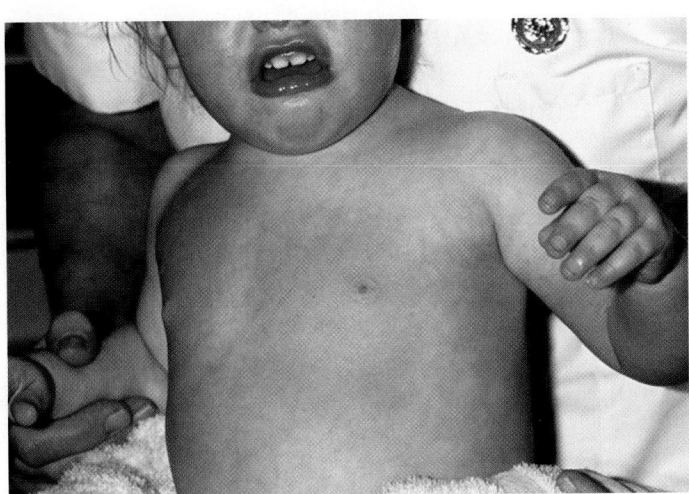

A

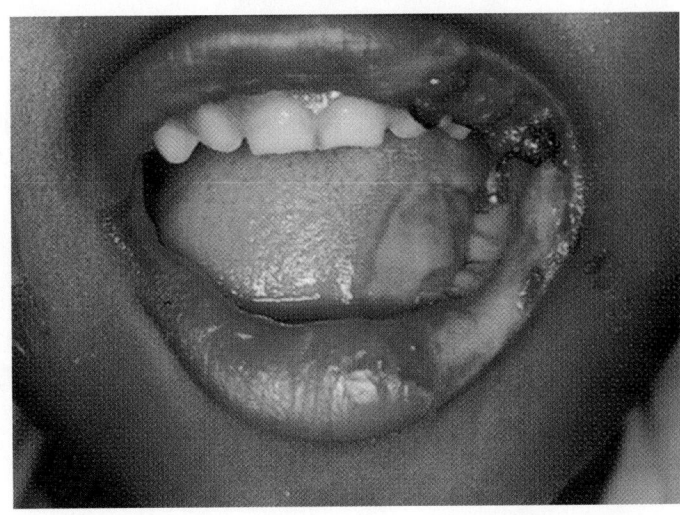

B

Figure 57–12 *A*, Scald injury from hot liquid is a common thermal burn injury in infants and toddlers. Notice the distribution of the burned skin, a wide area on the upper chest and arm where the hottest liquid fell, with a narrower area indicating the liquid cooled as it traveled down the chest. *B*, Electrical burn caused by biting on electrical cord. The burn is caused when the current arcs through the lips, often causing a full-thickness injury through the mucosa, muscle, nerves, and blood vessels. The labial artery may be injured and cause significant bleeding once the eschar falls off after 2 to 3 weeks.

SOURCE: *A*, Dr. P. Marazzi/Science Source. *B*, Dr. Lezley McIlveen / Children's National Medical Center.

The depth of the burn depends on the temperature and duration of the heat application, and on the ability of tissues to dissipate the transferred energy. Immediately after the burn, the cell membranes are altered, leading to increased capillary permeability and extracellular fluid loss. Fluid and plasma shift into the interstitial spaces, causing edema and decreased circulating volume in the blood vessels. Capillary perfusion to most capillaries is decreased because of myocardial depression, leading to tissue ischemia. The child loses increased water, electrolytes, and heat through the injured epidermis. A hypermetabolic state develops from the stress response, and severe alterations in glucose, lipid, and amino-acid metabolism may last for months after the burn injury (Jeschke & Herndon, 2014). A high number of calories are needed in an effort to maintain body temperature and begin healing. Immunosuppression also occurs, which increases the risk for infection.

SAFETY ALERT!

Coffee, tea, soup, and other hot beverages are often served at temperatures high enough to cause a serious scald injury. Adults should not hold infants in their laps while drinking hot beverages to prevent scald injuries.

CLINICAL MANIFESTATIONS

Burns are classified by the depth of penetration into the skin layers. Partial-thickness burns, in which the injured tissue can regenerate and heal, may be either first or second degree. Full-thickness burns, in which the injured tissue cannot regenerate, are also known as third-degree burns. See *Pathophysiology Illustrated: Classification of Burns by Depth* for clinical manifestations by burn depth.

Signs of infection include purulent drainage, swelling, erythema, discoloration of wound margins, and pain in the uninjured skin around the wound.

CLINICAL THERAPY

Assessment of Burn Severity. Burn severity is determined by the burn depth, percentage of body surface area (BSA) affected, and involvement of specific body parts. A Lund and Browder chart with BSA distributions for various body parts at different ages is used to calculate the area affected by the burn injury (Figure 57–13). The palm of a child's hand (without fingers and thumb) is 1% of the child's BSA and can be used to make a quick estimate of the burn size. Reassessment of the extent of burn injury is performed 24 to 48 hours after the injury. The true extent of BSA burned and depth of burns may not be apparent for several days.

Criteria for pediatric burns that should be referred to a specialized burn center include (American College of Surgeons, Committee on Trauma, 2014, p. 101):

- Partial-thickness burn greater than 10% BSA and full-thickness burns of any size
- Burns involving the hands, face, eyes, ears, feet, genitalia, perineum, and skin over major joints
- Electrical burns, including lightning injury
- Chemical or inhalation injury
- Burns in a child with another medical condition or additional trauma that increases the risk for death or increased morbidity
- Need for special social and emotional or long-term rehabilitation support, including cases of suspected child maltreatment

Initial Treatment. The first step is to ensure that the child has an airway, is breathing, and has a pulse. Then stop the burning process by removing jewelry and clothing. Moist soaks or ice (if a small surface area is affected) is used to stop the burning process and to relieve pain. A tetanus vaccine booster is given if more than

Pathophysiology Illustrated: **Classification of Burns by Depth**

| **SUPERFICIAL PARTIAL THICKNESS (FIRST DEGREE)** | **PARTIAL THICKNESS (SECOND DEGREE)** | **FULL THICKNESS (THIRD DEGREE)** |

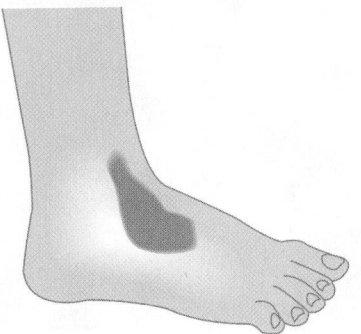 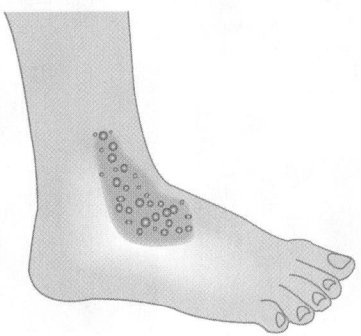 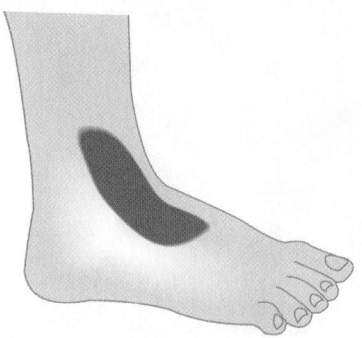

Damages only outer layer of skin; burn is painful and red; heals in a few days (e.g., sunburn)

Erythema, blanches on pressure, no bullae, peeling after a few days due to premature cell death

Involves epidermis and upper layers of dermis; may have sparing of sweat glands and sebaceous glands; heals in 10–14 days

Blisters or bullae, erythema, blanches on pressure, pain and sensitivity to cold air, minimal scar formation

Involves all of epidermis and dermis; may also involve underlying tissue; nerve endings usually destroyed; requires skin grafting

Skin may appear brown, black, deep cherry red, white to gray, waxy or translucent; usually no pain, injured area may appear sunken

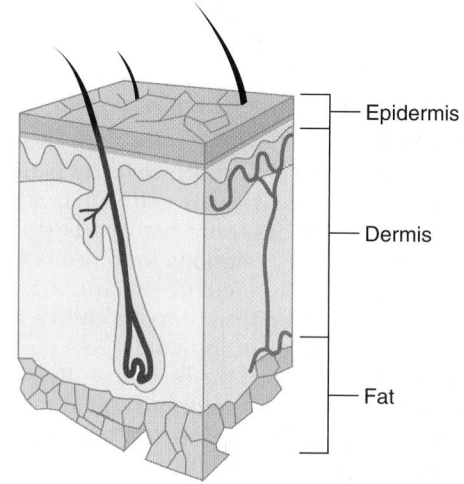

— Epidermis

— Dermis

— Fat

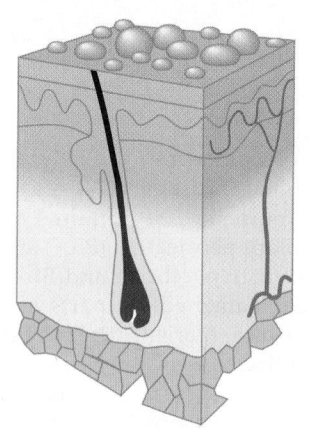 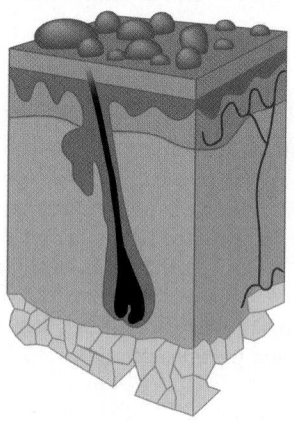

5 years have passed since the last vaccine, or when the child has not completed the full vaccine series.

Treatment of Major Burns. The goals of treatment include decreasing burn fluid losses, preventing infection, controlling pain, promoting nutrition, and salvaging all viable tissue. Fluid resuscitation is necessary to maintain the cardiovascular and renal systems. Fluid shifts from the vasculature to the interstitial spaces (third spacing) soon after the burn and can cause hypovolemic shock. Fluid replacement for the first 24 hours after the injury is based on a fluid volume formula calculated from the child's body weight, affected BSA, and normal maintenance needs (e.g., the Parkland and Galveston formulas):

- *Parkland formula:* 4 mL × body weight (kg) × percentage of total BSA burned = total 24-hour fluid requirement in milliliters. Maintenance fluids must be added to the amount of fluid calculated with this formula.

- *Galveston or Shriners Burn Hospital formula:* 5000 mL/m² burned area + 2000 mL/m² of total BSA = total 24-hour fluid requirement in milliliters.

Lactated Ringer or normal saline solution is the preferred IV fluid. Half of the total volume calculated for the 24-hour period is infused over the first 8 hours, starting at the time of the burn rather than emergency department arrival time. The remainder is distributed evenly over the next 16 hours. Urine output is used to monitor end-organ perfusion. When the urine output reaches 1 mL/kg/hr in children weighing less than 30 kg or 50 mL/kg/hr in heavier children, the fluid rate is reduced (Hazinski et al., 2014). Efforts are also focused on maintaining the child's temperature because heat is lost rapidly through burned skin.

A temperature elevation to 38.0°C (100.4°F) is expected because of the high metabolic rate, not always a sign of infection. A lower temperature is of concern as a possible sign of sepsis or physiologic reserves are exhausted for temperature maintenance (Hazinski et al., 2014). Infection is a frequent complication and wounds are cultured to identify specific organisms and sensitivities before prescribing antibiotic therapy.

Aggressive pain management with intravenous opioids is needed around the clock and for all procedures. The burns

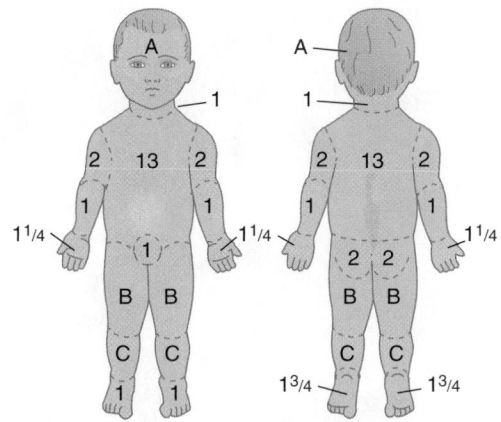

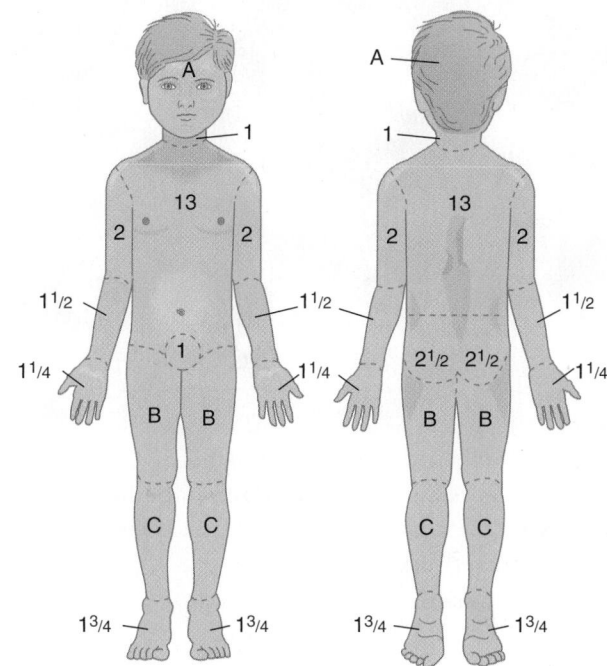

Relative Percentages of Areas Affected by Growth

Area	Age in years					
	0	1	5	10	15	Adult
A = $^1/_2$ of head	$9^1/_2$	$8^1/_2$	$6^1/_2$	$5^1/_2$	$4^1/_2$	$3^1/_2$
B = $^1/_2$ of one thigh	$2^3/_4$	$3^1/_4$	4	$4^1/_2$	$4^1/_2$	$4^3/_4$
C = $^1/_2$ of one lower leg	$2^1/_2$	$2^1/_2$	$2^3/_4$	3	$3^1/_4$	$3^1/_2$

Figure 57–13 Body surface area percentages for estimating pediatric burn injuries by age group.

SOURCE: Data from Artz, C. P., & Moncrief, J. A. (1969). *The treatment of burns* (2nd ed.). Philadelphia: Saunders; Fenlon, S., & Nene, S. (2007). Burns in children. *Continuing Education in Anaesthesia, Critical Care & Pain, 7*(3), 76–80; Tschudy, M. M., & Arcara, K. M. (2012). *The Harriet Lane handbook* (19th ed., p. 99). Philadelphia, PA: Elsevier Saunders.

cause a significant emotional distress that increases the perception of pain. See Chapter 40 for pain management information. Cimetidine or other H_2 blockers may be ordered to prevent a burn stress ulcer. Medications to help manage the hypermetabolic state may include propranolol, oxandrolone, and insulin (D'Cruz, Martin, & Holland, 2013).

Special consideration is needed when burns involve certain areas of the body:

- Deep partial-thickness and full-thickness burns develop **eschar** (the tough leathery scab that forms over severely burned areas) with no elasticity. When the burn is **circumferential** (surrounds the chest or an extremity), blood flow can become restricted as a result of edema, leading to tissue hypoxia. An **escharotomy** (incision into the constricting tissue) may be necessary to restore peripheral circulation.

- Facial burns usually cause significant edema. Care must be taken to ensure airway patency. An ophthalmologist should assess burns to the eye and prescribe treatment. If the lips are burned, an infant may be unable to suck.

- Burns of the hands require careful management to maintain function. Special splinting and physical therapy are usually necessary.

- Perineal burns are at higher risk for infection because of frequent contamination with urine and stool. Frequent dressing changes are required. A urinary catheter is usually inserted but is removed once hydration status is stable to minimize the risk of urinary tract infection.

Wound Management. Burn wound care has several goals: (1) to remove necrotic tissue and speed wound debridement, (2) to maintain moist wound conditions and adequate circulation, (3) to conserve body heat and fluids, (4) to protect from infection, and (5) to control scarring and prevent scar contracture. Several treatment regimens are used to achieve these goals.

When the burn is extensive, the entire body is bathed to initiate debridement. Sedation, pain management, and anesthesiology support are used during debridement sessions. Intact blisters provide a natural, pain-free, sterile dressing. However, some healthcare providers break blisters open, believing that the fluid provides a medium for bacterial infection. The tissues should be carefully cut away when the wound is being prepared for skin grafting.

Various options are used for wound management after debridement. Traditional burn care for a partial-thickness injury involved the application of antibacterial agents, such as silver sulfadiazine (Silvadene) or mafenide acetate (Sulfamylon) after initial cleansing, followed by a dressing that was changed once or twice daily. However, silver sulfadiazine was found to be cytotoxic (Kim, Martin, & Holland, 2012).

Silver-based antimicrobial dressings (e.g., Aquacel, Acticoat) provide a sustained-release delivery of silver, valued for its antimicrobial property. These dressings also absorb exudate from the wound and can be left in place several days (Figure 57–14). When the dressing is removed, a layer of eschar may also be debrided. These dressing changes are often painful, so pain management is needed (see Chapter 40).

Hydrotherapy (whirlpool bath or shower) may be used to cleanse extensive wounds before debridement, to increase vasodilation and circulation, and to speed healing. The water loosens exudate, topical medications, and dead tissue, and it may help soak off dressings that adhere to the skin. Gentle washing is necessary to protect new epithelial cells. Superficial partial-thickness burns reepithelialize within 3 weeks.

Skin grafting is necessary with any deep partial-thickness or full-thickness burn. Often a biologic dressing (e.g., Integra or Biobrane) or **allograft** (cadaver skin from a skin bank) is used to cover deep burns until an **autograft** (healthy skin taken from a nonburned area of the child's body) can be performed. The biologic dressing or allograft is effective in decreasing infection risk and pain, protecting against fluid loss, and promoting

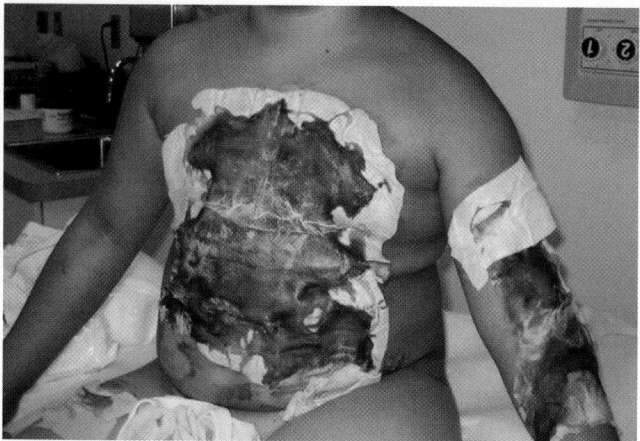

Figure 57–14 This child's scald burn is being treated with an Aquacel AG dressing, a silver-embedded dressing. Note the absorbed exudate that is visible through the burn dressing.

SOURCE: Courtesy of Martin Eichelberger, MD, and Lisa Ring, RN, PNP, Children's National Medical Center, Washington, DC.

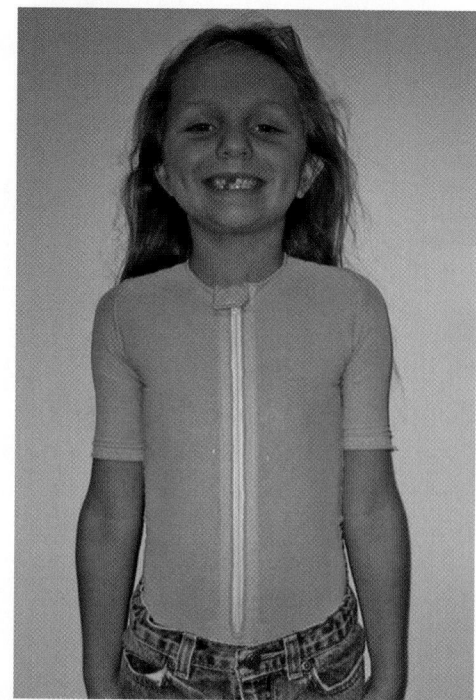

Figure 57–15 Pressure garment used to reduce hypertrophic scarring from a burn to the chest and upper arms.

SOURCE: Courtesy of Martin Eichelberger, MD, and Lisa Ring, RN, PNP, Children's National Medical Center, Washington, DC.

revascularization. An autograft is permanent. The autograft is placed after the wound is debrided in the operating room to reveal healthy, bleeding tissue. The donor site (where the autograft was harvested) is a new wound, causing pain and requiring close monitoring for signs of infection.

Vacuum-assisted wound closure (negative pressure wound therapy) is sometimes used for management of partial-thickness burns, graft sites, and other complex wounds. A pump generates a vacuum or suction to remove waste materials from the wound area. Once the burn site is debrided, a foam dressing is applied and sealed with adhesive before the device is attached. The vacuum over the surface of the wound draws out fluids, increases blood perfusion, decreases bacterial colonization, and draws wound edges together to speed healing. These devices are being used more often, but the U.S. Food and Drug Administration has not yet approved them for use in infants and children (U.S. FDA, 2014).

During the rehabilitation stage, pressure garments (e.g., Jobst) are used to reduce development of hypertrophic scarring and contractures. Such garments are worn 23 hours a day for 6 to 8 months to shorten the time of scar maturation and to reduce the thickness of the scars (Figure 57–15).

Severe morbidity is likely to occur with major burns. Significant scarring may occur despite the use of autografting and pressure garments. Contractures and loss of function are also possible. Children with major burns require comprehensive follow-up, sometimes involving repeated hospitalizations for surgery to release burn contractures or perform new grafting, or cosmetic surgery for scar revision.

Nursing Management

For the Child With a Burn Injury

Nursing Assessment and Diagnosis

Emergency assessment first focuses on the potential for life-threatening injuries that need immediate response. Assessment of the airway is necessary, especially when signs of smoke inhalation or burns to the face and neck are noted. Other potential injuries are important to identify when the mechanism of injury also includes a fall or explosion. Identify signs of respiratory distress and any potential bleeding source. A weak, thready pulse, tachycardia, and pallor are important signs of early shock that may provide clues to an internal injury.

Obtain information about the type of burn, when and how it happened, and first aid provided, along with a complete history. If a burn injury was preventable, parents may be emotionally stressed by feelings of guilt. Take care to avoid sounding accusatory when questioning parents about the injury. Be alert to signs of child abuse when the history does not match the injury (e.g., glove and stocking burns, popliteal or antecubital areas spared from burns where the child flexed the knees or elbows, contact burns from cigarettes or irons, and zebra burn lines from contact with a hot grate) (Figure 57–16). Photographs are often taken to document these injuries. Child neglect can be a factor in the burn of an inadequately supervised child.

Assess the extent of burn injury (BSA and depth). Frequently monitor the vital signs and pain control. Monitor the child's circulatory and respiratory status to identify signs of hypovolemia in the first 24 hours or fluid overload as capillary integrity is restored. A head-to-toe assessment is performed at the beginning of every shift, followed by system-specific assessments, depending on clinical findings and changes in the child's status. A urinary catheter may be inserted to enable close monitoring of urine output (see the *Clinical Skills Manual* SKILLS). Weigh the child daily, as the hypermetabolic state may result in weight loss if nutritional intake is inadequate. Be alert to signs of infection such as purulent drainage and edematous, red, or discolored wound margins.

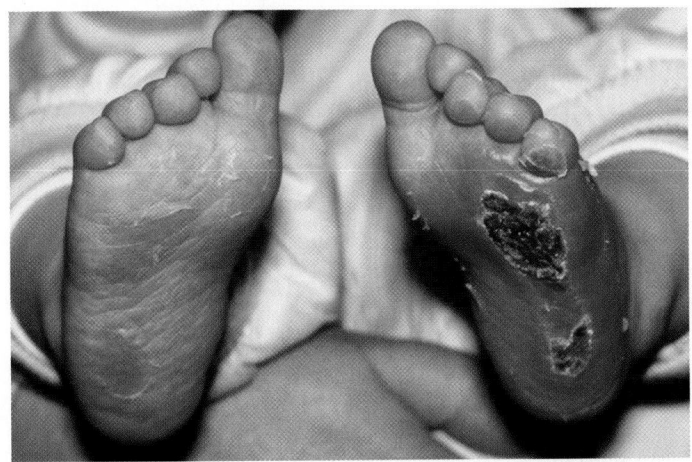

Figure 57–16 Burns of the hands or feet distributed like gloves or stockings are associated with child abuse. Contact burns on the soles of the feet in a pattern are also suspicious. Note the similar burn pattern on each foot.

SOURCE: SPL/Science Source.

SAFETY ALERT!

If a burn is circumferential, completely surrounding an extremity, compartment syndrome often occurs. Assess for an increase in cyanosis, deep tissue pain, capillary refill time, and a decreased pulse distal to the burn. If these signs are detected, notify the healthcare provider immediately.

Assess the child's concerns over appearance and the stress of hospitalization. Determine if the child has memories or nightmares about the burn and arrange psychologic support as needed. Identify any family stressors that might need to be addressed during the child's care.

Common nursing diagnoses for the child with a major burn injury are included in the accompanying *Nursing Care Plan*. Additional nursing diagnoses for the child with a major burn might include the following (NANDA-I © 2014):

- *Hyperthermia* related to hypermetabolic state
- *Body Image, Disturbed*, related to burn injury
- *Anxiety* related to situational crisis and threat of death or disfigurement

---

Nursing Care Plan: The Child With a Major Burn Injury

1. Nursing Diagnosis: *Pain, Acute,* related to physical injury agents (NANDA-I © 2014)

GOAL: The child will verbalize adequate relief from pain and will be able to perform activities of daily living (ADLs).

INTERVENTION	RATIONALE
• Assess the level of pain frequently using pain scales (see Chapter 40).	• Provides objective pain measurement. Changes in pain location and intensity may indicate complications.
• Cover burns as much as possible.	• Temperature change or air movement causes pain.
• Change the child's position frequently. Perform range-of-motion (ROM) exercises.	• Reduces joint stiffness and prevents contractures and increases comfort.
• Provide diversional activities.	• Helps lessen focus on pain.
• Promote uninterrupted sleep with use of medications and comfort measures.	• Sleep deprivation can increase pain perception.
• Use analgesics and sedation (as appropriate) before all dressing changes and burn care. Use sedation when appropriate for major debridement.	• Helps to reduce pain and decreases anxiety for subsequent dressing changes.

EXPECTED OUTCOME: Child will verbalize adequate relief from pain and be able to perform ADLs.

2. Nursing Diagnosis: *Infection, Risk for,* related to trauma and destruction of skin barrier (NANDA-I © 2014)

GOAL: The child will have reduced risk for infection or have secondary infection identified early.

INTERVENTION	RATIONALE
• Take vital signs frequently.	• Increased temperature may be an early sign of infection, but it is also common with the hypermetabolic state. A normal or decreased temperature may be a sign of sepsis.
• Use standard precautions (gown, gloves, mask) when wounds of a major burn are exposed. Do not allow anyone with an infectious disease to visit.	• Reduces risk of wound contamination.
• Clip hair around burns.	• Hair harbors bacteria and can irritate the wound.
• Keep burn dressing clean and intact.	• Helps reduce the number of bacteria introduced to the burned site.
• Do not place the IV in any burned area.	• Reduces risk of wound contamination.
• Administer oral or IV antibiotics for diagnosed infections as prescribed.	• Antibiotics help to clear the infection quickly.

EXPECTED OUTCOME: Child will have infection risk reduced, and secondary infections are diagnosed and treated promptly.

(continued)

Nursing Care Plan: The Child With a Major Burn Injury (*continued*)

3. Nursing Diagnosis: *Fluid Volume: Imbalanced, Risk for,* **related to loss of fluids through wounds and to subsequent excess fluid intake (NANDA-I © 2014)**

GOAL: The child will maintain adequate urine output.

INTERVENTION	RATIONALE
• Monitor vital signs, capillary refill time, and pulses.	• The child is initially at risk for hypovolemic shock and needs fluid resuscitation (see Chapter 47).
• Administer IV and oral fluids as ordered.	• Careful calculation of fluid needs and ensuring proper intake helps keep the child properly hydrated.
• Monitor intake and output.	• The child is initially at risk for hypovolemia and then overhydration during fluid resuscitation.
• Weigh child daily using the same scale and amount of clothing.	• Significant weight loss or gain can help determine fluid imbalances.
• Insert urinary catheter if prescribed.	• Helps maintain accurate output measurement during critical care stage.
• Monitor for hyponatremia and hypercalcemia (see Chapter 44).	• Sodium is lost with burn fluid and potassium is lost from damaged cells, causing electrolyte imbalances.

EXPECTED OUTCOME: Child will achieve the expected urine output for age during each stage of acute burn treatment.

4. Nursing Diagnosis: *Mobility: Physical, Impaired,* **related to joint stiffness due to burns (NANDA-I © 2014)**

GOAL: The child will maintain maximum range of motion.

INTERVENTION	RATIONALE
• Arrange physical and occupational therapy twice daily for stretching and ROM exercises. Splint as ordered.	• Positioning in alignment and ROM exercises help to prevent contractures.
• Encourage activities to promote range of motion (toss a bean bag, mimic animal movements).	• Fun activities help the child with diversion and provide movement.

EXPECTED OUTCOME: Child will maintain maximum range of motion without contractures.

5. Nursing Diagnosis: *Nutrition, Imbalanced: Less than Body Requirements,* **related to high metabolic needs (NANDA-I © 2014)**

GOAL: The child will maintain weight and demonstrate adequate serum albumin and hydration.

INTERVENTION	RATIONALE
• Provide an opportunity to choose meals and snacks. Offer a variety of high-protein and high-calorie foods. Provide small frequent feedings.	• Encourages intake. General malaise and anorexia lead to poor healing.
• Encourage the child to have meals with other children.	• Socialization improves intake.
• Provide a multivitamin supplement.	• Vitamin C aids zinc absorption; zinc aids in healing.
• Provide enteral feedings as needed.	• A child with a burn greater than 10% of BSA cannot usually meet nutrition requirements without assistance.
• Weigh the child daily.	• Provides objective evaluation.

EXPECTED OUTCOME: Child will maintain weight, adequate hydration, and normal serum albumin.

Planning and Implementation

Care of the burned child involves various treatments designed to promote healing and prevent complications. These include analgesia and comfort measures, wound management, infection control, fluid and nutrition management, physical therapy, and psychologic support. See the *Nursing Care Plan* for several of these topics.

PROMOTE COMFORT

Assess the child's pain frequently and provide pain management around the clock with intravenous opioids (see Chapter 40). To reduce stress on the child, begin pain and sedation management as soon as possible for the initial debridement. Promote the child's comfort during periods of elevated temperature while keeping burns covered to reduce pain. Fluids should be administered at the rate prescribed for resuscitation for the first 24 hours, and then adjusted as prescribed. Keep the room temperature at a comfortable level. Change bed linens as needed when the child perspires heavily.

PROVIDE WOUND CARE

The burned area is debrided and cleaned, often with a chemical enzyme in a whirlpool bath or shower. An antibacterial/antimicrobial dressing is applied. In some cases, a semipermeable wound membrane is applied to superficial partial-thickness burns. At each dressing change, the wound needs to be assessed for appearance, exudate, odor, appearance of surrounding tissue, and presence of granulation tissue.

Allografts or autografts may be put in place in the operating room after debridement to prepare the burned tissue for the graft. Following the grafting process, vacuum-assisted wound closure may be used over graft sites to maintain a moist environment for healing. Donor sites are treated as separate wounds. Splints may be required to promote healing when the skin over a joint is burned. The child may be kept on bed rest for several days following an autograft to protect the graft until it has a vascular supply.

PREVENT COMPLICATIONS

The healthcare team's goal is to prevent complications. Severe complications of burns include infections, pneumonia, and renal failure, as well as possible irreversible loss of function of the burned area. Significant scarring may occur regardless of autografting. Contractures and loss of function are also possible.

PROVIDE EMOTIONAL SUPPORT

Children with burns have received a profound insult to their body and their self-image. Fear and anxiety about disfigurement and scarring are common, especially among adolescents. The shock and pain of the injury cause increased stress, as do the unfamiliar surroundings and presence of healthcare providers.

Psychologic support is essential to the child's recovery. Continuity of healthcare providers is important in developing a trusting relationship with the child and family. Orient the child to their surroundings and give ample preparation for procedures, when possible. Encourage the child and parents to voice concerns, and show understanding and support for their concerns. Make appropriate referrals to social workers, chaplains, and child-life specialists to ensure that the child and family receive necessary services. See *Evidence-Based Practice: Psychologic Impact of Burn Injury.*

EVIDENCE-BASED PRACTICE | Psychologic Impact of Burn Injury

Clinical Question
How do the intensive treatments and long rehabilitation associated with a severe burn impact the child survivor and the family?

The Evidence
A qualitative review of 75 articles focused on the psychologic consequences of pediatric burns for the child and family. Findings revealed that injured children had anxiety, traumatic stress reactions, and behavior problems in the first months after the burn event, while parents had high rates of posttraumatic stress, depressive symptoms, and guilt feelings. After recovery, child survivors as a group had few differences (feelings of self-worth, body image, and social competence) from populations on which assessment tools were normalized. Some children had problems with social functioning and feeling stigmatized. A lower body image was noted more often in girls and those with more severe visible scarring. While family functioning was found to be comparable to norms, parental stress was apparent. Reviewed studies linked the psychologic responses of parents and family functioning as important factors in the child's psychologic outcome (Bakker, Maertens, Van Son, et al., 2013).

A study was conducted to determine the prevalence of posttraumatic stress disorder (PTSD), depression, anxiety, and stress among parents (n = 120) and the child in the first 6 months after the burn injury. Signs of PTSD in the child were determined from an interview with the parent and the Child Behavior Checklist. Tools administered to parents included the Posttraumatic Diagnostic Scale, Depression Anxiety Stress Scale-21, and a scale to assess coping styles used in stressful situations. During the first month after burn injury, parents scored in the moderate to extremely severe range for depression, anxiety, and stress, but these scores lowered to normal or to mild range 6 months after the injury. During the first month, 25 (22%) parents had a probable PTSD diagnosis, but at 6 months, 28 (24%) parents had moderate to moderately severe posttraumatic stress syndrome (PTSS) or impaired functioning. Presence of PTSS in the child was a factor associated with PTSS in parents at 1 month and 6 months postinjury (De Young, Hendrikz, Kenardy, et al., 2014).

A study of 98 child survivors of a burn injury greater than 30% BSA before age 16 years and treated in a Shriners' burn center investigated the potential for development of personality disorders after the injury (mean = 13.9 years later). A structured clinical interview tool and the 16 Personality Factor Fifth Edition Questionnaire were used to identify personality disorders. Half of the survivors (n = 49, 51%) did not have a personality disorder. The most common personality disorders found were paranoid (19.4%), passive aggressive (18.4% and more common in women [27.5%]), and antisocial personality disorder (17.3% and more common in men [22.4%]). Development of a personality disorder was not associated with age at time of burn, burn severity, or facial or other visible burn scars. However, the overall prevalence of personality disorders was higher in these burn survivors than in the general population (Thomas et al., 2012).

Best Practice
Concern about the parents' psychologic response to the child's acute burn is important because higher levels of distress may impact the parents' ability to be emotionally available to help their child manage distress. Young children may also model their responses to the parents' behavior. All children with severe burns and their families need psychologic support to improve coping during the acute and rehabilitation phases of care and to achieve the best social and psychologic functioning. Such support involves nurses, child-life therapists, and mental health professionals.

Clinical Reasoning
When caring for a child with burns in a clinic setting, investigate the resources available for ongoing mental health support for the child and parents. Is attention being paid to the child's behavioral symptoms? What support is provided to parents? What additional resources could help children with acute burn care in the clinic setting?

Play therapy is encouraged for children, even if they can only observe initially. Play therapy serves several purposes for the child with a major burn:

- It provides an outlet for frustration, independence, and creativity.
- It promotes activities that challenge range of motion.
- It normalizes the child's daily routine.
- It encourages the child, who sees the progress other children make day by day.

Families are at risk for emotional stress. Forewarn them about the expected edema and the changes in the child's body. Parents often feel guilty and responsible for the child's injury. Help parents focus on recovery rather than past actions. Anxiety usually results from lack of knowledge about the severity of the burn and the child's status, especially in the early stages of burn care and admission to the hospital ICU or burn center. Include the family in the child's care whenever possible. Involve parents in their child's care so they learn how to change dressings, assess for infection and dehydration, and perform range-of-motion exercises to aid in the child's recovery.

DISCHARGE PLANNING AND HOME CARE TEACHING

Identify and address home care needs well in advance of discharge. Discharge planning may include instructing parents in nutrition and diet needs, safety in the home, protection of the burned area, wound care, signs of infection and actions to take, use of pressure garments, and range-of-motion exercises to prevent contractures. Provide support and encouragement to parents as they learn how to care for the child with a burn injury.

COMMUNITY-BASED NURSING CARE

Care of the child with a serious burn requires long-term therapy and rehabilitation. Long-term care commonly occurs in the home. Many burn centers use silver-embedded burn dressings to reduce the frequency of dressing changes needed. After discharge, visits to the burn clinic are needed 2 to 3 times a week for dressing changes. Sedation may be necessary, depending on the extent of injury and debridement needed. Parents may be instructed to give pain medication prior to arrival at the clinic to ensure that the child has good pain management.

Children with extensive burns or with burns in locations where scarring may limit function must often wear a pressure garment, and sometimes a face mask if the face was burned. The garment is removed only for bathing and laundering. The pressure garment may present a threat to the child's body image, but it is an important way to decrease scarring. Help families understand the need for the special garments and masks, and how to clean and care for them.

Clinical Tip

Moisturizing creams can be used after burns heal to relieve drying. The healed skin is highly sensitive to sunburn, so cover the area or use a sunscreen. The sunscreen will also help prevent hyperpigmentation after burn healing.

Continued physical therapy and occupational therapy are often needed to regain strength and dexterity for self-care skills and to prevent contractures. Emphasis is placed on returning to normal activities of daily living as soon as possible, such as returning to school. Some children have home tutors or computer connections to school for a time to ensure opportunities for learning while decreasing their risk of exposure to infection.

School reentry is often a traumatic experience, especially for older children and adolescents, because of the fear of rejection, decreased self-esteem, and impaired body image. In some cases, the child's primary nurse may visit the school of a child with a burn injury before the child returns to school—bringing photographs of the child, pressure garments, or other items—to inform classmates and allow them to explore their feelings about the child's burn injury. Some communities may offer support groups for families and children with burn injuries. Referral to these groups may be beneficial.

A major role of nurses in the community is prevention. Provide burn prevention information to parents at each health promotion visit. Become involved with a Safe Kids coalition or with local firefighters to help educate families and caregivers about ways to prevent scald burns and house fires. Examples of prevention messages include the following:

- Appropriate temperature settings for hot water heaters
- Keeping the handles of pots on the stove turned toward the wall and dishes with hot liquids out of the toddler's reach
- Keeping infants and toddlers off the lap when drinking hot beverages or eating soup
- Keeping matches, lighters, and flammable materials away from children
- Installing smoke detectors and replacing the batteries annually

MANAGEMENT OF MINOR BURNS

Many children with minor burns are cared for at home after an initial visit to the emergency department or urgent care clinic. Discuss home remedies for minor burn care. For superficial burns covering a small area, use moist soaks to stop the burning process and to relieve pain. Any open blisters are debrided, and a thin layer of antibiotic medication (e.g., Bacitracin, silver sulfadiazine) is applied over the burn. Do not place this medication close to the eyes or mouth. The burn is then covered with one or two layers of gauze. Acetaminophen with codeine may be prescribed for burn dressing changes at home. Burn dressings should be changed twice daily. The child should be seen within 48 hours of initial treatment to monitor progress. Alternatively, a burn dressing may be applied and changed every few days in the clinical setting so the wound can be monitored. See *Teaching Highlights: Caring for Minor Burns.*

Evaluation

Examples of expected outcomes of nursing management are included in the *Nursing Care Plan.* Some additional outcomes include the following:

- The child expresses and shows signs of reduced anxiety.
- Effective pain management is provided for dressing changes.

Sunburn

Sunburn is a burn injury to the outer layer of skin caused by excess ultraviolet light exposure, or sun exposure after taking phototoxic drugs (acne medication, sulfonamides, tetracycline, nonsteroidal anti-inflammatory drugs, and birth control pills). Young children have less melanin to protect their skin against harmful ultraviolet (UV) rays. It is estimated more than 25% of a person's lifetime exposure to sunburns occurs before 18 years

TEACHING HIGHLIGHTS | Caring for Minor Burns

- Place burn under cool, running water to stop the burning process and to help reduce pain. Do not use ice, as it can cause more damage to the injured skin.
- Remove all clothing and jewelry from the burned area.
- Do not use butter or margarine on the burn as it may introduce bacteria into the wound.
- Topical application of gel from the leaf of an aloe vera plant may help promote healing (National Center for Complementary and Alternative Medicine [NCCAM], 2012).
- Apply a topical antibiotic such as bacitracin to the burned area and cover the area with a couple of layers of gauze. Keep the area clean and dry.
- Clean and change the dressing twice daily. The pain medication may be given about an hour before the dressing change is planned. The dressing may be saturated with sterile normal saline and gently removed if it adheres to the burn area. Reapply the antibiotic cream and cover.
- Monitor for signs of infection, such as odor, increased drainage, and increasing redness of the skin around the burn. Contact the healthcare provider if infection is suspected.

of age (Gupta & Cohen, 2012). A childhood sun exposure history that includes intense repeated sunburns and chronic overexposure to UV radiation for the purpose of tanning is strongly associated with the development of all three types of skin cancer (basal cell, squamous cell, and melanoma) in future years (Gupta & Cohen, 2012). Avoiding sunburn during childhood is believed to be more important than protecting skin during adulthood. Use of indoor tanning beds and facilities increases the risk for developing melanoma by 74% (Gupta & Cohen, 2012).

SAFETY ALERT!
Behaviors and skin characteristics that increase the risk for pediatric melanoma include light skin and eyes, freckling, skin with an inability to tan, family history of melanoma, immunosuppression, and ultraviolet radiation treatment for psoriasis (Gupta & Cohen, 2012). Other factors include intermittent intense sun exposure (e.g., blistering sunburns before 20 years of age) and frequent sun exposure without use of sunscreen.

Erythema, pain, skin tenderness, swelling, blistering, and itching usually develop between 3 and 5 hours after exposure to ultraviolet B (UVB) rays. Solar UVA rays penetrate more deeply into the skin. Increased vasodilation and vascular permeability result in the extravasation of fluid to the tissues (edema, vesicles, and bullae) and white blood cell migration to the damaged skin. The erythema peaks at 12 to 24 hours and subsides after 72 hours. Systemic complaints include malaise, poor sleep due to

Professionalism in Practice Sun Tanning
The American Academy of Pediatrics policy statement on ultraviolet radiation (UVR) states that the deliberate exposure to artificial sources of UVR (e.g., tanning beds and facilities) and overexposure to the sun to increase vitamin D concentrations should be avoided (AAP, 2011). Nurses have an important role in educating adolescents about the risks for skin cancer and damage to the eyes from UVR exposure. Nurses can also work with community leaders to develop local policies that ban adolescents under age 18 years from using tanning facilities or tanning beds.

skin tenderness, fatigue, headaches, and chilling resulting from rapid heat loss.

Treatment is generally supportive. Pain can be relieved by cool compresses, local anesthetic sprays or creams, and an emollient to help keep skin from drying out. Nonsteroidal anti-inflammatory drugs (NSAIDs) may be used for pain relief and to reduce inflammation. See Chapter 40 for information on NSAIDs. Skin exposed by broken blisters is gently washed 2 to 3 times a day and covered with clean clothing or a sterile dressing if the sunburned skin is limited to a small area.

Nursing Management

Educate parents and children about preventing sunburn. Advise parents and children that repeated sunburns may lead to permanent skin damage, skin cancer, cataracts, and premature aging of the skin. See *Teaching Highlights: Preventing Sunburn.*

Healthy People 2020

(C-20) Increase the proportion of persons who participate in behaviors that reduce their exposure to harmful ultraviolet (UV) irradiation and avoid sunburn

Hypothermia

Hypothermia is a condition in which the core body temperature falls below 35°C (95°F). This occurs when the heat produced by the body is less than the heat lost. Hypothermia is a life-threatening emergency that can occur in any season and any geographic location. Infants and young children are at risk because of immature temperature regulatory mechanisms, thinner skin, limited subcutaneous fat, and a high skin surface area-to-body mass ratio. Adolescents are at risk because of risk-taking behaviors such as drug and alcohol use and engaging in remote outdoor activities without proper equipment.

Primary hypothermia results from environmental exposure. As with newborns, heat is lost through radiation, conduction, convection, and evaporation. As the core body temperature falls, the body tries to conserve body heat and to rewarm the blood by vasoconstriction (to shunt blood to the body core). The body generates heat by increasing muscle tone and shivering. Hypothermia leads to increased blood viscosity, slower blood flow through the capillaries, and the potential for blood coagulation.

TEACHING HIGHLIGHTS | Preventing Sunburn

- Keep children out of direct sunlight as much as possible, especially between 10 a.m. and 4 p.m. Encourage children to play in the shade.
- Be aware that water, concrete, and sand reflect sunlight and increase exposure by reflecting UV rays up toward the skin.
- Minimize sun exposure by wearing a hat with a 3-inch brim, closely woven cotton long-sleeved clothing and pants, and wraparound UV blocking sunglasses with 99% UV blockage. Wear a T-shirt while swimming.
- Use sunscreen with a sun protection factor (SPF) of 30 or higher. Apply thickly to all exposed areas 30 minutes before sun exposure. Reapply 15 to 20 minutes after first sun exposure, and then again every 2 hours as needed. Reapply sooner if swimming, toweling off, or perspiring heavily.
- Use a waterproof sunscreen when swimming for protection in water that lasts 60 to 80 minutes. Then reapply. Avoid placing it near the eyes as it causes a chemical burn and pain. Call the poison control center immediately if eyes are exposed.
- Use UV blocking agents such as zinc oxide or titanium oxide for infants under 6 months of age because infants may absorb sunscreen chemical through their skin.
- If the child is taking any medications, check with the healthcare provider before exposure (some medications cause hypersensitivity to sunlight).
- Adolescents should avoid indoor tanning facilities and artificial tanning devices because the rays are as damaging to the skin as the sun.

Symptoms of mild hypothermia (32 to 35°C [89.6 to 95.0°F]) include slurred speech, poor coordination, poor judgment and inappropriate behavior, shivering, and muscle stiffness. Symptoms of moderate hypothermia (28 to 32°C [82.4 to 89.6°F]) include depressed respirations, slow pulse, low blood pressure, pale or cyanotic color, shivering, and dilated pupils. Lethargy, mental impairment, irrational thinking, hallucinations, and coma develop as the central nervous system becomes depressed. Profound hypothermia (body temperature below 28°C [82.4°F]) is characterized by apnea, no shivering, low blood pressure, ventricular fibrillation, dilated and unresponsive pupils, and coma.

Clinical therapy focuses on resuscitation, if necessary, and gradual core body rewarming. The child who has profound hypothermia should receive cardiopulmonary resuscitation until the body temperature returns to normal because the hypothermia may have preserved vital organs. Aggressive techniques for rewarming may include humidified, warm oxygen; warmed intravenous fluids; warm packs to the core circulation areas (axillae, groin, and neck); and peritoneal lavage and dialysis. Hypoglycemia is a common complication and is treated with IV glucose.

For mild hypothermia (temperature above 35°C [95°F]), external heat lamps, immersion in warm water, and an electric blanket are used.

Nursing Management

Monitor vital signs and urine output during rewarming. Educate parents to layer children's clothing in cold climates, recognize signs of hypothermia, decrease time of exposure to cold, and know how to treat mild hypothermia. Teach school-age children and adolescents who go on camping and hunting trips how to recognize and manage hypothermia in themselves and others. Teach preventive techniques such as to avoid riding snowmobiles or walking on ice that is not known to be deep enough to support the weight.

First aid for hypothermia includes moving the child to a dry area and removing any wet clothing. Replace with warm, dry clothing, and encourage the child to drink a warm, high-calorie liquid, if possible. If a child becomes hypothermic during a camping trip or other outing, a warm person should get into a sleeping bag (or under the blankets) next to the child after any wet or heavy clothing is removed. This action will trap heat the child's body generates and provide passive rewarming by the other person.

Frostbite

Frostbite is a cold injury in which the skin tissue is exposed to temperatures below freezing for more than an hour when environmental protection is inadequate. Areas of the body at high risk for frostbite include the hands, feet, cheeks, nose, and ears. Ice crystallizes in the tissues, resulting in dehydration of the cells and ischemic damage. Frostbite can also occur if a chemical cold pack used for first aid is left in contact with the skin for an extended period.

Clinical manifestations vary by the severity of injury. In mild or superficial frostbite, the skin appears reddened or mottled, edematous, and stiff, and transient tingling or burning is present. In severe or deeper frostbite, the skin is gray or mottled, edematous, hard with no rebounding, and numb.

With superficial injury, rapid rewarming causes a flush and the sensation of tingling, burning, or prickling in the affected area. With deeper injury, the skin may appear mottled and cyanotic followed by erythema, swelling, and burning pain with rewarming. Vesicles and bullae develop in 24 to 48 hours, which slowly heal. The extent of injury is not initially apparent.

If frostbite is suspected, get the child to a warmer environment and remove any wet clothes. Because the frostbitten area may be numb, protect it from trauma. Slowly rewarm the area to decrease the chance of cellular damage by immersing the affected part in warm water between 40°C and 42°C (104.0°F and 107.6°F) until thawed. Analgesics are given to treat pain caused by thawing. Gently clean the affected skin with saline and cover it with sterile dressings. Wound care may be similar to that provided to a child with burns. Physical therapy may be important to improve circulation and maintain function.

Nursing Management

As with hypothermia, the goal of management is prevention. Teach parents to layer children's clothing for warmth and to pack extra blankets and clothing if cold temperatures are expected during outdoor activities. Teach adolescents how to avoid frostbite during hunting and other cold weather expeditions. Wet clothing and gloves should be changed quickly.

Early care is instrumental in minimizing permanent injury. Severe frostbite requires hospitalization, fluid management, dressing changes, and careful attention to diet. Provide emotional support to the child and family while they wait to learn the full extent of injury and disability.

Bites

ANIMAL BITES

Dog bites accounted for nearly 134,000 emergency department visits in 2013 for children and youth less than age 20 years (National Center for Injury Prevention and Control, 2015). Children, and especially boys, ages 5 to 9 years have the highest rate of dog bites (CDC, 2014). In many cases, the dog or cat is known by the child, and most bites occur in the home or a familiar place. Bites are often associated with the child's inappropriate behavior, such as teasing, rough play, or interfering with feeding or care of puppies. Other animals that may bite include cats, birds, turtles, and wild animals such as bats, squirrels, and raccoons.

Assessment includes noting the location and number of puncture wounds, abrasions, lacerations, and crushing injuries; redness or swelling at entry sites; redness extending out from site (possible cellulitis); and any drainage related to the bite. Damage to nerves, muscles, tendons, and vascular structures is identified. Dog bites tend to be crushing rather than clean, sharp lacerations. Cat bites tend to be puncture wounds; 50% become infected (AAP, 2015, p. 205). Head and neck bites require radiographic examination to rule out any associated injury, such as trauma to the airway or a depressed skull fracture.

Initial treatment involves irrigation of the wound, removal of devitalized tissue, and application of a clean dressing. Povidone-iodine solution (a virucidal agent) may be used in some cases to irrigate the wound. Sedation and pain management may be needed for some children. Puncture wounds may be debrided in the operating room. Prophylactic antibiotics may be prescribed to reduce the risk for infections. A delay in seeking care after the bite is associated with a greater risk for infection.

Wounds may be closed with adhesive strips rather than suturing because of the potential for infection. Severe bites sometimes require surgical closure or reconstruction. Wounds over joints should be immobilized and elevated. The major complication of bites is infection (such as cellulitis, septic arthritis, or osteomyelitis), which may require hospitalization.

Dog bites should be reported to animal control, and the dog should be confined and observed for 10 days for signs of rabies. Cat bites are also dangerous because cats are less commonly immunized against rabies. If the animal develops rabies during that interval, human rabies immune globulin (HRIG) and rabies vaccine is administered immediately, followed by a rabies vaccine injection on days 3, 7, and 14 following the first injection. HRIG and rabies vaccine are given immediately to all children bitten by wild animals in which rabies cannot be excluded. See Chapter 43 for a description of rabies treatment.

Nursing Management

If a child is bitten by an animal, obtain information about the extent of the injury, circumstances surrounding the attack, present location of the animal, and attempts to assess the animal's health.

To decrease infection, the wound is gently washed with antibacterial soap and water followed by high-pressure irrigation (unless it is a puncture wound) with large quantities of sterile saline or lactated Ringer solution. An 18-gauge needle on a 60-mL syringe may be used to provide high-pressure irrigation. A clean dressing is applied and the affected body part is elevated to reduce bleeding. Check the child's immunization record to determine whether a tetanus booster is necessary. Teach parents how to care for the wound and signs of infection that indicate a need to return for care.

Prevention of animal bites is another important nursing role (see *Teaching Highlights: Preventing Animal Bites*).

HUMAN BITES

Human bites are more common than most people realize. Toddlers, young children, and adolescents often receive human bites during altercations. The skin may be broken, with erythema, abrasion, bruising, or laceration. Because the mouth harbors many bacteria, infection is fairly common. Assess the risk for hepatitis B and HIV infection. Initial treatment includes irrigating with sterile saline and debridement. Antibiotics may be prescribed to prevent systemic complications. Parents should be instructed about how to care for the wound and to observe for infection.

TEACHING HIGHLIGHTS | Preventing Animal Bites

General Guidelines for Pets in the Home

- Never leave a young child alone with an animal.
- Do not buy or adopt a pet unless you are confident of your child's ability to respect it.
- Spay or neuter the pet to reduce aggression.

Teach Children the Following Rules

- Avoid all unfamiliar animals and report them to a parent.
- Avoid contact with all wild animals. If an animal (wild or unknown) is sick or acting strangely, notify the health department.
- Do not touch an animal when it is eating, sleeping, or nursing.
- Never overexcite an animal, even in play. Do not roughhouse or play games that stimulate aggressive behavior. Do not tease or throw objects at an animal.
- Never put your face close to an animal. Seek permission before hugging or petting an animal.
- If approached by a dog, stay calm, stand still, talk softly, and back away slowly until the dog loses interest; do not run.
- If attacked, pretend to be a tree or a log and protect the face. If knocked down, curl into a ball and protect the face and neck.

INSECT BITES AND STINGS

Insect bites and stings occur frequently in children and usually are not a cause for concern. Exceptions include bites or stings by insects that carry parasites or communicable diseases (ticks, mosquitos), those of a venomous nature (spiders), and those that produce an allergic reaction. A small percentage of the population is sensitized to *Hymenoptera* (bee, wasps, fire ants) stings and has a generalized response. See Table 57–7 for clinical manifestations of insect bites and stings. For a discussion of communicable diseases carried by ticks and mosquitoes (e.g., Lyme disease, Rocky Mountain spotted fever, West Nile virus, malaria), see Chapter 43.

Nursing Management

The goal of nursing care is prevention. Become familiar with the harmful insects in your area, so you can identify them and recognize their effects. Teach children to avoid spiders and other biting or stinging insects. Teach children to stay calm when a bee or wasp approaches and to slowly walk away without swatting. Many commercial repellents (OFF, Cutter's, Deep Woods OFF) are available. Most products contain DEET (diethyltoluamide) or oil of lemon eucalyptus. They are effective against many insects, including mosquitoes, fleas, ticks, and chiggers, but do not repel stinging insects.

Warn parents against using heavily perfumed shampoos, powders, soaps, or lotions. Do not dress children in bright-colored or floral print clothing when outdoors, as these may attract insects. Avoid eating sweet foods and beverages outdoors as these will attract bees and wasps. Bees and wasps may crawl into a canned beverage and not be seen. Pour beverages into a cup rather than drinking from a can to prevent stings to the mouth and lips.

Household pets may be a source of fleas or ticks. Encourage frequent inspection of pets and preventive treatments against fleas and ticks before pets are allowed prolonged contact with children.

When a systemic reaction to *Hymenoptera* has occurred, the child should wear a medical alert identification and carry an emergency kit with epinephrine (see Chapter 48). Teach parents and school personnel how to administer epinephrine. Desensitization injections may be given.

SNAKE BITES

Venomous snakes are found in most areas of the country. During warm months, snakes are active and likely to bite if disturbed. Fortunately, many bites are dry, delivering no venom. Fatalities are rare.

Rattlesnake, copperhead, and cottonmouth venom is composed of enzymes and toxins that cause hemolysis and tissue necrosis. Coral snake venom causes neuromuscular paralysis that can affect breathing and lead to respiratory arrest (Wilbeck, & Gresham, 2013). The amount and toxicity of the venom injected has an impact on the consequences of the snakebite. Because children usually receive a higher amount of venom relative to body mass, their response may be greater than that of an adult.

Puncture marks, white wheal, and burning sensation appear at the site of the bite. With envenomation erythema, bruising and edema rapidly develop and extend from the site for up to 24 hours. Systemic signs include dizziness, tachycardia, nausea, vomiting, diarrhea, sweating, chills, and muscle twitching. Signs of a severe response may include hypotension, altered consciousness, bleeding from multiple sites (disseminated intravascular coagulation), pulmonary edema, and renal failure. Coral snake neurologic signs may include diplopia and ptosis, difficulty speaking and swallowing, hypersalivation, and altered mental status (lethargy, drowsiness, or euphoria).

Clinical therapy involves immobilization of the extremity and a cold compress to slow the spread of the venom. Laboratory studies include complete blood count, platelet count, coagulation studies, electrolytes, and renal function. Attempts to identify the snake causing the bite should be made to determine if it is venomous. A cell phone photograph of the snake is useful in identifying whether the snake is venomous. The poison control center is contacted to obtain treatment guidelines. Specific antivenom (often made with horse serum) is usually administered within 4 to 6 hours. CroFab, a newer antivenom used for cottonmouth, copperhead, and rattlesnake bites, has a lower rate of hypersensitivity reactions. Children at risk for severe hypersensitivity reaction are pretreated with antihistamines and corticosteroids. Monitor children treated with CroFab for thrombocytopenia, bleeding, or development of coagulopathy due to hemolytic effect of venom. Acetaminophen and codeine may be prescribed for pain management. A tetanus booster is given if vaccination status is unknown or the tetanus series is incomplete.

Nursing Management

Nursing care involves assessing the child for initial and progressive signs of envenomation. Try to keep the child calm to slow the circulation. First aid involves immobilizing the extremity, keeping it in a dependent position to slow the spread of venom, and cold compresses. Hands with a bite should be elevated after splinting in functional position. Ice should not be used. Rings or constricting items should be quickly removed from the injured extremity. Monitor the distal extremity's color, pulse, and sensation, and measure the circumference of the extremity above and below the affected extremity; reassess every 15 to 30 minutes to track progression of edema and response to treatment. Clean the wound with germicidal soap and water.

The child receiving antivenom may be cared for in the critical care unit. The antivenom is diluted in saline and slowly administered intravenously as ordered. Administer the antihistamines after tests for sensitivity to horse serum are completed. Have resuscitation equipment on hand in preparation for an anaphylactic reaction. Help locate additional antivenom if the hospital does not have an adequate supply. At time of discharge, educate parents of children who receive antivenom to monitor for unusual bleeding and to contact the health professional if noted. NSAIDs should not be used for 2 weeks after discharge because of increased bleeding risk.

Provide emotional support to the child and family. Teach children and their families to avoid future snakebites.

Contusions

Contusions are soft-tissue injuries that have a variety of causes. Often it is difficult to assess whether an injury has caused underlying tissue damage. An injury does not have to break the skin to result in internal damage. Radiographic examination may be necessary to rule out broken bones or further tissue damage. Signs and symptoms that indicate a need for treatment include swelling that does not subside within 72 hours, intense pain, inability to move the injured part, and infection. Elevate the injured extremity and apply ice as soon as possible after injury. This can reduce inflammation and swelling in the area.

Foreign Bodies

Many skin injuries result from penetration of foreign particles. Common substances include gravel from abrasions, bee

TABLE 57–7 Clinical Manifestations of Insect Bites and Stings

TYPE OF BITE AND CLINICAL MANIFESTATIONS	CLINICAL THERAPY
MOSQUITOES AND FLEAS	
Local inflammation results from injected foreign protein or chemicals. • Local reaction: discrete, red papules and edema at the bite site with itching, burning, pain, and hives; minimal discomfort; pruritic wheals and bullae tend to develop with repeat exposure. • Systemic reaction: wheezing, urticaria; laryngeal edema; shock	Local reactions: • Cold compresses or ice applied to the site • Antihistamine medication Systemic reactions need emergency medical treatment.
BED BUGS	
Local inflammation results from injected saliva, an anesthetic and anticoagulant. • Local reaction: numerous pruritic papules, often in pattern of three papules; child often wakes up with numerous lesions on exposed skin areas that were not present the night before. • Systemic reaction: rare severe allergic reaction	Local reactions: • Keep skin clean. • Topical corticosteroids may be applied. • Antihistamines may be prescribed. • Oral corticosteroids may be prescribed for severe allergic reaction. • Treat infested areas, and discard infested bedding.
BEE OR WASP STING	
Venoms contain enzymes that affect vascular tone and permeability. • Local reaction: mild, local pain; erythema and edema • Systemic reaction: generalized urticaria, flushing, angioedema, pruritus; wheezing; dizziness, hypotension; abdominal pain, vomiting, diarrhea; anaphylaxis is rare.	Local reactions: • Remove stinger as soon as possible. • Apply cold compresses and elevate extremity. • A dash of meat tenderizer (papain powder) and a drop of water massaged into the skin for 5 minutes to relieve pain. • Antihistamine medication Systemic reactions are treated with glucocorticoids and antihistamines or epinephrine. • Desensitization for severe reactions
FIRE ANTS	
Venom is hemolytic and neurotoxic, causing a histamine-like response. • Local reaction: a black center at the point of the bite, or trail of lesions across skin; initial wheal becomes a vesicle in a few hours; in 24 hr the fluid is cloudy, and the vesicle has a red halo; pruritus, erythema, edema, induration • Systemic and anaphylactic reactions can occur.	Local reactions: • Ice or cold compresses • Antihistamine medication • Elevate extremity. Systemic reactions—same as bees and wasps
BLACK WIDOW SPIDER	
Venom is neurotoxic. • Local reaction: stinging sensation at time of bite; localized edema and erythema, two fang marks, petechiae branching from site • Systemic reaction in 1–3 hr, symptoms peak in 3–12 hr, diminish in 72 hr; muscle rigidity of torso and abdomen, priapism, muscle cramps near the bite; malaise, sweating, nausea, vomiting, dizziness, restlessness, insomnia, and diaphoresis; hypertension and arrhythmias; oliguria	Ice Diazepam and opioids for pain management Antihistamine medication Hydrocortisone may decrease the inflammatory response. Antivenom IV is used in severe reactions after negative skin test for hypersensitivity to horse serum.
BROWN RECLUSE SPIDER	
Venom contains proteolytic enzymes and sphingomyelinase D, a cytotoxic factor. • Local reaction: within 2 hr, sinking blue macule with a halo of inflammation at the bite site; pain; a hemorrhagic blister forms in 1–2 days with a necrotic ulcer seen when it breaks. Most ulcers are 1–2 cm (0.4 to 0.8 in.) in diameter, but some progress to 15 cm (6 in.) in diameter with full-thickness injury. • Systemic reaction: fever, chills, nausea and vomiting, and hemolysis	Ice Cleanse the wound and good wound care Elevate extremity Analgesics Oral anti-inflammatory agent Antibiotics for secondary infection Excision and skin grafting in cases of severe necrosis

Source: Data from Krau, S. D. (2013). Bites and stings: Epidemiology and treatment. *Critical Care Nursing Clinics of North America, 25,* 143–150; Barnes, E. R., & Murray, B. S. (2013). Bedbugs: What nurses need to know. *American Journal of Nursing, 113*(10), 58–62; Camp, N. E. (2014). Black widow spider envenomation. *Journal of Emergency Nursing, 40*(2), 193–194.

stingers, and splinters. Treatment of superficial foreign bodies involves irrigating the wound to try to forcibly dislodge the debris. A deeply embedded foreign body is best removed under medical supervision to avoid permanent injury or scarring.

Lacerations

Lacerations are cuts or tears to the skin. In many cases, the cut is minor and can be managed at home with gentle cleansing, antibiotic ointment, and a bandage. More extensive lacerations and those on the face or over joints often need suturing to promote healing and reduce scarring. Laceration repair is performed after wound cleansing and appropriate local analgesia to control pain. Sutures or dermal adhesive may be used. Sutures are usually removed about 7 days later.

Focus Your Study

- Wound healing has three overlapping phases: hemostasis and inflammation, tissue formation, and maturation.

- Contact dermatitis is a skin inflammation that occurs following direct contact with an allergen that causes an immune response, or with an irritant that causes no immune response.

- Superabsorbent disposable diapers reduce the frequency and severity of diaper dermatitis because, when wet, a gel forms inside the diaper keeping moisture away from the skin.

- Seborrheic dermatitis is an inflammatory skin condition due to an overgrowth of *Malassezia furfur* yeast in areas of sebaceous gland activity. Lesions are commonly found on the scalp, nasolabial folds, behind the ears, and intertriginous areas.

- The classic impetigo lesion begins as a vesicle surrounded by edema and redness. The vesicle fluid turns cloudy and ruptures, leaving a honey-colored crust on an ulcerated base.

- Athletes are at high risk for community-acquired methicillin-resistant *Staphylococcus aureus* because of their potential for frequent skin-to-skin contact, cuts or abrasions, wound contact, and shared items.

- Folliculitis, a superficial inflammation of the pilosebaceous follicle, may be associated with *Pseudomonas* exposure in a poorly chlorinated pool or hot tub.

- Children with cellulitis appear ill with fever, chills, malaise, and enlarged lymph nodes. The infected site is red or lilac in color, warm, edematous, and tender with an indistinct border.

- Viral skin infections include molluscum contagiosum and warts (papillomavirus).

- Oral thrush (candidiasis), a fungal infection, is characterized by white patches that resemble coagulated milk on the oral mucosa and may bleed when removed.

- Children being treated for tinea capitis may develop an "id" hypersensitivity reaction rash to the fungal antigen, and this is not an allergic reaction to the medication.

- Drug reactions vary in severity from a simple allergic reaction and erythema multiforme minor to potential life-threatening conditions, such as Stevens–Johnson syndrome and toxic epidermal necrolysis.

- Treatment of atopic eczema involves hydration and lubrication of the skin by bathing followed by emollients to trap in skin moisture. Topical corticosteroids are used to treat skin flares and then discontinued.

- Acne medications, tretinoin or isotretinoin, are phototoxic, resulting in sunburn with even minimal exposure. Protection with sunscreen or protective clothing is important to prevent significant sunburn.

- Psoriasis is chronic skin condition with pruritic, thick, silvery, scaly erythematous plaques that have irregular borders surrounded by normal skin.

- Epidermolysis bullosa is a rare, autosomal dominant, severe chronic blistering skin disorder that occurs with minor trauma.

- Treatment for lice includes a pediculicide applied to the hair and combing the hair with a fine-toothed comb to remove all the nits. Depending on product used, a second treatment may be needed in 7 days.

- Scabies is a mite infestation in which the female mite burrows under the skin to lay eggs, which causes irritation and intense itching.

- Hemangiomas undergo a period of rapid growth during infancy before involuting. The rapid growth may cause significant complications, such as pressure on the airway, eye, or ear canal.

- Children at greatest risk for pressure ulcers are those with limited mobility, sensory deficits, or the inability to change positions. Tissue ischemia occurs when the soft tissues and capillary beds are compressed between a bony prominence and another surface.

- Of the four main types of burns (thermal, chemical, electrical, and radioactive), thermal burns are most common in children. Infants, toddlers, and preschool-age children most commonly suffer scald burns. Other types of thermal burns include flames and contact with a hot object.

- Initial treatment for a child with a significant burn injury includes emergency assessment of the airway, breathing, and circulation and stopping the burning process by removing jewelry and clothing, and applying moist soaks or ice.

- More than 25% of a person's lifetime exposure to the sun occurs by 18 years of age. Repeated blistering sunburns during childhood increase the risk for development of melanoma.

- Children are at greater risk for hypothermia because of their thinner skin, limited subcutaneous fat, and high surface area to body mass ratio. Body heat is lost more quickly in water or when clothing is wet.

- Frostbite occurs when ice crystallizes in the tissues, causing cellular dehydration and ischemic damage.

- Children at highest risk for dog bites are those 5 to 9 years old. Most children know the dog that bites them.

- Insects and spiders with venomous bites include bees, fire ants, black widow spiders, and brown recluse spiders.

- Venomous snakes living in the wild in the United States include rattlesnakes, copperheads, water moccasins, and coral snakes. Initial treatment includes calming the child, immobilization of the extremity, and applying cold compresses to slow the spread of the venom.

Clinical Reasoning in Action

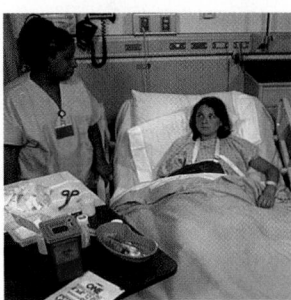

Twelve-year-old Rebecca is admitted to the burn unit with a scald burn from spilling a pot of boiling spaghetti water on her chest, abdomen, and legs. The burn is classified as a partial-thickness burn covering 12% of her body surface area (BSA) and full-thickness burn covering 3% of BSA. IV fluids are started in the emergency department and a continuous infusion of morphine is given for pain. Her temperature is 101.0°F (38.3°C). The initial debridement of the burns is performed in the operating room so that Rebecca is anesthetized and does not feel pain from the procedure. A silver-embedded dressing is applied to her partial-thickness burns, and a biologic dressing is placed over the full-thickness injury. Following debridement, Rebecca is put on a high-calorie, high-protein diet to help meet her increased nutritional requirements. Her parents are encouraged to bring in foods Rebecca enjoys to encourage her to eat. Wound care around the biologic dressing is performed twice a day, and all burn sites are inspected for signs of infection. The dressing over the partial-thickness burns is replaced every 3 days. Pain medication

for wound care is provided through the IV. After several days, Rebecca is scheduled for an autograft for the full-thickness injury. Rebecca's nutritional intake and urine output are carefully monitored while she is hospitalized. Physical therapy is initiated to maintain range of motion and to prevent contractures.

The nurse talks with Rebecca and her family about what to expect as the burns heal. Education of the family includes signs and symptoms of infection and the care of the graft donor site and the graft site. After a few days in the hospital, Rebecca is discharged with daily follow-up in the burn clinic for wound care.

1. Which IV fluid is most likely used to treat Rebecca when she is admitted to the emergency department? Why?

2. Why is it important to monitor Rebecca's urine output?

3. What are the advantages of the type of dressing used for Rebecca's partial-thickness burns?

4. What regular assessments of Rebecca's burn sites should be performed?

5. What are some high-protein, high-calorie foods that might appeal to Rebecca?

References

American Academy of Pediatrics Council on Environmental Health and Section on Dermatology. (2011). Policy statement—Ultraviolet radiation: A hazard to children and adolescents. *Pediatrics, 127*(3), 588–597.

American Academy of Pediatrics (AAP), Committee on Infectious Disease. (2015). *Red book: Report of the Committee on Infectious Disease* (30th ed.). Elk Grove Village, IL: Author.

American College of Surgeons, Committee on Trauma. (2014). *Resources for the optimal care of the injured patient, 2014*. Chicago, IL: Author.

Artz, C. P., & Moncrief, J. A. (1969). *The treatment of burns* (2nd ed.). Philadelphia, PA: Elsevier Saunders.

Bakker, A., Maertens, K. J. P., Van Son, M. J. M., & Van Loey, N. E. E. (2013). Psychological consequences of pediatric burns from a child and family perspective: A review of the empirical literature. *Clinical Psychology Review, 33*, 361–371.

Barnes, E. R., & Murray, B. S. (2013). Bedbugs: What nurses need to know. *American Journal of Nursing, 113*(10), 58–62.

Bhutani, T., Kamangar, F., & Cordoro, K. M. (2012). Management of pediatric psoriasis. *Pediatric Annals, 41*(1), e11–e17.

Block, S. L., & Blackmon, L. (2013). Treating infantile hemangiomatosis: A case study. *Pediatric Annals, 42*(6), 230–233.

Bowden, V. R. (2012). Losing the louse: How to manage this common infestation in children. *Pediatric Nursing, 38*(5), 253–254, 277.

Camp, N. E. (2014). Black widow spider envenomation. *Journal of Emergency Nursing, 40*(2), 193–194.

Centers for Disease Control and Prevention (CDC). (2014). *Dog bites*. Retrieved from http://www.cdc.gov /HomeandRecreationalSafety/Dog-Bites/index.html

Centers for Disease Control and Prevention (CDC). (2015). *Overall fire/burn nonfatal injuries and rates per 100,000, 2013, United States*. Retrieved from http://www.cdc.gov/injury/wisqars/nonfatal.html

Chen, X., Anstey, A. V., & Bugert, J. J. (2013). Molluscum contagiosum virus infection. *Lancet Infectious Diseases, 13*, 877–888.

Chung, J., & Cohen, B. A. (2014). Infant's growing birthmark causes blurry vision. *Contemporary Pediatrics, 31*(9), 58–59.

Cohen, B. A. (2014). Infant with a persistent nodular rash. *Contemporary Pediatrics, 31*(1), 32, 35.

Coulombe, P. A., & Lee, C. (2012). Defining keratin protein function in skin epithelia: Epidermolysis bullosa simplex and its aftermath. *Journal of Investigative Dermatology, 132*, 763–775.

D'Cruz, R., Martin, H. C. O., & Holland, A. J. A. (2013). Medical management of paediatric burn injuries: Best practice, Part 2. *Journal of Paediatrics and Child Health, 49*, e397–e404.

De Young, A. C., Hendrikz, J., Kenardy, J. A., Cobham, V. E., & Kimble, R. M. (2014). Prospective evaluation of parent distress following pediatric burns and identification of risk factors for young child and parent posttraumatic stress disorder. *Journal of Child and Adolescent Psychopharmacology, 24*(1), 9–17.

Eisenhower, C., & Farrington, E. A. (2012). Advancements in the treatment of head lice in pediatrics. *Journal of Pediatric Health Care, 26*(6), 451–461.

Feinberg, A. N., Shwayder, T. A., Ruqiya, T., & Therdpong, T. (2014). Pediatric dermatologic disorders. *Journal of Alternative Medicine Research, 6*(2), 95–137.

Fenlon, S., & Nene, S. (2007). Burns in children. *Continuing Education in Anaesthesia, Critical Care & Pain, 7*(3), 76–80.

Fonacier, L. S., Aquino, M. R., & Mucci, T. (2012). Current strategies in treating severe contact dermatitis in pediatric patients. *Current Allergy and Asthma Reports, 12*, 599–606.

Fritz, S. A., Hogan, P. G., Hyack, G., Eisenstein, K. A., Rodriguez, M., Epplin, E. K., ... Fraser, V. J. (2012). Household versus individual approaches to eradication of community-associated *Staphylococcus aureus* in children: A randomized trial. *Clinical Infectious Diseases, 54*, 743–751.

Gupta, A., & Cohen, B. (2012). Ultraviolet radiation exposure and melanoma. *Contemporary Pediatrics, 29*(5), 10–14.

Halloran, L. (2014). Developing dermatology detective powers: Allergic contact dermatitis. *Journal for Nurse Practitioners, 10*(4), 284–285.

Hazinski, M. F., Mondozzi, M. A., & Baker, R. A. U. (2014). Shock, multiple organ dysfunction syndrome, and burns in children. In K. L. McCance, S. E. Huether, V. L. Brashers, & N. S. Rote (Eds.), *Pathophysiology: The biologic basis for disease in adults and children* (7th ed., pp. 1699–1727). St. Louis, MO: Elsevier.

Jeschke, M. G., & Herndon, D. N. (2014). Burns in children: Standard and new treatments. *Lancet, 383*, 1168–1178.

Joyce, J. C. (2016). Vesiculobullous disorders. In R. M. Kliegman, B. F. Stanton, J. W. St. Geme, & N. F. Schor (Eds.), *Nelson textbook of pediatrics* (20th ed., pp. 3140–3150). St. Louis, MO: Elsevier.

Juern, A. M., & Drolet, B. A. (2016). Cutaneous bacterial infections. In R. M. Kliegman, B. F. Stanton, J. W. St. Geme, & N. F. Schor (Eds.), *Nelson textbook of pediatrics* (20th ed., pp. 3203–3213). Philadelphia, PA: Elsevier.

Kim, L. K. P., Martin, H. C. O., & Holland, A. J. A. (2012). Medical management of paediatric burn injuries: Best practice. *Journal of Paediatrics and Child Health, 48*, 290–295.

Kim, W., & Mancini, A. J. (2013). Acne in childhood: An update. *Pediatric Annals, 42*(10), 418–427.

Krau, S. D. (2013). Bites and stings: Epidemiology and treatment. *Critical Care Nursing Clinics of North America, 25*, 143–150.

Krowchuk, D. P., & Mancini, A. J. (2012). *Pediatric dermatology: A quick reference guide* (2nd ed.). Oak Grove, IL: American Academy of Pediatrics.

Kwan, J. M., & Jacob, S. E. (2012). Contact dermatitis in the atopic child. *Pediatric Annals, 41*(10), 422–428.

Lauren, C., & Garzon, M. C. (2012). Treatment of infantile hemangiomas. *Pediatric Annals, 41*(8), e167–e173.

McCann, S. A., & Huether, S. E. (2014). Structure, function, and disorders of the integument. In K. L. McCance, S. E. Huether, V. L. Brashers, & N. S. Rote (Eds.), *Pathophysiology: The biologic basis for disease in adults and children* (7th ed., pp. 1616–1652). St. Louis, MO: Elsevier.

National Center for Complementary and Alternative Medicine (NCCAM). (2012). *Aloe vera.* Retrieved from http://nccam.nih.gov/health/aloevera

National Center for Health Statistics, National Vital Statistics System. (2015). *Ten leading causes of unintentional injury deaths, United States, 2013, all races, both sexes.* Retrieved from http://www.cdc.gov/injury/wisqars/leading_causes_death.html

National Center for Injury Prevention and Control. (2015). *Overall dog bite nonfatal injuries and rates per 100,000, 2013, United States, all races, both sexes.* Retrieved from http://www.cdc.gov/injury/wisqars/nonfatal.html

Neville-Swensen, M., & Clayton, M. (2011). Outpatient management of community-associated methicillin-resistant *Staphylococcus aureus* skin and soft tissue infection. *Journal of Pediatric Health Care, 25*(5), 308–315.

Nicol, N. H., & Huether, S. E. (2014). Alterations in the integument in children. In K. L. McCance, S. E. Huether, V. L. Brashers, & N. S. Rote (Eds.), *Pathophysiology: The biologic basis for disease in adults and children* (7th ed., pp. 1653–1667), St. Louis, MO: Elsevier.

Ooi, E. T., & Tidman, M. J. (2014). Improving the management of seborrhoeic dermatitis. *The Practitioner, 258*(1768), 23–26.

Pariser, D. M., Meinking, T. L., Bell, M., & Ryan, W. G. (2012). Topical 0.5% ivermectin lotion for treatment of head lice. *New England Journal of Medicine, 367*(18), 1687–1693.

Reinke, J. M. & Sorg, H. (2012). Wound repair and regeneration. *European Surgical Research, 49*, 35–43

Roduit, C., Frei, R., Loss, G., Buchele, G., Weber, J., Depner, M., ... Lauener, R. (2012). Development of atopic dermatitis according to age of onset and association with early-life exposures. *Journal of Allergy and Clinical Immunology, 130*, 130–136.

Rolstad, B. S., Bryant, R. A., & Nix, D. P. (2012). Topical management. In R. A. Bryant & D. P. Nix (Eds.), *Acute & chronic wounds: Current management concepts* (4th ed., pp. 289–295). St. Louis, MO: Elsevier Mosby.

Rote, N. S., Huether, S. E., & McCance, K. L. (2014). Innate immunity: Inflammation. In K. L. McCance, S. E. Huether, V. L Brashers, & N. S. Rote (Eds.), *Pathophysiology: The biologic basis for disease in adults and children* (7th ed., pp. 191–223). St. Louis, MO: Elsevier.

Shulstad, R. M. (2012). Rash causing no fun in the sun. *Journal for Nurse Practitioners, 8*(9), 755–756.

Silverberg, J. I., & Silverberg, N. B. (2013). The US prevalence of common warts in childhood: A population-based study. *Journal of Investigative Dermatology, 133*, 2788–2790.

Simpson, E. L., Chalmers, J. R., Hanifin, J. M., Thomas, K. S., Cork, M. J.,McLean, W. H. I., ... Williams, H. C. (2014). Emollient enhancement of the skin barrier from birth offers effective atopic dermatitis prevention. *Journal of Allergy and Clinical Immunology, 134*, 818–823.

Stevens, D. L., Bisno, A. L., Chambers, H. F., Dellinger, E. P., Goldstein, E. J. C., Gorbach, S. L., ... Wade, J. C. (2014). *Practice guidelines for the diagnosis and management of skin and soft tissue infections: 2014 update by the Infectious Diseases Society of America.* Retrieved from http://cid.oxfordjournals.org/content/early/2014/06/14/cid.ciu296.full.pdf+html

Studor-Heikenfeld, J., & Colella, C. (2014). Isotretinoin: Reconsidering management of acne vulgaris in primary care. *Journal for Nurse Practitioners, 10*(9), 714–720.

Thomas, C. R., Russell, W., Robert, R. S., Holzer, C. E., Blakeney, P., & Meyer, W. J. (2012). Personality disorders in young adult survivors of pediatric burn injury. *Journal of Personality Disorders, 26*(2), 255–266.

Tollefson, M. M., Bruckner, A. L., & Section on Dermatology. (2014). Atopic dermatitis: Skin-directed management. *Pediatrics, 134*(6), e1735–e1744.

Tom, W. L. (2012). Atopic dermatitis: Recent findings and insights. *Pediatric Annals, 41*(1), e1–e5.

Tschudy, M. M., & Arcara, K. M. (2012). *The Harriet Lane handbook* (19th ed., p. 99). Philadelphia, PA: Elsevier Saunders.

Uihlein, L. C., Liang, M., G., & Mulliken, J. B. (2012). Pathogenesis of infantile hemangiomas. *Pediatric Annals, 41*(8), e154–e159.

U.S. Food and Drug Administration (FDA). (2014). *FDA safety communication: Update on serious complications associated with negative pressure wound therapy systems.* Retrieved from http://www.fda.gov/MedicalDevices/Safety/AlertsandNotices/ucm244211.htm#pediatric

Vloemans, A. F. P. M, Hermans, M. H. E., van der Wal, M. B. A., Liebregts J., & Middelkoop, E. (2014). Optimal treatment of partial thickness burns in children: A systematic review. *Burns, 40*, 177–190.

Weinstein, M. (2013). Acne and the adolescent: A practical approach to management. *Contemporary Pediatrics, 30*(5), 30–36.

Wilbeck, J., & Gresham, C. (2013). North American snake and scorpion envenomations. *Critical Care Nursing Clinics of North America, 25*, 173–190.

Wound Care Information Network. (2013). *Wound care product and category index.* Retrieved from http://www.medicaledu.com/prodindx.htm

Wound Educators. (2015). *Wound dressings.* Retrieved from http://woundeducators.com/resources/wound-dressings/

Wyatt, H. (2013). Common skin infections in children. *Nursing Standard, 27*(46), 43–48.

Yao, K., Bae, L., & Yew, W. P. (2013). Post-operative wound management. *Australian Family Physician, 42*(12), 867–870.

Yang, M., Kang, M., Jung, J., Song, W., Kang, H., Cho, S., & Min, K. (2013). Clinical features and prognostic factors in severe cutaneous drug reactions. *International Archives of Allergy and Immunology, 162*(4) 346–354.

Appendix A
Selected Maternal–Newborn Laboratory Values

Normal Maternal Laboratory Values*

TEST	NONPREGNANT VALUES	PREGNANT VALUES
Hematocrit	37%–47%	32%–42%
Hemoglobin	12–16 g/dL**	10–14 g/dL**
Platelets	150,000–350,000/mm^3	Significant increase 3–5 days after birth (predisposes to thrombosis)
Partial thromboplastin time (PTT)	12–14 seconds	Slight decrease in pregnancy and again in labor (placental site clotting)
Fibrinogen	250 mg/dL	400 mg/dL
Serum glucose		
Fasting	70–80 mg/dL	65 mg/dL
2-hour postprandial	60–110 mg/dL	Less than 140 mg/dL
Total protein	6.7–8.3 g/dL	5.5–7.5 g/dL
White blood cell total	4500–10,000/mm^3	5000–15,000/mm^3
Polymorphonuclear cells	54%–62%	60%–85%
Lymphocytes	38%–46%	15%–40%

*All maternal and newborn laboratory values are approximate. Consult your local laboratory for guidelines as to normal values.
**At sea level.

Normal Term Neonatal Cord Blood Laboratory Values*

TEST	NORMAL VALUES
Hematocrit	35%–60%**
Hemoglobin	14–20 g/dL
Platelets	150,000–350,000/mm^3
Reticulocyte	3%–7%
White blood cell total	16,200–31,500/mm^3
White blood cell differential	
Polymorphonuclear (segs)	40%–80%
Lymphocytes	20%–40%
Monocytes	3%–10%
Serum glucose	55–96 mg/dL**
Serum electrolytes	
Sodium	129–144 mEq/L**
Potassium	3.4–10.0 mEq/L**
Chloride	100–121 mEq/L**
Carbon dioxide	13–29 mmol/L
Bicarbonate	18–23 mEq/L
Calcium	8.2–11.1 mg/dL
Total protein	4.8–7.3 g/dL

Note: Data from Fanaroff, A. A., & Martin, R. J. (Eds.). (2015). *Neonatal–perinatal medicine* (10th ed.). Philadelphia, PA: Elsevier Saunders.
*All maternal and newborn laboratory values are approximate. Consult your local laboratory for guidelines as to normal values.
**At sea level.

Appendix B
Selected Pediatric Laboratory Values

All laboratory value intervals listed are approximate. Consult your local laboratory for guidelines as to normal values for the specific testing procedures used.

Normal Blood Chemistry and Hematology Value Intervals

Albumin (S)[1]

1 month–1 year:	2.8–4.8 g/dL
1–18 years:	3.2–4.7 g/dL

Alkaline Phosphatase (S)[1]

Age	Male Units/L	Female Units/L
1–30 days	75–316	48–406
1–3 years	104–345	108–317
4–6 years	93–309	96–297
7–9 years	86–315	69–325
10–12 years	42–362	51–332
13–15 years	74–390	50–162
16–18 years	52–171	47–119

α-Fetoprotein (AFP) (S)[1]

Newborn:	50–100,000 ng/mL
1–3 months:	40–1000 ng/mL
4 months–18 years:	0–12 ng/mL

Bilirubin (S)[1]

Conjugated	Newborn: Less than 0.6 mg/dL
Total	Birth–5 days: Less than 11.7 mg/dL

Blood Gases

CARBON DIOXIDE, PARTIAL PRESSURE (PCO_2) (B)[1]

Infant:	27–41 mmHg (3.6–5.5 kPa)
Children:	32–48 mmHg (4.3–6.4 kPa)

OXYGEN, PARTIAL PRESSURE (PO_2) (B)[1]

Greater than 1 day:	83–108 mmHg (11–14.4 kPa)

BICARBONATE, ACTUAL (P)[3]

22–29 mmol/L

pH (B)[1]

0–6 months:	7.18–7.50
6–12 months:	7.27–7.49
Children:	7.37–7.43
Adolescents:	7.35–7.41

BASE EXCESS (B)[1]

Infant:	–7 to –1 mmol/L
Child:	–4 to +2 mmol/L
Thereafter:	–3 to +3 mmol/L

OXYGEN SATURATION (B)[1]

Newborns:	85%–90%
Thereafter:	95%–99%

BUN—see Electrolytes, Urea Nitrogen

Coagulation Values[4]

Fibrinogen:	175–400 mg/dL
Partial thromboplastin time, activated (aPTT):	22.1–34.1 seconds
Prothrombin time (PT):	11.2–13.2 seconds
International normalized ratio (INR):	2–3

C-Reactive Protein (CRP) (P, S)[1]

0.08–1.8 mg/L

Creatinine (S, P)[1]

1–7 days:	0.7–1.2 mg/dL
7 days–1 year:	0.2–0.5 mg/dL
1–9 years:	0.2–0.8 mg/dL
10–18 years:	0.5–1.1 mg/dL

Electrolytes[1]

CALCIUM (S, P)

Newborn:	7.9–10.7 mg/dL
Thereafter:	8.7–10.7 mg/dL

CHLORIDE (S, P)

102–112 mmol/L

GLUCOSE, FASTING (S, P)[1]

Newborn:	55–117 mg/dL (3.1–6.4 mmol/L)
After 1 month of age:	70–126 mg/dL (3.9–7 mmol/L)

Key for type of specimen: S = serum; B = whole blood; P = plasma.

MAGNESIUM (P, S)
1.6–2.4 mg/dL (0.66–0.99 mmol/L)

OSMOLALITY (S)
280–300 mOsm/kg

PHOSPHORUS, INORGANIC (S, P)
2.8–5.6 mg/dL (0.91–1.8 mmol)

POTASSIUM (S, P)
3.7–5 mmol/L

SODIUM (P, S)
134–143 mmol/L

UREA NITROGEN (S, P)

1–13 years:	5–17 mg/dL (1.8–6 mmol/L)
14–19 years:	8–21 mg/dL (2.9–7.5 mmol/L)

Hematology Values (B)

Values are for children 2 to 12 years.

HEMATOCRIT (HCT)[1]
31.7%–39.8%

HEMOGLOBIN (HGB)[1]
10.2–13.4 g/dL

MEAN CORPUSCULAR HEMOGLOBIN (MCH)[1]
23.7–29.5 pg

MEAN CORPUSCULAR HEMOGLOBIN CONCENTRATION (MCHC)[1]
31.8%–34.9%

MEAN CORPUSCULAR VOLUME (MCV)[1]
71.3–87.6 mm^3

RED BLOOD CELL (RBC)[1]
3.89–5.03 × 10^{12}/L

WHITE BLOOD CELL (WBC)[1]
4.86–11.4 × 10^9/L

DIFFERENTIAL[1]

Neutrophils	22.4%–74.7%
Eosinophils	0%–4.7%
Basophils	0.1%–0.6%
Lymphocytes	18.1%–57.8%
Atypical lymphocytes	2%–4%
Monocytes	4.1%–12.3%

PLATELET COUNT[3]
202–367 × 10^9/L

RETICULOCYTE COUNT[1]
0.82%–1.49%

Erythrocyte Sedimentation Rate (Micro)[4]

1–13 mm/hr

Growth Hormone (P, S)[1]

0–6.9 years:	Less than 13.7 mcg/L
7–10.9 years:	Less than 16.5 mcg/L
11–14.9 years:	Less than 14.5 mcg/L
15–18.9 years:	Less than 13.5 mcg/L

Hemoglobin A$_{1c}$ (B)[1]

Normal:	4%–6%

Hemoglobin Fetal (B)[5]

1–30 days:	22.8%–92%
Decreases to adult levels by 12 months:	0%–0.9%

Iron-Related Values

FERRITIN (P, S)[1]

1–5 years:	6–24 ng/mL
6–9 years:	10–55 ng/mL
10–19 years:	Males: 23–70 ng/mL
	Females: 6–40 ng/mL

IRON (S, P)[1]

1–14 years:	22–136 mcg/dL (4–25 micromol/L)
14–19 years:	34–162 mcg/dL (6–29 micromol/L)

IRON-BINDING CAPACITY (S, P)[1]

1–5 years:	268–441 mcg/dL (48–79 micromol/L)
6–9 years:	240–508 mcg/dL (43–91 micromol/L)
10–19 years:	290–570 mcg/dL (52–102 micromol/L)

Lead (B)[3]

Less than 5 mcg/dL

Lipids (S)[2]

TOTAL CHOLESTEROL

Acceptable:	Less than 170 mg/dL
Elevated:	Greater than 200 mg/dL

HIGH-DENSITY LIPOPROTEIN

Acceptable:	Greater than 45 mg/dL or higher
Low:	Less than 40 mg/dL

Key for type of specimen: *S = serum; B = whole blood; P = plasma.*

LOW-DENSITY LIPOPROTEIN

Acceptable:	Less than 110 mg/dL
High:	130 mg/dL and higher

TRIGLYCERIDES

Acceptable	0 – 9 years: Less than 75 mg/dL
	10 – 19 years: Less than 90 mg/dL
High	0 – 9 years: Greater than 100 mg/dL
	10 – 19 years: Greater than 130 mg/dL

Thyroid Hormones

THYROID-STIMULATING HORMONE (TSH) (P, S)[1] (IN MILLI-INTERNATIONAL UNITS/L)

Age	Males	Females
1–30 days	0.7–16.1	1.0–13.7
1 month–5 years	0.8–7.5	0.7–8.6
6–18 years	0.6–6.4	0.6–6.2

THYROXINE (T_4) (S, P)[1]

1–5 years:	5–14.45 mcg/dL
6–20 years:	4.4–12.1 mcg/dL

THYROXINE, "FREE" (FREE T_4) (S, P)[1]

Under 1 year:	1.3–2.8 ng/dL (16.8–36.1 pmol/L)
1–18 years:	1.3–2.42 ng/mL (16.8–31 pmol/L)

THYROXINE-BINDING GLOBULIN (TBG) (P)[1] (IN MG/L)

Age	Males	Females
Cord blood	19–39	19–39
1–11 months	16–36	17–37
1–9 years:	12–28	15–27
10–19 years:	14–26	14–30

TRIIODOTHYRONINE (T_3) (S)[1]

1–5 years:	106–203 ng/dL
6–10 years:	104–183 ng/dL
11–14 years:	68–186 ng/dL
15–20 years:	71–175 ng/dL

Normal Value Ranges: Urine

Albumin[4]

Less than 1 mg/dL

Catecholamines (Norepinephrine, Epinephrine)[1]

(in mmol/mol creatinine)

Age	Norepinephrine	Epinephrine
0–24 months	0–0.28	0–0.46
2–4 years	0–0.8	0–0.035
5–9 years	0–0.059	0–0.022
10–19 years	0–0.055	0–0.021

Creatinine[1]

3–8 years:	0.11–0.68 g/24 hr
9–12 years:	0.17–1.41 g/24 hr
13–17 years:	0.29–1.87 g/24 hr
Adults:	0.63–2.5 g/24 hr

Osmolality[4]

500–800 mOsm/kg water

Should be higher than serum osmolality.

Protein[4]

Less than 150 mg/24 hr

Specific Gravity[4]

Birth – 2 years:	1.001–1.018
Over 2 years:	1.001–1.03

Normal Value Ranges: Sweat

Electrolytes[1]

Sodium and chloride: under 40 mmol/L

Normal Value Ranges: Cerebrospinal Fluid

Protein[1]

Under 1 month:	15–153 mg/dL
Over 1 month:	15–48 mg/dL

Glucose[1]

All ages: 41–84 mg/dL (60%–80% of blood glucose)

Key for type of specimen: S = serum; B = whole blood; P = plasma.
[1]Adapted from Soldin, S. J., Wong, E. C., Brugnara, C., & Soldin, O. P. (2011). Pediatric reference ranges (7th ed.). Washington, DC: American Association for Clinical Chemistry Press.
[2]National Heart Lung and Blood Institute. (2012). Expert panel on integrated guidelines for cardiovascular health and risk reduction in children and adolescents: Summary report. Retrieved from http://www.nhlbi.nih.gov/files/docs/peds_guidelines_sum.pdf
[3]Data from Kliegman, R. M., Stanton, B. F., St. Geme, J. W., & Schor, N. F. (2016). Nelson textbook of pediatrics (20th ed., Table 727-5). Philadelphia, PA: Elsevier Saunders.
[4]Data from Corbett, J. V. (2013). Laboratory tests and diagnostic procedures with nursing diagnoses (8th ed.). Upper Saddle River, NJ: Pearson Education.
[5] Data from Mayo Clinic Mayo Medical Laboratories. (2014). Test ID: Hemoglobin F. Retrieved from http://www.mayomedicallaboratories.com/test-catalog /Clinical + and + Interpretive/8269

Appendix C
Growth Charts

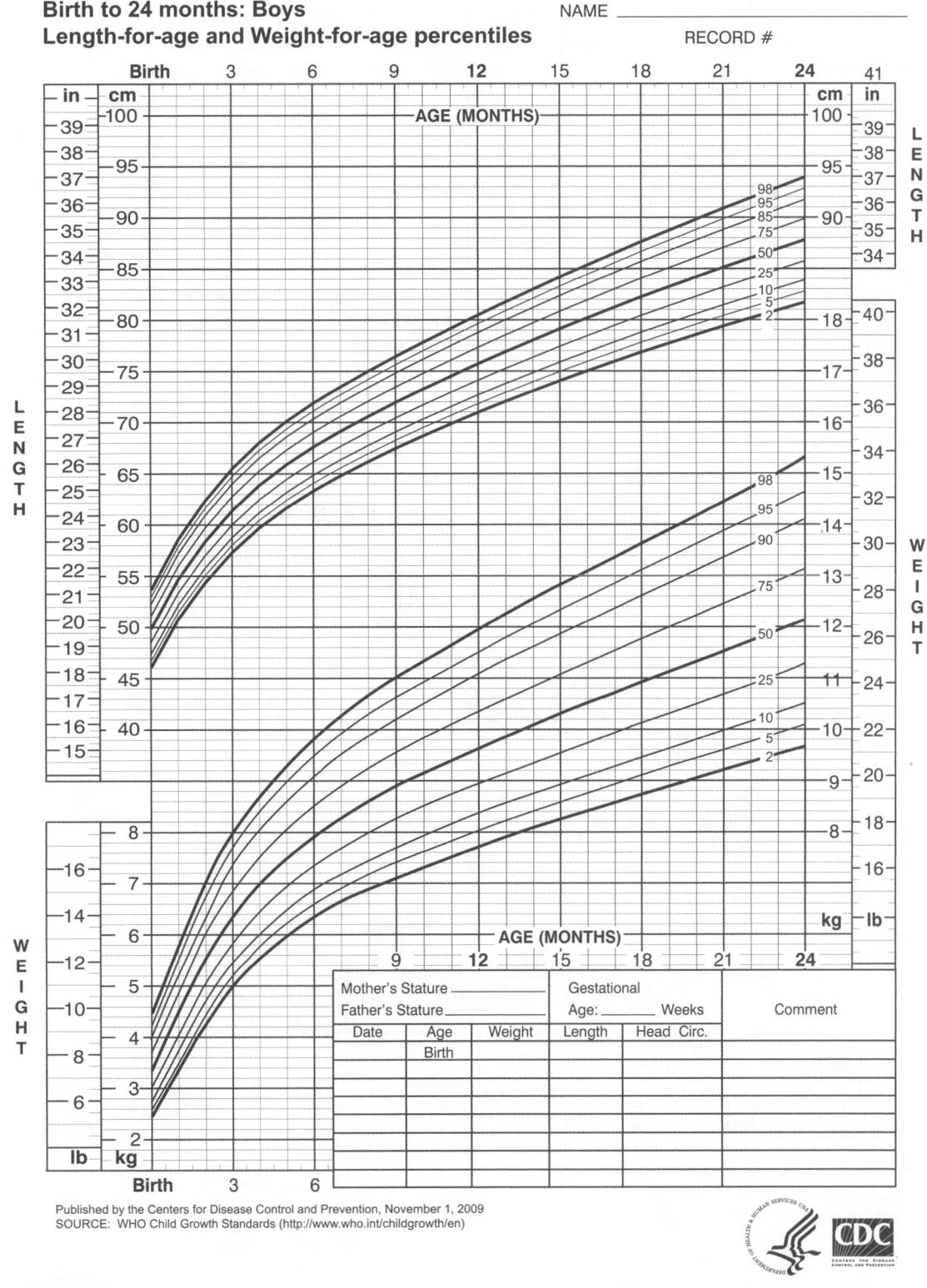

Birth to 24 months: Boys
Length-for-age and Weight-for-age percentiles

NAME _____

RECORD # _____

Published by the Centers for Disease Control and Prevention, November 1, 2009
SOURCE: WHO Child Growth Standards (http://www.who.int/childgrowth/en)

Figure C–1   Physical growth percentiles for length and weight—boys: birth to 24 months.

From WHO Child Growth Standards, http://www.who.int/childgrowth/en.

Birth to 24 months: Boys
Head circumference-for-age and
Weight-for-length percentiles

NAME _____

RECORD # _____

AGE (MONTHS)

Birth   3   6   9   12   15   18   21   24

HEAD CIRCUMFERENCE

98
95
90
75
50
25
10
5
2

LENGTH

| 64 66 68 70 72 74 76 78 80 82 84 86 88 90 92 94 96 98 100 102 104 106 108 110 | cm |
| 26 27 28 29 30 31 32 33 34 35 36 37 38 39 40 41 42 43 | in |

Date	Age	Weight	Length	Head Circ.	Comment

WEIGHT

| cm | 46 48 50 52 54 56 58 60 62 |
| in | 18 19 20 21 22 23 24 |

Published by the Centers for Disease Control and Prevention, November 1, 2009
SOURCE: WHO Child Growth Standards (http://www.who.int/childgrowth/en)

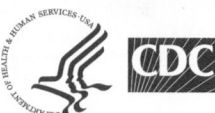

Figure C–2 Physical growth percentiles for head circumference, weight for length—boys: birth to 24 months.

From WHO Child Growth Standards, http://www.who.int/childgrowth/en.

Birth to 24 months: Girls
Length-for-age and Weight-for-age percentiles

NAME _____

RECORD # _____

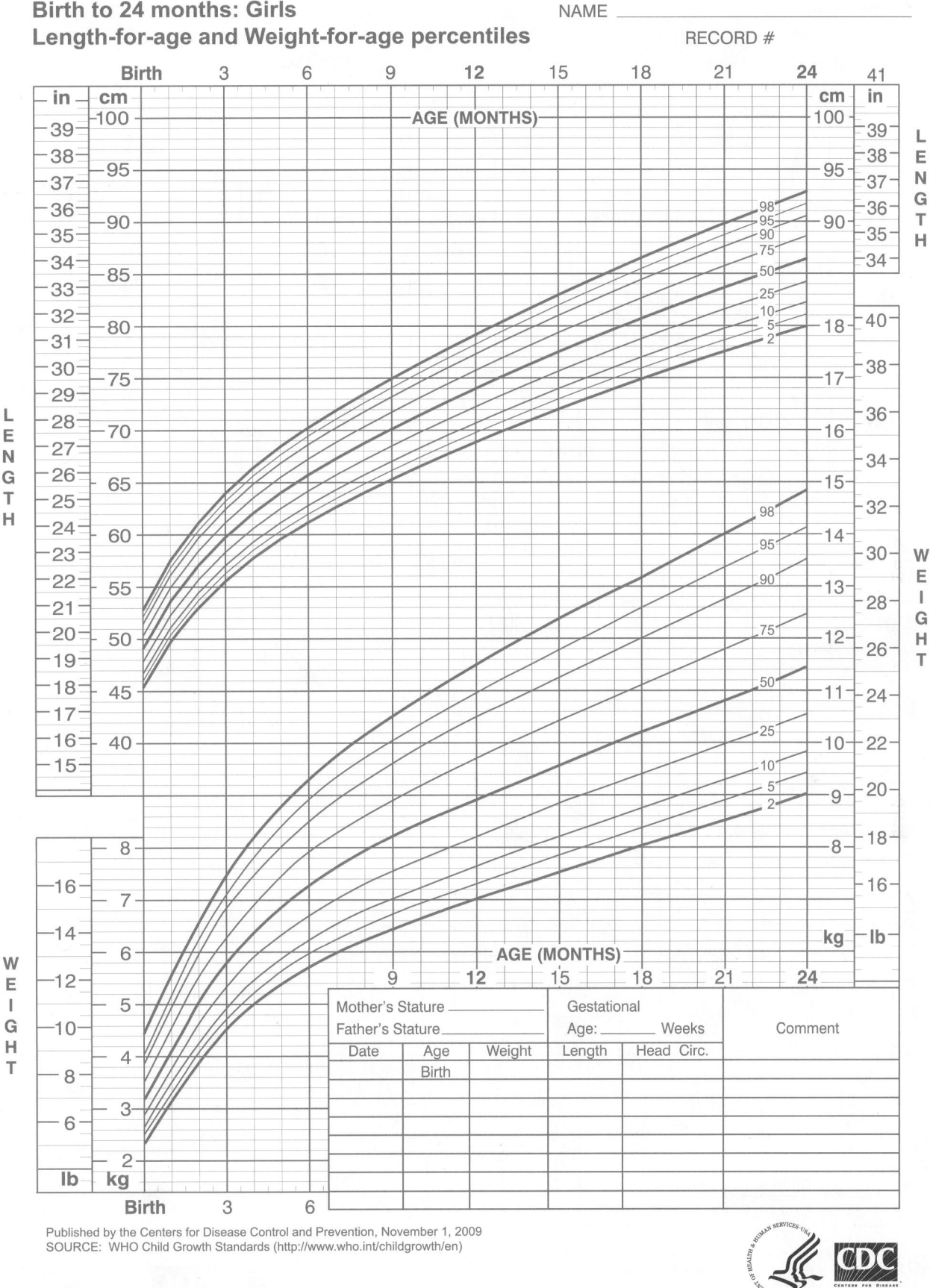

Published by the Centers for Disease Control and Prevention, November 1, 2009
SOURCE: WHO Child Growth Standards (http://www.who.int/childgrowth/en)

Figure C–3 Physical growth percentiles for length and weight—girls: birth to 24 months.

From WHO Child Growth Standards, http://www.who.int/childgrowth/en.

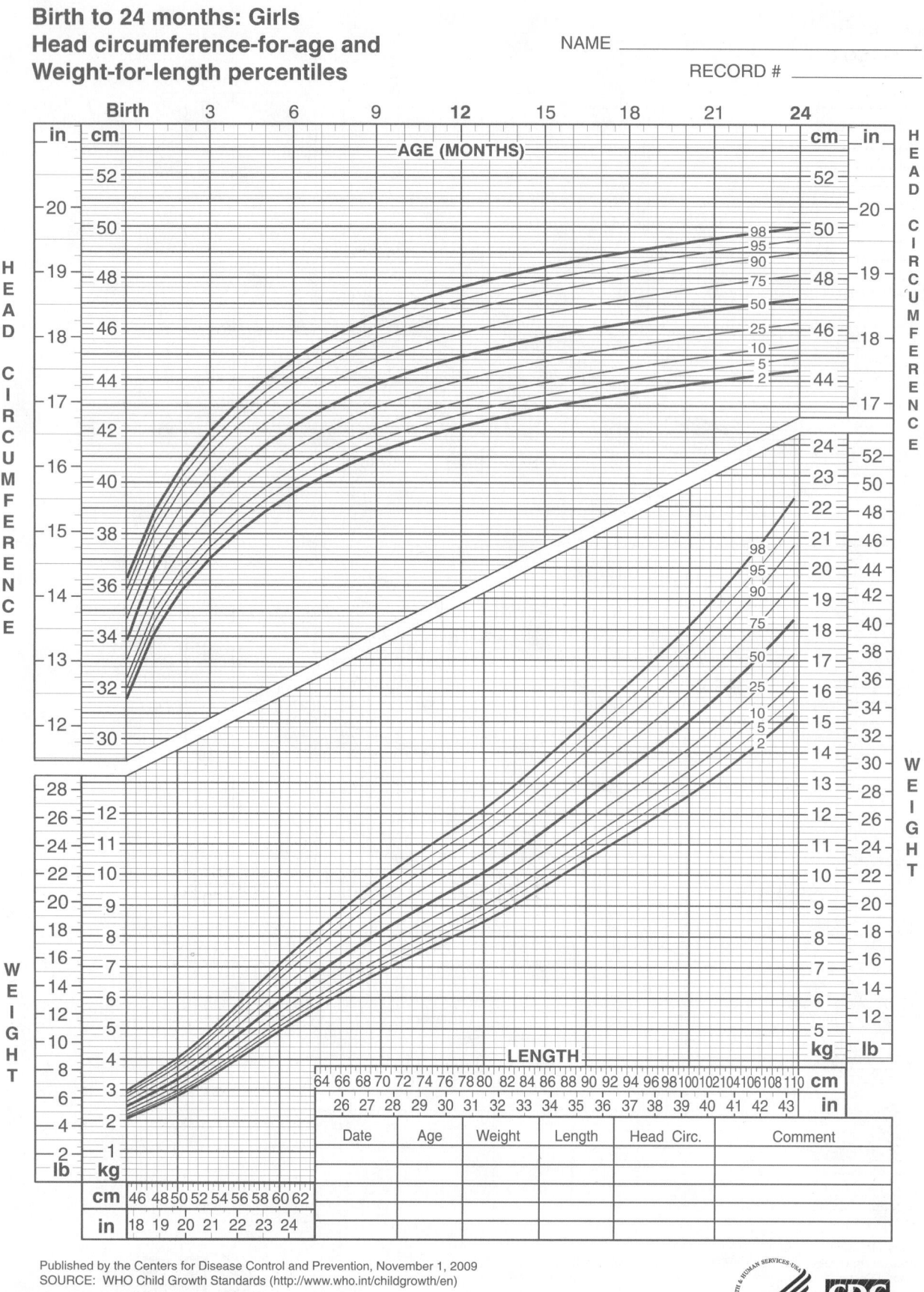

Birth to 24 months: Girls
Head circumference-for-age and
Weight-for-length percentiles

NAME _____

RECORD # _____

Published by the Centers for Disease Control and Prevention, November 1, 2009
SOURCE: WHO Child Growth Standards (http://www.who.int/childgrowth/en)

Figure C–4 Physical growth percentiles for head circumference, weight for length—girls: birth to 24 months.

From WHO Child Growth Standards, http://www.who.int/childgrowth/en.

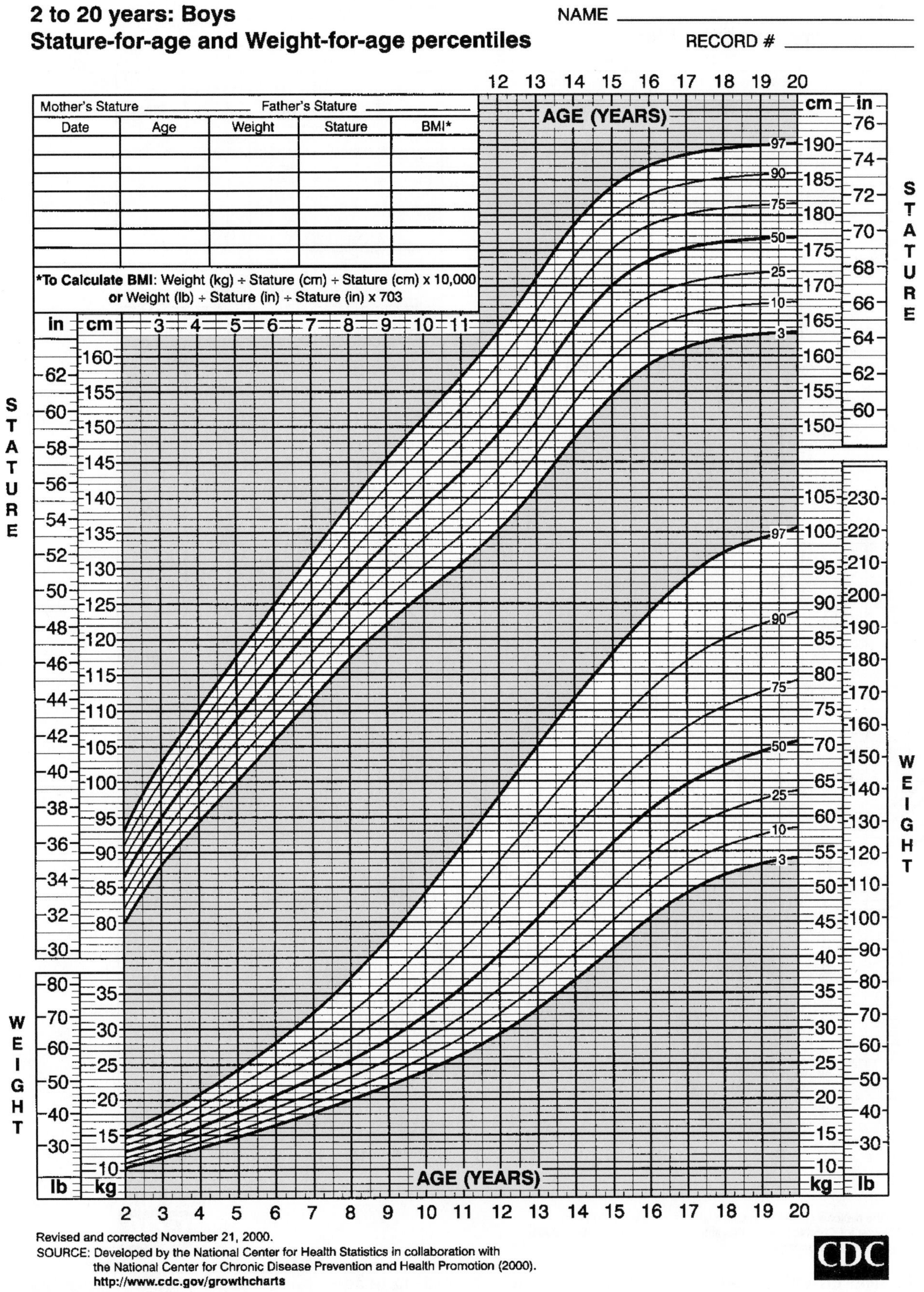

2 to 20 years: Boys
Stature-for-age and Weight-for-age percentiles

NAME _____

RECORD # _____

Revised and corrected November 21, 2000.

SOURCE: Developed by the National Center for Health Statistics in collaboration with
the National Center for Chronic Disease Prevention and Health Promotion (2000).
http://www.cdc.gov/growthcharts

CDC

Figure C–5 Physical growth percentiles for stature and weight according to age—boys: 2 to 20 years.

From CDC, 2001, http://www.cdc.gov/growthcharts.

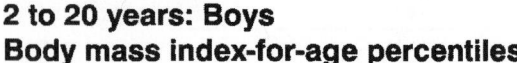

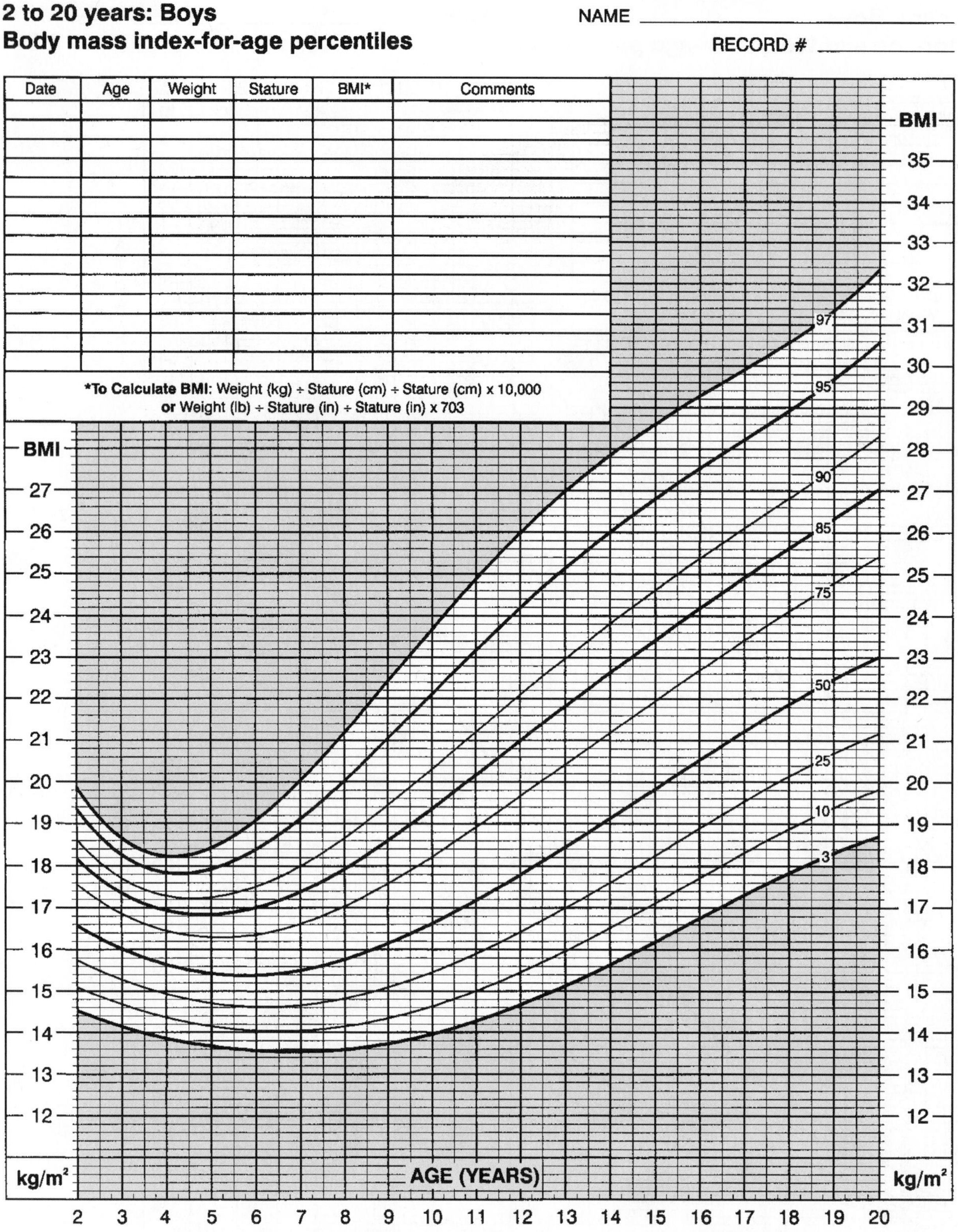
2 to 20 years: Boys
Body mass index-for-age percentiles
NAME
RECORD #
Date
Age
Weight
Stature
BMI*
Comments
*To Calculate BMI: Weight (kg) ÷ Stature (cm) ÷ Stature (cm) x 10,000
or Weight (lb) ÷ Stature (in) ÷ Stature (in) x 703
BMI
97
95
90
85
75
50
25
10
3
kg/m²
AGE (YEARS)
2
3
4
5
6
7
8
9
10
11
12
13
14
15
16
17
18
19
20
12
13
14
15
16
17
18
19
20
21
22
23
24
25
26
27
28
29
30
31
32
33
34
35

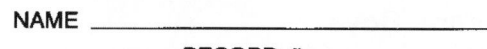

SOURCE: Developed by the National Center for Health Statistics in collaboration with the National Center for Chronic Disease Prevention and Health Promotion (2000). http://www.cdc.gov/growthcharts

CDC

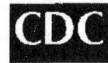

Figure C–6 Physical growth percentiles for body mass index according to age—boys: 2 to 20 years.

From CDC, 2001, http://www.cdc.gov/growthcharts.

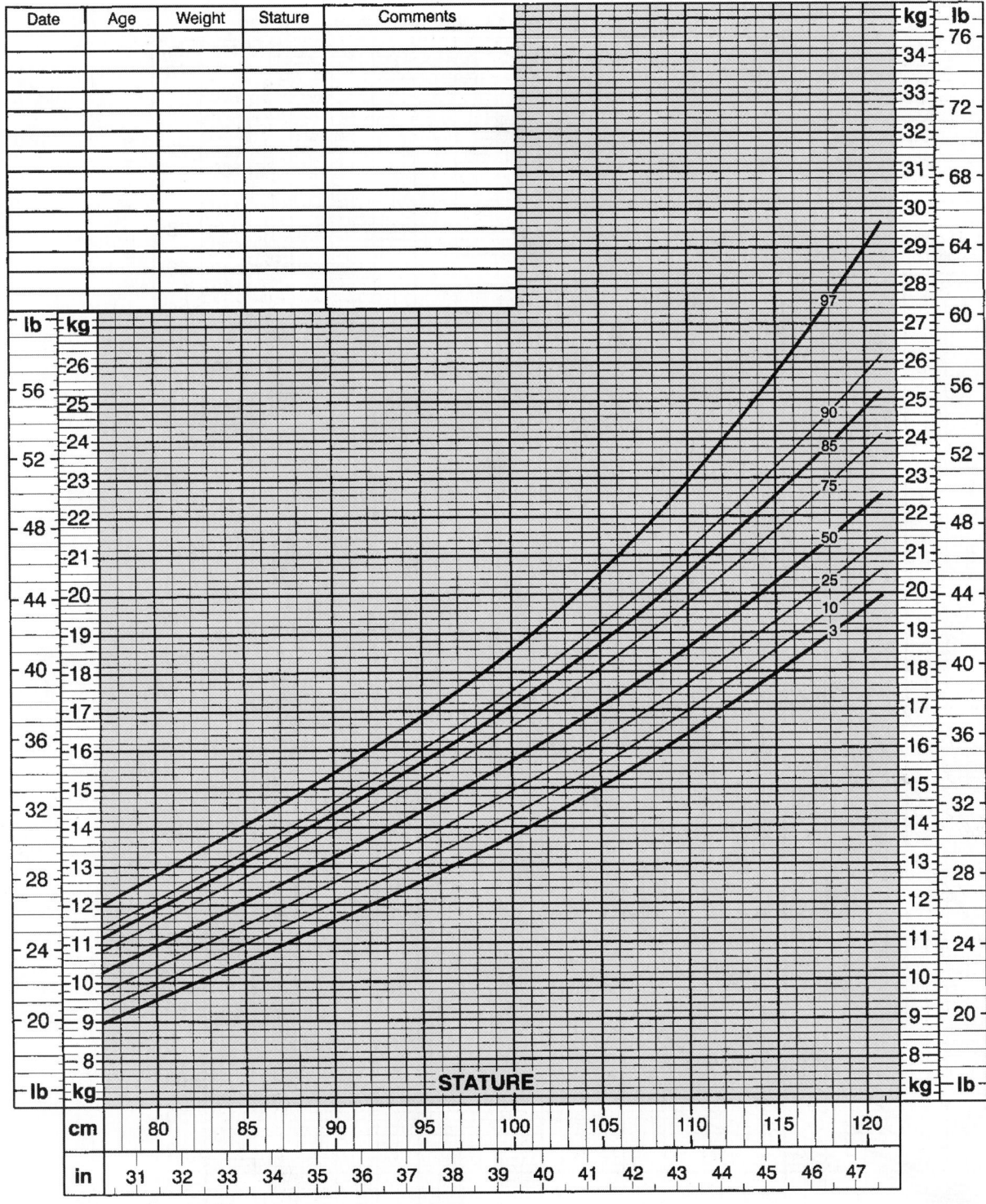

NAME _____

Weight-for-stature percentiles: Boys

RECORD # _____

Date	Age	Weight	Stature	Comments

STATURE

SOURCE: Developed by the National Center for Health Statistics in collaboration with the National Center for Chronic Disease Prevention and Health Promotion (2000). http://www.cdc.gov/growthcharts

CDC

Figure C–7 Physical growth percentiles for weight for stature—boys: 2 to 20 years.

From CDC, 2001, http://www.cdc.gov/growthcharts.

2 to 20 years: Girls
Stature-for-age and Weight-for-age percentiles

NAME _____

RECORD # _____

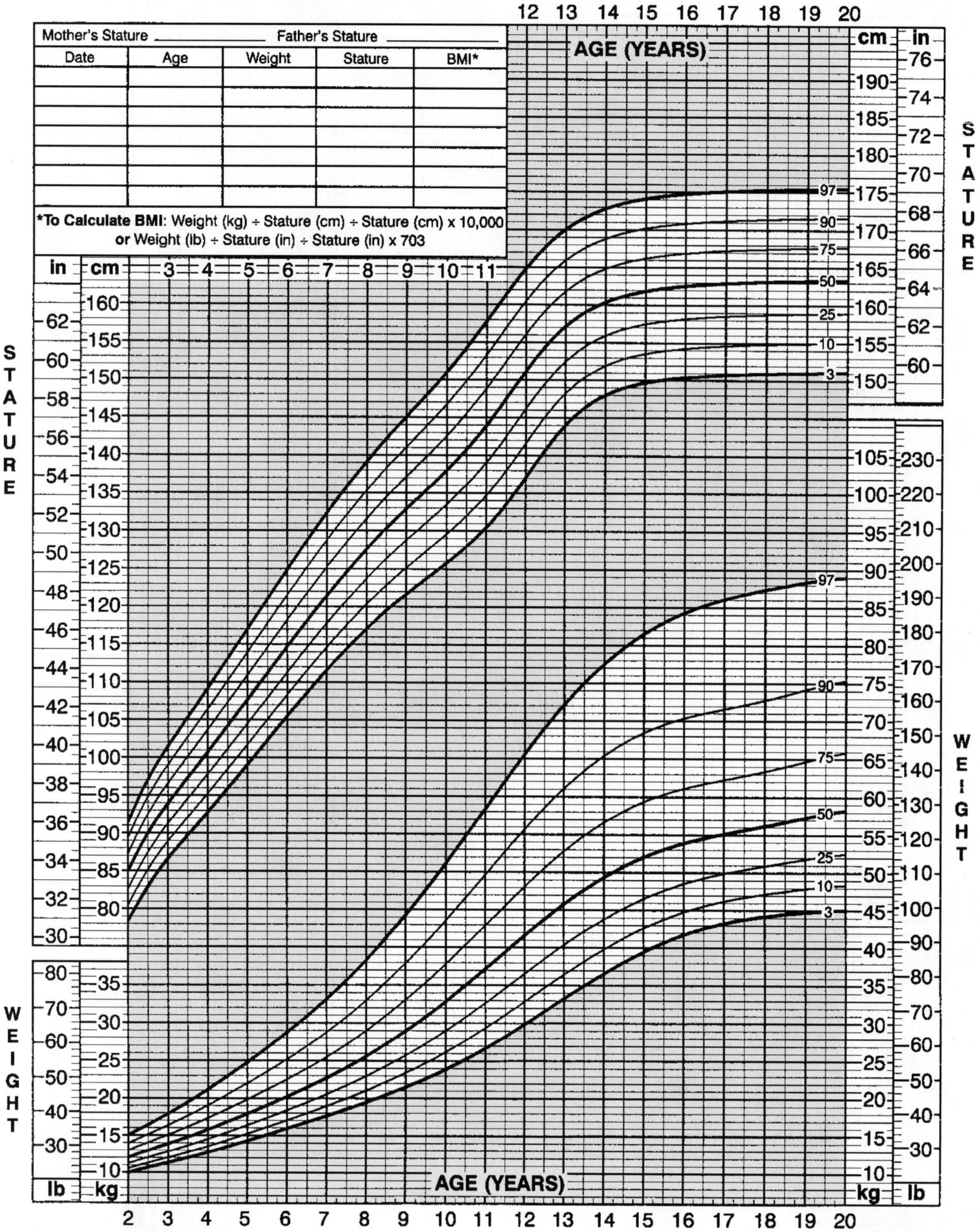

Mother's Stature _____ Father's Stature _____

Date	Age	Weight	Stature	BMI*

*To Calculate BMI: Weight (kg) ÷ Stature (cm) ÷ Stature (cm) x 10,000
or Weight (lb) ÷ Stature (in) ÷ Stature (in) x 703

AGE (YEARS)

AGE (YEARS)

STATURE

WEIGHT

Revised and corrected November 21, 2000.

SOURCE: Developed by the National Center for Health Statistics in collaboration with
the National Center for Chronic Disease Prevention and Health Promotion (2000).
http://www.cdc.gov/growthcharts

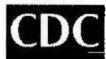

Figure C–8 Physical growth percentiles for stature and weight according to age—girls: 2 to 20 years.

From CDC, 2001, http://www.cdc.gov/growthcharts.

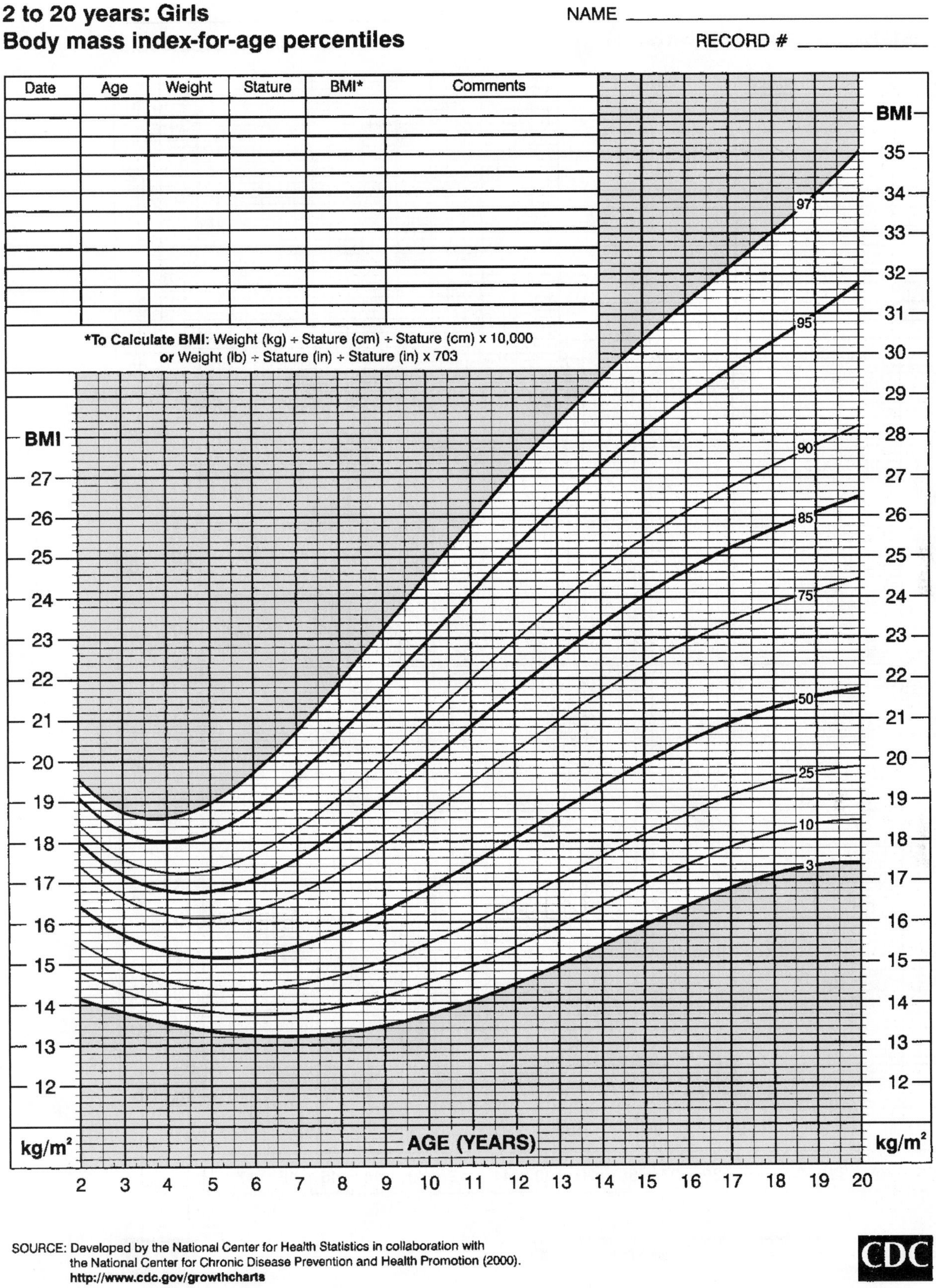
2 to 20 years: Girls
Body mass index-for-age percentiles
NAME
RECORD #
Date
Age
Weight
Stature
BMI*
Comments
*To Calculate BMI: Weight (kg) ÷ Stature (cm) ÷ Stature (cm) x 10,000
or Weight (lb) ÷ Stature (in) ÷ Stature (in) x 703
BMI
97
95
90
85
75
50
25
10
3
kg/m²
AGE (YEARS)
2 3 4 5 6 7 8 9 10 11 12 13 14 15 16 17 18 19 20
SOURCE: Developed by the National Center for Health Statistics in collaboration with the National Center for Chronic Disease Prevention and Health Promotion (2000).
http://www.cdc.gov/growthcharts
CDC

Figure C–9 **Physical growth percentiles for body mass index according to age—girls: 2 to 20 years.**

From CDC, 2001, http://www.cdc.gov/growthcharts.

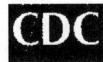

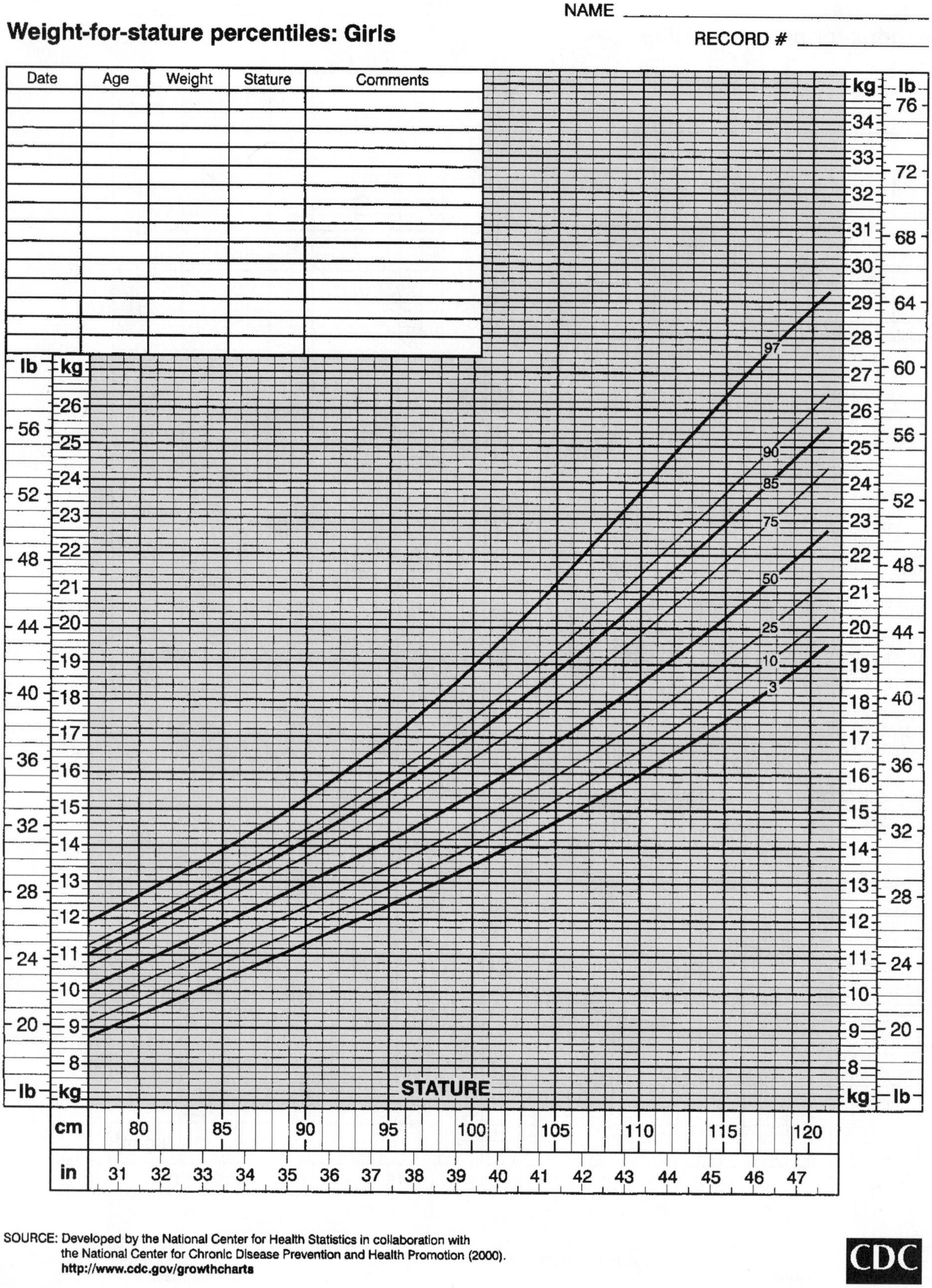
NAME
RECORD #
Weight-for-stature percentiles: Girls
Date
Age
Weight
Stature
Comments
kg
lb
97
90
85
75
50
25
10
3
STATURE
cm
in
SOURCE: Developed by the National Center for Health Statistics in collaboration with the National Center for Chronic Disease Prevention and Health Promotion (2000). http://www.cdc.gov/growthcharts
CDC

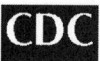

Figure C–10 **Physical growth percentiles for weight for stature—girls: 2 to 20 years.**

From CDC, 2001, http://www.cdc.gov/growthcharts.

Appendix D
Pediatric Blood Pressure Tables

TABLE D–1 Blood Pressure Levels for Boys by Age and Height Percentile

Use the child's height percentile for the age and gender from the standard growth charts found in Appendix C. A blood pressure value at the 50th percentile for the child's age, gender, and height percentile is considered the midpoint of the normal range. A reading at or above the 95th percentile indicates hypertension.

Age (Year)	BP Percentile	SYSTOLIC BP (MMHG) PERCENTILE OF HEIGHT							DIASTOLIC BP (MMHG) PERCENTILE OF HEIGHT						
		5th	10th	25th	50th	75th	90th	95th	5th	10th	25th	50th	75th	90th	95th
1	50th	80	81	83	85	87	88	89	34	35	36	37	38	39	39
	95th	98	99	101	103	104	106	106	54	54	55	56	57	58	58
2	50th	84	85	87	88	90	92	92	39	40	41	42	43	44	44
	95th	101	102	104	106	108	109	110	59	59	60	61	62	63	63
3	50th	86	87	89	91	93	94	95	44	44	45	46	47	48	48
	95th	104	105	107	109	110	112	113	63	63	64	65	66	67	67
4	50th	88	89	91	93	95	96	97	47	48	49	50	51	51	52
	95th	106	107	109	111	112	114	115	66	67	68	69	70	71	71
5	50th	90	91	93	95	96	98	98	50	51	52	53	54	55	55
	95th	108	109	110	112	114	115	116	69	70	71	72	73	74	74
6	50th	91	92	94	96	98	99	100	53	53	54	55	56	57	57
	95th	109	110	112	114	115	117	117	72	72	73	74	75	76	76
7	50th	92	94	95	97	99	100	101	55	55	56	57	58	59	59
	95th	110	111	113	115	117	118	119	74	74	75	76	77	78	78
8	50th	94	95	97	99	100	102	102	56	57	58	59	60	60	61
	95th	111	112	114	116	118	119	120	75	76	77	78	79	79	80
9	50th	95	96	98	100	102	103	104	57	58	59	60	61	61	62
	95th	113	114	116	118	119	121	121	76	77	78	79	80	81	81
10	50th	97	98	100	102	103	105	106	58	59	60	61	61	62	63
	95th	115	116	117	119	121	122	123	77	78	79	80	81	81	82
11	50th	99	100	102	104	105	107	107	59	59	60	61	62	63	63
	95th	117	118	119	121	123	124	125	78	78	79	80	81	82	82
12	50th	101	102	104	106	108	109	110	59	60	61	62	63	63	64
	95th	119	120	122	123	125	127	127	78	79	80	81	82	82	83
13	50th	104	105	106	108	110	111	112	60	60	61	62	63	64	64
	95th	121	122	124	126	128	129	130	79	79	80	81	82	83	83
14	50th	106	107	109	111	113	114	115	60	61	62	63	64	65	65
	95th	124	125	127	128	130	132	132	80	80	81	82	83	84	84
15	50th	109	110	112	113	115	117	117	61	62	63	64	65	66	66
	95th	126	127	129	131	133	134	135	81	81	82	83	84	85	85
16	50th	111	112	114	116	118	119	120	63	63	64	65	66	67	67
	95th	129	130	132	134	135	137	137	82	83	83	84	85	86	87
17	50th	114	115	116	118	120	121	122	65	66	66	67	68	69	70
	95th	131	132	134	136	138	139	140	84	85	86	87	87	88	89

Source: National Heart, Lung, and Blood Institute. (2004). *Blood pressure tables for children and adolescents from the fourth report on the diagnosis, evaluation, and treatment of high blood pressure in children and adolescents.* Retrieved from http://www.nhlbi.nih.gov/guidelines/hypertension/child_tbl.htm, accessed 6/11/2004.

Note: Key: BP, blood pressure.

*The 95th percentile is 1.645 SD over the mean.

TABLE D–2 Blood Pressure Levels for Girls by Age and Height Percentile

Use the child's height percentile for the age and gender from the standard growth charts found in Appendix C. A blood pressure value at 50th percentile for the child's age, gender, and height percentile is considered the midpoint of the normal range. A reading above the 95th percentile indicates hypertension.

Age (Year)	BP Percentile	SYSTOLIC BP (mmHg) PERCENTILE OF HEIGHT							DIASTOLIC BP (mmHg) PERCENTILE OF HEIGHT						
		5th	10th	25th	50th	75th	90th	95th	5th	10th	25th	50th	75th	90th	95th
1	50th	83	84	85	86	88	89	90	38	39	39	40	41	41	42
	95th	100	101	102	104	105	106	107	56	57	57	58	59	59	60
2	50th	85	85	87	88	89	91	91	43	44	44	45	46	46	47
	95th	102	103	104	105	107	108	109	61	62	62	63	64	65	65
3	50th	86	87	88	89	91	92	93	47	48	48	49	50	50	51
	95th	104	104	105	107	108	109	110	65	66	66	67	68	68	69
4	50th	88	88	90	91	92	94	94	50	50	51	52	52	53	54
	95th	105	106	107	108	110	111	112	68	68	69	70	71	71	72
5	50th	89	90	91	93	94	95	96	52	53	53	54	55	55	56
	95th	107	107	108	110	111	112	113	70	71	71	72	73	73	74
6	50th	91	92	93	94	96	97	98	54	54	55	56	56	57	58
	95th	108	109	110	111	113	114	115	72	72	73	74	74	75	76
7	50th	93	93	95	96	97	99	99	55	56	56	57	58	58	59
	95th	110	111	112	113	115	116	116	73	74	74	75	76	76	77
8	50th	95	95	96	98	99	100	101	57	57	57	58	59	60	60
	95th	112	112	114	115	116	118	118	75	75	75	76	77	78	78
9	50th	96	97	98	100	101	102	103	58	58	58	59	60	61	61
	95th	114	114	115	117	118	119	120	76	76	76	77	78	79	79
10	50th	98	99	100	102	103	104	105	59	59	59	60	61	62	62
	95th	116	116	117	119	120	121	122	77	77	77	78	79	80	80
11	50th	100	101	102	103	105	106	107	60	60	60	61	62	63	63
	95th	118	118	119	121	122	123	124	78	78	78	79	80	81	81
12	50th	102	103	104	105	107	108	109	61	61	61	62	63	64	64
	95th	119	120	121	123	124	125	126	79	79	79	80	81	82	82
13	50th	104	105	106	107	109	110	110	62	62	62	63	64	65	65
	95th	121	122	123	124	126	127	128	80	80	80	81	82	83	83
14	50th	106	106	107	109	110	111	112	63	63	63	64	65	66	66
	95th	123	123	125	126	127	129	129	81	81	81	82	83	84	84
15	50th	107	108	109	110	111	113	113	64	64	64	65	66	67	67
	95th	124	125	126	127	129	130	131	82	82	82	83	84	85	85
16	50th	108	108	110	111	112	114	114	64	64	65	66	66	67	68
	95th	125	126	127	128	130	131	132	82	82	83	84	85	85	86
17	50th	108	109	110	111	113	114	115	64	65	65	66	67	67	68
	95th	125	126	127	129	130	131	132	82	83	83	84	85	85	86

Source: National Heart, Lung, and Blood Institute. (2004). *Blood pressure tables for children and adolescents from the fourth report on the diagnosis, evaluation, and treatment of high blood pressure in children and adolescents.* Retrieved from http://www.nhlbi.nih.gov/guidelines/hypertension/child_tbl.htm, accessed 6/11/2004.

Note: *Key:* BP, blood pressure.

*The 95th percentile is 1.645 SD over the mean.

Appendix E
Conversions and Equivalents

Temperature Conversion

(Fahrenheit temperature − 32) × 5/9 = Centigrade temperature

(Centigrade temperature × 9/5) + 32 = Fahrenheit temperature

Selected Conversion to Metric Measures

KNOWN VALUE	MULTIPLY BY	TO FIND
inches	2.54	centimeters
ounces	28	grams
pounds	454	grams
pounds	0.45	kilograms

Selected Conversion From Metric Measures

KNOWN VALUE	MULTIPLY BY	TO FIND
centimeters	0.4	inches
grams	0.035	ounces
grams	0.0022	pounds
kilograms	2.2	pounds

Conversion of Pounds and Ounces to Grams

							OUNCES									
POUNDS	0	1	2	3	4	5	6	7	8	9	10	11	12	13	14	15
0	—	28	57	85	113	142	170	198	227	255	283	312	340	369	397	425
1	454	482	510	539	567	595	624	652	680	709	737	765	794	822	850	879
2	907	936	964	992	1021	1049	1077	1106	1134	1162	1191	1219	1247	1276	1304	1332
3	1361	1389	1417	1446	1474	1503	1531	1559	1588	1616	1644	1673	1701	1729	1758	1786
4	1814	1843	1871	1899	1928	1956	1984	2013	2041	2070	2098	2126	2155	2183	2211	2240
5	2268	2296	2325	2353	2381	2410	2438	2466	2495	2523	2551	2580	2608	2637	2665	2693
6	2722	2750	2778	2807	2835	2863	2892	2920	2948	2977	3005	3033	3062	3090	3118	3147
7	3175	3203	3232	3260	3289	3317	3345	3374	3402	3430	3459	3487	3515	3544	3572	3600
8	3629	3657	3685	3714	3742	3770	3799	3827	3856	3884	3912	3941	3969	3997	4026	4054
9	4082	4111	4139	4167	4196	4224	4252	4281	4309	4337	4366	4394	4423	4451	4479	4508
10	4536	4564	4593	4621	4649	4678	4706	4734	4763	4791	4819	4848	4876	4904	4933	4961
11	4990	5018	5046	5075	5103	5131	5160	5188	5216	5245	5273	5301	5330	5358	5386	5415
12	5443	5471	5500	5528	5557	5585	5613	5642	5670	5698	5727	5755	5783	5812	5840	5868
13	5897	5925	5953	5982	6010	6038	6067	6095	6123	6152	6180	6209	6237	6265	6294	6322
14	6350	6379	6407	6435	6464	6492	6520	6549	6577	6605	6634	6662	6690	6719	6747	6776
15	6804	6832	6860	6889	6917	6945	6973	7002	7030	7059	7087	7115	7144	7172	7201	7228
16	7257	7286	7313	7342	7371	7399	7427	7456	7484	7512	7541	7569	7597	7626	7654	7682
17	7711	7739	7768	7796	7824	7853	7881	7909	7938	7966	7994	8023	8051	8079	8108	8136
18	8165	8192	8221	8249	8278	8306	8335	8363	8391	8420	8448	8476	8504	8533	8561	8590
19	8618	8646	8675	8703	8731	8760	8788	8816	8845	8873	8902	8930	8958	8987	9015	9043
20	9072	9100	9128	9157	9185	9213	9242	9270	9298	9327	9355	9383	9412	9440	9469	9497
21	9525	9554	9582	9610	9639	9667	9695	9724	9752	9780	9809	9837	9865	9894	9922	9950
22	9979	10007	10036	10064	10092	10120	10149	10177	10206	10234	10262	10291	10319	10347	10376	10404

Appendix F
Dietary Reference Intakes

TABLE F–1 Dietary Reference Intakes (DRIs) for Nonpregnant Females and for Pregnant and Lactating Females

	Age	Vitamin A (mcg/d)	Vitamin D (mcg/d)	Vitamin E (mg/d α-tocopherol)	Vitamin K (mcg/d)	Vitamin C (mg/d)	Thiamine (mg/d)	Riboflavin (mg/d)
Females	9–13 years	600	15	11	60*	45	0.9	0.9
	14–18 years	700	15	15	75*	65	1.0	1.0
	19–30 years	700	15	15	90*	75	1.1	1.1
	31–50 years	700	15	15	90*	75	1.1	1.1
	50–70 years	700	15	15	90*	75	1.1	1.1
	>70 years	700	20	15	90*	75	1.1	1.1
Pregnancy	≤18 years	750	15	15	75*	80	1.4	1.4
	19–30 years	770	15	15	90*	85	1.4	1.4
	31–50 years	770	15	15	90*	85	1.4	1.4
Lactation	≤18 years	1200	15	19	75*	115	1.4	1.6
	19–30 years	1300	15	19	90*	120	1.4	1.6
	31–50 years	1300	15	19	90*	120	1.4	1.6

Source: Data from Otten, J. J., Hellwig, J. P., & Meyers, L. D. (Eds.). (2006). *Dietary reference intakes: The essential guide to nutrient requirements*. Washington, DC: National Academies Press; Wagner, C. L., Greer, F. R., & Section on Breastfeeding and Committee on Nutrition. (2008). Prevention of rickets and vitamin D deficiency in infants, children, and adolescents. *Pediatrics, 122*(5), 1142–1152; Institute of Medicine, Food and Nutrition Board. (2010). *Dietary reference intakes for calcium and vitamin D*. Washington, DC: National Academies Press.

*Values are Adequate Intakes (AIs) rather than Recommended Dietary Allowances (RDAs). All other values on chart are RDAs. See Chapter 11 for a discussion of nutrient requirements.

TABLE F–2 Dietary Reference Intakes for Infants, Children, and Adolescents

	Age	Vitamin A (mcg/d)	Vitamin D (mcg/d)	Vitamin E (mg/d α-tocopherol)	Vitamin K (mcg/d)	Vitamin C (mg/d)	Thiamin (mg/d)	Riboflavin (mg/d)	Niacin (mg/d)	Vitamin B₆ (mg/d)
Infants	0–6 months	400*	10*	4*	2.0*	40*	0.2*	0.3*	~0.2*	0.1*
	7–12 months	500*	10*	5*	2.5*	50*	0.3*	0.4*	~0.4*	0.3*
Children	1–3 years	300	15	6	30*	15	0.5	0.5	6	0.5
	4–8 years	400	15	7	55*	25	0.6	0.6	8	0.6
Males	9–13 years	600	15	11	60*	45	0.9	0.9	12	1.0
	14–18 years	900	15	15	75*	75	1.2	1.3	16	1.3
Females	9–13 years	600	15	11	60*	45	0.9	0.9	12	1.0
	14–18 years	700	15	15	75*	65	1.0	1.0	14	1.2

Source: Data from Otten, J. J., Hellwig, J. P., & Meyers, L. D. (Eds.). (2006). *Dietary reference intakes: The essential guide to nutrient requirements*. Washington, DC: National Academies Press; Wagner, C. L., Greer, F. R., & Section on Breastfeeding and Committee on Nutrition. (2008). Prevention of rickets and vitamin D deficiency in infants, children, and adolescents. *Pediatrics, 122*(5), 1142–1152; Ross, A. C., Taylor, C. L. O., Yaldine, A. L., & Del Valle, H. B. (Eds.). (2011). *Dietary reference intakes for calcium and vitamin D*. Washington, DC: Institute of Medicine.

*Values are Adequate Intakes (AIs) rather than Recommended Dietary Allowances (RDAs). All other values on chart are RDAs. See Chapter 32 for a discussion of nutrient requirements.

Niacin (mg/d)	Vitamin B6 (mg/d)	Folate (mcg/d)	Vitamin B12 (mcg/d)	Calcium (mg/d)	Phospho-rus (mg/d)	Magnesium (mg/d)	Iron (mg/d)	Zinc (mg/d)	Iodine (mcg/d)	Selenium (mcg/d)
12	1.0	300	1.8	1300	1250	240	8	8	120	40
14	1.2	400	2.4	1300	1250	360	15	9	150	55
14	1.3	400	2.4	1000	700	310	18	8	150	55
14	1.3	400	2.4	1000	700	320	18	8	150	55
14	1.5	400	2.4	1200	700	320	8	8	150	55
14	1.5	400	2.4	1200	700	320	8	8	150	55
18	1.9	600	2.6	1300	1250	400	27	12	220	60
18	1.9	600	2.6	1000	700	350	27	11	220	60
18	1.9	600	2.6	1000	700	360	27	11	220	60
17	2.0	500	2.8	1300	1250	360	10	13	290	70
17	2.0	500	2.8	1000	700	310	9	12	290	70
17	2.0	500	2.8	1000	700	320	9	12	290	70

Folate (mcg/d)	Vitamin B12 (mcg/d)	Calcium (mg/d)	Phosphorus (mg/d)	Magnesium (mg/d)	Iron (mg/d)	Zinc (mg/d)	Iodine (mcg/d)	Selenium (mcg/d)
65*	0.4*	200*	100*	30*	0.27	2*	110*	15*
80*	0.5*	260*	275*	75*	11*	3	130*	20*
150	0.9	700	460	80	7	3	90	20
200	1.2	1000	500	130	10	5	90	30
300	1.8	1300	1250	240	8	8	120	40
400	2.4	1300	1250	240	11	11	150	55
300	1.8	1300	1250	410	8	8	120	40
400	2.4	1300	1250	360	15	9	150	55

TABLE F–3 Recommended Dietary Allowances

	Age	Protein	Carbohydrate	Polyunsaturated Fatty Acids N-6	Polyunsaturated Fatty Acids N-3	Total Fat	Fiber
Infants	0–6 months	9.1 g/d or 1.52 g/kg/d*	60 g/d*	4.4 g/d	0.5 g/d	31 g/d	NE
	7–12 months	1.5 g/kg/d	95 g/d*	4.6 g/d	0.5 g/d	30 g/d	NE
Children	1–3 years	1.1 g/kg/d or 13 g/d	130 g/d	7 g/d (linoleic)	0.7 g/d (α-linolenic)	NE	19 g/d
	4–8 years	0.95 g/kg/d or 19 g/d	130 g/d	10 g/d (linoleic)	0.9 g/d (α-linolenic)	NE	25 g/d
Males	9–13 years	0.95 g/kg/d or 34 g/d	130 g/d	12 g/d (linoleic)	1.2 g/d (α-linolenic)	NE	31 g/d
	14–18 years	0.85 g/kg/d or 52 g/d	130 g/d	16 g/d (linoleic)	1.6 g/d (α-linolenic)	NE	38 g/d
Females	9–13 years	0.95 g/kg/d or 34 g/d	130 g/d	10 g/d (linoleic)	1.0 g/d (α-linolenic)	NE	26 g/d
	14–18 years	0.85 g/kg/d or 46 g/d	130 g/d	11 g/d (linoleic)	1.1 g/d (α-linolenic)	NE	26 g/d

Source: All data from Institute of Medicine. (2002). *Dietary reference intakes*. Washington, DC: National Academies Press.

*Values are Adequate Intakes (AIs) rather than Recommended Dietary Allowances (RDAs). All other values on charts are RDAs.

Key: NE, not established.

Appendix G
Body Surface Area Nomogram

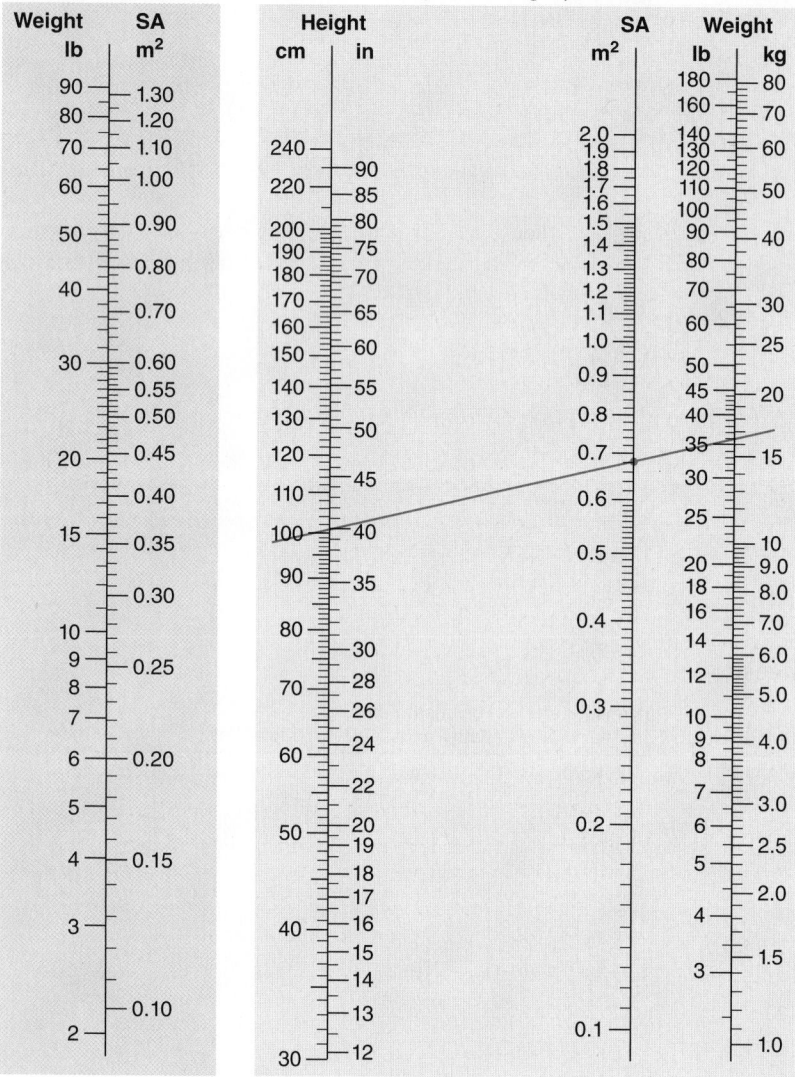

Nomogram
for child with proportional
height and weight

Weight	SA
lb	m²

Nomogram
for child with varied
height and weight percentiles

Height		SA	Weight	
cm	in	m²	lb	kg

The proportion between height and weight in children is different from the proportion in adults. These differences are most manifest in newborns, infants, and young children. Therefore, dosages of drugs that have been established for adults cannot simply be reduced and, correspondingly, be safe for young children. Weight is used as a better method of calculating drug dosage in children and is used when medications have a dose of drug recommended in mg/kg.

Weight alone, however, is not always accurate as a method of calculating a drug dosage for a child. Another more accurate method is that of body surface area (BSA). BSA is a relationship of height to weight and is measured in square meters. BSA increases about 7 times from birth to adulthood. It is a good reflection of many physiologic processes significant in metabolizing, transporting, and eliminating drugs, such as metabolic rate, extracellular fluid and total fluid volumes, cardiac output, and glomerular filtration rate. BSA is calculated by the formula:

$$\text{Surface area}(m^2) = \sqrt{\frac{\text{height(cm)} \times \text{weight(kg)}}{3600}}$$

A nomogram or graph has been developed to calculate BSA quickly and accurately. The nomogram on the left in Figure G–1 can be used when a child has height and weight in proportion, or in the same percentile range. (See Chapter 32 for a description of growth measurements and percentiles.) When the percentiles for height and weight differ, the nomogram on the right can be used. To calculate a child's BSA, draw a straight line from the height to the weight. The point at which the line intersects the surface area (SA) column is the BSA (measured in square meters, m²). Medications that are prescribed using the BSA system are dosed in mg/m².

Glossary

A

Abdominal effleurage   A light stroking movement made over the abdominal wall with the fingertips.

Abortion   Loss of pregnancy before the fetus is viable outside the uterus; miscarriage.

Abruptio placentae   Partial or total premature separation of a normally implanted placenta.

Abstinence   Refraining voluntarily, especially from indulgence in food, alcoholic beverages, or sexual intercourse.

Acanthosis nigricans   Hyperpigmentation and thickening of the skin associated with chronic hyperinsulinemia.

Accelerations   Periodic increases in the baseline fetal heart rate.

Accommodation   The process of changing one's cognitive structures to include data from recent experiences.

Acculturation   The process by which people adapt to a new cultural norm.

Acellular pertussis vaccine   A vaccine that uses pertussis proteins rather than the whole cell to stimulate active immunity.

Acidemia   Decreased blood pH.

Acidosis   Condition caused by excess acid in the blood.

Acme   Peak or highest point; time of greatest intensity (of a uterine contraction).

Acquaintance and date rape   Rape in which the assailant is someone with whom the victim has had previous nonviolent interaction (acquaintance rape) or which occurs between a dating couple. Date rape is a form of acquaintance rape.

Acquired immunity   Humoral (antibody-mediated) and cell-mediated immunity that is not fully developed until a child is about 6 years of age.

Acquired immunodeficiency syndrome (AIDS)   An immunologic disorder caused by infection with the human immunodeficiency virus (HIV) and characterized by increasing susceptibility to opportunistic infections and rare cancers.

Acrocyanosis   Cyanosis of the extremities.

Acrosomal reaction   Breakdown of hyaluronic acid in the corona radiata by enzymes from the heads of sperm; allows one spermatozoon to penetrate the ovum zona pellucida.

Active acquired immunity   Formation of antibodies by the pregnant woman or child in response to illness or immunization.

Active alert state   The awake state in which the newborn's eyes are open and motor activity is quite intense, with thrusting movements of the extremities.

Active immunity   Stimulation of antibody production without causing clinical disease.

Active management of labor (AMOL)   Medical protocol for augmentation of labor that includes (1) a strict criterion for labor admission, (2) early amniotomy, (3) high-dose oxytocin infusion for inefficient labor contractions, and (4) a commitment to provision of continuous nursing care.

Acupressure   Therapy using pressure from the fingers and thumbs to stimulate pressure points.

Acupuncture   Therapy using very fine (hairlike) stainless steel needles to stimulate specific acupuncture points depending on the client's medical assessment and condition.

Acute pain   Sudden pain of short duration, associated with a tissue-damaging stimulus.

Adaptation phase   Period during a crisis when the child and family meet the challenge and use resources effectively.

Adaptive functioning   The ability of individuals to meet the expected standards for their age by their cultural group.

Adequate intake (AI)   A value cited for a nutrient when there are not sufficient data to calculate an estimated average requirement.

Adjustment phase   Period just after a family is confronted by a crisis; characterized by disorganization and unsuccessful attempts to deal with the problem.

Adjustment reaction with depressed mood   A maternal adjustment reaction occurring in the first few postpartum days, characterized by mild depression, tearfulness, anxiety, headache, and irritability. Also called *postpartum blues*.

Adnexa   Adjoining or accessory parts of a structure, such as the uterine adnexa: the ovaries and fallopian tubes.

Adolescence   Period of human development initiated by puberty and ending with the attainment of young adulthood.

Adrenarche   The development of pubic and axillary sexual hair.

Advance directives   A client's living will or appointed durable power of attorney for healthcare decisions.

Adventitious   Breath sounds that are not normally heard, such as crackles and rhonchi.

Affect   Outward manifestation of feeling or emotion; the tone of a person's reaction or response to people or events.

Afterbirth   See *Placenta.*

Afterpains   Cramplike pains due to contractions of the uterus that occur after childbirth. They are more common in multiparas, tend to be most severe during nursing, and last 2 to 3 days.

Agoraphobia   Anxiety of being in places or situations from which escape may be difficult or embarrassing, or in which help may not be available.

Air hunger   The most severe form of dyspnea, when a person or child looks panicked, gasps for breath, and sits upright.

Airway remodeling   A thickening of the sub-basement membrane, subepithelial fibrosis, airway smooth muscle hypertrophy and hyperplasia, blood vessel proliferation and dilation, and mucous gland hyperplasia and hypersecretion. Decreased airway elasticity and decreased lung function result.

Airway resistance   The effort or force needed to move oxygen through the trachea to the lungs.

Alertness   The ability to react to stimuli.

Alkalemia   Increased blood pH.

Alkalosis   Condition caused by too little acid in the blood.

Alleles   Different forms of a gene or DNA occupying the same place on a pair of chromosomes; an allele for each gene is inherited from each parent.

Allergen   An antigen capable of inducing hypersensitivity.

Allergy   An abnormal or altered reaction to an antigen.

Allogeneic stem cell transplantation   A procedure in which a donor (often a sibling [related] or sometimes someone unrelated) with a compatible human leukocyte antigen (HLA) gives bone marrow to a child with an immune or hematologic disease needing restoration of normal cells.

Allograft   The use of cadaver skin from a skin bank in skin grafting; an allograft is used to cover a second-degree burn until healing occurs.

Allow natural death   Provision of ongoing care, pain management, and no initiation of cardiopulmonary resuscitation if the child stops breathing or the heart stops beating.

Alpha-fetoprotein (AFP)   A fetal protein produced in the yolk sac for the first 6 weeks of gestation and then by the fetal liver.

Alternative therapy   Usually considered a substance or procedure that has not undergone rigorous scientific testing in the United States, although it might have been thoroughly tested in other countries.

Alveoli   Small units of the breast tissue in which milk is synthesized by the alveolar secretory epithelium.

Amenorrhea   Suppression or absence of menstruation.

Amniocentesis   Removal of amniotic fluid by insertion of a needle into the amniotic sac; amniotic fluid is used to assess fetal health or maturity.

Amnioinfusion (AI)   Procedure used to infuse a sterile fluid (such as normal saline) through an intrauterine catheter into the uterus in an attempt to increase the fluid around the umbilical cord to decrease or prevent cord compression during labor contractions; also used to dilute thick meconium-stained amniotic fluid.

Amnion   The inner of the two membranes that form the sac containing the fetus and the amniotic fluid.

Amniotic fluid   The liquid surrounding the fetus in utero. It absorbs shocks, permits fetal movement, and prevents heat loss.

Amniotic fluid embolism   Amniotic fluid that has leaked into the chorionic plate and entered the maternal circulation. Also called *Anaphylactic syndrome of pregnancy*.

Amniotomy   The artificial rupturing of the amniotic membrane.

Ampulla   The outer two-thirds of the fallopian tube; fertilization of the ovum by a spermatozoon usually occurs here.

Anaphylactic syndrome of pregnancy   See *Amniotic fluid embolism*.

Anemia   Reduction in the number of red blood cells, the quantity of hemoglobin, and the volume of packed red cells per 100 mL of blood to below-normal levels.

Aneuploidy   An increase or decrease in chromosome number that is the result of an error during cell division, most often when nondisjunction occurs during meiosis.

Animal-assisted therapy   A form of therapy used in hospitals and certain units in which specially trained animals (commonly dogs) provide diversion, distraction, comfort, and relaxation during health care.

Antepartum   Time between conception and the onset of labor; usually used to describe the period during which a woman is pregnant.

Anthropometric measurement   The term used to refer to growth assessment of various parts of the body.

Antibodies   Proteins capable of responding to specific infectious agents.

Anticipation   The tendency for certain genetic disorders to display earlier onset and increased severity in successive generations of a family.

Anticipatory guidance   The process of understanding upcoming developmental needs and then teaching caretakers to meet those needs.

Antigen   A foreign substance that triggers an immune system response.

Anuria   Absence of urine output.

Anxiolysis   Minimal sedation by medication in which cognitive and motor functions may be impaired.

Aortocaval compression   See *Supine hypotensive syndrome*.

Apgar score   A scoring system used to evaluate newborns at 1 minute and 5 minutes after birth. The total score is achieved by assessing five signs: heart rate, respiratory effort, muscle tone, reflex irritability, and color. Each of the signs is assigned a score of 0, 1, or 2. The highest possible score is 10.

Apical impulse   Also called the point of maximum intensity, is located where the left ventricle taps the chest wall during contraction. The apical impulse is usually seen in thin children.

Apnea   Cessation of respiration lasting longer than 20 seconds.

Apoptosis   Programmed cell death. When the cell "realizes" something is wrong and destroys itself.

Areflexia   A lack of reflex response to verbal, sensory, or pain stimulation.

Areola   Pigmented ring surrounding the nipple of the breast.

Aromatherapy   The use of certain essential oils, derived from plants, whose odor or aroma is believed to have a therapeutic effect.

Arrhythmias   Abnormal rhythms or dysrhythmias.

Artificial rupture of membranes (AROM)   A procedure in which the amniotic membranes are ruptured by a healthcare provider, using an instrument called an amniohook. Also called an *amniotomy*.

Asplenia   An absent or dysfunctional spleen.

Assimilation   The process of incorporating new experiences into an individual's cognitive awareness.

Assisted reproductive technology (ART)   The term used to describe highly technologic approaches used to produce pregnancy. In vitro fertilization and embryo transfer (IVF-ET) is an example of ART.

Assistive technology   The process of incorporating new experiences into one's cognitive awareness.

Association   A group of abnormalities of unknown cause that is seen together more often than would be expected by chance.

Associative play   A type of play that emerges in preschool years when children interact with one another, engaging in similar activities and participating in groups.

Atopy   A hereditary allergic tendency.

Attachment   Enduring bonds or relationship of affection between persons.

Audiography   A test used to assess hearing in which sounds of various pitches and intensity are presented to children through earphones.

Aura   A visual, auditory, taste, or motor sensation that gives warning of an impending seizure or migraine headache.

Auscultation   The technique of listening to sounds produced by the airway, lungs, stomach, heart, and blood vessels to identify their characteristics. Auscultation is usually performed with the stethoscope to enhance the sounds heard.

Autografting   Use of healthy skin taken from a nonburned area of the child's body to cover an area with a full-thickness burn.

Autologous stem cell transplantation   A procedure in which the child's own marrow is taken, treated, stored, and reinfused after the child has received chemotherapy.

Automatism   Unusual body movements without purpose; e.g., lip smacking, lip chewing, sucking.

Autonomic dysreflexia   Condition in which hypertension, bradycardia, severe headaches, pallor below and flushing above the level of the spinal cord lesion, and seizures occurs because of an impaired autonomic nervous system, triggered by simultaneous sympathetic and parasympathetic activity.

Autosomes   Chromosomes other than the sex chromosomes.

Azotemia   Accumulation of nitrogenous wastes in the blood.

B

Babinski reflex   Reflex found normally in infants under 6 months of age in which the great toe dorsiflexes when the sole of the foot is stimulated.

Bacterial vaginosis   A bacterial infection of the vagina characterized by a foul-smelling, grayish vaginal discharge that exhibits a characteristic fishy odor when 10% potassium hydroxide (KOH) is added. Microscopic examination of a vaginal wet preparation reveals the presence of "clue cells" (vaginal epithelial cells coated with gram-negative organisms).

Bag of waters (BOW)   The membrane containing the amniotic fluid and the fetus.

Ballottement   A technique of palpation used to detect or examine a floating object in the body. In obstetrics, the fetus, when pushed, floats away and then returns to touch the examiner's fingers.

Barlow maneuver   Test designed to detect subluxation or dislocation of the hip. A dysplastic joint will be felt to be dislocated as the femur leaves the acetabulum.

Basal body temperature (BBT)   The lowest waking temperature.

Baseline fetal heart rate (BL FHR)   The average fetal heart rate observed during a 10-minute period of monitoring.

Baseline variability (BL VAR)   Changes in the fetal heart rate that result from the interplay between the sympathetic and the parasympathetic nervous systems.

Becoming a mother (BAM)   Alternative term for *maternal role attainment (MRA)*. The transitional process of becoming a mother that changes throughout the maternal–child relationship.

Behavior modification   A technique used to reinforce desirable behaviors, helping the child to replace maladaptive behaviors with more appropriate ones.

Benign   Describing a growth that does not endanger life or health.

Bereavement   To have suffered the event of loss.

Beta human chorionic gonadotropin (Beta hCG)   A product of the trophoblast or placenta that is detected through serum testing and is a very accurate marker of the presence of pregnancy and placental health.

Bilirubin encephalopathy   See *Kernicterus*.

Binge eating   A compulsion to consume large quantities of food in a short period of time.

Binocularity   Ability of the eyes to function together.

Biophysical profile (BPP)   Assessment of five variables in the fetus that help to evaluate fetal risk: breathing movement, body movement, tone, amniotic fluid volume, and fetal heart rate reactivity.

Biotherapy   A treatment that uses and/or enhances the body's abilities to fight disease, particularly by using biologic agents to promote immune response.

Birth center   A setting for labor and birth that emphasizes a family-centered approach rather than obstetric technology and treatment.

Birth plan   A written document prepared by expectant parents that is used to identify available options in the birth setting and aspects of the childbearing experience that are most important to them.

Birth rate   Number of live births per 1,000 population.

Birthing room   In hospitals or birthing centers, single rooms where the woman and her partner or other family members will stay for the labor, birth, recovery, and possibly the postpartum period. Also called *labor, delivery, recovery, and postpartum rooms or single-room maternity care.*

Bisexual   An adjective used to describe or refer to a person who is sexually attracted to both men and women.

Bishop score   A prelabor scoring system to assist in predicting whether an induction of labor may be successful. The total score is achieved by assessing five components: cervical dilatation, cervical effacement, cervical consistency, cervical position, and fetal station. Each of the components is assigned a score of 0 to 3, with the highest possible score being 13.

Blastocyst   The inner solid mass of cells within the morula.

Bloody show   Pink-tinged mucous secretions resulting from rupture of small capillaries as the cervix effaces and dilates.

Body fluid   Body water that has substances (solutes) dissolved in it.

Body image   The idea that one forms about one's body.

Body mass index (BMI)   A calculation (kilograms of weight/m^2 of height) used to determine the proportion between a child's or adult's height and weight.

Boggy uterus (uterine atony)   A term used to describe the uterine fundus when it is not firmly contracted after the birth of the baby and in the early postpartum period; excessive bleeding occurs from the placental site, and maternal hemorrhage may occur.

Bonding   Process of parent–newborn attachment occurring at or soon after birth.

Bone age   A radiographic image of the bones of the wrist used to evaluate the stage of bone ossification.

Brachial palsy   Partial or complete paralysis of portions of the arm resulting from trauma to the brachial plexus during a difficult birth.

Brachial plexus injury   Injury due to improper or excessive traction applied to the fetal head during birth that results in damage to the network of nerves that send signals from the spine to the shoulder, arm, and hand.

Brain death   The irreversible cessation of all functions of the brain, including the cerebral cortex and brainstem.

Braxton Hicks contractions   Intermittent painless contractions of the uterus that may occur every 10 to 20 minutes. They occur more frequently toward the end of pregnancy and are sometimes mistaken for true labor signs.

Brazelton Neonatal Behavioral Assessment Scale   A brief examination used to identify the newborn's behavioral states and responses.

Breakthrough pain   Pain that emerges as pain medication wears off, resulting in the loss of pain control.

Breast self-examination (BSE)   A manual examination conducted monthly by a woman to evaluate her own breasts for signs of masses, changes, nipple discharge, or evidence of abnormalities.

Breasts   Mammary glands.

Breech presentation   A birth in which the buttocks and/or feet are the presenting part rather than the head.

Broad ligament   A ligament that keeps the uterus centrally placed and provides stability within the pelvic cavity. It is a double layer that is continuous with the abdominal peritoneum. The broad ligament covers the uterus anteriorly and posteriorly and extends outward from the uterus to enfold the fallopian tubes.

Bronchophony   Change in vocal resonance in the presence of a lung consolidation, in which there is increased intensity and clarity of sounds while the words remain indistinct.

Brown adipose tissue (BAT)   Fat deposits in neonates that provide greater heat-generating activity than ordinary fat. Found around the kidneys, adrenals, and neck; between the scapulas; and behind the sternum. Also called *brown fat*.

Buffer   Related acid–base pair that gives up or takes up hydrogen ions as needed to prevent large changes in the pH of a solution.

Bullying   Repeatedly aggressive behavior intended to cause physical or emotional harm that exists in a relationship with an imbalance of power.

C

Calorie Amount of heat required to raise the temperature of 1 kg of water 1 degree Celsius.

Capacitation Removal of the plasma membrane overlying the spermatozoa's acrosomal area with the loss of seminal plasma proteins and the glycoprotein coat. If the glycoprotein coat is not removed, the sperm will not be able to penetrate the ovum.

Caput succedaneum Swelling or edema occurring in or under the fetal scalp during labor.

Carcinogens Chemicals or processes that, when combined with genetic traits and in interaction with one another, cause cancer.

Cardiac output Volume of blood ejected from the left ventricle each minute.

Cardinal ligaments The chief uterine supports, the cardinal ligaments suspend the uterus from the side walls of the true pelvis. Also called *Mackenrodt* or *transverse cervical ligaments*, they arise from the sides of the pelvic walls and attach to the cervix in the upper vagina. They prevent uterine prolapse and support the upper vagina.

Cardinal movements The positional changes of the fetus as it moves through the birth canal during labor and birth. The positional changes are descent, flexion, internal rotation, extension, restitution, and external rotation.

Cardiomegaly Enlargement of the heart muscle.

Cardiopulmonary adaptation Adaptation of the neonate's cardiovascular and respiratory systems to life outside the womb.

Care coordination The process of planning and integrating healthcare services among providers in an effort to achieve and promote good health in the child.

Caregiver burden The unrelenting pressure and anxiety related to providing daily care to a child with disabilities while meeting other family obligations.

Carrier Any individual who carries a single copy of an altered gene or mutation for a recessive condition on one chromosome of a chromosome pair and an unaltered form of that gene on the other chromosome. A carrier generally is not affected by the gene alteration; on the average, each person in the general population is a carrier of five or six gene mutations for recessive disorders.

Case management A process of coordinating the delivery of healthcare services in a manner that focuses on both quality and cost outcomes.

Case manager Person who coordinates health care to prevent gaps or overlaps.

Cell The basic unit of life and the working unit of all living systems.

Cell-free fetal DNA (cffDNA) testing A maternal screening blood test that can be obtained to test for trisomies 13, 18, and 21. The noninvasive test detects circulating fetal DNA within the maternal serum.

CenteringPregnancy® A model of prenatal health care designed to empower women to choose health-promoting behaviors and, as a result, improve prenatal care outcomes.

Cephalic presentation Birth in which the fetal head is presenting against the cervix.

Cephalocaudal development The process by which development proceeds from the head downward through the body and toward the feet.

Cephalohematoma Subcutaneous swelling containing blood found on the head of a neonate several days after birth; it usually disappears within a few weeks to 2 months.

Cephalopelvic disproportion (CPD) A condition in which the fetal head is of such a shape or size, or in such a position, that it cannot pass through the maternal pelvis.

Cerclage Surgical procedure in which a stitch is placed in the cervix to prevent a spontaneous abortion or premature birth.

Cerebral edema Increase in intracellular and extracellular fluid in the brain that results from anoxia, vasodilation, or vascular stasis.

Cerebral perfusion pressure Amount of pressure needed to ensure that adequate oxygen and nutrients will be delivered to the brain.

Certified nurse-midwife (CNM) A registered nurse who has received special training and education in the care of the family during childbearing and the prenatal, labor and birth, and postpartum periods. After a period of formal education, the nurse-midwife takes a certification test to become a CNM.

Certified registered nurse (RNC) A registered nurse who has shown expertise in a specific field by passing a national certification examination.

Cervical dilatation Process in which the cervical os and the cervical canal widen from less than 1 cm (0.4 in.) to approximately 10 cm (4 in.), allowing birth of the fetus.

Cervical insufficiency Painless dilatation of the cervix without contractions because of a structural or functional defect of the cervix. Also called *incompetent cervix*.

Cervical ripening Softening of the cervix; occurs normally as a physiologic process prior to labor or is stimulated to occur through the process of induction of labor.

Cervix The "neck" between the external os and the body of the uterus. The lower end of the cervix extends into the vagina.

Cesarean birth Birth of fetus accomplished by performing a surgical incision through the maternal abdomen and uterus.

Chadwick sign A blue-purple discoloration of the cervix caused by increased vascularization of the uterus during pregnancy is an objective change or probable sign of pregnancy.

Chelation A reaction in which an organic compound containing carbonyl (CO) and hydroxyl (OH) groups coordinates with a metal to form a firmly bound ringlike structure.

Chemical conjunctivitis Irritation of the mucous membrane lining of the eyelid; may be due to instillation of silver nitrate ophthalmic drops.

Chemotherapy Treatment to combat cancer that involves drugs taken orally, intravenously, intrathecally, or by injection, which kill both normal and cancerous cells.

Child-life specialist Trained professional who plans therapeutic activities for hospitalized children.

Child sexual abuse The exploitation of a child for the sexual gratification of an adult or older child.

Children with special healthcare needs (CSHCN) Children who have or are at increased risk for a chronic physical, developmental, behavioral, or emotional condition and who also require health and related services of a type or amount beyond that required by children generally.

Chlamydial infection A sexually transmitted infection caused by *Chlamydia trachomatis*.

Chloasma (melasma gravidarum) Brownish pigmentation over the bridge of the nose and the cheeks during pregnancy and in some women who are taking oral contraceptives. Also called *mask of pregnancy*.

Cholestasis Disruption of bile flow.

Chondrolysis The breaking down and absorption of cartilage.

Chordee A fibrous band of tissue on the penis causing downward bowing that is associated with hypospadias.

Chorion The fetal membrane closest to the intrauterine wall that gives rise to the placenta and continues as the outer membrane surrounding the amnion.

Chorionic villus sampling (CVS) Procedure in which a specimen of the chorionic villi is obtained from the edge of the developing placenta at about 8 weeks' gestation. The sample can be used for chromosomal, enzyme, and DNA tests.

Chromosomes The threadlike structures within the nucleus of a cell that carry the genes.

Chronic condition A health condition that lasts or is expected to last 3 months or more.

Chronic pain Persistent pain lasting longer than 3 months, generally associated with a prolonged disease process.

Chronic vomiting Low-grade nearly daily emesis.

Chvostek sign A spasm of facial muscles after tapping facial nerve. A positive Chvostek sign reveals hyperreflexia. It is used to assess for hypoparathyroidism.

Circumcision Surgical removal of the prepuce (foreskin) of the penis.

Circumferential Injury completely surrounding the thorax or an extremity.

Cleavage Rapid mitotic division of the zygote; cells produced are called *blastomeres*.

Clinical nurse specialist (CNS) A registered nurse possessing a master's degree and specialized knowledge and competence in a specific clinical area.

Clinical practice guidelines Outlines detailing specific medical and nursing assessments and interventions during specific time intervals for a specific condition. This guideline is often adopted in an institution for all healthcare providers to follow so that quality of care is increased and costs of care are minimized.

Clitoris Female organ homologous to the male penis; a small oval body of erectile tissue situated at the anterior junction of the vulva.

Clonic Alternating muscular contraction and relaxation; often used to describe seizure activity.

Clubbing A widening of the nail bed with an increased angle between the proximal nail fold and nail.

Cognition The change in thought, intelligence, and language that occurs from the mutual interaction of brain maturation with life experiences.

Cognitive power The ability to process data and respond either verbally or physically.

Cognitive therapy A therapeutic approach that attempts to help the person recognize automatic thought patterns that lead to unpleasant feelings.

Coitus interruptus Method of contraception in which the male withdraws his penis from the vagina prior to ejaculation.

Cold stress Excessive heat loss resulting in compensatory mechanisms (increased respirations and nonshivering thermogenesis) to maintain core body temperature.

Coloboma A keyhole-shaped pupil caused by a notch in the iris.

Colostrum Secretion from the breast before the onset of true lactation; contains mainly serum and white blood corpuscles. It has a high protein content, provides some immune properties, and cleanses the neonate's intestinal tract of mucus and meconium.

Colposcopy The use of an instrument inserted into the vagina to examine the cervical and vaginal tissues by means of a magnifying lens.

Coma State of unconsciousness in which the person cannot be aroused, even with powerful stimuli.

Combined oral contraceptives (COCs) Commonly called *birth control pills* or "the pill." A form of contraception that uses a combination of a synthetic estrogen and a progestin.

Comedone A plug of sebaceous and keratin material in a hair follicle; commonly called "whiteheads" and "blackheads."

Communicable disease An illness that is transmitted directly or indirectly from one person to another.

Compartment syndrome A condition of increased pressure in a limited space that compromises circulation and tissue function.

Complementary and alternative medicine (CAM) A group of diverse medical and healthcare systems, practices, and products that are not generally considered part of conventional medicine.

Complementary therapy May be defined as an adjunct to conventional medical treatment that has been through rigorous scientific testing, which shows that it has some reliability; approaches to health care that are usually not part of conventional Western medicine; sometimes called *alternative therapy*.

Compliance Amount of expansion the ventricles can achieve to increase stroke volume.

Conception Union of male sperm and female ovum; fertilization.

Condom A rubber sheath that covers the penis to prevent conception or disease.

Conduction Loss of heat to a cooler surface by direct skin contact.

Conductive hearing loss Hearing loss caused by inadequate conduction of sound from the outer to the middle ear.

Condylomata acuminata A common sexually transmitted infection caused by the human papillomavirus (HPV). Also called *venereal warts*.

Congenital dermal melanocytes Macular areas of bluish black or gray-blue pigmentation usually on the dorsal area and the buttocks but may be anywhere on the body. Also called *Mongolian blue spots*.

Conjugate Important diameter of the pelvis, measured from the center of the promontory of the sacrum to the back of the symphysis pubis. The diagonal conjugate is measured and the true conjugate is estimated.

Conjugate vera The true conjugate, which extends from the middle of the sacral promontory to the middle of the pubic crest.

Conjugated forms Forms of a vaccine against childhood diseases in the United States in which an altered organism is joined with another substance to increase the immune response.

Consanguinity Related by having a common ancestor; close blood relationship.

Consciousness The responsiveness to or awareness of sensory stimuli, involving alertness and cognitive power.

Conservation The knowledge that matter is not changed when its form is altered.

Constipation Difficult and infrequent defecation with passage of hard, dry stool.

Consultand A designated "index" patient who seeks genetic counseling without being known to have a given genetic disorder, around which a pedigree is often constructed.

Continuous epidural infusion (CEI) Postcesarean pain control technique in which the epidural catheter is left in place and medication is continually administered via an electric pump.

Contraception The prevention of conception or impregnation.

Contraction Tightening and shortening of the uterine muscles during labor, causing effacement and dilatation of the cervix; contributes to the downward and outward descent of the fetus.

Contraction stress test (CST) A method of assessing the reaction of the fetus to the stress of uterine contractions. This test may be utilized when contractions are occurring spontaneously or when contractions are artificially induced by an oxytocin challenge test (OCT) or breast self-stimulation test (BSST).

Convection Loss of heat from the warm body surface to cooler air currents.

Coombs test A test for antiglobulins in the red blood cells. The indirect test determines the presence of Rh-positive antibodies in maternal blood; the direct test determines the presence of maternal Rh-positive antibodies in fetal cord blood.

Cooperative play A type of play that emerges in school years when children join into groups to achieve a goal or play a game.

Coping The use of learned behavioral and cognitive strategies to manage or relieve perceived stress.

Copy number variation An additional source of human genetic variation in which stretches of DNA of variable size are replicated one or more times.

Cor pulmonale Obstruction of pulmonary blood flow that leads to right ventricular hypertrophy and heart failure.

Cordocentesis A technique used to obtain pure fetal blood from the umbilical cord while the fetus is in utero; used for diagnosis of hemophilias, hemoglobinopathies, fetal infections, chromosomal abnormalities, nonimmune hydrops, and isoimmune hemolytic disorders, as well as assessment of fetal hemoglobin and hematocrit for calculation of transfusion requirements in the second and third trimesters. Also called *percutaneous umbilical blood sampling (PUBS)*.

Cornua The elongated portion of the uterus where the fallopian tubes enter.

Corpus The upper two thirds of the uterus.

Corpus luteum A small yellow body that develops within a ruptured ovarian follicle; it secretes progesterone in the second half of the menstrual cycle and atrophies about 3 days before the beginning of menstrual flow. If pregnancy occurs, the corpus luteum continues to produce progesterone until the placenta takes over this function.

Cosleeping Practice whereby children and parents regularly sleep together in an adult bed.

Cotyledon One of the rounded portions into which the placenta's uterine surface is divided, consisting of a mass of villi, fetal vessels, and an intervillous space.

Couplet care A form of health care that is focused on keeping the mother and baby together as much as the mother desires. Also called *mother–baby care*, this type of care provides increased opportunities for parent–child interaction because the newborn shares the mother's room and they are cared for together. Mother–baby care enables the mother to have time to bond with her baby and learn to care for her newborn in a supportive environment.

Couvade In some cultures, the male's observance of certain rituals and taboos to signify the transition to fatherhood.

Crepitus A crinkly sensation palpated on the chest surface caused by air escaping into the subcutaneous tissues.

Crossing over A process that occurs during meiosis in which homologous maternal and paternal chromosomes break and exchange corresponding sections of DNA and then rejoin; this process can cause an exchange of alleles between chromosomes and provides human diversity.

Crowning Appearance of the presenting fetal part at the vaginal orifice during labor.

Cryotherapy The use of cold or cold agents to treat specific injuries or conditions. Often used for treating warts and other skin conditions.

Cultural competence Refers to the skills and knowledge necessary to appreciate, understand, and work with individuals from different cultures.

Culture Defined as the beliefs, values, attitudes, and practices that are accepted by a population, community, or an individual.

Cushing triad Reflex response associated with increased intracranial pressure or compromised blood flow to the brainstem; characterized by hypertension, increased systolic pressure with wide pulse pressure, bradycardia, and irregular respirations.

Cyberbullying A situation in which a child or adolescent is targeted by another via Internet posting or other digital technology, and threatened, tormented, harassed, humiliated, or embarrassed.

Cyclic vomiting Repeated severe vomiting of an episodic nature.

Cystocele The downward displacement of the bladder, which appears as a bulge in the anterior vaginal wall.

Cytogenetics The study of chromosomes and alterations to health caused by abnormalities in the number or structure of chromosomes.

D

Date rape A form of acquaintance rape that occurs between a dating couple.

Deamination Removal of an amino group from an amino compound.

Death anxiety A feeling of apprehension or fear of death.

Death imagery Any reference to death or death-related topics, such as going away, separation, funerals, and dying, given in response to a picture or story that would not usually stimulate other children to discuss death-related topics.

Debridement Enzyme action to clean a lesion and dissolve fibrin clots or scabs; or removal of dead tissue to speed the healing process.

Decelerations Periodic decreases in the baseline fetal heart rate.

Decibels Units used to measure the loudness of sounds.

Decidua Endometrium or mucous membrane lining of the uterus in pregnancy that is shed after childbirth.

Decidua basalis The part of the decidua that unites with the chorion to form the placenta. It is shed in lochial discharge after childbirth.

Decidua capsularis The part of the decidua surrounding the chorionic sac.

Decidua vera (parietalis) Nonplacental decidua lining the uterus.

Deciduous teeth Primary set of 20 teeth that is complete by about 2 years and will be lost during childhood, beginning at about 6 years.

Deep sedation A controlled state of depressed consciousness or unconsciousness in which the child may experience partial or complete loss of protective reflexes.

Deep sleep state State of sleep in which the infant will be nearly still except for occasional startles, twitches, and sucking.

Defense mechanism Technique used by the ego to unconsciously change reality, thereby protecting itself from excessive anxiety.

Dehydration The state of body water deficit.

Depo-Provera Trade name for a long-acting, injectable progestin contraceptive.

Dermatophytoses Fungal infections that affect primarily the skin, but also may affect the hair and nails.

Desaturated blood Blood with a lower than normal oxygen level resulting when a heart defect causes oxygenated and unoxygenated blood to mix.

Development The process of increasing capability or function.

Developmental delay A delay in mastering functions, such as motor coordination and behavioral skills.

Developmental disability Any of a variety of chronic conditions that are characterized by mental or physical impairments. Intellectual disability, pervasive developmental disorder, cerebral palsy, and sensory loss are examples of developmental disabilities.

Developmental surveillance A flexible, continuous process of skilled observations that also provides data about the child's capabilities, allows for early identification of any neurologic problems, and helps to verify that the home environment is stimulating.

Diagonal conjugate An anteroposterior diameter that extends from the subpubic angle to the middle of the sacral promontory and is typically 12.5 cm (5 in.). One of three diameters that are used to assess the size and shape of the pelvic inlet.

Dialysate The solution used in dialysis.

Diaphragm A flexible disc used to cover the cervix to prevent pregnancy.

Diarrhea Frequent passage of abnormally watery stool.

Diastasis recti abdominis Separation of the recti abdominis muscles along the median line. In women, it is seen with repeated childbirths or multiple gestations. In the newborn, it is usually caused by incomplete development.

Dietary Reference Intakes (DRIs) A set of nutrient values that can be used to assess and plan intake for individuals of different ages.

Diffusion Movement of molecules across a membrane from an area of higher concentration to lower concentration.

Digitalization Process of giving a higher than normal dose of digoxin initially to speed response to the drug.

Dilatation of the cervix Expansion of the external os from an opening a few millimeters in size to an opening large enough to allow the passage of the neonate.

Dilation and curettage (D&C) Stretching of the cervical canal to permit passage of a curette, which is used to scrape the endometrium to empty the uterine contents or to obtain tissue for examination.

Diploid number of chromosomes Containing a set of maternal and a set of paternal chromosomes; in humans, the diploid number of chromosomes is 46.

Direct transmission The passage of an infectious disease through physical contact between the source of the pathogen and a new host.

Disability Impairment in one or more of five categories of function: cognition, communication, motor abilities, social abilities, or patterns of interactions.

Disassociation relaxation A pattern of active relaxation in which the woman learns to tighten one area of the body and then relax other areas simultaneously. This relaxation pattern is very effective for some women during labor.

Disaster A serious and massive event that impacts many people and causes extensive damage, hardship, death, injuries, and psychologic trauma.

Disaster preparedness Planning and coordinated response readiness by a community to meet the personal safety, healthcare, emotional, and environmental needs of children and their families in the event of a natural or human-made disaster.

Disequilibrium syndrome Rapid changes in the body's water and electrolyte balance during treatment.

Dislocation Displacement of a bone from its normal articulation with a joint.

Distraction The ability to focus attention on something other than pain, such as an activity, music, or a story.

Domestic violence Defined as the collective methods used to exert power and control by one individual over another in an adult intimate relationship. Forms of abuse typically fall into three categories: psychologic abuse, physical abuse, and sexual abuse.

Dominant A characteristic or gene that is apparent even when the relevant gene is present in only one copy; a person with a dominant gene usually expresses that gene trait.

Doula A supportive companion who accompanies a laboring woman to provide emotional, physical, and informational support and acts as an advocate for the woman and her family.

Down syndrome An abnormality resulting from the presence of an extra chromosome number 21 (trisomy 21); characteristics include intellectual disability and altered physical appearance.

Dramatic play A type of play in which a child acts out the drama of daily life.

Drowsy or semidozing state A subcategory of the alert state of infants. Aspects of the drowsy state include open or closed eyes, fluttering eyelids, semidozing appearance, and slow, regular movements of the extremities. Mild startles may be noted from time to time.

Dubowitz tool A scoring tool to estimate gestational age of the newborn by maturity rating. It can be used from birth to 5 days of life.

Ductus arteriosus A communication channel between the main pulmonary artery and the aorta of the fetus. It is obliterated after birth by rising PO_2 and changes in intravascular pressure in the presence of normal pulmonary functioning. It normally becomes a ligament after birth but sometimes remains patent (patent ductus arteriosus, a treatable condition).

Ductus venosus A fetal blood vessel that carries oxygenated blood between the umbilical vein and the inferior vena cava, bypassing the liver; it becomes a ligament after birth.

Duncan mechanism Occurs when the maternal surface of the placenta rather than the shiny fetal surface presents upon birth.

Duration The time length of each contraction, measured from the beginning of the increment to the completion of the decrement.

Dwarfism A genetic condition usually resulting in an adult height of 58 inches (147 cm) or less. The most common cause of dwarfism is achondroplasia, which causes short arms and legs. The torso and head are approximately normal size, but decreased growth of long bones causes short stature.

Dysfunctional uterine bleeding (DUB) A condition characterized by anovulatory cycles with abnormal uterine bleeding that does not have a demonstrable organic cause.

Dysmenorrhea Painful menstruation.

Dysmorphology The study of human congenital defects or abnormalities of body structure that begin before birth.

Dyspareunia Painful intercourse.

Dysphagia Difficulty in swallowing.

Dysphonia Muffled, hoarse, or absent voice sounds.

Dysplasia Abnormal development resulting in altered size, shape, and cell organization.

Dyspnea Shortness of breath; difficulty breathing.

Dystocia Difficult labor due to mechanical factors produced by the fetus or the maternal pelvis or due to inadequate uterine or other muscular activity.

E

Early adolescence Refers to adolescents who are ages 14 years and under.

Early childhood caries (ECC) The presence of one or more decayed, lost, or filled tooth surfaces in primary teeth from birth to 71 months of age; frequently caused by drinking from a bottle or nursing for prolonged periods, especially when sleeping; previously referred to as *nursing bottle mouth syndrome* and *baby bottle tooth decay*.

Early deceleration A periodic decrease in fetal heart rate from the normal baseline.

Early intervention Special services provided by state or local education programs for infants and toddlers up to age 3 years who have developmental delay or are at risk for developmental delay in the hopes that these children will have a lowered total cost of educational services.

Early (primary) postpartum hemorrhage A loss of blood of greater than 500 mL following birth. The hemorrhage is classified as early if it occurs within the first 24 hours and late if it occurs after the first 24 hours.

Early-term birth   Births occurring between 37 weeks 0 days and 38 weeks 6 days.

Ecchymosis   A bruise.

Echolalia   A compulsive parroting of what is heard.

Eclampsia   A major complication of pregnancy. Its cause is unknown; it occurs more often in the primigravida and is accompanied by elevated blood pressure, albuminuria, oliguria, tonic and clonic convulsions, and coma. It may occur during pregnancy (usually after the 20th week of gestation) or within 48 hours after childbirth.

Ecologic theory   A theory of development that emphasizes the importance of interactions between the developing child and the settings in which the child lives.

Ecomap   An illustration of a family's relationships and social networks.

Ectoderm   Outer layer of cells in the developing embryo that gives rise to the skin, nails, and hair.

Ectopic pregnancy (EP)   Implantation of the fertilized ovum outside the uterine cavity; common sites are the abdomen, fallopian tubes, and ovaries. Also called *oocyesis*.

Edema   An accumulation of excess fluid in the interstitial spaces.

Effacement   Thinning and shortening of the cervix that occurs late in pregnancy or during labor.

Ejaculation   Expulsion of seminal fluids from the penis.

Electroanalgesia   A method of delivering electrical stimulation to the skin, to compete with pain stimuli for transmission to the spinal cord. Also called *transcutaneous electrical nerve stimulation* (TENS).

Electrolytes   Charged particles (ions) dissolved in body fluid.

Electronic fetal monitoring (EFM)   A method of placing a fetal monitor on the fetus in order to obtain a continuous tracing of the fetal heart rate (FHR), which allows many characteristics of the FHR to be observed and evaluated.

Emancipated minors   Minors who are legally considered to have assumed the rights of an adult. Adolescents may be considered emancipated if they are self-supporting and living away from home, married, pregnant, a parent, or in the military.

Embryo   The early stage of development of the young of any organism. In humans, the embryonic period is from about 2 to 8 weeks' gestation and is characterized by cellular differentiation and predominantly hyperplastic growth.

Embryonic membranes   The amnion and chorion.

Emergency contraception   Commonly called "Plan B" or the "morning after pill," this is a progestin-only approach (levonorgestrel) that is used within 72 hours of unprotected intercourse to eliminate the possibility of pregnancy.

Emergency preparedness   Readiness to manage a healthcare emergency that involves planning, equipment and supplies for responses, and provider training and guidelines for action when an emergency occurs.

Emollient   A topical product that soothes and softens the skin.

Emotional abuse   Shaming, ridiculing, embarrassing, or insulting a child.

Emotional neglect   A caretaker's inability to meet the psychosocial needs of a child.

En face   An assumed position in which one person looks at another and maintains the face in the same vertical plane as that of the other; direct face-to-face and eye-to-eye contact between two people.

Encephalopathy   Cerebral dysfunction resulting from an insult (toxin, injury, inflammation, or anoxic event) of limited duration; the tissue damage is often permanent, but the dysfunction may improve over time.

Endoderm   The inner layer of cells in the developing embryo that gives rise to internal organs such as the intestines.

Endogenous pyrogens   Pyrogens (chemicals) released in response to an invasive organism that travel through the circulatory system to the hypothalamus, where they trigger the production of prostaglandins.

Endometrial biopsy (EMB)   Procedure that provides information about the effects of progesterone produced by the corpus luteum after ovulation and endometrial receptivity.

Endometriosis   Ectopic endometrium located outside the uterus in the pelvic cavity. Symptoms may include pelvic pain or pressure, dysmenorrhea, dyspareunia, abnormal bleeding from the uterus or rectum, and sterility.

Endometritis (metritis)   An inflammation of the endometrial portion of the uterine lining.

Endometrium   The mucous membrane that lines the inner surface of the uterus.

Endorphins   Exogenous opioids.

End-stage renal disease (ESRD)   Irreversible kidney failure.

Engagement   The entrance of the fetal presenting part into the superior pelvic strait and the beginning of the descent through the pelvic canal.

Engorgement   Vascular congestion or distention. In obstetrics, the swelling of breast tissue brought about by an increase in blood and lymph supply to the breast, preceding true lactation.

Engrossment   Characteristic sense of absorption, preoccupation, and interest in the newborn demonstrated by fathers during early contact with their babies.

Enteral therapy   Nutrition introduced through the intestinal tract, including oral or tube feedings.

Enuresis   Involuntary micturition by a child who has reached the age at which bladder control is expected.

Environmental toxins   Chemical compounds found in air, food, and water, the bioaccumulation of which can lead to adverse health effects.

Epicanthal fold   An extra fold of skin covering all or part of the lacrimal caruncle of the medial canthus of the eye.

Epidural block   Regional anesthesia effective through the first and second stages of labor.

Epigenetic   Describes any factor that can affect gene function (usually by changing gene expression, or translation) without changing the DNA sequence.

Episiotomy   Incision of the perineum to facilitate birth and to avoid laceration of the perineum.

Epithelialization   The process by which epithelial cells grow into the wound from surrounding healthy tissue.

Epstein pearls   Small, white blebs found along the gum margins and at the junction of the hard and soft palates; commonly seen in the newborn as a normal manifestation.

Equianalgesic dose   The amount of a drug when administered orally that produces the same level of analgesia as when it is administered parenterally.

Equinus   A condition that limits dorsiflexion to less than normal; usually associated with clubfoot.

Erb-Duchenne paralysis (Erb palsy)   Paralysis of the arm and chest wall as a result of a birth injury to the brachial plexus or a subsequent injury to the fifth and sixth cervical nerves.

Ergogenic aids   Products that enhance physical performance.

Erythema toxicum   Innocuous pink papular rash of unknown cause with superimposed vesicles; it appears within 24 to 48 hours after birth and resolves spontaneously within a few days.

Erythroblastosis fetalis Hemolytic disease of the newborn characterized by anemia, jaundice, enlargement of the liver and spleen, and generalized edema. Caused by isoimmunization as a result of Rh incompatibility or ABO incompatibility.

Erythropoiesis Formation of red blood cells.

Eschar Slough or layer of dead skin or tissue.

Escharotomy Incision into constricting dead tissue of a burn injury to restore peripheral circulation.

Espiritistas A healer who communicates with spirits for the physical and emotional development of the client.

Estimated date of birth (EDB) During a pregnancy, the approximate date when childbirth will occur; the "due date."

Estrogens The hormones estradiol and estrone, produced by the ovary.

Ethnicity A social identity that is associated with shared beliefs, behaviors, and patterns.

Ethnocentrism An individual's belief that the values and practices of the individual's own culture are the best ones.

Euthyroid Normal thyroid state.

Evaporation Loss of heat incurred when water on the skin surface is converted to a vapor.

Evidence-based practice An approach to problem solving and decision making that is based on the consideration of data from research, statistical analysis, quality measures, risk management measurements, and other sources of reliable information.

Excoriation Scratches and abrasions of the skin.

Exophthalmos Prominent or bulging eyes.

Expressive jargon Use of unintelligible words with normal speech intonations as if truly communicating in words; common in toddlerhood.

External cephalic version (ECV) Procedure involving external manipulation of the maternal abdomen to change the presentation of the fetus from breech to cephalic.

External os The opening between the cervix and the vagina.

Extracellular fluid The fluid in the body that is outside the cells.

Extravasation Damage that occurs when a chemotherapeutic drug leaks into the soft tissue surrounding the infusion site.

F

Fallopian tubes Tubes that extend from the lateral angle of the uterus and terminate near the ovary; they serve as a passageway for the ovum from the ovary to the uterus and for the spermatozoa from the uterus toward the ovary. Also called *oviducts* and *uterine tubes*.

False labor Contractions of the uterus, regular or irregular, that may be strong enough to be interpreted as true labor but that do not dilate the cervix.

False pelvis The portion above the pelvic brim, or linea terminalis, that serves to support the weight of the enlarged pregnant uterus and direct the presenting fetal part into the true pelvis below.

Family Refers to two or more persons who are joined together by bonds of sharing and emotional closeness and who identify themselves as being part of a family.

Family assessment The process by which a nurse collects data regarding a family's current level of functioning, support systems, sociocultural influences, home and work environment, type of family, family structure, and needs.

Family crisis An event that causes problems for a family that for a time seem insurmountable and with which the family is unable to cope in its usual ways.

Family planning Actions an individual or a couple take to avoid a pregnancy, to space future pregnancies for a specific reason, or to gain control over the number of children conceived.

Family resilience The family's capacity to demonstrate a positive response to an adverse situation and to emerge from the situation feeling strengthened, more resourceful, and more confident.

Family strengths Relationships, processes, and resources that families can use during times of adversity and change to manage stressors.

Family-centered care A philosophy of care that integrates the family's values and potential contributions in the plans for and provision of care to the child.

Fecundability The ability to become pregnant.

Female condom A thin, disposable polyurethane sheath with a flexible ring at each end that is placed inside the vagina and serves to prevent sperm from entering the cervix, thus preventing conception.

Female genital mutilation (FGM) Also called *female genital cutting, female circumcision*, and *genital circumcision*, the practice of removing all or parts of a girl's or woman's genitalia for cultural reasons.

Female reproductive cycle (FRC) The monthly rhythmic changes in sexually mature women.

Ferning capacity Formation of a palm-leaf pattern by the crystallization of cervical mucus as it dries at midmenstrual cycle. Helpful in determining time of ovulation. Observed via microscopic examination of a thin layer of cervical mucus on a glass slide. This pattern is also observed when amniotic fluid is allowed to air dry on a slide and is a useful and quick test to determine whether amniotic membranes have ruptured.

Fertility awareness–based (FAB) methods Also called *natural family planning*, are based on an understanding of the changes that occur throughout a woman's ovulatory cycle. All these methods require periods of abstinence and recording of certain events throughout the cycle; cooperation of the partners is important.

Fertilization Impregnation of an ovum by a spermatozoon; conception.

Fetal acoustic stimulation test (FAST) A fetal assessment test that uses sound from a speaker, bell, or artificial larynx to stimulate acceleration of the fetal heart; may be used in conjunction with the non-stress test.

Fetal alcohol spectrum disorder (FASD) An umbrella term that includes all categories of prenatal alcohol exposure, including fetal alcohol syndrome (FAS). It is not meant to be used as a clinical diagnosis.

Fetal alcohol syndrome (FAS) Syndrome caused by maternal alcohol ingestion and characterized by microcephaly, intrauterine growth restriction, short palpebral fissures, and maxillary hypoplasia.

Fetal attitude Relationship of the fetal parts to one another. Normal fetal attitude is one of moderate flexion of the arms onto the chest and flexion of the legs onto the abdomen.

Fetal blood sampling A procedure to collect a small amount of blood from the umbilical cord or fetus during pregnancy to diagnose, treat, and monitor various fetal problems.

Fetal bradycardia Fetal heart rate less than 110 beats/min during a 10-minute period or longer.

Fetal breathing movements (FBM) Intrauterine practice respiratory movements that begin around the 17th to 20th week of gestation.

Fetal death Death of the developing fetus after 20 weeks' gestation. Also called *fetal demise*.

Fetal distress Evidence that the fetus is in jeopardy, such as a change in fetal activity or heart rate.

Fetal fibronectin (fFN) A glycoprotein that is produced by the trophoblast and fetal tissues whose presence between 20 and 34 weeks' gestation is a strong predictor of preterm birth associated with preterm spontaneous rupture of membranes.

Fetal heart rate (FHR) The number of times the fetal heart beats per minute; normal range is 110 to 160.

Fetal lie Relationship of the cephalocaudal axis (spinal column) of the fetus to the cephalocaudal axis (spinal column) of the woman. The fetus may be in a longitudinal or transverse lie.

Fetal movement count (FMC) A method for tracking fetal activity taught to pregnant women. Also called *fetal movement record (FMR)*.

Fetal position Relationship of the landmark on the presenting fetal part to the front, sides, or back of the maternal pelvis.

Fetal presentation The fetal body part that enters the maternal pelvis first. The three possible presentations are cephalic, shoulder, and breech.

Fetal tachycardia Sustained fetal heart rate of 161 beats/min or higher.

Fetoscope An adaptation of a stethoscope that facilitates auscultation of the fetal heart rate.

Fetus The child in utero from about the seventh to ninth week of gestation until birth.

Fever An increased body temperature of 38°C (100.4°F) or higher taken by rectal or tympanic route, and 37.8°C (100.0°F) or higher by the oral route.

Fibrocystic breast changes Benign breast changes characterized by bilateral, cyclic breast pain and breast nodularities that may be unilateral or bilateral, and often in the upper outer quadrants of the breasts.

Filtration Movement of fluid into or out of capillaries as the net result of several opposing forces.

Fimbria The funnel-like structure at the abdominal opening of the uterine tube that has many finger-like projections (fimbriae) reaching out to the ovary.

Fluorescene polarization (FP) Measures the surfactant-to-albumin ratio.

Focal Specific area of the brain; often used to describe seizures or neurologic deficits.

Folic acid A member of the vitamin B complex, required for amino acid metabolism, DNA synthesis, and production of red blood cells.

Follicle-stimulating hormone (FSH) Hormone produced by the anterior pituitary during the first half of the menstrual cycle, stimulating development of the graafian follicle.

Fontanelle In the fetus, unossified space, or soft spot, consisting of a strong band of connective tissue lying between the cranial bones of the skull.

Food allergy An immunoglobulin E (IgE)–mediated reaction to a given food that is potentially systemic, characteristically rapid in onset, and may be manifested as swelling of the lips, mouth, uvula or glottis, generalized urticaria, and, in severe reactions, anaphylaxis.

Food insecurity An inability or uncertainty that one will be able to acquire or consume adequate quality or quantity of foods in socially acceptable ways.

Food intolerance An abnormal physiologic response (flatulence, sweating, hives, indigestion) to a food that is not immunoglobulin E (IgE) mediated.

Food jags Eating only a few foods for several days or weeks.

Food security Access at all times to enough nourishment for an active, healthy life.

Foramen ovale Special opening between the atria of the fetal heart. Normally, the opening closes shortly after birth; if it remains open, it can be repaired surgically.

Forceps Obstetric instrument occasionally used to aid in childbirth.

Forceps marks Reddened areas over the cheeks and jaws caused by application of forceps. The red areas usually disappear within 1 or 2 days.

Forceps-assisted birth A birth in which a set of instruments, called *forceps*, is applied to the presenting part of the fetus to provide traction or to enable the fetal head to be rotated to an occiput-anterior position. Forceps-assisted birth is also called *instrumental delivery, operative delivery,* or *operative vaginal delivery.*

Foremilk Breast milk obtained at the beginning of the breastfeeding episode.

Frequency The time between the beginning of one contraction and the beginning of the next contraction.

Full-term birth Births occurring between 39 weeks 0 days and 40 weeks 6 days.

Functional residual capacity (FRC) The amount of air remaining in the lungs at the end of a normal expiration.

Fundus The upper portion of the uterus between the fallopian tubes.

G

Galactorrhea Nipple discharge.

Galant reflex See *Trunk incurvation.*

Gamete Female or male germ cell; contains a haploid number of chromosomes.

Gamete intrafallopian transfer (GIFT) procedure Retrieval of oocytes by laparoscopy; immediately combining oocytes with washed, motile sperm in a catheter; and placement of the gametes into the fimbriated end of the fallopian tube.

Gametogenesis The process by which germ cells are produced.

Gay An adjective used to describe or refer to a homosexual male.

Gene A sequence of DNA on a chromosome that represents a fundamental unit of heredity; occupies a specific spot on a chromosome (gene locus).

Gene expression When the protein product of a gene is visible (presence of a body structure or identifiable through biochemical tests such as insulin or phenylalanine levels).

General anesthesia A state of induced unconsciousness that may be achieved through intravenous injection, inhalation of anesthetic agents, or a combination of both methods.

Genogram A pedigree that displays information about a family's health history over at least three generations.

Genome-wide association study A rapid examination of many common genetic variations in DNA or genomes, in different individuals, to identify genetic variations associated with a certain disease.

Genomics The study of all the genes in the human genome together, including their interactions with each other, the environment, and the influence of other psychosocial and cultural factors.

Genotype The genetic composition of an individual.

Gestation The number of weeks of pregnancy since the first day of the last menstrual period.

Gestational age assessment tools Systems used to evaluate the newborn's external physical characteristics and neurologic and/or neuromuscular development to accurately determine gestational age. These replace or supplement the traditional calculation from the woman's last menstrual period.

Gestational diabetes mellitus (GDM) A form of diabetes of variable severity with onset or first recognition during pregnancy.

Gestational trophoblastic disease (GTD) Disorder classified into two types: benign (hydatidiform mole) and malignant.

Glucagon A hormone produced by the pancreas that helps release stored glucose from the liver.

Gluconeogenesis Formation of glycogen from noncarbohydrate sources such as protein or fat.

Glycosuria   Abnormal amount of glucose in the urine.

Goiter   Enlargement of the thyroid gland.

Gonadotropin-releasing hormone (GnRH)   A hormone secreted by the hypothalamus that stimulates the anterior pituitary to secrete FSH and LH.

Gonadotropins   Hormones that stimulate the gonads (ovaries in women or testes in men).

Gonorrhea   A sexually transmitted infection caused by the bacterium *Neisseria gonorrhoeae*.

Goodell sign   Softening of the cervix that occurs during the second month of pregnancy.

Graafian follicle   The ovarian cyst containing the ripe ovum; it secretes estrogens.

Graft-versus-host disease   A series of immunologic responses mounted by the host of a transplanted organ with the purpose of destroying the transplant cells.

Grasping reflex   Normal newborn reflex elicited by stimulating the palm with a finger or object, resulting in newborn firmly holding on to the finger or object.

Gravida   A pregnant woman.

Grief   An individual's reaction to loss, including physical symptoms, thoughts, feelings, functional limitations, and spiritual responses.

Grief work   The inner process of working through or managing the bereavement.

Growth   An increase in physical size.

Gynecoid pelvis   Typical female pelvis in which the inlet is round instead of oval.

H

Habituation   Infant's ability to diminish innate responses to specific repeated stimuli.

Haploid number of chromosomes   Half the diploid number of chromosomes. In humans, there are 23 chromosomes, the haploid number, in each germ cell.

Harlequin sign   A rare color change that occurs between the longitudinal halves of the newborn's body, such that the dependent half is noticeably pinker than the superior half when the newborn is placed on one side; it is of no pathologic significance.

Hazing   An activity that is forced on an individual that causes humiliation and is required for membership in an organization or group. It can sometimes be harmful.

Health   A state of complete physical, mental, and social well-being and not merely the absence of disease and infirmity.

Health maintenance (health protection)   Activities that preserve an individual's present state of health and prevent disease or injury occurrence.

Health promotion   Activities that increase well-being, enhance wellness or health, and lead to actualization of positive health potential; strategies that seek to foster conditions to allow populations to be healthy and to make healthy choices.

Health supervision   The process of health promotion services, growth and development monitoring, and disease and injury prevention throughout the child's life.

Heaving   Lifting of the chest wall during contraction.

Hegar sign   A softening of the lower uterine segment found upon palpation in the second or third month of pregnancy.

HELLP syndrome   A cluster of changes including *h*emolysis, *e*levated *l*iver enzymes, and *l*ow *p*latelet count; sometimes associated with severe preeclampsia.

Hemarthrosis   Bleeding into joint spaces.

Hematopoiesis   Blood cell production.

Hemodynamics   Pressures generated by blood and passage of blood through the heart and pulmonary system.

Hemoglobinopathy   Disease characterized by abnormal hemoglobin.

Hemolytic disease of the newborn   Hyperbilirubinemia secondary to Rh incompatibility.

Hemoptysis   Coughing up blood from the respiratory tract.

Hemosiderosis   Increased storage of iron in body tissues; associated with diseases involving the destruction of red blood cells.

Herd immunity   The protection provided by a large group of persons who have immunity to a disease and indirectly protect others without immunity by reducing the risk for exposure and infection.

Hernia   Protrusion or projection of a body part or structure through the muscle wall of the cavity that normally contains it.

Herniation   Protrusion of brain contents through the cranial vault at the base of the skull.

Herpes genitalis   A lifelong, recurrent sexually transmitted infection caused by the herpes simplex virus (HSV).

Heterozygous   Nonidentical copies of a particular gene (different alleles) on the paired chromosomes.

Hindmilk   Breast milk released after initial letdown reflex; high in fat content.

Homeopathy   Term derived from the Greek word *homos*, meaning "the same," and describing a healing system that uses as remedies minute dilutions of substances that, if ingested in larger amounts, would produce effects *similar* to the symptoms of the disorder being treated.

Homologous chromosomes   Chromosomes that are members of the same pair and normally have the same number and arrangement of genes; usually one copy is from the mother and the other copy is from the father.

Homosexuality   Sexual attraction to people of the same sex.

Homozygous   A genotypic situation in which two similar genes occur at a given locus on homologous chromosomes.

Hospice care   A philosophy of care that focuses on helping persons with short life expectancies to live their remaining lives to the fullest—without pain and with choices and dignity.

Huhner test   A test performed 1 or 2 days before the expected date of ovulation that evaluates the cervical mucus, the number of active sperm in the cervical mucus, and the length of sperm survival (in hours) after intercourse. Also called the *postcoital test*.

Human chorionic gonadotropin (hCG)   A hormone produced by the chorionic villi and found in the urine of pregnant women. Also called *prolan*.

Human genome   The entire DNA sequence of an individual.

Human immunodeficiency virus (HIV)   A virus that causes a progressive disease that ultimately results in the development of acquired immunodeficiency syndrome (AIDS).

Hydatidiform mole   Degenerative process in chorionic villi, giving rise to multiple cysts and rapid growth of the uterus, with hemorrhage.

Hydramnios   An excess of amniotic fluid, leading to overdistention of the uterus. Frequently seen in pregnant women who have diabetes, even if there is no coexisting fetal anomaly. Also called *polyhydramnios*.

Hydronephrosis   Collection of urine in the renal pelvis as a result of obstructed outflow.

Hydrops fetalis   Hemolytic disease of the newborn characterized by anemia, jaundice, enlargement of the liver and spleen, and generalized edema. Caused by isoimmunization as a result of Rh incompatibility or ABO incompatibility. See also *Erythroblastosis fetalis*.

Hydrotherapy   Type of therapy that makes use of hot or cold moisture in any form. Hydrotherapy is used to relax muscles, promote rest, decrease pain, reduce swelling, promote healing, cleanse wounds and burns, reduce fever, lessen cramps, and improve well-being.

Hyperbilirubinemia   Excessive amount of bilirubin in the blood; indicative of hemolytic processes due to blood incompatibility, intrauterine infection, septicemia, neonatal renal infection, and other disorders.

Hypercapnia   Greater than normal amounts of carbon dioxide in the blood.

Hyperemesis gravidarum   Excessive vomiting during pregnancy, leading to dehydration and starvation.

Hypersensitivity response   An overreaction of the immune system, responsible for allergic reactions.

Hypersplenism   A syndrome characterized by splenomegaly and blood cell deficiencies.

Hypertelorism   Widely spaced eyes.

Hypertonic dehydration (or hypernatremic dehydration)   Sodium loss that is proportionately greater than water loss.

Hypertonic saline   A solution that is more concentrated than body fluid. Used to rapidly increase body fluid concentration, but it must be monitored carefully because it can easily cause rebound hypernatremia.

Hyperventilation   Rapid breathing that occurs over a prolonged period of time resulting in an imbalance of oxygen and carbon dioxide that can result in tingling or numbness in the tip of nose, lips, fingers, or toes; dizziness; spots before the eyes; or spasms of the hands or feet (carpal-pedal spasms).

Hypoglycemia   Abnormally low level of sugar in the blood.

Hypoplastic   Small and nonfunctional.

Hypotonic dehydration (or hyponatremic dehydration)   Fluid loss characterized by a proportionately greater loss of sodium than water.

Hypotonic fluid   Fluid that is more dilute than normal body fluid.

Hypoxemia   Lower than normal amounts of oxygen in the blood.

Hypoxia   Lower than normal amounts of oxygen in the tissues.

Hysterectomy   Surgical removal of the uterus.

Hysterosalpingography (HSG)   Testing by instillation of radiopaque substance into the uterine cavity to visualize the uterus and fallopian tubes.

Hysteroscopy   Use of a special endoscope to examine the uterus.

I

Immunodeficiency   A state of the immune system in which it cannot cope effectively with foreign antigens.

Immunoglobulin   A protein that functions as an antibody. Immunoglobulins are responsible for humoral immunity.

In vitro fertilization (IVF)   Procedure during which oocytes are removed from the ovary, mixed with spermatozoa, fertilized, and incubated in a glass petri dish; then up to four viable embryos are placed in the woman's uterus.

Inborn error of metabolism   A hereditary deficiency of a specific enzyme needed for normal metabolism of specific chemicals.

Incarceration   Occurs when the presence of intestine in the groin causes constriction of the blood supply to the scrotal sac, leading to intestinal strangulation and testicular ischemia.

Incest   Sexual activity between family members close enough that marriage between them would be legally or culturally prohibited.

Incidental findings   Unanticipated, abnormal results of genetic testing that are not relevant to the diagnostic indication for which the test was ordered.

Incubation period   The time interval between infection exposure and development of symptoms.

Independent assortment   The random distribution of different combinations of parental genes to gametes.

Indirect transmission   The passage of an infectious disease involving survival of pathogens outside humans before they invade a new host.

Individualized approach   An assessment approach that involves measuring individual children seen in a clinic, sharing results with the family, and addressing appropriate teaching about weight control and nutritious intake.

Individualized education plan (IEP)   Formulation of a specific learning approach for a child with a physical or mental disability, following thorough assessment of the child's capabilities and areas of need.

Individualized family service plan (IFSP)   A form of education planning/intervention that is developed for early intervention with infants with special healthcare needs and their families. The IFSP contains information about the services required to support a child's development and enhance the family's capacity to facilitate the child's development. The family and education service providers work as a team to plan, implement, and evaluate services specific to the family's unique concerns, priorities, and resources.

Individualized health plan   A formal mechanism to ensure that the child's health needs are managed in the school setting.

Individualized transition plan   A plan that focuses on assisting the adolescent with special healthcare needs in moving successfully from school into the community.

Induction of labor   The process of causing or initiating labor by use of medication or surgical rupture of membranes.

Induration   An area of extra firmness on the skin with a distinct border.

Infant   A child between 29 days and 1 year of age.

Infant mortality rate   Number of deaths of infants under 1 year of age per 1000 live births in a given population per year.

Infant of a diabetic mother (IDM)   At-risk baby born to a woman previously diagnosed as being diabetic or who develops symptoms of diabetes during pregnancy.

Infant of a substance-abusing mother (ISAM)   Formerly called *infant of an addicted mother*. A baby who is born to a mother who abuses or is addicted to drugs or alcohol.

Infectious disease   Illness, caused by a microorganism, that is commonly communicated from one host (human or otherwise) to another.

Infertility   Diminished ability to conceive.

Informed consent   A legal concept that protects a person's rights to autonomy and self-determination by specifying that no action may be taken without that person's prior understanding and freely given consent.

Infundibulopelvic ligament   The ligament that suspends and supports the ovaries. It arises from the outer third of the broad ligament and contains the ovarian vessels and nerves.

Inguinal hernia   A painless inguinal or scrotal swelling of variable size that occurs when abdominal tissue, such as bowel, extends into the inguinal canal.

Insensible water loss   Water loss not directly measurable or observable, such as through skin and respirations.

Inspection   The technique of purposeful observation by carefully looking at the characteristics of the child's physical features and behaviors. Physical feature characteristics include size, shape, color, movement, position, and location.

Insulin deficiency   A condition in which the pancreas does not produce sufficient insulin (as in type 1 diabetes).

Insulin resistance   An alteration of the insulin receptor that signals the presence of insulin in the interior of cells.

Intellectual disability   Significant limitation in intellectual functioning and adaptive behavior, manifested by differences in conceptual, social, and practical adaptive skills, beginning before the age of 18 years.

Intensity   The strength of a uterine contraction during acme.

Internal os   An inside mouth or opening; the opening between the cervix and the uterus.

Internal version   Procedure used for the vaginal birth of a second twin. The obstetrician inserts a hand into the uterus, grasps the feet of the fetus, and changes the fetus from a transverse to a breech presentation.

Interstitial fluid   That portion of the extracellular fluid that is between the cells and outside the blood and lymphatic vessels.

Intertriginous (areas)   Skinfolds of the neck, axillae, and antecubital fossa.

Intimate partner violence (IPV)   A pattern of coercive behavior and methods used to exert power and control by one individual over another in an adult domestic or intimate relationship. Also called *domestic violence.*

Intracellular fluid   The fluid in the body that is inside the cells.

Intracranial pressure   Force exerted by brain tissue, cerebrospinal fluid, and blood within the cranial vault.

Intractable seizure   Seizures that continue to occur even with optimal medical management.

Intrapartum   The time from the onset of true labor until the birth of the baby and delivery of the placenta.

Intrathecal   A method of drug or medication delivery in which the drug is introduced into the spinal canal.

Intrauterine contraception (IUC)   The use of a device that is designed to be inserted into the uterus by a qualified healthcare provider and left in place for an extended period, providing continuous contraceptive protection for 3 to 10 years.

Intrauterine drug-exposed infants   Infants whose mothers used marijuana, alcohol, nicotine, or illicit drugs while pregnant.

Intrauterine fetal surgery   Surgery performed on a fetus to correct anatomic lesions that are not compatible with life if left untreated.

Intrauterine growth restriction (IUGR)   Fetal undergrowth due to any etiology, such as intrauterine infection, deficient nutrient supply, or congenital malformation. A term used to describe fetuses falling below the 10th percentile in ultrasonic estimation of weight at a given gestational age.

Intrauterine pressure catheter (IUPC)   A catheter that can be placed through the cervix into the uterus to measure uterine pressure during labor. Some types of catheters may be inserted for the purpose of infusing warmed saline to add additional intrauterine fluid when oligohydramnios is present.

Intrauterine resuscitation   Corrective measures used to optimize the oxygen exchange within the maternal–fetal circulation.

Intravascular fluid   That portion of the extracellular fluid that is in the blood vessels.

Intuitive touch   The use of physical contact with the laboring woman with the intent of helping her to slow down and regulate her breathing pattern and encouraging a reduction of anxiety and decrease of stress levels.

Inversion   A chromosomal alteration in which a gene or DNA sequence in a segment of a chromosome has been reversed.

Involution   Rolling or turning inward; the reduction in size of the uterus following childbirth.

Ischial spines   Prominences that arise near the junction of the ilium and ischium and jut into the pelvic cavity; used as a reference point during labor to evaluate the descent of the fetal head into the birth canal.

Isotonic dehydration (or isonatremic dehydration)   Fluid loss that is not balanced by intake; the loss of water and sodium are in proportion.

Isotonic fluid   Fluid that has the same osmolality as normal body fluid.

Isthmus   The straight, narrow part of the fallopian tube with a thick muscular wall and an opening (lumen) 2 to 3 mm in diameter; the site of tubal ligation. Also, a constriction in the uterus that is located above the cervix and below the corpus.

J

Jaundice   Yellow pigmentation of body tissues caused by the presence of bile pigments. See also *Physiologic jaundice.*

K

Karyotype   The set of chromosomes arranged in a standard order.

Kegel exercises   Perineal muscle tightening that strengthens the pubococcygeus muscle and increases its tone.

Keloid   Overdevelopment or hypertrophy of a scar that extends beyond the wound edges and above the skin line because of excess collagen.

Kerion   A large tender boggy mass on the scalp with drainage associated with tinea capitis.

Kernicterus   The yellow staining and degenerative lesions in basal ganglia associated with high levels of unconjugated bilirubin in newborns. Also called *bilirubin encephalopathy.*

Killed virus vaccine   A vaccine that contains a killed microorganism that is still capable of inducing the human body to produce antibodies to the disease.

Kilocalorie   Equivalent to 1000 calories, it is the unit used to express the energy value of food.

Kinesthesia   The sense of one's body position and movement.

Kussmaul respirations   Increased rate and depth of respirations (hyperventilation).

L

La Leche League International   A nonprofit organization that promotes breastfeeding and provides information on and assistance with breastfeeding.

Labor   The process by which the fetus is expelled from the maternal uterus. Also called *childbirth, confinement,* or *parturition.*

Labor augmentation   The stimulation of uterine contractions when spontaneous contractions have failed to result in progressive cervical dilatation or descent of the fetus.

Labor induction   The stimulation of uterine contractions before the spontaneous onset of labor, with or without ruptured fetal membranes, for the purpose of accomplishing birth.

Labor support   The emotional, physical, and informational support of the woman during childbirth.

Lactase deficiency (lactose intolerance)   A condition characterized by difficulty digesting milk and dairy products; results from an inadequate amount of the enzyme lactase, which breaks down the milk sugar lactose into smaller digestible substances.

Lactation The process of producing and supplying breast milk.

Lacto-ovovegetarians Vegetarians who include milk, dairy products, and eggs in their diets and occasionally fish, poultry, and liver.

Lactovegetarians Vegetarians who include dairy products but no eggs in their diets.

Lamaze method A method of childbirth preparation.

Lamellar body count (LBC) A fetal test to predict or establish the presence of fetal lung maturity.

Lanugo Fine, downy hair found on all body parts of the fetus, with the exception of the palms of the hands and the soles of the feet, after 20 weeks' gestation.

Laparoscopy Procedure that enables direct visualization of pelvic organs.

Large for gestational age (LGA) Excessive growth of a fetus in relation to the gestational time period.

Laryngospasm Spasmodic vibrations of the larynx, which create sudden, violent, unpredictable, involuntary contraction of airway muscles.

Last menstrual period (LMP) The last normal menstrual period experienced by the woman before pregnancy; sometimes used to calculate the infant's gestational age.

Late adolescence Refers to adolescents who are ages 18 to 19 years.

Late deceleration Symmetrical decrease in fetal heart rate beginning at or after the peak of the contraction and returning to baseline only after the contraction has ended, indicating possible uteroplacental insufficiency and potential that the fetus is not receiving adequate oxygenation.

Late preterm birth Births that occur between 34 weeks 0 days through 36 weeks 6 days' gestation.

Late preterm newborn Neonates born between 34 and 37 weeks' gestation. These babies are at greater risk for increases in mortality and morbidity because they are physically not mature and are more prone to have physiologic and metabolic complications.

Late (secondary) postpartum hemorrhage A loss of blood of greater than 500 mL following birth. The hemorrhage is classified as late if it occurs from 24 hours to 6 weeks after birth.

Late-term birth Births occurring between 41 weeks 0 days through 41 weeks 6 days.

Lecithin/sphingomyelin ratio (L/S ratio) Lecithin and sphingomyelin are phospholipid components of surfactant; their ratio changes during gestation. When the L/S ratio reaches 2:1, the fetal lungs are thought to be mature and the fetus will have a low risk of respiratory distress syndrome (RDS) if born at that time.

Leopold maneuvers A series of four maneuvers designed to provide a systematic approach whereby the examiner may determine fetal presentation and position.

Lesbian An adjective used to describe or refer to a homosexual woman.

Let-down reflex Pattern of stimulation, hormone release, and resulting muscle contraction that forces milk into the lactiferous ducts, making it available to the infant. Also called *milk ejection reflex.*

Leukocytosis A higher than normal leukocyte count.

Leukopenia A lower than normal white blood cell count.

Leukorrhea Mucous discharge from the vagina or cervical canal that may be normal or pathologic, as in the presence of infection.

Level of consciousness General description of cognitive, sensory, and motor response to stimuli.

Lichenification Thickening of the skin.

Life-threatening condition A condition in which there is a likelihood that the child will die prematurely.

Light sleep state State that makes up the highest proportion of newborn sleep and precedes awakening; characterized by some body movements, rapid eye movements (REM), and brief fussing or crying.

Lightening Moving of the fetus and uterus downward into the pelvic cavity.

Linea nigra The line of darker pigmentation extending from the umbilicus to the pubis noted in some women during the later months of pregnancy.

Live virus vaccine A vaccine that contains the microorganism in a live but attenuated, or weakened, form.

Local infiltration anesthesia Anesthesia accomplished by injecting an anesthetic agent into the intracutaneous, subcutaneous, and intramuscular areas of the perineum. Generally used at the time of birth, both in preparation for an episiotomy if one is needed and for episiotomy repair.

Lochia Maternal discharge of blood, mucus, and tissue from the uterus; may last for several weeks after birth.

Lochia alba White vaginal discharge that follows lochia serosa and that lasts from about the 10th to the 21st day after birth.

Lochia rubra Red, blood-tinged vaginal discharge that occurs following birth and lasts 2 to 4 days.

Lochia serosa Pink, serous, and blood-tinged vaginal discharge that follows lochia rubra and lasts until the 7th to 10th day after birth.

Luteinizing hormone (LH) Anterior pituitary hormone responsible for stimulating ovulation and for development of the corpus luteum.

Lymphangitis Inflammation of the lymphatic system draining the site of infection that is seen as tender erythematous streaks extending in a proximal direction.

M

Macronutrients The major building blocks of the body: carbohydrates, protein, and fat.

Macrosomia A condition seen in neonates of large body size and high birth weight (more than 4000 to 4500 grams [8 lb, 13 oz to 9 lb, 4 oz]), such as those born of mothers who are prediabetic and diabetic.

Major anomaly A serious structural defect present at birth that may have severe medical or cosmetic consequences that interfere with normal functioning of body systems, lead to a lifelong disability, or even cause early death.

Malignant The progressive growth of a tumor that will, if not checked by treatment, result in death.

Malposition An abnormal position of the fetus in the birth canal.

Malpresentations Presentations of the fetus into the birth canal that are not "normal"—that is, brow, face, shoulder, or breech presentation.

Mammogram A soft-tissue radiograph of the breast without the injection of a contrast medium.

Mastitis Inflammation of the breast.

Maternal mortality rate The number of maternal deaths from any cause during the pregnancy cycle per 100,000 live births.

Maternal role attainment (MRA) Process by which a woman learns mothering behaviors and becomes comfortable with her identity as a mother.

Maternal serum alpha-fetoprotein (MSAFP) Screening test performed between 16 and 22 gestational weeks that utilizes the multiple markers (the "triple screen") of alpha-fetoprotein (AFP), human chorionic growth hormone (hCG), and urine estriol (UE3) to screen pregnancies for neural tube defect, Down syndrome, and trisomy 18.

Maternal–child nursing Care of women during pregnancy, birth, and postpartum, as well as the care of newborns, infants, children, and adolescents.

Mature milk   Breast milk that contains 10% solids for energy and growth.

Mature minors   Adolescents of 14 and 15 years of age who are able to understand treatment risks and who in some states can consent to or refuse treatment.

McDonald sign   A probable sign of pregnancy characterized by an ease in flexing the body of the uterus against the cervix.

Meconium   Dark green or black material present in the large intestine of a full-term newborn; the first stools passed by the newborn.

Meconium aspiration syndrome (MAS)   Respiratory disease of term, postterm, and SGA newborns caused by inhalation of meconium or meconium-stained amniotic fluid into the lungs; characterized by mild to severe respiratory distress, hyperexpansion of the chest, hyperinflated alveoli, and secondary atelectasis.

Medical home   A consistent, continuous, comprehensive, family-centered, and compassionate source of primary health care. See *pediatric healthcare home*.

Medically fragile   Children who need skilled nursing care with or without medical equipment to support vital functions.

Meiosis   The process of cell division that occurs in the maturation of sperm and ova that decreases their number of chromosomes by one-half.

Melanin   Skin pigment.

Melasma gravidarum   See *Chloasma*.

Menarche   Beginning of menstrual and reproductive function in the female.

Mendelian inheritance   A major category of inheritance whereby a trait is determined by a pair of genes on homologous chromosomes. Also called *single-gene inheritance*.

Menopausal hormone therapy (MHT)   The administration of specific hormones, usually estrogen alone (ET) or a combination estrogen-progestogen (EPT), to alleviate menopausal symptoms. Formerly called *hormone replacement therapy (HRT)*.

Menopause   The permanent cessation of menses.

Menorrhagia   Increased menstrual bleeding.

Menstrual cycle   Cyclic buildup of the uterine lining, ovulation, and sloughing of the lining occurring approximately every 28 days in nonpregnant females.

Mental health   Foundational to a sense of personal well-being, it involves successful engagement in activities and relationships and the ability to adapt and cope with change.

Mesoderm   The intermediate layer of germ cells in the embryo that gives rise to connective tissue, bone marrow, muscles, blood, lymphoid tissue, and epithelial tissue.

Metastasis   The spread of cancer cells to other sites in the body.

Microcephaly   A small brain with a head circumference below the third percentile on growth curves.

Micronutrients   Substances needed in small quantities for healthy body functioning; vitamins and minerals are micronutrients.

Middle adolescence   Refers to adolescents who are ages 15 to 17 years.

Milia   Tiny white papules appearing on the face of a neonate as a result of unopened sebaceous glands; they disappear spontaneously within a few weeks.

Minor anomaly   An unusual morphologic feature that is of no serious medical or cosmetic concern.

Miscarriage   Abortion that occurs naturally; spontaneous abortion.

Mitosis   Process of cell division whereby both daughter cells have the same number and pattern of chromosomes as the original cell.

Mixed hearing loss   Hearing loss having a combination of conductive and sensorineural causes.

Modeling   Exhibiting appropriate behavior for someone else.

Moderate sedation   A lower sedative dose that enables the child to maintain protective reflexes, independently and continuously maintain a patent airway, and make an appropriate response to physical stimuli or verbal command.

Molding   Shaping of the fetal head by overlapping of the cranial bones to facilitate movement through the birth canal during labor.

Moniliasis   Yeastlike fungal infection caused by *Candida albicans*.

Monosomic (monosomy)   Genetic condition that occurs when a normal gamete unites with a gamete that is missing a chromosome.

Mons pubis   Mound of subcutaneous fatty tissue covering the anterior portion of the symphysis pubis.

Morning sickness   A term that refers to the nausea and vomiting that a woman may experience in early pregnancy. This lay term is sometimes used because these symptoms frequently occur in the early part of the day and disappear within a few hours.

Moro reflex   Flexion of the newborn's thighs and knees accompanied by fingers that fan, then clench, as the arms are simultaneously thrown out and then brought together, as though embracing something. This reflex can be elicited by startling the newborn with a sudden noise or movement. Also called the *startle reflex*.

Morula   Developmental stage of the fertilized ovum in which there is a solid mass of cells.

Mosaicism   Condition of an individual who has at least two cell lines with differing karyotypes.

Mother–baby care   A type of family health care that is focused on keeping the mother and baby together as much as the mother desires. Also called *couplet care*, it provides increased opportunities for parent–child interaction because the newborn shares the mother's room and they are cared for together. Mother–baby care enables the mother to have time to bond with her baby and learn to care for her newborn in a supportive environment.

Mottling   Discoloration of the skin in irregular areas; may be seen with chilling, poor perfusion, or hypoxia.

Mucous plug   A collection of thick mucus that blocks the cervical canal during pregnancy. Also called *operculum*.

Multifactorial   Health conditions determined by multiple factors, including genetic and environmental factors, each having an additive effect.

Multigravida   Woman who has been pregnant more than once.

Multipara   Woman who has had more than one pregnancy in which the fetus was viable.

Multiple gestation   More than one fetus in the uterus at the same time.

Murmur   Abnormal heart sounds produced by blood passing through a defective heart valve, great vessel, or other heart structure; heard by auscultation or palpated.

Mutation   A gene alteration that disrupts the order of amino acids in that gene's protein product.

Myelinization   Establishment of the myelin or fatty sheath on nerve fibers.

Myelodysplasia   Any malformation of the spinal cord and spinal canal.

Myelosuppression   A decreased production of blood cells in the bone marrow.

Myometrium   Uterine muscular structure.

Myringotomy   A procedure whereby an incision is made in the tympanic membrane to drain fluid.

N

Nadir   The lowest point.

Nägele's rule   A method of determining the estimated date of birth (EDB): After obtaining the first day of the last menstrual period, subtract 3 months and add 7 days.

Nasal flaring   A sign of respiratory distress; an effort the child makes to widen the airway.

Natural immunity   The defenses present at birth, such as intact skin, body pH, natural antibodies from the mother, and inflammatory and phagocytic properties.

Nature   The genetic or hereditary capability of an individual.

Neonatal morbidity   The number of potential cases per year of a disease, illness, or complication occurring in the neonatal period.

Neonatal mortality risk   The neonate's chance of death within the newborn period—that is, within the first 28 days of life.

Neonatal transition   The first few hours of life, in which the newborn stabilizes its respiratory and circulatory functions.

Neonatology   The specialty that focuses on the management of at-risk conditions of the newborn.

Neoplasms   Cancerous growths.

Nephrotic syndrome   An alteration in kidney function secondary to increased glomerular basement membrane permeability to plasma protein.

Neural tube defects   Malformation of embryonic tissue that develops into the central nervous system and includes anencephaly, encephalocele, spina bifida, and myelodysplasia.

Neurogenic bladder   The result of urinary tract obstruction related to an interrupted nerve supply to the bladder.

Neuropathic pain   A form of chronic pain, initiated or caused by a primary lesion or dysfunction of the nervous system.

Neutral thermal environment (NTE)   An environment that provides for minimal heat loss or expenditure.

Neutropenia   A low neutrophil count.

Nevus flammeus (port-wine stain)   A large, flat, pink to reddish purple vascular malformation usually found on the head and neck.

Nevus vasculosus (strawberry mark)   A raised, clearly delineated, dark-red, rough-surfaced birthmark commonly found in the head region.

New Ballard Score (NBS)   A postnatal gestational age assessment tool that is used within 12 hours of birth.

Newborn   Baby from birth through the first 28 days of life.

Newborn screening tests   Tests that detect inborn errors of metabolism that, if left untreated, cause intellectual and physical disabilities.

Nidation   Implantation of a fertilized ovum in the endometrium.

Night terrors (or sleep terrors)   A situation in which the child cries out and appears frightened while sleeping, but in contrast to nightmares, the child having a night terror is not fully awake and may appear disoriented.

Nightmares   Frightening dreams that awaken the child, who is often crying and upset.

Nipple   A protrusion about 0.5 to 1.3 cm in diameter in the center of each mature breast.

Nociceptive pain   The normal processing of pain stimuli caused by tissue injury or damage.

Nociceptors   Free nerve endings at the site of tissue damage.

Nondisjunction   An error in cell division in which a pair of homologous chromosomes does not separate as expected, resulting in monosomy or trisomy in gametes.

Nonmendelian (multifactorial) inheritance   The occurrence of congenital disorders that result from an interaction of multiple genetic and environmental factors.

Nonsteroidal anti-inflammatory drugs (NSAIDs)   Drugs used for the treatment of pain.

Non-stress test (NST)   An assessment method by which the reaction (or response) of the fetal heart rate to fetal movement is evaluated.

Nosocomial infection   An infection acquired in a health care agency, not present at the time of entrance to the agency.

Nuchal cord   Term used to describe the umbilical cord when it is wrapped around the neck of the fetus.

Nuchal folds   The accumulation of fluid between the posterior cervical spine and the overlying skin in the fetal neck identified during an ultrasound examination.

Nuchal rigidity   Resistance to neck flexion.

Nuchal translucency testing   A genetic screening test that uses ultrasound to scan the translucent or clear area on the back of the fetal neck, measuring the diameter of the area. Fetuses that have a nuchal translucency measurement of greater than 3 mm are at risk for trisomies 13, 18, and 21 and the mother should be offered an amniocentesis.

Nulligravida   A woman who has never been pregnant.

Nullipara   A woman who has not delivered a viable fetus.

Nurse practitioner   A professional nurse who has received specialized education in a master's degree program or doctor of nursing practice program and thus can function in an expanded role.

Nurse researcher   A nurse with an advanced doctoral degree (typically a Ph.D.) who assumes a leadership role in generating new research.

Nurture   The effects of environment on an individual's performance.

Nutrition   Taking in food and assimilating it metabolically for use by the body.

O

Object permanence   The knowledge that an object or person continues to exist when not seen, heard, or felt.

Obstetric conjugate   Distance from the middle of the sacral promontory to an area approximately 1 cm below the pubic crest.

Occult blood   Blood that is present in minute quantities and can be seen only on microscopic examination or through chemical testing.

Oligohydramnios   Decreased amount of amniotic fluid, which may indicate a fetal urinary tract defect.

Oliguria   Diminished urine output (less than 0.5 to 1 mL/kg/hr).

Oncogene   A portion of the DNA that is altered and, when duplicated, causes uncontrolled cellular division.

Oncotic pressure   The part of the blood osmotic pressure that is due to plasma proteins; also called *blood colloid osmotic pressure*.

Oocyte   Early primitive ovum before it has completely developed.

Oogenesis   Process during fetal life whereby the ovary produces oogonia, cells that become primitive ovarian eggs.

Operculum   See *Mucous plug*.

Opioids   Synthetic narcotic drugs used for the treatment of pain.

Opisthotonic position   Rigid hyperextension of the entire body.

Opisthotonos   Rigid hyperextension of the entire body.

Opportunistic infection   An infection that is often caused by normally nonpathogenic organisms in persons who lack normal immunity.

Oral contraceptives   Birth control pills that work by inhibiting the release of an ovum and by maintaining a type of mucus that is hostile to sperm.

Orchitis Inflammation of the epididymis, pain on testicular palpation, and scrotal swelling.

Organelle A small cellular structure such as a ribosome or mitochondria that performs specific cellular functions.

Orientation Infant's ability to respond to auditory and visual stimuli in the environment.

Ortolani maneuver A manual procedure performed to rule out the possibility of developmental dysplastic hip.

Osmolality The amount of concentration of a fluid; technically, the number of moles of particles per kilogram of water in the solution.

Osmosis Movement of water across a semipermeable membrane into an area of higher particle concentration.

Ossification Formation of bone from fibrous tissue or cartilage.

Osteodystrophy Defective mineralization of bone caused by renal failure and chronic hyperphosphatemia.

Osteoporosis A condition, more common in postmenopausal women, that is characterized by decreased bone strength related to diminished bone density and bone quality. Thought to be associated with lowered estrogen and androgen levels, osteoporosis puts an individual at increased risk for fractures of the hip, forearm, and vertebrae.

Osteotomy Surgical cutting of bone.

Ostomy An artificial abdominal opening into the urinary or gastrointestinal canal that provides an outlet for the diversion of urine or fecal matter.

Outcome expectancy What the person expects to get from performing a certain behavior.

Ovarian ligaments Ligaments that anchor the lower pole of the ovary to the cornua of the uterus. They are surrounded by muscle fibers that allow the ligaments to contract.

Ovaries The pair of almond-shaped female reproductive organs that contain the ova. The two structures lie just below the pelvic brim. One ovary is located on each side of the pelvic cavity.

Ovulation Normal process of discharging a mature ovum from an ovary approximately 14 days prior to the onset of menses.

Oxytocin Hormone normally produced by the posterior pituitary, responsible for stimulation of uterine contractions and the release of milk into the lactiferous ducts.

P

Pain An unpleasant sensory and emotional experience associated with actual or potential tissue damage. Pain exists when the client says it does.

Palliative care Active and compassionate therapies intended to comfort and support those with short life expectancies.

Palliative procedure Intervention used to preserve life in children with a potentially fatal or lethal condition.

Palmar grasping reflex A reflex elicited by stimulating the newborn's palm with a finger or object, causing the newborn to firmly grasp the finger or object.

Palpation The technique of touch to identify characteristics of the skin, internal organs, and masses. Characteristics include texture, moistness, tenderness, temperature, position, shape, consistency, and mobility of masses and organs.

Pancytopenia A decreased number of blood cell components.

Pandemic flu A worldwide influenza epidemic.

Papanicolaou (Pap) smear Procedure to detect the presence of cancer of the uterus by microscopic examination of cells gently scraped from the cervix.

Para A woman who has borne offspring who reached the age of viability.

Paradox breathing Severe respiratory distress in which the chest falls and the abdomen rises on inspiration.

Parallel play A type of play that emerges in toddlerhood when children play side by side with similar or different toys, demonstrating little or no social interaction.

Parametritis Inflammation of the parametrial layer of the uterus.

Parenteral Nutrition introduced outside of the intestinal tract, usually by the intravenous route.

Parent–newborn attachment Close affectional ties that develop between parent and baby. See also *Attachment*.

Partnership A relationship in which participants join together to ensure healthcare delivery in a way that recognizes the critical role and contribution of each partner in promoting health, preventing illness, and managing healthcare conditions.

Passive acquired immunity Transfer of antibodies (immunoglobulin G [IgG]) from the mother to the fetus in utero.

Passive immunity Immunity produced through introduction of specific antibodies to the disease, which are usually obtained from the blood or serum of immune persons and animals. Does not confer lasting immunity.

Patient-controlled analgesia (PCA) A method of pain control where anesthesia, usually morphine or meperidine, is initially administered by the anesthesiologist and subsequent doses are self-administered by pushing a button controlled by a special IV pump system.

Pediatric healthcare home The site of comprehensive, continuous, culturally sensitive, coordinated, and compassionate health care by a pediatric healthcare professional focused on the overall well-being of children and families.

Pedigree Graphic representation of a family tree.

Pelvic cavity The lower portion of the abdominopelvic cavity that contains the urinary bladder, the rectum, and internal parts of the reproductive system. The pelvic cavity is divided into the false pelvis and the true pelvis.

Pelvic cellulitis (parametritis) Inflammation of the parametrial layer of the uterus.

Pelvic diaphragm Part of the pelvic floor composed of deep fascia and the levator ani and the coccygeal muscles.

Pelvic floor Muscles and tissue that act as a buttress to the pelvic outlet.

Pelvic inflammatory disease (PID) An infection of the fallopian tubes that may or may not be accompanied by a pelvic abscess; may cause infertility secondary to tubal damage.

Pelvic inlet Upper border of the true pelvis.

Pelvic outlet Lower border of the true pelvis.

Pelvic tilt Exercise designed to reduce back strain and strengthen abdominal muscle tone. Also called *pelvic rocking*.

Penetrance The percentage or likelihood that an individual who has inherited a gene mutation will actually express the disease signs and symptoms in his or her lifetime.

Penis The male organ of copulation and reproduction.

Percussion The technique of striking the surface of the body, either directly or indirectly, to set up vibrations that reveal the density of underlying tissues and borders of internal organs.

Percutaneous umbilical blood sampling (PUBS) See *Cordocentesis*.

Perimenopause Refers to the period of time prior to menopause during which the woman moves from normal ovulatory cycles to cessation of menses.

Perimetrium The outermost layer of the corpus of the uterus. Also called the *serosal layer.*

Perinatal loss Death of a fetus or baby from the time of conception through the end of the newborn period 28 days after birth.

Perinatal mortality rate The number of neonatal and fetal deaths per 1000 live births.

Perineal body Wedge-shaped mass of fibromuscular tissue found between the lower part of the vagina and the anal canal.

Perineum The area of tissue between the anus and scrotum in a man or between the anus and vagina in a woman.

Periodic breathing Sporadic episodes of apnea, not associated with cyanosis, that last for about 10 seconds and commonly occur in preterm newborns.

Periods of reactivity Predictable patterns of neonate behavior during the first several hours after birth.

Peripartum major mood episodes A form of postpartum psychiatric disorder characterized by depressive moods that the mother experiences after the birth of a child. The periods of greatest risk occur around the fourth week, just before the initiation of menses, and upon weaning. Also called *postpartum depression.*

Peristalsis A progressive, wavelike muscular movement that occurs involuntarily throughout the gastrointestinal tract.

Peristaltic waves Visible rhythmic contractions of the intestinal wall smooth muscle, which moves food through the digestive tract.

Peritonitis Infection involving the peritoneal cavity.

Persistent occiput posterior position (POP position) Malposition of the fetus in which the fetal occiput is posterior in the maternal pelvis.

Persistent pulmonary hypertension of the newborn (PPHN) Respiratory disease resulting from right-to-left shunting of blood away from the lungs and through the ductus arteriosus and patent foramen ovale.

Pervasive developmental disorders Conditions that begin in early childhood and are characterized by impaired social interactions and communication, with restricted interests, activities, and behaviors.

Petechiae Pinpoint red lesions.

pH Negative logarithm of the hydrogen ion concentration; used to monitor the acidity of body fluid.

Pharmacogenomics The study of how an individual's genotype affects the individual's response to medications.

Phenotype The whole physical, biochemical, and physiologic makeup of an individual as determined both genetically and environmentally.

Phenylketonuria A common metabolic disease caused by an inborn error in the metabolism of the amino acid phenylalanine.

Phimosis A structural defect in which the foreskin over the glans penis cannot be retracted.

Phosphatidylglycerol (PG) A phospholipid in surfactant that appears when fetal lung maturity has been attained, at about 35 weeks' gestation. Because PG is not present in blood or vaginal fluids, its presence is reliable in predicting fetal lung maturity.

Phototherapy The treatment of jaundice by exposure to light.

Phototoxic A rapid nonimmunologic reaction of the skin when exposed to sunlight.

Physical abuse The deliberate maltreatment of another individual that inflicts pain or injury and may result in permanent or temporary disfigurement or even death.

Physical dependence The physiologic adaptation to an analgesic or sedative drug at the peripheral and central neurons.

Physical neglect The deliberate withholding of or failure to provide the necessary and available resources to a child.

Physiologic anemia of the newborn A harmless condition in which the hemoglobin level drops in the first 6 to 12 weeks after birth, then reverts to normal levels.

Physiologic anemia of pregnancy Apparent anemia that results because during pregnancy the plasma volume increases more than the erythrocytes increase.

Physiologic anorexia A decrease in appetite manifested when the extremely high metabolic demands of infancy slow to keep pace with the more moderate growth rate of toddlerhood.

Physiologic jaundice A harmless condition caused by the normal reduction of red blood cells, occurring 48 or more hours after birth, peaking at the 5th to 7th day, and disappearing between the 7th and 10th day.

Pica The eating of substances not ordinarily considered edible or to have nutritive value.

Pitting edema A "pit" or concave indentation that remains after an edematous area is pressed downward by the examiner's fingers.

Placenta Specialized disc-shaped organ that connects the fetus to the uterine wall for gas and nutrient exchange. Also called *afterbirth.*

Placenta accreta Partial or complete absence of the decidua basalis and abnormal adherence of the placenta to the uterine wall.

Placenta increta A high-risk condition that occurs when the placenta attaches to the uterine wall and invades or attaches itself within the myometrium.

Placenta percreta A high-risk condition that occurs when the placenta penetrates the myometrium, sometimes attaching to peritoneal structures within the abdominal cavity; the removal of the uterus (hysterectomy) is sometimes necessary when this condition is present.

Placenta previa Abnormal implantation of the placenta in the lower uterine segment. Classification of type is based on proximity to the cervical os: total—completely covers the os; partial—covers a portion of the os; marginal—is in proximity to the os.

Placental delivery Placenta and membranes expelled after the birth of the baby, during the third stage of labor.

Play therapy A therapeutic intervention often used with preschool and school-aged children. The child reveals conflicts, wishes, and fears on an unconscious level while playing with dolls, toys, clay, and other objects.

Podalic version Type of version used to turn a second twin during a vaginal birth.

Polycystic ovarian syndrome (PCOS) A complex endocrine disorder of ovarian dysfunction that is evidenced by amenorrhea or oligomenorrhea and clinical signs of androgen excess (typically hirsutism, acne) in the absence of other conditions that might have these same signs and symptoms.

Polycythemia Production of excessive red blood cells in response to chronic hypoxemia.

Polydactyly A developmental anomaly characterized by more than five digits on each hand or foot.

Polydipsia Excessive thirst.

Polyphagia Excessive or voracious eating.

Polypharmacy A term used to describe the act of taking multiple drugs to treat symptoms, when the etiology of the symptoms is actually a side effect from one or more prescribed medications.

Polysomnography A sleep study that simultaneously records the brain activity, eye movement, and respiration.

Polyuria Passage of a large volume of urine in a given period.

Population-based approach Health assessment and intervention performed with a group of children.

Positive signs of pregnancy Indications that confirm the presence of pregnancy.

Postcoital emergency contraception (EC) A form of combined hormonal contraception that is used when a woman is worried about pregnancy because of unprotected intercourse, rape, or possible contraceptive failure (e.g., broken condom, slipped diaphragm, missed oral contraceptives, or too long a time between Depo-Provera injections).

Postcoital test (PCT) An examination that evaluates the cervical mucus, sperm motility, sperm–mucus interaction, and the sperm's ability to negotiate the cervical mucous barrier. Also called *Sims-Huhner test*.

Postconception age periods Period of time in embryonic/fetal development calculated from the time of fertilization of the ovum.

Postictal period Period after seizure activity during which the level of consciousness is decreased.

Postmaturity See *Postterm newborn*.

Postpartum Describing the period after giving birth.

Postpartum blues See *Adjustment reaction with depressed mood*.

Postpartum depression See *Peripartum major mood episodes*.

Postpartum endometritis (metritis) A reproductive tract infection limited to the uterus and associated with childbirth that occurs at any time up to 6 weeks postpartum.

Postpartum hemorrhage A loss of blood of greater than 500 mL following birth. The hemorrhage is classified as *early* if it occurs within the first 24 hours and *late* if it occurs after the first 24 hours.

Postpartum home care Visits to postpartum families that occur in the home setting. This provides opportunities for expanding information and reinforcing self-care and infant care techniques initially presented in the birth setting.

Postpartum mood episodes with psychotic features Relatively rare but serious psychiatric disorder of the postpartum woman that can result in infanticide or suicide. Also called *postpartum psychosis*.

Postpartum psychosis See *Postpartum mood episodes with psychotic features*.

Postterm labor Labor that occurs after 42 weeks' gestation.

Postterm newborn Any baby born after 42 weeks' gestation.

Postterm pregnancy Pregnancy that lasts beyond 42 weeks' gestation.

Posttraumatic stress disorder (PTSD) Intense psychologic distress resulting from a traumatic event and evidenced by recurrent, intrusive thoughts; flashbacks, persistent avoidance of stimuli associated with the trauma; a generalized feeling of "numbness"; and persistent signs of arousal.

Posturing Abnormal position assumed after injury or damage to the brain that may be seen as extreme flexion or extension of the limbs.

Prebiotic A nondigestible food ingredient that can stimulate growth or activity of probiotic bacteria.

Precipitous birth (1) Unduly rapid progression of labor. (2) A birth in which no physician or certified nurse-midwife is in attendance.

Precipitous labor Unduly rapid progression of labor.

Preeclampsia Toxemia of pregnancy, characterized by hypertension, albuminuria, and edema. See also *Eclampsia*.

Preload Volume of blood in the ventricle at the end of diastole that stretches the heart muscle before contraction.

Premature newborn See *Preterm newborn*.

Premature labor See *Preterm labor (PTL)*.

Premature rupture of membranes (PROM) Rupture may be PROM (premature), SROM (spontaneous), or AROM (artificial). Some clinicians may use the abbreviation RBOW (rupture of bag of waters).

Premenstrual syndrome (PMS) Cluster of symptoms experienced by some women, typically occurring from a few days up to 2 weeks prior to the onset of menses.

Prenatal education Programs offered to expectant families, adolescents, women, or partners to provide education regarding the pregnancy, labor, and birth experience.

Presentation The fetal body part that enters the maternal pelvis first. The three possible presentations are cephalic, shoulder, and breech.

Presenting part The fetal part present in or on the cervical os.

Presumptive signs of pregnancy Symptoms that suggest but do not confirm pregnancy, such as cessation of menses, quickening, Chadwick sign, and morning sickness.

Preterm newborn Any baby born before 38 weeks' gestation.

Preterm labor (PTL) Labor occurring between 20 and 38 weeks of pregnancy. Also called *premature labor*.

Primary immune deficiency Congenital immunodeficiency.

Primary immune response The process in which B lymphocytes produce antibodies specific to a particular antigen on first exposure.

Primigravida A woman who is pregnant for the first time.

Primipara A woman who has given birth to her first child (past the point of viability), whether or not that child is living or was alive at birth.

Probable signs of pregnancy Manifestations that strongly suggest the likelihood of pregnancy, such as a positive pregnancy test, enlarging abdomen, and positive Goodell, Hegar, and Braxton Hicks signs.

Proband The family member around whom a family history is collected.

Probiotic A food supplement containing live microorganisms that alter the balance of gut microflora, thereby providing a health benefit.

Prodrome The phase of early manifestations of the infection until the development of the overt clinical syndrome.

Progesterone A hormone produced by the corpus luteum, adrenal cortex, and placenta whose function is to stimulate proliferation of the endometrium to facilitate growth of the embryo.

Progressive relaxation A relaxation technique that involves relaxing first one portion of the body and then another portion, until total body relaxation is achieved; may be used during labor.

Projectile vomiting Vomiting in which the stomach contents are ejected with great force.

Prolactin A hormone secreted by the anterior pituitary that stimulates and sustains lactation in mammals.

Prolapsed umbilical cord Umbilical cord that becomes trapped in the vagina before the fetus is born.

Prolonged decelerations Decelerations in which the fetal heart rate decreases from the baseline for 2 to 10 minutes.

Prolonged labor Labor lasting more than 24 hours.

Prostaglandins (PGs) Complex lipid compounds synthesized by many cells in the body. Protective factors Characteristics of a child and family that provide strength and assistance when dealing with a crisis.

Protocol A plan of action for chemotherapy that is based on the type of cancer, its stage, and the particular cell type.

Proto-oncogene A gene that regulates cellular growth and development but can become an oncogene, capable of causing cancerous growth.

Proximodistal development The process by which development proceeds from the center of the body outward to the extremities.

Pseudohermaphroditism Ambiguous development of the external genitalia.

Pseudohypertrophy Enlargement of the muscles as a result of infiltration by fatty tissue.

Pseudomenstruation In female newborns, a vaginal discharge composed of thick, whitish mucus that can become tinged with blood; caused by the withdrawal of maternal hormones.

Psychodrama Being assigned and playing out roles spontaneously in a therapeutic setting to assist in better understanding of the dynamics of the situation.

Psychologic disorders Abnormal mental or emotional conditions characterized by alterations in thinking, mood, or behavior.

Ptyalism Excessive salivation.

Puberty The developmental period between childhood and attainment of adult sexual characteristics and functioning.

Pubic Pertaining to the pubes or pubis.

Pubis Pertaining to the pubes or pubic area.

Pudendal block Injection of an anesthetizing agent at the pudendal nerve to produce numbness of the external genitals and the lower one third of the vagina, to facilitate childbirth and permit episiotomy if necessary.

Puerperal infection Infection of the reproductive tract associated with childbirth; occurs any time up to 6 weeks postpartum.

Puerperal morbidity A maternal temperature of 38.0°C (100.4°F) or higher on any 2 of the first 10 postpartum days, excluding the first 24 hours. The temperature is to be taken by mouth at least 4 times per day.

Puerperium The period after completion of the third stage of labor until involution of the uterus is complete, usually 6 weeks.

Purpura Bleeding into the tissues, particularly beneath the skin and mucous membranes, causing lesions that vary from red to purple.

Pyeloplasty Removal of an obstructed segment of the ureter and reimplantation into the renal pelvis.

Q

Quadruple screen Prenatal test of amniotic fluid or blood that assesses for appropriate levels of alpha-fetoprotein (AFP), human chorionic gonadotropin (hCG), unconjugated estriol (UE3), and the substance dimeric inhibin-A. It is used to screen for Down syndrome (trisomy 21), trisomy 18, and neural tube defects (NTDs). A more sensitive and accurate detector of trisomy 21 than the triple screen.

Quickening The first fetal movements felt by the pregnant woman, usually between 16 and 18 weeks' gestation.

Quiet alert state An alert state characterized by a brightening of the eyes and face. Babies are most attentive to their environment in this state and provide positive feedback to caregivers.

R

Race A group of people who share biologic similarities such as skin color, bone structure, and genetic traits. Examples of races include White (sometimes called Caucasian or European American), Black (sometimes called African American in the United States), Hispanic, Natives (such as Native Americans, Alaskan Native, Hawaiian Native, and First Nation people of Canada), and Asian.

Radiation Heat loss incurred when heat transfers to cooler surfaces and objects not in direct contact with the body.

Radioallergosorbent test (RAST) A technique in which radioimmunoassay is used to measure the presence in the blood of immunoglobulin E (IgE) antibodies to certain antigens.

Radiofrequency ablation The use of radioenergy to destroy a very small section of the myocardium through which an accessory conduction pathway passes.

Rape Sexual activity, often intercourse, against the will of the victim.

Recessive A characteristic that is apparent only when two copies of the gene encoding it are present, one from the mother and one from the father.

Reciprocity An interactional cycle that occurs simultaneously between mother and baby. It involves mutual cuing behaviors, expectancy, rhythmicity, and synchrony.

Recombinant form Type of vaccine in which an organism has been genetically altered.

Rectocele A condition that results when the posterior vaginal wall is weakened. The anterior wall of the rectum can then sag forward, ballooning into the vagina, pushing the weakened posterior wall of the vagina in front of it.

Recurrent pregnancy loss (RPL) Three or more consecutive pregnancy losses before 24 weeks' gestation.

Red reflex The orange-red glow of the vascular retina as the light travels through the cornea, aqueous humor, lens, and vitreous humor to the retina.

Regional analgesia The temporary and reversible loss of sensation produced by injecting an anesthetic agent (called a local anesthetic) into an area that will bring the agent into direct contact with nervous tissue.

Regional anesthesia Injection of local anesthetic agents so that they come into direct contact with nervous tissue.

Regression Return to an earlier behavior. A defense mechanism that may be displayed by children during times of stress.

Rehabilitation Assisting children with physical or mental challenges to reach their fullest potential through therapy and education that considers the physiologic, psychologic, and environmental strengths and limitations of the children.

Relaxin A water-soluble protein secreted by the corpus luteum that causes relaxation of the symphysis and cervical dilatation.

Reliability Consistent results are obtained when measured by the same rater or other raters.

Relinquishing mothers Mothers who choose to give their babies up for adoption.

Renal insufficiency Any degree of renal failure in which the kidneys' ability to conserve sodium and concentrate the urine decreases.

Repression Involuntary forgetting. A defense mechanism often displayed by children with life-threatening or mortal illness.

Resilience The ability to function with healthy responses, even with significant stress and adversity.

Resiliency theory An assessment theory that holds that all individuals experience crises that lead to adaptation and development of inner strengths and the ability to handle future crises.

Respiratory depression Unresponsiveness and progressively decreasing respiratory rate that may progress to respiratory arrest.

Respiratory distress syndrome (RDS) Respiratory disease of the newborn characterized by interference with ventilation at the alveolar level, thought to be caused by the presence of fibrinoid deposits lining the alveolar ducts. Formerly called *hyaline membrane disease.*

Respite care Short-term home care to relieve the primary caregiver and allow time away from home.

Retained placenta Retention of the placenta beyond 30 minutes after birth.

Retinopathy of prematurity (ROP) Formation of fibrotic tissue behind the lens; associated with retinal detachment and arrested eye growth, seen with hypoxemia in preterm newborns.

Retractions A visible drawing in of the skin of the neck and chest, which occurs on inspiration in infants and young children in respiratory distress.

Rh factor Antigens present on the surface of blood cells that make the blood cell incompatible with blood cells that do not have the antigen.

Rh immune globulin (RhoGAM) An anti-Rh(D) gamma globulin given after delivery to an Rh-negative mother of an Rh-positive fetus or neonate. Prevents the development of permanent active immunity to the Rh antigen.

Risk factors   Any findings that suggest the pregnancy may have a negative outcome, for either the woman or her unborn child.

Room sharing   An arrangement in which the baby sleeps in the same room in proximity to the parents, but has own bed.

Rooming in   Practice in which parents stay in the child's hospital room and care for the child.

Rooting reflex   A baby's tendency to turn the head and open the lips to suck when one side of the mouth or cheek is touched.

Round ligaments   Ligaments that arise from the sides of the uterus near the fallopian tube insertions. They extend outward between the folds of the broad ligament, passing through the inguinal ring and canals and eventually fusing with the connective tissue of the labia majora.

Rugae   Transverse ridges of mucous membranes lining the vagina that allow the vagina to stretch during the descent of the fetal head.

Rupture of membranes (ROM)   Rupture may be PROM (premature), SROM (spontaneous), or AROM (artificial). Some clinicians may use the abbreviation RBOW (rupture of bag of waters).

S

Sacral promontory   A projection into the pelvic cavity on the anterior upper portion of the sacrum; serves as an obstetric guide in determining pelvic measurements.

Saline   A mixture of salt and water; *normal saline* refers to the mixture of salt and water in equal concentration in body fluids.

Scalp stimulation   A test used during labor to assess fetal well-being by pressing a fingertip on the fetal scalp. A fetus not under excessive stress will respond to the digital stimulation with heart rate accelerations.

Scarf sign   The position of the elbow when the hand of a supine newborn is drawn across to the other shoulder until it meets resistance.

Schultze mechanism   Expulsion of the placenta with the shiny, or fetal, surface presenting first.

Scoliosis   A lateral spine curvature.

Screening   Procedures used to detect the presence of a health condition before symptoms are apparent.

Secondary cancers   Cancers (most commonly solid tumors) that appear subsequent to the primary cancer and treatment but are of a different histologic type. Also called *second malignant neoplasms (SMNs)*.

Secondary immune deficiency   Acquired immunodeficiency.

Secondary immune response   The body's response to an antigen at any time other than the initial exposure.

Secondary infertility   Condition in which couples are unable to conceive after one or more successful pregnancies.

Sedation   A medically controlled state of depressed consciousness used for painful diagnostic and therapeutic procedures.

Self-concept   Evaluation of the self in certain specific areas, such as those related to academic achievement, athletic ability, physical appearance, and social interactions.

Self-efficacy   A person's belief that he or she can change behavior to produce a desired outcome.

Self-esteem   The feelings and beliefs of children about their competence and worth as individuals, ability to meet challenges, and ability to learn lessons from success and failure.

Self-quieting ability   Infant's ability to use personal resources to quiet and console self.

Self-regulation   Infant's ability to maintain state and self-console, for example, by sucking on the fingers to stay calm instead of crying.

Semen   Thick whitish fluid ejaculated by the male during orgasm and containing spermatozoa and their nutrients.

Sensible water loss   Water loss that is measurable and observable, such as urine and drainage from tubes.

Sensorineural hearing loss   Hearing loss caused by damage to the inner ear structures or the auditory nerve.

Separation anxiety   Distress behaviors observed in young children separated from familiar caregivers.

Sepsis neonatorum   Infections experienced by a neonate during the first month of life.

Sequence   A cascade of events that are initiated by a single factor and lead to birth defects or congenital abnormalities.

Serosal layer   See Perimetrium.

Sex chromosomes   The X and Y chromosomes, which are responsible for sex determination.

Sexual assault   Involuntary sexual contact with another person.

Sexuality   A person's view of himself or herself as a sexual being.

Sexually transmitted infection (STI)   Refers to an infection ordinarily transmitted by direct sexual contact with an infected individual. Also called *sexually transmitted disease*.

Shaken baby injuries   A collection of symptoms that are caused by vigorously shaking an infant. Shaking can cause brain hemorrhage, spinal cord injury, retinal hemorrhage or detachment, long-term developmental problems, intellectual disability, or even death.

Shaman   In the Native American culture, a man or woman who enters an altered state of consciousness, at will, to contact and utilize another type of reality to acquire knowledge and power and to help other people.

Shock   An acute, complex state of circulatory dysfunction resulting in failure to deliver sufficient oxygen and other nutrients to meet cell and tissue demands.

Shunt   Movement of blood between heart chambers through an abnormal anatomic or surgically created opening.

Simian line   A single palmar crease frequently found in children with Down syndrome. Also called *transverse palmer crease*.

Sims-Huhner test   See *Postcoital test (PCT)*.

Single nucleotide polymorphism (SNP)   A variation in DNA sequence in which a single nucleotide base (A, T, C, or G) is substituted for another.

Skin turgor   Elasticity of skin; provides information on hydration status.

Skin-to-skin contact   Physical contact between the mother and newborn whereby the naked baby is placed prone on the mother's chest during the first 24 hours. Also called *kangaroo care*.

Sleep hygiene   Behaviors that foster a regular and sufficient sleep pattern and daytime alertness.

Small for gestational age (SGA)   Inadequate weight or growth for gestational age; birth weight below the 10th percentile.

Solitary play   When infants play by themselves.

Spermatogenesis   The process by which mature spermatozoa are formed, during which the number of chromosomes is halved.

Spermatozoa   Mature sperm cells of the male animal, produced by the testes.

Spermicides   A variety of creams, foams, jellies, and suppositories that, when inserted into the vagina prior to intercourse, destroy sperm or neutralize any vaginal secretions and thereby immobilize sperm.

Spinal block   Injection of a local anesthetic agent directly into the spinal fluid in the spinal canal to provide anesthesia for vaginal and cesarean births.

Spinal shock   A spinal cord concussion resulting in a transient suppression of nerve function below the level of the acute injury.

Spinnbarkeit   The elasticity of the cervical mucus that is present at ovulation.

Spiritual dimension   Belief in a connection with a greater power that guides a person to strive for inspiration, respect, meaning, and purpose in life.

Spiritual health   The ability to develop a spiritual nature, including awareness of a life purpose and fulfillment.

Spirituality   A belief in a transcendent power pertaining to the spirit or soul.

Spontaneous abortion   Abortion that occurs naturally. Also called *miscarriage.*

Spontaneous rupture of membranes (SROM)   The breaking of the "water" or membranes marked by the expulsion of amniotic fluid from the vagina.

Sprain   A tearing of ligaments usually caused when a joint is twisted or otherwise traumatized.

Station   Relationship of the presenting fetal part to an imaginary line drawn between the pelvic ischial spines.

Status epilepticus   A continuous seizure or recurrent seizures that last for more than 20 minutes without return to baseline.

Stenosis   Narrowing of a valve or below the valve, or in the blood vessel.

Stent   A device used to maintain patency of the urethral canal after surgery.

Stepping reflex   A reflex elicited by holding a newborn up with one foot touching a flat surface; the newborn will put one foot in front of the other and "walk." Pronounced at birth, this reflex disappears between 4 and 8 weeks of age.

Stereotyping   The assumption that all members of a cultural, ethnic, or racial group are alike and share the same attitudes and beliefs.

Stereotypy   Repetitive, obsessive, machine-like movements, commonly seen in autistic or schizophrenic children.

Sterilization   An inclusive term that refers to surgical procedures that permanently prevent pregnancy. In men, sterilization is achieved through a procedure called vasectomy. In women, sterilization is done by tubal ligation.

Stillbirth   The delivery of a dead baby.

Stoma   An opening, commonly in the abdominal wall, to provide for drainage from the intestinal or urinary systems.

Stranger anxiety   Wariness of strange people and places, often shown by infants between 6 and 18 months of age.

Striae   Stretch marks; shiny reddish lines that appear on the abdomen, breasts, thighs, and buttocks of pregnant women as a result of stretching the skin.

Stridor   An abnormal, high-pitched musical respiratory sound caused when air moves through a narrowed larynx or trachea.

Stroke volume   The amount of blood ejected with each ventricular contraction.

Subconjunctival hemorrhage   Hemorrhage on the sclera of a newborn's eye, usually caused by changes in vascular tension during birth.

Subdermal implants   A subdermal progestin contraceptive that is implanted in a woman's arm and provides contraceptive protection for up to 5 years.

Subfertility   A couple who have difficulty conceiving because both partners have reduced fertility.

Subinvolution   Failure of a part to return to its normal size after functional enlargement, such as failure of the uterus to return to normal size after pregnancy.

Subluxation   Partial or complete dislocation of a joint.

Sucking reflex   Normal newborn reflex elicited by inserting a finger or nipple in the newborn's mouth, resulting in forceful, rhythmic sucking.

Sudden infant death syndrome (SIDS)   The sudden death of an infant with no identifiable cause identified after autopsy and review of circumstances of the death; the primary cause of infant death beyond the neonatal period in the United States.

Supine hypotensive syndrome   Refers to a condition that can develop during pregnancy when the enlarging uterus puts pressure on the vena cava when the woman is supine. This pressure interferes with returning blood flow and produces a marked decrease in blood pressure with accompanying dizziness, pallor, and clamminess, which can be corrected by having the woman lie on her left side. Also called *vena caval syndrome* or *aortocaval compression.*

Support systems   The extended network of family, friends, and religious and community contacts that provide nurturance, emotional support, and direct assistance to parents.

Surfactant   A surface-active mixture of lipoproteins secreted in the alveoli and air passages that reduces surface tension of pulmonary fluids and contributes to the elasticity of pulmonary tissue.

Suture   Fibrous connection of opposed joint surfaces, as in the skull.

Symphysis pubis   A firm joint between the two pelvic bones.

Syncope   Transient loss of consciousness and muscle tone.

Syndactyly   Malformation of the fingers or toes in which there may be webbing or complete fusion of two or more digits.

Syndrome   A collection of anomalies that occur in a consistent pattern and have a common cause.

Syphilis   A chronic, sexually transmitted infection caused by the spirochete *Treponema pallidum.*

T

Taboos   Behaviors or objects that are avoided by individuals or groups.

Tachypnea   An abnormally rapid rate of respiration.

Tactile fremitus   Producing vibrations by either crying or talking that can be palpated on the chest.

Technology-assisted   State of depending on a medical device that is required to sustain life (mechanical ventilators, intravenous nutrition or drugs, tracheostomy, suctioning, oxygen, or nutritional support with tube feedings).

Telangiectasia   Permanent dilation of superficial capillaries and venules.

Telangiectatic nevi (stork bites)   Small clusters of pink-red spots appearing on the nape of the neck and around the eyes of newborns; localized areas of capillary dilation.

Teratogens   Nongenetic factors that can produce malformations of the fetus.

Term   The normal duration of pregnancy.

Testes   The male gonads, in which sperm and testosterone are produced.

Testosterone   The male hormone; responsible for the development of secondary male characteristics.

Tetraplegia   The loss of sensation and function in the head and neck and upper and lower extremities.

Thelarche   Breast development.

Therapeutic abortion   Medically induced termination of pregnancy when a malformed fetus is suspected or when the woman's health is in jeopardy.

Therapeutic insemination   A procedure to produce a pregnancy in which sperm obtained from a woman's husband or from a donor is deposited in the woman's vagina. Process by which semen is deposited at the cervical os or in the uterus by mechanical means.

Therapeutic play   Planned play techniques that provide an opportunity for children to deal with their fears and concerns related to illness or hospitalization.

Therapeutic touch   Complementary therapy grounded in the belief that people are a system of energy with a self-healing potential. The therapeutic touch practitioner, often a nurse, unites his or her energy field with that of the client, directing it in a specific way to promote well-being and healing.

Thermogenesis   The newborn's physiologic mechanisms that increase heat production.

Thrill   A vibration on the anterior chest caused by turbulent blood flow from a defective heart valve and a heart murmur.

Thrombocytopenia   A low platelet count.

Thrombophlebitis   Inflammation of a vein wall, resulting in thrombus.

Thrush   A fungal infection of the oral mucous membranes caused by *Candida albicans*. Most often seen in newborns and infants; characterized by white plaques in the mouth.

Thyrotoxicosis   A condition that can occur when thyroid hormone is suddenly released into the bloodstream during surgery. The child experiences fever, diaphoresis, and tachycardia, progressing to shock and, if untreated, death.

Tinnitus   Ringing in the ears.

Tocolysis   Use of medications to arrest preterm labor.

Tolerance   Adaptation to an opioid dosage that results in a shorter duration of drug effectiveness over time.

Tonic   Continuous muscular contraction; often used to describe seizure activity.

Tonic neck reflex   Postural reflex seen in the newborn. When the supine baby's head is turned to one side, the arm and leg on that side extend while the extremities on the opposite side flex. Also called the *fencing position*.

TORCH   An acronym used to describe a group of infections that represent potentially severe problems during pregnancy: *to*xoplasmosis; *r*ubella; *c*ytomegalovirus; *h*erpesvirus.

Torticollis   Persistent head tilting.

Total parenteral nutrition   A feeding regimen accomplished entirely by intravenous injection or other nongastrointestinal route.

Total serum bilirubin   Sum of conjugated (direct) and unconjugated (indirect) bilirubin.

Toxic appearance   Lethargy, poor perfusion, hypoventilation or hyperventilation, and cyanosis.

Toxic shock syndrome (TSS)   Infection caused by *Staphylococcus aureus*, found primarily in women of reproductive age.

Toxicants   Harmful natural or synthetic chemicals not metabolically produced by an organism.

Toxins   Harmful or poisonous chemicals produced by metabolism or an organism (e.g., ricin).

Toxoid   A toxin that has been treated (by heat or chemical) to weaken its toxic effects but retain its antigenicity.

Tracheostomy   Creation of a surgical opening into the trachea through the anterior neck at the cricoid cartilage; performed when long-term airway management is needed.

Traditional Chinese medicine   System of medicine developed more than 3000 years ago in China that seeks to ensure the balance of energy, which is called *chi* or *qi* (pronounced "chee"). Chi is thought to maintain health and vitality and enable the body to carry out its physiologic functions.

Transgendered   An adjective used to describe or refer to someone who feels compelled to (and does) dress and act like a member of the opposite sex.

Transitional milk   Breast milk produced from the end of colostrum production until about 2 weeks postpartum.

Translocation   The joining of a part of or a whole chromosome to another separate chromosome.

Transplacental immunity   Passive immunity that is transferred from mother to baby.

Transvaginal ultrasound   A follicular monitoring test that is used in women undergoing induction cycles, for timing ovulation for insemination and intercourse, for retrieving oocytes for in vitro fertilization, and for monitoring early pregnancy.

Transverse diameter   The largest diameter of the pelvic inlet; helps determine the shape of the inlet.

Transverse lie   A lie in which the fetus is positioned crosswise in the uterus.

Treatment room   In a hospital or medical center, a room designated for performing treatments such as intravenous starts, blood drawing, and lumbar punctures to promote the child's sense of security that this room is a "safe" and relatively pain-free site.

Trial of labor after cesarean (TOLAC)   An attempt to have a vaginal birth after a previous cesarean birth.

Trichomoniasis   A sexually transmitted infection caused by *Trichomonas vaginalis*, a microscopic motile protozoan that thrives in an alkaline environment.

Trigger   A stimulus that initiates an asthmatic episode; a substance or condition, including exercise, infection, allergy, irritants, weather, or emotions.

Trimester   Three months, or one third of the gestational time for pregnancy.

Tripod position   Sitting forward with arms on knees for support and extending the neck.

Trisomic (trisomy)   The presence of three homologous chromosomes rather than the normal two.

Trophoblast   The outer layer of the blastoderm that will eventually establish the nutrient relationship with the uterine endometrium.

True pelvis   The portion that lies below the linea terminalis, made up of the inlet, cavity, and outlet.

Trunk incurvation   Reflex resulting from the stroking of the spine, which causes the pelvis to turn to the stimulated side. Also called *Galant reflex*.

Tubal embryo transfer (TET)   Procedure in which eggs are retrieved and incubated with the man's sperm and then transferred back into the women's body at the embryo stage.

Tubal ligation   Sterilization of a woman accomplished by transecting or occluding the fallopian tubes.

Tummy time   Prone positioning of the infant while awake. Important for all babies because it assists them with learning developmentally appropriate skills and builds muscle strength for their shoulders, neck, and back.

Tumor suppressor genes   Genetic material that controls the growth of cells, decreasing the effects of oncogenes.

Turner syndrome   A number of anomalies that occur when a woman has only one X chromosome. Characteristics include short stature; little sexual differentiation; webbing of the neck, with a low posterior hairline; and congenital cardiac anomalies.

Tympanogram   A graph showing the ability of the middle ear to transmit sound energy; measured by inserting an airtight probe into the external ear entrance and emitting a tone.

Tympanometry   A hearing evaluation test that measures middle ear pressure and tympanic membrane movement.

Tympanostomy tubes   Pressure-equalizing tubes inserted to drain fluid from the middle ear.

U

Ultrasound High-frequency sound waves that may be directed, through the use of a transducer, into the maternal abdomen. The ultrasonic sound waves reflected by the underlying structures of varying densities allow identification of various maternal and fetal tissues, bones, and fluids.

Umbilical cord The structure connecting the placenta to the umbilicus of the fetus and through which nutrients from the woman are exchanged for wastes from the fetus.

Umbilical velocimetry A noninvasive ultrasound test that measures blood flow changes that occur in maternal and fetal circulation in order to assess placental function.

Uremia Toxicity resulting from the buildup of urea and nitrogenous waste in the blood.

Urinary tract infection (UTI) Significant bacteriuria in the presence of symptoms.

Uterine atony Relaxation of uterine muscle tone following birth.

Uterine inversion Prolapse of the uterine fundus through the cervix into the vagina; may occur just before or during expulsion of the placenta; associated with massive hemorrhage, requiring emergency treatment.

Uterine rupture A nonsurgical disruption of the uterine cavity.

Uterosacral ligaments Ligaments that provide support for the uterus and cervix at the level of the ischial spines. They arise on each side of the pelvis from the posterior wall of the uterus and sweep back around the rectum to insert on the sides of the first and second sacral vertebrae.

Uterus The hollow muscular organ in which the fertilized ovum is implanted and in which the developing fetus is nourished until birth.

Uveitis Inflammation of the middle layer of the eye.

V

Vacuum extraction An obstetric procedure used to assist in the birth of a fetus by applying suction to the fetal head with a soft suction cup attached to a suction bottle (pump) by tubing; the device is placed against the occiput of the fetal head.

Vacuum-assisted wound closure Negative-pressure wound therapy.

Vagina The musculomembranous tube or passageway located between the external genitals and the uterus of a woman.

Vaginal birth after cesarean (VBAC) Practice of permitting a trial of labor and possible vaginal birth for women following a previous cesarean birth for nonrecurring causes such as fetal distress or placenta previa.

Validity Accurately measures the concept it was designed to measure.

Variability Baseline fluctuations of two cycles per minute or greater in the fetal heart rate (FHR) and classified by the visually quantified amplitude of peak-to-trough in beats per minute.

Variable decelerations Periodic change in fetal heart rate caused by umbilical cord compression; decelerations vary in onset, occurrence, and waveform.

Varus A condition in which the hindfoot turns inward; usually associated with clubfoot.

Vasectomy Surgical removal of a portion of the vas deferens (ductus deferens) to produce infertility.

Vaso-occlusion Blockage of a blood vessel.

Vegan Strict vegetarian who eats absolutely no animal products.

Vegetarian One who eats no poultry, meat, or fish.

Vena caval syndrome See *Supine hypotensive syndrome.*

Vernix caseosa A protective, cheeselike, whitish substance made up of sebum and desquamated epithelial cells that is present on the fetal skin.

Version Turning of the fetus in utero.

Vertex The top or crown of the head.

Vertical transmission The passage of disease from the mother to the fetus during the period of pregnancy.

Vesicoureteral reflux The backflow of urine from the bladder into the ureters during voiding.

Viability The potential for the pregnancy to result in a live birth.

Vibroacoustic stimulation (VAS) Application of device delivering 90 dB of sound and vibration for 1 to 3 seconds to the mother's abdomen to stimulate movement in the fetus, thereby accelerating the fetal heart rate. (Also called *FAST for fetal acoustic stimulation test* or *VST* for *vibroacoustic stimulation test.*)

Violence Threatened or actual use of physical force that leads to potential or actual physical or emotional trauma.

Virilization The production of masculine secondary sexual characteristics in females.

Vision A complex process of acquiring meaning from what is seen, involving the eye, brain, and related neurologic and physiologic structures.

Visual acuity Measurement of the ability to discriminate a letter or other object to test sight.

Visualization Complementary therapy in which a person goes into a relaxed state and focuses on or "visualizes" soothing or positive scenes such as a beach or a mountain glade. Visualization helps reduce stress and encourage relaxation.

Vocal resonance How well voice sounds are transmitted over the chest.

Vulva The external structure of the female genitals, lying below the mons veneris.

Vulvovaginal candidiasis (VVC) A genital infection most often caused by *Candida albicans.* Also called *moniliasis or yeast infection.*

W

Water intoxication An abnormal proportion of water to sodium in the extracellular fluid.

Weaning The process of discontinuing breastfeeding and accustoming an infant to another feeding method.

Wharton jelly Yellow-white gelatinous material surrounding the vessels of the umbilical cord.

Wheezing A noise resulting from the passage of air through mucus or fluids in a narrowed lower airway.

Withdrawal The physical signs and symptoms that occur when a sedative or pain drug is suddenly stopped in a client who is physically tolerant.

X

Xerosis Generally dry skin that is likely to crack and fissure.

X-linked Any gene found on the X chromosome, or traits determined by such genes; also refers to the specific mode of inheritance of such genes; one altered gene on an X chromosome in a male fetus can produce disease, such as hemophilia.

Z

Zona pellucida Transparent inner layer surrounding an ovum.

Zygote A fertilized egg.

Zygote intrafallopian transfer (ZIFT) Retrieval of oocytes under ultrasound guidance, followed by in vitro fertilization and laparoscopic replacement of fertilized eggs into the fimbriated end of the fallopian tube.

Index

Note: Page numbers followed by f, t, and b indicate figures, tables, and boxes, respectively.

A

Abandoned infants, 1029
Abdomen
  assessment of, 835–836, 835f
    in newborn, 506–507, 519–520
    postpartum, 661–662
  landmarks of, 835f
Abdominal bleeding, in ectopic pregnancy, 296
Abdominal exercises, for childbirth, 212–213, 213f, 320
Abdominal hysterectomy, 121–122
Abdominal movement, 835
Abdominal pain, in appendicitis, 1342, 1343
Abdominal palpation
  intrapartum
    of contractions, 346, 347
    Leopold maneuvers in, 348, 349, 349f
    in newborn, 507
    postpartum, 661–662, 662f
Abdominal trauma, 1359–1360
Abducens nerve, assessment of, 846t
Abduction (joint movement), 1515f
Abduction (kidnapping), of newborn, 384
ABO incompatibility, 316
  hyperbilirubinemia and, 626–627, 628
Abortion, 91
  induced
    adolescent pregnancy and, 241
    legal/ethical aspects of, 12
    methods of, 91
    nursing management of, 91
    prenatal testing and, 48
    for stillbirth, 441
  spontaneous
    after amniocentesis, 263
    causes of, 293
    after chorionic villus sampling, 263
    clinical therapy for, 294
    cultural aspects of, 294b
    definition of, 292
    nursing management of, 294–295
    recurrent, 130, 445–446
    types of, 293–294, 293f
Abrasions
  corneal, 1127t
  ear, 1138t
Abruptio placentae, 344t, 412–416, 413f, 413t
Abscess
  breast, 727
  ear, 1138t
  pelvic, 116–117
  peritonsillar, 1140–1141, 1141t
  retropharyngeal, 1140–1141, 1141t
  skin, in MRSA infections, 1559–1560
  tubo-ovarian, pelvic inflammatory disease and, 116–117

Absence seizures, 1443t
Absolute neutrophil count, in cancer, 1282t
Abstinence, sexual, 84
Abuse. *See* Child abuse and neglect
Acanthosis nigricans, 1425, 1426f
Accessory (supernumerary) nipples, 505, 832
Accidents. *See* Safety concerns; Trauma
Accommodation, in cognitive development, 748
Acculturation, 20
Accutane (isotretinoin), for acne, 1568–1569
ACE inhibitors, for congestive heart failure, 1213
Acellular pertussis vaccine, 1046
Acetabulum, 65
Acetaminophen (Tylenol)
  dosage of, 1074
  overdose of, 1036t
  for pain, in children, 971
Acetylsalicylic acid, for pain, in children, 971, 972
Achilles reflex, 838t
Achondroplasia, 38t, 1535–1537
Acid burns, oropharyngeal, 1036t
Acid-base balance
  buffers in, 1104–1106, 1107
  kidney in, 1106, 1107
  in labor
    cord blood analysis for, 358
    in fetus, 337, 609
    in mother, 336–337
  liver in, 1106
  lung in, 1106
  physiology of, 1104–1106
Acid-base imbalances, 1106–1112, 1108t
  acidosis
    definition of, 1106
    metabolic, 336–337, 358, 609, 1110–1111, 1110t. *See also* Metabolic acidosis
    respiratory, 614, 615–616, 1106–1109, 1107–1109, 1108t
  alkalosis
    definition of, 1106
    respiratory, 1109–1110, 1110t
  arterial blood gases in, 1106, 1108t–1110t, 1112t
  mixed, 1112
Acidemia, 1104
Acidosis. *See* Acid-base imbalances, acidosis
Acne, 1554t, 1567–1571
  neonatal, 1568
  nursing care plan for, 1570
Acoustic nerve, assessment of, 846t
Acoustic stimulation tests, 258–259
Acquaintance rape, 101
Acquired immunity, 1233
Acquired immunodeficiency syndrome. *See* HIV/AIDS
Acrocyanosis, in newborn, 498–499, 499f
Acrosomal reaction, 138
ACTH (adren+ocorticotropic hormone), 1399t
Active immunity, 483, 1045
Active management of labor, 426
Activity and exercise. *See* Physical activity
Actonel (risedronate), for osteoporosis, 98

Special Features

EVIDENCE-BASED PRACTICE